This book is due for return on or before the last date shown below.

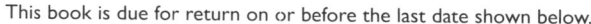

Surgery of the Hip

Surgery of the Hip

Daniel J. Berry, MD
L.Z. Gund Professor and Chairman
Department of Orthopedic Surgery
Mayo Clinic
Rochester, Minnesota

Jay R. Lieberman, MD
Director
New England Musculoskeletal Institute
Professor and Chairman
Department of Orthopaedic Surgery
University of Connecticut Health Center
Farmington, Connecticut

With 917 illustrations

ELSEVIER
SAUNDERS

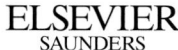

ELSEVIER
SAUNDERS

1600 John F. Kennedy Blvd.
Ste. 1800
Philadelphia, PA 19103-2899

Surgery of the Hip   ISBN: 978-0-4430-6991-8

Library of Congress Cataloging-in-Publication Data
Surgery of the hip / [edited by] Daniel J. Berry, Jay R. Lieberman.
    p. ; cm.
Includes bibliographical references and index.
ISBN 978-0-443-06991-8 (hardcover : alk. paper)
I. Berry, Daniel J. II. Lieberman, Jay R.
[DNLM: 1. Hip–surgery. 2. Hip Injuries–surgery. 3. Hip Joint–surgery. WE 855]
617.5′81059–dc23
                                        2012020970

Senior Content Strategist: Don Scholz
Senior Content Development Specialist: Ann Anderson
Publishing Services Manager: Catherine Jackson
Senior Project Manager: Rachel E. McMullen
Design Direction: Steve Stave

Working together to grow
libraries in developing countries

www.elsevier.com | www.bookaid.org | www.sabre.org

ELSEVIER   BOOK AID International   Sabre Foundation

Printed in China

Last digit is the print number: 9 8 7 6 5 4 3 2 1

To my father, John Berry, and my late mother, Elizabeth Berry, who provided me with remarkable opportunities and encouraged hard work and professional commitment alloyed with worthy goals.
To my wife, Camilla Berry, and my children, Charlotte Berry and John Berry, who provide the joys so important to sustain an academic life and practice and the occasional reality checks needed to maintain perspective.
Daniel J. Berry

To my wife Laura and my children, Danielle, Sam, and Jordan, whose love and unwavering support have allowed me to pursue an academic career committed to patient care, research, and education.
To my parents, Sol and Edith Lieberman, whose commitment to education and scholarship fostered my intellectual curiosity through the years.
Jay R. Lieberman

Section Editors

John Clohisy, MD
Daniel C. and Betty B. Viehmann Distinguished Professor, of Orthopaedic Surgery, Department of Orthopaedic, Surgery, Washington University School of Medicine, St. Louis, Missouri

Craig J. Della Valle, MD
Associate Professor, Orthopaedic Surgery, Rush University, Medical Center, Chicago, Illinois

George Haidukewych, MD
Professor of Orthopedic Surgery, University of Central Florida; Co-Director of Orthopedic Trauma, Chief of Complex Adult Reconstruction, Orlando Health, Orlando, Florida

Tad M. Mabry, MD
Assistant Professor of Orthopedic Surgery, Department of Orthopedic Surgery, Mayo Clinic, Rochester, Minnesota

Steven J. MacDonald, MD, FRCSC
Professor of Orthopaedic Surgery, University of Western Ontario; Chief of Orthopaedics & Chief of Surgery, University Hospital, London, Ontario, Canada

Bassam A. Masri, MD, FRCSC
Professor and Chairman, Department of Orthopaedics, University of British Columbia; Head of Orthopaedics and Surgeon-in-Chief, Vancouver Acute Health Services, Vancouver, British Columbia, Canada

R. Michael Meneghini, MD
Director of Joint Replacement, Indiana University Health Saxony Hospital; Assistant Professor of Clinical Orthopaedic Surgery, Department of Orthopaedic Surgery, Indiana University School of Medicine, Indianapolis, Indiana

Michael B. Millis, MD
Professor of Orthopaedic Surgery, Harvard Medical School Adolescent and Young Adult Hip Unit, Children's Hospital Boston, Boston, Massachusetts

Philip C. Noble, PhD
John S. Dunn Professor of Orthopedic Research, Center for Orthopedic Surgery, The Methodist Hospital; Professor, Joseph Barnhart Department of Orthopedic Surgery, Baylor College of Medicine; Director of Research, Institute of Orthopedic Research and Education, Houston, Texas

Vincent Pellegrini, Jr., MD
James L. Kernan Professor and Chair, Department of Orthopaedics, University of Maryland School of Medicine, Baltimore, Maryland

Peter S. Rose, MD
Assistant Professor, Mayo Clinic College of Medicine, Consultant Surgeon, Musculoskeletal Oncology Fellowship Director, Mayo Clinic, Rochester, Minnesota

Robert T. Trousdale, MD
Chairman, Division of Adult Reconstruction, Department of Orthopedic Surgery; Professor of Orthopedics, Mayo School of Graduate Medical Education, Rochester, Minnesota

Contributors

Derek F. Amanatullah, MD, PhD
Resident, Department of Orthopaedic Surgery, University of California, Davis, Davis Medical Center, Sacramento, California

Phillip J. Andersen, PhD
Principal, Andersen Metallurgical LLC, Madison, Wisconsin

David J. Backstein, MD, MEd, FRCS(C)
Associate Professor, Department of Surgery, University of Toronto; Head of the Division of Orthopedic Surgery, Mount Sinai Hospital, Toronto, Ontario, Canada

C. Lowry Barnes, MD
Professor, Department of Orthopaedic Surgery, University of Arkansas for Medical Sciences; Medical Director, HipKnee Arkansas Foundation, Arkansas Specialty Orthopaedics, Little Rock, Arkansas

Paul E. Beaulé, MD, FRCSC
Associate Professor, University of Ottawa; Head of Adult Reconstruction, The Ottawa Hospital, Ottawa, Ontario, Canada

Edward H. Becker
Orthopaedic Resident; University of Maryland Orthopaedic Department, Baltimore, Maryland

Hany Bedair, MD
Instructor, Orthopaedic Surgery, Harvard Medical School; Clinical, Department of Orthopaedic Surgery, Massachusetts General Hospital, Boston, Massachusetts

Keith R. Berend, MD
Associate, Joint Implant Surgeons, Inc., New Albany; Associate Professor, Department of Orthopaedic Surgery, The Ohio State University, Columbus, Ohio

Michael E. Berend, MD
Center for Hip and Knee Surgery, Joint Replacement Surgeons of Indiana, St. Francis Hospital—Mooresville, Mooresville, Indiana; Orthopaedic Biomedical Engineering Laboratory, Rose Hulman Institute of Technology, Terre Haute, Indiana

Georg Bergmann, MD
Professor, Julius Wolff Institute, Charité – Universitätsmedizin Berli, Berlin, Germany

Brett Bolhofner, MD
Diector of Orthopedic Tauma, Orthopedic Surgery, Bayfront Medical Center, St. Petersburg; Clinical Assistant Professor, Orthopedic Surgery, University of South Florida, Tampa, Florida

Mathias P.G. Bostrom, MD
Professor of Orthopaedic Surgery, Hospital for Special Surgery, New York, New York

Robert B. Bourne, MD, FRCSC
Past Chair/Chief, Division of Orthopaedic Surgery, University Hospital, Western University, London, Ontario, Canada

Kevin Bozic, MD, MBA
Associate Professor and Vice Chair, Department of Orthopaedic Surgery, Core Faculty, Philip R. Lee Institute for Health Policy Studies, University of California, San Francisco, San Francisco, California

Karen K. Briggs, MPH
Steadman Philippon Research Institute, Vail, Colorado

Joel D. Bumgardner, PhD
Professor, Biomedical Engineering, University of Memphis; Professor, Department of Orthopaedic Surgery and Biomedical Engineering, University of Tennessee Health Science Center, Memphis, Tennessee

Dennis W. Burke, MD
Attending Orthopaedic Surgeon, Massachusetts General Hospital; Instructor in Orthopaedics, Harvard Medical School, Boston, Massachusetts

R. Stephen J. Burnett, MD, FRCS(C), Dipl ABOS
Division of Orthopaedic Surgery—Adult Reconstructive Surgery, Vancouver Island Health—South Island, Royal Jubilee Hospital, University of British Columbia Island Medical School, Victoria, British Columbia, Canada

J.W. Thomas Byrd, MD
Nashville Sports Medicine & Orthopaedic Center; Nashville Sports Medicine Foundation, Nashville, Tennessee

Miguel E. Cabanela, MD
Emeritus Professor of Orthopedics, College of Medicine, Orthopedic Surgery, Mayo Clinic, Rochester, Minnesota

John J. Callaghan, MD
Lawrence & Marilyn Dorr Chair, Orthopaedics & Rehabilitation, University of Iowa; Orthopaedics, VA Medical Center, Iowa City, Iowa

Patricia A. Campbell, PhD
Adjunct Professor, Orthopaedic Surgery, University of California, Los Angeles, Los Angeles, California

William N. Capello, MD
Professor Emeritus, Orthopaedic Surgery, Indiana University, Indianapolis, Indiana

Michael L. Caravelli, MD
Orthopaedic Surgeon, The Center for Orthopaedic and Neurosurgical Care and Research, Bend, Oregon

Aaron Carter, MD, MS
Research Fellow, Orthopaedics, The Rothman Institute, Philadelphia, Pennsylvania

Yeukkei Cheung, MD
Fellow, Department of Orthopaedic Surgery, University of California Davis Medical Center, Sacramento, California

Ian C. Clarke, PhD
Professor in Research, Director of Peterson Tribology Laboratory, Department of Orthopedics, Loma Linda University Medical Center, Loma Linda; Co-Director, DARF Retrieval Center, Colton, California

John Clohisy, MD
Daniel C. and Betty B. Viehmann Distinguished Professor of Orthopaedic Surgery, Department of Orthopaedic Surgery, Washington University School of Medicine, St. Louis, Missouri

Adam M.M. Cohen, MBBS, FRCS (Tr & Orth), MSc (Orth Eng), Dipl (Tr & Orth)
Consultant Orthopaedic Surgeon, The James Paget University Hospital (lead clinician) and Spire Norwich Hospital, Norfolk, United Kingdom

Clifford W. Colwell, Jr., MD
Clinical Professor of Orthopaedic Surgery and Rehabilitation, University of California, San Diego, San Diego, California; Medical Director, Shiley Center for Orthopaedic Research and Education at Scripps Clinic, Orthopaedic Surgeon, Scripps Clinic, La Jolla, California

Ryan Cordry, DO
Orthopedic Surgeon, OrthoSports Associates, Birmingham, Alabama; Adult Reconstruction Fellow, Orthopedic Surgery, University of California, San Diego, San Diego, California

Kristoff Corten, MD
Young Adult Hip Unit and Reconstructive Surgery of the Hip, Orthopaedic Department, University Hospital Leuven, Leuven, Belgium

Michael B. Cross, MD
Orthopaedic Surgery Resident, Hospital for Special Surgery, New York, New York

James A. D'Antonio, MD
Associate Professor of Orthopaedic Surgery, University of Pittsburgh, Pittsburgh, Pennsylvania

Darin Davidson, MD, MHSc, FRCSC
Assistant Professor, Department of Orthopaedics and Sports Medicine, University of Washington, Seattle, Washington

Craig J. Della Valle, MD
Associate Professor, Orthopaedic Surgery, Rush University Medical Center, Chicago, Illinois

Douglas A. Dennis, MD
Adjunct Professor, Department of Biomedical Engineering, University of Tennessee, Knoxville, Tennessee; Adjunct Professor of Bioengineering, University of Denver; Director, Rocky Mountain Musculoskeletal Research Laboratory, Denver, Colorado

Paul E. Di Cesare, MD
Professor, Department of Orthopaedic Surgery, University of California, Davis Medical Center, Sacramento, California

Lawrence D. Dorr, MD
Director, Arthritis Institute, Los Angeles, California

Georg N. Duda, PhD
Professor Doctor, Julius Wolff Institute of Biomechanics and Musculoskeletal Regeneration, Charité-Universitätsmedizin Berlin; Center for Musculoskeletal Surgery, Charité-Universitätsmedizin Berlin; Director of the Berlin-Brandenburg Center for Regenerative Therapies and Spokesperson of the Berlin-Brandenburg School for Regenerative Therapies; Center for Sports Science and Sports Medicine Berlin, Berlin, Germany

Michael J. Dunbar, MD, FRCSC, PhD
Professor of Surgery, Dalhousie University; Professor of Biomedical Engineering, Dalhousie University; Professor of Community Health and Epidemiology, Dalhousie University; Adult Reconstruction Surgeon, QE II Health Sciences Centre; Director of Orthopaedic Research, Dalhousie University, Halifax, Nova Scotia, Canada

Clive P. Duncan, MD, MSc, FRCSC
Professor and Emeritus Chair, Department of Orthopaedic Surgery, University of British Columbia; Consultant and Emeritus Chair, Department of Orthopaedic Surgery, Vancouver General and University Hospitals, Vancouver, British Columbia, Canada

C. Anderson Engh, Jr., MD
Orthopaedic Surgeon, Anderson Orthopaedic Research Institute, Alexandria, Virginia

Charles A. Engh, Sr., MD
Orthopaedic Surgeon, Anderson Orthopaedic Research Institute, Alexandria, Virginia

Thomas Fehring, MD
OrthoCarolina Hip and Knee Center, Charlotte, North Carolina

Stephen Ferguson, PhD
M. E. Müller Institute for Surgical Technology and Biomechanics, University of Bern, Bern, Switzerland

John Fisher, CBE, PhD, DEng
Professor, Director, Institute of Medical and Biological Engineering, Centre of Excellence in Medical Engineering, WELMEC, University of Leeds; Co-Director, NIHR Leeds Musculoskeletal Biomedical Research Unit, Leeds Teaching Hospital Trust; NIHR, National Institute of Health Research Senior Investigator, Leeds, United Kingdom

Steven J. Fitzgerald, MD
Assistant Professor, Department of Orthopaedic Surgery, University Hospitals, Case Medical Center, Case Western Reserve University, Cleveland, Ohio

Bruno Fuchs, MD, PhD
Professor of Orthopedics, Director of the Sarcoma Service, University of Zurich, Zurich, Switzerland

Rajiv Gandhi, MD, MS, FRCSC
Assistant Professor, Division of Orthopedic Surgery, University of Toronto, Toronto, Ontario, Canada

Donald S. Garbuz, MD, MHSc, FRCSC
Associate Professor and Head, Division of Lower Limb Reconstruction and Oncology, Department of Orthopaedics, University of British Columbia, Vancouver, British Columbia, Canada

Kevin L. Garvin, MD
Professor and Chair, Department of Orthopaedic Surgery & Rehabilitation, University of Nebraska Medical Center, Omaha, Nebraska

Jeffrey A. Geller, MD
Associate Professor of Orthopedic Surgery, Associate Chief, Division of Hip & Knee Reconstruction, Director, Research Fellowship, Center for Hip & Knee Replacements, Department of Orthopedic Surgery, Columbia University Medical Center, New York, New York

Graham A. Gie, MBChB, FRCS (Ed), FRCSEd (Orth)
Emeritus Consultant Orthopaedic Surgeon, Exeter Hip Unit, Princess Elizabeth Orthopaedic Centre, Exeter, Devon, United Kingdom

Christopher R. Gooding, BSc, MD, FRCS (Tr & Orth)
Fellow in Lower Limb Reconstructive Orthopaedic Surgery, Department of Orthopaedic Surgery, University of British Columbia, Vancouver, British Columbia, Canada

Stuart Goodman, MD, PhD, FRCSC, FACS, FBSE
Ellenburg Professor of Surgery and (by courtesy) Bioengineering, Attending Orthopaedic Surgeon, Stanford University Medical Center, Fellowship Director, Adult Reconstruction, Department of Orthopaedic Surgery, Stanford University, Affiliated Faculty, Department of Biomechanical Engineering, Stanford University; Consultant Orthopaedic Surgeon, Lucile Salter Packard Children's Hospital at Stanford, Stanford, California

William L. Griffin, MD
OrthoCarolina Hip and Knee Center, Charlotte, North Carolina

Allan E. Gross, MD, FRCSC, O Ont
Division of Orthopaedic Surgery, Mount Sinai Hospital; Professor of Surgery, Faculty of Medicine, University of Toronto, Toronto, Ontario, Canada

Sandor Gyomorey, MD, MSc, FRCSC
Associate Staff, Orthopaedic Surgery, William Osler Health Center, Etobicoke General Hospital, Toronto, Ontario, Canada

Fares S. Haddad, BSc, MCh (Orth), FRCS (Orth), FFSEM
Professor of Orthopaedic Surgery, Divisional Clinical Director—Surgical Specialties, University College Hospital; Professor of Orthopaedic Surgery, Director—Institute of Sport, Exercise, and Health, Division of Surgery and Interventional Science, University College London, London, United Kingdom

Warren O. Haggard, PhD
Professor, Biomedical Engineering, University of Memphis; Professor, Department of Orthopaedic Surgery and Biomedical Engineering, University of Tennessee Health Science Center, Memphis, Tennessee

George Haidukewych, MD
Professor of Orthopedic Surgery, University of Central Florida; Co-Director of Orthopedic Trauma, Chief of Complex Adult Reconstruction, Orlando Health, Orlando, Florida

Armin Aalami Harandi
Orthopedic Surgeon, Otsego Memorial Hospital, Gaylord, Michigan

Markus O.W. Heller, PhD
Doctor, Julius Wolff Institute of Biomechanics and Musculoskeletal Regeneration, Charité-Universitätsmedizin Berlin; Center for Musculoskeletal Surgery, Charité-Universitätsmedizin Berlin; Center for Sports Science and Sports Medicine Berlin, Berlin, Germany

Terese T. Horlocker, MD
Professor of Anesthesiology and Orthopedics, Mayo Clinic, Rochester, Minnesota

Francis J. Hornicek, MD, PhD
Chief, Orthopaedic Oncology Service, Co-Director, Center for Sarcoma and Connective Tissue Oncology, Massachusetts General Hospital; Director, Stephan L. Harris Chordoma Center; Associate Professor, Harvard Medical School; Co-Leader, Dana Farber/Harvard Cancer Center Sarcoma Program, Boston, Massachusetts

Jonathan R. Howell, MBBS, MSc, FRCS (Tr & Orth)
Consultant Orthopaedic Surgeon, Exeter Hip Unit, Princess Elizabeth Orthopaedic Centre, Exeter, Devon, United Kingdom

William J. Hozack, MD
Professor, Rothman Institute; Medical Doctor, Thomas Jefferson University Hospital, Philadelphia, Pennsylvania

Matthew J.W. Hubble, FRCSI, FRCS (Tr & Orth)
Consultant Orthopaedic Surgeon, Exeter Hip Unit, Princess Elizabeth Orthopaedic Centre, Exeter, Devon, United Kingdom

James I. Huddleston III, MD
Assistant Professor, Department of Orthopaedic Surgery, Stanford University School of Medicine; Director, Center for Joint Replacement, Stanford University Medical Center, Stanford, California

Devyani Hunt, MD
Assistant Professor, Section of Physical Medicine and Rehabilitation, Department of Orthopaedic Surgery, Washington University School of Medicine, St. Louis, Missouri

Michael H. Huo, MD
Professor of Orthopedic Surgery, University of Texas Southwestern Medical Center, Dallas, Texas

Conor J. Hurson, MB, BCh, MCh, FRCSI (Trauma & Orth)
Fellow in Lower Limb Reconstructive Surgery, QE II Health Sciences Centre, Halifax, Nova Scotia, Canada

Stephen J. Incavo, MD
Professor of Clinical Orthopaedic Surgery, Weill Cornell College of Medicine, New York, New York; Section Chief Adult Reconstructive Surgery, The Methodist Hospital, Methodist Center for Orthopaedic Surgery, Houston, Texas

Richard Iorio, MD
Senior Attending Orthopaedic Surgeon, Director of Adult Reconstruction, Department of Orthopaedic Surgery, Lahey Clinic, Burlington; Professor of Orthopaedic Surgery, Department of Orthopaedic Surgery, Boston University School of Medicine, Boston, Massachusetts

J. Benjamin Jackson III, MD
Chief Resident, Department of Orthopaedic Surgery, Carolinas Medical Center, Charlotte, North Carolina

William A. Jiranek, MD
Professor of Orthopaedics; Chief of Adult Reconstruction, Department of Orthopaedic Surgery, Virginia Commonwealth University Health System, Richmond, Virginia

Derek R. Johnson, MD
Denver-Vail Orthopedics PC; Director of Joint Replacement, Parker Adventist Hospital; Assistant Clinical Professor of Surgery, Rocky Vista University College of Osteopathic Medicine, Parker; Adjunct Associate Professor of Bioengineering, University of Denver, Denver, Colorado

Deanne T. Kashiwagi, MD
Consultant, Hospital Internal Medicine, Mayo Clinic, Rochester, Minnesota

Joseph J. Kavolus, BA
Medical Student, Medical University of South Carolina, Charleston, South Carolina

E. Michael Keating, MD
Center for Hip and Knee Surgery, Mooresville, Indiana

James Keeney, MD
Assistant Professor, Department of Orthopaedic Surgery, Washington University School of Medicine, St. Louis, Missouri

A. Scott Keller, MD, MS
Assistant Professor, Division of Hospital Medicine, Mayo Clinic, Rochester, Minnesota

Catherine F. Kellett, BSc, BM, BCh, FRCS (Tr & Orth)
Consultant Orthopaedic Surgeon, Golden Jubilee National Hospital, Glasgow, United Kingdom

Saurabh Khakharia, MD, DNB, FICS
Clinical Fellow, Adult Reconstruction, Virginia Commonwealth University, Richmond, Virginia

Harry Kim, MD, MS
Director of Research, Texas Scottish Rite Hospital for Children; Associate Professor, Department of Orthopedic Surgery, University of Texas Southwestern Medical Center, Dallas, Texas

Raymond H. Kim, MD
Adjunct Associate Professor of Bioengineering, Department of Mechanical and Materials Engineering, University of Denver; Colorado Joint Replacement, Porter Center for Joint Replacement; Co-Director Rocky Mountain Musculoskeletal Research Laboratory, Denver, Colorado

Young-Jo Kim, MD, PhD
Associate Professor of Orthopaedic Surgery, Orthopaedic Surgery, Children's Hospital-Boston, Boston, Massachusetts

Gregg R. Klein, MD
Vice Chairman, Department of Orthopaedic Surgery, Hackensack University Medical Center, Hackensack; Hartzband Center for Hip and Knee Replacement, Paramus, New Jersey

Christian König, PhD
Doctor, Julius Wolff Institute of Biomechanics and Musculoskeletal Regeneration, Charité-Universitätsmedizin Berlin; Center for Musculoskeletal Surgery, Charité-Universitätsmedizin Berlin; Center for Sports Science and Sports Medicine Berlin, Berlin, Germany

Sandra L. Kopp, MD
Assistant Professor, Department of Anesthesiology, Mayo Clinic, Rochester, Minnesota

Kenneth J. Koval, MD
Professor, Department of Orthopaedics, Orlando Regional Medical Center, Orlando, Florida

Philip J. Kregor
Director, Hip and Fracture Institute-Nashville, Nashville, Tennessee

Richard F. Kyle, MD
Professor, Orthopedic Surgery, University of Minnesota; Chair, Department of Orthopaedic Surgery, Hennepin County Medical Center, Minneapolis, Minnesota

Brent A. Lanting, BESc, MD, FRSCS
Assistant Professor, Orthopaedic Surgery, London Health Sciences Center, London, Ontario, Canada

Brian Larkin, MD
Orthopaedic Surgeon, Orthopedic Associates, Denver, Colorado

Michel P. Laurent, PhD, MS
Scientist, Department of Orthopedic Surgery, Rush University Medical Center, Chicago, Illinois

Paul Tee Hui Lee, MB, MA, FRCS (Eng), FRCS (Trauma & Orth)
Consultant Trauma and Orthopaedic Surgeon, Barts and the London NHS Trust, London, United Kingdom

Michael Leunig, MD, PD
Head of Orthopaedics, Department Orthopaedics Surgery, Schulthess Klinik, Zürich, Switzerland

David G. Lewallen
Professor, Mayo Clinic College of Medicine, Consultant, Department of Orthopedic Surgery, Mayo Clinic, Rochester, Minnesota

Stephen Li, PhD
President, Medical Device Testing and Innovations, LLC; Biomedical Materials Consultant, Sarasota, Florida

Adolph V. Lombardi, Jr., MD, FACS
Clinical Assistant Professor, Department of Orthopaedics, Department of Biomedical Engineering, The Ohio State University, Columbus; Senior Associate, Joint Implant Surgeons, Inc.; Attending Surgeon, Mount Carmel Health System, New Albany, Ohio

Thuan V. Ly, MD
Assistant Professor, Department of Orthopaedic Surgery—Regions Hospital, University of Minnesota, Minneapolis, Minnesota

Ting Ma, MD MSc
Stanford University School of Medicine; Stanford, California

Tad M. Mabry, MD
Assistant Professor of Orthopedic Surgery, Department of Orthopedic Surgery, Mayo Clinic, Rochester, Minnesota

Steven J. MacDonald, MD, FRCSC
Professor of Orthopaedic Surgery, University of Western Ontario; Chief of Orthopaedics & Chief of Surgery, University Hospital, London, Ontario, Canada

Nizar Mahomed, MD, ScD, FRCSC
Nicki and Bryce Douglas Chair in Orthopaedic Surgery, Smith and Nephew Chair in Orthopaedic Surgery, Professor, Department of Surgery, University of Toronto; Head, Division of Orthopaedics, Director, Arthritis Program, Managing Director, Altum Health, Toronto Western Hospital, Toronto, Ontario, Canada

Henrik Malchau, MD, PhD
Professor, Harvard Medical School; Co-Director, Harris Orthopaedic Laboratory, Vice Chief of Orthopedics (Research), Attending Physician Adult Reconstructive Unit, Department of Orthopedics, Massachusetts General Hospital, Massachusetts General Hospital, Boston, Massachusetts

William J. Maloney, MD
Professor and Chairman, Department of Orthopaedic Surgery, Stanford University School of Medicine, Stanford, California

Carlos B. Mantilla, MD, PhD
Associate Professor, Anesthesiology and Physiology, College of Medicine, Consultant, Department of Anesthesiology, Mayo Clinic, Rochester, Minnesota

David R. Marker, MD
Radiology Resident, Department of Radiology, The Johns Hopkins Hospital, Baltimore, Maryland

Hal David Martin, DO
Sports Medicine and Hip Disorders Specialist, Orthopaedic Surgeon, The Hip Clinic, Oklahoma Sports Science and Orthopaedics; Research Director, Oklahoma Musculoskeletal Research Center, Oklahoma City, Oklahoma

Contributors

Thomas G. Mason, MD
Rheumatology, Mayo Clinic, Rochester, Minnesota

John L. Masonis, MD
OrthoCarolina Hip & Knee Center, OrthoCarolina; Adult Hip and Knee Reconstruction, Department of Orthopaedic Surgery Residency Program, Carolinas Medical Center, Charlotte, North Carolina

Bassam A. Masri, MD, FRCSC
Professor and Chairman, Department of Orthopaedics, University of British Columbia; Head of Orthopaedics and Surgeon-in-Chief, Vancouver Acute Health Services, Vancouver, British Columbia, Canada

Wadih Y. Matar, MD, MSc, FRCSC
Adult Reconstruction Fellow, Rothman Institute; Adult Reconstruction Fellow, Thomas Jefferson University Hospital, Philadelphia, Pennsylvania

Robert E. Mayle, Jr., MD
Resident, Department of Orthopaedics, Stanford University Medical Center, Stanford, California

Edward F. McCarthy
Professor of Pathology Professor of Orthopaedic Surgery, Department of Pathology, The Johns Hopkins Medical Institutions, Baltimore, Maryland

Brian J. McGrory, MD, MS
Clinical Associate Professor, Orthopaedic Surgery and Rehabilitation, University of Vermont School of Medicine, Burlington, Vermont; Co-Director, Maine Joint Replacement Institute; Director, Joint Replacement Center, Division of Orthopaedics, Maine Medical Center, Portland, Maine

R. Michael Meneghini, MD
Director of Joint Replacement, Indiana University Health Saxony Hospital; Assistant Professor of Clinical Orthopaedic Surgery, Department of Orthopaedic Surgery, Indiana University School of Medicine, Indianapolis, Indiana

Andrew M. Michael, MD
Rush University Medical Center, Chicago, Illinois

Michael A. Mont, MD
Director, Center for Joint Preservation and Replacement, Rubin Institute for Advanced Orthopedics, Sinai Hospital of Baltimore, Baltimore, Maryland

Michael J. Morris, MD
Associate, Joint Implant Surgeons, Inc., New Albany, Ohio

Bryan Nestor, MD
Associate Professor, Orthopaedics, Hospital for Special Surgery; Associate Professor Clinical Orthpaedics, Orthopaedics, Weill Cornell Medical College, New York, New York

Philip C. Noble, PhD
John S. Dunn Professor of Orthopedic Research, Center for Orthopedic Surgery, The Methodist Hospital; Professor, Joseph Barnhart Department of Orthopedic Surgery, Baylor College of Medicine; Director of Research, Institute of Orthopedic Research and Education, Houston, Texas

Philip A. O'Connor, M. Med. Sci., FRCSI (Tr & Orth)
Clinical Fellow, University of Western Ontario, London, Ontario, Canada

Douglas E. Padgett, MD
Chief, Adult Reconstruction, Hospital for Special Surgery, New York, New York

Mark W. Pagnano, MD
Professor of Orthopaedics, Consultant, Division of Adult Reconstruction, Department of Orthopaedic Surgery, Mayo College of Medicine, Rochester, Minnesota

Wayne G. Paprosky, MD
Associate Professor, Rush University Medical Center, Chicago, Illinois

Javad Parvizi, MD, FRCS
Professor, Vice Chair for Research, Orthopedic Surgery, Thomas Jefferson University, Philadelphia, Pennsylvania

Jay Patel, MD, MS
Resident, Orthopaedic Surgery, University of California, Irvine; Orthopaedic Surgeon, Orthopaedic Specialty Institute, Orange, California

Ronak M. Patel, MD
Department of Orthopaedic Surgery, Northwestern University Feinberg School of Medicine, Chicago, Illinois

Vincent Pellegrini, Jr., MD
James L. Kernan Professor and Chair, Department of Orthopaedics, University of Maryland School of Medicine, Baltimore, Maryland

Carsten Perka, MD
Professor of Orthopedic Surgery, Center for Musculoskeletal Surgery, Department of Orthopedics, Charité-Universitätsmedizin Berlin, Berlin Free and Humboldt-University of Berlin, Berlin, Germany

Giuseppe Pezzotti, PhD
Professor, Ceramic Physics, Kyoto Institute of Technology, Kyoto; Invited Professor, The Center for Advanced Medical Engineering and Informatics, Osaka University, Osaka, Japan; Adjunct Professor, Orthopaedic Research Center, Department of Orthopaedics, Loma Linda University, Loma Linda, California

Marc Philippon, MD
Steadman Philippon Research Institute, Vail, Colorado; Clinical Associate Professor, Department of Surgery, McMaster University, Hamilton, Canada; Adjunct Clinical Associate Professor, Department of Orthopaedic Surgery, University of Pittsburgh Medical Center, Pittsburgh, Pennsylvania

Trevor R. Pickering, MD, MA
Orthopaedic Surgeon, Mississippi Sports Medicine and Orthopaedic Center, Jackson, Mississippi

Robert M. Pilliar, BASc, PhD
Professor Emeritus, Faculty of Dentistry and Institute of Biomaterials & Biomedical Engineering, University of Toronto, Toronto, Ontario, Canada

Heidi Prather, DO
Associate Professor, Section of Physical Medicine and Rehabilitation, Department of Orthopaedic Surgery, Washington University School of Medicine, St. Louis, Missouri

Kawan S. Rakhra, MD
Assistant Professor, Radiology, University of Ottawa; Musculoskeletal Radiologist, Department of Medical Imaging, The Ottawa Hospital, Ottawa, Ontario, Canada

Michael D. Ries, MD
Professor of Orthopaedic Surgery, Chief of Arthroplasty, University of California, San Francisco, San Francisco, California

Andrew W. Ritting, MD
Resident, Department of Orthopaedics, University of Connecticut Health Center, Farmington, Connecticut

Randy Rizek, MD
Resident, Division of Orthopaedics, University of Toronto, Toronto, Ontario, Canada

Peter S. Rose, MD
Assistant Professor, Mayo Clinic College of Medicine, Consultant Surgeon, Musculoskeletal Oncology Fellowship Director, Mayo Clinic, Rochester, Minnesota

Oleg A. Safir, MD, MEd, FRCS(C)
Assistant Professor, Department of Surgery, University of Toronto, Mount Sinai Hospital, Toronto, Ontario, Canada

Richard Santore, MD
Clinical Professor, Orthopaedic Surgery, University of California, San Diego; Senior Orthopaedic Surgeon, Orthopaedic Surgery, Sharp Memorial Hospital, San Diego, California

Thierry Scheerlinck, MD, PhD
Professor of Orthopaedic Surgery and Traumatology, Vrije Universiteit Brussel; Professor and Head of Department, Department of Orthopaedic Surgery and Traumatology, Universitair Ziekenhuis Brussel, Brussels, Belgium

Thomas P. Schmalzried, MD
Medical Director, Joint Replacement Institute, Los Angeles, California; Physician Specialist, Harbor-UCLA Medical Center, Torrance, Califonia

Andrew H. Schmidt, MD
Professor, Orthopedic Surgery, University of Minnesota; Faculty, Orthopedic Surgery, Hennepin County Medical Center, Minneapolis, Minnesota

Perry L. Schoenecker, MD
Professor of Orthopaedic Surgery, Department of Orthopaedic Surgery, St. Louis Shriners Hospital and St. Louis Children's Hospitals, Washington University School of Medicine, St. Louis, Missouri

Bruno G. Schroder e Souza, MD, MS
Former International Scholar in Hip Arthroscopy and Biomechanics, Steadman Philippon Research Institute, Vail, Colorado; Orthopaedic Surgeon, Hospital de Misericórdia de Santos Dumont, Santos Dumont; Orthopaedic Surgeon, Hospital Monte Sinai, Juiz de Fora, MG, Brazil

Joseph H. Schwab, MD, MS
Instructor, Orthopedic Surgery, Division of Orthopaedic Oncology, Division of Spine Surgery, Massachusetts General Hospital, Boston, Massachusetts

S. Andrew Sems, MD
Chair, Division of Orthopaedic Trauma Surgery, Assistant Professor, Orthopedic Surgery, Consultant, Department of Orthopaedic Surgery, Mayo Clinic, Rochester, Minnesota

Thorsten M. Seyler, MD
Physician Scientist, Department of Orthopaedic Surgery, Wake Forest University Health Sciences, Winston-Salem, North Carolina

Peter F. Sharkey, MD
Professor, Thomas Jefferson University Hospital, Philadelphia, Pennsylvania

Adnan M. Sheikh, MD
Assistant Professor, Radiology, University of Ottawa; Musculoskeletal Radiologist, Department of Medical Imaging, The Ottawa Hospital, Ottawa, Ontario, Canada

Neil P. Sheth, MD
Orthopaedic Surgery Resident, University of Pennsylvania, Philadelphia, Pennsylvania

Rafael J. Sierra, MD
Associate Professor, Consultant, Department of Orthopedic Surgery, Mayo Clinic, Rochester, Minnesota

Eric A. Silverstein, MD
Academic Director of Orthopaedic Surgery and Director of Musculoskeletal Oncology, Orthopedic Surgery, Orthopaedic Oncology, Musculoskeletal Oncology, Saint Francis Medical Group, Inc., Cancer Center, Hartford, Connecticut

Ernest L. Sink, MD
Associate Professor of Orthopedic Surgery, Co-Director, Center for Hip Preservation, Hospital for Special Surgery, Weill-Cornell Medical College, New York, New York

Mark J. Spangehl, BSc, MD
Assistant Professor of Orthopaedic Surgery, Mayo Clinic College of Medicine, Mayo Clinic Arizona, Phoenix, Arizona

Scott M. Sporer, MD, MS
Associate Professor, Orthopaedic Surgery, Rush University Medical Center, Chicago; Attending Physician, Orthopaedic Surgery, Central Dupage Hospital, Winfield, Illinois

Bryan P. Springer, MD
OrthoCarolina Hip and Knee Center, Charlotte, North Carolina

Drew N. Stal
Research Fellow, Institute of Orthopedic Research and Education, Houston, Texas

Anthony A. Stans, MD
Chair, Division Pediatric Orthopedics, Department of Orthopedic Surgery, Mayo Clinic, Rochester, Minnesota

S. David Stulberg, MD
Professor of Clinical Orthopaedic Surgery, Orthopaedic Surgery, Northwestern University Feinberg School of Medicine; Director, Joint Reconstruction and Implant Service, Northwestern Memorial Hospital; Co-Founder and Co-Director, Northwestern Arthritis and Rehabilitation Institute; Director, Northwestern Orthopaedic Institute, Chicago, Illinois

Daniel J. Sucato, MD, MS
Staff Orthopaedic Surgeon, Orthopaedics, Director— Sarah M. and Charles Seay/Martha and Pat Beard Center of Excellence in Spine Research, Texas Scottish Rite Hospital for Children; Associate Professor— Department of Orthopaedic Surgery, Orthopaedics, University of Texas Southwestern Medical Center, Dallas, Texas

Nobuhiko Sugano, MD, PhD
Professor, Department of Orthopaedic Medical Engineering, Osaka University Graduate School of Medicine, Osaka, Japan

Dale R. Sumner, PhD
Mary Lou Bell McGrew Presidential Professor for Medical Research and Chair, Department of Anatomy & Cell Biology, Rush University Medical Center, Chicago, Illinois

Megan A. Swanson, MD
Orthopaedic Surgeon, Randolph Hospital, Asheboro, North Carolina

Marc F. Swiontkowski, MD
Professor, Department of Orthopaedic Surgery, University of Minnesota, Minneapolis, Minnesota

Khalid Syed, MD
Staff Orthopaedic Surgeon, University Health Network, Toronto, Canada

Karren Takamura, BA
Medical Student, David Geffen School of Medicine at University of California, Los Angeles, Los Angeles, California

Oliver O. Tannous, MD
Resident, Department of Orthopaedics, University of Maryland School of Medicine, Baltimore, Maryland

Dylan Tanzer, DEC
Jo Miller Orthopaedic Research Lab, Division of Orthopaedic Surgery, McGill University, Montreal, Quebec, Canada

Michael Tanzer, MD, FRCSC
Professor of Surgery, McGill University; Vice Chair (Clinical) Department of Surgery and Jo Miller Chair, Division of Orthopaedic Surgery, McGill University, Montreal, Quebec, Canada

Rupesh Tarwala, MD
Adult Reconstruction Fellow, Lenox Hill Hospital, New York, New York

Michael J. Taunton, MD
Clinical Instructor, Mayo Clinic College of Medicine, Department of Orthopedic Surgery, Mayo Clinic, Rochester, Minnesota Department of Orthopedic Surgery, Mayo Clinic, Rochester, Minnesota

Christi J. Sychterz Terefenko, MS
Orthopaedic Research Consultant, Arthritis & Joint Replacement Center of Reading, Wyomissing, Pennsylvania

John F. Tilzey, MD, PhD
Assistant Professor Orthopaedic Surgery, Orthopaedic Surgery, Lahey Clinic, Burlington, Massachusetts

Andrew J. Timperley, MB, ChB, FRCS (Ed), D Phil (Oxon)
Consultant Orthopaedic Surgeon, Exeter Hip Unit, Princess Elizabeth Orthopaedic Centre, Exeter, Devon, United Kingdom

Stephan Tohtz, MD
Center for Musculoskeletal Surgery, Charité-Universitätsmedizin Berlin, Berlin, Germany

Robert T. Trousdale, MD
Chairman, Division of Adult Reconstruction, Department of Orthopedic Surgery; Professor of Orthopedics, Mayo School of Graduate Medical Education, Rochester, Minnesota

Thomas Parker Vail, MD
Professor and Chairman, Department of Orthopaedic Surgery, University of California, San Francisco, San Francisco, California

Jean-Pierre Vidalain, MD
Surgeon, Executive Secretary, Artro Group Institute, Orthopaedic Surgery, Annecy, France

Amarjit S. Virdi, PhD
Associate Professor, Anatomy & Cell Biology and Orthopedic Surgery, Rush University Medical Center, Chicago, Illinois

Elizabeth Weber, MD, MS
Assistant Professor, Orthopaedic Surgery, University of Connecticut School of Medicine; Orthopaedic Surgery, Connecticut Children's Medical Center, Hartford, Connecticut

Sarah L. Whitehouse, PhD
Senior Research Fellow/Biostatistician, Orthopaedic Research Unit, Institute of Health and Biomedical Innovation, Queensland University of Technology, The Prince Charles Hospital, Brisbane, Australia

Daniel H. Williams, MBBCh, MSc, FRCS (Tr & Orth)
Consultant Orthopaedic Surgeon, Royal Cornwall Hospital, Truro, United Kingdom

Sophie Williams, PhD
Senior Lecturer, Institute of Medical and Biological Engineering School of Mechanical Engineering, University of Leeds, Leeds, United Kingdom

Matthew J. Wilson, MBBS, FRCS (Tr & Orth)
Consultant Orthopaedic Surgeon, Exeter Hip Unit, Princess Elizabeth Orthopaedic Centre, Exeter, Devon, United Kingdom

Markus A. Wimmer, PhD, Dipl Ing
Associate Professor, Director—Section of Tribology, Orthopedic Surgery, Rush University Medical Center, Chicago, Illinois

Geoffrey Wright, MD
Bone and Joint, Sports Medicine Institute, Naval Medical Center Portsmouth, Portsmouth, Virginia; Assistant Professor, Uniformed Services University of the Health Sciences, Bethesda, Maryland

Ira Zaltz, MD
Pediatric Orthopaedics Surgery, William Beaumont Hospital, Royal Oak; Senior Staff, Department of Orthopaedic Surgery, Henry Ford Health Systems, Detroit, Michigan

Adam Zierenberg, MD
Fellow, Physical Medicine and Rehabilitation, Orthopaedic Surgery, Washington University School of Medicine, St. Louis, Missouri; Physical Medicine and Rehabilitation, Providence St. Mary Medical Center, Walla Walla, Washington

Michael G. Zywiel, MD
Division of Orthopaedic Surgery, University of Toronto, Toronto, Ontario, Canada

Foreword

Hip surgery is one of the best examples of the explosion of knowledge and technology that has occurred in the past 30 years. However, the progress has not been linear. As in all fields of human endeavor, some missteps and backward steps have been taken, but I think it is fair to say that this field has reached a certain level of maturity. The book you have in your hands is a superb compilation of established practices and the latest advances in the field of hip surgery.

Meant as a companion to the classic *Insall and Scott Surgery of the Knee*, this book covers in 12 parts and 107 chapters the entire realm of hip surgery from cradle to grave and from laboratory bench to operating room. The editors, Drs. Berry and Lieberman, have assembled a cadre of experts that reads like a Who's Who in the world of hip surgery. Obviously, arthroplasty, the "queen" of all hip operative procedures, is given extraordinary coverage, and the reader should be able to find here answers to any questions that may be posed about routine or unique special primary procedures, as well as complications of arthroplasty and revision surgery. The hip surgeon today must have reasonable knowledge of biomechanics and biomaterials; both are covered in the first part of the book. The increasingly popular area of nonarthroplasty, so-called *conservative hip preservation surgery,* is given ample attention. Sections on anatomy, operative approaches, and perioperative management include the classic information along with the latest topics related to surgical approaches, anesthesia, and pain management. Sections on traumatic, pediatric, and tumorous disorders are also included.

Given its content and its visually appealing format, this book is destined to become a classic in the overcrowded field of hip surgery textbooks. Those interested in the hip will be enriched by reading it and will gain a greater appreciation of many of the evolving topics. The editors and their authors should be congratulated for their efforts on behalf of so many of us.

Miguel E. Cabanela, MD
Emeritus Professor
Department of Orthopedic Surgery
Mayo Clinic
Past President Hip Society
President International Hip Society

Preface

Hip surgery continues to evolve as a discipline. Although many of our procedures are established and successful, some are still in their infancy, and in other areas, further work clearly needs to be done. This text is divided into six sections and provides the reader with a comprehensive review of all aspects of the hip. The basic science section of this book explains how our enhanced understanding of tribology, the body's response to wear debris, and advances in material science have had a major impact on hip surgery. Although anatomy clearly has not changed, our development of new operative approaches has continued to evolve and has caught the attention of the public over the past 10 years. Perioperative management has undergone a true revolution, and many of our hip procedures today can be done with decreased discomfort for our patients and with less morbidity and recovery time. Advanced imaging techniques have transformed our ability to make accurate diagnoses and have facilitated our execution of surgical procedures. Pediatric hip surgery has benefited from long-term follow-up of well-known procedures and the implementation of new interventions. Hip surgery for trauma has seen an evolution in the use of fixation devices for proximal femoral fractures and the development of advanced fixation techniques in both the acetabulum and the pelvis. Oncologic surgery around the hip continues to consist of some of the most challenging procedures in orthopedic surgery and has benefited from advances with respect to imaging and new surgical techniques. Hip preservation surgery has exploded as a discipline unto itself. Our improved understanding of femoral acetabular impingement and the successful adoption of hip arthroscopy have revolutionized care of the nonarthroplasty patient. Hip arthroplasty has attained a high level of success with respect to longevity and durability and has benefited from continued advances in surgical technique, materials, and perioperative management. Revision total hip arthroplasty has become far more reliable over the past two decades, and our ability to solve difficult bone loss problems has clearly advanced. Finally, our proficiency in preventing and successfully managing complications related to hip surgery continues to improve.

However, in the midst of all these advances, hip surgeons have experienced the disconcerting realization that in an era in which our patients want us to implement new technology, not everything new may benefit our patients. The problems with metal-on-metal bearings and increased complication rates associated with some minimally invasive operative approaches are cautionary tales.

This book benefits from being a sister publication to the well-established and successful text, *Insall Scott's Surgery of the Knee*, which is now in its sixth edition. This book, which would not be possible without the tremendous academic community of hip surgeons who have made hip surgery one of the premier academic disciplines in all of orthopedic surgery, has been designed to take advantage of advances in electronic technology and information access. For selected procedures, illustrated videos are available. Owners of the book have access to its entire contents—in searchable form—on the Internet. It is our hope that this text will be of value to established practitioners who continue to seek the latest information related to hip surgery from experts in the field. This book also has also been written for those in training who require comprehensive exposure to hip surgery or just knowledge related to a specific area of this subspecialty of orthopedic surgery. On behalf of all section editors and authors, it is our hope that you and your patients will benefit from your reading and using of this text.

Daniel J. Berry
Jay R. Lieberman

Acknowledgments

A book of this scope requires the collective work of many individuals. First, we would like to thank the section editors and authors for sharing their time, expertise, and insights in creating this comprehensive textbook. We are incredibly fortunate to have a terrific staff—Karen Fasbender, Norma Mundt, and Erika Ivanov—all of whom spent a great amount of time editing and collating the contents of this book and corresponding with the publisher and authors.

We are indebted to Ann Ruzycka Anderson and Rachel E. McMullen for their constant efforts to provide a text of the highest quality and to keep a project of this size on task. We appreciate the efforts and vision of Dan Pepper and Don Scholz, who have overseen the project and provided the resources needed to make this a first-rate publication.

Finally, we are most grateful to our families, who provide us with tremendous support and grant us time to participate in these projects.

Contents

Contents

Contents

SECTION I

BASIC SCIENCE

CHAPTER 1

Biomechanics of the Natural Hip Joint

Drew N. Stal, Stephen Ferguson,
Stephen J. Incavo, and Philip C. Noble

KEY POINTS

- The physiologic range of motion (ROM) of the hip is affected by numerous morphologic and soft tissue factors that are not well understood. Clearly, systemic factors such as age and joint degeneration impair motion, but ethnicity, gender, and culture are also important as remodeling changes occur over time to accommodate the demands of customary activities of daily living (ADLs).
- The acetabular labrum plays a vital role in the function and lubrication of the hip. Because of its role as a mechanical seal, the labrum restricts the egress of synovial fluid from the joint under load. However, it is not known whether this normal physiologic mechanism is restored after labral resection and refixation, although clinical results of this procedure are superior to those of resection alone.
- Bony deformities of the proximal femur and acetabular margin have a dramatic impact on ROM of the hip and are implicated in the occurrence of coxarthrosis secondary to impingement. Many dysmorphic conditions can cause loss of abduction and a marked reduction in internal rotation of the hip in flexion. These conditions include SCFE, reduced femoral and acetabular anteversion, increased acetabular coverage, and asphericity of the femoral head. In active individuals, this may lead to pathologic changes at the labral-chondral junction and articular degeneration; however, the connection between morphologic abnormalities and coxarthrosis remains controversial.
- Instrumented prostheses and three-dimensional computer models play an essential role in measuring hip-joint reaction forces, especially during gait and stair climbing. During normal activities, the peak value of the joint force averages 2.1 to 5.5 body weight (BW), and they may reach values in excess of 8 BW during accidental stumbling.
- In normal hips, the distribution of contact pressure has shown to be almost even over the joint surface, whereas in the dysplastic hip joint, pressure is concentrated on the anterolateral edge of the acetabulum. Peak contact pressures for dysplastic and asymptomatic hips range from approximately 3 to 10 MPa.

INTRODUCTION

The hip joint plays a significant role in the human osteo-articular system, both in terms of locomotion and as a load-bearing joint for the torso by transmitting weight to different areas of the pelvis.[1,2] In an effort to improve the diagnosis and treatment of various pathologic and structural abnormalities of the hip, it is essential to acquire a basic understanding of hip biomechanics. This includes the anatomy of the hip joint, its normal range of motion (ROM), and the function of the hip musculature during gait.

Advances in this field have included the development of more effective methods of evaluating joint function and understanding pathologic conditions, the scientific investigation of alternative surgical approaches for hip reconstruction, and the development of methods for measuring joint forces and moments developed in vivo. In addition, the application of biomechanical principles has helped shed new light on dysmorphic conditions compromising normal hip motion, whether they stem from acquired abnormalities (e.g., post-traumatic deformities, Perthes disease, slipped capital femoral epiphysis [SCFE]), developmental abnormalities (e.g., congenital dysplasia of the hip [CDH], developmental dysplasia of the hip [DDH]), or abnormalities of unknown origin (e.g. cam deformity of the femoral head–neck junction, and pincer deformities of the acetabular margin). Ongoing investigations of the biomechanics of the capsule, labrum, and femoroacetabular impingement (FAI) hold the promise of revealing the underlying mechanism of "idiopathic" coxarthrosis.

KINEMATICS OF THE NORMAL AND DISEASED HIP

Any review of the biomechanics of the hip should address both the kinematics and the kinetics of normal hip function. *Joint kinematics* is the study of angular or translational motion of the hip in response to applied forces. *Kinetics* is the study of forces and moments acting on the joint, most commonly during stance, gait, or functional activities. Typically, these forces are created by the balance between gravity, acting to pull the body to the ground, and muscle contraction, which serves to keep the skeleton aloft. This balance relies on the transmission of load by intermediate structures such as tendons, ligaments, the hip capsule, and the articular tissues.

The study of hip biomechanics can be approached in several ways. Motion analysis can be used to quantify joint kinematics, especially in correlation with analytical models of the musculoskeletal system. Consequently, joint force calculations can be made using data obtained from gait and force platform measurements, in conjunction with analytical models that simulate the force of contraction and the line of action of the corresponding musculature.

The hip joint is classified as an enarthrodial ball and socket joint that allows for polyaxial articulation between the body and the lower extremity. The femoral head comprises nearly two-thirds of a sphere, whereas the mating acetabulum forms a hemisphere of the same diameter. The cartilaginous surfaces of the femur and the acetabulum are not perfectly conforming, in that the femoral head corresponds more to a conchoid than a sphere.[3] This permits the hip joint to undergo movement in an assortment of motion axes that allow flexion-extension, abduction-adduction, and internal-external rotation. Despite a sturdy articular capsule and ligamentous stability, the hip joint allows a great deal of mobility of the femur with respect to the pelvis. Joint motion is greatest in the sagittal plane, with the femur flexing and extending around a left-right axis.[4] With the knee flexed, the hip can be actively flexed to approximately 120 degrees before further motion if limited by the joint capsule; flexion of the hip with the knee fully extended is limited to only 90 degrees because of hamstring tension.[2,4,5] Passive hip flexion reaches 140 degrees when the knee is flexed.[6] Overall, existing data for maximum ROM values include 120 degrees for flexion, 20 degrees for extension, 45 degrees for abduction, 30 degrees for adduction, and 40 degrees for internal and external rotation.[6,7]

Gender/Racial Differences

In discussing normal hip kinematics, it is important to note ROM variations due to age, gender, ethnicity, and geographic location. It is difficult to establish an all-encompassing set of hip ROM values because of the subjectivity of a given population. By and large, studies have shown that females walk with higher cadence and with a shorter stride length, as well as with similar comfortable ambulatory rates, compared with men.[8,9] These findings were corroborated in a study by Kerrigan and associates,[10] who found females to exhibit a statistically significant increase in peak hip flexion but a decrease in hip extension compared with male subjects, yet overall kinematic and kinetic joint patterns were similar between genders.[10] In a comprehensive retrostudy by the First National Health and Nutrition Examination Survey, as reported by Roach and colleagues,[11] hip ROM measurements were recorded from a sample of 1683 subjects broken down by age (25-39, 40-59, and 60-74 years), sex, and ethnicity (white and African American).[11] Upon comparison of age alone, hip flexion, extension, abduction, and internal-external rotation all decreased with age, but not significantly. Additional measurements are shown in Table 1-1.

A majority of normal hip ROM investigation involves subjects from the Western hemisphere. This has led to accepted values for hip ROM, yet these values cannot necessarily pertain to subjects from non-Western cultures, who participate in different ADLs. In many Middle Eastern and Asian countries, ADLs involve postures that necessitate a larger range of flexion at the hip, knee, and ankle joints.[12] For instance, cross-legged sitting posture is popular in Asia during dining, as is kneeling during prayer in the Middle East and Japan, and can be maintained easily for hours.[12] Activities such as stretching,

Table 1-1. Difference in Mean Active Range of Motion (in Degrees) for Ages 25–39 Years Compared With Ages 60–74 Years by Sex and Race Groups

Motion	Combined Group	White Men	White Women	Black Men	Black Women
Hip Flexion					
Ages 25-39 yr	122	123	123	115	116
Ages 60-74 yr	118	118	119	118	106
Hip Extension					
Ages 25-39 yr	22	22	22	19	17
Ages 60-74 yr	17	17	16	16	12
Hip Abduction					
Ages 25-39 yr	44	46	44	41	38
Ages 60-74 yr	39	39	40	38	37
Hip Internal Rotation					
Ages 25-39 yr	33	34	33	32	27
Ages 60-74 yr	30	31	29	27	25
Hip External Rotation					
Ages 25-39 yr	34	33	36	32	32
Ages 60-74 yr	29	27	32	27	28

From Roach KM: Normal hip and knee active range of motion: the relationship to age. Phys Ther 71:656–664, 1991.

kneeling, and gardening are more common in North America.[12] In a study by Ahlberg and co-workers,[13] joint ROM was measured among 50 Saudi Arabian males, who exhibited greater hip flexion, abduction, and external rotation compared with normative data (130.8 degrees, 50.8 degrees, and 72.9 degrees, respectively), and less hip extension, adduction, and internal rotation (13.9 degrees, 30.1 degrees, 36.7 degrees, respectively).[13] This increase can be correlated with differences in repeated habitual activities involving squatting and kneeling compared with Western cultures. Similar findings were reported by Hoaglund and associates while examining Chinese subjects versus white subjects in Hong Kong, China.[14]

Because of geographic variation in ADLs such as squatting, kneeling, and sitting cross-legged, many studies have measured hip ROM in non-Western cultures in these corresponding positions to accompany normal ROM values. In a study of the range-of-motion of the joints of nonwestern subjects conducted by Mulholland and colleagues,[15] hip flexion reached 130 degrees during full squat and 90 to 100 degrees while sitting cross-legged; hip external rotation ranged from 5 to 36 degrees for full squat and from 35 to 60 degrees while sitting cross-legged, and hip abduction ranged from 10 to 30 degrees for full squat and from 40 to 45 degrees while sitting cross-legged.[15] Measurements of ROM of the hip during these activities are reported in Table 1-2 for a group of Indian subjects.[12]

Structures Controlling Hip Motion

To understand the basic kinematics of the hip joint, it is instructive to review in detail the basic anatomy of passive stabilizers of the hip, including the capsular ligaments, the acetabular labrum, and the ligamentum teres.

The Hip Capsule and Ligaments

During abduction and adduction, limb movement occurs around an anteroposterior axis, as well as in the frontal plane. Average hip abduction has been estimated at 50 degrees.[4] The hip capsule (capsular ligament) is critical to the stability of the joint during abduction and adduction and serves as a constraint in preventing dislocation at the extremes of motion.[16,17]

The capsule is a complex structure formed by three discrete ligaments: iliofemoral, femoral arcuate (pubofemoral), and ischiofemoral ligaments. The anteriorly located iliofemoral ligament, the largest and one of the strongest ligaments of the hip joint, serves to restrict extension and limit internal rotation. The ligament itself consists of two bands extending from the anterior-inferior iliac spine medially to two insertion sites along the intertrochanteric line laterally. The femoral arcuate ligament is located anteromedially and is attached to the superior ramus of the pubis; it connects to the femoral neck, helping to limit abduction and external rotation. Last, the ischiofemoral ligament is situated posteriorly and runs horizontally across the posterior surface of the femoral neck from the acetabular rim and the labrum to the inner surface of the greater trochanter. It serves to limit internal rotation and adduction during hip flexion. Several studies have demonstrated through mechanical testing that the ischiofemoral ligament is the weakest of the capsular ligaments,[17] which makes the joint susceptible to posterior dislocation.[18]

The Acetabular Labrum

The acetabular labrum, a fibrocartilaginous lip attached to the bony margin of the acetabulum, deepens the acetabular socket, substantially extending coverage of the femoral head. The labrum is characterized by a three-layer structure, with the inner layer at the articular surface covered by a fine mesh of type II collagen fibrils, below which one finds a lamellar collagen structure and finally an outer periphery composed of dense connective tissue with fibers oriented circumferentially. In an extensive histomorphologic study, Won and co-workers[19] identified several key features at the anterior portion of the labrum, which other studies have reported as the predominant area for labral tears, including a tall triangular shape with apex heights of up to 7 mm and sublabral clefts, perpendicular to the articular surface, at the interface between the labrum and the acetabular rim. The labrum is an avascular tissue with only limited blood supply in the peripheral third of the tissue from the adjacent capsule.[20,21] Mechanical properties of the labrum are highly anisotropic, with preferential stiffness in the circumferential direction[22] and strong dependence of its mechanical competence on gender, anatomic location, and the degenerative state of the hip.[23,24] Labral tears were first cited as a potential source of hip pain by Altenberg more than 30 years ago.[25] Labral tears may result from trauma, hypolaxity of the capsule, dysplasia, or impingement.

Although a link between labral pathology and joint degeneration has been proposed, only recently has the biomechanical function of the labrum been well understood. In the normal hip joint, the labrum contributes

Table 1-2. Range of Motion of the Hip During Functional Activities*

	Squatting Heels Down	Squatting Heels Up	Kneeling Dorsiflexed	Kneeling Plantar-Flexed	Sitting Cross-Legged
Flexion	95.4 ± 26.2	91.3 ± 17.1	73.9 ± 29.4	58.8 ± 9.7	85.4 ± 34.2
Abduction	28.2 ± 13.9	31.7 ± 11.2	25.3 ± 15.3	27.6 ± 12.5	36.5 ± 15
External rotation	25.7 ± 11.8	33.7 ± 12.7	28.1 ± 12.8	34 ± 14.9	40.3 ± 18.4

*All values are expressed as the average ± standard deviation; units are degrees.
From Hemmerich A, et al: Hip, knee, and ankle kinematics of high range of motion activities of daily living. J Orthop Res 24:770–781, 2006.

very little in the way of direct mechanical resistance to joint loading, despite its position and prominence at the acetabular rim.[26] However, the compliant and elastic labrum serves as a mechanical seal around the periphery of the joint, enhancing lubrication by effectively blocking passage of synovial fluid into and out of the joint.[27-29] This sealing property is readily demonstrated by the well-known suction effect observed during distraction or dislocation of the hip in surgery and has been proven to increase joint stability and to distribute compressive loads in a more uniform manner, thereby decreasing surrounding cartilage stress[30-32] (Figs. 1-1 and 1-2). In a series of computer simulations and in vitro experiments,[29,31,33] we have shown that the labrum allows a layer of synovial fluid to be maintained between the femur and the acetabulum, thus preventing direct contact of the articulating surfaces during short-term loading. With this sealing effect, loads are transferred across the joint predominantly by uniform pressurization of interstitial fluid of the cartilage layers, not by direct solid-on-solid contact stresses. In the absence of this seal, deformation of the solid matrix of the cartilage is substantially greater. However, in vitro experiments have shown that both sealing mechanisms are highly dependent on the fit of the compliant labrum against the femoral head.[31]

It has been proposed that the labrum may enhance retention of a boundary layer of lubricant even after fluid film depletion.[34] Over long-term loading (i.e., the diurnal cycle), the labrum contributes an important source of resistance to the flow of interstitial fluid that is expressed from the cartilage layers of the joint under load. Cartilage layer consolidation, in principle similar to the wringing out a sponge, is up to 40% faster following labral excision. This, in turn, has a dramatic influence on internal stresses within the cartilage layers, as

the center of pressure is shifted toward the acetabular rim, and subsurface shear strains are increased at the subchondral interface, which may contribute to delamination.[29]

Damage to the labrum through injury or pathology can compromise its sealing function, resulting in subtle but critical destabilization of the hip (Fig. 1-3). This may lead to a shift in the center of rotation of the joint, thereby increasing acetabular rim loading and potentially hastening the onset of early osteoarthritis (OA) and joint disease caused by sustained cartilage erosion.[27,28,35,36] Despite early descriptions of the labrum as a continuous structure connecting to the articular cartilage throughout the acetabulum, studies have shown that the anterior aspect makes minimal contact

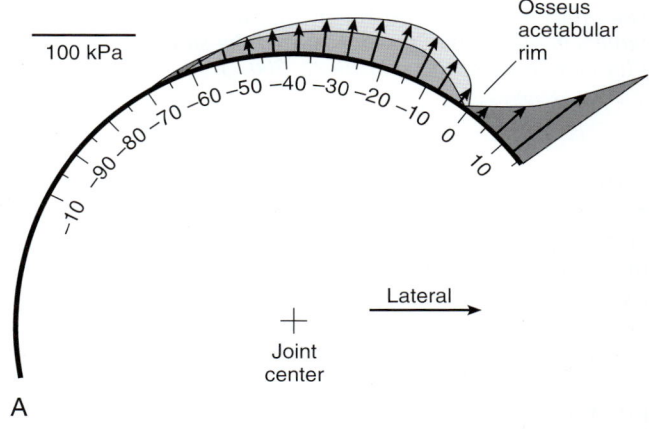

A

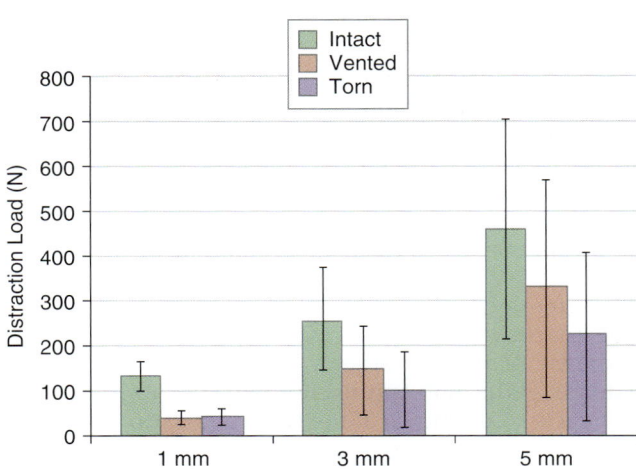

Figure 1-1. Average load required to distract the femur a distance of 1 mm, 3 mm, and 5 mm with the labrum intact, vented to release the partial vacuum, and incised to simulate a full-thickness tear. *(Redrawn from Crawford MJ, et al: The 2007 Frank Stinchfield Award: the biomechanics of the hip labrum and the stability of the hip. Clin Orthop Relat Res 465:16–22, 2007.)*

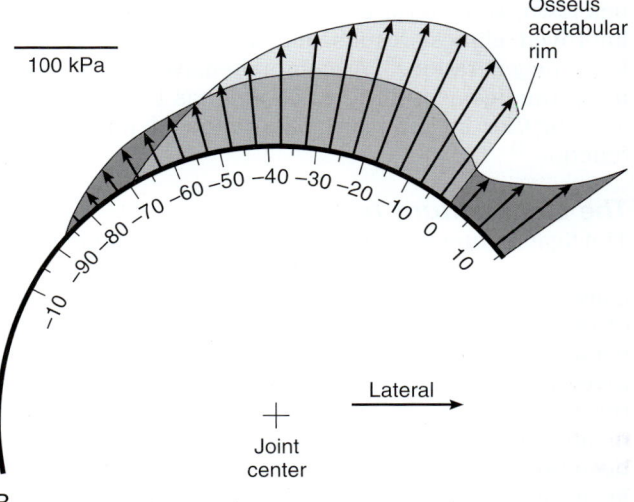

B

Figure 1-2. Predicted distribution of cartilage contact stresses at **(A)** 1000 seconds, and **(B)** 10,000 seconds after load application with the labrum *(dark gray)* and without the labrum *(light gray)*. *(Redrawn from Ferguson SJ, et al: The influence of the acetabular labrum on hip joint cartilage consolidation: a poroelastic finite element model. J Biomech 33:953–960, 2000.)*

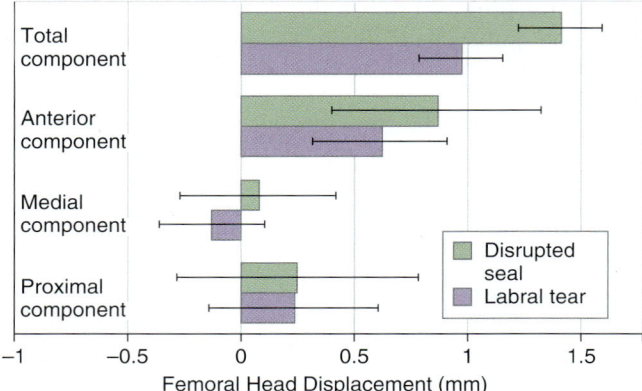

Figure 1-3. Change in displacement of the femoral head within the acetabulum when loaded with an abduction moment in 20 degrees of external rotation for hip joints tested with the labrum intact, then vented, then torn. (*Redrawn from Crawford MJ, Dy CJ, Alexander JW, et al: The biomechanics of the hip labrum and the stability of the hip. Clin Orthop Relat Res 465:16–22, 2007.*)

with the acetabular cartilage compared with the posterior aspect.[27,37] Consequently, tearing of the acetabular labrum will occur predominantly anteriorly as the result of inferior mechanical properties leading to hip instability, as well as watershed labral lesions, which ultimately can lead to degenerative joint disease.[27,28,35,36]

Reattachment of the damaged labrum has been suggested to partially restore its original function. This procedure is intended to avoid compromising the biomechanical function of the labrum caused by surgical débridement, which may otherwise lead to degenerative changes associated with OA. Although the long-term results of labral reattachment are still unknown, short-term follow-up is positive,[38] with both improved clinical results and less prevalent signs of joint degeneration.[39] A comprehensive labral repair using the ligamentum teres capitis has been proposed as a further step toward restoration of normal joint function.[40]

The Ligamentum Teres

The ligamentum teres is an intra-articular ligament that attaches the acetabulum and the femoral head. Specifically, two bands connect to the ischial and pubic sides of the acetabular notch in congruence with the transverse ligament of the acetabulum, and insert into the fovea capitis femoris.[41,42] To date, a paucity of investigative studies have explored the exact function of the ligamentum teres and its role in stability of the hip. It has been postulated that the ligamentum teres plays a role in stability, but corroborative data are scarce. It is known that the structure is taut during hip adduction, flexion, and external rotation—positions in which the joint is least stable—which demonstrates its potential role in hip stability.[43] A biomechanical study of immature porcine ligaments conducted by Wenger and colleagues[42] showed that ligaments followed a stepwise stress-strain curve.[42] The mode of failure was

discovered to be ligamentous disruption from the acetabulum, then avulsion from the femoral head with signs of mid- or intraligamentous tears.[41,42] Additional clinical and biomechanical studies of adult ligamentum teres are needed to conclusively determine the nature of its role in hip stability.

Hip Joint Motion During Normal Gait

The form of the hip joint permits motion of the lower extremity under the control of specific muscles. Researchers are particularly interested in examining the motion of the natural hip joint in basic locomotion. Gait analysis is also convenient because this process of motor development is fully integrated in hip patients, which simplifies comparison of gait parameters between individuals.[4]

During gait activities, the hip joint plays a crucial role in advancement of the lower extremity. Typically, one gait cycle commences when the heel of the reference limb makes contact with the ground, and it concludes when the toe of the same limb leaves the ground (i.e., measuring one full stride length of the reference limb).[2,4,44] The gait cycle is divided into two phases: stance (60% gait cycle) and swing (40% gait cycle).[2,4] Stance phase is subdivided into initial contact, loading response, midswing, terminal stance, and preswing. During stance phase, the body is propelled forward while being supported by the limb touching the ground. Because the supporting limb is ahead of the body at heel-strike (i.e., the hip is flexed) and is behind the body at toe-off (i.e., the hip is extended), the center of gravity of the body moves in an epicyclical pattern. Swing phase is subdivided into initial swing, midswing, and terminal swing, and occurs when the supporting limb is lifted free of the ground and is driven forward ahead of the body in preparation for the next cycle of weight-bearing support. During this phase, an open-chain loading configuration is present, as the foot is not constrained through ground contact, so that the extremity can rotate freely.

In a standard stride in the sagittal plane, the hip traverses two arcs of motion: flexion to extension during stance phase, and extension to flexion during swing phase. During each gait cycle, the average arc of motion of the hip is 40 degrees in the sagittal plane, ranging from 30 degrees of flexion to 10 degrees of hyperextension with respect to the neutral standing position (zero flexion).[2,45] At initial limb contact, the thigh is already in 20 degrees of flexion and is relatively stable.[2] Hip adduction reaches a maximum of 5 degrees in the loading response of the late stance phase.[4] The hip gradually extends as the limb approaches mid stance (10% to 30% gait cycle). Continuing at the same ambulatory rate, the thigh reaches the zero position at 38% of the gait cycle.[2] The femur then enters preswing (50% to 60% gait cycle), aligning in a posterior position with peak hip extension at 10 degrees.[2,4] The hip reaches a maximum abduction angle of 5 to 7 degrees as medial rotation occurs at the closing stages of the loading response.[4]

At the end of the stance period (60% gait cycle), the hip enters flexion and reaches neutral hip position, although the thigh is still in several degrees of extension.[2] The hip attains maximum flexion of 30 to 35 degrees at approximately 85% of the gait cycle in the terminal swing phase as the hip rotates laterally,[2,4,46] before returning to the beginning of the gait cycle. In the coronal plane, a small amount of adduction and abduction of the hip occurs as the non–weight-bearing portion of the pelvis moves through the gait cycle. During stance, the hip is initially 10 degrees adducted; as the load increases, the hip shifts to 5 degrees adduction until terminal stance is attained. At the onset of the swing phase, the hip abducts minimally at around 5 degrees.[2] In the transverse plane, the hip exhibits both internal and external rotation throughout the gait cycle, with peak internal rotation occurring at the conclusion of the loading response, and maximum external rotation at the launch of the swing phase (end of preswing). The net transverse internal-external hip motion is 8 degrees, with total thigh rotation of around 15 degrees.[2]

The Role of Muscles in Hip Motion

Extension
The hip extensor muscles, primarily the hamstrings, adductor magnus, and gluteus maximus, operate from the late midswing phase through the loading response. At the end of the midswing phase, the semimembranosus, semitendinosus, and long biceps femoris all simultaneously begin gradual contraction before peaking in early terminal swing. Semirelaxation of these muscles ensues before complete relaxation at the end of the swing phase. The adductor magnus initiates contraction at the end of the terminal swing, which increases during initial contact; it remains active during the loading response before tapering off. The lower half of the gluteus maximus contracts at the end of the terminal swing and increases its strength of contraction through heel-strike until the end of the loading response. Contraction of the gluteus maximus acts as a brake in slowing down the momentum of the lower limb in the terminal swing phase, in preparation for the stance phase. Because the action of body weight is to extend the hip joint, the gluteus maximus plays a critical role in enabling individuals to walk up an incline or a set of stairs, and to run and jump.[47]

Abduction
Hip abduction is more pronounced during the first half of the stance phase and involves the action of the gluteus medius, tensor fascia lata, and upper gluteus maximus. By acting medially, these muscles compensate for the contralateral drop of the pelvis caused by the force of overall body weight. The gluteus medius and the upper gluteus maximus initiate contraction at the end of terminal swing (95% gait cycle); this peaks after initial contact and then continues throughout midstance. Variation in the activity of the tensor fascia lata muscle is noted, as the posterior portion of the muscle contributes most during the loading response, while the anterior portion is only active during terminal stance.

Flexion and Adduction
The flexor muscles play a critical role in the function of the hip in normal gait and are active from late terminal stance to early in midswing as the hip is elevated free of the ground and carried through. Specific muscles contributing to this function are the adductor longus, rectus femoris, gracilis, pectineus, tensor fasciae latae, sartorius, and iliacus muscles. The chief flexor is the iliopsoas, which stems from the ventral surface of the transverse processes and the sides of the lumbar vertebrae and connects to the iliac portion, inserting immediately below the lesser trochanter.[47] Key muscles in the anterior aspect of adduction include the pectineus, adductor magnus, longus, brevis, and gracilis; the posterior aspect includes the gluteus maximus, quadratus femoris, obturator externus, and hamstrings.

Pelvic Motion
The pelvis acts similar to a stationary unit with coordinated motion occurring between the lumbar spine and the hip joint as the result of muscle coordination. Pelvic motion at the hip consists of anteroposterior pelvic tilting, lateral pelvic tilting, and pelvic rotation. Anterior pelvic tilting occurs via the hip flexors and trunk extensors as the result of contraction of the iliopsoas, which pulls the pelvis anteriorly and inferiorly; the extensors of the lumbar spine pull the pelvis superiorly.[47] This causes inferior movement of the symphysis pubis, increasing the lordotic curve of the lumbar spine. An opposite event is the decrease in the lordotic curve of the lumbar spine, which results in posterior pelvic tilt; this brings the posterior aspect of the pelvis closer to the posterior surface of the femur, resulting in hip extension as the hip extensor muscles work with the trunk flexors (rectus and obliquus muscles).[47] Lateral flexion and rotation of the vertebral spine cause lateral pelvic tilting, resulting in hip adduction or abduction.

Joint Motion, Gait, and Functional Adaptations

As individuals pursue more demanding ADLs, it is reasonable to predict that any limitations in hip function and range of motion will tend to compromise each individual's expectations and physical activities. Whether as the result of pathologies such as premature wear and tear of the hip joint and degenerative arthritis or artificial joint replacement, individuals will ultimately alter their normal functional movements to compensate for joint pain, muscle weakness, or instability. The Trendelenburg gait pattern, for example, occurs when patients experience a decrease in function of their abductor muscles as a result of reduced muscle strength or abductor moment arm length.[48] This leads to a compensatory gait pattern to reduce the demand placed on the abductor muscles by moving the trunk closer to the affected hip. Femoroacetabular impingement, which can cause pain and may lead to OA,[49,50] can significantly affect normal hip biomechanics during gait as the result of jamming of the femoral head into the acetabulum.[51,52]

Patients with FAI have demonstrated decreased frontal and sagittal hip ROM during gait.[52]

Impediments to normal gait, function, and range of motion often lead to total hip replacement (THR) or hip resurfacing in an attempt to restore daily functional activities.[53] Preoperatively, THR patients exhibit slower ambulatory speeds, decreased cadence, and shortened stride length as a result of reduced hip flexion during contact, and reversal of motion during extension at the end of the stance phase.[48,54-56] This reversal is caused by flexion contracture, which could reflect enhanced lumbar lordosis and lack of overall hip extension, as well as serving as a method to avoid pain by decreasing hip joint force.[48] Hip extension failure during late stance also contributes to decreased step length during gait. Changes in joint geometry can alter muscle strength and the ability of muscles to generate moments.[1] The head-neck angle, neck length, and joint center position play a significant role in abductor muscle function, with a varus hip (decreased head-neck angle) providing greater abductor muscle strength, decreasing contact forces, and increasing femoral head and acetabular congruency.[1,57] Increased femoral neck length and a more distal greater trochanter position have been shown to clinically increase abductor/adductor strength.[58]

Adding to these adaptations, the disease process itself alters properties of the hip joint with thickening of the capsule and hip joint effusion, leading to increased intracapsular pressure[59] with flexion, stretching of the joint capsule, and significant joint pain.[59-61] Further degeneration of the capsule increases stress on surrounding articular cartilage and continues OA-related pain. Studies also suggest that progressive loss of hip extensor strength leads to pathophysiologic complications such as muscle atrophy, buildup of connective tissue and adipocytes in muscles, and potential changes in hip torque-angle relationships.[61,62] Consequently, OA consistently remains a source of limitation in hip motion during gait, and studies have well documented the debilitating effects of OA through the impact of pain on physical function.[7,61,63]

PATHOLOGIC IMPEDIMENTS TO JOINT MOTION

Femoroacetabular Impingement

The natural range of motion of the hip joint is limited by a combination of kinematic constraints imposed by the flexibility of bounding soft tissues of the joint (i.e., capsule, ligaments, and surrounding musculature) and hard limits defined by the potential endpoint interference of bony structures. Impingement is a well-understood limitation of the motion of hip prostheses, and considerable effort has been directed toward understanding the process and consequences of femoroacetabular impingement (FAI) in the natural joint. In an early three-dimensional computational study of SCFE in the pediatric hip, impaction or inclusion of the metaphysis was shown to limit joint motion, with

consequent rim damage,[64] hinting already at future findings on the contribution of impingement to degenerative changes in the adult hip.

Acetabular impingement in nondysplastic hips, in which the femoral neck abuts against the acetabular labrum, or a nonspherical femoral head is pressed into the labrum and adjacent cartilage, was described in a magnetic resonance imaging (MRI)–based quantitative anatomic study by Ito and associates (Fig. 1-4).[51] Two mechanisms based on anatomic variations of normal bony anatomy were identified. These are now well known as "cam-type" and "pincer-type" impingements, in which an aspherical portion of the head-neck junction is pressed into the normal acetabulum, or the normal femoral neck abuts against a deep acetabular rim, respectively (Figs. 1-5 and 1-6). Cam FAI typically is characterized by an abnormally large femoral head jamming into the acetabulum during motion, particularly in flexion and internal rotation.[49,50,65] The source of abutment is a nonspherical extension of the femoral head, otherwise known as a "pistol grip" deformity,

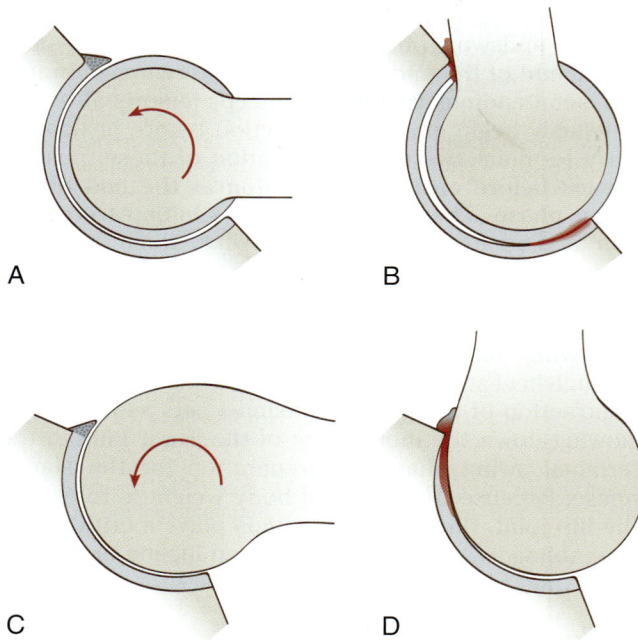

A   B

C   D

Figure 1-4. Diagrammatic representation of mechanisms for joint damage secondary to femoroacetabular impingement, as proposed by Ganz and associates. In "pincer impingement" (**A** and **B**), direct impact between the femoral neck and the acetabular labrum is observed as the result of overcoverage limiting hip motion. This can lead to labral damage and cyst formation at the site of impingement and contrecoup damage of the posterior-inferior chondral surface. In cam impingement (**C** and **D**), the enlarged area of the head-neck junction is jammed into the mouth of the acetabulum in flexion and internal rotation, leading to chondral and labral damage. (*Redrawn from Ganz R, et al: The etiology of osteoarthritis of the hip: an integrated mechanical concept. Clin Orthop Relat Res 466:264–272, 2008.*)

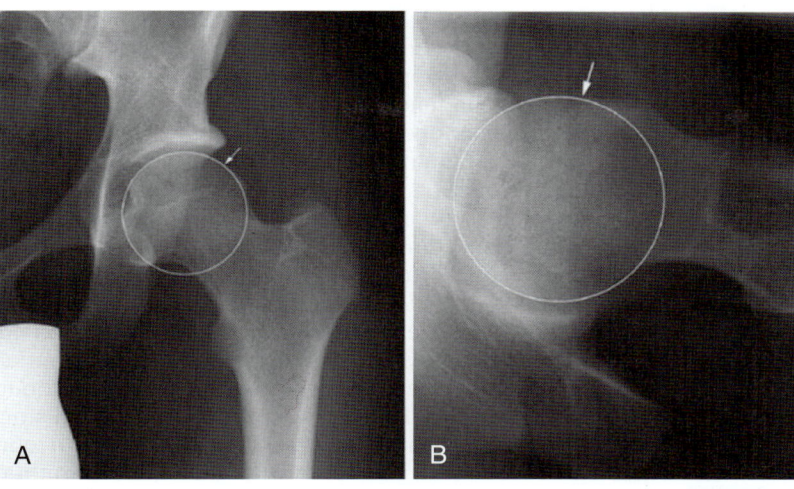

Figure 1-5. Radiographs of a hip with cam impingement presenting as a "pistol grip" deformity. **A,** Anteroposterior view showing asphericity of the femoral head as the area that extrudes from the circle laterally *(arrows)*. **B,** Lateral cross-table view showing asphericity of the femoral head extending from the circle *(arrows)*. *(From Beck M, Kalhor M, Leunig M, Ganz R: Hip morphology influences the pattern of damage to the acetabular cartilage: femoroacetabular impingement as a cause of early osteoarthritis of the hip. J Bone Joint Surg Br 87:1012–1018, 2005.)*

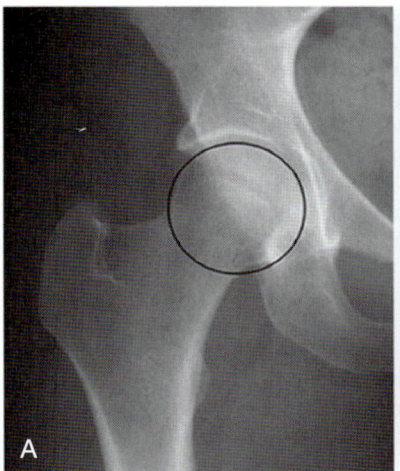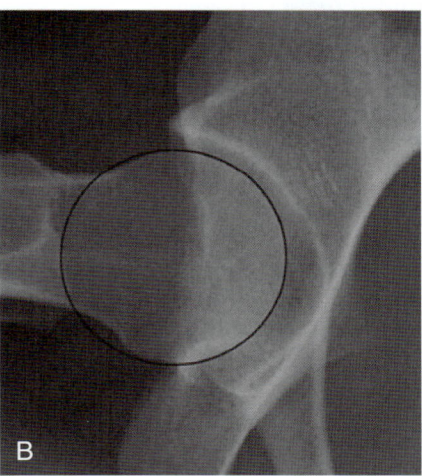

Figure 1-6. Radiographs of a hip with pincer impingement showing coxa profunda with ossification of the acetabular labrum. **A,** Anteroposterior and **(B)** lateral views. The head is spherical in both planes. *(From Beck M, Kalhor M, Leunig M, Ganz R: Hip morphology influences the pattern of damage to the acetabular cartilage: femoroacetabular impingement as a cause of early osteoarthritis of the hip. J Bone Joint Surg Br 87:1012–1018, 2005.)*

which is not always visible on standard anteroposterior radiographs and often can remain undiagnosed during initial evaluation.[50] Cam FAI produces shear forces that cause abrasion of the acetabular cartilage, avulsion of the anterosuperior rim of the acetabulum from the labrum and subchondral bone, or both. Over time, further destruction of the acetabular cartilage forces the femoral head to drift into the deficient area, which is recognized as joint space narrowing on MRI and radiographs.[49,50] This allows for overuse of the weight-bearing aspect of the femoral head cartilage, which results in surface damage to the non–weight-bearing cartilage.[50] It is also observed that cysts develop on the head or head-neck junction as the result of consistent jamming caused by cam FAI.

Physical limitations in joint motion arising from abnormalities of the head-neck junction have been extensively studied using three-dimensional computed tomography (CT)–based models. In a study by Kubiak-Langer and colleages,[66] clear reductions in flexion, internal rotation, and abduction were shown for hips with cam, pincer, and combined pathologies. Furthermore, in the impinging hip, internal rotation has been shown to decrease dramatically with increasing flexion and adduction. The authors also simulated surgical

correction of joint anatomy and demonstrated that this led to restoration of normal values of hip ROM (Table 1-3). In a more extensive study, ROM of the normal hip was predicted from CT reconstructions of a cohort of 150 patients and was compared with 31 consecutive hips of patients with FAI.[67] Findings similar to those of the previous study were reported; however, the mechanism of impingement was examined in greater detail. When the impingement subgroups (cam, pincer, and combined) were compared, it was shown that cam and pincer hips had significantly decreased abduction compared with combined pathologies, and that cam hips allowed greater extension. A further interesting observation from the study was that many current orthopedic textbooks may overestimate the normal range of hip motion.

Although imaging-based methods can provide detailed and accurate predictions of joint motion in the research setting, their routine clinical use is, of course, not always warranted. Indeed, a standardized anterior impingement test, with the leg flexed and interiorly rotated, can provide valuable insight into motion limits and joint status, with most impinging hips provoking pain at similarly limited motion (e.g., 97 degrees flexion and 9 degrees internal rotation[68]). Most recently, Leunig and colleagues proposed a standardized test of internal rotation with hip flexion.[69] Lamontagne and coworkers recommended the inclusion of deep squatting as a potential diagnostic exercise, and demonstrated characteristic differences in sagittal pelvic ROM and hip motion during squatting for FAI patients.[70] Kennedy and associates recently reported significant differences in several kinematic parameters during gait, although they propose that this may be due to a compensatory strategy developed over time, rather than being a direct consequence of impingement during gait.[52]

The hypothesized pathomechanical link between FAI, labral lesions, and cartilage degeneration at the acetabular rim has been strengthened by a comprehensive selection of clinical, anatomic, and biomechanical studies. Most labral lesions are associated with cartilage fraying,[35,36] predominantly in the superior acetabular margin.[71] Intraoperative observation has shown a clear correspondence of local cartilage damage zones with sites of impingement.[72] In most cases, a bony deformity or spatial malorientation of the femoral head, the head-neck junction, or the acetabulum is present in patients with reduced hip motion secondary to impingement. However, supraphysiologic motion or high impact can also cause labral injury, without impingement as an intermediary factor. For example, Dy and colleagues[73] have shown that external rotation and abduction in extension or modest flexion can generate substantial tensile strains in the anterior part of the labrum without impingement (Fig. 1-7). This supports the conclusion that injury to the anterior part of the labrum may occur from recurrent twisting or pivoting of the hip rather than direct impingement.[73]

In our own computational study of the biomechanical consequences of FAI, we investigated the relationship between morphologic variations of the hip and resultant stresses within the soft tissues of the joint during routine daily activities.[74] Three-dimensional computational models of normal and pathologic joints were developed based on variations in morphologic parameters of the femoral head (alpha angle) and acetabulum (center edge [CE] angle). Dynamic loads and motions for various activities were applied to all joint configurations. For impinging joints, the motion from standing to sitting was critical, with high loads applied during flexion and internal rotation, inducing excessive distortion and shearing of the tissue-bone interface (Fig. 1-8). However, stresses during simulated walking were similar to those in the normal joint, underlying the conclusion that impingement is a dynamic, motion-related problem —not one of static overload.[74] The results of these simulations correlate well with the clinically observed association between high alpha angles and the occurrence of chondral defects of the acetabular rim,

Table 1-3. Hip Motion Predicted by Computer Simulation of Patient-Specific Computed Tomography Reconstructions*

Parameter	Normal Hips	FAI Hips (preop)	FAI Hips (postop)
Flexion	$122.0 \pm 16.3^\dagger$	$105.2 \pm 12.2^\dagger$	$125.4 \pm 9.7^\dagger$
Extension	56.5 ± 20.1	61.1 ± 31.8	71.1 ± 26.4
Abduction	$63.3 \pm 10.9^\dagger$	$51.7 \pm 12.2^\dagger$	63.6 ± 7.5
Adduction	32.7 ± 12.3	34.6 ± 12.3	35.8 ± 15.3
Internal rotation (90 degrees of flexion)	$35.2 \pm 6.9^\dagger$	$11.1 \pm 6.9^\dagger$	35.8 ± 15.3
External rotation (90 degrees of flexion)	102.5 ± 14.2	83.0 ± 33.7	93.9 ± 32.7

*Values are reported for normal individuals compared with patients with femoroacetabular impingement, both at diagnosis and following surgical treatment. All values are expressed as the average ± standard deviation; units are degrees.
$^\dagger P < .05.$
From Kubiak-Langer M, et al: Range of motion in anterior femoroacetabular impingement. Clin Orthop Relat Res 458:117–124, 2007.

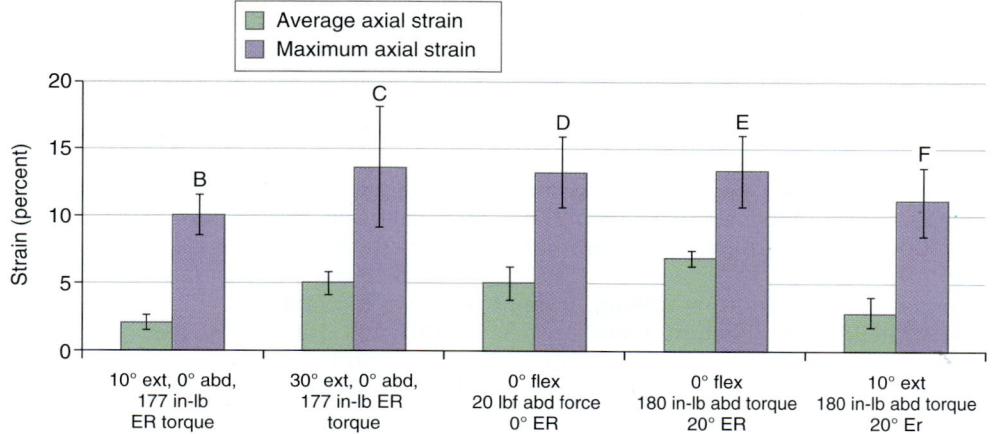

Figure 1-7. Bar graph showing maximum and average axial (medial-lateral) strains observed within the anterior labrum during a range of loading maneuvers (**B, C, D, E,** and **F**) performed by abducting the hip in extension and slight flexion. *abd,* Abduction; *ER,* external rotation; *ext,* extension. (*Redrawn from Dy CJ, Thompson MT, Crawford MJ, et al: Tensile strain in the anterior part of the acetabular labrum during provocative maneuvering of the normal hip. J Bone Joint Surg Am 90:1464–1472, 2008.*)

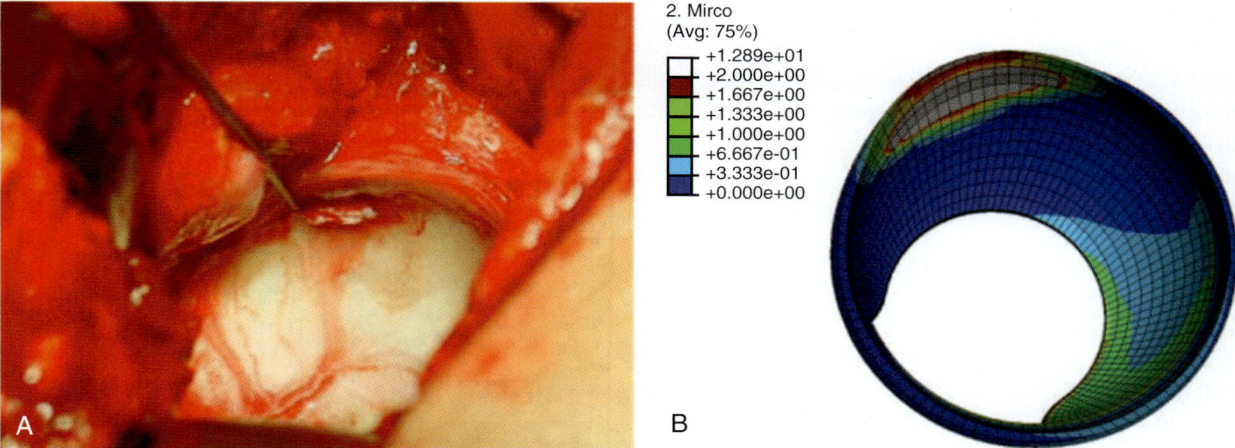

Figure 1-8. Damage patterns: **A,** Observed intraoperatively at the anterior-superior acetabular rim for a typical cam impingement. **B,** von Mises stress distribution in a typical cam-type ($\alpha = 80$ degrees) joint for deep flexion in the standing-to-sitting motion (anterior = left). *(From Chegini S, Beck M, Ferguson SJ: The effects of impingement and dysplasia on stress distributions in the hip joint during sitting and walking: a finite element analysis. J Orthop Res 27:195–201, 2009.)*

full-thickness delamination of the acetabular cartilage, and detachment of the labrum at its chondral junction.[75]

Early diagnosis and behavior modification and/or joint preservation surgery may reduce the rate of osteoarthrosis due to FAI.[76] Surgery is the treatment of choice, with open or arthroscopic bony resection to improve femoral head-neck clearance with resection or refixation of the damaged labrum. Both the femoral head-neck junction and the acetabular rim may require bony resection. Such surgery yields good relief of symptoms; however, the long-term efficacy of limiting degeneration remains an open question.[77,78] Suggested correction of the alpha angle to restore internal rotation to 20 to 25 degrees (with 90 degrees of flexion)[79] corresponds well with biomechanical prediction of an optimal alpha angle to within 50 degrees.[74] However, the study of Mardones and colleagues[80] provides strong evidence of an upper limit on surgical resection at the head-neck junction, with up to 30% resection being tolerable without significantly altering the load-bearing capacity of the proximal part of the femur.

Acetabular Retroversion

Historically, acetabular dysplasia has been characterized by the presence of a shallow acetabulum, but more recent attention has focused on the associated abnormality in version, given the association between acetabular retroversion and posterior hip OA.[81-83] In a retroverted hip, the proximal rim and the opening of the acetabulum typically lie at a retroverted angle when viewed in the sagittal plane, compared with the anteversion present in the normal hip. This causes anterior edge of the acetabulum to shift laterally and the posterior edge medially compared with the normal joint, indicating that retroversion is caused by an alteration in the orientation of the whole socket, rather than just the superior edge.[84] As this condition progresses, noticeable fragmentation of the acetabular edge can occur as

the result of impingement between the anterosuperior edge of the acetabulum and the anterior surface of the femoral head and neck, causing anterolateral overcoverage of the femoral head.[84,85] This decreased clearance can cause contact between the acetabular rim and the femoral head during internal rotation and adduction/abduction during hip flexion.[51,86] Posterior wall deficiency or excessive anterior coverage places an increased load on the cartilage of the posterior aspect of the acetabulum that can instigate degeneration.[83] Studies have shown a correlation between FAI and acetabular retroversion, but other explanations account for the role of the pelvis and the spine. Hips that have pelvic extension at the lumbosacral junction, as is the case with lumbar lordosis, have a greater chance for acetabular retroversion.[84]

A recent focus on quantifying acetabular version (AV) has emerged; this undertaking proved difficult in the past because of the lack of standard diagnostic techniques, as both anteroposterior pelvic radiography and CT are commonly used.[86] Because patients with AV are often predisposed to FAI, assessing AV early is critical in the treatment of FAI. Part of this assessment includes measuring the crossover sign (COS), which, when anteroposterior pelvic radiographs are used, displays the most proximal anterior aspect of the acetabular rim appearing lateral to the posterior rim, creating a figure-of-eight, a common sign of retroversion.[84] In a study by Dandachli and associates,[87] CT scans of patients showing signs of FAI were taken to investigate the correlation between the presence of COS and acetabular retroversion. Investigators concluded that although 92% of cases showed the COS, only 55% of those were retroverted, and the other 37% were wrongly labeled as anteverted.[87] These results differed from those of Jamali and colleagues,[86] who found the COS in 90% of cases and in 95% of those showing retroversion.[86] Because of variability in pelvic tilt, the reliability of COS in determining the presence of retroversion is questionable and

Table 1-4. Summary of Values of the Peak Joint Reaction Force Reported by Different Investigators Using Instrumented Hip Prostheses

Activity	Typical Peak Force, BW	Total Number of Patients	Time Since Surgery, mo	References
Walking, slow	1.6-4.1	9	1-30	10, 11, 12
Walking, normal	2.1-3.3	6	1-31	10
Walking, fast	1.8-4.3	7	2-30	10, 11, 12, 70
Jogging/running	4.3-5.0	2	6-30	11, 12
Ascending stairs	1.5-5.5	8	6-33	10, 12, 70
Descending stairs	1.6-5.1	7	6-30	10, 12, 70
Standing up	1.8-2.2	4	11-31	10
Sitting down	1.5-2.0	4	11-31	10
Standing/2-1-1 legs	2.2-3.7	3	11-14	10
Knee bend	1.2-1.8	3	11-14	10
Stumbling	7.2-8.7	2	4-18	11, 13

demands further investigation. Quantitative assessment is also difficult because version often varies with the proximal-distal level of the observation. Most authors agree that the more distal the occurrence of the COS, the greater is the magnitude of acetabular retroversion.

KINETICS OF THE NORMAL HIP

Any review of the biomechanics of the hip must address both the kinematics and the kinetics of normal hip function. Kinetics relates the forces and moments acting on the joint, most commonly during stance, gait, or functional activities. Typically, these forces are created by the balance between gravity, acting to pull the body to the ground, and muscle contraction, which serves to keep the skeleton aloft. This balance relies on the transmission of load by intermediate structures such as tendons, ligaments, the hip capsule, and articular tissues.

FORCES ACTING ACROSS THE HIP JOINT

The durability of the native hip is critically affected by the magnitude and direction of forces acting on the femoral head and acetabulum during functional activities. Because there is no standard method for measuring forces transmitted across the intact hip joint, some of the most useful data have been derived from hip prostheses instrumented with internal transducers that are able to transmit signals to external recording equipment. Over the past 40 years, several investigators have reported measurements of forces or pressures recorded using this method (Table 1-4). Exhaustive investigations of Bergmann and his research team have documented that joint reaction forces vary between 2.1 and 4.3 BW during gait[88-90] and between 2.3 and 5.5 BW during stair climbing,[88,89] and reach values in excess of 8 BW during accidental incidents of stumbling (Figs. 1-9 and 1-10).[88,91]

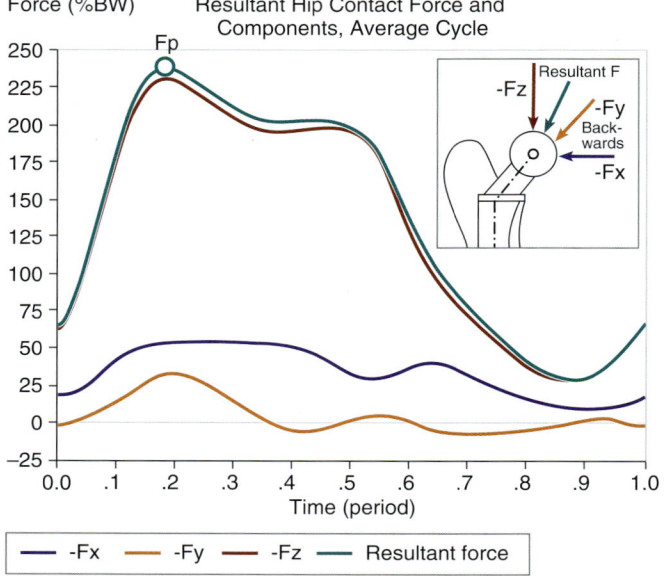

Figure 1-9. Typical hip contact force (F) developed during normal walking. Components of the force are shown.

The force acting on the head of the femur is directed laterally and inferiorly throughout the stance phase of the gait cycle, while simultaneously changing direction from posterior at heel-strike to anterior at toe-off. During gait, peak values of the mediolateral, anteroposterior, and superoinferior components of the joint reaction force vary extensively from 0.4 to 1.7 BW, from 0.2 to 1.0 BW, and from 1.4 to 4.1 BW, respectively. This variability is attributable to differences in the age, gender, height, and gait velocity of individual subjects and the length of the recovery period after implantation of the instrumented prosthesis.

Recordings from instrumented hip prostheses confirm that during common functional activities, transient pressures over the articular surface may exceed static values by fivefold. For example, peak articular pressures during gait average 5.6 MPa and occur early in the

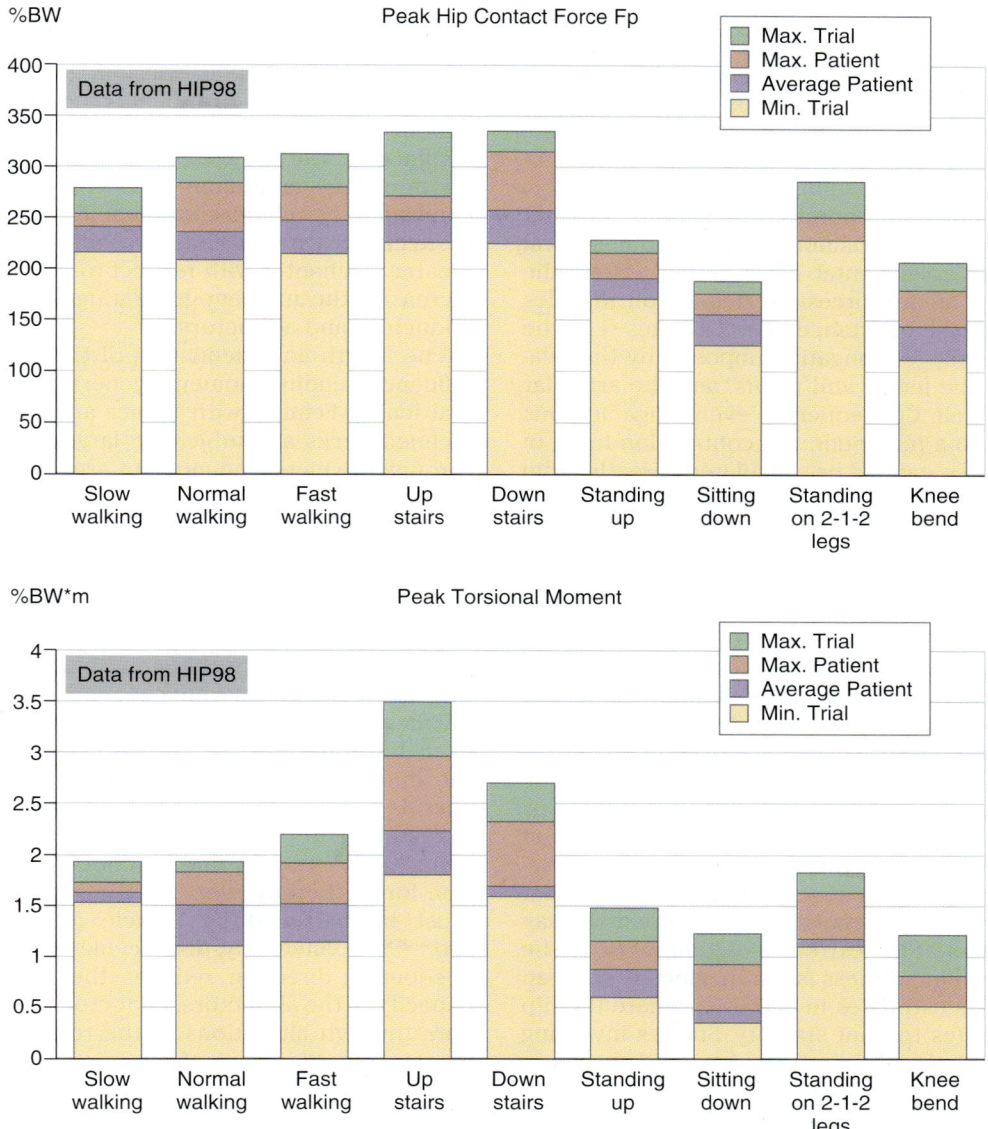

Figure 1-10. Average, minimum, and maximum peak values of *(top)* the hip contact force (in units of percentage of body weight [%BW]) and *(bottom)* the hip torsional moment (in units of % of body weight × height of subject in meters [%BW.m]). Values are shown for nine activities. *(Redrawn from Bergmann G, Deuretzbacher G, Heller M, et al: Hip contact forces and gait patterns from routine activities. J Biomech 34:859–871, 2001.)*

gait cycle (15%) over the superior-anterior surface of the femoral head and the superior acetabular dome.[92] In rising from a chair, articular pressures triple to values of 9 to 15 MPa on the apex of the femoral head and superior-posterior aspects of the acetabulum, which are common sites of degenerative changes observed in cadaver specimens.[93] Functional activities also generate substantial torsional and shear forces in the proximal femur.[88-90,92,94] During stair climbing, the anterior-posterior component of the hip reaction force reaches 20% to 25% of the force in the frontal plane load.[89] When climbing stairs, the peak twisting moment and the first peak contact force were 18% and 14% lower than normal.[95] Conversely, the axial torques recorded during descending stairs and walking were of similar magnitude.[88,89,95]

The number of subjects that can be studied using instrumented prostheses is limited by the cost and complexity of the instrumentation required; therefore, conclusions drawn from these studies suffer from some lack of generalizability caused by the idiosyncrasies of individual patients. Data recorded after THR are of reduced applicability to the intact hip joint. Because of these limitations, hip joint forces from larger populations of subjects have been estimated from kinematic and kinetic data collected during gait studies after incorporation into biomechanical models. External forces acting on the body can be measured with force platforms, and inertial forces generated by segmental motion can be readily derived from knowledge of the motion of each limb segment. This can provide great insight into forces generated at the hip joint during each stage of the gait cycle and at the extremes of motion. However, only the net force acting across the hip joint can be measured, rather than the contributions of individual muscles acting on the hip joint.

Contributions of the Hip Muscles

Although instrumented prostheses record contact forces acting between the acetabulum and the femoral head, the net intersegmental force acting across the joint is the sum of the forces exerted by all muscles crossing the hip, the resistance of soft tissues (i.e., the capsular ligaments) to elongation imposed by the relative position of the femur and pelvis, and the articular reaction force itself. Consequently, even if ligamentous forces are kept to a minimum, the contraction force of individual muscles cannot be calculated directly from the net joint reaction force. For this purpose, muscle force estimates are often based on quantitative electromyography (EMG), normalized to the signal generated during maximum voluntary contraction (MVC) of each muscle.

Another popular method is to distribute the net muscle force between active muscles on the basis of optimization criteria such as the minimum force per cross-sectional area of each muscle, or the energy required for contraction. These have been used to estimate muscle and contact forces based on externally measured forces during gait, stair climbing, and chair rising.[96-100] Because these methods distribute the **net** muscle force or moment generated by muscle contraction, they are unable to allow for the potential effect of co-contraction of antagonistic muscles, which may become significant at the extremes of joint motion. The influence of capsular stiffness is also neglected; this can lead to erroneous estimates in activities where the hip capsule contributes to joint stability. Studies involving both analytical estimates and in vivo load measurements have shown promising comparisons between the two: Heller and associates[101] showed mean peak force differences of 12% during walking and 14% during stair climbing; Stansfield and colleagues[102] demonstrated load differences of approximately 16% during activities such as walking and sit-to-stand.

Factors Affecting the Hip Reaction Force

The force acting between joint surfaces and hence intra-articular stresses developed during weight bearing are critically influenced by the effective moment arms of forces balanced about the hip fulcrum, primarily muscles crossing the joint and the center of gravity of the supported body. Consequently, alterations in joint anatomy, whether due to surgical intervention or a disease process, can dramatically affect hip loading and the health of articular tissues. A decrease in the head-neck angle (varus hip) increases the torque-generating capacity of the abductors and thereby reduces the muscle force needed to generate a given moment. This means that for a given neck length, the joint contact force decreases as the femoral neck becomes more horizontal and the medial head offset increases.[57] More horizontal inclination of the femoral neck also leads to increased joint stability through enhanced acetabular coverage of the femoral head. The mechanical advantage of the abductors may be increased also by lateral displacement of the greater trochanter, or by increased depth of the acetabulum. These predictions have been confirmed by clinical studies in which an increase in neck length and a more distal position of the greater trochanter with respect to the joint center have increased the moment-generating capacity of the hip abductors and adductors.[58,103]

The length and inclination of the femoral neck also influence bending moments generated within the proximal femur. Femurs with longer and more horizontally inclined necks are subject to larger bending moments through the increased moment arm of the joint reaction force. Conversely, when the femoral neck is shorter or more vertically inclined, the bending moment is reduced, although larger abductor forces are needed to balance the weight of the body, leading to an increase in the joint reaction force.

Mathematical models have been used to calculate the effects of changes in the anatomic position of the hip center on the torque imposed on the musculature in balancing the hip and the force-generating capacity of each hip muscle.[57,104-107] These calculations show that the minimum value of the joint reaction force corresponds to translation of the joint center medially, inferiorly, and anteriorly. In this position, the joint center is brought closer to the line of action of the foot-floor reaction force, thereby reducing the external moment that must be balanced by muscle forces acting at the hip.[57,104,105] Conversely, displacement of the hip center in a superior direction reduces the moment-generating capacity of the abductors, adductors, flexors, and extensors through alterations in the resting length of each muscle.[105,106] Elevation of hip joint forces after superolateral displacement of the joint center has been demonstrated experimentally in a loading fixture simulating loading of the hip via abductors, adductors, and extensors during single-legged stance and stair climbing. Using this simulation, superior displacement of the joint center alone did not substantially increase the hip joint force.[108] These theoretical and experimental simulations are all based on the assumption that subjects will not alter their kinematics in performing activities in response to changes in joint forces and muscle demands. Simulations have also assumed that the contributions of antagonistic muscle contractions are insignificant.

THE PATHOMECHANICS OF COXARTHROSIS

Hip arthrosis is typified by flattening the anterolateral surface of the femoral head and its corresponding acetabular support surface. Because normal contact between the femur and the acetabulum is disrupted, concentric or eccentric overload on the joint surfaces is increased; over time, this causes deterioration of local cartilaginous tissue.[49,71] With the native hip, as opposed to a prosthetic hip, the joint is under significant constraint, making it more difficult to avoid the detrimental effects of contact and shear forces, which results in decreased motion, causing abutment around the hip.[49] This is often a source for hip dysplasia, which ultimately leads to OA. However, only recently has conclusive evidence emerged relating FAI to arthritis, especially in younger patients with seemingly normal ROM, joint structure, and intra-articular pressure.[50]

The origin of hip coxarthrosis has been a subject of great interest and investigation, especially within the last decade. The focus has shifted not just to treatment of the osteoarthritic hip joint, but also to the study of abnormalities in hip-fortifying structures, such as soft tissue, tendons, and periarticular bone, which may serve as precursors to degenerative changes caused by loss of joint stability and proper biomechanics.[35] A working hypothesis explored by Ganz and co-workers[49] has emerged to demonstrate that a number of previously classified cases of idiopathic OA in fact were cases of secondary OA caused by "minor developmental deformities" that were not appreciated with the use of conventional diagnostic and radiographic modalities.[49] Studies are beginning to show initial support of this hypothesis, most notably that these deformities play a significant role later in the development of arthritis from FAI. Additional studies have revealed correlations between labral lesions and acetabular retroversion and arthritis.[35,36,82,83]

Effects of Deformities on Forces and Articular Stresses

Diarthrodial joints rely on a broad distribution of applied joint forces to evenly distribute pressure across articulating surfaces, thereby minimizing internal stresses within the cartilage. Peripheral structures of the joint (e.g., the acetabular labrum in the hip) tend to deepen the joint and thus distribute contact evenly around the periphery of the joint rather than focally. This modest incongruence has a significant effect on cartilage pressures and stresses and is beneficial from a load-bearing perspective.[109] However, strong deviations from normal joint morphology are associated with substantial changes in internal pressure and stress magnitudes and distributions and have been implicated in the development of OA. A logical focus of attention is the biomechanics of the dysplastic hip, because intuition dictates that a shallow and more vertically oriented acetabulum is in a compromised position for fulfilling the goal of a broad load distribution.

The influence of acetabular dysplasia on contact pressure has been studied using a variety of computer simulation and experimental methods. In early work by Genda and associates,[110] contact pressure was calculated and compared for a large number of normal and dysplastic hip joints, using a three-dimensional rigid body spring model. Rigid body spring models have the advantage of providing an efficient and robust prediction of local contact pressures, at the expense of a slight oversimplification of the true mechanical response of cartilage. In normal hips, the distribution of contact pressure was shown to be almost even over the joint surface, whereas in the dysplastic hip joint, pressure was concentrated on the anterolateral edge of the acetabulum. A strong negative correlation was predicted between contact pressure and both anterior and lateral coverage. Further refinement of such rigid body spring models, based on patient-specific CT data, was reported by Tsumura and colleagues.[111] These models predicted peak pressures at the acetabular rim of 2.5 MPa and 5.3 MPa for normal and dysplastic hips, respectively. It is enlightening to remind the reader that normal atmospheric pressure is approximately 0.1 MPa. Similarly, computer-assisted planning for hip surgery has evolved to include functional predictions. Hipp and co-workers showed contact pressures up to 25% higher for the dysplastic hip[112] and highlighted the complex influence of three-dimensional acetabular orientation on joint pressures (e.g., reorientation to minimize stresses in walking can increase stresses in stair climbing).

More recently, three-dimensional finite element models have been developed that allow more accurate prediction of surface contact pressures and internal cartilage stresses. Using patient-specific models, Russell and associates[113] completed an extensive study of accumulated pressure exposure over an entire gait cycle. Peak contact pressures for dysplastic and asymptomatic hips ranged from approximately 3 to 10 MPa (Fig. 1-11). A unique feature of this study was the prediction of pressure accumulation over a simulated lifetime of loading. In the dysplastic hip, substantial differences in accumulated pressure were demonstrated, providing a potential pathomechanical link to the chronic overload and degeneration hypothesis for OA. This study

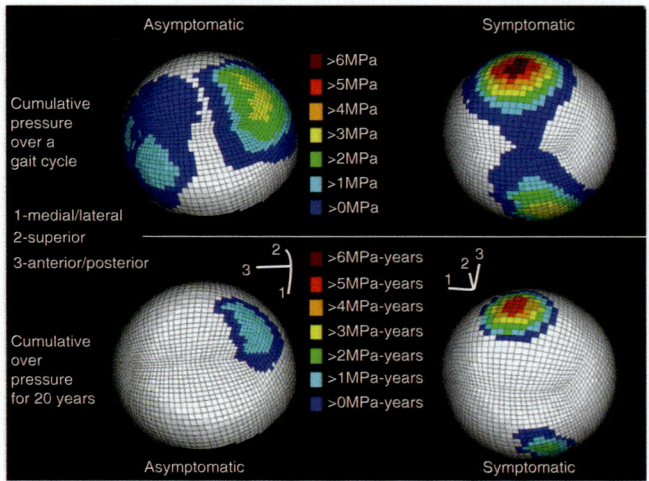

Figure 1-11. Predicted spatial distribution of cumulative contact pressure within the hip joint for symptomatic and asymptomatic subjects. Values are calculated over the course of one gait cycle *(top)* and are expressed as accumulated "over-pressure" (damage threshold = 2 MPa) over a period of 20 years *(bottom)*. *(From Russell ME, Shivanna KH, Grosland NM, Pedersen DR: Cartilage contact pressure elevations in dysplastic hips: a chronic overload model. J Orthop Surg Res 1:6, 2006.)*

also highlighted that, beyond gross morphologic differences, small bone irregularities can cause localized pressure elevations.[113] Subsequent computational models have provided further insight into the relationship between joint morphology, daily loading, and cartilage contact pressures and stresses.

Potential factors contributing to elevated stresses in the dysplastic hip—up to 100% higher—include decreased lateral coverage of the femoral head, larger horizontal separation of joint centers, a wider pelvis, and the medial position of the greater trochanter.[74] Daniel and associates[114] studied the effects of lateral coverage and anteversion on hip pressures during level walking and stair descent, and demonstrated that, compared with level walking, during stair descent contact stresses are dramatically increased by up to 70% and 115% for normal and dysplastic hips, respectively. This highlights the need to evaluate a variety of daily loading scenarios in our efforts to fully understand internal loading of the hip joint. The reader is encouraged to explore an extensive and fascinating public access database of in vivo joint load data, collected over the past 2 decades by researchers at the former Biomechanics Laboratory of the Oskar-Helene-Heim at the Free University of Berlin, now the Julius Wolff Institute of the Charité–Universitätsmedizin Berlin (http://www.orthoload.com).

Soft tissue damage with degeneration is an unavoidable consequence of dysplasia and related focal overload of the acetabular rim. In contrast to the impinging hip, in which the labrum is damaged through repetitive impaction and compaction, the labrum in the dysplastic hip must withstand high shearing and tensile stresses. The labrum is often the "last defense" for the joint and provides some residual resistance to lateral subluxation. As a consequence, labral hypertrophy is often observed in dysplastic hips,[115] although no direct correlation with acetabular coverage has been reported. Within the dysplastic hip, labral damage is most frequently observed in the anterior-superior region of the acetabular rim[116]; this corresponds well with computer predictions of focal rim overload for such joints.[74] Clinical observations have provided strong evidence that acetabular rim overload leads directly to cartilage degeneration and labral rupture.[85,117] Thinning of the anterior cartilage has been observed in 80% of dysplasia patients, with the biomechanical consequence of forward and upward mobility of the femoral head.[118] Ultimately, the peripheral soft tissues of the joint are an inadequate substitute for the stability afforded by a congruent acetabulum with good lateral coverage; hence surgery for acetabular reorientation remains a biomechanically justifiable treatment for the dysplastic hip.

REFERENCES

1. Callaghan J, Rosenberg A, Rubash H: The adult hip. In Hurwitz D, Andriacchi T (eds): Biomechanics of the hip, vol 1, Philadelphia, 1998, Lippincott-Raven, p 11.
2. Perry J (ed): Gait analysis: normal and pathological function, Thorofare, NJ, 1992, Slack Inc.
3. Balderston R, et al: The hip. In Parke W (ed): The anatomy of the hip, Philadelphia, 1992, Lea & Febiger.
4. Fagerson TL (ed): The hip handbook, Woburn, Mass, 1998, Butterworth-Heinemann.
5. Frankel VH (ed): Basic biomechanics of the skeletal system, vol XV, Philadelphia, 1980, Lea & Febiger.
6. Reese N, Bandy W (eds): Joint range of motion and muscle length testing, Philadelphia, 2002, WB Saunders.
7. Pua YH, et al: Intrarater test-retest reliability of hip range of motion and hip muscle strength measurements in persons with hip osteoarthritis. Arch Phys Med Rehabil 89:1146–1154, 2008.
8. Oberg T, Karsznia A, Oberg K: Basic gait parameters: reference data for normal subjects, 10-79 years of age. J Rehabil Res Dev 30:210–223, 1993.
9. Richard R, et al: Spatiotemporal gait parameters measured using the Bessou gait analyzer in 79 healthy subjects: influence of age, stature, and gender. Study Group on Disabilities due to Musculoskeletal Disorders (Groupe de Recherche sur le Handicap de l'Appareil Locomoteur, GRHAL). Rev Rhum Engl Ed 62:105–114, 1995.
10. Kerrigan DC, Todd MK, Della Croce U: Gender differences in joint biomechanics during walking: normative study in young adults. Am J Phys Med Rehabil 77:2–7, 1998.
11. Roach KM: Normal hip and knee active range of motion: the relationship to age. Phys Ther 71:656–664, 1991.
12. Hemmerich A, et al: Hip, knee, and ankle kinematics of high range of motion activities of daily living. J Orthop Res 24:770–781, 2006.
13. Ahlberg A, Moussa M, Al-Nahdi M: On geographical variations in the normal range of joint motion. Clin Orthop Relat Res 234:229–231, 1988.
14. Hoaglund FT, Yau AC, Wong WL: Osteoarthritis of the hip and other joints in southern Chinese in Hong Kong. J Bone Joint Surg Am 55:545–557, 1973.
15. Mulholland SJ, Wyss UP: Activities of daily living in non-Western cultures: range of motion requirements for hip and knee joint implants. Int J Rehabil Res 24:191–198, 2001.
16. Hewitt JD, et al: The mechanical properties of the human hip capsule ligaments. J Arthroplasty 17:82–89, 2002.
17. Stewart KJ, et al: Spatial distribution of hip capsule structural and material properties. J Biomech 35:1491–1498, 2002.
18. Offierski CM: Traumatic dislocation of the hip in children. J Bone Joint Surg Br 63:194–197, 2001.
19. Won YY, et al: Morphological study on the acetabular labrum. Yonsei Med J 44:855–862, 2003.
20. Kelly BT, et al: Vascularity of the hip labrum: a cadaveric investigation. Arthroscopy 21:3–11, 2005.
21. Kelly BT, et al: Arthroscopic labral repair in the hip: surgical technique and review of the literature. Arthroscopy 21:1496–1504, 2005.
22. Ferguson SJ, Bryant JT, Ito K: The material properties of the bovine acetabular labrum. J Orthop Res 19:887–896, 2001.
23. Ishiko T, Naito M, Moriyama S: Tensile properties of the human acetabular labrum—the first report. J Orthop Res 23:1448–1453, 2005.
24. Smith CD, et al: A biomechanical basis for tears of the human acetabular labrum. Br J Sports Med 43:574–578, 2009.
25. Altenberg AR: Acetabular labrum tears: a cause of hip pain and degenerative arthritis. South Med J 70:174–175, 1977.
26. Konrath GA, et al: The role of the acetabular labrum and the transverse acetabular ligament in load transmission in the hip. J Bone Joint Surg Am 80:1781–1788, 1998.
27. Beaule PE, O'Neill M, Rakhra K: Acetabular labral tears. J Bone Joint Surg Am 91:701–710, 2009.
28. Crawford MJ, et al: The 2007 Frank Stinchfield Award: the biomechanics of the hip labrum and the stability of the hip, Clin Orthop Relat Res 465:16–22, 2007.
29. Ferguson SJ, et al: The influence of the acetabular labrum on hip joint cartilage consolidation: a poroelastic finite element model. J Biomech 33:953–960, 2000.
30. Eijer HL: Cross-table lateral radiographs for screening of anterior femoral head-neck offset in patients with femoro-acetabular impingement. Hip Int 11:37–41, 2001.

31. Ferguson SJ, et al: An in vitro investigation of the acetabular labral seal in hip joint mechanics. J Biomech 36:171–178, 2003.

32. Takechi H, Nagashima H, Ito S: Intra-articular pressure of the hip joint outside and inside the limbus. Nippon Seikeigeka Gakkai Zasshi 56:529–536, 1982.

33. Ferguson SJ, et al: The acetabular labrum seal: a poroelastic finite element model. Clin Biomech 15:463–468, 2000.

34. Hlavacek M: The influence of the acetabular labrum seal, intact articular superficial zone and synovial fluid thixotropy on squeeze-film lubrication of a spherical synovial joint. J Biomech 35:1325–1335, 2002.

35. McCarthy JC, et al: The Otto E. Aufranc Award: the role of labral lesions to development of early degenerative hip disease. Clin Orthop Relat Res 393:25–37, 2001.

36. McCarthy JC, et al: The watershed labral lesion: its relationship to early arthritis of the hip. J Arthroplasty 16(Suppl 8 1):81–87, 2001.

37. Cashin M, et al: Embryology of the acetabular labral-chondral complex. J Bone Joint Surg Br 90:1019–1024, 2008.

38. Murphy KP, et al: Repair of the adult acetabular labrum. Arthroscopy 22:567e1–567e3, 2006.

39. Espinosa N, et al: Treatment of femoro-acetabular impingement: preliminary results of labral refixation. J Bone Joint Surg Am 88:925–935, 2006.

40. Sierra RJ, Trousdale RT: Labral reconstruction using the ligamentum teres capitis: report of a new technique. Clin Orthop Relat Res 467:753–759, 2009.

41. Bardakos NV, Villar RN: The ligamentum teres of the adult hip. J Bone Joint Surg Br 91:8–15, 2009.

42. Wenger D, et al: The mechanical properties of the ligamentum teres: a pilot study to assess its potential for improving stability in children's hip surgery. J Pediatr Orthop 27:408–410, 2007.

43. Kelly BT, Williams RJ 3rd, Philippon MJ: Hip arthroscopy: current indications, treatment options, and management issues. Am J Sports Med 31:1020–1037, 2001.

44. Cichy B, Wilk M, Sliwinski Z: Changes in gait parameters in total hip arthroplasty patients before and after surgery. Med Sci Monit 14:CR159–169, 2008.

45. Kadaba MP, et al: Repeatability of kinematic, kinetic, and electromyographic data in normal adult gait. J Orthop Res 7:849–860, 1989.

46. Oatis CA (ed): Biomechanics of the hip, New York, 1990, Churchill Livingstone.

47. Nicholas J, Hershman E: The lower extremity and spine in sports medicine, vol 2, St Louis, 1995, Mosby-Year Book.

48. Johnston RC, Noble PC, Hurwitz DE, Andriacchi TP: Biomechanics of the hip. In Callaghan JJ, Rosenberg AG, Rubash HE (eds): The adult hip, ed 2, Baltimore, 2007, Lippincott Williams & Wilkins.

49. Ganz R, et al: The etiology of osteoarthritis of the hip: an integrated mechanical concept. Clin Orthop Relat Res 466:264–272, 2008.

50. Ganz R, et al: Femoroacetabular impingement: a cause for osteoarthritis of the hip. Clin Orthop Relat Res 417:112–120, 2003.

51. Ito K, et al: Femoroacetabular impingement and the cam-effect: a MRI-based quantitative anatomical study of the femoral head-neck offset. J Bone Joint Surg Br 83:171–176, 2001.

52. Kennedy MJ, Lamontagne M, Beaule PE: Femoroacetabular impingement alters hip and pelvic biomechanics during gait: walking biomechanics of FAI. Gait Posture 30:41–44, 2009.

53. Morrey BF: Joint replacement arthroplasty. In Morrey BF, Zong-Ping L (eds): Biomechanics, Philadelphia, 2003, Elsevier Science.

54. Kerrigan DC, et al: Reduced hip extension during walking: healthy elderly and fallers versus young adults. Arch Phys Med Rehabil 82:26–30, 2001.

55. Kirkwood R, Gomes H, Sampaio RF, et al: Biomechanical analysis of hip and knee joints during gait in elderly subjects. Acta Ortop Bras 15:267–271, 2007.

56. Murray MP, Gore DR, Clarkson BH: Walking patterns of patients with unilateral hip pain due to osteo-arthritis and avascular necrosis. J Bone Joint Surg Am 53:259–274, 1971.

57. Johnston RC, Brand RA, Crowninshield RD: Reconstruction of the hip: a mathematical approach to determine optimum geometric relationships. J Bone Joint Surg Am 61:639–652, 1979.

58. Gore DR, et al: Roentgenographic measurements after Muller total hip replacement: correlations among roentgenographic measurements and hip strength and mobility. J Bone Joint Surg Am 59:948–953, 1977.

59. Bierma-Zeinstra SM, et al: Sonography for hip joint effusion in adults with hip pain. Ann Rheum Dis 59:178–182, 2000.

60. Goddard NJ, Gosling PT: Intra-articular fluid pressure and pain in osteoarthritis of the hip. J Bone Joint Surg Br 70:52–55, 1988.

61. Pua YH, et al: Hip flexion range of motion and physical function in hip osteoarthritis: mediating effects of hip extensor strength and pain. Arthritis Rheum 61:633–640, 2009.

62. Rasch A, et al: Reduced muscle radiological density, cross-sectional area, and strength of major hip and knee muscles in 22 patients with hip osteoarthritis. Acta Orthop 78:505–510, 2007.

63. Arokoski MH, et al: Physical function in men with and without hip osteoarthritis. Arch Phys Med Rehabil 85:574–581, 2004.

64. Leunig M, et al: Slipped capital femoral epiphysis: early mechanical damage to the acetabular cartilage by a prominent femoral metaphysis. Acta Orthop Scand 71:370–375, 2000.

65. Bardakos NV, Villar RN: Predictors of progression of osteoarthritis in femoroacetabular impingement: a radiological study with a minimum of ten years follow-up. J Bone Joint Surg Br 91:162–169, 2009.

66. Kubiak-Langer M, et al: Range of motion in anterior femoroacetabular impingement. Clin Orthop Relat Res 458:117–124, 2007.

67. Tannast M, et al: Noninvasive three-dimensional assessment of femoroacetabular impingement. J Orthop Res 25:122–131, 2007.

68. Clohisy JC, et al: Clinical presentation of patients with symptomatic anterior hip impingement. Clin Orthop Relat Res 467:638–644, 2009.

69. Reichenbach S, Jüni P, Nüesch E, et al: An examination chair to measure internal rotation of the hip in routine settings: a validation study. Osteoarthritis Cartilage 18:365–371, 2010.

70. Lamontagne M, et al: Gait and motion analysis of the lower extremity after total hip arthroplasty: what the orthopedic surgeon should know. Orthop Clin North Am 40:397–405, 2009.

71. Leunig M, et al: Acetabular rim degeneration: a constant finding in the aged hip. Clin Orthop Relat Res 413:201–207, 2003.

72. Tannast M, et al: Hip damage occurs at the zone of femoroacetabular impingement. Clin Orthop Relat Res 466:273–280, 2008.

73. Dy CJ, et al: Tensile strain in the anterior part of the acetabular labrum during provocative maneuvering of the normal hip. J Bone Joint Surg Am 90:1464–1472, 2008.

74. Chegini S, Beck M, Ferguson SJ: The effects of impingement and dysplasia on stress distributions in the hip joint during sitting and walking: a finite element analysis. J Orthop Res 27:195–201, 2009.

75. Johnston TL, et al: Relationship between offset angle alpha and hip chondral injury in femoroacetabular impingement, Arthroscopy 24:669–675, 2008.

76. Leunig M, Huff TW, Ganz R: Femoroacetabular impingement: treatment of the acetabular side. Instr Course Lect 58:223–229, 2009.

77. Lavigne M, et al: Anterior femoroacetabular impingement: part I. Techniques of joint preserving surgery. Clin Orthop Relat Res 418:61–66, 2004.

78. Parvizi J, Leunig M, Ganz R: Femoroacetabular impingement. J Am Acad Orthop Surg 15:561–570, 2007.

79. Neumann M, et al: Impingement-free hip motion: the "normal" angle alpha after osteochondroplasty. Clin Orthop Relat Res 467:699–703, 2009.

80. Mardones RM, et al: Surgical treatment of femoroacetabular impingement: evaluation of the effect of the size of the resection. J Bone Joint Surg Am 87:273–279, 2005.

81. Kalberer F, et al: Ischial spine projection into the pelvis: a new sign for acetabular retroversion. Clin Orthop Relat Res 466:677–683, 2008.

82. Kim WY, et al: The relationship between acetabular retroversion and osteoarthritis of the hip. J Bone Joint Surg Br 88:727–729, 2006.

83. Kiyama T, et al: Postoperative acetabular retroversion causes posterior osteoarthritis of the hip. Int Orthop 33:625–631, 2009.

84. Reynolds D, Lucas J, Klaue K: Retroversion of the acetabulum: a cause of hip pain. J Bone Joint Surg Br 81:281–288, 1999.

85. Klaue K, Durnin CW, Ganz R: The acetabular rim syndrome: a clinical presentation of dysplasia of the hip. J Bone Joint Surg Br 73:423–429, 1991.

86. Jamali AA, et al: Anteroposterior pelvic radiographs to assess acetabular retroversion: high validity of the "cross-over-sign." J Orthop Res 25:758–765, 2008.

87. Dandachli W, et al: Three-dimensional CT analysis to determine acetabular retroversion and the implications for the management of femoro-acetabular impingement. J Bone Joint Surg Br 91:1031–1036, 2009.

88. Bergmann G, et al: Hip contact forces and gait patterns from routine activities. J Biomech 34:859–871, 2001.

89. Bergmann G, Graichen F, Rohlmann A: Is staircase walking a risk for the fixation of hip implants? J Biomech 28:535–553, 1995.

90. Bergmann G, Graichen F, Rohlmann A: Hip joint contact forces during stumbling. Langenbecks Arch Surg 389:53–59, 2004.

91. Bergmann G, et al: Realistic loads for testing hip implants. Biomed Mater Eng 20:65–75, 2010.

92. Tackson SJ, Krebs DE, Harris BA: Acetabular pressures during hip arthritis exercises. Arthritis Care Res 10:308–319, 1997.

93. Hodge WA, Andriacchi TP, Galante JO: A relationship between stem orientation and function following total hip arthroplasty. J Arthroplasty 6:229–235, 1991.

94. Hurwitz D, Chertack C, Andriacchi T: How gait changes in preoperative and postoperative patients with total hip replacements. Proceedings of the Second North American Congress on Biomechanics, Chicago, August 24–28, 1992, pp 313–314.

95. Foucher KC, Hurwitz DE, Wimmer MA: Do gait adaptations during stair climbing result in changes in implant forces in subjects with total hip replacements compared to normal subjects? Clin Biomech 23:754–761, 2008.

96. Stansfield BW, Nicol AC: Hip joint contact forces in normal subjects and subjects with total hip prostheses: walking and stair and ramp negotiation. Clin Biomech 17:130–139, 2002.

97. Paul JP: Force actions transmitted by joints in the human body. Proc R Soc Lond B Biol Sci 192:163–172, 1976.

98. Seireg A, Arvikar RJ: The prediction of muscular lad sharing and joint forces in the lower extremities during walking. J Biomech 8:89–102, 1975.

99. Crowninshield RD, et al: A biomechanical investigation of the human hip. J Biomech 11:75–85, 1978.

100. Duda GN, Schneider E, Chao EY: Internal forces and moments in the femur during walking. J Biomech 30:933–941, 1997.

101. Heller MO, et al: Musculo-skeletal loading conditions at the hip during walking and stair climbing. J Biomech 34:883–893, 2001.

102. Stansfield BW, et al: Direct comparison of calculated hip joint contact forces with those measured using instrumented implants: an evaluation of a three-dimensional mathematical model of the lower limb. J Biomech 36:929–936, 2003.

103. Amaro A, et al: Radiographic geometric measures of the hip joint and abductor muscle function in patients after total hip replacement. Eur J Orthop Surg Traumatol 17:437–443, 2007.

104. Delp SL, Komattu AV, Wixson RL: Superior displacement of the hip in total joint replacement: effects of prosthetic neck length, neck-stem angle, and anteversion angle on the moment-generating capacity of the muscles. J Orthop Res 12:860–870, 1994.

105. Delp SL, Maloney W: Effects of hip center location on the moment-generating capacity of the muscles. J Biomech 26:485–499, 1993.

106. Delp SL, et al: How superior placement of the joint center in hip arthroplasty affects the abductor muscles. Clin Orthop Relat Res 328:137–146, 1996.

107. Lenaerts G, et al: Subject-specific hip geometry affects predicted hip joint contact forces during gait. J Biomech 41:1243–1252, 2008.

108. Doehring TC, et al: Effect of superior and superolateral relocations of the hip center on hip joint forces: an experimental and analytical analysis. J Arthroplasty 11:693–703, 1996.

109. Adeeb SM, et al: Congruency effects on load bearing in diarthrodial joints. Comput Methods Biomech Biomed Engin 7:147–157, 2004.

110. Genda E, et al: A computer simulation study of normal and abnormal hip joint contact pressure. Arch Orthop Trauma Surg 114:202–206, 1995

111. Tsumura H, Miura H, Iwamoto Y: Three-dimensional pressure distribution of the human hip joint–comparison between normal hips and dysplastic hips. Fukuoka Igaku Zasshi 89:109–118, 1998.

112. Hipp JA, et al: Planning acetabular redirection osteotomies based on joint contact pressures. Clin Orthop Relat Res 364:134–143, 1999.

113. Russell ME, et al: Cartilage contact pressure elevations in dysplastic hips: a chronic overload model. J Orthop Surg Res 1:6, 2006.

114. Daniel M, Iglic A, Kralj-Iglic V: Hip contact stress during normal and staircase walking: the influence of acetabular anteversion angle and lateral coverage of the acetabulum. J Appl Biomech 24:88–93, 2008.

115. Horii M, et al: Coverage of the femoral head by the acetabular labrum in dysplastic hips: quantitative analysis with radial MR imaging. Acta Orthop Scand 74:287–292, 2003.

116. Noguchi Y, et al: Cartilage and labrum degeneration in the dysplastic hip generally originates in the anterosuperior weight-bearing area: an arthroscopic observation. Arthroscopy 15:496–506, 1999.

117. Haene RA, Bradley M, Villar RN: Hip dysplasia and the torn acetabular labrum: an inexact relationship. J Bone Joint Surg Br 89:1289–1292, 2007.

118. Kawabe K, Konishi N: Three-dimensional modeling of cartilage thickness in hip dysplasia. Clin Orthop Relat Res 289:180–185, 1993.

CHAPTER 2

Biomechanics of the Artificial Hip Joint

Georg N. Duda, Christian König, Georg Bergmann, *Stephan Tohtz, Carsten Perka, and Markus O.W. Heller*

KEY POINTS

- Muscle forces play an integral role in the loading environment of the joint. If the mechanical role of major muscles is neglected in biomechanical analysis, joint contact forces tend to be underestimated, tensile and compressive strains in the femur are often overestimated, and torsional effects are most often underestimated.
- Restoring the hip center to its anatomic location, specifically its mediolateral position, is essential for minimizing contact forces in the hip joint and avoiding adverse effects.
- The orientation of femoral stems is essential for long-term performance in vivo. Femoral anteversion plays a more important role than prosthesis offset in determining cement mantle stresses and therefore may be considered a more influential parameter in the long-term clinical outcome of primary THA. Changes in femoral implant orientation and design are capable of causing substantial increases in cement stresses, most importantly in critical regions such as the calcar.
- A combination of increased offset and anteversion of the femoral stem can produce critical cement stresses, especially during stair climbing activities. Thus, care should be taken to avoid increases in femoral anteversion, particularly when cemented stems with a large offset are used, with which large femoral anteversion angles should be avoided.
- Use of a short-stemmed implant may facilitate minimally invasive surgical approaches, but despite the concept of proximal anchoring, some stress shielding can occur even with short-stemmed implants.
- Malplacement of a cementless short-stemmed implant leads to only small changes in internal loads within the proximal femur, provided that moderate changes occur in the anteversion or effective offset of the femoral stem. Much larger changes in cortical strains generally result from implantation of the prosthesis.
- In cases of dysplasia-associated secondary coxarthrosis with pathologic anteversion of the femoral neck, the use of short-stemmed implants can be—from a biomechanical point of view—somewhat critical, in that the possibilities for anatomic reconstruction of the anteversion are limited, possibly favoring high hip contact forces and large loads in the femur.

INTRODUCTION

Long-term survival of the artificial hip joint is influenced by several factors, including prosthesis design,[1,2] quality of surrounding bone stock,[3] degree of patient activity,[4] and surgical aspects such as orientation of the implant.[5] Furthermore, it is accepted that modifications in joint geometry secondary to hip arthroplasty have an impact on joint function,[6] primary stability,[7] and bone remodeling.[8]

To improve the long-term survival of joint replacements and to minimize rehabilitation time, a fundamental understanding of the biomechanics of the joint is necessary. This becomes even more relevant in revision cases. Such an understanding is important because the geometry of the artificial hip can differ from the preoperative condition, and this may lead to significantly altered mechanical boundary conditions in the joint. During total hip arthroplasty (THA), surgeons often aim to optimize function and loading conditions through specific geometric alteration of the musculoskeletal structures. However, without detailed knowledge regarding in vivo musculoskeletal loading, neither the short-term nor the long-term consequences of these intraoperative alterations can be accurately predicted.

This chapter aims to provide a basic explanation of the biomechanics of the artificial hip and to assess possible consequences when the geometry of the joint is altered. Even though the complex biomechanical analyses introduced in this chapter may be difficult to perform in daily clinical practice, an understanding of basic musculoskeletal mechanisms may help the clinician to incorporate biomechanical principles in the individual treatment of patients. This chapter also aims to raise awareness of the importance of preoperative planning for joint replacement. Although it is common to consider geometric aspects of joint reconstruction, planning tools or even navigation systems that consider the biomechanics of the artificial joint are not now a routine component of clinical practice of THA.

To fully comprehend the biomechanical consequences of changes in joint geometry, an appreciation of the internal loading conditions of the joint must be gained. Load transmission via the joints and in long bones has long been considered of importance for clinical evaluation and biomechanical analysis.[9] However, illustrations of loading conditions in the femur have often been oversimplified by displaying only the hip contact force acting on the femoral head. This tends to leave the impression that forces are transmitted through the bone and "leave" the bone at its distal end. This concept has widely influenced the design of experimental apparatus used in fatigue testing,[10] evaluation of the primary stability of implants,[11] and remodeling analyses.[12] As described in greater detail in the following pages, in vivo measurements and numeric analyses of musculoskeletal loading show that load transfer is modified along the entire length of the bone through continuous action of muscles. To understand the femoral load state, the original misconception should therefore be revised to reflect the close relationship between joint contact forces and muscle action.

THE BASIC SCIENCE OF THE HIP JOINT

Musculoskeletal Loading Conditions at the Hip

Background

Knowledge of external loads on the body and their corresponding internal counterparts is essential for gaining more detailed information on the loads that an artificial hip joint has to bear. Because these internal and external loads define mechanical boundary conditions in the joint, this knowledge also provides the basis for investigating and understanding biological processes that occur during bone healing and remodeling.[13,14]

In 1870, Julius Wolff described, for the first time, the interrelationship between loading, stress, and strain in anatomic structures; he later manifested this description in the so-called *Wolff's laws*.[15] Based on Wolff's investigations, Koch published the first analytical determination of loading conditions in long bones.[16] The remarkable role that muscles play in the loading scenario of long bones was first described later by Pauwels.[17] Using the abductors and the iliotibial tract, Pauwels illustrated the way in which muscle forces reduced internal loading within the bone. In numerous examples, Pauwels also described how muscles and tendons counteracted bending moments generated at the hip through the action of body weight by examining areas of tensile and compressive strain within the cross-section of long bones.[18]

Although it is now known that the contributions of muscles are essential in the mechanical loading of bones, the actual forces occurring in vivo are hardly accessible. Direct measurement of the coordinated action of all muscle forces in vivo is impossible, as ethical considerations discourage the use of invasive methods in humans. Therefore, the only opportunity to estimate the complex distribution of muscle forces is offered by computer analysis.

In various studies, optimization algorithms were used to solve the distribution problem and to simulate loading conditions at the hip.[19-30] A common approach to validating these models was comparison of muscle activation patterns obtained from simulation versus measured muscle activities as determined by electromyography (EMG). However, this method does not allow quantitative validation of musculoskeletal loading conditions. Instrumented implants provide hip contact forces for different activities for individual patients in vivo.[31-37] An additional method of validating predicted musculoskeletal loading conditions is comparison of calculated hip contact forces versus in vivo measured forces. Hip contact forces measured with instrumented prostheses have been compared with results of computer modeling in the same patients by Heller and coworkers[38] and Brand and coworkers.[34] The latter study measured hip contact forces 58 days postoperatively, and gait analysis was performed 90 days postoperatively. Therefore, a cycle-to-cycle comparison of measured and calculated hip contact forces was not possible. Heller and coworkers[38] used a cycle-to-cycle comparison of measured and calculated hip contact forces to attain a basic understanding of the biomechanics of the artificial hip joint.

Determination of Internal Loading Conditions

To analytically describe musculoskeletal loading conditions within the body, the movement of the extremities and the external loads must be known. This information can be gained through gait analysis, whereby movement of the lower extremity and ground reaction forces on the feet can be measured, even for large patient cohorts.[39] Based on this individual measurement of movement and external loads, resulting joint reaction forces can be calculated using an inverse dynamics approach.[40] Here, joint loads represent the sum of all forces and moments at the joint generated by muscular activity. With the use of optimization algorithms, a "reasonable" solution can be found for a pattern of muscular activity that can balance these forces and moments.[19,41] However, it is necessary to validate these mathematical analyses against in vivo data to verify the plausibility of the results.[34] One option for gaining such in vivo data is the use of telemetric implants as, for example, developed by Bergmann and colleagues.[42]

Heller and coworkers[38] followed such an approach in their study and verified their results calculated with a musculoskeletal model by using hip contact forces measured with telemetric hip implants. A full description of the musculoskeletal model of the lower limb,[38] muscle and joint contact force calculations,[43] and collection of gait data[42] can be found in greater detail in the literature and is briefly summarized here. Four THA patients with telemetric prostheses (11 to 31 months postoperatively) were considered in the study. For all four patients, individual anatomic measures were determined from computed tomography (CT) scans and radiographic findings (pelvic width and depth; femoral, tibial, and foot length). In addition, neck length, neck stem, and cervicodiaphyseal and anteversion angles were recorded. Gait analysis data for walking and stair climbing[42] (i.e., ground reaction forces, limb segment positions, velocities, and accelerations) were determined simultaneously with the use of in vivo hip contact forces. A computer model of the human lower extremity (CT data; Visible Human Project, National Library of Medicine), including bone surfaces and muscles, was developed (Fig. 2-1). Where appropriate, muscles were wrapped around bony contours. This model was then scaled to match the individual anatomies of the four different patients. Muscle and joint contact forces were calculated throughout the gait cycle for both walking and stair climbing using an optimization algorithm that minimized the sum of muscle forces. For validation, hip contact forces calculated for individual gait cycles were compared directly

with corresponding in vivo measurements, revealing good agreement.

With the use of such validated musculoskeletal models, the biomechanics of the artificial hip can be explored in greater detail. Variations in numerous parameters describing the anatomically reconstructed artificial hip can be simulated using the computer model, including, for example, variations in prosthesis placement and orientation. Furthermore, although in

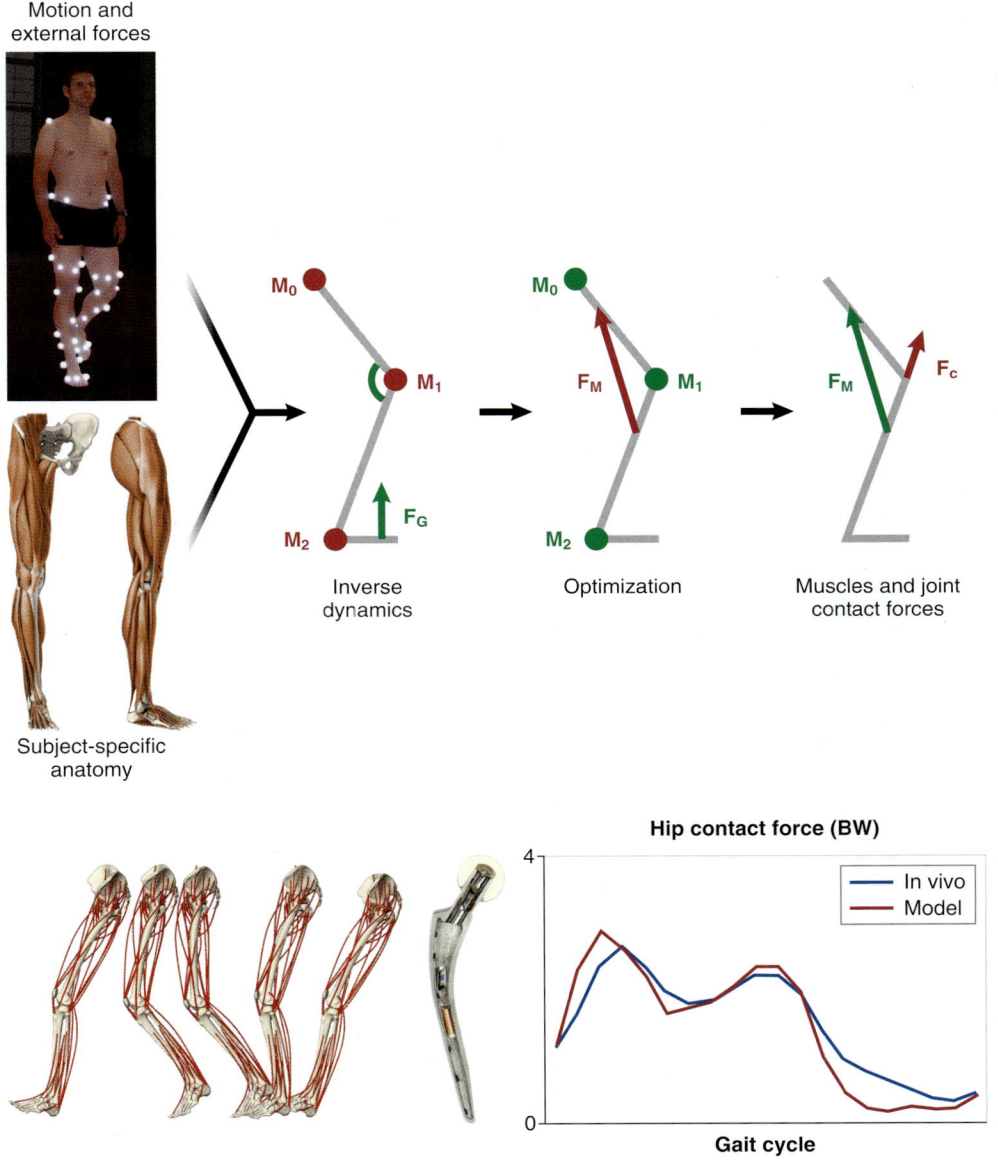

Figure 2-1. Schematic representation of patient-specific determination of internal loading conditions. Gait analysis data are recorded for a subject (i.e., ground reaction forces and moments), together with limb segment positions from which velocities and accelerations are determined *(upper left)*. Using key anatomic measures of the patient's anatomy (pelvic width and depth; femoral, tibial, and foot length; femoral neck length; cervicodiaphyseal and anteversion angles), which can be derived from medical imaging data, a patient-specific musculoskeletal model is generated *(lower left)*. Combining these data in an inverse dynamics approach provides access to intersegmental resultant joint moments. Muscle and joint contact forces are then calculated using an optimization algorithm, which minimizes the sum of muscle forces to balance these moments *(upper right)*. To validate the predictions of the musculoskeletal model, hip contact forces calculated for individual gait cycles of four patients were compared directly with corresponding in vivo forces measured with telemetric hip implants *(lower right)*.

vivo measurements provide limited data, describing internal forces acting at a single location, musculoskeletal models that predict muscle and joint forces throughout the entire extremity provide a means to analyze and better understand loading conditions throughout the entire bone.

Biomechanics of the Proximal Femur

The musculoskeletal model has revealed[44] that internal loading of the femur is predominantly characterized by axial compression (F_z), with small mediolaterally (F_x)

and anteroposteriorly (F_y) oriented shear forces (Fig. 2-2). During walking, both compressive and shear forces are largest at the femoral head and decrease distally toward the diaphysis. This is related to the relatively large activity of the abductors during gait.[45-47] Bending moments in the femur are dominated by the frontal plane bending moment (M_y), and axial torsion (M_z) is the smallest of all moments (see Fig. 2-2).

Even though patterns differed over time because of patients' individual gait characteristics,[48] combined with their postoperative rehabilitation, load magnitudes

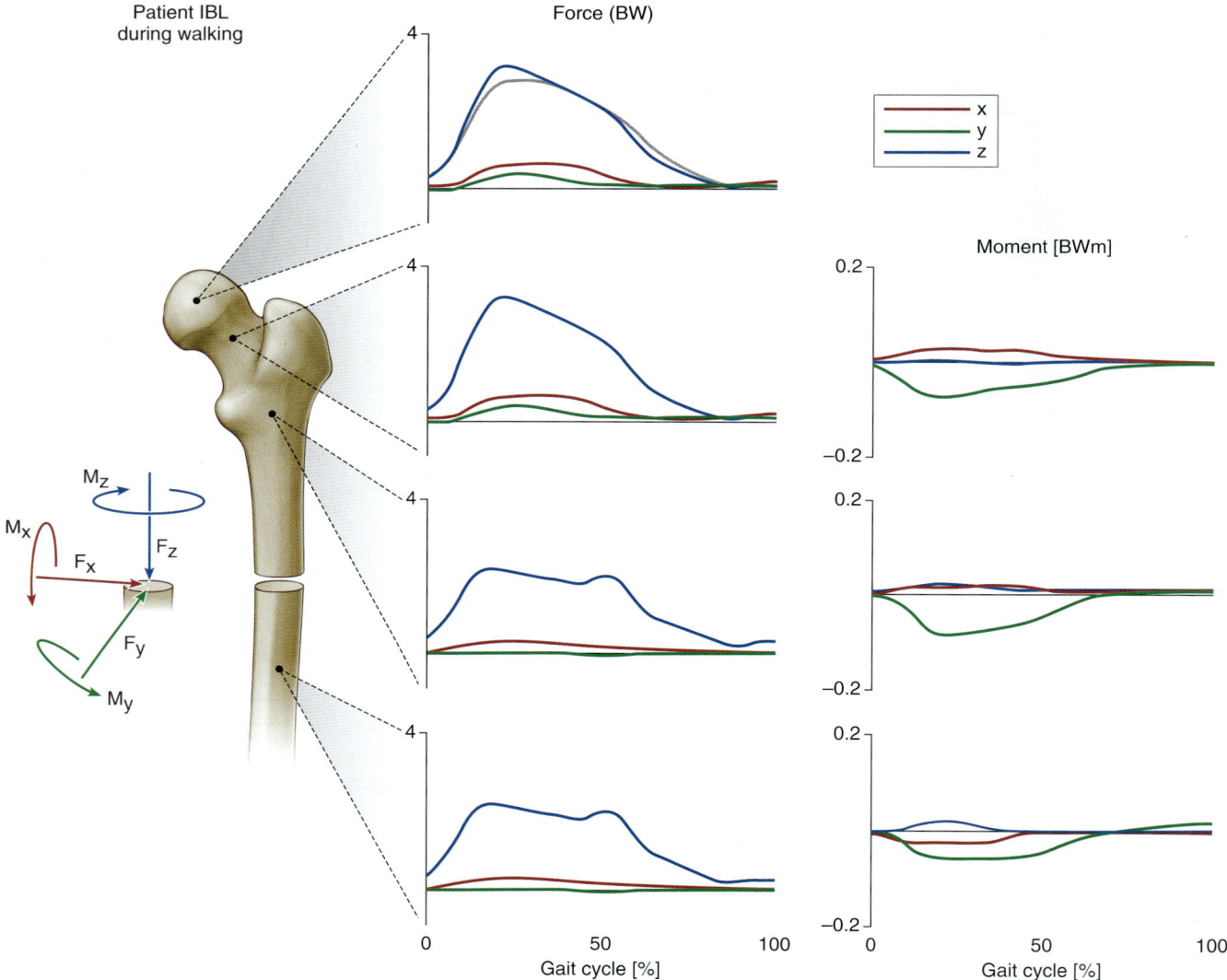

Figure 2-2. Internal loads at four levels of the femur during the walking cycle are shown for one specific subject. Forces are given in multiples of body weight (BW), moments in body weight meters (BWm), and time in percent of walking cycle, starting with heel strike. **Dark graphs,** F_x is the shear force from medial to lateral; F_y is the shear force from anterior to posterior; and F_x is the axial compression force from proximal to distal. M_x is the backward acting bending moment in the sagittal plane, M_y is the inward acting bending moment in the frontal plane, and M_z is the torsional moment in the transverse plane. The moments at the head center are zero. **Light graph,** In vivo measured hip contact force component is F_z. All signs are reversed for the proximal sides. (Redrawn from Heller MO, Bergmann G, Deuretzbacher G, et al: Influence of femoral anteversion on proximal femoral loading: measurement and simulation in four patients. Clin Biomech [Bristol, Avon] 8:644–649, 2001.)

appeared to be comparable between the four patients during walking (Fig. 2-3) and stair climbing (Fig. 2-4). However, large differences were found in the magnitude of compressive forces acting down the femur (F_z), where, during stair climbing, forces peaked in the diaphyseal part of the bone because of contraction of the vasti.[49,50] In addition to observed general patterns of forces and moments acting within the femur,

patient-specific loading characteristics were apparent. Variation was noted, not only in the head, but throughout the length of the bone. The importance of considering the muscle contribution when analyzing mechanical loading is underlined by the fact that the bending moments determined were considerably smaller than those predicted by previous analyses, which neglected muscle forces.[16,18,51]

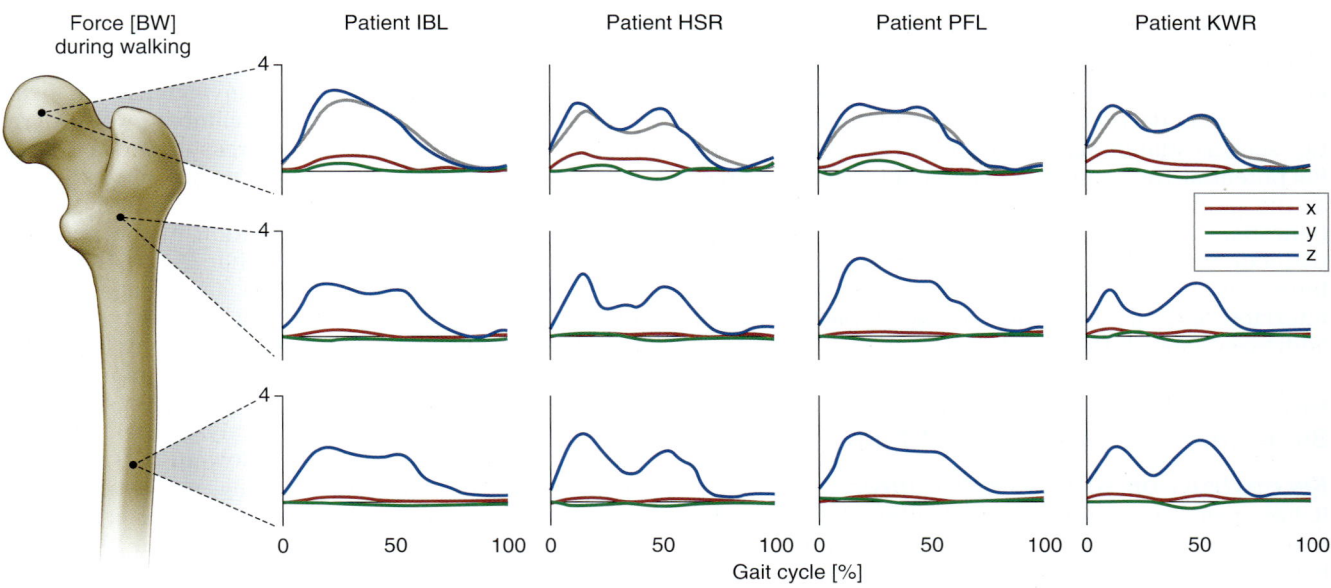

Figure 2-3. Internal forces at three levels of the femur, values in body weight (BW). Results are shown for four patients during walking (for further explanation, see Fig. 2-2). *(Redrawn from Heller MO, Bergmann G, Deuretzbacher G, et al: Influence of femoral anteversion on proximal femoral loading: measurement and simulation in four patients. Clin Biomech [Bristol, Avon] 8:644–649, 2001.)*

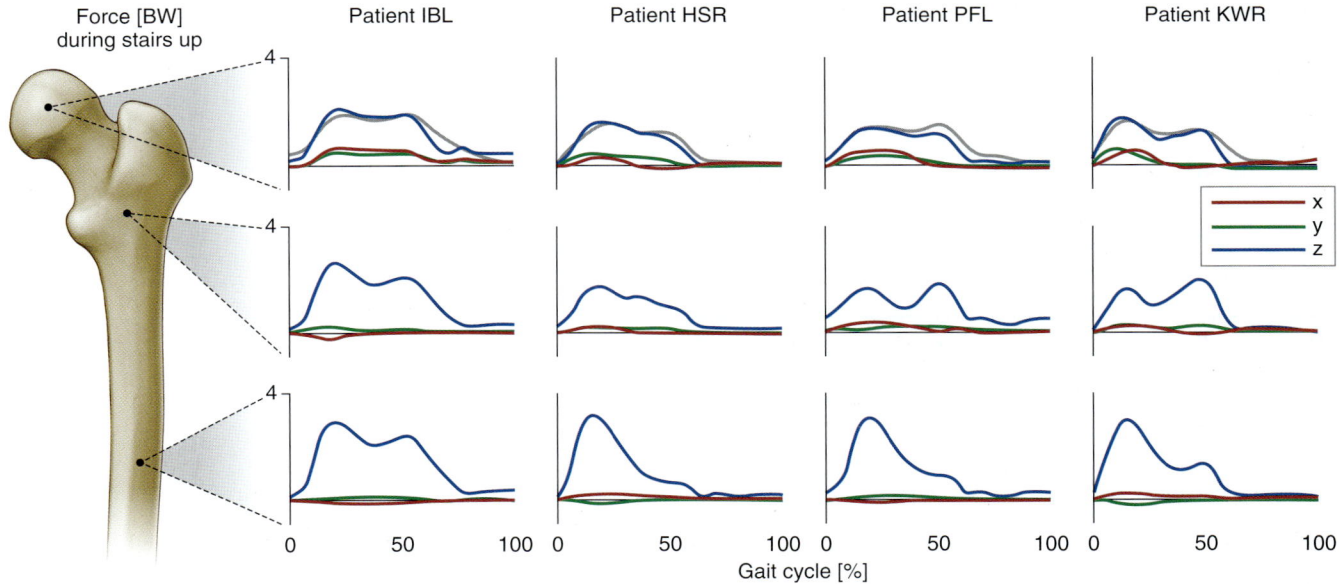

Figure 2-4. Internal forces at three levels of the femur, values in body weight (BW). Results are shown for four patients during stair climbing (for further explanation, see Fig. 2-2). *(Redrawn from Heller MO, Bergmann G, Deuretzbacher G, et al: Influence of femoral anteversion on proximal femoral loading: measurement and simulation in four patients. Clin Biomech [Bristol, Avon] 8:644–649, 2001.)*

Generally, analyses revealed that higher hip contact forces occurred during stair climbing activities than during level gait in all four patients,[42] corresponding to larger internal forces and moments. It has to be kept in mind, however, that fast walking causes forces at the hip joint that are higher than during stair climbing.[31] The general ratio of compression to shear forces and of bending to torsional moment remained similar throughout. The literature suggests that specific situations such as stumbling are capable of causing excessive hip contact forces.[32] Analysis of musculoskeletal interaction suggests that under these conditions, muscle activity alone is capable of generating extreme joint forces. Similarly, all other bony regions spanned by activated muscles may become excessively loaded during activities such as stumbling.[52] If muscles are activated to their full potential, they may produce not only maximal forces at the joints and extreme compression forces in the bone but also excessive bending and shear forces. In patients with joint arthroplasty, such high contact forces and bony loads may endanger the bone implant interface and the longevity of the implants; this is addressed later in the chapter.

Influence of Joint Reconstruction on Biomechanics of the Artificial Joint

Reconstruction of the Joint Center

It has been suggested that implanting the acetabular cup of the artificial joint in a cranialized position will lead to unfavorable loading conditions in the joint,[53] which are associated with disadvantageous long-term clinical results.[54,55] These observations led to additional studies evaluating the influence of acetabular cup placement on loading conditions at the hip, as well as on the long-term polyethylene wear of the cup itself.[56]

In a musculoskeletal model, the acetabular cup was translated up to 10 mm in the medial, lateral, anterior,

posterior, cranial, or caudal position. For these altered positions of the hip center, the mean joint contact force during the whole gait cycle and peak hip joint contact forces were determined during walking and stair climbing activities and were compared with those forces occurring in an anatomically reconstructed acetabulum.

This analysis revealed that mediolateral deviation from the anatomic location of the hip center has the greatest influence on loading conditions in the hip (Fig. 2-5). The mean joint contact force, which summarizes the net change in joint loading over the full cycle, decreased when the joint center was medialized, while lateralization by 10 mm led to an increase in mean contact forces (walking, 8%; stair climbing, 7%). A cranialized joint center slightly decreased and a 10-mm caudalized joint center increased mean contact forces by 1% during a cycle of normal walking, and by 2% for a stair climbing gait cycle. Deviation in the anterior-posterior direction resulted in changes to the mean contact forces, which stayed below 3%. Changes in peak hip contact forces during the gait cycle were greater than those noted in mean contact forces over the entire cycle, and the largest increase in peak joint contact force was seen in a lateralized hip center (+14%).

Among 109 retrospectively analyzed primary hip replacements with an average follow-up of 9.3 years,[57] the joint center was anatomically reconstructed in 61% (n = 66) (group I). The joint center was cranialized in 29 patients (27%) (group II), medialized in 10 patients (group III), and caudalized in 4 patients (group IV). Although no significant difference was observed between any of the groups in terms of Harris hip scores, and no difference in the linear polyethylene wear rate was found between groups I and II, the group with the medialized joint center (group III) and with lower joint contact forces exhibited significantly lower wear (0.077 mm³/year) than the group with an anatomically

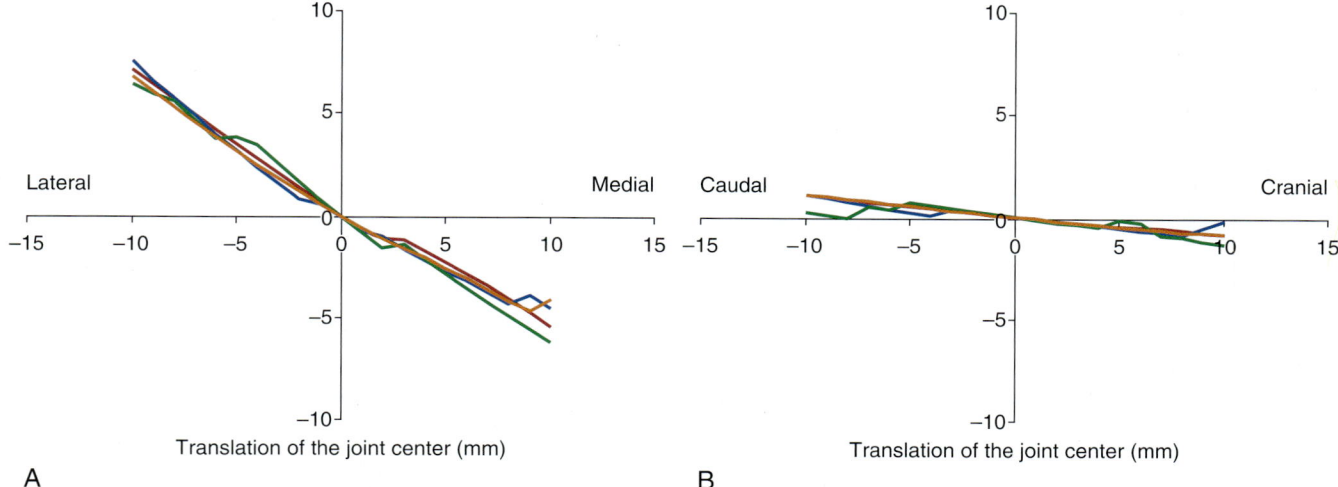

Figure 2-5. Influence of cranial-caudal **(A)** and mediolateral **(B)** translation of the hip center on joint contact forces in the hip. Displayed is the change in mean hip contact forces during a walking cycle in relation to values in the anatomically reconstructed joint. *(Modified from Heller MO, Schroder JH, Matziolis G, et al: [Musculoskeletal load analysis: a biomechanical explanation for clinical results—and more?]. Orthopade 3:188, 190–194, 2007.)*

reconstructed joint (group I; $P = .018$). Analyses[56] therefore revealed an interrelation between the location of the artificial hip joint center, joint contact forces acting in the artificial hip, and wear of the polyethylene inserts.

Femoral Anteversion

Anteversion is considered a possible factor in the onset of joint degeneration.[58,59] It has been suggested that femoral anteversion plays an important role in load transfer from implant to bone and hence may alter the outcome of a THA.[32]

Unfavorable modification of anteversion during surgery may lead to increased loading of the hip, which would be most prominent during repetitive daily activities, such as walking and stair climbing,[60] potentially leading to implant loosening.[31]

Using the validated numeric model of musculoskeletal loading conditions in the proximal femur, Heller and coworkers tested the hypothesis that femoral anteversion influences musculoskeletal loading conditions throughout normal activities.[44] In four patients in whom stems were implanted at anteversion angles of –2 degrees, +4 degrees, +14 degrees, and +23 degrees, changes in stem anteversion to an angle of 5 degrees of retroversion and to an angle of 30 degrees of anteversion were simulated, and the loads developed were compared with values for the actual implantation. In all four patients, an increase in anteversion to an angle of 30 degrees led to an increase in hip contact forces (Fig. 2-6) and the moment acting in the frontal plane (M_y;

Fig. 2-7). Decreasing stem anteversion to an angle of –5 degrees resulted in little or no change in the hip contact force. The effect of increased anteversion was most pronounced in patients with initially small anteversion (see Fig. 2-6), in whom large increases in hip contact force were found during walking (maximum, +24%) and stair climbing (maximum, +23%).

The overall conclusion of this analysis was that if anteversion is increased during joint replacement by less than 15 degrees, loading of the proximal femur may not be drastically altered. However, if anteversion is increased by more than 20 degrees, a considerable increase in femoral loading may occur. Moreover, the additional increase in bending moments within the proximal femur may influence bone remodeling and the long-term performance of implants.[32,61] However, this mechanical analysis suggests that large modifications of anteversion, compared with the preoperative situation, appear to be detrimental and should be avoided.

Strains and Stresses in the Artificial Hip Joint

Influence of Muscle Forces on Femoral Strain Distribution

Musculoskeletal loading generates stresses and strains within the human femur and thereby influences the processes of bone modeling and remodeling. As mentioned earlier in this chapter, bone in healthy subjects adapts to its mechanical environment.[15] Therefore, it is essential for implant design and simulations of bone modeling processes that locally high or low strain values that may lead to bone resorption, potentially affecting clinical outcome, are identified. In some patients with endoprosthetic joint replacement or fracture fixation devices, local strains and stresses may exceed biological limits,[62,63] leading to bone resorption or remodeling and possible implant loosening.[64,65]

Finite element analysis provides a convenient way to determine strains and stresses in the femur before and after joint replacement. An important precondition in these analyses is the correct definition of boundary conditions, specifically, loads applied to the bone. In most published studies on finite element analysis of the human femur, physiologic loading is approximated using the abductor muscles and the iliotibial band.[66-70] The particular importance of the iliotibial tract and the abductors to the femoral loading condition was described by Pauwels[17] and was later confirmed by a continuum mechanics approach.[71] However, given the relative contribution of muscle activity to the loading situation,[51,72] it may be important to consider the contributions of more muscles than only the abductors and the iliotibial band.[73] Duda and coworkers[74] determined the strain distribution within the femur during gait using a simulation that included all muscles of the thigh. They compared resulting cortical strain distributions with those obtained using simplified load regimes. This allowed them to determine which muscle forces should be included in analytical investigations for appropriate simulation of loading conditions for the proximal femur with maximal physiologic relevance.

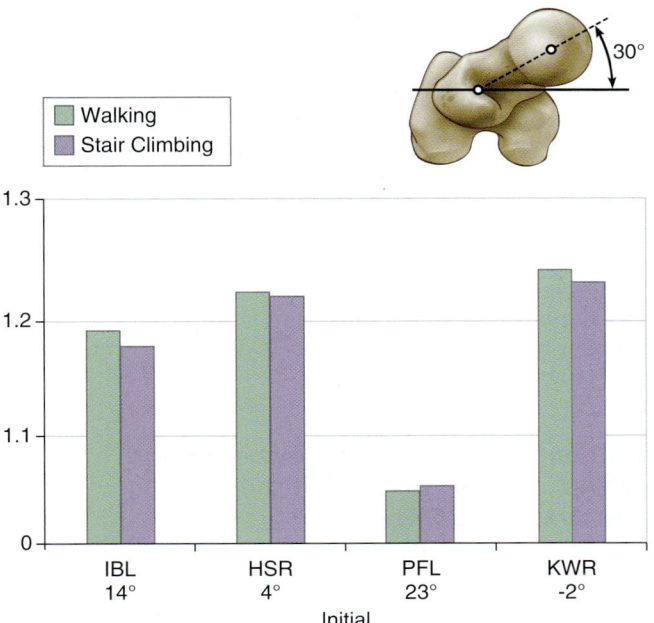

Figure 2-6. Ratio of maximal hip contact force with increased anteversion of +30 degrees to hip contact force with initial anteversion. Data for four patients and two activities are given. (*Redrawn from Heller MO, Bergmann G, Deuretzbacher G, et al: Influence of femoral anteversion on proximal femoral loading: measurement and simulation in four patients. Clin Biomech [Bristol, Avon] 8:644–649, 2001, Fig. 5.*)

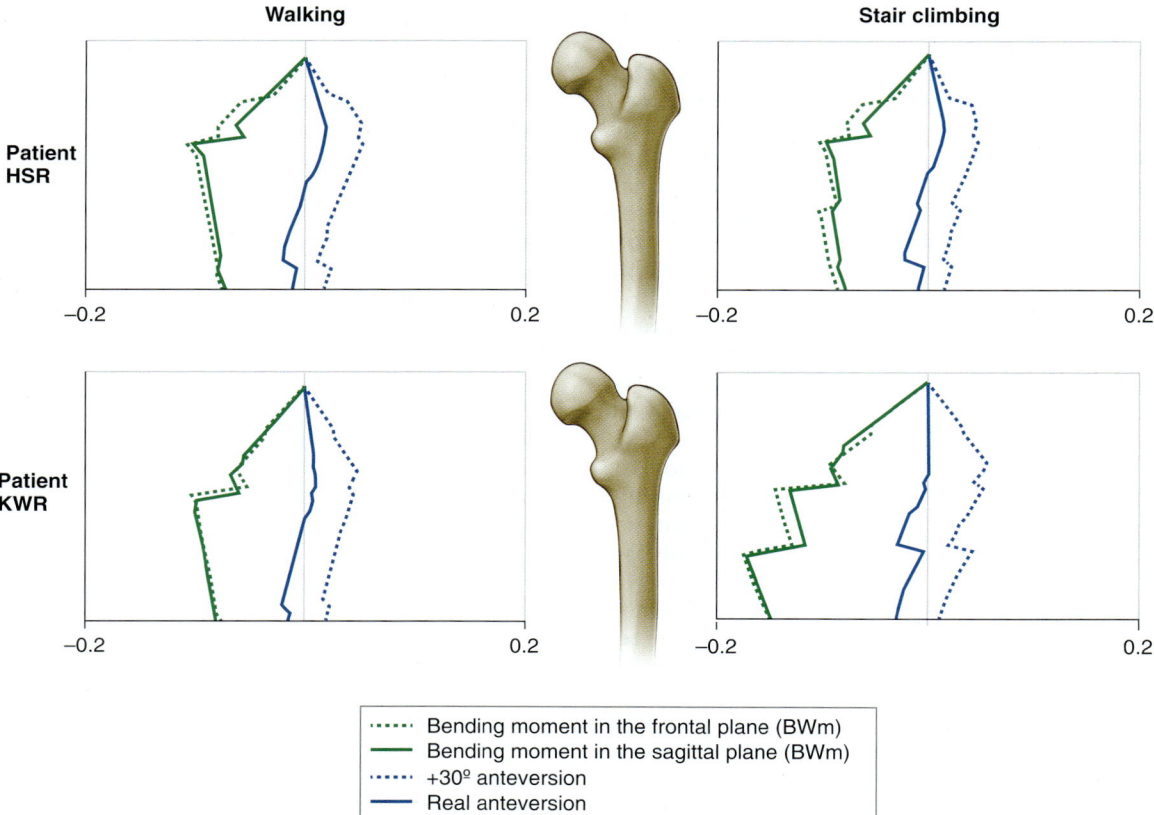

⋯⋯	Bending moment in the frontal plane (BWm)
——	Bending moment in the sagittal plane (BWm)
⋯⋯	+30º anteversion
——	Real anteversion

Figure 2-7. Internal loads at the proximal femur at the moment of maximum contact force for two patients during walking and stair climbing. Bending moments are given in body weight times meter (BWm). *Blue lines* show the bending moment in the sagittal plane (M_x), *green lines* show the bending moment in the frontal plane (M_y). *Solid lines* represent real anteversion; *dashed lines* simulate an increase in anteversion to an angle of 30 degrees. *(Modified from Heller MO, Bergmann G, Deuretzbacher G, et al: Influence of femoral anteversion on proximal femoral loading: measurement and simulation in four patients. Clin Biomech [Bristol, Avon] 8:644–649, 2001.)*

Even though finite element analysis was limited to four selected stages within the gait cycle, and thus the muscle and joint contact loads used represent only a rough approximation of the in vivo situation, this analysis nonetheless reveals the large influence of thigh loading on strain distribution. Bone loaded with all thigh muscles experienced a more or less homogeneous strain distribution (Fig. 2-8). The orientation of strains showed bending and torsion superimposed on compressive strains acting along the shaft of the femur. The use of simplified load cases, especially those involving only the abductors, the iliotibial band, and hip contact, led to the development of a large bending moment distally. This occurred because muscle contraction compensates for shear forces and bending moments developed within bone. If muscles are neglected, the effects of shear forces and bending moments on cortical strains will be overestimated.

If the appropriate muscle groups are considered, strain magnitudes and orientations similar to those reported from in vivo measurements may be obtained.

If major muscles are neglected, tensile and compressive strains are overestimated, and torsional effects are underestimated. This may significantly influence the predictions of mathematical simulations of bone remodeling or modeling processes, as well as interpretation of stress shielding effects.

Influence of Altered Anteversion and Offset on Stresses and Strains in the Artificial Joint

Aseptic loosening of artificial hip joints is believed to be influenced by the design[1,75] and orientation[5] of the implant. It is hypothesized that variations in implant anteversion[53] and offset[76-78] lead to changes in loading of the proximal femur, causing critical conditions in both bone and cement. Although these critical conditions in bone loading can lead to bone remodeling,[8] possibly causing degeneration,[79] it is known that initiation of cement failure correlates with applied loads and cement interface and integrity.[80,81]

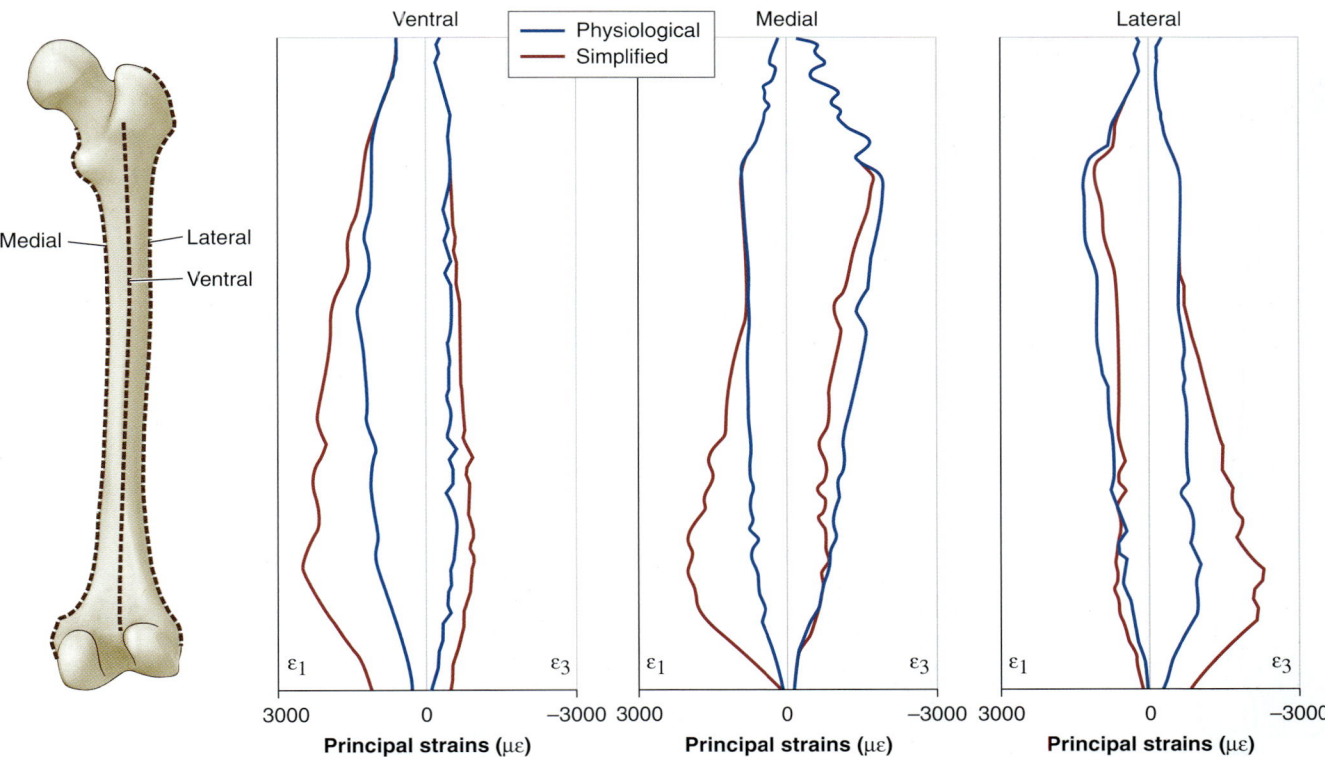

Figure 2-8. Principal strains ε_1 (maximal) and ε_3 (minimal) along lines on the ventral, medial, and lateral aspects of the human femur at 45% gait cycle with all thigh muscles included *(dark lines)*. For comparison, strains are given for simplified load regimes with only the hip contact, abductors, and iliotibial band included *(light lines)*. *(Redrawn from Duda GN, Heller M, Albinger J, et al: Influence of muscle forces on femoral strain distribution. J Biomech 9:841–846, 1998.)*

Although increased anteversion causes an increase in bending moments and hip contact forces,[44] an increase in offset could raise the stability of the joint[78] and reduce the hip contact force caused by the longer lever arm of the abductor muscles.[76-78] However, offset alterations cause ambivalent results. On one hand, a reduction in muscle forces is to be seen as a positive effect on the primary and long-term stability of the artificial hip joint. On the other hand, this same increase in offset might cause higher bending and torsion loads despite lower joint contact forces in the artificial joint.[76,82] In addition, prosthesis offset seems to influence the wear of the artificial hip joint: in patients with bilateral THA, significantly higher polyethylene wear has been found on the side of decreased postoperative offset compared with the side on which the offset was maintained.[78] The explanation given was that similar femoral offset before and after surgery tended to restore preoperative hip biomechanics more closely.

Anatomically Reconstructed Joint. Because the findings referenced earlier indicate that femoral anteversion and femoral offset contribute to loading conditions at the hip, and therefore probably influence the outcome of THA, Kleemann and coworkers[83] used a finite element model to further analyze the role of anteversion and offset in loading, bone strains, and cement stresses in cemented primary THA.

After the artificial joint was implanted at 4 degrees anteversion with a standard prosthesis offset, principal surface bone strains of the proximal femur were reduced in comparison with the intact femur (Fig. 2-9, *bottom*). Maximum surface bone strains of up to 3800 microstrain ($\mu\varepsilon$) were found in the posteromedial region during both walking and stair climbing exercises. The smallest strains were observed in the anterior region. The magnitudes of stresses in the cement mantle were analyzed and examined for peak tensile stresses over the assumed cement fatigue strength of 8 MPa.[5] The stress range of 3 to 10 MPa was examined in particular, as this is assumed to be responsible for cement crack initiation and damage accumulation under cyclic loading.[84] After implantation of the artificial hip joint, more than 80% of the elements modeled as cement in the finite element analysis were found in the 0 to 3 MPa range (Fig. 2-10). Almost 18% of the elements were found in the range 3 to 10 MPa, and only a small percentage (≈2%) were above 10 MPa.

Joint Reconstruction With Increased Femoral Offset and Anteversion. In modeling the effects of femoral offset and anteversion, Kleemann and associates varied the anteversion of the implanted prosthesis from 4 to 24 degrees, which is the difference between preoperative and postoperative femoral anteversion as clinically measured.[85] Furthermore, femoral offset was increased

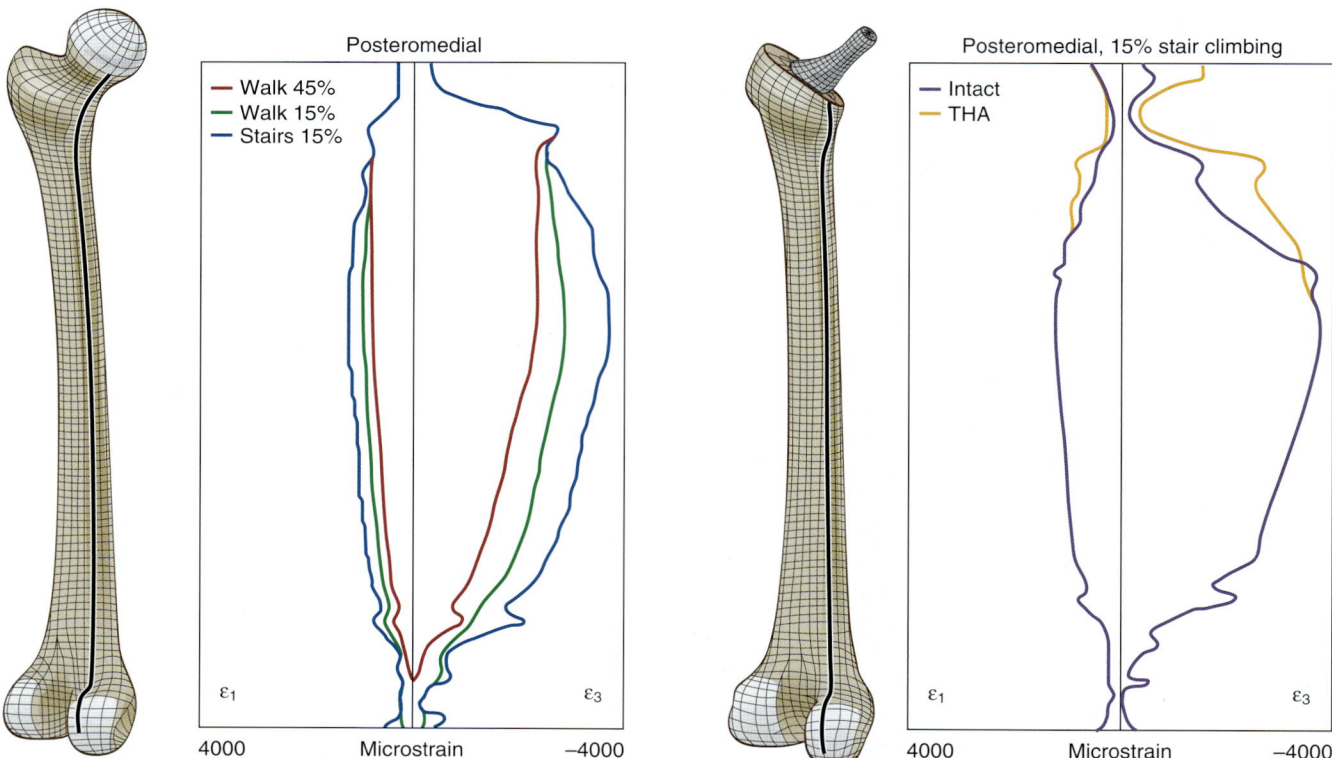

Figure 2-9. Principal strains ε_1 (tensile) and ε_3 (compressive) in microstrain of the posteromedial aspect of the human femur at 15% and 45% of the gait cycle during walking, and at 15% of the gait cycle during stair climbing *(top)*. Tensile and compressive strains of the implanted femur at 15% of the gait cycle demonstrate unloading of the proximal bone *(bottom)*. *(Redrawn from Kleemann RU, Heller MO, Stoeckle U, et al: THA loading arising from increased femoral anteversion and offset may lead to critical cement stresses. J Orthop Res 5:767–774, 2003.)*

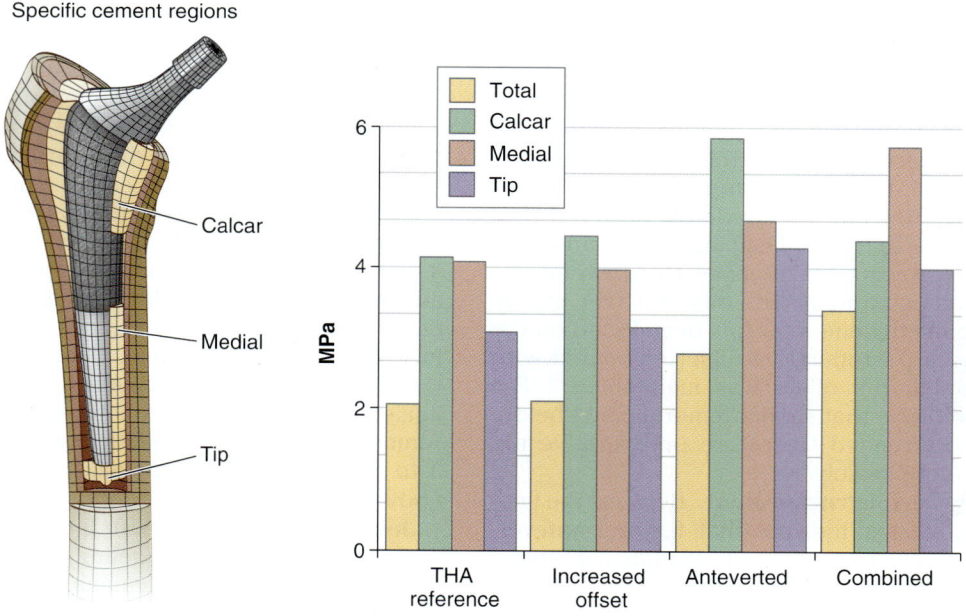

Figure 2-10. The 3 to 10 MPa range is considered critical for cement damage accumulation. Stresses in specific regions of interest within the cement mantle are shown for different loading configurations. *(Redrawn from Kleemann RU, Heller MO, Stoeckle U, et al: THA loading arising from increased femoral anteversion and offset may lead to critical cement stresses. J Orthop Res 5:767–774, 2003.)*

by 4.8 mm medially, corresponding to the difference between the normal neck and the long neck of a standard implant system (Fig. 2-11). Increasing the prosthesis anteversion from 4 to 24 degrees alone caused higher muscle and joint contact forces, resulting in an increase in bone strain of up to 16%.[83] Maximum strains in the proximal bone shifted from posteromedial to medial. At the same time, average cement stresses were increased by approximately 52% during walking and by 35% during stair climbing (see Fig. 2-10). Despite lower muscle and joint contact forces, increased offset caused a minor increase in strains at the bone surface (up to +5%). Only small changes were noted in the magnitude (up to +9%) and distribution of cement stresses (see Fig. 2-10).

The combination of increased femoral anteversion and offset during walking had an effect similar to that of increased anteversion alone: the number of cement elements that were stressed to the range of 3 to 10 MPa was almost doubled compared with the THA reference case and the case with increased offset alone (see Fig. 2-10). During stair climbing, however, increased loads caused substantial rises in cement stresses (up to +67% mean cement stress) and a minor increase in bone strains (up to +19%). The combination of increased offset and anteversion also raised the percentage of elements with cement stresses in the range responsible for damage accumulation (3 to 10 MPa) from 19% in the reference implantation to 51%. Three main regions of high stresses were identified: (1) around the tip of the stem, (2) at the calcar, and (3) at the distal-medial aspect of the stem (see Fig. 2-10, *left*). The mean stress recorded in these regions was almost 50% greater than

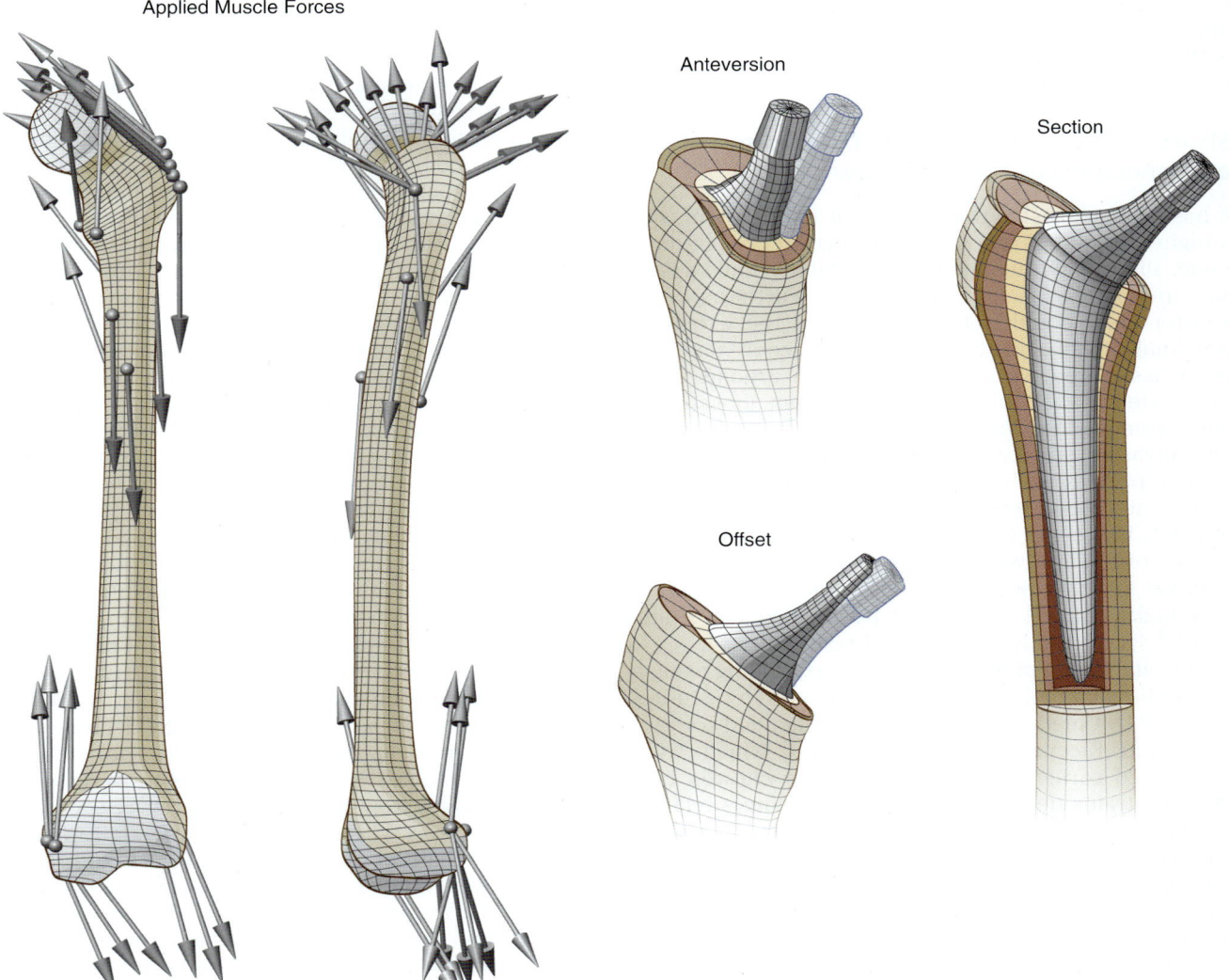

Applied Muscle Forces

Anteversion

Section

Offset

Figure 2-11. Finite element mesh, including all muscle forces and total hip arthroplasty (THA) reconstruction with a cemented polished tapered stem (MS-30, Sulzer Orthopedics Ltd., Baar, Switzerland). Vectors show the orientation of applied muscle forces. Views of anteverted (4 degrees and 24 degrees) and increased offset (+4.8 mm mediolateral) configurations are detailed, together with an open section of the proximal bone. (*Redrawn from Kleemann RU, Heller MO, Stoeckle U, et al: THA loading arising from increased femoral anteversion and offset may lead to critical cement stresses. J Orthop Res 5:767–774, 2003.*)

the mean stress computed for all elements of the cement mantle. When combined effects of large anteversion and increased offset were analyzed, nearly 80% of elements in these highly stressed regions of the mantle were found to be within the 3 to 10 MPa range.

These results indicate that increasing the anteversion of the stem, particularly in combination with greater offset, generates cement stresses that have been linked to damage accumulation under cyclic loading and increased risk of mantle failure.[86]

Clinically, the orientation of femoral stems seems to be essential for long-term performance in vivo. Here, anteversion plays a more important role in determining cement mantle loading than prosthesis offset. Femoral anteversion therefore may be considered a more influential parameter than offset in the long-term clinical outcome of THA, but their combination, especially during stair climbing activities, can produce critical cement stresses. In the clinical situation, these undesirable effects should be considered, and when an implant with a large offset is to be used, the surgeon should be careful to avoid large angles of femoral anteversion.

Short-Stemmed Implants in THA from a Biomechanical Point of View

It has been suggested that the use of a short stem with a higher proximal osteotomy could conserve proximal bone, allowing more bone to be available should a revision procedure become necessary.[87] Furthermore, a shorter stem could potentially reduce the extent of proximal stress shielding[88]—a phenomenon that has been associated with bone resorption around traditional stems,[89] which can lead to implant loosening.[90] Short-stemmed implants may also facilitate the use of a less invasive surgical approach. Morrey and associates[87] reported less blood loss, shorter operating times, and greater bone retention with a short-stemmed hip implant. This could potentially lead to faster postoperative recovery,[91] as well as improved long-term implant survival rates. However, the less invasive procedure may make optimal component positioning more difficult,[92,93] leading to inferior clinical results.[94]

The effects of femoral component positioning using a conventional stem have been examined by studies reported by Umeda and colleagues,[95] Heller and coworkers,[44] and Kleemann and associates,[83] which were introduced earlier in this chapter. They showed that in vitro strains decreased in implanted femurs relative to the intact, that increasing anteversion increased strains anteriorly and posteriorly near the distal tip of the implant,[95] that the hip contact force and internal loads in the femur are increased in such cases,[44] and that an increase in effective anteversion or offset of the implant increases proximal femur strains in the case of a traditional cemented stem.[83] Therefore, surgical placement of conventional stems can affect loading of the proximal femur, which could influence long-term bone remodeling[89,96] and possibly implant survival.[90] To investigate the influence of stem position and orientation on loading of the femur when a short stem is used, Speirs and associates[97] used a finite element approach.

In a first model, the implant was aligned with the femur (a solid model of the standardized femur, created by Marco Viceconti, Istituti Ortopedici Rizzoli, Bologna, Italy) such that the joint center was unchanged relative to the intact femur. In the second model, the implant was displaced 6 mm medially, 2 mm posteriorly, and 4 mm superiorly to retain more cortical bone in the neck area and increase the offset (Fig. 2-12, *left*). Further displacement of the stem would have resulted in resection through the femoral head. Both stem positions were approximately aligned with the neck axis of the femur to reproduce the anteversion of the intact femur. The third model was created by rotating the implant of the first model about the femoral shaft axis by 7 degrees, resulting in an anteversion angle of 11 degrees (Fig. 2-12, *middle*). This rotation was the maximum that could be achieved without overlap of the implant with the inner cortical surface of the standardized femur at the resection level. The three models are referred to as *reference, medialized,* and *anteverted* stems, respectively.

Speirs[97] found that stress shielding occurred even when a short-stemmed implant was used, and that this was relatively insensitive to changes to implant offset or anteversion. Results showed that proximal cortical strains varied by up to 500 microstrain (22%) in relation to implant position and were highest for the medialized stem. Strain energy density differences of up to 6.2 kJ/m^3 (33%, Gruen zone V) were related to implant position and orientation, although large relative differences of up to 45% were seen in the proximal zones (I and VII), where bone resorption is often seen radiographically with traditional[98] and conservative implants.[87] Increased strains in the medialized model are likely due to increased offset of the femoral shaft axis from the reconstructed hip center compared with the reference implanted model, because hip force magnitudes are approximately the same (1% difference). Increased strains in the anteverted model, relative to the reference model, are most often explained by the increase in hip contact force (6% increase).

Differences in strains between implanted models, however, were generally small when compared with overall change from the intact femur. For example, strain differences between implanted and intact femurs of up to 95% of the intact value were seen at the neck resection level. This difference generally decreased distally, and strain magnitudes returned to normal levels near the distal extent of the ingrowth surface. The largest changes from the intact femur were seen in the proximal cortex, with greater decreases on the medial side (95%) than on the lateral side (36%), and relative changes were similar under walking and stair climbing loads. Changes in cortical strain patterns caused by introduction of the stem were similar to those measured on cadaveric femurs. Although Umeda and colleagues[95] used a conventional stem and lower loads, minimum principal strains in the medial cortex at the neck resection level decreased by 79% from the intact femur, compared with a 95% reduction in the osseointegrated models used in this study, but strains were unchanged distal to the implant. The in vitro study is effectively a primary stability situation, and the integrated situation

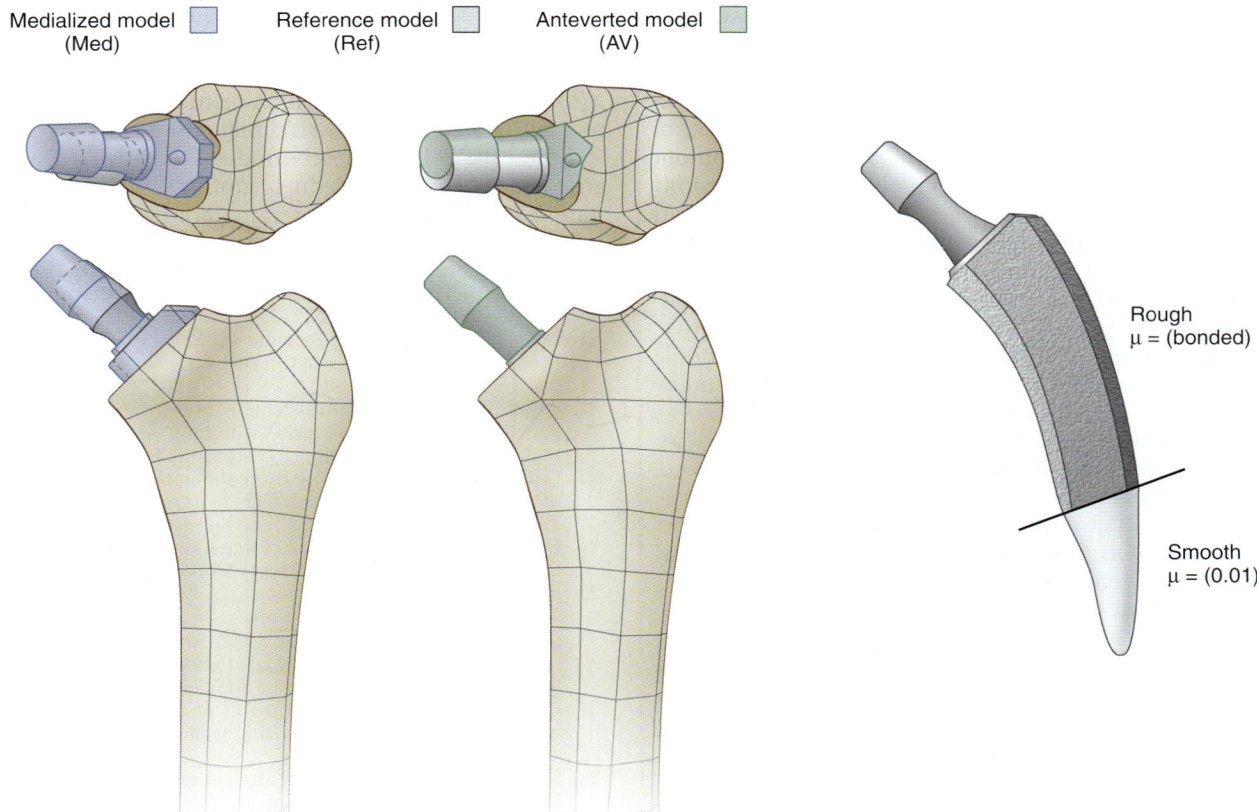

Medialized model (Med) Reference model (Ref) Anteverted model (AV)

Rough
μ = (bonded)

Smooth
μ = (0.01)

Figure 2-12. Left, Superior and anterior views showing reference ("Ref," *opaque*) and medialized ("Med," *transparent*) stem positions. **Middle,** Superior and anterior views showing reference ("Ref," *opaque*) and anteverted ("AV," *transparent*) stem positions. Finite element models of each of these configurations were constructed separately, each using the same mesh for the distal portions (≈three fourths) of the femur. **Right,** Implant surfaces and interface conditions used in the finite element model, simulating a fully osseointegrated implant over the proximal two thirds of the stem. *(Redrawn from Speirs AD, Heller MO, Taylor WR, et al: Influence of changes in stem positioning on femoral loading after THR using a short-stemmed hip implant. Clin Biomech [Bristol, Avon] 4:431–439, 2007.)*

would likely produce a further reduction in proximal strains.

Surgically induced variation in stem offset or anteversion (e.g., due to limited exposure provided by minimally invasive surgery) is therefore expected to have only a small influence on overall changes in proximal femoral loading and therefore on remodeling, within the limits studied by Speirs and colleagues.[97]

Short-stemmed implants are often used in cases of coxarthrosis secondary to femoral dysplasia, which commonly presents with pathologic anteversion of the proximal femur.[87,99,100] Because of the small dimension of the endosteal cavity of many dysplastic patients,[101] implantation of a short-stemmed implant is bound to constraints imposed by the dysmorphic cortical anatomy. The possibilities for an anatomic reconstruction of the anteversion are therefore limited.

Tohtz and colleagues[102] showed that small changes in antetorsion of the short-stemmed implant can increase hip contact forces by 22.5%. When changes in joint contact force were further analyzed, anterior-posterior directed forces on the artificial acetabular cup were found to be affected most. This is considered critical in

patients with dysplastic coxarthrosis, in whom ventral areas of the acetabulum are commonly deficient.[57,103] When effects on the femur and effects on the acetabulum are considered together, it is therefore not advisable to use short-stemmed implants in dysplastic coxarthrosis; use of stems of conventional length should be considered. These components enable correction of excessive anteversion, leading to reduction in hip contact forces and peak loads generated within the femur.[83]

CURRENT CONTROVERSIES AND FUTURE DIRECTIONS

- Although many new implant designs, including short-stemmed femoral components, are being introduced into the marketplace, stress shielding still occurs, but with few clinical sequelae. It remains to be seen how far new implants will be able to reproduce the excellent long-term results of more conventional stem designs. An integrated concept for THA that allows for muscle-sparing implantation might be key to optimal restoration of musculoskeletal loading conditions and provision of long-lasting function.

- To ensure that THA meets the heightened demands of increased life expectancy and ever-increasing expectations for normal postoperative function, a detailed understanding of the musculoskeletal interactions that define the mechanics of the joint is essential.

- Future efforts will be directed toward assessing the musculoskeletal competence of individual patients and the outcomes of specific reconstructions that are available as part of clinical practice. Quantitative information about the risks of overload and instability with the use of routine clinical imaging and simple yet specific tests of individual musculoskeletal competence would be useful to many joint surgeons. This information could form the basis of personalized treatment plans that would enable optimal restoration of dynamic joint function and longevity of the reconstruction. Such a plan could be defined in terms of specific target parameters for optimal joint reconstruction that could be monitored intraoperatively.

REFERENCES

1. Mann KA, Bartel DL, Ayers DC: Influence of stem geometry on mechanics of cemented femoral hip components with a proximal bond. J Orthop Res 5:700–706, 1997.
2. Mann KA, Bartel DL, Wright TM, Burstein AH: Coulomb frictional interfaces in modeling cemented total hip replacements: a more realistic model. J Biomech 9:1067–1078, 1995.
3. Ornstein E, Atroshi I, Franzen H, et al: Results of hip revision using the Exeter stem, impacted allograft bone, and cement. Clin Orthop Relat Res 389:126–133, 2001.
4. Sutherland CJ, Wilde AH, Borden LS, Marks KE: A ten-year follow-up of one hundred consecutive Muller curved-stem total hip-replacement arthroplasties. J Bone Joint Surg Am 7:970–982, 1982.
5. Chang PB, Mann KA, Bartel DL: Cemented femoral stem performance: effects of proximal bonding, geometry, and neck length. Clin Orthop Relat Res 355:57–69, 1998.
6. Hodge WA, Andriacchi TP, Galante JO: A relationship between stem orientation and function following total hip arthroplasty. J Arthroplasty 3:229–235, 1991.
7. Cheal EJ, Spector M, Hayes WC: Role of loads and prosthesis material properties on the mechanics of the proximal femur after total hip arthroplasty. J Orthop Res 3:405–422, 1992.
8. Weinans H, Huiskes R, Grootenboer HJ: Effects of fit and bonding characteristics of femoral stems on adaptive bone remodeling. J Biomech Eng 4:393–400, 1994.
9. Pauwels F: Gesammelte Abhandlungen zur funktionellen Anatomie des Bewegungsapparates, Berlin, 1965, Springer.
10. Baleani M, Cristofolini L, Viceconti M: Endurance testing of hip prostheses: a comparison between the load fixed in ISO 7206 standard and the physiological loads. Clin Biomech 5:339–345, 1999.
11. Monti L, Cristofolini L, Viceconti M: Methods for quantitative analysis of the primary stability in uncemented hip prostheses. Artif Organs 9:851–859, 1999.
12. Huiskes R, van Rietbergen B: Preclinical testing of total hip stems: the effects of coating placement. Clin Orthop Relat Res 319:64–76, 1995.
13. Claes L, Augat P, Suger G, Wilke HJ: Influence of size and stability of the osteotomy gap on the success of fracture healing. J Orthop Res 4:577–584, 1997.
14. Van Rietbergen B, Huiskes R, Weinans H, et al: ESB Research Award 1992. The mechanism of bone remodeling and resorption around press-fitted THA stems. J Biomech 4-5:369–382, 1993.
15. Wolff J: Das Gesetz der Transformation der Knochen, Berlin, 1892, A. Hirschwald.
16. Koch JC: The law of bone architecture. Am J Anat 21:177–298, 1917.
17. Pauwels F: Über die Bedeutung der Bauprinzipien des Stütz und Bewegungsapparates für die Beanspruchung des Röhrenknochens. Acta Anat (Basel) 12:207–227, 1951.
18. Pauwels F: Atlas zur Biomechanik der gesunden und kranken Hüfte, Berlin, 1973, Springer Verlag.
19. Brand RA, Pedersen DR, Friederich JA: The sensitivity of muscle force predictions to changes in physiologic cross-sectional area. J Biomech 8:589–596, 1986.
20. Collins JJ: The redundant nature of locomotor optimization laws. J Biomech 3:251–267, 1995.
21. Davy DT, Audu ML: A dynamic optimization technique for predicting muscle forces in the swing phase of gait. J Biomech 2:187–201, 1987.
22. Fuller JJ, Winters JM: Assessment of 3-D joint contact load predictions during postural/stretching exercises in aged females. Ann Biomed Eng 3:277–288, 1993.
23. Glitsch U, Baumann W: The three-dimensional determination of internal loads in the lower extremity. J Biomech 11-12:1123–1131, 1997.
24. Herzog W: Individual muscle force estimations using a nonlinear optimal design. J Neurosci Methods 2-4:167–179, 1987.
25. Pedersen DR, Brand RA, Cheng C, Arora JS: Direct comparison of muscle force predictions using linear and nonlinear programming. J Biomech Eng 3:192–199, 1987.
26. Pedersen DR, Brand RA, Davy DT: Pelvic muscle and acetabular contact forces during gait. J Biomech 9:959–965, 1997.
27. Rohrle H, Scholten R, Sigolotto C, et al: Joint forces in the human pelvis-leg skeleton during walking. J Biomech 6:409–424, 1984.
28. Seireg A, Arvikar RJ: A mathematical model for evaluation of forces in lower extremities of the musculo-skeletal system. J Biomech 3:313–326, 1973.
29. Seireg A, Arvikar RJ: The prediction of muscular load sharing and joint forces in the lower extremities during walking. J Biomech 2:89–102, 1975.
30. Siebertz K, Baumann W: [Biomechanical stress analysis of the lower extremity]. Biomed Tech 9:216–221, 1994.
31. Bergmann G, Graichen F, Rohlmann A: Is staircase walking a risk for the fixation of hip implants? J Biomech 5:535–553, 1995.
32. Bergmann G, Graichen F, Rohlmann A: Hip joint loading during walking and running, measured in two patients. J Biomech 26:969–990, 1993.
33. Bergmann G, Graichen F, Siraky J, et al: Multichannel strain gauge telemetry for orthopaedic implants. J Biomech 2:169–176, 1988.
34. Brand RA, Pedersen DR, Davy DT, et al: Comparison of hip force calculations and measurements in the same patient. J Arthroplasty 1:45–51, 1994.
35. Davy DT, Kotzar GM, Brown RH, et al: Telemetric force measurement across the hip after total hip arthroplasty. J Bone Joint Surg Am 70:45–50, 1988.
36. English TA, Kilvington M: In vivo records of hip loads using a femoral implant with telemetric output (a preliminary report). J Biomed Eng 1:111–115, 1979.
37. Rydell NW: Forces acting in the femoral head-prosthesis: a study on strain-gauge supplied prostheses in living persons. Acta Orthop Scand 37(Suppl 88):1–132, 1966.
38. Heller MO, Bergmann G, Deuretzbacher G, et al: Musculoskeletal loading conditions at the hip during walking and stair climbing. J Biomech 7:883–893, 2001.
39. Andriacchi TP, Alexander EJ: Studies of human locomotion: past, present and future. J Biomech 10:1217–1224, 2000.
40. Chao EY, Rim K: Application of optimization principles in determining the applied moments in human leg joints during gait. J Biomech 5:497–510, 1973.
41. Crowninshield RD: Use of optimization techniques to predict muscle forces. J Biomech Eng 100:88–92, 1978.
42. Bergmann G, Deuretzbacher G, Heller M, et al: Hip contact forces and gait patterns from routine activities. J Biomech 7:859–871, 2001.

43. Duda GN, Eckert-Hubner K, Sokiranski R, et al: Analysis of inter-fragmentary movement as a function of musculoskeletal loading conditions in sheep. J Biomech 3:201–210, 1998.

44. Heller MO, Bergmann G, Deuretzbacher G, et al: Influence of femoral anteversion on proximal femoral loading: measurement and simulation in four patients. Clin Biomech (Bristol, Avon) 8:644–649, 2001.

45. Winter DA, Yack HJ: EMG profiles during normal human walking: stride-to-stride and inter-subject variability. Electroencephalogr Clin Neurophysiol 5:402–411, 1987.

46. Wootten ME, Kadaba MP, Cochran GVB: Dynamic electromyography. II. Normal patterns during gait. J Orthop Res 2:259–265, 1990.

47. Ericson MO, Nisell R, Ekholm J: Quantified electromyography of lower-limb muscles during level walking. Scand J Rehabil Med 4:159–163, 1986.

48. Andriacchi TP, Ogle JA, Galante JO: Walking speed as a basis for normal and abnormal gait measurements. J Biomech 4:261–268, 1977.

49. Nadeau S, McFadyen BJ, Malouin F: Frontal and sagittal plane analyses of the stair climbing task in healthy adults aged over 40 years: what are the challenges compared to level walking? Clin Biomech 10:950–959, 2003.

50. Cowan SM, Bennell KL, Hodges PW, et al: Delayed onset of electromyographic activity of vastus medialis obliquus relative to vastus lateralis in subjects with patellofemoral pain syndrome. Arch Phys Med Rehabil 2:183–189, 2001.

51. Finlay JB, Chess DG, Hardie WR, et al: An evaluation of three loading configurations for the in vitro testing of femoral strains in total hip arthroplasty. J Orthop Res 5:749–759, 1991.

52. Bergmann G, Graichen F, Rohlmann A: Hip joint loading during walking and running, measured in two patients. J Biomech 8:969–990, 1993.

53. Johnston RC, Brand RA, Crowninshield RD: Reconstruction of the hip: a mathematical approach to determine optimum geometric relationships. J Bone Joint Surg Am 5:639–652, 1979.

54. Callaghan JJ, Salvati EA, Pellicci PM, et al: Results of revision for mechanical failure after cemented total hip replacement, 1979 to 1982: a two- to five-year follow-up. J Bone Joint Surg Am 7:1074–1085, 1985.

55. Pagnano MW, Hanssen AD, Lewallen DG, Shaughnessy WJ: The effect of superior placement of the acetabular component on the rate of loosening after total hip arthroplasty: long-term results in patients who have Crowe type-II congenital dysplasia of the hip. J Bone Joint Surg Am 7:1004–1014, 1996.

56. Heller MO, Schroder JH, Matziolis G, et al: [Musculoskeletal load analysis: a biomechanical explanation for clinical results—and more?]. Orthopade 3:188, 190–194, 2007.

57. Perka C, Fischer U, Taylor WR, Matziolis G: Developmental hip dysplasia treated with total hip arthroplasty with a straight stem and a threaded cup. J Bone Joint Surg Am 2:312–319, 2004.

58. Halpern AA, Tanner J, Rinsky L: Does persistent fetal femoral anteversion contribute to osteoarthritis? A preliminary report. Clin Orthop Relat Res 145:213–216, 1979.

59. Reikeras O, Bjerkreim I, Kolbenstvedt A: Anteversion of the acetabulum in patients with idiopathic increased anteversion of the femoral neck. Acta Orthop Scand 6:847–852, 1982.

60. Morlock M, Schneider E, Bluhm A, et al: Duration and frequency of every day activities in total hip patients. J Biomech 7:873–881, 2001.

61. Harrigan TP, Harris WH: A three-dimensional non-linear finite element study of the effect of cement-prosthesis debonding in cemented femoral total hip components. J Biomech 11:1047–1058, 1991.

62. Frost HM: The laws of bone structure, Springfeld, Ill, 1964, Charles C. Thomas.

63. Cowin SC, Hart RT, Balser JR, Kohn DH: Functional adaptation in long bones: establishing in vivo values for surface remodeling rate coefficients. J Biomech 9:665–684, 1985.

64. Harrigan TP, Biegler FB, Reuben JD: Bone adaptation to total hip femoral components: effects of multiple loads and comparison to clinical follow-up. In Transactions of the ORS, Atlanta, 1996, 42nd Annual Meeting of the Octhopedic Research Society.

65. van Rietbergen B, Müller R, Ulrich D, et al: Quantitative assessment of tissue loading in a proximal femur, using a full scale microstructura FE-model. In Transactions of the ORS, San Francisco, 1997, 43rd Annual Meeting of the Orthopedic Research Society.

66. Rybicki EF, Simonen FA, Weis EB Jr: On the mathematical analysis of stress in the human femur. J Biomech 2:203–215, 1972.

67. Crowninshield RD, Brand RA, Johnston RC, Milroy JC: An analysis of femoral component stem design in total hip arthroplasty. J Bone Joint Surg Am 1:68–78, 1980.

68. Huiskes R, Weinans H, Grootenboer HJ, et al: Adaptive bone-remodeling theory applied to prosthetic-design analysis. J Biomech 11-12:1135–1150, 1987.

69. Huiskes R: The various stress patterns of press-fit, ingrown, and cemented femoral stems. Clin Orthop Relat Res 261:27–38, 1990.

70. Lu Z, Ebramzadeh E, McKellop H, Sarmiento A: Stable partial debonding of the cement interfaces indicated by a finite element model of a total hip prosthesis. J Orthop Res 2:238–244, 1996.

71. Rohlmann A, Mossner U, Bergmann G, Kolbel R: Finite-element-analysis and experimental investigation of stresses in a femur. J Biomed Eng 3:241–246, 1982.

72. Duda GN, Schneider E, Chao EYS: Internal forces and moments in the femur during walking. J Biomech 9:933–941, 1997.

73. Taylor ME, Tanner KE, Freeman MA, Yettram AL: Stress and strain distribution within the intact femur: compression or bending? Med Eng Phys 2:122–131, 1996.

74. Duda GN, Heller M, Albinger J, et al: Influence of muscle forces on femoral strain distribution. J Biomech 9:841–846, 1998.

75. Mann KA, Ayers DC, Damron TA: Effects of stem length on mechanics of the femoral hip component after cemented revision. J Orthop Res 1:62–68, 1997.

76. Davey JR, O'Connor DO, Burke DW, Harris WH: Femoral component offset: its effect on strain in bone-cement. J Arthroplasty 1:23–26, 1993.

77. McGrory BJ, Morrey BF, Cahalan TD, et al: Effect of femoral offset on range of motion and abductor muscle strength after total hip arthroplasty. J Bone Joint Surg Br 6:865–869, 1995.

78. Sakalkale DP, Sharkey PF, Eng K, et al: Effect of femoral component offset on polyethylene wear in total hip arthroplasty. Clin Orthop Relat Res 388:125–134, 2001.

79. Reikeras O, Bjerkreim I, Kolbenstvedt A: Anteversion of the acetabulum and femoral neck in normals and in patients with osteoarthritis of the hip. Acta Orthop Scand 1:18–23, 1983.

80. Bauer TW, Schils J: The pathology of total joint arthroplasty. II. Mechanisms of implant failure. Skeletal Radiol 9:483–497, 1999.

81. Rice J, Prenderville T, Murray P, et al: Femoral cementing techniques in total hip replacement. Int Orthop 5:308–311, 1998.

82. Steinberg B, Harris W: The "offset" problem in total hip arthroplasty. Contemp Orthop 5:556–562, 1992.

83. Kleemann RU, Heller MO, Stoeckle U, et al: THA loading arising from increased femoral anteversion and offset may lead to critical cement stresses. J Orthop Res 5:767–774, 2003.

84. Harrigan TP, Kareh JA, O'Connor DO, et al: A finite element study of the initiation of failure of fixation in cemented femoral total hip components. J Orthop Res 1:134–144, 1992.

85. Schidlo C, Becker C, Jansson V, Refior J: [Change in the CCD angle and the femoral anteversion angle by hip prosthesis implantation]. Z Orthop Ihre Grenzgeb 3:259–264, 1999.

86. Verdonschot N, Huiskes R: The effects of cement-stem debonding in THA on the long-term failure probability of cement. J Biomech 8:795–802, 1997.

87. Morrey BF, Adams RA, Kessler M: A conservative femoral replacement for total hip arthroplasty: a prospective study. J Bone Joint Surg Br 7:952–958, 2000.

88. Thomas W, Lucente L, Mantegna N, Grundei H: [ESKA (CUT) endoprosthesis]. Orthopade 11:1243–1248, 2004.

89. Kerner J, Huiskes R, van Lenthe GH, et al: Correlation between pre-operative periprosthetic bone density and post-operative bone loss in THA can be explained by strain-adaptive remodelling. J Biomech 7:695–703, 1999.

90. Wilkinson JM, Hamer AJ, Rogers A, et al: Bone mineral density and biochemical markers of bone turnover in aseptic loosening after total hip arthroplasty. J Orthop Res 4:691–696, 2003.

91. Howell JR, Masri BA, Duncan CP: Minimally invasive versus standard incision anterolateral hip replacement: a comparative study. Orthop Clin North Am 2:153–162, 2004.

92. Hartzband MA: Posterolateral minimal incision for total hip replacement: technique and early results. Orthop Clin North Am 2:119–129, 2004.

93. Woolson ST, Mow CS, Syquia JF, et al: Comparison of primary total hip replacements performed with a standard incision or a mini-incision. J Bone Joint Surg Am 7:1353–1358, 2004.

94. Noble PC, Sugano N, Johnston JD, et al: Computer simulation: how can it help the surgeon optimize implant position? Clin Orthop Relat Res 417:242–252, 2003.

95. Umeda N, Saito M, Sugano N, et al: Correlation between femoral neck version and strain on the femur after insertion of femoral prosthesis. J Orthop Sci 3:381–386, 2003.

96. Lengsfeld M, Burchard R, Gunther D, et al: Femoral strain changes after total hip arthroplasty—patient-specific finite element analyses 12 years after operation. Med Eng Phys 8:649–654, 2005.

97. Speirs AD, Heller MO, Taylor WR, et al: Influence of changes in stem positioning on femoral loading after THR using a short-stemmed hip implant. Clin Biomech (Bristol, Avon) 4:431–439, 2007.

98. Wick M, Lester DK: Radiological changes in second- and third-generation Zweymuller stems. J Bone Joint Surg Br 8:1108–1114, 2004.

99. Ender SA, Machner A, Pap G, et al: Cementless CUT femoral neck prosthesis: increased rate of aseptic loosening after 5 years. Acta Orthop 5:616–621, 2007.

100. Hube R, Zaage M, Hein W, Reichel H: [Early functional results with the Mayo-hip, a short stem system with metaphyseal-intertrochanteric fixation]. Orthopade 11:1249–1258, 2004.

101. Noble PC, Kamaric E, Sugano N, et al: Three-dimensional shape of the dysplastic femur: implications for THR. Clin Orthop Relat Res 417:27–40, 2003.

102. Tohtz SW, Heller MO, Taylor WR, et al: [On the biomechanics of the hip: relevance of femoral anteversion for hip contact force and loading using a short-stemmed prostheses]. Orthopade 37:923–929, 2008.

103. Paavilainen T, Hoikka V, Solonen KA: Cementless total replacement for severely dysplastic or dislocated hips. J Bone Joint Surg Br 2:205–211, 1990.

CHAPTER 3

Tribology of the Artificial Hip Joint

Markus A. Wimmer and Michel P. Laurent

INTRODUCTION

Tribology is the science and technology of interacting surfaces in relative motion. It includes the study and application of the principles of friction, wear, and lubrication. Friction is a natural phenomenon in our daily lives and causes wear of bodies in contact. Although Leonardo da Vinci (1452–1519) and Guillaume Amontons (1663–1705) already recognized and formulated the basic principles of friction, the underlying mechanisms of many effects of friction and wear are poorly understood. Lubrication of contacting bodies helps to reduce and control detrimental consequences of friction and wear. In this chapter, we will present the current understanding of tribology in the context of prosthetic wear, with a focus on hip implants. However, the principles also apply to any other articulating joint replacement.

In the artificial hip, wear and the consequences of wear continue to be an important cause of implant failure. Billions of wear particles generated annually can migrate to the periprosthetic tissue and cause localized chronic inflammation and resorption of bone adjacent to the implant.[1,2] This mechanism, called *osteolysis,* may lead to subsequent implant loosening and failure and is discussed in detail in Chapters 11 and 12.

Because of the biological complications of wear debris generated by prosthetic joints, it is important to identify precise and purposeful measures for wear reduction. Knowledge of the multifactorial nature of wear and accurate modeling of in vivo conditions within the laboratory will allow us to overcome the simple trial-and-error methods of the past and will help reduce risks for the patient.

Therefore, it is essential to analyze surfaces that have been worn under the actual "operating conditions" to learn about the influencing factors of the system and replicate them satisfactorily in a bench test.

This chapter covers the major aspects of tribology related to the articulating surfaces of hip prostheses. First, the definitions of terms associated with a tribological system are given, with particular emphasis on the various wear mechanisms, wear modes, and lubrication regimes. The hip bearing is then presented as a tribological system, with specific wear modes and mechanisms, outputs (material loss, heat, and sometimes sound), and lubrication regimes. The wear characteristics of hip bearing couples as a function of geometry and bearing materials are discussed. This is followed by a section on wear testing procedures, covering screening tests for materials, and full-fledged tests of hip bearings in simulators. The chapter ends with a list of current concerns and future directions associated with hip wear, which include uncertainties in the long-term wear behavior of highly cross-linked polyethylenes, improving the wear of metal-on-metal bearings, developing new materials and coatings for bearing surfaces, improving wear testing of prosthetic hip joints, and developing virtual wear testing that would complement actual wear testing.

BASIC SCIENCE

Definition of Terms

A *tribosystem* consists of four principal elements: a body, a counterbody, an interfacial medium, and an environment (Fig. 3-1). The relative kinematics of the bodies, the contact load and loading profile, and the ambient temperature define the input variables of the system. The mechanical function of motion with load bearing that characterizes every tribosystem is

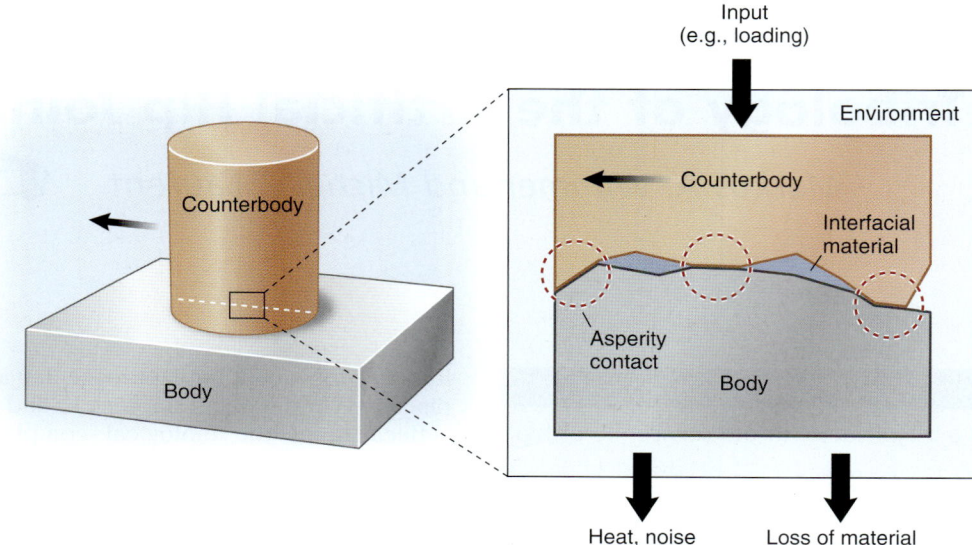

Figure 3-1. General description of a tribosystem, which consists of four elements: the two bodies in contact, the interfacial material, and the environment. All these elements can affect each other and change the mechanism of interaction.

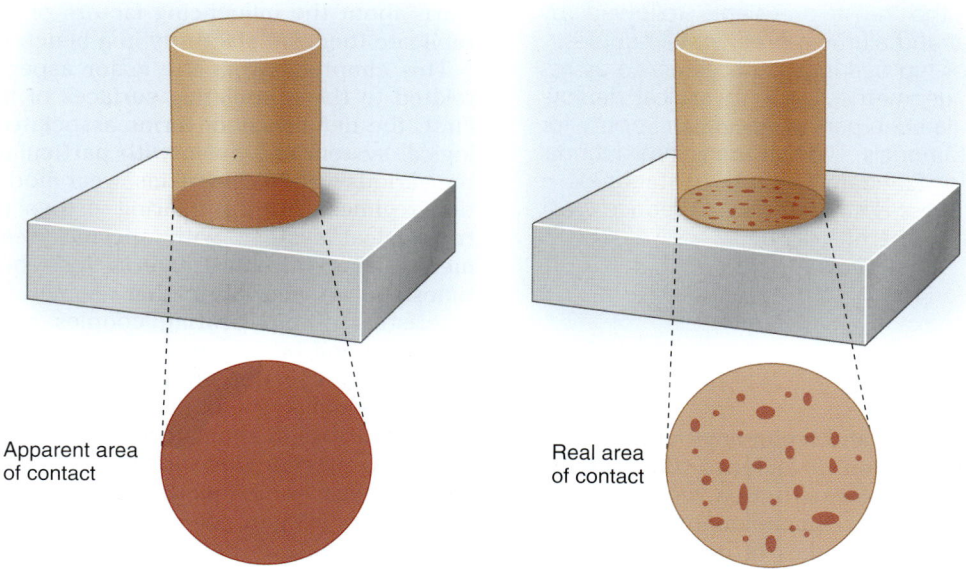

Figure 3-2. Apparent and real areas of contact established on asperities.

always accompanied by some loss of energy, mostly in the form of heat ($\approx$90% of the introduced energy), sound, and wear. Loss of material generated by the wear component is influenced by many factors, including general bulk properties of the articulating bodies, their surface characteristics (e.g., roughness, hardness, surface energy), and system conditions, such as the lubricant, the relative motion of the bodies, and the loads transmitted.

Knowledge of the *contact conditions* between interacting bodies is important for the understanding of wear mechanisms. On the microscopic level, all surfaces have an intrinsic roughness, even those that appear perfectly smooth (see Fig. 3-1). Hence, contact between

articulating surfaces is established only on asperities, yielding many tiny contact spots, so that the real contact area is significantly smaller than the apparent contact area (Fig. 3-2). This distinction between real and apparent contact areas is a key concept in tribology. During motion, these tiny contact locations are deformed elastically and/or plastically within a chemically challenging environment. Particles are then created by mechanically or chemically dominated wear mechanisms.

Currently, four major *wear mechanisms* are known and distinguished: (1) *abrasion;* (2) *surface fatigue,* which involves microscopic crack initiation and propagation; (3) *adhesion;* and *(4) tribochemical reactions,* which involve primarily chemical processes. These four mechanisms are described in greater detail in Box 3-1. Depending on the chemical reactivity of the bearing material, chemical bonding between articulating materials (adhesion) or with surrounding agents (tribochemical reaction) can occur. In simulating the wear of hip prostheses within the laboratory, it is essential to replicate the in vivo wear mechanisms, not just the observed *wear rates* (the wear loss per cycle or unit time). Key indicators of the validity of laboratory simulations include the surface appearance and morphology of the worn surfaces, which must resemble those of explanted components, and the shapes, size distributions, and chemistry of wear particles generated during laboratory testing, which must duplicate those collected from periprosthetic fluid and tissue.

The *wear mode* is the particular dynamic configuration of body, counterbody, lubricant, and environment that generates wear in the tribosystem. Eight common wear modes are depicted and defined in Figure 3-3, including sliding wear, rolling wear, and three-body abrasive wear. In the hip joint, for example, wear between the head and the cup occurs as the result of sliding wear. In the presence of bone cement particles, the wear mode shifts to three-body abrasive wear. These two-wear modes trigger profoundly different wear mechanisms, and thus generate different types of wear, which will be explained in detail later. As a consequence, a difference in volume loss is generated. Knowledge of the wear mode is important for proper replication of the wear situation in the laboratory (e.g., in the case of the hip joint, the daily activity profile of a patient must be emulated). It should be noted that a wear mode is not a steady-state condition, and that a shift between

modes may occur. For example, worn carbides generated from metal-on-metal sliding wear may change the wear mode to three-body abrasion, as the particles released from the bearing surfaces actively participate in the tribological process.

Each wear mechanism generates a characteristic *wear appearance,* also known as a "wear pattern" or "wear damage," observed through visible changes in surface structure (texture and shape) that occur as a consequence of wear. Examples are shown in Figure 3-4.

Friction is the introduction, transformation, and dissipation of energy. Surface asperities become elastically or plastically deformed when they come in contact (or interlock) with asperities of the countersurface (see Fig. 3-1). Another contribution comes from the adhesion of surface atoms and molecules of the body and counterbody.

Lubrication can reduce wear and friction. Both deformation and adhesion contributions to friction can be significantly reduced by lubrication. The extent of fluid film formation plays an important role in the wear process of artificial joints and has been described for technical bearings using a partial differential equation known as the *Reynolds equation,* derived from the general Navier-Stokes equations for laminar fluid flow.[3] Richard Stribeck (1861-1950) developed the groundwork for a quantity known as the *lambda ratio* (λ), which is the thickness of the lubricating fluid film relative to the surface roughness of the contacting materials.[4] The higher the value of lambda, the greater the thickness of the fluid film relative to the height of the asperities. The value of λ increases with the viscosity of the lubricant and the sliding velocity, and decreases with the load on the interface and the roughness of the

BOX 3-1 THE FOUR MAJOR WEAR MECHANISMS	
Abrasion	• Mechanical cutting or plowing process • Induced by asperities of the counterbody, foreign particles (contaminants from outside the wear system [e.g., bone cement] or particles generated within the system itself [e.g., fractured carbides, wear debris]) • Four different submechanisms of abrasion exist, depending on the properties of the bodies in contact: microplowing, microcutting, microcracking, and microfatigue, reflecting the cyclical elastic and/or plastic nature of the contact
Surface fatigue	• Repeated sliding or rolling over the same wear track • Initiation and propagation of microcracks parallel and orthogonal to the bearing surfaces for mechanical or material-related reasons • Wear appearance: shallow pits and delaminations
Adhesion	• Materials from both surfaces adhere to each other (similar to friction welding). • During mechanical action, these microjunctions are torn off and fragments become particles that are transferred from body to counterbody (and vice versa). • Wear appearance: adhering material flakes and pits. In severe cases, generated flakes and particles act abrasively, leaving severe scratches and grooves behind. The latter may cause joint seizure.
Tribochemical reactions	• Surfaces in mechanical contact become activated and react with the interfacial medium and/or environment. • Results in the alternating formation and removal of reaction products at the surfaces, which change the material characteristics of the surface • Wear appearance: often microscopically visible as a patchy layer

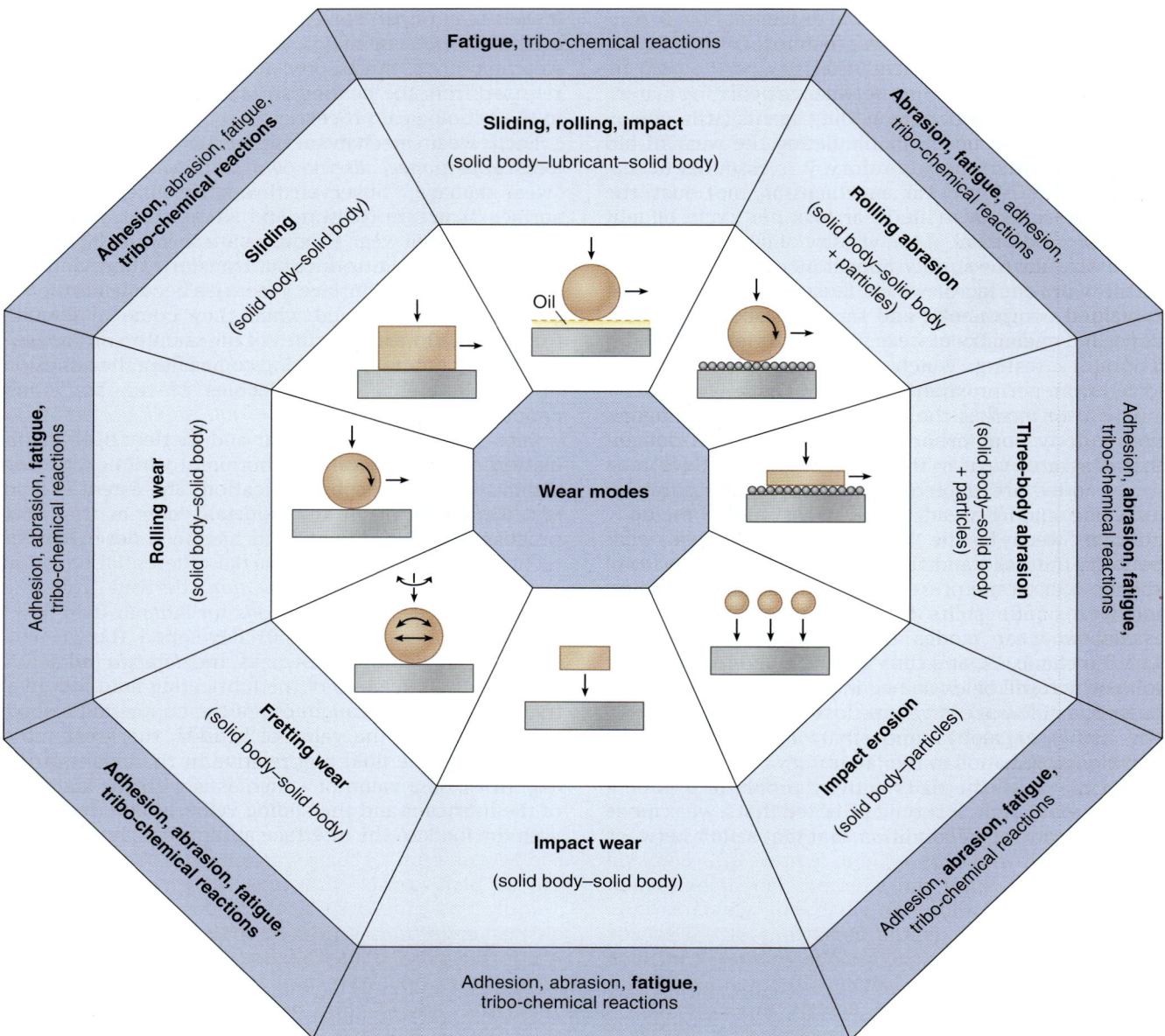

Figure 3-3. Schematic diagram of different wear modes and possible wear mechanisms in a tribological system. Tribological operating conditions are shown pictographically, followed by a description of the wear mode. Possible wear mechanisms are listed in the outer boxes for each mode, with the prevalent ones shown in bold.

mating surfaces. The value of λ also depends on the local gap geometry, because formation of a fluid film during sliding motion requires that the mating surfaces form a convergent gap (i.e., a slight wedge). During sliding, the fluid is entrained into the wider end of the wedge and gets partially trapped, forming a pressurized film that supports load. In a hip bearing, the slight difference in the head and cup radii will naturally produce such a convergent gap. The λ ratio is used to estimate the occurrence of three distinct lubrication regimes, as shown in Figure 3-5. These include (1) $\lambda < 1$, a region of boundary lubrication in which the asperities of the two articulating surfaces are in contact and the lubricant reduces resistance to relative motion between counterfaces by chemical and physical

processes; (2) $1 < \lambda < 3$, a region of mixed lubrication where parts of the surfaces are separated by the lubricant but isolated surface points are still in contact. In this context, the importance of well-polished surfaces is apparent: the higher a single large asperity protrudes through the lubricating film, the longer it will remain in contact with the other surface; and (3) $\lambda > 3$, a region of hydrodynamic lubrication where a full fluid film covers the asperities, completely separating the articulating surfaces. Although the friction coefficient is relatively low in this region, it increases with film thickness because the ability of the film to support load (F_N) decreases faster than the corresponding reduction in viscous drag (F_T), so the friction coefficient, which equals F_T/F_N, increases.

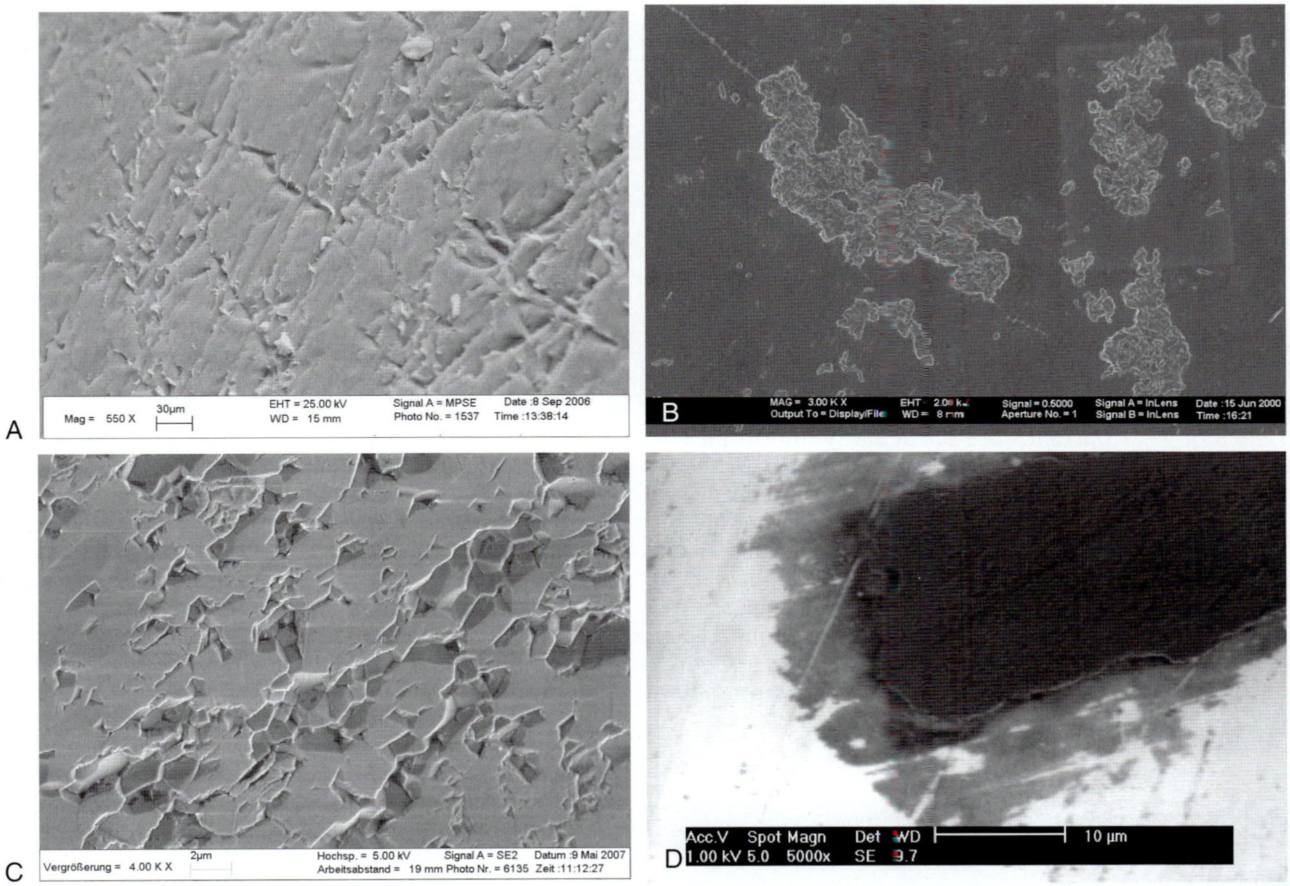

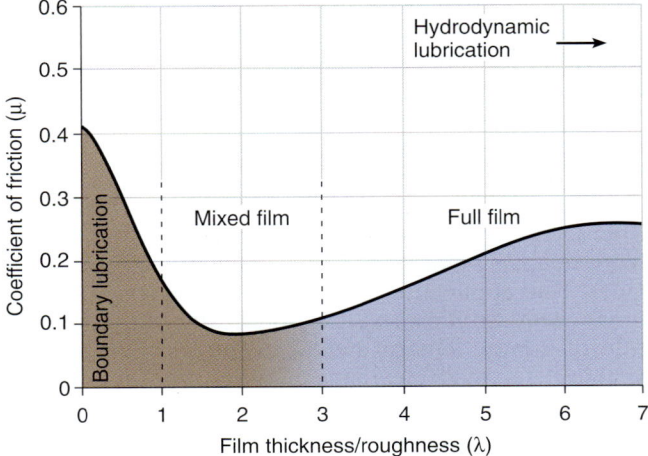

Figure 3-4. Typical appearances of the four major wear mechanisms *(from left to right)*. **A,** Abrasion: scratches and grooves on a polyethylene cup. **B,** Adhesion: transferred polyethylene flakes. **C,** Surface fatigue: intergranular fracture in the high wear region of a ceramic cup. **D,** Tribochemical reactions: organo-metallic deposit on the head of a metal/metal articulation.

Figure 3-5. Coefficient of friction in sliding contact as a function of the specific lubricant film thickness.

The Hip Bearing as a Tribological System

In this section, we will apply the terms explained previously to the artificial hip joint. Because of the complex nature of tribology, wear at the hip cannot be reduced

to a material property but is determined by the characteristics of the system. Such a system (compare with Fig. 3-1) consists of the acetabular liner and the femoral head, which are the contacting bodies, the fluid that interacts between the two bodies, and the surrounding soft tissue, with the latter defining environmental conditions such as ambient temperature and gas concentrations. These characteristics of the system, as well as the loads and motions that occur during daily activities, should be known for proper understanding and modeling of wear processes.

Wear Mode and Mechanisms

The wear mode in the human hip joint can be designated as multidirectional sliding wear—*multidirectional* because the wear tracks form quasi-elliptical paths, which cross each other during the cyclical motion of gait.[5] Crossing of wear tracks accelerates the formation of particulate debris[6] and thus is an important concept of hip wear. In addition, McKellop[7] has defined four modes of hip wear based on the conditions under which the joint functions in vivo: (1) regular (sliding) wear; (2) impingement (impact) wear; (3) three-body abrasive wear; and (4) backside (fretting) wear. They are briefly described under "Testing Procedures" (Box 3-3, Item 5). During regular sliding wear, all known major wear mechanisms—adhesion, abrasion, surface fatigue, and tribochemical reactions—may act at the same time (see Fig. 3-3). Therefore, to tribologically improve an artificial bearing, it is important to identify the mechanisms that dominate the wear behavior. This has been done through retrieval analysis and identification of characteristic wear appearances. Based on the observed wear types, all four major wear mechanisms are found to be acting, and this has been documented in an extensive body of literature. Examples are presented in Figure 3-4.

System Output

Material loss is the most relevant system output (see Fig. 3-1) for orthopedic applications. The characteristics of wear particles are particularly important in the context of wear-induced osteolysis. It has been shown that the tissue reaction depends on the size, shape, and composition of the particles generated.[8,9] A comparison of particle images (Fig. 3-6) reveals that different types of polyethylene result in different particle size distributions.[10] For instance, in some cases, significantly more particles are released even though the overall quantity of wear debris may be smaller. Conversion of current wear rates and particle sizes predicts

that $0.2 - 2.0 \times 10^{12}$ particles are generated per milligram of debris, corresponding to the generation of approximately one hundred million (!) wear particles per step.[11]

Despite the relevance of wear, most of the dissipated energy of the system is transformed into *heat*. The clinically observed heat generation of hip endoprostheses[12] is a direct result of the described microscopic process. In cases of couples with very small contact areas, as in metal-on-metal bearings, local temperatures can reach between 60° C and 80° C for a few milliseconds.[13] These temperature changes can initiate chemical reactions that generate reaction products and films on the acetabular and femoral bearing surfaces.[14] This phenomenon explains the higher starting torque measured for these metal-on-metal pairings,[15] which stresses the prosthesis-bone interface. In large diameter prostheses, this start-up torque can reach clinically relevant values and in unfortunate circumstances can contribute to loosening of the artificial device.[16] From a wear perspective, tribochemical reactions are positive. Transformation of the original surface into a hybrid material consisting of nanometer-sized metal crystals, oxidized wear debris, and organic matter from the interfacial synovial fluid[17] may be similar to the action of antiwear additives in high-performance lubricants used in race car engines. Here, additives form surface films that protect the underlying material, making them more durable and reducing their wear rates.[18]

Lately, audible *sound* as a system output has come under scrutiny for hip arthroplasty applications. Cases of "squeaking" of ceramics/ceramics pairings[19-21] have made their appearance in the orthopedic literature. The squeaky noise has been related to stick slip phenomena,[22] which occur as the result of roughening of bearing surfaces. The exact cause of hip squeaking, however, remains unclear and is presumably a multifactorial phenomenon that could involve component neck-cup impingement, microseparation, and subluxation. Debate over whether squeaking in ceramic hips is a cause for concern is ongoing.

Lubrication Regime

Ideally, as reviewed in Figure 3-5, the lubricating film completely separates the two articulating elements. This scenario requires a large contact area, sufficiently high relative velocities, and sufficiently smooth surfaces. One application of these effects is the so-called *large diameter prosthesis*. Theoretically, the combination of a large femoral head (leading to high relative velocity), a small clearance between ball and socket (yielding a large lubricated area), and smooth bearing surfaces will facilitate hydrodynamic lubrication and thus yield a long-life implant without wear. However, theoretical calculations by Dowson[23] showed that these effects are limited to the geometries of very few of the prostheses that are currently available. Nevertheless, clinical studies by Daniel and associates did not report significant differences in whole blood and urinary levels of cobalt and chromium between a theoretically low-friction group and a control group.[24] It is possible that the daily activity profile of patients, low walking speeds, and many start/stop activities could have masked

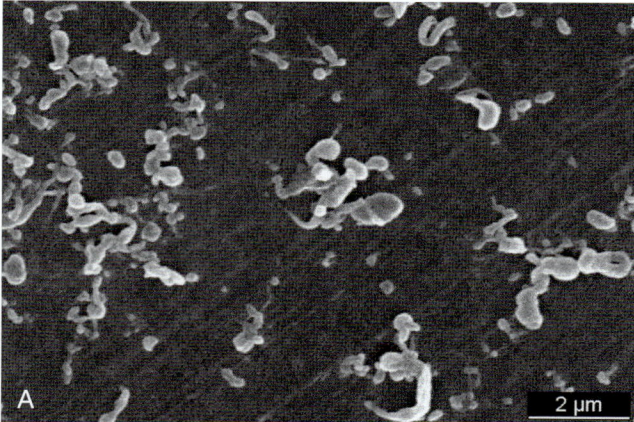

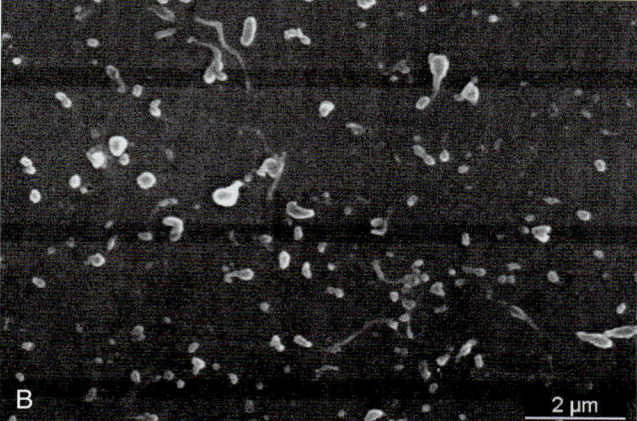

Figure 3-6. Typical polyethylene wear particles from **(A)** conventional and **(B)** cross-linked ultra-high-molecular-weight polyethylene (UHMWPE).

differences between groups in terms of wear under steady-state conditions.[15]

In addition, a small but significant deformation of the relatively thin metal socket may occur during implantation and physiologic loading of the pelvis (e.g., pinching effects around the equator). These deformations are considered in theoretical calculations[25,26] but are not simulated in wear tests. These observations could explain a study conducted by DeHaan and colleagues[27] on a marathon runner who had received a large diameter prosthesis: during the competition phase, a distinct increase in chromium urine concentration was found, which can occur only when the articulating components are moving in the mixed lubrication regime. Higher pelvis deformation and loads during running compared with those during walking may be responsible for this observation. Consequently, it must be assumed that all currently available implants interact under boundary or mixed lubrication conditions during physiologic loading to generate wear particles. The biological reactions that these particles elicit within the host will be reviewed in Chapters 11 and 12.

In this context, the question arises as to why in a natural hip joint, which is exposed to similar biomechanical boundary conditions, such wear processes do not occur. In the past, this difference was attributed primarily to elastohydrodynamic (EHD) processes. It was assumed that, in contrast to hard implant materials, the relatively soft cartilage is smoothed by the pressure of the lubricating film, reducing the effective height of protruding peaks. Under these conditions, it was assumed that a thinner lubricant film would be sufficient to separate the articulating layers without contact between the underlying surfaces. However, recent studies by Caligaris and coworkers[28] have shown that the interstitial fluid pressure of cartilage is sufficient to reduce friction and wear substantially, which is especially important during starting processes in which EHD does not apply. Glycosaminoglycan is particularly important for this phenomenon. This molecule prevents rapid diffusion of fluid from the cartilage matrix, forcing 90% of the joint contact load to be carried by water molecules. In addition, special proteins, such as lubricin, within the synovium and the lamina splendens of the articular cartilage contribute to the absence of cartilage wear even in regions of mixed friction. Despite significant progress made in the understanding of articular cartilage performance, the development of comparable artificial materials remains challenging.

Wear in Hip Bearings

Because of the multifactorial nature of tribology, the relevance of results obtained in wear experiments using wear simulators should always be interpreted with great care. Nevertheless, the importance of tribological experiments for the development of new materials and revolutionary implant geometries is without question. For instance, Harry Craven[29] was able to convince his boss, Sir John Charnley, who had considered the experiments a waste of time, of the suitability of ultra-high-molecular-weight polyethylene (UHMWPE) as a gliding component material and to replace the material Teflon.[30]

Craven used a pin-on-disk testing device manufactured from scrap, a device that would now be considered outdated. Nevertheless, use of this device facilitated the development of a milestone in endoprosthetics.

Approximately 5 years later (1966), Duff-Barclay started using the first hip simulator. Via several developmental stages, including Stanmore simulators (MKI and MKII), Munich simulators (Ungethüm 1 and 2[31]), and Leeds simulators,[32] new hip simulators were developed that meet current testing norms of the ISO (Standards 12424-1 and 14242-3). Although these tests exclusively simulate a normalized walking gait cycle (1 to 1.5 million movement cycles are assumed to reflect 1 year in vivo[33]), they have nonetheless provided major insights into wear processes in hip implants. Other activities of daily living, such as stair climbing or rising from a chair, are not considered, nor are events entailing high loads such as subluxation, start-stop movements, and neck-cup impingement.

In general, polyethylene wear increases by approximately 3% to 10% with each additional 1 mm in ball diameter because of increasing sliding distance and frictional area.[34,35] Consequently, the risk of revision for a 33-mm ball size has been regarded as threefold compared with that for a 22-mm ball size for conventional polyethylene.[36] Taking into consideration all ceramic-polyethylene pairings with a 28-mm diameter tested by a certified testing laboratory (Endolab GmbH, Rosenheim, Germany) into 12 groups of 3 pairings each during the past decade resulted in a median wear rate of 19.4 mg per million movement cycles (Fig. 3-7). The standard deviation was 6.8 mg per one million cycles, with values ranging from 7.8 to 29.8 mg per million cycles. Still, the worst 28-mm diameter pairing had a lower wear rate than the best 55-mm diameter pairing.

Wear rates of cross-linked polyethylene are in the range of 10% to 50% of those of conventional polyethylene.[37,38] These low wear rates have been confirmed in many clinical studies.[39-41] Likewise, studies by Endolab have shown wear in the range of a few milligrams per million loading cycles (see Fig. 3-7). In simulation experiments, all types of polyethylene absorb relatively large amounts of fluid from the surroundings, resulting in underestimation of weight loss through wear. In the past, these underestimations gave rise to the euphoric but scientifically unsound assumption that cross-linked polyethylenes are completely resistant to wear.[37]

Since the development of first-generation cross-linked polyethylenes, second-generation cross-linked polyethylenes have included additives such as vitamin E and altered manufacturing parameters. These additives primarily act as radical traps and allow the quenching of free radicals generated by irradiation without the need for thermal processing at temperatures that degrade the strength of the polymer. Removal of free radicals is beneficial in decreasing the rate of oxidation of polyethylene components and the risk of catastrophic embrittlement in vivo. Each group of polyethylenes with additives can be separated into subgroups[42] with a range of possible material parameters. Because of these variations, large variability in wear rates is observed for cross-linked polyethylenes, and generalization of wear

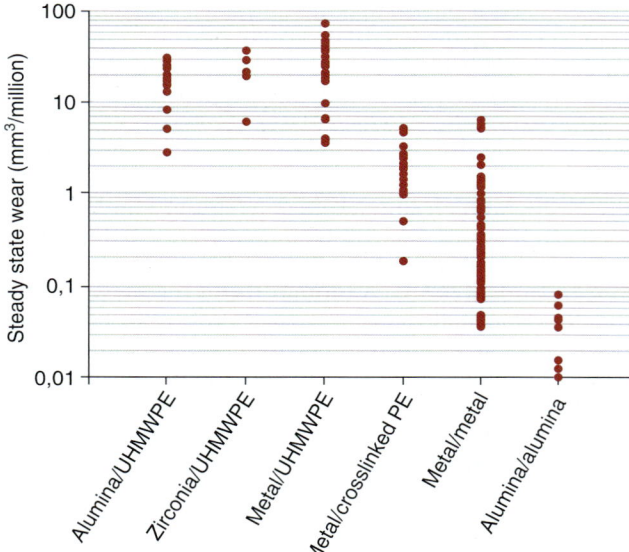

Figure 3-7. Steady-state wear rates of the most commonly used material combinations in hip bearing couples. Each dot represents the average of three bearings of the same design and manufacturer on a hip simulator according to the International Organization for Standardization (ISO) 14242-1. *(Data from repository of Endolab.)*

rates for these materials is not possible. In addition, aspects of the in vivo long-term stability of these materials cannot be generally addressed. However, because of the reduced fracture toughness of some formulations of cross-linked polyethylenes, enhanced protection against in vivo oxidation is especially important.

As was discussed previously, the "squeaking" of ceramic/ceramic pairings might be related to a subluxation problem with specific implant geometries. Subluxation was initially recognized in revised pairings[43] and later included microseparation as an add-on for hip simulator tests.[44] This helped to re-create areas of "stripe wear" in simulator testing that resembled those of ceramic/ceramic retrievals, namely, elongated zones with a dull appearance due to roughening of the surface. It is no surprise that such microseparation conditions produced considerably higher wear rates (typically one magnitude above those values shown in Fig. 3-7). Squeaking noises, however, could not be generated in the laboratory consistently. The reasons for this are currently under close investigation.[22,45]

Metal-on-metal bearings have regained popularity during the past decade. Until recently, 30% of all newly implanted hip joints in the United States were metal/metal articulations. Worldwide, its market share is approximately 10%. Although this material combination is attractive because of its low volumetric wear rate (see Fig. 3-7), it gained its popularity primarily because it provided new possibilities in surgical procedures using hip resurfacing rather than total hip replacement. Proper tribological behavior of metal-on-metal joints relies on the establishment of tribochemical reaction films.[17] The creation of such films is sensitive to surface chemistry and texture, as well as contact pressure and lubricant constituents (i.e., organic molecules

that adhere to surfaces). Hence, alloy microstructure, bearing dimensions, tolerances, and machining quality all may contribute to the large variability in wear rate seen with this combination (see Fig. 3-7). In vivo, surgical variation in implant positioning and the biomechanics of the patient are additional factors that need to be addressed. Also, variation in synovial fluid composition, as seen after osteoarthritic disease and/or menopause, may contribute to the wear outcome. This complex dependence on multiple factors may explain the variability in wear performance of metal-on-metal joints, including recent reports of higher than expected clinical wear rates and complications.[46-48] Therefore, to make this bearing combination more reliable for clinical use, strategies should be developed to control and stabilize the formation of tribochemical reaction films. Because these films are the result of the combined action of corrosion and wear, their study is best performed within the scope of the newly established field of tribocorrosion.[49,50]

Testing Procedures

New materials and designs involving the articulating surfaces of hip prostheses must undergo tribological testing before they are released for clinical use. As a matter of efficiency, tribological testing of materials is hierarchical, starting with screening tests of various degrees of sophistication and ending with wear tests in hip joint simulators. In discussing testing procedures, it is easy to lose sight of the overall picture in the details. An overall prospective on the subject is therefore given in Box 3-2.

Screening Wear Tests

Screening tests are relatively low cost, simple, and fast, and are performed primarily to rank materials with respect to wear and friction. Here we will concentrate on three screening wear tests that are particularly relevant to orthopedic applications:

1. Pin-on-flat: the most prevalent
2. Pin-on-disk: the simplest; appropriate for measuring basic tribological properties
3. Biaxial pin-on-ball: intermediate in sophistication between pin-on-flat and hip simulators

Pin-on-Flat Wear Test. The pin-on-flat (POF) wear test, also called the *pin-on-plate test,* is used extensively to screen polymeric materials sliding against metal, but it also may be used for hard-on-hard combinations, such as metal on metal. The test configuration entails the end of a cylindrical pin sliding against a flat counterface. The end of the pin may be flat, rounded, or hemispheric (Fig. 3-8). The typical configuration for testing polymers for use in joint prostheses consists of a flat-faced cylindrical pin sliding against a flat metal counterface, the metal usually being a Co-Cr-Mo orthopedic alloy. Because of its importance, this test has been standardized with ASTM Standard F-732, "Wear Testing of Polymeric Materials Used in Total Joint Prostheses."[51] This standard specifies three variants of the test: (1) for linear reciprocation wear motion applications, such as hinged knees; (2) for "hip-type motion"; and (3) for linear

BOX 3-2 KEY POINTS FOR WEAR TESTING

1. Wear testing of prostheses is an essential step in the development of new designs and materials. It is usually required for submissions to regulatory agencies such as the Food and Drug Administration (FDA) to gain approval for clinical use of a device that involves changes in design or material of the articular surfaces.
2. Wear testing is complex because it entails a tribological system—bearing surfaces articulating in a given lubricant and subjected to applied forces and motions.
3. Material combinations for hip bearing surfaces are evaluated for wear, using screening tests that entail simplified specimen geometries, loading, and motions. The most commonly performed screening test is the pin-on-flat wear test, based on American Society for Testing and Materials (ASTM) Standard F-732.
4. Hip wear tests are typically performed in multistation hip simulators. They are expensive because they are often lengthy and labor- and capital-intensive. A 12-station simulator typically costs several hundred thousand dollars.
5. Two broad types of hip simulators are commercially available: biaxial rocking motion simulators and simulators capable of applying the three rotations: flexion-extension, adduction-abduction, and internal-external rotation.
6. A hip wear test is deemed representative if it produces wear values (head penetration, weight loss) that are of the same order of magnitude as observed clinically. In addition, particle size distribution and shape and wear surface morphology should be comparable to what is observed clinically.
7. Standards related to hip wear testing have been developed by the ASTM and the ISO (see Table 3-3).
8. Although hip wear testing has evolved considerably in the past two decades, there is still plenty of room for improvements, such as the use of better characterized lubricants; simulation of activities other than walking, such as stair climbing and descent; and improved protocols for testing wear under severe conditions such as three-body wear.
9. A significant recent advance in hip wear testing is the inclusion of microseparation or lateralization, in which the head and the cup separate slightly during the swing phase of each walking gait cycle and recombine with slight cup edge impingement. Microseparation is important to reproduce clinically relevant wear rates for ceramic-on-ceramic bearings.
10. Hip wear testing most often yields relative results, in which designs or materials are ranked or compared with a control that is tested alongside. Internal controls are essential in any test because of the effects of factors that are hard to control and may change from test to test and from laboratory to laboratory.
11. There is reasonably good correlation between the wear rates predicted from modern hip simulators and clinically observed wear rates. Microseparation is required to reproduce clinically relevant wear rates for ceramic-on-ceramic bearings.

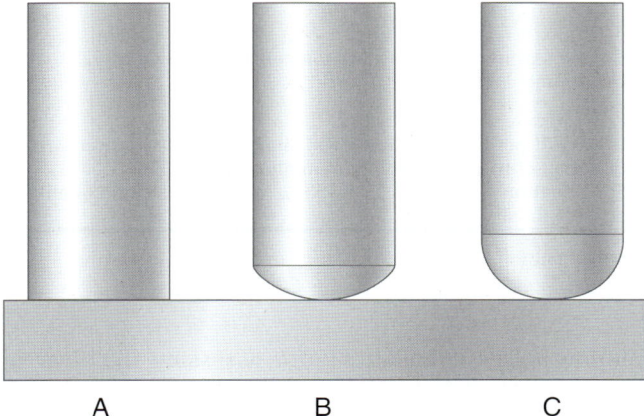

Figure 3-8. Typical pin geometries for the pin-on-flat test. The pins are cylindrical with a flat **(A)**, rounded **(B)**, or hemispheric end **(C).** The flat end sometimes is slightly beveled circumferentially to decrease edge effects.

motion delamination wear applications, mainly applicable to incongruent metal-polymer contact as encountered in knee prostheses. Motions and configurations for variants 1 and 2 are shown in Figure 3-9A and B, respectively. Variant 2 emulates the multidirectional motion found at the bearing surfaces of hip prostheses, determined to be essential for proper evaluation of UHMWPE for hip applications[6] because this material is susceptible to shear softening.[52] This enhancement of the wear rate of a polymer by "cross-shearing" had been reported earlier for high-density polyethylene.[53] Test conditions for the Trip-type motion are given in Table 3-1.

Pin-on-Disk Configuration. In its simplest form, the pin-on-disk (POD) configuration entails a pin subjected to a constant vertical force, sliding on the flat face of a rotating disk, describing a circular, unidirectional path (Fig. 3-10). The main advantage of this configuration is that it offers simple conditions for friction and wear measurements. Guidance for this test is given by ASTM Standard G-99.[54] Measurement of friction is readily accomplished by measuring the side force required to keep the pin in place on the rotating disk. Although the tip geometry is typically spherical, rounded and flat tip geometries are also possible. For a pin with a spherical tip, the wear scar is approximately circular as long as the disk wear is sufficiently small. Wear of the pin can then be determined directly from the mean diameter of the wear scar:

$$\text{Wear} = \pi d^4/32\, D$$

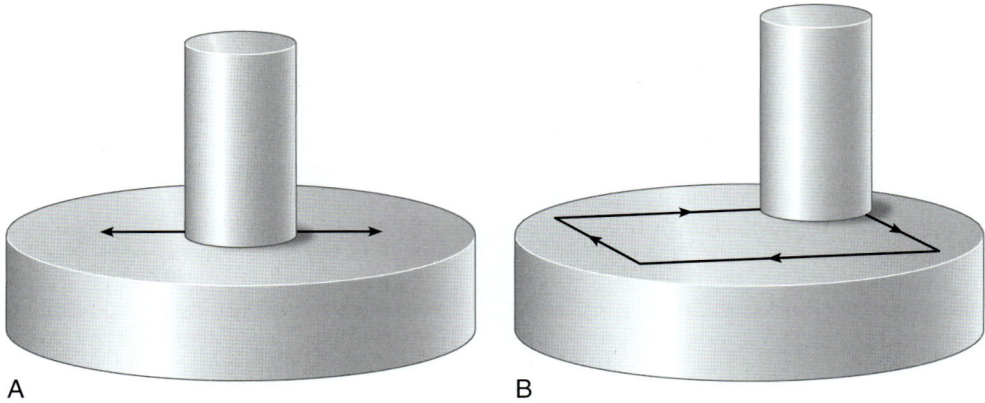

Figure 3-9. Pin-on-flat test paths. **A,** Linearly reciprocating, without crossing motion. **B,** Rectangular, with crossing motion.

Table 3-1. Test Conditions for the Pin-on-Flat Test per ASTM Standard F-732	
Condition	**Requirement**
Motion	Multidirectional (e.g., rectangular)
Pin geometry	Flat-ended circular cylinder
Pin dimensions	13 mm length × 9 mm diameter
Contact area, mm^2	63.6
Counterface geometry	Flat
Test load, N	130 to 640
Nominal stress, MPa	2 to 10
Load profile	Constant or variable
Load profile maximum deviation	±3%
Stroke, mm	N/A
Frequency, Hz	0.5 to 2
Average sliding speed, mm/sec	12.5 to 75
Polymer cross-shear	60 to 90 degrees
Test minimum duration, cycles	2,000,000
Minimum number of measurements, subsequent to the initial one	4
Lubricant	Bovine serum, diluted with deionized water down to ≥25% by volume
Lubricant replacement interval, max	2 weeks
Reference couple	UHMWPE per Specification F-648 sliding against counterfaces of cobalt-chromium-molybdenum alloy (per ASTM Specification F-75, F-799, or F-1537), having prosthetic quality surface finish

ASTM, American Society for Testing and Materials; *UHMWPE,* ultra-high-molecular-weight polyethylene.

where d and D are the wear scar and the tip diameter, respectively. Wear of the disk can be determined by weight loss or by profilometry. The POD method is suitable for obtaining friction and wear information on any type of material combination (e.g., polymer-metal, metal-metal). For a polymer-metal or polymer-ceramic couple, the pin can be chosen to be made of either of these materials, depending on the information sought. A good application of the method is to determine the frictional interaction between material couples as a function of lubricant type and composition, as might be used to compare materials (e.g., various polyethylenes) and lubricants (synovial fluid vs. bovine serum-based lubricants). However, lack of cross-shearing in the motion makes it unsuitable for assessing the wear of polymers, such as UHMWPE, subject to cross-shearing wear effects.

Biaxial Pin-on-Ball Wear Test. Intermediate in sophistication between pin-on-flat and hip simulator tests, this test was explicitly conceived as a method to screen and analyze bearing surfaces used in total hip arthroplasty (THR).[55] It entails a conforming and equatorial contact between the concave end of a cylindrical pin and a ball that oscillates rotationally about mutually perpendicular axes (Fig. 3-11). With appropriate input from rotational waveforms, the resulting biaxial motion yields wear tracks of desired shapes, from almost linear (Fig. 3-12a) to loops with crossing paths that

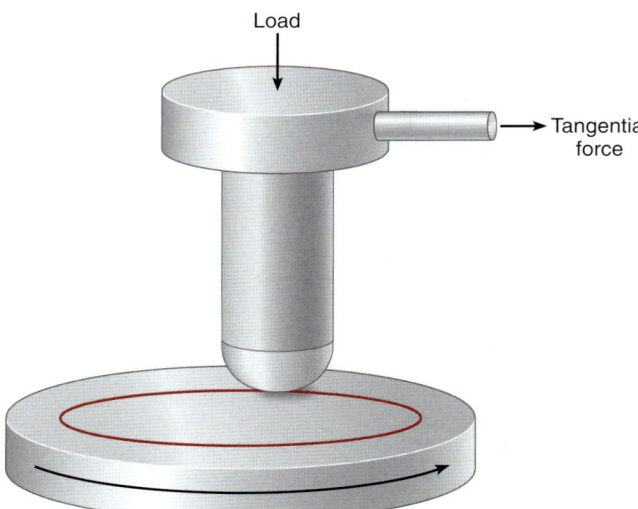

Figure 3-10. Pin-on-disk configuration. The circular, unidirectional path is shown in red.

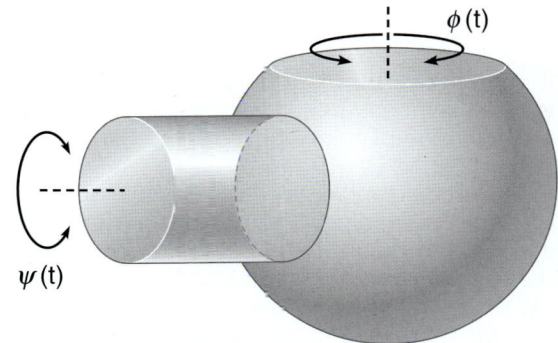

Figure 3-11. Biaxial pin-on-ball configuration. Pin rotation $\psi(t)$ and ball rotation $\phi(t)$ are controlled independently to yield arbitrary motion trajectories between pin and ball. *(Redrawn from Wimmer MA, Nassutt R, Lampe F, et al: A new screening method designed for wear analysis of bearing surfaces used in total hip arthroplasty. In Jacobs J, Cendrowska T, Speiser P [eds]: Alternative bearing surfaces in total joint replacement, STP 1346, West Conshohocken, Pa, 1998, American Society for Testing and Materials, pp 30–43.)*

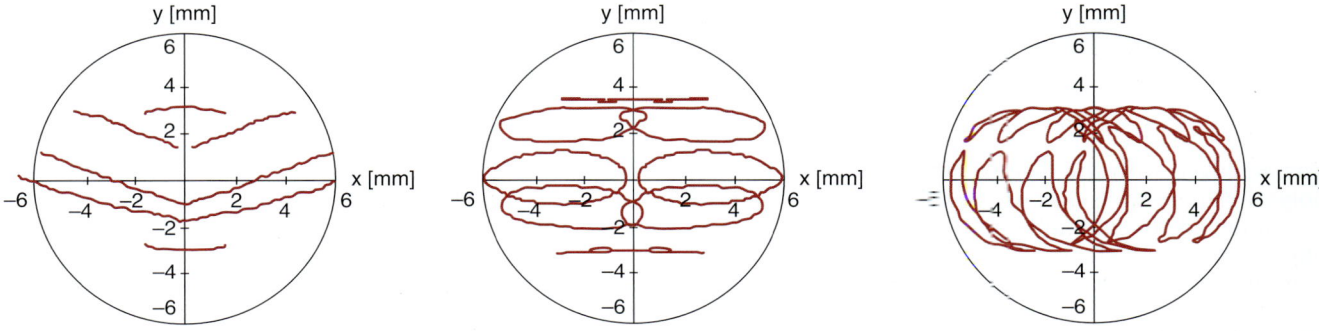

Figure 3-12. Trajectories plotted on the surface of a 12-mm-diameter pin obtained with the pin-on-ball configuration. **A,** Nearly linear paths obtained with biaxial oscillatory motion with no phase and frequency difference. **B,** Elliptical trajectories. *(Redrawn from Wimmer MA, Nassutt R, Lampe F, et al: A new screening method designed for wear analysis of bearing surfaces used in total hip arthroplasty. In Jacobs J, Cendrowska T, Speiser P [eds]: Alternative bearing surfaces in total joint replacement, STP 1346, West Conshohocken, Pa, 1998, American Society for Testing and Materials, pp 30–43.)*

approximate wear tracks observed in vivo for hips (Fig. 3-12*b* and *c*). This flexibility allows evaluation of the impact of motion trajectory on the wear of different candidate materials. The load is applied along the pin axis and can be kept constant or can be varied cyclically to correspond to various parts of the motion trajectory. Arbitrary combinations of materials can be tested, such as soft on hard (e.g., a UHMWPE pin against a Co-Cr-Mo ball) and hard on hard (e.g., metal against metal, ceramic against ceramic). The pin-on-ball assembly is immersed in a chamber that contains the lubricant, such as diluted bovine calf serum. Friction between pin and ball is determined from the torque used to rotate the ball. Linear wear and deformation are measured using a linear variable differential transformer (LVDT) displacement sensor aligned with the pin. For UHMWPE, the effects of creep and swelling may be reduced by loading and soaking the wear couple for a predetermined time before starting the wear test. Wear may also be determined gravimetrically. No standards are currently associated with this biaxial pin-on-ball test.

Hip Joint Wear Simulators

As useful and indispensable as the screening tests may be, ultimately it is essential that wear tests be performed using the prosthetic components themselves in a manner that simulates as closely as possible the relevant physiologic conditions in vivo. This is the role of a hip joint wear simulator. Such a simulator should possess the attributes listed in Box 3-3.

The design and use of hip simulators have evolved considerably over past decades, particularly after the mid-90s, when it became clear that simulators that applied only flexion-extension (FE) rotation, the dominant hip motion, produced wear rates well below clinical wear rates for polyethylene articulating against a metal cup. Those interested in the earlier history of hip wear testing are directed to Dumbleton's monograph,[56] which provides a comprehensive review of joint simulators up to 1980, and to Saikko's assessment of hip wear testing in the early 90s.[57] A comprehensive rundown of historical hip joint simulators is also given by Affatato and associates.[58] A significant breakthrough

---

BOX 3-3   ATTRIBUTES OF THE IDEAL HIP SIMULATOR

1. It reproduces the wear mechanisms observed in vivo, as demonstrated by:
   - Magnitude of the wear rates and proper ranking of materials
   - Microscopic appearance of the wear surfaces
   - Debris morphology and size distribution
2. It is able to duplicate all key physiologic motions, namely, flexion-extension (F-E), adduction-abduction (A-A), and internal-external rotation (I-E), reproducing the pertinent characteristics of wear tracks observed on explanted components.
3. It accepts a variety of applied motion and load profiles to simulate the desired activity (e.g., walking, running, stair climbing, stair descent). Load and motions applied to the joint closely follow the input.
4. It permits anatomic positioning of the joint (e.g., cup above the head).
5. It is able to simulate the four modes of hip wear defined by McKellop[7]:
   - Mode 1, regular wear, typically through reciprocating sliding, stemming from intended contact between bearing surfaces

- Mode 2, microseparation and subluxation, whereby a bearing surface is wearing against a nonbearing surface (e.g., the head impinges against the edge of the cup)
- Mode 3, as Mode 1, but abrasive particles interposed between the bearing surfaces, leading to three-body abrasive wear
- Mode 4, backside wear between the cup and the shell, typically in fretting mode

6. Test chambers are constructed of materials inert to the lubricant and are sealed to prevent lubricant evaporation and ingress of contaminants.
7. The machine is able to run unattended 24 hours a day, 7 days a week, except for occasional checks and periodic processing of the specimens for cleaning and measuring wear.
8. The machine is robust enough to withstand the many millions of cycles entailed in most hip wear tests without a breakdown.

---

was achieved with the discovery that the wear rate of polyethylene increases considerably when this material is subjected to multidirectional motion, as occurs physiologically, instead of reciprocating unidirectional motion as would occur with simple FE or linked flexion-extension–internal-external (FE–IE) rotations.[6,59] This effect of multidirectional motion on the wear of polyethylene is attributed to orientation softening from deformation-induced structural anisotropy in this semicrystalline high-molecular-weight linear polymer.[52]

Modern hip simulators can be divided into three broad classes based on their head-cup kinematics:
1. Biaxial rocking motion (BRM) simulators.
2. Two-axis simulators that apply two independent rotations: FE plus adduction-abduction (AA) or IE rotations.
3. Three-axis simulators that apply all three independent rotations: FE, AA, and IE rotations.

Biaxial rocking motion simulators are probably the most popular simulators because they are mechanically simple and compact, yet they generate clinically relevant wear rates.[37,60] With this clever and elegant design, a wedge rotates under a cup that itself is prevented from rotating, generating a rocking motion of the cup as it articulates against the head. A diagram of the mechanism is shown in Figure 3-13. The rocking motion is equivalent to FE and AA sinusoidal motions with a phase difference of 90 degrees and amplitude equal to the angle of the underlying wedge, typically 22.5 degrees. It thus simulates someone walking with normal FE but with a very large AA angle. Although the motion pattern is fixed, the load waveform may be changed at will.

Two- and three-axis simulators differ from BRM simulators in that arbitrary rotation waveforms may be

input, within the specifications of the simulator. For a three-axis simulator, all three rotations may be varied arbitrarily, permitting maximum flexibility to simulate various types of gaits. The disadvantage is that they are more costly and more complex, and therefore perhaps less robust, than BRM simulators. This complexity is evident in the cup rotation mechanism illustrated for the AMTI hip simulator (Advanced Mechanical Technology, Inc., Watertown, Mass) in Figure 3-14.

A list of current simulators, most of them commercially available, is given in Table 3-2. All yield multidirectional head-cup motion and cross-shearing on contacting sliding surfaces. However, in a detailed study of eight hip simulators, Calonius and Saikko[61] demonstrated that slide tracks on the articular surfaces differ substantially across simulators, a slide track being defined as the path drawn on the counterface by a point on the surface of the head or cup. As an illustration, the slide tracks they computed for walking gait[62] are shown in Figure 3-15, and those for the BMR, AMTI, and ProSim simulators, and per the ISO 14242-1 Standard,[61] are shown in Figure 3-16. Moreover, none of the slide tracks produced by the simulators match those computed for walking gait. Despite differences in their motions, a study indicated that AMTI and BRM simulators produce comparable polyethylene wear rates.[63] Therefore, it appears that the multidirectionality of the motion may be an even more important factor than the specific shape and dimensions of the slide tracks. Although current hip simulators are able to predict clinical wear behavior with some accuracy,[64-66] some specific limitations of hip simulator testing should be noted. Such testing does not sufficiently address the chance of fatigue failure, as was evident in some claims with

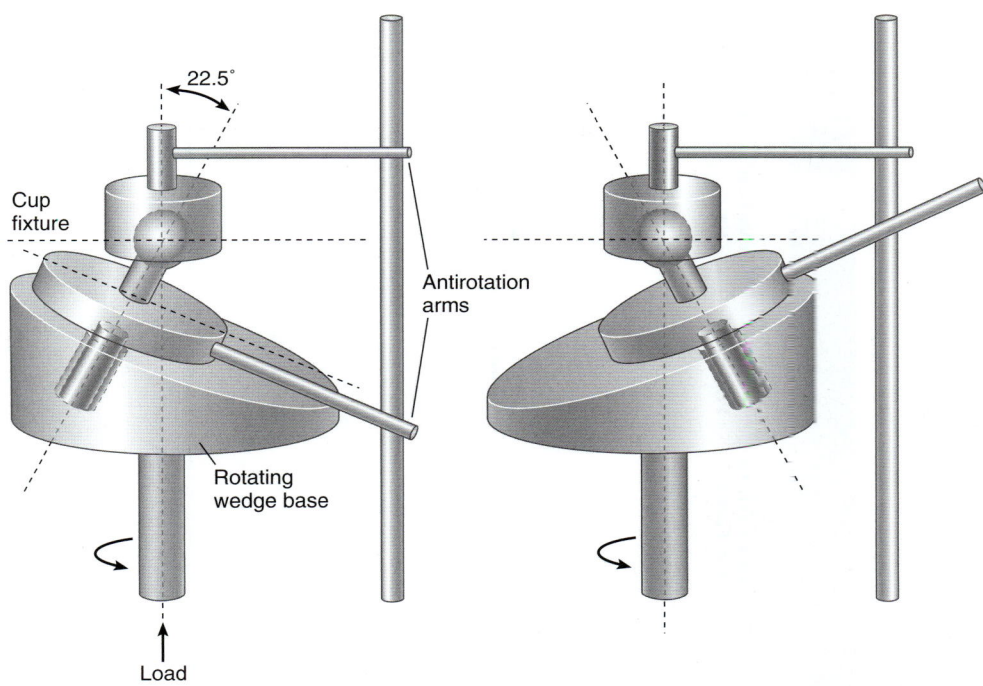

22.5°

Cup
fixture

Antirotation
arms

Rotating
wedge base

Load

Figure 3-13. Diagram illustrating the design principle of a biaxial rocking motion hip simulator.

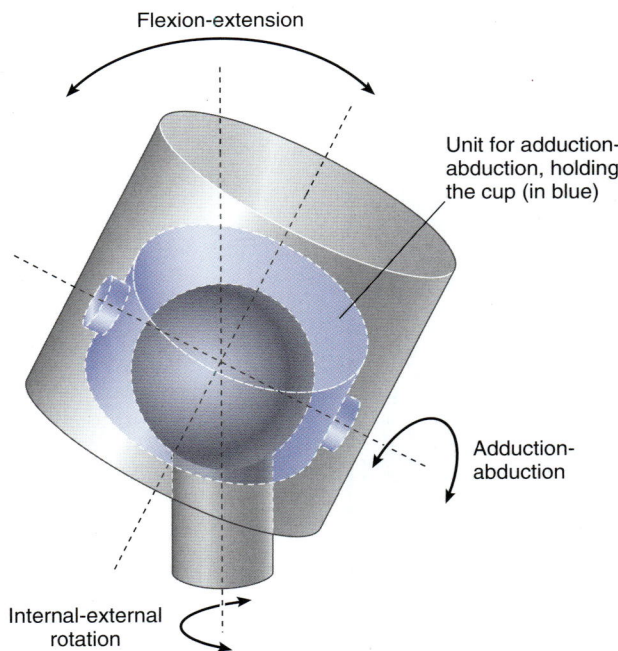

Flexion-extension

Unit for adduction-
abduction, holding
the cup (in blue)

Adduction-
abduction

Internal-external
rotation

Figure 3-14. Three-axis cup rotation mechanism in the AMTI (Boston, Mass) hip simulator.

first-generation cross-linked polyethylenes.[67,68] These aspects must be addressed using complementary material and design-specific methods. For example, testing the effects of head-neck impingement on an acetabular cup made from a new UHMWPE formulation is best performed in a test setup designed specifically for this purpose.

Load Profiles. Modern hip simulators generally accept load waveforms defined by the user, but simulator capabilities can be a limiting factor. A standardized load profile is specified in ISO 14242-1 that has double peaks of 3000 N and a minimum load of 300 N. This waveform, along with the corresponding motion curves, is shown in Figure 3-17. Also commonly used are the so-called *Paul curve*[59] and profiles based on Bergmann's in vivo instrumented hip prosthesis studies.[70]

The Lubricant. As one of the key components of the hip prosthesis tribosystem, the lubricant deserves special attention, even though in the past it seemed to be overlooked. Lubricant properties play a major role in the wear of UHMWPE in prosthetic hips.[71-73] Total protein concentration, the albumin-to-globulin ratio, the lubricant volume turnover rate, and the protein precipitation rate all have been found to affect the polyethylene wear rate.[72] Synovial fluid, the lubricant of choice, is much too expensive to be used in simulators, where tests often require many liters of lubricant. At the other extreme, water is inadequate as a lubricant because it lacks the proteins that provide boundary lubrication and are associated with triboreactions. Its rheologic properties are considerably different from those of synovial fluid, which has a markedly higher viscosity and exhibits shear thinning. The compromise has been to use some form of bovine serum, usually bovine calf serum, but also other forms such as fetal bovine serum. ISO Standard 14242-1 specifies bovine calf serum diluted with deionized water to 25% and a protein mass concentration of no less than 17 g/L (the revised standard will state 30 g/L). Ongoing research is seeking to enhance our understanding of the role of the components of the lubricant. A recent study reported marked lowering of

Table 3-2. List of Current Hip Simulators

Simulator Designation	Origin and Availability	Motions	Power	Maximum Load, N	Load Direction	Component Relative to Which Load Is Fixed	Head—Cup Position	Frequency, Hz	Test Stations
Shore Western	United States, commercial	Biaxial rocking motion, ±23 degrees	Hydraulic	4500	Vertical	Cup or head	Anatomic or inverted	1.5	9 to 12
MTS-Bionix	United States, commercial	Biaxial rocking motion, ±23 degrees	Hydraulic	2450	Vertical	Cup	Anatomic	1	12
ProSim	United Kingdom, commercial	FE: +30 to −15 degrees, IE: ±10 degrees	Pneumatic	2780	Vertical	Head	Anatomic	1	10
Leeds Mark II	United Kingdom, custom-made	FE: +30 to −15 degrees, IE: +8 to −20 degrees	Pneumatic	2000	Vertical	Cup	Anatomic	NS	5
HUT-4	Finland, commercial (Phoenix Tribology)	FE: ±23 degrees, AA: ±6 degrees	Pneumatic	3000	Vertical	Cup	Anatomic	1	12
AMTI	United States, commercial	FE: ±50 degrees, AA: ±20 degrees, IE: ±20 degrees	Hydraulic	4500	Vertical	Head	Anatomic	2	12
Endolab	Germany, semicommercial	FE: +30 to −20 degrees, AA: +10 to −20 degrees, IE: 17 degrees	Hydraulic	3000	Vertical	Cup	Anatomic	1	6

Data from manufacturer literature and from Affatato S, Spinelli M, Zavalloni M, et al: Tribology and total hip joint replacement: current concepts in mechanical simulation. Med Eng Phys 30:1305–1317, 2008.
NS, Not specified.

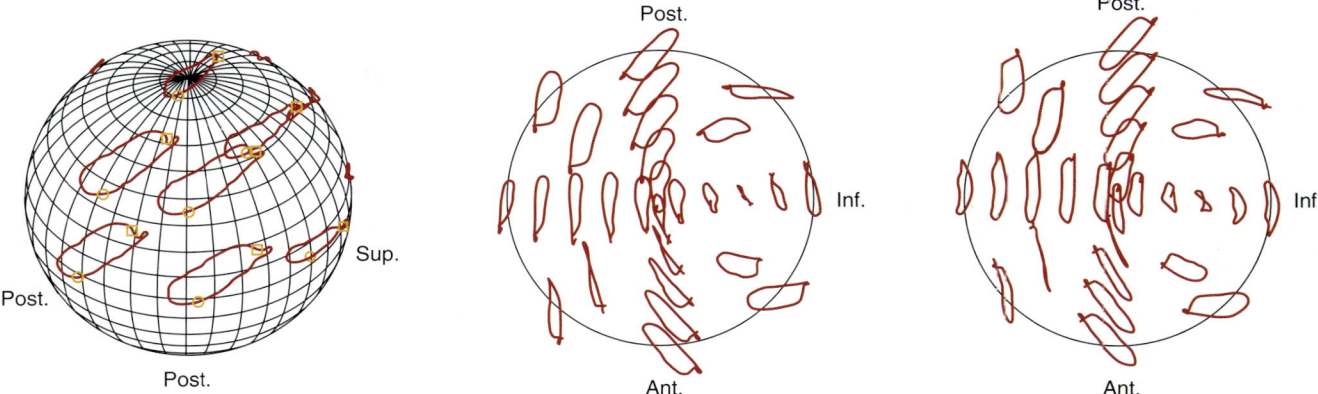

Figure 3-15. Slide tracks on the cup of selected points computed for walking gait waveforms from Johnston and Smidt (1969). The *large circle* represents the equator. (*Redrawn from Saikko V, Ahlroos T, Calonius O, Keränen J: Wear simulation of total hip prostheses with polyethylene against CoCr, alumina and diamond-like carbon. Biomaterials 22:1507–1514, 2001, with permission.*)

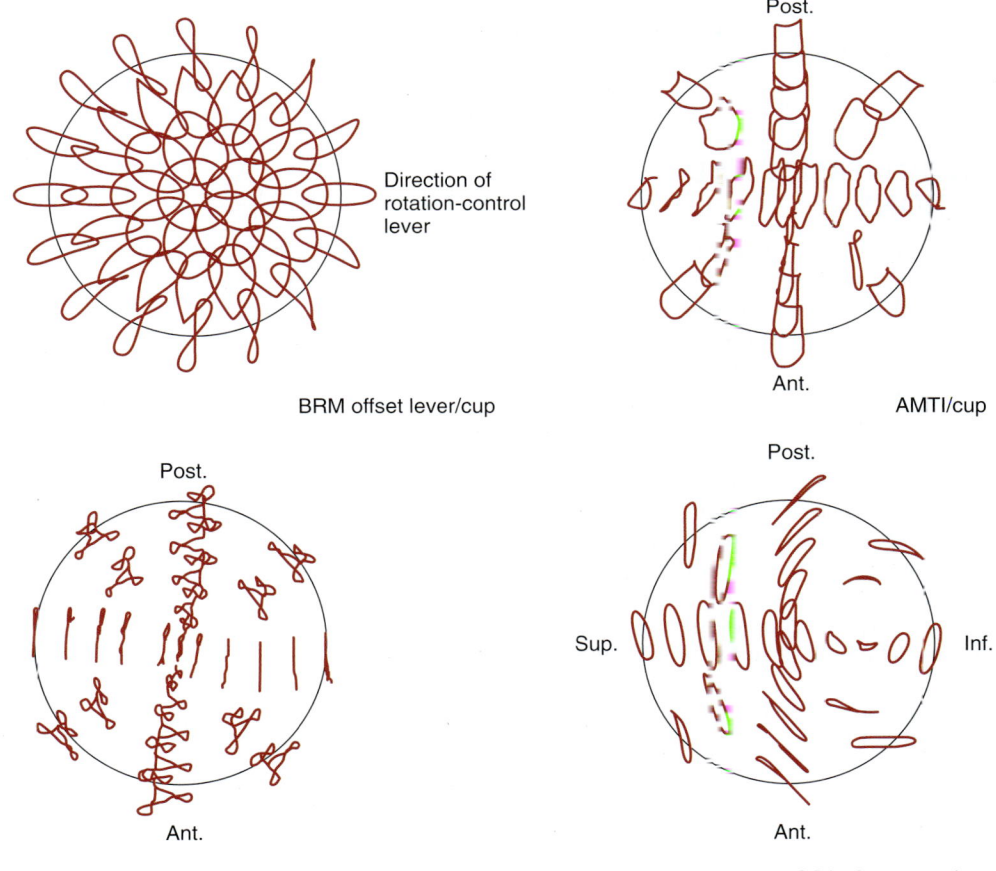

Figure 3-16. Slide tracks on the cup computed for the biaxial rocking motion (BRM), AMTI, and ProSim simulators, and based on the International Organization for Standardization (ISO) Standard 14242-1. (*Redrawn from Calonius O, Saikko V: Slide track analysis of eight contemporary hip simulator designs. J Biomech 35:1439–1450, 2002, with permission.*)

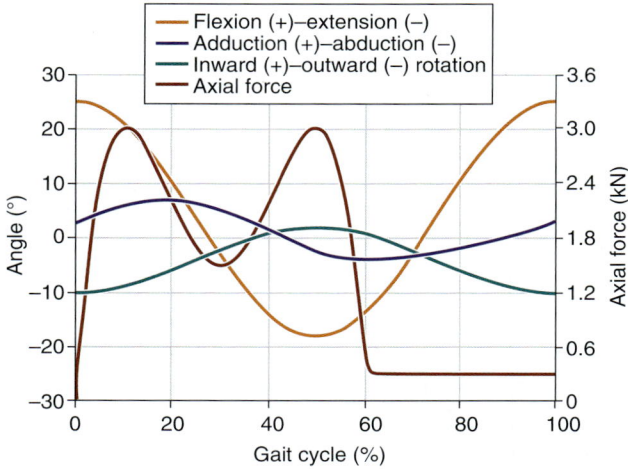

Figure 3-17. Axial force and motion curves for hip wear testing per International Organization for Standardization (ISO) Standard 14242-1.

the wear rate of UHMWPE with cleavage of albumin, and that the morphology of the wear surface greatly depended on the albumin concentration.[74] These results suggest that a standardized lubricant made from known base ingredients that would include purified proteins is needed to further increase the reproducibility of wear results on hip joint materials.

Standards. In an effort to permit a better comparison of hip wear results across laboratories for research and regulatory purposes, both the ISO and the ASTM have introduced standards applicable to hip wear testing. They are listed in Table 3-3.

CURRENT CONTROVERSIES AND FUTURE DIRECTIONS

With the advent of the new generation of polyethylenes with greatly enhanced wear resistance, the development of tougher ceramics, more advanced Co-Cr-Mo alloys, and better machining techniques, the wear issue in prosthetic joints may appear to have lost some of its former urgency. However, with the use of prosthetic joints in ever younger and more active patients, the expected considerable increase in procedures as the baby boomer generation ages, and the desire to have an artificial joint outlast the patient, the bar has been raised, keeping wear at the forefront in orthopedics. Here are the major controversies and proposed future directions as seen by the authors:
- The long-term mechanical and wear behavior of highly cross-linked UHMWPE is unknown. Therefore, there is a need:
  - To develop tests to gauge the long-term stability of UHMWPE with respect to its mechanical properties and wear performance
  - To continue to perform clinical studies monitoring the in vivo performance of cross-linked UHMWPE
- In view of current issues with metal-on-metal bearings, the following questions must be addressed:
  - Why are some modern metal-on-metal bearings performing less well than anticipated?

Standard Designation	Standard Title
ISO/TR 9325:1989	Implants for surgery; Partial and total hip joint prostheses; Recommendations for simulators for evaluation of hip joint prostheses
ISO 14242-1:2002	Implants for surgery; Wear of total hip joint prostheses; Part 1: Loading and displacement parameters for wear testing machines and corresponding environmental conditions for test
ISO 14242-2:2000	Implants for surgery; Wear of total hip joint prostheses; Part 2: Methods of measurement
ISO 14242-3:2009	Implants for surgery; Wear of total hip joint prostheses; Part 3: Loading and displacement parameters for orbital bearing-type wear testing machines and corresponding environmental conditions for test
ISO 7206-1:2008	Implants for surgery; Partial and total hip joint prostheses; Part 1: Classification and designation of dimensions
ASTM F-1714-96 (reapproved 2008)	Standard Guide for Gravimetric Wear Assessment of Prosthetic Hip Designs in Simulator Devices
ASTM F-2025-06	Standard Practice for Gravimetric Measurement of Polymeric Components for Wear Assessment

Table 3-3. ISO and ASTM Standards Applicable to Hip Wear Testing

- How can they be made more consistently wear resistant?
- To advance the use of ceramic components, it is important that we understand the origin of squeaking in alumina-on-alumina bearings and eliminate it.
- New materials and coatings are still needed for bearing surfaces.

- Materials are needed that can directly articulate against cartilage without causing damage to this tissue, thus simplifying joint repair.
- There is a fundamental need to develop effective and durable methods of cartilage repair that are biological or semibiological in nature. Developments in this area will greatly reduce the need for metal and plastic in joint repair. Such biologically created tissue still needs to be evaluated for its tribological and mechanical properties.
- Improvements in the wear testing of hip prosthetic joints should include:
  - Routine implementation of more realistic wear testing conditions entailing multiple activities, and updating of wear standards to that effect
  - Simulation of adverse conditions, in particular three-body wear (e.g., form loose bone or bone cement particles), malalignment, and impingement
- Increased understanding of the effects of the lubricant and its degradation on wear test results during testing may lead to improved formulations of test lubricants for use in wear tests.
- Reliable numeric methods are needed for modeling wear and lubrication, leading to the creation of "virtual" joint wear simulators to complement physical simulations.
- Greater insight into implant performance in service will enable more relevant laboratory testing. This knowledge can be gained through expansion of joint replacement registries.

Acknowledgment

The authors want to thank Christian Kaddick, Endolab GmbH, Rosenheim, Germany, for providing testing data and discussion.

REFERENCES

1. Jacobs JJ, Hallab NJ: Loosening and osteolysis associated with metal-on-metal bearings: a local effect of metal hypersensitivity? J Bone Joint Surg Am 88:1171–1172, 2006.
2. Catelas I, Jacobs JJ: Biologic activity of wear particles. Instr Course Lect 59:3–16, 2010.
3. Hamrock BJ, Schmid SR, Jacobson BO: Fundamentals of fluid film lubrication, ed 2, West Palm Beach, Fla, 2004, CRC Press.
4. Stribeck R: Die wesentlichen Eigenschaften der Gleit-und Rollenlager, Zeitschrift des Vereins Deutscher Ingenieure, 1902, Nr. 36, Band 46, p. 1341–1348, 1432–143.
5. Saikko V, Calonius O: Slide track analysis of the relative motion between femoral head and acetabular cup in walking and in hip simulators. J Biomech 35:455–464, 2002.
6. Bragdon CR, O'Connor DO, Lowenstein JD, et al: The importance of multidirectional motion on the wear of polyethylene. J Eng Med 210:157–165, 1996.
7. McKellop HA: The lexicon of polyethylene wear in artificial joints. Biomaterials 28:5049–5057, 2007.
8. Brown C, Fisher J, Ingham E: Biological effects of clinically relevant wear particles from metal-on-metal hip prostheses. Proc Inst Mech Eng H 220:355–369, 2006.
9. Galvin AL, Tipper JL, Jennings LM, et al: Wear and biological activity of highly cross-linked polyethylene in the hip under low serum protein concentrations. Proc Inst Mech Eng H 221:1–10, 2007.
10. Laurent MP, Johnson TS, Crowninshield RD, et al: Characterization of a highly cross-linked ultrahigh molecular-weight polyethylene in clinical use in total hip arthroplasty. J Arthroplasty 23:751–761, 2008.
11. Scott M, Morrison M, Mishra SR, Jani S: Particle analysis for the determination of UHMWPE wear. J Biomed Mater Res B Appl Biomater 73:325–337, 2005.
12. Bergmann G, Graichen F, Rohlmann A, et al: Frictional heating of total hip implants. Part 1. Measurements in patients. J Biomech 34:421–428, 2001.
13. Wimmer MA, Loos J, Nassutt R, et al: The acting wear mechanisms on metal-on-metal hip joint bearings: in vitro results. Wear 250:129–139, 2001.
14. Wimmer MA, Sprecher C, Hauert R, et al: Tribochemical reaction on metal-on-metal hip joint bearings—a comparison between in-vitro and in-vivo results. Wear 255:1007–1014, 2003.
15. Nassutt R, Wimmer MA, Schneider E, Morlock MM: The influence of resting periods on friction in the artificial hip joint. Clin Orthop Relat Res (407):127–138, 2003.
16. Bishop NE, Waldow L, Morlock MM: Friction moments of large metal-on-metal hip joint bearings and other modern designs. Med Eng Phys 30:1057–1064, 2008.
17. Wimmer MA, Fischer A, Büscher R, et al: Wear mechanisms in metal-on-metal bearings: the importance of tribochemical reaction layers. J Orthop Res 28:436–443, 2010.
18. Mosey NJ, Müser MH, Woo TK: Molecular mechanisms for the functionality of lubricant additives. Science 307:1612–1615, 2005.
19. Walter WL, O'Toole CC, Walter WK, et al: Squeaking in ceramic-on-ceramic hips: the importance of acetabular component orientation. J Arthroplasty 22:496–503, 2007.
20. Keurentjes JC, Kuipers RM, Wever DJ, Schreurs BW: High incidence of squeaking in THAs with alumina ceramic-on-ceramic bearings. Clin Orthop Relat Res 466:1438–1443, 2008.
21. Laurent MP, Pourzal R, Fischer MSA, et al: In vivo wear of a squeaky alumina-on-alumina hip prosthesis: a case report. J Bone Joint Surg Am, Accepted for publication, 2010.
22. Weiss C, Gdaniec P, Hoffmann NP, et al: Squeak in hip endoprosthesis systems: an experimental study and a numerical technique to analyze design variants. Med Eng Phys 32:604–609, 2010.
23. Dowson D: Friction and wear of medical implants and prosthetic devices. In ASM handbook: friction, lubrication, and wear technology, vol 18, Materials Park, Ohio, 1992, American Society for Metals, pp 656–664.
24. Daniel J, Ziaee H, Salama A, et al: The effect of the diameter of metal-on-metal bearings on systemic exposure to cobalt and chromium. J Bone Joint Surg Br 88:443–448, 2006.
25. Lin ZM, Meakins S, Morlock MM, et al: Deformation of press-fitted metallic resurfacing cups. Part 1. Experimental simulation. Proc Inst Mech Eng H 220:299–309, 2006.
26. Yew A, Jin ZM, Donn A, et al: Deformation of press-fitted metallic resurfacing cups. Part 2. Finite element simulation. Proc Inst Mech Eng H 220:311–319, 2006.
27. DeHaan R, Campbell P, Reid S, et al: Metal ion levels in a triathlete with a metal-on-metal resurfacing arthroplasty of the hip. J Bone Joint Surg Br 89:538–541, 2007.
28. Caligaris M, Ateshian GA: Effects of sustained interstitial fluid pressurization under migrating contact area, and boundary lubrication by synovial fluid, on cartilage friction. Osteoarthritis Cartilage 16:1220–1227, 2008.
29. Waugh W: John Charnley: the man and the hip, Berlin, 1990, Springer Verlag.
30. Charnley J: Low friction principle. In Low friction arthroplasty of the hip: theory and practice, Berlin, 1979, Springer Verlag.
31. Ungethüm M, Hinterberger J: Second generation of the Munich hip-joint-simulator. Arch Orthop Trauma Surg 91:233–237, 1978.
32. Dowson D, Jobbins B: Design and development of a versatile hip joint simulator and a preliminary assessment of wear and creep in Charnley total replacement hip joints. Eng Med 17:111–117, 1988.
33. Morlock M, Schneider E, Bluhm A, et al: Duration and frequency of everyday activities in total hip patients. J Biomech 34:873–881, 2001.
34. Clarke C, Gustafson A: Hip-simulator ranking of polyethylene wear. Acta Orthop Scand 67:128–132, 1996.

35. Hermida JC, Bergula A, Chen P, et al: Comparison of the wear rates of twenty-eight and thirty-two-millimeter femoral heads on cross-linked polyethylene acetabular cups in a wear simulator. J Bone Joint Surg Am 85:2325–2331, 2003.

36. Tarasevicius S, Kesteris U, Robertsson O, Wingstrand H: Femoral head diameter affects the revision rate in total hip arthroplasty: an analysis of 1,720 hip replacements with 9-21 years of follow-up. Acta Orthop 77:706–709, 2006.

37. McKellop HA, Campbell P, Park SH, et al: The origin of submicron polyethylene wear debris in total hip arthroplasty. Clin Orthop Relat Res (311):3–20, 1995.

38. Geerdink CH, Grimm B, Ramakrishnan R, et al: Cross-linked polyethylene compared to conventional polyethylene in total hip replacement: pre-clinical evaluation, in-vitro testing and prospective clinical follow-up study. Acta Orthop 77:719–725, 2006.

39. Röhrl SM, Li MG, Nilsson KG, Nivbrant B: Very low wear of non-remelted highly cross-linked polyethylene cups: an RSA study lasting up to 6 years. Acta Orthop 78:739–745, 2007.

40. Digas G, Kärrholm J, Thanner J, et al: The Otto Aufranc Award. Highly cross-linked polyethylene in total hip arthroplasty: randomized evaluation of penetration rate in cemented and uncemented sockets using radiostereometric analysis. Clin Orthop Relat Res 429:6–16, 2004.

41. Salineros MJ, Crowninshield RD, Laurent M, et al: Analysis of retrieved acetabular components of three polyethylene types. Clin Orthop Relat Res (465):140–149, 2007.

42. Kurtz SM: The UHMWPE handbook, ed 2, Amsterdam, 2009, Elsevier.

43. Nevelos JE, Ingham E, Doyle C, et al: Analysis of retrieved alumina ceramic components from Mittelmeier total hip prostheses. Biomaterials 20:1833–1840, 1999.

44. Nevelos JE, Ingham E, Doyle C, et al: Wear of HIPed and non-HIPed alumina-alumina hip joints under standard and severe simulator testing conditions. Biomaterials 22:2191–2197, 2001.

45. Rosneck J, Klika A, Barsoum W: A rare complication of ceramic-on-ceramic bearings in total hip arthroplasty. J Arthroplasty 23:311–313, 2008.

46. Garbuz DS, Tanzer M, Greidanus NV, et al: The John Charnley Award. Metal-on-metal hip resurfacing versus large-diameter head metal-on-metal total hip arthroplasty: a randomized clinical trial. Clin Orthop Relat Res 468:318–325, 2010.

47. Langton DJ, Jameson SS, Joyce TJ, et al: Early failure of metal-on-metal bearings in hip resurfacing and large-diameter total hip replacement: a consequence of excess wear. J Bone Joint Surg Br 92:38–46, 2010.

48. Kwon YM, Ostlere SJ, McLardy-Smith P, et al: "Asymptomatic" pseudotumors after metal-on-metal hip resurfacing arthroplasty prevalence and metal ion study. J Arthroplasty June 28 2010. [Epub ahead of print]

49. Hodgson AW, Mischler S, Von Rechenberg B, Virtanen S: An analysis of the in vivo deterioration of Co-Cr-Mo implants through wear and corrosion. Proc Inst Mech Eng H 221:291–303, 2007.

50. Mathew MT, Srinivasa Pai P, Pourzal R, et al: Significance of tribocorrosion in biomedical applications: overview and current status. [Review] Advances in Tribology, Article ID 250986, doi:10.1155/2009/250986.

51. American Society for Testing and Materials (ASTM): F742-00. Standard test method for wear testing of polymeric materials used in total joint prostheses, West Conshohocken, Pa, 2006, ASTM.

52. Wang A, Sun DC, Yau SS, et al: Orientation softening in the deformation and wear of ultra-high molecular weight polyethylene. Wear 203:230–241, 1997.

53. Pooley CM, Tabor D: Friction and molecular structure: the behaviour of some thermoplastics. Proc R Soc Med 329:251–274, 1972.

54. American Society for Testing and Materials (ASTM): G 99-05. Standard test method for wear testing with a pin-on-disk apparatus, West Conshohocken, Pa, 2010, ASTM.

55. Wimmer MA, Nassutt R, Lampe F, et al: A new screening method designed for wear analysis of bearing surfaces used in total hip arthroplasty. In Jacobs J, Cendrowska T, Speiser P (editors): Alternative bearing surfaces in total joint replacement, STP 1346, West Conshohocken, Pa, 1998, American Society for Testing and Materials, pp 30–43.

56. Dumbleton JH: Tribology of natural and artificial joints, Tribology Series 3, Amsterdam, The Netherlands, 1981, Elsevier.

57. Saikko V: Tribology of total replacement hip joints studied with new hip joint simulators and a materials-screening apparatus. Acta Polytech Scand Mech Eng Ser 110:1–44, 1993.

58. Affatato S, Spinelli M, Zavalloni M, et al: Tribology and total hip joint replacement: current concepts in mechanical simulation. Med Eng Phys 30:1305–1317, 2008.

59. Saikko V: A multidirectional motion pin-on-disk wear test method for prosthetic joint materials. J Biomed Mater Res 41:58–64, 1998.

60. Saikko V, Ahlroos T, Calonius O, Keränen J: Wear simulation of total hip prostheses with polyethylene against CoCr, alumina and diamond-like carbon. Biomaterials 22:1507–1514, 2001.

61. Calonius O, Saikko V. Slide track analysis of eight contemporary hip simulator designs. J Biomech 35:1439–1450, 2002.

62. Johnston RC, Smidt GL: Measurement of hip-joint motion during walking: evaluation of an electrogoniometric method. J Bone Joint Surg Am 51:1083–1094, 1969.

63. Laurent MP, Yao JQ, Gilbertson LN, Crowninshield RD: Comparison of the AMTI and Shore Western hip simulators for wear testing UHMWPE acetabular liners, 27th Annual Meeting Transactions, Society for Biomaterials, 2001, p 358.

64. Kaddick C, Wimmer MA: Hip simulator wear testing according to the newly introduced standard ISO 14242. Proc Inst Mech Eng H 215:429–442, 2001.

65. Wang A, Essner A, Cooper J: The clinical relevance of hip simulator testing of high performance implants. Semin Arthropathy 17:49–55, 2006.

66. McKellop HA, D'Lima D: How have wear testing and joint simulator studies helped to discriminate among materials and designs. J Am Acad Orthop Surg 16(Suppl 1):S111–S119, 2008.

67. Halley D, Glassman A, Crowninshield RD: Recurrent dislocation after revision total hip replacement with a large prosthetic femoral head: a case report. J Bone Joint Surg Am 86:827–830, 2004.

68. Tower SS, Currier JH, Currier BH, et al: Rim cracking of the cross-linked longevity polyethylene acetabular liner after total hip arthroplasty. J Bone Joint Surg Am 89:2212–2217, 2007.

69. Paul JP: Forces transmitted by joints in the human body. Proc Instn Mech Engr 181:8–15, 1966.

70. Bergmann G, Graichen F, Rohlmann A: Hip joint loading during walking and running, measured in two patients. J Biomech 26:969–990, 1993.

71. Liao YS, Benya PD, McKellop HA: Effect of protein lubrication on the wear properties of materials for prosthetic joints. J Biomed Mater Res 48:465–473, 1999.

72. Wang A, Essner A, Schmidig G. The effects of lubricant composition on in vitro wear testing of polymeric acetabular components. J Biomed Mater Res B Appl Biomater 68:45–52, 2004.

73. Mazzucco D, Spector M: The role of joint fluid in the tribology of total joint arthroplasty. Clin Orthop Relat Res (429):17–32, 2004.

74. Dwivedi Y, Laurent MP, Schmid T, Wimmer MA: Cleavage of albumin affects the wear of UHMWPE, 54th Annual Meeting Transactions, Orthopaedic Research Society, 2008, p 2318.

SUGGESTED READING

Gohar R: Fundamentals of tribology, London, 2008, Imperial College Press.
Recently published, this book is a comprehensive presentation of the fundamentals of tribology. It covers nano-triboley and biotribology. Geared toward readers with an engineering or scientific background.

Hutchings I: Tribology: friction and wear of engineering materials, New York, 1992, Butterworth Heinemann.
The basics of friction, boundary and fluid film lubrication, sliding, and abrasive wear are developed from fundamental principles in this information-dense, lucidly written book. Provides numerous citations to the research literature.

Rabinowicz E: Friction and wear of materials, ed 2, New York, 1995, Wiley-Interscience.

This book is a classic from one of the foremost authorities on surface interactions and friction. Excellent coverage of adhesive wear, abrasive wear, and boundary lubrication.

Wright TM, Goodman SB: Implant wear in total joint replacement: clinical and biologic issues. Material and design considerations, Rosemont, Ill, 2001, American Academy of Orthopaedic Surgeons.

The result of a symposium held in 2000, this monograph is an eclectic compendium of topics relevant to implant wear (http://web.archive.org/web/20020605163356/http://www3.aaos.org/implant/implant.cfm).

CHAPTER 4

Materials in Hip Surgery: Polymethylmethacrylate

Thierry Scheerlinck

KEY POINTS

- Bone cement acts as a "grout" and not as a "glue." Measures to improve cement-bone interdigitation (pressure lavage, cement pressurization) are recommended.
- Bone cement is more resistant to compression loading than to tension or shear loading. Whenever possible, the cement mantle should be loaded in compression and should be supported by strong cortical bone.
- Bone cement generates heat during polymerization. Heat can cause thermal bone necrosis and is a potential hazard, especially on the femoral side, in hip resurfacing.
- Bone cement is an effective drug carrier. Antibiotic-loaded cement can be used in the prevention and the treatment of hip arthroplasty infections.
- Bone cement has different mechanical properties compared with the stem. Therefore, micromotion at the cement-stem interface is difficult to avoid. For this, a polished stem with the same design, which tolerates better micromotions, performs generally better or similarly compared with rougher equivalents.

INTRODUCTION

Polymethylmethacrylate (PMMA) is a methylmethacrylate polymer, better known outside orthopedics by its trade name Plexiglas or Perspex. PMMA has numerous industrial applications, is easy to manufacture, can be made transparent, and has attractive chemical and mechanical properties. In orthopedic surgery and more particularly in hip surgery, PMMA is widely used to fix femoral and acetabular hip implants to bone,[1] to fill bone defects,[2] to improve the hold of fracture fixation devices in poor quality bone,[2,3] and to deliver high local doses of antibiotics[4-7] or antitumoral drugs.[8]

In orthopedic procedures, polymethylmethacrylate or "bone cement" is prepared intraoperatively by mixing a powder and a liquid. The powder (40.0-49.7 g/package[9]) contains methylmethacrylate polymers and/or copolymers, an initiator, and often additives (dye, radiopacifier, antibiotics).[1,9-11] The liquid (14.1-20.8 mL/package[9]) contains methylmethacrylate monomers, an activator, often a stabilizer, and sometimes a dye[1,9-11]

(Table 4-1). By combining the initiator in the powder and the activator in the liquid, free radicals are generated and the polymerization reaction is initiated (Fig. 4-1A). During polymerization, the reaction is sustained by the formation of new free radicals from methylmethacrylate (MMA) molecules. This allows the PMMA chains to grow rapidly and to combine. The polymerization reaction ends when the free radicals get depleted by mutual recombination[1,9] (Fig. 4-1B). During the polymerization process, the viscosity of the cement increases progressively and limits the mobility of the MMA monomers. As such, just after curing, the polymerized cement still contains 2% to 6% of residual MMA monomer. The monomer may elute from the polymerized mass and be eliminated into the bloodstream, or it may continue to polymerize slowly over the subsequent 2 to 4 weeks.[9,12]

The use of bone cement for fixation of hip implants varies widely between geographic regions. In Scandinavia, in European Anglo-Saxon countries, and in New Zealand, most stems and cups are fixed with cement (Sweden: stems 88%, cups 89%[13]; Norway: stems 73%, cups 82%[14]; United Kingdom: stems 73%, cups 59%[15]; New Zealand: stems 73%, cups 40%[16]). This choice is often justified by data from the literature and from hip registries.[17] In Southern Europe, North America, and Australia, cement fixation is much less popular (Canada: stems 29%, cups 3%[18]; Australia: stems 40%, cups 8%[19]), and a majority of hip replacements are implanted using "cementless" prosthesis designs. In general, cement is used in the "older, less active population with poor bone quality," whereas cementless implants are used more often in "young and active patients."[17] However, no consensus has been reached on the exact definition of both these populations.

Despite the excellent long-term survival rates of cemented total hip arthroplasty (THA) (>90% at 10 years and >80% at 15 years postoperatively[14,20]), the use of bone cement in hip arthroplasty is declining.[13,14,18-20] Nevertheless, PMMA continues to be widely used in hip surgery and is unlikely to be replaced in the near future.

This chapter describes the different types of bone cement in terms of their thermal and mechanical properties and the effects of cement shrinkage during polymerization. Then, the effects of additives in bone cement (radiopacifiers, antibiotics, pores) are discussed. Finally, phenomena occurring at the cement-bone and cement-stem interfaces are analyzed. Throughout the chapter, experimental and basic science concepts are described,

Table 4-1. Composition of the Powder and Liquid Components of Bone Cement

Powder	Liquid
Polymer	Monomer
• Polymethylmethacrylate (PMMA) and/or • Polymethylacrylate (PMA) and/or • Polybutylmethacrylate (PBUMA)	• Methylmethacrylate monomer (MMA) and/or • Butylmethacrylate (BUMA)
Copolymer*	Activator
• Methylacrylate (MA) and/or • Ethylacrylate (EA) and/or • Styrene	• *N,N*-dimethyl-*p*-toluidine (DMPT) or • 2-(4-[dimethylamino] phenyl)ethanol (DMAPE)
Initiator	Stabilizer (radical catcher)*
• Dibenzoyl peroxide (BPO)	• Ascorbic acid (vitamin C) or • Hydroquinone (benzene-1,4-diol)
Dye*	Dye*
• Chlorophyllin or • FD&C Blue N 2	• Chlorophyllin
Radiopacifier*	
• Barium sulfate or • Zirconium dioxide	
Antibiotics*	
• Gentamicin or • Tobramycin or • Clindamycin or Erythromycin/Colistin	
Plasticizer*	
• Dicyclohexylphtalate	
Other*	
• Hydroxyapatite (HA)	

*Optional.

with an overriding emphasis on practical implications for the orthopedic surgeon. This chapter ends with a list of current controversies and future directions.

CEMENT POLYMERIZATION AND TYPES OF BONE CEMENT

Although polymerization of PMMA bone cement is a continuous phenomenon, it can be divided into four phases: mixing, waiting, application, and setting phases[9] (Fig. 4-2). In the mixing phase, the liquid and the powder are mixed until a homogeneous putty is formed. In the waiting phase, the viscosity of the putty continuously increases until it no longer sticks to a gloved finger (dry powder-free latex glove). When the cement is no longer sticky, the application phase has been reached. At this stage, cement dough is delivered to the bone and the implants are inserted.[1,9] The application phase lasts until the dough cannot be joined back into a homogeneous mass when kneaded. In the setting phase, the cement hardens progressively and finally maintains a fixed shape. In this phase, shrinkage is commonly observed, and the cement reaches its maximum temperature as a result of the exothermic polymerization reaction. In the setting phase, the implant should be held still to avoid cement cracking or separation of the implant from the cement mantle.

The rate of polymerization of acrylic cement depends on both the temperature and the humidity. The higher the temperature of the cement and/or the ambient atmosphere,[1,9,21] the faster the rate of polymerization; the lower the humidity, the longer the application phase.[9] For this reason, the International Organization for Standardization (ISO) 5833 standard requires that the working properties of cement be measured at $23°$ C $\pm 1°$ C and 50% $\pm$ 10% humidity. The setting time

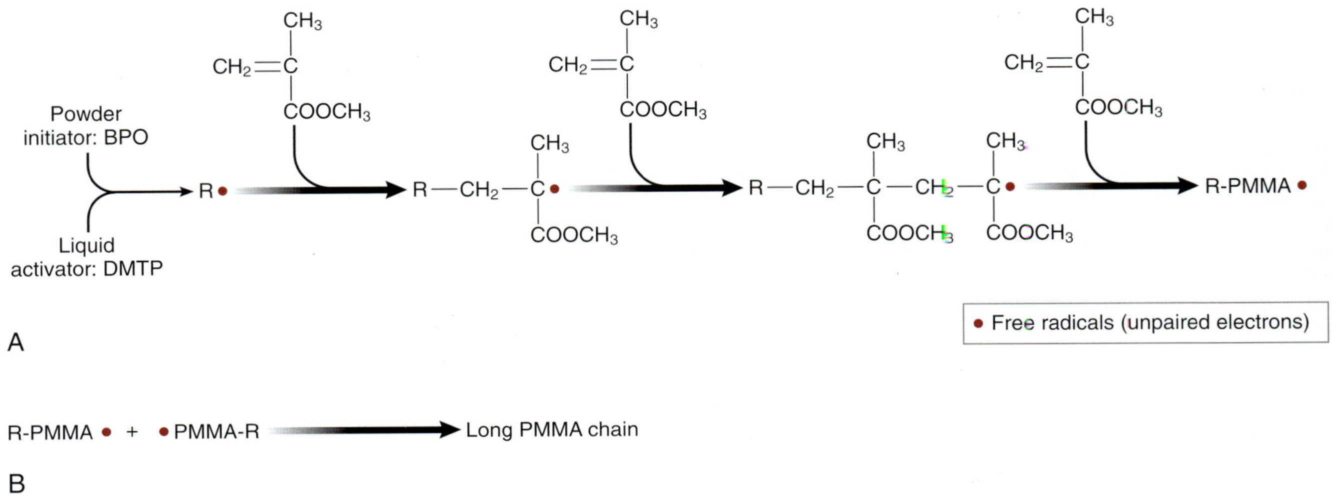

Figure 4-1. A, When the initiator (BPO) within the powder is mixed with the activator (mostly DMPT) in the liquid, benzoate radicals (R•) containing "unpaired electrons" are created. These radicals start the polymerization reaction by breaking up the C=C bond of methylmethacrylate (MMA), generating new radicals within the MMA molecules. The highly reactive "unpaired electrons" of the MMA molecules combine with new MMA molecules to create large (10^5-10^6 g/mol or more) polymethylmethacrylate (PMMA) chains. **B,** When two PMMA chains containing a free radical combine, the overall quantity of free radicals decreases. The polymerization reaction ends when free radicals are depleted.

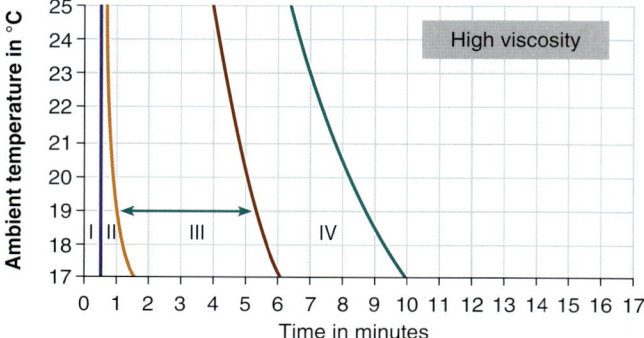

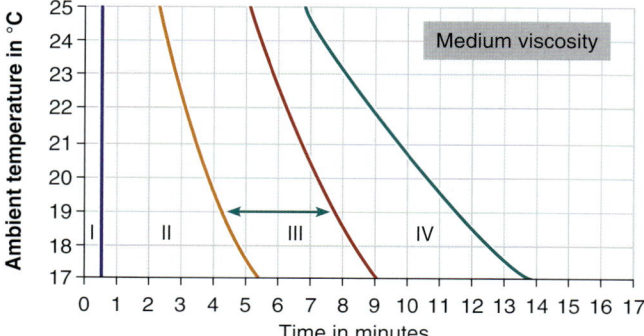

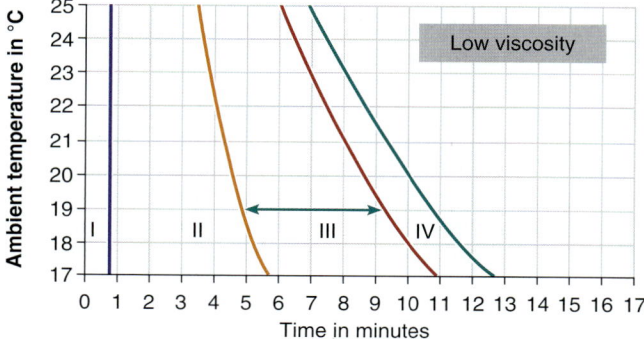

Figure 4-2. The temperature-working curve of high- (Palacos R, Heraeus Medical GmbH, Wehrheim, Germany *[top]*), medium- (Surgical Simplex P, Stryker, Mahwah, NJ *[middle]*), and low-viscosity cement (CMW 3, DePuy CMW, Blackpool, UK *[bottom]*). I, Mixing phase. II, Waiting phase. III, Application phase. IV, Setting phase. The *green arrow* shows the duration of the application phase at an ambient temperature of 19° C. *(Data from Heraeus Medical GmbH and from Kühn KD: Bone cements: up-to-date comparison of physical and chemical properties of commercial materials, ed 1, Berlin, 2000, Springer-Verlag, Fig. 97, p 128, and Fig. 51, p 75.[9])*

of a PMMA formulation is typically measured using a disk-shaped cement specimen (diameter: 60 mm; thickness: 6 mm) and is defined as the time elapsed between the start of the cement mixing and the moment the temperature within the center of the cement mass reaches half of the peak polymerization temperature.[9,21] The duration of each polymerization phase, in relation to the ambient temperature, is specific for each

formulation and is represented in temperature-working curves (see Fig. 4-2).

Large variations in the working properties of acrylic cements exist between formulations and between batches of the same formulation, depending on environmental factors. This may explain why surgeons often complain of faulty cement handling properties.[9,22] In view of this variability, it is important that joint surgeons become familiar with one formulation of acrylic cement and do whatever is necessary to standardize environmental conditions within the operating theater and the room designated for cement storage. These parameters are often neglected by surgeons, even in countries where cementing is common practice.[22]

The working properties of cement depend on the chemical composition and the proportions of powder and liquid.[9] Currently, three types of PMMA bone cement are used in hip surgery: high-, medium-, and low-viscosity cement (see Fig. 4-2):

- High-viscosity cement has a short waiting phase, as it quickly loses its stickiness after cement mixing. The application phase is long, and cement viscosity starts to increase progressively only toward the end of that phase. The setting phase lasts at least 1.5 to 2 minutes. Therefore, high-viscosity cement is easy to mix in a bowl, to knead manually, and to apply with a "finger packing technique" in the shaft or as a "cement ball" in the acetabulum. However, at room temperature, vacuum mixing and delivery with a syringe are difficult. Precooling the cement to lengthen the various polymerization phases can facilitate this process.[1]

- Medium-viscosity cement has a low viscosity in the waiting phase and therefore can be vacuum-mixed and delivered with a syringe easily. After approximately 3 minutes, the cement loses its stickiness, and in the application phase, it behaves like a high-viscosity cement. Initially, the viscosity remains almost constant, and at the end of the application phase, it starts to increase progressively. The setting phase lasts at least 1.5 to 2.5 minutes. Thus, medium-viscosity cement combines the convenience of low-viscosity cement for vacuum mixing and syringe delivery at room temperature with the user friendliness of a longer and less constraining application phase.[1]

- Low-viscosity cement has a long waiting phase in which it remains liquid for a long time. Once the application phase sets in, the temperature and viscosity of the cement increase rapidly, and the setting phase lasts only 1 to 2 minutes. Low-viscosity cement is easy to mix and to apply with a syringe. In the liquid phase, the cement can be pressurized into the cancellous bone. However, it produces a less stable stem-cement-bone construct[23] and a weaker cement-bone interface[24] compared with high-viscosity cement. This can be attributed to back-bleeding from the shaft, which displaces the low-viscosity dough and contaminates the cement mantle.[25] Moreover, liquid cement is difficult to contain, and because of the short application phase, correct timing and control of environmental factors are critical.[1] This might explain why low-viscosity cement, in combination with a Charnley stem, has a higher revision rate than high-viscosity cement.[26] In past years, interest in low-viscosity cement to fix femoral resurfacing implants has increased. The long liquid phase allows pressurizing of large quantities of cement into the reamed femoral head and facilitates seating of the implant when an implant-filling cementing technique is used.[27-29]

PROPERTIES OF POLYMETHYLMETHACRYLATE BONE CEMENT

Heat Generation

Polymerization of MMA monomer is an exothermic reaction that generates 52 kJ (31-71 kJ) (13 kcal [7-17 kcal]) of energy per mole MMA.[9,30] This means that, under the conditions specified by the ISO 5833 standard ($23 \pm 1° C$, $50 \pm 10\%$ humidity), the temperature within a cement cylinder of 60 mm diameter and 6 mm thickness can exceed $80° C$ ($52-90° C$) during polymerization.[9,30] In vivo, the implant, the bone, and the circulation dissipate the heat, and most cement mantles measure less than 6 mm in thickness.[31,32] Therefore, lower temperatures have been measured (stem: $40° C$ [$29-56° C$]; cup: $43° C$ [$38-52° C$])[33] or calculated at the bone-cement interface (stem: $45-55° C$[30]; cup: $57° C$[34]). Because a temperature of $50° C$ for 1 minute or $47° C$ for 5 minutes can cause bone necrosis,[35] the acetabular bone is at risk when a cup is cemented,[34] and the endomedullary bone is at risk when cement thickness exceeds 5 mm.[30] To avoid thermal bone necrosis, a copolymer cement with a lower curing temperature (Boneloc, Polymers Reconstructive A/S, Farum, Denmark) has been developed.[36] However, Boneloc cement has poor mechanical properties,[36,37] which caused high failure rates during clinical use.[36,38] Today, bone cements advertising a low polymerization temperature are still available (Cemex, Tecres, Italy). However, the gain in curing temperature is small,[9,39] and no clinical advantage has been demonstrated.[39]

Because large quantities of cement can be pressurized into the reamed femoral head, thermal bone necrosis could be an important issue in hip resurfacing.[40,41] Finite element analysis predicts peak temperatures up to $54° C$ for 6 mm of cement penetration, but $74° C$ for a thick cement mantle associated with a 1-cm³ cyst.[42] In vitro, temperatures have been reported to reach median values of $45.4° C$ ($41.6-56.5° C$) for thick and $37.2° C$ ($26.6-39.3° C$) for thin cement mantles,[43] but up to $90° C$ when cysts were simulated.[44] In vivo, temperatures of $68° C$ have been recorded during hip resurfacing, but pressure lavage, intramedullary suction, and cooling of the resurfaced head allowed adequate temperature control.[45] Further research should focus on optimizing the cementing technique to avoid cement congestion of the reamed femoral head during resurfacing procedures.

Cement Shrinkage

During polymerization, the volume of PMMA shrinks by 20.6% compared with the initial volume of liquid MMA.[46] However, because bone cement contains only a fraction ($\pm\frac{1}{3}$) of MMA as a result of the use of prepolymerized powder, the maximal theoretical volumetric shrinkage is 6% to 8%.[46] In practice, cement mixed under vacuum will shrink between 4% and 7%.[46,47] When hand-mixed, more air gets trapped within the cement, and volumetric shrinkage tends to decrease.[46]

Shrinkage during polymerization is important because it can be a source of cement porosity. When cement is constrained during polymerization (i.e., when the outer dimensions of the cement cannot be modified), polymerization shrinkage will induce pores within the cement mantle.[46] These pores will compensate for the volumetric shrinkage that could not occur by contraction of the external dimensions of the cement. This particular situation occurs in vivo when cement is inserted into the proximal femur at body temperature while the implant is at room temperature. In this case, cement will start to polymerize at the higher temperature interface (i.e., close to the bone) and will proceed toward the implant. Because the outer layer of cement cures first, it constrains the doughy cement located more centrally and creates shrinkage-induced or type I interfacial defects close to the implant.[48] These interfacial pores can act as initiators of fatigue cracks during repeated implant loading and can compromise long-term stem fixation.[49] This problem can be solved by reversing the polymerization direction by heating the implant[50] or by cooling the bone[51] prior to cementation. Our preference is to precool the femoral shaft with saline at $4° C$ during pressure lavage.

Mechanical Properties

The mechanical properties of PMMA bone cement can be divided into static and dynamic properties. *Static properties* include the behavior and the resistance of the material when subjected to a pure compressive, tensile, or shear load. *Dynamic properties* describe the fatigue resistance of bone cement when subjected to repeated loading cycles.

The Static Properties of Bone Cement

Strength and Elasticity. Three types of static loads can be applied to bone cement: compression, tension, and shear. Under any of these loading conditions, the material first will deform and finally will fail. How bone cement deforms and the ultimate load at which the material fails (ultimate strength [US]) depend on the shape of the specimen, the temperature, the loading regime (compression, tension, shear), the strain rate, the cement composition, the mixing procedure and mixing duration, the duration of aging, and the storage conditions (Table 4-2).[9,37,52-56] The ultimate strength of bone cement is about twice as great in compression as in tension or shear. This means that hip implants should be designed to load the cement

Table 4-2. Mechanical Properties of Bone Cement Under Static Loading Conditions

	Ultimate Strength (US), MPa	Elastic Modulus (E), GPa	Strain at Fracture Point (E_{max}), %
Compression load	72.6-117.0[52]	1.94-3.18[52]	5.0-7.5[52]
	45.6-129.0[55]*	1.87-3.00[55]*	—
	94.9-114.7[54]	—	—
	100.0-117.0[53]	—	—
	AB−: 75.4-112.9[9]	—	—
	AB+: 78.9-100.8[9]	—	—
	GI: 117.6[56]	GI: 2.51[56]	GI: 6.7[56]
	ETO: 118.2[56]	ETO: 2.65[56]	ETO: 6.46[56]
Tensile load	23.6-49.2[52]	1.58-4.12[52]	0.86-2.49[52]
	31.7-51.4[37]	2.26-3.53[37]	1.36-2.48[37]
	24.7-52.9[55]*	—	—
	44.3-52.2[54]	—	—
	GI: 45.1[56]	GI: 2.28[56]	GI: 3.16[56]
	ETO: 47.5[56]	ETO: 2.22[56]	ETO: 3.43[56]
Shear load	DST: 42.7-50.2[52]	—	—
	D732: 32.0-69.0[52]	—	
Flexural load	3-pt: 49.9-125.0[52]	3-pt: 1.29-2.92[52]	—
	3-pt: 61.0-79.2[55]*	3-pt: 2.52-3.00[55]*	—
	4-pt: 12.1-90.5[52]	4-pt: 1.95-3.16[52]	—
	4-pt: 51.0-81.7[54]	4-pt: 1.39-2.84[54]	—
	4-pt AB−: 45.6-78.7[9]	4-pt AB−: 1.76-3.09[9]	—
	4-pt AB+: 59.6-72.8[9]	4-pt AB+: 2.16-2.77[9]	—

*Mechanical testing performed under various conditions.
AB−, Without antibiotics; *AB+,* with antibiotics; *D732,* according to the ASTM D732 testing specifications; *DST,* according to a double shear test; *ETO,* sterilized by ethylene oxide gas; *GI,* sterilized by γ-irradiation; *3-pt,* 3-point bending test; *4-pt,* 4-point bending test.

mantle in compression and to avoid tensile and shear forces.[57]

In predefined circumstances, the relation between the applied load (stress) and the deformation of the material (strain) can be expressed in a stress-strain curve[55,58] (Fig. 4-3). Under low compressive and tensile loads, bone cement behaves elastically. This means that deformation of a cement specimen is almost proportional to the load applied, and the stress-strain curve is almost linear (see Fig. 4-3). The slope of the tangent to the initial section of the stress-strain curve is called the *modulus of elasticity* (E) or *Young's modulus.*[55] The elasticity modulus of bone cement in compression is similar to that of bone cement in tension (see Table 4-2). The strain at fracture point (e_{max}) represents the degree of deformation (elongation or compression) of the material at failure and is much larger for tensile than for compressive loading.

In practice, bone cement samples are often tested in three-point (e.g., ASTM D790, DIN 53435) or four-point (e.g., ISO 5833) bending. These protocols explore the *flexural properties* of bone cement (i.e., the combination of compression, tensile, and shear properties). For bone cement, the ultimate flexural or bending strength and the flexural or bending modulus depend on the loading pattern (three- or four-point bending), the cement

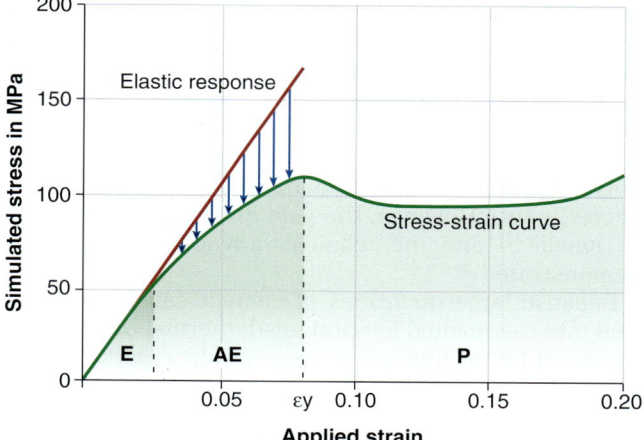

Figure 4-3. Simulated extension stress-strain curve of polymethylmethacrylate (PMMA) bone cement *(green curve* [temperature: 54.85° C; strain rate: 0.001/sec]). At low strains, PMMA behaves almost as an elastic material (E), and the slope of the tangent to the initial section of the stress-strain curve *(red line)* is the elastic modulus. At higher strains, PMMA behaves as an anelastic material (AE), and the stress drops as the result of relaxation *(blue arrows).* Past the yield strain (ε_y), PMMA undergoes plastic deformation (P). *(Data from Stachurski ZH: Strength and deformation of rigid polymers: the stress-strain curve in amorphous PMMA. Polymer 44:6067–6076, 2003, Fig. 5, p 6072.[58])*

composition, the mixing modalities, and the duration and storage conditions (see Table 4-2).[9,52]

Creep and Stress Relaxation. *Creep* is defined as "the time-dependent and irreversible deformation of a material under continuous static or dynamic loading"; *stress relaxation* describes "the time-dependent decrease in stress within a material under constant strain."[1,12,55] Both properties are typical of viscoelastic materials. The amount of stress relaxation is related to the degree of cement polymerization and decreases over the first 4 weeks after cement mixing.[12]

Bone cement behaves as a brittle viscoelastic material. The initial deformation of PMMA is almost elastic (i.e., reversible and proportional to the load applied) (see Fig. 4-3). However, as the load and the time of exposure to load increase, PMMA behaves as an *anelastic* material. Under these circumstances, constriction points between PMMA molecules break apart, motion between and within PMMA molecules occurs (molecular relaxation), and stress within the material dissipates (stress relaxation).[58] At low strain, when minimal deformation has occurred, the situation is reversible. However, higher loads cause irreversible molecular rearrangements, resulting in a permanent plastic deformation and further stress relaxation. Finally, as the proportion of oriented polymer chains increases, the degree of stress relaxation decreases and the material becomes stiffer again, before it finally fails.[58]

Creep and stress relaxation are thought to be important for cemented collarless polished and tapered femoral hip implants such as the Exeter (Stryker, Mahwah, NJ) or the CPT (Zimmer, Warsaw, Ind) stem. These stems are designed to subside within the cement mantle and act as a loaded taper.[1,57,59,60] Because of creep and plastic deformation of the cement under repetitive load, some subsidence can occur without fracture of the cement mantle. Therefore, the stem transforms axial load into compressive and hoop stresses within the cement. These stresses are transferred to the cortical bone that constrains the cement mantle.[1,60] Such a constrained construct seems very effective in resisting both static[55] and dynamic loading,[60,61] emphasizing the need for the surgeon to achieve cement pressurization up to the inner cortex of the femur. As patients are unloading the cement mantle at night, stress relaxation of PMMA could occur during such periods of inactivity. It has been hypothesized that this might reduce stresses within the cement mantle and thereby may decrease the risk of mechanical failure.[1,59,60]

Dynamic Properties of Bone Cement

When PMMA bone cement is subjected to repeated loading below its ultimate strength, it can fail progressively by fatigue, as cracks are initiated within the material and propagate to adjacent interfaces. This process is important for hip arthroplasty because (1) in vivo, cement is most often subjected to cyclical loading below its ultimate strength; (2) in vivo fatigue failure patterns can be reproduced in vitro by dynamic mechanical testing below ultimate strength[62]; and (3) fractographic analysis of retrieved bone cement[63,64] indicates

that fatigue failure of PMMA and fatigue crack propagation are important failure mechanisms.

The number of cycles needed to fracture a specimen depends on the amount of load applied (i.e., the stress within the material), the loading pattern, the cement composition,[65] and the cement porosity (and thus the mixing modalities used for cement preparation).[66] The fatigue characteristics of PMMA bone cement can be represented in an S-N curve,[52,65,67] which expresses the relationship between the magnitude of the cyclical stress (S) and the number of cycles (N) needed to achieve a given probability of failure (P). The higher the stress, the fewer the number of cycles needed to create fatigue failure (Fig. 4-4).

In clinical practice, hip implants generate repeated stresses within the cement mantle, which cause fatigue cracks within the material and stem-cement debonding. Generally, cement cracks set off at the cement-stem interface[49,61] proximally,[61] within the metaphyseal region, whereas stem-cement debonding starts around the stem tip distally.[64] During the patient's lifetime, accumulated cement damage and stem-cement debonding will progress toward the middle section of the stem and the implant until the component becomes macroscopically loose.[64] This failure mechanism can be reproduced in vitro during mechanical testing[62] and simulated with finite element analysis (FEA) models.[68] Such models allow differentiation between designs of femoral implants displaying different levels of survivorship in

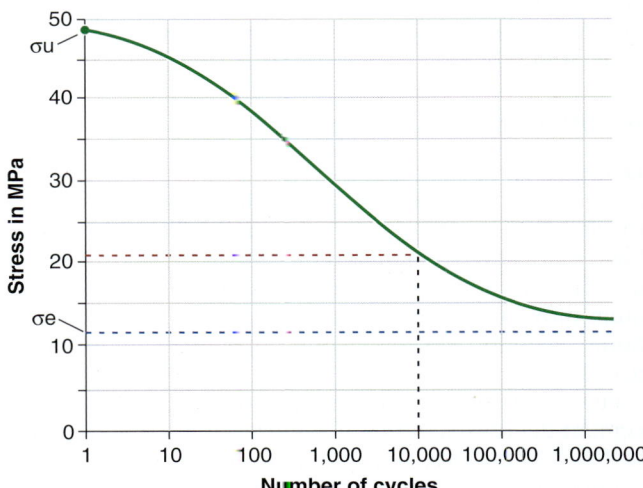

Figure 4-4. Estimated S-N curve of Surgical Simplex P bone cement for tension loading (temperature: 37° C, sinusoidal loading at 10 Hz). The *green dot* represents the stress needed to fracture 50% of the specimens after one cycle (i.e., the ultimate strength [σ_u]) with a fracture probability of 0.50. The stress at the lower asymptote of the S-N curve (*blue line*) is the endurance limit (σ_e). Stresses below this limit can be applied "indefinitely" without cement fracture. According to the graph (*red line*), 10,000 tension loading cycles of 21 MPa are needed to fracture 50% of the specimens. *(Data from Krause W, Mathis RS, Grimes LW: Fatigue properties of acrylic bone cement: S-N, P-N, and P-S-N data. J Biomed Mater Res 22:221–244, 1988, Fig. 7, p 23.[67])*

clinical practice.[68] FEA modeling can also be used to evaluate the impact of stem design[68] and implantation technique[61] on device performance, and the contribution to fatigue failure of cement porosity within the bulk of the material[66,69] and at the cement-stem interface.[49] On the acetabular side, a few studies have reported the results of mechanical fatigue testing[70] and dynamic FEA modeling[70,71] of cemented cups. These studies predict cup loosening at the cement-bone interface in the superior and posterosuperior regions of the acetabulum[70] and increased cement damage with a ceramic cup compared with a polyethylene cup.[71] This should encourage the clinician to enhance cemented cup fixation in the posterosuperior region of the acetabulum and to avoid cementing very stiff ceramic[72] or metal-backed components.[73]

Effects of Sterilization on Mechanical Properties of Bone Cement

The liquid constituent of bone cement is always sterilized by membrane filtration; this is not an issue. However, the powder constituent can be sterilized using ethylene oxide gas or γ-irradiation.[9,56] In contradiction to ethylene oxide gas sterilization, γ-irradiation causes chain scission of PMMA and can reduce the molecular weight of both the polymer powder and the fully polymerized cement by at least 50%.[9,56] Although this has no major impact on the static mechanical properties of cement (see Table 4-2), it does significantly reduce its resistance to fatigue loading.[56] This might be relevant, as the dynamic mechanical properties of bone cement are thought to be important for long-term implant survival. Thus, the way bone cement has been sterilized merits consideration when a cement brand is chosen in clinical practice.

Additives in Bone Cement

Opacifiers

Pure PMMA bone cement is radiolucent and is difficult to visualize on standard radiographs. To allow radiologic follow-up of cemented hip implants, 8% to 15%[9] of inorganic radiopaque powder (barium sulfate or zirconium dioxide) is added to most commercially available bone cements. However, both opacifiers have major drawbacks.

First, chemically unbound powder within bone cement decreases ultimate compression strength by 5% to 8%.[55] Therefore, the minimum amount of opacifier needed to attain proper radiographic visualization should be used. Because barium sulfate imparts less resistance to x-ray penetration than zirconium dioxide, more barium sulfate must be added to the powder to achieve the same degree of radiopacity.[9] In vitro, barium sulfate might increase the fatigue resistance of bone cement,[74] especially when nanoparticles are used.[75] In vivo, this effect remains controversial[63] but merits further investigation.

Second, when added to monocytic cells in conjunction with PMMA particles, barium sulfate or zirconium dioxide has the ability to stimulate production of cytokines,[76] to cause osteoblast-like cells to differentiate into osteoclasts,[77,78] and to induce bone or dentine resorption in vitro[77,78] and in vivo.[79] In both settings, barium sulfate was more deleterious to bone than zirconium dioxide or than PMMA alone.[77-79] These findings suggest that barium sulfate and, to a lesser extent, zirconium dioxide could favor bone destruction when used as radiopacifiers in PMMA cement.

Third, particles of barium sulfate or zirconium dioxide have the potential to scratch metallic surfaces and cause third-body wear if released from the cement.[76,80] Because zirconium dioxide is harder and more abrasive than barium sulfate, it causes more damage when rubbed against a metallic counterface. This can occur at the cement-stem interface or, when particles get embedded in a polyethylene cup, at the articular surface.[76,80]

In light if these drawbacks, other bone cement opacifiers have been investigated. Iodixanol and iohexol are water-soluble nonionic contrast agents used in angiography. Both can be mixed as a powder with the methylmethacrylate polymer.[78,81] Optimizing the concentration and particle size of these additions results in a PMMA formulation of comparable ultimate tensile strength with current cements but with a higher ultimate strain and a lower modulus of elasticity (Young's modulus).[81] Nonionic contrast media are well tolerated in vivo,[78] are less abrasive than barium sulfate or zirconium dioxide, and have the advantage of dissolving when released into the tissues or into the joint space.[81] Moreover, in contrast to barium sulfate, zirconium dioxide, and iodixanol, the addition of iohexol to PMMA particles does not boost osteoclast differentiation or bone resorption in vitro.[78] This makes iohexol an interesting alternative to classic bone cement opacifiers, at least in patients without iodine allergy. However, no clinical data are available at present.

Another alternative is to add organic iodine-containing methacrylate monomers such as IPMA (4-IEMA), TIBMA, or DISMA[74,82-84] into the cement. Unlike iodixanol and iohexol, I-monomers are not water soluble, and iodine is chemically bonded to the I-copolymer. The static[82-84] and dynamic[74,83,84] mechanical properties of the three I-copolymers are comparable with or superior to those of barium sulfate–containing PMMA. Moreover, I-cement has a more homogeneous dispersion of the contrast agent[83] and does not contain abrasive particles. In vivo studies with I-copolymers suggest good biocompatibility and a lower inflammatory response than with barium sulfate–containing cement.[82] However, further research is needed before this approach can be introduced into clinical practice.

Antibiotics

Antibiotics are added to PMMA bone cement both to prevent and to treat infection (Table 4-3).[5,7,11,85-97] Some antibiotics are premixed into the cement during manufacturing, while others can be mixed during surgery. When mixed during surgery, the antibiotic power is best blended with the powder component of the cement first, before the monomer is added in a second stage. Antibiotics elute better when added to the cement mix as a liquid than as a powder,[94,97] and liquid antibiotics

Table 4-3. Antibiotics Used In Bone Cement*

Antibiotic Class	Antibiotic Name	Dosage / 40 g PMMA
Beta-lactams	Penicillin[7]	—
	Methicillin[7,87,95]	T: 1.5 g[‡]
	Oxacillin[7]	—
	Cloxacillin[5,87]	T: 0.5-1.0 g
	Dicloxacillin[87,91]	T: 0.5 g
	Ampicillin[85,87]	T: 1.0 g
	Amoxicillin[7]	—
	Ticarcillin[7,92]	T: up to 12.0 g[‡]
	Cephalothin[87,95]	T: up to 3.0 g
	Cefazolin[7,89,92,94]	T: 2.0-6.0 g[‡]
	Cefazedone[85,91]	T: 0.5-2.0 g
	Cefuroxime[7,86]	P: 2.0 g, T:1.5-3.0 g
	Cefamandole[7,87]	—
	Cefoperazone[85]	T: 2.0 g
	Cefotaxime[85,87,90]	T: 1.0 g
	Cefuzonam[7]	—
	Imipenem-cilastatin[89,94]	T: 2.0-2.5 g
	Monobactam[89]	T: 2.0 g
Aminoglycosides	Streptomycin[7]	—
	Neomycin[5,87,91,95]	T: 1.0-3.0 g[‡]
	Kanamycin[5,95]	T: 1.0-3.0 g
	Gentamicin powder[85,87,88,90,93]	P: 0.5-1.0 g[†], T: 1.0 g
	Gentamicin liquid[97]	T: 480 mg (12 mL)[§]
	Tobramycin[87,88,92-94]	P: 1.0 g[†], T: up to 9.8 g
	Amikacin[7,85,87,94]	T: 2.0 g
Glycopeptides	Vancomycin[85,87,90,92]	P[¶] and T: 1.0-4.0 g
	Teicoplanin[96]	T: 0.2 g
Oxazolidinones	Linezolid[94]	T: 1.2 g
Lincosamines	Lincomycin[5,91]	T: 0.5 g or more
	Clindamycin[85,91,92,95]	T: up to 6.0 g
Fluoroquinolones	Ofloxacin[85]	T: 1.0 g
	Ciprofloxacin[7,92]	T: 6.0 g[‡]
Macrolides + Polymixins	Erythromycin + colistin[11,91]	P: 0.24 g + 0.73 g[†] T: 0.5-1.0 g[‡]
Tetracyclines	Tetracycline[5,7,87,91,95]	T: 1.0 g[‡]
Fusidic acid	Fusidic acid[5,87,91,94]	T: 0.5-1.0 g[‡]
Thiazolopeptides	Bacitracin[7,87,91]	T: 0.5 g[‡]
Lipopeptides	Daptomycin[7]	—
Coumarin antibiotics	Novobiocin[7]	—

*For implant fixation, no more than 4 g of antibiotic powder should be added to 40 g of cement. For cement spacers and beads, higher doses can be considered.
[†]Premixed antibiotic-loaded cement commercially available.
[‡]Less favorable elution from PMMA cement.
[§]Not suited for implant fixation.
[¶]Used as prevention in revisions following gentamicin or tobramycin-loaded cement.
P, Prevention of infection; T, treatment of infection in cement spacer.

boost the release of other antibiotics present within the cement.[97] However, liquid antibiotics impair cement curing and have a larger negative impact on the mechanical properties of PMMA, with strength reductions of 30% to 50%.[5,7,85,94,97] Therefore, bone cement prepared through the addition of liquid antibiotics is not suitable for implant fixation.

To be effective, antibiotic additions to PMMA should be thermally stable, should easily leach out of the cured cement, and should be present in a bactericidal concentration in the vicinity of the cement for a prolonged time. Finally, they should be active against the most common pathogens and/or against a specific infecting organism.[4,11,97] Some antibiotics are unsuitable or are less suitable for addition to bone cement because of thermal instability (flucloxaciline,[98] chloramphenicol,[5] tetracycline[7]) or suboptimal elution characteristics (see Table 4-3). In the rare case of a fungal implant infection, bone cement impregnated with amphotericin B or fluconazole can be used.[6]

Although only 10% of antibiotics leach out from cracks, from voids, and from the surface of the cement, antibiotic-loaded cement can achieve high local concentrations with minimal systemic absorption.[11,88] Because elution of antibiotics increases with cement porosity,[93] hand-mixed bone cement containing many voids has some advantage compared with vacuum-mixed cement.[94] The combination of two antibiotics in bone cement can have a synergistic effect and can improve the elution of both antibiotics.[94,97,99]

Mechanical Properties of Antibiotic-Loaded Cement. Overall, antibiotic-loaded cement has inferior static mechanical properties[9,55,97] (see Table 4-2) and increased creep properties[10] compared with plain cement. The ultimate strength of antibiotic-loaded cement is inversely proportional to the quantity of antibiotics used.[55] At doses given for prophylaxis (up to 1 g per 40 g cement), reduction of the ultimate compression strength is limited (5%-6%[55]) and fatigue resistance of the material is unaffected.[65] However, as the antibiotic concentration increases, the ultimate compressive strength tends to decrease further (2 g/40 g: −17% to −18%; 5 g/40 g: −19% to −26%[55]). In providing clinical guidance, several authors have claimed that up to 4 g of antibiotic powder can be added to 40 g cement (10% weight) without compromising implant fixation.[85,87,94]

Infection Prevention With Antibiotic-Loaded Cement. It is clear that cement containing gentamicin, tobramycin, or cefuroxime is effective against infection of joint replacements.[88,100,101] However, routine use of these formulations remains controversial. In the United States, only 11% of surgeons use antibiotic-loaded cement in primary surgery,[88] and although the Food and Drug Administration (FDA) approves antibiotic-loaded cement for the treatment of infection, it remains unapproved as a prophylactic measure in primary cases. A recent review[88] advocates against the preventive use of antibiotic-loaded cement in patients who are not at high risk for infection. The main arguments include lack of proven efficacy in patients who do not present a high risk of infection, especially in the long term,[102] lower mechanical strength, higher cost, lack of cost-effectiveness, possible local toxicity (seen only in vitro and at high doses), risk of allergic reaction (undocumented today), increased risk of antimicrobial resistance due to low-dose antibiotic release in the long term,[103] and difficulty with the detection of low-grade infection in cases of implant loosening.[103] In Europe, the preventive use of antibiotic-loaded cement in primary cases is well accepted (Norway: 48%; Britain: 69%-94%; Sweden: 85% of cemented hip arthroplasties[22,88,104]) and has proved cost-effective.[105] The main argument is a clear decrease in the revision rate and the incidence of infection in large patient populations, especially in operations performed before 1995.[100,101]

Today, strong arguments have been put forth for the use of antibiotic-loaded cement in patients at high risk of infection, including those undergoing revision surgery and prolonged operative duration (>150 minutes), patients with previous joint infection or previous steroid injection, and those with immunosuppression, inflammatory arthropathies, obesity (body mass index >30 kg/m²), insulin-dependent diabetes, malnourishment, malignant tumor, hemophilia, or organ transplantation.[88] In patients without these risk factors, the individual potential benefit of a decreased revision rate must be balanced against potential drawbacks for the patient and for the community in terms of cost and antibiotic resistance.

Infection Treatment With Antibiotic-Loaded Cement. Antibiotic-loaded cement has become a standard in the treatment of infected arthroplasty because of the high local concentrations of antibiotics that can be achieved at the site of infection. In the United States, this is the only FDA-approved application for antibiotic-loaded cement.[88] Two different strategies can be used: a single- or a two-stage procedure. The choice depends on the infecting agent, the local situation after implant removal, and the experience of the team.

- In a single-stage procedure, removal of the infected hip arthroplasty, extensive débridement of the implantation site, and reimplantation of new implants are performed in a single sitting. This strategy has been advocated when the patient is not immunocompromised, and when the infecting agent is known and is not very aggressive or difficult to eradicate (i.e., when the germ is not very virulent and is sensitive to antibiotics). Moreover, after implant removal and extensive débridement, reconstruction with cemented implants must be feasible.[85] In these cases, up to 10% (maximum 4 g per 40 g cement) of a well-selected antibiotic, or a combination of antibiotics, is mixed in the cement in powder form (see Table 4-3), and both the cup and the stem are cemented. The selection of antibiotic should take into account the susceptibility of the infecting agent and possible sensitivity reactions of the patient. Treatment should be supplemented with systemic antibiotics for several weeks or months.[7]

- In the two-stage procedure, implant removal, extensive débridement, and implantation of antibiotic-loaded "PMMA beads" or an antibiotic-loaded "cement spacer" are performed during a first procedure. When the infection is controlled, most often after several weeks of systemic antibiotic treatment, another débridement and reimplantation of a cemented or uncemented implant are performed during a second procedure.[89,90]

Antibiotic-loaded beads are available from the shelf at least in Europe (Septopal, Biomet Merck, Darmstadt, Germany) and contain 4.5 mg of gentamicin per bead. Because of their large contact area, antibiotic release is very satisfactory.[93] Most cement spacers are produced during the surgical procedure with a mold (e.g., StageOne Hip Cement Spacer Mold, Biomet, Warsaw, Ind) or are simply formed by hand. Some spacers are reinforced with a metallic component to avoid breakage when in situ. Up to 6 to 9 g of antibiotic powder[6,90,99] per 40 g cement can be used without systemic side effects. To produce cement spacers or beads, it is possible to add liquid antibiotics (up to 12 mL per 40 g cement[97]) to the monomer before mixing with the powder. However, both liquid antibiotics and high doses of antibiotic powder impair the curing of the cement and its ultimate mechanical properties.[55,97] With more than 8 g of antibiotic powder per 40 g PMMA, the cement becomes more difficult to handle,[6] but this is not a major problem, at least when used only to fabricate beads and spacers.

Cement spacers have two advantages compared with beads. First, because they can be adapted to the patient's morphology, spacers can better maintain the separation of the femur and the acetabulum by limiting retraction of the scar tissue and the action of the muscles. This facilitates the reimplantation of a new prosthesis during the second stage of the procedure. Second, spacers allow administration of the best antibiotic for treating each infection, based on the results of susceptibility testing[85] (see Table 4-3). However, the antibiotic elution from cement spacers is inferior to that from beads because of their smaller total surface area.[93]

Two-stage revision is still regarded as the gold standard for treatment of infected hip replacements[6] and should always be considered when the infecting agent is unknown prior to surgery, when it is virulent and/or multiresistant to antibiotics, when the patient is immunocompromised, and in the presence of major soft tissue or bone defects.[7] Two-stage procedures should also be considered when the local situation, after implant removal and débridement, compromises reconstructions with cemented implants.[6,89]

Cement Defects and Pores

The presence of pores or defects within the cement mantle or at the cement-stem interface has multiple origins.[48] First, cement porosity can arise from air trapped within the cement powder before mixing, or it can be introduced during cement mixing or cement transfer to the cartridge. Second, heating of the cement during polymerization expands the trapped air and can favor monomer vaporization in exiting voids or in small, newly created pores. Third, blood, bone, and fat can contaminate the cement mantle during cementation.[25] Finally, interfacial gaps can arise at the cement-stem interfacial from air dragged down along the implant during stem insertion,[48] and interfacial pores can develop as the result of cement shrinkage during polymerization, as described in the section on cement shrinkage in this chapter.

Most sources of cement porosity can be controlled. Centrifugation[106,107] or vacuum mixing[1,106] can reduce the amount of air trapped within the bulk of the cement. However, in a situation that mimics intraoperative conditions, vacuum mixing did not improve overall cement porosity.[108] Indeed, the porosity reduction in the bulk of the cement was counterbalanced by the presence of larger pores, especially at the cement-stem interface.[108] Cooling the femoral shaft with a cold pressure lavage can reduce interfacial porosity and control the temperature during cement curing.[51] Blood and fat contamination can be reduced by performing pressure lavage and drying the femoral canal before cement insertion, by introducing the cement in a more viscous state and pressurizing the cement to avoid back-bleeding,[25] and

by inserting the stem after the upper surface of the cement-filled proximal femur has been cleaned.[109] Finally, interfacial gaps can be reduced by using polished stems, by inserting the stem through a diaphragm, and by prewetting the implant with cement.[48]

The effect of cement porosity remains controversial. It is clear that pores decrease both the static[107] and the fatigue strength[69,106,107] of PMMA. However, pore location and distribution, rather than level of porosity, could be important.[66,69] Pores located within the cement mantle can act as fatigue crack initiators, crack promoters, and crack deviators, but also as crack stoppers, depending on their size and location.[69] Interfacial gaps act as fatigue crack initiators or promoters and could be deleterious in all cases.[49] However, reduced cement porosity does not seem to improve stem survival.[110] Therefore, it remains questionable whether porosity reduction is clinically relevant.[111,112]

Cement Interfaces

Both the cement-bone interface and the cement-implant interface play an important role in the load transfer between implant and bone. At both interfaces, the cement acts as a "grout" and not as a "glue."[112] It fills up the space between the bone and the implant and can resist traction forces only by interlocking on the implant or the bony surface. Because the two surfaces have different structures, the behaviors of the cement-bone and cement-implant interfaces are different.

The Cement-Bone Interface

The interlock between cement and bone occurs through interdigitation of cement between the trabeculae of the cancellous bone in the medullary canal or the pelvis.[112,113] To achieve good cement anchorage, sufficient cancellous bone must be present,[114] and the cement must be pressurized before implant insertion and during cement curing (Fig. 4-5). Although low-viscosity cement could improve cement penetration, particularly within the proximal femur,[23] it is more readily displaced from the bony surface through back-bleeding from the bone, leading to disruption of the cement-bone interface[24,25] and to increased prevalence of interfacial defects.[23] On the femoral side, some authors suggest that as much cancellous bone as possible should be preserved to allow proper cement interdigitation.[1] However, cement-free cancellous bone, interposed between the cement mantle and the cortical bone, is a weak link[61] and should be avoided, especially in high-stress areas such as the calcar region.[115] Because cement can be pressurized easily to a depth of 3 to 4 mm,[31] retention of only 3 to 4 mm of cancellous bone (but no more) within the proximal femur allows the surgeon to pressurize cement to the extent that it fills the cancellous layer through to the endomedullary cortex. From a mechanical point of view, support of the cement mantle by strong cortical bone is important for the mechanical integrity of both thin and thick cement layers[61,112] (Fig. 4-6).

In clinical practice, radiostereometric analysis has shown that very limited migration occurs between the cement mantle and the bone.[116,117] This suggests that the

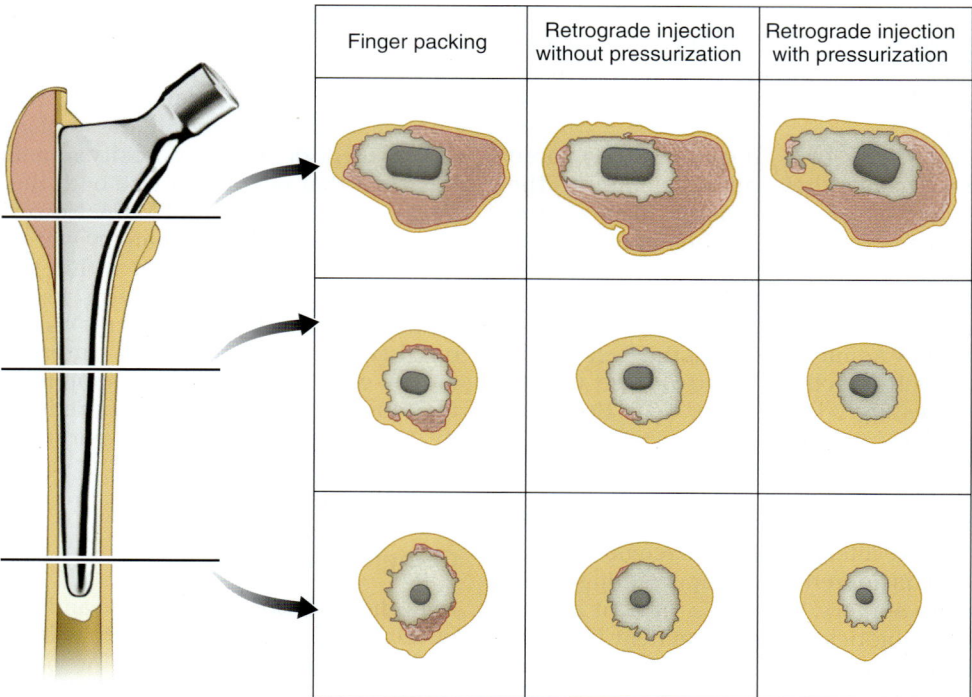

	Finger packing	Retrograde injection without pressurization	Retrograde injection with pressurization

Figure 4-5. Effects of the cementing technique on the amount of cement-bone interdigitation at different levels of the proximal femur. Finger packing allows pressurization of a limited amount of cement into the cancellous bone. Large quantities of weak cement-free cancellous bone persist between the cement mantle and the cortex in the proximal and middle parts of the upper femur. Retrograde cement injection without pressurization allows filling up of the distal and middle parts of the upper femur. In the proximal part, the cement mantle is rather thin and has limited support by cortical bone. Retrograde cement injection combined with pressurization allows attainment of a thicker cement mantle and better cortical support proximally. (Unpublished data provided by the author based on the analysis of computer tomography scans of cemented CPT-stems [Zimmer] in a cadaver model.)

large amount of cement-bone interdigitation that is generally present in the cemented femur[118] provides good stability at the cement-bone interface. However, improving the strength of the cement-stem bond by porous coating, grit blasting, or precoating the stem surface with PMMA (precoated stems) can result in transfer of loads that exceed the mechanical strength of the cement-bone interface. This might result in failure, especially in the presence of a suboptimal cementing technique.[119,120]

The Cement-Implant Interface

Because of high repetitive implant loading and because of differences in elasticity between the three components of the stem-cement-bone construct, cement-stem debonding and stem migration are often inevitable.[57,116,117,119] Two strategies have been developed to deal with this phenomenon.[57,59,112] First, implants were designed to accommodate stem migration (e.g., Exeter, Stryker; CPT, Zimmer). Such implants are collarless and tapered and have a polished surface finish that allows stem subsidence within the cement mantle. Implant subsidence occurs until a stable position is reached and favors compressive load transfer to the cement mantle and adjacent bone (loaded-taper principle).[60,116] Generally, with this type of stem, no migration occurs at the cement-bone interface.[116] Second, implants have been developed with the goal of

improving stem stability by providing direct cortical contact or by enhancing cement-stem fixation (composite beam principle). Such stems may be polished or satin canal-filling stems (e.g., Kerboull, Mathys Ltd, Bettlach, Switzerland; Müller, Zimmer) or undersized stems with a roughened or precoated surface finish (e.g., Spectron, Smith & Nephew, Memphis, Tenn; Harris Precoat, Zimmer). Composite beam stems can debond and migrate at both cement-stem and cement-bone interfaces.[116,117,119] Although good results have been reported with both strategies and with many different types of surface finish and stem design, roughening, porous coating, or precoating of implants with PMMA to improve cement-stem bonding could be counterproductive. Therefore, the survivorship of most cemented stems is insensitive to surface finish or is improved when a smoother surface is present.[57]

CURRENT CONTROVERSIES AND FUTURE DIRECTIONS

- Should the ideal cement mantle be thick or thin? What is the ideal quantity of cement within a femoral resurfacing head or surrounding a femoral stem? In clinical practice, how can cement mantle thickness be controlled?

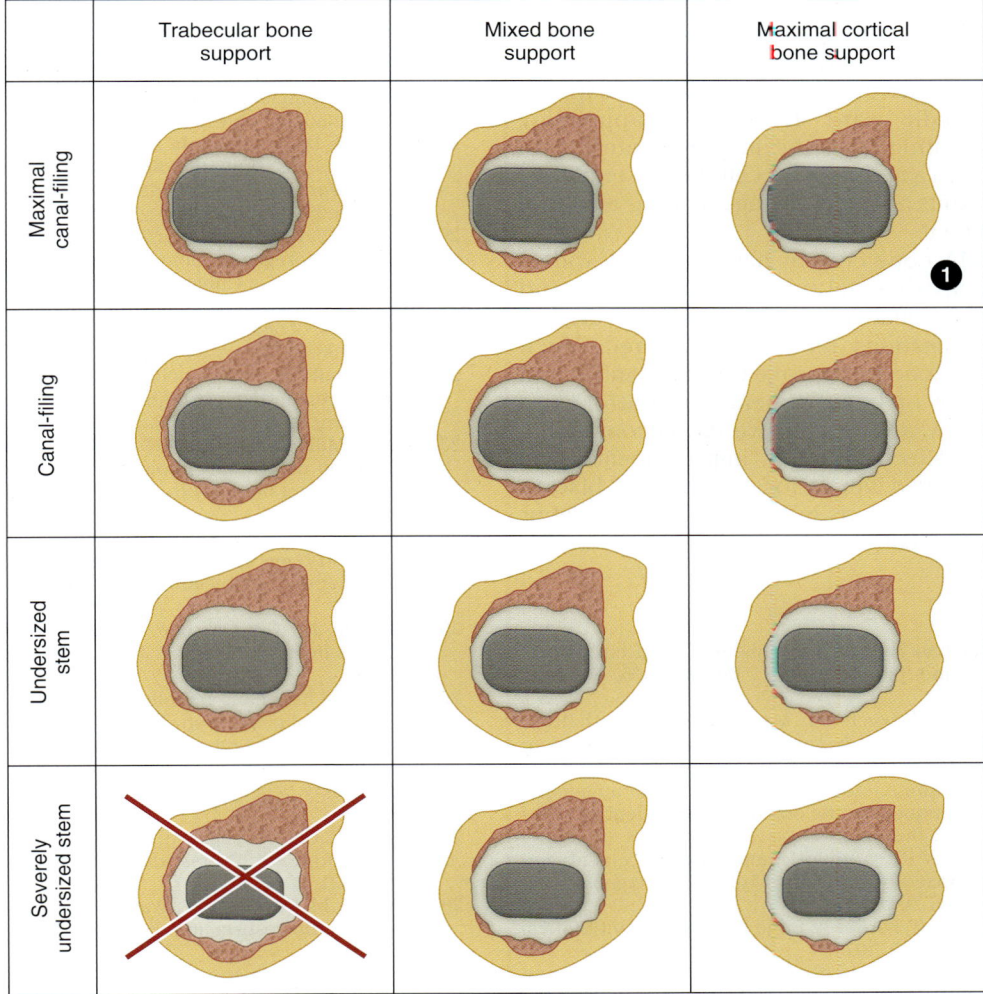

Figure 4-6. Finite element analysis models used to evaluate the impact of stem size *(vertical axis)* and cement mantle support *(horizontal axis)* on the mechanical stability of the cement mantle during cyclical loading in rotation. Maximal canal filling stems associated with a cement mantle that is well supported by cortical bone *(upper right corner)* show the fewest fatigue cracks within the cement mantle and the best rotational stability. A severely undersized stem with a cement mantle that is supported only by cancellous bone *(lower left corner)* is a poor mechanical construct. *(Redrawn from Janssen D, van Aken J, Scheerlinck T, Verdonschot N: Finite element analysis of the effect of cementing concepts on implant stability and cement fatigue failure. Acta Orthop 80:319–324, 2009, Fig. 2, p 320.[61])*

- How can mechanical properties of bone cement be improved without compromising biocompatibility? Addition of "reinforcing materials" or alteration in the chemical composition of bone cement should be further explored.
- How can drug release from bone cement be controlled without impairing the mechanical properties? Ideally, antibiotic release for infection prevention should be limited to the first days or weeks to avoid antimicrobial resistance; for infection, treatment with high doses and long-term release are mandatory.
- Because traditional radiopacifiers have major drawbacks, what are the alternatives?
- How can bone cement be made *bioactive* to control particle-induced osteolysis or to favor bone apposition at the cement-bone interface? Bioresorbable

cements or "gap fillers" that can be replaced by bone over time could be very useful in revisions and primary cases. However, actual formulations do not provide sufficient mechanical resistance.

CONCLUSION

Polymethylmethacrylate bone cement is still very commonly used for the fixation of hip arthroplasty implants, especially at the femoral side. Combining a well-designed stem with an adequate cementing technique will result in excellent long-term implant survival. Because bone cement is very versatile, it can be applied in situations where cementless implants might be more difficult to use (e.g., hip arthroplasties in nonstandard anatomic situations, graft impaction revision techniques, in combination with acetabular cages). Moreover, bone cement is an excellent drug carrier and can be used successfully to prevent and treat hip arthroplasty infection. For these reasons, PMMA is not due to disappear from the orthopedic ward. However, disappointing results, often resulting from the inappropriate use of cement, have led to a shift toward cementless implants, especially in regions without a long-standing tradition in the use of cement.

Although PMMA bone cement has been very widely investigated in experimental settings both in vitro and in vivo, with mathematical modeling and in clinical practice, many questions remain unanswered. Much work needs to be done to improve the mechanical and thermal properties of bone cement, to control drug release from PMMA, and to improve its biocompatibility. However, the effects of such "improvements" will have to be monitored very closely, because history shows that many alterations in the original material or in its use have been counterproductive.

REFERENCES

1. Breusch S, Malchau H: The well-cemented total hip arthroplasty: theory and practice, ed 1, Berlin, 2005, Springer Medizin Verlag.
2. Jacofsky DJ, Haidukewych GJ: Management of pathologic fractures of the proximal femur: state of the art. J Orthop Trauma 18:459–469, 2004.
3. Moroni A, Hoang-Kim A, Lio V, Giannini S: Current augmentation fixation techniques for the osteoporotic patient. Scand J Surg 95:103–109, 2006.
4. Wininger DA, Fass RJ: Antibiotic-impregnated cement and beads for orthopaedic infections. Antimicrob Agents Chemother 40:2675–2679, 1996.
5. Ger E, Dall D, Miles T, Forder A: Bone cement and antibiotics. S Afr Med J 51:276–279, 1977.
6. Cui Q, Mihalko WM, Shields JS, et al: Antibiotic-impregnated cement spacers for the treatment of infection associated with total hip or knee arthroplasty. J Bone Joint Surg Am 89:871–882, 2007.
7. Joseph TN, Chen AL, Di Cesare PE: Use of antibiotic-impregnated cement in total joint arthroplasty. J Am Acad Orthop Surg 11:38–47, 2003.
8. Rosa MA, Maccauro G, Sgambato A, et al: Acrylic cement added with antiblastics in the treatment of bone metastases: ultrastrctural and in vitro analysis. J Bone Joint Surg Br 85:712–716, 2003.
9. Kühn KD: Bone cements: up-to-date comparison of physical and chemical properties of commercial materials, ed 1, Berlin, 2000, Springer-Verlag.
10. Webb JCJ, Spencer RF: The role of polymethylmethacrylate bone cement in modern orthopaedic surgery. J Bone Joint Surg Br 89:851–857, 2007.
11. Hendriks JGE, Van Horn JR, van der Mei HC, Busscher HJ: Backgrounds of antibiotic-loaded bone cement and prosthesis-related infection. Biomaterials 25:545–556, 2004.
12. Eden OR, Lee AJ, Hooper RM: Stress relaxation modelling of polymethylmethacrylate bone cement. Proc Inst Mech Eng [H] 216:195–200, 2002.
13. Kärrholm J, Garellick G, Lindahl H, Herberts P: Improved analyses in the Swedish hip arthroplasty register, San Diego, 2007, AAOS.
14. Helse-Bergen HF: The Norwegian arthroplasty register: report 2007, Bergen, Norway, 2007, Haukeland University Hospital.
15. Sibanda N, Copley LP, Lewsey JD, et al: Revision rates after primary hip and knee replacement in England between 2003 and 2006. PLoS Med 5:e179, 2008.
16. Rothwell A, Hobbs T: New Zealand national joint registry: seven year report, Christchurch, New Zealand, 2007, Christchurch Hospital.
17. Scheerlinck T, Casteleyn PP: The use of primary total hip arthroplasties in university hospitals of the European Union. Acta Orthop Belg 70:231–239, 2004.
18. Kersteci M, Marin M, de Guia N, Shi E: Hip and knee replacements in Canada, 2006 report. Toronto, Ontario, Canada, 2006, Canadian Joint Replacement Registry.
19. Graves S, Davidson D, de Steiger R, et al: Australian Orthopaedic Association national joint replacement registry: annual report 2008, Adelaide, SA, Australia, 2008, Australian Orthopaedic Association.
20. Kärrholm J, Garellick G, Herberts P: The National Swedish hip arthroplasty register: annual report 2005, Göteborg, Sweden, 2006, Sahlgrenska University Hospital.
21. Meyer PR Jr, Lautenschlager EP, Moore BK: On the setting properties of acrylic bone cement. J Bone Joint Surg Am 55:149–156, 1973.
22. Nedungayil SK, Mehendele S, Gheduzzi S, Learmonth ID: Femoral cementing techniques: current trends in the UK. Ann R Coll Surg Engl 88:127–130, 2006.
23. Race A, Miller MA, Clarke MT, et al: The effect of low-viscosity cement on mantle morphology and femoral stem micromotion: a cadaver model with simulated blood flow. Acta Orthop 77:607–616, 2006.
24. Miller MA, Race A, Gupta S, et al: The role of cement viscosity on cement-bone apposition and strength: an in vitro model with medullary bleeding. J Arthroplasty 22:109–116, 2007.
25. Benjamin JB, Gie GA, Lee AJ, et al: Cementing technique and the effects of bleeding. J Bone Joint Surg Br 69:620–624, 1987.
26. Havelin LI, Espehaug B, Vollset SE, Engesaeter LB: The effect of the type of cement on early revision of the Charnley total hip prosthesis: a review of eight thousand five hundred and seventy-nine primary arthroplasties from the Norwegian arthroplasty register. J Bone Joint Surg Am 77:1543–1550, 1995.
27. Bitsch RG, Heisel C, Silva M, Schmalzried TP: Femoral cementing technique for hip resurfacing arthroplasty. J Orthop Res 25:423–431, 2007.
28. Chandler M, Kowalski RS, Watkins ND, et al: Cementing techniques in hip resurfacing. Proc Inst Mech Eng (H) 220:321–331, 2006.
29. Beckmann J, Goldapp C, Ringleff K, et al: Cementing technique in femoral resurfacing. Arch Orthop Trauma Surg 129:1317–1325, 2008.
30. Quarini G, Learmonth I, Gheduzzi S: Numerical predictions of the thermal behaviour and resultant effects of grouting cements while setting prosthetic components in bone. Proc Inst Mech Eng (H) 220:625–634, 2006.
31. Scheerlinck T, de Mey J, Deklerck R, Noble PhC: CT analysis of defects of the cement mantle and alignment of the stem: in vitro comparison of Charnley-Kerboul femoral hip implants inserted line-to-line and undersized in paired femora. J Bone Joint Surg Br 88:19–25, 2006.
32. Valdivia GG, Dunbar MJ, Parker DA, et al: Three-dimensional analysis of the cement mantle in total hip arthroplasty. Clin Orthop Relat Res 393:38–51, 2001.
33. Toksvig-Larsen S, Franzen H, Ryd L: Cement interface temperature in hip arthroplasty. Acta Orthop Scand 62:102–105, 1991.
34. Huiskes R: Heat-generation and conduction analyses of acrylic bone cement in situ. Acta Chir Scand (Suppl) 185:43–108, 1980.
35. Eriksson AR, Albrektsson T: Temperature threshold levels for heat-induced bone tissue injury: a vital-microscopic study in the rabbit. J Prosthet Dent 50:101–107, 1983.
36. Thanner J, Freij-Larsson C, Karrholm J, et al: Evaluation of Boneloc: chemical and mechanical properties, and a randomized clinical study of 30 total hip arthroplasties. Acta Orthop Scand 66:207–214, 1995.
37. Harper EJ, Bonfield W: Tensile characteristics of ten commercial acrylic bone cements. J Biomed Mater Res B Appl Biomater 53:605–616, 2000.
38. Nilsen AR, Wiig M: Total hip arthroplasty with Boneloc: loosening in 102/157 cases after 0.5-3 years. Acta Orthop Scand 67:57–59, 1996.

39. Nivbrant B, Karrholm J, Rohrl S, et al: Bone cement with reduced proportion of monomer in total hip arthroplasty: preclinical evaluation and randomized study of 47 cases with 5 years' follow-up. Acta Orthop Scand 72:572–584, 2001.

40. Scheerlinck T, Delport H, Kiewitt T: Influence of the cementing technique on the cement mantle in hip resurfacing: an in vitro computed tomography scan-based analysis. J Bone Joint Surg Am 92:375–387, 2010.

41. Falez F, Favetti F, Casella F, Panegrossi G: Hip resurfacing: why does it fail? Early results and critical analysis of our first 60 cases. Int Orthop 32:209–216, 2008.

42. Beaulé PE, Lu Z, Campbell P: Bone thermal necrosis and cement penetration in femoral head resurfacing. J Bone Joint Surg Br 90(Suppl 1):97, 2005.

43. Little JP, Gray HA, Murray DW, et al: Thermal effects of cement mantle thickness for hip resurfacing. J Arthroplasty 23:454–458, 2008.

44. Hsieh PH, Tai CL, Liaw JW, Chang Y-H: Thermal damage potential during hip resurfacing in osteonecrosis of the femoral head: an experimental study. J Orthop Res 26:1206–1209, 2008.

45. Gill HS, Campbell PA, Murray DW, De Smet KA: Reduction of the potential for thermal damage during hip resurfacing. J Bone Joint Surg Br 89:16–20, 2007.

46. Gilbert JL, Hasenwinkel JM, Wixson RL, Lautenschlager EP: A theoretical and experimental analysis of polymerization shrinkage of bone cement: a potential major source of porosity. J Biomed Mater Res 52:210–218, 2000.

47. Kwong FNK, Power M: A comparison of the shrinkage of commercial bone cements when mixed under vacuum. J Bone Joint Surg Br 88:120–122, 2006.

48. Scheerlinck T, Vandenbussche P, Noble PhC: Quantification of stem-cement interfacial gaps: in vitro CT analysis of Charnley-Kerboul and Lubinus SPII femoral hip implants. J Bone Joint Surg Br 90:107–113, 2008.

49. Scheerlinck T, Broos J, Janssen D, Verdonschot N: Mechanical implications of interfacial defects between femoral hip implants and cement: a finite element analysis of interfacial gaps and interfacial porosity. Proc Inst Mech Eng (H) 222:1037–1047, 2008.

50. Bishop NE, Ferguson S, Tepic S: Porosity reduction in bone cement at the cement-stem interface. J Bone Joint Surg Br 78:349–356, 1996.

51. Hsieh PH, Tai CL, Chang YH, et al: Precooling of the femoral canal enhances shear strength at the cement-prosthesis interface and reduces the polymerization temperature. J Orthop Res 24:1809–1814, 2006.

52. Lewis G: Properties of acrylic bone cement: state of the art review. J Biomed Mater Res 38:155–182, 1997.

53. Baleani M, Cristofolini L, Toni A: Temperature and ageing condition effects on the characterization of acrylic bone cement. Proc Inst Mech Eng (H) 215:113–118, 2001.

54. Liu C, Green S, Watkins N, et al: Some failure modes of four clinical bone cements. Proc Inst Mech Eng (H) 215:359–366, 2001.

55. Lee AJC, Ling RSM, Vangala SS: Some clinically relevant variables affecting the mechanical behaviour of bone cement. Arch Orthop Trauma Surg 92:1–18, 1978.

56. Lewis G, Mladsi S: Effect of sterilization method on properties of Palacos R acrylic bone cement. Biomaterials 19:117–124, 1998.

57. Scheerlinck T, Casteleyn PP: Review article: the design features of cemented femoral hip implants. J Bone Joint Surg Br 88:1409–1418, 2006.

58. Stachurski ZH: Strength and deformation of rigid polymers: the stress-strain curve in amorphous PMMA. Polymer 44:6067–6076, 2003.

59. Shen G: Femoral stem fixation: an engineering interpretation of the long-term outcome of Charnley and Exeter stems. J Bone Joint Surg Br 80:754–756, 1998.

60. Kaneuji A, Yamada K, Hirosaki K, et al: Stem subsidence of polished and rough double-taper stems. Acta Orthop 80:270–276, 2009.

61. Janssen D, van Aken J, Scheerlinck T, Verdonschot N: Finite element analysis of the effect of cementing concepts on implant stability and cement fatigue failure. Acta Orthop 80:319–324, 2009.

62. Cristofolini L, Erani P, Savigni P, et al: Preclinical assessment of the long-term endurance of cemented hip stems. Part 2: in-vitro and ex-vivo fatigue damage of the cement mantle. Proc Inst Mech Eng (H) 221:585–599, 2007.

63. Topoleski LDT, Ducheyne P, Cuckler JM: A fractographic analysis of in vivo poly(methyl methacrylate) bone cement failure mechanisms. J Biomed Mater Res 24:135–154, 1990.

64. Jasty M, Maloney WJ, Bragdon CR, et al: The initiation of failure in cemented femoral components of hip arthroplasties. J Bone Joint Surg Br 73:551–558, 1991.

65. Baleani M, Cristofolini L, Minari C, Toni A: Fatigue strength of PMMA bone cement mixed with gentamicin and barium sulphate vs pure PMMA. Proc Inst Mech Eng (H) 217:9–12, 2003.

66. Coultrup OJ, Browne M, Hunt C, Taylor M: Accounting for inclusions and voids allows the prediction of tensile fatigue life of bone cement. J Biomech Eng 131:051007, 2009.

67. Krause W, Mathis RS, Grimes LW: Fatigue properties of acrylic bone cement: S-N, P-N, and P-S-N data. J Biomed Mater Res 22:221–244, 1988.

68. Stolk J, Janssen D, Huiskes R, Verdonschot N: Finite element-based preclinical testing of cemented total hip implants. Clin Orthop Relat Res 456:138–147, 2007.

69. Janssen D, Aquarius R, Stolk J, Verdonschot N: The contradictory effects of pores on fatigue cracking of bone cement. J Biomed Mater Res B Appl Biomater 74:747–753, 2005.

70. Zant NP, Heaton-Adegbile P, Hussell JG, Tong J: In vitro fatigue failure of cemented acetabular replacements: a hip simulator study. J Biomech Eng 130:021019, 2008.

71. Janssen D, Stolk J, Verdonschot N: Finite element analysis of the long-term fixation strength of cemented ceramic cups. Proc Inst Mech Eng (H) 220:533–539, 2006.

72. Riska EB: Ceramic endoprosthesis in total hip arthroplasty. Clin Orthop Relat Res 297:87–94, 1993.

73. Chen FS, Di Cesare PE, Kale AA, et al: Results of cemented metal-backed acetabular components: a 10-year-average follow-up study. J Arthroplasty 13:867–873, 1998.

74. Manero J, Ginebra M, Gil F, et al: Propagation of fatigue cracks in acrylic bone cements containing different radiopaque agents. Proc Inst Mech Eng (H) 218:167–172, 2004.

75. Bellare A, Fitz W, Gomoll A, et al: Using nanotechnology to improve the performance of acrylic bone cements. Orthop J Harvard Medical School 4:93–96, 2002.

76. Shardlow DL, Stone MH, Ingham E, Fisher J: Cement particles containing radio-opacifiers stimulate pro-osteolytic cytokine production from a human monocytic cell line. J Bone Joint Surg Br 85:900–905, 2003.

77. Sabokbar A, Fujikawa Y, Murray DW, Athanasou NA: Radio-opaque agents in bone cement increase bone resorption. J Bone Joint Surg Br 79:129–134, 1997.

78. Wang JS, Diaz J, Sabokbar A, et al: In vitro and in vivo biological responses to a novel radiopacifying agent for bone cement. J R Soc Interface 2:71–78, 2005.

79. Wimhurst JA, Brooks RA, Rushton N: The effects of particulate bone cements at the bone-implant interface. J Bone Joint Surg Br 83:588–592, 2001.

80. Isaac GH, Atkinson JR, Dowson D, et al: The causes of femoral head roughening in explanted Charnley hip prostheses. Eng Med 16:167–173, 1987.

81. Kjellson F, Wang JS, Almén T, et al: Tensile properties of a bone cement containing non-ionic contrast media. J Mater Sci Mater Med 12:889–894, 2001.

82. Artola A, Gurruchaga M, Vázquez B, et al: Elimination of barium sulphate from acrylic bone cements: use of two iodine-containing monomers. Biomaterials 24:4071–4080, 2003.

83. van Hooy-Corstjens CSJ, Govaert LE, Spoelstra AB, et al: Mechanical behaviour of a new acrylic radiopaque iodine-containing bone cement. Biomaterials 25:2657–2667, 2004.

84. Lewis G, van Hooy-Corstjens CSJ, Bhattaram A, Koole LH: Influence of the radiopacifier in an acrylic bone cement on its mechanical, thermal, and physical properties: barium sulfate-containing cement versus iodine-containing cement. J Biomed Mater Res B Appl Biomater 73:77–87, 2005.

85. Walenkamp GHIM, Murray DW: Bone cements and cementing technique, ed 1, Berlin, 2001, Springer-Verlag.

86. Chiu FY, Lin CF, Chen CM, et al: Cefuroxime-impregnated cement at primary total knee arthroplasty in diabetes mellitus: a prospective, randomised study. J Bone Joint Surg Br 83:691–695, 2001.

87. Breusch SJ, Kühn K-D: Knochenzemente auf basis von polymethylmethacrylat. Orthopade 32:41–50, 2003.

88. Jiranek WA, Hanssen AD, Greenwald AS: Antibiotic-loaded bone cement for infection prophylaxis in total joint replacement. J Bone Joint Surg Am 88:2487–2500, 2006.

89. Diwanji SR, Kong IK, Park YH, et al: Two-stage reconstruction of infected hip joints. J Arthroplasty 23:656–661, 2008.

90. Koo KH, Yang JW, Cho SH, et al: Impregnation of vancomycin, gentamicin, and cefotaxime in a cement spacer for two-stage cementless reconstruction in infected total hip arthroplasty. J Arthroplasty 16:882–892, 2001.

91. Wahlig H, Dingeldein E: Antibiotics and bone cements: experimental and clinical long-term observations. Acta Orthop 51:49–56, 1980.

92. Adams K, Couch L, Cierny G, et al: In vitro and in vivo evaluation of antibiotic diffusion from antibiotic-impregnated polymethylmethacrylate beads. Clin Orthop Relat Res 278:244–252, 1992.

93. Moojen DJ, Hentenaar B, Charles VH, et al: In vitro release of antibiotics from commercial PMMA beads and articulating hip spacers. J Arthroplasty 23:1152–1156, 2008.

94. Anagnostakos K, Kelm J: Enhancement of antibiotic elution from acrylic bone cement. J Biomed Mater Res B Appl Biomater 90:467–475, 2009.

95. Levin PD: The effectiveness of various antibiotics in methyl methacrylate. J Bone Joint Surg Br 57:234–237, 1975.

96. Anagnostakos K, Kelm J, Regitz T, et al: In vitro evaluation of antibiotic release from and bacteria growth inhibition by antibiotic-loaded acrylic bone cement spacers. J Biomed Mater Res B Appl Biomater 72:373–378, 2005.

97. Hsieh PH, Tai CL, Lee PC, Chang YH: Liquid gentamicin and vancomycin in bone cement: a potentially more cost-effective regimen. J Arthroplasty 24:125–130, 2009.

98. Armstrong M, Spencer RF, Lovering AM, et al: Antibiotic elution from bone cement: a study of common cement-antibiotic combinations. Hip Int 12:23–27, 2002.

99. Penner MJ, Masri BA, Duncan CP: Elution characteristics of vancomycin and tobramycin combined in acrylic bone-cement. J Arthroplasty 11:939–944, 1996.

100. Engesaeter LB, Espehaug B, Lie SA, et al: Does cement increase the risk of infection in primary total hip arthroplasty? Revision rates in 56,275 cemented and uncemented primary THAs followed for 0-16 years in the Norwegian Arthroplasty Register. Acta Orthop 77:351–358, 2006.

101. Josefsson G, Lindberg L, Wiklander B: Systemic antibiotics and gentamicin-containing bone cement in the prophylaxis of postoperative infections in total hip arthroplasty. Clin Orthop Relat Res 159:193–200, 1981.

102. Josefsson G, Kolmert L: Prophylaxis with systematic antibiotics versus gentamicin bone cement in total hip arthroplasty: a ten-year survey of 1688 hips. Clin Orthop Relat Res 292:210–214, 1993.

103. Fletcher MDA, Spencer RF, Langkamerd VG, Lovering AM: Gentamicin concentrations in diagnostic aspirates from 25 patients with hip and knee arthroplasties. Acta Orthop Scand 75:173–176, 2004.

104. Malik MHA, Gambhir AK, Bale L, et al: Primary total hip replacement: a comparison of a nationally agreed guide to best practice and current surgical technique as determined by the North West Regional Arthroplasty Register. Ann R Coll Surg Engl 86:113–118, 2004.

105. Persson U, Persson M, Malchau H: The economics of preventing revisions in total hip replacement. Acta Orthop Scand 70:163–169, 1999.

106. Wixson RL: Do we need to vacuum mix or centrifuge cement? Clin Orthop Relat Res 285:84–90, 1992.

107. Burke DW, Gates EI, Harris WH: Centrifugation as a method of improving tensile and fatigue properties of acrylic bone cement. J Bone Joint Surg Am 66:1265–1273, 1984.

108. Messick KJ, Miller MA, Damron LA, et al: Vacuum-mixing cement does not decrease overall porosity in cemented femoral stems: an in vitro laboratory investigation. J Bone Joint Surg Br 89:1115–1121, 2007.

109. Noble PC, Collier MS, Maltry JA, et al: Pressurization and centralization enhance the quality and reproducibility of cement mantles. Clin Orthop Relat Res 355:77–89, 1998.

110. Hernigou PH, Le Mouël S: Do voids in a femoral cement mantle affect the outcome? J Arthroplasty 14:1005–1010, 1999.

111. Ling RS, Lee AJ: Porosity reduction in acrylic cement is clinically irrelevant. Clin Orthop Relat Res 355:249–253, 1998.

112. Hernigou P, Daltro G, Lachaniette CH, et al: Fixation of the cemented stem: clinical relevance of the porosity and thickness of the cement mantle. Open Orthop J 3:8–13, 2009.

113. Mann KA, Ayers DC, Werner FW, et al: Tensile strength of the cement-bone interface depends on the amount of bone interdigitated with PMMA cement. J Biomech 30:339–346, 1997.

114. Robinson RP, Lovell TP, Green TM, Balley GA: Early femoral component loosening in DF-80 total hip arthroplasty. J Arthroplasty 4:55–64, 1989.

115. Ayers D, Mann K: The importance of proximal cement filling of the calcar region: a biomechanical justification. J Arthroplasty 18:103–109, 2003.

116. Alfaro-Adrian J, Gill HS, Murray DW: Cement migration after THR: a comparison of Charnley Elite and Exeter femoral stems using RSA. J Bone Joint Surg Br 81:130–134, 1999.

117. Catani F, Ensini A, Leardini A, et al: Migration of cemented stem and restrictor after total hip arthroplasty: a radiostereometry study of 25 patients with Lubinus SP II stem. J Arthroplasty 20:244–249, 2005.

118. Maher S, McCormack B: Quantification of interdigitation at bone cement/cancellous bone interfaces in cemented femoral reconstructions. Proc Inst Mech Eng (H) 213:347–354, 1999.

119. Ong A, Wong KL, Lai M, et al: Early failure of precoated femoral components in primary total hip arthroplasty. J Bone Joint Surg Am 84:786–792, 2002.

120. Gardiner RC, Hozack WJ: Failure of the cement-bone interface: a consequence of strengthening the cement-prosthesis interface? J Bone Joint Surg Br 76:49–52, 1994.

CHAPTER 5

Materials in Hip Surgery: Ultra-High-Molecular-Weight Polyethylene

Stephen Li

KEY POINTS

- Not one, but many, ultra-high-molecular-weight polyethylene (UHMWPE) materials have serviced the orthopedic community. From the beginning, variations in the material and in manufacturing had clinical consequences. Unfortunately, in many cases, the relationship of material variables to clinical outcome was not known at the time of introduction of new products.
- UHMWPE has been continuously evolving over the past 60 years, mirroring the continued increase in knowledge that bridges clinical results with basic science and engineering. Some care must be taken to fully evaluate new technology to ensure that, in solving old problems, we have not created new ones.
- Today's highly cross-linked UHMWPE materials are the result of a 60-year evolution of technologies. An understanding of this evolution will lead to a better understanding of today's products.
- The highly cross-linked UHMWPE materials in surgical use today provide different trade-offs between wear resistance, oxidation resistance, and fracture toughness. Because the longest clinical experience with these materials is still less than 10 years, the long-term survivorship of these products is not yet known.
- Several technologies, including metal-on-metal and ceramic-on-ceramic total hip replacements, provide zero laboratory wear. This means that clinical performance will be the only way to determine which technology will provide the best long-term survivorship.

INTRODUCTION

Ultra-high-molecular-weight polyethylene (UHMWPE) has been the bearing material of choice in total hip replacement for over 50 years. It is the goal of this chapter to provide the practicing surgeon with basic knowledge and science of UHMWPE and to discuss key issues of UHMWPE as they apply to clinical performance.

UHMWPE has been the bearing material of choice in total hip replacement since its first use by Sir John Charnley in 1962. In this chapter, we will review the history of UHMWPE in joint replacement, the current status of the technology, and possible future directions.

THE HISTORY OF BEARING MATERIALS

Since the advent of total hip replacement, relatively few polymeric materials have been actually used in total joint replacement. Scales provided the early history of bearing materials in total hip replacements in 1967. One of the first attempts at joint replacement was undertaken in 1890 by Berliner Professor Themistocles Glück (1853-1942). Glück produced an ivory ball and socket joint that he fixed to bone with nickel-plated screws. During this same period, Sir Robert Jones (1855-1933) used a strip of gold foil to cover reconstructed femoral heads. One amazing report indicated that one patient retained effective motion at the joint.[4] In 1936, brothers Robert (1901-1980) and Jean (1905-1995) Judet introduced polymethylmethacrylate as the first synthetic polymeric material used as replacement for the femoral head. However, these acrylic devices became loose quickly because of high wear rates.

The first total hip replacement is credited to Philip Wiles (1899-1966), who developed a stainless steel, metal-on-metal device in 1938. In 1940, Austin Moore (1899-1963) and Harold Bohlman (1873-1979) first implanted Vitallium (cobalt-chrome-molybdenum alloy; Dentsply Austenal, York, Pa) in a 46-year-old, 250-pound male patient. The metal implant was made from molds, which were based on radiographic measurements. The implant was approximately 12 inches long and was bolted to the external surface of the femur.

In the 1940s through the 1960s, the development of metal-on-metal hip replacements continued with the McKee-Farrar and Ring prostheses. However, these devices fell out of favor with the introduction of the Charnley device. However, the metal-on-metal devices went through a renaissance starting in the 1980s and, once again, are used extensively.

Charnley initially chose polytetrafluoroethylene (PTFE) as a bearing material based on its general chemical inertness and low coefficient of friction. The first Charnley design to use PTFE was what we now refer to as a *surface replacement prosthesis.* The femoral head was covered with a "cup" of PTFE, and the acetabulum was lined with another layer of PTFE. This was a polymer-against-polymer total hip replacement. He next developed a procedure that replaced the femoral head and neck with a Moore femoral stem and a 42-mm ball to articulate against the PTFE cup. Last, he introduced the 22.225[12,13]-mm ($\frac{7}{8}$ ″) acetabular head and the use of acrylic bone cement for fixation. The (PTFE) materials that Charnley used are widely and incorrectly referred to as *Teflon,* the most familiar name in PTFE materials. Although it appears that Teflon may have been used for a short period, in private correspondence, Charnley identified the actual materials specifically as Fluon G1 and Fluon G2, products of Imperial Chemical Industries.[14] Clinical failures with Fluon PTFE acetabular cups generally occurred within 1 to 2 years and were attributed to the low creep and abrasive wear resistance of PTFE resins. Charnley found that the wear of PTFE against a stainless steel head provided 7 to 10 mm of wear in less than 3 years. Charnley's results were first reported in 1972.

Credit is provided to Harry Craven, an engineer who worked with Charnley, who tested a material termed *high-molecular-weight polyethylene* (UHMWPE) that was given to him by a plastic gear salesman. This selection was remarkable given that the first hips using this material were implanted in 1962, and it has been the material of choice ever since.[1] As will be discussed, UHMWPE had just been discovered a few years before, and it had only recently become commercially available for industrial applications.

UHMWPE

In the early literature, UHMWPE is often incorrectly called *high-density polyethylene* (HDPE). To make matters more confusing, HDPE was actually used in a few rare instances. Significant property and performance differences between UHMWPE and HDPE have been observed. HDPE would be a poor bearing material for joint replacement, because it has less wear resistance and lower resistance to fracture and fatigue.[17] With a few known exceptions, which will be discussed later, very few implants were actually made of HDPE.

The polymeric bearing material of choice remains UHWMPE. Fabricated sheet and bar forms of UHMWPE were first introduced during the K-fair in Dusseldorf in 1955 under the name of RCH (Ruhrchemie) 1000. The original polymer resin (particles) from which these forms were made were named *GUR (granular UHMWPE Ruhrchemie)* resins. The material was invented at the site of Ruhrchemie in Oberhausen, Germany, where the first pilot plant was built in 1955, followed by the first commercial scale production plant in 1960.

UHMWPE is synthesized from the polymerization of ethylene. This is done via Ziegler-Natta catalysis, which allows the polymer to form linear chains. The Ziegler-Natta catalyst is made from $TiCl_4$ and an aluminum alkyl compound; hence the small amounts of Ti, Cl, and Al that are always found in elemental analysis of UHMWPE. The reaction is typically conducted at low polymerization pressures and temperatures, typically between 4 and 6 Bar pressures and between 66° C and 80° C. These mild conditions maximize the molecular weight (long chains) of the polymer and minimize branching. With some grades, a very fine calcium stearate powder can be added to serve as an oxidant that minimizes yellowing of the material during subsequent fabrication processes.

UHMW RESINS

Since 2002, the main supplier of the UHMWPE materials used in orthopedics is Ticona (Auburn Hills, NJ), a business unit of Celanese. However, the history of suppliers and grades of UHMWPE is somewhat confusing. Before approximately 2002, there were two major suppliers of UHMWPE for medical implants, and each supplier also provided several grades of GUR resins.

As stated previously, Ruhrchemie first introduced RCH1000 in the 1950s. The first products fabricated from RCH1000 were made from GUR 412 resin. When the material was sold for medical applications, it was called *RCH1000C* and was made from GUR 112 resin. Although the physical properties of RCH1000 and RCH1000C were much the same, RCH1000C had lower levels of extraneous contaminants, and the final shaped material was ultrasonically checked to ensure that there were no unsintered areas. As the market for medical applications grew, fabricated forms of UHMWPE for medical applications were named *Chirulen,* and powder sold for medical applications of RCH1000C was renamed *Chirulen P.* In 1988, Ruhrchemie merged with the Hoechst/Celanese Corporation, which included operations in the United States in Bishop, Texas. In 1999, Celanese and another wholly owned company by Hoechst—Ticona—were separated from the Hoechst/Celanese Corporation. Ticona is now part of the Celanese Corporation and manufactures GUR UHMWPE for use in medical applications. This sequence of business changes had direct influence on the grades of materials sold to the medical community.

In the early 1990s, Hoechst/Celanese developed a four-number naming system for GUR resins (e.g., 4150 GUR) based on the manufacturing location, the molecular weight, and the presence of additives:
- The first digit of the code indicated whether the resin was made in Germany (1) or the United States (4).
- The second digit indicated the presence (1) or absence (0) of calcium stearate.
- The third digit indicated a molecular weight of 2 million (2) or 5 million (5).
- The fourth digit was always 0, and its meaning is not generally known.

For example, the designation "GUR 4120" indicates that the resin was manufactured in the United States (4) with the addition of calcium stearate (1), and it has a molecular weight of approximately 2 million. In the literature, the last "0" is often omitted in material descriptions; thus GUR 4120 resin is termed "*GUR 412.*" At this time, sheets sold for medical applications in Europe were termed "*Chirulen P.*" In the 1990s, the United States produced resins for medical applications that had "HP"

Table 5-1. Available UHMWPE Resins, 1995

Resin Name	Supplier
1900	Himont (Montel)
412 GUR	Hoechst Celanese (Texas)
415 GUR	
4050 HP	
4150 HP	
1020 HP	Hoechst (Germany)
1120 HP	
1050 HP	
1150 HP	

UHMWPE, Ultra-high-molecular-weight polyethylene.

Table 5-2. Names for Non–Highly CrossLinked UHMWPE Resins and Products

Enduron	415 GUR		DePuy
Hylamer, Hylamer M	415 GUR	Increased crystallinity	DePuy/Du Pont
Sulene	1020 GUR	Gamma sterilized, vacuum packed	Zimmer
Duramer	415 GUR	Ram extruded	Wright Medical Technology, Inc.
Arcom	1900	Hot isostatic pressed	Biomet
Duration	1020	Post irradiated heated 50C 144 hours	Stryker

UHMWPE, Ultra-high-molecular-weight polyethylene.

added to their GUR name to indicate *high purity*. Thus, GUR 4150 sold for medical applications was designated "GUR 4150HP." However, in 1998, the names of all the resins were consolidated. All medical resins now started with the number 1. The other three numbers still have their original meaning. The four available resins are now designated 1150, 1050, 1120, and 1020. However, because of market-driven purchasing, 1050 and 1020, the calcium stearate–free grades, are the major resins sold for medical applications.

1900 Resins

The other UHMWPE resin used in joint replacement was originally sold under the name "Hifax 1900," then "Himont 1900," and now, simply, "1900 resin." No 1900 resins have been sold to U.S. manufacturers since 2002. However, both Zimmer Orthopedics and Biomet made large purchases of 1900 just before it became unavailable for use in orthopedics, which allowed both companies to continue for several years the manufacture of implants traditionally made from 1900.

Similar to the GUR resins, several grades of 1900 were sold. They were designated "Hifax 1900," "Hifax 1900H," "Hifax 1900L," and "Hifax 1900CM." The differences in these grades were seen in their average molecular weight.

The grades of UHMWPE that were being supplied or used by orthopedic companies in 1995 are listed in Table 5-1. By this time, names containing "RCH1000" and "Chirulen" were no longer used. In 2010, the only resins available to orthopedic surgeons are GUR 1050 and GUR 1020 from Ticona. In addition to these resin names, in some instances, manufacturers have provided separate trade names to identify their products. These names have been used in the literature to describe different implants for correlation with clinical and laboratory performance, and are described more fully in Table 5-2.

Characteristics and Properties of UHMWPE

Molecular Weight

A key material property for UHMWPE is its molecular weight, because this property distinguishes UHMWPE from the other forms of polyethylene and determines the properties and behavior of the polymer. The molecular weight of UHMWPE is generally determined

experimentally by measuring the *relative* viscosity of solutions of the material at different concentrations. However, the higher the molecular weight of UHMWPE, the more difficult it is to dissolve in suitable solvents. For this reason, it is difficult to determine the molecular weight of any polymer when the value exceeds 1,000,000.

The specific method used to determine the molecular weight of UHMWPE is described in American Society for Testing and Materials (ASTM) Standard D-4020. In this method, a dilute solution of UHMWPE is made by dissolving a small amount of UHMWPE powder in decahydronapthalene.

The relative viscosity of the solution is determined with a capillary viscometer, which measures the rate of flow of the solution through a small orifice. The measured value of the relative viscosity is then used to estimate the average molecular weight of the polymer using the Mark-Houwink equation:

$$[\eta] = KM^a$$

where η is the intrinsic viscosity, M is the average molecular weight, and K and a are constants that vary with the solvent used and the temperature at which the measurements are made.

Once the value for $[\eta]$, is determined, the molecular weight can be estimated using the following equation:

Nominal viscosity molecular weight $= 5.37 \times 10^4 [\eta]^{1.37}$

Care must be taken in comparing molecular weight values from different sources, because it is possible that different equations were used, resulting in the possibility of different molecular weight values from the same viscosity measurements.

Physical Properties

The standards for physical properties are provided in ASTM DF-648, Standard Specification for Ultra-High-Molecular-Weight Polyethylene Powder and Fabricated Form for Surgical Implants. In this standard, requirements are given for the powdered resins provided for three types of UHMWPE, designated types 1,

Table 5-3. ASTM F648 UHMWPE Specifications

Property	Type 1	Type 2	Type 3
Viscosity number, mL/g	2000-3200	>3200	>3200
Elongation stress	.20	.42	.42
Ash (max mg/kg)	125	125	300
Ti	40	40	150
Al	20	20	100
Cl	30	30	90

Resin type spans Type 1, Type 2, Type 3.

UHMWPE, Ultra-high-molecular-weight polyethylene.

2, and 3, where type 1 comprises GUR resins with molecular weight of approximately 2 million (1020), type 2 GUR resins with molecular weights of approximately 5 (e.g., 1150), and type 3 1900 resins. Requirements for the powder resin of these three types are presented in Table 5-3.

Fabrication Methods

As described previously, UHWMPE is synthesized as a powder, which is formed into solid shapes by one of three methods: extrusion and machining, sheet compression molding and machining, and direct compression molding.

Extrusion and Machining. In this process, powder is continuously fed into a heated chamber. A ram pushes this powder into a heated cylindrical barrel, retracts, leaving the chamber empty, and waits for the next fixed amount of powder. The process is continuous, and each push of the ram advances the polyethylene through the heated barrel. In this manner, the powder is consolidated into a continuous cylindrical rod, which is then cut into 10-foot lengths for sale. Implants are machined from this cylindrical bar stock.

Sheet Compression Molding. In this process, the UHMWPE powder is introduced into a large rectangular container, typically measuring 4′ × 8′. A platen large enough to cover the entire container is used to apply pressure to the heated container. In this manner, sheets are formed that are up to 8 inches thick and measure up to 8 feet in length and width. Implants can be machined from these molded sheets.

Direct Compression Molding. Powder is placed into a mold in the shape of the final component and then is heated under pressure to achieve consolidation. After the mold has cooled, the net shape implant is removed and packaged. Devices formed in this fashion have no external machining lines and often exhibit a highly glossy surface finish. The properties of directly molded components are different from those of components produced by extrusion or compression molded sheet. This will be discussed in a subsequent section. The production advantages of direct compression molding are that it is possible to make very complicated geometries in a single step, the surface finish of the polyethylene is extremely smooth, and the process imparts beneficial properties to the UHMWPE. Disadvantages are that the process is relatively slow (e.g., expensive),

and individual molds must be made for each product. Reports indicate that direct molded components have lower wear rates than their corresponding extruded bar/compression molded sheet and machining components. Bankston and associates reported a 50% reduction in the average clinical wear rate of directly molded components compared with machined components (.05 mm/yr vs .11 mm/yr, respectively). These same differences in wear rates were noted in hip simulation wear studies.

As a final processing step, some suppliers anneal their bars after ram extrusion to presumably remove any residual stresses. The conditions of the annealing are proprietary, but they involve heating the material, which complicates the thermal history of the bar.

Sterilization Methods and Oxidation

Since it became commercially available in the late 1960s, the dominant method used for sterilization of UHMWPE components has been gamma irradiation from a Co^{60} source. In addition to sterilizing the material, the gamma rays create free radicals within the UHMWPE that can react with other free radicals within the polymer, and with oxygen from the atmosphere. These reactions are generally described as oxidation reactions. As will be seen, over the past 10 years, the issue of oxidation has greatly influenced methods of sterilization and methods used to improve the performance of UHMWPE.

The mechanisms of oxidation have been discussed at length elsewhere and will only be summarized here. Exposure of UHMWPE to gamma rays or electron beams can cause rupture of the carbon-carbon or carbon-hydrogen bonds. In either case, two free radicals are formed for each bond that is broken. These free radicals generally are very reactive and will undergo one of the following reactions:

1. Free radicals can extract a hydrogen atom from another carbon atom on the polymer and thus form another free radical.
2. Free radicals can break a bond within the polymer chain. This will reduce the molecular weight of the material and increase its density.
3. Free radicals can react with oxygen or any other molecules dissolved within the part, forming new chemical moieties, including carbonyls, ketones, and esters with carbon-oxygen double bonds.
4. Free radicals can combine to make a "cross-link" between polymer molecules, whether different molecules or even different sites within the same molecule.
5. Free radicals can, through atomic rearrangement, form double bonds within single polymer chains.

These different reaction pathways lead to chemical changes that can be measured in a variety of ways. Infrared spectroscopy can be used to detect the presence of chemical moieties such as carbonyl groups and double bonds, which appear after oxidation has occurred. In 1990, Fourier transform infrared (FTIR) was introduced as an updated form of the dispersive infrared method used by Eyerer. FTIR provided more sensitive than traditional infrared methods and allowed determination of the relative amounts of oxidative products as a function of depth from the surface of a sample.[27] This method is now described in ASTM 1421. It is important to note that values of oxidation measured with FTIR can be highly variable, with differences between test laboratories exceeding 129% under certain conditions. This large variability indicates that care must be taken in comparing values of the oxidation index of UHMWPE samples tested in different laboratories or at different times.

Oxidation also leads to increases in density of the UHMWPE, hence the reported change in density of UHMWPE samples with shelf aging in air after gamma irradiation with a dose of 25 to 40 KGy. The change in density is a slow process, with change of approximately 0.003 g/mL/yr noted. Density is measured with the use of a density gradient column and a protocol provided in ASTM D-1505. It should be noted that quality defects such as subsurface white bands and nonconsolidated particles appear at density values >0.95 g/mL.

It has been known since the late 1970s from the study of retrieved implants that UHMWPE oxidizes after gamma sterilization, and that physical properties may be adversely affected. However, UHMWPE oxidation was not considered a major clinical factor in limiting the performance of total hip replacement at that time. It was not until the early 1990s that interest in oxidation was rekindled, as factors that could influence the generation of particulate debris were sought out. If postirradiation aging is severe enough, the quality of a polyethylene component can be adversely affected, as is evidenced by the presence of nonconsolidated particles or by polyethylene exhibiting subsurface white bands on cross-sectioning. Collier and coworkers reported that 20% of acetabular components implanted for 4 years or longer exhibited signs of fracture and fatigue due to oxidation. Further, it was demonstrated that, over time, the mechanical properties of gamma-sterilized UHWMPE components that were not implanted were also reduced through the effects of oxidation. These reports and others showed that oxidation of UHWMPE after gamma irradiation in air could reduce its strength and fracture resistance, and that this process began immediately after irradiation and continued for years. However, because the rate of this process was relatively slow, guidelines were adopted that recommended that UHMWPE components exposed to gamma irradiation in air should be implanted within 5 years of sterilization. By 1996, most manufacturers had modified the gamma sterilization process or had abandoned gamma sterilization in favor of alternative methods in an attempt to minimize the effects of postirradiation oxidation. Common methods that did not employ ionizing radiation included sterilization with ethylene oxide or gas plasma; however, because these methods did not provide any cross-linking, they did not lead to improvement in the wear properties of UHMWPE.

It now appears that in the vast majority cases, oxidation does not significantly or adversely influence the clinical wear rate of UHMWPE components. This view is based on the following considerations.

The rate of postirradiation aging of UHMWPE outside the body is very slow. Typically, components must be stored for longer than 4 years under ambient conditions for visible signs of degradation to appear, such as the development of unconsolidated polyethylene particles and subsurface bands of embrittled material as observed in sectioned components. Because most devices are implanted within 4 years of sterilization, the amount of oxidation is generally low. Although ex vivo oxidation of UHMWPE has been well studied, in vivo oxidation is a more controversial topic. The conclusions of literature reports range from claims that little or no oxidation occurs in vivo to the assertion that oxidation is actually faster in vivo than ex vivo.[44] This subject has been difficult to elucidate because the oxidation state of retrieved implants is not known prior to implantation. Moreover, it has been reported that other factors such as mechanical loading, wear, and the polyethylene manufacturing process can significantly influence the rate of oxidation of UHMWPE in vivo.

Few reports convincingly correlate oxidation of UHMWPE to increased wear rate. Hip simulation studies of acetabular cups with postirradiation aging times ranging up to 10 years showed that significant oxidation of UHMWPE did not adversely affect the rate of wear.[46] In a report on the analysis of wear and oxidation level of 100 retrieved Charnley acetabular cups, it was noted that there was no correlation ($r^2 < 0.1$) between degree of oxidation of the polyethylene and radiographically or directly measured wear.[48]

In three reports on hip simulator tests, the wear of acetabular inserts was reduced by 30% to 46% after gamma irradiation (both in air and in an inert atmosphere) in comparison with rates after sterilization with ethylene oxide gas.[50] This was due primarily to the beneficial effects of cross-linking on the mechanical properties of UHMWPE, which is a by-product of gamma ray exposure, in addition to increased wear resistance and embrittlement with aging.

Dramatic loss of fracture toughness and fatigue resistance of UHMWPE with oxidation has led to catastrophic failure of some designs of implants that had regions of exceedingly high stress concentration. A well-publicized example is the acetabular cup system (ACS) liner, which was recalled by DePuy Orthopaedics (Warsaw, Ind) in 1989 because of rim fractures. This component was designed with a metal-backed shell that provided support only for the polyethylene insert around the rim. The liners that fractured in clinical service had a wall thickness of only 2.5 mm, which, in combination with high levels of oxidation, led to rim fractures in a small percent of cases.

The current view is that high-energy irradiation is the preferred method of sterilization of UHMWPE. Adverse effects of postirradiation aging are limited to decreases in fracture and fatigue resistance, without reduced wear resistance. Postirradiation issues can be minimized by irradiating components in a low-oxygen environment (e.g., vacuum, nitrogen, argon). The use of nonirradiation methods such as ethylene oxide gas has provided products that will not oxidize as the result of irradiation but have higher wear rates caused by lack of cross-linking. The issue of oxidation, however, has greatly influenced the adoption of methods of treatment of UHMWPE with higher doses of radiation used to minimize wear. This will be discussed in detail later under the section, "Highly Cross-Linked UHMWPE."

Modifications to Ultra-High-Molecular-Weight Polyethylene

Several notable efforts have been undertaken to improve the clinical performance of UHMWPE through material modifications. Four of these efforts will be reviewed here: carbon fiber reinforcement, increased crystallinity of UHMWPE, cross-linking of UHMWPE, and the addition of antioxidants.

Carbon-Reinforced

In the late 1970s, in an effort to reduce creep (cold flow) of UHMWPE and to decrease wear, Zimmer Inc. (Mendham, NJ) developed a material called *Poly II,* which was a reinforced composite of UHMWPE and carbon fibers. This composite was made by directly molding short carbon fibers and polyethylene powder into tibial inserts, patellar buttons, and acetabular components. The addition of carbon fibers led to increased compressive and flexural yield strength, tensile properties, and creep resistance, and to improved wear resistance. The magnitude of these changes in properties increased with the amount of fiber added.[56] However, after these materials had been introduced for clinical use, they were found to have lower fatigue resistance than UHMWPE. Additionally, the materials suffered from manufacturing problems associated with incomplete molding. This led to poor adhesion of fibers to the polyethylene matrix, as evidenced by apparent fiber pull-out during in vivo use. Efforts to improve adhesion between fibers and matrix, such as changing the geometry of the fibers or the use of coatings, did lead to significant clinical improvement. Surface damage scores of retrieved Poly II components were also higher than those of unreinforced UHMWPE components. Its use was discontinued approximately 7 years after its introduction into the marketplace. It is interesting to note that no reports have described the long-term clinical performance of these devices.

Highly Crystalline

Since Charnley's first use of UHMWPE in the 1960s, no purposeful changes have been made to the UHMWPE resin itself to improve clinical performance. Different grades of UHWMPE were available, as was the choice of UHWMPE over calcium stearate, but these variations were largely due to the general commercial use of UHWMPE, and the variations were not introduced for the benefit of the medical applications.

In the early 1990s, a new of form of UHMWPE, called *Hylamer* (Dupont, Wilmington, Del), was specifically developed for use in orthopedic implants. This material was manufactured by subjecting fabricated shapes of UIHMWPE, such as extruded GUR 415, to very high pressures (>235 MPa) and high temperatures (>300° C),

followed by cooling at a slow, controlled rate. This process increased the crystallinity of UHMWPE from normal values of 50% to 60% to 60% to 90%. The two commercial products made from this process were called *Hylamer* and *Hylamer M.* Hylamer had a crystallinity of approximately 70% and was used in acetabular liners and glenoid shoulder components. Hylamer M had a crystallinity of approximately 60% and was used in the production of tibial inserts. In general, increasing crystallinity through the Hylamer process led to a material with higher yield strength, tensile strength, creep resistance, impact resistance, and modulus. However, it was subsequently reported that no improvement in wear resistance was seen in hip simulator tests.[63]

Early clinical results of Hylamer inserts implanted in Duraloc cups (DePuy) were not promising. Chmell reported that after a minimum follow-up time of 2 years, 5 of 143 acetabular components were revised (4.2%) for severe eccentric wear. The 4-year survivorship was estimated to be as low as 86%. In a second study of 191 patients with 28-mm Hylamer liners, Livingston reported average wear rates more than double those of conventional UHMWPE (0.27 vs 0.12 mm/yr, respectively). However, during the same period, Sychertz and associates reported no differences in clinical wear rates in a comparative study of Hylamer against conventional UHMWPE liners. Subsequently, it was recognized that variations in reported Hylamer wear rates were due to several factors in addition to the choice of bearing material, including patient age, the combination of heads and cups from different manufacturers, and the choice of material for the femoral head. Another factor that adversely affected Hylamer performance was oxidation. Hylamer components appeared to oxidize just as rapidly as UHMWPE components after shelf aging for 3 or more years postirradiation, leading to loss of mechanical properties and fracture resistance. The use of Hylamer as a bearing material decreased rapidly in the late 1990s.

Highly Cross-Linked

Highly cross-linked UHMWPE products are currently in widespread use. The concept of using high dosages of irradiation to improve the wear rate of UHMWPE was first introduced in the early 1970s. Between 1971 and 1978, Oonishi implanted acetabular liners made from high-density UHMWPE that had been irradiated at 100 Mrads. This dosage was determined via laboratory wear measurements of polyethylene components irradiated at many different doses from 30 to 1000 Mrads (3 to 100 Mrads). In one work, Oonishi refers to three different materials described as Hizex Million, Hizex Million 340M, and RCH1000. Hizex is the name of a family of polyethylene products sold by the Mitsui Petrochemical Company Ltd. (Tokyo, Japan). The value of the molecular weight of Hizex Million is not clear without additional grade information, but it is possibly a high-density polyethylene (Table 5-4). The original prosthesis developed in 1971 was named *SOM* for Dr. Shikita, Dr. Oonishi, and Mizuho Co. Ltd. (Tokyo, Japan). The SOM prosthesis had femoral components made from COP

Table 5-4. Hizex UHMWPE Resins	
Grade	Molecular Weight (millions)
Hizex Million 145M	.7
Hizex Million 240	1.9
Hizex Million 340M	2.7

UHMWPE, Ultra-high-molecular-weight polyethylene.

alloy (stainless steel and 20% cobalt) measuring 28 or 32 mm diameter.

Several clinical series were conducted to compare the wear of unirradiated UHMWPE versus highly irradiated polyethylene against stainless steel and ceramic femoral heads. It is unclear which specific form of polyethylene was used in these clinical evaluations. It could have been a high-density polyethylene or one of the Hizex Million grades, or both. It should be noted that many cases were excluded from the evaluation. Excluded cases included cases where the acetabular or femoral component was loosened or migrated, or where it comprised metal-backed components and those not having acceptable radiographs.

The wear rate of the highly cross-linked (100 Mrads) polyethylene (0.076 mm/yr) was less than that of unirradiated UHMWPE (0.25 mm/yr). However, the value of 0.076 mm/yr is not much lower than the 0.1 mm/yr reported in other studies for UHMWPE irradiated at 2.5 to 4 Mrads.

Because Oonishi irradiated his components in the air, oxidation is expected. This has been confirmed by Sugano and colleagues, who reported that retrieved cups that had been irradiated at 100 Mrads in air demonstrated increased oxidation levels. An interesting and potentially important finding of this work was the presence of a fracture in the bearing surface of a retrieved cup after 24 years of implantation. This fracture possibly occurred because of sudden changes in joint loading that accompanied mechanical failure of the femoral stem, but was not associated with any changes in the radiographic appearance of the component. This liner fracture is consistent with the reduction in fracture resistance that accompanies the use of increased dosages of gamma irradiation. This will be discussed in detail in the following section.

Acetylene Cross-Linked: Grobbelar and Weber

In 1978, Grobbelaar and co-workers reported that the wear and mechanical properties of UHMWPE could be improved by the use of gamma irradiation in an atmosphere containing cross-linking agents such as acetylene and chlorotrifluoroethylene (CTFE). These cross-linking agents were used to increase the level of surface cross-linking at lower dosages of irradiation.

The process used to prepare acetabular cups with this method consisted of the following steps:

1. Machine acetabular cups into their final dimensions from extruded bars of RCH1000.
2. Gamma irradiate the cups to a dose of 100 KGy (10 Mrads) in a stainless steel container in the presence of an undisclosed amount of acetylene gas.
3. Package the irradiated cups and sterilize with gamma irradiation at 25 KGy (2.5 Mrads).[78]

This process yielded a material with a highly cross-linked outer layer with a thickness of 300 microns. The material measuring less than 300 microns was described as having eight times less cross-linking than the outer 300-micron layer. Femoral components consisted of a modified Charnley-type prosthesis made from stainless steel. The femoral head was 30 mm in diameter.

Between 1977 and 1982, 650 of these acetylene cross-linked components were implanted in Pretoria South Africa by Dr. C.J. Grobbelaar. An additional 409 components were implanted in Johannesburg, South Africa, by Dr. F.A. Weber. Although more than 1000 of these components were implanted, only 10% of patients had long-term follow-up. Sixty-four of the 650 Pretoria implanted patients and 39 of the Johannesburg patients were followed for an average of 15 years. Unfortunately, the long-term performance of more than 90% of these components is not known. However, of the 10% for which long-term follow-up of an average of 15.5 years was available, 83% demonstrated no measurable wear on the basis of conventional radiographs. The average wear rate of the 17% that demonstrated measurable wear was 0.09 mm/yr. Use of this acetylene cross-linked UHMWPE was resumed in the late 1990s; it is manufactured by Barc (Johannesburg, South Africa) and continues to be used in South Africa today.

In 1996, Wroblewski reported the clinical performance of material named *XLP*, which was UHWMPE that had been cross-linked using a Silane coupling agent. He implanted 19 XLP cups in 17 patients with a Charnley femoral stem and found that there was a "bedding-in period," during which femoral head penetration into the liner ranged between 0.2 and 0.4 mm and averaged 0.29 mm/yr. After 2 years, average wear rate decreased to 0.022 mm/yr. This was in contrast to the steady-state wear rate of 0.07 mm/yr that was observed in bearing couples with gamma sterilized (2.5 to 4 Mrads) acetabular cups. No reports have described the implantation of additional total hip replacements using XLP.

CONTEMPORARY MATERIALS: HIGHLY CROSS-LINKED UHMWPE

As described previously, UHMWPE components were initially sterilized by gamma irradiation in air, as used by Charnley since 1968. This was followed by a period from approximately 1990 to 1996, during which UHMWPE components were packaged in a vacuum or in an inert environment prior to gamma sterilization, in an attempt to minimize oxidation and increase cross-linking. This led to reduction in laboratory wear rates of 15% to 30%. The next approach used to improve the performance of UHMWPE was to increase the gamma irradiation dose.

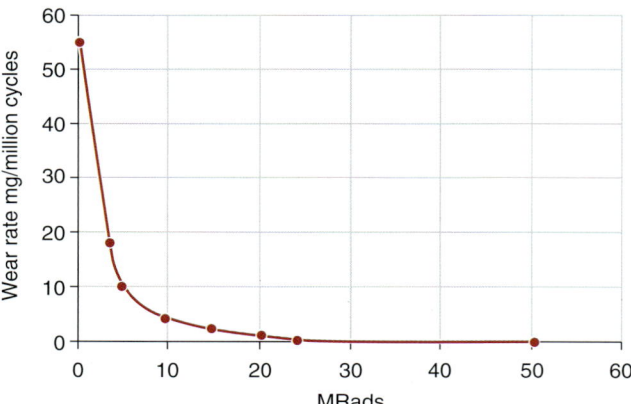

Figure 5-1. Hip simulator wear rate (mg/million cycles) versus gamma irradiation dose (MRads).

Table 5-5. Association of Wear Rate and Osteolysis

Clinical Wear Rate, mm/yr	Incidence of Osteolysis at 10 Years,%
>.3	100
.2-.3	80
.1-.2	43
<.1	0

Data from Wilkinson JM, Hamer AJ, Stockley I, Eastell R: Polyethylene wear rate and osteolysis: critical threshold versus continuous dose-response relationship. J Orthop Res 23:520–525, 2005.

Although it was known since the work of Oonishi that increasing gamma dosage would decrease wear (e.g., increase wear resistance), developments in the 1990s sought to optimize wear reduction and minimize oxidation. McKellop reported the results of hip simulator wear rates as a function of irradiation dose (Fig. 5-1). From the figure, it is clear that wear rates decrease as irradiation dose increases, and little benefit, in terms of wear resistance, is derived if the dose exceeds 100 KGy (10 Mrads). However, it was also known that irradiation generates free radicals, potentially leading to oxidation and thus to reduced resistance to fracture. To address this, some manufacturers subjected the UHMWPE to a postirradiation heating step to "quench" the free radicals and increase the number of cross-links. The result was the establishment of three different postirradiation heating regimes: (1) no postirradiation heat treatment, (2) postirradiation heat treatment below the melting point of the UHMWPE, and (3) postirradiation heating of the UHMWPE to above the melting point of UHMWPE. As will be described later, no two formulations of highly cross-linked UHMWPE used in the manufacture of implants are the same. They differ in terms of starting resin, type of irradiation, temperature at which irradiation occurs, irradiation dose, postirradiation heat treatment, and method of sterilization. Characteristics of various commercially available highly cross-linked types of UHMWPE are summarized in Appendix 5-2.

How Much Wear Resistance Do You Need?

The goals of the latest forms of highly cross-linked UHMWPE were to reduce the wear rate and to provide oxidation resistance to UHMWPE. By all accounts, it appears that these goals have been met. However, it is not clear how much clinical benefit these material improvements will provide, that is, will the reduction in wear offered by these new materials eliminate the problem of osteolysis and provide total hip replacement with improved survivorship?

All of the commercially available highly cross-linked forms of UHMWPE (irradiated at dosages greater than 60 KGy) show zero wear in hip simulator testing, that is, the wear rate is below the detection limit of wear simulation studies. However, in every clinical study undertaken since Oonishi introduced the 1000-KGy (100-Mrad) irradiated UHMWPE in 1978, true wear rates observed in clinical use have exceeded those predicted by laboratory testing. In this sense, laboratory wear simulations cannot distinguish one form of UHMWPE from another, nor precisely predict the clinical wear rate of these materials. The wear rates of some types of highly cross-linked UHMWPE observed in clinical studies are provided in Table 5-5. These wear rates (highly cross-linked vs. control, respectively) are derived from the head penetration rates. Despite differences noted in comparative controls, femoral heads, and so forth, it is clear that highly cross-linked UHMWPE materials provide a significant reduction in wear in vivo. It is also interesting to note that the clinical wear rate of Marathon is essentially the same as that of Longevity, Durasul, Crossfire, XLPE, and X3, despite the fact that Marathon is irradiated at 50 KGy, and the others are irradiated above 90 KGy.

CURRENT CONTROVERSIES OF HIGHLY CROSS-LINKED UHMWPE

Although currently available highly cross-linked products all exhibit wear properties superior to those of UHMWPE irradiated at dosages less than 40 KGy (4 Mrads), some associated potential disadvantages and controversies have been identified.

Controversy 1. Will Highly Cross-Linked UHMWPE Eliminate or Reduce the Incidence of Osteolysis Over the Long Term?

From Table 5-6, it is clear that reported wear results for all highly cross-linked UHMWPE with up to 7 years follow-up time are very good. However, the true long-term performance of these materials will not be truly known until significant numbers of these components reach 15-year, 20-year, and longer time periods. Lower wear rates would be expected to lower the incidence of

Table 5-6. Clinical Wear Rates of Highly Cross-Linked UHMWPE (Head Size: 28 mm)

Study	Material	Wear Rate (mm/yr)		Reduction, %
		XLPE	Control	
Dorr, 2005	Durasul	0.029	0.065	55
D'Antonio, 2005	Crossfire	0.036	0.13	72
Engh, 2006	Marathon	0.01	0.19	95
Leung, 2007	Marathon	0.06	0.2	70
Olyslaegers, 2008	Longevity	0.05	0.1	50
Garcia-Rey, 2008	Durasul	0.006	0.038	84
Bitsch, 2008	Marathon	0.039	0.1	61
Glyn Jones, 2008	Longevity	0.03	0.07	57
Geerdink, 2009	Duration	0.088	0.14	37
Average values				
	All grades	0.039	0.11	66
	Marathon	0.036	0.163	78
	Non-Marathon	0.040	0.091	56

UHMWPE, Ultra-high-molecular-weight polyethylene.

osteolysis, but an interesting question is how much reduction in osteolysis will actually be achieved.

Dowd and associates reported on a study of 48 32-mm total hip replacements with a minimum 10-year follow-up. The UHMWPE was gamma in air sterilized at a dosage between 25 and 40 KGy. Investigators found no incidences of osteolysis when the 10-year wear rate was less than 0.1 mm/yr of femoral head penetration into the UHMWPE liner. Data from this study are summarized in Table 5-5.

These results suggest that if the average rate is less than 0.1 mm/yr for a non–highly cross-linked UHMWPE, no osteolysis would be expected for at least 10 years. This is important because wear rates less than 0.1 mm/yr have been reported for non–highly cross-linked acetabular liners.[105,106,108] Lower wear rates reported for highly cross-linked products to 7 years strongly suggest that the incidence of osteolysis will be lower, but these values indicate that improvement in osteolysis rates may require long evaluation times.

In a larger study, Wilkinson examined the relationship between osteolysis and wear in 230 patients with acetabular cups made from non–highly cross-linked UHMWPE by studying equal numbers of patients with and without osteolysis (115 in each group). Average wear in the osteolysis group was 0.12 mm/yr versus 0.07 mm/yr in the nonosteolysis group (*P* <.001). Although this appears to support the concept of a threshold value for osteolysis, 9% of patients who exhibited osteolysis had wear rates less than 0.05 mm/yr. Important conclusions from this work are that osteolysis is more prevalent when the radiographic wear rate is greater than 0.1 mm/yr, but reduction of wear rates to below 0.1 mm/yr does not eliminate osteolysis. Similar results were reported from another study comparing the average 5-year clinical wear of 36 highly cross-linked UHMWPE cups (Marathon, DePuy) against 40 cups fabricated from conventional UHMWPE (no irradiation, gas plasma sterilized; Enduron, DePuy). In this

case, it was found that 11 of 40 (28%) patients with conventional UHMWPE and 3 of 36 (8%) patients with XLPE components exhibited radiographic changes interpreted as osteolysis.

There is no question that highly cross-linked UHMWPE acetabular liners have significantly lower rates than components that were irradiated at dosages less than 40 KGy. However, clinical results at 5-year follow-up indicate that osteolysis is not eliminated, even when wear rates are very low. The incidence of osteolysis at 10 years and longer for these highly cross-linked components is not yet known.

Controversy 2. Highly Cross-Linked UHMWPE Is More Prone to Fracture and Fatigue

To review some concepts introduced earlier in this chapter, oxidation of UHMWPE occurs slowly within the body and reduces the fracture and fatigue resistance of UHMWPE.

Irradiation of UHMWPE components with doses exceeding 40 KGy (4 Mrads) creates additional free radicals, which potentially can lead to additional oxidation of UHMWPE over time. To address this issue, most, but not all, of the commercially available UHMWPE products have used a postirradiation heating step to eliminate free radicals and increase the level of cross-linking. Postirradiation melting significantly alters the fracture resistance of highly cross-linked polyethylene. It is important to note that not all commercially available highly cross-linked materials undergo postirradiation melting. However, at the time of this writing, Longevity, Durasul, Marathon, and XLPE all undergo a postirradiation melting procedure.

Numerous reports have indicated that both increased irradiation dosage and postirradiation melting of UHMWPE reduce fracture and fatigue resistance of the material. Because products not treated with postirradiation melting retain their fracture toughness, a tradeoff between short- and long-term properties must be accepted if oxidation is to be eliminated. The question is, which have greater clinical consequences—materials with reduced fracture toughness as a consequence of postirradiation melting, or materials that exhibit slow loss of fracture toughness via oxidative pathways? To answer this question, the incidence of fracture in non–highly cross-linked liners will be reviewed. This would set the minimum incidence of fracture that we would expect to see in highly cross-linked products, if it is assumed that the decrease in fracture toughness of highly cross-linked material does not result in increased fracture incidence.

In a study by Birman and associates of 120 retrieved acetabular liners, 40% showed the presence of fracture or fatigue damage. Similarly, Furman and colleagues reported that 58% of 165 retrieved acetabular liners exhibited fracture and fatigue damage. In many cases, the presence of fracture or fatigue phenomena was associated with high levels of oxidation and/or impingement. Shon and coworkers reported that 56% of 162 retrieved implants exhibited clear signs of impingement. It was also important to note that impingement of the liner was seen in 94% of cases when revision was performed after dislocation of the hip. It is clear that a significant number of acetabular liners made from non–highly cross-linked UHWMPE exhibit fracture and fatigue phenomena. Fracture and fatigue are also associated with the presence of impingement and oxidation.

Given that the fracture and fatigue resistance of highly cross-linked UHMWPE is less than that of non–cross-linked UHMWPE, the incidence and perhaps severity of fracture damage to highly cross-linked liner would be expected to be higher. Unfortunately, this concern has been demonstrated by several reports of fracture of highly cross-linked UHMWPE liners at short implant times. Halley reported a fracture longevity liner revised at 10 months. Moore reported a fractured 36-mm-diameter Longevity liner that was revised at 33 months. Tower and coworkers reported on two fractured longevity liners retrieved at 7 and 27 months. Furmanski and associates described four fractured liners made from Longevity (fractured in 12 months), XLPE (3 months), Durasul (29 months), and Marathon (65 months) highly cross-linked UHMWPE. All four of these highly cross-linked types of UHMWPE were processed through a postirradiation melting step.

In a broader study, Bradford and colleagues studied 24 retrieved highly cross-linked acetabular liners (Durasul, Zimmer) that had been implanted for periods ranging from 10 to 24 months. These liners were removed in conjunction with the 2000 Device Recall of mating acetabular shells caused by contamination of their porous coating during manufacture. A significant incidence of fracture and fatigue-related damage was noted in these retrieved components, namely, 79% (19/24) of liners had areas of pitting, and 71% (17/24) exhibited surface cracking or delamination. These were all "silent fractures," in that none of these retrievals were

undertaken because of failure of the UHMWPE liner. However, the concern is that the high prevalence of fracture and fatigue-related damage observed after these short periods of implantation may be predictive of an increased prevalence of catastrophic failure at longer times. These fractures are often associated with malposition of the acetabular shell. High degrees of cup abduction angle and anteversion can lead to impingement, which can result in fracture and device failure. The overall, long-term effects of postirradiation melting will not be known until clinical reviews have been performed after longer periods of implantation.

VITAMIN E–DOPED HIGHLY CROSS-LINKED UHMWPE

Recognition that postirradiation melting leads to reduced fracture toughness and reduced risk of mechanical failure of cross-linked bearing components has led to the introduction of new methods to eliminate free radicals. One such technology involves the addition of vitamin E (α-tocopherol) as a radical scavenger to react with free radicals within the UHMWPE before they can undergo oxidation reactions. Vitamin E is a liquid at room temperature with a melting point of 2° C to 3° C and a boiling point of about 210° C. It was long thought that vitamin E was a "natural" antioxidant that, among other benefits, prevented oxidation of cell membranes. However, more recently, the role of vitamin E has become less clear, and its role as an antioxidant may be secondary to its role as a signaling molecule for biological processes.

The process of adding vitamin E to UHMWPE begins by submerging a fabricated form of 1050 GUR UHMWPE in vitamin E at 120° C for 5 hours. The UHMWPE is then annealed with argon gas at 120° C for another 64 hours. UHMWPE components treated by this process are reported to have lower wear rates, greater resistance to oxidation, and greater fracture toughness than those fabricated from irradiated and melted UHMWPE.[109] It is interesting to note that this process involves postirradiation heat treatment of treated parts below the melt temperature, similar to that used in the manufacture of some other highly cross-linked UHMWPE products. It is difficult to assign a relative contribution to properties from 120° C treatments for a total of 71 hours versus the presence of vitamin E. No clinical evaluations of vitamin E UHWMPE have been performed at the time of this writing. However, further development of this product requires recognition of the adverse effects of postirradiation melting.

Recent advancements in highly cross-linked UHMWPE have led to the development of materials that have demonstrated unprecedented clinical reductions in wear for periods less than 10 years. As discussed previously, along with these improvements, some trade-offs were made that allow room for future improvements.

Future grades of highly cross-linked UHMWPE will be developed through optimization of process variations to find the best balance of wear, oxidation resistance, and fracture resistance. Although the very low wear rates of all types of highly cross-linked UHMWPE give good reason for optimism, early 5-year results have clearly established several issues that could limit the long-term survivorship of these products. It is not known why some studies of highly cross-linked UHMWPE have reported the presence of osteolysis at wear rates and implant times where osteolysis would not be expected even for non–highly cross-linked UHMWPE. Some highly cross-linked UHMWPE materials have been post irradiation melted in an attempt to avoid oxidation. However, this melting step also significantly reduces the fracture resistance of the material. It does seem to be clear that the use of highly cross-linked UHMWPE should be avoided when dislocation and impingement may occur. Highly cross-linked UHMWPE products that are post irradiation heated below the melt are trying to balance maintaining a certain level of fracture toughness with knowing that some oxidation will be likely. Because the absence of post irradiation melting does not affect the wear rate, the concept is that these materials will have the same low wear rates, but will be less susceptible to fracture and fatigue as long as the materials do not become significantly oxidized.

Given these concerns, close inspection of long-term clinical results and prudence in choosing when to use and not use a highly cross-linked UHMWPE should be adopted.

APPENDIX 5-1

Commercial Formulations of Conventional UHMWPE Used in THR

- **Arcom.** Arcom is a name that Biomet (Warsaw, Ind) applies to UHMWPE that has been consolidated by a hot isostatic molding process or by direct compression molding. In the hot isostatic molding process, 1900 powder is cold compacted into cylinders and then is heated and consolidated under isostatic pressure in an argon gas atmosphere. The resulting cylindrical bars are then machined into the final product. Arcom is also used to name the material resulting from direct compression molding of UHMWPE components, initially using 1900 powder, and later using GUR 1050.
- **Duramer.** Duramer is GUR 415 ram-extruded by Wright Medical Technology, Inc. (Arlington, Tenn) under proprietary conditions. No claims have been made for any physical property differences from other ram-extruded GUR 415 products, apart from increased consolidation of UHMWPE.
- **Duration.** Duration is manufactured by Stryker (Mahwah, NJ) from ram-extruded 4150 GUR UHMWPE.

Acetabular liners are machined from the bars, packed in an inert atmosphere, and irradiated at between 25 and 40 KGy. The product is then heated at 50° C for 144 hours.
- **Enduron.** DePuy (Warsaw, Ind) did not make its own polyethylene but trademarked Enduron as a name for the extruded GUR 415 polyethylene that it purchased.
- **Hylamer.** Hylamer and Hylamer M (Dupont, Wilmington, Del) are made from GUR UHMWPE that has been processed at very high temperatures and pressures to increase its crystallinity. These materials have significantly different mechanical properties from UHMWPE that has been processed by molding or extrusion processes and will be discussed in detail in a later section.
- **Sulene.** Sulene is manufactured by Zimmer (Warsaw, Ind). It is made from a 1020 GUR compression molded sheet that is machined into acetabular cups. The cups are irradiated in a nitrogen atmosphere package by gamma irradiation between 25 and 40 KGy.

Commercially Available Formulations of Highly Cross-Linked UHMWPE

- **Arcom XL.** Arcom XL is manufactured by Biomet (Warsaw, Ind). The manufacturing process for Arcom XL is significantly different from that for other highly cross-linked UHMWPE materials. The process begins with isostatically compressing 1050 GUR UHMWPE with argon gas into cylindrical bars. These bars are then irradiated at 50 KGy with gamma irradiation. The bar is heated to 130° C and then is extruded through a circular die with a compression ratio of 1.5:1. The bar is reheated to 130° C. Final parts are then machined from this bar. The complexity of the process makes it difficult to determine the relative contributions of predeformation heating, the deformation process, and postdeformation heating to the final properties.

- **Marathon and AltrX.** Marathon and AltrX cross-linked UHWMPE by DePuy/Johnson & Johnson are similarly manufactured. Marathon was introduced first and is made by irradiating ram-extruded bars of 1050 GUR at 50 KGy. These bars are then heated at 150° C for 24 hours. The final product is machined from the bar. AltrX is similar, except that the UHMWPE used is 1020 GUR, and 75 KGy of gamma irradiation is used. Postirradiation heat treatment is the same.

- **Longevity and Durasul.** Longevity and Durasul are manufactured by Zimmer (Warsaw, Ind) and are processed similarly. In each case, bars of 1050 GUR are irradiated by electron beam at dosages of 95 (Durasul) and 100 KGy (Longevity). Longevity is produced from 1050 GUR UHMWPE. The bars are heated to approximately 40° C prior to electron beam irradiation at 100 KGy. They are then heated past the melting point (150° C) for 6 hours. Acetabular cups are machined from these bars and sterilized with gas plasma. Durasul is also prepared from 1050 GUR UHMWPE bars. The bars are heated to 120° C prior to electron beam irradiation at 95 KGy. They are then heated to above the melting point (150° C) for 2 hours. Acetabular liners are machined from the bars and are sterilized with ethylene oxide.[93,98]

- **XLPE.** XLPE is manufactured by Smith and Nephew (Memphis, Tenn). XLPE is prepared by electron beam irradiation of 1050 GUR bars at a dosage of 100 KGy. The bars are then heated to above the melt temperature (150° C) for an unreported length of time. They are machined, and sterilization is provided by ethylene oxide.[98]

- **Crossfire.** Crossfire is manufactured by Stryker Orthopaedics (Mahwah, NJ). Crossfire is prepared by gamma irradiation of 1050 GUR extruded rod at 75 KGy. The bars are subjected to a heat treatment below the melt of the UHMWPE. The final part is machined and sterilization is accomplished with gamma irradiation at 25 KGy. The total irradiation dosage received by the UHMWPE is 100 KGy. This final sterilization step, without any postheat treatment, creates free radicals in the UHMWPE. As will discussed, this makes Crossfire susceptible to oxidation. However, below the melt heat treatment, in contrast to melting treatments, does not reduce the mechanical properties of the UHMWPE.

- **X3.** X3 cross-linked UHMWPE is manufactured by Stryker (Mahwah, NJ). In this process, bars of 1050 GUR are irradiated and below the melt annealed three times, that is, the bar is irradiated at 30 KGy and then is heat treated below the melt. This is repeated three times so that the UHMWPE receives 90 KGy of total irradiation. Acetabular cups are machined from the bars and sterilized with gas plasma. This process is claimed to provide wear resistance from the 90 KGy irradiation and oxidation resistance and minimum loss of mechanical properties via multiple below the melt heat treatments.

- **Connexion GXL.** Connexion GXL is manufactured by Exactech (Gainesville, Fla). GXL is made by irradiating bars of 1020 GUR at 28 KGy with gamma irradiation. Acetabular liners are then made from the bars. Sterilization is attained with another gamma irradiation at 28 KGy. Postirradiation heat treatment is avoided to preserve fracture toughness and other mechanical properties. The total irradiation dose received by the UHMWPE is 56 KGy. Because there is no heat treatment, it is possible that oxidation of UHMWPE can occur. The GXL process is directed at maintaining initial fracture toughness over oxidation resistance.

- **Aeonian and Barc.** Aeonian (Kyocera, Kyoto, Japan) and Barc cross-linked types of UHMWPE (Barc, Johannesburg, South Africa) are not available in the United States. However, they are being used in significant quantities in Japan and South Africa, respectively. Both of these products utilize a postirradiation heat treatment below the melting point of the UHMWPE. As stated previously, Barc cross-linked UHWMPE is made by gamma irradiation, in the presence of acetylene gas, of the finished acetabular cup. **Aeonian is made** from irradiation of 1050 GUR at 35 KGy. This is followed by a heat treatment below the melting point (110° C for 10 hours) of UHMWPE. Final sterilization is done with gamma irradiation at doses between 25 and 40 KGy. The total irradiation received by the UHMWPE is between 60 and 75 KGy. Because both the Barc material and Aeonian have gamma sterilization as the last process step, there are free radicals in the UHMWPE.

REFERENCES

1. Waugh W: John Charnley: the man and the hip, Berlin, 1990, Springer Verlag.
2. Scales JT: Arthroplasty of the hip using foreign materials: a history. Proc Inst Mech Eng 181:63–89, 1967.
3. Rang M: Anthology of orthopaedics, Edinburgh, London, New York, 1966, Churchill Livingstone.
4. Jones ES: Joint lubrication. The Lancet 1:1426–1427, 1936.
5. Jones R, Lovett RW: Orthopaedic, Baltimore, 1929, Wm Wood.
6. Judet J, Judet R: The use of an artificial femoral head for arthroplasty of the hip joint. J Bone Joint Surg Br 32:166–173, 1950.
7. Wiles P: The surgery of the osteoarthritic hip. Br J Surg 45:488–497, 1958.
8. Thompson FR: Vitallium intramedullary hip prosthesis: preliminary report. N Y State J Med 52:3011–3020, 1952.
9. Moore AT, Bohlman HR: Metal hip joint: a case report. J Bone Joint Surg Am 25:688–692, 1943.
10. McKee GK, Watson-Farrar J: Replacement of arthritic hips by the McKee-Farrar prosthesis. J Bone Joint Surg Br 48:245–259, 1966.
11. Ring PA: Replacement of the hip joint. Ann R Coll Surg Engl 48:344–355, 1971.
12. The diameter of the Charnley femoral head was 7/8″, which is 22.225 mm. This conversion of inches to centimeters is often incorrectly reported as 22.25 mm.
13. Charnley J: Private correspondence with C. Homsy.
14. Trail IA, Frank PL, Minns RJ: Fluon interposition arthroplasty of the knee. Clin Mater 1:275–279, 1986.
15. Charnley J: The long-term results of low-friction arthroplasty of the hip performed as a primary intervention. J Bone Joint Surg Br 54:61, 1972. (Reedited in Clin Orthop Relat Res [319]:4, 1995.)
16. Kurtz SM: UHMWPE biomaterials hand book, ed 2, Burlington, Mass, 2009, Elsevier Press, p 3.
17. The density of HDPE is above .95 g/cc, and the density of UHMWPE is typically less than .94 g/cc. The IZOD impact strength for HDPE versus UHMWPE is 4 versus 20.
18. Rainer Walkenhorst: private communication, Ticona, May 18, 2010.
19. Stein HL: Personal communication, Product Manager, Hoechst/Celanese, Bishop, Tex.
20. American Society for Testing and Materials: D 4020. Standard specification for ultra high molecular weight polyethylene molding and extrusion materials. In: 1993 annual book of standards, vol 8.02, Philadelphia, 1993, ASTM Press, pp 612–614.
21. American Society for Testing and Materials: D F648-07. Standard specification for ultra high molecular weight polyethylene powder and fabricated form for surgical implants. In: Annual book of ASTM standards, vol 13.01 (Medical devices), Philadelphia, Pa, 2007, ASTM Press.
22. Bankston AB, Keating EM, Ranawat C, et al: Comparison of polyethylene wear in machined versus molded polyethylene. Clin Orthop Relat Res 317:37–43, 1995.
23. Li S, Ranawat CS, Furman B: Effect of direct molding acetabular cups on the clinical and hip simulator wear rates of UHMWPE. J Bone Joint Surg Br 86(Suppl 4):491, 2004.
24. Ploskonka J: Personal communication, Product manager, Westlake Plastics, Lenni, Pa.
25. Bhateja SK, Andrews EH, Yarbrough SM: Radiation induced crystallinity changes in linear polyethylenes: long term aging effects. Polymer Journal 21:739–750, 1989.
26. Nagy EV, Li S: Fourier transform infrared spectroscopy techniques for the evaluation of polyethylene orthopaedic bearing surfaces. Trans Soc Biomater 13:109, 1990.
27. Li S, Nagy EV: Analysis of retrieved components via Fourier transform infrared spectroscopy. Trans Soc Biomater 13:274, 1990.
28. American Society for Testing and Materials: F 2102-0. Standard guide for evaluating the extent of oxidation in ultra high molecular weight polyethylene fabricated forms intended for surgical implants, West Conshohocken, Pa, ASTM International.
29. Kurtz SM, Muratoglu OK, Buchanan F, et al: Interlaboratory reproducibility of standard accelerated aging methods for oxidation of UHMWPE. Biomaterials 23:1731–1737, 2001.
30. Furman BD, Lelas J, McNulty D, et al: Kinetics, chemistry and calibration of UHMWPE accelerated aging methods. Trans ORS 44:102, 1998.
31. American Society for Testing and Materials: D 1505-03. Standard test method for density of plastics by the density-gradient technique, Philadelphia, 2003, ASTM Press.
32. Nagy EV, Li S: Fourier transform infrared spectroscopy techniques for the evaluation of polyethylene orthopaedic bearing surfaces. Trans Soc Biomater 13:109, 1990.
33. Li S, Nagy EV: Analysis of retrieved components via Fourier transform infrared spectroscopy. Trans Soc Biomater 13:274, 1990.
34. Rimnac CM, Wright TM, Klein RW, et al: Characterization of material properties of ultra high molecular weight polyethylene molecular weight polyethylene before and after implantation. Trans Soc Biomater Implant Retrieval Symposium 15:16, 1992.
35. Jahan MS, Wang C, Schwartz G, Davidson JA: Combined chemical and mechanical effects of free radicals in UHMWPE joints during implantation. J Biomed Mater Res 25:1005–1017, 1991.
36. Li S: The identification of defects in ultra high molecular weight polyethylene molecular weight polyethylene. Trans Orthop Res Soc 587, 1994.
37. Li S, Saum K, Collier JP, Kazprzak D: Oxidation of UHMWPE over long time periods. Trans Soc Biomater 425, 1994.
38. Mayor MB, Wrona M, Collier JP, Jensen RE: The role of polyethylene quality in the failure of tibial knee components. Trans Orthop Res Soc 292, 1993.
39. Sutula LC, Collier JP, Saum KA, et al: Impact of sterilization on clinical performance of polyethylene in the hip. Clin Orthop Relat Res 319:28–40, 1995.
40. Currier BH, Currier JH, Collier JP, et al: Shelf life and in vivo duration. Clin Orthop Relat Res 342:111–122, 1997.
41. Kurtz SM (ed): UHMWPE biomaterials handbook, Philadelphia, 2009, Elsevier, section 3.7, p 28.
42. Schroeder DW, Pozorski KM: Hip simulator testing of isostatically molded UHMWPE: effect of EtO and gamma sterilization. Trans 42nd Orthop Res Soc 478, 1996.
43. Li S, Chang JD, Barrena EG, et al: Nonconsolidated polyethylene particles and oxidation in Charnley acetabular cups. Clin Orthop Relat Res 319:54–63, 1995.
44. Gómez-Barrena E, Medel F, Puértolas JA: Polyethylene oxidation in total hip arthroplasty: evolution and new advances. Open Orthop J 3:115–120, 2009.
45. Sommerich R, Flynn T, Schmidt MB, Zalenski E: The effects of sterilization on contact area and wear rate of UHMWPE. Trans 42nd Orthop Res Soc 486, 1996.
46. Wang A, Polineni VK, Essner A, et al: Effect of shelf aging on the wear of ultra high molecular weight polyethylene molecular weight polyethylene acetabular cups: a 10 million cycle hip simulator study. Trans Orthop Res Soc 139, 1997.
47. Li S, Chang JD, Barrena EG, et al: Nonconsolidated polyethylene particles and oxidation in Charnley acetabular cups. Clin Orthop Relat Res 319:54–63, 1995.
48. Gomez-Barrena E, Masri BA, Salvati EA, Li S: Polyethylene wear in Charnley acetabular components: the interaction between clinical factors and material properties. Trans 63rd Meeting AAOS 380, 1996.
49. Sun DC, Schmidg G, Yau SS, et al: Correlations between oxidation, cross linking and wear performance of UHMWPE. Trans 43rd Orthop Res Soc 783, 1997.
50. Furman BD, Lefebvre FK, Li S: Gamma irradiation does not adversely effect wear in total hip arthroplasty. Trans Soc Biomater 21:499, 1998.
51. Bono J, Sanford L, Toussaint J: Polyethylene wear in total hip arthroplasty: observations from retrieved AML plus hip implants with ACS polyethylene liner. J Arthroplasty 9:119–125, 1994.
52. Walsh HA, Furman BD, Naab S, Li S: Role of oxidation in the clinical fracture of acetabular cups. Trans ORS 45:845, 1999.
53. Williams IR, Mayor MB, Collier JP: The impact of sterilization method on wear in knee arthroplasty. Clin Orthop Relat Res 356:170–180, 1998.

54. Burstein AH: Structural mechanical properties of polyethylene. Proceedings of the 9th Open Scientific Meeting of the Hip Society 293–297, 1981.
55. Ainsworth R, Farling G, Bardos D: An improved bearing material for joint replacement prostheses: carbon fiber reinforced UHMWPE. Trans Orthop Res Soc 23:120, 1977.
56. Zimmer Technical Report: Poly two carbon polyethylene composite: a carbon fiber-reinforced molded UHMWPE, Zimmer Research and Development Division, January 1977, Zimmer Orthopaedics Company.
57. Connelly GM, Rimnac CM, Wright TM, et al: Fatigue crack propagation behavior of ultra high molecular weight polyethylene. J Orthop Res 2:119–125, 1984.
58. Wright TM, Rimnac CM, Faris PM, Bansal M: Trans Orthop Res Soc 13:263, 1987.
59. Wright TM, Fukubayshi T, Burstein AH: The effect of carbon reinforcement on contact area, contact pressure and time-dependent deformation in polyethylene tibial components. J Biomed Mater Res 15:719–730, 1981.
60. Howard EG, Li S: Process of manufacturing ultra high molecular weight polyethylene shaped articles, U.S. Patent 5,037,928, August 1991.
61. McKellop HA, Liu B, Li S: Wear of acetabular cups of conventional and modification UHMWPE compared on hip joint simulator. Trans Orthop Res Soc 17:356, 1992.
62. McKellop HA, Liu B, Li S: Wear of acetabular cups of conventional and modification UHMWPE compared on hip joint simulator. Trans Orthop Res Soc 17:356, 1992.
63. Chmell MJ, Poss R, Thomas WH, Sledge CB: Early failure of Hylamer acetabular inserts due to eccentric wear. J Arthroplasty 11:351–353, 1996.
64. Livingston BJ, Chmell MJ, Spector M, Poss R: Complications of total hip arthroplasty associated with the use of an acetabular component with a Hylamer 7 liner. J Bone Joint Surg Am 79:1529–1538, 1997.
65. Sychertz CJ, Shah N, Engh CA: Examination of wear in Duraloc acetabular components: two to five year evaluation of Hylamer and Enduron liners. J Arthroplasty 13:508–514, 1998.
66. Schmalzried TP, Dorey FJ, McKellop H: The multifactorial nature of polyethylene wear in vivo. J Bone Joint Surg Am 80:1234–1242, 1998.
67. Reggiani M, Tinti A, Visentin M, et al: Vibrational spectroscopy study of the oxidation of Hylamer UHMWPE explanted acetabular cups sterilized differently. J Mol Struct 834:129–135, 2007.
68. Wroblewski BM, Siney PD, Fleming PA: Wear of enhanced ultra-high molecular-weight polyethylene (Hylamer) in combination with a 22.225 mm diameter zirconia femoral head. J Bone Joint Surg Br 85:376–379, 2003.
69. Oonishi H, Igaka T, Takayama Y: Wear resistance of gamma-ray irradiated UHMW polyethylene socket in total hip prosthesis. Transactions of 3rd World Biomaterials Congress, Kyoto, Japan, April 21–25, 1988.
70. Oonish H, Takayama Y, Tsuji E: Improvements of polyethylene by irradiation in artificial joints. Radiat Phys Chem 39:495–504, 1992.
71. Oonishi H, Kuno M, Tsuji E, Fujisawa A: The optimum dose of gamma irradiation: heavy doses to low wear polyethylene in total hip prosthesis. J Mater Sci Mater Med 8:11–18, 1997.
72. Oonishi H, Kadoya Y: Wear resistance of gamma-ray irradiated UHMW polyethylene socket in total hip prostheses: wear test and long-term clinical results. MRS International Meeting on Advanced Materials, vol 1, Materials Research Society, 1989.
73. Oonishi H, Ishimaru H, Kato A: Effect of cross-linkage by gamma irradiation in heavy doses to low wear polyethylene in total hip prostheses. J Mater Sci Mater Med 7:753–763, 1996.
74. Oonishi H, Takayama Y, Tsuji E: The low wear of cross-linked polyethylene socket in total hip prostheses. In: Encyclopedic handbook of biomaterials and engineering. Part A. Materials, New York, 1995, Marcel Dekker, pp 1853–1868.
75. Grobbelaar CJ, DuPlessis TA, Maris F: The radiation improvement of polyethylene prostheses. J Bone Joint Surg Br 60:370–374, 1978.
76. Weber FA: Personal communication.
77. Grobbelaar CJ, Weber FA, Spirakis A, et al: Clinical experience with gamma irradiation-crosslinked polyethylene: a 14 to 20 year follow-up report. South Afr Bone Joint Surg 9:140–145, 1999.
78. Wroblewski BM: Prospective clinical and joint simulator studies of a new total hip arthroplasty using alumina ceramic heads and cross linked polyethylene cups. J Bone Joint Surg Br 78:280–285, 1996.
79. McKellop H, Shen FW, Lu B, et al: Effect of sterilization method and other modifications on the wear resistance of acetabular cups made of ultra-high molecular weight polyethylene: a hip-simulator study. J Bone Joint Surg Am 82:1708–1725, 2000.
80. McKellop H, Shen F-W, Lu B, et al: Development of an extremely wear-resistant ultra high molecular weight polyethylene for total hip replacements. J Orthop Res 17:160, 1999.
81. Ries MD, Pruitt L: Effect of crosslinking on the microstructure and mechanical properties of ultra high molecular weight polyethylene. Clin Orthop Relat Res 440:149–156, 2005.
82. Greenwald AS, Bauer TW, Ries MD: New polys for old: contribution or caveat? J Bone Joint Surg Am 83:27–31, 2001.
83. Furman BD, Bhattacharyya S, Hernoux C, et al: Independent evaluation of wear properties of commercially available cross linked UHMWPE. Trans 27th Annual Meeting Soc Biomater 33, 2001.
84. Dowd JE, Sychertz CJ, Young AM, Engh CA: Characterization of long-term femoral-head-penetration rates: association with and prediction of osteolysis. J Bone Joint Surg Am 82:1102–1107, 2000.
85. Wilkinson JM, Hamer AJ, Stockley I, Eastell R: Polyethylene wear rate and osteolysis: critical threshold versus continuous dose-response relationship. J Orthop Res 23:520–525, 2005.
86. Leung SB, Egawa H, Stepniewski A, et al: Incidence and volume of pelvic osteolysis at early follow-up with highly cross-linked and noncross-linked polyethylene. J Arthroplasty 22(Suppl 2):134–139, 2007.
87. Gillis AM, Schmieg JJ, Bhattacharya S, Li S: An independent evaluation of the mechanical, chemical and fracture properties of UHMWPE cross linked by 34 different methods. Trans ORS 45:908, 1999.
88. Walsh HA, Furman BD, Naab S, Li S: Determination of the role of oxidation in the clinical and in vitro fracture of acetabular cups. Trans Soc Biomaterials 22:50, 1999.
89. Duus LC, Walsh HA, Gillis AM, et al: A comparison of the fracture toughness of cross linked UHMWPE made from different resins, manufacturing methods and sterilization conditions. Trans Soc Biomater 384, 2000.
90. Walsh HA, Furman BD, Li S: The effects of cross linking on the fracture and fatigue properties of UHMWPE acetabular cups. Trans 27th Annual Meeting Soc Biomater 592, 2001.
91. Pruitt LA: Deformation, yielding, fracture and fatigue behavior of conventional and highly cross-linked ultra high molecular weight polyethylene. Biomaterials 26:905–915, 2005.
92. Bistolfi KS, Bellare A, Pruitt LA: The combined effects of crosslinking and high crystallinity on the microstructural and mechanical properties of ultra high molecular weight polyethylene. Biomaterials 27:1688–1694, 2006.
93. Bradford L, Baker D, Ries MD, Pruitt LA: Fatigue crack propagation resistance of highly crosslinked polyethylene. Clin Orthop Relat Res 429:68–72, 2004.
94. Rimnac C, Pruitt L: How do material properties influence wear and fracture mechanisms? J Am Acad Orthop Surg 16(Suppl 1):S94–S100, 2008.
95. Baker DA, Hastings RS, Pruitt L: Study of fatigue resistance of chemical and radiation crosslinked medical grade ultrahigh molecular weight polyethylene. J Biomed Mater Res 46:573–581, 1999.
96. Gencur SJ, Rimnac CM, Kurtz SM: Fatigue crack propagation resistance of virgin and highly crosslinked, thermally treated ultra-high molecular weight polyethylene. Biomaterials 27:1550–1557, 2006.
97. Pascaud RS, Evans WT, McCullagh PJ, FitzPatrick DP: Influence of gamma irradiation sterilization and temperature on the fracture toughness of ultra-high-molecular-weight polyethylene. Biomaterials 18:727–735, 1997.

98. Birman MV, Noble PC, Conditt MA, et al: Cracking and impingement in ultra-high-molecular-weight polyethylene acetabular liners. J Arthroplasty 20(7 Suppl 3):87–92, 2005.

99. Furman B, Callander P, Statz A, et al: Fracture related damage is common in retrieved UHMWPE acetabular cups. Trans 48th Orthop Res Soc 1039, 2002.

100. Sutula LC, Collier JP, Saum KA, et al: Impact of gamma sterilization on clinical performance of polyethylene in the hip. Clin Orthop Relat Res 319:28–40, 1995.

101. Shon WY, Baldini T, Petersen MG, et al: Impingement in total hip arthroplasty: a study of retrieved acetabular components. J Arthroplasty 20:427–435, 2005.

102. Halley D, Glassman A, Crowninshield RD: Recurrent dislocation after revision total hip replacement with a large prosthetic femoral head: a case report. J Bone Joint Surg Am 86:827–830, 2004.

103. Moore KD, Beck PR, Petersen DW, et al: Early failure of a cross linked polyethylene acetabular liner, a case report. J Bone Joint Surg Am 90:2499–2504, 2008.

104. Tower SS, Currier JH, Currier BH, et al: Rim cracking of the crosslinked polyethylene acetabular liner after total hip arthroplasty. J Bone Joint Surg Am 89:2212–2217, 2007.

105. Furmanski J, Anderson M, Bal S, et al: Clinical fracture of cross-linked UHMWPE acetabular liners. Biomaterials 30:5572–5582, 2009.

106. Orala E, Rowella SL, Muratoglua OK: The effect of α-tocopherol on the oxidation and free radical decay in irradiated UHMWPE. Biomaterials 27:5580–5587, 2006.

107. Atkinson J, Epand RF, Epand RM: Tocopherols and tocotrienols in membranes: a critical review. Free Rad Biol Med 44:739–764, 2008.

108. Azzi A: Molecular mechanism of alpha-tocopherol action. Free Rad Biol Med 43:16–21, 2007.

109. Zingg JM, Azzi A: Non-antioxidant activities of vitamin E. Curr Med Chem 11:1113–1133, 2004.

110. Arcom processed polyethylene, Biomet Orthopaedics Inc, 2002, Warsaw. Form No. Y-BMT-791/113002/M.

111. Wang XY, Li SY, Salovey R: Processing of ultra high molecular weight polyethylene. J Appl Poly Sci 35:2165–2171, 1988.

112. Kurtz SM (ed): UHMWPE handbook, Oxford, United Kingdom, 2000, Elsevier, section 14.2.1, p 206.

113. Saikko V, Calonius O, Keränen J: Effect of counterface roughness on the wear of conventional and crosslinked ultra-high molecular weight polyethylene studied with a multi-directional motion pin-on-disk device. J Biomed Mater Res 57:506–512, 2001.

114. Kurtz SM, Mazzucco D, Rimnac CM, Schroeder D: Anisotropy and oxidative resistance of highly cross lined UHMWPE after deformation processing by solid state ram extrusion. Biomaterials 27:24–34, 2006.

115. Oonishi H, Kim SC, Takao Y, et al: Wear of highly cross-linked polyethylene acetabular cup in Japan. J Arthroplasty 21:944–949, 2006.

116. Harris WH, Muratoglu OK: A review of current cross linked polyethylenes used in total joint arthroplasty. Clin Orthop Relat Res 430:46–52, 2005.

117. Miller G: Exactech, Gainesville, Fla, private communication.

CHAPTER 6

Materials in Hip Surgery: Metals for Cemented and Uncemented Implants

Warren O. Haggard, Joel D. Bumgardner, and Phillip J. Andersen

KEY POINTS

- Atomic, molecular, and crystalline structures provide and influence the mechanical, wear, and corrosion properties of metals used in total hip arthroplasty (THA).
- Smaller grain size and alloying elements increase the strength of THA metals.
- General or uniform corrosion occurs with all THA implant metals at a very low rate and is not generally a biological or mechanical concern. Accelerated corrosion processes, such as galvanic, pitting, crevice, fretting, and fatigue, result in significant release of metal ions and can present both biological and mechanical concerns.
- Fatigue strength testing is required to determine the endurance limit for new THA metal alloys, revised THA designs, and altered manufacturing processing.
- Through substitution of existing alloying elements with new alloying elements, new THA metal alloys are being developed with the goal of enhancing biocompatibility and mechanical strength.

INTRODUCTION

Hip arthroplasty started with the implantation of interpositional layers of various biological materials in the joint, including fascia, skin, and even pig bladder.[1] In the 1930s, these materials were replaced with shells of stainless steel and an early cobalt-chromium alloy, Vitallium.[1,2] The use of metals in interpositional and total hip joint replacement implants (THAs) continued through the 1930s and 1940s until the 1950s, when British orthopedic surgeon Sir John Charnley developed the lower friction bearing couple and enhanced fixation for THA. With improved survivorship of this procedure, stemming from the designs of Charnley, among others, total hip replacement has been referred to as "the orthopedic procedure" of the last century.[1] Improved survivorship for all THA systems resulted from enhanced surgical techniques, improved implant designs, and more

advanced materials and processing. The transition from stainless steel to cobalt-chromium (Co-Cr), titanium (Ti), and advanced stainless steel alloys has continued efforts to improve THA. This chapter provides a brief overview of the structure, mechanical properties, strengthening mechanisms, and advantages and disadvantages of metals used in THA.

BASIC SCIENCE

The performance of metals and alloys used in orthopedic implants and devices depends in part on atomic bonding and structures for bulk properties, as well as surface properties for material-host interactions. In this chapter, we review the bonding and crystal structure of metallic implant materials as they relate to the bulk physical and mechanical properties of these materials, along with the surface properties of orthopedic metals, as they affect corrosion resistance within the body.

Metallic Structures

Metals and alloys derive their classical characteristics of formability, toughness, and high heat and electrical conductance from primary bond formation called *metallic bonding*. In metallic bonding, the atoms share their outermost (valence) electrons, which create a "sea" or "cloud" of electrons surrounding the positive nuclear core of the metal atoms (Fig. 6-1). Charge neutrality is maintained because the negative electrons act as a thick paste between positive nuclear cores. Because of delocalization of the electrons around atom cores, metallic bonds are often referred to as *nondirectional* and *nonspecific*, and the mobility of the electrons in the metal is what leads to their high heat and electrical conductivity. Additionally, the delocalization enables individual metal atoms or planes of atoms to "slide" relatively easily with respect to each other, which gives metals and alloys their typical ductile and malleable characteristics.

Nondirectional and nonspecific bonding also allows metal atoms to arrange themselves in regular, long-range, repetitive patterns or crystal structures. Amorphous materials lack long-range order, although some

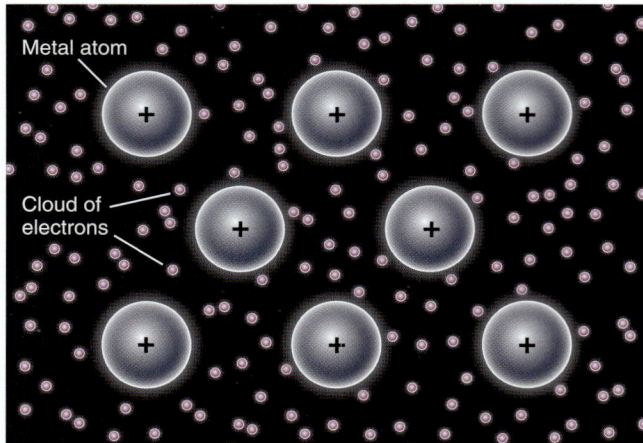

Figure 6-1. Schematic of metal bonding. Outer shell electrons are shared between positively charged nuclear cores of metal atoms, such that the atoms are bonded to each other via a "sea" or "cloud" of electrons.

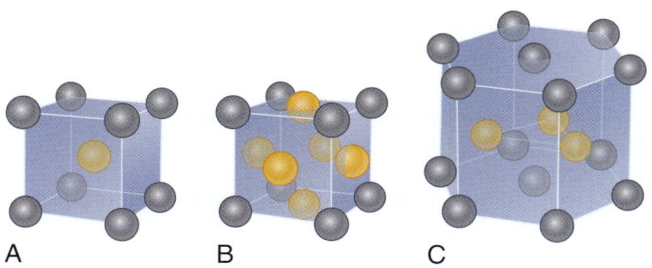

A   B   C

Figure 6-2. Schematic of crystal lattice systems common to implant alloys. **A,** Body-centered cubic (BCC). **B,** Face-centered cubic (FCC). **C,** Hexagonal close packed (HCP).

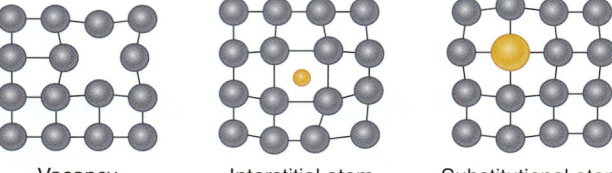

Vacancy   Interstitial atom   Substitutional atom

Figure 6-3. Schematic of point defects in metal crystal structures.

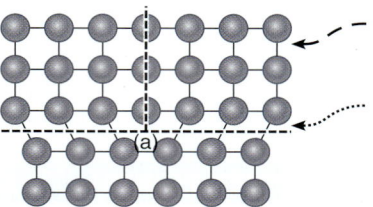

Figure 6-4. Schematic of a dislocation (⊥) in metal crystal structures. **a,** Increased lattice strain. This makes it relatively easy to break and re-form bonds, one at a time, along the edge of the dislocation *(dashed arrow)* as compared with a complete plane of atoms *(hyphened arrow)* and results in the ability of metals to be deformed at lower forces than might be predicted for a perfect crystalline metal.

short-range structures may be present. The crystalline patterns or structures are represented by three-dimensional space lattices based on a repeating unit cell. There are 14 distinct space lattices, called *Bravais lattices,* based on the relative lengths of the unit cell edges, the angles between edges, and the position of atoms within the cell. The atoms in implant metals are most commonly arranged in cubic or hexagonal structures (Fig. 6-2). In the body-centered cubic (BCC) arrangement, an atom is located in the center and at each corner of the cube. Iron, molybdenum, chromium, and tantalum are common metals that arrange in the BCC crystal structure. In the face-centered cubic (FCC) arrangement, an atom is located at each corner of the cube, and an atom is present in the center of each face of the cube. Aluminum, nickel, platinum, and silver are common metals that arrange in the FCC crystal structure. In the hexagonal, close-packed (HCP) arrangement, an atom is located at each corner of the hexagon and in the center of the top and bottom faces; three atoms are found within the center. Titanium, cobalt, and zinc arrange in the HCP structure. Using a hard-sphere model and simple geometry, the density of atoms per unit cell volume or the packing factor may be calculated as 0.76 for FCC and HCP unit cells and 0.68 for BCC unit cells. These crystalline arrangements are important for

overall mechanical and corrosion properties and the ability of metals to be mixed to form alloys.

Defects in Crystal Structures and Alloying

Although metal atoms readily assume crystalline structures, defects arise in the crystal arrangements as a result of the natural thermodynamics of crystal formation. The two major types of defects are point defects and line defects.

Point defects involve missing atoms or vacancies in crystal lattice positions, or impurity atoms, which can occupy spaces in between atoms in the lattice structure (i.e., *interstitial positions*) or in a normal lattice position (i.e., *substitutional positions*) (Fig. 6-3). The most common line defects are dislocations. Dislocation defects occur as the result of uneven completion of rows of atoms in a crystal, such that an extra half-plane of atoms appear in regular packing arrangements (Fig. 6-4). Grain boundaries also arise because of the thermodynamics of crystal formation and occur where two growing crystals meet but at slightly different orientations such that crystal lattices do not match up (Fig. 6-5). Except under some very special conditions, all metals and alloys have a grain structure.

In general, the presence of defects greatly reduces the strength of crystal structures from theoretical values based on perfect, defect-free crystal structures. In the case of dislocation defects, the energy required to break the metallic bond along the plane of the dislocation is much less than the energy required to break all of the bonds on an entire plane of a perfect crystal lattice. The

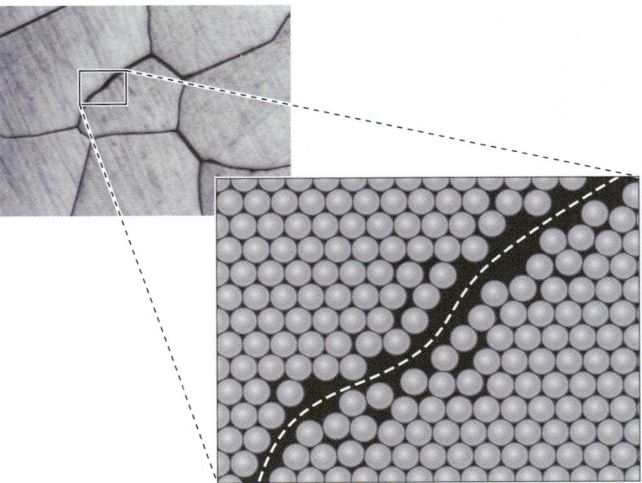

Figure 6-5. Schematic of grain boundary highlighting the mismatch in crystal lattices due to small changes in orientation between grains.

result is that a half-plane of atoms is moved and the metal is deformed in response to a lower mechanical force by breaking and reforming a line of bonds, one or a few at a time, as compared with the force needed to break bonds in an entire plane of atoms (see Fig. 6-4).

However, the purposeful introduction of interstitial or substitutional point defect atoms into crystal structures creates lattice strain, which makes it harder for dislocations to move, thus increasing the stress required to cause permanent changes in shape (i.e., the yield strength of the material). This is the basis of alloying metals together to impart greater strength and related properties. Interstitial alloys are formed when solute atoms are much smaller than the solvent atom (e.g., B, C, N, O are often used to form interstitial alloys with Fe, Co, and Ti metals). For example, enhanced grades of stainless steel are manufactured for orthopedic applications in which nitrogen has been added to iron alloys to occupy interstitial sites in the FCC lattice. Substitutional alloys are favored when the following conditions, also known as the *Hume-Rothery rules*, are satisfied:

- The difference in size of atomic radii of the solvent and solute atoms is less than 15%.
- Both elements have the same crystal structures (especially with a large proportion of solute atoms).
- Atoms exhibit similar electronegativities (i.e., close to each other in the periodic table).
- The two atoms have similar valence charges.

These rules are a result of the fact that if substitution necessitates a large change in the size of an atom in the matrix, the crystal structure, or the lengths and strengths of the bonds present, there will be too much strain in the lattice for atoms to remain in the normal equilibrium positions. In cobalt-chromium alloys used to manufacture hip prostheses, chromium can substitute into lattice positions normally occupied by cobalt atoms.

When these rules are not satisfied, some segregation of the atomic species into two or more phases is seen. For example, the Ti-6Al-4V (Titanium [Ti], Aluminum

[Al], Vandium [V]) alloy is a two-phase alloy containing an aluminum-rich HCP phase (α) and a vanadium-rich BCC phase (β).

Strengthening Mechanisms

In general, metals can be strengthened by making it more difficult for dislocations to move through the crystal lattice. This can be done in several basic ways, including developing fine grains in the metal, adding alloying elements that distort the crystal structure (solid solution strengthening), deforming the metal at low temperatures to increase the number of dislocations within the crystal lattice (work hardening or cold working), and creating fine dispersions of a second phase to interfere with dislocation motion (heat treatments to "age" the material are a common way to do this).

Grain Size Effects

In general terms, a metal with small grains is stronger than the same metal with coarse grains at temperatures of interest for implants. At room temperature, grain boundaries are significant barriers to dislocation motion. A classic description of this effect is given by the Hall-Petch equation: $\sigma_y = \sigma_o + kD^{-(1/2)}$, where σ_Y is the yield stress of the metal, σ_o is a frictional stress required to move dislocations, k is the Hall-Petch slope, and D is the grain size.[3] A variety of metals, including some stainless steels[3] and commercially pure (CP) titanium (Ti),[4] exhibit yield strength versus grain size relationships that follow this relationship.

Solid Solution Strengthening

High-purity metals typically are soft and ductile, and are very expensive to produce. This combination means that the uses for high-purity metals are limited. Metals used for orthopedic implants are alloys that have a major constituent (also referred to as the *solvent*) and a number of alloying ingredients (the solute atoms). Some of these elements are present at low levels because of impurities in the raw materials, but the main alloying elements are added for specific reasons (e.g., Cr is added to stainless steel and cobalt base alloys to enable formation of a passive film for corrosion protection and to increase strength). In general, the atoms of metallic alloying elements such as Cr, Ni, and Mo replace solvent atoms at random sites within the matrix. Because the size of atoms of the substrate and of alloying elements is not the same, distortions occur within the crystal lattice, which increase resistance to dislocation motion. As a result, strength increases but ductility decreases.

Small atoms such as nitrogen, carbon, and oxygen fit into the interstitial sites. The addition of interstitial alloying elements has a very large effect on the properties of some alloys used in medical devices. Nitrogen additions to stainless steel greatly increase strength and improve corrosion resistance. The strength of CP titanium also increases dramatically with iron and oxygen content. Whereas the tensile strength of grade 1 CP Ti (maximum, 0.18% O and 0.20% Fe) is only 240 MPa, grade 4 CP Ti, with more than twice the

Table 6-1. Mechanical Properties of Some Annealed and Cold-Worked Implantable Alloys

Alloy	Material Condition	Ultimate Tensile Strength, MPa	Yield Strength, MPa	% Elongation	10^7 Cycle Fatigue Endurance Limit, MPa	Reference
316L	Annealed	550	240	55	180	6
316L	60% cold-worked	1240	1000	12	450	6
BioDur108	Annealed	827-930	517-605	30-50	380	7, 8
BioDur108	35% cold-worked	1580	1350	15		8
BioDur108	65% cold-worked	2000	1790	5		8
L 605 (cobalt base)	Annealed or solution treated	950	455	60		6
L 605	30% cold-worked	1200	950	18		6

interstitial content (0.40% O and 0.50% Fe), has a strength of 550 MPa.[5]

Work Hardening/Cold Working

The response of metals to deformation depends on the temperature at which the deformation takes place. Deformed metallic structures contain large numbers of dislocations, which increase the total energy of the system. This energy provides a driving force to form new grains with low numbers of dislocations, but enough atomic mobility must be present to allow the new grains to form. This requires elevated temperatures. The temperature at which new grain formation occurs is referred to as the *recrystallization temperature,* but this usually is not a specific fixed temperature. The recrystallization temperature depends primarily on the alloy in question, but other factors (e.g., amount of deformation, hold time at temperature, presence of second-phase particles) influence recrystallization behavior. For Ti-6Al-4V, recrystallization temperatures are in the range of 800° C to 850° C.[4]

When metals are deformed at "low" temperatures (below the recrystallization temperature), additional dislocations are formed within the crystal lattice. With an increase in the number (or density) of dislocations within the lattice, interactions occur between dislocations, causing them to become less mobile. This increases the strength of the metal while decreasing its ductility. Work-hardened metals are often described by the amount of deformation that was involved in the production of the material (e.g., a 30% cold-worked, stainless steel). Work hardening (also known as *cold working*) is routinely used to increase the strength of stainless steel and cobalt base alloys for a variety of applications. In the case of the austenitic stainless steels used as implant materials (316L, BioDur 108, etc.), initial strengthening is attained through the addition of alloying elements to the iron substrate (termed *solid solution alloying*). Additional increases in strength occur only through work hardening treatments. If a work-hardened alloy is heated sufficiently (i.e., by processes such as welding or sintering a porous coating onto the surface), recrystallization will take place, and the new metal grains that form will not be in a work-hardened state. Consequently, any metal within the recrystallized region will have significantly reduced

strength and increased ductility. Table 6-1 shows the impact of work hardening on the strength and ductility of several common implantable alloys.

Precipitation Dispersion Strengthening

Alloys may be strengthened by a mechanism termed *precipitation dispersion,* which involves the formation of a large number of fine precipitates within the microstructure to increase resistance to the motion of dislocations, thus increasing strength. The necessary precipitation reactions are not possible in every alloy system. For example, the austenitic stainless steels, such as 316L, do not respond to this process because no desirable precipitates can be formed. In practice, precipitation dispersion strengthening generally is performed by rapidly cooling (quenching) a metal alloy that has been held at an elevated temperature (this is often referred to as a *solution treatment*), followed by a lower temperature exposure (the aging treatment). At elevated temperatures, alloying elements are in a solid solution within the alloy. Rapid cooling prevents the alloy from forming the structure that would be formed under slower, more equilibrium conditions. When the quenched alloy is then held at an intermediate temperature, small particles of second phases can form (precipitate) within the solution. The solution and aging treatment temperatures depend on the alloy in question. This approach can be used for β-titanium alloys, such as Ti-15Mo, cold-worked Co-Cr alloys (MP35N), and several of the stainless steels used to produce surgical instruments.

Orthopedic Implant Alloy Compositions and Microstructures

The major types of alloys used in orthopedics are the stainless steel, cobalt-chromium alloys (Co-Cr) and titanium (Ti) alloys (Table 6-2).

The most common type of stainless steel is 316L. It is a single-phase, iron-base alloy in an FCC crystal arrangement called the γ-phase or *austenite.* The "L" designation refers to the low (less than 0.03 wt%) carbon content of the alloy in comparison with the conventional 316 grade (0.08% C). The addition of chromium enables the development of a corrosion-resistant, chromium-oxide surface layer, and the addition of molybdenum enhances

Table 6-2. Composition of Some Common Orthopedic Implant Alloys

Material	ASTM Designation/ISO Designation	Common/Trade Name	Composition, % Major Metals	Minor Metals	Notes
Stainless steel	F 138[10] ISO 5832 Part 1[11]	316L	Cr 17.00-19.00 / Ni 13.00-15.00 / Mo 2.25-3.0 / Balance Fe	Mn max 2.0 / Cu max 0.5 / C max 0.03 / N max 0.1 / P max 0.025 / Si max 0.75 / S max 0.01	
Nitrogen-strengthened stainless steel	F 1586[12] ISO 5832 Part 9[13]	Rex 734 / Ortron 90	Cr 19.5-22.0 / Ni 9.0-11.0 / Mo 2.0-3.0 / Mn 2.00-4.25 / Balance Fe	N 0.25-0.50 / Nb 0.25-0.80 / Cu max 0.25 / Si max 0.75 / C max 0.08 / P max 0.025 / S max 0.01	
Low-nickel stainless steel	F 2229[7]	BioDur 108 Alloy	Mn 21.0-24.0 / Cr 19.0-23.0 / Mo 0.5-1.5 / N 0.85-1.1 / Balance Fe	C max 0.08 / P max 0.03 / Si max 0.75 / Ni max 0.10 / Cu max 0.25 / S max 0.01	
Investment cast Co-28Cr-6Mo	F 75[14] ISO 5832 Part 4[15]	Vitallium Haynes-Stellite 21 / Protasul-2	Cr 27.0-30.0 / Mo 5.0-7.0 / Balance Co	Mn max 1.0 / Si max 1.0 / Ni max 0.5 / Fe max 0.75 / C max 0.35 / N max 0.25	
Wrought Co-28Cr-6Mo	F 1537[16] ISO 5832 Part 12[17]	High-Strength Zimalloy	Cr 26.0-30.0 / Mo 5.0-7.0 / Balance Co	Ni 1.0 max / Si 1.0 max / Mn 1.0 max / Carbon, nitrogen, aluminum, and lanthanum content is dependent on alloy type.	There are 3 versions of this alloy in the ASTM specification and 2 ISO versions: alloy 1 is low carbon (0.14 max), alloy 2 contains more carbon (0.15-0.35), and alloy 3 is dispersion strengthened. Alloy 3 is not in the ISO standard.
Ti	F 67[5] ISO 5832 Part 2[18]	CP Ti	Balance Ti	C max 0.10 / Fe max 0.5 / H max 0.0125-0.015 / N max 0.05	Four grades based on oxygen content: grade I has 0.18% max O, grade II has 0.25% max O, grade III has 0.35% max O, grade IV has 0.40% max O. ISO standard also has a 0.10 max O grade.
Ti-6Al-4V	F 136[19] ISO 5832 Part 3[20]	Ti-6Al-4V	Al 5.5-6.5 / V 3.5-4.5 / Balance Ti	C max 0.08 / H max 0.0125 / Fe max 0.25 / N max 0.05 / O max 0.13	The ISO standard allows higher oxygen content, which is comparable with ASTM F 1472.

the oxide's resistance to corrosion, especially in chloride environments such as the body. Nickel is added to help stabilize the austenitic structure. The single-phase, stainless steel structure, along with the more densely packed FCC crystal arrangement, tends to provide greater corrosion resistance than the BCC-based stainless steels. The low carbon content also promotes corrosion resistance by preventing the formation of chromium carbides, which precipitate at grain boundaries and reduce corrosion resistance. Steels in which chromium carbides have formed are "sensitized" and may fail from corrosion-assisted fractures that arise at the weakened chromium-depleted grain boundaries.

The austenitic nitrogen-manganese–strengthened stainless steel known by the names Ortron 90 and Rex 734 alloy is in use to produce hip stems outside of the United States. This alloy can be processed to offer higher fatigue strength and corrosion resistance than 316L. A similar stainless steel, BioDur 108, is a low-nickel, austenitic alloy that has been developed to address concerns over the potential of nickel ions released from corrosion products of 316L to induce metal hypersensitivity reactions. In this low-nickel alloy, 0.85% to 1.10% nitrogen is added to stabilize the austenitic microstructure and to maintain high strength and corrosion resistance. The addition of large amounts of manganese (21%-24%) also aids in austenite stabilization.[8,9]

The cobalt (Co)-based alloy most commonly used for hip prostheses contains approximately 28 weight % chromium (Cr) and 6 weight % molybdenum (Mo). The use of cobalt-based alloys dates back to the 1930s, when this material was used by Smith-Peterson as an implant to cover the femoral head and prevent bone-to-bone contact. Several variations of the chemical compositions of this alloy are known; different manufacturing techniques result in significantly different mechanical properties.

The initial Co-Cr-Mo implants were made by investment casting. This process starts with a wax replica of the desired product, which is dipped in a ceramic slurry and then dried. With multiple applications of the ceramic coating, sufficient strength is built up for the ceramic shell to act as a mold without internal support. At this stage, the wax is melted out and the mold is preheated and then filled with molten metal to form an implant. After the metal solidifies, the mold materials are removed and the cast parts are further processed to achieve the dimensions and finish of the final product.

The resulting microstructure of the cast Co-Cr-Mo alloy is complex and is dependent on exact casting conditions, but it generally can be described as a cobalt-rich matrix (α-phase) with precipitated carbides (primarily $M_{23}C_6$, where M represents Co, Cr, or Mo). The carbides contribute to the alloys' excellent wear resistance. The casting process also results in an alloy with large grains comprising approximately 85% α-phase and 15% carbides. Casting conditions must be closely monitored to avoid casting defects, such as porosity and entrapment of foreign materials. Many cast products receive additional heat treatments to alter the carbide

morphology; the use of hot isostatic pressing (HIP'ing) to close internal porosity is also common.

Stronger femoral hip stems can be produced from the same basic Co-Cr-Mo alloy by using forging or by machining parts from warm-worked bar stock. Forging involves using dies with shaped cavities that are mounted in various types of presses or hammers. The shape of the final die cavity approximates the desired product shape. Metal bars are deformed in the die cavities by forces applied by the press. In most cases, the metal is heated before it is deformed, and a series of cavities must be used because the desired shape cannot be formed in a single step. Conventional bar stock is produced from large cast ingots through a series of deformation processes (open die forging, rolling, etc.) at elevated temperatures. These processes lead to much finer grain size than as-cast metals, improved chemical homogeneity, and, in many alloys including Co-Cr-Mo, the development of a complex, work-hardened structure. The term *wrought* is often applied to metal products that start as large cast ingots and are worked down to usable sizes through processes such as forging or rolling. Thus, the microstructures of cast and wrought Co-Cr-Mo alloys are dramatically different, as can be seen in Figure 6-6. The mechanical properties of wrought

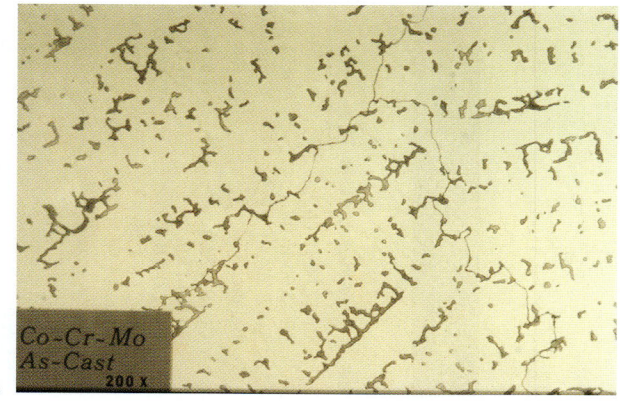

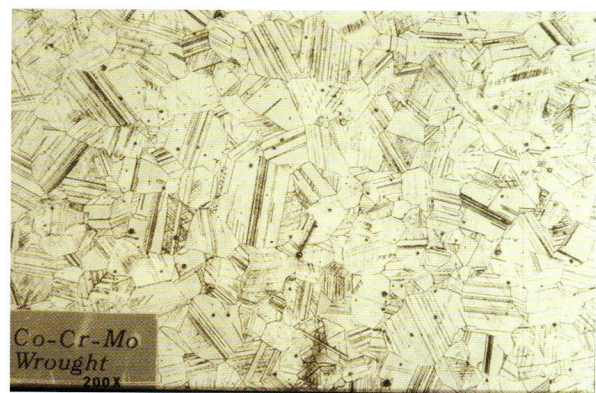

Figure 6-6. Microstructures of Co-Cr-Mo alloy in **(A)** as-cast and **(B)** forged conditions. Note the large carbides *(dark particles)* in the as-cast material. The forged specimen in this example is made with a Co-Cr-Mo composition that uses small additions of nitrogen instead of carbon. The grain size of the forged specimen is much smaller than that of the cast material. (Original magnification ×200.)

or forged Co-Cr-Mo are substantially greater than the cast material.

An alloy known as *MP35N* was once used widely to produce femoral hip stems, but it is no longer widely used for this application. The nominal composition of the alloy is 35 weight % Co and nickel (Ni), 20 weight % Cr, and 10 weight % Mo. This alloy can be processed to very high fatigue mechanical strengths, but it has been replaced by forged Co-Cr-Mo and Ti alloy hip stems.

The major types of titanium alloys are commercially pure (CP) Ti (α or HCP structure), α+β alloys such as Ti-6Al-4V, and β alloys such as Ti-12Mo-6Zr-2Fe. The crystal structure of Ti alloys depends on composition and processing parameters, such as the amount of deformation, the temperature at which deformation takes place, and the cooling rate after forging. In the case of Ti-6Al-4V, the addition of the alloying elements aluminum and vanadium has a stabilizing effect on the α- (HCP) structure and the β- (BCC) structure, respectively. Hence, the Ti-6Al-4V alloy is called an *α+β alloy*, in which the relationship of the α and β phases to each other depends on details of the processing methods used to produce the material. Carefully controlled hot working and annealing processes result in fine dispersion of the α and β phases, which results in superior, high-cycle fatigue properties.

CP Ti is commonly used to produce acetabular components; the higher-strength α+β or β alloys are used to produce femoral hip stems. Ti has a high affinity for oxygen, and CP Ti actually may be thought of as a single-phase alloy of titanium and oxygen, with the oxygen atoms occupying interstitial sites in the HCP lattice of the α phase. The high affinity of titanium for oxygen also results in the formation of a titanium oxide surface layer, which provides all Ti alloys with their exceptional corrosion resistance. The oxygen content of the alloy has a great impact on mechanical properties and forms the basis of the four grades of CP Ti, which range in oxygen content from 0.18% to 0.40% (see Table 6-2). CP

Ti is commonly used to produce acetabular components; the higher-strength α+β or β alloys are used to produce femoral hip stems.

MECHANICAL PROPERTIES

Several key attributes describe the overall performance of materials used in hip surgery, including biocompatibility, corrosion resistance, wear behavior, fatigue strength, and static mechanical properties. Biocompatibility, corrosion resistance, and wear behavior are the subjects of separate chapters of this book.

Mechanical properties critically affect the performance of all implantable devices and depend on the design of the device, as well as the materials and processes used to produce it. Different applications require different mechanical properties. Metal wire used for suture applications must be extremely ductile but heavily loaded devices, such as hip stems, that require high fatigue strength, because they will be subjected to millions of loading cycles over the life of the implant. The mechanical properties of interest for implantable materials can be separated into two categories: static properties, such as ultimate tensile strength, and dynamic properties, such as fatigue strength.

Static Mechanical Properties

When metal samples loaded in tension are tested, resistance of the sample to elongation is expressed in terms of stress and strain. Stress, denoted by σ, is defined as the applied force divided by the cross-sectional area of the sample; strain, denoted by ε, as the change in sample length divided by the original length. The relationship between these quantities over the range of elongation from the original, undeformed state until failure for a typical metal sample is shown in Figure 6-7. In a standard tensile test, the applied load is increased until the

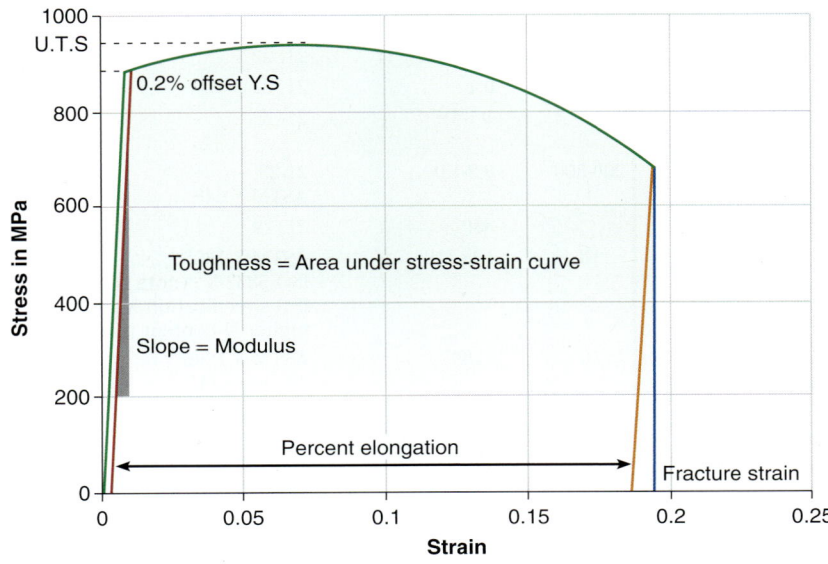

Figure 6-7. Typical tensile testing stress-strain diagram of ASTM F 136 Ti-6Al-4V alloy. The area under the stress-strain curve is an indicator of the material's toughness. (*Data from Mike Carroll, Wright Medical Technology.*)

sample fractures. At the start of loading, the deformation of the sample is elastic, meaning that the sample will return to its original dimensions when the load is removed. In the initial, elastic portion of the test, the strain (ε) or elongation of the sample increases linearly with applied stress (σ), according to the relationship $\sigma = E\varepsilon$, where E is termed *Young's modulus* or the *elastic modulus* (a measure of the inherent stiffness of the material). When the sample is loaded beyond a certain threshold, often referred to as the *yield stress*, permanent (or plastic) deformation results, meaning that the sample does not fully return to its original dimensions when unloaded. The maximum stress that the specimen supports is known as the *ultimate stress* (often referred to as the *ultimate tensile strength* [UTS], if the specimen is tested in tension).

In broad terms, metals are much stronger and stiffer than cortical or trabecular bone. Metals are also stronger and stiffer than ultra-high-molecular-weight polyethylene (UHMWPE) but are also less ductile. Ceramics, typified by alumina (aluminum oxide), have the highest elastic moduli of the materials used in THA, but exhibit low ductility and toughness. Table 6-3 shows approximate values for yield and ultimate tensile strength, elongation (where available), and elastic modulus for some commonly implanted metals, along with cortical and trabecular bone, UHMWPE, and bone cement (PMMA).

Dynamic Mechanical Properties

A common cause of failure of metal components that are exposed to cyclical (or dynamic) loading conditions is fatigue. In broad terms, fatigue is a result of cumulative damage to the material as it experiences a large number of loading cycles. The fatigue process consists of three basic steps: (1) initiation of a crack in the component, (2) growth of the crack, and (3) final failure of the component by overload. Overload and final failure occur when the cross-sectional area is reduced to the point that the load is sufficient to cause stress within the remaining material that exceeds the ultimate tensile strength. Figure 6-8 shows an overall view of a 316L screw that failed as the result of bending fatigue, along with images showing multiple initiation sites and fatigue striations.

Crack initiation, or nucleation, is the most critical step in the fatigue resistance of many medical implants because these products may experience enough load cycles to lead to fracture, if a crack initiates. Initiation sites for cracks may result from material, design, or surface finish issues. Discontinuities in the material, such as inclusion or second-phase particles, are representative of material issues; abrupt transitions in cross-section and sharp radii at corners are examples of design issues, and nicks and gouges in a surface from manufacturing and damage during handling are possible causes of surface damage. Repeated loading cycles may create microscopic discontinuities on the surface of the implant that can act as initiation sites.

Appropriate materials selection, design, and manufacturing processes are required to minimize the possibility of fatigue failure in hip stems and other permanent implants. This is especially critical in THA because loading conditions on the hip joint are high, with femoral head loads up to 3 to 8.5 times body weight during normal daily activities.[27]

To determine the fatigue properties of a material, a number of samples are tested at various stress levels; the results are plotted to show the stress (S) at which each sample failed and the number of cycles (N) the sample survived before it failed plotted on a logarithmic scale. Figure 6-9 shows a generalized S/N (or Wöhler) curve. Many metal alloys (including the alloys commonly used to make implants) exhibit an endurance

---

Table 6-3. Mechanical Properties of Selected Materials Relevant to Hip Replacement Surgery

Material	Yield Strength, MPa	Ultimate Strength, MPa	% Elongation	Tensile Modulus, GPa	Reference
Cortical bone		130		17	21, 22
Trabecular bone		50		0.1	21, 22
Bone cement (PMMA)		23-45 (tension) 85-110 (compression)		1.1-4.1	21, 22
UHMWPE	19-21	40	200-300	0.8-1.0	21-23 ASTM F 648
Al$_2$O$_3$				380	21, 22
Ti-6Al-4V (ELI)	795	860	10	105-110	ASTM F 136[19] ISO 5832-3[20] (note that the ISO specification includes higher O content material)
Ti-6Al-7Nb	800	900	10	≈100	ASTM F 1295[24] ISO 5832-11[25]
Ti-12Mo-6Zr-2Fe (solution annealed)	897	931	12	≈80	ASTM F 1813[26]
Co-Cr-Mo (warm-worked)	827	1192	12	225-240	ASTM F 1537[16] ISO 5832-12[17]
Rex 734 (medium hard condition)	700	1000	20	≈200	ISO 5832-9[13] ASTM F 1586[12]

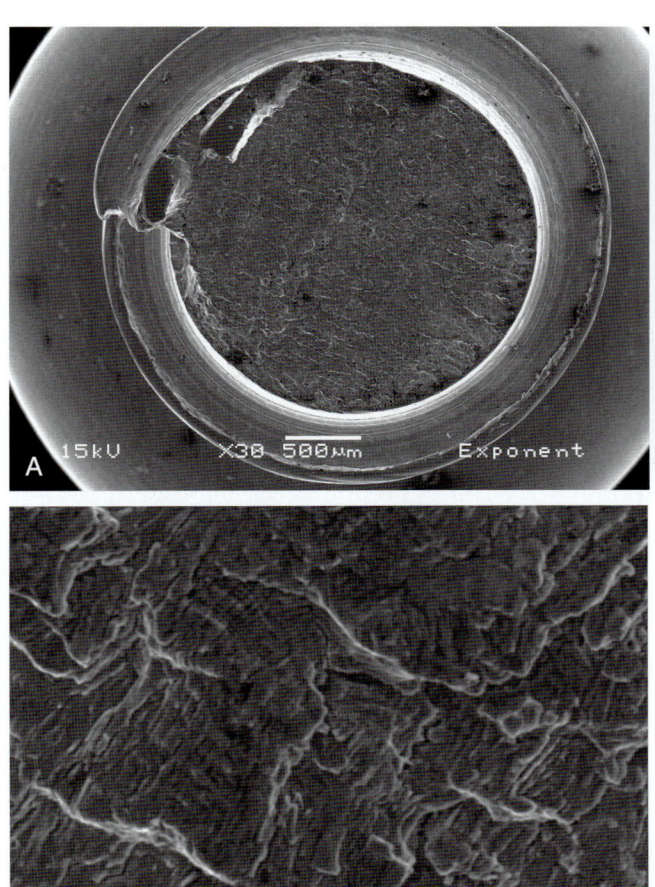

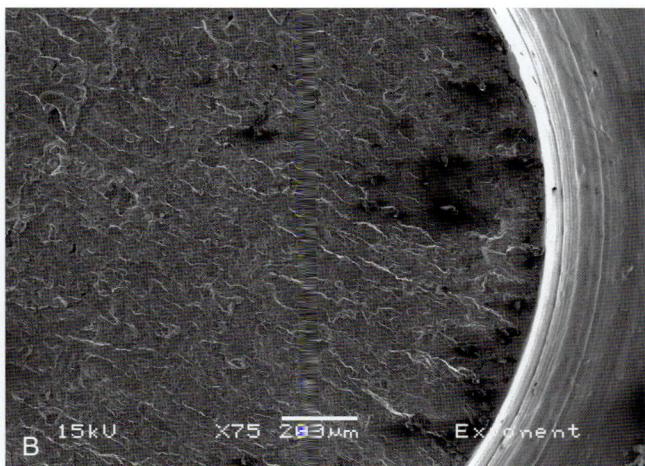

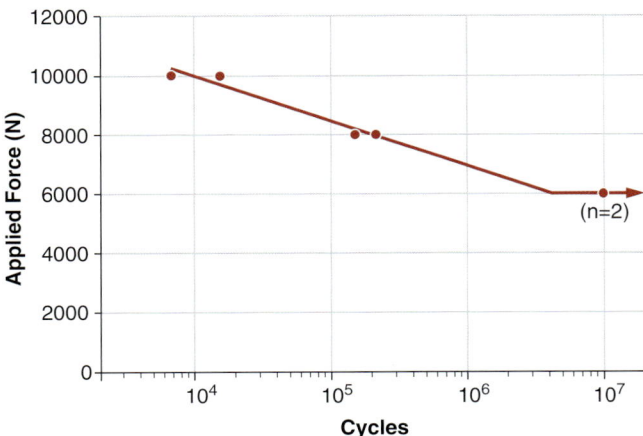

Figure 6-8. A, Overall view of a fractured 316L stainless steel screw. Multiple initiation sites are evident on the right side of the screw; the crack then grew by fatigue until the small region at the left of the image failed as the result of overload. **B,** A higher magnification view of the initiation sites. **C,** Fatigue striations. *(Images provided by B. James, PhD, Exponent.)*

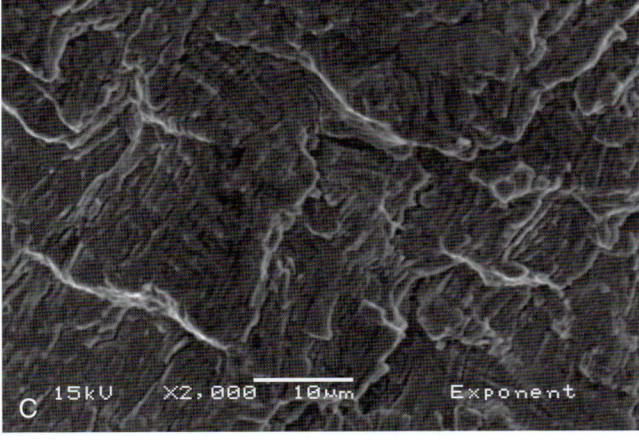

Figure 6-9. S/N curve for a material exhibiting an endurance limit. *(Data from Mike Carroll, Wright Medical Technology.)*

limit, sometimes referred to as the *fatigue limit* or *fatigue strength*, which is the maximum stress level that a material may withstand for an infinite number of loading cycles without failure. It is common practice to define the fatigue strength of a material at 10^7 million

cycles as the endurance limit, because the rate of decay in strength is very low beyond this point, and the testing time becomes an issue.

The fatigue resistance of an implant also depends on the nature of the loading cycle that it experiences. Fatigue tests are often performed in which peak loads alternate around zero (i.e., tension-compression or reverse bending) or the loads fluctuate in one fixed direction (i.e., tension or bending in one direction). Fatigue tests in which the sample is always in tension are common. These types of tests are performed on laboratory samples that have been machined out of actual hip implants or have been prepared from raw material, such as bars or forged coupons. Standard tests are used to measure the fatigue performance of actual hip stems. Examples of these tests are found in ISO specifications 7206 Part 4[28] and 7206 Part 6[29] and in ASTM specification F 1612.[30] In these tests, the stress state is more complex because both torsion and bending loads are applied during each loading cycle. In comparison with fatigue tests performed on laboratory specimens, testing of complete devices is advantageous in that observed fatigue strength reflects any effects of actual manufacturing processes and may reveal unexpected issues with the design of the product.

It is important to realize that a significant amount of variability in fatigue test results may be noted. Many factors can lead to variation, including small surface discontinuities (nicks or marks made by instruments during implant insertion, etc.), flaws within the metal (oxide particles), and variations in the processes used to produce the metal specimen. Different test methods may also result in somewhat different results. To understand the range of fatigue properties for a given material, it is useful to test large numbers of samples that have been made over a period of time (as opposed to testing one group of samples made at the same time). Figure 6-10 shows the range of fatigue behavior that has been observed in cast, cast+HIP, and wrought Ti-6Al-4V test specimens. Table 6-4 lists fatigue endurance limits for various hip implant materials.

The fatigue strength of implants is also influenced by processes commonly used in implant production. Control of raw material quality is a crucial first step, and all subsequent processes must be well understood and controlled, or the strength and durability of the implant may be compromised. Examples of some specific issues follow.

- Clinical failures of forged Co-Cr and Ti-6Al-4V hip stems have been associated with laser marking.[38,39] Laboratory tests of wrought Co-Cr and Ti-6Al-7Nb specimens show reductions in the endurance limit of approximately 60% and 70%, respectively, due to laser etching.[31,40] Laboratory tests used four-point bending with the laser-marked surface placed in tension.
- Ti alloys are notch sensitive; the presence of notches or surface discontinuities on the surface results in significant reductions in fatigue strength. Reported values for notched endurance limits of Ti-6Al-4V are in the range of 150[35] to 290 MPa.[41] The beta Ti alloy, Ti-12Mo-6Zr-2Fe, is somewhat less notch sensitive, with a reported endurance limit of 410 MPa versus smooth fatigue results of 585 MPa.[34] Fatigue strength reductions due to notch sensitivity can result from

surface damage during manufacture or during implantation at surgery. Notches may also be created at the interface of a porous layer with the underlying implant surface.

- Hip implants are manufactured with a variety of porous surfaces. The technique used to apply the porous coating can have significant effects on fatigue strength. The elevated temperatures used to sinter "bead" coatings result in significant structure and property changes for both Co-Cr and Ti alloy implants. In the case of Co-Cr implants, published fatigue strengths of sintered porous-coated samples range from 150 to 207 MPa for investment cast material[33]

Table 6-4. Approximately 10⁷ Million Cycle Fatigue Strength of Some Metals Used in THA

Material	Material Condition	10⁷ Cycle Endurance Limit, MPa	Reference
Co-Cr-Mo (ASTM F 75[14], ISO 5832-4[15])	Investment cast	345-480	31
Co-Cr-Mo (ASTM F 1537[16], ISO 5832-12[17])	Forged or warm worked	656-930	31-33
Ti-6Al-4V (ASTM F 136[19], ISO 5832-3[20])	Wrought	585-700	34, 35
Ti 6Al-7Nb (ASTM F 1295[24], ISO 5832-11[25])	Wrought	540-750	35, 36
Ti-12Mo-6Zr-2Fe (ASTM F 1813[26])	Wrought	585	34
Fe-21Cr-10Ni-3Mn-2.5Mo (Rex 734 ASTM F 1586[12], ISO 5832-9[13])	Forged Annealed	587 269	33, 37

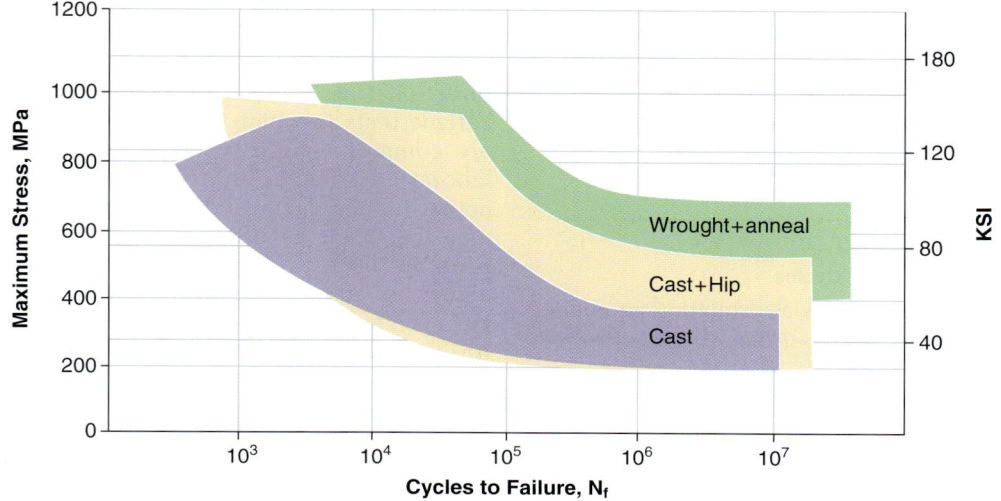

Figure 6-10. The range of fatigue results observed in cast, cast + Hot Isostatic Pressed (HIP), and wrought Ti-6Al-4V. All test data were generated using axial fatigue testing. *(Courtesy of F.H. [Sam] Froes and D. Eylon.)*

to 345 MPa[42] for forged, dispersion-strengthened samples. In nonporous Co-Cr sintered samples, fatigue strength can range from 345 to 930 MPa for specimens fabricated from cast and wrought material. For Ti implants, porous coating effects may be due to a number of factors. As in the case of Co-Cr implants, high-temperature sintering of Ti alloys leads to significant changes in microstructure and properties. Sintered coatings on Ti-6Al-4V exhibit reduced fatigue strengths in the range of 140 to 200 MPa.[33] Coatings applied at lower temperatures (e.g., diffusion bonding) still exhibit a notch effect whereby the coating is bonded to the implant. Plasma-sprayed coatings rely on a mechanical interlock between the implant and the coating. The implant experiences very little temperature increase during the coating operation, but the aggressive grit blast operation before plasma spraying can roughen the surface enough to cause reduced fatigue strength. In all of these cases, the implant design must take into account the changes in fatigue strength that result from use of the coating.

CORROSION PROPERTIES

The human physiologic environment is complex, involving salts (Na^+, Cl^-, K^+ PO_4^{2-}, SO_4^{2-}, OH^-), dissolved gases (O_2, H_2O_2, O_2, CO_2), proteins, cells, and mechanical and electrical loads. This environment causes the degradation or corrosion of most metals and alloys used in orthopedic applications. Corrosion of the metal implant is of great concern, not only because loss of material from the alloy may compromise mechanical and electrical integrity, but also because many of the metal ions released from the alloys (e.g., Ni, Cr, V) may have acute or chronic effects on local or systemic tissues. For example, Ni- and Cr-rich corrosion products formed from ions released by 316L stainless steel and Co-Cr implants have been associated with hypersensitivity reactions, and metal ion corrosion products have been associated with impaired bone cell function and bone resorption.[43-51]

Corrosion is an electrochemical process involving a pair of oxidation and reduction reactions in which electrons released by a metal react with entities within the surrounding solution (e.g., H_2O). For example, under acidic conditions, titanium can dissolve through the following chemical reactions:

Oxidation reaction:

$$Ti \rightarrow Ti^{+2} + 2e^- \qquad \text{[Equation 1]}$$

Reduction reaction:

$$2H^+ + 2e^- \rightarrow H_2 \text{ and } O_2 + 4H^+ + 4e^- \rightarrow 2H_2O \qquad \text{[Equation 2]}$$

Under neutral/basic conditions, the reduction reaction becomes

$$O_2 + 2H_2O + 4e^- \rightarrow 4(OH)^-$$

When this occurs, the metal ions go into solution (Equation 1), unless they form complex oxides/hydroxides. They also may become bound to proteins or other biological molecules, which may be distributed throughout the body via the lymph nodes and vasculature. The site where oxidation occurs is called the *anode,* and the site where reduction occurs is called the *cathode.* The type of reduction reaction that occurs is dependent in part on the environment such that in acidic environments, such as in inflammatory conditions, H^+ ions are reduced to H_2 gas, and O_2 may be reduced to water (Equation 2). In neutral or basic conditions, O_2 is reduced to OH^-.

The susceptibility of orthopedic implants to corrosion may be evaluated using an electrochemical cell (Fig. 6-11) in which the electrical potential of the alloy in a test electrolyte (e.g., saline) is monitored with respect to a reference electrode (e.g., a saturated calomel electrode). Corrosion potentials are an indication of the tendency of a metal or alloy to corrode in a given environment. The more positive the potential of the alloy, the lower is the driving force for the alloy to undergo oxidation or corrode; the more negative the potential, the higher is the driving force for the alloy to undergo corrosion. Metals and alloys with a relatively high potential are referred to as *inert* or *low reactive,* and those with a relatively low potential are referred to as *active.* However, corrosion potentials do not provide information about the rate of corrosion, which can be greatly influenced by the formation of a surface oxide film and other factors such as pH, proteins, and the availability of oxygen.

The rate of corrosion of an implant metal in a test environment can also be assessed using an electrochemical cell by measuring the amount of current (amps) generated by the oxidation-reduction reaction. The magnitude of the corrosion current can be converted into a corrosion penetration rate ($\mu m/yr$) using the following formula:

$$\mu m/yr = (0.129)[(ai)/(nD)]$$

where a is the atomic weight of the metal, i is current normalized to surface area ($\mu amps/cm^2$), n is the number of electrons lost (valence charge), and D is the density of the metal in g/cm. Table 6-5 gives a range of values of corrosion potentials and corrosion rates for orthopedic alloys in physiologic environments.[52] Note that in general, 316L stainless steel has the most active corrosion potentials and the highest corrosion rates, followed by the Co-Cr alloys, with Ti and Ti alloys exhibiting the most positive corrosion potentials and the lowest corrosion rates.

Orthopedic alloys derive their corrosion resistance from the formation of a protective surface oxide film or layer (Fig. 6-12), typically chromium oxide (stainless steels and Co-Cr alloys) or titanium oxide (Ti and Ti alloys). These surface oxides function as an insulating or nonconductive layer that prevents dissolution of the underlying metal atoms and the transfer of electrons in oxidation-reduction reactions. The development of the protective surface oxide is referred to as *passivation* because it makes the alloys appear to be unreactive or *passive* when exposed to chloride environments. The development of a robust oxide layer may be facilitated by passivation treatments, such as immersion in 20% to 45% nitric acid (ASTM F 86).[53] This process not only

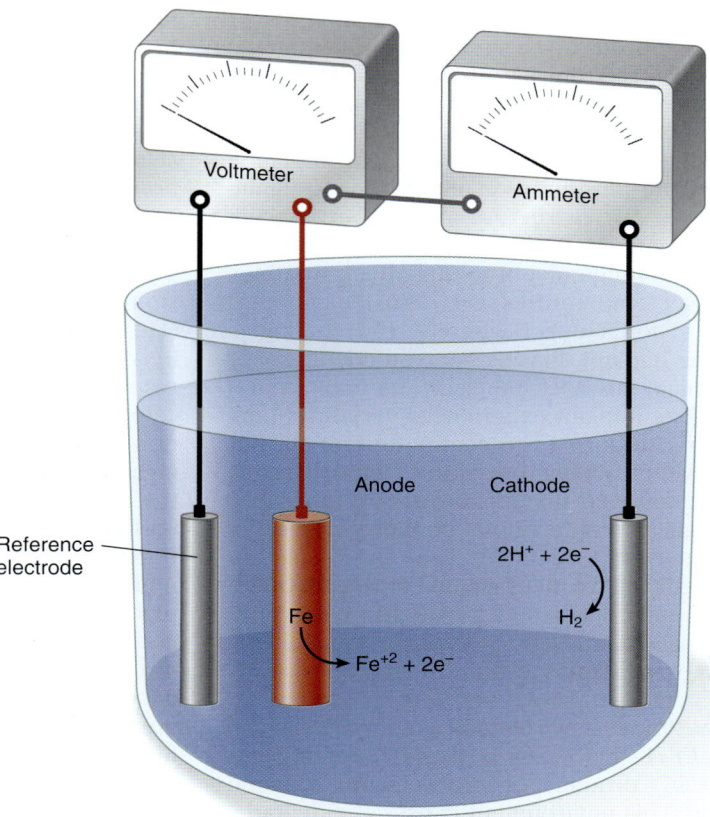

Figure 6-11. Simplified schematic of electrochemical corrosion cell. Corrosion potential is measured between reference electrode and test metal or anode, and corrosion rate is measured based on the flow of current between anode and cathode.

Table 6-5. Range of Corrosion Potentials and Rates Reported for Selected Orthopedic Alloys

Alloy	Corrosion Potential, mV vs. SCE	Corrosion Current, nA/cm²
316L	−400 to +400	2-2000
Co-Cr-Mo	−531 to +260	0.3-3000
CP Ti	−520 to +208	1-9000
Ti-6Al-4V	−540 to +260	0.01-5700

Data from Bundy KJ: Corrosion and other electrochemical aspects of biomaterials. Crit Rev Biomed Eng 22:139–251, 1994.

facilitates the development of the surface oxide, it can also remove foreign materials that may be present from previous processing steps.[53]

The stability of the surface oxide film is dependent on the presence of oxygen in the local environment and can change with implantation time.[54,55] Surface oxides for the most part can re-form (i.e., re-passivate) after being damaged (e.g., if scratched during implant placement), although if damage is severe or occurs under anaerobic conditions, corrosion resistance may be reduced. If the oxide layer breaks down or is unable to re-form after damage, the underlying metal may undergo active or accelerated corrosion.

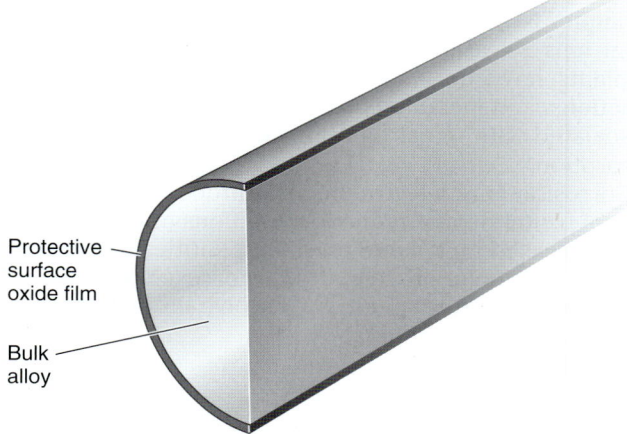

Figure 6-12. Schematic of protective surface oxide on implant alloy. For stainless steel and Co-Cr alloys, the surface oxide is predominantly a chromium oxide layer, and for CP Ti and Ti alloys, it is a titanium oxide layer.

Although orthopedic alloys have been selected to be highly corrosion resistant, no alloy is inert in the body but will release metal ions through slow dissolution to local tissues. This is referred to as *general* or *uniform corrosion* and occurs more or less over the entire metallic surface of the implant. Although uniform corrosion does not affect the mechanical integrity of the component, it may result in unwanted tissue reactions in some patients who show hypersensitivity to released metal ions, such as Ni or Cr from stainless steel or cobalt-based alloys.[44,45,56] Of greater concern in terms of both mechanical and host tissue reactions are the accelerated processes of galvanic pitting and crevice corrosion, as well as the electromechanical forms of degradation that involve combinations of corrosion with fretting, wear, and fatigue. These forms of corrosion are highly localized and (1) can result in the significant release of metal ions that may be matters of biological/toxicity concern, or (2) may compromise the mechanical integrity of the component itself.

Galvanic or two-metal corrosion occurs when two dissimilar metals or alloys are in electrical contact in the environment. The alloy with the more positive corrosion potential will act as the cathode in the electrochemical cell and will become protected, while the alloy with the more negative corrosion potential will act as the anode and will have its corrosion rate increased. The larger the difference between the potentials of the two metals, the greater is the driving force for corrosion, whereas the smaller or more similar the potentials, the less is the driving force. For example, if a K-wire, which is made from stainless steel, is in close proximity to be in electrical contact with or touching a titanium screw, or a stainless steel screw is used with a titanium fracture plate, then the stainless steel device will undergo accelerated corrosion. In modular hips with a Co-Cr-Mo femoral head and a Ti-6Al-4V stem, the difference in electrochemical corrosion potentials is considered small, such that coupling of the two alloys usually is not a matter of concern.[57,58] In general, the coupling of 316L stainless steels with Co-Cr or Ti alloys is not recommended, and the coupling of Co-Cr and Ti alloys is considered not to be a matter of concern.[52,59,60]

Pitting corrosion takes place on the surface of implant alloys in the presence of aggressive ions, such as chlorides. Chlorides damage the passive layer at grain boundaries, dislocations, inclusions, and other small surface defect/impurity sites. Once the oxide layer has been compromised, pits form at the sites of localized damage and grow through active corrosion, which occurs rapidly as the result of an autocatalytic process involving a reduction in oxygen concentration, an influx of chloride ions, and a decrease of pH in the pit. The initiation of a corrosion pit on the implant surface can take a long time because the conditions (locally high concentrations of chloride and hydrogen ions) are unstable and may be quickly removed through fluid flow. This type of corrosion is particularly destructive in that the pit can go unnoticed on the surface, leading to a reduction in the cross-sectional area of the device with relatively little loss of material and development of cracks at the corrosion pit tip, both of which can lead to sudden device fracture. The 316L stainless steel alloy is susceptible to pitting attack, and Co-Cr and Ti alloys are highly resistant.[52,59,60]

Crevice corrosion may occur where narrow gaps or spaces exist, such as within a modular junction or between screws and fixation plates, or when similar geometric conditions arise.[60-62] Crevice corrosion occurs when the fluid within the crevice becomes depleted in oxygen, leading to acidification of the fluid within the crevice. In a chloride environment, this sets up an autocatalytic mechanism similar to pitting corrosion. The 316L stainless steel alloy is susceptible to crevice corrosion, in part because of the lower stability of its chromium oxide film. Conversely, the surface oxides of the Co-Cr and Ti alloys are more stable and have very high resistance to crevice corrosion. Other factors that affect crevice corrosion are hydrodynamic conditions and size of the crevice.

Fretting or wear corrosion occurs because of the relative cyclical movement of two surfaces with respect to each other. This type of corrosion has been observed between femoral head and stem components of total hip implants.[63-65] This corrosion may also occur between screws and plates. Because fretting corrosion occurs when the protective surface oxide layer is removed by mechanical means, all implant alloys (stainless steel, Co-Cr, and Ti alloys) are susceptible to this form of degradation. The surface oxide layer may re-form only to be removed or destroyed by subsequent cycles. Removed oxides can further aggravate the process by acting as third-body wear particles.

Stress corrosion cracking occurs when some biomaterials are loaded in tension in a corrosive environment. The result is failure of the device under conditions where neither the stress nor the environment alone would normally be detrimental. It is believed that the combined action of the tensile stress and the corrosion environment leads to the breakdown of surface oxide and the initiation of small cracks perpendicular to applied load.[52,59] Once formed, the crack tip continues to grow, leading quickly to brittle fracture. The initiation period for stress corrosion cracking can be long, but once initiated, crack growth can be rapid and may lead to catastrophic failure. Austenitic stainless steels and some aluminum alloys, such as those used as components in external fixation devices, are susceptible to stress corrosion cracking in the aggressive, chloride-containing physiologic environment.[52,59,66]

Fatigue corrosion is the combined action of applied cyclical stresses and a corrosive environment. Repeated loading can initiate cracks in the protective oxide at surface defects, at areas of high surface roughness, or even at surface pits. The result is that cracks quickly grow in repeated cycles, dramatically diminishing the fatigue life of the device. Fatigue corrosion has been reported in the failure of stainless steel, Co-Cr, and Ti implants.[52,59]

Intergranular corrosion occurs by preferential attack of the corrosive environment along the grain boundaries of the material, with the result that the alloy disintegrates through progressive grain loss. Attack occurs along the grain boundaries under conditions that make them more reactive than the interior part of the grains. Intergranular corrosion can occur as the result of impurities, which tend to locate/segregate to grain boundaries and/or to depletion of alloying elements. This occurs in Co-Cr alloys in the cast condition when complex chromium carbides precipitate along grain boundaries, depleting the adjacent matrix of elements imparting corrosion resistance. This tendency caused failure of earlier hip stems fabricated in the cast condition but has been virtually eliminated through the use of lower carbon compositions and/or homogenizing heat treatments. 316L stainless steel also shows susceptibility to intergranular corrosion, but only under conditions in which the alloy has become sensitized, as described in the section, "Orthopedic Implant Alloy Compositions and Microstructures." This type of corrosion is easily prevented through careful control of alloy compositions (e.g., use of low carbon alloys) and manufacturing conditions.

Corrosion of orthopedic implants is prevented mainly through alloy selection, surface treatments, implant design, and handling during surgical use. 316L stainless steel, Co-Cr, and Ti alloys all have been empirically selected and have a long history of success as implant devices. These alloys are easy to passivate (via nitric acid) to impart corrosion resistance; numerous other experimental surface treatments use heat, chemicals, and/or coating technologies that can enhance the properties of the surface oxide layer.[52,59] In choosing the best manufacturing process for each alloy, the quest for optimal mechanical properties must be balanced with the impact of microstructure and composition on corrosion resistance. For example, the stainless steels should not be used with excessive cold work, and inclusions and pores should be avoided for the cast Co-Cr alloys. The design of implants and implant components should minimize stress-concentrating geometries and discontinuities, as well as unnecessary interfaces. Finally, care should be exercised during implantation to minimize/avoid damaging the surface oxides and introducing excessive deformation.

CURRENT CONTROVERSIES AND FUTURE DIRECTIONS

Many of the current controversies related to metals and alloys for cemented and uncemented hip implants will be discussed in other chapters within this book. Most of the current concerns or controversies involving THA metal alloys are a continuation of known material and design issues. Loss of metal ions through wear or corrosion continues to be a matter of concern, especially in metal-on-metal bearings and in patients with heightened metal sensitivity. New metal alloys with potentially more compatible alloying elements are being developed and commercialized. Hip stems fabricated

in smaller sizes and components with multiple modular taper connections can potentially create situations of reduced mechanical strength, especially under fatigue conditions. Diligence in the testing of existing and new metal alloys, in simulations that accurately mimic clinical applications, will continue to be a challenge in the evaluation of new and improved implant designs.

FUTURE DIRECTIONS

Possible directions for metallic THA implants include removing the nickel from stainless steels and improving both smooth and notched fatigue strength (and possibly reducing elastic modulus) of titanium alloys.

Stainless Steels

For several decades, 316L stainless steel was commonly used to produce hip implants. Although 316L is still in use today, the high chromium-manganese-nitrogen alloys (ASTM 1586, also marketed as Ortron-90 or Rex 734) are stronger and more corrosion resistant and have been used for approximately 20 years in the United Kingdom and Europe for the manufacture of hip prostheses, and in the United Sates for the production of hip fracture fixation devices. Improvements in strength and corrosion resistance in this alloy and a similar material known as *22-13-5* result primarily from the addition of (0.2%-0.50%) nitrogen. These alloys also contain more chromium (19.5%-23.5%, depending on the alloy) and manganese (2.0%-6.0%, depending on the alloy) than 316L.

Because the issue of nickel sensitivity causes concern for some patients, several stainless steels have been developed that contain essentially no nickel. A key reason for the presence of nickel in 316L is that it stabilizes the nonmagnetic austenite phase. Manganese and nitrogen also stabilize austenite, so the "nickel-free" stainless steels contain large quantities of these elements.

BioDur 108 is an example of a nickel-free stainless alloy. It is now being used in some fracture fixation products, but not to produce femoral hip stems. If a market is developed for nickel-free, stainless steel hip stems, BioDur 108 could be a candidate material.

Table 6-6 lists the chemical compositions of these alloys. Recent data show that the trend in implantable stainless steels is toward increased levels of nitrogen, chromium, and manganese with decreased levels of nickel.

Table 6-6. Chemical Compositions of 316L, Rex 734, 22-13-5, and BioDur 108 Alloys

Alloy Designation	Wt Percent Cr	Wt Percent Ni	Wt Percent Mn	Wt Percent Mo	Wt Percent N
316L (ASTM F 138[10])	17.00-19.00	13.00-15.00	2.00 max	2.25-3.00	0.10 max
Rex 734 (ASTM F 1586[12])	19.5-22.0	9.0-11.0	2.00-4.25	2.0-3.0	0.25-0.50
22-13-5 (ASTM F 1314[67])	20.50-23.50	11.50-13.50	4.00-6.00	2.00-3.00	0.20-0.40
BioDur 108 (ASTM F 2229[7])	19.00-23.00	0.05 max	21.00-24.00	0.50-1.50	0.85-1.10

Titanium Alloys

Although Ti-6Al-4V (an $\alpha+\beta$ alloy) continues to be used for a large number of hip stems, a number of other Ti alloys have been put into service for this demanding application. These alloys may be $\alpha+\beta$ alloys with different alloying elements (i.e., substituting Nobium [Nb] for V in the case of Ti-6Al-7Nb), or they may be β alloys.

Type β titanium alloys rely on large quantities of β-stabilizing elements, such as Mo, and rapid cooling to retain the β structure; rapid cooling of $\alpha+\beta$ alloys such as Ti-6Al-4V results in a nonequilibrium (also known as *martensitic*) transformation. In the martensitic condition, titanium alloys lack the appropriate mechanical properties for use in implants. The β alloys are sometimes referred to as *metastable β alloys* because they would revert to $\alpha+\beta$ structures under true equilibrium conditions, such as very slow cooling from elevated temperatures.

Several potential advantages of β alloys have been identified:

- High strengths can be achieved by heat treatments that precipitate fine α phase particles within the β phase; 10^7 cycle fatigue endurance limits of ≈ 700 MPa have been reported for aged Ti-15Mo and Ti-15Mo-5Zr-3Al.[68,69]
- Some experimental β alloys can be deformed extensively at room temperature.[70] This could lead to more cost-effective ways of producing implants. Mechanical properties may also improve as the result of work hardening.
- Because β alloys are less notch sensitive than $\alpha+\beta$ alloys, they may be better suited to porous coating applications whereby junctions between the porous layer and the implant act as notches.[34]
- Unlike $\alpha+\beta$ alloys, β alloys containing large amounts of alloying elements (e.g., 35 weight %Nb, 7 weight %Zr, 5 weight %Ta) may utilize large oxygen additions without becoming brittle, leading to ultimate strengths greater than 1050 MPa.[71]
- Finally, the elastic modulus of some β alloys can be very low ($\approx \frac{1}{2}$ the modulus of Ti-6Al-4V); unfortunately, at the lowest modulus condition, mechanical properties are reduced. A paper by Niinomi offers an excellent review of some current research into β titanium alloys.[72]

Currently, two β alloys are the subject of ASTM standards: Ti-12Mo-6Zr-2Fe (ASTM F 1813)[26] and Ti-15Mo (ASTM F 2066).[73] The Ti-15Mo-5Zr-3Al alloy is covered by ISO 5832-14.[74] The Ti-12Mo-6Zr-2Fe and Ti-15Mo-5Zr-3Al alloys are used to produce hip stems, and the Ti-15Mo alloy has been used to produce fracture fixation devices.[75] It is likely that additional β titanium alloys will be used in THAs in the future.

Acknowledgments

This chapter was prepared in part with the assistance of the Biomaterials Applications of Memphis (BAM) research group at the University of Memphis–University of Tennessee Health Science Center joint program in biomedical engineering. The authors acknowledge Sarah Stroupe, Benjamin Reves, Jared Cooper, and Marvin Mecwar for their assistance in preparing figures and tables and in formatting references.

REFERENCES

1. Learmonth ID, Young C, Rorabeck C: The operation of the century: total hip replacement. Lancet 370:1508–1519, 2007.
2. Cuckler JM: The rationale for metal-on-metal total hip arthroplasty. Clin Orthop Rela Res 441:132–136, 2005.
3. Meyers M, Chawla K: Mechanical behavior of materials, New York, NY, 2006, Cambridge University Press, pp 270–271.
4. Lutrjerung G, Williams J: Titanium, Berlin, 2007, Springer.
5. ASTM Standard F 67.200G: Standard specification for unalloyed titanium for surgical implant applications, West Conshohocken, Pa, 2006, ASTM International.
6. Shetty R, Ottersberg W: Metals in orthopedic surgery: encyclopedic handbook of biomaterials and bioengineering: part B, applications, New York, NY, 1995, Marcel Decker, pp 509–540.
7. ASTM Standard F 2229.2002: Standard specification for wrought, nitrogen strengthened 23manganese-21chromium-1molybdenum low-nickel stainless steel alloy bar and wire for surgical implants, West Conshohocken, Pa, 2007, ASTM International.
8. Technical Data Sheet BioDur108, Volume 2008.
9. Gebeau RC, Brown RS: Biomedical implant alloy. Adv Mater Proc 159:46–48, 2001.
10. ASTM Standard F 138.197: Standard specification for wrought 18chromium-14nickel-2.5molybdenum stainless steel bar and wire for surgical implants, West Conshohocken, Pa, 2008, ASTM International.
11. ISO Standard 5832-1.1997 Implants for surgery: metallic materials. Part 1. Wrought stainless steel, Geneva, Switzerland, 2007, International Organization for Standardization.
12. ASTM Standard F 1586.1995: Standard specification for wrought nitrogen strengthened 21chromium-10nickel-3manganese-2.5molybdenum stainless steel alloy bar for surgical implants, West Conshohocken, Pa, 2008, ASTM International.
13. ISO Standard 5832-9.1992: Implants for surgery: metallic materials. Part 9. Wrought high nitrogen stainless steel, Geneva, Switzerland, 2007, International Organization for Standardization
14. ASTM Standard F 75.1998 Standard specification for cobalt-28 chromium-6 molybdenum alloy castings and casting alloy for surgical implants, West Conshohocken, Pa, 2007, ASTM International.
15. ISO Standard 5832-4.1978 Implants for surgery: metallic materials. Part 4. Cobalt-chromium-molybdenum casting alloy, Geneva, Switzerland, 1996, International Organization for Standardization.
16. ASTM Standard F 1537.2000: Standard specification for wrought cobalt-28chromium-6molybdenum alloys for surgical implants, West Conshohocken, Pa, 2007, ASTM International.
17. ISO Standard 5832-12.1996: Implants for surgery: metallic materials. Part 12. Wrought cobalt-chromium-molybdenum alloy, Geneva, Switzerland 2007, International Organization for Standardization.
18. ISO Standard 5832-2.1993: Implants for surgery: metallic materials. Part 2. Unalloyed titanium, Geneva, 1999, International Organization for Standardization.
19. ASTM Standard F 136.1998e1: Standard specification for wrought titanium-6 aluminum-4 vanadium ELI (extra low interstitial) alloy for surgical implant applications, West Conshohocken, Pa, 2008, ASTM International.
20. ISO Standard 5832-3.1990: Implants for surgery: metallic materials. Part 3. Wrought titanium 6-aluminium 4-vanadium alloy, Geneva, 1996, International Organization for Standardization.
21. Mow V, Flatow E, Ateshia G: Biomechanics. In Buckwater J, Einhorn T, Simon S (eds): Biomechanics of the musculoskeletal system, Rosemont, Ill, 2000, American Academy of Orthopaedic Surgeons, pp 133–180.
22. Wright T, Li S: Biomaterials. In Buckwater J, Einhorn T, Simon S (eds): Biomechanics of the musculoskeletal system,

Rosemont, Ill, 2000, American Academy of Orthopaedic Surgeons, pp 181–215.

23. ASTM Standard F 648.2000: Standard specification for ultra-high-molecular-weight polyethylene powder and fabricated form for surgical implants, West Conshohocken, Pa, 2007, ASTM International.

24. ASTM Standard F 1295.1997a: Standard specification for wrought titanium-6 aluminum-7 niobium alloy for surgical implant applications, West Conshohocken, Pa, 2005, ASTM International.

25. ISO Standard 5832-11: Implants for surgery: metallic materials. Part 11. Wrought titanium 6-aluminium 7-niobium alloy, Geneva, Switzerland, 1994, International Organization for Standardization.

26. ASTM Standard F 1813.1997e1: Standard specification for wrought titanium-12 molybdenum-6 zirconium-2 iron alloy for surgical implant, West Conshohocken, Pa, 2006, ASTM International.

27. Simon S. Kinesiology. In Buckwater J, Einhorn T, Simon S (eds): Biomechanics of the musculoskeletal system, Rosemont, Ill, 2000, American Academy of Orthopaedic Surgeons, p 790.

28. ISO Standard 7206-4.1989: Implants for surgery: partial and total hip joint prostheses. Part 4. Determination of endurance properties of stemmed femoral components, Geneva, Switzerland, 2007, International Organization for Standardization.

29. ISO Standard 7206-6.1992: Implants for surgery: partial and total hip joint prostheses. Part 6. Determination of endurance properties of head and neck region of stemmed femoral components, Geneva, Switzerland, 1992, International Organization for Standardization.

30. ASTM Standard F 1612.1995: Standard practice for cyclic fatigue testing of metallic stemmed hip arthroplasty femoral components with torsion, West Conshohocken, Pa, 2005, ASTM International.

31. Berlin R, Gustavson L, Wang K: Influence of post processing on the mechanical properties of investment cast and wrought Co-Cr-Mo alloys. In Disegi J, Kennedy R, Pilliar R (eds): Cobalt-base alloys for biomedical applications, West Conshohocken, Pa, 1999, ASTM International, pp 62–70.

32. Del Corso G: Effect of cold drawing and heat treating on powder metallurgy processed ASTM F 1537 alloy 1 and alloy 2 barstock. In Shrivastava S (ed): Proceedings from the Materials and Processes for Medical Devices Conference 2003, Materials Park, Ohio, 2004, ASM International, pp 314–319.

33. Pilliar R: Metals and orthopaedic implants: past successes, present limitations, future challenges. In Shrivastava S (ed): Proceedings from the Materials and Processes for Medical Devices Conference 2003, Materials Park, Ohio, 2004, ASM International, pp 8–22.

34. Murray N, Jablokov V, Freese H: Mechanical and physical properties of titanium-12 molybdenum-6 zirconium-2 iron beta titanium alloy. In Zardiackas L, Kraay M, Freese H (eds): Titanium, niobium, zirconium, and tantalum for medical and surgical applications, ASTM STP 1471, West Conshohocken, Pa, 2006, American Society for Testing and Materials, pp 3–15.

35. Roach M, Williamson R, Zardiackas L: Comparison of the corrosion fatigue characteristics of CP Ti Grade 4, Ti-6Al-4V ELI, Ti-6Al-7Nb, and Ti-15Mo. In Zardiackas L, Kraay M, Freese H (eds): Titanium, niobium, zirconium, and tantalum for medical and surgical applications, ASTM STP 1471, West Conshohocken, Pa, 2006, American Society for Testing and Materials, pp 183–201.

36. Technical Data Sheet, ATI Titanium-6Al-7Nb Alloy.

37. Windler M, Steger R: Mechanical and corrosion properties of forged hip stems made of high-nitrogen stainless steel. In Winters G, Nutt M (eds): Stainless steels for medical and surgical applications, ASTM STP 1438, West Conshohocken, Pa, 2003, American Society for Testing and Materials, pp 39–49.

38. Woolson ST, Milbauer JP, Bobyn JD, et al: Fatigue fracture of a forged cobalt-chromium-molybdenum femoral component inserted with cement: a report of ten cases. J Bone Joint Surg Am 79:1842–1848, 1997.

39. Grivas TB, Savvidou OD, Psarakis SA, et al: Neck fracture of a cementless forged titanium alloy femoral stem following total hip arthroplasty: a case report and review of the literature. J Med Case Reports 1:174, 2007.

40. Robert Mathys Stiftung Newsletter, No. 02/07, September 2007.

41. Davis J (ed): Handbook of materials for medical devices, Materials Park, Ohio, 2003, ASM International, p 42.

42. Wang K, Berlin R, Gustavson L: Dispersion strengthened Co-Cr-Mo alloy for medical implants. In Disegi J, Kennedy R, Pilliar R (eds): Cobalt-base alloys for biomedical applications, ASTM STP 1365, West Conshohocken, Pa, 1999, American Society for Testing and Materials, pp 89–97.

43. Blumenthal NC, Cosma V: Inhibition of apatite formation by titanium and vanadium ions. J Biomed Mater Res 23(Suppl A1):13–22, 1989.

44. Granchi D, Cenni E, Trisolino G, et al: Sensitivity to implant materials in patients undergoing total hip replacement. J Biomed Mater Res B Appl Biomater 77:257–264, 2006.

45. Hallab NJ, Anderson S, Stafford T, et al: Lymphocyte responses in patients with total hip arthroplasty. J Orthop Res 23:384–391, 2005.

46. Jacobs JJ, Hallab NJ: Loosening and osteolysis associated with metal-on-metal bearings: a local effect of metal hypersensitivity? J Bone Joint Surg Am 88:1171–1172, 2006.

47. Jost-Albrecht K, Hofstetter W: Gene expression by human monocytes from peripheral blood in response to exposure to metals. J Biomed Mater Res B Appl Biomater 76:449–455, 2006.

48. Niki Y, Matsumoto H, Suda Y, et al: Metal ions induce bone-resorbing cytokine production through the redox pathway in synoviocytes and bone marrow macrophages. Biomaterials 24:1447–1457, 2003.

49. Patterson SP, Daffner RH, Gallo RA: Electrochemical corrosion of metal implants. AJR Am J Roentgenol 184:1219–1222, 2005.

50. Queally JM, Devitt BM, Butler JS, et al: Cobalt ions induce chemokine secretion in primary human osteoblasts. J Orthop Res 27:855–864, 2009.

51. Thompson GJ, Puleo DA: Effects of sublethal metal ion concentrations on osteogenic cells derived from bone marrow stromal cells. J Appl Biomater 6:249–258, 1995.

52. Bundy KJ: Corrosion and other electrochemical aspects of biomaterials. Crit Rev Biomed Eng 22:139–251, 1994.

53. ASTM Standard F 86.2000: Standard practice for surface preparation and marking of metallic surgical implants, West Conshohocken, Pa, 2004, ASTM International.

54. Sundgren JE, Bodo P, Lundstrom I: Auger-electron spectroscopic studies of the interface between human-tissue and implants of titanium and stainless-steel. J Colloid Interface Sci 110:9–20, 1986.

55. Sundgren JE, Bodo P, Lundstrom I, et al: Auger electron spectroscopic studies of stainless-steel implants. J Biomed Mater Res 19:663–671, 1985.

56. Park YS, Moon YW, Lim SJ, et al: Early osteolysis following second-generation metal-on-metal hip replacement. J Bone Joint Surg Am 87:1515–1521, 2005.

57. Lucas LC, Buchanan RA, Lemons JE: Investigations on the galvanic corrosion of multialloy total hip prostheses. J Biomed Mater Res 15:731–747, 1981.

58. Mueller Y, Tognini R, Mayer J, Virtanen S: Anodized titanium and stainless steel in contact with CFRP: an electrochemical approach considering galvanic corrosion. J Biomed Mater Res A 82:936–946, 2007.

59. Singh R, Dahotre NB: Corrosion degradation and prevention by surface modification of biometallic materials. J Mater Sci Mater Med 18:725–751, 2007.

60. Virtanen S, Milosev I, Gomez-Barrena E, et al: Special modes of corrosion under physiological and simulated physiological conditions. Acta Biomater 4:468–476, 2008.

61. Charles AE, Ness MG: Crevice corrosion of implants recovered after tibial plateau leveling osteotomy in dogs. Vet Surg 35:438–444, 2006.

62. Hol PJ, Molster A, Gjerdet NR: Should the galvanic combination of titanium and stainless steel surgical implants be avoided? Injury 39:161–169, 2008.

63. Cohen J, Lindenbaum B: Fretting corrosion in orthopedic implants. Clin Orthop Relat Res 61:167–175, 1968.

64. Gilbert JL, Mehta M, Pinder B: Fretting crevice corrosion of stainless steel stem-Co-Cr femoral head connections: comparisons of materials, initial moisture, and offset length. J Biomed Mater Res B Appl Biomater 88:162–173, 2009.

65. Maurer AM, Brown SA, Payer JH, et al: Reduction of fretting corrosion of Ti-6Al-4V by various surface treatments. J Orthop Res 11:865–873, 1993.
66. Cartner JL, Haggard WO, Ong JL, Bumgardner JD: Stress corrosion cracking of an aluminum alloy used in external fixation devices. J Biomed Mater Res B Appl Biomater 86:430–437, 1988.
67. ASTM Standard F 1314.1995: Standard specification for wrought nitrogen strengthened 22 chromium-13 nickel-5 manganese-2.5 molybdenum stainless steel alloy bar and wire for surgical implants, West Conshohocken, Pa, 2007, ASTM International.
68. Marquardt B, Shetty R: Beta titanium alloy processed for high strength orthopaedic applications. In Zardiackas L, Kraay M, Freese H (eds): Titanium, niobium, zirconium, and tantalum for medical and surgical applications, ASTM STP 1471, West Conshohocken, Pa, 1006, American Society for Testing and Materials, pp 71–82.
69. Nishimura T: Ti-15M0-5Zr-3Al. In Welsch G, Boyer R, Collings E (eds): Materials properties handbook, titanium alloys, Materials Park, Ohio, 1994, ASM International, pp 949–956.
70. Matsumoto H, Watanabe S, Hanada S: Strengthening of low modulus beta Ti-Nb-Sn alloys by thermomechanical processing. In Venugopalan R, Wu M (eds): Medical device materials III: proceedings from the Materials and Processes for Medical Devices Conference 2005, Materials Park, Ohio, 2006, ASM International, pp 9–14.
71. Jablokov V, Murray N, Lack H, Freese H: Influence of oxygen content on the mechanical properties of titanium-35 niobium-7 zirconium-5 tantalum beta titanium alloy. In Zardiackas L, Kraay M, Freese H (eds): Titanium, niobium, zirconium, and tantalum for medical and surgical applications, ASTM STP 1471, West Conshohocken, Pa, 2006, American Society for Testing and Materials, pp 40–51.
72. Niinomi M: Mechanical biocompatibilities of titanium alloys for biomedical applications. J Mech Behav Biomed Mater 1:30–42, 2008.
73. ASTM Standard F 2066.200: Standard specification for wrought titanium-15 molybdenum alloy for surgical implant applications, West Conshohocken, Pa, 2007, ASTM International.
74. ISO Standard 5832-14 2007: Implants for surgery: metallic materials. Part 14. Wrought titanium 15-molybdenum 5-zirconium 3-aluminium alloy, Geneva, Switzerland, 2007, International Organization for Standardization.
75. J, Zardiackas L: Metallurgical features of Ti-15Mo beta titanium alloy for orthopaedic trauma applications, Anaheim, Calif, 2003, ASM International, pp 337–342.

CHAPTER 7

Materials in Hip Surgery: Mechanical Properties That Influence Design and Performance of Ceramic Hip Bearings

Ian C. Clarke, Giuseppe Pezzotti, and Nobuhiko Sugano

KEY POINTS

- Ceramics currently used in total hip replacement (THR) include monolithic materials, alumina (ALX), magnesia-stabilized zirconia (m-ZR), and zirconia-reinforced alumina (AMC).
- The AMC ceramic now provides a 60% greater strength alternative to ALX.
- In Europe, ALX ceramic balls combined with both PE and ALX cups have a continuing history of 40 years' duration.
- CPE designs using ALX or AMC ceramic balls (diameter, 28 to 44 mm) are approved by the U. S. Food and Drug Administration (FDA) (for use with polyethylene cups and have a 20-year history in the United States.
- Only 28- and 32-mm diameters of the ALX/ALX ceramic combination have FDA approval to be marketed in the United States.
- The AMC ball used in conjunction with a ceramic cup of ALX or AMC has not yet gained FDA approval for market.
- In terms of ceramic ball designs, the short-neck ball is twice as strong as the long-neck design.
- In terms of diameters, the 32-mm ceramic ball is 60% stronger than the 28-mm ball of equivalent design.
- y-ZR ceramic balls were used with polyethylene liners from 1985 to 2000 and then were abandoned because of manufacturing problems accompanied by high fracture rates.
- m-ZR ceramic balls with polyethylene cups are still in use in the United States.

INTRODUCTION

Properties of Ceramic Implants

From a materials science point of view, the broad classification of ceramics includes all nonmetallic and nonorganic materials. For orthopedic implants, this includes forms of pure carbon and silicon along with carbides, oxides, and nitrides of base metals such as aluminum, magnesium, and zirconium. Ceramic materials are typically suitable for tasks that would be very difficult for survival of plastic and metal bearings. For example, pure alumina is an inert ceramic that is classed as 10 on the Mohr hardness scale, where the hardest known material diamond is ranked at Mohr 11. This property of high hardness makes a ceramic bearing extremely resistant to third-body abrasive wear. Alumina ceramic also has the highest rigidity of any implant material. Its elastic modulus (450 GPa) represents twice the stiffness of the nearest metal alloy (CoCr: 210 Ga). Thus ceramics are called into play when adverse combinations of temperature, pressure, stress, lubrication, and abrasion resistance are required. Thus the benefit of ceramic for total hip replacement (THR) is primarily that of a bearing that is dimensionally stable and chemically inert and possesses exceptionally high wear resistance.

Oxide ceramics may include two or more types of atoms. Oxygen ions typically are closely packed around the metal ions and thus shield reactive metals from the external environment. The major oxide ceramic used over a 40-year history in Europe and elsewhere has been pure alumina (Fig. 7-1).[1] Alumina is the oxide of the base metal aluminum; it has been extensively studied as an implant material and ranks highest in terms of physical and chemical inertness and biological compatibility. The strength of alumina implants has been steadily increasing (Table 7-1). The mating of ceramic with metal components has generally involved taper-locking geometries to smooth the transfer of interfacial stresses. Therefore, this is a critical component of design, materials selection, and quality control. Note that mating a ceramic liner with a flexible polyethylene sheath represents the most extreme example of adverse modulus and strength mismatches.[2] This will be discussed in a later section.

Improved processing of ceramic implants has included as most relevant a "hipping" process by which fully dense alumina implants could be obtained while grain growth was limited. This was an important limitation because abnormal shapes or sizes of ceramic grains would act as crack sites and so could lower the inherent

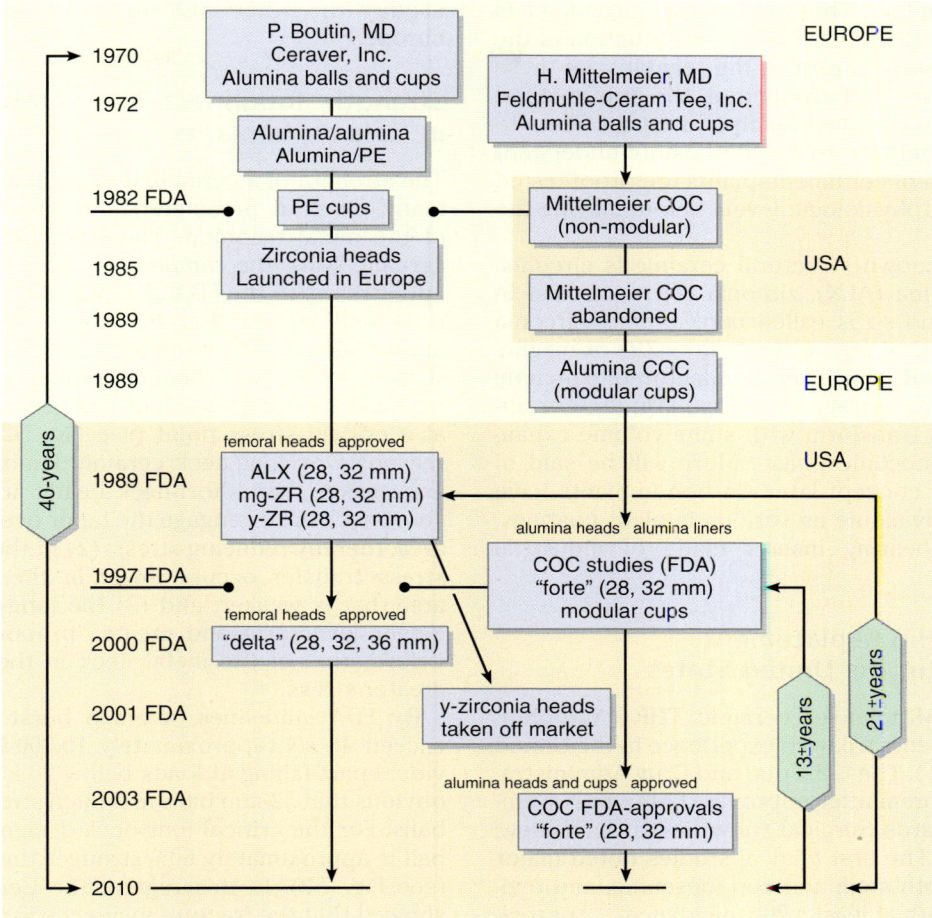

Figure 7-1. The 40-year history of ceramic hips.

Table 7-1. Mechanical and Physical Properties of Ceramics Used in Hip Bearings

Material Properties	Al_2O_3	ZTA	Mg-PSZ	Y-TZP	CoCr
Composition	99.9% Al_2O_3	Al_2O_3 20 vol %ZrO_2	ZrO_2 8 mol% MgO	ZrO_2 3 mol% Y_2O_3	
Grain size, μm	1-5	1-2	50	0.1-1.0	NA
Density, g/cm³	>3.97	4.4	5.75	6.05	8.5
Hardness, Hv	1800-2000	1600-1800	1250	1250	300-400
Elastic modulus, GPa	400-450	300-350	200-250	200-250	210-250
Fracture toughness Kc, MPa.m$^{\frac{1}{2}}$	4-5	6-10	6-10	6-12	50-100
Bending strength, MPa	300-500	700-1000	600-700	1000-1500	800-1000
Weibull's modulus	5	13	22	10	NA
Poisson's ratio	0.23	0.22	0.32	0.3	0.3
Thermal conductivity, Wm^{-1} K^{-1}	30	17	2-3	2-3	100
Thermal expansion coefficient, 10^{-6} K^{-1}	8	8.5	7-10	11	14
Water absorption, %	0	0	0	0	NA
Wetting angle, degrees	Water: 45 Ringer's: 5	Ringer's: 2.5	Water: >50	Water: >50 Ringer's: 10	Water: 86

strength of the implant. Thus hot-isostatic pressing has been in use since 1975 to 1977. The introduction of the *proof test* significantly improved the reliability of these components. Before its introduction, the only method of strength testing involved loading of components to fracture, so that only 2% to 3% of implants underwent testing. Now 100% of ceramic implants are proof-tested at stresses above physiologic levels before leaving the factory.[3]

The next well-known structural ceramic is zirconia. Unlike pure alumina (ALX), zirconia (ZR) can exist in several phases and so is called *polymorphic*. Zirconia implant grades are alloyed with yttria (y-ZR) or magnesia (m-ZR). The y-ZR ceramic is manufactured to include predominantly the tetragonal phase. Under certain conditions, it can transform with some volume expansion into the monoclinic phase. More will be said of this "toughening" concept later. Carbon implants have also been made available as various implant coatings, and even with bearing inserts made of industrial diamond.

Ceramic Total Hip Replacement Developments in the United States

The pioneering Mittelmeier ceramic THR (Autophor, Xenophor) represents a flawed experience in the United States (see Fig. 7-1). The U.S. Food and Drug Administration (FDA) gave premarket approval (PMA) in November 2002 to Richards Surgical (now Smith & Nephew, Memphis, Tenn). The first clinical studies noted major problems from both stem and cup loosening, and revisions appeared with at least a 20% incidence.[4-6] Approximately 3500 Mittelmeier THRs were implanted in the United States prior to their voluntary removal from the market. However, this first ceramic THR experience did pave the way for the FDA down-classification of alumina implants with the approval of ceramic/polyethylene combinations (CPE) in 1989 (see Fig. 7-1). All-ceramic bearings (ALX/ALX; 28 and 32 mm) were granted approval some 14 years later. Thus three key FDA actions controlling the sale of ceramic hips occurred in 1982, 1989, and 2003 (see Fig. 7-1). Marketing approvals also included the ceramic called *zirconia* in both magnesia-stabilized (m-ZR) and yttria-stabilized (y-ZR) forms.[7]

The introduction of ceramic liners with modular acetabular shells in 1989 represented another European innovation (see Fig. 7-1). Three companies launched FDA-monitored clinical studies a decade later with this modular cup design,[8,9] and FDA approvals to market began in January 2003. Note that because of FDA marketing requirements, these ceramic-on-ceramic (COC) developments were exclusive to products from one vendor.

The year 2000 saw the introduction of a composite alumina ceramic that had small zirconia grains interspersed between larger alumina grains. This ceramic has been referred to as an *alumina matrix composite* (AMC).[10] At the present time, the FDA has approved only AMC balls for use with polyethylene (PE) cups (diameter, 28 to 44 mm), although AMC balls can be used with either ALX or AMC cups in Asia and Europe.[11]

Strength, Toughness, and Safety Issues in Ceramic Implants

The strength of a ceramic femoral ball is dependent on many material parameters, but primarily the design of the metal trunnion. The standard strength test of ceramic balls, the *compressive burst test,* is used in all applications to the FDA (ASTM F2345).[12-14] For example, it is well known that the short-neck ball design is approximately 50% stronger than the long-neck design (Fig. 7-2) of the same diameter, which is counterintuitive because the long-neck ball has greater wall thickness at a critical stress point (see Fig. 7-2, *insert;* T_L). The reasons why long-neck ceramic femoral heads in fact are weaker than short-neck heads are as follows: (1) short-neck heads engage the taper over a larger surface area, thereby reducing stress; (2) in the long-neck head, stress transfer occurs lower in the ball taper in an area that is weaker; and (3) the long-neck head has a longer lever arm and creates proportionately higher deformation of the metal neck in the taper and thus greater stress.

By FDA guidelines, average burst strength should exceed 46 kN (approximately 10,000 lb), with no individual part failing at loads below 20 kN (5000 lb).[15] It is obvious that 32-mm balls are much stronger than 28-mm balls. For the critical long-neck design, the 32-mm ALX ball is approximately 60% stronger than the 28-mm ball (see Fig. 7-2). In this regard, the CeramTec database showed that the fracture incidence for 32-mm balls was 0.007% compared with 0.03% risk for 28-mm balls (i.e., a fourfold reduction in risk) (see Fig. 7-1).

The most direct path to increasing the strength and reliability of a ceramic lies in increased fracture toughness, as observed with zirconia (m-ZR, y-ZR) or zirconia-reinforced alumina (AMC; see later). Yttria-stabilized, zirconia polycrystalline ceramic (y-ZR) represents an extremely strong and fatigue-resistant material. This ceramic has the ability to transform from the as-manufactured tetragonal phase into the stable monoclinic phase. The tetragonal-to-monoclinic transformation produces a net 4% volume expansion of the zirconia grains. Thus, when a crack tries to propagate through a matrix composed of tetragonal grains, the sudden loss of matrix constraint allows spontaneous expansion from the tetragonal to the monoclinic phase. Resulting compressive stresses inhibit growth of the crack; this effect is termed *transformation toughening*. However, this could become a negative effect if transformation takes place spontaneously on the bearing surface as the result of the resulting increase in surface roughness.

Implant designers initially welcomed the introduction of zirconia ceramics, given the prospect of increased reliability, strength, and toughness compared with ALX (see Table 7-1). The zirconia saw widespread use in CPE bearings and in a few cases with y-ZR/y-ZR and y-ZR/ALX combinations.[16] However, the emergent problem observed with zirconia components partially stabilized with yttrium oxide (y-ZR) was lack of inherent stability.

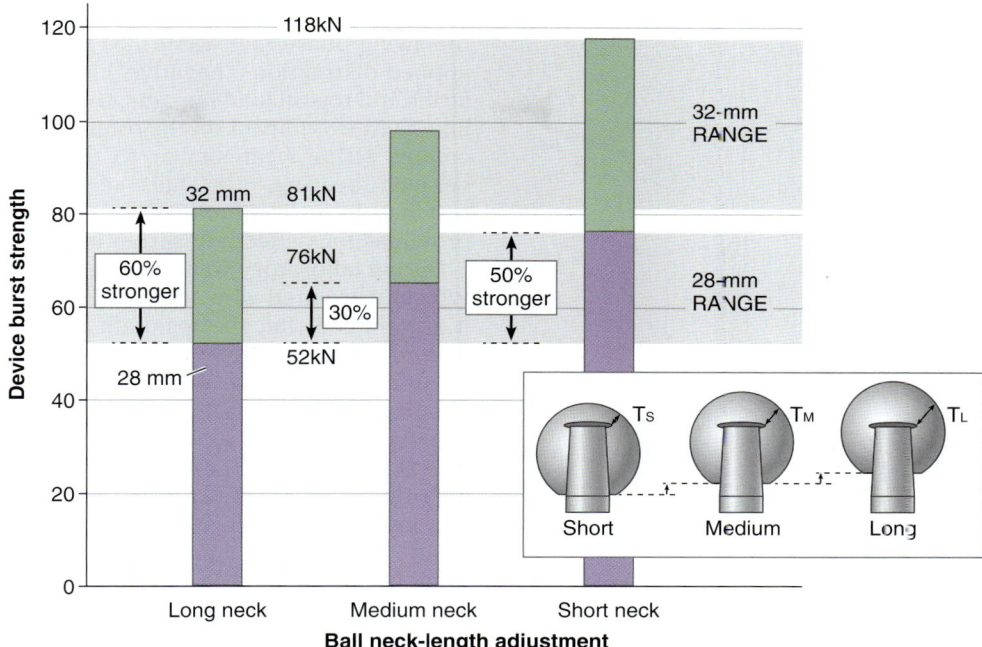

Figure 7-2. Range of burst strengths with varied neck lengths and diameters of ALX balls. *Inset depicts the wall thickness* (T) increasing with longer neck lengths (inset cartoon depicts wall thicknesses; $T_S < T_M < T_L$). *(Biolox-Forte data courtesy of CeramTec AG, Plochingen, Germany.)*

Table 7-2. Comparison of Hardness, Strength, and Toughness Properties for Biolox-Forte (ALX) and Biolox-Delta (AMC)

Property	Biolox-Forte	Biolox-Delta	Ratio
Hardness, Hv10	2100	1760	0.84
4-pt bend strength, MPa	580	1250	2.16
Weibull's modulus	5	13	2.60
Fx toughness, MPa.m$^{0.5}$	4.3	6.5	1.51

distribution of chromium inside the alumina lattice gives components a purple hue. The hardness of the resulting material is thus greater than that of the y-ZR ceramic, but still is not as great as that of alumina (see Tables 7-1 and 7-2). However, in terms of safety, the toughness of zirconia-reinforced alumina (AMC) is increased approximately 50% to 60% compared with that of pure alumina (see Table 7-2). In terms of the critical long-neck design, the *burst test* showed that AMC balls achieved 60% higher loads than alumina (Fig. 7-3). Here, the long-neck 28-mm AMC ball was as strong as the 36-mm ALX. Thus from the point of view of the AMC ceramic, the alumina phase externally provided the ideal bearing surface, while the zirconia phase internally contributed to strength and toughness.[18]

CERAMIC TRIBOLOGICAL PROPERTIES

Mechanics in the Tribology of Ceramic Cups

The hip simulator has been the dominant tool for assessing wear in THR bearings (science of tribology). The Standard Procedures specified by the International Organization for Standardization (ISO) and the American Society for Testing and Materials (ASTM) for hip simulators provide guidelines for testing actual implants; however, these were developed specifically for metal and polyethylene bearings.[19-22] Existing guidelines omit important test details relevant to ceramic tribology and provide no specific warnings with regard

This "metastability" resulted in significant and unforeseen degradation in mechanical properties in vivo when implants were manufactured under suboptimal conditions. Thus an unfortunate process change by one manufacturer in France resulted in a very high incidence of y-ZR ball fractures. Subsequent product recalls ended the life cycle of y-ZR ceramic balls by the year 2001 (see Fig. 7-1). Note that Mg-stabilized zirconia balls (m-ZR) are still in use.[7,17]

A ceramic composite material was developed to combine the superior bearing properties of alumina while exploiting the superior strength and toughness of zirconia (Table 7-2). In this concept, the toughening effect of zirconia is used to enhance the strength of alumina (see Table 7-2). However, zirconia also reduces the hardness of the composite ceramic. This can be alleviated by alloying alumina with chromium oxide, creating a solid solution within the alumina matrix. This

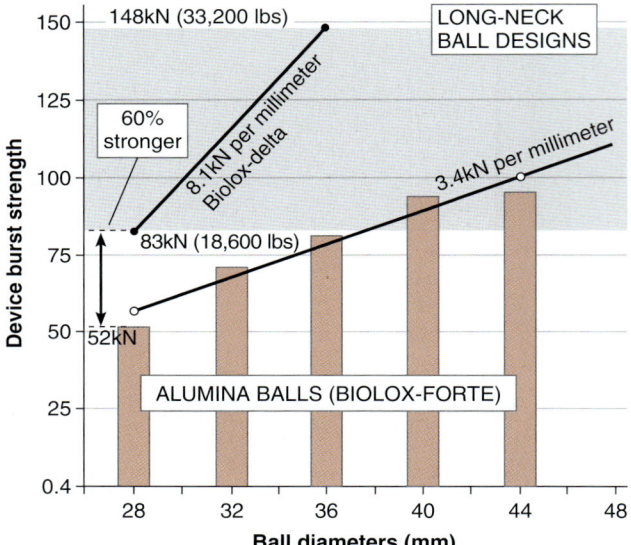

Figure 7-3. Burst strengths with varied diameters of long-neck (LN) ball design. Strength of two diameters of AMC balls (28 mm; 36 mm) indicated for comparison. *(Data courtesy of CeramTec AG, Plochingen, Germany.)*

Table 7-3. Comparison of Standard (STD) and Microseparation (MSX) Test Modes

ID	Simulator Parameters	STD	MSX
1	Serum lubrication	Similar	Similar
2	Hip kinetics (2D, 3D)	Similar	Similar
3	Anatomic setup	Similar	Similar
4	Cup inclination	35 degrees	50 degrees
5	Typical peak load, kN	2500	2500
6	Main wear zone, 12-mm diameter	Yes	Yes
7	Typical minimum load, kN	250	−250
8	Ball permitted to sublux from cup	No	Yes
9	Bearings separated each cycle	No	Yes
10	Boundary/fluid-film lubrication	Possible	Not likely
11	Abrasion of cup rim on ball	No	Yes
12	Stripe wear on ball and cup	No	Yes

to interpreting ceramic wear phenomena (as discussed in later sections).[11,23-31] In addition, available hip standards specify only what will be termed the *standard simulator test* (ASTM F1714; ISO 14242-3). In this mode, a predominantly compressive load is applied during both stance and swing phases (Table 7-3). Little or no separation of bearing surfaces is noted in the standard test mode, and the wear zone typically never crosses the cup rim (Fig. 7-4). This is a very conservative test under ideal lubrication conditions. It is likely that more adverse conditions are commonly present in the patient's hip joint (discussed in later sections). In contrast, the microseparation test mode permits the

femoral head to slightly subluxate from the cup during the swing phase (see Table 7-3) under the action of an applied distraction ("negative") load. Thus during heel-strike and toe-off load impacts, the rim of the acetabular liner is free to impact on the rotating femoral head. This creates stripe wear similar to that seen on retrieved ceramic bearings.[32,33] This "severe" microseparation test has little likelihood of being confounded by the proteinaceous effects of serum lubricants.

During laboratory wear testing, the acetabular cup is typically oriented with 40 degrees of lateral inclination. It is assumed that the resultant load (R) is located 20 degrees medial to the vertical and oscillates ±20 degrees, as indicated (see Fig. 7-4A). For a 12-mm contact zone (28-mm ceramic ball), cyclical translation to the medial side (see Fig. 7-4A, R_M) occurs into the safe zone. On the lateral side (see Fig. 7-4A, R_L), translation of the contact area does not cross the bevel of the ceramic liner. In this example, a 19-degree arc represents the *margin of safety*. However, in the hip simulator, there is no anatomic meaning for the terms *medial* and *lateral*. The simulator's resultant load is aligned in the vertical plane (see Fig. 7-4B). Thus the 40-degree cup inclination in the patient (see Fig. 7-4A) corresponds to a 20-degree cup angle in the simulator (see Fig. 7-4B), while the 50-degree cup position (see Fig. 7-4C) would correspond to a 70-degree inclination in the patient. In such a case, there is no margin of safety, because the contact wear zone can translate across the rim of the liner during every cycle. This is a severe but clinically relevant test. Note that no regulatory or standard guidelines have been provided for such clinically relevant microseparation test modes.

Validating Laboratory Wear Performance With Ceramic Clinical Results

Hip simulators require liters of lubricant to run the standard test of 5 million cycles, believed to represent 3 to 5 years of use in the patient.[1,34] Because no ready supply of synovial fluid is available, diluted bovine serum has been the lubricant of choice for decades.[35] To prove a point about water lubrication being nonphysiologic, the Peterson Tribology Laboratory ran studies with various material combinations (CoCr/PTFE, CoCr/PE, ALX/PTFE, and ALX/PE) with both water and serum lubrication. Compared with serum, water reduced ALX/PE wear rates to close to zero. With the CoCr/PE combination, wear also decreased, but less so. This phenomenon was clearly explained as an artifact of water lubrication.[23,24] Thus serum proteins are necessary to promote physiologically relevant PE wear. However, as discussed later, a review of the salient clinical history reveals that confounding artifacts were introduced into laboratory studies of ceramics. In the simulator laboratories, turning wear data into clinically relevant predictions can be a major challenge. Laboratory wear studies are only as good as their predictive power. Therefore it is important to validate simulator data wherever possible using good clinical and retrieval data.

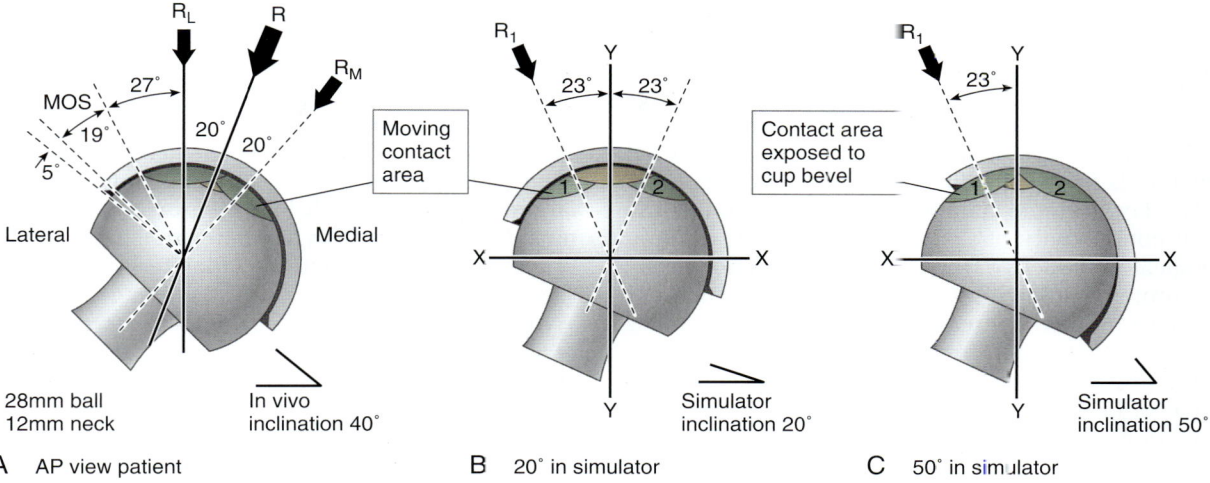

Figure 7-4. Contact areas under the path of the resultant load (R). These are compared for cups inclined at 40-degrees in the patient **(A)** and 20 degrees **(B)**, and 50 degrees **(C)** in the hip simulator (i.e., representative of standard and microseparation tests, respectively).[57]

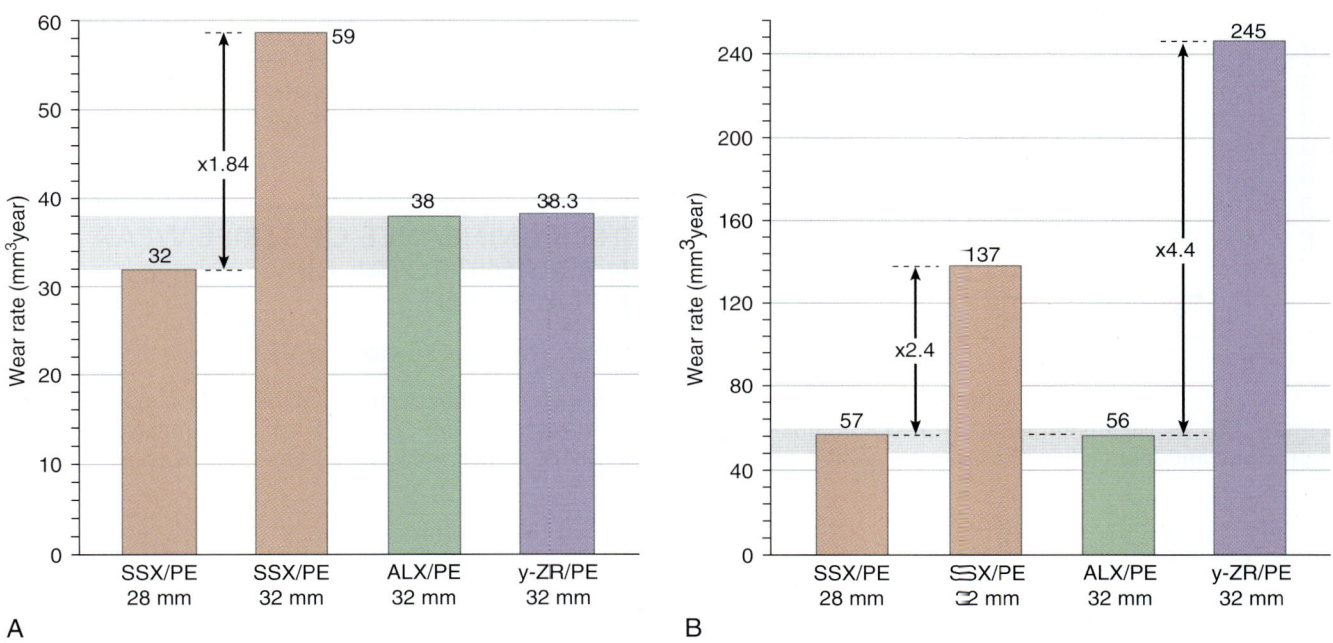

Figure 7-5. Clinical and radiographic studies of polyethylene (PE) wear with different femoral heads at **(A)** 5 years' follow-up, and **(B)** 12 years' follow-up.[44] Note that the Y-scale in the longer-term study (Fig. 7-5*B*) is fourfold larger than in the short-term study (Fig. 7-6*A*). Also note that data from retrieval studies provide an assessment of "overall" wear.

With a strong history of alumina in Europe, a review of CPE clinical performance noted that ALX balls conferred approximately 40% wear reduction compared with CoCr balls.[11] However, the first warning of monoclinic transformation in the y-ZR/PE combination used in Europe came from a retrieval report on two Japanese cases in which a 20% to 30% phase change was detected.[16,39] A French study also revealed 20% to 30% monoclinic transformation occurring 4 to 11 years post implantation.[36,37] The ominous report at 12 years was that the short-term wear rate had quadrupled for 28-mm ZR/PE, which now was fivefold higher than the rate for the larger-diameter ALX/PE combination

(Fig. 7-5*B*). These and other studies showed that y-ZR phase transformations could climb to over 80%.[38] A clinical study of y-ZR balls (6 years' follow-up) noted that PE wear rates showed an average 43% increase compared with CoCr balls. This zirconia series had 7% revisions, whereas CoCr revisions were reported as zero. The longer-term French study[36] compared PE wear with y-ZR balls versus that with stainless steel and ALX balls.[37] At 5 years' follow-up (see Fig. 7-5*A*), PE wear with 32-mm stainless steel balls averaged 50% higher than with 32-mm ALX. By 12 years (see Fig. 7-5*B*), this disparity had increased 2.4-fold. In terms of osteolytic changes, the 18-year report[40,45] revealed that the y-ZR/PE combination was now much inferior to ALX/PE.

In the simulator laboratories, various studies consistently predicted that (1) ALX/PE wear would be greater than M/PE wear,[40] and (2) y-ZR/PE wear would be less than M/PE wear.[40-42] It is important to note that varied ball materials have very different thermal conductivity (Fig. 7-6). For example, alumina ceramic has double the thermal conductivity of CoCr alloy (Fig. 7-7A). From a tribological perspective, the confounding factor is the use of protein-containing lubricants. In terms of wear phenomena, such increased bearing conductivity lowers lubricant temperatures and thus reduces damage to serum proteins. This one feature greatly accentuates the wear of PE liners.[43] Thus in the laboratory, ALX/PE combinations generally have produced 10% more wear than CoCr/PE combinations.[40,43] The Peterson Tribology Laboratory ran a comparative wear study for three types of ceramic balls using CoCr balls as controls.[44] A linear increase in PE wear rates was clearly seen as thermal conductivity increased from 2.5 to 28 $W \bullet m^{-1} \bullet K^{-1}$ (see Fig. 7-7B; high regression coefficient, R = 0.99). This wear ranking was identical to that noted in previous laboratory data (i.e., ZR/PE<<MPE<ALX/PE). However, it must be noted that this simulator ranking is exactly the opposite of that predicted by long-term clinical studies (see Fig. 7-5).

Another challenge lies in the fact that retrieval data of y-ZR/PE implants revealed surface cratering due to transformation to the monoclinic phase. Surface roughness increased from approximately 10 nm to 100 to 250 nm (Ra) as the result of ceramic cratering on surfaces with habitual polyethylene contact.[36,46,47] In direct contrast, simulator studies provided no evidence of such zirconia transformation or surface roughening. Clearly, the metastability of the y-ZR was not challenged by tribological conditions in hip simulators.[48] Such contradictory data indicate how little is known of tribological-hydrothermal events occurring between a zirconia ball and a PE liner. Thus laboratory studies have revealed at least four confounding interactions attributable to the use of protein-containing lubricants.

THE SIGNIFICANCE OF STRIPE WEAR IN CERAMIC TOTAL HIP REPLACEMENT

Wear Stripes Created In Vivo

Although well-functioning COC bearings can show linear wear rates as low as 0.005 to 0.025 mm/year,[49,50] the depth of linear wear in some cases was as great as

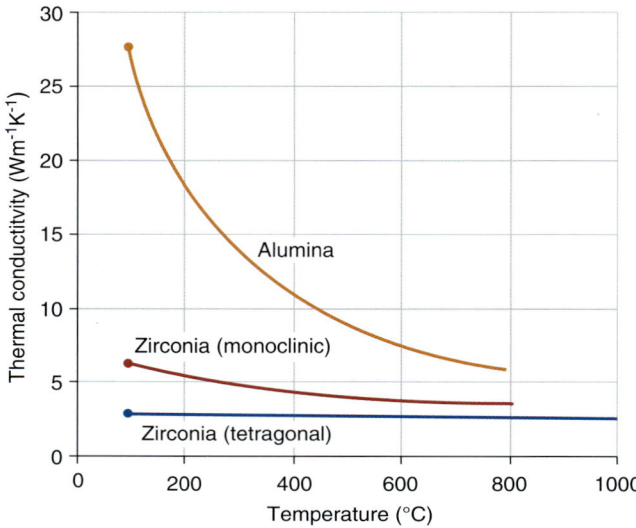

Figure 7-6. Thermal conductivity for ALX compared with tetragonal and monoclinic phases in the y-ZR ceramic.

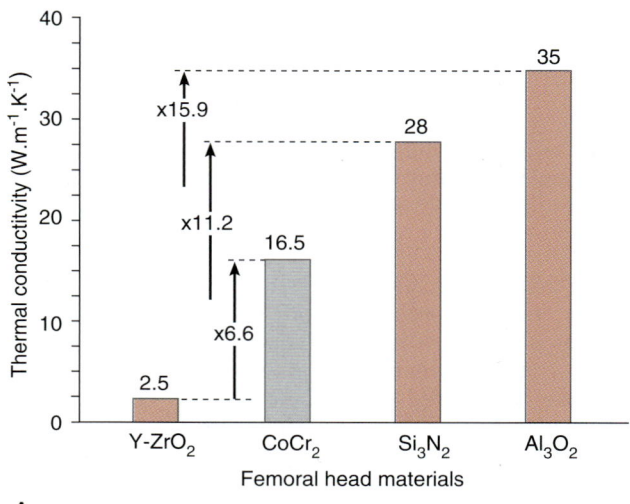

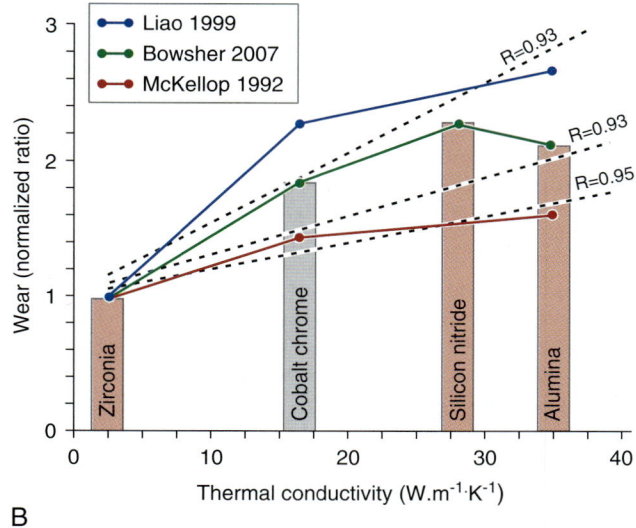

Figure 7-7. Ranking of thermal conductivity for metal and ceramic femoral heads: **A,** Divergence of zirconia and alumina ceramic.[37] **B,** Ranking of polyethylene (PE) wear performance with respect to thermal conductivity of ball materials (y-ZR<<CoCr<ALX). Here, the wear rates in three simulator studies[37,48,51] were normalized with respect to the y-ZR/PE combination.

3 mm.[27,51] Corresponding volumetric wear ranged up to 260 mm³/year. One detailed retrieval study[52] described six cases in which ceramic cups had worn at a rate exceeding 0.04 mm/year (Fig. 7-8), averaging 0.22 mm/year. In one patient with a steep cup, apparent wear was measured at 0.96 mm in 1 year (see Fig. 7-8; M8). Thus loosening of a rigid ceramic cup is a pathway to greatly accelerated wear.[53,54] Historical risks for adverse wear of these devices include (1) cups implanted too vertically, (2) tilting and migration of loosened cups, and (3) patients walking on malpositioned (or loose) ceramic cups for lengthy periods before revision.[55-57]

Stripe wear has been reported over the years as a dull, lunar area on the highly polished ceramic balls and a narrow circumferential area adjacent to the beveled edge of the bearing surface of the cup.[26,50,58-61] Stripe wear is also observed in approximately 50% of contemporary COC designs within 3 years of surgery.[61] Such wear scars have a rough appearance caused by pull-out of the ceramic grains. In contrast, the main wear area generally is so finely polished that unless it is stained gray by a transfer layer of metal debris, microscopic analysis is required for visualization.[59,60] Stripe wear has been attributed to various factors, including negative clearance between ball and cup, vertically inclined cups, loose cups, microseparation, and impingement effects.[18] It is intuitively obvious that stripe wear is one of the consequences of using rigid cups, as this leads to stress concentration effects.[11,53,54,62-64] One retrieval study documented that wear on ceramic balls showing visible stripes averaged approximately 1 mm³/year (Fig. 7-9).

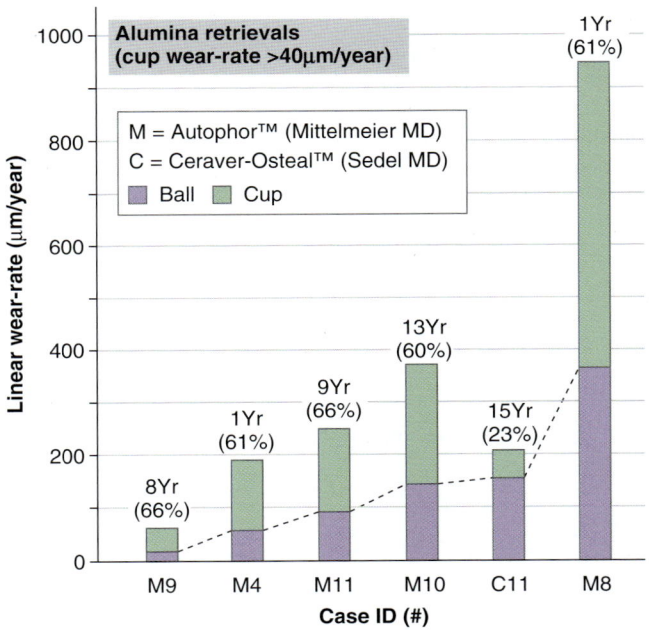

Figure 7-8. Six ceramic bearings ranked (data redrawn from that presented by Nevelos[34]) in order of increasing ball wear (for linear wear >0.04 mm). *Key: Black shading,* Cup wear; *C,* THR of Ceraver-Osteal design; *M,* THR of Autophor design; *Yr,* follow-up times indicated in years; *%,* ratio of cup to THR wear indicated.

Wear Stripes Created in the Laboratory

Boutin first described the wear of COC bearings during the "run-in" phase as very low.[65] Linear wear was measured as only 10 μm after 1 million simulator cycles, while "steady-state" wear was undetectable (Fig. 7-10). Steady-state wear is a true performance indicator because the transition into steady-state phase should represent a large reduction in wear rates. Among "standard" simulator tests reported over the decades, COC run-in wear typically averaged 0.5 mm³/Mc (Table 7-4).[65a] The steady-state wear rate was much more difficult to measure, with one estimate (>14 million cycles) as low as 0.02 mm³/Mc.[66] A meta-analysis of standard simulator tests showed that COC run-in and steady-state wear averaged 1.1 and 0.05 mm³/Mc, respectively (Fig. 7-11). These low wear magnitudes likely were typical of retrieval cases with no or mild stripe wear.[61]

The microseparation (MSX) test mode has been used to produce stripe wear similar to that seen on ceramic retrievals.[18,27,32,39,67] Under mild MSX test conditions,[68] run-in and steady-state wear was seen to increase two- to fivefold (Fig. 7-12). However, the severe MSX test increased run-in and steady-state wear by 36- and 26-fold, respectively (see Tables 7-4 and 7-5). For comparative purposes, it is advantageous to characterize the combination of run-in and steady-state trends by an "overall" wear rate (see Fig. 7-11), such as would be estimated in retrieval studies.[61,68] Thus the microseparation mode increased ALX wear by an order of magnitude to 1.8 mm³/Mc overall (see Fig. 7-12). This was also in the clinical range for retrievals with stripe wear (see Fig. 7-9 and Table 7-6).[61]

Unlike the standard simulator test, the microseparation method has provided good discrimination between the tribological performance of ALX and AMC ceramics. The four material combinations (36-mm ball:cup: ALX:ALX, ALX:AMC, AMC:ALX, AMC:AMC) all demonstrated the stripe wear phenomenon within 100,000 cycles.[39,69] Typically, two narrow stripes were created on the ceramic balls, corresponding to high impacts in the load profile: one narrow stripe at 45 to 60 degrees, and one at 75 to 90 degrees (as measured from the pole). Liners showed a narrow stripe along the rim bevel, beginning with an approximately 20- to 40-degree arc. Given the many differences represented by the test parameters, the two MSX studies were remarkably similar (see Fig. 7-12 and Tables 7-5 and 7-6). Thus overall, the hybrid AMC/ALX combination wore almost threefold higher than AMC/AMC, and the ALX/ALX combination appeared eightfold higher.

OVERALL RISKS AND BENEFITS OF CERAMIC TOTAL HIP REPLACEMENT

Fracture Risk of Ceramic Total Hip Replacement

Risk of ceramic fracture has always been a concern.[70] A recent meta-analysis of major journals and congresses included 35,000 cases for review and documented 24

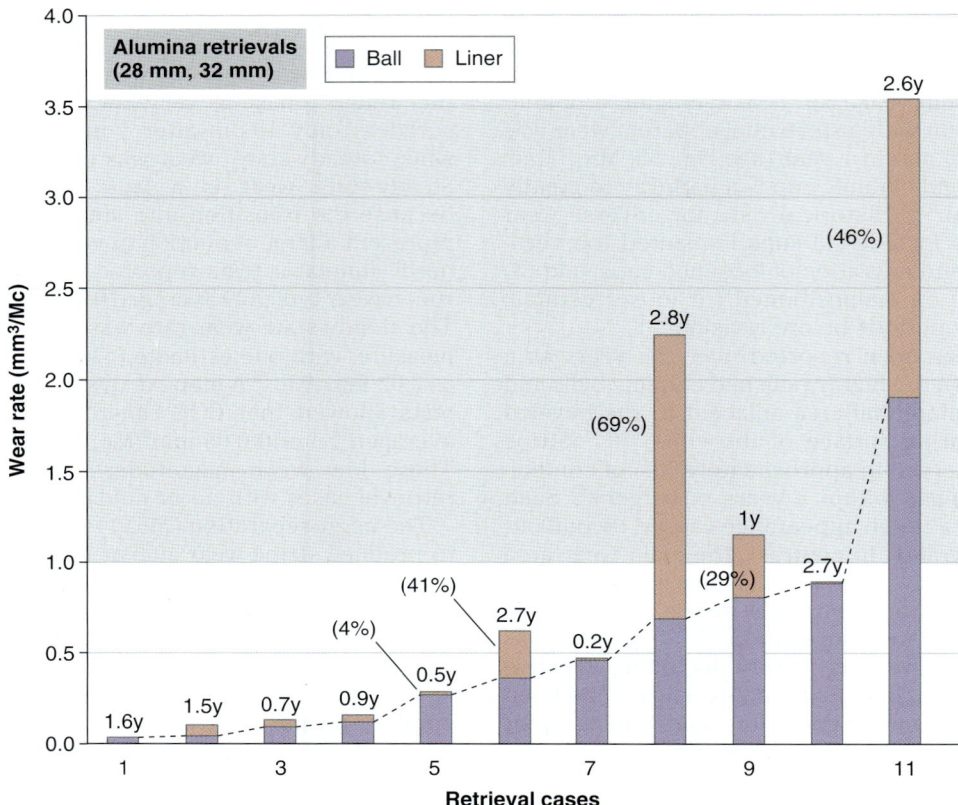

Figure 7-9. Contemporary alumina retrievals ranked in order of increasing volumetric wear of balls (N = 11; redrawn from data presented in Walter et al[65]). The authors noted that cases #5 and #8 had neck-cup impingement damage opposite the stripe area on the cup rim. *Key: Black shading,* Cup wear; *Yr,* follow-up times indicated in years; %, ratio of cup to THR wear indicated.

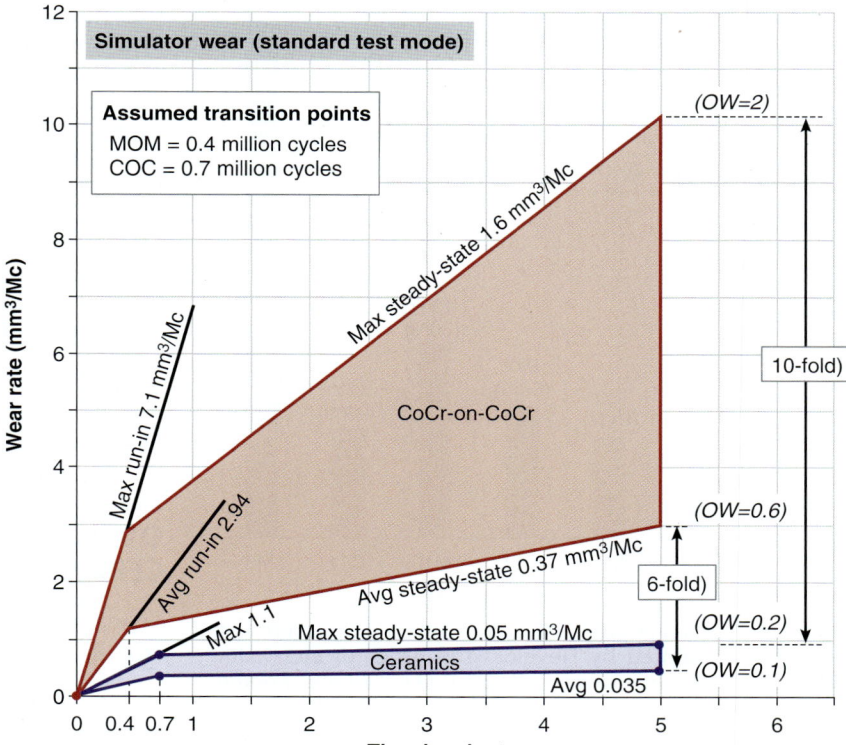

Figure 7-10. Representative wear trends in "standard" simulator test, showing run-in and steady-state phases for ALX/ALX.[3] The minimum (min), average (avg), maximum (max), and overall wear (OW) values are indicated.

Table 7-4. Meta-Analysis of Ceramic Wear Run in the Standard (STD) Simulator Mode[11]

Wear Rate	Min, mm³/Mc	Avg, mm³/Mc	Max, mm³/Mc
Run-in	0.020	0.500	1.10
Steady-state	0.015	0.035	0.05
Overall	0.016	0.128	0.26

fracture cases (i.e., a ratio of 1 in 1500).[71] Among FDA-monitored studies now approaching 10 years' follow-up, the clinical series in the United States generally noted a fracture incidence of zero to 0.5% (1 in 500) (Table 7-7). The manufacturer reported a ratio of 3 per 10,000 cases in its own internal database (Table 7-8). The risks of fracture are also accentuated for certain novel designs or in certain cultural activities, as will be discussed later.

With the modular alumina liner, one of the risks has been malseating the liner in the metal shell at surgery.

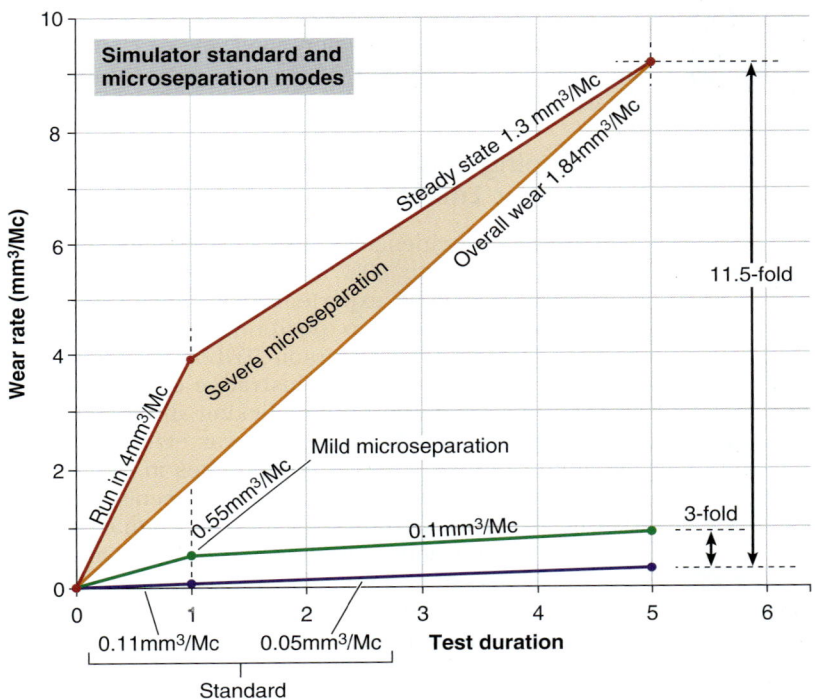

Figure 7-11. Representative wear trends in microseparation simulator test, showing run-in and steady-state phases for ALX/ALX with comparisons of "mild" and "severe" MSX modes to the "standard" test. (*Redrawn from data by Stewart et al.*[73])

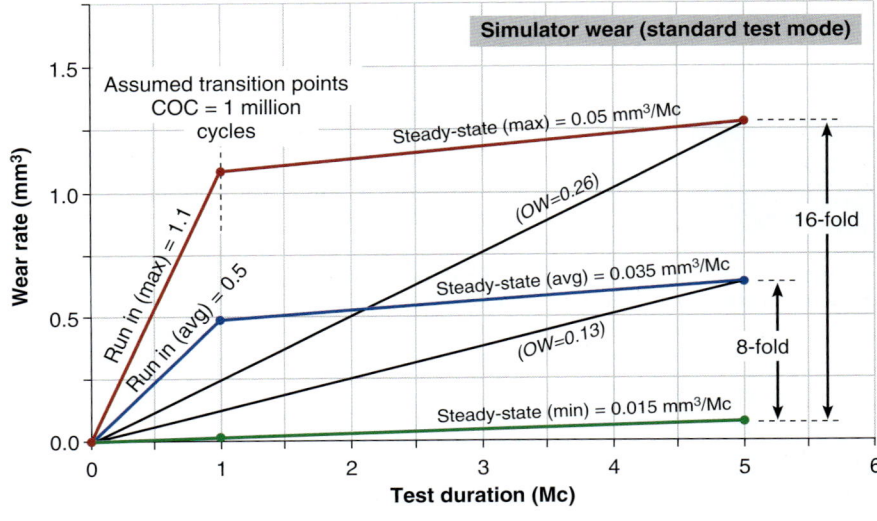

Figure 7-12. Comparison of ceramic-on-ceramic (COC) and metal-on-metal (MOM) wear from simulator studies run in "standard" test modes. Linear wear trends shown for minimum (min), average (avg), maximum (max), and overall wear rate (OW) values.

Table 7-5. Comparison of 28-mm ALX Bearings Run Under Standard (STD) and Microseparation (MSX) Modes[68]

Simulator Parameters	Run-in, mm³/Mc	Steady State, mm³/Mc	Overall Wear, mm³/Mc	Ratio Run-in to Steady State
Standard test mode	0.11	0.05	0.07	2.2
"Mild" microseparation	0.55	0.1	0.2	5.5
"Severe" microseparation	4	1.3	1.84	3.1
Ratio "severe" to standard	36.4	26.0	26.3	

Table 7-6. Generalized Wear Rates for Wear of 28- to 36-mm ALX and AMC Combinations Run Under Standard and Microseparation Modes*

Wear Phase	STD (ALX/ ALX)	MSX (ALX/ ALX)	MSX (ALX/ ZRA)	MSX (ZRA/ ALX)	MSX (ZRA/ ZRA)
Run-in	0.5	4.5	1	1	0.4
Steady-state	0.035	1.1	0.5	0.5	0.15
Overall (5 Mc)	0.13	1.8	0.6	0.6	0.2
Overall ALX/ALX ratio	Reference	14			
Overall MSX ratio		9	3	3	Reference

*Summarized from Figure 7-6.

Table 7-7. Summary of COC Performance Over 10 Years in FDA-Monitored Studies

Study	FU, y	Cases	Fractures	Incidence
Bierbaum, 2002	4	2313	0	0
Capello, 2008	8	380	2	0.5%
Murphy, 2006	4	194	1	0.5%
D'Antonio, 2005	4	328	0	0
Garino 2007[8]	3	333	0	0

Table 7-8. Comparison of Ceramic Fractures Reported Relative to the Numbers of Devices Sold Worldwide

Device	Sold	Fractures	Fractures per 10,000 Units Sold	Rate
Balls (ALX)	2,420,000	484	2	0.020%
Liners (ALX)	520,000	135	2.6	0.026%
Balls (ZRA)	570,000	11	2	0.002%
Liners (ZRA)	150,000	36	2.4	0.024%
Overall totals	3,660,000	667	1.8	0.018%

Data from CeramTec AG, Plochingen, Germany, March 2010.

In addition, some metal shells may have become deformed during the insertion procedure. The resulting malalignment may result in rim chipping, squeaking, or a loose or even fractured liner (see Table 7-7).[72] Recessed liner designs appeared more at risk, with estimates of up to 3%.[8,73]

Cup Impingement as a Risk to Ceramic Liners

The reported incidence of neck-cup impingement has varied from 40% to 80% in retrieved 28-mm THRs.[74] Impingement can be experienced in flexion or extension, depending on cup position,[72] and may create severe damage. The Peterson Tribology Laboratory encountered a particularly illustrative case in which a COC patient exhibited both a clicking and a squeaking while ambulating.[75] At revision, it was evident that the metal cup rim had created two notches in the femoral neck, while the posterior cup rim had been worn away (see Fig. 7-14). Metal transfer layers on ceramic surfaces revealed the presence of both equatorial and basal wear stripes. Thus such impingement with metal-backed cups can produce severe wear (Figs. 7-13 through 7-16).

A serious, design-related issue emerged for cups incorporating a ceramic liner factory-assembled inside a polyethylene sheath. This "sandwich" design offered no protection to the ceramic liner and proved extremely vulnerable. Any impingement has the potential to destabilize the femoral head, which then will be impacted against the opposing ceramic rim because of the action of the large hip muscles (see Figs. 7-14 and 7-15).[61,62] Clinical studies of a Japanese design using the PE-sandwich concept began in January 1998 (28-mm diameter; ABS, Kyocera Corporation, Kyoto, Japan). More than 5400 ABS cases had been recorded when sales were voluntarily discontinued in August 2000.[76,77] Subsequent follow-up studies showed approximately 12% of liner problems among three failures types.[63,64] Included were liner dissociation in approximately 60% of cases, disassembly of ceramic inlays in 20%, and fracture of ceramic liners in 14%. Neck-cup impingement and head-rim impact forces appeared to be the dominant problem (see Figs. 7-14 and 7-15). Similar short-term failures were encountered in the United States during an FDA-approved clinical study using a ceramic liner in a polyethylene sheath molded inside a trabecular metal shell. The initial report (1999-2002) described 4% of ceramic liners dissociated, with 12 of

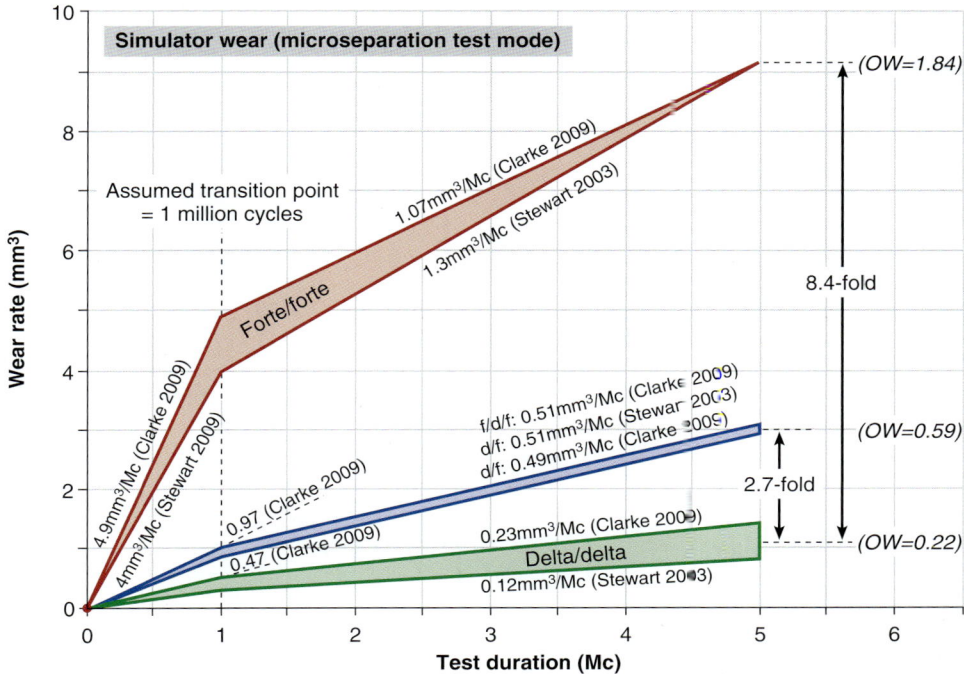

Figure 7-13. ALX and AMC wear trends in two microseparation simulator studies (28-mm diameter in Stewart et al[73]; 36-mm diameter in Clarke et al[26]). *Key: d/f,* ZRA ball in ALX cup; *f/d,* ALX ball in ZRA cup; *OW,* overall wear rate.

14 liners fractured. Anteversion of the femoral neck may also be a significant risk to ceramic liner impingement but seldom is well detailed.[78]

Squeaking and Osteolytic Risks With Ceramic Total Hip Replacement

The incidence of squeaking of ceramic THR can range from zero up to 20%.[79-81] Many of the underlying causes appear to be design related. Eicker and associates (2008) reported an incidence of 0.6% squeaking with flush-mounted liners (4/700 cases) in contrast to 3% (10/321 cases) with recessed liners.[79] When such cases featured a thin β-titanium femoral stem, the incidence rose to 7% (9/118 cases). This brand effect was confirmed in a separate study.[82] Squeaking has also been attributed to several other factors, including metal transfer onto the ceramic articulation, the use of thin metal shells that deformed during insertion, and failure to properly lock inserts into their metal backings during implantation.[83-86]

With 10 years of clinical monitoring in the United States, most COC cases appear to have few or no osteolytic changes.[8,73,87] However, clinical and retrieval reports have documented osteolysis proposed to be due to "ceramic debris." Extensive osteolysis has been documented with Mittelmeier THRs and with some contemporary THRs.[88,89] However, common features included short-term failures, black metallic staining of surfaces, and histologic evidence of "abundant metal debris" (Table 7-9). Thus the most likely reason for these early revisions (28-mm diameter THR) was neck-cup impingement (see Fig. 7-14). Similar findings were noted for

metal-on-metal (MOM) bearings, where rim contact accelerated the formation of stripe wear, greatly increasing CoCr wear.[54,74] As previously emphasized, wear discussions for hard-on-hard bearings must consider effects of microseparation (Mode 2: rim contact) and impingement/subluxation damage (Mode 4). Mode 4 can produce metallic debris from both the femoral stem and the acetabular shell (see Fig. 7-14). It is to be noted that black discoloration has generally been conspicuous in such ceramic retrievals (see Table 7-9).

Cultural practices also come into play, for example, the squatting position common among Asian patients presents a known risk. Hyperflexion with hip abduction was a common cause of fracture in Korean cases with the novel "sandwich" cup design. Also, cups in the fracture group (males) generally were more anteverted than those in the nonfracture group.[62] All showed superoposterior damage to the PE sandwich cups, and all had metal transfer onto the ceramic balls. Impingement occurred at 95 to 100 degrees flexion with 40 to 45 degrees abduction (see Figs. 7-14 and 7-15). Thus optimization of implant position is an important but challenging task with 28-mm diameter THR.

Phase Transformation Studies in Retrieved Alumina Matrix Composite Implants

Studies exploring the clinical performance of AMC bearings are scarce. Two trials reported use of AMC femoral heads with ALX liners.[90] In addition, two retrieval studies of AMC femoral heads showed monoclinic transformation ranging from 10% to 46%. Roughness studies

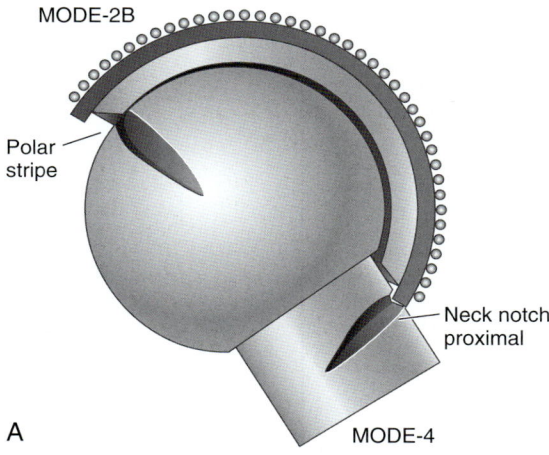

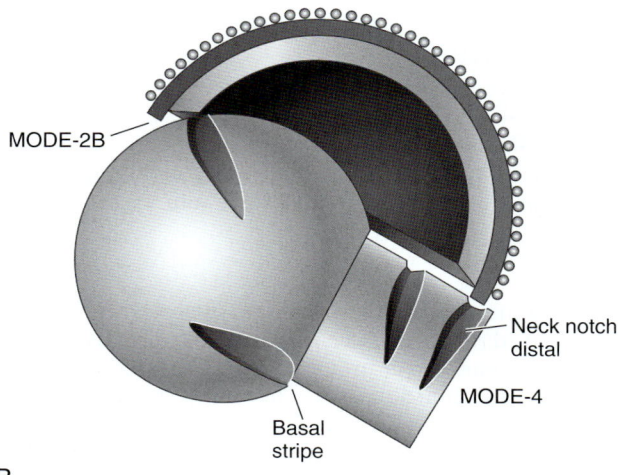

Figure 7-14. Schematic of cup impingement (as shown in Fig. 7-3) with damage to the cup rim cause by the hip muscles forcing the ball against the opposing cup edge to create stripe wear: **A,** First neck notch due to impingement; **B,** second more distal notch due to subluxation with impingement and new wear stripe.

showed retention of an excellent surface finish (<5 nm Ra) in the main wear zone. However, at the sites of stripe wear, roughness rose to 140 nm.[18,91]

The Peterson Tribology Laboratory compared the metastability of AMC femoral heads using autoclave conditioning combined with simulator wear studies.[92] Phase transformations and surface roughening were compared for (1) accelerated aging alone, and (2) simulated aging followed by hip wear simulation. AMC bearings were autoclaved by the manufacturer for 5, 10, and 30 hours (theoretically equivalent to 20, 40, and 120 years in vivo). The monoclinic phase on as-received balls phase averaged 7% ± 3%. After aging, the monoclinic phase increased linearly with autoclave time and averaged 19% by 10 hours. The roughness of AMC balls in the as-received conditions, as measured by atomic force microscopy (AFM) averaged 3 nm. With autoclave treatments, only a very minor increase to 5 nm was reported, even after 30 hours of autoclaving.

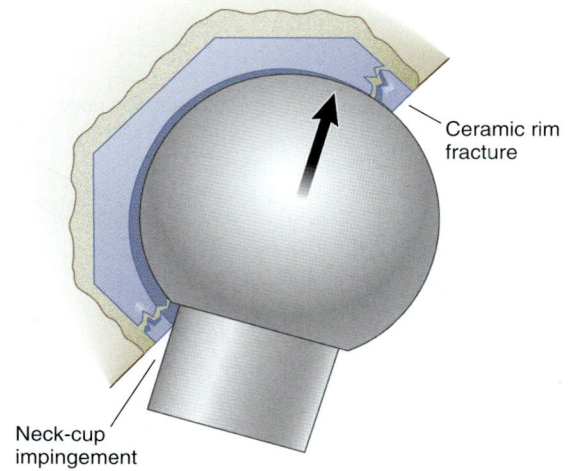

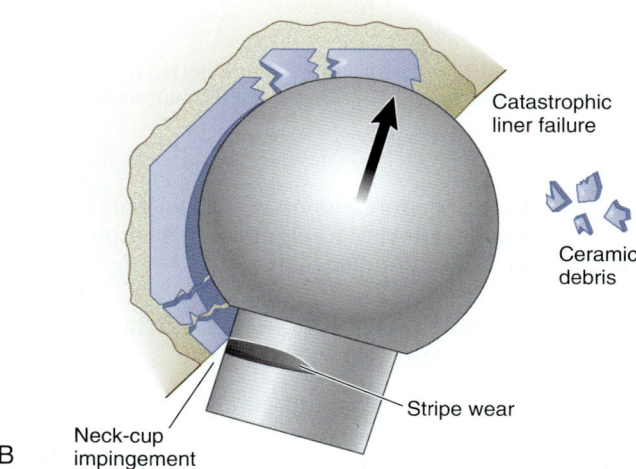

Figure 7-15. Schematic illustration of neck-cup impingement that destabilizes the femoral head, allowing impaction against the opposite cup rim. With low-stiffness polyethylene (PE) backing, risk is high for fracture of the ALX rim followed by catastrophic failure and release of ceramic, polyethylene, and metal debris. *(Redrawn from Figure 5, Ha et al.)*

The microseparation simulator wear study produced the expected main-wear zone (area of habitual contact) and stripe-wear zones. After 5 million cycles, nontreated AMC balls demonstrated 12% monoclinic phase, whereas autoclave-aged balls had up to 18%. The surface roughness of the main-wear zone was unchanged (<6 nm), whereas stripe sites increased to 50 nm (Ra). Thus AMC surfaces reacted to both tribological and microseparation effects.

A recent AMC retrieval study included six cases with ceramic liners and two with PE liners[92] (follow-up <3 years). Bearing surfaces featured highly polished surfaces marred only by black metallic transfer. Visual attempts to define any stripe wear zones were

Table 7-9. Studies Reporting Osteolysis With the ALX/ALX Combination

Study	Implant	Details	Follow-up, months	Impingement	Metal/Black
Murali, 2008[78]	32-mm Stryker	Excessive AV-stem (32 f)	34 (yoga)	Three sites (Ti fence)	Stripes, abundant metal debris, osteolysis
Murali, 2008[78]	32-mm Stryker	Squeak, clunk (48 m)	NA	Posterior (Ti fence)	Abundant black metallic debris
Nam, 2007	28-mm Aesculap	Osteolysis (63 f)	96	None	Black Ti-metal transfer, stripe wear, abundant ceramic debris
Ha, 2006	28-mm Lima	6 liner Fxs (25-68 m); sandwich cups	24-48	Flexed and 45-ABD	Rim chipping, black smears, PE rim damage; ALX debris
Yoon, 1998	Mittelmeier	22% osteolysis, loose cups (21-66 years)	60-125	79% cups loose	Bearing cracks, grooving, smearing, ceramic/metal debris, 22% osteolysis
Wirganowicz 1997[89]	32-mm Mittelmeier	Distal femoral cyst and Fx (66 f)	111	NA	THR and ORIF, extensive "metal staining"

NA, Not applicable; *ORIF*, open reduction internal fixation; *THR*, total hip replacement.

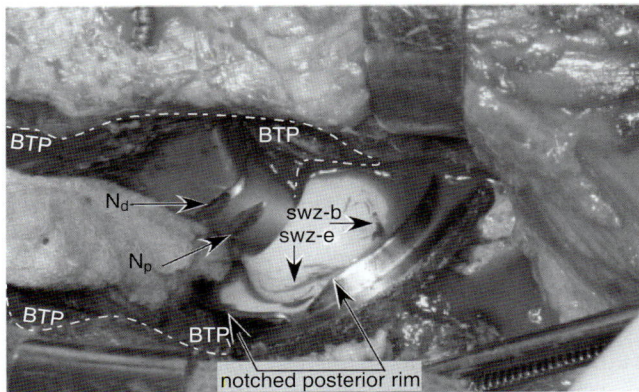

Figure 7-16. Revision photograph of 28-mm ceramic total hip replacement (THR) revealing titanium cup rim impinging onto titanium femoral neck, creating proximal (Np) and distal notches (Nd) with black-stained tissue planes (BTPs). The elevated metal fence has been eroded on the posterior rim of the cup. Stripe wear zones of equatorial (SWZe) and basal types (SWZb) are seen by black transfer on the ceramic. *(From Eickmann et al.[82])*

unsuccessful. In confirmation of the two previous retrieval reports, the surface monoclinic content varied from 14% to 38%, with AMC/PE combinations appearing no different from the AMC/AMC surfaces. Such retrievals demonstrated higher percentages in the monoclinic phase than in the accelerated aging study alone or following the microseparation wear test. Even with this degree of surface transformation, retrieved AMC surfaces retained an exceptional finish (<6 nm Ra). Thus transformation of surface zirconia grains had little effect on the bearing surface (i.e., the alumina ceramic was contributing the dominant wear resistance). Thus both the simulator and the retrieved AMC bearings appeared to show a self-limiting effect following monoclinic transformation of the zirconia. This was very much in contrast to studies of retrieved zirconia (y-ZR) balls, which had revealed 30% to 80% monoclinic transformation.[92]

Acknowledgments

Simulator wear studies were supported by CeramTec AG (Plochingen, Germany), the Peterson Foundation at Loma Linda University, and the Department of Orthopedics, Loma Linda University Medical Center. Grateful thanks are also due to R. Heros and T. Pandorf (CeramTec AG) for access to company R&D information, and to P. Williams and A. Clarke for editorial assistance with the manuscript.

REFERENCES

1. Clarke IC, Willmann G: Structural ceramics in orthopedics. In Cameron HU (ed): Bone implant interface, St Louis, 1994, Mosby, pp 203–252.
2. Poggie RA, Turgeon TR, Coutts RD: Failure analysis of a ceramic bearing acetabular component. J Bone Joint Surg Am 89:367–375, 2007.
3. Willmann G, Pfaff HG, Richter HG: [Increasing the safety of ceramic femoral heads for hip prostheses]. Biomed Tech (Berl) 40:342–346, 1995.
4. Miller EH, Heidt RS, Welch MC, et al: Self-bearing, uncemented, ceramic total hip replacement arthroplasty. Instr Course Lect 35:188–202, 1986.
5. Mahoney OM, Dimon JH 3rd: Unsatisfactory results with a ceramic total hip prosthesis. J Bone Joint Surg Am 72:663–671, 1990.
6. Huo MH, Martin RP, Zatorski LE, Keggi KJ: Total hip replacements using the ceramic Mittelmeier prosthesis. Clin Orthop 332:143–150, 1996.
7. Roy BR, Nevelos AB, Ingham E, et al: Comparison of ceramic on ceramic to ceramic on polyethylene total hip replacement. In Bioceramics, Zurich-Uetikon, 2007, Trans Tech Publications Ltd, pp 991–994.
8. Garino JP: Clinical experience with ceramic on ceramic in the USA. In Bioceramics and alternative bearings in joint arthroplasty, Seoul, Korea, 2007, Steinkopff, pp 169–171.
9. D'Antonio J, Sutton K: Ceramic materials as bearing surfaces for total hip arthoplasty. J AAOS 17:63–68, 2009.
10. Willmann G: New generation ceramics. In Willmann G, Zweymuller K (eds): Bioceramics in hip joint replacement, Stuttgart, 2000, Georg Thieme Verlag, pp 127–135.
11. Clarke IC, Gustafson A: Chapter 5. The design of ceramics for joint replacement. In Kokubo T (ed): Bioceramics and their clinical applications, Osaka, Japan, 2008, Woodhead, pp 106–132.

12. American Society for Testing and Materials (ASTM): ASTM 2345-2303. Standard test methods for determination of static and cyclic fatigue strength of ceramic modular femoral heads, Conshohocken, Pa, 2008, ASTM International.

13. International Organization for Standardization (ISO): ISO-7206-10. Implants for surgery—partial and total hip-joint prostheses. Part 10. Determination of resistance to static load of modular femoral heads, Geneva, Switzerland, 2003, ISO.

14. Morrell R, Hughes S: Factors influencing the reliability of ceramic femoral components. J Eur Ceramic Soc 27:1535–1541, 2007.

15. U.S. Food and Drug Administration: Guidance document for the preparation of premarket notifications for ceramic ball hip systems, Silver Springs, Md, 1995, FDA.

16. Clarke IC, Manaka M, Green DD, et al: Current status of zirconia used in total hip implants, Bone Joint Sung Am 85 (4):73–84, 2003.

17. Piconi C, Maccauro G: Review: zirconia as a ceramic biomaterial. Biomaterials 20:1–25, 1999.

18. Clarke IC, Green DD, Williams PA, et al: Hip-simulator wear studies of an alumina-matrix composite (AMC) ceramic compared to retrieval studies of AMC balls with 1-7 years follow-up. Wear 267:702–709, 2009.

19. International Organization for Standardization (ISO): ISO-14242-1. Implants for surgery—wear of total hip-joint prostheses. Part 1. Loading and displacement parameters for wear-testing machines and corresponding environmental conditions for test, Geneva, Switzerland, 2002, ISO.

20. International Organization for Standardization (ISO): ISO-14242-2. Implants for surgery—wear of total hip-joint prostheses. Part 2. Methods of measurement, Geneva, Switzerland, 2000, ISO.

21. International Organization for Standardization (ISO): ISO-14242-3. Implants for surgery—wear of total hip-joint prostheses. Part 3. Loading and displacement parameters for orbital bearing type wear testing machines and corresponding environmental conditions for test, Geneva, Switzerland, 2009, ISO.

22. American Society for Testing and Materials (ASTM): ASTM1714. Standard guide for gravimetric wear assessment of prosthetic hip designs in simulator devices, Conshohocken, Pa, 2008, ASTM International.

23. Phipatanakul WP, Johnson SA, Good V, Clarke IC: The fallacy of evaluating biomaterial wear-rates with water as lubricant: a hip simulator study of alumina-PTFE and CoCr-PTFE combinations. J Biomed Mater Res 39:229–233, 1998.

24. Good VD, Clarke IC, Anissian L: Water and bovine serum lubrication compared in simulator PTFE/CoCr wear model. J Biomed Mater Res 33:275–283, 1996.

25. Good V: The tribological significance of the joint fluid analog in a hip joint simulator. In Engineering, Glasgow, Scotland, 2001, University of Strathclyde, p 163.

26. Nevelos JE, Ingham E, Doyle C, et al: Analysis of retrieved alumina ceramic components from Mittelmeier total hip prostheses. Biomaterials 20:1833–1840, 1999.

27. Nevelos J, Ingham E, Doyle C, et al: Micro-separation in vitro produces clinically relevant wear of ceramic-ceramic total hip replacements. In Bioceramics, Zurich-Uetikon, 2000, Trans Tech Publications Ltd, pp 529–532.

28. Wang A, Essner A, Stark C, Dumbleton JH: Comparison of the size and morphology of UHMWPE wear debris produced by a hip joint simulator under serum and water lubricated conditions. Biomaterials 17:865–871, 1996.

29. Bowsher J, Clarke I: Thermal conductivity of femoral ball strongly influenced UHMWPE wear in a hip simulator study, Anaheim, Calif, 2007, Orthopedic Research Society, p 278.

30. Clarke IC, Green DD, Pezzotti G, et al: The bio-lubrication (proteins) phenomena may control the wear performance of zirconia hip joints, Nashville, 2003, American Ceramics Society.

31. Clarke IC, Oonishi H, Anissian L, et al: Serum protection important for all-metal and all-ceramic (rigid-on-rigid) bearings in hip simulator studies. Paper presented at the 48th Meeting of the Orthopaedic Research Society, Dallas, February 9–13, 2002, p 1017.

32. Nevelos J, Ingham E, Doyle C, et al: Microseparation of the centers of alumina-alumina artificial hip joints during simulator testing produces clinically relevant wear rates and patterns. J Arthroplasty 15:793–795, 2000.

33. Nevelos JE, Ingham E, Doyle C, et al: Wear of hiped and non-hiped alumina-alumina hip joints under standard and severe simulator testing conditions. Biomaterials 22:2191, 2001.

34. Clarke I, Donaldson T, Jobe C: Total joint replacement: effects of materials and designs on osteolysis. In Garino JP, Beredjiklian PK (eds): Total hip arthroplasty, St Louis, 2007, Mosby, pp 1–28.

35. McKellop H, Clarke I, Markolf K, Amstutz H: Friction and wear properties of polymer, metal, and ceramic prosthetic joint materials evaluated on a multichannel screening device. J Biomed Mater Res 15:619–653, 1981.

36. Chevalier J: What future for zirconia as a biomaterial? Biomaterials 27:535–543, 2006.

37. Hernigou P, Bahrami T: Zirconia and alumina ceramics in comparison with stainless-steel heads: polyethylene wear after a minimum ten-year follow-up. J Bone Joint Surg Br 85:504–509, 2003.

38. Green DD, Williams P, Donaldson T, Clarke IC: Biolox-forte vs. Biolox-delta under micro separation test mode in the USA, Washington, DC, 2005, Orthopaedic Research Society.

39. Haraguchi K, Sugano N, Nishii T, et al: Phase transformation of a zirconia ceramic head after total hip arthroplasty. J Bone Joint Surg Br 83:996–1000, 2001.

40. McKellop H, Lu B, Benya P: Friction lubrication and wear of cobalt-chromium, alumina, and zirconia hip prostheses compared on a joint simulator. Presented at the 38th Annual Meeting of the Orthopaedic Research Society, Washington, DC, February 19, 1992, p 402.

41. Saikko V: A simulator study of friction in total replacement hip joints. Proc Inst Mech Eng (H) 206:201–211, 1992.

42. Derbyshire B, Fisher J, Dowson D, et al: Comparative study of the wear of UHMWPE with zirconia ceramic and stainless steel femoral heads in artificial hip joints. Med Eng Phys 16:229–236, 1994.

43. Liao YS, Benya PD, McKellop HA: Effect of protein lubrication on the wear properties of materials for prosthetic joints. J Biomed Mater Res 48:465–473, 1999.

44. Bowsher JG, Clarke I: Thermal conductivity of femoral ball strongly influenced UHMWPE wear in a hip simulator study. Paper presented at the 53rd Annual Meeting of the Orthopaedic Research Society, San Diego, February 11–14, 2007, p 278.

45. Hernigou P, Nogier A, Poignard A, Filippini P: Alumina ceramic against polyethylene: a long term follow up. In Lazennec JY, Dietrich M (eds): Bioceramics in joint arthroplasty: 9th Biolox Symposium, Steinkopff, 2004, Darmstadt, pp 41–42.

46. Green DD, Pezzotti G, Sakakura S, et al: Zirconia ceramic femoral heads in the USA. Paper presented at the 49th Annual Meeting of the Orthopaedic Research Society, New Orleans, La, February 2–5, 2003, p 1392.

47. Walter WL, Skyrme AD, Richards S, et al: Polyethylene wear rates with zirconia and cobalt chrome heads. Paper presented at the 51st Annual Meeting of the Orthopaedic Research Society, Washington, DC, February 20–23, 2005.

48. Brown SS, Green DD, Pezzotti G, et al: Possible triggers for phase transformation in zirconia hip balls. J Biomed Mater Res B Appl Biomater 85:444–452, 2008.

49. Mittelmeier H, Heisel J: Sixteen-years' experience with ceramic hip prostheses. Clin Orthop 282:64–72, 1992.

50. Dorlot JM: Long-term effects of alumina components in total hip prostheses. Clin Orthop 282:47–52, 1992.

51. Kummer FJ, Stuchin SA, Frankel VH: Analysis of removed autophor ceramic-on-ceramic components. J Arthroplasty 5:28–33, 1990.

52. Nevelos JE, Prudhommeaux F, Hamadouche M, et al: Comparative analysis of two different types of alumina-alumina hip prosthesis retrieved for aseptic loosening. J Bone Joint Surg Br 83:598–603, 2001.

53. Clarke IC, Manley MT: How do alternative bearing surfaces influence wear behavior? J Am Acad Orthop Surg 16:S86–S93, 2008.

54. Morlock M, Nassutt R, Janssen R, et al: Mismatched wear couple zirconium oxide and aluminum oxide in total hip arthroplasty. J Arthroplasty 16:1071–1074, 2001.

55. Hamadouche M, Boutin P, Daussange J, et al: Alumina-on-alumina total hip arthroplasty: a minimum 18.5-year follow-up study. J Bone Joint Surg Am 84:69–77, 2002.

56. Sedel L: Evolution of alumina-on-alumina implants: a review. Clin Orthop Relat Res 379:48–54, 2000.

57. Sedel L: Recent clinical experience of all-alumina THR. Paper presented at the XXII SICOT World Congress, San Diego, August 23–30, 2002.

58. Griss P: Four- to eight-year postoperative results of the partially uncemented lindenhof-type ceramic hip endoprosthesis. In Morscher E (ed): The cementless fixation of hip endoprostheses, Berlin, 1984, Springer-Verlag, pp 220–224.

59. Manaka M, Clarke IC, Yamamoto K, et al: Stripe wear rates in alumina THR—comparison of microseparation simulator study with retrieved implants. J Biomed Mater Res 69B:149–157, 2004.

60. Shishido T, Clarke IC, Williams P, et al: Clinical and simulator wear study of alumina ceramic THR to 17 years and beyond. J Biomed Mater Res 67B:638–647, 2003.

61. Walter WL, Insley GM, Walter WK, Tuke MA: Edge loading in third generation alumina ceramic-on-ceramic bearings: stripe wear. J Arthroplasty 19:402–413, 2004.

62. Ha YC, Kim SY, Kim HJ, et al: Ceramic liner fracture after cementless alumina-on-alumina total hip arthroplasty. Clin Orthop Relat Res 458:106–110, 2007.

63. Hasegawa M, Sudo A, Uchida A: Alumina ceramic-on-ceramic total hip replacement with a layered acetabular component. J Bone Joint Surg Br 88:877–882, 2006.

64. Kawate K, Ohmura T, Kawahara I, et al: Tragedy of polyethylene backed ceramic on ceramic articulation. In Chang J-D, Billau K (eds): Proceedings of ceramics in orthopaedics: bioceramics and alternative bearings in joint arthroplasty, 12th Biolox Symposium, Seoul, Korea, 2007, Steinkopff, pp 299–301.

65. Boutin P: [Total arthroplasty of the hip by fritted aluminum prosthesis: experimental study and 1st clinical applications]. Rev Chir Orthop Reparatrice Appar Mot 58:229–246, 1972.

65a. Clarke IC, Manaka M, Shishido T, et al: Tribological and material properties for all-alumina THR: convergence with clinical retrieval data. In Zippel H, Dietrich M (eds): Bioceramics in joint arthroplasty, Berlin, 2003, Steinkopff Verlag, pp 3–18.

66. Oonishi H, Clarke IC, Good V, et al: Alumina hip joints characterized by run-in wear and steady-state wear to 14 million cycles in hip-simulator model. J Biomed Mater Res 70A:523–532, 2004.

67. Green DD, Pezzotti G, Sakakura S, et al: 2 and 10 year retrievals of zirconia femoral heads: xrd, sem, and raman spectroscopy studies, Nashville, 2003, American Ceramic Society.

68. Stewart T, Tipper J, Streicher R, et al: Long-term wear of hiped alumina on alumina bearings for THR under microseparation conditions. J Mater Sci Mater Med 12:1053–1056, 2001.

69. Green DD, Williams P, Pezzotti G, Clarke IC: Simulator investigation of al-doped zirconia in water for THR. In Ben-Nissan B, Sher D, Walsh W (eds): Bioceramics-15, Sydney, Australia, 2002, Trans Tech Pub.

70. Heros RJ, Willmann G: Ceramic in total hip arthroplasty: history, mechanical properties, clinical results, and current manufacturing state of the art. Semin Arthroplasty 3:114–122, 1998.

71. Tateiwa T, Clarke IC, Williams PA, et al: Ceramic total hip arthroplasty in the United States: safety and risk issues revisited. Am J Orthop 37: E26–E31, 2008.

72. Walter WL, Waters TS, Gillies M, et al: Squeaking hips. J Bone Joint Surg Am 90:102–111, 2008.

73. D'Antonio JA, Sutton K: Ceramic materials as bearing surfaces for total hip arthroplasty. J Am Acad Orthop Surg 17:63–68, 2009.

74. Kubo K, Clarke I, Lazennec JY, et al: Wear mapping analysis with retrieval of 28 mm CoCr-CoCr hip bearings: 11 years experience. Presented at Wear of Materials Conference, Las Vegas, April 19–22, 2009.

75. Eickmann T, Manaka M, Clarke I, Gustafson A: Squeaking and neck-socket impingement in a ceramic total hip arthroplasty. Bioceramics 240:849–852, 2003.

76. Hasegawa M, Sudo A, Hirata H, Uchida A: Ceramic acetabular liner fracture in total hip arthroplasty with a ceramic sandwich cup. J Arthroplasty 18:658–666, 2003.

77. Suzuki K, Matsubara M, Morita S, et al: Fracture of a ceramic acetabular insert after ceramic-on-ceramic THA—a case report. Acta Orthop Scand 74:101–103, 2003.

78. Murali R, Bonar SF, Kirsh G, et al: Osteolysis in third-generation alumina ceramic-on-ceramic hip bearings with severe impingement and titanium metallosis. J Arthroplasty 23:13–19, 2008.

79. Eicker TM, Robbins C, van Flandern G, et al: Squeaking in total hip replacement: no cause for concern. Orthopedics 31:875–877, 2008.

80. Keurentjes JC, Kuipers RM, Wever DJ, Schreurs BW: High incidence of squeaking in THAs with alumina ceramic-on-ceramic bearings. Clin Orthop Relat Res 466:1438–1443, 2008.

81. Walter WL, O'Toole GC, Walter WK, et al: Squeaking in ceramic-on-ceramic hips: the importance of acetabular component orientation. J Arthroplasty 22:496–503, 2007.

82. Restrepo C, Matar WY, Parvizi J, et al: Natural history of squeaking after total hip arthroplasty. Clin Orthop Relat Res (published online January 2010).

83. Langdown J, Pickard R, Hobbs C, et al: Incomplete seating of the liner with the trident system: a cause for concern? J Bone Joint Surg Br 89:291–295, 2006.

84. Miller ANS, Edwin P, Bostrom MPG, et al: Incidence of ceramic liner malseating in Trident acetabular shell. Clin Orthop Relat Res 467:1552–1556, 2009.

85. Rodriguez JA: The squeaking hip is a multifactorial concern: rim impingement, microseparation, subluxation are all suspects in the sound generation. Orthopedics Today 28–92, 2008.

86. Rodríguez JA, DelaValle AG, McCook N: Squeaking in total hip replacement: a cause for concern. Orthopedics 31:874–878, 2008.

87. Kim YH, Choi Y, Kim JS: Cementless total hip arthroplasty with ceramic-on-ceramic bearing in patients younger than 45 years with femoral-head osteonecrosis. Int Orthop 34:1123–1127, 2010.

88. Yoo JJ, Kim YM, Yoon KS, et al: Contemporary alumina-on-alumina total hip arthroplasty performed in patients younger than forty years: a 5-year minimum follow-up study. J Biomed Mater Res B Appl Biomater 78:70–75, 2006.

89. Wirganowicz PZ, Thomas BJ: Massive osteolysis after ceramic on ceramic total hip arthroplasty a case report. Clin Orthop Relat Res 338:100–104, 1997.

90. Lombardi AV Jr, Berend KR, Seng BE, et al: Delta ceramic-on-alumina ceramic articulation in primary THA: prospective, randomized FDA-IDE study and retrieval analysis. Clin Orthop Relat Res 468:367–374, 2010.

91. Medel FJ, Shah P, Kurtz SM: Retrieval anlaysis of contemporary alternative femoral head materials oxinium and biolox delta. Paper presented at the 55th Annual Meeting of the Orthopaedic Research Society, Las Vegas, February 22–24, 2009.

92. Clarke IC, Manaka M, Green DD, et al: Current status of zirconia used in total hip implants. J Bone Joint Surg Am 85(Suppl 4):73–84, 2003.

SUGGESTED READING

Bansal N, Zhu D: Thermal conductivity of zirconia-alumina composites. Ceram Int 31:911–916, 2001.

Bierbaum BE, Nairus J, Kuesis D, et al: Ceramic-on-ceramic bearings in total hip arthroplasty. Clin Orthop Relat Res 405:158–163, 2002.

Capello W, D'Antonio J, Feinberg JR, et al: Ceramic-on-ceramic total hip arthroplasty: update. J Arthroplasty 23:39–43, 2008.

Clarke I, Donaldson T, Bowsher J, et al: Current concepts of metal-on-metal hip resurfacing. Orthop Clin North Am 36:143–162, 2005.

Clarke IC, Keggi KJ, Kegg J, et al: 38-year tracking of ceramic science and results in hip joints. In Bellosi A, Babini GN (eds):

Global roadmap for ceramics: proceedings of B-ICC2, Verona, Italy, 2008, Litografica Faenza Srl, pp 87–96.

Clarke IC, Williams P, Shishido T, et al: Hip simulator validations of alumina THR wear rates for run-in and steady-state wear phases. In Garino J, Willmann G (eds): Proceedings of the 7th International Biolox Symposium, Thieme, 2002, Verlag, pp 20–26.Ha Y, Koo H, Jeong S, et al: Ten-year survivorship of cemented ceramic-ceramic total hip prosthesis. J Bone Joint Surg Am 88:780–787, 2006.

D'Antonio JA, Capello WN, Manley MT, et al: A titanium-encased alumina ceramic bearing for total hip arthroplasty: 3- to 5-year results. Clin Orthop Relat Res 441:151–158, 2005.

Murphy SB, Ecker TM, Timo M, Tannast M: Two to 9 year clinical results of alumina ceramic-on-ceramic THA. Clin Orthop Relat Res 453:97–102, 2006.

Nam KW, Yoo JJ, Kim YL, et al: Alumina-debris-induced osteolysis in contemporary alumina-on-alumina total hip arthroplasty: a case report. J Bone Joint Surg Am 89:2499–2503, 2007.

Raghavan S, Wang H, Dinwiddie R, et al: The effect of grain size, porosity and yttria content on the thermal conductivity of nano-crystalline zirconia. Scrip Mater 39:1119–1125, 1998.

Yoon TR, Rowe SM, Jung ST, et al: Osteolysis in association with a total hip arthroplasty with ceramic bearing surfaces. J Bone Joint Surg Am 80:1459–1468, 1998.

CHAPTER 8

Materials in Hip Surgery: Metals as a Bearing Material

Sophie Williams and John Fisher

KEY POINTS

- Metal (usually >0.2% carbon cobalt chromium molybdenum) is used as a bearing material in MOM hip replacements and surface replacements; manufacturing processes have little effect on the alloy's wear characteristics.
- Design variables (such as diameter, clearance, and inclusion angle) will influence the wear performance of metal-on-metal (MOM) prostheses in optimal conditions.
- Wear behavior will be affected by nonoptimal component positioning (e.g., steeply inclined cups).
- Concern exists regarding some clinical failures of MOM bearings.
- Aspheric bearings, ceramic-on-metal articulations, and the use of coatings may offer alternatives to current MOM designs in the future.

INTRODUCTION

Metal-on-metal (MOM) bearings are used worldwide in conventional hip replacements and hip resurfacing designs. In Australia, approximately 19% of all hip prostheses implanted in 2008 were MOM (of which approximately 12% were conventional designs).[1] In the United Kingdom in 2008, 6% of implanted hip prostheses were surface replacements (data for numbers of conventional MOM hip replacements implanted were not available).[2]

Metal-on-metal hip replacements gained early prominence in the 1960s; usage then declined following reports of early failures in initial series and the success of metal-on-polyethylene bearings. With these early bearings, a number of configurations were used; in some cases, they were existing components intended for use in hemiarthroplasty such as the McBride/Moore, Urist/Moore, and Urist Thompson systems. Observed problems were primarily impingement, loss of range of motion, and the presence of a stress riser in the stem portion of the acetabular component. More widely used was the McKee-Farrar design, which used a standard Thompson femoral component (later modified to reduce impingement). Clinical experience with early devices yielded less than satisfactory results in many cases; however, there were exceptions.[3]

The observation that a small number of patients with first-generation MOM prostheses exhibited good clinical and radiologic results after 20 years in vivo led to the development of second-generation MOM hip prostheses.[4] In 1988, the Metasul prosthesis was introduced into clinical practice; early experience demonstrated low wear rates, and few prostheses required revision. More recently, MOM hip resurfacing has been offered as an alternative, in particular to young, active patients. Clinical results of MOM resurfacing are generally favorable; however, some variation in outcome is dependent on a number of factors. Clinical wear rates of MOM vary up to 40-fold.[5,6] Factors effecting wear have been cited as design, component geometry (diameter and clearance), metallurgy of the alloy, component positioning, and prosthesis use. There is a drive to reduce MOM wear and ion release, following observations that some patients have increased cobalt and chromium blood/serum and/or urine levels. Long-term consequences of elevated levels of ions and effects of metal particles are not known.

BASIC SCIENCE

Metallurgy

Cobalt-based alloys dominate the material selection for bearing surfaces of MOM prostheses, because of their high wear resistance and corrosion resistance. The composition is specified by American Society for Testing and Materials (ASTM) F-1537 (Table 8-1); carbon content can vary (carbon is responsible for the generation of carbides, which strengthen the material and affect the wear resistance[7]). Additionally, processing (wrought or cast; with or without heat treatment) can affect the microstructure of the alloy. This has generated much debate in terms of effects on wear rate, production of wear particles, and ultimately the release of metal ions, all of which will be affected by the altered distribution of carbides.

High-carbon (>0.2% w/w) CoCr alloy has a biphasic structure; small grains of CoCr are surrounded by embedded, hard, scratch-resistant carbides, which restrict grain size. Low-carbon (<0.05% w/w) CoCr alloys are softer than high-carbon alloys (because of the lack of carbides) and comprise a single-phase structure of larger grain size. Low carbon content alloys produce significantly higher wear rates than high carbon content

Table 8-1. Composition of CoCr Alloy as Specified by ASTM F-1537 Low and High Carbon

	ASTM F-1537 (low carbon) Forged	ASTM F-1537 (high carbon) Forged
Chromium	26-30	26-30
Molybdenum	5-7	5-7
Carbon	0.14 max	0.15-0.35
Nickel	1 max	1 max
Iron	0.75 max	0.75 max
Manganese	1 max	1 max
Silicon	1 max	1 max
Tungsten	n/s	n/s
Phosphorus	n/s	n/s
Sulfur	n/s	n/s
Nitrogen	0.25 max	0.25 max
Aluminium	n/s	n/s
Titanium	n/s	n/s
Boron	n/s	n/s
Lanthanum	n/s	n/s
Cobalt	Balance	Balance

ASTM, American Society for Testing and Materials; *max*, maximum; *n/s*, not significant.

alloys in both simple configuration wear tests and hip joint wear simulator tests.[3,8-10] Hence, the pairing of low carbon cups with low carbon femoral heads is not recommended. High carbon/high carbon pairings show the lowest wear rates in hip joint simulator tests.[10]

The wear rates of cast and wrought CoCrMo alloys with and without various heat treatments have been compared and are the subject of debate. Dowson and associates[11] reported no significant differences between wear volumes of wrought and cast high carbon CoCrMo materials. Heat treatments and hot isostatic pressing have been shown to have little effect on the wear rate of MOM hip prostheses. The effect of the method of manufacture on the wear resistance of MOM bearings has been further studied under adverse wear conditions in hip simulator studies. Bowsher and colleagues[12] investigated the wear of double–heat-treated and as cast large diameter MOM hip bearings using standard and "severe" gait simulations. High carbon MOM bearings (40 mm diameter) were manufactured and were subjected to hot isostatic pressing and solution annealing, or to no heat treatment, after casting. No differences between the two groups under running-in and steady-state conditions were observed, and the authors concluded that changes in alloy microstructure (due to manufacturing route) do not appear to influence the wear behavior of high carbon cast MOM articulations with similar chemical compositions.

Wear Mechanisms

The low wear rates recorded for metal-on-metal articulations are surprising in the context of traditional engineering terms, which presume that like-on-like materials do not produce low wearing surfaces. In recent years, several mechanisms have been suggested to explain this observation.[13] Abrasion is commonly suggested as a wear mechanism, because scratches and grooves are obvious on in vitro tested samples and MOM retrievals.[14-16] Abrasion may be induced by foreign particles (contaminants from outside the system) or most likely by inherent particles in the system, such as fractured carbides, compacted wear debris, and plastically deformed parts of the metal matrix.

In theory, fluid film lubrication is a potential mechanism for generating low wear in like-on-like bearings.[17] However, hydrodynamic lubrication is unlikely to be achieved in practice, because surfaces generally are roughened through the effects of third-body particles, and the articulations are subjected to conditions ranging from loaded static to cyclical motion, with frequent changes in load, velocity, and direction of relative motion. Wear mechanisms previously discussed include boundary lubrication by proteins, lipids, and even calcium phosphate deposits, and high carbon content carbides acting as ceramic/metal composites.[8] Following pin-on-plate testing of CoCr on CoCr articulations, Tipper and co-workers[8] suggested further alternative mechanisms: that multidirectional motion and its polishing action may act as a mechanism for reducing wear, and that nanometer-sized spherical wear particles may act as self-lubricating ball bearings, acting as third bodies between bearing surfaces, rolling, deforming, and acting as sites for motion and velocity accommodation, thereby minimizing the wear of the actual bearing surfaces. Later, Wimmer and associates[7] carried out in vitro studies to assess the acting wear mechanisms. It was concluded that tribolayers (also seen on ex vivo samples[13]) are derived from protein buildup on surfaces due to a combination of mechanical and thermal contact stresses generated between the surfaces. These layers act as solid lubricants and act to reduce wear.

The wear mechanism of MOM bearings has been further considered with investigation of biotribocorrosion processes. A series of studies have demonstrated that depassivation of CoCr materials occurs as a result of contact between metallic counterfaces,[18] and that ion release is dominated by the production of Co ions, but not in the ratio of the base alloy.[19] In tribometer studies, corrosion can contribute up to 44% of the total damage,[19,20] as reported by other authors.[7,13] Yan and colleagues[21,22] reported on the production of a protein-assisted tribofilm; it is believed that this is responsible for the wear-induced passivation seen in polarization studies. Corrosion also plays a significant role in ion release; corrosion enhanced by wear and wear debris dissolution are the two main sources, each having very different kinetics.[23]

Wear Performance

MOM prostheses have been estimated to have 40 to 100 times less wear than metal-on-polyethylene bearings[24]; this is critical in extending the life of MOM bearings. However, much in vitro evidence suggests that the wear of MOM prostheses is highly dependent on the materials, the tribological design, and the finishing technique. Clinical studies of retrieved first- and second-generation MOM hip prostheses have shown linear penetrations of approximately 5 μm/yr[25] and volumetric measures of approximately 0.33 mm^3/yr.[15] However, large levels of variation have been observed.

The wear of hard-on-hard bearings such as MOM hip prostheses has two distinct phases: (1) a period of initially elevated bedding-in wear that lasts approximately 1 million cycles, or the first year in vivo, followed by (2) a lower steady-state wear period, once the bearing surfaces have been subjected to the self-polishing action of metal wear particles, which may act as a solid-phase lubricant. This phenomenon is reported in numerous in vitro hip simulator tests[9-12,26,27] and has been studied in greater detail than the clinical situation described by Heisal and co-workers.[28] In vitro hip simulator testing of MOM implants and a parallel study assessing clinical serum metal ion concentration were conducted with the aim of characterizing the early running-in period in vivo and in vitro by assessing metal ion levels. Hip resurfacing prostheses were implanted in 15 consecutive patients, and serum metal ion concentrations were determined preoperatively and at 1, 6, 12, 24, and 52 weeks; also, the number of walking cycles was measured. In vitro, five similar components were investigated for three million cycles in a hip simulator; wear was assessed by quantifying wear particles and ions in serum samples. Serum chromium and cobalt levels of patients continuously increased during the first 6 months and showed an insignificant decrease thereafter. In contrast, simulator measurements showed a different wear pattern with a high-wear running-in period and a low-wear steady-state phase. The running-in period was delayed by 300,000 cycles and lasted up to 1 million cycles. In contrast, clinical data showed a slow increase in measured ion concentrations. The difference in wear patterns was attributed to the effects of distribution, accumulation, and excretion of particles and ions in vivo.

Implant Design Factors

Diameter

The head diameter of total hip replacements has long been recognized as a factor affecting the stability and range of motion of the articulation because of the basic premise that the larger the head, the larger the distance must be displaced to dislocate from the cup.[29]

In terms of MOM bearings, the diameter of the head and cup and the clearance between them have been cited as design factors affecting the tribological performance of the bearing and so will be considered in this section. The premise that head diameter will affect wear is driven by theoretical predictions of lubrication conditions at the bearing surfaces. These analyses suggest that increasing the diameter will lead to reductions in wear rates caused by increased entrainment velocity of the surrounding fluid for a given angular velocity of the extremity, which, in turn, is predicted to improve lubrication and reduce friction.[17]

The effect of diameter has become increasingly important with resurfacing prostheses, as these cover the reamed femoral head (rather than replacing it) and therefore are of large diameter (average, approximately 54 mm). In hip simulator testing of MOM (CoCrMo on CoCrMo) prostheses with femoral heads of 16, 22.225, and 28 mm diameter, increasing the head size from 16 mm to 22.225 mm increased the mean volumetric wear rate (4.85 mm^3/mill on cycles for 16-mm-diameter bearings and 6.30 mm^3/million cycles for 22.225-mm bearings). When the diameter was further increased to 28 mm, it was observed that the average wear rate dropped to 1.6 mm^3/million cycles.[30] Dowson and colleagues[31] further considered 36-mm total hip replacements and 54-mm resurfacing prostheses in a hip simulator study; steady-state wear rates were quickly established as the head diameter increased from 28 to 36 mm and then to 54 mm. In agreement with previous studies, as head diameter increased, wear volume decreased markedly, with steady-state values of 0.17 mm^3/10^6 cycles for the 54-mm-diameter bearings.

Direct comparison has been made of surface replacements of different diameters (approximately 39 mm and 55 mm).[32] Again, two distinct phases of wear were observed for both bearing sizes: bedding-in (up to 1 million cycles), during which the wear rate was elevated, and steady state (beyond 1 million cycles), where the wear rate was reduced. The bedding-in wear rate of the 39-mm bearings was significantly greater (123%) than that of the 55-mm bearings. It is interesting to note that this difference ceased to be significant between 1 and 15 million cycles, again showing the wear of surface replacements to be biphasic with bedding-in and steady-state wear phases, consistent with previous findings for MOM total hip replacements.[9-12,27,28,30-32]

A theoretical study by Jin and associates[17] and previously discussed experimental studies all confirm that increasing head diameter wear in MOM bearings decreases overall wear rate.[30,31] However, a study by Leslie and colleagues,[32] comparing 39-mm and 55-mm bearings of the same type, was the first to report that the bedding-in period (as demonstrated by measurements of ion levels from the lubricating serum, in addition to gravimetric wear assessment) was shorter for the larger bearing. This suggests the possibility that the 55-mm bearings had a similar initial wear rate to the 39-mm bearings but a shorter bedding-in period, resulting in reduced wear in the first million cycles—a conclusion that is consistent with the geometric analysis of Hu and co-workers.[33] As the volume of material that must be removed for bedding-in decreases with head diameter, the duration of the bedding-in period and the total wear volume generated are less with larger bearings, even if the actual rate of wear remains constant.

The work of Leslie and associates[32] has also demonstrated that bearing size has no influence on the steady-state wear of larger bearings. Previous theoretical studies of lubrication have predicted differences in wear rates on the assumption that the wear process itself would not change the geometry of contact between counterfaces. However, as bedding-in occurs, the contact area increases and contact pressures decrease. Theoretical analysis indicates that the worn contact area (and therefore contact pressure) following bedding-in (after 1 million cycles) is similar for 39- and 55-mm bearings, despite the fact that the initial contact area is less (and contact pressures higher) for the smaller, 39-mm bearing. At the end of 15 million cycles of simulator testing, contact pressures and contact areas were similar for the 39-mm- and 55-mm-diameter bearings. So the importance of the conventional lubrication theory in determining wear of MOM bearings is mainly evident during the initial bedding-in stage. However, after the bedding-in stage, it appears that wear is determined largely by improved conformity of the bearing surfaces generated by bedding-in wear, as well as by the corresponding contact mechanics. The fact that little difference is observed in the measured wear volume of 39-mm and 55-mm bearings appears to be the result of two competing effects: the higher entraining velocity of the larger size, leading to improved fluid film lubrication, versus the shorter sliding distance of the smaller size.

The effect of the bearing diameter of MOM prostheses has also been studied clinically. Antoniou and associates[34] compared blood ion levels (cobalt, chromium, and molybdenum) of patients with metal-on-metal total hip prostheses versus a 28- or 36-mm-diameter femoral head, and patients with hip resurfacing prostheses. Variations between groups with MOM bearings of different diameter were noted 6 months postoperatively (e.g., the median cobalt level was significantly lower in the 36-mm hip replacement group than in the 28-mm hip replacement group). However, neither median cobalt levels nor median chromium levels were significantly different among the three MOM groups at 12 months. These findings reflect in vitro findings[32] where the most significant differences in wear were observed in the bedding-in period.

Langton and colleagues[35] considered a series of 76 consecutive patients after resurfacing arthroplasty and measured chromium and cobalt ion concentrations in whole blood. They found that patients with smaller (≤51 mm) femoral components had ion levels that were significantly higher than those with larger (≥53 mm) components at a mean of 26 months postoperatively. These findings contrast with those from the study by Antoniou and co-workers.[34] Langton and associates[35] also reported the effects of variations in cup positioning on ion levels. Cup position is important because it affects bedding-in wear and may possibly explain the differences between published studies.

The trend widely observed with MOM bearings where wear decreases with increasing diameter contrasts with that reported for conventional ultra-high-molecular-weight polyethylene (UHMWPE)-on-metal hip prostheses, where the wear of the UHMWPE acetabular cups was shown to be proportional to the sliding distance,[36] as predicted by basic engineering principles.[37] Therefore, reducing the femoral head diameter in polyethylene bearings should lead to a reduction in wear volume and extension of prosthesis life. Charnley demonstrated

the validity of this relationship and showed that the maximum wear life of hip replacements could be achieved by making the head diameter half the acetabular socket diameter.[38] The Charnley low-friction arthroplasty, appropriately regarded as the "gold standard" of hip replacement, falls within this range, with a standard femoral head diameter of 22.225 mm.

Clearance

The diametral clearance of an MOM bearing couple is defined as the diameter of the acetabular cup minus the diameter of the femoral head. A direct relationship between clearance and lubrication has been noted,[37] and because MOM bearings are lubrication sensitive, clearance would be expected to have a direct effect on wear. It has been reported for both 36-mm and 54-mm MOM bearings that bedding-in wear increases significantly as diametral clearance is increased.[37] For resurfacing components of 54- to 54.5-mm head diameter, couples with smaller diametral clearances (83 to 129 microns) exhibited running-in wear rates that were fourfold lower and steady-state wear rates that were twofold lower than components with larger clearances (254 to 307 microns).[37] However, there does appear to be an optimal band of clearance, which produces favorable wear rates under optimal conditions. Farrar and Schmidt[39] were the first to show reducing wear rates with reducing clearance down to approximately 80 microns with 28-mm MOM hip prostheses.

However, reduction of clearance to less than 30 microns causes wear to increase substantially. This was thought to be due to geometric errors, which are inevitable with any manufactured part. Whenever values of the diametral clearance become so small that they approach the magnitude of cumulative geometric errors, contacts may develop much closer to the equator, and the possibility of a local negative clearance exists. These authors found that it was possible to simulate the wear of equatorial bearing devices, such as those described for the pre-1970 McKee-Farrar and Ring prostheses, with modern MOM prostheses in a hip simulator by having negative or very low clearances. During testing, these devices with low clearances reached approximately 20,000 cycles and exhibited extremely high wear before seizing completely.

Other predictions that have been made suggest a third phase of wear in the life cycles of MOM bearings[40]; this is related to the endpoint and failure, as well as to low clearance bearings, where it is predicted that in the third phase, the large contact area (potentially up to 80% of the bearing surface area) could increase torque during motion and exceed implant fixation strength, leading to failure. However, these predictions have not been supported by experimental data.

Inclusion Angle

Hip replacements and, in particular, surface replacements vary in design in terms of the coverage they give (i.e., they are usually, and to varying extents, less than a full hemisphere), which is specified by the inclusion angle (or subtended acetabular component angle, alpha [Fig. 8-1]).[41] The inclusion angles of designs vary,

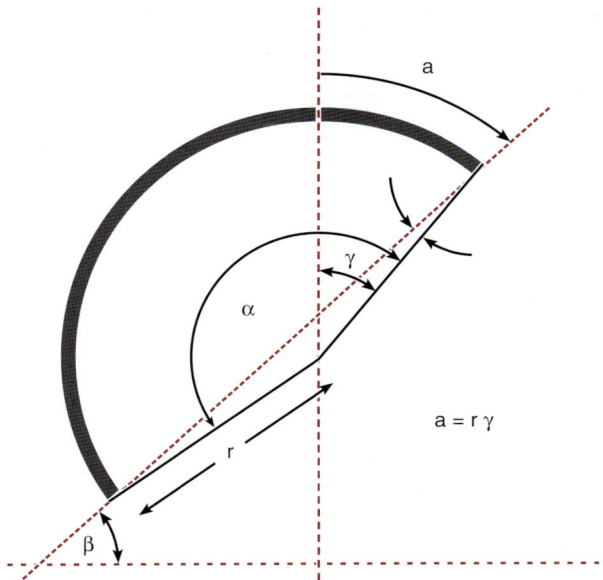

Figure 8-1. Diagram showing calculation of the arc of cover (a) using the equation a = r.α (with α measured on the radiograph). *(Redrawn from De Haan R, Pattyn C, Gill H, et al: Correlation between inclination of the acetabular component and metal ion levels in metal-on-metal hip resurfacing replacement. J Bone Joint Surg Br 90:1291–1297, 2008.)*

for example, Conserve (Wright Medical Technology, Memphis, Tenn), 170 degrees; BHR (Birmingham Hip Resurfacing, Smith and Nephew, Memphis, Tenn), 164 degrees. In terms of clinical performance, the parameter of greatest interest is the extent of coverage of the proximal pole of the femoral head by the lateral edge of the acetabular component (the angle gamma; see Fig. 8-1). This quantity is directly linked to the cup position in vivo (and inclination in particular) and indicates the risk of edge-loading. The circumferential portion of this cover in the frontal plane is termed the *arc of cover* (a) and can be calculated for each patient (assuming that the version of the acetabular component is neutral) as the product of the component radius (r) and the angle (in radians) subtended between the vertical and lateral acetabular component edges (γ). Additionally, as diameter decreases, it becomes more difficult to achieve adequate coverage (i.e., an arc of cover of 10 mm), and cup positioning becomes even more critical. However, lower-profile cups are less likely to suffer from head-neck impingement.

De Haan and associates[41] examined the relationships between serum levels of chromium and cobalt ions and the inclination angle of the acetabular component and the arc of cover. Arcs of cover of less than 10 mm (a combination of cup size and designs with differing inclusion angles) were correlated with a greater risk of high concentrations of serum metal ions. The arc of coverage was also related to the design of the component and to size, as well as to the abduction angle of the acetabular component. Steeply inclined acetabular components with abduction angles greater than 55 degrees, combined with a small component, are likely to give rise to higher serum levels of cobalt and chromium ions. This is probably due to greater risk of edge-loading.

Effects of Patient Activity

The wear rate of polyethylene has long been associated with the amount of use,[42] and because MOM components have been increasingly used in younger and more active patients, the relationship between use and wear of these prostheses must be understood. Several studies, starting with the work of Heisel and colleagues[43] published in 2005, have examined the impact of patient activity on ion levels within the body. In this study, eight subjects were followed: seven patients with well-functioning metal-on-metal bearing hip prostheses and one control subject with no implants. All had normal renal function, and serum levels of cobalt and chromium ions were monitored for 2 weeks, as was activity. During the first week, subjects were requested to limit physical activity; they then completed an hour-long treadmill test, followed by a week during which they were encouraged to be as physically active as practically possible.

Regardless of activity (patients were on average 28% more active the second week), serum ion levels for a given patient were essentially constant, and no correlation was found between patient activity and serum levels of cobalt and chromium. The treadmill test provided an average increase in activity of 1621% and was associated with increases of only 3.0% in the average level of serum cobalt and 0.8% in serum chromium. All results fell within the variability for measurement accuracy, and it was concluded that serum cobalt and chromium ion levels were not acutely affected by patient activity. De Haan and colleagues[41] also observed no correlation between level of activity and serum levels of chromium and cobalt ions in 214 patients implanted with a metal-on-metal resurfacing hip replacement at least 1 year after surgery.

When in vivo and in vitro volumetric wear rates are compared, much variation is seen (Table 8-2). It is important to note that in most hip simulator studies, only one walking waveform is repeatedly applied, and load and motion regimes that better represent patterns of daily living, such as intermittent motion,[44] jogging,[12] and variations in load,[26] are likely to lead to increased wear rates. The ideal hip simulator would provide a mix of these.

In hip simulator studies, increasing the joint load during the swing phase has increased wear and friction of MOM hip replacements.[26,45] Average values for the overall wear rate increased approximately 10-fold (0.06 mm³/million cycles to 0.58 mm³/million cycles), and this was stated to be due to depletion of lubricating film during the stance phase—a theory that was supported by later computational predictions.[46] This effect is also consistent with the findings of Roter and co-workers,[42] who observed an increase in the wear of metal bearings under a stop-start testing regime in hip simulator experiments. During these tests, the hip simulator was restarted after each dwell period at the maximum load (3400 N). This intermittent motion

Table 8-2. Comparison of Mean Volumetric Wear Rates From In Vitro Simulator and Ex Vivo Retrieval Studies

Author	Sample	Wear Rate (mm³/yr)*
Bowsher et al, 2002[12]	MTS simulator, normal walking (as cast CoCr)	Overall, 0.41
	Fast jogging (as cast CoCr)	Overall, 3.95
Roter et al, 2002[42]	MATCO simulator Continuous motion	Overall, 0.14
	Intermittent motion (peak load at restart)	Overall, 0.20
Clarke et al, 2000[45]	Stop-start motion every 300 cycles (low load at restart)	Bedding-in, 2.68 Steady-state, 0.98
	Standard conditions (ISO load)	Bedding-in, 2.03 Steady-state, 0.22
Williams et al, 2004[27]	Load swing phase load	Bedding-in, 0.13 Steady-state, 0.05
	Microseparation	Bedding-in, 2.70 Steady-state, 1.30
Sieber et al, 1999[15]	In vivo, study of 118 explanted metal-on-metal prostheses	Steady-state, 0.31
Morlock et al, 2008[5]	Ex vivo study of 12 resurfacing prostheses	Overall, 1.1

*1 million cycles has historically been assumed to equate to 1 year of in vivo activity; however, a recent investigation found activity levels ranging from 1.01 to 3.21 million cycles per year.[29]

ISO, International Organization for Standardization.

caused a breakdown in the protective lubricant film, resulting in higher wear results. Higher wear rates have also been observed in simple geometry pin-on-plate testing,[8] which was conducted under constant load with increased contact stresses. This increase in wear rate was also attributed to poor lubricant film protection of the surfaces, because the pin was statically loaded.

It has been observed that the femoral head of hip prostheses can migrate laterally and superiorly from the cup center (0.5 to 2 mm) during normal walking.[47] This phenomenon, termed *joint separation*, has been linked to tension in the ligaments and soft tissues following joint replacement surgery and led to the development of microseparation studies in hip simulators. Head separation has also been observed during swing phase and has led to stripe wear in simulator tests of ceramic-on-ceramic bearings, which mimic the observations of clinical retrievals.[48] When MOM hip replacements were tested under microseparation conditions, wear increased because of high stresses generated when the head contacted the insert rim at heel strike. This caused a wear stripe on the femoral head and corresponding insert rim damage. Reports of such wear patterns observed on retrieved metal-on-metal explants are limited. However, it is postulated that this may be due to a self-polishing mechanism between metal components in gait (i.e., in vivo microseparation does not occur with every step, as it does in the hip simulator), and this may mask the stripe wear in vivo, unlike ceramics, where microseparation causes grain fracture and pull-out in the region that is subjected to these high stresses.[45]

Bowsher and associates[12] reported an increase in wear rate when moving from a walking to a jogging gait cycle in vitro. MOM hip bearings 40 mm in diameter were subjected to normal walking and fast jogging simulations in an orbital hip joint simulator. Fast jogging simulations generated a sevenfold increase in volumetric wear, a 33% increase in mean wear particle size, and a threefold increase in the number of larger (needle) particles compared with walking simulations. This resulted in a 20-fold increase in total surface area of wear particles per million cycles of fast jogging compared with walking.

These reports demonstrate the importance of testing MOM bearings under appropriate conditions in vivo.

Effects of Component Positioning

Acetabular components of hip arthroplasties implanted with more than 50 degrees of inclination in the frontal plane have been shown to increase wear in metal-on-polyethylene bearings.[49,50] Manufacturers of ceramic-on-ceramic bearings recommend that the cup should be positioned in less than 50 degrees of abduction to avoid the risk of fracture.[51] Metal-on-metal articulations have been implanted in increasing numbers during the past decade, and mounting information is being gathered about the effects of positioning the cup in various inclination angles.

Retrieval studies on current designs of MOM surface replacements have shown a large (40-fold) variation in wear rate.[5,52] A study by Morlock and colleagues[5] included 267 components from hip resurfacings retrieved worldwide. Devices were analyzed in terms of patient demographics, radiographic positioning, and wear. Specimens were grouped into four different failure types: (1) fractures involving the implant rim, (2) fractures inside the femoral head, (3) cup loosening, and (4) failures not due to fracture or loosening. Retrievals were also grouped into rim-loaded and non–rim-loaded groups, and failures were assessed in terms of the effect of the surgeon learning curve. Time to failure was significantly different between the four revision-type groups: specimens with fractures involving the implant rim were most common (46%) and failed earliest after surgery (mean, 99 days), followed by fractures inside the femoral head (20%, 262 days) and loose cups (9%, 423 days). Revisions not due to fracture or cup loosening (25%) occurred at a mean of 722 days after surgery. Rim-loaded implants exhibited an average 21- to 27-fold higher wear rate than implants without rim loading. Rim-loaded implants also showed a steeper mean cup inclination than their non–rim-loaded counterparts (59 degrees compared with 50 degrees). Most failures occurred during the learning curve of the surgeon (the first 50 to 100 implantations). Morlock and co-workers[5] concluded that failure on the femoral side usually occurred within the first 9 months after surgery and appeared to be most directly related to the implantation technique or to patient selection. Most failures that occurred later involved the acetabular component, with a dramatic increase in component wear or poor cup anchorage. Improper cup anteversion may be similar to or more important than cup inclination in producing excessive wear.

A correlation between inclination angle and patient ion levels has been demonstrated in a series of studies. De Haan and colleagues[41] examined the relationships between serum levels of chromium and cobalt ions and the inclination angle of the acetabular component and the level of activity in 214 patients implanted with MOM resurfacing prostheses at least 1 year after surgery. The inclination of the acetabular component was considered to be steep if the abduction angle was greater than 55 degrees. Significantly higher levels of metal ions were noted in patients with steeply inclined components; these increased even further in cases performed with an acetabular component of a lower inclusion angle.

Brodner and co-workers[53] investigated the relationship between cup inclination and serum levels of cobalt and chromium after MOM total hip arthroplasty. Sixty patients in a consecutive series were divided into three groups of equal size, according to their cup inclination angle: greatest inclination (55 to 63 degrees; mean, 58 degrees), intermediate inclination (44 to 46 degrees; mean, 45 degrees), and smallest inclination (23 to 37 degrees; mean, 33 degrees). No significant differences in serum cobalt or chromium levels were observed between the three groups. However, three patients with cup inclinations of 58, 63, and 61 degrees exhibited 9.8- to 53.6-fold elevated cobalt and 9.5- to 30.5-fold elevated chromium levels when compared with median concentrations in this study. It was recommended that accurate cup placement was vital for MOM articulations.

It should be noted that in these studies, some bearings implanted with a moderate cup inclination angle (35 to 45 degrees) have shown high wear, and not all bearings implanted with a high cup angle have had high wear rates, suggesting that other factors such as head position, joint laxity (both may cause a microseparation-type action between the head and the cup), impingement, or version angle may also influence wear.

In vitro hip simulator tests have replicated the elevated wear rates observed with increased cup angles clinically. In a hip simulator study, Leslie and colleagues[54] tested 39-mm metal-on-metal surface replacements with combinations of increased cup inclination angle and microseparation. Increasing cup inclination to 60 degrees resulted in a ninefold increase in wear rate; the combination of increased cup inclination angle and microseparation resulted in a 17-fold increase in wear rate compared with a study using standard gait (i.e., without microseparation) and a cup inclination of 45 degrees.

CURRENT CONTROVERSIES AND FUTURE DIRECTIONS

Current Controversies

Effects of Elevated Wear

Reports of cases of adverse soft tissue reactions to MOM hip resurfacings have come to the fore. One of the first reports[55] details a group of 20 resurfaced hips (17 patients; all female mean, 17 months postoperatively; range, 0 to 60 months) with a mass associated with various symptoms (most commonly, discomfort in the hip region and, on occasion, spontaneous dislocation, nerve palsy, and rash). All patients had a mass (stated as neither malignant nor infective in nature), which the authors called a *pseudotumor*. At the time the paper was published, 13 of 20 hips had required revision to a conventional hip replacement. Histology was undertaken, and a common feature was extensive necrosis and lymphocytic infiltration. The authors estimated that approximately 1% of patients who have a metal-on-metal resurfacing develop a pseudotumor within 5 years and concluded that the cause is unknown and probably multifactorial. A toxic reaction to an excess of particulate metal wear debris or a hypersensitivity reaction to a normal amount of metal debris may be noted. Case reports of non-MOM hip replacements have cited swelling granulomatous lesions, cysts, and related masses (similar to what has been described recently as pseudotumor).[56-58]

However, growing evidence[59,60] suggests that small diameter MOM hip resurfacings may cause adverse soft tissue reactions, particularly in certain subgroups of patients. Further analysis has focused on the incidence and cause of soft tissue reactions or pseudotumors following MOM resurfacing. Asymptomatic patients with a minimum 2-year follow-up were recruited (with BHR, Cormet, Conserve Plus, and Recap Hip Resurfacing systems), and pseudotumors were detected using ultrasound; these were confirmed by magnetic resonance imaging (MRI). It was concluded that reported pseudotumors were almost exclusively confined to females (ratio of 5 female to 1 male) and smaller cup sizes. Soft tissue reactions appeared to be related to abnormal wear caused by component malpositioning, because pseudotumors were not reported in patients with "normal" ion levels. The overall incidence of pseudotumor in the series of 16 revisions was as follows: males, 0.5%; females over 40 years, 6%; and females younger than 40 years, 25%. The authors recommended using

MOM resurfacings in females with caution and avoiding their use in females younger than 40 years. Data reported in the Australian Orthopaedic Association National Joint Replacement Registry[1] also demonstrate clearly that revision rates for hip resurfacings are significantly higher for female patients and for femoral components smaller than 49 mm in diameter.

It is important to note that these soft tissue reactions have not been reported frequently, at least as yet, in modular MOM bearings. It has been postulated that this is so because modular MOM THRs have greater bearing coverage, in that conventional acetabular cups used in the THR have inclusion angles of approximately 180 degrees versus 164–170 degrees for hip resurfacing components. In comparison with hip resurfacing, MOM THRs offer more options for better fixation, better visibility when positioning implants, and increased ease of implantation, which is expected to lead to a lower incidence of cup malpositioning.

Future Directions

Increasing concerns about MOM bearings and the in vivo effects of cobalt and chromium ions have led to investigation of alternative hard-on-hard bearings.

Ceramic-on-Metal Hip Replacements

A novel combination of a ceramic head articulating against a metal acetabular liner (COM) was first reported in 2001.[61] This showed significant reduction in terms of metal wear when COM bearings were compared with MOM bearings in a hip simulator. More recent data[62] additionally show reduced wear and friction under adverse conditions in hip simulator testing. Lower wear has been attributed to a reduction in corrosive wear, smoother surfaces, improved lubrication, and differential hardness, reducing adhesive wear.[62,63] A randomized prospective clinical trial has also been reported, comparing COM, MOM, ceramic-on-polyethylene, and ceramic-on-ceramic bearings in an otherwise identical THR procedure[64]; whole blood metal ion levels were measured. Among COM components, median increases in chromium and cobalt levels at 12 months were 0.08 µg/L and 0.22 µg/L, respectively. Comparable values for MOM bearings were 0.48 µg/L and 0.32 µg/L. Chromium levels were significantly lower in COM than in MOM bearings. Cobalt levels were lower, but the difference was not significant. The COM bearing is now available for clinical use.

Aspheric Bearings

The use of aspheric bearings has been proposed.[65] Such bearings have variable clearance, with conforming geometry in the contact zone and large clearances at the equator of the bearing. Hip simulator testing demonstrated bearings of this design to have greater than 80% reduction in wear compared with clinically available MOM bearings.

Surface Coatings

Surface-engineered coatings were investigated by Fisher and associates[66,67] in an effort to examine their potential in reducing the volume of wear, the concentration of metal debris, and the levels of cobalt, chromium, and molybdenum ions released. Thick (8 to 12 microns) surface-engineered coatings, chromium nitride (CrN), and chromium carbonitride (CrCN) were deposited by arc evaporative physical vapor deposition (AEPVD) on cobalt-chrome-molybdenum heads and cups and tested in a hip simulator. Overall wear of CrN-on-CrN and CrCN-on-CrCN bearing couples was at least 22-fold lower than metal-on-metal. Additionally, the cytotoxicity of CrN and CrCN wear particles was assessed by coculture with macrophages; CrN wear particles were found to be less toxic than clinically relevant CoCr wear particles. These initial findings support further development and additional clinical trials of surface-engineered metal-on-metal bearings. In particular, surface-engineered coatings may offer an alternative to metal-on-metal surface replacement designs, because of reduced wear and ion release compared with metal-on-metal, and enhanced design flexibility compared with ceramics.

REFERENCES

1. Australian Orthopaedic Association National Joint Replacement Registry, Annual Report, 2009.
2. National Joint Registry for England and Wales, 5th Annual Report, 2008.
3. St John KR, Zardiackas LD, Poggie RA: Wear evaluation of cobalt-chromium alloy for use in a metal-on-metal hip prosthesis. J Biomed Mater Res B 68:1–14, 2004.
4. Streicher R, Semlitsch M, Schon R, et al: Metal on metal articulation for artificial joints: laboratory study and clinical results. Proceedings of the Institution of Mechanical Engineers, 210, part H, 223, 1996.
5. Morlock MM, Bishop N, Zustin J, et al: Modes of implant failure after hip resurfacing: morphological and wear analysis of 267 retrieval specimens. J Bone Joint Surg Am 90(Suppl 3):89–95, 2008.
6. Campbell P, Beaule PE, Ebramzadeh E, et al: The John Charnley Award. A study of implant failure in metal-on-metal surface arthroplasties. Clin Orthop Relat Res 453:35–46, 2006.
7. Wimmer M, Loos J, Nassutt R, et al: The acting wear mechanisms on metal-on-metal hip joint bearings: in vitro results. Wear 250:129–139, 2001.
8. Tipper JL, Firkins PJ, Ingham E, et al: Quantitative analysis of wear and wear debris for high and low carbon content cobalt chrome alloys used in metal on metal hip replacements. J Mater Sci Mater Med 10:353–362, 1999.
9. Firkins PJ, Tipper JL, Saadatzadeh MR, et al: Quantitative analysis of wear and wear debris from metal-on-metal hip prostheses tested in a physiological hip joint simulator. Biomed Mater Eng 11:143–157, 2001.
10. Farrar R, Schmidt M, Hamilton J, Greer K: The development of low wear articulations. In Stein H (ed): Sivot 97 Haifa Intermeeting, Scientific Proceedings, 1999.
11. Dowson D, Hardaker C, Flett M, Isaac GH: A hip joint simulator study of the performance of metal-on-metal joints. Part I. The role of materials. J Arthroplasty 19:118–123, 2004.
12. Bowsher JG, Nevelos J, Williams PA, Shelton JC: "Severe" wear challenge to "as-cast" and "double heat-treated" large-diameter metal-on-metal hip bearings, Proceedings of the Institution of Mechanical Engineers, part H. J Eng Med 220:135–143, 2006.
13. Wimmer M, Sprecher C, Hauert R, et al: Tribochemical reaction on metal-on-metal hip joint bearings: a comparison between in vitro and in vivo results. Wear 255:1007–1014, 2003.
14. Pourzal R, Theissmann R, Williams S, et al: Subsurface changes of a MoM hip implant below different contact zones. J Mech Behav Biomed Mater 2:186, 2009.
15. Sieber H, Reiker C, Kottig P: Analysis of 118 second-generation metal-on-metal retrieved hip implants. J Bone Joint Surg Br 81:46, 1999.

16. McKellop H, Park S, Chiesa R, et al: In vivo wear of 3 types of metal on metal hip prostheses during two decades of use. Clin Orthop Relat Res 329:S128, 1996.

17. Jin ZM, Dowson D, Fisher J: Analysis of fluid film lubrication in artificial hip joint replacements with surfaces of high elastic modulus. Proc Inst Mech Eng H 211:247–256, 1997.

18. Yan Y, Neville A, Dowson D: Biotribocorrosion—an appraisal of the time dependence of wear and corrosion interactions. Part 1. The role of corrosion. J Phys D Appl Phys 39:3200–3205, 2006.

19. Yan Y, Neville A, Dowson D: Biotribocorrosion—an appraisal of the time dependence of wear and corrosion interactions. Part 2. Surface analysis. J Phys D Appl Phys 39:3206–3211, 2006.

20. Yan Y, Neville A, Dowson D: Understanding the role of corrosion in the degradation of metal-on-metal implants. Proc IMechE, Part H. J Eng Med 220:173–180, 2006.

21. Yan Y, Neville A, Dowson D, Williams S: Tribocorrosion in implants: assessing high carbon and low carbon Co-Cr-Mo alloys by in-situ electrochemical measurements. Tribol Int 39:1509–1517, 2006.

22. Yan Y, Neville A, Dowson D: Tribo-corrosion properties of cobalt-based medical implant alloys in simulated biological environments. Wear 263:1105–1111, 2007.

23. Yan Y, Neville A, Dowson D: Biotribocorrosion of CoCrMo orthopaedic implant materials: assessing the formation and effect of the biofilm. Tribol Int 40:1492–1497, 2007.

24. Amstutz HC, Grigoris P: Metal on metal bearings in hip arthroplasty. Clin Orthop Relat Res 329:11–34, 1996.

25. Ebied A, Journeaux S: Metal-on-metal hip resurfacing. Curr Orthop 16:420–425, 2002.

26. Williams S, Stewart T, Ingham Stone M, Fisher J: Metal-on-metal bearing wear with different swing phase loads. J Biomed Mater Res B Appl Biomater 70:233–239, 2004.

27. Anissian HL, Stark A, Good V, et al: The wear pattern in metal-on-metal hip prostheses. J Biomed Mater Res 58:673–678, 2001.

28. Heisel C, Streich N, Krachler M, et al: Characterization of the running-in period in total hip resurfacing arthroplasty: an in vivo and in vitro metal ion analysis. J Bone Joint Surg Am 90(Suppl 3):125–133, 2008.

29. Kelley SS, Lachiewicz PF, Hickman JM, Paterno SM: Relationship of femoral head and acetabular size to the prevalence of dislocation. Clin Orthop Relat Res 355:163–170, 1998.

30. Smith SL, Dowson D, Goldsmith AAJ: The effect of femoral head diameter upon lubrication and wear of metal-on-metal total hip replacements. Proc Inst Mech Engr H 215:161–170, 2001.

31. Dowson D, Hardaker C, Flett M, Isaac GH: A hip joint simulator study of the performance of metal-on-metal joints. Part II. Design. J Arthroplasty 19:124–130, 2004.

32. Leslie I, Williams S, Brown C, et al: Effect of bearing size on the long-term wear, wear debris, and ion levels of large diameter metal-on-metal hip replacements: an in vitro study. J Biomed Mater Res B Appl Biomater 87:163–172, 2008.

33. Hu XQ, Isaac GH, Fisher J: Changes in the contact area during the bedding-in wear of different sizes of metal on metal hip prostheses. Biomed Mater Eng 14:145–149, 2004.

34. Antoniou J, Zukor D, Mwale F, et al: Metal ion levels in the blood of patients after hip resurfacing: a comparison between twenty-eight and thirty-six-millimeter-head. J Bone Joint Surg Am 90:142–148, 2008.

35. Langton DJ, Jameson SS, Joyce TJ, et al: The effect of component size and orientation on the concentrations of metal ions after resurfacing arthroplasty of the hip. J Bone Joint Surg Br 90:1143–1151, 2008.

36. Livermore J, Ilstrup D, Morrey B: Effect of femoral head size on wear of the polyethylene acetabular component. J Bone Joint Surg Am 72:518–528, 1990.

37. Fisher J, Dowson D: Tribology of total artificial joints. Proceedings of the Institution of Mechanical Engineers, part H. J Eng Med 205:73–79, 1991.

38. Charnley J, Kamanger A, Longfield M: The optimum size of prosthetic heads in relation to the wear of plastic sockets in total replacement of the hip. Med Biol Eng 7:31–38, 1969.

39. Farrar R, Schmidt MB: The effect of diametral clearance on wear between head and cup for metal on metal articulations. Trans 43rd Orthop Res Soc 71, 1997.

40. Tuke M, Scott G, Roques A, et al: Design considerations and life prediction of metal-on-metal bearings: the effect of clearance. J Bone Joint Surg Am 90(Suppl 3):134–141, 2008.

41. De Haan R, Pattyn C, Gill H, et al: Correlation between inclination of the acetabular component and metal ion levels in metal-on-metal hip resurfacing replacement. J Bone Joint Surg Br 90:1291–1297, 2008.

42. Schmalzried TP, Shepherd EF, Dorey FJ, et al: The John Charnley Award. Wear is a function of use, not time. Clin Orthop Relat Res 381:36–46, 2000.

43. Heisel C, Silva M, Skipor A, et al: The relationship between activity and ions in patients with metal-on-metal bearing hip prostheses. J Bone Joint Surg Am 87:781–787, 2005.

44. Roter G, Medley J, Cheng N, et al: Intermittent motion: a clinically significant protocol for metal-metal hip simulator testing. Trans 48th Annual Meeting Orthop Res Soc 100, 2000.

45. Clarke I, Good V, Williams P, et al: Ultra-low wear rates for rigid-on-rigid bearings in total hip replacements. Proceedings of the Institution of Mechanical Engineers, part H, 331, 2000.

46. Williams S, Jalali-Vahid D, Brockett C, et al: Effect of swing phase load on metal-on-metal hip lubrication, friction and wear. J Biomech 39:2274–2281 2006.

47. Lombardi AV, Mallory TH, Dennis DA, et al: An in-vivo determination of total hip arthroplasty pistoning during activity. J Arthroplasty 15:702–709, 2000.

48. Nevelos J, Ingham E, Doyle C, et al: Microseparation of the centers of alumina-alumina artificial hip joints during simulator testing produces clinically relevant wear and patterns. J Arthroplasty 15:793–795, 2000.

49. Schmalzried TP, Guttmann D, Grecula M, Amstutz H: The relationship between the design, position, and articular wear of acetabular components inserted without cement and the development of pelvic osteolysis. J Bone Joint Surg Am 76:677, 1994.

50. Kennedy JG, Rogers WB, Soffe KE, et al: Effect of acetabular component orientation on recurrent dislocation, pelvic osteolysis, polyethylene wear, and component migration. J Arthroplasty 13:530, 1998.

51. Willmann G: The evolution of ceramics in total hip replacement. Hip Int 10:193, 2000.

52. Campbell P, Beaule PE, Ebramzadeh E, et al: The John Charnley Award. A study of implant failure in metal-on-metal surface arthroplasties. Clin Orthop Relat Res 453:35–46, 2006.

53. Brodner W, Grubl A, Jankovsky A, et al: Cup inclination and serum concentration of cobalt and chromium after metal-on-metal total hip arthroplasty. J Arthroplasty 19(Suppl 3):66–70, 2004.

54. Leslie IJ, Williams S, Isaac CH, et al: High cup angle and microseparation increase the wear of hip surface replacements. Clin Orthop Relat Res 467:2259–2265, 2009.

55. Pandit H, Glyn-Jones S, McLardy-Smith P, et al: Pseudotumours associated with metal-on-metal hip resurfacings. J Bone Joint Surg Br 90:847–851, 2008.

56. Wang JW, Lim CC: Pelvic mass caused by polyethylene wear after uncemented hip arthroplasty. J Arthroplasty 14:771, 1999.

57. Korkala O, Syrajanen KJ: Intrapelvic cyst formation after hip arthroplasty with a carbon fibre reinforced polyethylene socket. Arch Orthop Trauma Surg 118:113–115, 1998.

58. Howie DW, Cain CM, Cornish EL: Pesudo-abscess of the psoas bursa in a failed double cup arthroplasty of the hip. J Bone Joint Surg Br 73:29–32, 1991.

59. Kwon YM, Ostlere S, McLardy-Smith P, et al: Metal ion levels in asymptomatic pseudo-tumours associated with metal-on-metal hip resurfacing, vol 34, Oxford, United Kingdom, 2009, ORS.

60. Kwon YM, Ostlere S, Thomas P, et al: Lymphocyte proliferation responses in patients with pseudo-tumours following metal-on-metal hip resurfacing, vol 34, Oxford, United Kingdom, 2009, ORS.

61. Firkins PJ, Tipper JL, Ingham E, et al: A novel low wearing differential hardness, ceramic-on-metal hip joint prostheses. J Biomech 34:1291–1298, 2001.

62. Williams S, Schepers A, Isaac G, et al: Aufranc Award. Ceramic-on-metal hip replacements: a comparative in vitro and in vivo study. Clin Orthop Relat Res 465:23–32, 2007.

63. Figueiredo-Pina CG, Yan Y, Neville A, Fisher J: Understanding the differences between the wear of metal-on-metal and ceramic-on-metal total hip replacements. Proc Inst Mech Eng H 222:285–296, 2008.

64. Isaac GH, Brockett CL, Breckon A, et al: Ceramic-on-metal bearings in total hip replacement: whole blood metal ion levels and analysis of retrieved components. J Bone Joint Surg Br 91:1134–1141, 2009.

65. Ernsberger C, Frazee E: Low ion release aspheric metal on metal hip design. Trans 54th Annual Meeting of the Orthopaedic Research Society, San Francisco, 2008, p 1788.

66. Fisher J, Hu X, Williams S, et al: New bearing surfaces: what does the future hold? Semin Arthroplasty 14:131, 2003.

67. Fisher J, Hu X, Stewart T, et al: Wear of surface engineered metal on metal hip prostheses. J Mater Sci Mater Med 15:225, 2004.

CHAPTER 9

Materials in Hip Surgery: Porous Metals for Implant Fixation

Robert M. Pilliar

- *Rationale for cementless hip implants:* The goal of developing cementless hip implant components has been to achieve "biological fixation" by bone ingrowth (into porous surface structures) or ongrowth (into irregular surface features) as a preferred alternative to using acrylic bone cement for implant fixation (especially for younger, physically active patients).
- *Necessary requirements for success with cementless implants include the following:*
  - For implants intended for bone ingrowth, formation of interconnected pore networks with pore size sufficient to allow bone ingrowth (i.e., pore openings preferably greater than 100 microns)
  - For implants intended for bone ongrowth, surface features of suitable size and quantity to allow secure biological fixation, resulting in interface strength sufficient to prevent breakdown during normal activities
  - For both ongrowth and ingrowth designs, limited relative movement of implant and host bone during the healing period to allow rapid formation of new bone and development of secure fixation in as short a time as possible
  - The use of biocompatible and corrosion-resistant material for surface coatings and underlying substrates
  - Adequate strength of the surface coating and the coating-substrate interface
  - Overall implant strength following processing (fatigue strength, in particular)
  - Minimal stress shielding through appropriate implant design

INTRODUCTION

Porous metals serve two major uses in musculoskeletal reconstruction surgery, namely, constructs for replacing or augmenting bone, and implant surface coatings to allow implant fixation by bone ingrowth. Open-pored structures are used when needed for bone augmentation, an example being reconstruction of the acetabulum to allow acetabular cup placement. Such implants typically are highly porous with volume percent porosity in the 60% to 85% range, and have large pore openings to promote vascularity and bone ingrowth throughout. These scaffold-like structures can be formed in a variety of shapes and sizes. They may or may not serve a significant load-bearing role and typically are intended to substitute for or replace cancellous bone. Structures made of porous tantalum (Ta) or titanium (Ti) are available and are used clinically for this purpose, as are other nonmetallic implants (ceramic and polymeric). Their major role is to replace or augment bone rather than achieve fixation per se as a result of bone ingrowth, although this invariably happens. This article does not deal to any great extent with this class of porous implants, but rather with those designed to achieve secure fixation of joint replacements, hip replacements specifically, without the use of acrylic bone cement (i.e., so-called *cementless implants*). Other earlier reviews of this subject are recommended to the reader.[1-3]

The development of cementless designs for hip implants in the 1970s, formed with a porous coating with three-dimensional interconnected porosity through which new bone could form (referred to herein as bone *ingrowth*), or with an irregular surface with protrusions and recesses that allowed implant fixation by *bone ongrowth* and mechanical anchorage, was an indirect result of success in the 1960s with cemented low-friction arthroplasties.[4] Bone cement as a medium for hip implant fixation was designed initially for treatment of the very elderly and of less physically active individuals suffering from debilitating joint degeneration (hip primarily) in that era. Early success of the procedure with this patient population resulted in its application to younger patients. Its use in younger, physically more active individuals tested the limits of bone cement for secure, long-term implant fixation. With consequent longer periods of use and more aggressive functional loading, the implant-supporting cement broke down more frequently as a result of microcracks, resulting in implant loosening in many cases. As a result, an unacceptably high number of failed implants requiring revision surgery were reported in the 1970s. This resulted in the search for and subsequent use of alternative methods for implant fixation and the development of strategies for forming cementless implants (initially hip replacements) that could be fixed in situ by bone *ingrowth* or bone *ongrowth*.

Early studies explored the use of fully porous metallic[5] and ceramic systems[6]; however, the need for implant fatigue strength (for highly loaded devices such as femoral stem components) led to the development of dual-structured designs. These consisted of a strong (fully dense) metal core, which provided the required fracture and fatigue resistance, and surface zones suitable for achieving reliable fixation by mechanical interlock of newly formed bone and implant through bone *ingrowth* (with porous-coated implants) or *ongrowth* (with plasma-sprayed implants) (so-called *biological fixation*). Porous polymers (polyethylene,[7] polysulfone[8]), ceramics (alumina,[9] calcium aluminate[6]), and composites (carbon-reinforced Teflon[10]) were also investigated. However, the need for the porous layer to be sufficiently stiff to resist excessive distortion on loading and yet strong enough not to fracture or de-bond from the substrate upon repeated loading over many millions of loading cycles led to metals as the preferred choice for surface preparation of hip implant components. These were formed using CoCrMo alloy, Ti, or Ti alloy.[11-13] These metals continue to be used for currently available porous-coated or plasma-sprayed hip implant components. Tantalum scaffold-like acetabular components (described later) have become available recently.[14] Although stainless steel was considered initially for use in forming porous structures,[15] its use in such implant designs was not pursued because of the greater susceptibility of that alloy to crevice corrosion compared with the other metals noted previously. Porous-coated implants with surface coatings made by sintering metal powders (CoCrMo and cp Ti primarily), diffusion bonding Ti wires (or fibers), and plasma-spraying Ti layers became available for clinical use in the 1980s; these surface designs continue to the present for cementless implant components. Currently, these cementless designs represent the preferred choice of many surgeons for use in younger patients.

In vivo animal studies throughout the 1970s and 1980s identified certain necessary conditions for successful design and use of cementless implants. In addition to being biocompatible, these included the following requirements to ensure adequate and timely bone ingrowth or ongrowth:

1. Need for initial implant stability to avoid significant movement of the implant relative to surrounding bone following placement (a snug press-fit was recommended, or in situations in which this is not sufficient, use of ancillary anchorage devices such as screws provides initial stability).
2. Provision of suitable pore openings or surface recesses to allow uninhibited bone ingrowth or ongrowth to an extent sufficient to ensure rigid fixation during functional loading for the patient's lifetime.
3. Adequate local vascularity and the ability of the patient to form new bone.
4. An infection-free site during and after bone formation.

In addition, to ensure long-term reliability of these load-bearing implants, the following engineering design requirements were recommended:

1. Sufficient coating strength to avoid its fracture.
2. A strong coating-to-substrate interfacial strength to prevent coating debonding from the substrate.

3. Coatings that would not corrode at unacceptable rates that could result in release of toxic degradation products and/or weakening of the coating structures.
4. Adequate fatigue and fracture strength of the substrate metal following processing to form the surface coating.

It is also desirable to have the implant stiffness similar to that of adjacent host bone to avoid undesirable bone loss due to stiffness mismatch of implant and bone. Such mechanical mismatch can lead to zones of very high stress in regions of surrounding bone (e.g., at the distal tip region of a femoral stem), increasing susceptibility of bone to fracture, and zones of very low stress in other regions, causing bone loss over time due to disuse atrophy (stress shielding), also resulting in bone that is more fracture prone. A clinical follow-up study using a novel lower modulus composite stem (wrought CoCrMo core surrounded by a polymer, polyaryletherketone, and a Ti surface mesh to allow bone ingrowth—Epoch stem) placed in patients for periods out to 7 years has been reported, indicating significant reduction in bone loss compared with conventional metallic-stemmed implants (CoCrMo or Ti based), at least for the period studied.[16] The need for longer-term studies was noted by investigators. A concern associated with using lower-stiffness stems, particularly in younger, active patients in whom long-term active loading is expected, is the fatigue resistance of such designs.

IMPLANT SURFACE DESIGN FOR CEMENTLESS FIXATION

Hip implant components currently used for cementless fixation are predominantly made with either:

1. Plasma spray-deposited irregular surface layers that allow mechanical interlock of bone and implant through bone *ongrowth* (grit-blasted surfaces offer another means of achieving this), or
2. Sintered coatings to form porous structures allowing three-dimensional bone *usually involving* multilayered arrangements of particles or fibers, although single-layer particle designs have also been reported.[17]

Following successful bone ongrowth, implant-bone interfaces formed by plasma-sprayed layers (similar to grit-blasted surfaces) can resist shear forces as a result of the physical interlock of bone with surface features. However, these surfaces do not provide resistance against interfacial tensile forces. This contrasts with porous surface coatings with three-dimensional pore networks that do provide significant resistance to interface shear and tensile forces following bone ingrowth. A number of articles in the past have described as "porous" plasma spray-deposited layers nominally formed with no intended internal porosity, but such a description is misleading. For femoral stem components, which primarily are exposed to interfacial shear forces, this difference may not be clinically significant—a fact that attests to the successful and wide use of plasma spray-coated femoral stem components. However, for acetabular components, in which more complex force components may act and in which interfacial tensile stresses can develop, implants designed for bone ingrowth are preferred because they are expected to provide better long-term stability in this location compared with ongrowth designs.

As discussed later, results of in vivo animal studies have indicated a significant difference between plasma-sprayed and porous-coated surfaces (i.e., irregular surfaces vs. three-dimensional interconnected porous structures) with regard to rate of osseointegration resulting in development of secure fixation.[18-20] This study is briefly summarized later and represents one of the few investigations that have focused on very early healing phenomena (i.e., within days) for bone-interfacing implants with specific focus on the effect of implant surface design on rate of osseointegration.

FACTORS INFLUENCING BONE INGROWTH/ONGROWTH

The development of as rapid as possible bone ingrowth or ongrowth to achieve secure implant fixation represents a primary goal in the design and use of cementless implants, because this increases the likelihood that successful biological fixation will occur. A number of factors have been shown to influence the rate of bone formation and development of implant fixation. These include relative micromovement of implant and bone during early healing, vascularity at the implant site, implant surface geometry, pore size and possibly shape for porous-coated implants, closeness of fit of implant relative to bone, and the effects of mechanical stimulation on bone formation.

SURFACE DESIGN—*INGROWTH* VERSUS *ONGROWTH:* THE EFFECTS OF LOCAL TISSUE STRAIN ON OSTEOGENESIS

A significant difference exists between plasma-sprayed or grit-blasted (ongrowth) and sintered porous-coated (ingrowth) implants in terms of rate of development of rigid implant fixation. This conclusion is based on a study using a rabbit implant model to determine the nature of tissues forming within the implant-bone interface zone and the interface strength and stiffness at very early periods following implant placement (e.g., 4 to 16 days following implantation).[18] Press-fitted implants (porous-coated or plasma-sprayed) were placed with a snug initial fit transversely in rabbit femoral condyle sites. The healing response for sintered porous-coated and plasma-sprayed implants was compared. Tapered truncated conical-shaped implants were used with a 300-micron (approximate)-thick porous coating formed by sintering Ti6Al4V alloy powders (45- to 150-micron size range) or Ti plasma-sprayed deposit of approximately 30 microns in thickness. The sintered porous coating had approximately 35 volume percent porosity and consisted of two to three layers of particles sintered to form 50- to 200-micron interconnected pores. The tapered implants (5-degree taper) were self-seating and allowed a good press-fit on placement. The taper shape minimized friction effects at the implant-host bone interface during pull-out testing, so that a sensitive assessment of the mechanical characteristics of interface zone fixation by newly formed tissues was possible. Animals were sacrificed at 4-, 8-, and 16-day periods. Implant fixation after these periods (as well as an initial zero time period that allowed confirmation of the effectiveness and similarity of the initial press-fit anchorage for the two designs) was compared by mechanical pull-out testing (to determine interface shear strength and interface stiffness, as indicated by the slope of the load-displacement curve), histology, and SEM examination (secondary and back-scattered electron imaging).

Mechanical pull-out tests indicated that despite similar initial (time-zero) pull-out resistance (due to snug press-fitting), sintered porous-coated implants exhibited significantly higher pull-out forces and higher interface stiffness at day 4 and day 8. No significant difference was noted at the 16-day period. Examination of interface zones by light microscopy, back-scattered SEM imaging of ground and polished sections, and secondary electron emission imaging of the surface of pulled-out implants indicated localized bone formation within some of the pores of the sintered coating by day 8. This contrasted with the absence of any new bone interlocking with the surface features of plasma-sprayed implants at that time period. The day 4 porous-coated samples (prior to formation of any mineralized tissue) showed a collagen matrix network interwoven throughout the porous structure, which is consistent with the higher pull-out strength and interface stiffness observed at day 4 and may have contributed to earlier bone formation by day 8.

Finite element models representing the two interface zone geometries were then developed to enable prediction of local tissue strains.[19,20] According to Carter's tissue differentiation hypothesis, predicted strain states corresponded to significant differences in the osteogenic potential of the two designs.[21] This analysis suggested that three-dimensional open-pored coatings offer an advantage in terms of rate of fixation by ingrowth when compared with ongrowth onto plasma-sprayed surfaces. In addition to the strain state, other factors such as vascularity and local biochemical and biological environment may differ significantly. Nevertheless, the effects of biomechanics as determined by implant surface design appeared to significantly influence cellular events during the healing process. Lower distortional strains were predicted within some pore regions compared with tissues next to the plasma-sprayed layer. It was proposed that pore architecture protected tissues that initially formed at the interface region (i.e., clot, collagen fibers, and cell infiltrate) from imposed forces, thereby resulting in lower distortional strains that, according to the tissue differentiation hypothesis, would favor osteogenesis. This suggests a preferred peri-implant stress/strain environment for rapid bone formation, which is consistent with the concept that mechanical stimulation under controlled levels of imposed cyclical forces promotes osteogenesis. Studies have also indicated the potential benefits of a three-dimensional porous network for enhanced osteoinduction.[22,23]

Relative Micromovement and Bone Ingrowth/Ongrowth

Bone ingrowth into the porous surfaces of cementless implants has been compared with bone formation during primary fracture healing. A necessary condition for successful bone ingrowth (as with primary fracture healing) is mechanical stability at the implant-bone junction. Reported animal studies have showed that with excessive relative movement at the implant-bone interface, bone ingrowth does not occur, but, rather, fibrous tissue develops.[24] This may result in fixation through a pseudoligamentous attachment if a collagen fiber structure forms throughout the porous network.[25] With very large relative movement, however, fibrous tissue encapsulation of the implant results.[26] Studies to determine the quantitative limits of relative movement causing bone or fibrous tissue attachment or fibrous tissue encapsulation have been reported. In a canine model study using porous-surfaced Ti6Al4V implants (average pore size ≈100 microns with 35 volume percent porosity) placed in healed mandibular premolar sites, it was shown that bone ingrowth occurred if imposed shear displacement at the implant interface was less than 50 microns. With relative displacement of approximately 150 microns, fibrous tissue encapsulation resulted, while fibrous tissue ingrowth and development of a pseudoligamentous attachment were observed for relative displacements between 50 and 150 microns.[26,27] The findings of other studies[28,29] using Ti fiber mesh-coated implants appear consistent with these results. The different structures (fixation by bone ingrowth, pseudoligamentous attachment, and fibrous encapsulation) are readily distinguished radiographically,[30] and images observed in animal studies have been related to light microscopy (histology) and scanning electron microscopic assessments.[25]

Although excessive movement under load can inhibit and even prevent bone ingrowth, some level of mechanical stimulation during the postimplantation healing period may be beneficial for faster bone formation. This is consistent with observations of enhanced osteosynthesis during application of controlled levels of repeated mechanical force during fracture healing.[31]

For successful biological fixation of cementless implants, it is essential to achieve secure initial implant stabilization to minimize risk of disruption of the implant-bone interface, preventing or slowing osteogenesis. Several different strategies may be used to achieve this condition, including achievement of a snug press-fit followed by limited loading for an appropriate period (i.e., 3 to 4 months), or protection of the interface through use of an adjuvant method of implant fixation such as screws—the most common method used for initial stabilization of acetabular cup components. Recent porous-coated implant designs have attempted to improve initial press-fit fixation by using more irregularly shaped (asymmetrical) powder particles to form porous coatings that more firmly grip initially when press-fitted into a prepared site (see Fig. 9-3C).

Pore Geometry Effect

Pore Size

Pore size is known to affect bone ingrowth rate. As the discussion on relative movement suggests, prevention of excessive relative movement of porous-coated and plasma-sprayed implants is a necessary condition for bone formation. Thus, the influence of implant design on rate of bony ingrowth is noted because this determines the potential length of exposure of the cementless interface to disruptive forces that could result in excessive relative movement. Early studies by Bobyn and associates[32] showed that pore size affects the rate of bone ingrowth. Porous-coated implants formed by sintering CoCrMo alloy particles of four different pore sizes were implanted transversely across the cortex of canine femurs, and fixation strengths and interface structures were assessed by mechanical push-out testing and histology at 4-, 8-, and 12-week periods. In these studies, resistance to push-out developed most rapidly for samples having pores in the 50- to 400-micron size range. For finer pore-sized samples (20 to 50 microns), bone ingrowth was inhibited and maximum interface shear strength (as measured by push-out testing) was lower at all time points. Samples with coatings with pore size of 400 to 800 microns, although eventually approaching fixation strength similar to the 50- to 200- and the 200- to 400-micron samples, required a significantly longer time to do so (longer than 12 weeks versus 8 weeks for the 50- to 200- and 200- to 400-micron pore-sized coatings). This pore size dependence of the rate of bone ingrowth may be related to the different microenvironments present within pores of different sizes and the effect that this has on osteogenesis.

Clemow and colleagues[33] investigated the effects of pore size on implant fixation in cortical and cancellous bone using porous-coated Ti6Al4V rods implanted in canine femurs. Three different coatings of equivalent porosity (36% to 40% by volume) with average pore size of 175, 225, or 375 microns were investigated. Implants were placed for a 6-month period, after which pull-out force was measured. Results for implants interfacing both cortical and cancellous bone showed that strength of fixation increased with decreasing pore size. This dependence correlated with measured volume of bone ingrowth. Investigators concluded that decreasing pore size beyond the minimum pore size necessary for bone ingrowth resulted in higher interfacial shear strength.

Pore Shape/Surface Morphology

Micron- and nano-sized surface features have effects on both osteoconduction and osteoinduction. A study by Fujibayashi and co-workers[22] showed that more complex pore shapes (i.e., porous Ti structures formed by plasma spraying compared with pressure-bonded Ti fibers) resulted in enhanced osteoinduction if the implants were appropriately chemically and thermally treated to make the Ti "bioactive." Others have reported no significant effects of pore shape on bone ingrowth[34] (for those coatings included in the study).

Materials for Forming Porous Structures

Although sintered porous coatings made from polymers, ceramics, and metals have been investigated in animal studies, only metals are commonly used currently for making implants because of the superior fracture and fatigue resistance of metals, their acceptable corrosion resistance and biocompatibility, and their ability to readily form porous-coated structures over substrates with a number of fairly straightforward techniques. Of the metallic biomaterials available for use in orthopedics, 316-L stainless steel, although it is considered suitable for some other implants, is not recommended for forming cementless implants (either sintered porous-coated or plasma spray-coated) because of its greater susceptibility to crevice corrosion with the more complex surface geometry of the coatings. Currently, porous-coated hip implant components are made from CoCrMo, cpTi, or Ti6Al4V alloy powders and Ti short wires/fibers. For plasma spray-coated implants, Ti coatings are most common. Because of their greater osseointegration potential,[35,36] Ti and Ti alloys are presently favored. Tantalum is also used for making some implants for fixation by bone ingrowth. Surface modification resulting in the deposit of calcium phosphate films and layers onto Ti substrates has been shown to promote osteoconduction.[37-40] A calcium phosphate surface layer combined with a three-dimensional pore structure has been suggested as enhancing osteoinduction.[22]

STRESS SHIELDING AND IMPLANT FIXATION

Stress shielding with rigidly fixed implants can occur if (1) bone and implant of sufficient length are appropriately aligned parallel to the direction of an applied force, (2) they are rigidly fixed to each other over a sufficient length for significant force transfer from bone to implant, and (3) the implant is much stiffer than adjacent bone. Resulting bone loss due to reduced stresses acting in bone over periods of months or years makes the bone more susceptible to fracture. To minimize stress shielding with porous-coated implants, some femoral stem components are designed with porous-coated regions limited to the proximal portions of the stems. Judicious limitations on the extent of porous coating do not compromise implant fixation and long-term stability following bone ingrowth.[28] Stress shielding can also be avoided by using lower-stiffness stems. Selection of Ti alloys with their lower modulus compared with CoCrMo alloys (110 GPa c.f. 220 GPa) has been rationalized in this way, but it is unlikely that this results in a significant difference. This is supported by results of a canine study comparing bone loss due to stress shielding by stainless steel onlay plates (E =

200 GPa, similar to CoCrMo) versus Ti alloy plates (E = 110 GPa). After 6-month implantation periods, the structure of bone next to the two implants was virtually the same, displaying significant bone loss under the plates.[41] Composite-structured and hollow tubular stems have been suggested as possible ways of avoiding stress shielding.[42] However, the fatigue characteristic of such designs is a concern. This continues to be an area of active investigation. As previously noted, clinical investigation of a novel CoCrMo + polyaryletherketone + Ti mesh composite femoral stem having lower stiffness (≈50% of that of an equivalently dimensioned Ti stem) revealed that it has been shown to significantly reduce bone loss, yielding encouraging results, at least over a 7-year patient follow-up period.[16]

CLOSENESS OF FIT: EFFECT OF INTERFACE GAP

Direct apposition of implants to a bone surface is preferred because this provides the greatest initial resistance to implant-bone relative movement and minimizes the distance over which bone must form to achieve fixation and the time needed to do so. If it is assumed that excessive relative movements can be avoided, new bone should form across existing gaps in a manner similar to gap healing during primary fracture healing. Although slower rates of fixation will be seen with larger gaps,[43] gaps as wide as 2 mm eventually can be bridged.[44]

FABRICATION OF CEMENTLESS IMPLANTS

Preparation of implants for fixation by bone ingrowth or ongrowth involves the use of processing techniques that can result in significant alteration of implant material mechanical properties. It is important that potential changes are considered in the selection and design of cementless implants. Currently, most hip implant components designed for cementless fixation are made by adding surface layers/coatings made of CoCrMo, Ti, or Ti alloy in forms suitable for uninhibited bone ingrowth or ongrowth, as described earlier. Such coatings are made primarily by (1) gravity sintering or pressure bonding of metal powders, fibers, or wire mesh structures to a solid substrate or (2) plasma spray deposition of layers of particles. Implants are designed to provide the necessary stiffness, strength, and fracture resistance for long-term repeated loading. As previously noted, stainless steel alloys are not used to form such surface layers because of their greater susceptibility to crevice corrosion. In addition to Co- and Ti-based systems, a Ta scaffold-like structure is used to make some implants designed for cementless use.

Outlined here are some of the processes used currently in preparing cementless implants, along with descriptions of the microstructural and property changes that may result and may compromise implant characteristics and, therefore, must be considered during cementless implant fabrication.

CoCrMo Powder–Made Porous Coatings

The use of metal powder sintering to form porous coatings on cast CoCrMo implant substrates was reported in the early 1970s.[45,46] Spherical atomized alloy powders made by inert gas atomization or spun electrode processes were sintered to form porous coatings over bone-interfacing surfaces of alloy substrates (Fig. 9-1). Methods used for coating the preparation have been described in some detail in earlier papers.[47,48] Alloy powders of selected size fractions are applied onto the substrate surface as a single layer or as multiple layers of powder, using an organic binder to initially hold the particles next to each other and to the substrate. For CoCrMo coatings, parts are heated in a nonoxidizing environment at a suitable rate to (1) burn off the binder without disruption of the powder particle arrangement (burn-off occurs at between 300° C and 400° C), and (2) develop metallic bonding at particle-particle and particle-substrate contacts, allowing sinter necks to form and grow as temperature is increased to and is held at the final sinter temperature. Crucial for the coating process is the selection of an organic binder of appropriate viscosity to allow initial particle adherence while allowing particle-particle contact to develop as the binder burns off. Coating strength is achieved through sinter neck development during the high temperature sintering phase of the operation (for CoCrMo, parts are held at 1300° C for 1 hour or so). Typically, multilayered coatings having 35 to 50 volume percent interconnected porosity result, with average pore size dependent on the particle size range used for commercially available implants, usually in the 100- to 500-micron range.

Sintering CoCrMo alloy particles to form a well-bonded, open-pored surface coating, as shown in Figure 9-1, involves a sintering anneal at temperatures well above the normal temperature used to heat-treat conventional cast CoCrMo implants. These are normally given a solution anneal at 1200° C to 1220° C, which is intended to at least partially homogenize the "cored" structure that forms on casting a compositionally heterogeneous structure with interdendritic regions enriched in Cr, Mo, and C. For CoCrMo alloys, the sintering anneal (1 hour or so at a temperature of ≈1300° C) is approximately 100° C above the "solution anneal" treatment. Localized Cr-, Mo-, and C-enriched zones invariably remain following the 1-hour solution anneal. These solute-enriched regions melt at approximately 1235° C (eutectic melting temperature for the Co, [Mo]-Cr-C system[49]), so that during the sintering anneal, localized incipient melting occurs in these solute-enriched zones. This causes two major effects: one beneficial and the other detrimental. First, the liquid phase enhances particle-to-particle and particle-to-substrate bonding as a result of liquid phase sintering. Examination of sinter neck regions clearly reflects the solidification of a prior liquid phase on cooling (Fig. 9-1*B* and *C*). Also seen on the sintered particle surfaces in Figure 9-1*B* are features resulting from liquid phase run-out along grain boundaries that occurs during the sinter anneal. Examination of a polished and etched cross-section through the particles and the substrate shows long, continuous secondary phase regions along grain boundaries, as well as along sinter neck junctions (Fig. 9-2*A* through *C*). These result from resolidification of the eutectic liquid phase. Grain boundary formations consist of mixed Co-rich γ-phase and carbides (primarily $M_{23}C_6$, where M = Cr and Mo) (see Fig. 9-2*C*) and represent brittle regions along

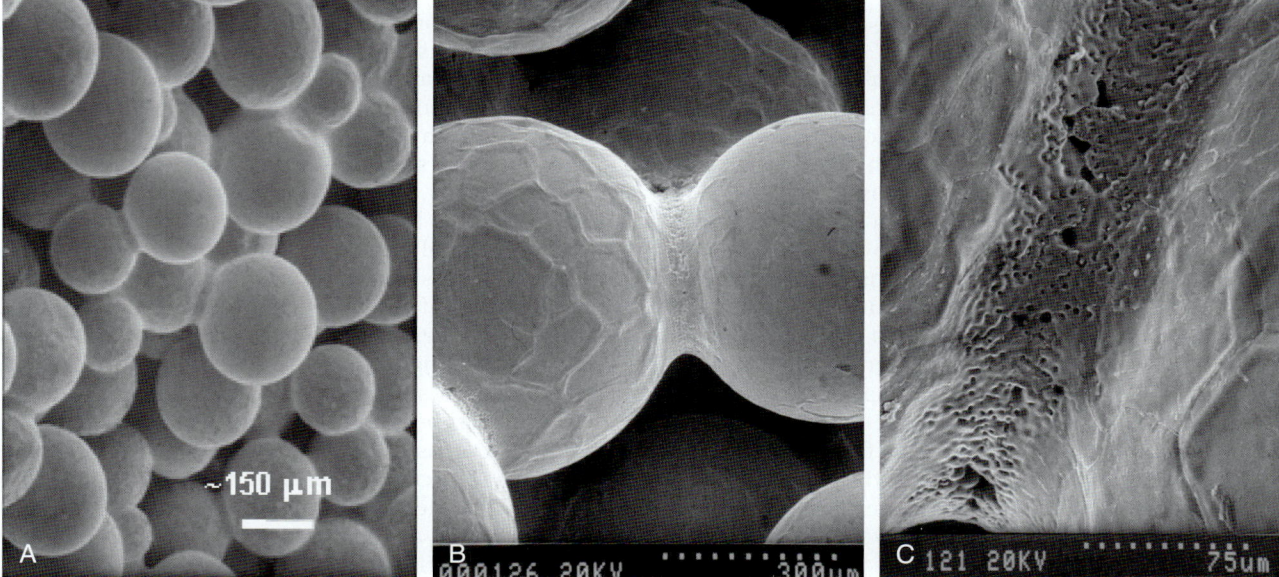

Figure 9-1. Secondary electron imaging (SEM) of sintered CoCrMo porous coating. **A,** Overview showing interconnected pore structure. **B,** Sinter neck region showing surface features where localized liquid phase formed during the 1300° C sinter anneal has run out along grain boundary regions (refer to Fig. 9-2). **C,** High-magnification image of sinter neck showing the structure produced by rapid solidification on cooling of the locally melted interdendritic eutectic.

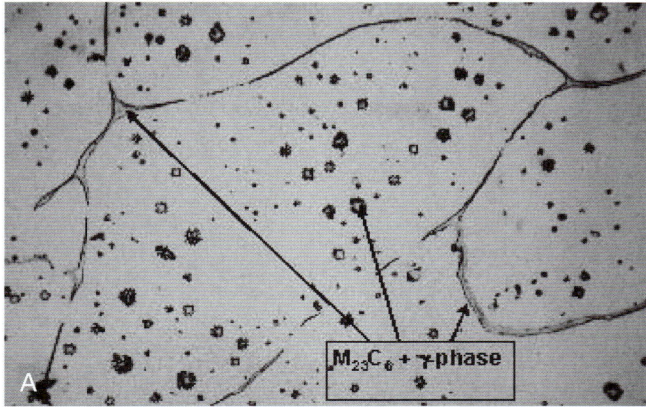

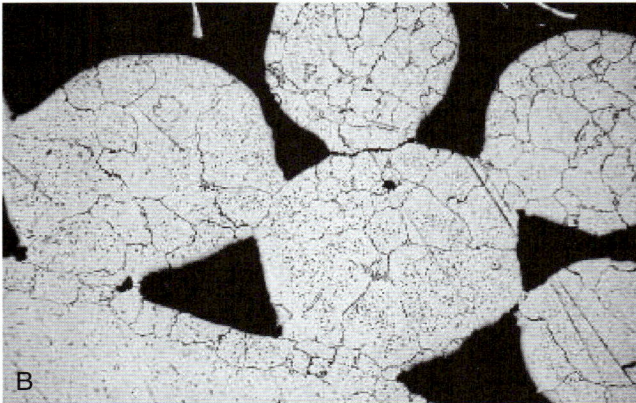

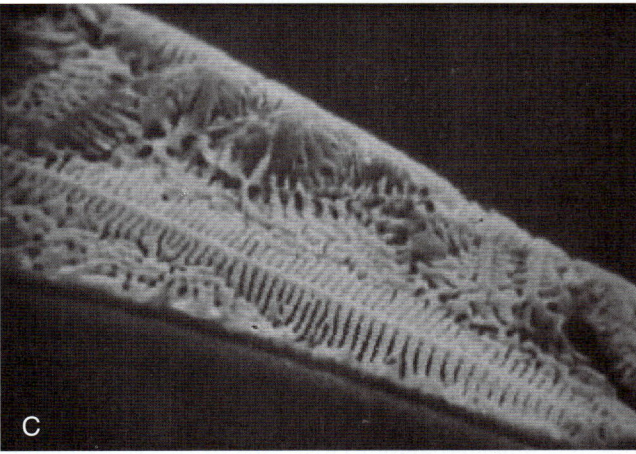

Figure 9-2. Light and scanning electron microscopic images showing microstructures that developed **(A)** within the CoCrMo substrate and **(B)** at the particle-substrate interface region, following sintering and normal cooling to room temperature. **C,** Secondary electron imaging (SEM) showing a grain boundary region with the eutectic γ phase + carbide structure clearly shown. This undesirable structure results in unacceptable low ductility.

which cracks can readily propagate, thereby resulting in limited implant ductility and unacceptable mechanical properties. Both the solid substrate and the interparticle and particle-substrate connections are susceptible to easy fracture (resulting in possible debonding of particles) because of the presence of these long, continuous eutectic structures.

The number of brittle, carbide-containing grain boundary regions can be minimized by using a controlled slow cool from the sintering temperature to below the 1235° C eutectic temperature,[50] or by reducing the carbon content of the alloy, thereby limiting the amount of liquid phase that forms.[51] The latter solution, unfortunately, also lowers the yield and fatigue strength of the Co-based alloy because, for the cast CoCrMo alloy, strengthening is primarily due to carbides ($M_{23}C_6$ mainly) dispersed throughout the structure. This would be especially detrimental to wear properties, although increasing use of modular implant designs in which femoral components can be designed with wear-resistant femoral head components for coupling to high-strength wrought stems overcomes this concern.

The issue of increased stem fracture susceptibility of porous-coated implants is a significant concern because removal and revision of fractured component parts represents a difficult surgical procedure f bony ingrowth has occurred. In theory, wrought CoCrMo alloys would offer an advantage in this regard because of their higher strength. However, the beneficial mechanical properties of these alloys are sacrificed during the high-temperature annealing process that is used to form the porous coating; this allows recrystallization and grain growth to occur within the body of the implant. A procedure performed to allow strength retention following sinter annealing has been reported.[52] This involves the development of dispersion-hardened CoCrMo alloys formed by hot consolidation of nitrogen atomized high-carbon CoCrMo alloy powders containing trace amounts of La and Al added to the melt during atomization. The La and Al minor additives form fine oxides dispersed throughout the powders during atomization; these act to inhibit grain growth during the sinter anneal. Powders are fabricated in bars and then are consolidated to their full density by hot forging or hot isostatic pressing in vacuum. This process is termed *gas atomized dispersion strengthened (GADS)*. Because of their fine microstructure, (fine grain size and dispersed fine carbides), GADS alloys are suitable for further shaping to final implant form. The fine dispersed oxides inhibit grain growth during sintering, so that relatively fine-grained, porous-coated implants with high fatigue strength approaching that of wrought CoCrMo alloys can be made.

These studies indicate that formation of CoCrMo alloys able to maintain high strength following a sinter treatment is possible; however, Ti and Ti alloys (mainly Ti6Al4V) have become more popular for load-bearing cementless implant fabrication because of the osseointegration characteristics of Ti and Ti alloys—a feature related to the passive oxide film that develops on the surfaces of these metals.[53]

Ti and Ti Alloy Powder-Made Porous Coatings

Sintered porous coatings of cp Ti or Ti6Al4V (Fig. 9-3A through E), unlike CoCrMo alloy powders, are formed by solid-state sintering of metal powders (i.e., no localized melting or liquid phase formation contributes to sinter neck formation). Gravity-sintered porous Ti

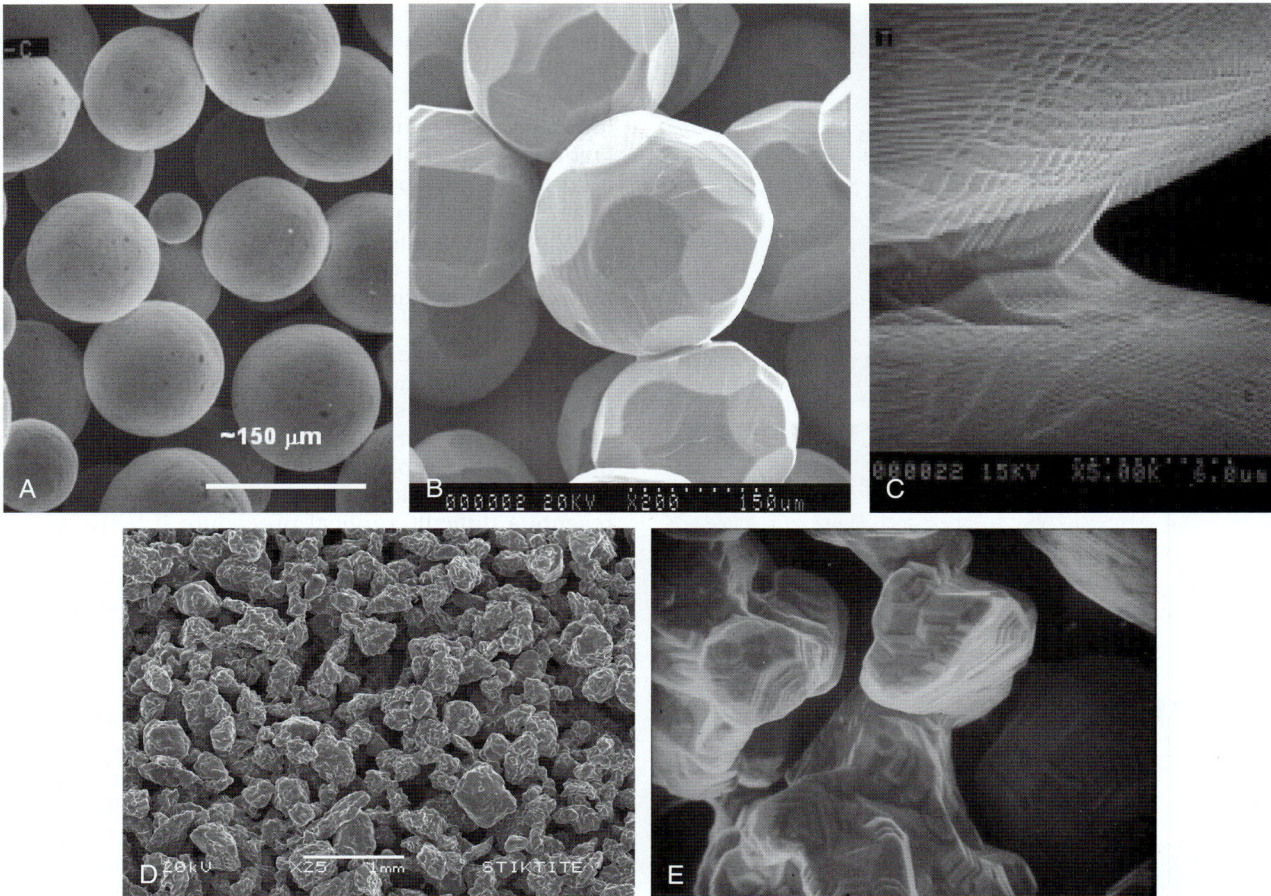

Figure 9-3. Secondary electron imaging (SEM) of **(A)** sintered Ti6Al4V, **(B)** sintered (regular-shaped) Ti powders, **(C)** sinter neck region of a Ti6Al4V sample showing thermal etch lines that form during sintering, **(D)** irregular sintered Ti ("asymmetrical") powder used to give better initial "grip" of implant at the implantation site. **E,** Sintered Ti formed from TiH$_2$ powder. (**D** *Courtesy Smith & Nephew Orthopaedics, Fort Washington, Pa.*)

coatings are formed by sintering Ti or Ti alloy powders at 1250° C, or slightly higher temperatures, for approximately 1 hour in a nonoxidizing furnace atmosphere (high-vacuum 10^{-6} mm Hg or higher, or partial pressure inert gas atmosphere) (see Fig. 9-3*A* through *D*). During the sintering operation, particularly during high-vacuum sintering, characteristic submicron-spaced features develop over Ti or Ti alloy particle surfaces (see Fig. 9-3*C*). These are due to thermal etching that occurs during the high-temperature sintering operation. (It has been suggested that these features may be beneficial for bone formation by providing surface features for osteoblast attachment and enhanced osteoconductivity[54]).

Porous Ti coatings can also be made from TiH$_2$ starting powders (see Fig. 9-3*E*).[55] After TiH$_2$ particles are applied to the substrate surface using a binder, the powders are annealed and decompose to Ti and H$_2$ at 1000° C. Continued heating to 1250° C results in the formation of a porous coating but with angular Ti particle shapes, as shown in Figure 9-3*E*.

The high sintering temperature used during gravity sintering is well above the β-transus temperature (the temperature above which the bcc β-phase transforms to the hcp α-phase, ≈1000° C for the Ti alloys). Furnace cooling of the Ti alloy results in microstructural modification, with the so-called *mill-annealed* α + β structure characterized by equiaxed α-grains surrounded by fine β-phase regions (the preferred structure for high fatigue strength) being transformed to a β-annealed structure, with lamellar α- and β-phase regions forming in colonies (Fig. 9-4*A* and *B*).[56] This microstructural change causes the mill-annealed alloy to lose 10% to 20% of its fatigue strength when tested using smooth polished fatigue specimens. However, a greater drop in fatigue strength occurs for Ti porous-coated samples (or other Ti samples with significant surface topographic irregularities) because of the formation of stress concentrators along the substrate surface (e.g., at sinter neck regions, as seen in Fig. 9-3*B* and *C*). Ti and Ti alloys are notch fatigue sensitive, so that easier fatigue crack initiation can occur at these points. Thus, fatigue strength (10^7 endurance strength) is reduced from approximately 625 MPa for smooth-surfaced, mill-annealed Ti6Al4V samples to below 200 MPa for porous-coated Ti alloy samples, regardless of whether they form mill-annealed or β-annealed microstructures. Measures that have been explored to minimize these notch effects include sintering below the β-transus temperature to prevent

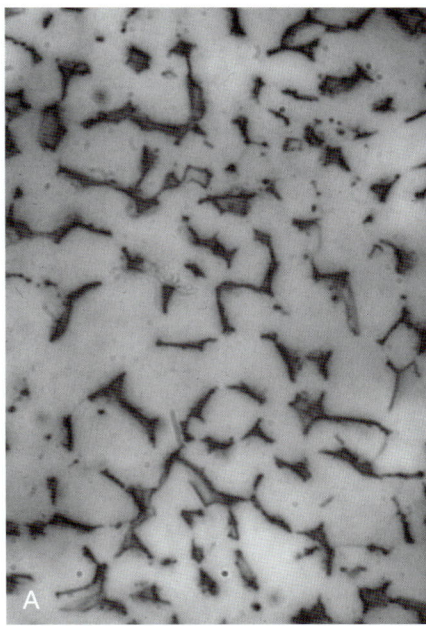 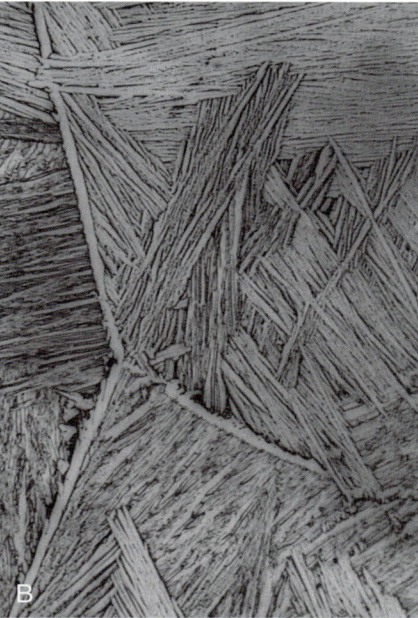

Figure 9-4. Microstructures of **(A)** mill-annealed Ti5Al4V (α-phase etched light, β-phase etched dark) and **(B)** the β-annealed structure resulting after high-temperature sintering, showing the colony structures formed by α and β lamellae.

transformation to the β-annealed microstructure, and the use of pressure during sintering to enhance sinter neck formation and the development of increased bond strength. However, a large reduction in fatigue strength is still observed because of the stress concentration at the sinter neck regions. This effect is not unique to sintered porous-coated Ti alloys but, as noted, also occurs with any Ti alloy component lacking a smooth, polished surface (i.e., plasma-sprayed and grit-blasted surfaces, pressure-bonded Ti fiber coatings, and other structures intended to allow fixation by bone ingrowth or ongrowth will result in similar fatigue strength reduction).

To reduce the probability of fatigue failure of femoral stems due to these effects, porous-coated Ti alloy implants can be designed to avoid stress risers in expected high tensile stress regions. Thus, the lateral aspect of femoral stem components can be left uncoated because the highest tensile stress is expected to develop along this surface during functional implant loading. Unfortunately, this limits the effectiveness of bone ingrown regions to act as barriers to migration of wear debris particles formed at bearing surfaces. Presently, endosteal osteolysis due to wear debris is considered the major cause of hip implant failure. It is suggested that bone ingrown regions represent an effective barrier to debris migration.[57] Thus, a coating that covers only a portion of the implant periphery will be less effective in this regard than a coating that completely covers the proximal implant surface.

Ti Fiber Metal Composite Coatings

Porous Ti fiber metal coatings (Fig. 9-5A) were also developed in the late 1960s and early 1970s.[12] The method described by its developers in their early studies involved the use of short kinked wires (or fibers) of 190- to 300-micron diameter and 6.35 mm in length

that were compacted within molds and sintered at 1093° C for 2 hours in vacuum. The porous structure formed by this process has an interconnected porosity of approximately 50 volume percent, with 200- to 400-micron openings for bone ingrowth. This process was modified by pressure sintering of longer Ti fibers at temperatures just below the β-transus temperature (≈882° C for commercial purity Ti) to securely bond the fibers while retaining the Ti6Al4V mill-annealed microstructure of the substrate.[53] The high-temperature pressure bonding/sintering process required the use of nonreactive pressure pads for compressing the Ti wire during the pressure bonding/sintering operation. High-density, high-purity graphite and certain other refractory materials were found to be suitable for this purpose. Pressure bonding to curved surfaces, however, presented difficulties, so the application of Ti fiber mesh structures was further limited to flat regions of the implant surface (Fig. 9-5B). The final density of fiber compacts is dependent on wire/fiber diameter, applied pressure used during wire compaction, and the time and temperature used for diffusion bonding. As with the powder metal sintering process, secure interfiber and fiber-substrate bonding occurs through sinter neck development.

Orderly Oriented Wire Mesh (OOWM) Coatings

Orderly oriented wire mesh (OOWM) structures formed using woven Ti wire mesh were developed in the 1980s as a method of forming a regular porous coating structure of predictable pore size.[59] In addition, the interwoven wires forming the structures were considered an improvement over the Ti metal fiber coatings with regard to prevention of debonding and release of loose wire fragments. To achieve bonding at the wire-wire and wire-substrate contact points, pressure sintering at just

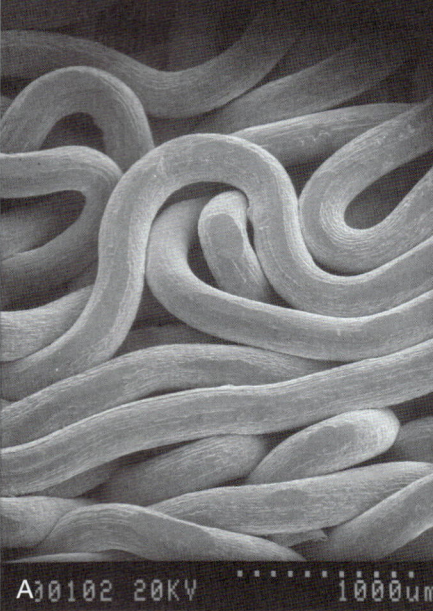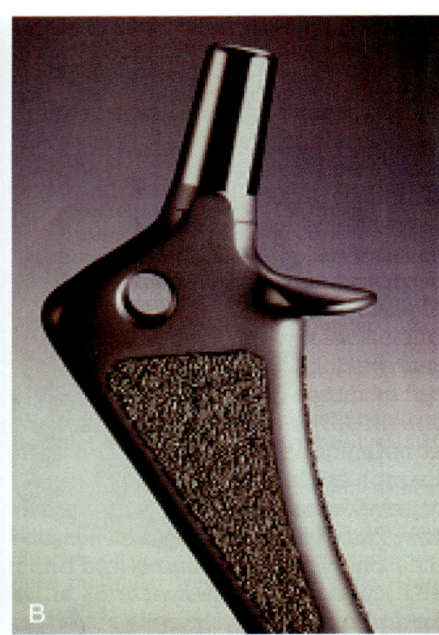

Figure 9-5. A, Ti fiber metal-sintered structure. **B,** Femoral hip stem showing the Ti fiber mesh bonded to flat recesses within the stem and devoid of coating on the lateral aspect.

below the β-transus temperature (800° C to 900° C) was used. Selection of appropriate weave patterns allowed formation of porous coatings with well-controlled pore networks. A disadvantage of OOWM coatings, as with Ti fiber composite coatings, is that the porous mesh can be applied conveniently and effectively only to flat regions of a substrate.

Cast CoCrMo structures

Porous-coated implants (even OOWN coatings) are susceptible to delamination of particles, wires, or fibers with release of fragments into surrounding tissues. This source of particulate debris can cause a foreign body host response and increased rates of wear due to third-body abrasion of articulating surfaces. One strategy for increasing the integrity of ingrowth coatings is to form an open-pored surface structure as an integral part of the implant during casting rather than as a separate coating bonded to the substrate. Cast CoCrMo alloy implants made by investment casting to form surfaces suitable for bone *ongrowth* (not *ingrowth*)[60,61] were made and clinically used in the 1970s. Presently, a CoCrMo alloy implant formed with a structure suitable for bone ingrowth is available (Fig. 9-6*A* and *B*). The cast CoCrMo has open-pored, crucifix-like features on its surface (see Fig. 9-6*B*), forming a scaffold-like architecture for bone ingrowth. Acceptable follow-up results have been reported for this implant.[62]

Novel Open-Pored Hip Implant Components: Porous Scaffold Designs

Novel acetabular implant designs with scaffold-like regions for fixation by bone ingrowth have been made available. They are fabricated by methods developed for making fully porous parts for bone substitute and bone augmentation procedures, and involve deposition

of Ti or Ta onto reticulated skeleton structures. The skeleton structure typically consists of a foam template that decomposes during subsequent thermal annealing processes (for organic materials, such as polyurethane) or is retained in the final part (fine vitreous carbon fiber cores within Ta trabecular metal struts). Fabrication of some acetabular components with such porous structures has been reviewed elsewhere.[63] In view of their proprietary nature, only limited information is available on methods for forming some commercial products. In common with all approaches, however, is the formation of a highly porous surface structure featuring three-dimensional interconnected pore networks with volume percent porosity in the 60% to 85% range.

One such product that has been described in some detail is Hedrocel (trabecular metal[64]), which was originally developed as a bone augment material and was later incorporated into a monoblock acetabular cup consisting of a polyethylene bearing surface integrally bonded with a trabecular metal tantalum shell (Fig. 9-7*A* and *B*).[65] Trabecular metal is made by forming a porous Ta structure through chemical vapor deposition of Ta onto a reticulated vitreous carbon scaffold. The carbon scaffold itself is formed by pyrolysis of a precursor polyurethane foam.[14,63] The porosity of the final scaffold and the size of the openings available for bone ingrowth are controlled by varying the thickness of the deposited tantalum layer. To form the acetabular component, the polyethylene liner is compressed against the tantalum shell until the liner becomes embedded in the shell, with part of the Ta scaffold remaining exposed for implant fixation.

Other novel approaches for forming fully porous structures may be possible for making joint replacement components in future implant designs. An example of a metal foam structure formed by mixing Ti (or Ti alloy) powders with a polymeric binder and a foaming agent and subjecting the mixture to three-step thermal

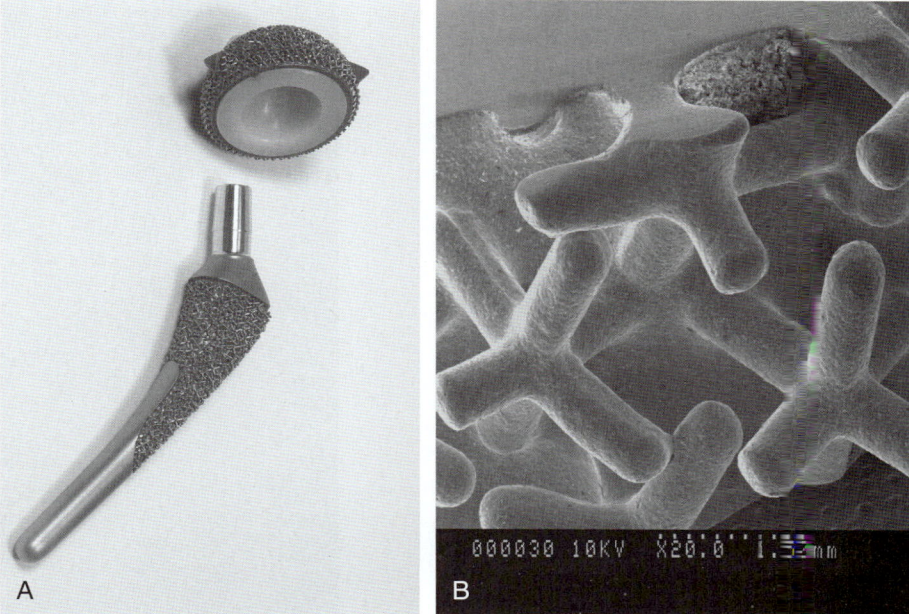

Figure 9-6. **A,** CoCrMo cast implant components and **(B)** with integrally cast scaffold-like structure for bone ingrowth.

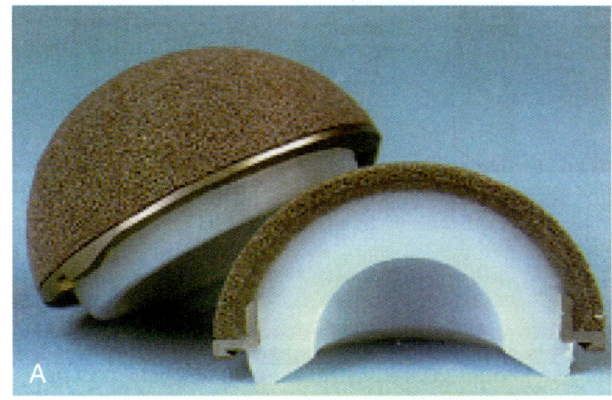

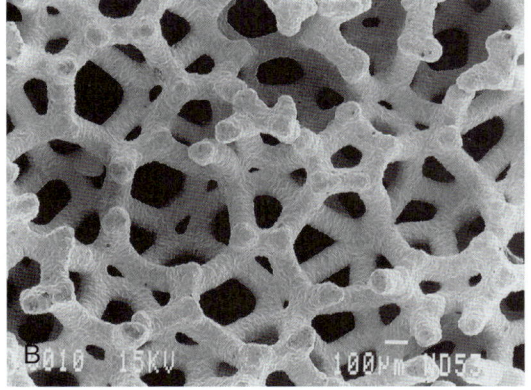

Figure 9-7. **A,** Acetabular cup made with **(B)** trabecular metal (Ta) scaffold embedded in the polyethylene bearing material and providing an open-pored structure suitable for bone ingrowth. *(Courtesy Dr. J. D. Bobyn, McGill University, Montreal, Quebec, Canada.)*

treatment is shown in Figure 9-8*A* through *C*.[66] This structure, to the best of the author's knowledge, has yet to be used clinically. It also displays the thermal etch features referred to previously (see Fig. 9-8*C*).

Bone Ongrowth Structures

Modification of implant surfaces to facilitate bone ongrowth has primarily involved application of plasma-sprayed Ti. Plasma spray deposition of Ti results in the formation of very irregular surfaces with recesses and outcroppings that are suitable for anchoring newly formed bone. Studies have also explored methods of texturing Ti or Ti alloy implant surfaces, especially in the development of dental implants aimed at achieving more rapid osseointegration. These methods have included grit blasting, acid etching, laser ablation, anodizing, and ion beam etching processes. With the exception of grit-blasted surfaces, the effectiveness of these surface preparations in enhancing fixation of cementless orthopedic implants has not been investigated. However, these surface configurations do appear to significantly enhance osteoconductivity and hence might promote increased rates of bone ingrowth or ongrowth in attachment of cementless orthopedic implants.

Plasma Spray Deposition

For plasma spray deposition of a Ti surface layer onto a Ti or Ti alloy substrate, powders are injected into a hot plasma flame (≈20,000° C in its hottest zone) created by ionization of a carrier gas in a nonoxidizing atmosphere, typically a mixture of hydrogen and argon. The high-speed plasma jet sweeps the wholly or partially

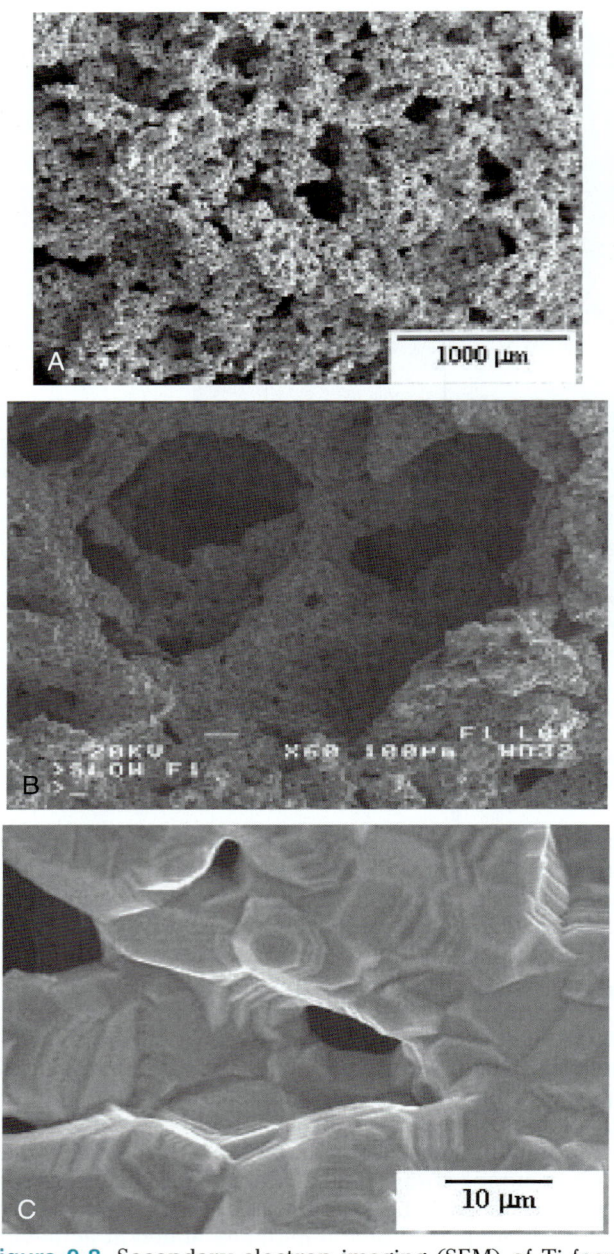

Figure 9-8. Secondary electron imaging (SEM) of Ti foam structure for bone ingrowth. **A,** Low magnification, **(B)** intermediate magnification, and **(C)** high magnification showing thermal etch features. *(Courtesy Dr. Lefevbre, NRC-CSNR, IMI, Boucherville, Quebec, Canada.)*

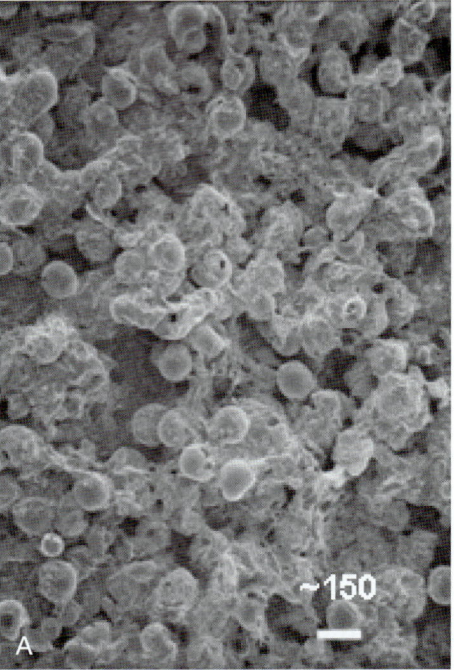

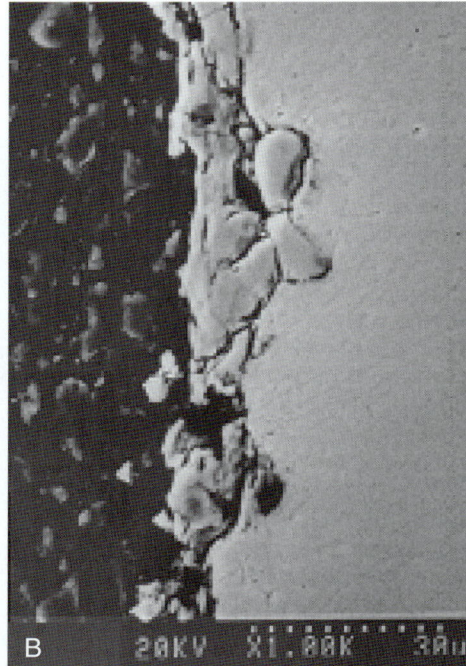

Figure 9-9. Back-scattered electron imaging (SEM) of Ti plasma-sprayed coating. **A,** Surface appearance showing wholly and partially melted particles, and **(B)** ground and polished section normal to the coating-substrate interface showing the irregular structure of the plasma-sprayed coating.

melted powders onto the surface of the implant being coated. Ti compounds may also be injected into the flame. In early studies reported by Hahn and Pahlich,[13] TiH_2 powders injected into plasma decomposed to Ti and H_2 during the spraying operation, thereby enhancing the reducing atmosphere while depositing molten Ti droplets. On deposition, the molten Ti droplets impact onto the workpiece surface (the implant substrate) and rapidly solidify (solidification rate approaching $10^{6°}$ C/sec). This results in a very fine microstructured deposit

of metal with an irregular surface topography (Fig. 9-9). The plasma flame is rastered back and forth across the workpiece to deposit layers of particles to the desired thickness (typically ≈50 to 100 microns). Although spraying conditions can be controlled to allow porosity and even the formation of graded porosity,[13,67] to ensure a more fracture-resistant plasma-sprayed layer, fully dense coatings with minimum porosity or inclusion content have been the usual goal. Some internal isolated voids may develop, as well as entrainment of some nonmetallic inclusions within the deposited layers. A post–plasma spraying anneal can be used to partially eliminate some of the internal voids, thereby forming a more fracture-resistant layer. This also serves to round off any sharp surface asperities that may form at the irregular outer coating surface. Such sharp asperities could stimulate an inflammatory response. In general, during plasma spraying, the workpiece is maintained at a low temperature as a consequence of the very rapid solidification of the deposited molten (or partially molten) metal particles, thereby avoiding phase transformations within Ti alloy substrates. However, as already noted, significant reduction in fatigue strength with the alloy is due to the introduction of stress concentrators at the implant surface—features that develop on plasma spray–coated implants. The resulting irregular surface topography is effective for achieving fixation by bone ongrowth.

FUTURE CONSIDERATIONS

Some suggested directions for future studies are presented here. These include studies on enhancing osteoconduction or osteoinduction, adapting novel processing currently being implemented to form fully porous structures for bone augment and void filler applications, and developing more infection-resistant porous-coated structures. In addition, there is a need to develop an understanding of the microenvironment (physical, mechanical, and chemical) within pores and recesses and its influence on osteogenesis. This information should be useful in guiding the design of surface structures for future cementless implants.

1. Increasing Osteoconductivity

With the goal of increasing the rate of bone ingrowth (or ongrowth), as well as increasing the possibility for successful ingrowth/ongrowth in patients with compromised bone-forming ability, a number of studies have focused on modifying surfaces to make them more osteoconductive. Approaches have included the following:

1. Addition of calcium phosphate surface layers (by deposition from solution,[68] by formation of sol gel-formed calcium phosphate films,[69,70] or by electrochemical deposition[71]).
2. Use of biomimetic strategies with surfaces modified through chemical/thermal treatment (alkali or hydrogen peroxide soaking plus annealing) to promote apatite layer formation in vivo.[72-75]
3. Radiofrequency (RF) magnetron sputtering.[76]
4. Formation of micron and submicron surface textures.[77]

2. Increasing Osteoinductivity

Enhancing osteoinductivity of porous coatings through incorporation of growth factors or other biologicals within porous surface structures has been studied.[78] The results of one such study suggest that Ti fiber metal composite–coated implants with calcium phosphate (HA/TCP) plasma–sprayed overlayers soaked in transforming growth factor (TGF-β–containing solutions for prolonged periods ($\approx$18 hours) display a significant increase in rate of bone ingrowth. However, this approach may not be practical at this time because of the added costs associated with the use of presently available growth factors and biologicals.

Studies with fully porous structures (foams and scaffolds) have suggested that a three-dimensional microenvironment, as presented by porous structures in combination with a microtextured and calcium phosphate surface layer, results in enhanced osteoinduction.[22,23] From these studies, a macroscopic pore structure (pore size $\approx$100 to 500 microns) promoting osteoinduction with microscopic (or nanoscopic) features on pore wall surfaces is suggested for achieving more rapid osteogenesis and bone ingrowth. It is not known whether a similar effect will occur with porous-coated implants because the solid substrate underlying the porous coating may significantly affect pore microenvironment. Additional studies using porous-coated implants are suggested to determine whether additional benefits of microtexturing and nanotexturing are observed. This underscores the need for a fundamental understanding of the microenvironment within pores and recesses and how this might affect osteogenesis. Studies on surface topography and its effects on cellular response at implant surfaces have been reported.[79-82] These findings should be useful in designing model studies aimed at defining any significant differences in local microenvironments within the confined regions of pores and deep recesses.

3. Scaffold-Like Implants for Joint Replacements

Ryan and associates[83] reviewed fabrication methods for forming porous metallic structures for orthopedic applications. This review focused on the formation of fully porous structures, but some of the methods outlined might be applicable to forming novel porous coatings for joint replacement implants. Rapid manufacturing techniques using solid free form (SFF) fabrication of Ti structures, either selective laser melting or selective laser sintering,[84-87] may be suitable for forming implants for fixation by bone ingrowth. The advantage of SFF processing is that the surface zone structure can be closely controlled to produce whatever structure is deemed most suitable, including structures with graded porosities.[86] In addition to regular formations, it is possible to design and produce structures with an architecture more closely mimicking natural cancellous bone. Whether this would offer an advantage for more rapid bone ingrowth is not known but could be studied by forming such structures.

4. Infection Resistance

Infection resistance is related to implant surface area; the greater the area, as is the case with all cementless implants, the greater is the probability for implant-related infection. This has been a concern with cementless implants since they were first proposed. Further study on the effectiveness of antibactericidal additive incorporation into these structures is desirable.

SUMMARY

Cementless implants offer an advantage in the treatment of younger, physically active individuals. Optimal structures for forming the most reliable implants for specific uses remain to be defined. Based on information garnered from animal studies, there appears to be an advantage of implants formed with porous coatings having three-dimensional interconnected porous networks for bone *ingrowth* and formed with appropriate surface structure and chemistry for some applications. The ultimate choice for design and manufacture of implants, however, depends on the cost of manufacture to achieve an acceptable outcome. This may be the predominant factor in determining the design of future devices.

In terms of our current understanding of fundamental factors influencing bone *ingrowth* or *ongrowth* to achieve fixation, much is yet unknown. The region within a pore or recess may present a local environment that differs significantly from that of regions outside these zones. The specific surface area, stress distribution acting on ingrown tissues, accumulation of factors promoting osteogenesis, and degradation products that may inhibit bone formation in these regions may significantly affect cellular response during early postimplantation healing and at later times may represent poorly understood issues. Studies are needed to clarify the influence of these matters on osteogenesis to serve as a guide for future cementless implant design.

REFERENCES

1. Spector M: Bone ingrowth into porous metals. In Williams DF (ed): Biocompatibility of clinical implant materials, Boca Raton, Fla, 1981, CRC Press, pp 89–128.
2. Pilliar RM: Porous-surfaced metallic implants for orthopaedic applications. J Biomed Mater Res 21:1–33, 1987.
3. Kienapfel H, Sprey C, Wilke A, Griss P: Implant fixation by bone ingrowth. J Arthroplasty 14:355–367, 1999.
4. Pilliar RM: Cementless implant fixation: towards improved reliability. Orthop Clin North Am 36:113–119, 2005.
5. Hirschhorn JS, Reynolds JT: Powder metallurgy fabrication of cobalt alloy surgical implant materials. In Korostoff E (ed): Research in dental and medical materials, New York, 1969, Plenum Press, pp 137–150.
6. Hulbert SF, Klawitter JJ, Talbert CD, Fitts CT: Materials of construction for artificial bone segments. In Korostoff E (ed): Research in dental and medical materials, New York, 1969, Plenum Press, pp 19–67.
7. Spector M, Flemming WR, Kreutner A: Bone growth into porous high density polyethylene. J Biomed Mater Res 10:595–603, 1976.
8. DeMane M, Beals NB, McDowell DL, et al: Porous polysulfone-coated femoral stems. In Lemons JE (ed): Quantitative characterization and performance of porous implants for hard tissue applications, ASTM 953, Philadelphia, 1987, American Society for Testing and Materials, pp 315–329.
9. Hulbert SF, Matthews JR, Klawitter JJ, et al: Effect of stress on tissue ingrowth into porous aluminum oxide. J Biomed Mater Res 8:85–97, 1974.
10. Homsy CA, Cain TE, Kessler FB, et al: Porous systems for prosthesis stabilization. Clin Orthop Relat Res 89:220, 1972.
11. Pilliar RM, Cameron HU, Macnab I: Porous surface layered prosthetic devices. Biomed Eng J 10:126–131, 1975.
12. Galante J, Rostoker W, Lueck R, Ray R: Sintered fiber metal composites as a basis for attachment of implants to bone. J Bone Joint Surg Am 53:101–114, 1971.
13. Hahn H, Palich W: Preliminary evaluation of porous metal surfaced titanium for orthopedic implants. J Biomed Mater Res 4:571–577, 1970.
14. Bobyn JD, Stackpool GJ, Hacking SA, et al: Characteristics of bone ingrowth and interface mechanics of a new porous tantalum biomaterial. J Bone Joint Surg Br 81:907–914, 1999.
15. Nunamaker DM, Black J: Tissue responses associated with ingrowth into porous stainless steel. Trans Orthop Res Soc 3:160, 1978.
16. Akhavan S, Matthiesen MM, Schulte L, et al: Clinical and histologic results related to a low-modulus composite total hip replacement stem. J Bone Joint Surg Am 88:1308–1314, 2006.
17. Engh CA, Bobyn JD: Biological fixation in total hip arthroplasty, Thorofare, NJ, 1988, Slack Inc, p 15.
18. Simmons CA, Valiquette N, Pilliar RM: Osseointegration of sintered porous-surfaced and plasma-spray coated implants: an animal model study of early post-implantation healing response and mechanical stability. J Biomed Mater Res 47:127–138, 1999.
19. Simmons CA, Meguid SA, Pilliar RM: Mechanical regulation of localized and appositional bone formation around bone-interfacing implants. J Biomed Mater Res 55:63–71, 2001.
20. Simmons CA, Pilliar RM: A biomechanical study of early tissue formation around bone-interfacing implants: the effect of implant surface geometry. In Davies JE (ed): Bone engineering, Toronto, Ontario, Canada, 1999, Em Squared Inc, pp 369–380.
21. Carter DR, Beaupre GS, Giori NJ, Helms JA: Mechanobiology of skeletal regeneration. Clin Orthop Relat Res 355(Suppl 1):S41–S55, 1998.
22. Fujibayashi S, Neo M, Kim HM, et al: Osteoinduction of porous bioactive titanium metal. Biomaterials 25:443–450, 2004.
23. Habibovic P, Yuan H, van der Valk CM, et al: 3D microenvironment as essential for osteoinduction by biomaterials. Biomaterials 26:3565–3575, 2005.
24. Spector M: Bone ingrowth into porous polymers. In Williams DF (ed): Biocompatibility of orthopedic implants, Boca Raton, Fla, 1982, CRC Press, p 55.
25. Szivek JA, Weatherly GC, Pilliar RM, Cameron HU: A study of bone remodelling using metal-polymer laminates. J Biomed Mater Res 15:853–865, 1981.
26. Pilliar RM, Lee JM, Maniatopoulos C: Observations on the effect of movement on bone ingrowth into porous-surfaced implants. Clin Orthop Relat Res 208:108–113, 1986.
27. Pilliar RM, Deporter DA, Watson PA: Tissue-implant interface: micromovement effects. In Vincenzini P (ed): Materials in clinical applications, Faenza, Italy, 1995, Techna, pp 569–579.
28. Jasty M, Krushnell R, Zalenski E, et al: The contribution of the nonporous distal stem to the stability of proximally porous-coated canine femoral components. J Arthroplasty 8:33–41, 1993.
29. Burke DW, Bragdon CR, Lowenstein L: Mechanical aspects of the bone porous surface interface under known amounts of implant motion. Trans Orthop Res Soc 18:470, 1993.
30. Engh CA, Bobyn JD: Radiographic study of biological fixation. In Biological fixation in total hip arthroplasty, Thorofare, NJ, 1985, Slack Inc, Chap 6.
31. Goodship AE, Kenwright J: The influence of induced micromovement upon the healing of experimental tibial fractures. J Bone Joint Surg Br 67:650–655, 1985.

32. Bobyn JD, Pilliar RM, Cameron HU, Weatherly GC: The optimum pore size for fixation of porous surfaced metal implants by the ingrowth of bone. Clin Orthop Relat Res 149:291–298, 1980.

33. Clemow AJ, Weinstein AM, Klawitter JJ, et al: Interface mechanics of porous titanium implants. J Biomed Mater Res 15:73–82, 1981.

34. Turner TM, Sumner DR, Urban RM, et al: A comparative study of porous coatings in weight-bearing total hip arthroplasty model. J Bone Joint Surg Am 68:1396–1409, 1986.

35. Ellingsen JE: On the properties of surface-modified titanium. In Davies JE (ed): Bone engineering, Toronto, Ontario, Canada, 1999, Em Squared Inc, Chap 15, pp 183–189.

36. Head WC, Bauk DJ, Emerson RH Jr: Titanium as the material of choice for cementless femoral components in total hip arthroplasty. Clin Orthop Relat Res 311:85–90, 1995.

37. Rivero DP, Fox J, Skipor AK, et al: Calcium phosphate-coated porous titanium implants for enhanced skeletal fixation. J Biomed Mater Res 22:191–201, 1988.

38. Thomas KA, Kay JF, Cook SD, Jarcho M: The effect of surface microtexture and hydroxylapatite coating on the mechanical strengths and histologic profiles of titanium implant materials. J Biomed Mater Res 21:1395–1414, 1987.

39. Soballe K, Hansen ES, Brockstedt-Rasmussen H, et al: Hydroxy-apatite coating enhances fixation of porous coated implants. Acta Orthop Scand 61:299–306, 1990.

40. Cook SD, Thomas KA, Dalton JE, et al: Hydroxylapatite coating of porous implants improves bone ingrowth and interface attachment strength. J Biomed Mater Res 26:989–1001, 1992.

41. Szivek JA, Weatherly GC, Pilliar RM, Cameron HU: A study of bone remodelling using metal-polymer laminates. J Biomed Mater Res 15:853–865, 1981.

42. Bobyn JD, Mortimer ES, Glassman AH, et al: Producing and avoiding stress shielding: laboratory and clinical observations of non-cemented total hip arthroplasty. Clin Orthop Relat Res 274:79–96, 1992.

43. Dalton JE, Cook SD, Thomas KA, Kay JF: The effect of operative fit and hydroxyapatite coating on the mechanical and biological response to porous implants. J Bone Joint Surg Am 72:97–110, 1995.

44. Bobyn JD, Pilliar RM, Cameron HU, Weatherly GC: Osteogenic phenomena across endosteal bone-implant spaces with porous surfaced intramedullary implants. Acta Orthop Scand 52:145–153, 1981.

45. Welsh PR, Pilliar RM, Macnab I: The role of surface porosity in fixation to bone and acrylic. J Bone Joint Surg Am 53:963–977, 1971.

46. Pilliar RM, Cameron HU, Macnab I: Porous surface layered prosthetic devices. Biomed Eng 10:126–131, 1975.

47. Pilliar RM: P/M processing of surgical implants: sintered porous surfaces for tissue-to-implant fixation. Int J Powder Metallurgy 34:33–45, 1998.

48. Pilliar RM: Porous-surfaced metallic implants for orthopaedic applications. J Biomed Mater Res 21:1–33, 1987.

49. Kilner T, Pilliar RM, Weatherly GC: Phase identification and incipient melting in a cast Co-base surgical implant alloy. J Biomed Mater Res 16:63–79, 1982.

50. Pilliar RM: Metals and orthopaedic implants: past successes, present limitations, future challenges. In Shrivastava S (ed): Medical device materials. Proceedings of Materials and Processes for Medical Devices Conference, September 2003, pp 8–22.

51. Kilner T, Laanamae M, Pilliar RM, et al: Static mechanical properties of cast and sinter annealed cobalt-chromium surgical-implants. J Mater Sci 21:1349–1356, 1986.

52. Wang KK, Berlin RM, Gustavson LJ: A dispersion strengthened Co-Cr-Mo alloy for medical implants. In Disegi JA, Kennedy RL, Pilliar RM: Cobalt-base alloys for biomedical applications, ASTM STP 1365, West Conshohocken, Pa, 1999, American Society for Testing and Materials, pp 89–97.

53. Thomsen P, Esposito M, Gretzer C, Liao H: Inflammatory response to implanted materials. In Davies JE (ed): Bone engineering, Toronto, Ontario, Canada, 1999, Em Squared Inc, Chap 10, pp 119–136.

54. Pilliar RM, Davies JE, Smith DC: The bone-biomaterial interface for load-bearing implants. MRS Bulletin 16:55–61, 1991.

55. Pilliar RM: Powder metal-made orthopaedic implants with porous surface for fixation by tissue ingrowth. Clin Orthop Relat Res 176:42, 1983.

56. Yue S, Pilliar RM, Weatherly GC: The fatigue strength of porous-coated Ti-6Al-4 V implant alloy. J Biomed Mater Res 18:1043–1058, 1984.

57. von Knoch M, Engh CA, Sychterz C, et al: Migration of polyethylene wear debris in one type of uncemented femoral component with circumferential porous coating: an autopsy study of 5 femurs. J Arthroplasty 15:72–78, 2000.

58. Andersen P, Levine DL: Adhesion of fiber metal coatings. In Lemons JE (ed): Quantitative characterization and performance of porous implants for hard tissue applications, ASTM 953, Philadelphia, 1987, American Society for Testing and Materials, pp 7–15.

59. Ducheyne P, Martens M: Orderly oriented wire meshes as porous coatings on orthopaedic implants. I. Morphology. Clin Mater 1:59–67, 1986.

60. Judet R, Siguer M, Brump B, Judet T: A non-cemented total hip prosthesis. Clin Orthop Relat Res 137:76–84, 1978.

61. Lord G, Bancel P: The madreporic cementless total hip prosthesis. Clin Orthop Relat Res 176:67–76, 1978.

62. Matsui M, Nakata K, Masuhara K, et al: The metal-cancellous cementless Lubeck total hip arthroplasty: five to nine year results. J Bone Joint Surg Br 80:404–410, 1998.

63. Levine B: A new era in porous metals: applications in orthopaedics. In Lefebvre LP, Banhart J, Dunand DC (eds): Porous metals and metallic foams, Lancaster, Pa, 2008, DEStech Publications Inc, pp 251–254.

64. Zardiackas LD, Parsell DE, Dillon LD, et al: Structure, metallurgy, and mechanical properties of a porous tantalum foam. J Biomed Mater Res Appl Biomater 58:180–187, 2001.

65. Mulier M, Rys B, Moke L: Hedrocel trabecular metal monoblock acetabular cups: mid-term results. Acta Orthop Belg 72:326–331, 2006.

66. Gauthier M, Menini R, Bureau MN, et al: Properties of novel titanium foams for biomedical applications. In Shrivastava S (ed): Medical device materials. Proceedings Materials and Processes for Medical Devices Conference, September 2003, pp 382–387.

67. Yang YZ, Tian JM, Chen ZQ, et al: Preparation of graded porous titanium coatings on titanium implant materials by plasma spraying. J Biomed Mater Res 52:333–337, 2000.

68. Wen HB, de Wijn JR, Cui FZ, de Groot K: Preparation of calcium phosphate coatings on titanium implant materials by simple chemistry. J Biomed Mater Res 41:227–236, 1998.

69. Nguyen HQ, Deporter DA, Pilliar RM, et al: The effect of sol-gel-formed calcium phosphate coatings on bone ingrowth and osteoconductivity of porous-surfaced Ti alloy implants. Biomaterials 25:865–876, 2004.

70. Gan L, Wang J, Tache A, et al: Calcium phosphate sol-gel-derived thin films on porous-surfaced implants for enhanced osteoconductivity. II. Short-term in vivo studies. Biomaterials 25:5313–5321, 2004.

71. Becker P, Neumann HG, Nebe B, et al: Cellular investigation on electrochemically deposited calcium phosphate composites. J Mater Sci Mater Med 15:437–440, 2004.

72. Nishiguchi S, Kato H, Neo M, et al: Alkali- and heat-treated porous titanium for orthopaedic implants. J Biomed Mater Res 54:198–208, 2001.

73. Miyazaki T, Kim HM, Miyaji F et al: Apatite formation on chemically treated tantalum metal in body environment. In Kokubo T, Nakamura T, Miyaji F (eds): Bioceramics, vol 9, Oxford, United Kingdom, 1996, Elsevier Science, pp 317–320.

74. Barre F, Layrolle P, van Blitterswijk CA: Biomimetic coatings on titanium: a crystal growth study of octacalcium phosphate. J Mater Sci Mater Med 12:529–534, 2001.

75. Li P: Biomimetic nano-apatite coating capable of promoting bone ingrowth. J Biomed Mater Res 66:79–85, 2003.

76. Vehof JW, Spauwen Janser JA: Bone formation in calcium-phosphate-coated titanium mesh. Biomaterials 21:2003–2009, 2000.

77. Klokkevold PR, Nishimura RD, Adachi M, Caputo AM: Osseo-integration enhanced by chemical etching of the titanium

surface: a torque study in the rabbit. Clin Oral Implants Res 8:442–447, 1997.

78. Sumner DR, Turner TM, Purchio AF, et al: Enhancement of bone ingrowth by transforming growth factor-beta. J Bone Joint Surg Am 77:1135–1147, 1995.

79. Davies JE: Mechanisms of endosseous integration. Int J Prosthodont 11:391–401, 1998.

80. Kieswetter K, Schwartz Z, Hummert TW, et al: Surface roughness modulates the local production of growth factors and cytokines by osteoblast-like MG-63 cells. J Biomed Mater Res 32:55–63, 1996.

81. Boyan BD, Schwartz T: Modulation of osteogenesis via implant surface design. In Davies JE (ed): Bone engineering, Toronto, Ontario, Canada, 1999, Em Squared Inc, pp 232–239.

82. Zhao G, Raines AL, Wieland M, et al: Requirement for both micron- and submicron scale structure for synergistic responses of osteoblasts to substrate surface energy and topography. Biomaterials 28:2821–2829, 2007.

83. Ryan G, Pandit A, Apatsidis PD: Fabrication methods of porous metals for use in orthopaedic applications. Biomaterials 27:2651–2670, 2006.

84. Mullen L, Stamp RC, Brooks WK, et al: Selective laser melting: a regular unit cell approach for the manufacture of porous, titanium, bone in-growth constructs, suitable for orthopedic applications. J Biomed Mater Res B Appl Biomater 89:325–334, 2009.

85. Lin C-Y, Wirtz T, LaMarca F, Hollister SJ: Structural and mechanical evaluations of a topology optimized titanium interbody fusion cage fabricated by selective laser melting process. J Biomed Mater Res 83:272–279, 2007.

86. Melican MC, Zimmerman MC, Dhillon MS, et al: Three-dimensional printing and porous metallic surfaces: a new orthopedic application. J Biomed Mater Res 55:194–202, 2001.

87. Traini T, Mangano C, Sammons RL, et al: Direct laser metal sintering as a new approach to fabrication of an isoelastic functionally graded material for manufacture of porous titanium dental implants. Dent Mater 24:1525–1533, 2008.

CHAPTER 10

Materials in Hip Surgery: Bioactive Coatings for Implant Fixation

Dale R. Sumner and Amarjit S. Virdi

KEY POINTS

- Bioactive implant coatings are designed to improve long-term fixation, but even reduction in the time needed to obtain fixation in the absence of long-term effects would be beneficial. Important characteristics of these coatings include topography (surface roughness) and chemistry.
- The use of bioactive coatings is not likely to alter the basic principles needed to attain cementless fixation, such as initial mechanical stability and close fit to host bone, but may improve the likelihood of successful fixation when these conditions are not perfectly met.
- Implant surfaces can be functionalized in specific ways with biologically active agents such as growth factors, peptide fragments, or antibiotic drugs, which then can influence bone attachment, implant fixation strength, and susceptibility to bacterial colonization.
- Calcium phosphates are the major class of bioactive coatings tested in clinical orthopedics. These surface treatments, which often are referred to as *hydroxyapatite* because of their similarity to bone mineral, have been used for over 20 years.
- Very few well-controlled trials have compared the clinical outcomes of different implant surface treatments or bioactive coatings in orthopedics because of the long observation times needed. The use of surrogate endpoints such as roentgen stereophotogrammetric analysis (RSA) to assess implant migration could significantly shorten the development time for scientific innovations. Long-term data from implant registries and implant retrieval programs will also be critical.

The nature of the implant surface and the health status of the host affect the biological response and the ability to attain secure implant fixation. Currently, it is not clear if it would be helpful to use different bioactive coatings to maximize the response from different patients (personalized medicine).

INTRODUCTION

The need to replace and restore diseased tissues has paralleled the increase in longevity of the general population. This is particularly true in dentistry and orthopedics, where structure and function have been restored by prosthetic implants. These procedures have been enormously successful and have improved the quality of life of a large number of people. This success, for the most part, can be attributed to the body's own capacity to integrate with the implants. In return, implant materials and surface characteristics have been adopted that most efficiently elicit body responses. The surface of the implants can be modified in a variety of ways, either directly or by placing a coating to support fixation to the host bone.

Here, we review bioactive coatings for implant fixation. The term *bioactive* suggests a biological effect on surrounding tissue. The term *coating* implies the presence of a covering layer. Thus, a bioactive coating is a treatment for an implant that creates a surface layer meant to impart a biological effect. Some of the early references to bioactive coatings refer to bioglass in 1978[1] and to hydroxyapatite[2] coating of metal implants in 1980. For our purposes, the most important biological effect of a bioactive coating is one that leads to improved long-term mechanical fixation of the implant to the host. Primary mechanisms include enhanced bone-implant contact, improved architecture of peri-implant bone, and reduced chance of infection (Fig. 10-1).

The focus on enhanced long-term mechanical fixation of the implant as the desired goal is based on the supposition that secure coupling of the implant and the host bone will contribute to long-term clinical success. Even if a bioactive coating does not allow an implant to perform its intended function for a longer period (i.e., improve survivorship), decreasing the time needed to obtain fixation would be beneficial.

In the most general sense, the implant surface can vary by topography, chemistry, and surface energy.[3] In Chapter 9 of this text, considerable attention is given to topography at the macro level, as that chapter focuses on the use of porous metal coatings for implant fixation. Here we focus on various means of altering surface topography at the micrometer and nanometer scale, altering the surface chemistry, and functionalizing the surface through the addition of peptide motifs, growth

145

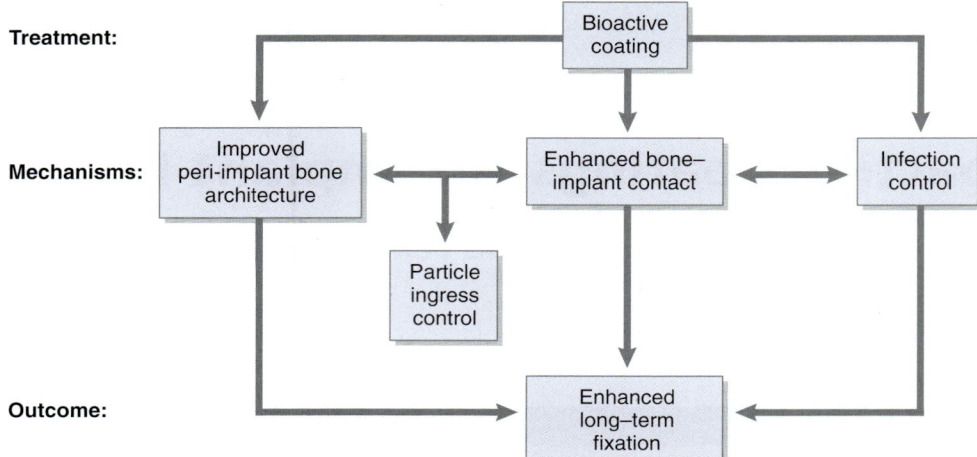

Figure 10-1. Potential mechanisms of action of bioactive coatings.

factors, or other agents to modify the response of local cells and tissues.

BASIC SCIENCE OF BIOACTIVE COATINGS

Definitions

Bioactive coatings have one major long-term function: to ensure long-term mechanical fixation of the implant to the host skeleton. The primary mechanisms by which this can happen include enhanced bone regeneration, increased bone-implant contact (even in the absence of enhanced bone regeneration), and inhibition of bacterial colonization of the implant surface. As depicted in Figure 10-1, these mechanisms are not mutually exclusive. Although it is possible to impart antibacterial properties directly to implant coatings, it is also likely that enhanced bone-implant contact indirectly inhibits infection by reducing the chance of bacterial colonization. Experimental data demonstrate that improved bone-implant contact impedes ingress of particles along the bone-implant interface.[4-6] Therefore, improved bone-implant contact not only provides stability to the implant, it also reduces the risk of implant loosening by preventing wear particle debris from migrating along the implant and causing peri-implant osteolysis.

Three key terms defining the interaction between bioactive coatings and bony tissues are *osteoinduction, osteoconduction,* and *osteointegration.*[7]

1. *Osteoinduction* refers to the ability of an agent to bring about the formation of bone tissue; it is classically assessed through observation of the ability of a putative osteoinductive agent to cause bone formation at a heterotopic site such as a subcutaneous or muscle pouch. The best known osteoinductive agents are the bone morphogenetic proteins (BMPs). Osteoinduction also occurs in bone tissue when mesenchymal cells are induced to differentiate into bone-forming osteoblasts. This process, which occurs in fracture

healing and in response to the surgical placement of implants, is discussed in greater detail later.

2. *Osteoconduction* refers to bone growth on the surface of the implant, although the term has also been defined as the ability to facilitate angiogenesis and new bone formation in the context of bone graft substitutes.[8]

3. *Osteointegration* was originally defined as direct bone-implant contact at the light microscopic level (i.e., a static result of the dynamic process of osteoconduction), but more recent definitions refer to rigid mechanical fixation of the implant in the face of functional loading.[7] For implants lacking a porous surface or other surface topography that can impart resistance to shear and tensile forces, direct bone-to-implant contact is presumably important for attaining mechanical fixation. For implants with a porous surface, interlocking of bone tissue with the porous surface can provide rigid mechanical fixation even in the absence of direct contact between the bone and the underlying implant surface.

Biological Response to Implants

All implants are perceived by the body as foreign objects; therefore, they elicit a biological response as a "nonself" material to counter any adverse effects. This reaction is based on factors related to the implant and factors related to the host. We discuss here implant-related factors that are dependent on the physical, chemical, and biological characteristics of the implant surface. We do not discuss in any detail tissue-related factors such as the implant site, patient gender and age, tissue integrity, and systemic conditions. However, the reader should appreciate that the biological response to a given implant should not be assumed to be uniform across all patients.

In general, the body's reaction to an implant is determined by the characteristics of its material of manufacture. The term *bioinert* implies that the reaction to the implant is absent. In actuality, the introduction of bioinert materials causes an interaction with surrounding tissue that can result in a minimal response. The outcome is the formation of a fibrous membrane that encapsulates the implant with no effective bonding. *Bioactive* materials, on the other hand, trigger a reaction with adjacent tissue to initiate a cascade of events leading to synthesis of new extracellular matrix, which under the best circumstances forms in close contact with the implant and leads to mechanical fixation. It is worth noting that if the implant elicits an adverse reaction, such as causing cell death in surrounding tissue, it is referred to as a *toxic* material.

In Situ Modification of Implant Surfaces

Introduction of biomaterials at the site of implantation initiates a series of events that occur on varying time scales and length scales. These events play critical roles in the eventual outcome that may result in acceptance or rejection of the biomaterial. In the orthopedic field, experience is sufficient to allow the design of materials with minimal chance of rejection, but an appreciable knowledge gap has been noted in the conditions required to maximize osseointegration and the long-term success of joint replacements. To this end, it is important to understand interactions between the implant and cells and tissues in immediate proximity to the implant.

Even before an orthopedic implant is placed in the body, the implantation site is subjected to local trauma during surgical preparation. This process causes mechanical disturbance of tissue organization and to some extent cell death due to shear stress and heat generation. It is also inevitable that the surgical procedure breaks blood vessels and results in bleeding. Therefore, this process triggers an inflammatory response that influences the implant through changes in cytokine/chemokine status and cell kinetics in the area. In addition, at this stage, there exists an opportunity for microbial infection that would adversely alter the healing process. Overall, the implant surface encounters a hostile environment that challenges its biocompatibility.

In simple terms, we can consider bioactive implant coatings as ex vivo modifications of surfaces to enhance osseointegration; however, it is worth bearing in mind that these surfaces are subject to additional changes in vivo that may lower or elevate this bioactivity. It is nearly impossible to study the relevant contributions of initial ex vivo modifications and subsequent changes due to in vivo events. Let's consider the earliest events that occur on the implant surface following implantation. According to Kasemo and colleagues, the surface is subject to modification almost immediately after placement at the surgical site.[9,10] Water molecules present in the physiologic fluid interact immediately with the implant surface and form a double layer. This interaction happens within a few nanoseconds after the implant surface is exposed to body fluid and depends on the hydrophilic/hydrophobic properties of the surface (i.e., its wettability). The aqueous layer then attracts cations and anions to form a complex that adsorbs protein biomolecules from the surroundings.

The interaction of endogenous proteins with the implant surface depends on its geometric, chemical, and electrical characteristics.[11] For example, rough surfaces provide greater area for proteins to adsorb than smooth surfaces. The local surface charge due to the distribution of cations and anions determines the adsorption of proteins with corresponding charges. The complexity of the physiologic fluid indicates a very heterogeneous distribution of proteins on the implant surface. Once a protein is adsorbed, its conformation may change, thereby exposing active sites for cell binding and intracellular signaling. The composition and organization of this protein layer determine the specificity of this interaction. The scenario described here implies that uniform cell response occurs at the implant-tissue interface once the protein layer is deposited and the cells have become attached. In fact, the composition of this protein layer is very dynamic and may change constantly over the whole process of tissue neogenesis adjacent to the implant. The composition of this layer is determined by many factors, including possible degradation of the surface material or adsorbed proteins and arrival of new proteins during the repair process and competitive binding.

Bone Repair and Regeneration

It is useful to briefly review the regenerative context in which implant fixation is seen (Fig. 10-2). Implant fixation occurs via the intramembranous pathway.[12] Careful ultrastructural examination of the titanium-bone interface in a rat model has shown that mineralized bone begins to form de novo a short distance from the implant surface at day 5.[13] Bone formation is not initiated on the implant surface or from existing bone surfaces. These early bone spicules are later encased by lamellar bone, which achieves direct contact with the titanium surface by day 14. It is possible that bioactive coatings may promote direct initial bone formation on the implant surface, but studies at this level of detail are not yet available.

The marrow ablation model provides a relatively simple means of investigating the intramembranous pathway and is typically performed in the mouse or rat.[14] In this model, medullary space in the long bones is accessed by drilling a hole in the cortical bone or the condyle. The marrow content is then mechanically removed by vacuum or is flushed out with sterile saline. Although other models can be used to study implant fixation,[15,16] the rat ablation model has proved particularly useful because it allows investigation of the reparative cascade in detail. The response to marrow ablation surgery typically is divided into three major overlapping phases: (1) inflammation, (2) repair, and (3) remodeling,[14,17,18] paralleling the concepts of fracture healing.[19] Although we will not describe details here, some agents or bioactive coatings affect only one of these phases, while other agents or coatings may have more pervasive effects. Although our understanding of the histologic changes characterizing these phases is well

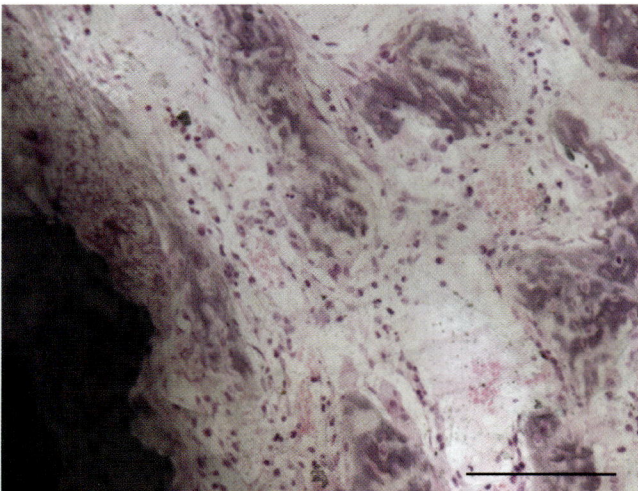

Figure 10-2. Photomicrograph at an early time point following placement of a hydroxyapatite-coated titanium implant in a rat model (7 days). Note the presence of woven bone near the implant, which is an integral part of the reparative stage of the regenerative response following surgery. This is an undecalcified plastic-embedded section, ground to approximately 50 μm and stained with basic fuchsin and toluidine blue (scale bar = 100 μm).

established, more information on the molecular and cellular mechanisms is now being gathered, including temporal and, to a limited degree, spatial patterns of gene and protein expression following marrow ablation.[17-20] It is likely that the bioactive coatings manipulate or alter these cascades, but this is a relatively unexplored area.[21] One of the important concepts is that bone repair mimics embryonic development. This is not exactly the case[19,22]; however, parallels are evident, and it does seem likely that improvements in understanding of the bone regeneration response in both the absence and presence of an implant[23] will ultimately lead to novel strategies for improving implant fixation.

Surface Topography

Surface structure is known to influence the long-term mechanical fixation of implants. Chapter 9 in this volume covers millimeter scale surface structures as provided by porous metals. Here, we describe surface topography at the micrometer and nanometer scale. Most studies have been performed in the context of dental implants[24-26]; thus, a majority of the work has been performed on commercially pure titanium. Less information is available on titanium alloys and cobalt-based alloys, which are frequently used in orthopedics.

Implant surface topography is manipulated by using subtractive processes such as polishing, blasting, acid etching, or oxidation, and by using additive processes such as coating with calcium phosphates, use of titanium via plasma spray, and ion deposition.[24] These treatments alter various quantitative characteristics defining the implant's surface roughness and

topography, including the arithmetic mean deviation of a profile (R_a) or surface (S_a)—the most frequently reported characterization parameter. In an extensive review of the literature, Wenneberg and Albrektsson[24] reached the following conclusions:

- The orientation of surface features does not determine the amount of new bone formation that has occurred (isotropic vs. anisotropic surface treatments).
- Moderately rough surfaces (R_a or S_a values of approximately 1 μm) have better bone integration than smoother or rougher surfaces (in the micrometer scale range).
- Blasted, etched, blasted+etched, and oxidized surfaces all tend to have better bone integration than machined (i.e., relatively smooth) surfaces in animal experiments, but the only clear improvement in clinical studies has been observed with oxidized surfaces.
- Plasma-sprayed titanium surfaces have better integration than smoother surfaces.
- Changes in surface topography at the nanometer level appear to affect early bone healing responses in a positive way but may not have persistent long-term effects.

It should be noted that changes in surface roughness are often accompanied by changes in surface chemistry such as charge or wettability, and it is often difficult to determine which factor is responsible for the observed effect.[25] Despite this limitation, a growing body of literature examines the response of various cell types to biomaterial surfaces in vitro.[3,27,28] These studies are often designed to answer one of two basic questions:

1. What surface characteristic will lead to the best osteointegration?
2. Which cell or molecular pathway is involved in how cells interact with surfaces?

For the first question, there is often an underlying assumption that a particular in vitro endpoint such as cell adhesion, migration, or proliferation will predict the in vivo behavior. In some cases, correlative studies now involve both in vitro and in vivo work. Variation in a number of experimental details, including characterization of the implant surface, the cell population(s) studied, the culture media used, the timing of observations, and the plating density, makes it difficult to compare individual studies. Nonetheless, a considerable amount has been learned about how cells interact with artificial materials. It is becoming clear that topographic features, surface chemistry, and surface energy affect protein attachment to the implant and, therefore, influence cell attachment, shape, proliferation, and differentiation.[3] Because of their important role in cell attachment, the integrins are key players through which cells transfer information from the implant surface to influence cell behavior.[29]

The reported experience with roughened surfaces in orthopedics is meager. In a comparison of porous coated and grit-blasted femoral stems in THA in which both types of components were further treated with a hydroxyapatite coating, the authors reported no differences in fixation or peri-implant bone remodeling at 2 years.[30] Because of the use of the hydroxyapatite coating, it is not possible to make a direct comparison of the roughened surface performance versus the porous coating performance.

Surface Chemistry

In terms of alterations in surface chemistry, we include discussions of many treatments that are meant to act through mechanisms not related to surface topography, although, as already noted, it is not always clear that these two variables can be considered independently. These surface alterations include calcium phosphate coatings, bioactive glass coatings, oxidation, and surfaces functionalized with other bioactive agents such as peptides, growth factors, and antibacterial materials. The term *biomimetic* deserves definition because it sometimes is used to describe a particular way of creating a calcium phosphate coating and sometimes is used to describe the more general concept of creating a surface that demonstrates particular functional characteristics. In orthopedics, the best investigated and most frequently used means of altering surface chemistry is to apply a calcium phosphate surface to the implant.

Calcium Phosphate Surfaces

Interest in using calcium phosphates (CaPs) as bone graft substitutes and for implant coatings has been considerable[26,31] (Fig. 10-3). The term *hydroxyapatite* (HA) refers to a particular form of CaP found in bone, and some CaPs mimic the structure and composition of bone HA. Thus, not all CaPs are HAs. CaP coatings are

bioactive because they are osteoconductive and have been shown to improve bone-implant contact and mechanical fixation of implants in the presence of interface gaps of up to 2 mm.[32] CaPs are attractive as coatings for joint replacement implants because of lack of toxicity, lack of an inflammatory response even to particulates, and direct bone bonding.[33] Some concern has arisen that pieces of CaP coatings can reach the joint surface and cause third-body wear.

Hydroxyapatite coatings seem to induce direct bone-implant bonding even in the presence of some micromotion at the interface, and low-crystallinity HA coatings may be more beneficial for early bone ingrowth. Improved bone ingrowth is associated with inhibited migration of polyethylene particles along the interface.[6] When these HA coatings are resorbed, no loss of implant fixation is apparent.

The plasma flame spray method is the most commonly used technique commercially for coating implants; it results in coating thickness in the range of 20 to 250 μm. A limitation of the plasma spray technique for applying CaP coatings is that the method is "line-of-site," meaning that surfaces not facing the source remain uncoated; there is also concern about occluding the openings of porous coated surfaces. CaP coatings can be created by a biomimetic process in which CaP nucleates from supersaturated solutions called *simulated body fluids*.[34] This technique creates thinner CaP coatings of varying composition that can cover all surfaces of implants with more complex surface topographies (i.e., porous coatings).

In vitro studies have shown that CaP surfaces promote osteogenic differentiation of human mesenchymal stem and MG-63 cells (a model of osteoblasts) even in the absence of osteogenic additives to the media.[35] These authors found elevated alkaline phosphatase activity and gene expression and increased gene expression of a key osteogenic transcription factor, Runx2.[35] Because of the importance of cell interaction with the substrate (which might mimic cell–extracellular matrix interactions in vivo), these authors investigated focal adhesions and found that the number and size of cellular structures were reduced, but their mobility was increased, when MG-63 cells were cultured on a calcium phosphate surface rather than tissue culture plastic or titanium.[35] Although it is not possible to attribute the response definitively to surface chemistry as opposed to topography, the ability to direct differentiation of cells without using exogenous growth factors is potentially very significant.

An extensive in vitro study examined the response of three cell types to different formulations of calcium phosphate in the presence and absence of adsorbed BMP-2. All formulations were of similar composition (80% hydroxyapatite and 20% β-tricalcium phosphate), with varying microstructure (pore size and porosity), crystal size, specific surface area, ability to adsorb proteins, and surface roughness. Experiments showed that the ability to concentrate proteins with increased surface area improved the ability to differentiate cells along the osteogenic lineage.[36] Cell function was not dependent upon micropore size, crystal size, or surface

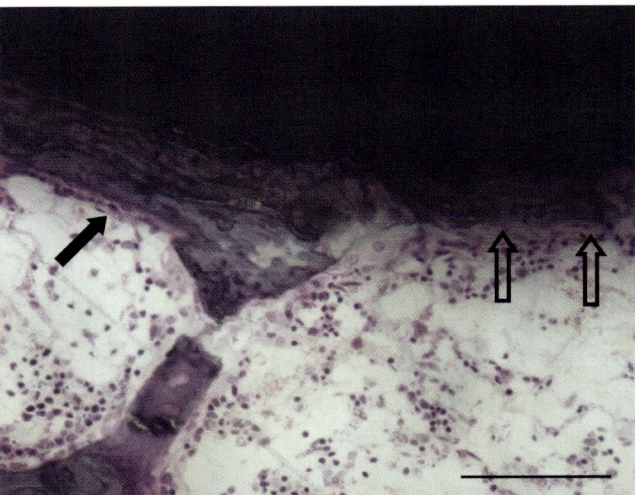

Figure 10-3. Photomicrograph at 4 weeks following placement of a hydroxyapatite-coated titanium implant in a rat model. Note the presence of lamellar bone with a row of osteoblasts *(closed arrow)* and a region of bone resorption that appears to extend into the hydroxyapatite coating *(open arrows)*, underscoring the dynamic nature of the bone-implant interface. This is an undecalcified plastic-embedded section, ground to approximately 50 μm and stained with basic fuchsin and toluidine blue (scale bar = 100 μm).

roughness. Although the conclusions are valid only for the conditions studied, this paper nicely demonstrates the complexity of sorting out factors involved in controlling cell behavior and the caution that needs to be applied when extrapolating to other surface types or cells. Some of these conditions have been associated with the ability of these different materials to promote bone attachment or to induce bone formation in vivo.[36]

Here, we briefly review the clinical data because there is now a 20+-year history of use of CaP as a bioactive coating in joint replacement. We are aware of nine studies in which the in vivo fixation of calcium phosphate–treated tibial components of total knee arthroplasty was compared with fixation of similar untreated components (Table 10-1). In all of these studies, implant fixation was assessed with roentgen stereophotogrammetric analysis (RSA), a technique that allows the study of implant migration and inducible motion at much finer sensitivity than is attained with conventional radiographic analysis. Findings tend to show that calcium phosphate coatings were associated with less implant migration, although the differences were not always statistically significant. In addition, it has been reported that HA-coated tibial components without adjuvant screw fixation had a much lower incidence of radiolucent lines at the bone-implant interface than did comparable uncoated tibial components that had adjuvant screw fixation.[37]

In general, the published literature has reported a positive clinical experience with CaP-coated implants, with survival rates typically 90% or better at 10- to 15-year follow-up.[38-43] Some reports have described high failure rates in prostheses with CaP coatings,[44] although the cause of failure was not always evident. It is interesting to note that use of an HA coating apparently was not sufficient to "protect" the interface from osteolysis in an implant system with considerable polyethylene wear.[45] Clinically, the use of HA coatings did not lead to better outcomes in knee arthroplasty at 5 years[46] or in hip arthroplasty at 10 years,[47] although in the hip study, the authors reported a lower incidence of radiolucent lines at the interface, implying improved osseointegration with the HA coating. In primary hip replacement in which patients were randomized to a proximally HA coated porous-coated femoral stem or the same stem without HA, no clinical differences in terms of Harris Hip Score or stem survivorship were noted at 4.6-year follow-up, although some slight differences were evident in radiographic findings.[48] In a paired prospective design, femoral stems with an HA coating had fewer radiolucent zones at the bone-implant interface than identical components without the HA coating at 6 years.[49] In acetabular cups with an HA coating compared with the same cups without the HA coating, less implant migration and fewer radiolucent lines were seen at the bone-implant interface as assessed radiographically, although wear rates and clinical outcomes were similar.[50] A 2-year retrospective study of the femoral component in THR showed no differences as a function of the presence of an HA coating in any of the radiographic or clinical outcomes.[51]

Other studies have found lack of evidence that HA coatings affect clinical or radiographic outcomes.[52,53] Two studies showed early enhancement of femoral stem

Table 10-1. RSA Studies of Tibial Component Migration in Total Knee Arthroplasty

Test Bioactive Coating	Control	Findings	Year Reported (Reference)
HA coated by plasma spray (Interax, Howmedica) (n = 10)	Similar implants (n = 10)	Less subsidence and transverse plane migration in HA group	1998 (107)
MG II HA/TCP coated (n = 18)	Noncoated MG II (n = 18)	Improved stability, fewer radiolucent zones	1998 (108)
HA coated (Osteonics) (n = 16), HA coated (Duracon) (n = 16)	Noncoated Osteonic (n = 15)	Reduced migration in HA groups	2000 (109)
HA coated (Freeman-Samuelson) (n = 25 knees)	Porous-coated Miller Galante II (n = 26 knees)	Less migration in HA components at 5 years and less inducible displacement at 1 year	2000 (110)
Plasma-sprayed HA-coated MG II (n = 24 knees)	Similar untreated implants (n = 27 knees)	Slight trend toward less migration in HA components at 2 years	2003 (111)
Plasma-sprayed HA (CAM implants) on a Johnson and Johnson implant) (n = 37)	Similar untreated implants (n = 40)	HA-coated implants migrated less at 2 years, but difference was not significant at 5 years	2005 (112,113)
Solution-deposited HA coating (Duracon knee, Stryker) (n = 11 [14 knees])	Similar untreated implants (n = 10 [12 knees])	Trend toward less migration, finding of less variance in HA group up to 2 years	2006 (114)
HA (plasma spray or periapatite, Howmedica) (n = 7)	Similar untreated implants (n = 7)	Trend of less migration, finding of less variance in HA group	2008 (115)
Peri-Apatite (solution-deposited HA) (n = 30)	Similar untreated implants (n = 30)	Less early subsidence in the Peri-Apatite group, but no difference at 24 months	2008 (116)

HA, Hydroxyapatite; *MG,* Miller-Galante; *RSA,* roentgen stereophotogrammetric analysis; *TCP,* tricalcium phosphate.

stability with HA coating.[54,55] At 1-year follow-up, HA-coated femoral stems had fewer proximal radiolucencies at the bone-implant interface and more evidence of proximal load transfer than non–HA-coated implants, suggesting to the authors that the HA coating was beneficial.[56] A recent report from the Swedish Hip Replacement Registry associates the use of hydroxyapatite coating with higher risk of revision of the acetabular cup for aseptic loosening,[57] and a report from the Danish Hip Arthroplasty Registry provided no clear evidence of reduced aseptic loosening for components with hydroxyapatite coatings,[58] although a trend in that direction was evident. In revision hip replacement, retrospective analysis indicated that bone fixation was improved with the use of CaP coatings, but only in the presence of Paprosky type III bone defects.[59]

With dental implants, thin CaP coatings have shown effectiveness in animal models, but lack of clinical studies leaves open the question of whether this additional surface modification offers any advantage over a simple roughened surface.[25]

Some experience with histologic analysis of calcium phosphate–coated components retrieved at revision or at autopsy has been described. In one report, the CaP coating was no longer evident, but this degradation did not negatively affect bone-implant contact in the authors' opinion.[60] In a second report, consistent bone ingrowth, degradation of the CaP coating (especially in those implants in place for longer periods), and evidence of osteoclastic resorption of the coating without adverse tissue reactions were described.[61] In a third study of HA-coated femoral stems from THR, the authors report that the histology was consistent with that of mechanically stable implants and noted that peri-implant macrophages had ingested HA particles, and that evidence showed osteoclast-mediated resorption of the HA coating.[62] A report of excessive polyethylene wear has been ascribed to migration of HA particles from an implant coating to the articulating surface.[63]

Major disadvantages of plasma-sprayed CaP coatings include inability to deposit carbonate apatite, potential for particle release and delamination, nonuniform crystallinity, inconsistent coating thickness and surface topography, line-of-site application, and inability to incorporate organic phases into the coating during application.[31] These potential limitations have motivated research into other methods of application of calcium phosphate coatings, especially in dentistry.[25] These other methods include sol-gel deposition, pulsed laser deposition, radiofrequency magnetron sputtering, ion beam–assisted deposition, electrophoretic deposition, discrete crystalline deposition, grit blasting with biocompatible bioceramics, electrospray deposition, hot isostatic pressing, dip coating, and biomimetic deposition.[26,31] The resulting coating thickness varies over several orders of magnitude (from <1 μm to 500 μm); some of the techniques are line-of-site, while others can coat complex geometries. Considerable differences have also been noted between coating methods in terms of the adhesive strength of the coating to the base metal and the inherent strength of the coating itself, the Ca/P ratio and composition of the coating,

and the cost of manufacture.[3] Each of these methods offers potential advantages and disadvantages.[31] Another study showed no difference in implant fixation in a canine model in the presence of a 1-mm interface gap between plasma spray HA, electrochemical-assisted deposition of HA, and the same coating with a collagen type I superficial layer, although all three were better than the Ti plasma spray control.[64] A recent report of an alkaline heat treatment method for applying a thin CaP coating reported a 100% implant survival rate at approximately 6 years.[38]

Bioactive Glasses

Bioactive glasses belong to the family of synthetic bioceramics that includes hydroxyapatite. These materials possess excellent osteoconductive properties and are far more bioactive than hydroxyapatite. Bioactive glasses were discovered 4 decades ago by Larry Hench and colleagues.[65-67] The original glasses consisted of four components: SiO_2, Na_2O, CaO, and P_2O_5. Since that time, combinations of other oxides (Na_2O-K_2O-CaO-MgO-P_2O_5-SiO_2) have been reported with similar properties. The bioactivity of bioactive glasses depends on their chemical composition, with the content of SiO_2 being the main determinant. To maintain bioactivity, it is critical that the content of SiO_2 is <60% (w/w) in the whole material. By keeping the content of P_2O_5 constant at 6%, varying the content of SiO_2, Na_2O, CaO has been shown to yield materials with distinct properties. Based on earlier work, 45S5 Bioglass with composition of 45% (w/w) SiO_2, 24.5% (w/w) Na_2O, 24.5% (w/w) CaO, and 6% (w/w) P_2O_5 is the most studied and best characterized bioactive glass that shows binding to bone.[65-67]

The bioactivity of bioglasses is related to the surface chemistry on the material and the effect on local cells. The chemical nature of the surface plays an immediate role by initiating a reaction on the surface when the material comes in contact with aqueous media such as body fluid.[68] This causes a rapid exchange of Na^+ or K^+ ions from the bioglass with H^+ or H_3O^+ ions from the solution, leading to dissolution of the bioglass network and loss of soluble silica (as Si^{4+}) and Ca^{2+} to the surroundings. A silica-rich layer is formed on the surface as the result of condensation of hydroxylated silica groups, and it attracts Ca^{2+} and PO_4^{3-} to form an amorphous calcium phosphate layer that later crystallizes to form a bonelike mineral. It is noteworthy that this is a physical-chemical process that precedes any of the biochemical processes associated with bone formation and takes place in the absence or with the involvement of cells. The calcium phosphate layer in itself can act as a bioactive coating by absorbing local proteins and directing new bone formation.

The other mode of action of bioglasses is the direct stimulation of cells. A number of in vitro studies have reported that bioactive glasses stimulate osteoblast growth and differentiation. This is achieved by direct contact with the bioglass or by ionic dissolution from the material.[69,70] The exact mechanism of bioglass-released Si on bone cells is not known, but gene expression studies using microarrays have revealed that a number of pathways involved in osteoblast function are affected by ionic dissolution.[71,72] These pathways include cell surface ligands and receptors, apoptosis, signal transduction, transcription and cell cycle regulation, growth factors and cytokines, and extracellular matrix components. Together, these molecular events control all aspects of osteoblast proliferation and differentiation and may explain the stimulatory effects of bioglasses in new bone formation.

With all known bioactive osteogenic and osseointegration properties of bioglasses, it is reasonable to assume that they would serve as ideal candidates for orthopedic applications, especially implant fixation. Because of their very low mechanical strength, bioglasses are not suitable for load-bearing allocations. Coating the metallic implants with a thin layer of bioactive glass would present the option of using their biological activity with mechanical strength provided by the core implant. This can be achieved by formulating the composition so that the main characteristics are retained during the enameling process. However, the problem of the coating cracking or delaminating remains. Current research is focused on improving coating composition to minimize these problems. Thus, although bioglasses may find a place as bioactive coatings for joint replacement implants in the future, very few studies related to this application can be found within the orthopedic literature. One rare study involved a canine hip replacement model that showed better early implant fixation with the use of apatite- and wollastonite-containing glass-ceramic, but no long-term differences.[73]

Oxidized Surfaces

Oxidized surfaces on titanium implants have a thicker oxide layer than is normally found with this material. These surfaces are created through heat treatments or with the implant serving as an anode in a galvanic bath, in which case the oxide layer can grow from the normal 5 nm to as large as a millimeter.[24] Other surface treatments that affect the oxide layer include enhancing the fluoride content of this layer or making it hydrophilic.[26] All of these treatments appear to have beneficial effects on early wound healing, but it is not yet clear whether these early effects will translate into stronger mechanical fixation and better clinical results.

Functionalized (Biomimetic) Surfaces

As mentioned previously, once an implant is placed in vivo, its surface is coated by a number of endogenous proteins present in the surrounding physiologic fluid. The chemical and electrical characteristics of the implant determine the types of proteins that interact with the surface and thus have an effect on the local environment. Because some of the proteins may have neutral or even negative effects on bone growth, attention has been focused on preferential attachment of molecules that promote cell attachment and activation to enhance tissue regeneration. Surfaces have been functionalized with full-length growth factors (which include the complete amino acid sequence of the factor), peptides (which include only the active motif of the

factor), antiresorptive agents, enzymes, and antibiotic agents.

Full-length growth factors are most frequently delivered via CaP coatings. For instance, our laboratory has been active in this area and has demonstrated that transforming growth factor-beta (TGF-β),[74-76] BMP-2,[77] and a combination of TGF-β and BMP-2[78] can lead to enhanced bone ingrowth into a porous coating or improved mechanical fixation. It is interesting to note that when used in combination, TGF-β and BMP-2 had additive effects, suggesting that cocktails of growth factors may be needed to maximize the biological response. CaP coatings have also been used for local delivery of antiresorptive agents, which otherwise are administered systemically. An example is the use of alendronate in a canine hip replacement model,[79] although no effect on initial implant fixation or peri-implant bone remodeling was noted. In another study, elution of zolendronate from a CaP coating was associated with elevated peri-implant bone volume and bone ingrowth in a canine model[80] and with elevated peri-implant bone volume and implant fixation strength in a rat model.[81] Studies incorporating other agents into CaP coatings are now being reported, including lithium, with the rationale being that lithium ions stimulate the Wnt signaling pathway.[82]

Small fragments of some proteins (peptides) that still retain the bioactivity of the native protein and other biomolecules have been used to mimic the biological situation. Short peptides are more stable (less susceptible to biodegradation), less likely to elicit an immune response, and more easily synthesized chemically in a cost-effective manner than full-length proteins. Perhaps one of the best studied peptide motifs is the arginine-glycine-aspartic acid (RGD) sequence for cell attachment.[83-85] This sequence signals the adhesion of cells via integrins and is present in a number of major bone extracellular matrix components such as type I collagen, osteopontin, and bone sialoprotein, as well as in other extracellular molecules (ECM) such as fibronectin, laminin, vitronectin, and fibrinogen. Modification of material surfaces with RGD-containing peptides has been shown to increase the strength of adhesion and the spreading of osteoblasts in vitro.[86,87] The use of similar modifications for in vivo studies has shown more bone regeneration around the implant but not necessarily higher implant fixation strength.[88] Other bioactive agents are currently under investigation, including coating with DNA because of its potentially beneficial biomaterial properties[89] and coating with alkaline phosphatase because of its role in mineralization.[90]

Studies in which growth factors or other noncollagenous proteins had only a marginally positive effect or no effect have been reported.[91,92] Many of these reports lack dose-response curves and have limited information on the release kinetics and bioactivity of the adsorbed protein, making it difficult to interpret the findings.

Antibacterial Surface Treatments

Silver has antibacterial properties and has been used recently in experimental models. An in vitro study showed that doping of an HA surface with silver did not adversely affect the behavior of preosteoblasts, but did inhibit the ability of bacteria to adhere to the implant.[93] A second in vitro study showed that doping a CaP surface with silver did not adversely affect formation of HA in simulated body fluid, but did have strong antibacterial activity.[94] Another in vitro study has shown that bioglass can be doped with silver ions, can maintain its biocompatibility profile, and can impart antibacterial properties.[95] Similar findings have been reported for a nanoscale titanium surface.[96] A wollastonite coating doped with silver ions showed a slight depression in the ability to form HA in simulated body fluids and strong antibacterial properties in vitro.[97] Another approach to inhibiting bacterial colonization is coating the implant with dextran.[98] These antibacterial surfaces have not yet been tested in in vivo models.

CURRENT CONTROVERSIES AND FUTURE DIRECTIONS

Some very significant gaps in knowledge are related to clinical effects and mechanisms. In both orthopedics and dentistry, well-controlled clinical trials are lacking.[99] Accordingly, it often is not clear that new surface treatments will make a difference clinically, although they may have effects in vitro and in preclinical animal studies. Part of the problem is the long lag time between initiation of treatment (i.e., placement of the implant) and the clinical endpoint of interest (e.g., failure rates at 5 or 10 years). Thus, accurate surrogate outcomes that predict long-term clinical findings are needed.

One such surrogate measurement in orthopedics may be to use RSA, which is a very sensitive method of tracking implant migration and inducible micromotion in three dimensions.[100] The method is approximately 20-fold more sensitive than planar radiographs. Based on RSA, it has been argued that early migration of the implant (1-2 mm during the first 2 years) is a good predictor of late loosening.[101,102] As reviewed previously, RSA has been used in several studies to examine implant migration following placement of joint replacement implants with bioactive coatings. Additional studies of this type should prove useful in shortening the evaluation period for novel surface treatments in the clinic.

Considerable interest has been expressed in the use of biomarkers to assess implant fixation. Imaging biomarkers such as the presence and extent of radiolucent zones at the bone-implant interface have been used. In addition, serum biomarkers may prove useful. However, in both cases, these must be considered as investigational, because it is not yet clear whether they are well validated.

Most of the preclinical in vivo studies are phenomenologic and are designed to answer a seemingly simple question—Does the surface treatment under question enhance implant fixation? In some cases, implant fixation itself is not studied, but a surrogate marker such as bone-implant contact is investigated. Lack of thorough characterization of the implant surfaces and inherent difficulties involved in altering one variable at a time (e.g., surface topography without altering surface chemistry) often make it difficult to draw conclusions about which aspects of the bioactive coating are responsible for the observed effect.[24,26]

Another limitation in developing a more thorough understanding of how bioactive coatings affect the local biology is that few in vivo studies have explored mechanisms at the tissue, cell, or molecular level. At the tissue level, a handful of reports have described how a given bioactive coating alters bone remodeling kinetics at the interface or in the peri-implant bone. Even fewer studies have explored how implant treatments affect cellular or molecular effects, such as characterizing cell types present at the interface and examining alterations in gene or protein expression. Studies that do exist have found that bioactive coatings affect the mechanical properties[103] and rates of bone remodeling of the peri-implant bone[104] and patterns of gene expression.[21]

Some work has been done to investigate the correlation between the effects of surface treatments and implant fixation and bone-implant contact or bone ingrowth, peri-implant bone volume and architecture, and peri-implant mechanical properties. Typically, about 50% of the variance in implant fixation strength is associated with variations in implant-bone contact and in peri-implant bone volume and architecture.[78] This implies that other factors, such as the material properties of the bone, are important. One recent study performed in a rat model showed that bone adjacent to acid-etched titanium implants was considerably harder and had a higher elastic modulus than bone adjacent to machined surfaces.[103] Once these relationships are better understood, there will be better treatment targets (i.e., it will be clear if it is simply a matter of increasing bone volume, or if coatings associated with bone that has enhanced intrinsic material properties are a key consideration).

Many in vitro studies have examined how alterations in implant surfaces affect the behavior of cells grown on these surfaces. In vitro cell culture performance can give information on biocompatibility and cell behavior, but these types of studies are not necessarily predictive of in vivo performance.[26] Some of these studies are based on the presumption that a robust in vivo response with a particular cell type will be predictive of the outcome of clinical applications. This is often not the case, although studies have been described in which in vitro findings were related to in vivo performance.[105,106] More of this type of work is needed so that hypotheses about mechanisms can be developed and tested. Focused investigations would also facilitate the development of robust in vitro screening assays to predict the clinical behavior of new implants and materials.

The mechanisms of action of bioactive coatings at the tissue level are not well understood (see Fig. 10-1). Potential factors include how the surface treatment affects the initial mechanical stability of the implant, how the treatment influences the "battle" between bone tissue and infectious agents in colonizing the surface, the ingress of particles along the interface, and how the surface treatment affects bone-implant contact. Bone-implant contact would, in turn, appear to be affected by several variables, including the amount of bone formation that is stimulated by the implant and the ability of the bone cells or bone matrix to attach to the implant. Molecular and cellular mechanisms will need to be correlated with these tissue level mechanisms. Although the body of in vitro studies on cell and molecular mechanisms is growing, very few in vivo studies have gone beyond tissue level effects.

Because of the clinical success of implant fixation in relatively uncomplicated cases and the relatively poor results in more challenging environments such as revision surgery and patients with significant comorbidities affecting wound healing, such as diabetes, osteoporosis, and previous chemotherapy or radiation therapy, it is likely that indications for implants depending on osseointegration will expand in the future.[25] Thus, novel animal models will be needed,[16] as will more fundamental studies exploring the underlying mechanisms of action and well-controlled clinical trials.

Despite these knowledge gaps, clinical success rates with orthopedic and dental implants are very high.[26] Improved scientific knowledge regarding underlying mechanisms is likely to yield future improvements in the clinic. The fortunate situation is that bone implants work well. Future work will lead to additional improvements, will be likely to reduce the time needed to attain secure mechanical fixation, and will provide novel means of addressing the vexing clinical problem of placing an implant in a compromised site, as often occurs in revision surgery.

REFERENCES

1. Strunz V, Bunte M, Gross UM, et al: [Coating of metal implants with the bioactive glass ceramics Ceravital]. Dtsch Zahnarztl Z 33:862–865, 1978.
2. Ducheyne P, Hench LL, Kagan A, et al: Effect of hydroxyapatite impregnation on skeletal bonding of porous coated implants. J Biomed Mater Res 14:225–237, 1980.
3. Boyan BD, Schwartz Z: Response of musculoskeletal cells to biomaterials. J Am Acad Orthop Surg 14:S157–S162, 2006.
4. Coathup MJ, Blackburn J, Goodship AE, et al: Role of hydroxyapatite coating in resisting wear particle migration and osteolysis around acetabular components. Biomaterials 26:4161–4169, 2005.
5. Bobyn JD, Jacobs JJ, Tanzer M, et al: The susceptibility of smooth implant surfaces to periimplant fibrosis and migration of polyethylene wear debris. Clin Orthop Relat Res 311:21–39, 1995.
6. Rahbeck O, Overgaard S, Soballe K: Calcium phosphate coatings for implant fixation. In Epinette JA, Manley MT (eds): Fifteen years of clinical experience with hydroxyapatite coatings in joint arthroplasty, Paris, 2004, Springer, pp 35–51.
7. Albrektsson T, Johansson C: Osteoinduction, osteoconduction and osseointegration. Eur Spine J 10(Suppl 2):S96–S101, 2001.
8. Greenwald AS, Boden SD, Goldberg VM, et al: Bone-graft substitutes: facts, fictions, and applications. J Bone Joint Surg Am 83(Suppl 2 Pt 2):98–103, 2001.
9. Kasemo B, Lausmaa J: The biomaterial-tissue interface and its analogues in surface science and technology. In The bone-biomaterial interface, Toronto, University of Toranto Press, 1991, pp 19–32.
10. Kasemo B, Gold J: Implant surfaces and interface processes. Adv Dent Res 13:8–20, 1999.
11. Dettin M: Bioactive surfaces using peptide grafting in tissue engineering. In Di Silvio L (ed): Cellular response to biomaterial, Cambridge, 2009, Woodhead Publishing Limited, pp 479–507.
12. Sumner DR, Virdi AS, Leven RM, Healy KE: Enhancing cementless fixation. In Shanbhag A, Rubash HE, Jacobs JJ (eds): Joint replacements and bone resorption: pathology, biomaterials and clinical practice, New York, NY, 2006, Taylor & Francis, pp 727–754.
13. Morinaga K, Kido H, Sato A, et al: Chronological changes in the ultrastructure of titanium-bone interfaces: analysis by light microscopy, transmission electron microscopy, and micro-computed tomography. Clin Implant Dent Relat Res 11:59–68, 2009.
14. Bab IA: Postablation bone marrow regeneration: an in vivo model to study differential regulation of bone formation and resorption. Bone 17:437S–441S, 1995.
15. Sumner DR, Turner TM, Urban RM: Animal models relevant to cementless joint replacement. J Musculoskelet Neuronal Interact 1:333–345, 2001.
16. Muschler GF, Raut VP, Patterson TE, et al: The design and use of animal models for translational research in bone tissue engineering and regenerative medicine. Tissue Eng Part B Rev 16:123–145, 2010.
17. Suva LJ, Seedor JG, Endo N, et al: Pattern of gene expression following rat tibial marrow ablation. J Bone Miner Res 8:379–388, 1993.
18. Kuroda S, Virdi AS, Dai Y, et al: Patterns and localization of gene expression during intramembranous bone regeneration in the rat femoral marrow ablation model. Calcif Tissue Int 77:212–225, 2005.
19. Bais M, McLean J, Sebastiani P, et al: Transcriptional analysis of fracture healing and the induction of embryonic stem cell-related genes. PLoS ONE 4:e5393, 2009.
20. Gerstenfeld LC, Cho TJ, Kon T, et al: Impaired intramembranous bone formation during bone repair in the absence of tumor necrosis factor-alpha signaling. Cells Tissues Organs 169:285–294, 2001.
21. De Ranieri A, Virdi AS, Kuroda S, et al: Local application of rhTGF-beta2 modulates dynamic gene expression in a rat implant model. Bone 36:931–940, 2005.
22. Bahar H, Benayahu D, Yaffe A, Binderman I: Molecular signaling in bone regeneration. Crit Rev Eukaryot Gene Expr 17:87–101, 2007.
23. Colnot C, Romero DM, Huang S, et al: Molecular analysis of healing at a bone-implant interface. J Dent Res 86:862–867, 2007.
24. Wennerberg A, Albrektsson T: Effects of titanium surface topography on bone integration: a systematic review. Clin Oral Implants Res 20(Suppl 4):172–184, 2009.
25. Junker R, Dimakis A, Thoneick M, Jansen JA: Effects of implant surface coatings and composition on bone integration: a systematic review. Clin Oral Implants Res 20(Suppl 4):185–206, 2009.
26. Coelho PG, Granjeiro JM, Romanos GE, et al: Basic research methods and current trends of dental implant surfaces. J Biomed Mater Res B Appl Biomater 88:579–596, 2009.
27. Bachle M, Kohal RJ: A systematic review of the influence of different titanium surfaces on proliferation, differentiation and protein synthesis of osteoblast-like MG63 cells. Clin Oral Implants Res 15:683–692, 2004.
28. Meyer U, Buchter A, Wiesmann HP, et al: Basic reactions of osteoblasts on structured material surfaces. Eur Cell Mater 9:39–49, 2005.
29. Olivares-Navarrete R, Raz P, Zhao G, et al: Integrin alpha-2beta1 plays a critical role in osteoblast response to micron-scale surface structure and surface energy of titanium substrates. Proc Natl Acad Sci USA 105:15767–15772, 2008.
30. Won YY, Dorr LD, Wan Z: Comparison of proximal porous-coated and grit-blasted surfaces of hydroxyapatite-coated stems. J Bone Joint Surg Am 86:124–128, 2004.
31. de Jonge LT, Leeuwenburgh SC, Wolke JG, Jansen JA: Organic-inorganic surface modifications for titanium implant surfaces. Pharm Res 25:2357–2369, 2008.
32. Dalton JE, Cook SD, Thomas KA, Kay JF: The effect of operative fit and hydroxyapatite coating on the mechanical and

biological response to porous implants. J Bone Joint Surg Am 77:97–110, 1995

33. Manley MT, Sutton K, Dumbleton J: Calcium phosphates: a survey of the orthopaedic literature. In Epinette J-A, Manley MT (eds): Fifteen years of clinical experience with hydroxyapatite coatings in joint arthroplasty, Paris, 2004, Springer, pp 9–26.

34. Barrere F, Habibovic P, DeGroot K: Biological activities of biomimetic calcium phosphate coatings. In Epinette JA, Manley MT: Fifteen years of clinical experience with hydroxyapatite coatings in joint arthroplasty, Paris, 2004, Springer, pp 55–65.

35. Muller P, Bulnheim U, Diener A, et al: Calcium phosphate surfaces promote osteogenic differentiation of mesenchymal stem cells. J Cell Mol Med 12:281–291, 2008.

36. Li X, van Blitterswijk CA, Feng Q, et al: The effect of calcium phosphate microstructure on bone-related cells in vitro. Biomaterials 29:3306–3316, 2008.

37. Gejo R, Akizuki S, Takizawa T: Fixation of the NexGen HA-TCP-coated cementless, screwless total knee arthroplasty: comparison with conventional cementless total knee arthroplasty of the same type. J Arthroplasty 17:449–456, 2002.

38. Kawanabe K, Ise K, Goto K, et al: A new cementless total hip arthroplasty with bioactive titanium porous-coating by alkaline and heat treatment: average 4.8-year results. J Biomed Mater Res B Appl Biomater 90:476–481, 2009.

39. Epinette JA, Manley MT: Is hydroxyapatite a reliable fixation option in unicompartmental knee arthroplasty? A 5- to 13-year experience with the hydroxyapatite-coated unix prosthesis. J Knee Surg 21:299–306, 2008.

40. Baltopoulos P, Tsintzos C, Papadakou E, et al: Hydroxyapatite-coated total hip arthroplasty: the impact on thigh pain and arthroplasty survival. Acta Orthop Belg 74:323–331, 2008.

41. Epinette JA, Manley MT: Uncemented stems in hip replacement—hydroxyapatite or plain porous: does it matter? Based on a prospective study of HA Omnifit stems at 15-years minimum follow-up. Hip Int 18:69–74, 2008.

42. Cross MJ, Parish EN: A hydroxyapatite-coated total knee replacement: prospective analysis of 1000 patients. J Bone Joint Surg Br 87:1073–1076, 2005.

43. Shetty AA, Slack R, Tindall A, et al: Results of a hydroxyapatite-coated (Furlong) total hip replacement: a 13- to 15-year follow-up. J Bone Joint Surg Br 87:1050–1054, 2005.

44. Kim SY, Kim DH, Kim YG, et al: Early failure of hemispheric hydroxyapatite-coated acetabular cups. Clin Orthop Relat Res 446:233–238, 2006.

45. Gallo J, Landor I, Cechova I, Jahoda D: Comparison of hydroxyapatite-coated stems in total hip arthroplasty after a minimum 10-years follow-up. Acta Chir Orthop Traumatol Cech 75:339–346, 2008.

46. Beaupre LA, al Yamani M, Huckell JR, Johnston DW: Hydroxyapatite-coated tibial implants compared with cemented tibial fixation in primary total knee arthroplasty: a randomized trial of outcomes at five years. J Bone Joint Surg Am 89:2204–2211, 2007.

47. Landor I, Vavrik P, Sosna A, et al: Hydroxyapatite porous coating and the osteointegration of the total hip replacement. Arch Orthop Trauma Surg 127:81–89, 2007.

48. Yee AJ, Kreder HK, Bookman I, Davey JR: A randomized trial of hydroxyapatite coated prostheses in total hip arthroplasty. Clin Orthop Relat Res 366:120–132, 1999.

49. Dorr LD, Wan Z, Song M, Ranawat A: Bilateral total hip arthroplasty comparing hydroxyapatite coating to porous-coated fixation. J Arthroplasty 13:729–736, 1998.

50. Moilanen T, Stocks GW, Freeman MA, et al: Hydroxyapatite coating of an acetabular prosthesis: effect on stability. J Bone Joint Surg Br 78:200–205, 1996.

51. Rothman RH, Hozack WJ, Ranawat A, Moriarty L: Hydroxyapatite-coated femoral stems: a matched-pair analysis of coated and uncoated implants. J Bone Joint Surg Am 78:319–324, 1996.

52. McPherson EJ, Dorr LD, Gruen TA, Saberi MT: Hydroxyapatite-coated proximal ingrowth femoral stems: a matched pair control study. Clin Orthop Relat Res 315:223–230, 1995.

53. Ciccotti MG, Rothman RH, Hozack WJ, Moriarty L: Clinical and roentgenographic evaluation of hydroxyapatite-augmented and nonaugmented porous total hip arthroplasty. J Arthroplasty 9:631–639, 1994.

54. Karrholm J, Malchau H, Snorrason F, Herberts P: Micromotion of femoral stems in total hip arthroplasty: a randomized study of cemented, hydroxyapatite-coated, and porous-coated stems with roentgen stereophotogrammetric analysis. J Bone Joint Surg Am 76:1692–1705, 1994.

55. Huracek J, Spirig P: The effect of hydroxyapatite coating on the fixation of hip prostheses: a comparison of clinical and radiographic results of hip replacement in a matched-pair study. Arch Orthop Trauma Surg 113:72–77, 1994.

56. Abrahams TG, Crothers OD: Radiographic analysis of an investigational hydroxyapatite-coated total hip replacement. Invest Radiol 27:779–784, 1992.

57. Lazarinis S, Karrholm J, Hailer NP: Increased risk of revision of acetabular cups coated with hydroxyapatite. Acta Orthop 81:53–59, 2010.

58. Paulsen A, Pedersen AB, Johnsen SP, et al: Effect of hydroxyapatite coating on risk of revision after primary total hip arthroplasty in younger patients: findings from the Danish Hip Arthroplasty Registry. Acta Orthop 78:622–628, 2007.

59. Bolognesi MP, Pietrobon R, Clifford PE, Vail TP: Comparison of a hydroxyapatite-coated sleeve and a porous-coated sleeve with a modular revision hip stem: a prospective, randomized study. J Bone Joint Surg Am 86:2720–2725, 2004.

60. Aebli N, Krebs J, Schwenke D, et al: Degradation of hydroxyapatite coating on a well-functioning femoral component. J Bone Joint Surg Br 85:499–503, 2003.

61. Tonino A, Oosterbos C, Rahmy A, et al: Hydroxyapatite-coated acetabular components: histological and histomorphometric analysis of six cups retrieved at autopsy between three and seven years after successful implantation. J Bone Joint Surg Am 83:817–825, 2001.

62. Bauer TW, Geesink RC, Zimmerman R, McMahon JT: Hydroxyapatite-coated femoral stems: histological analysis of components retrieved at autopsy. J Bone Joint Surg Am 73:1439–1452, 1991.

63. Bloebaum RD, Dupont JA: Osteolysis from a press-fit hydroxyapatite-coated implant: a case study. J Arthroplasty 8:195–202, 1993.

64. Daugaard H, Elmengaard B, Bechtold JE, et al: The effect on bone growth enhancement of implant coatings with hydroxyapatite and collagen deposited electrochemically and by plasma spray. J Biomed Mater Res A 92:913–921, 2010.

65. Hench LL, Paschall HA: Direct chemical bond of bioactive glass-ceramic materials to bone and muscle. J Biomed Mater Res 7:25–42, 1973.

66. Hench LL: Biomaterials. Science 208:826–831, 1980.

67. Hench LL, Wilson J: Surface active biomaterials. Science 226:630–636, 1984.

68. Valimaki VV, Aro HT: Molecular basis for action of bioactive glasses as bone graft substitute. Scand J Surg 95:95–102, 2006.

69. Silver IA, Deas J, Erecinska M: Interactions of bioactive glasses with osteoblasts in vitro: effects of 45S5 Bioglass, and 58S and 77S bioactive glasses on metabolism, intracellular ion concentrations and cell viability. Biomaterials 22:175–185, 2001.

70. Bielby RC, Christodoulou IS, Pryce RS, et al: Time- and concentration-dependent effects of dissolution products of 58S sol-gel bioactive glass on proliferation and differentiation of murine and human osteoblasts. Tissue Eng 10:1018–1026, 2004.

71. Bombonato-Prado KF, Bellesini LS, Junta CM, et al: Microarray-based gene expression analysis of human osteoblasts in response to different biomaterials. J Biomed Mater Res A 88:401–408, 2009.

72. Jell G, Stevens MM: Gene activation by bioactive glasses. J Mater Sci Mater Med 17:997–1002, 2006.

73. Ido K, Matsuda Y, Yamamuro T, et al: Cementless total hip replacement: bio-active glass ceramic coating studied in dogs. Acta Orthop Scand 64:607–612, 1993.

74. Sumner DR, Turner TM, Purchio AF, et al: Enhancement of bone ingrowth by transforming growth factor beta. J Bone Joint Surg Am 77:1135–1147, 1995.

75. Sumner DR, Turner TM, Urban RM, et al: Locally delivered rhTGF-beta$_2$ enhances bone ingrowth and bone regeneration at local and remote sites of skeletal injury. J Orthop Res 19:85–94, 2001.

76. Sumner DR, Turner TM, Cohen M, et al: Aging does not lessen the effectiveness of TGF-β$_2$ enhanced bone regeneration. J Bone Miner Res 18:730–736, 2003.

77. Sumner DR, Turner TM, Urban RM, et al: Locally delivered rhBMP-2 enhances bone ingrowth and gap healing in a canine model. J Orthop Res 22:58–65, 2004.

78. Sumner DR, Turner TM, Urban RM, et al: Additive enhancement of implant fixation following combined treatment with rhTGF-beta2 and rhBMP-2 in a canine model. J Bone Joint Surg Am 88:806–817, 2006.

79. Mochida Y, Bauer TW, Akisue T, Brown PR: Alendronate does not inhibit early bone apposition to hydroxyapatite-coated total joint implants: a preliminary study. J Bone Joint Surg Am 84:226–235, 2002.

80. Tanzer M, Karabasz D, Krygier JJ, et al: The Otto Aufranc Award: bone augmentation around and within porous implants by local bisphosphonate elution. Clin Orthop Relat Res 441:30–39, 2005.

81. Suratwala SJ, Cho SK, Van Raalte JJ, et al: Enhancement of periprosthetic bone quality with topical hydroxyapatite-bisphosphonate composite. J Bone Joint Surg Am 90:2189–2196, 2008.

82. Wang J, de Groot K, Van Blitterswijk C, De Boer J: Electrolytic deposition of lithium into calcium phosphate coatings. Dent Mater 25:353–359, 2009.

83. Dettin M, Conconi MT, Gambaretto R, et al: Effect of synthetic peptides on osteoblast adhesion. Biomaterials 26:4507–4515, 2005.

84. Massia SP, Hubbell JA: Covalently attached GRGD on polymer surfaces promotes biospecific adhesion of mammalian cells. Ann N Y Acad Sci 589:261–270, 1990.

85. Xiao SJ, Textor M, Spencer ND, et al: Immobilization of the cell-adhesive peptide Arg-Gly-Asp-Cys (RGDC) on titanium surfaces by covalent chemical attachment. J Mater Sci Mater Med 8:867–872, 1997.

86. Rezania A, Thomas CH, Branger AB, et al: The detachment strength and morphology of bone cells contacting materials modified with a peptide sequence found within bone sialoprotein. J Biomed Mater Res 37:9–19, 1997.

87. Rezania A, Healy KE: Biomimetic peptide surfaces that regulate adhesion, spreading, cytoskeletal organization, and mineralization of the matrix deposited by osteoblast-like cells. Biotechnol Prog 15:19–32, 1999.

88. Barber TA, Ho J, De Ranieri A, et al: Peri-implant bone formation and implant integration strength of peptide-modified p(AAm-co-EG/AAc) IPN coated titanium implants. J Biomed Mater Res A 80:306–320, 2007.

89. Schouten C, van den Beucken JJ, Meijer GJ, et al: In vivo bioactivity of DNA-based coatings: an experimental study in rats. J Biomed Mater Res A 92:931–941, 2010.

90. Schouten C, van den Beucken JJ, de Jonge LT, et al: The effect of alkaline phosphatase coated onto titanium alloys on bone responses in rats. Biomaterials 30:6407–6417, 2009.

91. Schouten C, Meijer GJ, van den Beucken JJ, et al: Effects of implant geometry, surface properties, and TGF-beta1 on peri-implant bone response: an experimental study in goats. Clin Oral Implants Res 20:421–429, 2009.

92. O'Toole GC, Salih E, Gallagher C, et al: Bone sialoprotein-coated femoral implants are osteoinductive but mechanically compromised. J Orthop Res 22:641–646, 2004.

93. Chen W, Oh S, Ong AP, et al: Antibacterial and osteogenic properties of silver-containing hydroxyapatite coatings produced using a sol gel process. J Biomed Mater Res A 82:899–906, 2007.

94. Noda I, Miyaji F, Ando Y, et al: Development of novel thermal sprayed antibacterial coating and evaluation of release properties of silver ions. J Biomed Mater Res B Appl Biomater 89:456–465, 2009.

95. Verne E, Miola M, Vitale BC, et al: Surface silver-doping of biocompatible glass to induce antibacterial properties. Part I. Massive glass. J Mater Sci Mater Med 20:733–740, 2009.

96. Feng Y, Cao C, Li BE, et al: [Primary study on the antibacterial property of silver-loaded nano-titania coatings]. Zhonghua Yi Xue Za Zhi 88:2077–2080, 2008.

97. Li B, Liu X, Cao C, et al: Biological and antibacterial properties of plasma sprayed wollastonite/silver coatings. J Biomed Mater Res B Appl Biomater 91:596–603, 2009.

98. Shi Z, Neoh KG, Kang ET, et al: Titanium with surface-grafted dextran and immobilized bone morphogenetic protein-2 for inhibition of bacterial adhesion and enhancement of osteoblast functions. Tissue Eng Part A 15:417–426, 2009.

99. Esposito M, Murray-Curtis L, Grusovin MG, et al: Interventions for replacing missing teeth: different types of dental implants. Cochrane Database Syst Rev (4):CD003815, 2007.

100. Selvik G: Roentgen stereophotogrammetry: a method for the study of the kinematics of the skeletal system. Reprint from the original 1974 thesis. Acta Orthop Scand 60(Suppl 232):1–51, 1989.

101. Kärrholm J, Borssen B, Lowenhielm G, Snorrason F: Does early micromotion of femoral stem prostheses matter? J Bone Joint Surg Br 76:912–917, 1994.

102. Ryd L, Albrektsson BEJ, Carlsson L, et al: Roentgen stereophotogrammetric analysis as a predictor of mechanical loosening knee prostheses. J Bone Joint Surg Br 77:377–383, 1995.

103. Butz F, Aita H, Wang CJ, Ogawa T: Harder and stiffer bone osseointegrated to roughened titanium. J Dent Res 85:560–565, 2006.

104. Suzuki K, Aoki K, Ohya K: Effects of surface roughness of titanium implants on bone remodeling activity of femur in rabbits. Bone 21:507–514, 1997.

105. Schwartz Z, Raz P, Zhao G, et al: Effect of micrometer-scale roughness of the surface of Ti6Al4V pedicle screws in vitro and in vivo. J Bone Joint Surg Am 90:2485–2498, 2008.

106. Oron A, Agar G, Oron U, Stein A: Correlation between rate of bony ingrowth to stainless steel, pure titanium, and titanium alloy implants in vivo and formation of hydroxyapatite on their surfaces in vitro. J Biomed Mater Res A 91:1006–1009, 2009.

107. Nelissen RG, Valstar ER, Rozing PM: The effect of hydroxyapatite on the micromotion of total knee prostheses: a prospective, randomized, double-blind study. J Bone Joint Surg Am 80:1665–1672, 1998.

108. Regner L, Carlsson L, Karrholm J, Herberts P: Ceramic coating improves tibial component fixation in total knee arthroplasty. J Arthroplasty 13:882–889, 1998.

109. Toksvig-Larsen S, Jorn LP, Ryd L, Lindstrand A: Hydroxyapatite-enhanced tibial prosthetic fixation. Clin Orthop Relat Res 370:192–200, 2000.

110. Regner L, Carlsson L, Karrholm J, Herberts P: Tibial component fixation in porous- and hydroxyapatite-coated total knee arthroplasty: a radiostereometric evaluation of migration and inducible displacement after 5 years. J Arthroplasty 15:681–689, 2000.

111. Hildebrand R, Trappmann D, Georg C, et al: [What effect does the hydroxyapatite coating have in cementless knee arthroplasty?]. Orthopade 32:323–330, 2003.

112. Carlsson A, Bjorkman A, Besjakov J, Onsten I: Cemented tibial component fixation performs better than cementless fixation: a randomized radiostereometric study comparing porous-coated, hydroxyapatite-coated and cemented tibial components over 5 years. Acta Orthop 76:362–369, 2005.

113. Onsten I, Nordqvist A, Carlsson AS, et al: Hydroxyapatite augmentation of the porous coating improves fixation of tibial components: a randomised RSA study in 116 patients. J Bone Joint Surg Br 80:417–425, 1998.

114. van der Linde MJ, Garling EH, Valstar ER, et al: Periapatite may not improve micromotion of knee prostheses in rheumatoid arthritis. Clin Orthop Relat Res 448:122–128, 2006.

115. Therbo M, Lund B, Jensen KE, Schroder HM: Effect of bioactive coating of the tibial component on migration pattern in uncemented total knee arthroplasty: a randomized RSA study of 14 knees presented according to new RSA-guidelines. J Orthop Traumatol 9:63–67, 2008.

116. Hansson U, Ryd L, Toksvig-Larsen S: A randomised RSA study of Peri-Apatite HA coating of a total knee prosthesis. Knee 15:211–216, 2008.

CHAPTER 11

Biological Responses to Particle Debris

Stuart Goodman and Ting Ma

KEY POINTS

- Periprosthetic osteolysis is an adverse biological reaction due to wear particles from joint replacements. Other contributory factors include increased intra-articular pressure and contamination of particles with bacterial or cellular by-products.
- Excessive wear particle production stimulates a nonspecific chronic inflammatory reaction that results in increased bone degradation and decreased bone formation.
- Interactions among many cell types, including macrophages, foreign body giant cells, osteoclasts, fibroblasts, osteoblasts, and their precursors, are important to the development of osteolytic reactions. Lymphocytes and other immune cells may modulate these biological processes.
- Cytokines, chemokines, prostanoids, nitric oxide and superoxide metabolites, receptor activator of nuclear factor kappa B (NFκB) (RANK), and other factors are the main biological mediators of osteolysis.
- Particle characteristics, including type of material, number (particle load), shape, surface area, surface energy, and other factors, determine the response of cells to particles. Individual patient characteristics may also modulate the extent of the adverse response to wear particles.
- Improved bearing couples that decrease the overall particle load will undoubtedly decrease the incidence and consequences of periprosthetic osteolysis. Increased understanding of the cellular and molecular biological principles underlying particle disease may facilitate the development of novel pharmacologic approaches to treatment of this problem.

INTRODUCTION

Overview

Wear—loss of material from the surfaces of the bearing couple—inevitably occurs with use of total joint replacements, leading to the production of particulate debris. According to McKellop, hundreds of thousands to millions of particles are produced from a metal-on-conventional-polyethylene total hip replacement with

each step.[1] The body normally distributes this debris locally and regionally via phagocytosis of particles by macrophages and other cells, leading to activation of cells to produce proinflammatory mediators. Despite the ongoing generation of small amounts of particulate debris, a state of homeostasis normally exists in the joint and surrounding tissues, and the minor localized biological reaction to wear debris has minimal consequences.[2] However, when the host reaction to wear debris and associated by-products is excessive and persistent (state of decompensation), chronic inflammation can lead to periprosthetic bone loss by biological processes that increase bone degradation and inhibit bone formation. This pathologic process is called *particle-associated periprosthetic osteolysis* or, among joint replacement surgeons and researchers, simply *osteolysis*. Although we normally think of osteolysis as a radiologic phenomenon (loss of bone on a radiograph of a joint replacement on follow-up), osteolysis is a complex pathophysiologic process with potentially major adverse clinical implications. This chapter will review the basic science underlying the biological reactions to wear debris from polymeric, metallic, and ceramic implants.

BASIC SCIENCE

The Bone-Implant Interface: Histology, Cell, and Molecular Biology

Regardless of whether a hip prosthesis is cemented or cementless, or contains a bioactive surface coating, long-term implant stability within bone is a prerequisite for optimal pain-free function. During the "surgical trauma" of prosthesis implantation, an inflammatory response is initiated in which proinflammatory mediators are released locally. This begins a cascade of events resulting in the resorption of dead bone and marrow contents, and the accretion of new bone immediately surrounding the implant.[3] Over the ensuing weeks to months, the prosthesis becomes surrounded by a network of bony trabeculae, which undergo remodeling according to local biological influences and mechanical loads. Thus, the bone-implant interface is a dynamic structure that matures and remodels over time, long after the prosthesis is implanted. Long-term prosthesis stabilization is possible whether the method of fixation is cemented or cementless.[4-6] However, if the cement

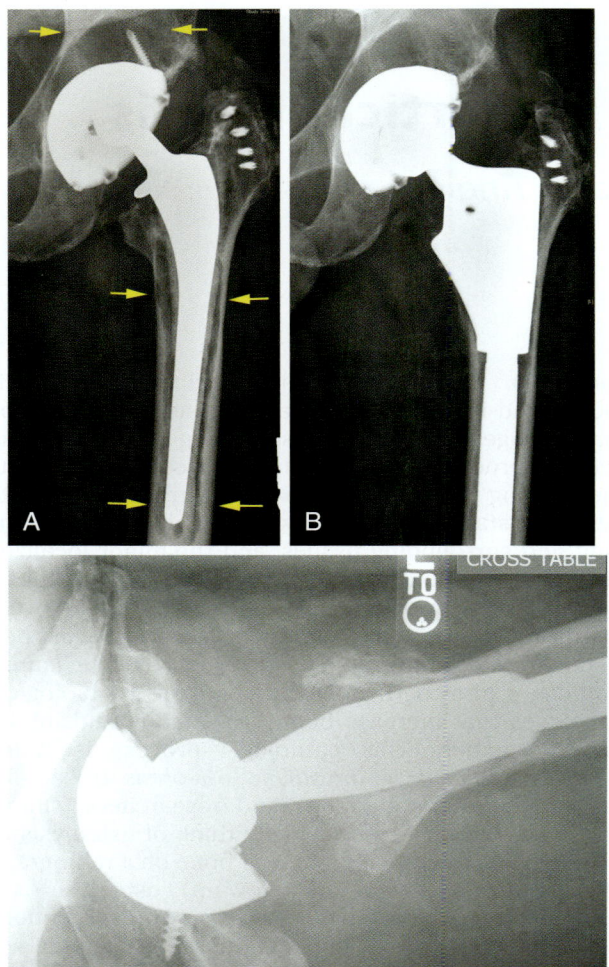

Figure 11-1. Total hip replacement with polyethylene wear, acetabular osteolysis, and loosening and osteolysis around the cemented femoral component. **A,** Preoperative radiograph. The *upper arrows* point to the acetabular osteolysis. Note the eccentrically positioned femoral head indicating wear of the plastic. The cemented femoral component is loose, and the prosthesis has subsided within the bone. The cement mantle has fragmented. Cement debris has led to scalloping of the surrounding bone *(lower arrows).* Postoperative anteroposterior **(B)** and lateral **(C)** radiographs of the revised hip replacement. The osteolytic areas in the acetabulum were bone grafted, and the acetabular plastic liner and femoral component were changed.

mantle fractures and degrades, or if excessive amounts of wear debris are produced from articulating and nonarticulating interfaces, an aggressive chronic inflammatory reaction can develop in response to foreign bodies, which may result in periprosthetic osteolysis[7-13] (Fig. 11-1).

Examination of periprosthetic tissues retrieved at surgery has allowed identification of some of the key histologic characteristics and biological mediators of bone destruction and remodeling. If the prosthesis is well fixed to bone, there little tissue is often found at the interface. This is true whether the prosthesis is cemented or cementless.[6] The fibrohistiocytic tissues surrounding loose implants (with or without radiographic osteolysis) usually contain debris from various materials implanted in the operative site[9,14,15] (Fig. 11-2). These particles vary in size from the submicron (exceeding the visual capabilities of the light microscope) to larger shards of particles often several hundreds of microns in length. As we will see later, particles in the phagocytosable range, up to about 10 microns in size, and especially those around 1 micron in size or smaller, appear to be most stimulatory to cells.

Willert and associates first described the biology of prosthetic stabilization and recognized that continuous production of wear particles involved many cell types from hematopoietic and mesenchymal cell lineages. Normally, a state of prosthesis-tissue homeostasis exists, and the particle load that is generated is dealt with by normal clearance mechanisms without adverse consequences.[2] However, if these mechanisms are overwhelmed (state of decompensation) as the result of excessive production of debris or other causes, osteolysis due to cellular activation and bone resorption will ensue. It is interesting to note that Willert described the pathophysiology of prosthetic loosening long before others postulated more widespread distribution of particles into an "effective joint space," or that increased hydraulic pressure with loading of the limb resulted in fluid flow around the prosthesis, distributing inflammatory cells and factors more extensively.[13,16-18] Charnley first believed that areas of osteolysis around hip replacements were the result of low-grade infection.[5]

Cemented metal-on-polyethylene hip implants that are still well functioning may already demonstrate histologic findings consistent with excessive wear particle production.[9] In autopsy specimens, the density of macrophages and foreign body giant cells in periprosthetic tissues was found to correlate with time after prosthetic implantation, membrane thickness, and polyethylene particle density. Wear particles in the joint gain access to the edges of the prosthesis interface, and then migrate in centripetal fashion through the fibrous interface and the cancellous bone.[13,19] Examination of tissues harvested from cemented implants has revealed that the most critical factor associated with radiologic osteolysis was the concentration of polyethylene (PE) particles in the membranous tissue interface.[20] In cementless implants, fibrous tissue present at the prosthetic interface functions as a conduit for migration of particles from the joint articulation into immediate periprosthetic tissues.[21]

Goldring and colleagues were among the first to apply the techniques of cell biology to tissues retrieved from revised implants.[14,15] Using histologic, cell, and organ culture methods, they showed that tissue around loose cemented prostheses contained a pseudosynovial layer adjacent to the cement. Particles of polymethylmethacrylate (PMMA) bone cement within the membrane were found to be surrounded and engulfed by mononucleated and multinucleated macrophages and foreign body giant cells in a fibrovascular stroma. Lymphocytes were

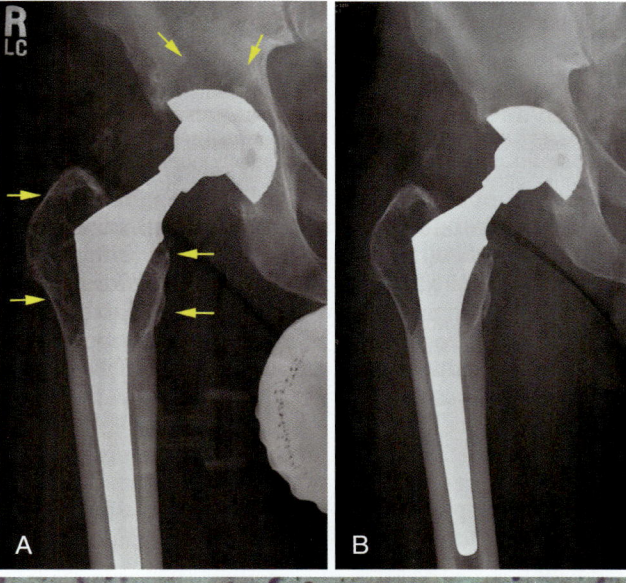

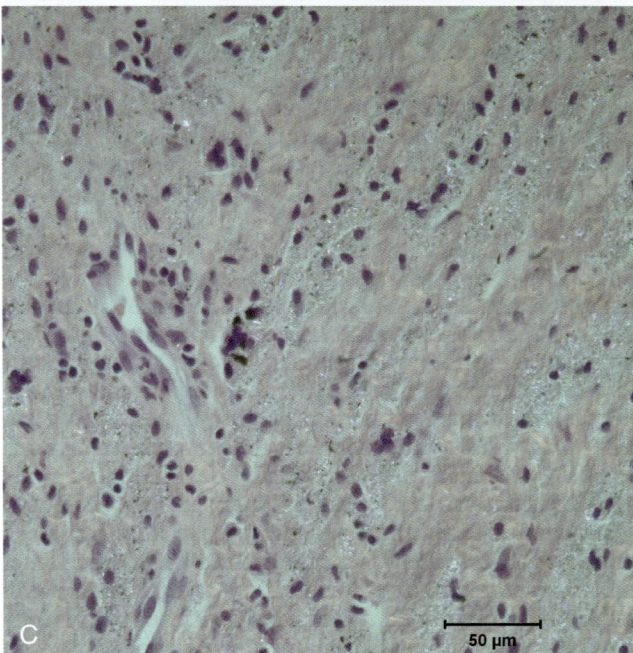

Figure 11-2. Total hip replacement with polyethylene wear and osteolysis. **A,** This metal-on-polyethylene cementless total hip replacement demonstrates eccentricity of the head within the polyethylene liner, indicating substantial wear of the plastic. Extensive osteolysis is seen around the metal socket and in the proximal femur *(arrows)*. **B,** Postoperative radiograph after polyethylene liner and femoral head exchange. The osteolytic lesions were débrided and then filled with bone graft. The acetabular shell and the femoral component were well fixed and in satisfactory position. **C,** Photomicrograph of histologic section from tissue retrieved from granulomatous synovial capsular tissues demonstrates sheets of macrophages in a fibrovascular stroma. Abundant granular white specks of polyethylene and black metal particles are seen (hematoxylin and eosin stain, polarized light, ×40 magnification).

seen more rarely. Culture and analysis of the membrane showed that it had the capacity to produce large amounts of prostaglandin (PG)E_2 and collagenase and enhanced bone-resorbing activity. Since these seminal studies were conducted, numerous investigators have shown that osteolytic membranes from failed prostheses express numerous degradative enzymes, cytokines, chemokines, nitrogen oxide and superoxide metabolites, and other proinflammatory and anti-inflammatory molecules[22-31] (Fig. 11-3).

In rare cases, an aggressive granulomatous reaction develops, with localized, progressively expanding areas of bone lysis containing activated macrophages, fibroblasts, and other cells. It is postulated that these cases may be due to an uncoupling of events that normally lead to monocyte-macrophage clearance of wear particles via the nonspecific foreign body reaction and fibroblast-mediated formation and remodeling of the extracellular tissue matrix.[32-34] However, the periprosthetic tissues are heterogeneous; biopsies from different areas may yield different histologic and cytokine profiles.[35] It is interesting to note that the bony interface surrounding loose hip and knee prostheses presents histologic evidence of both bone destruction and active bone formation, which implies that even during osteolysis, an active reparative process is ongoing.[36] Thus, heightened alkaline phosphatase activity, a marker of bone formation, has been noted at the bony surface surrounding areas of osteolysis.[36]

NFκB is a transcription factor that regulates numerous proinflammatory and anti-inflammatory pathways. Tumor necrosis factor-alpha (TNF-α) and interleukin-1β are two proinflammatory cytokines that play an important role in particle-associated periprosthetic osteolysis; they are under the regulatory control of NFκB. RANK (receptor activator of NFκB), a membrane-bound receptor on the surface of osteoclasts, activates the transcription factor NFκB. Receptor activator of nuclear factor kappa-B ligand (RANKL), a member of the TNF superfamily, is a receptor ligand that is released from osteoblasts, stromal cells, and other activated cells in the inflammatory process. RANKL interacts with RANK, which, together with macrophage colony-stimulating factor (M-CSF), is essential for the differentiation and maturation of tissue monocytes/macrophages into bone-resorbing osteoclasts RANKL is inhibited by the soluble decoy protein receptor antagonist osteoprotegerin (OPG). Studies have shown increased expression of RANKL and M-CSF and decreased OPG in the synovial fluid and periprosthetic tissues of revised prostheses exhibiting radiographic osteolysis.[37-44]

The host reaction to metal-on-polyethylene implants is generally thought to be both a nonspecific foreign body reaction and a chronic inflammatory reaction. Although attempts have been made to demonstrate an important role for T and B lymphocytes, it would appear that lymphocytes play an immunomodulatory rather than a primary role. Nevertheless, evidence of antigen presentation to lymphocytes has been reported in metal-on-polyethylene joint replacements.[45,46] These biological pathways should be distinguished from the T cell–mediated, antigen-associated type IV allergic

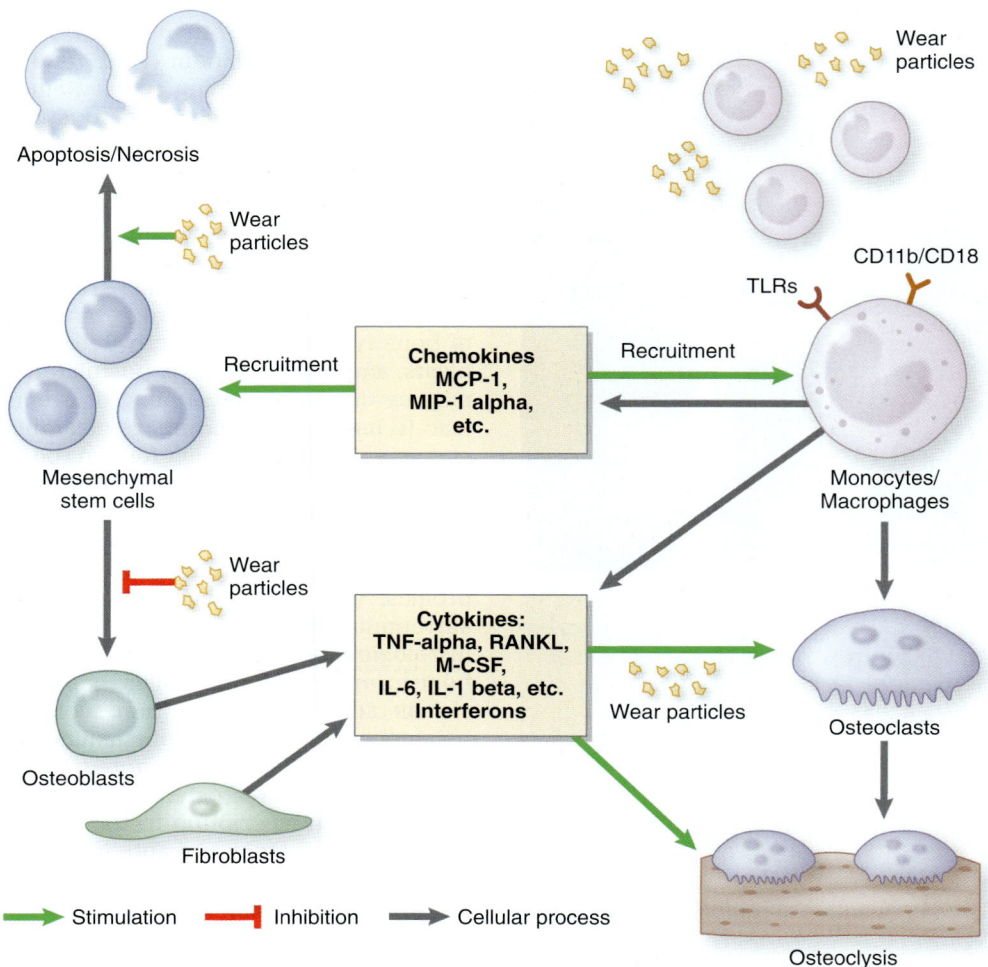

Figure 11-3. Diagram of the biological reactions associated with wear particles.

reactions seen in cases of metal-on-metal implants, which are discussed in Chapter 12.[47-52]

In Vivo Animal Models and In Vitro Studies

In Vivo Studies

Numerous in vivo animal models and in vitro studies have attempted to simulate the biological processes associated with particle-induced osteolysis and to identify the critical variables and mechanisms underlying particulate disease. Animal models have included various small and large species, with and without weight-bearing implants, particles with different material properties and characteristics, and harvest periods that have varied from hours to many months. Many of these in vivo models have been summarized in recent review articles[22,31,53-56] (Table 11-1). It is often difficult to make definitive statements about particle-induced osteolysis on the basis of in vivo animal models because of the different variables used in each model and the relatively short duration of animal studies (weeks and months) compared with the period required for development of clinical and radiologic osteolysis in humans

Table 11-1. Animal Models Currently Used to Study Wear Debris–Induced Inflammation

Species	Type of Model	Key References
Mouse	Calvarial	148, 188, 189
Mouse	Air pouch	127, 128, 190
Mouse	Intramedullary implant with particles—femur	119-121
Rat	Intra-articular or intramedullary—femur	116, 118, 166, 191
Rabbit	Intramedullary—femur	192-194
Rabbit	Harvest chamber—tibia	62, 195, 196
Dog	Pistoning implant - femoral condyle	107
Dog	Intramedullary–hip replacement	175, 197, 198
Sheep	Intra-articular injection–hip replacement	199

(years). However, experiments performed in animal models have provided some useful concepts that can be generalized to periprosthetic reactions in humans.

The biological pathways involved in foreign body and chronic inflammatory reactions are complex, redundant, and difficult to inhibit completely. As mentioned previously, numerous cellular constituents and inflammatory factors participate in this reaction. Furthermore, various characteristics, including the material, number, size, shape, surface area, topography, and surface chemistry of particulate debris, have been shown to influence the cellular and inflammatory profile.[25,57-62] In general, bulk materials produce a more benign interface compared with the same volume of material in particulate form. Smaller particles that are phagocytosable, especially those around 1 micron or smaller, appear to be the most reactive. However, very small particles, less than about 0.3 microns, do not appear to activate cells as they undergo pinocytosis rather than phagocytosis. Smaller particles may agglomerate together and therefore become much larger than the individual particles. This is especially true for polymers such as polyethylene. Irregularly shaped particles are more activating than rounder particles. In general, excluding the type IV cell-mediated immune reactions that are sometimes seen with metals, particulate materials such as alumina ceramics evoke less of a foreign body and chronic inflammatory reaction compared with metals (e.g., titanium alloy, cobalt chrome alloy, tantalum) at the same dose.[63]

Particulate polymers such as polyethylene and polymethylmethacrylate evoke the most exuberant reactions. In one study in which PE particles incited an inflammatory response, the same concentration of cobalt chrome alloy particles caused cell necrosis.[62] These experiments are controversial though because of difficulties involved in obtaining and exposing cells to particles of similar doses, shapes, surface areas, surface chemistries, and so forth. For example, highly cross-linked PE particles have been found to be more bioreactive (i.e., they produce more inflammatory cytokines) than similar particles of conventional polyethylene in vitro.[58,60] However, in vivo wear of highly cross-linked polyethylene is far less than that of conventional polyethylene, thereby presenting a much lower particle load to the body. It is clear that there is a need for standardized in vitro and in vivo models using standardized particles with known characteristics to more clearly delineate the biological effects of particles.

In Vitro Studies

In vitro studies performed over the past 20 years have clearly shown that wear particles can activate cells, resulting in the production of proinflammatory cytokines, chemokines, prostanoids, nitrogen oxide and superoxide metabolites, degradative enzymes, and other molecules. Indeed, the production of proinflammatory and anti-inflammatory factors is determined by the local presence of sufficient numbers of wear particles. In other words, there is a dose-response relationship between the amount of debris and the degree of cell activation. The type and magnitude of the reaction are also governed by the particle material, size, and shape, as well as by topography, surface area, surface chemistry and energy, contamination with other ligands, and other factors.* Indeed, particles do not necessarily have to be phagocytosed to activate cells; the particle-protein complex is able to activate cells by interacting with the cell surface integrins.[71]

In past experiments performed in vitro to study particle-induced cell activation, much emphasis was placed on traditional proinflammatory cytokines, such as TNF-α, interleukin (IL)-1 beta (IL-1β), and IL-6.[78-80] However, the list of proinflammatory and anti-inflammatory mediators released from particle-exposed cells is almost endless. Furthermore, although macrophages have generally been used for in vitro cell stimulation studies, mediator release has been documented for other cell types, including fibroblasts,[31,56,81-87] osteoblasts,[85,88-94] and other cells. Indeed, some particles appear to be more toxic for macrophages than fibroblasts.[95]

Osteoblasts are derived from mesenchymal stem cells (MSCs), which become osteoprogenitors after further cellular differentiation. Recent research has shown that MSCs and osteoprogenitors are adversely affected by orthopedic materials in particulate form.[25,96] These adverse effects have been shown for particles of titanium, cobalt chrome, polymethylmethacrylate and polyethylene.[97-102] In general, particles in sufficient doses suppress MSC proliferation, differentiation, and maturation. This is reflected in decreased total DNA, decreased expression of osteoblastic markers such as osteocalcin and osteoblast-specific transcription factors, and decreased calcified matrix as seen in the von Kossa stain.

Pressure. Although it is beyond the scope of this chapter to review the effects of pressure on cells in general, in the context of implant fixation, pressure can also cause alterations in local bone remodeling, including new bone formation and osteolysis.[103] This fact has been known for some time: clinical cases in which implants have subsided during loading are often associated with pressure-induced widening of the medullary canal, thinning of the cortices, and the presence of a bony pedestal distal to the implant. During each step, hip and knee implants are loaded in a way that is dependent on the magnitude and direction of the loads, the anatomic shape, the mechanical characteristics, and the material properties of the bone and prosthesis.

Normally, a thin layer of synovial fluid bathes the natural or replaced joint articulation; this fluid is pumped into contiguous accessible areas of the joint, also known as the *effective joint space,* during loading of the limb, much like a hydraulic piston. Increased fluid production within the joint (synovitis) will cause increased intra-articular pressure during loading; this pressure will be transmitted to the joint space and contiguous areas. An increased number of wear particles may overwhelm the local homeostatic mechanisms, resulting in transport of fluid laden with wear particles,

---

*References 22, 31, 59, 60, and 64-77.

cellular infiltrates, proinflammatory factors, and other molecules into the effective joint space.[2,13] This may lead to osteolysis remote from the source of particle generation, as is seen in cases of polyethylene wear with widespread osteolysis around the femoral stem.

In vivo animal studies have confirmed that pressure alone can lead to bone remodeling, mostly in an adverse fashion.[16-18,104,105] Indeed particles and cyclical loading, pressure, and mechanical strain have been shown to be synergistic.[106-108] Although these animal models are somewhat different from the clinical situation, they do illustrate the point that pressure can induce adverse bone remodeling in the absence of wear particles.

Particles, Endotoxin, and Bacterial By-products

When particles are generated, they are immediately coated with specific serum proteins.[109,110] Bacteria and their by-products may also attach to particles. Many of the earlier in vitro and in vivo studies probably were performed with particles unknowingly contaminated with bacterial by-products. This is a serious problem because endotoxin and other bacterial antigens attached to orthopedic particles are powerful stimuli for cell activation and proinflammatory cytokine release.[75,111-114] Studies have also shown that retrieved wear particles that have been processed to rid particles of endotoxin have blunted stimulatory effects on macrophages. When endotoxin-coated particles were introduced to the same cells, the cells became activated as evidenced by heightened proinflammatory cytokine release. One may criticize these studies on the grounds that strong acids and bases, substances that surely would alter the surface chemistry and energy of the particles, were used to rid the particle surface of endotoxin. As a result, particle-protein surface interaction with cells would be changed, possibly resulting in attenuated cellular activation. Nevertheless, the issue of implant contamination by bacterial by-products has gained increasing interest because of recent reports that lipopolysaccharide (LPS) has been detected on failed retrieved implants that were revised for supposed aseptic loosening.[115] Whether remote bacterial contamination induced prosthetic loosening (despite the absence of overt bacterial infection at retrieval) or loosening preceded bacterial colonization of the prosthesis is currently unknown.

RECENT DEVELOPMENTS IN PARTICLE DISEASE: NEW MODELS AND NEW CONCEPTS

Clinically, ongoing production of excessive wear debris may be asymptomatic or may result in chronic synovitis with pain, swelling, and compromised joint function, periprosthetic osteolysis with pathologic fracture, or other local symptoms. Although newer alternative bearing surfaces will decrease the particle load delivered to local tissues, presently no successful nonsurgical pharmacologic methods are available to treat the adverse effects of wear particles. This fact has spawned new research into the pathogenesis of particle disease in the hope that early nonsurgical intervention may mitigate the clinical symptoms and signs and may delay revision surgery. Several new in vitro and in vivo models have further delineated the biological pathways involved in wear particle disease. Furthermore, new preclinical pharmacologic treatments for osteolysis have been proposed and tested in the laboratory.

Models of Continuous Delivery of Particles In Vivo

In humans, wear particles are produced continuously with use of the joint. Therefore, local tissues are exposed to wear debris over prolonged periods of time, despite the body's attempts to rid itself of the particles. Most animal models have incorporated a single application of particles or multiple periodic injections of particles to an anatomic site, which is unlike the clinical situation. Kim and colleagues used a diffusion pump to deliver PE particles to the knee joint containing an intramedullary femoral Kirschner wire in rats, simulating continuous particle exposure.[116-118] This novel model showed that continuous high-density PE particle infusion was associated with formation of an inflammatory periprosthetic membrane lined with osteoclasts, increased expression of TNF-α mRNA, and radiographic osteolysis around the rod.

Our group has optimized and validated a similar model using bench-top experiments, a murine femoral intramedullary infusion explant model, and in vivo murine infusion experiments.[119-122] In the first experiment, we suspended two types of particles in mouse serum: polystyrene particles (dyed blue) and particles of ultra-high-molecular-weight polyethylene (UHMWPE) that had been retrieved from clinical cases. This suspension was then loaded into Alzet miniosmotic pumps (Durect Corporation, Cupertino, Calif) attached to hollow titanium rods via vinyl tubing.[120] The number of particles delivered to a collection vessel was evaluated over 2- and 4-week time periods. Infusion of UHMWPE particles at clinically relevant dose levels yielded significantly more bone loss compared with controls, in which only mouse serum was infused. Finally, we infused clinically derived UHMWPE particles into the intramedullary space of the mouse femur for 4 weeks using a subcutaneous osmotic pump[122] (Fig. 11-4). Infusion of UHMWPE for 4 weeks was associated with reduced bone volume and altered alkaline phosphatase expression. Continuous infusion of particles using the murine femoral implant model appeared to simulate the human clinical scenario of wear particle generation and delivery. This model has proved useful in studying the biological processes associated with wear debris.

Cell Migration (Trafficking) in the Presence of Wear Particles

Macrophages, foreign body giant cells, and osteoclasts are derived from monocytes in the blood circulation. Foreign body giant cells and osteoclasts result from

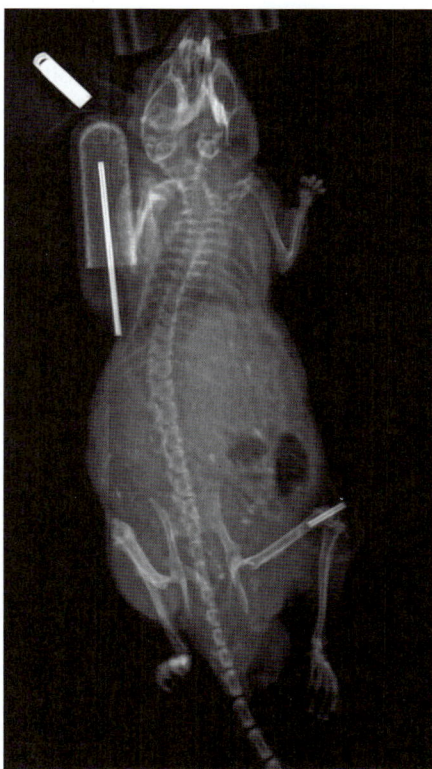

Figure 11-4. This radiograph of a mouse demonstrates a hollow intramedullary rod in the distal right femur to which is attached radiolucent tubing connected to an osmotic pump containing a solution of polyethylene particles *(upper left of figure)*. The particles are driven from the pump into the tubing through the hollow rod into the distal femur.

fusion of macrophages and differentiate down their particular functional pathways to accomplish primarily phagocytosis and bone resorption, respectively. It has been assumed that macrophages at the site of particle generation are locally derived. In other words, there has been a paucity of evidence to suggest that local wear debris causes systemic migration of macrophages to the site of particle generation. To test the hypothesis that polymer particles induce systemic migration of macrophages, the distal femurs of nude mice were injected with suspensions of simplex bone cement (BC) or UHMWPE particles or saline controls.[123] One week later, reporter murine RAW 264.7 macrophages, which stably expressed the bioluminescent reporter gene *fluc,* and the fluorescence reporter gene *gfp* were injected intravenously through the tail vain. Bioluminescence imaging was performed immediately and periodically at 2-day intervals until day 14. Compared with the nonoperated contralateral femurs, the bioluminescent signal of femurs injected with BC or UHMWPE particle suspensions increased significantly at days 6 to 8, whereas the saline controls did not show this effect. Histologic study confirmed the large numbers of reporter macrophages within the medullary canal of mice that received the particles. Thus, BC and UHMWPE particles implanted in the mouse femur stimulated the systemic recruitment

of macrophages during an early time course. Interference with systemic macrophage trafficking may be a therapeutic strategy to mitigate particle-induced periprosthetic osteolysis.

Yang and associates developed a clever mouse-human (SCID-Hu) chimera model to study the role of human periprosthetic tissue in osteolysis.[124] Human periprosthetic tissues harvested from patients during revision arthroplasty for aseptic loosening were transplanted into the quadriceps and paravertebral muscles of severe combined immunodeficient (SCID) mice. Engrafted tissues, recovered up to 30 days after implantation, expressed high levels of IL-1, TNF. and IL-6. Incubation of periprosthetic tissues with retroviruses encoding for the human IL-1 receptor antagonist (hIL-1Ra) prior to implantation in the mouse decreased the total number of inflammatory cells and expression of IL-1 and TNF. This novel model laid the foundation for the potential clinical application of gene therapy in aseptic loosening.

To enhance our understanding of the biological pathways associated with osteolysis, other studies by this group have explored the usefulness of gene therapy using various animal models.[125-128] This group used the mouse-human chimera model to confirm that human circulating blood monocytes will migrate to implanted human periprosthetic tissues and bone.[129] Periprosthetic tissue and bone specimens were harvested from patients undergoing revision surgery for aseptic prosthetic loosening. Tissue specimens were implanted into the muscles of immune-deficient SCID mice that had undergone periodic intraperitoneal injection of anti–asialo GM1 rabbit sera (ASGM1) to deplete the mouse of host macrophages. Thereafter. the patient's peripheral blood monocytes (PBMCs) were labeled with PKH2 fluorescent dye and were injected into the peritoneum of the same mice. Fourteen days later, the mice were sacrificed, and the implanted tissues and bone were harvested. The injected fluorescent PBMCs migrated to the xenografts, which were associated with increased expression of IL-1, IL-6, TNF-α. and RANK within the periprosthetic tissue. This experiment confirmed that systemically delivered blood monocytes migrate systemically to an area of particle-induced inflammation.

POTENTIAL NONSURGICAL TREATMENTS FOR PARTICULATE DISEASE

Despite the introduction of new bearing surfaces with improved wear characteristics, wear debris is continuously produced with use of the joint. Two additional factors have led to increased demand on joint replacements: (1) patients are living longer and remain more physically active with advancing age, and (2) joint replacement is being performed on younger, more robust, and more active patients. Revision joint replacement surgery is more complex than primary replacement, the complications are greater, and the outcomes are not as favorable as with the first prosthesis.

Therefore, if the prosthesis and bearing surfaces are still functional, there exists an opportunity to extend the lifetime of a joint replacement even in the face of continued production of wear particles, chronic inflammation, and osteolysis. The strategies discussed in the following paragraphs show promise for the treatment of particulate disease.

Modulation of Inflammatory Factors

Wear debris activates macrophages, fibroblasts, and other cells to produce a host of proinflammatory factors. In vitro and in vivo studies have proven the efficacy of specific agents that interfere with the inflammatory cascade; however, to date, no pharmacologic treatment has been approved for particle-associated chronic inflammation and osteolysis.[130] This may be due to one or more of the following reasons: issues related to safety and potential toxicity of the treatments, the fact that the treatments are not specific to particle disease and might interfere with biological processes that are vital to general immune surveillance and homeostasis, issues related to timing and dosing of pharmacologic agents that probably would have to continue indefinitely, and questions of efficacy given the fact that the inflammatory cascade is redundant with numerous interacting and branching pathways. For these reasons, local delivery of a particular agent probably would prove to be more favorably regarded compared with systemic treatment.

Inhibition of Eicosanoids

Eicosanoids are proinflammatory molecules that are composed of unsaturated C20 fatty acids. The lipoxygenase subgroup includes leukotrienes and lipoxins, and the prostanoid subgroup includes prostaglandins, prostacyclin, and thromboxane. In vitro studies using mouse bone marrow cells exposed to particles of UHMWPE, PMMA, and hydroxyapatite have been reported. Inhibition of leukotriene production through administration of the drug ICI 230487 led to decreased bone resorption and nonspecific esterase staining, compared with cultures without the drug.[131] ICI 230487 also diminished the adverse effects of particulates on osteoblasts.

PGE_2 is an important eicosanoid whose synthesis is controlled by the cyclo-oxygenase (COX) enzyme. COX-1 is the isoenzyme that regulates normal homeostatic functions and is present in all tissues. COX-2 is a more tightly controlled but rapidly inducible isoenzyme that is upregulated during inflammation, infection, tissue injury, and other unfavorable situations. Nonsteroidal anti-inflammatory drugs (NSAIDs) and COX-2 inhibitors have been used in vitro, in vivo, and in tissue retrieval studies to reduce the inflammation and bone loss associated with particulate debris[84,132-136]; however, the efficacy of a pharmaceutical agent is time dependent and varies with the drug, dose, and experimental model used. Misoprostol is a PGE_1 analogue that inhibits cellular degranulation and the release of eicosanoids, cytokines, and other proinflammatory mediators. The addition of misoprostol was shown to reduce

in a dose-dependent manner cytokine release by neutrophils exposed to cement particles in vitro.[137] Thus, it appears that the judicious use of inhibitors of eicosanoids may decrease the chronic inflammatory reaction associated with excessive production of wear debris.

Modulation of Cytokines

The key role of cytokines in particle-induced inflammation and osteolysis is well established in tissue retrieval, in vitro, and in vivo models.[25,138,139] A logical extension of this work is the inhibition of proinflammatory cytokines such as TNF-α, IL-1, and others. Many of these cytokines have autocrine and paracrine effects on nearby cells, thereby modulating the release of other inflammatory factors.

Inhibition of the effects of particles has been carried out using (1) soluble inhibitors of TNF-α given systemically in vivo, (2) gene delivery of a soluble inhibitor of TNF-α (sTNFR:FC, a fusion protein containing the extracellular domain of human type I TNF receptor fused to the Fc region of mouse immunoglobulin), and (3) small interfering RNAs (siRNAs) targeted at TNF.[79,140-142] However, anti-TNF therapy has not been demonstrated to alter the degree of radiographic osteolysis in a human trial.[143] Inhibition of the proinflammatory effects of IL-1 and enhancement of the anti-inflammatory effects of IL-4 and IL-10 have also shown promise.[125,144-148] IL-4 and IL-10 downregulate the expression of human leukocyte antigen (HLA) class II on human monocytes and decrease secretion of the proinflammatory cytokines IL-1, IL-6, IL-8, TNF-α, and granulocyte macrophage–colony-stimulating factor (GM-CSF) by macrophages; increase the production of the anti-inflammatory cytokine IL-1ra; and inhibit the production of PGE_2 and reactive oxygen (H_2O_2) and nitrogen oxide (NO) intermediates after macrophage activation. Anti-inflammatory cytokines such as IL-4 and IL-10 may prove to be more effective because they target a broader array of inflammatory processes.

NFκB and NF-IL-6 are two key transcription factors that regulate inflammatory cytokine pathways.[71] RANK (receptor activator of NFκB) is a membrane-bound receptor on the osteoclast surface that activates the transcription factor NFκB. RANKL is a receptor ligand released from osteoblasts, stromal cells, and other activated cells during inflammation. RANKL interacts with RANK, which, together with M-CSF, is essential for the differentiation and maturation of monocytes/macrophages into osteoclasts. Interference with the function of specific tyrosine and serine/threonine kinases decreases the activity of the transcription factors NFκb and NF-IL-6, thereby decreasing proinflammatory cytokine release.[71,149] Other studies have demonstrated that interference with the RANK/OPG axis can diminish cytokine release and osteolysis.[25,130,150,151]

Erythromycin is a macrolide antibiotic that inhibits the transcription factor NFκB. In a mouse air pouch model containing a section of a syngeneic calvarium and PE particles, intraperitoneal injection of erythromycin at a dose of 2 mg/kg/day led to several positive changes. These included reduced thickness and cellularity of the inflammatory membrane; gene expression of TNF-α, IL-1β, RANK, and RANKL; and a reduction in the number of osteoclast-like cells and in the mRNA levels of cathepsin K.[152]

Pentoxifylline, an alkylxanthine derivative, inhibits phosphodiesterase, thereby interfering with cytokine-macrophage interactions such as adherence, shape change, oxidative burst, degranulation, and chemotactic movement.[153] In so doing, pentoxifylline reduces the production of proinflammatory cytokines such as IL-1, IL-6, and TNF. Pentoxifylline synergizes with adenosine, another anti-inflammatory mediator. In vitro studies using macrophages exposed to titanium particles have shown that pentoxifylline or active analogues (agonists) of cyclical adenosine monophosphate (cAMP), dibutyryl cAMP, and Sp cAMP (a thiophosphate analogue of cAMP) can inhibit the production of proinflammatory cytokines.[136,154,155] Ciprofloxacin, a fluoroquinolone, also has been shown to inhibit prostanoid and inflammatory cytokine production.[149]

Modulation of Growth Factor Expression

Growth factors can also modulate the inflammatory cascade. Although the effects of different growth factors are time and dose dependent, they do not necessarily follow a simple dose-response curve (i.e., they are pleiotropic). Specific growth factors enhance the proliferation and differentiation of osteoprogenitor cells and therefore might prove useful in diminishing the adverse effects of wear debris on bone formation.[156] In this regard, the addition of a single 1.5 μg dose of recombinant transforming growth factor beta (rTGF-β) or the continuous infusion of 50 ng/day of fibroblast growth factor 2 (FGF-2) has been shown to increase new bone formation in the presence of PE particles placed in a rabbit harvest chamber. Infusion of bone morphogenetic protein-7 at 110 ng/day had similar positive effects on bone ingrowth despite particle exposure.[157]

Vascular endothelial growth factor (VEGF) is highly expressed in periprosthetic tissues, in cell culture, and in local tissues in animal models with particle exposure.[158-161] Blockade of VEGF has been shown to attenuate the inflammatory response to particles and osteolysis using the mouse calvarial model.[158]

Bisphosponates

Bone resorption is affected by multinucleated osteoclasts and mononuclear osteoclast-like cells derived from the monocyte-macrophage cell lineage. These cells are integral players in the bone remodeling unit or cutting cone, which comprises osteoclasts and related cells, osteoblasts and their precursors, and endothelial cells and vascular structures. Together, this unit removes older bone from the exposed surface and lays down osteoid that subsequently becomes calcified.

Bisphosphonates are medications used primarily to treat osteoporosis and conditions characterized by excessive bone resorption. These drugs become incorporated into the bone matrix, making it resistant to resorption by osteoclasts.[162] The mechanism by which

this is accomplished is controversial; however, it has been shown that bisphosphonates suppress the differentiation of osteoclast precursors into mature osteoclasts, induce apoptosis of macrophages, and decrease cytokine production in the presence of a normally proinflammatory stimulus, although the latter finding has been controversial.[151,162,163] At normal doses, bisphosphonates have few effects on osteoblasts.[164]

In vitro and in vivo studies have shown that bisphosphonates decrease particle-induced bone resorption.* However, in at least one animal model, bisphosphonates had no effect on the characteristics of the inflammatory infiltrate or on the number of proinflammatory cytokines released when particles were added to an implant, although osteolysis was inhibited.[175] Bisphosphonates have also been shown to enhance bone stock in the presence of pressure-induced osteolysis in animals.[177]

Systemic treatment with bisphosphonates seems logical in the elderly patient with periprosthetic osteolysis, given the high prevalence of osteoporosis in this age group. Some evidence suggests that bisphosphonate therapy may preserve bone stock around joint replacements.[178] However, some of the bisphosphonates have half-lives of up to 10 years, and there are issues with respect to patient compliance and adverse effects. Furthermore, whether the effect of treatment is sustained once the drug is stopped is unknown. One unreported multicenter study in humans was terminated because of the lack of an effect of bisphosphonate therapy on radiographic osteolysis around hip replacements. This has piqued interest in the local application of bisphosphonates, which has been shown to enhance initial osseointegration of implants and to decrease subsequent component migration, while possibly occluding access of particles to the bone-implant interface.[179-181] The positive effects of local bisphosphonate treatment have been confirmed in a model of pressure-induced osteolysis.[182] Nevertheless, local bisphosphonate treatment will not enhance the incorporation of an unstable implant that has not obtained initial fixation,[183] although this effect may be achieved with very high systemic doses.[184]

Drugs That Modulate Other Cellular Functions

By interfering with critical cellular functions, some drugs may render the cell less able to mount an inflammatory reaction to particle exposure. Such drugs have been shown to reduce proinflammatory factor release. These drugs or approaches include those that prevent a drop in pH within phagosomes, inhibit phagocytosis (cytochalasin B), inhibit macrophage receptors (using integrin-specific antibodies to macrophage CD11b/CD18 receptors), and inhibit RNA (actinomycin D) or protein (cycloheximide) synthesis.[71,149,156,185]

Statins are drugs that inhibit 3-hydroxy-3-methylglutaryl-coenzyme A (CoA) reductase (HMG-CoA reductase), the rate limiting enzymatic step in the mevalonate

---

*References 31, 56, 118, 130, 151, and 165-176.

pathway, which is important in the synthesis of sterols, isoprenoids, and other lipids such as cholesterol. Statins have been shown to have anti-inflammatory properties. In vitro and in vivo studies have shown that statins reduce TNF-α and MCP-1 production and particle-induced osteolysis using the mouse calvarial model.[186,187]

SUMMARY

Particles from the bearing surfaces and prosthetic interfaces of all artificial joint replacements are generated with daily use. These particles circulate in the synovial fluid and are engulfed by cells that normally populate the joint. Phagocytosis of particles and subsequent biological events involve the interaction and activation of many cell types that communicate through paracrine and autocrine pathways. Cytokines, chemokines, and other proinflammatory factors released from cells induce an inflammatory and foreign body response that is dependent on the characteristics of the particles, the patient, and the local biological and biomechanical milieu. Wear particles and their by-products also induce a systemic reaction that results in migration of cells to the area of particle generation. In most cases, the patient is asymptomatic until periprosthetic osteolysis is well advanced. Novel bearing couples that reduce wear and thus the overall particle burden are being developed to minimize the adverse effects of wear debris. Pharmacologic approaches have been developed on the basis of a clear understanding of the pathogenesis of particle-induced inflammation and osteolysis and may offer alternative nonsurgical treatment options if the joint implant is still functional.

REFERENCES

1. McKellop HA: Wear modes, mechanisms, damage, and debris: separating cause from effect in the wear of total hip replacements. In Galante JO, Rosenberg AG, Callaghan JJ (eds): Total hip revision surgery, New York, 1995, Raven Press, pp 21–39.
2. Willert HG: Reactions of the articular capsule to wear products of artificial joint prostheses. J Biomed Mater Res 11:157–164, 1977.
3. Draenert K: The John Charnley Award Paper. Histomorphology of the bone-to-cement interface: remodeling of the cortex and revascularization of the medullary canal in animal experiments. Hip 71–110, 1981.
4. Charnley J: The reaction of bone to self-curing acrylic cement: a long-term histological study in man. J Bone Joint Surg Br 52:340–353, 1970.
5. Charnley J: Low friction arthroplasty of the hip, New York, 1979, Springer-Verlag.
6. Maloney WJ, Sychterz C, Bragdon C, et al: The Otto Aufranc Award. Skeletal response to well fixed femoral components inserted with and without cement. Clin Orthop Relat Res 333:15–26, 1996.
7. Willert HG, Bertram H, Buchhorn GH: Osteolysis in alloarthroplasty of the hip: the role of ultra-high molecular weight polyethylene wear particles. Clin Orthop Relat Res 258:95–107, 1990.
8. Willert HG, Bertram H, Buchhorn GH: Osteolysis in alloarthroplasty of the hip: the role of bone cement fragmentation. Clin Orthop Relat Res 258:108–121, 1990.
9. Fornasier V, Wright J, Seligman J: The histomorphologic and morphometric study of asymptomatic hip arthroplasty: a postmortem study. Clin Orthop Relat Res 271:272–282, 1991.
10. Maloney WJ, Jasty M, Harris WH, et al: Endosteal erosion in association with stable uncemented femoral components. J Bone Joint Surg Am 72:1025–1034, 1990.
11. Maloney WJ, Jasty M, Rosenberg A, Harris WH: Bone lysis in well-fixed cemented femoral components. J Bone Joint Surg Br 72:966–970, 1990.
12. Maloney WJ, Peters P, Engh CA, Chandler H: Severe osteolysis of the pelvic in association with acetabular replacement without cement. J Bone Joint Surg Am 75:1627–1635, 1993.
13. Schmalzried TP, Kwong LM, Jasty M, et al: The mechanism of loosening of cemented acetabular components in total hip arthroplasty: analysis of specimens retrieved at autopsy. Clin Orthop Relat Res 274:60–78, 1992.
14. Goldring SR, Jasty M, Roelke MS, et al: Formation of a synovial-like membrane at the bone-cement interface: its role in bone resorption and implant loosening after total hip replacement. Arthritis Rheum 29:836–842, 1986.
15. Goldring SR, Schiller AL, Roelke M, et al: The synovial-like membrane at the bone-cement interface in loose total hip replacements and its proposed role in bone lysis. J Bone Joint Surg Am 65:575–584, 1983.
16. Aspenberg P, Herbertsson P: Periprosthetic bone resorption: particles versus movement. J Bone Joint Surg Br 78:641–646, 1996.
17. Aspenberg P, van der Vis H: Fluid pressure may cause periprosthetic osteolysis: particles are not the only thing. Acta Orthop Scand 69:1–4, 1998.
18. Aspenberg P, Van der Vis H: Migration, particles, and fluid pressure: a discussion of causes of prosthetic loosening. Clin Orthop Relat Res 352:75–80, 1998.
19. Schmalzried TP, Maloney WJ, Jasty M, et al: Autopsy studies of the bone-cement interface in well-fixed cemented total hip arthroplasties. J Arthroplasty 8:179–188, 1993.
20. Kobayashi A, Freeman MA, Bonfield W, et al: Number of polyethylene particles and osteolysis in total joint replacements: a quantitative study using a tissue-digestion method. J Bone Joint Surg Br 79:844–848, 1997.
21. Cook S: Clinical, radiographic and histologic evaluation of retrieved human noncemented porous coated implants. J Long Term Eff Med Implants 1:11–51, 1991.
22. Goodman SB, Lind M, Song Y, Smith RL: In vitro, in vivo, and tissue retrieval studies on particulate debris. Clin Orthop Relat Res 352:25–34, 1998.
23. Goodman SB, Huie P, Song Y, et al: Cellular profile and cytokine production at prosthetic interfaces: study of tissues retrieved from revised hip and knee replacements. J Bone Joint Surg Br 80:531–539, 1998.
24. Goodman SB, Gomez Barrena E, Takagi M, Konttinen YT: Biocompatibility of total joint replacements: a review. J Biomed Mater Res A 90:603–618, 2009.
25. Tuan RS, Lee FY, Konttinen Y, et al: What are the local and systemic biologic reactions and mediators to wear debris, and what host factors determine or modulate the biologic response to wear particles? J Am Acad Orthop Surg 16:S33–S38, 2008.
26. Kim KJ, Rubash HE, Wilson SC, et al: A histologic and biochemical comparison of the interface tissues in cementless and cemented hip prostheses. Clin Orthop Relat Res 287:142–152, 1993.
27. Jiranek WA, Machado M, Jasty M, et al: Production of cytokines around loosened cemented acetabular components: analysis with immunohistochemical techniques and in situ hybridization. J Bone Joint Surg Am 75:863–879, 1993.
28. Chiba J, Rubash HE, Kim KJ, Iwaki Y: The characterization of cytokines in the interface tissue obtained from failed cementless total hip arthroplasty with and without femoral osteolysis. Clin Orthop Relat Res 300:304–312, 1994.
29. Goodman SB, Chin RC, Chiou SS, et al: A clinical-pathologic-biochemical study of the membrane surrounding loosened and nonloosened total hip arthroplasties. Clin Orthop Relat Res 244:182–187, 1989.
30. Holt G, Murnaghan C, Reilly J, Meek RM: The biology of aseptic osteolysis. Clin Orthop Relat Res 460:240–252, 2007.

31. Purdue PE, Koulouvaris P, Potter HG, et al: The cellular and molecular biology of periprosthetic osteolysis. Clin Orthop Relat Res 454:251–261, 2007.

32. Tallroth K, Eskola A, Santavirta S, et al: Aggressive granulomatous lesions after hip arthroplasty. J Bone Joint Surg Br 71:571–575, 1989.

33. Santavirta S, Hoikka V, Eskola A, et al: Aggressive granulomatous lesions in cementless total hip arthroplasty. J Bone Joint Surg Br 72:980–984, 1990.

34. Santavirta S, Konttinen YT, Bergroth V, et al: Aggressive granulomatous lesions associated with hip arthroplasty: immunopathological studies. J Bone Joint Surg Am 72:252–258, 1990.

35. Goodman SB, Knoblich G, O'Connor M, et al: Heterogeneity in cellular and cytokine profiles from multiple samples of tissue surrounding revised hip prostheses. J Biomed Mater Res 31:421–428, 1996.

36. Kadoya Y, Revell PA, Al-Saffar N, et al: Bone formation and bone resorption in failed total joint arthroplasties: histomorphometric analysis with histochemical and immunohistochemical technique. J Orthop Res 14:473–482, 1996.

37. Andersson MK, Lundberg P, Ohlin A, et al: Effects on osteoclast and osteoblast activities in cultured mouse calvarial bones by synovial fluids from patients with a loose joint prosthesis and from osteoarthritis patients. Arthritis Res Ther 9:R18, 2007.

38. Horiki M, Nakase T, Myoui A, et al: Localization of RANKL in osteolytic tissue around a loosened joint prosthesis. J Bone Miner Metab 22:346–351, 2004.

39. Crotti TN, Smith MD, Findlay DM, et al: Factors regulating osteoclast formation in human tissues adjacent to peri-implant bone loss: expression of receptor activator NFkappaB, RANK ligand and osteoprotegerin. Biomaterials 25:565–573, 2004.

40. Veigl D, Niederlova J, Krystufkova O: Periprosthetic osteolysis and its association with RANKL expression. Physiol Res 56:455–462, 2007.

41. Al-Saffar N, Khwaja HA, Kadoya Y, Revell PA: Assessment of the role of GM-CSF in the cellular transformation and the development of erosive lesions around orthopaedic implants. Am J Clin Pathol 105:628–639, 1996.

42. Mandelin J, Li TF, Liljestrom M, et al: Imbalance of RANKL/RANK/OPG system in interface tissue in loosening of total hip replacement. J Bone Joint Surg Br 85:1196–1201, 2003.

43. Mandelin J, Liljestrom M, Li TF, et al: Pseudosynovial fluid from loosened total hip prosthesis induces osteoclast formation. J Biomed Mater Res B Appl Biomater 74:582–588, 2005.

44. Haynes DR, Crotti TN, Potter AE, et al: The osteoclastogenic molecules RANKL and RANK are associated with periprosthetic osteolysis. J Bone Joint Surg Br 83:902–911, 2001.

45. Bainbridge JA, Al-Saffar N: Co-stimulatory molecule expression following exposure to orthopaedic implants wear debris. J Biomed Mater Res 54:328–334, 2001.

46. Farber A, Song Y, Huie P, Goodman SB: Chronic antigen-specific immune system activation may potentially be involved in the loosening of cemented acetabular components. J Biomed Mater Res 55:433–441, 2001.

47. Lohmann CH, Nuechtern JV, Willert HG, et al: Hypersensitivity reactions in total hip arthroplasty. Orthopedics 30:760–761, 2007.

48. Willert HG, Buchhorn GH, Fayyazi A, et al: Metal-on-metal bearings and hypersensitivity in patients with artificial hip joints: a clinical and histomorphological study. J Bone Joint Surg Am 87:28–36, 2005.

49. Hallab NJ, Caicedo M, Finnegan A, Jacobs JJ: Th1 type lymphocyte reactivity to metals in patients with total hip arthroplasty. J Orthop Surg 3:6, 2008.

50. Hallab NJ, Anderson S, Caicedo M, et al: Immune responses correlate with serum-metal in metal-on-metal hip arthroplasty. J Arthroplasty 19:88–93, 2004.

51. Goodman SB: Wear particles, periprosthetic osteolysis and the immune system. Biomaterials 28:5044–5048, 2007.

52. Revell PA: The combined role of wear particles, macrophages and lymphocytes in the loosening of total joint prostheses. J R Soc Interface 5:1263–1278, 2008.

53. Bostrom M, O'Keefe R: What experimental approaches (e.g., in vivo, in vitro, tissue retrieval) are effective in investigating the biologic effects of particles? J Am Acad Orthop Surg 16(Suppl 1):S63–S67, 2008.

54. Jacobs JJ, Roebuck KA, Archibeck M, et al: Osteolysis: basic science. Clin Orthop Relat Res 393:71–77, 2001.

55. Goodman SB, Trindade M, Ma T, et al: Pharmacologic modulation of periprosthetic osteolysis. Clin Orthop Relat Res 430:39–45, 2005.

56. Purdue PE, Koulouvaris P, Nestor BJ, Sculco TP: The central role of wear debris in periprosthetic osteolysis. HSS J 2:102–113, 2006.

57. Warashina H, Sakano S, Kitamura S, et al: Biological reaction to alumina, zirconia, titanium and polyethylene particles implanted onto murine calvaria. Biomaterials 24:3655–3661, 2003.

58. Illgen RL 2nd, Forsythe TM, Pike JW, et al: Highly crosslinked vs conventional polyethylene particles—an in vitro comparison of biologic activities. J Arthroplasty 23:721–731, 2008.

59. Ingham E, Fisher J: The role of macrophages in osteolysis of total joint replacement. Biomaterials 26:1271–1286, 2005.

60. Ingram JH, Stone M, Fisher J, Ingham E: The influence of molecular weight, crosslinking and counterface roughness on TNF-alpha production by macrophages in response to ultra high molecular weight polyethylene particles. Biomaterials 25:3511–3522, 2004.

61. Yang SY, Ren W, Park Y, et al: Diverse cellular and apoptotic responses to variant shapes of UHMWPE particles in a murine model of inflammation. Biomaterials 23:3535–3543, 2002.

62. Goodman SB: The effects of micromotion and particulate materials on tissue differentiation: bone chamber studies in rabbits. Acta Orthop Scand Suppl 258:1–43, 1994.

63. Catelas HO, Petit A, Zukor DJ, et al: Flow cytometric analysis of macrophage response to ceramic and polyethylene particles: effects of size, concentration, and composition. J Biomed Mater Res 41:600–607, 1998.

64. Nakashima Y, Sun DH, Trindade MC, et al: Induction of macrophage C-C chemokine expression by titanium alloy and bone cement particles. J Bone Joint Surg Br 81:155–162, 1999.

65. Matthews JB, Besong AA, Green TR, et al: Evaluation of the response of primary human peripheral blood mononuclear phagocytes to challenge with in vitro generated clinically relevant UHMWPE particles of known size and dose. J Biomed Mater Res 52:296–307, 2000.

66. Matthews JB, Green TR, Stone MH, et al: Comparison of the response of three human monocytic cell lines to challenge with polyethylene particles of known size and dose. J Mater Sci Mater Med 12:249–258, 2001.

67. Mitchell W, Bridget Matthews J, et al: Comparison of the response of human peripheral blood mononuclear cells to challenge with particles of three bone cements in vitro. Biomaterials 24:737–748, 2003.

68. Green TR, Fisher J, Matthews JB, et al: Effect of size and dose on bone resorption activity of macrophages by in vitro clinically relevant ultra high molecular weight polyethylene particles. J Biomed Mater Res 53:490–497, 2000.

69. Ingham E, Fisher J: Biological reactions to wear debris in total joint replacement. Proc Inst Mech Eng H 214:21–37, 2000.

70. Shanbhag AS, Jacobs JJ, Black J, et al: Macrophage/particle interactions: effect of size composition and surface area. J Biomed Mater Res 28:81–90, 1994.

71. Nakashima Y, Sun DH, Trindade MC, et al: Signaling pathways for tumor necrosis factor-alpha and interleukin-6 expression in human macrophages exposed to titanium-alloy particulate debris in vitro. J Bone Joint Surg Am 81:603–615, 1999.

72. Lind M, Trindade MC, Nakashima Y, et al: Chemotaxis and activation of particle-challenged human monocytes in response to monocyte migration inhibitory factor and C-C chemokines. J Biomed Mater Res 48:246–250, 1999.

73. Lind M, Trindade MC, Schurman DJ, et al: Monocyte migration inhibitory factor synthesis and gene expression in particle-activated macrophages. Cytokine 12:909–913, 2000.

74. Lind M, Trindade MC, Yasay B, et al: Effects of particulate debris on macrophage-dependent fibroblast stimulation in coculture. J Bone Joint Surg Br 80:924–930, 1998.

75. Bi Y, Seabold JM, Kaar SG, et al: Adherent endotoxin on orthopedic wear particles stimulates cytokine production and osteoclast differentiation. J Bone Miner Res 16:2082–2091, 2001.

76. Nakashima Y, Sun DH, Maloney WJ, et al: Induction of matrix metalloproteinase expression in human macrophages by orthopaedic particulate debris in vitro. J Bone Joint Surg Br 80:694–700, 1998.

77. Baumann B, Rader CP, Seufert J, et al: Effects of polyethylene and TiAlV wear particles on expression of RANK, RANKL and OPG mRNA. Acta Orthop Scand 75:295–302, 2004.

78. Schwarz EM, Lu AP, Goater JJ, et al: Tumor necrosis factor-alpha/nuclear transcription factor-kappaB signaling in periprosthetic osteolysis. J Orthop Res 18:472–480, 2000.

79. Peng X, Tao K, Cheng T, et al: Efficient inhibition of wear debris-induced inflammation by locally delivered siRNA. Biochem Biophys Res Commun 377:532–537, 2008.

80. Glant TT, Jacobs JJ, Mikecz K, et al: Particulate-induced, prostaglandin- and cytokine-mediated bone resorption in an experimental system and in failed joint replacements. Am J Ther 3:27–41, 1996.

81. Manlapaz M, Maloney WJ, Smith RL: In vitro activation of human fibroblasts by retrieved titanium alloy wear debris. J Orthop Res 14:465–472, 1996.

82. Bukata SV, Gelinas J, Wei X, et al: PGE2 and IL-6 production by fibroblasts in response to titanium wear debris particles is mediated through a COX-2 dependent pathway. J Orthop Res 22:6–12, 2004.

83. Tsutsumi R, Xie C, Wei X, et al: PGE2 signaling through the EP4 receptor on fibroblasts upregulates RANKL and stimulates osteolysis. J Bone Miner Res 24:1753–1762, 2009.

84. Wei X, Zhang X, Zuscik MJ, et al: Fibroblasts express RANKL and support osteoclastogenesis in a COX-2-dependent manner after stimulation with titanium particles. J Bone Miner Res 20:1136–1148, 2005.

85. Shanbhag AS, Jacobs JJ, Black J, et al: Effects of particles on fibroblast proliferation and bone resorption in vitro. Clin Orthop Relat Res 342:205–217, 1997.

86. Yao J, Glant TT, Lark MW, et al: The potential role of fibroblasts in periprosthetic osteolysis: fibroblast response to titanium particles. J Bone Miner Res 10:1417–1427, 1995.

87. Koreny T, Tunyogi-Csapo M, Gal I, et al: The role of fibroblasts and fibroblast-derived factors in periprosthetic osteolysis. Arthritis Rheum 54:3221–3232, 2006.

88. O'Connor DT, Choi MG, Kwon SY, Paul Sung KL: New insight into the mechanism of hip prosthesis loosening: effect of titanium debris size on osteoblast function. J Orthop Res 22:229–236, 2004.

89. Shida J, Trindade MC, Goodman SB, et al: Induction of interleukin-6 release in human osteoblast-like cells exposed to titanium particles in vitro. Calcif Tissue Int 67:151–155, 2000.

90. Atkins GJ, Welldon KJ, Holding CA, et al: The induction of a catabolic phenotype in human primary osteoblasts and osteocytes by polyethylene particles. Biomaterials 30:3672–3681, 2009.

91. Choi MG, Koh HS, Kluess D, et al: Effects of titanium particle size on osteoblast functions in vitro and in vivo. Proc Natl Acad Sci U S A 102:4578–4583, 2005.

92. Lohmann CH, Dean DD, Bonewald LF, et al: Nitric oxide and prostaglandin E2 production in response to ultra-high molecular weight polyethylene particles depends on osteoblast maturation state. J Bone Joint Surg Am 84:411–419, 2002.

93. Pioletti DP, Kottelat A: The influence of wear particles in the expression of osteoclastogenesis factors by osteoblasts. Biomaterials 25:5803–5808, 2004.

94. Granchi D, Ciapetti G, Amato I, et al: The influence of alumina and ultra-high molecular weight polyethylene particles on osteoblast-osteoclast cooperation. Biomaterials 25:4037–4045, 2004.

95. Olivier V, Duval JL, Hindie M, et al: Comparative particle-induced cytotoxicity toward macrophages and fibroblasts. Cell Biol Toxicol 19:145–159, 2003.

96. Goodman SB, Ma T, Chiu R, et al: Effects of orthopaedic wear particles on osteoprogenitor cells. Biomaterials 27:6096–6101, 2006.

97. Chiu R, Ma T, Smith RL, Goodman SB: Kinetics of polymethylmethacrylate particle-induced inhibition of osteoprogenitor differentiation and proliferation. J Orthop Res 25:450–457, 2007.

98. Schofer MD, Fuchs-Winkelmann S, Kessler-Thones A, et al: The role of mesenchymal stem cells in the pathogenesis of Co-Cr-Mo particle induced aseptic loosening: an in vitro study. Biomed Mater Eng 18:395–403, 2008.

99. Wang ML, Nesti LJ, Tuli R, et al: Titanium particles suppress expression of osteoblastic phenotype in human mesenchymal stem cells. J Orthop Res 20:1175–1184, 2002.

100. Wang ML, Tuli R, Manner PA, et al: Direct and indirect induction of apoptosis in human mesenchymal stem cells in response to titanium particles. J Orthop Res 21:697–707, 2003.

101. Chiu R, Ma T, Smith RL, Goodman SB: Polymethylmethacrylate particles inhibit osteoblastic differentiation of bone marrow osteoprogenitor cells. J Biomed Mater Res A 77:850–856, 2006.

102. Chiu R, Ma T, Smith RL, Goodman SB: Polymethylmethacrylate particles inhibit osteoblastic differentiation of MC3T3-E1 osteoprogenitor cells. J Orthop Res 26:932–936, 2008.

103. Greenfield EM, Bechtold J: What other biologic and mechanical factors might contribute to osteolysis? J Am Acad Orthop Surg 16(Suppl 1):S56–S62, 2008.

104. Van der Vis HM, Aspenberg P, Marti RK, et al: Fluid pressure causes bone resorption in a rabbit model of prosthetic loosening. Clin Orthop Relat Res 350:201–208, 1998.

105. Skoglund B, Aspenberg P: PMMA particles and pressure—a study of the osteolytic properties of two agents proposed to cause prosthetic loosening. J Orthop Res 21:196–201, 2003.

106. McEvoy A, Jeyam M, Ferrier G, et al: Synergistic effect of particles and cyclic pressure on cytokine production in human monocyte/macrophages: proposed role in periprosthetic osteolysis. Bone 30:171–177, 2002.

107. Bechtold JE, Kubic V, Soballe K: Bone ingrowth in the presence of particulate polyethylene: synergy between interface motion and particulate polyethylene in periprosthetic tissue response. J Bone Joint Surg Br 84:915–919, 2002.

108. MacQuarrie RA, Fang Chen Y, Coles C, Anderson GI: Wear-particle-induced osteoclast osteolysis: the role of particulates and mechanical strain. J Biomed Mater Res B Appl Biomater 69:104–112, 2004.

109. Maloney WJ, Sun DH, Nakashima Y, et al: Effects of serum protein opsonization on cytokine release by titanium-alloy particles. J Biomed Mater Res 41:371–376, 1998.

110. Sun DH, Trindade MC, Nakashima Y, et al: Human serum opsonization of orthopedic biomaterial particles: protein-binding and monocyte/macrophage activation in vitro. J Biomed Mater Res A 65:290–298, 2003.

111. Bi Y, Collier TO, Goldberg VM, et al: Adherent endotoxin mediates biological responses of titanium particles without stimulating their phagocytosis. J Orthop Res 20:696–703, 2002.

112. Ragab AA, Van De Motter R, Lavish SA, et al: Measurement and removal of adherent endotoxin from titanium particles and implant surfaces. J Orthop Res 17:803–809, 1999.

113. Akisue T, Bauer TW, Farver CF, Mochida Y: The effect of particle wear debris on NFkappaB activation and pro-inflammatory cytokine release in differentiated THP-1 cells. J Biomed Mater Res 59:507–515, 2002.

114. Cho DR, Shanbhag AS, Hong CY, et al: The role of adsorbed endotoxin in particle-induced stimulation of cytokine release. J Orthop Res 20:704–713, 2002.

115. Nalepka JL, Lee MJ, Kraay MJ, et al: Lipopolysaccharide found in aseptic loosening of patients with inflammatory arthritis. Clin Orthop Relat Res 451:229–235, 2006.

116. Kim KJ, Kobayashi Y, Itoh T: Osteolysis model with continuous infusion of polyethylene particles. Clin Orthop Relat Res 352:46–52, 1998.

117. Kobayashi Y, Kim KJ, Itoh T: Gene expression of bone-resorbing cytokines in rat osteolysis model. J Orthop Sci 10:62–69, 2005.

118. Iwase M, Kim KJ, Kobayashi Y, et al: A novel bisphosphonate inhibits inflammatory bone resorption in a rat osteolysis model with continuous infusion of polyethylene particles. J Orthop Res 20:499–505, 2002.

119. Ortiz SG, Ma T, Regula D, et al: Continuous intramedullary polymer particle infusion using a murine femoral explant model. J Biomed Mater Res B Appl Biomater 87:440–446, 2008.

120. Ortiz SG, Ma T, Epstein NJ, et al: Validation and quantification of an in vitro model of continuous infusion of submicron-sized particles. J Biomed Mater Res B Appl Biomater 84:328–333, 2008.

121. Ma T, Ortiz SG, Huang Z, et al: In vivo murine model of continuous intramedullary infusion of particles—a preliminary study. J Biomed Mater Res B Appl Biomater 88:250–253, 2009.

122. Ma T, Huang Z, Ren PG, et al: An in vivo murine model of continuous intramedullary infusion of polyethylene particles. Biomaterials 29:3738–3742, 2008.

123. Ren PG, Lee SW, Biswal S, Goodman SB: Systemic trafficking of macrophages induced by bone cement particles in nude mice. Biomaterials 29:4760–4765, 2008.

124. Yang SY, Nasser S, Markel DC, et al: Human periprosthetic tissues implanted in severe combined immunodeficient mice respond to gene transfer of a cytokine inhibitor. J Bone Joint Surg Am 87:1088–1097, 2005.

125. Yang SY, Wu B, Mayton L, et al: Protective effects of IL-1Ra or vIL-10 gene transfer on a murine model of wear debris-induced osteolysis. Gene Ther 11:483–491, 2004.

126. Yang SY, Yu H, Gong W, et al: Murine model of prosthesis failure for the long-term study of aseptic loosening. J Orthop Res 25:603–611, 2007.

127. Yang SY, Mayton L, Wu B, et al: Adeno-associated virus-mediated osteoprotegerin gene transfer protects against particulate polyethylene-induced osteolysis in a murine model. Arthritis Rheum 46:2514–2523, 2002.

128. Sud S, Yang SY, Evans CH, et al: Effects of cytokine gene therapy on particulate-induced inflammation in the murine air pouch. Inflammation 25:361–372, 2001.

129. Zhang K, Jia TH, McQueen D, et al: Circulating blood monocytes traffic to and participate in the periprosthetic tissue inflammation. Inflamm Res 58:837–844, 2009.

130. Schwarz EM: What potential biologic treatments are available for osteolysis? J Am Acad Orthop Surg 16(Suppl 1):S72–S75, 2008.

131. Anderson GI, MacQuarrie R, Osinga C, et al: Inhibition of leukotriene function can modulate particulate-induced changes in bone cell differentiation and activity. J Biomed Mater Res 58:406–414, 2001.

132. Goodman SB, Lee JS, Chin RC, Chiou SS: Modulation of the membrane surrounding particulate cement and polyethylene in the rabbit tibia. Biomaterials 12:194–196, 1991.

133. Goodman SB, Chin RC, Chiou SS, Lee JS: Suppression of prostaglandin E2 synthesis in the membrane surrounding particulate polymethylmethacrylate in the rabbit tibia. Clin Orthop Relat Res 271:300–304, 1991.

134. Herman JH, Hess EV: Nonsteroidal antiinflammatory drug modulation of prosthesis pseudomembrane induced bone resorption. J Rheumatol 21:338–343, 1994.

135. Zhang X, Morham SG, Langenbach R, et al: Evidence for a direct role of cyclo-oxygenase 2 in implant wear debris-induced osteolysis. J Bone Miner Res 16:660–670, 2001.

136. Sun JS, Lin FH, Tsuang YH, et al: Effect of anti-inflammatory medication on monocyte response to titanium particles. J Biomed Mater Res 52:509–516, 2000.

137. Papatheofanis FJ, Barmada R: Misoprostol inhibits polymethylmethacrylate-stimulated lysosomal degranulation and IL-1 release from neutrophils. Am J Ther 3:21–26, 1996.

138. Jacobs JJ, Campbell PA: How has the biologic reaction to wear particles changed with newer bearing surfaces? J Am Acad Orthop Surg 16(Suppl 1):S49–S55, 2008.

139. Bauer TW, Shanbhag AS: Are there biological markers of wear? J Am Acad Orthop Surg 16(Suppl 1):S68–S71, 2008.

140. Childs LM, Goater JJ, O'Keefe RJ, Schwarz EM: Effect of anti-tumor necrosis factor-alpha gene therapy on wear debris-induced osteolysis. J Bone Joint Surg Am 83:1789–1797, 2001.

141. Peng X, Zhang X, Zeng B: Locally administered lentivirus-mediated siRNA inhibits wear debris-induced inflammation in murine air pouch model. Biotechnol Lett 30:1923–1929, 2008.

142. Childs LM, Goater JJ, O'Keefe RJ, Schwarz EM: Efficacy of etanercept for wear debris-induced osteolysis. J Bone Miner Res 16:338–347, 2001.

143. Schwarz EM, Looney RJ, O'Keefe RJ: Anti-TNF-alpha therapy as a clinical intervention for periprosthetic osteolysis. Arthritis Res 2:165–168, 2000.

144. Trindade MC, Nakashima Y, Lind M, et al: Interleukin-4 inhibits granulocyte-macrophage colony-stimulating factor, interleukin-6, and tumor necrosis factor-alpha expression by human monocytes in response to polymethylmethacrylate particle challenge in vitro. J Orthop Res 17:797–802, 1999.

145. Im GI, Han JD: Suppressive effects of interleukin-4 and interleukin-10 on the production of proinflammatory cytokines induced by titanium-alloy particles. J Biomed Mater Res 58:531–536, 2001.

146. Pollice PF, Hsu J, Hicks DG, et al: Interleukin-10 inhibits cytokine synthesis in monocytes stimulated by titanium particles: evidence of an anti-inflammatory regulatory pathway. J Orthop Res 16:697–704, 1998.

147. Trindade MC, Lind M, Nakashima Y, et al: Interleukin-10 inhibits polymethylmethacrylate particle induced interleukin-6 and tumor necrosis factor-alpha release by human monocyte/macrophages in vitro. Biomaterials 22:2067–2073, 2001.

148. Carmody EE, Schwarz EM, Puzas JE, et al: Viral interleukin-10 gene inhibition of inflammation, osteoclastogenesis, and bone resorption in response to titanium particles. Arthritis Rheum 46:1298–1308, 2002.

149. Haynes DR, Rogers SD, Howie DW, et al: Drug inhibition of the macrophage response to metal wear particles in vitro. Clin Orthop Relat Res 323:316–326, 1996.

150. von Knoch F, Heckelei A, Wedemeyer C, et al: Suppression of polyethylene particle-induced osteolysis by exogenous osteoprotegerin. J Biomed Mater Res A 75:288–294, 2005.

151. Ren W, Markel DC, Schwendener R, et al: Macrophage depletion diminishes implant-wear-induced inflammatory osteolysis in a mouse model. J Biomed Mater Res A 85:1043–1051, 2008.

152. Ren W, Li XH, Chen BD, Wooley PH: Erythromycin inhibits wear debris-induced osteoclastogenesis by modulation of murine macrophage NF-kappaB activity. J Orthop Res 22:21–29, 2004.

153. Mandell G: Cytokines, phagocytes, and pentoxifylline. J Cardiovasc Pharmacol 2:S20–S22, 1995.

154. Blaine TA, Pollice PF, Rosier RN, et al: Modulation of the production of cytokines in titanium-stimulated human peripheral blood monocytes by pharmacological agents: the role of cAMP-mediated signaling mechanisms. J Bone Joint Surg Am 79:1519–1528, 1997.

155. Pollice PF, Rosier RN, Looney RJ, et al: Oral pentoxifylline inhibits release of tumor necrosis factor-alpha from human peripheral blood monocytes: a potential treatment for aseptic loosening of total joint components. J Bone Joint Surg Am 83:1057–1061, 2001.

156. Vermes C, Chandrasekaran R, Jacobs JJ, et al: The effects of particulate wear debris, cytokines, and growth factors on the functions of MG-63 osteoblasts. J Bone Joint Surg Am 83:201–211, 2001.

157. Ma T, Nelson ER, Mawatari T, et al: Effects of local infusion of OP-1 on particle-induced and NSAID-induced inhibition of bone ingrowth in vivo. J Biomed Mater Res A 79:740–746, 2006.

158. Ren W, Zhang R, Markel DC, et al: Blockade of vascular endothelial growth factor activity suppresses wear debris-induced inflammatory osteolysis. J Rheumatol 34:27–35, 2007.

159. Spanogle JP, Miyanishi K, Ma T, et al: Comparison of VEGF-producing cells in periprosthetic osteolysis. Biomaterials 27:3882–3887, 2006.

160. Ren WP, Markel DC, Zhang R, et al: Association between UHMWPE particle-induced inflammatory osteoclastogenesis and expression of RANKL, VEGF, and Flt-1 in vivo. Biomaterials 27:5161–5169, 2006.

161. Miyanishi K, Trindade MC, Ma T, et al: Periprosthetic osteolysis: induction of vascular endothelial growth factor from human monocyte/macrophages by orthopaedic biomaterial particles. J Bone Miner Res 18:1573–1583, 2003.

162. Aspenberg P: Bisphosphonates and implants: an overview. Acta Orthop 80:119–123, 2009.

163. Petit A, Mwale F, Antoniou J, et al: Effect of bisphosphonates on the stimulation of macrophages by alumina ceramic

particles: a comparison with ultra-high-molecular-weight polyethylene. J Mater Sci Mater Med 17:667–673, 2006.

164. Peter B, Zambelli PY, Guicheux J, Pioletti DP: The effect of bisphosphonates and titanium particles on osteoblasts: an in vitro study. J Bone Joint Surg Br 87:1157–1163, 2005.

165. Horowitz SM, Algan SA, Purdon MA: Pharmacologic inhibition of particulate-induced bone resorption. J Biomed Mater Res 31:91–96, 1996.

166. Millett PJ, Allen MJ, Bostrom MP: Effects of alendronate on particle-induced osteolysis in a rat model. J Bone Joint Surg Am 84:236–249, 2002.

167. Tsutsumi R, Hock C, Bechtold CD, et al: Differential effects of biologic versus bisphosphonate inhibition of wear debris-induced osteolysis assessed by longitudinal micro-CT. J Orthop Res 26:1340–1346, 2008.

168. Suzuki Y, Nishiyama T, Hasuda K, et al: Effect of etidronate on COX-2 expression and PGE(2) production in macrophage-like RAW 264.7 cells stimulated by titanium particles. J Orthop Sci 12:568–577, 2007.

169. von Knoch F, Eckhardt C, Alabre CI, et al: Anabolic effects of bisphosphonates on peri-implant bone stock. Biomaterials 28:3549–3559, 2007.

170. Wedemeyer C, von Knoch F, Pingsmann A, et al: Stimulation of bone formation by zoledronic acid in particle-induced osteolysis. Biomaterials 26:3719–3725, 2005.

171. Huk OL, Zukor DJ, Antoniou J, Petit A: Effect of pamidronate on the stimulation of macrophage TNF-alpha release by ultra-high-molecular-weight polyethylene particles: a role for apoptosis. J Orthop Res 21:81–87, 2003.

172. Thadani PJ, Waxman B, Sladek E, et al: Inhibition of particulate debris-induced osteolysis by alendronate in a rat model. Orthopedics 25:59–63, 2002.

173. Schwarz EM, Benz EB, Lu AP, et al: Quantitative small-animal surrogate to evaluate drug efficacy in preventing wear debris-induced osteolysis. J Orthop Res 18:849–855, 2000.

174. Sabokbar A, Fujikawa Y, Murray DW, Athanasou NA: Bisphosphonates in bone cement inhibit PMMA particle induced bone resorption. Ann Rheum Dis 57:614–618, 1998.

175. Shanbhag AS, Hasselman CT, Rubash HE: The John Charnley Award. Inhibition of wear debris mediated osteolysis in a canine total hip arthroplasty model. Clin Orthop Relat Res 344:33–43, 1997.

176. Pandey R, Quinn JM, Sabokbar A, Athanasou NA: Bisphosphonate inhibition of bone resorption induced by particulate biomaterial-associated macrophages. Acta Orthop Scand 67:221–228, 1996.

177. Astrand J, Skripitz R, Skoglund B, Aspenberg P: A rat model for testing pharmacologic treatments of pressure-related bone loss. Clin Orthop Relat Res 409:296–305, 2003.

178. Kinov P, Tivchev P, Doukova P, Leithner A: Effect of risedronate on bone metabolism after total hip arthroplasty: a prospective randomised study. Acta Orthop Belg 72:44–50, 2006.

179. Xing Z, Hasty KA, Smith RA: Administration of pamidronate alters bone-titanium attachment in the presence of endotoxin-coated polyethylene particles. J Biomed Mater Res B Appl Biomater 83:354–358, 2007.

180. Suratwala SJ, Cho SK, van Raalte JJ, et al: Enhancement of periprosthetic bone quality with topical hydroxyapatite-bisphosphonate composite. J Bone Joint Surg Am 90:2189–2196, 2008.

181. Hilding M, Aspenberg P: Local preoperative treatment with a bisphosphonate improves the fixation of total knee prostheses: a randomized, double-blind radiostereometric study of 50 patients. Acta Orthop 78:795–799, 2007.

182. Astrand J, Aspenberg P: Topical, single dose bisphosphonate treatment reduced bone resorption in a rat model for prosthetic loosening. J Orthop Res 22:244–249, 2004.

183. Astrand J, Aspenberg P: Alendronate did not inhibit instability-induced bone resorption: a study in rats. Acta Orthop Scand 70:67–70, 1999.

184. Astrand J, Aspenberg P: Reduction of instability-induced bone resorption using bisphosphonates: high doses are needed in rats. Acta Orthop Scand 73:24–30, 2002.

185. Fritz EA, Glant TT, Vermes C, et al: Titanium particles induce the immediate early stress responsive chemokines IL-8 and MCP-1 in osteoblasts. J Orthop Res 20:490–498, 2002.

186. von Knoch F, Heckelei A, Wedemeyer C, et al: The effect of simvastatin on polyethylene particle-induced osteolysis. Biomaterials 26:3549–3555, 2005.

187. Laing AJ, Dillon JP, Mulhall KJ, et al: Statins attenuate polymethylmethacrylate-mediated monocyte activation. Acta Orthop 79:134–140, 2008.

188. Merkel KD, Erdmann JM, McHugh KP, et al: Tumor necrosis factor-alpha mediates orthopedic implant osteolysis. Am J Pathol 154:203–210, 1999.

189. Ren W, Wu B, Mayton L, Wooley PH: Polyethylene and methyl methacrylate particle-stimulated inflammatory tissue and macrophages up-regulate bone resorption in a murine neonatal calvaria in vitro organ system. J Orthop Res 20:1031–1037, 2002.

190. Wooley PH, Morren R, Andary J, et al: Inflammatory responses to orthopaedic biomaterials in the murine air pouch. Biomaterials 23:517–526, 2002.

191. Howie DW, Vernon-Roberts B, Oakeshott R, Manthey B: A rat model of resorption of bone at the cement-bone interface in the presence of polyethylene wear particles. J Bone Joint Surg Am 70:257–263, 1988.

192. Im GI, Kwon BC, Lee KB: The effect of COX-2 inhibitors on periprosthetic osteolysis. Biomaterials 25:269–275, 2004.

193. Lalor PA, Namba R, Mitchell SL, et al: Migration of polyethylene particles around stable implants in an animal model. J Long Term Eff Med Implants 9:261–272, 1999.

194. Sundfeldt M, Widmark M, Johansson CB, et al: Effect of submicron polyethylene particles on an osseointegrated implant: an experimental study with a rabbit patello-femoral prosthesis. Acta Orthop Scand 73:416–424, 2002.

195. Goodman SB, Song Y, Chun L, et al: Effects of TGFbeta on bone ingrowth in the presence of polyethylene particles. J Bone Joint Surg Br 81:1069–1075, 1999.

196. Goodman SB, Song Y, Yoo JY, et al: Local infusion of FGF-2 enhances bone ingrowth in rabbit chambers in the presence of polyethylene particles. J Biomed Mater Res A 65:454–461, 2003.

197. Jones LC, Frondoza C, Hungerford DS: Effect of PMMA particles and movement on an implant interface in a canine model. J Bone Joint Surg Br 83:448–458, 2001.

198. Kraemer WJ, Maistrelli GL, Fornasier V, et al: Migration of polyethylene wear debris in hip arthroplasties: a canine model. J Appl Biomater 6:225–230, 1995.

199. Coathup MJ, Blackburn J, Goodship AE, et al: Role of hydroxyapatite coating in resisting wear particle migration and osteolysis around acetabular components. Biomaterials 26:4161–4169, 2005.

CHAPTER 12

Biological Responses to Metal Debris and Metal Ions

Patricia A. Campbell and Karren Takamura

KEY POINTS

- Metal wear products are substantially smaller and more bioreactive than polyethylene wear particles. This makes the study of their local and distant effects more complex.
- Unlike polyethylene particles, which stimulate a mostly nonspecific foreign body reaction, metal wear products elicit an immune system response.
- ALVAL is a term that describes histologic features that occur in response to metal wear products. Disruption of the synovial lining, lymphocyte infiltration, and loss of normal tissue organization are the key features.
- Adverse tissue reactions in the form of masses (pseudotumors) can occur in response to hypersensitivity but more typically appear to be a reaction to abundant wear products.
- Lymphocytic infiltration typically is more pronounced in tissues from patients with metal hypersensitivity.

INTRODUCTION

Metal-on-metal (MOM) bearings were reintroduced in the late 1980s with the goal of reducing polyethylene (PE)-induced osteolysis and aseptic loosening, thus improving implant longevity, particularly in young and active patients. MOM articulations produce significantly less volumetric wear compared with metal-on-polyethylene bearings, but the particles are much smaller (nanometer-sized) and much more numerous. These wear products have the potential to cause locally aggressive biological responses that may be a major limiting factor to the long-term success of MOM implants. Biological reactions to metal particles and ionic corrosion products are the focus of this chapter.

BASIC SCIENCE OF WEAR DEBRIS

Polyethylene Wear and Osteolysis

It is useful to discuss metal wear debris reactivity from the context of what has been learned from studies of PE debris. Debate is ongoing as to which factor is most important for the cellular response to wear particles,

but it is generally accepted that for PE particles, their submicron to micron size the nondegradable nature of the polymer, and the high volumes that are typically produced are the characteristics that, when combined, lead to an aggressive local response that results in bone resorption and implant loosening.[1-5] The more subtle particle characteristics, such as aspect ratio, surface roughness, and the composition of absorbed proteins, may also determine bioreactivity, but these are less well understood.[2] Much work on the bioreactivity of wear particles has been performed using particles of commercial polymers, including the powder form of ultra-high-molecular-weight polyethylene that is used as the base material for fabrication of bearing inserts for hip or knee implants. In these studies, this material was chosen to simulate the debris produced by metal-polyethylene hip replacements, because the primary goal of these studies was to understand and thus prevent polyethylene-induced osteolysis. It is more difficult to perform comparable studies to understand the biological mechanisms involved in reactions to metal particles, because, as discussed later, several aspects of metal debris present special challenges for the study of their bioreactivity.

HISTORICAL BACKGROUND

The late Professor Hans Willert proposed a possible biological mechanism of aseptic loosening, namely, that continuous release of large volumes of particles quickly overwhelms the joint clearance mechanisms, and accumulated particles induce a foreign body reaction.[7] According to his proposed mechanism, the particles were ingested by macrophages, which triggered the production of inflammatory cytokines, leading to bone resorption and implant loosening. At one point, bone cement was thought to be the main source of debris,[8] but the introduction of cementless devices did not solve the problem of aseptic loosening or osteolysis.[9]

Retrieval analysis of hip resurfacing components with osteolysis of the femoral neck and the resurfaced head contributed to the understanding that polyethylene rather than cement or titanium was the culprit.[10] In contrast to stemmed prostheses, which generally are removed from the bone and any osteolytic membranes at the time of revision, hip resurfacings retain the bone-membrane interfaces and facilitate their histologic evaluation. By using a special stain that showed intracellular aggregates of PE particles that otherwise were invisible at the light microscope level, we showed the extensive distribution of PE particles even when titanium metallosis was present.[4,10]

CELLULAR MECHANISMS OF OSTEOLYSIS

Improved understanding of the process of wear debris–induced osteolysis came when methods to isolate and characterize PE wear particles from tissues and hip simulator lubricants were developed by our group and others.[3,6] We reported that the particles were predominantly micron to submicron in size, with both elongated and rounded shapes, and that these features appeared to make them particularly attractive to macrophage phagocytosis.

Molecular details of the processes involved in macrophage phagocytosis, cytokine production, and osteoclast activation have been investigated over the ensuing years, and our understanding has greatly improved. Several excellent reviews document those studies.[11-13] The characteristic periprosthetic tissue response to particulate polyethylene can be summarized as follows:

1. The response involves a nonspecific foreign body reaction reminiscent of a granulomatous response (i.e., where the nondegradable material is sequestered by macrophages and fibrous tissue) that does not require active participation of T lymphocytes and generally does not lead to tissue necrosis.
2. The biological reaction is strongly determined by the concentration, size, material, and form of the wear particles; although individual variability in the extent of osteolysis has been noted, a threshold amount of wear related to risk for osteolysis has been established (0.3 mm/yr).[14]

It is on the basis of this knowledge that we have come to realize how much local and systemic reactions to cobalt-chromium (Co-Cr) wear products differ from all that we have learned about the periprosthetic tissue response to particulate debris of polyethylene, as the following sections will demonstrate.

ANALYSIS OF FIRST-GENERATION METAL-ON-METAL TOTAL HIPS

Radiographic and retrieval analyses of long-term surviving first-generation MOM bearings have shown very low annual wear of the bearings and minimal osteolysis.[15] In comparison with the histiocytic inflammation typifying metal-polyethylene hip tissues, we reported that the local tissue response to well-functioning MOM bearings was markedly less inflammatory, with mostly fibrous tissue containing few macrophages.[16] This was especially clear from postmortem analysis of a hip joint implanted with a McKee-Farrar hip for 30 years. A thorough histopathologic examination of tissues was performed.[17] Samples from periprosthetic capsule, interface membrane, inguinal lymph nodes, kidney, spleen, and

liver were examined for the amount and type of wear debris and any associated tissue pathology.

Despite 30 years of use and loosening of the cemented femoral stem, tissues around the loose implant showed only a small amount of metal staining (Fig. 12-1). Histologically, a mild histiocytic response and minimal apparent metal and minimal lymphocytes were noted in the periprosthetic tissues (Fig. 12-2). In the

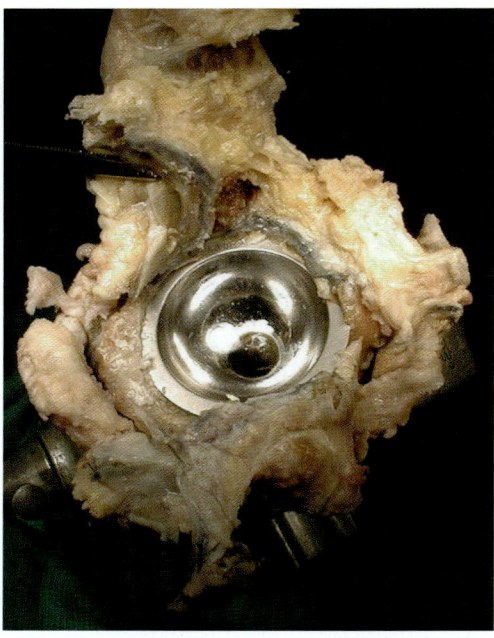

Figure 12-1. The removed acetabular component from an autopsy-retrieved McKee-Farrar, 30 years postoperatively. Note the small amount of metal staining (metallosis) within the inner capsule. Overall wear amounted to a few microns per year.

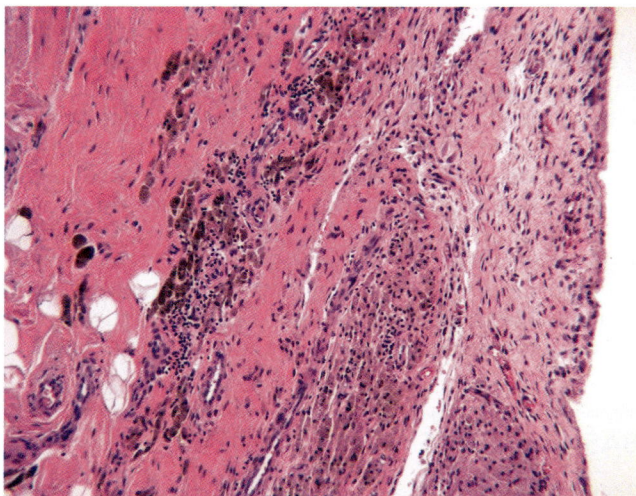

Figure 12-2. Light micrograph of periprosthetic tissue from Figure 12-1 showing mild histiocytic infiltration of the synovial lining. Phagocytic cells contain dark hematin pigment and occasional metal particles. Only a minimal lymphocyte response is seen (hematoxylin and eosin [H&E], ×200).

reticuloendothelial tissues, cobalt- and/or chromium-based particles large enough to be visible at the light microscope level were rarely seen, although particles of environmental origin were present. With the use of energy-dispersive x-ray analysis (EDAX), none of the particles in any of the organ tissues could be identified as cobalt-chromium alloy, except for one particle in a phagocytic cell within the liver. Lymphocytes and plasma cells were rare, and polymorphonuclear leukocytes were absent. No abnormalities were noted in any of the organ samples, despite the presence of high levels of cobalt (average of the four specimens was 119 ng/g; control tissue 27 ng/g) and chromium (average 105 ng/g; control undetectable) ions in the liver.

If it is presumed that sampled tissues were representative of the particle burden of the organ as a whole, absence of detectable particles suggested that (1) migration away from the joint was limited, (2) particles that had migrated were too small to be detected using the methods employed, or (3) they had already dissolved. It was thought initially that benign effects seen in this case were a result of the greatly reduced volume of debris alone. However, because cobalt-chromium particles are significantly smaller than PE particles, these particles most likely enter cells without inducing the inflammatory cytokine pathways associated with phagocytosis of particles of polyethylene. This is just one of the ways that biological responses to cobalt-chromium wear debris are more complicated than those involved with polyethylene.

HOW COBALT-CHROMIUM PRODUCTS ARE FORMED

Examination of particles produced under the ideal bearing conditions found in a hip simulator reveals that cobalt-chromium particles are both globular and needle shaped.[18] Electron microscopic studies have suggested that globular wear particles result from torn-off nanocrystals, and that needle-shaped particles are generated by fractured epsilon-martensite structures within the outermost layers of the metal component.[19] Wear particles comprise the alloy material and oxides from the articulating surface, particularly chromium-rich oxides of the outer passivation layer and organometallic phosphates, which are deposited from the synovial fluid.[20] Wimmer and colleagues described a tribolayer less than 200 nm thick that consisted of a nanocrystalline mixture of metal and organic material.[21]

Metal wear particles are known to be nanometer-sized, and recent improvements in isolation and examination techniques have shown that their size is affected by the specific wear mechanism responsible for their production.[22] Adhesive and abrasive wear processes release billions of particles per year into the synovial tissues and fluid.[23] In some conditions, this can lead to tissue staining (metallosis) (see Figs. 12-1 and 12-3). Under more severe wear conditions, such as edge loading, the stable protective chromium oxide layers found on the outermost surfaces can be damaged or removed, producing larger particles and leading to local crevice corrosion, pitting, and dissolution of metal in areas of damage.[24,25]

Although most of the particles entering the joint are produced from the bearing, it must be remembered that nonarticulating surfaces can contribute to the particle burden. For example, the taper connections of modular total joint replacements can be an important source of metal wear and corrosion products (Fig. 12-4).[26] Collier and coworkers[27] examined the tapered interface between the head and neck of total hip replacements and reported that in 91 cases in which the same alloy was used for the femoral head and stem, no corrosion products were found. In contrast, corrosion products were detected in 25 of 48 prostheses with a titanium alloy stem coupled with a cobalt-chromium head. The potentially inflammatory nature of these corrosion products has also been noted.[28,29]

THE FATE OF PARTICLES ENTERING THE JOINT

Wear particles are released into the joint fluid, where they may come into contact with phagocytic cells, primarily of the macrophage lineage, and become internalized by phagocytosis or pinocytosis, depending on their size. Although some particle-laden cells may be distributed away from the joint via the vascular and lymphatic systems,[30,31] many remain in the local tissues.[32] This results in the accumulation of particles within synovial phagocytic cells and histiocytes in the tissues lining the joint (Fig. 12-5). Particles can also be stored freely in the interstitial fluids, in synovial fluid, and in fluids that can accumulate within tissue bursae. Additionally, particles can be bound up in fibrin-lining bursae, in joint tissues, or within bone cysts.

When ingested by phagocytes, Co-Cr particles are exposed to the aggressive intracellular environment of lysosomes and phagosomes, where pH values can be as low as 4.6.[33] This will accelerate corrosion of metallic debris, locally increasing cobalt and chromium ions to potentially toxic levels. When the cell dies, particles are spilled back into joint tissues, where they may enter joint fluid or be rephagocytosed to continue the cycle locally, if the cell remains in the joint or at a distant site, if the cell migrates through the vascular or lymphatic system.

Metal particle migration from total hip replacements with metal-polyethylene bearings was studied in a group of 30 autopsy retrievals collected after an average of 5.8 years (range, 3.6 to 14.3 years) from patients ranging in age from 43 to 91 years.[34] Light and electron microscopy and identification of particle species through x-ray microanalysis demonstrated submicrometer metal particles within macrophages in the liver and/or the spleen in 11 of 15 patients with a revised arthroplasty and in 2 of 15 patients with a primary hip replacement.

Among patients with a revised hip replacement, particles were present in the spleen alone in five patients, in both the liver and spleen in another four patients, and in the liver alone in two. Particles had been generated from nonbearing surfaces such as loosened

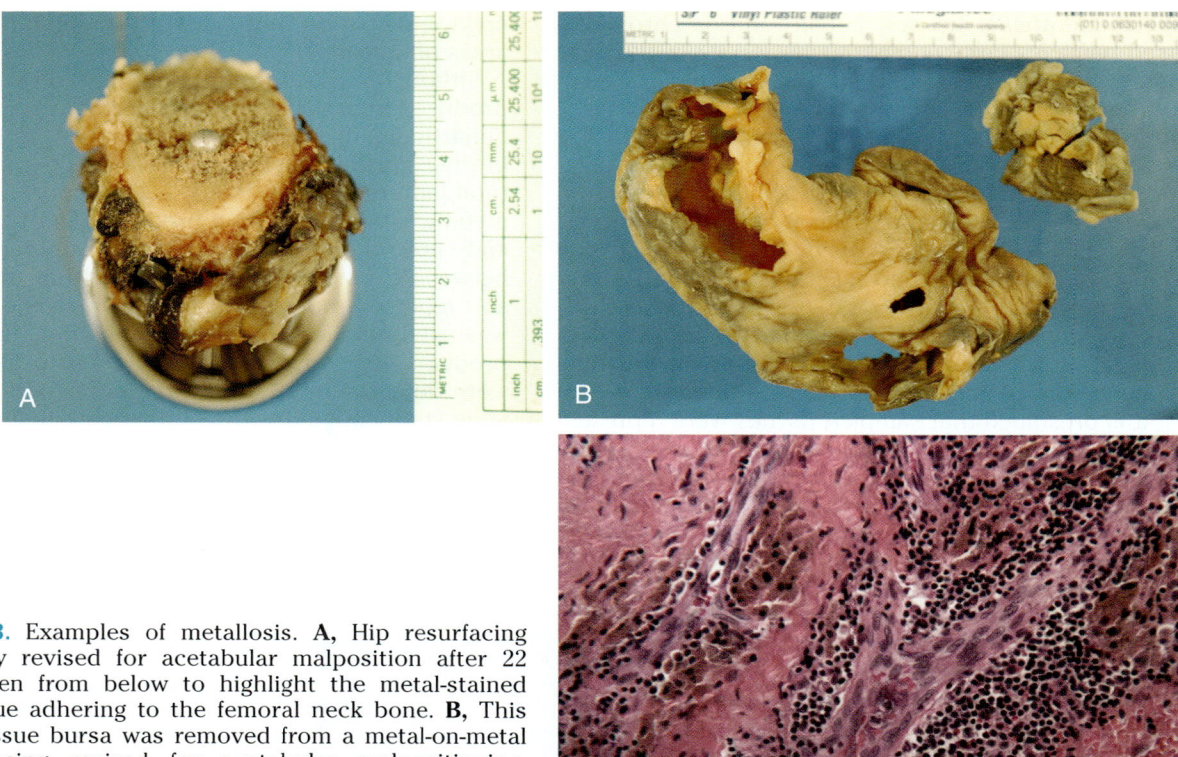

Figure 12-3. Examples of metallosis. **A,** Hip resurfacing arthroplasty revised for acetabular malposition after 22 months, seen from below to highlight the metal-stained villous tissue adhering to the femoral neck bone. **B,** This enlarged tissue bursa was removed from a metal-on-metal hip resurfacing revised for acetabular malpositioning, femoral osteolysis, and pain after 56 months. This bursa contained several hundred milliliters of brown fluid under pressure. **C,** Histology of this bursa tissue shows a mix of dark macrophages containing hematin and metal, and lymphocyte aggregates containing plasma cells (hematoxylin and eosin [H&E], ×200).

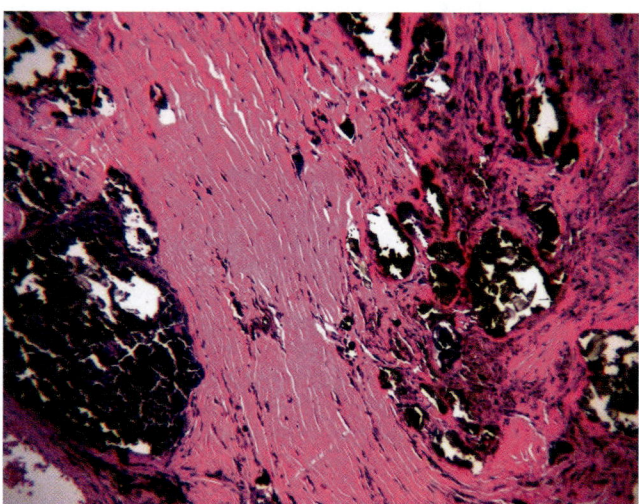

Figure 12-4. Histologic micrograph of solid corrosion products in periprosthetic tissue taken from a modular total hip replacement with signs of corrosion on the stem taper. Only a mild histiocytic response to this material is noted (hematoxylin and eosin [H&E], ×200).

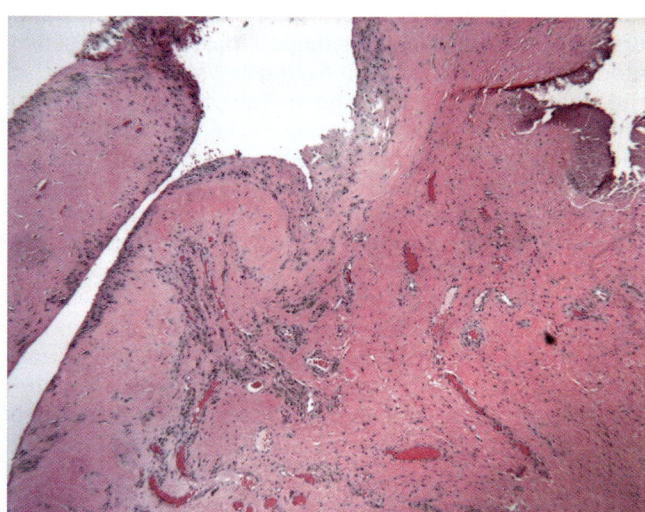

Figure 12-5. Histologic micrograph of synovial tissue from a case revised with metallosis shows discolored macrophages containing metal particles at the tissue edge. In this example, no lymphocytic response is obvious (hematoxylin and eosin [H&E], ×100).

components, ancillary fixation wires, plates or screws, and a well-fixed acetabular component and its fixation screws. In patients with primary hip replacement, metal particles generated between nonbearing surfaces were detected in the liver of one patient and in the spleen of another patient. The size of disseminated particles ranged from 0.1 to 8 μm, with most particles measuring less than 1 μm.

Particles were phagocytosed by macrophages, which formed focal aggregates in the organs without apparent toxicity. In the spleen, macrophages containing metal particles were found primarily within the lymphatic sheaths surrounding arterial vessels, where they formed foreign body granulomas. In the liver, metal particles were found in focal clusters in macrophages of the portal tracts and were distributed around venules in the parenchyma. These particles were commonly mixed with particles from environmental origins such as silicates and particles containing titanium or aluminum.

From these observations, it is clear that both local and systemic effects of cobalt-chromium particles must be considered. The following discussion will review what is known about cobalt and chromium wear and corrosion products in the context of patients with MOM hip replacements. In particular, important factors influencing the measurement of metal ions and the effects of large quantities of wear products will be discussed.

COBALT AND CHROMIUM IONS IN PATIENTS WITH METAL-ON-METAL IMPLANTS

The billions of nanometer-sized metal particles have an extremely high surface area, facilitating corrosion processes producing products that become detectable in blood, urine, and other bodily fluids as cobalt and chromium ions. Depending on the chemistry of the periparticulate fluid, various corrosion products can be produced, including soluble and insoluble forms of various salts and metal-protein complexes, free radicals, and reactive oxygen species.[35,36] These will vary in size, stability, and solubility, and consequently in their bioavailability.[37-39] However, when a sample of blood and urine is tested using atomic absorption or inductively coupled plasma mass spectrometry, these circulating corrosion products are detected as cobalt and chromium ions.

Systemic responses to circulating ions and nanometer-sized metallic particles debris are still not well understood, but concerns have been raised that the long-term consequences may be dire.[40] Since the time that cobalt-chromium alloy bearings were first implanted, long-term local and systemic effects of the particulate, and of ionic forms of the resulting wear debris or corrosion products, have been matters of concern.[41,42] Reports of sustained elevations in circulating metal levels and of the presence of chromosomal aberrations in joint tissues from MOM patients added to this concern.[43,44] A small-scale epidemiologic study that looked for associations between cancer rates and MOM bearings reported slight elevations in certain types of cancers.[45] Later follow-up involving comparison of the causes of death among 579 patients with McKee-Farrar MOM components and Brunswick or Lubinus metal-polyethylene prostheses noted that cancer mortality in the McKee group was similar to that of the general population,[46] although it was recognized that any detectable increase in cancer would require a large-scale survey for several decades to account for the anticipated 20- to 30-year latency period.[47]

Metal Wear Products and Cancer

Concern that cobalt-chromium wear products could cause cancer in patients is based on the known carcinogenic potential of these metals, particularly chromium in the hexavalent form (CrVI), and observations that exposure to cobalt and chromium ions can cause aberrations in cellular DNA.[44,48,49] It is extremely difficult to determine whether particles produced in an MOM bearing exist in the trivalent or hexavalent form. Chromium in its hexavalent form can enter cells much more readily than in its trivalent form. It is thought to bind mostly to nucleoproteins.[50] The intracellular process of reduction of hexavalent chromium to the more stable trivalent form is thought to be harmful to chromosomes and other intracellular organelles.[48]

Chromosomal changes have been demonstrated in patients with various types of joint replacements, including metal-on-polyethylene and MOM devices.[48,51] A statistically significant increase in both chromosome translocations (relocation of a chromosomal segment in a different position in the genome) and aneuploidy (chromosome loss and gain) was noted in the peripheral blood lymphocytes of 95 patients with Metasul MOM (Zimmer, Warsaw, Ind) total hips at 6, 12, and 24 months after surgery.[49] No statistically significant correlations between chromosome translocation indices and cobalt or chromium concentrations were reported, but they did correlate with molybdenum levels despite their low levels. Similar aberrations were shown to occur with titanium; the clinical implications of this and other studies are as yet unclear, as no case of an implant-induced cancer has been confirmed to date.[52-54] The multifactorial nature of DNA damage makes linking the results of these studies to a clinical problem very difficult.[55]

Metal Hypersensitivity (Allergy)

Another concern with MOM bearings was that some patients would have an allergic reaction to the nickel content (typically trace to 2%) or, more likely, to the cobalt (typically 60%), which has a tendency to elicit a comparable response to nickel in some individuals. Isolated reports described apparent metal sensitivity reactions that took the form of painful periprosthetic effusions, local necrosis, or, rarely, skin urticaria in a small number of patients with first-generation MOM total hip replacements (THRs). However, these reactions often were attributed to excessive wear (metallosis), which was a common finding with these early devices.[56] Histologic evaluation of tissues derived from revised second-generation MOM THRs and hip resurfacings by our group and others indicated a generally bland periprosthetic response with greatly reduced presence of macrophages and minimal wear debris, which was attributed to manufacturing improvements.[57,58] At a symposium held in 1995 to evaluate the reintroduction of MOM implants in the United States, it was estimated that less than 1% of patients would be affected by metal allergy. However, the more widespread benefits of reduced osteolysis and long-term durability would far outweigh this potential adverse event.[59]

ALVAL: A Unique Form of Metal Allergy?

As the number of patients with MOM THRs increased, concerns over metal allergy or hypersensitivity re-emerged. Reports of well-fixed implants revised for pain and, in some cases, osteolysis noted that pain was not relieved when the patient received a second MOM hip.[60,61] Tissues from these suspected metal hypersensitivity cases showed histologic features consistent with metal allergy (prominent, perivascular, and/or diffuse lymphocyte and plasma cell infiltrates, fibrin deposition, and extensive necrosis).[61] These features had not been seen in metal-on-polyethylene hip tissues, which were widely reported to be dominated by macrophages with few, if any, lymphocytes present[62,63] and were also rare in first-generation MOM implants.[64]

Predominant T lymphocytes, coupled with a clinical presentation of pain in the absence of loosening, infection, or high wear of the bearings, were interpreted to represent a form of type IV delayed-type hypersensitivity (DTH) response to metal.[61] Other features of this reaction included a distinct tissue layering wherein perivascular lymphocytes were located behind a tidemark of dense fibrin or necrosis, which replaced the synovial surface.[65] Because important differences from classical DTH histology were noted, particularly the presence of B lymphocytes, this phenomenon was termed an *aseptic lymphocytic vasculitis-associated lesion (ALVAL)*.[61,66] The term is now used in a more general sense as a name for painful soft tissue reactions around MOM hips, although it was coined to describe histologic features. Examples of ALVAL features are shown in Figure 12-6.

Cellular and Immune System Reaction to Metal Wear Debris and Ions

The host defense against bacterial, viral, or chemical challenges relies on the concerted action of both antigen (Ag)-nonspecific innate immunity and Ag-specific adaptive immunity. Both arms of the host defense systems are elicited in the reaction to biomaterial wear debris. Polyethylene debris was dealt with by the innate system in a nonspecific reaction that did not require the active participation of lymphocytes.[62,63] Because metal implants produce corrosion products in addition to discrete particles, they elicit a variety of immune responses.[2] It has been established with in vitro and in vivo studies that particulate cobalt-chromium can engage the innate immune system through monocyte-macrophage activation and secretion of proinflammatory cytokines that can upregulate transcription factor nuclear factor kappa B (NFκB) and downstream proinflammatory cytokines.[67] Caicedo and associates determined that metal ions and particles can activate inflammasome-mediated interleukin (IL)-1β secretion in macrophages[67] (the *inflammasome* is a multiprotein complex in cells such as macrophages that participates in the processing and secretion of inflammatory cytokines). Additionally, it has been shown that cobalt-chromium alloy degradation products in ionic and nanoparticulate forms can act as haptens, which, when complexed with local proteins and altering their confirmation, elicit an adaptive immune response analogous to a DTH reaction.[68]

Hallab and his team at Rush University have conducted extensive research on immune responses to metal wear particles and ions.[69] Their in vitro studies have shown lymphocyte proliferation in response to high concentrations of certain metal challenge agents, but in patients, the dose response is less clearly seen.[70] Despite the confusion between histologic and clinical differentiation of tissue reactions caused by excessive metal and those that are the result of a metal allergy,[71] it is clear that a small number of patients will suffer from a form of allergy or hypersensitivity to constituents of MOM bearings even in the absence of high wear.[38,72-74]

Toxicity and Necrosis

It has been shown that cobalt and chromium cytotoxicity of macrophages in vitro is dose dependent.[75] Other in vitro studies have shown that ion type, concentration, and time of exposure determine the type of cell response. Specifically, apoptosis was shown to be predominant at low concentrations, while necrosis occurred at elevated concentrations of metal ions.[76] Even more specifically, elevated chromium concentration has been linked to apoptotic phenomena rather than to necrosis. At low cobalt concentrations, apoptosis prevails, while high concentrations of cobalt may be able to produce cell necrosis.[77] Chromium is more cytotoxic than cobalt when it is present as the hexavalent form, which is taken up more easily by cells.[78,79] However, hexavalent chromium is extremely unstable and is reduced rapidly to the trivalent form. Cobalt enters readily into the intracellular environment and has been found to be more toxic than chromium.[76,80] However, it is still a matter of discussion whether cobalt or chromium plays a fundamental role in eliciting adverse periprosthetic reactions, especially in view of the fact that cobalt is excreted from the body rapidly, and detectable amounts of chromium are normally found in serum and urine because of dietary and environmental exposure.[47] It may not be a coincidence that malpositioned implants are associated with an elevation in systemic and local concentrations of cobalt, and that these hips have also been associated with extensive necrosis of joint tissues (Fig. 12-7). Extensive necrosis around MOM joints is one of the current concerns about this type of bearing.[81-83]

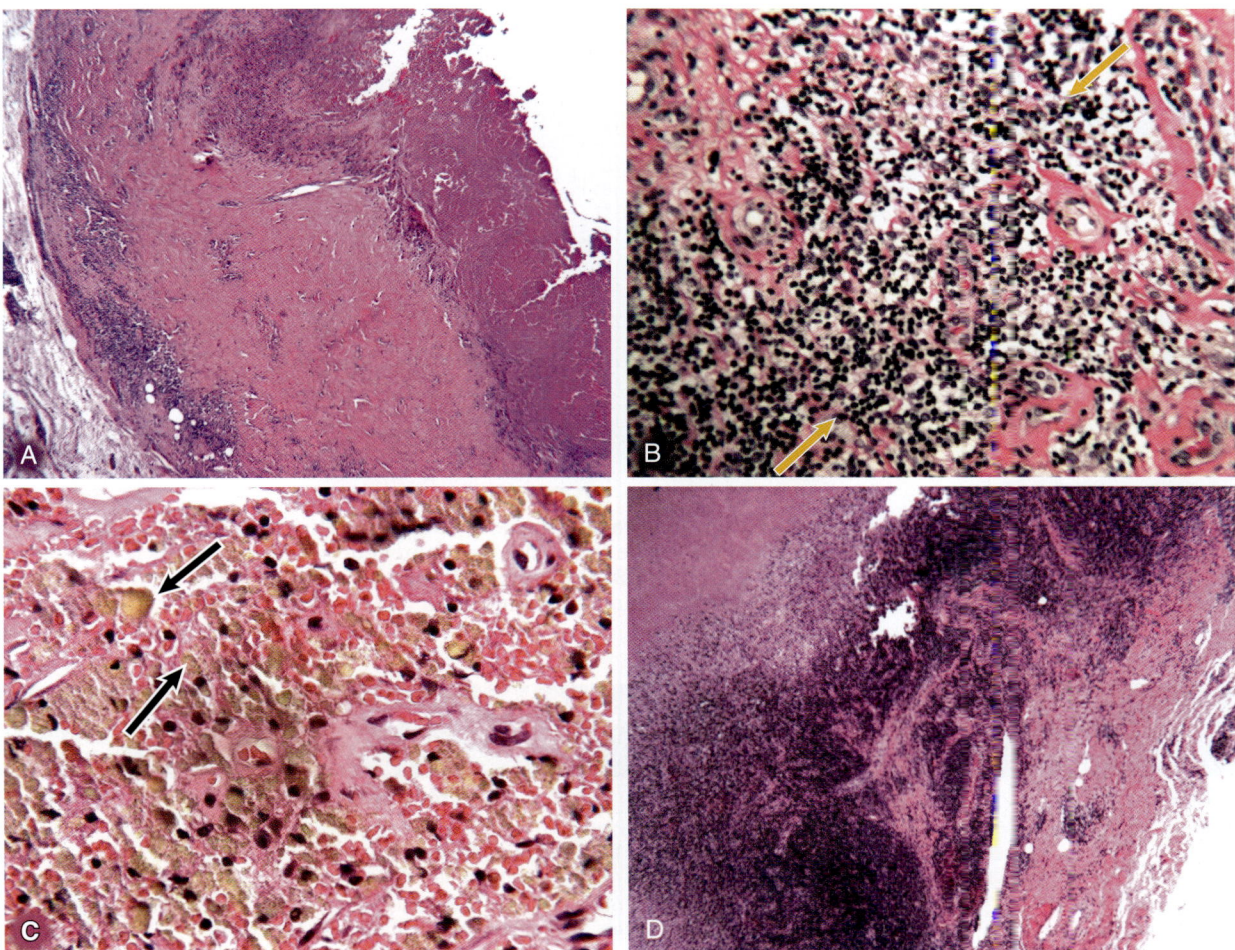

Figure 12-6. Examples of ALVAL (aseptic lymphocytic vasculitis-associated lesion) features. **A,** Adherent fibrin and lymphocytic infiltrates are common features (hematoxylin and eosin [H&E], ×40). **B,** This dense aggregate of predominantly lymphocytes also contains plasma cells *(arrows)* (H&E, ×200). **C,** Droplike inclusions *(arrows)* in macrophages have also been described in ALVAL, although they are not a common feature (H&E, ×400). **D,** In contrast to Figure 12-6*A,* this tissue contains very dense lymphocytic infiltrates, which are typical of cases revised for metal hypersensitivity (H&E, ×40).

Pseudotumors: Allergy or Wear?

Reports from a large-volume teaching hospital in England described painful "pseudotumors" forming in the hip joints of female patients with MOM THRs.[82] These were initially attributed to metal hypersensitivity due to the presence of extensive lymphocytic infiltrates in the tissues and their occurrence only in female patients.[84] Another large hip resurfacing arthroplasty (HRA) series reported a high incidence of revisions for elevated serum cobalt and chromium ions in patients with steep acetabular components, which are at risk for a severe type of wear known as *edge-loading*.[85] At revision, these joints were characterized by metallosis, the formation of enlarged, fluid-filled bursae, (see Fig. 12-3*B*), and tissue histology that included abundant debris-filled macrophages and often also extensive lymphocyte infiltrations (see Fig. 12-3*C*).[86] These failures were attributed to the effects of high wear. Other studies have similarly reported a high failure rate associated with edge-loading, elevated metal ions, and adverse soft tissue reactions.[87-89]

Our group semiquantitatively examined the histologic features of 32 cases of unusual periprosthetic tissue reactions from cases with known high wear and also with suspected metal hypersensitivity.[71] We found common histologic features in both groups, most notably lymphocyte aggregates, macrophage infiltrates, fibrin adherence, and necrosis, but these tended to differ in quantity and in distribution such that larger and more extensive lymphocyte aggregates were seen in tissues from patients with metal hypersensitivity, and more macrophages with metal in patients with high wear (Table 12-1). However, diagnosing the cause of a periprosthetic reaction on the basis of histology alone is not recommended. To assess the role of high wear in the origin of periprosthetic masses and pseudotumors, it is recommended that prerevision metal ion levels and/or postrevision component wear measurements be obtained.[87]

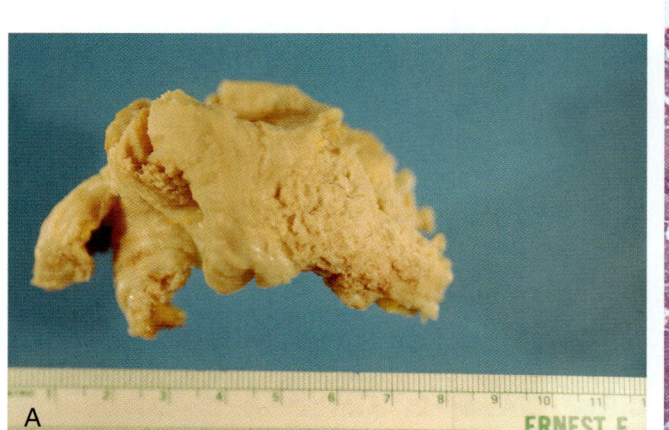

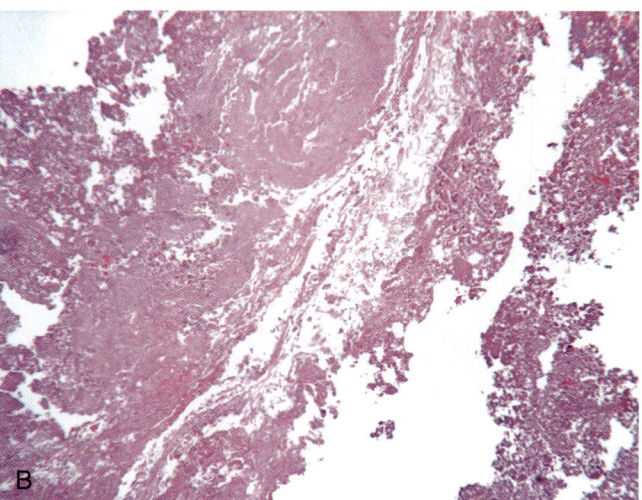

Figure 12-7. A, Gross tissue from metal-on-metal hip resurfacing revised after 11 months for pain and suspected metal hypersensitivity. This is part of a larger periprosthetic tissue mass that was removed. Note the caseous (cottage cheese–like) appearance and the lack of color, indicating necrosis. **B,** Histologic micrograph of tissue from Figures 12-7**A,** which consists primarily of fibrin and necrotic fibrous tissue (hematoxylin and eosin [H&E], ×40).

Table 12-1. Results of Histologic Comparison Between Cases Revised for Wear-Related Problems Versus Pain and Suspected Metal Sensitivity

Group	Lymphocytes	Macrophages	Fibrin
High wear–related cases	Diffuse and/or perivascular; predominantly B cells with T cells; plasma cells may be present	Predominant cells, scattered throughout; often plump with hematin and metal	Variable amounts
Low wear, suspected metal sensitivity	Typically perivascular and extensive; often a mix of T and B cells; plasma cells may be abundant	Located around lymphocyte aggregates or interposed between lymphocytes	Often large amounts
Nonmetal-metal control tissues	Very few lymphocytes and plasma cells are rare	Scattered, or close to subsynovial vessels	Typically minimal

Why cobalt-chromium wear products elicit almost no clinically relevant response in some patients, while pseudotumors, necrosis, and effusions occur in other patients, is unclear, but factors that determine the biological response to wear debris are beginning to be defined (Fig. 12-8).[2,90,91] Further work in this area will continue to provide important insights into biological reactions to metal from hip implants.

COBALTISM

Cobalt poisoning from excessive wear of joint arthroplasty devices is an exceedingly rare event, and to date, the orthopedic literature reports only a handful of cases.[88-95] Clinical symptoms include blindness, deafness, neuropathy, cardiopathy, fatigue, and headaches. In all but one of these reports, the levels of cobalt were extraordinarily high and were the result of rare and catastrophic wear events. For example, Steens and colleagues[94] reported finding a cobalt-chromium ball worn down to a cylinder following fracture of the mated ceramic liner. The serum cobalt in that patient at the time of revision was 398 µg/L. A similar case involving severe destruction of the Co-Cr revision component femoral head after ceramic component fracture reported a serum level greater than 600 µg/L in a patient suffering from neurologic and cardiac problems.[93] Another report captured wide attention because one of the two patients it describes had serum cobalt levels of 20 µg/L at the time of revision of a hip replacement.[95] Although 20 µg/L represents an outlier level in many MOM patient series, it is considerably lower than the extreme levels described in the other reports of cobalt poisoning. The patient reported cognitive decline, vertigo, hearing loss, groin pain, rashes, and dyspnea. The author of the report, who himself suffered cobalt-related anxiety, headaches, irritability, fatigue, hearing loss, and cognitive decline with serum cobalt levels of 83 µg/L from a failed total hip, recommended that revision should be considered for patients with neurologic or cardiac impairment linked to elevated serum cobalt levels. In all of these reports, systemic symptoms progressively improved and metal ion levels in serum declined upon removal of the source of the cobalt. Therefore, timely revision is recommended.[92,95]

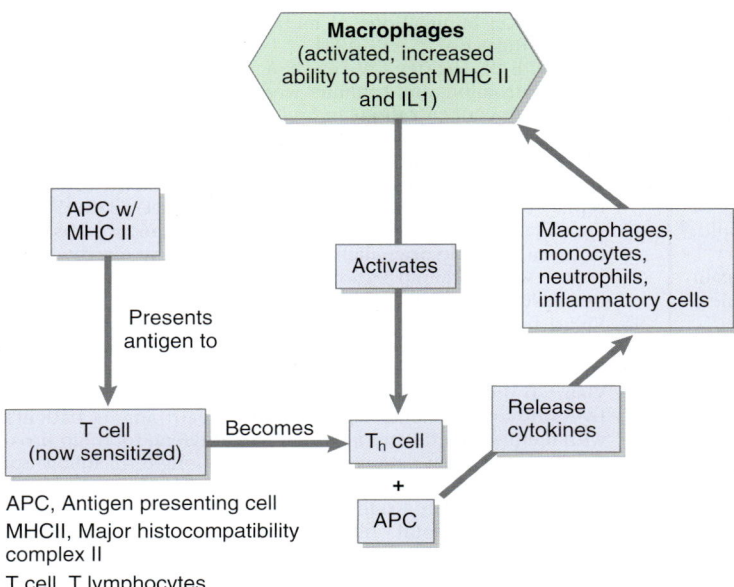

Figure 12-3. Model showing biological response to wear debris produced by metal-on-metal hip replacements as a delayed-type hypersensitivity (DTH) response. (*Adapted from Hallab NJ, Caicedo M, Epstein R, McAllister K, Jacobs JJ: In vitro reactivity to implant metals demonstrates a person-dependent association with both T-cell and B-cell activation. J Biomed Mater Res A 92(2):667–682, 2009.*)

APC, Antigen presenting cell
MHCII, Major histocompatibility complex II
T cell, T lymphocytes
T$_h$ cell, Helper T lymphocyte

SUMMARY

Biological reactions to cobalt-chromium particles have been less thoroughly studied than reactions to polyethylene particles, but what is presently known can be summarized and compared with reactions to polymeric debris as follows:

1. Although the volume of debris is reduced by MOM bearings, the nanometer-sized particles provide an enormous surface area for corrosion; thus, in addition to particulate debris, corrosion products with varying biostability and bioavailability are formed.
2. Local responses to these wear products involve the immune system, and both macrophages and lymphocytes are common features in these tissues.
3. Systemic effects over the long term are not well known, but isolated autopsy retrieval studies suggest that normal quantities of metal wear products are well tolerated.
4. In contrast, excessive wear products can result in a variety of painful soft tissue problems, sometimes termed *pseudotumors,* and may lead to revision surgery.
5. Allergic responses to cobalt and chromium affect a small percentage of patients; these reactions share similar clinical and histologic features with the reaction to wear debris.

REFERENCES

1. Jacobs JJ, Shanbhag AS, Glant TT, et al: Wear debris in total joint replacements. J Am Acad Orthop Surg 2:212, 1994.
2. Jacobs JJ, Campbell PA: How has the biologic reaction to wear particles changed with newer bearing surfaces? J Am Acad Orthop Surg 16(Suppl 1):S49, 2008.
3. Shanbhag AS, Jacobs JJ, Black J, et al: Human monocyte response to particulate biomaterials generated in vivo and in vitro. J Orthop Res 13:792, 1995.
4. Amstutz HC, Campbell P, Clarke IC, Kossovsky N: Mechanism and clinical significance of wear debris-induced osteolysis. Clin Orthop Relat Res 276:7, 1992.
5. Schmalzried TP, Jasty M, Harris WH: Periprosthetic bone loss in total hip arthroplasty: polyethylene wear debris and the concept of the effective joint space. J Bone Joint Surg Am 74:849, 1992.
6. Campbell P, Ma S, Yeom B, et al: Isolation of predominantly submicron-sized UHMWPE wear particles from periprosthetic tissues. J Biomed Mater Res 29:127, 1995.
7. Willert HG: Reactions of the articular capsule to wear products of artificial joint prostheses. J Biomed Mater Res 11:157, 1977.
8. Jones L, Hungerford D: Cement disease. Clin Orthop Relat Res 225:191, 1987.
9. Hungerford DS, Jones LC: The rationale for cementless total hip replacement. Orthop Clin North Am 24:617, 1993.
10. Nasser S, Campbell PA, Kilgus D, et al: Cementless total joint arthroplasty prostheses with titanium-alloy articular surfaces: a human retrieval analysis. Clin Orthop Relat Res 261:171, 1990.
11. Archibeck MJ, Jacobs JJ, Roebuck KA, Glant TT: The basic science of periprosthetic osteolysis. Inst Course Lect 50:185, 2001.
12. Ingham E, Fisher J: Biological reactions to wear debris in total joint replacement. Proc Inst Mech Eng (H) 214:21, 2000.
13. Revell PA, al-Saffar N, Kobayashi A: Biological reaction to debris in relation to joint prostheses. Proc Inst Mech Eng (H) 211:187, 1997.
14. McKellop HA: Wear assessment. In Callaghan JJ, Rosenberg AG, Rubash HE (eds): The adult hip, Philadelphia, 1998, Lippincott Raven Publishers, p 231.
15. McKellop H, Park S-H, Chiesa R, et al: In vivo wear of three types of metal on metal hip prostheses during two decades of use. Clin Orthop Relat Res (329)(Suppl):S128, 1996.
16. Doorn PF, Mirra JM, Campbell PA, Amstutz HC: Tissue reaction to metal on metal total hip prostheses. Clin Orthop Relat Res (329)(Suppl):S187, 1996.
17. Campbell P, Urban RM, Catelas I, et al: Autopsy analysis thirty years after metal-on-metal total hip replacement: a case report. J Bone Joint Surg Am 85:2218, 2003.

18. Catelas I, Medley JB, Campbell PA, et al: Comparison of in vitro with in vivo characteristics of wear particles from metal-metal hip implants. J Biomed Mater Res B 70:167, 2004.

19. Buscher R, Tager G, Dudzinski W, et al: Subsurface microstructure of metal-on-metal hip joints and its relationship to wear particle generation. J Biomed Mater Res B Appl Biomater 72:206, 2005.

20. Lewis AC, Kilburn MR, Heard PJ, et al: The entrapment of corrosion products from CoCr implant alloys in the deposits of calcium phosphate: a comparison of serum, synovial fluid, albumin, EDTA, and water. J Orthop Res 24:1587, 2006.

21. Wimmer MA, Fischer A, Buscher R, et al: Wear mechanisms in metal-on-metal bearings: the importance of tribochemical reaction layers. J Orthop Res 28:436, 2010.

22. Billi F, Benya P, Ebramzadeh E, McKellop H: An accurate and extremely sensitive method to isolate and display nanoparticulate metallic wear debris for morphometric analysis. Presented at the 54th Annual Meeting of the Orthopaedic Research Society, San Francisco, Calif, March 2-5, 2008. Poster No. 1929.

23. Doorn PF, Campbell PA, Worrall J, et al: Metal wear particle characterization from metal on metal total hip replacements: transmission electron microscopy study of periprosthetic tissues and isolated particles. J Biomed Mater Res 42:103, 1998.

24. Willert HG, Buchhorn GH, Gobel D, et al: Wear behavior and histopathology of classic cemented metal on metal hip endoprostheses. Clin Orthop Relat Res 329(Suppl):S160, 1996.

25. Jacobs JJ, Gilbert JL, Urban RM: Corrosion of metal orthopaedic implants. J Bone Joint Surg Am 80:268, 1998.

26. Gilbert JL, Buckley CA, Jacobs JJ: In vivo corrosion of modular hip prosthesis components in mixed and similar metal combinations: the effect of crevice, stress, motion and alloy coupling. J Biomed Mater Res 27:1533, 1993.

27. Collier JP, Surprenant VA, Jensen RE, et al: Corrosion between the components of modular femoral hip prostheses. J Bone Joint Surg Br 74:511, 1992.

28. Urban RM, Jacobs JJ, Gilbert JL, Galante JO: Migration of corrosion products from modular hip prostheses: particle microanalysis and histopathological findings. J Bone Joint Surg Am 76:1345, 1994.

29. Huber M, Reinisch G, Trettenhahn G, et al: Presence of corrosion products and hypersensitivity-associated reactions in periprosthetic tissue after aseptic loosening of total hip replacements with metal bearing surfaces. Acta Biomater 5:172, 2009.

30. Case CP, Langkamer VG, James C, et al: Widespread dissemination of metal debris from implants. J Bone Joint Surg Br 76:701, 1994.

31. Urban RM, Jacobs JJ, Tomlinson MJ, et al: Dissemination of wear particles to the liver, spleen, and abdominal lymph nodes of patients with hip or knee replacement. J Bone Joint Surg Am 82:457, 2000.

32. Lewis CG, Belniak RM, Hopfer SM, et al: Cobalt in periprosthetic soft tissue. Acta Orthop Scand 62:447, 1991.

33. Thiele L, Reszka R, Merkle HP, Walter E: Competitive adsorption of serum proteins at microparticles affects phagocytosis by dendritic cells. Biomaterials 24:1409, 2003.

34. Urban RM, Tomlinson MJ, Hall DJ, Jacobs JJ: Accumulation in liver and spleen of metal particles generated at nonbearing surfaces in hip arthroplasty. J Arthroplasty 19:94, 2004.

35. Hallab NJ, Jacobs JJ, Skipor A, et al: Systemic metal-protein binding associated with total joint replacement arthroplasty. J Biomed Mater Res 49:353, 2000.

36. Papageorgiou I, Brown C, Schins R, et al: The effect of nano- and micron-sized particles of cobalt-chromium alloy on human fibroblasts in vitro. Biomaterials 28:2946, 2007.

37. Venezia C, Karol MH: Comparison of cobalt and chromium binding to blood elements. Toxicology 30:125, 1984.

38. Hallab N, Merritt K, Jacobs JJ: Metal sensitivity in patients with orthopaedic implants. J Bone Joint Surg Am 83:428, 2001.

39. Beyersmann D: Interactions in metal carcinogenicity. Toxicol Lett 72:333, 1994.

40. Black J: Metal on metal bearings: a practical alternative to metal on polyethylene total joints? Clin Orthop Relat Res (329) (Suppl):S244, 1996.

41. Wapner KL: Implications of metallic corrosion in THA. Clin Orthop Relat Res 271:12, 1991.

42. Shahgaldi BF, Heatley FW, Dewar A, et al: In vivo corrosion of cobalt-chromium and titanium wear particles: nickel-, chrom- and cobalt-concentrations in human tissue and body fluids of hip prosthesis patients. J Bone Joint Surg Br 77:962, 1995.

43. Jacobs JJ, Skipor AK, Doorn PF, et al: Cobalt and chromium concentrations in patients with metal on metal total hip replacements. Clin Orthop Relat Res 329(Suppl):S256, 1996.

44. Case CP, Langkamer VG, Howell RT, et al: Preliminary observations on possible premalignant changes in bone marrow adjacent to worn total hip arthroplasty implants. Clin Orthop Relat Res 329(Suppl):S269, 1996.

45. Visuri T, Pukkala E, Paavolainen P, et al: Cancer risk after metal on metal and polyethylene on metal total hip arthroplasty. Clin Orthop Relat Res 329(Suppl):S280, 1996.

46. Visuri T, Borg H, Pulkkinen P, et al: A retrospective comparative study of mortality and causes of death among patients with metal-on-metal and metal-on-polyethylene total hip prostheses in primary osteoarthritis after a long-term follow-up. BMC Musculoskelet Disord 23:11, 2010.

47. MacDonald SJ: Can a safe level for metal ions in patients with metal-on-metal total hip arthroplasties be determined? J Arthroplasty 19:71, 2004.

48. Doherty AT, Howell RT, Ellis LA, et al: Increased chromosome translocations and aneuploidy in peripheral blood lymphocytes of patients having revision arthroplasty of the hip. J Bone Joint Surg Br 83:1075, 2001.

49. Ladon D, Doherty A, Newson R, et al: Changes in metal levels and chromosome aberrations in the peripheral blood of patients after metal-on-metal hip arthroplasty. J Arthroplasty 19:78, 2004.

50. Yang J, Black J: Competitive binding of chromium, cobalt and nickel to serum proteins. Biomaterials 15:262, 1994.

51. Case CP: Chromosomal changes after surgery for joint replacement. J Bone Joint Surg Br 83:1093, 2001.

52. Visuri T: Cancer risk after metal on metal hip prosthesis. In Rieker C, Windler M, Wyss U (eds): METASUL: a metal-on-metal bearing, Bern, 1998, Hans Huber, p 149.

53. Tharani R, Dorey FJ, Schmalzried TP: The risk of cancer following total hip or knee arthroplasty. J Bone Joint Surg Am 83:774, 2001.

54. Shimmin A, Beaule PE, Campbell P: Current concept review: metal-on-metal hip resurfacing arthroplasty. J Bone Joint Surg Am 90:637, 2008.

55. Paustenbach DJ, Finley BL, Kacew S: Biological relevance and consequences of chemical- or metal-induced DNA cross-linking. Proc Soc Exp Biol Med 211:211, 1996.

56. Evans EM, Freeman MA, Miller AJ, Vernon-Roberts B: Metal sensitivity as a cause of bone necrosis and loosening of the prosthesis in total joint replacement. J Bone Joint Surg Br 56:626, 1974.

57. Doorn PF, Campbell PA, Amstutz HC: Metal versus polyethylene wear particles in total hip replacements: a review. Clin Orthop Relat Res 329(Suppl):S206, 1996.

58. Campbell P, Mirra J, Doorn P, et al: Histopathology of metal-on-metal hip joint tissues. In Rieker C, Oberholzer S, Wyss U (eds): World tribology forum in arthroplasty, Gottingen, 2000, Hans Huber, p 167.

59. Amstutz HC, Campbell P, McKellop H, et al: Metal on metal total hip replacement workshop consensus document. Clin Orthop Relat Res 329(Suppl):S297, 1996.

60. Willert H, Buchhorn G, Fayaayazi A, Lohmann C: Histopathological changes around metal/metal joints indicate delayed type hypersensitivity: preliminary results of 14 cases. Osteologie 9:2, 2000.

61. Willert HG, Buchhorn GH, Fayyazi A, et al: Metal-on-metal bearings and hypersensitivity in patients with artificial hip joints: a clinical and histomorphological study. J Bone Joint Surg Am 87:28, 2005.

62. Goodman SB: Wear particles, periprosthetic osteolysis and the immune system. Biomaterials 28:5044, 2007.

63. Sandhu J, Waddell JE, Henry M, Boynton EL: The role of T cells in polyethylene particulate induced inflammation. J Rheumatol 25:1794, 1998.

64. Willert H-G, Buchhorn GH, Semlitsch M: Particle disease due to wear of metal alloys: findings from retrieval studies. In Morrey BF (ed): Biological, material, and mechanical considerations of joint replacement, Bristol-Myers Squibb/Zimmer Orthopaedic Symposium Series, New York, 1993, Raven Press, p 129.

65. Davies AP, Willert HG, Campbell PA, et al: An unusual lymphocytic perivascular infiltration in tissues around contemporary metal-on-metal joint replacements. J Bone Joint Surg Am 87:18, 2005.

66. Campbell P, Mirra J: Lymphocytic vasculitis associated lesions around metal-metal total hips. Presented at Society for Biomaterials 28th Annual Meeting, Tampa, April 24-29, 2002.

67. Caicedo MS, Desai R, McAllister K, et al: Soluble and particulate Co-Cr-Mo alloy implant metals activate the inflammasome danger signaling pathway in human macrophages: a novel mechanism for implant debris reactivity. J Orthop Res 27:847–854, 2009.

68. Hallab NJ, Caicedo M, Finnegan A, Jacobs JJ: Th1 type lymphocyte reactivity to metals in patients with total hip arthroplasty. J Orthop Surg 3:6, 2008.

69. Hallab NJ, Jacobs JJ: Biologic effects of implant debris. Bull NYU Hosp Jt Dis 67:182, 2009.

70. Hallab N, Anderson S, Caicedo M, et al: Immune responses correlate with serum-metal in metal-on-metal hip arthroplasty. J Arthroplasty 19:88, 2004.

71. Campbell P, Ebramzadeh E, Nelson S, et al: Histological features of pseudotumor-like tissues from metal-on-metal hips. Clin Orthop Relat Res 468:2321, 2010.

72. Gawkrodger DJ: Metal sensitivities and orthopaedic implants revisited: the potential for metal allergy with the new metal-on-metal joint prostheses. Br J Dermatol 148:1089, 2003.

73. Campbell P, Shimmin A, Walter L, Solomon M: Metal sensitivity as a cause of groin pain in metal-on-metal hip resurfacing. J Arthroplasty 23:1080, 2008.

74. Hallab NJ, Caicedo M, Epstein R, et al: In vitro reactivity to implant metals demonstrates a person-dependent association with both T-cell and B-cell activation. J Biomed Mater Res A 92(2):667–682, 2009.

75. Kwon YM, Xia Z, Glyn-Jones S, et al: Dose-dependent cytotoxicity of clinically relevant cobalt nanoparticles and ions on macrophages in vitro. Biomed Mater 4:025018, 2009.

76. Catelas I, Petit A, Vali H, et al: Quantitative analysis of macrophage apoptosis vs. necrosis induced by cobalt and chromium ions in vitro. Biomaterials 26:2441, 2005.

77. Granchi D, Cenni E, Ciapetti G, et al: Cell death induced by metal ions: necrosis or apoptosis? J Mater Sci Mater Med 9:31, 1998.

78. O'Brien TJ, Ceryak S, Patierno SR: Complexities of chromium carcinogenesis: role of cellular response, repair and recovery mechanisms. Mutat Res 533:3, 2003.

79. Wise SS, Holmes AL, Wise JP Sr: Hexavalent chromium-induced DNA damage and repair mechanisms. Rev Environ Health 23:39, 2008.

80. Yamamoto A, Honma R, Sumita M: Cytotoxicity evaluation of 43 metal salts using murine fibroblasts and osteoblastic cells. J Biomed Mater Res 39:331, 1998.

81. Boardman DR, Middleton FR, Kavanagh TG: A benign psoas mass following metal-on-metal resurfacing of the hip. J Bone Joint Surg Br 88:402, 2006.

82. Pandit H, Glyn-Jones S, McLardy-Smith P, et al: Pseudotumours associated with metal-on-metal hip resurfacings. J Bone Joint Surg Br 90:847, 2008.

83. Ollivere B, Darrah C, Barker T, et al: Early clinical failure of the Birmingham metal-on-metal hip resurfacing is associated with metallosis and soft-tissue necrosis. J Bone Joint Surg Br 91:1025, 2009.

84. Pandit H, Vlychou M, Whitwell D, et al: Necrotic granulomatous pseudotumours in bilateral resurfacing hip arthroplasties: evidence for a type IV immune response. Virchows Arch 453:529, 2008.

85. De Haan R, Pattyn C, Gill HS, et al: Correlation between inclination of the acetabular component and metal ion levels in metal-on-metal hip resurfacing replacement. J Bone Joint Surg Br 90:1291, 2008.

86. De Haan R, Campbell PA, Su EP, De Smet KA: Revision of metal-on-metal resurfacing arthroplasty of the hip: the influence of malposition of the components. J Bone Joint Surg Br 90:1158, 2008.

87. De Smet K, De Haan R, Calistri A, et al: Metal ion measurement as a diagnostic tool to identify problems with metal-on-metal hip resurfacing. J Bone Joint Surg Am 90:202, 2008.

88. Glyn-Jones S, Pandit H, Kwon YM, et al: Risk factors for inflammatory pseudotumour formation following hip resurfacing. J Bone Joint Surg Br 91:1566, 2009.

89. Langton DJ, Jameson SS, Joyce TJ, et al: Early failure of metal-on-metal bearings in hip resurfacing and large-diameter total hip replacement: a consequence of excess wear. J Bone Joint Surg Br 92:38, 2010.

90. Jacobs JJ, Urban RM, Hallab NJ, et al: Metal-on-metal bearing surfaces. J Am Acad Orthop Surg 17:69, 2009.

91. Catelas I, Jacobs JJ: Biologic activity of wear particles. Instr Course Lect 59:3, 2010.

92. Jacobs J: Commentary on tower S. J Bone Joint Surg, October 29, 2010 (http://www.ejbjs.org/cgi/content/full/JBJS.J.00125v1/DC1).

93. Oldenburg M, Wegner R, Baur X: Severe cobalt intoxication due to prosthesis wear in repeated total hip arthroplasty. J Arthroplasty 24:825.e15-e20, 2009.

94. Steens W, von Foerster G, Katzer A: Severe cobalt poisoning with loss of sight after ceramic-metal pairing in a hip—a case report. Acta Orthop 77:830, 2006.

95. Tower S: Arthroprosthetic cobaltism: neurological and cardiac manifestations in two patients with metal-on-metal arthroplasty: a case report. J Bone Joint Surg 92A:2847–2851, 2010 (http://www.ejbjs.org/cgi/doi/10.2106/JBJS.J.00125).

CHAPTER 13

Bone Grafts in Hip Surgery

*Paul Tee Hui Lee, Sandor Gyomorey,
Oleg A. Safir, David J. Backstein,
and Allan E. Gross*

KEY POINTS

- Autologous bone graft is osteogenic, osteoinductive, and osteoconductive, with complete histocompatibility and no risk of infectious disease transmission. It is considered the gold standard for bone graft and is the most favored graft material in musculoskeletal reconstruction.
- Advantages of bone allograft use include availability of materials and avoidance of donor site morbidity associated with autograft harvesting. Disadvantages of bone allograft use include lack of osteogenic cells, decreased osteoinductive factors, host immune response, and risk of infection.
- Impaction bone grafting is generally excellent for treating patients with small to moderate-sized contained cavitary defects but poor with regard to implant fixation stability for patients with large uncontained segmental defects.
- For such large uncontained segmental bone defects, structural bulk allograft can provide adequate support for primary implant fixation stability with relatively reasonable long-term outcomes, despite mixed concerns over long-term resorption.
- The success of graft incorporation depends on several factors, principally graft revascularization, new bone formation (around and within the graft), and healing at the graft-host interface. These in turn depend on a combination of the biological activity of the graft, the vascularity of the host bed, and the mechanical stability of the graft-host interface.

INTRODUCTION

Historical Perspective

Bone grafting is an ancient art. Anthropologist A. Jagharian at Erivan Medical Centre in Armenia examined a prehistoric Khuritic skull from the ancient Centre of Ishtkun and found a piece of animal bone filling a 7-mm defect with bony regrowth around the grafted bone.[4] It has been suggested that the ancient Egyptians and Greeks attempted bone transplantation. In the modern age, the first documented bone graft was successfully performed in 1668 by a Dutch surgeon named Job Van Meekeren, who successfully inserted a fragment of a dog bone into the skull of an injured soldier.[5] The first documented successful autograft transplant was performed in Germany in 1821 by Philips von Walter in experimentally created animal bone defects.[7] The first documented allograft transplant was performed in 1879 by Sir William MacEwen in Scotland, who replaced the infected proximal two thirds of a humerus in a 4-year-old boy with the tibia from another child with rickets.[6] In 1915, F. H. Albee published his work on autologous bone graft in the United States, which promoted the use of bone transplantation.[8] In 1942, Inclan reported his experience in a large number of operations using autograft and allograft.[9] Similar to other surgeons, Inclan considered the difficulties of finding suitable grafts for operations. When met with supply difficulties for autologous bone transplant, he used homologous bone graft between living patients of the same blood group. He did this because immune-related problems were known then, and graft from cadaver was prohibited on religious and sentimental grounds. Modern-day bone banks emerged in the 1960s and 1970s with improvements in cooling techniques combined with allograft processing; this led to the relative immunogenic impunity of allografts after transplantation. Several reports have helped to define safety and techniques in bone banking, thereby facilitating increased use of bone allografts.[10-12] In recent times, despite its limitations, allogeneic bone graft is the most commonly used graft tissue.[13] Several important clinical applications include restoration of bone stock in tumor surgery and in revision hip arthroplasty.

In hip surgery, the use of bone graft includes autografts, allografts, and bone substitutes. We will focus our discussion on the use of autologous and allogeneic bone grafts and will include various grafting techniques, their clinical applications and results, the basic scientific basis of these materials, current controversies, and future directions.

Bone Autograft

Clinical indications for the use of bone autograft include primary total hip replacement for hip dysplasia and protrusio to treat bone defects and achieve primary implant fixation stability and restore the center of rotation for the joint.[1-3] Femoral head osteonecrosis can also be treated by vascularized and nonvascularized autologous bone grafts. Morselized autografts generally are used for treating smaller contained defects, and structural autografts are used for larger defects that may be uncontained. The resected host femoral head is the most frequently used form of autograft bone. It is readily available, adequate in size, cheap, biomechanically compatible, and easy to contour to fit defects, and it does not need processing. Total hip replacements performed in dysplastic hips using femoral head autograft have shown graft incorporation in most cases, with generally good clinical outcomes over the short term to midterm.[1,17-27] Longer-term results have been mixed. Harris and associates reported a 10% revision rate (n = 47) at a mean of 7.1 years,[1] a 20% revision rate (n = 46) at a mean of 11.8 years,[19] and a 29% revision rate (n = 55) at a mean of 16.5 years.[20] The authors expressed concern regarding low stem offset and posterior cup uncoverage in this cohort. Gross and colleagues[21] reported a revision rate of 13% (n = 15) at a mean of 8.4 years' follow-up and later, Nousiainen and co-workers[27] reported a revision rate of 32% (n = 31) at a mean of 14 (8 to 18) years' follow-up. Inao and associates[22] reported 0% revision rate (n = 20) at a mean of 8.4 years; however, Iida and colleagues[25] reported a 4% revision rate (n = 133) at a mean of 12.3 (8 to 24) years, and Akiyama and associates[26] reported a 4% revision rate (n = 147) at a mean of 11.8 (6.3 to 15.4) years. Note that mean patient weight was 51 (29 to 78) kg in Iida's cohort and 51.6 ± 7.9 kg in Akiyama's. With regard to resorption of the autologous graft, results from various series were similarly mixed.[17,19,21,27] Nevertheless, there is consensus among most authors that the bulk autograft incorporated well, restored pelvic bone stock, and facilitated revision surgery.

Allograft

Allografts, morselized or structural, have been used mainly to address significant bone loss in revision hip arthroplasty and post tumor resection.

Impaction Bone Grafting

Impaction bone grafting is used because it is considered a biological technique for restoring host bone stock. Metal wire meshes are used to enclose segmental bone defects, which then are filled with morselized bone allograft that is densely impacted before cementing of the acetabular or femoral component. Studies have indicated that the success of the construct depends upon graft incorporation, which relies on the quality of the host bone bed.

The choice of bone graft is controversial. A systematic review performed by the Cochrane Database demonstrated insufficient evidence to suggest differences between processed (freeze dried or irradiated) and unprocessed (fresh-frozen) bone for impaction grafting.[119] However, it is recommended that the graft be used in the form of cancellous cubes that are 7 to 10 mm in width.

Results

Acetabular Side

The results of acetabular reconstructions using this technique for contained cavitary defects have generally been good, with survivorship approaching 85% to 90% at 20 years.[28,29] Buma and colleagues[31] took core biopsies from 8 patients after 1 to 72 months from surgery to show the different stages of graft incorporation. At 4 months after surgery, histologic analysis showed revascularization of the graft. Osteoclasts had removed parts of the graft, and woven bone had formed on the remnants of the graft and in the stroma that was invading the graft (Fig. 13-1). Between 8 and 28 months after surgery, the mixture of graft and new bone showed remodeling with time into normal trabecular bone structure with viable bone marrow that contained few or no remnants of the original graft (Fig. 13-2). Although some specimens showed the presence of graft-cement interface and local apposition of vital bone with the cement layer, a soft tissue interface predominated (see Fig. 13-2B and D).

For uncontained segmental defects, concerns with impaction bone grafting include early mechanical failure, mesh rupture, frequent significant cup migration, and poor survivorship.[2,33] Reports suggest that this technique is excellent for patients with small to moderate-sized contained cavitary defects, but poor for those with large uncontained segmental defects.

Femoral Side

Published reports have shown good clinical success in patients with significant cavitary femoral bone loss treated with impaction grafting[34-37] and radiographic and histologic evidence of revascularization of impacted allograft.[38]

In a retrieval study of a well-fixed stem with good radiographic graft incorporation (Fig. 13-3), Ling and co-workers[39] showed at 3.5 years' follow-up that the grafted bone had become organized into three zones (Fig. 13-4): a newly regenerated cortical surface, an interface zone, and a deep zone. In the regenerated cortical surface, the bone was fully mineralized and revascularized. The fatty bone marrow was normal looking with no fibrosis. The zone was generally viable, as shown by more than 90% of filled osteocyte lacunae (Fig. 13-5), but occasional islands of dead bone were evident. The interface zone was irregular with direct contact between bone cement and osteoid. Foreign body giant cells were visible, and in some areas, there was a thin soft tissue lining (Fig. 13-6). No direct contact occurred between viable mineralized bone and cement. The deep layer included trabeculae of dead bone, entombed in cement at the time of its insertion. These trabeculae had empty lacunae but were linked to surrounding viable bone by bridges of soft tissue, osteoid, and bone (see Fig. 13-6)

In cases with substantial and fully circumferential bone loss of the proximal femur, concerns with impaction grafting techniques remain because of the risk of prosthetic migration and periprosthetic fracture.[40,41] Some would consider this a contraindication

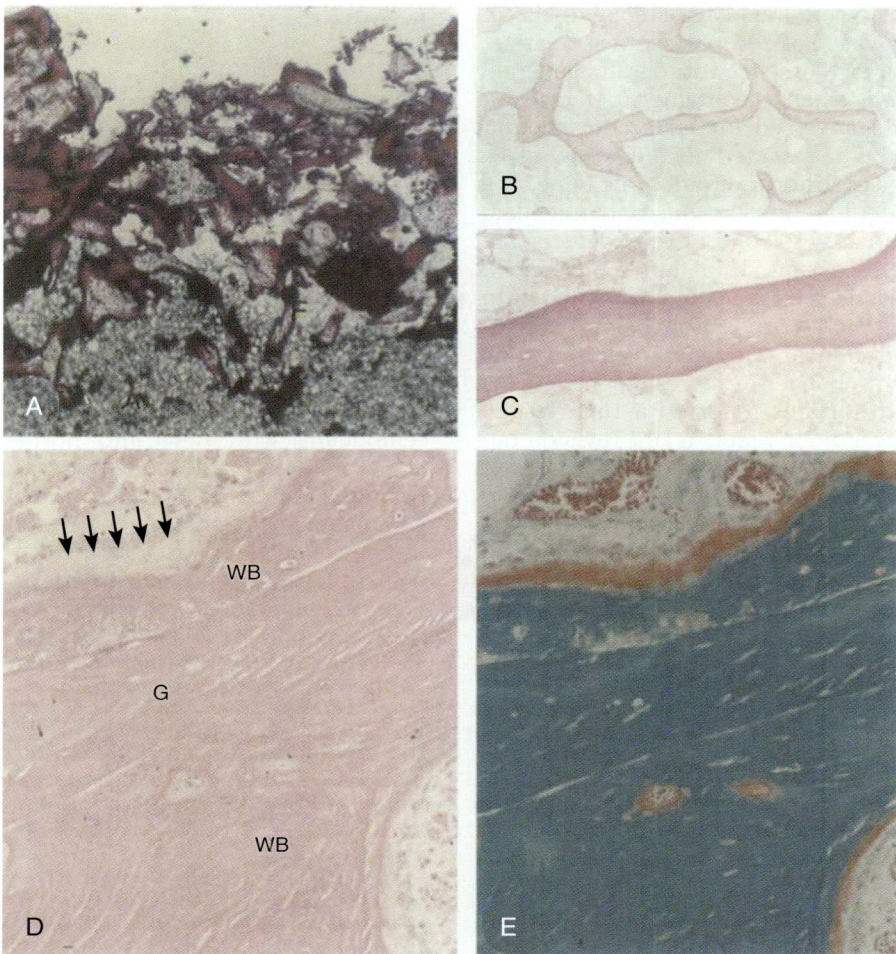

Figure 13-1. A through C, One month post acetabular reconstruction. **A,** Graft-cement interface in fuchsin-stained thick section. Note penetration of cement into the graft. **B and C,** No incorporation of graft in hematoxylin and eosin (H&E)-stained section. Note acellular medullary tissue in **C** (**A** and **B,** ×20; **C,** ×90). **D** and **E,** Case 2.4 months postoperatively. New woven bone (We) is formed on the remnants of the graft (G) by active osteoblasts *(arrows)*. (**D,** H&E-stained section; **E,** Goldner-stained adjacent section.) Note red-stained osteoid indicating active bone formation (×225). *(From Buma P, Lamerigts N, Schreurs BW, et al: Impacted graft incorporation after cemented acetabular revision: histological evaluation in 8 patients. Acta Orthop Scand 67:536–540, 1996, Fig. 2.)*

for impaction bone grafting. Few studies have shown reasonable results in this situation. Buttaro and associates[42] reported the use of this technique for 15 cases of severe proximal femoral bone defects averaging 12 cm in length that were followed for an average of 43.2 months (range, 20 to 72 months). The Merle d'Aubigné and Postel score improved from a mean of 4.8 to 14.4 points, and implant survivorship was 100% at 1 year and 87% at 72 months. However, a high incidence of severe complications was reported, including 2 (13%) fractures, 3 (20%) dislocations, and 3 (20%) deep infections.

Structural Allografts

Structural allograft can provide adequate support for primary implant fixation stability in revision surgery with large uncontained segmental bone loss.

Disadvantages include lack of universal availability, technical difficulties, and concerns over long-term graft resorption and collapse.

Acetabular Side

A minor column or shelf allograft is a structural graft that provides 50% or less support to the new acetabular component. The bulk graft is shaped intraoperatively, is snug-fitted into the defect, and is held with compression screws with washers (Fig. 13-7). Midterm results for treatment of uncontained segmental defects involving <50% of the acetabulum have been around 80% for cup survivorship at 10 years, with aseptic loosening as the endpoint.[43,44] Similar results have been reported with the use of bulk femoral head and acetabular and distal femur allografts.[43,44]

Despite concerns about long-term graft resorption, collapse, and failure, mid- to long-term studies have short-term to midterm survivorships of 45% to 60%.[45,46] Treatment of the same defects with cemented cups supported by reconstruction cages securely fixed to the ilium and ischium in conjunction has led to more encouraging midterm results, with survivorships of 77% to 87%.[47,48] The cage protects the structural graft by providing pelvic stability in spanning across the ilium and ischium and by offloading the graft until bony interdigitation occurs.

Hooten and colleagues[49] examined two acetabuli that were revised with femoral head structural allografts and cementless cups at 25 and 48 months' follow-up. Both grafts were functioning well at revision and were radiographically stable without evidence of graft collapse, cup loosening, or failure of union at the graft-host interface. Histologic examination showed that vascularity was increased at the host-graft interface, but evidence of bone union between the graft and the host was limited, in contrast to the radiographic appearance (Figs. 13-9 and 13-10). In areas where union had occurred, revascularization extended to 2 mm beyond the graft-host interface. Within the body of the graft, revascularization and remodeling were limited; the trabecular matrix appeared acellular, but the structural integrity was maintained at 48 months after surgery. In areas where the allograft was adjacent to an implant, fibrous tissue was oriented parallel to the implant surface. Bony ingrowth was limited to areas of porous coating that were in contact with viable host bone but did not occur between the ingrowth coating and the graft (Fig. 13-11).

Femoral Side

Uncontained fully circumferential proximal femur segmental defects may be addressed with the use of a proximal femoral structural allograft in conjunction with a long-stem prosthesis. The stem is cemented into the proximal femur allograft to form an allograft-prosthesis composite. Fixation of the prosthesis to the host distal femur is maintained by a stem extension, which is implanted into the medullary canal and augmented with a step or oblique cut at the graft-host junction, multiple cerclage wires at the graft-host junction, and the optional addition of cortical (fibular or ulnar) strut grafts.

This method of treatment has shown good long-term survivorship and functional outcomes.[50-53] Safir and associates[54] reported 82% survivorship (n = 93) at a mean follow-up of 16 years (range, 15 to 22 years) with stem revision as the endpoint. Two (4%) infections, 6 (11%) aseptic loosenings, 3 (5%) nonunions, and 4 (7%) dislocations were reported. Complication rates were considered acceptable in view of the complexity of the clinical condition.

The main advantages of treatment with proximal femoral allografts over distally fixed proximal femoral replacements (cementless) include lower dislocation rates,[55,56] better abductor function, less frequent Trendelenburg limp,[57] and better survivorship with a lower rate of loosening of the distal stem.[57,58]

Hamadouche and colleagues,[59] in a case report, showed the histologic appearance of a proximal femoral allograft via biopsies taken during stem revision for

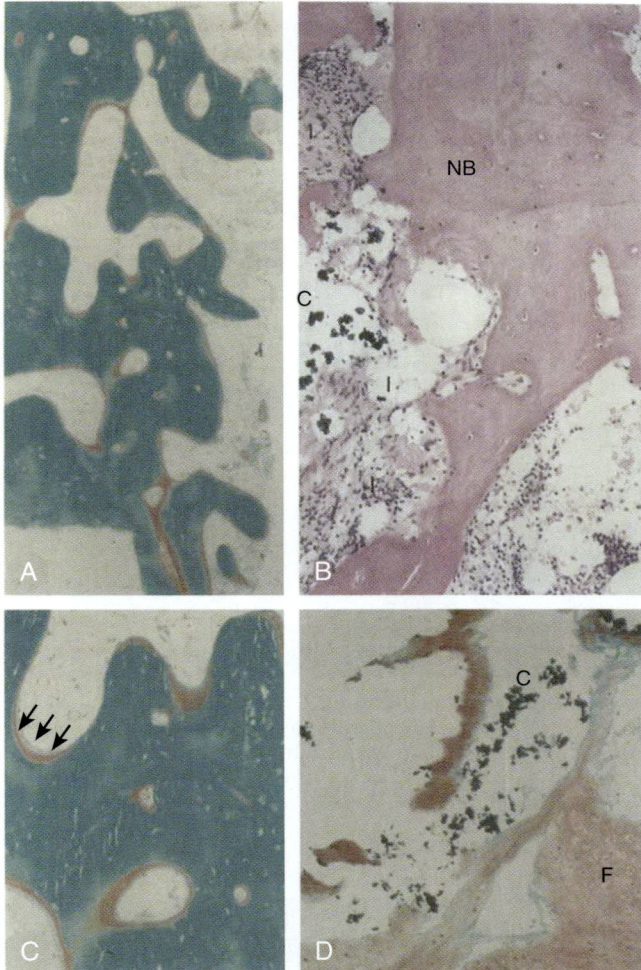

Figure 13-2. A through **C**, Eight months postacetabular reconstruction. The graft is incorporated into a new trabecular structure. If inspected with polarized light, the structure mainly consists of woven bone, with many active bone remodeling sites indicated by red osteoid staining (Goldner staining, ×30). **C**, Magnification of part of Figure 13-2A. Note active osteoblasts *(arrows)* (×55). **B** and **D**, 28 months postoperatively. At the graft-cement (C) interface, new bone (NB) is locally present, graft remnants are absent, and locally a soft tissue interface (I) and/or fibrocartilage (F) is present (hematoxylin and eosin [H&E] and Goldner staining, ×140). *(From Buma P, Lamerigts N, Schreurs BW, et al: Impacted graft incorporation after cemented acetabular revision: histological evaluation in 8 patients. Acta Orthop Scand 67:536–540, 1996, Fig. 3.)*

shown that during rerevision surgery, most of the bulk allograft remained intact with host-graft boundaries obscured, enabling cup-only exchanges.[43,44]

A major column allograft is a structural graft that provides more than 50% support to the new acetabular component (Fig. 13-8). These allografts are used in revision cases with uncontained segmental defects involving more than 50% of the acetabulum and both columns, with or without pelvic discontinuity. The use of major column allografts without support by an anti–protrusio ilioischial cage has met with poor results, with

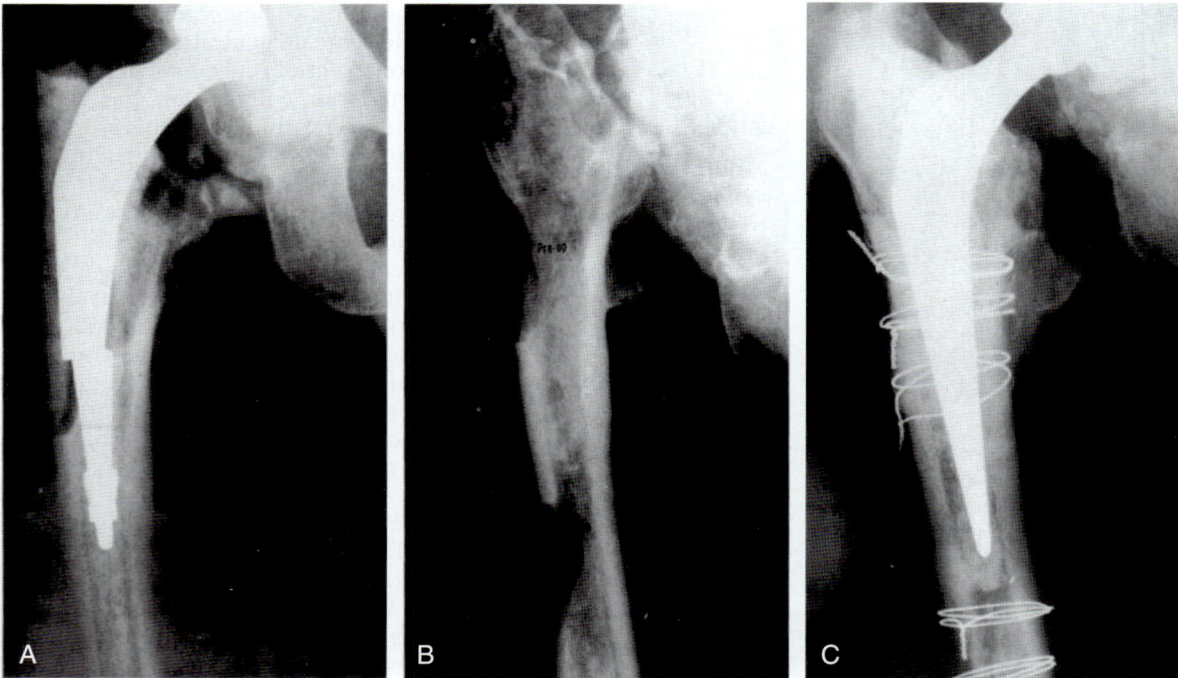

Figure 13-3. A, The fractured femoral stem with an adjacent cortical defect. **B,** The femur 1 year after removal of the prosthesis and cement. Two cortical defects are present: the distal one was created surgically to remove the distal cement. **C,** Two years after revision arthroplasty with impaction cancellous grafting. Cerclage wires, which secure the wire mesh, mark the levels of cortical defects; these appear to be filled by bone. *(From Ling RS, Timperley AJ, Linder L: Histology of cancellous impaction grafting in the femur: a case report. J Bone Joint Surg Br 75:693–696, 1993, Fig. 1.)*

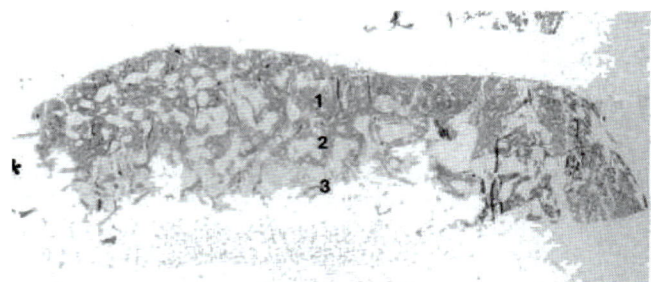

Figure 13-4. Low-power view of a histologic section taken at the level of the upper cortical window. Cement has been dissolved out, and staining indicates mineralized bone. At one point (*), cement has protruded between the cortex and the graft. The three zones of interest are shown: (1) cortical bone; (2) interface between living tissue and cement; and (3) bone trabeculae buried in the cement (Goldner stain, ×4). *(From Ling RS, Timperley AJ, Linder L: Histology of cancellous impaction grafting in the femur: a case report. J Bone Joint Surg Br 75:693–696, 1993, Fig. 5.)*

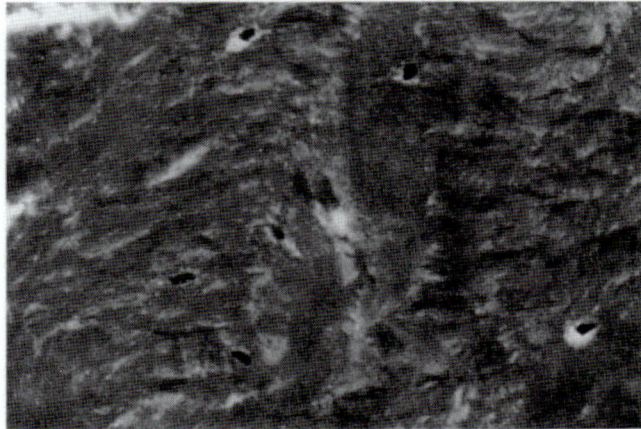

Figure 13-5. High-power view of regenerated bone showing filled osteocyte lacunae in a mineralized stroma with all the histologic characteristics of normal cortical bone (Goldner stain, ×600). *(From Ling RS, Timperley AJ, Linder L: Histology of cancellous impaction grafting in the femur: a case report. J Bone Joint Surg Br 75:693–696, 1993, Fig. 6.)*

loosening after 10 years following surgery. Three layers were seen within the allograft: inner, intermediate, and superficial layers. The inner layer of the bone graft consisted of the zone of contact between the graft and bone cement and was composed of trabeculae of dead bone and cellular debris without evidence of remodeling (Fig. 13-12). The superficial or interfacial layer, corresponding to the region of contact between the graft and the host bone, was composed of areas of remodeling bone and osteoclasts, osteoblasts, and fatty bone marrow (see Fig. 13-8). Evidence of creeping substitution was noted with new bone and osteoid formation. Revascularization occurred through the formation of woven bone to a depth of 5 mm. Between inner and superficial

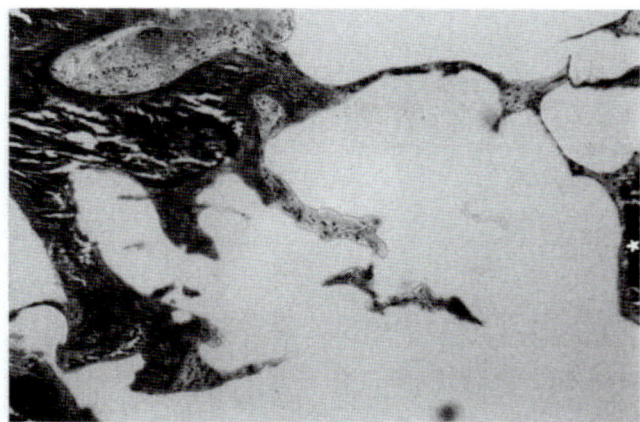

Figure 13-6. The interface between viable tissue and bone cement that has been dissolved out. Viable bone has been capped with osteoid, which is in direct contact with the (absent) cement surface. Some dead bone trabeculae (*) are probably remnants of the graft. Bridges of soft tissue and osteoid connect these trabeculae to living bone. Multinucleated giant cells are also seen in contact with the cement surface (Goldner stain, ×120). *(From Ling RS, Timperley AJ, Linder L: Histology of cancellous impaction grafting in the femur: a case report. J Bone Joint Surg Br 75:693–696, 1993, Fig. 7.)*

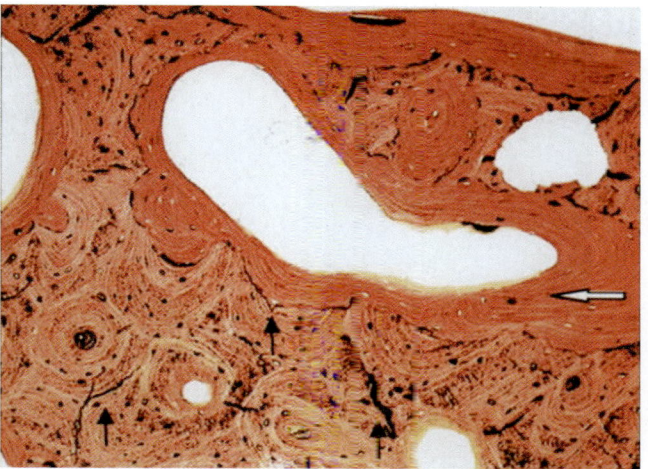

Figure 13-8. Low-power magnification photomicrograph of the allograft-host junction. Newly formed bone *(white arrow)* was present on the allograft surface and bridging to host. The microfractures *(black arrows)* are parallel or perpendicular to the newly formed osteons (van Gieson picrofuchsin, ×40). *(From Hamadouche M, Blanchat C, Meunier A, et al: Histological findings in a proximal femoral structural allograft ten years following revision total hip arthroplasty: a case report. J Bone Joint Surg Am 84:269–273, 2002, Fig. 4.)*

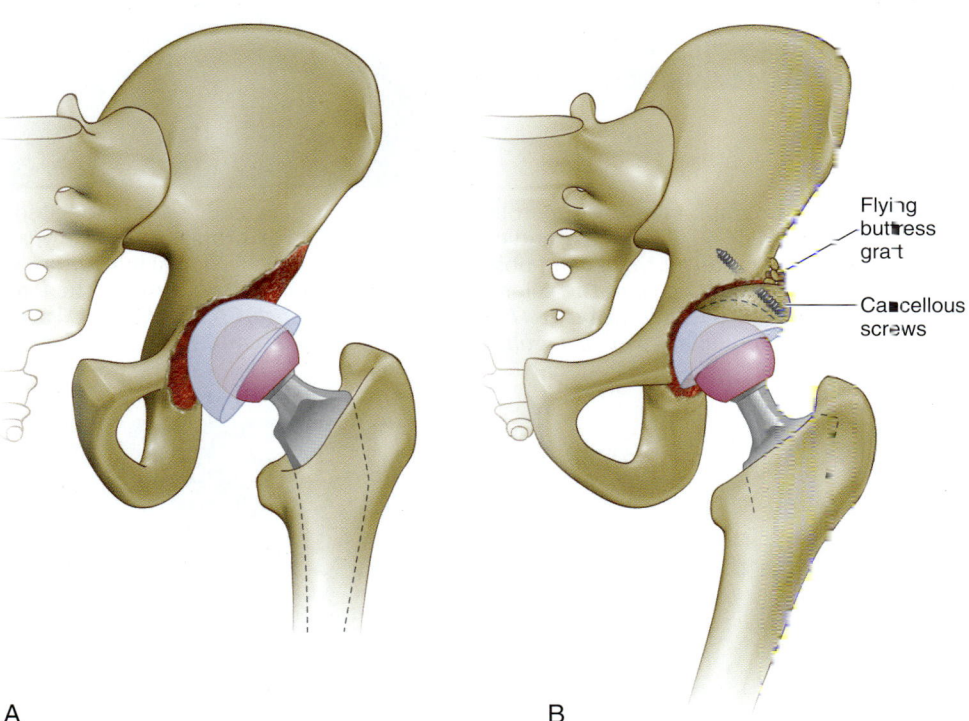

A   B

Figure 13-7. A, An uncontained defect involving less than 50% of the acetabulum. **B,** A minor column (shelf) graft supporting less than 50% of the cup is held with two cancellous screws. The flying buttress graft is cancellous autograft bone. *(Redrawn from Gross AE, Duncan CP, Garbuz D, Mohamed MZ: Revision arthroplasty of the acetabulum in association with loss of bone stock. J Bone Joint Surg Am 80:440–451, 1998.)*

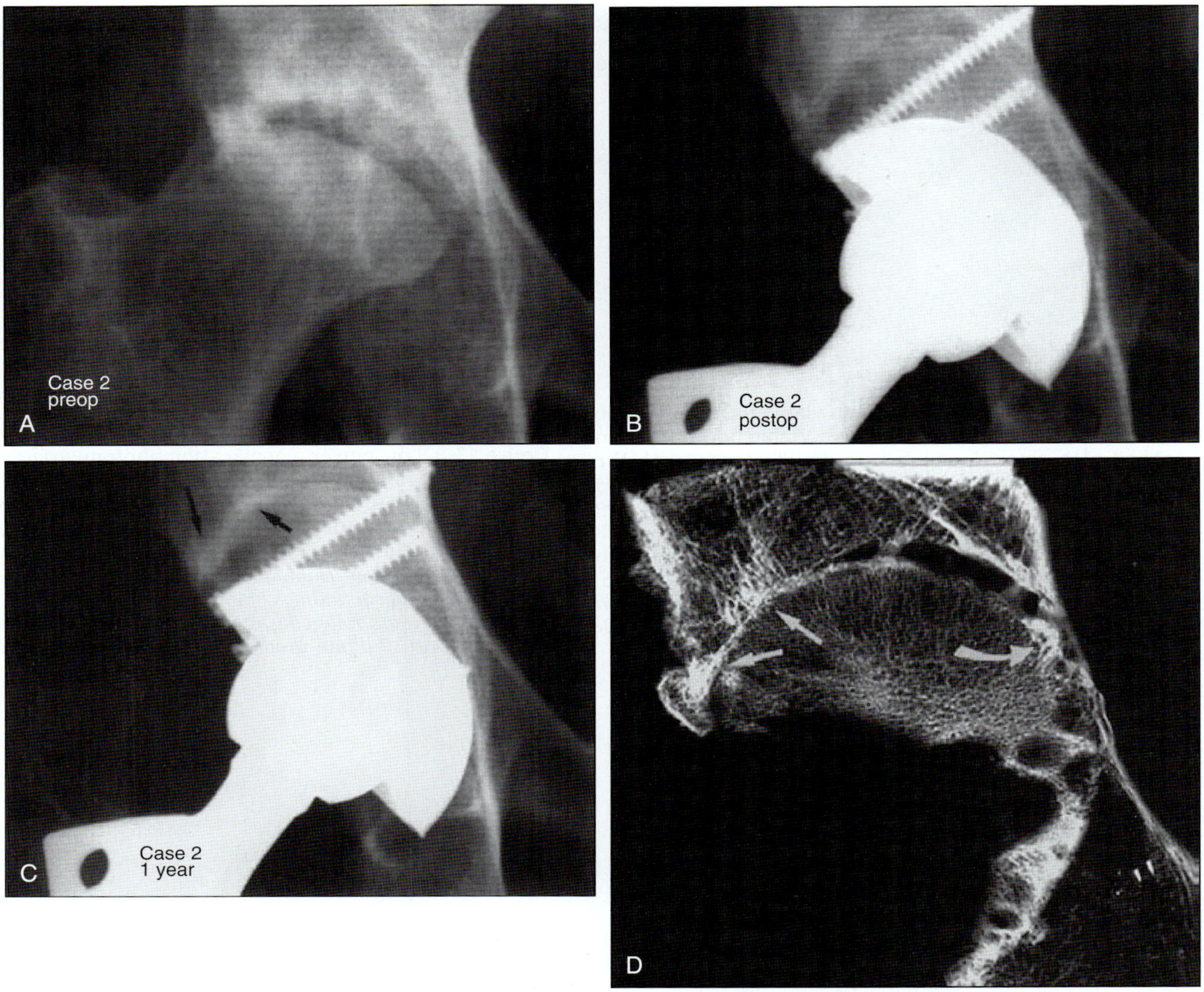

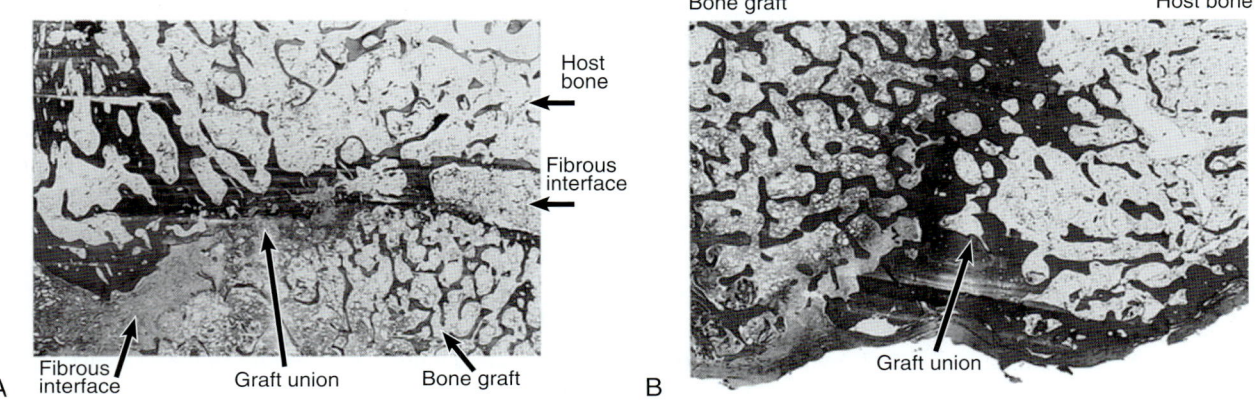

Figure 13-9. A, Preoperative radiograph showing superolateral acetabular deficiency with associated femoral head deficiency. **B,** Radiograph after femoral head allografting and cementless total hip arthroplasty. **C,** One year after surgery with trabecular bridging superolaterally *(black arrows)* and obscured interface medially, consistent with partial incorporation. **D,** Specimen radiograph showing persistence of the sclerotic border circumferentially around the femoral head allograft with partial graft healing in two areas *(white arrows). (From Hooten JP Jr, Engh CA, Heekin RD, Vinh TN: Structural bulk allografts in acetabular reconstruction: analysis of two grafts retrieved at post-mortem. J Bone Joint Surg Br 78:270–275, 1996, Fig. 2A-D.)*

Figure 13-10. A, Appearance of the superolateral graft-host junction *(area depicted by white arrows in Fig. 13-12D).* **B,** Appearance of the superomedial graft-host junction *(area depicted by black arrow in Fig. 13-12D)* (hematoxylin and eosin, ×1.5). *(From Hooten JP Jr, Engh CA, Heekin RD, Vinh TN: Structural bulk allografts in acetabular reconstruction: analysis of two grafts retrieved at post-mortem. J Bone Joint Surg Br 78:270–275, 1996, Fig. 4A and B.)*

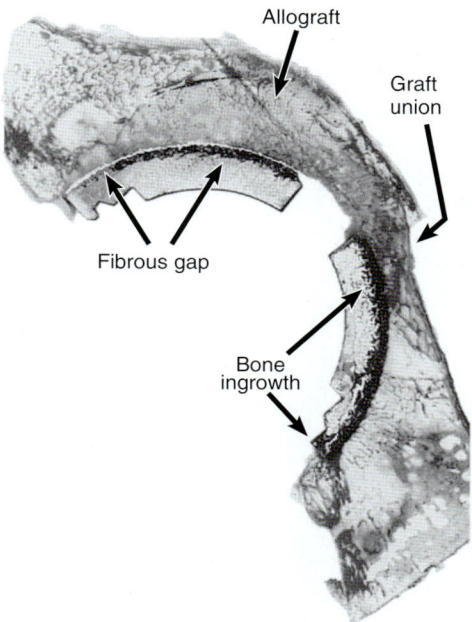

Figure 13-11. Graft-host junction (25-μm methylmethacrylate section, hematoxylin and eosin). *(From Hooten JP Jr, Engh CA, Heekin RD, Vinh TN: Structural bulk allografts in acetabular reconstruction: analysis of two grafts retrieved at post-mortem. J Bone Joint Surg Br 78:270–275, 1996, Fig. 5.)*

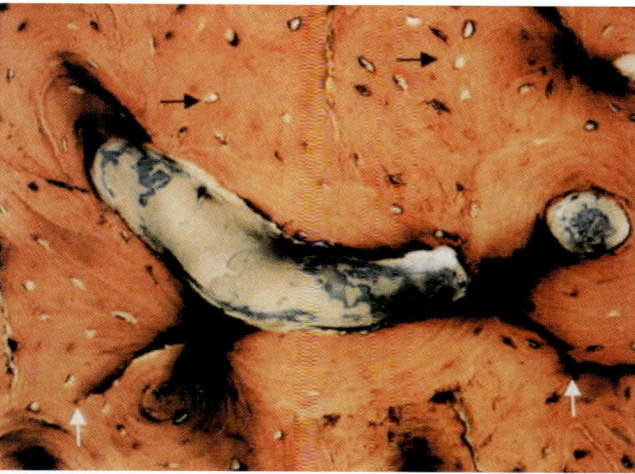

Figure 13-12. Photomicrograph of an unremodeled area of the allograft, showing empty lacunae *(black arrows)* and microfractures *(white arrows)*. Cellular debris is present in the middle of the image (Stevenel blue and van Gieson picrofuchsin, ×100). *(From Hamadouche M, Blanchat C, Meunier A, et al: Histological findings in a proximal femoral structural allograft ten years following revision total hip arthroplasty: a case report. J Bone Joint Surg Am 84:269–273, 2002, Fig. 3.)*

layers within the substance of the graft lay the intermediate layer, which consisted of a sparsely cellular area with resorption and no remodeling. Of note, numerous microfractures were seen in the unremodeled area of the allograft, especially under high magnification, but not in the remodeled area. These microfractures were parallel or perpendicular to the bone lamellae and bypassed newly formed osteons at the level of the cement line.

No fibrous membrane was seen between the allograft and the host femur. Radiologically, the graft appeared united (Fig. 13-13). Macroscopically, the allograft appeared as viable bleeding bone surrounded by host bone. It had united to the host bone but remained distinguishable from the recipient bone as it appeared denser. This was confirmed by microradiographic analysis, which showed that the allograft was more densely mineralized with smaller pore size than the host bone (Fig. 13-14).

BASIC SCIENCE

Autograft Bone

General Biology

Autologous bone graft is bone that is taken from an individual and transplanted into another site of the same individual. Several advantages have been noted with the use of autologous bone graft. It is osteogenic, as it contains marrow-derived preosteoblastic precursor cells and osteoblastic cells that are involved in new bone synthesis. It is osteoinductive, as it contains noncollagenous bone matrix proteins, including growth factors that modulate the recruitment of mesenchymal stem cells and differentiation into chondroblasts and osteoblasts. It is osteoconductive, as it is a three-dimensionally ordered scaffold of bone mineral and collagen that facilitates ingrowth of capillaries, perivascular tissue, and mesenchymal stem cells; this allows the formation of new bone in an organized fashion. In addition, complete histocompatibility occurs without the potential for immune-related problems, and there is no risk for infectious disease transmission. As a result, autograft is considered the gold standard for bone graft and is the most favored graft material in musculoskeletal reconstruction. However, several potential disadvantages to autograft use have been identified. These include an insufficient amount of graft material, donor site morbidity, increased surgical time, and increased blood loss. Potentially significant post-surgical donor site morbidity includes infection, pain, hemorrhage, muscle weakness, and nerve injury.[14] Donor site morbidity is relatively common, and complication rates from harvesting range from 10% to 25%.[15,16]

Cancellous Autograft

Cancellous autograft is highly osteogenic and promotes rapid revascularization and incorporation into host bone, because it has a large surface area lined with numerous osteoblasts. However, its poor initial mechanical strength often necessitates the use of early mechanical protection to allow graft-induced formation of new bone to provide early anchorage to the recipient bed.

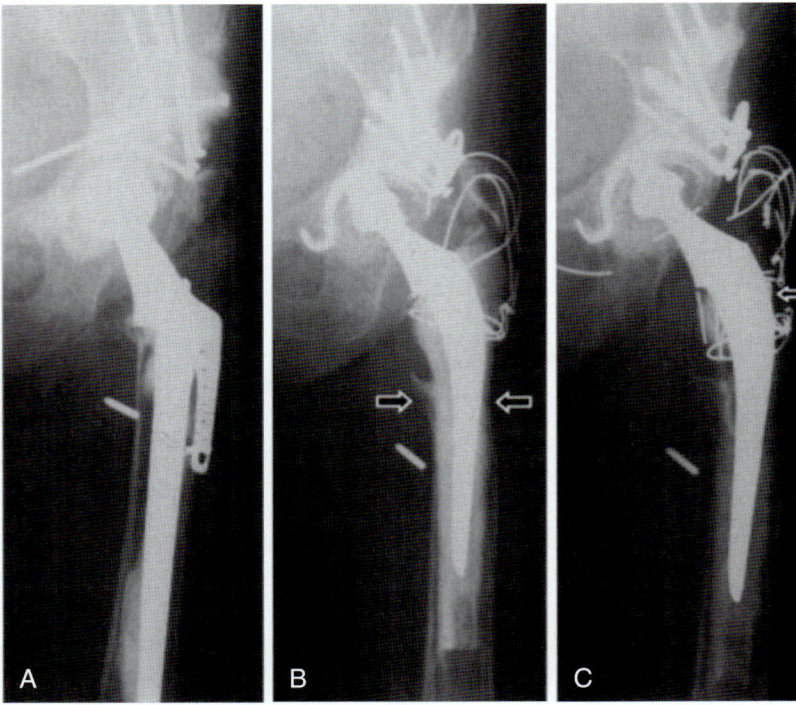

Figure 13-13. Serial anteroposterior radiographs of the patient in Figure 13-12. **A,** Preoperative radiograph showing major structural bone loss on the femoral side with deficient proximal part of the femur. **B,** One year after arthroplasty, the graft has healed to the host *(arrows)*. **C,** At 10 years, resorption of the proximal portion of the allograft is seen *(arrow)*. No migration of the femoral stem is seen. *(From Hamadouche M, Blanchat C, Meunier A, et al: Histological findings in a proximal femoral structural allograft ten years following revision total hip arthroplasty: a case report. J Bone Joint Surg Am 84:269–273, 2002, Fig. 1.)*

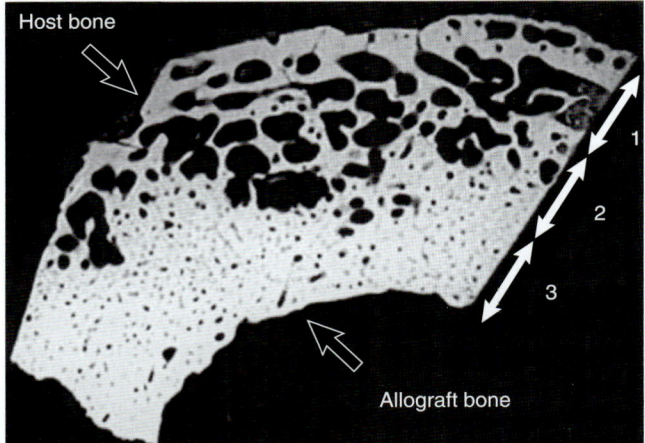

Figure 13-14. Microradiograph of a transverse section at the graft-host junction. Differences in pore size and density are evident between the host bone *(1)* and the allograft *(3)*. No demarcation line is present, indicating that the graft has healed to the host. However, remodeling has not proceeded more than a few millimeters into the graft *(2)*. *(From Hamadouche M, Blanchat C, Meunier A, et al: Histological findings in a proximal femoral structural allograft ten years following revision total hip arthroplasty: a case report. J Bone Joint Surg Am 84:269–273, 2002, Fig. 2.)*

In the primary phase of graft incorporation, immediately after bone grafting, inflammation[117] and hematoma formation lead to coagulation. Infiltration of vascular buds into the recipient bed begins and neovascularization promptly occurs over the next few days. In the first week, the graft is bathed by a soup of lymphocytes, plasma cells, osteoclasts, mononuclear cells, and polynuclear cells. Some early fibrous tissue forms. In the second week, fibrous granulation tissue is predominant and osteoclastic activity increases. Macrophages arrive to remove necrotic debris within the haversian canals of the graft. Mediators released by the macrophages, combined with low oxygen tension and low pH, have a chemotactic effect on undifferentiated mesenchymal stem cells, which migrate from the host to the graft, subsequently repopulating the marrow. These primitive cells differentiate into osteogenic cells under the influence of osteoinductive agents such as cytokines, growth factors, and prostaglandins. By the fourth week, osteoblastic bone formation and osteoclastic resorption occur in a coordinated fashion.

In the secondary phase of graft incorporation, the osteoblasts cover the edges of the dead trabeculae and lay down osteoid around central cores of dead bone.[77] This is followed by osteoclastic resorption, formation of hematopoietic marrow cells within the new marrow of the graft, and remodeling at the graft-host junction.

Radiographically, an initial increase in radiodensity is due to osteoblastic activity. This gradually decreases as necrotic bone undergoes osteoclastic resorption. Evidence of graft interdigitation can be seen radiographically by the blurring of margins between graft and host bone. This is due to bone remodeling at the graft-host junction, which may take several months to complete.[91]

Biomechanically, cancellous autografts have increased initial strength as the result of new bone formation on a necrotic bed. Subsequently, resorption of the necrotic bed causes a decrease in mechanical strength. With remodeling of the graft-host junction, the strength of the interface between graft and host bone eventually improves.

Cortical Autograft

Incorporation of nonvascularized cortical grafts involves slower revascularization and a lesser degree of osteoinduction than cancellous grafts[118] (see Fig. 13-14). However, the process is similar during early stages of hematoma formation and inflammation. The cortical graft has a dense architecture that impairs revascularization and has fewer endosteal cells to promote neovascularization.[91] Unlike cancellous autograft, incorporation is initiated by osteoclasts instead of osteoblasts.

At about 2 weeks after grafting, extensive resorption begins and increases until about 6 months, before it gradually decreases to normal levels over the following 6-month period. Initial revascularization and resorption follow along peripheral haversian canals and interstitial lamellae. Resorption of inner cortical material occurs at a much slower rate. When the central osteonal canal reaches a certain size, osteoblastic new bone formation replaces osteoclastic bone resorption, which is further impaired by appositional bone growth. Eventually, creeping substitution occurs when the entire graft is resorbed and replaced by new living bone. Creeping substitution is most evident at the graft-host junction and progresses in a parallel manner along the longitudinal axis of the graft toward its middle.[60]

Radiographically, increasing radiolucencies are seen at irregular peripheral bony margins between 6 months and 1 year.[120] With continuing osteogenesis, a gradual increase in radiodensity occurs, initially at the graft-host junction, and progresses into the middle of the graft. The cortical autograft remains as a composite of necrotic and new bone for prolonged periods.

Biomechanically, the remodeling process initiated by osteoclastic activity leads to initial bone loss and a decrease in mechanical strength of up to 75%.[83] In vascularized cortical autografts, the graft heals much more rapidly at the graft-host junction, as the remodeling process is similar to normal bone and virtually no residual weakness is noted.[83]

Allograft

General Biology

Because of limitations in the use of bone autograft, such as lack of availability and donor site morbidity, bone allograft has been used as an alternative. Bone allografting is the process by which bone is transferred from one individual to another individual within the same species. Most commonly, bone is procured from patients who underwent primary hip arthroplasty or postmortem from organ donors. It is available as fresh or preserved specimens. Preserved specimens are frozen or freeze dried. Fresh specimens elicit a higher level of immunologic response[62] and are reserved for tumor reconstruction or joint resurfacing.[63] Advantages of bone allograft use include availability and avoidance of donor site morbidity associated with autograft harvesting. Disadvantages of bone allograft use include lack of osteogenic cells, decreased osteoinductive factors, host immune response, and infection risks.[74,75,?] Morselized and structural cancellous allografts are commonly used in revision hip arthroplasty for acetabular and femoral bone defects. Structural allografts are used primarily to support mechanical loads and resist failure at sites where structural support is desired.

Bone Banks

The development of modern tissue banks has resulted in a supply of high-quality allogeneic tissue for reconstructive orthopedic surgery. More than 50 tissue banks in the United States are accredited by the American Association of Tissue Banks (AATB). The success of allografting in recent years may be directly related to stringent measures to ensure the safety of transplanted tissue and to improvements in processing technology.[61] Combined efforts of the U.S. Food and Drug Administration (FDA) and the AATB have helped ensure that tissue donors are adequately screened, and that allograft material is properly processed, labeled, and distributed. Screening of cadaveric donors begins with a detailed medical, social, and sexual history questionnaire completed by the life partner or next of kin. Any of the following automatically disqualifies the individual as a donor: positive history of exposure to specific communicable disease, unprotected sexual contact, drug use, neurologic disease, autoimmune disease, collagen disorder, or metabolic disease.

Infection Risks and Sterilization Methods

The risk of viral disease transmission with allograft use is very small. Primary concerns include hepatitis C, hepatitis B, and human immunodeficiency virus (HIV).[73] Two reported cases of HIV transmission in the 1980s were due to bone allograft[74] but none since that time, because of implementation of strict donor screening programs by the AATB and mandatory screening of blood tests for all donors. Blood tests required by the FDA for all tissue transplants include HIV-1 and HIV-2 antibody, hepatitis B surface antigen, hepatitis B core antibody, hepatitis C antibody, syphilis, human T-lymphotropic virus I antibody, and HIV p24 antigen.[75,76]

Bone harvested for use as allograft is subjected to rigorous processing to remove all antigenic components to decrease the host immune response and ensure sterility while desirable biological and biomechanical properties are retained. Processing methods include low-dose (<20 kGy) irradiation, physical débridement, ultrasonic or pulsatile water washes, ethanol treatment, and antibiotic soaking (4° C for >1 hour).[77]

Terminal sterilization by gamma irradiation, electron beam irradiation, or ethylene oxide treatment may be performed when contamination is anticipated. These have an adverse dose-dependent effect on the mechanical strength of the graft.[78]

A fatal clostridial infection associated with implantation of a femoral condyle allograft[79] was reported in 2002. An investigation by the Centers for Disease Control and Prevention determined that the likely source of contamination was hematogenous seeding from bowel flora before harvesting. Twenty-six patients with allograft-associated infections were identified (13 with clostridial infections); 14 infections were associated with a single tissue-processing unit. The time interval between death of the donor and tissue retrieval, delays in refrigeration, and the mechanism of death (i.e., trauma) were likely factors that contributed to contamination from the bowel. Of note, cultures obtained before and after processing in antibiotic/antifungal solution by the tissue processor were negative. This showed that bacteriostasis was unsatisfactory and sterilization must include methods that can kill bacterial spores such as gamma irradiation. When a sporicidal method is unavailable, tissue should be cultured before soaking in antimicrobial solutions, and if bowel flora is isolated, all tissue from that particular donor should be discarded.[79]

Immune Response and Graft Processing

It is unclear what relationship exists between cells and cytokines of the immune system and cells of the bone remodeling and repair system. A variety of antigens present in allograft bone elicit a host immune response. This is primarily a cell-mediated response to major histocompatibility complex class I and II antigens on specialized antigen-presenting cells. Horowitz and Friedlander[67] reported that allogeneic bone cells activate host T cells of the suppressor phenotype and induce their proliferation.

In a prospective multicenter study on large fresh-frozen structural allograft used in revision hip arthroplasty, Ward and colleagues[64] showed that donor and recipient human leukocyte antigen (HLA) mismatches and recipient antibody responses to donor HLA antigens did not affect union rates at the graft-host junction. Donor-specific HLA sensitization occurred in 57% of patients but had no demonstrable effect on graft incorporation or union. The type of host-allograft junction did have a major effect on graft incorporation. Cortical-cortical allograft-host junctions healed more slowly (mean, 542 days) than corticocancellous allograft-host junctions (mean, 243 days), although most healed allografts survived for the minimum 3-year follow-up period, and no correlation was noted between HLA status and the prevalence of other complications, revisions, or articular deterioration. It is our view that longer-term follow-up is required to determine if there is an association between HLA sensitization and long-term graft survival.

Measures to further minimize or modulate HLA sensitization or response are not indicated at present to improve the union of reconstructions using structural bone allografts. However, other benefits could be derived from minimizing the rate of HLA sensitization. One drawback for sensitized patients is the greater difficulty in finding suitably matched organs should they ever need a living tissue organ transplantation such as a kidney or heart transplant.[68] At the present moment, allograft bone procedures are performed without HLA matching because tissue matching of bone between donors and recipients currently is considered unnecessary by the Musculoskeletal Transplant Foundation.

Although immunologic reaction to bone allografts has been recognized in patients and in animal models,[65-70] it has been reduced by deep-freezing and, to a larger extent, by freeze-drying (lyophilizing).[71,72]

Fresh allografts incorporate unsatisfactorily, and processing of allografts is favored for clinical use. Processing involves removal of antigenic cells and proteins by removal of the periosteal sleeve and other immunogenic soft tissues such as donor marrow.[82] Preservation techniques include deep-freezing at −70° C and freeze-drying. Deep frozen grafts retain their mechanical properties and may be implanted after thawing. Freeze-drying diminishes immunogenicity to a greater extent but causes deterioration in the biomechanical properties of the graft.[81] Rehydration (reconstitution) of the allograft before implantation improves the biomechanical properties, but the allografts remain weak and are vulnerable to mechanical failure in torsion and bending.

Cancellous Bone Allograft

Allogeneic cancellous bone is a poor promoter of bone healing compared with autologous cancellous bone. With fresh allografts, an aggressive host immune response occurs[121] in the first 2 weeks of grafting with high lymphocyte and macrophage activity. This impairs the efficiency of osteoinductive growth factors to promote union at the graft-host interface. A delay in neovascularization occurs in the presence of adjacent inflammatory cells, which cause vessel occlusion and graft necrosis. By about 2 months, the necrotic allograft is surrounded by fibrous tissue. This prompts the use of fresh-frozen or freeze-dried allografts in an attempt to reduce immunogenicity and improve incorporation.[80]

Allograft cancellous chips are incorporated more completely and more rapidly than cortical bone allografts because they are more easily revascularized.[122] Cancellous grafts act as a scaffold to allow the host to lay down new bone. However, they usually do not undergo complete osteoclastic resorption by the host, and necrotic graft remnants are usually trapped within host bone.[77]

Cortical Bone Allograft

During attempts at revascularization, the host inflammatory response against graft-derived cellular antigens leads to occlusion of invading host vessels, graft necrosis, and invasion by granulation tissue. Cortical allograft incorporates by sporadic appositional bone formation. Poor vascularization is seen in larger cortical allografts as the result of increased density of cortical bone, lack of construct stability, and immune response to the grafts.

Factors Affecting Graft Incorporation

The success of graft incorporation depends on several factors, principally, graft revascularization, new bone formation (around and within the graft), and healing at the graft-host interface. These in turn depend on a combination of biological activity of the graft, vascularity of the host bed, and mechanical stability of the graft-host interface (Table 13-1).

Revascularization of the Substance of the Graft

The principal determinant of the rate, pattern, and amount of revascularization is the availability of a vascular pedicle. Animal studies with dogs showed that vascularized autografts exhibited minimal disruption of osteonal remodeling patterns, osteocyte death, and peripheral resorption or centripetal vessel ingrowth.[83] The nonvascularized bone graft is totally dependent on the condition of the host bed for its revascularization, which occurs at a much slower rate via centripetal vessel ingrowth.

Factors that have been associated with impaired revascularization of cortical grafts include freezing,[84,85] histocompatibility discrepancy,[84-86] and treatments that interfere with biological properties of the graft and surrounding tissue, such as irradiation.[87]

New Bone Formation

The rate and amount of new bone formation in and around grafts are mainly dependent on the availability of viable osteoblasts. The pattern of new bone formation is determined by the availability of a vascular pedicle. Fresh vascularized autografts, whether cortical or cancellous, show rapid bone formation. In nonvascularized bone grafts, the living cells that are needed to form new bone must be derived from host tissues, and so new bone formation is delayed. In cancellous autografts, new bone forms on the surface of trabeculae, but in cortical autografts, new bone forms on the periosteum.[83,86,87]

Host-Graft Union

The principal determinants of host-graft union include stability of the construct and contact between host bone and graft.[69,70] In animal studies, healing has occurred when host-graft interfaces are intimately apposed and stably fixed, regardless of whether the grafts were autogenous or allogeneic, or fresh or frozen.[86] When intimate contact between host bed and graft was absent, healing was very severely impaired despite stable graft fixation. Local and systemic interference with the biological activity of the graft and surrounding tissue secondary to irradiation or chemotherapy (e.g., cisplatin) severely impairs graft healing.[69] A mismatch in immunohistocompatibility and deep-freezing of the graft during preparation or storage have been shown to impair graft healing to a certain extent.[69] Freezing muted the effects of mismatch in immunohistocompatibility but simultaneously reduced the biological activity of the graft by killing viable cells.[88]

Clinically, the frozen or processed mismatched allograft is the most commonly implanted graft, and it has a less predictable process of incorporation. However, the effects of freezing and mismatch in immunohistocompatibility on impairment of graft healing have not been shown to be sufficiently clinically significant to warrant routine tissue-antigen matching and the use of fresh-matched cortical bone grafts—a practice that would be challenging from a feasibility standpoint.

Impairment of Bone Graft Healing

Several factors may impair bone graft incorporation. Smoking inhibits cellular proliferation and causes vasoconstriction. Systemic steroid use inhibits differentiation of progenitor cells into osteoblasts. Nonsteroidal anti-inflammatory drugs inhibit prostaglandin formation and lead to diminished local blood flow and delay in graft resorption. They are contraindicated during the acute healing phase because they reduce inflammatory responses and inhibit osteoblasts at endosteal surfaces. Malnutrition, especially deficiency of calcium and phosphorus, has been associated with delayed mineralization of new bone.[89]

CURRENT CONTROVERSIES AND FUTURE DIRECTIONS

The use of bone graft material in hip surgery still presents major challenges. The most commonly used materials are autograft, allograft, and synthetic materials. The gold standard, however, is still considered to be autogenous bone graft, as it provides all three elements necessary to generate and maintain bone: a scaffold for osteoconduction, growth factors for osteoinduction, and progenitor cells for osteogenesis. However, autograft is in limited supply, and its harvesting can result in significant donor site morbidity.

Processed allograft and synthetic bone graft substitutes are more readily available and do not pose an additional insult to the patient. However, they lack living

Table 13-1. Local and Systemic Factors Influencing Graft Incorporation

Factor	Positive	Negative
Local	Good vascular supply at the graft site	Radiation
	Large surface area	Tumor
	Mechanical stability	Mechanical instability
	Mechanical loading	Local bone disease
	Growth factors	Denervation
	Electrical stimulation	Infection
Systemic	Growth hormone	Corticosteroids
	Thyroid hormone	Nonsteroidal anti-inflammatory drugs*
	Somatomedins	Chemotherapy
	Vitamins A and D	Smoking
	Insulin	Sepsis
	Parathyroid hormone	Diabetes
		Malnutrition
		Metabolic bone disease

*The effect of new selective cyclo-oxygenase (COX)-2 inhibitors is unknown. From Khan SN, Cammisa FP Jr, Sandhu HS, et al: The biology of bone grafting. J Am Acad Orthop Surg 13:77–86, 2005, Table 2.

cells and thus only function as an osteoconductive scaffold for bone ingrowth.[90,91] Therefore, in the recent past, an explosion has occurred in the development of bone substitutes and growth factors that have made their way to the medical market and into operating rooms.[92,93]

The biology of allograft incorporation is poorly understood; most studies lack histologic support and are based on radiographic data alone, which may not reflect true incorporation. Analysis of retrieved allografts demonstrates that incorporation is very slow, irregular, and incomplete. Cortical-cortical union is observed from internal cancellous-cancellous interfaces but is confined to only 20% of the superficial surface and the ends of the graft at 5 years post implantation.[94,95] This leads to graft fracture and implant failure in the short to medium term in up to 35% of cases.[48,96,97] Moreover, massive allografts are estimated to have a 10-year survival rate of between 40% and 60% because of accumulation of unremodeled microfractures, which decrease their torsional properties, leading to catastrophic failure.[99-101] Nonetheless, mechanical strength provided by large structural allografts is probably the main reason why they are used in difficult reconstructions in an attempt to avoid early mechanical failures. Thus the race is ongoing between incorporation of the graft and failure of the implant.

Biological advantages of particulate grafts over structural grafts are well documented and include better revascularization, incorporation, and remodeling as a consequence of the increased surface area between implant and host bone.[29,101] Because particulate grafts lack the mechanical support required for many applications, several adjuvants have been proposed to enhance the biological response and incorporation of structural allografts. One strategy is to add factors to the host bed to stimulate angiogenesis and bone formation around massive allografts; these factors include bone morphogenic proteins, mesenchymal stem cells, and the use of gene therapy.

Recombinant human bone morphogenic proteins (rhBMPs) offer the potential of accelerating the incorporation of structural grafts, as they have been used successfully clinically in combination with cancellous allograft in spinal fusion, and also in the treatment of fractures.[102-105] Improved incorporation with an rhBMP addition has been reported in several animal models.[106-108] In more recent accounts, healing of cortical strut allografts to the rabbit femur was significantly accelerated after implantation of an rhBMP-2/gelatin device at the allograft-host junction. In this work, grafts treated with rhBMP showed great improvement in terms of quality, quantity, and time required for new bone formation and graft healing.[108] In fact, strut healing at 4 weeks postoperatively was shown to be superior to healing when compared with controls at 8 weeks. Although the use of BMPs in hip surgery is limited to case studies, findings do support the conclusions of animal studies. Cook and associates[109] reported on the use of BMPs in conjunction with a proximal femoral allograft at the site of a failed proximal femoral allograft, with a proximal femoral strut allograft, a bulk femoral head allograft in an acetabular reconstruction, and a morselized allograft for reconstitution of an area of absent femoral cortex. In each case, the authors concluded that new bone formed earlier and graft incorporation was more rapid than they would have expected in the absence of BMPs. However, clinical trials are still lacking, and reports remain anecdotal.

Mesenchymal stem cells have been shown experimentally to be involved in bone graft healing through activation of osteogenesis and angiogenesis.[110-112] Multipotent mesenchymal stem cells found in periosteum can differentiate into bone as well as cartilage, but the molecular mechanisms involved are poorly understood.

Genetically engineered human mesenchymal stem cells have been used as a platform for the delivery of osteogenic factors (BMPs) and have proved effective in vitro in enhancing proliferation and osteogenic differentiation. They have also demonstrated the ability to engraft and form bone and cartilage in ectopic sites and to regenerate bone defects when transplanted into mice.[113,114]

Studies have also been performed to look at the use of freeze-dried recombinant adeno-associated viruses (rAAVs) carrying angiogenic, osteogenic, and remodeling signals to stimulate graft incorporation through mediation of in vivo gene transfer. Addition of the freeze-dried virus to the cortical surface of allografts led to marked revascularization and new bone formation in mice.[115,116]

Although the therapies discussed here have not as yet been expanded to the clinical setting, good evidence suggests that allograft incorporation, bone formation, and remodeling may be enhanced by using several of these emerging adjuvant therapies, as our understanding of the mechanism of osteoinduction and osteogenesis expands.

REFERENCES

1. Gerber SD, Harris WH: Femoral head allografting to augment acetabular deficiency in patients requiring total hip replacement. J Bone Joint Surg Am 68:1241–1248, 1986.
2. Harris WH, Crothers O, Oh I: Total hip replacement and femoral head bone grafting for severe acetabular deficiency in adults. J Bone Joint Surg Am 59:752–759, 1977.
3. McCollum DE, Nunley JA, Harrelson JM: Bone grafting in total hip replacement for acetabular protrusion. J Bone Joint Surg Am 62:1065–1073, 1980.
4. Flati G, Di Stanisloa C: Chirurgia nella Preistoria. Parte I. Provincia Med Aquila 2:8–11, 2004.
5. van Meekeren J: Heel en geneeskonstige aanmerkingen, Amsterdam, 1668, Commelijin.
6. MacEwen W: Observation concerning transplantation of bone: illustrated by a case of interhuman osseous transplantation whereby over two thirds of a shaft of a humerus was restored. Proc R Soc London 32:232–247, 1881.
7. von Walter PH: Wiedereinheilung der bei der Trapanation ausgebohrten Knochenscheibe. J Chir Augen-Heilkunde 2:671, 1821.
8. Albee FH: Bone graft surgery, Philadelphia, 1915, WB Saunders.
9. Inclan A: The use of preserved bone graft in orthopaedic surgery. J Bone Joint Surg Am 24:81, 1942.
10. Doppelt SH, Tomford WW, Lucas AD, Mankin HJ: Operational and financial aspects of a hospital bone bank. J Bone Joint Surg Am 63:244, 1981.

11. Friedlaender GE, Mankin HJ: Bone banking: current methods and suggested guidelines. In Murray D (ed): AAOS instructional course lecture, vol 30, St Louis, 1981, CV Mosby.

12. Tomford WW, Doppelt SH, Mankin HJ, Friedlaender GE: 1983 bone bank procedures. Clin Orthop Relat Res 174:15–21, 1983.

13. Warwick RM, Eastland T, Fehily D: Role of blood transfusion service in tissue banking. Vox Sang 71:71–77, 1996.

14. Younger EM, Chapman MW: Morbidity at bone graft donor sites. J Orthop Trauma 3:192–195, 1989.

15. Ahlmann E, Patzakis M, Roidis N, et al: Comparison of anterior and posterior iliac crest bone grafts in terms of harvest-site morbidity and functional outcomes. J Bone Joint Surg Am 84:716–720, 2002.

16. Summers BN, Eisenstein SM: Donor site pain from the ilium: a complication of lumbar spine fusion. J Bone Joint Surg Br 71:677–680, 1989.

17. Rodriguez JA, Huk OL, Pellicci PM, Wilson PD Jr: Autogenous bone graft from the femoral head for the treatment of acetabular bone deficiency in primary hip arthroplasty with cement: long term results. J Bone Joint Surg Am 77:1227–1233, 1995.

18. Biant LC, Bruce WJM, Assini JB, et al: Primary total hip arthroplasty in severe developmental dysplasia of the hip: ten-year result using a cementless modular stem. J Arthrop 24:27–32, 2009.

19. Mulroy RD, Harris WH: Failure of acetabular autogenous grafts in total hip arthroplasty: increasing incidence: a follow-up note. J Bone Joint Surg Am 72:1536–1540, 1990.

20. Shinar AA, Harris WH: Bulk structural autogenous and grafts and allografts for reconstruction of the acetabulum in total hip replacement: sixteen-year-average follow-up. J Bone Joint Surg Am 79:159–168, 1997.

21. Gross AE, Catre MG: The use of femoral head autograft shelf reconstruction and cemented acetabular components in the dysplastic hip. Clin Orthop Relat Res 298:60–66, 1994.

22. Inao S, Gotoh E, Ando M: Total hip replacement using femoral neck bone to graft the dysplastic acetabulum: follow-up study of 18 patients with old congenital dislocation of the hip. J Bone Joint Surg Br 76:735–739, 1994.

23. Morsi E, Garbuz D, Gross AE: Total hip arthroplasty with shelf grafts using uncemented cups: a long term follow-up study. J Arthroplasty 11:81–85, 1996.

24. Hintermann B, Morscher EW: Total hip replacement with solid autologous femoral head autograft for hip dysplasia. Arch Orthop Trauma Surg 114:137–144, 1995.

25. Iida H, Matsusue Y, Kawanabe K, et al: Cemented total hip arthroplasty with acetabular bone graft for developmental dysplasia: long term result and survivorship analysis. J Bone Joint Surg Br 82:176–184, 2000.

26. Akiyama H, Kawanabe K, Iida H, et al: Long-term results of cemented total hip arthroplasty in developmental dysplasia with acetabular bulk bone graft after improving operative techniques. J Arthroplasty 25:716–720, 2010.

27. Nousiainen MT, Maury AC, Alhoulei A, et al: Long term outcome of shelf grafts in total hip arthroplasty for developmental hip dysplasia. Orthopedics 32:9, 2009.

28. Schreurs BW, Bolder SB, Gardeniers JW, et al: Acetabular revision with impacted morselized cancellous bone grafting and a cemented cup: a 15 to 20 year follow-up. J Bone Joint Surg Br 86:492–497, 2004.

29. Schreurs BW, Slooff TJ, Gardeniers JW, Buma P: Acetabular reconstruction with bone impaction grafting and a cemented cup: 20 years' experience. Clin Orthop Relat Res 393:202–215, 2001.

30. Spandehl MJ, Berry DJ, Trousdale RT, Cabanela ME: Uncemented acetabular components with bulk femoral head autograft for acetabular reconstruction in developmental dysplasia of the hip. J Bone Joint Surg Am 83:1484–1489, 2001.

31. Buma P, Lamerigts N, Schreurs BW, et al: Impacted graft incorporation after cemented acetabular revision: histological evaluation in 8 patients. Acta Orthop Scand 67:536–540, 1996.

32. Buttaro MA, Comba F, Pusso R, Piccaluga F: Acetabular revision with metal mesh, impaction bone grafting, and a cemented cup. Clin Orthop Relat Res 466:2482–2490, 2008.

33. Van Haaren EH, Heyligers IC, Alexander FG, Wuisman PI: High rate of failure of impaction grafting in large acetabular defects. J Bone Joint Surg Br 89:296–300, 2007.

34. Halliday BR, English HW, Timperley AJ et al: Femoral impaction grafting with cement in revision total hip replacement: evolution of the technique and results. J Bone Joint Surg Br 85:809–817, 2005.

35. Lind M, Krarup N, Mikkelsen S Horyck E: Exchange impaction allografting for femoral revision hip arthroplasty: results in 87 cases after 3.6 years' follow-up. J Arthroplasty 17:158–164, 2002.

36. van Biezen FC, ten Have BL, Verhaar JA: Impaction bone grafting of severely defective femora in revision total hip surgery: 21 hips followed for 41–85 months. Acta Orthop Scand 71:135–142, 2000.

37. Pekkarinen J, Alho A, Lepistö J, et al: Impaction bone grafting in revision hip surgery: a high incidence of complications. J Bone Joint Surg Br 82:103–107, 2000.

38. Linder L: Cancellous impaction grafting in the human femur: histological and radiographic observations in 6 autopsy femurs and 8 biopsies. Acta Orthop Scand 71:543–552, 2000.

39. Ling RS, Timperley AJ, Linder L: Histology of cancellous impaction grafting in the femur: a case report. J Bone Joint Surg Br 75:693–696, 1993.

40. Masterson EL, Duncan CP: Subsidence and the cement mantle in femoral impaction allografting. Orthopedics 20:821–822, 1997.

41. Meding JB, Ritter MA, Keating EM, Faris PM: Impaction bone grafting before insertion of a femoral stem with cement in revision total hip arthroplasty: a minimum two-year follow-up study. J Bone Joint Surg Am 79:1834–1841, 1997.

42. Buttaro MA, Comba F, Piccaluga F: Proximal femoral reconstructions with bone impaction grafting and metal mesh. Clin Orthop Relat Res 467:2325–2334, 2009.

43. Woodgate I, Gross AE: Minor column structural acetabular allografts in revision hip arthroplasty. Clin Orthop Relat Res 371:75–85, 2000.

44. Sporer SM, O'Rourke M, Chong P, Paprosky WG: The use of structural distal femoral allografts for acetabular reconstruction: average ten-year follow-up. J Bone Joint Surg Am 87:760–765, 2005.

45. Garbuz D, Morsi E, Mohamed N, Gross AE: Classification and reconstruction in revision acetabular arthroplasty with bone stock deficiency. Clin Orthop Relat Res 323:98–107, 1996.

46. Sporer S, O'Rourke M, Paprosky W: The treatment of pelvic discontinuity during acetabular revision. J Arthroplasty 20:79–84, 2005.

47. Regis D, Magnan B, Sandri A, Bartolozzi P: Long-term results of anti-protrusio cage and massive allografts for the management of periprosthetic acetabular bone loss. J Arthroplasty 23:826–832, 2008.

48. Saleh KJ, Jaroszynski G, Woodgate I, et al: Revision total hip arthroplasty with the use of structural acetabular allograft and reconstruction ring: a case series with a 10-year average follow-up. J Arthroplasty 15:951–958, 2000.

49. Hooten JP Jr, Engh CA, Heekin RD, Vinh TN: Structural bulk allografts in acetabular reconstruction: analysis of two grafts retrieved at post-mortem. J Bone Joint Surg Br 78:270–275, 1996.

50. Blackley HR, Davis AM, Hutchison CR, Gross AE: Proximal femoral allografts for reconstruction of bone stock in revision arthroplasty of the hip: a nine- to fifteen-year follow-up. J Bone Joint Surg Am 83:346–354, 2001.

51. Graham NM, Stockley I: The use of structural proximal femoral allografts in complex revision hip arthroplasty. J Bone Joint Surg Br 86:337–343, 2004.

52. Haddad FS, Garbuz DS, Masri BA, Duncan CP: Structural proximal femoral allografts for failed total hip replacements: a minimum review of five years. J Bone Joint Surg Br 82:830–836, 2000.

53. Haddad FS, Spangehl MJ, Masri BA, et al: Circumferential allograft replacement of the proximal femur: a critical analysis. Clin Orthop Relat Res 371:98–107, 2000.

54. Safir O, Kellett CF, Flint M, et al: Revision of the deficient proximal femur with a proximal femoral allograft. Clin Orthop Relat Res 467:206–212, 2009.

55. Zehr R, Enneking W, Scarborough M: Allograft-prosthesis composite versus megaprosthesis in proximal femoral reconstruction. Clin Orthop Relat Res 322:207–223, 1996.

56. Mankin HJ, Gebhardt MC, Jennings LC, et al: Long-term results of allograft replacement in the management on bone tumors. Clin Orthop Relat Res 324:86–97, 1996.

57. Farid Y, Lin PP, Lewis VO, Yasko AW: Endoprosthetic and allograft-prosthetic composite reconstruction of the proximal femur for bone neoplasms. Clin Orthop Relat Res 442:223–229, 2006.

58. Anract P, Coste J, Vastel L, et al: Proximal femoral reconstruction with megaprosthesis versus allograft prosthesis composite: a comparative study of functional results, complications and longevity in 41 cases. Rev Chir Orthop Reparatrice Appar Mot 86:278–288, 2000.

59. Hamadouche M, Blanchat C, Meunier A, et al: Histological findings in a proximal femoral structural allograft ten years following revision total hip arthroplasty: a case report. J Bone Joint Surg Am 84:269–273, 2002.

60. Stevenson S: Enhancement of fracture healing with autogenous and allogeneic bone grafts. Clin Orthop Relat Res 355 (Suppl):S239–S246, 1998.

61. Voggenreiter G, Ascherl R, Blumel G, Schmit-Neuerburg KP: Effects of preservation and sterilization on cortical bone grafts: a scanning electron microscopic study. Arch Orthop Trauma Surg 113:294–296, 1994.

62. Stevenson S, Horowitz M: The response of bone allograft. J Bone Joint Surg Am 74:939–950, 1992.

63. Gazdag AR, Lane JM, Glaser D, Forster RA: Alternatives to bone autogenous bone graft: efficacy and indication. J Am Acad Orthop Surg 3:1–8, 1995.

64. Ward WG, Gautreaux MD, Lippert DC II, Boles C: HLA sensitization and allograft bone graft incorporation. Clin Orthop Relat Res 466:1837–1848, 2008.

65. Aho AJ, Eskola J, Ekfors T, et al: Immune responses and clinical outcome of massive human osteoarticular allografts. Clin Orthop Relat Res 346:196–206, 1997.

66. Freidlander GE: Immune responses to osteochondral allografts: current knowledge and future directions. Clin Orthop Relat Res 174:58–68, 1983.

67. Horowitz MC, Friedlander GE: Induction of specific T-cell responsiveness to allogeneic bone. J Bone Joint Surg Am 73:1157–1168, 1991.

68. Lee MY, Finn HA, Lazda VA, et al: Bone allografts are immunogenic and may preclude subsequent organ. Clin Orthop Relat Res 340:215–219, 1997.

69. Stevenson S, Emery DW, Goldberg VM: Factors affecting bone graft incorporation. Clin Orthop Relat Res 323:66–74, 1996.

70. Stevenson S, Qing X, Davy DT, et al: Critical biological determinants of incorporation of non-vascularized cortical bone grafts. J Bone Joint Surg Am 79:1–16, 1997.

71. Friedlander GE, Strong DM, Sell KW: Studies on the antigenicity of bone. I: freeze-dried and deep frozen allografts in rabbits. J Bone Joint Surg Am 58:854–858, 1976.

72. Friedlaender GE: The antigenicity of preserved allografts. Transplant Proc 8(Suppl 1):195–200, 1976.

73. Tomford WW, Mankin HJ: Bone banking: update on methods and materials. Orthop Clin North Am 30:565–570, 1990.

74. Transmission of HIV through bone transplantation: case report and public health recommendations. MMWR Morb Mortal Wkly Rep 37:597–599, 1988.

75. Tomford WW: Transmission of disease through transplantation of musculoskeletal allografts. J Bone Joint Surg Am 77:1742–1754, 1995.

76. U.S. Department of Health and Human Services (FDA): Human tissue intended for transplantation. Fed Reg 62:40429–40447, 1997.

77. Stevenson S: Biology of bone grafts. Orthop Clin North Am 30:543–552, 1999.

78. Jinno T, Miric A, Feighan J, et al: The effects of processing and low dose irradiation on cortical bone grafts. Clin Orthop Relat Res 375:275–285, 2000.

79. Update: allograft-associated bacterial infections: United States, 2002. MMWR Morb Mortal Wkly Rep 51:207–210, 2002.

80. Boyce T, Edwards J, Scarborough N: Allograft bone: the influence of processing on safety and performance. Orthop Clin North Am 30:571–581, 1999.

81. Thorén K, Aspenberg P: Ethylene oxide sterilization impairs allograft incorporation in a conduction chamber. Clin Orthop Relat Res 318:259–264, 1995.

82. Guo MZ, Xia ZS, Lin LB: The mechanical and biological properties of demineralised cortical bone allografts in animals. J Bone Joint Surg Br 73:791–794, 1991.

83. Goldberg VM, Stevenson S, Shaffer JW, et al: Biological and physical properties of autogenous vascularized fibular grafts in dogs. J Bone Joint Surg Am 72:801–810, 1990.

84. Stevenson S, Frederick RW, Li XQ, et al: Together, the host bed and the properties of the graft determine the outcome of graft incorporation. Trans Orthop Res SOC 14:463, 1989.

85. Stevenson S, Frederick RW, Zart DJ, et al: The interaction and effects of freezing and histocompatibility on the incorporation of allogeneic cortical graft in rats. Trans Orthop Res SOC 14:269, 1989.

86. Stevenson S, Li XQ, Martin B: The fate of cancellous and cortical bone after transplantation of fresh and frozen tissueantigen-matched and mismatched osteochondral allografts in dogs. J Bone Joint Surg Am 73:1143–1156, 1991

87. Emery SE, Brazinski MS, Koka A, et al: The biological and biomechanical effects of irradiation on anterior spinal bone grafts in a canine model. J Bone Joint Surg Am 97:504–548, 1994.

88. Stevenson S, Li XQ, Davy DT, et al: Critical biological determinants of incorporation of non-vascularized cortical bone grafts: quantification of a complex process and structure. J Bone Joint Surg Am 79:1–16, 1997.

89. Boden SD, Sumner DR: Biologic factors affecting spinal fusion and bone regeneration. Spine 20(Suppl 24):102S–112S, 1995.

90. Burchardt H: The biology of bone graft repair. Clin Orthop Relat Res 174:28–42, 1983.

91. Burchardt H: Biology of bone transplantation. Orthop Clin North Am 18:187–196, 1987.

92. Johnson KD, Frierson KE, Keller TS, et al: Porous ceramics as bone graft substitutes in long bone defects: a biomechanical, histological, and radiographic analysis. J Orthop Res 14:351–369, 1996.

93. Marchetti DG: Spinal lesions: bone and bone substitutes. Eur Spine J 9:372–378, 2000.

94. Enneking WF, Campanacci DA: Retrieved human allografts: a clinicopathological study. J Bone Joint Surg Am 83:971–986, 2001.

95. Enneking WF, Mindell ER: Observations on massive retrieved human allografts. J Bone Joint Surg Am 73:1123–1142, 1991.

96. Udomkiat P, Dorr LD, Won YY: Technical factors for success with metal ring acetabular reconstruction. J Arthroplasty 16:961–969, 2001.

97. Gamradt SC, Lieberman JR: Bone graft for revision hip arthroplasty: biology and future applications. Clin Orthop Relat Res 417:183–194, 2003.

98. Matejovsky Z Jr, Matejovsky Z, Kofranek I: Massive allografts in tumor surgery. Int Orthop 30:478–483, 2006.

99. Wang J, Temple HT, Pitcher JD, et al: Salvage of failed massive allograft reconstruction with endoprosthesis. Clin Orthop Relat Res 443:296–301, 2006.

100. Wheeler DL, Enneking WF: Allograft bone decreases in strength in vivo over time. Clin Orthop Relat Res 435:36–42, 2005.

101. Shatzker J, Wong M: Acetabular revision: the role of rings and cages. Clin Orthop Relat Res 369:187–197, 1999.

102. Boden SD, Kang J, Sandhu H, Heller JG: Use of recombinant human bone morphogenetic protein-2 to achieve posterolateral lumbar spine fusion in humans: a prospective, randomized clinical pilot trial: 2002 Volvo Award in clinical studies. Spine 27:2662–2673, 2002.

103. Burkus JK, Sandhu HS, Gornet MF, Longley MC: Use of rhBMP-2 in combination with structural cortical allografts: clinical and radiographic outcomes in anterior lumbar spinal surgery. J Bone Joint Surg Am 87:1205–1212, 2005.

104. Govender S, Csimma C, Genant HK, et al: Recombinant human bone morphogenetic protein-2 for treatment of open tibial

fractures: a prospective, controlled, randomized study of four hundred and fifty patients. J Bone Joint Surg Am 84:2123–2134, 2002.

105. Jones AL, Bucholz RW, Bosse MJ, et al: Recombinant human BMP-2 and allograft compared with autogenous bone graft for reconstruction of diaphyseal tibial fractures with cortical defects: a randomized, controlled trial. J Bone Joint Surg Am 88:1431–1441, 2006.

106. Pluhar GE, Manley PA, Heiner JP, et al: The effect of recombinant human bone morphogenetic protein-2 on femoral reconstruction with an intercalary allograft in a dog model. J Orthop Res 19:308–317, 2001.

107. Zabka AG, Pluhar GE, Edwards RB 3rd, et al: Histomorphometric description of allograft bone remodeling and union in a canine segmental femoral defect model: a comparison of rhBMP-2, cancellous bone graft, and absorbable collagen sponge. J Orthop Res 19:318–327, 2001.

108. Li-Dong W, Yan X, Hua-Chen Y: Effects of rhBMP-2 on cortical strut allograft healing to the femur in revision total hip arthroplasties: an experimental study. Int Orthop 31:605–611, 2007.

109. Cook SD, Barrack RL, Shimmin A, et al: The use of osteogenic protein-1 in reconstructive surgery of the hip. J Arthroplasty 16(Suppl 1):88–94, 2001.

110. Tsuchida H, Hashimoto J, Crawford E, et al: Engineered allogeneic mesenchymal stem cells repair femoral segmental defect in rats. J Orthop Res 21:44–53, 2003.

111. Xie C, Reynolds D, Awad H, et al: Structural bone allograft combined with genetically engineered mesenchymal stem cells as a novel platform for bone tissue engineering. Tissue Eng 13:435–445, 2007.

112. Zhang X, Xie C, Lin AS, et al: Periosteal progenitor cell fate in segmental cortical bone graft transplantations: implications for functional tissue engineering. J Bone Miner Res 20:2124–2137, 2005.

113. Gazit D, Turgeman G, Kelley P, et al: Engineered pluripotent mesenchymal cells integrate and differentiate in regenerating bone: a novel cell-mediated gene therapy. J Gene Med 1:121–133, 1999.

114. Turgeman G, Pittman DD, Muller R, et al: Engineered human mesenchymal stem cells: a novel platform for skeletal cell mediated gene therapy. J Gene Med 3:240–251, 2001.

115. Ito H, Koefoed M, Tiyapatanaputi P, et al: Remodeling of cortical bone allografts mediated by adherent rAAV-RANKL and VEGF gene therapy. Nat Med 11:291–297, 2005.

116. Koefoed M, Ito H, Gromov E, et al: Biological effects of rAAV-caAlk2 coating on structural allograft healing. Mol Ther 12:212–218, 2005.

117. ten Cate JW, van der Poll T, Levi M, et al: Cytokines: triggers of clinical thrombotic disease. Thromb Haemost 78:415–419, 1997.

118. Burchardt H: The biology of bone graft repair. Clin Orthop Relat Res 174:28–42, 1983.

119. Board TN, Brunskill S, Doree C, et al: Processed versus fresh frozen bone for impaction bone grafting in revision hip arthroplasty. Cochrane Database Syst Rev (4):CD006351, 2009.

120. Nigro N, Grace D: Radiographic evaluation of bone grafts. J Foot Ankle Surg 35:378–385, 1996.

121. Elves MW, Ford CHJ: A study of the humoral immune response to massive osteoarticular allografts in sheep. Clin Exp Immunol 23:360–366, 1976.

122. Judas F, Figueiredo MH, Cabrit AM, Proença A: Incorporation of impacted morselised bone allograft in rabbits. Transplant Proc 37:2802–2804, 2005.

SECTION II

ANATOMY AND OPERATIVE APPROACHES

CHAPTER 14

Normal Hip Embryology and Development

Elizabeth Weber and Andrew W. Ritting

KEY POINTS

- Lower limb development occurs in utero in its entirety during the fetal stage of development.
- The primordium of the hip joint is an amorphous cartilage model in which the two sides of the joint are indistinct until the autolytic process at the inter-zone creates a "joint space" during the seventh week post conception.
- Developmental dysplasia occurs when the intimate fit between the developing femoral head and the developing acetabulum is disrupted; if untreated, this may lead to poor hip joint congruity and early arthritis.
- Legg-Calvé-Perthes disease results from a vascular insult in the immature femoral epiphysis. Depending on the age of the child at presentation and the degree to which the lateral epiphysis is involved, significant residual deformity may lead to early arthritis. Slipped capital femoral epiphysis may result when shear forces across the adolescent physis overwhelm its strength. The resultant deformity may cause significant alterations in gait and joint mechanics and may lead to early arthritis.

INTRODUCTION

Normal hip development is the result of a carefully orchestrated series of prenatal events, which act in concert to form the acetabulum, the femoral head, intra-articular structures of the hip, and the blood supply to the hip joint. After birth, the hip joint remains immature and the intimate relationship between the femoral head and the acetabulum is crucial for appropriate postnatal development. This chapter will elucidate normal hip embryology and some of the postnatal pathology that can influence the ultimate shape and motion of the mature adult hip.

Intrauterine life is divided into three phases: blasto-cystic, embryonic, and fetal. The *blastocyst phase* refers to fertilization through the end of the second week post conception. Following blastocyst, the period of primary tissue differentiation is weeks 2 through 8. During this *embryonic phase,* the entire musculoskeletal system develops in the following ways: both upper and lower limb buds appear, along with the cartilaginous anlage of the osseous limbs; joints, longitudinal growth plates, and vascular supply to the bones are formed; and, ultimately, the complex articulated human mobility system is fully differentiated and formed. Vascular insults, confining pathology, and teratogens, which act during this phase, have the greatest likelihood of interfering with the development of healthy functional symmetric lower extremities. The *fetal phase,* from 8 weeks to birth, consists of refinement of the vascular supply, ossification of the diaphysis of long bones, and formation of intra-articular structures. The hip joint is fully mature at 35 weeks post conception. The complex genetic code and signaling pathways, which direct the development of the human hip, are mostly unknown.

THE EMBRYONIC PHASE OF PRENATAL DEVELOPMENT

At the end of the third week of development, the three primary germ layers—ectoderm, endoderm, and mesoderm—have formed and will give rise to all tissues in the developing embryo.[1] After the formation of the notochord and neural tube, the mesodermal tissue alongside forms the paraxial mesoderm, which subsequently divides into 38 paired somites. These are the primordia of the future axial skeleton and all associated muscles.[1] The mesoderm is also responsible for most of the structures in the appendicular skeleton. Cartilage, connective tissue, striated muscle, bone, and blood vessels all take their origins from the mesoderm. The appendicular skeleton begins at day 26 with upper limb buds, which appear as paired outpouchings along the lateral wall of the developing embryo. More caudal, at the level of the lumbar and first sacral elements,[2] lower limb bud swellings appear at day 28. At this time, a cellular template for the future femur exists. Chondroblasts aggregate and condense, and through chondrification, the separate aggregates condense to form the femoral anlage.[3] At the same time, a similar process is defining the future innominate.[3]

Development and refinement of the limbs are continuous during the embryonic period, with the upper extremities preceding the lower at all points. Between 37 and 40 days, foot plates are formed, and by 46 days, the digital rays are visible. The limbs continue to elongate ventrally toward each other. By 55 days, the toe webbing has disappeared and the toes are distinct.[1]

Within the lower limb bud, cells are dividing and differentiating into specific tissues. The bones, which will form the articulating hip joint, begin as a solid mass of chondroblasts. The first recognizable structure to appear is the cartilage model of the femoral diaphysis during the sixth week. Precartilage is present at the future site of the femoral head, which is indistinguishable at this time from the acetabulum. Undifferentiated mesenchymal cells called *blastemal cells* appear as the trochanteric projection.[4] Blastemal cells will form apophyses, precartilage will form the covering at the articulations of long bones, and cartilage will form the anlagen for the osseous structures.[2]

During the seventh week, an interzone appears, which will distinguish the sides of the hip joint. Proximally, the acetabulum appears as a shallow depression that must deepen from 65 to 180 degrees during its development.[2] Distally, the femoral head and the overlying articular cartilage are forming. In the middle, autolytic degeneration occurs by programmed cell death in this interzone to separate the two structures and form the actual joint space.[5] This is the first time the hip joint could theoretically be "dislocated." The hip is well protected from dislocating in all directions except for inferiorly because the transverse acetabular ligament is poorly defined.[2] The beginnings of synovial tissue and the ligamentum teres are found at this time in the middle layer of the interzone. Blastemal cells at the periphery of the acetabulum condense to begin to form the acetabular labrum.[4] At the end of the embryologic stage, the secondary center of ossification appears in the ilial portion of the pelvis. No secondary center of ossification is present in the femur, but the neck of the femur has elongated.

right.[3] As the vascular supply matures, a distinction is made between the metaphyseal supply and the epiphyseal supply. Retinacular vessels enter the head and neck.[2] At 20 weeks' gestation, the spherical femoral head is 7 mm and anteversion is 25 to 30 degrees. At 32 weeks, the shaft ossification has reached the level of the greater trochanter. Both the ilium and the ischium are ossified[4] (Table 14-1; Figs. 14-1 through 14-7).

Table 14-1. Prenatal Lower Extremity Development		
Time Post Conception	**Embryonic Development**	**Hip Development**
28 days	Lower limb bud appears	
37 days	Foot plates appear	
46 days	Digital rays are visible	
55 days	Toe webbing is gone	
6th week	Cartilage model of femoral diaphysis appears	Trochanteric projection (blastemal cells) and nonarticulating hip joint (cartilage)
7th week		Interzone appears, which separates the acetabulum from the femoral head
8th week		Secondary center of ossification in the ilium

THE FETAL PHASE OF PRENATAL DEVELOPMENT

From 8 weeks post conception until birth is the fetal phase. The vital organs and the appendicular skeleton are completely formed. This phase is focused on ossification, vascularization, and maturation. Ossification in the femur proceeds proximally and distally from the center. The labrum has coalesced as a triangular structure in coronal section. The lower limb bud begins to internally rotate so the knee joint moves from lateral to anterior.[3] In the 11th week, the femur is characterized by a 2-mm spherical head and 5 to 10 degrees of anteversion, which will continue to increase to 45 degrees at 36 weeks' gestation.[6] The limb is characterized by knee flexion and hip flexion and adduction. By the 16th week, the muscles investing the hip joint and the hip capsule are formed. The joint capsule joins distally with the femoral perichondrium.[2] Internally, the acetabular labrum, the ligamentum teres, and the transverse acetabular ligament are now formed. Mature hyaline cartilage covers the articulating surfaces of both the femoral head and the acetabulum. The femoral shaft is fully ossified, and the ossification center of the ischium is now evident.[4] Muscles are formed and attached and can actively move the hip; the left leg comes to override the

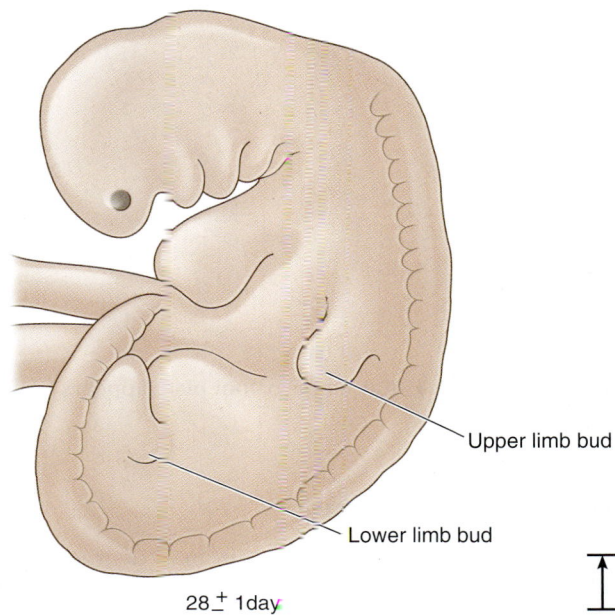

Upper limb bud

Lower limb bud

28 ± 1day

Figure 14-1. The 28-day embryo: the first appearance of the lower limb bud (length, 4 mm).

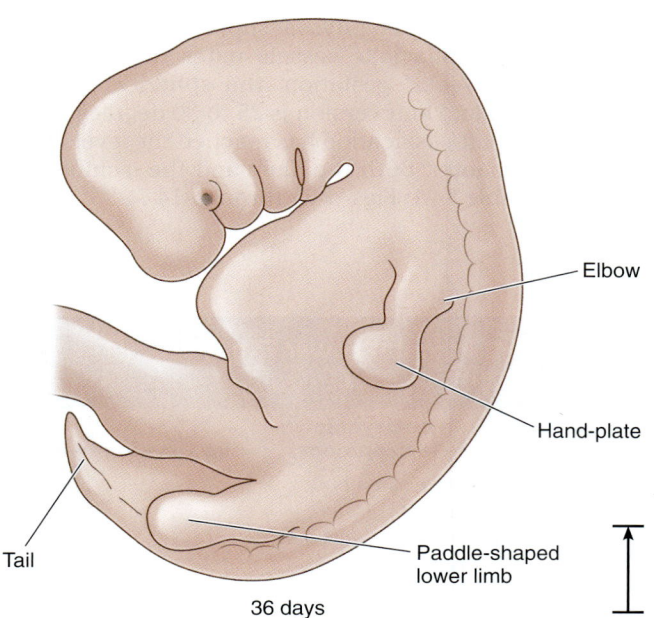

Figure 14-2. The 36-day embryo: paddle-shaped limb (length, 9 mm).

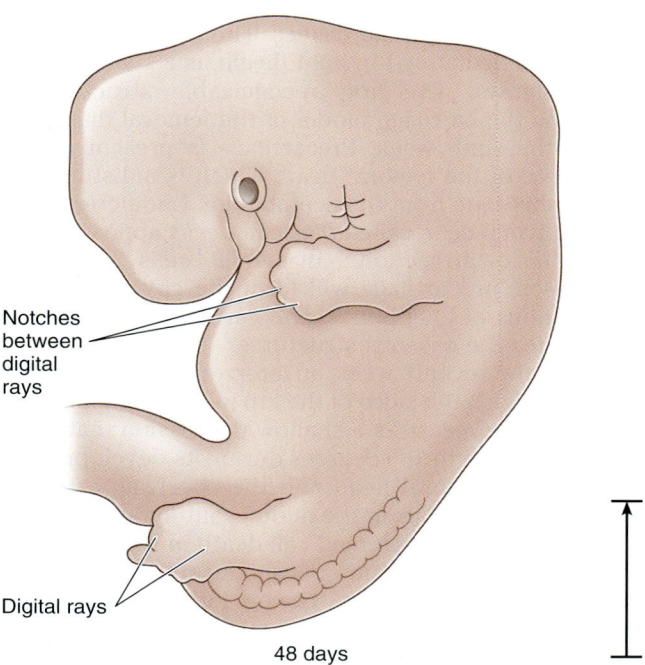

Figure 14-4. The 48-day embryo: digital rays are distinguishable (length, 15 mm).

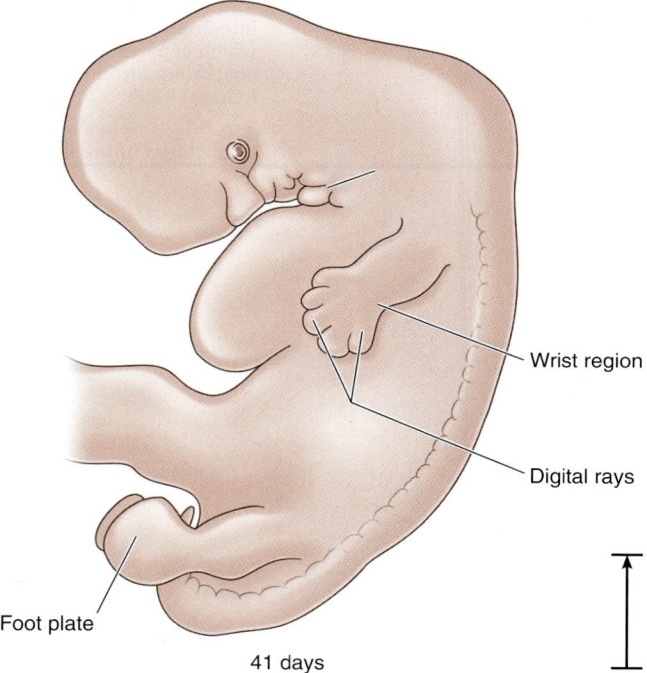

Figure 14-3. The 41-day embryo: foot plate appears (length, 10 mm).

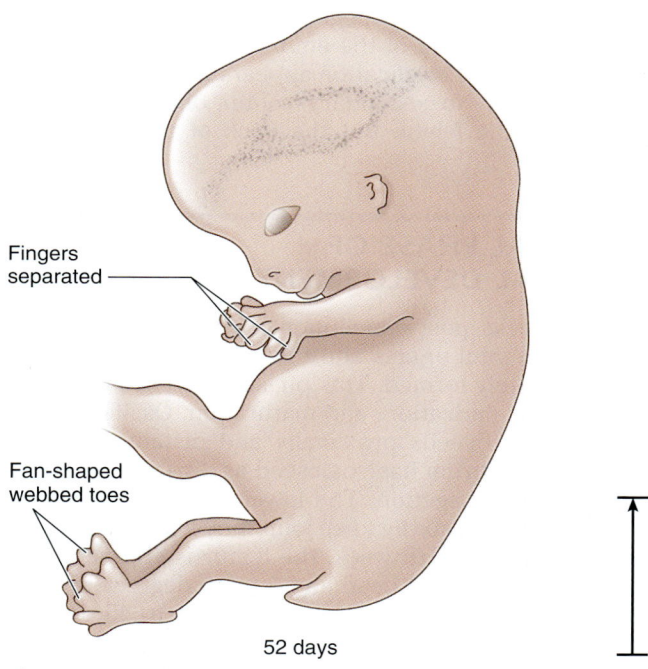

Figure 14-5. The 52-day embryo: fan-shaped foot with webbed toes (length, 19 mm).

Femoral Anteversion

Femoral anteversion increases from 5 degrees in the 11th week to 45 degrees at 36 weeks' gestation. Postnatally, femoral anteversion begins to decrease as the result of muscle forces acting across the hip joint.[5] Normal postnatal femoral anteversion is approximately 30 degrees at 1 year and 15 degrees at skeletal maturity.[7]

Neck Shaft Angle

The neck shaft angle is very valgus in early development, decreasing from 145 degrees in the 15th week to

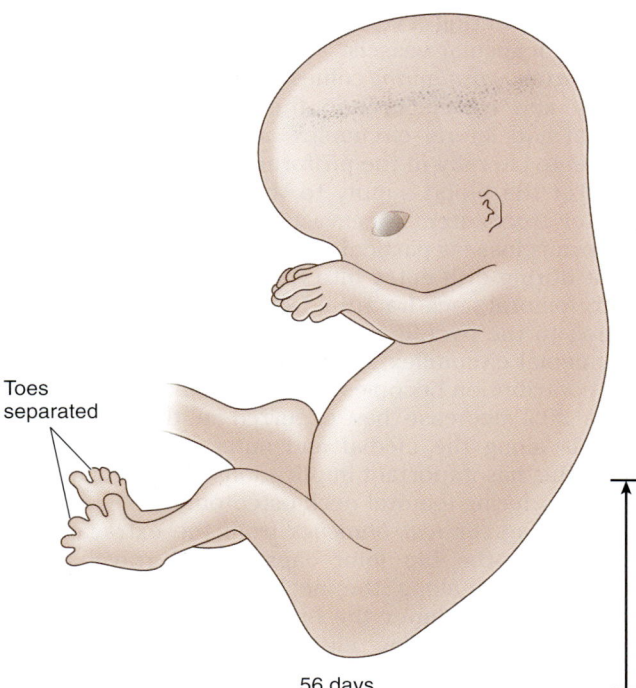

Toes
separated

56 days

Figure 14-6. The 56-day embryo: toes are separated (length, 27 mm).

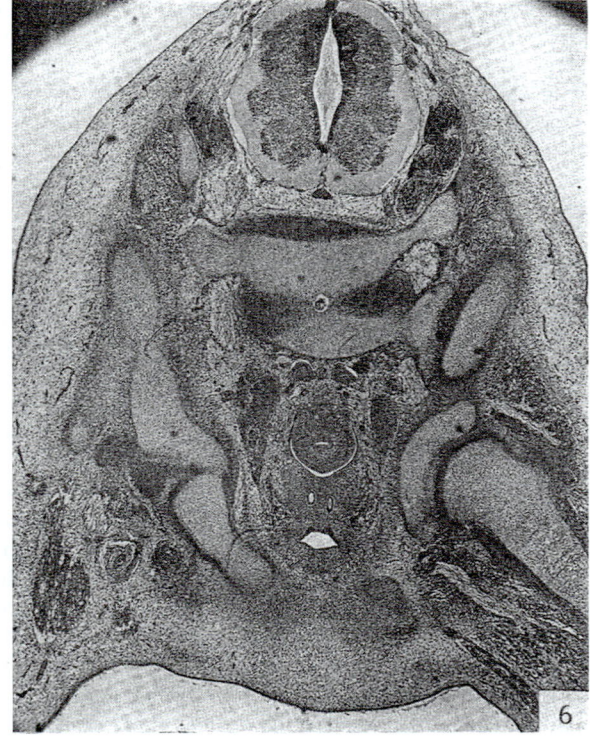

6

Figure 14-7. Human hip at the end of embryonic development. Note that the femoral head is completely distinct from the acetabulum. This is the first time the joint could conceivably dislocate. *(From Strayer LM: The embryology of the human hip joint. Yale J Biol Med 16:13–26, 1943.)*

130 degrees at 36 weeks' gestation.[6] Postnatally, with normal muscle forces acting across the hip joint, a further decrease in the neck shaft angle to approximately 127 degrees occurs at 18 months.[8]

Both femoral anteversion and the neck shaft angle are found to remain constant postnatally in cerebral palsy patients, suggesting that abnormal muscle forces inhibit normal postnatal development of the hip.[9]

POSTNATAL DEVELOPMENT

Acetabulum

At birth, the acetabulum is immature, consisting of a cartilaginous ring surrounding the femoral head. At its depth, the ring is confluent with a Y-shaped triradiate cartilage. Eventually, with growth, the arms of the triradiate cartilage coalesce to form the medial, nonarticular acetabulum. Growth of the triradiate cartilage is interstitial. During this same period, the ring of cartilage investing the femoral head enlarges to become the load-bearing acetabulum, which grows at pace with the developing femoral head by apposition. The triradiate cartilage develops from three primary centers of ossification. The os acetabuli is the pubic contribution. It is the largest center of ossification and eventually will form the anterior wall of the mature acetabulum. The superior dome is formed from the iliac contribution, and the posterior wall is formed by the ischial contribution. The shape and depth of the adult acetabulum are heavily dependent on the dynamic interaction of the mature femoral head. A preponderance of acetabular shape and depth has been established by the appearance of ossification centers at 8 or 9 years of age. This is the watershed age, after which very little acetabular remodeling can be expected; t therefore defines the prognosis in many pediatric hip disorders. Ossification centers of the acetabulum fuse between 17 and 18 years of age.[10]

Femur

At birth, the ossified portion of the femur has progressed proximally to the level of the greater trochanter and the femoral neck. Three separate growth plates define the cartilaginous proximal femur: the longitudinal growth plate (LGP) of the femoral neck, the growth plate of the greater trochanter (TGP), and the connecting growth plate on the lateral neck called the *femoral neck isthmus* (FNI) (Fig. 14-8). The LGP and the TGP have divergent growth vectors that additively create longitudinal growth of the proximal femur along the axis of the femoral shaft. Alterations in growth of either of these physes result in angular deformities of the mature hip. Additionally acting on the LGP is contact pressure from the acetabulum, which forces spherical appositional growth within the socket. The mature shape of the femoral head and that of the acetabulum are interrelated and rely heavily on the dynamic and continuous reciprocal relationship of the round head in the round socket. Disruptions in this relationship result in failures

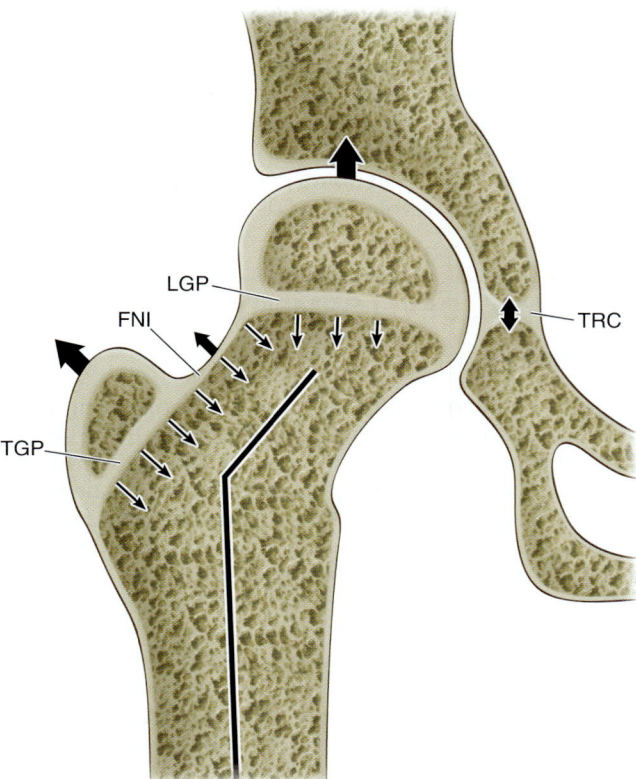

Figure 14-8. Growth plates at the hip joint. On the femoral side, the trochanteric growth plate (TGP) grows by traction, and the longitudinal growth plate (LGP) grows by apposition. The femoral neck isthmus (FNI) connects the two and allows widening of the femoral neck with growth. On the acetabular side, the triradiate cartilage (TRC) allows the socket to expand by interstitial growth.

of formation and imperfect adult hip joints. For example, if developmental hip dysplasia is unrecognized and untreated, the resultant acetabulum is shallow and steep from inconsistent pressure from the femoral head within the developing socket.

BLOOD SUPPLY

Femoral

The first evidence of vascularity to the femur occurs at 8 weeks post conception, as capillaries break into the cartilage model of the femur in the middle third of the diaphysis, at the site of the primary ossification center. This eventually will become the nutrient artery in the mature bone. By the 14th week, a ring of vessels has encircled the femoral neck to form primitive retinacular vessels. These vessels invade the cartilage model. This primitive femoral model of vascularity does not change appreciably from week 14 to skeletal maturity.[11] The postnatal vascularity of the proximal femur can be broken down into three distinct supplies: an extracapsular ring of vessels, ascending cervical vessels, and intracapsular vessels.

The *extracapsular ring* comes directly from the femoral artery and travels around the femoral neck as the medial and lateral circumflex arteries. These vessels converge laterally in the piriformis fossa. They provide most of the blood supply to the proximal femur and greater trochanter.[11] The vascular anastomosis in the piriformis fossa is particularly vulnerable to embarrassment during drill entry into the femoral canal, as well as to femoral neck fracture. During growth, the contribution to the overall supply of the proximal femur by the medial circumflex increases, as the lateral circumflex contribution becomes less significant. By the age of 10, a 50% decrease has occurred in the number of vessels along the medial and anterior aspect of the neck; this has important implications for vascular preservation during femoral neck osteotomy.

Ascending cervical branches from the extracapsular ring pierce the hip joint capsule and travel under the synovium along the neck inside the hip joint. These branches enter the bone and travel distally in the metaphysis; they either anastomose with the ascending diaphyseal vessels or travel lateral or medial to supply the greater trochanter or the femoral neck, respectively.

The *intracapsular synovial ring* of vessels ascend superficial to the perichondrial ring and supply the epiphysis. In this way, the physis serves as a barrier between the blood supplies of the primary and secondary centers of ossification until the two supplies coalesce at skeletal maturity.[12] An orderly pattern of blood supply to the epiphysis occurs such that each penetrating vessel defines an autonomous vascular zone. Until this system matures, the femoral head is susceptible to patterned necrosis should any vascular territory suffer an occlusion.

Acetabular

The blood supply to the acetabular portion of the hip joint is completely defined before birth. The incidence of acetabular side avascular necrosis, either idiopathic or iatrogenic, is very low. From the internal iliac artery within the pelvis, the acetabular supply arises from three different branches, which arborize in such a way that they allow circumferential supply to the socket. The posterior division of the internal iliac terminates as the superior gluteal after giving off the iliolumbar and lateral sacral arteries. It supplies the superior portion of the acetabulum and the weight-bearing dome.[13] Most of the inferior acetabulum is supplied by the posterior branch of the obturator artery. A small watershed area in the posterior acetabulum is redundantly supplied by the inferior gluteal artery. If the right acetabulum is seen as a clock face, superior and inferior gluteal arteries exit the pelvis at the greater sciatic notch at 10 o'clock. They diverge to supply an area superior and anterior (10-4 o'clock) and an area posterior (8-10 o'clock), respectively. The obturator artery exits the pelvis through the obturator foramen at 6 o'clock and supplies the acetabulum inferiorly (4-8 o'clock).[14]

DEVELOPMENTAL DYSPLASIA OF THE HIP

Developmental dysplasia of the hip (DDH) is a disease process that affects primarily very young children and has the ability to interfere with early postnatal hip development. Its course is variable, ranging from full resolution with or without treatment to frank hip dislocation; therefore its true incidence is unknown.[15] An intimate dynamic relationship between the spherical femoral head in the reciprocal acetabulum is crucial for appropriate postnatal development of a congruent hip joint. The primary disturbance in DDH is loss of femoral head congruency within the acetabulum, resulting in abnormal development of the femoral head and acetabular concavity.[16] As many as 95% of cases of subluxation or frank dislocation can be successfully treated with conservative abduction devices such as the Pavlik harness.[17] However, intra-articular pathology such as hypertrophied acetabular cartilage (neolimbus) or accessory centers of ossification may develop concurrently.[18-20] If the young hip has been dislocated for any length of time, pressure against the ilium, superior to the actual acetabulum, may lead to the formation of a false acetabulum, the presence of which markedly increases the risk of future osteoarthritis.[21] If persistent, these changes may require operative management, including closed reduction and casting, open reduction with or without femoral shortening, a variety of acetabuloplasties, and ultimately total hip arthroplasty. "Successful" treatment of DDH carries a risk of later avascular necrosis, which, depending on severity and on the age of the patient, may result in radiographic features that challenge the adult arthroplasty surgeon and may mimic changes seen in Legg-Calvé-Perthes disease.[22]

Initial radiographic findings in the infant with DDH include delayed presentation of the ossific nucleus, increased acetabular index for age, poorly formed teardrop or sourcil, a break in Shenton's line, and the presence of an acetabular notch and a false acetabulum[23] (Fig. 14-9). Often, the earliest radiographic finding in DDH with subluxation is increased sclerosis in the weight-bearing dome at the point of greatest contact. Osteoblastic activity is thought to be activated in response to increased forces born in this area, resulting in sclerosis.[24] A definite association of dysplasia with roentgenographic degenerative joint disease has been noted, especially in females.[10,15] Several other radiographic findings unique to DDH evolve over time. Children with dysplastic hips fall into a broad continuum of congruency at skeletal maturity. Moderate to severe arthritis is not seen in Severin I hips but is evident in 22% of Severin II, 35% of Severin III, and 76% of hips that are subluxated or dislocated at maturity[25] (Table 14-2). These hips were thought to have valgus proximal femurs related to selective lateral growth arrest, which does not manifest radiographically until the adolescent growth spurt.[25] However, more critical review suggests that persistent femoral anteversion gives the radiographic appearance of increased valgus (>135 degrees), and

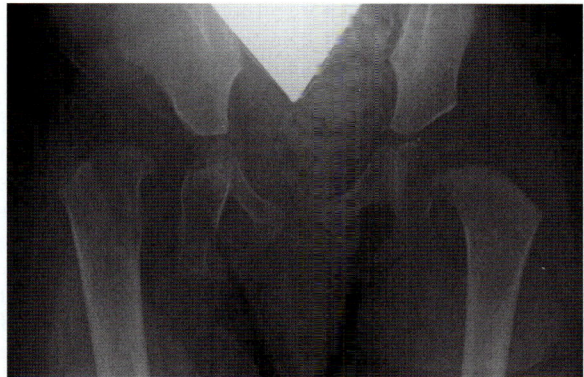

Figure 14-9. Anteroposterior (AP) radiograph of a dysplastic right hip. On the left, the acetabular sourcil is well defined and sclerotic. An ossific nucleus (secondary center of ossification at the femoral epiphysis) is present, along with a developing teardrop. Shenton's line (a continuation of the curvature of the medial femoral neck as it relates to the inferior aspect of the superior pubic ramus) is intact. In the right, dysplastic hip, these features are absent.

Table 14-2. Severin Classification of Hip Dysplasia

Class	Radiographic Appearance	Center Edge Angle, degrees
I	Normal	
IA		>19 (6-13 yo), >25 (>14 yo)
IB		15-19 (6-13 yo), 20-25 (>14 yo)
II	Moderate femoral head; neck and acetabular deformity	
IIA		>19 (6-13 yo), >25 (>14 yo)
IIB		>15-19 (6-13 yo), 20-25 (>14 yo)
III	Dysplasia without subluxation	<15 (6-13 yo), <20 (>14 yo)
IVA	Moderate subluxation	>0
IVB	Severe subluxation	<0
V	Femoral head pseudoarticulation with acetabulum	
VI	Redislocation	

that the true incidence of femoral valgus in DDH is no greater than that in the general population.[22]

Clinical symptoms may lag substantially behind radiographic findings. Risk factors for adult degenerative joint disease include increasing age at reduction and increasing head height at the time of reduction. Of children with reductions occurring before the age of 1 year, 21% have adult arthritis, but those undergoing reductions after 3 years carry a 36% chance of adult arthritis. Patients with low dislocations have only an 18% chance of moderate to severe arthritis in adulthood, whereas those who have high-riding dislocations carry a 48% chance.[25] Patients with radiographic subluxation are most likely to have early clinical symptoms, with severe subluxation manifesting clinically in the second decade of life and moderate subluxation in the third or fourth decade.[15] The prognosis for patients with frank dislocations is better than for the group with subluxations and depends primarily on bilaterality and the presence of a false acetabulum. Bilateral posterosuperior hip dislocation causes hyperlordotic compensation in the low back, the long-term implication of which is early lumbar degenerative joint disease. If a well-developed false acetabulum forms whereon the femoral head articulates with the bony ilium, the chance of a good clinical result is only 24% versus a 52% chance if the false acetabulum is only moderately developed.[21] In unilateral complete dislocations, limb length discrepancies, knee pain, deformity, and scoliosis become clinically relevant, and the issues of development of a false acetabulum are the same.[10] In adolescents with radiographically silent arthritis and known DDH, symptoms are thought to result from cartilage lesions and labral tears. These are seen at arthroscopy nearly 78% of the time in conjunction with one another, primarily in the anterosuperior portion of the acetabulum.[26]

Surgery in the patient with failed conservative treatment or late diagnosis of DDH generally consists of femoral osteotomy before age 4 or acetabular osteotomy at a later age. When relocation fails, or when these methods are unsuccessful in producing appropriate further development and hip articulation, the adolescent or adult patient may ultimately need total hip arthroplasty for progressive osteoarthritis. Radiographic findings of concern are common in the DDH child who has failed conservative treatment, but the correlation between radiographic findings and the development of osteoarthritis is unclear. As the patient ages, radiographic findings correlate well with functional ability.[25]

When arthroplasty is indicated in a DDH patient, a variety of anatomic deformities can present many challenges to the surgeon. Femoral changes include a reduced mediolateral and anteroposterior femoral intramedullary canal diameter of 9.3 to 9.7 mm and 12.6 to 13.6 mm, respectively, in Crowe stage I to IV hip subluxation, compared with 11.2 and 14.2 mm in normal hips[27] (Table 14-3). The proximal medial curvature is straighter and the neck is shorter than in normal femurs.[28,29] Greater degrees of subluxation correlate with greater abnormalities in femoral canal size and anteversion.[30] A progressive decrease in medial head offset is seen with increased Crowe classification; this must be addressed with the extramedullary portion of the prosthesis to restore an appropriate abductor lever arm.[27] Anteversion ranges from 36.4 to 43.6 degrees in DDH hips versus 22.9 in normal hips.[27] "Normal" contralateral hips have been shown to have increased anteversion.[31] The femoral neck is progressively foreshortened in proportion to the severity of involvement. A significant subtrochanteric deformity or retained implants from previous surgery may be noted; this further adds to the need for fastidious preoperative planning.[22] Finally, an increase in relative avascular necrosis on the weight-bearing portion of the femoral head exists[32] and

Type	Description	Dislocation Rate
I	Femur and acetabulum show minimal abnormalities	<50%
II	Acetabular abnormalities	50%-75%
III	Inadequate roof development with superior subluxation of femur	75%-100%
IV	Insufficient acetabular development and high-riding dislocation	100%

Table 14-3. Crowe Classification of Hip Dysplasia

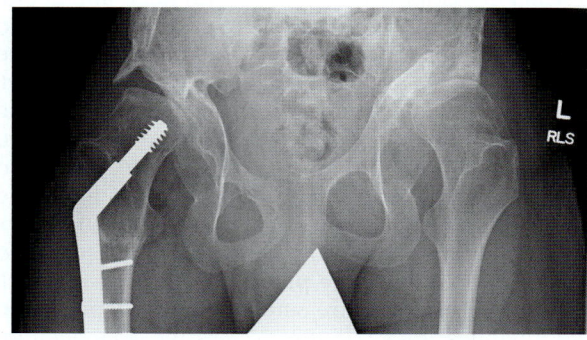

Figure 14-10. Anteroposterior (AP) radiograph of a 17-year-old boy who had a late diagnosis of bilateral hip dysplasia. Surgical reductions and right-sided pelvic osteotomy were performed at 4 years of age. Note the very dysplastic acetabula and the misshapen femoral heads.

may precipitate the need for early arthroplasty. With the culmination of these anatomic changes, authors have noted the necessity to use a smaller and straighter femoral component during arthroplasty, often requiring custom implants[33,34] or concurrent femoral osteotomy.[35] Intraoperative fracture during stem insertion has been reported in as many as 27% of cases.[34]

Acetabular changes in DDH include shallow cup formation and early degeneration at the superolateral aspect of the acetabulum,[36] resulting in an elevated acetabular index[37] and an abnormal center edge angle.[38] A significant decrease in medial acetabular bone stock correlates with acetabular depth, and a greater degree of subluxation is inversely related to increased medial bone stock.[39] Therefore, acetabular components in arthroplasty commonly require abundant use of bone graft, both for the initial procedure and for facilitation of subsequent revision procedures.[40] The goal is to obtain complete coverage of the socket and appropriate seating at the site of the original triradiate cartilage.[34] The surgeon should be cognizant that the dysplastic acetabulum may have altered orientation in all three planes. In the coronal plane, the socket may be translated superolateral with excessive verticality; in the sagittal plane, variable anteroposterior positioning occurs; and in the transverse plane, anteversion may be altered[22] (Fig. 14-10).

Soft tissue and alignment abnormalities are also present in the DDH patient, including malalignment of the ipsilateral knee and leg length discrepancy.[40] The dislocated or subluxated hip is predictably shorter than the contralateral side, with associated shortening of the adductors, hamstrings, and quadriceps. Additionally, the abductors have assumed a relatively horizontal position and are susceptible to damage at the time of surgery.[41] Therefore, to equalize pelvic obliquity, lengthening may be necessary. Safe lengthening ranges between 4 and 6 cm[42]; greater lengthening may result in sciatic nerve palsy. Arthroplasty patients with a preoperative diagnosis of DDH have a significantly increased odds ratio for postoperative motor nerve palsy.[43,44] Difficult procedures, defined as those performed in patients who (1) have undergone previous surgery, (2) have severe deformity, (3) have defects in the acetabular roof, or (4) have flexion deformities, have been shown to have a higher incidence of postoperative nerve palsy.[45] Soft tissue procedures such as tenotomy of contracted muscles and physical therapy for atrophied abductors are essential for arthroplasty success.[40] Abductor weakness is common after childhood surgery for DDH owing to the combination of an inadequate lever arm secondary to proximal femoral deformity and to multiple insults secondary to the surgical approach. Deficits may range from a subtle limp with fatigue to significant disability and pain on activity known as the *gluteus medius syndrome.*[22]

Failure of total hip arthroplasty in DDH patients is more common from stem or acetabular socket loosening than from the common particle wear or infection seen in primary arthroplasty due to idiopathic osteoarthritis.[40,44] Acetabular loosening is increasingly problematic when cup placement is outside the true acetabular region, especially inferiorly and medially.[46-48] Results are typically inferior to those of arthroplasty for idiopathic osteoarthritis, especially in more advanced Crowe staging,[49] and dislocation rates are higher in DDH patients.

PERTHES DISEASE

The cause of Legg-Calvé-Perthes disease (Perthes) is currently unknown, and many studies have supported or refuted claims of elevated intracapsular pressure, increased blood viscosity, defective chondrogenesis, or endocrine disorders playing a role in its development.[50-52] Theories converge at a vascular insult in the immature proximal femoral blood supply. The lateral ascending cervical artery gives rise to both metaphyseal and epiphyseal branches, which supply the majority of blood to the epiphysis. This parent vessel is particularly vulnerable to compression in its course through the trochanteric notch in the immature femur. After age 2, a gradual decrease occurs in the blood supply along the anterior and medial neck. The intracapsular arterial supply is commonly incomplete in males more often than in females.[11] These observations of vascular development support what little we know about Perthes in that it is a disease of vascular embarrassment seen

most commonly in 4- to 8-year-old boys. Whatever the cause, a progressive sequence of ischemia, resorption, collapse, and repair describes the natural history of the disease.[53] When identified early and treated appropriately, children can commonly function at a normal level into the sixth decade, but if left untreated, 50% may have arthritis, ultimately requiring total hip arthroplasty by the age of 55.[54]

The disease includes an initial period of bone necrosis, usually from the anterior physis to the subchondral bone, which is followed by a stage of resorption[53] (Fig. 14-11). The final stage involves osteoblastic remodeling and revascularization and is essential to healing[55] but can lead to coxa magna in 57% to 86% of patients, defined as a 10% increase in femoral head diameter.[54,56-58] Collapse of the lateral epiphysis without subsequent remodeling results in flattening of the femoral head, which ultimately may require arthroplasty. Several theories have been put forth to explain the development of coxa magna, including decreased epiphyseal height early in the disease process, increased local blood supply, broadening of the epiphysis due to plasticity, and adaptive broadening of the femoral neck to attempt to restore normal sphericity.[5] Secondary to coxa magna, morphologic changes are noted in the acetabulum as it fails to keep pace with the rapidly enlarging femoral head. The initial consequence of this phenomenon is focal pressure on the acetabular labrum, likely with subsequent tear and dysfunction.[5] Indicators of the need for arthroplasty include higher-grade head-at-risk signs, femoral head-size ratio, and age of onset of disease.[54] Head-at-risk signs refer to Caterall staging of head involvement, with group I as anterior involvement without metaphyseal reaction, group II as anterolateral involvement of 50% with metaphyseal lesions, group III with 75% involvement and lateral involvement, and group IV as complete head involvement.[59]

The more contemporary classification system is based on the integrity of the lateral pillar on anteroposterior radiography. Maintenance of the lateral pillar, as well as age of onset of the disease, guides treatment options and is prognostic of future hip joint symptoms. In this system, group A shows maintenance of the lateral

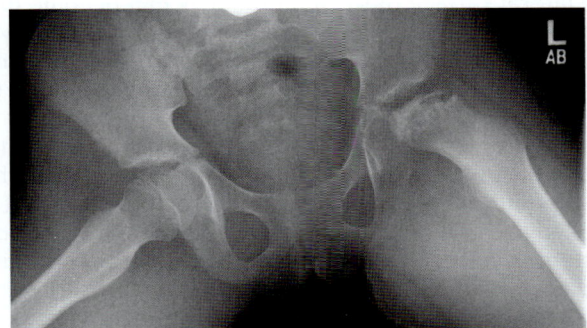

Figure 14-11. Anteroposterior (AP) radiograph of a 9-year-old boy with lateral pillar C Legg-Calvé-Perthes disease. Note the nearly normal appearance of the acetabulum. Significant lateral epiphyseal collapse, metaphyseal cysts, and some femoral neck widening are evident.

Table 14-4. Lateral Pillar Classification of Perthes Disease

Grade	Features
A	Lateral pillar maintained
B	>50% lateral pillar maintained
B/C	≥50% maintained but thin or poorly ossified lateral pillar
C	<50% lateral pillar maintained

Table 14-5. Stulberg Classification

Class	Features
I	Normal hip joint; spherical head in spherical acetabulum
II	Spherical head with
	a. Enlarged head
	b. Shortened femoral neck
	c. Steep acetabulum
III	Nonspherical head; ovoid head
IV	Flat femoral head + any features (a, b, or c)
V	Flat head

pillar with fragmentation at the center of the head, group B shows greater than 50% of the lateral pillar maintained with possible extrusion of the lateral head, and group C shows less than 50% of the lateral pillar maintained with the lateral pillar lower than the central segment[60] (Table 14-4). Nonsurgical treatment is recommended in children younger than 8 at presentation and in children with lateral pillar A disease, because these children do uniformly well regardless of treatment. In children older than 8 at presentation, with lateral pillar C disease, the prognosis is poor, and surgery has not been shown to improve prognosis. Surgical treatment, such as soft tissue procedures, varus-producing femoral osteotomy, acetabular osteotomy, or hip distraction, may be warranted in the watershed group consisting of children older than 8 years at presentation with lateral pillar B or B/C disease.[60] Some authors believe in early containment and advocate for femoral varus osteotomy when the condition is diagnosed at 6 years of age or older.[61] In the face of progressive arthritis from Perthes disease, total hip arthroplasty may be required at a young age. The sequelae of Perthes disease account for an estimated 1.3% of all total hip arthroplasties.[62]

Challenges to the arthroplasty surgeon in Perthes disease are related to significant changes in the femoral head. Coxa magna, coxa plana, and varus and valgus deformities in the femoral head and neck regions have been repeatedly described, and subsequent osteotomies in conjunction with total hip arthroplasty may be necessary.[63] When the head is removed during arthroplasty, most of the deformity is removed, thus making arthroplasty following Perthes typically less technically demanding than in patients with DDH or SCFE. However, the lateral surface of the femoral neck can become flattened and can progress to a pistol-grip deformity,[64] which may produce difficulties in cutting, sizing, and selecting the appropriate femoral component, similar to arthroplasty in the setting of an SCFE patient.

If severe femoral head deformity exists before final acetabular development, the subsequent shape of the acetabulum may be deformed, and this may present a challenge to the adult hip surgeon. In the classification system described by Stulberg, a dysplastic acetabulum correlates with the amount of femoral head congruency; class I and II hips have a spherical congruency, class III and IV hips have an aspherical congruency, and class V hips have an aspherical incongruency[58] (Table 14-5). Acetabular retroversion is present in 42% of Perthes cases,[65] and a more deformed femoral head likely has a cause-and-effect relationship to retroversion.[66,67] A study

by Thillemann and associates indicated Perthes with resultant acetabular dysplasia as a significant risk factor for revision within 0 to 6 months, mainly as a result of dislocation.[68]

Finally, in the case of the patient who has previously undergone osteotomy, additional difficulties include retained metalwork and dysfunction of the abductors as muscle lever arms are manipulated with surgery to unload the femoral head.[22] Although the procedure is more technically demanding, patients requiring total hip arthroplasty after previous osteotomy do not have a higher rate of complications.[69] Therefore, although Perthes is a disease defined by femoral head involvement, changes on the acetabular side of the joint can present challenges to the arthroplasty surgeon.

SLIPPED CAPITAL FEMORAL EPIPHYSIS

Slipped capital femoral epiphysis (SCFE) is a hip disorder that affects primarily obese adolescents and demonstrates regional variation in its incidence, affecting as few as 0.2 per thousand children in parts of Japan and more than 10 per thousand in the northeastern United States.[70,71] SCFE is seen more commonly among Polynesians, blacks, and Hispanics, and less commonly in children of Asian and Indo-Mediterranean ancestry.[72-74] SCFE is most commonly seen in children between the ages of 9 and 16.[73] Risk factors for SCFE include obesity, endocrinopathy, renal osteodystrophy, and a history of radiation therapy.

Under certain conditions, the adolescent physis is overcome with shear and/or torsional forces, allowing the metaphysis to displace, most commonly anteriorly and externally relative to the epiphysis, which is held fixed by the ligamentum teres within the acetabulum.[75] The cause is thought to be a combination of mechanical and chemical factors that weaken the physis. Primary mechanical factors influencing the physis include obesity, femoral retroversion, and relative verticality of the physis.[76-79] These factors cause an increase in the shear force felt at the physis with weight bearing. Chemical factors associated with idiopathic SCFE are related to puberty. Testosterone and growth hormone have been proven to weaken the growth plate. The adolescent growth spurt causes the growth plate to widen at a time when the protective influence of the perichondrial ring is diminishing.[75]

The traditional classification system qualifies the slip as a pre-slip—acute, chronic, or acute on chronic. This is based on the history of knee, thigh, or groin pain of more or less than 3 weeks' duration, physical examination findings of loss of hip internal rotation, obligate external rotation with hip flexion, and substantiation of radiographic findings.[75] This classification system has little prognostic value and has been generally replaced with a newer system, which qualifies the slip as stable or unstable based on whether the child is able to walk with or without crutches.[80] Unstable SCFE is much less common but carries up to a 50% risk of subsequent avascular necrosis[80] (Fig. 14-12). This is thought to be due to an acute vascular insult at the time of the initial metaphyseal displacement.[81] This type of slip behaves like a Salter-Harris fracture of the proximal femur, with the child presenting with exquisite groin pain, and resists any attempts at passive motion.[75]

Radiographs show early evidence of slip as a widened growth plate (Fig. 14-13). The lateral view is likely to show subtle slips earlier than the AP image. Klein's line drawn along the anterior or superior neck should intersect the head, but in early slips, the epiphysis may be level with or below this line. Over time, metaphyseal remodeling anteriorly and superiorly occurs with new bone formation posteriorly and inferiorly, resulting in an increasingly varus and extended orientation of the neck (Fig. 14-14). The magnitude of the slip is characterized by measuring the amount of displacement of the epiphysis on the metaphysis. In a mild slip, epiphyseal displacement is less than one-third the width of the metaphysis. A moderate slip is classified by one third to one half of the metaphyseal width, and greater slippage is quantified as severe.[82] This method assumes that the landmarks used to measure metaphyseal width are clearly defined, which may not be the case with a chronic slip that has undergone substantial remodeling. Alternatively, the epiphyseal shaft angle of Southwick can be more consistently applied to quantify the severity of slip. On the lateral image, the perpendicular to a line drawn between the anterior physis and the posterior physis is measured against a line drawn down the shaft of the femur. This angle is compared with the normal side, or 12 degrees if both sides are involved (Fig. 14-15).[83] A mild slip is one in which the difference

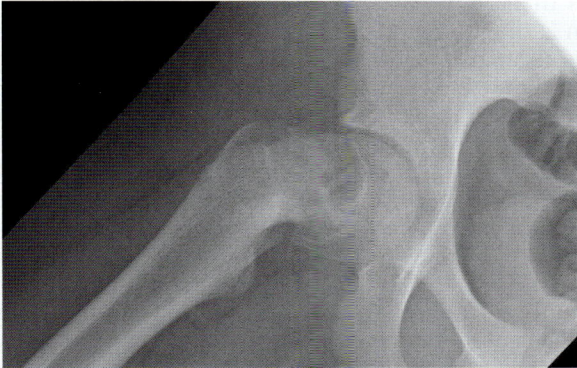

Figure 14-14. Lateral radiograph of a chronic slipped capital femoral epiphysis. Note the classic "pistol-grip" deformity resulting from remodeling.

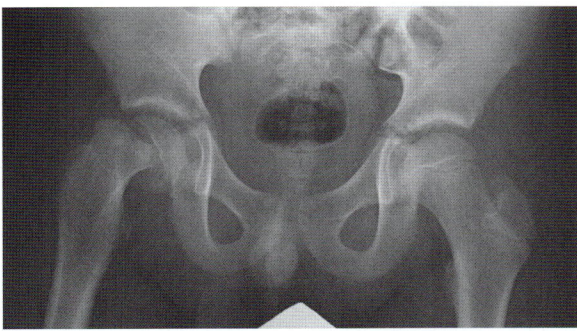

Figure 14-12. Anteroposterior (AP) radiograph of an acute, unstable slipped capital femoral epiphysis (SCFE). This uncommon presentation behaves more like a femoral neck fracture than a chronic SCFE. The risk of vascular compromise and subsequent avascular necrosis is very high with this pattern.

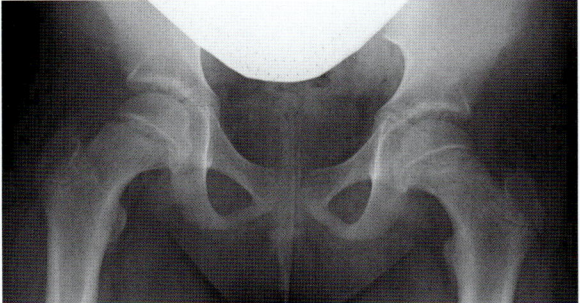

Figure 14-13. Anteroposterior (AP) radiograph of subtle, bilateral slipped capital femoral epiphysis. Widening of both physes is noted.

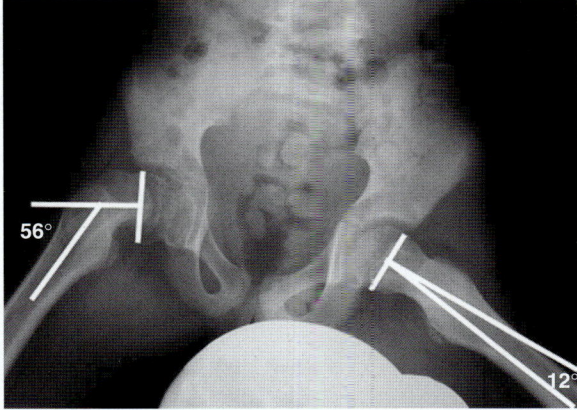

Figure 14-15. Epiphyseal shaft angle of Southwick. A reference line is drawn between the anterior physis and the posterior physis on the lateral radiograph. The perpendicular to this line is measured against the femoral shaft. The normal side is subtracted from the slipped side. A measurement of 12 degrees is used if both sides are slipped. (*From Aronsson DD, Loder RT, Breur GJ, Weinstein SL: Slipped capital femoral epiphysis: current concepts. J Am Acad Orthop Surg 14:666–679, 2006.*)

between these angles is less than 30 degrees, moderate is 30 to 50 degrees, and severe is greater than 50 degrees.[84]

Most commonly, the initial slip results in an extension, varus, and external rotation deformity. Over time, the radiographic hallmarks of SCFE include flattening of the acetabulum, pistol-grip deformity of the femoral neck, and cystic degeneration in the metaphyseal-epiphyseal region.[85] Many patients with the diagnosis of primary osteoarthritis may have radiographic tilt of the femoral head, which suggests SCFE as the true cause,[64] although other authors believe this to be a normal finding in primary osteoarthritis.[86]

In the patient with untreated SCFE, the progression to degenerative joint disease is highly dependent on the grade of the SCFE.[87,88] In the treated population, instability at presentation is highly correlated with progression to osteoarthritis.[89] Natural history studies suggest that the prognosis for mild slips is generally good.[90] A favorable functional outcome has been seen with in situ screw fixation of slips with epiphyseal shaft angles of less than 40 degrees.[91] The more challenging presentation is that of a moderate or severe slip. The significant alteration in proximal femoral anatomy causes changes in hip joint biomechanics, and this can result in femoroacetabular impingement. This phenomenon can cause two distinct patterns: impaction and inclusion. Initially, the anterior neck prominence contacts the anterior acetabulum (impaction) (Fig. 14-16); this is compensated for by obligate external rotation. As remodeling occurs over time, the metaphyseal prominence becomes increasingly able to fit into the acetabulum, and range of motion in flexion improves (inclusion). The consequences of metaphyseal bone articulating with the acetabulum without the protective covering of articular cartilage are labral tears and progressive arthritis.[92] Several proximal femoral procedures, ranging from arthroscopic or open neck osteoplasty to subtrochanteric, basicervical, and cuneiform osteotomies, are designed to correct these altered mechanics before the development of significant osteoarthritis.[81,93] Depending on the severity of the slip and the alteration of hip mechanics, total hip arthroplasty may be necessary in the SCFE patient at an early age. The risk of osteoarthritis seems to be related to the magnitude of residual deformity.[90]

The surgeon contemplating total hip arthroplasty in an SCFE patient should be aware that the femur will show loss of neck-head offset, acetabular neck impingement, loss of superior peripheral articular cartilage adjacent to the superior neck,[94] and a hook of bone at the junction of the head and neck caused by osteophytic changes and remodeling.[64] As increased external rotation of the femur becomes necessary to restore normal range of motion in response to impingement, both increased head-neck offset and a metaphyseal prominence will develop.[95] In SCFE hips, femoral anteversion averages 7 degrees, and the femoral neck shaft angle averages 134.2 degrees.[96] Additionally, osteonecrosis can develop secondary to vascular insult at the time of onset of symptoms in the setting of an acute unstable slip or attempted treatment. Iatrogenic causes of avascular necrosis (AVN) include reduction or over-reduction of a slip and errant pin placement in the superolateral quadrant of the femoral head at the time of initial fixation[81] (Fig. 14-17). Also, in a patient who has undergone a compensatory osteotomy to restore mechanical parameters, a complex, multiplanar deformity may develop; this will add to the difficulty of fitting a femoral prosthesis into the medullary canal at the time of joint replacement[22] (Fig. 14-18).

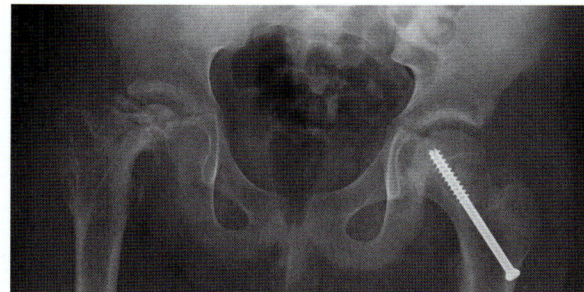

Figure 14-17. Avascular necrosis of the femoral head after surgical treatment for slipped capital femoral epiphysis.

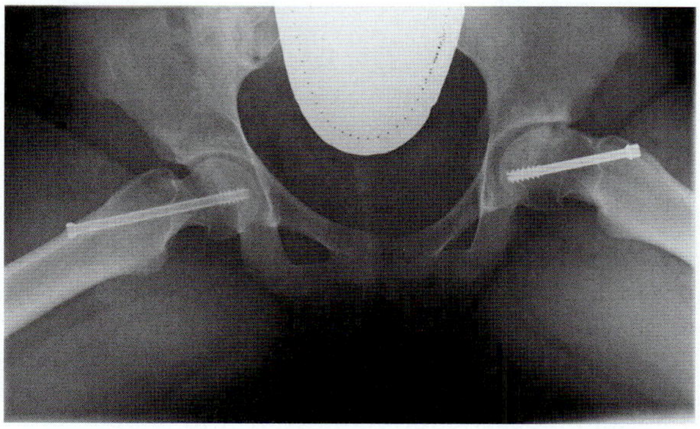

Figure 14-16. Femoroacetabular impingement is noted on the left hip anteriorly, where the altered shape of the femoral neck causes impaction at the anterior acetabulum with hip flexion.

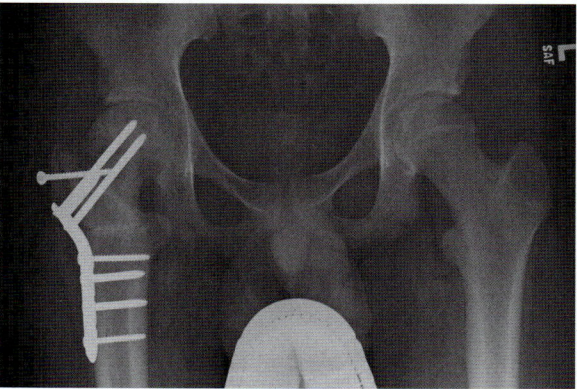

Figure 14-18. Triplanar osteotomy of Imhäuser done to improve hip mechanics. This is a flexion, valgus, and internal rotation osteotomy.

Acetabular changes typically are those related to arthritic wear, secondary to impingement by the dysmorphic femur. The superior neck of the femur impinges on the acetabular rim, resulting in increased wear and arthritic changes in response to the functional increase in external rotation.[92] Computed tomography imaging has revealed no differences between an SCFE and a non-SCFE acetabulum, and no correlation between acetabular changes and the degree of slip.[97]

REFERENCES

1. Moore KL, Persaud TVN: Before we are born: essentials of embryology and birth defects, Philadelphia, 1993, WB Saunders.
2. Strayer LM: The embryology of the human hip joint. Yale J Biol Med 16:13–26, 1943.
3. Lee MC, Eberson CP: Growth and development of the child's hip. Orthop Clin North Am 37:119–132, 2006.
4. Bowen JR, Kotzias-Neto A: Developmental dysplasia of the hip, ed 5, Brooklandville, Md, 2006, Data Trace Publishing Company.
5. Watanabe RS: Embryology of the human hip. Clin Orthop Relat Res 98:8–26, 1974.
6. Jouve JL, Glard Y, Garron E: Anatomical study of the proximal femur in the fetus. J Bone Joint Surg Br 14:105–110, 2005.
7. Fabry G, MacEwen GD, Shands AR: Torsion of the femur: a follow-up study in normal and abnormal conditions. J Bone Joint Surg Am 55:1726–1738, 1973.
8. Zippel H: Normal development of the structural elements of the hip joint in adolescence. Beitr Orthop 18:255–270, 1971.
9. Bobroff ED, Chambers HG, Saroris DJ: Femoral anteversion and neck-shaft angle in children with cerebral palsy. Clin Orthop Relat Res 364:194–204, 1999.
10. Weinstein SL, Mubarak SJ: Developmental hip dysplasia and dislocation: part I. AAOS Instr Course Lect 53:523–530, 2004.
11. Chung SM: The arterial supply of the developing proximal end of the human femur. J Bone Joint Surg Am 58:961–970, 1976.
12. Crock HV: An atlas of the arterial supply of the head and neck of the femur in man. Clin Orthop Relat Res 152:17–27, 1980.
13. Netter FH: Pelvis. In Colacino S (ed): Atlas of human anatomy, Summit NJ, 1994, Ciba-Geigy Corporation.
14. Beck M, Leunig M, Ellis T, et al: The acetabular blood supply: implications for periacetabular osteotomies. Surg Radiol Anat 25:361–367, 2003.
15. Weinstein S: Natural history of congenital hip dislocation (CDH) and hip dysplasia. Clin Orthop Relat Res 225:62–76, 1987.
16. Coleman CR, Slager RF, Smith WS: The effect of environmental influence on acetabular development. Surg Forum 9:75, 1958.
17. Mubarak S, Garfin S, Vance R: Pitfalls in the use of the Pavlik harness for treatment of congenital dysplasia, subluxation and dislocation of the hip. J Bone Joint Surg Am 63:1239, 1981.
18. Lindstrom J, Ponseti I, Wenger DR: Acetabular development after reduction in congenital dislocation of the hip. J Bone Joint Surg Am 61:112, 1979.
19. Osborne D, Effmann E, Broda K: The development of the upper end of the femur with special reference to its internal architecture. Radiology 137:71–76, 1980.
20. Ponseti I: Morphology of the acetabulum in congenital dislocation of the hip: gross, histological and roentgenographic studies. J Bone Joint Surg Am 60:586–591, 1978.
21. Wedge J, Wasylenko M: The natural history of congenital disease of the hip. J Bone Joint Surg Br 61:334–338, 1979.
22. Gent E, Clarke NMP: Joint replacement for sequelae of childhood hip disorders. J Pediatr Orthop 24:235–240, 2004.
23. Greenspan A: Anomalies of the upper and lower limbs. In Palumbo R (eds): Orthopedic radiology: a practical approach, Philadelphia, 2000, Lippincott, Williams & Wilkins.
24. Bombelli R: Osteoarthritis of the hip, Heidelberg, 1983, Springer.
25. Angliss R, Fujii G, Pickvance E, et al: Surgical treatment of late developmental displacement of the hip: results after 33 years. J Bone Joint Surg Br 87:384–394, 2005.
26. Fujii M, Nakashima Y, Jingushi S, et al: Intraarticular findings in symptomatic developmental dysplasia of the hip. J Pediatr Orthop 29:9–13, 2009.
27. Argenson JN, Ryembautl E, Flecher X, et al: Three-dimensional anatomy of the hip in osteoarthritis after developmental dysplasia. J Bone Joint Surg Br 87:1192–1196, 2005.
28. Noble PC, Amaric E, Sugano N, et al: Three-dimensional shape of the dysplastic femur: implications for THR. Clin Orthop Relat Res 417:27–40, 2003.
29. Robertson DD, Essinger JR, Imura S, et al: Femoral deformity in adults with developmental hip dysplasia. Clin Orthop Relat Res 327:196–206, 1996.
30. Sugano N, Nobel PC, Kamari E, et al: The morphology of the femur in developmental dysplasia of the hip. J Bone Joint Surg Br 80:711–719, 1998.
31. Cyvin KB: A follow-up study of children with instability of the hip joint at birth: clinical and radiological investigations with special reference to the anteversion of the femoral neck. Acta Orthop Scand Suppl 166:1–62, 1977.
32. Gage JR, Winter RB: Avascular necrosis of the capital femoral epiphysis as a complication of closed reduction of congenital dislocation of the hip. J Bone Joint Surg Am 54:373–388, 1972.
33. Crowe JF, Mani VJ, Ranawat CS: Total hip replacement in congenital dislocation and dysplasia of the hip. J Bone Joint Surg Am 61:15–23, 1979.
34. Dunn HK, Hess W: Total hip reconstruction in chronically dislocated hips. J Bone Joint Surg Am 58:838–845, 1976.
35. Saglam N, Sener M, Beksac B, Tozun IR: Total hip arthroplasty and problems encountered in patients with high-riding developmental dysplasia of the hip. Acta Orthop Traumatol Turc 36:187–194, 2002.
36. Hartofilakidis G, Karachalios T, Stamos KG: Epidemiology, demographics and natural history of congenital hip disease in adults. Orthopedics 23:823–827, 2000.
37. Kleinberg S, Lieberman HS: The acetabular index in infants in relation to congenital dislocation of the hip. Arch Surg 32:1049–1054, 1936.
38. Tonnis D, Brunken D: Differentiation of normal and pathological acetabular roof angle in the diagnosis of hip dysplasia: evaluation of 2294 acetabular roof angles of hip joints in children. Arch Orthop Unfallchir 64:197–228, 1968.
39. Liu RY, Wang KZ, Wang CS, et al: Evaluation of medial acetabular wall bone stock in patients with developmental dysplasia of the hip using helical computed tomography multiplanar reconstruction technique. Acta Radiol 50:791–797, 2009.
40. Mendes DG: Total hip arthroplasty in congenital dislocated hips. Clin Orthop Relat Res 161:163–179, 1981.
41. Haddad FS, Masri BA, Garbuz DS: Primary total replacement of the dysplastic hip. AAOS Instr Course Lect 49:23–39, 2000.
42. Ai J, Sun Y, Han Y, Li P: Treatment of osteoarthritis secondary to acetabular dysplasia by total hip arthroplasty. Chin J Repar Reconstruct Surg 22:653–656, 2008.
43. Farrell CM, Springer BD, Haidukewych GJ, Morrey BF: Motor nerve palsy following primary total hip arthroplasty. J Bone Joint Surg Am 87:2619–2625, 2005.
44. Schmalzried TP, Noordin S, Amstutz HC: Update on nerve palsy associated with total hip replacement. Clin Orthop Relat Res 334:188–204, 1997.
45. Eggli S, Hankemayer S, Muller ME: Nerve palsy after leg lengthening in total replacement arthroplasty for developmental dysplasia of the hip. J Bone Joint Surg Br 81:843–845, 1999.
46. Garcia-Cimbrelo E, Munuera L: Low-friction arthroplasty in severe acetabular dysplasia. J Arthroplasty 8:459–469, 1993.
47. Numair J, Joshi AB, Murphy JC, et al: Total hip arthroplasty for congenital dysplasia or dislocation of the hip: survivorship analysis and long-term results. J Bone Joint Surg Am 79:1352–1360, 1997.
48. Pagnano W, Hanssen AD, Lewallen DG, Shaughnessy WJ: The effect of superior placement of the acetabular component on the rate of loosening after total hip arthroplasty. J Bone Joint Surg Am 78:1004–1014, 1996.
49. Cameron HU, Botsford DJ, Park YS: Influence of the Crowe rating on the outcome of total hip arthroplasty in congenital hip dysplasia. J Arthroplasty 11:582–587, 1996.

50. Gregosciewicz A, Okonski M, Stolecka D, et al: Ischemia of the femoral head in Perthes' disease: is the cause intra- or extravascular? J Pediatr Orthop 9:160–162, 1989.

51. Guerado E, Garces G: Perthes disease: a study of constitutional aspects in adulthood. J Bone Joint Surg Br 83:569–571, 2001.

52. Neidel J, Boddenberg B, Zander D, et al: Thyroid function in Legg-Calve-Perthes disease: cross-sectional and longitudinal study. J Pediatr Orthop 13:592–597, 1993.

53. Skaggs DL, Tolo VT: Legg-Calve-Perthes disease. J Am Acad Orthop Surg 4:9–16, 1996.

54. McAndrew MP, Weinstein SL: A long-term follow-up of Legg-Calve-Perthes disease. J Bone Joint Surg Am 66:860–869, 1984.

55. Catterall A, Pringle J, Byers PD, et al: A review of the morphology of Perthes' disease. J Bone Joint Surg Br 64:269–275, 1982.

56. Bowen JR, Foster BK, Hartzell CR: Legg-Calve-Perthes disease. Clin Orthop Relat Res 185:97–108, 1984.

57. Rowe SM, Moon ES, Song EK, et al: The correlation between coxa magna and final outcome in Legg-Calve-Perthes disease. J Pediatr Orthop 25:22–27, 2005.

58. Stulberg SD, Cooperman DR, Wallensten R: The natural history of Legg-Calve-Perthes disease. J Bone Joint Surg Am 63:1095–1108, 1981.

59. Catterall A: The natural history of Perthes disease. J Bone Joint Surg Br 53:37–53, 1971.

60. Herring JA, Kim HT, Browne R: Legg-Calve-Perthes disease. Part II. Prospective multicenter study of the effect of treatment on outcome. J Bone Joint Surg Am 86:2121–2134, 2004.

61. Wiig O, Terjesen T, Svenningsen S: Prognostic factors and outcome of treatment in Perthes disease: a prospective study of 368 patients with five-year follow-up. J Bone Joint Surg Br 90:1364–1371, 2008.

62. Engesaeter LB, Furnes O, Espehaug B, et al: Survival of total hip arthroplasty after previous paediatric hip disease. Eur Paediatr Orthop 85B:258, 2003.

63. Boyd HS, Ulrich SD, Seyler TM, et al: Resurfacing for Perthes disease: an alternative to standard hip arthroplasty. Clin Orthop Relat Res 465:80–85, 2007.

64. Harris WH: Etiology of osteoarthritis of the hip. Clin Orthop Relat Res 213:20–33, 1986.

65. Ezoe M, Naito M, Inoue T: The prevalence of acetabular retroversion among various disorders of the hip. J Bone Joint Surg Am 88:372–379, 2006.

66. Meurer A, Bohm B, Decking J, Heine J: Analysis of acetabular changes in Morbus Perthes disease with radiomorphometry. Z Orthop Ihre Grenzgeb 143:100–105, 2005.

67. Sankar WN, Flynn JM: The development of acetabular retroversion in children with Legg-Calve-Perthes disease. J Pediatr Orthop 28:440–443, 2008.

68. Thillemann TM, Pederson AB, Johnssen SP, Soball EK: Danish Hip Arthroplasty registry: implant survival after primary total hip arthroplasty due to childhood hip disorders: results from the Danish Hip Arthroplasty Registry. Acta Orthop 79:769–776, 2008.

69. Boos N, Krushell R, Ganz R, Muller ME: Total hip arthroplasty after previous proximal femoral osteotomy. J Bone Joint Surg Br 79:247–253, 1997.

70. Kelsey J, Keggi K, Southwick W: The incidence and distribution of slipped capital femoral epiphysis in Connecticut and southwestern United States. J Bone Joint Surg Am 52:1203–1216, 1970.

71. Ninomiya S, Nagasaka Y, Tagawa H: Slipped capital femoral epiphysis: a study of 68 cases in the eastern half area of Japan. Clin Orthop Relat Res 119:172–176, 1976.

72. Lehmann C, Arons R, Loder R, Vitale M: The epidemiology of slipped capital femoral epiphysis: an update. J Pediatr Orthop 26:286–290, 2006.

73. Loder R: The demographics of slipped capital femoral epiphysis: an international multicenter study. Clin Orthop Relat Res 322:8–27, 1996.

74. Stott S, Bidwell T: Epidemiology of slipped capital femoral epiphysis in a population with a high proportion of New Zealand Maori and Pacific children. N Z Med J 116:647, 2003.

75. Loder R, Aronsson D, Weinstein S, et al: Slipped capital femoral epiphysis. AAOS Instr Course Lect 57:473–498, 2008.

76. Galbraith R, Gelberman R, Hajek P: Obesity and decreased femoral anteversion in adolescence. J Orthop Res 5:523–528, 1987.

77. Gelberman R, Cohen M, Shaw B, et al: The association of femoral retroversion with slipped capital femoral epiphysis. J Bone Joint Surg Am 68:1000–1007, 1986.

78. Mirkopulos N, Weiner D, Askew M: The evolving slope of the proximal femoral growth plate relationship to slipped capital femoral epiphysis. J Pediatr Orthop 8:268–273, 1988.

79. Pritchett J, Perdue K: Mechanical factors in slipped capital femoral epiphysis. J Pediatr Orthop 8:385–388, 1988.

80. Loder R, Richards B, Shapiro P, et al: Acute slipped capital femoral epiphysis: the importance of physeal stability. J Bone Joint Surg Am 75:1134–1140, 1993.

81. Aronsson D, Loder R: Treatment of the unstable (acute) slipped capital femoral epiphysis. Clin Orthop Relat Res 322:99–110, 1996.

82. Jacobs B: Diagnosis and natural history of slipped capital femoral epiphysis. Instr Course Lect 21:167–173, 1972.

83. Aronsson DD, Loder RT, Breur GJ, Weinstein SL: Slipped capital femoral epiphysis: current concepts. J Am Acad Orthop Surg 14:666–679, 2006.

84. Southwick W: Osteotomy through the lesser trochanter for slipped capital femoral epiphysis. J Bone Joint Surg Am 1967;807–835, 1967.

85. Goodman DA, Feighan JE, Smith AD, et al: Subclinical slipped capital femoral epiphysis: relationship to osteoarthrosis of the hip. J Bone Joint Surg Am 79:1489–1497, 1997.

86. Resnick D: The "tilt deformity" of the femoral head in osteoarthritis of the hip: a poor indicator of previous epiphysiolysis. Clin Radiol 27:355–363, 1976.

87. Joplin RJ: Slipped capital femoral epiphysis: the still unsolved adolescent hip lesion. JAMA 188:379–381, 1964.

88. Oram V: Epiphysiolysis of the head of the femur: a follow-up examination with special reference to the end results and the social prognosis. Acta Orthop Scand 23:100–120, 1953.

89. DeLullo JA, Thomas E, Cooney TW, et al: Femoral remodeling may influence patient outcomes in slipped capital femoral epiphysis. Clin Orthop Relat Res 457:163–170, 2006.

90. Carney BT, Weinstein SL: Natural history of untreated slipped capital femoral epiphysis. Clin Orthop Relat Res 322:43–47, 1996.

91. Morrissy RT: Slipped capital femoral epiphysis. J Am Acad Orthop Surg 23:5–7, 2002.

92. Rab GT: The geometry of slipped capital femoral epiphysis: implications for movement, impingement and corrective osteotomy. J Pediatr Orthop 19:419–424, 1999.

93. Roy DR: Arthroscopy of the hip in children and adolescents. J Child Orthop 3:89–100, 2009.

94. Abraham E, Gonzalez MH, Pratap S, et al: Clinical implications of anatomical wear characteristics in slipped capital femoral epiphysis and primary osteoarthritis. J Pediatr Orthop 27:788–795, 2007.

95. Mamisch TC, Kim YJ, Richolt JA, et al: Femoral morphology due to impingement influences the range of motion in slipped capital femoral epiphysis. Clin Orthop Relat Res 467:692–698, 2009.

96. Kordelle J, Millis M, Jolesz FA, et al: Three-dimensional analysis of the proximal femur in patients with slipped capital femoral epiphysis based on computed tomography. J Pediatr Orthop 21:179–182, 2001.

97. Kordelle J, Richolt JA, Millis M, et al: Development of the acetabulum in patients with slipped capital femoral epiphysis: a three-dimensional analysis based on computed tomography. J Pediatr Orthop 21:174–178, 2001.

CHAPTER 15

Anatomy of the Hip

Raymond H. Kim and Douglas A. Dennis

INTRODUCTION

Although commonly referred to as a "*simple ball-and-socket joint,*" the hip is a beautifully architectured joint that is worthy of appreciation for its form and function. Knowledge of hip anatomy is critical to perform surgical approaches and to avoid potential complications. This chapter describes the surface anatomy, the osseous anatomy, the musculature, the vasculature, and the neuroanatomy as they pertain to the hip surgeon.

SURFACE ANATOMY

The superficial landmarks are clinically relevant for describing areas of pain on physical examination and are surgically significant for determining incision placement.

Anteriorly, the anterior superior iliac spine (ASIS) is easily palpable and represents the anterior prominence of the iliac crest (Fig. 15-1). The sartorius and the tensor fascia lata rely on the ASIS for their proximal attachments. At the anterior midline of the pelvis, the pubic symphysis is buttressed by the pubic tubercles, which represent the medial ends of the superior pubic rami. The ASIS and the pubic symphysis define the coronal plane of the pelvis. The ASIS and the pubic tubercle are bridged by the inguinal ligament. The femoral artery can be palpated midway between the ASIS and the pubic tubercle, just distal to the inguinal ligament.

Laterally, the iliac crest can be traced from the ASIS arching posteriorly, and it ends posteriorly at the posterior superior iliac spine (PSIS). The greater trochanter is an easily palpable lateral prominence that serves as the muscular insertion for the gluteus medius and minimus laterally and the piriformis, obturator internus, and gemelli medially; the trochanteric ridge distally serves as the origin for the vastus lateralis.

Posteriorly, the PSIS is easily palpable and provides part of the origin of the gluteus maximus, as well as the posterior sacroiliac ligaments (Fig. 15-2). The PSIS is often identifiable by a characteristic dimpling of the skin. Inferior to the lower border of the gluteus maximus, the ischial tuberosity can be palpated.

OSSEOUS AND LIGAMENTOUS ANATOMY

The hemipelvis comprises the ilium, the ischium, and the pubis, which developmentally unite after fusion of the triradiate cartilage within the acetabulum (Fig. 15-3). The ilium is the superior flattened portion of the pelvis with the superficial anatomy described previously. The greater sciatic notch is a major landmark on

Figure 15-1. The anterior superior iliac spine represents the anterior prominence of the iliac crest. The femoral triangle is bordered superiorly by the inguinal ligament, laterally by the sartorius, and medially by the adductor longus, and the floor by the iliopsoas, the pectineus, and the adductor brevis. Within the triangle, the artery is positioned adjacent to the femoral nerve laterally and the femoral vein medially.

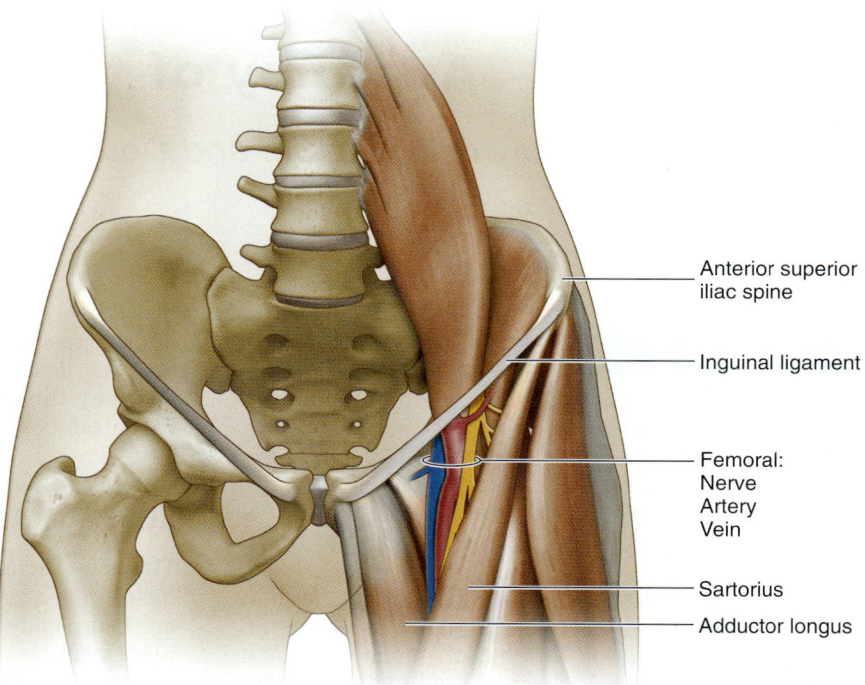

Anterior superior
iliac spine

Inguinal ligament

Femoral:
Nerve
Artery
Vein

Sartorius

Adductor longus

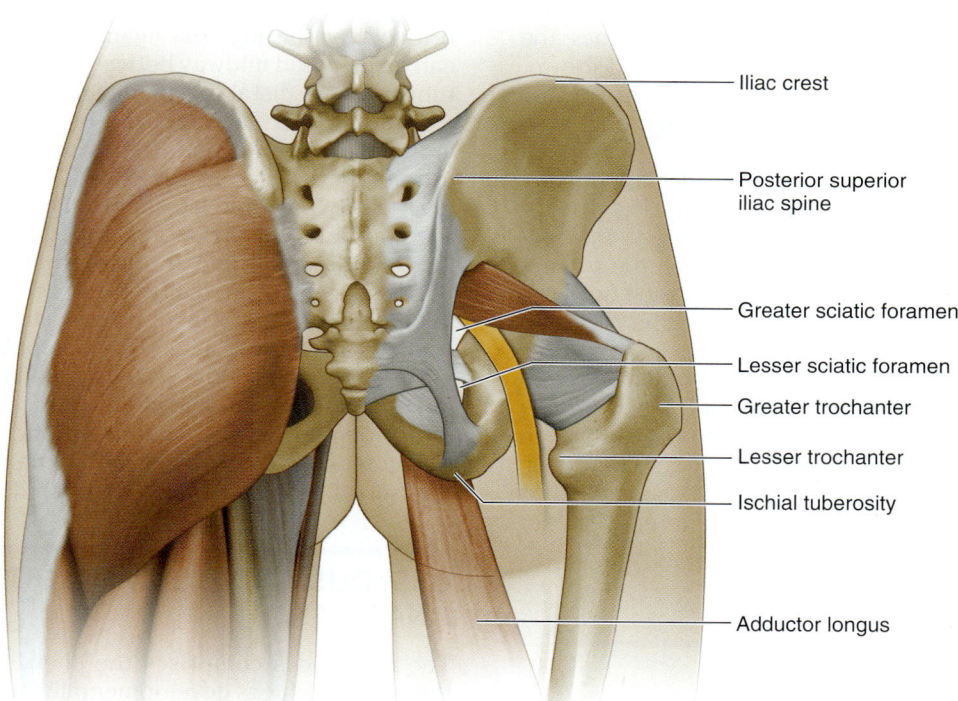

Iliac crest

Posterior superior
iliac spine

Greater sciatic foramen

Lesser sciatic foramen

Greater trochanter

Lesser trochanter

Ischial tuberosity

Adductor longus

Figure 15-2. The posterior superior iliac spine provides part of the origin of the gluteus maximus and the posterior sacroiliac ligaments.

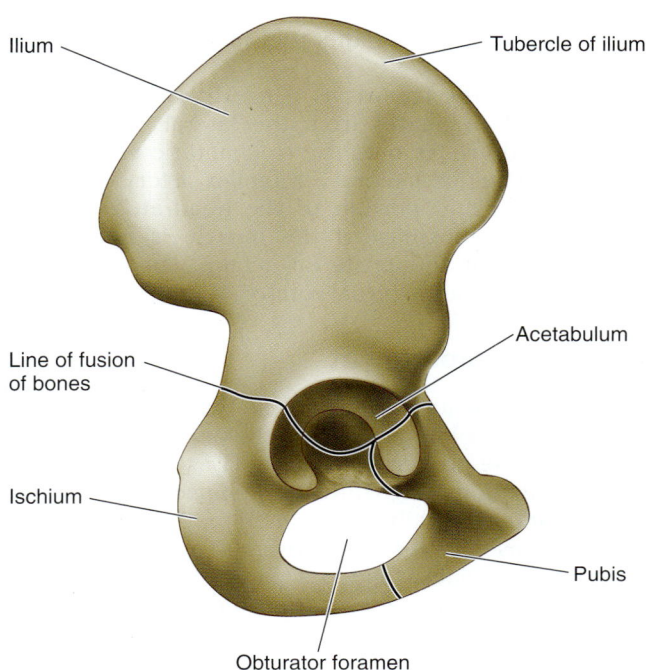

Figure 15-3. The hemipelvis comprises the ilium, the ischium, and the pubis.

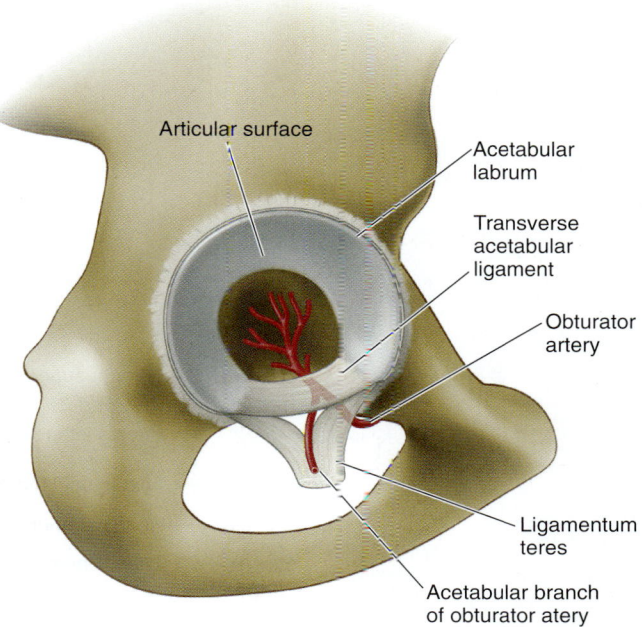

Figure 15-4. The acetabulum consists of a lunate-shaped articular region of hyaline cartilage and a central nonarticular fossa. From the inferior aspect of the fossa, the ligamentum teres carries the acetabular branches of the posterior division of the obturator vessels.

the ilium and is located posterior and superior to the acetabulum. The ischium is an L-shaped bone that comprises the inferior portion of the pelvis. The pubis is composed of a body and a superior and inferior ramus. The rami in conjunction with the ischium form a window called the *obturator foramen.* The bodies of the pubis articulate at the midline anteriorly at the pubic symphysis.

The acetabulum consists of a lunate-shaped articular region of hyaline cartilage and a central nonarticular fossa (Fig. 15-4). From the inferior aspect of the fossa, the ligamentum teres carries the acetabular branches of the posterior division of the obturator vessels over to the fovea capitis, which is a small depression on the medial aspect of the femoral head. The acetabulum is deepened by the labrum, a fibrocartilaginous rim, which becomes the transverse acetabular ligament inferiorly as it bridges the cotyloid notch.

The acetabulum articulates with the femoral head in a ball-and-socket configuration and allows a wide range of motion. The joint is circumferentially enclosed by the hip capsule, which attaches to the labrum medially. Intimately associated with the capsule are ligaments, which also surround the hip joint. Anteriorly, the hip joint is covered by an inverted Y–shaped iliofemoral ligament and by the pubofemoral ligament (Fig. 15-5). Posteriorly, the iliofemoral and ischiofemoral ligaments attach the pelvis to the femur (Fig. 15-6).

The femoral head tapers down to the femoral neck, which bridges the hip joint to the shaft of the femur (Fig. 15-7). The neck shaft angle averages 127 degrees with

an anteversion averaging 14 degrees. The greater and lesser trochanters are prominences about the proximal femur that serve as attachment sites for various tendons and are connected by the intertrochanteric line. The femoral diaphysis has a gentle anterior bow as it extends distally toward the knee. Posteriorly, the diaphysis has a ridge called the *linea aspera,* which provides an attachment site for muscles and the intermuscular septa.

MUSCULATURE

The muscles of the hip serve to abduct, adduct, flex, extend, externally rotate, and internally rotate the femur relative to the pelvis.

Gluteal Musculature

Posteriorly the gluteus maximus is the largest muscle in the body; it originates from the posterior gluteal line, the iliac crest, the posterior surface of the sacrum and coccyx, and the sacrotuberous ligament (Figs. 15-8 and 15-9). Most of the muscle fibers insert into the iliotibial tract, and a small portion of fibers insert into the gluteal tuberosity of the femur. The gluteus maximus is innervated by the inferior gluteal nerve and functions to extend and externally rotate the hip.

The gluteus medius is a fan-shaped muscle that arises from both the lateral surface of the ilium and the undersurface of the tensor fascia lata. The insertion is on the

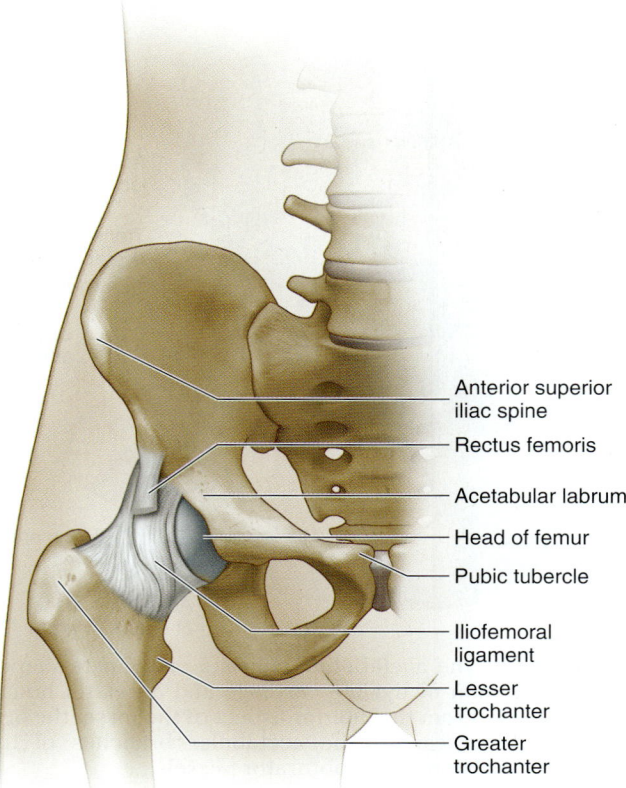

Anterior superior
iliac spine

Rectus femoris

Acetabular labrum

Head of femur

Pubic tubercle

Iliofemoral
ligament

Lesser
trochanter

Greater
trochanter

Figure 15-5. Anteriorly, the hip joint is covered by an inverted Y–shaped iliofemoral ligament and the pubofemoral ligament.

lateral aspect of the greater trochanter. The gluteus medius is a powerful abductor that internally rotates the hip with its anterior muscle fibers. Innervation is supplied by the superior gluteal nerve.

The gluteus minimus lies just deep to the gluteus medius and also abducts the hip. The muscle fibers originate from the ilium and insert into the hip capsule, as well as the anterior aspect of the greater trochanter. The gluteus minimus receives innervation from the superior gluteal nerve.

The tensor fascia lata lies over the abductors and originates from the anterior iliac crest. The fibers insert onto the iliotibial tract. The tensor fascia lata provides traction to the iliotibial band and is innervated by the superior gluteal nerve.

The piriformis originates within the pelvis, exits through the greater sciatic notch, and inserts into the piriformis fossa on the greater trochanter. The anatomic position of the pirformis is significant because the sciatic nerve travels deep to the muscle. The piriformis also separates the superior and inferior neurovascular bundles as they exit the greater sciatic notch. The piriformis is an external rotator of the hip joint.

The obturator internus originates from within the pelvis, exits via the lesser sciatic notch, and inserts just

distal to the piriformis on the greater trochanter. The obturator internus is shouldered by the superior and inferior gemelli, and together they function to externally rotate the hip.

The quadratus femoris is a quadrilaterally shaped muscle that originates from the lateral edge of the ischium and inserts onto the trochanteric crest of the femur. The medial femoral circumflex artery lies anterior to the distal portion of the quadratus femoris, which will hemorrhage if the muscle is completely released off of the posterior femur. The quadratus femoris is another external rotator of the hip.

Anterior Compartment

The sartorius is a straplike muscle that originates from the ASIS, runs obliquely across the anterior thigh, and inserts on the proximal medial tibia as one of the pes anserine tendons (Fig. 15-10). The muscle acts to flex, abduct, and externally rotate the hip.

The iliopsoas muscle represents a fusion of two muscles, the iliacus and the psoas. The iliacus is a broad-based muscle arising from the medial aspect of the ilium; it tapers as it joins the psoas muscle. The psoas is fusiform shaped and originates from the transverse processes, the vertebral bodies, and the disks from T12 through L5. The conjoined tendon of the iliopsoas inserts on the lesser trochanter of the proximal femur, and the muscle functions as a powerful hip flexor and externally rotates the hip.

The pectineus is a broad muscle that arises from the superior pubic ramus and inserts on the linea aspera on the proximal femur. Contraction of the pectineus performs hip flexion and adduction.

The quadriceps femoris is a combination of four muscles: rectus femoris, vastus lateralis, vastus medialis, and vastus intermedius. All four muscles insert onto the patella via the quadriceps tendon. The rectus femoris has two heads: one originating from the anterior inferior iliac spine, and a reflected head arising from the anterior acetabular rim. The vastus lateralis arises from the base of the greater trochanter, the linea aspera, and the iliotibial tract. The vastus medialis originates from the supracondylar line and the linea aspera. The anterolateral femoral diaphysis gives rise to the vastus intermedius. The quadriceps muscle works as a powerful knee extensor. Because the rectus femoris originates above the hip joint, it also works as a hip flexor.

Medial Compartment

The gracilis is a strap-shaped muscle that arises from the inferior pubic ramus and the ischium and runs down the medial thigh until it inserts on the proximal medial aspect of the tibia as one of the pes anserine tendons (Fig. 15-11). The gracilis is a hip adductor that flexes the knee.

The adductor longus is a triangular muscle that arises from the anterior pubic body and fans out as it inserts on the linea aspera. The adductor longus primarily adducts the hip but also contributes to external rotation.

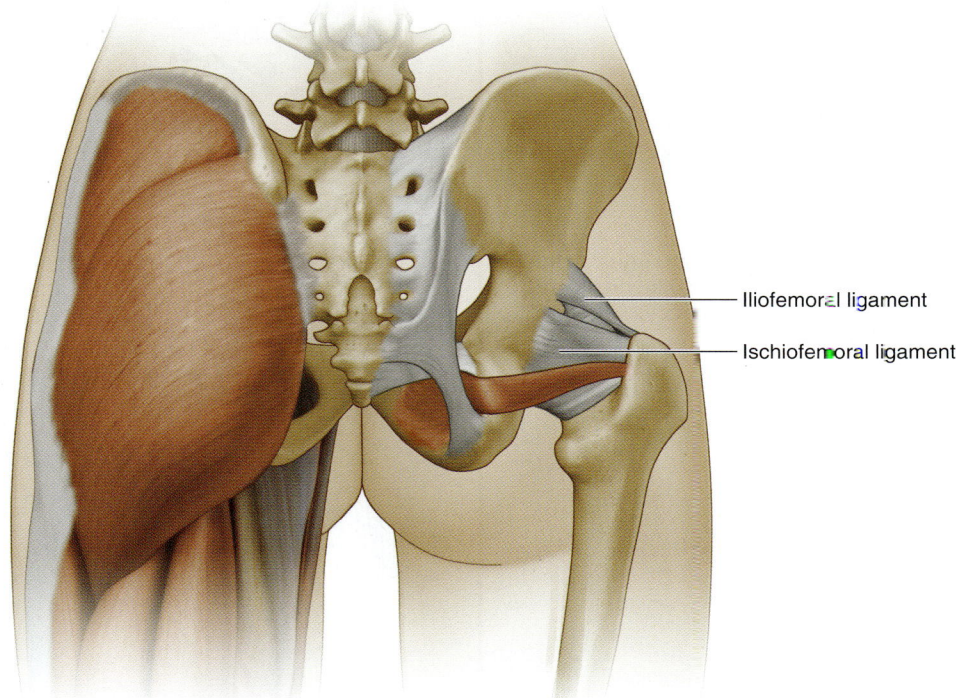

Figure 15-6. Posteriorly, the iliofemoral and ischiofemoral ligaments attach the pelvis to the femur.

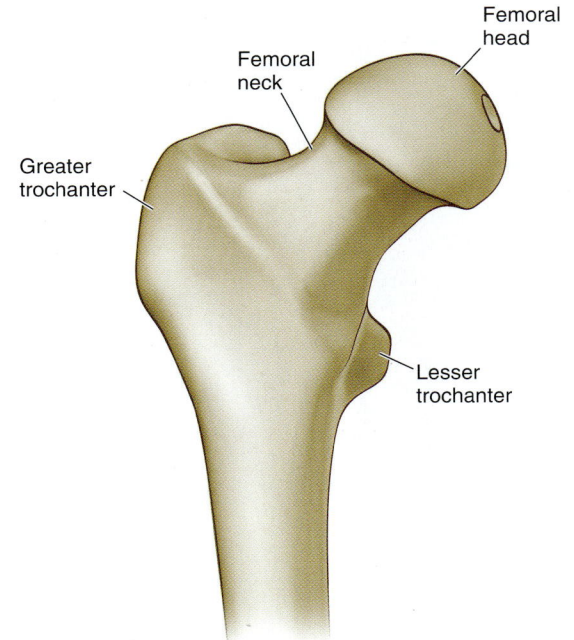

Figure 15-7. The femoral head tapers down to the femoral neck, which bridges the hip joint to the shaft of the femur. The greater and lesser trochanters are prominences about the proximal femur that serve as attachment sites for various tendons.

The adductor brevis originates from the inferior pubic ramus and also inserts onto the linea aspera. Similar to the adductor longus, the adductor brevis is a hip adductor and external rotator.

The adductor magnus has two heads, one from the inferior pubic ramus and one from the ischial tuberosity. The muscle inserts on the linea aspera and the adductor tubercle. The adductor hiatus is a defect in the muscle that allows passage of the femoral vessels into the popliteal space. The adductor magnus adducts and externally rotates, and the hamstring portion extends the hip.

The obturator externus arises from the outer surface of the obturator membrane and inserts onto the medial aspect of the greater trochanter. The muscle serves to externally rotate the hip.

Posterior Compartment

The biceps femoris has two heads: the long head originating from the ischial tuberosity, and the short head arising from the linea aspera and the lateral intermuscular septum (Fig. 15-12). The insertion is on the fibular head, and the muscle functions to extend the hip and to flex the knee and externally rotate the leg.

The semitendinosus originates on the ischial tuberosity and inserts on the proximal medial tibia as one of the pes anserine tendons. The semitendinosus extends the hip, flexes the knee, and internally rotates the leg.

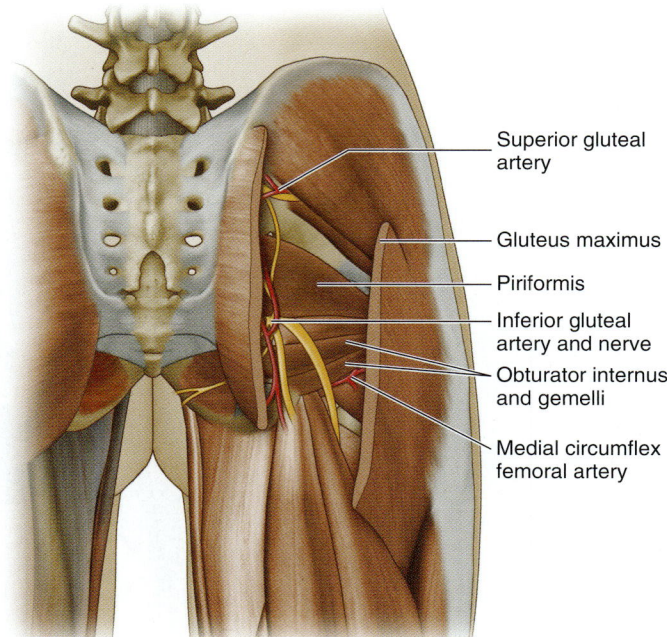

Figure 15-8. Posteriorly, the gluteus maximus originates from the posterior gluteal line, the iliac crest, the posterior surface of the sacrum and coccyx, and the sacrotuberous ligament.

Figure 15-9. The gluteus medius arises from both the lateral surface of the ilium and the undersurface of the tensor fascia lata. The gluteus minimus originates from the ilium and inserts into the hip capsule, as well as the anterior aspect of the greater trochanter. The sciatic nerve exits the greater sciatic foramen deep to the piriformis and travels distally superficial to the superior gemellus, the obturator internus, the inferior gemellus, and the quadratus femoris.

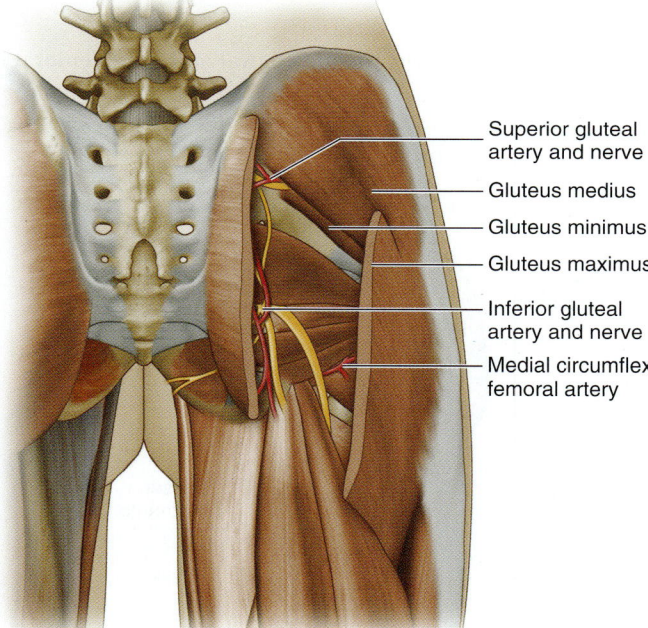

The semimembranosus also arises from the ischial tuberosity and inserts on the posterior medial tibia. Similar to the semitendinosus, the semimembranosus extends the hip, flexes the knee, and internally rotates the leg.

The ischial tuberosity gives rise to the adductor magnus, which inserts on the adductor tubercle of the femur and acts as a hip extender.

VASCULAR ANATOMY

The common iliac artery divides into the internal and external iliac arteries anterior to S1 (Fig. 15-13). The posterior division of the internal iliac artery gives rise to the superior gluteal artery, which exits the pelvis through the greater sciatic notch above the piriformis,

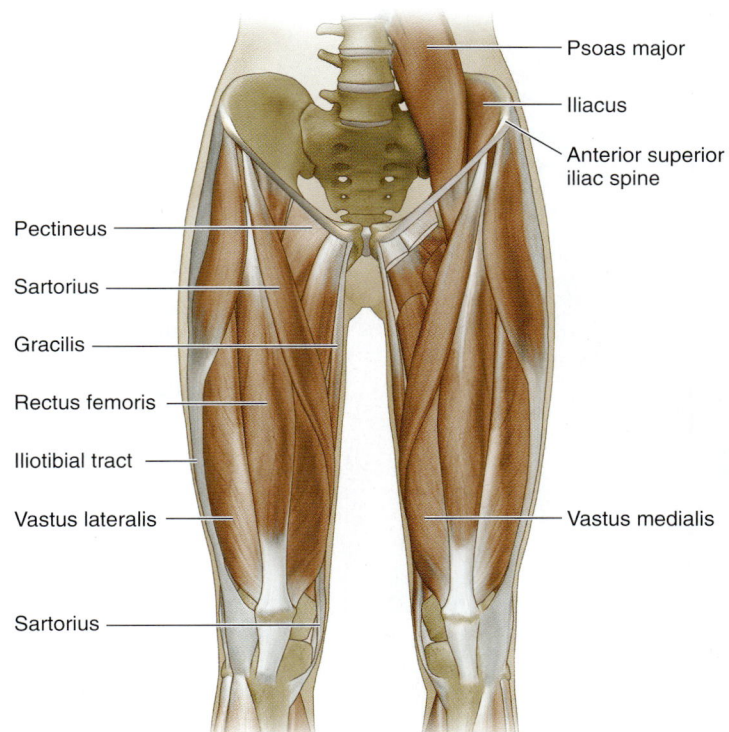

Pectineus

Sartorius

Gracilis

Rectus femoris

Iliotibial tract

Vastus lateralis

Sartorius

Psoas major

Iliacus

Anterior superior
iliac spine

Vastus medialis

Figure 15-10. The sartorius originates from the anterior superior iliac spine (ASIS) and inserts on the proximal medial tibia. The iliacus arises from the medial aspect of the ilium and joins the psoas muscle. The psoas originates from the transverse processes, the vertebral bodies, and the disks from T12 through L5. The pectineus arises from the superior pubic ramus and inserts on the linea aspera. The quadriceps femoris is a combination of four muscles: rectus femoris, vastus lateralis, vastus medialis, and vastus intermedius. The rectus femoris has two heads: one originating from the anterior inferior iliac spine, and a reflected head arising from the anterior acetabular rim.

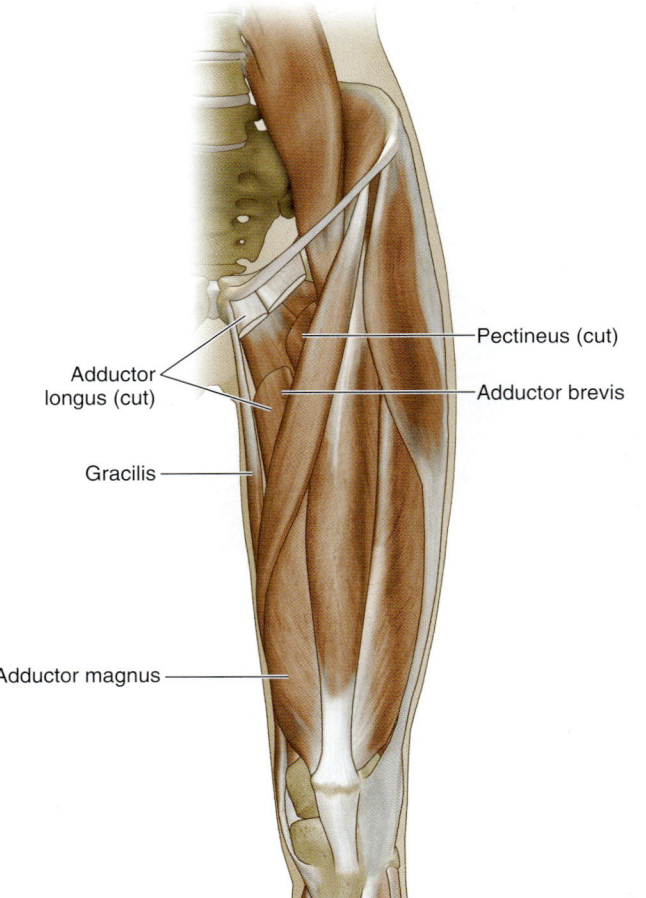

Adductor
longus (cut)

Gracilis

Adductor magnus

Pectineus (cut)

Adductor brevis

Figure 15-11. The gracilis arises from the inferior pubic ramus and the ischium and runs down the medial thigh until it inserts on the proximal medial aspect of the tibia. The adductor longus arises from the anterior pubic body and fans out as it inserts on the linea aspera. The adductor brevis originates from the inferior pubic ramus and also inserts onto the linea aspera. The adductor magnus has two heads: one from the inferior pubic ramus, and one from the ischial tuberosity. The muscle inserts on the linea aspera and the adductor tubercle. The obturator externus arises from the outer surface of the obturator membrane and inserts onto the medial aspect of the greater trochanter.

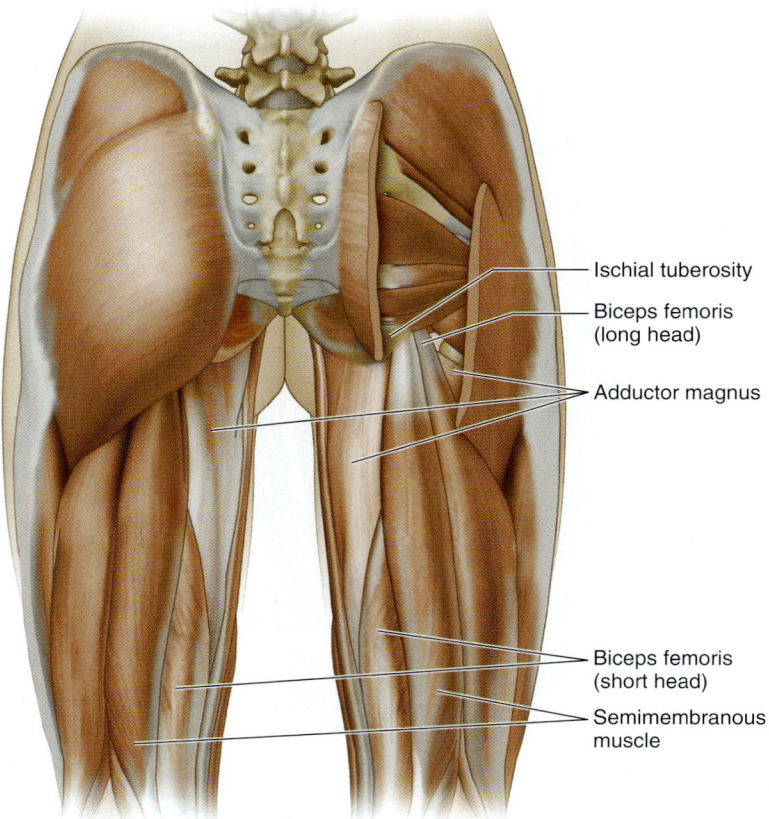

Figure 15-12. The biceps femoris has two heads: the long head originating from the ischial tuberosity, and the short head arising from the linea aspera and the lateral intermuscular septum; the insertion is on the fibular head. The semitendinosus originates on the ischial tuberosity and inserts on the proximal medial tibia. The semimembranosus also arises from the ischial tuberosity and inserts on the posterior medial tibia. The ischial tuberosity gives rise to the adductor magnus, which inserts on the adductor tubercle.

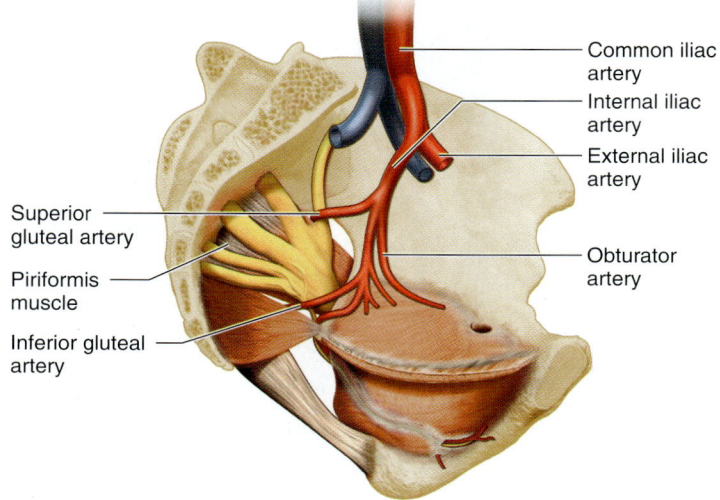

Figure 15-13. The common iliac artery divides into the internal and external iliac arteries anterior to S1. The posterior division of the internal iliac artery gives rise to the superior gluteal artery, which exits the pelvis through the greater sciatic notch above the piriformis. The inferior gluteal artery arises from the anterior division of the internal iliac artery and exits below the piriformis. The obturator artery, which is a branch off of the anterior division of the internal iliac artery, courses along the inner pelvic wall just medial to the acetabulum and exits through the obturator foramen.

and serves as a blood supply to the gluteus maximus, medius, and minimus, as well as the tensor fascia muscle. The inferior gluteal artery arises from the anterior division of the internal iliac artery and exits below the piriformis to supply the gluteus maximus and the short external rotators.

The obturator artery, which is a branch off of the anterior division of the internal iliac artery, courses along the inner pelvic wall just medial to the acetabulum and exits through the obturator foramen. The artery then divides into anterior and posterior branches, which supply the medial muscles, and provides an acetabular branch that enters the hip joint deep to the transverse acetabular ligament and courses through the ligamentum teres to supply the femoral head.

The external iliac artery continues as the femoral artery after it passes deep to the inguinal ligament and

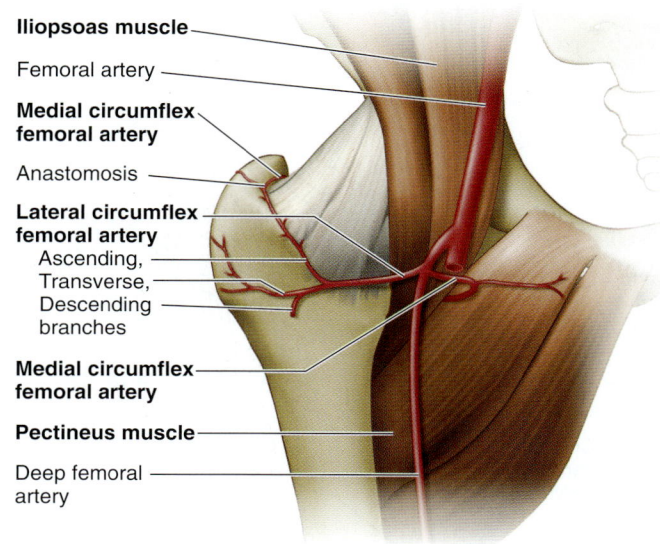

Iliopsoas muscle
Femoral artery
Medial circumflex femoral artery
Anastomosis
Lateral circumflex femoral artery
  Ascending,
  Transverse,
  Descending
  branches
Medial circumflex femoral artery
Pectineus muscle
Deep femoral artery

Figure 15-14. The medial femoral circumflex artery travels between the pectineus and the iliopsoas, then between the obturator externus and the adductor brevis, then between the adductor brevis and magnus, and then distal to the quadratus femoris. The lateral femoral circumflex artery divides into ascending, descending, and transverse branches.

enters the "femoral triangle." The femoral triangle is defined superiorly by the inguinal ligament, laterally by the sartorius, and medially by the adductor longus, and the floor by the iliopsoas, the pectineus, and the adductor brevis (see Fig. 15-1). Within this triangle, the artery is positioned adjacent to the femoral nerve laterally, and the femoral vein medially.

The profunda femoris branches off of the femoral artery within the femoral triangle and branches into the medial and lateral femoral circumflex arteries, as well as four perforating arteries that supply the muscles.

The medial femoral circumflex artery travels between the pectineus and iliopsoas, then between the obturator externus and adductor brevis, then between the adductor brevis and magnus, and then distal to the quadratus femoris (Fig. 15-14). The medial femoral circumflex provides the primary blood supply to the femoral head. The transverse branch anastomoses with the transverse branch of the lateral femoral circumflex artery, the descending branch of the inferior gluteal artery, and the ascending branch of the first perforating artery.

The lateral femoral circumflex artery divides into ascending, descending, and transverse branches. The transverse branch contributes to the cruciate anastomosis, as was previously mentioned. The ascending branch travels deep to the tensor fascia lata along the rectus femoris toward the trochanteric region and is at risk for hemorrhaging in anterior approaches.

NEUROANATOMY

The lower limb is entirely innervated by the lumbar (T12 to L4) and sacral (L4 and L5, S1, S2, and S3) plexuses. The lumbar plexus is formed from the anterior rami of the subcostal nerve (T12) and the first four lumbar nerves (L1, L2, L3, and L4). Its roots emerge lateral to the intervertebral foramina, and its branches course distally to pierce the psoas muscle to provide

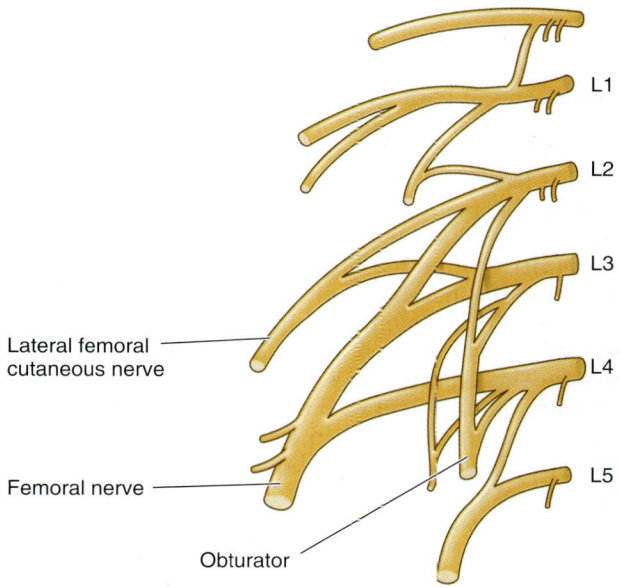

Lateral femoral cutaneous nerve

Femoral nerve

Obturator

L1
L2
L3
L4
L5

Figure 15-15. The lateral femoral cutaneous nerve arises from L2 and L3. The femoral nerve originates from L2, L3, and L4. The obturator nerve also emerges from L2, L3, and L4.

motor and sensory innervation to various lower limb structures. The branches of the lumbar plexus that are clinically relevant to the orthopedic surgeon are the lateral femoral cutaneous nerve (L2 and L3), the femoral nerve (L2, L3, and L4), and the obturator nerve (L2, L3, and L4) (Fig. 15-15).

The lateral femoral cutaneous nerve (L2 and L3) pierces the psoas muscle approximately at its middle, crosses anteriorly over the iliacus muscle, and travels obliquely toward the ASIS. It exits the pelvic area just medial to the anterior iliac spine, coursing under the inguinal ligament via the lateral muscular lacuna. The

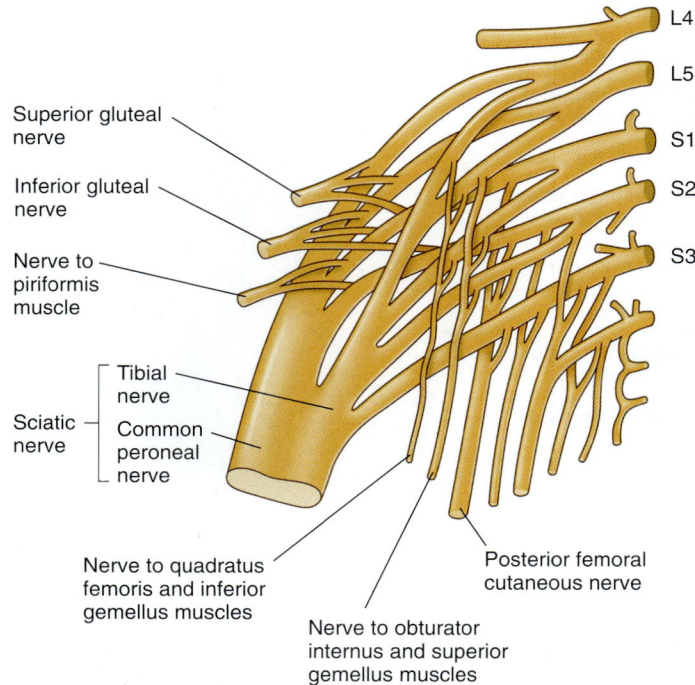

Figure 15-16. The sacral plexus is located anterior and lateral to the sacrum and includes the anterior rami of L4 to S3. The anterior divisions of the sacral plexus give rise to the superior gluteal nerve, the inferior gluteal nerve, and the nerve to the piriformis, and combine to form the common peroneal portion of the sciatic nerve. The posterior divisions give rise to the posterior femoral cutaneous nerve, nerves to the obturator internus, superior and inferior gemelli, and the quadratus femoris, and combine to form the tibial portion of the sciatic nerve.

lateral femoral cutaneous nerve then courses over the sartorius muscle just distal to its origin at the anterior iliac spine, emerges approximately 10 cm below the inguinal ligament, and provides sensory innervation to the lateral aspect of the thigh.

The femoral nerve, the largest branch of the lumbar plexus, arises from L2, L3, and L4. It travels between the psoas and the iliacus and enters the anterior thigh deep to the inguinal ligament. Within the femoral triangle, the femoral nerve is positioned lateral to the femoral vessels. The femoral nerve innervates all muscles of the anterior compartment of the thigh.

The obturator nerve also arises from L2, L3, and L4 and travels along the medial border of the psoas muscle, traverses over the pelvic brim anterior to the sacroiliac joint, and exits the pelvis through the obturator foramen into the thigh. The obturator nerve separates into anterior and posterior divisions. The anterior division innervates the gracilis, the adductor longus, the adductor brevis, and the pectineus, and provides an articular branch to the hip joint. The posterior division supplies the obturator externus and the posterior portion of the adductor magnus.

The sacral plexus is located anterior and lateral to the sacrum and includes the anterior rami of L4 to S3. The anterior divisions of the sacral plexus give rise to the superior gluteal nerve, the inferior gluteal nerve, and the nerve to the piriformis, and combine to form the common peroneal portion of the sciatic nerve. The posterior divisions give rise to the posterior femoral cutaneous nerve, nerves to the obturator internus, superior and inferior gemelli, and the quadratus femoris, and combine to form the tibial portion of the sciatic nerve (Fig. 15-16).

The posterior femoral cutaneous nerve arises from S1, S2, and S3 of the sacral plexus, travels out through the greater sciatic foramen and inferior to the piriformis, and provides cutaneous innervation to the lower buttock and the posterior thigh.

The sciatic nerve, the largest nerve in the body, is a branch of the sacral plexus (L4 and L5, and S1, S2, and S3). The sciatic nerve exits the pelvis through the lower part of the greater sciatic foramen deep to the piriformis and travels distally superficial to the superior gemellus, the obturator internus, the inferior gemellus, and the quadratus femoris (see Fig. 15-9). The sciatic nerve has two portions: the common peroneal and tibial nerves. The short head of the biceps femoris is innervated by the common peroneal portion of the sciatic nerve, and the long head of the biceps femoris and the semitendinosus, the semimembranosus, and the adductor magnus all receive innervation from the tibial portion of the sciatic nerve.

The superior gluteal nerve arises from L4, L5, and S1, and exits the pelvis through the upper part of the greater sciatic foramen superior to the piriformis. It travels deep to the gluteus medius and innervates the gluteus medius, the gluteus minimus, and the tensor fascia lata.

The inferior gluteal nerve is formed from L5, S1, and S2, and leaves the pelvis through the lower part of the greater sciatic foramen inferior to the piriformis to supply the gluteus maximus.

FURTHER READING

Agur AMR: Grant's atlas of anatomy, ed 9, Baltimore, 1991, Williams & Wilkins.
Netter FH: Atlas of human anatomy, Summit, NJ, 1989, Ciba-Geigy Corporation.
Snell RS: Clinical anatomy for medical students, ed 6, Baltimore, 2000, Lippincott, Williams & Wilkins.

CHAPTER 16

Exposures of the Acetabulum

S. Andrew Sems

ILIOINGUINAL APPROACH

The ilioinguinal approach allows access to visualize the entire anterior column of the acetabulum, as well as palpable access to portions of the posterior column.[1-3] Multiple neurovascular structures must be identified, mobilized, and carefully protected during this exposure. Modifications to this exposure allow full access to the quadrilateral surface of the acetabulum as well.[4-9] This exposure involves opening portions of the abdominal wall, and careful closures are required to prevent the formation of hernias.

Indications

1. Anterior column fractures of the acetabulum
2. Both-column fractures of the acetabulum
3. In conjunction with other approaches or for use alone:
   - Transverse fractures of the acetabulum
   - Anterior column–posterior hemitransverse fractures of the acetabulum
   - T-type fractures of the acetabulum
   - Anterior wall fractures of the acetabulum

Positioning

The ilioinguinal approach is performed with the patient in the supine position (Fig. 16-1). The arms of the patient may be tucked at the side, but placing them in an abducted position may facilitate exposure of the lateral window and may improve the ability to obtain intraoperative oblique radiographs of the operative region. A radiolucent fracture table with a perineal post and leg traction can be used with this approach to assist in obtaining reduction of the fracture. A urethral catheter should be placed in the patient's bladder before the surgical site is prepared, to decompress the bladder.

Landmarks

The iliac crest is palpated from the anterior superior iliac spine posteriorly. Additionally, the pubic symphysis is palpated and the midline of the abdomen is located. The operative field is prepared from an area proximal to the superolateral portion of the iliac crest to the superior portion of the introitus or the top of the penis. The umbilicus can be carefully draped out of the field. Care should be taken to note scars from previous herniorrhaphies or surgeries in the inguinal region and prior Pfannenstiel incisions from gynecologic/urologic surgery; previous cesarean sections should be noted, and these can be incorporated into the surgical incision.

Technique

1. The skin over the lateral aspect of the iliac crest is incised from the anterior superior iliac spine posteriorly 10 to 15 cm depending on the size of the patient (Fig. 16-2). Dissection is carried through the skin subcutaneous tissue with hemostasis gained along the way. The fascia over the hip abductors and the fascia over the abdominal musculature are identified. These fasciae come together into an aponeurosis over the proximal lateral aspect of the iliac crest. This aponeurosis is incised in line with its fibers along the iliac crest (Fig. 16-3).
2. Subperiosteal dissection along the superolateral aspect of the iliac crest elevates the abdominal aponeurosis into the inner table of the ilium.
3. A large periosteal elevator is utilized to elevate the iliacus muscle from its origin on the inner table of the ilium. Nutrient vessels encountered at this time

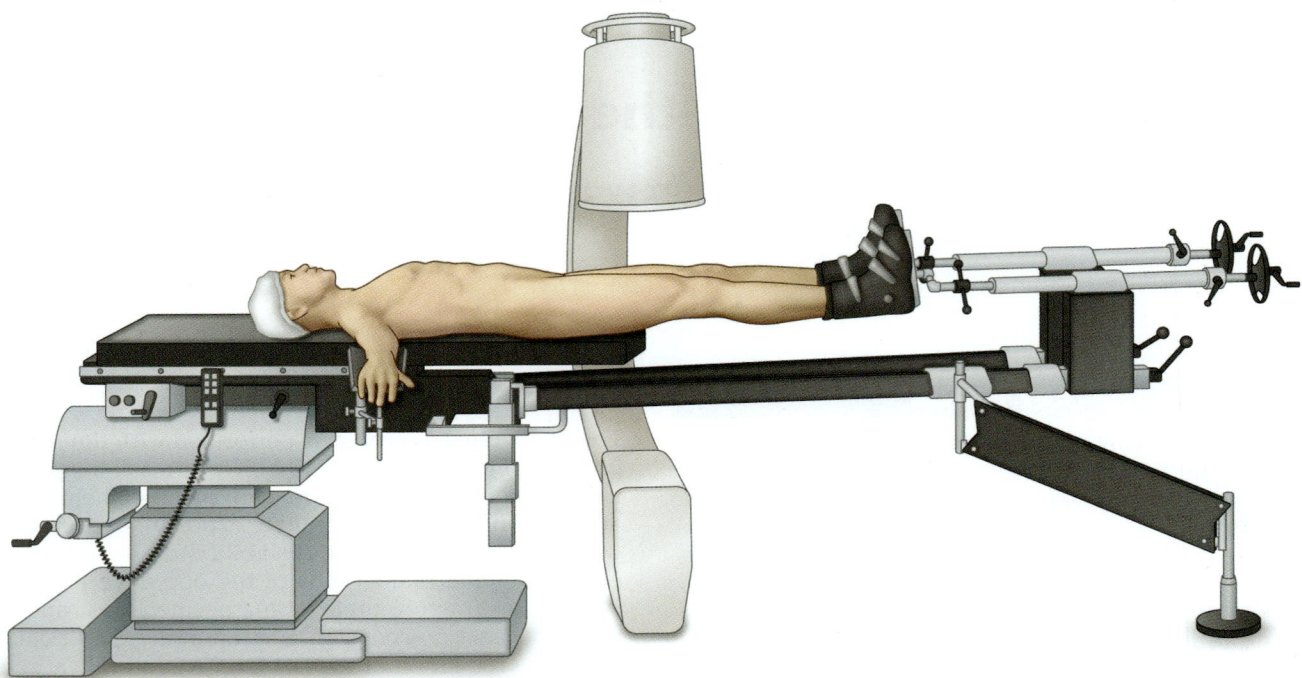

Figure 16-1. The patient is positioned supine on a radiolucent fracture table. The arms are abducted and intraoperative image intensification is positioned on the contralateral side.

can contribute to a significant hemorrhage in this region. Care should be taken to identify these vessels and coagulate when possible. In certain instances, these coagulations may not be possible, and the use of bone wax in this region may help with hemorrhage control.

4. Once the iliac fossa has been exposed, a sponge is placed into this wound to pack it off while further dissection is performed distally.

5. The skin incision is extended from the anterior superior iliac spine to a point approximately 2 cm proximal to the pubic symphysis. The skin incision needs to be extended beyond the midline by 3 to 5 cm to gain full exposure of the rectus abdominis.

6. Once the incision is carried to the level of the abdominal fascia, the fascia of the external abdominal oblique is identified as it courses toward the external inguinal ring. The inguinal ligament is identified coursing from the anterior superior iliac spine to the pubic tubercle. The spermatic cord or round ligament should be identified exiting from the superficial inguinal ring. A Penrose drain or surgical tape can be placed around this structure for control and mobilization (Fig. 16-4). The external abdominal oblique is dissected in line with its fibers and is incised 3 to 5 mm proximal to the inguinal ligament, leaving tendon on each side for later repair (Fig. 16-5). The external abdominal oblique can be split to a point just distal to the superficial inguinal ring, allowing this ring to be maintained in place to decrease the potential for the development of postoperative inguinal hernias.

7. The conjoined tendon of the transversus abdominis and the internal abdominal oblique is identified. Before this is split, care should be taken to identify the lateral femoral cutaneous nerve of the thigh. This nerve courses over the iliopsoas muscle and exits laterally near the anterior superior iliac spine. This nerve may not be able to be preserved in all cases, and careful preoperative discussion with the patient should include the potential for postoperative lack of sensation in the distribution of the lateral femoral cutaneous nerve. Once the lateral femoral cutaneous nerve has been identified, the conjoined tendon of the transversus abdominis and the internal abdominal oblique is incised in line with its fibers (Fig. 16-6). This should be done 2 to 4 mm proximal to its insertion on the inguinal ligament. This will allow later repair of this fascia in two separate layers to decrease the chance of postoperative hernia.

8. Circumferential control of the iliopsoas with the femoral nerve should be obtained (Fig. 16-7). Care should be taken to make sure that the nerve and the psoas stay together as a single unit. A large, curved clamp can be advanced behind and around the psoas and used to guide a Penrose drain or surgical tape around the neuromuscular unit of the psoas and femoral nerve for retraction and control.

9. Careful dissection along the iliopectineal fascia is necessary to mobilize the external iliac vessels. These vessels can be identified by palpation of the pulse, and careful dissection mobilizes the vessels medially. With constant protection of the external

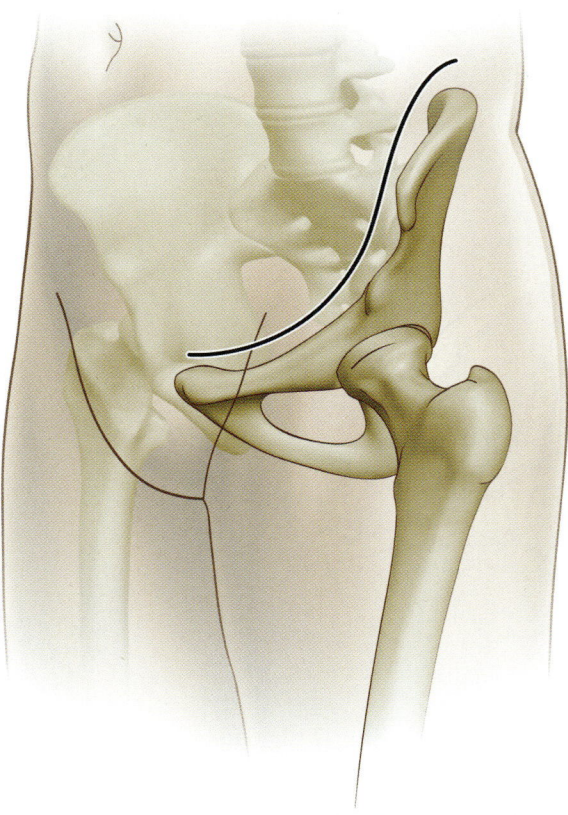

Figure 16-2. The skin incision courses along the proximal aspect of the iliac crest, extending to a point 2 cm above the pubic symphysis and then continued 3 to 5 cm past the midline of the abdomen.

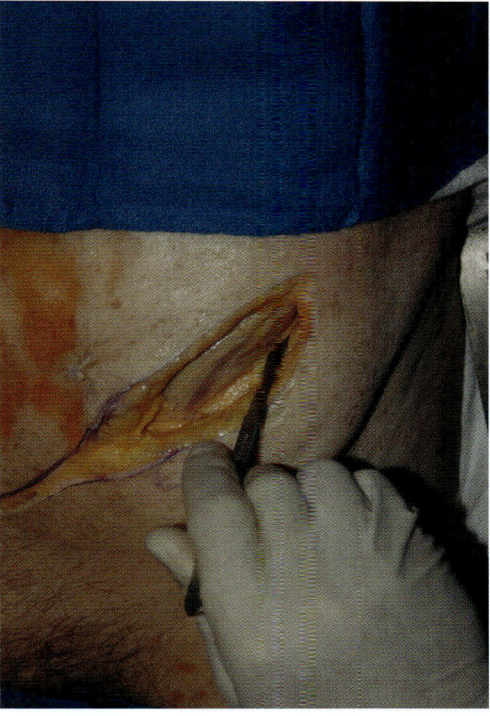

Figure 16-3. The aponeurosis of the abdominal musculature and hip abductors is identified and split along the edge of the iliac crest.

iliac vessels, the iliopectineal fascia can be split down to the pelvic brim (Fig. 16-8).

10. The fascia of the rectus abdominis is identified as it inserts onto the pubic tubercle (Fig. 16-9). This can be incised in a transverse direction to gain access in the space of Retzius. The rectus abdominis should be transected so that the fascial incision is in continuity with the release of the external iliac oblique, as well as the conjoined tendon of the transversus abdominis and the internal abdominal oblique.

11. Once the iliopectineal fascia and the rectus abdominis are released, circumferential control of the external iliac vessels can be obtained, and a large, curved clamp can be advanced behind the vessels and used to guide a Penrose drain or surgical tape to maintain control of the vessels (Fig. 16-10). At this point, the three windows of the ilioinguinal approach have been exposed, and the desired surgical procedure can be performed.

12. Following internal fixation, closure is performed in multiple layers. The transected rectus abdominis fascia is reapproximated using no. 0 nonabsorbable suture.

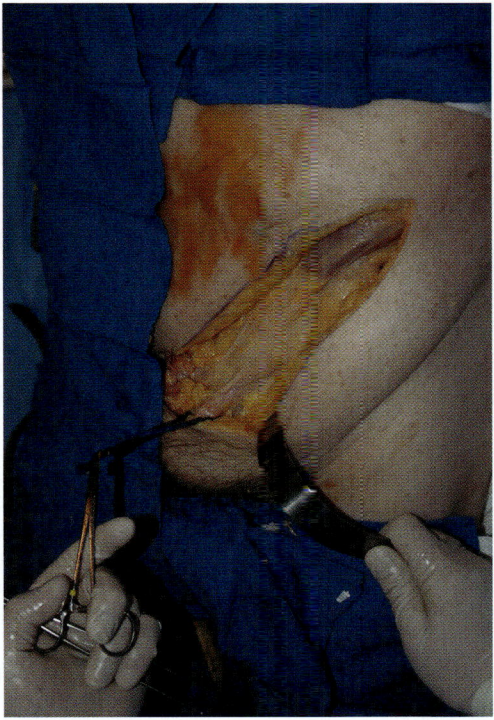

Figure 16-4. The skin incision is carried distally; the spermatic cord is identified and circumferential control is gained with a tape or Penrose drain. The fibers of the external abdominal oblique and inguinal ligaments are identified.

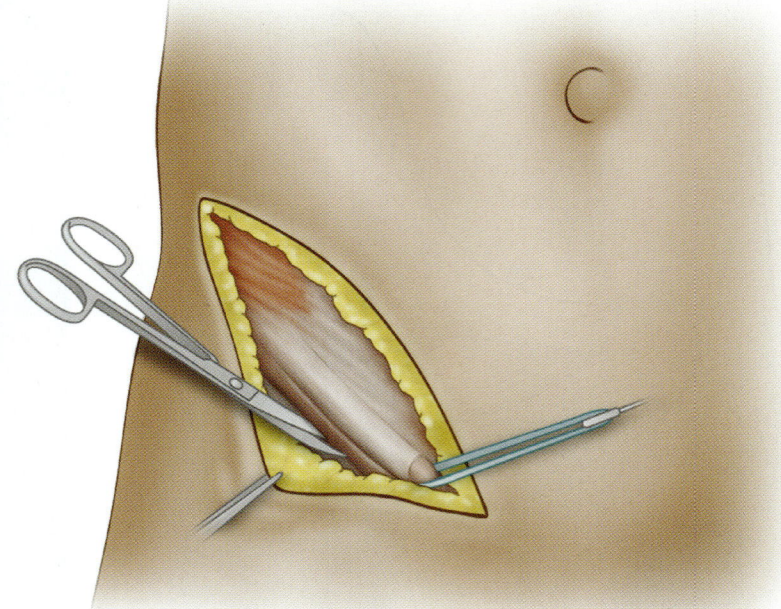

Figure 16-5. The fibers of the external abdominal oblique are split 4 to 5 mm proximal to their insertion on the inguinal ligament distally to a point just distal to the external inguinal ring.

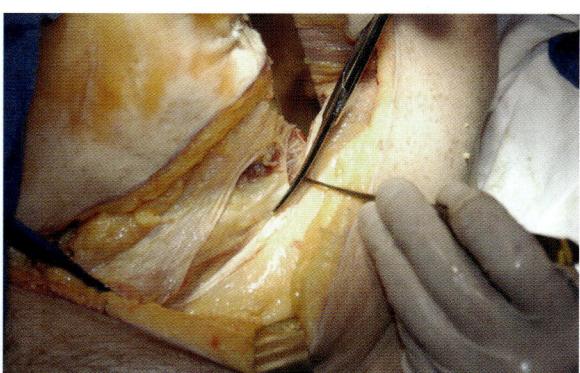

Figure 16-6. The conjoined tendon of the transversus abdominis and the internal abdominal oblique is incised 2 to 3 mm from their insertion on the inguinal ligament, leaving an adequate amount of tendon on each side for repair during closure.

13. The conjoined tendon of the transversus abdominis and the internal oblique is closed with multiple non-absorbable sutures with less than 1 cm spacing between sutures. Additionally, an absorbable suture can be used to overrun this repair to further reinforce the inguinal region.

14. The external abdominal oblique is then repaired using no. 0 nonabsorbable suture. Drains can be placed deep into the wound, including one drain in the iliac fossa. The aponeurosis of the abdominal musculature is then reapproximated to the aponeurosis of the abductor musculature over the iliac crest. Subcutaneous tissue can be closed in layers

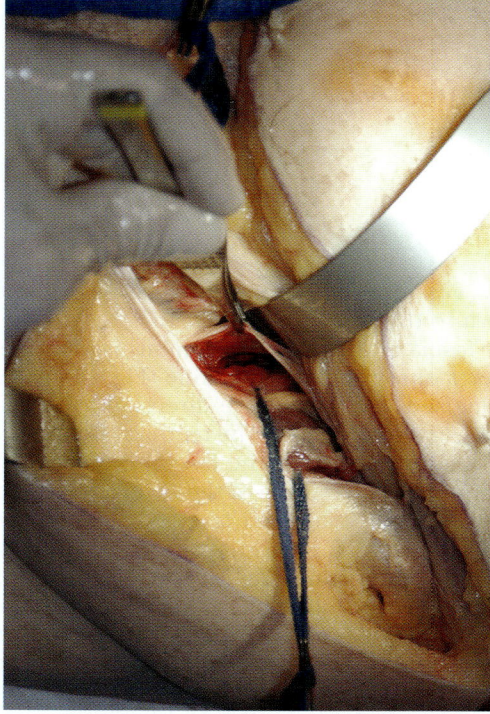

Figure 16-7. The femoral nerve and the psoas muscle have been mobilized and a tape or Penrose drain passed behind these structures for circumferential control. The iliopectineal fascia is identified medial to the psoas and the femoral nerve. The iliopectineal fascia is being held by forceps.

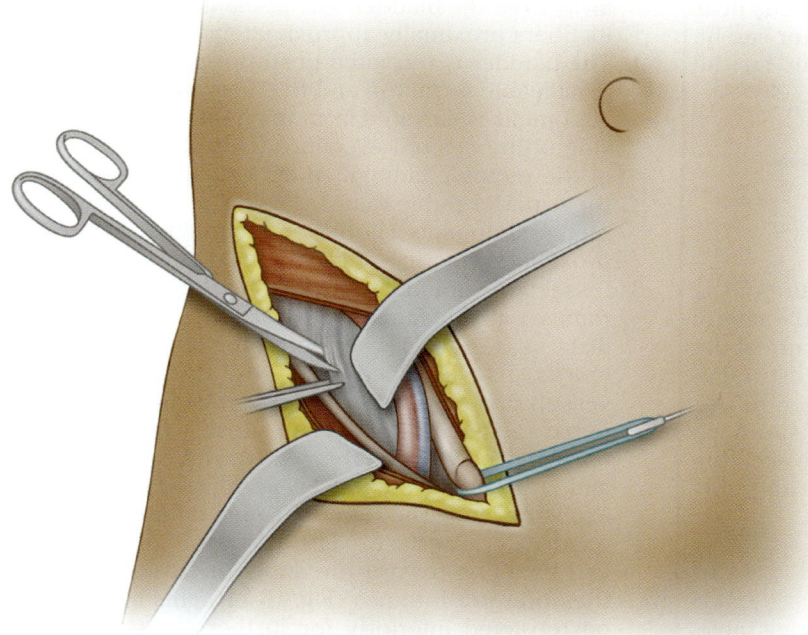

Figure 16-8. Dissection medial to the iliopectineal fascia mobilizes the external iliac vessels, and a Deaver retractor is used to retract the vessels as the iliopectineal fascia is split to the pelvic brim.

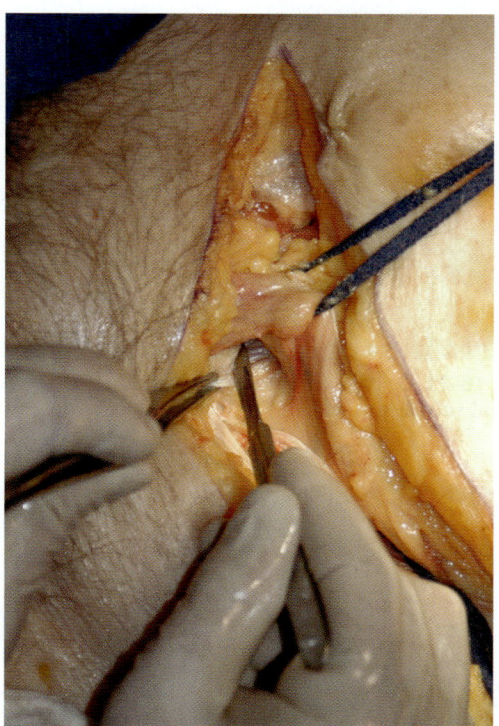

Figure 16-9. Dissection beneath the spermatic cord allows transection of the rectus abdominis tendon on the operative side.

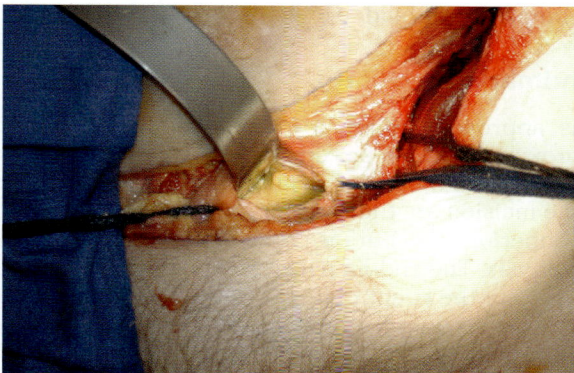

Figure 16-10. Circumferential control of the external iliac vessels and the spermatic cord allows exposure of the medial window and bladder and access into the space of Retzius.

using absorbable suture, and the skin can be closed with sutures or staples.

Helpful Hints

1. Malleable retractors can be used to retract the iliacus and psoas medially in the lateral window, and then can be moved to the middle window to retract the external iliac vessels medially. The edges of these retractors can be acute, and torque must be maintained on the retractor while in the middle window to prevent it from rotating and the edge from injuring or occluding the vessels

2. A pointed lever-type retractor like a Homan can be used in the lateral window to retract the iliacus near the sacroiliac joint. The point of the retractor can be gently introduced into the sacroiliac joint so the entire iliac wing is visualized.

STOPPA APPROACH

Indications

The Stoppa approach can be used for exposure of the anterior pelvic ring and in conjunction with the lateral window of the ilioinguinal approach for exposure of the acetabular region. This exposure utilizes an extraperitoneal approach with retraction of the bladder, bowel, and external iliac vessels.[10-12] The Stoppa approach gives access to the quadrilateral surface of the acetabulum and to the low anterior column, the superior pubic ramus, and the pubic symphysis.[13,14]

Positioning

The patient is positioned supine on the operating table. The arms can be tucked at the side, although an abducted position may make intraoperative oblique imaging easier, because the arms will not obscure the images. A urethral catheter should be placed in the patient's bladder before the surgical site is prepared, to decompress the bladder.

Landmarks

This approach utilizes a Pfannenstiel incision based approximately 2 cm proximal to the superior aspects of the pubis and the superior pubic ramus. The landmarks of the incision are the anterior superior iliac spines and the superior aspect of the pubic tubercles and the pubic symphysis. The abdominal area should be prepped into the field in the event of injury to the bladder or bowel, which may require laparotomy. The patient is prepped distally from the top of the introitus or penis, and laterally past the iliac crests.

Technique

1. The incision is centered over the pubic symphysis and extends laterally in both directions 5 to 8 cm based on the size of the patient (Fig. 16-11). The incision is in line with the abdominal crease and is directed toward the anterior superior iliac spine. Dissection is carried through the skin and subcutaneous tissue with hemostasis obtained through the subcutaneous fat.
2. The midline fascia over the rectus abdominis is identified. It can be identified by observing the decussation of the fibers of the fascia, as they tend to cross in the midline.
3. At the proximal aspect of the pubic symphysis, the rectus abdominis is split over a small distance just enough to get a right angle clamp beneath it. The right angle clamp is placed point proximally and is

retracted anteriorly to elevate the rectus abdominis away from the bladder. The fascia is split in line with its fibers proximally approximately 8 cm (Fig. 16-12).
4. The bladder is retracted posteriorly with a finger or a malleable retractor, and the insertion of the rectus abdominis is elevated from the pubic tubercle on the side of the desired exposure. This allows retraction of the rectus abdominis anteriorly and exposure of the superior pubic ramus. The distal insertion of the rectus abdominis should be maintained to prevent proximal retraction of the rectus.
5. Dissection should continue along the superior pubic ramus until an anastomosis between the external iliac vessels and the obturator vessels (corona mortis) is identified (Fig. 16-13). Anastomosing vessels cross over the superior edge of the superior pubic ramus. Multiple small vessels or a few large ones may be found in this region, and careful ligation and transection should be performed to allow for exposure along the superior pubic ramus toward the quadrilateral surface.[15] The obturator nerve is identified coursing toward the superior lateral aspect of the obturator foramen (Fig. 16-14). This may have to be retracted inferiorly for further exposure of the quadrilateral surface. A thick periosteal covering over the superior pubic ramus and the pelvic rim is

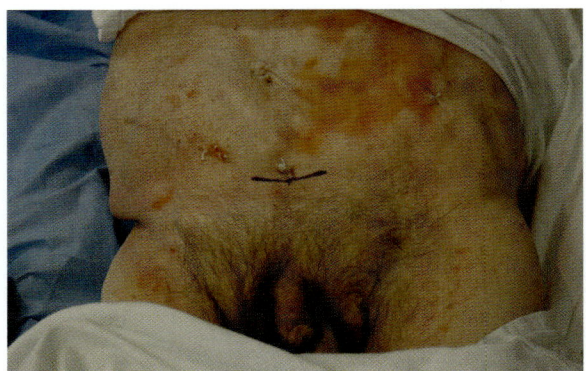

Figure 16-11. A Pfannenstiel incision is based 1 to 2 cm proximal to the top of the pubic symphysis.

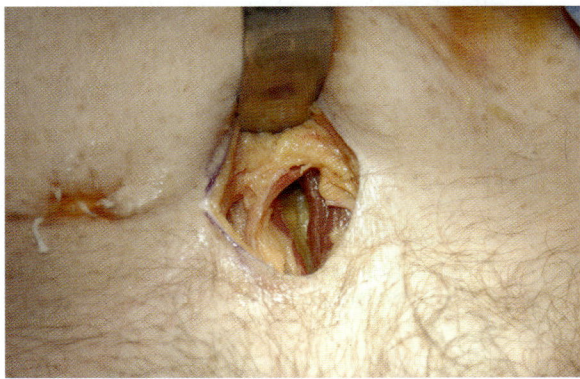

Figure 16-12. The fascia over the rectus abdominis is split longitudinally, allowing access to the prevesicular area and the space of Retzius.

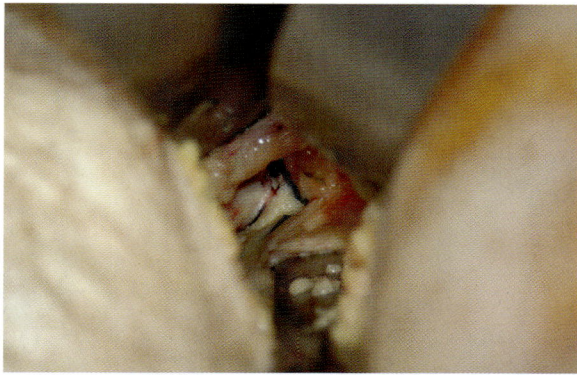

Figure 16-13. Dissection along the superior pubic ramus behind the rectus abdominis allows identification of the corona mortis, an anastomosis between the external iliac and obturator vessels.

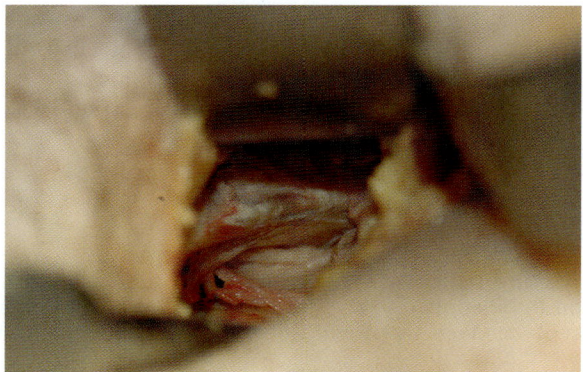

Figure 16-14. After ligation of any anastomosing vessels, dissection continues along the superior pubic ramus and the pelvic brim, exposing the quadrilateral surface of the acetabulum and the obturator nerve.

identified. It may have to be split and elevated for further exposure of the fracture segments if the fracture extends into the superior pubic ramus.

6. A large Deaver or malleable retractor can be placed below the external iliac vessels to retract them superiorly and allow visualization of the pelvic brim.

7. After the surgical procedure through the Stoppa approach, the rectus abdominis fascia is closed with no. 0 suture. Great care should be taken to protect the bladder during repair of this fascia because it will tend to protrude through the split in the rectus abdominis. Subcutaneous tissue can be closed in standard fashion with absorbable sutures and staples, or nylon sutures may be used to close the skin.

Helpful Hints

1. The quadrilateral surface of the acetabulum is visualized several centimeters deep in the wound, so the use of a headlamp may be necessary to get enough light into the area to visualize the structures adequately.

2. Malleable retractors can be helpful to retract the bladder away from the superior pubic ramus and to

retract the iliacus and external iliac vessels superiorly away from the pelvic brim.

3. The Stoppa approach may be combined with the lateral window of the ilioinguinal approach (modified ilioinguinal approach) to gain access to the more superior aspects of the anterior column and sacroiliac joint.

APPROACH TO THE POSTERIOR PELVIS (KOCHER-LANGENBECK APPROACH)

Indications

1. Open reduction and internal fixation of acetabular fractures[16-18]
   a. Posterior wall
   b. Posterior column
   c. Transverse posterior wall
   d. Posterior column–posterior wall
   e. Transverse
   f. T-type
2. Open irrigation and débridement of the hip joint

Positioning

The patient can be placed in a lateral or prone position during a Kocher-Langenbeck approach.[19] The operative knee should be maintained in 90 degrees of flexion at all times to minimize tension from the sciatic nerve and to allow for retraction of the nerve and the posterior flap. By using a special fracture table that accommodates prone positioning, the patient's knee can be maintained in the flexed position with a table attachment that can also apply traction to the femur to distract the hip joint (Fig. 16-15). Traction applied through a distal femoral traction pin can allow precise control of the amount of hip joint distraction. Sequential compression devices can continue to be utilized intraoperatively when the patient is in the prone position.

Landmarks

The posterior superior iliac spine and the greater trochanter and the lateral aspect of the femur are identified. The gluteal crease generally approximates the level of insertion of the gluteus maximus tendon on the femur.

Technique

1. The incision is directed along a line from the posterior superior iliac spine toward the center of the greater trochanter and then is extended distally on the lateral aspect of the femur (Fig. 16-16). The incision can be curved gently at the corner, but it may be preferable in more obese patients to keep it sharp. In the larger patient, the center of the greater trochanter may be difficult to identify until some of the subcutaneous adipose tissue has been dissected. By maintaining the corner of the incision as an angle, the posterior portion of the skin incision (from the

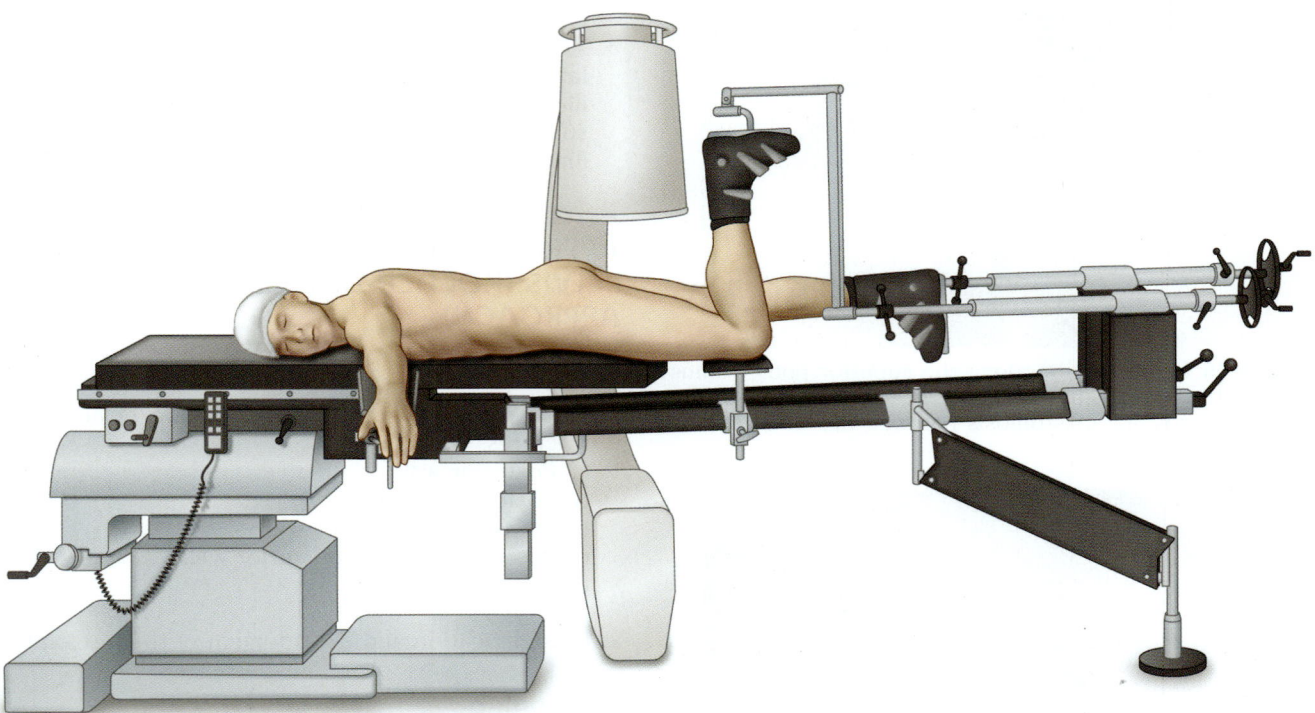

Figure 16-15. The patient is positioned prone of a radiolucent fracture table with a distal femoral traction pin on the operative side. The specialized table allows intraoperative traction to be applied to the hip while the knee is maintained in 90 degrees of flexion. Sequential compression devices are kept in place to provide deep vein thrombosis (DVT) prophylaxis.

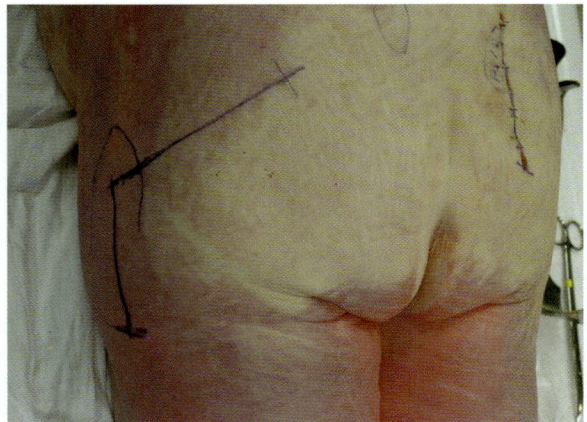

Figure 16-16. The incision follows a line from the posterior superior iliac crest to the center of the greater trochanter. At the center of the greater trochanter, the incision is extended distally in line with the femoral shaft to a level of the inferior gluteal fold.

posterior superior iliac spine toward the center of the greater trochanter) may be extended anteriorly to the level of the femur, once the correct level is identified by palpation. Once the posterior limb is extended to the desired level, the longitudinal portion of the incision (in line with the femoral shaft) is made.

2. The fascia over the gluteus maximus, the gluteal muscle fibers, and the iliotibial band and the lateral thigh fascia are identified. The fascial incision is started over the center of the greater trochanter. The fascia is opened in line with the skin incision over a 3- to 4-cm length, enough to slide a finger beneath the fascia distally and identify the tendon of the gluteus maximus inserting on the femur.

3. The iliotibial band and the lateral thigh fascia are split in line with their fibers distally to a point just anterior to the insertion of the sling of the gluteus maximus on the femur. The fascial incision usually extends distally to a level equal to the inferior gluteal fold of the skin, because this is the location that corresponds with the tendinous sling of the gluteus maximus. This tendon may have to be incised as it inserts on the femur to allow sufficient posterior retraction of the flap. If the gluteus maximus tendon is transected to allow posterior retraction, it should be repaired during closure.

4. The fascia over the gluteus maximus is then split in line with the underlying muscle fibers, and the muscle fibers of the gluteus maximus are split by blunt finger dissection (Fig. 16-17). The gluteus maximus may be split two thirds of the distance from the greater trochanter to the posterior superior iliac spine before damage to the superior gluteal neurovascular bundle is encountered. Once the posterior flap is created by splitting the gluteus maximus and the iliotibial band,

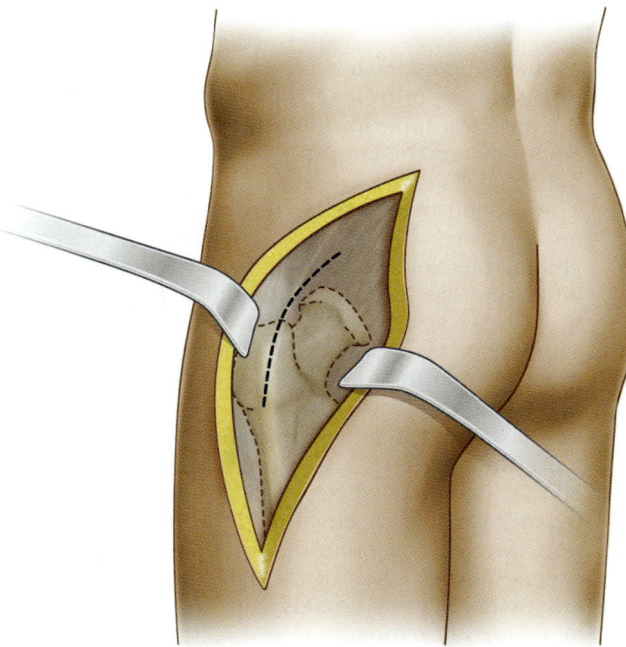

Figure 16-17. The fascia over the gluteus maximus and the iliotibial band and the lateral thigh are split to create a posterior flap.

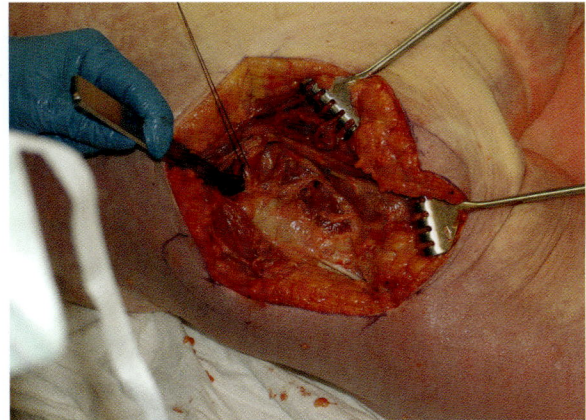

Figure 16-18. The short external rotators are identified inserting on the femur. The rotators are tagged and incised more than 1 cm from their insertion on the femur to protect the medial circumflex femoral vessels coursing to the femoral head.

it can be held in place with large no. 5 Ethibond sutures tacked to the posterior skin.

5. The short external rotators are then identified, beginning superiorly with the piriformis. The muscle and tendon of the piriformis are tagged and incised approximately 1 cm from its insertion onto the femur and retracted posteriorly (Fig. 16-18). The combined tendon of the gemellae and the obturator internus is then identified and tagged. The tendinous portions of these muscles tend to form anteriorly along the surface adjacent to the capsule. Tagging sutures

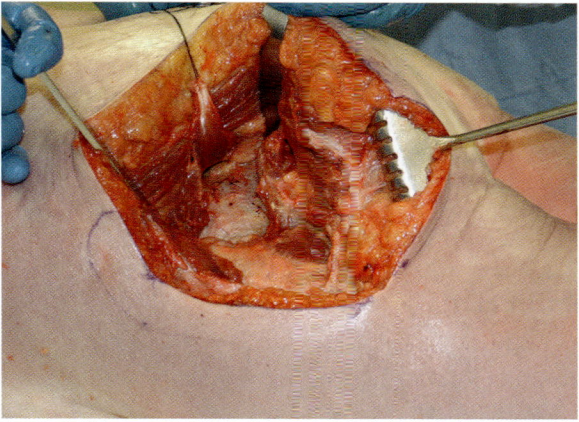

Figure 16-19. The short external rotators are elevated from the hip capsule, and dissection continues to the greater and lesser sciatic notches. A retractor is placed in front of the obturator internus muscle into the lesser sciatic notch. The entire retroacetabular surface is now exposed.

should be placed deep into the muscle to gain control of the tendinous portion, but not so deep that the suture passes through the capsule. These muscles should not be incised closer than 1 cm from the insertion on the femur to protect the blood supply to the femoral head. Dissection should stop at the inferior border of the inferior gemellus muscle and should not be carried into the quadratus femoris because the risk of damage to the ascending branch of the medial circumflex femoral artery and the subsequent femoral head blood supply is encountered.

6. Following transection and retraction of the short external rotators, dissection continues in a subperiosteal plane along the retroacetabular surface. The piriformis muscle is mobilized and elevated to the greater sciatic notch, and the obturator internus and gemellae muscles are elevated back to their insertions near the lesser sciatic notch (Fig. 16-19). The obturator internus passes anterior to the sciatic nerve, so that posterior retraction of the tagging sutures in the obturator internus will form a sling around the sciatic nerve and will retract it posteriorly. A retractor may be safely placed into the lesser sciatic notch once it is then exposed, so long as tension is kept on the obturator internus tag suture to protect the sciatic nerve at all times. Anterior dissection beneath the gluteus minimus and the remainder of the hip abductor muscle provides exposure of the posterior-superior aspect of the posterior wall and ilium. A retractor can be placed beneath the hip abductors to expose the superior aspect of the acetabulum for placement of hardware in this region.

7. After the surgical procedure, the short external rotators are reapproximated to the greater trochanter. In the prone position on the fracture table, the leg may be externally rotated to reduce the distance to the greater trochanter for the short external rotators, allowing a tension-free repair. Permanent sutures are used to repair the short external rotators through a

drill hole in the trochanter or by sewing into the tendinous portion of the hip abductors as they insert on the greater trochanter. The posterior flap is then closed by a side-to-side reapproximation of the fascia both laterally and posteriorly over the gluteus maximus. The subcutaneous tissue is closed in multiple layers, with care taken to avoid leaving large dead spaces in the adipose tissue. The skin is then closed with sutures or staples.

Helpful Hints

1. If performed in the prone position, initial internal rotation of the leg during exposure will place the short external rotators in a stretched position and will allow easier identification and exposure of the tendinous portions of these muscles.
2. Incision of a portion of the gluteus maximus tendinous sling that inserts on the femur may be required in extremely muscular patients or obese patients in whom further posterior retraction of the muscle flap is necessary.
3. Placing the patient in a prone position with a distal femoral traction pin and perineal post traction may facilitate exposure of the hip. Traction can be applied using the table's traction mechanism and the hip joint can be distracted to allow débridement of any intra-articular fragments, and to assess the femoral head for articular cartilage injury.

EXTENDED ILIOFEMORAL APPROACH

Indications

Routine use of the extended iliofemoral approach in the treatment of most acetabular fractures is rare. Most complex fractures can be managed through combined Kocher-Langenbeck and ilioinguinal approaches, obviating the need for the extended iliofemoral approach.[20] However, certain T-type or transtectal transverse acetabular fractures with acetabular dome impaction or associated fractures of the posterior wall are still appropriately treated through the extended iliofemoral approach.[21-23] This approach may also be useful for treatment of malunited fractures or fractures that are several weeks or months old.

Positioning

The patient is positioned in the lateral decubitus position, with the entire leg free and prepped in the field. Surgical prepping should be carried out to the midline of the posterior sacrum, and the entire region around the iliac crest and the inguinal region should be included.

Landmarks

The entire iliac crest from the anterior superior iliac spine to the posterior superior iliac spine should be identified, as well as the lateral edge of the patella.

Technique

1. A curvilinear incision is made beginning over the posterior superior iliac spine and extending toward the anterior superior iliac spine, then continuing in a line toward the lateral border of the patella to the midthigh (Fig. 16-20).
2. The aponeurosis between the abdominal and gluteal musculature is identified along the iliac crest. The gluteal muscles are released from their origin on the ilium, and elevation is continued subperiosteally to the greater sciatic notch (Fig. 16-21).
3. The tensor fascia is released from its origin on the ilium by continued subperiosteal elevation anteriorly along the iliac crest.
4. The fascia of the anterior thigh is incised longitudinally on the lateral border of the sartorius (Fig. 16-22). The interval between the sartorius and the tensor fascia lata is developed through blunt dissection. Vessels encountered in this area represent ascending branches of the lateral femoral circumflex artery. These vessels can be ligated safely to allow further exposure (Fig. 16-23).

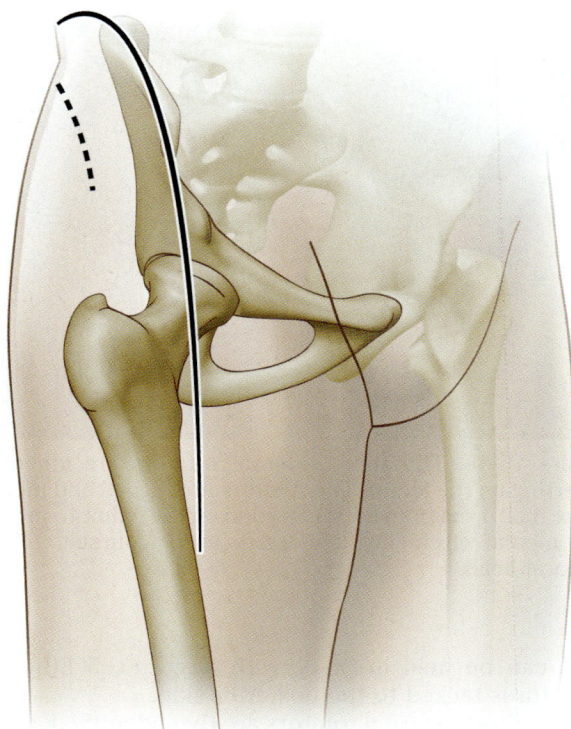

Figure 16-20. In the lateral position, the surgical field is prepared from an area proximal to the iliac crest to include the entire thigh to the knee. The incision parallels the iliac crest from the posterior superior iliac spine to the anterior superior iliac spine. Distally, the incision is made along a line from the anterior superior iliac spine to the lateral border of the patella.

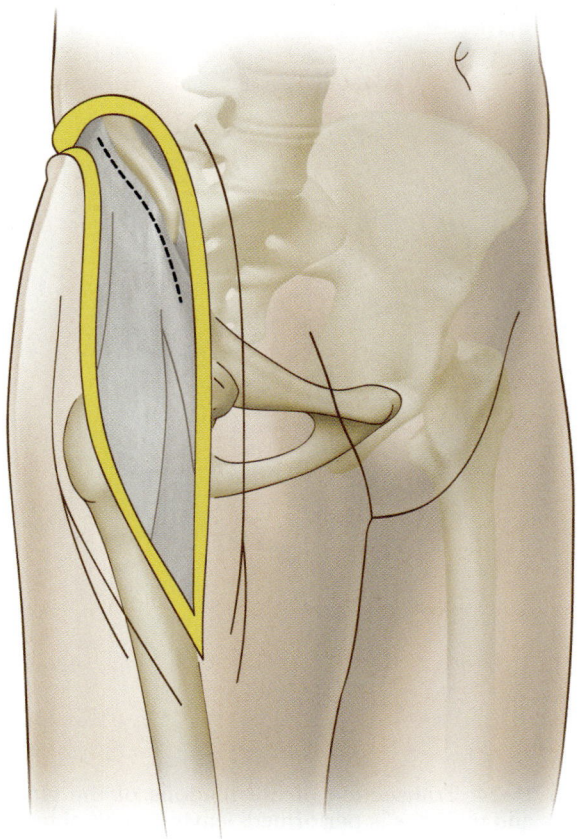

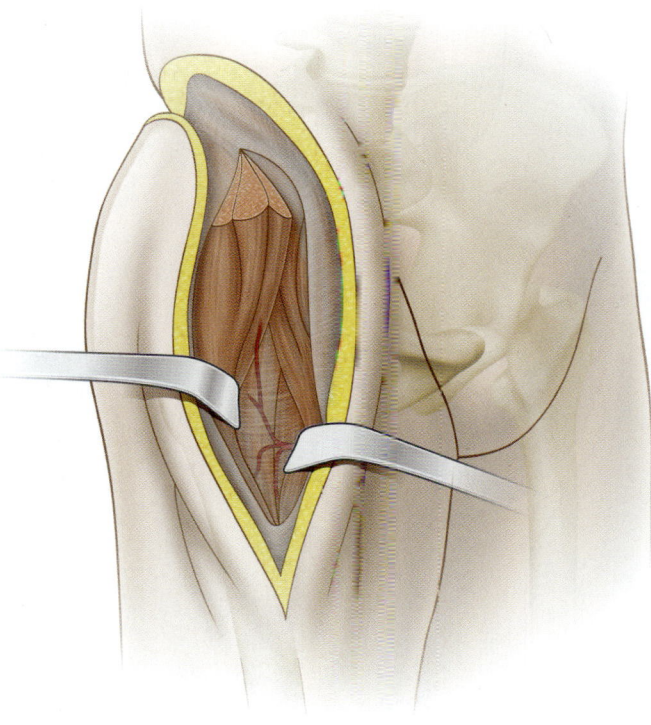

Figure 16-21. The junction of the aponeuroses of the abdominal musculature and the hip abductors is identified and split along the iliac crest. Subperiosteal dissection is used to elevate the hip abductors from the ilium.

Figure 16-22. The interval between the sartorius and the tensor fascia lata is identified, and the thigh fascia is split following this interval. Retraction of the tensor fascia lata and the sartorius exposes the ascending branches of the lateral femoral circumflex artery.

5. Retract the tensor fascia lata laterally and the sartorius medially to continue dissection between the gluteus medius laterally and the rectus femoris medially. Release the origin of the reflected head of the rectus femoris tendon from the supra-acetabular ilium.

6. Elevate the gluteus minimus from the ilium and the hip capsule, and incise the tendon near its insertion on the greater trochanter. Take care to leave a cuff of tendon on the greater trochanter for later repair. Next, incise the tendon of the gluteus medius near its insertion on the greater trochanter, again leaving a tendinous cuff on the greater trochanter for later repair (Fig. 16-24).

7. Dissect posteriorly on the greater trochanter, and release the insertion of the short external rotators in order: piriformis, superior gemellae, obturator internus, and inferior gemellae. Maintain at least 1 cm of tendon on the femoral side to protect branches of the medial circumflex femoral artery that supply the femoral head. Next, dissect beneath the external rotators, elevating them off the posterior capsule and the retroacetabular surface of the ilium back to the greater and lesser sciatic notches (Fig. 16-25).

8. The sciatic nerve courses posterior to the obturator internus, so retraction of the obturator internus posteriorly will create a protective sling in front of the sciatic nerve. With the sciatic nerve protected by the obturator internus, retractors may be carefully placed into the greater or lesser sciatic notches. The tendon of the gluteus maximus may need to be transected near its insertion on the femur to allow further posterior retraction of the posterior flap. This tendon should be transected to leave a cuff of tendon on the femur for later repair.

9. The anterior column may be exposed further by releasing the origin of the sartorius and the inguinal ligament from the anterior superior iliac spine. The insertion of the abdominal muscles on the iliac crest can be elevated to gain access to the iliac fossa in the same manner as the lateral window of the ilioinguinal approach. The iliopsoas can be elevated subperiosteally to the pelvic brim. Osteotomizing the iliac crest is an alternative to complete release of all structures from the anterior superior iliac spine. If this is desired, the inguinal ligament, the sartorius, and abdominal musculature insertions and origins on the ilium are maintained, and the ilium is osteotomized in a line parallel to the iliac

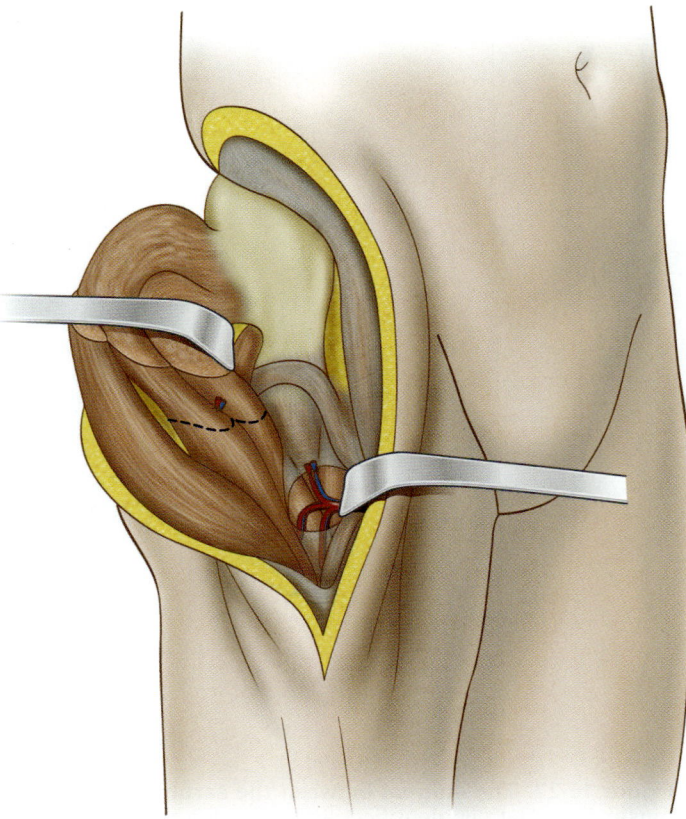

Figure 16-23. Ligation of the ascending branches of the lateral femoral circumflex artery allows further retraction and exposure of the hip capsule. The gluteus medius and minimus tendons inserting on the femur are identified so they can be transected.

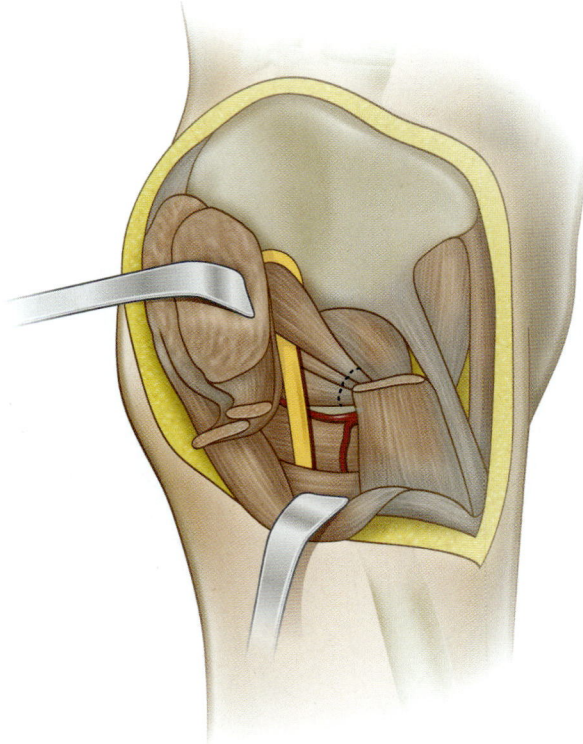

Figure 16-24. Transection of the tendons of the gluteus medius and minimus is performed, leaving a cuff of tendon on the femur for later repair. The short external rotators are identified, as is the sciatic nerve.

crest, creating a 2- to 3-cm segment of iliac crest that can be mobilized for intrapelvic exposure. Easier reduction and fixation during closure may be facilitated by predrilling the osteotomy.

10. After the surgical procedure, multiple tendons must be repaired to their insertions. Closure begins with reapproximation of the common tendon of the obturator internus and gemellae muscles. The piriformis is repaired to the cuff of tendon remaining on the femur. Closure is carried anteriorly on the greater trochanter by repairing the gluteus medius tendon and the gluteus minimus tendons. Next, the reflected head of the rectus femoris is sewn back to the tendon stump on the supra-acetabular ilium. The hip is moved into an abducted position, and the abductors are repaired by sewing them to the abdominal aponeurosis and the lumbodorsal fascia. Side-to-side repair of the fascia over the sartorius completes the deep closure. The subcutaneous tissues and the skin are closed to complete the procedure. Postoperative restriction of hip motion is

recommended to protect repairs of the hip abductors on both the femur and the ilium. A hip abduction pillow is useful during the initial postoperative period, and transition to a hip abduction brace for the first several weeks may be desired. Active abduction of the hip is not recommended for at least 6 weeks postoperatively.

Helpful Hints

1. This exposure requires the release of multiple tendons. Time taken to carefully release the tendons and to tag both ends with a matching suture pattern will facilitate repair in the correct position.
2. Release the gluteus medius from a posterior-to-anterior direction along the ilium, all the way to the anterior superior iliac spine. Exposure of the anterior superior iliac spine will make identifying the interval between the sartorius and the tensor fascia lata easier. It is occasionally necessary to dissect distally along the sartorius until the interval between the sartorius and the tensor fascia lata can be determined.

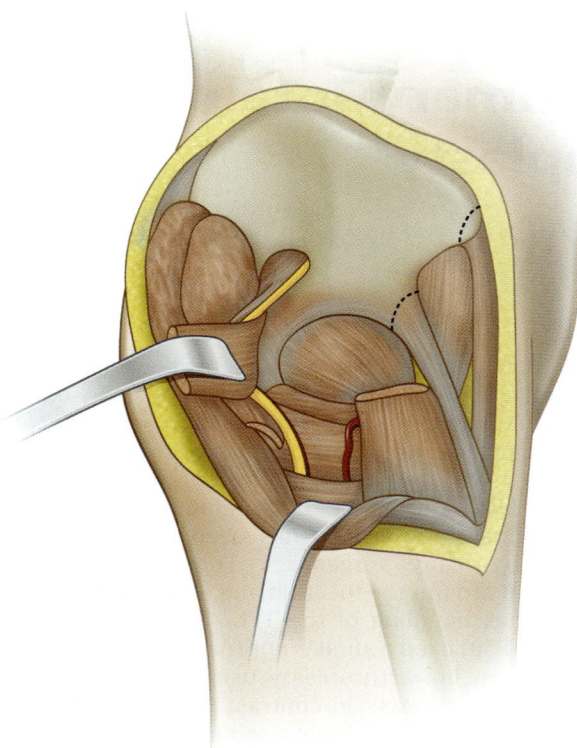

Figure 16-25. The short external rotators are tagged, released, and elevated from the retroacetabular surface back to the greater and lesser sciatic notches. Homan retractors may be placed in the notches for exposure of the posterior column of the acetabulum. The tendon of the gluteus maximus may have to be transected near the femur to allow further retraction of the posterior flap.

REFERENCES

1. Letournel E: The treatment of acetabular fractures through the ilioinguinal approach. Clin Orthop 292:62–76, 1993.
2. Matta JM: Operative treatment of acetabular fractures through the ilioinguinal approach: a 10-year perspective. J Orthop Trauma 20(Suppl 1):S20–S29, 2006.
3. Letournel E. The treatment of acetabular fractures through the ilioinguinal approach. Clin Orthop Relat Res 292:62–76, 1993.
4. Wolf H, Wieland T, Pajenda G, et al: Minimally invasive ilioinguinal approach to the acetabulum. Injury 38:1170–1176, 2007.
5. Jakob M, Droeser R, Zobrist R, et al: A less invasive anterior intrapelvic approach for the treatment of acetabular fractures and pelvic ring injuries. J Trauma 60:1364–1370, 2006.
6. Karunakar MA, Le TT, Bosse MJ: The modified ilioinguinal approach. J Orthop Trauma 18:379–383, 2004.
7. Kloen P, Siebenrock KA, Ganz R: Modification of the ilioinguinal approach. J Orthop Trauma 16:586–593, 2002. Review.
8. Farid YR: The subinguinal retroperitoneal approach for fractures of the acetabulum: a modified ilioinguinal approach. Orthop Trauma 22:270–275, 1988.
9. Weber TG, Mast JW: The extended ilioinguinal approach for specific both column fractures. Clin Orthop Relat Res 305:106–111, 1994.
10. Sagi HC, Afsari A, Dziadosz D: The anterior intra-pelvic (modified Rives-Stoppa) approach for fixation of acetabular fractures. J Orthop Trauma 24:263–270, 2010.
11. Ponsen KJ, Joosse P, Schigt A, et al: Internal fracture fixation using the Stoppa approach in pelvic ring and acetabular fractures: technical aspects and operative results. J Trauma 61:662–667, 2006.
12. Qureshi AA, Archdeacon MT, Jenkins MA, et al: Infrapectineal plating for acetabular fractures: a technical adjunct to internal fixation. J Orthop Trauma 18:175–178, 2004.
13. Andersen RC, O'Toole RV, Nascone JW, et al: Modified Stoppa approach for acetabular fractures with anterior and posterior column displacement: quantification of radiographic reduction and analysis of interobserver variability. J Orthop Trauma 24:271–278, 2010.
14. Guy P, Al-Otaibi M, Harvey EJ, Helmy N: The 'safe zone' for extra-articular screw placement during intra-pelvic acetabular surgery. J Orthop Trauma 24:279–283, 2010.
15. Darmanis S, Lewis A, Mansoor A, Bircher M: Corona mortis: an anatomical study with clinical implications in approaches to the pelvis and acetabulum. Clin Anat 20:433–439, 2007.
16. Borrelli J Jr, Goldfarb C, Ricci W, et al: Functional outcome after isolated acetabular fractures. J Orthop Trauma 16:73–81, 2002.
17. Jimenez ML, Vrahas MS: Surgical approaches to the acetabulum. Orthop Clin North Am 28:419–434, 1997.
18. Moed BR, McMichael JC: Outcomes of posterior wall fractures of the acetabulum: surgical technique. J Bone Joint Surg Am 90(Suppl 2 Pt 1):87–107, 2008.
19. Negrin LL, Benson CD, Seligson D: Prone or lateral? Use of the Kocher-Langenbeck approach to treat acetabular fractures. J Trauma 69:137–141, 2010.
20. Harris AM, Althausen P, Kellam JF, Bosse MJ: Simultaneous anterior and posterior approaches for complex acetabular fractures. J Orthop Trauma 22:494–497, 2008.
21. Griffin DB, Beaulé PE, Matta JM: Safety and efficacy of the extended iliofemoral approach in the treatment of complex fractures of the acetabulum. J Bone Joint Surg Br 87:1391–1396, 2005.
22. Helfet DL, Schmeling GJ: Management of complex acetabular fractures through single nonextensile exposures. Clin Orthop Relat Res 305:58–68, 1994.
23. Stöckle U, Hoffmann R, Südkamp NP, et al: Treatment of complex acetabular fractures through a modified extended iliofemoral approach. J Orthop Trauma 16:220–230, 2004.

CHAPTER 17

Direct Anterior Primary Total Hip Arthroplasty

Wadih Y. Matar and William J. Hozack

KEY POINTS

- The DA approach provides a safe approach to the hip joint with the advantage of being intermuscular without abductor muscle disruption; it allows for patients' early mobilization and fast recovery.
- Setup in the supine position is easy.
- The DA approach allows for intraoperative hip stability and accurate leg length measurements.
- No special operating room table is needed.

INTRODUCTION

Total hip arthroplasty (THA) can be performed through various approaches to the hip. The direct anterior (DA) approach has recently gained some popularity because it provides a safe approach to the hip joint with the advantage of being intermuscular without abductor muscle disruption, and it can allow for patients' early mobilization and fast recovery. Critics of the DA approach argue that the specialized table (e.g., Judet traction table) advocated as a means of performing this procedure is awkward and expensive and can lengthen operative time. We present here the direct anterior approach performed in the supine position but on a regular operative table. Advantages of performing THA through the DA approach in this manner (on a regular table) include easier setup time compared with the lateral position, lack of need for a specialized table, and an easy way to check for intraoperative hip stability and leg length discrepancy compared with the DA approach with a traction table.

Smith-Petersen was the first to describe the anterior approach to the hip in 1917 for congenital hip reduction, and subsequently in 1949, when he used the approach for mold arthroplasty.[1,2] The incision spanned from the middle of the iliac crest to the anterior superior iliac spine (ASIS) and then deviated slightly laterally along the medial border of the tensor fascia lata (TFL). Distally, the interval between the sartorius and the TFL is used, whereas proximally, the interval between the abdominal and gluteal muscles is developed down to bone, resulting in medial reflection of the abdominal muscles, the sartorius, and Poupart's ligament, and lateral reflection of the gluteus medius, the gluteus minimus, and the TFL. Smith-Petersen also advocated that motor nerve fibers to the rectus femoris originating from the femoral nerve must always be exposed before the rectus muscle and the acetabular origin of the iliacus muscle are incised. Finally, the approach also included an osteotomy of the anterior inferior iliac spine (AIIS) and the anterior acetabular wall.

This classic approach has been modified over the years by many surgeons.[3-8] These variations have revolved around the location and length of the incision, as well as handling of the TFL.[8] In France, Judet and Judet (1950) used a similar approach credited to Hueter to perform hip arthroplasty using a polymethylmethacrylate prosthesis.[5] In contrast to the Smith-Petersen approach, Judet and Judet used a traction table, allowing hip dislocation with traction, extension, and external rotation of the hip. Surgically, this approach included only the lower half of the Smith-Petersen approach and was vertical from the ASIS, passing between the TFL and sartorius muscles. Unlike the traditional Smith-Petersen approach, which detached the TFL from the iliac crest, Hueter's approach left the insertion of this muscle intact and allowed access to the hip by retraction of this muscle laterally.

During the latter part of the 20th century, the DA approach regained popularity among arthroplasty surgeons as they looked for tissue-sparing incisions that provided a safe way to perform THA with little muscle or tendon disruption.[9-11] The contemporary DA approach most resembles that described by Hueter. However, as surgeons became more comfortable with the approach, specialized retractors were developed, allowing the incision size to be decreased from the classic 15 cm to 6 to 8 cm.[12] The smaller incision is more aesthetically appealing to the patient; however, it is important to note that the underlying dissection remains the same as one would expect with a larger incision, and that, if needed, surgeons should not hesitate to enlarge the incision if exposure is compromised by the smaller incision. That being stated, the DA approach remains an acceptable tissue-sparing approach to THA.

INDICATIONS AND CONTRAINDICATIONS

All patients scheduled for THA according to its classic indications are candidates to undergo their replacement via the DA approach. The easiest patient from a technical standpoint is one who is thin, flexible, and nonmuscular with good bone quality and femoral head offset. It is imperative that the surgeon have expertise with hip replacement, along with different approaches to the hip, and that he or she can work with a knowledgeable and dedicated team to avoid unnecessary complications. Of course, this is true of all surgical procedures.

Few absolute contraindications are known; they include skin irritation or active infection over the incision site, abnormal proximal femoral anatomy requiring correction, and retained hardware that needs removal via the lateral approach. Lack of availability of specialized instruments should be considered as a relative contraindication, because the DA approach is performed more easily and less traumatically with the help of these instruments.[12-15] Patients with a high body mass index (BMI) should be evaluated individually because it may be significantly easier to perform THA through a DA approach. The depth of adipose tissue is significantly less anteriorly as compared with lateral or posterior locations, especially in female patients. Roue and associates prospectively compared two groups of patients: one with BMI less than 25, and the second with BMI of 25 or greater, who underwent THA through a 7-cm DA incision with the use of a Judet traction table.[16] Results showed that bleeding and operative time correlated with BMI, and that incision extension and abrasions were noted in the group with BMI of 25 or greater, possibly owing to stronger traction and reamer injury. Socket position was unaffected by BMI, and the authors did not find a higher complication rate related to skin breakdown or infection in the group with BMI greater than 25. Our only concern is the obese patient with abdominal tissue that overhangs the incision area, which may affect wound healing in these patients. Muscular patients pose the biggest technical challenge for the DA approach to THA (but this is true for the other approaches as well). Surgeons should start with a longer incision and should decrease its length as they become more comfortable with the approach, to a length that allows the surgery to be carried out safely.

PREOPERATIVE PLANNING

Preoperative workup of patients undergoing THA through the DA approach is similar to the workup conducted for a standard THA. Preoperative clinical evaluation consists of an examination for range of motion (ROM), abductor strength, and leg length, and complete neurovascular evaluation of both lower extremities. The patient's body habitus should be considered because central obesity around the abdomen can render the procedure more difficult during femoral canal preparation. On the other hand, increased adipose tissue around the thighs can affect the lateral and posterior approach to the hip but not necessarily the DA approach, prompting the surgeon to favor this approach.

Preoperative radiographs include an anteroposterior (AP) view of the pelvis showing both hips and the proximal two thirds of the femur, along with a cross-table or a frog-leg lateral of the affected hip. Radiographs are

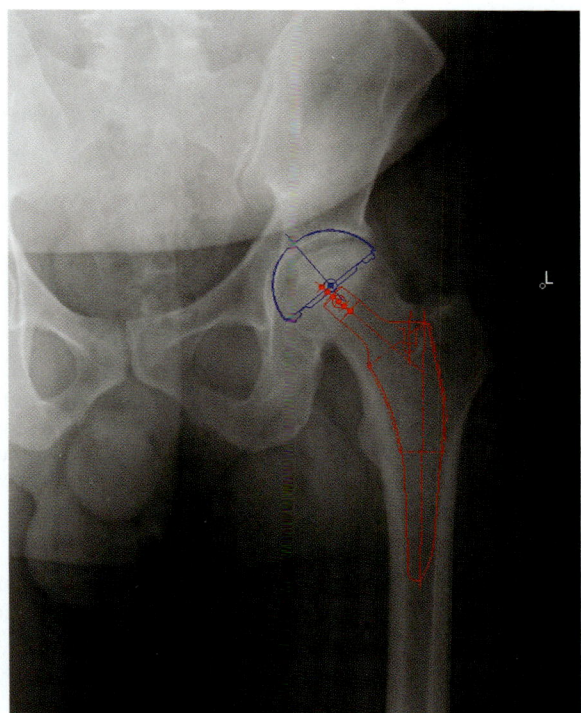

Figure 17-1. Preoperative anteroposterior (AP) view of a left hip after templating. The AP view is examined for appropriate implant fit, and the level of resection should be marked out. The varus/valgus angle should be chosen to closely match normal anatomy and reestablish the patient's femoral head offset. The acetabular implant is positioned at 45 degrees of abduction against the medial wall at the level of the teardrop.

examined for proximal femur anatomic abnormalities. Femoral offset should be evaluated carefully because decreased femoral offset or significant femoral retroversion can increase the technical difficulty of the DA approach. Preoperative templating is done in similar fashion to that carried out for a standard THA (Fig. 17-1). We are currently using relatively short femoral implants that require no reaming and have a recessed lateral shoulder, which makes their insertion through the DA approach easier.

OPERATIVE TECHNIQUE

The patient is placed in the supine position on a regular operative table with care taken to ensure that all bony prominences of the upper extremity are well padded. The supine position places the pelvis in a neutral position, facilitating cup placement, and permits more accurate intraoperative evaluation of hip stability and leg length. An additional arm board is placed longitudinally on the nonoperative lower aspect of the table, allowing abduction of the contralateral side and adduction of the operative side during femoral preparation. A 1-inch-high rectangular bump is placed under the pelvis, and the hip is positioned along the axis of flexion of the

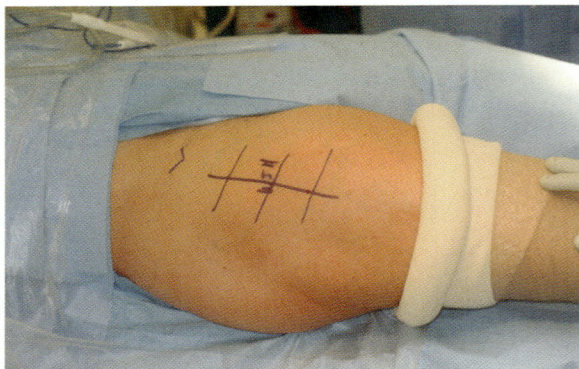

Figure 17-2. Starting 3 cm laterally and 3 cm distally to the anterior superior iliac spine (ASIS), a 10- to 12-cm straight incision is centered over the tensor fascia lata (TFL) and is directed in an oblique fashion laterally toward the lateral aspect of the distal femur.

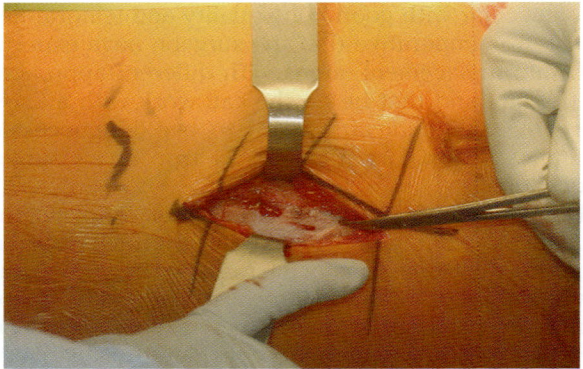

Figure 17-3. Perforating vessels (held with hemostat) through the fascia covering the tensor fascia lata (TFL). These vessels can be used to identify the TFL and are usually oriented from lateral to medial.

operative table. Before proceeding, the surgeon should verify that table flexion results in proper hip extension because this is helpful during femoral preparation. The limb is then prepped and draped to include the lower abdominal quadrant of the operative side.

The hip is approached through a 10- to 12-cm straight incision starting approximately 3 cm laterally and 3 cm distally to the ASIS; the starting point of this incision is approximately halfway between the ASIS and the greater trochanter (Fig. 17-2). The ASIS is easily identified from distal to proximal to avoid placing the incision too proximal. The incision is centered over the TFL and is directed laterally toward the lateral aspect of the distal femur. The placement of this incision makes it more lateral than the classic incision described by Smith-Peterson. Incision length can be increased as needed: Proximal extension improves femoral exposure, and distal extension facilitates acetabular exposure. Superficial dissection is then carried down to the fascia covering the TFL. The surgeon should properly identify the TFL to avoid injury to the lateral femoral cutaneous nerve (LFCN). This can be carried out by feeling for the muscle belly of the TFL between the surgeon's two thumbs. Also, the fascia covering the TFL is thicker and whiter medially along the interval between the TFL and the sartorius. Finally, this fascia is usually perforated by several blood vessels coming from lateral to medial. These vessels should be identified and cauterized before proceeding (Fig. 17-3).

To avoid injury to the LCFN, which lies on the sartorius muscle, the fascia overlying the TFL is incised longitudinally along its fibers at a distance 1 cm lateral to the TFL/sartorius interval represented by the thicker and whiter fascia medially. The medial fascial flap is then separated from the underlying fibers of the TFL in a parallel fashion to the muscle fibers (Fig. 17-4). A subfascial exposure is performed by retracting the fibers of the TFL laterally to expose adipose tissue that is covered by a thin layer of deeper fascia overlying the vastus muscles. The surgeon then may use his index finger to find the space proximal to the neck of the femur superior to the hip capsule at the proximal end of the

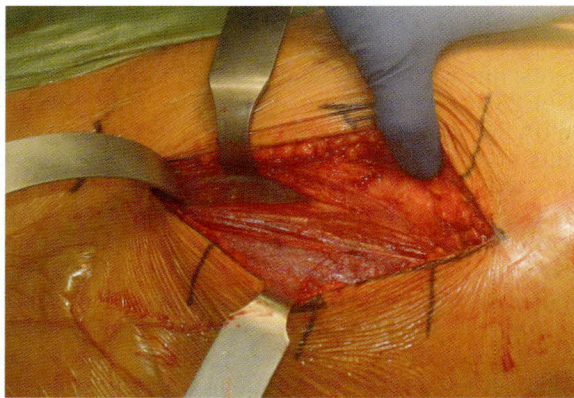

Figure 17-4. The fascia of the tensor fascia lata (TFL) is incised longitudinally 1 to 2 cm lateral to the TFL/sartorius interval, and the muscle fibers are retracted laterally to expose the deeper fascia covering the rectus femoris and vastus medialis muscles.

incision; the first narrow blunt Cobra superior retractor is introduced into that space and is used to retract the gluteus minimus and the superior part of the TFL muscle. A second sharp Hohmann lateral retractor is introduced lateral to the greater tuberosity through the lateral intramuscular septum and is used to retract the TFL muscle fibers laterally. The sartorius muscle is retracted medially with a Hibbs retractor to expose the deep thin fascia. Cautery is then used in a superficial fashion to release the fascia; the fascial release can be extended over the rectus femoris to improve visualization distally. Caution should be taken to avoid penetration of the underlying pericapsular fat with the cautery, because this area contains the ascending branches of the lateral circumflex vessels (Fig. 17-5). These should be dissected from the surrounding fat and cauterized individually before proceeding. After homeostasis is achieved, the remaining pericapsular adipose tissue may be removed with a rongeur, exposing the anterior hip capsule.

The inferior capsule should now be visualized, and an infracapsular space can be found by the surgeon's index finger. The third narrow blunt Cobra inferior retractor is placed inferior to the neck. This retractor is used to retract the rectus femoris muscle fibers medioinferiorly. A Cobb is then used to find a space anterior to the hip capsule along the anterior column inferior to the iliopsoas muscle. The Cobb is introduced and lifted anteriorly; cautery can be used to dissect any remaining muscle fibers from the anterior capsule. The fourth sharp Hohmann anterior retractor is placed anteriorly as the Cobb is removed; this should be done carefully to avoid injury to the femoral neurovascular bundle. A light attachment can be added to this retractor to improve acetabular visualization. With the four retractors in place, the hip capsule is fully exposed. An anterior capsulectomy is then performed with the use of cautery, exposing the femoral neck and head (Fig. 17-6). The distal extent of the capsulectomy is the vastus muscle; cautery into the vastus muscle can cause bleeding and should be avoided. The superior and inferior retractors are then moved intra-articularly and are used to retract the remaining superior and inferior capsule. They also protect the posterior structures when the femoral neck is osteotomized. Although a T-shaped capsulotomy can be performed and ultimately repaired at the end of the procedure, we have found that a capsulectomy provides greater visualization with minimal risk of dislocation.

The femoral saddle (area medial to the greater trochanter) is then exposed using cautery. The femoral neck osteotomy is performed in situ without dislocation of the femoral head. Internally rotating the leg ensures an even osteotomy along the anterior and posterior femoral cortices. The definitive osteotomy is marked out along the origin of the vastus medialis fibers spanning from the femoral saddle to an area 1 cm proximal to the lesser trochanter along the inferior femoral neck. A second osteotomy is marked 1 cm proximal and parallel to the definitive osteotomy. A narrow 1-cm-wide saw blade is then used to perform the osteotomies, starting with the proximal osteotomy. The narrow saw blade minimizes the potential for damage to the muscular structures in the area. The two osteotomies should be parallel to facilitate subsequent removal of the osteotomized disk between the two osteotomies (Fig. 17-7). The femoral head is then removed with a corkscrew. In some cases, overhanging large anterior osteophytes should be removed to facilitate femoral head removal.

After femoral head removal, the surgeons should ensure that the anterior retractor is placed directly onto

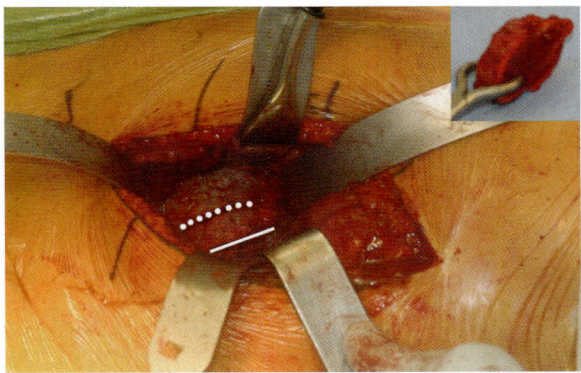

Figure 17-7. Double osteotomy is carried out with a narrow 1-cm saw. The definitive osteotomy *(solid white line)* is carried out along the origin of the vastus medialis from the femoral saddle to an area 1 cm proximal to the lesser trochanter on the femoral neck. A second osteotomy is carried out 1cm proximal to the definitive osteotomy *(dashed line)*. The osteotomized disk is then removed *(inset)*.

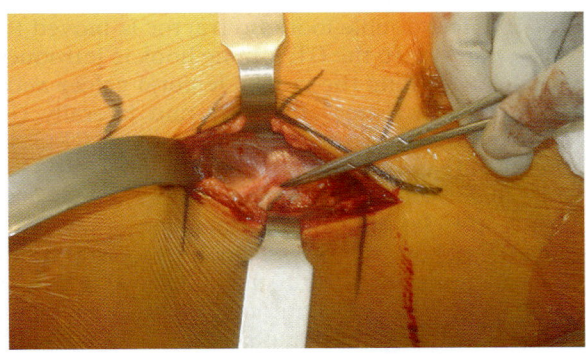

Figure 17-5. Once the deep fascia is released, cautery should be used to coagulate branches of the lateral circumflex artery and vein after their dissection from surrounding adipose tissue.

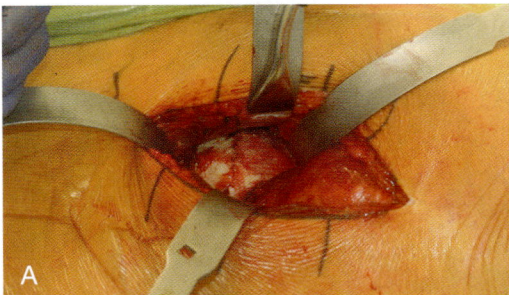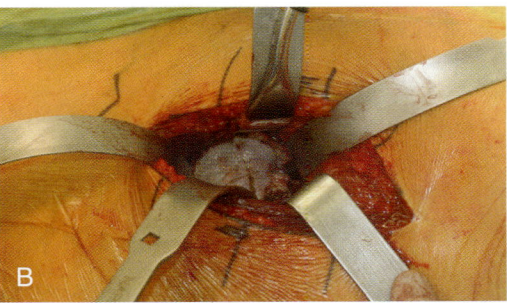

Figure 17-6. A, The anterior hip capsule is exposed by placing the superior, lateral, inferior, and anterior retractors. **B,** An anterior capsulectomy is then performed with cautery, exposing the anterior neck and the femoral head.

bone along the anterior column. The superior retractor is removed. The sharp lateral retractor is then moved along the posterior acetabular wall at 180 degrees opposite from the anterior retractors. The inferior blunt retractor is also moved to an area between the inferior capsule and the transverse acetabular ligament; this retractor should be placed 90 degrees opposite to the anterior retractor (Fig. 17-8). With the edges of the acetabulum properly exposed, the labrum, ligamentum teres, and transverse acetabular ligaments are excised. Any inferior or central osteophytes should be removed before reaming. Acetabular reaming is then carried out using a double-offset reamer handle by 2-mm increments until the desired size is reached. The double-offset reamer makes it easier to ream in the proper orientation and avoids injury to the muscles (i.e., the TFL or vastus), which can be encountered with the use of a straight reamer, as was demonstrated in a cadaveric

study by Meneghini and colleagues.[17] We find it easier to place the reamer inside the acetabulum and then connect it to the reamer handle; the latter avoids the soft tissue injury usually encountered by introducing a pre-mounted reamer (Fig. 17-9). We disengage the reamer from the handle before removing it manually with a kocher to minimize soft tissue damage. The last reamer is left in situ to verify coverage and acetabular position; we use the teardrop for acetabular height and the bottom of the cotyloid fossa for cup depth. We aim for 15 to 20 degrees of anteversion and 45 degrees of inclination. The acetabular implant is then put into place with the use of a double-offset inserter. Although a straight inserter can be used, the chance of excessive cup anteversion and abduction is increased when the double-offset inserter is not used.

After the acetabular component is implanted, all acetabular retractors are removed except the anterior lighted retractor. The operative table is then extended to 30 degrees as the operative leg is adducted 25 degrees and the opposite leg is abducted onto the previously added longitudinally placed arm board. An assistant then holds the extended adducted limb in maximal external rotation as the proximal femur is delivered through the wound. The latter is done by first placing a double-footed retractor between the remaining supero-posterior capsule and the glutei muscles. The sharp, lateral double-angled retractor is once again placed lateral to the greater trochanter (GT) to improve visualization. The remaining superoposterior capsule, which is shaped like a triangle, is then excised using cautery (Fig. 17-10). The double-footed retractor is moved to a position posterior to the GT. A bone hook is introduced intramedullarly along the medial femoral calcar and is used to pull the femur anteriorly and laterally (Fig. 17-11); the surgeon should ensure that the GT is not caught on the rim of the acetabulum. In some cases, to facilitate femoral delivery, cautery is used to release the piriformis muscle, and an assistant can apply gentle push on the posteriorly placed double-footed retractor to assist in translating the femur anteriorly. Once the femur is delivered, the anteriorly lighted acetabular retractor is removed and is replaced by a double-footed retractor along the medial aspect of the femur. The femoral neck cut is then assessed, and re-cut is performed if needed.

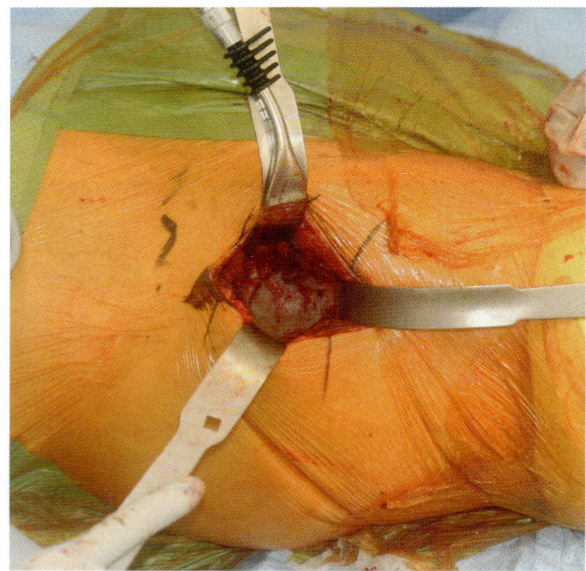

Figure 17-8. To ensure proper acetabular exposure, a sharp lateral retractor is placed along the posterior acetabular wall and an inferomedial blunt retractor is placed between the inferior capsule and the transverse acetabular ligament.

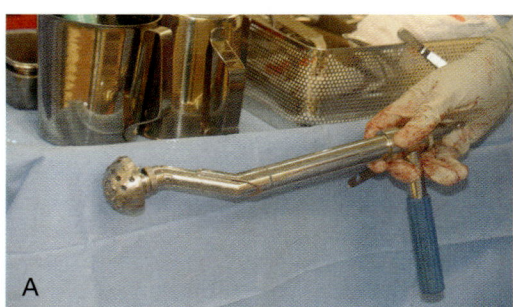
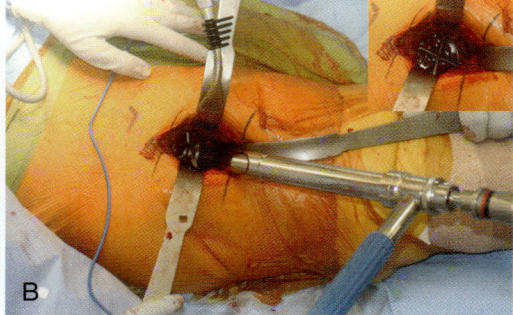

Figure 17-9. A, A double-offset reamer is used for acetabular preparation. **B,** The reamer is placed inside the acetabulum (*inset*) and then is hooked onto the reamer handle.

A small curette is used to find the orientation of the femoral canal. The femur is then broached sequentially until the desired broach fit is achieved. A double-offset broach handle makes broaching easier by avoiding medial soft tissue or the need to excessively extend the

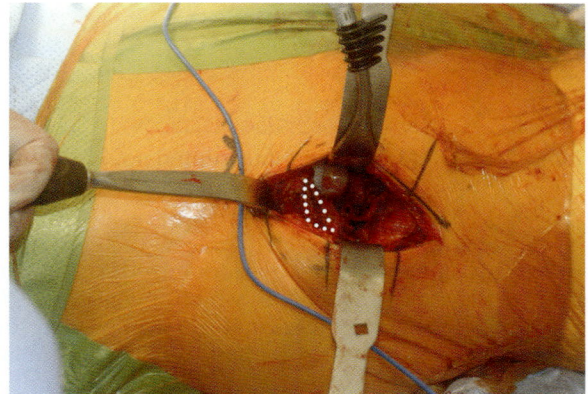

Figure 17-10. Before the proximal femur is delivered, a double-footed retractor is placed between the remaining superoposterior capsule and the glutei muscles. The remaining capsule, which is shaped like a triangle *(dotted triangle),* is then excised by using cautery.

hip[15] (Fig. 17-12). It is important to lateralize with the initial broach to avoid varus malposition of the implant. Both cemented and uncemented prostheses can be implanted. Once the desired broach size is attained, a trial neck and head are placed on the broach (see Fig. 17-12). Retractors are then removed, and the hip is reduced using traction and internal rotation. The hip is checked for stability and appropriate leg length. The latter is carried out by having the assistant hold both legs together in line with the patient's body. The trials are then removed, and the appropriate prosthesis is implanted. This should be carried out by placing the final implant by hand into the prepared femur with a nonlocking impact, while applying force laterally to avoid possible calcar fracture. The hip is then reduced. After a stability check, the operating table is returned to its starting position, and the hip is irrigated thoroughly. Before closure, meticulous homeostasis, especially of the coagulated vessels at the beginning of the case, is obtained. Closure is done by using interrupted no. 1 Monocryl suture through the fascia overlying the TFL (Fig. 17-13). Surgeons should avoid taking big bites to avoid injury to the LCFN. The subcutaneous layer is again lavaged before its closure with no. 1 Vicryl and then with a no. Monocryl suture placed in the subcuticular location. Staples are used for the skin, and the incision is covered with a sterile dressing.

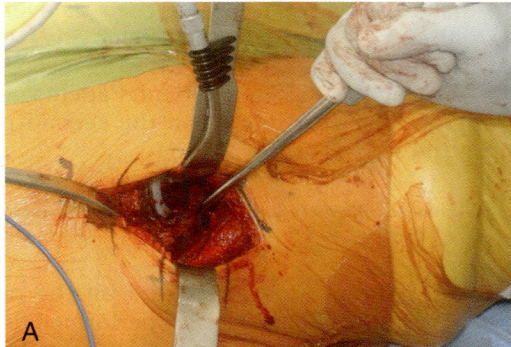
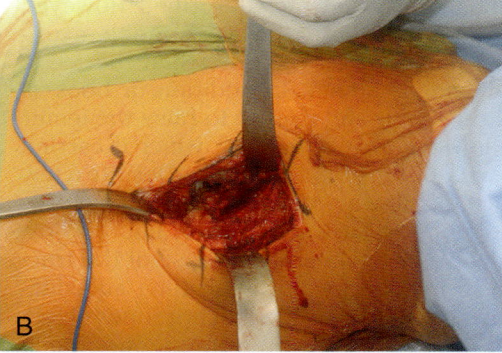

Figure 17-11. A, The femur is pulled anteriorly with a bone hook as a double-footed retractor is placed posterior to the greater trochanter (GT). In some cases, the piriformis muscle needs to be released to facilitate the anterior translation of the femur. **B,** The femur is delivered anteriorly as the leg is maintained in adduction, extension, and external rotation.

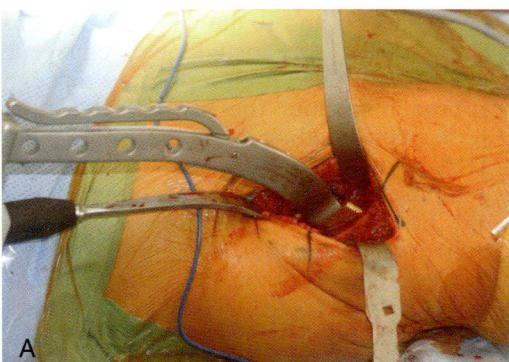
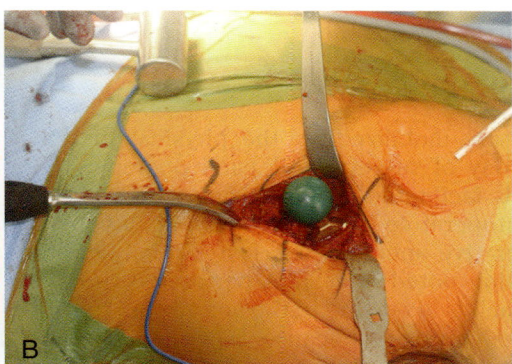

Figure 17-12. A, An offset broach handle is used during femoral preparation. **B,** With the final broach left in situ, a trial femoral head and trial are placed on the broach, and the hip is reduced.

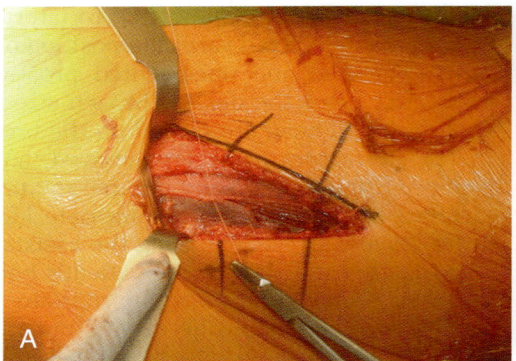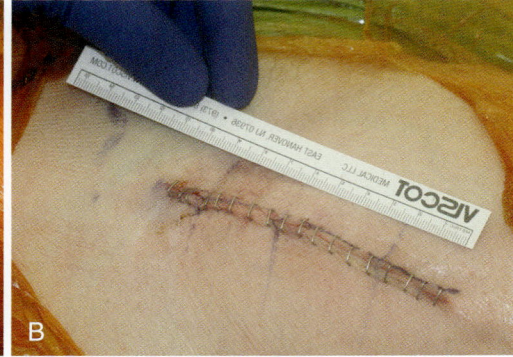

Figure 17-13. A, The fascia covering the tensor fascia lata (TFL) is closed using figure-of-eight interrupted no. 1 Monocryl. **B,** Staples are used for the skin.

VARIATIONS/UNUSUAL SITUATIONS

Several variations of the DA approach have been described, including the use of additional mini-incisions for femoral and acetabular preparation,[9,13] along with different setup positions such as placing the patient in the lateral decubitus position[18] or in the supine position with the use of a traction table, as described by Matta and co-workers.[11,12,19] The patient is placed on the traction table and has boot traction applied to both feet. Acetabular preparation and implantation are done using a similar method to the one already described. However, femoral preparation differs by having the table externally rotate the femur by 90 degrees while the leg is hyperextended and adducted. In addition, a hook is placed behind the femur and is used to raise the femur anteriorly to allow femoral preparation, which is carried out with the use of offset broach handles. Despite a few advantages such as allowing the surgeon to verify cup position intraoperatively with the use of fluoroscopy, we have found several limitations with use of the traction table. These include longer setup time and difficulty testing hip stability and leg length intraoperatively unless the feet are disengaged from the traction table or fluoroscopy is used, which subjects the patient and the surgeon to undue radiation. Furthermore, a few reports of intraoperative femoral and ankle fractures are alarming, discouraging us from using the traction table.[11,19]

POSTOPERATIVE CARE

Our patients are mobilized by the physical therapy team on the day of surgery. This early postoperative mobilization is facilitated by optimizing pain management and postoperative hemodynamics (e.g., hypotension, postoperative anemia). The faster rehabilitation and mobilization noted after THA performed through the DA approach is likely due to the soft tissue–sparing nature of the approach because the major muscle groups, especially the abductors, are not violated throughout the procedure.[14,19,20] We no longer use any postoperative hip precaution because of findings reported by the prospective randomized study conducted by Peak and associates, which investigated the role of postoperative functional restrictions in our direct lateral approach THA patient population.[21] When looking at dislocation within the first 6 postoperative months as the endpoint, they found only one dislocation in the entire cohort in a patient from the "restricted" group during transfer from the operating room table to the bed with an abduction pillow in place. Furthermore, patients in the "unrestricted" group returned to side-sleeping sooner, driving automobiles more often, returning to work sooner, and having a higher level of satisfaction with the pace of their recovery than those in the "restricted" group. Removing the functional restrictions was associated with a cost savings of approximately $655 per patient. Patients usually are discharged the next day or on the second postoperative day, directly to home.

RESULTS

Several authors have reported on the outcomes and clinical results following THA performed through the DA approach[9-13,22]; others have performed comparative studies.[14,20,23] After using the traction table, Matta and colleagues reported on a consecutive series of 494 THAs performed through the DA approach, whereas Siguier and co-workers described 1037 THAs performed through a mini-DA approach, in which the skin incision was between 5 cm and 10 cm.[11,12] On the other hand, Kennon and associates reported on a consecutive series of more than 2132 THAs performed through the anterior approach without the use of a traction table.[13] This series consisted of both cemented and uncemented THAs and included procedures performed in "complex" patients such as those with congenital hip dysplasia, old fractures, and previous osteotomies. Although they were very thorough in describing the surgical procedures and associated complications, all of these investigators failed to report any clinical outcome measurements.

Hozack and colleagues randomized 122 THA patients to a DA approach, without the use of a traction table, or to a direct lateral approach.[14] The same postoperative and pain control protocols were used in both groups. The authors did not find a statistical difference between the two groups with regard to analgesic need, estimated blood loss, drop in hemoglobin, need for transfusion, surgical time, or length of hospital stay. However, they did report early (up to 1 year) postoperative statistically significant improvements in clinical outcome scores among the DA group, as measured by the Short Form-36, the Western Ontario McMaster Osteoarthritis Index, and linear analog scale assessment. The reported advantage of the DA group was lost in the 2-year follow-up group.

Early improvements in the DA group were corroborated by Nakata and co-workers in a comparison with a group of patients who underwent THA through a minimally invasive posterior approach to the hip.[20] The DA group could perform a single-leg 5-second stance for a shorter time, a lower percentage of group members exhibited persistent Trendelenburg sign at 3 weeks (29% versus 67%), and patients in this group showed better functional recovery, as measured by their ability to walk and by Merle d'Aubigné and Postel scores. However, these noted clinical outcome improvements in the DA group were no longer statistically better at 2 and 6 months.

CURRENT CONTROVERSIES AND FUTURE CONSIDERATIONS

The DA approach can be used to perform hip resurfacing arthroplasty with specific modifications in surgical steps and instrumentation design. However, independent of current controversies regarding metal-on-metal bearings, performing resurfacing arthroplasty through the DA approach is quite challenging, because surgeons have to dislocate the hip and perform the whole procedure while making sure to avoid compromising the blood supply to the hip (i.e., posterior circumflex artery)—a problem that is not an issue with conventional THA.

In the hands of experienced surgeons, the DA approach can be used to perform revision THA. However, the variety of possible cases is limited to liner exchange and simple cup revision on the acetabular side and simple stem revision on the femoral side. The DA approach does not provide full exposure to the acetabulum, especially the posterior column, when complex acetabular reconstruction is performed. On the femoral side, revision surgical exposure can be achieved through limited extension of the DA approach distally, or via a separate lateral approach to the femur; however, we favor the direct lateral approach for these cases owing to its ease of completion and its excellent acetabular exposure if needed.

COMPLICATIONS

In addition to expected systemic complications following THA, few complications inherent to the DA approach have been described. On the other hand, it is important to note that the risk of dislocation, which can be elevated with other, more traditional approaches to the hip (2% to 10%),[24-28] actually is lower following the DA approach, with reported rates ranging from 0.61% to 1.5%.[11-13,29]

With regard to inherent complications due to the approach, injury to the LCFN remains at the forefront for consideration. The applied anatomy of this nerve has been studied extensively, and different areas of danger to the common trunk, as well as the gluteal and femoral branches of the LCFN, have been identified.[30,31] These areas of danger can be avoided by placing the incision more lateral than the traditional sartorius/TFL interval and as distal from the ASIS as possible. After applying these recommendations, Hozack reported on the incidence of LCFN injury in an initial 52 cases. He found that 82.7% of patients had no symptoms, whereas 9.6% had peri-incisional paresthesia and 7.7% had temporary anterior paresthesia. All symptoms had resolved by the time of the 2-year follow-up.

CONCLUSION

The DA approach is a safe approach for performing THA; it offers the advantage of being intermuscular without substantial compromise of any muscular attachment. This approach can be performed easily with the patient in the supine position without the use of a traction table, allowing intraoperative hip stability and leg length measurement checks. In addition, it may offer a lower risk of dislocation than the more traditional THA approaches, and with proper incision placement, the risk of LCFN is significantly reduced.

REFERENCES

1. Smith-Petersen MN: A new supra-articular subperiosteal approach to the hip joint. Am J Orthop Surg 15:592, 1917.
2. Smith-Petersen MN: Approach to and exposure of the hip joint for mold arthroplasty. J Bone Joint Surg Am 31:40, 1949.
3. Cubbins WR, Callahan JJ, Scuderi CS: Fractures of the neck of the femur. Surg Gynecol Obstet 68:87, 1939.
4. Fahey JJ: Surgical approaches to bones and joints. Surg Clin North Am 29:65, 1949.
5. Judet J, Judet R: The use of an artificial femoral head for arthroplasty of the hip joint. J Bone Joint Surg Br 32:166, 1950.
6. Kirkaldy-Willis WH: Ischio-femoral arthrodesis of the hip in tuberculosis; an anterior approach. J Bone Joint Surg Br 32:187, 1950.
7. Luck JV: A transverse anterior approach to the hip. J Bone Joint Surg Am 37:534, 1955.
8. Lowell JD, Aufranc OE: The anterior approach to the hip joint. Clin Orthop Relat Res 61:193, 1968.
9. Light TR, Keggi KJ: Anterior approach to hip arthroplasty. Clin Orthop Relat Res 152:255, 1980.
10. Keggi KJ, Huo MH, Zatorski LE: Anterior approach to total hip replacement: surgical technique and clinical results of our first one thousand cases using non-cemented prostheses. Yale J Biol Med 66:243, 1993.
11. Matta JM, Shahrdar C, Ferguson T: Single-incision anterior approach for total hip arthroplasty on an orthopaedic table. Clin Orthop Relat Res 441:115, 2005.
12. Siguier T, Siguier M, Brumpt B: Mini-incision anterior approach does not increase dislocation rate: a study of 1037 total hip replacements. Clin Orthop Relat Res 426:164, 2004.

13. Kennon RE, Keggi JM, Wetmore RS, et al: Total hip arthroplasty through a minimally invasive anterior surgical approach. J Bone Joint Surg Am 85(Suppl 4):39, 2003.

14. Hozack WJ: A randomized, prospective study comparing two surgical techniques. The Hip Society, 2005.

15. Nogler M, Krismer M, Hozack WJ, et al: A double offset broach handle for preparation of the femoral cavity in minimally invasive direct anterior total hip arthroplasty. J Arthroplasty 21:1206, 2006.

16. Roué J, de Thomasson E, Carlier AM, Mazel C: [Influence of body mass index on outcome of total hip arthroplasty via a minimally invasive anterior approach]. Rev Chir Orthop Reparatrice Appar Mot 93:165, 2007.

17. Meneghini RM, Pagnano MW, Trousdale RT, Hozack WJ: Muscle damage during MIS total hip arthroplasty: Smith-Petersen versus posterior approach. Clin Orthop Relat Res 453:293, 2006.

18. Michel MC, Witschger P: MicroHip: a minimally invasive procedure for total hip replacement surgery using a modified Smith-Peterson approach. Orthop Traumatol Rehabil 9:46, 2007.

19. Paillard P: Hip replacement by a minimal anterior approach. Int Orthop 31(Suppl 1):S13–S15, 2007.

20. Nakata K, Nishikawa M, Yamamoto K, et al: A clinical comparative study of the direct anterior with mini-posterior approach: two consecutive series. J Arthroplasty 24:698–704, 2009.

21. Peak EL, Parvizi J, Ciminiello M, et al: The role of patient restrictions in reducing the prevalence of early dislocation following total hip arthroplasty: a randomized, prospective study. J Bone Joint Surg Am 87:247, 2005.

22. Masonis J, Thompson C, Odum S: Safe and accurate: learning the direct anterior total hip arthroplasty. Orthopedics 31(12 Suppl 2), 2008.

23. D'Arrigo C, Speranza A, Monaco E, et al: Learning curve in tissue sparing total hip replacement: comparison between different approaches. J Orthop Traumatol 10:47, 2009.

24. Coventry MB: Late dislocations in patients with Charnley total hip arthroplasty. J Bone Joint Surg Am 67:832, 1985.

25. McCollum DE, Gray WJ: Dislocation after total hip arthroplasty: causes and prevention. Clin Orthop Relat Res 261:159, 1990.

26. Kelley SS, Lachiewicz PF, Hickman JM, Paterno SM: Relationship of femoral head and acetabular size to the prevalence of dislocation. Clin Orthop Relat Res 355:163, 1998.

27. Robbins GM, Masri BA, Garbuz DS, et al: Treatment of hip instability. Orthop Clin North Am 32:593, 2001.

28. DeWal H, Su E, DiCesare PE: Instability following total hip arthroplasty. Am J Orthop 32:377, 2003.

29. Sariali E, Leonard P, Mamoudy P: Dislocation after total hip arthroplasty using Hueter anterior approach. J Arthroplasty 23:266, 2008.

30. Chen LH, Huang QW, Wang WJ, et al: The applied anatomy of anterior approach for minimally invasive hip joint surgery. Clin Anat 22:250, 2009.

31. Ropars M, Morandi X, Huten D, et al: Anatomical study of the lateral femoral cutaneous nerve with special reference to minimally invasive anterior approach for total hip replacement. Surg Radiol Anat 31:199, 2009.

CHAPTER 18

Anterolateral Approach for Primary Total Hip Replacement

Michael E. Berend

KEY POINTS

- The anterolateral approach to the hip retains the posterior capsule and the external rotators, which may enhance hip stability.
- The anterolateral approach reduces hip dislocation compared with the posterior approach.
- Patients at higher risk for postoperative dislocation such as those with spasticity, high range of motion, small socket sizes, abductor deficiencies, and compliance issues such as alcohol abuse may benefit from an anterolateral approach.
- Repair of the anterior portion of the abductors is critical to gait recovery after an anterolateral approach to total hip arthroplasty (THA).
- The anterolateral approach facilitates repair of partial gluteus medius/minimus tendinous avulsions in patients with hip arthritis.

INTRODUCTION AND HISTORY

The anterolateral approach to the hip for total hip replacement (THR) was described and popularized by Hardinge in 1970.[1] It offers an extensile approach for both primary and revision THR. Traditionally, it involved a split in the anterior portion of the abductor musculature and hip capsule. Modifications have been made in the trajectory and extent of the abductor split over the past three decades.[2,3] Exposure of the acetabulum involves retractor insertion to achieve posterior displacement of the femur. In general, advantages have traditionally been ascribed to extensibility and reduction of postoperative dislocation in primary[3-6] and revision THR[7]; proposed disadvantages have included postoperative limp and abductor weakness.

PATIENT SELECTION

Most patients who are indicated for a total hip arthroplasty are amenable to an anterolateral surgical approach. Patients who are at higher risk for postoperative dislocation such as femoral neck fracture,[8] neuromuscular disorders,[9] high range of motion (ROM),[10] abductor tendon tears,[11] and rotational deformities may benefit from an anterolateral surgical approach.

POSITIONING

The patient is placed in the lateral decubitus position with the use of a padded pegboard. Attention to ensure that the pelvis is perpendicular to the table is important before skin preparation and draping. Special attention should be focused on posterior stability of the pelvis because femoral retraction to achieve acetabular exposure tends to retrovert the pelvis.

An axillary roll is inserted to help protect the brachial plexus. The leg is positioned anterior to the table during femoral preparation, and leg sterility must be ensured. This may be accomplished with multiple stockinettes or a leg bag, in which the distal extent of the leg may be placed during femoral preparation.

SURGICAL ANATOMY

The incision for an anterolateral approach to the hip is placed over the greater trochanter. With smaller incisions, approximately two thirds of the incision should be proximal to the tip of the trochanter and one third distal. An oblique incision (proximal extent posterior and distal extent anterior) may permit a smaller incision, and skin mobility permits a mobile window during acetabular preparation through the distal extent of the incision. Similarly the proximal extent may be mobilized during femoral preparation and implant insertion.

The tensor fascia and the gluteus maximus are split in line with their fibers centered over the greater trochanter, exposing the gluteus medius insertion. The tendinous portion of the gluteus medius is covered superiorly by muscular fibers and must be included in the final repair. The proximal portion of the vastus lateralis inserts into the vastus ridge at the inferior portion of the greater trochanter. Approximately 2 cm of the anterior one third of the vastus lateralis is split in line with its fibers and is extended superiorly over the anterior portion of the trochanter and obliquely at a 70- to 90-degree angle, spreading the fibers of the gluteus medius; this exposes the gluteus minimus and hip capsule (Fig. 18-1). Over the anterior-superior femoral neck, the gluteus minimus and capsule are split in one layer; this facilitates subsequent repair in a tenodesis fashion. A retractor can be placed into the hip joint at this point, and the femoral insertion of the anterior hip

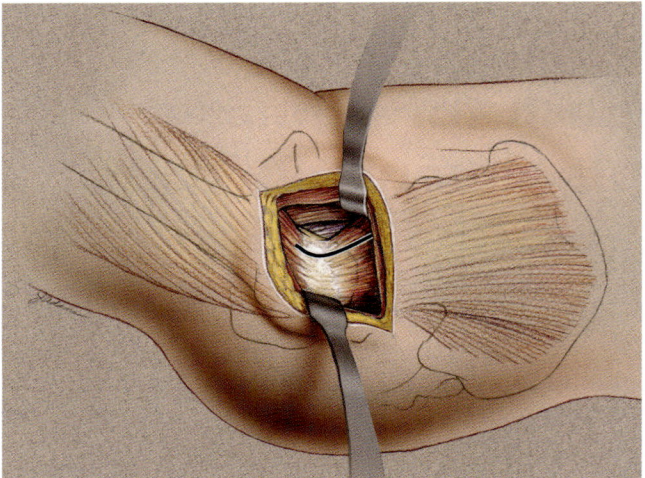

Figure 18-1. Graphical representation of the deep dissection of the abductors for an anterolateral approach to the hip shown in the operative photograph. (Used with permission from JIS, Inc. Joanne Adams.) *(Krenzel BA, Berend ME, Malinzak RA, et al: High preoperative range of motion is a significant risk factor for dislocation in primary total hip arthroplasty, J Arthroplasty 25(6 Suppl):31–35, 2010; Epub 2010 Jun 11.)*

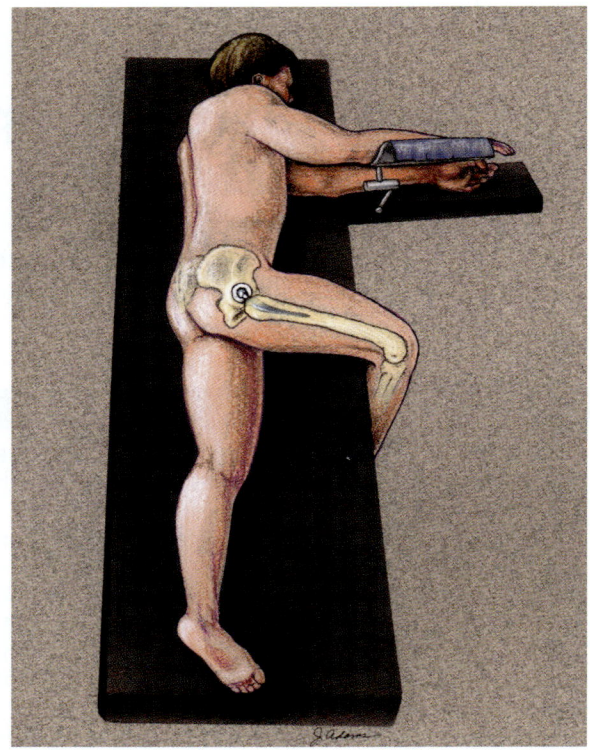

Figure 18-2. Graphic representation of leg position utilized during anterolateral approach to the hip. (Used with permission from JIS, Inc. Joanne Adams.)

capsule and the iliofemoral or Y ligament are released off the femur with external rotation of the leg. The release is continued down to the level of the lesser trochanter and the iliopsoas insertion. The superior dissection is carried cephalad to the level of the acetabular rim. Care should be taken to not extend the abductor split more than 4 cm superior to the tip of the greater trochanter because the superior gluteal nerve may be at risk of injury.[11]

The opportunity for recognition and repair of attritional abductor tears has been described with this approach.[12] Often the superior-most superficial layer of the gluteal medius fibers is intact, and after they are incised, a significant tear of the insertion of the gluteal medius is noted. In these cases, a large osteophyte with a sclerotic cortex is present on the anterior portion of the trochanter. This is similar in appearance to a rotator cuff tear and the changes noted in the humeral head. This osteophyte is removed at the completion of the case to expose cancellous bone and to facilitate healing of the repaired abductor attritional tear.

The hip can be dislocated with external rotation of the leg (Fig. 18-2). A bone hook or hip skid may be a useful adjunct if soft tissue contracture or osteophytes inhibit dislocation. Alternatively, a neck cut can be made in situ, as in cases of acetabular protrusio or significant deformity. Retractors should be placed around the femoral neck and a "napkin ring" of bone removed; this allows femoral head visualization and removal with a corkscrew. Alternatively, after dislocation, retractors are placed around the superior and inferior femoral neck, while the femoral neck osteotomy is completed at the level based on preoperative templating with reference to the lesser trochanter. The femoral head is then removed.

With external rotation of the leg, the inferior hip capsule is placed under tension and can be divided, which further facilitates posterior displacement of the femur and enhances acetabular exposure. Anterior and posterior acetabular retractors are placed between the capsule and the acetabular rim. The anterior retractor is placed under the iliopsoas and anterior capsule, while the posterior retractor is placed into the ischium at a 4 and 8 o'clock positions, respectively. A superior "Hohmann-type" retractor is placed beneath the capsule and the gluteal muscles. Acetabular reaming and component insertion are then undertaken.

Acetabular implantation and positioning are based on preoperative templating. In general, 5 to 10 degrees less acetabular anteversion is recommended with the anterolateral approach in comparison with the posterior surgical approach, which divides the posterior capsule. Following acetabular implantation, residual osteophytes, which protrude beyond the cup and liner, are removed. Attention should be focused on the anterior-superior and posterior-inferior osteophytes, which may limit range of motion through extra-articular impingement.

Following acetabular implantation, attention is turned to the femur. Acetabular retractors are removed and the proximal femur is exposed with flexion of the hip and external rotation of the limb. Positioning of the tibia may be referenced to determine femoral anteversion. Alternatively, native femoral neck orientation may be reproduced in hips without femoral, acetabular, or combination rotational deformities. A curved Bennett-type retractor, which provides posterior soft tissue retraction and femoral elevation, is placed beneath the greater trochanter. A sharp Hohmann is placed in the piriformis fossa; it retracts the remaining portion of the hip capsule and abductors that are inserting into the proximal femur. The femur is prepared with reamers or broaches for whatever stem design is to be implanted. Most often, the femoral neck anteversion is replicated with the femoral implant. In cases of severe dysplasia, femoral anteversion must be carefully assessed because it can be significantly increased, which may lead to anterior instability in cases of excessive combined acetabular and femoral anteversion.

Based on preoperative templating and limb length correction necessary during THA, the femoral implant position may be determined by measurement from the lesser trochanter or from the tip of the greater trochanter. Often a line drawn perpendicular to the longitudinal axis of the femur from the tip of the greater trochanter passes through the center of the femoral head. This is a helpful starting point for femoral positioning and restoration of the hip center of rotation.

Next, a trial reduction is performed. The assistant who is positioning the limb should provide simultaneous longitudinal traction and internal rotation, which will permit reduction. Assessment of the force required to perform the reduction is often an early indication of leg length and appropriate modifications required to achieve a stable articulation. A so-called *shuck test* is used to assess soft tissue tension about the hip. This is qualitative rather than quantitative and provides feedback; results may vary based on overall patient laxity, head size, offset, and implant position. In the anterolateral approach, whereby posterior soft tissues including the capsule, external rotators, and gluteal sleeve are intact, soft tissue tension may be helpful in assessing offset and leg length. Range of motion (ROM) should include flexion and internal rotation with examination for anterior-superior impingement and subluxation, followed by extension and external rotation. ROM before impingement varies according to implant femoral head size, femoral offset, cup size, and soft tissue laxity. Modifications in length and offset may correct soft tissue laxities and impingement patterns observed during trialing. Leg length is assessed in the context of all aspects of trialing, and a Gallizzi-type examination is performed with the thighs parallel to compare the patella of the operative leg with that of the nonoperative down leg.

Following femoral implantation and femoral head insertion, an abductor repair is performed. Numerous repair techniques have been described. We have utilized two drill holes in the proximal femur—one for the capsule and one for the gluteus medius tendon. The superior capsule is closed in the same layer as the gluteus minimus with a running nonabsorbable polyester suture. The suture is passed through the proximal drill hole, which allows soft tissue to bone repair. A second nonabsorbable suture, in a horizontal mattress fashion, is utilized to repair the vastus lateralis and the superior gluteus medius in one layer. The second portion of the repair begins with the anterior border of the vastus lateralis reapproximated to the posterior portion. The suture is passed out and back through the gluteus medius tendon, then through the proximal bone tunnel through the greater trochanter. The mattress suture is placed through the tendinous portion of the medius insertion and finally is tied to the distal end of the suture. The entire repair is then oversewn with a running absorbable suture from the proximal to the distal portion of the medius and vastus split. The fascia and remaining soft tissues are closed in a standard fashion.

Postoperative hip precautions most likely are not as necessary with the anterolateral approach as with the posterior approach.[13] Peak and associates demonstrated early return to activities and greater patient satisfaction with few restrictions. Similar findings have not been demonstrated with the posterior approach.

SPECIAL CONSIDERATIONS

1. The superior gluteal nerve is at risk during abductor musculature splitting and must be carefully protected.[11]
2. Functional repair of the abductors and the capsule to the proximal femoral bone is critical at the completion of the case. This can involve soft tissue to soft tissue or soft tissue to bone.
3. Preoperatively, consider the influence of patient factors such as diagnosis, preoperative range of motion,[10] surgical approach,[4] and head size on restrictions and dislocation. Higher-risk patients may benefit from an anterolateral surgical approach.[7-9]

LIMITATIONS

Potential drawbacks of the anterolateral approach include possible compromised return of abductor function, more challenging acetabular exposure in cases of pelvic defects and discontinuity of treatments, heterotopic ossification, and can be associated with increased risk of intraoperative femoral fracture.[14,15] Abductor weakness and persistent limp have been reported with the anterolateral approach.

SUMMARY OF BENEFITS

The anterolateral approach to the hip offers excellent exposure of the acetabulum and proximal femur. It preserves the posterior capsule and short external rotators; this reduces rates of postoperative instability following THR, which has been described by many authors with both primary and revision THR. We have stratified our dislocation data according to surgical approach, prosthetic femoral head size, and patients' preoperative range of motion.[10] We reported an overall dislocation rate of 2.8% for a cohort of THR patients from our center. A significant reduction in postoperative dislocation was noted with the anterolateral approach (0.37% versus 3.6% for the posterior approach) (Fig. 18-3).

Patients with significant flexion contracture of the hip may benefit from this surgical exposure because the anterior capsule can be readily released off both the femoral side and the acetabular side through this

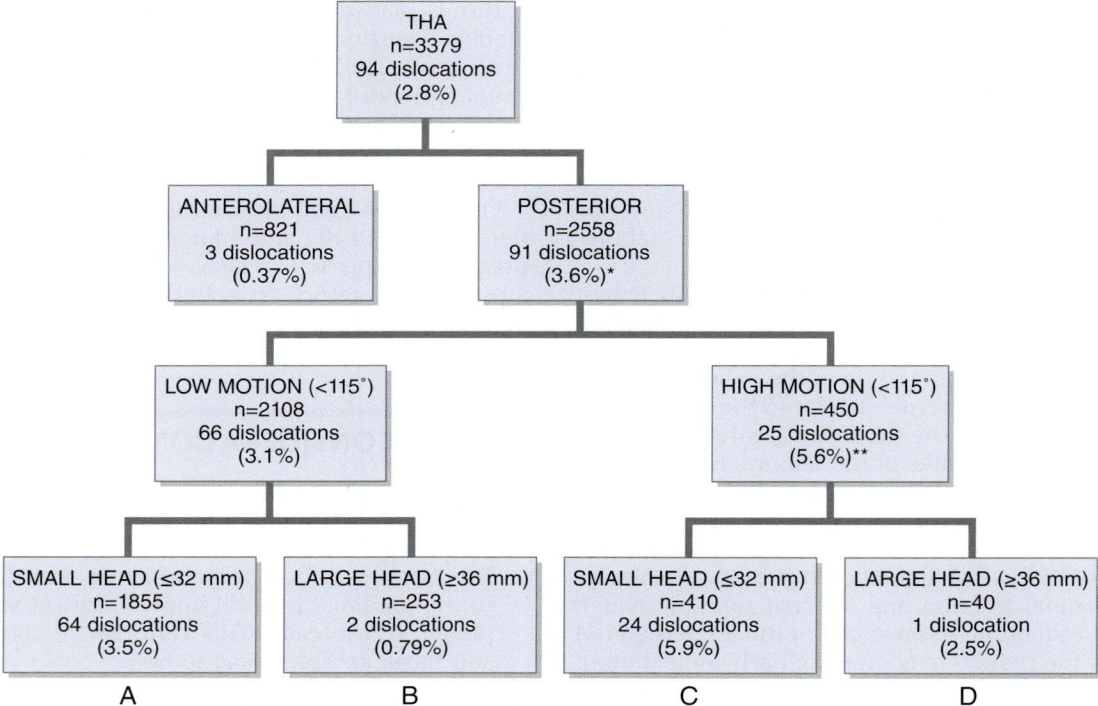

Figure 18-3. Influence of preoperative range of motion, surgical approach, and head size on dislocation following primary total hip replacement (THR). The overall dislocation rate for all THRs was 2.8%. A significant reduction in postoperative dislocation was noted with the anterolateral approach (0.37% vs. 3.6% for the posterior approach). *(Redrawn from Krenzel BA, Berend ME, Malinzak RA, et al: High preoperative range of motion is a significant risk factor for dislocation in primary total hip arthroplasty. J Arthroplasty 25[6 Suppl]:31–35, 2010.)*

approach. Patients with neuromuscular conditions such as Parkinson's disease, post cerebrovascular accident (CVA), or dementia may benefit from the protective effect of the anterolateral surgical approach in reducing dislocation. Finally, patients with lower extremity spasticity, as occurs after cerebrovascular events or Parkinson's disease, may significantly benefit from an anterolateral approach with preservation of posterior capsular structures, reducing the risk of postoperative instability.

REFERENCES

1. Hardinge K: The direct lateral approach to the hip. J Bone Joint Surg Br 64:17–19, 1982.
2. Frndak PA, Mallory TH, Lombardi AV Jr: Translateral surgical approach to the hip: the abductor muscle "split." Clin Orthop Relat Res 295:135–141, 1993.
3. Lombardi AV Jr, Mallory TH, Fada RA: Surgical technique in total hip arthroplasty utilizing the anterolateral approach. Surg Technol Int IX:291–294, 2000.
4. Berry DJ, von Knoch M, Schleck CD, Harmsen WS: Effect of femoral head diameter and operative approach on risk of dislocation after primary total hip arthroplasty. J Bone Joint Surg Am 87:2456–2463, 2005.
5. Masonis JL, Bourne RB: Surgical approach, abductor function, and total hip arthroplasty dislocation. Clin Orthop Relat Res 405:46–53, 2002.
6. Mulliken BD, Rorabeck CH, Bourne RB, Nayak N: A modified direct lateral approach in total hip arthroplasty: a comprehensive review. J Arthroplasty 13:737–747, 1998.
7. Smith TM, Berend KR, Lombardi AV Jr, et al: Isolated liner exchange using the anterolateral approach is associated with a low risk of dislocation. Clin Orthop Relat Res 441:221–226, 2005.
8. Enocson A, Hedbeck CJ, Tidermark J, et al: Dislocation of total hip replacement in patients with fractures of the femoral neck. Acta Orthop 80:184–189, 2009.
9. Queally JM, Abdulkarim A, Mulhall KJ: Total hip replacement in patients with neurological conditions. J Bone Joint Surg Br 91:1267–1273, 2009.
10. Krenzel BA, Berend ME, Malinzak RA, et al: High preoperative range of motion is a significant risk factor for dislocation in primary total hip arthroplasty. J Arthroplasty 25(6 Suppl):31–35, 2010.
11. Ramesh M, O'Byrne JM, McCarthy N, et al: Damage to the superior gluteal nerve after the Hardinge approach to the hip. J Bone Joint Surg Br 78:903–906, 1996.
12. Howell GE, Biggs RE, Bourne RB: Prevalence of abductor mechanism tears of the hips in patients with osteoarthritis. J Arthroplasty 16:121–123, 2001.
13. Peak EL, Parvizi J, Ciminiello M, et al: The role of patient restrictions in reducing the prevalence of early dislocation following total hip arthroplasty: a randomized, prospective study. J Bone Joint Surg Am 87:247–253, 2005.
14. Berend ME, Bertrand T: Intraoperative fractures: rising problems. Orthopedics 30:750–751, 2007.
15. Berend ME, Smith A, Meding JB, et al: Long-term outcome and risk factors of proximal femoral fracture in uncemented and cemented total hip arthroplasty in 2551 hips. J Arthroplasty 21(6 Suppl 2):53–59, 2006.

CHAPTER 19

Posterior Approaches to the Hip

Bryan P. Springer

KEY POINTS

- The posterior approach to the hip allows excellent exposure of the femur and acetabulum for total hip arthroplasty.
- The extensile nature of the posterior approach makes it an important tool for primary and revision surgery.
- Minimally invasive surgery has yet to show any clinical advantage over standard posterior approaches to the hip.
- The posterior approach to the hip preserves the hip abductor mechanism.
- Posterior capsular repair is associated with reduced dislocation rates, similar to those of other approaches.

INTRODUCTION

The basic fundamentals of total hip arthroplasty begin with the surgical approach. A complete understanding of anatomy and the surgical approach is critical to a successful outcome. It is clear that one surgical approach may not satisfy all patients, and different situations may require an alternative approach, such as extensile approaches or osteotomies. Although most surgeons choose a surgical approach based on experience and training, it is important that they be familiar with multiple exposures.

Much debate and controversy have arisen in the past decade regarding the ideal surgical approach. Surgical approaches that require specialized instruments and even modified implants have been developed. Minimally invasive surgery gained popularity by promoting less muscle damage, faster recovery, and improved clinical outcomes.[1-4] To date however, little evidence exists to support these claims, and concern continues regarding associated complications.[5-9] The direct anterior approach is now gaining attention and is touting many of the same benefits of minimally invasive surgery. Likewise, however, few data currently show the superiority of one approach over another.

This chapter focuses on the posterior approach to the hip for total hip arthroplasty. The purpose is to review the historical background, pertinent anatomy, and surgical techniques. In addition, extensile exposures and current controversies regarding the posterior approach are reviewed.

HISTORICAL BACKGROUND OF THE POSTERIOR APPROACH TO THE HIP

This procedure was initially described as a surgical approach to the hip joint for the treatment of infection and war wounds. Bernhard von Langenbeck is credited with the first description in 1867 of what he termed "the longitudinal incision to the hip."[10,11] With the hip in a flexed position, he fashioned an incision "from above the ischiadic notch to the middle of the greater trochanter that reaches the joint passing between the bundles of the gluteal muscles." Langenbeck applied this surgical approach for resection of the femoral head (what he called "hip joint resection") and used hooks or "ball-screw" devices to extract the femoral head after cutting the ligamentum teres.

Kocher modified Langenbeck's approach by extending it in a caudal direction. He stated, "The incision is an angular (or curved) one, extending from the base of the outer surface of the great trochanter upwards to its anterior superior angle, and from thence obliquely upwards and backwards in the direction of the gluteus maximus."[12] Division of the gluteus maximus tendon and anterior reflection of the gluteus medius and minimus were followed by internal rotation of the hip and detachment of the piriformis and the other short external rotators. Regarding this approach, Kocher said that "it is a further development of Langenbeck's method by the oblique incision."

Melham and associates, in their 2000 article entitled "Hyphenated-History: The Kocher-Langenbeck Surgical Approach," stated as follows:

> "The Kocher-Langenbeck surgical approach continues to be widely used today by both orthopaedic trauma surgeons and reconstructive hip surgeons. By many it is considered to be a workhorse approach for posterior wall fractures of the acetabulum, femoral neck fractures treated via hemiarthroplasty, and total hip replacement. The durability of an idea born in the nineteenth century on the battlefields of Europe and refined in the operating theaters of Bern is indeed impressive. If he were around today, Kocher's humility would certainly be challenged by the widespread use of his particular portion of hyphenated-history."[13]

Dr. Alexander Gibson and Dr. A.T. Moore are largely credited with popularization of the posterior approach, often referred to as the "Southern approach," which is used today for total hip arthroplasty.[14,15] Although their initial description of the posterior approach has undergone several modifications since its initial description in 1950, the fundamentals of the exposure remain largely intact. Many of the modifications involve different placement and size of the skin incision, preferential detachment of the short external rotators, and posterior capsular repair. The usefulness of this approach can be appreciated by the diverse surgical procedures that can be performed through the posterior approach. These include hemiarthroplasty and total hip arthroplasty of the hip, hip resurfacing, open reduction and internal fixation of acetabular fractures, and arthrotomy and drainage of the hip joint for infection.

SURGICAL ANATOMY OF THE POSTERIOR APPROACH TO THE HIP

Muscular Anatomy

The muscles covering the posterior aspect of the hip joint are divided into deep and superficial layers. Henry described the outer layer as the "deltoid" muscle of the hip, similar to the deltoid of the shoulder.[16] This layer consists of the gluteus maximus, the fascia lata, and the tensor fascia lata, which together form the outer sheath of the hip musculature (Fig. 19-1).

The deep layer of the hip encountered during the posterior approach consists of the short external rotators. From cephalad to caudad, they include the piriformis, the superior gemelli, the obturator internus, the

inferior gemelli, the obturator externus, and the quadratus femoris (Fig. 19-2). The musculotendinous insertions of the gluteus medius and minimus insert at the tip of the greater trochanter and are not disturbed during the posterior approach to the hip. Table 19-1 lists the origins and insertions of pertinent muscles of the posterior approach, along with their neurologic innervation.

Neurovascular Anatomy

All neurologic and vascular structures pertinent to the posterior approach to the hip enter the hip from the pelvis through the sciatic notch. The piriformis tendon defines the pathway for the neurovascular anatomy of the hip. Ten structures enter the hip through the sciatic notch, passing superior or inferior to the tendon to supply their given muscles. Box 19-1 lists the neurovascular structures of the hip relative to the piriformis tendon.

The superior gluteal nerve and artery enter the pelvis above the piriformis to supply the gluteus medius and minimus muscles. Although not frequently encountered during the posterior approach to total hip arthroplasty, the superior gluteal artery and nerve tether the gluteus medius and minimus musculature to the ilium, preventing complete mobilization of these muscles and limiting

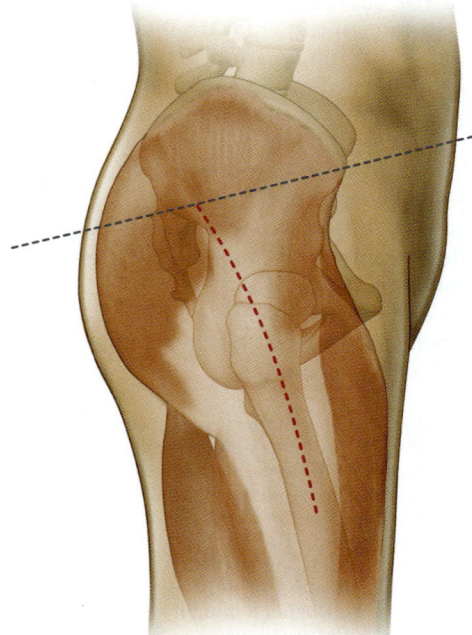

Figure 19-1. Picture demonstrates the "outer sheath" of the hip joint muscles, including the gluteus maximus, fascia lata, and tensor fascia lata.

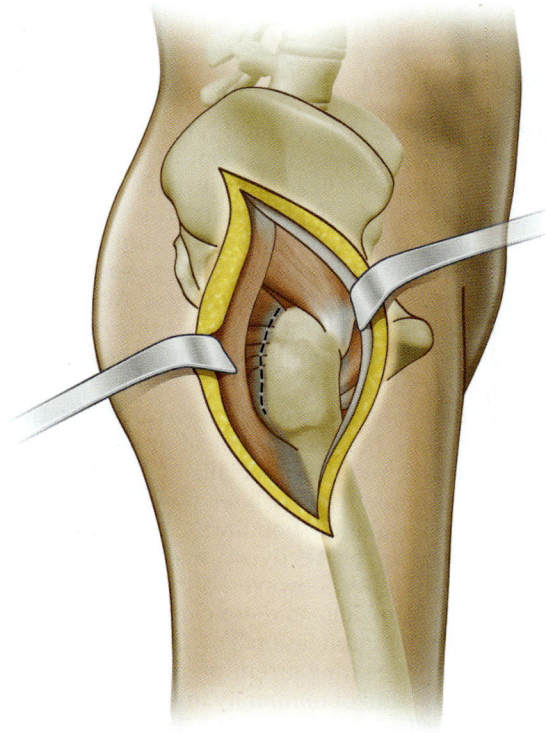

Figure 19-2. The "deep layer" of the hip includes the short external rotators: piriformis, superior gemelli, obturator internus, inferior gemelli, obturator externus, and quadratus femoris.

Table 19-1. Anatomic, Functional, and Nervous Innervation of Posterior Structures of the Hip

Muscle	Origin	Insertion	Function	Innervation
	Posterior Ilium	Iliotibial band	Hip extension and external rotation	Inferior gluteal nerve
Gluteus Maximus	Sacrum and coccyx	Gluteal tuberosity		
	Sacrum	Upper border greater trochanter	Hip abduction and external rotation	1st and 2nd sacral nerves
Piriformis				
Superior Gemelli	Inner aspect obturator foramen	Medial surface greater trochanter	Hip external rotation	Sacral plexus
Obturator Internus				
Inferior Gemelli				
Obturator Externus	Upper border ischial tuberosity	Linea quadrata of femur	Hip external rotation	Sacral plexus
Quadratus Femoris				
Gluteus Medius	Outer surface of ilium	Anterior border of greater trochanter	Hip abduction and internal rotation	Superior gluteal nerve
Gluteus Minimus				

BOX 19-1. NEUROVASCULAR STRUCTURES OF THE HIP RELATIVE TO THE PIRIFORMIS TENDON

Above Piriformis
- Superior gluteal nerve
- Superior gluteal artery

Below Piriformis
- Inferior gluteal nerve
- Inferior gluteal artery
- Pudendal nerve
- Inferior pudendal artery
- Nerve to obturator internus
- Sciatic nerve
- Posterior femoral cutaneous nerve
- Nerve to quadratus femoris

exposure of the ilium. Damage to the superior gluteal nerve can lead to denervation of these muscles, resulting in abductor muscle dysfunction. Injury to the superior gluteal artery can result in brisk pelvic bleeding and is difficult to control because the artery may retract into the pelvis during injury, making identification and ligation difficult. In these circumstances, an extraperitoneal approach to the pelvis may be required to control the internal iliac artery, which is the feeding branch to the superior gluteal artery.

The inferior gluteal nerve and artery reach the hip below the piriformis tendon. They provide the neurovascular supply to the gluteus maximus. Because they enter the muscle almost immediately, they remain well medial and are not encountered during a routine posterior approach to the hip.

The sciatic nerve enters the hip below the piriformis and traverses between the superficial (gluteus maximus) and deep (short external rotators) layers of the hip. During the posterior approach to the hip, it is generally protected by the muscular flaps of the short external rotators but may be injured during errant posterior

retractor placement, surgical reduction and dislocation of the prosthetic hip joint, or excessive leg lengthening.

SURGICAL TECHNIQUE

Patient Positioning (Fig. 19-3)

The patient is positioned in the lateral decubitus position. All bony prominences should be well padded and an axillary roll placed in the downside axilla to prevent undue pressure on the brachial plexus during surgery. The down leg should be padded to ensure minimal pressure on the peroneal nerve at the knee. Various positioners are available to stabilize the pelvis for surgery. These should allow for stable fixation of the pelvis and free mobilization of the operative extremity to allow adequate testing of the stability of the prosthesis during surgery. A mobile pelvis may affect exposure and positioning of the acetabular component during surgery. In general, the pelvis should be fixed perpendicular to the floor or slightly tilted in a posterior direction.

Incisions

Gaining adequate exposure to the hip joint through the posterior approach requires an accurately placed incision. The skin incision should be placed to maximize exposure and allow unhindered views of the femur and acetabulum. Previous incisions should be used when possible; however, the use of prior incisions should not compromise adequate exposure. Unlike the subcutaneous and fragile vascular anatomy of the knee, old incisions over the hip can be crossed or made parallel with little if any consequence. The size of the incision should not be limited in any way to compromise exposure of the hip. To date, no prospective randomized data show that the length of the surgical incision has any effect on patient recovery and outcome.

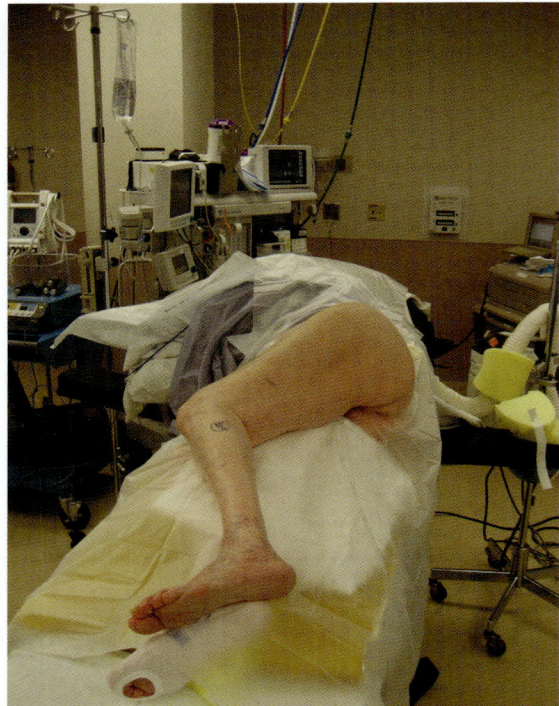

Figure 19-3. Patient positioning before total hip arthroplasty.

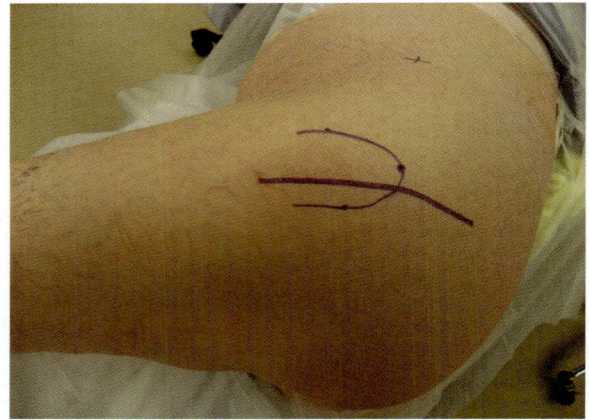

Figure 19-4. The incision is centered over the posterior one third of the trochanter and curves posteriorly in line with the fibers of the gluteus maximus and distally in line with the femur.

With the hip flexed approximately 45 degrees, a straight incision is made over the posterior one third of the trochanter. Distally, the incision travels in line with the lateral aspect of the femur. Proximally, the skin incision travels in line with the underlying fibers of the gluteus maximus, curving slightly and gently in a posterior direction (Fig. 19-4). The dissection is then carried deep through the subcutaneous tissue to expose the deep fascia of the thigh (Fig. 19-5). The deep fascia is split in line with the incision, extending proximally to split the fibers of the gluteus maximus. A deep retractor is placed to retract the fascia, exposing the deep layer

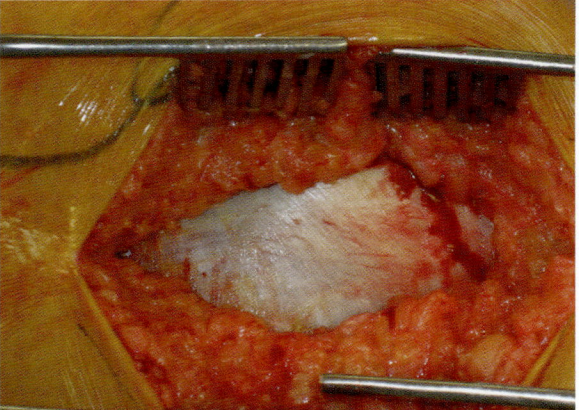

Figure 19-5. Dissection through subcutaneous tissue reveals the fascia overlying the gluteus maximus.

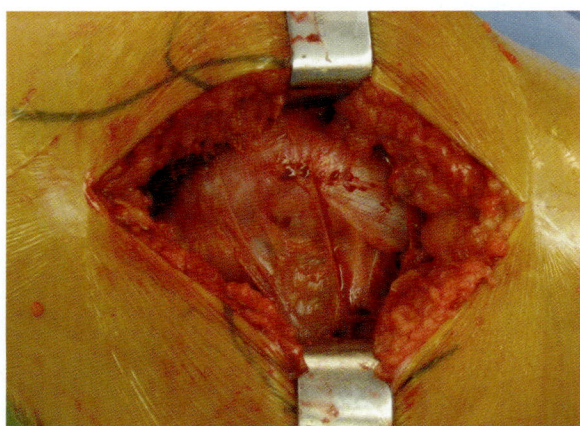

Figure 19-6. Trochanteric bursae overlying the short external rotators.

of the hip joint along with the trochanteric bursa overlying the short external rotators (Fig. 19-6). The posterior approach to the hip has no internervous plane because the fibers of the gluteus maximus, supplied by the inferior gluteal nerve, are split along its fibers.

The interval between the posterior border of the gluteus medius and the piriformis tendon is identified and dissected free. A retractor may be placed in this interval to assist with superior retraction of the gluteus medius (Fig. 19-7). The short external rotators are removed from the posterior aspect of the greater trochanter and femoral neck and are tagged with a suture for later repair. Below the short external rotators, the thick posterior capsule runs from the posterior wall of the acetabulum to the femoral neck. The capsule should be removed from the posterior aspect of the femoral neck and preserved for later repair. This posterior flap, which consists of the short external rotators and the posterior hip capsule, is reflected posterior to protect the sciatic nerve (Fig. 19-8). The femoral head, neck, and posterior wall are then visualized (Fig. 19-9). On occasion in hips that are stiff, or when extensile exposures are required, the tendon of the gluteus maximus may

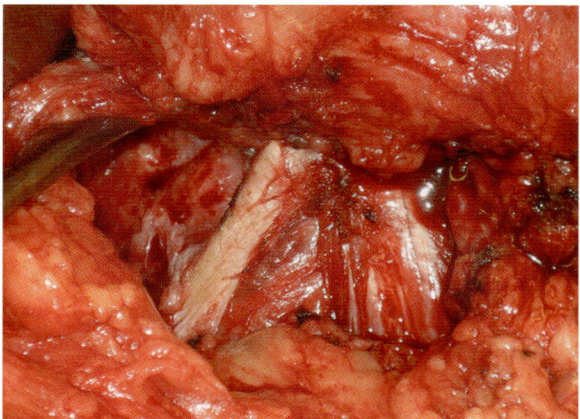

Figure 19-7. Interval between gluteus minimus and piriformis tendon and short external rotators. The gluteus medius has been retracted superiorly.

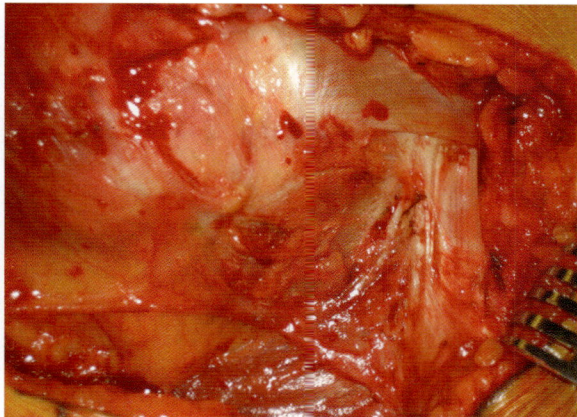

Figure 19-10. Gluteus maximus tendon.

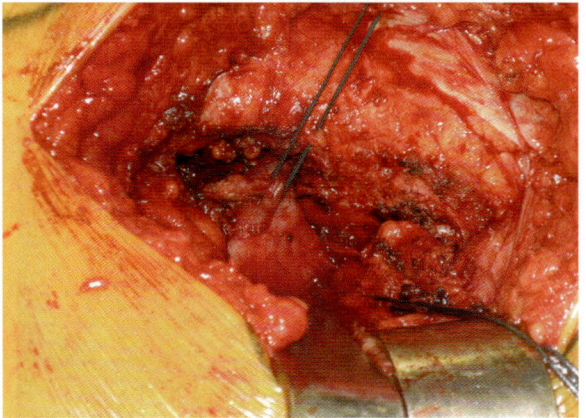

Figure 19-8. The posterior capsule has been tagged and dissected free.

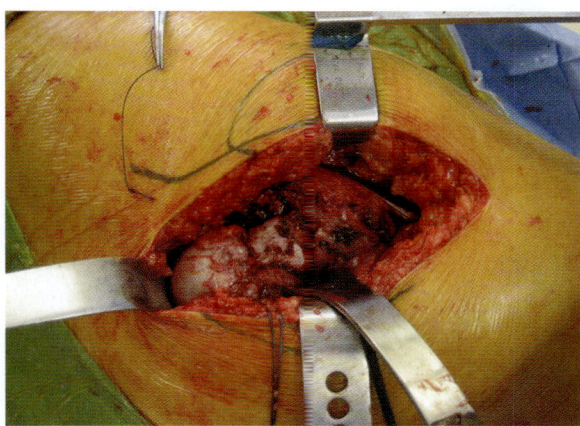

Figure 19-11. Posterior dislocation of the hip.

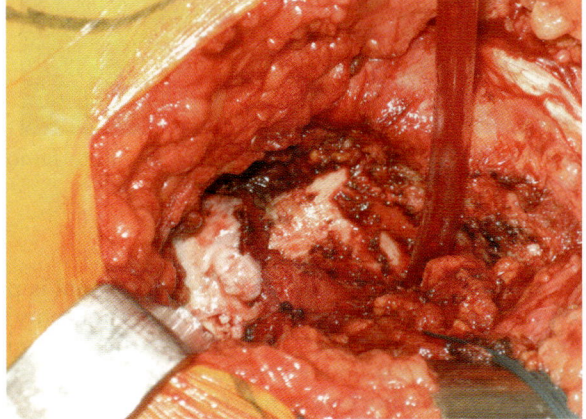

Figure 19-9. Reflection of the posterior capsule reveals the femoral head and neck.

need to be released to allow anterior mobilization of the femur for acetabular exposure (Fig. 19-10). Care should be taken when the gluteus maximus tendon is released, because the sciatic nerve traverses just below the tendon.

The hip is then flexed and internally rotated to allow posterior dislocation of the femoral head from the acetabulum (Fig. 19-11). In patients with ankylosis of the hip joint from prior surgery, heterotopic bone, and so forth, it may be necessary to perform an in situ osteotomy of the femoral neck before dislocation. This allows dislocation of the femur without undue stress that may risk fracture of the femoral shaft. The femoral neck is then exposed and is cut in accordance with preoperative templating.

Acetabular Exposure

The posterior approach allows excellent visualization of the acetabulum but requires anterior translation of the femur in front of the acetabulum. This is achieved by the use of an anterior retractor placed at the level of the anterior inferior iliac spine (Fig. 19-12A and B). Care should be taken when placing this retractor to ensure that it stays in direct contact with the anterior pelvis. Aggressive placement can put the femoral artery and nerve at risk. Slight hip flexion and external rotation of the hip allow for anterior translation of the femur and

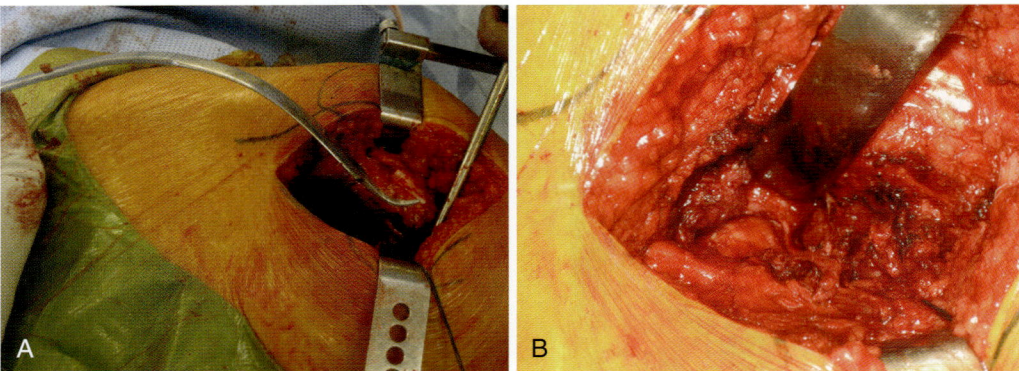

Figure 19-12. A and **B,** An anterior retractor is placed at the level of the anterior inferior iliac spine to assist in translation of the femur forward to expose the anterior acetabulum.

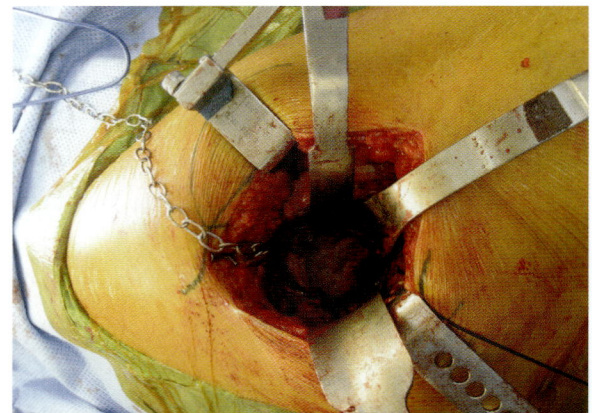

Figure 19-13. Circumferential exposure of the acetabulum.

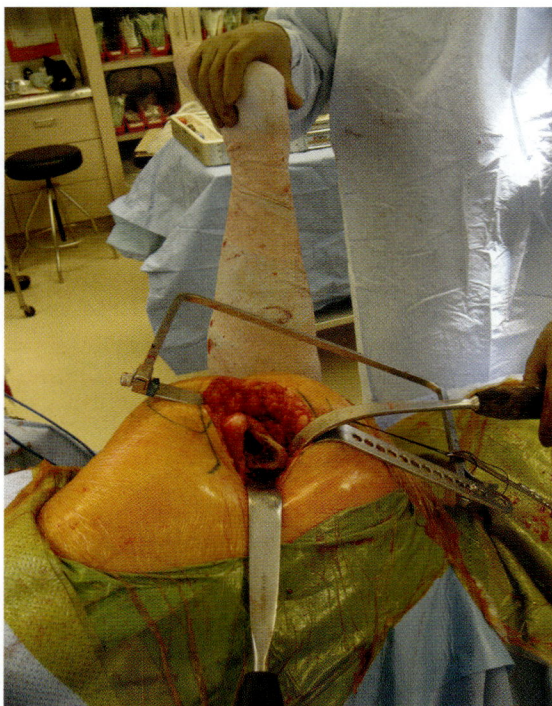

Figure 19-14. The position of the leg to facilitate femoral canal preparation.

circumferential exposure of the acetabulum. A posteriorly based retractor placed at the level of the ischium and the posterior column enhances visualization. A superior retractor may be placed into the ilium to retract the gluteus medius superior to improve visualization of the superior aspect of the acetabulum. The acetabulum then can be prepared with hemispherical reamers with excellent visualization of the entire acetabulum (Fig. 19-13).

Femoral Exposure

Femoral exposure for placement of the femoral component during total hip arthroplasty is easily visualized through the posterior approach with minimal retraction and assistance. The assistant places the leg in hip flexion and internal rotation so the lower portion of the leg is perpendicular to the floor (Fig. 19-14). This allows for unhindered placement of the stem and provides an accurate check for femoral anteversion. Retractors are placed at the level of the lesser trochanter to retract the medial soft tissue and anteriorly to elevate the femur out of the wound for better visualization (Fig. 19-15). A posterior starting point in the femur is attained, and lateralization of the broaches is necessary to avoid

varus positioning of the stem. The femoral canal is prepared via direct visualization of the femoral anatomy for placement of the stem (Fig. 19-16). Upon completion of the arthroplasty, it is imperative to repair the posterior capsule and the short external rotators. Figure 19-17 demonstrates anatomic closure of the hip capsule and short external rotators.

Extensile Exposures

One of the many advantages of the posterior approach to the hip is its ability to be readily extensile in both primary and revision settings. The standard posterior approach can be easily extended to include a standard

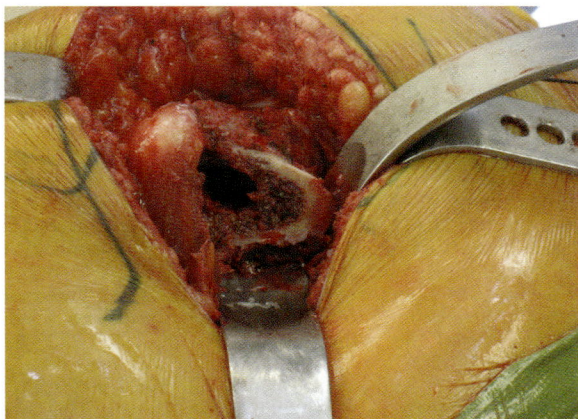

Figure 19-15. Exposure of the upper portion of the femur for canal preparation.

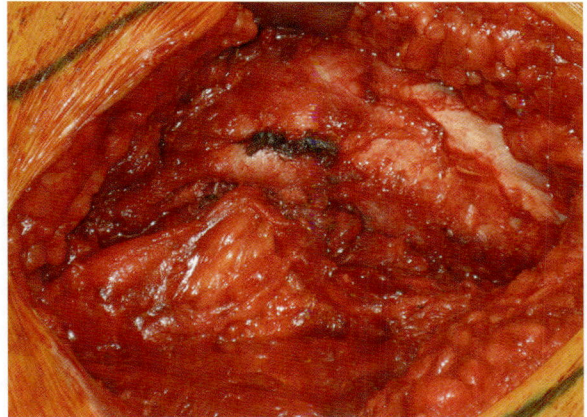

Figure 19-17. Anatomic closure of the hip capsule and short external rotators.

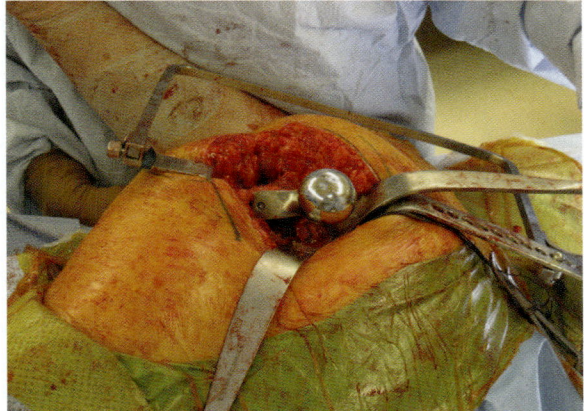

Figure 19-16. Final femoral component in place.

trochanteric osteotomy, a trochanteric slide osteotomy, and a posteriorly based extended trochanteric osteotomy. Extensile exposures of the hip are addressed in Chapters 20 and 21.

CURRENT CONTROVERSIES AND FUTURE DIRECTIONS

No consensus has been reached on the optimal surgical approach for every patient. However, the posterior approach to the hip provides a versatile option that can be used to deal with most issues encountered in primary and revision total hip arthroplasty. Its ability to be readily converted to an extensile exposure makes it an essential part of the armamentarium of the arthroplasty surgeon.

The main concern with the posterior approach to the hip has been its association with a higher incidence of dislocation compared with other anteriorly based surgical approaches. The dislocation rate after total hip arthroplasty performed through a posterior approach ranges from 0.2% to 9.5%.[17-30] Many variables other than surgical approach affect the rate of dislocation; these include patient factors and implant design and femoral head size.[31-35] These variables make it difficult to ascertain the sole influence of approach on dislocation.

Preservation and repair of the posterior capsule and the short external rotators constitute an important step in reducing dislocation after total hip arthroplasty. Initial descriptions of the posterior approach did not include repair or even preservation of the posterior structures. Charnley advocated advancement of the greater trochanter to maintain soft tissue tension.[36] Hedley and Pellicci advocated posterior capsular repair and reduced dislocation rates to below 1%.[37,38] Multiple studies now confirm reduced dislocation rates with capsular repair and rates of dislocation comparable with those of anterolateral surgical approaches.[39-46]

Abductor dysfunction can lead to pain, prolonged rehabilitation, postoperative limp, and patient dissatisfaction after total hip arthroplasty. A major advantage of the posterior approach to the hip is preservation of the abductor mechanism. This approach stays posterior to and thus preserves the abductor muscles. Comparative functional outcome data have shown improved strength with less limp during the initial postoperative period with the posterior approach compared with anterolaterally based approaches.[47-50]

Advances in surgical techniques, instruments, implants, anesthesia techniques, and rehabilitation protocols will continue to improve patient outcomes following total hip arthroplasty. Through a better understanding of anatomy and biomechanics, improvement will continue to limit the amount of muscular damage and dislocation rates. Because of its versatility, its extensile nature, and preservation of the abductor mechanism, the posterior approach to the hip will continue to be a mainstay in surgical approaches to total hip arthroplasty.

REFERENCES

1. Nakamura S, Matsuda K, Arai N, et al: Mini-incision posterior approach for total hip arthroplasty. Int Orthop 28:214–217, 2004.

2. Bottner F, Delgado S, Sculco TP: Minimally invasive total hip replacement: the posterolateral approach. Am J Orthop 35:218–224, 2006.

3. Ward SR, Jones RE, Long WT, et al: Functional recovery of muscles after minimally invasive total hip arthroplasty. Instr Course Lect 57:249–254, 2008.

4. Sculco TP, Boettner F: Minimally invasive total hip arthroplasty: the posterior approach. Instr Course Lect 55:205–214, 2006.

5. Sharma V, Morgan PM, Cheng EY: Factors influencing early rehabilitation after THA: a systematic review. Clin Orthop Relat Res 467:1400–1411, 2009.

6. Ogonda L, Wilson R, Archbold P, et al: A minimal-incision technique in total hip arthroplasty does not improve early postoperative outcomes: a prospective, randomized, controlled trial. J Bone Joint Surg Am 87:701–710, 2005.

7. Meneghini RM, Pagnano MW, Trousdale RT, Hozack WJ: Muscle damage during MIS total hip arthroplasty: Smith-Petersen versus posterior approach. Clin Orthop Relat Res 453:293–298, 2006.

8. Meneghini RM, Smits SA, Swinford RR, Bahamonde RE: A randomized, prospective study of 3 minimally invasive surgical approaches in total hip arthroplasty: comprehensive gait analysis. J Arthroplasty 23(6 Suppl 1):68–73, 2008.

9. Pagnano MW, Leone J, Lewallen DG, Hanssen AD: Two-incision THA had modest outcomes and some substantial complications. Clin Orthop Relat Res 441:86–90, 2005.

10. Langenbeck B: Chirurgische beobachtungen aus dem kriege, Berlin, 1874, Hirschwald.

11. Langenbeck B: Ueber die schussfracturen der gelenke und ihre behandlung, Berlin, 1868, A. Hirschwald.

12. Kocher T: Operative surgery, 3rd English ed, transl by Siles HJ, Paul CB, London, 1911, Black.

13. Mehlman CT, Meiss L, DiPasquale TG: Hyphenated-history: the Kocher-Langenbeck surgical approach. J Orthop Trauma 14:60–64, 2000.

14. Gibson A: Posterior exposure of the hip joint. J Bone Joint Surg Br 32:183–186, 1950.

15. Moore AT: The self-locking metal hip prosthesis. J Bone Joint Surg Am 39:811–827, 1957.

16. Henry A: Extensile exposures, ed 2, Edinburgh and London, 1966, Livingstone, pp 180–197.

17. Sherk HH: Posterior exposure of the hip joint. Clin Orthop Relat Res 429:3–5, 2004.

18. Mullins MM, Norbury W, Dowell JK, Heywood-Waddington M: Thirty-year results of a prospective study of Charnley total hip arthroplasty by the posterior approach. J Arthroplasty 22:833–839, 2007.

19. Masonis JL, Bourne RB: Surgical approach, abductor function, and total hip arthroplasty dislocation. Clin Orthop Relat Res 405:46–53, 2002.

20. Barber TC, Roger DJ, Goodman SB, Schurman DJ: Early outcome of total hip arthroplasty using the direct lateral vs the posterior surgical approach. Orthopedics 19:873–875, 1996.

21. Hedlundh U, Ahnfelt L, Hybbinette CH, et al: Surgical experience related to dislocations after total hip arthroplasty. J Bone Joint Surg Br 78:206–209, 1996.

22. McCollum DE, Gray WJ: Dislocation after total hip arthroplasty: causes and prevention. Clin Orthop Relat Res 261:159–170, 1990.

23. Patiala H, Lehto K, Rokkanen P, Paavolainen P: Posterior approach for total hip arthroplasty: a study of postoperative course, early results and early complications in 131 cases. Arch Orthop Trauma Surg 102:225–229, 1984.

24. Woo RY, Morrey BF: Dislocations after total hip arthroplasty. J Bone Joint Surg Am 64:1295–1306, 1982.

25. Gore DR, Murray MP, Sepic SB, Gardner GM: Anterolateral compared to posterior approach in total hip arthroplasty: differences in component positioning, hip strength, and hip motion. Clin Orthop Relat Res 165:180–187, 1982.

26. Gristina AG, Rovere GD, Nicastro JF, Burke JG: Posterior approach for total hip arthroplasty. South Med J 73:51–54, 1980.

27. Hovelius L, Hussenius A, Thorling J: Posterior versus lateral approach for hip arthroplasty. Acta Orthop Scand 48:47–51, 1977.

28. Blaimont P, Dieu N, Baillon JM: On approaches to total hip arthroplasty: presentation of instruments facilitating the posterior approach. Acta Orthop Belg 39:649–657, 1973.

29. Robinson RP, Robinson HJ Jr, Salvati EA: Comparison of the transtrochanteric and posterior approaches for total hip replacement. Clin Orthop Relat Res 147:143–147, 1980.

30. Roberts JM, Fu FH, McClain EJ, Ferguson AB Jr: A comparison of the anterolateral approaches to total hip arthroplasty. Clin Orthop Relat Res 187:205–210, 1984.

31. Peters CL, McPherson E, Jackson JD, Erickson JA: Reduction in early dislocation rate with large-diameter femoral heads in primary total hip arthroplasty. J Arthroplasty 22(6 Suppl 2):140–144, 2007.

32. Lachiewicz PF, Soileau ES: Dislocation of primary total hip arthroplasty with 36 and 40-mm femoral heads. Clin Orthop Relat Res 453:153–155, 2006.

33. Hedlundh U, Ahnfelt L, Hybbinette CH, et al: Dislocations and the femoral head size in primary total hip arthroplasty. Clin Orthop Relat Res 333:226–233, 1996.

34. Berry DJ: Unstable total hip arthroplasty: detailed overview. Instr Course Lect 50:265–274, 2001.

35. Sanchez-Sotelo J, Berry DJ: Epidemiology of instability after total hip replacement. Orthop Clin North Am 32:543–552, 2001.

36. Charnley J, Cupic Z: The nine and ten year results of the low-friction arthroplasty of the hip. Clin Orthop Relat Res 95:9–25, 1973.

37. Hedley AK, Hendren DH, Mead LP: A posterior approach to the hip joint with complete posterior capsular and muscular repair. J Arthroplasty 5(Suppl):S57–S66, 1990.

38. Pellicci PM, Bostrom M, Poss R: Posterior approach to total hip replacement using enhanced posterior soft tissue repair. Clin Orthop Relat Res 355:224–228, 1998.

39. Jolles BM, Bogoch ER: Posterior versus lateral surgical approach for total hip arthroplasty in adults with osteoarthritis. Cochrane Database Syst Rev 2006;3:CD003828.

40. Kwon MS, Kuskowski M, Mulhall KJ, et al: Does surgical approach affect total hip arthroplasty dislocation rates? Clin Orthop Relat Res 447:34–38, 2006.

41. Jolles BM, Bogoch ER: Surgical approach for total hip arthroplasty: direct lateral or posterior? J Rheumatol 31:1790–1796, 2004.

42. Dixon MC, Scott RD, Schai PA, Stamos V: A simple capsulorrhaphy in a posterior approach for total hip arthroplasty. J Arthroplasty 19:373–376, 2004.

43. Suh KT, Park BG, Choi YJ: A posterior approach to primary total hip arthroplasty with soft tissue repair. Clin Orthop Relat Res 418:162–167, 2004.

44. Weeden SH, Paprosky WG, Bowling JW: The early dislocation rate in primary total hip arthroplasty following the posterior approach with posterior soft-tissue repair. J Arthroplasty 18:709–713, 2003.

45. van Stralen GM, Struben PJ, van Loon CJ: The incidence of dislocation after primary total hip arthroplasty using posterior approach with posterior soft-tissue repair. Arch Orthop Trauma Surg 123:219–222, 2003.

46. Chiu FY, Chen CM, Chung TY, et al: The effect of posterior capsulorrhaphy in primary total hip arthroplasty: a prospective randomized study. J Arthroplasty 15:194–199, 2000.

47. Mihalko WM, Whiteside LA: Hip mechanics after posterior structure repair in total hip arthroplasty. Clin Orthop Relat Res 420:194–198, 2004.

48. Downing ND, Clark DI, Hutchinson JW, et al: Hip abductor strength following total hip arthroplasty: a prospective comparison of the posterior and lateral approach in 100 patients. Acta Orthop Scand 72:215–220, 2001.

49. Navarro RA, Schmalzried TP, Amstutz HC, Dorey FJ: Surgical approach and nerve palsy in total hip arthroplasty. J Arthroplasty 10:1–5, 1995.

50. Weale AE, Newman P, Ferguson IT, Bannister GC: Nerve injury after posterior and direct lateral approaches for hip replacement: a clinical and electrophysiological study. J Bone Joint Surg Br 78:899–902, 1996.

CHAPTER 20

Trochanteric Osteotomy

Brian J. McGrory

INTRODUCTION

Leopold Ollier initially described trochanteric osteotomy (TO) as part of the lateral approach to the hip for surgeries such as joint excision and hip arthrodesis,[1] and Charnley popularized TO for total hip arthroplasty (THA) exposure.[2,3] Because first-generation implants were monolithic and were available only in limited sizes, trochanteric advancement was a usual part of the standard procedure.

Once a commonplace surgical technique for primary and revision THA, TO has become a tool that is rarely needed. The trochanteric flip osteotomy and the extended trochanteric osteotomy are used much more regularly today (for specific purposes), but each is the subject of its own chapter. Specific advantages of TO include exposure and soft tissue tensioning. The decision to proceed with osteotomy must balance the need for these benefits with associated increased surgical time, postoperative limitations, and risk of complications.

An orthopedic surgeon should be able to perform a TO and reliably repair it. A plethora of specific osteotomy techniques and fixation methods are described in the literature, but no one method has been conclusively shown to be advantageous. This chapter will review indications and contraindications and preoperative planning and will highlight major osteotomy variations and fixation techniques; postoperative care and recognition and treatment of TO complications will also be discussed.

INDICATIONS/CONTRAINDICATIONS

Contemporary THA accentuates a streamlined approach to surgery and recovery while maximizing long-term success. Present-day exposure techniques and modular implants make the routine use of osteotomy obsolete. In 1984, Hamblin[4] estimated that 10% to 20% of hips require TO for restoration of normal joint anatomy, but this estimate is likely high by today's standards. Rates of TO reflect geographic trends and surgeon preferences. In my single-surgeon practice, the incidence of trochanteric osteotomy in primary hip replacement is only 0.3% (5/1720) over the past 10 years. The incidence during the same time period is higher for conversion to THA (1.2%, 2/172) and is even higher for revision THA (2.1%, 9/420, excluding extended trochanteric osteotomy). Current indications for trochanteric osteotomy are limited to cases of difficult surgical exposure and soft tissue tensioning.

In the infrequent THA that requires enhanced exposure, osteotomy may be extremely useful. Examples include cases in which a very complex acetabular reconstruction is performed, as in severe developmental dysplasia of the hip (DDH), pelvic discontinuity, and tumor removal. Ankylosis linked to take-down of a prior fusion or marked rigidity due to heterotopic ossification may also require TO. Severe protrusio acetabuli is sometimes associated with inability to dislocate the hip; osteotomy may be a useful tool in these cases. Striking femoral malformations found in some cases of DDH, Paget's disease, and post-traumatic or postsurgical abnormalities may also lend themselves to TO.

Many of these deformities require appropriate soft tissue balancing, as well as exposure. In a situation with a marked hip varus deformity or one in which it is necessary to correct unacceptable laxity of the abductors for any reason, osteotomy and trochanteric advancement may be quite useful. Although contemporary implants allow the ability to modify soft tissue balance, trochanteric advancement is sometimes necessary in cases of leg length inequality (Fig. 20-1A and B) or of revision surgery with a nonmodular femoral component. It is also useful in cases of osteotomy in which the femur is shortened or the hip is unstable because of a high hip center.

Osteotomy is not indicated today in most cases of THA because adequate exposure and tensioning of the hip can be reliably achieved without associated

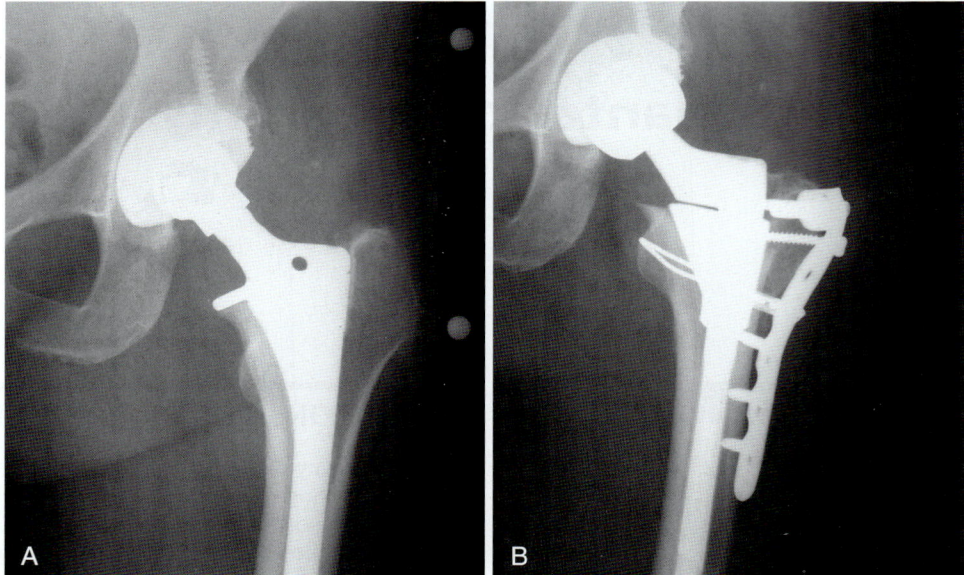

Figure 20-1. Anteroposterior radiographs of a hip replacement with unacceptable leg lengthening **(A)** before and **(B)** after revision surgery with trochanteric osteotomy and advancement. Internal fixation using a locking plate with cable augmentation.

increased risks, increased surgical time, and postoperative restrictions of this procedure. Even when TO appears indicated, osteotomy is contraindicated in some circumstances. Alternative methods of exposure, such as myofascial flap,[5] should be strongly considered in cases of pathologic bone (e.g., fibrous dysplasia of the proximal femur). In revision surgery with severe trochanteric osteolysis, extending the trochanteric osteotomy to an area of thicker and more viable bone (distally) should be considered. Another option in this scenario is the bulk allograft and locking plate technique introduced for trochanteric fracture through osteolytic bone.[6] In cases of ankylosis with abductor scarring, the surgeon should be prepared to release the abductors (the so-called *abductor slide technique*[7]). Surgeries that leave a large proximal prosthesis or bone cement in the greater trochanteric bed are likely to lead to nonunion and are relative contraindications to TO. If exposure is not attainable by other means, the potential consequences of a nonunited trochanter must be accepted or trochanteric osteoplasty considered.[8]

PREOPERATIVE PLANNING

The one factor that a surgeon has greatest control over in attaining an excellent outcome is a well-executed surgical strategy. In hip replacement surgery, this is best achieved through preoperative planning. A trochanteric osteotomy (and subsequent fixation) must be part of that plan in some circumstances.

If an osteotomy is anticipated, the optimal type and fixation method are chosen to maximize healing, minimize postoperative restriction, and allow an efficient surgery. These plans should be included in the consent process discussion with the patient. Preoperative radiographs should be used to anticipate the precise location of the

osteotomy and whether advancement is needed. Any special tools or implants can then be made available.

OSTEOTOMY TECHNIQUES

TO techniques can be generally divided into standard, slide, and repeat osteotomy groups. Multiple variations of the standard and slide categories have been developed; these will be highlighted.

Standard

The standard TO was originally popularized for use in hip arthroplasty by Charnley,[2,9] and later was optimized by many surgeons, including Harris.[10,11] After exposure of the hip, a Cushing elevator is inserted from anterior to posterior in the interval between the tendon of the gluteus minimus and the superior part of the hip capsule. Next, the origin of the vastus lateralis is elevated from the vastus tubercle. The osteotomy cut traverses the sulcus between the lateral portion of the origin of the vastus intermedius muscle and the insertions of the gluteus medius and minimus. The osteotomy is started 1 cm distal to the vastus tubercle and is performed with an oscillating saw or osteotome, which is aimed at the Cushing elevator (Fig. 20-2). Once the trochanter has been cut, it is retracted proximally, and the short external rotators are released from the trochanteric fragment. This enhances mobilization of the trochanter proximally. Healing rates of the standard osteotomy vary, but in one large study of 804 cases (725 primary and 79 revision), 8 osteotomies (1%) did not heal. Delayed union of the osteotomized trochanter (defined as that occurring more than 6 months after the procedure) was noted in 17 (2.3%) primary cases and 6 (7.6%) revision cases.[10]

Modifications of the Standard Osteotomy

Chevron. Bi-plane, dihedral, or chevron osteotomy (CO) was first described by Debeyre and Duliveux[12] and was later popularized by Weber and Stuhmer.[13] This

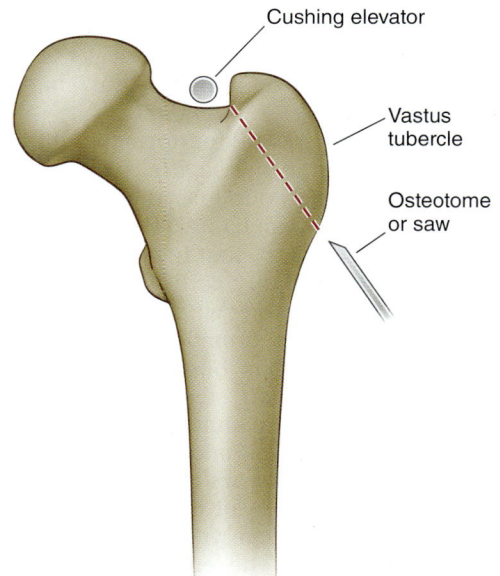

Figure 20-2. Standard trochanteric osteotomy. *(Redrawn from McGrory BJ, Bal BS, Harris WH: Trochanteric osteotomy for total hip arthroplasty: six variations and indications for their use. J Am Acad Orthop Surg 4:258, 1996.)*

technique is said to allow immediate rotatory stability and at the same time permits near-anatomic replacement of the trochanteric fragment. It is not indicated in cases of trochanteric advancement. Weber compared two groups of 69 patients with standard and chevron osteotomies and noted a nonunion prevalence of 11% in the standard group and 1.5% in the chevron group.[14] Berry and Muller reported trochanteric union rates of 98% for primary surgery (53 hips) and 97% for revision surgery (74 hips) with this technique.[15] These results were confirmed by Wroblewski and Shelley in a larger group of 222 primary and revision surgeries.[16]

Several technical variations are available for the CO. Similar to the flat standard osteotomy, the CO starts 1 cm distal to the vastus tubercle. The anterior and posterior limbs are equal in size and the thickness of the apex adequate to avoid fracture. The limbs are angled approximately 30 degrees from the apex; the trochanteric cancellous surface is concave and the femur surface convex (the "chevron" is in the sagittal plane). Cuts can be made with a narrow oscillating saw, a straight or chevron-shaped[17] osteotome, or a Gigli saw. The Gigli saw method, as presented by Wroblewski and Shelley,[16] starts by passing a 4-mm smooth Steinmann pin into the center of the trochanter, directing it 45 degrees to the shaft of the femur. The saw is then passed craniad to the femoral neck at the junction of the greater trochanter with the superior part of the femoral neck. The saw lies proximal to the pin and is directed distally, cutting anteriorly and posteriorly, creating a CO (Fig. 20-3).

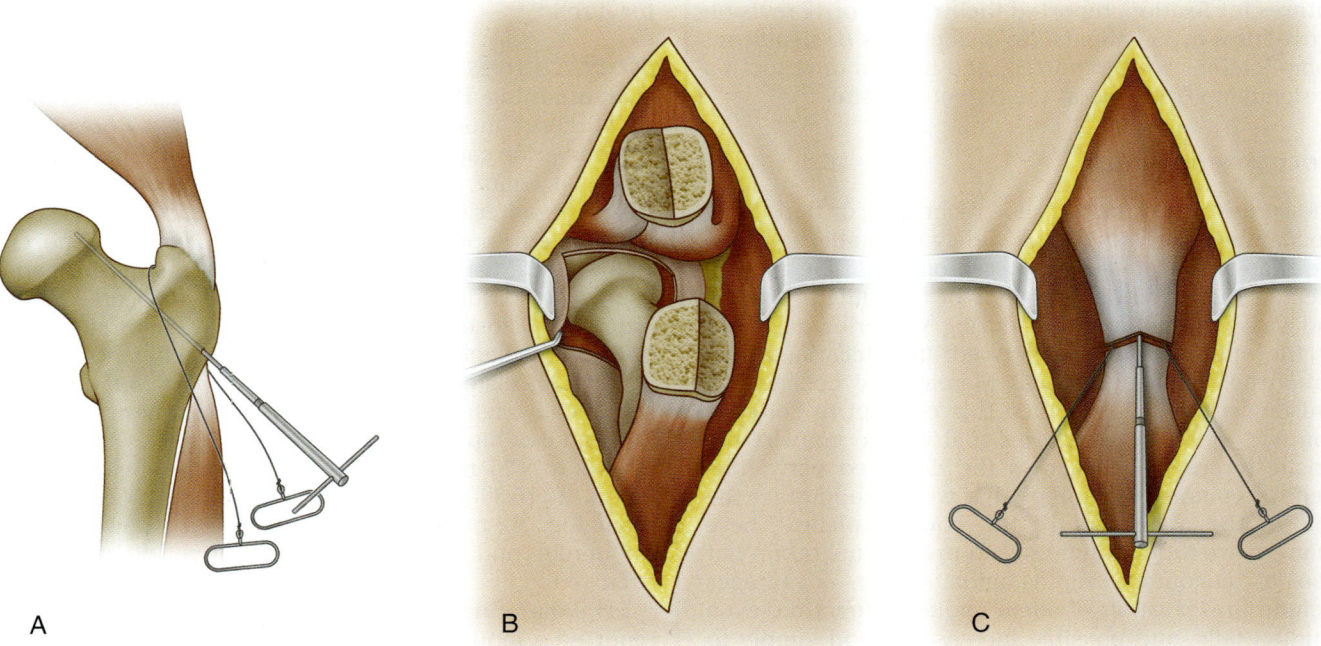

A   B   C

Figure 20-3. Chevron osteotomy. This specific technique was described by Wroblewski and Shelly.[16] *(Redrawn from Wroblewski BM, Shelley P: Reattachment of the greater trochanter after total hip replacement. J Bone Joint Surg Br 67:736, 1985.)*

Oblique

McGrory, Bal, and Harris described a partial osteotomy that was devised to increase the somewhat limited exposure that is sometimes attained with a direct lateral approach for primary total hip replacement while minimizing the risk of posterior dislocation.[11] The anterior portion of the osteotomy begins over the palpable sharp ridge that is the limiting structure of the anterior aspect of the insertion of the abductors. The anterior portion of the osteotomy is similar to, but slightly craniad to, that used for a standard TO. The posterior bone cut remains superficial to the intertrochanteric ridge and the insertion of the short external rotators (which are left attached to the femur). Thus the fragment is wider anteriorly than posteriorly but contains all of the insertion of the gluteus medius and gluteus minimus. The trochanter is reflected proximally, and an anterior capsulotomy is performed. The hip is dislocated anteriorly. In 26 consecutive cases, the authors reported a nonunion rate of 4% (1/26) using this approach, with no postoperative instability.[11]

Posterior

Several authors have reported variations of a technique credited to Iyer[18] for THA with modification of a limited posterior trochanteric osteotomy. The osteotomized bone fragment includes the posterior insertions of the short external rotators and the posterior capsule. Similar to the oblique osteotomy, this variation was designed to enhance postoperative stability. Sanchez-Sotelo and associates reported that radiographic union was achieved in 94% (64/66) of primary hip replacements, with two cases of postoperative instability.[19] Stuchin and Millman,[20] after adapting this technique for revision surgery and using heavy, nonabsorbable sutures for fixation, reported their results of 47 revision procedures in 35 patients. No dislocations or significant complications were reported, and no loss of reduction or nonunion occurred at the osteotomy site.

Trochanteric Slide

The anterior trochanteric slide technique, or the sliding trochanteric osteotomy, is a widely used alternative to the standard trochanteric osteotomy.[21-24] The idea of keeping the tendinous portions of the gluteus medius and vastus lateralis intact during posterior exposure of the hip was first described by McFarland and Osbourne,[25] although it was Mercati and colleagues[26] and English[22] who described this concept in conjunction with an osteotomy. The goal was to convert the tensile forces placed across the detached bony fragment to compressive forces that would counteract the pull of the abductors in the coronal plane. These changes are thought not only to prevent migration but also to encourage rapid union. Other advantages include preservation of some abductor function, even if union fails, and possible increased blood supply to the trochanteric fragment.[27] Glassman described this approach in detail in 1987 and popularized its use in revision surgery.[21]

The skin incision with this osteotomy diverges anteriorly from the course usually taken with a posterior approach. It parallels the anterior border of the greater trochanter before continuing posteriorly, along with the fibers of the gluteus maximus. The gluteus medius muscle is isolated anteriorly and posteriorly, and the fascia overlying the vastus lateralis is incised for 10 to 15 cm distal to the vastus ridge and 1 cm anterior to the intermuscular septum. The vastus lateralis is then elevated subperiosteally from the femoral shaft and is retracted anteriorly.

The osteotomy cut, usually performed with an oscillating saw, is oriented in the sagittal plane and begins just medial to the tendinous insertions of the gluteus medius into the greater trochanter. The osteotomy exits distal to the vastus ridge, so that the origin of the lateralis is preserved in continuity with the bony wafer. The osteotomy fragment is somewhat thinner than for a standard trochanteric osteotomy (Fig. 20-4).

Once the trochanter has been osteotomized, it is retracted with its muscular sleeve craniad and commonly is held with a self-retaining retractor. The external rotators and the gluteus minimus are then divided close to their insertion and are preserved for reattachment after reapproximation of the trochanter. Dislocation is usually accomplished with the hip in adduction and external rotation, and the leg is placed anteriorly in a sterile bag. Alternatively, the hip can be dislocated posteriorly, but in this case, a posterior incision is needed.

Glassman and colleagues reported on slide osteotomy for 90 THAs, of which 88 were revision cases. Nine osteotomies (10%) resulted in nonunion, and seven of the nine had proximal migration of the osteotomy fragment. No cases of instability were reported; however, 23 hips (28%) were noted to have an abductor lurch.[21]

Modifications of the Trochanteric Slide

Maintaining Posterior Attachments. Goodman and co-workers[28] modified the slide technique to preserve the posterior capsule and the external rotators on the proximal femur, with translation of the osteotomized fragment anteriorly. This change imparts increased resistance to posterior hip dislocation. In their report, 14.8% (4/27) of the acetabular revisions performed using a traditional trochanteric slide dislocated and required a closed reduction within 1 year of surgery. With maintenance of the posterior attachments, only 3.3% (1/30) dislocated. This difference was found to be statistically significant. When this technique was used for complex hip arthroplasty in 83 surgeries followed for up to 126 months, 77 (84.4%) healed with bony union, 9 (10.8%) had fibrous union, and 4 (4.8%) had nonunion. Six patients (7.2%) developed a new abductor lurch, and 4 (4.8%) postoperative dislocations occurred.[29]

Triplanar Slide. Ackerman and Trousdale recently reported a modification of the trochanteric slide osteotomy, which they call a *triplanar trochanteric osteotomy*.[30] This variation not only preserves the posterior structures, it also adds further stability through a triplanar or chevron geometric contour. The "chevron" in this case, however, is in the coronal plane (Fig. 20-5).

After exposure of the trochanter, the interval between the gluteus medius and the gluteus minimus is developed, and the medius is retracted anteriorly. The minimus, short external rotators, and piriformis remain posterior to the retractor. A point is then identified along the posterior border of the greater trochanter, approximately equidistant from the tip of the trochanter and the vastus ridge. The thickness is estimated, and a goal of 2 cm is marked with electrocautery (outlining

the apex of the chevron-shaped osteotomy). With care taken to leave the vastus lateralis in continuity distally, the osteotomy is carried 90% to 95% of the way and then is levered and fractured anteriorly (leaving an anterior vertical ridge). This ridge resists anteriorly directed forces after reduction, allowing for anatomic reduction.

Step. Schoeniger and associates have proposed another modification of the slide osteotomy that consists of similar soft tissue attachments but with a unique bony contour, again to add stability during bony

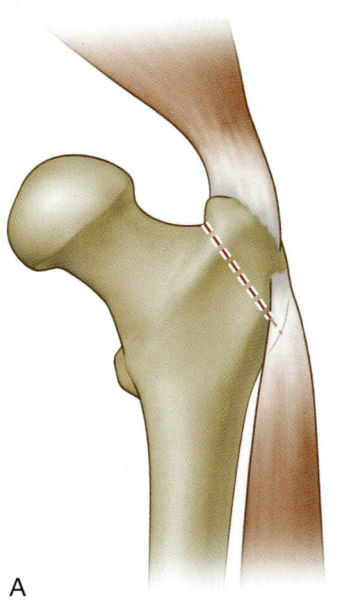 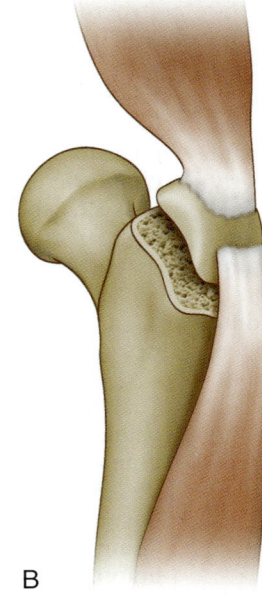

A   B

Figure 20-4. Anterior trochanteric slide osteotomy. (*Redrawn from Harris WH: Traumatic arthritis of the hip after dislocation and acetabular fractures: treatment by mold arthroplasty. J Bone Joint Surg Am 51:737, 1969.*)

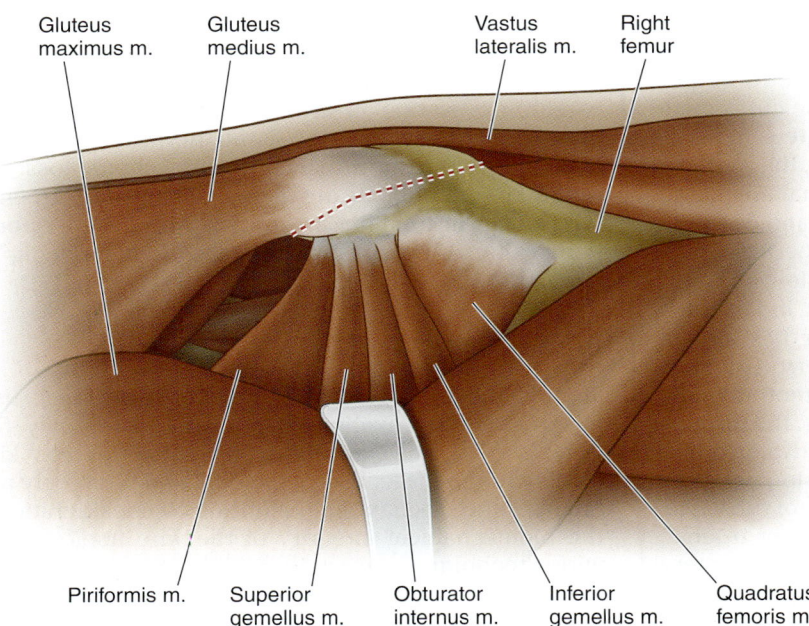

Gluteus maximus m.   Gluteus medius m.   Vastus lateralis m.   Right femur

Piriformis m.   Superior gemellus m.   Obturator internus m.   Inferior gemellus m.   Quadratus femoris m.

Figure 20-5. Chevron modification of the trochanteric slide osteotomy as described by Ackerman and Trousdale.[30] (*Redrawn from Ackerman DB, Trousdale RT: Triplanar trochanteric osteotomy: a modified anterior trochanteric slide osteotomy. J Arthroplasty 23:459, 2008.*)

reattachment.[31] The superior cut of the step osteotomy is performed similarly to the traditional slide, but a diagonal step is added. The step is inclined 20 to 30 degrees inferiorly on the anterior side, with a 5-mm step depth. This osteotomy has been shown by in vitro testing to be a more stable construct than the commonly performed slide osteotomy.

Anterior Trochanter Only. Dall[32] is credited with a technique of slide osteotomy that is based on the transgluteal approach of Hardinge.[33] The gluteus minimus is split for 2 cm proximal to the tip of the greater trochanter, and the vastus lateralis is split distally in line with its muscle fibers. A Gigli saw is then passed superficial to the capsule anteriorly, but deep to the anterior one half of the gluteus medius and gluteus minimus. A partial (anterior) osteotomy is then performed with the hip adducted, slightly flexed, and internally rotated. The saw is directed as far posteriorly as possible to avoid making the osteotomy fragment too small. The triangular bone fragment that is created carries the anterior one half of the gluteus medius, gluteus minimus, and anterior vastus lateralis. The hip is dislocated anteriorly by this approach.

Split Trochanter (Stracathro). McLaughlin has described the Stracathro Hospital technique, which splits the trochanter into anterior and posterior fragments.[34] Two wafers of trochanter are created by first dividing the gluteus medius and vastus lateralis. The short external rotators remain attached to the posterior fragment. After hip implantation, the trochanteric fragments fall back into place and are anchored with sutures to the soft tissues. This type of osteotomy may not be advisable for revision surgery.

Repeat Osteotomy

Horizontal/Vertical

The description of specific revision osteotomies (i.e., the short oblique or horizontal osteotomy and the vertical osteotomy) is credited to Harris.[11] The horizontal osteotomy is used when the proximal femoral anatomy is such that no cancellous bed would be available for reattachment if a standard osteotomy were to be performed. A short oblique or horizontal bone cut is made as far proximally as possible while the gluteus minimus and maximus are protected. After revision, the resultant fragment is advanced to reach the remaining intact lateral cortex for reattachment (Fig. 20-6A and B). In one study in which horizontal osteotomy was performed, 25 of 28 osteotomies (89%) had healed at follow-up.[35]

The vertical osteotomy (Fig. 20-6C) is indicated in revision surgery in which the trochanter has already been advanced during a previous surgery. Examples include cases of prior horizontal osteotomy and advancement, revision of hips following the original Charnley technique with trochanteric advancement,[9] and prior surgeries with abductor tensioning. Wide exposure is recommended with full release of the vastus intermedius and lateralis, distal to the greater trochanter. The vertical bone cut is performed 3 to 5 mm lateral to the lateral femoral cortex so that a sufficient lateral bed is left for reattachment. All ten horizontal osteotomies in the previously discussed study healed after fixation, and rates of union after horizontal, vertical, and standard osteotomy did not differ.[35]

With advancement to the lateral femur in both horizontal and vertical osteotomies, friction contact between the fragment and the cortex is decreased. Metallic mesh was commonly utilized in the aforementioned reports to distribute forces evenly on the trochanteric fragment, and wire reattachment was recommended.

Repeat Trochanteric Slide

Lakstein and colleagues reported results of the modified trochanteric slide procedure (leaving the posterior structures attached to the proximal femur) on greater trochanters that previously had osteotomies and were healed.[36] At a minimum follow-up of 13 months, 33 (87%) osteotomies healed with bony union, 4 (11%) had fibrous union, and one (3%) had nonunion. Two patients had new-onset abductor lurch, persistent trochanteric pain, and dislocation. The authors concluded that this technique is reliable, and that it has similar clinical outcome and complication rates as primary osteotomy.

FIXATION TECHNIQUES

Techniques for fixation of the greater trochanter after osteotomy are varied and have changed over time. The type of osteotomy performed has a strong influence on the exposure gained and the ability to tension the soft tissues. Fixation technique, on the other hand, has more of an influence on surgical complications such as nonunion, bursitis, and hardware-related issues. Although historical data can be gathered through the myriad wiring methods published until a decade ago, today's surgeons are more likely to use simpler techniques.

To achieve stable fixation and eventual union, the technique employed must counteract the destabilizing forces associated with pull of the peritrochanteric musculature.[37] Additional challenges are encountered with osteotomy fixation in arthroplasty versus nonarthroplasty hip surgery, as well as further issues with revision surgery with proximal femoral bone loss. For example, screws alone are not usually used for trochanteric repair in total hip arthroplasty because less bone is available for purchase compared with resurfacing[24] or nonarthroplasty surgery.[30,31]

Wiring

Monofilament surgical wires have long been used for trochanteric fixation, specifically, osteotomy fixation.[2,9,11,32,38,39] However, monofilament wires can kink, leading to breakage, loss of fixation, and ultimately nonunion of the trochanter. In addition to consideration of the biomechanical integrity of the wire itself, various wiring techniques vary in their ability to resist displacement. Markoff and associates[40] reported on an experimental evaluation of techniques popular at the time and

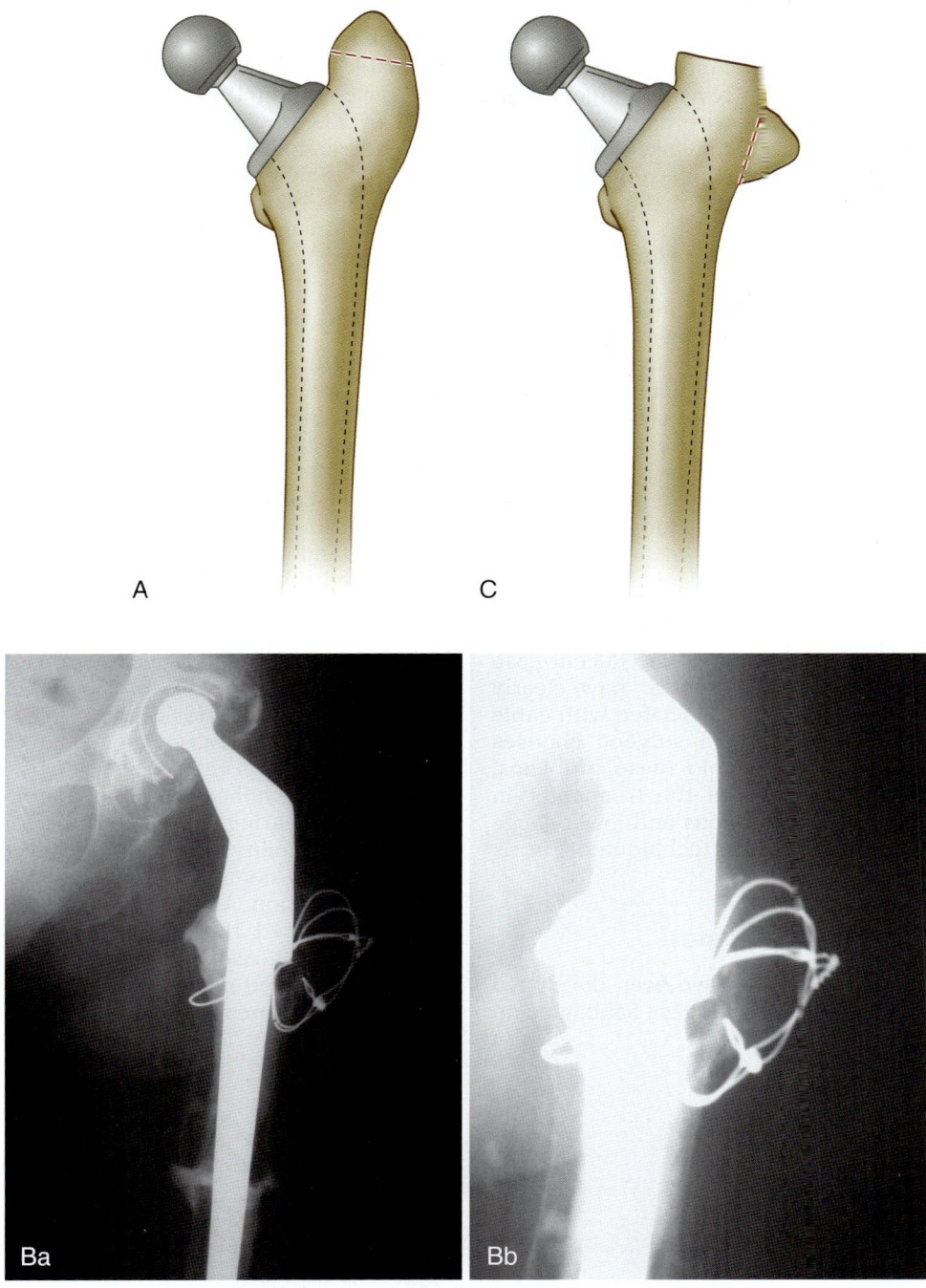

Figure 20-6. A, Horizontal trochanteric osteotomy. **B,** Anteroposterior radiograph showing healed osteotomy. **C,** Vertical osteotomy on a femur in which the greater trochanter was advanced to the lateral femoral cortex in a previous procedure with trochanteric advancement. *(A and B redrawn from Harris WH: Traumatic arthritis of the hip after dislocation and acetabular fractures: treatment by mold arthroplasty. J Bone Joint Surg Am 51:737, 1969.)*

found that Charnley[2] and Harris[39] techniques resulted in the least displacement after simulation of the proximal pull of the hip abductors after standard osteotomy.

The ultimate strength of a wire construct is dependent on both the wire diameter and the type of knot used. Bostrum examined the load capabilities of different wire sizes and knot types and determined that the square knot and the knot twist were preferable to the

uniform symmetrical twist method.[41] They also found, as did Shaw and Daubert,[42] that lower-gauge wire performed better.[41] If monofilament wire is used, 16-gauge wire secured with a knot twist or a square knot leads to the best result. In addition, special tools are convenient and are preferable in knot tying.[11]

Jarit and colleagues compiled survey data over a 25-year period ending in 1993 that demonstrate an overall wire breakage rate of 22% in 2910 THAs using various wiring techniques.[37] Nonunion occurs less frequently and ranges from 0 to 7.9% in primary surgery.[37] Wire breakage, which is more common in trochanteric nonunion,[39,43] is associated with revision surgery, uniplanar osteotomies, and simple wire configurations.[44] Other characteristics that have been linked to trochanteric nonunion or wire breakage include surgical experience,[43,45] osteoporosis,[45] small size of the fragment,[45] poor apposition of bone surfaces,[45,46] contact with cement[45,46] or cortical bone,[45] and failure to tighten wire loops.[45]

Today, trochanteric osteotomy is much more frequently employed in revision than primary total hip replacement. Surgical technique may be even more important in these cases, as was exemplified by Schutzer and Harris,[44] who found that technical error (e.g., poor wire or mesh placement) explained most of the nonunions in their study of 188 hips. Similarly, Hodgkinson and co-workers[47] were able to improve union using a modified wiring technique in their study of revision THA and osteotomy.

Although wiring techniques have decreased in popularity in the United States because of the availability of cables, cable-grip systems, and plate constructs, wire fixation may be preferred in some cases. Recent case reports[48] and long-term follow-up studies[49] have clearly demonstrated the complications associated with cable fraying and debris generation. If a surgeon chooses monofilament wire fixation to avoid these problems, the literature supports fixation of the trochanter in two planes, using knot configurations and lower-gauge alloy steel.[37] I prefer the four-wire technique of Harris (Fig. 20-7).

Bolts and First-Generation Plates

Newer internal fixation methods have been developed in the setting of historical techniques. Sabbagh and associates presented a plate and cable system that attached to the femur and used two vertical passes of the cable.[50] Volz and Turner reported the results of a bolt assembly in 1975, along with a nonunion rate of 1.3% of 229 trochanters.[51] Gottschalk and colleagues designed a similar mechanical system but had poorer results.[52] Scher designed a short plate based on the tension band principle for revision arthroplasty,[53] and Courpied and Postel used a similar device with wires.[54]

Cable Fixation

Multifilament cables were introduced by Dall and Miles in 1977[55] and are now available in several different compositions and configurations. These variations were introduced to provide better resistance to deforming forces and to allow better compression at the osteotomy site. Early biomechanical comparison studies favored the use of cables over wires for construct strength and compression, but current studies have questioned the long-term ramifications of cables vis-à-vis early revision and debris formation.[48,49,56-58] Data are mixed regarding the results of cable fixation, but results reported by Kelley and Johnston are a matter of concern. Upon reviewing a series of 322 THAs, they noted a breakage rate of 43% for cables versus 12% for wires.[58] In addition, Hop and associates found that cables led to a higher nonunion rate: 19.7% versus 14% for wires.[57] Both studies implicated cable debris in accelerated wear of the bearing surface. For these reasons, as well as the availability of more advanced technologies, cables are not commonly used alone for proximal trochanteric fixation. A novel isoelastic cable has recently been introduced that may circumvent some of the issues of metallic cables, but to date this has been used only for extended osteotomy, intraoperative and periprosthetic fractures, and allograft strut fixation.[59,60]

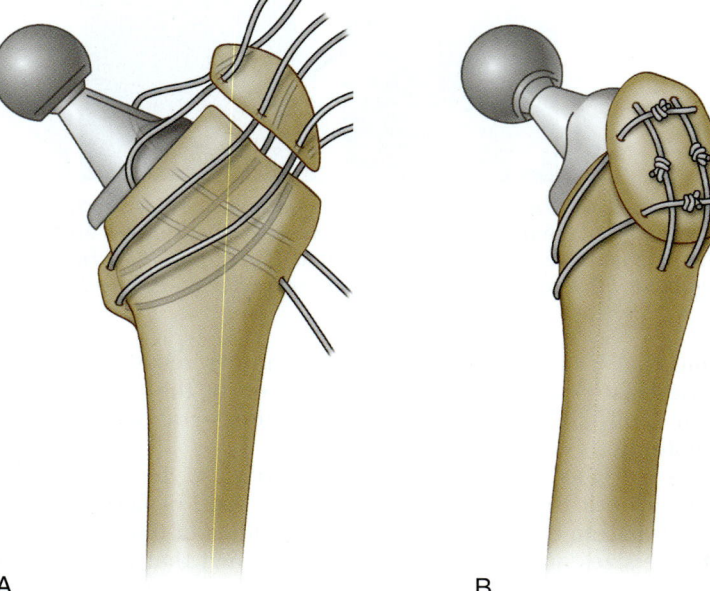

Figure 20-7. The four-wire technique of fixation of the trochanteric osteotomy. (*Redrawn from McGrory BJ, Bal BS, Harris WH: Trochanteric osteotomy for total hip arthroplasty: six variations and indications for their use. J Am Acad Orthop Surg 4: 258, 1996.*)

A   B

Cable Grip System

In addition to multifilament cables, Dall and Miles introduced an H-shaped trochanteric grip system that was touted to supplement these cables and was said to be better at resisting destabilizing forces[55] (Fig. 20-8A). Over time, innovators reported less breakage with 2-mm compared with the original 1.6-mm cables. Furthermore, the cable grip system withstood more load compared with cables or wires alone when tested in vitro.[61] Ultimately, the cable grip system did not offer better outcomes compared with wires, but its application was said to be more convenient. Dall and Miles reported a nonunion rate of 1.5% and a fibrous union rate of 3.1% with a horizontal 2.0-mm cable construct.[55] In contrast, Ritter and associates reported a 38% nonunion rate in 40 hip replacements,[62] and Koyama and colleagues described a 30.6% nonunion rate in their study of the cable grip system as used in revision surgery.[63] Silverton and colleagues, who also reported a high rate of nonunion (25%), found no better results using four versus two cables, and warned of a 47% incidence of cable fraying and fragmentation with a 17% chance of debris migration.[64]

McCarthy and co-workers reported on 223 hip replacements (available at 1 to 8 years' follow-up) using a cable grip system. Two multifilament cables were passed medially through drill holes in the lesser trochanter in 67% (149/223) of cases. Thirteen percent (30/223) had a prior trochanteric nonunion. Cable breakage was noted in 10% of cases and unraveling of the cable in 18%. Nineteen nonunions occurred (9%), although only 4% occurred when bone-to-bone apposition was achieved. Based on multiple analyses, the authors recommended use of the slide osteotomy technique when possible, employing vitallium cables and placing the cables medially through the lesser trochanter, while trying to achieve bone-to-bone apposition.[46]

Compared with cable systems, monofilament wire has been shown to yield significantly less metallic debris and reduced migration.[65] Although Hop and co-workers found no increase in the revision rate using cables versus wire,[57] evidence now indicates that revisions are more common.[49] I currently recommend removal of the cable grip after 1 year if this construct is employed, whether or not bony bridging occurs (Fig. 20-8B).

Claw Plate

The next generation of trochanteric reattachment devices introduced after the cable grip was the claw plate system. One style (Zimmer Inc., Warsaw, Ind) uses a denser pattern of multifilament cable and proximally has a contour that fits better over the greater trochanter. Plates of different lengths are available, and they have the ability to cerclage the femur and theoretically better distribute deforming forces. For enhanced proximal fixation, I have sometimes added a proximal screw through the impaction hole (Fig. 20-9). This particular system allows pretensioning of the cable, which in my experience decreases the frequency of cable loosening. Barrack and Butler demonstrated less wire breakage and lower nonunion rates with this system compared with the cable grip.[66] A trend toward less limp and stronger abduction was noted in this study.

Another style of claw plate (Biomet Inc., Warsaw, Ind) was described by Zarin, Zarakowski, and Burke for fixation of seven trochanteric osteotomies.[67] A major

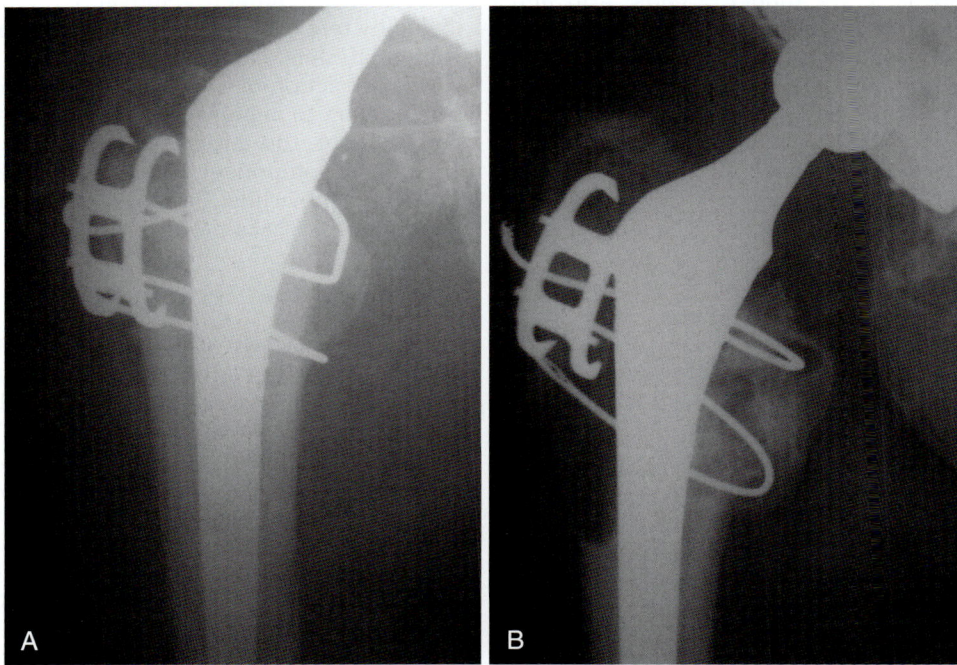

Figure 20-8. A, Anteroposterior radiograph showing use of cable grip system after revision surgery. **B,** Nonunion of the trochanter and failure of the multifilament cables. Note marked lateral femoral osteolysis associated with debris and polyethylene wear.

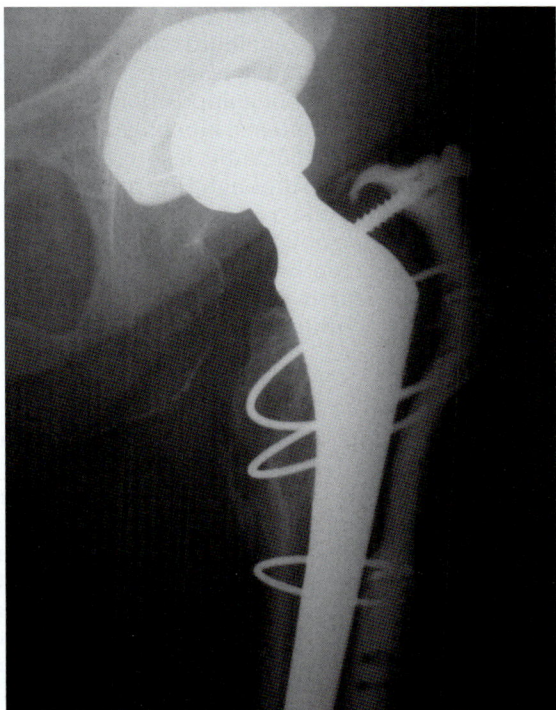

Figure 20-9. Fixation of trochanteric osteotomy with a claw plate system. Note added fixation with proximal cortical screw.

advantage of this system is that a monofilament wire is used for distal fixation; therefore the risk of significant debris formation postoperatively is theoretically decreased.

Disadvantages of the claw plate construct include the fact that the plate is larger than the cable grip and therefore requires more dissection for application. Likewise, potential soft tissue irritation and bursitis may be more common. Therefore, claw plates may be more appropriate for fractures and trochanteric nonunions than for osteotomies.[37,68] Poor bone stock or osteolysis common in revisions may require a longer osteotomy (below the vastus tubercle) to bypass thin, avascular bone. In these cases, the claw plate may be an excellent option for fixation.

Locking Plate

Use of a tibial locking plate for trochanteric osteotomy fixation was recently reported by McGrory and Lucas.[6] Similar to the claw plate construct, the locking plate may be best used in difficult osteotomy cases. Potential benefits include rigid fixation and limited need for cerclage wires or cables. The technique involves provisional fixation of the trochanter with the leg abducted, as well as application of a contoured locking-type plate to capture the trochanteric fragment. Longer locking screws are employed in the proximal fragment, and unicortical locking and/or bicortical nonlocking screws are used distally. Cable or wire augmentation may be used, if additional fixation is warranted (see Fig. 20-1A and B). Precontoured plates designed specifically

for the proximal femur are currently in development, but I presently use a proximal tibial plate (a right tibial plate for a right femur) or humeral plate to capture the relatively posterior trochanter. Biomechanical and clinical studies are lacking, but this technique holds promise in my opinion.

VARIATIONS/UNUSUAL SITUATIONS

Myriad techniques for trochanteric osteotomy and selected results have been described. However, in some instances, osteotomy is difficult or impossible. The surgeon must be prepared for these situations.

Osteoplasty and Trochanteric Excision

Attarian and Bolognesi reported on a technique of osteoplasty (reshaping and partially resecting the greater trochanteric tip) performed through a modified direct lateral approach.[8] Based on two case reports with successful outcomes, the authors conclude that this technique is useful in situations of proximal migration of the greater trochanter to avoid impingement and potential osteotomy and reattachment complications. The surgeon must plan this approach from the beginning as a soft tissue dissection while skeletonizing the trochanter; however, maintaining proximal-distal continuity of supporting soft tissues is necessary. The soft tissue sleeve is then reattached to the modified proximal lateral femur (Fig. 20-10A-C).

Capello and Feinberg have shown that removal of a trochanteric fragment following persistent nonunion is likewise possible; their technique may also be applied in cases in which osteotomy cannot be repaired.[69] Complete or near-complete removal of the trochanter is followed by tenodesis of the gluteus medius tendon to the vastus lateralis. A small wafer of bone is left in cases where retraction of the tendon is significant. Tenodesis is necessary to minimize limp, according to the authors. Furthermore, the authors suggest using a constrained acetabular component, an abductor brace (worn at all times except while bathing), and protected weight bearing for 8 weeks postoperatively.

Myofascial Flap Techniques

In 1991 McMinn and associates described a myofascial flap technique[5] (a variation of the Hardinge[33] technique) that may be useful in cases where osteotomy or fixation is not advisable. With this method, a V-shaped flap of the gluteus minimus, gluteus medius, and proximal vastus lateralis is reflected proximally. The authors, who report that this technique was used in 25 difficult revision THAs, conclude that their exposure and postoperative results are similar to those attained with TO, but without risks of nonunion and migration. Soft tissue reattachment was accomplished in all but one case, and if lengthening was needed, a V-Y advancement could be achieved. However, the postoperative course is protracted: The authors recommend 3 weeks of bed rest with the leg in abduction. Functional assessment after

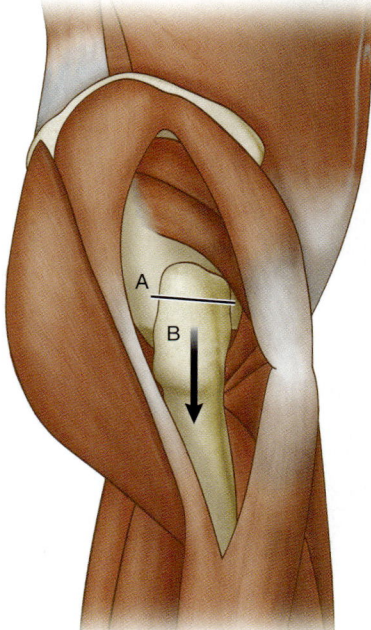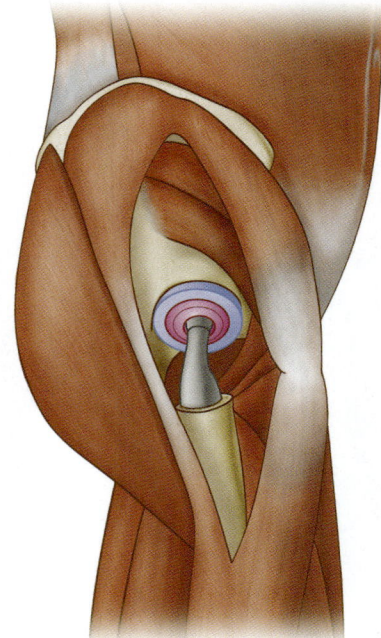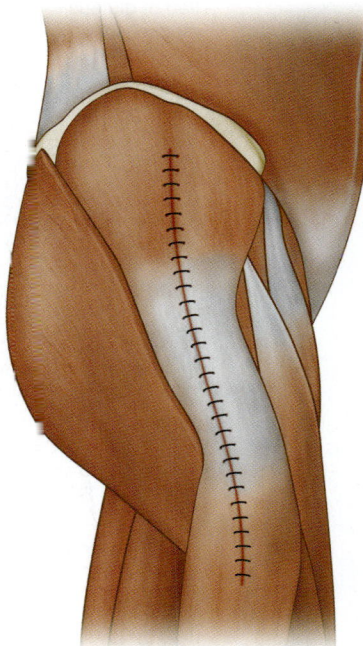

Figure 20-10. A through **C,** Attarian and Bolognesi osteoplasty technique for overriding the trochanter in revision surgery. *(Redrawn from Attarian, D, Bolognesi M: Greater trochanteric osteoplasty in revision hip arthroplasty: two case reports. Am J Orthop 40: E1, 2011.)*

6 months noted no patient with decreased abductor power or function.

Whiteside and associates demonstrated successful results in a situation in which a trochanteric osteotomy could not be advanced to viable bone.[70] This is most common in cases of advanced proximal femur loss and so-called *trochanteric escape*, but may also occur after an osteotomy is performed. The technique involves raising a triangular flap of gluteus maximus muscle and sewing this to the gap between the greater trochanter and the lateral cortex of the femur. It is secured to the inner surface of the anterior capsule of the hip. With the hip abducted 10 to 15 degrees, the gluteus maximus is closed over the flap and the greater trochanter (Fig. 20-11). Upon comparing a group of five patients in whom this technique was used with a group of patients who had the trochanter left unrepaired (five hips), and also with a group with trochanteric excision (four hips), the authors found that the flap group had less pain, lower risks of limp and Trendelenburg sign, and less need for support than the other two groups.

Abductor Advancement

Brick and Chin presented a technique that may be useful in particularly difficult cases of osteotomy repair in which abductor scarring or deformity is severe.[7] The "abductor slide" technique was described for reattaching migrated trochanters in nonunion surgery but may also be considered in very difficult osteotomy repairs. Advancement of the abductor muscles is based on the

superior gluteal neurovascular pedicle and is achieved through a separate transverse curvilinear incision over the iliac crest. Subperiosteal release of the entire origins of the gluteus minimus, medius, and maximus muscles is said to allow safe advancement of the trochanter. However, some authors have expressed concern over the trochanteric blood supply if osteotomy is also performed.[32,71]

POSTOPERATIVE CARE

Sir John Charnley predicated widespread use of the transtrochanteric approach on a high rate of union within 3 weeks of surgery without imposing restrictions that would impede rehabilitation.[2,3,9] Because anteroposterior shearing forces are as high as four times body weight,[3] some postoperative restrictions are appropriate. Most patients are able to stand after surgery and can walk with the aid of a walker or crutches. However, they must be limited to only partial weight bearing until the trochanter has healed; the surgeon should be guided by the radiographic appearance. The patient should not start abduction exercises against gravity until the radiographs confirm union. Recovery and healing can be aided with the use of an abduction orthosis in special cases of tenuous repair or high risk if instability occurs.

I currently recommend removal of multifilament cables at 1 year, whether or not bony union has been achieved. This decreases the chance that metallic debris will be generated and may protect against

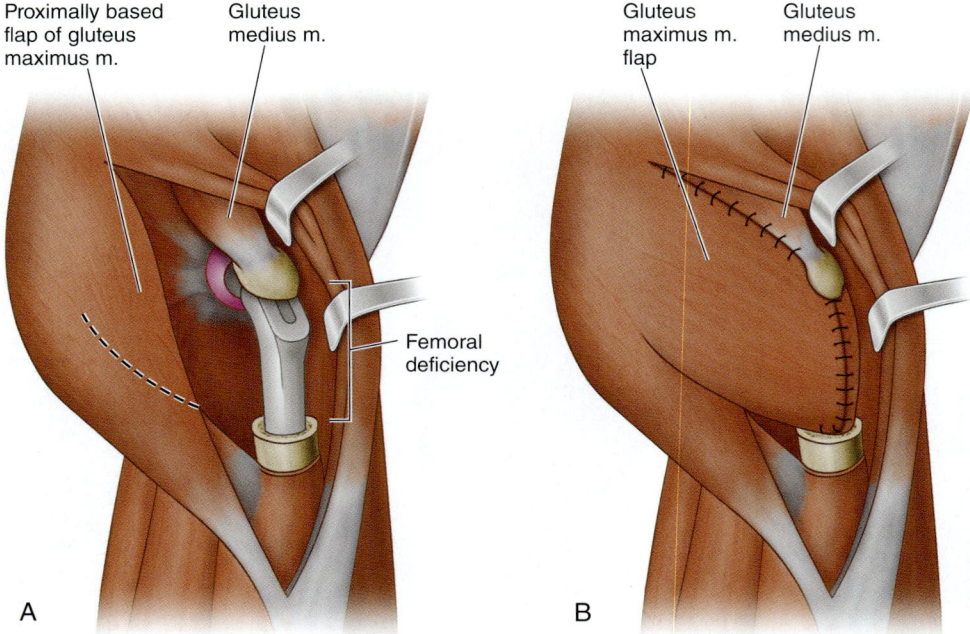

Figure 20-11. A and **B,** Technique of Whitesides and colleagues[70] for reconstruction when trochanteric osteotomy cannot be repaired. *(Redrawn from Whitesides LA, Nayfeh T, Katerberg BJ: Gluteus maximus flap transfer for greater trochanter reconstruction in revision THA. Clin Orthop Relat Res 453:203, 2006.)*

third-body–mediated wear of the bearing surface, as well as osteolysis (see Fig. 20-8*B*).

COMPLICATIONS

Complications of trochanteric osteotomy can be divided into two broad categories: those related to osteotomy healing and those related to the mode of fixation. Nonunion or a fibrous union of the trochanter is not necessarily a complication with clinical significance.[2,72] If the trochanter does not heal by bony bridging (Fig. 20-12), however, associated issues of pain, hardware breakage, or abductor dysfunction may manifest as impaired gait, Trendelenburg lurch, subluxation, or dislocation of the hip replacement. Even when union of the trochanter occurs, the patient may still have problems. Trochanteric pain and bursitis may be related to a prominent trochanter or to irritating hardware. Fraying and breakage of hardware can lead not only to pain, but also to wear and the need for early revision.[48,49,56,57]

Pain after hip replacement with trochanteric osteotomy should be approached in a systematic way. If sufficient time has passed to allow for healing, and other causes of pain have been ruled out,[32] attention can be directed to the trochanter. If trochanteric pain occurs with palpation, if crepitation is noted over the lateral hip, and if the patient temporarily responds to a diagnostic anesthetic injection, surgery is warranted. Permanent pain relief is by no means guaranteed[73]; this should be discussed with the patient. If there are no other issues such as gait abnormality, removal of the hardware and débridement of the bursa make sense.

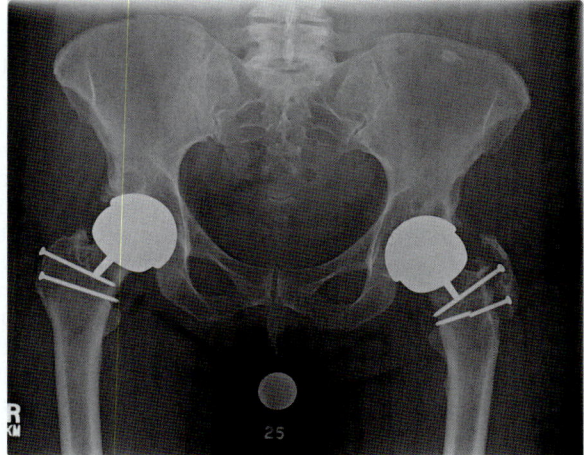

Figure 20-12. Nonunion and fragmentation of trochanteric slide osteotomy (left hip) and well-healed osteotomy (right hip) in contemporary resurfacing hip replacement. The patient had left lateral hip pain and a left-sided Trendelenburg limp.

Bernard and Brooks found no difference in pain relief after hardware removal in trochanters with union or with nonunion.[73] If instability or gait abnormalities are present, in addition to pain, and if there is a fibrous union or nonunion, then repeat fixation is the most appropriate intervention. A low-profile device that allows rigid fixation and appropriate soft tissue tensioning should be pre-formed. Autologous bone grafting can be considered but has not definitively been shown to be helpful.[74]

A patient who presents with an isolated gait abnormality after trochanteric osteotomy introduces a more challenging problem. If a trochanteric nonunion or fibrous union occurs, and if the patient has a positive Trendelenburg sign, both surgical[72] and nonsurgical treatment should be considered. If trochanteric migration is greater than 1 cm, abductor power is likely impaired[45,75] and surgery is the preferred treatment. On the other hand, if the trochanter is healed without migration, abduction strengthening and physical therapy focusing on gait training should be considered before surgery is undertaken. Hardware removal and appropriate soft tissue débridement should be considered if hardware breakage occurs, or if significant pain is attributable to the trochanter, and the patient does not respond to strengthening.

Hip replacement instability is multifactorial, but nonunion and migration of the trochanter can be implicated in some cases. Nonunion of the trochanter is said to occur in 5% of cases of trochanteric osteotomy, and of these, approximately 15% will be unstable.[32] If instability occurs in conjunction with trochanteric nonunion, the surgeon should consider surgery. At surgery, biomechanical parameters (i.e., femoral offset, leg length, cup and stem position, head size) should be optimized. Next, internal fixation of the trochanter should be attained, with tensioning of the greater trochanter. Kaplan and colleagues showed that if union is achieved in these cases, instability is eliminated in the vast majority.[76] Postoperatively, in addition to protected weight bearing, an abduction orthosis may be worn to minimize risk of dislocation during the recovery period.

CURRENT CONTROVERSIES

- Greater trochanteric osteotomy is rarely used in contemporary hip replacement, and its application is likely related to both the type of surgery and the surgeon's predisposition.
- Although the indications of exposure and soft tissue tensioning are well accepted, the exact application of these indications is somewhat controversial.
- Some surgeons apply the approach more liberally than others. Likewise, the type of internal fixation needed to maximize healing is not universally agreed upon.
- Various options are available, and surgeon preference dominates their application.
- Based on newly available literature, I would recommend avoiding or removing multifilament cables; this advice will likely be considered controversial.
- Also, newer unproven technologies such as locking plates and nonmetallic tensioning wire may prove beneficial, but objective studies will be required if their usage is to be endorsed.

REFERENCES

1. Ollier L: Traité des résections et des opérations conservatives qúont peut practiquere sur le système osseux, Paris, 1885, G. Masson.
2. Charnley J: The long-term results of low-friction arthroplasty of the hip performed as a primary intervention. J Bone Joint Surg Br 54:61, 1972.
3. Charnley J: Low friction arthroplasty of the hip: theory and practice, Berlin, 1979, Springer-Verlag.
4. Hamblin DL: Complications of trochanteric osteotomy. In Ling RSM (ed): Complications of total hip replacement, New York, 1984, Churchill Livingstone.
5. McMinn DJ, Roberts P, Forward GR: A new approach to the hip for revision surgery. J Bone Joint Surg Br 73:899, 1991.
6. McGrory BJ, Lucas R: The use of locking plates for greater trochanteric fixation. Orthopaedics 32:917, 2009.
7. Chin KR, Brick GW: Reattachment of the migrated ununited greater trochanter after revision hip arthroplasty: the abductor slide technique. A review of four cases. J Bone Joint Surg Am 82:401, 2000.
8. Attarian D, Bolognesi M: Greater trochanteric osteoplasty in revision hip arthroplasty: two case reports. Am J Orthop 40: E1, 2011.
9. Charnley J: Arthroplasty of the hip: a new operation. Lancet 1:1129, 1961.
10. Jensen NF, Harris WH: A system for trochanteric osteotomy and reattachment for total hip arthroplasty with a ninety-nine percent union rate. Clin Orthop Relat Res 208:174, 1986.
11. McGrory BJ, Bal BS, Harris WH: Trochanteric osteotomy for total hip arthroplasty: six variations and indications for their use. J Am Acad Orthop Surg 4:258, 1996.
12. Debeyre J, Duliveux P: Les arthroplasties de la hanche: études critique à propos de 200 cas opérés, Paris, 1954, Editions Medicales Flammarion.
13. Weber BG, Stuhmer G: Improvements in total hip prosthesis implantation technique: a cement-proof seal for the lower extremity medullary cavity and a dihedral self-stabilizing trochanteric osteotomy. Arch Orthop Trauma Surg 93:185, 1979.
14. Weber BG: Osteotomy of the greater trochanter in total hip replacement: conventional versus dihedral technique. Orthopade 18:540, 1989.
15. Berry DJ, Muller ME: Chevron osteotomy and single wire reattachment of the greater trochanter in primary and revision total hip arthroplasty. Clin Orthop Relat Res 294:155, 1993.
16. Wroblewski BM, Shelley P: Reattachment of the greater trochanter after total hip replacement. J Bone Joint Surg Br 67:736, 1985.
17. Sochart DH, Paul AS, Kurdy WM: A new osteotome for performing chevron trochanteric osteotomy. Acta Orthop Scand 66:445, 1995.
18. Iyer K: A new posterior approach to the hip joint. Injury 13:76, 1981.
19. Sanchez-Sotelo J, Gipple J, Berry D, et al: Primary hip arthroplasty through a limited posterior trochanteric osteotomy. Acta Orthop Belg 71:548, 2005.
20. Stuchin SA, Millman J: Oblique posterior trochanteric osteotomy in revision total hip arthroplasty. J Arthroplasty 26:472, 2011.
21. Glassman AH, Engh CA, Bobyn JD: A technique of extensile exposure for total hip arthroplasty. J Arthroplasty 2:11, 1987.
22. English TA: The trochanteric approach to the hip for prosthetic replacement. J Bone Joint Surg Am 57:1128, 1975.
23. Fulkerson JP, Crelin ES, Keggi KJ: Anatomy and osteotomy of the greater trochanter. Arch Surg 114:19, 1979.
24. Pitto R: The trochanter slide osteotomy approach for resurfacing hip arthroplasty. Int Orthop 33:387, 2009.
25. McFarland B, Osborne G: Approach to the hip: a suggested improvement on Kocher's technique. J Bone Joint Surg Br 36:364, 1954.
26. Mercati E, Guary A, Myquel C, et al: A postero-external approach to the hip joint: value of the formation of a digastric muscle [in French]. J Chir (Paris) 103:499, 1972.
27. Engh CA, Bobyn JD: Biological fixation in total hip replacement, Thorofare, NJ, 1985, Slack.
28. Goodman GS, Pressman A, Saastamoinen H: Modified sliding trochanteric osteotomy in revision total hip arthroplasty. J Arthroplasty 19:1039, 2004.
29. Lakstein D, Backstein D, Safir O, et al: Modified trochanteric slide for complex hip arthroplasty: clinical outcomes and complication rates. J Arthroplasty 25:363, 2010.

30. Ackerman DB, Trousdale RT: Triplanar trochanteric osteotomy: a modified anterior trochanteric slide osteotomy. J Arthroplasty 23:459, 2008.

31. Schoeniger R, LaFrance AE, Oxland TR, et al: Does trochanteric step osteotomy provide greater stability than classic slide osteotomy? A preliminary study. Clin Orthop Relat Res 467:775, 2009.

32. Silverton CD, Rosenberg AG: Management of the trochanter. In Callaghan JJ, Rosenberg AG, Rubash HE (eds): The adult hip, New York, 1998, Lippincott-Raven, p 1269.

33. Hardinge K: The direct lateral approach to the hip. J Bone Joint Surg Br 64:17, 1982.

34. McLauchlan J: The Stracathro approach to the hip. J Bone Joint Surg Br 66:30, 1984.

35. Bal BS, Maurer BT, Harris WH: Trochanteric union following revision total hip arthroplasty. J Arthroplasty 13:29, 1998.

36. Lakstein D, Kosashvili Y, Backstein D, et al: Trochanteric slide osteotomy on previously osteotomized greater trochanters. Clin Orthop Relat Res 468:1630, 2010.

37. Jarit GJ, Sathappan SS, Panchal A, et al: Fixation systems of greater trochanteric osteotomies: biomechanical and clinical outcomes. J Am Acad Orthop Surg 15:614, 2007.

38. Harris WH: Traumatic arthritis of the hip after dislocation and acetabular fractures: treatment by mold arthroplasty. J Bone Joint Surg Am 51:737, 1969.

39. Harris WH, Crothers OD: Reattachment of the greater trochanter in total-hip arthroplasty: a new technique. J Bone Joint Surg Am 1978:211, 1978.

40. Markoff KL, Hirschowitz DL, Amstutz HC: Mechanical stability of the greater trochanter following osteotomy and reattachment by wiring. Clin Orthop Relat Res 141:111, 1979.

41. Bostrom MP, Asnis SE, Ernberg JJ, et al: Fatigue testing of cerclage stainless steel wire fixation. J Orthop Trauma 8:422, 1994.

42. Shaw JA, Daubert HB: Compressive capability of cerclage fixation systems: a biomechanical study. Orthopaedics 11:1169, 1988.

43. Boardman KP, Bocco F, Charnley J: An evaluation of a method of trochanteric fixation using three wires in the Charnley low friction arthroplasty. Clin Orthop Relat Res 132:31, 1978.

44. Schutzer SF, Harris WH: Trochanteric osteotomy for revision total hip arthroplasty: 97% union rate using a comprehensive approach. Clin Orthop Relat Res 227:172, 1988.

45. Amstutz HC, Maki S: Complications of trochanteric osteotomy in total hip replacement. J Bone Joint Surg Am 60:214, 1978.

46. McCarthy J, Bono JV, Turner RH, et al: The outcome of trochanteric reattachment in revision total hip arthroplasty with a cable grip system: mean 6-year follow-up. J Arthroplasty 14:810, 1999.

47. Hodgkinson JP, Shelley P, Wroblewski BM: Re-attachment of the ununited trochanter in Charnley low friction arthroplasty. J Bone Joint Surg Br 71:523, 1989.

48. Bauer TW, Ming J, D'Antonio JA, et al: Abrasive three-body wear of polyethylene caused by broken multifilament cables of a total hip prosthesis: a report of these cases. J Bone Joint Surg Am 78:1244, 1996.

49. Altenburg AJ, Callaghan JJ, Yehyawi TM, et al: Cemented total hip replacement cable debris and acetabular construct durability. J Bone Joint Surg Am 91:1664, 2009.

50. Sabbagh MA, Galline Y, Soria C: Osteosynthese du grand trochanter par plaque et cables dans les arthroplasties totales de hanche. J Chir (Paris) 127:230, 1990.

51. Voltz RG, Turner RH: Reattachment of the greater trochanter in total hip arthroplasty by use of a bolt. J Bone Joint Surg Am 57:129, 1975.

52. Gottschalk FA, Morein G, Weber F: Effect of the position of the greater trochanter on the rate of union after trochanteric osteotomy for total hip arthroplasty. J Arthroplasty 3:235, 1988.

53. Scher MA, Jakim I: Trochanter reattachment in revision hip arthroplasty. J Bone Joint Surg Br 72:435, 1990.

54. Courpied JP, Postel M: Pseudarthroses trochanteriennes apres arthroplastie totale de hanche: leur fixation par une nouvelle plaque-griffe. Rev Chir Orthop 72:583, 1986.

55. Dall DM, Miles AW: Re-attachment of the greater trochanter: the use of the trochanter cable-grip system. J Bone Joint Surg Br 65:55, 1983.

56. Langlais FL, Thomazeau H: Abrasive three-body wear of polyethylene caused by broken multifilament cables of a total hip prosthesis: a report of three cases. J Bone Joint Surg Am 79:1892, 1997.

57. Hop JD, Callaghan JJ, Olejniczak JP, et al: The Frank Stinchfield Award. Contribution of cable debris generation to accelerated polyethylene wear. Clin Orthop Relat Res 344:20, 1997.

58. Kelley S, Johnston RC: Debris from cobalt-chrome cable may cause acetabular loosening. Clin Orthop Relat Res 285:140, 1992.

59. Sarin VK, Mattchen TM, Hack B: A novel iso-elastic cerclage cable for treatment of fractures. Presented at the 51st Annual Meeting of the Orthopaedic Research Society, Washington, DC, 2005.

60. Ting N, Wera G, Levine B, et al: Early experience with a novel nonmetallic cable in reconstructive hip surgery. Clin Orthop Relat Res 468:2382, 2010.

61. Hersh CK, Williams RP, Trick LW, et al: Comparison of the mechanical performance of trochanteric fixation devices. Clin Orthop Relat Res 329:317, 1996.

62. Ritter MA, Eizember LE, Keating EM, et al: Trochanteric fixation by cable grip in hip replacement. J Bone Joint Surg Am 73:580, 1991.

63. Koyama K, Higuchi F, Kubo M, et al: Reattachment of the greater trochanter using the Dall-Miles cable grip system in revision hip arthroplasty. J Orthop Sci 6:22, 2001.

64. Silverton CD, Jacobs JJ, Rosenberg AG, et al: Complications of a cable grip system. J Arthroplasty 11:400, 1996.

65. Kelley S, Johnston RC: Debris from cobalt-chrome cables may cause acetabular loosening. Clin Orthop Relat Res 285:140, 1992.

66. Barrack RL, Butler RA: Current status of trochanteric reattachment in complex total hip arthroplasty. Clin Orthop Relat Res 441:237, 2005.

67. Zarin J, Zurakowski D, Burke D: Claw plate fixation of the greater trochanter in revision total hip arthroplasty. J Arthroplasty 24:272, 2008.

68. Hamadouche M, Zniber B, Dumaine V, et al: Reattachment of the ununited greater trochanter following total hip arthroplasty: the use of a trochanteric claw plate. J Bone Joint Surg Am 85:1330, 2003.

69. Capello WN, Feinberg JR: Trochanteric excision following persistent nonunion of the greater trochanter. Orthopedics 31:711, 2008.

70. Whitesides LA, Nayfeh T, Katerberg BJ: Gluteus maximus flap transfer for greater trochanter reconstruction in revision THA. Clin Orthop Relat Res 453:203, 2006.

71. Naito M, Ogata K, Emoto G: The blood supply to the greater trochanter. Clin Orthop Relat Res 323:294, 1996.

72. Ritter MA, Gioe JJ, Stringer EA: Functional significance of nonunion of the greater trochanter. Clin Orthop Relat Res 159:177, 1981.

73. Bernard AA, Brooks S: The role of trochanteric wire revision after total hip replacement. J Bone Joint Surg 69:352, 1987.

74. Stefanich R, Jabbur M: Autogeneic cancellous bone grafting following transtrochanteric hip arthroplasty: an attempt to facilitate union of the greater trochanter. Clin Orthop Relat Res 228:141, 1988.

75. Nutton RW, Checketts RG: The effects of trochanteric osteotomy on abductor power. J Bone Joint Surg Br 66:180, 1984.

76. Kaplan SJ, Thomas WH, Poss R: Trochanteric advancement for recurrent dislocation after total hip arthroplasty. J Arthroplasty 2:119, 1987.

CHAPTER 21

Extensile Approaches for Revision Total Hip Arthroplasty

R. Stephen J. Burnett

KEY POINTS

- Always plan for an extensile exposure on the femoral side, and template that plan preoperatively.
- Isolated acetabular revision with retention of a well-fixed femoral component requires extensile exposure.
- Femoral revision for removal of well-fixed implants and femoral canal cement and for varus remodeling of the proximal femur is the primary indication for extended trochanteric osteotomy.
- Extended trochanteric osteotomy may be performed via an anterolateral or posterolateral extensile exposure.

INTRODUCTION

Surgical exposure in revision total hip arthroplasty (THA) requires careful preoperative planning and attention to detail. The most common surgical exposures utilized for revision THA surgery include posterolateral and anterolateral/direct lateral exposures. These exposures are the mainstay of revision THA surgery and are useful when acetabular revision alone is required, or when an uncomplicated revision of a femoral component is necessary, without more extensive bone defects. The decision of which surgical exposure to use will depend on factors that include surgeon experience and preference, patient body habitus (i.e., obesity), patient anatomic factors, location and type of prior surgical incisions over the hip, and implant selection. The most important aspect to consider is surgeon experience and preference. The two most commonly used *routine* surgical revision exposures utilized are the anterolateral and posterolateral approaches to the hip.

The anterolateral exposure is an abductor splitting approach that requires removal and repair of the anterior 30% to 40% of the gluteus medius and minimus. This approach may also be utilized for revision total hip replacement (THR) surgery. Disadvantages of this exposure include (1) an increase in limp due to splitting of the abductor muscle (also likely due to traction injury to anterior branches of the superior gluteal nerve during surgery); (2) an increase in formation of heterotopic

bone within the abductor muscles and anteriorly over the capsule and greater trochanter; (3) a greater incidence of trochanteric complications (e.g., intraoperative fracture, postoperative fracture or "escape" of the greater trochanter, trochanteric pain usually secondary to failure of the abductor to heal back following repair); and (4) a tendency to insert the femoral component angled from anterior to posterior within the femoral canal (i.e., nonanatomic femoral component placement). Many surgeons select this approach on the basis of the potential for a reduced dislocation rate and are willing to accept the "disadvantages" already discussed. With the popularity of less invasive surgery, the posterolateral exposure has again gained prominence. Disadvantages of the posterolateral approach include (1) a slightly higher risk of dislocation, although with experience this is minimized, and (2) careful attention to component orientation, so that implants are inserted in proper anteversion. In Canada between 2008 and 2009,[1] the direct lateral approach (60%) and the posterolateral approach (36%) were combined for more than 95% of all surgical exposures in primary and revision THA surgery.

More extensile exposures may be required to access the hip to address bone defects and exposure of acetabular or femoral periprosthetic fractures, as well as for removal of well-fixed implants (e.g., removal of a well-fixed femoral component) and those in the previously multiply operated hip. The ideal extensile exposure should satisfy several objectives. It should provide satisfactory exposure of both components. It should allow preservation of healthy bone and soft tissue for exposure and closure. Ideally, this exposure would incorporate previously healed incisions and soft tissue planes from prior exposures. Finally, extensile exposures should preserve the blood supply to bone and soft tissues, which will be incorporated into the reconstruction. The objectives of this chapter are to discuss extensile exposures to the hip (femoral and acetabular) in revision THA, while discussing the most common extensile exposures utilized, which the surgeon should be familiar with, along with indications for their use.

A detailed description focusing on the extended trochanteric femoral osteotomy extensile exposure will highlight the chapter, including pearls and technique recommendations.

INDICATIONS/CONTRAINDICATIONS FOR EXTENSILE EXPOSURE OF THE HIP IN REVISION TOTAL HIP ARTHOPLASTY

The most common revision indications include polyethylene liner wear with or without periprosthetic osteolysis, aseptic loosening of one or more components, recurrent instability, and infection (chronic or acute). Not all of these indications will require extensile exposure of the hip. If one or more components are loose and no cement is retained distal to the femoral component, then extensile exposure may not be required. If varus remodeling of the proximal femur occurs, then careful preoperative templating is required to determine the reconstructive options and whether an extensile exposure is required on the femoral side. If an isolated acetabular revision is required with retention of a well-fixed femoral component, then a more extensile exposure is required to expose the acetabulum and at the same time retract the femoral component out of the field, so that it does not prevent adequate acetabular exposure. Removal of a well-fixed (cemented) or cementless femoral component may require an extended trochanteric osteotomy; this should be planned for preoperatively. More extensile exposure of the acetabulum, which may include the outer table of the ilium or the ischium, is required if the surgeon is planning to use a reconstruction cage or porous metal augments, or to stabilize a pelvic discontinuity. Both standard trochanteric osteotomy and the trochanteric slide osteotomy provide useful extensile exposures of the acetabulum; their limitations include fixation of the osteotomy and the risk of nonunion.

Contraindications to utilizing an extensile exposure to the hip include when the hip may be approached safely by one of the previously discussed standard approaches, when there is significant risk to neurovascular structures with the extensile exposure, and when the surgeon is unfamiliar with extensile exposure techniques and options.

PREOPERATIVE PLANNING

Old Incisions and Previous Surgical Exposure

Prior incisions should be noted by the surgeon for incision length, location over the hip, scarring, and mobility of underlying deep soft tissues, and should be considered for their utility in revision surgery (Fig. 21-1). The preoperative history should include questions about wound healing or breakdown along one or more of the old incision(s), wound problems such as infection, and any required intervention for the wound beyond routine wound care. In addition, a history of any postoperative transient neurologic symptoms should heighten surgeon awareness of a nerve injury, transient or permanent, and may have implications for selection of a revision exposure. Frequently, patients may be unable to recall

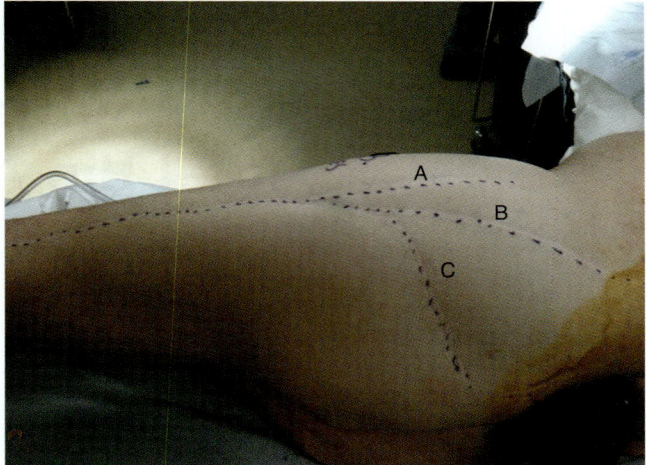

Figure 21-1. A, Direct lateral incision. This incision is centered longitudinally over the greater trochanter and is an abductor muscle splitting approach. **B,** Posterolateral incision. This approach distally is similar to the anterolateral, curving from the tip of the greater trochanter slightly posteriorly and entering the hip posterior to the abductor musculature. **C,** Southern posterior approach incision. This approach is done even farther posteriorly and limits exposure to the superior-lateral acetabulum.

which of several incisions was used for which procedure if more than one old incision is present. Obtaining previous operating room (OR) reports, in addition to the implant record, should be imperative to determine prior exposure and to identify whether any problems were present at the time of the previous procedure(s). Incisions from childhood pelvic osteotomy procedures should be noted, particularly the ilioinguinal and iliofemoral approaches, which are not commonly utilized in revision THA surgery. The significance of these prior incisions is that there may be significant scarring in the anterior aspect of the hip, including the acetabulum and the femur, and neurovascular structures in these areas may be tethered form these prior exposures. Similarly, if a prior Southern exposure (far posterior approach at the proximal aspect) has been utilized, the surgeon should beware that the sciatic nerve may be similarly scarred or tethered within the soft tissues posteriorly.

The type of prior incision should alert the surgeon to component orientation factors, which should be noted preoperatively. For example, if the prior exposure was a direct lateral (or anterolateral) approach, the acetabular and femoral components most likely will have been implanted in anatomic orientation (i.e., matching the native acetabular and the native femoral neck anteversion). In contrast, if the prior exposure used a posterolateral approach, then the components likely will have been implanted with increased femoral and acetabular anteversion. This may have implications in the selection of your exposure at revision. If the prior incision has utilized a transgluteal approach, then careful physical examination should be performed to assess side-lying abduction strength, because weakness or pain in the region of a prior abductor splitting exposure may be associated with abductor pull-off, nonhealed abductor repair (Fig. 21-2), or a dysfunctional superior gluteal nerve. If an isolated revision is being performed on the femoral side and the prior exposure was direct lateral, then if the surgeon elects to use a revision posterolateral approach, the acetabular component will have limited anteversion, and this may have implications for postoperative instability concerns.

Prior incisions should be considered whenever possible, depending on the procedure to be performed, to avoid the issues surrounding multiple incisions in close proximity over the hip. It is not uncommon for surgeons who use the direct lateral approach to the hip in primary THA to extend the incision slightly posterior at the proximal aspect, allowing less skin tension during femoral preparation while the leg is in the sterile leg bag. Thus, the surgeon should seek the prior OR report to identify the deep exposure because this may be confused as a prior posterolateral exposure (Fig. 21-3).

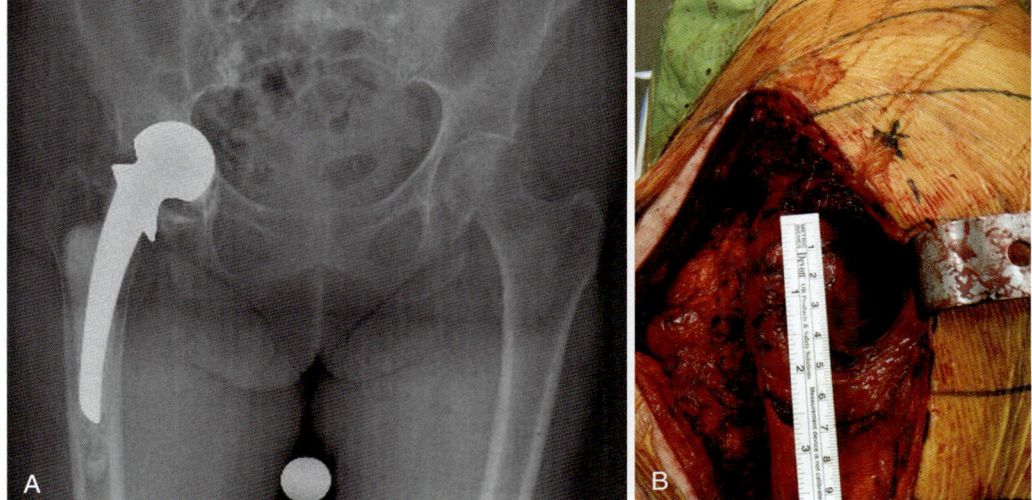

Figure 21-2. The previous hip exposure used at the time of hemiarthroplasty **(A)** for hip fracture was a direct lateral abductor splitting approach. At revision **(B),** the anterior 60% of the hip abductor musculature was absent with failure of the previous repair and the "bald eagle" sign of a bare trochanter, along with a large anterior defect of abductors and hip capsule.

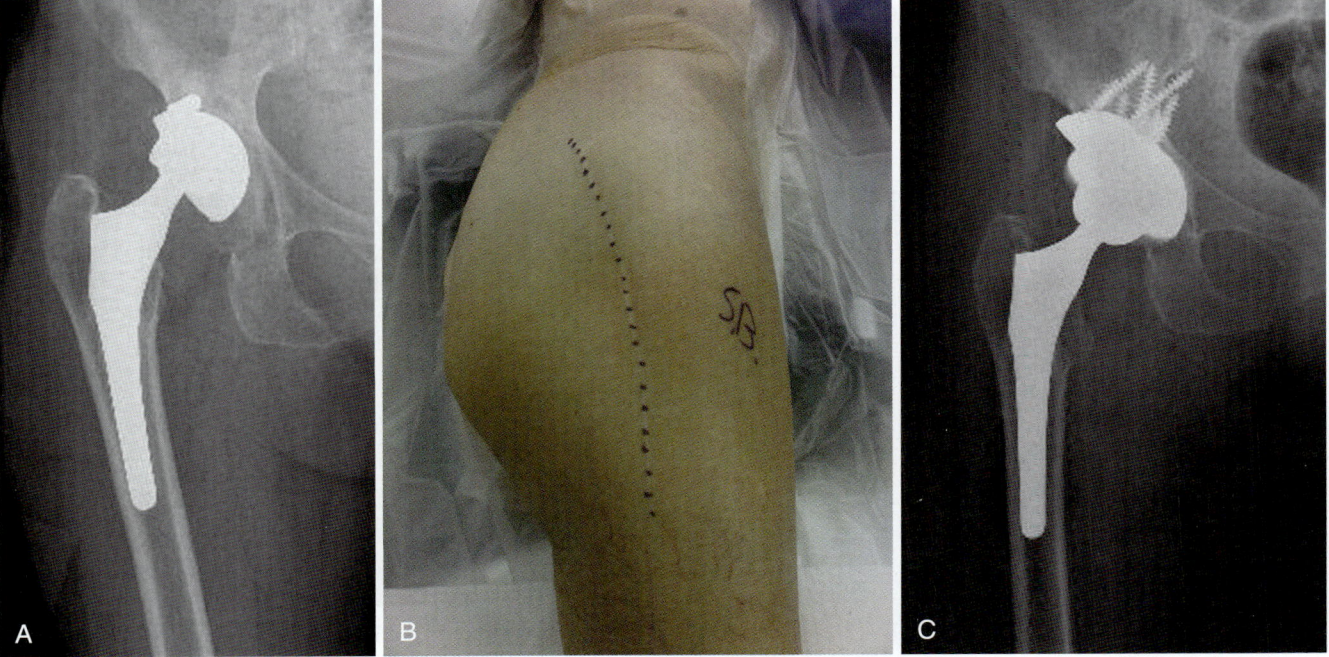

Figure 21-3. A, Preoperative right total hip arthroplasty (THA) acetabular revision for aseptic loosening and a type 3A Paprosky acetabular defect. **B,** The prior hip incision appears to resemble a posterolateral exposure. Review of the operating room (OR) report indicates a direct lateral abductor splitting deep exposure. The same incision was utilized for an extensile posterolateral approach for the acetabular revision. **C,** Postoperative x-ray of acetabular reconstruction utilizing a porous metal acetabular structural augment.

Incorporating the distal aspect of an old incision that extends down the thigh is most commonly utilized, even if it is slightly anterior or posterior to the mid axial line. If the surgeon changes the direction of that old incision proximally, attempts should be made to minimize acute angles when extending off an old incision. This will help minimize wound edge necrosis. If surgery has been performed recently over the hip, the surgeon should strongly consider using the recent incision, with distal and proximal extension as needed. Performing a new parallel incision adjacent to a recent incision will place the wound at risk for wound necrosis in the bridge between these two incisions, and thus is contraindicated in the setting of a recent hip incision. If a new parallel incision is utilized in close proximity (and with a narrow skin bridge) to a remote incision, there is still concern for wound healing problems in the skin bridge (Fig. 21-4). If in doubt about old incisions and wound problems, a preoperative consultation with a plastic surgeon may be useful, especially in the multiply operated hip with scarring of the soft tissues.

Deep dissection is preferred along the route of prior surgical exposure, when possible and when the surgeon is familiar with the prior deep exposure. Deep exposure for direct lateral, posterolateral, and transtrochanteric exposures may be performed utilizing a laterally based skin incision, provided the incision is long enough and is in the midline. Attempting to perform a direct lateral (anterolateral) exposure utilizing a posteriorly based skin incision is difficult because exposure of the abductors anteriorly is very difficult.

Selecting which approach to use will be dependent on surgeon experience and familiarity. Although surgeons typically perform one approach for primary and uncomplicated revision THA surgery, the surgeon who is performing revision surgery must be familiar with multiple exposures, so that the most appropriate exposure is selected.

Radiographs and Templating for Extensile Exposures

Typical radiographs obtained before revision THA surgery include low-centered anteroposterior (AP) pelvis, AP hip, and lateral of the femur. Additional views may be helpful, such as Judet views to assess the potential for pelvic discontinuity, and cross-table lateral to assess the acetabular component version. Digital templating has emerged as a useful tool that utilizes radiographic markers to calibrate accurate implant sizes and preoperative templating (Fig. 21-5). In revision surgery for osteolysis involving the femur or the acetabulum or both, computed tomography (CT) scanning may provide useful information regarding the location and degree of osteolysis, as routine radiographs may underestimate the degree of osteolysis of the pelvis and acetabulum.

It is critical to plan and template for an extensile exposure in advance, specifically, on the femoral side when an extended trochanteric osteotomy is considered. Assessment and planning for radiographic bone defects, the length of a retained femoral implant or distal cement mantle, and the implant selected for the femoral reconstruction must all be considered. On the acetabular side, if there is suspicion for pelvic discontinuity or a periprosthetic acetabular fracture, this must be considered preoperatively. Wide and extensile

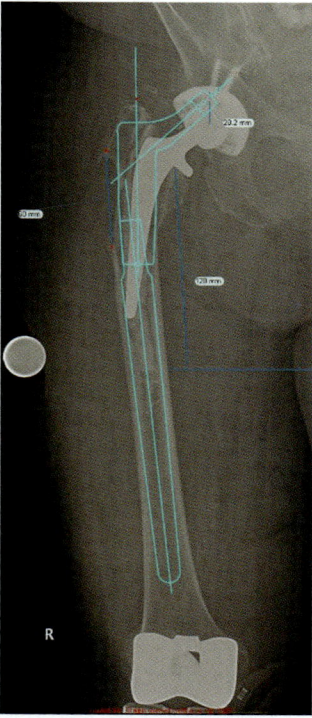

Figure 21-5. Digital templating for a revision femoral component. The radiograph must be a long film to include the femur and must be of sufficient length for revision femoral component templating so the component, as well as the acetabular component, can be revised. A ball marker of known dimension (2.54 cm) or the known femoral head diameter allows for size calibration.

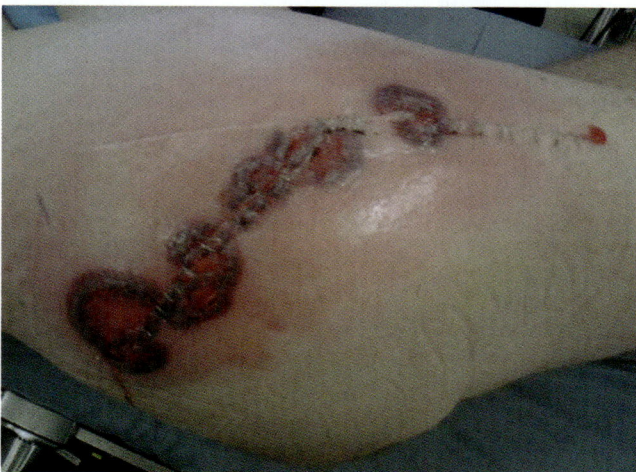

Figure 21-4. The hip exposure used previously was a direct lateral approach. At revision, the surgeon elected to incorporate a posterolateral incision with a narrow skin bridge, resulting in wound healing problems, most notably in the skin bridge between the prior incisions.

exposure of the posterior column of the acetabulum, ilium, and ischium is a specialized exposure, with the sciatic nerve and superior gluteal neurovascular structures at risk. If the surgeon is unfamiliar with this exposure, we recommend asking a surgeon with complex pelvic and acetabular trauma surgery experience to be involved in that aspect of the exposure and reconstruction.

The presence and severity of heterotopic ossification (HO) of bone around the hip on radiographs (Fig. 21-6) should alert the surgeon to the possibility of a difficult exposure, and to the fact that recurrence of heterotopic bone may occur. If the heterotopic bone is extensive and is causing impingement of the hip, this may affect the decision about surgical exposure and resection of this bone, which is rarely necessary. In the presence of heterotopic bone on a preoperative radiograph, the surgeon should consider utilizing HO prophylaxis, a single dose of preoperative or postoperative radiotherapy to the field, or postoperative indomethacin oral prophylaxis for 6 weeks.

DECRIPTION OF EXTENSILE EXPOSURE TECHNIQUES: FEMORAL

Extended Trochanteric Osteotomy

The extended trochanteric osteotomy (**ETO**) is the most widely utilized extensile exposure for the femoral canal and is a useful exposure in revision THA surgery. Originally described by Wagner,[2] this technique and its results have been reported and popularized by Paprosky and associates[3-9]; this approach is indicated for exposure of the femur to remove a well-fixed femoral component (and cement mantle), direct femoral canal access for femoral revision difficult dislocation secondary to significant HO or protrusion, excellent access for acetabular revision, and correction of proximal femoral deformity in the setting of proximal femoral varus remodeling. The osteotomy may be performed via the posterolateral and the anterolateral exposure. The principle of the approach is that the greater trochanter with

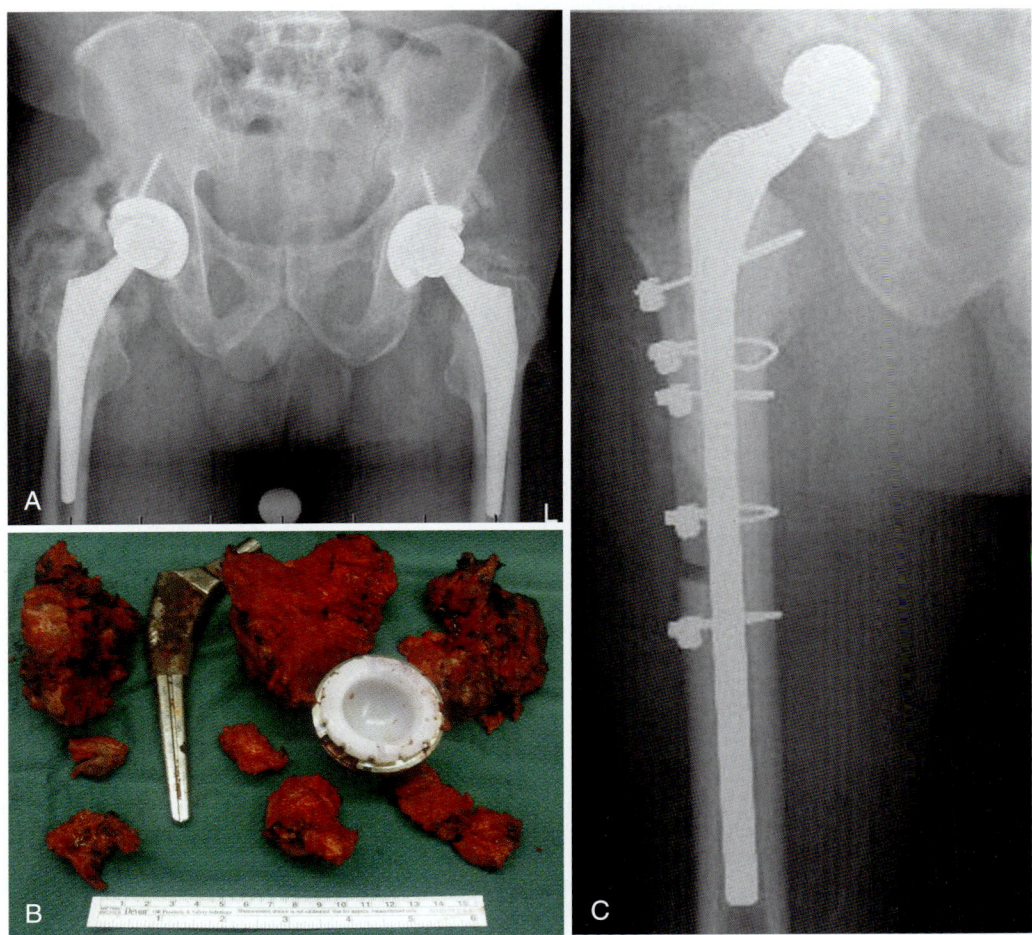

Figure 21-6. A, Preoperative x-ray showing severe heterotopic ossification (HO) of the right hip. This patient has an infected total hip arthroplasty (THA) with a draining sinus. **B,** Removal of the extensive HO, exposure of the hip, and removal of the cementless femoral component were facilitated by an extended trochanteric osteotomy. **C,** Postoperative x-ray following revision to a prosthesis of antibiotic-loaded cement (PROSTALAC, DePuy, Warsaw, Ind). Indomethacin was used postoperatively for HO prophylaxis for 6 weeks.

abductor attachments remains in continuity with a femoral shaft osteotomy with attached vastus lateralis musculature. The osteotomy, when performed postero-laterally, incorporates the lateral one third to one half of the femoral cortical shaft, and the vastus lateralis is elevated posteriorly off the intermuscular septum. Most of the vastus muscle remains attached to the cortical fragment, preserving its vascularity. When performed via the direct lateral approach, the vastus is divided at its midsubstance, and the osteotomy is hinged posteri-orly. The difference between these two approaches and

their muscular intervals is depicted in Figure 21-7. In addition, the ETO is useful when a standard trochan-teric osteotomy may be unfavorable, as with osteolysis of the greater trochanter. With attention to surgical technique, preservation of the blood supply to the oste-otomy fragment, and rigid fixation, the results of this osteotomy have been very favorable.[10]

Preoperative planning for an ETO requires careful templating. Assessment of leg length differences, com-ponents to be removed, and bone defects/osteolysis are identified. The length of the osteotomy is templated to

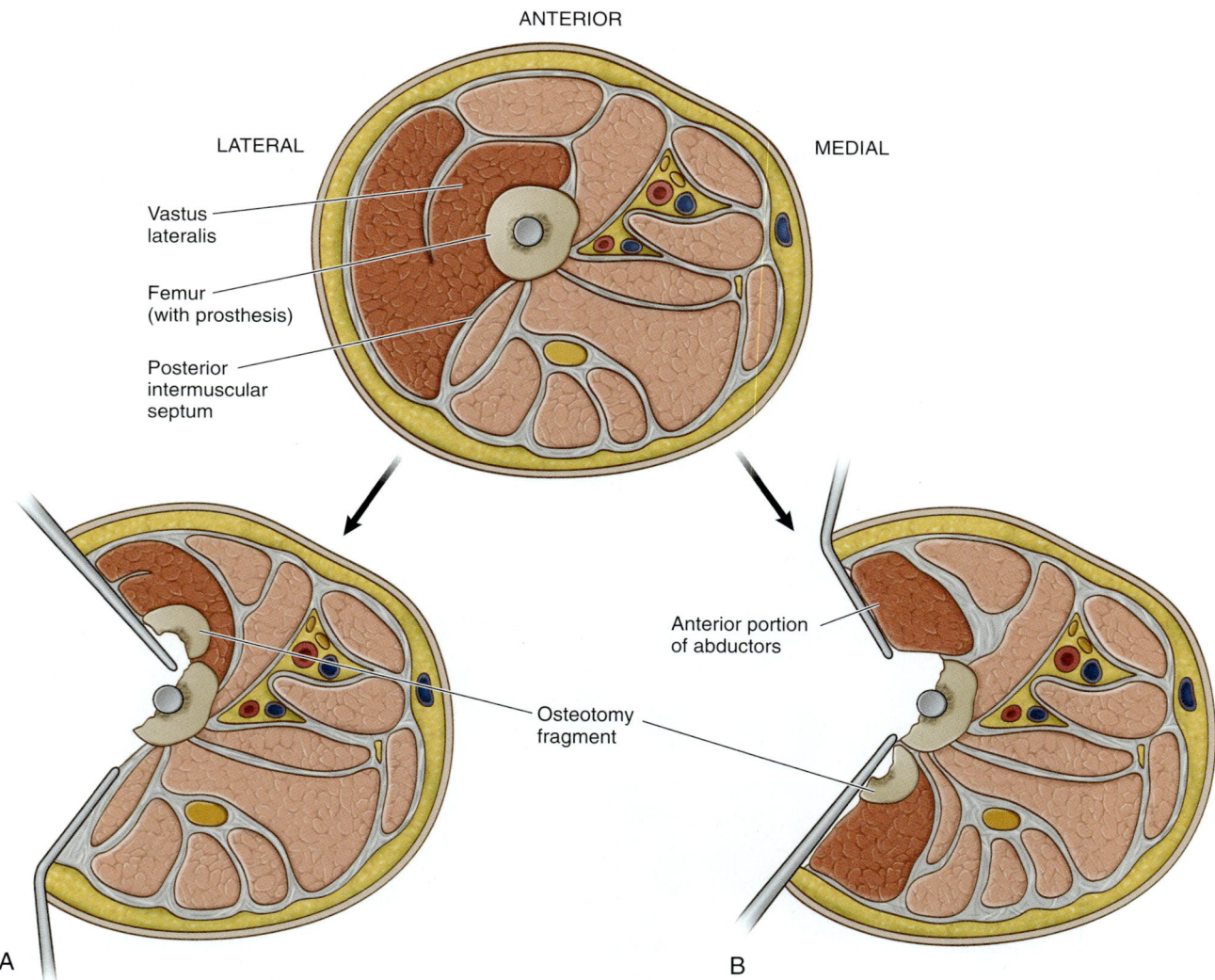

Figure 21-7. Cross-section of the proximal femur below the level of the greater trochanter demonstrating anatomic differ-ences between the extended trochanteric osteotomy (ETO) performed via a posterolateral approach versus a modified direct lateral approach. **A,** When performed through a posterolateral approach, the vastus lateralis is elevated off the posterior intermuscular septum and is retracted anteriorly. The posterior limb of the osteotomy is created first, and after the remaining anterior and distal cuts are completed, the osteotomy fragment is hinged anteriorly. Most of the vastus muscle substance remains attached to the cortical fragment and helps preserve its vascularity. **B,** When performed through a direct lateral approach, the vastus lateralis is divided in midsubstance. The anterior portion of the vastus is retracted anteriorly in continuity with the anterior third of the abductors. The anterior limb of the osteotomy is created first, and after the remaining posterior and distal cuts are completed, the osteotomy fragment is hinged posteriorly. The posterior portion of the vastus muscle substance remains attached to the cortical fragment, which helps preserve its vascularity.

allow component removal and to preserve distal bone for the revision implant. Generally, the minimum osteotomy length is 10 cm (a shorter osteotomy may be performed) measured from the tip of the greater trochanter or 7 to 8 cm from the lesser trochanter. To remove a cemented implant with a distal cement mantle and plug, the surgeon must consider that it may not be simple to remove distal cement and the plug if the osteotomy has been performed above the cement mantle and plug. Although specialized instruments such as ultrasonic cement removal tools and cement osteotomes are helpful,[11] removal of cement from above remains a challenge and is time-consuming. When possible, the osteotomy should be long enough to remove the implant along with any cement mantle, with awareness of the principle that 4 to 6 cm of scratch-fit endosteal contact may be required beyond the osteotomy for

a porous-coated cylindrical revision stem. To remove an ingrown fully porous-coated cylindrical primary THA straight stem, the osteotomy should extend distal below the metaphyseal flare of the implant, to the level of the cylindrical portion of the stem. The stem may then be cut with a metal cutting wheel, and the distal stem removed with trephines[3] (Fig. 21-8). If the stem is a revision bowed fully porous-coated implant, the osteotomy will not span the entire length of the implant, rather the surgeon must perform the ETO to the junction of the middle and distal one third of the implant, section the implant using a metal disk–cutting wheel, and then use trephines to trephine over the distal remaining portion of the stem.

A word of caution about removing cementless titanium stems with a proximal ingrowth surface combined with a distally roughened or even smooth surface. Do

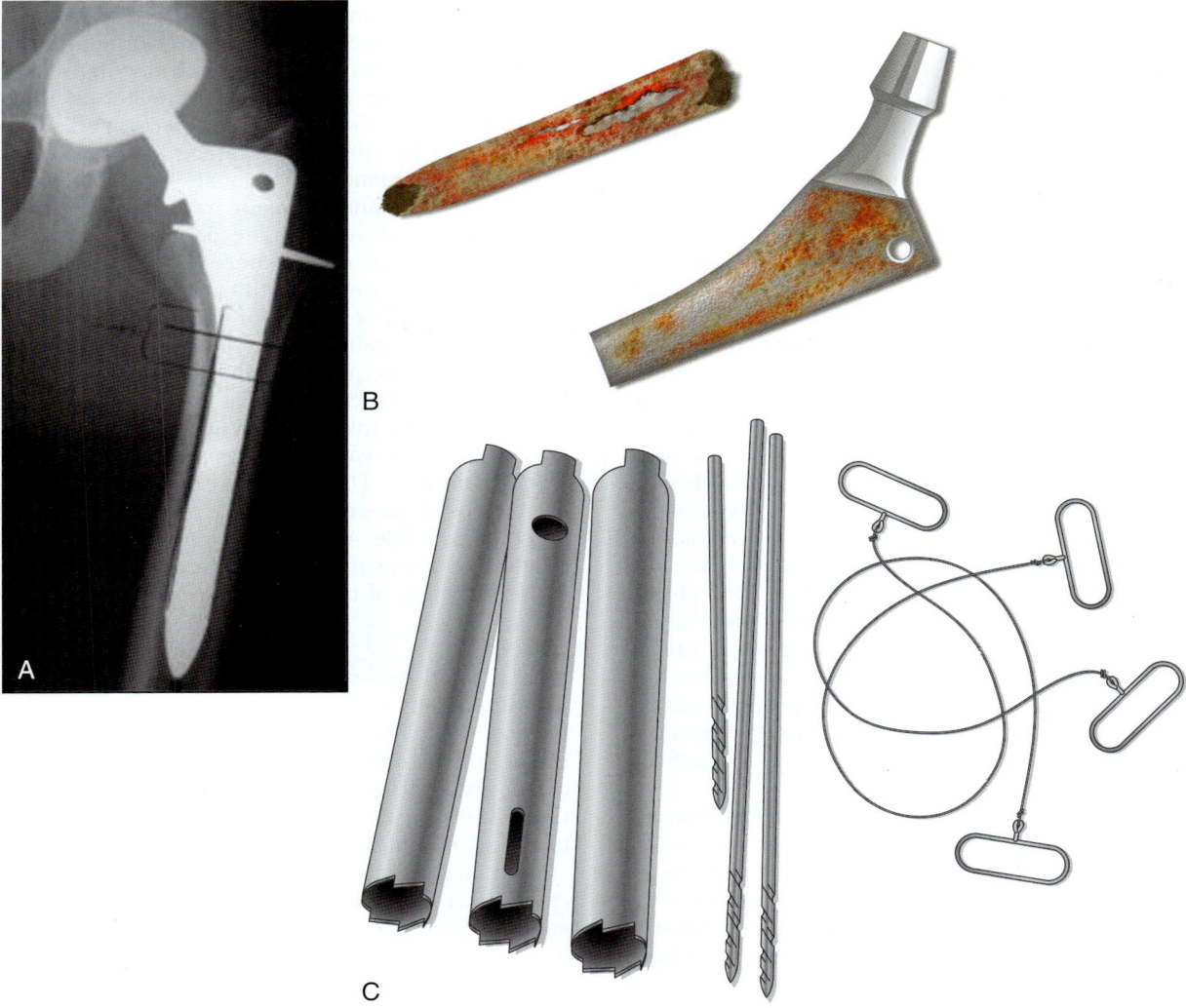

Figure 21-8. A, Removal of a cementless cobalt chrome cylindrical fully porous-coated stem requires preoperative planning and templating. The stem is cut below the metaphyseal flare of the implant with a metal cutting burr (diamond wheel disk or burr). **B,** The proximal metaphyseal portion is removed with Gigli saw assistance (multiple Gigli saws are necessary because they overheat and break during the procedure). Cylindrical hollow trephines are then used to trephine over the retained distal cylindrical portion of the stem. Several trephines of the same diameter are recommended because the trephine frequently cracks at the head because of fatigue and heat damage during trephining. **C,** Femoral implant after removal.

not expect the implant to be removed by just performing the osteotomy to the level of the porous ingrowth on the proximal aspect of the stem. These femoral components are often utilized for minimally invasive surgery. In our experience, performing an osteotomy that is longer, including toward the distal aspect of the stem, may be useful and should be considered and templated for. Significant bone ongrowth may occur even onto the smooth surfaces of these titanium stems, making removal difficult. Similarly, "working from above" to remove cementless titanium femoral implants using thin flexible osteotomes to work in the bone ingrowth interface may be time-consuming and associated with trochanteric fracture and surgeon frustration; it may eventually require an extended trochanteric osteotomy. In these instances, while attempting to remove the implant from above, we frequently perform an ETO to facilitate stem removal.

Extended Trochanteric Osteotomy Performed Via the Posterolateral Exposure

Exposure

The patient is positioned in the lateral decubitus position, and a posterolateral skin incision is utilized. It is not advantageous to extend the incision far posterior (i.e., Southern exposure), rather it should be extended in a posterolateral direction. Distally, the incision is ideally in the mid axial line or is slightly posterior off the midline. The deep fascia lata is identified and carefully exposed; identifying the normal fascia beyond the previous incision is helpful. Careful attention is required at this stage to not dissect through the subcutaneous layer and the fascia as one because this will make identification of the fascial plane difficult at the time of closure. The leg is then abducted by an assistant or onto a padded mayo stand, which relieves tension on the fascia. The fascia lata is incised distally in-line with the skin incision. Proximally, the fascia and gluteus maximus fibers are split in-line with the skin incision. It is preferable to not split the gluteus maximus quickly because vessels that may be identified during the split may be easily coagulated, and this may occur posteriorly and toward the distal third of the tendon insertion. Failure to control these vessels will result in significant blood loss throughout the procedure.

The fascia is then developed and separated from the vastus lateralis, trochanteric bursa, and gluteus medius. Frequently, the gluteus medius and the tensor fascia lata are conjoined, and separation may cause bleeding. The leg is then brought out of the abducted position and is internally rotated, to put tension on the piriformis and short external rotators. It is important to remember to keep the hip extended; this keeps tension off the sciatic nerve. The posterior border of the gluteus medius is identified and retracted anteriorly, and the piriformis tendon is identified. The sciatic nerve is palpated in the field posteriorly for reference and tension but is not dissected out, to avoid devascularization of the nerve. The gluteus minimus is elevated off of the

posterosuperior hip capsule to expose the intact capsule. In every revision THA case at our institution, a needle on a syringe is inserted into the hip joint capsule just posterior to the greater trochanter into the joint to obtain fluid for nucleated cell count, differential, and cultures before the capsulotomy is performed. A posterior trapezoidal capsulotomy is performed beginning parallel to the superior border of the piriformis, extending to the posterior border of the greater trochanter (GT), along the posterior undersurface of the trochanter, and releasing the capsule, piriformis, short rotators, and quadrates as a single flap. Release is carried to the lesser trochanter (LT), maintaining the iliopsoas insertion onto the lesser trochanter when possible.

If needed, the tendon may be elevated off the LT. Dissection continues along the posterior border of the vastus lateralis. At the gluteus maximus tendon insertion, dissection continues through the posterior border of the vastus, leaving a cuff of fascia for closure. At this stage, the gluteus maximus tendon and the vastus lateralis may be elevated from the posterior femur together, releasing the gluteus maximus and decompressing the sciatic nerve. The hip may be dislocated at this stage or after the osteotomy has been performed. We prefer to dislocate the hip at this stage and to remove the femoral component if it is loose. The vastus lateralis (VL) is retracted under tension from its posterior border in an anterior direction. The posterior border of the intermuscular septum is where the VL inserts. The VL fascia is then incised along its posterior border, leaving a posterior cuff of fascia for later repair. The muscle fibers are then split carefully posteriorly and longitudinally the length required for the osteotomy. At this stage it is important to coagulate or control any perforating vessels, and to take time to identify and ligate. Frequently, we use vascular clips because these vessels may be sizable. The posterolateral femoral cortex is then exposed, preserving the VL attachment laterally as much as possible. At the distal aspect of the osteotomy length, the vastus must be reflected off the lateral femur for preparation of the distal aspect of the osteotomy.

Osteotomy

After the soft tissues have been appropriately exposed, it is important to place a cerclage cable distal to the proposed osteotomy site to prevent unexpected stress riser or distal extension of the osteotomy during femoral canal preparation, trialing, and component insertion (Fig. 21-9). The osteotomy is then marked on the bone using a marking pen or electrocautery. This marking should incorporate one third to one half of the femoral canal laterally and should be anterior to the linea aspera. The osteotomy angles slightly at the GT to incorporate the GT fragment. The longitudinal portion of the osteotomy is then performed with a thin saw blade angling from posterior to anterior. The saw begins mid osteotomy and extends proximally. At this stage, the distal aspect of the osteotomy is prepared, using a pencil-tipped burr to create a smooth round arc from posterior to anterior. Externally rotating the leg facilitates completion of the anterior aspect of the curve. The saw is then used beginning in the mid portion of

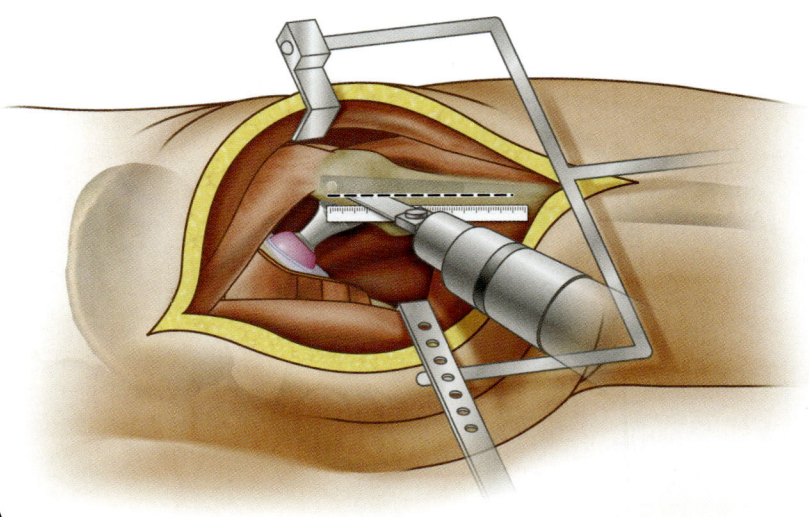

A

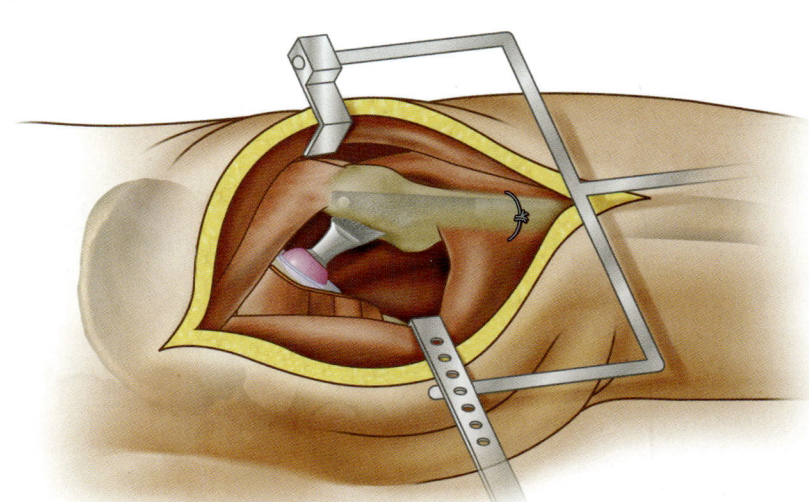

B

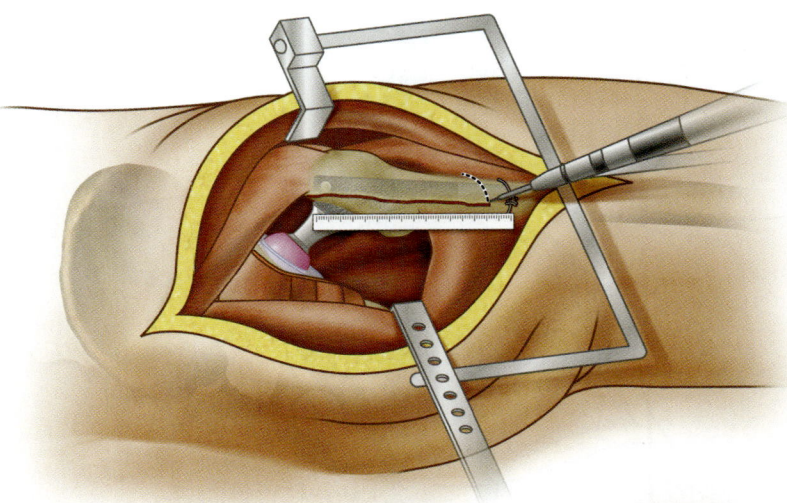

C

Figure 21-9. Extended trochanteric oste-otomy (ETO) performed via the postero-lateral approach. **A,** The length and direction of the osteotomy are marked; then the longitudinal osteotomy is per-formed with a thin oscillating saw from posterior to anterior. Note that the proxi-mal aspect of the osteotomy angles slightly medially at the level of the vastus ridge. **B,** Before the distal aspect of the osteotomy is performed, a cable (or double-looped cerclage wire in this case of infected total hip arthroplasty [THA]) is passed distal to the osteotomy and is tightened, to protect against osteotomy stress riser distal propagation. **C,** The distal end of the osteotomy is performed with a fine pencil-tipped burr rounding the osteotomy from posterior to anterior at the distal aspect, creating a smooth rounded osteotomy at the distal aspect.

Continued

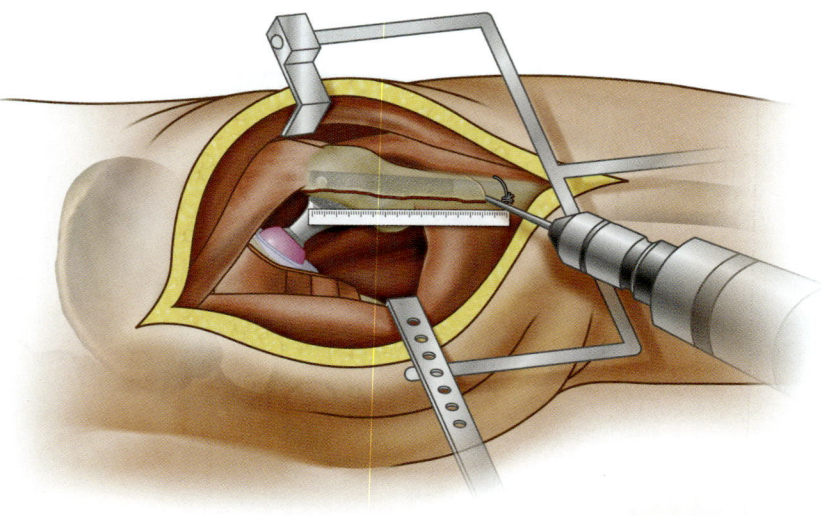

D

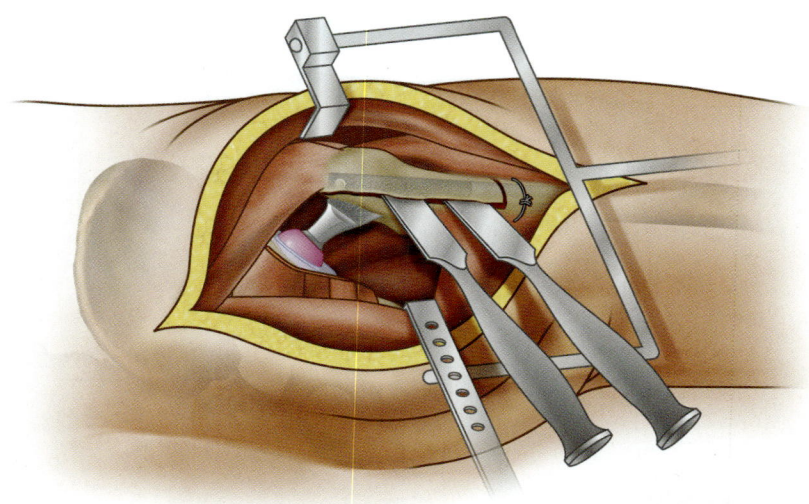

E

Figure 21-9, cont'd D, The anterior longitudinal limb of the osteotomy is then completed by drilling through the anterior cortex. A 2 mm drill bit may be used similarly to perforate the anterior cortex along the anterior osteotomy. **E,** The osteotomy is gently levered open from posterior to anterior with two or three broad straight osteotomes. **F,** The proximal anterior capsule *(white arrow)* and soft tissue must be released longitudinally to retract the proximal portion of the ETO anteriorly.

F

the osteotomy and extending distally to join the distal aspect, which has been prepared with the burr. The saw may be used to pass through the anterior cortical bone to complete the osteotomy along its length. Alternatively, multiple small 2.0 mm drill holes are made while passing the drill from posterior through the osteotomy site and perforating the anterior cortex. If the femoral component is well fixed, the osteotomy may be performed by extending the saw down to bone and then having the saw deflect lateral to the stem.

Alternatively, we will accept an osteotomy segment measuring slightly less than one third of the canal, if the stem is canal filling. However, this does risk fragmentation of the osteotomy fragment. A one-quarter inch straight osteotome is then passed from posterior to anterior to complete any anterior perforation. Two or more broad osteotomes are inserted across the osteotomy, and the fragment is elevated from posterior to anterior. At this stage, if the osteotomy is tethered or incomplete, the surgeon must stop and complete the osteotomy with the saw or drill along its anterior length, if necessary. Attempting to lever open an incomplete osteotomy typically will result in fracture of the osteotomy at its thinnest location, which is at the vastus ridge portion of the fragment. One important caveat is that to mobilize the proximal (GT) portion of the ETO anteriorly, a portion of the anterolateral capsule must be released at this time. Two blunt-tipped Bennett retractors are placed beneath the fragment, allowing it to be retracted anteriorly.

Osteotomy Fixation

After the reconstruction is completed, the osteotomy may be reapproximated to the femur. To facilitate this, abduct and internally rotate the leg. The osteotomy fragment may then be brought down to its bed. Provisional fixation of the fragment with a pointed reduction tenaculum along the distal osteotomy is useful for determining the appropriate location for fixation. If tensioning of the abductors is indicated, then the osteotomy fragment may be advanced. If varus remodeling of the proximal segment has occurred, the osteotomy fragment may not reduce anatomically. Burring the GT bed on the osteotomy fragment may allow contouring of the ETO fragment, facilitating a more anatomic fragment reduction back to the femur. If the fragment does not reduce anatomically and a gap is present posteriorly, longitudinally this may be accepted. In this instance, cancellous bone graft (obtained from femoral canal preparation) may be packed into the gap. Alternatively, if the bone of the osteotomy fragment or proximal femur is poor, an onlay cortical strut allograft may be used. We typically place the strut posterolaterally, secured with cables, at the time of osteotomy fixation. The strut also serves to protect the proximal femoral host bone from cables cutting though bone. Cables are passed from posterior to anterior, staying subperiosteal at the linea aspera, and staying directly on bone using cable passers. These cables are placed beneath the vastus lateralis.

We do not recommend anterior-to-posterior passage of cables because the sciatic nerve and profunda vessels

and perforating vessels may be at risk. The cables (usually two to three cables) are tightened[12] for the diaphyseal portion of the osteotomy. One cable should be passed just distal to the LT. If the osteotomy is a short segment, without 4 to 6 cm of cortical bone distally, we often use a trochanteric cable grip plate for fixation. A combination of vertical trochanteric and horizontal metaphyseal cable fixation has been reported with excellent results.[13]

Postoperative Care

Following ETO and cementless femoral revision, patients are kept protected while weight bearing 30% for 6 to 8 weeks. Similarly, during this period no active abduction of the hip is permitted, although passive hip abduction is allowed. Limited flexion of 70 to 90 degrees is used. When the revision is performed via the posterolateral approach, limitation in adduction combined with internal rotation is recommended.

Extended Trochanteric Osteotomy Performed Via Direct Lateral Exposure

Exposure

The technique and results[14-16] of this osteotomy were described most recently by MacDonald and associates[17] for the direct lateral approach to the hip in revision THA. The patient is positioned in the direct lateral position, with a direct lateral skin incision centered over the greater trochanter. The fascia is incised, and the interval between the tensor fascia lata (TFL) and the gluteus maximus muscles is split. The abductor gluteus medius is identified, and the posterior and anterior borders are palpated. A modified Hardinge exposure is then performed by splitting through the medius, minimus, and capsule as a single layer, while distally maintaining continuity with the vastus lateralis. Distally, the deep dissection is continued longitudinally by splitting the vastus 2 cm anterior to the posterior intermuscular septum and inserting the gluteus maximus. The anterior one half of the longitudinally split vastus is then retracted anteriorly in continuity with the abductor split as a single soft tissue sleeve (Fig. 21-10A).

Osteotomy

The osteotomy may be performed before or after dislocation, as necessary. Cerclage cable should be placed distal to the proposed osteotomy site for protection against stress riser during femoral preparation. The femur is extended and externally rotated. The osteotomy length is marked. The oscillating saw is used similarly, passing anterior to posterior. At the distal end, the osteotomy is rounded with a pencil-tipped burr. The osteotomy is completed posteriorly with the saw, with care taken to not extend the blade into the posterior soft tissues and sciatic nerve. A drill may be used to complete the anterior perforation. Broad osteotomes are used to elevate the osteotomy and retract it posteriorly (Fig. 21-10B). The osteotomy fragment maintains its soft tissue attachments and vascularity from the posterior two thirds of the abductors proximally and the

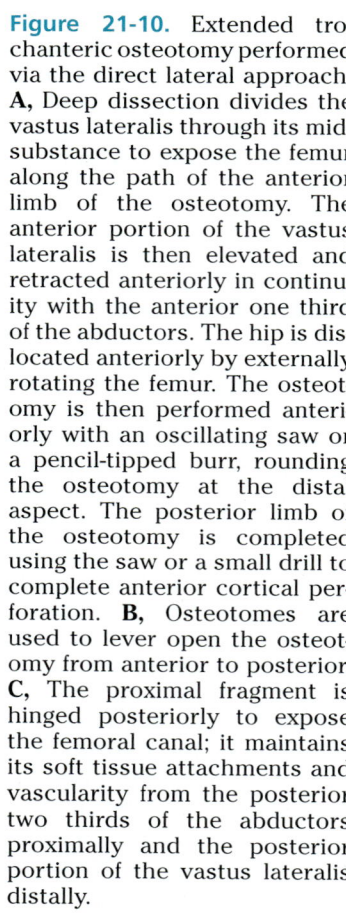

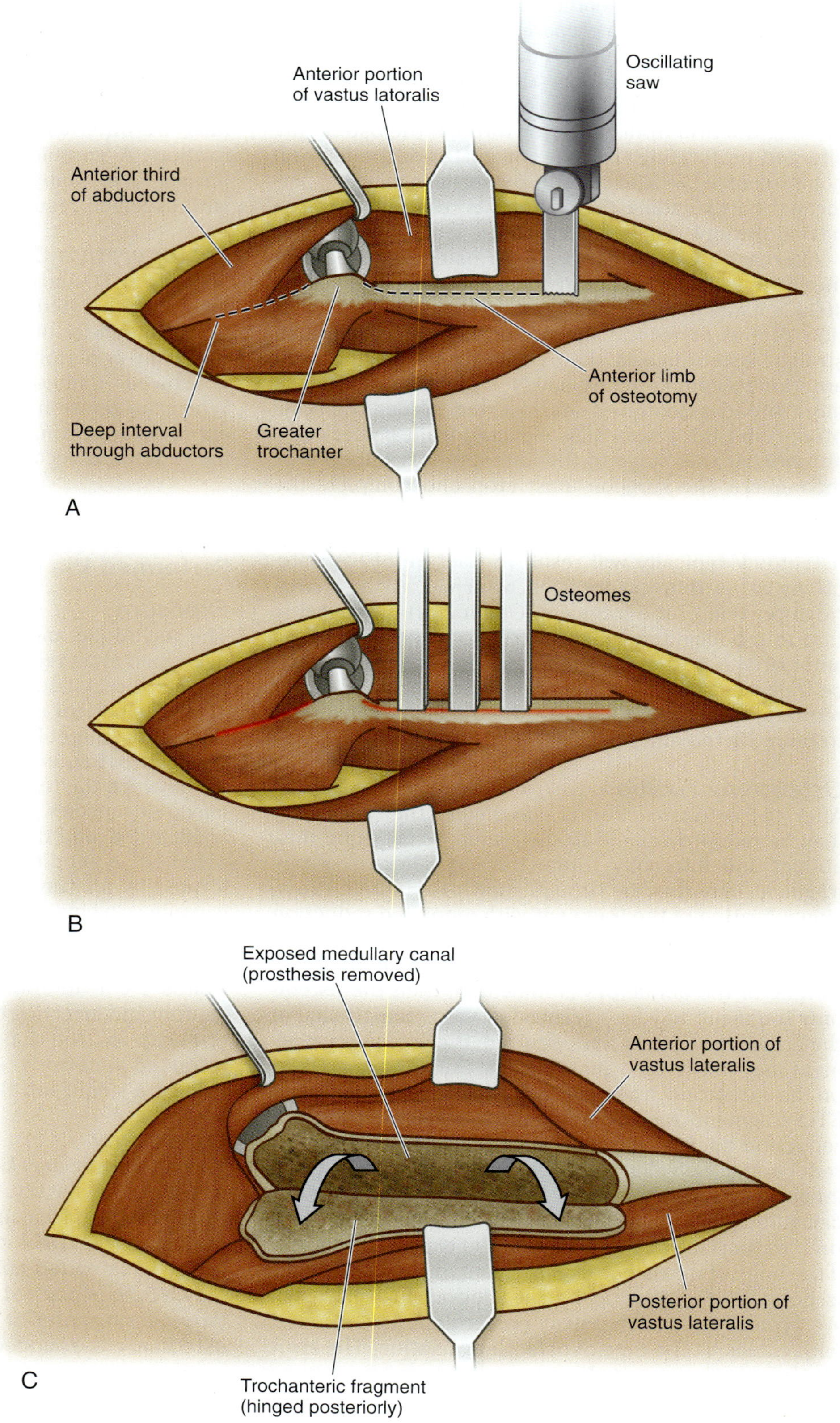

Figure 21-10. Extended trochanteric osteotomy performed via the direct lateral approach. **A,** Deep dissection divides the vastus lateralis through its midsubstance to expose the femur along the path of the anterior limb of the osteotomy. The anterior portion of the vastus lateralis is then elevated and retracted anteriorly in continuity with the anterior one third of the abductors. The hip is dislocated anteriorly by externally rotating the femur. The osteotomy is then performed anteriorly with an oscillating saw or a pencil-tipped burr, rounding the osteotomy at the distal aspect. The posterior limb of the osteotomy is completed using the saw or a small drill to complete anterior cortical perforation. **B,** Osteotomes are used to lever open the osteotomy from anterior to posterior. **C,** The proximal fragment is hinged posteriorly to expose the femoral canal; it maintains its soft tissue attachments and vascularity from the posterior two thirds of the abductors proximally and the posterior portion of the vastus lateralis distally.

posterior portion of the vastus lateralis distally (Fig. 21-10*C*).

Fixation

Osteotomy fixation is similar to that for the ETO performed posterolaterally. However, passage of cerclage wires is different. When the ETO is performed via the direct lateral approach, cerclage wires are passed from anterior to posterior. This requires care to protect the sciatic nerve. Fixation principles, bone grafting, and the use of strut allograft onlay grafts are otherwise similar to the posterolateral ETO.

Postoperative Care

Weight-bearing and flexion restrictions are the same as for the posterolateral approach. When the revision is performed via the direct lateral approach, limitation in adduction combined with external rotation in extension is recommended.

Rates of trochanteric nonunion or escape and the time to union with this osteotomy performed via the anterolateral approach are slightly greater than with that performed via the posterolateral approach. This may be a function of the difficulties involved in maintaining the same soft tissue envelope through the direct lateral approach in comparison with the posterior approach. The vastus lateralis stripping is greater, and more significant disruption of the blood supply to the greater trochanter may occur (Fig. 21-11).[18] The dislocation rate when the ETO is performed via the direct lateral approach[17] appears to be lower in revision surgery when compared with the dislocation rate when the posterolateral approach is used.[6]

Trochanteric Slide Osteotomy

The trochanteric slide osteotomy (TSO) is a modification of the standard trochanteric osteotomy. The three methods of trochanteric osteotomy—standard trochanteric, trochanteric slide, and extended trochanteric—differ in the extent of osteotomy and in the muscles left attached to the trochanteric fragment (Fig. 21-12). Note that the trochanteric slide and the ETO incorporate the origin of the vastus lateralis muscle, but the standard trochanteric osteotomy does not. The advantage of this osteotomy is excellent exposure of the acetabulum for revision, while preserving the continuity of the gluteus medius–trochanteric osteotomy–vastus lateralis complex, with a lower nonunion rate than standard trochanteric osteotomy. A modified TSO has been described by Ganz[19] for femoroacetabular impingement (FAI) and also may be used for acetabular trauma and revision THA. This osteotomy has recently been reported for both short and longer osteotomy with favorable results,[20-22] which preserves the posterior hip capsule and short external rotators to enhance stability. This osteotomy has been described for revision THA, femoroacetabular impingement, and acetabular trauma. Contraindications to this exposure include a preexisting trochanteric nonunion, irradiated hips, and abductor rupture from the trochanter. A planned plane of osteotomy, from posterior to anterior, is used. The plane is

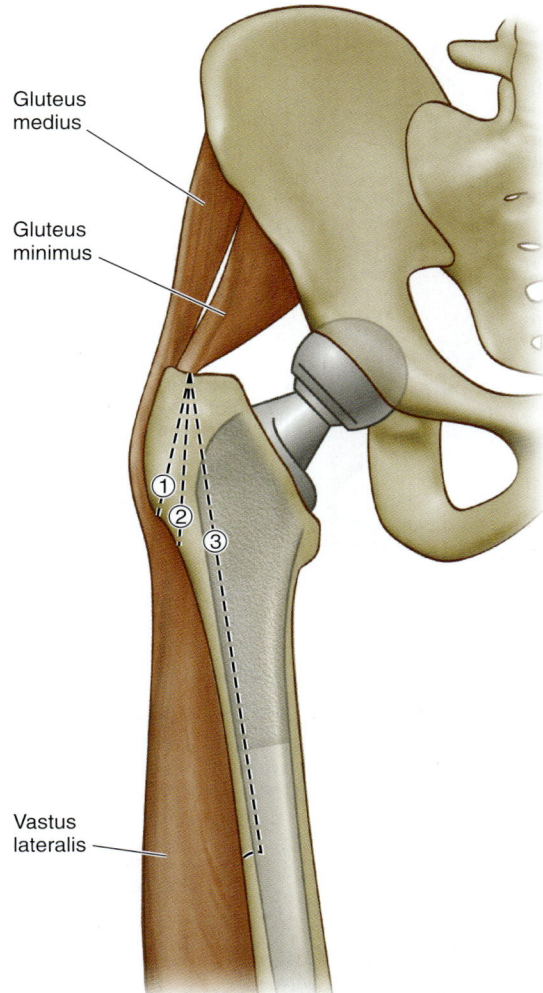

Figure 21-11. Relative extents of cortical fragments for the standard trochanteric osteotomy *(1)*, trochanteric slide osteotomy (TSO) *(2)*, and extended trochanteric osteotomy (ETO) *(3)*. TSO and ETO fragments maintain the origin of the vastus lateralis muscle, whereas the standard trochanteric osteotomy has no distal soft tissue attachments.

between the posterior border of the gluteus medius and minimus anteriorly, and the piriformis and short external rotators posteriorly. The distal extent of the osteotomy is just distal to the origin of the vastus lateralis. The osteotomized trochanter is retracted anteriorly, the capsule is incised, and the hip is dislocated anteriorly. The femur is then retracted posteriorly to expose the acetabulum. Reattachment of the osteotomy is performed with two or three double-looped cerclage wires. Postoperative care is the same as for direct lateral ETO exposure.

FEMORAL CORTICAL WINDOWS

In instances of extensive retained distal cement in the femur, working proximally from above will not allow

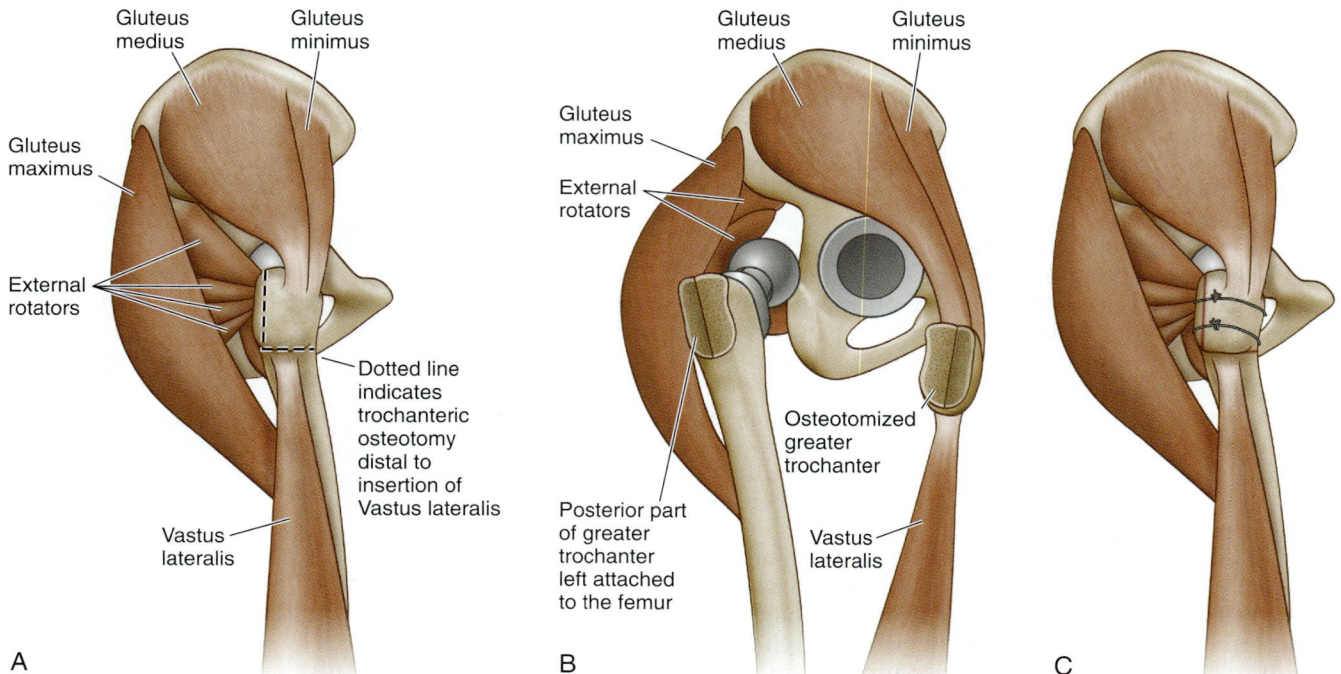

Figure 21-12. Trochanteric slide osteotomy right hip. **A,** Planned plane of osteotomy, immediately anterior to the insertion of the short external rotators, exiting just distal to the origin of the vastus lateralis. **B,** Dislocation of the hip anteriorly after the osteotomy is performed. Note that the osteotomized fragment is retracted anteriorly with the vastus and the abductors attached. **C,** Fixation of the osteotomy with two horizontal cerclage wires through drill holes.

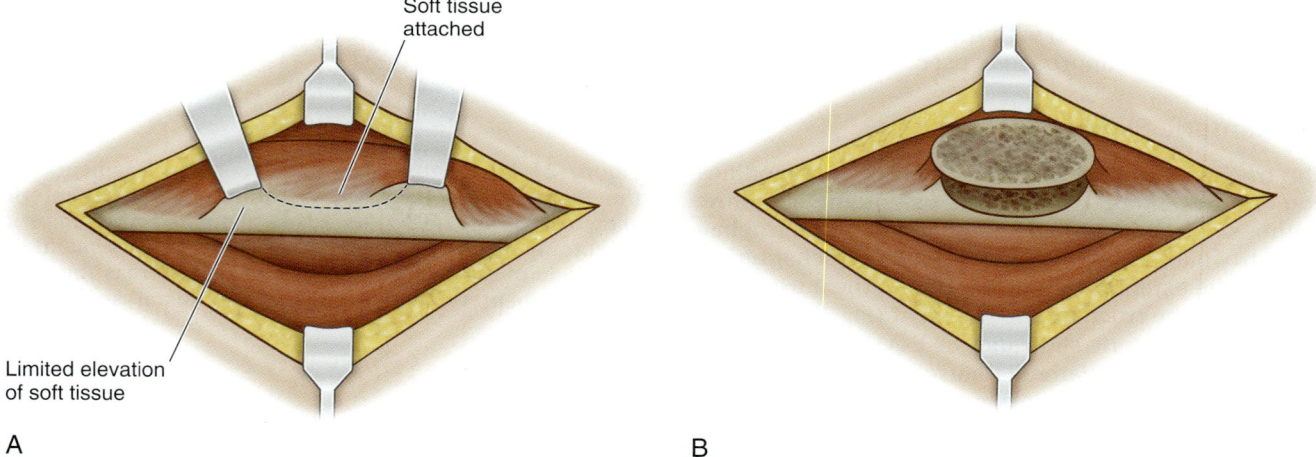

Figure 21-13. The pencil box osteotomy. **A,** The lateral femoral cortex is exposed at the appropriate level, avoiding stripping of soft tissue attachments. An oval osteotomy is created with a pencil-tipped burr. **B,** The cortical windowed fragment is hinged forward with attached soft tissues to provide access to the intramedullary canal and cement.

adequate exposure to remove the distal cement. Frequently, the cement may extend into the bow of the femur, making removal techniques from above dangerous, with risks of canal perforation and fracture. Instead, controlled perforation(s) of the anterior femur has been described.[23-25] This technique involves making one or more 9 mm drill holes in the anterior femur after subperiosteal mobilization of the vastus lateralis. Two full diameters between adjacent perforations are recommended, to minimize stress riser and fracture. The

"pencil box osteotomy" as described by Duncan and colleagues[25] is another technique whereby the lateral femoral shaft is osteotomized in an oval fashion (pencil burr or oscillating saw), osteotomizing one third of the shaft circumference while maintaining attachment of the vastus lateralis to the osteotomized fragment (Fig. 21-13). Following cement or plug removal, the oval fragment is reattached with cerclage wires or cables (see Fig. 21-13). This technique is rarely utilized owing to the extensile nature of the extended trochanteric osteotomy, although it may be indicated in removal of extremely long cement mantles in the distal isthmus of the femur.

DECRIPTION OF EXTENSILE EXPOSURE TECHNIQUES: ACETABULAR

Isolated Revision of the Acetabular Component

Isolated revision of the polyethylene[26] or acetabular component for polyethylene wear with acetabular loosening and acetabular osteolysis is the most commonly performed revision THA procedure. The principles of this procedure include an exposure, which will allow for extensile acetabular exposure, while a well-fixed femoral component is retained and managed.[27] The hip is approached typically via direct lateral or posterolateral exposure. The decision of which exposure to select will depend on several factors, including the previous exposure, acetabular defects, osteolysis, or pelvic discontinuity. If the polyethylene is simply being exchanged (with or without curettage of contained osteolytic defects), then the surgeon may utilize the prior surgical approach. If the acetabular component requires revision, then the surgeon's approach will be directed by the location of bone defects. Preoperative CT scan will help confirm the location of defects. If posterior column defects are present, the posterolateral approach will provide more extensile access to these defects.

If the hip is approached posterolaterally, the exposure is performed and the hip dislocated. Anteversion of the retained femoral component should be noted at this time. The modular head is disengaged and the taper is examined. If the stem is a monoblock component or has a ceramic head, then the component is protected and retracted anteriorly. Alternatively, if it is a modular ceramic head, the implant company may provide new trunion sleeves, which are placed over the existing trunion and allow placement of a new ceramic head. If the head is a fixed monoblock 22, 26, or 28 head, the surgeon should plan to have bipolar heads 40 and 44 mm, which may fit over the monoblock femoral head, provided that the acetabulum may accept a matching diameter polyethylene liner. One useful technique is to use a plastic chest tube sleeve to cover the exposed trunion of the femoral component, protecting it during retraction from damage from metal retractors. The leg is internally rotated and a cobra retractor placed over the anterosuperior acetabulum. This places the anterosuperior capsule under tension; this capsule may then be reflected off the anterosuperior acetabulum. Repositioning this retractor or using an additional right angle retractor to retract the abductors superiorly will allow an anterosuperior pocket to place the femoral neck of the retained femoral component. If the femur remains difficult to retract anteriorly, release of the gluteus maximus tendon from the femur will aid retraction.

If the exposure is being performed via the direct lateral approach, the hip is dislocated anteriorly. To expose the acetabulum, the femoral neck of the implant must be retracted posterosuperiorly, over the posterosuperior wall (Fig. 21-14). To facilitate this, a retractor is placed over the posterior wall to retract the femoral neck. Release of the posterosuperior capsule may facilitate retraction of the femoral neck. TSO allows retraction of the femur posteriorly, similar to the direct lateral approach. Transtrochanteric osteotomy allows extensile exposure of the acetabulum, with retraction of the retained femoral component in the anterior or posterior direction.

Exposure for Reconstruction Cages and Posterior Column Fractures

In rare instances, exposure of the acetabulum may be more extensile to allow for complex reconstructions. This includes the use of bulk structural allograft, structural porous metal augments (including column augments), and reconstruction rings. This procedure may be performed via several surgical exposures. Standard trochanteric osteotomy with proximal reflection of the greater trochanter and abductors, including elevation of the abductors from the iliac wing, may be considered and requires release of the anterior and posterior capsule to reflect the trochanter and abductor musculature proximally. The direct lateral approach[28] does not permit safe exposure for these reconstructions because the abductor musculature must be split further proximally to the iliac wing, which may excessively denervate the gluteus medius and minimus muscles, especially their anterior portions. The direct lateral approach should not be extended more than 3 cm proximal to the tip of the greater trochanter within the abductor musculature to avoid injury to the inferior branch of the superior gluteal nerve. When the abductors are split proximal to this, injury to the branches of the superior gluteal nerve will result in denervation and abductor dysfunction. Our preferred method of exposure for extensive acetabular defects is via the posterolateral approach. This allows for exposure of the posterior column to address pelvic discontinuity and plating from the ilium to the ischium. It also allows for exposure of the ischium, and for ischial fixation of a reconstruction ring.[29] The posterolateral approach allows for excellent superolateral acetabular exposure and posterior column iliac exposure, allowing for reconstruction of ring flanges, columns, and acetabular porous metal augments. The gluteus medius and minimus may be safely elevated subperiosteally in a superior direction, while their superior gluteal nerve and blood supply is maintained as a pedicle from the sciatic notch. The use of sharp spiked Taylor retractors aids in retracting the muscle safely with retractor fixation in the iliac bone. Excessive anterior retraction of the abductors will result in traction injury to the superior gluteal nerve and vessels; thus caution is required when performing this exposure. If bleeding from the superior gluteal artery occurs (which can be excessive), the surgeon must be prepared to consult a vascular surgeon, requiring a retroperitoneal approach to access the internal iliac artery for ligation or

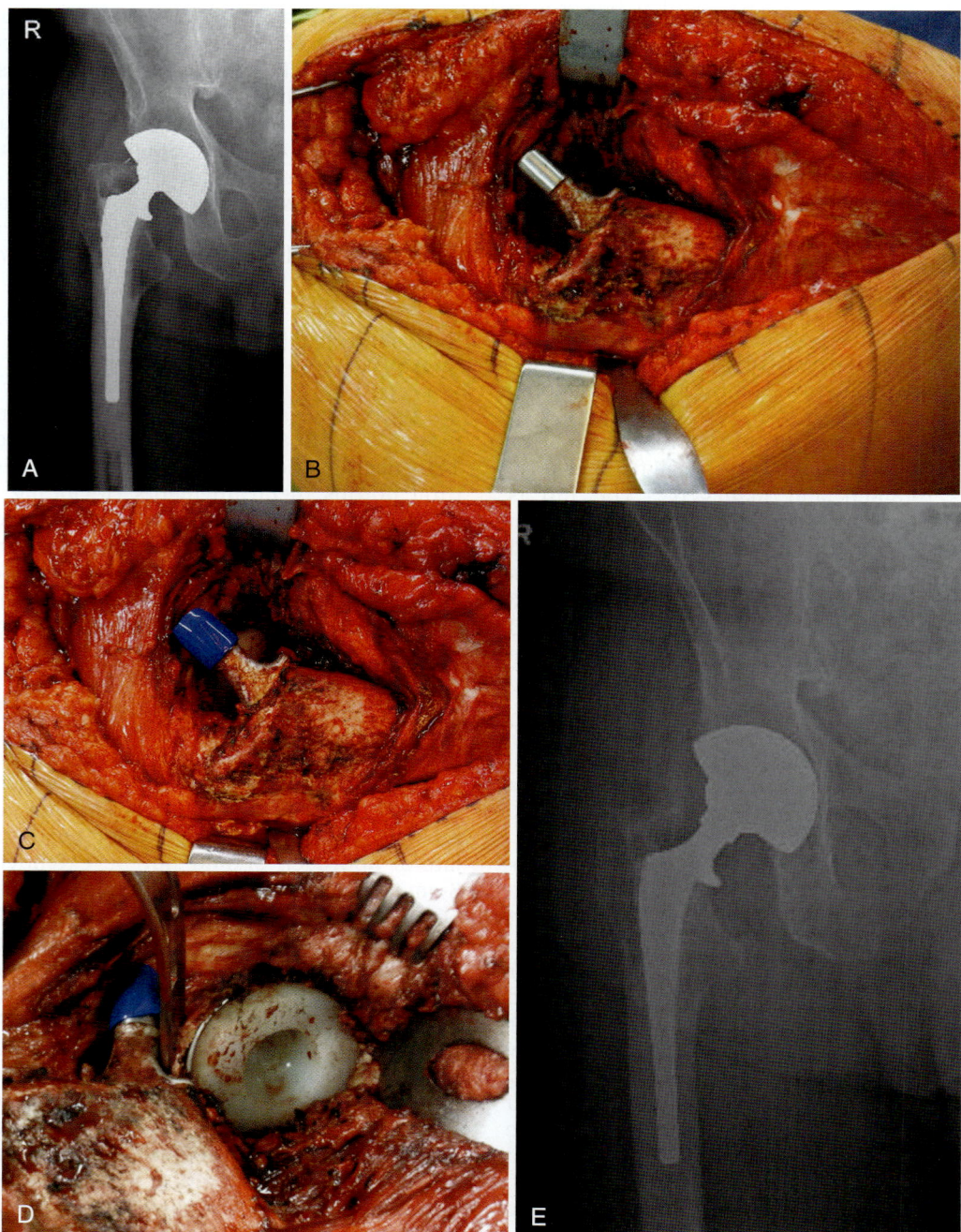

Figure 21-14. Exposure for isolated acetabular polyethylene revision with retention of a well-fixed femoral component **(A)** and preoperative x-ray showing modular polyethylene wear. **B,** Exposure to the right hip has been performed via the direct lateral approach. The modular head has been removed. The cemented femoral component is well fixed. **C,** An end cap from a chest tube has been placed over the trunion of the femoral component to protect the neck during retraction. **D,** The hip is slightly flexed and externally rotated. The trunion is retracted posterosuperiorly, and the acetabulum is exposed. **E,** Postoperative x-ray following polyethylene liner and femoral head exchange/upsizing.

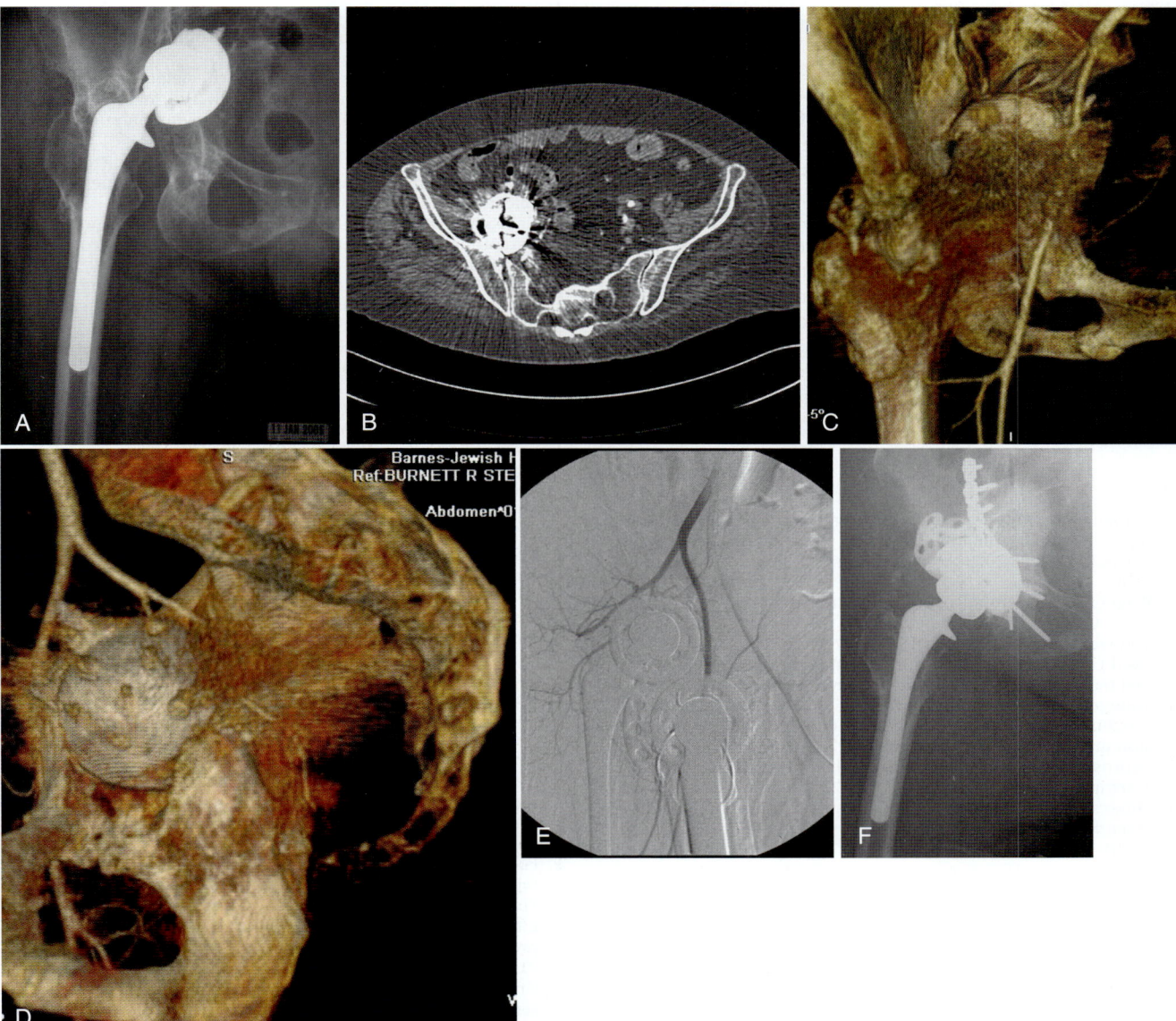

Figure 21-15. Exposure for intrapelvic implants, pelvic discontinuity, and complex acetabular reconstruction. **A,** Right total hip arthroplasty (THA) with migration of the intrapelvic acetabular component and associated pelvic discontinuity. **B,** Preoperative axial computed tomography. **C** and **D,** Three-dimensional (3D) anatomic reconstruction views. The acetabular component and screw are located against the internal iliac vessels and immediately adjacent to bowel. **E,** Preoperative angiogram confirms the close proximity of the screw and the cup to the internal iliac vessels. No vessel distortion or compression is noted. **F,** Postoperative x-ray. The implant was removed after the vascular surgeon approached and protected the vessels via a separate exposure. The hip was approached via a posterolateral extensile exposure, and the acetabular component and screw were removed from the acetabular side, without injury to vascular or visceral structures. The posterior column was plated to stabilize pelvic discontinuity. The acetabulum was reconstructed with a porous metal cup and a reconstruction cage over the cup (cup-cage construct).

embolization of the superior gluteal artery and its branches.

RETAINED INTRAPELVIC IMPLANTS, CEMENT

Removal of an intrapelvic acetabular component that has migrated medially or cement from a cemented acetabular reconstruction is a challenging problem that has been associated with intrapelvic visceral and neurovascular injuries.[30-32] The iliac vessels, bladder, sigmoid colon, cecum, and rectum are in close proximity to the inner wall of the true acetabulum. The most common reason for removal is revision for periprosthetic infection, acetabular component loosening, or periprosthetic acetabular fracture with subsequent intrapelvic implant migration. When an acetabular component is loosened and shows gradual medial migration beyond the ilioischial line (Kohler's line) with an intact medial wall and bone remodeling (protrusion with intact bone), removal may be straightforward. However, if the implant or cement is intrapelvic, fibrous and osteolytic granulomas attached to the implant material with adhesions to viscera and vascular structures must be anticipated.[33] Preoperative contrast imaging of the colon and genitourinary and vascular structures must be performed to assess their proximity to the implants. CT angiography provides vascular information and allows for three-dimensional (3D) reconstruction to evaluate the proximity of these structures to the implants. Use of an additional ilioinguinal[34] or retroperitoneal approach may be considered if the implants require safe intrapelvic removal and dissection from visceral intrapelvic structures. Consultation with a vascular or general surgeon in advance to plan for safe intrapelvic component removal is recommended.[35]

REFERENCES

1. Canadian Institute for Health Information (CIHI): Hip and knee replacements in Canada—Canadian Joint Replacement Registry (CJRR) 2008-2009 Annual Report, Ottawa, Ontario, 2009, CIHI.
2. Wagner H: [Revision prosthesis for the hip joint in severe bone loss]. Orthopade 16:295–300, 1987.
3. Younger TI, Bradford MS, Paprosky WG: Removal of a well-fixed cementless femoral component with an extended proximal femoral osteotomy. Contemp Orthop 30:375–380, 1995.
4. Younger TI, Bradford MS, Magnus RE, Paprosky WG: Extended proximal femoral osteotomy: a new technique for femoral revision arthroplasty. J Arthroplasty 10:329–338, 1995.
5. Paprosky WG, Sporer SM: Controlled femoral fracture: easy in. J Arthroplasty 18(3 Suppl 1):91–93, 2003.
6. Miner TM, Momberger NG, Chong D, Paprosky WL: The extended trochanteric osteotomy in revision hip arthroplasty: a critical review of 166 cases at mean 3-year, 9-month follow-up. J Arthroplasty 16(8 Suppl 1):188–194, 2001.
7. Levine BR, Della Valle CJ, Lewis P, et al: Extended trochanteric osteotomy for the treatment of Vancouver B2/B3 periprosthetic fractures of the femur. J Arthroplasty 23:527–533, 2008.
8. Levine BR, Della Valle CJ, Hamming M, et al: Use of the extended trochanteric osteotomy in treating prosthetic hip infection. J Arthroplasty 24:49–55, 2009.
9. Aribindi R, Paprosky W, Nourbash P, et al: Extended proximal femoral osteotomy. Instr Course Lect 48:19–26, 1999.
10. Mardones R, Gonzalez C, Cabanela ME, et al: Extended femoral osteotomy for revision of hip arthroplasty: results and complications. J Arthroplasty 20:79–83, 2005.
11. Fletcher M, Jennings GJ, Warren PJ: Ultrasonically driven instruments in the transfemoral approach—an aid to preservation of bone stock and reduction of implant length. Arch Orthop Trauma Surg 120:559–561, 2000.
12. Schwab JH, Camacho J, Kaufman K, et al: Optimal fixation for the extended trochanteric osteotomy: a pilot study comparing 3 cables vs 2 cables. J Arthroplasty 23:534–538, 2008.
13. Huffman GR, Ries MD: Combined vertical and horizontal cable fixation of an extended trochanteric osteotomy site. J Bone Joint Surg Am 85:273–277, 2003.
14. Peters PC Jr, Head WC, Emerson RH Jr: An extended trochanteric osteotomy for revision total hip replacement. J Bone Joint Surg Br 75:158–159, 1993.
15. Head WC, Mallory TH, Berklacich FM, et al: Extensile exposure of the hip for revision arthroplasty. J Arthroplasty 2:265–273, 1987.
16. Cameron HU: Use of a distal trochanteric osteotomy in hip revision. Contemp Orthop 23:235–238, 1991.
17. MacDonald SJ, Cole C, Guerin J, et al: Extended trochanteric osteotomy via the direct lateral approach in revision hip arthroplasty. Clin Orthop Relat Res 417:210–216, 2003.
18. Najima H, Gagey O, Cottias P, Huten D: Blood supply of the greater trochanter after trochanterotomy. Clin Orthop Relat Res 349:235–241, 1998.
19. Ganz R, Gill TJ, Gautier E, et al: Surgical dislocation of the adult hip: a technique with full access to the femoral head and acetabulum without the risk of avascular necrosis. J Bone Joint Surg Br 83:1119–1124, 2001.
20. Lakstein D, Backstein DJ, Safir O, et al: Modified trochanteric slide for complex hip arthroplasty: clinical outcomes and complication rates. J Arthroplasty 25:363–368, 2010.
21. Lakstein D, Kosashvili Y, Backstein D, et al: Trochanteric slide osteotomy on previously osteotomized greater trochanters. Clin Orthop Relat Res 468:1630–1634, 2010.
22. Lakstein D, Kosashvili Y, Backstein D, et al: The long modified extended sliding trochanteric osteotomy. Int Orthop 35:13–17, 2011.
23. Sydney SV, Mallory TH: Controlled perforation: a safe method of cement removal from the femoral canal. Clin Orthop Relat Res 253:168–172, 1990.
24. Moreland JR, Marder R, Anspach WE Jr: The window technique for the removal of broken femoral stems in total hip replacement. Clin Orthop Relat Res 212:245–249, 1986.
25. Masterson EL, Masri BA, Duncan CP: Surgical approaches in revision hip replacement. J Am Acad Orthop Surg 6:84–92, 1998.
26. O'Brien JJ, Burnett RS, McCalden RW, et al: Isolated liner exchange in revision total hip arthroplasty: clinical results using the direct lateral surgical approach. J Arthroplasty 19:414–423, 2004.
27. Neil MJ, Solomon MI: A technique of revision of failed acetabular components leaving the femoral component in situ. J Arthroplasty 11:482–483, 1996.
28. Mulliken BD, Rorabeck CH, Bourne RB, Nayak N: A modified direct lateral approach in total hip arthroplasty: a comprehensive review. J Arthroplasty 13:737–747, 1998.
29. Berry DJ: Antiprotrusio cages for acetabular revision. Clin Orthop Relat Res 420:106–112, 2004.
30. Slater RN, Edge AJ, Salman A: Delayed arterial injury after hip replacement. J Bone Joint Surg Br 71:699, 1989.
31. Roberts JA, Loudon JR: Vesico-acetabular fistula. J Bone Joint Surg Br 69:150–151, 1987.
32. Feeney M, Masterson E, Keogh P, Quinlan W: Risk of pelvic injury from femoral neck guidewires. Arch Orthop Trauma Surg 116:227–228, 1997.
33. Eftekhar NS, Nercessian O: Intrapelvic migration of total hip prostheses: operative treatment. J Bone Joint Surg Am 71:1480–1486, 1989.
34. Grigoris P, Roberts P, McMinn DJ, Villar RN: A technique for removing an intrapelvic acetabular cup. J Bone Joint Surg Br 75:25–27, 1993.
35. Archibeck MJ, Rosenberg AG, Berger RA, Silverton CD: Trochanteric osteotomy and fixation during total hip arthroplasty. J Am Acad Orthop Surg 11:163–173, 2003.

FURTHER READING

Archibeck MJ, Rosenberg AG, Berger RA, Silverton CD: Trochanteric osteotomy and fixation during total hip arthroplasty. J Am Acad Orthop Surg 11:163–173, 2003.

Cabanela ME: Revision hip arthroplasty: surgical approaches. In Sedel L, Cabanela ME (eds): Hip surgery: materials and developments, London, 1998, Martin Dunitz, pp 173–175.

Glassman AH: Exposure for revision: total hip replacement. Clin Orthop Relat Res 420:39–47, 2004.

Jando VT, Greidanus NV, Masri BA, et al: Trochanteric osteotomies in revision total hip arthroplasty: contemporary techniques and results. Instr Course Lect 54:143–155, 2005.

Masterson EL, Masri BA, Duncan CP: Surgical approaches in revision hip replacement. J Am Acad Orthop Surg 6:84–92, 1998.

Meek RM, Greidanus NV, Garbuz DS, et al: Extended trochanteric osteotomy: planning, surgical technique, and pitfalls. Instr Course Lect 53:119–130, 2004.

CHAPTER 22

Minimally Invasive Hip Arthroplasty

R. Michael Meneghini and Mark W. Pagnano

KEY POINTS

- The risks and benefits of minimally invasive surgical approaches for total hip arthroplasty (THA) remain controversial.
- There is no single definition of "minimally invasive" THA, but the term has been used for approaches with a shorter skin incision and for approaches that spread rather than transect muscles.
- Most prospective, randomized trials have shown little long-term demonstrable benefit of "minimally invasive" THA approaches.
- Some studies of "minimally invasive" THA have suggested more rapid early functional recovery with certain minimally invasive methods.
- Some studies of "minimally invasive" THA have identified increased complication rates, especially early in the surgical learning curve.

INTRODUCTION AND BACKGROUND

Minimally invasive surgical (MIS) approaches to hip arthroplasty remain controversial and have gained the attention of patients and surgeons alike. Some investigators report that MIS techniques result in faster rehabilitation and rapid recovery after total hip arthroplasty (THA).[1-8] However, an increased rate of complications has been reported with minimally invasive techniques,[9-13] and significant learning curves have been associated with the various MIS surgical approaches.[9,14,15] It has been reported that total hip replacements performed via MIS techniques may have a substantially higher early failure rate compared with THAs performed through a standard surgical approach.[12]

The exact meaning and definition of "minimally invasive" as it relates to surgical approaches in total hip arthroplasty remain ill defined. It has been reported that the skin incision size itself does not appear to affect early functional outcomes of total hip arthroplasty, with both the mini-posterior approach[16] and the mini-direct lateral approach.[17] More recently, the term "minimally invasive" is being used for approaches that claim to avoid muscle damage by performing THA through an internervous plane, such as the direct anterior approach, which avoids directly transecting or cutting muscles. This concept was originally popularized by proponents of the MIS two-incision approach. However, both direct anterior and two-incision procedures in THA have been shown to damage muscle,[18,19] despite claims to the contrary.

This chapter will discuss available research and evidence surrounding various minimally invasive surgical approaches for total hip arthroplasty. It is beyond the scope of this chapter to discuss details of the various surgical approaches or surgical techniques. Rather, our intent is to present available evidence on clinical results, patient rehabilitation, and recovery outcomes and potential complications of MIS approaches. Comparative clinical studies, cadaveric studies, and gait analyses are presented to compare and contrast the relative merits and potential drawbacks of MIS surgical approaches for THA.

MINIMALLY INVASIVE SURGICAL APPROACHES

Posterior Approach

The posterior, or posterolateral, surgical approach to total hip arthroplasty is one of the most commonly employed approaches for hip replacement. It provides the benefit of relative sparring of the abductors along with rapid recovery of gait with a minimal incidence of residual limp. A randomized, prospective study utilizing an MIS technique that minimizes soft tissue and muscle trauma during surgery reports that the mini-posterior approach results in improved early pain and early function after THA.[20] The authors reported a shorter hospital stay, less postoperative pain in the hospital, and less reliance on an assist device in the mini-posterior group; however, no clinical difference in pain or function was noted between MIS and standard groups after hospital discharge.[20] In a recent prospective cohort study, MIS and standard posterior approach THA were compared for recovery and muscle trauma postoperatively.[21] Muscle-derived enzymes and pain and function scores were documented preoperatively and postoperatively. The MIS approach group exhibited significantly less loss of blood, less pain at rest, and a faster rate of recovery, but clinical chemistry values and other clinical parameters were comparable, and no difference could be discerned.[21] Chimento and associates reported on 60 patients who underwent THA via MIS or standard surgical approaches.[22] Authors reported less blood loss and fewer patients who limped at 6 weeks following the MIS posterior approach compared with those who underwent the traditional posterior approach. However, operative time, transfusion requirements, narcotic usage, length of hospital stay, achievement of rehabilitation milestones, cane usage, and complications were similar in the two groups, and no difference was reported between the groups at 1- and 2-year follow-up.[22]

Contrary to the reports just described, published reports fail to demonstrate any substantial advantage for an MIS posterior approach compared with a traditional posterior approach. In a scientifically rigorous study, Ogonda and associates reported on 219 THAs performed through an MIS (less than 10 cm) or traditional posterior approach.[16] All patients and staff were blinded to the size of the incision for the duration of the hospital stay, and identical perioperative pain and physical therapy protocols were used to minimize confounding variables. No significant difference was detected with respect to postoperative hematocrit, blood transfusion requirements, pain scores, or analgesic use, and the authors found no difference in early walking ability or length of hospital stay, component placement, cement-mantle quality, or functional outcome scores at 6 weeks. The authors concluded that the MIS posterior approach offers no significant benefit in the early postoperative period compared with a standard incision.[16]

Further studies have corroborated these findings, demonstrating minimal benefit of the MIS posterior approach over the traditional approach. In a prospective comparative cohort study of 42 MIS posterior approach THAs of shorter incision length versus 42 traditional posterior THAs, the authors reported no difference in preoperative Harris hip score (HHS), estimated blood loss, or length of hospital stay ($P > .05$).[23] Authors reported that those patients undergoing MIS THA in this study expressed considerable enthusiasm regarding the cosmetic appearance of the surgical incisions, and their postoperative HHS was slightly higher than that of group 2 ($P = .042$). The authors concluded that total hip arthroplasty through a smaller MIS incision offers no dramatic clinical benefit other than cosmetic appeal.[23] In a study with similar conclusions, Woolson and colleagues reported a consecutive series of patients who underwent 135 consecutive THAs with MIS (less than 10 cm in incision length) and traditional posterior approaches.[24] The authors found no significant difference between the groups with respect to average surgical time, intraoperative blood loss, in-hospital transfusion rate, length of hospital stay, or patients' disposition after discharge. The mini-incision group was found to have a significantly higher risk of a wound complication ($P = .02$), a higher percentage of acetabular component malposition ($P = .04$), and poor fit and fill of femoral components inserted without cement ($P = .0036$).[24] The authors concluded that no evidence was available to support the use of a small incision when THA is performed through a posterior approach.

Anterolateral (or Direct Lateral) Approach

The anterolateral (or direct lateral or modified Hardinge) approach is a long-standing and well-popularized surgical approach for total hip arthroplasty. The downside of this approach is the inevitable muscle damage with occasional persistent limp that occurs secondary to splitting of the gluteus medius and minimus muscles; the benefit is the well-documented stability inherent in the approach because of preservation of the posterior capsule and short external rotators. In comparative studies, no conclusive evidence has suggested that an MIS anterolateral approach offers benefit in terms of recovery. A recent double-blind randomized controlled trial compared 120 consecutive primary uncemented THAs performed through MIS or through a traditional anterolateral or posterolateral approach.[25] For patients in the MIS groups (average 7.8 cm incision length), minimally improved functional scores (HSS) were seen compared with the traditional approach groups at 6 weeks and 1 year, mainly caused by favorable results of the MIS posterior approach. In the MIS groups, surgical time was longer and a learning curve was observed based on operation time and complication rates. The authors also noted an excessively high perioperative complication rate in the anterolateral MIS group and concluded that MIS surgical approaches did not result in substantial benefit in the first postoperative year.[25] In further support, a study of 60 THAs was undertaken to evaluate clinical advantages of performing THA through a single-incision, MIS (less than 10 cm) direct lateral approach compared with a standard-length skin incision.[17] The authors failed to demonstrate any significant difference with regard to operative time, in-hospital opioid consumption, blood loss, complications, hospital length of stay, or functional scores at 6 weeks. They concluded that the MIS direct lateral approach does not appear to afford any clinical advantage to the patient in the short term and may create technical challenges that have the potential to adversely affect long-term outcome.[17]

Direct Anterior Approach

The direct anterior approach has been promoted as an intermuscular and internervous MIS approach to THA that provides the potential for early recovery and pain minimization as a result of decreased muscle damage. Analogous to the anterolateral approach, the direct anterior approach maintains inherent hip stability through relative avoidance of posterior structures, including the hip capsule. However, during the technically challenging aspect of the procedure, mobilization and exposure of the femur may necessitate release of the piriformis and the posterior capsule.[19] Additional technical issues related to this approach include whether or not a specific (and frequently costly) operating table is required to perform the approach, the increased incidence of lateral femoral cutaneous nerve palsy,[13] and the learning curve associated with minimizing complications.[14,15] Regardless, the direct anterior approach is currently gaining interest and acceptance from surgeons and patients as a true MIS approach alike owing to claims of early recovery and return to function.

The direct anterior approach is currently gaining interest and acceptance from surgeons and patients alike as a true MIS approach. In a prospective, randomized trial comparing a single-incision modified Smith-Peterson approach versus a direct lateral approach, 100 patients were followed through the same perioperative protocol.[26] No difference was demonstrated between the two groups in operative time, estimated blood loss, analgesia requirement, transfusions, or length of stay. The authors reported that up to 1-year follow-up, the direct anterior approach group demonstrated significantly better improvement in the mental and physical health dimensions of Short Form-36 and the Western Ontario McMaster Osteoarthritis Index compared with the direct lateral approach group; however, at 2 years, the results in these groups were the same.[26] These early functional benefits have been supported with gait analysis. In a comparative report of 33 patients undergoing THA via a traditional anterolateral or MIS direct anterior approach, gait analysis was performed preoperatively and postoperatively.[27] The authors reported that MIS direct anterior approach patients improved in a larger number of gait parameters than patients receiving the traditional anterolateral approach, and most improvements occurred between the 6- and 12-week follow-ups.[27]

In a recent prospective, comparative study of 57 patients treated with MIS THA through a direct anterior approach or a posterior approach, serum creatine kinase (CK) levels and inflammatory markers were measured preoperatively and postoperatively.[28] The rise in the CK level in the posterior approach group was significantly higher than that in the anterior approach group postoperatively. The authors concluded that the anterior total hip arthroplasty approach caused significantly less muscle damage than was caused by the posterior surgical approach, as indicated by serum CK levels. However, the overall physiologic burden, as demonstrated by measurement of inflammation marker levels, appears to be similar between the anterior and posterior approaches.[28]

Two-Incision Approach

The two-incision MIS approach for total hip arthroplasty was developed and popularized as a novel technique that minimized soft tissue trauma via elimination of muscle and tendon transection.[1,8] In a retrospective investigation of 100 consecutive THAs performed through a two-incision approach, Berger and co-workers reported that 97% of the surgeries were performed on an outpatient basis, and that patients demonstrated rapid recovery of function.[8] However, this cohort was a nonconsecutive series of highly selected patients who were relatively younger, thinner, and more active compared with most patients undergoing THA. Furthermore, the investigation failed to compare results against a control group of traditional THA patients to assess what effect rapid rehabilitation protocols, perioperative pain protocols, and patient selection factors had on early functional outcomes. Conversely, Pagnano and associates reported an increased rate of complications and only modest improvement in early functional recovery in patients undergoing the two-incision approach THA.[11] Authors reported a consecutive series of 80 hip

replacement procedures performed through a two-incision MIS approach and documented a 14% rate of complications, including three postoperative femoral fractures requiring revision and four intraoperative femoral calcar fractures requiring application of a cerclage cable.[11] In a prospective, randomized study by Della Valle and colleagues, investigators examined the mini-incision posterior approach and the two-incision approach.[29] Preoperative teaching, anesthetic protocols, implants used, and rehabilitation pathways were identical for the two groups. At a minimum of 1 year postoperatively, the authors found no differences in perioperative outcomes between the two approaches, as well as no differences in component position or complication rates. They further stated that variables other than the surgical approach, including perioperative protocols, patient expectations, and general health of the patient, likely have a greater effect on outcomes such as pain during the early postoperative period, functional recovery, and length of hospital stay.[29] Furthermore, even in comparative studies that reported a shorter hospital stay with MIS approaches,[20,30] the differences are described in hours, which is not particularly relevant among the many factors related to patient discharge.

As previously mentioned, cadaveric studies have demonstrated that muscle damage may actually be greater with minimally invasive techniques.[18,19] Mardones and co-workers reported significantly greater damage to the gluteus minimus and medius with the two-incision MIS technique compared with the mini-posterior approach, using an accepted muscle grading system in cadaveric specimens.[18] However, the functional implications of this muscle damage and its effect on early functional recovery, postoperative pain levels, and gait biomechanics are not currently known. In a study of 26 patients who underwent staged bilateral hip replacements through a two-incision MIS approach on one side and a mini-posterior approach on the contralateral side, the authors reported no difference in time to reach early functional milestones.[31] In addition, 16 of the 26 patients preferred the mini-posterior approach over the two-incision approach.[31]

Reports have described increased complication rates of periprosthetic fracture and component malposition using the two-incision approach.[9-11] Along with failure to demonstrate viable scientific evidence for more rapid recovery and return of function,[31-33] early enthusiasm for the MIS two-incision approach has virtually disappeared, and it is questioned whether long-term results will equal those of single-incision MIS or traditional approaches.

GAIT STUDIES

Gait analysis has been shown to be an objective way to assess patient recovery and muscle function before and after total hip arthroplasty,[34-40] and studies have demonstrated improvement in multiple measured gait parameters after total THA.[20,35,38,40] Despite significant interest in MIS techniques, few studies have utilized gait analysis to evaluate and compare hip muscle function and recovery after THA performed through MIS approaches.[2,20,41,42] A prospective, randomized study was conducted to assess early pain and function following total hip arthroplasty performed through a mini-posterior approach or a standard posterior approach. Functional gait analysis was performed preoperatively and at 6 weeks postoperatively in 13 mini-posterior patients and 12 standard incision group patients utilizing office-based gait analysis to determine kinematic parameters of gait such as velocity, cadence, and single-leg support. All patients showed improvement in measured gait parameters compared with preoperative values; however, no difference in any of the measured gait parameters was noted between the two groups at the 6-week postoperative visit.[20] In a prospective, blinded gait analysis study of 17 patients (9 mini-posterior approach, 8 standard incision posterior approach), Bennett and co-workers found no difference between the groups at 6 weeks postoperatively in joint kinematics, such as velocity, step length, stride length, or duration of stance phase.[41] These study results were reinforced by the same authors in a larger study cohort in a subsequent published report.[43] Despite these published reports, both studies do not report in the gait analysis kinetic or force data, which have been shown to be an effective means of quantifying antalgic gait after total hip arthroplasty.[37]

In a randomized, prospective study comparing two-incision MIS and mini-posterior approaches, Pagnano and associates examined strength testing and the gait analysis parameters of velocity, cadence, step length, stride length, and single-leg stance, as well as hip joint moments derived from force plate data.[42] Authors measured these parameters preoperatively and 8 weeks postoperatively and found that the mini-posterior approach demonstrated greater hip extension strength, improvement in single-leg stance time, and greater improvement in hip flexor moments when compared with the two-incision MIS approach.[42] No statistical difference was observed between the two groups with respect to all other measured strength and gait parameters, and the authors concluded that no evidence supports the notion that early functional outcomes of the two-incision MIS approach are superior to those of other MIS approaches in THA.[42]

Meneghini and colleagues reported on 24 consecutive hips that were randomized to total hip arthroplasty through one of three MIS approaches: two-incision, mini-posterior, or mini-anterolateral.[32] Despite the fact that all three approaches demonstrated overall improvement in gait parameters at 6 weeks postoperatively, the anterolateral approach patients showed a decrease in the vertical ground reaction force at midstance, which was not seen in the two-incision and posterior approaches. The authors failed to demonstrate any significant advantage of the two-incision approach over the posterior approach in kinetic gait parameters, and the anterolateral approach demonstrated a gait pattern consistent with abductor muscle injury in the early recovery period, despite the MIS approach.[32] Further

elucidating the effects of abductor injury with the MIS anterolateral approach, Madsen and co-workers performed a comparative gait analysis on patients who underwent THA performed with a standard anterolateral or posterior approach.[36] The authors described increased trunk inclination and greater loading asymmetry at 6 months postoperatively for anterolateral approach patients over those who underwent a posterior approach, supporting the concern of persistent abductor dysfunction 6 months after THA with an approach that splits the gluteus minimus and medius.[36] This supports the expected notion that the mini-anterolateral approach continues to demonstrate greater hip abductor muscle injury in the early postoperative period compared with the other two MIS approaches, which do not intentionally violate the abductors in their respective techniques. Finally, a comparative gait analysis study compared MIS Watson-Jones and traditional direct lateral Hardinge approaches at up to 12 weeks postoperatively.[44] No significant differences were noted between the two groups with regard to the temporospatial variables of velocity, cadence, step length, and stride length at any tested time point. The authors concluded that in the early postoperative period up to 12 weeks, no significant benefits were derived by patients who underwent total hip arthroplasty through a minimally invasive Watson-Jones approach in comparison with those who were managed with a standard anterolateral approach.[44]

CONCLUSION

It is essential that these MIS surgical approaches continue to be subjected to strict scientific study to determine whether more rapid recovery is truly achieved, so that an informed decision, arrived at by weighing risks and potential benefits, can be made between the patient and the surgeon. Although evidence is emerging that minimizing muscle damage in surgical approaches may lead to less pain and an expedited recovery, little evidence currently supports the idea that a certain MIS surgical approach provides faster recovery and return to function after total hip replacement surgery. Finally, because of numerous reports in the literature that support a clear surgical learning curve for these techniques,[9,14,15,25,27] each surgeon who embarks on performing them should discuss with the patient the potential risks and benefits of such approaches, and should consider his or her own training and experience in performing the surgical techniques as it relates to that learning curve.

REFERENCES

1. Berger RA: Total hip arthroplasty using the minimally invasive two-incision approach. Clin Orthop Relat Res 417:232–241, 2003.
2. Berry DJ, Berger RA, Callaghan JJ, et al: Minimally invasive total hip arthroplasty: development, early results, and a critical analysis. Presented at the Annual Meeting of the American Orthopaedic Association, Charleston, South Carolina, June 14, 2003. J Bone Joint Surg Am 85:2235–2246, 2002.

3. DiGioia AM 3rd, Plakseychuk AY, Levison TJ, Jaramaz B: Mini-incision technique for total hip arthroplasty with navigation. J Arthroplasty 18:123–128, 2003.
4. Hartzband MA: Posterolateral minimal incision for total hip replacement: technique and early results. Orthop Clin North Am 35:119–129, 2004.
5. Kennon RE, Keggi JM, Wetmore RS, et al: Total hip arthroplasty through a minimally invasive anterior surgical approach. J Bone Joint Surg Am 85(Suppl 4):39–48, 2003.
6. Sculco TP: Minimally invasive total hip arthroplasty: in the affirmative. J Arthroplasty 19(4 Suppl 1):78–80, 2004.
7. Wenz JF, Gurkan I, Jibodh SR: Mini-incision total hip arthroplasty: a comparative assessment of perioperative outcomes. Orthopedics 25:1031–1043, 2002.
8. Berger RA, Jacobs JJ, Meneghini RM, et al: Rapid rehabilitation and recovery with minimally invasive total hip arthroplasty. Clin Orthop Relat Res 429:239–247, 2004.
9. Archibeck MJ, White RE Jr: Learning curve for the two-incision total hip replacement. Clin Orthop Relat Res 429:232–238, 2004.
10. Bal BS, Haltom D, Aleto T, Barrett M: Early complications of primary total hip replacement performed with a two-incision minimally invasive technique. J Bone Joint Surg Am 87:2432–2438, 2005.
11. Pagnano MW, Leone J, Lewallen DG, Hanssen AD: Two-incision THA had modest outcomes and some substantial complications. Clin Orthop Relat Res 441:86–90, 2005.
12. Graw BP, Woolson ST, Huddleston HG, et al: Minimal incision surgery as a risk factor for early failure of total hip arthroplasty. Clin Orthop Relat Res 468:2372–2376, 2010.
13. Bhargava T, Goytia RN, Jones LC, Hungerford MW: Lateral femoral cutaneous nerve impairment after direct anterior approach for total hip arthroplasty. Orthopedics 33:472, 2010.
14. Bhandari M, Matta JM, Dodgin D, et al: Outcomes following the single-incision anterior approach to total hip arthroplasty: a multicenter observational study. Orthop Clin North Am 40:329–342, 2009.
15. Masonis J, Thompson C, Odum S: Safe and accurate: learning the direct anterior total hip arthroplasty. Orthopedics 31(12 Suppl 2), 2008.
16. Ogonda L, Wilson R, Archbold P, et al: A minimal-incision technique in total hip arthroplasty does not improve early postoperative outcomes: a prospective, randomized, controlled trial. J Bone Joint Surg Am 87:701–710, 2005.
17. de Beer J, Petruccelli D, Zalzal P, Winemaker MJ: Single-incision, minimally invasive total hip arthroplasty: length doesn't matter. J Arthroplasty 19:945–950, 2004.
18. Mardones R, Pagnano MW, Nemanich JP, Trousdale RT: The Frank Stinchfield Award. Muscle damage after total hip arthroplasty done with the two-incision and mini-posterior techniques. Clin Orthop Relat Res 441:63–67, 2005.
19. Meneghini RM, Pagnano MW, Trousdale RT, Hozack WJ: Muscle damage during MIS total hip arthroplasty: Smith-Petersen versus posterior approach. Clin Orthop Relat Res 453:293–298, 2006.
20. Dorr LD, Maheshwari AV, Long WT, et al: Early pain relief and function after posterior minimally invasive and conventional total hip arthroplasty: a prospective, randomized, blinded study. J Bone Joint Surg Am 89:1153–1160, 2007.
21. Fink B, Mittelstaedt A, Schulz MS, et al: Comparison of a minimally invasive posterior approach and the standard posterior approach for total hip arthroplasty: a prospective and comparative study. J Orthop Surg Res 5:46, 2010.
22. Chimento GF, Pavone V, Sharrock N, et al: Minimally invasive total hip arthroplasty: a prospective randomized study. J Arthroplasty 20:139–144, 2005.
23. Wright JM, Crockett HC, Delgado S, et al: Mini-incision for total hip arthroplasty: a prospective, controlled investigation with 5-year follow-up evaluation. J Arthroplasty 19:538–545, 2004.
24. Woolson ST, Mow CS, Syquia JF, et al: Comparison of primary total hip replacements performed with a standard incision or a mini-incision. J Bone Joint Surg Am 86:1353–1358, 2004.
25. Goosen JH, Kollen BJ, Castelein RM, et al: Minimally invasive versus classic procedures in total hip arthroplasty: a double-blind randomized controlled trial. Clin Orthop Relat Res 469:200–208, 2011.
26. Restrepo C, Parvizi J, Pour AE, Hozack WJ: Prospective randomized study of two surgical approaches for total hip arthroplasty. J Arthroplasty 25:671–679, e671, 2010.
27. Mayr E, Nogler M, Benedetti MG, et al: A prospective randomized assessment of earlier functional recovery in THA patients treated by minimally invasive direct anterior approach: a gait analysis study. Clin Biomech 24:812–818, 2009.
28. Bergin PF, Doppelt JD, Kephart CJ, et al: Comparison of minimally invasive direct anterior versus posterior total hip arthroplasty based on inflammation and muscle damage markers. J Bone Joint Surg Am 93:1392–1398, 2011.
29. Della Valle CJ, Dittle E, Moric M, et al: A prospective randomized trial of mini-incision posterior and two-incision total hip arthroplasty. Clin Orthop Relat Res 468:3348–3354, 2010.
30. Duwelius PJ, Burkhart RL, Hayhurst JO, et al: Comparison of the 2-incision and mini-incision posterior total hip arthroplasty technique: a retrospective match-pair controlled study. J Arthroplasty 22:48–56, 2007.
31. Pagnano MW, Trousdale RT, Meneghini RM, Hanssen AD: Patients preferred a mini-posterior THA to a contralateral two-incision THA. Clin Orthop Relat Res 453:156–159, 2006.
32. Meneghini RM, Smits SA, Swinford RR, Bahamonde RE: A randomized, prospective study of 3 minimally invasive surgical approaches in total hip arthroplasty: comprehensive gait analysis. J Arthroplasty 23(6 Suppl 1):68–73, 2008.
33. Pagnano MW, Trousdale RT, Meneghini RM, Hanssen AD: Slower recovery after two-incision than mini-posterior-incision total hip arthroplasty: a randomized clinical trial. J Bone Joint Surg Am 90:1000–1006, 2008.
34. Hodge WA, Andriacchi TP, Galante JO: A relationship between stem orientation and function following total hip arthroplasty. J Arthroplasty 6:229–235, 1991.
35. Long WT, Dorr LD, Healy B, Perry J: Functional recovery of noncemented total hip arthroplasty. Clin Orthop Relat Res 288:73–77, 1993.
36. Madsen MS, Ritter MA, Morris HH, et al: The effect of total hip arthroplasty surgical approach on gait. J Orthop Res 22:44–50, 2004.
37. McCrory JL, White SC, Lifeso RM: Vertical ground reaction forces: objective measures of gait following hip arthroplasty. Gait Posture 14:104–109, 2001.
38. Murray MP, Brewer BJ, Zuege RC: Kinesiologic measurements of functional performance before and after McKee-Farrar total hip replacement: a study of thirty patients with rheumatoid arthritis, osteoarthritis, or avascular necrosis of the femoral head. J Bone Joint Surg Am 54:237–256, 1972.
39. Perron M, Malouin F, Moffet H, McFadyen BJ: Three-dimensional gait analysis in women with a total hip arthroplasty. Clin Biomech 15:504–515, 2000.
40. Stauffer RN, Smidt GL, Wadsworth JB: Clinical and biomechanical analysis of gait following Charnley total hip replacement. Clin Orthop Relat Res 99:70–77, 1974.
41. Bennett D, Ogonda L, Elliott D, et al: Comparison of gait kinematics in patients receiving minimally invasive and traditional hip replacement surgery: a prospective blinded study. Gait Posture 23:374–382, 2006.
42. Pagnano MW, Meneghini RM, Kaufman K, et al: No benefit of the two-incision technique over the mini-posterior total hip arthroplasty: a comprehensive gait analysis and strength testing study. Paper presented at American Association of Hip and Knee Surgeons 17th Annual Meeting, Dallas, Tex, November 2–4, 2007.
43. Bennett D, Ogonda L, Elliott D, et al: Comparison of immediate postoperative walking ability in patients receiving minimally invasive and standard-incision hip arthroplasty: a prospective blinded study. J Arthroplasty 22:490–495, 2007.
44. Pospischill M, Kranzl A, Attwenger B, Knahr K: Minimally invasive compared with traditional transgluteal approach for total hip arthroplasty: a comparative gait analysis. J Bone Joint Surg Am 92:328–337, 2010.

PERIOPERATIVE MANAGEMENT IN HIP SURGERY

CHAPTER 23

Blood Management

E. Michael Keating and Trevor R. Pickering

KEY POINTS

- Preoperative evaluation and treatment of anemia are essential.
- Preoperative hemoglobin of less than 13 g/dL indicates a high risk for postoperative blood transfusion.
- Preoperative treatment with erythropoietin (EPO)-α can be a cost-effective way to reduce the need for postoperative allogeneic blood transfusion.
- Intraoperative techniques and the use of perioperative blood salvage tools can further reduce the risk of postoperative allogeneic blood transfusion.
- Use of a comprehensive blood conservation algorithm reduces the need for blood transfusion following total hip replacement.

INTRODUCTION

Primary hip replacement and revision hip replacement surgery are often associated with significant blood loss and risk of allogeneic transfusion. Although this risk has changed dramatically over the past 15 years,[1] a certain minimum amount of blood loss will always be due to the nature of hip replacement surgery, as bone bleeding is unsuitable for conventional cautery. The risk of blood loss is particularly high in areas consisting of inflammatory tissues. Furthermore, hip arthroplasty procedures are often performed on geriatric patients whose vessels are fragile, and who may be less tolerant of acute blood loss anemia. Blood loss from primary total hip replacement surgery has been reported to range from 500 to 2000 mL, with an average drop in hemoglobin of 4.0 ± 1.5 g/dL reported in the literature; this has not improved in recent years.[1-5] Blood loss of this magnitude indicates that careful planning is required to decrease transfusion risk.[6]

BASIC SCIENCE

In a multicenter study, Bierbaum and associates described blood usage in 9482 patients undergoing total joint replacement surgery.[7] They found greater blood loss in patients who were in the revision joint replacement category. A total of 5741 patients (61%) had predonated autologous blood, of which 45% (4464 units) was not used and was discarded. In this study, patients undergoing primary hip or knee arthroplasty had the greatest number of wasted units. Also noted were 503 patients (9%) who predonated blood and received their autologous units, yet still required an additional allogeneic blood transfusion.[7] Patients with a preoperative hemoglobin of 13 g/dL or less and those undergoing revision total joint replacement had the highest allogeneic transfusion risk.[7] An Orthopaedic Surgery Transfusion Hemoglobin European overview study of 3945 patients in Europe showed similar results. In this study, 75% of patients received transfusions, 35% received only autologous blood, and 26% received only allogeneic blood.[8] In the European study, allogeneic transfusions were associated with an increased wound infection rate of 4.2% versus 1%.[8] Findings in both of these studies showed that patients requiring allogeneic transfusion had a longer hospital stay. Both studies also found that preoperative hemoglobin levels less than 13 g/dL increased allogeneic transfusion risk by about four times.[7,8]

Generally, the public has expressed its concerns regarding the safety of the blood supply with respect to the risk of human immunodeficiency virus (HIV) transmission through blood transfusion (Table 23-1).[9-11] In the United States, transmission of disease through blood transfusion is less than it has ever been. An estimate of the risk is 1 in 1.6 million units for hepatitis C transmission and 1 in 1.8 million units for HIV transmission.[10] However, in a national telephone survey, a substantial portion of responders did not consider the U.S. blood supply safe.[9] Beyond the risks related to viral disease transmission, it is known that exposure to leukocytes in allogeneic blood can cause immunosuppression. The importance of this has not yet been clearly defined.[12] The most serious immediate risks following allogeneic blood transfusion include ABO mismatch secondary to administrative error and transfusion-related lung injury.

CURRENT CONTROVERSIES AND FUTURE DIRECTIONS

Preoperative Evaluation

Because of the significant blood loss associated with hip replacement surgery, application of a blood management program is appropriate.[1] This program should

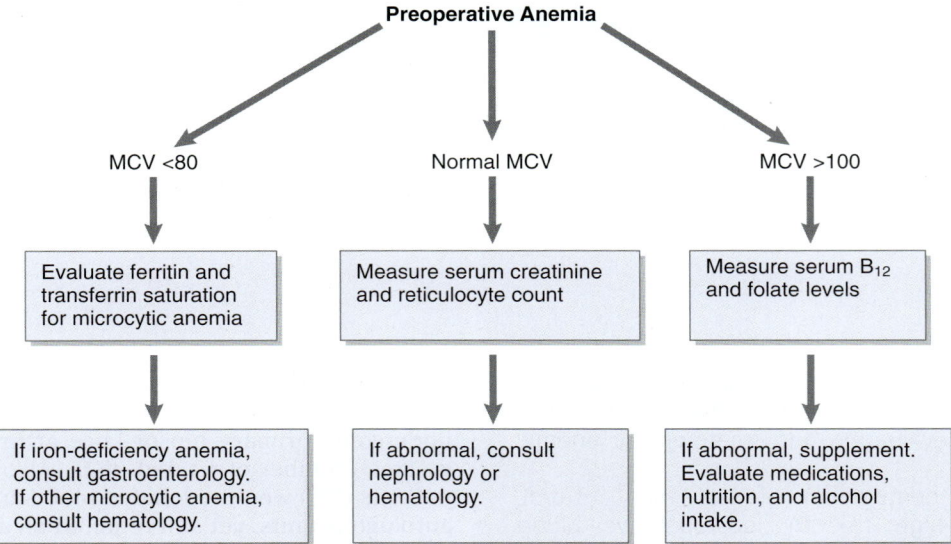

Figure 23-1. A simplified algorithm for evaluating common causes of anemia from a routine preoperative blood laboratory test. Abnormalities without a clear cause require additional workup and may indicate significant illness or chronic disease.

Table 23-1. Risk of Infection From Blood Transfusion

Agent	Risk
Virus	
HIV	1 in 1,800,00010
HCV	1 in 1,600,00010
HBV	1 in 220,00010
Bacteria	
Red cells	1 in 500,00011
Platelets	1 in 200011
Acute hemolytic reaction	1 in 250,00011
Delayed	1 in 100011
Transfusion lung injury	1 in 800011

HBV, Hepatitis B virus; *HCV,* hepatitis C virus; *HIV,* human immunodeficiency virus.
Data from Busch MP, Kleinman SH, Nemo GJ: Current and emerging infectious risks of blood transfusions. JAMA 289:959–962, 2003; Goodnough LT: Risks of blood transfusion. Crit Care Med 31(Suppl):S678–686, 2003.

encompass areas such as preoperative evaluation protocols, surgical techniques, and intraoperative interventions, where appropriate. Most surgeons would not think of taking a patient to the operating room for major surgery without performing a thorough evaluation of the heart and lungs. Likewise, a clinical care pathway for the detection, evaluation, and treatment of preoperative anemia in surgical patients would involve a hemoglobin level test done a minimum of 30 days before the scheduled surgical procedure. This would allow for evaluation and management of anemia before surgery. It should be kept in mind that anemia can be a symptom of significant illness that may preclude elective surgery (e.g., infection, hepatic or renal disease, cancer). Patients with a hemoglobin level below the normal range should undergo additional testing. Although any number of workup algorithms can be adopted, the surgeon should be comfortable recognizing basic patterns of major anemias on blood tests, so that a referral can be made as needed for further evaluation. This testing should include serum B_{12} and folate levels if the mean corpuscular volume (MCV) is greater than 100. If the MCV is found to be less than 80, additional testing should be performed to measure ferritin and transferrin saturation levels to identify iron deficiency or other causes of microcytic anemia. In the presence of iron deficiency, a gastrointestinal evaluation is recommended. If the patient has a low hemoglobin level and a normal MCV, the reticulocyte count and serum creatinine should be measured. If either is abnormal, then appropriate consultation should be obtained (Fig. 23-1). Anemia of chronic disease is a diagnosis of exclusion.[1]

Preoperative Autologous Donation

Preoperative autologous donation is a blood conservation strategy that is widely used before elective orthopedic surgery is performed.[13] However, evidence suggests that this practice is declining.[1] The popularity of autologous donation can be partially attributed to its perceived safety and acceptance by the patient population, especially in light of public perception of the safety of the blood supply.[13] Autologous blood does not eliminate all of the risks of blood transfusion. The risk of an untoward reaction from the transfusion is seen as an incidence of 20,000 to 30,000 units.[14] The chance that autologous blood may be transfused to the wrong recipient is possible. The American College of Pathologists reporting that 1% of institutions surveyed issued allogeneic blood to the wrong patient on at least one occasion in 1 year, and half of those facilities had transfused autologous blood to the wrong patient. Other adverse events can occur in recipients of autologous blood, including febrile transfusion reactions and volume overload.[15-17]

Another problem with the use of preoperative autologous donation is preoperative anemia.[18,19] When the patient donates blood, typically 2 units within 42 days of surgery, this donation has been shown to lower the patient's preoperative hemoglobin and hematocrit levels by approximately 1.2 to 1.5 g/dL per donated unit.[20] This preoperative anemia independently increases the need for perioperative transfusion.[18-20] Hatzidakis and associates analyzed the risk factors of allogeneic transfusion in patients who had donated autologous blood.[20] They reviewed 489 patients, 207 of whom underwent total hip replacement. They found that preoperative autologous donation reduced the need for allogeneic blood. They also reported that preoperative hemoglobin levels greater than 15 and patients with hemoglobin levels between 13 and 15 who were younger than 65 were at low risk for requiring allogeneic blood and did not benefit from preoperative donation.[20] Billote and colleagues[21] performed a randomized prospective study of preoperative autologous donations. These investigators found that an autologous donation was of no benefit for the nonanemic patient (preoperative hemoglobin >12) undergoing primary total hip replacement.

The cost-effectiveness of preoperative autologous donation has been questioned in large part as a result of the underuse of predeposited blood. Between 50% and 70% of predeposited blood is discarded; therefore, treatment of preoperative anemia may be more cost-effective than autologous donation.[7]

Preoperative Hematopoiesis

Preoperative hematopoiesis can be stimulated in total hip arthroplasty (THA) patients with the use of iron therapy and erythropoietin-α. Iron therapy has been used for many years; however, oral iron is poorly absorbed in the gut, is very slow-acting for hematopoiesis, and is much less effective than erythropoietin-α.[13] Oral iron preparations are inexpensive; however, many patients do not tolerate these medications over the long term because of gastrointestinal side effects. Intravenous iron preparations, although very effective, have been associated with significant allergic reactions.

In patients with anemia of chronic disease, preoperative administration of erythropoietin-α has been shown to be a very effective means of improving the starting hemoglobin level before elective total hip replacement surgery. This preparation was initially used as an adjunctive method to improve autologous donation.[22] It has been shown to be safe and effective in the treatment of preoperative anemia in orthopedic patients with anemia of chronic disease and a preoperative hemoglobin level between 10 and 13.[3,22-25] In one randomized prospective study of 490 patients undergoing total hip replacement arthroplasty that compared preoperative autologous donation (PAD) with epoetin-α therapy, a smaller proportion of patients required allogeneic transfusion—12.9% compared with 19.2% in the PAD only group.[26] This difference was not statistically significant ($P = .078$); however, it approached significance. When PAD, EPO, and the combination were studied, Bezwada and associates found that PAD and EPO combined were more effective in reducing allogeneic risk than was PAD or EPO alone.[27] Despite its effectiveness, erythropoietin-α has been considered inconvenient because of its dosing regimen. Medicare fiscal intermediaries have approved the use of erythropoietin-α in patients undergoing elective surgery, with the following restrictions[28]: (1) the operation must be expected to cause loss of greater than 2 units of blood, (2) preoperative hemoglobin must be between 10 and 13 g/dL, (3) the patient must be unwilling or unable to donate autologous blood, and (4) the preoperative evaluation must suggest the presence of anemia of chronic disease.[28] These stringent reimbursement requirements have made it more difficult for orthopedic surgeons to effectively treat preoperative anemia with erythropoietin-α. Studies have shown that the use of a blood conservation algorithm designed to predict which patients would likely need allogeneic transfusions, combined with use of a lower transfusion threshold, has been able to decrease the allogeneic risk of hip replacement patients to 2.8% without the use of an autologous donation program.[6]

Hemodilution

Acute normovolemic hemodilution (ANH) has been considered as an alternative to preoperative autologous donation. ANH involves simultaneous removal of whole blood from the patient immediately before surgery is begun and replacement of blood with fluid such as crystalloid or colloid to maintain normovolemia. Because the technique is time consuming and labor intensive, it is often impractical in many orthopedic procedures that are of short duration.[29] In contrast to PAD, ANH does not require testing to screen for transfusion-related viral disease, and there is virtually no risk of bacterial contamination or administrative error. A recent meta-analysis comparing ANH with other blood conservation methods concluded that only modest benefits could be attained, and so widespread use should not be encouraged.[30] However, ANH is a technique that is useful among Jehovah's Witnesses and other patients whose beliefs forbid the use of allogeneic blood transfusion.

Intraoperative Blood Management Strategies

The use of regional anesthesia has resulted in a measurable reduction in blood loss when compared with general anesthesia.[31-33] Hypotensive epidural anesthesia has led to a further decrease and has lowered surgical times.[33-37] Incision location and patient position are related to blood loss, with the lateral position allowing gravity to reduce venous engorgement and intraoperative blood loss in THA.[38] This was evaluated by Nelson and Bowen, who compared blood loss in patients in the lateral or supine position and found less intraoperative bleeding among patients in the lateral position.[36] They also showed a 15% reduction in blood loss attributed to shorter surgical time.

Hemostatic Agents

Fibrin glues, platelet gels, and thrombin sprays have been used to decrease blood loss.[14,39] Fibrin glue has decreased drainage in total knee replacement from 878 mL to 360 mL. Use of these agents is somewhat controversial because most are made from allogeneic blood products or bovine thrombin, and their efficacy reports have been largely anecdotal. Antifibrinolytic drugs such as aprotinin and tranexamic acid have been used in other types of surgery and with success in heart surgery.[41] More recently tranexamic acid has been tested in orthopedic surgery and seems to be effective in reducing postoperative bleeding and transfusion risk in knee arthroplasty.[40-47] Tranexamic acid competitively inhibits the conversion of plasminogen to plasmin. It is typically given intravenously at a dose of 20 mg per kilogram of the patient's body weight 10 minutes before incision (total hips) or just prior to release of the tourniquet (total knees). These studies report a 15% to 30% reduction in the need for postoperative blood transfusion and, in the study by Railey et al, a resultant savings of $65,000 (Canadian) in a population of 1000 total joint arthroplasties.[46] Wong et al described the topical application of tranexamic acid to the wound bed at the end of total joint replacement and reports a decrease in postoperative bleeding of 20% to 25%.[48] The use of tranexamic acid has not been found to increase the incidence of postoperative deep vein thrombosis.

Intraoperative Blood Salvage

Intraoperative blood salvage is the collection of blood during orthopedic surgery with retrieval of red blood cells for reinfusion back to the patient. This salvages about 60% of the red blood cells lost in surgery.[49] A recent study by Colwell analyzed red blood cell viability, which was found to be as high as 88%.[50] Therefore, erythrocytes retrieved with cell salvage are of comparable viability to the erythrocytes found in fresh autologous blood. Zerin and associates reported that intraoperative collection and reinfusion significantly reduced net perioperative blood loss among patients who had undergone revision of the acetabular and femoral components, or the femoral component alone.[51,52] Grosvenor and colleagues analyzed the effectiveness of postoperative salvage and reported that it was effective in post–total hip replacement patients, irrespective of their preoperative blood donation status.[53] Patients without blood salvage collection were approximately 10 times more likely to require allogeneic transfusions then those who had been reinfused.[53]

Transfusion Thresholds

In 1988, the National Institutes of Health (NIH) held a consensus conference on perioperative red blood cell transfusion.[54] The recommendation put forth by the NIH was to drop the old 10/30 rule advocated since 1942, and instead use a guideline associated with clinical needs and symptoms in individual patients. The recommended transfusion threshold was a hemoglobin concentration of 7 g/dL in most patients. Although the medical community at large has been slow to embrace this more stringent standard, its use has resulted in dramatic reductions in red cell transfusions without added medical morbidity.[6]

Pierson focused on the preoperative treatment of anemia in conjunction with this more stringent transfusion threshold.[6] The lowest predicted postoperative hemoglobin value was determined preoperatively by subtracting from the preoperative value the expected hemoglobin loss (4.0 g/dL for THA and 3.8 g/dL for total knee arthroplasty [TKA]), and then subtracting an additional standard deviation. If the lowest predicted postoperative hemoglobin was less than 7.0 g/dL, epoetin-α was given prior to surgery; if the value was greater than 7.0 g/dL, no treatment was initiated. All patients received aggressive fluid volume replacement after surgery. No preoperative blood donation, intraoperative blood salvage or hemostatic agents, or postoperative drains were used. With use of this algorithm in treating preoperative anemia, the rate of postoperative allogeneic blood transfusion decreased from 16.4% to 1.4% in TKA and to 2.8% in THA, thus providing a cost-effective method for blood management in elective orthopedic hip and knee replacement patients.[6]

In summary, preoperative autologous donation and intraoperative and postoperative use of cell washing or blood salvage tools, as well as good surgical technique and anesthesia choices, can effectively decrease surgical blood loss and allogeneic transfusion risk. However, this effect is minor when compared with the effects of educating physicians and patients in blood conservation and evaluating and treating patients preoperatively for anemia (Table 23-2). Adhering to the guidelines of the NIH consensus conference on red cell transfusion and treatment of preoperative anemia has a larger effect on decreasing allogeneic transfusion risk than most other interventions, potentially lowering the risk to less than 3% in primary THA.

Table 23-2. Summary of Interventions to Reduce the Risk of Postoperative Blood Transfusion

Highly Effective	Moderately Effective	Minimally Effective
Algorithm to identify and treat preoperative anemia with epoetin-α	Combined use of • Preoperative autologous donation • Hemodilution • Anesthesia choice • Operative technique • Intraoperative blood salvage, cell washing, hemostatic agents • Postoperative reinfusion drain	Individual use of • Preoperative iron therapy • Preoperative autologous donation • Hemodilution • Anesthesia choice • Operative technique • Intraoperative blood salvage, cell washing, hemostatic agents • Postoperative reinfusion drain

REFERENCES

1. Keating EM, Meding JB: Perioperative blood management practices in elective orthopaedic surgery. J Am Acad Orthop Surg 10:393–400, 2002.
2. Nuttal GA, Santrach PJ, Oliver WC Jr, et al: The predictors of red cell transfusions in total hip arthroplasties. Transfusion 36:144–149, 1996.
3. Keating EM, Meding JB, Faris PM, Ritter MA: Predictors of transfusion risk in elective knee surgery. Clin Orthop Relat Res 357:50–59, 1998.
4. Keating EM, Faris PM, Meding JB, Ritter MA: Comparison of the midvastus muscle-splitting approach with the median parapatellar approach in total knee arthroplasty. J Arthroplasty 14:29–32, 1999.
5. Keating EM, Ritter MA: Transfusion options in total joint arthroplasty. J Arthroplasty 17(Suppl 1):125–128, 2002.
6. Pierson JL, Hannon TJ, Earles DR: A blood-conservation algorithm to reduce blood transfusion after total hip and knee arthroplasty. J Bone Joint Surg Am 86:1512–1518, 2004.
7. Bierbaum BE, Callaghan JJ, Galante JO, et al: An analysis of management in patients having a total hip or knee arthroplasty. J Bone Joint Surg Am 81:2–10, 1999.
8. Rosencher N, Kerkkamp HE, Macheras G, et al: Orthopedic Surgery Transfusion Hemoglobin European Overview (OSTHEO) study: blood management in elective knee and hip arthroplasty in Europe. Transfusion 43:459–469, 2003.
9. Finucane ML, Slovic P, Mertz CK: Public perception of the risk of blood transfusion. Transfusion 40:1017–1022, 2000.
10. Busch MP, Kleinman SH, Nemo GJ: Current and emerging infectious risks of blood transfusions. JAMA 289:959–962, 2003.
11. Goodnough LT: Risks of blood transfusion. Crit Care Med 31(Suppl):S678–S686, 2003.
12. Goodnough LT, Brecher ME, Kanter MH, AuBuchon JP: Transfusion medicine: first of two parts—blood transfusion. N Engl J Med 340:438–447, 1999.
13. Clark C: Perioperative blood management in total hip arthroplasty. AAOS Instruct Course Lect 58:167–172, 2009.
14. Sculco TP, Baldini A, Keating EM: Blood management in total joint arthroplasty. AAOS Instruct Course Lect 54:51–66, 2005.
15. Klein HG: Transfusion safety: avoiding unnecessary bloodshed. Mayo Clin Proc 75:5–7, 2000.
16. Linden JV, Kruskall MS: Autologous blood: always safer? Transfusion 37:455–456, 1997.
17. Linden JV: Errors in transfusion medicine: scope of the problem. Arch Pathol Lab Med 123:563–565, 1999.
18. Pola E, Papaleo P, Santoliquido A, et al: Clinical factors associated with an increased risk of perioperative blood transfusion in nonanemic patients undergoing total hip arthroplasty. J Bone Joint Surg Am 86:57–61, 2004.
19. Salido JA, Marin LA, Gomez LA, et al: Perioperative hemoglobin levels and the need for transfusion after prosthetic hip and knee surgery. J Bone Joint Surg Am 84:216–220, 2002.
20. Hatzidakis AM, Mendlick RM, McKillip T, et al: Preoperative autologous donation for total joint arthroplasty: an analysis of risk factors for allogenic transfusion. J Bone Joint Surg Am 82:89–100, 2000.
21. Billote DB, Glisson SN, Green D, Wixson RL: A prospective randomized study of preoperative autologous donation for hip replacement surgery. J Bone Joint Surg Am 84:1299–1304, 2002.
22. Goodnough LT, Price TH, Rudnick S, et al: Preoperative red cell production in patients undergoing aggressive autologous blood phlebotomy with and without erythropoietin therapy. Transfusion 32:441–445, 1992.
23. Faris PM, Ritter MA, Abels RI, for the American Erythropoietin Study Group: The effects of recombinant human erythropoietin on perioperative transfusion requirements in patients having a major orthopedic operation. J Bone Joint Surg Am 78:62–72, 1996.
24. de Andrade JR, Jove M, Landon G, et al: Baseline hemoglobin as a predictor of risk of transfusion and response to epoetin alfa in orthopedic surgery patients. Am J Orthop 25:533–542, 1996.
25. Goldberg MA, McCutchen JW, Jove M, et al: A safety and efficacy comparison study of two dosing regimens of epoetin alfa
26. in patients undergoing major orthopedic surgery. Am J Orthop 25:544–552, 1996.
26. Stowell CP, Chandler H, Jove M, et al: An open-label, randomized study to compare the safety and efficacy of perioperative epoetin alfa with preoperative autologous blood donation in total joint arthroplasty. Orthopedics 22(Suppl):S105–S112, 1999.
27. Bezwada HP, Nazarian DG, Henry DH, Booth RE Jr: Preoperative use of recombinant human erythropoietin before total joint arthroplasty. J Bone Joint Surgery Am 85:1795–1800, 2003.
28. Administer Medicine Fiscal Intermediary: CMS program memorandum 60AB, Transmittal AB-00-76, Change request 1243, August 16, 2000, Modification of EPO policy.
29. Keating EM: Preoperative evaluation and methods to reduce blood use in orthopedic surgery. Anesth Clin N Am 23:305–313, 2005.
30. Srgal JB, Blasco-Colmenares E, Norris EJ, et al: Preoperative acute normovolemic hemodilution: a meta-analysis. Transfusion 44:632–644, 2004.
31. Flordal PA, Neander G: Blood loss in total hip replacement: a retrospective study. Arch Orthop Trauma Surg 111:34–38, 1991.
32. Sculco TP, Ranawat C: The use of spinal anesthesia for total hip-replacement arthroplasty. J Bone Joint Surg Am 57:173–177, 1975.
33. Sharrock NE, Mineo R, Urquhart B, Salvati EA: The effect of two levels of hypotension on intraoperative blood loss during total hip arthroplasty performed under lumbar epidural anesthesia. Anesth Analg 76:580–584, 1993.
34. An HS, Mikhail WE, Jackson WT, et al: Effects of hypotensive anesthesia, nonsteroidal anti-inflammatory drugs, and polymethylmethacrylate on bleeding in total hip arthroplasty patients. J Arthroplasty 6:245–250, 1991.
35. Mallory TH: Hypotensive anesthesia in total hip replacement. JAMA 224:248, 1973.
36. Nelson CL, Bowen WS: Total hip arthroplasty in Jehovah's Witnesses without blood transfusion. J Bone Joint Surgery Am 68:350–353, 1986.
37. Davis NJ, Jennings JJ, Harris WH: Induced hypotensive anesthesia for total hip replacement. Clin Orthop Relat Res 101:93–98, 1974.
38. Nelson CL, Fontenot HJ: Ten strategies to reduce blood loss in orthopedic surgery. Am J Surg 1709(Suppl 6A):64S–68S, 1995.
39. Levi O, Martinowitz U, Oran A, et al: The use of fibrin tissue adhesive to reduce blood loss and need for blood transfusion after total knee arthroplasty: a prospective, randomized, multicenter study. J Bone Joint Surg Am 81:1580–1588, 1999.
40. Benoni G, Fredin H: Fibrinolytic inhibition with tranexamic acid reduces blood loss and blood transfusion after knee arthroplasty: a prospective, randomized, double-blind study of 86 patients. J Bone Joint Surg Br 78:434–440, 1996.
41. Howes JP, Sharma V, Cohen AT: Tranexamic acid reduces blood loss after knee arthroplasty. J Bone Joint Surg Br 78:995–996, 1996.
42. Ido K, Neo M, Asada Y, et al: Reduction of blood loss using tranexamic acid in total knee and hip arthroplasties. Arch Orthop Trauma Surg 120:518–520, 2000.
43. Jansen AJ, Andreica S, Claeys M, et al: Use of tranexamic acid for an effective blood conservation strategy after total knee arthroplasty. Br J Anaesth 83:596–601, 1999.
44. Tanaka N, Sakahashi H, Sato E, et al: Timing of the administration of tranexamic acid for maximum reduction in blood loss in arthroplasty of the knee. J Bone Joint Surg Am 83:702–705, 2001.
45. Zohar E, Fredman B, Ellis M, et al: A comparative study of the postoperative allogeneic blood-sparing effect of tranexamic acid versus acute normovolemic hemodilution after total knee replacement. Anesth Analg 89:1382–1387, 1999.
46. Railey FE, Berta D, Binns V, et al: One intraoperative dose of tranexamic acid for patients having primary hip or knee arthroplasty. Clin Orthop Relat Res 468:1905–1911, 2010.
47. MacGillivray RG, Tarabichi SB, Hawari MF, et al: Tranexamic acid to reduce blood loss after bilateral total knee

arthroplasty: A prospective, randomized double blind study. J Arthroplasty 26:24–28, 2011.

48. Wong J, Abrishami A, Beheiry H, et al: Topical application of tranexamic acid reduces postoperative blood loss in total knee arthroplasty: A randomized, controlled trial. J Bone Joint Surg Am 92:2503–2513, 2010.

49. Williamson KR, Taswell HF: Intraoperative blood salvage: a review. Transfusion 31:662–675, 1991.

50. Colwell CW Jr, Beutler E, West C, et al: Erythrocyte viability in blood salvaged during total joint arthroplasty with cement. J Bone Joint Surg Am 84:23–25, 2002.

51. Zarin J, Grosvenor D, Schurman D, Goodman S: Efficacy of intraoperative blood collection and reinfusion in revision total hip arthroplasty. J Bone Joint Surg Am 85:2147–2151, 2003.

52. Garvin KL, Feschuk CA, Sekundiak TD, Lyden ER: Blood salvage and allogenic transfusion needs in revision hip arthroplasty. Clin Orthop Relat Res 441:205–209, 2005.

53. Grosvenor D, Goyal V, Goodman S: Efficacy of postoperative blood salvage following total hip arthroplasty in patients with and without deposited autologous units. J Bone Joint Surg Am 82:951–954, 2000.

54. Perioperative red cell transfusion: NIH Consensus Development Statement. Consens Statement 7:1–17, 1988.

SUGGESTED READING

Bierbaum BE, Callaghan JJ, Galante JO, et al: An analysis of management in patients having a total hip or knee arthroplasty. J Bone Joint Surg Am 81:2–10, 1999.
This article reviews a large number of patients from multiple centers undergoing hip and knee arthroplasty. The most important predictors of allogeneic transfusion included a low baseline hemoglobin concentration (<13 g/dL) and lack of preoperative autologous donation. Complications associated with allogeneic blood transfusion included infection, fluid overload, and prolonged hospitalization.

Carson JL, Hill S, Carless P, et al: Transfusion triggers: a systematic review of the literature. Transfus Med Rev. 16:187–199, 2002.
This review offers a comparison of clinical outcomes in patients randomized to restrictive versus liberal transfusion thresholds.

Faris PM, Ritter MA, Abels RI, for the American Erythropoietin Study Group: The effects of recombinant human erythropoietin on perioperative transfusion requirements in patients having a major orthopedic operation. J Bone Joint Surg Am 78:62–72, 1996.
This study reviews the safety and efficacy of preoperative erythropoietin in the setting of orthopedic surgery. Patients with preoperative anemia were noted to receive the greatest benefit from this intervention.

Keating EM, Meding JB: Perioperative blood management practices in elective orthopedic surgery. J Am Acad Orthop Surg 10:393–400, 2002.
This recent review article discusses pertinent issues related to a comprehensive perioperative blood conservation program.

Pierson JL, Hannon TJ, Earles DR: A blood-conservation algorithm to reduce blood transfusion after total hip and knee arthroplasty. J Bone Joint Surg Am 86:1512–1518, 2004.
This study reviews a simple and effective blood conservation algorithm for elective hip and knee arthroplasty. Patients with preoperative anemia are identified and treated with erythropoietin-α. Postoperatively, patients are managed with aggressive volume resuscitation, with allogeneic blood reserved for patients with hemoglobin values less than 7.0 g/dL. Patients following this algorithm were noted to have a 2.8% allogeneic transfusion rate after unilateral primary total hip arthroplasty.

CHAPTER 24

Anesthesia for Hip Surgery: Options and Risks

Carlos B. Mantilla

KEY POINTS

- Patients undergoing hip surgery pose specific challenges to the anesthesiologist. Anesthetic options for hip surgery include general and regional techniques, but options will vary depending on patient and procedure-specific characteristics.
- Patients undergoing hip surgery commonly suffer from arthritis and other musculoskeletal disorders that demand great care in airway management and patient positioning.
- Regional anesthesia such as neuraxial (spinal or epidural) and peripheral techniques may offer specific advantages for hip surgery, including reduced intraoperative risk and superior postoperative analgesia.
- Risk factors for increased morbidity and mortality include older age and comorbidities common in patients undergoing hip surgery, including cardiac, pulmonary, and renal pathology.

INTRODUCTION

Patients undergoing hip surgery pose specific challenges to the anesthesiologist. Old arthritic and young trauma patients may require hip surgery. The breadth of the patient population with its diverse comorbid conditions demands detailed preoperative preparation. Ambulatory or inpatient procedures and multistage surgeries add particular anesthetic requirements. Furthermore, the varied surgical techniques, treatment approaches, and positioning needs, as well as the assortment of postoperative analgesic and rehabilitation strategies, are important perioperative considerations that are best approached in a comprehensive way, starting with the anesthetic plan.

Health care practitioners providing anesthesia for orthopedic surgery, including hip surgery, must keep pace with the growing number of surgical techniques while maintaining a broad range of skills in advanced airway management, regional anesthesia, intraoperative blood salvage, and invasive physiologic monitoring of hemodynamic and neurologic function. Perioperative thromboprophylactic strategies require detailed knowledge of their interaction with anesthetic agents and

techniques. It is important to note that the number of hip surgeries performed annually has continually risen over the past several decades,[1,2] and this number is expected to increase further with the aging of the population, and as improved perioperative care of the hip surgery patient allows ever older patients to undergo surgery.

This chapter reviews the options and risks associated with anesthesia for hip surgery. Specific consideration is given to patient and procedural characteristics that may influence perioperative care and long-term outcomes. Available evidence is discussed, and areas of uncertainty are highlighted as they relate to anesthetic options and risks. Related topics such as perioperative transfusion, analgesic and medical management, and morbidity and mortality after hip surgery are addressed in other chapters of this book.

ANESTHETIC TECHNIQUES FOR HIP SURGERY: OPTIONS

Surgery of the hip lends itself to regional anesthetic techniques, and the relative risks and benefits of regional versus general anesthesia have been the subject of intense debate. General anesthesia is safe and universally effective, whereas regional anesthesia offers advantages in specific surgical populations and is associated with a low failure rate in expert hands (Table 24-1). When combined in a postoperative multimodal analgesic regimen, regional anesthesia can provide additional benefits, minimizing patient discomfort while permitting early rehabilitation and hospital discharge in a cost-effective manner.[3,4]

Preoperative evaluation of the patient scheduled for hip surgery must address a number of specific and important factors present in this surgical population.[5,6] Underlying pathology and conditions necessitating surgery will affect preoperative preparation of the orthopedic patient. For instance, preparation for emergency surgery in a young, presumably healthy patient with traumatic hip fracture clearly differs from that for elective joint replacement in an elderly patient with multiple comorbidities. Identifying patient-specific conditions that may place the patient at higher risk for perioperative complications is particularly important in formulating the anesthetic plan.

Table 24-1. Anesthetic Options and Perioperative Management Considerations for Patients Undergoing Hip Surgery

Intraoperative		Postoperative	
Options	**Considerations**	**Options**	**Considerations**
General anesthesia	Airway management (arthritis) Difficult assessment of exercise tolerance Patient positioning Preexisting comorbidities	**Continuous neuraxial analgesia** Epidural catheter	Anticoagulation Infection (systemic or localized) Preexisting spinal stenosis Rehabilitation strategies
Neuraxial anesthesia Subarachnoid anesthesia Epidural anesthesia	Anticoagulation Failure rate (low; epidural > subarachnoid) Infection (systemic or localized) Patient positioning Preexisting spinal stenosis or nerve injury	**Peripheral nerve blockade** Lumbar plexus compartment block Fascia iliaca compartment block	Anticoagulation Infection (systemic or localized) Preexisting nerve injury Rehabilitation strategies

The presence of arthritis (e.g., rheumatoid arthritis, osteoarthritis, ankylosing spondylitis) may indicate potential difficulties in airway management and patient positioning. In particular, involvement of the cervical spine and the temporomandibular joint may limit cervical range of motion and mouth opening, respectively, requiring adjunct airway management strategies beyond direct laryngoscopy (e.g., use of a fiberoptic bronchoscope, videolaryngoscopy). Laryngeal involvement may predispose patients to vocal cord dislocation with intubation or placement of laryngeal airway devices (e.g., laryngeal mask airway). Limited shoulder or contralateral hip range of motion may limit the ability of a patient to tolerate lateral decubitus or other positions (e.g., lithotomy) needed for a specific surgical approach. These positioning requirements are not circumvented with the use of general anesthesia because both neurologic and vascular injuries may occur if patients are positioned in ways that they would not tolerate while awake.

The functional impact of cardiovascular disease (e.g., coronary artery disease) may be difficult to ascertain in patients who are limited by joint pain and who do not routinely exert themselves physically. These patients may necessitate specific cardiac evaluation, including imaging studies (e.g., dobutamine stress echocardiography), or beta blocker therapy for control of intraoperative heart rate, depending on the presence of cardiovascular risk factors.[7] Risk factors include (1) history of myocardial infarction (longer than 1 month before surgery) or abnormal Q waves on electrocardiogram; (2) history of prior or compensated congestive heart failure; (3) diabetes mellitus requiring insulin treatment; (4) renal insufficiency (serum creatinine >2 mg/dL); and (5) history of cerebrovascular disease (defined as transient ischemic attack or stroke).[7,8] Although advanced age is no longer included as a clinical risk factor for cardiovascular risk, patients older than 70 years of age commonly have coexisting diseases that may place them at higher risk for perioperative complications[9-11] and may affect long-term outcomes after hip arthroplasty.[12,13]

General Anesthesia

General anesthesia provides safe and effective anesthesia for surgical procedures around the hip. Adult patients are commonly induced using intravenous agents and are maintained with a combination of inhaled volatile anesthetic agents and intravenous opioid analgesics with optional neuromuscular blocking agents. Deep levels of muscle relaxation are possible with the use of general anesthesia and are sometimes necessary for final reduction of the hip joint. General anesthesia is universally effective and thus may be resorted to after failed regional anesthesia. Induction of general anesthesia can be accomplished in a short time, although in patients with suspected difficult airways (e.g., cervical spine or temporomandibular joint arthritis), additional time may be required. Although regional anesthesia may avoid issues related to airway manipulation in such patients, the low rate of failed regional blocks may require that the airway be secured. In this sense, patient positioning and accessibility may dictate pre-emptive airway management and use of general anesthesia despite the possible use of a regional technique. For instance, obese patients with a suspected difficult airway may be best approached by using general anesthesia with awake fiberoptic intubation rather than risking failed regional anesthesia and emergent intraoperative airway management in the lateral decubitus position. These considerations must be weighed individually on the basis of patient and surgery-specific conditions.

Newer general anesthetic agents offer significant advantages for short procedures in that their effects can be closely titrated; thus general anesthesia is now commonly employed for outpatient surgical procedures. Furthermore, laryngeal airway devices that avoid laryngoscopy and endotracheal tube placement may allow safe general anesthesia to be provided with ease in multiple settings.[14] Aggressive perioperative management of nausea, vomiting, and pain may facilitate discharge and minimize unanticipated hospital admissions.[15,16]

Regional Anesthesia

Regional anesthesia can be performed at the level of the central neuraxis or peripheral nerves. Regional anesthetic techniques offer several advantages over general anesthetic techniques, including reduced intraoperative blood loss, respiratory or cardiac derangements, and analgesic requirements, as well as a decreased incidence of postoperative nausea or vomiting.[3,17-20] The use of regional anesthesia should be considered in the absence of absolute contraindications (e.g., patient refusal, infection at the site of needle puncture or its path, ongoing systemic anticoagulation).

A large, systematic review of 141 clinical trials that included 9559 patients (of which 43 trials and 3617 patients underwent lower extremity orthopedic surgery) compared outcomes of patients randomized to neuraxial blockade versus general anesthesia.[17] Overall, patients randomized to neuraxial blockade experienced fewer adverse events, including deep venous thrombosis, pulmonary embolism, and death. Patients in the neuraxial block group had less blood loss and reduced requirement for transfusion of two or more units. These effects were similar in the orthopedic surgery subgroup. In keeping with these findings, a meta-analysis of 10 studies involving 678 patients after elective total hip arthroplasty reported that the risk for deep venous thrombosis and pulmonary embolism was reduced in patients randomized to neuraxial blockade (odds ratio [OR], ≈0.26).[18] Intraoperative blood loss was also significantly reduced in patients undergoing neuraxial blockade (on average, by 275 mL per case). Furthermore, substantially similar results were recently reported in a meta-analysis of total knee and hip replacement surgeries[21] and in a systematic review of total hip arthroplasty patients designed to reflect contemporary practice by including only studies conducted from 1990 onward.[22] Regional anesthesia (including neuraxial and peripheral nerve blockade) reduced postoperative pain scores, systemic opioid requirements, and nausea and vomiting.[22]

Regional anesthetic techniques can be used in concert with general anesthesia. It is important to note that regional anesthesia should be avoided in the anesthetized patient because intraneural needle or catheter placement may go unnoticed. Thus, any regional anesthetic techniques should be performed before induction of general anesthesia. This aspect is particularly relevant to the pediatric practice, where performance of regional anesthesia may not be possible in unanesthetized patients. A recent report including 2236 regional anesthetic procedures performed in 1809 children under general anesthesia (1169 between the ages of 6 months and 12 years) described only two complications possibly related to peripheral nerve blocks.[23] The relative safety of performing regional anesthetic procedures in children while anesthetized may reflect the type of anesthetic blocks selected. Central neuraxial blocks may be associated with a very small risk for neurologic complications in these patients.[24,25] However, future studies should explore whether differences in the risk of performing regional anesthesia in anesthetized

patients may depend on patient age and the regional anesthetic procedure selected, and whether nerve stimulation or ultrasound guidance might affect this risk.

Central Neuraxial Anesthesia

Sensory innervation of the hip and thigh is provided by branches of the lumbar plexus and the sacral plexus.[26-28] Thus neuraxial anesthesia above this level can provide adequate conditions for surgery around the hip joint. Spinal (subarachnoid) anesthesia can be performed safely with high success rates in most patients. However, in some patients, the onset of sympathetic block might result in dangerous reductions in blood pressure and venous return, and even death.[29] The use of subarachnoid catheters to permit gradual titration of local anesthetic agents was stopped because of safety concerns after reports of neurologic complications, including cauda equina syndrome, with small-diameter catheters (24-gauge).[30] Although placement of large-bore catheters (e.g., 18- or 19-gauge) is possible, their use for continuous spinal anesthesia is associated with a high rate of postdural puncture headache. Placement of an indwelling epidural catheter might allow gradual dosing and incremental titration of local anesthetic agents to achieve the desired anesthetic level. Most anesthesiologists are expert at placement of spinal or epidural anesthesia, and these techniques are used extensively for orthopedic surgery of the lower extremities.

Several major issues must be appraised when neuraxial blockade is considered. Infectious and hemorrhagic complications may occur as a result of needle placement.[31] Therefore patients must be screened for signs or symptoms of systemic or localized infection at the site of needle puncture, as well as for anticoagulant use. Sympathetic blockade may result in significant reductions in blood pressure, which are compounded by concomitant general anesthesia.[32] In addition, anesthesia of the contralateral (nonsurgical) extremity and urinary retention may delay discharge from the postanesthesia care unit. In this regard, concomitant use of peripheral nerve blocks (e.g., psoas or fascia iliaca compartment block) and neuraxial anesthesia may permit substantial reductions in the dose of local anesthetic necessary to provide an adequate level of surgical anesthesia.[19] The addition of subarachnoid opioids may permit the use of lower doses of local anesthetic agents.[33,34] Unfortunately, although undesirable effects of neuraxial blockade can be minimized by reductions in the dose of local anesthetic, they cannot be prevented entirely. The choice and dose of local anesthetic agent (e.g., bupivacaine, ropivacaine) must be tailored individually according to patient, surgeon, and procedural characteristics. If adequate surgical anesthesia must be ensured (e.g., in an obese patient with suspected difficult airway), then larger anesthetic doses may be needed, even if this results in delayed discharge from the postanesthesia care unit. Additional studies into the safety and efficacy of short-acting local anesthetic agents for use in the central neuraxis are needed, because significant, even transient, neurologic symptoms have been reported with subarachnoid lidocaine.[30,35]

Combined spinal-epidural techniques are possible that combine the near-complete success rate of spinal anesthesia with the flexibility of additional dosing provided by the epidural catheter. Prolonged intraoperative anesthesia is possible, and if desired, postoperative analgesia can be provided via an epidural infusion.

Peripheral Nerve Blockade

The lumbar plexus is located within the psoas muscle and is formed by the ventral rami of segmental lumbar nerves from L2 to L4.[26,36] Branches of the lumbar plexus include the lateral femoral cutaneous nerve of the thigh (formed by L2 and L3 nerves), the obturator nerve (L2 to L4), and the femoral nerve (L2 to L4). The lumbar plexus also contributes to the genitofemoral nerve (with L1, L2, and sometimes T12 nerves) and the sciatic nerve (with L4 and L5 nerves, and sacral nerves S1 through S3).

The lumbar plexus provides near-complete sensory innervation to the hip joint. In a detailed anatomic study of the innervation of the hip joint,[27] anterior and medial portions of the joint capsule were found to be innervated by articular branches of the femoral and obturator nerves, and it was noted that the posteromedial capsule is innervated at least in part by articular branches from nerves to the quadratus femoris. However, the posterior capsule is also innervated by articular branches from the sciatic nerve, and the posterolateral capsule receives innervation from the superior gluteal nerve (L5-S1 nerves). Therefore surgical anesthesia requires anesthesia of both the lumbar plexus and the sacral plexus.[31]

Peripheral nerve blockade for hip surgery can thus be performed by a posterior approach to the lumbar plexus within the psoas compartment (Fig. 24-1) or by an anterior approach at the fascia iliaca or femoral

compartment (Fig. 24-2). These approaches have been shown to enhance postoperative analgesia and reduce opioid analgesic requirements during the perioperative period,[37-40] but some studies suggest that the functional benefit may be limited.[41-44] Some anterior approaches do not consistently produce anesthesia of the obturator or lateral femoral cutaneous nerve.[45] In this sense, a posterior approach seems more reliable in producing anesthesia of all three nerves, although epidural spread may not be uncommon (≈10%).[38] However, neither approach to the lumbar plexus resulted in sacral plexus anesthesia in a small prospective study involving 80 patients.[45] At this point, definitive, multicenter, randomized studies involving a large number of patients are lacking. It seems that the choice of peripheral nerve blockade must reflect the surgical approach, the expected surgical duration, and the specific technique. Future studies should address these issues directly.

Psoas compartment blockade can be achieved via different landmark-based approaches (see Fig. 24-1). In general, these are performed with the patient in a lateral decubitus position,[26,36] with the use of a nerve stimulator and a needle with an uninsulated tip. The intercristal line (between the iliac crests bilaterally) and a line parallel to the lumbar spinous processes passing through the ipsilateral posterior superior iliac spine are used as general landmarks. Needle placement is such that a perpendicular path results in contact with the L5 transverse process. In this regard, careful examination of routine hip x-rays that include this anatomic area is useful in determining the exact needle entry site relative to the cutaneous landmarks. A motor response is sought using peripheral nerve stimulation (starting current ≈1.2 to 2.0 mA, depending on patient comfort), and once a "twitch" in the appropriate distribution (anterior thigh) is elicited, current is gradually reduced to approximately 0.5 mA. A twitch in both the anterior and the posterior thigh would suggest stimulation of lumbosacral roots epidurally and necessitates needle redirection. An indwelling catheter is usually placed within the belly of the psoas muscle.

Fascia iliaca compartment blockade can be accomplished easily in most patients while supine, without the need for repositioning (see Fig. 24-2). Needle insertion occurs 1 cm inferior to the point between the lateral and middle thirds of a line between the anterior superior iliac spine and the pubic tubercle.[39,46,47] Resistance is felt upon passing first the fascia lata and subsequently the fascia iliaca, at which point a single injection of 20 to 40 mL of local anesthetic solution and/or insertion of an indwelling catheter can be performed. Ultrasound-guided visualization may improve the reliability of block placement.[48] In a randomized, double-blind, placebo-controlled study of 44 patients scheduled for hip arthroplasty surgery,[39] fascia iliaca compartment blocks were associated with reduced morphine consumption for up to 24 hours postoperatively. Fascia iliaca blocks may also facilitate patient positioning and improve comfort following hip fracture before surgery. In a randomized, placebo-controlled trial involving 48 patients with suspected hip fracture upon emergency room admission,[47]

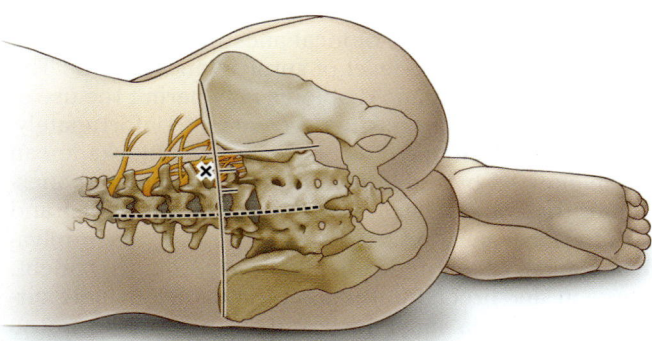

Figure 24-1. Anatomic landmarks for blockade of the lumbar plexus at the psoas compartment. (Redrawn from Hebl JR, Lennon RL: Mayo Clinic atlas of regional anesthesia and ultrasound-guided nerve blockade, Rochester, Minn, 2010, Mayo Clinic Scientific Press, p 373.)

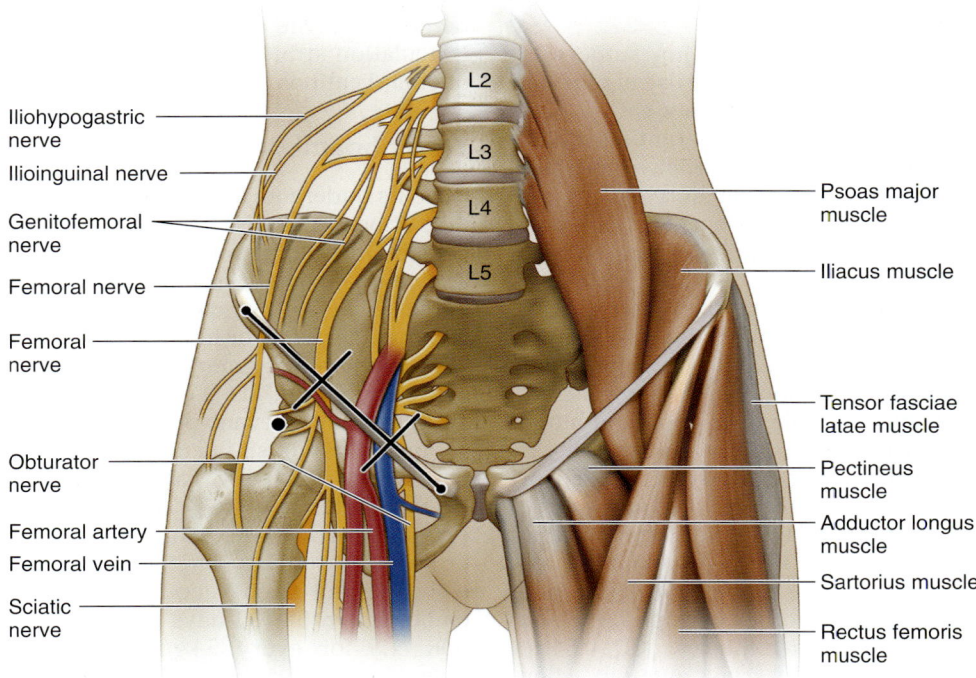

Iliohypogastric nerve
Ilioinguinal nerve
Genitofemoral nerve
Femoral nerve
Femoral nerve
Obturator nerve
Femoral artery
Femoral vein
Sciatic nerve

L2
L3
L4
L5

Psoas major muscle
Iliacus muscle
Tensor fasciae latae muscle
Pectineus muscle
Adductor longus muscle
Sartorius muscle
Rectus femoris muscle

Figure 24-2. Anatomic landmarks for fascia iliaca compartment block. (Redrawn from Hebl JR, Lennon RL: Mayo Clinic atlas of regional anesthesia and ultrasound-guided nerve blockade, Rochester, Minn, 2010, Mayo Clinic Scientific Press, p 339.)

patients randomized to a single-injection fascia iliaca compartment block with 40 mL of 1% mepivacaine reported superior analgesia at rest and with movement compared with those given 0.1 mg/kg intramuscular morphine.

Although a more traditional, paravascular approach to the femoral nerve ("3-in-1" block) has been advocated in some studies,[41,49] this anterior approach commonly results in sparing of the obturator and lateral femoral cutaneous nerves.[45,46] However, it seems that failure to provide adequate anesthesia with this approach is related to difficulty in controlling the final position of the indwelling catheter (if one is used). In a prospective study of 100 patients receiving a continuous paravascular nerve block, the course of the catheter could not be predicted, and only 23 catheters were documented with the use of fluoroscopy and contrast injection as placed in direct proximity to the lumbar plexus.[50] In this sense, use of a stimulating catheter (a special indwelling catheter that permits continuous stimulation via the catheter and thus fine-tuning of the position of the tip) may improve the quality of the anesthetic block.[51] Additional studies are needed to evaluate the clinical implications of using stimulating catheters in the perioperative management of patients undergoing hip surgery.

ANESTHETIC TECHNIQUES FOR HIP SURGERY: RISKS

Cardiovascular Complications

In general terms, hip surgery would be considered to present "intermediate risk," given reported rates of cardiovascular events or death of between 0.3% and 2.4%.[9,52,53] Clearly, specific cardiovascular and mortality risk depends on the surgical procedure. Higher event rates have been reported for fracture repair than for elective arthroplasty. For instance, of 5233 patients who underwent primary total hip arthroplasty during a 10-year period,[9] 108 (2.1%) patients had one or more clinically relevant cardiopulmonary adverse event. Overall, 24 (0.5%) patients experienced myocardial infarction, and 29 (0.6%) patients died within 30 days of surgery. Both myocardial infarction and death increased in frequency with older age, particularly for patients aged 70 years or older. Myocardial infarction also occurred more frequently in male patients. Among 7774 patients who underwent surgery for acute hip fracture during a 28-year period,[53] 186 (2.4%) patients died within 30 days of surgery. Similar to the elective hip arthroplasty cohort, patients aged 70 years or older were at increased risk of death. However, the risk of death among female patients was greater than that among male patients (3.1% in females vs. 1.8% in males; $P < .003$).

Hemodynamic derangements during hip surgery in elderly patients might be mitigated by the use of regional anesthetic techniques. Among 40 patients with a high risk of ischemic heart disease who were randomly allocated to receive spinal or general anesthesia for elective hip arthroplasty or peripheral vascular surgery,[54] spinal anesthesia provided greater stability in a heart rate variability index of sympathovagal balance compared with general anesthesia.

Preoperative anemia has been associated with increased risks of cardiovascular morbidity and mortality in large series of patients. Anemia is common in patients undergoing major orthopedic surgery, including hip surgery. However, the role of anemia (and blood transfusion) in perioperative morbidity and mortality is controversial. In a recent 20-year study of 391 hip or knee arthroplasty patients who experienced myocardial infarction or death within 30 days of surgery,[55] anemia (Hb <12.0 g/dL for females and <13.0 g/dL for males) was not a significant independent risk factor for these complications after adjustment for other perioperative risk factors (OR, 0.81; 95% confidence interval [CI], 0.54 to 1.20; $P = .286$). The outcome was not different when preoperative hemoglobin was treated as a continuous variable (OR, 0.98; 95% CI, 0.81 to 1.19 per 1.0 g/dL decrease below 13.0 g/dL; $P = .868$). Indeed, preexisting cardiovascular, cerebrovascular, or pulmonary disease and history of recent malignancy were the most important risk factors.

Early administration of appropriate analgesia in patients with hip fracture may have an impact on their risk of cardiac complications. Use of regional anesthetic techniques may be particularly helpful in these patients because the quality of analgesia can be substantially improved compared with standard parenteral opioid agents.[47] For instance, in a prospective, randomized study involving 68 patients with hip fracture who were considered to be at high cardiac risk,[56] patients who were administered an epidural infusion experienced significantly fewer preoperative adverse cardiac events compared with the control group receiving parenteral opioid analgesics (7 of 34 vs. 0 of 34, respectively; $P = .01$). Four patients died (three with myocardial infarction and one with congestive heart failure), one experienced new-onset congestive heart failure, and two new-onset atrial fibrillation. The frequency of intraoperative or postoperative cardiac events was not different between the two groups (2 of 34 in the epidural group vs. 4 of 30 in the control group). In a similar study involving 77 patients with hip fracture who were monitored with Holter recordings,[57] patients receiving a preoperative epidural infusion experienced fewer intraoperative and postoperative ischemic episodes compared with those given a standard parenteral opioid regimen. No myocardial infarctions were reported in this study. The clinical implications of these studies remain unclear, because differences in the timing of operative repair following admission to the emergency room may influence perioperative adverse events,[58]

especially in patients with comorbid conditions.[59] Finally, the use of regional anesthetic techniques must be placed in the context of thromboprophylactic anticoagulation strategies that have an impact on the risk of complications.

Thromboembolic Complications

Patients undergoing hip surgery are known to be at high thromboembolic risk.[60] Multiple embolic sources are possible, including fat, bone marrow, cement, air, and thrombus. Venous thromboembolism is a major cause of death in orthopedic patients undergoing surgery, whether electively or following trauma. Of 5233 patients who underwent primary total hip arthroplasty during a 10-year period,[9] 0.6% died within 30 days of surgery, and clinically relevant pulmonary embolism and deep venous thrombosis occurred in 0.6% and 1.3% of patients, respectively. Fatal pulmonary embolism has been reported in up to 8% of patients undergoing lower extremity orthopedic surgery.[60] In primary elective hip or knee arthroplasty, independent risk factors for clinically relevant deep venous thrombosis or pulmonary embolism within 30 days of surgery included obesity (OR, 1.5 for every 5-kg/m² increase in body mass index) and American Society of Anesthesiologists physical status classification[61] consistent with systemic disease (≥3).[62]

Cognitive Dysfunction

Patients undergoing regional anesthesia commonly receive fewer medications that affect the function of the central nervous system. Thus it stands to reason that these patients would experience fewer cognitive disturbances postoperatively. However, several studies have not substantiated this notion.[63,64] In fact, patients commonly receive sedative medications to help them tolerate the procedure comfortably, and these can contribute to cognitive problems, especially in the elderly.[65] In a review of 12 different studies, hip fracture surgery was associated with an average incidence of postoperative delirium of 35%.[66] Embolization of surgical material (e.g., methylmethacrylate), bone marrow, or medullary fat is commonly cited as a possible mechanism for postoperative cognitive decline.[67] Surgical embolization likely occurs independently of anesthetic technique.[68,69] Whether microemboli correlate with cognitive outcomes, however, remains controversial.[70] Regardless, postoperative cognitive dysfunction is an important source of morbidity and mortality. Future studies should directly address whether specific perioperative interventions can successfully reduce the risk of delirium in the elderly patient undergoing hip surgery.[65]

Nerve Injury

Nerve injuries, including motor palsy, are recognized complications of hip surgery. Injury occurs most commonly to the peroneal division of the sciatic nerve, but the femoral, obturator, and superior gluteal nerves can also be injured.[71,72] In a 30-year series of 27,004 patients undergoing primary total hip arthroplasty, 47 (0.17%) patients experienced incomplete or complete motor nerve dysfunction postoperatively.[73] Risk factors for motor palsy included a preoperative diagnosis of developmental hip dysplasia or post-traumatic arthritis, as well as surgery via a posterior approach, involving lengthening of the extremity or use of an uncemented femoral implant.[72,73] The underlying pathophysiologic mechanisms for these associations, however, remain unclear. It seems plausible that lengthening of the surgical extremity or a history of developmental abnormalities may result in traction and thus mechanical or ischemic injury to peripheral nerves. How other documented risk factors (e.g., not using cement for the femoral implant) contribute to increased risk of motor nerve injury is not straightforward.

Major neurologic complications following regional anesthesia are rare.[29,74] Patients with preexisting pathology of the lumbosacral spinal canal (e.g., spinal stenosis) seem to be at greater risk of neurologic complications after neuraxial blockade. Hebl and colleagues recently reported that patients with a history of spinal stenosis or lumbar radiculopathy who underwent neuraxial anesthesia are at greater risk of new or progressive neurologic deficits.[75] In their 15-year study, the rate of neurologic complications (i.e., new or worsening deficits) following neuraxial anesthesia in 937 patients with a history of spinal stenosis or lumbar radiculopathy was 1.1% (95% CI, 0.5% to 2.0%). This rate was believed to be substantially higher than expected based on prospective epidemiologic investigations reporting neurologic complications in the order of 1:1000 to 1:10,000.[29,74,76] Clearly, a thorough preoperative evaluation with specific attention paid to a history of radicular symptoms and complicated back pain should raise awareness of possible spinal canal pathology that may place patients at higher risk of neurologic complications.

Similarly, patients with peripheral neuropathy may be at higher risk of neurologic complications following major orthopedic surgery. In a retrospective study of 567 patients with a preoperative diagnosis of peripheral neuropathy (sensorimotor deficits or diabetic polyneuropathy) who underwent neuraxial anesthesia, the rate of neurologic complications was 0.4% (95% CI, 0.1% to 1.3%).[77] Once again, this rate was thought by investigators to be higher than expected, suggesting that preexisting distal nerve pathology may predispose patients to subsequent injury with anatomically remote, neuraxial anesthesia. Although preexisting pathology may theoretically make a nerve more vulnerable to subsequent injury, this assumption may not hold true. In a series of 360 patients undergoing ulnar nerve transposition surgery, patients who received axillary blockade experienced a comparable rate of new or worsening neurologic symptoms compared with patients who underwent general anesthesia alone (6% in both groups).[78] In addition, a recent 20-year study involving 12,329 patients undergoing total knee arthroplasty reported an overall incidence of neurologic injury of 0.79% (95% CI, 0.64% to 0.96%).[79] Nerve injury was not

associated with the use of regional anesthesia, either peripheral nerve or neuraxial blockade. However, for those rare patients who experienced a perioperative nerve injury, complete recovery was less likely if they had received peripheral, but not neuraxial, blockade. Future studies are needed to more clearly elucidate the role, if any, of peripheral nerve versus neuraxial blockade in the risk of neurologic complications in the context of major orthopedic surgery, including hip surgery.

MANAGEMENT CONSIDERATIONS

Choice of general or regional anesthesia will be based on careful consideration of patient and surgery-specific characteristics, as has been discussed. In addition, several other issues must be appraised in deciding upon the best course of action. Integration of the anesthetic plan into the overall perioperative care of the hip surgery patient is paramount.

Positioning

Patients are commonly placed in the lateral decubitus position for hip surgery. This position provides convenient access, and in patients undergoing neuraxial and/or psoas compartment blockade, these regional anesthetic procedures can be performed without the need to move the patient further. Discomfort in assuming this position can usually be alleviated by judicious use of intravenous opioid analgesics or ketamine.[80] In transferring from supine to lateral positioning, care must be taken to protect the neck and upper extremities.[6] For instance, a small roll or an inflatable pillow can be placed under the upper chest just distal to the axilla to avoid compression of the neurovascular bundle to the dependent extremity.[81] Achieving a comfortable position for a patient with extensive arthritis involving the spine or shoulders while lightly sedated might not be possible; in such cases, general anesthesia may be warranted. Similarly, in deciding whether to proceed with general versus neuraxial anesthesia in a patient with a suspected or known difficult airway, the clinician must carefully appraise the likelihood and possibility of emergently securing the airway in a particular position.

Fracture tables can be used to help maintain traction on the injured extremity while improving access for radiographic examination.[82] Their use requires sufficient personnel to aid in the safe transfer and positioning of patients. In addition, hemodynamic stability during transfer must be monitored carefully. If it is difficult for a patient to become comfortable in these devices, general anesthesia might be necessary.

Pain

Regional anesthetic techniques, neuraxial or peripheral, can be extended into the postoperative period if a catheter is placed at the time of the procedure. The benefit of regional anesthetic techniques in postoperative analgesia has been consistently substantiated across clinical studies.[3,19,22,83-85] The use of continuous psoas compartment blocks or epidural catheters, for example, reduces postoperative opioid consumption and opioid-related side effects.[20,37] However, some studies have reported short-term gains limited to the first 24 hours postoperatively,[42,43] thus calling into question the relative effectiveness of continuous plexus blockade. These issues are discussed in much greater detail elsewhere in this book (see Chapter 27).

One important consideration in formulating the anesthetic plan is the postoperative pain management strategy. Anticipated analgesic needs may also influence the choice of anesthetic technique.[84] For instance, in patients undergoing hip fracture repair, the surgical procedure influences the postoperative pain experience. In a prospective evaluation of 117 hip fracture patients treated with continuous epidural analgesia and a standard rehabilitation program,[86] patients who received dynamic or intramedullary hip screws reported significantly higher pain scores compared with those who underwent arthroplasty surgery.

Blood Transfusion

Multiple studies show that the use of regional anesthesia is associated with reduced blood loss and requirements for blood transfusion following major orthopedic surgery, including hip surgery.[17,18,21,22,38,87] Although it is not clear whether this effect results from reduced intraoperative duration,[18] improved hemodynamic stability,[32] or reduced venous pooling in the operative limb,[38,88] current transfusion practices are conservative because of increasing evidence that transfusion itself may negatively influence patient outcomes.[89-93] In fact, physicians are more likely to tolerate lower hemoglobin levels in orthopedic patients before transfusing. For instance, at the Mayo Clinic, the transfusion threshold decreased from 11.8 g/dL to 10.5 g/dL from 1981-1982 to 1993-1994.[94] This is an important consideration given the prevalence of anemia in elderly patients,[95,96] including orthopedic patients. Patients undergoing elective orthopedic surgery, especially patients with fractured hips, show a high frequency of preoperative anemia (>21%).[55,97-99] The change in transfusion practice has not been associated with major changes in the frequency of adverse perioperative outcomes (e.g., stroke, myocardial infarction [MI], death).[9,100-102] These issues are discussed in much greater detail elsewhere in this book (see Chapter 23).

Perioperative Anticoagulation

An important consideration in patients receiving regional anesthesia is the choice and timing of thromboprophylactic agents. Hip surgery patients are recognized as being at high risk of thromboembolic complications, and routine perioperative anticoagulation is recommended. Other risk factors for bleeding complications in patients undergoing regional anesthesia include advanced age, traumatic needle placement, and the presence of underlying anatomic abnormalities (e.g., spinal pathology) or coagulation abnormalities. These issues are reviewed in great detail in the evidence-based guidelines published by the American Society of Regional Anesthesia and Pain Medicine, now in its third edition.[103] Practitioners are urged to review the most recent update.

The timing of regional anesthesia after systemic anticoagulation is critically important, and the interval considered safe varies, depending on the thromboprophylactic agent and the regional technique. Protocols for thromboprophylaxis that include preoperative administration of systemic anticoagulants should be reviewed by all stakeholders, including the orthopedic surgery and anesthesia teams. Continuous peripheral and neuraxial catheters should be removed at a time that minimizes bleeding risk. This is particularly important for neuraxial (e.g., epidural) and lumbar compartment catheters because bleeding sites are not compressible, neurologic complications can be devastating, and large amounts of bleeding can occur before symptoms become evident. Unfortunately, many thromboprophylactic agents are not amenable to laboratory testing, and/or their anticoagulant effect is incompletely evaluated by available tests. Thus, the safe levels of systemic anticoagulation at which catheter removal can be performed remain controversial. Indeed, some proponents suggest that patients are being unnecessarily deprived of adequate analgesia by early removal of continuous perineural catheters in accordance with current guidelines.[104] However, the possibility of major neurologic injury in the context of scant information regarding a specific patient's hemorrhagic risk warrants caution. Strict institutional protocols that incorporate pharmacy and nursing may help prevent undesirable complications by avoiding catheter removal at unintended times.

CURRENT TOPICS AND FUTURE DIRECTIONS

Patients undergoing hip surgery pose specific challenges to the anesthesiologist, which demand updated review when new surgical procedures and advanced techniques are introduced. Anesthetic options for hip surgery include general and regional techniques, but options will vary depending on patient and procedure-specific characteristics. Patients undergoing hip surgery commonly suffer from arthritis and other musculoskeletal disorders that demand great care in airway management and patient positioning. Regional anesthesia such as neuraxial (spinal or epidural) and peripheral techniques may offer specific advantages for hip surgery, including reduced intraoperative blood loss and cardiovascular risk, and superior postoperative analgesia with fewer side effects. However, these benefits must be evaluated in the context of complex perioperative care that includes thromboprophylactic anticoagulation strategies that are continually revised. For instance, the recent introduction of direct factor Xa inhibitors and the oral direct thrombin inhibitor, dabigatran, requires careful consideration and study of their use in the context of neuraxial and psoas compartment blockade.[105,106] Older age and comorbidities, which are common in patients undergoing hip surgery, place them at risk for increased morbidity and mortality. Studies appropriately designed to help identify those patients at highest risk and to evaluate strategies used to mitigate the negative impact of these risk factors on patient outcomes are needed.

REFERENCES

1. Baron JA, Barrett J, Katz JN, Liang MH: Total hip arthroplasty: use and select complications in the US Medicare population. Am J Public Health 86:70–72, 1996.
2. Mahomed NN, Barrett JA, Katz JN, et al: Rates and outcomes of primary and revision total hip replacement in the United States Medicare population. J Bone Joint Surg Am 85:27–32, 2003.
3. Hebl JR, Dilger JA, Byer DE, et al: A pre-emptive multimodal pathway featuring peripheral nerve block improves perioperative outcomes after major orthopedic surgery. Reg Anesth Pain Med 33:510–517, 2008.
4. Duncan CM, Hall Long K, Warner DO, Hebl JR: The economic implications of a multimodal analgesic regimen for patients undergoing major orthopedic surgery: a comparative study of direct costs. Reg Anesth Pain Med 34:301–307, 2009.
5. Urban MK: Anesthesia for orthopedic surgery. In Miller RD (ed): Miller's anesthesia, ed 7, Philadelphia, 2010, Churchill Livingstone-Elsevier, pp 2241–2259.
6. Horlocker TT, Wedel DJ: Anesthesia for ortrhopaedic surgery. In Barash PJ, Cullen BF, Stoelting RK (eds): Clinical anesthesia, ed 5, Philadelphia, Lippincott, Williams & Wilkins, 2006, pp 1112–1128.
7. Fleisher LA, Beckman JA, Brown KA, et al, ACC/AHA 2007 guidelines on perioperative cardiovascular evaluation and care for noncardiac surgery: executive summary: a report of the American College of Cardiology/American Heart Association Task Force on Practice Guidelines (Writing Committee to Revise the 2002 Guidelines on Perioperative Cardiovascular Evaluation for Noncardiac Surgery) developed in collaboration with the American Society of Echocardiography, American Society of Nuclear Cardiology, Heart Rhythm Society, Society of Cardiovascular Anesthesiologists, Society for Cardiovascular Angiography and Interventions, Society for Vascular Medicine and Biology, and Society for Vascular Surgery. J Am Coll Cardiol 50:1707–1732, 2007.
8. Lee TH, Marcantonio ER, Mangione CM, et al: Derivation and prospective validation of a simple index for prediction of cardiac risk of major noncardiac surgery. Circulation 100:1043–1049, 1999.
9. Mantilla CB, Horlocker TT, Schroeder DR, et al: Frequency of myocardial infarction, pulmonary embolism, deep venous thrombosis, and death following primary hip or knee arthroplasty. Anesthesiology 96:1140–1146, 2002.
10. Higuera CA, Elsharkawy K, Klika AK, et al: 2010 Mid-America Orthopaedic Association Physician in Training Award: predictors of early adverse outcomes after knee and hip arthroplasty in geriatric patients. Clin Orthop Relat Res 469:1391–1400, 2011.
11. Alfonso DT, Howell RD, Strauss EJ, Di Cesare PE: Total hip and knee arthroplasty in nonagenarians. J Arthroplasty 22:807–811, 2007.
12. de Thomasson E, Caux I, Guingand O, et al: Total hip arthroplasty for osteoarthritis in patients aged 80 years or older: influence of co-morbidities on final outcome. Orthop Traumatol Surg Res 95:249–253, 2009.
13. Röder C, Parvizi J, Eggli S, et al: Demographic factors affecting long-term outcome of total hip arthroplasty. Clin Orthop Relat Res 417:62–73, 2003.
14. Casati A, Aldegheri G, Vinciguerra E, et al: Randomized comparison between sevoflurane anaesthesia and unilateral spinal anaesthesia in elderly patients undergoing orthopaedic surgery. Eur J Anaesthesiol 20:640–646, 2003.
15. Wu CL, Berenholtz SM, Pronovost PJ, Fleisher LA: Systematic review and analysis of postdischarge symptoms after outpatient surgery. Anesthesiology 96:994–1003, 2002.
16. Fleisher LA, Pasternak LR, Lyles A: A novel index of elevated risk of inpatient hospital admission immediately following outpatient surgery. Arch Surg 142:263–268, 2007.
17. Rodgers A, Walker N, Schug S, et al: Reduction of postoperative mortality and morbidity with epidural or spinal anaesthesia: results from overview of randomised trials. BMJ 321:1493, 2000.
18. Mauermann WJ, Shilling AM, Zuo Z: A comparison of neuraxial block versus general anesthesia for elective total hip replacement: a meta-analysis. Anesth Analg 103:1018–1025, 2006.
19. Horlocker TT, Kopp SL, Pagnano MW, Hebl JR: Analgesia for total hip and knee arthroplasty: a multimodal pathway featuring peripheral nerve block. J Am Acad Orthop Surg 14:126–135, 2006.
20. Hebl JR, Kopp SL, Ali MH, et al: A comprehensive anesthesia protocol that emphasizes peripheral nerve blockade for total knee and total hip arthroplasty. J Bone Joint Surg Am 87(Suppl 2):63–70, 2005.
21. Hu S, Zhang ZY, Hua YQ, et al: A comparison of regional and general anaesthesia for total replacement of the hip or knee: a meta-analysis. J Bone Joint Surg Br 91:935–942, 2009.
22. Macfarlane AJ, Prasad GA, Chan VW, Brull R: Does regional anaesthesia improve outcome after total hip arthroplasty? A systematic review. Br J Anaesth 103:335–345, 2009.
23. DeVera HV, Furukawa KT, Matson MD, et al: Regional techniques as an adjunct to general anesthesia for pediatric extremity and spine surgery. J Pediatr Orthop 26:801–804, 2006.
24. Giaufre E, Dalens B, Gombert A: Epidemiology and morbidity of regional anesthesia in children: a one-year prospective survey of the French-Language Society of Pediatric Anesthesiologists. Anesth Analg 83:904–912, 1996.
25. Horlocker TT, Abel MD, Messick JM Jr, Schroeder DR: Small risk of serious neurologic complications related to lumbar epidural catheter placement in anesthetized patients. Anesth Analg 96:1547–1552, 2003.
26. Chayen D, Nathan H, Chayen M: The psoas compartment block. Anesthesiology 45:95–99, 1976.
27. Birnbaum K, Prescher A, Eessler S, Heller KD: The sensory innervation of the hip joint—an anatomical study. Surg Radiol Anat 19:371–375, 1997.
28. Hanna MH, Peat SJ, D'Costa F: Lumbar plexus block: an anatomical study. Anaesthesia 48:675–678, 1993.
29. Auroy Y, Benhamou D, Bargues L, et al: Major complications of regional anesthesia in France: the SOS Regional Anesthesia Hotline Service. Anesthesiology 97:1274–1280, 2002.
30. Moore JM: Continuous spinal anesthesia. Am J Ther 16:289–294, 2009.
31. Capdevila X, Zetlaoui P, Mannion S: Neural blockade for orthopedic surgery. In Cousins MJ, Bridenbaugh PO, Carr DB, Horlocker TT (eds): Cousins & Bridenbaugh's neural blockade in clinical anesthesia and pain medicine, ed 4, Philadelphia, 2009, Lippincott, Williams & Wilkins, pp 566–583.
32. Borghi B, Casati A, Iuorio S, et al: Frequency of hypotension and bradycardia during general anesthesia, epidural anesthesia, or integrated epidural-general anesthesia for total hip replacement. J Clin Anesth 14:102–106, 2002.
33. Olofsson C, Nygards EB, Bjersten AB, Hessling A: Low-dose bupivacaine with sufentanil prevents hypotension after spinal anesthesia for hip repair in elderly patients. Acta Anaesthesiol Scand 48:1240–1244, 2004.
34. Ben-David B, Frankel R, Arzumonov T, et al: Minidose bupivacaine-fentanyl spinal anesthesia for surgical repair of hip fracture in the aged. Anesthesiology 92:6–10, 2000.
35. Pollock JE, Neal JM, Stephenson CA, Wiley CE: Prospective study of the incidence of transient radicular irritation in patients undergoing spinal anesthesia. Anesthesiology 84:1361–1367, 1996.
36. Capdevila X, Macaire P, Dadure C, et al: Continuous psoas compartment block for postoperative analgesia after total hip arthroplasty: new landmarks, technical guidelines, and clinical evaluation. Anesth Analg 94:1606–1613, 2002.
37. Becchi C, Al Malyan M, Coppini R, et al: Opioid-free analgesia by continuous psoas compartment block after total hip

arthroplasty: a randomized study. Eur J Anaesthesiol 25:418–423, 2008.

38. Stevens RD, Van Gessel E, Flory N, et al: Lumbar plexus block reduces pain and blood loss associated with total hip arthroplasty. Anesthesiology 93:115–121, 2000.

39. Stevens M, Harrison G, McGrail M: A modified fascia iliaca compartment block has significant morphine-sparing effect after total hip arthroplasty. Anaesth Intensive Care 35:949–952, 2007.

40. Marino J, Russo J, Kenny M, et al: Continuous lumbar plexus block for postoperative pain control after total hip arthroplasty: a randomized controlled trial. J Bone Joint Surg Am 91:29–37, 2009.

41. Fournier R, Van Gessel E, Gaggero G, et al: Postoperative analgesia with "3-in-1" femoral nerve block after prosthetic hip surgery. Can J Anaesth 45:34–38, 1998.

42. Biboulet P, Morau D, Aubas P, et al: Postoperative analgesia after total-hip arthroplasty: comparison of intravenous patient-controlled analgesia with morphine and single injection of femoral nerve or psoas compartment block: a prospective, randomized, double-blind study. Reg Anesth Pain Med 29:102–109, 2004.

43. Bogoch ER, Henke M, Mackenzie T, et al: Lumbar paravertebral nerve block in the management of pain after total hip and knee arthroplasty: a randomized controlled clinical trial. J Arthroplasty 17:398–401, 2002.

44. Siddiqui ZI, Cepeda MS, Denman W, et al: Continuous lumbar plexus block provides improved analgesia with fewer side effects compared with systemic opioids after hip arthroplasty: a randomized controlled trial. Reg Anesth Pain Med 32:393–398, 2007.

45. Parkinson SK, Mueller JB, Little WL, Bailey SL: Extent of blockade with various approaches to the lumbar plexus. Anesth Analg 68:243–248, 1989.

46. Dalens B, Vanneuville G, Tanguy A: Comparison of the fascia iliaca compartment block with the 3-in-1 block in children. Anesth Analg 69:705–713, 1989.

47. Foss NB, Kristensen BB, Bundgaard M, et al: Fascia iliaca compartment blockade for acute pain control in hip fracture patients: a randomized, placebo-controlled trial. Anesthesiology 106:773–778, 2007.

48. Dolan J, Williams A, Murney E, et al: Ultrasound guided fascia iliaca block: a comparison with the loss of resistance technique. Reg Anesth Pain Med 33:526–531, 2008.

49. Winnie AP, Ramamurthy S, Durrani Z: The inguinal paravascular technic of lumbar plexus anesthesia: the "3-in-1 block." Anesth Analg 52:989–996, 1973.

50. Capdevila X, Biboulet P, Morau D, et al: Continuous three-in-one block for postoperative pain after lower limb orthopedic surgery: where do the catheters go? Anesth Analg 94:1001–1006, 2002.

51. Salinas FV, Neal JM, Sueda LA, et al: Prospective comparison of continuous femoral nerve block with nonstimulating catheter placement versus stimulating catheter-guided perineural placement in volunteers. Reg Anesth Pain Med 29:212–220, 2004.

52. Parvizi J, Johnson BG, Rowland C, et al: Thirty-day mortality after elective total hip arthroplasty. J Bone Joint Surg Am 83:1524–1528, 2001.

53. Parvizi J, Ereth MH, Lewallen DG: Thirty-day mortality following hip arthroplasty for acute fracture. J Bone Joint Surg Am 86:1983–1988, 2004.

54. Backlund M, Toivonen L, Tuominen M, et al: Changes in heart rate variability in elderly patients undergoing major noncardiac surgery under spinal or general anesthesia. Reg Anesth Pain Med 24:386–392, 1999.

55. Mantilla CB, Wass CT, Goodrich KA, et al: Risk for perioperative myocardial infarction and mortality in patients undergoing hip or knee arthroplasty: the role of anemia. Transfusion 51:82–91, 2011.

56. Matot I, Oppenheim-Eden A, Ratrot R, et al: Preoperative cardiac events in elderly patients with hip fracture randomized to epidural or conventional analgesia. Anesthesiology 98:156–163, 2003.

57. Scheinin H, Virtanen T, Kentala E, et al: Epidural infusion of bupivacaine and fentanyl reduces perioperative myocardial ischaemia in elderly patients with hip fracture—a randomized controlled trial. Acta Anaesthesiol Scand 44:1061–1070, 2000.

58. Shiga T, Wajima Z, Ohe Y: Is operative delay associated with increased mortality of hip fracture patients? Systematic review, meta-analysis, and meta-regression. Can J Anaesth 55:146–154, 2008.

59. Moran CG, Wenn RT, Sikand M, Taylor AM: Early mortality after hip fracture: is delay before surgery important? J Bone Joint Surg Am 87:483–489, 2005.

60. Geerts WH, Bergqvist D, Pineo GF, et al: Prevention of venous thromboembolism: American College of Chest Physicians evidence-based clinical practice guidelines (8th edition). Chest 133:381S–453S, 2008.

61. American Society of Anesthesiologists: New classification of physical status. Anesthesiology 24:111, 1963.

62. Mantilla CB, Horlocker TT, Schroeder DR, et al: Risk factors for clinically relevant pulmonary embolism and deep venous thrombosis in patients undergoing primary hip or knee arthroplasty. Anesthesiology 99:552–560, discussion 555A, 2003.

63. Williams-Russo P, Sharrock NE, Mattis S, et al: Cognitive effects after epidural vs general anesthesia in older adults: a randomized trial. JAMA 274:44–50, 1995.

64. Wu CL, Hsu W, Richman JM, Raja SN: Postoperative cognitive function as an outcome of regional anesthesia and analgesia. Reg Anesth Pain Med 29:257–268, 2004.

65. Sanders RD, Maze M: Contribution of sedative-hypnotic agents to delirium via modulation of the sleep pathway. Can J Anaesth 58:149–156, 2011.

66. Bitsch MS, Foss NB, Kristensen BB, Kehlet H: Acute cognitive dysfunction after hip fracture: frequency and risk factors in an optimized, multimodal, rehabilitation program. Acta Anaesthesiol Scand 50:428–436, 2006.

67. Sauer AM, Kalkman C, van Dijk D: Postoperative cognitive decline. J Anesth 23:256–259, 2009.

68. Ereth MH, Weber JG, Abel MD, et al: Cemented versus noncemented total hip arthroplasty—embolism, hemodynamics, and intrapulmonary shunting. Mayo Clin Proc 67:1066–1074, 1992.

69. Koessler MJ, Fabiani R, Hamer H, Pitto RP: The clinical relevance of embolic events detected by transesophageal echocardiography during cemented total hip arthroplasty: a randomized clinical trial. Anesth Analg 92:49–55, 2001.

70. Patel RV, Stygall J, Harrington J, et al: Cerebral microembolization during primary total hip arthroplasty and neuropsychologic outcome: a pilot study. Clin Orthop Relat Res 468:1621–1629, 2010.

71. DeHart MM, Riley LH Jr: Nerve injuries in total hip arthroplasty. J Am Acad Orthop Surg 7:101–111, 1999.

72. Oldenburg M, Muller RT: The frequency, prognosis and significance of nerve injuries in total hip arthroplasty. Int Orthop 21:1–3, 1997.

73. Farrell CM, Springer BD, Haidukewych GJ, Morrey BF: Motor nerve palsy following primary total hip arthroplasty. J Bone Joint Surg Am 87:2619–2625, 2005.

74. Moen V, Dahlgren N, Irestedt L: Severe neurological complications after central neuraxial blockades in Sweden 1990-1999. Anesthesiology 101:950–959, 2004.

75. Hebl JR, Horlocker TT, Kopp SL, Schroeder DR: Neuraxial blockade in patients with preexisting spinal stenosis, lumbar disk disease, or prior spine surgery: efficacy and neurologic complications. Anesth Analg 111:1511–1519, 2010.

76. Auroy Y, Narchi P, Messiah A, et al: Serious complications related to regional anesthesia: results of a prospective survey in France. Anesthesiology 87:479–486, 1997.

77. Hebl JR, Kopp SL, Schroeder DR, Horlocker TT: Neurologic complications after neuraxial anesthesia or analgesia in patients with preexisting peripheral sensorimotor neuropathy or diabetic polyneuropathy. Anesth Analg 103:1294–1299, 2006.

78. Hebl JR, Horlocker TT, Sorenson EJ, Schroeder DR: Regional anesthesia does not increase the risk of postoperative neuropathy in patients undergoing ulnar nerve transposition. Anesth Analg 93:1606–1611, 2001.

79. Jacob AK, Mantilla CB, Sviggum HP, et al: Perioperative nerve injury after total knee arthroplasty: regional anesthesia risk during a 20-year cohort study. Anesthesiology 114:311–317, 2011.

80. Sandby-Thomas M, Sullivan G, Hall JE: A national survey into the peri-operative anaesthetic management of patients presenting for surgical correction of a fractured neck of femur. Anaesthesia 63:250–258, 2008.

81. Gonzalez Della Valle A, Salonia-Ruzo P, Peterson MG, et al: Inflatable pillows as axillary support devices during surgery performed in the lateral decubitus position under epidural anesthesia. Anesth Analg 93:1338–1343, 2001.

82. Flierl MA, Stahel PF, Hak DJ, et al: Traction table-related complications in orthopaedic surgery. J Am Acad Orthop Surg 18:668–675, 2010.

83. Ilfeld BM, Ball ST, Gearen PF, et al: Ambulatory continuous posterior lumbar plexus nerve blocks after hip arthroplasty: a dual-center, randomized, triple-masked, placebo-controlled trial. Anesthesiology 109:491–501, 2008.

84. Foss NB, Kristensen MT, Kristensen BB, et al: Effect of postoperative epidural analgesia on rehabilitation and pain after hip fracture surgery: a randomized, double-blind, placebo-controlled trial. Anesthesiology 102:1197–1204, 2005.

85. Choi PT, Bhandari M, Scott J, Douketis J: Epidural analgesia for pain relief following hip or knee replacement. Cochrane Database Syst Rev (3):CD003071, 2003.

86. Foss NB, Kristensen MT, Palm H, Kehlet H: Postoperative pain after hip fracture is procedure specific. Br J Anaesth 102:111–116, 2009.

87. Rashiq S, Finegan BA: The effect of spinal anesthesia on blood transfusion rate in total joint arthroplasty. Can J Surg 49:391–396, 2006.

88. Borghi B, Casati A, Iuorio S, et al: Effect of different anesthesia techniques on red blood cell endogenous recovery in hip arthroplasty. J Clin Anesth 17:96–101, 2005.

89. Vincent JL, Baron JF, Reinhart K, et al: Anemia and blood transfusion in critically ill patients. JAMA 288:1499–1507, 2002.

90. Corwin HL, Gettinger A, Pearl RG, The CRIT Study: Anemia and blood transfusion in the critically ill—current clinical practice in the United States. Crit Care Med 32:39–52, 2004.

91. Moore FA, Moore EE, Sauaia A: Blood transfusion: an independent risk factor for postinjury multiple organ failure. Arch Surg 132:620–624, discussion 624–625, 1997.

92. Hebert PC, Wells G, Blajchman MA, et al, Transfusion Requirements in Critical Care Investigators, Canadian Critical Care Trials Group: A multicenter, randomized, controlled clinical trial of transfusion requirements in critical care. N Engl J Med 340:409–417, 1999.

93. Rao SV, Jollis JG, Harrington RA, et al: Relationship of blood transfusion and clinical outcomes in patients with acute coronary syndromes. JAMA 292:1555–1562, 2004.

94. Warner DO, Warner MA, Schroeder DR, et al: Changing transfusion practices in hip and knee arthroplasty. Transfusion 38:738–744, 1998.

95. Zakai NA, Katz R, Hirsch C, et al: A prospective study of anemia status, hemoglobin concentration, and mortality in an elderly cohort: the Cardiovascular Health Study. Arch Intern Med 165:2214–2220, 2005.

96. Landi F, Russo A, Danese P, et al: Anemia status, hemoglobin concentration, and mortality in nursing home older residents. J Am Med Dir Assoc 8:322–327, 2007.

97. Goodnough LT, Vizmeg K, Sobecks R, et al: Prevalence and classification of anemia in elective orthopedic surgery patients: implications for blood conservation programs. Vox Sang 63:90–95, 1992.

98. Carson JL, Terrin ML, Magaziner J, et al: Transfusion trigger trial for functional outcomes in cardiovascular patients undergoing surgical hip fracture repair (FOCUS). Transfusion 46:2192–2206, 2006.

99. Shander A, Knight K, Thurer R, et al: Prevalence and outcomes of anemia in surgery: a systematic review of the literature. Am J Med 116(Suppl 7A):58S–69S, 2004.

100. Waggoner JR 3rd, Wass CT, Polis TZ, et al: The effect of changing transfusion practice on rates of perioperative stroke and myocardial infarction in patients undergoing carotid endarterectomy: a retrospective analysis of 1114 Mayo Clinic patients. Mayo Perioperative Outcomes Group. Mayo Clin Proc 76:376–383, 2001.

101. Wass CT, Long TR, Faust RJ, et al: Changes in red blood cell transfusion practice during the past two decades: a retrospective analysis, with the Mayo database, of adult patients undergoing major spine surgery. Transfusion 47:1022–1027, 2007.

102. Long TR, Curry TB, Stemmann JL, et al: Changes in red blood cell transfusion practice during the turn of the millennium: a retrospective analysis of adult patients undergoing elective open abdominal aortic aneurysm repair using the Mayo Database. Ann Vasc Surg 24:447–454, 2010.

103. Horlocker TT, Wedel DJ, Rowlingson JC, et al: Regional anesthesia in the patient receiving antithrombotic or thrombolytic therapy: American Society of Regional Anesthesia and Pain Medicine evidence-based guidelines (3rd edition). Reg Anesth Pain Med 35:64–101, 2010.

104. Chelly JE, Szczodry DM, Neumann KJ: International normalized ratio and prothrombin time values before the removal of a lumbar plexus catheter in patients receiving warfarin after total hip replacement. Br J Anaesth 101:250–254, 2008.

105. Levy JH, Key NS, Azran MS: Novel oral anticoagulants: implications in the perioperative setting. Anesthesiology 113:726–745, 2010.

106. Eriksson BI, Dahl OE, Huo MH, et al: Oral dabigatran versus enoxaparin for thromboprophylaxis after primary total hip arthroplasty (RE-NOVATE II): a randomised, double-blind, non-inferiority trial. Thromb Haemost 105:721–729, 2011.

CHAPTER 25

Mortality After Total Hip Arthroplasty

Wadih Y. Matar, Armin Aalami Harandi, and Javad Parvizi

INTRODUCTION

Although total hip arthroplasty (THA) is generally considered to be a safe and effective procedure, it can be associated with a number of complications. Perioperative mortality is the most devastating and feared of these complications.[1-5] Most of these deaths occur during the early postoperative period and most are the result of cardiorespiratory complications such as myocardial infarction and pulmonary embolism. Intraoperative death can also occur and represents the most dramatic event facing the adult reconstructive hip surgeon.[6] Cementing during THA has traditionally been considered to be the main factor associated with intraoperative death.[6-8] However, with more contemporary cementing techniques, the incidence of cement-related intraoperative deaths has decreased drastically.[9,10]

MORTALITY RATES

In the United States, rates of primary and revision THA are projected to increase significantly over the coming decades.[11,12] Improvements in surgical and anesthesia techniques, including better perioperative monitoring and postoperative protocols, allow the arthroplasty surgeon to offer THA to the older patient, who is at higher risk for perioperative complications.[13] Theoretically, this could lead to a higher mortality rate if not offset by the expected concomitant increase in demand for THA in the younger, healthier patient population.[14,15]

Most studies show that the immediate postoperative period represents the highest risk of death following THA.[1-3,5,16-19] Studies looking at 30-day mortality report rates between 0.24% and 0.95%. Studies looking at 90-day mortality report rates between 0.3% and 1.0% (Table 25-1).

Over the long term, the survival rates of patients who have undergone THA are generally better than those reported for the general population, suggesting a possible beneficial effect of the procedure in prolonging patients' lives.[5,18,20-22] Barrett and associates investigated whether improved survival was directly attributable to THA, or whether it was due to other factors.[23] By studying 28,469 primary THA Medicare patients over a 6-year period and matching them 5:1 to a control group, the authors used proportional hazards regression analysis for three postoperative periods. THA patients had a higher mortality rate in the immediate postoperative period; however, by 3 months, THA patients had a lower mortality rate than matched controls. From 3 months to 5 years, the mortality rate of THA patients was only two-thirds that of the control group after adjustments were made for sex, age, Medicaid eligibility, and other comorbidities. Beyond 5 years, mortality rates started to converge.

In a more recent study, Aynardi and colleagues reported on the mortality rate following 7478 consecutive elective primary and revision THAs between 2000 and 2006.[5] The overall reported mortality rate at 30 days was 0.24% (18 of 7478), with the vast majority of deaths occurring in the hospital (13 of 18). The 90-day mortality rate was 0.55% (41 of 7478). The authors noted that death rates increased with increasing age in this patient cohort. Patients younger than 65 years undergoing primary THA had the lowest death rate (0.03%), and patients older than 85 years had the highest death rate (4.91%). These findings have been corroborated by other authors.[2,5,18] After studying mortality rates in elective THA in nonfracture patients, Whittle and coworkers showed an 11-fold increase in the mortality rates of older patients (age 85 years or older) when compared with a group of patients between the ages of 66 and 69 years.[18]

In addition to age at the time of surgery, the type of surgery performed seems to have an impact on perioperative mortality. Aynardi and coworkers reported

Table 25-1. Sample Studies of Early Mortality After Total Hip Arthroplasty

Author	Number of THA	Study Period	30-Day	90-Day
Aynardi et al (2008)[5]	7478	2000-2006	0.24	0.55
Blom et al (2006)[16]	1727	1993-1996	0.41*	1.00*
Lie et al (2002)[3]	67,548	1987-1999	0.41	0.93
Parvizi et al (2001)[6]	30,714	1969-1997	0.29	
Dearborn et al (1998)[2]	2736	1969-1996		0.3
Whittle et al (1993)[18]	5078	1983-1985	0.95	
Seagroatt et al (1991)[19]	11,607	1976-1985		0.8
Coventry et al (1974)[1]	2012	1969-1973	0.4*	

*Included only primary hip arthroplasty surgery.

higher mortality rates following revision THA compared with primary THA (1.24% vs. 0.41%).[5] In fact, patients older than 85 years undergoing revision THA had the highest death rate among all groups at 6.25%. Using 2003 nationwide U.S. data, Zhan and associates reported on death rates among 200,000 primary THAs and 36,000 revision THAs.[24] The in-hospital death rate was 0.33% for primary and 0.84% for revision THA. The authors associated advanced age and comorbidities with worse outcomes.

Simultaneous bilateral THA has been associated with increased perioperative complications, prompting the arthroplasty surgeon to reserve this procedure for a select group of young and healthy patients. Tsiridis and associates performed a meta-analysis of all studies that compared the results of THA in unilateral and simultaneous bilateral THA and reported no statistically significant difference in the rate of pulmonary embolism, deep venous thromboembolism (DVT), or instability between the two groups.[25] Simultaneous bilateral THA had a shorter overall hospital stay when compared with staged unilateral THA, but the bilateral group required more blood transfusions. The reported mortality rate following simultaneous bilateral THA appears to be as low as that reported for unilateral THA.[26,27] However, the selection bias of younger patients without major comorbidities poses a challenge in extrapolating these results.[26]

CAUSES OF DEATH FOLLOWING TOTAL HIP ARTHROPLASTY

Causes of mortality following THA can be separated into those that occur intraoperatively and those that occur postoperatively.*

Intraoperative Mortality

Sudden intraoperative death is the most feared complication of THA. The occurrence of this phenomenon has greatly diminished over time with advancements in anesthesia techniques, cementing techniques, and the use of uncemented femoral stems.[5,6,9,10,31] Parvizi and colleagues reported 23 intraoperative deaths in a series of more than 29,000 patients undergoing hip arthroplasty.[6] All deaths occurred in cemented arthroplasties. Although approximately half of these cases occurred in elderly hip fracture patients with preexisting cardiovascular disease undergoing hemiarthroplasty, the other half of these cases occurred in the setting of elective THA. The authors identified irreversible cardiorespiratory disturbance during cementing as the cause of death in all patients. Microemboli were identified in the lungs of 11 of 13 patients during autopsy. Notably, no intraoperative deaths were reported in more than 15,000 patients undergoing uncemented arthroplasties performed in the same time period, suggesting that cementing is a major risk factor for sudden intraoperative death during THA.

Several causes of intraoperative mortality during cementation have been proposed. These include bone marrow and fat emboli,[9,32] polymethylmethacrylate (PMMA)-induced myocardial depression,[33] vasodilatation secondary to PMMA,[34,35] autonomic reflexation effects,[36] thromboplastin generation,[37] and prostaglandin-induced vasodilatation.[38] The term *bone cement implantation syndrome,* which can encompass varying degrees of systemic hypotension, pulmonary hypertension, cardiogenic shock, hypoxemia, cardiac arrhythmias, and even cardiac arrest, has been used to describe events that can occur within minutes of cementing of prosthetic components.[6,10,32,39] Embolization of fat and marrow contents during THA can be detected and quantified using transesophageal echocardiography.[9] Even though embolization of marrow occurs with impaction of uncemented components, emboli following cementation can be greater in number, size, and duration, probably because of the higher intramedullary pressures produced by cementing the stem.[32,39,40]

Postoperative Mortality

Many studies have investigated the causes of postoperative death following THA.* As noted previously, age has been shown to be a significant risk factor, as perioperative mortality rates increase with increasing age.[2,5,18] Conditions afflicting the cardiovascular system

---

*References 2, 5, 10, 16, 17, 23, 26, and 28-30.

*References 2, 17, 23, 26, 28, and 30.

such as acute coronary syndrome, cardiopulmonary arrest, stroke, arrhythmia, and pulmonary embolism are the leading causes of mortality following THA.[5,16,26,30] Respiratory conditions, sepsis, and malignancy are the other common conditions that may be responsible for early postoperative mortality.

PREVENTION OF DEATH

Overall improvements in perioperative care for THA patients in terms of surgical techniques, anesthesia care, and postoperative pain control have resulted in a marked decrease in mortality rate following THA.[4,6,17] In most centers, total joint arthroplasty patients are seen preoperatively by an internal medicine or cardiology consultant along with an anesthesiologist for assessment and optimization of health prior to the procedure. The American College of Cardiology/American Heart Association (ACC/AHA) publishes perioperative cardiac assessment guidelines that can be used during preoperative assessment of THA patients.[41] The goal of these guidelines is to perform a thorough evaluation of the patient's medical status preoperatively and to make recommendations regarding appropriate testing that is likely to influence patient treatment and aid in management of the cardiac patient during the perioperative period. Salerno and coworkers showed that these guidelines accurately predicted perioperative cardiac risk in the orthopedic patient.[42]

Currently, the authors routinely ask for a detailed preoperative assessment of THA patients by an internal medicine consultant. During this assessment, a detailed history and physical examination is carried out with special emphasis on potential high-risk comorbidities. Routine testing is also done, including blood work, electrocardiography, and chest x-rays. More invasive testing is carried out as needed according to the patient's condition. At the authors' institution, THA patients are followed by the same internist in the postoperative period. Patients considered at high risk for cardiovascular complications are admitted to the intensive care unit or a step-down unit with available continuous monitoring. Low-risk patients are admitted to the regular surgical floor, where the vitals are monitored closely and any abnormalities are further investigated. Daily blood work includes complete blood count, serum chemistries, and coagulation studies.

Deep vein thrombosis prophylaxis (chemical and mechanical) is provided to all patients in an effort to prevent sudden death resulting from pulmonary embolism. We currently favor Coumadin (warfarin) with a target international randomized ratio of 1.5 to 2.0 for a period of 6 weeks. Prophylactic antibiotics, which are started preoperatively, are continued for a period of 24 hours postoperatively to decrease the perioperative risk of infection.

The benefits of performing THA in a specialized high-volume hospital have been reported in several studies. It is believed that a higher case load along with greater surgeon experience can lead to a lower overall mortality rate and a lower rate of in-hospital death.[43-46] Performing the procedure with a trained and skilled team results in shorter operative time, which may lead to less blood loss, reduced infection, and fewer intraoperative adverse events.[5,26] Equally important is the use of standardized anesthesia and pain management protocols concentrating on hypotensive, neuraxial anesthesia to reduce cardiorespiratory complications.[13,47,48] Advances in multimodal anesthesia administered during the early rehabilitation period have led to improved functional scores and faster mobilization, which may further decrease thromboembolic-related deaths.[49,50]

While analyzing fatal or near-fatal complications around total joint replacements, Parvizi and colleagues showed that 6% of 1636 patients sustained at least one life-threatening medical complication in the postoperative period.[4] More important, 90% of these complications occurred during the first 4 postoperative days following the index procedure. In more than half of patients, the complication could not have been predicted based on the patient's medical history. Further analysis of these data revealed that if these complications occurred outside the hospital, 20 to 25 patients may have died as a result of the complications. This fact stresses the importance of postoperative monitoring and warns against early hospital discharge as advocated by the proponents of minimally invasive surgery.[51,52]

CURRENT CONTROVERSIES AND FUTURE CONSIDERATIONS

Bhandari and co-workers compared patient mortality rates following femoral neck fractures treated with arthroplasty (partial and total) versus those treated with internal fixation.[53] Despite a greater infection rate, increased perioperative blood loss, extended operative time, and potentially increased early mortality, treatment of displaced femoral neck fracture with arthroplasty led to a significantly lower revision rate when compared with internal fixation.[53-55] Bhandari concluded that larger trials are needed to find out whether non-elective THA performed for displaced femoral neck fracture might truly have a higher mortality rate compared with elective THA.

CONCLUSION

Death following THA remains the most feared complication. Despite recent trends toward uncemented THA and advances in anesthesia, perioperative monitoring, and postoperative rehabilitation protocols, 90-day mortality rates remain between 0.2% and 1.0%. It remains the responsibility of the surgeon and the perioperative team to ensure that patients are appropriately selected and optimized for surgery and are carefully monitored postoperatively, while set protocols aimed at decreasing morbidity and mortality are followed.

REFERENCES

1. Coventry MB, Beckenbaugh RD, Nolan DR, Ilstrup DM: 2,012 total hip arthroplasties: a study of postoperative course and early complications. J Bone Joint Surg Am 56:273–284, 1974.

2. Dearborn JT, Harris WH: Postoperative mortality after total hip arthroplasty: an analysis of deaths after two thousand seven hundred and thirty-six procedures. J Bone Joint Surg Am 80:1291–1294, 1998.

3. Lie SA, Engesaeter LB, Havelin LI, et al: Early postoperative mortality after 67,548 total hip replacements: causes of death and thromboprophylaxis in 68 hospitals in Norway from 1987 to 1999. Acta Orthop Scand 73:392–399, 2002.

4. Parvizi J, Mui A, Purtill JJ, et al: Total joint arthroplasty: when do fatal or near-fatal complications occur? J Bone Joint Surg Am 89:27–32, 2007.

5. Aynardi M, Pulido L, Parvizi J, et al: Early mortality after modern total hip arthroplasty. Clin Orthop Relat Res 467:213–218, 2009.

6. Parvizi J, Holiday AD, Ereth MH, Lewallen DG: The Frank Stinchfield Award. Sudden death during primary hip arthroplasty. Clin Orthop Relat Res 369:39–48, 1999.

7. Ereth MH, Weber JG, Abel MD, et al: Cemented versus noncemented total hip arthroplasty—embolism, hemodynamics, and intrapulmonary shunting. Mayo Clin Proc 67:1066–1074, 1992.

8. Cohen CA, Smith TC: The intraoperative hazard of acrylic bone cement: report of a case. Anesthesiology 35:547–549, 1971.

9. Pitto RP, Koessler M, Kuehle JW: Comparison of fixation of the femoral component without cement and fixation with use of a bone-vacuum cementing technique for the prevention of fat embolism during total hip arthroplasty: a prospective, randomized clinical trial. J Bone Joint Surg Am 81:831–843, 1999.

10. Sierra RJ, Timperley JA, Gie GA: Contemporary cementing technique and mortality during and after Exeter total hip arthroplasty. J Arthroplasty 24:325–332, 2009.

11. Kurtz S, Ong K, Lau E, et al: Projections of primary and revision hip and knee arthroplasty in the United States from 2005 to 2030. J Bone Joint Surg Am 89:780–785, 2007.

12. Bozic KJ, Kurtz SM, Lau E, et al: The epidemiology of revision total hip arthroplasty in the United States. J Bone Joint Surg Am 91:128–133, 2009.

13. Sharrock NE, Cazan MG, Hargett MJ, et al: Changes in mortality after total hip and knee arthroplasty over a ten-year period. Anesth Analg 80:242–248, 1995.

14. Kurtz SM, Lau E, Ong K, et al: Future young patient demand for primary and revision joint replacement: national projections from 2010 to 2030. Clin Orthop Relat Res 467:2606–2612, 2009.

15. Bozic KJ, Kurtz S, Lau E, et al: The epidemiology of bearing surface usage in total hip arthroplasty in the United States. J Bone Joint Surg Am 91:1614–1620, 2009.

16. Blom A, Pattison G, Whitehouse S, et al: Early death following primary total hip arthroplasty: 1,727 procedures with mechanical thrombo-prophylaxis. Acta Orthop 77:347–350, 2006.

17. Parvizi J, Johnson BG, Rowland C, et al: Thirty-day mortality after elective total hip arthroplasty. J Bone Joint Surg Am 83:1524–1528, 2001.

18. Whittle J, Steinberg EP, Anderson GF, et al: Mortality after elective total hip arthroplasty in elderly Americans: age, gender, and indication for surgery predict survival. Clin Orthop Relat Res 295:119–126, 1993.

19. Seagroatt V, Tan HS, Goldacre M, et al: Elective total hip replacement: incidence, emergency readmission rate, and postoperative mortality. BMJ 303:1431–1435, 1991.

20. Lie SA, Engesaeter LB, Havelin LI, et al: Mortality after total hip replacement: 0-10-year follow-up of 39,543 patients in the Norwegian Arthroplasty Register. Acta Orthop Scand 71:19–27, 2000.

21. Visuri T, Pulkkinen P, Turula KB, et al: Life expectancy after hip arthroplasty: case-control study of 1018 cases of primary arthrosis. Acta Orthop Scand 65:9–11, 1994.

22. Holmberg S: Life expectancy after total hip arthroplasty. J Arthroplasty 7:183–186, 1992.

23. Barrett J, Losina E, Baron JA, et al: Survival following total hip replacement. J Bone Joint Surg Am 87:1965–1971, 2005.

24. Zhan C, Kaczmarek R, Loyo-Berrios N, et al: Incidence and short-term outcomes of primary and revision hip replacement in the United States. J Bone Joint Surg Am 89:526–533, 2007.

25. Tsiridis E, Pavlou G, Charity J, et al: The safety and efficacy of bilateral simultaneous total hip replacement: an analysis of 2063 cases. J Bone Joint Surg Br 90:1005–1012, 2008.

26. Tarity TD, Herz AL, Parvizi J, Rothman RH: Ninety-day mortality after hip arthroplasty: a comparison between unilateral and simultaneous bilateral procedures. J Arthroplasty 21:60–64, 2006.

27. Parvizi J, Tarity TD, Herz A, et al: Ninety-day mortality after bilateral hip arthroplasty. J Arthroplasty 21:931–934, 2006.

28. Miller KA, Callaghan JJ, Goetz DD, Johnston RC: Early postoperative mortality following total hip arthroplasty in a community setting: a single surgeon experience. Iowa Orthop J 23:36–42, 2003.

29. Nunley RM, Lachiewicz PF: Mortality after total hip and knee arthroplasty in a medium-volume university practice. J Arthroplasty 18:278–285, 2003.

30. Paavolainen P, Pukkala E, Pulkkinen P, Visuri T: Causes of death after total hip arthroplasty: a nationwide cohort study with 24,638 patients. J Arthroplasty 17:274–281, 2002.

31. Parvizi J, Sullivan T, Duffy C, Cabanela ME: Fifteen-year clinical survivorship of Harris-Galante total hip arthroplasty. J Arthroplasty 19:672–677, 2004.

32. Herndon JH, Bechtol CO, Crickenberger DP: Fat embolism during total hip replacement: a prospective study. J Bone Joint Surg Am 56:1350–1362, 1974.

33. Mir GN, Lawrence WH, Autian J: Toxicological and pharmacological actions of methacrylate monomers: effects on respiratory and cardiovascular functions of anesthetized dogs. J Pharm Sci 63:376–381, 1974.

34. McMaster WC, Bradley G, Vaugh TR: Blood pressure lowering effect of methylmethacrylate monomer: potentiation by blood volume deficit. Clin Orthop Relat Res 98:254–257, 1974.

35. Peebles DJ, Ellis RH, Stride SD, Simpson BR: Cardiovascular effects of methylmethacrylate cement. Br Med J 1:349–351, 1972.

36. Rudigier J, Scheuermann H, Kotterbach B, Ritter G: [Release and diffusion of methylmethacrylic monomers after the implantation of self curing bone cements: study on laboratory specimens and animal experiments (author's transl)]. Unfallchirurgie 7:132–137, 1981.

37. Modig J, Busch C, Waernbaum G: Effects of graded infusions of monomethylmethacrylate on coagulation, blood lipids, respiration and circulation: an experimental study in dogs. Clin Orthop Relat Res 113:187–197, 1975.

38. Byrick RJ: Cement implantation syndrome: a time limited embolic phenomenon. Can J Anaesth 44:107–111, 1997.

39. Breed AL: Experimental production of vascular hypotension, and bone marrow and fat embolism with methylmethacrylate cement: traumatic hypertension of bone. Clin Orthop Relat Res 102:227–244, 1974.

40. Kallos T, Enis JE, Gollan F, Davis JH: Intramedullary pressure and pulmonary embolism of femoral medullary contents in dogs during insertion of bone cement and a prosthesis. J Bone Joint Surg Am 56:1363–1367, 1974.

41. Fleisher LA, Beckman JA, Brown KA, et al: ACC/AHA 2007 guidelines on perioperative cardiovascular evaluation and care for noncardiac surgery: a report of the American College of Cardiology/American Heart Association Task Force on Practice Guidelines (Writing Committee to Revise the 2002 Guidelines on Perioperative Cardiovascular Evaluation for Noncardiac Surgery): developed in collaboration with the American Society of Echocardiography, American Society of Nuclear Cardiology, Heart Rhythm Society, Society of Cardiovascular Anesthesiologists, Society for Cardiovascular Angiography and Interventions, Society for Vascular Medicine and Biology, and Society for Vascular Surgery. Circulation 116:e418–e499, 2007.

42. Salerno SM, Carlson DW, Soh EK, Lettieri CJ: Impact of perioperative cardiac assessment guidelines on management of orthopedic surgery patients. Am J Med 120:185–186, 2007.

43. Charnley J: Sub-specialization or super-specialization in surgery? Br Med J 2:719–722, 1970.

44. Lavernia CJ, Guzman JF: Relationship of surgical volume to short-term mortality, morbidity, and hospital charges in arthroplasty. J Arthroplasty 10:133–140, 1995.

45. Shervin N, Rubash HE, Katz JN: Orthopaedic procedure volume and patient outcomes: a systematic literature review. Clin Orthop Relat Res 457:35–41, 2007.

46. Doro C, Dimick J, Wainess R, et al: Hospital volume and inpatient mortality outcomes of total hip arthroplasty in the United States. J Arthroplasty 21:10–16, 2006.

47. Keith I: Anaesthesia and blood loss in total hip replacement. Anaesthesia 32:444–450, 1977.

48. Lieberman JR, Huo MM, Hanway J, et al: The prevalence of deep venous thrombosis after total hip arthroplasty with hypotensive epidural anesthesia. J Bone Joint Surg Am 76:341–348, 1994.

49. Andersen LJ, Poulsen T, Krogh B, Nielsen T: Postoperative analgesia in total hip arthroplasty: a randomized double-blinded, placebo-controlled study on preoperative and postoperative ropivacaine, ketorolac, and adrenaline wound infiltration. Acta Orthop 78:187–192, 2007.

50. Nuelle DG, Mann K: Minimal incision protocols for anesthesia, pain management, and physical therapy with standard incisions in hip and knee arthroplasties: the effect on early outcomes. J Arthroplasty 22:20–25, 2007.

51. Berger RA, Jacobs JJ, Meneghini RM, et al: Rapid rehabilitation and recovery with minimally invasive total hip arthroplasty. Clin Orthop Relat Res 429:239–247, 2004.

52. Berry DJ, Berger RA, Callaghan JJ, et al: Minimally invasive total hip arthroplasty: development, early results, and a critical analysis. J Bone Joint Surg Am 85:2235–2246, 2003.

53. Bhandari M, Devereaux PJ, Swiontkowski MF, et al: Internal fixation compared with arthroplasty for displaced fractures of the femoral neck: a meta-analysis. J Bone Joint Surg Am 85:1673–1681, 2003.

54. Parker MJ, Pryor G, Gurusamy K: Hemiarthroplasty versus internal fixation for displaced intracapsular hip fractures: a long-term follow-up of a randomised trial. Injury 41:370–373, 2009.

55. Dai Z, Li Y, Jiang D: Meta-analysis comparing arthroplasty with internal fixation for displaced femoral neck fracture in the elderly. J Surg Res 165:68–74, 2010.

SUGGESTED READING

Barrett J, Losina E, Baron JA, et al: Survival following total hip replacement. J Bone Joint Surg Am 87:1965–1971, 2005.

In a study of more than 28,000 primary Medicare THAs, Barrett and associates showed that mortality rates following THA are lower than controls after adjustment for sex, age, Medicaid eligibility, and other comorbidities.

Paavolainen P, Pukkala E, Pulkkinen P, Visuri T: Causes of death after total hip arthroplasty: a nationwide cohort study with 24,638 patients. J Arthroplasty 17:274–281, 2002.

Using the Finnish National Register of Arthroplasty from 1980 to 1995, these authors calculated that the standardized mortality ratio (SMR) is lower following THA in 33,694 THAs, signifying that fewer deaths occurred during the study period than calculated.

Parvizi J, Holiday AD, Ereth MH, Lewallen DG: The Frank Stinchfield Award. Sudden death during primary hip arthroplasty. Clin Orthop Relat Res 369:39–48, 1999.

Reporting on 23 intraoperative THA deaths in a series of 29,000, these authors show that these deaths occurred in cemented cases as the result of irreversible cardiorespiratory failure.

Parvizi J, Mui A, Purtill JJ, et al: Total joint arthroplasty: when do fatal or near-fatal complications occur? J Bone Joint Surg Am 89:27–32, 2007.

These authors showed that 6% of 1636 patients sustained at least one life-threatening medical complication in the early postoperative period, prompting the recommendation for careful postoperative monitoring.

CHAPTER 26

Perioperative Medical Management of Hip Surgery Patients

A. Scott Keller and Deanne T. Kashiwagi

KEY POINTS

- The pathophysiologic surgical stress response causes widespread changes in organ function and can lead to postoperative complications. Perioperative care should be aimed at minimizing the stress response.
- Preoperative assessment should include careful review of each patient's past medical history, given that most adverse outcomes are due to an exacerbation of underlying medical problems rather than to surgical or anesthetic complications.
- Patients should be medically optimized to the extent possible before undergoing surgery, with appropriate treatment of any acute illness or chronic disease exacerbation.
- The most important aspect of the preoperative evaluation is the cardiac assessment, which includes functional status. Patients with no acute illness who have a good functional capacity (>4 metabolic equivalents [METs]) with no cardiopulmonary symptoms and those with no cardiac risk factors regardless of functional status can proceed directly with hip surgery.
- Coronary ischemia is the most feared postoperative complication. In keeping with current American College of Cardiology/American Heart Association preoperative guidelines, controlling hemodynamics and providing appropriate beta blockade can decrease the risk of ischemia.

INTRODUCTION

Orthopedic hip surgeries are becoming more common as our population ages. Approximately 200,000 total hip replacements, 100,000 partial hip replacements (90% of which were performed for fractures of the neck of the femur), and 36,000 revision hip replacements were performed in the United States in 2003, with in-hospital mortality rates of 0.33%, 3.04%, and 0.84%, respectively.[1] In 2006 alone, 330,000 hip fractures were reported.[2] Although surgical techniques have continually been refined and improved and modern anesthesia is extremely safe, with an estimated mortality of 1 in 250,000,[3] patients still may suffer from medical complications. Most of these complications occur after surgery because of the significant surgical stress response,

which may lead to an acute exacerbation of underlying chronic disease, especially in older patients who have diminished organ reserve capacity and comorbid medical conditions.

This chapter explains the surgical stress response, reviews the components of the preoperative evaluation, discusses techniques to help medically optimize patients, and provides a symptom-based approach to diagnosis and treatment of postoperative medical complications.

BASIC SCIENCE

The Surgical Stress Response

The human body responds to the stress of an injury through a remarkable physiologic process that activates the sympathetic nervous and endocrine systems and promotes an increased inflammatory response with decreased immune function (despite initially increased production of reparative leukocytes).[4-7] The magnitude and duration of these effects are directly proportional to the degree of injury,[6,8] with overall goals of maintaining intravascular volume for cardiovascular homeostasis and increasing catabolism to provide energy sources.[4] Although the stress response is appropriate and can prolong survival following accidental injury, it can be counterproductive following the "controlled injury" of surgery.

Many of the initial surgical stress response effects are attenuated by anesthesia and opioids but may manifest postoperatively. As a result, most postoperative complications are due to subsequent increased demands on organ function[6,9,10] in the setting of preexisting comorbid conditions,[6,11,12] rather than to anesthetic[13] or surgical effects. The overall stress response may persist for up to 7 days,[7] and knowledge of the duration of individual organ or system changes can be helpful in distinguishing expected physiologic changes from pathologic complications. For example, Dorman and associates[14] showed that interleukin-6, which contributes to postoperative fever,[15] peaks at 24 hours but still is slightly elevated at 72 hours. So, although a postoperative fever of 38° C may be expected within the first 48 hours, prolonged fevers warrant further workup. Awareness of the surgical stress response can be helpful in diagnosing complications based on when they are most likely to occur. For example, catecholamines are increased for 24 to 48 hours following surgery and are associated with an increased incidence of myocardial infarction.[16]

A multimodal approach may help decrease complications related to the stress response through the use of techniques such as minimally invasive surgery, neural blocks with local anesthetics, intraoperative body heat conservation, early enteral nutrition and ambulation, and minimal use of surgical drains and nasogastric tubes.[6] Adequate postoperative pain control may help attenuate the effects of the stress response.[6] The authors use a simple regimen of scheduled acetaminophen and as-needed oxycodone to help control pain with few adverse effects. More severe pain can be treated with patient-controlled analgesia.

The Preoperative Evaluation

The preoperative evaluation, an important aspect of any surgical procedure, should assess the patient's current medical status and provide risk identification, as well as recommendations to reduce risk. This evaluation also provides an opportunity to ensure that acute conditions/exacerbations are treated and chronic medical conditions optimized. The preoperative evaluation is not done to simply declare the patient "clear for surgery," but is a multidisciplinary effort that includes input from the surgeon, the anesthesiologist, and possibly a medical consultant. The evaluation should be performed before the day of surgery for patients with very severe disease and for patients with less severe disease undergoing highly invasive surgical procedures.[17]

The history and physical examination serve as the cornerstone of the preoperative evaluation. Information should focus on pertinent past medical history, current review of systems/symptoms, physical examination findings (including airway evaluation), and current medications and drug allergies. The most important aspect of the history and physical is the cardiac assessment, which includes functional status. Patients with no acute illness or exacerbation who have good functional capacity with no cardiopulmonary symptoms can proceed directly with hip surgery.[18] Patients with poor functional capacity require further evaluation and, depending on cardiac risk factors, may need preoperative cardiac stress testing if it will change management. Patients with no cardiac risk factors, even if they have poor or unknown functional status, can proceed directly with hip surgery.[18]

The preoperative evaluation should also include any recommendations for testing before surgery; preoperative tests should not be ordered routinely, but rather should be obtained for purposes of guiding or optimizing perioperative management.[17] As emphasized in the American College of Cardiology/American Heart Association (ACC/AHA) 2007 Guidelines on Perioperative Cardiovascular Evaluation and Care for Noncardiac Surgery, "intervention is rarely necessary to simply lower the risk of surgery unless such intervention is indicated irrespective of the preoperative context."[18] The benefits of any testing or medical treatment must be weighed against the risks of delays in surgical treatment, especially for hip fracture patients requiring urgent surgery. Recent study results have been conflicting,[19-25] but operative repair of hip fracture likely should be performed within 48 hours.

It is unclear which type of anesthesia—general or neuraxial (spinal or epidural)—leads to better outcomes following hip surgery. This topic remains controversial, and decisions about the specific type of anesthesia to be used should be made by the anesthesiologist.

History

Past Medical History and Review of Systems. Review the patient's known medical problems and assess each for optimization/stability, including new and chronic symptoms. A mnemonic ("The ABCs," Box 26-1), adapted from guidelines taught at Mayo Clinic,[26] can serve as a reminder of the most important questions to ask each patient.

Patients who need emergency surgery should proceed directly to the operating room with testing only as allowed by their clinical condition, such as vital signs and possible baseline laboratory tests (see later). On the other hand, patients who are undergoing elective hip surgery and who have an active cardiac condition should undergo evaluation and treatment before surgery is performed.[18] Active cardiac conditions include unstable coronary syndromes, decompensated heart failure, significant arrhythmias (including high-grade atrioventricular block, symptomatic ventricular arrhythmias, supraventricular arrhythmias with ventricular tachycardia, and symptomatic bradycardia), and severe valvular disease such as severe aortic stenosis. Likewise, any symptoms suggestive of acute infection or disease exacerbation (e.g., asthma) also require further evaluation and treatment before elective surgery is undertaken.

Special attention should be given to the patient's airway and to any previous anesthesia complications or adverse reactions. For patients with a history of penicillin allergy, consider referral for formal allergy consultation and penicillin skin testing if beta-lactam therapy is being considered. Always review the patient's alcohol history, and be alert for alcohol withdrawal postoperatively. For patients who use tobacco products, smoking cessation 4 to 8 weeks before surgery is important to decrease the risk of postoperative complications.[27-29] Of note, severe obesity (body mass index [BMI] ≥ 40 kg/m^2) is not associated with increased mortality but is associated with increased length of hospital stay and greater likelihood of renal failure and prolonged assisted ventilation.[30] Also, these patients have been found to require longer operating times for total hip arthroplasty.[31]

Physical Examination

A focused review of systems and a preoperative physical examination should be performed on all patients. Important findings that may require further evaluation are listed in the following sections.

Vital Signs. Measure and document current vital signs, including temperature, blood pressure, heart rate and rhythm, respiratory rate and pattern, oxygen saturation, and height and weight.

BOX 26-1. THE ABCS OF PREOPERATIVE MEDICAL HISTORY

A

Activity level (functional status in metabolic equivalents [METs])
Airway concerns
Alcohol use/abuse
Allergies (drugs, latex)
Anesthesia complications (malignant hyperthermia, postoperative nausea/vomiting, other reactions)

B

Bleeding disorder (inherited or acquired thrombophilia, long-term antiplatelet or anticoagulation therapy)

C

Cardiac history (coronary disease, valvular disease, heart failure, pacemaker)
Cervical spine instability
Clots (deep vein thrombosis or pulmonary embolism)
Consent for blood transfusion, if indicated
Corticosteroid use that could lead to adrenal suppression

D

Deficit (preexisting neurologic disease such as focal limb weakness or seizure disorder)
Dementia
Diabetes mellitus
Drug abuse

E

Embolic history (stroke or transient ischemic attack)

F

Family history of anesthesia complications (malignant hyperthermia)
Fetus (pregnant)

G

Gastroesophageal reflux disease
Glaucoma

H

Height and weight
Hypoxia (pulmonary disease, pulmonary hypertension, obstructive sleep apnea)

Airway. Patients with a small mouth, micrognathia, limited neck range of motion, or a poorly visualized posterior oropharynx (Mallampati class III or IV; as shown in Fig. 26-1) may be more difficult to intubate and establish an airway, so the anesthesiologist should be alerted to a potential "difficult airway." Patients who are edentulous or who have a full beard may be difficult to oxygenate with a face mask, so these conditions should be noted as well.

Cardiac. Ask patients if they have any chest pain/pressure or dyspnea at rest or with activity, palpitations, orthopnea, or syncope. Assess the heart rate and rhythm, paying particular attention to bradycardia or tachycardia and any irregularity that could indicate atrial fibrillation or a conduction block. Listen for significant cardiac murmurs. Aortic stenosis, which typically causes a harsh systolic murmur (occurring between the first and second heart sounds), poses the highest risk for noncardiac surgery; evaluation is required before surgery is undertaken. This murmur characteristically radiates to one or both carotid arteries. Note that the physical examination often underestimates cardiac dysfunction in severely obese patients (BMI ≥ 40 kg/m^2).[30]

Respiratory. Ask patients if they have dyspnea, cough with sputum, or wheezing, and whether these symptoms are baseline, worse than baseline, or new. Listen for inspiratory crackles (rales), which could indicate pulmonary edema or infection, and wheezes, which can be found in asthma, chronic obstructive pulmonary disease (COPD), and pulmonary edema. Patients with COPD commonly have decreased breath sounds and a prolonged expiratory phase of respiration.

Gastrointestinal. Ask patients if they have nausea, vomiting, abdominal pain, constipation, or diarrhea. The abdomen should be soft, nontender, and nondistended with normal bowel sounds. Special note should be made of findings suggestive of liver disease, including ascites.

Vascular. Look for evidence of elevated jugular venous pressure and lower extremity edema, which could indicate increased intravascular volume related to right heart failure. Diminished peripheral pulses may be due to peripheral vascular disease that could impair wound healing.

Neurologic/Psychiatric. Any preexisting neurologic deficit should be documented, along with conditions such as a seizure disorder, dementia, or a history of delirium.

Skin. Any skin ulcers should be documented and may need treatment before the time of surgery, particularly if evidence of infection is noted.

Functional Status

Patients who are highly functional and asymptomatic are at low risk for perioperative cardiac complications.[18] Functional status is quantified in terms of metabolic equivalents (METs), as shown in Table 26-1.

Patients who can achieve at least 4 METs without cardiopulmonary symptoms have adequate functional capacity and may proceed directly to hip surgery without preoperative cardiac testing, assuming no acute symptoms.

However, it is often difficult to estimate functional capacity in orthopedic patients, who may have joint pain that limits ambulation. In this case, ask about other activities as listed in Table 26-1,[18] such as the ability to perform housework. Patients who cannot achieve 4 METs should be further assessed in terms of clinical cardiac risk factors derived from the Revised Cardiac Risk Index (diabetes mellitus treated with insulin, chronic kidney disease with creatinine greater than 2, ischemic heart disease, cerebrovascular disease, or heart failure).

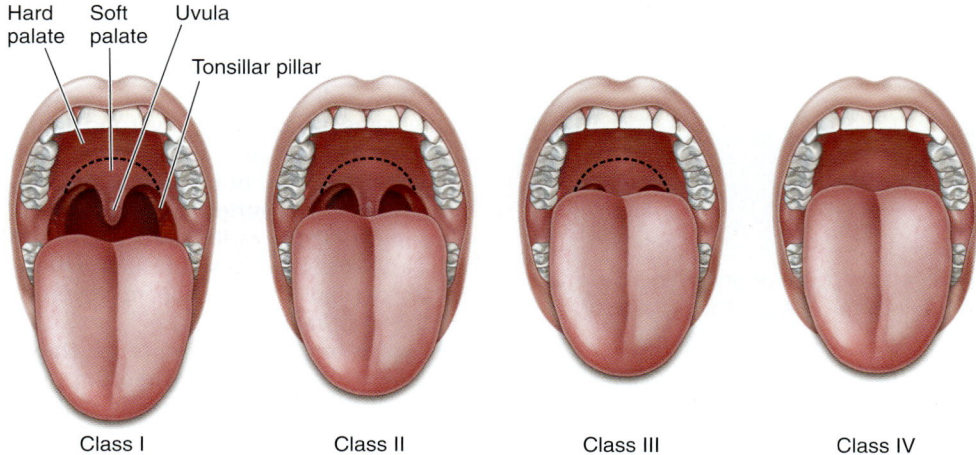

Hard palate   Soft palate   Uvula
Tonsillar pillar

Class I   Class II   Class III   Class IV

Figure 26-1. Mallampati Classification. Class I: Full visibility of tonsils, uvula, and soft palate. Class II: Visibility of hard and soft palate, upper portion of tonsils, and uvula. Class III: Soft and hard palate and base of the uvula are visible. Class IV: Only hard palate visible.

Table 26-1. Metabolic Equivalents (METs) for Various Physical Activities

Estimated Energy	Activity
1 MET	Self-care Eating, dressing, or using the toilet Walking indoors and around the house Walking one to two blocks on level ground at 2 to 3 mph
4 METs	Light housework (e.g., dusting, washing dishes) Climbing a flight of stairs or walking up a hill Walking on level ground at 4 mph Running a short distance Heavy housework (e.g., scrubbing floors, moving heavy furniture) Moderate recreational activities (e.g., golf, dancing, doubles tennis, throwing a baseball or football)
>10 METs	Strenuous sports (e.g., swimming, singles tennis, football, basketball, skiing)

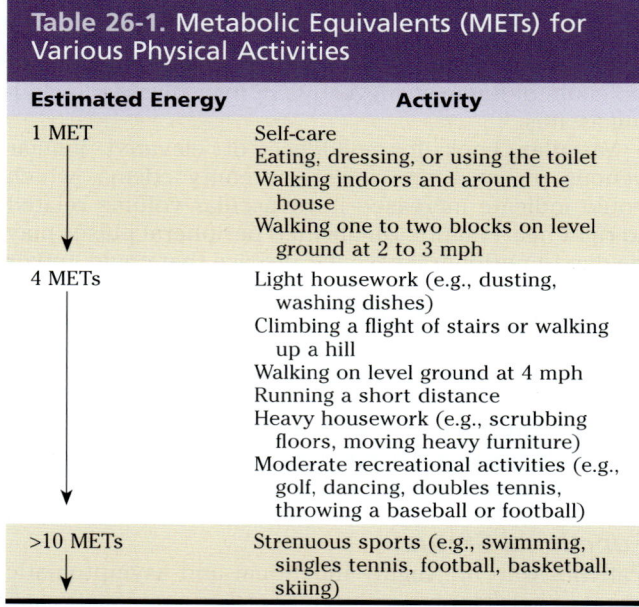

Adapted from Fleisher LA, Beckman JA, Brown KA, et al: ACC/AHA guidelines on perioperative cardiovascular evaluation and care for noncardiac surgery: a report of the American College of Cardiology/American Heart Association Task Force on Practice Guidelines. Circulation 116:e425, 2007. *MET,* Metabolic equivalent; *mph,* miles per hour.

Patients with no cardiac risk factors may proceed directly to hip surgery without preoperative cardiac testing, assuming no acute symptoms.

Consideration can be given for preoperative cardiac testing in patients with at least one risk factor *if it will change management, or if the patient would need testing independent of hip surgery.*[18] Always ask whether a patient has had a recent cardiac stress test, especially if he or she is nonambulatory or is minimally active. Certain patients may benefit from starting a beta blocker, as discussed in the section, "Current Controversies and Future Directions."

Current Medications

Obtain an accurate list of all medications, dosing, and schedules, including over-the-counter and herbal medications. In general, most prescription medications should be continued perioperatively, especially drugs with known withdrawal syndromes (such as beta blockers, clonidine, or benzodiazepines), and should be taken with sips of water on the morning of surgery. However, certain drugs should be held the morning of surgery, and herbal medications should be held for at least 1 week because of possible drug-drug interactions with anesthetic agents and concerns for increased bleeding risk (among others, bleeding can be potentiated by the "G" herbal medications: garlic, ginger, ginkgo biloba, and ginseng).[32] Aspirin and clopidogrel each can increase the risk of surgical bleeding, but they provide essential treatment for patients with a recent coronary stent (especially drug-eluting stents) and may be given for other indications, including stroke. In cases in which aspirin and clopidogrel must be stopped because of high risk of surgical bleeding, aspirin should be held for 7 to 10 days and clopidogrel for 5 to 10 days before surgery. However, because of the high mortality associated with in-stent coronary thrombosis, the surgical team should consult with a cardiologist for patients with recent coronary stent placement (within 1 year for drug-eluting stents) before these medications are stopped. If clopidogrel must be stopped, aspirin should be continued if at all possible.

Table 26-2 provides suggestions regarding which medications should be taken and which should be held the morning of surgery.[32,33] Some of these recommendations are based on expert opinion at the authors' institution, and practitioners should be aware of local preferences and recommendations.

Preoperative Testing

Preoperative testing should be limited to those tests that may change the risk of surgery, especially if the underlying disease can be treated, or that provide a

Table 26-2. Recommendations for Medication Dosing the Morning of Orthopedic Surgery

Drug Class	Take	Hold
Cardiac	Beta blockers	Diuretics
	α_2-Agonists (e.g., clonidine)	ACE inhibitor[1]
	Calcium channel blockers	ARB[1]
	Digoxin	Fibrates (hold the night before)
	Isosorbide mononitrate and dinitrate	Niacin (hold the night before)
	Statins	
Pulmonary	Nebulizer/MDI	
	Leukotriene inhibitors	
GI	Proton pump inhibitors	
	H$_2$-blockers	
	Stool softeners	
GU	α_1-Antagonists (e.g., tamsulosin)	Tolterodine
		Oxybutynin
Endocrine	Levothyroxine	Sulfonylureas
	Corticosteroid[2]	Metformin[3]
		Insulin[4]
		Thiazolidinediones
		Hormone replacement therapy (hold 4 weeks preop)
Psychiatric	SSRI unless high bleeding risk	MAOI (hold 2 weeks preop[5])
	Benzodiazepines	
	Tricyclic antidepressants	
	Antipsychotics	
	Lithium	
Neurologic	Antiepileptic drugs	
	Carbidopa/levodopa[5]	
Rheumatologic	Methotrexate[6]	Leflunomide (hold 2 weeks preop)
	Hydroxychloroquine	
	Azathioprine	
	Sulfasalazine	
	NSAIDs	(hold 3 days preop)
Pain	Opioids	
	NSAIDs	
	Tylenol	

1. Hold if the indication is hypertension and current blood pressure is <140/90, or if the indication is heart failure.
2. Patients taking long-term steroids may benefit from perioperative stress-dose steroids.
3. Metformin should be held starting 1 day before surgery and resumed on postop day 2 to 3, assuming adequate kidney function and no heart failure exacerbation.
4. Insulin dose should be adjusted the morning of surgery, depending on time of day and duration of surgery; typically one-half the usual morning dose is given for patients taking NPH insulin, and the usual dose of glargine is given the night before surgery.
5. Discuss with the anesthesiologist; it may be safe to continue.
6. Methotrexate should be held for 2 weeks preoperatively in patients with chronic kidney disease, but otherwise should be continued.

ACE, Angiotensin-converting enzyme; *ARB,* angiotensin receptor blocker; *GI,* gastrointestinal; *GU,* genitourinary; *MAOI,* monoamine oxidase inhibitor; *MDI,* metered dose inhaler; *NSAID,* nonsteroidal anti-inflammatory drug; *SSRI,* selective serotonin reuptake inhibitor.

baseline that will be used to monitor a clinical condition or treatment perioperatively. Because of the risk of false-positive results or minor abnormalities that will not influence surgical outcome, tests should be ordered selectively rather than routinely. Indications for tests should be documented, and any abnormal test result must be addressed. Laboratory tests obtained within the previous 4 months should safely provide adequate information unless there is an interim change in clinical status[34] or in medications that could affect electrolytes has occurred.

Laboratory Tests. A complete blood count (CBC) with hemoglobin, white cell count, and platelet count should be obtained in patients with a history or symptoms of anemia or infection or a history of bleeding diathesis, or if the surgical procedure may lead to blood loss requiring a transfusion. A baseline platelet count may be helpful for patients who will be on heparin perioperatively. Kidney function (creatinine) should be checked in all persons undergoing hip surgery. Electrolytes should be checked in patients with chronic kidney disease or heart failure, and in those taking digoxin or medications that affect electrolytes, such as diuretics, angiotensin-converting enzyme (ACE) inhibitors, and angiotensin receptor blockers (ARBs). An international normalized ratio (INR) can be obtained in persons on warfarin therapy and in those with a history of bleeding diathesis, liver disease, or malnutrition. Low albumin is predictive of 30-day mortality[35]; therefore, albumin should be measured if it is likely to be low, such as in patients with liver disease or malnutrition, given that oral protein and calorie supplementation may be of benefit in hip fracture patients.[36] Fasting glucose should be checked in diabetic individuals and in persons at high risk for diabetes. A pregnancy test should be considered for all female patients of childbearing age. Urinalysis and culture should be checked in patients with symptoms of a urinary tract infection who will have a prosthetic hip implant.

Electrocardiogram. Obtain a preoperative electrocardiogram (ECG) in patients with a history of coronary artery disease (CAD), peripheral arterial disease, or cerebrovascular disease undergoing intermediate-risk procedures such as hip surgery.[18] It is also reasonable to obtain an ECG for severely obese patients.[30] Consideration can be given to an ECG for persons with risk factors for coronary disease or for asymptomatic men over 40 years old and women over 50 years old.

Chest X-rays and Spirometry. These tests should not be used routinely for predicting risk for postoperative pulmonary complications, but they may be appropriate in patients with a previous diagnosis of COPD or asthma,[37] and they may be helpful in assessing the status of known lung disease, especially when the history and physical examination do not lead to a firm conclusion.[38] It is also reasonable to obtain a chest x-ray for severely obese patients.[30]

Cervical Spine X-rays. Patients with long-standing rheumatoid arthritis have a high prevalence of cervical spine subluxation.[39] These patients, as well as those with ankylosing spondylitis or Down syndrome, should have preoperative flexion and extension x-rays of the cervical spine to look for evidence of subluxation or other instability.

RISK REDUCTION AND MEDICAL OPTIMIZATION

Identification of risk factors for postoperative complications can help guide preoperative evaluation and risk reduction strategies. Likewise, it is important to assess each patient's history and symptoms before surgery to help determine whether a new, acute process or an exacerbation of a chronic illness is under way. Patients undergoing surgery should be at their best baseline regarding comorbid medical conditions, functional status, and nutritional status. This does not mean that each chronic condition must be "cured," but if an acute process or exacerbation is present, elective procedures may need to be deferred. On the other hand, for urgent procedures such as repair of hip fracture, the important question is whether surgery should be delayed (and for how long) to allow medical optimization.

Memtsoudis and associates found that advanced age is the single most important risk factor for postoperative complications following hip and knee arthroplasty,[40] along with comorbid medical conditions. Bhattacharyya and colleagues identified five preoperative medical risk factors for inpatient mortality after any orthopedic surgery: chronic renal failure, congestive heart failure, COPD, hip fracture, and patient older than 70 years.[41] Maxwell and colleagues[42] noted a number of independent predictors of 30-day mortality for hip fracture patients: age older than 65 years, male sex, at least two comorbidities, low mini-mental test score, admission hemoglobin concentration less than 10 g/dL, living in an institution, and the presence of malignant disease.

Cardiac

Postoperative cardiac complications include myocardial ischemia/infarction, congestive heart failure, hemodynamic instability, and arrhythmias. The key points are to distinguish acute or unstable conditions from those that are chronic and stable, and to estimate a patient's risk of severe cardiac disease.

Risk Factors

Approximately 30% of adults undergoing surgery each year in the United States have CAD or risk factors such as advanced age, male gender, hypertension, hypercholesterolemia, diabetes mellitus, cigarette smoking, obesity, sedentary lifestyle, family history of premature CAD (men younger than 55 and women younger than 65 years old), and psychosocial stress.[43]

Recommendations

- Continue current cardiac medications perioperatively, although ACE inhibitors and ARBs should be held the morning of surgery if blood pressure is less than 140/90, or if recommended by the local institution.
- Strive to minimize effects of the surgical stress response and conditions that may lead to coronary ischemia, including hypertension, tachycardia, pain, anxiety, hypoxemia, anemia, volume depletion or overload, fever, urine retention, or constipation.
- Consider the use of continuous epidural analgesia, which is associated with a lower incidence of adverse cardiac events in at-risk elderly patients with hip fracture.[44]
- Be vigilant for withdrawal syndromes that may lead to increased cardiac stress.
- Patients at high risk for cardiac complications may benefit from perioperative beta blockade, further preoperative evaluation, and/or postoperative care in a monitored setting.
- Patients with decompensated heart failure should be diuresed and at their baseline volume status before orthopedic surgery is performed.
- Patients with symptomatic severe aortic stenosis may benefit from aortic valve replacement before undergoing orthopedic surgery.
- Patients with chronic arrhythmias should be hemodynamically stable and rate controlled (<100 beats/

min). Patients with stable atrial arrhythmias such as atrial fibrillation may be on anticoagulation, which should be discontinued and/or bridged with heparin based on cardioembolic risk. Patients with ventricular arrhythmias should be evaluated preoperatively by a cardiologist.

- Any unstable patient should be hospitalized preoperatively for evaluation and treatment.

Pulmonary

Postoperative pulmonary complications include atelectasis, hypoxemic or hypercarbic respiratory failure, pneumonia, COPD exacerbation, aspiration, and prolonged mechanical ventilation.

Risk Factors

Patient-related risk factors include COPD, age older than 60 years, American Society of Anesthesiologists (ASA) class II or greater, functional dependence, congestive heart failure, and a low serum albumin level (<35 g/L).[37] Use of cigarettes is associated with a modest increase in risk, but obesity and mild to moderate asthma are not associated with increased pulmonary risk.[37] Although most orthopedic procedures are not as high risk for postoperative pulmonary complications as aortic, thoracic, or upper abdominal surgery, factors such as prolonged surgery (>3 hours) do increase risk.[45] Risk factors for aspiration, which occurs in up to 0.01% to 0.06% of anesthetized patients at the time of anesthesia induction and intubation, include advanced age, gastroesophageal reflux disease (GERD)/hiatal hernia, obesity, pregnancy, and conditions such as diabetes that may predispose to delayed gastric emptying.[46] Of note, aspiration related to anesthesia induction or intubation may lead to pulmonary complications, but complications are unlikely if no signs or symptoms are seen within 2 hours of the aspiration event.[47]

Obstructive sleep apnea (OSA) is another risk factor that may lead to hypoxemia, hypercarbia, and cardiovascular dysfunction. Patients with OSA may have difficulty with airway management, including intubation. A presumptive diagnosis of OSA can be made in patients with obesity (BMI ≥ 35 kg/m^2), large neck circumference (>17 inches [43 cm] in men or 16 inches [40.6 cm] in women), snoring, congenital airway abnormalities, daytime hypersomnolence, inability to visualize the soft palate, and tonsillar hypertrophy.[48]

Recommendations

- Patients who smoke should quit at least 4 to 8 weeks before surgery.[27-29]
- Patients with acute respiratory symptoms such as chest tightness or wheezing should be given aggressive bronchodilator therapy with the option of preoperative systemic corticosteroid therapy. A short course of steroids is unlikely to increase perioperative infection risk or to hinder wound healing.[49]
- Patients with evidence of a pulmonary infection may need treatment with antibiotics.
- All patients with increased risk for postoperative pulmonary complications should perform deep breathing

exercises or use incentive spirometry. Early ambulation may also be helpful.

- Avoid placing nasogastric tubes if possible, although they may be used selectively for postoperative nausea or vomiting, inability to tolerate oral intake, or symptomatic abdominal distention.
- Postoperative epidural pain control has been shown to reduce the risk of pulmonary complications.[50]
- Patients with GERD/hiatal hernia should be given acid-blocking medications before surgery to decrease aspiration risk.
- Patients with suspected OSA ideally should undergo evaluation long enough before scheduled surgery for the clinician to develop a perioperative management plan, including possible formal polysomnography. Preoperative initiation of continuous positive airway pressure (CPAP) should be considered for these patients, although the literature is insufficient to evaluate its impact.[48]
- Patients who have previously been diagnosed with OSA and who use positive-pressure airway devices should bring their units to the hospital or should know their device settings, to allow hospital personnel to set up a comparable unit.
- Patients with suspected OSA should have continuous pulse oximetry while in bed for as long as they remain at increased risk. These patients should be given supplemental oxygen until they are able to maintain their baseline oxygen saturation while breathing room air.[48]
- Patients with hypercarbia should be monitored closely for symptoms such as somnolence that could indicate worsening carbon dioxide (CO_2) retention; supplemental oxygen may need to be minimized while avoiding hypoxemia. Opioid pain medications should be used cautiously in these patients, and continuous opioid basal infusions (for patient-controlled analgesia) probably should be avoided. If possible, patients at risk for OSA should be placed in nonsupine positions during their recovery.

Gastrointestinal

Gastrointestinal complications following hip surgery include postoperative nausea and vomiting (PONV), postoperative ileus (POI), and acute colonic pseudo-obstruction (Ogilvie's syndrome).

Risk Factors

Risk factors for PONV include female sex, prior history of PONV or motion sickness, nonsmoking status, prolonged surgery, volatile anesthetics or nitrous oxide, and intraoperative or postoperative opioid use.[51] Pain, anxiety, and dehydration may also increase the incidence of PONV.[52] Risk factors for POI include the surgical stress response (sympathetic hyperactivity, systemic endocrine response, and production of endogenous opioids and inflammatory cytokines), increased surgical blood loss (possibly contributing to a heightened inflammatory response), and factors related to perioperative care, such as general anesthesia and the use of opioid medications.[53] Preexisting gastrointestinal disease such as Crohn's and decreased perioperative physical activity can contribute to POI, which can cause abdominal symptoms and increased hospital length of stay.[54] Significant risk factors for acute colonic pseudo-obstruction include advanced age, male sex, and medications that affect bowel motility (including opioids, phenothiazines, tricyclic antidepressants, calcium channel blockers, H_2-receptor blockers, and anticholinergics).[55] Slow postoperative mobility and revision hip arthroplasty were also found to be significant risk factors in a study by Petrisor and associates.[56] Other risk factors may include prior abdominal surgery, hypothyroidism, diabetes mellitus, and preexisting gastrointestinal disease.[55]

Patients with known liver disease deserve special mention given their increased risk of perioperative complications and mortality. Acute hepatitis (viral or drug-induced) may present with symptoms of nausea, vomiting, anorexia, jaundice, and dark urine. Elective surgery should be deferred until patients demonstrate symptomatic and biochemical improvement. Patients should be advised to avoid strenuous activity, alcohol, and acetaminophen. Chronic liver disease is often diagnosed before surgery is performed, but it may present undiagnosed with fatigue, malaise, abdominal pain, and abnormal liver tests, especially in advanced disease and cirrhosis.[57] Patients are at high risk for early complications[58] and limited prosthesis longevity.[59] Surgery should be delayed in patients with decompensated cirrhosis, which may manifest with encephalopathy and/or ascites.

Recommendations

- Give patients at high risk for PONV one or more antiemetics, such as droperidol, metoclopramide, ondansetron, cyclizine, or dexamethasone, before or during anesthesia.[60] A single preoperative dose of dexamethasone 40 mg intravenous (IV) was shown to decrease PONV in a small study of total hip arthroplasty patients without causing adverse outcomes, including wound complications, deep infection, or osteonecrosis in the contralateral hip.[61] However, even with multiple drug treatment, more than 30% of high-risk patients had postoperative emetic symptoms in a large prospective observational study.[62]
- Apply P6 acupoint stimulation in patients at risk for PONV. (The P6 acupoint is located between the tendons of the palmaris longus and flexor carpi radialis muscles, 4 cm proximal to the wrist crease.[63])
- Although it has been reported that "little can be done preoperatively to reduce the risk for POI,"[54] the medical team should strive to minimize both the surgical stress response and opioid medications as tolerated.
- Patients with chronic constipation should be on an appropriate bowel regimen and ideally should have a bowel movement before surgery, given that anesthesia and opioid pain medications can worsen constipation.
- Medications that increase the risk for acute colonic pseudo-obstruction should be carefully reviewed and decreased or stopped if possible.

- Medical conditions associated with acute colonic pseudo-obstruction should be optimized.
- Patients with advanced liver disease may require perioperative evaluation by a gastroenterologist.
- Patients with advanced liver disease who require emergent surgery should be hydrated and given oral vitamin K if they have an increased INR. They may need a platelet transfusion, depending on the platelet count. Those with a history of significant alcohol consumption may be at risk for alcohol withdrawal and should be closely monitored perioperatively.

Genitourinary

Urinary complications following hip surgery include urine retention and infection.

Urine retention itself can lead to urinary tract infection[64]; bladder catheterization, which is used to treat urine retention, can also lead to infection, especially in the setting of prolonged catheterization. Each day of catheter use is associated with an approximately 5% increase in bacteriuria, which is usually asymptomatic.[65] However, even catheter-associated urinary tract infections (CA-UTIs) are rarely symptomatic.[66] According to current guidelines from the Infectious Diseases Society of America,[67] "signs and symptoms compatible with CA-UTI include new onset or worsening of fever, rigors, altered mental status, malaise, or lethargy with no other identified cause; flank pain; costovertebral angle tenderness; acute hematuria; pelvic discomfort; and, in those whose catheters have been removed, dysuria, urgent or frequent urination, or suprapubic pain or tenderness." Of note, a study by Koulouvaris and associates suggests that no clear evidence has linked preoperative or postoperative urinary tract infection with prosthetic joint infection.[68]

Risk Factors

Risk factors for urinary tract infection include female sex and poor preoperative medical condition.[69] Risk factors for postoperative urine retention include age greater than 50, male sex, preexisting obstructive urinary symptoms (benign prostatic hyperplasia [BPH]), previous pelvic surgery, neurologic disease (cerebral or spinal lesions, diabetic or alcoholic neuropathy), surgery of long duration, spinal or epidural anesthesia, postoperative sedative medications like midazolam, and continuous epidural analgesia.[70]

Recommendations

- David and Vrahas[71] recommend that patients undergoing total joint arthroplasty should have a preoperative urinalysis if they have "irritative" voiding symptoms. If results show more than 10,000 white blood cells (WBCs) per milliliter (greater than 4 WBCs per high-powered field), a urine culture should be performed, and surgery should be delayed for antibiotic treatment if more than 1000 colony-forming units per milliliter are detected. The authors note that data were insufficient for recommendations if fewer than 10,000 WBCs per milliliter were found on urinalysis, or fewer than 1000 colony-forming units per milliliter on culture. They recommend obtaining a preoperative urine culture in asymptomatic patients and then proceeding with surgery, but treating positive cultures with a 10-day course of antibiotics. Hanssen and colleagues recommend that patients with urinary tract difficulties should be identified and managed before total joint arthroplasty is performed.[72]

- Infectious Diseases Society of America guidelines state that pyuria accompanying asymptomatic bacteriuria (≥100,000 colony-forming units per milliliter [diagnosis requires two consecutive specimens for women, one for men] with a clean-catch specimen, or ≥100 colony-forming units per milliliter with a catheterized specimen) is not an indication for antimicrobial treatment.[73] However, these guidelines do not discuss patients with prosthetic implants.
- Likewise, Infectious Diseases Society of America guidelines state that pyuria in the catheterized patient is not diagnostic of catheter-associated bacteriuria or CA-UTI, and pyuria accompanying catheter-associated asymptomatic bacteriuria should not be interpreted as an indication for antimicrobial treatment.[67] These guidelines do not discuss patients with prosthetic implants.
- Urinary catheters, if required, should be used only for a short duration (≤24 hours). In-and-out catheterization is preferred over indwelling bladder catheters.
- Patients with an indwelling bladder catheter who have a CA-UTI should be treated with antibiotics for 7 days if they have prompt resolution of symptoms, and for 10 to 14 days if they have a delayed response, regardless of whether they remain catheterized.[67] A 5-day regimen of levofloxacin may be considered in patients with CA-UTI who are not severely ill, and a 3 day antimicrobial regimen may be considered for women 65 years of age or younger who develop CA-UTI without upper urinary tract symptoms after an indwelling catheter has been removed.[67]
- A study of patients undergoing abdominal surgery who had an indwelling urinary catheter for 1 week showed a significant reduction in symptomatic urinary tract infections and bacteriuria when antibiotic prophylaxis was given with trimethoprim-sulfamethoxazole at the time of catheter removal.[74]

Renal

Postoperative acute kidney injury and failure may occur after surgery and increase mortality and length of stay.[75] Note that decreased urine output is common in the first 12 to 24 hours after surgery; it does not necessarily imply kidney failure, but mostly reflects an increase in antidiuretic hormone due to the surgical stress response.

Risk Factors

Risk factors for perioperative acute kidney injury or failure include age greater than 55 years, preexisting kidney dysfunction, perioperative cardiac dysfunction, hypertension, diabetes, sepsis, liver failure, COPD, obesity, anemia, nephrotoxic medications, and IV contrast agents.[76-79] No preventive measure other than maintaining normal intravascular volume appears to be effective in decreasing risk.[80]

Recommendations
- Hold diuretics the morning of surgery.
- For patients who are normotensive, hold ACE inhibitors and ARBs the morning of surgery.
- Provide IV hydration postoperatively until patients have improving oral intake (typically at least 500 mL).
- Strive to maintain euvolemia, and avoid hypotension/decreased kidney perfusion pressure.[76]

Psychiatric

Psychiatric complications following orthopedic surgery include delirium, unexpected chronic postoperative pain, and alcohol withdrawal. Delirium after hip fracture is associated with prolonged hospital stay, higher cost, poor outcome, and the need for nursing home placement.[81]

Risk Factors

Underlying dementia is a primary risk factor for postoperative delirium and may not be evident until the episode of delirium occurs. Other risk factors include advanced age, lower education level, sensory impairment, decreased functional status, comorbid medical conditions, malnutrition, depression,[82] general anesthesia,[83] and a history of delirium.[84] Preoperative use of opioid medications and/or benzodiazepines has also been identified as a risk factor.[84] Precipitating factors include hemodynamic instability, hypoxemia, electrolyte disturbance, transfusion requirement, sleep deprivation, urinary catheterization, immobility, poorly controlled pain, and polypharmacy, especially with anticholinergics such as diphenhydramine (Benadryl) and benzodiazepines.[82] Patients with preoperative anxiety and depression may be more likely to have persistent long-term discomfort after total hip arthroplasty.[85] Alcohol abuse is an important risk factor even if there is no overt alcohol-related organ dysfunction, because it can lead to immunosuppression, subclinical cardiac dysfunction, and an amplified hormonal response to surgery.[86]

Recommendations
- Patients at high risk for delirium (older adult hip fracture patients and those with underlying dementia) should have a preoperative baseline mental status assessment such as the Folstein Mini-Mental Status Exam or the clock drawing test (ask the patient to draw a clock and place the hands at 11:10; if normal, then likely dementia).
- Diagnose delirium using the Confusion Assessment Method[87] (see later under "Postoperative Medical Complications"), noting that many patients may have the hypoactive form rather than the hyperactive/agitated form, either of which can cause hallucinations and delusions.
- Geriatric consultation has been shown to reduce the incidence of delirium and should be considered for patients at high risk for delirium.[88]

- Strive to balance pain control and opioid use. Consider opioid-sparing analgesia as tolerated, including acetaminophen and regional nerve blocks.
- Prophylactic low-dose haloperidol (0.5 mg by mouth three times daily) may be helpful in patients at high risk for postoperative delirium, assuming they have a normal QTc interval on their ECG. In a study by Kalisvaart, this dose reduced the severity and duration of delirium episodes and reduced the length of hospital stay in hip surgery patients, but made no difference in the incidence of delirium.[89]
- Patients with preoperative anxiety and depression may need appropriate treatment before surgery to help decrease the likelihood of persistent pain following surgery.
- Patients with a history of alcohol abuse should be monitored for withdrawal and should have electrolytes, including potassium and magnesium, checked perioperatively and replaced as needed. They should be given thiamine 100 mg daily for 3 days (one intramuscular dose and two oral doses) and a daily multivitamin.

POSTOPERATIVE MEDICAL COMPLICATIONS

Postoperative medical complications are most commonly related to the surgical stress response, which can lead to exacerbations of underlying medical conditions, although patients may have untoward problems directly related to the surgery itself. This section provides an overview of eight symptoms that patients commonly experience following hip surgery, along with diagnostic and treatment recommendations. Figure 26-2

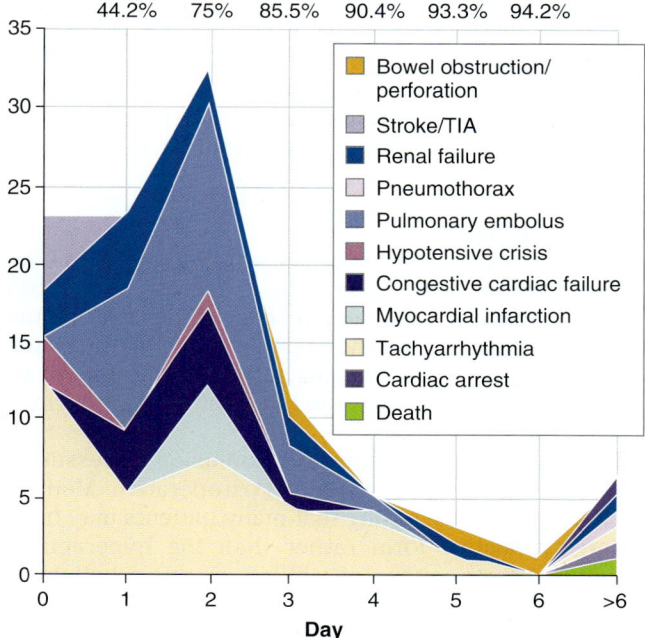

Figure 26-2. Incidence and timing of major complications following hip surgery. *TIA,* Transient ischemic attack.

shows the typical incidence and timing of major medical complications that may occur after hip surgery, based on a study by Parvizi and coworkers.[90] This study found that complications could not have been predicted on the basis of medical history for 58% of patients who had a major medical complication.

Hypertension

Postoperative hypertension is common and may lead to cardiovascular complications (ischemia, myocardial infarction, arrhythmia, congestive heart failure [CHF] with pulmonary edema), neurologic complications (cerebral ischemia or hemorrhagic stroke, encephalopathy), and surgical site bleeding. A previous history of hypertension is the most important risk factor for developing postoperative hypertension.

Definition

Hypertension is any blood pressure reading above 140/90 mm Hg. Hypertensive <u>emergency</u> is severe hypertension (usually greater than 180/120) with evidence of target organ damage.[91] Although no threshold blood pressure is associated with developing hypertensive emergency, target organ damage is uncommon if the diastolic blood pressure is less than 130.[92] In contrast, hypertensive <u>urgency</u> is severe hypertension without symptoms.

Differential Diagnosis/Causes
- Bladder distention
- Chronic untreated hypertension
- Constipation
- Drug withdrawal (clonidine, opioids, cocaine, alcohol, benzodiazepines)
- Hypercarbia
- Hypoxemia
- Intravascular volume depletion
- Intravascular volume overload
- Missed dose(s) of usual medication(s)
- Pain or anxiety
- Sympathetic nervous system stimulation from surgery and anesthesia

Evaluation
General assessment: Review vital signs, particularly blood pressure and heart rate, preferably in both arms and while the patient is seated. Evaluate general clinical status to ensure that additional assistance or a higher level of care is not immediately needed.

Symptoms: Patients with hypertension may be asymptomatic or may have symptoms suggestive of the underlying cause, including surgical site pain or bladder distention. Patients with hypertensive emergency have evidence of target organ damage, including such symptoms as encephalopathy, chest pain, shortness of breath, or acute kidney injury.

Examination: Somnolence or confusion causes concern regarding neurologic complications or hypercarbia. Cardiac examination should assess for third or fourth heart sound (S3 or S4), pulmonary crackles, or unequal peripheral pulses. High blood pressure can cause surgical site bleeding with increased drain output. Decreased urine output may signal urine retention or may indicate intravascular volume depletion due to bleeding or inadequate volume replacement.

Laboratory evaluation/testing: Depending on the clinical situation, consider CBC, electrolytes and creatinine, troponin, urinalysis, ECG, and chest x-ray.

Management

First, determine whether the patient has a hypertensive emergency and needs treatment in an intensive care setting. Then, identify and treat potentially reversible causes of hypertension as listed previously. In noncardiac surgery patients, no consensus has been reached regarding the threshold for treatment; this is usually a clinical decision based on blood pressure elevation, the nature of the surgery, patients' comorbidities, and risks of treatment.[92] Unless the patient has findings worrisome for aortic dissection, which requires immediate blood pressure reduction, blood pressure should not be lowered too much too soon because of concern for organ hypoperfusion and ischemia. For hypertensive emergencies, the initial goal of therapy is to reduce mean arterial pressure (MAP; see below) by no more than 25% within the first hour, then, if stable, to 160/100 to 110 mm Hg within the next 2 to 6 hours.[91] For patients with hypertensive urgency, blood pressure should be reduced gradually over 24 to 48 hours with oral medications.

$$MAP = (Systolic\ blood\ pressure + 2 \times Diastolic\ blood\ pressure)/3$$

Various medications are available for patients who require treatment of hypertension. Aside from hypertensive emergencies, which require IV medications, oral antihypertensives are preferable and should be selected on the basis of the suspected underlying cause of hypertension and known comorbid conditions. For example, patients with evidence of intravascular volume overload may benefit from a diuretic, but those with a history of coronary disease should be given a beta blocker, assuming they are not bradycardic (heart rate <60). Also, if a patient is already taking an antihypertensive, consider increasing the dose before adding a new agent. Other medications that can be given to lower blood pressure acutely include labetalol, clonidine, and captopril, although ACE inhibitors should be used cautiously in patients with kidney disease. Avoid hydralazine because it can cause reflex tachycardia that could lead to increased myocardial demand.

Hypotension

The most common cause of hypotension following hip surgery, intravascular volume depletion, can be treated by giving IV fluids and selectively holding antihypertensive medications.

Definition

Hypotension is a systolic blood pressure (SBP) of less than 90 mm Hg or any decrease in SBP of 40 mm Hg from baseline.[93]

Differential Diagnosis/Causes

- Adrenal insufficiency
- Bleeding
- Cardiac dysrhythmias
- Coronary ischemia
- Intravascular volume depletion
- Medication effect
- Pneumothorax
- Pulmonary embolus
- Sepsis syndrome

Evaluation

General assessment: Review vital signs and confirm blood pressure and heart rate. Evaluate general clinical status to ensure that additional assistance or a higher level of care is not immediately needed.

Symptoms: Altered mentation, dizziness, and syncope may be caused by low blood pressure. Cardiac causes of hypotension can present with chest pain and palpitations, whereas dyspnea and pleuritic pain may indicate a pulmonary cause. Fever and chills suggest underlying infection.

Examination: Somnolence and confusion may be consequences of low blood pressure. Focal examination findings such as tachycardia or bradycardia, diminished or unequal breath sounds, pulmonary crackles, surgical site bleeding, increased drain output, or decreased urine output help delineate the cause of hypotension.

Laboratory evaluation/testing: CBC to evaluate for evidence of bleeding (also consider coagulation studies) or infection; electrolyte panel to evaluate renal and adrenal function; cardiac biomarkers and ECG for evidence of coronary ischemia and dysrhythmias; and chest x-ray to look for infiltrates, pulmonary edema, or pneumothorax. Perform chest computed tomography (CT) angiogram or lung ventilation/perfusion (V/Q) scan if concern for pulmonary embolus (PE) arises, although be aware of possible contrast nephropathy in patients with known kidney disease (these patients should be given IV hydration and N-acetylcysteine to decrease the risk of kidney injury). Check a morning cortisol level if adrenal insufficiency is suspected; these patients may benefit from corticosteroids. Obtain blood cultures along with a serum lactate level if sepsis is a concern.

Management

IV fluid therapy with 0.9% normal saline is the cornerstone of treatment. The rate of fluid resuscitation is based on severity of symptoms, presumed origin, and concern for heart failure. Patients who are largely asymptomatic may need to receive only gentle fluid boluses of 250 mL over 1 hour and to hold their antihypertensive agents. In contrast, those who are septic need aggressive fluid resuscitation, usually several liters, along with broad-spectrum antibiotic therapy, and should be managed in an intensive care setting. Patients with hypotension and altered mental status should be placed in the Trendelenburg (head lower than heart) position. Patients with ongoing bleeding may require a transfusion. Supplemental oxygen should be administered as needed.

Antihypertensive medications should be held selectively, although patients taking beta blockers or clonidine are at risk for rebound effects (tachycardia or hypertension). Holding diuretics first is preferred, then holding medications such as ACE inhibitors and ARBs, alpha blockers, and calcium channel blockers. If the patient is severely or symptomatically hypotensive, hold all antihypertensives initially, and resume one at a time as the patient recovers. These medications may need to be held until outpatient follow-up. Additional therapies should be directed at the underlying cause of hypotension.

Hypoxia

Postoperative hypoxia is a common effect of anesthesia but may represent an acute cardiopulmonary problem or an exacerbation of a chronic condition. Always ask patients if they use oxygen at home, and look for baseline preoperative oxygen saturation readings in the medical record for comparison.

Definitions

Hypoxia, a general term referring to impaired oxygen delivery to tissues, takes into account cardiac output and oxygen uptake at the tissue level. By comparison, hypoxemia refers to low oxygen in the blood.

Differential Diagnosis/Causes

- Acute lung injury/acute respiratory distress syndrome (ALI/ARDS)
- Anesthesia effects (reduced functional residual capacity, depressed respiratory drive, and neuromuscular blockade)
- Aspiration
- Atelectasis
- Asthma
- COPD
- Congestive heart failure with pulmonary edema
- Coronary ischemia/myocardial infarction
- Fat embolism syndrome
- Negative-pressure pulmonary edema (caused by forceful inspiration against a closed glottis during extubation)
- OSA
- Pain that may limit adequate respirations
- Pneumonia
- PE
- Sepsis syndrome
- Transfusion-related acute lung injury (TRALI)

Evaluation

General assessment: Review vital signs, including respiratory rate and oxygen saturation. Evaluate general clinical status to ensure that additional assistance or a higher level of care is not immediately needed.

Symptoms: Dyspnea and/or tachypnea are common findings, but patients may not be symptomatic. Other symptoms may include chest pain, pleuritic pain, orthopnea, wheezing, a productive cough, fevers, chills, hemoptysis, altered mental status, or somnolence.

Examination: Worrisome findings include somnolence or confusion, pulmonary crackles, diminished breath sounds, wheezing, or a pleural friction rub. A petechial rash on the head, subconjunctivae, chest, and axillae is characteristic of fat embolism syndrome.

Laboratory evaluation/testing: CBC, electrolytes and creatinine, brain natriuretic peptide (if concern for heart failure), troponin and ECG (if concern for coronary ischemia), and chest x-ray. Check arterial blood gas in patients with suspected CO_2 retention, but this test is usually not necessary otherwise because of the accuracy and convenience of pulse oximetry. Consider blood cultures in febrile patients with findings consistent with pneumonia or sepsis syndrome. Perform chest CT angiogram or V/Q scan if concern for PE, although be aware of possible contrast nephropathy in those with known kidney disease (these patients should be given IV hydration and *N*-acetylcysteine to decrease the risk of kidney injury).

Management

Provide supplemental oxygen as necessary to keep oxygen saturation at least 90%. Patients with known CO_2 retention should have a goal oxygen saturation of 88% to 93% if they are at risk of worsening hypercarbia; these patients should still be given oxygen if they are hypoxemic. Patients with respiratory distress who are not able to maintain adequate oxygen saturation despite supplemental oxygen, or who are acidemic with acute hypercarbia, should be treated in an intensive care setting, possibly with noninvasive positive-pressure ventilation or intubation and mechanical ventilation.

Patients with an acute asthma or COPD exacerbation should be given nebulizer therapy and possibly corticosteroids. Patients with findings suggestive of infection should be started on antibiotic therapy; a sputum specimen can be obtained for culture to help determine the causative organism. Empirical therapy should be started in accordance with local bacterial resistance patterns. Levofloxacin may be an appropriate first choice, although patients who have been previously hospitalized or who are otherwise at risk for methicillin-resistant *Staphylococcus aureus* should also be given vancomycin.

Patients with evidence of heart failure should be treated with diuretic therapy. As a general rule of thumb, give IV furosemide at the same or a higher dose than the outpatient oral dose (e.g., patients who take 40 mg of oral furosemide can be given 40 mg IV). Monitor urine output, fluid balance, electrolytes (primarily potassium and magnesium), and kidney function. Patients who take furosemide long term should resume their usual oral dose as symptoms improve.

Patients with chest pain worrisome for coronary ischemia should have a priority ECG and may need cardiology consultation or transfer to a monitored cardiac unit. Immediately give these patients four chewable 81 mg aspirin (or a single chewable 325 mg aspirin). They may also need sublingual nitroglycerin (avoid if systolic blood pressure less than 90 mm Hg, or if known aortic stenosis) or morphine (if they have ongoing pain), beta blockade, and anticoagulation with heparin or low-molecular-weight heparin (LMWH).

Patients with dyspnea, hypoxemia, tachypnea, and tachycardia should be assumed to have a PE, although these symptoms are not specific for PE. However, some patients with PE may be largely asymptomatic. Consider empirically starting anticoagulation with heparin or LMWH in patients who are hemodynamically unstable or who appear acutely ill, while taking measures to minimize surgical site bleeding. Otherwise, if chest CT angiogram or V/Q scan is positive for PE, then start anticoagulation. Warfarin should be started along with heparin/LMWH. Note that warfarin typically takes 3 to 4 days to become therapeutic—even if the INR rises quickly above 2.0—because of different half-lives of the vitamin K–dependent clotting factors. Heparin/LMWH therefore should be given concurrently with warfarin for at least 5 days, and until the INR has been at least 2.0 for 24 hours. Because most PEs result from lower extremity deep vein thrombosis (DVT), patients should be prescribed knee-high compression stockings (30 to 40 mm Hg) to be worn for 2 years whenever they are upright, to help decrease the risk of post-thrombotic syndrome.

Patients with OSA should continue their positive-pressure airway devices. Those with suspected OSA should have continuous pulse oximetry while in bed for as long as they remain at increased risk. These patients should be given supplemental oxygen until they are able to maintain their baseline oxygen saturation while breathing room air. They may need to start empirical positive-pressure therapy with an autotitrating CPAP device.

All patients with hypoxia or hypoxemia should be encouraged to use lung expansion techniques such as incentive spirometry. Patients with a productive cough may benefit from a flutter valve device (i.e., Acapella [Smiths Medical, Norwell, Maine]) to help break up and mobilize pulmonary secretions.

Decreased Urine Output

Urinary retention and acute kidney injury (AKI) are causes of decreased urine output that may occur after hip surgery. Urine retention has a reported incidence of 10.7% to 84% following joint arthroplasty.[70] Postoperative acute kidney injury and failure are common after surgery and increase mortality and length of stay.[75] Acute tubular necrosis (ATN) is the most common cause of postoperative AKI.[80] Other causes of decreased urine output include an absolute decrease in intravascular volume from blood loss or third-spacing, a relative decrease in intravascular volume from vasodilation (due to anesthetic agents, sepsis, liver disease, or nephrotic syndrome), and decreased kidney perfusion from structural causes such as thromboembolism.[94]

Definitions

Urinary retention, the inability to void despite a full bladder,[66] is commonly related to the effects of anesthesia and medications. Acute kidney injury indicates a twofold increase in serum creatinine or a decrease in glomerular filtration rate (GFR) greater than 50% (or urine output less than 0.5 mL/kg/hour for 12 hours), and acute kidney failure is defined by a threefold increase in creatinine, a decrease in GFR of 75%, or a creatinine greater than or equal to 4 (or urine output less than 0.3 mL/kg/hour for 24 hours or anuria for 12 hours).[95]

Differential Diagnosis/Causes
- Urinary retention
  - Bladder dysfunction (anesthetic or medication effect)
  - Urethral obstruction (BPH, stone)
- Acute kidney injury
  - Prerenal (hypovolemia, hypotension)
  - Intrinsic renal (hypotension leading to acute tubular necrosis; nephrotoxins such as nonsteroidal anti-inflammatory drugs [NSAIDs], antibiotics, or IV contrast)
  - Postrenal (urinary tract obstruction)

Evaluation

General assessment: Review vital signs. Evaluate general clinical status to ensure that additional assistance or a higher level of care is not immediately needed. Confirm urine output and bladder catheter patency.

Symptoms: Generalized fatigue, dizziness, lower abdominal pain or discomfort, nausea, vomiting, and anorexia may be manifestations of urinary retention and acute kidney injury or failure. Patients who are volume depleted may be orthostatic.

Examination: Patients with urinary retention may be asymptomatic or may present with abdominal distention and a palpable bladder. Confusion, a cardiac rub, flank pain, or edema may be present in patients with acute kidney injury or failure.

Laboratory evaluation/testing: Bladder ultrasound helps to diagnose urinary retention and should be the first step in evaluation if the patient's urine output has decreased. Check electrolytes, blood urea nitrogen (BUN), creatinine, urinalysis with microscopy, and urine culture and sensitivity to further evaluate kidney function. Consider renal ultrasound for patients with urinary retention or urinary tract obstruction to determine whether hydronephrosis is present, and as a step in evaluation of acute kidney injury.

Management

Surgical stress incites the increased secretion of antidiuretic hormone with the overall effect of impaired water and sodium excretion.[80] Decreased urine output after surgery may signal the body's attempt to conserve fluids or may indicate potential derangements at any of multiple sites along the genitourinary tract. Oliguria (urine output <500 mL/24 hr) and anuria (urine output <50 mL/24 hr) deserve immediate attention. Bladder ultrasound helps distinguish whether urine production is decreased, suggesting acute kidney injury or failure, or whether urinary obstruction or retention is the underlying problem, as indicated by a large volume of urine on ultrasound.

If urinary retention is the cause of decreased urine output, intermittent catheterization should be performed for bladder ultrasound volumes greater than 300 to 400 mL.[96] Risk factors for urinary retention include age greater than 50 years, male sex, preexisting obstructive urinary symptoms such as BPH, previous pelvic surgery, neurologic disease, perioperative beta blockers, long surgery duration, neuraxial anesthesia, postoperative sedating medications, and continuous epidural analgesia.[70] Removing or minimizing causative medications, such as anticholinergic drugs and opioids, quickly mobilizing the patient, and resuming BPH medications postoperatively help prevent urinary retention. For male patients with a history of BPH who are not already treated, consider initiation of tamsulosin.

Those with chronic kidney disease are at highest risk to develop AKI postoperatively.[77] Maintaining normal intravascular volume appears to be the only effective preventive measure to decrease risk of AKI.[80] Avoiding hypotension is important, and diuretics, ACE inhibitors, and ARB medications should be held the morning of surgery. Reports have described AKI after placement of tobramycin-impregnated cement in patients with preexisting renal dysfunction.[97]

If AKI develops, the underlying cause should be identified and corrected. Correct volume status, and maintain euvolemia. Evaluate for metabolic and electrolyte derangements, and correct as needed. Dose medications according to renal function, and remove or minimize nephrotoxic medications.

Acute Altered Mental Status

Acute altered mental status (delirium) can occur in 16% to 62% of patients following hip fracture repair,[98] but it is commonly missed (nondetection rate of 33% to 66%),[99] largely because it may manifest in hyperactive, hypoactive, or mixed forms. In a prospective study by de Jonghe and associates, patients most commonly developed delirium on the second postoperative day.[100] Common causes include medication effects and metabolic derangements, although delirium may unmask previously undiagnosed dementia. Ischemic stroke is an uncommon cause of delirium, but women are more likely than men to have mental status changes following ischemic stroke.[101] Because delirium may be caused by a serious underlying medical condition, prompt recognition and evaluation are essential.

Definition
Delirium is diagnosed using the Confusion Assessment Method (CAM)[87] as an acute change in mental status with a fluctuating course and inattention, with evidence of disorganized thinking or altered level of consciousness.

Differential Diagnosis/Causes
The mnemonic DELIRIUM is a useful tool in recalling the differential diagnosis and identifying causes of delirium (Figure 26-3).

Evaluation
General assessment: Review vital signs. Evaluate general clinical status to ensure that additional assistance or a higher level of care is not immediately needed.
Symptoms: Patients present with an acute change in mental status and may have hyperactive, hypoactive, or mixed features. Other symptoms may or may not be present or identifiable based on the patient's behavior and ability to communicate.
Examination: Somnolence or confusion deserves prompt attention in the postoperative patient. Focal neurologic deficits raise concern for intracranial events. Assess for dysrhythmias, pulmonary crackles, abdominal pain, surgical site pain, or decreased urine output to help focus the evaluation of a patient with delirium.
Laboratory evaluation/testing: CBC, electrolytes, glucose, and urinalysis. Depending on the clinical situation, consider troponin, ECG, and chest x-ray. Drug levels and drug screening may also be indicated. Obtain head CT if the patient has an evident neurologic deficit.

Management
First identify and treat any possible precipitating causes based on symptoms and physical findings and after review of medications and laboratory values. Strive to optimize acute and comorbid medical conditions, ensure adequate pain control, remove urinary catheter

D	**D**rug effects or withdrawal, **D**ehydration, **D**eprivation (sleep)
E	**E**lectrolytes, **E**motion (psychiatric), **E**mbolism (thrombotic or fat)
L	**L**ow oxygen, **L**ow hemoglobin
I	**I**nfection (urinary tract, pneumonia, meningitis/encephalitis), **I**mmobility
R	**R**etained carbon dioxide, **R**educed sensory input
I	**I**schemia, **I**nfarct (coronary or cerebrovascular), **I**ctal
U	**U**remia, **U**rine retention/constipation, **U**ncontrolled pain
M	**M**etabolic (glucose, thyroid, B_{12}, ammonia)

Figure 26-3. The mnemonic DELIRIUM helps with recall of differential diagnoses and identifying causes of delirium.

(if present), encourage early ambulation, and provide a calm and supportive environment. Gentle, frequent reorientation is important, and having family members or sitters in the room can help in this regard. Maintain appropriate sensory stimulation by having patients wear their glasses and hearing aids. Help normalize the sleep-wake cycle by keeping window shades open during the daytime and lights off at night.

For patients who are agitated and at risk to harm themselves or care providers, consider antipsychotics if supportive care is not effective; avoid physical restraints, if possible. The first-line medication is low-dose haloperidol, typically 0.25 to 1 mg, although this is a non–U.S. Food and Drug Administration (FDA)-labeled indication. Oral haloperidol is preferable, but the intramuscular (IM) form should be used if the patient is unwilling or unable to take a pill. The IV form of haloperidol has a rapid onset of action, but it also has a limited duration of about 20 minutes. Patients who have persistent agitation after the initial dose should not be given a repeat dose for at least 30 minutes after an IV or IM dose, and at least 60 minutes after an oral dose. Do not give haloperidol to patients who have Parkinson's disease or a prolonged QTc interval of more than 460 milliseconds. Patients should not receive more than 5 mg in a 24 hour period—the level at which the dopamine D2 receptors are saturated—because higher doses will only increase the risk of side effects. Patients receiving haloperidol should have daily ECGs to monitor the QTc interval.

Benzodiazepines paradoxically may worsen delirium and generally should not be used unless the delirium is due to alcohol or benzodiazepine withdrawal. However, a short-acting benzodiazepine such as lorazepam 0.5 mg may be helpful to treat severe agitation if there has been no response to haloperidol and additional sedation is needed.

Chest Pain

Although cardiopulmonary causes of postoperative chest pain are worrisome, there is a broad differential diagnosis underlying chest pain. Risk factors for cardiac ischemia or pulmonary events should be considered, but the past medical history of a patient with chest pain should be elicited. Those with peptic ulcer disease, cholelithiasis, or GERD may describe upper abdominal pain as chest pain.

The frequency of myocardial infarction after hip arthroplasty ranged from 0.1% to 2.2%, depending on age and gender, at one academic center.[102] Similarly, 2% of patients manifested serious cardiac complications after hip fracture repair in a large, multicenter retrospective study.[103] The prevalence of postoperative pulmonary embolus in hip fracture patients has been reported at 3% to 11%.[104]

Definition

Angina is chest pain caused by myocardial ischemia. Inflammation of the lung pleura causes pleuritic chest pain. Dyspepsia describes pain or discomfort in the epigastric area.

Differential Diagnosis/Causes
Cardiac
- Acute coronary syndrome
- Aortic dissection
- Pericarditis/myocarditis

Pulmonary
- Pleuritic pain
- Pneumonia
- Pneumothorax
- Pulmonary embolus

Musculoskeletal
- Chest wall

Gastrointestinal
- Cholelithiasis/cholecystitis
- GERD
- Peptic ulcer disease

Evaluation

General assessment: Review vital signs. Evaluate general clinical status to ensure that additional assistance or a higher level of care is not immediately needed. Heart rhythm monitors should be in place if the underlying cause of chest pain is believed to be cardiac in nature.

Symptoms: Shortness of breath, diaphoresis, palpitations, dizziness, syncope, or intrascapular pain suggests cardiac causes of chest pain. Pain that is similar to prior angina/myocardial infarction, chest pressure, pain that radiates to the arms or shoulders, or exertional pain is more likely to result from an acute coronary syndrome.[105] Conversely, pain that is sharp/stabbing, positional, reproducible with palpation, pleuritic, or localized to a small area of the chest is less likely to be caused by an acute coronary syndrome.[105] Upper abdominal pain or worsening of pain with oral intake may indicate a gastrointestinal (GI) source of chest pain. Nausea and vomiting can accompany both cardiac and GI sources of pain. Pain that is worsened with deep inspiration may represent pleuritic pain or musculoskeletal chest wall pain. Fever and chills signal infectious or inflammatory causes of chest pain.

Examination: A thorough cardiac examination is warranted, although abnormalities may not be auscultated despite underlying cardiac ischemia. Pulmonary examination findings of concern include crackles, unequal or absent breath sounds, and pleural friction rub. Chest wall tenderness with palpation supports musculoskeletal pain. An abdominal examination should be performed with attention to the upper abdomen, as pain originating here may be described as chest pain.

Laboratory evaluation/testing: Check troponin and ECG if coronary ischemia is a matter of concern. Obtain a chest x-ray to evaluate lung fields for pneumonia or pneumothorax. Perform chest CT angiogram if PE or aortic dissection is of concern, although be aware of possible contrast nephropathy in patients with known kidney disease (these patients should be given IV hydration and *N*-acetylcysteine to decrease the risk of kidney injury).

Management

If coronary ischemia is suspected or diagnosed, oxygen and four chewable 81 mg aspirin or a single 325 mg chewable tablet should be given immediately. Sublingual nitroglycerin should also be given unless the patient is hypotensive (systolic blood pressure <90 mm Hg) or has a history of aortic stenosis. Morphine may be needed for pain relief. Beta blockade and anticoagulation with heparin/LMWH may be needed.

For inflammatory causes of chest pain such as pericarditis, pleuritic pain, or musculoskeletal chest wall pain, NSAIDs can be used if the chance of increased bleeding risk is acceptable and there are no concerns regarding bone healing or kidney function. Dyspepsia may be relieved with antacids, H_2-receptor blockers, or proton pump inhibitors.

Note that standard postoperative pain control regimens may actually mask chest pain, and a heightened level of awareness is needed to detect adverse events. Also, patients with diabetes may not feel chest pain.

Nausea, Vomiting, and Abdominal Pain

Postoperative nausea and vomiting (PONV) is a common occurrence after surgery. Frequently, it is a side effect of anesthesia or opioid medications, particularly in the immediate postoperative period. However, other causes should not be overlooked, especially if nausea or vomiting is accompanied by abdominal pain, abdominal distention, or other focal symptoms.

Definition

Nausea is a subjective feeling of the urge to vomit with the absence of expulsive muscular movements. Vomiting is the forcible expulsion of gastric contents through the mouth.[51] Postoperative paralytic ileus is defined as the functional inhibition of propulsive bowel activity lasting longer than 3 days after surgery.[106] Colonic pseudo-obstruction (Ogilvie's syndrome) is a functional colonic obstruction that leads to progressive dilatation of the large bowel[55] without underlying mechanical cause.[107]

Differential Diagnosis/Causes

- Anesthesia side effect
- Bowel obstruction
- Bowel perforation
- Cardiac ischemia
- Cholelithiasis/cholecystitis
- Constipation
- Gastrointestinal bleeding
- GERD
- Ileus
- Infection (*Clostridium difficile* colitis, urinary tract infection, pneumonia)
- Medication adverse effect (narcotics, NSAIDs)
- Metabolic derangements (hypoglycemia, hypokalemia, hypomagnesemia)
- Pancreatitis
- Peptic ulcer disease
- Pseudo-obstruction (Ogilvie's syndrome)

Evaluation

General assessment: Review vital signs. Evaluate general clinical status to ensure that additional assistance or a higher level of care is not immediately needed.

Symptoms: Chills, sweats, and rigors may signal systemic infection. The character of emesis (hematemesis, bilious) and the location of abdominal pain can help focus the differential diagnosis. Diarrhea may be copious, may overflow with constipation, or may be indicative of infection such as *C. difficile* colitis. Focal symptoms of infection such as cough or dysuria should be elicited from the patient. Hematemesis, melena, or hematochezia, an acutely ill-appearing patient, or peritoneal signs on abdominal examination should prompt aggressive, rapid evaluation and treatment.

Examination: The abdominal examination should focus on the presence and nature of bowel sounds (hypoactive, high-pitched, or "tinkling"), distention, masses, and tenderness. Assess for peritoneal signs such as rigidity, guarding, or rebound tenderness.

Laboratory evaluation/testing: Check electrolytes, including magnesium, and blood glucose if the patient is diabetic. Obtain lipase, hepatic transaminases, alkaline phosphatase, and total bilirubin if pancreatitis, liver disease, or gallbladder disease is in the differential diagnosis. CBC, along with urinalysis, urine culture and sensitivity, chest x-ray, and stool sample for *C. difficile*, can help evaluate for infection. Plain x-rays of the abdomen should be obtained if abdominal distention or peritoneal signs are noted on examination. CT imaging helps differentiate between mechanical obstruction and pseudo-obstruction.

Management

Support patients with nausea, vomiting, and abdominal pain postoperatively with antiemetics and pain medications, adequate hydration, and replacement of electrolytes. Keep patients fasting until the cause of symptoms is delineated, and consider alternate forms of nutrition if a prolonged fast is required. An H_2-receptor blocker or proton pump inhibitor should be provided to those patients with peptic ulcer disease, gastroesophageal reflux, or gastrointestinal bleeding. Acupressure at the P6 point may help with PONV.[63] Chewing gum three times daily[108] or direct abdominal massage[109] may help decrease the duration of ileus.

For patients in whom medications are believed to be the cause of symptoms, as a direct side effect or through their slowing of GI motility, eliminate or minimize offending medications (opioids, calcium channel blockers, anticholinergics). Provide an adequate regimen of stool softeners or laxatives, particularly if the patient is on opioids, to prevent constipation and ileus. Other pain medications, such as NSAIDs, may be used as alternates or adjuncts to opioids to help minimize narcotic use.

Electrolyte depletion, especially hypokalemia and hypomagnesemia, in patients with ileus may be both a cause and an effect of gastrointestinal dysmotility. Nasogastric tubes may be selectively (rather than routinely) placed to decrease symptoms of ileus.[110] Promotility agents have not shown benefit in the treatment of postoperative ileus.[111]

Given the risk of colonic perforation, the goal of therapy for Ogilvie's syndrome is prompt colonic decompression. In one study of patients undergoing total joint arthroplasty, 1.6% of those who underwent total hip arthroplasty developed postoperative Ogilvie's syndrome.[55] Neostigmine, an anticholinesterase inhibitor, or decompressive colonoscopy may be considered[55] to achieve decompression. Laxatives in this case are contraindicated because they may increase gas production by promoting bacterial fermentation.[107]

Postoperative Fever

Patients commonly develop a self-limited fever of over 38° C following orthopedic surgery. This is usually a cytokine-mediated process due to surgical inflammation and tends to peak on postoperative day 1 or 2.[112] However, fevers occurring after postoperative day 3 or at greater than 40° C, or patients with worrisome symptoms, warrant further evaluation. Note that atelectasis does <u>not</u> cause fever.

Definition

An oral temperature greater than 38° C is generally considered to be a fever.

Differential Diagnosis/Causes[113]

- Noninfectious
  - Acalculous cholecystitis
  - Adrenal crisis
  - Alcohol or drug withdrawal
  - Aspiration chemical pneumonitis
  - Bowel infarction
  - Cytokine-mediated surgical inflammation
  - DVT or PE
  - Fat embolism
  - Gout or pseudogout
  - Malignancy
  - Medication effect
  - Myocardial infarction
  - Pancreatitis
  - Stroke
  - Surgical hematoma
  - Thyrotoxicosis or thyroid storm
  - Transfusion reaction
- Infectious
  - Cellulitis
  - C. difficile (in patients with recent or current antibiotic use)
  - Intravenous catheter-related infection
  - Pulmonary infection
  - Sepsis syndrome
  - Sinusitis
  - Surgical site infection
  - Toxic shock syndrome
  - Urinary tract infection

Evaluation

General assessment: Review vital signs, especially the temperature trend and maximum value. Evaluate general clinical status to ensure that additional assistance or a higher level of care is not immediately needed.

Symptoms: Chills, rigors, and delirium frequently accompany fevers. Symptoms that help localize the source of fever after hip surgery include neurologic deficits, nasal/sinus congestion or drainage, cough with sputum, dyspnea, chest pain, abdominal pain, nausea or vomiting, diarrhea, dysuria or increased urine frequency, joint pain or swelling, calf or thigh pain or swelling, and surgical site pain.

Examination: Assess for somnolence or confusion. Focal neurologic deficits are matters of concern for stroke or central nervous system infection. Sinus tenderness, pulmonary crackles, abdominal or suprapubic tenderness, and joint erythema, swelling, or tenderness are findings that can help localize the source of fever. A deep vein thrombus may present with calf or thigh swelling and/or tenderness. Skin or surgical site erythema and/or drainage suggests cellulitis or surgical site infection.

Laboratory evaluation/testing: None needed if fever is most likely due to surgical inflammation. Otherwise, consider CBC, electrolytes and creatinine, urinalysis with Gram stain and culture, and chest x-ray. Obtain blood cultures only if there is a high suspicion for bacteremia. Obtain lower extremity ultrasound or chest CT angiogram if concern for DVT/PE arises, but be aware of possible contrast nephropathy in patients with known kidney disease (these patients should be given IV hydration and *N*-acetylcysteine to decrease the risk of kidney injury). Consider abdominal x-ray or CT if findings are suggestive of an intra-abdominal pathology. Other tests can be performed as indicated based on the suspected illness, including troponin, thyroid tests, liver and pancreatic enzymes, uric acid, cortisol level, and stool *C. difficile* toxin. Finally, for patients with concern for severe sepsis or bowel infarction, obtain a serum lactate level.

Management

Observation is safe for patients who have an immediate moderate postoperative fever who otherwise look well with no worrisome findings. However, if the fever persists or occurs beyond postoperative day 3, patients should undergo a focused investigation, as outlined earlier. Empirical antibiotics should be reserved for patients who clearly have an infectious process, but broad-spectrum antibiotics should be started immediately in patients who may have sepsis syndrome. Be aware that DVT/PE can occur despite appropriate prophylaxis.

CURRENT CONTROVERSIES AND FUTURE DIRECTIONS

Perioperative beta blocker therapy has been the subject of a number of clinical trials (and some controversy), although none has focused specifically on hip surgery patients. Intuitively, beta blockers should be cardioprotective because they help attenuate the sympathetic response of surgical stress. Indeed, some studies suggest that beta blockers reduce perioperative coronary ischemia and may reduce the risk of myocardial infarction and cardiovascular death in high-risk patients. However, not all studies have shown improved outcomes,[114-117] possibly because of varying beta blocker formulations, dosing, and duration of therapy. Furthermore, beta blockers may cause perioperative hypotension and bradycardia, as evidenced by the recent POISE (Perioperative Ischemic Evaluation) trial,[117] which showed higher risk of stroke and death in patients taking a beta blocker, despite fewer primary cardiac events. Of note, orthopedic patients made up 21% of the study population. One important concern with this trial, however, was that each patient received the same high dose of extended-release metoprolol succinate (100 mg 2 to 4 hours before surgery, and 200 mg daily thereafter), which was higher than the starting dose that many clinicians would use. By comparison, the recent DECREASE-IV trial,[118] which used bisoprolol, showed a significant reduction in 30 day cardiac death and nonfatal myocardial infarction; orthopedic patients made up 16% of this study population.

So which patients should be given perioperative beta blockers, and when? The 2009 Focused Update from the American College of Cardiology Foundation (ACCF)/ American Heart Association (AHA) provides class recommendations for perioperative beta blockers (see below).[119] This Update, which was prompted by results of the POISE trial, emphasizes that perioperative beta blockers are associated with risk, and "routine administration of perioperative beta blockers, particularly in higher fixed-dose regimens begun on the day of surgery, cannot be advocated." Beta blockers should be considered in the context of each patient's clinical and surgical risk and, if used, should be titrated throughout the preoperative, intraoperative, and postoperative periods to maintain heart rate control (60 to 80 beats/min) while avoiding hypotension and bradycardia.[119] If indicated, beta blockers should be started well in advance (days to weeks) before elective surgery. Indications and contraindications to beta blocker therapy should be assessed throughout the postoperative period.

Class I Indication ("Should Be Performed")

- Beta blockers should be continued in patients undergoing surgery who are receiving beta blockers for treatment of conditions with ACCF/AHA Class I guideline indications for the drugs, including angina, symptomatic arrhythmias, or hypertension.

Class IIa Indication ("Reasonable to Perform")

- Beta blockers titrated to heart rate and blood pressure are reasonable for patients in whom preoperative assessment identifies coronary artery disease or high cardiac risk, as defined by the presence of more than one clinical risk factor (history of ischemic heart disease, history of compensated or prior heart failure, history of cerebrovascular disease, diabetes mellitus on insulin, or renal insufficiency [serum creatinine > 2mg/dL]) who are undergoing intermediate-risk surgery such as orthopedic surgery.

Class IIb Indication ("May Be Considered")

- The usefulness of beta blockers is uncertain for patients who are undergoing intermediate-risk procedures or vascular surgery, in whom preoperative assessment identifies a single clinical risk factor in the absence of coronary artery disease.

Class III Indications ("Should Not Be Performed")

- Beta blockers should not be given to patients undergoing surgery who have absolute contraindications to beta blockade.
- Routine administration of high-dose beta blockers in the absence of dose titration is not useful and may be harmful to patients not currently taking beta blockers who are undergoing noncardiac surgery.

What about hip fracture patients who require urgent surgical intervention? Some of these patients may have coronary artery disease or high cardiac risk and potentially could benefit from beta blocker therapy, especially if they have a high resting heart rate or hypertension. However, clinicians do not have the luxury of starting beta blockers well in advance of surgery to allow for dose titration, and, as noted earlier, significant concerns are associated with starting fixed high-dose beta blocker therapy on the day of surgery. A reasonable approach to treating these patients is based on the authors' experience and the large retrospective review by Lindenauer and colleagues. This study[120] showed that patients with at least <u>three</u> clinical risk factors (as defined previously, but NOT including heart failure) had improved outcomes when given perioperative beta blockers, and for patients with <u>two</u> risk factors, perioperative beta blockers appeared to be beneficial.

For patients with an elevated heart rate, first identify and treat possible causative factors, including pain, anxiety, anemia, intravascular volume depletion, hypoxia, and drug withdrawal. If the patient is not hypotensive, has at least two clinical risk factors, and has a heart rate greater than 100 beats per minute, consider starting short-acting metoprolol at least 1 day before surgery, if possible. A suggested starting dose is 12.5 to 25 mg by mouth twice daily, depending on patient age, heart rate, and blood pressure. Increase the metoprolol gradually by 12.5 to 25 mg per dose if the heart rate and/or blood pressure remains elevated and other causative factors have been identified and treated. Stop the metoprolol if the heart rate decreases to below 60 beats per minute, or if the systolic blood pressure drops below 100 mm Hg. Otherwise, continue the beta blocker for at least 30 days (or longer if the patient has other indications). If the beta blocker is to be stopped at that time, it should be gradually tapered to avoid rebound effects.

REFERENCES

1. Zhan C, Kaczmarek R, Loyo-Berrios N, et al: Incidence and short-term outcomes of primary and revision hip replacement in the United States. J Bone Joint Surg Am 89:526–533, 2007.
2. DeFrances CJ, Lucas CA, Buie VC, Golosinskiy A: National Health Statistics Reports, Number 5, July 30, 2008. United States Department of Health and Human Services, Centers for Disease Control and Prevention, National Center for Health Statistics. http://www.cdc.gov/nchs/data/nhsr/nhsr005.pdf (accessed on August 2, 2009).
3. Stoelting RK, Miller RD: History and scope of anesthesia. In Stoelting RK, Miller RD (eds): Basics of anesthesia, ed 4, Philadelphia, 2000, Churchill Livingstone.
4. Desborough JP: The stress response to trauma and surgery. Brit J Anaesth 85:109–117, 2000.
5. Guyton AC, Hall JE: The autonomic nervous system and the adrenal medulla. In Guyton AC, Hall JE (eds): Textbook of medical physiology, ed 11, Philadelphia, 2006, Elsevier Saunders.
6. Kehlet H: Multimodal approach to control postoperative pathophysiology and rehabilitation. Brit J Anaesth 78:606–617, 1997.
7. Kohl BA, Deutschman CS: The inflammatory response to surgery and trauma. Curr Opin Crit Care 12:325–332, 2006.
8. Chernow B, Alexander HR, Smallridge RC, et al: Hormonal responses to graded surgical stress. Arch Intern Med 147:1273–1278, 1987.
9. Kehlet H: The surgical stress response: should it be prevented? Can J Surg 34:565–567, 1991.
10. Hahnenkamp K, Herroeder S, Hollmann MW: Regional anaesthesia, local anaesthetics and the surgical stress response. Best Pract Res Clin Anaesth 18:509–527, 2004.
11. Parvizi J, Pour AE, Keshavarzi NR, et al: Revision total hip arthroplasty in octogenarians: a case-control study. J Bone Joint Surg Am 89:2612–2618, 2007.
12. Roche JJW, Wenn RT, Sahota O, Moran CG: Effect of comorbidities and postoperative complications on mortality after hip fracture in elderly people: prospective observational cohort study. BMJ 331:1374–1379, 2005.
13. Cohen MM, Duncan PG, Tate RB: Does anesthesia contribute to operative mortality? JAMA 260:2859–2863, 1998.
14. Dorman T, Clarkson K, Rosenfeld B, et al: Effects of clonidine on prolonged postoperative sympathetic response. Crit Care Med 25:1147–1152, 1997.
15. Andres BM, Taub DD, Gurkan I, Wenz JF: Postoperative fever after total knee arthroplasty: the role of cytokines. Clin Orthop Relat Res 415:221–231, 2003.
16. Weissman C: Chapter 95: Nutrition and metabolic control. In Miller RD (ed): Miller's anesthesia, ed 7, Philadelphia, Pa, 2009, Churchill Livingstone.
17. Pasternak LR, Arens JF, Caplan RA, et al: Practice advisory for preanesthesia evaluation: a report by the American Society of Anesthesiologists Task Force on Preanesthesia Evaluation. Anesthesiology 96:485–496, 2002.
18. Fleisher LA, Beckman JA, Brown KA, et al: ACC/AHA 2007 guidelines on perioperative cardiovascular evaluation and care for noncardiac surgery: a report of the American College of Cardiology/American Heart Association Task Force on Practice Guidelines. J Am Coll Cardiol 50:e159–e241, 2007.
19. Novack V, Jotkowitz A, Etzion O: Does delay in surgery after hip fracture lead to worse outcomes? A multicenter survey. Int J Qual Health Care 19:170–176, 2007.
20. Sircar P, Godkar D, Mahgerefteh S, et al: Morbidity and mortality among patients with hip fractures surgically repaired within and after 48 hours. Am J Ther 14:508–513, 2007.
21. Radcliff TA, Henderson WG, Stoner TJ, et al: Patient risk factors, operative care, and outcomes among older community-dwelling male veterans with hip fracture. J Bone Joint Surg Am 90:34–42, 2008.
22. Moran CG, Wenn RT, Sikand M, Taylor AM: Early mortality after hip fracture: is delay before surgery important? J Bone Joint Surg Am 87:483–489, 2005.
23. Smektala R, Endres HG, Dasch B, et al: The effect of time-to-surgery on outcome in elderly patients with proximal femoral fractures. BMC Musculoskel Disord 9:171, 2008.
24. Majumdar SR, Beaupre LA, Johnston DWC, et al: Lack of association between mortality and timing of surgical fixation in elderly patients with hip fracture: results of a retrospective population-based cohort study. Med Care 44:552–559, 2006.
25. Grimes JP, Gregory PM, Noveck H, et al: The effects of time-to-surgery on mortality and morbidity in patients following hip surgery. Am J Med 112:702–709, 2002.
26. Schultz HJ, et al: PAME (Pre-Anesthetic Medical Evaluation), 1999-2000 Mayo Clinic Department of Internal Medicine orientation manual, Rochester, Minn, 1999, Mayo Graduate School of Medicine, Mayo Press.
27. Lindstrom D, Sadr Azodi O, Wladis A, et al: Effects of a perioperative smoking cessation intervention on postoperative complications: a randomized trial. Ann Surg 248:739–745, 2008.
28. Moller AM, Villebro N, Pedersen T, Tønnesen H: Effect of preoperative smoking intervention on postoperative complications: a randomised clinical trial. Lancet 359:114–117, 2002.
29. Sadr Azodi O, Bellocco R, Eriksson K, Adami J: The impact of tobacco use and body mass index on the length of stay in hospital and the risk of postoperative complications among patients undergoing total hip replacement. J Bone Joint Surg Br 88:1316–1320, 2006.
30. Poirier P, Alpert MA, Fleisher LA, et al: Cardiovascular evaluation and management of severely obese patients undergoing surgery: a science advisory from the American Heart Association. Circulation 120:86–95, 2009.
31. Andrew JG, Palan J, Kurup HV. et al: Obesity in total hip replacement. J Bone Joint Surg Br 90:424–429, 2009.
32. Mercado DL, Petty BG: Perioperative medication management. Med Clin N Am 87:41–57, 2003.
33. Cohn SL, Macpherson DS: Chapter 7A: Perioperative medication management. In Cohn SL, Smetana GW, Weed HG (eds): Perioperative medicine: just the facts, New York, NY, 2006, McGraw-Hill.
34. Smetana GW, Macpherson DS: The case against routine preoperative laboratory testing. Med Clin N Am 87:7–40, 2003.
35. Gibbs J, Cull W, Henderson W, et al: Preoperative serum albumin level as a predictor of operative mortality and morbidity: results from the National VA Surgical Risk Study. Arch Surg 134:36–42, 1999.
36. Avenell A, Handoll HHG: Nutritional supplementation for hip fracture aftercare in older people. Cochrane Database Syst Rev (3):CD001880, 2009.
37. Qaseem A, Snow V, Fitterman N, et al: Risk assessment for and strategies to reduce perioperative pulmonary complications for patients undergoing noncardiothoracic surgery: a guideline from the American College of Physicians. Ann Intern Med 144:575–580, 2006.
38. Grant PJ, Wesorick DH: Perioperative medicine for the hospitalized patient. Med Clin N Am 92:325–348, 2008.
39. Neva MH, Häkkinen A, Mäkinen H, et al: High prevalence of asymptomatic cervical spine subluxation in patients with rheumatoid arthritis waiting for orthopaedic surgery. Ann Rheum Dis 65:884–888, 2006.
40. Memtsoudis SG, Rosenberger P, Walz JM: Critical care issues in the patient after major joint replacement. J Intensive Care Med 22:92–104, 2007.
41. Bhattacharyya T, Iorio R, Healy WL: Rate of and risk factors for acute inpatient mortality after orthopaedic surgery. J Bone Joint Surg Am 84:562–572, 2002.
42. Maxwell MJ, Moran CG, Moppett IK: Development and validation of a preoperative scoring system to predict 30 day mortality in patients undergoing hip fracture surgery. Br J Anaesth 101:511–517, 2008.
43. Shamsuddin A: Chapter 1: Ischemic heart disease. In Hines EL, Marschall KE (eds): Stoelting's anesthesia and co-existing disease, ed 5, Philadelphia, 2008, Churchill Livingstone.
44. Matot I, Oppenheim-Eden A, Ratrot R, et al: Preoperative cardiac events in elderly patients with hip fracture randomized to epidural or conventional analgesia. Anesthesiology 98:156–163, 2003.

45. Smetana GW, Lawrence VA, Cornell JE: Preoperative pulmonary risk stratification for noncardiothoracic surgery: systematic review for the American College of Physicians. Ann Intern Med 144:581–595, 2006.
46. Asai T: Editorial II. Who is at increased risk of pulmonary aspiration? Brit J Anaesth 93:497–500, 2004.
47. Sakai T, Planinsic RM, Quinlan JJ, et al: The incidence and outcome of perioperative pulmonary aspiration in a university hospital: a 4-year retrospective analysis. Anesth Analg 103:941–947, 2006.
48. Gross JB, et al: Practice guidelines for perioperative management of patients with obstructive sleep apnea. Anesthesiology 104:1081–1093, 2006.
49. Pien LC, Grammer LC, Patterson R: Minimal complications in a surgical population with severe asthma receiving prophylactic corticosteroids. J Allergy Clin Immunol 82:696–700, 1988.
50. Ballantyne JC, Carr DB, deFerranti S, et al: The comparative effects of postoperative analgesic therapies on pulmonary outcome: cumulative meta-analysis of randomized, controlled trials. Anesth Analg 86:598–612, 1998.
51. Gan TJ: Risk factors for postoperative nausea and vomiting. Anesth Analg 102:1884–1898, 2006.
52. Gan TJ: Postoperative nausea and vomiting—can it be eliminated? JAMA 287:1233–1236, 2002.
53. Artinyan A, Nunoo-Mensah JW, Balasubramaniam S, et al: Prolonged postoperative ileus—definition, risk factors, and predictors after surgery. World J Surg 32:1495–1500, 2008.
54. Senagore AJ: Pathogenesis and clinical and economic consequences of postoperative ileus. Am J Health-System Pharm 64:S3–S7, 2007.
55. Nelson JD, Urban JA, Salsbury TA, et al: Acute colonic pseudo-obstruction (Ogilvie syndrome) after arthroplasty in the lower extremity. J Bone Joint Surg Am 88:604–610, 2006.
56. Petrisor BA, Petruccelli DT, Winemaker MJ, de Beer JV: Acute colonic pseudo-obstruction after elective total joint arthroplasty. J Arthroplasty 16:1043–1047, 2001.
57. Marschall KE: Chapter 11: Diseases of the biliary tract and liver. In Hines EL, Marschall KE (eds): Stoelting's anesthesia and co-existing disease, ed 5, Philadelphia, 2008, Churchill Livingstone.
58. Moon YW, Kim YS, Kwon SY, et al: Perioperative risk of hip arthroplasty in patients with cirrhotic liver disease. J Korean Med Sci 22:223–226, 2007.
59. Hsieh PH, Chen LH, Lee MS, et al: Hip arthroplasty in patients with cirrhosis of the liver. J Bone Joint Surg Br 85:818–821, 2003.
60. Carlisle JB, Stevenson CA: Drugs for preventing postoperative nausea and vomiting. Cochrane Database Syst Rev (3): CD004125, 2006.
61. Bergeron SG, Kardash KJ, Huk OL, et al: Perioperative dexamethasone does not affect functional outcome in total hip arthroplasty. Clin Orthop Related Res 467:1463–1467, 2009.
62. White PF, O'Hara JF, Roberson CR, et al: The impact of current antiemetic practices on patient outcomes: a prospective study on high-risk patients. POST-OP Study Group. Anesth Analg 107:452–458, 2008.
63. Lee A, Fan LT: Stimulation of the wrist acupuncture point P6 for preventing postoperative nausea and vomiting. Cochrane Database Syst Rev (2):CD003281, 2009.
64. Iorio R, Whang W, Healy WL, et al: The utility of bladder catheterization in total hip arthroplasty. Clin Orthop Relat Res 432:148–152, 2005.
65. Maki DG, Tambyah PA: Engineering out the risk for infection with urinary catheters. Emerg Infect Dis 7:342–347, 2001.
66. Tambyah PA, Maki DG: Catheter-associated urinary tract infection is rarely symptomatic: a prospective study of 1,497 catheterized patients. Arch Intern Med 160:678–682, 2000.
67. Hooten TM, Bradley SF, Cardenas DD, et al: Diagnosis, prevention, and treatment of catheter-associated urinary tract infection in adults: 2009 international clinical practice guidelines from the Infectious Diseases Society of America. Clin Infect Dis 50:625–663, 2010.
68. Koulouvaris P, Sculco P, Finerty E, et al: Relationship between perioperative urinary tract infection and deep infection

after joint arthroplasty. Clin Orthop Relat Res 467:1859–1867, 2009.
69. Hedström M, Gröndal L, Ahl T: Urinary tract infection in patients with hip fractures. Injury 30:341–343, 1999.
70. Baldini G, Bagry H, Aprikian A, Carli F: Postoperative urinary retention: anesthetic and perioperative considerations. Anesthesiology 110:1139–1157, 2009.
71. David TS, Vrahas MS: Perioperative lower urinary tract infections and deep sepsis in patients undergoing total joint arthroplasty. J Am Acad Orthop Surg 8:66–74, 2000.
72. Hanssen AD, Osmon DR, Nelson CL: Patients with difficulties related to the urinary tract should be identified and managed before total joint arthroplasty. Instructional Course Lectures, The American Academy of Orthopaedic Surgeons, Prevention of Deep Periprosthetic Joint Infection. J Bone Joint Surg Am 78:458–471, 1996.
73. Nicolle LE, Bradley S, Colgan R, et al: Infectious Diseases Society of America guidelines for the diagnosis and treatment of asymptomatic bacteriuria in adults. Clin Infect Dis 40:643–654, 2005.
74. Pfefferkorn U, Sanlav L, Moldenhauer J, et al: Antibiotic prophylaxis at urinary catheter removal prevents urinary tract infections: a prospective randomized trial. Ann Surg 249:573–575, 2009.
75. Bihorac A, Yavas S, Subbiah S, et al: Long-term risk of mortality and acute kidney injury during hospitalization after major surgery. Ann Surg 249:851–858, 2009.
76. Mahon P, Shorten G: Perioperative acute renal failure. Curr Opin Anaesthesiol 19:332–338, 2006.
77. Kheterpal S, Tremper KK, Englesbe MJ, et al: Predictors of postoperative acute renal failure after noncardiac surgery in patients with previously normal renal function. Anesthesiology 107:892–902, 2007.
78. Kheterpal S, Tremper KK, Heung M, et al: Development and validation of an acute kidney injury risk index for patients undergoing general surgery: results from a national data set. Anesthesiology 110:505–515, 2009.
79. Karkouti K, Wijeysundera DN, Yau TM, et al: Acute kidney injury after cardiac surgery: focus on modifiable risk factors. Circulation 119:495–502, 2009.
80. Sear JW: Kidney dysfunction in the postoperative period. Brit J Anaesth 95:20–32, 2005.
81. Robertson BD, Robertson TJ: Postoperative delirium after hip fracture. J Bone Joint Surg Am 88:2060–2068, 2006.
82. Bagri AS, Rico A, Ruiz JG: Evaluation and management of the elderly patient at risk for postoperative delirium. Clin Geriatr Med 24:667–686, 2008.
83. Edelstein DM, Aharonoff GB, Karp A, et al: Effect of postoperative delirium on outcome after hip fracture. Clin Orthop Relat Res 422:195–200, 2004.
84. Litaker D, Locala J, Franco K, et al: Preoperative risk factors for postoperative delirium. Gen Hosp Psychiatry 23:84–89, 2001.
85. Rolfson O, Dahlberg LE, Nilsson JÅ, et al: Variables determining outcome in total hip replacement surgery. J Bone Joint Surg Br 91:157–161, 2009.
86. Tønnesen H, Petersen KP, Højgaard L, et al: Postoperative morbidity among symptom-free alcohol misusers. Lancet 340:334–337, 1992.
87. Inouye SK, Van Dyck CH, Horwitz RI, et al: Clarifying confusion: the Confusion Assessment Method. Ann Intern Med 113:941–948, 1990.
88. Marcantonio ER, Flacker JM, Wright RJ, Resnick NM: Reducing delirium after hip fracture: a randomized trial. J Am Geriatr Soc 49:516–522, 2001.
89. Kalisvaart KJ, de Jonghe JF, Bogaards MJ, et al: Haloperidol prophylaxis for elderly hip-surgery patients at risk for delirium: a randomized placebo-controlled study. J Am Geriatr Soc 53:1658–1666, 2005.
90. Parvizi J, Mui A, Purtill JJ, et al: Total joint arthroplasty: when do fatal or near-fatal complications occur? J Bone Joint Surg Am 89:27–32, 2007.
91. Chobanian AV, Bakris GL, Black HR, et al, and the National High Blood Pressure Education Program Coordinating Committee: Seventh report of the Joint National Committee on

Prevention, Detection, Evaluation, and Treatment of High Blood Pressure. JAMA 42:1206–1252, 2003.

92. Marik PE, Varon J: Perioperative hypertension: a review of current and emerging therapeutic agents. J Clin Anesth 21:220–229, 2009.

93. Bone RC, Balk RA, Cerra FB, et al: Definitions for sepsis and organ failure and guidelines for the use of innovative therapies in sepsis. The ACCP/SCCM Consensus Conference Committee. American College of Chest Physicians/Society of Critical Care Medicine. Chest 101:1644–1655, 1992.

94. Subramanian S, Ziedalski TM: Oliguria, volume overload, Na+ balance, and diuretics. Crit Care Clin 21:291–303, 2005.

95. Bellomo R, Ronco C, Kellum JA, et al: Acute renal failure—definition, outcome measures, animal models, fluid therapy and information technology needs: the Second International Consensus Conference of the Acute Dialysis Quality Initiative (ADQI) Group. Crit Care 8:R204–R212, 2004.

96. Stevens E: Bladder ultrasound: avoiding unnecessary catheterizations. MEDSURG Nursing 14:249–253, 2005.

97. Curtis JM, Sternhagen V, Batts D: Acute renal failure after placement of tobramycin-impregnated bone cement in an infected total knee arthroplasty. Pharmacotherapy 25:876–880, 2005.

98. Bitsch MS, Foss NB, Kristensen BB, et al: Pathogenesis of and management strategies for postoperative delirium after hip fracture: a review. Acta Orthop Scand 75:378–389, 2004.

99. Meagher DJ: Delirium: optimising management. BMJ 322:144–149, 2001.

100. de Jonghe JFM, Kalisvaart KJ, Dijkstra M, et al: Early symptoms in the prodromal phase of delirium: a prospective cohort study in elderly patients undergoing hip surgery. Am J Geriatr Psych 15:112–121, 2007.

101. Lisabeth LD, Brown DL, Hughes R, et al: Acute stroke symptoms: comparing women and men. Stroke 40:2031–2036, 2009.

102. Mantilla CB, Horlocker TT, Schroeder DR, et al: Frequency of myocardial infarction, pulmonary embolism, deep venous thrombosis, and death following primary hip or knee arthroplasty. Anesthesiology 96:1140–1146, 2002.

103. Lawrence VA, Hilsenbeck SG, Noveck H, et al: Medical complications and outcomes after hip fracture repair. Arch Intern Med 162:2053–2057, 2002.

104. Geerts WH, Bergqvist D, Pineo GF, et al: Prevention of venous thromboembolism. American College of Chest Physicians Evidence-Based Clinical Practice Guidelines (8th edition). Chest 133:381S–453S, 2008.

105. Swap CJ, Nagurney JT: Value and limitations of chest pain history in the evaluation of patients with suspected acute coronary syndromes. JAMA 294:2623–2629, 2005.

106. Livingston EH, Passaro EP: Postoperative ileus. Dig Dis Sci 35:121–131, 1990.

107. DeGiorgio R, Knowles CH: Acute colonic pseudo-obstruction. Brit J Surg 96:229–239, 2009.

108. Asao T, Kuwano H, Nakamura J, et al: Gum chewing enhances early recovery from postoperative ileus after laparoscopic colectomy. J Am Coll Surg 195:30–32, 2002.

109. Le Blanc-Louvry I, Costaglioli B, Boulon C, et al: Does mechanical massage of the abdominal wall after colectomy reduce postoperative pain and shorten the duration of ileus? Results of a randomized study. J Gastrointest Surg 6:43–49, 2002.

110. Cheatham ML, Chapman WC, Key SP, Sawyers JL: A meta-analysis of selective versus routine nasogastric decompression after elective laparotomy. Ann Surg 221:469–478, 1995.

111. Luckey A, Livingston E, Tache Y: Mechanisms and treatment of postoperative ileus. Arch Surg 138:206–214, 2003.

112. Shaw JA, Chung R: Febrile response after knee and hip arthroplasty. Clin Orthop Relat Res 367:181–189, 1999.

113. Pile JC, Weed HG: Chapter 50: Fever. In Cohn SL, Smetana GW, Weed HG (eds): Perioperative medicine: just the facts, New York, NY, 2006, McGraw-Hill.

114. Juul AB, Wetterslev J, Gluud C, et al, DIPOM Trial Group: Effect of perioperative beta blockade in patients with diabetes undergoing major non-cardiac surgery: randomised placebo controlled, blinded multicentre trial. BMJ 332:1482, 2006.

115. Yang H, Raymer K, Butler R, et al: The effects of perioperative beta-blockade: results of the Metoprolol after Vascular Surgery (MaVS) study, a randomized controlled trial. Am Heart J 152:983–990, 2006.

116. Brady AR, Gibbs JS, Greenhalgh RM, et al, POBBLE Trial Investigators: Perioperative beta-blockade (POBBLE) for patients undergoing infrarenal vascular surgery: results of a randomized double-blind controlled trial. J Vasc Surg 41:602–609, 2005.

117. Devereaux PJ, Yang H, Yusuf S, et al, for the POISE Study Group: Effects of extended-release metoprolol succinate in patients undergoing non-cardiac surgery (POISE trial): a randomised controlled trial. The Lancet 371:1839–1847, 2008.

118. Dunkelgrun M, Boersma E, Schouten O, et al, for The Dutch Echocardiographic Cardiac Risk Evaluation Applying Stress Echocardiography Study Group. Bisoprolol and fluvastatin for the reduction of perioperative cardiac mortality and myocardial infarction in intermediate-risk patients undergoing noncardiovascular surgery: a randomized controlled trial (DECREASE-IV). Ann Surg 249:921–926, 2009.

119. Fleischmann KE, Beckman JA, Buller CE, et al: 2009 ACCF/AHA focused update on perioperative beta blockade. J Am Coll Cardiol 54:1–29, 2009.

120. Lindenauer PK, Pekow P, Wang K, et al: Perioperative beta-blocker therapy and mortality after major noncardiac surgery. N Engl J Med 353:349–361, 2005.

FURTHER READING

Cohn SL, Smetana GW, Weed HG (eds): Perioperative medicine: just the facts, New York, 2006, McGraw-Hill.
Excellent and concise reference for perioperative medical management.

Hines RL, Marschall KE (eds): Stoelting's anesthesia and co-existing disease, ed 5, Philadelphia,, 2008, Saunders Elsevier.
Disease-specific perioperative management from the anesthesia perspective.

Marshall SA, Ruedy J: On call: principles and protocols, ed 4, Philadelphia, 2004, Saunders.
Concise reference for on-call house physicians for evaluating and treating common emergencies.

Wachter RM, Goldman L, Hollander H (eds): Hospital medicine, ed 2, Philadelphia, 2005, Lippincott Williams & Williams.
Standard reference textbooks for hospitalists that include sections on perioperative medical management.

Williams MV (ed): Comprehensive hospital medicine: an evidence-based approach, Philadelphia, 2007. Saunders Elsevier.
Standard reference textbooks for hospitalists that include sections on perioperative medical management.

CHAPTER 27

Perioperative Pain Management

Terese T. Horlocker and Sandra L. Kopp

KEY POINTS

- Multimodal analgesia, including regional blockade and nonopioid medication, reduces opioid requirements and side effects.
- Lumbar plexus blockade is superior to neuraxial analgesia for patients undergoing major hip surgery.
- Psoas compartment block provides anesthesia/analgesia to the complete lumbar plexus.
- Femoral and fascia iliacus techniques consistently block the femoral nerve, but unreliably block the lateral femoral cutaneous and obturator nerves.
- Deep venous thrombosis (DVT) chemoprophylaxis may affect management of peripheral and neuraxial catheters.

INTRODUCTION

Pain after major hip surgery is severe. Failure to provide adequate analgesia impedes aggressive physical therapy and rehabilitation and potentially delays hospital dismissal. Traditionally, postoperative analgesia following total joint replacement was provided by intravenous patient-controlled analgesia (PCA) or epidural analgesia. However, each technique has distinct advantages and disadvantages. For example, opioids do not consistently provide adequate pain relief and often cause sedation, constipation, nausea/vomiting, and pruritus. Epidural infusions containing local anesthetics (with or without an opioid) provide superior analgesia but are associated with hypotension, urinary retention, motor block–limiting ambulation, and spinal hematoma secondary to anticoagulation.[1] Single-dose and continuous peripheral nerve techniques that block the lumbar plexus (fascia iliaca, femoral, psoas compartment blocks) with/without sciatic nerve blockade have been used with success for total hip replacement patients.[1-4] Appreciation of the indications, benefits, and side effects associated with both conventional and novel analgesic approaches is paramount in maximizing rehabilitative efforts and improving patient satisfaction. This chapter will discuss the analgesic techniques unique to patients undergoing hip surgery, with a focus on those undergoing primary total or revision total hip arthroplasty.

MULTIMODAL ANALGESIA

Multimodal analgesia is a multidisciplinary approach to pain management, with the aim of maximizing the positive aspects of treatment while limiting associated side effects. Because many of the negative side effects of analgesic therapy are opioid related (and dose dependent), limiting perioperative opioid use is a major principle of multimodal analgesia. Anti-inflammatory medications and acetaminophen are valuable adjuvants to systemic opioids. The addition of nonopioid analgesics reduces opioid use, improves analgesia, and decreases opioid-related side effects. The use of peripheral or neuraxial regional anesthetic techniques and a combination of opioid and nonopioid analgesic agents for breakthrough pain results in superior pain control, attenuation of the stress response, and decreased opioid requirements.

SYSTEMIC ANALGESICS

Opioid Analgesics

Adequate analgesia achieved with systemic opioids is frequently associated with side effects, including sedation, nausea, and pruritus. However, despite these well-defined side effects, opioid analgesics remain an integral component of postoperative pain relief. Systemic opioids may be administered by intravenous, intramuscular, and oral routes. Current analgesic regimens typically employ intravenous PCA for 24 to 48 hours postoperatively, with subsequent conversion to oral agents. The PCA device may be programmed for several variables, including bolus dose, lockout interval, and background infusion (Table 27-1). The optimal bolus dose is determined by the relative potency of the opioid; insufficient dosing results in inadequate analgesia, whereas excessive dosing increases the potential for side effects, including respiratory depression. Likewise, the lockout interval is based on the onset of analgesic effects; too short of a lockout interval allows the patient to self-administer additional medication before achieving the full analgesic effect (and may result in accumulation/overdose of the opioid). A prolonged lockout interval will not allow adequate analgesia. The optimal bolus dose and lockout interval are not known, but ranges have been determined. Varying settings

Table 27-1. Intravenous Opioids for Patient-Controlled Analgesia

Agent	Bolus	Lockout Interval	Four-Hour Maximum Dose	Infusion Rate*
Fentanyl, 10 mcg/mL	10-20 mcg	5-10 min	300 mcg	20-100 mcg/hr
Hydromorphone (Dilaudid), 0.2 mg/mL	0.1-0.2 mg	5-10 min	3 mg	0.1-0.2 mg/hr
Morphine sulfate, 1 mg/mL	0.5-2.5 mg	5-10 min	30 mg	1-10 mg/hr

*A background infusion rate is not recommended for opioid-naive patients.
From Lennon RL, Horlocker T: Mayo Clinic analgesic pathway: peripheral nerve blockade for major orthopedic surgery, Rochester, Minn, 2006, Mayo Clinic Scientific Press, Table 1, p 109, with permission.

within these ranges appears to have little effect on analgesia or side effects. Although most PCA devices allow the addition of a background infusion, routine use in adult opioid-naive patients is not recommended; however, a background opioid infusion may have a role in the treatment of opioid-tolerant patients. Because of variation in patient pain tolerance, PCA dosing regimens may have to be adjusted to maximize the benefits and minimize the incidence of side effects.

Adverse effects of opioid administration can cause serious complications in patients undergoing major orthopedic procedures. In a systematic review, Wheeler and associates[5] reported gastrointestinal issues (nausea, vomiting, ileus) in 37%, cognitive effects (somnolence and dizziness) in 34%, pruritus in 15%, urinary retention in 16%, and respiratory depression in 2% of patients receiving PCA opioid analgesia.

Oral opioids (Table 27-2) are available in immediate-release and controlled-release formulations. Although immediate-release oral opioids are effective in relieving moderate to severe pain, they must be administered as often as every 4 hours. When these medications are prescribed "as needed" (prn), there may be a delay in administration and a subsequent increase in pain. Furthermore, interruption of the dosing schedule, particularly during the night, may lead to an increase in the patient's pain. Adverse effects of oral opioid administration are considerably less compared with those of intravenous administration and are mainly gastrointestinal in nature.[5]

A controlled-release formulation of oxycodone (Oxy-Contin) has been shown to provide therapeutic opioid concentrations and sustained pain relief over an extended time period. Combined with prn oxycodone for breakthrough pain, scheduled administration of controlled-release oxycodone maximizes the analgesia and decreases associated side effects. However, because pain decreases substantially over the first 24 to 36 hours, sustained-release formulations should be limited to the early postoperative period in most cases.

Tramadol (Ultram) is a centrally acting analgesic that is structurally related to morphine and codeine (but is not truly an opioid). Its analgesic effect is manifest through binding to the opioid receptors and blocking the reuptake of both norepinephrine and serotonin. Tramadol should be used with caution in patients taking certain antidepressant medications (e.g., selective serotonin reuptake inhibitors) affecting the levels of these two neurotransmitters. Tramadol has gained popularity because of the low incidence of adverse effects, specifically, respiratory depression, constipation, and abuse potential. Thus, tramadol may be used as an alternative to opioids in a multimodal approach to postoperative pain, specifically in patients who are intolerant to opioid analgesics.

Nonopioid Analgesics (Acetaminophen and Nonsteroidal Anti-Inflammatory Drugs)

The addition of nonopioid analgesics reduces opioid use, improves analgesia, and decreases opioid-related side effects. The multimodal effect is maximized through selection of analgesics that have complementary sites of action. For example, acetaminophen acts predominantly centrally, while other nonsteroidal anti-inflammatory drugs (NSAIDs) exert their effects peripherally.

The mechanism of analgesic action of acetaminophen has not been fully determined. Acetaminophen may act predominantly by inhibiting prostaglandin synthesis in the central nervous system. Acetaminophen has very few adverse effects and is an important addition to the multimodal postoperative pain regimen, although the total daily dose must be limited to 4000 mg. It is important to note that many oral analgesics are an opioid-acetaminophen combination. In these preparations, the total dose of opioid will be restricted to the acetaminophen ingested.

NSAIDs have a mechanism of action through the cyclooxygenase (COX) enzymatic pathway and ultimately block two individual prostaglandin pathways. The COX-1 pathway is involved in prostaglandin E_2–mediated gastric mucosal protection and thromboxane effects on coagulation. The inducible COX-2 pathway is mainly involved in the generation of prostaglandins included in the modulation of pain and fever but has no effect on platelet function or the coagulation system. In general, NSAIDs block both COX-1 and COX-2 pathways. Traditionally, NSAIDs have been viewed as peripherally acting agents. However, a central analgesic effect may occur through inhibition of spinal COX.

The introduction of specific COX-2 inhibitors represented a breakthrough in the treatment of pain and inflammation. However, despite their efficacy, two (rofecoxib [Vioxx]; valdecoxib [Bextra]) of three COX-2 inhibitors were voluntarily removed from general use because of an increased relative risk for confirmed

Table 27-2. Oral Analgesics

Drug	Analgesic Dose	Dosing Interval	Maximum Daily Dose	Comments
Acetaminophen	500-1000 mg PO	q 4-6 h	4000 mg	As effective as aspirin; 1000 mg more effective than 650 mg in some patients
Nonsteroidal Anti-Inflammatory Drugs				
Celecoxib (Celebrex)	400 mg initially, then 200 mg PO	q 12 h		Celecoxib is the only cyclooxygenase (COX)-2 inhibitor available in North America. Valdecoxib and rofecoxib were removed from general use because of concerns regarding cardiovascular risk.
Aspirin	325-1000 mg PO	q 4-6 h	4000 mg	Most potent antiplatelet effect
Ibuprofen (Advil, Motrin, Nuprin, others)	200-400 mg PO	q 4-6 h	3200 mg	200 mg equal to 650 mg of aspirin or acetaminophen
Naproxen (Aleve, Naprosyn, others)	500 mg PO	q 12 h	1000 mg	250 mg equal to 650 mg of aspirin, but with longer duration
Ketorolac (Toradol)	15-30 mg IM/IV	q 4-6 h	60 mg (>65 years); 120 mg (<65 years)	Comparable with 10 mg morphine; reduce dose in patients <50 kg or with renal impairment; total duration of administration is 5 days
Opioids				
Extended-release oxycodone (OxyContin)	10-20 mg PO	q 12 h		Limit to total of four doses to avoid accumulation and opioid-related side effects
Extended-release morphine (MS Contin)	15-30 mg PO	q 8-12 h		Limit to total of four doses to avoid accumulation and opioid-related side effects
Oxycodone (Roxicodone)	5-10 mg PO	q 4-6 h		Combination products* of oxycodone/acetaminophen (Percocet, Tylox) and oxycodone/aspirin (Percodan) are also available.
Hydromorphone (Dilaudid)	2-4 mg PO	q 4-6 h		Also available as Dilaudid suppository (3 mg) with effect of 6 to 8 hours
Hydrocodone (Lortab, Vicodin, Zydone)	5-10 mg PO	q 4-6 h		All preparations contain acetaminophen.*
Codeine	30-60 mg PO	q 4 h		Combination products* of codeine/acetaminophen (Tylenol #2, Tylenol #3, Tylenol #4) and codeine/aspirin (Empirin with codeine) are also available.
Propoxyphene (Darvon)	50-100 mg PO	q 4-6 h	600 mg propoxyphene	Combination products* of propoxyphene/acetaminophen (Darvocet, Propoxacet, Tylenol #4) and propoxyphene/aspirin are also available.
Tramadol (Ultram)	50-100 mg PO	q 6 h	400 mg; less in cases of renal or hepatic disease	Combination product of tramadol/acetaminophen (Ultracet) is also available.

*Dose in combination products limited by total acetaminophen or aspirin ingestion.[54]
IM, Intramuscularly; *IV,* intravenously; *PO,* orally.
From Lennon RL, Horlocker T: Mayo Clinic analgesic pathway: peripheral nerve blockade for major orthopedic surgery, Rochester, Minn, 2006, Mayo Clinic Scientific Press, Table 2, pp 110–111, with permission.

cardiovascular events, such as heart attack and stroke, after 18 months of treatment. Celecoxib (Celebrex) is currently the only COX-2 inhibitor available in the United States, although the Food and Drug Administration (FDA) has requested that safety information be included regarding potential cardiovascular and gastrointestinal risks of all selective and nonselective NSAIDs *except* aspirin.*

Although numerous NSAIDs have been used in the perioperative management of pain, ketorolac is the only NSAID that can be given parenterally. An intravenous dose of ketorolac 10 to 30 mg was found to have similar efficacy to 10 to 12 mg of intravenous morphine. In surgical patients, ketorolac reduces opioid consumption by 36%. Because of the potential for serious side effects, ketorolac should be used for 5 or fewer days in the adult population with moderate to severe acute pain.[6]

Major side effects limiting NSAID use to postoperative pain control (renal failure, platelet dysfunction, and gastric ulcers or bleeding) are related to nonspecific

*FDA Public Health Advisory. The FDA announces important changes and additional warnings for COX-2 selective and nonselective NSAIDs (http://www.fda.gov/cder/drug/advisory/COX2.htm, April 7, 2005).

inhibition of the COX-1 enzyme.[6] Advantages of COX-2 inhibitors include lack of platelet inhibition and a decreased incidence of gastrointestinal effects. All NSAIDs have the potential to cause serious renal impairment. Inhibition of the COX enzyme may have only minor effects in the healthy kidney, but unfortunately can lead to serious side effects in elderly patients and those with a low-volume condition (blood loss, dehydration, cirrhosis, or heart failure). Therefore, NSAIDs should be used cautiously in patients with underlying renal dysfunction, specifically in the setting of volume depletion due to blood loss.[6] Similar to the COX-2 inhibitors, NSAIDs interfere with the inhibitory COX-1 effect of aspirin on platelet activity and may counter its cardioprotective effects.[7]

The effects of NSAIDs on bone formation and healing are of concern to the orthopedic population. Although data are conflicting, evidence from animal studies suggests that COX-2 inhibitors may inhibit bone healing.[8] Thus, adverse effects of COX-2 inhibitors must be weighed against the benefits. Until definitive human trials are performed, it is reasonable to be cautious with the use of COX-2 inhibitors, especially when bone healing is critical.

NEURAXIAL ANALGESIA

A variety of single-dose and continuous infusion neuraxial techniques may be performed to provide analgesia following major hip surgery. A single dose of neuraxial opioid may be efficacious as a sole analgesic agent for moderate pain of limited duration, such as that associated with primary hip arthroplasty.[9] However, the prolonged moderate to severe pain associated with revision arthroplasty typically necessitates supplemental oral or intravenous analgesic agents or a continuous neuraxial infusion.

SINGLE-DOSE SPINAL AND EPIDURAL OPIOIDS

Neuraxial opioids provide superior analgesia compared with systemic opioids. The onset and duration of neuraxial opioids are determined by the lipophilicity of the drug. For example, lipophilic opioids, such as fentanyl, provide a rapid onset of analgesia, limited spread within the cerebrospinal fluid (and less respiratory depression), and rapid clearance/resolution. Conversely, hydrophilic opioids, including morphine and hydromorphone, have a longer duration of action but are associated with a higher frequency of side effects such as pruritus, nausea and vomiting, and delayed respiratory depression (Table 27-3). A new sustained-release formulation of epidural morphine (Depodur) has been released. Limited information exists regarding its efficacy following orthopedic surgery.[10] The analgesic effect is present for approximately 48 hours. Unfortunately, Depodur is not to be administered in the presence of local anesthetics (i.e., an epidural anesthetic may not be converted to provide epidural analgesia). It is important to note that the central side effects of opioid administration are much more common (and more prolonged) following neuraxial administration than with all other routes. For example, in a large series, the frequency of pruritus, nausea and vomiting, and respiratory depression was 37%, 25%, and 3% with an intrathecal morphine injection.[11] Therefore, patients who exhibit sensitivity to an opioid when administered systemically should not receive that opioid neuraxially.

EPIDURAL ANALGESIA

Epidural analgesia may consist of an opioid, a local anesthetic, or a combination local anesthetic–opioid infusion (see Table 27-3). The combination of a local anesthetic–opioid creates a synergistic analgesic effect and allows a lower concentration of each component of the solution. For example, without an opioid adjuvant, the concentration of a local anesthetic solution may be sufficiently high to result in a dense sensory and motor block; the patient may be unable to ambulate or void.[12] Likewise, a pure opioid epidural infusion may not provide adequate analgesia.[13] As a result, most epidural solutions consist of dilute concentrations of both local anesthetic and opioid. Use of this combination results in superior analgesia, minimal sensory and motor block (allowing ambulation and mobilization), and a decreased incidence of opioid-related side effects (nausea/vomiting

Table 27-3. Dosing Regimens for Neuraxial Opioids*

| Drug | Single Injection | | | Epidural Continuous Infusion[†] | |
	Intrathecal	Epidural	Duration of Analgesia	Opioid Concentration[‡]	Epidural Infusion Rate
Fentanyl	5-25 mcg	25-100 mcg	2-4 hr	5-10 mcg/mL	40-80 mcg/hr
Hydromorphone	0.04-0.08 mg	0.5-1 mg	12-18 hr	5-10 mcg/mL	0.04-0.08 mg/hr
Morphine (Duramorph)	0.2-0.3 mg	1-5 mg	18-24 hr	100 mcg/mL	400-800 mcg/hr
Extended-Release Epidural Morphine (Depodur)		5-25 mg	48 hr		

*Note units vary across agents for single dosing (mcg, mg).
[†]Epidural solutions for major orthopedic surgery are typically local anesthetics (ropivacaine 0.2% or bupivacaine 0.0625% to 0.125%) with an opioid adjuvant. Only preservative-free solutions may be used.
[‡]The concentration of the opioid is selected to achieve an infusion rate of 6 to 10 mL/hr. Lower infusion rates may not deliver adequate analgesia, and higher infusion rates will be associated with motor block and inability to ambulate.

and pruritus). Although epidural analgesia provides excellent analgesia, the associated risk of spinal hematoma in (anticoagulated) patients with indwelling epidural catheters led to a search for alternative methods of providing postoperative analgesia following major orthopedic surgery.

PERIPHERAL REGIONAL ANESTHETIC TECHNIQUES

Lower extremity peripheral techniques, which allow complete unilateral blockade, have traditionally been underutilized.[14] In part, this is a result of the widespread acceptance and safety of spinal and epidural anesthesia. Furthermore, unlike the brachial plexus, nerves supplying the lower extremity are not anatomically clustered, where they can be easily blocked with a relatively superficial injection of local anesthetic. Because of anatomic considerations, lower extremity blocks are technically more difficult and require more training and practice before expertise is acquired. Many of these blocks were classically performed using paresthesia, loss of resistance, or field block technique; success was variable. Advances in needles, catheters, and nerve stimulator technology have facilitated localization of neural structures and have improved success rates. These blocks are safe and have certain advantages, such as postoperative pain relief and lack of complete sympathectomy, which make them ideal for selected patients. Although single-injection techniques have been used, the duration of effect is not sufficient to result in major improvements in analgesia or outcome.[15,16]

Over the past decade, applications have focused on prolonged postoperative analgesia (with an indwelling catheter) to assist rehabilitation and hospital dismissal.[2,3,17,18] Several studies have demonstrated that unilateral peripheral block provided a quality of analgesia and surgical outcomes similar to those of continuous epidural analgesia, but with fewer side effects.[4] Recent innovations emphasize continuous peripheral nerve blocks with scheduled (acetaminophen and tramadol) and prn (oxycodone) analgesics; no intravenous opioids are administered. In accordance with strict criteria, 90% of patients undergoing *minimally invasive* hip (or knee) replacement using a comprehensive, preemptive, multimodal analgesic regimen emphasizing peripheral nerve block achieved readiness for hospital discharge within 48 hours.[2] When a similar regimen was applied to patients undergoing standard total joint replacement, significantly improved perioperative outcomes were reported, along with fewer adverse events, compared with patients receiving traditional intravenous opioids during the initial postoperative period. Improved perioperative outcomes include a shortened hospital length of stay and a significant reduction in postoperative urinary retention and ileus formation.[19] Finally, because hospital costs appear to be directly related to the length of hospital stay, analgesic techniques associated with improved recovery and reduced complications may decrease total direct medical costs among these patients. The reduction in mean cost is

primarily associated with lower hospital-based (Medicare Part A) costs, with the greatest overall cost difference reported among patients with significant comorbidities.[17] These studies support the movement toward continuous peripheral technique as the optimal analgesic method following total knee and hip arthroplasty.

Protocols used at the Mayo Clinic and other centers with respect to preoperative, intraoperative (pain injection cocktail), and postoperative multimodal pain regimens are shown in Table 27-4. It is important to note that no formal comparison between clinical pathways has been performed. Likewise, critical elements within a given clinical pathway are not easily determined because of the large numbers of component and system adaptations that typically occur during implementation of a new practice model. Institutions proposing to initiate a recovery/rehabilitation pathway should consider the critical concepts of a multimodal approach: limit opioid administration and thereby reduce the frequency/severity of opioid-related side effects (through administration of nonopioid analgesics, performance of regional techniques and local infiltration, and use of other nonpharmacologic therapies such as ice application), and

Table 27-4. Mayo Clinic Total Joint Regional Anesthesia Clinical Pathway	
Preoperative holding area	• Extended-release oxycodone (OxyContin) 20 mg PO for patients <60 years old or 10 mg PO for patients 60-74 years old. Do not administer OxyContin to patients 75 years of age or older. • Celecoxib 400 mg PO • Gabapentin 600 mg PO
Anesthesia procedure room	• Lumbar plexus continuous peripheral nerve catheter • Total knee arthroplasty: femoral continuous nerve catheter • Total hip arthroplasty: posterior lumbar plexus (psoas) continuous nerve catheter • Sciatic nerve blockade (total knee arthroplasty patients)
PACU	• Lumbar plexus continuous peripheral nerve catheter • Bolus 10 mL 0.2% bupivacaine upon arrival in PACU • Begin continuous infusion bupivacaine 0.2% at 10 mL/hr • Oxycodone 5 mg and acetaminophen 500 mg (Tylox) prn VAS ≥4. One capsule for patients 70 years of age or older; two capsules for patients <69 years of age.
Patient care unit	• Ketorolac 15 mg IV q 6 h prn × 4 doses • Acetaminophen 1000 mg PO TID (8 AM, noon, 4 PM) • Oxycodone 5 mg PO q 4 h prn VAS ≥4 (10 mg PO q 4 h prn VAS ≥6) • Lumbar plexus continuous peripheral nerve catheter: change infusion on POD 1 (6 AM) to bupivacaine 0.1% at 12 mL/hr for 24 hours

BID, Twice a day; *IV,* intravenous; *PACU,* postanesthesia care unit; *PO,* per os; *POD,* postoperative day; *prn,* as necessary; *TID,* three times a day; *VAS,* verbal analogue pain score.

adapt them to the institution's practice model. For example, the local anesthetic infusion concentration/infusion rate in patients with peripheral nerve catheters may be adjusted according to the amount of weight bearing desired.

Potential side effects of single-injection and continuous peripheral blocks include nerve injury (which is rare and occurs less frequently than with neuraxial block),[20] bleeding,[21] and infection.[22] In addition, the presence of a lower extremity block may make ambulation difficult and may lead to patient falls.[23] A knee immobilizer is sometimes placed to decrease the risk of quadriceps buckling in the presence of a femoral block.

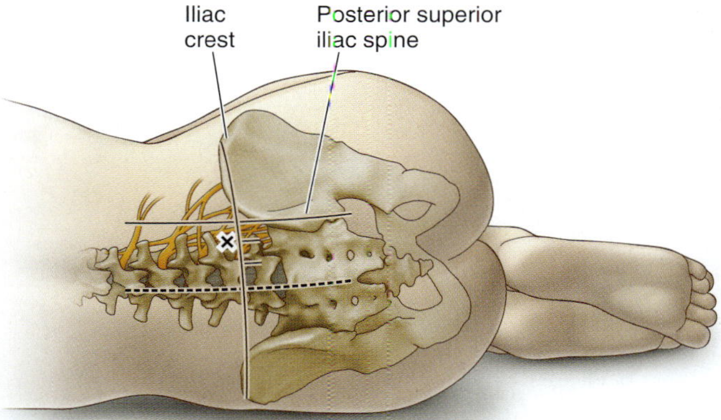

LUMBAR PLEXUS BLOCK

The lumbar plexus may be blocked via three distinct approaches. Block of the full lumbar plexus (femoral, lateral femoral cutaneous, obturator) is accomplished with the psoas block.[14,24,25] In comparison, the fascia iliaca and femoral approaches reliably block the femoral but not the lateral femoral, cutaneous, and/or obturator nerves.[24,25] Selection of regional analgesic technique is dependent on the surgical site (Table 27-5). For example, the psoas compartment approach to the lumbar plexus (Fig. 27-1) is preferable for surgery of the hip because it is the most proximal lumbar plexus technique and provides complete block of the lumbar plexus, and the needle/catheter insertion site is distant from the surgical incision (allowing preoperative placement). However, should a psoas approach be contraindicated because of infection or existing coagulopathy, a more distal femoral (Fig. 27-2) or fascia iliaca (Fig. 27-3) blockade is warranted. It is important to note that the proximity of the

Figure 27-1. Lumbar plexus block: psoas compartment approach. A horizontal line is drawn parallel to the posterior superior iliac spine (PSIS), while a vertical line is drawn at the L4-L5 level. The distance from midline to the PSIS horizontal is divided into thirds, and the junction of the lateral third and the medial two thirds is identified. Needle insertion is 1 cm cephalad to this point. A 10-cm (4-inch) stimulating needle is advanced until the transverse process of L4 is contacted. The needle is redirected caudad and is advanced behind the transverse process. Approximately 2 cm deep to the transverse process, the lumbar plexus is identified (through elicitation of a quadriceps motor response), and 25 mL of local anesthetic is injected incrementally. (Redrawn from Lennon RL, Horlocker T: Mayo Clinic analgesic pathway: peripheral nerve blockade for major orthopedic surgery, Rochester, Minn, 2006, Mayo Clinic Scientific Press, with permission.)

Table 27-5. Peripheral Regional Analgesic Techniques for Major Hip Surgery

Peripheral Technique	Technique of Neural Localization	Area of Blockade	Duration of Blockade*	Perioperative Outcomes†
Lumbar plexus			12-18 hr	
Femoral	Neural stimulation, paresthesia	Femoral, partial lateral femoral cutaneous, and obturator		Improved analgesia and joint range of motion, decreased hospital stay compared with PCA; fewer technical problems and less urinary retention and hypotension than with epidural analgesia
Fascia iliaca	Loss of resistance	Femoral, partial lateral femoral cutaneous, obturator, and sciatic (S1)		Improved analgesia compared with PCA
Psoas compartment	Neural stimulation, loss of resistance	Complete lumbar plexus; occasional spread to sacral plexus or neuraxis		Reduced morphine consumption, pain at rest compared with PCA; reduced blood loss
Sciatic	Neural stimulation, paresthesia	Posterior thigh and leg (except for saphenous area)	18-30 hr	Proximal approach necessary for hip (compared with knee) procedures

*Duration of block performed with long-acting local anesthetic (bupivacaine or ropivacaine), intermediate-acting agents (lidocaine or mepivacaine) will resolve after 4 to 6 hours.
†Outcomes most marked in patients who receive a *continuous* lumbar plexus catheter with infusion of 0.1% to 0.2% bupivacaine or ropivacaine at 6 to 12 mL/hr for 48 to 72 hours.
PCA, Patient-controlled analgesia.

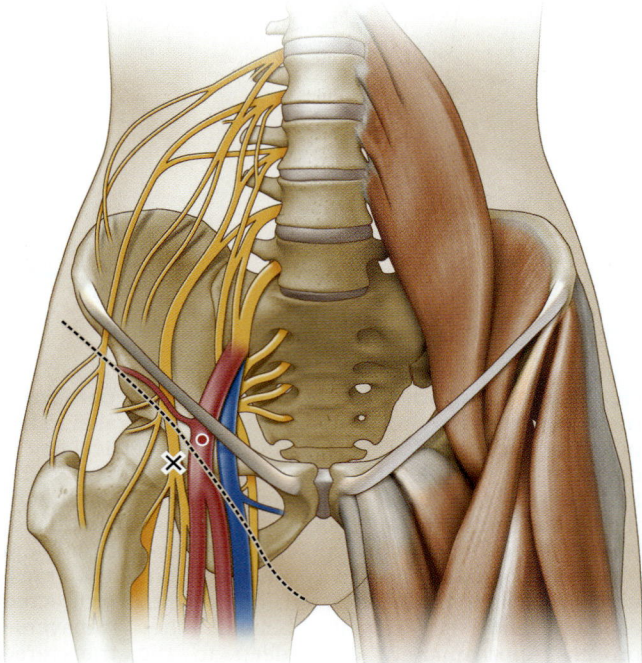

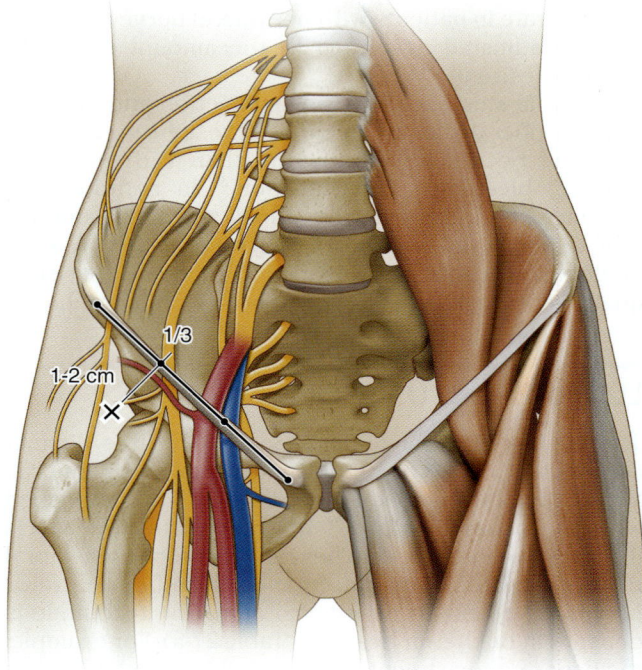

Figure 27-2. Lumbar plexus block: femoral approach. The *dotted line* corresponds to the inguinal crease. Needle insertion site is 1 to 2 cm lateral to the femoral arterial pulsation at this level. A 5-cm (2-inch) needle is advanced until a quadriceps response is noted, and 25 mL of local anesthetic is injected incrementally. (Redrawn from Lennon RL, Horlocker T: Mayo Clinic analgesic pathway: peripheral nerve blockade for major orthopedic surgery, Rochester, Minn, 2006, Mayo Clinic Scientific Press, with permission.)

Figure 27-3. Lumbar plexus block: fascia iliaca approach. The inguinal ligament is identified and divided into thirds. The junction of the lateral one third and the medial two thirds is determined. A 17-gauge Tuohy needle is inserted 1 cm below this point. An initial loss of resistance is noted as the needle penetrates the fascia lata. The second loss of resistance is felt as the needle penetrates the fascia iliaca, and 30 mL of local anesthetic is injected incrementally. (Redrawn from Lennon RL, Horlocker T: Mayo Clinic analgesic pathway: peripheral nerve blockade for major orthopedic surgery, Rochester, Minn, 2006, Mayo Clinic Scientific Press, with permission.)

insertion site to the surgical incision with these approaches precludes catheter placement *pre*operatively for patients undergoing hip replacement, but not necessarily for those undergoing hip fracture repair.

PSOAS COMPARTMENT BLOCK

The psoas compartment block was first described by Chayen in 1976.[26] It can be performed as a single-injection technique or with a catheter placed for prolonged analgesia. It has been used to provide anesthesia for thigh surgery. In combination with parasacral nerve block, it has been used for hip fracture repair,[27] to provide analgesia following total hip arthroplasty (THA), and in the treatment of chronic hip pain.[28]

Continuous psoas techniques have been described to provide analgesia following a variety of operations, including THA, open reduction and internal fixation (ORIF) of acetabular fractures, and ORIF of femoral fractures.[3,18,29,30] Interest in this block developed as practitioners sought alternatives to neuraxial techniques that

could provide consistent analgesia following hip and femur surgery.

Technique: Psoas Compartment Block

Several descriptions of the needle entry site for psoas compartment blocks have been put forth. All rely on bony contact with the transverse process as a guide to depth of needle placement. The patient is placed in the lateral position with hips flexed and operative extremity uppermost. Based on anatomic imaging studies, Capdevila and associates[3] modified the classic psoas technique. The needle insertion site is at the junction of the lateral third and the medial two thirds of a line between the spinous process of L4 and a line parallel to the spinal column passing through the posterior superior iliac spine (PSIS). (The spinous process of L4 was estimated to be approximately 1 cm cephalad to the upper edge of the iliac crests.) The needle is advanced perpendicularly to the skin until contact with the transverse process of L4 is obtained and is advanced caudad off the transverse process until quadriceps femoris muscle twitches are elicited (see Fig. 27-1). (In traversing from posterior to anterior at the level of L4-L5, the following structures would be encountered: posterior lumbar fascia, paraspinous muscles, anterior lumbar fascia, quadratus lumborum, and the psoas muscle.) The common iliac artery and vein are situated anterior to the psoas muscle. The lumbar plexus is identified by elicitation of a quadriceps motor response, and 30 mL of solution is injected. Despite a difference between men and women in the depth of the lumbar plexus (median values, 8.5 and 7.0 cm, respectively), the distance from the L4 transverse process to the lumbar plexus was comparable (median value, 2 cm) in the two sexes. Thus, the authors stressed the importance of achieving contact with the L4 transverse process to establish appropriate needle depth and position.

Complications of Psoas Compartment Block

Deep needle placement with the psoas compartment approach increases the risk of possible renal hematoma and retroperitoneal hematoma.[31,32] To ensure proper position of the needle during these deep techniques and to avoid excessive needle insertion, it is recommended that the transverse process be intentionally sought. Peripheral nerve damage is another potential risk with this technique. A side effect of the paravertebral approach to the lumbar plexus is the development of a sympathetic block secondary to the spread of local anesthetic. However, this unilateral sympathectomy usually is of little consequence.

Epidural spread of local anesthetic is another common side effect of psoas compartment block, occurring in 9% to 16% of adult patients.[33,34] This side effect is usually attributed to retrograde diffusion of local anesthetic to the epidural space when large volumes of local anesthetic are used (greater than 20 mL). In most cases, residual lumbar plexus blockade is apparent after resolution of the contralateral block. However, case reports have described total spinal anesthesia during lumbar plexus blockade, and vigilance must be maintained during management of this block.[35]

FEMORAL NERVE BLOCK

Indications for femoral nerve block include analgesia for femoral shaft fractures, as well as for major hip and knee surgery.[36-40]

Technique: Femoral Nerve Block

The patient lies supine with the anesthesiologist standing next to the side that is to be blocked. After careful palpation, a skin wheal is raised just lateral to the femoral artery, where it emerges distal to the inguinal ligament (see Fig. 27-2). A 22-gauge 5-cm insulated needle is inserted just over the tip of the palpating finger in a cephalad direction. Commonly, the anterior branch of the femoral nerve will be identified first.

Stimulation of this branch leads to contraction of the sartorius muscle on the medial aspect of the thigh and should not be accepted, as the articular and muscular branches derive from the posterior branch of the femoral nerve. The needle should be redirected slightly laterally and with a deeper direction to encounter the posterior branch of the femoral nerve. Stimulation of this branch is identified by *patellar ascension* as the quadriceps contract. The needle is then fixed, and 25 to 30 mL of local anesthetic is injected.

It has been advocated to use a higher volume of local anesthetic and apply firm pressure just distal to the needle during and a few minutes after injection to block the femoral, lateral femoral cutaneous, and obturator nerves, the so named "3-in-1 block." However, despite many efforts to consistently produce a 3-in-1 block, the effectiveness of these maneuvers has not been demonstrated. In most reports, the femoral nerve is the only nerve consistently blocked with this approach. Blockade of the lateral femoral cutaneous nerve occurs through lateral diffusion of local anesthetic and not through proximal spread to the lumbar plexus.[41] The obturator nerve is anesthetized less frequently than the lateral femoral cutaneous nerve; this is not surprising, given the number of fascial barriers between these structures at the level of the inguinal ligament.

Technique: Modified Femoral (Fascia Iliacus) Block

Indications for the fascia iliacus block are the same as those for femoral nerve block.[25,42] Advocates believe its usefulness lies in the double pop technique for applying this block. The double pop refers to the sensation felt as the needle traverses the fascia lata, then the fascia iliaca. Penetration of both layers of fascia is important for successful fascia iliacus blockade. To facilitate appreciation of the "clicks" or "pops," use of a short bevel or pencil-tipped needle has been advocated to obtain more tactile feedback than is obtained with cutting needles. This technique does not require a nerve stimulator; however, confirmatory motor responses may be sought. The needle entry site for the fascia iliacus block is determined by drawing a line between the pubic tubercle and the anterior superior iliac crest and dividing this line into thirds. The needle entry point is 1 cm caudal to the intersection of the medial two thirds and lateral one third along this line. This site is well away from the femoral artery, making it useful for patients in whom femoral artery puncture is contraindicated (see Fig. 27-3).

Complications of Femoral and Fascia Iliacus Block

Intravascular injection and hematoma are possible because of the close proximity of vascular structures throughout the course of the nerve. However, anatomically, the nerve and the femoral artery are located in separate sheaths approximately 1 cm apart (Fig. 27-4). In most patients with normal anatomy, the femoral artery can be easily palpated, allowing correct, safe

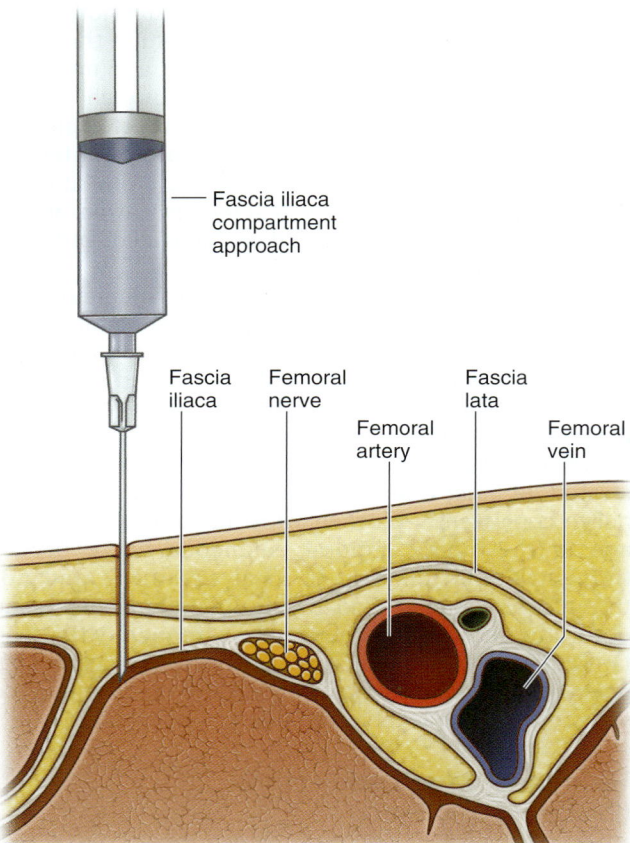

Figure 27-4. The neurovascular bundle and fascia iliacus block. The needle insertion site is lateral to that of the femoral nerve block. Note that the femoral nerve is also under the fascia iliaca. (Redrawn from Lennon RL, Horlocker T: Mayo Clinic analgesic pathway: peripheral nerve blockade for major orthopedic surgery, Rochester, Minn, 2006, Mayo Clinic Scientific Press, with permission.)

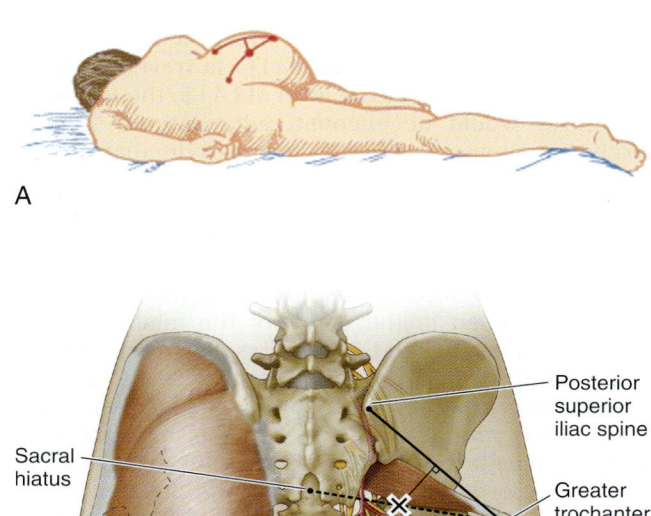

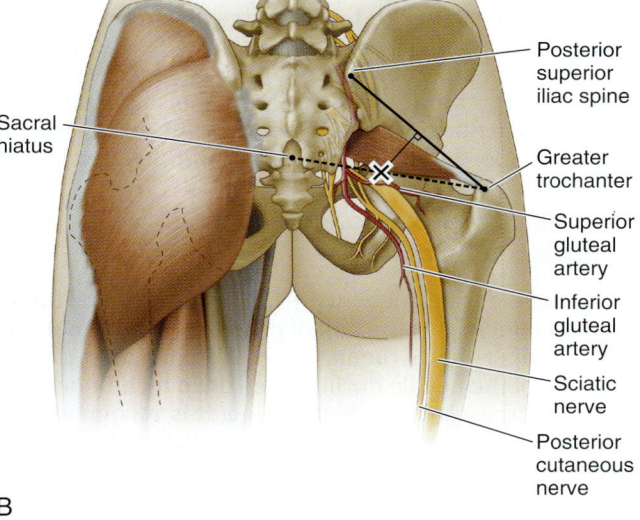

Figure 27-5. Sciatic nerve block: classic posterior approach of Labat. A, Patient positioning. **B,** Block technique. Needle insertion is 5 cm along the perpendicular that bisects a line connecting the greater trochanter and the posterior superior iliac spine. A 10-cm (4-inch) stimulating needle is advanced until a tibial or peroneal motor response is elicited; then 20 to 30 mL of local anesthetic is injected incrementally. (**A,** From Wedel DJ, Horlocker T: Nerve blocks. In Miller RD, ed: Miller's anesthesia, ed 7, Philadelphia, 2010, Elsevier, pp 1639–1674. **B,** Redrawn from Lennon RL, Horlocker T: Mayo Clinic analgesic pathway: peripheral nerve blockade for major orthopedic surgery, Rochester, Minn, 2006, Mayo Clinic Scientific Press, with permission.)

needle positioning lateral to the pulsation. The presence of femoral vascular grafts is a relative contraindication to femoral block; however, the fascia iliacus approach may be used in these patients because of the lateral needle insertion site. Nerve damage is rare with this technique. Both local inflammation and proximal abscess have been reported with indwelling catheters. Finally, the presence of femoral or combined femoral-sciatic block may lead to lateral gait instability, resulting in difficulty with pivoting maneuvers and patient falls.[43]

SCIATIC NERVE BLOCK

Complete unilateral lower extremity blockade is achieved by combining a lumbar plexus technique with a proximal sciatic block[2,14] (Fig. 27-5). However, because most of the innervation to the hip is provided by the lumbar plexus, adequate analgesia may be achieved with a continuous lumbar plexus technique alone.[18,44]

Technique: Classic Approach of Labat

The classic approach to the sciatic nerve block involves the patient lying on the side opposite the one to be blocked, rolled forward onto the flexed knee, with the heel in opposition to the knee of the outstretched dependent leg (see Fig. 27-5A). A line is drawn between points made over the upper aspect of the greater trochanter of the femur and the PSIS. This line should coincide with the upper border of the piriformis muscle and with the upper border of the sacrosciatic foramen (sciatic notch). A line perpendicular and bisecting this is drawn downward 3 cm and represents the needle insertion point. Verification of this point may be made by projecting a line from the greater trochanter to a point 1 to 2 cm below the sacral cornua. This line crosses the perpendicular at about 3 cm and also represents a point overlying the sciatic nerve where it exits from the pelvis (see Fig. 27-5B). A 10- to 15-cm needle is inserted through a wheal made at this point in a direction perpendicular to the skin. The needle may enter the sciatic notch and localize the nerve on the first needle advance. If bone is encountered, the needle is redirected medially. If blood is aspirated (superior gluteal artery), the needle is redirected laterally. Motor responses must be elicited in the leg *below* the level of the thigh to assure complete sciatic blockade.

Surface landmarks can be difficult to identify accurately in sciatic nerve blockade, because of the variable amount of subcutaneous tissue overlying the bony landmarks. Use of vascular imaging guides (e.g., ultrasound, Doppler) may provide a more consistent landmark—the superior gluteal artery. The superior gluteal artery, the largest branch of the internal iliac artery, passes between L5 and S1 and emerges from the upper border of the piriformis muscle at the upper aspect of the sciatic notch. The artery is typically located 1 to 2 cm medial to Labat's line and usually slightly cephalad to Labat's point, with the nerve slightly inferior and lateral to the artery.

Complications

Serious complications of sciatic nerve block are rare. However, theoretical concerns regarding muscle trauma and puncture of a variety of vascular structures must be considered. Sciatic nerve block is primarily a somatic nerve block. It does carry some sympathetic fibers to the extremity, however, and therefore may allow pooling of small quantities of blood—usually insufficient to cause significant hypotension. Residual dysesthesias for periods of 1 to 3 days are not uncommon but usually resolve within several months.[35] It is important to note that many orthopedic surgical procedures are associated with neurapraxia to one or both components of the sciatic nerve. Thus, thoughtful application of this technique is required to optimize neurologic outcome for patients considered to be at high risk of perioperative nerve injury from surgery or preexisting neurologic dysfunction.

NEURAXIAL ANESTHESIA AND ANALGESIA IN THE ORTHOPEDIC PATIENT RECEIVING DVT CHEMOPROPHYLAXIS

Venous thromboembolism is a major cause of death after surgery or trauma to the lower extremities. Without prophylaxis, venous thrombosis develops in 40% to 80% of orthopedic patients, and 1% to 28% show clinical or laboratory evidence of pulmonary embolism. Fatal pulmonary embolism occurs in 0.1% to 8% of patients.[45] Guidelines for antithrombotic therapy, including selection of pharmacologic agent, degree of anticoagulation desired, and duration of therapy, continue to evolve.[45] For patients undergoing major lower extremity surgery, administration of low-molecular-weight heparin (LMWH), warfarin, or fondaparinux is recommended.

Several studies have showed a decrease in the incidence of both DVT and pulmonary embolism (PE) in patients undergoing hip surgery under epidural and spinal anesthesia.[46-48] Proposed mechanisms for this effect include (1) rheologic changes resulting in hyperkinetic lower extremity blood flow, thereby reducing venous stasis and preventing thrombus formation; (2) beneficial circulatory effects from epinephrine added to local anesthetic solutions; (3) altered coagulation and fibrinolytic responses to surgery under central neural blockade, resulting in a decreased tendency for blood to clot and better fibrinolytic function; (4) absence of positive-pressure ventilation and its concomitant effects on circulation; and (5) direct local anesthetic effects such as decreased platelet aggregation. It is important to note that most studies examining the value of epidural and spinal anesthesia in preventing DVT and PTE involved patients who were not receiving currently recommended pharmacologic prophylaxis.

Despite the advantages of neuraxial techniques, patients receiving perioperative anticoagulants and antiplatelet medications often are not considered candidates for spinal or epidural anesthesia/analgesia because of the risk of neurologic compromise from expanding spinal hematoma. The actual incidence of neurologic dysfunction resulting from hemorrhagic complications associated with neuraxial blockade is unknown; however, the incidence cited in the literature is estimated to be less than 1 in 150,000 epidural and less than 1 in 220,000 spinal anesthetics.[49] The frequency of spinal hematoma is increased in patients who receive perioperative anticoagulation.[21,50,51]

Spinal hematoma was considered a rare complication of neuraxial blockade until the introduction of LMWH as a thromboprophylactic agent in the 1990s. The calculated incidence (approximately 1 in 3000 epidural anesthetics), along with the catastrophic nature of spinal bleeding (only 30% of patients had good neurologic recovery), warranted an alternate approach to analgesic management following total hip and knee replacement.[52] Although the psoas compartment and femoral catheters are suitable (if not superior) alternatives to neuraxial infusions, no investigations have examined the frequency and severity of hemorrhagic complications following plexus or peripheral blockade in anticoagulated patients. It is reassuring that few serious complications following *intentional* neurovascular sheath cannulation for surgical, radiologic, or cardiac indications have been reported. For example, during interventional cardiac procedures, large-bore catheters are placed within brachial or femoral vessels, and heparin, LMWH, antiplatelet medications, and/or thrombolytics are subsequently administered. Despite significant vessel trauma and coagulation deficiencies, neurologic complications are rare, although patients occasionally require a blood transfusion. In addition, all cases of major bleeding (significant decrease in hemoglobin and/or blood pressure) with non-neuraxial techniques occurred after psoas compartment or lumbar sympathetic blockade and involved heparin, LMWH,

Table 27-6. Neuraxial* Anesthesia and Analgesia in the Orthopedic Patient Receiving Antithrombotic Therapy

LMWH

Needle placement should occur 10 to 12 hours after a dose. Indwelling neuraxial catheters are allowed with once-daily (but not twice-daily) dosing of LMWH. In general, it is optimal to place/remove indwelling catheters in the morning and administer LMWH in the evening to allow normalization of hemostasis to occur before catheter manipulation is performed.

Warfarin

Adequate levels of all vitamin K–dependent factors should be present during catheter placement and removal. Patients on warfarin long term should have normal INR prior to performance of regional technique. Monitor prothrombin time and INR daily. Remove catheter when INR <1.5.

Fondaparinux

Neuraxial techniques are not advised in patients anticipated to receive fondaparinux perioperatively.

Nonsteroidal Anti-inflammatory Drugs

No significant risk of regional anesthesia-related bleeding is associated with aspirin-type drugs. However, for patients receiving warfarin or LMWH, combined anticoagulant and antiplatelet effects may increase the risk of perioperative bleeding. In addition, other medications affecting platelet function such as thienopyridine derivatives and glycoprotein IIb/IIIa platelet receptor inhibitors should be avoided.

*Similar management is warranted for psoas compartment and sciatic blockade.
INR, International normalized ratio; *LMWH*, low-molecular-weight heparin. Adapted from Horlocker TT, Wedel DJ, Benzon H, et al: Regional anesthesia in the anticoagulated patient: defining the risks (the second ASRA Consensus Conference on Neuraxial Anesthesia and Anticoagulation), Reg Anesth Pain Med 28:172–197, 2003.

warfarin, and thienophyridine derivatives. These cases suggest that significant blood loss, rather than neural deficits, may be the most serious complication of non-neuraxial regional techniques in the anticoagulated patient. Additional information is needed to allow definitive recommendations. Current information focuses on neuraxial blocks and anticoagulants (Table 27-6).[53] These neuraxial guidelines should be applied to deep lumbar plexus and sciatic techniques.

Thus, thromboembolism is a serious complication of total joint replacement. Neuraxial and peripheral techniques, which allow for early ambulation and earlier hospital dismissal, may prove to be an integral component of patient care. However, at this time, they do not replace the need for pharmacologic thromboprophylaxis.

In summary, analgesic approaches that minimize opioids through the use of peripheral nerve blocks and a combination of analgesic agents allow early mobilization, facilitate rehabilitation, and decrease hospital stay and costs. Continued collaborations between orthopedic surgeons and anesthesiologists are necessary to further advance the perioperative management of these complex patients.

CURRENT CONTROVERSIES AND FUTURE CONSIDERATIONS

- Critical elements in multimodal analgesia remain undetermined. Future research is needed to define the relative roles of preoperatively administered medications, peripheral nerve block, and postoperative analgesics (both nonopioid and opioid).
- The relative risk of poor bone formation/healing following NSAID administration is unclear. However, these medications are associated with a significant opioid-sparing effect.
- Although peripheral nerve block is associated with superior analgesia and improved surgical and enhanced economic outcomes, these techniques are not universally performed or taught. Training programs and future research should be directed toward improving ease of performance, success, and safety.
- As hospital dismissal occurs earlier and rehabilitation continues to move from inpatient to outpatient settings, analgesic pathways will continue to evolve.

REFERENCES

1. Choi PT, Bhandari M, Scott J, Douketis J: Epidural analgesia for pain relief following hip or knee replacement. Cochrane Database Syst Rev (3):CD003071, 2003.
2. Hebl JR, Kopp SL, Ali MH, et al: A comprehensive anesthesia protocol that emphasizes peripheral nerve blockade for total knee and total hip arthroplasty. J Bone Joint Surg Am 87(Suppl 2):63–70, 2005.
3. Capdevila X, Macaire P, Dadure C, et al: Continuous psoas compartment block for postoperative analgesia after total hip arthroplasty: new landmarks, technical guidelines, and clinical evaluation [see comment]. Anesth Analg 94:1606–1613, 2002.
4. Singelyn FJ, Gouverneur JM: Postoperative analgesia after total hip arthroplasty: i.v. PCA with morphine, patient-controlled epidural analgesia, or continuous "3-in-1" block? A prospective evaluation by our acute pain service in more than 1,300 patients. J Clin Anesth 11:550–554, 1999.
5. Wheeler M, Oderda GM, Ashburn MA, Lipman AG: Adverse events associated with postoperative opioid analgesia: a systematic review. J Pain 3:159–180, 2002.
6. Stephens JM, Pashos CL, Haider S, Wong JM: Making progress in the management of postoperative pain: a review of the cyclooxygenase 2-specific inhibitors. Pharmacotherapy 24:1714–1731, 2004.
7. Capone ML, Sciulli MG, Tacconelli S, et al: Pharmacodynamic interaction of naproxen with low-dose aspirin in healthy subjects [see comment]. J Am Coll Cardiol 45:1295–1301, 2005.
8. Gajraj NM: Cyclooxygenase-2 inhibitors. Anesth Analg 96:1720–1738, 2003.
9. Rathmell JP, Pino CA, Taylor R, et al: Intrathecal morphine for postoperative analgesia: a randomized, controlled, dose-ranging study after hip and knee arthroplasty. Anesth Analg 97:1452–1457, 2003.
10. Gambling D, Hughes T, Martin G, et al: A comparison of Depodur, a novel, single-dose extended-release epidural morphine, with standard epidural morphine for pain relief after lower abdominal surgery. Anesth Analg 100:1065–1074, 2005.
11. Gwirtz KH, Young JV, Byers RS, et al: The safety and efficacy of intrathecal opioid analgesia for acute postoperative pain: seven years' experience with 5969 surgical patients at Indiana University Hospital. Anesth Analg 88:599–604, 1999.
12. Pettine KA, Wedel DJ, Cabanela ME, Weeks JL: The use of epidural bupivacaine following total knee arthroplasty. Orthop Rev 18:894–901, 1989.
13. Weller R, Rosenblum M, Conard P, Gross JB: Comparison of epidural and patient-controlled intravenous morphine

following joint replacement surgery. Can J Anaesth 38:582–586, 1991.

14. Enneking FK, Chan V, Greger J, et al: Lower-extremity peripheral nerve blockade: essentials of our current understanding. Reg Anesth Pain Med 30:4–35, 2005.
15. Allen HW, Liu SS, Ware PD, et al: Peripheral nerve blocks improve analgesia after total knee replacement surgery. Anesth Analg 87:93–97, 1998.
16. Stevens RD, Van Gessel E, Flory N, et al: Lumbar plexus block reduces pain and blood loss associated with total hip arthroplasty [see comment]. Anesthesiology 93:115–121, 2000.
17. Duncan CM, Hall Long K, Warner DO, Hebl JR: The economic implications of a multimodal analgesic regimen for patients undergoing major orthopedic surgery: a comparative study of direct costs. Reg Anesth Pain Med 34:301–307, 2009.
18. Pagnano MW, Hebl J, Horlocker T: Assuring a painless total hip arthroplasty: a multimodal approach emphasizing peripheral nerve blocks. J Arthroplasty 21:80–84, 2006.
19. Hebl JR, Dilger JA, Byer DE, et al: A pre-emptive multimodal pathway featuring peripheral nerve block improves perioperative outcomes after major orthopedic surgery. Reg Anesth Pain Med 33:510–517, 2008.
20. Auroy Y, Narchi P, Messiah A, et al: Serious complications related to regional anesthesia: results of a prospective survey in France. Anesthesiology 87:479–486, 1997.
21. Horlocker TT, Wedel DJ, Rowlingson JC, et al: Regional anesthesia in the patient receiving antithrombotic or thrombolytic therapy: American Society of Regional Anesthesia and Pain Medicine evidence-based guidelines, ed 3. Reg Anesth Pain Med 35:64–101, 2010.
22. Capdevila X, Pirat P, Bringuier S, et al: Continuous peripheral nerve blocks in hospital wards after orthopedic surgery: a multicenter prospective analysis of the quality of postoperative analgesia and complications in 1,416 patients. Anesthesiology 103:1035–1045, 2005.
23. Ilfeld BM, Ball ST, Gearen PF, et al: Ambulatory continuous posterior lumbar plexus nerve blocks after hip arthroplasty: a dual-center, randomized, triple-masked, placebo-controlled trial. Anesthesiology 109:491–501, 2008.
24. Awad IT, Duggan EM: Posterior lumbar plexus block: anatomy, approaches, and techniques. Reg Anesth Pain Med 30:143–149, 2005.
25. Capdevila X, Coimbra C, Choquet O: Approaches to the lumbar plexus: success, risks, and outcome. Reg Anesth Pain Med 30:150–162, 2005.
26. Chayen D, Nathan H, Chayen M: The psoas compartment block. Anesthesiology 45:95–99, 1976.
27. Ho AM, Karmakar MK: Combined paravertebral lumbar plexus and parasacral sciatic nerve block for reduction of hip fracture in a patient with severe aortic stenosis. Can J Anaesth 49:946–950, 2002.
28. Goroszeniuk T, di Vadi PP: Repeated psoas compartment blocks for the management of long-standing hip pain. Reg Anesth Pain Med 26:376–378, 2001.
29. Matheny JM, Hanks GA, Rung GW, et al: A comparison of patient-controlled analgesia and continuous lumbar plexus block after anterior cruciate ligament reconstruction. Arthroscopy 9:87–90, 1993.
30. Turker G, Uckunkaya N, Yavascaoglu B, et al: Comparison of the catheter-technique psoas compartment block and the epidural block for analgesia in partial hip replacement surgery. Acta Anaesthesiol Scand 47:30–36, 2003.
31. Aida S, Takahashi H, Shimoji K: Renal subcapsular hematoma after lumbar plexus block. Anesthesiology 84:452–455, 1996.
32. Aveline C, Bonnet F: Delayed retroperitoneal haematoma after failed lumbar plexus block. Br J Anaesth 93:589–591, 2004.
33. Farny J, Girard M, Drolet P: Posterior approach to the lumbar plexus combined with a sciatic nerve block using lidocaine. Can J Anaesth 41:486–491, 1994.
34. Parkinson SK, Mueller JB, Little WL, Bailey SL: Extent of blockade with various approaches to the lumbar plexus. Anesth Analg 68:243–248, 1989.
35. Auroy Y, Benhamou D, Bargues L, et al: Major complications of regional anesthesia in France: the SOS Regional Anesthesia Hotline Service. Anesthesiology 97:1274–1280, 2002.
36. Singelyn FJ, Gouverneur JM: Extended "three-in-one" block after total knee arthroplasty: continuous versus patient-controlled techniques. Anesth Analg 91:176–180, 2000.
37. Capdevila X, Barthelet Y, Biboulet P, et al: Effects of perioperative analgesic technique on the surgical outcome and duration of rehabilitation after major knee surgery [see comment]. Anesthesiology 91:8–15, 1999.
38. Fletcher AK, Rigby AS, Heyes FL: Three-in-one femoral nerve block as analgesia for fractured neck of femur in the emergency department: a randomized, controlled trial. Ann Emerg Med 41:227–233, 2003.
39. Singelyn FJ, Deyaert M, Joris D, et al: Effects of intravenous patient-controlled analgesia with morphine, continuous epidural analgesia, and continuous three-in-one block on postoperative pain and knee rehabilitation after unilateral total knee arthroplasty [see comment]. Anesth Analg 87:88–92, 1998.
40. Williams BA, Kentor ML, Vogt MT, et al: Femoral-sciatic nerve blocks for complex outpatient knee surgery are associated with less postoperative pain before same-day discharge: a review of 1,200 consecutive cases from the period 1996-1999. Anesthesiology 98:1206–1213, 2003.
41. Marhofer P, Nasel C, Sitzwohl C, Kapral S: Magnetic resonance imaging of the distribution of local anesthetic during the three-in-one block. Anesth Analg 90:119–124, 2000.
42. Lopez S, Gros T, Bernard N, et al: Fascia iliaca compartment block for femoral bone fractures in prehospital care. Reg Anesth Pain Med 28:203–207, 2003.
43. Muraskin SI, Conrad B, Zheng N, et al: Falls associated with lower-extremity-nerve blocks: a pilot investigation of mechanisms. Reg Anesth Pain Med 32:67–72, 2007.
44. Horlocker TT, Kopp SL, Pagnano MW, Hebl JR: Analgesia for total hip and knee arthroplasty: a multimodal pathway featuring peripheral nerve block. J Am Acad Orthop Surg 14:126–135, 2006.
45. Geerts WH, Bergqvist D, Pineo GF, et al: Prevention of venous thromboembolism: American College of Chest Physicians evidence-based clinical practice guidelines, ed 8. Chest 133:381S–453S, 2008.
46. Modig J, Borg T, Bagge L, Saldeen T Role of extradural and of general anaesthesia in fibrinolysis and coagulation after total hip replacement. Br J Anaesth 55:625–629, 1983.
47. Modig J, Borg T, Karlstrom G. et al: Thromboembolism after total hip replacement: role of epidural and general anesthesia. Anesth Analg 62:174–180, 1983.
48. Davis FM, Laurenson VG, Gillespie WJ, et al: Deep vein thrombosis after total hip replacement: a comparison between spinal and general anaesthesia. J Bone Joint Surg Br 71:181–185, 1989.
49. Tryba M: [Epidural regional anesthesia and low molecular heparin: Pro]. Anasthesiol Intensivmed Notfallmed Schmerzther 28:179–181, 1993.
50. Moen V, Dahlgren N, Irestedt L: Severe neurological complications after central neuraxial blockades in Sweden 1990-1999. Anesthesiology 101:950–959, 2004.
51. Vandermeulen EP, Van Aken H, Vermylen J: Anticoagulants and spinal-epidural anesthesia. Anesth Analg 79:1165–1177, 1994.
52. Horlocker T, Wedel DJ: Neuraxial blockade and low molecular weight heparin: balancing perioperative analgesia and thromboprophylaxis. Reg Anesth Pain Med 23:164–177, 1998.
53. Horlocker TT, Wedel DJ, Benzon H, et al: Regional anesthesia in the anticoagulated patient: defining the risks (the second ASRA Consensus Conference on Neuraxial Anesthesia and Anticoagulation). Reg Anesth Pain Med 28:172–197, 2003.

CHAPTER 28

Prevention of Venous Thromboembolism in Surgery of the Hip

Clifford W. Colwell, Jr.

KEY POINTS

- Assess all patients for factors increasing the risk of venous thromboembolic events (VTE).
  - Having total hip arthroplasty (THA) puts patient in a high-risk group.
  - THA patients are often older, with comorbidities that increase the risk of VTE.
- Multiple methods of VTE prophylaxis are available.
  - Chemoprophylactic
    - Low-molecular-weight heparin (LMWH)
    - Fondaparinux
    - Vitamin K antagonist (VKA) (warfarin)
    - Aspirin
  - Mechanical
    - Calf length
    - Thigh length
    - Boots
    - Portable or stationary pump
- Bleeding is a concern for all types of prophylaxis.
- Continue to assess clinically for VTE during hospitalization and at follow-up.
- Regulations (Surgical Care Improvement Project [SCIP], Joint Commission on Accreditation of Healthcare Organization (JCAHO) mandate that some type of prophylaxis must be prescribed for THA patients.

INTRODUCTION

Prophylaxis for venous thromboembolic events (VTE) for total hip arthroplasty (THA) patients is an accepted fact. However, the method of prophylaxis is the topic of ongoing controversy. The incidence of VTE, including deep venous thrombosis (DVT) and pulmonary embolism (PE), is unacceptably high without any type of prophylaxis (Table 28-1). Although prophylaxis has been recommended since 1986,[1] more is known about the epidemiology and risk factors, and methods for determining the presence of VTE and methods of prophylaxis have evolved. Low-molecular-weight heparins (LMWHs) have been available since 1993, and new oral anticoagulants. Compression devices have also been available for many years, but a recently developed portable compression device may alter nonpharmacologic prophylaxis. Various guidelines are available; confusion often surrounds which guidelines should be followed for

optimal patient outcomes. A government agency and the accreditation body for hospitals have mandated that THA patients must be assessed and provided with prophylaxis after surgery. In this chapter, we will discuss all of these issues.

EPIDEMIOLOGY AND RISK FACTORS

Thromboprophylaxis in THA begins with assessment of each patient's risk for VTE. Given that surgery and orthopedic surgery of the lower extremity, specifically, automatically place our patients in the high-risk category, initial assessment for other factors that put the patient at even higher risk of VTE is done during preparation for surgery. This assessment may affect the type of prophylaxis prescribed and the length of time prophylaxis should be continued by the patient. Many available assessment tools[8-13] provide checklists for risks and often suggest prophylaxis based on these risks (Box 28-1). Patients should be assessed perioperatively and during recovery for any signs or symptoms of VTE, in addition to receiving prophylaxis. Assessments should be documented in patients' records to communicate with other healthcare professionals regarding assessment findings. Patients should be educated about clinical VTE signs and symptoms, so they can appropriately report these findings to their physician. Clinical signs alone, however, are notoriously flawed with respect to an accurate diagnosis and should be adjudicated by objective tests, which are almost universally carried out by duplex ultrasound.

Evidence suggests that proximal DVT is more important than distal DVT in terms of its sequelae and risk of development of subsequent PE.[14] Proximal DVT occurs in veins above the knee, from the popliteal upward. Because these vessels are larger, the thrombosis is usually more significant and, if dislodged, could cause a larger PE. Studies have shown, however, that between 20% and 30% of thromboses that originate in the distal veins propagate to proximal veins and can cause PE.[15-17] Calf vein thrombi are not totally benign: a high proportion leave residual venous abnormalities, including persistent occlusion and/or venous valvular incompetence,[18] and post-thrombotic syndrome (PTS) develops in 5% of patients after total knee arthroplasty (TKA) and THA.[19] Therefore, prophylaxis to prevent proximal and distal DVT, as well as PE, appears to be important.

Table 28-1. VTE Prevalence After THA and Hip Fracture Surgery (HFS) Based on Mandatory Venography in Patients Who Received Placebo or No Prophylaxis

	DVT Prevalence	Proximal DVT Prevalence	PE Prevalence	Fatal PE Prevalence
THA	42%-57%	18%-36%	0.9%-28%	0.1%-2.0%
HFS	46%-60%	23%-30%	3%-11%	0.3%-7.5%

DVT, Deep vein thrombosis; *PE,* pulmonary embolism; *THA,* total hip arthroplasty; *VTE,* venous thromboembolism.
From Geerts WH, Pineo GF, Heit JA, et al: Prevention of venous thromboembolism: the Seventh ACCP Conference on Antithrombotic and Thrombolytic Therapy. Chest 127:2297–2298, 2005.

BOX 28-1   CLINICAL RISK FACTORS FOR VTE

- Institutionalization (hospital/nursing home)
- Trauma (pelvic, lower extremity)
- Major orthopedic surgery
- Antiphospholipid syndrome
- Malignancy with chemotherapy or radiotherapy
- Stroke
- Malignancy with no therapies
- Inherited thrombophilia/hypofibrinolysis
- Limited mobility, including lower extremity paresis
- History of VTE
- Tamoxifen or raloxifene therapy
- ASA score—3
- Oral contraceptives or hormone replacement therapy (HRT)
- Advanced age
- Obesity
- Diabetes mellitus
- Coronary artery disease
- Congestive heart disease
- Varicose veins
- Smoking, current/former

ASA, American Society of Anesthesiologists; *VTE,* venous thromboembolism.
From Beksac B, Gonzalez Della Valle A, et al: Thromboembolic disease after total hip arthroplasty: who is at risk? Clinical Orthopaedics and Related Research 453:211, 2006.

Genetics and Clotting Factors

Genetic factors, including mutations of factor V Leiden, prothrombin gene *G20210A,* have been reported to increase the risk of VTE in the population. One study of TKA or THA patients indicated that the prothrombin gene mutation *G20210A* was significantly represented in those in this group with symptomatic VTE ($P = .0002$).[20] A tendency toward increased risk of VTE was found with factor V Leiden mutation ($P = .09$).[20] However, because 90% of the population who had these genetic risk factors did not have a VTE, general preoperative genotype screening is of questionable value.

Clotting factors, which have been associated with VTE, include increased levels of factor VIII[21] and fibronectin.[22] However, these factors have not been examined in relation to orthopedic surgery patients and VTE. Also implicated is a low level of high-density lipoprotein (HDL),[23] although this has not been studied in the orthopedic surgical patient. Another study reports a positive relationship between plasma cholesterol ester transfer proteins and increased coagulability in young males,[24] although again, whether this would transfer to surgical patients is not known.

Recently, two genetic variants of the enzyme that metabolizes warfarin, cytochrome P-450 2C9 (CYP2C9) and vitamin K epoxide reductase (VKORC1), have been associated with differences in patient response to warfarin doses.[25] One study of this genetic-based dosing in TKA and THA has been reported.[26] This study of 92 patients proposed an algorithm for warfarin dosing after orthopedic surgery that took into consideration genetic type, clinical variables, current medication, and preoperative and postoperative laboratory values. With validations, a safer, more effective process for initiating warfarin therapy could be provided.

PATHOPHYSIOLOGY

In discussing thrombosis, the difference between venous thrombosis and arterial thrombosis needs clarification. Thrombosis in arteries is usually triggered by underlying arteriosclerosis and is composed mainly of platelets that deposit in the sclerotic rough area. Venous thrombosis is composed mainly of clotting proteins, with platelets playing a very minor role. Therefore, the methods used to prevent one type of thrombosis do not necessarily work for the other type of thrombosis. The essence of this chapter is the occurrence of venous thrombosis following THA.

CLINICAL FEATURES AND DIAGNOSIS

Diagnosis

Doppler duplex ultrasound is a major tool used in practice and in research to detect DVT in patients with joint arthroplasty of the lower extremities. Because venous ultrasound is noninvasive, has almost no contraindications, and can be used as a repeated measure, it has become the most widely used test for clinical detection of symptomatic and asymptomatic DVT.[27] Doppler ultrasound is also used by some surgeons as a screening tool to determine whether any thrombi are present at the time of hospital discharge. Screening has not been shown to be effective in changing an existing protocol because of short hospital stays after THA.[28] Although compression venous Doppler ultrasound has been shown to have high specificity in the thigh in almost all institutions,[27,29] this specificity is not maintained in the calf by all institutions.

Because no standardized documentation procedure exists for Doppler ultrasound that allows central adjudication, venography is still considered the "standard"

Table 28-2. Pharmacologic Prophylaxis Options for THA

Drug	Manufacturer/Type of Drug	Dosing	Start Time
enoxaparin (Lovenox)	Sanofi-Aventis (Bridgewater, NJ)/LMWH	30 mg subcutaneous; 40 mg subcutaneous may be used for extended prophylaxis	Start 12-24 hours after surgery, then twice daily for 7-10 days; may extend prophylaxis for 35 days after initial 7-10 days
dalteparin (Fragmin)	Pfizer (Brooklyn, NY)/LMWH (FDA approved only for total hip arthroplasty)	2500 U (half dose) subcutaneous 5000 U (full dose) subcutaneous	May start within 2 hours before surgery with half dose or start 4-8 hours after surgery with half dose, then full dose once daily; may extend to 14 days
fondaparinux (Arixtra)	GlaxoSmithKline (Research Park, NC)/synthetic pentasaccharide	2.5 mg subcutaneous	Start approximately 6-8 hours after surgery or the next day, then once daily for 7-10 days; may extend for 35 days
warfarin (Coumadin)	Bristol-Myers Squibb (Princeton, NJ)/VKA	2-10 mg oral to maintain INR of 2-2.5	Start 1-12 hours before or after surgery; may extend for 35 days

INR, International normalized ratio; *LMWH*, low-molecular-weight heparin; *THA*, total hip arthroplasty; *VKA*, vitamin K antagonist.

for large VTE prophylaxis studies of new anticoagulants seeking approval by the United States (U.S.) Food and Drug Administration (FDA). Venograms are rarely done in clinical practice to detect symptomatic DVT because of the invasiveness of the procedure, exposure to radiation and contrast agents, the cumbersome nature of the procedure, and resultant pain.

After lower extremity orthopedic surgery, 50% of deaths are caused by vascular events[30] and death may occur within a matter of minutes, making prophylaxis critical. Diagnosis of symptoms of PE, after a check for an elevated D-dimer blood test, is currently done most often by computed tomographic pulmonary angiography (CTPA), although some institutions continue to use ventilation-perfusion (V-P) lung scans. Lung scans are categorized as normal, low probability, and high probability. An angiography study is done as follow-up to confirm the PE after an intermediate probability V-P scan. A study comparing these two techniques found that the procedures were similar in diagnosing PE and determined that 0.4% (2/561) of patients who had CTPA and 1.0% (6/611) of patients who had a V-P lung scan later developed a PE.[31] Either method appears to be acceptable in diagnosing PE; however, a few failures with both screening methods have been reported.

TREATMENT

Pharmacologic Prophylaxis

The category of drugs most commonly used worldwide for VTE prophylaxis is LMWHs. These drugs are given subcutaneously in different doses with different timing, depending on the particular drug, but do not require laboratory monitoring or dose adjustment. Extensive data have shown that this category of drugs is safe and effective, although concern still exists about related bleeding. Fondaparinux, also given subcutaneously, is a synthetic pentasaccharide used for prophylaxis. Another drug commonly used is warfarin, a VKA, which is given orally. Warfarin is dosed by checking the prothrombin time using the international normalized ratio (INR) to adjust the warfarin dose (Table 28-2). The point at which each of these agents provides inhibition in the coagulation cascade is shown in Figure 28-1. Aspirin is prescribed in various doses and often is used as part of a multimodal approach. Meta-analysis has shown low-dose unfractionated heparin or aspirin prophylaxis to be more effective than no prophylaxis, but both are less effective than other prophylactic regimens in this high-risk THA patient group. Each of these drugs has the potential to cause unwanted bleeding.

Oral anticoagulation with adjusted-dose warfarin sodium is the most common and the longest practiced prophylaxis protocol by a majority of orthopedic surgeons in North America. Adjusted-dose warfarin has the potential advantage of allowing continued prophylaxis after hospital discharge provided the infrastructure is available to continue home therapy effectively and safely. Oral anticoagulation should be administrated in a dose sufficient to prolong the INR to a target of 2.5 (range, 2 to 3) (see Table 28-2). The half-life of warfarin is 36 to 42 hours, and its effects can be reversed with vitamin K. The initial oral anticoagulant dose may be administered before surgery or as soon after surgery as possible. However, even with early initiation of oral anticoagulation therapy, the INR does not usually reach the target range until the third postoperative day. The effectiveness of adjusted-dose warfarin is shown in Table 28-3.

The safety of using warfarin prophylaxis requires that patients understand the benefits and the risks of this medication. Clinical studies report a major bleeding event similar to that seen with placebo (Table 28-4). Many factors, including medications, smoking, alcohol, foods, and changes in activity, may interact with warfarin. Because many patients are discharged with warfarin prophylaxis, patients must be made aware of these interactions and must monitor themselves for any symptoms of over-anticoagulation. Optimal use of warfarin requires consideration of the time frame of its effects, use of the INR for close monitoring of effects and interacting factors, patient education, and a systematic approach.

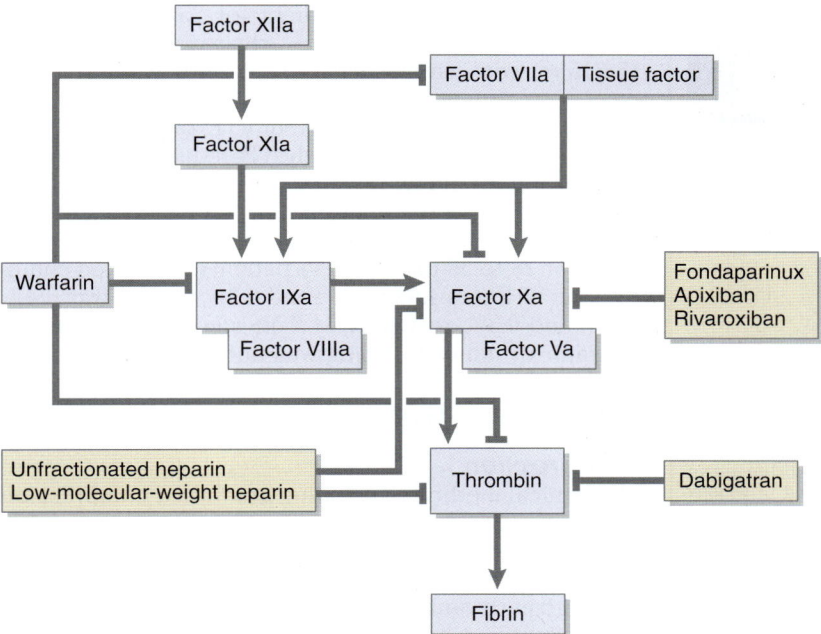

Figure 28-1. The points at which each VTE prophylactic drug agents provide inhibition in the coagulation cascade. (Redrawn from Colwell CW Jr: Prophylaxis for deep vein thrombosis after total knee arthroplasty. In Lieberman JR, Berry DJ, Azar FM [eds]: Advanced reconstruction: knee, Rosemont, Ill, 2010, American Academy of Orthopaedic Surgeons.)

Table 28-3. Major Randomized Trial Results

Agent	Number of Studies/Patients	PE, % (95% CI)	Proximal DVT, % (95% CI)	Total DVT, % (95% CI)
Placebo	13/947	1.5 (0.8-2.6)	25.8 (21-31)	48.5 (43-54)
Pneumatic compression	5/431	0.3 (0.01-1.4)	13.3 (10-18)	20.7 (15-29)
Warfarin	12/1493	0.2 (0.02-0.6)	6.3 (5-8)	23.2 (19-28)
Low-dose unfractionated heparin	11/1859	1.4 (0.9-2.0)	19.0 (13-27)	31.1 (23-41)
Aspirin	8/687	1.3 (0.6-2.5)	11.4 (7-18)	30.6 (21-42)
LMWH	21/5512	0.4 (0.2-0.6)	7.7 (6-10)	17.7 (15-21)
Fondaparinux[1,2]	2/2255	0.3 (0.2-0.4)	1.2 (1-2)	4.7 (4-6)

CI, Confidence interval; DVT, deep vein thrombosis; LMWH, low-molecular-weight heparin; PE, pulmonary embolus.
Data from Turpie AG, Bauer KA, Eriksson BI, Lassen MR: Postoperative fondaparinux versus postoperative enoxaparin for prevention of venous thromboembolism after elective hip-replacement surgery: a randomised double-blind trial. Lancet 359:1721–1726, 2002; Lassen MR, Bauer KA, Eriksson BI, Turpie AG: Postoperative fondaparinux versus preoperative enoxaparin for prevention of venous thromboembolism in elective hip-replacement surgery: a randomised double-blind comparison. Lancet 359:1715–1720, 2002; Freedman KB, Brookenthal KR, Fitzgerald RH Jr, et al: A meta-analysis of thromboembolic prophylaxis following elective total hip arthroplasty. J Bone Joint Surg Am 82:929–938, 2000.

Low-molecular-weight heparins were approved for prophylactic use for THA in 1993 and have been adopted in practice by many clinicians. The LMWHs most commonly used in North America are enoxaparin and dalteparin (see Table 28-2). LMWHs have been studied extensively and are highly effective and generally safe. Pooled results from clinical trials are shown in Table 28-3.

LMWHs are pharmacologically different from unfractionated heparin. LMWHs bind less to proteins and endothelial cells, resulting in

• A more predictable dose response
• A dose-independent mechanism of clearance
• A longer plasma half-life

With highly predictable pharmacokinetic properties and high bioavailability, LMWHs have the ability to target factor Xa while affecting factor IIa to a lesser extent (see Fig. 28-1) and are associated with a lower incidence of thrombocytopenia than unfractionated heparin. The half-life of LMWH is 4.5 hours, and its effects can be reversed by protamine sulfate. Their propitious pharmacokinetics allows LMWH administration subcutaneously once or twice daily without requisite monitoring of drug levels or activity.

However, the possibility of increased bleeding remains a concern with LMWH prophylaxis (see Table 28-4). One trial showed an increase in bleeding complications. Another trial reported greater blood loss.

Fondaparinux, a synthetic pentasaccharide that anticoagulates through inhibition of factor Xa (see Fig. 28-1), has been shown to provide effective prophylaxis in a once-daily dose in THA and hip fracture surgery (see Table 28-2). This pentasaccharide has a half-life of 18 hours with no known antidote. The reported total incidence of DVT in THA is shown in Table 28-3. The bleeding rate is reported in Table 28-4.

Table 28-4. Major and Minor Bleeding As Defined by Study for Anticoagulant Treatment Type

Agent	Number of Patients	Major	Minor
Placebo	713	0.6%	3.0%
Pneumatic compression	388	0	4.1%
Warfarin	1381	1.7%	5.7%
Low-dose unfractionated heparin	1992	3.5%	13.5%
Aspirin	687	0.7%	1.2%
LMWH	5412	2.2%	10.5%
Fondaparinux	2268	0.3%	2.7%

LMWH, Low-molecular-weight heparin.
Data from Turpie AG, Bauer KA, Eriksson BI, Lassen MR: Postoperative fondaparinux versus postoperative enoxaparin for prevention of venous thromboembolism after elective hip-replacement surgery: a randomised double-blind trial. Lancet 359:1721–1726, 2002; Lassen MR, Bauer KA, Eriksson BI, Turpie AG: Postoperative fondaparinux versus preoperative enoxaparin for prevention of venous thromboembolism in elective hip-replacement surgery: a randomised double-blind comparison. Lancet 359:1715–1720, 2002; Freedman KB, Brookenthal KR, Fitzgerald RH Jr, et al: A meta-analysis of thromboembolic prophylaxis following elective total hip arthroplasty. J Bone Joint Surg Am 82:929–938, 2000.

Differences in efficacy between LMWHs, pentasaccharide, and adjusted-dose warfarin prophylaxis were relatively small (see Table 28-3). Pooled rates for major and minor bleeding are presented in Table 28-4. In general, bleeding rates should be compared with placebo bleeding rates.

From these data, it can be seen that LMWHs, as well as pentasaccharide, are more effective than warfarin in preventing asymptomatic and symptomatic in-hospital VTE. An increase in surgical site bleeding and in wound hematoma is noted with both the LMWH and the pentasaccharide, but bleeding in both is not statistically different from the placebo bleeding rate. The more rapid onset of anticoagulation activity with LMWH and pentasaccharide compared with warfarin accounts for the increase in bleeding. Based on issues of cost, convenience, availability of an infrastructure to provide safe oral anticoagulation, potential bleeding and thrombosis risks, and duration of planned prophylaxis, the selection of LMWH, pentasaccharide, or warfarin prophylaxis is best made at the specific hospital level or, on occasion, at the individual patient level.

New oral anticoagulant drugs have recently been approved by the FDA for VTE prophylaxis after THA. Two of these are oral anti–factor Xa drugs (apixaban, Bristol-Myers Squibb, Princeton, NJ; rivaroxaban, Bayer Health-Care, Seattle, Wash), and one is an oral direct thrombin inhibitor (dabigatran, Boehringer Ingelheim, Ingelheim, en Rhein, Germany) (see Fig. 28-1). These drugs have the advantages of being given orally and do not require monitoring of blood levels or adjustment of dosing.

Apixaban clinical trials for prophylaxis in THA using the drug for 10 to 14 days compared with enoxaparin reported VTE of 0.5% (10/2199) for apixaban and 1.1% (25/2195) for enoxaparin with similar bleeding events.[31a] Rivaroxaban has been reported in two clinical trials after THA, both comparing rivaroxaban with enoxaparin. One with treatment for 35 days reported VTE of 1.1% (18/1595) with rivaroxaban and 3.7% (58/1558) with enoxaparin.[32] The other with 31 to 39 days of treatment with rivaroxaban and 10 to 14 days of enoxaparin treatment reported VTE of 2.0% (17/864) and 9.3% (81/869), respectively.[33] Bleeding was reported as similar with the two treatments in both studies. Dabigatran 220 mg and 150 mg orally once daily was compared with enoxaparin 40 mg subcutaneously once daily for 28 to 35 days in THA patients. Reported symptomatic VTE was 4.6%, 7.2%, and 6.3%, and PE was 0.4%, 0.1%, and 0.3%, respectively.[32] No significant difference in major or minor bleeding was noted.

Nonpharmacologic Prophylaxis

Compression

Mechanical methods, including graduated compression stockings (GCS), intermittent pneumatic compression (IPC) of the calf or calf and thigh, and venous foot pumps (VFP), are reported to be effective in combination with early ambulation. Compression devices appear to be effective when used properly; however, fewer data are available for devices compared with antithrombotic agents. Two key concerns when these devices are used are proper fit and the percentage of time used each day. Drawbacks to use of these devices are that patients find them too warm or uncomfortable to wear, IPC devices and VFPs require a larger motorized pump, which can be noisy and cumbersome, and the devices have to be disconnected when the patient is ambulating, making compliance an issue for both patient and staff.

A study evaluating use of above-the-knee and below-the-knee GCS found no reduction of DVT rates with either type of GCS compared with a control group that received no form of prophylaxis.[50] A further study of GCS revealed that 98% of the stockings failed to produce the "ideal" pressure gradient from the ankle to the knee.[34]

An observational study by Hooker and associates evaluated the number of VTE events after hip revision and THA and found an overall incidence of VTE of 6.1% (26/425), including 3.8% proximal DVT and 0.6% PE.[35] A similar observational study reported an overall VTE incidence of 2.1% (31/1492), including 1% DVT, 0.94% nonfatal PE, and 0.13% fatal PE.[36]

Of the various types of compression devices available, a mobile compression device has been studied. Its portability allows the patient to use the device at home, as well as in the hospital, and allows use of the device when the patient is out of bed without disconnecting the device, which increases compliance. In addition, this portable device contains a sensor that monitors respiratory-related venous phasic flow and times compression during the expiratory phase, when thoracic pressure is low and right heart filling is maximal. Studies of this device have shown that the incidence of DVT with this device ranges from 4.0% to 14.3% compared with incidence with enoxaparin, which ranges from 4.1% to 20%.[37-39] A study comparing the mobile compression device with LMWH reported a significant (0 vs. 6%) increase in major bleeding with LMWH and similar rates of VTE.[39]

Compression devices are difficult to compare because no standardization exists; therefore, results from a study of one device cannot be applied to another device.[40] Most studies of compression devices cannot be blinded, which leaves open the question of investigator bias. With decreasing hospital stays for THA patients, the effectiveness of compression agents for prophylaxis after discharge has not been demonstrated.

Multimodal

Multimodal prophylaxis, combining nonpharmacologic methods and/or pharmacologic methods, has not been well studied. One of the difficulties of examining multimodal prophylaxis is that the same combinations are seldom used in more than one study, not allowing any kind of meta-analysis. Although the use of layered modalities or multimodal prophylaxis is a matter of considerable interest, no prospective randomized trials presently indicate that multimodal prophylaxis is more effective than single-modality therapy.

Regional Anesthesia

Hypotensive regional anesthesia (spinal or epidural) has shown a significantly reduced incidence of postoperative DVT in the absence or presence of other prophylaxis for THA.[41] VTE prevalence after regional anesthesia, although reduced, remains substantial. Regional anesthesia alone has not been documented to match primary prophylaxis with other agents.

IVC Filter

Inferior vena cava (IVC) filter placement continues to be suggested as a prophylaxis option for patients at extremely high risk for both postoperative VTE and bleeding. Only one randomized trial has reported using IVC filter prophylaxis alone compared with LMWH or unfractionated heparin prophylaxis. After 12 days, filter recipients had significantly fewer PEs (symptomatic and asymptomatic), but filters were not associated with reduction of symptomatic PE. The IVC filter did not reduce mortality and revealed significantly more recurrent DVTs on follow-up.[42] A population-based observational study showed no association with significant reduction in the incidence of rehospitalization for PE at 1 year and increased the incidence of rehospitalization for DVT.[43] Thus, prophylactic IVC filter placement may reduce the immediate risk of postoperative PE in THA patients but will increase the risk of future DVT. Prophylactic IVC filter placement should be relegated to individuals who have failed previous adequate pharmacologic prophylaxis.

Treatment of Diagnosed Vascular Thromboembolic Events

Treatment regimens for established DVT or PE most often are carried out by internal medicine or pulmonary medicine, depending on the institution. Overall, the most consistently used treatment program is warfarin with an INR of 2 to 3 continued for a minimum of 3 months and often continued for 6 months. Warfarin therapy may be preceded by short-term treatment for about 5 days with LMWH, unfractionated heparin (UFH), or fondaparinux subcutaneously or UFH intravenously because of lag time to achieve therapeutic warfarin levels.[44] Treatment programs vary depending on the protocol adopted by each institution.

Treatment programs often are individualized to the patient, with customization depending on the area of the DVT and/or the area and amount of involvement of the PE. Treatment protocols may differ significantly with respect to distal DVT versus proximal DVT. These protocols also may differ in the treatment of acute PE, depending on whether the patient has a prior history of VTE.

CURRENT CONTROVERSIES AND FUTURE CONSIDERATIONS

Prophylaxis Length

Historically, prophylaxis has been continued during hospitalization of 7 to 14 days, but with the length of hospital stays now 5 days or less, the period of hospital prophylaxis may be inadequate. Some studies suggest that the risk of DVT may persist for as long as 3 months after THA.[45-47] A study continuing warfarin prophylaxis for 4 weeks after hospital discharge reported a 5.1% symptomatic confirmed DVT prevalence in the non-treated group and a 0.5% prevalence in the warfarin-treated group.[48] Analysis of six THA studies that used LMWH extended prophylaxis versus placebo reveals that the prevalence of DVT in the placebo group was 22.5% and in the LMWH group was 7.9% (relative risk ratio [RRR], 41%). The prevalence of proximal DVT was 11.2% in the placebo group and 3.0% in the LMWH group (RRR, 31%).[49] Results from studies of extended LMWH for up to 35 days demonstrate that prolonged LMWH prophylaxis is beneficial and is significantly superior to conventional prophylaxis of 7 to 10 days, with a 50% reduction in DVT over placebo.[50] Extended prophylaxis is recommended to reduce the number of thrombosis events after THA hospital discharge.

Bridging Therapy for Patients Receiving Vitamin K Antagonist

Many patients are on continuous anticoagulation therapy because of atrial fibrillation, a mechanical heart valve, or repeated VTE episodes. In patients who must have their VKA therapy interrupted while undergoing THA, bridging therapy is often used. Bridging therapy consists of discontinuing the VKA approximately 7 days before surgery and beginning LMWH or UFH approximately 5 days before surgery. Because of the shorter half-life of these subcutaneous anticoagulants, they can be stopped 5 to 24 hours before surgery and resumed as soon as hemostasis has been achieved, usually 12 to 24 hours after surgery.[51-53] This bridging therapy usually is done in conjunction with VKA therapy prescribed by the physician. VKA therapy is restarted after surgery, and LMWH or UFH is discontinued when VKA reaches a therapeutic INR. The timing may vary from institution to institution and from physician to physician.

Surveillance

Withholding primary prophylaxis in favor of case findings by noninvasive screening techniques or by serial techniques has not demonstrated effectiveness as an alternative to primary prophylaxis. Many screening trials have demonstrated lack of sensitivity, specificity, and accuracy, particularly for calf thrombi, and variable detection of proximal thrombi.[27, 54] Clinical trials and cohort studies indicate that screening for proximal DVT with predischarge color duplex ultrasound is also ineffective.[55] Consequently, primary prophylaxis continues to be recommended for all THA patients.

Economics of Thromboprophylaxis

Because of changing costs of prophylaxis agents, variation in costs of prophylaxis not only by region but by facility, depending on the contracts negotiated, use of monitoring for oral anticoagulation, and use of extended prophylaxis, cost-effectiveness continues to be an elusive issue. The cost of treating patients who fail prophylaxis or who have a bleeding event and the cost of long-term treatment of those patients who develop post-thrombotic syndrome and chronic pulmonary hypertension also affect the economics of VTE prophylaxis. Despite these problems, reports comparing costs and economic efficacy of the various methods of prophylaxis are available. A retrospective analysis of inpatient billing data determined that fondaparinux was

---

BOX 28-2   JCAHO-APPROVED VTE CORE MEASURES

VTE-1: Venous Thromboembolism Prophylaxis
Numerator: Patients who received VTE prophylaxis or have documentation why no VTE prophylaxis was given:
- The day of or the day after hospital admission
- The day of or the day after surgery end date for surgeries that start the day of or the day after hospital admission

Denominator: All patients

VTE-2: Intensive Care Unit Venous Thromboembolism Prophylaxis
Numerator: Patients who received VTE prophylaxis or have documentation why no VTE prophylaxis was given:
- The day of or the day after ICU admission (or transfer)
- The day of or the day after surgery end date for surgeries that start the day of or the day after ICU admission (or transfer)

Denominator: Patients directly admitted or transferred to ICU

VTE-3: Venous Thromboembolism Patients With Anticoagulation Overlap Therapy
Numerator: Patients who received overlap therapy
Denominator: Patients with confirmed VTE who received warfarin

VTE-4: Venous Thromboembolism Patients Receiving Unfractionated Heparin With Dosages/Platelet Count Monitoring by Protocol or Nomogram
Numerator: Patients who have their IV UFH therapy dosages AND platelet counts monitored according to

defined parameters such as a nomogram or protocol
Denominator: Patients with confirmed VTE receiving IV UFH therapy

VTE-5: Venous Thromboembolism Discharge Instructions
Numerator: Patients with documentation that they or their caregivers were given written discharge instructions or other educational material about warfarin addressing all of the following:
1. Compliance issues
2. Dietary advice
3. Follow-up monitoring
4. Potential for adverse drug reactions and interactions

Denominator: Patients with confirmed VTE discharged on warfarin therapy

VTE-6: Incidence of Potentially Preventable Venous Thromboembolism
Numerator: Patients who received no VTE prophylaxis prior to the VTE diagnostic test order date
Denominator: Patients who developed confirmed VTE during hospitalization

---

ICU, Intensive care unit; *IV,* intravenous; *JCAHO,* Joint Commission on Accreditation of Healthcare Organizations; *UFH,* unfractionated heparin; *VTE,* venous thromboembolism.
Joint Commission Perspectives®, April 2009, Volume 29, Issue 4, Copyright 2009.

lower in cost and resulted in a lower number of VTEs than LMWH or unfractionated heparin.[56] A Canadian study looked at the value of extended prophylaxis in THA with LMWH and warfarin. They identified a net gain in quality-adjusted life-years for both drugs but were unclear on whether economic evidence was sufficient to support extended prophylaxis in THA.[57]

Guidelines and National Mandates for Prophylaxis

Guidelines for thromboprophylaxis are available to assist in the practice of evidence-based medicine. The American College of Chest Physicians released its 8th edition of antithrombotic and thrombotic therapy guidelines in 2008.[44] These guidelines are based on current literature reporting on the effectiveness and safety of various types of thromboprophylaxis.

The American Academy of Orthopaedic Surgeons released guidelines in 2007 for prevention of symptomatic PE in patients undergoing total hip or knee arthroplasty.[58] Most studies with symptomatic PE as the endpoint were underpowered to evaluate the benefit of prophylaxis. Therefore these recommendations allow for multiple as well as additive protocols, because no evidence is available to suggest that any one protocol is more or less effective.

The National Institute of Health Excellence (NICE) has published prophylaxis guidelines in Britain, but they do not contain guidelines for TKA.[59] Current reports indicate that these guidelines are being redrafted for orthopedic surgery with assistance from the British Orthopaedic Association. The International Consensus Statement (ICS),[60] published in 2001, recommended LMWH for THA patients, recognizing that residual DVT frequency remains high, and suggesting that further studies of compression devices in THA are needed.

In the United States, prevention of thrombosis after THA has been mandated by several regulatory agencies. SCIP Venous Thromboembolism Measures state the following:

- SCIP VTE 1: Surgery patients with recommended venous thromboembolism prophylaxis ordered.
- SCIP VTE 2: Surgery patients who received appropriate venous thromboembolism prophylaxis within 24 hours prior to surgery to 24 hours after surgery.[59]

The SCIP Website also contains tools to assist in achieving these measures, such as a sample order set, a nursing assessment guide, a pocket reminder card, and an education module.

The Nation Quality Forum (NQF) released six measures in 2008 that "target the most common preventable cause of hospital death—venous thromboembolism." These measures are directed at all hospital patients, not just surgery patients, and include appropriately documented risk of VTE, prescribed and received prophylaxis, and provided discharge instructions. The measures also discuss reporting the incidence of potentially preventable VTE.

The National Consensus Standards for the Prevention and Care of Deep Vein Thrombosis (DVT) is a project between the JCAHO and the NQF that began in 2005.

The JCAHO approved six VTE core measures (Box 28-2) that are available for data collection and reporting for discharges that occurred in late 2009.[61]

CONCLUSIONS

THA has become an excellent surgical procedure with long-term pain relief and return to normal function. Risks, however, accompany any major surgical procedure such as THA. VTE and its sequelae have been identified as a significant surgical risk. Many recommended guidelines are available, and the surgeon has the opportunity and the responsibility to choose that protocol that gives his patient the best risk/benefit ratio. VTE prophylaxis in THA is a changing field, with new agents and devices currently being tested that may be available in the near future. Physicians should remain current and willing to adopt new protocols when evidence-based medicine shows that a new modality produces better risk/benefit ratios than are produced by older protocols.

REFERENCES

1. NIH Consensus Development: Prevention of venous thrombosis and pulmonary embolism. JAMA 256:744–749, 1986.
2. Kurtz S, Ong K, Lau E, et al: Projections of primary and revision hip and knee arthroplasty in the United States from 2005 to 2030. J Bone Joint Surg Am 89:780–785, 2007.
3. Eriksson BI, Kalebo P, Anthymyr BA, et al: Prevention of deep-vein thrombosis and pulmonary embolism after total hip replacement: comparison of low-molecular-weight heparin and unfractionated heparin. J Bone Joint Surg Am 73:484–493, 1991.
4. Dahl OE: Cardiorespiratory and vascular dysfunction related to major reconstructive orthopedic surgery. Acta Orthop Scand 68:607–614, 1997.
5. Planes A, Vochelle N, Darmon JY, et al: Risk of deep-venous thrombosis after hospital discharge in patients having undergone total hip replacement: double-blind randomised comparison of enoxaparin versus placebo. Lancet 348:224–228, 1996.
6. Dahl OE, Andreassen G, Aspelin T, et al: Prolonged thromboprophylaxis following hip replacement surgery—results of a double-blind, prospective, randomised, placebo-controlled study with dalteparin (Fragmin). Thromb Haemost 77:26–31, 1997.
7. Caprini JA, Botteman MF, Stephens JM, et al: Economic burden of long-term complications of deep vein thrombosis after total hip replacement surgery in the United States. Value Health 6:59–74, 2003.
8. Caprini JA, Arcelus JI, Reyna JJ: Effective risk stratification of surgical and nonsurgical patients for venous thromboembolic disease. Semin Hematol 38(2 Suppl 5):12–19, 2001.
9. Motte S, Samama CM, Guay J, et al: Prevention of postoperative venous thromboembolism: risk assessment and methods of prophylaxis. Can J Anaesth 53(6 Suppl):S68–S79, 2006.
10. McCaffrey R, Bishop M, Adonis-Rizzo M, et al: Development and testing of a DVT risk assessment tool: providing evidence of validity and reliability. Worldviews on Evidence-Based Nursing/Sigma Theta Tau International, Honor Society of Nursing 4:14–20, 2007.
11. Muntz JE: Deep vein thrombosis and pulmonary embolism in the perioperative patient. Am J Manag Care 6(Suppl 20):S1045–S1052, 2000.
12. Caprini JA: Thrombosis risk assessment as a guide to quality patient care. Dis Mon 51:70–78, 2005.
13. McLafferty RB, Passman MA, Caprini JA, et al: Increasing awareness about venous disease: the American Venous Forum

expands the National Venous Screening Program. J Vasc Surg 48:394–399, 2008.

14. Markel A: Origin and natural history of deep vein thrombosis of the legs. Semin Vasc Med 5:65–74, 2005.

15. Grady-Benson JC, Oishi CS, Hanson PB, et al: Postoperative surveillance for deep venous thrombosis with duplex ultrasonography after total knee arthroplasty. J Bone Joint Surg Am 76:1649–1657, 1994.

16. Lohr JM, James KV, Deshmukh RM, et al: Karmody Award. Calf vein thrombi are not a benign finding. Am J Surg 170:86–90, 1995.

17. Lohr JM, Kerr TM, Lutter KS, et al: Lower extremity calf thrombosis: to treat or not to treat? J Vasc Surg 14:618–623, 1991.

18. Prandoni P, Lensing AW, Cogo A, et al: The long-term clinical course of acute deep venous thrombosis. Ann Intern Med 125:1–7, 1996.

19. Ginsberg JS, Turkstra F, Buller HR, et al: Postthrombotic syndrome after hip or knee arthroplasty: a cross-sectional study. Arch Intern Med 160:669–672, 2000.

20. Wahlander K, Larson G, Lindahl TL, et al: Factor V Leiden (G1691A) and prothrombin gene G20210A mutations as potential risk factors for venous thromboembolism after total hip or total knee replacement surgery. Thromb Haemost 87:580–585, 2002.

21. Kyrle PA, Minar E, Hirschl M, et al: High plasma levels of factor VIII and the risk of recurrent venous thromboembolism. N Engl J Med 343:457–462, 2000.

22. Pecheniuk NM, Elias DJ, Deguchi H, et al: Elevated plasma fibronectin levels associated with venous thromboembolism. Thromb Haemost 100:224–228, 2008.

23. Eichinger S, Pecheniuk NM, Hron G, et al: High-density lipoprotein and the risk of recurrent venous thromboembolism. Circulation 115:1609–1614, 2007.

24. Deguchi H, Fernandez JA, Griffin JH: Plasma cholesteryl ester transfer protein and blood coagulability. Thromb Haemost 98:1160–1164, 2007.

25. Schwarz UI, Ritchie MD, Bradford Y, et al: Genetic determinants of response to warfarin during initial anticoagulation. N Engl J Med 358:999–1008, 2008.

26. Millican EA, Lenzini PA, Milligan PE, et al: Genetic-based dosing in orthopedic patients beginning warfarin therapy. Blood 110:1511–1515, 2007.

27. Schellong SM, Beyer J, Kakkar AK, et al: Ultrasound screening for asymptomatic deep vein thrombosis after major orthopaedic surgery: the VENUS study. J Thromb Haemost 5:1431–1437, 2007.

28. Robinson KS, Anderson DR, Gross M, et al: Ultrasonographic screening before hospital discharge for deep venous thrombosis after arthroplasty: the post-arthroplasty screening study. A randomized, controlled trial. Ann Intern Med 127:439–445, 1997.

29. Grady-Benson JC, Oishi CS, Hanson PB, et al: Routine postoperative duplex ultrasonography screening and monitoring for the detection of deep vein thrombosis: a survey of 110 total hip arthroplasties. Clin Orthop Relat Res 307:130–141, 1994.

30. Dahl OE, Caprini JA, Colwell CW Jr, et al: Fatal vascular outcomes following major orthopedic surgery. Thromb Haemost 93:860–866, 2005.

31. Anderson DR, Kahn SR, Rodger MA, et al: Computed tomographic pulmonary angiography vs ventilation-perfusion lung scanning in patients with suspected pulmonary embolism: a randomized controlled trial. JAMA 298:2743–2753, 2007.

31a. Lassen MR, Gallus A, Raskob CE, Pineo G, Chen D, Ramirez LM. Apixaban versus enoxaparin for thromboprophylaxis after hip replacement. N Engl J Med 363(26):2487, 2010.

32. Eriksson BI, Borris LC, Friedman RJ, et al: Rivaroxaban versus enoxaparin for thromboprophylaxis after hip arthroplasty. N Engl J Med 358:2765–2775, 2008.

33. Kakkar AK, Brenner B, Dahl OE, et al: Extended duration rivaroxaban versus short-term enoxaparin for the prevention of venous thromboembolism after total hip arthroplasty: a double-blind, randomised controlled trial. Lancet 372:31–39, 2008.

34. Best AJ, Williams S, Crozier A, et al: Graded compression stockings in elective orthopaedic surgery: an assessment of the in vivo performance of commercially available stockings in patients having hip and knee arthroplasty. J Bone Joint Surg Br 82:116–118, 2000.

35. Hooker JA, Lachiewicz PF, Kelley SS: Efficacy of prophylaxis against thromboembolism with intermittent pneumatic compression after primary and revision total hip arthroplasty. J Bone Joint Surg Am 81:690–696, 1999.

36. Sarmiento A, Goswami AD: Thromboembolic prophylaxis with use of aspirin, exercise, and graded elastic stockings or intermittent compression devices in patients managed with total hip arthroplasty. J Bone Joint Surg Am 81:339–346, 1999.

37. Edwards JZ, Pulido P, Ezzet KA, et al: Portable compression device and low-molecular-weight heparin compared with low-molecular-weight heparin for thromboprophylaxis following total joint arthroplasty. J Arthroplasty 23:1122–1127, 2008.

38. Gelfer Y, Tavor H, Oron A, et al: Deep vein thrombosis prevention in joint arthroplasties: continuous enhanced circulation therapy vs low molecular weight heparin. J Arthroplasty 21:206–214, 2006.

39. Colwell CW Jr, Froimson MI, Mont MA, et al: Thrombosis prevention after total hip arthroplasty: a prospective, randomized trial comparing a mobile compression device with low-molecular-weight heparin. J Bone Joint Surg Am 92:527–535, 2010.

40. Morris RJ, Woodcock JP: Evidence-based compression: prevention of stasis and deep vein thrombosis. Ann Surg 239:162–171, 2004.

41. Westrich GH, Farrell C, Bono JV, et al: The incidence of venous thromboembolism after total hip arthroplasty: a specific hypotensive epidural anesthesia protocol. J Arthroplasty 14:456–463, 1999.

42. Decousus H, Leizorovicz A, Parent F, et al: A clinical trial of vena caval filters in the prevention of pulmonary embolism in patients with proximal deep-vein thrombosis. Prevention du Risque d'Embolie Pulmonaire par Interruption Cave Study Group. N Engl J Med 338:409–415, 1998.

43. White RH, Zhou H, Kim J, Romano PS: A population-based study of the effectiveness of inferior vena cava filter use among patients with venous thromboembolism. Arch Intern Med 160:2033–2041, 2000.

44. Geerts WH, Bergqvist D, Pineo GF, et al: Prevention of venous thromboembolism: American College of Chest Physicians evidence-based clinical practice guidelines (8th edition). Chest 133(Suppl 6):381S–453S, 2008.

45. Bjornara BT, Gudmundsen TE, Dahl OE: Frequency and timing of clinical venous thromboembolism after major joint surgery. J Bone Joint Surg Br 88:386–391, 2006.

46. White RH, Romano PS, Zhou H, et al: Incidence and time course of thromboembolic outcomes following total hip or knee arthroplasty. Arch Intern Med 158:1525–1531, 1998.

47. Phillips CB, Barrett JA, Losina E, et al: Incidence rates of dislocation, pulmonary embolism, and deep infection during the first six months after elective total hip replacement. J Bone Joint Surg Am 85:20–26, 2003.

48. Prandoni P, Bruchi O, Sabbion P, et al: Prolonged thromboprophylaxis with oral anticoagulants after total hip arthroplasty: a prospective controlled randomized study. Arch Intern Med 162:1966–1971, 2002.

49. Hull RD, Pineo GF, Stein PD, et al: Extended out-of-hospital low-molecular-weight heparin prophylaxis against deep venous thrombosis in patients after elective hip arthroplasty: a systematic review. Ann Intern Med 135:858–869, 2001.

50. Dahl OE, Bergqvist D, Cohen AT, et al: Low-molecular-weight heparin prophylaxis against thromboembolism after total hip replacement—the never-ending story? Acta Orthop Scand 72:199–204, 2001.

51. Kovacs MJ, Kearon C, Rodger M, et al: Single-arm study of bridging therapy with low-molecular-weight heparin for patients at risk of arterial embolism who require temporary interruption of warfarin. Circulation 110:1658–1663, 2004.

52. Dunn AS, Spyropoulos AC, Turpie AG: Bridging therapy in patients on long-term oral anticoagulants who require surgery: the prospective perioperative enoxaparin cohort trial (PROSPECT). J Thromb Haemost 5:2211–2218, 2007.

53. Jaffer AK, Ahmed M, Brotman DJ, et al: Low-molecular-weight-heparins as periprocedural anticoagulation for patients on

long-term warfarin therapy: a standardized bridging therapy protocol. J Thromb Thrombolysis 20:11–16, 2005.

54. Robinson KS, Anderson DR, Gross M, et al: Accuracy of screening compression ultrasonography and clinical examination for the diagnosis of deep vein thrombosis after total hip or knee arthroplasty. Can J Surg 41:368–373, 1998.

55. Anderson DR, Gross M, Robinson KS, et al: Ultrasonographic screening for deep vein thrombosis following arthroplasty fails to reduce posthospital thromboembolic complications: the Postarthroplasty Screening Study (PASS). Chest 114(Suppl Evidence 2):119S–122S, 1998.

56. Shorr AF, Sarnes MW, Peeples PJ, et al: Comparison of cost, effectiveness, and safety of injectable anticoagulants used for thromboprophylaxis after orthopedic surgery. Am J Health Syst Pharm 64:2349–2355, 2007.

57. Skedgel C, Goeree R, Pleasance S, et al: The cost-effectiveness of extended-duration antithrombotic prophylaxis after total hip arthroplasty. J Bone Joint Surg Am 89:819–828, 2007.

58. Johanson NA, Lachiewicz PF, Leberman JR, et al: Prevention of symptomatic pulmonary embolism in patients undergoing total hip or knee arthroplasty. J Am Acad Orthop Surg 17:183–196, 2009.

59. The Surgical Care Improvement Project (SCIP), 2008. Available at: http://www.premierinc.com/safety/topics/scip/index.jsp. Accessed December 1, 2008.

60. Nicolaides AN, Breddin HK, Fareed J, et al: Prevention of venous thromboembolism. International Consensus Statement: guidelines compiled in accordance with the scientific evidence. Int Angiol 20:1–37, 2001.

61. JCAHO: Approved: more options for hospital core measures, April 2009. Available at: http://www.jointcommission.org/NR/rdonlyres/AD24B9CB-57F6-4EDC-86DD-5DA0576AC15E/0/S4JCP0409.pdf. Accessed August 24, 2009.

CHAPTER 29

Rehabilitation After Hip Surgery

Robert E. Mayle, Jr. and James I. Huddleston III

KEY POINTS

- The goal of rehabilitation is to maximize functional outcomes and improve an individual's ability to perform activities of daily living in a timely fashion after treatment has been rendered.
- Surgical treatment options for hip pathology include total hip arthroplasty, resurfacing arthroplasty, arthroscopy, osteotomies, and fracture care.
- To be discharged home after hip surgery, a patient must be able to ambulate approximately 50 to 100 feet with an assistive device, use a toilet, perform transfers, perform activities of daily living, demonstrate understanding of and compliance with hip precautions, independently perform home exercises, and be medically stable. It may be beneficial to have additional help at home in the perioperative period.
- Following THA, functional improvement, patient satisfaction, and walking ability at the time of discharge were better in patients who received the accelerated rehabilitation protocol, regardless of the size of the incision.
- The postoperative rehabilitation program following hip arthroscopy will be based on the patient's diagnosis, the procedure performed, and patient characteristics. Typically, 10 to 12 weeks of supervised therapy is to be expected. Hip range of motion is permitted in the perioperative period to prevent labral-capsular adhesions. Patients who undergo cheilectomy are usually advised to be partial weight-bearing for 4 to 6 weeks postoperatively.
- Following acetabular reorientation and proximal femoral osteotomy procedures, a period of restricted weight bearing is required. Focus should be placed on mobilization, gait training, and isolated exercises with strict observance of weight-bearing restrictions. Once allowed, patients should work with their therapists on gait training, range of motion, and strengthening exercises.

INTRODUCTION

Surgical treatment options for hip pathology include arthroplasty, resurfacing, arthroscopy, osteotomies, and fracture care. Rehabilitation after hip surgery is a crucial part of a patient's recovery. In this chapter, we will focus on key components of rehabilitation of the patient following arthroplasty, arthroscopy, and osteotomy.

Rehabilitation is the field of medicine that focuses on return of function after illness or injury. Rehabilitation is coordinated by a team consisting of physical and occupational therapists, orthopedic surgeons, physical medicine and rehabilitation physicians, nurses, and ancillary staff. Successful rehabilitation addresses the physical and psychological challenges faced by the patient. Rehabilitation should not be limited to activities that occur postoperatively, as events and activities that occur preoperatively may influence outcomes. The goal of rehabilitation is to maximize functional outcomes and improve an individual's ability to perform activities of daily living in a timely fashion after treatment has been rendered.

HIP ARTHROPLASTY

Hip arthroplasty is one of the most successful and cost-effective operations performed, reliably leading to pain relief, increased function, and return to activity. Rehabilitation is directly related to the success of the procedure, as it allows a patient to gain maximal functional performance and improves his or her ability to perform activities of daily living. Common impairments that patients face following arthroplasty include pain, range-of-motion limitations, muscular weakness, and postoperative protective restrictions (positional and weight-bearing precautions). Maximal beneficial effects of rehabilitation are seen by 3 to 6 months following surgery, yet some patients are able to make continued improvement up to 2 years postoperatively.

Projected demands for total hip arthroplasty (THA) are expected to increase by 174% by the year 2030.[1] Although the average length of stay in the acute hospital setting has decreased substantially over the past 15 years to average 4.2 days after hip arthroplasty,[2] demands to discharge patients earlier are increasing.

Components of Rehabilitation
Education

Preoperative education of patients undergoing THA is effective in preventing early dislocation, deep venous thrombosis, and pulmonary embolism, and in decreasing preoperative anxiety.[3,4] However, as noted by a review conducted and published in 2004 by the Cochrane Database, although preoperative education led to a decrease in preoperative anxiety, no benefit was derived in terms of functional outcomes, postoperative pain, reduction in length of hospital stay, or change in postoperative anxiety level.[3]

Patients' concerns and expectations vary widely.[5] Anxiety prior to THA is common and can be reduced by making the unknown familiar.[6] This can be accomplished by allowing patients to meet the staff that will care for them, introducing them to the hospital environment, and addressing the experiences that the patient will encounter postoperatively.[6] This can also include a discussion of the surgeon's approach to obstacles that may be encountered in the perioperative period.

The patient's preoperative concerns may differ from those of the surgeon.[5] Although a positive correlation of preoperative with postoperative functional outcomes may be lacking, patients' expectations should not be underestimated, as they are linked to requests for elective, costly procedures and correlated with assessments of outcome.[7]

Preoperative Exercise

Osteoarthritic hips are painful and lead to reduced muscle strength, difficulty with performance of activities of daily living, and a decline in preoperative function.[8] In a study conducted by Lavernia and associates, a correlation between preoperative function and postoperative function was noted in patients undergoing total hip or knee arthroplasty.[9] Specifically, patients who had more extreme functional limitations preoperatively did not fare as well as those whose functional levels were better.

The goal of a preoperative exercise program is to enhance range of motion, muscle strength, and overall physical function.[10] Despite this, the effectiveness of a preoperative physiotherapy program remains controversial. Grocen and associates,[11] Wijman and coworkers,[12] and Ferrara and colleagues[13] published reports noting no significant difference in Harris Hip Scores, Barthel Index, SF-36 scores, Western Ontario and McMaster Universities Arthritis Index (WOMAC) scores, hip abduction, pain, length of hospital stay, and time to stand/walk/climb a stair. To the contrary, Wang and associates[14] and Rooks and colleagues[15] reported significant differences in preoperative strength and functional status following a short preoperative exercise protocol. Additionally, significant postoperative differences were observed in gait velocity, stride length, and walking distance, along with a reduction in the odds for discharge to inpatient rehabilitation. As proposed by D'Lima and coworkers,[16] this discrepancy may be due to three issues: (1) the duration of preoperative physical therapy may be insufficient for any substantial gains to be seen, (2) the dramatic improvement in symptoms following surgery may overshadow any small gains made preoperatively, and (3) the act of surgery deconditions the function of the extremity and erases any preoperative improvement. Additional studies are required to quantify the potential benefits of a preoperative exercise program.

Surgical Exposure

In recent years, an increase has been seen in patient and market demand for the least invasive form of THA.[17] Procedures performed using a certain technique or with a skin incision <10 cm are often defined as less invasive.[10] Advocates of less invasive procedures purport that a patient's rehabilitation is expedited, along with a reduction in soft tissue trauma, shorter intraoperative time, less perioperative blood loss, less postoperative pain, improved cosmetic appearance, and earlier discharge from the hospital.[1] Despite this, there is a paucity of studies that support expedited rehabilitation. In a review performed by Sharma and associates,[10] five studies were identified that pertained to the effects of a less invasive approach to THA on rehabilitation. Dorr and colleagues[18] and Pagnano and coworkers[19] noted that patients who underwent a less invasive approach had better pain control, earlier discharge home, earlier discontinuation and less usage of assistive devices, and faster return to activities of daily living. In contrast, Ogonda and associates[20] identified no significant difference in early walking ability, length of hospital stay, and functional outcome. Pour and colleagues[21] performed a randomized study of 100 patients undergoing the anterolateral approach for THA and evaluated the effects of an accelerated rehabilitation protocol and the length of the incision. Functional improvement at time of discharge, patient satisfaction, and walking ability at the time of discharge were better in patients who received the accelerated rehabilitation protocol, regardless of the size of the incision.

Perioperative Pain Management

Pain management directly correlates with patient satisfaction following THA.[2] Effective perioperative management of pain is critical to the recovery of a patient following hip surgery. Consequences of uncontrolled postoperative pain include prolonged hospital stay, increased incidence of readmission, decreased range of motion, arthrofibrosis, potential for medicolegal action, and increased opioid use with possible side effects of nausea and vomiting.[23] Currently, no gold standard exists for perioperative management of pain following THA. In recent years, the development of a multimodal approach to pain management has gained much attention. Maheshwari and associates defined multimodal analgesia as a multidisciplinary approach to pain management with goals to maximize analgesic effects and minimize potential side effects of medications.[23] Analgesic methods for perioperative pain control include general or regional anesthesia, neuraxial analgesia, intraoperative periarticular injection, intravenous and oral narcotics, and preemptive analgesia. Preemptive analgesia effectively limits the sensitization of the nervous system to noxious stimuli by producing dense blockade of the transmission of a noxious afferent stimulus from the peripheral to the central nervous system for the appropriate duration.[24] Effective multimodal perioperative analgesia has been demonstrated by Peters and colleagues[25] to cause a significant reduction in rest pain scores, total narcotic consumption, and hospital length of stay, along with improvements in distance ambulated and time to achieve therapy goals.

Functional Activities

Dislocation

Dislocation following primary THA is a common complication and an important problem, occurring in 0.2% to 7% of patients. Instability is also an important mode of THA failure, with 10% to 25% of patients undergoing revision THA for this complication.[26,27] Fifty percent of dislocations following primary THA occur within 3 months of the index procedure, and 75% may occur within 1 year.[28] Surgical factors affecting the potential for dislocation include approach, implant selection and position, soft tissue tension, and experience of the surgeon. Patient factors include neuromuscular disorders, alcoholism, cognitive disorders, noncompliance, and history of previous hip surgery.

In the rehabilitation phase preceding and following THA, education and instruction regarding hip precautions can help to reduce the risk of dislocation. A surgical approach to the hip dictates these precautions. The surgical approach is classified on the basis of its location relative to the anatomy of the hip. Most THAs are performed from a posterolateral approach. This approach leads to minimal trauma to the abductor complex. Implantation of larger femoral heads and repair of posterior soft tissue structures are believed to reduce the risk of dislocation.[29-32] Patients in whom the posterolateral approach was used must be instructed not to internally rotate, adduct, or flex their hips more than 70 to 90 degrees. The most common scenarios in which dislocations occur after a posterolateral approach to the hip include bending down from a seated position to tie shoes, getting off a low toilet or chair with the hip adducted and internally rotated, and twisting the trunk toward the operative side with the feet planted in sitting and standing positions.[33] A direct lateral approach to the hip requires partial takedown of the glutei musculature. This has been associated with prolonged postoperative weakness of the abductor complex. A transtrochanteric osteotomy approach through the greater trochanter will require that patients avoid active abduction of the hip while the osteotomy heals. Patients who undergo an anterior or anterolateral approach to the hip, in which the anterior capsule is violated, should be instructed to avoid hyperextension, adduction, and external rotation to prevent dislocation.

Preoperative and postoperative education regarding hip precautions is crucial for patients' understanding and compliance. The duration of hip precautions varies and depends on both the surgeon and the patient. Uncomplicated patients should adhere to precautions for 6 weeks; more complicated patients who are at higher risk for dislocation should observe precautions for 12 weeks.[34]

In an attempt to prevent patients' operative extremities from moving into a position that would make them vulnerable to dislocation, many physicians advocate functional restrictions, in addition to hip range-of-motion precautions. Functional restrictions include placing an abduction wedge or pillows between the legs when in bed, using a knee immobilizer placed on the operative extremity,[35] as well as higher chairs and toilet seats, and avoiding getting into and out of an automobile with low seats. Few studies, however, have evaluated the efficacy of the use of aids in helping to prevent dislocation. A recently published randomized prospective study, conducted to assess the efficacy of functional restrictions in preventing dislocation following THA from an anterolateral approach, revealed no increased benefit of functional restrictions.[23] In addition, patients reported a higher level of satisfaction when functional restrictions were not placed.

Weight Bearing

Historically, full weight bearing on the operative extremity was permitted in patients who underwent THA with a cemented femoral component, while patients receiving cementless femoral components were restricted to partial weight bearing for 6 weeks. Restricted weight bearing in cementless femoral component fixation was thought to decrease micromotion of the stem, which may interfere with osseointegration. Early investigations examining immediate weight bearing following bilateral THAs with cementless femoral components, however, revealed that bone ingrowth can occur despite initial subsidence of the femoral stem.[35,36] Woolson and associates reported their results following implantation of cementless, fully porous-coated collared femoral components, noting excellent bone ingrowth in patients allowed to bear weight immediately following THA.[37] In this series, no patients exhibited evidence of radiographic subsidence of the femoral component at last follow-up (minimum of 2 years). In addition, at final follow-up, patients who were allowed to immediately bear full weight had a higher Harris Hip Score compared with patients who had restricted weight bearing immediately following surgery. Similar results were demonstrated in a recent study by Klein and coworkers with a minimum of 5-year follow-up using the Fiber Metal Taper Stem (Zimmer Inc., Warsaw, Ind), a cementless, collarless, proximally coated, distally tapered femoral implant.[38] Duration of hospital stay and postoperative rehabilitation were significantly decreased when patients were allowed to bear weight immediately after surgery.[39] Partial weight bearing for a 6-week period is not a benign limitation and may slow and prolong a patient's rehabilitation.[36] Partial weight-bearing status leads to muscle atrophy of the operative limb and increased stresses placed on the upper extremities and the contralateral lower extremity.

Restriction of weight-bearing status may be unavoidable in instances where a fracture in the greater trochanter, femoral calcar, or shaft is observed intraoperatively, or when a trochanteric osteotomy is performed. In these instances, weight bearing should be restricted until the fracture or osteotomy site has healed. Patients should be allowed toe-touch weight-bearing status during this period. Non–weight bearing should be avoided, as this action requires the patient to hold the affected limb off the ground. This may place as much, if not more, force across the implants, as does full body weight.[40]

Assistive Devices

Restoration of balance and gait is a primary goal of any postoperative rehabilitation program following THA. Sensory input and functional changes that contribute to instability of the hip following surgery include excision of the capsule with damage to proprioceptors, abductor weakness, altered abductor lever arms, restricted range of motion, and potential changes in leg length.[41] Assistive devices are a routine component of a patient's postoperative rehabilitation, as they provide stability and promote restoration of gait. Canes, crutches, and walkers are examples of ambulatory assistive devices. They provide stability, augment muscle action, and allow for joint and soft tissue unloading. Assistive devices have a direct effect on a patient's physical and psychological well-being. Improvement in confidence and safety allows for enhanced levels of activity and independence. Increased activity leads to prevention of cardiorespiratory deconditioning, enhanced circulation, and improved renal function.[42] Selection of an assistive device should be based on evaluation of the patient's balance, coordination, mental status, strength, age, weight-bearing status, other joint impairments, and purpose for use.

The cane is the most commonly used assistive device. A cane is lightweight and versatile and can be used to improve balance, transmit sensory input from the floor/ground surface, decrease joint reaction force on an arthritic hip, and reduce force on the prosthetic hip and incised abductor muscles.[43,44] Use of a cane requires good upper body strength; a cane can support only 15% to 20% of body weight. A cane is most beneficial when there is unilateral lower extremity involvement or when physical impairment is mild. Correct use of a cane requires that it be held by the contralateral upper extremity. This can reduce the hip contact force by 60%.[45] Ajemian and associates noted a decrease in the abduction moment by 26% and 28% on operative and nonoperative sides, respectively, when a cane was used on the contralateral side. In addition, they noted a decrease in the duration of contraction of the hip abductor musculature during gait.[44] Proper fit of a cane requires that it come up to the ulnar styloid with the shoulder and elbow in a neutral position. Once held, the elbow should be flexed 15 to 20 degrees.[43]

Axillary crutches are versatile, allow for easy maneuvering of stairs, are associated with increased gait velocity, and can support full body weight. Disadvantages include balance instability leading to a fall and the potential for neurologic palsy if direct pressure is applied to the brachial plexus. Their use is often better tolerated in younger patients, who are more agile and are better able to control/maneuver the operative extremity. Proper sizing of axillary crutches should allow 2 inches between the armpit and the top of the crutch. This places the elbow in approximately 15 degrees of flexion.

Walkers are commonly used in the immediate period following hip arthroplasty. They provide a wide base to enhance stability with ambulation. Walkers are commonly used for patients with bilateral lower extremity weakness, balance disorders, or when greater body weight support is needed than can be provided by a cane alone. Walkers may come with two, four, or no wheels. Walkers without wheels provide the greatest support; however, they require more energy to use. The two-wheeled walker is the most commonly used model. The sizing of a walker is analogous to that of a cane.

In the early postoperative period, gait training should be provided with the use of a walker under the direction of a physical therapist. As strength, balance, and mobility improve, patients should be transitioned from a walker to crutches or a cane. Patients may expect to use a walker for 2 to 4 weeks or longer if needed. Delay in progression is often attributed to advanced age, multiple medical comorbidities, lack of work with physical therapy, lack of support at home, or the inability to control the operative extremity with less supportive assistive devices. Additional assistive devices that should be considered for a patient who has undergone THA include raised seats for a chair, a toilet, and the shower.[43]

Brace Wear

Dislocation after revision THA has a reported incidence of 10% to 25%.[27] In an effort to mobilize patients immediately and safely following revision THA, a hip abduction orthosis may be prescribed. Efficacy of brace wear and prevention of dislocation continue to be controversial.

Hip abduction orthoses (Fig. 29-1) are customized for each patient, with consideration given to height, weight, waist size, widest part of the hip, and circumference of the affected thigh. Settings for patients at risk for posterior dislocation include a hip abduction angle of 15 degrees and allowance of 70 degrees for forward flexion of the hip. Patients at risk for anterior dislocation should be allowed hip flexion from 40 to 70 degrees. A knee-ankle-foot orthosis may be added to control and prevent rotation of the extremity.[27]

Hip abduction orthoses should be worn for 6 to 12 weeks, whenever a patient is out of bed. Comfort level, familiarity, and ease of application will directly influence a patient's compliance with brace wear.

Postoperative Exercise

The postoperative rehabilitation of a patient after THA begins immediately in the acute hospital setting. However, the intensity and setting of rehabilitation will vary between patients. The nursing staff, physical therapists, and occupational therapists should begin to work with patients immediately postoperatively. Initial assessments should be performed once patients are medically stable. If a patient undergoes surgery in

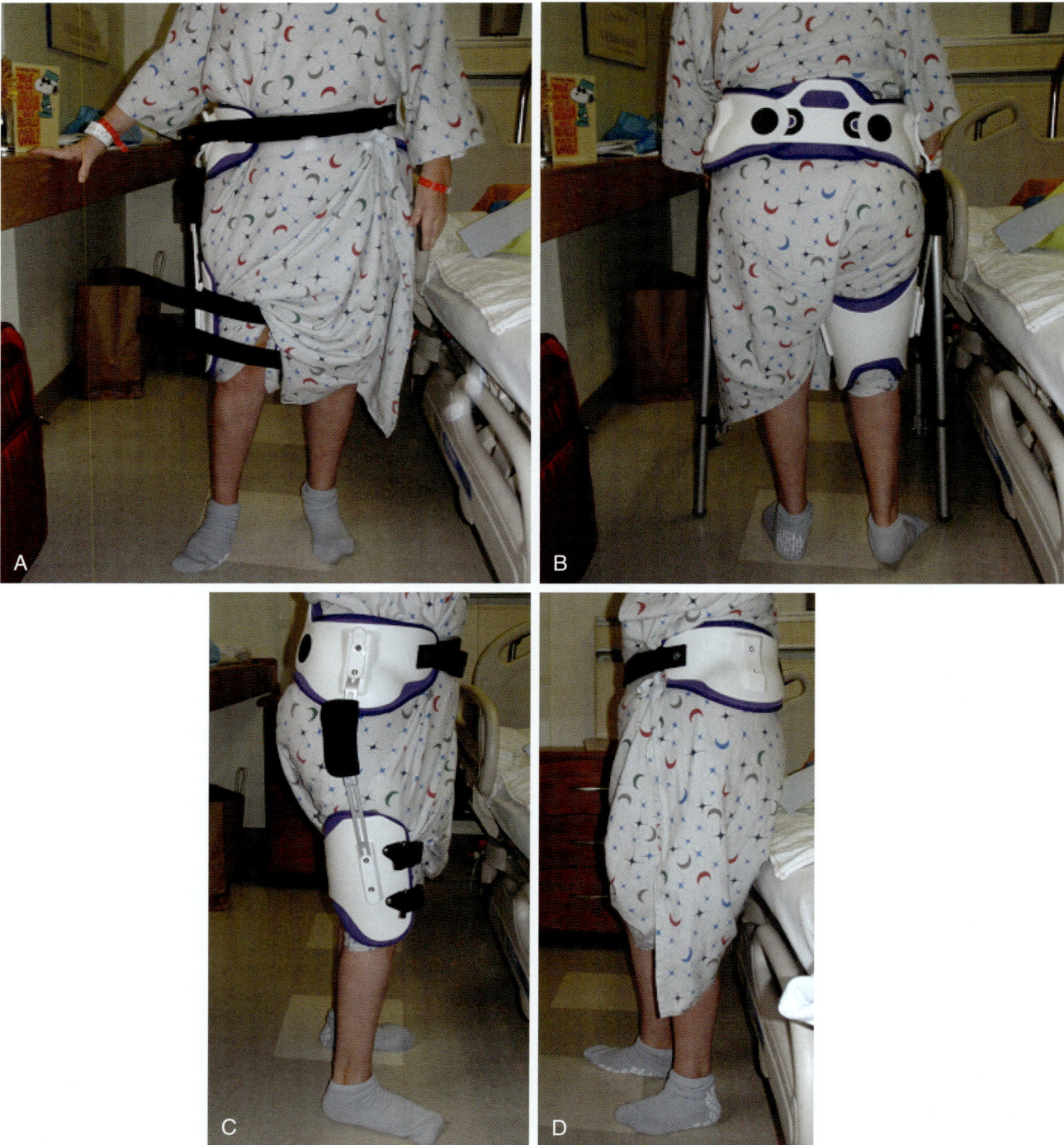

Figure 29-1. A through D, Hip abduction orthosis.

the morning, physical therapists may begin to mobilize the patient as early as the afternoon on the day of surgery. The nursing staff should encourage patients to get out of bed and sit in a chair at least two times per day for 30 minutes at a time. Occupational therapists may begin to work with patients to instruct and advise on proper maneuvers to perform activities of daily living.

Following hip surgery, physical activity and goals of therapy should consist of a graduated series of events (Table 29-1). In the immediate postoperative period, range of motion of the hip, knee, ankle, and foot of the operative extremity should be instituted (Figs. 29-2 and 29-3). Patients may begin with simple exercises such as foot/ankle pumps and ankle rotations. These can be followed by gluteal contractions, bed-supported knee

Table 29-1. Exercises After Total Hip Arthroplasty*

Exercise	Description	Frequency
Abduction	While supine, abduct hip and then return to neutral	10 times, 3-4 times per day
Ankle pumps	Plantar/dorsiflexion of ankle	Ad lib
Ankle rotations	Internal/external rotation of ankle	5 times each direction, 3-4 times per day
Bed-supported knee bends	Slide heel toward buttocks while lying in bed; avoid internal rotation of the knee	10 times, 3-4 times per day
Buttock contractions	Tighten gluteal muscles and hold contraction for 5 seconds	10 times, 3-4 times per day
Exercycling	While seated with no resistance, pedal backward; once a comfortable motion has been established, pedal forward; increase resistance once strength builds (4-6 weeks)	10-15 minutes, 2 times per day; increase to 30-40 minutes 3-4 times per week
Quadriceps set	While supine, tighten quadriceps in attempts to straighten knee; hold for 5-10 seconds	10 times, 3-4 times per day
Resistive hip flexion†	Stand with feet slightly apart, flex hip then return to neutral	10 times, 3-4 times per day
Resistive hip abduction†	Abduct operative hip to one side, then return to neutral	10 times, 3-4 times per day
Resistive hip extension†	Extend the operative hip, then return to neutral	10 times, 3-4 times per day
Stair climbing/descending	Use a side rail for assistance; lead with nonoperated extremity going up the stairs; descend stairs with operated leg first	
Standing	Transition from supine to standing position	Ad lib
Standing hip abduction	With hip, knee, and foot pointing straight forward, abduct hip; slowly return to neutral	10 times, 3-4 times per day
Standing hip extension	Keeping back straight, extend hip while keeping knee straight; hold for 2-5 seconds; slowly return to neutral	10 times, 3-4 times per day
Standing knee raises	Flex hip and knee (avoid lifting knee higher than your waist); hold for 2-5 seconds; lower slowly	10 times, 3-4 times per day
Straight-leg raise	While supine, tighten quadriceps, flex hip and keep knee straight while lifting extremity off bed; hold for 5-10 seconds; lower slowly	10 times, 3-4 times per day
Walking‡	Stand erect and comfortably, attempt to walk smoothly; cadence: heel-strike, foot flat, toe-off; aim to spend same amount of time on each lower extremity	5-10 minutes, 3-4 times per day

*Please adhere to postoperative restrictions imparted by your surgeon.
†Resistive exercises performed with an elastic tubing around the ankle of the operative extremity and attached to a stationary object; a chair should be used to help maintain balance.
‡Please adhere to any weight-bearing restriction imparted by your surgeon.

bends, and abduction exercises. Once ready, patients should be encouraged to sit outside of the bed in a chair and/or to stand with assistance. Muscle strengthening of the operative extremity should focus on the hip abductors/extensors and the quadriceps, and can be performed in the supine or standing position. The goal of these exercises is to increase muscle strength and gain control of the limb. Gait training should focus on teaching patients to stand erect and walk comfortably. A walker should be used to aid in balance, support, and coordination. Assistive devices should be required until the patient is able to ambulate with a minimal Trendelenburg lurch and/or antalgic gait. Patients should be instructed on navigation of stairs. A side rail should be used with stair ascent and descent. Patients should always ascend stairs leading with their "good" or nonoperated leg and should descend stairs leading with their operative leg. Stairs higher than the standard height of 7 inches should be avoided.

In the subacute phase following surgery, goals of therapy should include continued strengthening of the lower extremity musculature, proprioceptive training to improve spatial awareness, endurance training to increase cardiovascular fitness, and functional training to promote independence in activities of daily living. Throughout the postoperative period, patients should be encouraged to work diligently with their therapists. Poor participation in therapy is associated with poorer functional outcomes.

Levels of Rehabilitation Care

Discharge from an acute care hospital following THA is to one of three venues: home, an inpatient rehabilitation facility, or a skilled nursing facility. Seventy-five percent of patients who have undergone a lower extremity total joint arthroplasty will receive rehabilitation care through a home health agency, an inpatient rehabilitation facility, or a skilled nursing facility.[46] Establishment of clinical care pathways and Medicare's Inpatient Prospective Payment Systems by Diagnosis Related Group have led to increased pressure on acute care hospitals to decrease patients' length of stay following surgery. As a result, the average length of stay following total joint arthroplasty decreased from 8.0 days in 1993 to 4.4 days in 2003, with an increase in discharge to extended care facilities (skilled nursing or inpatient rehabilitation) from 17.1% in 1993 to 54.6% in 2003.[47] Implementation of clinical pathways has demonstrated effectiveness in reducing a patient's length of stay in the acute care hospital, reducing costs, and reducing or maintaining rates of perioperative complications, with improvement or no change in clinical outcomes.[48,49] Clinical pathways are hospital and procedure specific and aim to coordinate the activities of physicians, nurses, therapists, and ancillary staff in an effort to reduce cost and improve quality.

Anticipating postoperative care requirements in the preoperative period can decrease length of the stay in the acute care hospital and increase discharge directly home.[1] Oldmeadow and associates[50] identified seven factors subjected to univariate analysis that were significantly related to discharge destination, including age, gender, preoperative walking distance, use of a gait aid, community supports, patient expectations, and presence of a caregiver on return home. Using these factors, they developed a risk assessment and predictor tool (RAPT) that was found to have an 89% accuracy rate for predicting patients who were most likely at risk for being discharge to an extended care facility. Bozic and colleagues[47] evaluated 7818 consecutive patients from three high-volume total joint arthroplasty centers using a stepwise linear regression model to identify baseline patient characteristics that are predictive of discharge to an extended care facility. They noted that older age, higher American Society of Anesthesiologist class, Medicare insurance, and female gender were associated with a higher probability of being discharged to an extended care facility. Significant differences were observed among practice patterns with respect to discharge disposition among the three institutions studied. In their assessment, the acute care hospital of origin was the most powerful predictor of discharge disposition following total joint arthroplasty.

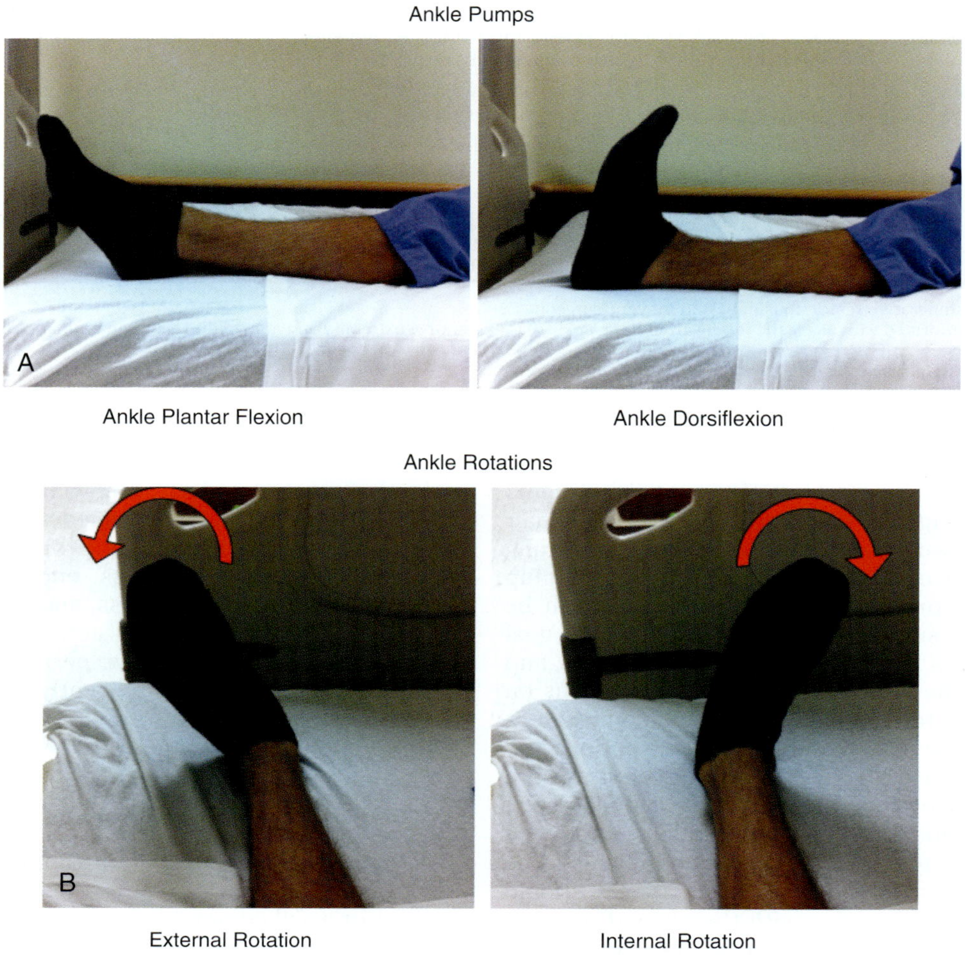

Figure 29-2. **Postoperative range-of-motion exercises performed supine. A,** Ankle pumps. Plantar flexion *(left)* and dorsiflexion *(right)*. **B,** Ankle rotations. External rotation *(left)* and internal rotation *(right)*.

Supine Exercise

Supine Abduction Exercises

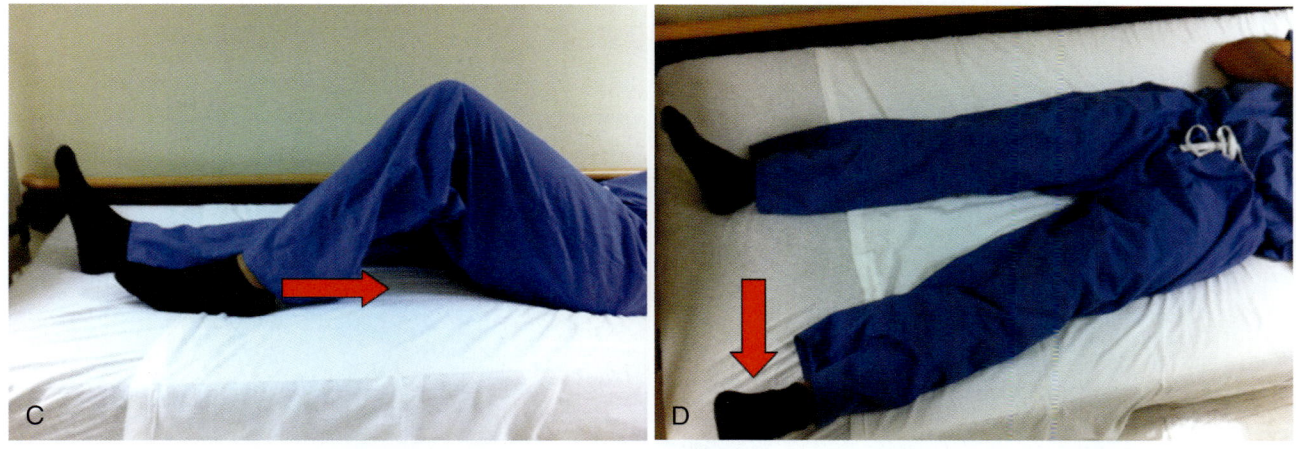

Bed-Supported Knee Bends

Quadricep Contractions

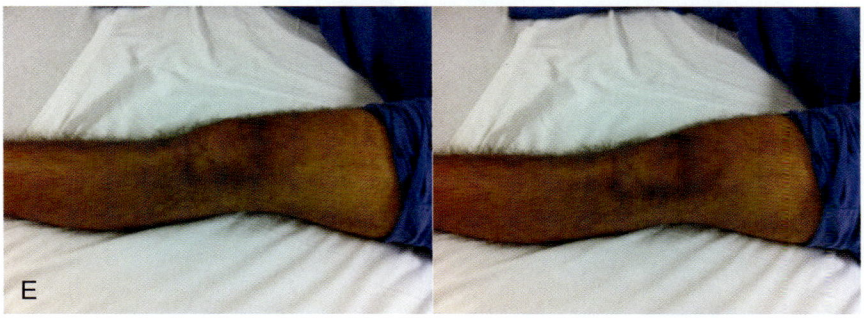

Straight Leg Raise

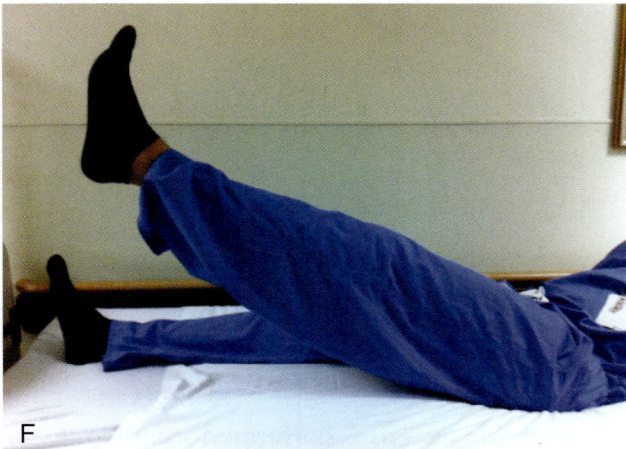

Figure 29-2, cont'd C, Bed-supported knee bends. **D,** Abduction. **E,** Quadriceps contractions. **F,** Straight-leg raise.

Discharge Home

The decision to discharge a patient home following THA is based on clinical goals. To be discharged home, a patient must be able to ambulate approximately 50 to 100 feet with an assistive device, use a toilet, perform transfers, perform activities of daily living, demonstrate understanding of and compliance with hip precautions, and independently perform home exercises, and the patient must be medically stable[34] (Fig. 29-4). Motivated patients who work with a physical therapist soon after surgery and who have familial support are more likely to be discharged home.

Inpatient Rehabilitation Facilities

Inpatient rehabilitation facilities provide intensive inpatient rehabilitation services. In 2007, more than 60% of patients discharged from inpatient rehabilitation facilities were paid for by Medicare, totaling $6 billion

Standing Exercises

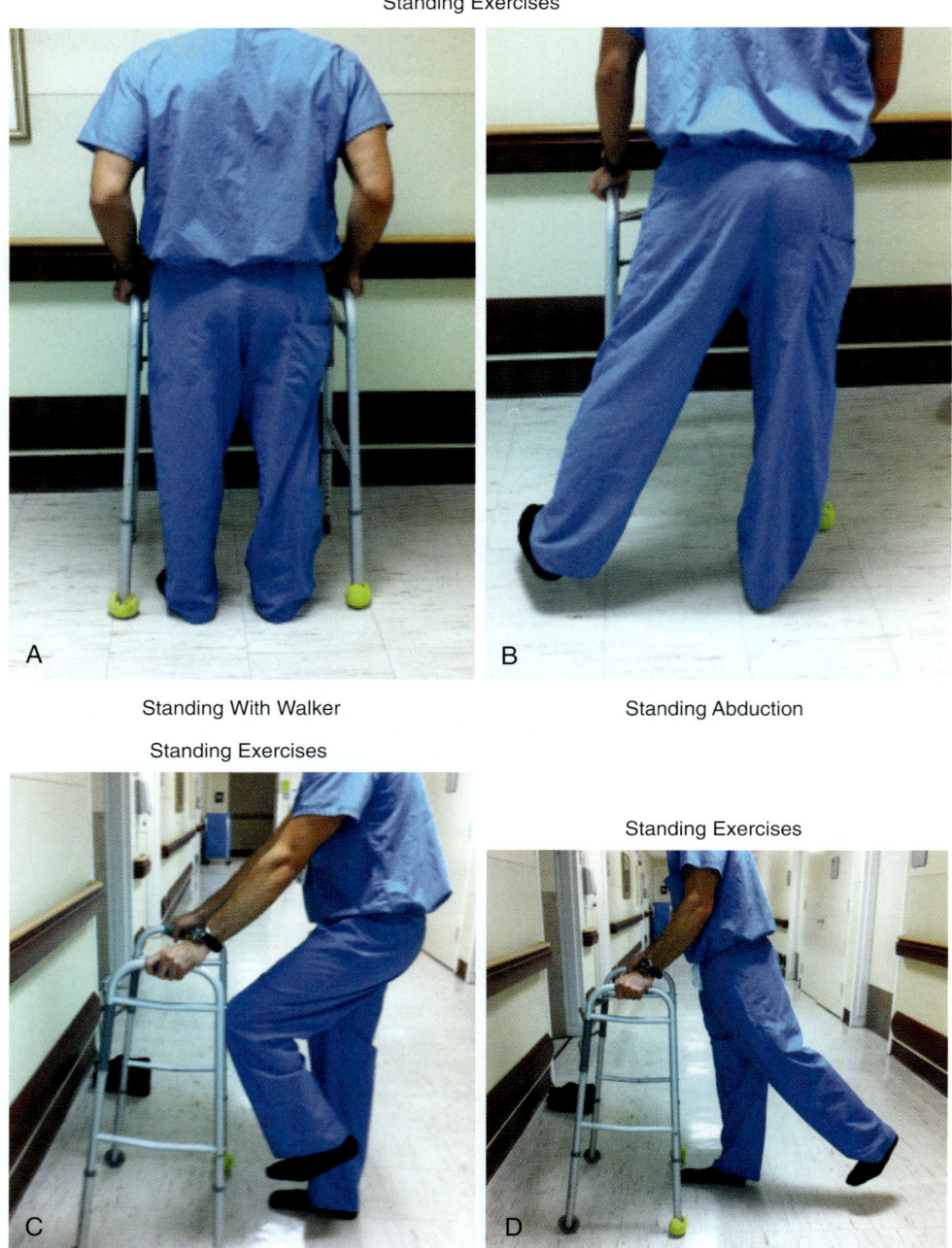

A   Standing With Walker

B   Standing Abduction

Standing Exercises

Standing Exercises

C   Standing Knee Raises

D   Standing Leg Extension

Figure 29-3. **Postoperative range-of-motion exercises performed standing. A,** Standing with walker. **B,** Abduction. **C,** Knee raises. **D,** Leg extension.

dollars.[51] Facilities that provide these services receive a higher Medicare reimbursement. Regulatory changes by the Center for Medicare and Medicaid Services adopted the "75-percent" rule, where at least 75% of patients in an inpatient rehabilitation facility must present with 1 of 13 conditions. Patients admitted after total joint arthroplasty must be able to participate in at least 3 hours of therapy per day and be over 85 years

old, must have a body mass index (BMI) of 50 or greater, or must have undergone bilateral total joint arthro-plasty.[51] The new regulatory changes resulted in a decrease in the number of total joint arthroplasty patients admitted to inpatient rehabilitation facilities from 28% in 2004 to 16% in 2007.[51] It is not surprising that the numbers of patients discharge to skilled nursing facilities and to home have increased.

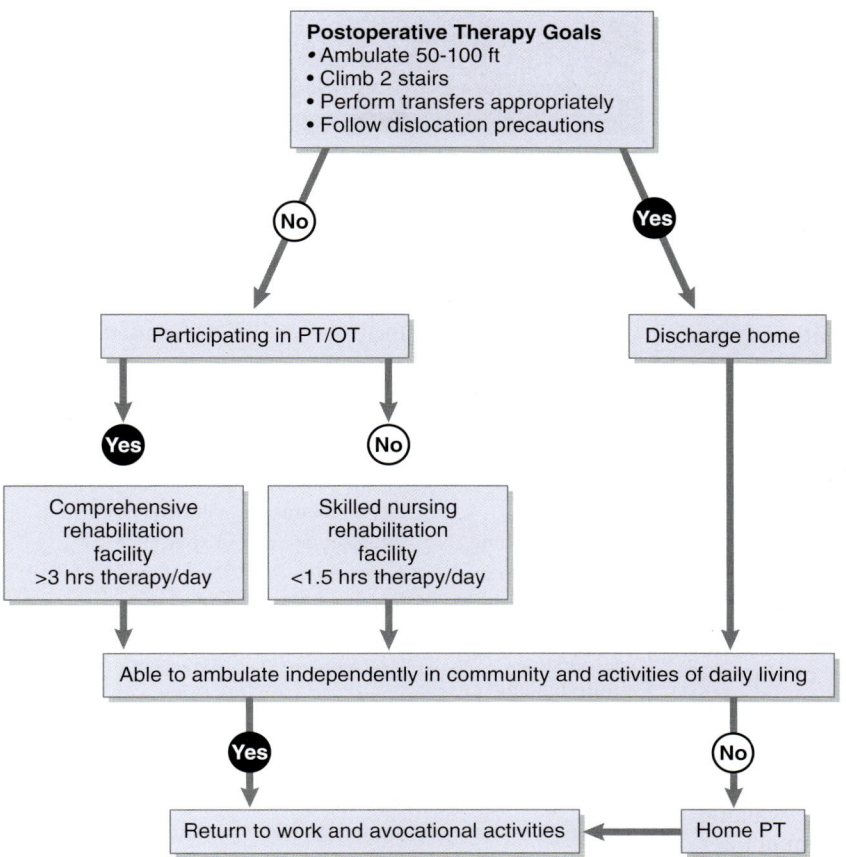

Figure 29-4. Clinical goals of therapy and algorithm for determining readiness for discharge home following rehabilitation.

Skilled Nursing Facility

Patients who do not meet the clinical criterion to be discharged home and cannot participate in 3 hours of physical therapy per day or do not qualify for admission to an inpatient rehabilitation facility may be candidates for admission to a skilled nursing facility. Skilled nursing facilities have been considered a complement to inpatient rehabilitation facilities[52] and are more cost-effective than continued admission to an acute care hospital. Total joint arthroplasty patients constitute a majority of patients admitted to a skilled nursing facility.[46] A study by DeJong and colleagues[46] aimed to characterize rehabilitation services for patients who have undergone hip and knee arthroplasty. Using a multisite prospective observational cohort study, they noted that although total hours of physical and occupational therapy were similar, inpatient rehabilitation facilities had more intensive therapy and shorter lengths of stay compared with free-standing skilled nursing facilities. A separate study by DeJong and coworkers[53] performed 7.5 months following admission to a skilled nursing facility or to an inpatient rehabilitation facility examined potential differences in functional and health status outcomes after hip or knee arthroplasty. Outcome measures were assessed with the Functional Independent Measure and Short-Form 12-Item Health Survey (SF-12). At follow-up, patients who had been admitted to an independent rehabilitation facility showed better motor outcomes on the Functional Independent Measure. No difference was noted between the two groups in terms of SF-12 outcomes. Overall, study findings did not decisively favor one setting over the other.

Home Therapy

Numerous studies have consistently demonstrated the benefits of home therapy, including improvements in function, quality of life, lower limb strength, and walking speed, as well as a reduction in the chance of accidental falls.[35,54,55] Furthermore, a home-based therapy rehabilitation program with supervision is more cost-effective than center-based rehabilitation programs.[35] In a randomized controlled trial, Galea and associates[35] demonstrated that a supervised home exercise program that focuses on functional tasks, daily living tasks, balance, strength, and endurance is as effective as a center-based program.

Long-Term Home Therapy

Despite the overall satisfaction of patients and physicians noted in outcome studies following THA, long-term studies indicate persistent impairment and functional limitation. Reported impairments and limitations include decreased muscle strength, postural stability, flexibility, and walking speed, along with reduced ratings on assessment tools to measure ability to function. Weakness of muscles surrounding the hip, especially the hip abductors, has been associated with joint instability and potential implant failure. Home exercise programs or formal outpatient therapy is crucial to combat functional decline. Jan and colleagues[56] showed that patients who comply with a home exercise program 1.5 years following THA are able to show significant improvement in muscle strength of the operative hip, faster walking speeds, and higher functional scores when compared with controls. Trudelle-Jackson and coworkers[57] demonstrated statistically significant improvement in self-perceived function, postural stability, and muscle strength among patients who participated in an 8-week home exercise program 4 to 12 months following THA.

Avocational Activities

Patient expectations following hip arthroplasty encompass pain relief, psychological well-being, and restoration of function.[58] Currently, no prospective randomized studies have delineated guidelines for safe and appropriate activities following THA.[59] Klein and associates[59] conducted a survey of active members of the American Hip Society and the American Association of Hip and Knee Surgeons (AAHKS) to evaluate joint arthroplasty surgeons' preferences for the return to sporting activity following THA. The consensus of the 549 responses suggests waiting 3 to 6 months before returning to sporting activity. Recommended activities include walking, golf, swimming, speedwalking, bowling, low-impact aerobics, weight machines, hiking, stairclimber, elliptical machines, stationary and road cycling, treadmill, and doubles tennis. Activities allowed with experience include cross-country skiing, ice skating, rollerblading, weightlifting, dancing, and downhill skiing. High-impact activities may lead to decreased longevity of the prosthetic hip or early failure and are not recommended following THA (Table 29-2). These activities include jogging, contact sports, baseball, softball, high-impact aerobics, racquetball, and squash.

Driving a car is an important activity of daily living and a necessity for independent living. The question of timing of the return to driving following hip arthroplasty is common. Factors that must be considered before a patient is cleared to drive include operative side, ability to maintain hip precautions while entering and exiting the car, and transmission and type of automobile the patient is driving. Historically, physicians have recommended abstinence from driving for 4 to 6 weeks postoperatively to allow soft tissue healing and patient recuperation. These recommendations were not based on scientific data. Driving reaction time is an objective measure of a patient's driving capability. Ganz and colleagues[60] used an automatic brake reaction timer to assess 90 patients in terms of driving reaction time before and after THA. Patients were tested 24 hours before undergoing surgery and at postoperative weeks 1, 4 to 6, 26, and 52. Results revealed a difference in driving reaction time between patients based on the operative side. Driving reaction times for patients who underwent a left THA were quicker at every time point tested postoperatively when compared with

Table 29-2. Activities as Classified by Clifford and Mallon and Recommended Guidelines Based on AAHKS/HS Survey*

Activity	Impact Level	Recommendation
Racquetball/squash	High	Not allowed
Jogging	High	Not allowed
Contact sports	High	Not allowed
Baseball/softball	High	Not allowed
High-impact aerobics	High	Not allowed
Martial arts	High	Undecided
Singles tennis	Intermediate	Undecided
Doubles tennis	Intermediate	Allowed
Stairclimber	Intermediate	Allowed
Hiking	Intermediate	Allowed
Downhill skiing	Intermediate	Experience
Snowboarding	*Intermediate*	Not allowed
Weight machines	Intermediate	Allowed
Weightlifting	Intermediate	Experience
Ice skating/rollerblading	Intermediate	Experience
Low-impact aerobics	Intermediate	Allowed
Bowling	Potentially low	Allowed
Road cycling	Potentially low	Allowed
Rowing	Potentially low	Allowed
Speedwalking	Potentially low	Allowed
Cross-country skiing	Potentially low	Experience
Dancing	Potentially low	Allowed
Pilates	*Potentially low*	Allowed
Golf	Low	Allowed
Swimming	Low	Allowed
Walking	Low	Allowed
Stationary skiing	Low	Allowed
Treadmill	*Low*	Allowed
Stationary bicycle	Low	Allowed
Elliptical machine	*Low*	Allowed

*Italicized text indicates impact level not previously described by Clifford and Mallon.
AAHKS/HS, American Association of Hip and Knee Surgeons/Hip Society.
From Klein GR, Levine BR, Hozack WJ, et al: Return to athletic activities after total hip arthroplasty. J Arthroplasty 22:171–175, 2007, based on data from Clifford PE, Mallon WJ: Sports after total joint replacement. Clin Sports Med 24:175, 2005.

preoperative times. For patients who underwent right THA, driving reaction time worsened at the 1 week postoperative time point compared with before surgery. However, at all subsequent evaluations, driving reaction times were improved compared with preoperative times. The authors noted that it would seem prudent to recommend that patients who have undergone a right THA should wait 4 to 6 weeks after surgery before returning to driving. Patients who have undergone left THA may resume driving sooner. Some patients may require formal assessment of driving reaction time by an occupational therapist.

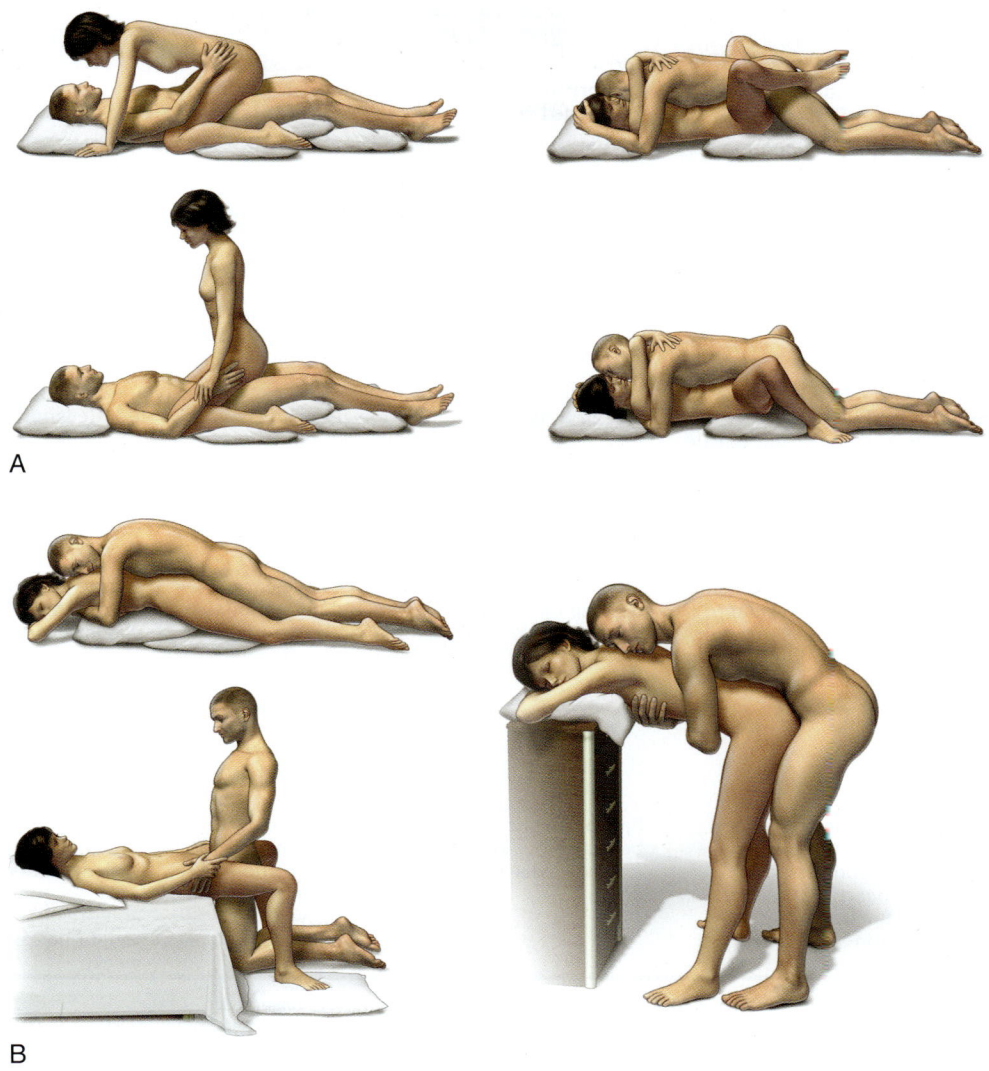

Figure 29-5. A and **B,** Sexual positioning for the post–total hip arthroplasty (THA) patient.

Chronic hip pain can have an impact on sexual activity; 60% to 75% of patients indicate that arthritis has caused sexual difficulty in their lives.[61,62] Sexual difficulty experienced by patients with hip osteoarthrosis is due to loss of mobility and hip pain, and is not attributed to loss of libido. According to a survey of 135 patients conducted by Laffossee and coworkers, 19% of patients consider their difficulties with sexual activity to be severe to extreme, causing unhappiness or tension in their relationship in 7% of these patients.[63] Significant improvement in sexual function can occur following THA. Surveys have revealed relief from preoperative symptoms in 60% to 75% of patients.[61,62] Delay in return to sexual activity following THA allows for healing of pericapsular tissue, muscles, and wounds, thereby improving comfort and reducing the risk of hip instability.[26] In a survey of members of AAHKS, most responding members (67%) indicated that patients can safely resume sexual activity within 1 to 3 months following THA.[26] Upon resumption of sexual activities, patients should be encouraged to play a more passive role, to utilize the supine position, and to avoid extremes of motion (Fig. 29-5). Women may find the supine position or side lying on the nonoperative side to be more comfortable. Once comfortable with resumption of sexual activity, males may attempt the prone position 2 to 3 months postoperatively.[61] Discussion of sexual activity is a sensitive topic. It has been reported that although less than 10% of patients discuss this topic with their surgeon, 89% would welcome information (in the form of a discussion or an educational brochure) regarding sexual activity following THA.[61]

HIP ARTHROSCOPY

Improvement in understanding and diagnosis of intra-articular and extra-articular hip pathology, including femoral-acetabular impingement, acetabular labral tears, capsular laxity, and chondral lesions, has led to

Table 29-3. Rehabilitation Guidelines After Selected Arthroscopic Procedures of the Hip Joint*

Surgical Procedure	Rehabilitation Concerns	Weight-Bearing Precautions	Range-of-Motion Precautions	Strength Issues
Labral resection	Avoid initiation of joint inflammation	Partial weight bearing for 10-14 days	Avoid excessive early flexion and abduction to prevent inflammation of affected tissue; full passive range of motion (PROM) by 2 weeks	Gentle isometrics on day 2; active range of motion (AROM) at 2 weeks; weight-bearing progressive resisted exercises (PREs) as tolerated after full weight bearing
Labral repair	Avoid initiation of joint inflammation	Partial weight bearing for 10-28 days	Avoid excessive early flexion and abduction to prevent inflammation of affected tissue; full PROM by 2 weeks	Gentle isometrics on day 2; AROM at 2 weeks; weight-bearing PREs as tolerated after full weight bearing
Osteoplasty/rim trimming procedure	Avoid excessive compressive and tensile forces to femoral neck and head-neck junction, protecting exposed bone	Partial weight bearing (≈9.1 kg) for 4-6 weeks	Avoid excessive early flexion and abduction to prevent inflammation of affected tissue; full PROM by 2 weeks	Gentle isometrics on day 2; AROM at 2 weeks; caution with sagittal plane straight-leg raise secondary to increased compressive forces; gentle weight-bearing PREs by 4-6 weeks
Capsular modification: thermal assisted, plication	Avoid excessive tension of affected capsular tissue (usually anterior region); avoid capsular inflammation	Partial weight bearing for 10-14 days	Avoid excessive early flexion and abduction; avoid forced external rotation and extension for 3-4 weeks to protect anterior capsule; progress external rotation and extension after 3 weeks; full PROM allowed by 4 weeks	Gentle isometrics on day 2; limited AROM at 3 weeks; weight-bearing PREs as tolerated after full weight bearing
Microfracture	Avoid reinitiation of inflammatory response and protect early fibrocartilage formation by limiting early compression and shear forces	Partial weight bearing (≈9.1 kg) for 4-6 weeks	Avoid excessive early flexion and abduction to prevent inflammation of affected tissue; full PROM allowed by 2 weeks	Gentle isometrics on day 2; AROM at 2 weeks; caution with sagittal plane straight-leg raise secondary to increased compressive forces; gentle weight-bearing PREs by 4-6 weeks

*For combined procedures, the most conservative guidelines for each aspect of rehabilitation are observed.
From Enseki KR, Martin RL, Draovitch P, et al: The hip joint: arthroscopic procedures and postoperative rehabilitation. J Orthop Sports Phys Ther 36:516–525, 2006.

the development of arthroscopic procedures to address these pathologies. Arthroscopic techniques beyond diagnostic arthroscopy include osteoplasty of the acetabulum and/or femur, chondroplasty, labral débridement/repair, microfracture, and capsular modification. As arthroscopic treatment for intracapsular and extracapsular hip pathologies evolves, so must postoperative rehabilitation protocols. Diagnosis and specific treatment options are outside the scope of this review.

Patients undergoing hip arthroscopy tend to be younger and more active than those undergoing THA; some patients are competitive, elite athletes. Goals of hip arthroscopy and rehabilitation include returning the patient to his or her level of preinjury activity, including competitive sports or strenuous labor. Several concerns have been raised regarding postoperative rehabilitation following arthroscopic procedures of the hip, including control of pain and swelling, soft tissue healing, weight-bearing precautions, range-of-motion

limitations, initiation of strengthening activities, and sports-specific training.[64,65]

The postoperative rehabilitation program following hip arthroscopy will be based on the patient's diagnosis, the procedure performed, and patient characteristics (Table 29-3). Typically, 10 to 12 weeks of supervised therapy is to be expected. Hip range of motion is permitted in the perioperative period but should allow for soft tissue healing. A hip brace may be used during periods of ambulation for the first 10 postoperative days. The brace is set to allow 80 degrees of flexion in the sagittal plane. External rotation should be avoided after certain procedures, such as anterior capsular plication, as this motion places anterior capsuloligamentous structures under increased tension. Antirotation boots may be issued to prevent rotation in the supine position. Labral-capsular adhesions can be avoided by early range of motion. Patients who undergo cheilectomy are usually advised to be partial weight-bearing for 4 to 6 weeks postoperatively.

OSTEOTOMIES

Proximal Femoral Osteotomy

Before the advent of THA, osteotomy of the proximal femur was an attractive therapeutic option for the treatment of hip pain.[66] Despite the success of THA, the problem of wear remains a significant issue, especially in the young patient. In this subgroup, proximal femoral osteotomy remains a viable option for certain patients, as it may delay or even eliminate the need for THA. Osteotomies can be categorized by technique as angulation, displacement, or rotational. Alteration in alignment of the proximal femur has been noted to reduce peak joint force by 10% to 25%, depending on the degree of osteotomy.[67-69] The efficacy of proximal femoral osteotomies has been attributed to an increase in the weight-bearing area, reduction of joint force by division of muscles or alteration of the lever arm, and reduction in intramedullary pressure.[70] Reconstructive osteotomies can be performed when the primary problem is malalignment of the proximal femur. These procedures are performed most often in younger patients with progressive symptoms and near-normal motion and function. Salvage osteotomies can be performed for patients with moderate to severe symptoms and changes in motion, function, and articular surfaces. The goal of the salvage osteotomy is to reduce pain and delay the need for THA. Rigid internal fixation of the osteotomy allows maintenance of fragments in proper position, early ambulation, and prevention of complications following prolonged hip and knee immobilization.

Postoperative rehabilitation following proximal femoral osteotomy includes a period of non–weight bearing for 4 to 6 weeks to allow healing of the osteotomy. With radiographic evidence of healing, weight bearing is gradually increased.

Acetabular Reorientation

Acetabular dysplasia is a common cause of osteoarthritis of the hip and can lead to joint destruction in 25% to 50% of patients by the age of 50 years. The dysplastic acetabulum typically is shallow, lateralized, anteverted, and deficient anteriorly and superiorly.[71] Timely surgical intervention with realignment of the congruous dysplastic acetabulum can reduce or eliminate symptoms.[72] Multiple types of osteotomies of the pelvis have been described for treatment of acetabular dysplasia, including single innominate, double innominate, triple innominate, spherical periacetabular, Chiari, and the Bernese periacetabular osteotomy. The Bernese periacetabular osteotomy is preferred by many surgeons. Part of its appeal is that the posterior column is left intact. This allows minimal internal fixation of the osteotomized and reoriented acetabulum, no requirement for postoperative casting or bracing, and relatively early ambulation.

Postoperative care generally requires a period of partial weight bearing for 6 to 10 weeks. Once radiographic bone healing becomes apparent, progressive weight bearing is allowed. Abduction exercises, use of a stationary bicycle, and water exercises may be encouraged 4 weeks postoperatively.[71] By 3 months postoperatively, patients usually are ambulatory without assist devices and can resume activities as tolerated. After this point, decreases in range of motion or persistent strength deficits may be addressed by a physical therapist.

CURRENT CONTROVERSIES AND FUTURE CONSIDERATIONS

- The efficacy of preoperative exercise programs continues to be debated. Although some authors[11-13] identify no significant improvement from preoperative physical therapy as measured by Harris Hip Scores, Barthel Index, SF-36 scores, and WOMAC scores, others note improvement in postoperative gait velocity, stride length, and walking distance, and a reduction in the odds of discharge to inpatient rehabilitation.[14,15]

- Debate over the benefits of various surgical approaches to THA continues. Short-term benefits of decreased blood loss, postoperative pain, hospital stay, and incision length have been reported by some.[73,74] Other studies refute these findings, reporting higher complication rates and worse cosmetic appearance of the incision.[75-77] Ultimately, it may be decided that the approach has no significant long-term benefit.[78]

- Analgesic methods for perioperative pain control include general or regional anesthesia, neuraxial analgesia, intraoperative periarticular injection, intravenous and oral narcotics, and preemptive analgesia. Effective multimodal perioperative analgesia has been demonstrated to lead to a significant reduction in rest pain scores, total narcotic consumption, and hospital length of stay, with improvements in distance ambulated and time to achieve therapy goals. In conjunction with multimodal perioperative pain control, advancements in the surgical approach and in initiation of rapid rehabilitation protocols have decreased the duration of hospitalization and subsequent length of recovery following elective THA.[79] Effective application of these methods in select patients has led to the ability to perform THA in an outpatient setting.

- Currently, physical exercise protocols most frequently used following THA in the early postoperative phase are neither supported nor denied by clinical trials.[80] Wide variation in physical therapy protocols has been reported, due in part to lack of evidence-based literature.[10] Therapy routines vary between institutions and surgeons. However, therapeutic exercise, transfer and gait training, education on hip precautions, and instruction in activities of daily living are consistent themes in any routine. Poor participation in inpatient therapy is associated with longer hospital stays and a reduced likelihood of discharge to home.[81] Additionally, frequent poor participation in therapy is associated with poorer functional outcomes.

- Establishment of clinical care pathways and Medicare's Inpatient Prospective Payment System have led to increased pressure for acute care hospitals to decrease patients' length of stay following surgery. As a result, the average length of stay following total joint arthroplasty decreased from 8.0 days in 1993 to 4.4 days in 2003, with an increase in discharge to extended care facilities (skilled nursing or inpatient rehabilitation) from 17.1% in 1993 to 54.6% in 2003.[47] Implementation of clinical pathways has demonstrated effectiveness in reducing a patient's length of stay in the acute care hospital, reducing costs, and reducing or maintaining rates of perioperative complications, with improvement or no change in clinical outcomes.[48,49] Given the expected increase in demand for primary THA and total knee arthroplasty in ensuing years, pressure to streamline the care of these patients and to decrease their length of hospital stay will be increased.

REFERENCES

1. Barsoum WK, Murray TG, Klika AK, et al: Predicting patient discharge disposition after total joint arthroplasty in the United States. J Arthroplasty 25:885–892, 2010.
2. Zhan C, Kaczmarek R, Loyo-Berrios N, et al: Incidence and short-term outcomes of primary and revision hip replacement in the United States. J Bone Joint Surg Am 89:526–533, 2007.
3. McDonald S, Hetrick S, Green S: Pre-operative education for hip and knee replacement. Cochrane Database Syst Rev (1):CD003526, 2004.
4. Brady OH, Masri BA, Garbuz DS, Duncan CP: Rheumatology: joint replacement of the hip and knee: when to refer and what to expect. Can Med Assoc J 163:1285–1291, 2000.
5. Wright JG, Rudicel S, Feinstein AR: Ask patients what they want: evaluation of individual complaints before total hip replacement. J Bone Joint Surg Br 76:229–234, 1994.
6. Spalding NJ: Reducing anxiety by pre-operative education: make the future familiar. Occup Ther Int 10:278–293, 2003.
7. Mancuso CA, Sculco TP, Wickiewicz TL, et al: Patients' expectations of knee surgery. J Bone Joint Surg Am 83:1005–1012, 2001.
8. Lugade V, Klausmeier V, Jewett B, et al: Short-term recovery of balance control after total hip arthroplasty. Clin Orthop Relat Res 466:3051–3058, 2008.
9. Lavernia C, D'Apuzzo M, Rossi MD, Lee D: Is postoperative function after hip or knee arthroplasty influenced by preoperative functional levels? J Arthroplasty 24:1033–1043, 2009.
10. Sharma V, Morgan PM, Cheng EY: Factors influencing early rehabilitation after THA: a systematic review. Clin Orthop Relat Res 467:1400–1411, 2009.
11. Gocen Z, Sen A, Unver B, et al: The effect of preoperative physiotherapy and education on the outcome of total hip replacement: a prospective randomized controlled trial. Clin Rehabil 18:353–358, 2004.
12. Wijgman AJ, Dekkers GH, Waltje E, et al: No positive effect of preoperative exercise therapy and teaching in patients to be subjected to hip arthroplasty. Ned Tijdschr Geneeskd 138:949–952, 1994.
13. Ferrara PE, Rabini A, Maggi L, et al: Effect of pre-operative physiotherapy in patients with end-stage osteoarthritis undergoing hip arthroplasty. Clin Rehabil 22:977–986, 2008.
14. Wang AW, Gilbey HJ, Ackland TR: Perioperative exercise programs improve early return of ambulatory function after total hip arthroplasty: a randomized, controlled trial. Am J Phys Med Rehabil 81:801–806, 2002.
15. Rooks DS, Huang J, Bierbaum BE, et al: Effect of preoperative exercise on measures of functional status in men and women undergoing total hip and knee arthroplasty. Arthritis Rheum 55:700–708, 2006.
16. D'Lima DD, Colwell CW Jr, Morris BA, et al: The effect of preoperative exercise on total knee replacement outcomes. Clin Orthop Relat Res 326:174–182, 1996.
17. Ciminiello M, Parvizi J, Sharkey PF, et al: Total hip arthroplasty: is smaller incision better? J Arthroplasty 21:484–488, 2006.
18. Dorr LD, Maheshwari AV, Long WT, et al: Early pain relief and function after posterior minimally invasive and conventional total hip arthroplasty. J Bone Joint Surg Am 89:1153–1160, 2007.
19. Pagnano MW, Trousdale RT, Meneghini RM, Hanssen AD: Slower recovery after two-incision than mini-posterior-incision total hip arthroplasty: a randomized clinical trial. J Bone Joint Surg Am 90:1000–1006, 2008.
20. Ogonda L, Wilson R, Archbold P, et al: A mini-incision technique in total hip arthroplasty does not improve early postoperative outcomes: a prospective, randomized, controlled trial. J Bone Joint Surg Am 87:701–710, 2005.
21. Pour AE, Parvizi J, Sharkey PF, et al: Minimally invasive hip arthroplasty: what role does patient preconditioning play? J Bone Joint Surg Am 89:1920–1927, 2007.
22. Lieberman JR, Dorey F, Shekelle P, et al: Differences between patients' and physicians' evaluations of outcome after total hip arthroplasty. J Bone Joint Surg 78:835–838, 1996.
23. Maheshwari AV, Blum YC, Shekhar L, et al: Multimodal pain management after total hip and knee arthroplasty at the Ranawat Orthopaedic Center. Clin Orthop Relat Res 467:1418–1423, 2009.
24. Horlocker TT, Kopp SL, Pagnano MW, Hebl JR: Analgesia for total hip and knee arthroplasty: a multimodal pathway featuring peripheral nerve block. J Am Acad Orthop Surg 14:126–135, 2006.
25. Peter CL, Shirley B, Erickson J: The effect of a new multimodal perioperative anesthetic regimen on postoperative pain, side effects, rehabilitation, and length of hospital stay after total joint arthroplasty. J Arthroplasty 21(6 Suppl 2):132–138, 2006.
26. Dahm DL, Jacofsky D, Lewallen DG: Surgeons rarely discuss sexual activity with patients after THA: a survey of members of the American Association of Hip and Knee Surgeons. Clin Orthop Relat Res 428:237–240, 2004.
27. Lima D, Magnus R, Paproksy WG: Team management of hip revision patients using a post-op hip orthosis. J Prosthet Orthop 6:20–24, 1994.
28. Woo RY, Morrey BF: Dislocations after total hip arthroplasty. J Bone Joint Surg Am 64:1295–1306, 1982.
29. Berry DJ, von Knoch M, Schleck CD, Harmsen WS: Effect of femoral head diameter and operative approach on risk of dislocation after primary total hip arthroplasty. J Bone Joint Surg Am 87:2456–2463, 2005.
30. Weeden SH, Paprosky WG, Bowling JW: The early dislocation rate in primary total hip arthroplasty following the posterior approach with posterior soft tissue repair. J Arthroplasty 18:709–713, 2003.
31. Suh KT, Roh HL, Moon KP, et al: Posterior approach with posterior soft tissue repair in revision total hip arthroplasty. J Arthroplasty 23:1197–1203, 2008.
32. Soong M, Rubash HE, Macaulay W: Dislocation after total hip arthroplasty. J Am Acad Orthop Surg 12:314–321, 2004.
33. Bitar A, Kaplan RJ, Stitik TP, et al: Rehabilitation of orthopaedic and rheumatologic disorders: total hip arthroplasty rehabilitation. Arch Phys Med Rehabil 86:S56–S60, 2005.
34. Brander VA, Stulberg SD: Rehabilitation after hip- and knee-joint replacement: an experience- and evidence-based approach to care. Am J Phys Med Rehab 85(Suppl):S98–S118, 2006.
35. Galea MP, Levinger P, Lythgo N, et al: A targeted home- and center-based exercise program for people after total hip replacement: a randomized clinical trial. Arch Phys Med Rehabil 89:1442–1447, 2008.
36. Rao RR, Sharkey PF, Hozack WJ, et al: Immediate weightbearing after uncemented total hip arthroplasty. Clin Orthop Relat Res 349:156–162, 1998.
37. Woolson ST, Adler NS: The effect of partial or full weight bearing ambulation after cementless total hip arthroplasty. J Arthroplasty 17:820–825, 2002.

38. Klein GR, Levine HB, Nafash SC, et al: Total hip arthroplasty with a collarless, tapered, fiber metal proximally coated femoral stem. J Arthroplasty 24:579–585, 2009.
39. Kishida Y, Sugano N, Sakai T, et al: Full weight-bearing after cementless total hip arthroplasty. Int Orthop 25:25–28, 2001.
40. Davy DT, Kotzar GM, Brown RH, et al: Telemetric force measurements across the hip after total arthroplasty. J Bone Joint Surg Am 70:45–50, 1988.
41. Nallegowda M, Singh U, Bhan S, et al: Balance and gait in total hip replacement: a pilot study. Am J Phys Med Rehabil 82:669–677, 2003.
42. Bateni H, Maki BE: Assistive devices for balance and mobility: benefits, demands, and adverse consequences. Arch Phys Med Rehabil 86:134–145, 2005.
43. Hoenig H: Assistive technology and mobility aids for the older patient with disability. Ann Long-Term Care 12:12–19, 2004.
44. Ajemian S, Thon D, Clare P, et al: Cane assisted gait biomechanics and electromyography after total hip arthroplasty. Arch Phys Med Rehabil 85:1966–1971, 2004.
45. Brand RA, Crowninshield RD: The effect of cane use on hip contact force. Clin Orthop Relat Res 147:181–184, 1980.
46. DeJong G, Hsieh CH, Gassaway J, et al: Characterizing rehabilitation services for patients with knee and hip replacement in skilled nursing facilities and inpatient rehabilitation facilities. Arch Phys Med Rehabil 90:1269–1283, 2009.
47. Bozic KJ, Wagie A, Naessens JM, et al: Predictors of discharge to an inpatient extended care facility after total hip or knee arthroplasty. J Arthroplasty 21(Suppl 2):151–156, 2006.
48. Kim S, Losina E, Solomon DH, et al: Effectiveness of clinical pathways for total knee and total hip arthroplasty: literature review. J Arthroplasty 18:69–74, 2003.
49. Walter FL, Bass N, Bock G, Markel DC: Success of clinical pathways for total joint arthroplasty in a community hospital. Clin Orthop Relat Res 457:133–137, 2007.
50. Oldmeadow LB, McBurney H, Robertson VJ: Predicting risk of extended inpatient rehabilitation after hip or knee arthroplasty. J Arthroplasty 18:775–779, 2003.
51. Medicare Payment Advisory Commission (MedPAC): Report to the Congress: Medicare payment policy, Washington, DC, 2009, MedPAC, pp 207–227.
52. Salcido R, Moore RW: Acute and subacute rehabilitation [letter]. Arch Phys Med Rehabil 77:100–101, 1996.
53. DeJong G, Tian W, Smout RJ, et al: Long-term outcomes of joint replacement rehabilitation patients discharged from skilled nursing and inpatient rehabilitation facilities. Arch Phys Med Rehabil 90:1306–1316, 2009.
54. Hauer K, Specht N, Schuler M, et al: Intensive physical training in geriatric patients after severe falls and hip surgery. Age Ageing 21:49–57, 2002.
55. Gilbey HJ, Ackland TR, Wang AW, et al: Exercise improves early functional recovery after total hip arthroplasty. Clin Orthop Relat Res 408:193–200, 2003.
56. Jan MH, Hung JY, Lin JC, et al: Effects of a home program on strength, walking speed, and function after total hip replacement. Arch Phys Med Rehabil 85:1943–1951, 2004.
57. Trudelle-Jackson E, Smith SS: Effects of a late-phase exercise program after total hip arthroplasty: a randomized controlled trial. Arch Phys Med Rehabil 85:1056–1062, 2004.
58. Ghandi R, Davey JR, Mahomed N: Patient expectations predict greater pain relief with joint arthroplasty. J Arthroplasty 24:716–721, 2009.
59. Klein GR, Levine BR, Hozack WJ, et al: Return to athletic activities after total hip arthroplasty. J Arthroplasty 22:171–175, 2007.
60. Ganz SB, Levin AZ, Peterson MG, Ranawat CS: Improvement in driving reaction time after total hip arthroplasty. Clin Orthop Relat Res 413:192–200, 2003.
61. Stern SH, Fuchs MD, Ganz SB, et al: Sexual function after total hip arthroplasty. Clin Orthop Relat Res 269:228–235, 1991.
62. Todd RC, Lightowler CDR, Harris J: Low friction arthroplasty of the hip joint and sexual activity. Acta Orthop Scand 44:690, 1973.
63. Laffosse JM, Tricoire JL, Chiron P, Puget J: Sexual function before and after primary total hip arthroplasty. Joint Bone Spine 75:189–194, 2008.
64. Enseki KR, Martin RL, Draovitch P, et al: The hip joint: arthroscopic procedures and postoperative rehabilitation. J Orthop Sports Phys Ther 36:516–525, 2006.
65. Stalzer S, Wahoff M, Scanlan M: Rehabilitation following hip arthroscopy. Clin Sports Med 25:337–357, 2006.
66. Brand RA: Hip osteotomies: a biomechanical consideration. J Am Acad Orthop Surg 5:282–291, 1997.
67. Pauwels F: Biomechanics of the normal and diseased hip: theoretical foundation, technique and results of treatment—an atlas, Berlin, 1976, Springer-Verlag, pp 55, 129–272.
68. Bombelli R: Structure and function in normal and abnormal hips: how to mechanically jeopardized hips, ed 3, Berlin, 1993, Springer-Verlag, pp 3–9, 24–55.
69. Brand RA, Pedersen DR: Computer modeling of surgery and a consideration of the mechanical effects of proximal femoral osteotomies. In Welch RB (ed): The hip: proceedings of the Twelfth Open Scientific Meeting of the Hip Society, St Louis, 1984, CV Mosby, pp 193–210.
70. D'Souza SR, Sadiq S, New AMR, Northmore-Ball MD: Proximal femoral osteotomy as the primary operation for young adults who have osteoarthrosis of the hip. J Bone Joint Surg Am 80:1428–1438, 1998.
71. Sanchez-Sotelo J, Trousdale RT, Berry DJ, Cabanela ME: Surgical treatment of developmental dysplasia of the hip in adults. I. Non-arthroplasty options. J Am Acad Orthop Surg 10:321–333, 2002.
72. Matheney T, Kim YJ, Zurakowski D, et al: Intermediate to long-term results following the Bernese periacetabular osteotomy and predictors of clinical outcome. J Bone Joint Surg Am 91:2113–2123, 2009.
73. Sculco TP: Minimally invasive total hip arthroplasty: in the affirmative. J Arthroplasty 19(4 Suppl 1):78, 2004.
74. Dorr LD, Maheshwari AV, Long WT, et al: Early pain relief and function after posterior minimally invasive and conventional total hip arthroplasty: a prospective, randomized, blinded study. J Bone Joint Surg Am 89:1153–1160, 2007.
75. de Beer J, Petruccelli D, Zalzal P, et al: Single-incision, minimally invasive total hip arthroplasty: length doesn't matter. J Arthroplasty 19:945, 2004.
76. Woolson ST, Mow CS, Syquia JF, et al: Comparison of primary total hip replacements performed with a standard incision or a mini-incision. J Bone Joint Surg Am 86:1353, 2004.
77. Woolson ST, Pouliot MA, Huddleston JI: Primary total hip arthroplasty using an anterior approach and a fracture table: short-term results from a community hospital. J Arthroplasty 24:999–1005, 2009.
78. Restrepo C, Parvizi J, Pour AE, Hozack WJ: Prospective randomized study of two surgical approaches for total hip arthroplasty. J Arthroplasty 25:671–679, 2010.
79. Berger RA, Sanders SA, Thill ES, et al: Newer anesthesia and rehabilitation protocols enable outpatient hip replacement in selected patients. Clin Orthop Relat Res 467:1424–1430, 2009.
80. Di Monaco M, Vallero F, Tappero R, Cavanna A: Rehabilitation after total hip arthroplasty: a systemic review of controlled trials on physical exercise programs. Eur J Phys Rehabil Med 45:1–15, 2009.
81. Lenze EJ, Munin MC, Quear T, et al: Significance of poor patient participation in physical and occupational therapy for functional outcome and length of stay. Arch Phys Med Rehabil 85:1599–1601, 2004.

SUGGESTED READING

Berger RA, Sanders SA, Thill ES, et al: Newer anesthesia and rehabilitation protocols enable outpatient hip replacement in selected patients. Clin Orthop Relat Res 467:1424–1430, 2009.
Authors review their experience with the application of a comprehensive perioperative management protocol to allow THA to be performed on an outpatient basis in select patients.
Bozic KJ, Wagie A, Naessens JM, et al: Predictors of discharge to an inpatient extended care facility after total hip or knee arthroplasty. J Arthroplasty 21(Suppl 2):151–156, 2006.
The authors review baseline characteristics that are predictive of discharge to an inpatient extended care facility for patients undergoing elective total joint arthroplasty.

Enseki KR, Martin RL, Draovitch P, et al: The hip joint: arthroscopic procedures and postoperative rehabilitation. J Orthop Sports Phys Ther 36:516–525, 2006.

Recent advancements in the treatment of hip pathology with arthroscopic techniques have led to a greater number of surgical procedures, including labral tear resection, labral repair, capsular modification, osteoplasty, and microfracture procedures. Postoperative rehabilitation following these procedures differs from that following THA because of concern regarding range of motion, weight-bearing precautions, and initiation of strength activities.

Joyce BM, Kirby RL: Canes, crutches, and walkers. Am Fam Physician 43:535–542, 1991.

A review of the biomechanical aids prescribed to assist patients with an unstable gait.

Walter FL, Bass N, Bock G, Markel DC: Success of clinical pathways for total joint arthroplasty in a community hospital. Clin Orthop Relat Res 457:133–137, 2007.

A review of the successful application of clinical pathways following elective primary total joint arthroplasty in a community teaching hospital.

Woolson ST, Adler NS: The effect of partial or full weight bearing ambulation after cementless THA. J Arthroplasty 17:820–825, 2002.

An early, retrospective evaluation of the senior author's experience with permitting full weight bearing following cementless THA.

SECTION IV

HIP EVALUATION, DIAGNOSIS, AND PATHOLOGY

CHAPTER 30

History and Physical Examination of the Hip

Hal David Martin

INTRODUCTION

The goal of the clinical examination of the hip is to assess the four layers: the osseous, capsulolabral, musculotendinous, and neurovascular. It is important to understand the balance and interrelationship that each system has with the other in a static and dynamic fashion, as the hip assumes an essential role in most activities. Not only is the hip responsible for distributing weight between the appendicular and axial skeletons, it is also the joint from which motion is initiated and executed. During running and jumping, forces upon the hip joint can reach three to five times body weight.[1] Hip pain often stems from a sports-related injury,[2] and some athletes are prone to hip injury and secondary degenerative hip disease.[3,4]

Currently, 60% of intra-articular disorders are misdiagnosed initially.[5] An organized physical examination is designed to assess the hip, the back, and abdominal, neurovascular, and neurologic systems. Comorbidities often coexist with complex hip pathology; therefore it is important that physical examination of the hip be inclusive enough to rule out other joints as a dominant cause of complaint. The hip is recognized early as the source of pain when a consistent method of interpreting the history and clinical examination of the hip is followed. The goals of this chapter are (1) to review pertinent information required for a detailed patient history, (2) to describe how clinical examination of the hip are performed, and to explain why these tests are important, and (3) to discuss current controversies and future considerations related to physical examination of the hip.

HISTORY AND PHYSICAL EXAMINATION

History

A complete patient history is obtained before physical examination of the hip is performed. The first factors in consideration of treatment are the age of the patient and the presence or absence of trauma.[1] A description of the present condition is documented, including date of onset, mechanism of injury, pain location, and factors that increase or decrease the pain.[6,7] Previous consultations, surgical interventions, and injuries are documented. Treatments to date, such as rest, physical therapy, ice, heat, nonsteroidal anti-inflammatories, surgery, injections, orthotics, and the use of support aids, must be delineated. Limitations to patient function are detailed; these may involve getting into or out of the bathtub or car, performing activities of daily living, jogging, walking, or climbing stairs. Symptoms related to the back, the neurologic system, or the abdomen and lower extremity complaints must be recognized.[7] Lumbar problems occasionally are confused with problems in the hip as a partial or dominant cause of complaint. Associated complaints, such as pain in the abdomen or back, numbness, weakness, cough, or sneeze exacerbation, help the clinician to identify lumbar issues.[7]

The vascular supply to the femoral head and any possible sources of disruption are screened, including metabolic disorders such as abnormalities in lipids, thyroid, homocysteine, and clotting mechanisms.[7] The social history of the patient is reviewed to identify the presence or use of tobacco, alcohol, steroids, or altitude issues, all of which can affect the blood supply to the femoral head. A history of sports and recreational activities helps to reveal the type of injury.[3,6,7] Rotation sports, such as golf, tennis, ballet, and martial arts, have been commonly associated with injury to the intra-articular structures, including the labrum, iliofemoral ligament, and ligamentum teres.

The history and physical examination of the hip will direct the differentiation of intra-articular versus extra-articular sources of pain, along with location of the presenting pain and the presence or absence of popping/locking. Extra-articular sources of pain often respond well to nonoperative treatment, and intra-articular sources require further workup, which may include x-rays,[8-13] magnetic resonance imaging (MRI),[14,15] MRI arthrogram,[16-19] or injection tests. Patient goals and realistic expectations of treatment are discussed. Communication, understanding, empathy, and compassion are important in obtaining an accurate history. Figure 30-1 provides an example of a complete hip history form.

Several questionnaires that provide quantitative and qualitative descriptions of a patient's functional ability are available. The modified Harris Hip Score[20] (HHS), the most documented and standardized functional score to date, is a quantitative score based on pain and function. Other hip scores that have been outlined with quantification in more specific patient populations include Merle d'Aubigné[21] (MDA), the Non-Arthritic Hip Score[22] (NAHS), the Musculoskeletal Function Assessment[23] (MFA), Short Form-36[24] (SF-36), and the Western Ontario and McMaster University Osteoarthritis Index (WOMAC).[25] A verbal analogue score is also subjectively useful.

Physical Examination of the Hip

A consistent hip examination is performed quickly and efficiently to screen the hip, the back, and abdominal, neurovascular, and neurologic systems. It is important that physical examination of the hip is inclusive enough to rule out other joints as a dominant cause of complaint. The technique of physical examination is dependent on the examiner's experience and efficiency. Interobserver consistency and practice account for some of the most important aspects of the evaluation.[26] Figure 30-2 shows an example of a physical examination of the hip intake form.

The physical examination consists of a variety of tests involving wide ranges of motion and palpation; therefore loose-fitting clothing about the waist is needed. A trained assistant provides accurate documentation by recording the examination on a written form. The order of the examination is designed to be easy on the patient and to flow for the physician; it begins with standing tests, which are followed by seated, supine, lateral, and prone tests. A comprehensive assessment requires scheduling adequate time with the patient. For international clarification among clinicians, each test is given a descriptive functional title.

Standing Examination

The general area of pain is noted by having the patient point with one finger. The groin region directs suspicion of an intra-articular problem, and laterally based pain is primarily associated with both intra-articular and extra-articular aspects. A characteristic sign of patients with hip pain is the "C sign."[26] The patient holds his or her hand in the shape of a C and places it above the greater trochanter, with the thumb positioned posterior to the trochanter and fingers extending into the groin.[26] This can be misinterpreted as lateral soft tissue pathology such as trochanteric bursitis or the iliotibial band; however, the patient may often describe deep interior hip pain.[26] Posterior-superior pain necessitates a complete evaluation for differentiating hip and back pain.

Table 30-1. Standing Examination Assessment

Examination	Assessment/Association
Abductor deficient gait	Abductor strength, proprioception mechanism
Antalgic gait	Trauma, fracture, synovial inflammation
Pelvic rotational wink	Intra-articular pathology, hip flexion contracture, increased femoral anteversion, anterior capsular laxity
Foot progression angle with excessive external rotation	Femoral retroversion, increased acetabular anteversion, torsional abnormalities, effusion, ligamentous injury
Foot progression angle with excessive internal rotation	Increased femoral anteversion or acetabular retroversion, torsional abnormalities
Short leg limp	Iliotibial band pathology, true/false leg length discrepancy
Single-leg stance phase test	Abductor strength, proprioception mechanism
Spinal alignment	Shoulder/iliac crest height, lordosis, scoliosis, leg length
Laxity	Ligamentous laxity in other joints: thumb, elbows, shoulders, or knee

Often, back issues are noted, along with musculotendinous hip pathology.[7]

As the patient stands (Table 30-1), general body habitus is assessed, and shoulder height and iliac crest heights are evaluated for leg length discrepancies. Placing incremental wooden blocks under the short-side heel will aid in orthotic considerations. Issues of ligamentous laxity are determined by the thumb test or by hyperextension of the elbows or knees. Forward bending allows assessment of spinal alignment and differentiation of structural versus nonstructural scoliosis. The degree of flexion at the waist is recorded, and side-to-side bending is helpful.

An understanding of mechanical load transfer in the hip in both static and dynamic situations is essential for assessment and diagnosis of hip pathology. Comprehensive knowledge of normal gait will aid the physician in discriminating between normal and abnormal gait patterns. Abnormal gait patterns can indicate where abnormal transfer of load is applied across the hip joint; this can result in improper force load transfer to the lower back and knee joints.[27] Irregularities in gait are derived most often by compensating for pain perceived in stride. The musculature of the lower limbs produces the forces required for ambulation, and the ligamentous capsule maintains hip stability.[27] This relationship emphasizes the importance of adequate postoperative rehabilitation, especially with connective tissue disorders and improper osseous alignment.

Adequate space such as a hallway is needed, so that a full gait of six to eight stride lengths can be assessed. Gait evaluation includes observation of foot rotation (internal/external progression angle), pelvic rotation in

Complete Hip History Form

NAME: _____ DATE: _____ AGE: _____

EMPLOYMENT: _____

REFERRED BY: _____

CHIEF COMPLAINT: L HIP   R HIP   OTHER:_____

HISTORY OF PRESENT ILLNESS:

• Date of onset _____

• Traumatic/nontraumatic

• Mechanism of injury _____

• Pain location _____

• Pain increased with _____

• Pain decreased with _____

• Have you ever been diagnosed with AVN? If yes, do you have a family history of heart disease, stroke, or clotting disorders?_____

Alcohol use_____   Tobacco use_____   Steroid use_____

Labs: Homocysteine_____   Factor V Leiden_____   Lipid profile_____   Thyroid profile_____

• Pain AM/PM   Popping/Locking

TREATMENT TO DATE:

Rest   Ice   Heat   NSAIDS_____

PT _____

Surgery_____

Chiropractic tx_____

Injections_____

Support (cane, crutch)_____

Orthotics_____

TESTS AND EVALUATIONS:

MRI   MRI Arthrogram   X-rays   Lab   Biometrics   Consults_____

PAST INJURIES: _____

LIMITATIONS:

    • Sitting   Length of time able to sit_____

    • Getting in or out of car

    • Getting in or out of tub

    • Sports

    • Jogging

    • Walking

    • Stairs

    • Work

    • ADLs

    • Household activities

FUNCTION:

HHS_____   VAS: Pain at rest (0-10)

Pain With Activity

ASSOCIATED

    • Back   L   R

    • Night pain awakening

    • Numbness

    • Weakness

SPORTS AND ACTIVITIES: _____

GOAL IN TREATMENT:_____

HHS: Harris Hip Score

VAS: Visual Analogue Scale

Figure 30-1. Complete hip history form.

Physical Examination of the Hip Intake Form

PHYSICAL EXAMINATION: HT:_____ WT:_____ T:_____ R:_____ P:_____ BP:_____

Gait/Posture:
- Shoulder height: Equal   Not equal
- Iliac crest height: Equal   Not equal
- Active forward bend: Degrees
- Spine: Straight
          Scoliosis: Structural   Nonstructural
- Recurvatum: Thumb test   Elbows   Knees   >5 degrees
- Lordosis: Normal   Increased   Paravertebral muscle spasms
- Gait: Normal   Antalgic   Abductor deficient (Trendelenburg)
                 Pelvic wink   Arm swing   Short stride length, short stance phase
    Foot progression angle: External   Neutral   Hyperpronation
- Single leg stance phase test (Trendelenburg test):   R _____   L _____

Seated Piriformis Stretch Test:
- Neurologic Findings:
    Motor: _____
    Sensory: _____
    DTR: Achilles   Patella
- Circulation: DP   PT
- Skin inspection: _____
- Lymphatic: Lymphedema   No lymphedema   Pitting edema: 1+ 2+
- Straight leg raise: R _____ L _____
- Range of motion: Internal rotation: External rotation:
                       R _____ L _____   R _____ L _____

Supine Examination:
- Leg lengths: R_____ cm L_____ cm Equal/Not equal
- ROM: Right leg   Left leg
    Flexion: 80 100 110 120 130 140   80 100 110 120 130 140
    Abduction: 10   20   30 45   50   10   20   30 45 50
    Adduction: 0   10   20 30   0   10   20 30
- Hip flexion contracture test (Thomas test):   R + -   L + -
- FADDIR: R + -   L + -
- DIRI: R + -   L + -
- DEXRIT: R + -   L + -
- Posterior rim impingement test: R + -   L + -
- Abduction extension external rotation (Instability sign):   R + -   L + -
- Palpation:
    Musculature: Tender   Non-tender
    Adductor tubercle: Tender   Non-tender
    Pubic symphysis/Adductor   Tender   Non-tender
- Tinels—emoral nerve   R + -   L + -
- FABER (Patrick test):   R + -   L + -
- Straight leg raise against resistance (Stitchfield test):   R + -   L + -
- Passive supine rotation test (Log roll test):   R + -   L + -
- Heel strike: R + -   L + -

Lateral Examination (Active Piriformis Test)
- Palpation:
    SI joint   Tender   Non-tender
    Ischium   Tender   Non-tender
    Greater trochanter   Tender   Non-tender
    ASIS   Tender   Non-tender
    Piriformis   Tender   Non-tender
    Tinels—sciatic nerve
    G. Max insertion into ITB   Tender   Non-tender
    Sciatic nerve   Tender   Non-tender
    Gluteus medius   Tender   Non-tender
- Abductor strength: Straight leg _____ Gluteus maximus _____ Gluteus medius _____
- Tensor fascia lata contracture test: Grade(1-3)
- Gluteus medius contracture test: Grade (1-3)
- Gluteus maximus contracture test: Grade (1-3)
- Lateral rim impingement test: R + -   L + -
- FADDIR test: R + -   L + -

Prone Examination:
- Rectus contracture test (Ely's test):   R + -   L + -
- Femoral anteversion test (Craig's test): _____ degrees anteversion
- Palpation:
    Spinous processes   + -
    SI joints   R + -   L + -
    Bursae ischium

Figure 30-2. Physical examination of the hip intake form.

the coronal and sagittal planes, stance phase, and stride length. The foot progression angle will indicate osseous or static rotatory malalignment, which occurs with increased or decreased femoral anteversion, versus a capsular or musculotendinous problem. Simultaneous observation of the knee and thigh is critical in assessment of rotatory parameters. Secondary abnormal hip rotation may be caused by holding the knee in internal or external rotation in an effort to maintain proper patellofemoral joint alignment. This abnormal motion or battle between the hip and the knee for a comfortable position will affect the gait; this is usually seen in cases of severe increased femoral anteversion. In cases of a painful gait, it is important to document the anatomic location of pain and the phase within the gait cycle during which pain is experienced. Pain alleviated with an abducted gait raises suspicion for the possibility of dysplasia.

Careful observation of iliac crest rotation and terminal hip extension will assess pelvic rotation. On average, normal gait requires 8 degrees of hip rotation and 7 degrees of pelvic rotation, equaling a total rotation of 15 degrees.[28] Excessive rotation in the axial plane toward the affected hip is demonstrative of a pelvic wink. The pelvic wink produces extension and rotation through the lumbar spine to attain terminal hip extension. The winking gait can be associated with laxity or hip flexion contracture, which can be exacerbated by increased lumbar lordosis or a forward-stooping posture. Ischiofemoral impingement can also produce a lumbar pelvic flexion to gain hip extension. Spinal function and mechanics can be affected by gait abnormalities. In cases of excessive femoral anteversion, the patient will try to create greater anterior coverage with a rotated pelvis to achieve terminal hip extension. Anterior capsular injury or laxity can also attribute to a winking gait.

During the stance phase, body weight must be supported by a single leg, with the gluteus maximus, gluteus medius, and gluteus minimus providing the majority of support forces.[27,28] Heel strike occurs at 30 degrees of hip flexion, thus generating maximum ground reactive forces to the hip.[28] Neuromuscular abnormalities, trauma, and leg length discrepancies can be indicated by a shortened stance phase. Abductor weakness or disrupted proprioception can be attributed to abductor deficient gait (common nomenclature, Trendelenburg gait or abductor lurch). The abductor deficient gait is an unbalanced stance phase, which may present in two ways: a pelvic shift away from the body ("dropping out" of the hip on the affected side), or a weight shift over the adducted leg (shift of the upper body "over the top" of the affected hip). Antalgic gait, a self-protecting limp caused by pain, is characterized by a shortened stance phase on the painful side, limiting the duration of weight bearing. Differentiation of a short leg gait involves a drop of the shoulder in the direction of the short leg.

The single-leg stance phase test (traditionally known as the *Trendelenburg test*) is an assessment of hip joint function that simulates the single-leg stance phase with load on the examined hip. The single-leg stance phase test is performed bilaterally, with the nonaffected side examined first and serving as a baseline reference for the affected side (Fig. 30-3). The examiner observes the single-leg stance phase test from behind and in front of the patient, while carefully assessing the bony

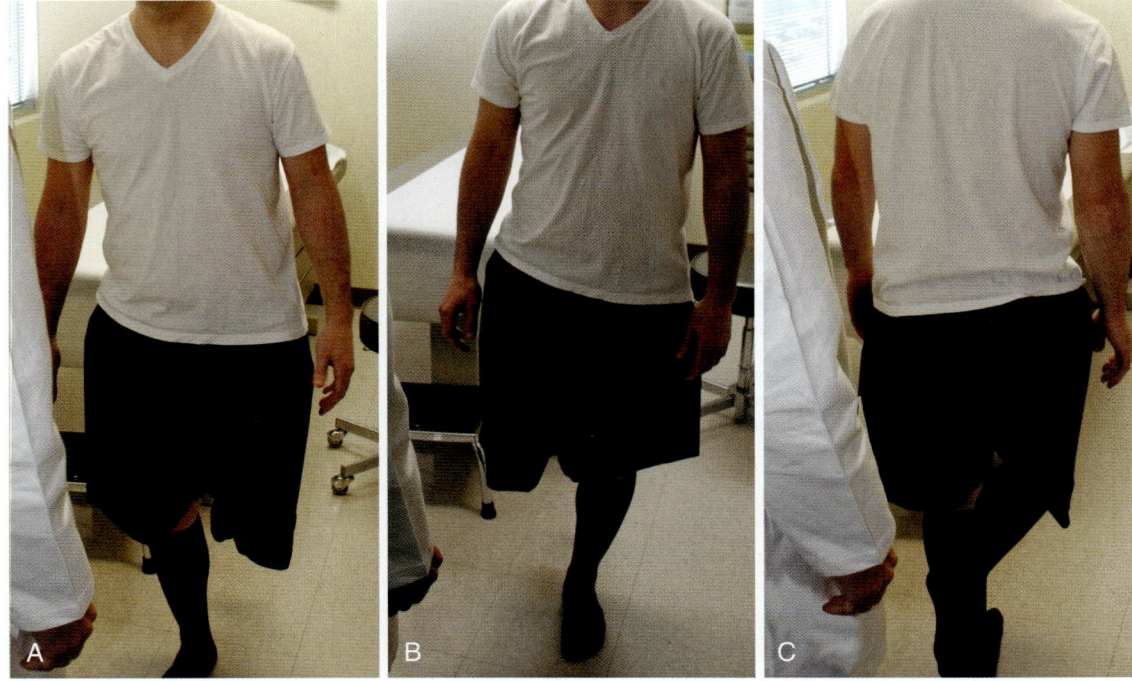

Figure 30-3. The single-leg stance phase test. The single-leg stance phase test is performed bilaterally and is observed from behind and in front of the patient. The patient holds this position for 6 seconds. A pelvic shift of greater than 2 cm is a positive, indicating abductor weakness or proprioception disruption. **A,** Right leg, front view. **B,** Left leg, front view (note the positive pelvic shift). **C,** Left leg, rear view.

landmarks of the iliac crests, shoulder heights, knees, and ankles. The patient stands with feet shoulder width apart and brings one leg forward by flexing the leg to 45 degrees at the hip and 45 degrees at the knee. The single-leg stance phase position is held for 6 seconds. As the patient lifts and holds one foot off the ground, the contralateral hip abductor musculature and the neural loop of proprioception are being evaluated. If the musculature is weak, or if the neural loop of proprioception is disrupted, the pelvis will tilt toward or away from the unsupported side. Normal dynamic midstance translocation is 2 cm during a normal gait pattern,[28] and a shift in either direction of greater than 2 cm constitutes a positive shift. This test is also performed in a dynamic fashion.

Seated Examination

A thorough neurologic and vascular examination is performed during the seated hip examination (Table 30-2). Criteria for the care of the patient, as well as for coding, are available; therefore it is important to check the basics even in apparently healthy individuals.[7] The posterior tibial pulse is checked first, any swelling of the extremity is noted, and inspection of the skin is performed at this time. A straight-leg raise test is performed by the examiner by passively extending the patient's knee into full extension; this will detect any radicular neurologic symptoms, such as stretching of an entrapped nerve root.

Loss of internal rotation is one of the first signs of the possibility of intra-articular disorder[29-34]; therefore one of the most important assessments is that of internal and external rotation in the seated position. The seated

position ensures that the ischium is square to the table, thus providing sufficient stability at 90 degrees of hip flexion and a reproducible platform for accurate rotational measurement. Gently perform passive internal and external rotation until a firm endpoint or pain is involved, and compare bilaterally (Fig. 30-4). Seated rotation range of motion is also compared and contrasted with extended hip position during the prone examination.

Musculotendinous, ligamentous, and osseous control of internal and external rotation is complex; therefore any differences in seated versus extended positions may raise the question of ligamentous versus osseous abnormality. For proper hip function, sufficient internal rotation is needed. At the midstance phase of normal

Table 30-2. Seated Examination Assessment

Examination	Assessment/Association
Neurologic	Sensory nerves originating from the L2-S1 levels, DTR of patella (L2-L4 spinal nerves and femoral nerve) and Achilles (L5-S1 sacral nerves)
Straight-leg raise	Radicular neurologic symptoms
Vascular	Pulses of the dorsalis pedis and posterior tibial artery
Lymphatic	Skin inspection for swelling, scarring, or side-to-side asymmetry
Internal rotation	Normal between 20 and 35 degrees
External rotation	Normal between 30 and 45 degrees

DTR, Deep tendon reflex.

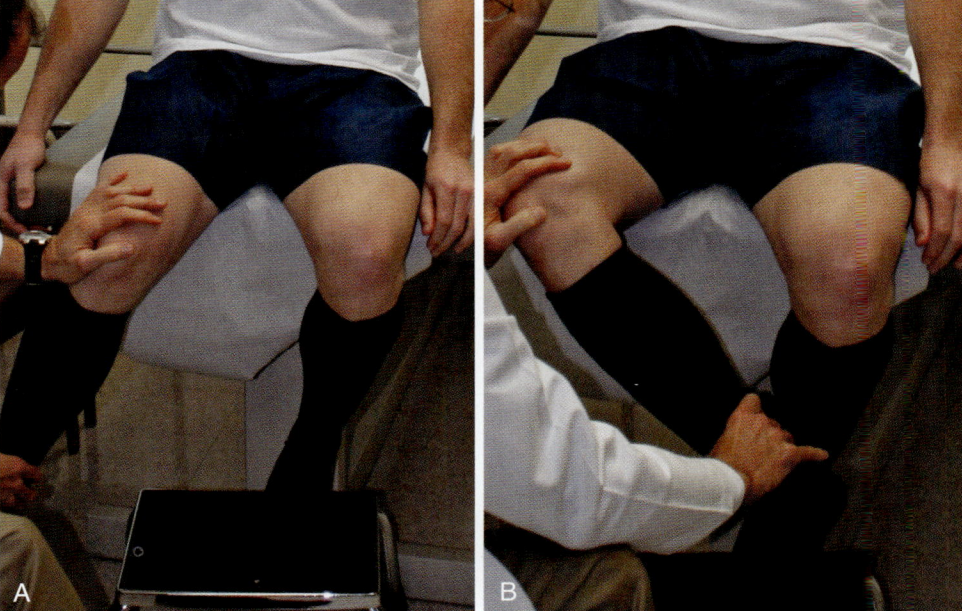

Figure 30-4. Seated internal and external rotation range of motion. Passive internal and external rotation testing is compared from side to side. In the seated position, the ischium is square to the table, thus providing sufficient stability at 90 degrees of hip flexion. Internal and external rotation in the seated position offers a reproducible platform for accurate rotational measurement.

Table 30-3. Summary of Supine Examinations and Assessment

Examination	Assessment/Association
Range of motion	Flexion, abduction, adduction
FADDIR	Anterior femoroacetabular impingement, torn labrum
Hip flexion contracture test (Thomas test)	Hip flexor contracture (psoas), femoral neuropathy, intra-articular pathology, abdominal origin
FABER (Patrick/Faber)	Distinguish between back and hip pathology, specifically, sacroiliac joint pathology
Dynamic internal rotatory impingement test (similar to McCarthy test)	Anterior femoroacetabular impingement, torn labrum
Dynamic external rotatory impingement test (similar to McCarthy test)	Superior femoroacetabular impingement, torn labrum
Posterior rim impingement test	Posterior femoroacetabular impingement, torn labrum
Passive supine rotation test (log roll)	Trauma, effusion, synovitis
Heel strike	Trauma, femoral fracture
Straight-leg raise against resistance (Stitchfield)	Hip flexor strength
Palpation	
1. Abdomen	Fascial hernia, associated Gastrointestinal/genitourinary pathology
2. Pubic symphysis	Osteitis pubis, calcification, fracture, trauma
3. Adductor tubercle	Adductor tendinitis

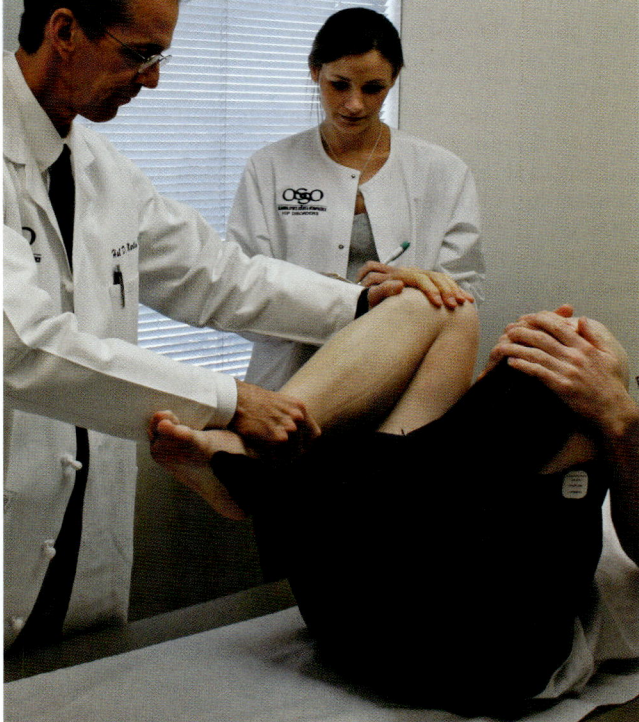

Figure 30-5. Supine examination, starting position. Zero set point of the pelvis is achieved by having the patient hold the contralateral leg in full flexion, thus establishing neutral pelvic inclination.

gait should be at least 10 degrees of internal rotation; however, less than 20 degrees is poorly tolerated for normal activity. Diagnoses such as arthritis, effusion, internal derangement, slipped capital femoral epiphysis, femoroacetabular impingement, and muscular contracture can be related to loss of internal hip rotation.[7] Significant side-to-side differences can be related to femoroacetabular impingement or to rotational constraint from increased or decreased femoral acetabular anteversion. Increased internal rotation combined with decreased external rotation may indicate excessive femoral anteversion, although hip capsular function will require further radiographic and biometric assessment.[14,35]

Supine Examination

The supine position (Table 30-3) helps to further distinguish internal from extra-articular sources of hip symptoms. The supine position allows assessment of any leg length discrepancies with the hip in an unloaded state. Passive hip flexion range of motion is assessed as both knees are brought up to the chest, and the degree of flexion is recorded (Fig. 30-5). It is important to note the pelvic position, as the hip may stop early in flexion with the end range of motion being predominantly pelvic

rotation. From this position, the hip flexion contracture test (also known as the *Thomas test*) is performed by having the patient extend and relax one leg down toward the table. Any lack of terminal hip extension, noted by inability of the thigh to reach the table, demonstrates a hip flexion contracture. Both sides are assessed for comparison of the difference. An important aspect of the hip flexion contracture test is obtaining the zero set point for the lumbar spine. Patients with hyperlaxity or connective tissue disorder could receive a false negative. In these patients, the zero set point can be established with an abdominal contraction. The hip flexion contracture test could be falsely negative if lumbar spine hyperlordosis due to previous spinal fusion is present.

During the course of the supine examination, any pop in this plane can sometimes be related to a snapping iliopsoas tendon. A fan test (the patient circumducts and rotates the hip in rotatory fashion) can help delineate the presence of the snapping iliopsoas tendon over the femoral head or the iliopectineal eminence. Often this can be eliminated with an abdominal contraction, which will decrease lumbar lordosis, thus affecting the innominate ridge on the anterior wall and eliminating the pop of coxa sultans internus. A hula hoop maneuver, in which the patient stands and twists, or a bicycle test (performed in the lateral position) can help to distinguish the pop internally from the external pop of coxa sultans externus caused by the subluxing iliotibial band over the greater trochanter.

The flexion/abduction/external rotation test (FABER), also known as the *Patrick test*, is helpful in determining hip versus nonhip complaints. A positive re-creation of pain directed to the hip can be associated with musculotendinous or osseous posterior lateral acetabular incongruence or ligamentous injury. In cases of a coup contrecoup injury, in which the mechanism of injury is initiated posteriorly, pain may be referred to the anterior secondarily.

Tests such as flexion/adduction/internal rotation are used to detect impingement or intra-articular pathology. The degree of flexion required in this position of adduction/internal rotation depends on the degree of impingement and the type and location of impingement. The degree of hip flexion with the amount of pressure of internal rotation is taken on a case-by-case basis, depending on the function required of the patient, as well as the patient complaint.

Dynamic Internal Rotatory Impingement Test. For the dynamic internal rotatory impingement (DIRI) test, the patient, in the supine position, is instructed to hold the nonaffected leg in flexion beyond 90 degrees, thus establishing a zero pelvic set point and eliminating lumbar lordosis. The examined hip is then brought into 90 degrees of flexion or beyond and is passively taken through a wide arc of adduction and internal rotation (Fig. 30-6). A positive test is noted with re-creation of the complaint pain. DIRI can also be performed in the operating theater for direct visualization of femoral neck and acetabular congruence. DIRI is similar to the traditional McCarthy's test, which elicits a pop.[26]

Dynamic External Rotatory Impingement Test. With the dynamic external rotatory impingement (DEXRIT) test, the zero pelvic set point is maintained as the patient holds the nonaffected leg in flexion beyond 90 degrees, which will eliminate lumbar lordosis. The examined hip is then brought into 90 degrees of flexion or beyond and is dynamically taken through a wide arc of abduction and external rotation (Fig. 30-7). A positive test is noted with re-creation of the complaint pain. DEXRIT can be performed in the operating theater for direct visualization of femoral neck and acetabular congruence.

Passive abduction and adduction range of motion is easily assessed in the supine position. Palpation of the abdomen is performed and any abdominal tenderness appreciated. Abdominal tenderness is differentiated from a fascial hernia and/or adductor tendinitis. Resisted torso flexion with palpation of the abdomen will differentiate a fascial hernia from other complaints. Palpation of the adductor tubercle with active testing will detect adductor tendinitis. Common physical examination findings associated with athletic pubalgia include inguinal canal tenderness, pubic crest/tubercle tenderness, adductor origin tenderness, pain with resisted sit-ups or hip flexion, and a tender, dilated superficial ring.

Another useful test is Tinel's test of the femoral nerve. Tinel's test is found to be positive with hip flexion contractures presenting at greater than 25 degrees because of the proximity of the psoas tendon and the femoral nerve. A heel strike is performed by striking the heel abruptly, which is indicative of some type of trauma and/or stress fracture. The passive supine rotation test (commonly known as the *leg roll*) involves passive internal and external rotation of the femur, with the leg lying in an extended or slightly flexed position. The passive supine rotation test is performed bilaterally, and any side-to-side differences in this maneuver can alert the examiner to the presence of laxity, effusion, or internal derangement. The straight-leg raise against resistance test (also known as the *Stitchfield test*) is an assessment of the psoas labral interface. The patient performs an active straight-leg raise with knee extension to 45 degrees; the examiner's hand is placed distal to the knee while downward force is applied. A positive

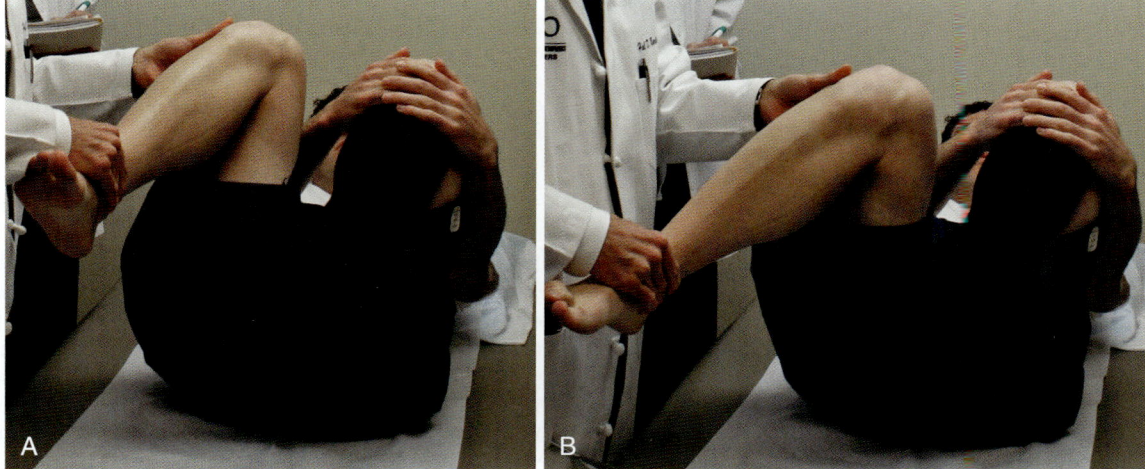

Figure 30-6. The dynamic internal rotatory impingement test (DIRI). DIRI begins with the hip at 90 degrees of flexion or beyond. It is passively taken through a wide arc of adduction and internal rotation while flexion is decreased to about 80 degrees.

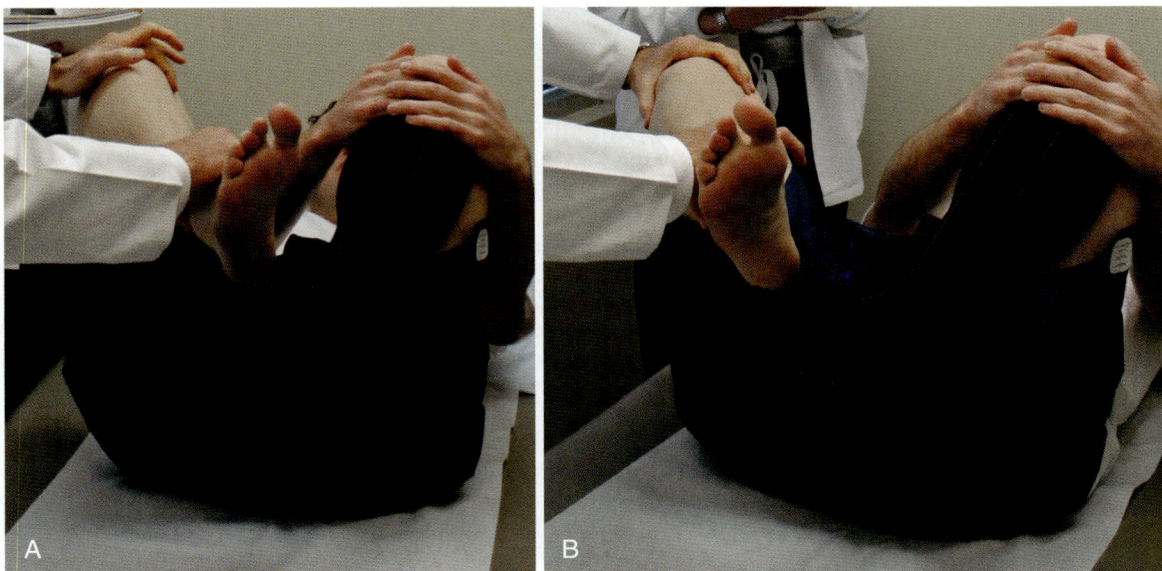

Figure 30-7. The dynamic external rotatory impingement test (DEXRIT). DEXRIT begins with the hip at 90 degrees of flexion or beyond. It is dynamically taken through a wide arc of abduction and external rotation.

test is noted with re-creation of the complaint pain or weakness.

The importance of multiple examinations for the detection of intra-articular pathology has been recognized. Even in the presence of normal internal and external rotation, further delineation is needed of the relationships that exist between musculotendinous, osseous, and ligamentous structures. No single test is sensitive enough to be used exclusively in the detection of subtle pathology. Furthermore, the ligamentous contribution to range of motion varies with flexion and rotation.[36]

The posterior rim impingement test can be performed in the supine position. The patient is positioned at the edge of the examining table, so that the examined leg hangs freely at the hip, and the patient draws up both legs into the chest, thus eliminating lumbar lordosis. The affected leg is then extended off the table, allowing for full extension of the hip, and is abducted and externally rotated (Fig. 30-8). The posterior rim impingement test takes the hip into extension while assessing the congruence of the posterior acetabular wall and femoral neck. A variation of this test is the lateral rim impingement test, which is explained in the "Lateral Examination" section.

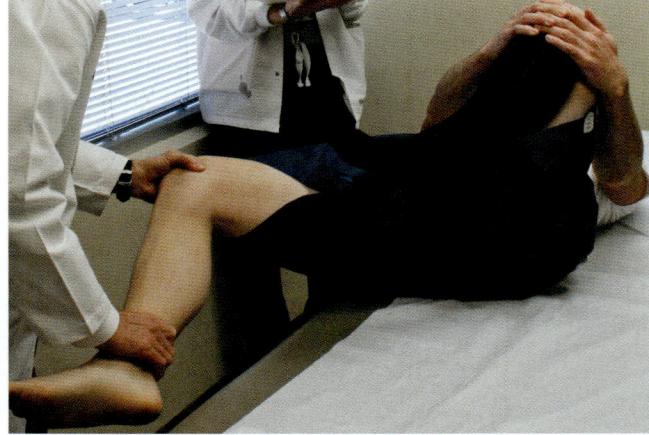

Figure 30-8. The posterior rim impingement test. The posterior rim impingement test is performed with the patient at the edge of the examining table. The leg should hang freely at the hip while the patient holds the contralateral leg in full flexion. The examined leg is then brought into full hip extension and is abducted and externally rotated.

Lateral Examination

The lateral examination (Table 30-4) places the hip in an excellent position for additional musculotendinous, ligamentous, and osseous evaluations. The lateral examination begins with the patient on the contralateral side by palpating areas of the supra-sacroiliac (SI) and SI joints, muscles of abduction, and, in particular, the origin of the gluteus maximus as it inserts along the lateral border of the sacrum, as well as the most posterior aspect of the ilium. The next point of palpation is

the ischium for detection of avulsions or bursitis. Finally, the piriformis and the sciatic nerve are palpated for any sign of tenderness, along with the abductor musculature, which includes the gluteus maximus, gluteus medius, gluteus minimus, and tensor fascia lata. An active piriformis test is performed when the patient pushes the heel down into the table and abducts and externally rotates the leg against resistance, while the examiner monitors the piriformis. The active piriformis test is similar to the pace test, which assesses pain and weakness on resisted abduction and external rotation

Table 30-4. Summary of Lateral Examinations and Assessment

Examination	Assessment/Association
Flexion, adduction, internal rotation	Anterior femoroacetabular impingement, torn labrum
Lateral rim impingement	Lateral femoroacetabular impingement, torn labrum, instability
Tensor fascia lata contracture test (Ober's test)	Tensor fascia lata contracture
Gluteus medius Contracture test (Ober's test)	Gluteus medius contracture/tear (decreased strength with knee flexion, suspect tear)
Gluteus maximus Contracture test	Gluteus maximus contracture, contribution to iliotibial band
Palpation	
1. Greater trochanter	Greater trochanter bursitis, iliotibial band contracture
2. Sacroiliac joint	Distinguish between hip and back pathology
3. Maximus origin	Gluteus maximus origin tendinitis
4. Ischium	Biceps femoris tendinitis, avulsion fracture, ischial bursitis

of the thigh in the seated position.[37] A set of passive adduction tests (most like Ober's test) are performed with the leg in three positions (Fig. 30-9): extension (tensor fascia lata contracture test), neutral (gluteus medius contracture test), and flexion (gluteus maximus contracture test). Evaluation of gluteus medius tension is achieved by release of the iliotibial band with knee flexion, and the hip should be able to be adducted down toward the table. Any restrictions of these motions are recorded. When the gluteus maximus contracture test is performed, the shoulder is rotated toward the side of the table with the hip flexed and the knee extended. If adduction cannot occur in this position, the gluteus maximus portion is contracted. The hip should be able to move freely into a fully adducted position, and any restriction of the gluteus maximus is recognized. The gluteus maximus is balanced with the tensor fascia lata anteriorly. If the hip does not move beyond the midline in the longitudinal axis of the torso, this is graded as 3+ restriction above torso, 2+ at the midline, and 1+ restriction below. Clear delineation of the exact area of restriction will help to direct physical therapy and peritrochanteric treatment options.

Strength is assessed with any type of laterally based hip complaint. The gluteus medius strength test is performed with the knee in flexion to remove the iliotibial

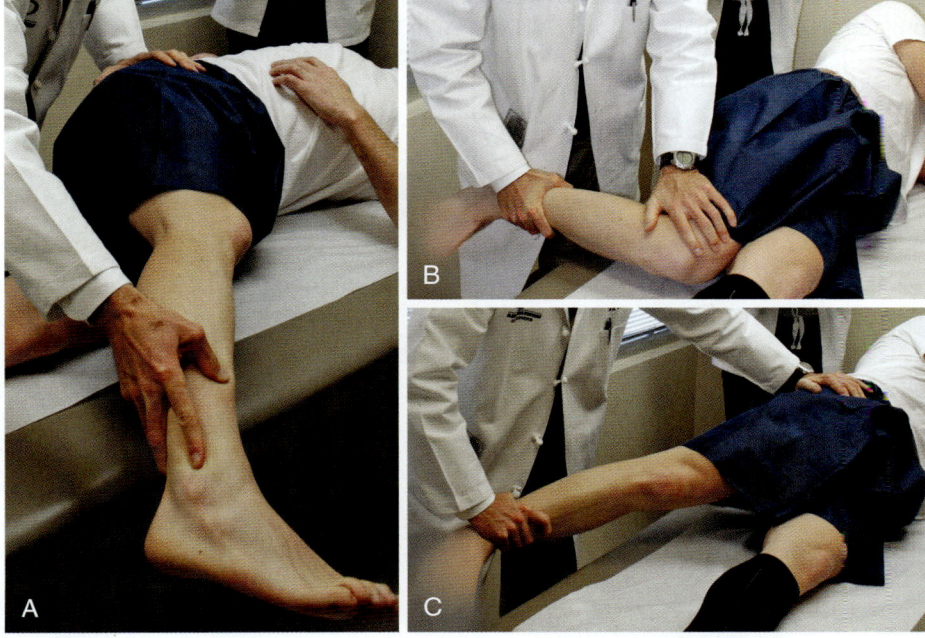

Figure 30-9. Passive adduction tests. **A,** The gluteus maximus contracture test is performed with the ipsilateral shoulder rotated toward the examination table. The examined leg is held in knee extension as the examiner passively brings the hip into flexion, then adduction. **B,** The gluteus medius contracture test is performed with knee flexion, thus eliminating contributions of the iliotibial band and zero flexion. The examiner passively adducts the hip toward the examination table. **C,** The tensor fascia lata contracture test is performed with knee extension. The examiner passively brings the hip into extension, then adduction.

band contribution. Each muscle group is graded in traditional fashion on a 5-point scale.

Next is passive assessment of flexion/adduction/internal rotation (FADDIR), which is performed in a dynamic manner (Fig. 30-10). The examiner holds the monitoring hand in and about the superior aspect of the hip with the lower leg cradled on the forearm and with the knee upon the hand. The hip is then brought into flexion and adduction and is internally rotated. Any reproduction of the patient's complaint and the degree of impingement are noted. FADDIR is commonly performed as part of the supine assessment.[38] The difference is the position of the pelvis. The supine position eliminates lumbar lordosis, whereas the lateral position tests the normal dynamic pelvic inclination. Pelvic inclination may affect testing, and both positions are helpful in evaluation.

The lateral rim impingement test is performed with the hip passively abducted and externally rotated (Fig. 30-11). The examiner cradles the patient's lower leg with one arm and monitors the hip joint with the opposing hand. The examiner passively brings the affected hip through a wide arc from flexion to extension in continuous abduction while externally rotating the hip.

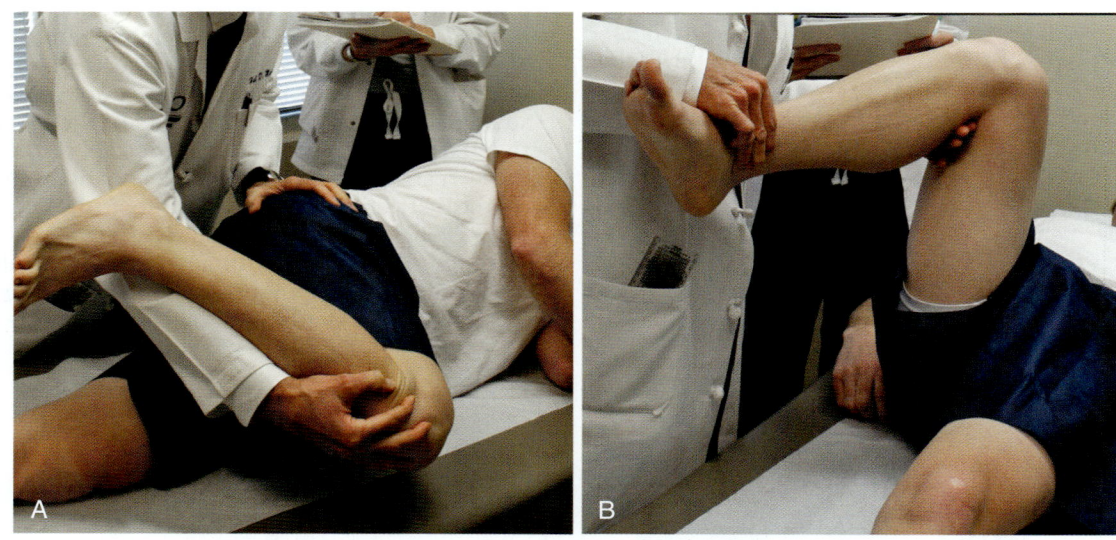

Figure 30-10. Flexion, adduction, internal rotation (FADDIR). **A,** In the lateral position, the examiner brings the examined hip into flexion, adduction, and internal rotation, while monitoring the superior aspect of the hip. **B,** FADDIR is traditionally performed in the supine position. However, both are helpful.

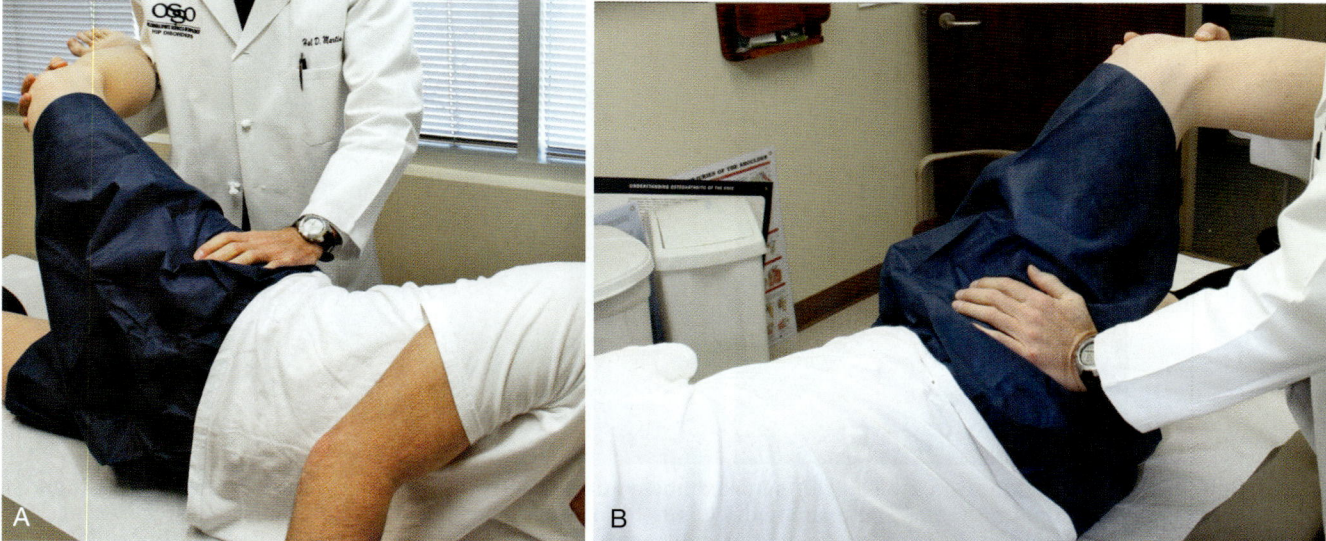

Figure 30-11. The lateral rim impingement test. The lateral rim impingement test is performed in the lateral position and can be taken into extension to assess the posterior wall. The examiner cradles the patient's lower leg with one arm and monitors the hip joint with the opposing hand. The examiner passively brings the affected hip through a wide arc from flexion to extension in continuous abduction while externally rotating the hip. **A,** Front view. **B,** Rear view.

Reproduction of the patient's pain is scored positively. If the feeling of guarding or the feeling of instability is present, the test is positive for apprehension, which is not to be confused with coup contrecoup. The traditional Patrick test performed in the supine position is good for differentiating hip and back pain; however, when performed in the lateral position, the lateral rim impingement test is useful for detection of posterior or lateral impingement issues. Any type of re-creation of a posterior or lateral rim complaint specific to the hip or impingement can be precipitated in this position. Lateral rim impingement, FABER, and posterior rim impingement tests all place the hip into positions of posterior and lateral impingement. The lateral rim impingement test establishes a functional lumbar lordosis with a clear ability to comfortably monitor sites of impingement; this aids in separation of posterior and lateral points of impingement.

Prone Examination

The prone examination (Table 30-5) focuses predominantly on palpation of four distinct areas—the supra-SI, the SI, the gluteus maximus origin, and the spine (facet)—thus identifying the exact area of complaint. Should the pain be identified in the supra-SI joint region or about the facet, a lumbar hyperextension test can help to identify the exact location of suspected pain. If this test is positive, the patient can be placed into a supine position with the knees flexed. If this helps to alleviate the pain, the back should be further evaluated.

The femoral anteversion test (traditionally known as *Craig's test*) gives the examiner a generalized idea of femoral anteversion/retroversion (Fig. 30-12). With the patient in the prone position, the knee is flexed to 90 degrees and the examiner manually rotates the leg while palpating the greater trochanter. The examiner positions the greater trochanter so that it protrudes most laterally, thereby placing the femoral head into the center portion of the acetabulum. Femoral anteversion/retroversion is assessed by noting the angle between the axis of the tibia and an imaginary vertical line. Normally, femoral anteversion is between 10 and 20 degrees.[39] This test will help to identify cases of retroversion. If a significant difference between internal rotation in extended and seated flexed positions is noted, an osseous versus ligamentous origin should be differentiated. The rectus contracture test (also known as *Ely's test*) is performed with the patient in the prone position and the lower extremity flexed toward the gluteus maximus. Any elevation of the pelvis or restriction of hip flexion motion is indicative of a rectus femoris contracture.

Table 30-5. Prone Examination

Examination	Assessment/Association
Rectus contracture test (Ely's test)	Rectus femoris contracture
Femoral anteversion test (Craig's test)	Detect increased femoral anteversion or retroversion, ligamentous injury, hyperlaxity
Palpation	
1. Supra-SI	Mechanical transverse process ilial conflict
2. SI	Sacroiliitis
3. Glut max insertion	Gluteus maximus tendinitis
4. Spine	Detect spinal mechanical pathology
5. With lumbar hyperextension	Rule out spine as a prominent or secondary issue

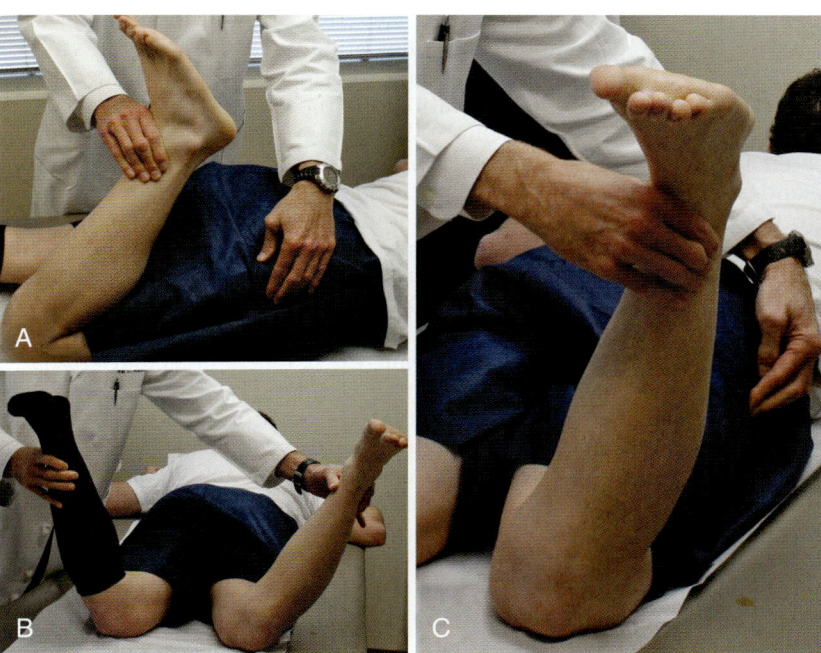

Figure 30-12. Femoral anteversion test, prone external rotation, and the rectus contracture test. **A,** The rectus contracture test. The lower extremity is flexed toward the gluteus maximus. Any raise of the pelvis or restriction of hip flexion motion is indicative of rectus femoris contracture. **B,** Internal rotation in the extended position. Note any differences from the seated flexed position. **C,** The femoral anteversion test. The knee is flexed to 90 degrees, and the examiner manually rotates the leg while palpating the greater trochanter. The examiner positions the greater trochanter so that it protrudes most laterally, noting the angle between the axis of the tibia and an imaginary vertical line.

Specific Tests

McCarthy Test. The McCarthy Test maneuver is associated with McCarthy's sign, a reproducible pop or click.[26] The McCarthy test is performed with the contralateral leg held in flexion. The examined hip is brought to 90 degrees of flexion, then is abducted, externally rotated, and extended. The hip is brought to 90 degrees of flexion, then is adducted, internally rotated, and extended. A positive McCarthy's sign is helpful in detecting anterior femoroacetabular impingement or a torn labrum.

Scour. This test is performed in the same manner as DIRI; however, the examiner applies pressure at the knee, thereby increasing pressure at the hip joint. It is helpful in assessing intra-articular congruence.

Foveal Distraction Test. Intra-articular pressure is alleviated by gently pulling the leg away from the body while the patient is in the supine position. Both relief of pain and re-creation of pain will help to delineate extra-articular versus intra-articular pathology.

Bicycle Test. This is performed with the patient in the lateral position. The patient mimics a bicycle pedaling pattern while the examiner monitors the iliotibial band to detect coxa sultans externus.

Fulcrum Test. The examiner's knee is placed under the patient's knee and acts as the fulcrum. The patient then performs a straight-leg test against resistance.

Seated Piriformis Stretch Test. The seated position offers a stable and reproducible platform with the hip at 90 degrees of flexion. The examiner extends the knee and passively moves the flexed hip into adduction with internal rotation while palpating 1 cm lateral to the ischium (middle finger) and proximally at the sciatic notch (index finger). A positive test is the re-creation of posterior pain. Freiberg has described sciatic nerve entrapment by the piriformis[40]; however, the nerve may be entrapped in other areas, and this is best described as deep gluteal syndrome.[41] Palpation of the involved anatomy, along with a physical examination that includes the straight-leg raise test, the seated piriformis stretch test, and the pace test, will aid in the differential diagnosis of deep gluteal syndrome.

Abduction/Extension/External Rotation Test. The abduction/extension/external rotation (ABDEER) test is performed in the lateral position. The affected leg is passively brought into abduction, extension, and external rotation as forward pressure is applied to the posterior aspect of the hip. Re-creation of the patient's complaint pain is a positive test. As with the apprehension test performed on the shoulder, ABDEER is helpful in the detection of any type of anterior capsular laxity, instability, or injury. Of note, current research suggests that this position specifically releases the teres ligament.

Resisted Sit-up Test. The athletic hernia (sports hernia), or athletic pubalgia, results in chronic pain in the groin that may refer to other surrounding areas and is exacerbated by activity.[42] Diagnosis of the athletic hernia may be difficult because the pain may mimic pain associated with hip labral tears or other hip pathologies. Common physical examination findings include inguinal canal tenderness, pubic crest/tubercle tenderness, adductor origin tenderness, pain with resisted sit-ups or hip flexion, and a tender, dilated superficial ring.[42]

Pudendal Nerve Block Test. Four clinical features must be present for a diagnosis of pudendal nerve entrapment according to Nantes criteria.[43] The Nantes criteria include pain in the urogenital area, pain increased with sitting, pain that does not wake the patient at night, and loss of sensation of the genitalia.[43] If these essential criteria are met, a diagnostic anesthetic pudendal nerve block should be performed, and relief of symptoms strongly supports these elements of clinical possibilities. This test is best performed by a radiologist with experience in this complex area of anatomy.

CURRENT CONTROVERSIES AND FUTURE DIRECTIONS

One pitfall within the literature reporting clinical findings of various hip pathologies is the lack of a standardized functional outcome score. For example, the HHS is useful within the general population; however, the high-performing athletic population may best be evaluated by the Athletic Hip Score.[2] Internationally, the Merle d'Aubigné[21] (MDA) is often used. Currently, the MAHORN (Multicenter Arthroscopy of the Hip Outcomes Research Network) Group is producing the International Hip Outcome Score (IHOT) which will provide an internationally accepted score and will be useful for the athletic population. However, there is still a need for consensus regarding optimal hip outcome measures for distinct patient populations. Clohisy and associates described the clinical presentation of patients with anterior hip impingement and provided functional measures such as the HHS for hip function, the SF-12 for overall health, and the Baecke and UCLA scores for activity.[44] Also in this report was a comprehensive clinical history characterizing pain according to onset (acute/traumatic/insidious), location, severity, and duration, along with aggravating and alleviating factors.[44] Future studies require such detailed information for continued progress in the evaluation of hip pathologies.

The MAHORN (Multicenter Arthroscopy of the Hip Outcomes Research Network) Group identified common trends among hip specialists in physical examination of the hip.[45] In the standing position, common tests included gait analysis, single-leg stance phase test, and laxity. In the supine position, common tests included range of motion (ROM) of hip flexion, internal and external hip ROM, DIRI, DEXRIT, FADDIR, palpation, FABER, straight-leg raise against resistance, muscular strength, passive supine rotation, and the posterior rim impingement test. Common lateral position tests included palpation, passive adduction tests, and abductor strength. In the prone position, the femoral anteversion test was commonly performed. The sensitivity and specificity of this battery of tests need further study. High accuracy and sensitivity to the presence of a labral lesion have been reported for FADDIR, loss of internal rotation, and posterior rim impingement tests.[44,46-49] However, some physical examination tests of the hip have been reported

Table 30-6. Physical Examination Findings and Related Pathology

	History	Dominant Positive Physical Exam Findings	Radiographic
Labral tear	Groin pain C Sign Clicking/Popping Pain with llexion and rotatory motions	Loss of IR FADDJR (ant. tear) 01 RI (ant. tear) LRI (sup. tear) FABER (sup. tear) PRI (post. tear) DEXRIT	CAM Pincer Alpha angle >50° abnormal rotatory alignment Contreccup
FAI CAM			
Atraumatic	Pain exacerbated with deep flexion ,ll1d rotation	Loss of IR FADDIR DIRI DEXRIT	Reduced Head-Neck offset Prominence Alpha > 50° Asymmetry
Traumatic	Repetitive flexion with internal rotation		Herniation Pit MRI or CT–rotatory impingcment
FAI pincer			
Anterior	Anterior based pain	Loss of IR FADDIR DJRI DEXRIT	Acetabular Retroversion
Lateral	Lateral based pain	LRI Decreased ER FABER DEXRIT	Overhanging lip on acetabulum AI > 50°
Posterior	Posterior based pain	Decreased ER PRI FABER (coup-contracoup)	Coxa Profunda Posterior Rim outside center axis
Hip instability			
Osseous	Difficulty-down stairs/hill "Giving Way" Chronic pain after excessive activity	In-Toeing Gait + Femoral Anteversion Test ABDEER	Upsloped Acetabular Roof AI >10° Cephalad Coxa Valga >143° Femoral Version >20°
Ligamentous	Laxity Recurvatum of other joints	Recurvatum/Laxity ABDEER PSR FABER w/apprehension PRI w/apprehension Hyperinstability	
Musculotendonous	Musuclar complaints Tendonpathies	+Contracture Tests Passive Adduction test Weak Abductor strength Weak Core strength	
Chondral lesion			
Acute	Traumatic Event	Decreased IR/ER	Decreased Joint Space Width (Standing AP)
Chronic	Hip pain with long standing pathology or OA	FADDIR D1RI LRI FABER PRI DEXRIT Scour (acute lesion)	
GT pain	Lateral based pain Difficulty sleeping on side	Restricted ROM Pain with palpation specific to anatomical location + Passive Adduction Tests Abductor Weakness	
Snapping hip			
Psoas	"Snap/Pop" Weak Core Strength	+ Fan test Restricted Abd/Add Abductor Weakness	
Iliotibial Band	"Clunk"	+ Bicycle test Restricted Abd/Add Abductor Weakness	

ABDEER indicates abduction extension external rotation; AI, acetabular inclination; AP, anteroposterior; CAM, cam-type; DEXRIT, Dynamic External Rotatory Impingement Test; DIRI, Dynamic Internal Rotatory Impingement Test; ER, External Rotation; FABER, flexion Abduction External Rotation; FADDIR, Flexion Adduction Internal Rotation; FAI, femoroacetabular impingement; GT, greater trochanter; IR, Internal Rotation; LRI, Lateral Rim Impingement; OA, osteoarthritis; PRI, Posterior Rim Impingement; PSR, passive supine rotation; ROM, range of motion.
From Martin HD, Shears SA, Palmer IJ: Evaluation of the hip. *Sports Med Arthrosc Rev* 18(2):63–75, 2010.

to have only a fair level of agreement[50] and lack specificity, which should improve with standardization.[51]

The diagnostic value of clinical tests of the hip joint must be evaluated, as has been done for tests in other joints such as the knee[52-54] and the shoulder.[55] A standardized physical examination will facilitate and improve multicenter studies, thus increasing sensitivity and specificity, as well as interobserver and intraobserver reliability. Current best evidence for the diagnostic value of the physical examination test is embedded within the literature specific to particular hip pathologies such as labral tears, femoroacetabular impingement, ligamentous injury, or patient populations.

Labral tears and cam impingement have been diagnosed clinically by FADDIR,[38] DEXRIT (McCarthy's test),[55,56] passive supine rotation (log roll),[26] loss of internal rotation,[44,46-57] passive abduction tests (Ober's test),[6,7,12,55-58] and the single-leg stance phase test (Trendelenburg).[44] Restricted internal rotation is a classic physical examination finding related to femoroacetabular impingement (FAI).[29-32] It has been accepted that ROM assessment, especially with pain, is an important physical test associated with labral tears.[33,34] The clinical presentation of patients with anterior hip impingement was reported by Clohisy and colleagues, who detailed bilateral hip ROM and used provocative tests of the FABER test, the passive supine rotation test, the straight-leg against resistance test, the FADDIR test, and the posterior rim impingement test.[44]

The biomechanical function of the ligamentum teres is not well understood. However, reports of ligamentum teres (LT) tears are on the rise.[2,59-65] In an in-house study of 19 patients with arthroscopically confirmed complete LT tears, more than 70% of patients exhibited gait abnormalities, positive FADDIR, and positive DEXRIT. FAI was present in all cases, and the patient population was highly active, with individuals involved in professional athletics, sports instruction, or military/police duties. Byrd and Jones reported on 23 patients with LT tears, all of whom had pain with maximal flexion with internal rotation; 15 patients had pain with log roll, and 6 patients averaged loss of 24 degrees of range of motion.[59] Hyperabduction case reports by Kusma and associates[62] and Delcamp and colleagues[60] described pain with abduction and internal rotation.

Philippon and coworkers[2] reviewed 45 professional athletes with FAI, of whom 49% had cam FAI, 7% had pincer FAI, and 47% had cam and pincer FAI. Partial ligamentum teres tears were identified in 58% of these patients, and 7% had complete ligamentum teres tears. Physical examination criteria included a positive FADDIR or a positive FABER.

Current advancements in the understanding of posterior hip pathology have helped develop the recognition of posterior hip pain etiology. Posterior hip pain can be confused with the lumbar spine and pelvic (genitourinary and abdominal) pathology emphasizing the importance of a comprehensive history and physical examination. The complexity of this region requires a thorough understanding of the anatomy, biomechanics and pathokinematics. There are four sources of posterior extra-articular hip pain for which the surgeon

should be aware: deep gluteal syndrome, hamstring pathology, pudendal nerve, and ischiofemoral impingement.

Biases regarding physical examination findings may still be found in single-center studies; however, use of a consistent protocol and a detailed report will expand our knowledge of physical examination of the hip. Table 30-6 is a list of common physical examination findings and related pathology.

SUMMARY/CONCLUSIONS

This chapter has (1) reviewed pertinent information required for a detailed patient history, (2) described how to perform clinical examination of the hip and explained why these tests are important, and (3) discussed current controversies and future considerations related to physical examination of the hip. As our understanding of hip pathology advances, physical examination of the hip continues to evolve. The physical examination of the hip is an assessment of the four layers of the hip, the osseous, capsulolabral, musculotendinous, neurovascular, and their interrelationships. To fully understand the findings of the physical examination, one must be familiar with the anatomy and biomechanics of the hip joint. Use of a formalized, reproducible physical examination will help the clinician to identify and distinguish osseous, musculotendinous, and ligamentous abnormalities and their comorbidities in a timely fashion.

Acknowledgments

I would like to thank Shea A. Shears, R.N., B.S.N.; Ian J. Palmer, Ph.D., and all members of the MAHORN (Multicenter Arthroscopy of the Hip Outcomes Research Network) Group, who were very instrumental in the development of this chapter.

REFERENCES

1. Scopp JM, Moorman CT 3rd: The assessment of athletic hip injury. Clin Sports Med 20:647–659, 2001.
2. Philippon M, Schenker M, Briggs K, Kuppersmith D: Femoroacetabular impingement in 45 professional athletes: associated pathologies and return to sport following arthroscopic decompression. Knee Surg Sports Traumatol Arthrosc 15:908–914, 2007.
3. DeAngelis NA, Busconi BD: Assessment and differential diagnosis of the painful hip. Clin Orthop Relat Res 406:11–18, 2003.
4. Kujala UM, Kaprio J, Sarna S: Osteoarthritis of weight bearing joints of lower limbs in former elite male athletes. BMJ 308:231–234, 1994.
5. Boyd KT, Peirce NS, Batt ME: Common hip injuries in sport. Sports Med 24:273–288, 1997.
6. Braly BA, Beall DP, Martin HD: Clinical examination of the athletic hip. Clin Sports Med 25:199–210, vii, 2006.
7. Martin HD: Clinical examination of the hip. Oper Tech Orthop 15:177–181, 2005.
8. Clohisy JC, Nunley RM, Otto RJ, Schoenecker PL: The frog-leg lateral radiograph accurately visualized hip cam impingement abnormalities. Clin Orthop Relat Res 462:115–121, 2007.
9. Eijer H, Leunig M, Mahomed M, Ganz R: Cross-table lateral radiograph for screening of anterior femoral head-neck offset

in patients with femoroacetabular impingement. Hip Int 11:37–41, 2001.

10. Clohisy JC, Carlisle JC, Beaule PE, et al: A systematic approach to the plain radiographic evaluation of the young adult hip. J Bone Joint Surg Am 90(Suppl 4):47–66, 2008.

11. Murphy SB, Ganz R, Muller ME: The prognosis in untreated dysplasia of the hip: a study of radiographic factors that predict the outcome. J Bone Joint Surg Am 77:985–989, 1995.

12. Notzli HP, Wyss TF, Stoecklin CH, et al: The contour of the femoral head-neck junction as a predictor for the risk of anterior impingement. J Bone Joint Surg Br 84:556–560, 2002.

13. Tannast M, Siebenrock KA, Anderson SE: Femoroacetabular impingement: radiographic diagnosis—what the radiologist should know. AJR Am J Roentgenol 188:1540–1552, 2007.

14. Beall DP, Martin HD, Mintz DN, et al: Anatomic and structural evaluation of the hip: a cross-sectional imaging technique combining anatomic and biomechanical evaluations. Clin Imaging 32:372–381, 2008.

15. Tonnis D, Heinecke A: Acetabular and femoral anteversion: relationship with osteoarthritis of the hip. J Bone Joint Surg Am 81:1747–1770, 1999.

16. Petersilge CA: From the RSNA refresher courses, Radiological Society of North America. Chronic adult hip pain: MR arthrography of the hip. Radiographics 20(Spec No):S43–S52, 2000.

17. Millis MB, Murphy SB: Use of computed tomographic reconstruction in planning osteotomies of the hip. Clin Orthop Relat Res 274:154–159, 1992.

18. Keeney JA, Peelle MW, Jackson J, et al: Magnetic resonance arthrography versus arthroscopy in the evaluation of articular hip pathology. Clin Orthop Relat Res 429:163–169, 2004.

19. Kim YJ, Jaramillo D, Millis MB, et al: Assessment of early osteoarthritis in hip dysplasia with delayed gadolinium-enhanced magnetic resonance imaging of cartilage. J Bone Joint Surg Am 85:1987–1992, 2003.

20. Byrd JW, Jones KS: Prospective analysis of hip arthroscopy. Arthroscopy 16:578–587, 2000.

21. D'Aubigné RM, Postel M: Functional results of hip arthroplasty with acrylic prosthesis. J Bone Joint Surg Am 36:451, 1954.

22. Christensen CP, Althausen PL, Mittleman MA, et al: The nonarthritic hip score: reliable and validated. Clin Orthop Relat Res 406:75–83, 2003.

23. Martin DP, Engelberg R, Agel J, Swiontkowski MF: Comparison of the Musculoskeletal Function Assessment questionnaire with the Short Form-36, the Western Ontario and McMaster Universities Osteoarthritis Index, and the Sickness Impact Profile health-status measures. J Bone Joint Surg Am 79:1323–1335, 1997.

24. Ware J Jr, Kosinski M, Keller SD: A 12-item short-form health survey: construction of scales and preliminary tests of reliability and validity. Med Care 34:220–233, 1996.

25. Bellamy N, Buchanan WW, Goldsmith CH, et al: Validation study of WOMAC: a health status instrument for measuring clinically important patient relevant outcomes to antirheumatic drug therapy in patients with osteoarthritis of the hip or knee. J Rheumatol 15:1833–1840, 1988.

26. Byrd JW: Physical examination. In Byrd JW (ed): Operative hip arthroscopy, New York, 2005, Springer, pp 36–50.

27. Torry MR, Schenker ML, Martin HD, et al: Neuromuscular hip biomechanics and pathology in the athlete. Clin Sports Med 25:179–197, vii, 2006.

28. Perry J: Gait analysis: normal and pathological function, Thorofare, NJ, 1992, Slack Inc.

29. Fitzgerald RH Jr: Acetabular labrum tears: diagnosis and treatment. Clin Orthop Relat Res 311:60–68, 1995.

30. Ito K, Minka MA 2nd, Leunig M, et al: Femoroacetabular impingement and the cam-effect: an MRI-based quantitative anatomical study of the femoral head-neck offset. J Bone Joint Surg Br 83:171–176, 2001.

31. Lavigne M, Parvizi J, Beck M, et al: Anterior femoroacetabular impingement: part I. Techniques of joint preserving surgery. Clin Orthop Relat Res 418:61–66, 2004.

32. Troum OM, Crues JV 3rd: The young adult with hip pain: diagnosis and medical treatment, circa 2004. Clin Orthop Relat Res 418:9–17, 2004.

33. Farjo LA, Glick JM, Sampson TG: Hip arthroscopy for acetabular labral tears. Arthroscopy 15:132–137, 1999.

34. Santori N, Villar RN: Acetabular labral tears: result of arthroscopic partial limbectomy. Arthroscopy 16:11–15, 2000.

35. McKibbin B: Anatomical factors in the stability of the hip joint in the newborn. J Bone Joint Surg Br 52:148–159, 1970.

36. Martin HD, Savage A, Braly BA, et al: The function of the hip capsular ligaments: a quantitative report. Arthroscopy 24:188–195, 2008.

37. Pace JB, Nagle D: Piriform syndrome. Western J Med 124:435–439, 1976.

38. Klaue K, Durnin CW, Ganz R: The acetabular rim syndrome: a clinical presentation of dysplasia of the hip. J Bone Joint Surg Br 73:423–429, 1991.

39. Reider B, Martel J: Pelvis, hip and thigh. In Reider B, Martel J (eds): The orthopedic physical examination, Philadelphia, 1999, WB Saunders, pp 159–199.

40. Freiberg A: Sciatic pain and its relief by operations on muscle and fascia. Arch Surg 34:337–350, 1937.

41. McCrory P, Bell S: Nerve entrapment syndromes as a cause of pain in the hip, groin and buttock. Sports Med 27:261–274, 1999.

42. Swan KG Jr, Wolcott M: The athletic hernia: a systematic review. Clin Orthop Relat Res 455:78–87, 2007.

43. Labat JJ, Riant T, Robert R, et al: Diagnostic criteria for pudendal neuralgia by pudendal nerve entrapment (Nantes criteria). Neurourol Urodyn 27:306–310, 2008.

44. Clohisy JC, Knaus ER, Hunt DM, et al: Clinical presentation of patients with symptomatic anterior hip impingement. Clin Orthop Relat Res 467:638–644, 2009.

45. Martin HD, Kelly BT, Leunig M, et al: The pattern and technique in the clinical evaluation of the adult hip: the common physical examination tests of hip specialists. Arthroscopy 26:161–172, 2010.

46. Beaule PE, Zaragoza E, Motamedi K, et al: Three-dimensional computed tomography of the hip in the assessment of femoroacetabular impingement. J Orthop Res 23:1286–1292, 2005.

47. Ito K, Leunig M, Ganz R: Histopathologic features of the acetabular labrum in femoroacetabular impingement. Clin Orthop Relat Res 429:262–271, 2004.

48. Leunig M, Werlen S, Ungersbock A, et al: Evaluation of the acetabular labrum by MR arthrography. J Bone Joint Surg 79:230–234, 1997.

49. Martin RL, Sekiya JK: The interrater reliability of 4 clinical tests used to assess individuals with musculoskeletal hip pain. J Orthop Sports Phys Ther 38:71–77, 2008.

50. Martin RL, Irrgang JJ, Sekiya JK: The diagnostic accuracy of a clinical examination in determining intra-articular hip pain for potential hip arthroscopy candidates. Arthroscopy 24:1013–1018, 2008.

51. Malanga GA, Andrus S, Nadler SF, McLean J: Physical examination of the knee: a review of the original test description and scientific validity of common orthopedic tests. Arch Phys Med Rehabil 84:592–603, 2003.

52. Noyes FR, Cummings JF, Grood ES, et al: The diagnosis of knee motion limits, subluxations, and ligament injury. Am J Sports Med 19:163–171, 1991.

53. Noyes FR, Grood ES, Cummings JF, Wroble RR: An analysis of the pivot shift phenomenon: the knee motions and subluxations induced by different examiners. Am J Sports Med 19:148–155, 1991.

54. King GJ, Richards RR, Zuckerman JD, et al: A standardized method for assessment of elbow function. Research Committee, American Shoulder and Elbow Surgeons. J Shoulder Elbow Surg 8:351–354, 1999.

55. Busconi BD, Owens BD: Differential diagnosis of the painful hip. In McCarthy JC (ed): Early hip disorders, New York, 2003, Springer-Verlag, pp 7–16.

56. McCarthy JC, Busconi BD, Owens BD: Assessment of the painful hip. In McCarthy JC (ed): Early hip disorders, New York, 2003, Springer, pp 3–6.

57. Murphy S, Tannast M, Kim YJ, et al: Débridement of the adult hip for femoroacetabular impingement: indications and preliminary clinical results. Clin Orthop Relat Res 429:178–181, 2004.

58. McCarthy JC, Noble PC, Schuck MR, et al: The Otto E. Aufranc Award. The role of labral lesions to development of early degenerative hip disease. Clin Orthop Relat Res 393:25–37, 2001.

59. Byrd JW, Jones KS: Traumatic rupture of the ligamentum teres as a source of hip pain. Arthroscopy 20:385–391, 2004.

60. Delcamp DD, Klaaren HE, Pompe van Meerdervoort HF: Traumatic avulsion of the ligamentum teres without dislocation of the hip: two case reports. J Bone Joint Surg Am 70:933–935, 1988.

61. Gray AJ, Villar RN: The ligamentum teres of the hip: an arthroscopic classification of its pathology. Arthroscopy 13:575–578, 1997.

62. Kusma M, Jung J, Dienst M, et al: Arthroscopic treatment of an avulsion fracture of the ligamentum teres of the hip in an 18-year-old horse rider. Arthroscopy 20(Suppl 2):64–66, 2004.

63. Michaels G, Matles AL: The role of the ligamentum teres in congenital dislocation of the hip. Clin Orthop Relat Res 71:199–201, 1970.

64. Rao J, Zhou YX, Villar RN: Injury to the ligamentum teres: mechanism, findings, and results of treatment. Clin Sports Med 20:791–799, vii, 2001.

65. Yamamoto Y, Usui I: Arthroscopic surgery for degenerative rupture of the ligamentum teres femoris. Arthroscopy 22:e1–e3, 2006.

CHAPTER 31

Imaging of the Hip

Kawan S. Rakhra and Adnan M. Sheikh

KEY POINTS

- A broad spectrum of radiologic investigations can be used to provide the orthopedic surgeon with important information regarding hip anatomy and pathology, hence facilitating diagnosis, monitoring, and treatment planning for hip disease.
- Radiography is the first line of imaging in investigating the hip; various techniques and projections are used to optimize visualization of select structures and regions of the hip joint.
- Femoroacetabular impingement (FAI) results from anatomic abnormalities of the acetabulum (pincer) and/or the femoral head-neck junction (cam). Radiography and magnetic resonance imaging (MRI) can effectively demonstrate the primary anatomic deformities, as well as the secondary joint derangements that ensue with FAI.
- Developmental dysplasia of the hip (DDH) is characterized by an underdeveloped acetabular fossa, which predisposes to hip instability and osteoarthritis (OA). Radiography is the primary modality for characterizing and quantifying the degree of dysplasia and in evaluating for OA.
- MRI is a robust imaging modality for detecting and characterizing a broad spectrum of hip pathologies, including ischemic, traumatic, inflammatory, arthritic, and neoplastic causes.

INTRODUCTION

Radiologic investigation of the hip has rapidly evolved through advances in technology and in knowledge about the causes and physiology of hip disease. In situations where the clinical history and physical examination findings are equivocal, orthopedic diagnosis and management of hip disorders often require adjuvant radiologic evidence of disease before treatment and intervention are begun. Today, several imaging modalities are available to physicians; each modality has a multitude of variations and protocols that can be optimized according to the patient profile, the clinical scenario, and the nature of the hip pathology. It is important for the orthopedic surgeon, radiologist, rheumatologist, and physiatrist, and all other allied musculoskeletal specialists, to understand the basic principles of hip imaging. Knowledge of the strengths and limitations of the various available radiologic modalities can facilitate and expedite efficient diagnosis and management of hip pathology.

IMAGING MODALITIES

The various imaging modalities are compared in Table 31-1.

Conventional Radiography

Radiography is the first line of imaging for investigation of all hip pathologies, as it can demonstrate gross osseous alignment, morphology, and integrity. Advantages of plain radiography include ease of access, rapid acquisition, lack of any post processing, and flexibility in patient positioning. However, the shape, contour, and spatial relationships of bones may not be demonstrated by radiography to the same degree as by cross-sectional modalities such as computed tomography (CT) and magnetic resonance imaging (MRI).[1-3] Radiography is also limited by its inability to demonstrate internal joint structures, including cartilage, labrum, capsule, and surrounding periarticular soft tissues.[4-6]

Many radiographic projections can be used in investigation of the hip; these are variably selected depending on the nature of the pathology and on the anatomic regions of concern. Standard imaging protocols have been established to ensure consistent positioning and optimal visualization of regions of interest.[7-9]

Anteroposterior (PA) Pelvis
(Fig. 31-1)
Positioning: Patient supine (standing for dysplasia); feet internal rotation 15 degrees
X-ray technique: x-ray beam perpendicular to table, centered at the midpoint between the superior margin of the symphysis pubis and at the midpoint between the anterior superior iliac spines (ASISs)
Structures of interest: bilateral hips, sacrum, innominate bones, proximal femurs, anterior column, posterior column, anterior and posterior acetabular rims, medial acetabular wall, acetabular version, dysplasia
Indications: all pathologies, including trauma, congenital dysmorphisms, and arthritis

Table 31-1. Comparison of Modalities

	Conventional Radiography	Computed Tomography	Magnetic Resonance Imaging	Ultrasound	Nuclear Medicine
Flexibility in position	H	I	L	H	L
Patient tolerance (claustrophobia)	H	H	I	H	I
Radiation	L	H	None	None	I
Spatial resolution	H	H	I	H	L
Contrast resolution	L	I	H	L	L
Evaluation of bone, mineralized structures	H	H	I	L	H
Evaluation of soft tissues	L	I	H	I	L
Accessibility	H	H	I	H	I
Relative cost	L	I	H	I	H
Acquisition time	L	I	H	I	H

H, High; *I*, intermediate; *L*, low.

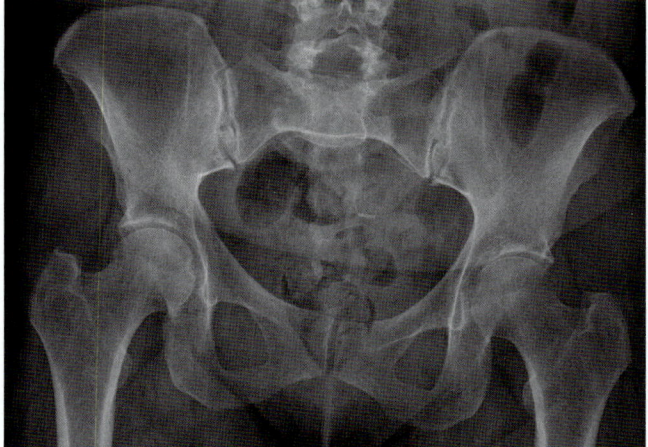

Figure 31-1. Anteroposterior (AP) view of the pelvis. The femurs are held in 15 degrees of internal rotation, and the x-ray beam is centered at the midpoint between the superior margin of the symphysis pubis and at the midpoint between the anterior superior iliac spines (ASISs).

Judet (Oblique) Views

Positioning: anterior oblique 45 degrees/posterior oblique 45 degrees

X-ray technique: x-ray beam directed perpendicular to the table centered at the hip joint

Structures of interest: anterior (iliopubic) column and posterior acetabular rim/posterior (ilioischial) column, anterior acetabular rim, quadrilateral plate

Indications: trauma, fracture

Frog-Leg Lateral

Positioning: patient supine, knee flexed 30 degrees, thigh abducted 45 degrees

X-ray technique: x-ray beam directed perpendicular to the table centered at the midpoint between the

ipsilateral ASIS and the superior margin of the symphysis pubis

Structures of interest: proximal femur (head, neck, shaft)

Indications: trauma, fracture

Cross-Table Lateral

Positioning: patient supine; femur of hip of interest internally rotated 15 degrees, contralateral hip and knee flexed beyond 80 degrees

X-ray technique: x-ray beam directed parallel to table, oriented 45 degrees cephalad from inferomedial to superolateral, centered at the femoral head

Structures of interest: femoral neck and head in lateral projection

Indications: trauma, fracture, when patient unable to position for frog-leg lateral

Dunn View

(Fig. 31-2)

Positioning: patient supine; symptomatic hip flexed 45 or 90 degrees, abducted 20 degrees, neutral rotation

X-ray technique: x-ray beam in AP direction, centered at midpoint between ASIS and superior margin of symphysis pubis

Structures of interest: femoral head, neck; optimally evaluates head-neck junction for cam femoroacetabular impingement (FAI) deformity; anterosuperior hip joint space

Indications: FAI (cam)

False Profile View

(Fig. 31-3)

Positioning: patient standing; pelvis rotated 65 degrees with hip of interest against cassette and ipsilateral foot parallel to cassette

X-ray technique: x-ray beam perpendicular to cassette, centered at femoral head

Structures of interest: acetabular coverage of femoral head anteriorly, posterior joint space

Indications: FAI (pincer)

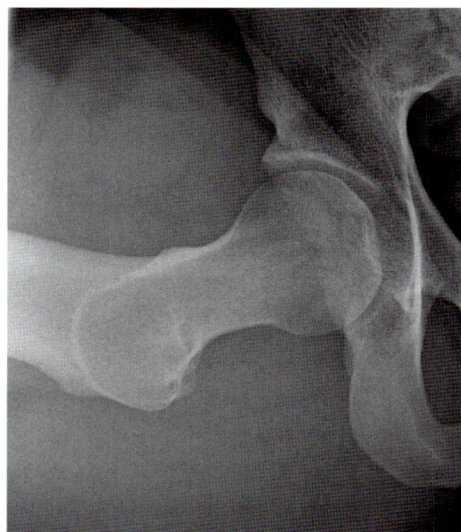

Figure 31-2. Dunn projection, 45 degrees. The hip is held in 45 degrees of flexion and 20 degrees of abduction with the x-ray beam centered and the midpoint between the anterior superior iliac spine (ASIS) and the symphysis pubis.

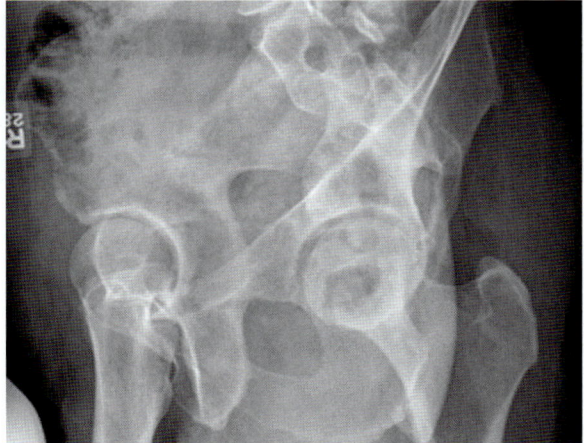

Figure 31-3. False profile view of the right hip. The patient is standing with the body rotated 65 degrees, with the right side rotated posteriorly toward the cassette. The x-ray beam is centered at the femoral head.

Computed Tomography

Computed tomography (CT) is a modality that allows accurate depiction of hip joint anatomy and many pathologies. It can provide very high spatial resolution images, revealing detailed information on osseous morphology, alignment, and integrity. CT acquires images in the axial plane, although images in the coronal, sagittal, and other oblique planes can be secondarily constructed by software reformation. Three-dimensional (3D) volume surface shaded images, models, and rotational series can be generated using advanced computer software algorithms. These postprocessing algorithms and filters can be applied to selectively optimize evaluation of the bones or soft tissues. Various structures, including bone, soft tissue, and even hardware, can be subtracted or emphasized with postprocessing techniques. The acquisition time of a CT scan is very short; thus motion artifacts are not significant.

Indications for CT evaluation of the hip include acute trauma (fracture, dislocation, intra-articular bodies, preoperative planning), treatment follow-up (healing assessment, joint congruity, hardware fixation devices), characterization of mineralized components of bone and soft tissue tumors and neoplasms, and characterization of congenital/developmental abnormalities.

In certain situations and pathologies, CT can be used to diagnose and characterize hematomas, fluid collections, and gross changes of inflammation and infection. However, it should be noted that compared with MRI, CT has relatively lower contrast resolution, which can limit evaluation of nonosseous and nonmineralized articular and periarticular structures and soft tissues of the hip. A potential concern with CT is the radiation dose that patients receive, especially to the gonads. Therefore, CT parameters should be optimized to minimize the radiation dose to the patient, with consideration of the degree of detail required given the clinical situation.

CT may be combined with intra-articular injection of iodinated contrast agents (CT arthrography) to assess labral and chondral integrity and to detect intra-articular bodies,[6,10,11] although this is done only when MRI is contraindicated.

Magnetic Resonance Imaging

MRI offers exquisite contrast resolution, allowing optimal characterization of nonosseous and nonmineralized articular and periarticular structures, including labrum, cartilage, joint space, capsule, marrow space, and regional soft tissues.[3,12,13] It can assess compact and cancellous bone as well, although sometimes not as accurately as CT.

MRI has multiplanar image acquisition capability. Images in standard axial, sagittal, coronal, or any oblique planes can be directly acquired or secondarily constructed with the use of postprocessing reformation software. Recent technological advances in MRI field strength and sequence protocols allow the preparation of 3D sequences with fairly high resolution. It is important to note that MRI does not involve ionizing radiation.

Indications for MRI of the hip are broad because of its ability to evaluate both osseous and regional soft tissue structures. Indications include trauma (detection of radiograph and CT occult fractures and stress or insufficiency fractures), avascular necrosis (AVN), bone marrow edema syndromes (transient osteoporosis, migratory osteoporosis), oncology (detection and characterization of lesions), arthritis (detailed cartilage assessment), internal joint derangement (labral evaluation), osseous deformity (femoroacetabular impingement, hip dysplasia), infection (joint, bone, surrounding soft tissues), myotendinous injury, and soft tissue inflammation (bursitis).

The combination of MRI with intra-articular injection of gadolinium-based contrast agents—direct magnetic resonance arthrography (MRA)—is often used to facilitate evaluation of small structures in the hip joint, including labrum, hyaline cartilage, and intra-articular bodies. The distention effect of the arthrogram may cause separation of capsular, labral, and osteochondral structures, resulting in increased spatial resolution. Injected contrast solution outlines both normal anatomic structures and abnormal pathologies, further improving contrast resolution and increasing the conspicuity of intra-articular pathology (Fig. 31-4A–C).[14,15]

Indirect MRA involves intravenous injection of gadolinium contrast, followed by a variable delay and/or physical activity regimen. Gadolinium contrast will distribute within the joint space, diffusely enhancing the synovial fluid.[16] This will provide greater contrast resolution between joint fluid and labrum, cartilage, and capsule. The benefit of indirect MRA is that it is less invasive for the patient and does not require fluoroscopically guided joint injection. However, the distention effect that direct MRA provides is not realized. Enhancement of background extra-articular soft tissues and vascular structures, both normal and pathologic,

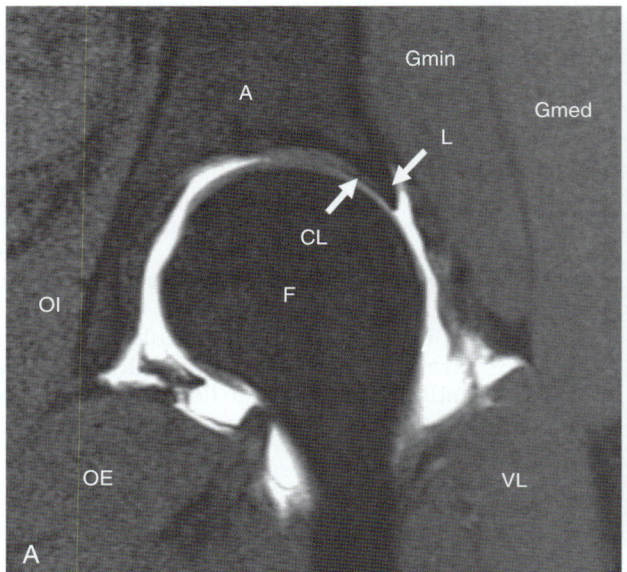
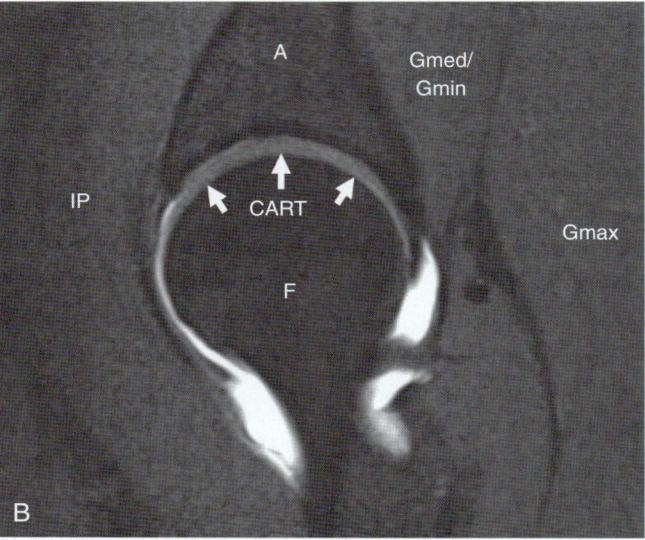
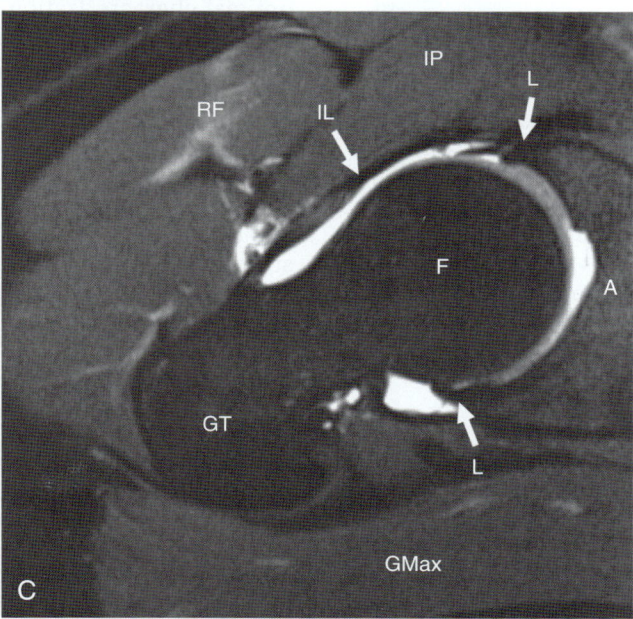

Figure 31-4. A through **C,** Direct magnetic resonance arthrography (MRA) T1-weighted images with fat suppression in the **(A)** oblique coronal, **(B)** oblique sagittal, and **(C)** oblique axial planes, with key anatomic structures labeled. *A,* Acetabulum; *CART,* hyaline cartilage; *CL,* chondrolabral junction; *F,* femoral head; *Gmax,* gluteus maximus; *Gmed,* gluteus medius; *Gmin,* gluteus minimus; *IL,* iliofemoral ligament/anterior capsule; *IP,* iliopsoas; *L,* labrum; *OE,* obturator externus; *OI,* obturator internus; *RF,* rectus femoris; *VL,* vastus lateralis.

will also be noted. This may make articular pathology less conspicuous.

MRI pulse sequence selection depends on the technique used; multiple, variable combinations of sequence classes can provide equally diagnostic studies. Spin echo, fast spin echo, and gradient recalled echo sequences can be used in the MRI investigation of hip pathology. Three-dimensional volume and isotropic voxel acquisitions with multiplanar reformations have become feasible in terms of time and imaging quality and can be applied to MRI and MRA of the hip.[3] Multiplanar imaging with at least one sequence or reformation in each plane should be standard.

For nonarthrographic MRI, the protocol should include T1-weighted (T1W) imaging without fat suppression to demonstrate anatomy, joint alignment, marrow abnormality, or fracture. A fluid-sensitive sequence (T2W or proton density[PD]W) with fat suppression, or short tau inversion recovery (STIR), should always be part of any protocol to detect abnormal edema within marrow and soft tissues, as well as periarticular fluid collections or cysts.[17] In addition, fluid-sensitive sequences increase the contrast between joint fluid and adjacent labrum, cartilage, bone, and capsule. With nonarthrographic MRI studies, higher resolution and an increased number of sampling averages[13,18] are used; this may offset the lower contrast and spatial resolution of MRI compared with MRA.

With direct MRA, the most commonly used sequence is T1W, with or without fat suppression, in addition to fluid-sensitive sequences.[16] With indirect MRA, the same sequence selection as for direct MRA is adequate, although with a few caveats. Fat suppression is strongly advised for maximal contrast resolution because the concentration of gadolinium within the joint may not be as high as with direct injection. As well, multiphasic imaging may be considered to understand the vascular physiology of the joint.[16]

Drawbacks of MRI include relatively longer acquisition times, susceptibility to motion artifacts, magnetic susceptibility artifacts due to regional metal prostheses, and/or postsurgical artifacts, along with several other absolute and relative contraindications (claustrophobia, non–MRI-compatible prostheses, some makes of electronic implanted devices and cardiac pacer equipment, orbital metal bodies).

Ultrasound

Ultrasound (US) is not as widely used as other modalities in radiologic investigation of the adult hip. It is very important in the pediatric hip for evaluation of developmental dysplasia. US is limited to assessment of soft tissues, fluid structures, and nonmineralized structures. It can detect the presence of an effusion, synovitis, and capsular thickening. As well, tendon abnormalities such as tendinosis, tenosynovitis, or tears can be diagnosed. US may also assess regional soft tissues for muscle tears, fluid collections, and bursitis. US is unique in that it allows dynamic, real-time visualization of periarticular structures with patient feedback. No parameters for US of the hip have been defined, although a high-frequency linear transducer should be used for high-resolution imaging of periarticular soft tissues. It is important to note that no ionization radiation is associated with US. However, US may be limited by patient habitus such as obesity, it can be operator dependent, and, unlike other modalities, it does not provide any gross information on regional osseous structures.

Nuclear Medicine

Nuclear medicine studies may be useful in providing insight into the physiologic state of the hip joint. A radioactive compound is injected into the bloodstream; this is followed by a variable imaging regimen. Several protocols and various radiotracers can used in isolation or in combination to generate images that track the flow and accumulation of tracers. Although traditionally two-dimensional (2D) images were acquired, 3D datasets can be obtained with the use of multiple rotational detectors, yielding greater spatial information. Indications for nuclear medicine studies include trauma (detection of occult acute and stress fractures), AVN, infection, and oncologic workup.

FEMOROACETABULAR IMPINGEMENT

Femoroacetabular impingement (FAI) has become a well-recognized pathogenic factor in the evolution of hip osteoarthritis (OA). The impingement is secondary to anatomic abnormalities of the femoral head-neck junction and/or the acetabulum. These dysmorphisms lead to impaired, pathologic interaction of the femur with the acetabulum during motion of the hip joint, resulting in altered biomechanics and premature degeneration of hyaline cartilage, and eventually to OA.[19-23] Given that the impingement results from underlying structural aberrations, radiologic imaging is essential in the investigation of FAI. Imaging provides a visual presentation of the primary deformities, as well as the secondary joint derangements, that can result from FAI in both cam and pincer forms. It is known that most patients with FAI in fact have a variable combination of both forms of impingement. Radiography,[19,24,25] CT,[23] and MRI[13,14,22,26,27] are validated modalities for imaging the hip in the setting of FAI. Characteristic radiographic morphologic features of both the femur and the acetabulum can facilitate, expedite, or confirm the diagnosis of clinically suspected FAI, even before gross osteoarthritic changes evolve.

Primary Anatomic Abnormalities of Femoroacetabular Impingement

Cam Femoroacetabular Impingement

In the cam form of FAI, the main dysmorphism is of the femoral head-neck junction. An excess of bone and/or cartilage bulk at the anterosuperior femoral head-neck junction results in reduced offset of the femoral head over the neck and femoral head asphericity.[19,20,22,28,29] The abnormality can also be described as an osteochondral bump or excrescence, lack of head-neck concavity, diminished offset, or reduced wasting of the head-neck junction.[21]

The cam deformity can be identified on several radiographic projections. The optimal projection is the flexion abduction view (Dunn), which demonstrates the anterosuperior femoral head-neck junction in profile, followed by the cross-table lateral. The AP view may underestimate or even miss a cam deformity.[24] Depending on the size and location of the cam deformity, and on the position of the femur, it may manifest on AP radiograph as an abnormal convexity along the lateral femoral head-neck junction, resembling the hand grip of a pistol.[25]

CT and MRI with their multiplanar capabilities are more sensitive than radiography in the detection of subtle osseous deformities.[1-3] The oblique axial plane, parallel to the long axis of the femoral neck, is the imaging plane most frequently used to evaluate the femoral head-neck junction. This plane optimally images the anterior contour of the femoral head-neck junction. However, several studies have reported that, although present anteriorly, diminished offset is most pronounced anterosuperiorly and potentially at any location within the anterosuperior quadrant.[27,28,30] Thus radial images, obtained using the femoral neck as the axis of rotation, have been recommended as a method for evaluating the femoral head-neck junction over its full circumference, as opposed to just anteriorly, as occurs when the more conventional oblique axial plane method is used.[13,22,23,27,30] Radial images are based on a rotating plane such that each image is orthogonal to the femoral surface and visualizes the head-neck junction in profile. A clock face nomenclature can be applied for localization around the femoral head-neck junction, with superior and anterior locations designated 12 o'clock and 3 o'clock, respectively.

The alpha angle is a parameter used to qualify and quantify the cam deformity.[14,26] Previous studies show that an elevated alpha angle is associated with symptomatic impingement.[14,23,26,27] It can be measured on radiography, CT, or MRI on any plane. The alpha angle is determined by first drawing a best-fit circle around the perimeter of the femoral head. The first arm of the angle is the long axis of the femoral neck, defined as the line drawn between the center of the femoral neck at its narrowest point and the center of the best-fit circle. The second arm of the angle is drawn from the center of the circle anteriorly to the point where the head extends beyond the margin of the circle.[26] Larger cam deformities will yield larger alpha angle values (Fig. 31-5).

Several studies have proposed absolute thresholds (ranging from 50 to 55 degrees) for calling an alpha angle abnormal.[23,26] In symptomatic cam-type FAI patients, the mean alpha angle value found in several studies ranges from 66.4 to 74.0 degrees.[14,23,26,28] There is a range of normal values for the alpha angle. In asymptomatic patients, the alpha angle ranges from 39.3 to

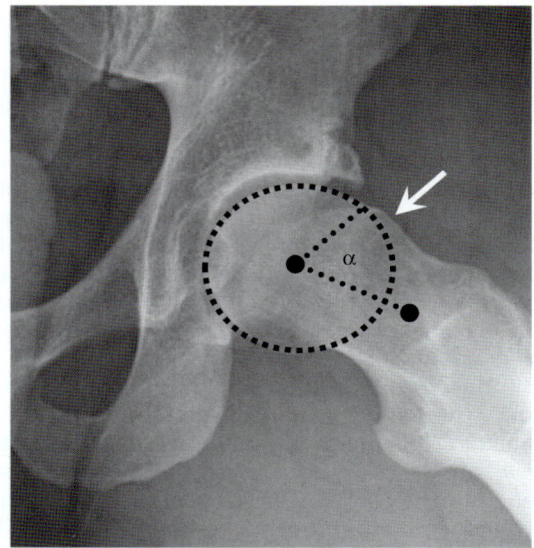

Figure 31-5. Dunn view (45 degrees) demonstrating a cam deformity with an elevated alpha angle of 74 degrees.

48.3 degrees.[23,26,31,32] In the normal hip, the mean alpha angle value in males and females, anteriorly, has been reported to be 44.0 degrees and 38.1 degrees, respectively, while anterosuperiorly, it was 54.1 degrees and 47.0 degrees, respectively.[32] Thus, depending on which location around the femoral head-neck junction is being evaluated, and on the gender of the patient, threshold values for the alpha angle considered to be abnormal may have to be varied.

Anterior offset is another validated parameter for quantifying reduced offset of the femoral head on the neck. It is best measured on a cross-table lateral radiograph or on any radial CT or MRI view. A line is drawn parallel and tangential to the anterior cortex of the femoral neck. A second, parallel line is drawn tangential to the most anterior aspect of the femoral head. The perpendicular distance between these two lines is the anterior offset. In asymptomatic hips, the mean offset is 11.6 mm, and in cam FAI hips, offset is reduced to 7.2 mm. To normalize for patient size, the offset ratio can be calculated; this is the ratio between the anterior offset and the femoral head diameter. The mean offset ratio is 0.21 in asymptomatic hips; in cam FAI hips, it is 0.13.[25,33]

Pincer Femoroacetabular Impingement

In the pincer form of FAI, the primary abnormality is of the acetabulum. The impingement is the result of overcoverage of the femoral head by the acetabulum. This may be related to acetabular retroversion, coxa profunda, or acetabular protrusion.[19,20,22]

Acetabular retroversion causes focal overcoverage of the femoral head, and coxa profunda and acetabular protrusio result in more global overcoverage. All result in relative deepening of the acetabular fossa. These dysmorphisms lead to abnormal abutment of the femoral neck against the overcovering acetabulum, resulting in a linear zone of impingement anterosuperiorly, and shifting of the femoral head posteriorly.[20,21] This latter phenomenon may lead to a predilection for posteroinferior joint space narrowing and OA.

The version of the acetabulum refers the orientation of the opening of the acetabular fossa relative to the sagittal plane. In the normal hip, the opening of the acetabular fossa is directed anteriorly, or is anteverted. With retroversion, the acetabular fossa is oriented posteriorly.[21,34,35] Although this abnormality is best evaluated with the use of cross-sectional modalities such as CT or MRI, radiographs can detect gross morphologic features of the acetabulum that predispose to pincer impingement. On an AP pelvis radiograph, with acetabular retroversion, the superoanterior acetabular rim abnormally sits more lateral than the posterior rim. Crossing of the anterior rim margin laterally over the posterior rim gives a figure-of-eight density, referred to as the *crossover sign*.[25] Retroversion may also manifest as a deficient posterior wall, where, on an AP radiograph, the posterior rim of the acetabulum projects medial to the center of the femoral head[25] (Fig. 31-6).

Acetabular version is best evaluated on axial plane images,[36] whether by MRI or CT. CT, with its better depiction of compact bone, may allow more accurate delineation of the exact margins of osseous landmarks. The entire transverse dimension of the osseous pelvis, with both hips in the field of view, is required to correct for any positional tilt of the pelvis.

The normal acetabulum is anteverted by 20 to 23 degrees,[34,37,38] with 15 to 25 degrees generally considered to be within normal limits. On axial images through the retroverted acetabulum, the anterior acetabular rim sits more lateral than the posterior rim.[34] The orientation of the acetabular version is not fixed at all levels. A natural decrease in the degree of anteversion is noted, progressing from superior to inferior.[34,36,39] It has been suggested that the version of the acetabulum should be evaluated at the level through the mid femoral head, on the image where the diameter of the femoral head is largest,[34,36] or on the image where the head is most congruent with the acetabulum.[39]

Acetabular overcoverage can be global, resulting from increased depth of the acetabular fossa. Normally, the medial acetabular fossa line should be lateral to the ilioischial line. Coxa profunda is present when the fossa acetabuli line lies medial to the ilioischial line (Fig. 31-7A). Acetabular protrusio occurs when any portion of the femoral head sits medial to the ilioischial line[25] (Fig. 31-7B).

Secondary Abnormalities of Femoroacetabular Impingement

The repetitive mechanical trauma of impingement results in structural changes to various components of the joint, including labrum, hyaline cartilage, and bone. In cam FAI, injury occurs preferentially in the anterosuperior quadrant of the joint. With pincer FAI, the joint injury can start anterosuperiorly, but later on, also posteriorly, eventually leading to more circumferential global changes to the joint.[19,20]

Labrum

A spectrum of morphologic labral injury may be seen with FAI, including degeneration, disruption of the chondrolabral junction, and labral tears, most commonly occurring in the anterosuperior quadrant. A high prevalence of labral degeneration and tearing is known to exist in the setting of FAI.[14]

MRA is the test of choice for evaluation of the acetabular labrum.[40-44] Specifically, it is an excellent investigation for detecting labral tears; studies comparing it with arthroscopy have reported sensitivity and accuracy values ranging from 92% to 100% and from 93% to 96%, respectively.[43-45] However, more recent studies have demonstrated that high-resolution, nonarthrographic MRI is adequate for evaluation of the labrum and cartilage.[13,18] With rapidly improving MRI technology, higher field strengths, and newer sequences, MRA may become antiquated in the future.

Normally, the labrum has a pointed, triangular shape with sharp margins and very low signal intensity across most MRI sequences. A firm, continuous attachment of the labrum to the osseous acetabular rim and the acetabular cartilage has been noted.[46] This interface between hyaline cartilage and labrum is referred to as the *chondrolabral junction*.

The degenerate labrum may manifest on MRI with increased size, globularization, increased intrasubstance signal, and surface irregularity[47] (Fig. 31-8).

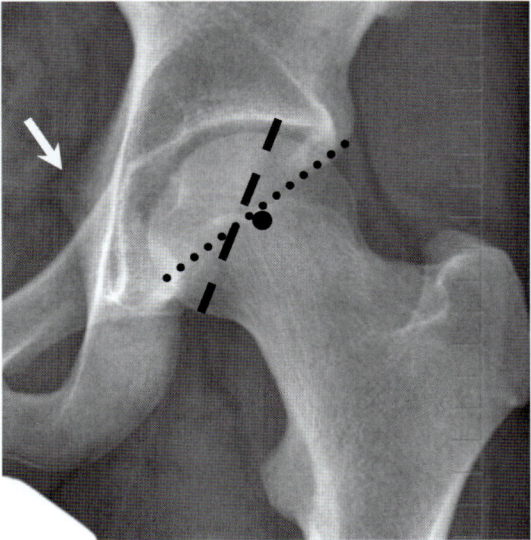

Figure 31-6. Anteroposterior (AP) view of the left hip with signs of acetabular retroversion. The superior portion of the anterior rim of the acetabulum *(dotted line, more horizontal)* abnormally projects lateral to the superior portion of the posterior rim *(dashed line, more vertical)*, resulting in "crossover." Note that the posterior rim of the acetabulum lies medial to the center of the femoral head *(solid dot).* Retroversion also results in medialization and a prominent profile of the ischial spine *(white arrow).*

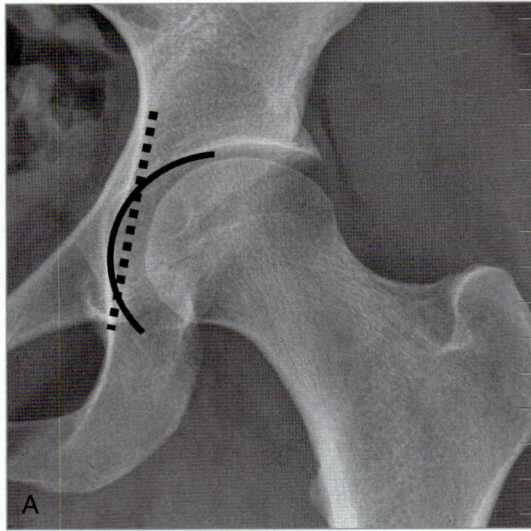

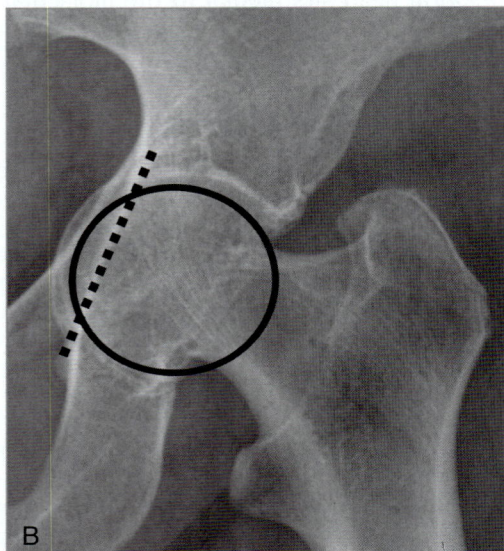

Figure 31-7. Anteroposterior (AP) radiographs of the hip demonstrate **(A)** coxa profunda—the fossa acetabuli line *(solid line)* lies medial to the ilioischial line *(dashed line),* and **(B)** acetabular protrusio—the femoral head *(solid line circle)* lies medial to the ilioischial line *(dashed line).*

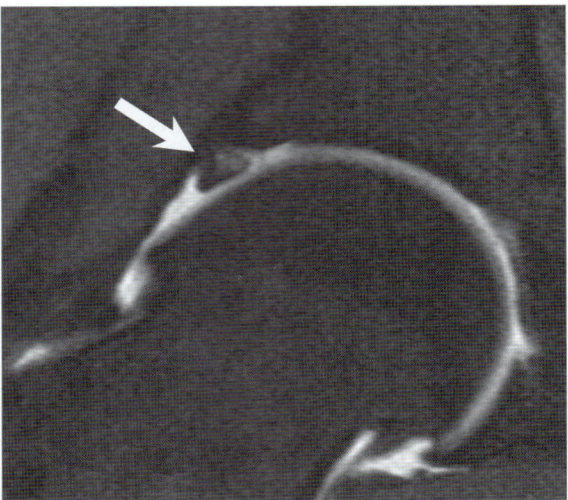

Figure 31-8. Degenerate labrum on magnetic resonance arthrography (MRA), oblique coronal T1W image with fat suppression. Note that the triangular labrum *(white arrow)* is slightly globular, with a blunted rounded free edge, and centrally, the normal low signal *(black)* has been replaced with a higher, intermediate signal *(gray),* consistent with myxoid degenerative change.

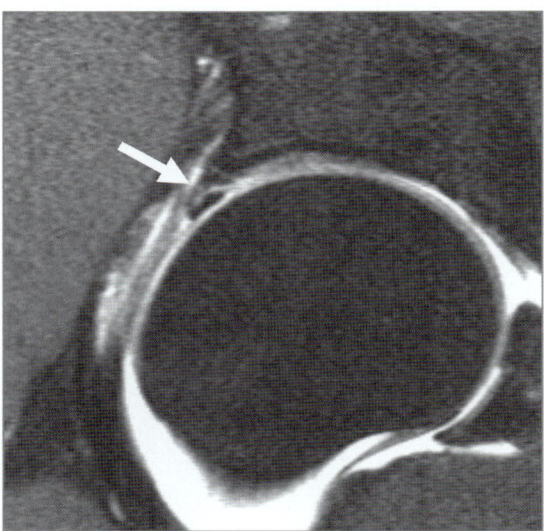

Figure 31-9. Labral tear on magnetic resonance arthrography (MRA), oblique coronal T1W image with fat suppression. Note that the triangular labrum *(white arrow),* normally with diffuse low signal *(black),* now demonstrates an abnormal linear cleft of high-signal *(white)* gadolinium, extending into the substance of the labrum from the deep articular surface, from medial to lateral.

Labral tears will be demonstrated by extension of contrast solution into the substance of the labrum and are most commonly seen in the anterosuperior quadrant[18,42,43,45,48] (Fig. 31-9).

With labral detachments, the contrast will undermine the base of the labrum at the chondrolabral and acetabular-labral junctions. Paralabral cysts are small, fluid-filled cysts that can develop secondary to labral degeneration, tears, and detachments. Although theoretically they may fill with gadolinium, most will not and thus are most conspicuous on fluid-sensitive sequences.[49]

Although the aforementioned labral changes in cam and pincer FAI can be similar, some features are more commonly seen in each of the two forms. In cam

FAI, labral injury is initiated at the chondrolabral junction anterosuperiorly, where repetitive shear trauma occurs,[20,47] resulting in focal separation of the labrum from the cartilage along the deep, articular margin.[13,50] This will manifest as imbibition of fluid into the defect at the chondrolabral junction.[47] In pincer FAI, abutment of the anterior acetabular rim onto the femoral neck results in focal impaction on the labrum,[21] most frequently occurring anterosuperiorly.[19] Labral fissuring with prominent intralabral cyst formation is seen more frequently in pincer than cam FAI.[20,21]

Over time, the traumatized labrum can become ossified, leading to increased depth of the rigid component of the acetabulum. This in turn will lead to further increased coverage of the femoral head. Ossification of the labrum/acetabular rim can occur in both cam and pincer forms of FAI and is seen most often in the anterosuperior quadrant.[27]

Cartilage

Both cam and pincer types of FAI are known to result in significant cartilage abnormality, with almost all patients demonstrating varying degrees of chondral injury.[14,19,27] Chondral morphologic changes may be seen in the form of surface fraying, fissuring, partial- or full-thickness loss of cartilage, and delamination. However, the dominant pattern of damage to the cartilage can vary between cam and pincer forms.

MRI is the optimal radiologic modality for evaluation of cartilage status.[51] In FAI, chondral abnormality can manifest with signal and morphologic changes. Both routine MRI[13,18] and MRA[11,14,47,52,53] can be used to detect chondral defects of femoral and acetabular articular surfaces. Various MRI sequences have been used to evaluate cartilage morphology in the hip. These include proton density, gradient echo, and T1-weighted sequences, with or without fat suppression, and with or without arthrographic technique. More quantitative techniques such as delayed gadolinium-enhanced MRI of cartilage (dGEMRIC) and T2- and T1-rho mapping have been introduced in the hope of detecting biochemical changes in cartilage before gross morphologic damage occurs.[3] In situations where MRI is contraindicated, CT arthrography may allow evaluation of gross cartilage morphology and thickness.[10,11]

The initial chondral insult in cam FAI occurs at the chondrolabral junction anterosuperiorly, with disruption of the normally continuous interface between the two structures. With repetitive impingement of the cam deformity against the acetabulum, the damage extends more medially, into the hyaline cartilage.[47] With cam FAI, chondral injury preferentially occurs along the peripheral margin of the acetabulum anterosuperiorly, tending to be more focal and deeper than with pincer FAI.[19,27] The insult may begin as fissuring or thinning, and eventually may evolve to a full-thickness chondral defect (Fig. 31-10).

One form of chondral injury, specifically seen in cam FAI, is delamination, whereby a focal area of cartilage detaches from the acetabular subchondral compact bone. This debonding manifests as signal change within the substance of the cartilage, typically focal, linear hypointensity paralleling the articular surface on various sequences, including gradient echo, proton density, and intermediate weighted images.[53,54] When debonding coexists with a full-thickness chondral fissure or defect, a flap is created. On MRI, a flap is identified by fluid interposition between cartilage and

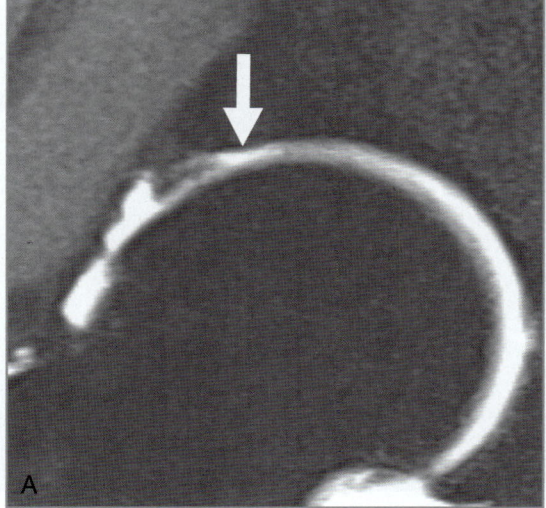

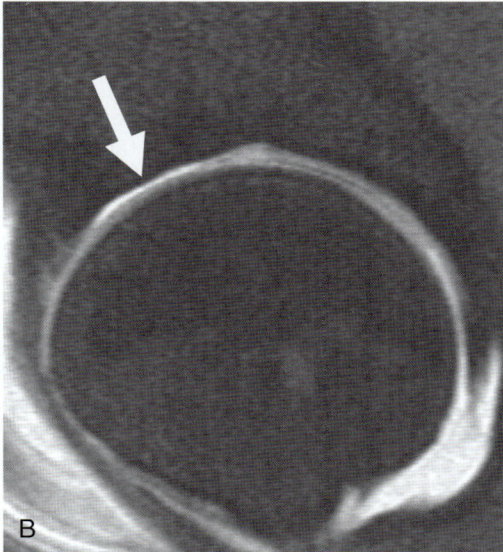

Figure 31-10. Full-thickness chondral defect *(white arrows)* noted along the periphery of the anterosuperior acetabular roof on **(A)** oblique coronal and **(B)** oblique sagittal magnetic resonance arthrography (MRA) T1W image with fat suppression. Note the degenerate and frayed labrum on **(A)** just adjacent to the chondral defect.

subchondral compact bone[53] (Fig. 31-11). The sensitivity, specificity, and accuracy of routine high-resolution MRI in detecting chondral injury in the hip range from 86% to 100%, from 72% to 82%, and from 82% to 88%, respectively.[13,18] The sensitivity, specificity, and accuracy of MRA in detecting chondral injury in the hip range from 58% to 79%, from 69% to 100%, and from 69% to 81%, respectively.[52,55]

With pincer FAI, repetitive impaction of the anterosuperior acetabular rim on the femoral neck initially results in a narrow band of injury to the acetabular cartilage. Chondral lesions tend to be more diffuse and shallower than with cam FAI.[19,27] With chronic pincer impingement, contrecoup chondral lesions may be seen along the posteroinferior acetabular surface. This is

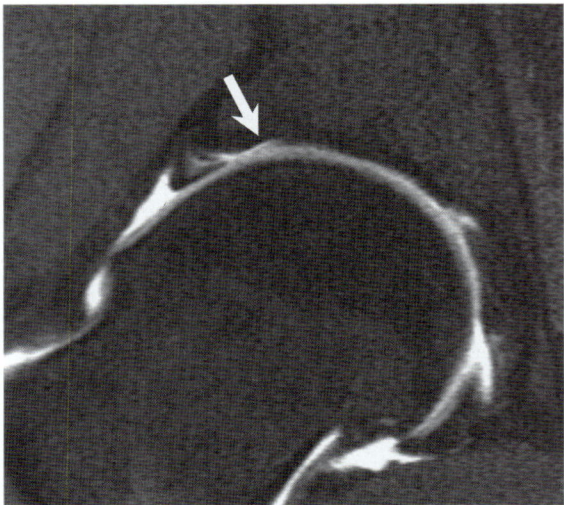

Figure 31-11. Focal chondral delamination along the periphery of the superior acetabular roof *(white arrow)* on magnetic resonance arthrography (MRA), oblique coronal T1W image with fat suppression. Note the very fine, linear, high signal of gadolinium *(white)* interposed between the dark signal of subchondral compact bone *(black)* and the intermediate signal of hyaline cartilage *(gray)*. A thin cleft of gadolinium is seen extending into the substance of the labrum, consistent with a labral tear.

related to reduced excursion of the femoral head anteriorly caused by acetabular overcoverage and leads to a secondary posterior shift of the femoral head with greater pressure against the posterior cartilage.[19] Preferential posterior joint cartilage thinning can be evaluated on MRI on the false profile radiograph.

Bone

Fibrocysts are known to be associated with both cam and pincer FAI[27,56] and can be demonstrated on both CT[51,57] and MRI.[14,27,51,57,58] Although the general population prevalence of fibrocysts has long been presumed to be approximately 5%, a recent CT-based study found the prevalence to be 43%.[57] In patients with FAI, reported prevalence ranges from 4% to 24% with the use of MRI[13,14,27] and is 52% with MRA.[56]

Fibrocysts vary in size, ranging from 2 to 15 mm,[56-58] and may be unilocular or multilocular.[51] It has been reported that small fibrocysts may progressively evolve into larger cysts with continuing impingement.[59]

On CT, fibrocysts appear as lucent lesions just deep to the cortex. They typically are well defined with sclerotic margins, although the overlying cortex may be thinned and irregular. The attenuation value varies from that of fluid to that of soft tissue, depending on the composition of the internal contents.[57] On MRI, fibrocysts appear as well-defined lesions that peripherally are of low T1 and T2 signals, and centrally are of variable T1 and T2 signals, again depending on the internal composition.[56]

A spatial relationship between the location of fibrocysts and the site of impingement has been established.[56] They are most commonly seen along the anterosuperior femoral neck, just at the margin of the articular surface.[19] Fibrocysts may be associated with local marrow edema as seen on MRI.[51] Fibrocysts have been noted to be associated with higher alpha angles.[57] Given their prevalence, location, and association with higher alpha angle values, fibrocysts may be a radiologic marker of FAI.[56]

Marrow edema may be seen at a subchondral location as the result of chondropathic changes. Nonsubchondral, or marginal, marrow edema may develop as a result of the focal contact of impingement. Edema can occur on femoral and acetabular sides of the joint.[12]

Impingement leads to increased stress along the anterosuperior acetabular rim. This may cause focal osseous fracture or fragmentation, or chronic nonfusion of the normal epiphysis in this area, referred to as the *os acetabuli*.[60] Os acetabuli can be seen with both cam and pincer forms of FAI.[14] A focal linear zone of depression along the anterior femoral neck, just below the head-neck junction, may be seen with pincer FAI secondary to contact with the anterosuperior acetabular rim.

Joint

In both cam and pincer types of FAI, primary morphologic abnormalities of the hip, along with secondary derangement of articular structures, result in altered biomechanics, leading to OA. The variable constellation of OA findings, including chondral loss, osteophytosis, synovitis, effusion, capsular thickening, and intraarticular bodies, can be seen on MRI. However, these findings are nonspecific and can be seen in a variety of arthritides in the absence of FAI.

DEVELOPMENTAL DYSPLASIA OF THE HIP

Developmental dysplasia of the hip results from a shallow acetabulum with relative undercoverage of the femoral head, leading to joint instability and premature OA. Joint instability results in anterolateral migration of the femoral head with abnormal chronic shear and stress loading along the rim of the acetabulum anterosuperiorly. This leads to focal premature chondral thinning and OA.[61] The diagnosis can be made with the use of radiography, by measuring the acetabular index and the lateral and vertical center edge (CE) angles.[7]

The acetabular index, or inclination angle, is drawn on an AP pelvis radiograph (Fig. 31-12). The angle is subtended by a line drawn laterally from the inferiormost portion of the sourcil (the sclerotic weight-bearing portion of the acetabulum), parallel to the transverse axis of the pelvis, and by a line drawn from the inferior sourcil to the lateral-most margin of the sourcil. Hips with angle values greater than 10 degrees may be at increased risk of structural instability.[7]

The lateral CE angle and the vertical CE angle reflect the degree of femoral head coverage by the acetabulum. Angle values for either measuring less than 25 degrees suggest inadequate femoral head coverage.[7] As drawn on an AP pelvis radiograph, the lateral CE angle is

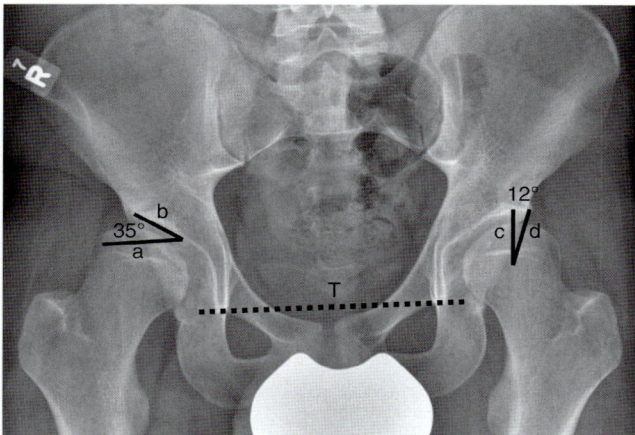

Figure 31-12. Anteroposterior (AP) radiograph demonstrating bilateral hip dysplasia with measurements of the **(1)** acetabular inclination angle on the right hip, and **(2)** lateral center edge (CE) angle on the left hip. Both measurements first require determination of the true transverse axis of the pelvis by drawing a line *(T)* through the inferior margins of both teardrops **(1).** The acetabular inclination angle is formed by a line drawn laterally from the inferior-most portion of the sourcil *(a),* parallel to line T, and a line drawn from the inferior sourcil to the lateral-most margin of the sourcil *(b).* The acetabular inclination angle in the right hip is 35 degrees. **(2)** The lateral CE angle is subtended by a line extended superiorly from the femoral head center *(c),* perpendicular to the transverse axis of the pelvis *(T),* and a line from the center of the femoral head to the superolateral rim of the acetabulum *(d).* The lateral CE angle in the left hip is 12 degrees.

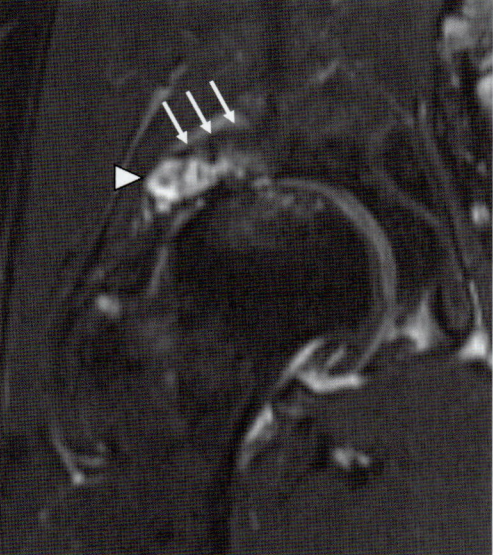

Figure 31-13. Developmental dysplasia of the hip (DDH) coronal T2W image with fat suppression demonstrates an enlarged, globular, degenerate labrum *(small arrows),* partially detached and displaced superiorly. A complex paralabral cyst *(arrowhead)* is also present. Note the undercovered femoral head, with chronic remodeling resulting in mild superolateral flattening, chondral thinning, and mild subchondral marrow edema.

subtended by a line that extends superiorly from the femoral head center, perpendicular to the transverse axis of the pelvis, and a line from the center of the femoral head to the superolateral rim of the acetabulum[7] (see Fig. 31-12). As drawn on the false profile view, the vertical CE angle is subtended by a line that extends superiorly from the femoral head center, perpendicular to the transverse axis of the pelvis, and a line from the center of the femoral head to the anterior rim of the acetabulum.[7]

MRI can demonstrate other associated soft tissue abnormalities such as labrum hypertrophy, degeneration, or tearing and chondral damage (Fig. 31-13).[61]

OTHER COMMON HIP PATHOLOGIES

Avascular Necrosis

Avascular necrosis (AVN) of the femoral head, an increasingly common cause of musculoskeletal disability, results from interruption of the blood supply leading to cellular death of bone components.[62] The diagnosis of AVN of the femoral head depends on the combination of clinical symptoms and evaluation of radiography and/or MRI views. The Ficat classification

and the Association Research Circulation Osseous (ARCO) classification are commonly used to assess both imaging modalities.[63]

By convention, the term *avascular (ischemic) necrosis* generally is applied to areas of epiphyseal or subarticular involvement, whereas *bone infarct* usually is reserved for metaphyseal and diaphyseal involvement. The cause of AVN is multifactorial. Although the pathophysiology of AVN is not fully understood, it typically affects bones with a single, terminal blood supply such as the femoral head, carpal bones, talus, and humerus. In clinical practice, AVN is most commonly encountered in the hip.[63]

Pathophysiology

AVN has many causes, including trauma, hemoglobinopathies, Cushing syndrome, exogenous steroid use, alcoholism, pancreatitis, human immunodeficiency virus, Gaucher disease, and Caisson disease, although the condition may also be idiopathic. Age of onset depends on the underlying cause. Primary AVN most often occurs during the fourth or fifth decade and is bilateral in 40% to 80% of cases. It has no racial predilection except in cases associated with sickle cell disease and hemoglobin S, which predominantly occur in people of African and Mediterranean descent.

Imaging. Conventional radiography, CT, nuclear medicine study, and MRI can identify AVN. MRI has the greatest sensitivity of all modalities.

Radiography. Radiographs may be normal in the earliest stages of the disease. One of the earliest radiographic findings is a subchondral lucency (crescent sign), which reflects collapse of necrotic trabeculae. Later findings include sclerosis, possible collapse and fragmentation of the head, and subsequent OA.[64] The Ficat staging system is commonly used to classify the radiographic appearances of AVN in the hip.[63]

Radionuclide Imaging. With radionuclide imaging, specifically, a Tc99m-MDP multiphase bone scan, early AVN will manifest with reduced radiotracer uptake. Thereafter, an area of increased uptake surrounds the central area of decreased uptake; this "doughnut" sign indicates a reactive zone surrounding the necrotic area. However, the bone scan has limitations. In early AVN, findings are less sensitive than those obtained on MRI.[65]

Computed Tomography. CT scan cannot reliably demonstrate early vascular and marrow abnormalities. In the later stages of AVN, CT will demonstrate the sclerotic margins of the infarction, thus revealing its distribution and size, and will detect subtle areas of head flattening or osteoarthritis.[64]

Magnetic Resonance Imaging. MRI has evolved as the most sensitive modality in the early detection of AVN. It has a sensitivity of 97% and a specificity of 98% in the diagnosis of AVN of the hip.[66] The high frequency of bilateral avascular necrosis supports large field-of-view sequences of the entire pelvis.[66]

In early AVN, diffuse bone marrow edema is seen as decreased signal intensity with poorly defined margins on T1W, and as high signal intensity on fluid-sensitive sequence images. A serpiginous line of low signal intensity is seen on T1W images. A variable degree of marrow edema can surround, or may be found within, the area of necrosis. A classic appearance of AVN—the "double line" sign—occurs later in the disease process, after the start of osseous repair.[65] This describes a focal area of high or intermediate signal intensity surrounded by a rim of low signal intensity on both T1 and T2W images (Fig. 31-14). A high signal intensity line may represent hypervascular granulation, and a low signal intensity line may correlate with the reactive zone at the outer margin of a necrotic lesion. The "double line" sign is seen in up to 80% of cases. Osseous collapse and sclerosis are seen as focal areas of low signal on T1W images and of variable signal on T2W images.[66]

MRI findings of AVN of the hip may be classified according to a system proposed by Mitchell[66]:

Class A lesion: signal intensity characteristics analogous to those of fat on T1W images and intermediate signal intensity on T2W images

Class B lesion: signal intensity characteristics similar to those of blood, which has high signal intensity on both T1- and T2-weighted images

Class C lesion: signal intensity properties similar to those of fluid, that is, low signal intensity on T1-weighted images and high signal intensity on T2-weighted images

Class D lesion: signal similar to that of fibrous tissue, which has low signal intensity on both T1- and T2-weighted images

MRI helps to quantify the percentage of involvement of the femoral head and the extent of articular cartilage involvement, along with femoral head collapse, joint effusion, and degenerative changes in the hip joint.[67,68]

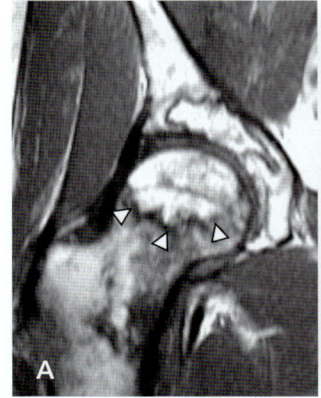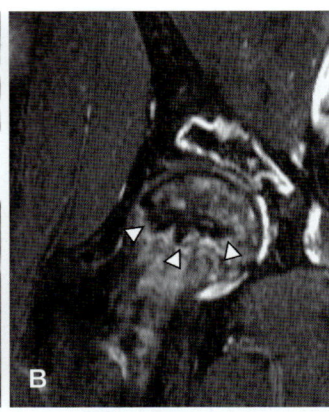

Figure 31-14. A, Magnetic resonance imaging (MRI) coronal T1W image, and **(B)** T2W image with fat suppression of the hip with avascular necrosis (AVN). Both demonstrate a subchondral well-marginated geographic area with a thin rim of uniform thickness, together showing a "double line" sign *(white arrowheads)*. **B,** T2W image with fat suppression demonstrates high signal both in the subchondral region within the infarction and surrounding it and extending into the femoral neck. Note also another area of infarction in the acetabular roof.

Differential Diagnosis for AVN

Transient Osteoporosis of the Hip. Transient osteoporosis of the hip (TOH) is a self-limiting condition that resolves over time. Although it was first described in women in the third trimester of pregnancy, it primarily affects middle-aged men.[69] Radiographic evidence of osteopenia extends from the head to the intertrochanteric region. Bone scintigraphy shows increased uptake, reflecting increased bone turnover and inflammatory change, but this is nonspecific.[70] MRI shows diffuse bone marrow edema involving the femoral head, starting in the subchondral region and extending distally across the femoral neck region (Fig. 31-15).[71] In contrast to AVN, TOH does not result in a well-marginated geographic zone of signal abnormality, and marrow edema tends to be diffuse and more homogeneous. TOH resolves within 4 to 10 months and does not progress to AVN.

Subchondral Stress Fracture. In addition to surrounding marrow edema, a subchondral, linear low-signal area on T1 or PDW sequences can be seen paralleling the articular surface, reflecting a subchondral fracture.[72,73]

Fractures

Fractures of the hip are relatively common in adults and often lead to devastating consequences. Hip fractures are associated with substantial morbidity and mortality, particularly in the older population. Fractures involving the hip can be classified as traumatic, stress, or insufficiency fractures.[74]

Acute traumatic proximal femur fractures are most common and may be capital, subcapital, transcervical, basicervical, intertrochanteric, or subtrochanteric. The obvious fracture can often be easily identified on AP

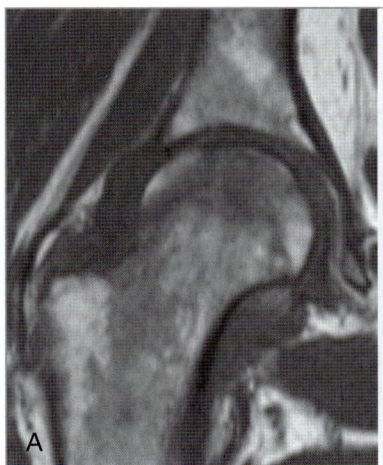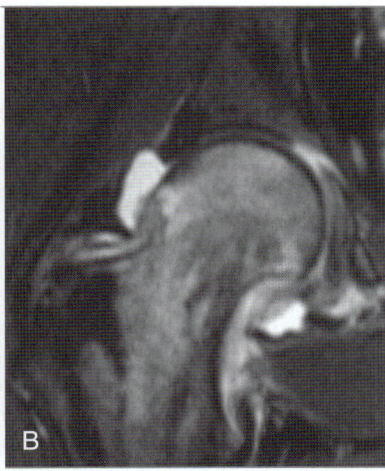

Figure 31-15. Transient osteoporosis of the hip in a 31-year-old female at 34 weeks' gestation. Magnetic resonance imaging (MRI) coronal **(A)** T1W image and **(B)** T2W image with fat suppression. The T2W image demonstrates diffuse, continuous marrow with increased signal extending from the subchondral femoral head into the femoral neck, without well-defined margins. Note also the reactive, moderate-sized joint effusion.

and lateral radiographs. Although the displaced hip fracture can be visualized easily on plain radiography, the nondisplaced fracture may be radiographically occult and may require different imaging modalities for detection. CT is better for detecting and delineating a fracture.[75] Occult fractures in the elderly result from trauma or chronic stress and are often seen in the femoral neck, the greater trochanter, and the acetabulum. In an osteoporotic patient, the radiograph may not demonstrate the fracture. CT is less sensitive in detecting fracture in the osteoporotic patient. Nuclear scintigraphy may show increased uptake at the fracture site, albeit only days after trauma.[76] MRI has evolved as an imaging modality that has the ability to detect the fracture line and surrounding edema.[75] MRI is particularly useful in detecting incomplete femoral neck fractures, which may not be evident on radiographs. Detection of these fractures is important in that they can progress to complete and displaced fractures if the patient continues to bear weight.[77]

Although some studies have shown that a coronal T1 sequence is sufficient to identify a fracture, the addition of a coronal fat-suppressed PD T2 or a STIR sequence, permits superior visualization of surrounding marrow edema and soft tissue injury.[75]

Stress fractures are seen more frequently in adults who participate in strenuous activity. They are common among military recruits and athletes. These fractures result from the inability of bony trabeculae to withstand physical stresses. Unusually high physical demands on normal bone over the long term can lead to mechanical failure of bony trabeculae. Pertaining to the hip, these types of stresses can result in a compression type of fracture involving the cancellous bone of the medial inferior femoral neck without disruption of cortical bone.[72-74]

Insufficiency fractures of the femoral neck are the result of normal stresses of everyday activity placed on structurally compromised bone. Insufficiency fractures can be seen in the supra-acetabular region.[72,77]

Both stress and insufficiency fractures manifest on MRI as linear bands of low signal intensity on T1- or PDW

images, reflecting the fracture line, with surrounding high signal on fluid-sensitive sequences in the marrow and surrounding soft tissues. Similar insufficiency fractures can be seen in the supra-acetabular region.[72,77]

Soft Tissue Abnormalities

Greater use of MRI has allowed us to better assess soft tissue injury around the hip joint, in particular musculotendinous unit injuries. The most commonly strained muscles around the hip are the rectus femoris and the iliopsoas.

MRI characteristics of musculotendinous injuries have been graded as follows[78,79]:

Grade I: diffuse or focal high signal around the myotendinous junction on fluid-sensitive sequences secondary to edema and hemorrhage. This edema and hemorrhage may track along the muscle fascicles, creating a feathery pattern.

Grade II: depending on the timeline of the tear, acute and chronic grade II injuries can manifest differently.

Acute: partial tear of the musculotendinous junction has surrounding feathery signal or hematoma (Fig. 31-16).

Chronic: diminished caliber of the musculotendinous junction. Low signal on T2W images at the myotendinous junction is related to hemosiderin and fibrosis.

Grade III: complete tear of the musculotendinous junction with or without retraction.

Hematomas are common after musculotendinous junction injury. They can be intramuscular or intermuscular and usually resolve 6 to 8 weeks after injury. MRI findings vary because blood products are in different stages of degradation. In the acute stage (deoxyhemoglobin), hematoma appears as intermediate signal on T1 and dark on T2W sequences. In the subacute stage, the blood (methemoglobin) appears bright on both T1 and T2W sequences; a chronic hematoma (hemosiderin) can appear dark on both T1 and T2W sequences. Not infrequently, it may be difficult to differentiate a hematoma from a hemorrhagic neoplasm. In these

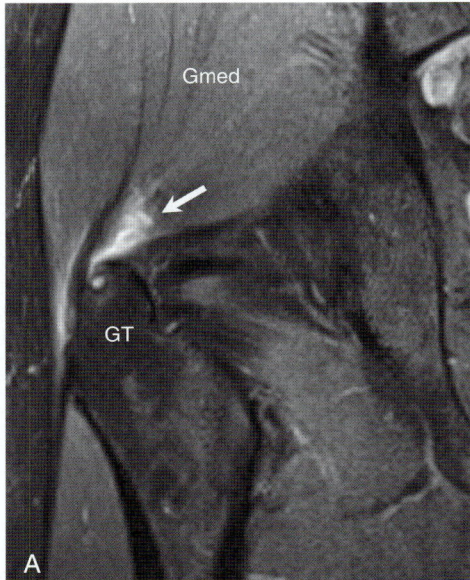

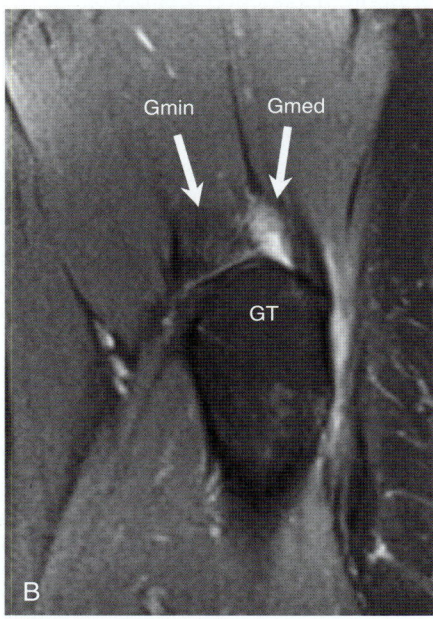

Figure 31-16. Gluteus medius partial-thickness tear at the greater trochanteric insertion. Magnetic resonance imaging (MRI) T2W images with fat suppression in the **(A)** coronal and **(B)** sagittal planes demonstrate irregularity and mild attenuation of the tendon with intratendinous and peritendinous edema.

cases, administration of gadolinium may be helpful in the search for enhancing nodules suggestive of neoplasm.[78]

Bursitis

Bursae are synovial lined, saclike structures located between bone and soft tissue structures such as tendons or ligaments, often with adjacent osseous prominences. Inflammation of a bursa may be seen secondary to trauma, infection, arthritis, friction, and surgery. Greater trochanteric and iliopsoas bursae are the most commonly inflamed bursae around the hip joint. Radiographs are typically normal. Enthesopathic changes at the tendon insertion site or calcification within the bursa is seen less frequently.[80] Ultrasound is an important modality in the diagnosis of bursitis and is used to guide therapeutic injections.[81] Greater trochanteric bursitis will manifest as a rim of hypoechoic fluid adjacent to the greater trochanter.[81] Coronal T2W or STIR MRI sequences will demonstrate a peritrochanteric high-signal fluid collection. In addition, MRI may reveal marrow edema and associated edema in the gluteus minimus and medius tendon insertions.[80]

The iliopsoas bursa is present in 98% of hips and communicates with the hip joint in 15% of the population. In addition to overuse and inflammatory conditions, snapping of the iliopsoas tendon over the iliopectineal eminence may lead to iliopsoas bursitis. The iliopsoas bursa is seen as an elongated fluid collection anterior to the hip joint, medial and posterior to the iliopsoas muscle, and lateral to the femoral vessels.[81] Ultrasound demonstrates hypoechoic fluid collection within the distended iliopsoas bursa. Complex fluid may also be seen in pigment villonodular synovitis, hematoma, and infection. Doppler imaging is useful in differentiating iliopsoas bursitis from a pseudoaneurysm of the femoral vessels. On MRI, the distended bursa shows low T1 and high T2W signals.[82,83]

Tumor and Tumor-Like Lesions Around the Hip

Multiple tumor and tumor-like conditions can occur around the hip (Box 31-1).[84] In most cases, imaging findings will be nonspecific and image-guided biopsy may be required for a histologic diagnosis. Patient age, anatomic location of the lesion, and characteristic imaging findings of some osseous, soft tissue, and synovial-based lesions can facilitate making a definitive diagnosis through a combination of radiography, CT, and MRI. The workup of a suspected hip mass should begin with a radiograph, although it may be normal. Chondroid matrix in an enchondroma, phleboliths in a hemangioma, and peripheral mature ossification in myositis ossificans are examples in which radiographs may allow a definitive diagnosis to be made.[84] Periosteal reaction, bone remodeling, and bone destruction can also be assessed with a conventional radiograph. CT can complement the radiograph. It may be helpful in detecting and characterizing calcifications not visualized on radiographs and is superior in the delineation of osseous details. Disadvantages of CT include poor soft tissue contrast and ionizing radiation.[84,85] MRI has evolved as the modality of choice in the assessment of masses around the hip by providing information for diagnosis and staging. MRI provides superior marrow and soft tissue contrast and enables better assessment of the internal architecture of the lesion when compared with CT and radiography. It also allows multiplanar image acquisitions to be obtained.[85]

When a mass lesion is imaged, a few basic principles should be followed. A marker should be placed over the area of concern to ensure that it is completely included within the field of view. The lesion should be imaged in two orthogonal planes using T1W and fluid-sensitive imaging sequences; the joint closest to the lesion should be included in at least one sequence. Fat suppression on T2W increases lesion-to-background signal intensity differences for high signal intensity lesions within marrow or fatty soft tissue. Use of contrast in assessment of a mass lesion is controversial. It can be useful in evaluating hematomas and in excluding an underlying tumor. It is also helpful in differentiating a solid from a cystic lesion and in identifying necrotic areas within a lesion.[86-88]

CURRENT CONTROVERSIES AND FUTURE CONSIDERATIONS

MRI is a powerful noninvasive tool used to evaluate hip joint hyaline cartilage. Traditional MRI techniques have been effective in identifying macroscopic changes to cartilage. These MRI protocols can detect chondral injury such as focal or global, partial- or full-thickness defects and delaminations. However, these gross structural alterations often manifest later in the OA pathway, at a point where treatment options may be limited to invasive surgical procedures. Thus advanced MRI cartilage mapping techniques are being explored in the hope of interrogating the hyaline cartilage at the molecular level. The goal is to detect compositional and biochemical changes in the macromolecular matrix (proteoglycan, collagen, water) before gross morphologic cartilage damage occurs. dGEMRIC and T2- and T1-rho cartilage mapping have been performed in the hip at basic science and clinical levels; these approaches will receive increasing attention in the future by those conducting global research activity in the area of arthritis.

Although MRA has been the test of choice in the investigation of internal derangement of the hip, nonarthrographic protocols eventually may replace it. Nonarthrographic, or routine, MRI of the hip has traditionally been used to assess only large extra-articular joint structures, including muscle, bone, and the marrow space. However, the use of higher field strength MRI scanners (3.0 T and higher) will allow higher-resolution imaging and faster scan times. With increases in commercially available MRI field strength over the past decade (from 1.5 to 3.0T), and with improvements in MRI hardware and software and sequence technologies, nonarthrographic MRI protocols may obviate the need for arthrogram-based protocols. A nonarthrographic MRI protocol of the hip would be ideal because it would allow comprehensive evaluation of the joint with no radiation or gadolinium contrast exposure, and thus would be less resource intense and less costly.

REFERENCES

1. Clohisy JC, et al: Radiographic evaluation of the hip has limited reliability. Clin Orthop Relat Res 467:666–675, 2009.
2. Dudda M, et al: Do normal radiographs exclude asphericity of the femoral head-neck junction? Clin Orthop Relat Res 467:651–659, 2009.
3. Mamisch TC, et al: Magnetic resonance imaging of the hip at 3 Tesla: clinical value in femoroacetabular impingement of the hip and current concepts. Semin Musculoskelet Radiol 12:212–222, 2008.
4. Petersilge CA, from the RSNA Refresher Courses, Radiological Society of North America: Chronic adult hip pain: MR arthrography of the hip. Radiographics 20(Spec No):S43–S52, 2000.
5. McCarthy JC, Busconi B: The role of hip arthroscopy in the diagnosis and treatment of hip disease. Orthopedics 18:753–756, 1995.
6. Yamamoto Y, et al: Usefulness of radial contrast-enhanced computed tomography for the diagnosis of acetabular labrum injury. Arthroscopy 23:1290–1294, 2007.
7. Clohisy JC, et al: A systematic approach to the plain radiographic evaluation of the young adult hip. J Bone Joint Surg Am 90(Suppl 4):47–66, 2008.
8. Greenspan A: Lower limb 1: pelvic girdle and proximal femur. In Greespan A (ed): Orthopaedic radiology: a practical approach, Philadelphia, 2004, Lippincott Williams & Wilkins, pp 197–225.
9. Llopis E, Ferrer P, Aparisi F: Pelvis-hip: technical aspects, normal anatomy, common variants, and basic biomechanics. In Pope TL, et al (eds): Imaging of the musculoskeletal system, Philadelphia, 2008, Saunders-Elsevier, pp 405–433.
10. Nishii T, et al: Disorders of acetabular labrum and articular cartilage in hip dysplasia: evaluation using isotropic high-resolutional CT arthrography with sequential radial reformation. Osteoarthritis Cartilage 15:251–257, 2007.
11. Wyler A, et al: Comparison of MR-arthrography and CT-arthrography in hyaline cartilage-thickness measurement in radiographically normal cadaver hips with anatomy as gold standard. Osteoarthritis Cartilage 17:19–25, 2008.
12. Bredella MA, Stoller DW: MR imaging of femoroacetabular impingement. Magn Reson Imaging Clin N Am 13:653–664, 2005.
13. James SL, et al: MRI findings of femoroacetabular impingement. AJR Am J Roentgenol 187:1412–1419, 2006.
14. Kassarjian A, et al: Triad of MR arthrographic findings in patients with cam-type femoroacetabular impingement. Radiology 236:588–592, 2005.
15. Hodler J, et al: MR arthrography of the hip: improved imaging of the acetabular labrum with histologic correlation in cadavers. AJR Am J Roentgenol 165:887–891, 1995.
16. Steinbach LS, Palmer WE, Schweitzer ME: Special focus session: MR arthrography. Radiographics 22:1223–1246, 2002.

17. Kassarjian A, Brisson M, Palmer WE: Femoroacetabular impingement. Eur J Radiol 63:29–35, 2007.

18. Mintz DN, et al: Magnetic resonance imaging of the hip: detection of labral and chondral abnormalities using noncontrast imaging. Arthroscopy 21:385–393, 2005.

19. Beck M, et al: Hip morphology influences the pattern of damage to the acetabular cartilage: femoroacetabular impingement as a cause of early osteoarthritis of the hip. J Bone Joint Surg Br 87:1012–1018, 2005.

20. Ganz R, et al: The etiology of osteoarthritis of the hip: an integrated mechanical concept. Clin Orthop Relat Res 466:264–272, 2008.

21. Ganz R, et al: Femoroacetabular impingement: a cause for osteoarthritis of the hip. Clin Orthop Relat Res 417:112–120, 2003.

22. Ito K, et al: Femoroacetabular impingement and the cam-effect: a MRI-based quantitative anatomical study of the femoral head-neck offset. J Bone Joint Surg Br 83:171–176, 2001.

23. Beaule PE, et al: Three-dimensional computed tomography of the hip in the assessment of femoroacetabular impingement. J Orthop Res 23:1286–1292, 2005.

24. Meyer DC, et al: Comparison of six radiographic projections to assess femoral head/neck asphericity. Clin Orthop Relat Res 445:181–185, 2006.

25. Tannast M, Siebenrock KA, Anderson SE: Femoroacetabular impingement: radiographic diagnosis—what the radiologist should know. AJR Am J Roentgenol 188:1540–1552, 2007.

26. Notzli HP, et al: The contour of the femoral head-neck junction as a predictor for the risk of anterior impingement. J Bone Joint Surg Br 84:556–560, 2002.

27. Pfirrmann CW, et al: Cam and pincer femoroacetabular impingement: characteristic MR arthrographic findings in 50 patients. Radiology 240:778–785, 2006.

28. Rakhra KS, et al: Comparison of MRI alpha angle measurement planes in femoroacetabular impingement. Clin Orthop Relat Res 467:660–665, 2009.

29. Jager M, et al: Femoroacetabular impingement caused by a femoral osseous head-neck bump deformity: clinical, radiological, and experimental results. J Orthop Sci 9:256–263, 2004.

30. Siebenrock KA, et al: Abnormal extension of the femoral head epiphysis as a cause of cam impingement. Clin Orthop Relat Res 418:54–60, 2004.

31. Hack K, Rakhra K, Beaulé P: Prevalence of CAM type FAI morphology in 200 asymptomatic volunteers. J Bone Joint Surg (Am) 92:2436–2444, 2010.

32. Deleted in proof.

33. Eijer H, et al: Cross-table lateral radiographs for screening of anterior femoral head-neck offset in patients with femoroacetabular impingement. Hip Int 11:37–41, 2001.

34. Reynolds D, Lucas J, Klaue K: Retroversion of the acetabulum: a cause of hip pain. J Bone Joint Surg Br 81:281–288, 1999.

35. Siebenrock KA, Schoeniger R, Ganz R: Anterior femoroacetabular impingement due to acetabular retroversion: treatment with periacetabular osteotomy. J Bone Joint Surg Am 85:278–286, 2003.

36. Anda S, Terjesen T, Kvistad KA: Computed tomography measurements of the acetabulum in adult dysplastic hips: which level is appropriate? Skeletal Radiol 20:267–271, 1991.

37. Stem ES, et al: Computed tomography analysis of acetabular anteversion and abduction. Skeletal Radiol 35:385–389, 2006.

38. Murphy SB, et al: Acetabular dysplasia in the adolescent and young adult. Clin Orthop Relat Res 261:214–223, 1990.

39. Tonnis D, Heinecke A: Acetabular and femoral anteversion: relationship with osteoarthritis of the hip. J Bone Joint Surg Am 81:1747–1770, 1999.

40. Czerny C, et al: Lesions of the acetabular labrum: accuracy of MR imaging and MR arthrography in detection and staging. Radiology 200:225–230, 1996.

41. Leunig M, et al: Evaluation of the acetabular labrum by MR arthrography. J Bone Joint Surg Br 79:230–234, 1997.

42. Czerny C, et al: MR arthrography of the adult acetabular capsular-labral complex: correlation with surgery and anatomy. AJR Am J Roentgenol 173:345–349, 1999.

43. Chan YS, et al: Evaluating hip labral tears using magnetic resonance arthrography: a prospective study comparing hip arthroscopy and magnetic resonance arthrography diagnosis. Arthroscopy 21:1250, 2005.

44. Toomayan GA, et al: Sensitivity of MR arthrography in the evaluation of acetabular labral tears. AJR Am J Roentgenol 186:449–453, 2006.

45. Freedman BA, et al: Prognostic value of magnetic resonance arthrography for Czerny stage II and III acetabular labral tears. Arthroscopy 22:742–747, 2006.

46. Ito K, Leunig M, Ganz R: Histopathologic features of the acetabular labrum in femoroacetabular impingement. Clin Orthop Relat Res 429:262–271, 2004.

47. Werlen S: Magnetic resonance arthrography of the hip in femoroacetabular impingement. Oper Tech Orthop 15:191–203, 2005.

48. Blankenbaker DG, et al: Classification and localization of acetabular labral tears. Skeletal Radiol 36:391–397, 2007.

49. Magee T, Hinson G: Association of paralabral cysts with acetabular disorders. AJR Am J Roentgenol 174:1381–1384, 2000.

50. Eijer H, Myers SR, Ganz R: Anterior femoroacetabular impingement after femoral neck fractures. J Orthop Trauma 15:475–481, 2001.

51. James SL, et al: Femoroacetabular impingement: bone marrow oedema associated with fibrocystic change of the femoral head and neck junction. Clin Radiol 62:472–478, 2007.

52. Schmid MR, et al: Cartilage lesions in the hip: diagnostic effectiveness of MR arthrography. Radiology 226:382–386, 2003.

53. Beaule PE, Zaragoza E, Copelan N: Magnetic resonance imaging with gadolinium arthrography to assess acetabular cartilage delamination: a report of four cases. J Bone Joint Surg Am 86:2294–2298, 2004.

54. Pfirrmann CW, et al: MR arthrography of acetabular cartilage delamination in femoroacetabular cam impingement. Radiology 249:236–241, 2008.

55. Knuesel PR, et al: MR arthrography of the hip: diagnostic performance of a dedicated water-excitation 3D double-echo steady-state sequence to detect cartilage lesions. AJR Am J Roentgenol 183:1729–1735, 2004.

56. Leunig M, et al: Fibrocystic changes at anterosuperior femoral neck: prevalence in hips with femoroacetabular impingement. Radiology 236:237–246, 2005.

57. Panzer S, Augat P, Esch U: CT assessment of herniation pits: prevalence, characteristics, and potential association with morphological predictors of femoroacetabular impingement. Eur Radiol 18:1869–1875, 2008.

58. Nokes SR, et al: Herniation pits of the femoral neck: appearance at MR imaging. Radiology 172:231–234, 1989.

59. Gunther KP, et al: Large femoral-neck cysts in association with femoroacetabular impingement: a report of three cases. J Bone Joint Surg Am 89:863–870, 2007.

60. Klaue K, Durnin CW, Ganz R: The acetabular rim syndrome: a clinical presentation of dysplasia of the hip. J Bone Joint Surg Br 73:423–429, 1991.

61. Leunig M, et al: Magnetic resonance arthrography of labral disorders in hips with dysplasia and impingement. Clin Orthop Relat Res 418:74–80, 2004.

62. Vogler JB 3rd, Murphy WA: Bone marrow imaging. Radiology 168:679–693, 1988.

63. Ficat RP: Idiopathic bone necrosis of the femoral head: early diagnosis and treatment. J Bone Joint Surg Br 67:3–9, 1985.

64. Imhof H, et al: Imaging of avascular necrosis of bone. Eur Radiol 7:180–186, 1997.

65. Saini A, Saifuddin A: MRI of osteonecrosis. Clin Radiol 59:1079–1093, 2004.

66. Mitchell DG, et al: Femoral head avascular necrosis: correlation of MR imaging, radiographic staging, radionuclide imaging, and clinical findings. Radiology 162:709–715, 1987.

67. Beltran J, et al: Core decompression for avascular necrosis of the femoral head: correlation between long-term results and preoperative MR staging. Radiology 175:533–536, 1990.

68. Koo KH, Kim R: Quantifying the extent of osteonecrosis of the femoral head: a new method using MRI. J Bone Joint Surg Br 77:875–880, 1995.

69. Potter H, et al: Magnetic resonance imaging in diagnosis of transient osteoporosis of the hip. Clin Orthop Relat Res 280:223–229, 1992.

70. Grimm J, et al: MRI of transient osteoporosis of the hip. Arch Orthop Trauma Surg 110:98–102, 1991.

71. Guerra JJ, Steinberg ME: Distinguishing transient osteoporosis from avascular necrosis of the hip. J Bone Joint Surg Am 77: 616–624, 1995.

72. Daffner RH, Pavlov H: Stress fractures: current concepts. AJR Am J Roentgenol 159:245–252, 1992.

73. Dorne HL, Lander PH: Spontaneous stress fractures of the femoral neck. AJR Am J Roentgenol 144:343–347, 1985.

74. Devas MB: Stress fractures of the femoral neck. J Bone Joint Surg Br 47:728–738, 1965.

75. Verbeeten KM, et al: The advantages of MRI in the detection of occult hip fractures. Eur Radiol 15:165–169, 2005.

76. Holder LE, et al: Radionuclide bone imaging in the early detection of fractures of the proximal femur (hip): multifactorial analysis. Radiology 174:509–515, 1990.

77. Beltran J, Opsha O: MR imaging of the hip: osseous lesions. Magn Reson Imaging Clin N Am 13:665–676, vi, 2005.

78. Boutin RD, Fritz RC, Steinbach LS: Imaging of sports-related muscle injuries. Radiol Clin North Am 40:333–362, vii, 2002.

79. Gyftopoulos S, et al: Normal anatomy and strains of the deep musculotendinous junction of the proximal rectus femoris: MRI features. AJR Am J Roentgenol 190:W182–W186, 2008.

80. Lagier R, Vasey H: Calcium pyrophosphate dihydrate (CPPD) crystal deposition in the trochanteric bursa of a patient with hip osteoarthritis. J Rheumatol 13:473–474, 1986.

81. Cho KH, Park BH, Yeon KM: Ultrasound of the adult hip. Semin Ultrasound CT MR 21:214–230, 2000.

82. Wunderbaldinger P, et al: Imaging features of iliopsoas bursitis. Eur Radiol 12:409–415, 2002.

83. Shabshin N, Rosenberg ZS, Cavalcanti CF: MR imaging of iliopsoas musculotendinous injuries. Magn Reson Imaging Clin N Am 13:705–716, 2005.

84. Bancroft LW, Peterson JJ, Kransdorf MJ: MR imaging of tumors and tumor-like lesions of the hip. Magn Reson Imaging Clin N Am 13:757–774, 2005.

85. Kransdorf MJ, Murphey MD (eds): Imaging of soft tissue tumours, 2nd ed, Baltimore, 2006, Lippincott Williams & Wilkins.

86. Dalinka MK, et al: The use of magnetic resonance imaging in the evaluation of bone and soft-tissue tumors. Radiol Clin North Am 28:461–470, 1990.

87. Tehranzadeh J, et al: Comparison of CT and MR imaging in musculoskeletal neoplasms. J Comput Assist Tomogr 13:466–472, 1989.

88. Aisen AM, et al: MRI and CT evaluation of primary bone and soft-tissue tumors. AJR Am J Roentgenol 146:749–756, 1986.

SUGGESTED READING

Bredella MA, Stoller DW: MR imaging of femoroacetabular impingement. Magn Reson Imaging Clin N Am 13:653–664, 2005.

This article discusses hip MRI techniques and protocols for the investigation of FAI, with a review of common MRI findings and hip derangements associated with both cam and pincer forms.

Clohisy JC, et al: A systematic approach to the plain radiographic evaluation of the young adult hip. J Bone Joint Surg Am 90(Suppl 4):47–66, 2008.

This is a comprehensive review, appropriate for the orthopedic surgeon, radiologist, and technologist, of positioning and technical factors for image acquisition. Clinically relevant measurements in FAI and the dysplastic hip are highlighted.

Hong RJ, Hughes TH, Gentili A, Chung CB: J Magn Reson Imaging 27:435–445, 2008.

This article reviews the basic anatomy of the hip, as well as protocols and applications of MRI for the investigation of intra-articular and extra-articular causes of hip pain.

Pope TL, et al: Imaging of the musculoskeletal system, vol 1, Philadelphia, 2008, Saunders Elsevier, Section 2-B, Chapters 18-21, pp 405–521.

This reference textbook provides a comprehensive up-to-date review of multimodality radiologic imaging of all major pathologies of the hip.

Tannast M, Siebenrock KA, Anderson SE: Femoroacetabular impingement: radiographic diagnosis—what the radiologist should know. AJR Am J Roentgenol 188:1540–1552, 2007.

This review article compares the cam and pincer forms of FAI, with an emphasis on radiographic technique and pitfalls. Major morphologic features and quantitative parameters measurable with radiographs are presented.

CHAPTER 32

Osteoarthritis

Ira Zaltz and Brian Larkin

KEY POINTS

- Epidemiology and risk factors
  - Hip osteoarthritis affects up to one third of the population and has a varied clinical course, with a final degenerative pathway.
  - Plain radiographs are commonly used to diagnosis osteoarthritis, with joint space narrowing being the best predictor of symptomatic osteoarthritis (OA).
  - Newer imaging modalities, including magnetic resonance imaging (MRI) and delayed enhanced magnetic resonance imaging of cartilage (dGMERIC), assess hip joint integrity before conventional radiographic changes are apparent.
  - Risk factors for the development of end-stage hip OA include obesity, history of heavy manual labor, female gender, hip trauma, and anatomic abnormalities such as femoroacetabular impingement (FAI).
- Pathophysiology
  - Femoroacetabular impingement can present as cam-type or pincer-type impingement, but often is seen clinically as a combination of the two.
  - Articular cartilage is the tissue affected by hip OA, and cytokines produced by chondrocytes and synovial tissue alter the balance between anabolic and catabolic pathways.
  - Early changes in articular cartilage include increased water content, progressive collagen disorganization, and abnormal proteoglycan synthesis.
  - Bony changes in OA include an increase in subchondral bone thickness, advancement of the tidemark, osteophyte and cyst formation, and progressive bone marrow edema.
- Clinical features and diagnosis
  - Hip OA presents with groin pain, decreased range of motion, and gate alterations.
  - A thorough history and physical examination are essential in the correct diagnosis of hip pathology, and specialized physical examination tests are often utilized.
  - Initial plain radiographs should include anteroposterior (AP) and lateral projections of the hip and should be carefully scrutinized for bone and soft tissue abnormalities.

- Normal plain radiographs do not exclude hip pathology, and special radiographic views may be necessary for complete evaluation.
- To evaluate chondral and labral injuries, advanced imaging methods, including MRI-arthrogram using radial sequences and dGMERIC, are available.
- Treatment
  - First-line treatment includes medications such as nonsteroidal anti-inflammatory medications and acetaminophen to minimize pain and improve function.
  - Other modalities such as nontraditional medications, weight loss, exercise, and other alternative treatments may prove beneficial for hip OA but lack support in the literature.
  - Nonarthroplasty surgical options are often reserved for the young adult presenting with FAI and may include arthroscopic or open procedures aimed at addressing labral and chondral damage.
  - Hip arthrodesis is an option for the young patient with significant unilateral osteoarthritic changes but comes with adaptations in gait and load transfer to surrounding joints.
  - Total hip arthroplasty is the gold standard for the treatment of end-stage hip OA, and approaches, prosthetic design, and bearing surfaces continue to evolve.

INTRODUCTION

A comprehensive definition of osteoarthritis (OA) was agreed upon at a 1994 workshop entitled "New Horizons in Osteoarthritis," which was sponsored by the American Academy of Orthopaedic Surgeons; the National Institute of Arthritis, Musculoskeletal, and Skin Diseases; the National Institute on Aging; the Arthritis Foundation; and the Orthopaedic Research and Education Foundation:

"Osteoarthritic (OA) diseases are a result of both mechanical and biologic events that destabilize the normal coupling of degradation and synthesis of articular cartilage chondrocytes and extracellular matrix,

and subchondral bone. Although they may be initiated by multiple factors, including genetic, developmental, metabolic, and traumatic, OA diseases involve all of the tissues of the diarthrodial joint. Ultimately, OA diseases are manifested by morphologic, biochemical, molecular, and biomechanical changes of both cells and matrix which lead to a softening, fibrillation, ulceration, loss of articular cartilage, sclerosis and eburnation of subchondral bone, osteophytes, and subchondral cysts. When clinically evident, OA diseases are characterized by joint pain, tenderness, limitation of movement, crepitus, occasional effusion, and variable degrees of inflammation without systemic effects."[1]

OA, a common condition affecting millions of people, is associated with pain and disability that have a negative impact on quality of life, productivity, self-worth, and self-related health. The estimated cost of lost productivity and employment for American workers between the ages of 40 and 65 is greater than $7 billion.[2] Currently, approximately 27 million Americans older than age 25 are limited by OA.[3] As the population ages, the prevalence of OA is expected to increase substantially[4]; OA already trails only cardiovascular, cerebrovascular, and pulmonary disease in terms of disability in people older than age 65.[5]

Although the final clinical appearance and common pathway of hip OA may appear similar, multiple precipitating causes are known, including trauma, lower extremity misalignment, developmental abnormalities, synovial disease, infection, and crystalline arthropathy. It is now understood that subtle anatomic abnormalities that have different pathomechanical consequences and can be subclinical initially may initiate a continuum of disease that may not manifest until early adulthood or beyond. Thus the common pathway of OA leads to irreversible damage to the acetabular labrum and articular surface that causes joint dysfunction resulting in deformity, reduction in range of motion, and pain.

Many different treatment options are available to the clinician and patient; current accepted treatment goals are to improve function, decrease pain, and preserve the hip joint for as long as possible. Treatment modalities include a variety of medications, physical therapies and exercises, alternative modalities, and operative interventions ranging from arthroscopy to arthrotomy, osteotomy, arthrodesis, and arthroplasty.

This chapter will focus on the epidemiology and risk factors for osteoarthritis, the pathophysiology, the clinical features and diagnostic tests, the differential diagnosis, treatment options, and the prognosis of this common musculoskeletal disease.

EPIDEMIOLOGY AND RISK FACTORS

Hip osteoarthritis (OA) is a common condition that affects millions of people worldwide and is present in virtually all races. Although the clinical course, presentation, and patient demographics vary considerably, all patients share a common degenerative pathway.

Prevalence varies by race and regional population. In a population-based study in Finland, hip OA was found to affect 4.9% of people.[6] In South Korea, the prevalence of hip OA was estimated to be 1.2%, with men affected more frequently than women.[7] In England, the prevalence was 7% in males and 10% in females over the age of 45.[8] Within the United States, the prevalence of radiographic hip OA in population studies has varied, ranging from 7%[9] to 28%.[10] A systematic literature review found that the prevalence of radiographic hip OA ranges between 0.9% and 27%, depending on the population studied, with a mean of 8% and a standard deviation of 7%.[11]

Much of the difficulty involved in arriving at an accurate estimate for the prevalence of hip OA is explained by differing clinical and radiographic criteria used to define the disease. Many attempts have been made to quantify the radiographic changes noted at the onset of hip OA. Kellgren and Lawrence relied on assessing progressive radiographic changes seen in OA. They used the following criteria: formation of marginal joint osteophytes; periarticular ossicles; narrowing of joint cartilage associated with sclerosis of subchondral bone; small pseudocystic areas with sclerotic walls usually found in the subchondral bone; and altered shape of the bone ends, particularly in the head of the femur. Their grading system ranges from 0 to 4 as follows: 0—no findings, 1—equivocal findings, 2—minimal findings, 3—moderate findings, and 4—severe findings.[12] Tonnis used many of the same radiographic findings but defined his grades slightly differently.[13] Grade 0 has no changes. Grade 1 has increased sclerosis of the femoral head and acetabulum, a slight decrease in the height of the cartilage, and slight osteophytes. Grade 2 reveals small cysts in the femoral head or acetabulum, a marked decrease in the height of the cartilage, and slight deviation from the round form of the femoral head. Grade 3 shows large cysts in the femoral head and acetabulum, a severe decrease in cartilage up to complete absence of the joint cleft, severe deviation of the round form of the femoral head, or avascular necrosis.

Both descriptive grading systems start with the formation of osteophytes, progress to narrowed joint spaces and small cystic changes, and conclude with severe changes in the shape of the bone ends on either side of the joint. Croft compared seven radiographic indices of hip OA in an attempt to quantify the radiographic factor most strongly associated with the clinical picture of OA.[14] Four measures of the joint space, the maximum thickness of subchondral sclerosis, and the size of the largest osteophyte were analyzed; minimum joint space was determined to be the best predictor of symptomatic OA—a conclusion that has been supported in other studies.[15-17] It is now understood that once radiographic evidence of arthrosis is visible, chondral and labral damage is irreversible, and plain radiographic findings of arthritis probably underestimate the actual prevalence of hip joint disease. Newer imaging modalities such as magnetic resonance imaging (MRI) have been improved in terms of their ability to diagnose OA before the onset of plain radiographic changes and will be used in the future for grading early findings of

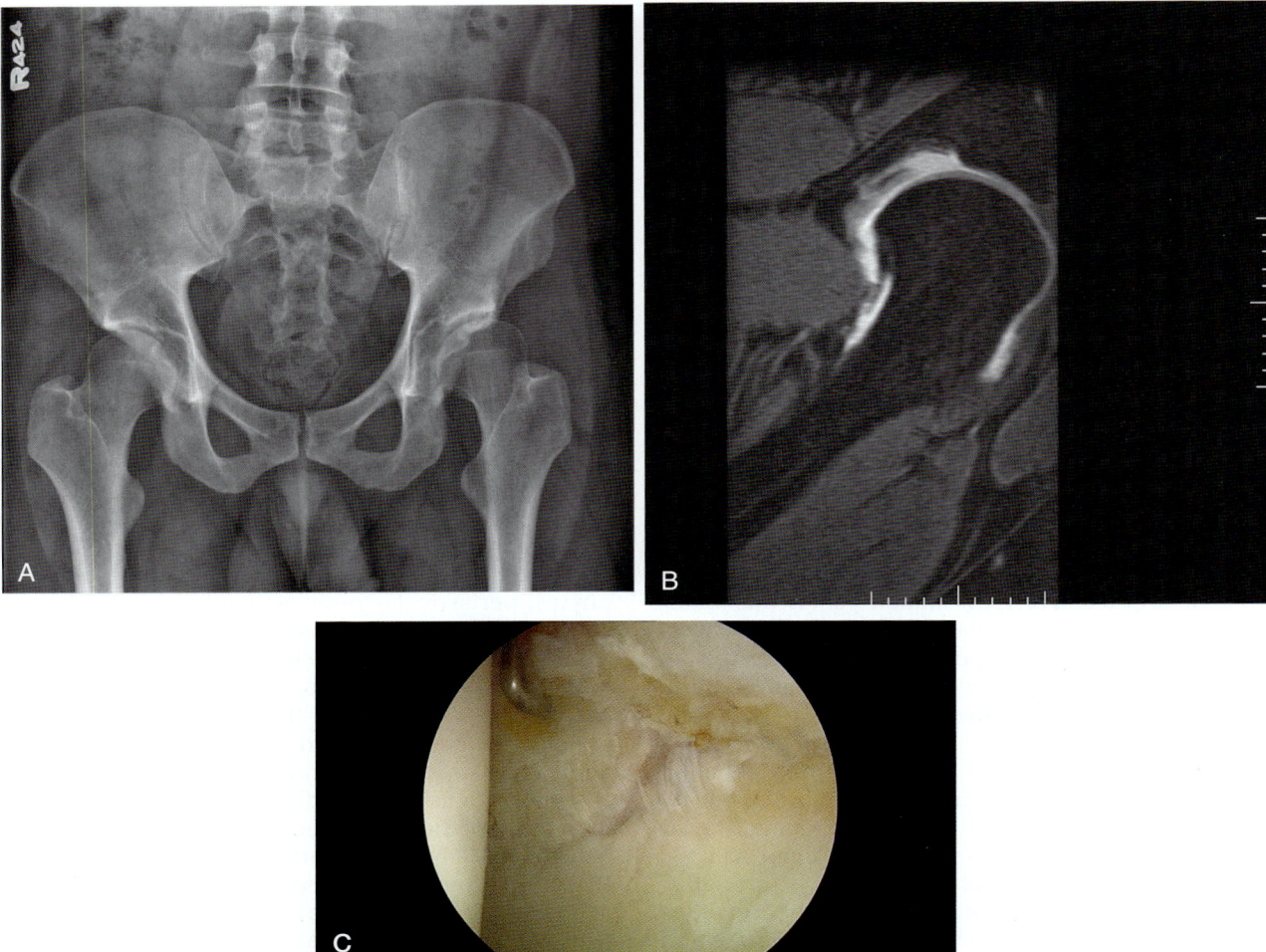

Figure 32-1. A, Anteroposterior (AP) pelvis demonstrating early arthritic changes in the left hip with sclerosis of the sourcil. **B,** Magnetic resonance imaging (MRI) arthrogram of the left hip demonstrating chondrolabral separation with paraganglion cyst formation. **C,** Hip arthroscopy images noting chondrolabral separation.

OA (Fig. 32-1). Newer biochemical imaging modalities such as delayed enhanced magnetic resonance imaging of cartilage (dGMERIC) are now used to estimate the quantity of negative charge within hyaline cartilage—a measure that correlates with chondral integrity.

Many proposed occupational and avocational risk factors for the development of OA are associated with repetitive or sustained mechanical joint overload. Any anatomic abnormality may potentiate the effects of excessive, sustained extrinsic and intrinsic joint overload. Accordingly, these individuals are at risk for developing end-stage OA at a younger age.

Obesity. The effect of body habitus on the development of OA has regional variations. In Australia, body weight, body mass index (BMI), fat mass, percentage fat, waist circumference, and waist-to-hip ratio have been correlated with increased risk of arthroplasty.[18] These factors are more highly correlated with knee OA than hip OA. A linear relationship has been noted between BMI and the risk of severe OA in Swedish construction workers.[19] Among the Dutch, obesity was associated with both self-reported OA and chronic pain; the higher the weight, the stronger was the association.[20] Compared with Caucasians, Asians presenting with end-stage OA have worse joint pain and dysfunction and present at a younger age with a lower BMI.[21] A systematic literature review for obesity as a specific risk factor for hip OA found moderate evidence of a positive association, with an odds ratio of approximately 2.[22]

Heavy manual labor. It is assumed that hips subjected to increased levels of stress are more likely to develop OA. A history of heavy manual labor seems to be associated with an increased prevalence of hip OA. A study evaluating occupational risk and hip OA in French workers showed that female cleaners had the greatest prevalence of OA with an odds ratio of 6.2, followed by women in the clothing industry (odds ratio 5.0), male construction workers (odds ratio 2.9), and agriculture workers (odds ratio 2.8). Early onset of OA was seen in those exposed to heavy labor jobs, and almost 40% reported initial symptoms before the age of 50.[23] A Finnish series demonstrated that the odds ratio of developing hip OA with a history of heavy manual labor was 6.7 compared with 5.0 for previous trauma to the hip.[24] A systematic literature review looking at 16 studies demonstrated a moderate association between previous heavy workload and the occurrence of hip OA, with an odds ratio of 3.[25]

Gender. In most series, women have a higher prevalence of hip OA than men.[26-28] Females are particularly at risk after menopause, showing a progressive postmenopausal decline in joint space compared with age-matched males.[15,29] The exact cause of this female preponderance is not known and is likely multifactorial. Alterations in hip joint biomechanics that increase the joint reactive forces in older females may cause joint overload.[30] The predilection for hip dysplasia in females and its potential to predispose to OA may contribute.

Trauma. A history of trauma to a joint surface increases the chance of developing late OA. Because the articular cartilage is avascular and has limited cellularity, its reparative capacity is limited. Consequently, trauma that alters the articular surface initiates the degenerative cascade. As the surface is exposed to physiologic joint forces, chondrocytes are unable to maintain a homeostatic environment. Consequently, degenerative changes develop and the degenerative biological cascade progresses.

Anatomic anomalies. Certain anatomic variants that have been described can predispose to the development of osteoarthritis. Subtle anatomic variations contribute to the development of femoroacetabular impingement (FAI), which has been associated with subsequent development of cartilage degeneration and osteoarthritis.[31,32] Certain conditions associated with abnormal acetabulum orientation, such as acetabular retroversion, coxa profunda, and coxa protrusion, predispose to FAI. Similarly, patients with acetabular dysplasia are at risk for damage to the chondrolabral junction and progressive development of OA. Murphy demonstrated that patients with a center edge angle of Wiberg measuring less than 16 degrees developed osteoarthritis by age 65.[33] Decreasing anterior center edge angle and the presence of a labral tear have also been associated with the development of osteoarthritis.[34] Other growth-related disorders such as Legg-Calvé-Perthes and slipped capital femoral epiphysis (SCFE) that alter the anatomy of the hip joint are associated with long-term hip dysfunction and development of osteoarthritis. The concept that FAI is a prearthritic condition has been suggested[31,32,35] and is consistent with anatomic conditions associated with repetitive abnormal contact between the proximal femur and the acetabulum. Retroverted acetabuli have been shown to be present in 20% of patients undergoing total hip arthroplasty compared with 5% of the general population.[36] Retroversion has been noted in 20% of patients with OA, 18% of patients with developmental dysplasia of the hip, 6% of patients with osteonecrosis, and 42% of patients with Legg-Calvé-Perthes.[37] Furthermore, variations in proximal femoral anatomy that decrease head-neck offset or produce aspherical femoral heads can contribute to the development of FAI and subsequent OA.

PATHOPHYSIOLOGY

Multiple anatomic and inflammatory factors predispose patients and contribute to the biomechanical environment associated with the development of hip arthritis. These may be inherited congenital anatomic variations or acquired abnormalities that may be cumulative over time. These factors eventually produce degenerative changes within the joint and the slow development of end-stage OA. Although each factor can affect the hip differently, if exposure is substantially injurious or of sufficient duration, the inflammatory cascade associated with the development of hip arthritis will follow.

Some of the early changes in hip OA are exemplified by femoroacetabular impingement. In anatomically predisposed hips, the proximal femur repetitively abuts the acetabular rim during normal range of motion or predisposing activities. Two primary pathomechanisms of FAI are predisposed: cam-type and pincer-type impingement. Cam-type impingement, a complex femoral-based deformity, results in impingement on a normal acetabulum. Resultant patterns of injury secondary to cam impingement include labral tears, chondral delamination, acetabular rim fracture, and proliferation of bone and fibrous tissue on the anterosuperior femoral neck.[31,38] Pincer-type impingement, secondary to an acetabular-based deformity, results in damage to the acetabular rim, labrum, and peripheral articular cartilage. Most commonly, patients presenting with impingement have a combination of cam and pincer features that lead to coexisting patterns of acetabular damage. The femoral head articular cartilage is generally relatively well preserved until late in the cascade of hip OA.

Articular cartilage is the primary degenerative tissue affected in hip OA. Articular cartilage is an aneural and avascular multilayered structure composed of chondrocytes, glycoproteins, matrix molecules, and water that absorbs stress and distributes loads evenly through a joint. Articular cartilage, when properly lubricated, minimizes friction between articulating surfaces and allows for pain-free range of motion. Water, adsorbed within the extracellular matrix, facilitates chondrocyte nutrition and assists in joint lubrication. Shifts in water allow cartilage to deform in response to stress. Type II collagen accounts for approximately 95% of collagen within the articular cartilage. Type II collagen functions as a framework for the cartilage and provides tensile strength. Proteoglycans provide compressive strength and are synthesized by chondrocytes in subunits called *glycosaminoglycans.*

Articular cartilage has three distinct layers: superficial, middle, and deep. The superficial layer is composed of collagen fibers arranged tangentially to the articular surface and is thought to resist shear forces. The middle layer, with fibers oriented obliquely, is thought to resist compressive forces; the deep layer, with fibers oriented vertically, resists compressive forces as well. The articular cartilage is adherent to the subchondral bone plate by the tidemark, which is a histologically unique layer of calcified cartilage that merges with the subchondral bone.

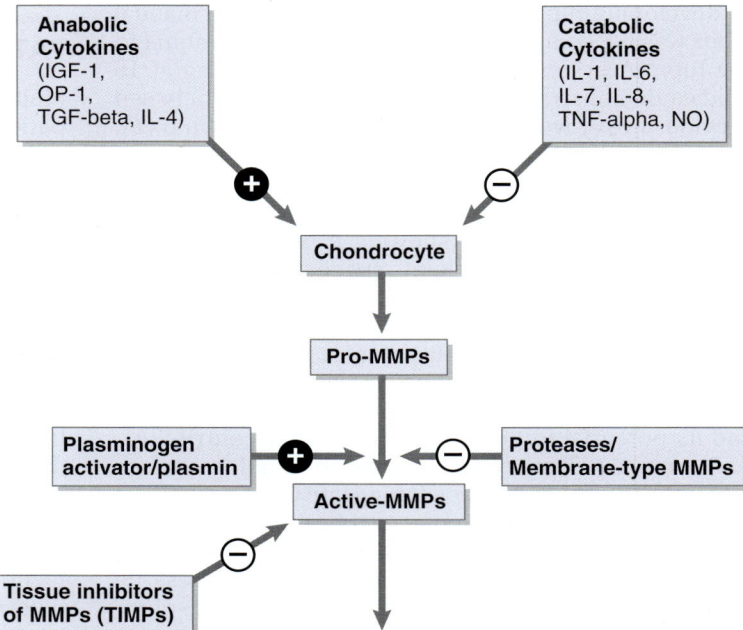

Figure 32-2. Competing anabolic and catabolic pathways leading to cartilage degradation.

In the arthritic hip, a combination of factors leads to end-stage OA. Articular cartilage depends on the integrity of its extracellular matrix for optimal function. Chondrocytes maintain a homeostatic environment by regulating competing catabolic and anabolic pathways (Fig. 32-2).[39] Biomechanical abnormalities and associated progressive chondral injury lead to damage that exceeds the capacity of the chondrocyte for repair.[40] These catabolic changes are mediated in part by cytokine production from both the synovium and the chondrocytes.[41] Cytokines act on the release of pro-matrix metalloproteinases (MMPs) by the chondrocyte. Pro-MMPs are turned into active MMPs by a process that is regulated by the plasminogen activator/plasmin system and other proteases. Active MMPs induce matrix degradation and cartilage damage, while tissue inhibitors of MMPs (TIMPs) are able to bind the active site of degradative MMPs and thus slow cartilage degradation.

Interleukin (IL)-1 and transforming growth factor-beta (TGF-β) are two of the known catabolic and anabolic stimuli for chondrocytes.[42] Catabolic cytokines such as IL-1, tumor necrosis factor-alpha (TNF-α), and inducible nitric oxide synthase (iNOS) have been localized within the superficial zone of arthritic cartilage.[43] These changes are thought to be caused by the biomechanical stresses seen in OA, as unloaded chondrocytes do not have iNOS present, whereas intermittent and static compression of chondrocytes can induce the upregulation of iNOS.[44] Chondrocyte senescence also plays a role in this balance. As the chondrocyte ages, it is less responsive to anabolic stimuli.[45] With continued improved detection of these inflammatory signaling pathways, a better understanding of this complex process will potentially guide future treatment options.

Early compositional changes seen in articular cartilage affected by osteoarthritis include an increase in water content and progressive disorganization of the collagen framework. As degeneration progresses, the articular surface becomes more susceptible to shear forces that aggravate cartilage degeneration. While proteoglycan synthesis increases, the overall content decreases and the chains become shorter secondary to marked increases in proteoglycan degradation.

As the articular surface is degenerating, changes in the subchondral bony architecture are noted. The cause of these changes is not clear, but the thickness of the subchondral bone plate increases and the trabecular architecture of the subchondral bone becomes disorderly as the layer of calcified cartilage begins to advance into the deep layer of hyaline cartilage. Subsequently, osteophytes begin to form at the articular margin, and subchondral cysts begin to form.[46] Progressive edema of the marrow is also noted.

The consequences of increased subchondral bone plate thickness have not been clearly resolved. Radin proposed that the progressive thickness and volume increase the stiffness of the subchondral bone, which negatively influences the biomechanical environment of the articular cartilage.[47] More recent contradictory studies[48-50] have demonstrated that the progressive volume of subchondral bone is associated with decreasing subchondral stiffness. Within the subchondral bone plate, an increase in the vertical orientation of trabeculae, as well as thinning of the normal trabeculae, is thought to make the area relatively osteoporotic and less able to tolerate loading.[51] Coincident with the increase in thickness of the subchondral bone plate, the zone of calcified cartilage, or the tidemark, advances.

Although the mechanism of this phenomenon has not been elucidated, progressive tidemark advancement further diminishes the thickness of the residual articular cartilage. This leads to increasing mechanical stresses in the deep zone, likely contributing to further degradation of the articular cartilage.[52]

Other pathologic changes noted include bone marrow edema, subchondral cyst formation, microfractures, and osteophyte formation. Analysis of areas of bone marrow edema revealed that 70% of patients had pseudocysts in regions of bone marrow edema with microfractures of the trabecular bone in various stages of healing. These pathologic changes correlated with the area of most severe damage of the overlying cartilage.[53] Studies of osteophyte formation in animal models have demonstrated initial proliferation of periosteal cells at the joint margin that differentiate into chondrocytes, which hypertrophy and ossify through endochondral ossification.[54] Local production of growth factors, including TGF-β and bone morphogenic proteins (BMPs), has been implicated in the formation of osteophytes.[55,56] Although osteophyte formation is ubiquitous and osteophytes are seen in areas of increased joint loading, the precise pathogenesis of osteophytes and their adaptive role remain unclear.

CLINICAL FEATURES AND DIAGNOSIS

The classic presentation of hip OA consists of gradual onset of pain in the groin, thigh, or peritrochanteric region. Initially, the pain may be activity related; however, as arthritis progresses, pain tends to increase in frequency and severity and eventually may become more consistent and easily provoked. With progression of OA, global hip range of motion typically decreases, and gait alterations may become visible.

History. A thorough history is essential in the initial evaluation of any patient presenting with hip pain; thus the patient's chief complaint is of utmost importance. Whether a patient has problems related to hip instability or impingement is often elucidated only by a careful history and physical examination. A thorough understanding of the patient's symptoms will ultimately guide treatment. A past history of developmental dysplasia of the hip (DDH), SCFE, Legg-Calvé-Perthes, malignancy, blood dyscrasia, or trauma may affect hip development. Onset of symptoms and any specific precipitating events such as a change in athletic training, as well as the nature and location of symptoms, is important. The physician should question the patient about walking tolerance and duration; sports participation; peritrochanteric, groin, buttock, thigh, or knee pain; mechanical symptoms; and night pain. A family history of hip osteoarthritis is often present. Symptoms of allied conditions such as spinal stenosis, disk herniation, lower abdominal disorders, and inflammatory disorders should be identified.

Physical examination. Physical examination is essential in the evaluation, diagnosis, and management of hip patients. Diagnoses suspected from historical assessment are often confirmed on the basis of physical examination. Patients should be inspected in standing and supine positions for limb length discrepancies, overall development, and muscular symmetry. The spine, abdomen, and pelvis should be evaluated with specific attention to palpation of the lower abdomen, inguinal region, pubis, trochanters, and anterior hips. A complete neurovascular examination should include assessment of hip muscle strength with side-lying assessment of gluteal and tensor fascia lata strength. Careful vascular assessment with palpation of lower extremity pulses is essential.

Gait should be observed with an unobstructed view of the lower extremities. Gait evaluation should record the presence of Trendelenburg and antalgic gait patterns, as well as foot progression angles. The presence of a single-leg Trendelenburg sign should be sought. The antalgic, or coxalgic, gait pattern is characterized by short strides on the affected side, so as to minimize loading of the hip joint, and a mild abductor lurch. Trendelenburg gait is characterized by an inability to sustain a level pelvis during the stance phase of the gait cycle. The hemipelvis shifts onto the affected side during stance, when the abductor lever arm is affected by joint derangement or by intrinsic muscle weakness.

Neurovascular testing should assess the motor, sensory, and vascular status of both lower extremities. This should include documentation of strength and sensation in all major muscles, and the presence and quality of lower extremity pulses should be documented. Provocative testing for lower extremity nerve tension signs should be sought if clinically indicated. Secondary signs of vascular insufficiency may indicate the presence of claudication.

Range-of-motion testing is an essential component of the physical examination. Loss of internal rotation has been shown to be the most predictive finding for hip OA in patients reporting hip pain.[57] Progressive loss of hip range of motion is a hallmark of end-stage hip OA, although the mechanism of motion loss is incompletely understood. Specific motions that should be documented include flexion in the sagittal plane, internal rotation at 90 degrees of flexion, external rotation at 90 degrees of flexion, abduction/external rotation, abduction in extension, and internal and external rotation in extension. Femoral version can be estimated with the patient in the prone position by palpating for a maximal trochanteric prominence while internally rotating the hip joint.[58]

Leg length assessment is performed with the patient in standing position. The iliac crests are palpated simultaneously to detect a pelvic obliquity and to estimate the degree of limb length inequality. Blocks of varying thickness placed beneath the short limb will assist the examiner in estimating the magnitude of leg length difference. Apparent limb lengths can be measured from the anterior superior iliac spine (ASIS) to the medial malleolus. The presence of a fixed pelvic obliquity secondary to a hip contracture or a lumbar spine abnormality is important to document, particularly when reconstructive surgery is contemplated.

Clinical signs of femoroacetabular impingement have been shown to be similar to those of hip OA.[59] In one series, pain was present in the groin 83% of the time. Most reliably, patients had pain with anterior impingement testing 88% of the time. The presence of an impingement sign is usually assessed with the patient supine by flexing, slightly adducting, and simultaneously internally rotating the hip to produce pain (Fig. 32-3). Posterior impingement should be tested by flexing, abducting, and externally rotating the hip joint, or by lying supine with the legs hanging off the end of the examining table and externally rotating the femur to elicit pain.[60]

Other provocative tests used in hip examination include the following:

- **Ober's test** may be associated with trochanteric bursitis or lateral snapping hip syndrome secondary to iliotibial band dysfunction. It is performed with the patient in the lateral decubitus position with the symptomatic side toward the examiner. The patient's knee is flexed to 90 degrees, and the hip is abducted maximally. The hip is then extended and the hip joint gradually adducted. Pain or the inability to get past neutral adduction is considered indicative of greater trochanteric pathology.
- **Patrick's test,** also known as the *FABER (flexion, abduction, external rotation) test,* for the position in which the test is performed, is classically a provocative test for the sacroiliac joint. The patient is positioned supine, and the limb to be examined is in the figure-of-four position, abducted and externally rotated. The examiner pushes posteriorly on the ipsilateral knee while stabilizing the contralateral anterior superior iliac spine. The production of pain may indicate sacroiliac dysfunction, posterior impingement, or anterior instability, depending on the location of perceived discomfort.
- **Stinchfield's test** is a nonspecific test for the presence of intra-articular hip pathology. The patient, in

supine position, is asked to maintain the knee in extension while flexing the hip against the examiner's resistance. Pain reported in the groin suggests the presence of intra-articular pathology.

Radiographic studies. Once a detailed history and physical examination have been completed, initial radiographs in the anteroposterior (AP) and lateral (cross-table or frog) directions should be obtained. An accurate AP pelvis x-ray is obtained by directing the beam orthogonal to the frontal plane, midway between the pubis and a line connecting the anterosuperior iliac spines to eliminate pelvic rotation and flexion.[61] Plain radiographs are assessed for soft tissue and bone abnormalities. Early radiographic signs of acetabular osteoarthritis include sclerosis of the subchondral bone plate, asymmetrical hip joint space narrowing, small radiolucent subchondral cysts, and a floor osteophyte. Early signs of femoral osteoarthritis include inferior head-neck junctional osteophyte, foveal osteophytes, and anterolateral herniation pits (subchondral cysts) (Fig. 32-4). Despite normal appearing radiographs, chondral and labral damage may be severe, and MRI studies have proved more sensitive in detecting early joint derangement.

Normal AP and cross-table lateral radiographs do not exclude abnormalities of the femoral head-neck junction,[62] and a combination of specialized plain x-rays and MRI arthrography can be used to completely evaluate patients with hip pain. In attempts to assess femoral head-neck sphericity in these patients, it has been demonstrated that a Dunn view in 45 or 90 degrees of hip flexion best evaluates the most common region of asphericity: the anterosuperior femoral head.[63] The Dunn view is obtained with the hip in neutral rotation and 20 degrees of abduction with 45 or 90 degrees of hip flexion. Anterior femoral head coverage and superoanterior hip joint space narrowing can be assessed using the false-profile radiograph performed with the patient standing 65 degrees oblique to the cassette with the contralateral hip rotated posteriorly to avoid superimposition of the two hips. The frog-lateral radiograph has been shown to accurately visualize the femoral head-neck offset in patients evaluated for FAI[64] and can also be useful in evaluation of posterior head-neck pathology.

Frequently, patients with normal appearing radiographs present with advanced stages of chondral and labral degeneration. Excessive osteoarthritis damage often precludes surgical preservation of the hip. Advanced imaging studies, including MRI arthrography and dGMERIC techniques, are useful in assessment of chondral damage. MRI obtained using a 3-Tesla magnet with a dedicated body or hip coil provides superior imaging.[65] Head-neck damage is best visualized using radial sequence images, which are reconstructions of axial views orthogonal to the acetabular plane and sagittal obliques parallel to the acetabular plane.[66] These image sequences are superior to standard orthogonal MRI in the diagnosis of labral pathology, associated chondral damage, and alterations in the head-neck junction that are not as well visualized on conventional radiographs.

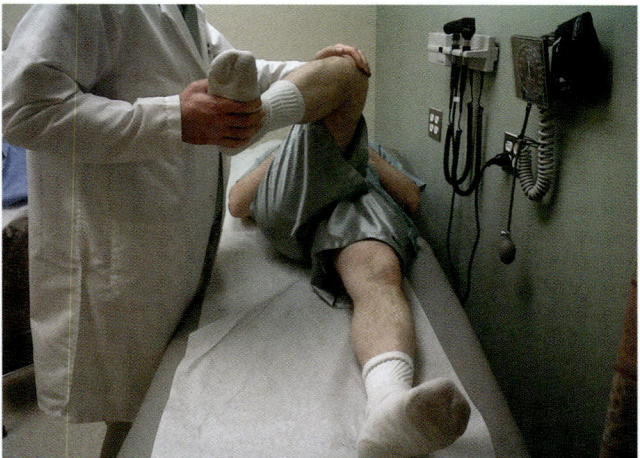

Figure 32-3. Impingement test. The involved lower extremity is flexed, internally rotated, and adducted to re-create symptoms of femoroacetabular impingement.

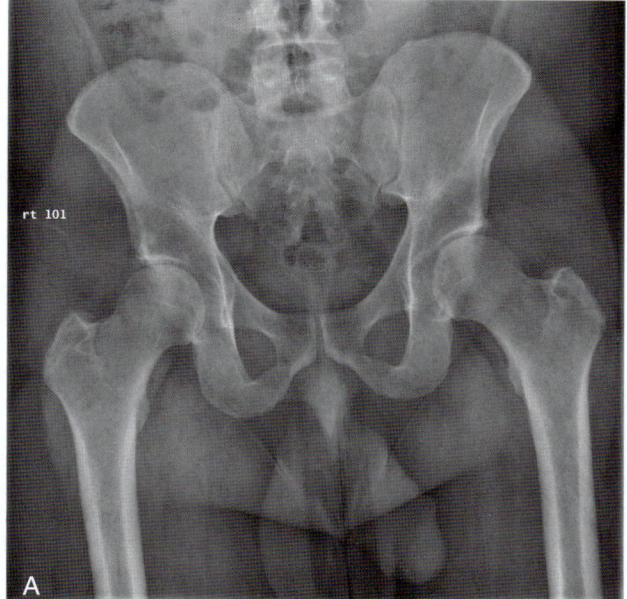

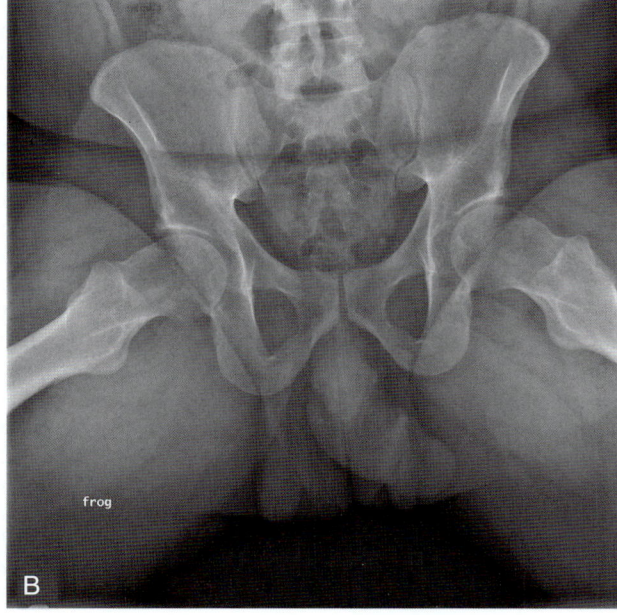

Figure 32-4. Early radiographic changes in osteoarthritis (OA). Anteroposterior (AP) and frog lateral radiographs demonstrate sclerosis of the subchondral bone plate, mild hip joint space narrowing, and inferior head-neck junctional osteophytes.

DIFFERENTIAL DIAGNOSIS

Accurate diagnosis of hip, pelvic, buttock, and lower back pain can be challenging. Variable contributions to hip joint sensation from the obturator, femoral, and sciatic nerves account for the diversity of symptoms that may originate in the hip joint. These include the following:

- Trochanteric bursitis
- Sacroiliitis

Table 32-1. Nonsurgical Treatment Options for Osteoarthritis of the Hip

Nonsurgical	Comments
Medical therapies	
• Nonsteroidal anti-inflammatory drugs (NSAIDs)	• Comparable pain relief to acetaminophen • Potential for gastrointestinal side effects • Some selective COX-2 inhibitors have been withdrawn from U.S. market because of cardiovascular side effects.
• Acetaminophen	• Comparable pain relief to NSAIDs • Potential for hepatic toxicity with greater than 4 g/day ingestion
• Glucosamine and chondroitin sulfate	• Unclear benefit, dosing has not been optimized • Potential for allergic reactions
Weight loss/exercise	• Marginal benefit for hip OA • More pronounced improvement with knee OA
Viscosupplementation	• Requires fluoroscopic guidance • Not currently FDA approved for the hip in the United States
Alternative therapies (acupuncture, massage, manipulations, etc.)	• No support in the literature for any long-lasting pain relief

COX, Cyclo-oxygenase; *FDA,* U.S. Food and Drug Administration; *OA,* osteoarthritis.

- Lateral femoral cutaneous nerve entrapment
- Lumbar spine degenerative disease
- Herniated lumbar disk
- Retroperitoneal disease
- Renal and collecting system diseases
- Abdominal wall hernia
- Femoral head osteonecrosis
- Bone or soft tissue tumor of pelvis or hip
- Peripheral vascular disease
- Piriformis syndrome
- Ischiogluteal bursitis
- Femoropelvic impingement
- Fracture
- Infection
- Inflammatory disease and crystalline arthropathy
- Snapping iliopsoas or tensor fascia lata
- Osteitis pubis
- Sports complex hernia

TREATMENT

Multiple modalities are available for the treatment of hip osteoarthritis (Tables 32-1 and 32-2). Selection of the most appropriate option is dependent on the stage of osteoarthritis, the severity of symptoms, occupation, avocation, body habitus, allied medical conditions, and desired level of activity.

Table 32-2. Surgical Treatment Options for Osteoarthritis of the Hip

Surgical	Comment
Surgical hip dislocation (SHD)	• Muscle-sparing approach • Allows complete visualization of the femoral head and acetabulum • Addresses chondral and labral damage and femoral head-neck junction remodeling
Periacetabular osteotomy (PAO)	• Addresses disorders of acetabular version and/or volume • Most effective in patients with no to minimal radiographic changes in OA
Hip arthroscopy	• Limitations in the ability to visualize and treat pathology • Anterior and lateral portions are well visualized, but posterior access is limited. • May be combined with anterior arthrotomy for osteochondroplasty
Arthrodesis	• Historically used for young patients with unilateral end-stage degenerative joint disease • Gait adaptations and energy expenditure are increased. • May require late conversion to THA, which is a more complex procedure
Arthroplasty	• Gold standard for end-stage degenerative joint disease • Optimal approach, bearing surface, and implants are controversial

OA, Osteoarthritis; *THA*, total hip arthroplasty.

Medical therapies. The first line of treatment for the relief of pain associated with hip osteoarthritis is medication. Many different classes of agents are available and have been used with varying effects. Initial treatment is typically an over-the-counter analgesic such as acetaminophen or a nonsteroidal anti-inflammatory drug (NSAID). Acetaminophen is effective in relieving mild to moderate pain from both knee and hip osteoarthritis.[67,68] Recent literature suggests that both acetaminophen and NSAIDs are more efficacious than placebo in randomized controlled trials. NSAIDs have been shown to be more effective than acetaminophen in achieving pain reduction and improvements in functional status.[69]

The overall safety profile of acetaminophen and those of NSAIDs are nearly equivalent. Acetaminophen dosing should not exceed 4 g/day because of potential hepatic toxicity. NSAID medications have a low risk profile, with gastrointestinal abnormalities ranging from dyspepsia to hemorrhage being the most frequently encountered side effects. The relative risk that an NSAID will cause a gastrointestinal effect is 1.47.[69]

NSAIDs work by inhibiting the production of prostaglandins in the cyclo-oxygenase (COX) pathway. One strategy that can diminish the frequency of gastrointestinal side effects is the use of selective COX-2 inhibitors, which do not interfere with the normal production of prostaglandins and thromboxane. COX-2 inhibitors are as clinically effective as nonspecific NSAIDs but have a reduced incidence of gastrointestinal side effects.[70] However, COX-2 inhibitors potentially cause both renal and cardiovascular side effects. In 2004, rofecoxib and valdecoxib were withdrawn from the market over concerns regarding their cardiovascular side effect profiles. Despite this, celecoxib remains on the market with a black box warning that it may increase the risk of serious and potentially fatal cardiovascular thrombotic events, myocardial infarction, and stroke. No statistically significant evidence shows that celecoxib has a higher risk profile for cardiovascular events than nonselective NSAIDs.[71]

Medications—glucosamine and chondroitin sulfate. Two over-the-counter nutritional supplements have received considerable attention for their ability to relieve pain associated with osteoarthritis. Glucosamine sulfate is a precursor to glycosaminoglycans, and chondroitin sulfate is the most prevalent glycosaminoglycan found in articular cartilage. Although the mechanisms of action are not clearly known, it has been proposed that supplementation with these molecules may slow cartilage degradation by stimulating chondrocyte synthesis of glycosaminoglycans and inhibiting degradative enzymes detrimental in OA.[72] This mechanism is thought to positively affect the structure of articular cartilage in the osteoarthritic joint.[73] Some studies have shown marginal clinical benefit in the short term for patients with moderate to severe OA.[73] The largest randomized trial has shown that these agents were no more effective than placebo.[72] Certain formulations of glucosamine, particularly the Rotta preparation, have been shown to be superior to placebo in terms of pain relief and functional improvement.[74] The optimal treatment duration is not known, and adverse allergic reactions have been reported.

Weight loss and exercise. Because mechanical joint overload is implicated in the pathogenesis of osteoarthritis, decreased loading is often a first-line recommendation. Weight loss and periarticular muscle strengthening have been shown to improve functional outcomes and pain scores for both hip and knee OA, with a more pronounced effect noted in knee patients.[75] Two systematic reviews concluded that exercise has a small beneficial effect in decreasing pain in the hip but is not beneficial for self-reported physical function.[76,77] Because no well-controlled trials have been designed to study the effect of exercise on OA, its role in management has not been precisely defined.

Viscosupplementation. Many different formulations of viscosupplementation are commercially available; however, these modalities are traditionally reserved for patients with knee OA. Especially outside the United States, interest in the use of intra-articular hyalurons to treat the symptoms of hip OA has increased. A systematic review of the literature identified 16 studies predominantly conducted in Europe that assessed the effectiveness of viscosupplementation in the hip. When performed under fluoroscopic or ultrasound guidance, viscosupplementation was effective for the treatment of hip OA.[78] Indications for and usage of viscosupplementation in hip OA will continue to evolve, but currently it is not approved by the U.S. Food and Drug Administration (FDA) for use in any joint except the knee. Potential complications include septic arthritis, injection site reactions, and pseudoseptic inflammatory arthritis.

Alternative treatments. Alternative therapies are often sought by the patient in an attempt to delay surgical intervention or to improve pain relief. Modalities such as acupuncture, massage, manipulation, and spa therapy are commonly advocated. Studies evaluating acupuncture report contradictory results. Acupuncture has been found to improve Western Ontario and McMaster Osteoarthritis Index (WOMAC) scores and quality-of-life assessments versus controls—an effect maintained for a period of 6 months.[79] Other reviews, however, have revealed moderate evidence that acupuncture does little for joint pain or function.[80] Selective European studies have supported the use of spa therapy,[81] although many of these studies lack sufficient follow-up to determine whether immediate effects on quality of life, pain, and self-esteem are long lasting.

Nonarthroplasty options. Multiple surgical procedures have been designed to reorient the acetabulum and/or the proximal femur. These are often performed in the young adult population to prevent or slow patients' progression to end-stage OA. The indications for nonarthroplasty procedures are not precisely defined at the present time. Most authors agree that for a joint to be preserved, it must be concentric with no asymmetrical narrowing of the joint space. Furthermore, secondary signs of osteoarthritis should not be present.

Patients with FAI are potential candidates for surgical dislocation or arthroscopy to address damaged labral and cartilage tissue and to remodel the upper femur and head-neck junction. Surgical hip dislocation[82,83] is performed through a muscle-preserving Gibson approach[84] using a trochanteric osteotomy to retract the gluteus medius and vastus lateralis. This procedure allows for dislocation of the femoral head without detachment of the short external rotators and is designed to protect the medial femoral circumflex artery and the vascular retinaculum. The procedure provides a full view of both the femoral head and the acetabulum and allows evaluation of all deformities, as well as dynamic assessment of the hip joint. The spectrum of pathology that has been implicated in the pathogenesis of osteoarthritis secondary to femoroacetabular impingement involves the acetabular hyaline cartilage, the acetabular labrum, the femoral head and head-neck junction, and the morphology of the upper femur. Relief of femoroacetabular impingement and repair of damaged tissue require proper preoperative and intraoperative assessment and access. Although arthroscopic techniques continue to develop, surgical dislocation currently provides superior joint visualization.

Periacetabular osteotomy (PAO) is currently utilized to address disorders of acetabular version and volume and is indicated in symptomatic individuals with preserved hyaline cartilage and concentric articular surfaces. It is contraindicated in patients with excessive posterior wall coverage, significant combined cam and pincer impingement, and advanced degeneration of the anterior aspect of the acetabulum.[66] Periacetabular osteotomy is most effective in patients who have no or minimal osteoarthritic changes on plain radiographs, as the risk of conversion to total hip arthroplasty increases with increasing Tonnis stage.[85] Preoperative characteristics predictive of poor postoperative outcome include age at surgery, low preoperative Merle d'Aubigné and Postel scores, presence of anterior impingement test, presence of a limp, advancing OA grade, and postoperative extrusion index.[86] Intermediate to long-term results are available for this procedure, with 76% of hips preserved at 9 years[87] and 60% of the first 75 hips originally treated by Professor Ganz preserved at 19 years.[86] Patients who have a periacetabular osteotomy on one side and a total hip arthroplasty on the other report higher satisfaction scores for PAO compared with arthroplasty at follow-up greater than 5 years.[88]

Hip arthroscopy is a developing technique for assessment and treatment of deformities associated with the development of hip OA. Its ability to visualize pathology and to adequately address labral and acetabular sided lesions is limited, but in the correctly selected patient, it can be a useful tool in treating the early arthritic hip. Anterior and lateral portions of the hip are well visualized, but access to posterior femoral neck and acetabular regions remains a challenge. Dynamic assessment of joint motion is incomplete, and radiographic views are utilized intraoperatively to evaluate the adequacy of femoral head-neck osteochondroplasty. Hip arthroscopy may be performed in conjunction with a small anterior arthrotomy for osteochondroplasty of the head-neck junction. This may allow more complete assessment of the head-neck junction than can be performed through the arthroscope with less morbidity than a surgical hip dislocation procedure. Precise indications for hip arthroscopy, anterior arthrotomy, and surgical dislocation continue to evolve.

Arthrodesis. Hip arthrodesis is an option for select young patients with developmental or acquired hip osteoarthritis. The optimal position for hip arthrodesis is 5 to 10 degrees of external rotation, 20 to 30 degrees of flexion, neutral to 5 degrees of adduction, and limb length discrepancy less than 2 cm.[89] Musculoskeletal adaptations necessary to accommodate a fused hip include an increase in lumbar lordosis to assist hip extension and a decrease in coronal plane motion to reduce joint loads.[90] Although pain relief following an arthrodesis is reproducible, energy expenditures in ambulation are approximately 30% higher than in patients without hip fusion. Complications include nonunion, malpositioning, and development of arthritis in adjacent joints, especially the knee and lumbar spine.[91] Late conversion to total hip arthroplasty is performed for pain in the lumbar spine, ipsilateral knee, or contralateral hip. Recovery from surgical conversion is longer and requires prolonged use of assistive devices for ambulation, and the surgery itself is more technically demanding with a higher infection rate.[89,92]

Arthroplasty. Total hip arthroplasty is the standard treatment for end-stage hip OA. Multiple anatomic approaches and prosthetic devices are available, each indicated by the specific clinical situation. Development of alternate bearing surfaces and prosthetic design continue to improve wear characteristics, implant fixation, and survivorship.

PROGNOSIS

An understanding of anatomic deformities associated with the development of hip arthritis and their pathomechanical consequences has improved our ability to treat patients during the early stages of hip arthritis. Imaging modalities, particularly those designed to evaluate chondral structures, are enabling detection of early-stage osteoarthritis and are helping is understand the natural history of hip OA. Improvements in prosthetic design and implantation techniques allow arthroplasty use in younger and more active individuals. The use of nonprosthetic procedures for relief of symptoms and prevention of arthritis is increasing as our understanding of the disease process improves.

CURRENT CONTROVERSIES AND FUTURE CONSIDERATIONS

- Improvement in chondral mapping sequences and evaluation of cartilage in early-stage OA
- Understanding the rate of hip joint deterioration
- Natural history of femoroacetabular impingement
- Impact of joint preservation surgery on disease natural history
- Prosthetic design and application
- Hip arthroscopy

REFERENCES

1. Keuttner KE, Goldberg VM (eds): Osteoarthritic disorders, Rosemont, Ill, 1995, American Academy of Orthopaedic Surgeons.
2. Ricci JA, Stewart WF, Chee E, et al: Pain exacerbation as a major source of lost productive time in US workers with arthritis. Arthritis Rheum 53:673–681, 2005.
3. Lawrence RC, Felson DT, Helmick CG, et al: Estimates of the prevalence of arthritis and other rheumatic conditions in the United States: part II. Arthritis Rheum 58:26–35, 2008.
4. Hootman JM, Helmick CG: Projections of US prevalence of arthritis and associated activity limitations. Arthritis Rheum 54:226–229, 2006.
5. Michaud CM, McKenna MT, Begg S, et al: The burden of disease and injury in the United States 1996. Popul Health Metr 4:11, 2006.
6. Juhaksoki R, Heliovaara M, Impivaara O, et al: Risk factors for the development of hip osteoarthritis: a population-based prospective study. Rheumatology (Oxford) 48:83–87, 2009.
7. Kim HA, Koh SH, Lee B, et al: Low rate of total hip replacement as reflected by a low prevalence of hip osteoarthritis in South Korea. Osteoarthritis Cartilage 16:1572–1575, 2008.
8. Birrell F, Lunt M, Macfarlane G, Silman A: Association between pain in the hip region and radiographic changes of osteoarthritis: results from a population-based study. Rheumatology (Oxford) 44:337–341, 2005.
9. Nevitt MC, Lane NE, Scott JC, et al: Radiographic osteoarthritis of the hip and bone mineral density. Arthritis Rheum 38:907–916, 1995.
10. Jordan JM, Helmick CG, Renner JB, et al: Prevalence of hip symptoms and radiographic and symptomatic hip osteoarthritis in African Americans and Caucasians: the Johnston County Osteoarthritis Project. J Rheumatol 36:809–815, 2009.
11. Dagenais S, Garbedian S, Wai EK: Systematic review of the prevalence of radiographic primary hip osteoarthritis. Clin Orthop Relat Res 467:623–637, 2009.
12. Kellgren JH, Lawrence JS: Radiological assessment of osteoarthrosis. Ann Rheum Dis 16:494–502, 1957.
13. Tonnis D: Normal values of the hip joint for the evaluation of x-rays in children and adults. Clin Orthop Relat Res 119:39–47, 1976.
14. Croft P, Cooper C, Wickham C, Coggon D: Defining osteoarthritis of the hip for epidemiologic studies. Am J Epidemiol 132:514–522, 1990.
15. Jacobsen S: Adult hip dysplasia and osteoarthritis: studies in radiology and clinical epidemiology. Acta Orthop Suppl 77:1–37, 2006.
16. Jacobsen S, Sonne-Holm S, Soballe K, et al: Radiographic case definitions and prevalence of osteoarthrosis of the hip: a survey of 4151 subjects in the Osteoarthritis Substudy of the Copenhagen City Heart Study. Acta Orthop Scand 75:713–720, 2004.
17. Reijman M, Hazes JM, Koes BW, et al: Validity, reliability, and applicability of seven definitions of hip osteoarthritis used in epidemiological studies: a systematic review. Ann Rheum Dis 63:226–232, 2004.
18. Wang Y, Simpson JA, Wluka AE, et al: Relationship between body adiposity measures and risk of primary knee and hip replacement for osteoarthritis: a prospective cohort study. Arthritis Res Ther 11:R31, 2009.
19. Jarvholm B, Lewold S, Malchau H, Vingard E: Age, bodyweight, smoking habits and the risk of severe osteoarthritis in the hip and knee in men. Eur J Epidemiol 20:537–542, 2005.
20. Tukker A, Visscher TL, Picavet HS: Overweight and health problems of the lower extremities: osteoarthritis, pain, and disability. Public Health Nutr 12:359–368, 2009.
21. Gandhi R, Razak F, Mahomed NN: Ethnic differences in the relationship between obesity and joint pain and function in a joint arthroplasty population. J Rheumatol 35:1874–1877, 2008.
22. Lievense AM, Bierma-Zeinstra SM, Verhagen AP, et al: Influence of obesity on the development of osteoarthritis of the hip: a systematic review. Rheumatology (Oxford) 41:1115–1162, 2002.
23. Rossignol M, Leclerc A, Allaert FA, et al: Primary osteoarthritis of hip, knee, and hand in relation to occupational exposure. Occup Environ Med 62:772–777, 2005.
24. Juhakoski R, Heliovaara M, Impivaara O, et al: Risk factors for the development of hip osteoarthritis: a population-based prospective study. Rheumatology (Oxford) 48:83–87, 2009.
25. Lievense A, Bierma-Zeinstra S, Verhagen A, et al: Influence of work on the development of osteoarthritis of the hip: a systematic review. J Rheumatol 28:2520–2528, 2001.
26. Scher DL, Belmont PJ Jr, Mountcastle S, Owens BD: The incidence of primary hip osteoarthritis in active duty US military service members. Arthritis Rheum 61:468–475, 2009.
27. Srikanth VK, Fryer JL, Zhai G, et al: A meta-analysis of sex differences prevalence, incidence and severity of osteoarthritis. Osteoarthritis Cartilage 13:769–781, 2005.
28. Arden NK, Lane NE, Parimi N, et al: Defining incident radiographic hip osteoarthritis for epidemiologic studies in women. Arthritis Rheum 60:1052–1059, 2009.
29. Lanyon P, Muir K, Doherty S, Doherty M: Age and sex differences in hip joint space among asymptomatic subjects without structural change: implications for epidemiologic studies. Arthritis Rheum 48:1041–1046, 2003.
30. Boyer KA, Beaupre GS, Andriacchi TP: Gender differences exist in the hip joint moments of healthy older walkers. J Biomech 41:3360–3365, 2008.
31. Ganz R, Parvizi J, Beck M, et al: Femoroacetabular impingement: a cause for osteoarthritis of the hip. Clin Orthop Relat Res 417:112–120, 2003.
32. Siebenrock KA, Schoeniger R, Ganz R: Anterior femoroacetabular impingement due to acetabular retroversion: treatment with periacetabular osteotomy. J Bone Joint Surg Am 85:278–286, 2003.

33. Murphy SB, Ganz R, Muller ME: The prognosis in untreated dysplasia of the hip: a study of radiographic factors that predict outcome. J Bone Joint Surg Am 77:985–989, 1995.

34. Jessel RH, Zurakowski D, Zilkens C, et al: Radiographic and patient factors associated with pre-radiographic osteoarthritis in hip dysplasia. J Bone Joint Surg Am 91:1120–1129, 2009.

35. Reynolds D, Lucas J, Klaue K: Retroversion of the acetabulum: a cause of hip pain. J Bone Joint Surg Br 81:281–288, 1999.

36. Giori NJ, Trousdale RT: Acetabular retroversion is associated with osteoarthrosis of the hip. Clin Orthop Relat Res 417: 263–269, 2003.

37. Ezoe M, Naito M, Inoue T: The prevalence of acetabular retroversion among various disorders of the hip. J Bone Joint Surg Am 88:372–379, 2006.

38. Ito K, Minka MA 2nd, Leunig M, et al: Femoroacetabular impingement and the cam-effect: an MRI-based quantitative anatomical study of the femoral head-neck offset. J Bone Joint Surg Br 83:171–176, 2001.

39. Aigner T, Soeder S, Haag J: IL-1 beta and BMPs—interactive players of cartilage matrix degeneration and regeneration. Eur Cell Mater 12:49–56, 2006.

40. Dieppe PA, Lohmander LS: Pathogenesis and management of pain in osteoarthritis. Lancet 365:965–973, 2005.

41. Abramson SB: Inflammation in osteoarthritis. J Rheumatol Suppl 70:70–76, 2004.

42. Lotz M, Blanco FJ, von Kempis J, et al: Cytokine regulation of chondrocyte functions. J Rheumatol Suppl 43:104–108, 1995.

43. Melchiorri C, Meliconi R, Frizziero L, et al: Enhanced and coordinated in vivo expression of inflammatory cytokines and nitric oxide synthase by chondrocytes from patients with osteoarthritis. Arthritis Rheum 41:2165–2174, 1998.

44. Fermor B, Weinberg JB, Pisetsky DS, et al: The effects of static and intermittent compression on nitric oxide synthase production in articular cartilage explants. J Orthop Res 19: 729–737, 2001.

45. Martin JA, Buckwalter JA: The role of chondrocyte senescence in the pathogenesis of osteoarthritis and in limiting cartilage repair. J Bone Joint Surg Am 85:106–110, 2003.

46. Goldring SR: The role of bone in osteoarthritis pathogenesis. Rhem Dis Clin N Am 34:561–571, 2008.

47. Radin EL, Rose RM: Role of subchondral bone in the initiation and progression of cartilage damage. Clin Orthop Relat Res 213:34–40, 1986.

48. Burr DB: Anatomy and physiology of the mineralized tissues: role in the pathogenesis of osteoarthritis. Osteoarthritis Cartilage 12(Suppl A):S20–S30, 2004.

49. Day JS, Ding M, Van der Linden JC, et al: A decreased subchondral trabecular bone tissue elastic modulus is associated with pre-arthritic cartilage damage. J Orthop Res 19:914–918, 2001.

50. Li B, Aspden RM: Mechanical and material properties of the subchondral bone plate from the femoral head of patients with osteoarthritis or osteoporosis. Ann Rheum Dis 56:247–254, 1997.

51. Karvonen RL, Miller PR, Nelson DA, et al: Periarticular osteoporosis in osteoarthritis of the knee. J Rheumatol 25:2187–2194, 1998.

52. Burr DB, Schaffler MB: The involvement of subchondral mineralized tissues in osteoarthrosis: quantitative microscopic evidence. Microsc Res Tech 37:343–357, 1997.

53. Taljanovic MS, Graham AR, Benjamin JB, et al: Bone marrow edema pattern in advanced hip osteoarthritis: quantitative assessment with magnetic resonance imaging and correlation with clinical examination, radiographic findings, and histopathology. Skeletal Radiol 37:423–431, 2008.

54. Van der Kraan PM, van den Berg WB: Osteophytes: relevance and biology. Osteoarthritis Cartilage 15:237–244, 2007.

55. Zoricic S, Maric I, Bobinac D, Vukicevic S: Expression of bone morphogenic proteins and cartilage-derived morphogenic proteins during osteophyte formation in humans. J Anat 202(Pt 3):269–277, 2003.

56. Blaney Davidson EN, van der Kraan PM, van den Berg WB: TGF-beta and osteoarthritis. Osteoarthritis Cartilage 15: 597–604, 2007.

57. Birrell F, Croft P, Cooper C, et al: Predicting radiographic hip osteoarthritis from range of movement. Rheumatology (Oxford) 40:506–512, 2001.

58. Ruwe PA, Gage JR, Ozonoff MB, DeLuca PA: Clinical determination of femoral anteversion: a comparison with established techniques. J Bone Joint Surg Am 74:820–830, 1992.

59. Clohisy JC, Knaus ER, Hunt DM, et al: Clinical presentation of patients with symptomatic anterior hip impingement. Clin Orthop Relat Res 467:638–644, 2009.

60. Leunig M, Beck M, Dora C, Ganz R: Femoroacetabular impingement: etiology and surgical concepts. Oper Tech Orthop 15:247–255, 2005.

61. Siebenrock KA, Karlbertmatten DF, Ganz R: Effect of pelvic tilt on acetabular retroversion: a study of pelves from cadavers. Clin Orthop Relat Res 407:241–248, 2003.

62. Dudda M, Albers C, Mamisch TC, et al: Do normal radiographs exclude asphericity of the femoral head-neck junction? Clin Orthop Relat Res 467:651–659, 2009.

63. Meyer DC, Beck M, Ellis T, et al: Comparison of six radiographic projections to assess femoral head/neck asphericity. Clin Orthop Relat Res 445:181–185, 2006.

64. Clohisy JC, Nunley RM, Otto RJ, Schoenecker PL: The frog-leg lateral radiograph accurately visualized hip cam impingement abnormalities. Clin Orthop Relat Res 462:115–121, 2007.

65. Mamisch TC, Bittersohl B, Hughes T, et al: Magnetic resonance imaging of the hip at 3 Tesla: clinical value in femoracetabular impingement of the hip and current concepts. Semin Musculoskelet Radiol 12:212–222, 2008.

66. Sierra RJ, Trousdale RT, Ganz R, Leunig M: Hip disease in the young, active patient: evaluation and nonarthroplasty surgical options. J Am Acad Orthop Surg 16:689–703, 2008.

67. Zhang W, Moskowitz RW, Nuki G, et al: OARSI recommendations for the management of hip and knee osteoarthritis. Part II: OARSI evidence-based, expert consensus guidelines. Osteoarthritis Cartilage 16:137–162, 2008.

68. Hochberg MC, Altman RD, Brandt KD, et al: Guidelines for the medical management of osteoarthritis. Part I. Osteoarthritis of the hip. American College of Rheumatology. Arthritis Rheum 38:1535–1540, 1995.

69. Towheed TE, Maxwell L, Judd MG, et al: Acetaminophen for osteoarthritis. Cochrane Database Syst Rev 25(1):CD004257, 2006.

70. Singh G, Fort JG, Goldstein JL, et al: Celecoxib versus naproxen and diclofenac in osteoarthritis patients: SUCCESS-1 study. Am J Med 119:255–266, 2006.

71. McGettigan P, Henry D: Cardiovascular risk and inhibition of cyclooxygenase: a systematic review of the observational studies of selective and nonselective inhibitors of cyclooxygenase 2. JAMA 296:1633–1644, 2006.

72. Clegg DO, Reda DJ, Harris CL, et al: Glucosamine, chondroitin sulfate, and the two in combination for painful knee osteoarthritis. N Engl J Med 354:795–808, 2006.

73. Bruyere O, Reginster JY: Glucosamine and chondroitin sulfate as therapeutic agents for knee and hip osteoarthritis. Drugs Aging 24:573–580, 2007.

74. Towheed TE, Maxwell L, Anastassiades TP, et al: Glucosamine therapy for treating osteoarthritis. Cochrane Database Syst Rev 18(2):CD002946, 2005.

75. Roddy E, Zhang W, Doherty M, et al: Evidence-based recommendations for the role of exercise in the management of osteoarthritis of the hip or knee: the MOVE consensus. Rheumatology (Oxford) 44:67–73, 2005.

76. Fransen M, McConnell S, Hernandz-Molina G, Reichenbach S: Exercise for osteoarthritis of the hip. Cochrane Database Syst Rev (3):CD007912, 2009.

77. McNair PJ, Simmonds MA, Boocock MG, Larmer PJ: Exercise therapy for the management of osteoarthritis of the hip joint: a systematic review. Arthritis Res Ther 11:R98, 2009.

78. van den Bekerom MP, Lamme B, Sermon A, Mulier M: What is the evidence for viscosupplementation in the treatment of patients with hip osteoarthritis? Systematic review of the literature. Arch Orthop Trauma Surg 128:815–823, 2008.

79. Witt CM, Jena S, Brinkhaus B, et al: Acupuncture in patients with osteoarthrosis of the knee or hip: a randomized,

controlled trial with an additional nonrandomized arm. Arthritis Rheum 54:3485–3493, 2006.

80. Moe RH, Haavardsholm EA, Christie A, et al: Effectiveness of nonpharmacological and nonsurgical interventions for hip osteoarthritis: an umbrella review of high-quality systematic reviews. Phys Ther 87:1716–1727, 2007.

81. Guillemin F, Virion JM, Escudier P, et al: Effect on osteoarthritis of spa therapy at Bourbonne-les-Bains. Joint Bone Spine 68:499–503, 2001.

82. Lavigne M, Parvizi J, Beck M, et al: Anterior femoroacetabular impingement. Part I. Techniques of joint preserving surgery. Clin Orthop Relat Res 418:61–66, 2004.

83. Ganz R, Gill TJ, Gautier E, et al: Surgical dislocation of the adult hip: a technique with full access to femoral head and acetabulum without the risk of avascular necrosis. J Bone Joint Surg Br 83:1119–1124, 2001.

84. Gibson A: Posterior exposure of the hip. J Bone Joint Surg Br 32:183–186, 1950.

85. Millis MB, Kain M, Sierra R, et al: Periacetabular osteotomy for acetabular dysplasia in patients older than 40 years: a preliminary study. Clin Orthop Relat Res 467:2228–2234, 2009.

86. Steppacher SD, Tannast M, Ganz R, Siebenrock KA: Mean 20-year followup of Bernese periacetabular osteotomy. Clin Orthop Relat Res 466:1633–1644, 2008.

87. Matheney T, Kim YJ, Zurakowski D, et al: Intermediate to long-term results following the Bernese periacetabular osteotomy and predictors of clinical outcome. J Bone Joint Surg Am 91:2113–2123, 2009.

88. Hsieh PH, Huang KC, Lee PC, Chang YH: Comparison of periacetabular osteotomy and total hip replacement in the same patient: a two- to ten-year follow-up study. J Bone Joint Surg Br 91:883–888, 2009.

89. Beaule PE, Matta JM, Mast JW: Hip arthrodesis: current indications and techniques. J Am Acad Orthop Surg 10:249–258, 2002.

90. Thambyah A, Hee HT, Das De S, Lee SM: Gait adaptations in patients with longstanding hip fusion. J Orthop Surg (Hong Kong) 11:154–158, 2003.

91. Kirkos JM, Papavasiliou KA, Kyrkos MJ, et al: The long-term effects of hip fusion on the adjacent joints. Acta Orthop Belg 74:779–787, 2008.

92. Joshi AB, Markovic L, Hardinge K, Murphy JC: Conversion of a fused hip to total hip arthroplasty. J Bone Joint Surg Am 84:1335–1341, 2008.

Femoroacetabular Impingement

Ernest L. Sink

INTRODUCTION

Femoroacetabular impingement (FAI) occurs when osseous abnormalities of the proximal femur and/or the acetabulum through the process of hip motion result in hip pain and eventual damage to the acetabular rim complex (labrum and acetabulum). Unlike dysplasia, which is a static overload of the acetabular rim, FAI is a dynamic process whereby overload occurs with motion. Two mechanisms of impingement have been identified: the *cam* mechanism is due to a proximal femoral deformity, and the *pincer* mechanism is due to acetabular overcoverage. Most hips with FAI have a combination of both pincer and cam mechanisms.[1] The end of physiologic hip flexion and rotation is the motion that is responsible for the process of impingement. Symptoms usually include groin pain exacerbated by flexion activities. The hip examination commonly reveals limited flexion and internal rotation. Patients have pain with hip flexion, adduction, and internal rotation, known as the *impingement test*.[2] Radiographs often reveal acetabular overcoverage and an abnormality of the proximal femur. Femoroacetabular impingement is one of the causes of degenerative osteoarthritis.[3] Retrospective studies have indicated that surgical treatment can improve pain and function on a short-term to midterm basis (Fig. 33-1*A* and *B*).

EPIDEMIOLOGY AND RISK FACTORS

The epidemiology of femoroacetabular impingement is still unknown. Patients who have FAI commonly have a history of performing athletic activities that require extremes of hip motion, particularly flexion and rotation, such as female dancers or a hurdler (rear leg). What is not clear is whether these activities lead to the osseous morphology of FAI, or if these patients have a predisposition that results in symptoms after activity. Patients who participate in activities with extremes of motion may have only a small osseous deformity and still may develop symptoms caused by repetitive trauma. Patients may not have symptoms despite evidence of the typical *cam* deformity on radiographs.[4] In one study on adolescents, females with the *pincer* mechanism were more common than males with cam lesions. Many of these adolescent females were competitive dancers; therefore repetitive extreme hip motion may occur, in contrast to their male cohorts in this age group.[5] What is unknown is exactly how hip morphology changes over time, and whether patients with large cam lesions in their third and fourth decades had less involved osseous abnormalities when they were younger.

In the skeletally immature hip, the physis of the anterior-lateral head and neck junction may grow anteriorly-inferiorly in response to different stresses and activities, resulting in an early cam lesion. Also, a femoral retroversion as seen in slipped capital femoral epiphysis (SCFE) over years of hip motion may impinge on the acetabular rim, resulting in a progressive cam lesion. In one study of cadaver bones, Goodman described that "post-slip morphology" is associated with hip osteoarthritis.[6] Therefore it is theoretically possible that the cam lesion or deficient offset between the femoral head and neck is a result of a silent subclinical SCFE in some adolescents. It has been reported that there might be a genetic predisposition to the osseous deformities that predispose the hip to FAI. Siblings had a risk 2.8 times that of a control group of having a cam deformity, and a risk 2.0 times that of the control group of having a pincer deformity.[7] In summary, acetabular deformities such as retroversion or overcoverage and proximal femoral deformities such as retroversion, a

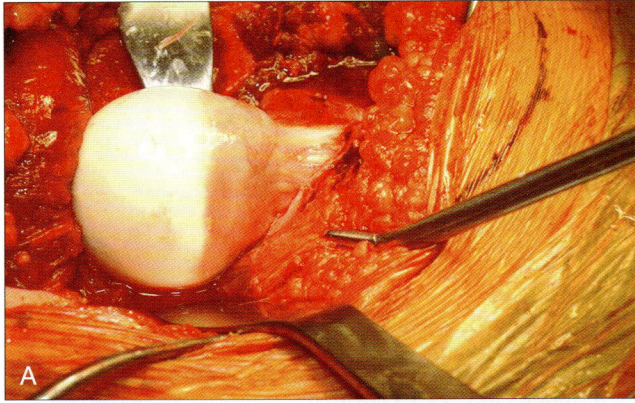

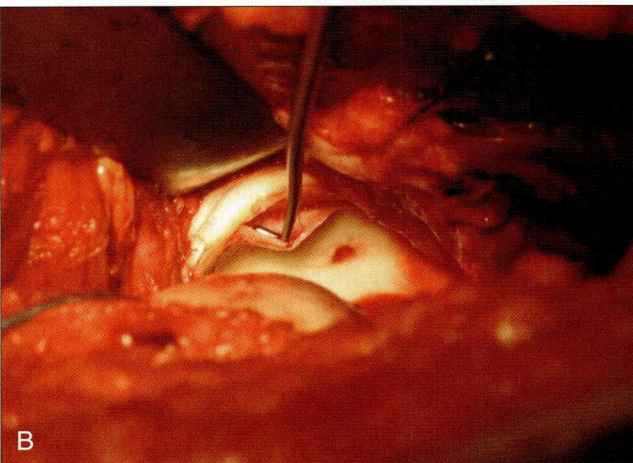

Figure 33-1. A, Femoral head deformity associated with hip impingement. **B,** Cartilage delamination as a result of hip impingement in a 19-year-old.

nonspherical femoral head, and deficient offset at the anterior-lateral head and neck junction likely predispose the hip to FAI. If a younger patient with these predispositions partakes in athletic activities in which repetitive nonphysiologic hip motion occurs, this may stimulate mild osseous abnormalities to worsen, or repetitive activities may result in symptoms at a young age without a severe deformity.

The prevalence of symptomatic FAI is unknown. Ochoa evaluated young patients with complaints of hip pain and noted radiographic signs of FAI in 87% of hips.[8] Early data indicate that hip impingement disorders may be the cause of hip osteoarthritis in 40% to 50% of patients.[9] Uncertainty about the prevalence of FAI continues, because many hips with the osseous abnormalities of FAI may be asymptomatic for decades, and some do not rapidly progress to osteoarthritis.[10] Allen and colleagues[4] analyzed the contra-lateral hip in patients with symptomatic FAI and found deformities suggestive of FAI, although the hip was asymptomatic in most cases. Why some hips with osseous abnormalities of FAI remain asymptomatic and some hips with rather mild radiographic abnormalities become symptomatic is still a mystery. Many hips will have advanced arthritis before becoming symptomatic. These realities make

clear knowledge of the incidence and natural history of FAI and the effects of treatment on the natural history perplexing.

PATHOPHYSIOLOGY

The pathophysiology of hip impingement is better understood. The basic principle is that through a process of hip motion, osseous deformities of the proximal femur and acetabulum lead to abnormal force on the acetabular rim complex, causing progressive labral and cartilage injury. Osseous deformities and how injury occurs were originally described by Ganz and coworkers.[3] On the femoral side, osseous deformities are defined as the *cam mechanism*. Osseous deformities on the acetabular side are known as the *pincer mechanism*. Most hips have some component of both a cam and a pincer deformity.[1]

The cam mechanism occurs when the proximal femur lacks sufficient offset between the femoral head and neck, or when the femoral head is not spherical. With hip motion, particularly flexion, clearance for the head and neck junction is not sufficient as it enters the acetabulum. Therefore, as the hip is flexed, an outside-to-inside increased shearing force occurs on the anterosuperior acetabular cartilage, beginning at the labral-chondral junction. The femoral head and neck will deflect the labrum as it enters the joint. This chronic, repetitive trauma may over time result in labral injury and articular cartilage injury. Injury to the cartilage and to the labral-chondral junction is more significant than labral pathology. This injury manifests as labral irritation, intrasubstance degeneration, and labral base tears. Greater cartilage injury is seen with the cam mechanism. The cartilage injury manifests as superficial degeneration followed by delamination of cartilage from the subchondral bone, eventual separation of the labral-chondral junction, and a flap tear of the cartilage into the acetabulum. Osseous deformity ranges from a femoral head that is not spherical, to a straight takeoff of the femoral neck from the anterior femoral neck, to an obvious "bump" or convexity at the proximal femoral neck. The cam deformity is commonly located anterolateral on the femoral neck, but it may also be direct anterior, anteromedial, or posterolateral. This deformity is more common among young males and has often been described as a silent undiagnosed SCFE deformity,[6] but it can be present with retroversion of the femoral neck or a short femoral neck when clearance with hip flexion is poor (Fig. 33-2).

The pincer mechanism is a result of acetabular overcoverage. The extreme of this would be protrusio acetabuli. With the pincer mechanism, as the hip reaches the physiologic end of motion, the femoral neck has a direct abutment on the acetabular rim, causing more direct labral trauma. The cartilage injury is usually contained to the rim, unlike in the cam mechanism, whereby the osseous abnormality enters the joint, causing greater cartilage injury. Because the femoral head has anterior abutment, the femoral head can be forced in a posterior direction, resulting in a posterior cartilage contrecoup injury adjacent to the fovea. Theoretically, this would be more likely to occur in those with greater laxity in their anterior hip capsule. Acetabular overcoverage is caused by global acetabular retroversion, a prominent anterior wall, and a deep acetabulum (protrusion or coxa profunda). Cartilage pathology in those with more of a pincer mechanism is isolated to the periphery of the acetabulum[1] (Fig. 33-3).

To conclude, osseous abnormalities that occur through the process of hip motion result in a dynamic process of labral and cartilage injury. The severity of the deformities, the level of activity of the patient, and likely the patient's ligamentous laxity all play a role in the development of symptomatic hip impingement. Many patients with significant osseous deformities do not have symptoms; other patients are highly symptomatic with minimal abnormalities. It remains a mystery why some hips even in the same patient will become symptomatic and why some will not.

CLINICAL FEATURES AND DIAGNOSIS

The diagnosis of femoroacetabular impingement is based largely on history and physical examination findings (Box 33-1). The most common symptom of patients with FAI is anterior groin pain. When asked the location of pain, patients commonly will point directly to the groin. This is often referred to as the *c-sign,* or *grab sign* (Fig. 33-4). Pain in the buttocks or the peritrochanteric region is possible, although it is less common than groin pain. Patients occasionally will point to the posterior trochanteric region. Hip pain does not radiate distal to the knee joint but may radiate down the anterior thigh. A spinal cause for the pain should be ruled out in patients with pain distal to the knee. Pain is often exacerbated by flexion activities and may be worse with sitting than with ambulation. Onset of symptoms usually is insidious and episodic at first. An increase in physical activity or a minor traumatic event can exacerbate or initiate symptoms. Symptoms may become more frequent with time or may remain intermittent, despite progressive hip osteoarthritis. It is poorly understood why some patients suffer more than others with similar radiographic findings. Allen showed in patients who underwent surgical treatment that the contralateral hip had cam deformities consistent with FAI in 77.8% of cases, but only 26.1% of these had bilateral pain.[4]

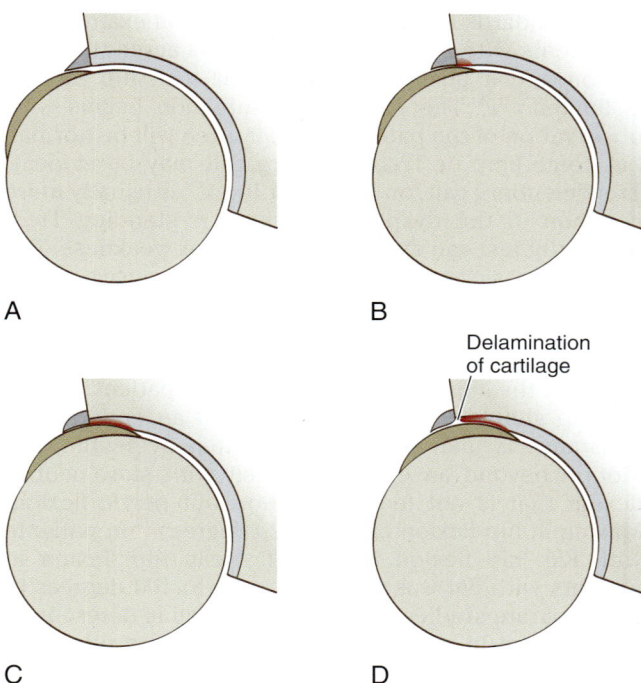

Delamination of cartilage

Figure 33-2. **A** through **D,** Illustration of the *cam mechanism.* As the hip is flexed, a dynamic abnormal force on the acetabular cartilage starts at the labral-chondral junction. (Redrawn from Beck M, et al: Hip morphology influences the pattern of damage to the acetabular cartilage: femoroacetabular impingement as a cause of early osteoarthritis of the hip. J Bone Joint Surg Br 87:1012–1018, 2005.)

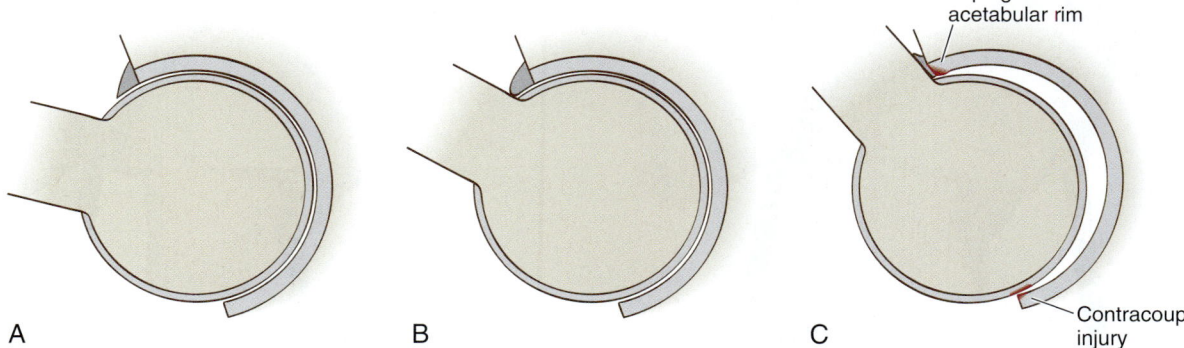

Impingement of acetabular rim

Contracoup injury

Figure 33-3. **A** through **C,** Illustration of the *pincer mechanism.* As the hip is flexed, the femoral neck abuts the rim of the acetabulum. Direct injury to the labrum and rim cartilage is evident. A contrecoup injury to the posterior acetabular cartilage also may occur. (Redrawn from Beck M, et al: Hip morphology influences the pattern of damage to the acetabular cartilage: femoroacetabular impingement as a cause of early osteoarthritis of the hip. J Bone Joint Surg Br 87:1012–1018, 2005.)

BOX 33-1.   DIAGNOSTIC FEATURES COMMON IN FEMOROACETABULAR IMPINGEMENT

History
- Anterior groin pain
  - Increased with flexion activities
- History of activities requiring extreme hip motion

Examination
- Limited hip flexion (<100 degrees)
- Limited hip internal rotation at 90 degrees flexion, <25 degrees
- Positive impingement test

Anteroposterior (AP) X-rays
- Acetabular overcoverage
- Lateral center edge (CE) angle greater than 35 degrees
- Crossover sign
- Post wall sign with or without crossover
- Ischial spine sign
- Coxa profunda
- Nonspherical femoral head (i.e., pistol grip deformity)

Lateral X-rays
- Nonspherical femoral head
- Deficient (flat or convex) offset between the femoral head and neck
- Alpha angle greater than 50 to 55 degrees

Magnetic Resonance Imaging (MRI)
- Labral tear
- Chondral delamination
- Alpha angle greater than 50 degrees

Patients with advanced symptoms will have a mild antalgic or Trendelenburg gait. Patients with dysplasia may complain of similar groin pain but often will have more of an abductor fatigue with activities. Pain with sitting and flexion activities is more associated with FAI than with dysplasia. Most patients will participate or have participated in an activity or sport that involves supraphysiologic hip motion such as dancing. They may have participated in these activities for years before the start of symptoms.

No standards have been set for physical examination of patients with FAI, but most surgeons agree that with flexion and a positive impingement test, hip motion is limited.[5,11,12] The physical examination begins with observation of the patient's gait. It often will be normal, but some limp or Trendelenburg gait may be evident. Trendelenburg gait, or "abductor lurch," is usually more common in the dysplastic patient. A standing Trendelenburg test can examine for abductor weakness. The foot progression angle should be noted because patients with retroversion of the proximal femur may have an external rotated gait. The critical component of the examination for FAI consists of hip flexion, internal rotation, and the impingement test. With the patient supine, the hip should be flexed slowly until an endpoint or resistance is met. Hip flexion is often overestimated. Motion beyond an endpoint is felt with slow neutral flexion that is not femoral motion but pelvic flexion. Maximum hip flexion is up to 120 degrees.[13] In patients with FAI, hip flexion is limited. Mean hip flexion in patients with FAI was reported as 90 to 100 degrees in two separate studies.[5,11] Internal rotation is determined with the leg in extension and, more important, at 90

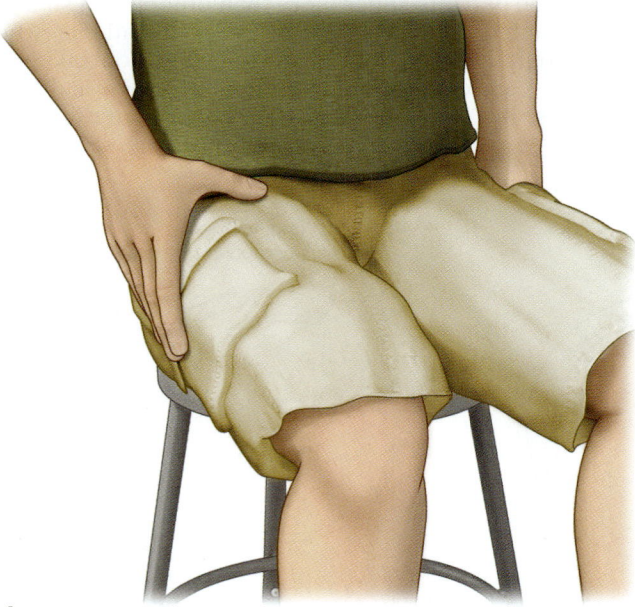 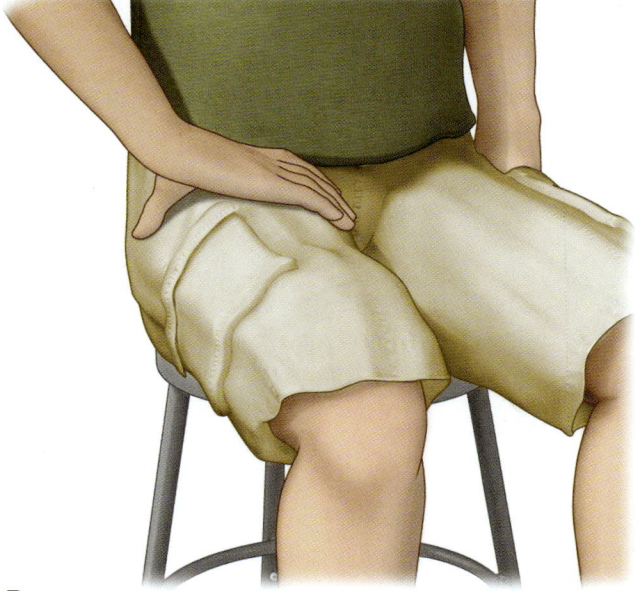

A   B

Figure 33-4. The hip "grab sign" also referred to as the "c-sign." A patient with femoroacetabular impingement (FAI) will often perform this when describing the location of pain. (From Sink EL, et al: Clinical presentation of femoroacetabular impingement in adolescents. J Pediatr Orthop 28:806–811, 2008.)

degrees of hip flexion. Hip internal rotation at 90 degrees of flexion is decreased; mean internal rotation of patients with symptomatic FAI has been reported to be 9 to 15 degrees versus 30 degrees[5,11,13] in asymptomatic patients.

Patients may have decreased external rotation. The impingement test is a sign of hip and labral irritation.[2] The test is performed with hip flexion and internal rotation and adduction (Fig. 33-5). Patients will state that this provocative maneuver reproduces their groin pain. Commonly, external rotation will resolve the pain. The author would rarely consider treatment for FAI if this test is negative, but would look for extra-articular causes of hip pain. The impingement test can be positive in patients with any sort of hip irritation such as developmental dysplasia of the hip (DDH). Those with hip dysplasia commonly will have greater hip flexion and internal rotation with the impingement test than patients with hip impingement. The examination should include looking for previous surgical scars, a good neurologic examination including straight-leg raise to rule out spinal pathology, leg length, and palpation of the abdomen, the trochanter, and the iliac crest. The bicycle test performed with the patient in the lateral position will assess for trochanteric bursitis.

The standard radiographic examination includes two views of the hip: an anteroposterior (AP) pelvic radiograph and a true lateral view of the proximal femur. Some surgeons prefer to take the AP pelvis supine, and others prefer standing. Whatever method is chosen, it is important to make sure the hips are centered on the radiographs without excessive sagittal or frontal plane rotation. If the pelvis is excessively rotated, the landmarks of acetabular version will be altered. The sacrum should be centered over the symphysis. The average distance between the sacrococcygeal joint and the symphysis should be around 3 mm in males and 4.5 mm in females. Siebenrock studied the effects of rotation on pelvic markers and found that 6 degrees of rotation resulted in an inaccurate assessment of the acetabular version.[14] Important measurements on AP radiographs include the lateral center edge angle of Wiberg, the Tonnis sourcil angle, Shenton's line, the anterior and posterior wall for the acetabulum, and the depth of the medial joint in relation to the ilioischial line. The proximal femur can be evaluated for femoral head sphericity on the AP radiograph.

The acetabular version should be analyzed when a diagnosis of hip impingement is considered. This is evaluated by looking at the relationship of the anterior and posterior walls of the acetabulum on a well-positioned anteroposterior radiograph. Normally, the anterior wall is medial and more horizontal than the posterior wall, and the posterior wall is more lateral and vertical than the anterior wall. The anterior and posterior walls should meet at the lateral aspect of the sourcil. When the anterior wall is projected lateral to the anterior wall, this is known as the *crossover sign*[15] (Fig. 33-6). This is a sign of global or cranial acetabular retroversion. If the posterior wall is medial to the center of the femoral head, this is known as the *posterior wall sign*. If a posterior wall sign and a crossover sign are noted, this would represent global acetabular retroversion. In this case, the ischial spine is often visualized on the radiograph (Fig. 33-7). If no posterior wall sign but

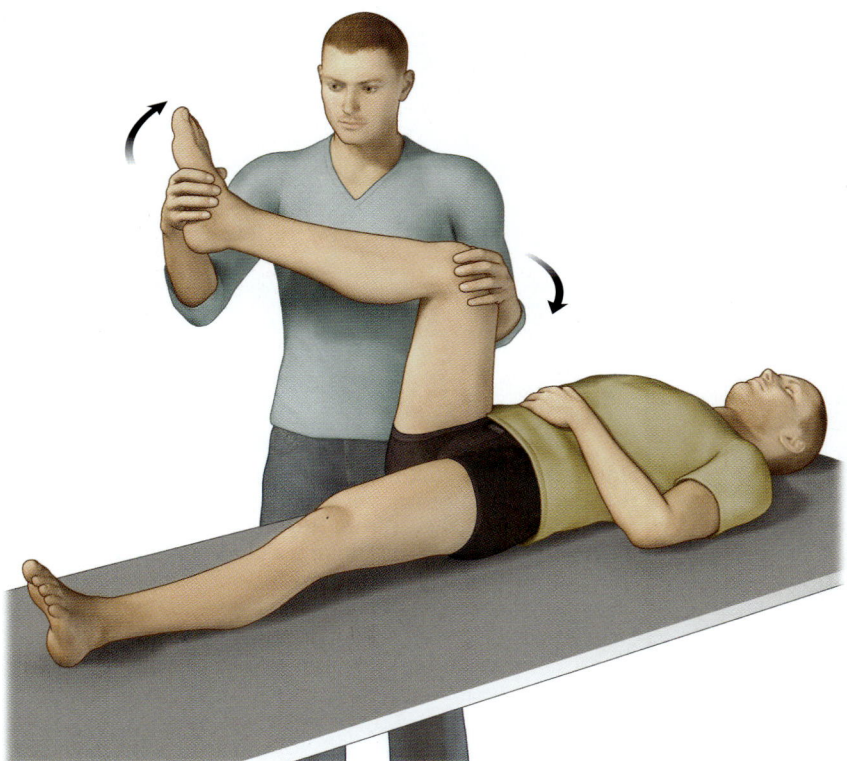

Figure 33-5. Drawing showing performance of the impingement test. (From Sink EL, et al: Clinical presentation of femoroacetabular impingement in adolescents. J Pediatr Orthop 28:806–811, 2008.)

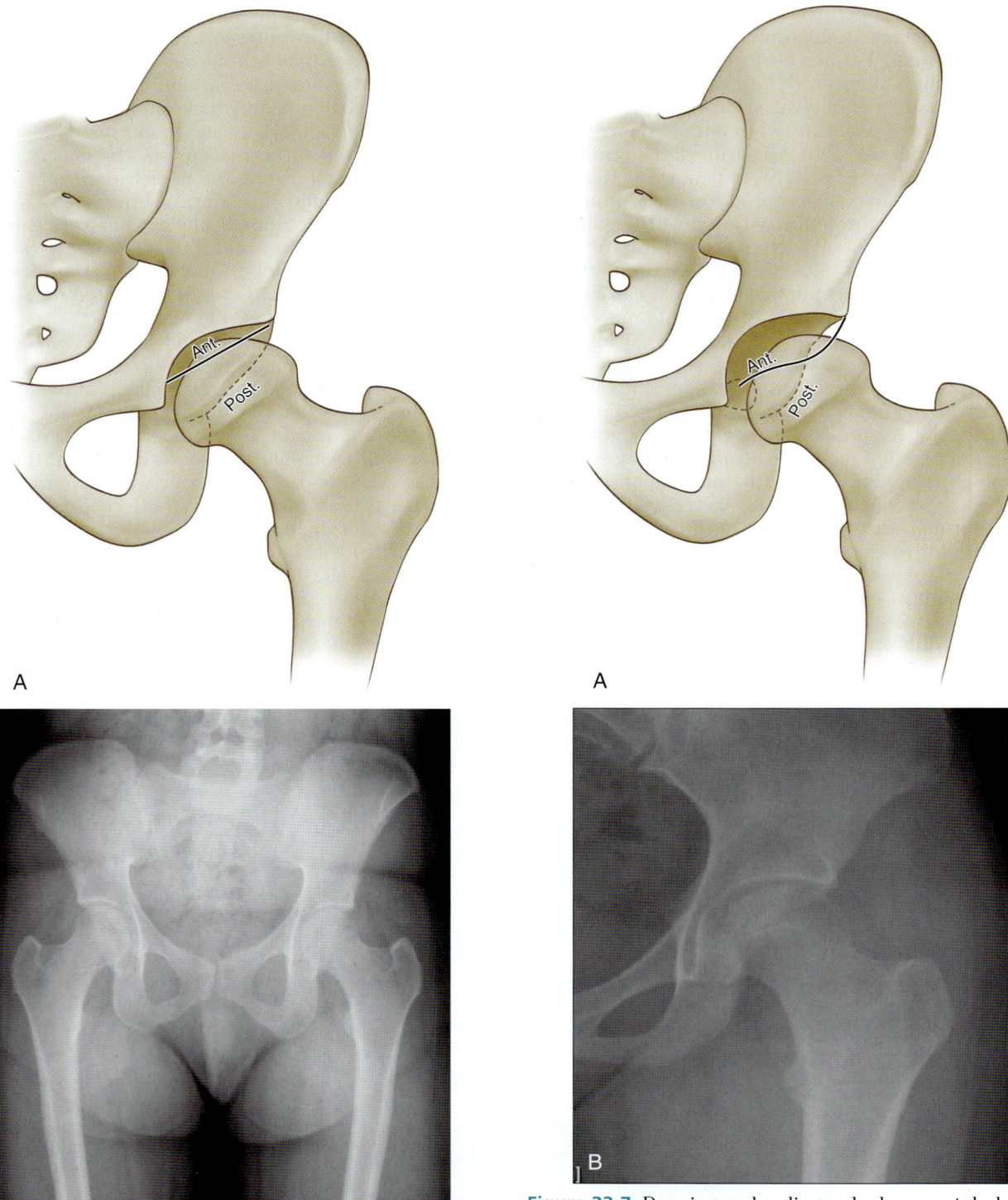

A

B

Figure 33-6. Normal acetabular version. (From Reynolds D, Lucas J, Klaue K: Retroversion of the acetabulum: a cause of hip pain. J Bone Joint Surg Br 81:281–288, 1999.)

A

B

Figure 33-7. Drawing and radiograph show acetabular retroversion with a crossover sign, a posterior wall sign, and an ischial spine sign. (From Reynolds D, Lucas J, Klaue K: Retroversion of the acetabulum: a cause of hip pain. J Bone Joint Surg Br 81:281–288, 1999.)

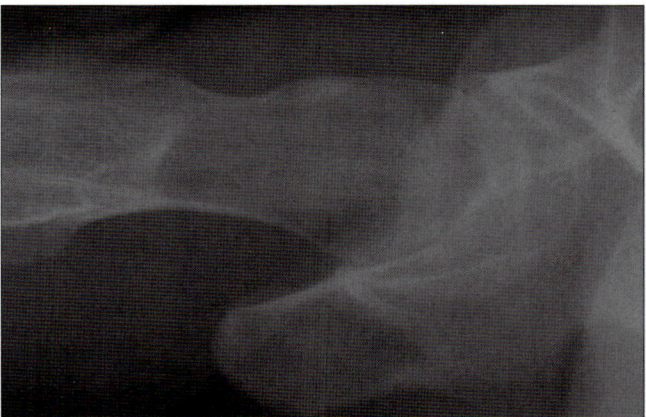

Figure 33-8. Lateral of the femoral neck with the leg internally rotated 15 degrees. A convexity is obvious at the region of the femoral head-neck junction.

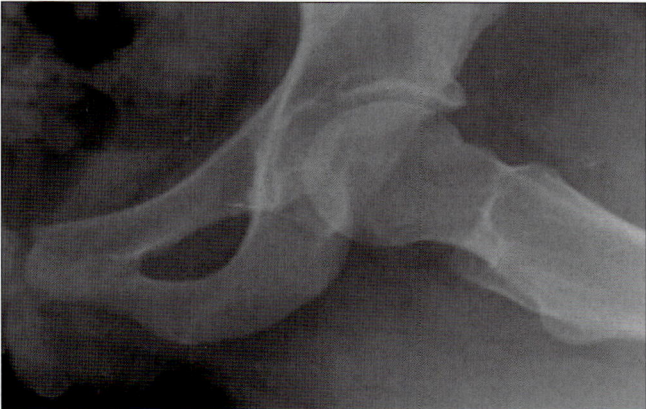

Figure 33-9. Lateral radiograph of the femoral neck illustrating an impingement trough from a prominent anterior rim. A crossover sign and an ischial spine sign can be seen.

a crossover sign is seen, anterior acetabular overcoverage is present. Another sign of FAI and acetabular overcoverage is a deep hip socket, or *coxa profunda.* When the floor of the acetabular fossa is medial to the ilioischial line, this is the criterion for coxa profunda.[16] Patients with borderline dysplasia (lateral center edge [CE] angle of 20 to 25 degrees) may have a retroverted acetabulum; therefore it is critical to consider this in the differential diagnosis when considering treatment.

The lateral radiograph should allow a view of the anterior and anterolateral head and neck junction. A few different techniques can be used to take the lateral; it is important to have the longest view of the femoral neck without interposition of the greater or lesser trochanters. These techniques include a true lateral of the hip (with the leg internally rotated 15 degrees), the Dunn lateral (an AP projection of the hip with the leg flexed and abducted), and the frog lateral. Important information from this view includes the sphericity of the femoral head and the degree of offset between femoral head and femoral neck. With FAI, this view will reveal no offset between femoral head and neck, a convexity, or a nonspherical femoral head (Fig. 33-8). Impingement lesions that appear like cysts on the anterior aspect of the femoral neck and impingement troughs have been described (Fig. 33-9). The alpha angle is measured on this radiograph. This angle, originally described by Notzli, is obtained by drawing a circle superimposed on the femoral head.[17] The angle comes from two lines: (1) a line drawn from the center of the circle, splitting the femoral neck, and (2) a second line drawn from the center of the head, to where the head and neck bone come outside the circle. This value can be obtained on the lateral radiograph or on magnetic resonance imaging (MRI) (Fig. 33-10). The normal value of the alpha angle has been reported as 40 to 45 degrees, and many authors have considered greater than 50 degrees to be abnormal.[17] The angle is highly dependent on technique and on femoral rotation.[18] If the nonspherical portion of the femoral head and neck is off plane, a normal alpha angle

and a cam lesion on the femoral head may be noted (see Fig. 33-10).

MRI is important for the diagnosis of hip impingement. The purposes of MRI are to evaluate the cartilage and labrum and to better define the three-dimensional anatomy of the femoral head and neck. Most surgeons will utilize a radial sequence MRI with cuts directed around the axis of the femoral neck. Radial sequencing allows 360-degree visualization of the femoral head and neck to obtain a better understanding of the anatomic morphology of the femoral head and neck junctions and of associated labral and chondral injury.[19] Traditional hip and pelvis MRI studies that do not perform radial sequencing often will be out of plane, allowing visualization of the deformity (Fig. 33-11).[20] An arthrogram with capsular distention will more clearly define injuries to the labrum and possible cartilage lesions. Recent studies indicate that indirect arthrography (delayed gadolinium-enhanced magnetic resonance imaging of cartilage [dGEMRIC] and subsequent three-dimensional T1 mapping) may improve the diagnostic ability of the MRI to detect early cartilage lesions.[21] The sensitivity of MRI in diagnosing labral and cartilage injury is still variable. The sensitivity of MRI in detecting labral injury is greater than its sensitivity in detecting articular cartilage injury. In the future, better techniques to evaluate the hip and to map cartilage injury will improve the diagnostic accuracy of MRI in detecting early cartilage lesions.

In conclusion, the diagnosis of FAI is based mostly on the history and physical examination. Groin pain and limited hip flexion and internal rotation, along with a positive impingement test, are common examination findings. An anteroposterior radiograph of the pelvis, lateral radiographs of the proximal femur, and radial sequence MRI are important in confirming the clinical examination in most cases of hip impingement. The use of computed tomography (CT) scanning is still debated, but many surgeons who perform the arthroscopic approach obtain a CT scan for preoperative planning.

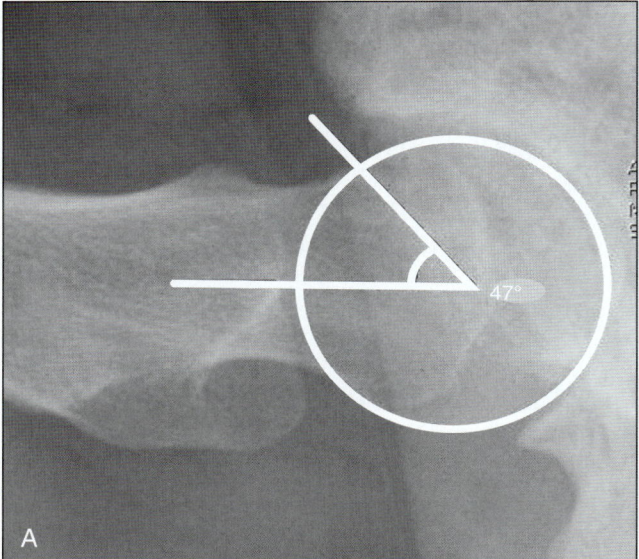

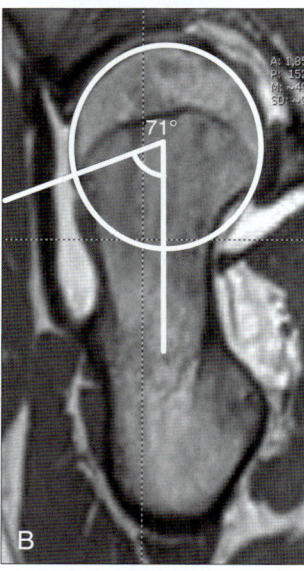

Figure 33-10. A, Illustration of the alpha angle on the lateral radiograph. **B,** The same hip with the alpha angle as seen on radial sequence magnetic resonance imaging (MRI). Because radial sequences allow for multiplanar imaging, the offset abnormality is viewed in a different plane than the lateral radiograph.

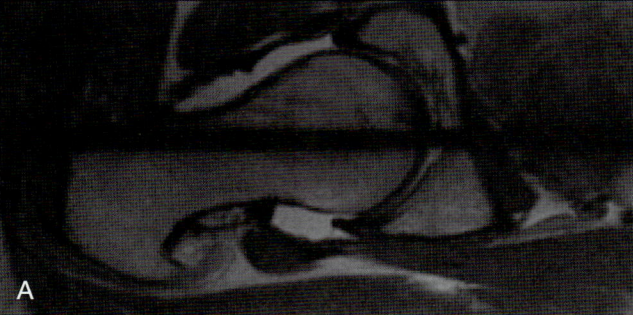

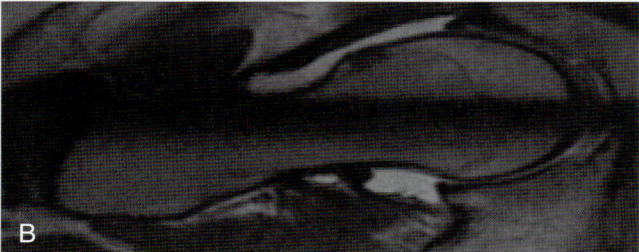

Figure 33-11. Radial sequences around the axis of the femoral neck allow better determination of the osseous abnormality by visualization of multiple planes, as illustrated in these two different views of the same patient.

DIFFERENTIAL DIAGNOSIS

The differential diagnosis of FAI consists of hip dysplasia, osteonecrosis, trochanteric bursitis, femoral neck stress fracture, snapping iliopsoas tendinitis, rectus femoris strain, adductor muscle strain, tumor, infection, SCFE, Perthes disease, other causes of hip arthritis such as rheumatoid arthritis, and lumbar disk herniation.

The greatest challenge is seen in patients with borderline dysplasia (lateral CE angle of 20 to 25 degrees). Many of these patients will have symptoms of dysplasia and impingement. The predominant pathomechanical process—instability or impingement—that is causing symptoms can be a diagnostic dilemma. Therefore, the physician needs to take into account the history, physical examination findings, and radiographs in deciding appropriate treatment. The patient with dysplasia more likely will have a history of activity-related abductor fatigue, a positive apprehension test, and greater hip flexion and internal rotation than are seen with FAI, in which symptoms are more associated with hip flexion, and hip flexion and internal rotation are decreased. MRI in dysplasia will show a hypertrophied labrum with cysts and some subchondral sclerosis (Fig. 33-12).

TREATMENT

Many different surgical options may be used to treat femoroacetabular impingement. With correct indications, different approaches have been reported to improve pain and function on a short-term to mid-term basis. Many single-institution retrospective studies indicate that pain and function are improved by surgery in most patients who do not already have advanced osteoarthritis.[22-28] Many of these studies have relatively short-term follow-up, so the effect of treatment on the natural history of the disease over the long term remains unknown.

Before a decision is made on surgical treatment, a trial of conservative management is recommended for most patients. Few data on the effectiveness of nonoperative management are available, but it consists of rest, activity limitation, and physical therapy. Physical therapy should include core strengthening, and the therapist should avoid attempting to increase range of motion, as this may exacerbate symptoms.

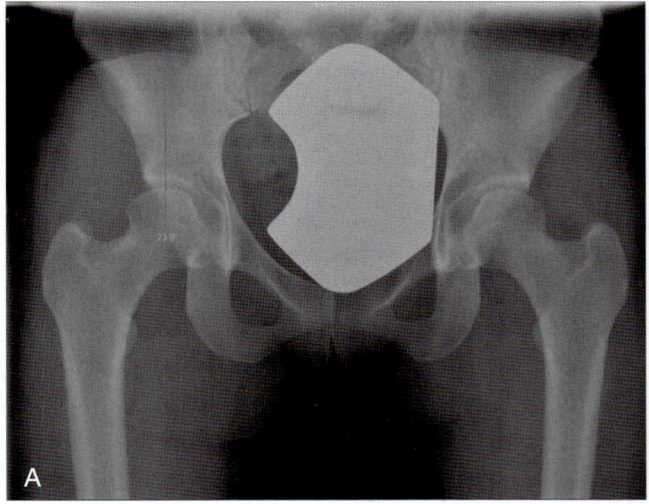

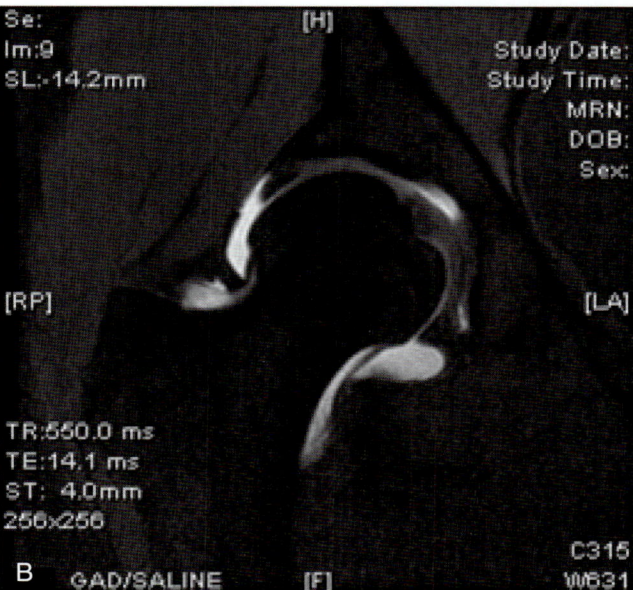

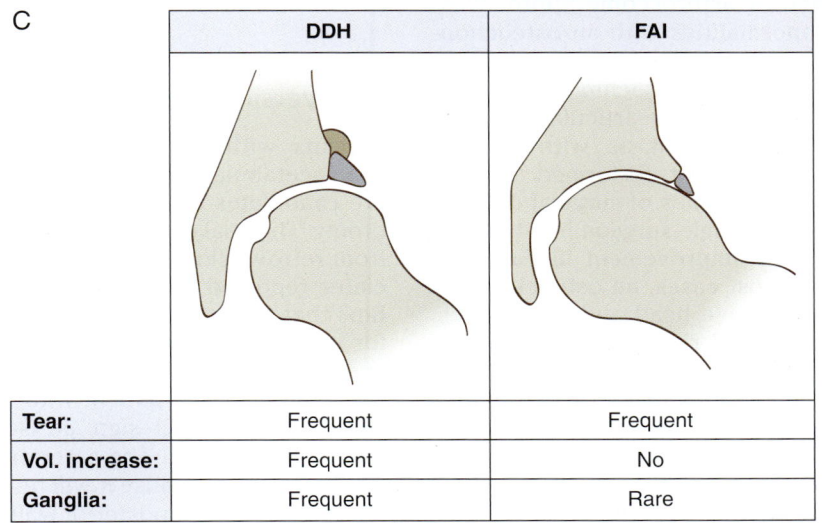

	DDH	FAI
Tear:	Frequent	Frequent
Vol. increase:	Frequent	No
Ganglia:	Frequent	Rare

Figure 33-12. A, Anteroposterior (AP) pelvic view with an anterior center edge (CE) angle of 23 degrees. **B,** Magnetic resonance imaging (MRI) shows a hypertrophied labrum that acts as a secondary stabilizer. This is consistent with instability (dysplasia). **C,** Illustration of different labral presentations on MRI for femoroacetabular impingement (FAI) and developmental dysplasia of the hip (DDH). (**C** Redrawn from Leunig M, Podeszwa D, Beck M, et al: Magnetic resonance arthrography of labral disorders in hips with dysplasia and impingement. Clin Orthop Relat Res [418]:74–80, 2004.)

Surgical treatment is recommended if symptoms are not improved with activity modification, medication, and/or therapy. The goals of treatment are to obtain a functional range of motion that is free of osseous impingement, and to repair any damage to the labrum and cartilage to improve the patient's pain and range of motion. A long-term goal of avoiding or delaying the onset of osteoarthritis is attained by restoring impingement-free motion of the hip joint.

Surgical techniques include surgical dislocation of the hip, anteversion, periacetabular osteotomy, arthroscopic methods, and a combination of arthroscopy and limited open procedures. Which treatment is chosen is entirely dependent on many factors, including surgeon preference and comfort with open or arthroscopic

approaches. There is no true comparison between different approaches. Results appear comparable, but all reported series have different surgical criteria and different reported outcome variables. The body of knowledge on which technique may be best for specific patient variables is increasing, but there remains a significant difference with respect to surgeon preference and opinion. We will briefly describe here each technique, its reported outcomes, and the pros and cons of each method.

Conservative

No data are available on the effectiveness of nonoperative treatment. For patients who are involved in activities that aggravate hip pain such as dancing, the recommendation would be to limit those activities. For patients whose hips do not have significant labral and chondral injury, there is some theoretical chance of symptom improvement once the repetitive extreme motion is modified.

Surgical Hip Dislocation

Safe hip dislocation is the most common open surgical approach used to treat hip impingement disorders. Much of the pathomechanics and many of the injury patterns in FAI have come to be understood through the visualization possible with this technique. This approach, originally described by Ganz and associates,[29] allows complete visualization of the proximal femur and acetabulum. Benefits of this approach include visualization of the pathologic process by hip motion at the time of surgery and the ability to get a three-dimensional assessment of hip damage. Conditions such as extra-articular impingement of the trochanter are more easily observed through this approach compared with limited open or arthroscopic approaches. Addressing osseous abnormalities with an osteochondroplasty is straightforward with this exposure. Acetabular rim resection and labral reattachment are less challenging with this approach. Extra-articular impingement evaluation and management as with relative femoral neck lengthening are best performed through this approach. Promising outcomes of surgical dislocation have been described in single-surgeon institutional retrospective reviews, with improvement in pain and function (Table 33-1). In most cases, an osteochondroplasty is performed to improve head and neck offset. The need for labral repair and rim resection depends on the magnitude of labral injury and the depth of the acetabulum. Outcome studies using this approach result in a good to excellent outcome in 68% to 96% with a minimum 2-year follow-up and "failure" of treatment in 1% to 10%. Negative aspects of the open procedure include the trochanteric osteotomy and the potential for trochanteric nonunion in 1% to 2% of patients. Reported complications of the procedure are trochanteric nonunion and heterotopic ossification, along with very rare neuropraxia.

Arthroscopic

The arthroscopic approach is being used more as surgeons come to understand hip impingement and become comfortable with the techniques. Because of the anatomy particular to the hip joint, there are challenges to both visualization and treatment. Which patients are perfect candidates for hip arthroscopy remains unknown. Through this approach, an osteochondroplasty can be performed. Performing an osteochondroplasty in close proximity and posterior to the retinacular vessels is difficult through an arthroscopic approach. Experienced hip arthroscopists can perform rim resection and labral repair. Single-surgeon reports have shown outcomes comparable with the open surgical dislocation approach. For those without large experience in arthroscopy, there is a steep learning curve.

Negative results have been reported in hip arthroscopy and labral repair in patients with hip dysplasia.[30] Because the arthroscopic approach allows less visualization, radiographic assistance both preoperatively and intraoperatively is helpful to ensure complete osteochondroplasty. With experience and additional comparative studies, indications and use of the arthroscopic approach will become more apparent.

Combined Arthroscopy With Limited Anterior Open Approach

Some authors have advocated a combined approach of intra-articular arthroscopy with a limited anterior open osteochondroplasty.[25,31] The anterior approach utilizes the interval between the sartorius and the tensor fascia. The benefit of this approach is direct visualization of the anterior head-neck junction while surgical dislocation and a trochanteric osteotomy are avoided. Arthroscopy allows intra-articular inspection and labral-chondral débridement and repair as necessary.

Anteversion Periacetabular Osteotomy

Patients with hip impingement symptoms primarily from acetabular retroversion and minimal joint damage are candidates for an anteversion periacetabular osteotomy. The goal of surgery is to reorient the acetabulum from retroversion to anteversion. Seibenrock and associates reported "good to excellent" results in 26 of 29 hips that had an anteversion periacetabular osteotomy for impingement from acetabular retroversion with an average follow-up of 30 months. This procedure should be considered in a patient with retroversion characterized by a crossover sign, an ischial spine sign, and a posterior wall sign. The anterior cartilage should have minimal injury because it will be in a more static weight-bearing position. A posterior wall sign is needed because posterior wall impingement has been reported as a side effect of the procedure.[32] An arthrotomy and an anterior osteochondroplasty may be performed concurrently. The procedure is slightly more challenging than the osteotomy for hip dysplasia.

PROGNOSIS

Outcome studies of surgical treatment for femoroacetabular impingement through a variety of methods indicate that pain and function are improved in most patients. Evidence is based on relatively short-term follow-up. Long-term follow-up is necessary to evaluate the effects of treatment on the natural history and survivorship of treated hips. Results of treatment are improved for those with minimal joint injury. Femoroacetabular impingement is a proven cause of secondary hip osteoarthritis in the young adult hip. How long hips will survive with and without treatment is unknown, but the improvement in symptoms and function is promising.

Table 33-1. Results of Open and Arthroscopic Approaches to Treatment of Hip Impingement

Study	Hips/ Patients	Clinical Outcome Scores	Clinically Good or Excellent Outcome, n (%)	Mean Change in Hip Score, Average Change	Failure Definition	Failure, n (%)	Complications Including Subsequent Surgery, n (%)	Complications, n (%)
Open Approach Studies								
Siebenrock et al (JBJS-A 2003)	29/22	Merle d'Aubigné Score	28 hips (96)	2.9 points	Fair results/ residual pain	1 hip (3)	4 hips (14)	1 hip (3)
Beck et al (CORR 2004)	19/19	Merle d'Aubigné Score	13 hips (68)	2.4 points	Conversion to THA	5 hips (26)	0 hips (0)	0 hips (0)
Murphy et al (CORR 2004)	23/23	Merle d'Aubigné Score	15 hips (65)	NA	Conversion to THA	7 hips (23)	1 hip (4)	0 hips (0)
Espinosa et al (JBJS-A 2006)	60/52	Merle d'Aubigné Score	52 hips (87)	4 points	Poor or moderate results	3 hips (5)	0 hips (0)	0 hips (0)
Peters et al (JBJS-A 2006)	30/29	Harris Hip Store	26 hips (87)	17 points	Pain and/or progressive arthrosis	4 hips (13)	0 hips (0)	0 hips (0)
Beaule et al (JBJS-A 2007)	37/34	WOMAC, UCLA, SF-12 Physical, SF-12 Mental	30 hips (81)	20.2 points, 2.7 points, 8.3 points, 4.8 points, respectively	Unsatisfactory outcome, no clinical improvement, and/or worsening WOMAC score	6 hips (16)	13 hips (35)	11 (30)
Arthroscopic Approach Studies								
Ilizaliturri et al (JBJS-Br 2007)	14/13	WOMAC	NA	7.7 points	NA	0 hips (0)	0 hips (0)	0 hips (0)
Ilizaliturri et al (J Arthroplasty 2008)	19/19	WOMAC	16 hips (84)	9.6 points	Advanced OA, recommended THA	1 hip (5)	0 hips (0)	0 hips (0)
Laude et al (CORR 2009)	100/97	NAHS	NA	29.1 points	Conversion to THA	11 hips (11)	33 hips (33)	18 hips (18)
Philippon et al (JBJS-Br 2009)	112/112	MHHS, HOS ADL, HOS Sport, NAHS	NA	24 points, 17 points, 24 points, 14 points, respectively	Conversion to THA	10 hips (9)	0 hips (0)	0 hips (0)
Brunner et al (AJSM 2009)	53/53	SFS, NAHS, VAS	NA	1.06 points, 31.3 points, 4.1 points	NA	NA	NR	NR

From Clohisy JC, St. John LC, Schutz AL: Surgical treatment of femoroacetabular impingement: a systematic review of the literature. Clin Orthop Relat Res 468:555–564, 2010.
ADL, Activities of daily living; *HOS,* Hip Outcome Score; *MHHS,* Modified Harris Hip Score; *NA,* not applicable; *NAHS,* Nonarthritic Hip Score; *NR,* not reported; *SF,* Short Form; *SFS,* XXX; *THA,* total hip arthroplasty; *UCLA,* University of California, Los Angeles; *VAS,* visual analogue scale; *WOMAC,* Western Ontario and McMaster Universities Arthritis Index.

CURRENT CONTROVERSIES AND FUTURE CONSIDERATIONS

- The effect of treatment on the natural history of hip impingement
- Comparing outcomes of hips treated via open surgical dislocation versus an arthroscopic approach
- What are the proven criteria by examination and radiographs for an accurate diagnosis?
- Which patients and their specific characteristics may benefit from one method of treatment over another?
- Which treatment is best when early osteoarthritis is already evident at the time of presentation?

REFERENCES

1. Beck M, et al: Hip morphology influences the pattern of damage to the acetabular cartilage: femoroacetabular impingement as a cause of early osteoarthritis of the hip. J Bone Joint Surg Br 87:1012–1018, 2005.
2. MacDonald SJ, Ganz R: Clinical evaluation of the symptomatic young adult hip. Semin Arthroplasty 8:3–9, 1997.
3. Ganz R, et al: Femoroacetabular impingement: a cause for osteoarthritis of the hip. Clin Orthop Relat Res 417:112–120, 2003.

4. Allen D, et al: Prevalence of associated deformities and hip pain in patients with cam-type femoroacetabular impingement. J Bone Joint Surg Br 91:589–594, 2009.

5. Sink EL, et al: Clinical presentation of femoroacetabular impingement in adolescents. J Pediatr Orthop 28:806–811, 2008.

6. Goodman DA, et al: Subclinical slipped capital femoral epiphysis: relationship to osteoarthrosis of the hip. J Bone Joint Surg Am 79:1489–1497, 1997.

7. Pollard TC, et al: Genetic influences in the aetiology of femoroacetabular impingement: a sibling study. J Bone Joint Surg Br 92:209–216, 2010.

8. Ochoa LM, et al: Radiographic prevalence of femoroacetabular impingement in a young population with hip complaints is high. Clin Orthop Relat Res 468:2710–2714, 2010.

9. Aronson J: Osteoarthritis of the young adult hip: etiology and treatment. Instr Course Lect 35:119–128, 1986.

10. Bardakos NV, Villar RN: Predictors of progression of osteoarthritis in femoroacetabular impingement: a radiological study with a minimum of ten years follow-up. J Bone Joint Surg Br 91:162–169, 2009.

11. Clohisy JC, et al: Clinical presentation of patients with symptomatic anterior hip impingement. Clin Orthop Relat Res 467:638–644, 2009.

12. Martin HD, et al: The pattern and technique in the clinical evaluation of the adult hip: the common physical examination tests of hip specialists. Arthroscopy 26:161–172, 2010.

13. Tannast M, et al: Noninvasive three-dimensional assessment of femoroacetabular impingement. J Orthop Res 25:122–131, 2007.

14. Siebenrock KA, Kalbermatten DF, Ganz R: Effect of pelvic tilt on acetabular retroversion: a study of pelves from cadavers. Clin Orthop Relat Res 407:241–248, 2003.

15. Reynolds D, Lucas J, Klaue K: Retroversion of the acetabulum: a cause of hip pain. J Bone Joint Surg Br 81:281–288, 1999.

16. Ruelle M, et al: [Introduction to the study of arthrosis of the elbow]. J Belge Rhumatol Med Phys 20:161–176, 1965.

17. Notzli HP, et al: The contour of the femoral head-neck junction as a predictor for the risk of anterior impingement. J Bone Joint Surg Br 84:556–560, 2002.

18. Beaule PE, et al: Three-dimensional computed tomography of the hip in the assessment of femoroacetabular impingement. J Orthop Res 23:1286–1292, 2005.

19. Plotz GM, et al: Magnetic resonance arthrography of the acetabular labrum: value of radial reconstructions. Arch Orthop Trauma Surg 121:450–457, 2001.

20. Rakhra KS, et al: Comparison of MRI alpha angle measurement planes in femoroacetabular impingement. Clin Orthop Relat Res 467:660–665, 2009.

21. Zlatkin MB, et al: Acetabular labral tears and cartilage lesions of the hip: indirect MR arthrographic correlation with arthroscopy—a preliminary study. AJR Am J Roentgenol 194: 709–714, 2010.

22. Beck M, et al: Anterior femoroacetabular impingement: part II. Midterm results of surgical treatment. Clin Orthop Relat Res 418:67–73, 2004.

23. Espinosa N, et al: Treatment of femoro-acetabular impingement: preliminary results of labral refixation. J Bone Joint Surg Am 88:925–935, 2006.

24. Peters CL, Erickson JA: Treatment of femoro-acetabular impingement with surgical dislocation and débridement in young adults. J Bone Joint Surg Am 88:1735–1741, 2006.

25. Laude F, Sariali E, Nogier A: Femoroacetabular impingement treatment using arthroscopy and anterior approach. Clin Orthop Relat Res 467:747–752, 2009.

26. Philippon MJ, et al: Outcomes following hip arthroscopy for femoroacetabular impingement with associated chondrolabral dysfunction: minimum two-year follow-up. J Bone Joint Surg Br 91:16–23, 2009.

27. Ilizaliturri VM Jr, et al: Arthroscopic treatment of cam-type femoroacetabular impingement: preliminary report at 2 years minimum follow-up. J Arthroplasty 23:226–234, 2008.

28. Beaule PE, Le Duff MJ, Zaragoza E: Quality of life following femoral head-neck osteochondroplasty for femoroacetabular impingement. J Bone Joint Surg Am 89:773–779, 2007.

29. Ganz R, et al: Surgical dislocation of the adult hip a technique with full access to the femoral head and acetabulum without the risk of avascular necrosis. J Bone Joint Surg Br 83: 1119–1124, 2001.

30. Parvizi J, et al: Arthroscopy for labral tears in patients with developmental dysplasia of the hip: a cautionary note. J Arthroplasty 24(Suppl 6):110–113, 2009.

31. Clohisy JC: Combined hip arthroscopy and limited open osteochondroplasty for the treatment of anterior femoroacetabular impingement. J Bone Joint Surg Am 92:1697–1706, 2010.

32. Siebenrock KA, Schoeniger R, Ganz R: Anterior femoroacetabular impingement due to acetabular retroversion: treatment with periacetabular osteotomy. J Bone Joint Surg Am 85:278–286, 2003.

CHAPTER 34

Dysplasia in the Skeletally Mature Patient

Perry L. Schoenecker

KEY POINTS

- Hip dysplasia commonly presents in adolescent and young adult patients with no known history of hip disease.
- Early diagnosis is essential to provide the opportunity for optimal hip preservation treatments.
- History, examination, and plain radiographs are the essential components of the diagnostic workup.
- Multiple hip preservation surgical treatments can be considered for the treatment of symptomatic hip dysplasia before established secondary osteoarthritis, yet acetabular reorientation is the most appropriate surgical intervention in most cases.
- Hip dysplasia with advanced secondary osteoarthritis should be managed with total hip arthroplasty when nonoperative management has failed.

INTRODUCTION

Instability secondary to hip dysplasia frequently does not become symptomatic until skeletal maturity. A history of previous treatment may be reported, as in an infant or young child with closed reduction with an orthosis or a spica cast; more often, no history of previous awareness or treatment of hip dysplasia is noted. Once an unstable hip has become symptomatic in the skeletally mature patient, surgical correction of existing acetabular dysplasia is necessary to arrest progressive pathologic processes.

DIFFERENTIAL DIAGNOSIS

Patients presenting with hip pain can be classified into many different categories. One early distinction is the site of the pain. Lateral hip pain often can be caused by a trochanteric bursitis, which can be related to abductor dysfunction. Low back pain or radiculopathy can also be present or can manifest as lateral hip pain. Most intra-articular hip pathology presents as groin pain. Patients with limited range of motion and pain may suffer from impingement about the hip with a femoral side "cam" lesion, an acetabular side "pincer" lesion, or both. They tend to report pain with sitting in low chairs or in a car for an extended period of time. Patients with hip dysplasia (and no impingement) typically exhibit a normal range of motion. They describe pain more with activities, walking, or running. Patients with either condition may experience labral tears and may have mechanical symptoms. Certainly other causes of adult hip pain are known, such as infection (septic arthritis or osteomyelitis), tumor, metabolic disease, avascular necrosis, trauma, or general osteoarthritis independent of dysplastic development. After a careful history and physical examination are performed, diagnostic imaging with plain radiographs is the next step in narrowing a differential diagnosis for hip pain in the adult. Figure 34-1 outlines a general algorithm for assessment of hip pain in the young adult.[1]

CLINICAL FINDINGS

History

Skeletally mature patients with symptomatic clinical instability secondary to hip dysplasia present with a history of variable hip pain and/or limp. This pain can be localized to various areas about the hip but primarily is reported as groin pain. The pain can be rather insidious, persisting for months to years before presentation. The pain is often accentuated with activity. A fatigue limp is often present. With this presentation, the pain initially may be localized to the hip abductors and/or the greater trochanter. This is attributed to lateralization of the hip center and increased load on the hip abductors. More active patients typically become symptomatic earlier in life given the same degree of dysplasia owing to increased demand placed on the hip. Other reports of mechanical symptoms such as catching, locking, or popping can accompany this, suggesting labral pathology or a chondral flap.

The level and character of pain, as well as its duration and associated symptoms, should be outlined; this can help in diagnosis and can guide treatment. Questions pertinent to hip joint function in daily activities used to calculate the Harris Hip Score are helpful for preoperative evaluation and can be used to assess the efficacy of treatment. Although typically used to evaluate outcomes of hip arthroplasty, this scoring system has also been used to assess hip preservation. Patients in studies of adult hip dysplasia treated with hip preservation techniques have preoperative scores that vary between 50 and 65 on a 100-point scale. If the patient had been treated as a child for hip dysplasia, a detailed history

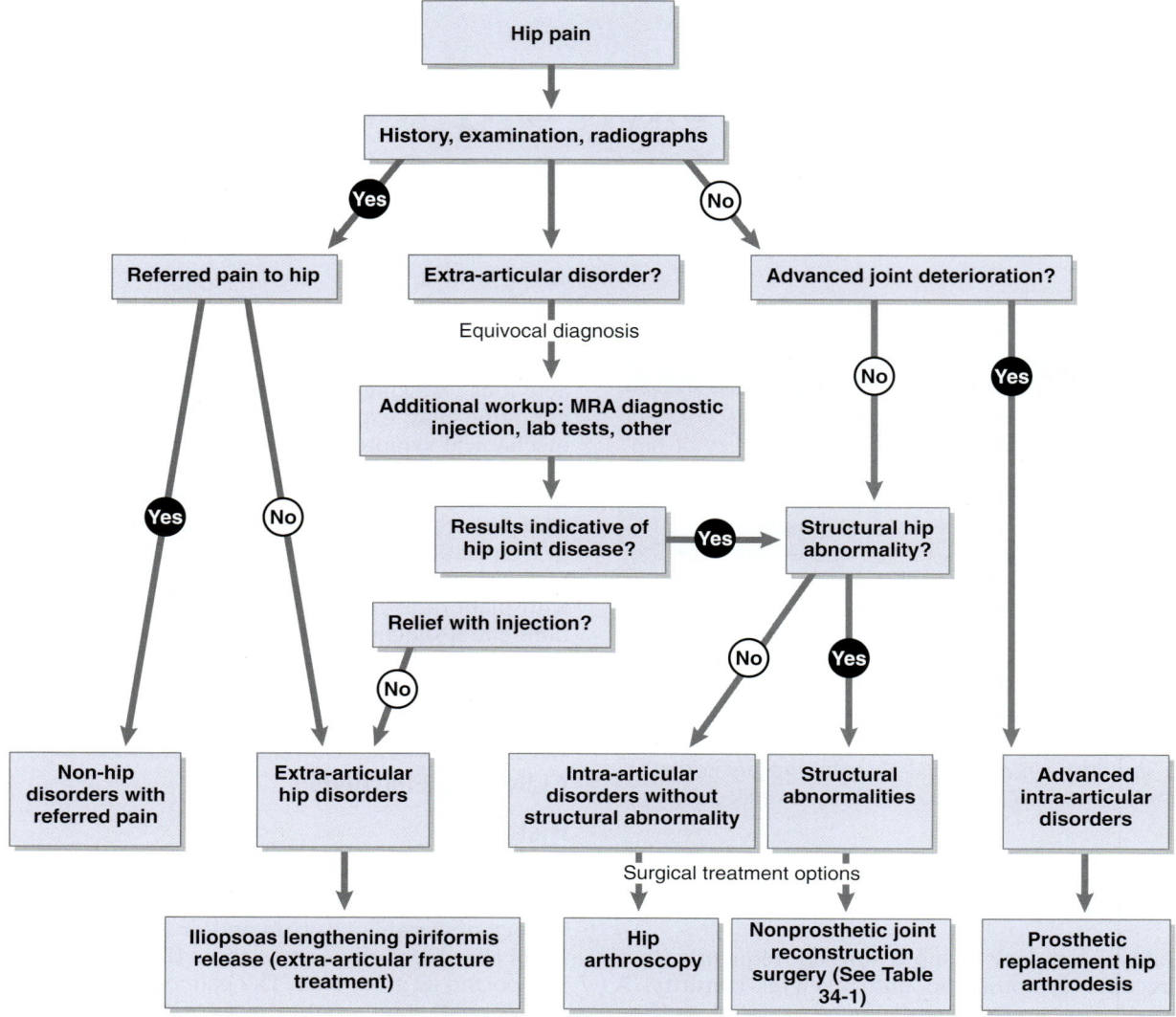

Figure 34-1. Algorithm for assessment and treatment of hip pain in the young adult. (Redrawn from Clohisy JC, Keeney JA, Schoenecker PL: Preliminary assessment and treatment guidelines for hip disorders in young adults. Clin Orthop Relat Res 441:168–179, 2005.)

of childhood treatment, both nonsurgical and surgical, must be obtained.

Physical Examination

The first step in examining a painful hip is to evaluate the patient's gait. Patients can present with an antalgic or a Trendelenburg gait. Patients with an antalgic gait may have significant labral pathology causing more acute pain or more involved degenerative changes from years of lateral point loading. Those with a Trendelenburg gait are exhibiting manifestations of a lateralized joint center and abductor weakness. If the hip joint is functionally unstable, the single-leg stance Trendelenburg test will be positive. Sometimes it is necessary to have the patient perform the test for several seconds. Occasionally, the patient will note reproduction of trochanteric hip pain while performing the Trendelenburg test.

Next, active and passive range of motion should be evaluated. Coupled with this is assessment of motor strength in the hip flexors, extensors, adductors, and abductors. Patients with pure acetabular dysplasia may have a normal passive range of motion. Occasionally, patients also have a femoral side osteochondral prominence or a cam-type lesion, leading to a positive impingement sign with the typical position of flexion, adduction, and internal rotation resulting in the reproduction of pain.

Radiographic Evaluation

Four standard radiographic views are helpful in evaluating dysplasia in the skeletally mature hip: a standing anteroposterior (AP) pelvis and false profile of both hips, a supine frog lateral, and a cross-table lateral[2] (Fig. 34-2A through D). Additionally, a flexion, abduction, and internal rotation (Von Rosen) view can be added to

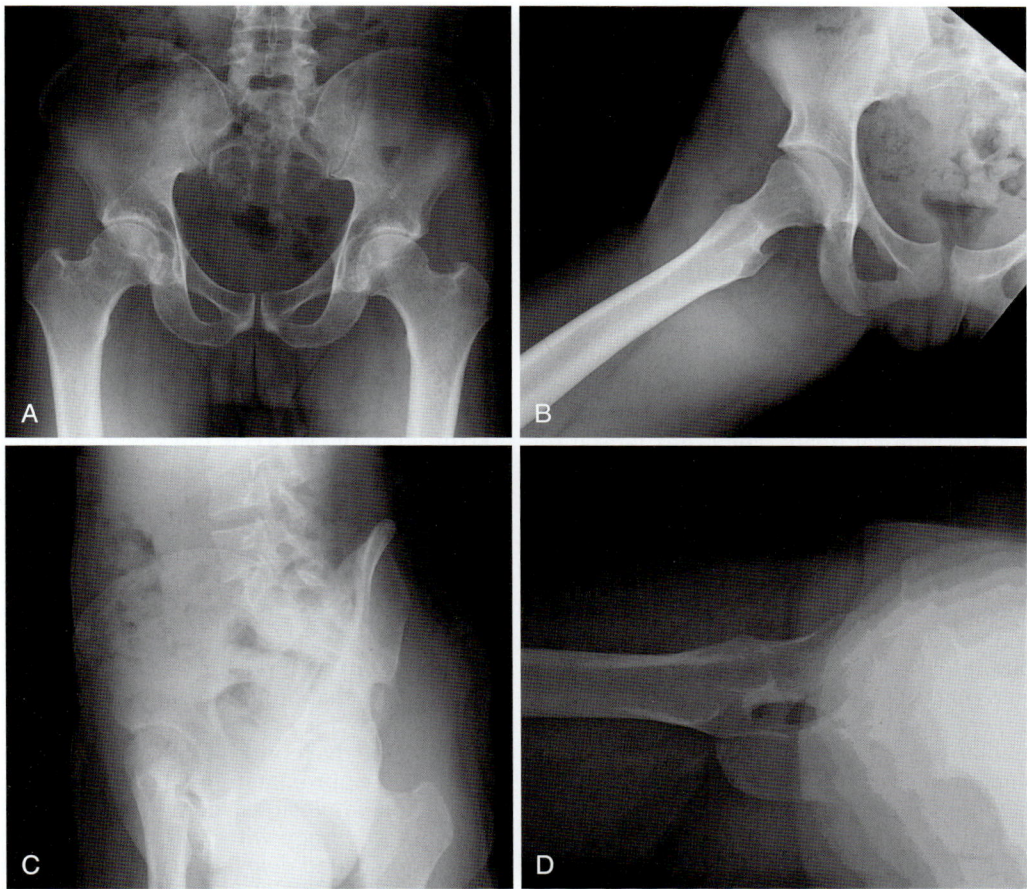

Figure 34-2. Normal examples of four initial radiographs taken in the evaluation of a young adult with a painful hip. **A,** Anteroposterior (AP) pelvis: beam centered between the pubic symphysis and the level of the anterosuperior iliac spine (ASIS), with both lower extremities in 15 degrees of internal rotation, to profile the proximal femur. **B,** Frog lateral: 45 degrees of hip abduction, 30 to 40 degrees of knee flexion, hip external rotation so that the sole of the foot faces the other leg. **C,** False profile (see Fig. 34-4A through C). **D,** Cross-table lateral. (From Clohisy JC, Carlisle JC, Beaule PE, et al: A systematic approach to the plain radiographic evaluation of the young adult hip. J Bone Joint Surg Am 90:47–66, 2008.)

show the coverage and congruence that can be obtained with pelvic and/or femoral osteotomies.

The AP pelvis provides perhaps the most information on the shape and orientation of the acetabulum and offers a comparison with the contralateral hip. Figure 34-3 details the important lines and measurements taken from this radiograph. Shenton's line, a curvilinear line connecting the obturator ring with the inferior border of the femoral neck, should be intact in a normal hip, and any discontinuity or irregularity is indicative of subluxation of the hip. A horizontal interteardrop line connecting the inferior aspect of the teardrop of each acetabulum provides a point of reference for further evaluation. This can serve as the reference for a parallel line drawn to connect the medial margins of the weight-bearing portion of the acetabular. The Tonnis angle, or acetabular index, is an angle created between this paral-lel line and its intersection with a second line outlining the weight-bearing portion of the acetabular dome. This

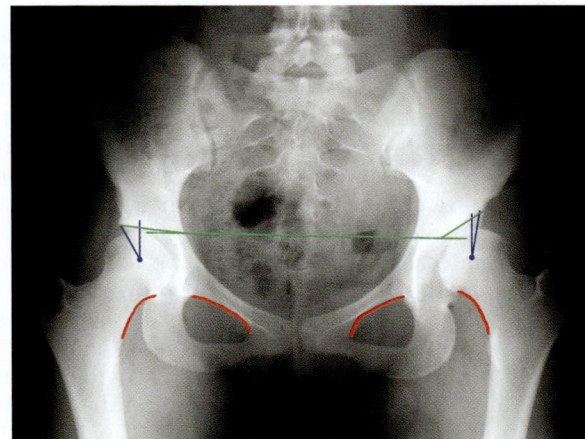

Figure 34-3. Standard anteroposterior (AP) pelvis radio-graph with important landmarks/measurements: Shenton's line, lateral center edge angle, Tonnis angle.

angle should measure 0 to 10 degrees. Angles greater than 10 degrees indicate dysplasia. The AP pelvis x-ray also provides a measurement of the lateral center edge angle. This angle is created between a vertical line through the center of the femoral head and a line connecting the center of the femoral head with the lateral edge of the acetabulum. The center of the femoral head in a normal hip should be well medial to the lateral edge of the acetabulum, producing a lateral center edge angle of 25 degrees or greater. However, in a dysplastic hip, the femoral head may be subluxated and lateralized and/or the acetabular weight-bearing dome (the sourcil) relatively short with resultant decreased femoral head coverage. Another measure of femoral head coverage is the lateral head *extrusion index*. This is represented as a percentage of the femoral head, which lies lateral to the lateral border of the acetabulum. This serves not only as an indicator of the degree of dysplasia but also as a postoperative marker predictive of success for hip preservation osteotomies.[3] The lateral center edge angle typically will be pathologically decreased, sometimes with a negative value (if the center of the head migrates lateral to the acetabulum). Direct measurement of hip joint lateralization relative to the pelvis can also be assessed on the AP view. A horizontal measurement in millimeters should be made from the ilioischial line to the medial aspect of the femoral head. This should be compared with the contralateral side if normal. An absolute value of less than 10 mm is considered normal.[2] Finally, the relative length of the lower extremities can be indirectly assessed on the standing AP pelvis radiograph by observing (and measuring) any tilt of the pelvis. The presence of a leg length discrepancy can relatively uncover the hip on the side of the longer leg, potentiating the development of a low-grade dysplastic hip—a condition known as *long leg arthropathy*.

Another important radiograph in the evaluation of adult hip dysplasia is the false profile view. This view is obtained with the patient standing 25 degrees off axis from a true lateral of the pelvis, with the affected hip centered on the film (Fig. 34-4A through C). On this view, the anterior center edge angle is measured, indicating the amount of anterior coverage that the acetabulum provides over the femoral head. The angle is formed between a vertical line drawn through the center of the femoral head and a line between the center of the femoral head and the anterior edge of the articular surface of the acetabulum. This value should be greater than 20 degrees. Undercoverage indicates a dysplastic hip, whereas overcoverage seen as increasing values causes impingement.

The frog lateral is taken as a supine AP projection with the hip and the knee each flexed approximately 45 degrees and the lower extremity externally rotated so that the sole of the foot touches the medial side of the opposite lower extremity. This position provides a variable lateral profile of the femoral head and the anterior and anterolateral head-neck junction. Typically, the anterior and anterolateral head and neck junction will be abnormally prominent and potentially will serve as a relative block to both flexion and internal rotation in

flexion.[2] The Von Rosen view is taken supine in the AP projection with the hip(s) positioned in approximately 25 to 30 degrees each of flexion, abduction, and internal rotation. This functional view demonstrates how congruently the femoral head reduces into the acetabulum and simulates coverage of the head following a redirective osteotomy, acetabular or femoral, or both. Three-dimensional (3D) imaging is not utilized routinely in the evaluation of hip dysplasia. In special circumstances, it can be helpful in obtaining a more definitive assessment of acetabular version, such as in pathologic retroversion, which is seen in up to 18% of acetabular dysplasia patients.[4-6]

Magnetic resonance imaging (MRI) with intra-articular gadolinium for contrast (i.e., magnetic resonance arthrography [MRA]) is the advanced imaging modality of choice for adult hip dysplasia. It provides additional and often helpful diagnostic information pertinent to intra-articular pathology. The acetabular labrum typically is enlarged with hip dysplasia, and symptomatic labral tears or chondral flap injuries can occur. In addition to symptoms secondary to hip dysplasia and resulting instability, patients with intra-articular pathology often present with position-related painful hip catching, locking, or snapping. In this clinical setting, MRA predictably provides more definitive information than MRI without the dye contrast. MRA yields 91% to 95% sensitivity and approximately 88% accuracy for identifying labrocapsular lesions, compared with 80% sensitivity and 65% accuracy with MRI alone.[7] A more recent MRI technique called *delayed gadolinium-enhanced magnetic resonance imaging of cartilage* (dGEMRIC) allows assessment of the relative quality of femoral head articular cartilage by measurement of glycosaminoglycans (GAGs). Initial reports indicate that low GAG scores on dGEMRIC reveal a poorer prognosis for hip preservation with osteotomy than do normal cartilage scores.[8] When dGEMRIC is not available, use of the Tonnis grade can aid treatment decision making. Grade 0 to 1 hips have no or very minimal joint space narrowing or evidence of degenerative changes such as sclerosis or marginal osteophytes. Tonnis grade 2 hips have moderate joint space narrowing with small cysts and can have mild loss of sphericity of the femoral head. In 2008, a report on periacetabular osteotomy patients from three different institutions revealed a 12% conversion to total hip arthroplasty (THA) by 5 years for Tonnis grade 0 or 1 hips versus 27% for grade 2 hips. Typically, grade 3 hips and those with advanced joint collapse or "bone-on-bone" arthritis are not candidates for hip preservation; patients should be counseled about other options such as arthroplasty.[9]

PATHOLOGY

Hip dysplasia begins even before birth as underdevelopment and/or imbalance of the hip joint. The development of a hip socket with a sufficiently covered femoral head requires a concentrically seated femoral head with balanced muscle forces about the hip throughout skeletal growth. Early in childhood, before age 3, simply

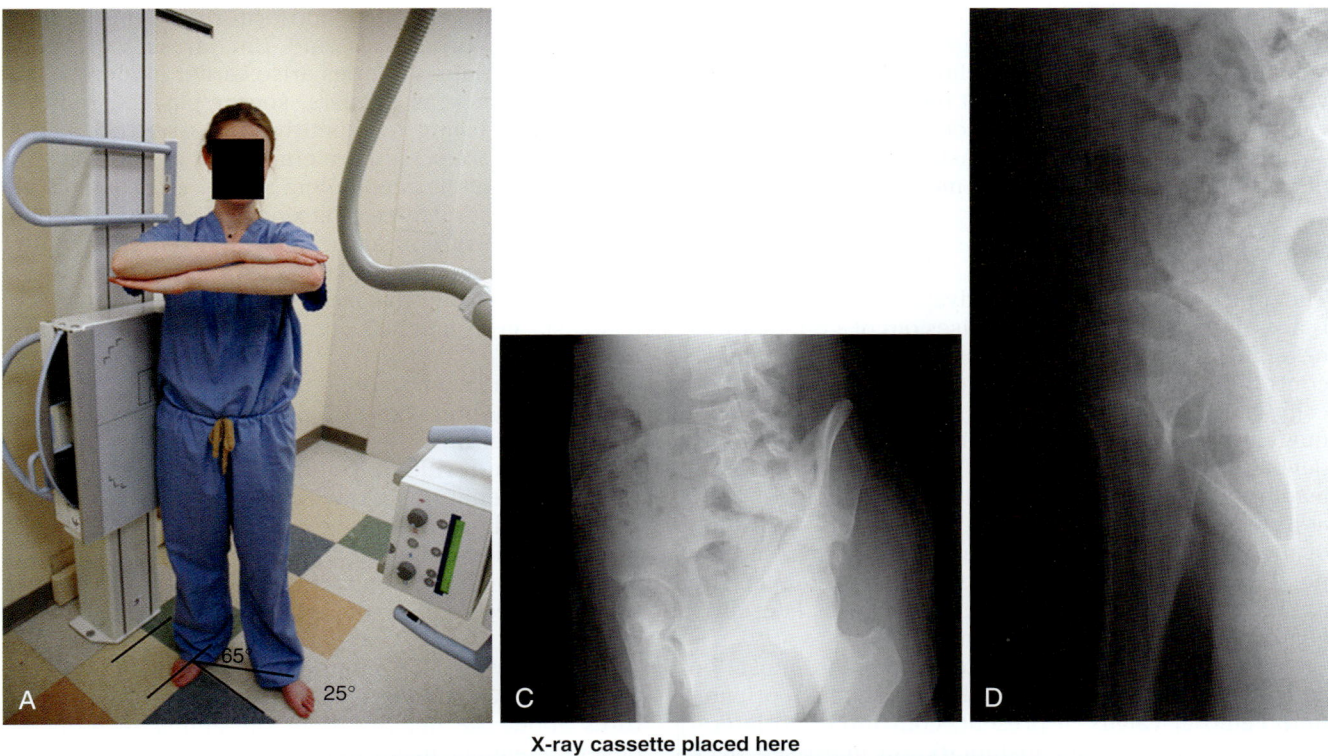

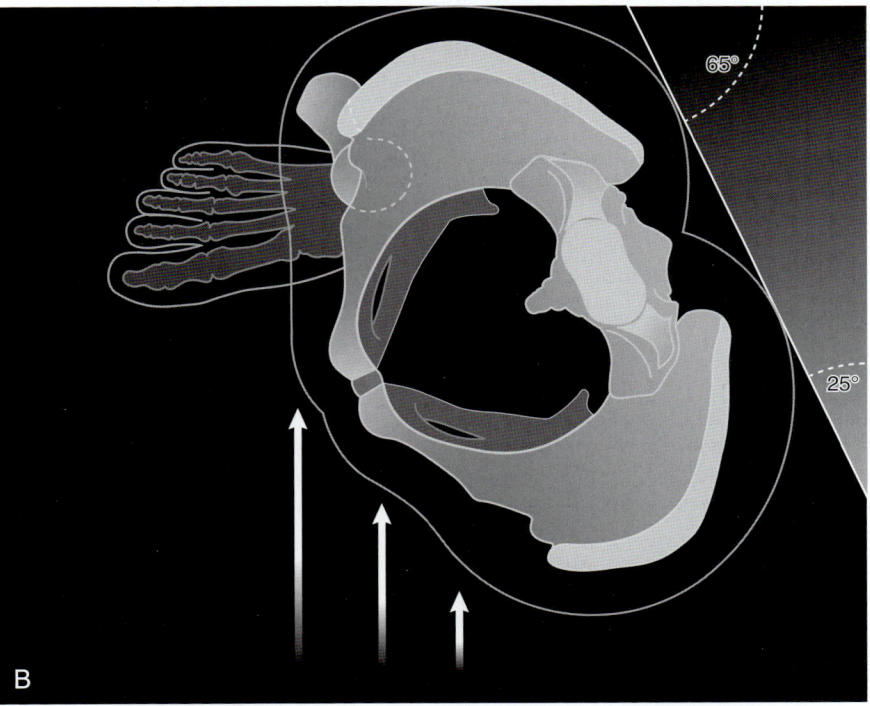

Figure 34-4. The false profile view. **A,** Patient is positioned standing with pelvis/torso rotated 25 degrees off the plane of a true lateral, producing a 65-degree oblique view of the imaged hip. The foot on the desired side is parallel to the cassette. **B,** Cross-sectional schematic of the same position. **C,** Example of a false profile view of a normal hip with measured anterior center edge angle. **D,** Example of a false profile view of a dysplastic acetabulum with anterior undercoverage. (Adapted from Clohisy JC, Carlisle JC, Beaule PE, et al: A systematic approach to the plain radiographic evaluation of the young adult hip. J Bone Joint Surg Am 90:47–66, 2008.)

balancing the femoral head within the acetabulum will deepen the socket as the hip grows and will improve stability. As acetabular remodeling potential decreases with age, the hip socket will not improve without surgical correction. Predictably, a poorly covered or imbalanced hip will progress toward instability with worsening of symptoms and radiographic measures.

Bony Pathology

The primary component of hip dysplasia with instability is acetabular deficiency. This arises out of a hip that was never fully seated or from one that has muscle imbalance contributing to instability during skeletal growth. Typically, once skeletal maturity is reached, a stable, adequately covered hip will remain stable; however, any degree of acetabular dysplasia can put the hip at risk, leading to progression of instability. An upsloping sourcil, as assessed by the Tonnis angle, allows lateral migration of the femoral head with weight bearing. This leads to point loading and increased stress at the acetabular rim as the femoral head pathologically migrates laterally.[10] Figure 34-5 illustrates this pathology.

Proximal femoral deformities at times must be addressed, in addition to acetabular surgical reorientation. Femoral valgus, if present, contributes to lateral extrusion and hip joint instability. An increased neck shaft angle translates forces laterally within the hip joint. If indicated, a proximal femoral varus/rotational osteotomy is combined with an acetabular redirection osteotomy to improve lateral coverage. Alternatively, residual proximal femoral varus may cause lateral impingement after an acetabular reorientation (periacetabular osteotomy [PAO]), requiring a valgus-producing proximal femoral osteotomy (PFO) to restore passive abduction. Frequently, an anterior arthrotomy is performed to address asphericity of the femoral head and the head-neck offset.[11,12]

Soft Tissue Pathology

In the setting of acetabular deficiency, the labrum responds in an effort to impart secondary stability. Dysplastic hips often have marked labral hypertrophy and redundancy. The abnormally large anterolateral labrum

can become degenerative and/or torn as femoral head lateralization progresses and rim stresses increase. Symptomatic labral injuries arise earlier in more active individuals such as dancers, soccer players, runners, and cyclists owing to repetitive rim overload. Labral injuries also are seen more commonly in patients with retroversion of the acetabulum as the result of impingement at a lesser degree of flexion and internal rotation. In 2005, Clohisy and associates reported that 36% of patients presenting with labral tears met radiographic parameters for hip dysplasia versus a 0% incidence of dysplasia in a matched control cohort without labral tears.[13]

Muscle imbalance about the hip potentiates symptoms of acetabular-based hip joint instability. Relative abductor weakness leads to increased joint reactive forces with a resultant Trendelenburg gait and a positive Trendelenburg sign. With subluxation and lateralization, the iliopsoas muscle can become shortened and further influence lateral proximal femoral migration. Muscle balance is essential in optimizing the outcomes of joint preservation or arthroplasty reconstructive operations.

At an early age, the anteromedial hip capsule and the transverse acetabular ligament are soft tissue structures about the hip that limit the ability to reduce a developmentally dislocated hip. In the child, incising both the contracted anteromedial capsule and the transverse acetabular ligament allows for expansion of a small acetabulum to accommodate the femoral head. In the adult, these structures typically are less of an issue in a reduced but dysplastic hip. Occasionally, when a surgical hip dislocation is performed as part of the hip preservation strategy, a pulvinar, similar to that seen in children, is appreciated and removed to allow the hip to seat fully.

TREATMENT OPTIONS

Nonoperative

All patients presenting for the first time with symptomatic hip pain as a result of hip instability secondary to acetabular dysplasia should be counseled as to the

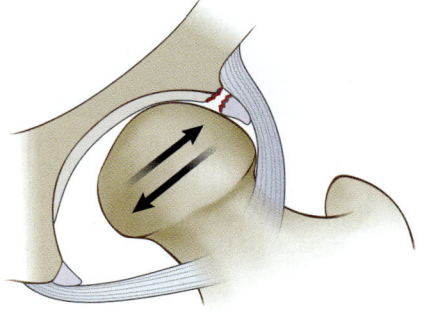
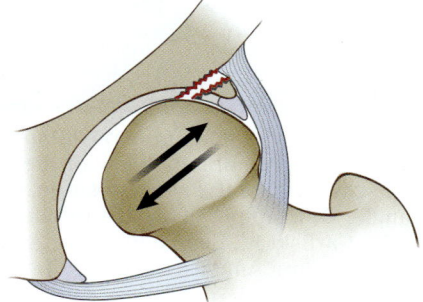

Figure 34-5. Schematic diagram of point loading and acetabular rim fracture seen with lateralization due to acetabular dysplasia. (Redrawn from Klaue K, Durnin CW, Ganz R: The acetabular rim syndrome. J Bone Joint Surg Br 73:423–429, 1991.)

biomechanical issues surrounding the disease. Patients who present with intermittent, mild symptoms and minimal radiographic evidence of hip dysplasia can be observed initially and treated with nonoperative measures. These include anti-inflammatory medications, goal-directed physical therapy, and activity modification that must be coupled with expectation management. Some patients who present with hip pain early in life with mild radiographic dysplasia do so because they are more active and place above average demands on undercovered or underdeveloped hip joints. As a result, the patient's level of activity should be determined; educating the patient about more favorable mechanics with more appropriate activities provides him or her with the opportunity to prolong the nonoperative life of the hip. Coupling activity modification with anti-inflammatory medications can provide needed relief early in the disease process. Adequate precautions should be taken with these medications, and they should not be used for long periods to mask hip pain that might be a sign of significant underlying pathology. In conjunction with these efforts, goal-directed physical therapy aimed at strengthening muscles around the hip can improve function. Abductor strengthening improves the ability for single-leg stance and can also improve gait. Strengthening these muscles can offset the loss of mechanical advantage caused by lateralization of the hip center. Coupling this with hip flexor, extensor, and core strengthening can improve a patient's hip endurance as well. Certainly younger patients with preserved joint space but with significant dysplasia should be educated early on with regard to joint preservation options that might prolong their need for an arthroplasty.

Arthroscopy

Symptomatic patients with a clinical history and findings of hip instability from more severe acetabular-based hip dysplasia will not appreciate lasting relief of their symptoms resulting from an arthroscopic surgical approach alone. A few selected patients with a lesser degree of acetabular dysplasia and hip pain associated with intra-articular pathology such as labral tears may be considered for arthroscopic treatment. Nevertheless, the long-term efficacy of arthroscopy in the setting of hip dysplasia remains unclear. Avulsion-type injuries often can be repaired, and small areas of chondromalacia can be treated arthroscopically as well. A recent study noted at least grade I chondral lesions in 78% of prearthritic hips, as well as labral tears in 78%. Concomitant lesions were noted in 56% of patients. A majority (72%) of chondral lesions were located on the acetabular side of the joint. Not all lesions are amenable to arthroscopic treatment; some require an open approach.[14]

In patients with significant dysplasia, it is essential to surgically correct the acetabular bony deficiency with a redirective pelvic osteotomy and, in turn, to restore critically needed functional hip joint stability. Arthroscopy can be incorporated into the treatment but as an adjunct to the necessary redirective pelvic osteotomy, not as standalone treatment. A report of 34 patients treated with hip arthroscopy for labral tears with documented dysplasia revealed that arthroscopy alone failed to provide relief for 24 patients, and 16 went on to undergo additional hip surgery.[15]

Joint Preservation

Patients with intact articular cartilage and significant dysplasia can anticipate notable prolonging of the life of their native hip after undergoing joint preservation procedures. Joint preservation surgery is potentially of optimal benefit for the patient when it is aimed at improving femoral head coverage and optimizing joint contact surface area. Most important, it optimizes congruency and motion. This is accomplished with an acetabular reorientation performed as a Bernese periacetabular osteotomy or a rotational acetabular or triple innominate osteotomy. The functional goal of acetabular reorientation is to restore joint stability. The acetabular dome (sourcil) is variably redirected so as to achieve optimal coverage of the femoral head both laterally and anteriorly. Radiographically, the lateral and anterior center edge angles will be restored to near or normal values as the deficient femoral head coverage is corrected. Increased upward lateral sloping of the acetabular dome (sourcil) will be turned to a more horizontal (stable) inclination after correction. The lateralized cup joint center is medialized, improving hip joint mechanics.[16-18] Figure 34-6 illustrates medialization of the hip center with a periacetabular osteotomy. For the moderate deformity and/or relatively younger patients, satisfactory correction can be achieved with a triple-type innominate osteotomy. For most acetabular-based deficiencies, more comprehensive correction can be attained with a Bernese-type PAO (Fig. 34-7).[3,16-18] Although more difficult to perform than a triple innominate osteotomy, the Bernese PAO has become the acetabular redirection osteotomy of choice. Its versatility makes it possible to correct all possible aspects of acetabular dysplasia (version and lateralization, as well as lateral and anterior femoral head coverage deficiency). Rehabilitation begins immediately, and the rate of delayed union or nonunion is relatively low. A concomitant arthrotomy is typically performed; if present, resection osteochondroplasty of the abnormally prominent anterolateral head and neck junction will potentially improve flexion and internal rotation in flexion.

Proximal Femoral Osteotomy

In addition to an acetabular reorientation osteotomy, a proximal femoral osteotomy (PFO) is needed occasionally to obtain satisfactory coverage and/or maintain optimal functional motion following acetabular reorientation in the treatment of hip joint instability.[10,11,18,20,21] An increased femoral neck shaft angle (valgus) may require some degree of varus-producing osteotomy so as to obtain satisfactory lateral femoral head coverage; the femoral head extrusion index should be less than 20% following joint-preserving surgery in addressing instability secondary to acetabular dysplasia.[3] Preoperative and intraoperative assessment of the patient's passive abduction and radiographic coverage gives an

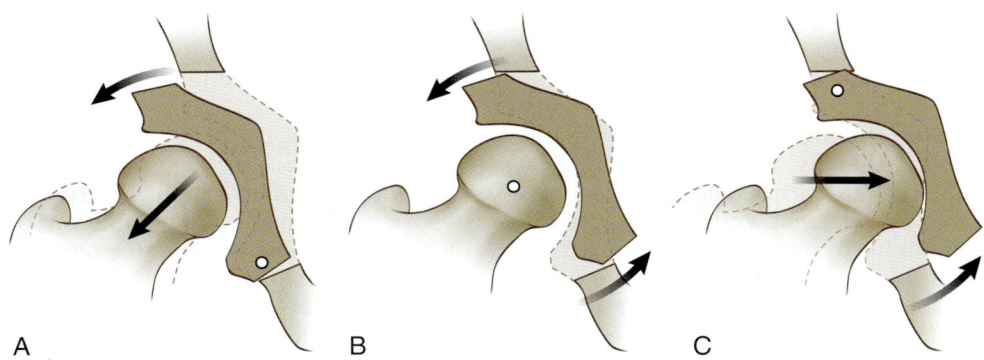

Figure 34-6. Schematic depiction of the medialization that can be achieved with a periacetabular osteotomy (PAO). (Redrawn from Clohisy JC, Barrett SE, Gordon JE, et al: Medial translation of the hip joint center associated with the Bernese periacetabular osteotomy. Iowa Orthop J 24:43–48, 2004.)

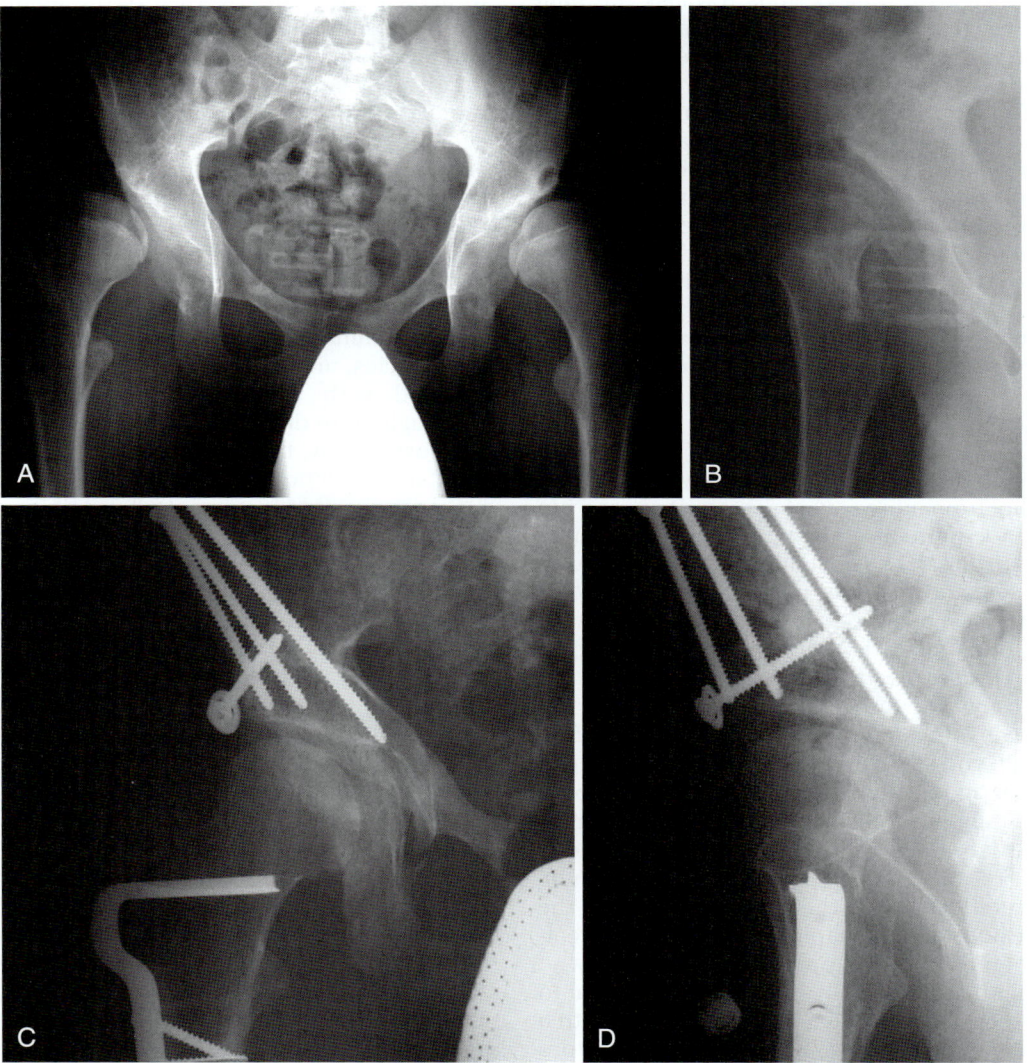

Figure 34-7. A 15-year-old male with a painful right hip and severe dysplasia demonstrated on **(A)** anteroposterior (AP) hip and **(B)** false profile images. Treated with a Bernese periacetabular osteotomy and a varus shortening proximal femoral osteotomy. At 3 years postoperative, he is pain free and has returned to full activity. **C** and **D,** Radiographs show improved anterior and lateral coverage, as well as improved acetabular inclination and medialization of the hip center with a congruent joint and well-maintained joint space.

indication of the amount of varus that can be introduced safely. Similarly, following acetabular reorientation, passive abduction may be limited; a valgus proximal femoral osteotomy may be indicated to restore essential hip abduction motion.[11] Again, the optimal degree of desirable valgus is determined by passive examination of the hip and is correlated with functional radiographs.

Arthroplasty

The eventual definitive treatment for most cases of adult hip dysplasia has been total hip arthroplasty. Many issues should be taken into account during planning for arthroplasty of a dysplastic hip. Previous surgical procedures alter the anatomy, both bony and soft tissue. These alterations can be helpful, such as an acetabular reorientation that would medialize the joint center and place the acetabulum in a more normal position.[22] In contrast, previous femoral osteotomies and resulting secondary deformities often present additional salvage challenges when THR is performed in a previously treated hip. Deforming proximal femoral osteotomies may necessitate the performance of additional and structurally compromising proximal femoral osteotomies to place the femoral component. Similarly, the necessity to remove retained proximal implants, such as a blade plate, concomitant with performing the THR, can compromise both the relative bony integrity of the proximal femur and the potential for achieving a stable and durable proximal femoral construct. Reviewing operative reports of previous procedures, such as the approach used and hardware that has been placed, can provide helpful preoperative THR planning. This may, in turn, be essential in planning a successful arthroplasty.

Proper placement of the acetabular shell and liner is essential for restoring hip biomechanics and producing a stable, long-lasting hip. Attempts should be made to place the shell in the position of the true acetabulum. Because the acetabulum is shallow by definition, the amount of remaining bone stock can be an issue in providing adequate support for an acetabular shell. Grafting with bulk allograft, femoral head autograft, or porous trabecular metal augments creates additional structural support for the acetabular component. Adjustments for limb length and version can also be made with placement of the femoral component.

CONCLUSION

Hip dysplasia in the adult population stems from undetected or undertreated dysplasia of childhood. This becomes symptomatic with time and with increased demands placed on the hip joint. Evaluation through history, physical examination, and proper radiographic imaging will reveal the source of the pathology and will guide management of the dysplastic hip.

REFERENCES

1. Clohisy JC, Keeney JA, Schoenecker PL: Preliminary assessment and treatment guidelines for hip disorders in young adults. Clin Orthop Relat Res 441:168–179, 2005.
2. Clohisy JC, Carlisle JC, Beaule PE, et al: A systematic approach to the plain radiographic evaluation of the young adult hip. J Bone Joint Surg Am 90:47–66, 2008.
3. Steppenbacker SD, Tannast M, Ganz R, Siebenrock KA: Mean 20-year follow-up of Bernese periacetabular osteotomy. Clin Orthop Relat Res 466:1633–1644, 2008.
4. Li PL, Ganz R: Morphologic features of congenital acetabular dysplasia: one in six is retroverted. Clin Orthop Relat Res 416:245–253, 2003.
5. Mast JW, Brunner RL, Zerback J: Recognizing acetabular version in the radiographic presentation of hip dysplasia. Clin Orthop Relat Res 418:48–53, 2004.
6. Ezoe M, Naito M, Inoue T: The prevalence of acetabular retroversion among various disorders of the hip. J Bone Joint Surg Am 88:372–379, 2006.
7. Keeney JA, Peelle MW, Jackson J, et al: Magnetic resonance arthrography versus arthroscopy in the evaluation of articular hip pathology. Clin Orthop Relat Res 429:163–169, 2004.
8. Cunningham T, Jessel R, Zurakowski D, et al: Delayed gadolinium-enhanced magnetic resonance imaging of cartilage to predict early failure of Bernese periacetabular osteotomy for hip dysplasia. J Bone Joint Surg 88:1540–1548, 2006.
9. Millis MB, Kain M, Sierra R, et al: Periacetabular osteotomy for acetabular dysplasia in patients older than 40 years: a preliminary study. Clin Orthop Relat Res 467:2228–2234, 2009.
10. Klaue K, Durnin CW, Ganz R: The acetabular rim syndrome. J Bone Joint Surg Br 73:423–429, 1991.
11. Clohisy JC, Nunley RM, Carlisle JC, Schoenecker PL: Incidence and characteristics of femoral deformities in the dysplastic hip. Clin Orthop Relat Res 467:128–134, 2009.
12. Clohisy JC, Nunley RM, Curry MC, Schoenecker PL: Periacetabular osteotomy for the treatment of acetabular dysplasia associated with major aspherical femoral head deformities. J Bone Joint Surg Am 89:1417–1423, 2007.
13. Peelle MW, Della Rocca GJ, Maloney WJ, et al: Acetabular and femoral radiographic abnormalities associated with labral tears. Clin Orthop Relat Res 441:327–333, 2005.
14. McCarthy JC, Lee JA: Acetabular dysplasia: a paradigm of arthroscopic examination of chondral injuries. Clin Orthop Relat Res 405:122–128, 2002.
15. Parvizi J, Bican O, Bender B, et al: Arthroscopy for labral tears in patients with developmental dysplasia of the hip: a cautionary note. J Arthroplasty 6(Suppl):110–113, 2009.
16. Clohisy JC, Beaule PE, Beck M: AOA Symposium. Hip disease in the young adult: current concepts of etiology and surgical treatment. J Bone Joint Surg Am 90:2267–2281, 2008.
17. Clohisy JC, Barrett SE, Gordon JE, et al: Medial translation of the hip joint center associated with the Bernese periacetabular osteotomy. Iowa Orthop J 24:43–48, 2004.
18. Leunig M, Siebenrock KA, Ganz R: Rationale of periacetabular osteotomy and background work. In Sim FH (ed): AAOS instructional course lectures, vol 50, Rosemont, Ill, 2001, American Academy of Orthopedic Surgeons, pp 229–238.
19. Clohisy JC, Barrett SE, Gordon JE, et al: Periacetabular osteotomy for the treatment of severe acetabular dysplasia. J Bone Joint Surg Am 87:254–259, 2005.
20. Hersche O, Casillas M, Ganz R: Indications for intertrochanteric osteotomy after periacetabular osteotomy for adult hip dysplasia. Clin Orthop Relat Res 347:19–26, 1998.
21. Sierra RJ, Trousdale RT, Ganz R, Leunig M: Hip disease in the young active patient: evaluation and non-arthroplasty options. J Am Acad Orthop Surg 12:689–703, 2008.
22. Parvizi J, Burmeister H, Ganz R: Previous Bernese periacetabular osteotomy does not compromise the results of total hip arthroplasty. Clin Orthop Relat Res 423:118–122, 2004.

CHAPTER 35

Osteonecrosis and Bone Marrow Edema Syndrome

*David R. Marker, Thorsten M. Seyler,
Michael A. Mont, and Edward F. McCarthy*

KEY POINTS

- As many as 10,000 to 20,000 new cases of osteonecrosis (ON) are reported each year in the United States. Bone marrow edema syndrome (BEMS) is a relatively rare disease.
- ON and BMES similarly present in young and middle-aged patients with hip or groin pain.
- Magnetic resonance imaging (MRI) is the most sensitive and specific diagnostic tool for both ON and BMES.
- ON progresses to end-stage arthritis in as many as 80% to 90% of patients. BMES has an excellent prognosis, typically resolving within 2 to 9 months.
- BMES should be treated nonoperatively with protected weight bearing, analgesics, and bisphosphonates. ON treatment is dependent on the stage of the disease. Early stages can be treated with pharmaceutical therapy, core decompression, and/or bone grafting. Later stages, with evidence of severe femoral head collapse and/or acetabular involvement, require total hip arthroplasty using resurfacing or stemmed components.

INTRODUCTION

Osteonecrosis of the hip (ON) and bone marrow edema syndrome (BMES), also called *transient osteoporosis of the hip (TOH),* are causes of hip pain in middle-aged patients who show evidence of bone morrow edema. Although some literature has suggested that BMES may be a reversible form of osteonecrosis rather than a disease entity of its own,[1,2] no definitive documentation is available to support this theory. The current general consensus is that BMES is a unique disease entity.[3] In contrast to ON, BMES is a transient but painful condition of the hip that is limited to marrow changes without associated joint space narrowing and arthritic changes. Because of the low incidence of BMES, few reports have described large series, making it difficult to further elucidate the pathophysiology of this disease. It was originally defined by Curtiss and Kincaid in 1959 as a syndrome of transient demineralization of the hip in the third trimester of pregnancy.[4] It has since been found to occur more frequently in young and middle-aged men.[5-7]

In contrast to the extremely low incidence of BMES, osteonecrosis is a more common condition that has existed for millennia; evidence of the disease has been found in Egyptian mummies.[8] ON is defined by compromise of bone blood circulation that leads to ischemic death of subchondral bone in the femoral head. The hallmark that separates these two entities is that most patients who are diagnosed with ON progress to advanced stages of the disease with femoral head collapse and painful arthritis that require total hip arthroplasty, in contrast to the usual self-limited nature of BMES (Fig. 35-1).

Differentiation of ON and BMES is complicated by various terms that have been used to describe these two diseases. Ultimately, it is important for orthopedic surgeons to understand this terminology so they can properly use the current literature in their diagnoses, decision making, and surgical management. Some of the descriptions that have been used are based on the underlying pathogenesis or the clinical nature of the disease, but others are outdated and are no longer commonly used. Lequesne and associates were the first to characterize the syndrome of transient demineralization of the hip as transient osteoporosis.[5] The usefulness of *transient osteoporosis of the hip* as a clinical term supplanted use of the original terminology of transient demineralization of the hip. In general, many investigators consider BMES and transient osteoporosis of the hip as the same disease. Because of its similarity to other transient clinical entities at other sites in the body, it is now included in the umbrella of diseases commonly referred to as *bone marrow edema syndromes.*[9] In cases of bone marrow edema characterized by concurrent or subsequent involvement of additional anatomic sites other than the primary hip, the overall syndrome may be referred to as *regional migratory osteoporosis.* Although it remains unclear whether regional migratory osteoporosis is the same entity as is seen in cases of isolated BMES that have no other sites of involvement, many clinician experts consider regional migratory osteoporosis a variant of BMES.[10]

Other authors initially postulated that BMES was a form of reflex sympathetic dystrophy (now called *complex regional pain syndrome, type 2*), but this theory has largely fallen out of favor.[11,12] Also, as previously noted, some authors have proposed that BMES may be a nonprogressive, reversible form of osteonecrosis.[1] Regardless of the proposed pathophysiology, BMES remains the most commonly used term to describe this

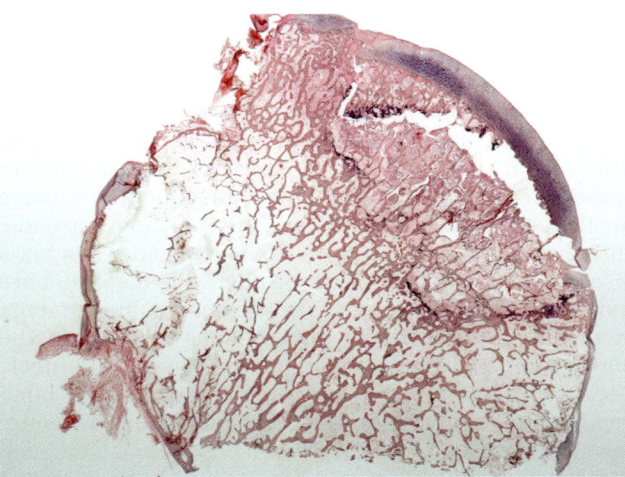

Figure 35-1. This macro-photomicrograph of a hip specimen demonstrates the subchondral fracture that corresponds with the "crescent sign" seen on radiographs in advanced-stage osteonecrosis. Patients who reach this stage of disease invariably require reconstructive total joint surgery. Because this degree of joint destruction does not occur in patients who have bone marrow edema syndrome, it is important that surgeons are able to distinguish these disease entities and provide appropriate treatment.

disease. In the case of ON, the terminology has been less variable. Initially, *avascular necrosis* was commonly used. This term was an accurate descriptor of this disease for cases with a known traumatic origin in which the vascular supply to the femoral head was directly compromised. However, this terminology was deemed inaccurate in its use when describing lesions in individuals who had associated risk factors such as corticosteroid usage, systemic lupus erythematosus, or Gaucher's disease, where bone marrow displacement and increased compartment pressure were considered to be the likely pathogenetic mechanisms. *Osteonecrosis* has subsequently become the preferred term. Although ON can be grouped with other diseases that cause bone marrow edema, it is typically studied as a distinct entity.

Part of the difficulty in differentiating ON from BMES may be that patients with these diseases can present with seemingly nonspecific groin pain and equivocal findings on physical and radiologic examination. Nevertheless, some progress has been made in understanding the underlying origins of these conditions and in examining the outcomes of various surgical and nonsurgical treatments. The present work will serve as a review of current knowledge about these conditions to assist clinicians in their management. This chapter begins by discussing the differences in epidemiology, risk factors, pathophysiology, and clinical and diagnostic features that can be used to distinguish these two diseases, while providing some of the arguments that have been put forth against this taxonomy. The second part of the chapter reviews various treatment options available for each condition and provides a discussion of their rationale and indications, along with a summary of results obtained when various techniques were used.

EPIDEMIOLOGY AND RISK FACTORS

The exact prevalence of ON and BMES remains undefined. It is estimated that approximately 10,000 to 20,000 new cases of ON are diagnosed in the United States each year.[13] In more than 10% of these cases, the disease will also involve the knee and the shoulder, and in less than 3% of patients, the disease will be multifocal and will affect more than three anatomic sites. These numbers are clinically more important when it is considered that more than 10% of hip arthroplasties performed in the United States are related to ON. The prevalence of BMES is considerably less than that of ON. Only several hundred cases of BMES have been reported in the literature, and the incidence is less than 1% of the number of ON cases each year.[14]

The prevalence of ON is higher in specific at-risk populations. Recent studies have evaluated the increased prevalence of ON associated with corticosteroid use, alcohol abuse, sickle cell disease, and genetic factors. Griffith and associates reported that 5% of patients (12 of 254) with systemic adult respiratory syndrome (SARS) first had evidence of osteonecrosis of the femoral head, and that the cumulative prednisolone-equivalent dose was the most important risk factor, with the risk being 0.6% for patients receiving a dose less than 3 g, and 13% for those receiving a dose greater than 3 g. For transplant patients on high doses of corticosteroids, the prevalence of ON has been reported to be between 3% and 23%.[15-17] Recognition of the association between ON and corticosteroids has led to preventative measures, and organ transplant patients on modern immunosuppressive drugs have a risk of ON that is likely at the lower end of the spectrum previously reported—near 5%.[18] The association of alcohol abuse with increased risk for ON was evaluated in separate studies by Hirota and associates and Matsuo and colleagues. Investigators found similar findings with a clear dose-response relationship. Hirota and coworkers reported a higher risk for development of ON in occasional drinkers (<8 mL of alcohol once a week, but not daily; relative odds = 3.2) and in regular drinkers (≥8 mL of alcohol daily; relative odds = 13.1) than in controls. The dose-response relationship reported in their study revealed relative odds for current drinkers of 2.8, 9.4, and 14.8 in association with ethanol intakes of <320, 320 to 799, and ≥800 g/wk, respectively. Matsuo and associates reported an elevated risk for regular drinkers (>8 mL of alcohol every day; relative risk = 7.8). They also described a dose-response relationship, with relative risks of 3.3, 9.8, and 17.9 for current drinkers consuming <400, 400 to 1000, and ≥1000 mL/wk of alcohol, respectively. The incidence of ON in sickle cell patients was recently studied in a cohort of 200 patients over a mean 15-year follow-up.[19] Osteonecrosis was greatest among groups with the SS genotype (43% developed multifocal disease), followed by those with the hemoglobin SC genotype (38%) and the Sβ⁺ thalassemia genotype (19%).

Genetic factors that may predispose individuals to ON remain poorly defined. Familial high plasminogen activator inhibitor and resulting hypofibrinolysis were initially associated with the development of ON by Glueck and colleagues,[20] who reported that, compared with control subjects, patients with osteonecrosis were more likely to have heterozygosity and homozygosity for the hypofibrinolytic 4G polymorphism of the plasminogen activator inhibitor-1 gene. Other studies have reported that genes affecting lipid transport and metabolism,[21] or production of increased catalase and decreased nitric oxide,[22,23] may increase the risk for ON.

Much less is known regarding the risk factors for BMES. Pregnancy was the first risk factor identified. Even in patients who are believed to be at risk, the incidence of BMES is low. It has been reported that middle-aged men are at higher risk.[24] However, early diagnosis of pregnant BMES patients remains important, because evidence suggests that they have a unique risk for femoral neck and stress fractures compared with their nonpregnant counterparts. Pregnant patients who develop BMES should be followed clinically until radiographic evidence (MRI) indicates that the hips have undergone adequate reconstitution of their bone mass.[25]

PATHOGENESIS

Although ON is a well-described clinical entity, its cause and pathogenesis have not been completely elucidated. The pathogenesis of BMES is even less well defined. In most cases, the cause of ON can be characterized by a final common pathway of (1) focal intravascular coagulation and subsequent thrombosis that affect the terminal arterioles or the postsinusoidal venules, and/or (2) increased intraosseous pressure that is postulated to compress the subchondral microvasculature. The predilection of the femoral head for coagulation and thrombosis may be based on the microanatomy of its blood supply. Minimal collateral circulation is seen, and end arterioles form vascular arcades that must make abrupt turns at the ends of cortical bone before returning venous blood from the femoral head.

The pathogenetic mechanism of osteonecrosis can also be characterized according to underlying causes or associated risk factors. ON is a multifactorial disease that is associated with various direct and indirect risk factors. Direct causes include trauma, Caisson's disease, chemotherapy, Gaucher's disease, and radiation. Indirect causes that have been associated with ON include alcohol and smoking abuse, coagulation abnormalities (thrombophilia, hypofibrinolysis), corticosteroid use, inflammatory bowel disease, organ transplants, pregnancy, and systemic lupus erythematosus.

In cases such as trauma or radiation, the pathogenetic mechanism directly causes necrosis. Other causes initiate events that lead to thrombosis and disruption of the microcirculation of the femoral head. For example, in sickle cell disease and Caisson's disease, direct restriction or occlusion of blood vessels is noted. Other factors that may contribute to risk in sickle cell patients include higher blood viscosity and bone marrow hyperplasia. Additionally, deformed erythrocytes may cause

microinfarcts in the subchondral bone.[26] In patients who develop osteonecrosis after corticosteroid use or alcohol abuse, intraosseous pressure is increased likely as the result of enlarged adipocyte size and proliferation. In addition, fat emboli may become trapped in the end arterioles and occlude these vessels in the subchondral bone. Subsequently, damage to the endothelium initiates the clotting cascade, and the microvasculature is compromised. Gaucher's disease, leukemia, and myeloproliferative disorders are thought to increase pressure in the bony compartments of the hip by displacing intraosseous marrow in the bony compartments of the femoral head and neck. Because the bone marrow cannot expand, the bone involved cannot compensate for increased pressure; this leads to collapse of vessels, ischemia, and cell damage. Systemic lupus erythematosus has been shown to be an independent risk factor in osteonecrosis. Recent reports have assessed whether patients who have systemic lupus erythematosus may be at increased risk for osteonecrosis if they also present with Raynaud's phenomenon, hyperlipidemia, and/or high levels of anticardiolipin or antiphospholipid antibodies, but additional studies with more patients are needed to further assess any correlation.[27,28] Controversy concerning the influence of antiphospholipid antibodies is ongoing, with some studies suggesting that there is an association,[29] while others suggest there is not.[30] Much recent research has been undertaken to explore the risk of development of osteonecrosis in patients who have inherited coagulation disorders. Associations have been shown between ON and thrombophilia and hypofibrinolysis because of an increase in blood clots and a decreased ability to lyse blood clots, respectively.[31-35]

The cause of BMES is unknown. Mechanisms such as demineralization, neurogenic compression, reflex sympathetic dystrophy, and obstruction of venous return with localized hyperemia have been proposed previously but are no longer widely accepted.[4,5,11,12] Currently, two pathogenetic mechanisms propose that BMES (1) results from sequelae of a subchondral insufficiency fracture at, or near, a weight-bearing surface,[36] or (2) is caused by subacute transient ischemia seen along the spectrum of osteonecrosis.[9] The postulate that a subchondral insufficiency fracture is associated with BMES is supported by recent research assessing regional accelerated phenomenon activation. When bone is exposed to noxious stimuli such as microfractures, it has been shown to undergo localized modeling and remodeling at rates of up to 10 times normal. Prolonged activation of this phenomenon may result in transient osteoporosis.[37] Imaging studies suggest that subchondral insufficiency fractures may eventually be detected in all BMES patients as the resolution and technology of advanced MRI continue to improve.[36,38]

Histopathology

Some of the histologic features of ON and BMES are similar. It has been suggested that changes such as marrow edema, dilated medullary sinuses, and fat vacuoles in the interstitial fluid are indicative of a common pathophysiologic entity.[39] Hofman and associates suggested that BMES is a precursor to osteonecrosis than can progress to advanced osteonecrosis or can improve if ischemic levels are subcritical.[40] However, key differences have been noted in the histopathologies of ON and BMES, the most notable being the continued presence of osteocytes in BMES. This finding is used in the argument that these are distinct entities.

The histopathologic process of ON is dynamic and nondiscrete but can be defined in terms of four key stages (Box 35-1). The first stage is marked by true necrosis with morphologic changes that occur in tissues after death (Fig. 35-2). These histologic changes do not begin until several days after death. Therefore, histologic study of bone immediately after an infarct will reveal no changes. The first change to occur is dissolution of hematopoietic cells. This begins approximately 2 to 3 days after death. Then, osteocytes drop out of lacunae anywhere from 2 days to 4 weeks after death.

BOX 35-1. CORRELATION OF HISTOPATHOLOGIC TO RADIOLOGIC STAGES OF OSTEONECROSIS

Histopathology	Ficat Classification
1. Early necrosis (fat necrosis and osteocyte dropout)	Stage I: no radiographic evidence
2. Appositional bone formation and marrow calcification	Stage II: mottled radiodensity
3. Osteoclastic resorption	Stage III: subchondral fracture
4. Cartilage failure	Stage IV: signs of osteoarthritis

Marrow fat begins to show necrotic changes about 5 days after the bone is dead. Therefore, bone may not be recognizably dead by histologic study until 5 or more days after irreversible cessation of cellular activity. These early histologic changes correlate with Ficat stage I.

After several weeks following tissue death, necrotic marrow begins to show dystrophic calcification (Fig. 35-3). This is a common morphologic change in fat necrosis in any location of the body. After several weeks, a reparative reaction begins at the margin of the bone infarct. Ingrowth of granulation tissue brings multipotential cells that begin to lay down new viable bone on dead trabeculae. This causes marked thickening of bone trabeculae in a process called *appositional new bone formation.* As time progresses, this front of reparative bone extends into the center of the infarct; this correlates with radiographic changes of radiodensity (Ficat stage II).

The next change that occurs is due to osteoclastic resorption at the viable/necrotic interface. Osteoclastic resorption begins to weaken trabeculae, and a subchondral fracture often occurs. This signals failure of the surface of the bone. It is visible histologically as a crack beneath the articular cartilage and radiographically as a "crescent sign" (Ficat stage III).

The final stage (Ficat stage IV) is the development of osteoarthritis. Histologic features are consistent with osteoarthritis in showing diminution of superficial chondrocytes and proliferation of deeper chondrocytes in broad capsule clusters, with capillary buds penetrating the layer of calcified cartilage in areas overlying the segment of bone that underwent necrosis and subsequent subchondral fracture.

The earliest change in BMES is a change in the marrow (Fig. 35-4). The marrow is filled with a faintly eosinophilic material that is edema fluid. This corresponds

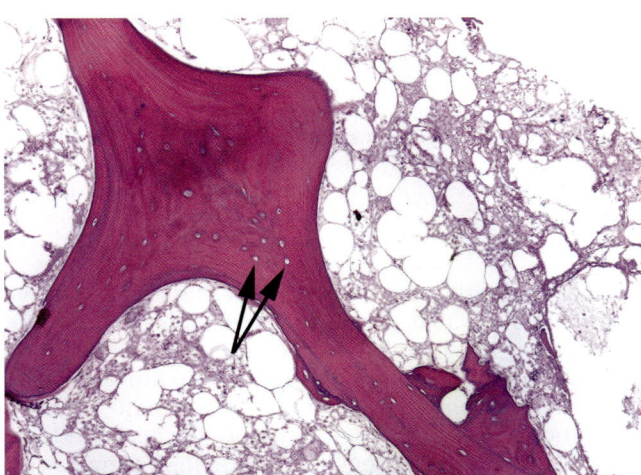

Figure 35-2. This histopathologic sample represents the first stage of osteonecrosis: cell death and necrosis. Bone death is evident by the absence of osteocytes in the trabecular bone lacunae *(black arrows).* The surrounding marrow is necrotic with almost complete absence of hematopoietic elements.

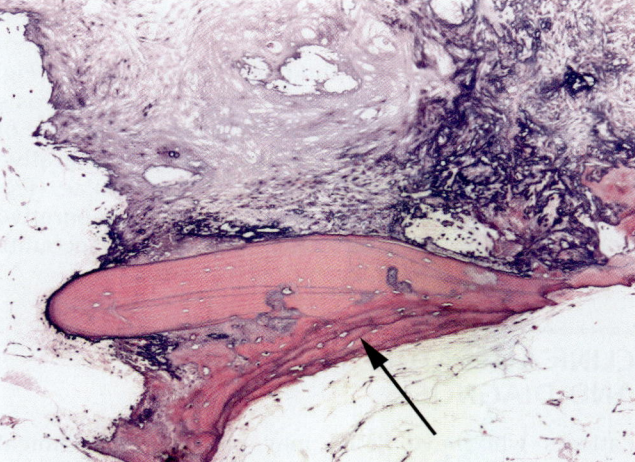

Figure 35-3. This photomicrograph demonstrates the reparative reaction that occurs in Ficat stage II osteonecrosis of the hip (ON). Granulation tissue at the margin of the bone infarct brings multipotential cells that begin to lay down new viable bone *(black arrow)* on the dead trabeculae. The surrounding fat in this sample has undergone focal dystrophic calcification changes.

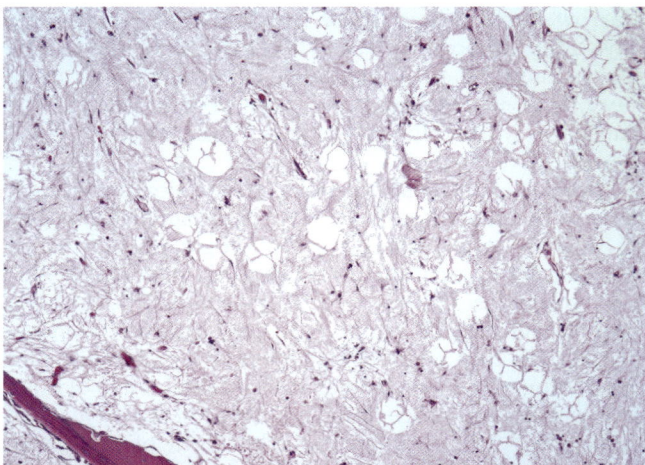

Figure 35-4. The histopathologic finding characteristic of bone marrow edema syndrome is edema in the fatty marrow. This slide demonstrates this edema as evidenced by amorphous material between fat cells.

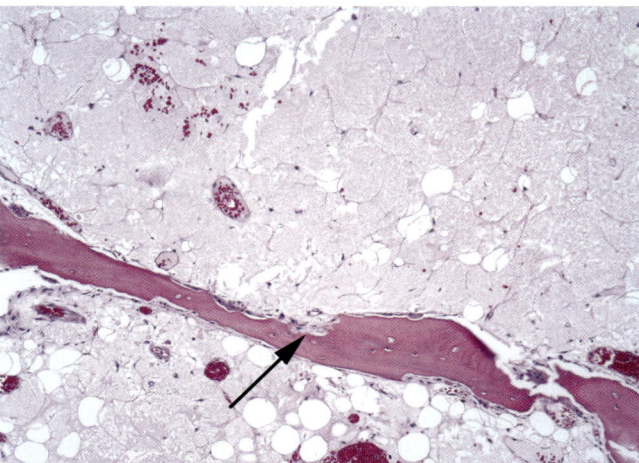

Figure 35-5. As bone marrow edema syndrome (BMES) progresses, osteoclasts begin to form resorption cavities *(black arrows)*. The degree of osteoporosis noted in the hip of the patient is a function of how extensive this resorptive process removes trabecular bone.

BOX 35-2. CORRELATION OF HISTOPATHOLOGIC TO RADIOLOGIC STAGES OF BONE MARROW EDEMA SYNDROME	
Histopathology	**Radiographic Findings**
1. Marrow edema fluid	Bright T2 magnetic resonance
2. Osteoclastic resorption	Diffuse, ill-defined osteoporosis on radiograph
3. Osteoblastic reparation	Radiodensity normalizes and marrow edema persists with slow resolution

radiographically to a bright signal on T2-weighted MRI images (Box 35-2). Mild fibrosis may be associated with vascular congestion. After about 3 weeks, teams of osteoclasts are activated and begin to resorb bone (Fig. 35-5). This will account for the changes of osteoporosis seen in cases that are several weeks old. Resolution of osteoporosis is signaled by ingrowth of reparative tissue with an osteoblastic lining of trabeculae (Fig. 35-6). Osteoblasts are able to deposit new reparative bone on the thinned trabeculae. This process accounts for the resolution of transient osteoporosis.

CLINICAL FEATURES AND DIAGNOSIS

Patients who have BMES may present with clinical symptoms that are similar to those experienced by ON patients. In both diseases, patients may have disabling hip pain with no known antecedent trauma (with the exception of trauma-associated osteonecrosis of the hip). The pain can be located in the inguinal area, buttocks, or anterior thigh. It is deep and throbbing, worse with ambulation, and marked at night. The patient may

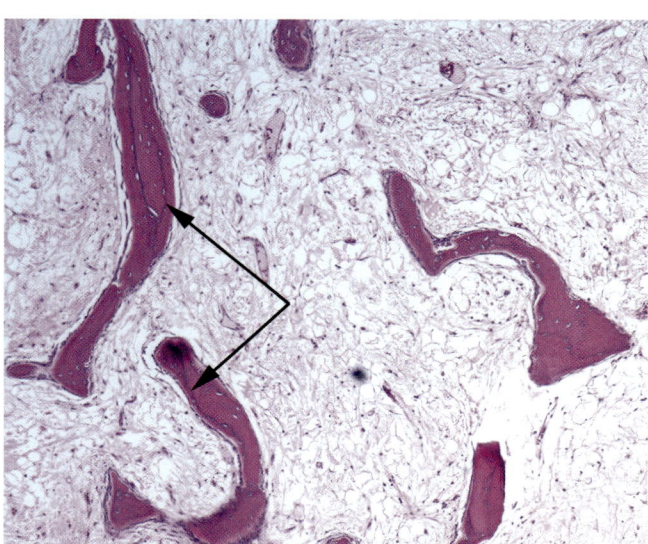

Figure 35-6. Seams of new woven bone *(black arrows)* are evident in this image of a sample taken from a patient with bone marrow edema syndrome (BMES). This osteoblastic activity restores trabecular bone in the hip back to pre-BMES levels.

have a limp with pain on weight bearing and a positive Trendelenburg sign. Physical examination may elicit nonspecific hip pain on extremes in range of motion that may limit the ability of the patient to move through a full range of motion. The most severe pain is felt in abduction and internal rotation. However, many patients with ON or BMES present with no pain. **Patients with these diseases experience a variety of different symptoms, and their diagnosis should be made with the use of MRI.**

Several clinical differences can be used to help differentiate between patients with ON and those with BMES (Table 35-1). Although the diseases are similarly

Table 35-1. Comparison of Osteonecrosis and Bone Marrow Edema Syndrome Clinical Assessments

Characteristic	Osteonecrosis of the Hip	Bone Marrow Edema Syndrome
Epidemiology	Approximately 20,000 new cases each year	Rare
Age, yr	Typically, 20 to 50	Men 40 to 50, women last trimester of pregnancy
Gender	♂>♂ with SLE as associated factor; ♂>♀ with alcohol as associated factor	3:1 ♀:♂
Onset of pain	Sudden	Sudden
Bilaterality	>70%	Rare
Number of lesions	Multiple	One
Femoral head involvement	Yes	Yes
Femoral neck involvement	No	Yes
Joint space	Narrowing in later stages	Preserved
Associated factors	Corticosteroids, alcohol, tobacco, other	Pregnancy
Associated diseases	SLE, sickle cell, Caisson's disease, Gaucher's disease, thrombophilia, hypofibrinolysis	None

SLE, Systemic lupus erythematosus.

Table 35-2. Comparison of Osteonecrosis and Bone Marrow Edema Syndrome Radiographic Assessments

Diagnostic Modality	Osteonecrosis of the Hip	Bone Marrow Edema Syndrome
Radiograph		
Key findings	Early: normal appearance to mottled radiodensity Mid: "crescent sign" Late: joint space narrowing, subchondral cysts, and osteophytes	Early: no changes to osteopenia at 4 to 6 weeks Mid: complete disappearance of osseous architecture in some cases, joint space preserved Late: resolution within months to 2 years
Utility	Poor sensitivity Used to stage disease and determine appropriate treatment Follow-up to assess for progression of disease	Early stages: poor sensitivity; late stages: pathognomonic Follow-up to ensure resolution of osteopenia
Bone Scan		
Key findings	Uptake localized to segment of femoral head	Diffuse, homogeneous uptake of whole femoral head
Utility	Not recommended for diagnosis of osteonecrosis	Sensitive for early-stage disease Usually returns to normal at 1 to 2 years
Magnetic Resonance Imaging		
Key findings	Focal lesion in superior, subchondral region Double-line sign Advanced disease shows cartilage loss and femoral head deformity	Diffuse bone marrow edema pattern No other pathologic changes Resolves after several months
Utility	Sensitive and specific; gold standard	Sensitive and specific; recommended standard
Dual Energy X-ray Absorptiometry		
Key findings	No known relationship between osteonecrosis and decreased bone density	Unlikely to discover systemic osteopenia
Utility	No usefulness	No usefulness

present in middle-aged patients and may affect pregnant women,[41,42] BMES rarely presents in women other than those who are in their third trimester of pregnancy. Evidence of bilateral disease can be used to exclude a diagnosis of BMES in most cases. However, there are exceptions to these rules, as some evidence suggests that bilateral, as well as early-trimester, BMES may occur on rare occasions.[42] In general, although clinical findings may be more suggestive of one of these diseases, physical examination findings are not very helpful in differentiating the two diagnoses; imaging is required.

ON and BMES have distinct imaging characteristics that serve as the primary tool for differentiating these diseases (Table 35-2). MRI is the imaging modality of choice because of its ability to demonstrate the distribution of bone marrow abnormalities. In both diseases, MRI shows low intensity on T1-weighted images and high intensity on T2-weighted images, with normal bone marrow on fat-suppressed T2-weighted images and short tau inversion recovery (STIR) images. Edema in BMES is extensive, involving the entire femoral head and often extending into the intertrochanteric region (Fig. 35-7A). Vande Berg and associates reported characteristics of MRI that can be used to identify patients who have BMES.[43,44] They described a positive predictive value of 100% for transient lesions when additional subchondral changes other than bone marrow edema are lacking on T2-weighted and contrast-enhanced T1-weighted images. Conversely, disruption of femoral head contour and the presence of subchondral areas of

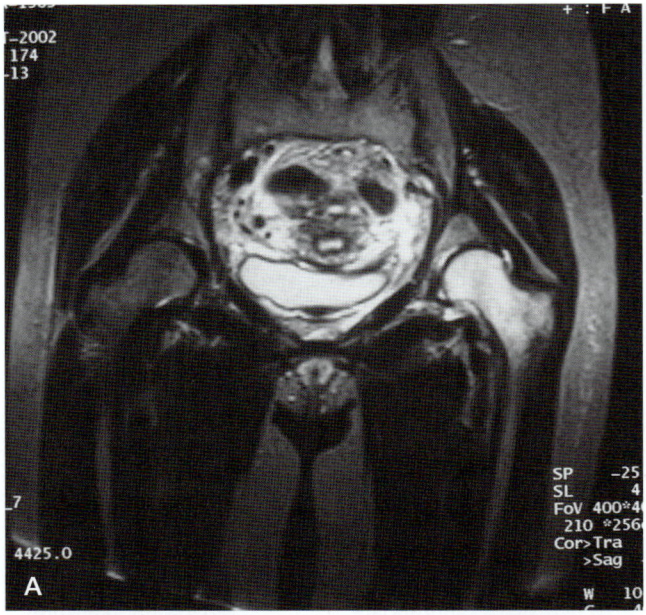

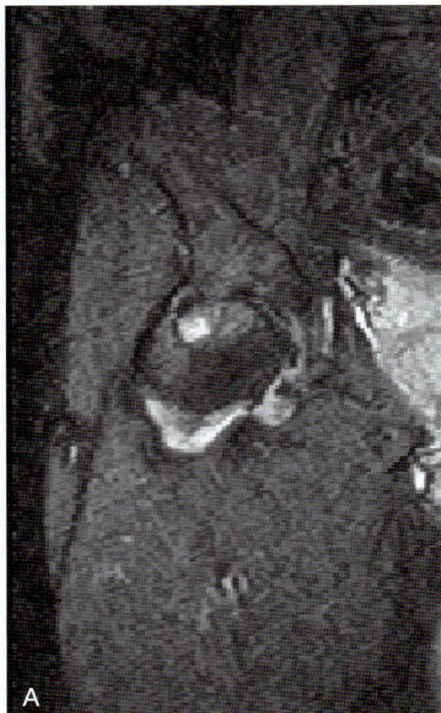

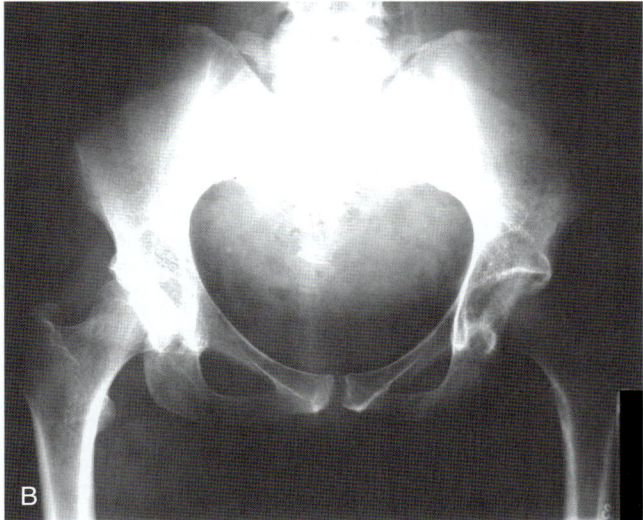

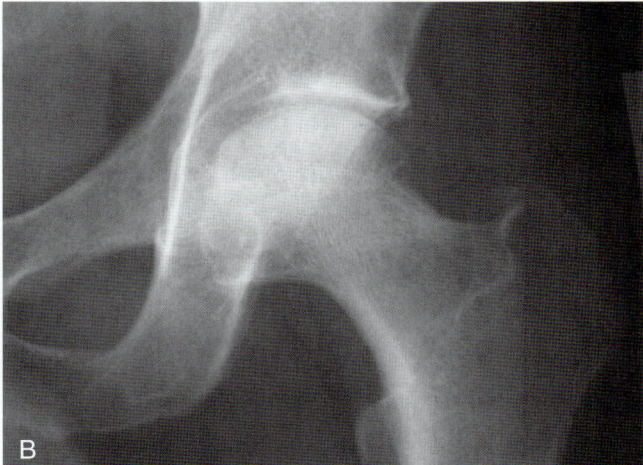

Figure 35-7. A, This T2 magnetic resonance image of a patient with bone marrow edema syndrome (BMES) shows increased signal that encompasses the entire femoral head and neck. This appearance is unique to BMES. **B,** This radiograph is of a female who had BMES of the left hip. Comparison of the left side with the normal right hip demonstrates the characteristic appearance of decreased bone density. As its name suggests, this decreased bone density is transient, and the patient will usually have a normal-appearing radiograph in less than 1 year.

Figure 35-8. A, Similar to bone marrow edema syndrome (BMES), osteonecrosis of the hip (ON) has increased signal on T2 magnetic resonance imaging. However, as shown in this image, the lesion is focal and typically is located at the superior portion of the femoral head. **B,** This radiograph shows some of the key characteristics of osteonecrosis, including sclerosis, mottled radiolucency, and the crescent sign that is indicative of subchondral fracture.

low signal intensity were predictive of irreversible lesions. Caution is still advised in managing patients diagnosed with BMES using these criteria; they should be followed to ensure that disease resolution occurs. MRI findings for ON are considered the gold standard in diagnosing this disease (Fig. 35-8A). Patients who have associated risk factors such as corticosteroid use or sickle cell disease and who present with signs of groin pain should be evaluated early with MRI. In addition,

patients who have a positive ON diagnosis based on MRI findings should be further evaluated for potential bilateral disease and other joint involvement. As many as 80% to 90% of patients will develop disease at other sites, such as the knees or the shoulders.[45,46]

Radiography is less sensitive than MRI for early stages of both ON and BMES, but it can often be used in later stages to differentiate these diseases. In addition, radiography is a low-cost modality that is useful for staging and follow-up. In BMES patients, radiographs progress to a focal osteopenic stage that usually begins within 2 months of clinical symptoms. Other bones in the patient have normal bone density. This localized osteopenia of the hip is distinct and is considered pathognomonic of BMES (Fig. 35-7B). Radiography should be used to verify that the BMES hip regains bone density similar to its prediseease state by comparison with the contralateral normal hip. In some cases, it may take longer than 2 years for the patient to have full resolution of the osteopenia seen on radiography. Signs of joint narrowing or osteophytes are not associated with BMES, and other diseases such as ON that cause osteoarthritis should be suspected. For ON patients, the hip should be followed radiographically for evidence of subchondral fracture and other signs of advanced disease (see Fig. 35-8B). Unlike BMES, ON rarely shows improvement and subsequent resolution of disease. Various systems have been proposed for staging ON using radiographic imaging. Most of these are derivatives of the original system proposed by Ficat and Arlet.[47] These stages are useful in choosing appropriate treatment for ON.

Historically, bone scans were used to evaluate patients who had suspected BMES or ON. MRI has supplanted bone scans as the gold standard for ON diagnosis.[46] Bone scanning is still used in early diagnosis of BMES because of its sensitivity for detecting early disease. The affected joint shows increased technetium-99 uptake within a few days after onset of symptoms. Some authors have suggested that bone scans may be useful for monitoring BMES and distinguishing it from clinical entities that cause more regional osteopenia.[48] However, the specificity of bone scans remains poorly defined, and additional studies are recommended to further assess the utility of bone scans versus MRI in BMES. Furthermore, bone scans are contraindicated in pregnancy.[49] In contrast, although MRI is not recommended in the first trimester, it is frequently used in patients during the second or third trimester.[50]

Differential Diagnosis

Several disease entities may present similarly to ON and BMES with hip pain and radiographic evidence of bone marrow edema. Some of the more common diagnoses that should be considered include regional migratory osteoporosis, complex regional pain syndrome type 2 (reflex sympathetic dystrophy), osteoarthritis, inflammatory and infectious arthritis, insufficiency fracture, and neoplasm. It is important to distinguish these diseases because differences in treatment and prognosis are considerable.

As previously noted, few studies have provided criteria for distinguishing BMES from regional migratory osteoporosis (RMO).[11,51] In general, RMO should be considered a variant of BMES. RMO occurs in the same patient population, commonly affecting middle-aged men, and patients have a similar clinical presentation to patients who have bone marrow edema limited to a single joint. The feature typically cited for distinguishing between RMO and BMES is the migratory nature of RMO.[52] Migration for RMO of the hip usually occurs to

the contralateral hip or to the ipsilateral knee.[53] Rather than considering BMES and RMO as separate entities, the clinician should consider the possibility of additional joint involvement for a patient who has been initially diagnosed with BMES. In terms of prognosis and treatment, most patients have excellent outcomes following nonoperative measures, regardless of whether a single joint or multiple joints are involved.

Complex regional pain syndrome type 2 (reflex sympathy dystrophy) is a disease that initially is observed as nonspecific findings of osteopenia and atrophy of soft tissue. Bone marrow edema on MRI is not always a finding for this disorder but may be present in some cases. Features that are often useful for distinguishing this disease include a history of trauma or changes such as skin atrophy, sensorimotor alterations, and contractures.[53] It commonly continues to progress to more advanced stages and thus should be distinguished from BMES.

Osteoarthritis (OA) of the hip generally can be recognized by involvement of the acetabulum and femoral head with the presence of subchondral cysts and subchondral bone sclerosis, and evidence of cartilage changes. In some cases, OA demonstrates bone marrow edema, which makes it difficult to distinguish from other diseases that lead to similar radiographic changes. This finding has been associated with cases of rapidly progressive OA, which is a destructive disease that typically requires early surgical intervention.[54] Although end-stage ON is defined as progression to OA, early-stage ON and BMES can be treated with less invasive joint-preserving interventions.

Other causes of arthritis, such as rheumatoid arthritis, gout, seronegative spondyloarthropathies, and infectious arthritis, may also present similarly to ON and BMES. Evaluation of joint fluid and serologic tests are diagnostic in most cases. If patients have low back pain or other clinical symptoms suggestive of HLA B-27–positive spondyloarthropathies, MRI is recommended to assess for early sacroiliitis that is not yet evident on plain films.[55] Infectious causes of arthropathy typically have MRI features of an effusion with synovitis and bone marrow edema on either side of the joint. The presence of fluid collections, sinus tracts, and osteomyelitis is indicative of septic arthritis. Unique algorithms devised for each of these arthritis entities and early diagnosis and differentiation from ON and BMES allow for optimal outcomes.

Insufficiency fractures are stress fractures that occur in bone that is unable to withstand the stresses of normal activity. Two morphologic changes are diagnostic clues of insufficiency fracture: (1) impaction fractures of the trabecular bone appear as thin low-signal intensity bands or lines, or more globular speckled areas of low-signal intensity, on T2- or enhanced T1-weighted spin echo (SE) images, and (2) subtle focal deformities of the subchondral bone plate are occasionally visible in the anterosuperior or lateral aspects of the femoral head, just below the acetabular roof margin.[44] Various disease processes may compromise the strength of the bone, leading to these fractures. Some cases of trabecular bone fracture of the femoral head may be found in ON and BMES. However, other underlying causes such as primary or secondary osteoporosis should be ruled out. Especially in elderly osteoporotic people, a sudden limp with antalgic gait and painful limitation of hip range of motion on clinical examination should raise suspicion of occult stress fracture, even if initial plain radiographs were normal or equivocal. When clinically appropriate, patients should undergo laboratory testing to assess for possible hyperparathyroidism, hypothyroidism, Hashimoto's disease, Cushing's disease, diabetes mellitus, and rheumatoid arthritis.

Primary and metastatic neoplasms may also mimic ON and BMES. Benign tumors such as osteoid osteoma, osteoblastoma, chondroblastoma, and Langerhans' cell histiocytosis, as well as malignant lesions such as leukemia, osteosarcoma, Ewing's sarcoma, and chondrosarcoma, have been reported to be associated with bone marrow edema.[56] If these lesions involve the metaphysis or diaphysis, they can be distinguished readily from ON and BMES based on location alone. In other cases, history, physical examination findings, and laboratory values, especially in cases of multiple myeloma and leukemia, are essential for diagnosing neoplastic entities. Malignant lesions require aggressive intervention that may include chemotherapy, radiation, and surgical intervention. A low threshold is recommended to further evaluate suspicious lesions that initially were considered to be possible cases of ON and BMES.

TREATMENT

Treatment approaches for ON and BMES are markedly different (Figs. 35-9 and 35-10). For both diseases, level 1 evidence for treatments options is lacking, and most treatment approaches are recommended on the basis of expert opinion or retrospective reviews. Early stages of BMES are treated similarly with nonoperative measures and treatment of symptoms. However, ON frequently progresses to more advanced stages of disease, and more invasive treatment modalities are often used early. Although extensive literature has reported the results of various types of treatment for ON, including pharmacotherapy, core decompression, less invasive surgical procedures such as bone grafting or osteotomy, and standard or resurfacing total hip arthroplasty, minimal scientific studies have assessed treatment modalities for BMES. In the early stage of ON, when the disease is detectable only on MRI and minimal or no sclerosis is present, nonoperative treatment or core decompression can be used. Some authors have suggested that nonoperative treatment is supported by evidence that lack of immobilization and continued weight bearing could eventually result in further displacement, subchondral collapse, and subsequent extension of necrosis.[57] However, other studies suggest that this approach is inadequate, in that many of these patients progress to more advanced stages of disease.[58] As another potential alternative to, or adjunct for,

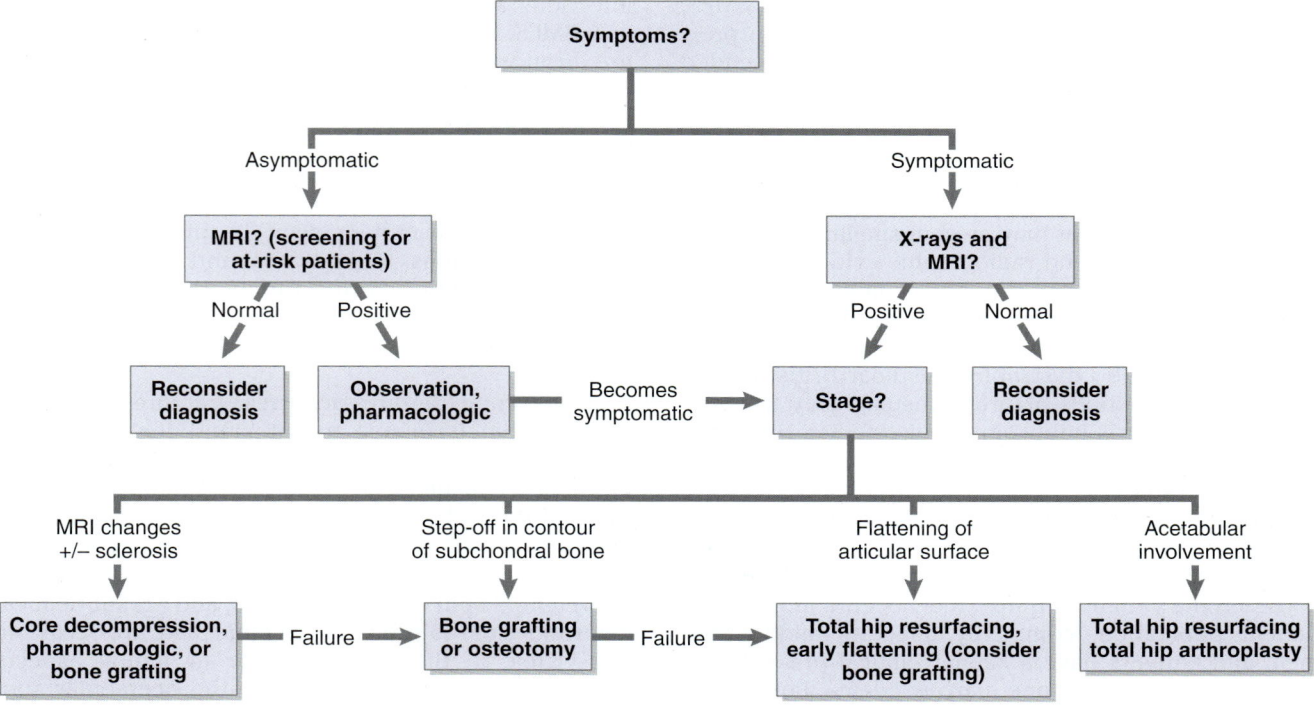

Figure 35-9. The treatment algorithm for osteonecrosis of the hip is based on the stage of disease. Bone grafting may be attempted in patients who initially fail core decompression, but many of these patients will require total hip arthroplasty. Because level 1 studies are currently lacking, this algorithm represents the preferences of the authors.

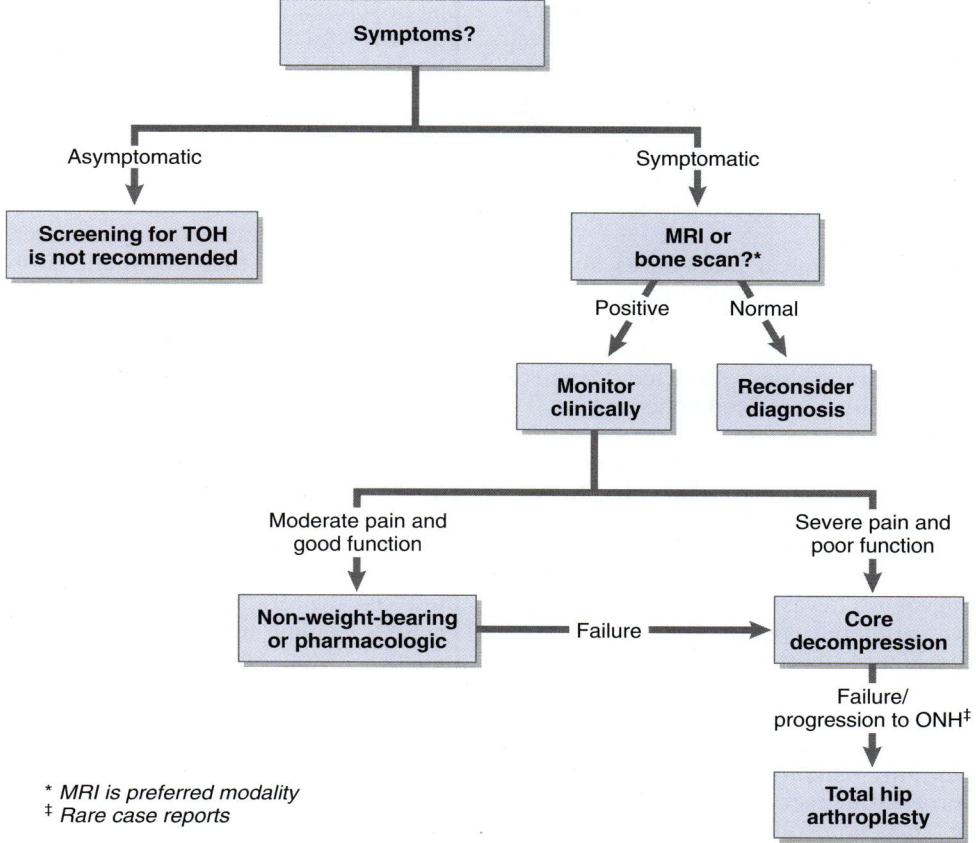

Figure 35-10. This algorithm depicts the recommended treatment approach for hip bone marrow edema syndrome. Most patients require only nonoperative treatment.

Table 35-3. Studies Assessing Medical Treatments for Osteonecrosis and Bone Marrow Edema Syndrome

Author	Year	Treatment	Proposed Mechanism
Osteonecrosis of the Hip			
Pritchett et al[60]	2001	Lipid-lowering agents	Reduce lipid levels that may lead to increased intraosseous pressure in patients with risk factors such as alcohol abuse or corticosteroid use
Disch et al[59]	2005	Prostacyclin analogues	Inhibit platelet aggregation and promote vascularization
Glueck et al[62]	2005	Anticoagulants	Reverse coagulation abnormalities associated with hypofibrinolysis or thrombophilia
Agarwala et al[61]	2005	Bisphosphonates	Decrease osteoclastic resorption of bone and promote bone growth
Bone Marrow Edema Syndrome			
Aginer et al[76]	2009	Prostacyclin analogues	Inhibit platelet aggregation and promote vascularization
Ringe et al[77]	2005	Bisphosphonates	Decrease osteoclastic resorption of bone and promote bone growth

surgery, recent reports have suggested that pharmacologic measures, such as lipid-lowering agents, bisphosphonates, or anticoagulants, may be used for early-stage ON (Table 35-3).[59-62] The theoretical benefit of these therapies is that they may correct or alleviate some of the pathophysiologic features of osteonecrosis.

Core decompression is often used in patients with precollapse disease. It is postulated that the therapeutic benefit is due to reduced bone marrow pressure and increased neovascularization in the bone surrounding the core track, which allows the formation of healthy bone. Early studies used a large-diameter trephine.

More recently, the technique of performing core decompression has varied in terms of surgical approaches, numbers of drillings, and the diameter of the trephines used. Some authors have supplemented core decompression with electrical stimulation[63] or growth and differentiation factors.[64-66] A number of authors have advocated the use of small-diameter percutaneous drilling as an even less invasive approach for treating patients.[67-69]

Other joint-preserving surgical procedures such as bone grafting or osteotomy can be used in an effort to save the joint. The rationale for bone grafting is to provide structural support to the subchondral bone and articular cartilage. Studies have reported the use of vascularized[70] and/or nonvascularized bone grafting.[71,72] For nonvascularized bone grafting, autologous and/or fresh-frozen allografts can be used. Autologous grafts are taken from healthy bone and are remodeled to substitute for necrotic bone. Surgical techniques for the three commonly used approaches—Phemister, trapdoor, and lightbulb techniques—have been described by Seyler and colleagues.[73] Vascularized bone grafting has been used in an attempt to restore the blood supply to the femoral head using harvesting of the fibula or ilium. This procedure is technically challenging and requires a dedicated surgical center with teams that are able to harvest bone and perform the graft placement. The goal of performing osteotomies is to redistribute weight-bearing forces from necrotic cartilage to healthy tissue. Although this procedure has been adopted widely in Asian countries, it has been used less frequently in other countries because results have been less than optimal. The higher success rate in Asia may be due to differences in the vascular supply or cartilage, or to increased numbers of patients who have a posterior capsule of the hip that is more lax and allows better rotation of the anterior portion of the neck.[74] Technical expertise may also serve as an explanation for the better results reported by Asian investigators.

Despite early operative and nonoperative modalities, many patients eventually progress to advanced stages of ON with femoral head collapse and osteoarthritic changes in the joint. Both standard total hip arthroplasty (THA) and resurfacing hip arthroplasty are used. Hemi-resurfacing has been used in cases that show signs of femoral head flattening without acetabular involvement, although this metal-on-cartilage interface typically is viewed as a temporizing procedure only.

BMES is typically a self-limiting disease. Clinical symptoms determine the approach selected for management (see Fig. 35-10). Most patients report improvement in pain and discomfort following treatment with protected weight bearing, mild analgesics, and nonsteroidal anti-inflammatory medications. The goal during management of BMES is to reduce associated pain while allowing time for bone remineralization. Periodic assessment of the bone mineral content may be useful for determining the length of treatment tailored to each case.[75] Although glucocorticoids were initially proposed as treatment, subsequent evidence has suggested that remineralization was inadequate with the use of this intervention.[10] Other studies have begun to assess the usefulness of

bisphosphonates or iloprost as a treatment option for patients who have migratory osteoporosis, but additional studies are required to assess this treatment in patients who have BMES (see Table 35-3).[52,76,77] Core decompression can be used as a treatment for BMES in patients who remain symptomatic despite taking protective weight-bearing measures.[78] However, treatment of BMES with core decompression is extremely controversial, and only limited evidence in small retrospective studies supports this treatment. More invasive joint-preserving procedures such as THA are used in patients who progress to end-stage osteoarthritis. However, it is likely that patients who develop end-stage OA were originally misdiagnosed with BMES or had concurrent disease of the joint due to another cause.

PROGNOSIS

The prognosis of osteonecrosis depends largely on the stage at which the disease was first diagnosed, associated risk factors, and the treatment modality used. Factors leading to the best prognosis include pre-collapse lesion, small lesion, less than 2 mm of head depression, and little or no acetabular involvement. Intervention prior to collapse is important, as poor results are associated with operative treatment for hips with collapse of the femoral head. Nonoperative measures have proved largely unsuccessful, with more than 80% of cases progressing to femoral head collapse within 4 years after diagnosis.[58] The efficacy of pharmacologic treatment is difficult to determine, as few studies with randomized, controlled trials are currently reported. A literature review assessing the outcomes of core decompression using various approaches indicated that studies from the last 15 years reported an average success rate of 70% (range, 39% to 100%) with surgery-free survival. A recent review of the various techniques used for bone grafting reported that the overall clinical success rate of the lightbulb technique was 79%, compared with 66% for the Phemister technique and 77% for the trapdoor technique.[73] Historically, results of standard THA in patients with osteonecrosis have not been as successful as outcomes reported in the overall THA population. However, recent advances in design and surgical technique have led to improved survival rates.[79] A number of recent studies have reported that osteonecrosis patients who are treated with THA or resurfacing arthroplasty have outcomes (survival greater than 90% at short to mid-term follow-up) that are similar to those of their counterparts who have OA or other degenerative joint diseases.[80-83] Long-term follow-up studies are necessary to determine whether these excellent early results will be maintained.

The clinical course of BMES is considerably more favorable than that of most cases of ON. The disease typically runs a course of 6 to 8 months. Pain is well controlled with the previously noted management of pain medications and adherence to non–weight-bearing recommendations. Patients show gradual improvement over the course of the disease and are weaned from pain medication within 8 months in most cases. Following this course, patients are able to return to their level of activity prior to the disease without limitations caused by pain or function. It is important to note that although bone marrow edema may resolve, continued compromise of full mechanical strength and caution should be used to ensure that pathologic fractures are avoided. In patients who undergo core decompression, improvement in pain is seen within 1 week of the procedure, and after 6 weeks of partial weight bearing, patients may be able to return to full activity.[40] However, additional studies are needed to further assess the efficacy of core decompression for the treatment of BMES. Although evidence is limited, patients who receive pharmacotherapy through interventions such as iloprost or alendronate may have excellent outcomes, with pain relief and restoration of full functional capacity.[76]

CURRENT CONTROVERSIES AND FUTURE CONSIDERATIONS

Current controversy concerning ON and BMES covers three areas: (1) new treatment modalities, (2) new imaging techniques, and (3) the use of novel biomarkers. With respect to cell-based therapies, Gangji and associates studied the implantation of autologous bone marrow mononuclear cells in patient who had precollapse ON, to determine its effects on clinical symptoms and disease progression. After 24 months, a marked reduction in pain and in joint symptoms was noted within the bone marrow graft group. Also at 24 months, five of eight hips in the control group had collapsed, whereas only one of 10 hips in the bone marrow graft group had progressed to this stage. Although these findings are promising, their interpretation is limited because of the small number of patients studied.[84]

In another study, Hernigou and colleagues used autologous bone marrow obtained from the iliac crest of patients operated on for osteonecrosis of the hip.[66] They reported that only 9 of 145 precollapse hips treated with core decompression and autologous bone marrow grafting went on to require THA at 5- to 10-year follow-up. Investigators used the fibroblast colony forming unit as an indicator of stromal cell activity to measure the number of osteoprogenitor cells transplanted. They reported that patients who had greater numbers of osteoprogenitor cells transplanted had better outcomes.

Platelet-rich plasma (PRP) is another cell-based therapeutic approach that has recently gained focus because platelets contain many growth factors that have the ability to accelerate angiogenesis and promote bone healing.[85,86] Again, reports of PRP in the treatment of osteonecrosis are mostly anecdotal, and one must be careful in interpreting results from case reports and case series.

New imaging techniques continue to gain in sophistication. Gadolinium-enhanced dynamic fast MRI appears to be a promising technique for evaluating vascularity and studying bone perfusion.[87,88] Another emerging imaging modality used to evaluate blood flow is F-18 fluoride positron emission tomography (PET) imaging,

Table 35-4. Potential Biochemical Biomarkers for Detection of Disease and Staging

Biochemical Markers of New Bone Formation		
Biochemical Marker	**Specimen**	**Detection Method**
Alkaline phosphatase, total (total ALP, tALP)	Serum	Colorimetry
Alkaline phosphatase, bone specific (bone ALP, BALP)	Serum	Colorimetry, EIA, IRMA
Osteocalcin (OC)	Serum	RIA, ELISA
C-terminal propeptide of type I procollagen (PICP)	Serum	RIA, ELISA
N-terminal propeptide of type I procollagen (PINP)	Serum	RIA, ELISA, ECLIA
Biochemical Markers of Bone Resorption		
Biochemical Marker	**Specimen**	**Detection Method**
Hydroxyproline, total and dialyzable (Hyp)	Urine	Colorimetry, HPLC
Hydroxylysine-glycosides (HLG)	Urine	HPLC
Pyridinoline, total (PYD)	Urine, serum	HPLC, ELISA
Pyridinoline, free (f-PYD)	Urine, serum	HPLC, ELISA
Deoxypyridinoline, total (DPD)	Urine, serum	HPLC, ELISA
Deoxypyridinoline, free (f-DPD)	Urine, serum	HPLC, ELISA
Serum carboxyterminal cross-linked telopeptide of type I collagen (ICTP, CTx-MMP)	Serum	RIA
Urine carboxyterminal cross-linked telopeptide of type I collagen (CTx-I)	Urine (α/β), serum ($\alpha\alpha/\beta\beta$)	RIA, ELISA
Aminoterminal cross-linked telopeptide of type I collagen (NTx-I)	Urine, serum	RIA, ELISA
Collagen I alpha 1 helicoidal peptide (HELP)	Urine	ELISA
Bone sialoprotein (BSP)	Serum	RIA, ELISA
Osteocalcin fragments (ufOC, U-Mid-OC, U-LongOC)	Urine	ELISA
Tartrate-resistant acid phosphatase (TRAcP)	Plasma, serum	RIA, ELISA, Colorimetry
Cathepsin K or L (CatK, CatL)	Plasma, serum	ELISA
Osteopontin (OPN)	Serum	ELISA

ECLIA, Electrochemiluminescence immunoassay; *ELISA,* enzyme-linked immunosorbent assay; *HPLC,* high-performance liquid chromatography; *IRMA,* immunoradiometric assay; *RIA,* radioimmunoassay.

which has been shown to be more sensitive in detecting ON when compared with MRI, single-photon emission computed tomography, and bone scans.[89]

Over the past decade, characterization of cellular and extracellular components of the skeletal matrix has resulted in the identification of biochemical markers that specifically reflect bone formation or bone resorption (Table 35-4).[90-92] In a histologic evaluation of signaling factors that control angiogenesis in core biopsies from ON patients, Radke and coworkers found that vascular endothelial growth factor (VEGF) and cysteine-rich protein (CYR61) were highly expressed in edematous areas, whereas connective tissue growth factor (CTGF) was noted in areas with marrow fibrosis and edema.[93] Berger and colleagues studied several biomarkers specific for bone turnover in patients with bone marrow edema syndrome. Bone-specific alkaline phosphatase, osteocalcin, procollagen type I N-terminal propeptide, and C-terminal cross-linking telopeptide were measured in aspirates from cancellous bone and in samples obtained simultaneously from peripheral blood. All markers of bone formation were increased, suggesting increased bone turnover. In addition, measurements of these markers not only correlated with each other in the serum and in aspirates from cancellous bone, they also matched the histopathologic findings of irregularly woven bone, osteoid seams, and lining cells. However, serum concentrations of all markers were not different from those in healthy individuals, and the authors concluded that these biomarkers did not provide a sensitive measure for the diagnosis of this disease histology.[94]

None of the biochemical markers of bone turnover have proved useful as a single diagnostic test, but a distinct combination of markers together with imaging studies may play an important role in diagnosis and monitoring of the disease course, as well as in response to treatment of both entities. However, none of these concepts has been proved in controlled prospective trials, and clinical use of these markers has not been sufficiently addressed.

REFERENCES

1. Harvey EJ: Osteonecrosis and transient osteoporosis of the hip: diagnostic and treatment dilemmas. Can J Surg 46:168–169, 2003.
2. McCarthy EF: The pathology of transient regional osteoporosis. Iowa Orthop J 18:35–42, 1998.
3. Balakrishnan A, Schemitsch EH, Pearce D, McKee MD: Distinguishing transient osteoporosis of the hip from avascular necrosis. Can J Surg 46:187–192, 2003.
4. Curtiss PH Jr, Kincaid WE: Transitory demineralization of the hip in pregnancy: a report of three cases. J Bone Joint Surg Am 41:1327–1333, 1959.
5. Rosen RA: Transitory demineralization of the femoral head. Radiology 94:509–512, 1970.
6. Bolland MJ: Bilateral transient osteoporosis of the hip in a young man. J Clin Densitom 11:339–341, 2008.
7. Grouwels P, Vandevenne J, Verswijvel G, Palmers Y: Transient osteoporosis of the hip in a 38-year-old man. JBR-BTR 90:188–189, 2007.
8. Hall FM, Harris AK: Case report 396: osseous sequelae of tuberculous spondylitis as demonstrated by computer tomography. Skeletal Radiol 15:589–592, 1986.
9. Hofmann S: The painful bone marrow edema syndrome of the hip joint. Wien Klin Wochenschr 117:111–120, 2005.
10. Banas MP, Kaplan FS, Fallon MD, Haddad JG: Regional migratory osteoporosis: a case report and review of the literature. Clin Orthop Relat Res 250:303–309, 1990.
11. Gil HC, Levine SM, Zoga AC: MRI findings in the subchondral bone marrow: a discussion of conditions including transient osteoporosis, transient bone marrow edema syndrome, SONK, and shifting bone marrow edema of the knee. Semin Musculoskelet Radiol 10:177–186, 2006.
12. Lequesne M: Transient osteoporosis of the hip: a nontraumatic variety of Sudeck's atrophy. Ann Rheum Dis 27:463–471, 1968.
13. Steinberg ME: The advantages of core decompression for treating avascular necrosis. University of Pennsylvania Orthopaedic Journal 13:84–88, 2000.
14. Schapira D: Transient osteoporosis of the hip. Semin Arthritis Rheum 22:98–105, 1992.
15. Hashikura Y, Kawasaki S, Matsunami H, et al: Immunosuppressant switching between cyclosporine and tacrolimus after liver transplantation. Transplant Proc 28:1034–1035, 1996.
16. Kubo T, Yamazoe S, Sugano N, et al: Initial MRI findings of nontraumatic osteonecrosis of the femoral head in renal allograft recipients. Magn Reson Imaging 15:1017–1023, 1997.
17. Torii Y, Hasegawa Y, Kubo T, et al: Osteonecrosis of the femoral head after allogeneic bone marrow transplantation. Clin Orthop Relat Res 382:124–132, 2001.
18. Mankin HJ: Nontraumatic necrosis of bone (osteonecrosis). N Engl J Med 326:1473–1479, 1992.
19. Flouzat-Lachaniete CH, Roussignol X, Poignard A, et al: Multifocal joint osteonecrosis in sickle cell disease. Open Orthop J 3:32–35, 2009.
20. Glueck CJ, Freiberg RA, Fontaine RN, et al: Hypofibrinolysis, thrombophilia, osteonecrosis. Clin Orthop Relat Res 386:19–33, 2001.
21. Hirata T, Fujioka M, Takahashi KA, et al: ApoB C7623T polymorphism predicts risk for steroid-induced osteonecrosis of the femoral head after renal transplantation. J Orthop Sci 12:199–206, 2007.
22. Glueck CJ, Freiberg RA, Oghene J, et al: Association between the T-786C eNOS polymorphism and idiopathic osteonecrosis of the head of the femur. J Bone Joint Surg Am 89:2460–2468, 2007.
23. Kim TH, Hong JM, Oh B, et al: Genetic association study of polymorphisms in the catalase gene with the risk of osteonecrosis of the femoral head in the Korean population. Osteoarthritis Cartilage 16:1060–1066, 2008.
24. Lakhanpal S, Ginsburg WW, Luthra HS, Hunder GG: Transient regional osteoporosis: a study of 56 cases and review of the literature. Ann Intern Med 106:444–450, 1987.
25. Guerra JJ, Steinberg ME: Distinguishing transient osteoporosis from avascular necrosis of the hip. J Bone Joint Surg Am 77:616–624, 1995.
26. Rao VM, Mitchell DG, Steiner RM, et al: Femoral head avascular necrosis in sickle cell anemia: MR characteristics. Magn Reson Imaging 6:661–667, 1988.
27. Zonana-Nacach A, Jimenez-Balderas FJ: Avascular necrosis of bone associated with primary antiphospholipid syndrome: case report and literature review. J Clin Rheumatol 10:214–217, 2004.
28. Cozen L, Wallace DJ: Risk factors for avascular necrosis in systemic lupus erythematosus. J Rheumatol 25:188, 1998.
29. Mont MA, Glueck CJ, Pacheco IH, et al: Risk factors for osteonecrosis in systemic lupus erythematosus. J Rheumatol 24:654–662, 1997.
30. Mok MY, Farewell VT, Isenberg DA: Risk factors for avascular necrosis of bone in patients with systemic lupus erythematosus: is there a role for antiphospholipid antibodies? Ann Rheum Dis 59:462–467, 2000.
31. Elishkewich K, Kaspi D, Shapira I, et al: Idiopathic osteonecrosis in an adult with familial protein S deficiency and hyperhomocysteinemia. Blood Coagul Fibrinolysis 12:547–550, 2001.
32. Etienne G, Mont MA, Ragland PS: The diagnosis and treatment of nontraumatic osteonecrosis of the femoral head. Instr Course Lect 53:67–85, 2004.

33. Ferrari P, Schroeder V, Anderson S, et al: Association of plasminogen activator inhibitor-1 genotype with avascular osteonecrosis in steroid-treated renal allograft recipients. Transplantation 74:1147–1152, 2002.

34. Lee JS, Koo KH, Ha YC, et al: Role of thrombotic and fibrinolytic disorders in osteonecrosis of the femoral head. Clin Orthop Relat Res 417:270–276, 2003.

35. Lieberman JR, Berry DJ, Mont MA, et al: Osteonecrosis of the hip: management in the 21st century. Instr Course Lect 52: 337–355, 2003.

36. Miyanishi K, Kaminomachi S, Hara T, et al: A subchondral fracture in transient osteoporosis of the hip. Skeletal Radiol 36:677–680, 2007.

37. Trevisan C, Ortolani S, Monteleone M, Marinoni EC: Regional migratory osteoporosis: a pathogenetic hypothesis based on three cases and a review of the literature. Clin Rheumatol 21:418–425, 2002.

38. Malizos KN, Zibis AH, Dailiana Z, et al: MR imaging findings in transient osteoporosis of the hip. Eur J Radiol 50: 238–244, 2004.

39. Plenk H Jr, Hofmann S, Eschberger J, et al: Histomorphology and bone morphometry of the bone marrow edema syndrome of the hip. Clin Orthop Relat Res 334:73–84, 1997.

40. Hofmann S, Engel A, Neuhold A, et al: Bone-marrow oedema syndrome and transient osteoporosis of the hip: an MRI-controlled study of treatment by core decompression. J Bone Joint Surg Br 75:210–216, 1993.

41. Ugwonali OF, Sarkissian H, Nercessian OA: Bilateral osteonecrosis of the femoral head associated with pregnancy: four new cases and a review of the literature. Orthopedics 31: 183, 2008.

42. Xyda A, Mountanos I, Natsika M, Karantanas AH: Postpartum bilateral transient osteoporosis of the hip: MR imaging findings in three cases. Radiol Med 113:689–694, 2008.

43. Vande Berg B, Lecouvet F, Koutaissoff S, et al: Bone marrow edema of the femoral head. JBR-BTR 90:350–357, 2007.

44. Vande Berg BC, Lecouvet FE, Koutaissoff S, et al: Bone marrow edema of the femoral head and transient osteoporosis of the hip. Eur J Radiol 67:68–77, 2008.

45. Symptomatic multifocal osteonecrosis: a multicenter study. Collaborative Osteonecrosis Group. Clin Orthop Relat Res 369:312–326, 1999.

46. Mont MA, Ulrich SD, Seyler TM, et al: Bone scanning of limited value for diagnosis of symptomatic oligofocal and multifocal osteonecrosis. J Rheumatol 35:1629–1634, 2008.

47. Mont MA, Marulanda GA, Jones LC, et al: Systematic analysis of classification systems for osteonecrosis of the femoral head. J Bone Joint Surg Am 88(Suppl 3):16–26, 2006.

48. Watson RM, Roach NA, Dalinka MK: Avascular necrosis and bone marrow edema syndrome. Radiol Clin North Am 42: 207–219, 2004.

49. Tan TX, Dardani M, Neal DJ, et al: Atypical findings of discordant bone scan and radiographs in transient osteoporosis of the hip: case report and review of the literature. Clin Nucl Med 23:160–162, 1998.

50. Nagayama M, Watanabe Y, Okumura A, et al: Fast MR imaging in obstetrics. Radiographics 22:563–580, 2002; discussion 80–82.

51. Doury P: Bone-marrow oedema, transient osteoporosis, and algodystrophy. J Bone Joint Surg Br 76:993–994, 1994.

52. Horiuchi K, Shiraga N, Fujita N, et al: Regional migratory osteoporosis: a case report. J Orthop Sci 9:178–181, 2004.

53. Korompilias AV, Karantanas AH, Lykissas MG, Beris AE: Bone marrow edema syndrome. Skeletal Radiol 38:425–436, 2009.

54. Boutry N, Paul C, Leroy X, et al: Rapidly destructive osteoarthritis of the hip: MR imaging findings. AJR Am J Roentgenol 179:657–663, 2002.

55. Guglielmi G, Scalzo G, Cascavilla A, et al: Imaging of the sacroiliac joint involvement in seronegative spondylarthropathies. Clin Rheumatol 28:1007–1019, 2009.

56. James SL, Panicek DM, Davies AM: Bone marrow oedema associated with benign and malignant bone tumours. Eur J Radiol 67:11–21, 2008.

57. Neumayr LD, Aguilar C, Earles AN, et al: Physical therapy alone compared with core decompression and physical therapy for femoral head osteonecrosis in sickle cell disease: results of a multicenter study at a mean of three years after treatment. J Bone Joint Surg Am 88:2573–2582, 2006.

58. Mont MA, Carbone JJ, Fairbank AC: Core decompression versus nonoperative management for osteonecrosis of the hip. Clin Orthop Relat Res 324:169–178, 1996.

59. Disch AC, Matziolis G, Perka C: The management of necrosis-associated and idiopathic bone-marrow oedema of the proximal femur by intravenous iloprost. J Bone Joint Surg Br 87:560–564, 2005.

60. Pritchett JW: Statin therapy decreases the risk of osteonecrosis in patients receiving steroids. Clin Orthop Relat Res 386:173–178, 2001.

61. Agarwala S, Jain D, Joshi VR, Sule A: Efficacy of alendronate, a bisphosphonate, in the treatment of AVN of the hip: a prospective open-label study. Rheumatology (Oxford) 44:352–359, 2005.

62. Glueck CJ, Freiberg RA, Sieve L, Wang P: Enoxaparin prevents progression of stages I and II osteonecrosis of the hip. Clin Orthop Relat Res 435:164–170, 2005.

63. Steinberg ME, Brighton CT, Corces A, et al: Osteonecrosis of the femoral head: results of core decompression and grafting with and without electrical stimulation. Clin Orthop Relat Res 249:199–208, 1999.

64. Simank HG, Brocai DR, Brill C, Lukoschek M: Comparison of results of core decompression and intertrochanteric osteotomy for nontraumatic osteonecrosis of the femoral head using Cox regression and survivorship analysis. J Arthroplasty 16:790–794, 2001.

65. Gangji V, Hauzeur JP: Treatment of osteonecrosis of the femoral head with implantation of autologous bone-marrow cells: surgical technique. J Bone Joint Surg Am 87(Suppl 1):106–112, 2005.

66. Hernigou P, Beaujean F: Treatment of osteonecrosis with autologous bone marrow grafting. Clin Orthop Relat Res 405: 14–23, 2002.

67. Marker DR, Seyler TM, Ulrich SD, et al: Do modern techniques improve core decompression outcomes for hip osteonecrosis? Clin Orthop Relat Res 466:1093–1103, 2008.

68. Mont MA, Ragland PS, Etienne G: Core decompression of the femoral head for osteonecrosis using percutaneous multiple small-diameter drilling. Clin Orthop Relat Res 429: 131–138, 2004.

69. Song WS, Yoo JJ, Kim YM, Kim HJ: Results of multiple drilling compared with those of conventional methods of core decompression. Clin Orthop Relat Res 454:139–146, 2007.

70. Yoo MC, Chung DW, Hahn CS: Free vascularized fibula grafting for the treatment of osteonecrosis of the femoral head. Clin Orthop Relat Res 277:128–138, 1992.

71. Plakseychuk AY, Kim SY, Park BC, et al: Vascularized compared with nonvascularized fibular grafting for the treatment of osteonecrosis of the femoral head. J Bone Joint Surg Am 85:589–596, 2003.

72. Kim SY, Kim YG, Kim PT, et al: Vascularized compared with nonvascularized fibular grafts for large osteonecrotic lesions of the femoral head. J Bone Joint Surg Am 87:2012–2018, 2005.

73. Seyler TM, Marker DR, Ulrich SD, et al: Nonvascularized bone grafting defers joint arthroplasty in hip osteonecrosis. Clin Orthop Relat Res 466:1125–1132, 2008.

74. Dean MT, Cabanela ME: Transtrochanteric anterior rotational osteotomy for avascular necrosis of the femoral head: long-term results. J Bone Joint Surg Br 75:597–601, 1993.

75. Trevisan C, Ortolani S: Bone loss and recovery in regional migratory osteoporosis. Osteoporos Int 13:901–906, 2002.

76. Aigner N, Meizer R, Meraner D, et al: Bone marrow edema syndrome in postpartal women: treatment with iloprost. Orthop Clin North Am 40:241–247, 2009.

77. Ringe JD, Dorst A, Faber H: Effective and rapid treatment of painful localized transient osteoporosis (bone marrow edema) with intravenous ibandronate. Osteoporos Int 16:2063–2068, 2005.

78. Aigner N, Schneider W, Eberl V, Knahr K: Core decompression in early stages of femoral head osteonecrosis—an MRI-controlled study. Int Orthop 26:31–35, 2002.

79. Seyler TM, Cui Q, Mihalko WM, et al: Advances in hip arthroplasty in the treatment of osteonecrosis. Instr Course Lect 56:221–233, 2007.

80. Kim YH, Choi Y, Kim JS: Cementless total hip arthroplasty with ceramic-on-ceramic bearing in patients younger than 45 years with femoral-head osteonecrosis. Int Orthop 34:1123–1127, 2010.
81. Mont MA, Seyler TM, Marker DR, et al: Use of metal-on-metal total hip resurfacing for the treatment of osteonecrosis of the femoral head. J Bone Joint Surg Am 88(Suppl 3):90–97, 2006.
82. Stulberg BN, Fitts SM, Zadzilka JD, Trier K: Resurfacing arthroplasty for patients with osteonecrosis. Bull NYU Hosp Jt Dis 67:138–141, 2009.
83. Yuan B, Taunton MJ, Trousdale RT: Total hip arthroplasty for alcoholic osteonecrosis of the femoral head. Orthopedics 32:400, 2009.
84. Gangji V, Hauzeur JP, Matos C, et al: Treatment of osteonecrosis of the femoral head with implantation of autologous bone-marrow cells: a pilot study. J Bone Joint Surg Am 86:1153–1160, 2004.
85. Badr MS, Oliver RJ: Platelet-rich plasma: an adjunctive treatment modality for bisphosphonate osteonecrosis? J Oral Maxillofac Surg 67:1357, 2009.
86. Yokota K, Ishida O, Sunagawa T, et al: Platelet-rich plasma accelerated surgical angiogenesis in vascular-implanted necrotic bone: an experimental study in rabbits. Acta Orthop 79:106–110, 2008.
87. Munk PL, Lee MJ, Janzen DL, et al: Gadolinium-enhanced dynamic MRI of the fractured carpal scaphoid: preliminary results. Australas Radiol 42:10–15, 1998.
88. Cova M, Kang YS, Tsukamoto H, et al: Bone marrow perfusion evaluated with gadolinium-enhanced dynamic fast MR imaging in a dog model. Radiology 179:535–539, 1991.
89. Dasa V, Adbel-Nabi H, Anders MJ, Mihalko WM: F-18 fluoride positron emission tomography of the hip for osteonecrosis. Clin Orthop Relat Res 466:1081–1086, 2008.
90. Berger CE, Kroner A, Thomas E, et al: Comparison of biochemical markers of bone metabolism in serum and femur aspirates. Clin Orthop Relat Res 395:174–179, 2002.
91. Looker AC, Bauer DC, Chesnut CH 3rd, et al: Clinical use of biochemical markers of bone remodeling: current status and future directions. Osteoporos Int 11:467–480, 2000.
92. Seibel MJ: Biochemical markers of bone remodeling. Endocrinol Metab Clin North Am 32:83–113, vi–vii, 2003.
93. Radke S, Battmann A, Jatzke S, et al: Expression of the angio-matrix and angiogenic proteins CYR61, CTGF, and VEGF in osteonecrosis of the femoral head. J Orthop Res 24:945–952, 2006.
94. Berger CE, Kroner AH, Minai-Pour MB, et al: Biochemical markers of bone metabolism in bone marrow edema syndrome of the hip. Bone 33:346–351, 2003.

CHAPTER 36

Synovial Diseases of the Hip

John Clohisy

INTRODUCTION

The hip is a synovial joint that functions as the primary link between the trunk and lower limbs, and provides bodily support and mobility in the upright position. Synovial joints are differentiated from cartilaginous and fibrous joints by the existence of capsules surrounding the articulating surfaces of the joint and the presence of lubricating synovial fluid within the capsule. The synovium is a thin, specialized tissue that lines noncartilaginous spaces within the joints (e.g., hips, knees, elbows). This tissue is a few cell layers thick and plays a major role in regulating the fluid and cellular environment within the joint.[1] A highly vascular capillary system within the synovium provides joint lubricating fluid containing hyaluronan and lubricin. The synovium mediates molecular and cellular changes within the joint and protects the joint from physiologic and biomechanical stresses. Additionally, the synovium provides macrophage access to the joint.[2] Activated macrophages perform several immunologic functions within the joint space and are important mediators of both joint homeostasis and certain disease states.

Primary disorders of hip synovium are relatively rare, even in a high-volume hip practice. The most common disorders include synovial chondromatosis and pigmented villonodular synovitis (PVNS). Both of these conditions are benign tumors of synovial origin. Successful orthopedic management of these conditions is dependent on a timely diagnosis and successful removal of the primary tumor. Failed treatment and recurrent disease can be associated with articular cartilage degeneration

and secondary osteoarthritis. This chapter will review the important concepts associated with diagnosing and treating these benign synovial disorders.

SYNOVIAL CHONDROMATOSIS

Overview

Synovial chondromatosis is a benign, monoarticular arthopathy that infrequently involves the hip. In fact, hips account for only 10% of diagnosed cases. Disease involving knees (50% to 65% of cases) and elbows (20% to 25%) is far more common. Males are affected twice as often as females. The disease process begins with metaplastic differentiation of mesenchymal cells in the synovial membrane of the joint. These cells mature into chondroblasts and form small nodules of cartilage in intimal layers of the synovial membrane. These nodules subsequently enlarge and detach to lie within the joint space, resulting in the formation of multiple intracapsular and extracapsular loose bodies.[3] These loose bodies continue to grow in diameter via multiplying chondrocytes and may calcify in their central zones, leading to the term *osteochondromatosis* (Fig. 36-1).

Villacin[4] described two forms of synovial chondromatosis. The primary form of synovial chondromatosis is characterized by numerous small, round loose bodies that are uniform in size. It is not precipitated by any identifiable joint pathology and likely occurs secondary to metaplasia. Lesions are often aggressive and are associated with a high incidence of recurrence. Conversely, the secondary form is characterized by fewer, larger, more variably sized cartilaginous masses. This form is more likely to occur in the setting of preexistent osteoarthritis, rheumatoid arthritis, osteonecrosis, osteochondritis dissecans, neuropathic osteoarthopathy, tuberculosis, or osteochondral fracture. The underlying disease process generates chondral fragments that implant into synovium, inducing metaplastic cartilage formation.

Milgram further described synovial chondromatosis as a self-limited intrasynovial process that occurs in three phases: early, transitional, and late.[5] In the early phase, only active intrasynovial disease is present, with no loose bodies. The transitional phase includes both active intrasynovial proliferation and free loose bodies. The late phase shows multiple free osteochondral bodies extruded in the joint space but no demonstrable

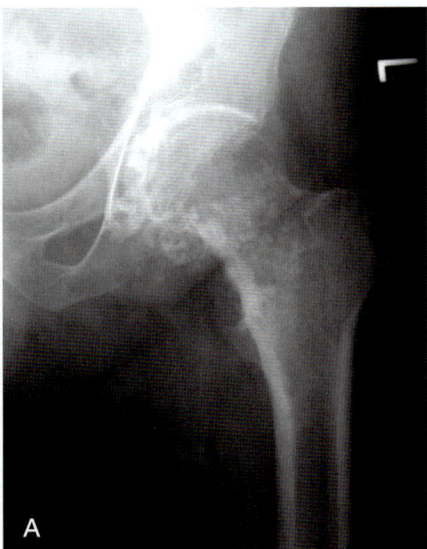

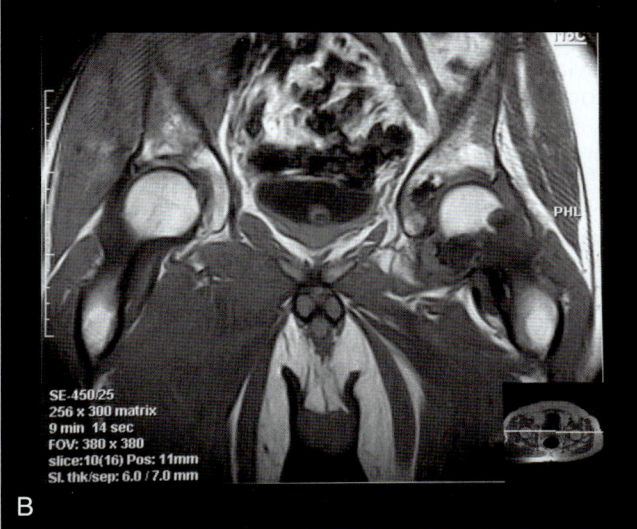

Figure 36-1. A, Anteroposterior (AP) radiograph of the left hip in a 63-year-old male. The radiograph shows numerous calcific densities within the hip joint. They surround the femoral neck and are seen within the acetabular notch. The pattern of calcification is typical for cartilage, and the lesions represent osteocartilaginous bodies within the joint and synovium. **B,** T1-weighted coronal magnetic resonance imaging (MRI) shows the thickened synovium surrounding the head and within the acetabular notch. The pattern is consistent with a primary intra-articular process. Together with the plain film, this represents synovial chondromatosis.

intrasynovial disease. These phases become important in clinical decision making in determining the necessity of performing synovectomy to treat symptoms and prevent disease recurrence.

Clinical Features and Diagnosis

Synovial chondromatosis of the hip can be challenging to diagnose. In contrast to disease presentation in other joints (knees and elbows), signs of synovial thickening,

crepitus, and palpable loose bodies usually are absent. Synovial chondromatosis of the hip most commonly presents with nonspecific and insidious symptoms such as pain, stiffness, and limitation of motion. Further complicating the diagnosis are plain radiographic images, which are normal in more than 50% of cases because tumorous lesions often are noncalcified and radiographically lucent. When clinical suspicion prompts further imaging, computed tomography (CT) and/or magnetic resonance imaging (MRI) studies usually identify chondral and/or osteochondral bodies in the joint. On CT, loose bodies form a soft tissue mass of water density that elevates the joint capsule. MRI may show three distinct patterns as described by Kramer and associates.[6] Pattern A (12%) is described as a lobulated homogeneous intra-articular signal isointense to muscle on T1-weighted images and hyperintense on T2-weighted images. Pattern B (80%) incorporates the features of pattern A with addition of signal void foci on all pulse sequences. Last, pattern C (8%) has features of patterns A and B plus foci of lesions with peripheral low signal surrounding a central fatlike signal. The diagnosis of synovial chondromatosis can be supplemented by magnetic resonance arthrography with gadolinium contrast, which shows multiple filling defects in the joint. Biopsy remains the gold standard in diagnosis. Histopathology shows a thickened synovium with loose bodies adherent to the synovium or floating freely in the joint.

Treatment

Recommended management of synovial chondromatosis consists of surgical removal of loose bodies combined with a partial or complete synovectomy.[7,8] Total excision of loose bodies is essential to optimize symptom relief and to theoretically protect the joint from additional articular cartilage damage. Historically, loose body removal was thought to be as efficacious as synovectomy for prevention of recurrence, but later studies showed a statistically lower recurrence rate with synovectomy.[7,8] Nevertheless, recurrence rates from 0% to 23% have been reported after synovectomy.[3,7,8]

The most established treatment remains complete synovectomy via surgical dislocation of the femoral head. Full exposure of the hip is achieved only by surgical dislocation. Postel and colleagues showed in 23 patients treated with open arthrotomy (11 hips left in situ and 12 dislocated) that recurrence rate and prevention of secondary arthrosis were more favorable with dislocation.[9] Lim and co-workers showed in 21 patients undergoing open arthrotomy and complete synovectomy (13 hips left in situ and 8 dislocated) that recurrence rates increased in patients treated without surgical dislocation.[10] The increase in recurrence rates was believed to stem from the persistence of pathologic synovium in the depth of the acetabular fossa.

Previously, surgical dislocation carried an unknown risk of avascular necrosis (AVN); it now is safe and carries minimal risk of AVN. Specifically, the approach introduced by Ganz and associates preserves the terminal branches of the medial circumflex femoral artery and has a very low risk of osteonecrosis.[11] Schoeniger and colleagues used the Ganz approach to avoid risk of osteonecrosis in eight patients with monoarticular synovial chondromatosis of the hip.[8] They performed joint débridement and a modified total synovectomy via surgical hip dislocation with a trochanteric flip osteotomy. After follow-up for at least 4 years (mean, 6.5 years), no patients had recurrence of disease. Furthermore, no patients developed complications secondary to osteonecrosis of the femoral head.

Arthroscopic management of synovial chondromatosis has become more acceptable for early management of the disease. Boyer and co-workers[12] showed that hip arthroscopy provided good or excellent outcomes in more than half of cases. Of 111 patients, 63 reported excellent (>75% subjective improvement) or good (>50% subjective improvement) outcomes. However, 38% of patients failed arthroscopic treatment and required open surgery. This high rate of treatment failure suggests that arthroscopic treatment has limitations in achieving complete tumor removal. The major advantage of an arthroscopic procedure is less invasive exposure of the hip joint performed without dislocation and/or trochanteric osteotomy. Nevertheless, these advantages are tempered by more restricted access to the joint and limitations with loose body removal and synovectomy. Although open procedures are better for preventing recurrence, the role of arthroscopic surgery needs to be better defined. Open procedures seem more appropriate for nonfocal disease patterns (Fig. 36-2), and arthroscopy may have a role in focal or less extensive disease patterns.

Prognosis

Early diagnosis and timely management of this disease are important in optimizing clinical results. When the disease is diagnosed before joint erosions develop,

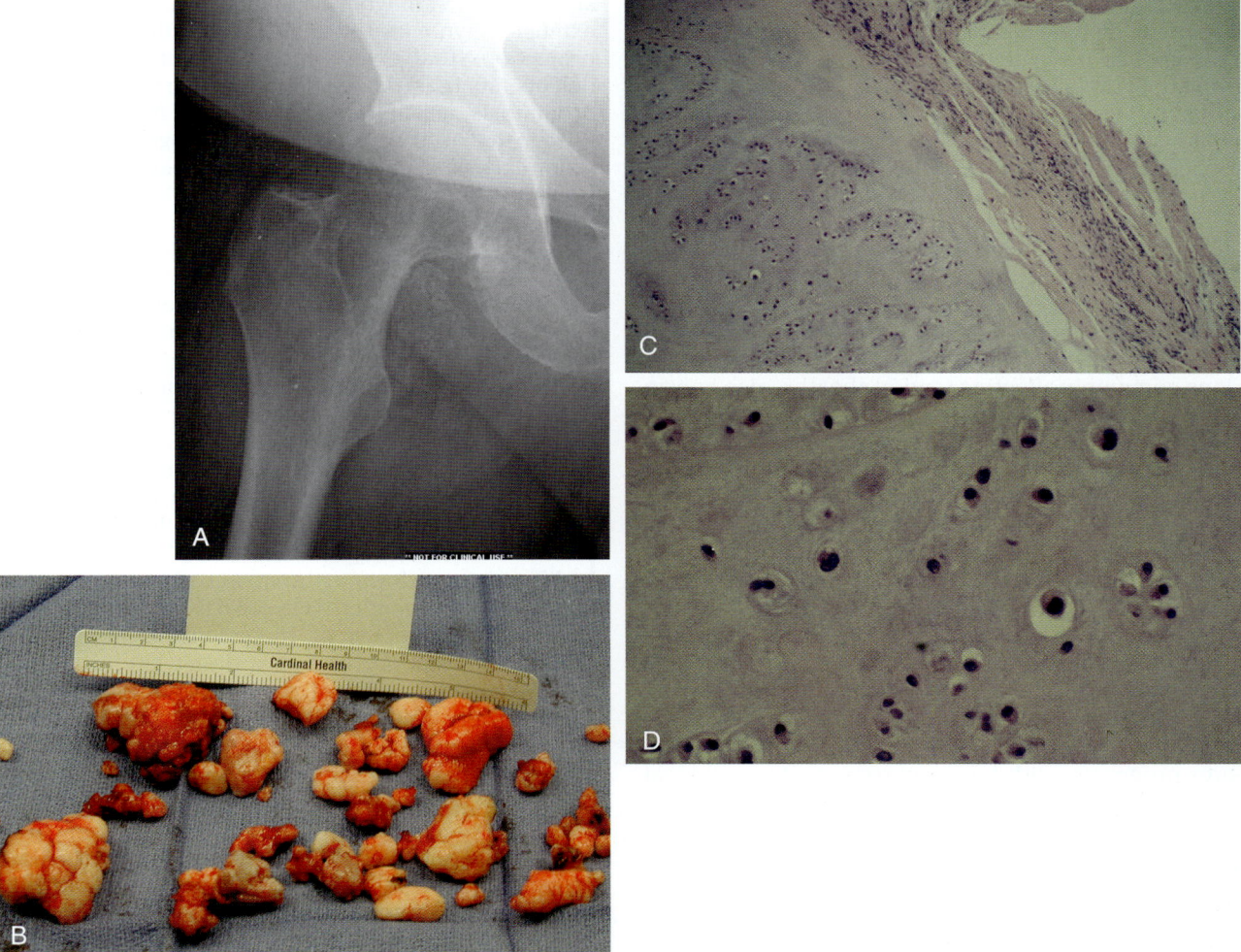

Figure 36-2. A, Anteroposterior (AP) radiograph of the right hip in a 61-year-old male with hip pain and stiffness. A large osteochondral body is inferior to the femoral neck, and numerous smaller osteocartilaginous lesions can be seen surrounding the femoral neck and the inferior acetabulum. **B,** Gross photograph of numerous osteocartilaginous loose bodies that were removed from within the joint and those embedded within the synovium. **C,** Low-power photomicrograph shows the edge of one of the osteochondral bodies with a benign pattern of cartilage proliferation. **D,** High-power photomicrograph illustrating benign chondrocytes with no nuclear atypia and abundant cartilaginous matrix.

surgical intervention is more likely to be successful. Extensive joint involvement and associated articular damage predispose the joint to secondary osteoarthritis. Progressive secondary osteoarthritis may be associated with worsening symptoms and the need for total joint replacement surgery. Malignant transformation of synovial chondromatosis is rare.

PIGMENTED VILLONODULAR SYNOVITIS

Overview

Pigmented villonodular synovitis is an idiopathic, benign proliferative disorder that can affect both extra-articular (bursa, tendons) and intra-articular structures. Most commonly, PVNS is found in the knees (80%), but it can involve hips, shoulders, and elbows.[13] This rare disease has an incidence of 1.8 cases per million people per year. Both men and women are affected, and the average age at presentation is 30 to 50 years.[14] The cause of the disease is attributed to a chronic inflammatory response or benign locally aggressive growth of fibrohistiocytic origin. Histologically, PVNS is a hypertrophic, hypervascular synovial process characterized by villous, nodular, and villonodular proliferation. The dark pigmentation is the result of hemosiderin deposits in the synovium, which also contains multinucleate giant cells and macrophages. These express local inflammatory cytokines, which stimulate osteoclastic bone resorption, leading to articular cartilage damage and erosion of periarticular bone.

PVNS occurs in two forms: localized (focal) and diffuse. Localized forms occur as discrete nodular lesions commonly affecting tendon sheaths, also known as *giant cell tumors of the tendon sheath*. These occur in approximately 75% of cases, affecting women more frequently than men in their fifth or sixth decades, and usually affect digits of the hands or feet. Nevertheless, localized PVNS can be intra-articular and can involve the hip joint. These tumors tend to be well-circumscribed lesions that are more easily managed than diffuse forms. Localized forms have a favorable prognosis and a very low recurrence rate. Conversely, diffuse forms affect the entire synovial membrane of a joint or bursa. Surgical management of these disease forms is more challenging because tumorous tissue is more diffuse and infiltrates surrounding tissue (Fig. 36-3). These lesions have a poorer prognosis, with high recurrence rates and local progression.

Clinical Features and Diagnosis

PVNS usually presents with nonspecific, insidious joint symptoms, including pain, mechanical locking, decreased range of motion, and stiffness. Cases usually are monoarticular and are not associated with other disorders. Localized PVNS usually presents as a painless, slow-growing mass, especially if extra-articular. Intra-articular lesions can result in effusion and joint irritability. Progression of the disease leads to persistent discomfort and mechanical impingement at the extremes of motion. Because of the inconsistent nature of the presentation, diagnosis is often significantly delayed.

Radiographs of advanced joint involvement will demonstrate bony erosions, subchondral cysts, and concentric loss of joint space. In early disease stages, radiographs are commonly normal. Therefore, further imaging with CT scan or MRI is indicated to diagnose early disease. CT commonly shows diffuse thickening of the tissue about the joint and increased attenuation of the lesion relative to that of muscle owing to the presence of hemosiderin. MRI also demonstrates key features such as joint effusions, elevation of the joint capsule, hyperplastic synovium, and low to intermediate signal intensity resulting from hemosiderin deposition in the synovium. These imaging studies assist in determining the extent of synovial disease, its location, and its anatomic relationship to other intra-articular and extra-articular structures.

Interventional imaging can further aid in the diagnosis of PVNS. A magnetic resonance arthrogram shows extensive synovial thickening with villous or nodular projections that extend into the joint. Multiple filling defects, such as those seen in primary synovial chondromatosis, are not an arthrographic finding of diffuse intra-articular PVNS. Definitive diagnosis of PVNS requires tissue pathology for histopathologic evaluation and confirmation.

Treatment

Early diagnosis and complete tumor removal are necessary to minimize the secondary effects of PVNS on the integrity of the joint articular cartilage. Surgical synovectomy, local or complete, is the standard treatment. Similar to the knee, localized disease can be managed with surgical resection alone because the risk of recurrence is low.[13-15] This may be done as an open procedure or arthroscopically. The diffuse form presents a challenging surgical problem with high local recurrence rates after incomplete removal. Complete synovectomy is difficult to perform arthroscopically, and open treatment is recommended (Fig. 36-4). Vastel and associates,[16] in their report of 16 patients treated with an anterior dislocation through a direct lateral approach with trochanteric osteotomy, showed that complete synovectomy is effective in preventing local recurrence of synovitis. With a mean follow-up of 16.7 years, none of the patients had radiographic or clinical evidence of recurrence. One patient, however, had asymptomatic recurrent or persistent PVNS 14 years after synovectomy, found at the time of total hip arthroplasty. Radiotherapy, as external beam or intra-articular radiocolloid injection, has a role for patients with recurrence or with high risk of recurrent disease. Low- to moderate-dose (16 to 25 Gy) external beam radiation has been used in combination with surgical synovectomy. Specific results for hip disease are lacking, but data from knee disease are useful. O'Sullivan and colleagues[18] showed in 14 patients that radiotherapy improved function of the limb and eradicated disease in 13 of 14 patients. Other

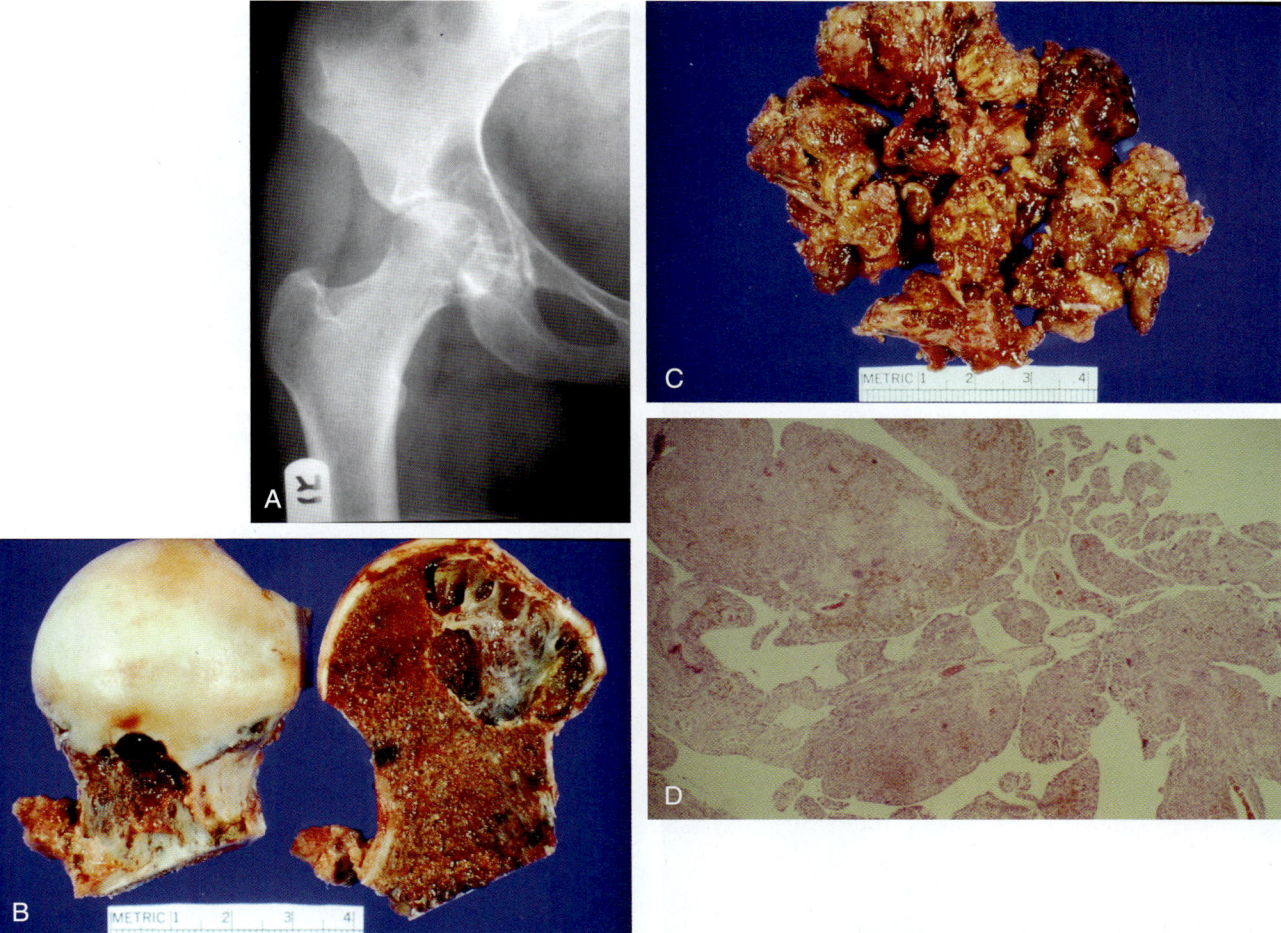

Figure 36-3. A, Anteroposterior (AP) radiograph of the right hip in a 29-year-old female. A large radiolucent defect is seen within the acetabulum, as is radiolucent cystic change within the femoral head. Cystic changes on both sides of a joint suggest a primary intra-articular process; in this case, pigmented villonodular synovitis is seen. **B,** Photograph of bi-valved femoral head showing erosive cystic changes in the head. **C,** Photograph of gross tissue removed, showing a reddish brown friable material consistent with PVNS. **D,** Photomicrograph at low power showing the villous nature of some of the tissue. A mixture of giant cell histiocytes and sheets of round cells is present. Abundant hemosiderin formation is evident.

authors have reported similar results with combined treatment, noting recurrence rates of 4% to 14%.[15,16]

Intra-articular radiosynovectomy with yttrium 90 or dysprosium 165 has been used in combination with surgery. Shabat and associates[17] reported on 10 patients treated with combined surgical synovectomy and yttrium 90 injection; one had hip disease. After a mean follow-up of 6 years, only one recurrence was noted. As beta emission colloids, their effects likely would be better on minimal residual disease because penetration through bulk disease would be limited to 8 to 12 mm. Other authors have reported less consistent results. Chin and colleagues[18] reported on 40 patients with disease of the knee treated with open synovectomy alone (5 patients), open synovectomy with intra-articular dysprosium 165 (30 patients), or open surgery and external beam radiotherapy (5 patients). Although good to excellent functional results were achieved in more than 90% of patients, 18% had recurrent disease regardless of the method of radiation given. The authors

believe that complete surgical synovectomy was the most important factor in preventing recurrent disease.

Primary or recurrent disease associated with significant bone erosion or articular cartilage damage is difficult to manage with joint preservation techniques. Joint arthroplasty is recommended for these patients and is effective in controlling disease and restoring function. Della-Valle and coworkers[19] reported their experience in seven patients with hip disease and provided a meta-analysis for an additional 55 patients with hip disease from the reported literature. Among their own seven patients, four patients had significant disease associated with arthritis and were treated with hip arthroplasty. No recurrences were noted at an average follow-up of 13 years. Meta-analysis revealed that 52 of 55 patients were treated surgically with synovectomy (26 patients) or total hip arthroplasty (24 patients), the most common procedures. Ten patients had recurrent disease—nine patients in the synovectomy group and none in the arthroplasty group. Although total hip

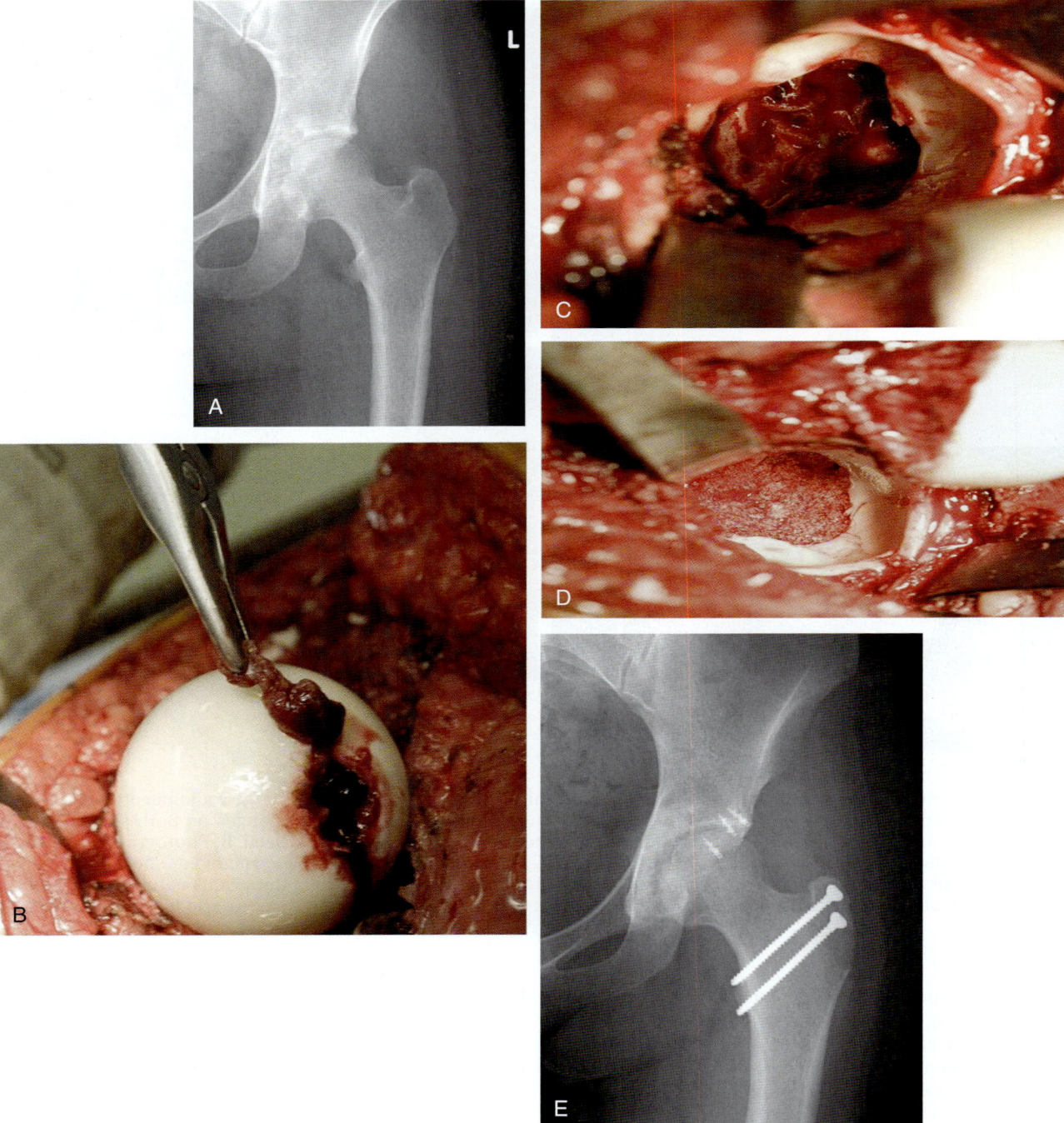

Figure 36-4. A, Anteroposterior (AP) radiograph of the left hip in a 23-year-old female with progressive hip pain. Erosion of the medial wall is evident and magnetic resonance imaging (MRI) reveals a soft tissue mass consistent with pigmented villonodular synovitis (PVNS). **B,** Because of the extent and location of the lesion, the hip was treated with surgical dislocation. The central femoral head had an erosive lesion treated with curettage and grafting. **C,** The acetabulum had a large erosive lesion that made up a major portion of the acetabular articular surface. **D,** The acetabular lesion was also treated with curettage and grafting. The hip had a large anterosuperior labral tear and femoroacetabular impingement treated with labral repair and femoral head-neck osteochondroplasty. **E,** Six months postoperatively, the trochanteric osteotomy had healed and the patient noted clinical improvement. This hip has a guarded prognosis because of the nonfocal disease pattern and the aggressive behavior of the tumor.

arthroplasty is effective in controlling PVNS, it should be reserved for patients with advanced disease because many of these patients are young adults.

CONCLUSION

Primary synovial disorders of the hip are uncommon and can be difficult to diagnose. Evaluation of patients presenting with an insidious onset of hip pain of unknown origin should include consideration of these disorders. Synovial chondromatosis and PVNS are the two most common synovial disorders. Definitive treatment focuses on complete tumor removal. The type of resection or ablation is dependent on the disease pattern, biological aggressiveness, the extent of the tumor, and the degree of secondary joint degeneration. When end-stage disease is present, total joint replacement surgery is considered.

CURRENT CONTROVERSIES AND FUTURE CONSIDERATIONS

- The comparative efficacy of open and arthroscopic treatments needs to be clarified.
- Improved imaging techniques may enhance the assessment of articular cartilage integrity and may impact treatment recommendations.
- The role of radiation therapy in the treatment of PVNS is promising but needs to be better defined.

REFERENCES

1. Barland P, Novikoff AB, Hamerman D: Electron microscopy of the human synovial membrane. J Cell Biol 14:207–220, 1962.
2. Burmester GR, Dimitriu-Bona A, Waters SJ, Winchester RJ: Identification of three major synovial lining cell populations by monoclonal antibodies directed to Ia antigens and antigens associated with monocytes/macrophages and fibroblasts. Scand J Immunol 17:69–82, 1983.
3. Maurice H, Crone M, Watt I: Synovial chondromatosis. J Bone Joint Surg Br 70:807–811, 1988.
4. Villacin AB, Brigham LN, Bullough PG: Primary and secondary synovial chondrometaplasia: histopathologic and clinicoradiologic differences. Hum Pathol 10:439–451, 1979.
5. Milgram JW: Synovial osteochondromatosis: a histopathological study of thirty cases. J Bone Joint Surg Am 59:792–801, 1977.
6. Kramer J, Recht M, Deely DM, et al: MR appearance of idiopathic synovial osteochondromatosis. J Comput Assist Tomogr 17:772–776, 1993.
7. Ogilvie-Harris DJ, Saleh K: Generalized synovial chondromatosis of the knee: a comparison of removal of the loose bodies alone with arthroscopic synovectomy. Arthroscopy 10:166–170, 1994.
8. Schoeniger R, Naudie DD, Siebenrock KA, et al: Modified complete synovectomy prevents recurrence in synovial chondromatosis of the hip. Clin Orthop Relat Res 451:195–200, 2006.
9. Postel M, Courpied JP, Augouard LW: [Synovial chondromatosis of the hip: value of dislocation of the hip for complete removal of pathological synovial membranes]. Rev Chir Orthop Reparatrice Appar Mot 73:539–543, 1987.
10. Lim SJ, Park YS: Operative treatment of primary synovial osteochondromatosis of the hip: surgical technique. J Bone Joint Surg Am 89(Suppl 2 Pt 2):232–245, 2007.
11. Ganz R, Gill TJ, Gautier E, et al: Surgical dislocation of the adult hip a technique with full access to the femoral head and acetabulum without the risk of avascular necrosis. J Bone Joint Surg Br 83:1119–1124, 2001.
12. Boyer T, Dorfmann H: Arthroscopy in primary synovial chondromatosis of the hip: description and outcome of treatment. J Bone Joint Surg Br 90:314–318, 2008.
13. Dorwart RH, Genant HK, Johnston WH, Morris JM: Pigmented villonodular synovitis of synovial joints: clinical, pathologic, and radiologic features. AJR Am J Roentgenol 143:877–885, 2004.
14. Flandry FC, Hughston JC, Jacobson KE, et al: Surgical treatment of diffuse pigmented villonodular synovitis of the knee. Clin Orthop Relat Res 300:183–192, 1994.
15. Blanco CE, Leon HO, Guthrie TB: Combined partial arthroscopic synovectomy and radiation therapy for diffuse pigmented villonodular synovitis of the knee. Arthroscopy 17:527–531, 2001.
16. Ustinova VF, Podliashuk EL, Rodionova SS: [Combined treatment of the diffuse form of pigmented villonodular synovitis]. Med Radiol (Mosk) 31:27–31, 1986.
17. Shabat S, Kollender Y, Merimsky O, et al: The use of surgery and yttrium 90 in the management of extensive and diffuse pigmented villonodular synovitis of large joints. Rheumatology (Oxford) 41:1113–1118, 2002.
18. Chin KR, Barr SJ, Winalski C, et al: Treatment of advanced primary and recurrent diffuse pigmented villonodular synovitis of the knee. J Bone Joint Surg Am 84:2192–2202, 2002.
19. Gonzalez Della Valle A, Piccaluga F, Potter HG, et al: Pigmented villonodular synovitis of the hip: 2- to 23-year followup study. Clin Orthop Relat Res 388:187–199, 2001.
20. Masih S, Antebi A: Imaging of pigmented villonodular synovitis. Semin Musculoskelet Radiol 7:205–216, 2003.
21. Vastel L, Lambert P, De Pinieux G, et al: Surgical treatment of pigmented villonodular synovitis of the hip. J Bone Joint Surg Am 87:1019–1024, 2005.
22. Yoo JJ, Kwon YS, Koo KH, et al: Cementless total hip arthroplasty performed in patients with pigmented villonodular synovitis. J Arthroplasty 25:552–557, 2010.
23. O'Sullivan B, Cummings B, Catton C, et al: Outcome following radiation treatment for high-risk pigmented villonodular synovitis. Int J Radiat Oncol Biol Phys 32:777–786, 1995.

CHAPTER 37

Acetabular Rim Damage

Paul E. Beaulé and Michael Leunig

INTRODUCTION

Klaue and coauthors[1] were the first to coin the term *acetabular rim syndrome,* which encompasses pathologic loading and resulting damage to the labrum, acetabular cartilage, and/or bony rim. In their study of acetabular dysplasia, a spectrum of pathologies ranging from a torn labrum to an acetabular rim fracture, as well as cysts within the acetabular bony rim or adjacent soft tissues, was described. Until recently, diagnosis and imaging of these lesions were difficult and often required operative intervention to confirm the diagnosis.[2-6] With the advent of more advanced surgical (open hip dislocation) and imaging techniques such as magnetic resonance arthrography,[7,8] the knowledge base and understanding of the origin of damage to the acetabular labral-chondral complex, as well as its role in degenerative arthritis, have greatly evolved over the past two decades. Despite recent advancements in imaging and in operative techniques, patients with acetabular rim damage still are often misdiagnosed.[9] This chapter will review the causes and pathomechanisms of acetabular rim damage, as well as its diagnosis and treatment.

ETIOLOGY

In hip dysplasia, Klaue and associates[1] introduced the term *acetabular rim syndrome* as a precursor of secondary osteoarthritis, wherein intrinsically normal intraarticular soft tissue structures are exposed to loading joint forces that physically exceed their tolerance level, resulting in hip damage. The frequently enlarged acetabular labrum in dysplastic hips[10] initially aids in maintaining the femoral head within the joint; however, the unstable femoral head potentially translates and eventually subluxes secondary to deficient coverage. If these chronic "inside-out" shear stresses do persist, labral soft tissue compensation will fail and the labrum can tear off the acetabular rim or can avulse with an osseous fragment; this is described as *rim fracture.*[1]

Although management of damage/degeneration to the acetabular rim is still evolving, consistency in the location of damage within the acetabular rim has been demonstrated in several studies, both cadaveric and in vivo. Peripheral damage to the hip joint was first brought to attention in the classic studies of osteoarthrosis conducted by Harrison and colleagues[11] and Byers and coworkers.[12] This was further supported by the work of Bullough and associates,[13] who emphasized the importance of the shape of the hip joint in the form of minor incongruencies leading to failure of articular cartilage at the acetabular rim within normal daily contact. Despite these early reports documenting the acetabular rim as an early site of hip damage, specific disorders such as hip instability due to dysplasia (Fig. 37-1) and, more recently, femoroacetabular impingement (FAI) (Fig. 37-2) were underappreciated as causative factors for hip osteoarthritis (OA). The acetabular labrum and adjacent cartilage are early structures to fail in acetabular rim disorders secondary to localized stresses. This notion was more recently confirmed by Leunig and colleagues,[14] who compared cadaveric findings and noted anterior acetabular quadrant damage with associated insufficient femoral head-neck offset. Seldes and coworkers[15] further characterized acetabular rim damage as two main types of rim degeneration correlating with our current understanding of FAI.[14]

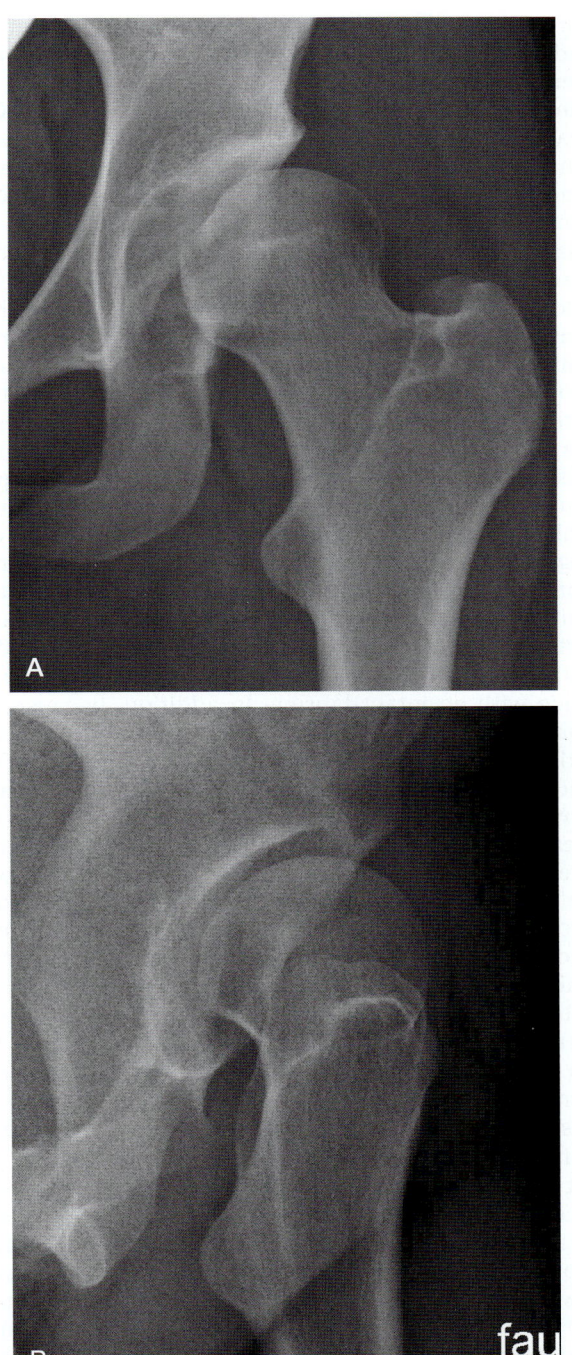

Figure 37-1. A, Acetabular rim damage as exemplified by an anteroposterior hip (taken from a correct anteroposterior [AP] pelvis) **(B)** and faux profile radiographs of classic anterolateral hip dysplasia. As the consequence of a short and steep acetabular roof, the femoral head translates anterolaterally, resulting in high "inside-out" shearing forces leading to secondary joint incongruity and static rim overload.

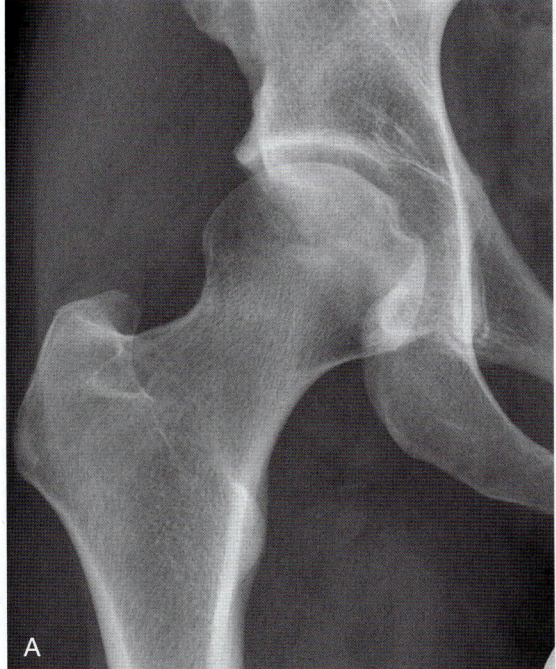

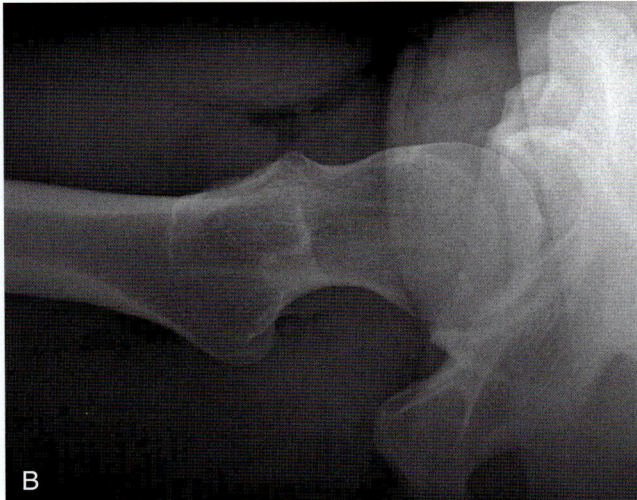

Figure 37-2. A, Acetabular rim damage exemplified by anteroposterior hip (taken from a correct anteroposterior [AP] pelvis) **(B)** and cross-table lateral radiographs of femoroacetabular impingement. As the consequence of primary incongruity of the hip caused by femoral head overcoverage and/or asphericity, hip motion with "outside-in" shearing forces will result in dynamic rim overload.

In FAI, the femoral head is well centered, but the free arc of hip motion is limited by a deep or malorientated acetabulum, producing pincer FAI or a misshaped proximal femur (insufficient head-neck offset, nonspherical head causing cam FAI). It is not uncommon that a combination of cam and pincer FAI exists. In FAI, articular damage initially occurs by point or regional loading of the femoral neck against the acetabular rim. The site of hip damage is similar to that of acetabular rim damage seen in hip dysplasia; however, failure mechanisms are almost the opposite. Furthermore, damage patterns of pincer and cam FAI differ substantially when one of these two types exists as an isolated deformity. In pincer FAI, pathology is more localized to the labrum, and in cam FAI, damage takes place at the cartilage with "outside-in" abrasion and/or delamination, with the occasional rim fracture.[16] An osseous rim fragment in FAI may be seen in athletes with a combined type and pronounced acetabular malorientation. Speed, force, and degree of hip motion, in addition to the quality of tissue at the labral-chondral junction, might contribute to enhanced vulnerability at the anterosuperior rim.[17]

To date, our knowledge indicates that hip dysplasia and FAI are the two major bony deformities associated with the development of osteoarthritis in the hip. Alterations in hip joint mechanics represent a continuum between "undercoverage" (dysplasia) as described by Klaue and associates[1] and, as introduced more recently, "overcoverage" (FAI). As our understanding of these morphologic alterations of the hip has improved, it has become clear that combinations of these mechanical factors frequently lead to reactive pain within the periarticular soft tissues such as trochanteric (abductors) and/or groin pain (hip flexors/adductors).

ACETABULAR RIM DAMAGE AND THE LABRUM

The acetabular labrum is triangular in cross-section, with the base applied to the acetabular rim and the apex being the free margin.[15] The joint capsule attaches to its external edge, creating a potential recess between the capsule and the labrum. The labrum can be subdivided into two distinct zones: the extra-articular side, consisting of dense connective tissue, is well vascularized at its junction with the joint capsule, whereas the intra-articular portion is largely avascular.[18] In addition, recent embryologic studies of the hip joint show that the anterior and posterior acetabular-labral chondral junctions have different morphologic appearances.[19,20] In a study of 11 human embryos, Cashin and associates[19] found that the anterior labrum has a rather marginal attachment to the acetabular cartilage with an intra-articular projection, whereas the posterior labrum is attached and continuous with the acetabular cartilage. In addition, anteriorly the labral-chondral transition zone is sharp and abrupt, while posteriorly it is gradual and interdigitated. These most recent findings contrast with those of Petersen and associates[21] and Seldes and colleagues,[15] who initially described the acetabular labrum as continuous with the articular cartilage throughout the acetabulum.[21] This abrupt anterior transition zone would make the labrum more susceptible to tearing and corresponds to some extent to the so-called *watershed lesion*.[22] Based on intraoperative observations of a large number of hip arthroscopies for labral tears, as well as cadaveric dissections, McCarthy and associates[22] described the anterior labrum as an at risk zone because of potentially inferior mechanical properties, higher mechanical demands, and relative hypovascularity, and proposed that a labral

tear alters the biomechanical environment of the hip, leading to degeneration of the articular cartilage and eventual osteoarthritis.[23]

In terms of its predilection for failure, Dorrell and Catterall[24] correlated the occurrence of a labral tear with abnormal shear stresses transmitted by the uncovered femoral head, as may occur in acetabular dysplasia. From this clinical situation, they postulated that the enlarged labrum contributes to stability of the femoral head within the acetabulum in adulthood. This aspect of load sharing was later supported by the work of Kim and associates,[25] who demonstrated that the labrum contributed to growth and development of the acetabular roof. Although a role of load sharing, similar to that of the meniscus in the knee, may be correct in cases of dysplasia, more recent work by Konrath and associates[26] shows that the labrum does not have an important load sharing role. Instead, based on a finite element analysis and cadaveric investigation, Ferguson and colleagues[27] found that the labrum acts as a seal, ensuring more constant fluid film lubrication within the hip and limiting the rate of fluid expression from the articular cartilage layers of the joint, as noted by greater hydrostatic fluid pressurization within the intra-articular space with an intact labrum. In addition, because the labrum adds extra resistance to the flow path for interstitial fluid expression, cartilage consolidation was significantly quicker without the labrum.[27,28] Consequently, disruption of the labral seal could be detrimental to the overall nutrition of the cartilage, leading to its premature degeneration.[29] Takechi and coworkers[30] showed the labrum contributing to stability of the hip joint through its valve effect and structure. Both of these mechanisms were dependent on the fit of the labrum against the femoral head.[28] Similarly, Crawford and associates[31] reported that loss of the labral seal is the critical event leading to destabilization of the hip, shifting the hip center of rotation and making the hip susceptible to increased impact loading and repetitive trauma through loss of the protective function provided by the intact labrum and its seal.

It is interesting to note that the morphologic appearance of the labrum can differ on the basis of its underlying mechanism of failure: dysplasia or femoroacetabular impingement.[32,33] Klaue and colleagues[1] and Leunig and coworkers[32] showed that in dysplasia, the labrum is distinctly hypertrophic with myxoid degeneration and/or detachment from the bony rim, whereas in femoroacetabular impingement, the labrum is more commonly characterized by an undersurface tear with no hypertrophy.[32] These findings can be helpful in establishing the dominating underlying bony abnormality when in the presence of mixed deformities such as dysplasia and FAI.

In terms of pincer-type FAI, Seldes and associates[15] described labral damage extending perpendicular to the surface of the labrum and in more severe cases to the subchondral bone with associated endochondral ossification within the labrum; this is consistent with operative findings seen in pincer impingement. With acetabular rim damage associated with cam-type FAI, Seldes and colleagues[15] described disruption of the transition zone between the fibrocartilaginous labrum and the acetabular cartilage perpendicular to the articular surface, leading to cleavage/disruption at the anterior labral-chondral junction.

Diagnosis

Clinical Evaluation

In most patients with acetabular rim damage, the chief complaint will be anterior groin pain made worse by long periods of standing, sitting, walking, or getting into and out of a car. The pain can be referred to the gluteal area or the trochanteric region. Although no specific clinical findings differentiate dysplasia from FAI, the vast majority of patients with dysplasia will have symptoms ranging from early fatigue to clear weakness of the abductors, with irritation over the greater trochanter. In addition, some patients may experience a catching phenomenon similar to that caused by meniscal disease of the knee; this occasionally requires manipulation of the lower limb, usually in the form of a "shaking-free" movement.[34] As symptoms increase in frequency, residual pain may result in a slight limp, whereas patients with FAI will complain of chronic/recurring "groin" injury, as well as limited hip flexibility, but with well-preserved muscle function. Onset of pain in most cases is insidious,[35] with patients often unable to recall a specific traumatic event.[5] Among patients with labral tears in general, Burnett and associates[9] found that only 9% (6 of 66 patients) had a major traumatic episode as a causative factor for acetabular rim damage. The pain was often sharp in nature and was aggravated by activity such as walking and pivoting on the affected side. Mechanical symptoms such as clicking and catching are highly variable and are not necessarily indicative of intra-articular hip pathology.[5] On history, it is critical to inquire about childhood hip diseases such as dysplasia,[25] Legg-Calvé-Perthes (LCP),[36] and slipped capital femoral epiphysis (SCFE),[37] all of which are known causes of osteoarthritis.[38,39]

On physical examination, the most reliable sign of labral pathology[35] is pain reproduced with flexion past 90 degrees, combined with internal rotation and adduction. This is referred to as the *impingement sign*.[1] Others have found that forced external rotation with hip extension can irritate the damaged rim[40] and is more commonly reported in patients with dysplasia. In addition, in dysplasia, Leunig and associates[34] describe the bicycle test, whereby trochanteric irritation reflects abductor muscle insufficiency. This test is performed with the affected hip up; a bicycle pedaling maneuver is then performed as the lateral and posterior margins of the trochanter are palpated. Increasing the load on the pedaling foot may exacerbate the pain. Tenderness is most commonly palpated along the posterior border of the gluteus medius muscle. As for patients with FAI, they typically will have limited internal rotation (usually less than 20 degrees) with the hip flexed at 90 degrees.

Although labral pathology is now recognized as a common cause of hip pain, it is important to include in the differential diagnosis other causes of hip pain such as osteonecrosis, stress fracture, and snapping psoas tendon. In cases of abnormal physical findings and normal or equivocal radiologic findings, an anesthetic block of the symptomatic hip may provide important diagnostic information in terms of delineating intra-articular versus extra-articular hip pathology. Temporary pain relief represents a positive finding for intra-articular hip pathology.[41]

Radiologic Evaluation

Because a large proportion of acetabular rim damage (i.e., labral-chondral pathology) is associated with a bony abnormality, initial investigation must include plain radiographs with a minimum of two views: anteroposterior pelvic and lateral radiographs (Dunn view or cross-table lateral radiographs),[42,43] as well as a false profile view.[44] For all of these views, proper patient positioning is critical for correct assessment of the bony anatomy. For the anteroposterior radiograph, the x-ray beam should be centered over the midline with collinear alignment of the symphysis and coccyx, and the distance between the symphysis and the sacrococcygeal junction should be 32 mm for men and 47 mm for women if acetabular version is assessed correctly.[45] The normal acetabulum should cover the femoral head with the anterior and posterior walls meeting at its most lateral edge.

In assessment of dysplasia, the three main radiographic parameters are the lateral center edge angle of Wiberg (normal greater than 25 degrees),[34] the acetabular roof inclination or Tonnis angle (normal less than 10 degrees),[46] and the anterior center edge angle measured on the false profile view (normal greater than 20 degrees[44]). In cases of acetabular retroversion, the anterior and posterior walls of the acetabulum will be seen to cross over the femoral head; a so-called *crossover* or *figure-of-eight sign*[47,48] is then present. Another sign of retroversion is the ischial sign: ischial tuberosity is seen on the anteroposterior pelvic view.[49] Coxa profunda is diagnosed on the anteroposterior pelvis x-ray when the medial wall of the acetabulum lies on or medial to the ilioischial line,[50] with protrusio representing the more severe form with the femoral head crossing the ilioischial line.[50] In assessment of cam-type impingement, insufficient head-neck offset and/or femoral head asphericity are best assessed on a lateral radiograph such as the cross-table with the leg in 10 to 15 degrees of internal rotation[51,52] or a Dunn view (anteroposterior view of hip in 90 degrees of flexion, 25 degrees of abduction, with no rotation).

Magnetic resonance imaging (MRI) is the preferred modality for the investigation of intra-articular hip pathology, providing exquisite resolution of the labrum, cartilage, and joint space, as well as regional soft tissues. In addition, MRI permits multiplanar image acquisition such as radial imaging. Magnetic resonance arthrography (MRA), which is the combination of MRI with intra-articular injection of gadolinium-based contrast agents, is the test of choice for evaluation of the acetabular labrum.[7,8,53-55] The arthrogram component distends the joint, causing separation of the labrum from the capsule and osteochondral structures, resulting in increased spatial resolution. The injected contrast solution outlines both normal anatomic structures and abnormal pathologies, further improving contrast resolution and increasing the conspicuity of labral pathology.[56,57] Labral tears will be demonstrated by extension of contrast solution into the substance of the labrum and are most commonly seen in the anterosuperior quadrant.[53,54,58-60]

With regard to sensitivity and accuracy of MRA for diagnosing labral pathology with hip arthroscopy as the definitive diagnosis, sensitivity and accuracy values range from 92% to 100% and from 93% to 96%, respectively.[54,55,59] Pitfalls that may lead to a false diagnosis of labral tear include a sublabral sulcus, an anteroinferior cleft at the labral–transverse ligament junction, cartilage undercutting of the labrum, and increased signal intensity at the chondral-labral junction.[55,58,61-63]

More recently, several centers have focused on identification of acetabular cartilage damage through erosion[64] or delamination[65] on MRA. Schmid and associates[64] reported gadolinium-enhanced MRA (GD-MRA) to be moderately sensitive and specific in detecting acetabulum articular cartilage defects with associated labral tears in patients who underwent surgical correction for FAI. In their investigation, defects were consistently found in the anterosuperior quadrant, which is consistent with the concept of acetabular rim damage.[14] Others have focused on the identification of cartilage delamination[66-68] (Fig. 37-3), which is an earlier stage of cartilage damage,[50,69] compared with full-thickness defects, as reported by Schmid and associates.[64] In our clinical series of 48 hips,[68] the sensitivity and specificity of GD-MRA for detecting acetabular cartilage delamination confirmed at surgery was 97% and 84%, respectively, with a positive predictive value of 90% and a negative predictive value of 94%. Anderson and associates,[66] looking at the same radiologic sign, found the inverted "oreo cookie" quite specific at 100% but to have very low sensitivity at 22%. They attributed the low sensitivity to lack of training of the radiologist.

In patients for whom MRI is contraindicated (claustrophobia, non–MRI-compatible prostheses, electronic implanted devices, cardiac pacing wires, orbital metal bodies), computed tomography (CT) arthrography is an acceptable alternative study with equally high sensitivity, specificity, and accuracy, although it involves gonadal radiation exposure.[70,71]

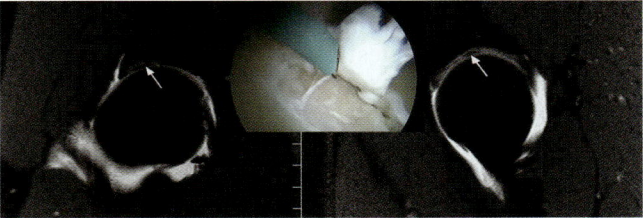

Figure 37-3. Cartilage delamination observed in gadolinium-enhanced magnetic resonance arthrography (GD-MRA) images was characterized as a linear intra-articular defect best seen on T1-weighted sagittal and coronal images. Inset shows arthroscopic view of delaminated cartilage in the same patient.

Treatment Options

Appropriate timing of surgical intervention for hip dysplasia is well established, but for FAI it is still evolving. Although physiotherapy and/or anti-inflammatory therapy remains the first line of treatment for most musculoskeletal injuries, its benefits in FAI and hip dysplasia are questionable. Of concern is the possible delay in surgical correction of symptomatic patients with bony abnormalities due to hip dysplasia or FAI, because the disease may progress to the point where joint preservation is no longer indicated. Therefore, clinical and radiographic diagnosed disease requires correction of the underlying bony abnormality, possible only through surgery.

In hip dysplasia, increasing evidence suggests that the hip's prognosis can be substantially improved by joint-preserving osteotomies with a recent shift in emphasis from the proximal part of the femur to the pelvis.[34] The goal of pelvic osteotomy is to change the pathologic mechanical environment that leads to secondary osteoarthrosis by improving femoral head coverage and/or acetabular congruity under certain conditions combined with correction of the femoral deformity. Soft tissue débridement as recommended by some arthroscopic surgeons will not optimize the mechanical environment and frequently only delays appropriate surgical treatment. Long-term results of periacetabular osteotomies are superior to those of proximal femoral osteotomies. The best results can be achieved when the rim-labrum complex is undamaged[72,73]; however, pelvic osteotomies are more technically demanding and have the potential for serious complications. As with femoral osteotomies, older patients with more advanced arthritis have a worse prognosis.

Open surgical dislocation of the hip was the first technique described for the treatment of FAI. Good to excellent short-term to mid-term results have been reported, with 70% to 80% of patients demonstrating clinical improvement.[74] Also, less invasive techniques such as arthroscopy have emerged.[75] Minor structural deformities and cam FAI have become the domain of arthroscopic or arthroscopically assisted mini open techniques. Mini open techniques without visualization of cartilaginous surfaces are surely limited because the surgeon can obtain no information about the condition of the cartilage. Several recent studies have confirmed that treatment of labral abnormalities with neglect of underlying bony pathology (FAI) is a major cause of treatment failure,[76,77] in that most, if not all, labral abnormalities occur in the presence of structural deformity.[78,79] Today, complex bony abnormalities such as extra-articular impingement, major deformities, and global pincer FAI still seem to be more precisely treated by open techniques. Furthermore, open techniques allow for femoral osteotomies at the level of the head-neck, the base of the neck, or the intertrochanteric region when appropriate.[80] In severe acetabular retroversion, acetabular reorientation may be required. This decision is based on the position of the posterior wall in relation to the center of rotation of the femoral head, and on the quality of cartilage in the superomedial area of the acetabulum.

Current indications for labral refixation are still evolving, but it appears that resecting the labrum from its bony attachment is to be avoided whenever possible.[81] In exposing the acetabular rim for trimming bony overgrowth, the labrum should be taken down as part of the approach and should be reattached to maintain an intact acetabular cartilage interface. Given its physiologic role,[27,82,83] reattachment of the intact portion of the labrum[84] appears logical, because absence of a labrum might lead to hip OA, as was similarly seen in previously meniscectomized knees. Successful refixation requires both a labral substance of sufficient quality and highly precise bony procedures to correct the underlying FAI.[81] This allows the labrum to regain its physiologic function (sealing, pressure distribution). Poor results of labral refixation follow suboptimal impingement treatment. Today, the technique of arthroscopic labral refixation is possible because of improved surgical technique and advanced instrumentation, but nonetheless, it remains difficult to perform.

CURRENT CONTROVERSIES

The site of hip damage is similar in hip dysplasia and FAI; however, the failure mechanisms are almost the opposite. In hip dysplasia, it is well established that the unstable femoral head migrates and subluxates in regions of least coverage of the femoral head, causing secondary joint incongruity and subsequent OA. In contrast, in FAI, the femoral head remains well centered, but the free arc of hip motion is limited by an acetabulum that is functionally excessive, by a malshaped proximal femur, or by a combination of the two. So far, the disease concept has been proposed mainly on the basis of clinical findings reported with surgical treatment of FAI, although mechanistic studies, in particular animal studies, to support this disease concept are lacking. In addition to experimental and mechanistic research is the need for further effort in the development of clinical and radiographic outcome instruments to allow assessment of the natural course of FAI disease, as well as the impact of nonsurgical and surgical treatment (open and arthroscopic). Only with these investments will new information concerning the significance of FAI disease and its potential treatment or even prophylaxis become attainable and comparable with today's accepted treatment of hip dysplasia.

REFERENCES

1. Klaue K, Durnin CW, Ganz R: The acetabular rim syndrome: a clinical presentation of dysplasia. J Bone Joint Surg Br 73:423–429, 1991.
2. Edwards DJ, Lomas D, Villar RN: Diagnosis of the painful hip by magnetic resonance imaging and arthroscopy. J Bone Joint Surg Br 77:374–376, 1995.
3. Lage LA, Patel JV, Villar RN: The acetabular labral tear: an arthroscopic classification. Arthroscopy 12:269–272, 1996.
4. Suzuki S, Awaya G, Okada Y, et al: Arthroscopic diagnosis of ruptured acetabular labrum. Acta Orthop Scand 57:513–515, 1996.
5. Byrd JW: Labral lesions: an elusive source of hip pain case reports and literature review. Arthroscopy 12:603–612, 1996.
6. Ikeda T, Awaya G, Suzuki S, et al: Torn acetabular labrum in young patients. J Bone Joint Surg Br 70:13–16, 1988.
7. Czerny C, Hofmann S, Neuhold A, et al: Lesions of the acetabular labrum: accuracy of MR imaging and MR arthrography in detection and staging. Radiology 200:225–230, 1996.
8. Leunig M, Werlen S, Ungersbock A, et al: Evaluation of the acetabular labrum by MR arthrography. J Bone Joint Surg Br 79:230–234, 1997.
9. Burnett SJ, Della Rocca GJ, Prather H, et al: Clinical presentation of patients with tears of the acetabular labrum. J Bone Joint Surg Br 88:327–333, 2006.
10. Ponseti IV: Morphology of the acetabulum in congenital dislocation of the hip: gross, histological and roentgenographic studies. J Bone Joint Surg Am 60:586–599. 1978.
11. Harrison MHM, Schajowicz F, Trueta J: Osteoarthritis of the hip: a study of the nature and evolution of the disease. J Bone Joint Surg Br 35:598–626, 1953.
12. Byers PD, Contepomi CA, Farkas TA: A post mortem study of the hip joint. Ann Rheum Dis 29:15–31, 1970.
13. Bullough PG, Goodfellow J: The relationship between degenerative changes and load-bearing in the human hip. J Bone Joint Surg Br 55:746–758, 1973.
14. Leunig M, Beck M, Woo A, et al: Acetabular rim degeneration: a constant finding in the aged hip. Clin Orthop Relat Res 413:201–207, 2003.
15. Seldes RM, Tan V, Hunt J, et al: Anatomy, histologic features and vascularity of the adult acetabular labrum. Clin Orthop Relat Res 382:232–240, 2001.
16. Martinez AE, Li SM, Ganz R, Beck M: Os acetabuli in femoroacetabular impingement: stress fracture or unfused secondary ossification centre of the acetabular rim? Hip Int 16:281–286, 2006.
17. Leunig M, Beaule PE, Ganz R: The concept of femoroacetabular impingement: current status and future perspectives. Clin Orthop Relat Res 467:616–622, 2009.
18. Kelly BT, Shapiro GS, Digiovanni CW, et al: Vascularity of the hip labrum: a cadaveric investigation. Arthroscopy 21:3–11, 2005.
19. Cashin M, Uhthoff HK, O'Neill M, Beaule PE: Embryology of the acetabular-labral complex. J Bone Joint Surg Br 90:1019–1024, 2008.
20. Walker JM: Histological study of the fetal development of the human acetabulum and labrum: significance in congenital hip disease. Yale J Biol Med 54:255–263, 1981.
21. Petersen W, Petersen F, Tillmann B: Structure and vascularization of the acetabular labrum with regard to the pathogenesis and healing of labral lesions. Arch Orthop Trauma Surg 123:283–288, 2004.
22. McCarthy JC, Noble PC, Schuck MR, et al: The watershed labral lesion. J Arthroplasty 16:81–87, 2001.
23. McCarthy JC, Noble PC, Schuck MR, et al: The role of labral lesions to development of early degenerative hip disease. Clin Orthop Relat Res 393:25–37, 2001.
24. Dorrell JH, Catterall A: The torn acetabular labrum. J Bone Joint Surg Br 68:400–403, 1986.
25. Kim YH: Acetabular dysplasia and osteoarthritis developed by an eversion of the acetabular labrum. Clin Orthop Relat Res 215:289–295, 1987.
26. Konrath GA, Hamel AJ, Olson SA, Sharkey NA: The role of the acetabular labrum and the transverse acetabular ligament in load transmission in the hip. J Bone Joint Surg Am 80A:1781–1788, 1998.
27. Ferguson SJ, Ganz R, Ganz R, Ito K: An in vitro investigation of the acetabular labral seal in hip joint mechanics. J Biomechanics 36:171–178, 2003.
28. Hlavacek M: The influence of the acetabular labrum seal, intact articular superficial zone and synovial fluid thixotropy on squeeze-film lubrication of a spherical synovial joint. J Biomechanics 35:1325–1335, 2002.
29. O'Driscoll SW: The healing and regeneration of articular cartilage. J Bone Joint Surg Am 80:1795–1812, 1999.
30. Takechi H, Nagashima H, Ito S: Intra-articular pressure of the hip joint outside and inside the limbus. J Japanese Orthop Assoc 56:529–536, 1982.

31. Crawford MR, Dy CJ, Alexander JW, et al: The 2007 Frank Stinchfield Award. The biomechanics of the hip labrum and the stability of the hip. Clin Orthop Relat Res 465:16–22, 2007.

32. Leunig M, Podeszwa D, Beck M, et al: Magnetic resonance arthrography of labral disorders in hips with dysplasia and impingement. Clin Orthop Relat Res 418:74–80, 2004.

33. Ganz R, Leunig M, Leunig-Ganz K, Harris WH: The etiology of osteoarthritis of the hip: an integrated mechanical concept. Clin Orthop Relat Res 466:264–272, 2008.

34. Leunig M, Siebenrock KA, Ganz R: Rationale of periacetabular osteotomy and background work. J Bone Joint Surg Am 83:438–448, 2001.

35. Fitzgerald RHJ: Acetabular labrum tears: diagnosis and treatment. Clin Orthop Relat Res 311:60–68, 1995.

36. Grossbard GD: Hip pain during adolescence after Perthes' disease. J Bone Joint Surg Br 63:572–574, 1981.

37. Leunig M, Casillas MM, Ganz R: Slipped capital femoral epiphysis: early mechanical damage to the acetabular cartilage by impingement of the prominent femoral metaphysis. Acta Othop Scand 71:370–375, 2000.

38. Stulberg SD, Cordell LD, Harris WH, et al: Unrecognized childhood hip disease: a major cause of idiopathic osteoarthritis of the hip. In Amstutz HC (ed): The hip, proceedings of the Third Open Scientific Meeting of the Hip Society, St Louis, 1975, CV Mosby, pp 212–228.

39. Goodman DA, Feighan JE, Smith AD, et al: Subclinical slipped capital femoral epiphysis. J Bone Joint Surg Am 79:1489–1497, 1997.

40. McCarthy JC, Noble PC, Aluisio FV, et al: Anatomy, pathologic features, and treatment of acetabular labral tears. Clin Orthop Relat Res 406:38–47, 2003.

41. Crawford RW, Gie GA, Ling RSM, Murray DW: Diagnostic value of intra-articular anaesthetic in primary osteoarthritis of the hip. J Bone Joint Surg Br 80:279–281, 1998.

42. Meyer DC, Beck M, Ellis T, et al: Comparision of six radiographic projections to assess femoral head/asphericity. Clin Orthop Relat Res 445:181–185, 2006.

43. Zaragoza EJ, Beaule PE: Imaging the painful nonarthritic hip. Oper Tech Orthop 14:42–48, 2004.

44. Garbuz DS, Masri BA, Haddad F, Duncan CP: Clinical and radiographic assessment of the young adult with symptomatic hip dysplasia. Clin Orthop Relat Res 418:18–22, 2004.

45. Siebenrock KA, Kalbermatten DF, Ganz R: Effect of pelvic tilt on acetabular retroversion: a study of pelves from cadavers. Clin Orthop Relat Res 407:241–248, 2003.

46. Tonnis D: Normal values of the hip joint for the evaluation of x-rays in children and adults. Clin Orthop Relat Res 119:39–47, 1976.

47. Reynolds D, Lucas J, Klaue K: Retroversion of the acetabulum: a cause of hip pain. J Bone Joint Surg Br 81:281–288, 1999.

48. Jamali AA, Maldenov K, Meyer DC, et al: Anteroposterior pelvic radiographs to assess acetabular retroversion: high validity of the "cross-over-sign." J Orthop Res 25:758–765, 2007.

49. Kalberer F, Sierra RJ, Madan SS, et al: Ischial spine projection into the pelvis: a new sign for acetabular retroversion. Clin Orthop Relat Res 466:677–683, 2008.

50. Beck M, Kalhor M, Leunig M, Ganz R: Hip morphology influences the pattern of damage to the acetabular cartilage: femoroacetabular impingement as a cause of early osteoarthritis of the hip. J Bone Joint Surg Br 87:1012–1018, 2005.

51. Eijer H, Leunig M, Mahomed N, Ganz R: Cross-table lateral radiographs for screening of anterior femoral head-neck offset in patients with femoro-acetabular impingement. Hip Int 11:37–41, 2001.

52. Ito K, Minka II MA, Leunig S, et al: Femoroacetabular impingement and the cam-effect. J Bone Joint Surg Br 83:171–176, 2001.

53. Czerny C, Hofmann S, Urban M, et al: MR arthrography of the adult acetabular capsular-labral complex: correlation with surgery and anatomy. AJR Am J Roentgenol 3:345–349, 1999.

54. Chan YS, Lien LC, Hsu HL, et al: Evaluating hip labral tears using magnetic resonance arthrography: a prospective study comparing hip arthroscopy and magnetic resonance arthrography diagnosis. Arthroscopy 21:1250e1–1250e8, 2005.

55. Toomayan G, Holman WR, Major NM, et al: Sensitivity of MR arthrography in the evaluation of acetabular labral tears. AJR Am J Roentgenol 186:449–453, 2006.

56. Hodler J, Yu J, Goodwin D, et al: MR arthrography of the hip: improved imaging of the acetabular labrum with histologic correlation in cadavers. AJR Am J Roentgenol 165:887–891, 1995.

57. Steinbach LS, Palmer WE, Schweitzer ME: Special focus session: MR arthrography. Radiographics 22:1223–1246, 2002.

58. Mintz DN, Hooper T, Connell D, et al: Magnetic resonance imaging of the hip: detection of labral and chondral abnormalities using noncontrast imaging. Arthroscopy 21:385–393, 2005.

59. Freedman BA, Potter BK, Dinauer PA, et al: Prognostic value of magnetic resonance arthrography for Czerny stage II and III acetabular labral tears. Arthroscopy 22:742–747, 2006.

60. Blankenbaker DG, De Smet AA, Keene JS, Fine JP: Classification and localization of acetabular labral tears. Skeletal Radiol 36:391–397, 2007.

61. Dinauer PA, Murphy KP, Carroll JF: Sublabral sulcus at the posteroinferior acetabulum: a potential pitfall in MR arthrography diagnosis of acetabular labral tears. AJR Am J Roentgenol 183:1745–1753, 2004.

62. Petersilge CA, Haque MA, Petersilge WJ, et al: Acetabular labral tears: evaluation with MR arthrography. Radiology 200:231–235, 1996.

63. Keene GS, Villar RN: Arthroscopic anatomy of the hip: an in vivo study. Arthroscopy 10:392–399. 1994.

64. Schmid MR, Notzli HP, Zanetti M, et al: Cartilage lesions in the hip: diagnostic effectiveness of MR arthrography. Radiology 226:382–386, 2003.

65. Beaule PE, Zaragoza EJ, Copelan N: Magnetic resonance imaging with gadolinium arthrography to assess acetabular cartilage delamination: a report of four cases. J Bone Joint Surg Am 86:2294–2298, 2004.

66. Anderson LA, Peters CL, Park BB, et al: Acetabular cartilage delamination in femoroacetabular impingement: risk factors and magnetic resonance imaging diagnosis. J Bone Joint Surg Am 91:305–313, 2009.

67. Pfirrmann CW, Duc SR, Zanetti M, et al: MR arthrography of acetabular cartilage delamination in femoroacetabular cam impingement. Radiology 249:236–241, 2008.

68. Zaragoza EJ, Lattanzio PJ, Beaule PE: Magnetic resonance imaging with gadolinium arthrography to assess acetabular cartilage delamination. Hip Int 19:18–23, 2009.

69. Buckwalter JA, Mankin HJ, Grodzinsky AJ: Articular cartilage and osteoarthritis. Instr Course Lect 54:465–480, 2005.

70. Yamamoto Y, Tonotsuka H, Ueda T, Hamada Y: Usefulness of radial contrast-enhanced computed tomography for the diagnosis of acetabular labrum injury. Arthroscopy 23:1290–1294, 2007.

71. Nishii T, Tanaka H, Sugano N, et al: Disorders of acetabular labrum and articular cartilage in hip dysplasia: evaluation using isotropic high-resolutional CT arthrography with sequential radial reformation. Osteoarthritis Cartilage 15:251–257, 2007.

72. Steppacher SD, Tannast M, Werlen S, et al: Femoral morphology differs between deficient and excessive acetabular coverage. Clin Orthop Relat Res 466:782–790, 2009.

73. Voos JE, Ranawat AS, Pellici PM, et al: Varus rotational osteotomies for adults with hip dysplasia: a 20-year followup. Clin Orthop Relat Res 457:138–143, 2009.

74. Clohisy JC, St John LC, Schutz AL: Surgical treatment of femoroacetabular impingement: a systematic review of the literature. Clin Orthop Relat Res 468:555–564, 2010.

75. Philippon MJ, Stubbs AJ, Schenker ML, et al: Arthroscopic management of femoroacetabular impingement: osteoplasty technique and literature review. Am J Sports Med 35:1571–1580, 2007.

76. Heyworth BE, Shindle MK, Voos JE, et al: Radiologic and intraoperative findings in revision hip arthroscopy. Arthroscopy 23:1295–1302, 2007.

77. Kim KC, Hwang DS, Lee CH, Kwon ST: Influence of femoroacetabular impingement on results of hip arthroscopy in patients

with early osteoarthritis. Clin Orthop Relat Res 456:128–132, 2007.

78. Kassarjian A, Yoon LS, Belzile E, et al: Triad of MR arthrographic findings in patients with cam-type femoroacetabular impingement. Radiology 236:588–592, 2005.

79. Wenger DE, Kendall KR, Miner M, Trousdale RT: Acetabular labral tears rarely occur in the absence of bony abnormalities. Clin Orthop Relat Res 426:145–150, 2004.

80. Ganz R, Huff TW, Leunig M: Extended retinacular soft-tissue flap for intra-articular hip surgery: surgical technique, indications, and results of application. Instr Course Lect 58:241–255, 2009.

81. Espinosa N, Rothenfluh D, Beck M, Ganz R: Treatment of femoro-acetabular impingement: preliminary results of labral refixation. J Bone Joint Surg Am 88:925–935, 2006.

82. Ferguson SL, Bryant JT, Ganz R, Ito K: The acetabular labrum seal: a poroelastic finite element model. Clin Biomech 15:463–468, 2000.

83. Ferguson SJ, Bryant JT, Ganz R, Ito K: The influence of the acetabular labrum on hip joint cartilage consolidation: a poroelastic finite element model. J Biomech 33:953–960, 2000.

84. Ito K, Leunig M, Ganz R: Histopathologic features of the acetabular labrum in femoroacetabular impingement. Clin Orthop Relat Res 429:262–271, 2004.

FURTHER READING

Cashin M, Uhthoff HK, O'Neill M, Beaule PE: Embryology of the acetabular-labral complex. J Bone Joint Surg Br 90:1019–1024, 2004.
Most recent work on the histomorphology of the acetabular labrum.

Ferguson SJ, Ganz R, Ganz R, Ito K: An in vitro investigation of the acetabular labral seal in hip joint mechanics. J Biomech 36:171–178, 2003.
Key paper on the biomechanical function of the labrum.

Klaue K, Durnin CW, Ganz R: The acetabular rim syndrome: a clinical presentation of dysplasia. J Bone Joint Surg Br 73:423–429, 1991.
First paper to introduce the term acetabular rim syndrome *into the literature in conjunction with hip dysplasia.*

Leunig M, Beaule PE, Ganz R: The concept of femoroacetabular impingement: current status and future perspectives. Clin Orthop Relat Res 467:616–622, 2009.
Most recent summary of the evolution of the FAI concept and current status and future directions of this disease.

Leunig M, Siebenrock KA, Ganz R: Rationale of periacetabular osteotomy and background work. J Bone Joint Surg Am 83:438–448, 2001.
Paper describing the pathomechanics of hip dysplasia including surgical treatment options focused on the acetabular side.

CHAPTER 38

Hip Joint Infection

James Keeney

KEY POINTS

- Septic arthritis of the hip, if untreated, can lead to significant joint destruction and disability, or systemic illness.
- Early diagnosis and treatment are important toward optimizing outcomes.
- Clinical history, physical examination, and joint aspiration identify most cases.
- Advanced imaging techniques (magnetic resonance imaging [MRI], nuclear medicine) may assist in the assessment of early or subclinical infection.
- Multiple surgical options, including arthroscopy, arthrotomy, arthroplasty and arthrodesis, may be beneficial in treatment.

INTRODUCTION

Septic arthritis is an uncommon, clinically significant condition that can rapidly produce hip joint destruction and physical impairment. If unrecognized or untreated, a septic joint can result in significant localized consequences, including chondrolysis, osteomyelitis, osteonecrosis, and leg length discrepancy[1] (Fig. 38-1). Severe systemic complications, including sepsis and death, may occur and have been noted with increased frequency in association with advanced age.[2] Early diagnosis and initiation of surgical intervention remain essential components of successful treatment. Although septic arthritis occurs most commonly in children or in adults with prosthetic joint replacements, it remains a significant diagnostic consideration in evaluating other adult patients presenting with hip pain.

EPIDEMIOLOGY AND RISK FACTORS

Epidemiology

The most common pathway for entry of infection into the nonreplaced adult hip joint is a hematogenous source.[3] Bacteria from the urinary tract, lungs, skin, or other distant sites have been postulated to enter the hip joint through inflamed or diseased synovial tissue. Although antegrade flow through the arterial system most likely contributes to most cases, the proximity of the hip to Batson's plexus provides the potential for retrograde venous introduction of bacteria from pelvic floor organs.

Direct introduction of bacteria into the hip joint can also occur through a variety of diagnostic and therapeutic procedures.[4] Although inoculation has historically contributed to a small percentage of cases, increasing use of arthrocentesis, arthroscopy, and open surgical approaches in the treatment of nonarthritic and prearthritic hip conditions may result in a higher future incidence of infection associated with these diagnostic and therapeutic interventions.

Regional extension of infection from the lumbar spine, genitourinary structures, and lower gastrointestinal tract can also cause hip joint infection. This may occur by direct communication or by extension of infection along the iliopsoas tendon.[5-8]

Risk Factors

Conditions that result in increased venous or arterial perfusion, capillary permeability, or synovial tissue inflammation elevate the potential for bacteria to enter into the hip (Box 38-1). Impaired immune system surveillance, caused by host factors, disease, or pharmacologic immunosuppression, further contributes to an individual's susceptibility for joint sepsis (Box 38-2).

Microbiology

The most common infecting organisms are similar to those encountered with other musculoskeletal infections. *Staphylococcus aureus* is the most frequently reported organism resulting in hip infection, accounting for between 30% and 60% of cases.[2,9-11] Group A streptococcal bacteria are the second most commonly identified, and an increasing number of infections have been reported with a variety of gram-negative and anaerobic organisms (Box 38-3). Recent trends indicate an zincreasing incidence of community-acquired methicillin-resistant strains of *S. aureus* (MRSA) in Western cultures.[5] Among patients with osteonecrosis or sickle cell disease, salmonella has been reported as an organism with a predisposition for the hip at a higher incidence than nonsalmonella infection, and it may be associated with a chronic carrier state within the necrotic bone in susceptible individuals.[12]

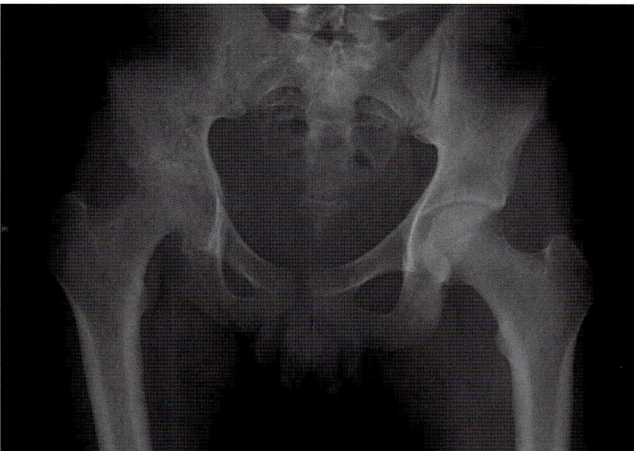

Figure 38-1. Loss of right hip cartilage and bone after septic hip.

BOX 38-1.   CONDITIONS PREDISPOSING TO JOINT INFECTION

Osteoarthritis
Post-traumatic arthritis
Inflammatory arthropathy
- Rheumatoid arthritis
- Spondyloarthropathy
- Crystalline arthropathy
Periarticular trauma
Osteonecrosis
Sickle cell disease
Charcot arthropathy
Hemophilia

BOX 38-2.   CONDITIONS THAT DIMINISH HOST RESPONSE TO INFECTION

Diabetes mellitus
Systemic lupus erythematosus
Connective tissue disease
Chronic alcoholism
Cirrhosis
Renal failure
Malignancy
Human immunodeficiency virus (HIV)
Radiation therapy
Immunosuppression
- Organ transplant
- Inflammatory arthropathy
Malnutrition
Advanced age

PATHOPHYSIOLOGY

Synovial tissue is highly vascularized and permeable. Synovial fluid, synthesized by cells within the synovial membrane, contributes to the nutrition of articular cartilage by active diffusion through the surface cartilage layers during physiologic joint loading.

BOX 38-3.   COMMON AND UNCOMMON HIP PATHOGENS

Gram-Positive Cocci (Common)
Staphylococcus aureus (MSSA/MRSA)
Staphylococcus epidermidis (coagulase-negative)
Streptococcus
- Group A
- Group B
- *Pneumococcus*
- *Enterococcus*

Gram-Negative Bacilli (Intermediate)
Escherichia coli
Klebsiella
Proteus
Enterobacter
Pseudomonas
Salmonella
Neisseria

Other Bacteria (Rare)
Brucella
Anaerobic bacteria

Mycobacteria (Rare)
M. tuberculosis, M. marinum, M. kansasii

Fungi (Rare)
Blastomycosis, coccidiomycosis, cryptococcosis, candidiasis, histoplasmosis, sporotrichosis

MRSA, Methicillin-resistant *Staphylococcus aureus;* *MSSA,* methicillin-susceptible *Staphylococcus aureus.*

Pyogenic Infection

Inflammation of the joint lining from local or systemic disease processes allows bacteria to enter the synovium and to enter the joint along with synovial fluid. After entry into the joint, bacterial growth occurs, inciting a localized inflammatory response and systemic activation of the host immune system. In pyogenic infection, immune complexes are formed, inflammatory mediators are secreted, and proteolytic enzymes are released into the joint, exerting nonselective actions that result in the degradation of articular cartilage. With prolonged exposure, articular cartilage loss can expose subchondral bone interfaces, which can be further weakened by direct effects of enzymatic activity and by inhibitory effects of limited weight bearing on maintenance of bone strength. Intra-articular pressure from an expanding joint effusion can potentially affect the vascular supply to the femoral head and, in rare cases, can produce osteonecrosis. Increased intra-articular pressure, when combined with erosive effects of intrasynovial inflammatory enzymes, can cause capsular disruption and can contribute to the formation of soft tissue abscesses, sinus tract formation, and hip joint subluxation or dislocation (Fig. 38-2).

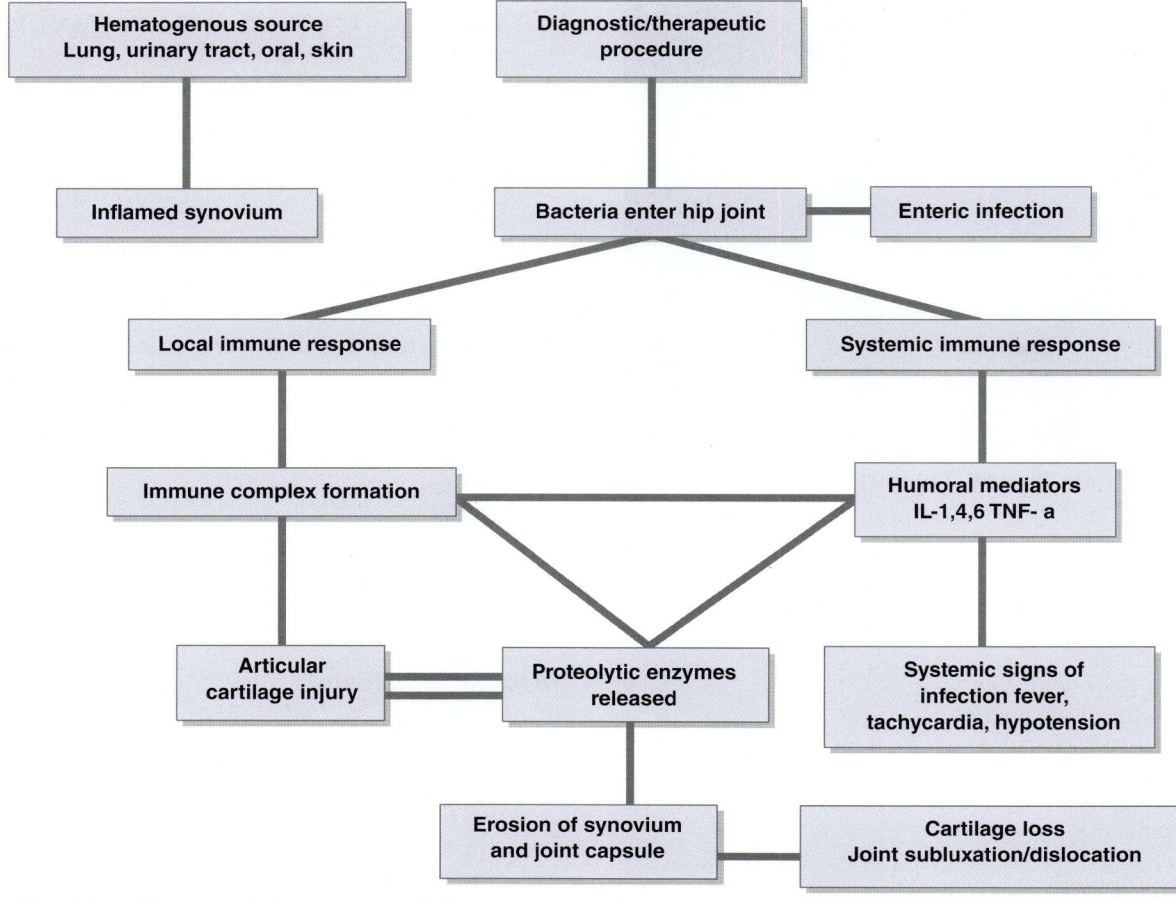

Figure 38-2. Flow diagram of the pathophysiology of septic joints.

Granulomatous Infection

Atypical bacteria and fungal organisms incite a T-cell–mediated granulomatous reaction in the synovium. The synovium thickens, producing fluid and an enlarging granuloma without the proteolytic enzymes that aggressively degrade articular cartilage in a pyogenic infection. Cartilage erosion results from direct effects of the granuloma at the periphery of the joint and extending throughout the joint and between the cartilage and bone. Soft tissue abscesses and sinus tracts may form, although these typically appear with a less aggressive time course.

CLNICAL FEATURES AND DIAGNOSIS

Patients with a septic joint may present with a variable combination of clinical features. Although each characteristic may independently suggest the presence of a septic joint, it is the combination of patient history with clinical examination and diagnostic testing that is most useful in establishing a diagnosis.

- *Pain:* Most patients will complain of pain in the region of their hip joint. Patterns for referred pain of the hip result in patients noting predominantly groin pain, pain radiating down the anterior thigh to the knee, or buttock pain. Pain may be present at rest, but typically will increase with joint movement and potentially with weight bearing. In the presence of an effusion, the hip will be most comfortable in a position of slight flexion, abduction, and external rotation, which places the capsular ligaments in a more relaxed posture. Host factors including pain perception, immune system health and response to infection, and specific organism characteristics may influence the time course and severity of pain reported by an individual patient. An insidious time course may occur with gram negative bacterial, atypical bacterial, or fungal infection; an immunocompromised state; neuropathy; or extension of infection from an anatomically contiguous site.
- *Fever:* Most patients without immune system impairment will develop a fever in response to infection. Although the presence of fever can be helpful in drawing attention to the potential for infection, its absence does not exclude the possibility of a septic joint.
- *Sepsis:* In severe, neglected, or advanced stages of infection, patients may present obtunded or in a state of hemodynamic collapse. Patients in septic shock require urgent intervention and a multidisciplinary approach to care.

Physical Examination

A systematic approach to physical examination is centrally important in patient assessment.

General physical appearance and vital signs recorded may suggest the presence of infection. Patients with significant synovial inflammation usually will be less willing to move the involved joint, and may appear fatigued or in a general state of discomfort or physical distress. Elevated temperature should raise suspicion for infection in a patient presenting with hip pain, although patients may be afebrile. Increased heart rate and decreased blood pressure may also be present, although it should be recognized that individual health status and the effects of medications may influence baseline heart rate and blood pressure, and physiologic response to infection.

Focused examination of the hip and adjacent joints including the lower back, sacroiliac joints, and the knee should be performed to identify the affected region and to differentiate between intra-articular and extra-articular sources of pain.

In the presence of a significant effusion or infection, the patient may place his/her hip in a position of flexion, abduction, and external rotation. Although range of motion of the hip is often limited and painful at extremes of flexion or extension for patients with noninfectious synovial inflammation, pain reproduced during passive range of motion through the midrange of hip motion should raise suspicion for the presence of infection. Pain with axial loading may be present, but is not independently specific for infection.

Radiographic Assessment

- *Plain radiographs:* An anteroposterior (AP) view of the pelvis, as well as AP and lateral projections of the affected hip, should be performed. Initial radiographs may demonstrate no visible abnormalities. As the intra-articular process progresses, radiographs may demonstrate joint space widening, erosive bony changes, and subluxation or dislocation of the hip. Because many patients with septic joints have preexisting hip disease, osteoarthritis or femoral head osteonecrosis will frequently be present and should not be presumed to exclude the diagnosis of septic hip.
- *Serology:* Systemic laboratory analysis is typically performed to assess the patient's health before undergoing surgical intervention. Inflammatory markers are typically elevated, but are not specific to the diagnosis of infection. The erythrocyte sedimentation rate (ESR) is elevated in a significant majority of patients. The C-reactive protein level (CRP) is frequently elevated and corrects more rapidly than the ESR with successful treatment. Peripheral blood cultures may be taken for patients to assist in identification of a causative organism.
- *Ancillary radiographic studies:* Advanced techniques may be helpful in the detection of infection early in the inflammatory process, although the relative cost of each study and the potential for establishing a diagnosis should be considered.

- *Ultrasonography* is a relatively inexpensive study that can demonstrate the presence of hip joint fluid and may be used successfully to direct a needle for arthrocentesis of the joint.
- *Computed tomography* (CT) scans are readily available in most hospital facilities. In the absence of erosive changes to surrounding bone, many of the signs of early septic involvement may not be readily visible. Soft tissue swelling adjacent to the hip joint or extending along the psoas tendon and psoas muscle may be an early visible sign and may help to identify an underlying source of infection. CT may also be used to guide needle aspiration of the hip joint.
- *Magnetic resonance imaging* (MRI) can be useful in identifying soft tissue inflammation around the hip joint, as well as intra-articular fluid. MRI is effective in differentiating joint, bone, and soft tissue involvement with enhanced sensitivity and specificity (Fig. 38-3). MRI can be useful in early identification of traumatic and nontraumatically acquired conditions affecting the hip, and may also be useful in cases of suspected infection, when a positive aspiration cannot be obtained.
- *Aspiration:* Joint aspiration is the primary means of confirming the presence of intra-articular infection. Aspiration should be performed with the assistance of imaging (fluoroscopy, ultrasound, CT) to confirm successful needle placement. Fluid from the hip should be assessed for cell count, cell differential, crystals, gram stain, and culture. Cell counts for non-inflammatory fluid are typically fewer than 2000 white blood cells (WBCs)/mL, cell counts between 2000 and 20,000 WBCs/mL usually indicate an inflammatory arthropathy, and cell counts greater than 50,000 WBCs/mL should be approached with suspicion of a septic joint. Cell counts between 20,000 and 100,000 WBCs/mL may be present with an inflammatory or an infectious arthropathy, so the complete clinical picture should be considered in conjunction with the synovial fluid count. Assessing the differential of white blood cells within the synovial fluid may be

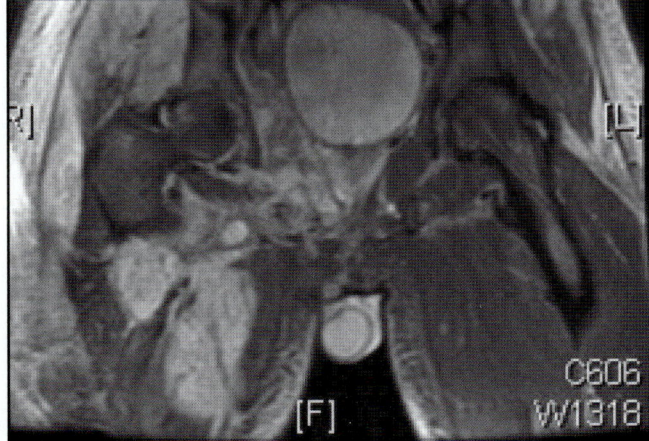

Figure 38-3. Magnetic resonance imaging (MRI) demonstrating soft tissue edema in soft tissues adjacent to infected hip and small fluid collection in hip joint.

helpful. A preponderance of neutrophils (≥60%) would be more suggestive of an acute infectious process, and a predominance of lymphocytes and macrophages would be more typical of a chronic inflammatory process. Gram stain and culture results should be utilized together to assist in identification of a specific infecting organism.

Initial cultures for most common aerobic and anaerobic organisms from purulent joint fluid may be acceptable. For individuals with delayed clinical presentation, an immunosuppressed condition, or history of travel or potential exposure to atypical infections, consideration should be given to assess for mycobacterial and fungal organisms.

DIFFERENTIAL DIAGNOSIS

The differential diagnosis for patients presenting with hip joint pain includes a wide variety of intra-articular and extra-articular processes (Box 38-4).

Because preexisting disease can contribute to the development of septic arthritis, it is important to differentiate the possibility of infection from the underlying clinical condition.

TREATMENT

Treatment of the septic hip should be undertaken to minimize the effects of proteolytic enzymes on hip cartilage. The patient's overall health should be considered, and medical interventions that can be safely performed to optimize the patient for surgery may be considered before anesthetic induction.

Surgical Drainage

A variety of procedural techniques have been advocated in the treatment of articular sepsis. Serial aspiration has been performed for patients with joint sepsis, although most orthopedic surgeons have preferred surgical intervention.[13,14] Surgical drainage of the hip has most commonly been an open procedure that facilitates drainage and synovial tissue sampling for biopsy and

culture. Although serial aspiration has been performed for other joints, it has been discouraged for use in the hip because of difficulty in confirming successful needle placement without radiographic support.[15] Open surgical drainage has been performed most commonly, although arthroscopic management is more frequent with increasing surgeon familiarity with arthroscopic portal placement and techniques. Arthroscopic lavage has become common for the treatment of septic knee, and increasing familiarity with hip arthroscopy will likely result in more widespread use of this approach over the next decade.[16,17] Resection of necrotic bone may still be considered for advanced states of infection, and may be considered as the first of a two-stage hip reconstruction procedure for individuals with advanced cartilage loss who may be candidates for hip replacement surgery after treatment.[18]

Antibiotic Therapy

Antibiotic treatment remains vitally important in the treatment of infection. Consultation with infectious disease staff should be strongly considered, particularly when bacteria with a significant antibiotic resistance pattern are identified. If the infecting organism has not been established before operative intervention, broad-spectrum antibiotics should be initiated to cover both gram-positive and gram-negative organisms. This is particularly the case among patients with immunocompromised states, among whom gram-negative and polymicrobial infections are more likely. A first-generation cephalosporin is usually the most appropriate initial antibiotic therapy for most gram-positive infections, although consideration should be given to local resistance patterns. Consideration should be given to the prevalence of community-acquired MRSA infections, as this may influence the choice of initial gram-positive coverage until definitive cultures have been obtained. Patients typically are discharged to home with successful completion of antibiotic therapy delivered by the individual or by a home health care provider.[19]

PROGNOSIS

Prognosis for successful treatment of hip sepsis is directly correlated with patient age, host immune status, duration of symptoms before presentation, and timely initiation of surgical treatment and antibiotic therapy.[2,20]

Gavet and associates reported a significant increase in mortality rate among patients with septic arthritis, increasing with age. Patients younger than 60 years had a 0.7% mortality rate. The rate increased to 4.8% for patients between 60 and 79 years of age, and to 9.5% for patients older than 80 years. The increase in mortality was positively correlated with a longer average time from symptom onset to diagnosis.[2]

Huang and colleagues noted a 10% mortality rate among 30 patients with systemic lupus erythematosus (SLE) who developed a septic joint. The mortality rate among patients with a septic hip joint was 6.5%.[12]

BOX 38-4. DIFFERENTIAL DIAGNOSIS FOR HIP PAIN

Osteoarthritis
Inflammatory arthropathies
Crystalline arthropathy
Osteonecrosis
Occult fracture
Stress/insufficiency fracture
Referred pain
- Lumbar radiculopathy
- Extra-articular tendinopathy
- Knee arthropathy

CURRENT CONTROVERSIES AND FUTURE CONSIDERATIONS

Differences in treatment approach in the management of a septic hip joint may persist among surgical and nonsurgical physicians. Concern among surgical specialists has focused on the importance of timely and maximal removal of bacterial and proteolytic enzymes from the joint. Recent pediatric orthopedic literature has suggested that serial aspirations may be effective in this patient group and may allow surgery to be avoided, but this approach has not been adequately established in an adult patient population; therefore this position cannot be advocated broadly.[21]

Although the primary concern in the treatment of septic hip is acute management of infection, the future need for reconstructive surgery may be a reasonable consideration. Because a septic hip joint frequently occurs in the setting of preexisting disease, staged joint replacement may be an option to consider during surgical management. Chen and coworkers reported on a series of 28 patients with septic hip who were managed with a two-stage revision protocol.[18] Although they noted a high rate of satisfaction among patients with successful reconstruction, reinfection occurred in 4 patients (14%). Further study will be beneficial in determining the value of this treatment approach in comparison with delayed reconstruction for individuals who remain symptomatic after successful treatment of infection before conversion to arthroplasty.[18,22]

REFERENCES

1. Ryan MJ, Kavanaugh R, Wall PG, Hazleman BL: Bacterial joint infections in England and Wales: analysis of bacterial isolates over a four year period. Br J Rheumatol 36:370–373, 1997.
2. Gavet F, Tournadre A, Soubrier M, et al: Septic arthritis in patients aged 80 and older: a comparison with younger adults. J Am Geriatr Soc 53:1210–1213, 2005.
3. Yeargan PJ, Kane TJ, Richardson AB: Hematogenous septic arthritis of the adult hip. Orthopedics 26:771–776, 2003.
4. Morshed S, Huffman GR, Ries MD: Septic arthritis of the hip and intrapelvic abscess following intra-articular injection of Hylan G-F 20: a case report. J Bone Joint Surg Am 86:823–826, 2004.
5. Ash N, Salai M, Aphter S, Olchovsky D: Primary psoas abscess due to methicillin-resistant *Staphylococcus aureus* concurrent with septic arthritis of the hip joint. South Med J 88:863–865, 1995.
6. Compain C, Michou L, Orcel P, et al: Septic arthritis of the hip with psoas abscess caused by non-typhi *Salmonella* infection in an immunocompetent patient. Joint Bone Spine 75:67–69, 2008.
7. Kumagai K, Ushiyama T, Kawasaki T, Matsusue Y: Extension of lumbar spine infection into osteoarthritic hip through psoas abscess. J Orthop Sci 10:91–94, 2005.
8. Yang SH, Yang RS, Tsai CL: Septic arthritis of the hip joint in cervical cancer patients after radiotherapy: three case reports. J Orthop Surg (Hong Kong) 9:41–45, 2001.
9. Al-Nammari SS, Bobak P, Venkatesh R: Methicillin resistant *Staphylococcus aureus* versus methicillin sensitive *Staphylococcus aureus* adult haematogenous septic arthritis. Arch Orthop Trauma Surg 127:537–542, 2007.
10. Arnold SR, Elias D, Buckingham SC, et al: Changing patterns of acute hematogenous osteomyelitis and septic arthritis: emergence of community-associated methicillin-resistant *Staphylococcus aureus*. J Pediatr Orthop 26:703–708, 2006.
11. Matthews PC, Dean BJ, Medagoda K, et al: Native hip joint septic arthritis in 20 adults: delayed presentation beyond three weeks predicts need for excision arthroplasty. J Infect 57:185–190, 2008.
12. Huang JL, Hung JJ, Wu KC, et al: Septic arthritis in patients with systemic lupus erythematosus: salmonella and nonsalmonella infections compared. Semin Arthritis Rheum 36:61–67, 2006.
13. Cleeman E, Auerbach JD, Klingenstein GG, Flatow EL: Septic arthritis of the glenohumeral joint: a review of 23 cases. J Surg Orthop Adv 14:102–107, 2005.
14. Donatto KC: Orthopedic management of septic arthritis. Rheum Dis Clin N Am 24:275–286, 1998.
15. Broy SB, Schmid FR: A comparison of medical drainage (needle aspiration) and surgical drainage (arthrotomy or arthroscopy) in the initial treatment of infected joints. Clin Rheum Dis 12:501–522, 1986.
16. Blizer CM: Arthroscopic management of septic arthritis of the hip. Arthroscopy 9:414–416, 1993.
17. Nusem I, Jabur MK, Playford EG: Arthroscopic treatment of septic arthritis of the hip. Arthroscopy 22:1–3, 2006.
18. Chen C, Want J, Juhn R: Total hip arthroplasty for primary septic arthritis of the hip in adults. Intern Orthop 32:573–580, 2008.
19. Matthews PC, Conlon CP, Berendt AR, et al: Outpatient parenteral antimicrobial therapy (OPAT): is it safe for selected patients to self-administer at home? A retrospective analysis of a large cohort over 13 years. J Antimicrob Chemother 60:356–362, 2007.
20. Wang CL, Wang SM, Yang YJ, et al: Septic arthritis in children: relationship of causative pathogens, complications and outcome. J Microbiol Immunol Infect 36:41–46, 2003.
21. Givon U, Liberman B, Schindler A, et al: Treatment of septic arthritis of the hip joint by repeated ultrasound-guided aspirations. J Pediatr Orthop 24:266–270, 2004.
22. Lustig S, Vaz G, Guyen O, et al: Total hip arthroplasty after hip arthrodesis performed for septic arthritis. Rev Chir Orthop Reparatrice Appar Mot 93:828–835, 2007.

SUGGESTED READING

Mathews CJ, Coakley G: Septic arthritis: current diagnostic and therapeutic algorithm. Curr Opin Rheumatol 20:457–462, 2008.
Palombarani S, Gardella N, Tuduri A, et al: Community-acquired methicillin-resistant *Staphylococcus aureus* infections in a hospital for acute diseases. Rev Argent Microbiol 39:151–155, 2007.
Zalavras CG, Dellamaggiora R, Patzakis MJ, et al: Septic arthritis in patients with human immunodeficiency virus. Clin Orthop Relat Res 451:46–49, 2006.
Zalavras CG, Rigopoulos N, Lee J, et al: Magnetic resonance imaging findings in hematogenous osteomyelitis of the hip in adults. Clin Orthop Relat Res 467:1688–1692, 2009.

CHAPTER 39

Soft Tissue Pathology: Bursal, Tendon, and Muscle Diseases

Heidi Prather, Devyani Hunt, and Adam Zierenberg

KEY POINTS

- Extra-articular hip disorders coexist with intra-articular hip disorders.
- Biomechanics of the pelvic girdle and its relationship to the hip and spine are complex.
- Some extra-articular hip disorders are diagnosed best by clinical presentation and exclusion of other diagnoses. The distribution of pain and pertinent findings on clinical examination are typically essential in finding the source of pain and dysfunction.
- It is important to differentiate specific pathophysiology by acuity and specific anatomic and biomechanical faults. This knowledge is essential for optimal treatment planning.

INTRODUCTION

Extra-articular hip pain originating from the pelvic girdle has many sources. Extra-articular disorders may be the primary source of hip pain in some cases; others are the result of adaptations or guarding mechanisms for intra-articular hip disorders. Recognizing and differentiating the two can be difficult. Nevertheless, we will attempt to describe extra-articular sources of hip pain by their region of distribution at clinical presentation. These regions include the anterior pelvis and groin, the lateral hip and thigh, and the posterior pelvis (Fig. 39-1).

EPIDEMIOLOGY AND RISK FACTORS

Hip pain occurs in any age group but is most prevalent between the ages of 40 and 60.[1] The prevalence of extra-articular pain differentiated from intra-articular pain is unknown, and it is likely that the two types commonly coexist. The most common site of soft tissue pathology in the hip region is found laterally over the greater trochanter. Reports indicate that the prevalence of greater trochanteric pain in adults ranges between 20% and 35%.[6-8] Posterior pelvic pain related to the sacroiliac joint (SIJ) ranges in prevalence between 13% and 62%.[9-13] Many reported variations in SIJ prevalence are related to the method of confirming the diagnosis by history

and physical examination alone or by image-guided intra-articular injection. Risk factors associated with extra-articular hip pain are many and variable. They include age, female gender, other lower extremity injuries or osteoarthritis, low back pain, previous lumbar spine surgery, and cumulative injury. Chou and colleagues reported that of patients who responded to intra-articular SIJ injection, 44% had a history of trauma and 21% had cumulative trauma. Although the specific mechanisms of cumulative trauma have not been studied, others have described these to include activities that require torsion, repetitive rotation, or single-leg stance.[14,15] Acute trauma with loading or a blow to the pelvic girdle is an obvious risk factor for the development of extra-articular hip pain and can be difficult to diagnose in the setting of normal diagnostic imaging.

PATHOPHYSIOLOGY

The pathophysiology of extra-articular hip pain is twofold. Some disorders occur as the result of acute overload or trauma. Others may be more insidious in onset and may be related to multiple factors, including guarding, biomechanical failure related to repetitive overuse or overload, biology, and adaptations to underlying articular disorders. The biomechanics about the pelvic girdle is complex, not only because of multidirectional loading and transmission of forces across the pelvic girdle, but also because of the load and transmission of forces through the spine and hip. Extra-articular soft tissue structures function to help reduce load at any one particular joint. Specifically, the pubic symphysis, the L5-S1 three-joint complex (disk and facet joints), the hip, and the sacroiliac joint must share and transfer load as efficiently as possible to decrease the presence of abnormal forces across any or all of these joints and associated soft tissue structures. Any bony disorder such as deformity, fracture, or cartilage injury can then overload the extra-articular structure, causing dysfunction and pain. The large body of work by researchers such as Vleeming, Snijders, and DonTigny has brought to light the complex biomechanics of the lumbar spine and pelvic girdle and the complexity of biomechanical dysfunction. Researchers have tied their findings to clinical implications.[16-25]

Figures 39-2 through 39-4 demonstrate the roles of muscles and ligaments when accepting an asymmetrical

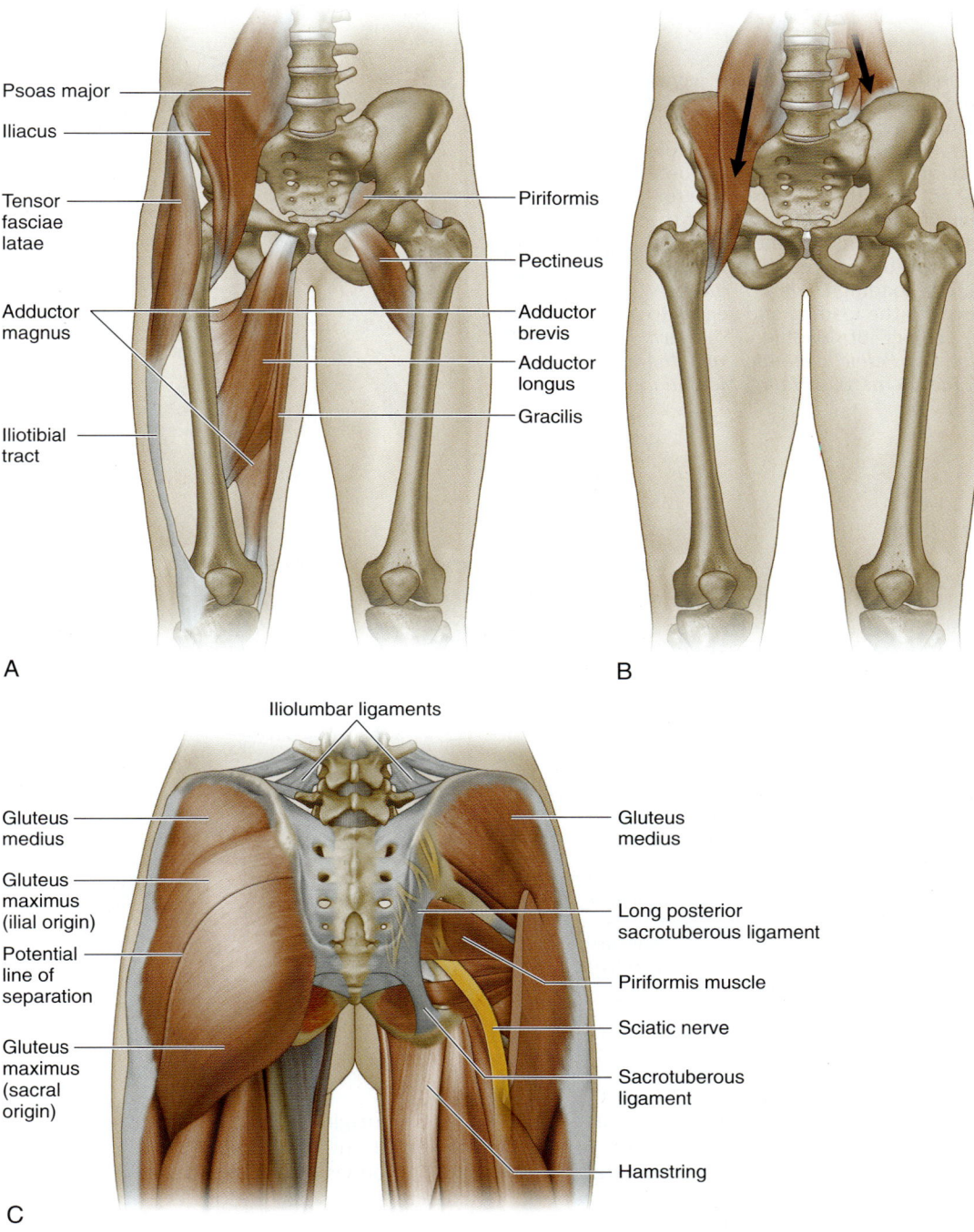

Figure 39-1. A, Muscles and tendons involved in pelvic, groin, and anterior pelvic pain. **B,** Orientation of activation of iliopsoas in relationship to the spine and the hip. *(Redrawn from DeRosa C: Functional anatomy of the lumbar spine and sacroiliac joint. Paper presented at 4th Interdisciplinary World Congress on Low Back and Pelvic Pain, Montreal, Canada, November 2001.)* **C,** Muscles, tendons, and ligaments associated with posterior pelvic girdle pain.

load across the pelvic girdle. A dysfunction in any one of the moving parts may result in secondary adaptations and potentially in painful syndromes. These are just a few examples that reinforce the importance of understanding the complex underlying reasons for extra-articular hip disorders.

CLINICAL FEATURES AND DIAGNOSIS

A common dilemma for a hip specialist is determining whether a patient's pain and dysfunction are caused by an intra-articular or extra-articular source.

Asymmetric pelvis at two-point support
Oblique sacral movement

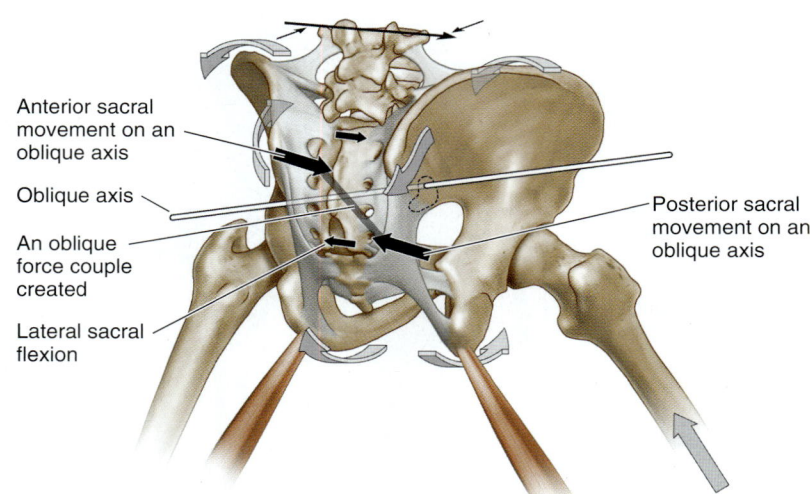

Figure 39-2. Oblique loading causing asymmetry in loading and movement. The longer the stride during the gait cycle, the greater is the asymmetry across the pelvic girdle causing an oblique force. An oblique force couple is created from the posterior interosseous ligament of the sacroiliac joint on the left to the sacrotuberous ligament on the right. The sacral rotation drives trunk rotation toward the side of loading *(here it is the right side);* this **precedes** the loading and serves to decrease the impact of loading. *(Redrawn from DonTigny RL: Pelvic dynamics and the subluxation of the sacral axis. Havre, Montana, CD-ROM, 2009.)*

Anterior sacral movement on an oblique axis

Oblique axis

An oblique force couple created

Lateral sacral flexion

Posterior sacral movement on an oblique axis

Muscle function on the asymmetric pelvis

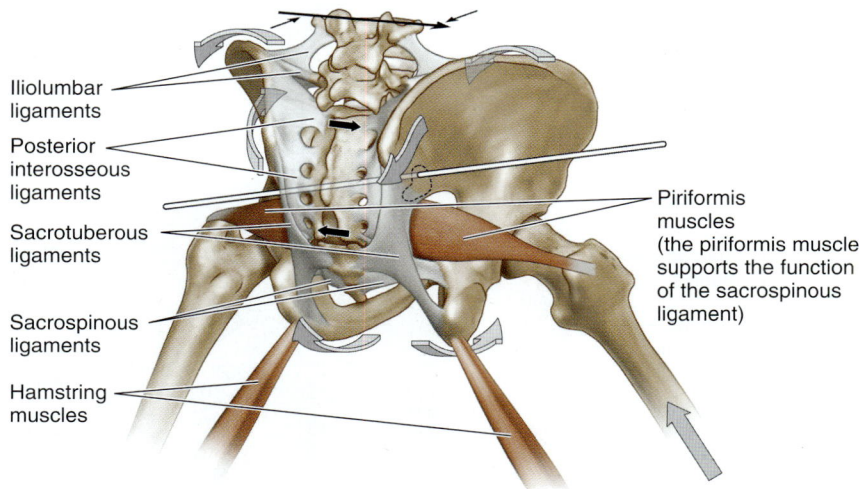

Figure 39-3. Function of the piriformis muscle The piriformis muscle functions to support and assist the sacrospinous ligament in restoring the sacrum to its resting position as the pelvis moves to a position of symmetry at midstep. *(Redrawn from DonTigny RL: Pelvic dynamics and the subluxation of the sacral axis. Havre, Montana, CD-ROM, 2009.)*

Iliolumbar ligaments

Posterior interosseous ligaments

Sacrotuberous ligaments

Sacrospinous ligaments

Hamstring muscles

Piriformis muscles (the piriformis muscle supports the function of the sacrospinous ligament)

The distribution of pain is a helpful place to start when formulating a differential diagnosis. Intra-articular hip pain is thought to cause anterior groin or lateral hip pain and occasionally posterior pelvic pain.[26-30] However, several soft tissue abnormalities may cause the same distribution of pain. The following is a brief description of the clinical features and diagnostic algorithms pertaining to soft tissue abnormalities of the hip (Fig. 39-5 through 39-7).

Extra-articular Anterior Hip Pain

Iliopsoas Muscle–Tendon Complex Disorders

The iliopsoas muscle–tendon complex consists of three muscles: the psoas major, the psoas minor, and the iliacus (Fig. 39-1A). The proximal fibers of the psoas

muscles originate on the bodies of the 12th thoracic vertebrae and the lumbar vertebrae; they then cross into the pelvis and join with the fibers of the iliacus to make the iliopsoas tendon. The fibers of the tendon hug the anterior aspect of the hip capsule, and the psoas portion rotates as it descends, so the ventral surface becomes the medial aspect. The conjoined tendons of the psoas and iliacus insert onto the lesser trochanter. The innervation of the psoas major is derived from the anterior nerves of the second and third lumbar roots. The psoas minor is innervated by the first lumbar nerve root, and the iliacus by the anterior branches of the second and third lumbar nerves through the anterior crural nerve. The iliopsoas not only functions as the prime mover of hip flexion, it also plays an essential role in the functional stability of the hip, the pelvis, and even the spine (Fig. 39-1B). Unilateral contraction of the iliopsoas muscle facilitates lateral flexion of the lumbar

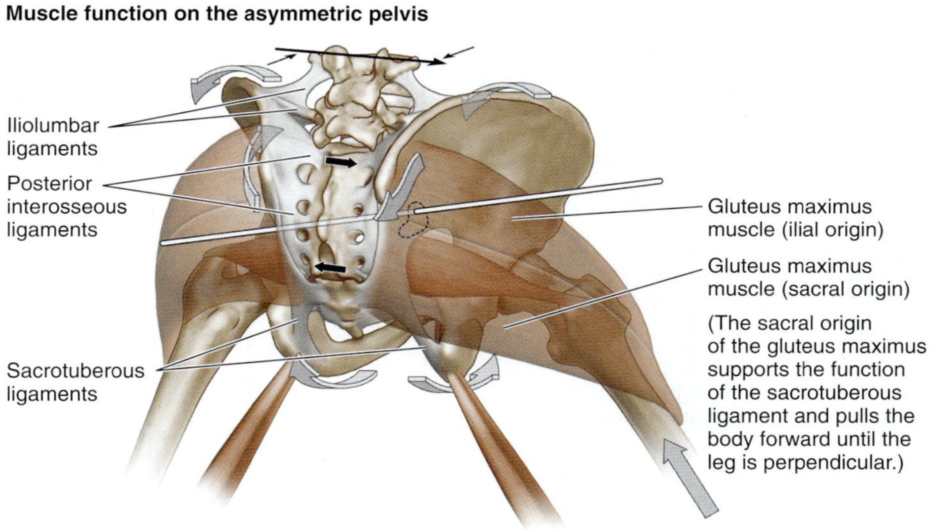

Muscle function on the asymmetric pelvis

Figure 39-4. Function of the gluteus maximus muscle. The sacral origin of the gluteus maximus serves to assist and support the function of the sacrotuberous ligament in bringing the distal sacrum anteriorly and laterally as the sacrum moves from lateral flexion to its resting position when the pelvis moves to symmetry at midstep. The sacral origin of the gluteus maximus and the piriformis must act as prime movers on the sacroiliac joint when the pelvis is asymmetrically loaded. The sacral origin of the gluteus maximus also functions to pull the pelvis anteriorly over the loaded side until the leg is perpendicular at midstep. The ilial origin of the gluteus maximus then undergoes an eccentric contraction to decrease loading forces on the contralateral side. *(Redrawn from DonTigny RL: Pelvic dynamics and the subluxation of the sacral axis. Havre, Montana, CD-ROM, 2009.)*

spine and external rotation of the hip. Dysfunction and injury to the complex can manifest as anterior hip pain and can cause compensatory biomechanical alterations in hip functioning and therefore secondary pain complaints. Owing to its close association with the spine, disorders of the iliopsoas are associated with low back pain.[31] Cumulative changes to the tendon can occur as the result of increased muscle firing related to guarding for a primary spine or hip dysfunction, or firing of the muscle in an inefficient manner, such as in a lengthened position that may occur secondary to a hip, pelvic girdle, or hip dysfunction. Any of these situations can lead to the development of bursitis in the acute setting and, later, to tendinosis. Iliopsoas muscle–tendon complex disorders are commonly seen in conjunction with an intra-articular hip problem. The pattern of a shortened, painful tendon can develop as the result of compensation for reduced hip internal rotation and extension, leading to pain with hip extension. This pattern is seen in patients with hip osteoarthritis or other intra-articular disorders. Acute injuries to the iliopsoas tendon, such as tears and avulsion injuries, may occur.[32,33] These injuries typically are associated with a traumatic event; however, repetitive overuse can predispose to this type of injury.

Patients with iliopsoas muscle tendon disorders present with anterior hip pain or groin pain that is worse with concentric or eccentric contraction of the hip flexor. Sports activities that require forceful hip flexion or adduction are painful, and even low-level activities such as walking or rising from a seated position can be painful.[32] Runners describe anterior groin pain when trying to lengthen their stride, during speed training, or with uphill running.[32,34]

Key features on examination include a tender tendon with palpation and pain with activation of the hip flexor. Hip range of motion (ROM) can also be painful owing to stretching of the tendon and most notably occurs with abduction and extension of the hip.[32] Special tests of the hip, including the flexion-abduction-external rotation (FABER) test, can be painful because of a relative stretch to the tendon that occurs in the position of testing. Caution should be taken in drawing conclusions from the examination because the presence of a painful tendon to palpation and pain with activation of the hip flexor does not rule out an intra-articular hip disorder. Secondary dysfunction of the hip flexor muscle–tendon complex commonly occurs as the result of an underlying intra-articular disorder. It is important to examine the hip in weight bearing during dynamic motion to further assess for abnormal motor patterns that contribute to repetitive overuse injuries. Matrix testing[35] in three planes of motion (frontal, sagittal, and transverse) has been found to be a reliable measure; it is not specific to the hip joint but gives a general assessment of side-to-side symmetry of motion.[30]

Snapping Hip Syndrome. Snapping hip syndrome is a complex of symptoms in which the key feature is an audible snap heard at or around the hip joint.[36] Three types of snapping hip have been identified: intra-articular, internal, and external. The most common type, external snapping hip, occurs when the gluteus maximus tendon or the iliotibial band snaps over the greater trochanter. The intra-articular type refers to an

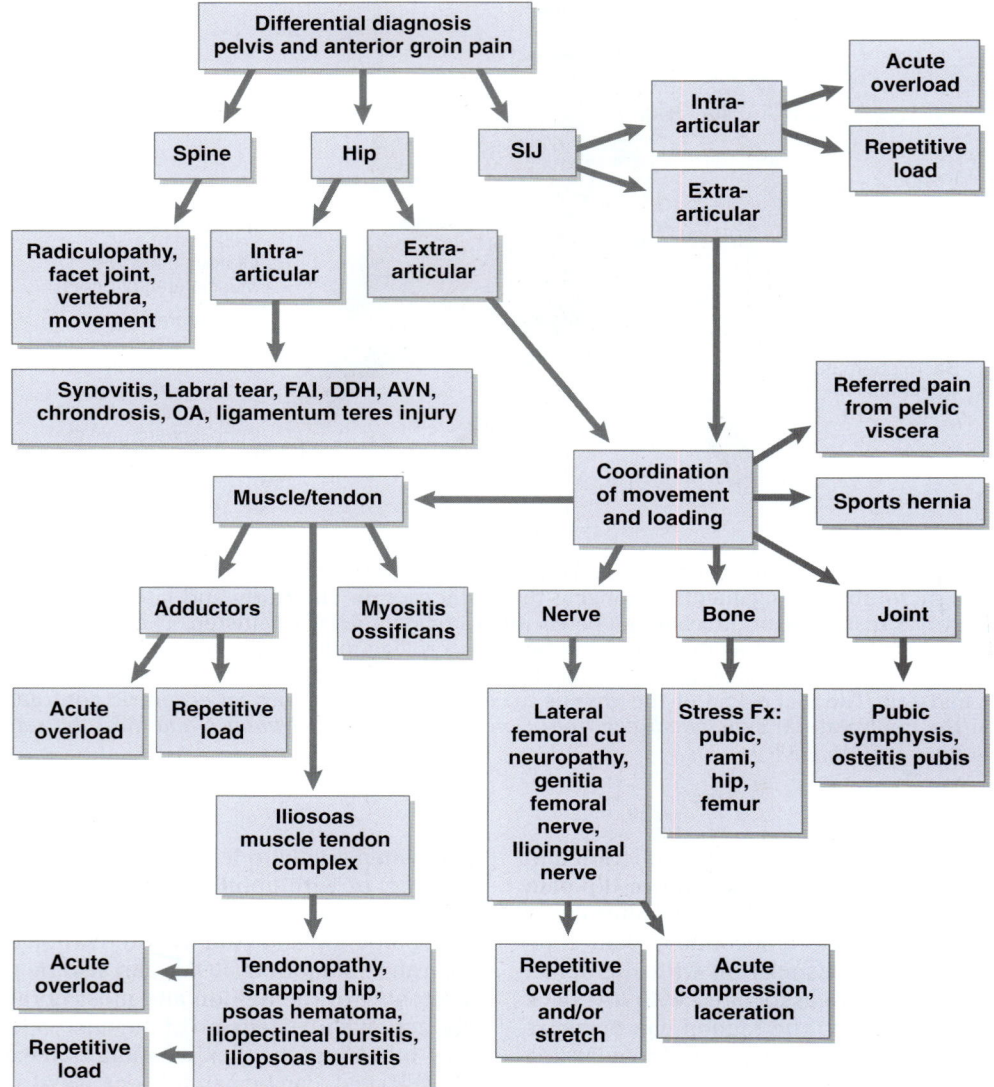

Figure 39-5. Differential diagnosis of pelvic and anterior groin pain.

abnormality of a structure inside the hip, which causes the "snapping" and typically is associated with pain. Causes include loose bodies, synovial osteochondromatosis, labral tears, cartilage flaps, osteochondral fractures, and transient hip subluxation.[34,36]

Internal snapping hip occurs when the iliopsoas tendon glides across the iliopectineal prominence, causing an audible snap.[37,38] It is usually painful, and the pop or snap occurs in the anterior aspect of the hip as the hip goes from flexion to extension. Snapping can also occur across the femoral head[39] or, less commonly, at the lesser trochanter.[32,36] The pathophysiology has been studied and numerous causes have been found, including an association with a thickened tendon.[34,40] More commonly, the tendon is structurally normal; however, it may not be at its optimal length. It is most likely a part of the continuum of chronic iliopsoas dysfunction. A shortened or lengthened tendon contributes to the development of iliopsoas tendinopathy and

snapping. It is important to assess for other soft tissue abnormalities or joint problems at the hip or spine when evaluating the iliopsoas tendon because they commonly occur together.

The clinical presentation of medial snapping hip is similar to those of iliopsoas muscle tendon disorders; however, the hallmark feature is a painful audible snap in the anterior aspect of the hip.[32,34] Painful hip ROM and pain with palpation of the iliopsoas muscle and tendon may not always occur. The painful snap can be reproduced by ranging the hip from the FABER position into extension, adduction, and internal rotation.[41]

Diagnostic Imaging. Diagnostic imaging for snapping hip pain does not always reveal objective indications for the source of pain and dysfunction in patients without hip deformity or degenerative changes. Radiographs may be normal. Ultrasound evaluation can provide good information regarding the integrity of the iliopsoas tendon and can be used to dynamically assess

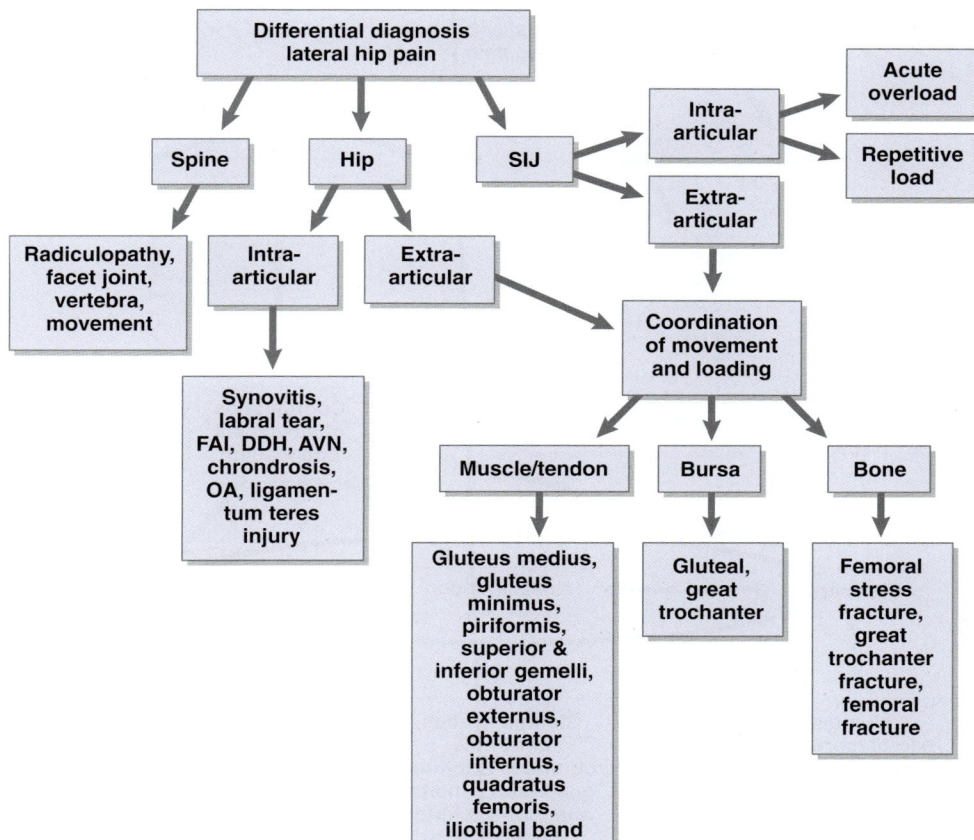

Figure 39-6. Differential diagnosis of lateral hip pain.

for a snapping tendon across the iliopectineal prominence.[42] MRI can be useful in evaluation of the muscle and tendon and to rule out an intra-articular abnormality.[42] Structural changes to the tendon are not always seen, and the diagnosis becomes one of exclusion with the clinician relying on the history and physical examination findings.

Diagnostic injections of anesthetic are useful when the diagnosis remains in question after imaging. The tendon or the bursa can be injected with anesthetic under image guidance (fluoroscopy or ultrasound).[42] A diagnostic intra-articular injection should also be considered if an intra-articular abnormality needs to be ruled out.

Specific Considerations for the Treatment of Iliopsoas Muscle–Tendon Complex Disorders. Initial treatment of iliopsoas muscle–tendon complex disorders consists of conservative measures. A period of rest can be very helpful to reduce acute pain. The rest period should be relative to the activity causing the dysfunction and should be variable in length as determined by evidence of reduction of symptoms and recovery. In chronic conditions that are associated with an abnormal pattern of movement, a relative rest period is necessary to break the cycle of pain. With acute injuries, a rest period is essential to allow the tendon to heal. A course of oral or topical anti-inflammatory medications is recommended.

Evidence suggests that physical therapy should be part of the initial treatment protocol.[39,43,44] Physical therapy should focus on the iliopsoas tendon with the goal of optimizing the length and strength of the muscle–tendon complex. The iliopsoas tendon typically is shortened or chronically "turned on" owing to a learned overuse pattern. It is important for physical therapy to address these abnormal movement patterns at the hip, pelvic girdle, and spine and to restore optimal functioning during everyday activities. Once this has been accomplished, advancing to higher-level activities, including sports-specific exercises, is essential for returning to full activity. Modalities such as ultrasound or iontophoresis can be used to decrease inflammation in the tendon or bursa.

If a 3-month period of conservative treatment fails, a lidocaine and corticosteroid steroid injection into the bursa should be considered for iliopsoas or iliopectineal bursitis. The literature also describes corticosteroid injection into the iliopsoas tendon sheath.[45] However, caution should be taken because tendon ruptures after steroid injections have been documented.[46,47] Injections should be performed under image guidance with fluoroscopy or ultrasound.[42,45]

Surgical Treatment for Painful Iliopsoas Muscle–Tendon Complex Disorders. Surgical release or lengthening of the iliopsoas tendon has been used successfully for recalcitrant cases of internal snapping hip. The

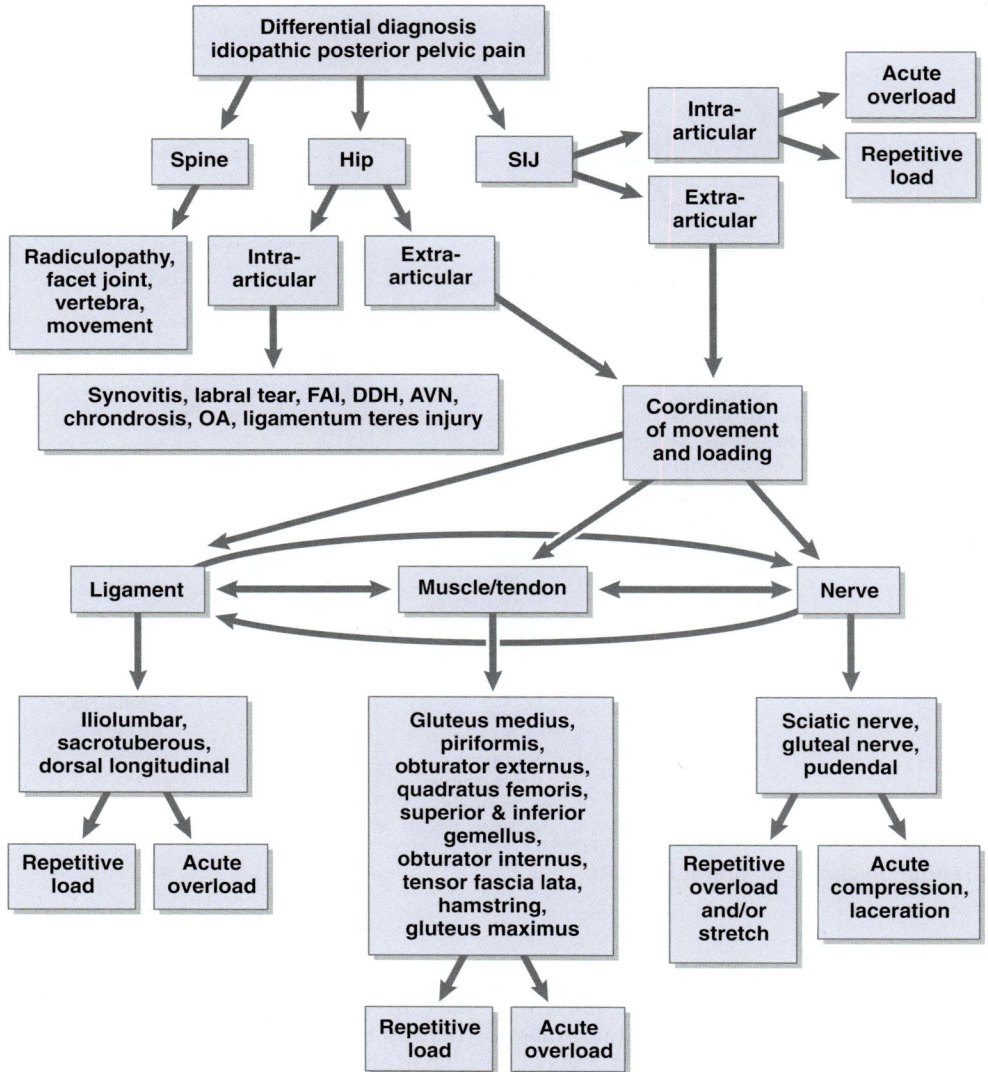

Figure 39-7. Differential diagnosis of idiopathic posterior pelvic pain.

response to a diagnostic injection of the tendon with lidocaine can predict the response to surgical release.[42]

Open procedures and arthroscopic approaches have been described.[39,48] No comparative data on open and endoscopic procedures are available. Arthroscopically, the tendon can be lengthened at the lesser trochanter, or the tendinous portion of the musculotendinous unit can be released using a transcapsular approach from the peripheral compartment. A study of 19 patients randomly assigned to either approach showed that both groups improved their Western Ontario and McMaster Universities Osteoarthritis Index (WOMAC) scores, and no difference in clinical improvement was noted between the groups.[49]

Postoperative management is patient specific with limitation of active hip flexion. Typically, no range-of-motion or weight-bearing restrictions are recommended. Patients have weak hip flexors postoperatively and require a program of graded strengthening. Return to full activity generally is allowed after 3 to 6 months.

Complications resulting from the operation include motor and sensory changes, swelling of the bursa, hematoma formation, heterotopic ossification, hip flexor weakness, and infection.[39,48,49]

Adductor Strains. The adductor muscle group consists of six muscles in the medial thigh and includes the adductor longus, adductor brevis, adductor magnus, gracilis, obturator externus, and pectineus. They originate at various points along the pubis and insert into the medial femur. The obturator nerve innervates this group of muscles, except for the pectineus, which is supplied by the femoral nerve. In the open chain, the primary function of this muscle group involves hip adduction. In the closed chain, along with lower abdominal muscles, the adductors stabilize the pelvis and the lower extremity during activity.[50] Individual muscles have secondary roles such as femoral flexion and rotation.[51,52] The adductor longus is the most commonly strained muscle owing to its poor mechanical advantage.[53]

Chronic muscle strains and associated pain have been attributed to myofascial trigger points (MTrPs). MTrPs are described as localized areas of tenderness and hyperirritability in a muscle tendon or ligament associated with a characteristic referral pattern.[58] Simons and associates[59] described the pain associated with MTrPs as stemming from hypersensitive taut bands of muscle, which may have sustained previous injury. Shah and colleagues[60] further demonstrated a change in the biochemical milieu surrounding MTrPs. Bradykinins, cytokines, catecholamines, prostaglandins, and other markers are elevated and bind to nociceptors, causing localized pain and tenderness.

Patients with adductor strains typically present with groin pain and or medial thigh pain that is worse with activity. In most cases, this event is insidious in onset, and occasionally it is associated with an inciting event. In these cases, acute rupture or osseous avulsion should be considered.[62] On examination, tenderness to palpation is noted, along with associated pain with passive stretch or activation of the adductors. Swelling of the muscle group and weakness of hip adduction have been described.[41,63]

As with other soft tissue disorders of the hip, radiographic evaluation is of low yield but can be helpful in discerning between this and other bony abnormalities of the hip such as osteitis pubis or pelvic stress fracture. Musculoskeletal ultrasound evaluation can enhance visualization of the tendon, enthesis, muscles, ligaments, and nerves[64] (Table 39-1). MRI should be used to confirm the diagnosis or to differentiate other potential soft tissue disorders of the hip.[65] Treatment initially consists of relative rest, liberal ice, and oral anti-inflammatory medication. Special rehabilitation considerations for adductor disorders include the importance of balancing muscle length and strength not just of the adductors but of other pelvic girdle muscles that contribute to counterforces across the pelvis. Any associated problems such as intra-articular hip disorders or spine disorders should be evaluated and treated. In recalcitrant cases, serial injections of lidocaine at the site of insertion or in the muscle belly can be helpful to interrupt the pain cycle and reduce symptoms. Surgical management should be considered in cases of acute rupture. Open repair with suture anchors has been described with good results for osseous avulsions.[62]

Sports Hernia. Another soft tissue cause of anterior groin pain is a sports hernia, which is also termed *athletic pubalgia* or *rectus abdominis injury.*[66] The exact cause is highly debated. Meyers and coworkers[67] described the cause as a hyperextension injury to the rectus abdominis insertion onto the pubic symphysis. Others describe it as an occult hernia of the posterior inguinal wall without signs of a visualized tear.[66,68] This is similar to Gilmore's groin, which is a tear in the external oblique aponeurosis and conjoint tendon.[66] Participants in activities and sports that require repetitive twisting and turning of the upper leg and torso, such as ice hockey, soccer, and rugby, are at risk for sports hernias.[66-68] Repetitive trunk hyperextension and thigh hyperabduction cause shearing at the pubic symphysis.[66] Another risk factor is muscle imbalance between strong proximal thigh muscles and relatively weaker abdominal muscles.[66]

Patients typically describe insidious onset of groin pain with activity, worsened by coughing or sneezing or by sudden movement such as sprinting or kicking. Patients can but do not always have tenderness to palpation of the superficial inguinal ring, posterior inguinal canal, pubic tubercle, or conjoined tendon. No hernia is palpable. Patients may have pain with resisted sit-ups, active hip adduction, or Valsalva. MRI is the recommended imaging study because of its good sensitivity and specificity.[69]

Surgical exploration and repair can be considered after failure of at least 6 to 8 weeks of conservative management consisting of relative rest, icing, nonsteroidal anti-inflammatory drugs (NSAIDs), and physical therapy, to address the muscle imbalances and improve core strengthening.[66,68] Both open and laparoscopic approaches are used with or without mesh.[66-69] Results of repair and return to play are generally good, and full activity is expected for most patients.[66-69]

Osteitis Pubis. The cause of osteitis pubis is debated, but most agree that it represents degenerative changes that occur at the pubic symphysis. The cause is not well understood but has been linked to trauma, pregnancy, rheumatologic disorders, and postinfectious sequelae. In idiopathic cases, musculoskeletal imbalances at the pelvis have been theorized to contribute. In a study of athletes,[70] a correlation was found between decreased hip ROM and the development of osteitis pubis. Sports activities that require repetitive and forceful twisting and kicking are associated with pubic symphysis disorders, as are chronic overuse injuries to the adductors and rectus abdominis muscles.[71,72]

Table 39-1. Ultrasound for Diagnosis of Extra-Articular Hip Disorders

Location	Benefit
Muscle	• Loss of normal fibers can be visualized after the first 24 hours.
Muscle–tendon junction	• Using dynamic stress at the junction, the operator can visualize partial tears.
Tendon	• Can analyze the amount of fluid in the tendon sheath, which is increased in tendinopathy • Can detect earlier changes than can be detected via MRI • Color Doppler U/S allows for diagnosis of neovascularization and visualization of blood vessels. • Direct visualization of split tendons and/or partial tears
Enthesis	• Can evaluate cortical irregularities; displays increased vascularity
Ligament	• Partial ruptures and neovascularization via repetitive injury can be detected.

MRI, Magnetic resonance imaging; *U/S,* ultrasound.
Reproduced from Borg-Stein JZJ, Hanford M: New concepts in the assessment and treatment of regional musculoskeletal pain and sports injury. 1:744–754, 2009.[117]

Patients report aching anterior pelvic pain that can radiate into the groin, medial or anterior thigh, or abdomen. The pain can be sharp with activity and worse with weight-bearing activities or sports activities that require twisting or pivoting. Motions that require activation of the lower abdominals or adductors can be painful. The pain can be debilitating and can have a significant effect on ambulation and therefore on activities of daily living.

Examination reveals pain over the pubic symphysis and/or pubic rami. Hip ROM, specifically, internal rotation, can be painful. Passive adduction is painful as is activation of the adductors.[71-73] Radiographic evaluation in acute cases of pubic symphysitis is usually normal. In the chronic setting, changes consistent with osteitis pubis may be seen.[71-73] These include a widened or narrowed symphysis, sclerosis, and cystic changes to the bone. Views of the pelvis during single-leg stance can be helpful in evaluating for instability or motion at the pubic symphysis.[41] Further imaging with nuclear bone scan can show increased uptake, but the clinician should consider that evidence of changes on the bone scan can lag weeks to months behind the development of symptoms.[41,71-73] MRI can show evidence of bone edema and is helpful in ruling out parasymphyseal stress fractures and other causes of anterior pelvic pain.[71]

Treatment options begin with a course of conservative measures. Specific considerations when treating osteitis pubis include addressing movement disorders of the pelvic girdle. A pelvic stabilizing belt such as a sacroiliac joint belt can be used to decrease shear stresses across the pubic symphysis. Image-guided injections with fluoroscopy or ultrasound can be helpful. Injection of anesthetic should be considered in cases in which radiographs do not show significant degenerative changes to the pubic symphysis, and the diagnosis of pubic symphysitis is in question. Corticosteroid injections, which should be considered for recalcitrant cases of osteitis pubis, yield varying results.[72,73] Surgical options have been described with mixed results.[72,73]

Extra-Articular Lateral Hip Pain

In the past, lateral hip pain has been diagnosed commonly as greater trochanteric bursitis. Current literature is beginning to refute that bursitis is the primary diagnosis. Intra-articular hip disorders that present with lateral hip pain include labral disorders, hip deformity, and osteoarthritis.[26-29] Extra-articular sources include referral pain from the SIJ and loading, as well as muscle length and strength disorders at the lateral hip crossing and insertion sites. The term *greater trochanter pain syndrome (GTPS)* is used to denote a clinical syndrome that consists of chronic intermittent pain and tenderness over the greater trochanter. GTPS has been called by some "the Great Mimicker" because it is often mistaken for or seen in conjunction with other sources of pain such as lumbar radiculopathy or intra-articular hip pathology.[2] Studies have found GTPS to be associated with a number of other conditions that can alter shearing and tension forces of the hip abductors caused by weakness or altered gait mechanics. These associated conditions include degenerative joint disease of the hip, degenerative conditions of the lumbar spine, obesity, fibromyalgia, iliotibial band syndrome, pes planus, knee osteoarthritis, and lower limb amputation.[1,6,7] Although it has been suggested by some that leg length discrepancy is also associated with GTPS, a recent study by Segal and associates refutes this finding.[74] GTPS involves the tendons and bursae of the lateral hip region. The gluteal muscle tendons, especially tendons of the gluteus medius and minimus, are involved in this syndrome (Fig. 39-8). Typically, two main bursae are present in the trochanteric region: the subgluteus medius bursa and the subgluteus maximus bursa. It is the subgluteus maximus bursa that is often implicated as the source of pain in trochanteric bursitis. According to a literature review performed by Dunn and colleagues,[75] a great deal of ambiguity can be found in the literature regarding the location and constancy of the trochanteric bursa. They performed anatomic dissection on 16 hips of subjects aged 63 to 91 to attempt

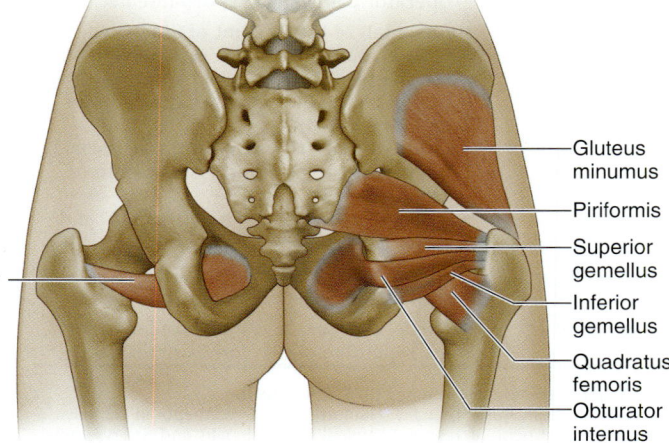

Figure 39-8. Orientation of the hip rotators associated with posterior pelvic girdle and lateral hip pain.

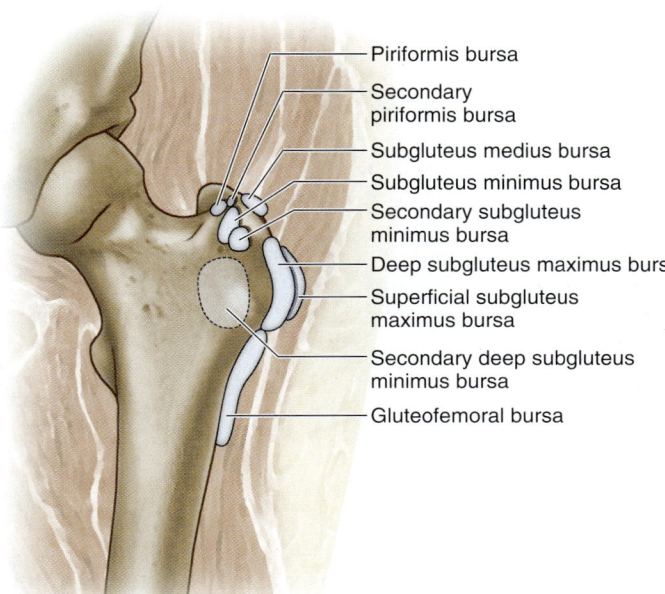

Piriformis bursa
Secondary piriformis bursa
Subgluteus medius bursa
Subgluteus minimus bursa
Secondary subgluteus minimus bursa
Deep subgluteus maximus bursa
Superficial subgluteus maximus bursa
Secondary deep subgluteus minimus bursa
Gluteofemoral bursa

Figure 39-9. Bursa of the left greater trochanter *(anterior view)*. The *dotted lines* indicate a posterior location.

to clarify the terminology and anatomic structure. Their findings showed a subgluteus maximus bursa in 13 hips. This "deep bursa" was found just superficial to the attachment of the gluteus medius, gluteus minimus, and vastus lateralis on the greater trochanter. Five hips showed a second "superficial" gluteus maximus bursa, and in two hips, a total of four bursae were found. Histologic analysis showed varying degrees of synovial development; this led the authors to conclude that bursae were acquired in response to friction.[75] Other smaller bursae may be present in the trochanteric region (Fig. 39-9).

Tears of the gluteus medius and to a lesser degree the gluteus minimus are increasingly recognized as a source of lateral hip pain. Bunker and Kagan independently described these tears as "rotator cuff tears of the hip." As the name implies, they compared the anatomy of the hip versus that of the shoulder, with tears of the gluteus medius and minimus being analogous to tears of the supraspinatus and infraspinatus, respectively.[76,77] We propose that specific changes in muscle tendon soft tissue structures at the greater trochanter occur in a continuum. These symptoms and dysfunctions continue as a result of biomechanical dysfunction and individual biological factors. In the initial overload phase, bursitis may occur as a result of unbalanced loads and shear forces. Without a change in this pattern of loading, bursitis evolves into tendinopathy, enthesopathy at the greater trochanter, tendon thinning, and eventual microtears and macrotears at the muscle–tendon junction. MRI may specifically detect where on the continuum the patient's disorder falls, thereby facilitating identification of appropriate treatment interventions.

Patients with GTPS often report discomfort when sleeping on the affected side and lateral hip pain when climbing stairs, getting up and down from a chair, crossing the affected leg, or single-leg weight bearing on the affected limb. The pain can radiate down along the outside of the hip to the knee, although it is unclear whether this is a result of the pathology in the trochanteric region itself, or whether it is caused by an associated condition. GTPS is more common in women, with approximately a 3:1 or 4:1 female-to-male predominance. It is more common in the fourth and sixth decades of life.[1,6,7]

On physical examination, patients note lateral hip pain with weight bearing, resisted hip abduction, palpation over the region of the greater trochanter, and passive hip internal rotation aimed at stretching the hip external rotators. Often, a Trendelenburg sign and an antalgic gait are present. In addition to the hip rotators and abductors, the iliotibial band (ITB) is a source of lateral hip pain. At times this dysfunction is associated with lateral hip snapping. As with other sources of lateral hip pain, lateral iliotibial band pain is associated with pain on palpation of the ITB, a short ITB, and pain with resisted hip abduction.

Diagnostic imaging studies are useful for assessing acute trauma and chronic repetitive overload but are not uniformly positive. In other words, patients with chronic lateral hip pain related to muscle tendon overload may have imaging that varies from normal to muscle/tendon tear. Radiographs of the pelvis are helpful in determining whether an underlying hip deformity or osteoarthritis is present; this may put the patient at increased risk for muscle tendon dysfunction and pain at the lateral hip. Further, stress reaction, stress fracture, and fracture must be eliminated from the differential diagnosis, especially in patients with acute direct trauma or chronic repetitive overload. This

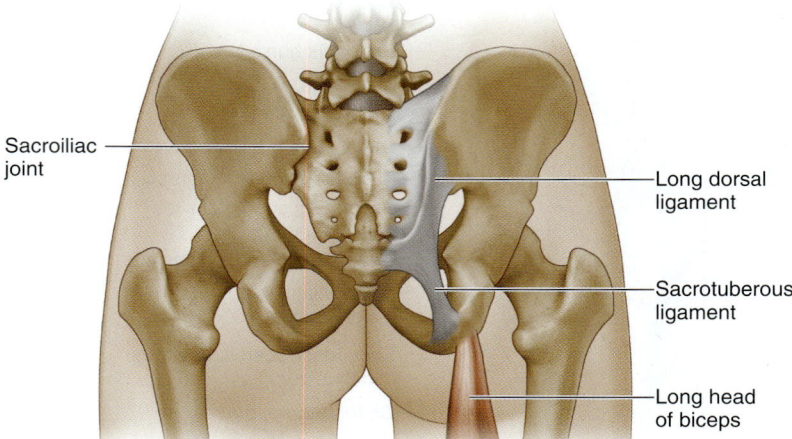

Sacroiliac joint

Long dorsal ligament

Sacrotuberous ligament

Long head of biceps

Figure 39-10. Ligaments of the sacroiliac joint (SIJ) associated with posterior pelvic girdle pain.

can be accomplished with the use of radiographs, three-phase bone scan, or MRI. Ultrasound (US) can assess dynamically for lateral snapping of the ITB or hip rotators at the greater trochanter. MRI and US can also be used to identify the stage of the continuum of the overuse injury. These studies[78-80] can show bursitis, tendinopathy, enthesopathy, thinning of the tendons, and partial and complete hip rotator and abductor tears. A more unusual diagnosis that includes denervation (from the lumbar spine or pelvic nerves) may present with increased muscle signal intensity on T2-weighted images.

Posterior Pelvic Pain

Patients who experience posterior pelvic pain present with a wide variety of complaints. No gold standard is available for diagnosis, and the specific diagnosis is often made by clinical presentation and exclusion of other sources. Commonly, patients with SIJ pain present with gluteal pain near or surrounding the posterior superior iliac spine, as described by Fortin.[81] Other symptoms include groin pain, pain radiating into the lower extremity, numbness, and clicking or popping in the posterior pelvis. Pain may be reported with popping and/or clicking with transitional activities such as getting up from a chair, or with sport-specific activities that require unilateral loading or torsion through the pelvis and lower extremity. In particular, patients who participate in activities that require single-leg stance and torsion are at risk. Examples of these activities include skating, step aerobics, stair stepper, elliptical trainers, and bowling. Two studies have been published regarding the risk of SIJ dysfunction in rowers related to the mechanics of rowing.[82,83] Trauma, including a direct fall onto or a blow to the pelvis, is an important historical point to note when a patient presents with posterior pelvic pain. Bernard[9] reported that 58% of those with SIJ pain by history and physical examination presented with a history of trauma. Similarly, Chou and colleagues[84] found that 44% of patients who experienced

pain relief with a fluoroscopically guided SIJ steroid injection had a history of trauma. Ligaments that support the SIJ work in a sling fashion anteriorly. Interosseous ligaments facilitate joint stiffness and force closure. The dorsal longitudinal ligament has been found to be a contributor to periarticular pain based on the presence of nociceptors and proprioceptors[19] (Fig. 39-10).

In addition to the SIJ, the piriformis muscle has been studied and reported to be a muscular and neurogenic source of posterior pelvic pain. Unfortunately, some nomenclature confusion is present in the literature. Yeoman[85] first described sciatic nerve entrapment at the piriformis; this was later coined by Robinson[86] as *piriformis syndrome*. Fishman and colleagues[87] confirmed these descriptions by describing an objective test, a prolonged H wave of the tibial nerve on a nerve conduction study performed with the hip in flexion, adduction, and internal rotation, to confirm the diagnosis of piriformis syndrome. Numerous studies have described a painful piriformis as a source of posterior pelvic pain.[88,89]

The latter may occur without documentation of nerve entrapment and can potentially be confirmed with anesthetic injection of the muscle under image guidance.[90,91] In addition to hip pain, low back pain (LBP) related to acute overload of soft tissues, intervertebral disks, and degenerative conditions can present in similar distributions. In caring for the patient with posterior pelvic pain, the history and pain distribution provide important information to guide the diagnostic evaluation and treatment. Because of the overlap in symptoms, the specialist must often rely on his or her individual experiences to direct care.

Diagnosis

The diagnosis for specific causes of posterior pelvic pain often involves a combination of exclusion, clinical suspicion based on history and physical examination findings, and, occasionally, objective testing (Boxes 39-1 and 39-2).

BOX 39-1.   PHYSICAL EXAMINATION FINDINGS FOR POSTERIOR PELVIC PAIN

Gait deviations
Pain with palpation at the sacral sulci
Movement asymmetries:
    Standing and seated flexion test
    Gillet's test
    Femoral or tibial rotation with single-leg stance
    Motion on weight bearing in sagittal, frontal, and transverse planes
Muscle strength
Muscle length
Normal muscle stretch reflexes
Provocative tests:
    FABER/Patrick's
    Active straight-leg raise
    Pain with end-range hip flexion and/or internal rotation

FABER, Flexion-abduction-external rotation test.

BOX 39-2.   DIAGNOSTICS FOR POSTERIOR PELVIC PAIN

Imaging often normal:
    X-ray, CT scan can show degenerative changes and can exclude invasive or inflammatory bone changes.
    Bone scan and MRI can assess fracture and age of fracture and inflammatory changes.
    Doppler ultrasound has shown an asymmetry in vibration across the joint in patients with SIJ pain.
Injections help confirm or exclude the diagnosis:
    Image-guided intra-articular SIJ injection
    Image-guided muscle (e.g., piriformis, obturator internus) injection
    Ligamentous injections less well studied
    Proposals for value of prolotherapy and platelet-rich plasma injections

CT, Computed tomography; *MRI*, magnetic resonance imaging; *SIJ*, sacroiliac joint.

BOX 39-3.   POSSIBLE DISORDERS PRESENTING AS HIP AND PELVIC GIRDLE PAIN

Fracture
Tumor
Infection
Inflammatory arthropathy
Iatrogenic
Pregnancy
Idiopathic*

*Idiopathic posterior pelvic pain differential diagnosis algorithm.

BOX 39-4.   ANATOMIC REGIONS REFERRING PAIN TO THE HIP

Anterior Hip Pain
• Lumbar spine
• Abdomen
• Hip
• Pelvic girdle

Lateral Hip Pain
• Lumbar spine
• Sacroiliac joint
• Hip

Posterior Pelvic Pain
• Lumbar spine
• Hip
• Sacroiliac joint

DIFFERENTIAL DIAGNOSIS

The differential diagnosis for extra-articular hip pain is varied and can be related to underlying trauma, infection, tumor, metabolic disorders, and pregnancy (Box 39-3). Further, several anatomic regions can refer pain to the hip region (Box 39-4). The algorithms that follow (see Figs. 39-5 through 39-7) are intended to help direct the diagnosis of patients presenting with idiopathic extra-articular anterior, lateral, and posterior pelvic pain.

TREATMENT

Therapeutics

Treatment for the patient with extra-articular hip pain should be individualized according to the mechanism of injury, biomechanical deficits, and the directional preference of pain-free motion with the ultimate goal of return to function, whether that is a work-related or home activity or sports and exercise. Rehabilitation should be approached in phases. Special treatment considerations for individual disorders are listed in Table 39-2. One example of an algorithm to direct treatment is listed as Figure 39-11.

Acute Phase (1 to 3 Days)

When an injury is acute in onset or is related to a specific trauma or event, it is often easier to identify the dysfunctional structures of movement patterns as compared with injuries that are insidious in onset. Acute injury often is associated with direct trauma or a marked increase in intensity, frequency, or duration of a specific activity. Often idiopathic extra-articular hip pain presents as a progressive problem with fluctuations in symptoms, so that the patient may experience symptoms only during certain activities, including sports and exercise. The usual principles of ice, relative rest, and

Table 39-2. Special Considerations for Treatment of Extra-Articular Disorders of the Hip

Diagnosis	Conservative Considerations	Surgical Considerations
Iliopsoas tendinitis/bursitis, snapping hip	• Modalities to consider include ultrasound or iontophoresis to the bursa or tendon. • Image-guided corticosteroid injection to the iliopsoas bursa, the iliopectineal bursa, or the peritendinous bursa[1]	• Surgery considered after 3 months of failed conservative care • Response to a diagnostic injection of the tendon can predict surgical outcome[2] • Open procedures • Lengthening or release with or without bursectomy[2a] • Arthroscopic procedures • Lengthening or release at lesser trochanter • Lengthening or release at level of the hip joint[3]
Adductor strain	• Serial injections of lidocaine at the enthesis or the muscle trigger point	• Surgical repair for acute ruptures • Open repair with suture anchors with good results[4]
Sports hernia	• Physical therapy must address core and rectus abdominis deficits	• Surgical exploration and repair indicated after 8 weeks of conservative care • Open and laparoscopic approaches generally produce good results. • Return to activity in 6 months after open repair • Return to activity 6 weeks after laparoscopic repair[5-8]
Osteitis pubis	• Physical therapy must address associated pelvic obliquity. • Image-guided corticosteroid injections to the pubic symphysis[10,11]	• Surgery considered after 3 months of failed conservative care • Surgical wedge resection[10] • Unpredictable results • Synthroidesis[10] • Unpredictable results • Curettage[11] • Complete to near complete resolution in 80% of athletes (n = X) • Mesh reinforcement[12] • Case series (n = X)
Greater trochanteric pain syndrome	• Physical therapy should address underlying hip movement and loading disorder. • Corticosteroid injections can reduce pain but should be used as an adjunct to treatment. Plasma-rich protein injection is an emerging adjunct treatment.	• Surgery considered after 3 months of failed conservative care • Surgical iliotibial band release or débridement of the bursa • Open and arthroscopic approaches[13]
SIJ intra-articular pain	• Image-guided SIJ injection should be used as adjunct treatment. • Radiofrequency ablation is an emerging adjunct treatment for patients with chronic conditions.	• Long-term surgical outcomes have mixed results. • Surgery ranges from percutaneous fixation to open reduction internal fixation.

analgesics should be implemented. Activities that provoke pain should be avoided during this phase. Correcting asymmetries in muscle length or stiffness should start as soon as possible and should be progressed within pain-free limits. Patients with significant muscle weakness and/or poor endurance may need to focus on stabilization and improved motor control rather than on stretching and recurrent joint mobilization. Although considerable focus is placed on gaining ROM during this phase and continuing into the recovery phase, it is important to differentiate hip ROM limits that are related to pain or soft tissue restrictions versus limitations related to bony deformity, such as femoroacetabular impingement (FAI) and developmental dysplasia of the hip (DDH). For example, continuously attempting to stretch hip internal rotators in patients with FAI not only

will be met with failure but may actually increase symptoms.

Recovery Phase (3 Days to 8 Weeks)

After pain control and relative rest are in place, correction of the functional biomechanical deficit and tissue overload complex[92] becomes the focus of rehabilitation. Balancing lower extremity muscle length and strength is important because of direct and indirect force transmission across the pelvic girdle. Muscle length must first be restored.

Neuromuscular re-education and facilitation techniques are helpful in restoring muscle function and strength. Closed kinetic chain strengthening should be attempted first and incorporated into the lumbopelvic stabilization program. As trunk strengthening improves,

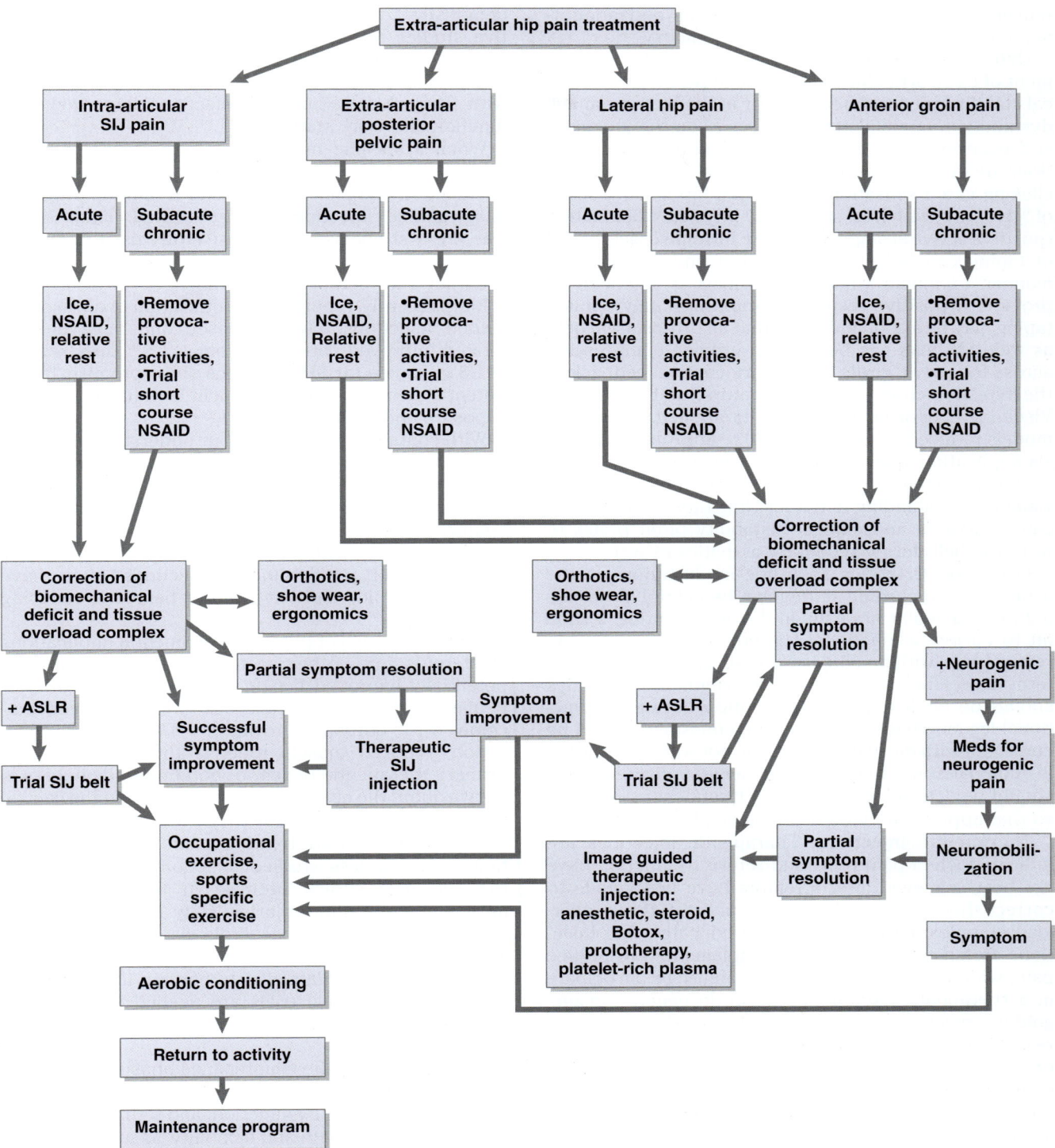

Figure 39-11. Treatment algorithm for extra-articular hip pain.

adding multiplanar strengthening exercises will facilitate return to functional activities. Although muscle flexibility and strength are important, retraining motor control groups with groups of muscles firing in coordination is key to a successful recovery. Lumbopelvic stabilization, advanced proprioceptive re-education, plyometrics, and occupational, exercise,

or sport-specific activities can serve as potential interventions to facilitate recovery. Education in proper ergonomics in activities of daily living and the work environment should be included. Return to occupational, sports, or exercise activities is recommended when a pain-free state without medications is achieved. Proper muscle balance in flexibility and strength should remain a part of the maintenance program, and monitoring during initial return can prevent reinjury.

Orthosis. An orthosis may have a role in the management of extra-articular hip pain when pelvic girdle clinical stability is considered a factor in the biomechanical dysfunction. Implementation is based on the judgment and experiences of the examiner. Most of the indications are drawn from the history (consistent popping or clicking catch sensation with active hip flexion, sense of "give way" with heel-strike) and physical examination (positive active straight-leg raise). In some cases, a trial of taping can be implemented first and applied in a manner to mimic what the orthosis is intended to provide. A positive response to appropriately applied taping may be a good indicator that an orthosis will help as well. SIJ belts can be used to provide compression across the pelvic girdle and proprioceptive feedback to the hip abductors, external rotators, and extenders. Vleeming[93] reported that SIJ belts applied to cadaver models reduced SIJ rotation by 30%. Appropriate orthosis application is key in ensuring the correct fit.

Patients often are advised to wear the belt during walking and standing activities, but those with significant weakness and clinical instability often prefer to wear the belt during sedentary activities as well.

Orthotics. Orthotics and shoe modifications in the acute through chronic setting can be helpful in managing extra-articular hip pain. In the acute setting, a shoe lift to correct a functional leg length discrepancy can reduce pain with weight bearing or ambulation. Long-term shoe lifts for functional leg length discrepancies should be implemented with caution because a functional leg length discrepancy, when possible, should be corrected with muscle rebalancing, not with an orthotic. In comparison, anatomic leg length discrepancies should be determined as early in treatment as possible so that appropriate modifications can be completed.

Therapeutic Injections. Therapeutic injections are indicated when pain relief and return to function have not been achieved after attempts have been made to correct the biomechanical deficit and the tissue overload complex. Patients should be educated that injections are an adjunct treatment implemented to reduce pain, which will lead to improved ability to participate in a therapeutic exercise program. In general, image-guided injections should be advocated for several reasons. First, confirming the specificity of a successful or unsuccessful injection directs future care. Second, confirmation of the structure injected followed by reduced pain, in some diagnoses, may be the only mechanism of confirming the diagnosis.

Injections can be used as an adjunct treatment when progress with recovery plateaus or the physical therapy program cannot be advanced because of pain provocation. Utilization of image (fluoroscopic, ultrasound, or computed tomography [CT]) guidance is important to ensure the accuracy of the placement of the medication and to avoid complications.

Rosenberg[94] reviewed the accuracy of blind placement of the needle presumably into the SIJ. Of 37 blind injections, 22% were placed within the SIJ confirmed on CT, 24% showed epidural flow of contrast, and 44%

demonstrated dorsal sacral foraminal flow. No prospective studies are available at this time regarding the therapeutic benefit of SIJ injections in patients with idiopathic SIJ pain. In a retrospective review of 31 patients with 94-week follow-up, SIJ injections improved pain function and work status.[95]

When a specific muscle (e.g., piriformis) or bursa (e.g., iliopsoas) has been determined to be part of the dysfunction and pain complex and is limiting progress, image-guided injections are advocated. Fluoroscopy was the first imaging tool consistently used in studies reporting intramuscular and peritendinous placement accuracy and therapeutic outcome.[91,96-98]

More recently, reports of the utilization of ultrasound-guided injections have increased and have demonstrated improved patient outcomes.[42,45,99] Early reports of US guidance for SIJ injections show promise.[100] The potential benefits of using US include reduced radiation exposure and reduced cost.

With continued advances in our understanding of biological factors associated with chronic painful muscle and tendon disorders, recommendations regarding what substance to inject will likely change. Historically, epidural infusion of phenol has been used to treat painful muscles with increased muscle tone.[102] Intramuscular and peritendinous injections often have included steroids and have shown benefit in reducing pain.[1,42,45,87,103-105]

With knowledge of potential detrimental implications of steroids,[46,47,106] other agents are being studied for potentially improved benefit and reduced risk. In particular, recent reports have described improved outcomes with botulinum toxin.[107-110] The mechanism of action, reduced muscle tone, is thought to be the primary therapeutic benefit of botulinum toxin. Less is known about the effect of botulinum toxin on the central nervous system, which may play a role in the beneficial effects derived from treating painful muscle conditions.[111] Other less studied injections such as prolotherapy have shown promise in the treatment of muscular and tendon injuries. Only a few studies are dedicated to general pelvic girdle disorders, and specifics regarding timing and utilization of the intervention are variable.[112,113] Platelet-rich plasma injections are controversial; clinical trials are needed to determine the specific indications and efficacy of these interventions.

Advancement to the maintenance phase of treatment begins with absence of pain, inflammation, functional joint and myofascial dysfunction, and return of approximately 75% of strength and flexibility, as judged per the patient's preinjury baseline. Normal activities of daily living, especially walking, should not provoke symptoms.[92]

Maintenance Phase

During this phase, the focus of the program is to devise concisely a series of activities that the patient will follow independently upon completion of therapy. This is a clear distinction from the end of "treatment." Patients need ongoing education to remain an active part of their recovery and prevention program. The exercise program should be concise and specific to the individual's functional requirements and should simulate the individual's activities. This is also a time to review specific exercises or activities that should be avoided. Athletes with reduced hip flexion due to hip deformity should not aggressively stretch the hip musculature in attempts to improve hip flexion. Even if the hip is asymptomatic, aggressive stretching across a joint with inherent bony limitation will increase stress across the SIJ and may initiate intra-articular hip pain. At this time, aerobic conditioning should be advanced while a return to usual occupational and sport/exercise activities is monitored. Emphasis is placed on the need for an exercise prescription to fit the individual.

CURRENT CONTROVERSIES AND FUTURE CONSIDERATIONS

Extra-articular Hip Pain: Current Controversies

- Extra-articular anterior hip pain
  - Pain with hip flexion: Is it related to primary muscle dysfunction or to the labrum, or is it a guarding mechanism for intra-articular disorders?
- Extra-articular lateral hip pain
  - Is all extra-articular lateral hip pain bursitis?
  - Is there a continuum of bursitis, tendinopathy, enthesopathy, intrasubstance microtears, and macrotears?
- Piriformis syndrome and piriformis pain
  - Piriformis syndrome includes muscle pain and entrapment of the sciatic nerve with neurogenic pain.
  - Painful hip rotators: The piriformis may not be the only hip rotator causing posterior pelvic pain.
  - What substance should be injected to best improve outcomes in painful hip rotators?
- SIJ
  - Motion at the joint occurs but is minimal and therefore should not significantly impact dysfunction.
  - Biomechanics of the SIJ integrated with hip and spine biomechanics is complex.
  - No gold standard of diagnosis is available, and therefore no gold standard for treatment is known.
  - Other sources of pain mimic or coexist with SIJ pain.
  - Intra-articular injections are useful in diagnosing intra-articular pain, but no consistencies have been noted in diagnosing extra-articular sources of pain.

Extra-Articular Hip Pain: Future Considerations

- Extra-articular anterior hip pain
  - Additional studies are needed to prognosticate which therapeutic intervention will best produce effective outcomes in patients with iliopsoas pain.
- Extra-articular lateral hip pain
  - Additional trials are needed regarding comparison and effectiveness of therapeutic injections.

- Posterior pelvic pain
  - Additional trials are needed for prognosticating and reporting the effectiveness of radiofrequency ablation.

REFERENCES

1. Shbeeb MI, Matteson EL: Trochanteric bursitis (greater trochanter pain syndrome). Mayo Clin Proc 71:565–569, 1996.
2. Stegemann H: Die chirurgische bedevtung paraartikularer kalkablagerungen. Arch Klin Chir 125:718–738, 1923.
3. Le Cocq E: Peritrochanteric bursitis. J Bone Joint Surg Br 13:872–873, 1931.
4. Leonard M: Trochanteric syndrome: calcareous and noncalcareous tendonitis and bursitis about the trochanter major. JAMA 168:175–177, 1958.
5. Karpinsky MR, Pigott H: Greater trochanteric pain syndrome. J Bone Joint Surg Br 67:762–763, 1985.
6. Collee G, Dijkmans BA, Vandenbroucke JP, et al: A clinical epidemiological study in low back pain. Description of two clinical syndromes. Br J Rheumatol 29:354–357, 1990.
7. Segal NA, Felson DT, Torner JC, et al: Greater trochanteric pain syndrome: epidemiology and associated factors. Arch Phys Med Rehabil 88:988–992, 2007.
8. Tortolani PJ, Carbone JJ, Quartararo LG: Greater trochanteric pain syndrome in patients referred to orthopedic spine specialists. Spine J 2:251–254, 2002.
9. Bernard TN Jr, Kirkaldy-Willis WH: Recognizing specific characteristics of nonspecific low back pain. Clin Orthop Relat Res 217:266–280, 1987.
10. Maigne JY, Aivaliklis A, Pfefer F: Results of sacroiliac joint double block and value of sacroiliac pain provocation tests in 54 patients with low back pain. Spine 21:1889–1892, 1996.
11. Schwarzer AC, Aprill CN, Bogduk N: The sacroiliac joint in chronic low back pain. Spine 20:31–37, 1995.
12. Aprill C, Bogduk N: High-intensity zone: a diagnostic sign of painful lumbar disc on magnetic resonance imaging. Br J Radiol 65:361–369, 1992.
13. Greenman PE: Manipulation with the patient under anesthesia. J Am Osteopath Assoc 92:1159–1160, 1167–1170, 1992.
14. Dreyfuss P, Dreyer SJ, Cole A, Mayo K: Sacroiliac joint pain. J Am Acad Orthop Surg 12:255–265, 2004.
15. Foley BS, Buschbacher RM: Sacroiliac joint pain: anatomy, biomechanics, diagnosis, and treatment. Am J Phys Med Rehabil 85:997–1006, 2006.
16. DonTigny RL: Function and pathomechanics of the sacroiliac joint: a review. Phys Ther 65:35–44, 1985.
17. DonTigny RL: Anterior dysfunction of the sacroiliac joint as a major factor in the etiology of idiopathic low back pain syndrome. Phys Ther 70:250–265, 1990; discussion 262–265.
18. Pool-Goudzwaard AL, Vleeming A, Stoeckart R, et al: Insufficient lumbopelvic stability: a clinical, anatomical and biomechanical approach to "a-specific" low back pain. Man Ther 3:12–20, 1998.
19. Vleeming A, Pool-Goudzwaard AL, Hammudoghlu D, et al: The function of the long dorsal sacroiliac ligament: its implication for understanding low back pain. Spine 21:556–562, 1996.
20. Vleeming A, Stoeckart R, Volkers AC, Snijders CJ: Relation between form and function in the sacroiliac joint. Part I: Clinical anatomical aspects. Spine 15:130–132, 1990.
21. Vleeming A, Volkers AC, Snijders CJ, Stoeckart R: Relation between form and function in the sacroiliac joint. Part II: Biomechanical aspects. Spine 15:133–136, 1990.
22. DonTigny RL: Critical analysis of the sequence and extent of the result of the pathological release of self-brasing of the sacroiliac joint. J Orthop Med 22:16–23, 2000.
23. DonTigny RL: Clinical analysis of the functional dynamics of the sacroiliac joints as they pertain to normal gait. J Orthop Med 27:3–10, 2005.
24. DonTigny RL: Pathology of the sacroiliac joint, its effect on normal gait and its correction. J Orthop Med 27:61–69, 2005.

25. DonTigny RL: A detailed and critical biomechanical analysis of the sacroiliac joints and relevant kinesiology: the implications for lumbopelvic function and dysfunction. In Vleeming A, Mooney V, Stoeckart R (eds): Movement, stability and lumbopelvic pain: integration of research and therapy, New York, 2007, Churchill Livingstone, pp 265–278.

26. Burnett RS, Della Rocca GJ, Prather H, et al: Clinical presentation of patients with tears of the acetabular labrum. J Bone Joint Surg Am 88:1448–1457, 2006.

27. Clohisy JC, Knaus ER, Hunt DM, et al: Clinical presentation of patients with symptomatic anterior hip impingement. Clin Orthop Relat Res 467:638–644, 2009.

28. Lesher JM, Dreyfuss P, Hager N, et al: Hip joint pain referral patterns: a descriptive study. Pain Med 9:22–25, 2008.

29. Nunley RM, Clohisy JC, Hunt D, et al: Early, symptomatic acetabular dysplasia: are we making the diagnosis? Paper presented at 75th Annual Meeting, American Academy of Orthopaedic Surgery, San Francisco, Calif, February 2008.

30. Prather H, Dugan S, Fitzgerald C, Hunt D: Review of anatomy, evaluation, and treatment of musculoskeletal pelvic floor pain in women. PMR 1:346–358, 2009.

31. Little TL, Mansoor J: Low back pain associated with internal snapping hip syndrome in a competitive cyclist. Br J Sports Med 42:308–309, 2008; discussion 309.

32. Blankenbaker DG, Tuite MJ: Iliopsoas musculotendinous unit. Semin Musculoskelet Radiol 12:13–27, 2008.

33. Nelson EN, Kassarjian A, Palmer WE: MR imaging of sports-related groin pain. Magn Reson Imaging Clin N Am 13:727–742, 2005.

34. Johnston CA, Wiley JP, Lindsay DM, Wiseman DA: Iliopsoas bursitis and tendinitis: a review. Sports Med 25:271–283, 1998.

35. Gray G: Total body functional profile, Adrian, Mich, 2001, Wynn Marketing.

36. Schaberg JE, Harper MC, Allen WC: The snapping hip syndrome. Am J Sports Med 12:361–365, 1984.

37. Lyons JC, Peterson LF: The snapping iliopsoas tendon. Mayo Clin Proc 59:327–329, 1984.

38. Rotini R, Spinozzi C, Ferrari A: Snapping hip: a rare form with internal etiology. Ital J Orthop Traumatol 17:283–288, 1991.

39. Jacobson T, Allen WC: Surgical correction of the snapping iliopsoas tendon. Am J Sports Med 18:470–474, 1990.

40. Janzen DL, Partridge E, Logan PM, et al: The snapping hip: clinical and imaging findings in transient subluxation of the iliopsoas tendon. Can Assoc Radiol J 47:202–208, 1996.

41. Tibor LM, Sekiya JK: Differential diagnosis of pain around the hip joint. Arthroscopy 24:1407–1421, 2008.

42. Blankenbaker DG, De Smet AA, Keene JS: Sonography of the iliopsoas tendon and injection of the iliopsoas bursa for diagnosis and management of the painful snapping hip. Skelet Radiol 35:565–571, 2006.

43. Gruen GS, Scioscia TN, Lowenstein JE: The surgical treatment of internal snapping hip. Am J Sports Med 30:607–613, 2002.

44. Taylor GR, Clarke NM: Surgical release of the "snapping iliopsoas tendon." J Bone Joint Surg Br 77:881–883, 1995.

45. Adler RS, Buly R, Ambrose R, Sculco T: Diagnostic and therapeutic use of sonography-guided iliopsoas peritendinous injections. AJR Am J Roentgenol 185:940–943, 2005.

46. Mikolyzk DK, Wei AS, Tonino P, et al: Effect of corticosteroids on the biomechanical strength of rat rotator cuff tendon. J Bone Joint Surg Am 91:1172–1180, 2009.

47. Wei AS, Callaci JJ, Juknelis D, et al: The effect of corticosteroid on collagen expression in injured rotator cuff tendon. J Bone Joint Surg Am 88:1331–1338, 2006.

48. Dobbs MB, Gordon JE, Luhmann SJ, et al: Surgical correction of the snapping iliopsoas tendon in adolescents. J Bone Joint Surg Am 84:420–424, 2002.

49. Ilizaliturri VM Jr, Chaidez C, Villegas P, et al: Prospective randomized study of 2 different techniques for endoscopic iliopsoas tendon release in the treatment of internal snapping hip syndrome. Arthroscopy 25:159–163, 2009.

50. Nicholas SJ, Tyler TF: Adductor muscle strains in sport. Sports Med 32:339–344, 2002.

51. Kendall F, McCreary E: Muscles: testing and function, ed 3, Baltimore, 1983, Williams and Wilkins.

52. Moore K: Clinically oriented anatomy, ed 3, Baltimore, 1992, Williams and Wilkins.

53. Renstrom P, Peterson L: Groin injuries in athletes. Br J Sports Med 14:30–36, 1980.

54. Strauss EJ, Campbell K, Bosco JA: Analysis of the cross-sectional area of the adductor longus tendon: a descriptive anatomic study. Am J Sports Med 35:996–999, 2007.

55. Maffey L, Emery C: What are the risk factors for groin strain injury in sport? A systematic review of the literature. Sports Med 37:881–894, 2007.

56. Ekstrand J, Gillquist J: The avoidability of soccer injuries. Int J Sports Med 4:124–128, 1983.

57. Sim FH, Chao EY: Injury potential in modern ice hockey. Am J Sports Med 6:378–384, 1978.

58. Hoffberg H, Rosen N: Myofascial pain and dysfunction syndrome. In Frontera W, Silver (eds): Essentials of physical medicine and rehabilitation, Philadelphia, 2002, Hanley and Belfus.

59. Simons DG, Travell J, Simon P: Travell and Simon's myofascial pain and dysfunction: the trigger point manual, ed 2, Baltimore, 1999, Williams and Wilkins.

60. Shah JP, Danoff JV, Desai MJ, et al: Biochemicals associated with pain and inflammation are elevated in sites near to and remote from active myofascial trigger points. Arch Phys Med Rehabil 89:16–23, 2008.

61. Deleted in proof.

62. Vogt S, Ansah P, Imhoff AB: Complete osseous avulsion of the adductor longus muscle: acute repair with three fiberwire suture anchors. Arch Orthop Trauma Surg 127:613–615, 2007.

63. Schilders E, Bismil Q, Robinson P, et al: Adductor-related groin pain in competitive athletes: role of adductor enthesis, magnetic resonance imaging, and entheseal pubic cleft injections. J Bone Joint Surg Am 89:2173–2178, 2007.

64. Smith JFJ: Diagnostic and interventional musculoskeletal ultrasound. Part 1. Fundamentals. PMR 1:64–75, 2009.

65. Cunningham PM, Brennan D, O'Connell M, et al: Patterns of bone and soft-tissue injury at the symphysis pubis in soccer players: observations at MRI. AJR Am J Roentgenol 188:W291–W296, 2007.

66. Farber AJ, Wilckens JH: Sports hernia: diagnosis and therapeutic approach. J Am Acad Orthop Surg 15:507–514, 2007.

67. Meyers WC, Foley DP, Garrett WE, et al: Management of severe lower abdominal or inguinal pain in high-performance athletes. PAIN (Performing Athletes with Abdominal or Inguinal Neuromuscular Pain Study Group). Am J Sports Med 28:2–8, 2000.

68. van Veen RN, de Baat P, Heijboer MP, et al: Successful endoscopic treatment of chronic groin pain in athletes. Surg Endosc 21:189–193, 2007.

69. Zoga AC, Kavanagh EC, Omar IM, et al: Athletic pubalgia and the "sports hernia": MR imaging findings. Radiology 247:797–807, 2008.

70. Verrall GM, Slavotinek JP, Barnes PG, et al: Hip joint range of motion restriction precedes athletic chronic groin injury. J Sci Med Sport 10:463–466, 2007.

71. Paajanen H, Hermunen H, Karonen J: Pubic magnetic resonance imaging findings in surgically and conservatively treated athletes with osteitis pubis compared to asymptomatic athletes during heavy training. Am J Sports Med 36:117–121, 2008.

72. Radic R, Annear P: Use of pubic symphysis curettage for treatment-resistant osteitis pubis in athletes. Am J Sports Med 36:122–128, 2008.

73. Mehin R, Meek R, O'Brien P, Blachut P: Surgery for osteitis pubis. Can J Surg 49:170–176, 2006.

74. Segal NA, Harvey W, Felson DT, et al: Leg-length inequality is not associated with greater trochanteric pain syndrome. Arthritis Res Ther 10:R62, 2008.

75. Dunn T, Heller CA, McCarthy SW, Dos Remedios C: Anatomical study of the "trochanteric bursa." Clin Anat 16:233–240, 2003.

76. Bunker TD, Esler CN, Leach WJ: Rotator-cuff tear of the hip. J Bone Joint Surg Br 79:618–620, 1997.

77. Kagan A 2nd: Rotator cuff tears of the hip. Clin Orthop Relat Res 368:135–140, 2009.

78. Krishnamurthy G, Connolly BL, Narayanan U, Babyn PS: Imaging findings in external snapping hip syndrome. Pediatr Radiol 37:1272–1274, 2007.

79. Pelsser V, Cardinal E, Hobden R, et al: Extraarticular snapping hip: sonographic findings. AJR Am J Roentgenol 176:67–73, 2001.

80. Winston P, Awan R, Cassidy JD, Bleakney RK: Clinical examination and ultrasound of self-reported snapping hip syndrome in elite ballet dancers. Am J Sports Med 35:118–126, 2007.

81. Fortin JD, Dwyer AP, West S, Pier J: Sacroiliac joint: pain referral maps upon applying a new injection/arthrography technique. Part I: Asymptomatic volunteers. Spine 19:1475–1482, 1994.

82. Rumball JS, Lebrun CM, Di Ciacca SR, Orlando K: Rowing injuries. Sports Med 35:537–555, 2005.

83. Timm KE: Sacroiliac joint dysfunction in elite rowers. J Orthop Sports Phys Ther 29:288–293, 1999.

84. Chou LH, Slipman CW, Bhagia SM, et al: Inciting events initiating injection-proven sacroiliac joint syndrome. Pain Med 5:26–32, 2004.

85. Yeoman W: The relation of arthritis of the sacroiliac joint to sciatica. Lancet 2:1119–1122, 1998.

86. Robinson D: Piriformis syndrome in relation to sciatic pain. Am J Surg 73:355–358, 1947.

87. Fishman LM, Dombi GW, Michaelsen C, et al: Piriformis syndrome: diagnosis, treatment, and outcome—a 10-year study. Arch Phys Med Rehabil 83:295–301, 2002.

88. Durrani Z, Winnie AP: Piriformis muscle syndrome: an underdiagnosed cause of sciatica. J Pain Symptom Manage 6:374–379, 1991.

89. Wyant GM: Chronic pain syndromes and their treatment. III. The piriformis syndrome. Can Anaesth Soc J 26:305–308, 1979.

90. Finnoff JT, Hurdle MF, Smith J: Accuracy of ultrasound-guided versus fluoroscopically guided contrast-controlled piriformis injections: a cadaveric study. J Ultrasound Med 27:1157–1163, 2008.

91. Gonzalez P, Pepper M, Sullivan W, Akuthota V: Confirmation of needle placement within the piriformis muscle of a cadaveric specimen using anatomic landmarks and fluoroscopic guidance. Pain Physician 11:327–331, 2008.

92. Herring SA: Rehabilitation of muscle injuries. Med Sci Sports Exerc 22:453–456, 1990.

93. Vleeming A, Buyruk HM, Stoeckart R, et al: An integrated therapy for peripartum pelvic instability: a study of the biomechanical effects of pelvic belts. Am J Obstet Gynecol 166:1243–1247, 1992.

94. Rosenberg JM, Quint TJ, de Rosayro AM: Computerized tomographic localization of clinically-guided sacroiliac joint injections. Clin J Pain 16:18–21, 2000.

95. Slipman CW, Lipetz JS, Plastaras CT, et al: Fluoroscopically guided therapeutic sacroiliac joint injections for sacroiliac joint syndrome. Am J Phys Med Rehabil 80:425–432, 2001.

96. Betts A: Combined fluoroscopic and nerve stimulator technique for injection of the piriformis muscle. Pain Physician 7:279–281, 2004.

97. Fishman SM, Caneris OA, Bandman TB, et al: Injection of the piriformis muscle by fluoroscopic and electromyographic guidance. Reg Anesth Pain Med 23:554–559, 1998.

98. Vaccaro JP, Sauser DD, Beals RK: Iliopsoas bursa imaging: efficacy in depicting abnormal iliopsoas tendon motion in patients with internal snapping hip syndrome. Radiology 197:853–856, 1995.

99. Peng PW, Tumber PS: Ultrasound-guided interventional procedures for patients with chronic pelvic pain: a description of techniques and review of literature. Pain Physician 11:215–224, 2008.

100. Pekkafahli MZ, Kiralp MZ, Basekim CC, et al: Sacroiliac joint injections performed with sonographic guidance. J Ultrasound Med 22:553–559, 2003.

101. Filler AG, Haynes J, Jordan SE, et al: Sciatica of nondisc origin and piriformis syndrome: diagnosis by magnetic resonance neurography and interventional magnetic resonance imaging with outcome study of resulting treatment. J Neurosurg Spine 2:99–115, 2005.

102. Loubser PG: Epidural phenol administration for iliopsoas hypertonicity. Anesth Analg 80:639–640, 1995.

103. Nunley RM, Wilson JM, Gilula L, et al: Iliopsoas bursa injections can be beneficial for pain after total hip arthroplasty. Clin Orthop Relat Res 2009.

104. Gordon EJ: Trochanteric bursitis and tendinitis. Clin Orthop Relat Res 20:193–202, 1961.

105. Krout RM, Anderson TP: Trochanteric bursitis: management. Arch Phys Med Rehabil 40:8–14, 1959.

106. Akpinar S, Hersekli MA, Demirors H, et al: Effects of methylprednisolone and betamethasone injections on the rotator cuff: an experimental study in rats. Adv Ther 19:194–201, 2002.

107. Childers MK, Wilson DJ, Gnatz SM, et al: Botulinum toxin type A use in piriformis muscle syndrome: a pilot study. Am J Phys Med Rehabil 81:751–759, 2002.

108. Fish DE, Chang WS: Treatment of iliopsoas tendinitis after a left total hip arthroplasty with botulinum toxin type A. Pain Physician 10:565–571, 2007.

109. Fishman LM, Anderson C, Rosner B: BOTOX and physical therapy in the treatment of piriformis syndrome. Am J Phys Med Rehabil 81:936–942, 2002.

110. Yoon SJ, Ho J, Kang HY, et al: Low-dose botulinum toxin type A for the treatment of refractory piriformis syndrome. Pharmacotherapy 27:657–665, 2007.

111. Porta M: A comparative trial of botulinum toxin type A and methylprednisolone for the treatment of myofascial pain syndrome and pain from chronic muscle spasm. Pain 85:101–105, 2000.

112. Fullerton BD: High-resolution ultrasound and magnetic resonance imaging to document tissue repair after prolotherapy: a report of 3 cases. Arch Phys Med Rehabil 89:377–385, 2008.

113. Paoloni JA, Orchard JW: The use of therapeutic medications for soft-tissue injuries in sports medicine. Med J Aust 183:384–388, 2005.

114. Hammond JW, Hinton RY, Curl LA, et al: Use of autologous platelet-rich plasma to treat muscle strain injuries. Am J Sports Med 37:1135–1142, 2009.

115. Lyras DN, Kazakos K, Verettas D, et al: The influence of platelet-rich plasma on angiogenesis during the early phase of tendon healing. Foot Ankle Int 30:1101–1106, 2009.

116. Virchenko O, Aspenberg P: How can one platelet injection after tendon injury lead to a stronger tendon after 4 weeks? Interplay between early regeneration and mechanical stimulation. Acta Orthop 77:806–812, 2006.

117. Borg-Stein J, Zaremski J, Hanford M: New concepts in the assessment and treatment of regional musculoskeletal pain and sports injury. PM R 1:744–754, 2009.

118. DeRosa C: Functional anatomy of the lumbar spine and sacroiliac joint. Paper presented at 4th Interdisciplinary World Congress on Low Back and Pelvic Pain, Montreal, Canada, November 2001.

119. Williams BS, Cohen SP: Greater trochanteric pain syndrome: a review of anatomy, diagnosis and treatment. Anesth Analg 108:1662–1670, 2009.

120. Vleeming A, de Vries HJ, Mens JM, van Wingerden JP: Possible role of the long dorsal sacroiliac ligament in women with peripartum pelvic pain. Acta Obstet Gynecol Scand 81:430–436, 2002.

BIBLIOGRAPHY

Akpinar S, Hersekli MA, Demirors H, et al: Effects of methylprednisolone and betamethasone injections on the rotator cuff: an experimental study in rats. Adv Ther 19:194–201, 2002.

Beatty RA: The piriformis muscle syndrome: a simple diagnostic maneuver. Neurosurgery 34:512–514, 1994; discussion 514.

Byrd JW, Jones KS: Diagnostic accuracy of clinical assessment, magnetic resonance imaging, magnetic resonance arthrography, and intra-articular injection in hip arthroscopy patients. Am J Sports Med 32:1668–1674, 2004.

Cohen SP, Narvaez JC, Lebovits AH, Stojanovic MP: Corticosteroid injections for trochanteric bursitis: is fluoroscopy necessary? A pilot study. Br J Anaesth 94:100–106, 2005.

Hallin RP: Sciatic pain and the piriformis muscle. Postgrad Med 74:69–72, 1983.

Prather H, Hunt D: Conservative management of low back pain. Part I. Sacroiliac joint pain. Dis Mon 50:670–683, 2004.

Prather H: Sacroiliac joint pain: practical management. Clin J Sport Med 13:252–255, 2003.

Snijders CJ, Slagter AH, van Strik R, et al: Why leg crossing? The influence of common postures on abdominal muscle activity. Spine 20:1989–1993, 1995.

SECTION V

PEDIATRIC HIP DISORDERS

CHAPTER 40

Hip Dysplasia in the Child and Adolescent

Darin Davidson and Young-Jo Kim

KEY POINTS

- Developmental dysplasia of the hip represents a spectrum of severity of involvement of the hip.
- A high degree of clinical suspicion can allow for early diagnosis of acetabular dysplasia.
- Early treatment of acetabular dysplasia can be effective in preventing later sequelae.
- Treatment of acetabular dysplasia in the older child or adolescent requires invasive treatment and is associated with a high risk of complications.

INTRODUCTION

Developmental dysplasia of the hip (DDH) is an idiopathic condition that presents as a continuum of hip instability, which may affect children and adolescents. Newborn or young DDH presents as a spectrum from hip joint laxity to dislocation (Fig. 40-1), which may be reducible or irreducible. In older children and adolescents, DDH is associated with variable components of acetabular dysplasia, proximal femoral abnormality, and ligamentous laxity. Acetabular dysplasia is characterized by a globally shallow acetabulum with a steep acetabular roof. Proximal femoral abnormalities consist of varying degrees of coxa valga and anteversion. Varying degrees of subluxation of the femoral head from the acetabulum are present. Some degree of ligamentous laxity in the affected hip joint is universal before treatment, and generalized ligamentous laxity is common. In addition to the primary anatomic abnormalities associated with DDH, a variety of secondary deformities may occur after local growth disturbances following treatment.

EPIDEMIOLOGY

Prevalence

The prevalence of DDH has been difficult to ascertain because of the wide spectrum of the disorder. The overall prevalence of dislocation has been reported to be 1.4 per 1000 live births, the prevalence of clinical findings consistent with acetabular dysplasia has been 2.3 per 1000 live births, and the prevalence of ultrasound abnormalities has been 8 per 100 live births.[1] In addition, wide variation in prevalence among various ethnic groups has been recognized, ranging from 0.1 per 1000 live births in a Hong Kong population[2] to 188.5 per 1000 live births in a Native Canadian population.[3] Further complicating these estimates are the cases of subtle acetabular dysplasia not presenting until adolescence or adulthood and, therefore, not included in prevalence studies of infant DDH.

Risk Factors

Risk factors associated with infant DDH have been well studied. This condition most likely is multifactorial in nature. Implicated predisposing factors include ligamentous laxity, prenatal positioning, postnatal positioning, and genetic factors. Additional implicated factors are first born, female sex, and a history of oligohydramnios.[4-6] The left hip has been affected more commonly in unilateral cases, possibly owing to left hip adduction in the most common intrauterine position of the occiput anterior.[5,6]

Prenatal positioning has been associated with DDH. Early studies demonstrated that 16% of newborns with DDH were born in a breech position,[7] and this risk increased to 20% in a frank breech position.[8] According to Dunn,[5,6] it is the intrauterine position, not necessarily the breech position during birth, that is responsible for elevated risk of DDH because the prevalence of DDH among those in a breech position born via cesarean section was not found to be decreased. Postnatal positioning of newborns has been demonstrated to increase the risk of DDH on the basis of increased prevalence among populations who use cradleboards.[9,10] Klisic and associates[11] reported a 65% decrease in DDH attributed to an intervention with positioning newborns in hip abduction, instead of adduction. Other postural abnormalities have been associated with DDH, with the underlying proposed mechanism of so-called *packaging disorders*. Torticollis has been thought to coexist with DDH in 15% to 20% of cases.[12] Metatarsus adductus has been associated with DDH in 1.5% to 10% of cases.[13,14] Contradicting these so-called *packaging phenomena* has been the lack of association between clubfoot and DDH.[15,16]

PATHOPHYSIOLOGY

Normal hip development is a complex process, both during the embryonic phase and postnatally. Its details

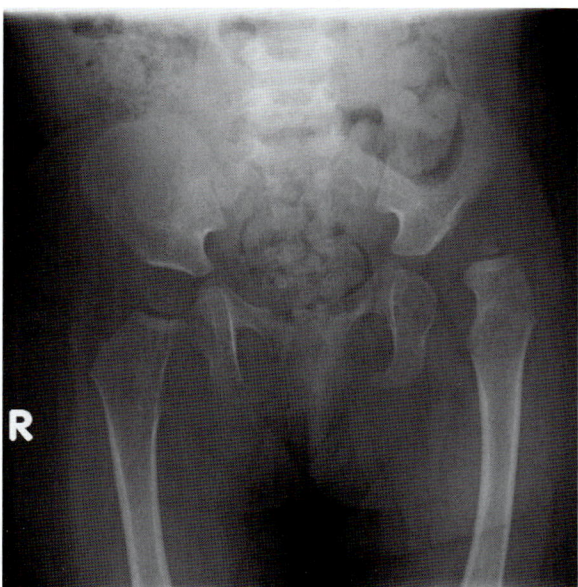

Figure 40-1. An anteroposterior radiograph demonstrating left hip dislocation in a 16-month-old female.

are beyond the scope of this chapter, and interested readers are directed to other sources.[1,17] Hip dysplasia represents a spectrum of pathophysiologic and anatomic abnormalities that, although initially potentially reversible, tend to become more severe and less correctable over time.[1,17] Bony deformity in infant DDH is believed to be due to lack of normal mechanical forces in and around the joint, plus the application of abnormal mechanical forces on the elements of a joint with varying degrees of instability and subluxation. In the newborn with DDH, the capsule is lax and the posterosuperior acetabular rim may be abnormal, allowing the femoral head to subluxate or dislocate. Over time, the rim can become thickened and develops into the so-called *neolimbus* as the result of pressure exerted by the femoral head.[18] If a newborn unstable hip becomes and remains persistently dislocated, secondary obstacles to reduction usually develop, including a fibrofatty pulvinar, hypertrophic ligamentum teres, a thickened transverse acetabular ligament, an inverted or hourglass labrum and cartilaginous acetabulum, and an interposed iliopsoas tendon. Complete reduction of the hip can allow for acetabular remodeling with further growth, with earlier improved restoration of normal containment. If, however, the hip is persistently dislocated or subluxated, certain characteristic bony changes tend to develop and become permanent, including the characteristic flattening of the acetabular roof, thickening of the medial acetabular wall, and, in the case of frank dislocation, development of a false acetabulum.

NATURAL HISTORY

The natural history of the unstable hip in the newborn is difficult to ascertain, in part because of the difficulty involved in defining an unstable hip. Barlow[19] initially suggested that 60% of subluxatable or dislocatable hips resolved by 1 week and 88% by 2 months. Coleman[9] reported resolution of only 5 of 23 unstable hips, illustrating a wide-ranging understanding of the natural history.

The natural history of persistent acetabular dysplasia includes progressive premature degeneration of the hip joint with the onset of osteoarthritis due to abnormal concentrations of mechanical hip joint forces on a decreased contact area. Wiberg[20] defined abnormal femoral coverage as a center edge angle less than 25 degrees, which would lead to eventual osteoarthritis. Cooperman and associates[21] reported that all dysplastic hips with a center edge angle less than 20 degrees developed osteoarthritis by 22 years' follow-up. However, the onset of osteoarthritis was difficult to predict unless the hip was subluxated. Subluxation clearly worsens the prognosis greatly, no matter what the degree of acetabular dysplasia. Murphy and colleagues[22] reported a study of the contralateral hip among 286 patients who were treated with total hip arthroplasty for osteoarthritis due to acetabular dysplasia. They found that all hips with good function at 65 years of age were associated with a center edge angle greater than 16 degrees.

CLINICAL FINDINGS/PHYSICAL EXAMINATION

Typical physical examination findings associated with DDH depend, to some extent, upon the age of the child and the degree of instability and deformity. In the newborn period, usually up to 2 to 3 months of age, Barlow and Ortolani tests are performed. The Barlow test is a gentle test of stability, performed by adducting each hip sequentially and applying a posteriorly directed force. This test assesses the ability to subluxate or dislocate the hip. The Ortolani test is a test that assesses reducibility. It attempts to reduce the dislocated hip, and for this reason it is best performed before the Barlow test. It is performed by abducting the flexed hip with an anteriorly directed force applied at the level of the greater trochanter. These signs usually are not detectable, even in an unstable hip, after the age of 2 to 3 months. Note that the absence of a Barlow or Ortolani sign is no guarantee that a hip is normal. An irreducible dislocated hip will show neither sign!!

In the child older than 2 or 3 months of age with an unstable or dislocated hip, the ipsilateral adductor muscles tend to shorten, and some limitation of abduction is often present. In the older than 3 month age group, often Barlow and Ortolani signs are absent, but the limitation of motion will remain. Asymmetrical range of motion is suggestive of an abnormality, but the possibility of bilateral involvement must always be considered.

The Galeazzi sign is elicited by noting limb length discrepancy while flexing both hips and knees to approximately 90 degrees and comparing the relative levels of the knees. It is present if shortening of one femur is apparent. It is important to be aware of the possibility of bilateral hip dislocations, in which case hip abduction can be decreased bilaterally but symmetrical and the Galeazzi sign negative. The Klisic test can be of use to delineate this situation and is performed by placement of the index finger on the anterior superior iliac spine and the middle finger on the greater trochanter. A line between these two points should intersect the umbilicus if the hip is reduced and will be inferior to this if dislocated.

In the older child with a complete hip dislocation or high-grade subluxation, physical findings may include a limb length discrepancy with the shorter leg being the affected side, a positive Galeazzi sign, increased lumbar lordosis, usually related to hip flexion contractures, and decreased range of hip abduction in the dislocated hip. The hip with a complete dislocation usually is hypermobile in childhood, especially in rotation.

By midchildhood, certain symptoms associated with hip dysplasia may occur and may be elicited by careful patient questioning. The earliest symptoms of hip dysplasia usual are reported as postactivity ache over the greater trochanter. Later symptoms often include activity-related groin pain as the overloaded acetabular rim and the labrum begin to fail. If the labrum tears, this could lead to mechanical symptoms of locking and catching, although this rarely occurs before the time of maturity. With the onset of osteoarthritis after maturity, the joint may have persistent aching pain as well as night pain.

IMAGING

Ultrasound

Ultrasound is the best imaging modality for assessing hip anatomy and stability during the first 6 months of life. Owing to the large cartilaginous component of the hip at this age, it is far superior to radiography. Graf[23] was the first to quantify measurements to describe the anatomy of the newborn hip. The alpha angle represents the angle between the bony acetabular roof and the aspect of the ilium where it intersects the bony and cartilaginous components of the acetabulum. A normal alpha angle is greater than 50 degrees from birth to about 3 months of age, and greater than 60 degrees after 3 months of physiologic age. The beta angle represents the intersection between the line along the lateral margin of the cartilaginous acetabulum and a line intersecting the bony and cartilaginous aspects of the acetabulum. A normal angle measures less than 55 degrees. With progressive severity of dysplasia, the alpha angle will decrease and the beta angle will increase. The percent of head coverage on the coronal image is another commonly measured parameter, with the fraction of the head medial to the iliac line read as a percent. Less than 40% coverage is subnormal. Ultrasonographic assessment is technician dependent both for clarity of images and for ensurance that the correct planes are scanned. Recent recommendations suggest that ultrasound is a useful modality for stratification of hips as normal, immature, having mild dysplasia, or having severe dysplasia[24] (Fig. 40-2).

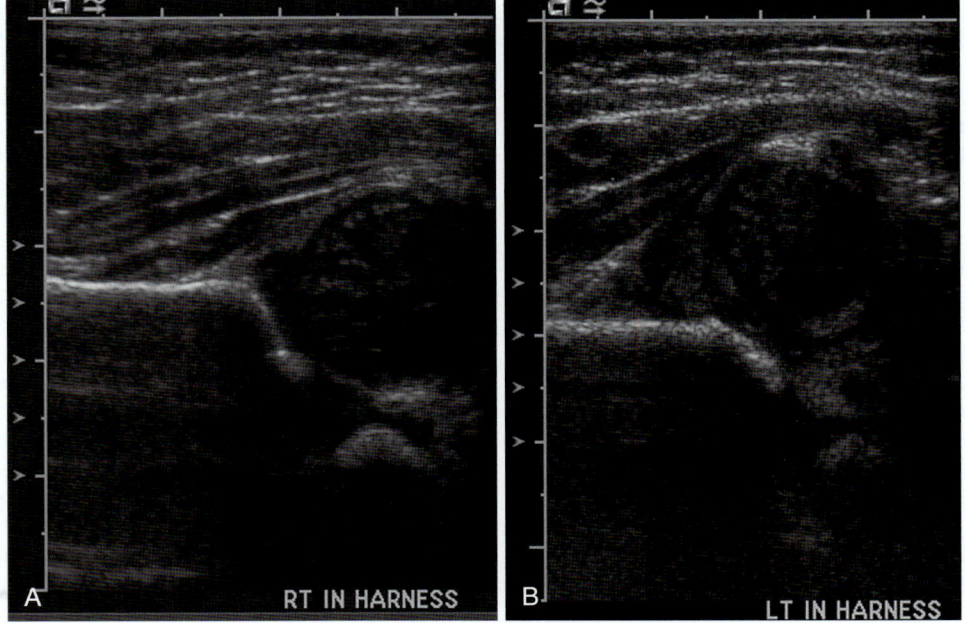

Figure 40-2. Ultrasound of both hips in a 7-week female. **A,** The right hip demonstrates a normal alpha angle and approximately 50% coverage of the femoral head. **B,** The left hip demonstrates a reduced alpha angle and a dislocated hip.

An alternative to the static ultrasound measurement of Graf is a dynamic ultrasound evaluation of the hip during performance of the Ortolani and Barlow tests with assessment of the extent of instability.[25] Using this method, 4 to 6 mm of motion is believed to be normal in the first few days of life; however, guidelines for normal motion in older children have not been developed.[25,26] Often, both static and dynamic methods are utilized. The general consensus in the literature is that ultrasound is a sensitive tool in assessment of the newborn hip.[24,27-29] The resulting concern is the potential for treatment of newborns who do not require treatment.

A current issue that has not received much attention in the literature concerns the ultrasound appearance and clinical assessment of the premature infant. Much has been reported regarding the natural history of improvement in clinical stability and ultrasound improvement of the newborn over the initial weeks of life; however, the natural history has been less well documented. Simic and associates[30] recently reported a study that attempted to investigate this issue. They studied 2045 newborns, 83% of whom were born prematurely at a mean gestational age of 34 weeks. They performed an ultrasound assessment and clinical evaluation of each hip and reported that 3.2% of all hips were unstable. They recommended early treatment of the unstable hip, even in the premature infant, by wide swaddling. No additional studies have explored the evaluation or treatment of premature infants.

Radiographs

Plain radiographs may demonstrate frank dislocation of the hips at any age, yet the largely cartilaginous nature of the hip before 6 months of age renders radiologic assessment generally inferior to ultrasound in this age group.[24] Typical radiographic evaluation of dysplasia requires a well-centered and nonrotated film to identify the following parameters: (1) Hilgenreiner's (horizontal) line between the triradiate cartilages bilaterally; (2) Perkin's line, represented by a vertical line at the lateral extent of the acetabulum; (3) Shenton's line along the inferior femoral neck and the inferior margin of the superior pubic ramus (Fig. 40-3) (Shenton's line should be smooth and should not be broken by more than a

millimeter); (4) the ossific nucleus of the femoral head, which, if present, should lie in the lower inner quadrant formed by the intersection of Hilgenreiner's and Perkin's lines; and (5) the acetabular teardrop, which is normally thinner centrally than proximally or distally. A V-shaped teardrop, which is wider proximally than distally, reflects abnormally deficient loading of the medial joint, which is a common component of the abnormal mechanics in a dysplastic hip.

Certain standard radiographic measures are important in describing the immature and mature hip. The acetabular index (AI) as a measure of the obliquity of the bony acetabular subchondral bone is useful to quantify the extent of dysplasia in the immature hip. The AI is the angle between Hilgenreiner's line, which is the horizontal line formed by connecting the triradiate cartilage, and a tangent to the acetabular articular surface (Fig. 40-4). The magnitude varies with age, with normal being less than 30 degrees in the newborn, less than 25 degrees by 1 year of age, and less than 20 degrees by 2 years of age.[1,17] The Tonnis angle, which is the analogue of the acetabular index in the skeletally mature hip, is the angle between the horizontal line formed by connecting the centers of both femoral heads and a tangent to the acetabular sourcil; a normal value is less than 15 degrees.[22,31] The lateral center edge angle of Wiberg is the angle between a vertical line from the center of the femoral head and a line from the center of the femoral head to the lateral edge of the acetabulum. A normal lateral center edge angle is greater than 20 degrees if the patient is younger than 13 years of age and is greater than 25 degrees in older patients.[1] The acetabular teardrop should be assessed and if widened is suggestive of abnormal loading of the acetabulum, as would occur in a subluxated or dislocated hip.

Arthrography

Arthrography employs contrast to outline the cartilaginous surfaces of the femoral head and acetabulum and to outline the labrum and the capsule. Radiopaque dye introduced percutaneously or during open surgery is usual, although air or carbon dioxide (CO_2) has been used in the past. The risks of gas embolism make the use of air or CO_2 relatively contraindicated. Arthrography is most commonly used intraoperatively for assessment of the quality of closed reduction. The so-called *rose thorn sign* represents the free border of the labrum

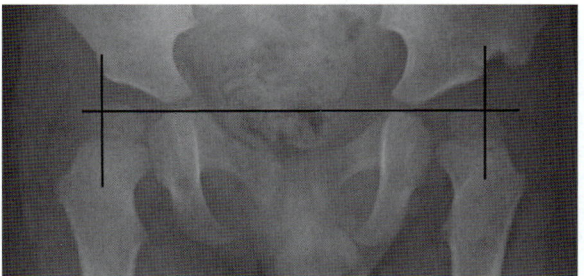

Figure 40-3. Radiographic demonstration of Hilgenreiner's line *(horizontal line)* and Perkin's line *(vertical line).* Note placement of the femoral heads in the lower inner quadrant, consistent with a reduced hip.

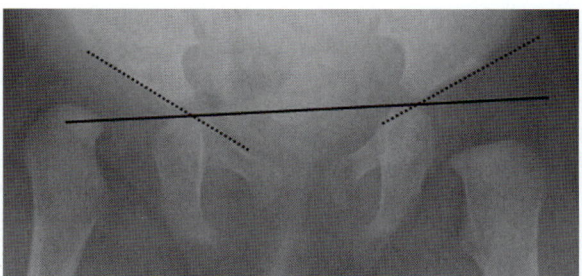

Figure 40-4. Radiographic demonstration of the acetabular index of both hips.

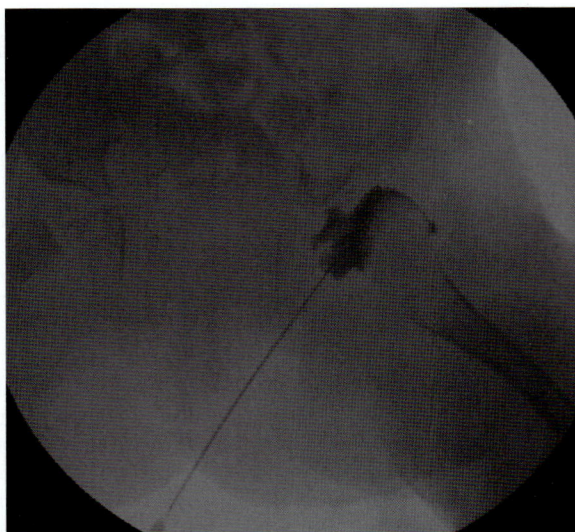

Figure 40-5. Arthrogram of a dislocated hip in a 17-month-old female. Note the increased medial dye pool, suggesting that the femoral head is not seated fully within the acetabulum.

and is a normal finding, if present.[1] Another feature visualized on the arthrogram is the depth of reduction. When the reduction is not sufficiently deep within the acetabulum, a medial dye pool will be seen. More than 6 mm of pooling[10] (Fig. 40-5) is considered abnormal.

Current recommendations for screening have been reported by the American Academy of Pediatrics.[33] The Academy has suggested, on the basis of available evidence, that each newborn should receive a physical examination of the hips performed by the pediatrician, and the child should be referred for orthopedic evaluation if any abnormality is detected. The Academy has recommended against routine screening with ultrasound. An ultrasound evaluation was recommended in the setting of a female infant with a history of breech positioning, and such an evaluation was determined to be optional in the setting of a female infant with a positive family history of DDH or a male baby with a history of breech presentation. In Germany, Austria, and Israel, every baby is screened routinely at 6 to 8 weeks of age with an ultrasound of the hips; this universal screening has reduced dramatically the incidence of later-presenting dislocations and the incidence of surgery in DDH, and it has been shown to be very cost-effective in those countries. Such universal infant hip screening by ultrasound has not been recommended in the general population in Canada and the United States.[24,34,35] Recently the benefits of any type of screening program for infant DDH have been questioned. Mahan and associates[35A] performed a decision analysis using the best evidence available and determined that the present universal physical examination screening with selective use of ultrasound screening was the optimal approach to minimizing the risk of development of hip osteoarthritis.

Screening studies have reported a prevalence of 7.7% with universal screening protocols, compared with 2.1%

with only a clinical screening program.[36,37] The recommendation in the literature is that universal screening does not impart additional benefit over selective screening because the prevalence of delayed acetabular dysplasia following selective screening was not found to be significantly greater than that following universal screening.[24,38,39]

TREATMENT

Stable Hip With Ultrasound Evidence of Dysplasia

Management of the hip that is clinically stable (Ortolani and Barlow negative) but has ultrasound evidence of dysplasia, in particular a borderline alpha angle of 50 to 60 degrees, has not been well described in the literature. Spontaneous improvement from deficient acetabular coverage diagnosed by ultrasound in the newborn period has been reported[1,19,40]; however, this has not translated into uniform recommendations regarding the time by which treatment should be instituted in the setting of a clinically stable hip with an abnormal ultrasound evaluation. Variation in recommendations regarding management of this clinical subgroup has been noted. Some clinicians institute treatment solely on the basis of the clinical evaluation without consideration of the ultrasound appearance; others advocate treatment, regardless of clinical stability, if the alpha angle is less than 50 degrees in the baby younger than 3 months old, and less than 60 degrees[1] in the child older than 3 months. Another option that has been suggested is to base treatment on the combination of clinical stability and the ultrasound appearance at 6 weeks of age, with treatment consisting of a Pavlik harness if any abnormality is observed at the time of this assessment.

Bialik and colleagues[40] studied the issue of overtreatment of initially abnormal hips in the newborn time period. Their study evaluated 8638 newborn hips by ultrasound soon after birth. Their protocol consisted of repeat clinical examination and ultrasound of those newborns with a stable hip at birth to 6 weeks of age. If the hips were unstable at birth, then the newborns were reassessed clinically and by ultrasound at 2 weeks of age. In either situation, a Pavlik harness was used for treatment if any abnormality was noted on assessment at the follow-up visit. Investigators reported that only 0.6% of hips studied required treatment. They did not encounter any complications as a result of delayed treatment using their protocol. This protocol has not been studied further in the literature.

Questions persist regarding patients with a clinically stable hip and an abnormal ultrasound. In particular, no definite recommendations have been put forth regarding management of the infant younger than 3 months of age with a borderline abnormal alpha angle of between 50 and 60 degrees. Similarly, whether treatment with a Pavlik harness or observation alone is necessary for the hip with an alpha angle less than 50 degrees or less than 30% acetabular coverage despite being clinically stable remains undetermined. It has been suggested, however, that if the hip is severely or moderately dysplastic with an alpha angle less than 50 degrees or with less than 30% coverage, then the hip should be treated with a Pavlik harness of an abduction brace. Furthermore, if the hip remains dysplastic beyond 3 months of life, then treatment should be initiated.

Serial imaging evaluation is extremely important in the dysplastic hip. Worsening of any abnormality and failure to improve with time represent relative indications to intervene or to change tactics.

Barlow-Positive Hip

Management of the Barlow-positive, Ortolani-negative hip in the newborn is controversial. Given the natural history of spontaneous improvement in the first few weeks of life,[1,19,40] variation has been seen in current practice regarding the need for immediate commencement of treatment in this population. Such newborns can be reassessed both clinically and with an ultrasound before bracing treatment is begun at 2 weeks[40] or 6 weeks.[1] If any persistent abnormality is observed clinically or on ultrasound, treatment is instituted.[1,40] The most common treatment recommendations include treatment with the Pavlik harness on a full-time basis until the hip stabilizes and the ultrasound normalizes, followed by a weaning period. Ongoing follow-up is then required to ensure both clinical and radiographic normalization of the hip. At present, the recommended follow-up period for these hips ranges from 1 year of life to skeletal maturity.

Ortolani-Positive Hip

If the hip is dislocated, a Pavlik harness usually is applied and close observation is required to ensure that the hip reduces. Initially, the child should be followed on a weekly basis to determine reduction of the hip, function of the femoral nerve, and proper fit of the Pavlik harness. The presence of femoral nerve dysfunction should be an indication for stopping the harness. If the hip does not reduce within 3 weeks of brace treatment, then the Pavlik harness should be stopped because of the risk of so-called *Pavlik harness disease*, caused by excessive pressure on the posterior acetabular wall.

The Pavlik harness is worn for a minimum of 6 weeks and generally is continued for 6 weeks after the hip is reduced, in cases where the hip is initially Ortolani positive. The success of harness treatment of a Barlow-positive hip has been correlated with a higher alpha angle on ultrasound, and irreducible hips were not treated successfully if the initial alpha angle measured less than 20 degrees.[41]

Results of treatment with the Pavlik harness have been generally good, with as high as 95% success[42] overall and of 80% with initially irreducible hips.[42] The overall proportion of avascular necrosis of the femoral head after Pavlik treatment of dislocated hips has been 2.4%,[42] ranging between 0 and 15%.[43,44] A recent study has suggested that factors associated with unsuccessful treatment with a Pavlik harness include an adduction contracture and high dislocation.[45] The predominant failures of Pavlik harness treatment include failure to reduce a dislocated hip and failure of stabilization of a subluxatable hip. Complications such as femoral nerve palsy and Pavlik harness disease[1,17] can occur, in addition to treatment failure. Pavlik harness disease was first described by Jones and colleagues[46] and consists of flattening of the posterosuperior acetabular wall caused by excessive pressure from the femoral head. This can be avoided by stopping use of the Pavlik harness if a dislocated hip does not reduce over a maximum of 3 to 4 weeks of treatment.

Failed Pavlik Treatment

In the situation of a dislocated hip that fails to reduce after 2 to 4 weeks, the Pavlik harness should be discontinued. Other treatment options should be considered, including closed reduction and hip spica casting. Alternatively, the use of abduction bracing has been advocated in this situation; one study reported successful outcomes in 13 of 15 hips (87%).[47] Before beginning treatment with an abduction brace, it is necessary to confirm reducibility of the hip by physical examination or by ultrasound. In the event that neither Pavlik harness nor abduction brace treatment is effective in obtaining or maintaining a reduction, formal closed or open reduction is necessary. The timing of closed reduction in this situation is affected by the risk of anesthesia in children younger than 4 to 6 months. Typically, if a general anesthetic is required, it can be delayed until this time to minimize the risk of general anesthesia.

Closed Reduction of a Dislocated Hip

Closed reduction has been associated with a higher general risk of osteonecrosis than is seen with brace treatment or open reduction. It is used less commonly than in the past, likely for several reasons. Diagnosis of DDH in most countries usually is made earlier than in the past because of increased awareness and improved screening, leading to greater numbers of dysplastic hips being managed successfully by bracing.

For the dislocated hip first diagnosed after the age of 6 months but before 1 year of age, closed reduction often is a first choice. Management with the Pavlik harness will not likely achieve reduction, and other methods of treatment are almost always necessary. Treatment options in this age group include closed or open reduction, usually accompanied by soft tissue releases. These treatment options are also necessary in the setting of failure to obtain or maintain reduction with a Pavlik harness or an abduction brace. Controversy continues regarding reduction before the appearance of the femoral head ossific nucleus. Some authors have advocated that reduction be delayed until its appearance owing to increased risk of avascular necrosis of the femoral head before its appearance.[48,49] Others have suggested that no increased risk of avascular necrosis of the femoral head is associated with reduction before the appearance of the ossific nucleus.[50,51] No consensus has been reached regarding the timing of reduction. Although used historically, traction before reduction is no longer recommended[52-54] by most authors.

The initial attempt at acute reduction should be performed in the operating room with the patient under a general anesthetic. With good muscular relaxation and with the baby placed supine on a radiolucent table, the surgeon should assess reducibility, stability, and the range of passive hip motion. Any tightness of the adductors, which is nearly universal, should be noted. The classic reduction maneuver is passive hip flexion to greater than 90 degrees, with abduction and anterior lifting of the greater trochanter with the fingers. The maneuver is identical to the Ortolani test.

Any sense of reduction must be confirmed by imaging because partial reduction or even reduction into a false acetabulum can be accompanied by an Ortolani-like clunk. An apparent flexion contracture of the ipsilateral knee may be noted after a true reduction because the ipsilateral hamstrings are commonly shortened. Well-recognized adductor longus tightness is more apparent if the hip is truly reduced.

The safe zone defined by the range between maximum abduction and the degree of adduction at which the hip re-dislocates[55] is the position of casting after reduction. Sometimes no "safe zone" exists; in these cases, the hip is irreducible and open reduction must be considered. A decreased safe zone, that is, less than 30 degrees, indicates the need for a percutaneous adductor longus tenotomy to improve the stability of the reduction. Note that the presence of an anatomic safe zone with the patient under anesthesia guarantees neither anatomic hip stability when muscle tone returns after the patient awakens nor that the precarious blood supply to the femoral head remains sufficient.

An arthrogram may be obtained to assess the quality and depth of reduction. A medial approach for spinal needle placement is preferred for the arthrogram, to minimize the risk of anterior obscuring of the quality of reduction by anterior extravasation of dye. In the best reduction, the femoral head lies below the labrum, and almost all contrast lies lateral to the head, with minimal medial dye pooling. Less than 5 mm of medial dye pool is usually present in association with a stable "deep concentric" reduction. More than 6 mm of medial dye pooling often indicates an unstable and incomplete reduction.[10] The so-called *rose thorn* sign, representing the free labral edge outlined with contrast, helps one to determine the important relationship of the femoral head to the labrum.[1]

The closed reduction must be anatomically adequate with regard to quality of reduction. It also must be mechanically stable, with a safe zone greater than 30 degrees but not requiring more than 50 degrees of abduction. Excessive hip abduction has been associated with the development of avascular necrosis.

If the closed reduction satisfies these stringent conditions, the child should be placed in a hip spica cast, with the hip carefully maintained in the "safe" position. This position usually is in approximately 100 or more degrees of flexion, neutral rotation, and abduction in the middle of the safe zone. The cast must be skillfully applied and well fitted. The best reduction may be lost if casting is suboptimal.

Biplanar imaging is essential, both before the child is awakened and afterward. Magnetic resonance imaging (MRI) is optimal because it can confirm the reduction in three dimensions and allow visualization of cartilage and labrum, and it can be used to assess the blood supply to the head. Some centers do the reduction in an operating room with MRI capability to confirm reduction (Fig. 40-6). A limited computed tomography scan can be used to confirm reduction of the hip, but MRI offers the advantages of avoiding ionizing radiation and providing additional information regarding the vascularity of the head.[56] In a recent important study, perfusion MRI was performed following closed reduction. On follow-up, 21% of hips developed clinically important avascular necrosis of the femoral head. Of these, 50% demonstrated globally decreased perfusion of the femoral head on MRI, whereas only 2 of 22 hips that did not develop avascular necrosis had similar changes. Although preliminary in nature, this study demonstrated an additional important use of MRI. The value of MRI in predicting residual acetabular dysplasia following hip reduction was reported in a study comparing 13 hips with resolved DDH by 4 years of age versus 5 that required pelvic osteotomy.[57] Although the study

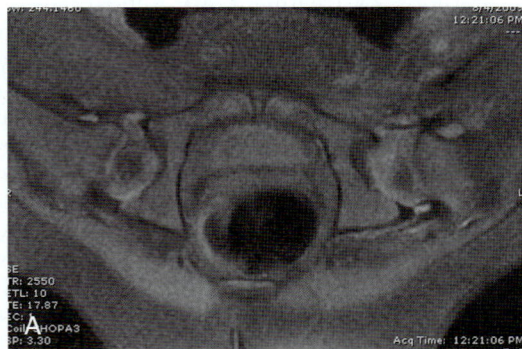
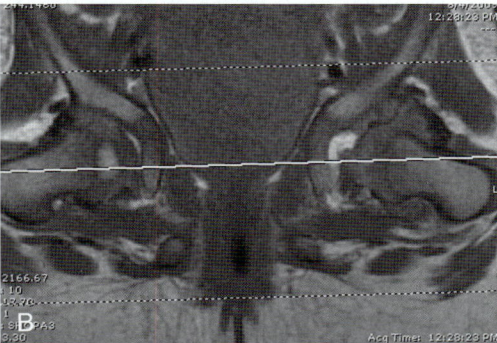

Figure 40-6. Magnetic resonance imaging following closed reduction of the left hip in a 16-month-old female, demonstrating reduction of the hip in **(A)** axial and **(B)** coronal planes.

was limited by small numbers, no MRI findings were predictive of the likelihood of residual dysplasia requiring future osteotomy.

The hip spica cast is utilized for a minimum of 3 months, with cast changes under general anesthesia provided at 4- to 6-week intervals. The spica cast is extended proximally at least to the nipple line and distally at least to the ankle on the dislocated side. Maintenance of satisfactory reduction must be confirmed at the time of each cast change while the child is still under anesthesia.

A rough rule of thumb used by some centers for judging the duration of immobilization after closed reduction involves the age in months at which the reduction is done, with a minimum of 3 months. Therefore if closed reduction is achieved at 5 months of age, the time of cast immobilization required may be as long as 5 months. Following the period of full casting, weaning to a bivalve cast, to part-time casting, or to abduction bracing is usual, although protocols vary widely.

Open Reduction

Open reduction offers the most direct way to eliminate obstacles to reduction. Open reduction also allows establishment of some soft tissue stability to supplement that which can come from bony realignment and from the external stability of a spica cast. Open reduction should be performed if a stable closed reduction cannot be obtained in the operating room, or if subsequent loss of reduction occurs while in the hip spica cast. In children of walking age, it should be considered strongly as a primary intervention because closed reduction in this age group is likely to be unsatisfactory.

Both medial and anterior approaches have been described and are used for open reduction. Whichever approach is used, the obstacles to reduction must be eliminated to allow a concentric and stable reduction. These anatomic obstacles may include fibrofatty pulvinar, hypertrophic ligamentum teres, a thickened transverse acetabular ligament, an inverted labrum, and an hourglass anteromedial capsular constriction with interposed psoas tendon. Each approach offers advantages and disadvantages.

The medial approach is used frequently in children younger than 1 year; it offers the advantage of more direct access to inframedial obstacles to reduction. Disadvantages of this approach include an inability to perform a formal capsulorrhaphy and the potentially higher risk of avascular necrosis. The classic anterior approach, through the sartorius-tensor interval of Smith-Petersen, is used typically in children older than 1 year, after failed open or closed surgery, or in any situation in which an extensile approach to the hip is required. Advantages of the anterior approach include an ability to perform a formal capsulorrhaphy and an ability to perform pelvic osteotomy through the same incision. A relative disadvantage of the extensive nature of the anterior approach compared with medial approaches consists of increased blood loss and less direct access to the inferomedial capsule and joint. If a concomitant pelvic osteotomy is to be performed, the anterior approach is highly preferred, except in the rare instance where some advantage may come from combining the two approaches.

Following open reduction, a hip spica cast for supplemental stability is applied for a minimum of 6 to 12 weeks, or longer, depending on the severity of the dysplasia and the degree of residual instability present at the end of the surgical procedure. The position of greatest stability is chosen—typically in slight flexion, abduction, and neutral to slight internal rotation. The results of open reduction have been reported as good in up to 76% of cases, and a secondary procedure was required in 26%.[58] A recent study of the medial approach for open reduction of the hip in 24 patients with a mean age of 4.8 months and with mean follow-up of 59 months was reported.[59] At the most recent follow-up, all hips were clinically normal, and the acetabular index was within normal limits. The authors reported that neither the age of the child nor the presence of the proximal femoral ossific nucleus affected the outcome (Fig. 40-7).

An important consideration in the child of walking age or older who requires open reduction is the frequent need for bony realignment of the proximal femur and/or acetabulum to correct secondary bony deformity. Leaving extensive bony deformity uncorrected can seriously compromise the stability of even the best open reduction, particularly in the older child with a long-standing dislocation. A proximal femoral shortening osteotomy may allow for a stable reduction of the hip while alleviating excessive pressure on the femoral head in the reduced position, which may be a causative factor of avascular necrosis. The need for both pelvic osteotomy and femoral osteotomy should be considered preoperatively and evaluated intraoperatively. If femoral anteversion is excessive, this can contribute to instability. In this situation, derotation can be combined with shortening at the time of osteotomy.

Treatment of children older than 2 years is more difficult because of generally more severe contractures, greater secondary bony deformity than in younger children with DDH, and decreased remodeling potential following reduction. Remodeling of the acetabulum after concentric reduction can continue up to approximately

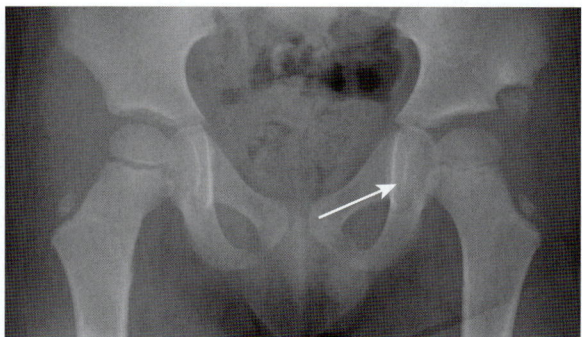

Figure 40-7. Radiographic demonstration of a successful outcome following open reduction of the left hip at 66 months following open reduction. Note the narrow teardrop *(arrow)* and the intact Shenton's line.

8 years of age, with the greatest improvement noted in the first 18 months following reduction but with continued remodeling for 4 years following reduction.[54,60,61] This potential for acetabular remodeling has led some to suggest femoral osteotomy as the first choice for osteotomy in the child who requires bony realignment at the time of open reduction. Others have proposed that pelvic osteotomy is necessary if open reduction is performed in a child older than 18 months, because of insufficient remodeling potential.[62-64] The most frequently utilized osteotomies in this setting are the Salter and the Pemberton. Potential complications of combined pelvic osteotomy and femoral shortening include posterior dislocation, particularly if the femur is derotated at the time of shortening.[1] Galpin and coworkers[65] reported good radiographic results in 66% of children, with a mean age of 4 years at the time of treatment and with avascular necrosis developing in 12%. Children who are older than 3 years at the time of open reduction frequently will require both acetabular and femoral osteotomy for several reasons. First, soft tissue contractures present in the older child with unreduced DDH usually render atraumatic reduction difficult without femoral shortening. Also, the severity of the dysplasia, caused by secondary deformity present in unreduced hips at this age and older, often makes stability difficult to achieve without realignment of both the acetabulum and the femur. Further, even if primary stability can be achieved in these older unreduced hips without primary osteotomy of both femur and pelvis, insufficient bony remodeling with open reduction alone almost always requires later osteotomy as a secondary procedure.

Controversy continues regarding the upper age limit for reduction of the dislocated hip. Current recommendations suggest that the unilateral hip dislocation should be reduced up to 9 to 10 years of age, and the bilateral dislocation up to 8 years of age.[1]

RESIDUAL ACETABULAR DYSPLASIA IN THE IMMATURE HIP

Even mild dysplasia can lead to osteoarthritis in adulthood, particularly if any subluxation is present. For this reason, every hip treated for developmental dysplasia must be followed though skeletal maturity, because recurrent dysplasia can occur even after early normalization of radiographic appearance, and mild, apparently resolving dysplasia can persist. As long as residual acetabular dysplasia is continuing to improve in the immature hip, it generally can be watched and treatment withheld. Any worsening of deformity in the older child should be treated by osteotomy, and any plateau in improvement of the residually dysplastic hip should put the treating physician on alert.

The acetabulum is thought to have the ability to remodel for up to 4 years after reduction, provided reduction occurred before 4 years of age.[66] After 4 years of age, the potential for acetabular remodeling is decreased, thereby increasing the likelihood for requirement of a pelvic osteotomy.[67-74] If acetabular dysplasia

is accompanied by major femoral deformity, consideration should be given to the need to address proximal femoral deformity with an osteotomy. It has been further suggested that an acetabular index greater than 35 degrees by 2 years after reduction is unlikely to sufficiently remodel.[75] Kim and associates[76] further noted that hip joint widening and an upsloping sourcil were predictive of the need for pelvic osteotomy in children older than 4 years. Residual acetabular dysplasia in the skeletally mature individual typically is characterized by the presence of anterolateral uncovering of the femoral head, coxa valga, and an anteverted proximal femur.[77] Furthermore, the magnitude of residual dysplasia exists on a spectrum and may include the presence of labral hypertrophy, labral tearing, and fatigue fracture of the acetabular rim.[77]

Evaluation of the skeletally immature child with residual acetabular dysplasia includes a complete physical examination and radiographic evaluation, including anteroposterior, false profile, and von Rosen views. Radiographic parameters that should be considered specifically include Shenton's line and the shape and degree of widening of the teardrop. A normal teardrop is only a few millimeters wide and has a thin waist. A V-shaped or diffusely widened teardrop is an indicator that the acetabulum has not been stimulated sufficiently by a well-reduced femoral head.

The attitude of the femoral head and neck and the alignment and condition of the capital femoral physis are important to hip function and prognosis. The presence of lateral proximal femoral growth arrest should be considered because this may lead to residual subluxation and a less than satisfactory outcome unless compensation is provided for its presence.

Treatment options for residual deformity in the previously reduced hip depend on the pathoanatomy of the acetabulum and the proximal femur. Proximal femoral deformity associated with DDH may cause anterior and or lateral subluxation due to coxa valga or excessive anteversion with resultant anterior undercoverage.[31,73,74] Femoral neck anteversion usually resolves following reduction[79]; however, if this does not occur, proximal femoral derotation, potentially combined with a varus-producing osteotomy, can be performed. The need for this is further suggested by disruption of Shenton's line.[17] Before a proximal femoral osteotomy is performed, it is necessary to confirm concentric hip reduction with an abduction, internal rotation radiograph.

Pelvic osteotomy for correction of residual acetabular dysplasia is performed not only to achieve or augment stability. It also is done to improve the biomechanics of the hip to correct and relieve mechanical overload of the acetabular rim to avoid or delay degenerative changes.[80] An increased acetabular index—greater than 28 degrees—particularly if it is not improving over time, suggests the need for a pelvic osteotomy. Pelvic osteotomy options depend on the age of the child and the extent of skeletal maturity. These osteotomies may be classified as complete or incomplete in extent and as redirectional or augmentation in type. Osteotomies that redirect the acetabulum consist of Salter, Dega-Pemberton, double pelvic, and triple

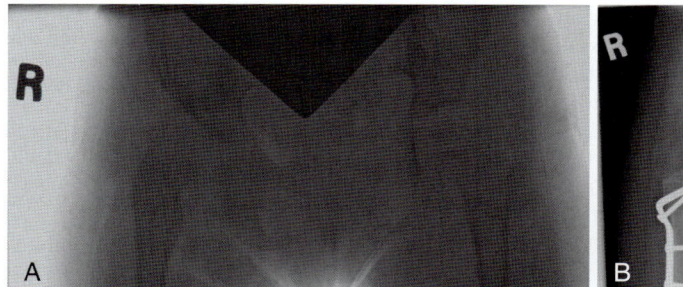
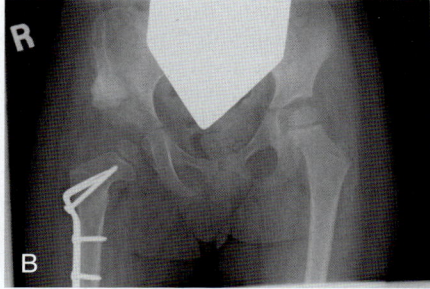

Figure 40-8. Dega osteotomy in the management of developmental hip dysplasia of the right hip. **A,** Preoperative antero-posterior radiograph in a 3-year-old female with a dislocated right hip and a dysplastic acetabulum. An open reduction with femoral varus osteotomy and Dega osteotomy was performed. **B,** Follow-up radiograph at 3 months of age shows reduction of the hip and healing of the Dega osteotomy in a position with an improved acetabular index.

pelvic osteotomies. Periacetabular and spherical oste-otomies are redirectional pelvic osteotomies, but they are contraindicated in the immature patient owing to the damage that these osteotomies would cause to the triradiate cartilage. The general principle is that oste-otomies closer to the joint have a greater corrective ability. Each of these requires a concentric hip reduc-tion, a congruous joint, and a sufficient hip range of motion. Each can be performed in skeletally immature hips. The Salter innominate osteotomy, which hinges on the pubic symphysis, is most likely to be of benefit in younger children with a center edge angle greater than 10 degrees.[17] Consideration of the extent and location of the acetabular deficiency is necessary as part of pre-operative planning and choosing the best osteotomy. The Salter osteotomy is more successful in younger children because of their increased remodeling poten-tial; 93% good to excellent results[81] were reported in one study, and in another study, 79% good results were reported among those younger than 3 years, but only 66% in those older than 4 years.[31] Some studies have reported less optimistic results, with one third of chil-dren with a subluxated hip and only one half of those with an initially dislocated hip experiencing a satisfac-tory result.[82] The long-term outcome following open reduction of the hip combined with a Salter osteotomy has been reported at 45-year follow-up.[83] In a series of 80 hips in 60 patients, survival, defined as conversion to total hip arthroplasty as the end point, was 99% at 30 years, 86% at 40 years, and 54% at 45 years. All patients were between the ages of 18 months and 5 years at the time of surgery, and the follow-up propor-tion was 79%. A total of 51 hips had available radio-graphs at the most recent follow-up, of which 38 (75%) had at least 2 mm of remaining joint space and 13 (25%) were indicative of osteoarthritis.

Complications following triple pelvic osteotomy and their impact on overall patient satisfaction have been investigated.[84] In a study of 61 hips treated at a median age of 23 years with a Tonnis triple pelvic osteotomy, good to excellent results were reported in 68% of the entire patient group; 8 hips (13%) required revision. Patient satisfaction was found to be influenced by the occurrence of complications, in particular, nonunion.

Complications were more common among older patients. The extent of acetabular correction did not influence overall patient satisfaction.

Incomplete osteotomies include Pemberton and Dega osteotomies, which hinge on the triradiate cartilage (Fig. 40-8). These offer the potential advantage of decreasing acetabular volume and increasing both ante-rior and lateral acetabular coverage. A further advan-tage of these osteotomies, in comparison with the Salter innominate osteotomy, is the ability to tailor to some degree the extent of anterior and lateral coverage to the location of the acetabular deficiency. A recent report on the Dega osteotomy in 26 hips with a DDH, of which 54% were dislocated and 31% subluxated, indicated a mean 22-degree improvement in the acetabular index.[85] Mean age at the time of surgery was 3 years, and complica-tions included lateralization of the femoral head in 8% and avascular necrosis of the femoral head in 8%. An MRI study of the acetabular volume of patients with a previous Dega osteotomy for treatment of DDH demon-strated an increase in the volume of the acetabulum following osteotomy,[86] which contrasts with the concept of decreased acetabular volume following Dega and Pemberton osteotomies.

The third group of pelvic osteotomies involve bony augmentation. They are considered as salvage proce-dures that rely upon cartilage metaplasia of the capsule under a shelf. This group includes the classic Shelf and Chiari osteotomies. These procedures are uncommonly performed in the primary management of acetabular dysplasia but may be considered in the salvage situation.

Complications

Serious complications associated with treatment of DDH include avascular necrosis (AVN) of the femoral head with related growth disturbances, re-dislocation, and osteoarthritis (OA), although it may be best to con-sider OA as a consequence of DDH itself, rather than of its treatment. AVN has been reported as occurring in less than 5% of cases.[1] The true incidence of AVN is dif-ficult to determine. Different studies have utilized various definitions of AVN. The risk of AVN has been reported to be as high as 73%[17] in some series. A commonly mentioned factor associated with AVN is excessive pressure on the femoral head following reduction. This factor is potentially preventable by avoiding extreme positions of immobilization and by using femoral shortening osteotomy if excessive transarticular pressure seems present in the hip position required to maintain reduction.[1] Tension on the sensitive extraosseous vasculature to the femoral head is clearly an additional related causative factor in AVN.

The diagnosis of AVN has been defined as any of the following: failure of femoral head ossification and growth by 1 year following reduction, widening of the femoral neck, abnormal bone density of the femoral head, and residual deformity, including lateral physeal arrest, which usually is apparent only in adolescents.[76,87-90] The most widely utilized classification was reported by Salter and colleagues[89] and combines these findings. Class 1 is characterized by failure of the ossific nucleus to appear by 1 year after reduction, class 2 is indicated by failure of growth of the femoral head by 1 year after reduction, class 3 by widening of the femoral neck by 1 year after reduction, class 4 by increased bone density of the femoral head and fragmentation, and class 5 by residual deformity after reossification. Although no specific treatment for avascular necrosis of the femoral head is known, several options are available for its sequelae. Epiphysiodesis of the greater trochanter can be performed to prevent overgrowth, usually at between 5 and 8 years of age.[91,92] An alternative approach consists of advancement of the greater trochanter if an abduction limp has developed and the child is older than 8 years.[93]

REFERENCES

1. Herring JA: Developmental dysplasia of the hip. In Herring JA (ed): Tachdjian's pediatric orthopaedics, ed 4, Philadelphia, 2008, Saunders, Elsevier, pp 637–770.
2. Hoaglund FT, Kalamchi A, Poon R, et al: Congenital hip dislocation and dysplasia in Southern Chinese. Int Orthop 4:243–246, 1981.
3. Walker J: A preliminary investigation of congenital hip disease in the Island Lake Reserve population, Manitoba. Winnipeg: University of Manitoba; 1973.
4. Carter CO, Wilkinson JA: Genetic and environmental factors in the etiology of congenital dislocation of the hip. Clin Orthop Relat Res 33:119–128, 1964.
5. Dunn PM: The anatomy and pathology of congenital dislocation of the hip. Clin Orthop Relat Res 119:23–27, 1976.
6. Dunn PM: Perinatal observations on the etiology of congenital dislocation of the hip. Clin Orthop Relat Res 119:11–22, 1976.
7. Muller GM, Seddon HJ: Late results of treatment of congenital dislocation of the hip. J Bone Joint Surg Br 35:342–362, 1953.
8. Suzuki S, Yamamuro T: Correlation of fetal posture and congenital dislocation of the hip. Acta Orthop Scand 57:81–84, 1986.
9. Coleman SS: Congenital dysplasia of the hip in the Navajo infant. Clin Orthop Relat Res 56:179–193, 1968.
10. Race C, Herring JA: Congenital dislocation of the hip: an evaluation of closed reduction. J Pediatr Orthop 3:166–172, 1983.
11. Klisic P, Zivanovic V, Brdar R: Effects of triple prevention of CDH, stimulated by distribution of "baby packages." J Pediatr Orthop 8:9–11, 1988.
12. Hummer CD, MacEwen GD: The coexistence of torticollis and congenital dysplasia of the hip. J Bone Joint Surg Am 54:1255–1256, 1972.
13. Ilfeld FW, Westin GW, Makin M: Missed or developmental dislocation of the hip. Clin Orthop Relat Res 203:276–281, 1986.
14. Kumar SJ, MacEwen GD: The incidence of hip dysplasia with metatarsus adductus. Clin Orthop Relat Res 164:234–235, 1982.
15. Westberry DE, Davids JR, Pugh LI: Clubfoot and developmental dysplasia of the hip: value of screening hip radiographs in children with clubfoot. J Pediatr Orthop 23:503–507, 2003.
16. Wynne-Davies R, Littlejohn A, Gormley J: Aetiology and interrelationship of some common skeletal deformities (talipes equinovarus and calcaneovalgus, metatarsus varus, congenital dislocation of the hip, and infantile idiopathic scoliosis). J Med Genet 19:321–328, 1982.
17. Weinstein SL: Developmental hip dysplasia and dislocation. In Morrissy RT, Weinstein SL (eds): Lovell and Winter's pediatric orthopaedics, ed 6, Philadelphia, 2006, Lippincott Williams & Wilkins, pp 987–1037.
18. Landa J, Benke M, Feldman DS: The limbus and the neolimbus in developmental dysplasia of the hip. Clin Orthop Relat Res 466:776–781, 2008.
19. Barlow TG: Early diagnosis and treatment of congenital dislocation of the hip. J Bone Joint Surg Br 44:292–301, 1962.
20. Wiberg G: Studies on dysplastic acetabula and congenital subluxation of the hip joint: with special reference to the complication of osteoarthritis. Acta Chir Scand 83(Suppl 58):28–38, 1939.
21. Cooperman DR, Wallensten R, Stulberg SD: Acetabular dysplasia in the adult. Clin Orthop Relat Res 175:79–85, 1983.
22. Murphy SB, Ganz R, Muller ME: The prognosis in untreated dysplasia of the hip: a study of radiographic factors that predict the outcome. J Bone Joint Surg Am 77:985–989, 1985.
23. Graf R: Classification of hip joint dysplasia by means of sonography. Arch Orthop Trauma Surg 102:248–255, 1984.
24. Keller MS, Nijs EL: The role of radiographs and US in developmental dysplasia of the hip: how good are they? Pediatr Radiol 39(Suppl 2):S211–S215, 2009.
25. Harcke HT, Kumar SJ: The role of ultrasound in the diagnosis and management of congenital dislocation and dysplasia of the hip. J Bone Joint Surg Am 73:622–628, 1991.
26. Keller MS, Weltin GG, Rattner Z, et al: Normal instability of the hip in the neonate: US standards. Radiology 169:733–736, 1988.
27. Clarke NM, Clegg J, Al-Chalabi AN: Ultrasound screening of hips at risk for CDH: failure to reduce the incidence of late cases. J Bone Joint Surg Br 71:9–12, 1989.
28. McEvoy A, Paton RW: Ultrasound compared with radiographic assessment in developmental dysplasia of the hip. J R Coll Surg Edinb 42:254–255, 1997.
29. Sochart DH, Paton RW: Role of ultrasound assessment and harness treatment in the management of developmental dysplasia of the hip. Ann R Coll Surg Engl 78:505–508, 1996.
30. Simic S, Vukasinovic Z, Samardzic J, et al: Does the gestation age of newborn babies influence the ultrasonic assessment of hip condition? Srp Arh Celok Lek 137:402–408, 1999.
31. Tonnis D: Congenital dysplasia and dislocation of the hip in children and adults. New York, 1987, Springer-Verlag.
32. Von Rosen S: Early diagnosis and treatment of congenital dislocation of the hip joint. Acta Orthop Scand 26:136–155, 1956.
33. Clinical practice guideline: early detection of developmental dysplasia of the hip. Committee on Quality Improvement, Subcommittee on Developmental Dysplasia of the Hip. American Academy of Pediatrics. Pediatrics 105(4 Pt 1):896–905, 2000.
34. Screening for developmental dysplasia of the hip: recommendation statement. Am Fam Physician 73:1992–1996, 2006.
35. Screening for developmental dysplasia of the hip: recommendation statement. Pediatrics 117:898–902, 2006.
35A. Mahan ST, Katz JN, Kim YJ: To screen or not to screen? A decision analysis of the utility of screening for developmental dysplasia of the hip. J Bone Joint Surg Am 91:1705–1719, 2009.
36. Dezateux C, Brown J, Arthur R, et al: Performance, treatment pathways, and effects of alternative policy options for screening for developmental dysplasia of the hip in the United Kingdom. Arch Dis Child 88:753–759, 2003.
37. Paton RW, Srinivasan MS, Shah B, Hollis S: Ultrasound screening for hips at risk in developmental dysplasia. Is it worth it? J Bone Joint Surg Br 81:255–258, 1999.

38. Eastwood DM: Neonatal hip screening. Lancet 361:595–597, 2003.

39. Holen KJ, Tegnander A, Bredland T, et al: Universal or selective screening of the neonatal hip using ultrasound? A prospective, randomised trial of 15,529 newborn infants. J Bone Joint Surg Br 84:886–890, 2002.

40. Bialik V, Bialik GM, Wiener F: Prevention of overtreatment of neonatal hip dysplasia by the use of ultrasonography. J Pediatr Orthop B 7:39–42, 1998.

41. Lerman JA, Emans JB, Millis MB, et al: Early failure of Pavlik harness treatment for developmental hip dysplasia: clinical and ultrasound predictors. J Pediatr Orthop 21:348–353, 2001.

42. Grill F, Bensahel H, Canadell J, et al: The Pavlik harness in the treatment of congenital dislocating hip: report on a multicenter study of the European Paediatric Orthopaedic Society. J Pediatr Orthop 8:1–8, 1998.

43. Bradley J, Wetherill M, Benson MK: Splintage for congenital dislocation of the hip. Is it safe and reliable? J Bone Joint Surg Br 69:257–263, 1987.

44. Kalamchi A, MacEwen GD: Avascular necrosis following treatment of congenital dislocation of the hip. J Bone Joint Surg Am 62:876–888, 1980.

45. Kitoh H, Kawasumi M, Ishiguro N: Predictive factors for unsuccessful treatment of developmental dysplasia of the hip by the Pavlik harness. J Pediatr Orthop 29:552–557, 2009.

46. Jones GT, Schoenecker PL, Dias LS: Developmental hip dysplasia potentiated by inappropriate use of the Pavlik harness. J Pediatr Orthop 12:722–726, 1992.

47. Hedequist D, Kasser J, Emans J: Use of an abduction brace for developmental dysplasia of the hip after failure of Pavlik harness use. J Pediatr Orthop 23:175–177, 2003.

48. Carney BT, Clark D, Minter CL: Is the absence of the ossific nucleus prognostic for avascular necrosis after closed reduction of developmental dysplasia of the hip? J Surg Orthop Adv 13:24–29, 2004.

49. Segal LS, Boal DK, Borthwick L, et al: Avascular necrosis after treatment of DDH: the protective influence of the ossific nucleus. J Pediatr Orthop 19:177–184, 1999.

50. Konigsberg DE, Karol LA, Colby S, O'Brien S: Results of medial open reduction of the hip in infants with developmental dislocation of the hip. J Pediatr Orthop 23:1–9, 2003.

51. Luhmann SJ, Bassett GS, Gordon JE, et al: Reduction of a dislocation of the hip due to developmental dysplasia: implications for the need for future surgery. J Bone Joint Surg Am 85:239–243, 2003.

52. Quinn RH, Renshaw TS, DeLuca PA: Preliminary traction in the treatment of developmental dislocation of the hip. J Pediatr Orthop 14:636–642, 1994.

53. Weinstein SL: Traction in developmental dislocation of the hip. Is its use justified? Clin Orthop Relat Res 338:79–85, 1997.

54. Weinstein SL, Ponseti IV: Congenital dislocation of the hip. J Bone Joint Surg Am 61:119–124, 1979.

55. Ramsey PL, Lasser S, MacEwen GD: Congenital dislocation of the hip: use of the Pavlik harness in the child during the first six months of life. J Bone Joint Surg Am 58:1000–1004, 1976.

56. Tiderius C, Jaramillo D, Connolly S, et al: Post-closed reduction perfusion magnetic resonance imaging as a predictor of avascular necrosis in developmental hip dysplasia: a preliminary report. J Pediatr Orthop 29:14–20, 2009.

57. Mitchell PD, Chew NS, Goutos I, et al: The value of MRI undertaken immediately after reduction of the hip as a predictor of long-term acetabular dysplasia. J Bone Joint Surg Br 89:948–952, 2007.

58. Morcuende JA, Meyer MD, Dolan LA, Weinstein SL: Long-term outcome after open reduction through an anteromedial approach for congenital dislocation of the hip. J Bone Joint Surg Am 79:810–817, 1997.

59. Di Mascio L, Carey-Smith R, Tucker K: Open reduction of developmental hip dysplasia using a medial approach: a review of 24 hips. Acta Orthop Belg 74:343–348, 2008.

60. Cherney DL, Westin GW: Acetabular development in the infant's dislocated hips. Clin Orthop Relat Res 242:98–103, 1989.

61. Lalonde FD, Frick SL, Wenger DR: Surgical correction of residual hip dysplasia in two pediatric age-groups. J Bone Joint Surg Am 84:1148–1156, 2002.

62. Gallien R, Bertin D, Lirette R: Salter procedure in congenital dislocation of the hip. J Pediatr Orthop 4:427–430, 1984.

63. Haidar RK, Jones RS, Vergroesen DA, Evans GA: Simultaneous open reduction and Salter innominate osteotomy for developmental dysplasia of the hip. J Bone Joint Surg Br 78:471–476, 1996.

64. Salter RB: Role of innominate osteotomy in the treatment of congenital dislocation and subluxation of the hip in the older child. J Bone Joint Surg Am 48:1413–1439, 1966.

65. Galpin RD, Roach JW, Wenger DR, et al: One-stage treatment of congenital dislocation of the hip in older children, including femoral shortening. J Bone Joint Surg Am 71:734–741, 1989.

66. Lindstrom JR, Ponseti IV, Wenger DR: Acetabular development after reduction in congenital dislocation of the hip. J Bone Joint Surg Am 61:112–118, 1979.

67. Clohisy JC, Barrett SE, Gordon JE, et al: Periacetabular osteotomy for the treatment of severe acetabular dysplasia. J Bone Joint Surg Am 87:254–259, 2005.

68. Faciszewski T, Coleman SS, Biddulph G: Triple innominate osteotomy for acetabular dysplasia. J Pediatr Orthop 13:426–430, 1993.

69. Ganz R, Klaue K, Vinh TS, Mast JW: A new periacetabular osteotomy for the treatment of hip dysplasias: technique and preliminary results. Clin Orthop Relat Res 232:26–36, 1988.

70. Guille JT, Forlin E, Kumar SJ, MacEwen GD: Triple osteotomy of the innominate bone in treatment of developmental dysplasia of the hip. J Pediatr Orthop 12:718–721, 1992.

71. Steel HH: Triple osteotomy of the innominate bone. J Bone Joint Surg Am 55:343–350, 1973.

72. Steel HH: Triple osteotomy of the innominate bone: a procedure to accomplish coverage of the dislocated or subluxated femoral head in the older patient. Clin Orthop Relat Res 122:116–127, 1977.

73. Tonnis D, Behrens K, Tscharani F: A modified technique of the triple pelvic osteotomy: early results. J Pediatr Orthop 1:241–249, 1981.

74. Tonnis D, Bruning KI, Heinecke A: Lateral acetabular osteotomy. J Pediatr Orthop B 3:40, 1994.

75. Albinana J, Dolan LA, Spratt KF, et al: Acetabular dysplasia after treatment for developmental dysplasia of the hip: implications for secondary procedures. J Bone Joint Surg Br 86:876–886, 2004.

76. Kim HT, Kim JI, Yoo CI: Acetabular development after closed reduction of developmental dislocation of the hip. J Pediatr Orthop 20:701–708, 2000.

77. Ganz R, Leunig M: Morphological variations of residual hip dysplasia in the adult. Hip Int 17(Suppl 5):22–28, 2007.

78. Oh CW, Joo SY, Kumar SJ, Macewen GD: A radiological classification of lateral growth arrest of the proximal femoral physis after treatment for developmental dysplasia of the hip. J Pediatr Orthop 29:331–335, 2009.

79. Doudoulakis JK, Cavadias A: Open reduction of CDH before one year of age: 69 hips followed for 13 (10-19) years. Acta Orthop Scand 64:188–192, 1993.

80. Millis MB, Kim YJ: Rationale of osteotomy and related procedures for hip preservation: a review. Clin Orthop Relat Res 405:108–121, 2002.

81. Salter RB, Dubos JP: The first fifteen years' personal experience with innominate osteotomy in the treatment of congenital dislocation and subluxation of the hip. Clin Orthop Relat Res 98:72–103, 1974.

82. Lehman WL, Grogan DP: Innominate osteotomy and varus derotational osteotomy in the treatment of congenital dysplasia of the hip. Orthopedics 8:979–986, 1985.

83. Thomas SR, Wedge JH, Salter RB: Outcome at forty-five years after open reduction and innominate osteotomy for late-presenting developmental dislocation of the hip. J Bone Joint Surg Am 89:2341–2350, 2007.

84. Hailer NP, Soykaner L, Ackermann H, Rittmeister M: Triple osteotomy of the pelvis for acetabular dysplasia: age at operation and the incidence of nonunions and other complications influence outcome. J Bone Joint Surg Br 87:1622–1626, 2005.

85. Karlen JW, Skaggs DL, Ramachandran M, Kay RM: The Dega osteotomy: a versatile osteotomy in the treatment of developmental and neuromuscular hip pathology. J Pediatr Orthop 29:676–682, 2009.

86. Ozgur AF, Aksoy MC, Kandemir U, et al: Does Dega osteotomy increase acetabular volume in developmental dysplasia of the hip? J Pediatr Orthop B 15:83–86, 2006.

87. Kim HW, Morcuende JA, Dolan LA, Weinstein SL: Acetabular development in developmental dysplasia of the hip complicated by lateral growth disturbance of the capital femoral epiphysis. J Bone Joint Surg Am 82:1692–1700, 2000.

88. Malvitz TA, Weinstein SL: Closed reduction for congenital dysplasia of the hip: functional and radiographic results after an average of thirty years. J Bone Joint Surg Am 76:1777–1792, 1994.

89. Salter RB, Kostuik J, Dallas S: Avascular necrosis of the femoral head as a complication of treatment for congenital dislocation of the hip in young children: a clinical and experimental investigation. Can J Surg 12:44–61, 1969.

90. Zadeh HG, Catterall A, Hashemi-Nejad A, Perry RE: Test of stability as an aid to decide the need for osteotomy in association with open reduction in developmental dysplasia of the hip. J Bone Joint Surg Br 82:17–27, 2000.

91. Gage JR, Cary JM: The effects of trochanteric epiphyseodesis on growth of the proximal end of the femur following necrosis of the capital femoral epiphysis. J Bone Joint Surg Am 62:785–794, 1980.

92. Langenskiold A, Salenius P: Epiphyseodesis of the greater trochanter. Acta Orthop Scand 38:199–219, 1967.

93. Bialik V, Rosenberg N: Transfer of greater trochanter. J Pediatr Orthop B 3:30, 1994.

Legg-Calvé-Perthes Disease

Harry Kim

INTRODUCTION

Legg-Calvé-Perthes disease (LCPD) is a complex pediatric hip disorder that affects children over a wide age range and produces variable outcomes even with treatment. Since the original reports of the disease in 1910 by Legg from the United States, Calvé from France, and Perthes from Germany, controversies regarding its causes, pathogenesis, natural history, and treatment have persisted. Various theories on its origin have been proposed, but none has yet to be conclusively substantiated. With limited understanding of the disease process, it is difficult at this time to reconcile various clinical features of the disease with one etiologic factor. Recent studies on the causes of Legg-Calvé-Perthes disease have described type II collagen mutation as a potential cause of the disease in a limited number of inherited, bilateral cases in Asian families. Although the cause of disruption of the blood supply to the femoral head remains unknown, further insight into the pathogenesis of a femoral head deformity has been gained through experimental studies using animal models of ischemic osteonecrosis. These studies reveal that mechanical and biological factors contribute to the pathogenesis of the femoral head deformity following ischemic necrosis. Long-term studies suggest that although femoral head deformity is relatively well tolerated over short and intermediate terms, 50% of patients develop disabling arthritis in the sixth decade of life.

Thus the overall goal of treatment should focus on preventing or minimizing the femoral head deformity. Along with recent large retrospective studies, two multicenter prospective cohort studies provide some guidance on treating this condition in patients of different age groups.

EPIDEMIOLOGY AND RISK FACTORS

The annual incidence of Perthes disease shows regional variability. Overall, the lowest incidences have been reported from Asian countries, with 1 case per 450,000 in South China and from 0.4 to 14.4 per 100,000 in South India.[1] In North America, an incidence of 5.1 per 100,000 was found in British Columbia and 5.7 per 100,000 in Massachusetts.[2,3] The cumulative incidence of Perthes disease appearing in children up to 15 years of age was 1 in 740 males and 1 in 3700 females in Massachusetts.[3] In Europe, reported incidences have ranged from 7.9 per 100,000 in Trent, England, to 16.9 per 100,000 in Liverpool. In contrast to these data from Liverpool obtained in the period from 1976 to 1981, subsequent study has shown a decrease in incidence to 8.7 in 1990 to 1995, indicating a significant decline in incidence within the region.[4] Improvements in socioeconomic status and nutritional deprivation have been proposed as factors associated with the decline in incidence. In other European countries, rates of 9.2 per 100,000 in Norway and 8.5 per 100,000 in Sweden have been reported.[1] A comparison of incidence from one region to another requires caution because some studies were performed more recently and others were performed more than 30 years ago. The older studies may or may not truly reflect the current incidence of the disease in the region because the demographics may have changed over time.

Perthes disease can affect children younger than 15 years, but it is most commonly seen in children between the ages of 4 and 9 years. The male-to-female ratio ranges from 3.3:1 in Norway to 5:1 in Massachusetts.[1,3] Bilateral disease occurs in about 10% to 15% of patients, and the presentation tends to be asynchronous in timing. In most studies, the reported incidence of a positive family history is less than 5%.[5,6]

Studies have reported an increased association between Perthes disease and congenital abnormalities (odds ratio = 2.0), including congenital hip dislocation, Down syndrome, undescended testicle, clubfoot, hypospadias, atrial septal defect (ASD), ventricular septal defect (VSD), and anomalies of skull and facial bones or upper extremities. Studies have also reported an increased association between very low birth weight or short body length at birth and Perthes disease, suggesting that genetic or early developmental factors may be linked to the disease. An increased association has also been reported with maternal smoking and second-hand smoke exposure.[7-9]

Since the original description of the condition was put forth in 1910, numerous theories on the origin of Perthes disease have been proposed (Box 41-1). A conceptual challenge has been to explain various clinical features, such as unilateral presentation in most patients, predilection for boys, delayed bone age, patient hyperactivity, and association with congenital anomalies in some patients, using a single etiologic theory. The prevailing view at this time is that Perthes disease is a multifactorial disease that is caused by a combination of genetic and environmental factors. It is postulated that genetic factors impart "susceptibility" to the disruption of blood supply to the femoral head, and environmental factors, such as repeated subclinical trauma or mechanical overloading, trigger the disease.

Of proposed etiologic factors, the hypothesis postulating alteration of the insulin-like growth factor 1 (IGF-1) pathway as a cause of Perthes disease merits attention because IGF-1 is known to be expressed in many tissues, including brain and skeleton, and affects postnatal development of these tissues. Because IGF-1 pathway dysfunction can influence brain and skeletal development, it can potentially explain the delayed skeletal maturity, hyperactive behavior, and minor congenital abnormalities seen in patients with Perthes disease. Low levels of serum IGF-1 have been reported in patients during the first 2 years after the diagnosis of Perthes disease in a cohort consisting of 59 consecutive patients.[10] In one study, the serum level of IGF-1 was reported to be normal and the level of its major binding protein, IGF-1 binding protein 3, was decreased.[11] These results conflict with those of another study, which reported normal IGF-1 binding protein levels.[12] Thus, the significance of the IGF-1 pathway in the origin of Perthes disease remains unclear.

BOX 41-1. PROPOSED ETIOLOGIES OF PERTHES DISEASE

- Genetic susceptibility with environmental trigger
- Type II collagen mutation or hereditary factors
- Hyperactivity with subclinical trauma to the femoral head vascularity
- Insulin-like growth factor 1 (IGF-1) pathway abnormality
- Coagulopathy/Thrombophilia
- Vasculopathy
- Inflammatory process
- Venous congestion
- Arterial occlusion
- Maternal or passive smoking

Recently, advances in our understanding of the origin of Perthes disease have come from genetic studies of Asian families with inherited bilateral avascular necrosis of the femoral head. Taiwanese, Japanese, and Chinese families with multiple members affected by femoral head osteonecrosis in an autosomal dominant fashion were found to have a missense mutation in the type II collagen gene (replacement of glycine with serine at codon 1170 of COL2A1).[13-15] What is noteworthy is that in contrast to skeletal dysplasias and other type II collagenopathies, affected individuals with this mutation in general did not appear to have skeletal abnormalities outside the hips. In affected individuals with open growth plates, radiographic changes typical of Perthes disease were observed[14,15] (Fig. 41-1). Although secondary structural consequences due to the mutation appeared minor in nature, it is speculated that the mutation may cause weakening of the cartilage matrix.[15] Given that the femoral head is a major weight-bearing structure, it is proposed that cartilage matrix weakening may compromise blood vessels within the cartilage as they traverse from the femoral neck to the bony epiphysis through the cartilage. Although these findings provide new insight into the pathophysiology of femoral head osteonecrosis, the type II collagen mutation may account for only a small number of patients with LCPD because it has yet to be reported in sporadic unilateral or nonfamilial bilateral cases of LCPD.[16] It also is not completely clear at this time whether this small number of cases in fact represents an ischemic condition, or whether it represents a subtle form of skeletal dysplasia.

Thrombophilia leading to thrombotic venous occlusion of the femoral head has been proposed as a cause of Perthes disease, but this theory remains controversial. In a case control study that reported on the association between Perthes disease and coagulation abnormalities, Glueck and associates found that 75% of the patients in the study had a coagulation abnormality.[17] Although some studies have reported an increased rate of coagulation abnormalities in patients with Perthes disease, others have not found any association at all. A prospective study of a random series of 50 consecutive patients with Perthes disease also did not find a difference in the prevalence of protein C, protein S, or antithrombin III deficiencies, or factor V Leiden mutation, between the study group and the estimated population frequency.[18] The authors of the study proposed that the high prevalence of coagulation abnormalities found in the study by Glueck and colleagues may be attributed to the less stringent reference range used to define the coagulation abnormalities. A recent case control study that included some of the investigators from the original study by Glueck and coworkers also found no increase in the prevalences of protein C, protein S, and antithrombin III deficiencies, hyperhomocysteinemia, and elevated plasminogen activator inhibitor-1 activity between 72 nonselected, consecutive series of patients with Perthes disease and 197 healthy controls.[19] However, this study did find a higher prevalence of factor V Leiden (8 of 72 in the study group compared with 7 of 197 in the control group) and

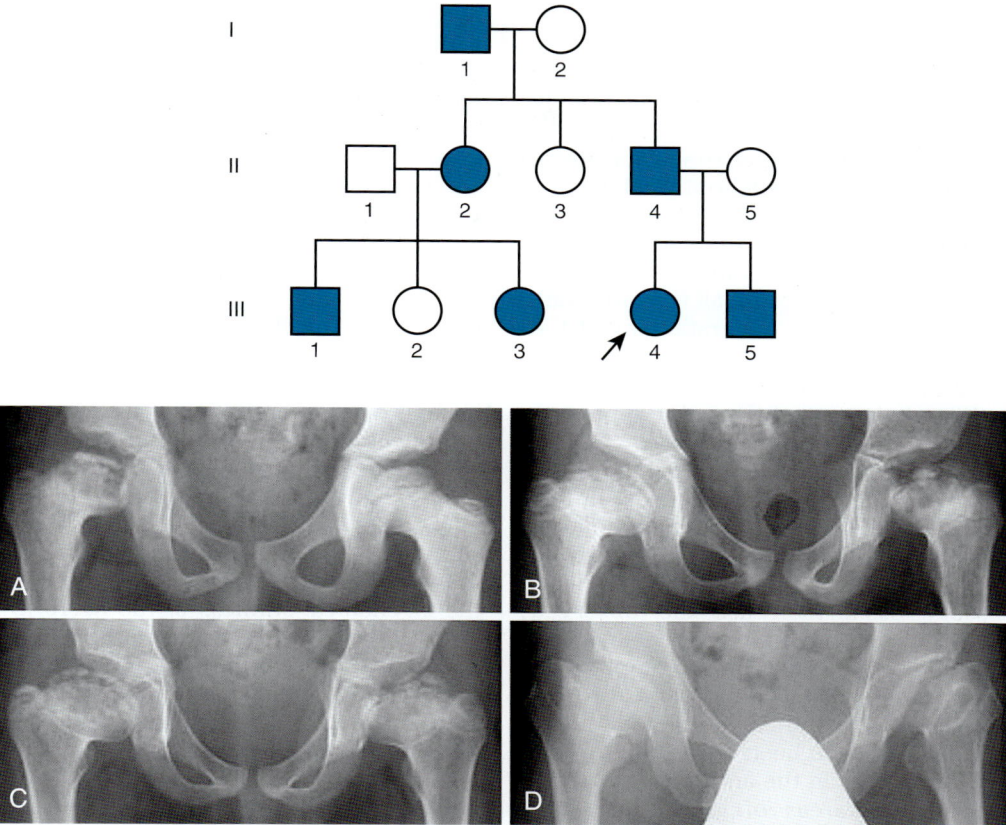

Figure 41-1. Pedigree of a Japanese family with Legg-Calvé-Perthes disease, and radiographs of subject II-4 at **(A)** age 7, **(B)** age 9, **(C)** age 11, and **(D)** age 45. *(From Miyamoto Y, Matsuda T, Kitoh H, et al: A recurrent mutation in type II collagen gene causes Legg-Calvé-Perthes disease in a Japanese family. Hum Genet 121:625–629, 2007.)*

anticardiolipin antibodies (19 of 72 in the study group compared with 22 of 197 in the control group) among patients with Perthes disease. Because thrombotic events are uncommon during childhood, even in those patients with inherited thrombophilia,[20] the significance of inherited or acquired thrombophilia in the pathogenesis of Perthes disease remains unclear at this time.

PATHOPHYSIOLOGY

Although the origin of Perthes disease remains unknown, clinical and experimental evidence supports the hypothesis that disruption of the blood supply to the femoral head is a key pathogenic event associated with the disease process. Selective angiography,[21-23] bone scintigraphy,[24] perfusion magnetic resonance imaging (MRI),[25] and biopsy studies[26] from early stages of the disease show evidence of disruption of perfusion and tissue damage consistent with ischemic necrosis. Furthermore, disruption of the blood supply to the femoral head in large animal models produced the histopathologic and radiographic changes observed in Perthes disease, including a fragmented appearance of the bony epiphysis and the coxa plana.[27]

It is debatable whether a single episode or multiple episodes of ischemia are necessary to produce Perthes disease. The second or multiple infarction theory is based on observations from an immature canine model in which a single surgical attempt at inducing femoral head infarction did not produce the femoral head deformity and histologic features of Perthes disease.[28,29] These findings were observed only after a second infarction surgery in some animals, leading to speculation that Perthes disease may be due to more than one episode of infarction.[28] In contrast, a single infarction surgery produced a femoral head deformity and histologic changes resembling Perthes disease in a piglet model of ischemic necrosis.[27] The finding of thickened trabeculae with multiple cement lines from the specimens of patients with Perthes disease has been proposed as supportive evidence for the multiple infarction theory.[30] An alternative interpretation of the finding, however, is that a single episode of ischemia produces the disease, but subsequent reinjury or injuries of the revascularized region occur as the result of repeated mechanical overloading and/or further collapse of the femoral head during a vascular repair phase. One implication of the latter theory is that femoral head overloading and deformation during the healing phase may hinder revascularization of the necrotic femoral head and may prolong the healing process.

A report describing histopathologic findings from six whole femoral heads constitutes the largest assembly of whole head samples of Perthes disease studied to date.[31] The small number underscores the major obstacle in attempts to understand the pathophysiology of a condition with very limited availability of tissue samples for research investigation. Findings from this study, a few isolated necropsy reports, and some studies based on surgical biopsy specimens[26,30-37] are all that are available at this time to enhance our understanding of the disease process. From these studies, it can be summarized that pathologic processes in Perthes disease affect the articular cartilage (also called the *epiphyseal cartilage*), bony epiphysis, physis, and metaphysis.

Articular cartilage changes are found mainly in the middle and deep layers of the cartilage. Necrosis in the deep layer of the cartilage, cessation of endochondral ossification, separation of cartilage from underlying subchondral bone, vascular invasion of the cartilage, and new accessory ossification are the observed changes (Fig. 41-2). In the bony epiphysis, necrosis of the marrow space and of trabecular bone, compression fracture of trabeculae, osteoclastic resorption, fibrovascular granulation tissue invasion of the necrotic head, and thickened trabeculae have been reported. Physeal changes are seen most often in the anterior part of the femoral head, with focal areas of growth cartilage columns extending below the endochondral ossification line. Premature growth arrest of the growth plate is seen in only 30% of patients with Perthes disease, suggesting that in most patients, the growth plate continues to function. Findings of a recent experimental study are consistent with clinical findings indicating that in most patients with Perthes disease, the growth plate remains functional.[38] Metaphyseal changes are commonly seen

during the early stages of Perthes disease and usually are found subjacent to or below the growth plate in the anterior aspect of the femoral head. The mechanisms responsible for the appearance of these lesions are unclear. Various tissue types have been reported, including columns of normal or degenerated cartilage extending down to the metaphysis, fibrocartilage, fat necrosis, vascular proliferation, and focal fibrosis.[31] Some have found an association between the presence of radiolucent metaphyseal changes and poor prognosis, but others have not.

The lack of availability of clinical samples for research has prompted alternative approaches, such as the use of animal models, to investigate the pathogenesis of Perthes disease. In particular, a piglet model of ischemic osteonecrosis has allowed more systematic and in-depth investigation of ischemic tissue damage, the repair process, and the pathogenesis of femoral head deformity following disruption of the epiphyseal blood supply. Key findings from this line of investigation are that the induction of ischemia produces a decrease in the mechanical stiffness of the necrotic femoral head, making it relatively soft in comparison with the normal femoral head, from the early avascular necrotic phase to the latter vascular repair phase of the model.[39] The mechanical properties of the two components of the femoral head—articular cartilage and trabecular bone from the bony epiphysis—were found to be decreased.[40] The mechanical compromise observed in the avascular necrotic phase may be due to necrosis of the deep layer of the articular cartilage,[41] changes in the material properties of calcified cartilage and trabecular bone in the infarcted head,[42] and possible accumulation of microfractures in the necrotic bone. Repetitive loading is known to produce microfractures or microcracks in the bone, which are detected and repaired by bone cells.[43] However, in necrotic bone, no cells are available to

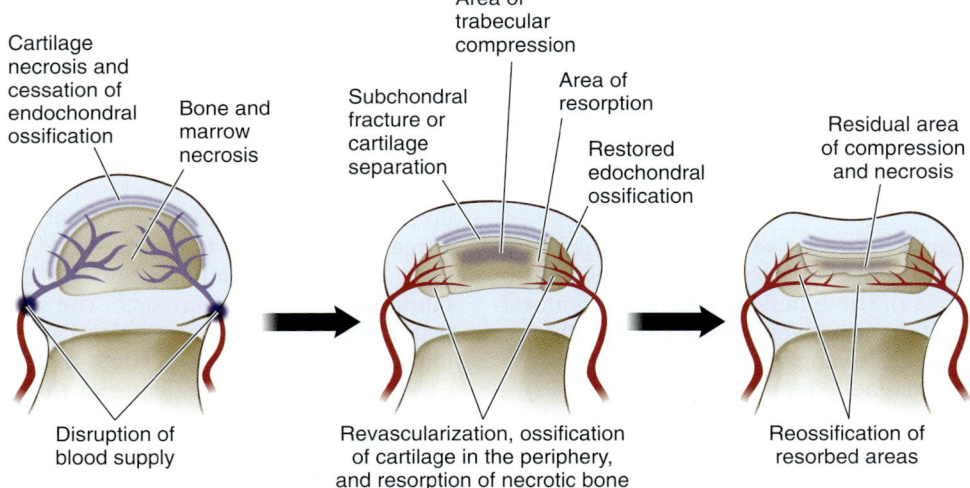

Figure 41-2. An illustration combining the described histopathologic changes from the necropsy and biopsy studies of Legg-Calvé-Perthes disease. Important pathologic processes include cartilage and bone necrosis, subchondral fracture and compaction of necrotic bone, revascularization from the periphery of the epiphysis with associated resorption of necrotic bone and further collapse, and asymmetrical restoration of endochondral ossification at the periphery, further contributing to the deformed, ovoid shape.

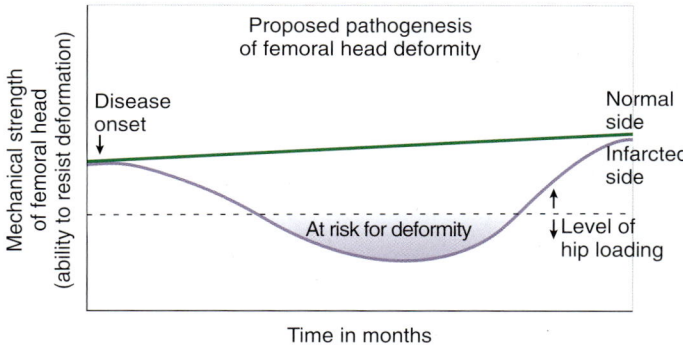

Figure 41-3. Line drawing depicting the proposed pathogenesis of the femoral head deformity following ischemic necrosis based on piglet mechanical studies. With the onset of ischemic osteonecrosis, the mechanical properties of the femoral head decrease over time owing to factors described in the text. It is proposed that when hip joint loading surpasses the mechanical strength of the femoral head, the deformity is initiated and progresses.

detect and repair the microdamage related to repetitive "wear-and-tear." Furthermore, it is proposed that a significant increase in the mineral content of necrotic trabecular bone makes it more brittle and prone to microdamage.[42] As a result, a subchondral fracture (crescent sign) or a compaction fracture may occur in the necrotic femoral head with repetitive overloading of the hip joint.

Vascular invasion and subsequent resorption of necrotic bone further compromise the mechanical properties of the infarcted head in the vascular repair phase.[39] The mismatch of bone resorption and formation produces a net bone loss, seen radiographically as a radiolucent area within the necrotic bone.[27] The predominance of bone resorption during the early vascular phase of the repair weakens the femoral head, predisposing it to flattening. It is postulated that the weakened femoral head begins to deform when its ability to resist deformation falls below a critical level surpassed by hip joint loading (Fig. 41-3). Inhibition of bone resorption using antiresorptive agents, such as bisphosphonates and receptor activator of nuclear factor (NF)κB ligand (RANKL) inhibitor, has been shown to decrease the deformity in animal studies, indicating that the resorptive process is an important component of the pathogenesis of femoral head deformity in these models.[44,45] Clinical studies are required to validate the significance of bone resorption and the efficacy of antiresorptive agents in decreasing femoral head deformity in Perthes disease. Further discussion on the development of medical treatment for Perthes disease is found in the treatment section.

Because the hip joint is a major load-bearing joint, it is important to consider the development of the femoral head deformity in the context of loading of the joint. This is one of the areas of Perthes disease research that has a paucity of data. The relationship between the magnitude and frequency of hip joint loading and the development of the femoral head deformity remains unclear. Basic data such as hip contact pressures associated with various activities of daily living are not available in children. In adults, a sophisticated femoral head prosthesis equipped with a strain gauge and telemetric data transmission capability has allowed real-time collection of these valuable data following total hip replacement, with patients performing various activities and positioning of the leg.[46] The measurements indicate that significant forces act on the femoral head with daily activities. Walking was associated with hip contact pressure reaching about 2.5 times the body weight. Running on a treadmill at a rate of 8 kilometers per hour increased the contact pressure to about 4.5 times the body weight. Some supine and prone activities were also associated with hip contact pressures elevated above the body weight. These measurements have provided insight into the magnitude of loading associated with various activities and leg positioning. A complete loading history and magnitude for an individual will likely depend on the list of activities the person performs, the frequency of each activity, and the body weight. In a disease where femoral head deformity is produced as the result of mechanical weakening, avoidance of activities that generate a significant increase in hip contact pressure would seem reasonable. At this time it is unknown what "significant" loading is, and what effect restricting activities has on preventing the deformity.

In contrast to femoral head weakening and hip joint loading, which promote the development of femoral head deformity, the healing or remodeling potential related to age at onset of the disease appears to offset the deformity. Clinical studies consistently show a better outcome in terms of femoral head shape in patients with early onset of Perthes disease.[47] It is unclear what factors determine the healing and remodeling potentials. Important biological factors to keep in mind are that Perthes disease affects a wide age range of children from preschool years to early teenage years, and that the age range represents a growth period when significant changes are taking place in terms of femoral head anatomy, size, and vasculature[48-51] (Fig. 41-4). The size of the bony epiphysis increases while the thickness of the articular cartilage and the growth potential of the bony epiphysis decrease with age. In addition, more subtle changes, such as regression of cartilage vascularity (presence of cartilage vascular canals) and changes in the vascular anatomy of the proximal femur, are taking place. Given these changes, onset of the disease at different ages implies that the disease is affecting a femoral head that may have significantly different growth and remodeling potentials. These factors are likely to affect the final outcome of the femoral head.

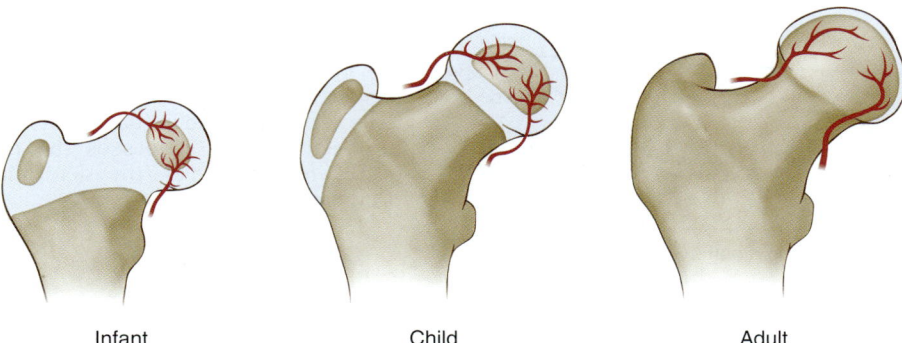

Infant   Child   Adult

Figure 41-4. A drawing showing significant developmental changes occurring in the proximal femur from infancy to maturity. Notable changes included decreased cartilage thickness and cartilage vascularity, increased size of the bony epiphysis, and regression of the growth plate. It is postulated that the onset of ischemic necrosis at different stages of femoral head development will have a significant implication in terms of the healing and remodeling potentials of the femoral head owing to these changes.

BOX 41-2. DIAGNOSTIC FEATURES OF PERTHES DISEASE

History
- Unilateral hip, thigh, or knee pain
- Insidious onset
- Absence of other causes of osteonecrosis

Physical Examination
- Mild limp
- Hip joint irritability
- Decreased range of motion
- Mild limb length discrepancy

Radiography
- Depends on the stage of the disease and the extent of head involvement

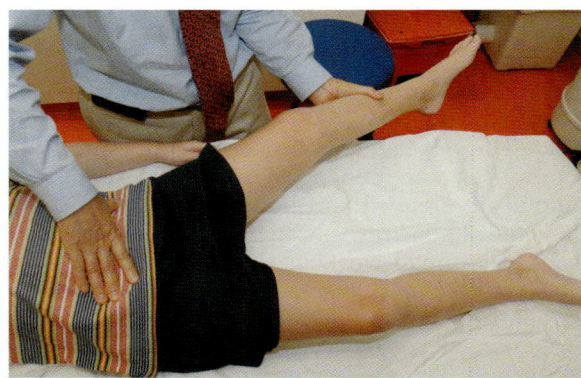

Figure 41-5. To assess hip abduction, a hand should be placed on the pelvis (anterior superior iliac spines) to ensure that the abduction is coming from the hip joint and not from the lateral pelvic rotation.

CLINICAL FEATURES AND DIAGNOSIS

Patients with Perthes disease generally present with pain, a mild limp, and limited hip motion (Box 41-2). In general, the pain is mild and does not restrict the child from daily activities. Often, the pain is not localized to the hip joint, misleading the unsuspecting physician to obtain radiographs or an MRI of the knee. In a study of 425 patients with Perthes disease, 50% of children had pain in the hip and thigh, 18% in the thigh and knee, 14% in the knee only, 8% in the hip, thigh, and knee, and 1% in other areas; 9% had no pain.[1] It is important to recognize that what is perceived as thigh or knee pain can be due to hip disease in a child. Occasionally, a patient may become symptomatic after a minor trauma or a fall during a sports activity.

Physical examination often reveals a mild limp at the time of presentation. The limitation of hip range of motion depends on the stage of the disease. Hip motion

may be good in the early stage, before the development of fragmentation or resorptive changes in the epiphysis. In those patients with marked synovitis, however, the motion may become restricted early. Gentle rotation of the affected hip with the leg extended often demonstrates restriction to the rolling maneuver, so-called *irritability of the hip.* During the stage of fragmentation, hip motion can decrease further and become severely limited. Hip abduction and internal rotation are the earliest motions to become restricted. When assessing passive hip abduction, it is important to stabilize or feel the pelvis to confirm that the leg abduction is coming from the hip joint, not from the lateral rotation of the pelvis (Fig. 41-5). Hip motion improves during the stage of reossification unless significant flattening or deformity of the femoral head that mechanically restricts hip abduction and rotation is present. Depending on the duration of the disease, hip adductor contracture, atrophy of thigh and calf muscles, and limb length discrepancy (0.5 to 1.5 cm) are observed in some patients.

The presence of hip adduction contracture or complete absence of passive abduction during the fragmentation stage of the disease should alert the examiner to the possibility of hinge abduction.

Imaging Studies

Plain radiography remains the main diagnostic and clinical assessment tool for Perthes disease. Anteroposterior (AP) and frog-leg lateral x-rays of the pelvis are used to determine the radiographic stage of the disease, the extent of head involvement, serial progression of the disease, and the development of head-at-risk signs such as lateral subluxation, metaphyseal reaction, Gage's sign, lateral calcification, and horizontal alignment of the growth plate[52] (Fig. 41-6). Some have found that lateral subluxation has greater prognostic importance than the other signs[53]; others have found that two or more head-at-risk signs are associated with a poor outcome.[54] The Catterall, Salter-Thompson, or lateral pillar classification can be applied to assist with treatment decision making when patients reach the stage of fragmentation. These classification systems are further discussed later in the natural history and treatment sections.

Waldenström (1922) described four radiographic stages during the active phase of the disease: the initial stage or the stage of increased radiodensity, the stage of fragmentation, the stage of reossification, and the healed stage, according to characteristic radiographic features of each stage (Fig. 41-7). The duration of each stage is variable from one patient to another. What determines the duration of each stage and the total duration of the active phase remains unknown. In general, older patients appear to have a longer duration than younger patients. According to one study, fragmentation staging lasts about 1 year and the reossification stage lasts from 3 to 5 years.[55] It is during the initial and fragmentation stages that femoral head deformity develops and progresses. During the reossification stage, the femoral head shape can improve, worsen, or remain unchanged. Herring and associates observed that the femoral head was more likely to undergo progressive flattening in older patients, in those with more severe lateral pillar involvement, and in those with prolonged ossification.[55] Although plain radiographs are useful in assessing the progression of the disease, they lack the sensitivity and specificity needed to reveal vascular and repair changes occurring within the bony epiphysis.

Bone scintigraphy can detect changes in bone perfusion in the early stage of Perthes disease, when radiographic changes are not apparent. On the basis of scintigraphic findings, Conway proposed that two distinct processes are involved with revascularization (i.e., recanalization and neovascularization), and that they carry different prognostic significance.[24] Bone scintigraphy has been used to assess femoral head revascularization with good correlation with MRI findings.[25] However, exposure to ionizing radiation and an inability to provide cross-sectional imaging are significant barriers to wide use of this technique.

The role of MRI in the management of Perthes disease is evolving. Like bone scintigraphy, MRI is a sensitive tool for detecting femoral head avascularity. As the techniques, resolution, and scanning time of MRI continue to improve, gadolinium-enhanced MRI may serve as a useful imaging tool to quantify the extent of femoral head avascularity at early stages of the disease and to quantify and compare the extent of revascularization of the femoral head that occurs over time[25] (Fig. 41-8). Because MRI is much more sensitive than plain radiography in visualizing vascular and repair changes that occur in the bony epiphysis, the possibility of using this technique as an early prognostic indicator before the development of deformity to guide treatment decision making requires investigation. Another future application of MRI in assessing Perthes disease consists of exploiting its ability to visualize the outline of the femoral head cartilage to assess the femoral head shape change. A three-dimensional MRI reconstruction technique has been shown to be able to quantify the extent of loss of femoral head sphericity in patients with Perthes disease.[56] Whether such a quantitative method is superior to a qualitative radiographic outcome system such as the Stulberg classification remains to be studied.

DIFFERENTIAL DIAGNOSIS

It is important to remember that Perthes disease is a diagnosis of exclusion. A careful history must be obtained to rule out known causes of femoral head osteonecrosis in children (Box 41-3). Past medical history may reveal neonatal sepsis, proximal femoral trauma, or a history of treatment for developmental dysplasia of the hip (DDH), which may have compromised the blood supply to the femoral head. Past medical history may also reveal use of a corticosteroid for treatment of various medical conditions such as asthma or inflammatory conditions. A high dose of corticosteroid is also used as part of a chemotherapeutic protocol to treat acute lymphoblastic leukemia and other cancers and is associated with femoral head osteonecrosis.

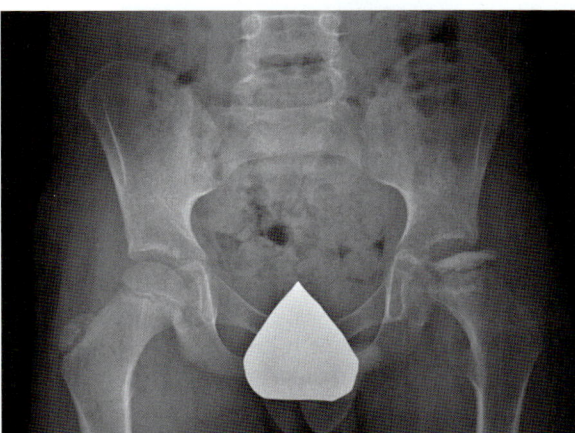

Figure 41-6. A radiograph demonstrating some Catterall's at-risk signs: lateral subluxation with a break in Shenton's line, metaphyseal reaction, lateral calcification, and horizontal alignment of the growth plate.

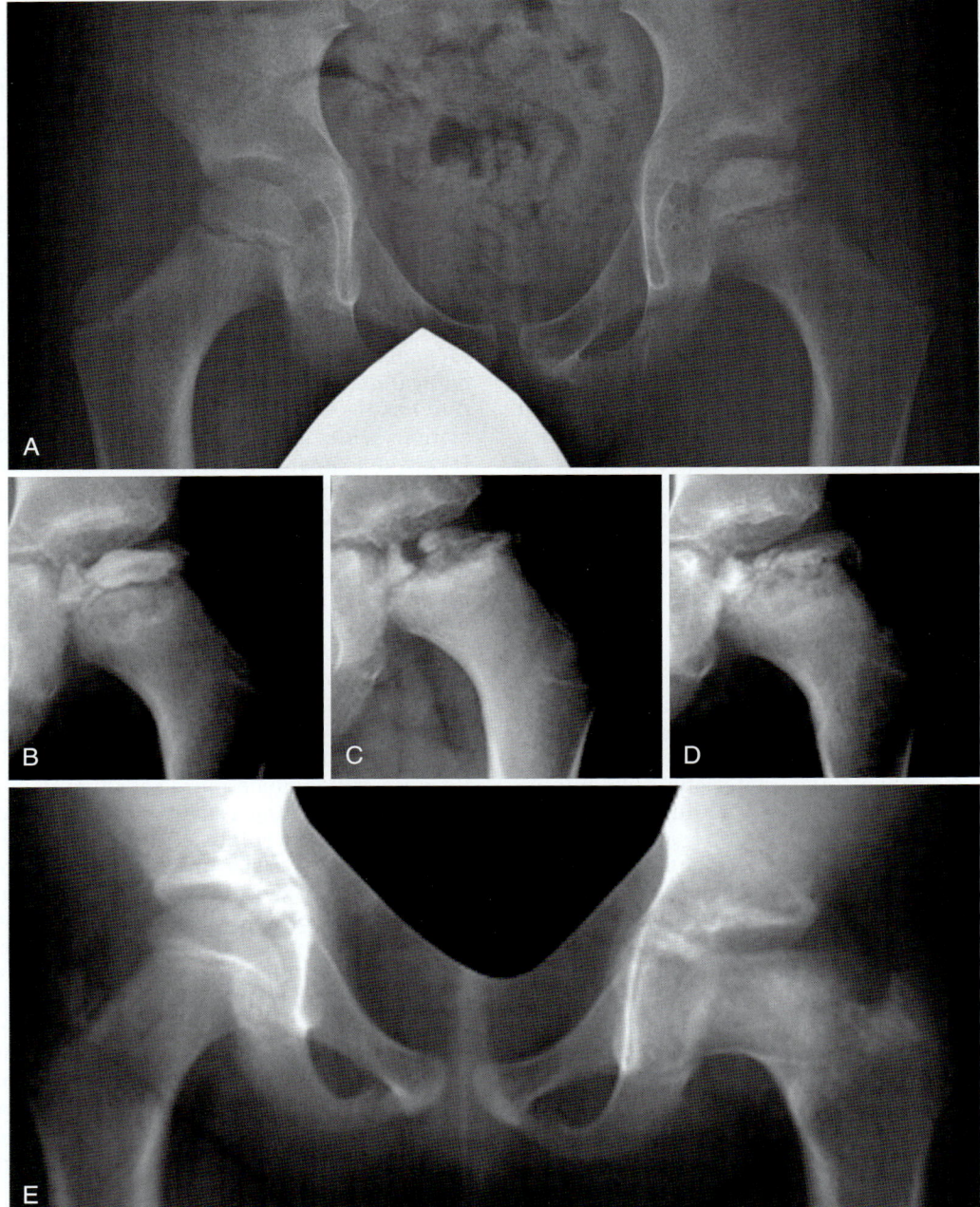

Figure 41-7. Radiographs demonstrating Waldenström's radiographic stages. **A,** Initial stage. This stage is also called the *stage of increased radiodensity.* Characteristic features of this stage include a smaller epiphysis compared with the unaffected side, increased radiodensity, and minimal flattening. A subchondral fracture (crescent sign) may or may not be present. **B** and **C,** Fragmentational stage. This stage is also called the *resorptive stage.* During this stage, resorptive and fragmented changes are seen in the epiphysis. This is the stage when most deformity occurs. **D,** Stage of reossification. Radiolucent areas in the epiphysis are filled in with new bone. Along with reossification of the epiphysis, remodeling of the epiphysis takes place, making the radiodensity of the epiphysis more homogeneous. **E,** Healed stage.

However, these patients present with multiple-site osteonecrosis. Other diseases associated with femoral head osteonecrosis such as sickle cell disease must also be ruled out through a thorough history taking. Inflammatory arthritides such as juvenile rheumatoid arthritis, reactive synovitis, and toxic synovitis can produce hip pain, hip irritability, and limping, which may mimic Perthes disease. Endocrinopathies and metabolic bone disorders such as hypothyroidism, Gaucher disease, and mucopolysaccharidosis can radiographically mimic Perthes disease. In patients presenting with bilateral disease, skeletal dysplasias such as multiple epiphyseal dysplasia should be considered. A positive family history and involvement of other skeletal sites will aid in distinguishing skeletal dysplasias from the isolated Perthes disease.

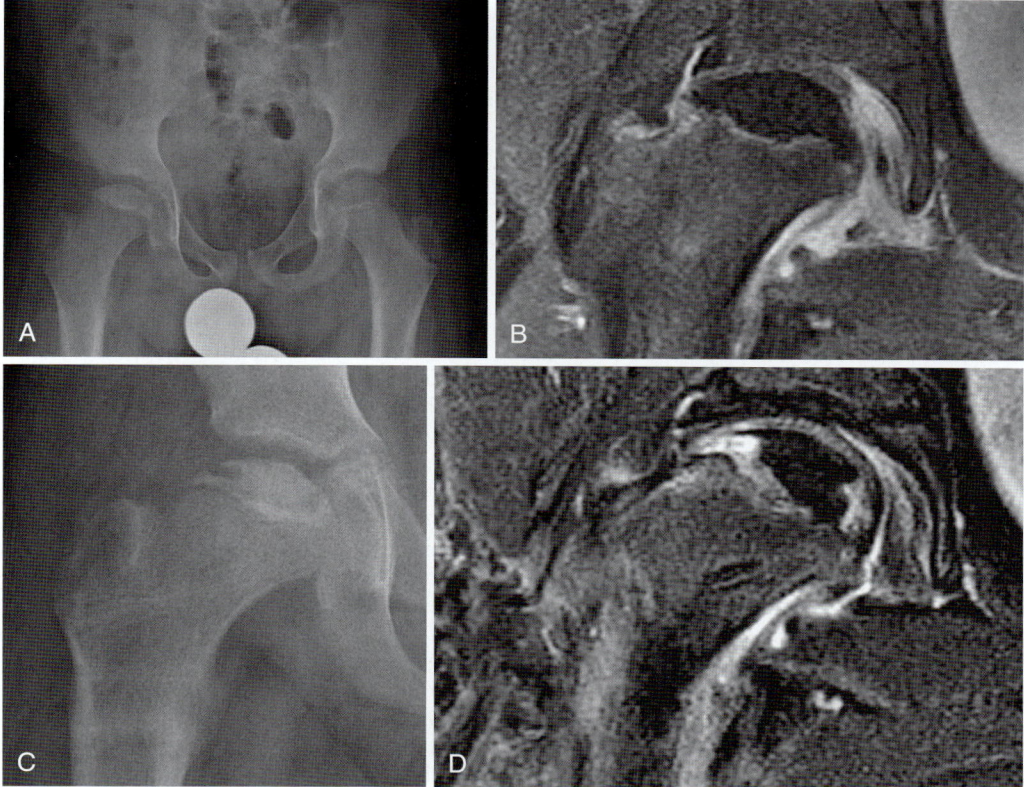

Figure 41-8. An 11-year-old male with right Legg-Calvé-Perthes disease. **A,** An anteroposterior (AP) pelvis radiograph showing the initial stage of the disease. Based on the radiograph, it is difficult to determine the extent of the femoral head necrosis. **B,** Dynamic subtraction magnetic resonance imaging (MRI) following an intravenous gadolinium administration showing complete absence of perfusion in the epiphysis, indicating a total disruption of perfusion. **C,** A radiograph obtained 7 months after a femoral varus osteotomy and subsequent removal of the fixation device showing maintenance of the femoral head shape with the presence of resorptive changes. **D,** A repeat gadolinium-enhanced MRI showing partial revascularization of the femoral head in the medial and lateral aspects of the epiphysis with the central region remaining avascular. Based on this information, the patient was maintained on non–weight-bearing status on the affected side.

BOX 41-3. DIFFERENTIAL DIAGNOSIS OF PERTHES DISEASE

- Corticosteroid-associated osteonecrosis
- Sickle cell disease and other hemoglobinopathies
- Septic arthritis/osteomyelitis
- Inflammatory arthritis
- Avascular necrosis related to treatment for DDH
- Traumatic causes—hip fracture or dislocation
- Metabolic disorders—Gaucher disease and mucopolysaccharidosis
- Endocrinopathy—hypothyroidism
- Skeletal dysplasia and type II collagenopathy
- Perthes disease associated with syndromes and dysplasia
  - Martsolf syndrome
  - Maroteaux-Lamy syndrome
  - Stickler syndrome
  - Trichorhinophalangeal dysplasia

DDH, Developmental dysplasia of the hip.

NATURAL HISTORY

Management of patients with Perthes disease requires an understanding of the natural history of the disease, prognostic factors that can assist with treatment decision making (Box 41-4), and the effectiveness of operative and nonoperative treatments. Although long-term studies on the natural history of the disease are few in number and have limitations related to small sample size, loss of follow-up, and inclusion of patients treated with various nonoperative treatments that may have positively or negatively influenced their outcome, this is the best information currently available to formulate management principles. In general, long-term studies with an average follow-up of less than 40 years show that most patients are asymptomatic and remain active despite having a deformed femoral head. A study cohort from Iowa described by Gower and Johnston with an average follow-up of 36 years (range, 30 to 48 years) shows that 6 of the 36 had undergone surgical procedure(s) as an adult (i.e., diagnostic biopsy, subtrochanteric osteotomy, bone grafting of the femoral head, or cup arthroplasty).[57] Among the remaining 30 patients, the typical patient had a mild limp, minimum shortening, absent or mild hip pain, and minimum or no functional impairment with respect to job and activities of daily living. The average Iowa hip rating score was 91 points for the cohort. Those with round femoral heads had better hip ratings than those with flattened heads (average, 97 points compared with 89 points). Despite good hip ratings, 25% of patients were found to have radiographic evidence of moderate to severe degenerative arthritis. In longer follow-up studies, noticeable deterioration of hip function has been reported. A study by McAndrew and Weinstein of the cohort from Iowa with an average follow-up of 47 years (range, 39 to 64 years) found that only 40% of patients maintained a good level of function (rating >80 points).[54] Although 40% already had undergone an arthroplasty at the time of follow-up, an additional 10% had disabling pain, and the remaining 10% had an Iowa hip rating of less than 80 points. Mose studied three groups of patients with Perthes: groups with an average follow-up of 17 years, 27 years, and 57 years.[58] Twelve percent, 22%, and 100% of femoral heads with irregular shapes at healing had severe radiographic evidence of osteoarthritis at an average of 17, 27, and 57 years' follow-up. In contrast to irregularly shaped femoral heads, flattened femoral heads did not show evidence of severe osteoarthritis at

17 and 27 years' follow-up, indicating that the degree of deformity affects the outcome.

The relationship between the shape of the femoral head at skeletal maturity and long-term risk for the development of premature osteoarthritis is reported in the study by Stulberg and colleagues.[59] Their five-class radiographic classification system based on the severity of the femoral head deformity and loss of hip joint congruence at maturity correlated with the development of radiographic signs of premature osteoarthritis at 40 years' follow-up (Table 41-1). These results show a significant decline in outcome from spherical femoral heads (class I or II), which are considered good results, and from nonspherical femoral heads (classes III to V), which are considered fair to poor results. The validity of the classification system has been questioned for having low to moderate intraobserver and interobserver reliability.[60] Additional studies show improvements in intraobserver and interobserver reliability by numerically defining the femoral head deformity as the original classification based on a qualitative description of the deformity, and do not provide quantitative parameters defining the groups.[61] Decreasing the number of categories from a five-class to a three-class system also improved interobserver reliability.[62] The need to wait many years before applying the Stulberg classification system in young patients (until skeletal maturity) remains a major limitation of this outcome system. Recently, the deformity index has been reported as a continuous outcome measure that can predict the Stulberg outcome 2 years into the disease.[63] It remains to be seen whether this method proves to be a reliable indicator of outcome for other investigators in large prospective studies.

BOX 41-4. PROGNOSTIC INDICATORS OF PERTHES DISEASE

- Extent of femoral head deformity and loss of hip joint congruity at maturity (Stulberg class)
- Age at onset
- Lateral pillar height at the fragmentation stage (Caterall's, pillar classification)
- Extent of head involvement at the fragmentation stage (Catterall's classification)
- Extent of subchondral fracture (Salter-Thompson classification)
- Two or more Catterall's head-at-risk signs (lateral subluxation, lateral calcification, diffuse metaphyseal reaction, horizontal growth plate, Gage's sign)
- Premature physeal closure

TREATMENT

General management of patients during the active stage of the disease requires clinical and radiographic assessments every 3 to 4 months to monitor the progression of the disease. During these visits, the patient's pain, activity level, range of motion, and radiographic changes should be assessed and compared with findings from previous visits. Based on increasing pain, loss of hip abduction, and development of at-risk signs, such as lateral subluxation and calcification of the femoral head,

---

Table 41-1. Stulberg Radiographic Classification and Osteoarthritis at Follow-up

Stulberg Class	Descriptive Features	Radiographic Signs of Osteoarthritis at Mean Follow-up of 40 Years	Radiographic Evidence of Joint Space Narrowing at Mean Follow-up of 40 Years
I	Normal hip joint	0	0
II	Spherical head with enlargement, short neck, or steep acetabulum	16%	0
III	Nonspherical head (ovoid, mushroom, or umbrella shaped)	58%	47%
IV	Flat head	75%	53%
V	Flat head with incongruent hip joint	78%	61%

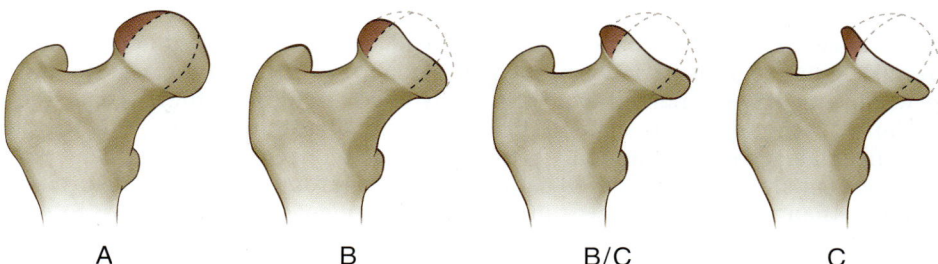

Figure 41-9. Lateral pillar classification.

symptomatic treatments (decrease in activities, restriction of weight bearing with crutches, wheelchair use, short-term use of anti-inflammatory drugs, and/or 1 to 2 days of bed rest) are instituted to decrease hip joint irritation and to improve motion.

Prolonged use of anti-inflammatory agents may be counterproductive based on their negative effects on bone healing, although no specific data on their effects on bone healing following osteonecrosis are available.[64] After weight bearing and activities are restricted, reassessment of hip motion is beneficial at 4 to 6 weeks to check whether hip motion is improving. If motion does not improve, compliance with treatment should be discussed. In addition, discussion regarding other methods of improving hip abduction and preventing hinge abduction, such as the use of Petrie casting, may be warranted.

A long-standing dilemma for the treating surgeon at the time of presentation has been discerning who will benefit from operative or nonoperative treatments and who will not. Three radiographic classification systems—Catterall's, Salter-Thompson, and lateral pillar—have been developed as predictors of outcome in active stages of the disease to aid in the decision-making process. Ideally, a prognostic indicator for the purpose of guiding treatment should be applicable at the time of clinical presentation; it should be applicable before the deformity occurs, easy to use, reliable, and reproducible between observers.

The Salter-Thompson classification is a two-category system (groups A and B) based on the extent of subchondral fracture (crescent sign).[65] Because the crescent sign can be observed in the early fragmentation stage of the disease, it offers the advantage of being applicable at an earlier time point than the other two systems. However, its application is restricted by absence of the crescent sign in many patients at the time of presentation and subsequent follow-up. The presence of the sign may be transient, providing a narrow window for detection.

The Catterall classification system is a four-category system (groups 1 to 4) that was the first to emphasize the relationship between extent of head involvement and outcome.[66] It was designed to be applied during the fragmentation stage, when the necrotic sequestrum becomes well demarcated from the viable segment of the femoral head. Along with his classification system, Catterall described head-at-risk signs associated with a poor outcome, as discussed previously.[52] The major

criticism of the Catterall classification system has involved its poor interobserver reliability. Recently, a modified Catterall classification system with two categories (groups 1 and 2 combined and groups 3 and 4 combined) has been shown to have better interobserver reliability.[67] Because groups 1 and 2 are often associated with good outcome and groups 3 and 4 with poor outcome, the simplification seems justified.

The lateral pillar classification was originally designed as a three-category system (groups A, B, and C) with recent addition of a group B/C border, making this a four-category system[61,68] (Fig. 41-9). It is based on the height of the lateral 15% to 30% of the epiphysis, termed the *lateral pillar*. Because the lateral aspect of the femoral head is a site of new ossification, it does pose uncertainty regarding what is actually being assessed anatomically in some cases—the collapsed lateral pillar or newly formed bone in the lateral aspect of the femoral head. Regardless of this uncertainty, the classification system does reflect the extent of the femoral head deformity, and the three-category lateral pillar classification has been shown to have better interobserver reliability than the Salter-Thompson and Catterall classification systems.[67,69] It has also been reported to be a better predictor of a Stulberg outcome than the Catterall classification.[69]

Both the Catterall and lateral pillar classification systems are applicable during the fragmentation stage when a femoral head deformity has occurred. This poses a dilemma for those patients who present at the initial stage or at the early fragmentation stage, when the femoral head cannot be correctly classified until a subsequent visit or visits. Furthermore, assignment of the lateral pillar classification based on initial presenting radiographs was found to be premature in 92 of 275 hips (33%), in that the hips showed worsening of lateral pillar height over time.[70] One treatment approach has been to wait until the patient can be classified into one of the guarded prognosis groups—Catterall's group III or IV or lateral pillar group B, B/C, or C—before instituting surgical treatments. Given that the main goal of treatment is to prevent deformity, the concept of "wait-to-classify" for femoral heads to declare the extent of lateral pillar involvement and allow the femoral head to deform before treatment is initiated has raised some concerns about this approach in patients who present early and who are in the older age group (>8 years old), known to have limited potential to remodel the deformed femoral head. An argument for the "wait-and-classify" approach is that it will prevent the likelihood of operating on patients who otherwise would not have needed the surgery (Catterall's group I or II or lateral pillar group A), or who would not have benefited from the surgery (lateral pillar C). An argument against this approach is that if the main goal of treatment is to prevent deformity, treatment should be instituted early in older patients rather than waiting for the head to deform, because older patients do not have as much remodeling potential as younger patients. These arguments underscore the limitations of these classification systems, which are not predictive of the prognosis of the femoral heads before development of the deformity. In addition, these classification systems may not be relevant for older patients (>12 years), whose femoral head collapse and lack of remodeling behave more like adult osteonecrosis.[71] Currently, an early prognostic indicator based on a sensitive imaging modality such as MRI is needed to guide treatment for older patients in the early stage of disease, before the deformity develops.

The natural history studies already discussed indicate that the degree of residual femoral head deformity and loss of congruity are key determinants of long-term outcome in Perthes disease. Given this understanding, the primary goal of treatment at the early stage of the disease (at the initial or early fragmentation stage) in patients with minimal deformity should be to prevent or minimize the deformity, so that a normal or near-normal hip (Stulberg class I or II hip) can be attained at skeletal maturity. In those patients who present at the fragmentation stage with femoral head flattening, the goal of treatment should be to minimize further

deformity and to improve the roundness of the femoral head, so that a flattened head with or without hip joint incongruity (Stulberg class IV and V hips) can be avoided. Achieving these goals requires appropriate timing of treatment before it is too late and availability of effective treatments that can prevent the deformity or restore roundness to the deformed head. At this time, no treatment has been shown to consistently produce these results. However, recent prospective studies do show better results with operative treatments than with nonoperative treatments in patients of a certain age group.

Evidence-based practice requires the use of "current best evidence" in making decisions about the care of individual patients. Two recent multicenter prospective cohort studies provide the highest level of evidence (level II) to date on operative and nonoperative treatments for Perthes disease.[72,73] The two studies differ considerably regarding their study design, age stratification, and follow-up period, but both studies show a beneficial effect of femoral osteotomy over nonoperative treatment for a select group of patients. Because many studies, including the two prospective studies, show differences in outcome depending on age at onset of the disease, it is useful to divide Perthes patients into three age groups for management purposes and for discussion (age at onset before 6, 6 to 8, and after 8). A treatment algorithm based on age at onset of the disease and findings from the two multicenter prospective studies should serve as a general guide (Fig. 41-10). It is important to note that the following treatment discussion pertains to patients who present during early stages of the disease, that is, at the stage of increased

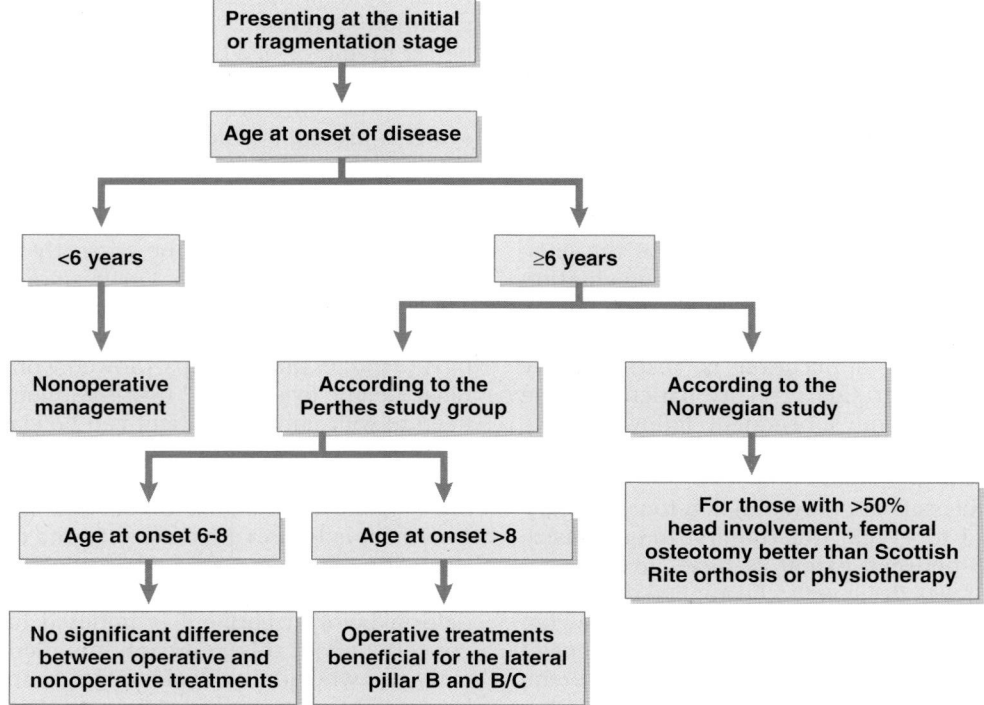

Figure 41-10. Treatment algorithm based on age at onset of the disease and current best evidence.

radiodensity or fragmentation. Patients who present well into the stage of reossification or the healed stage generally do not require active treatment unless the patient is symptomatic, has hinge abduction, or develops late sequelae, such as anterior femoroacetabular impingement[74] or central head osteochondritis dissecans.[75]

Onset Before Age 6

Decision making in this age group is relatively less controversial because most patients in this group have been shown to do well with symptomatic treatment. In a recent retrospective study of 172 patients, 80% were found to have good results (Stulberg class I/II hips) at skeletal maturity with symptomatic or nonoperative treatment.[47] A total of 114 patients received treatment for symptoms only, and 54 patients received brace or cast treatment. Less favorable outcomes were seen in the lateral pillar groups B/C and C.

Another recent retrospective study comparing the results of innominate osteotomy versus those of nonoperative treatment for Catterall's groups III and IV found no significant difference between treatments. About 80% and 50% of Catterall's groups III and IV, respectively, had Stulberg I/II hips.[76] In this study, however, a selection bias was noted, with more severely involved patients being treated with the innominate osteotomy.

The multicenter prospective study by Wiig and colleagues provides the current best level of evidence (level II prospective cohort study) for nonoperative management of patients in this age group.[77] Radiographic outcomes of three treatments (physiotherapy, Scottish Rite adduction orthosis, and proximal femoral varus osteotomy) in patients with greater than 50% head involvement (Catterall's III or IV) were compared at 5 years' follow-up. A total of 126 patients were treated with physiotherapy, 22 with Scottish Rite adduction orthosis (SRO), and 23 with proximal femoral varus osteotomy. Investigators found no significant differences between the three treatments. Physiotherapy, SRO, and femoral varus osteotomy produced 53%, 46%, and 52% of patients with Stulberg I/II hips, respectively. In contrast to the two retrospective studies already described, less than 60% of patients in this age group in this study had good results.

Not all patients in this age group have a good radiographic outcome (Stulberg I or II hip). One to two patients in five developed Stulberg class III or worse hips according to the previous studies. These results raise the question of how to select the subgroup of patients in the younger age group with a poor prognosis and how to treat them more effectively. Because these studies show no added benefit of instituting operative treatment in improving outcomes, it appears that patients in this age group are best managed nonoperatively for now.

Onset at Age 6 to 8

Treatment results for this age group are less clear because two prospective studies differ in their findings.

The Perthes Study Group results show no statistically significant difference between hips in the nonoperative group (no treatment, range of motion, and Scottish Rite orthosis groups combined) and those in the operative group (femoral and innominate osteotomy groups combined).[72] However, the rate of good outcomes varied noticeably between treatment groups (Table 41-2). Of note is the lower success rate in the no treatment group (27%) compared with a much higher success rate in the brace (62%) and operative groups (68% to 69%), raising the possibility of insufficient power of the study to demonstrate a significant difference between the no treatment group and the brace and operative groups.

The second arm of the prospective study by Wiig and colleagues compared radiographic outcomes of patients 6 years or older from the time of diagnosis treated with physiotherapy, SRO, or femoral osteotomy.[77] The femoral osteotomy group had significantly better radiographic results (43% Stulberg I or II hips) compared with the SRO (20%) and physiotherapy (33%) groups. A few obvious differences between this study and the study by the Perthes Study Group are noteworthy. This study did not stratify patients into 6 to 8 years and greater than 8 years groups, as was done in the study by the Perthes Study Group. Without such stratification, it is difficult to determine whether the low rate of good outcomes (43% in this study vs. 68% in the Perthes Study Group for femoral osteotomy) was caused by older patients pulling down results in the study. Another consideration is that treatment was initiated at the stage of fragmentation in this study compared with the stage of increased radiodensity or early fragmentation in more than 95% of patients in the study by the Perthes Study Group. It is argued that initiating a treatment after substantial flattening of the femoral head has occurred may not be as effective as initiating a treatment before

Table 41-2. Stulberg Outcome of Five Treatments Studied by the Perthes Study Group

	Stulberg Radiographic Outcome	
	I or II	III, IV, or V
Age 6 to 8 Years at Disease Onset		
No treatment	27%	73%
Range of motion	48%	52%
Brace	62%	38%
Innominate osteotomy	69%	11%
Femoral osteotomy	68%	12%
Age >8 Years at Disease Onset		
No treatment	25%	75%
Range of motion	30%	70%
Brace	36%	64%
Innominate osteotomy	41%	59%
Femoral osteotomy	62%	38%

From Herring JA, Kim HT, Browne R: Legg-Calve-Perthes disease. Part II. Prospective multicenter study of the effect of treatment on outcome. J Bone Joint Surg Am 86:2121–2134, 2004.

flattening. A large retrospective study of 640 patients conducted by Joseph and colleagues suggests that earlier intervention is associated with better results.[78,79] Finally, the final follow-up occurred at 5 years in this study, when the healed stage was reached, compared with skeletal maturity in the latter study. Because the shape of the deformed femoral head can improve from the stage of reossification to skeletal maturity,[55,58] it is possible that with longer follow-up, the deformed heads may have improved.

In summary, evidence from one prospective study favors femoral osteotomy over no treatment, physiotherapy, or SRO at the radiographic stage of fragmentation. However, femoral osteotomy had a modest effect on achieving Stulberg class I or II hips in this study. The other prospective study found no difference between nonoperative and operative treatments among cohorts who were treated early.

Onset After Age 8

According to the Perthes Study Group results, no treatment, range of motion, SRO, innominate osteotomy, and femoral osteotomy groups had 25%, 30%, 36%, 41%, and 62% good results, respectively. Although these results suggest superiority of operative treatments, especially the femoral osteotomy, the difference was not statistically significant.[72] Insufficient power of the study due to relatively small sample sizes cannot be ruled out. An analysis of the results based on the lateral pillar classification did show a beneficial effect of the operative group compared with the nonoperative group for the lateral pillar B and B/C border groups, but not for the C group. Clinical applicability of treatment recommendations based on the lateral pillar classification, however, has raised controversy because operative treatments in the study were rendered at the stage of increased radiodensity in most patients when lateral pillar classification could not be determined.[80,81] The possibility of different treatments affecting the lateral pillar height

differently when they are instituted early cannot be excluded. A recent study suggests that different nonoperative treatments can influence lateral pillar height, and that lateral pillar height may be an outcome variable of treatment.[82] These observations raise the question of whether patients in this age group should be treated with early surgery, as was done in this study, or whether they should be on hold until the lateral pillar classification can be determined. Similar to the 6 to 8 years age group, the effect of surgery on achieving Stulberg I or II hips in this age group appears to be modest, with 41% of the innominate osteotomy and 62% of the femoral osteotomy groups achieving Stulberg I or II hips.

While reviewing results of operative treatments, it is pertinent to discuss possible reasons why they produced good results (Stulberg I or II hips) in some cases and not in others. Both femoral and innominate osteotomies are based on the concept of containment. According to this concept, to prevent deformities of the affected femoral head, the head must be contained within the depth of the acetabulum, thereby equalizing pressure on the head and subjecting it to the molding action of the acetabulum.[83] This is a mechanical concept that does not directly address the pathobiology of the disease, such as the predominance of bone resorption and delayed bone formation, which occur during the repair process. Current operative treatments may be performed on the pelvic bone or in the intertrochanteric region of the femur, away from the femoral head where the pathology lies. Although the mechanical effects of the surgeries may be adequate for some patients, they may not be sufficient for older patients, who may have slower and impaired healing, and who may have limited potential to remodel the deformed head. To improve the outcomes of patients treated operatively with a femoral or pelvic osteotomy, some have advocated a longer period of protected weight bearing postoperatively and allowing return to normal weight bearing based on femoral head healing (Fig. 41-11).

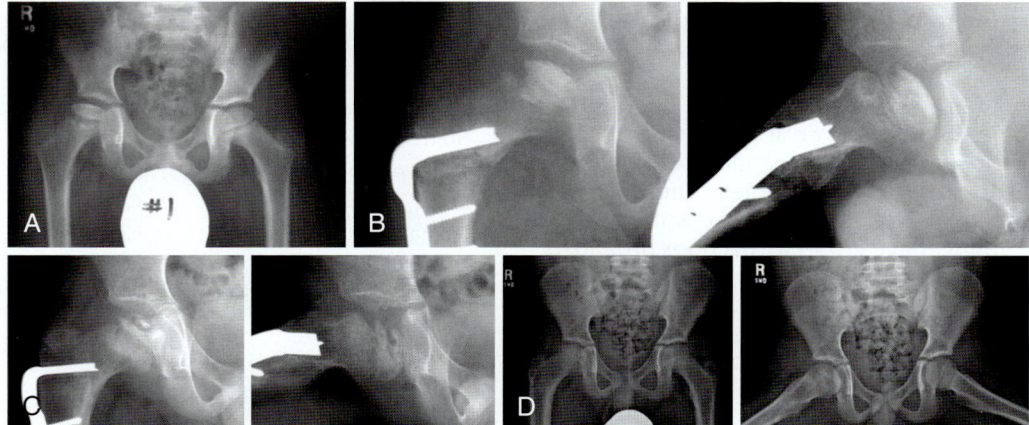

Figure 41-11. A, Radiograph of an 8-year-8-month-old male presenting at the initial stage of the disease. **B,** Radiographs obtained 1 month after the proximal femoral varus osteotomy showing resorptive changes in the epiphysis. **C,** Four- and 9-month follow-up radiographs showing that the femoral head was still in the resorptive stage. During this time, the patient was kept non–weight bearing on the affected hip. **D,** Three-year follow-up radiographs showing a spherical femoral head.

One important technical consideration regarding operative treatment is how much varus angulation or femoral head coverage is optimal for preserving the spherical shape of the femoral head. A recent study that reviewed 52 patients treated with proximal femoral varus osteotomy found that greater varus angulation did not necessarily produce better femoral head preservation.[84] Furthermore, 37% of the 52 patients showed no improvement in their postoperative varus neck shaft angle at maturity. Taken together, the authors recommended 10 to 15 degrees of varus correction when a proximal femoral varus osteotomy is performed in the early stages of Perthes disease. A greater degree of varus correction may be needed if the operation is performed in the later stages, when loss of containment is greater. Regarding Salter's innominate osteotomy, the possibility of placing too much anterior coverage or creating acetabular retroversion that may produce anterior femoroacetabular impingement is a concern,[85] especially given that acetabular retroversion appears to be relatively common among patients with LCPD.[86-88] At this time it is unclear how significant or prevalent the problem is after Salter's innominate osteotomy is performed; additional follow-up studies are needed.

Although some have advocated more extensive containment procedures such as combined femoral and innominate osteotomies or a triple pelvic osteotomy, at this time no evidence demonstrates that an aggressive mechanical approach produces better results. In a recent study in which investigators reviewed the radiographic outcomes of combined femoral and innominate osteotomies performed in patients older than age 8 at the onset of the disease, no Stulberg I hips were identified, 6 of 20 patients had Stulberg II hips, and the rest had Stulberg III to V hips.[89] After a triple pelvic osteotomy, 8 of 30 hips were found to have spherical femoral heads, and the rest had aspherical heads in one study, with a minimum follow-up of 3 years and mean age at surgery of 10 years.[90] Similar to Salter's innominate osteotomy, over-coverage and the possibility of femoroacetabular impingement are matters of concern after a triple pelvic osteotomy is performed.

The role of the Scottish Rite orthosis in the treatment of Perthes disease appears to be diminished at this time based on the results of two prospective studies and two retrospective studies, which have not shown the brace to be effective in producing a spherical femoral head.[91,92] The major limitation of the prospective and retrospective studies is their inability to confirm brace compliance, which could affect the outcome.

Other Nonoperative and Operative Treatments

A wide abduction weight-bearing cast introduced by Petrie and Bitenc in 1971 remains one of the nonoperative options still used to obtain femoral head containment.[93] In the original study, a bed rest or traction was used to relieve muscle spasm, and the cast was applied after 45 degrees of abduction was possible in each hip. The cast was changed every 3 to 4 months, and the knees were exercised before reapplication of the cast.

The average duration of treatment was 19 months. Over the years, several modifications have been made to the original treatment protocol, including application of the cast in the operating room with performance of hip adductor tenotomy and an arthrogram, if necessary; shortening of the duration of treatment; restriction of weight bearing in the cast; and using the cast treatment to improve abduction before performing an operative containment treatment. The effectiveness of this treatment has been reported only in retrospective studies.[94] These studies report that a Petrie cast is comparable with other treatments, including a pelvic or femoral osteotomy. At this time, there is no standard duration for a Petrie cast treatment, but shortening the duration of casting to 6 weeks can lead to recurrence of hip stiffness and hinge abduction.

A wide abduction brace called an *A-frame* has been advocated as an alternative method of maintaining femoral head containment following Petrie casting for 6 weeks (Fig. 41-12). An A-frame brace can be used as a weight-bearing or a non–weight-bearing brace to maintain femoral head containment. The recommended duration of brace wear is variable from center to center (8 to 20 hours per day), and a longer duration is recommended in the initial period of use. Proposed advantages of the A-frame treatment over operative treatment include that it avoids surgery-related problems such as limb shortening due to varus osteotomy, abductor muscle weakening, and creation of over-coverage, leading to femoral head impingement. In comparison with prolonged Petrie abduction casting, an A-frame brace allows part-time wearing of the brace and allows removal of the brace for range-of-motion exercises. Major disadvantages of this treatment include a prolonged duration of treatment (12 to 18 months), the cumbersome nature of the treatment, and loss of patient compliance over time.

A review of 253 patients (285 hips; age range, 2.2 to 11.3 years; mean age, 6.5 years) managed by a Petrie cast for 6 weeks followed by protected weight bearing in an A-frame brace for a prolonged period (20 hours per day for 6 to 9 months followed by part-time use during the day for 4 to 6 months) was reported.[95] Patients performed multi-plane hip range-of-motion exercises as part of the treatment protocol. This study showed good results, with Stulberg I and II outcomes at maturity in 85 of 97 lateral pillar class B hips and in 62 of 97 lateral pillar class C hips. In this study, the definition of Stulberg I outcome was a normal hip, and the Stulberg II hip outcome was spherical but with mild coxa magna with up to a 3 mm increase in maximum femoral head/neck width and a minimal (<5 mm) difference in epiphyseal height and/or neck length.

Other surgical procedures have been advocated for the treatment of Perthes disease. Shelf acetabuloplasty is used by some to improve acetabular coverage of the femoral head. This procedure may stimulate acetabular depth growth to a greater extent than the femoral osteotomy.[96] However, prospective studies examining results of this procedure are lacking. In a study that reviewed the results of patients with age at onset between 8 and 13 years, 14 of 27 hips were Stulberg I or II at maturity.[97]

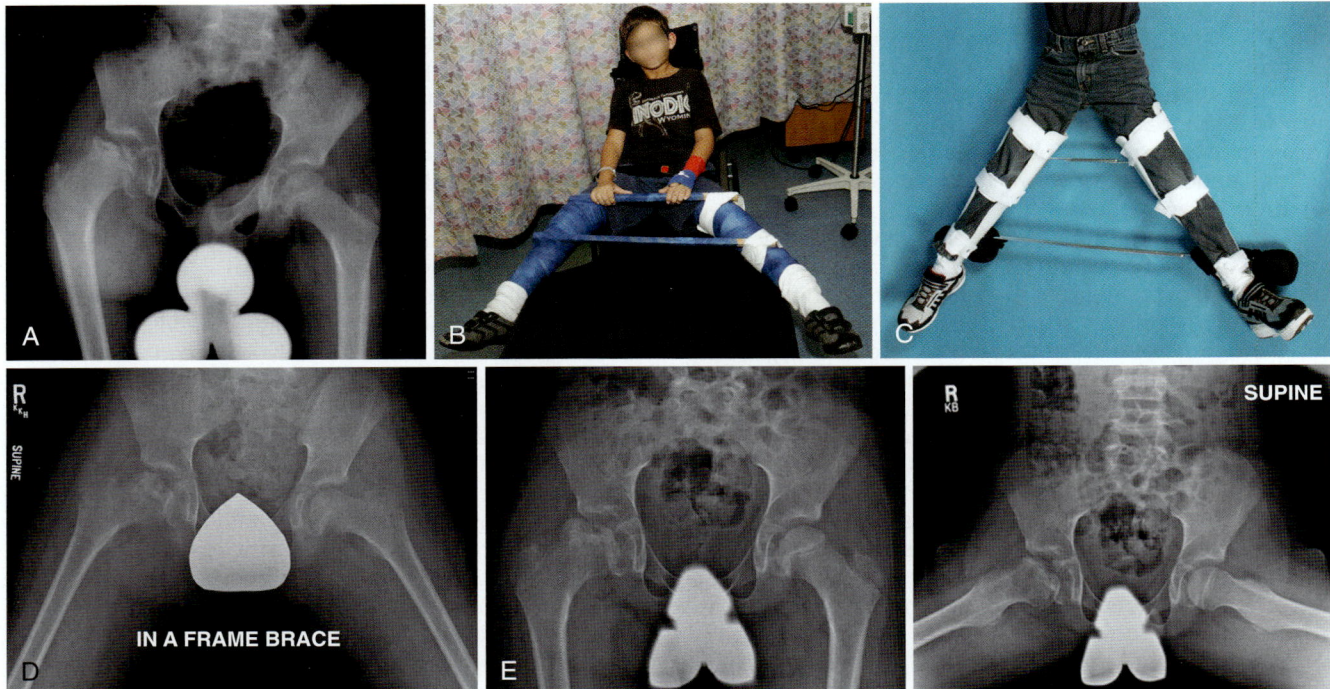

Figure 41-12. A, Radiograph of a 10-year-6-month-old male presenting with hip adduction contracture at the fragmentational stage of the disease. **B,** The patient underwent hip arthrography, hip adductor tenotomy, and application of a Petrie cast in the operating room. The cast was used for 6 weeks. **C** and **D** The patient in a nighttime (supine) wide abduction brace (A-frame), which was used 12 hours per day after removal of the Petrie cast, followed by weaning down to 8 hours per day as hip abduction was being maintained. **E,** Radiographs obtained at 4-month follow-up.

A recent study showed that those with less femoral head flattening and with reducible subluxation had more favorable acetabular remodeling and outcome.[98]

In preliminary studies, articulated hip distraction has been shown to have a protective effect on the femoral head when applied in early stages of the disease. or to have a restorative effect on femoral head height when applied at the fragmentation stage.[99,100] Follow-up studies on the outcomes of patients treated with this method are lacking. A recent intermediate follow-up study showed that femoral head height gained through the treatment was subsequently lost after removal of the distractor, with 7 of 10 poor results at maturity (Stulberg IV hips).[101] The remaining three patients had a Stulberg III hip. One of the limitations of this treatment is the duration of hip distraction (usually 4 to 5 months) that is being dictated by pin loosening, pin site infection, or patient tolerance, instead of the healing status of the femoral head.

For those patients presenting with femoral head deformity and hinge abduction, the best treatment remains undefined. In the active phase of the disease, a Petrie cast followed by an A-frame brace treatment or operative containment treatment remains an option, but it is unknown whether one form of treatment is superior to another. For those patients in the reossification or healed stage of the disease, a valgus femoral osteotomy has been shown to improve function and Iowa or Harris hip scores at an average follow-up of 5

to 7 years.[102-104] In a longer study consisting of 48 patients, 4 patients had a total hip replacement, 1 had an arthrodesis, and 6 had repeat valgus extension osteotomy for recurrence or fixed adduction at mean follow-up of 10 years.[105]

The role of trochanteric epiphysiodesis as a prophylactic procedure combined with femoral varus osteotomy, or as treatment for femoral varus deformity, remains controversial because it is difficult to predict who will benefit from the procedure. Its effectiveness appears to be dependent on multiple variables, including age at surgery and premature physeal growth arrest.[106,107] Prophylactic trochanteric osteotomy has been shown to normalize articulo-trochanteric and center-trochanteric distances in 60% of 62 patients studied to maturity, with the remaining 30% achieving undercorrection and 10% achieving overcorrection.[108] The size of the femoral head at healing and age at surgery were found to significantly influence the outcome in this study. Because varus angulation does improve spontaneously in some patients treated with femoral varus osteotomy, the true beneficial effect of the prophylactic procedure cannot be ascertained without a proper control, and such a comparative study is lacking. Results of trochanteric advancement to treat the overriding greater trochanter have been mixed, with one recent study reporting no beneficial effects on pain and limping[109] but older studies reporting beneficial effects.[110]

Femoroacetabular Impingement (FAI) in Adolescents and Young Adults With Perthes Disease

Recognition that femoroacetabular impingement (FAI) can be a source of hip pain and an etiologic factor in labral pathology and secondary osteoarthritis has extended clinical interest in assessing symptomatic adolescents and young adults with Perthes disease for the presence of this condition.[111,112] Currently, the number of studies specifically addressing patients with Perthes disease and FAI is limited, and our understanding of FAI as it relates to Perthes disease is still evolving. The subset of patients with residual deformity of the femoral head and FAI who become symptomatic as an adolescent or a young adult typically have groin pain, a positive impingement sign, and MRI findings of labral pathology.[74] Surgical dislocation to further define the pathology and to address impingement, labral pathology, and the overriding trochanter has led to improvement in hip pain and function in early studies with small numbers of patients.[74,113,114] In addition to addressing intra-articular pathology, some advocate addressing acetabular dysplasia with periacetabular osteotomy at the same time or as a staged procedure.[114] No long-term studies on the effects of these procedures are available at this time. It is also unclear why some adolescents with deformed femoral heads become symptomatic and some do not. Additional studies are needed to define patients who would benefit from surgical intervention, the best time to intervene, and which procedures are effective in preserving the hip joint.

Developing Medical Treatment for Perthes Disease

Appreciation of Perthes disease as having biological components that contribute to the deformity, such as a predominance of bone resorption or a delay in replacement of resorbed areas with new bone during the fragmentation stage, has led to investigation of the effects of modulating the pathologic repair process or preventing femoral head deformity. Preclinical studies using small and large animal models show that antiresorptive therapy using bisphosphonates can minimize the development of femoral head deformity in these models.[45,115,116] Although necrotic bone within the infarcted femoral heads of bisphosphonate-treated animals shows significantly better preservation, lack of new bone formation on the preserved necrotic bone remains a matter of concern. Although new appositional bone formation has been shown in rodent models, this process has not been demonstrated in a large animal model (piglet model).[45] Another concern is related to the possible effects of bisphosphonates on the growing skeleton because the drugs have a long half-life within bone. Early studies on the safety of bisphosphonates for the treatment of Perthes disease and other osteonecrotic conditions in a limited number of patients showed that the drug did not produce growth inhibition or significant complications over the short term.[117] Long-term effects of bisphosphonates on the growing skeleton remain to be studied. To decrease exposure of bisphosphonates to the rest of the skeleton, local intraosseous administration of bisphosphonates has been proposed to decrease the dose and the number of doses required to obtain a therapeutic effect. An experimental study using a radioactive bisphosphonate showed that local bioavailability of systemically administered bisphosphonate correlated with the vascular status of the femoral head and was limited in the avascular region of the infarcted head.[118] Local administration was shown to be an effective route for minimizing femoral head deformity while significantly decreasing the total amount of the drug administered in a large animal study.[119]

Clinical validation of animal studies on the use of bisphosphonates to treat Perthes disease is lacking at this time. A case series reporting on the effects of intravenous bisphosphonate therapy on traumatic femoral head osteonecrosis in adolescents constitutes the only study so far conducted in a pediatric population.[120] Because of lack of a control group, the efficacy of the treatment cannot be determined. In the adult population, oral bisphosphonate therapy has been shown to have a protective effect by preventing femoral head collapse in short-term studies.[121-123] In a longer follow-up study with a mean follow-up of 4 years, improvements and maintenance of pain and disability scores were observed in patients with Ficat stage I and II hips (precollapse stages).[121] However, radiologic progression in terms of femoral head collapse was observed in 12.6% of patients in Ficat stage I and in 55.8% of stage II hips with mean time to collapse of 3.1 years (2 to 6 years).

PROGNOSIS

The degree of femoral head deformity based on the Stulberg classification, age at onset of the disease, Catterall's head-at-risk signs, the extent of femoral head involvement based on Catterall's classification, and lateral pillar involvement are reported prognostic factors in Perthes disease.

CURRENT CONTROVERSIES

- For older patients (>8 years at the onset of disease), when is the best time to institute operative treatment? Is it better to institute treatment early (the initial stage) before the development of a significant femoral head collapse, or later, when the lateral pillar or Catterall's classification can be determined?
- Should return to full weight-bearing activities after femoral or innominate osteotomy be based on a predetermined time period (usually 6 weeks), or should it be based on the healing status of the necrotic femoral head?
- What is the role of core decompression or hip distraction in the treatment of late-onset Perthes disease?
- How does femoroacetabular impingement affect the natural course of Perthes disease, and do surgical treatments to address impingement and chondrolabral pathology improve the outcome?

FUTURE CONSIDERATIONS

Perthes disease remains a controversial topic in pediatric orthopedics. Several key questions related to its causes, pathogenesis, and treatment remain only partially answered. Improvements in gaps in knowledge have been gained through recent experimental and clinical studies. Going forward, there is a need to develop earlier prognostic indicators, which can be applied before development of the femoral head deformity. Biological treatments that specifically address the pathobiology of the disease and the mechanical compromise of the femoral head are needed to improve the outcomes of older patients with a poor prognosis. There is also a need to better define the contribution of femoroacetabular impingement to the pathogenesis of premature osteoarthritis in Perthes disease, and to determine how effective newer surgical treatments are in preserving the hip over the long term.

REFERENCES

1. Wiig O, Terjesen T, Svenningsen S, Lie SA: The epidemiology and aetiology of Perthes' disease in Norway: a nationwide study of 425 patients. J Bone Joint Surg Br 88:1217–1223, 2006.
2. Gray IM, Lowry RB, Renwick DH: Incidence and genetics of Legg-Perthes disease (osteochondritis deformans) in British Columbia: evidence of polygenic determination. J Med Genet 9:197–202, 1972.
3. Molloy MK, MacMahon B: Incidence of Legg-Perthes disease (osteochondritis deformans). N Engl J Med 275:988–990, 1966.
4. Margetts BM, Perry CA, Taylor JF, Dangerfield PH: The incidence and distribution of Legg-Calve-Perthes disease in Liverpool, 1982-95. Arch Dis Child 84:351–354, 2001.
5. Hall DJ: Genetic aspects of Perthes' disease: a critical review. Clin Orthop Relat Res 209:100–114, 1986.
6. Wynne-Davies R, Gormley J: The aetiology of Perthes' disease: genetic, epidemiological and growth factors in 310 Edinburgh and Glasgow patients. J Bone Joint Surg Br 60:6–14, 1978.
7. Bahmanyar S, Montgomery SM, Weiss RJ, Ekbom A: Maternal smoking during pregnancy, other prenatal and perinatal factors, and the risk of Legg-Calve-Perthes disease. Pediatrics 122:e459–e464, 2008.
8. Garcia Mata S, Ardanaz Aicua E, Hidalgo Ovejero A, Martinez Grandez M: Legg-Calvé-Perthes disease and passive smoking. J Pediatr Orthop 20:326–330, 2000.
9. Gordon JE, Schoenecker PL, Osland JD, et al: Smoking and socio-economic status in the etiology and severity of Legg-Calve-Perthes disease. J Pediatr Orthop B 13:367–370, 2004.
10. Neidel J, Zander D, Hackenbroch MH: Low plasma levels of insulin-like growth factor I in Perthes' disease: a controlled study of 59 consecutive children. Acta Orthop Scand 63:393–398, 1992.
11. Matsumoto T, Enomoto H, Takahashi K, Motokawa S: Decreased levels of IGF binding protein-3 in serum from children with Perthes' disease. Acta Orthop Scand 69:125–128, 1998.
12. Neidel J, Schönau E, Zander D, et al: Normal plasma levels of IGF binding protein in Perthes' disease: follow-up of previous report. Acta Orthop Scand 64:540–542, 1993.
13. Liu YF, Chen WM, Lin YF, et al: Type II collagen gene variants and inherited osteonecrosis of the femoral head. N Engl J Med 352:2294–2301, 2005.
14. Miyamoto Y, Matsuda T, Kitoh H, et al: A recurrent mutation in type II collagen gene causes Legg-Calve-Perthes disease in a Japanese family. Hum Genet 121:625–629, 2007.
15. Su P, Li R, Liu S, et al: Age at onset-dependent presentations of premature hip osteoarthritis, avascular necrosis of the femoral head, or Legg-Calve-Perthes disease in a single family, consequent upon a p.Gly1170Ser mutation of COL2A1. Arthritis Rheum 58:1701–1706, 2008.
16. Kenet G, Ezra E, Wientroub S, et al: Perthes' disease and the search for genetic associations: collagen mutations, Gaucher's disease and thrombophilia. J Bone Joint Surg Br 90:1507–1511, 2008.
17. Glueck CJ, Glueck HI, Greenfield D, et al: Protein C and S deficiency, thrombophilia, and hypofibrinolysis: pathophysiologic causes of Legg-Perthes disease. Pediatr Res 35(4 Pt 1):383–388, 1994.
18. Hresko MT, McDougall PA, Gorlin JB, et al: Prospective reevaluation of the association between thrombotic diathesis and Legg-Perthes disease. J Bone Joint Surg Am 84:1613–1618, 2002.
19. Balasa VV, Gruppo RA, Glueck CJ, et al: Legg-Calve-Perthes disease and thrombophilia. J Bone Joint Surg Am 86:2642–2647, 2004.
20. Martinelli I, Mannucci PM, De Stefano V, et al: Different risks of thrombosis in four coagulation defects associated with inherited thrombophilia: a study of 150 families. Blood 92:2353–2358, 1998.
21. Atsumi T, Yamano K, Muraki M, et al: The blood supply of the lateral epiphyseal arteries in Perthes' disease. J Bone Joint Surg Br 82:392–398, 2000.
22. de Camargo FP, de Godoy RM Jr, Tovo R: Angiography in Perthes' disease. Clin Orthop Relat Res 191:216–220, 1984.
23. Theron J: Angiography in Legg-Calve-Perthes disease. Radiology 135:81–92, 1980.
24. Conway JJ: A scintigraphic classification of Legg-Calve-Perthes disease. Semin Nucl Med 23:274–295, 1993.
25. Lamer S, Dorgeret S, Kharouni A, et al: Femoral head vascularisation in Legg-Calvé-Perthes disease: comparison of dynamic gadolinium-enhanced subtraction MRI with bone scintigraphy. Pediatr Radiol 32:580–585, 2002.
26. Jonsater S: Coxa plana: a histo-pathologic and arthrographic study. Acta Orthop Scand Suppl 12:5–98, 1953.
27. Kim HK, Su PH: Development of flattening and apparent fragmentation following ischemic necrosis of the capital femoral epiphysis in a piglet model. J Bone Joint Surg Am 84:1329–1334, 2002.
28. Sanchis M, Zahir A, Freeman MA: The experimental simulation of Perthes disease by consecutive interruptions of the blood supply to the capital femoral epiphysis in the puppy. J Bone Joint Surg Am 55:335–342, 1973.
29. Zahir A, Freeman AR: Cartilage changes following a single episode of infarction of the capital femoral epiphysis in the dog. J Bone Joint Surg Am 54:125–136, 1972.
30. Inoue A, Freeman MA, Vernon-Roberts B, Mizuno S: The pathogenesis of Perthes' disease. J Bone Joint Surg Br 58:453–461, 1976.
31. Catterall A, Pringle J, Byers PD, et al: A review of the morphology of Perthes' disease. J Bone Joint Surg Br 64:269–275, 1982.
32. Catterall A, Pringle J, Byers PD, et al: Perthes' disease: is the epiphyseal infarction complete? J Bone Joint Surg Br 64:276–281, 1982.
33. Dolman CL, Bell HM: The pathology of Legg-Calve-Perthes disease: a case report. J Bone Joint Surg Am 55:184–188, 1973.
34. McKibbin B, Ralis Z: Pathological changes in a case of Perthes' disease. J Bone Joint Surg Br 56:438–447, 1974.
35. Milgram JW: Idiopathic osteonecrosis of the juvenile femoral head (Legg-Calve-Perthes disease) in radiologic and histologic pathology of nontumorous diseases of bones and joints, New Berlin, Wis, 1990, Northbrook Publishing Company, pp 1093–1113.
36. Ponseti IV: Legg-Perthes disease; observations on pathological changes in two cases. J Bone Joint Surg Am 38:739–750, 1956.
37. Ponseti IV, Maynard JA, Weinstein SL, et al: Legg-Calvé-Perthes disease: histochemical and ultrastructural observations of the epiphyseal cartilage and physis. J Bone Joint Surg Am 65:797–807, 1983.
38. Kim HK, Stephenson N, Garces A, et al: Effects of disruption of epiphyseal vasculature on the proximal femoral growth plate. J Bone Joint Surg Am 91:1149–1158, 2009.

39. Pringle D, Koob TJ, Kim HK: Indentation properties of growing femoral head following ischemic necrosis. J Orthop Res 22:122–130, 2004.

40. Koob TJ, Pringle D, Gedbaw E, et al: Biomechanical properties of bone and cartilage in growing femoral head following ischemic osteonecrosis. J Orthop Res 25:750–757, 2007.

41. Kim HK, Su PH, Qiu YS: Histopathologic changes in growth-plate cartilage following ischemic necrosis of the capital femoral epiphysis: an experimental investigation in immature pigs. J Bone Joint Surg Am 83:688–697, 2001.

42. Hofstaetter JG, Roschger P, Klaushofer K, Kim HK: Increased matrix mineralization in the immature femoral head following ischemic osteonecrosis. Bone 46:379–385, 2010.

43. Seeman E, Delmas PD: Bone quality—the material and structural basis of bone strength and fragility. N Engl J Med 354:2250–2261, 2006.

44. Kim HK, Morgan-Bagley S, Kostenuik P: RANKL inhibition: a novel strategy to decrease femoral head deformity after ischemic osteonecrosis. J Bone Miner Res 21:1946–1954, 2006.

45. Kim HK, Randall TS, Bian H, et al: Ibandronate for prevention of femoral head deformity after ischemic necrosis of the capital femoral epiphysis in immature pigs. J Bone Joint Surg Am 87:550–557, 2005.

46. Bergmann G, Deuretzbacher G, Heller M, et al: Hip contact forces and gait patterns from routine activities. J Biomech 34:859–871, 2001.

47. Rosenfeld SB, Herring JA, Chao JC: Legg-Calve-Perthes disease: a review of cases with onset before six years of age. J Bone Joint Surg Am 89:2712–2722, 2007.

48. Chung SM: The arterial supply of the developing proximal end of the human femur. J Bone Joint Surg Am 58:961–970, 1976.

49. Meszaros T, Kery L: Quantitative analysis of the growth of the hip joint: a radiological study. Acta Orthop Scand 51:275–283, 1980.

50. Ogden JA: Changing patterns of proximal femoral vascularity. J Bone Joint Surg Am 56:941–950, 1974.

51. Trueta J: The normal vascular anatomy of the human femoral head during growth. J Bone Joint Surg Br 39:358–394, 1957.

52. Catterall A: Legg-Calve-Perthes syndrome. Clin Orthop Relat Res 158:41–52, 1981.

53. Mukherjee A, Fabry G: Evaluation of the prognostic indices in Legg-Calve-Perthes disease: statistical analysis of 116 hips. J Pediatr Orthop 10:153–158, 1990.

54. McAndrew MP, Weinstein SL: A long-term follow-up of Legg-Calve-Perthes disease. J Bone Joint Surg Am 66:860–869, 1984.

55. Herring JA, Williams JJ, Neustadt JN, Early JS: Evolution of femoral head deformity during the healing phase of Legg-Calve-Perthes disease. J Pediatr Orthop 13:41–45, 1993.

56. Pienkowski D, Resig J, Talwalkar V, Tylkowski C: Novel three-dimensional MRI technique for study of cartilaginous hip surfaces in Legg-Calve-Perthes disease. J Orthop Res 27:981–988, 2009.

57. Gower WE, Johnston RC: Legg-Perthes disease: long-term follow-up of thirty-six patients. J Bone Joint Surg Am 53:759–768, 1971.

58. Mose K: Methods of measuring in Legg-Calve-Perthes disease with special regard to the prognosis. Clin Orthop Relat Res 150:103–109, 1980.

59. Stulberg SD, Cooperman DR, Wallensten R: The natural history of Legg-Calve-Perthes disease. J Bone Joint Surg Am 63:1095–1108, 1981.

60. Neyt JG, Weinstein SL, Spratt KF, et al: Stulberg classification system for evaluation of Legg-Calve-Perthes disease: intra-rater and inter-rater reliability. J Bone Joint Surg Am 81:1209–1216, 1999.

61. Herring JA, Kim HT, Browne R: Legg-Calve-Perthes disease. Part I. Classification of radiographs with use of the modified lateral pillar and Stulberg classifications. J Bone Joint Surg Am 86:2103–2120, 2004.

62. Wiig O, Terjesen T, Svenningsen S: Inter-observer reliability of the Stulberg classification in the assessment of Perthes disease. J Child Orthop 1:101–105, 2007.

63. Nelson D, Zenios M, Ward K, et al: The deformity index as a predictor of final radiological outcome in Perthes' disease. J Bone Joint Surg Br 89:1369–1374, 2007.

64. Vuolteenaho K, Moilanen T, Moilanen E: Non-steroidal anti-inflammatory drugs, cyclooxygenase-2 and the bone healing process. Basic Clin Pharmacol Toxicol 102:10–14, 2008.

65. Salter RB, Thompson GH: Legg-Calve-Perthes disease: the prognostic significance of the subchondral fracture and a two-group classification of the femoral head involvement. J Bone Joint Surg Am 66:479–489, 1984.

66. Catterall A: The natural history of Perthes' disease. J Bone Joint Surg Br 53:37–53, 1971.

67. Wiig O, Terjesen T, Svenningsen S: Inter-observer reliability of radiographic classifications and measurements in the assessment of Perthes' disease. Acta Orthop Scand 73:523–530, 2002.

68. Herring JA, Neustadt JB, Williams JJ, et al: The lateral pillar classification of Legg-Calve-Perthes disease. J Pediatr Orthop 12:143–150, 1992.

69. Ritterbusch JF, Shantharam SS, Gelinas C: Comparison of lateral pillar classification and Catterall classification of Legg-Calve-Perthes disease. J Pediatr Orthop 13:200–202, 1993.

70. Lappin K, Kealey D, Cosgrove A: Herring classification: how useful is the initial radiograph? J Pediatr Orthop 22:479–482, 2002.

71. Joseph B, Mulpuri K, Varghese G: Perthes' disease in the adolescent. J Bone Joint Surg Br 83:715–720, 2001.

72. Herring JA, Kim HT, Browne R: Legg-Calve-Perthes disease. Part II. Prospective multicenter study of the effect of treatment on outcome. J Bone Joint Surg Am 86:2121–2134, 2004.

73. Wiig O: Perthes' disease in Norway: a prospective study on 425 patients. Acta Orthop Suppl 80:1–44, 2009.

74. Eijer H, Podeszwa DA, Ganz R, Leunig M: Evaluation and treatment of young adults with femoro-acetabular impingement secondary to Perthes disease. Hip Int 16:273–280, 2006.

75. Rowe SM, Moon ES, Yoon TR, et al: Fate of the osteochondral fragments in osteochondritis dissecans after Legg-Calve-Perthes disease. J Bone Joint Surg Br 84:1025–1029, 2002.

76. Canavese F, Dimeglio A: Perthes' disease: prognosis in children under six years of age. J Bone Joint Surg Br 90:940–945, 2008.

77. Wiig O, Terjesen T, Svenningsen S: Prognostic factors and outcome of treatment in Perthes' disease: a prospective study of 368 patients with five-year follow-up. J Bone Joint Surg Br 90:1364-1371, 2008.

78. Joseph B, Nair NS, Narasimha Rao KL, et al: Optimal timing for containment surgery for Perthes disease. J Pediatr Orthop 23:601–606, 2003.

79. Joseph B, Rao N, Mulpuri K, et al: How does a femoral varus osteotomy alter the natural evolution of Perthes' disease? J Pediatr Orthop B 14:10–15, 2005.

80. Little DG: Legg-Calve-Perthes disease: the effect of treatment on outcome. J Bone Joint Surg Am 87:1164–1165, 2005; author reply 1164–1165.

81. Price CT: The lateral pillar classification for Legg-Calve-Perthes disease. J Pediatr Orthop 27:592–593, 2007.

82. Kuroda T, Mitani S, Sugimoto Y, et al: Changes in the lateral pillar classification in Perthes' disease. J Pediatr Orthop B 18:116–119, 2009.

83. Harrison MH, Menon MP: Legg-Calve-Perthes disease: the value of roentgenographic measurement in clinical practice with special reference to the broomstick plaster method. J Bone Joint Surg Am 48:1301–1318, 1966.

84. Kim HK, da Cunha AM, Browne R, et al: How much varus is optimal with proximal femoral osteotomy to preserve the femoral head in Legg-Calve-Perthes disease? J Bone Joint Surg Am 93:341–347, 2011.

85. Dora C, Mascard E, Mladenov K, Seringe R: Retroversion of the acetabular dome after Salter and triple pelvic osteotomy for congenital dislocation of the hip. J Pediatr Orthop B 11:34–40, 2002.

86. Ezoe M, Naito M, Inoue T: The prevalence of acetabular retroversion among various disorders of the hip. J Bone Joint Surg Am 88:372–379, 2006.

87. Noelle Larson A, Stans AA, Sierra RJ: Ischial spine sign reveals acetabular retroversion in Legg-Calve-Perthes disease. Clin Orthop Relat Res 469:2012–2018, 2011.

88. Sankar WN, Flynn JM: The development of acetabular retroversion in children with Legg-Calve-Perthes disease. J Pediatr Orthop 28:440–443, 2008.

89. Javid M, Wedge JH: Radiographic results of combined Salter innominate and femoral osteotomy in Legg-Calve-Perthes disease in older children. J Child Orthop 3:229–234, 2009.

90. Vukasinovic Z, Pelillo F, Spasovski D, et al: Triple pelvic osteotomy in the treatment of Legg-Calve-Perthes disease. Int Orthop 33:1377–1383, 2009.

91. Martinez AG, Weinstein SL, Dietz FR: The weight-bearing abduction brace for the treatment of Legg-Perthes disease. J Bone Joint Surg Am 74:12–21, 1992.

92. Meehan PL, Angel D, Nelson JM: The Scottish Rite abduction orthosis for the treatment of Legg-Perthes disease: a radiographic analysis. J Bone Joint Surg Am 74:2–12, 1992.

93. Petrie JG, Bitenc I: The abduction weight-bearing treatment in Legg-Perthes disease. J Bone Joint Surg Br 53:54–62, 1971.

94. Grzegorzewski A, Bowen JR, Guille JT, Glutting J: Treatment of the collapsed femoral head by containment in Legg-Calve-Perthes disease. J Pediatr Orthop 23:15-19, 2003.

95. Rich MM, Schoenecker PL: Management of Perthes disease by protected weight-bearing in an A-frame orthosis and multiplane hip range of motion: twenty-five year experience. J Children Orthop, in press.

96. Domzalski ME, Glutting J, Bowen JR, Littleton AG: Lateral acetabular growth stimulation following a labral support procedure in Legg-Calve-Perthes disease. J Bone Joint Surg Am 88:1458–1466, 2006.

97. Daly K, Bruce C, Catterall A: Lateral shelf acetabuloplasty in Perthes' disease: a review of the end of growth. J Bone Joint Surg Br 81:380–384, 1999.

98. Yoo WJ, Choi IH, Cho TJ, et al: Shelf acetabuloplasty for children with Perthes' disease and reducible subluxation of the hip: prognostic factors related to hip remodelling. J Bone Joint Surg Br 91:1383–1387, 2009.

99. Maxwell SL, Lappin KJ, Kealey WD, et al: Arthrodiastasis in Perthes' disease: preliminary results. J Bone Joint Surg Br 86:244–250, 2004.

100. Segev E: Treatment of severe late onset Perthes' disease with soft tissue release and articulated hip distraction: early results. J Pediatr Orthop B 13:158–165, 2004.

101. Segev E, Ezra E, Wientroub S, et al: Treatment of severe late-onset Perthes' disease with soft tissue release and articulated hip distraction: revisited at skeletal maturity. J Child Orthop 1:229–235, 2007.

102. Myers GJ, Mathur K, O'Hara J: Valgus osteotomy: a solution for late presentation of hinge abduction in Legg-Calve-Perthes disease. J Pediatr Orthop 28:169–172, 2008.

103. Raney EM, Grogan DP, Hurley ME, Ogden MJ: The role of proximal femoral valgus osteotomy in Legg-Calve-Perthes disease. Orthopedics 25:513–517, 2002.

104. Yoo WJ, Choi IH, Chung CY, et al: Valgus femoral osteotomy for hinge abduction in Perthes' disease: decision-making and outcomes. J Bone Joint Surg Br 86:726–730, 2004.

105. Bankes MJ, Catterall A, Hashemi-Nejad A: Valgus extension osteotomy for "hinge abduction" in Perthes' disease: results at maturity and factors influencing the radiological outcome. J Bone Joint Surg Br 82:548–554, 2000.

106. Gage JR, Cary JM: The effects of trochanteric epiphyseodesis on growth of the proximal end of the femur following necrosis of the capital femoral epiphysis. J Bone Joint Surg Am 62:785–794, 1980.

107. Langenskiold A, Salenius P: Epiphyseodesis of the greater trochanter. Acta Orthop Scand 38:199–219, 1967.

108. Shah H, Siddesh ND, Joseph B, Nair SN: Effect of prophylactic trochanteric epiphyseodesis in older children with Perthes' disease. J Pediatr Orthop 29:889–895, 2009.

109. Joo SY, Lee KS, Koh IH, et al: Trochanteric advancement in patients with Legg-Calve-Perthes disease does not improve pain or limp. Clin Orthop Relat Res 466:927–934, 2008.

110. Macnicol MF, Makris D: Distal transfer of the greater trochanter. J Bone Joint Surg Br 73:838–841, 1991.

111. Leunig M, Beaule PE, Ganz R: The concept of femoroacetabular impingement: current status and future perspectives. Clin Orthop Relat Res 467:616–622, 2009.

112. Wenger DR, Kishan S, Pring ME: Impingement and childhood hip disease. J Pediatr Orthop B 15:233–243, 2006.

113. Anderson LA, Erickson JA, Severson EP, Peters CL: Sequelae of Perthes disease: treatment with surgical hip dislocation and relative femoral neck lengthening. J Pediatr Orthop 30:758–766, 2010.

114. Schoenecker PL, Clohisy JC, Millis MB, Wenger DR: Surgical management of the problematic hip in adolescent and young adult patients. J Am Acad Orthop Surg 19:275–286, 2011.

115. Little DG, McDonald M, Sharpe IT, et al: Zoledronic acid improves femoral head sphericity in a rat model of Perthes disease. J Orthop Res 23:862–868, 2005.

116. Little DG, Peat RA, Mcevoy A, et al: Zoledronic acid treatment results in retention of femoral head structure after traumatic osteonecrosis in young Wistar rats. J Bone Miner Res 18:2016–2022, 2003.

117. Johannesen J, Briody J, McQuade M, et al: Systemic effects of zoledronic acid in children with traumatic femoral head avascular necrosis and Legg-Calve-Perthes disease. Bone 45:898–902, 2009.

118. Kim HK, Sanders M, Athavale S, et al: Local bioavailability and distribution of systemically (parenterally) administered ibandronate in the infarcted femoral head. Bone 39:205–212, 2006.

119. Aya-ay J, Athavale S, Morgan-Bagley S, et al: Retention, distribution, and effects of intraosseously administered ibandronate in the infarcted femoral head. J Bone Miner Res 22:93–100, 2007.

120. Ramachandran M, Ward K, Brown RR, et al: Intravenous bisphosphonate therapy for traumatic osteonecrosis of the femoral head in adolescents. J Bone Joint Surg Am 89:1727–1734, 2007.

121. Agarwala S, Shah S, Joshi VR: The use of alendronate in the treatment of avascular necrosis of the femoral head: follow-up to eight years. J Bone Joint Surg Br 91:1013–1018, 2009.

122. Lai KA, Shen WJ, Yang CY, et al: The use of alendronate to prevent early collapse of the femoral head in patients with nontraumatic osteonecrosis: a randomized clinical study. J Bone Joint Surg Am 87:2155–2159, 2005.

123. Nishii T, Sugano N, Miki H, et al: Does alendronate prevent collapse in osteonecrosis of the femoral head? Clin Orthop Relat Res 443:273–279, 2006.

CHAPTER 42

Slipped Capital Femoral Epiphysis

Daniel J. Sucato

INTRODUCTION

Slipped capital femoral epiphysis (SCFE) is a primarily posterior migration of the epiphysis on the metaphysis in the skeletally immature patient. The clinical presentation of these patients is somewhat challenging because they often have painful symptoms in the thigh and knee region, which makes the diagnosis difficult and often delayed. Chronic or stable SCFE presents with discomfort and can lead to the more serious acute or unstable SCFE, which presents as a hip fracture with acute pain and an inability to bear weight and carries a high risk for developing avascular necrosis. The cause of SCFE is unknown; however, relative weakening of the physis compared with the size and activity of these patients is often a contributing factor. Treatment, especially for unstable SCFE, continues to evolve fairly rapidly with more aggressive surgical treatment to limit the incidence of avascular necrosis (AVN) and residual deformity, which can lead to femoroacetabular impingement (FAI).

This chapter describes the current perspective on slipped capital femoral epiphysis with traditional information on the incidence, origin, and classification. An up-to-date review of current surgical management and thinking behind these treatments will be discussed.

INCIDENCE AND EPIDEMIOLOGY

SCFE is estimated to occur in approximately 2 per 100,000 population and is somewhat dependent on race and geographic region. African Americans living in the Eastern United States are more prone to SCFE.[1] Males have a greater predisposition to developing SCFE than females, with some studies suggesting that it is up to five times more likely to occur in the male population. More current studies demonstrate a 2:1 or 3:2 ratio of males to females, suggesting a decrease in male prevalence over time.[2,3]

SCFE is more commonly seen in the summer months; June is a common month for this condition in North America,[4] and July is more common in Europe.[5] This is geographically determined because time-related incidence has not been seen in the Southern hemisphere.

Race is a characteristic feature of slipped capital femoral epiphysis; African Americans and Hispanics more commonly develop SCFE than Caucasians.[6] Increased prevalence of bilateral SCFE did not occur more commonly in black children.[6] Loder further analyzed Polynesian children, who demonstrated the highest prevalence of slipped capital femoral epiphysis.[3] The left hip is more commonly affected than the right side.

The cause of SCFE is unknown, although some have suggested that because children are more commonly right-handed, the sitting posture during school time predisposes the left hip to SCFE.[7] The most common age for the occurrence of SCFE is the adolescent period, which is generally considered the time of maximal skeletal growth. Boys are most commonly affected during the ages of 13 to 15 years; girls in the 11 to 13 year age group are more commonly affected.[2-6] SCFE can be seen in the younger patient (<10 years of age), and in this setting, a careful endocrinopathy workup, including thyroid function assessment, should be performed.[8] Bilateral involvement of slipped capital femoral epiphysis is generally regarded to be approximately 25%; this is important to realize when evaluating a patient who presents with a SCFE. It is mandatory that anteroposterior (AP) and frog-leg pelvis radiographs are performed to visualize both hips to ensure that bilateral SCFEs are not present.[2,9]

CLASSIFICATION

The most common classification utilized to date is the one described by Loder and coworkers in defining a stable versus an unstable slip (Fig. 42-1). This is an important classification because it predicts the incidence of avascular necrosis (AVN) in the setting of in situ pin fixation treatment. Loder and associates described 55 patients who presented with an acute SCFE and based their classification on the ability to bear weight. For those hip patients who could bear weight even with crutches, this was defined as a stable slip, and the incidence of AVN in their series was 0% (0 of 25 SCFEs). In stark contrast, patients who were unable to ambulate or get up with crutches were defined as having an unstable SCFE, and their incidence of AVN was 47% (14 of 30 patients).[10] This classification system has been adopted and is the most common classification utilized today because it does prognosticate the incidence of AVN and has been studied and confirmed by others.[11-14]

Older classifications include the one based on the chronicity of the SCFE. The acute SCFE is one in which symptoms have occurred for 3 weeks or less. This typically coincides with having an unstable SCFE in that the patient has an acute event leading to severe symptoms and usually the inability to ambulate. Acute SCFE is often difficult to distinguish from the Salter-Harris type 1 fracture, which also occurs through the physis;

however, it is generally agreed that the type 1 epiphyseal fracture occurs secondary to significant trauma in an otherwise normal patient without prodromal symptoms. This distinction is important because the Salter-Harris type 1 fracture often carries an incidence of AVN of nearly 100%.

Chronic SCFE is characterized by symptoms for longer than 3 weeks and is, by far, the more common slip, seen in up to 85% of cases of SCFE.[3] Traditionally, chronic SCFEs have been described with radiographic findings of proximal femoral neck morphologic changes with bending of the femoral neck and lipping inferiorly and posteriorly, suggesting chronicity.[15] Acute-on-chronic SCFE is a traditional classification in which prodromal symptoms have been present for longer than 3 weeks, and a sudden event led to the acute unstable situation. More recently, it has been thought that in all cases, SCFE is an acute event on chronic symptoms that has been confirmed by the recently advocated approach of open reduction of the unstable SCFE in which posterior and medial callus is seen.[16]

The most commonly used radiographic classification was reported by Southwick and describes the femoral head–to–femoral shaft angle on AP and frog-leg radiographs (Fig. 42-2).[17] Mild slips are ones in which the head-shaft angle is 30 degrees or less, moderate slips between 30 and 60 degrees, and severe slips greater than 60 degrees. These are all comparisons with the contralateral hip when it is normal. Certainly, challenges arise with this classification secondary to bilaterality in that no comparison can be made with adequate radiographs, difficulty is associated with positioning a painful hip, and a complex three-dimensional deformity is present in this condition.[18]

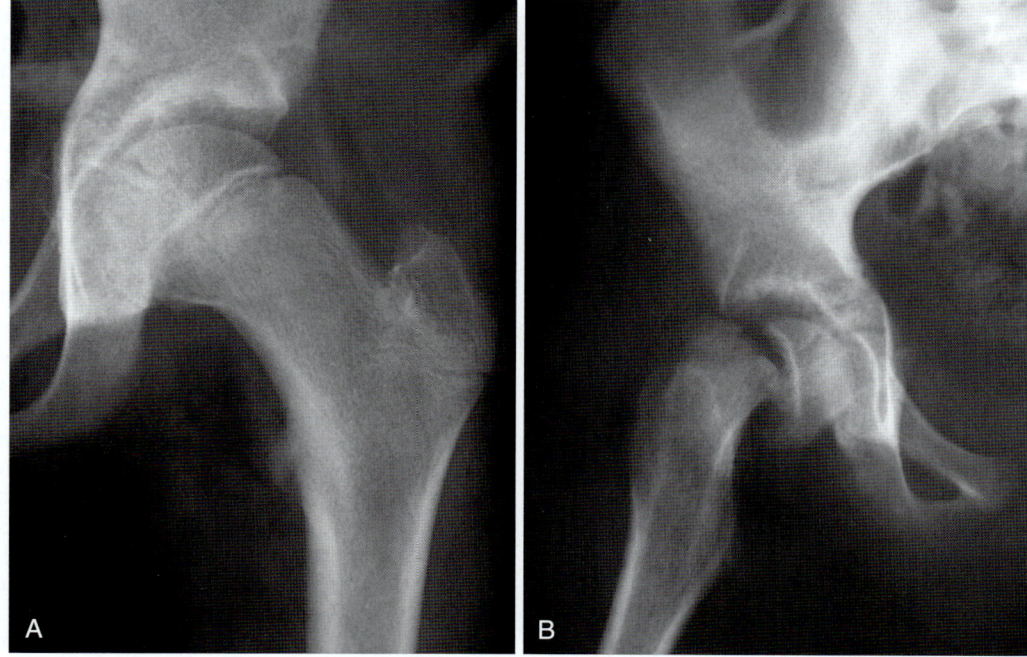

Figure 42-1. Stable and unstable slipped capital femoral epiphysis (SCFE). **A,** Stable: a mild slip with no loss of continuity between the epiphysis and the metaphysis. **B,** Unstable: note the significant displacement of the epiphysis with the appearance of an acute event.

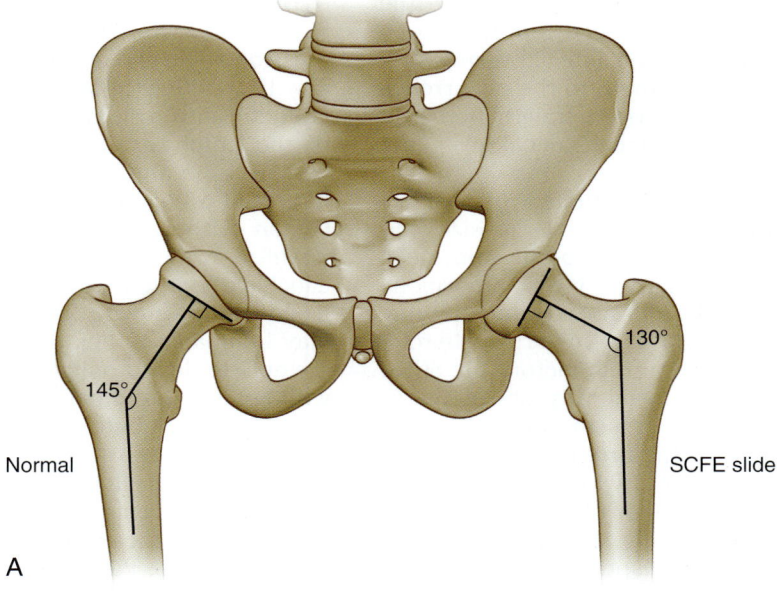

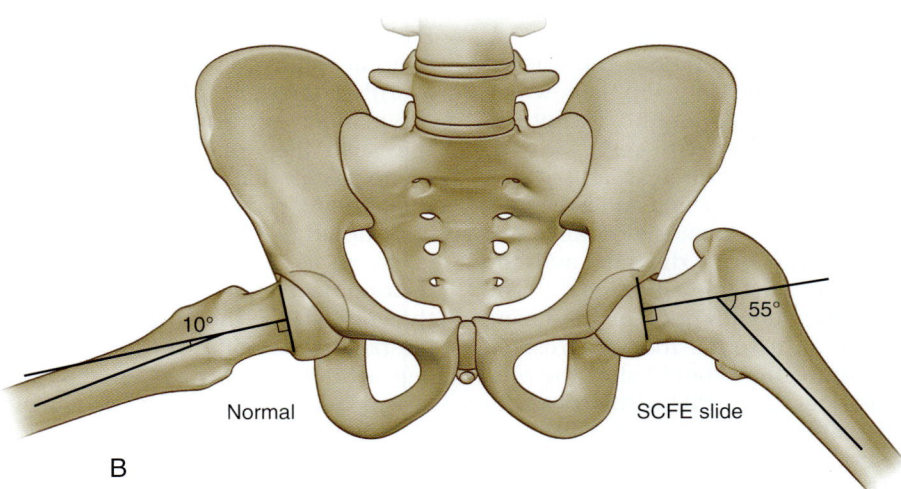

Figure 42-2. Southwick radiographic classification. This measures the angle between the axis of the femoral shaft and the axis of the epiphysis. **A,** On anteroposterior (AP) radiograph, the angle subtended by the anatomic axis of the femur and perpendicular to the base of the epiphysis is the slip angle. In this example, the slip angle is 145 – 130 degrees = 15 degrees. **B,** On the frog-leg pelvic radiograph, the same lines are drawn. In this example, the slip angle is 55 – 10 = 45 degrees. Mild is less than 30 degrees, moderate 30 to 60 degrees, and severe greater than 60 degrees.

CAUSES

Causes of SCFE are essentially unknown at this point; however, several features of SCFE provide some insight as to possible etiologic factors. Many of these patients have a high body mass index (BMI) along with clinical evidence of endocrinopathies. Mechanical factors that may play a role in this condition include the larger size of the patient relative to skeletal maturity. Some have proposed that the perichondrial ring, which encircles the physis at the cartilage-bone interface, is thin, and its resistance to shear forces is diminished.[19,20] Considerable study of version of both the proximal femur and the acetabulum has been performed using computed tomography (CT) imaging. Retroversion of the proximal femur has been reported as a more common finding in SCFE,[21] and acetabular version has been reported to be normal.[22] Other anatomic changes include an anecdotal observation by the author's group that protrusio is more commonly seen in these patients. Finally, the slope of the proximal femur has been reported to be greater than that of the unaffected side (11 degrees vs. 5 degrees), and this may contribute to the occurrence of SCFE.[23,24] All of these factors, together with increased size of these patients, may play a mechanical role in the development of SCFE.

Endocrine factors have been studied extensively because many patients present with large size and hypogonadal features. In addition, endocrine abnormalities such as hypothyroidism,[25-27] growth hormone administration,[28-31] renal failure[32,33] and panhypopituitarism with intracranial tumors,[8] and hyperparathyroidism[34] have been reported to be risk factors for SCFE. These patients typically present at 10 years of age or younger.[8] Many patients who present with SCFE at a young age are evaluated for the first time for endocrinopathies, and the diagnosis of hypothyroidism is the result. Patients younger than 10 or older than 16 years of age are four times more likely to have an atypical SCFE and endocrine workup, especially thyroid, and growth hormone deficiency is important.[35]

CLINICAL PRESENTATION

Patients with SCFE typically present in two main ways. In the first, more common presentation, the patient reports thigh, knee, or, less commonly, hip pain, which is insidious in onset and is often sporadic. Symptoms are worse with activity and better with rest, with the character of the pain typically described as aching-type symptoms, rather than sharp pain. Thigh and knee pain often contributes to the delay in diagnosis because this distracts the physician away from the hip, and the stable slip may become an unstable situation.[36,37] The presentation of any adolescent with thigh or knee pain, especially in the face of an external foot progression angle in an overweight individual, should alert the physician to this diagnosis (Fig. 42-3). This is the presentation of the patient with stable SCFE; making the diagnosis is critical because outcomes of in situ pinning for stable slips are significantly better than for the same treatment for unstable SCFE.

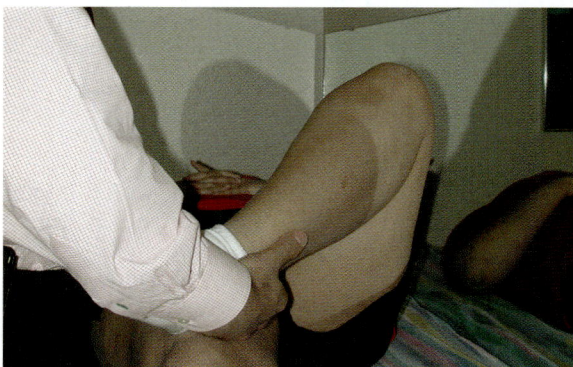

Figure 42-3. The typical patient presentation for a slipped capital femoral epiphysis (SCFE). Obligate external rotation is seen with hip flexion.

The physical examination of the patient with chronic SCFE is characteristic and reveals an external foot progression angle and often a Trendelenburg lurch secondary to relative abductor weakness from decreased abductor muscle length secondary to the posterior slip of the epiphysis. Examination of the hip while the patient is in the supine position reveals the classic finding of "obligate external rotation" during attempted flexion of the hip (see Fig. 42-3), that is, patients are unable to bring the hip to a neutral position, and instead can have marked external rotation of the hip during flexion. In the severe Southwick angle SCFE, the patient may be unable to flex the hip to 90 degrees and often are able to flex to only 60 degrees, which is associated with anterior groin pain.

Unstable or acute and chronic SCFE presents very similarly to a hip fracture, with the patient in acute distress and having significant hip symptoms. Any attempted movement of the affected lower extremity will cause significant apprehension by the patient and significant pain. Patients are unable to get up and can be transported only via stretcher and ambulance.

RADIOGRAPHIC FINDINGS

Patients presenting with a chronic slipped capital femoral epiphysis will have several key features seen on an AP radiograph. AP and frog-leg pelvis radiographs are mandatory to identify and confirm the diagnosis; they also allow one to fully visualize the contralateral hip to ensure that the SCFE is not occurring on that side.

On the AP radiograph, findings may be subtle. Klein's line should be utilized to assist in diagnosis.[38] This line is drawn as a tangent along the lateral aspect of the femoral neck and should intersect the lateral aspect of the epiphysis in the normal situation. When it does not intersect, this confirms the SCFE (Fig. 42-4). Other findings include a slightly widened physis with some irregularity.[39,40] The metaphyseal blanch sign as described by Steel is due to femoral neck and posteriorly displaced capital epiphysis overlap.[41] The frog-leg lateral radiograph is confirmatory for SCFE and demonstrates posterior migration of the epiphysis on the metaphysis; it is the best radiograph to identify this condition (Fig. 42-5). In a chronic situation, appositional bone is identified. Although other radiographs have been described, including the true lateral radiograph, these are not typically utilized and can often be difficult to obtain, especially when the patient is overweight.

Computed tomography is not typically utilized in the diagnosis of SCFE. However, it has great utility following treatment in several situations, including determining whether the physis has healed or whether there has been penetration of an implant following surgery, and in the setting of avascular necrosis.

Technetium bone scan is occasionally useful in the setting of delayed presentation of an unstable SCFE, to determine whether perfusion to the epiphysis is present. Ultrasonography has a limited role in North America; however, it has been utilized in Europe to help define instability of the epiphysis, defined by a joint effusion.[42]

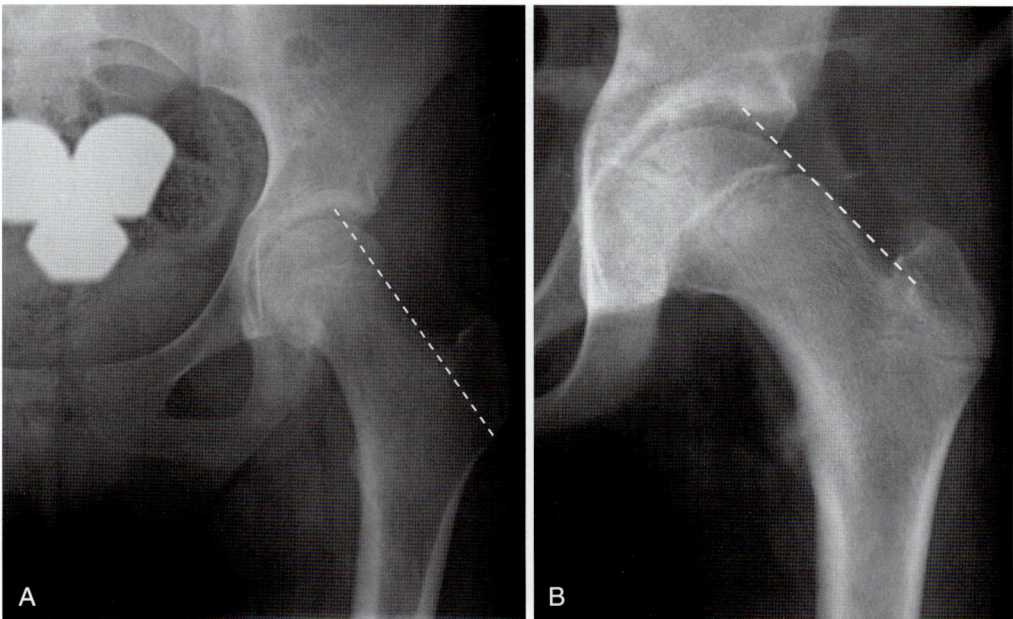

Figure 42-4. Klein's line: On the anteroposterior (AP) pelvic radiograph, a line tangential to the lateral aspect of the femoral neck is drawn. **A,** Intersection of the epiphysis by Klein's line is normal. **B,** When Klein's line does not intersect the epiphysis, a slipped capital femoral epiphysis (SCFE) is noted.

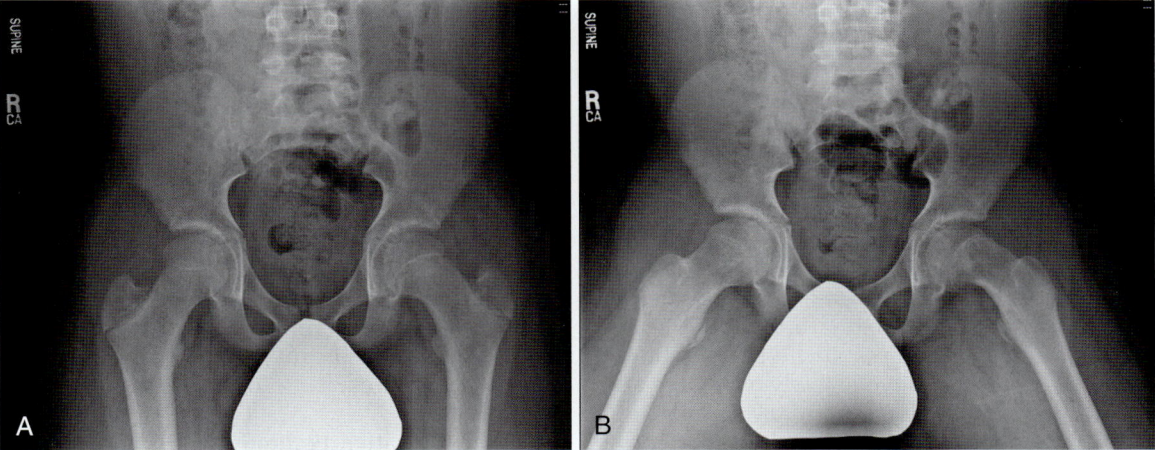

Figure 42-5. The utility of the frog-leg pelvic radiograph in identifying a slipped capital femoral epiphysis (SCFE) is noted. The anteroposterior (AP) radiograph suggests an SCFE; however, the posterior slip of the epiphysis seen on the frog-leg pelvic radiograph confirms the SCFE. Note that the posterior remodeled bone seen on this radiograph is due to the chronic nature of the SCFE.

Magnetic resonance imaging (MRI) has a limited role in the diagnostic workup for SCFE; however, it can be utilized in the situation where perfusion to the epiphysis is being evaluated, most commonly, in the author's practice, when there has been a delay in presentation of an unstable SCFE.

TREATMENT

The traditional treatment for stable slipped capital femoral epiphysis is in situ pinning. This method has

withstood the test of time and requires little surgical time; it generally yields overall good results with respect to the physis closing, and it maintains the position of the epiphysis relative to the metaphysis. Other methods include bone peg epiphysiodesis, casting, and open reduction. However, by far the most common treatment is in situ pinning.

For in situ pinning, the patient may lie on a flat-top radiolucent table or on a fracture table (author's preferred method). Imaging of the hip is then performed to identify the starting incision. If a fracture table is used, the patient is placed in the supine position, and the contralateral hip is fully abducted to allow access to the fluoroscopy unit (Fig. 42-6). An AP projection of the hip is used to draw a line on the skin in-line with the axis of the neck, with its trajectory in the center of the epiphysis.[43] A lateral radiograph is then performed and a guide wire is placed onto the skin in-line with a projected screw trajectory into the center of the femoral head. This usually begins in the anterior aspect of the femoral neck, especially when there is significant deformity. The intersection of these two lines on the skin is the point for the skin incision; a small skin incision measuring a centimeter in length is then made. A large hemostat can be placed through the soft tissues and onto the anterior femoral neck at the starting point and is visualized under fluoroscopy. The author usually utilizes the lateral radiograph to first identify this starting point, along with a guide wire from the 6.5 mm or 7.3 mm cannulated system placed in the center of the femoral neck relative to the superior and inferior femoral necks. The guide wire is advanced in-line with the skin line, which had been placed during the AP fluoroscopy image. The lateral radiograph is utilized to advance the guide wire into the center of the femoral head of the subchondral bone.

Next, the guide wire is confirmed to be in good placement in both AP and lateral projections. A measuring stick is used to determine the length of the screw. The anterior cortex can then be tapped. Next, a fully threaded, stainless steel 6.5 mm or 7.3 mm screw is advanced over the guide wire to the level of the subchondral bone. It should be placed in the center of the femoral head so that maximum purchase of the screw is attained; this allows one to place the screw in a safe manner. Four screw threads crossing the physis into the epiphysis should be the goal. After placement, the guide wire can be pulled back a bit to allow the tip of the screw to be visualized under fluoroscopy. Next, the hip is put through a range of motion to allow for the near-far-near technique, so that the screw is placed deep into the epiphysis without penetrating into the hip joint.[44]

A stable SCFE usually requires single screw fixation because the epiphysis has moved slowly over time and should be relatively stable. If a secondary screw is utilized, the initial screw should be placed in the central epiphysis; the second screw could then be placed more peripherally and preferably in the inferior aspect of the epiphysis to maintain blood flow to the epiphysis. If the bony anatomy is somewhat small, then a smaller-diameter screw (5.5 mm or 4.5 mm) can be utilized for the second screw.

Postoperative management of the patient varies across centers but usually includes a short time of using crutches while fully weight bearing, usually for 6 weeks. This is somewhat arbitrary, and the crutches most likely are not necessary; however, it does slow the child down, and healing occurs during this time. The length of time needed for the physis to heal is dependent on many factors, including the age of the patient and the slip angle with younger patients with more severe deformity that takes longer to heal. It is important that patients have significant improvement in their pain following in situ pinning because a properly secured epiphysis will become asymptomatic. If this does not occur postoperatively, one must be suspicious that there is not enough stability, or that loosening has occurred over time.

Stainless steel screws are preferred by the author because titanium screw heads can strip if they require removal. In situ pinning using cannulated screws demonstrates optimal results with screws in the center of the epiphysis[45] or again in the inferior-posterior position.[46] The number of pins is generally one, and several studies have demonstrated excellent results. In a review of 114 hips in which treatment with one, two, or three screws or pins was provided, the incidence of pin-related complications was directly related to the number of pins. Investigators suggest single pin fixation in the stable fracture.[47] A similar study demonstrated overall 91% good results with single screw fixation compared with 74% with multiple pins[48]; others have demonstrated similar results using single screws.[49-51]

Pin screw location has been studied in relation to subsequent further slip, and the central screw position is most ideal.[46] The eccentrically placed screw has been directly related to further slip progression.[45,49] Placement of screws can be associated with complications such as pin joint penetration, which can lead to chondrolysis as first described by Walters and Simon.[44] It is important to put the hip through a range of motion following screw placement to ensure that it is subchondral. Other methods used to ensure safe screw placement include injecting dye through the cannulated screw to see whether dye enters the joint indicating joint penetration[52] and endoscopic inspection of the drill hole.[53] Screws should not be placed distal to the lesser trochanter because this leads to a greater likelihood of femoral neck fracture, specifically subtrochanteric fracture,[49,54-56] which may lead to significant malunion or nonunion, as well as avascular necrosis. When the screw is placed too far proximally in the anterior position, screw impingement may occur,[57] so care should be taken to start the screw as distal as possible, especially when there is significant deformity, because the starting position requires it to be placed anteriorly on the femoral neck.

Other operative techniques for stable slips include bone peg epiphysiodesis, in which a portion of the residual physis is removed by drilling and curettage, and a peg of autologous bone graft from the iliac crest is placed across the physis to achieve fusion or healing (Fig. 42-7). This technique can be supplemented with screws and can be utilized in both the stable and the unstable situation. This technique has been described by many authors, including Heyman and Herndon.[58] Indications for this are somewhat limited but may include the patient with delayed union who has severe deformity in an attempt to get fusion across the physis. Generally, it is not utilized as a routine procedure for the typical stable SCFE.

The surgical technique for a bone peg epiphysiodesis includes an anterior-lateral surgical approach through which the joint capsule is open to allow access to the femoral neck. A guide wire is used to drill in a similar trajectory as the in situ pin, beginning in the anterior

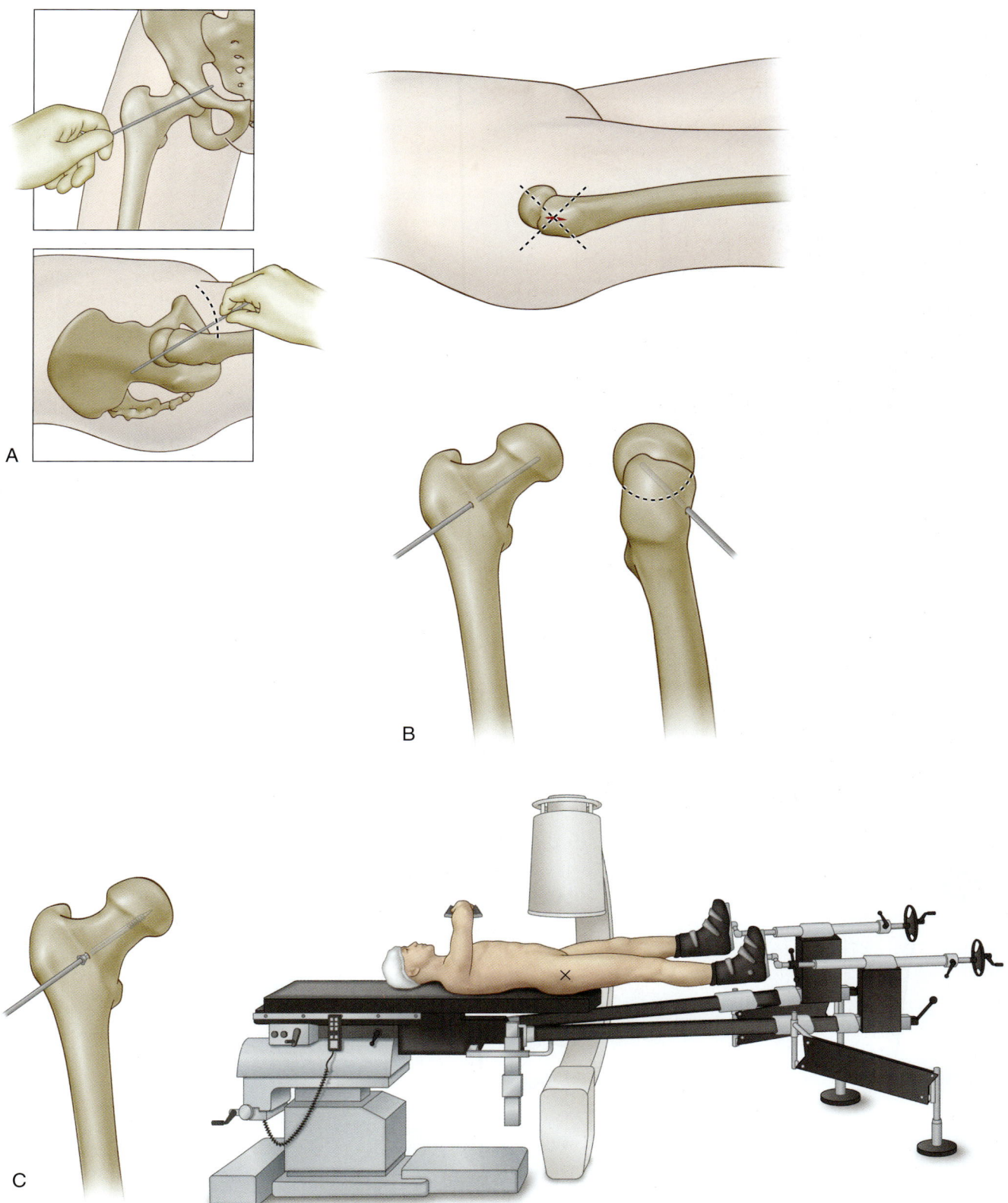

Figure 42-6. Technique for percutaneous pinning of a slipped capital femoral epiphysis (SCFE) on the fracture table. **A,** Skin markings are made on anteroposterior (AP) and lateral fluoroscopy images, and the intersection of the two lines marks the skin incision. **B,** The guide wire is placed onto the anterior femoral neck and is imaged on the lateral fluoroscopy image. The guide wire then is partially advanced using the lateral fluoroscopy image and following the anterior skin marking. The guide pin is advanced across the physis into the subchondral bone. **C,** After the appropriate length is measured, a fully threaded screw is placed across the physis into the epiphysis, with at least four threads crossing the physis.

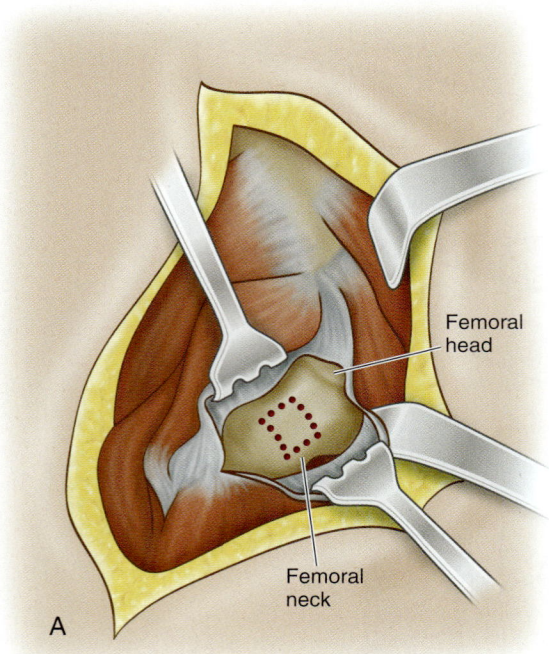

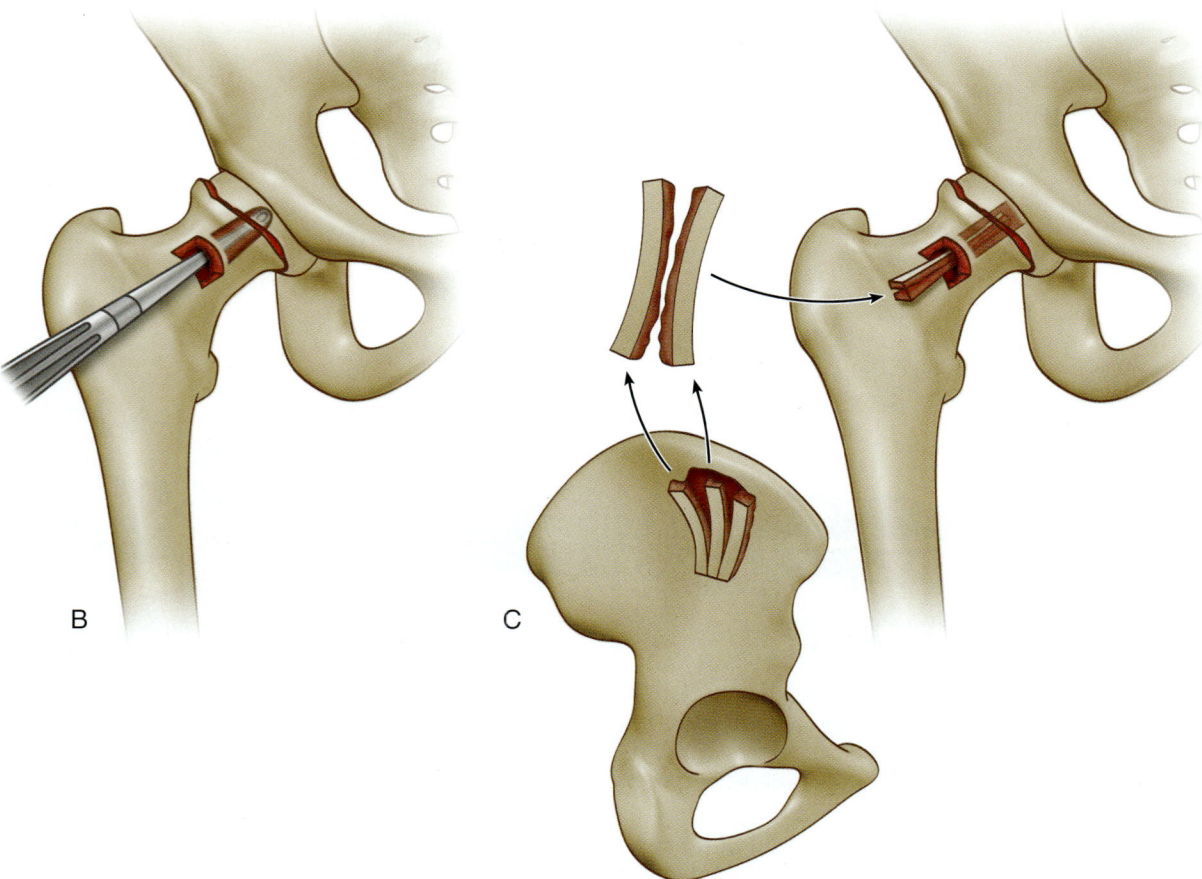

Figure 42-7. Bone peg epiphysiodesis. **A,** An anterior or anterolateral approach to the femoral neck is performed, a small capsulotomy is made, and a small cortical window is placed on the anterior neck. **B,** A larger cannulated drill is used to remove the central physis and create a tunnel for the bone graft. **C,** Tricortical autologous iliac crest bone graft is taken and is used to cross the physis into the femoral epiphysis. The anterior cortical window can then be replaced, and the joint capsule is closed.

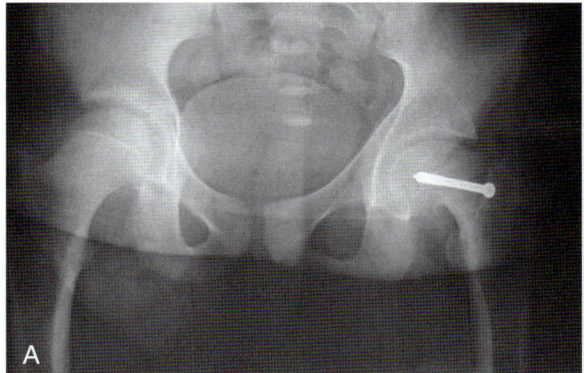
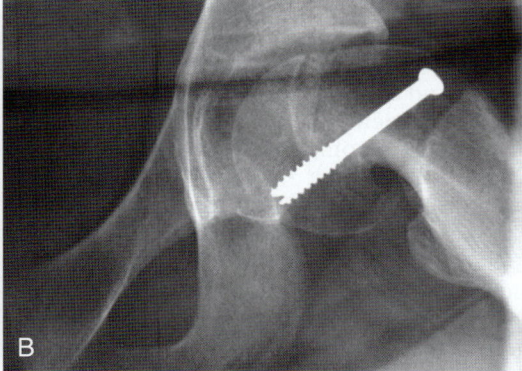

Figure 42-8. Femoroacetabular impingement (FAI) from slipped capital femoral epiphysis (SCFE). **A,** Following in situ pinning of the left SCFE, radiographs demonstrate the typical apparent alignment of the epiphysis on the metaphysis. Evidence of loss of femoral neck offset is seen at the metaphysis. **B,** The frog-leg lateral demonstrates the more characteristic lack of femoral head-neck offset.

femoral neck and traveling into the epiphysis. A hollow mill drill can be used, which is $\frac{3}{16}$ inch in diameter and is advanced over the guide wire into the epiphysis. The curette is utilized to enlarge a cylindrical bone tunnel and to create as much physeal exposure as possible. The corticocancellous bone is then harvested from the iliac crest and placed across the neck region. Most commonly, the bone peg epiphysis does not utilize implants for fixation, but a modification of the technique includes the use of freeze-dried allograft.

Overall results of bone peg epiphysiodesis are very good; a recent study demonstrated good results in 26 acute and 159 chronic slips.[59] A follow-up study of these patients and additional patients from the same center demonstrated excellent results 1 year from surgery. Chondrolysis was seen in one patient, and three cases of AVN were identified.[60] The incidence of nonunion can be high[61]; however, most patients experience good results when this technique is used.

Unstable Slipped Capital Femoral Epiphysis

The presentation for an unstable slipped capital femoral epiphysis is similar to that for a hip fracture in which the patient is unable to bear weight and is in acute distress secondary to pain. Any motion induced to the leg will cause significant apprehension and pain. The hip is typically positioned in external rotation with the patient supine, and log rolling the leg causes significant pain. Radiographs typically demonstrate a moderate or severe SCFE. On occasion, a frog-leg lateral has been attempted after an AP/pelvis radiograph was obtained and reduction of the epiphysis has occurred. This discrepancy in significant displacement on the AP and reduction on the frog-leg AP pelvis should not preclude the diagnosis of an SCFE.

Considerable controversy surrounds treatment of the unstable SCFE. The traditional treatment for this has been in situ pinning following positioning of the patient on the fracture table or the radiolucent table, which typically results in an incidental reduction of the

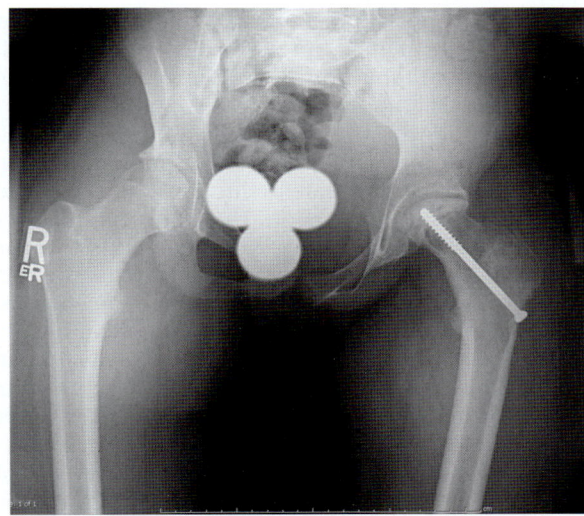

Figure 42-9. Avascular necrosis (AVN) from slipped capital femoral epiphysis (SCFE). Collapse of the femoral head is seen following pinning for an unstable SCFE. The second screw has already been removed to avoid screw penetration into the joint with collapse of the femoral head.

epiphysis. Although this typically leads to overall good results, the incidence of avascular necrosis can be high, and the more recently described femoroacetabular impingement (FAI) results in residual pain and can lead to early osteoarthritis (Fig. 42-8). Most recently, more aggressive surgical treatments have been proposed to safely reduce the epiphysis without tension on the blood vessels supplying the epiphysis and to decrease the incidence of residual deformity to prevent FAI.[16,42]

The main complication to avoid with the unstable SCFE is AVN (Fig. 42-9). The surgeon's decision regarding various factors that can minimize this involves timing of surgery and selection of surgical technique. Evaluation and treatment of the patient with an unstable SCFE as an urgent situation has been recognized; however, the level of urgency needed to take the patient to the operating room is somewhat controversial. In general, most believe that this earlier intervention and immediate surgical treatment are useful when the appropriate surgical team can perform in the operating room. Peterson and associates reported a 7% incidence of AVN when the patient was brought to the operating room within 24 hours compared with 20% when treatment began after 24 hours.[13] Similarly, Aadalen and colleagues had a 0% incidence of AVN within 24 hours and an 18% incidence after 24 hours.[62] In contrast, Loder and coworkers demonstrated no difference when patients were brought to the operating room within 48 hours compared with after 48 hours and in fact demonstrated improved AVN after 48 hours.[63] Several factors may be involved in these series, including relatively small numbers and various techniques with respect to reduction and surgical fixation. Evidence suggests that perfusion to the epiphysis is dependent on the amount of displacement of the epiphysis, and further that the risk for avascular necrosis is dependent on the management of reduction and tension on the vasculature. Maeda and associates demonstrated reperfusion of the epiphysis in a patient with an unstable SCFE who was studied with selective angiography both before and after reduction of the epiphysis.[64]

When one adopts the philosophy that the vascular supply to the epiphysis is intact at the time of SCFE, and that an organized and safe reduction should be performed to maintain perfusion, the opportunity for an open approach is warranted. When one adds the complication of FAI from an unreduced epiphysis, the argument becomes more compelling to reduce the epiphysis in a safe manner to avoid these two complications.

The question of when AVN occurs, its causes, and methods to avoid this potentially catastrophic complication have not been fully answered. Recent evidence would suggest that several factors play a role, many of which can be controlled by the surgeon. Herrera-Soto studied 13 patients with a unilateral unstable SCFE demonstrating increased intracapsular pressure of 48 mm on the affected hip compared with 23 mm on the unaffected hip and increased to 75 mm with manipulation.[65] The concept of decompression of the joint following in situ pinning with stable fixation has been adopted by some.

Closed reduction versus open reduction continues to be an important and timely topic. The traditional method of performing closed treatment with in situ fixation remains the gold standard, and all new techniques should compare with this. Advocates of in situ fixation argue that the technique is applicable to all surgeons, has been very useful for most patients without subsequent AVN, and may be more effective when used in combination with intracapsular decompression. Advocates for a more aggressive approach would suggest that anatomic or near-anatomic reduction using a safe open approach to the hip provides more controlled reduction to maintain epiphyseal blood flow while eliminating the risk for subsequent FAI.

In Situ Fixation

The traditional method of in situ fixation continues in North America as the most popular method

of treatment of SCFE. This is a simple straightforward surgical procedure that does not require significant time or equipment. Three important features of this technique should be considered. First is reduction of the epiphysis. In general, most would perform positioning of the leg on the operating room table without a formal reduction. Because of the instability of the epiphysis, some reduction of the acute component is indirectly achieved and prevents excessive traction to the retinacular vessels. The second component is the type and number of fixation that is necessary. It is generally considered that a single screw is inadequate to achieve stability of this epiphysis in the unstable SCFE. The authors and many others recommend two screws when performing in situ fixation. The first screw attempt should be placed in the center of the femoral head with the additional screw placed inferiorly (Fig. 42-10). Four screw threads should engage the epiphysis, which should be checked fluoroscopically to ensure that they are not going into the joint. Decompression of the hip joint using a large-bore needle or using a formal hip arthrotomy is most likely helpful in this scenario. Others have utilized various techniques to open the capsule following pin fixation and have demonstrated an overall decreased incidence of AVN. Gordon and associates, who performed an urgent closed reduction followed by in situ pinning using two screws and a concomitant arthrotomy, reported that only of 2 of 16 patients (12.5%) developed AVN. Their more recent study demonstrates a similarly low incidence of AVN (14.2%) in 28 consecutive patients.[66]

Open Reduction

Various techniques of open reduction have been proposed throughout the years and have taken on greater interest for pediatric hip surgeons in treatment of the unstable SCFE. One of the initial techniques was described by Dunn and colleagues, who used an open anterior approach that they described as a trapezoidal osteotomy of the femoral neck through a lateral approach[67] (Fig. 42-11). Dunn later described an open replacement of the displaced femoral head to reduce the epiphysis by resecting some femoral neck bone to allow reduction of the epiphysis without tension on the blood vessels.[68] Dunn reported on 11 (15.1%) patients with AVN and 13 (17.8%) patients with chondrolysis out of 73 patients treated in this way.[68] Others have described similar approaches to achieving the same goal with some femoral neck shortening to relieve tension on the vessels.[69-75]

The modified Dunn technique was developed by Ganz and coworkers in Switzerland, who recently reported on their series after combining their patients with the Boston group.[16] The theory behind this technique consists of the following: (1) blood flow to the epiphysis is intact following an SCFE; (2) preservation of this important blood flow is best performed through a controlled surgical dislocation approach, which allows removal of the posterior and medial callus or shortening of the femoral neck and reduction of the epiphysis; and (3) all unstable slips occur as an acute-chronic process, so that posterior and medial callus is present and requires

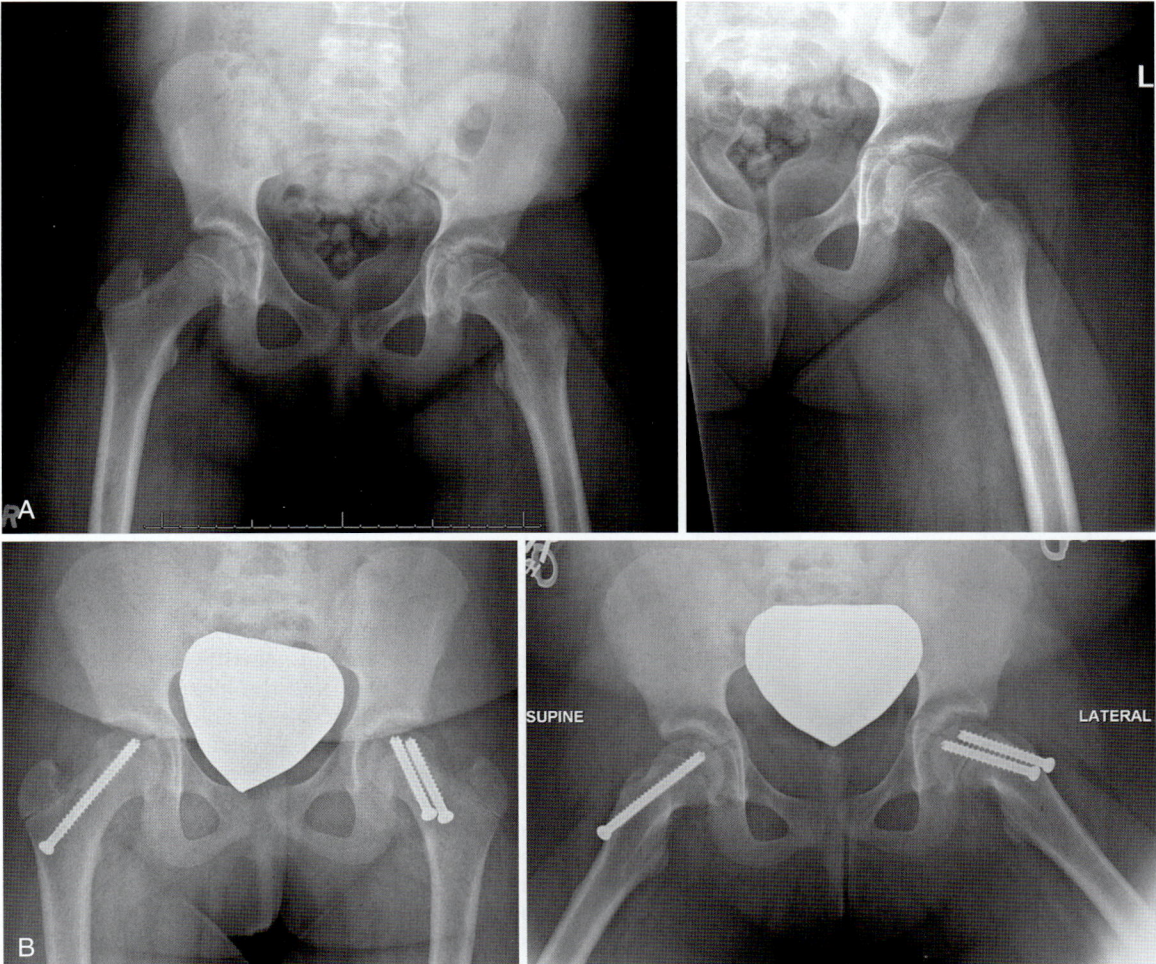

Figure 42-10. In situ pinning of unstable slipped capital femoral epiphysis (SCFE). **A,** Preoperative anteroposterior (AP) and frog-leg lateral demonstrating a left hip unstable SCFE. **B,** Following pinning of the left hip with two screws and contralateral prophylactic pinning of the right hip, no avascular necrosis (AVN) is seen at 6 months.

removal to prevent undo tension on the retinacular vessels during epiphyseal reduction. The authors combined their series of patients with a group of patients from Boston Children's and reported on a total of 40 patients with both stable and unstable SCFE with near-complete correction of the slip angle; no patients had developed AVN or chondrolysis.[16]

The surgical technique uses a surgical hip dislocation approach (Fig. 42-12A). The patient is placed in the lateral decubitus position with the affected hip up, and the standard surgical dislocation approach is performed.[76] The interval between the piriformis and the gluteus minimus is developed to preserve the blood flow to the epiphysis. A Z-capsulotomy is performed, at which point the epiphysis is pinned in situ to allow one to dislocate the proximal femur with the intact epiphysis and metaphysis from the acetabulum, after release of the ligamentum teres (Fig. 42-12B). Following dislocation, the epiphysis and the metaphysis are in full view, and access is provided. The pins are removed, and the epiphysis can be displaced posteriorly after careful surgical dissection.

Soft tissue dissection to allow for epiphysis mobility was described by Ganz; an extended retinacular flap was created to allow safe posterior displacement of the epiphysis by osteotomizing the proximal aspect of the stable trochanter at the level of the apophyseal line (Fig. 42-12C). This bony fragment is then sharply dissected off the periosteum. Incision of the periosteum on the anterior femoral neck begins the soft tissue dissection to allow the epiphysis to be translated posteriorly while maintaining its blood flow (Fig. 42-12D). This provides full access to the proximal femur. At this point, Ganz describes resecting the medial and posterior callus. This brings the neck down to its native morphology. The epiphysis can then be reduced to provide excellent position of the epiphysis without tension on the vessels.

The author has mildly amended this technique in two ways. First, if the epiphysis is mobile enough to allow access to the femoral neck, then only the medial periosteum is incised and stripped off circumferentially on the medial side of the femoral neck, while the lateral aspect of the periosteum is stripped just to the antero-lateral corner. The second difference is the additional

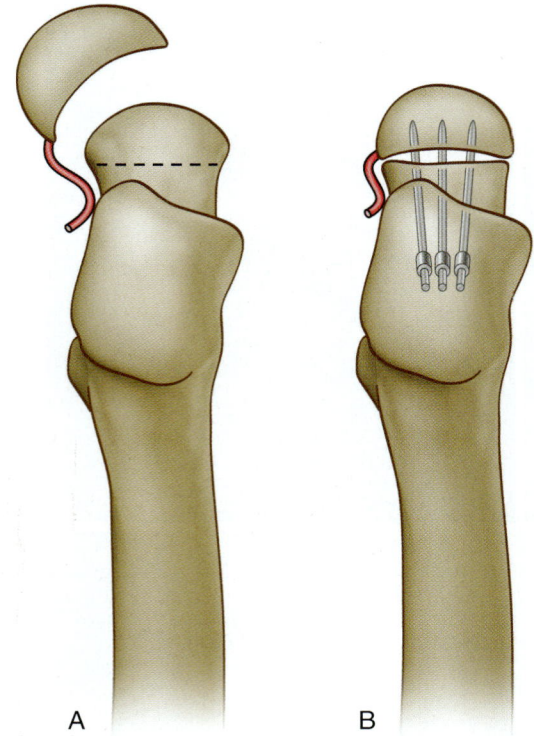

Figure 42-11. Dunn osteotomy. **A,** With the slipped capital femoral epiphysis (SCFE), the retinacular vessels *(arrow)* are intact posteriorly and have no tension. The *dotted line* denotes the level of resection of the proximal femoral neck, which takes tension off the blood vessels during reduction of the epiphysis. **B,** The vessels are under no tension during reduction of the epiphysis to an anatomic position.

step of shortening the femoral neck to allow the epiphysis to be reduced onto the neck without tension being placed on the epiphysis (Fig. 42-12F). This is the author's first step once the epiphysis has been displaced posteriorly. Excessive shortening has not occurred in the author's experience, and no evidence for subluxation has been found. The amount of shortening is generally 1.5 cm to start and can be increased depending on how much tension occurs across the soft tissues when reduction of the epiphysis is attempted.

Another method proposed to reduce the epiphysis without creating AVN is that put forth by Parsch and colleagues.[77] They described an open anterior arthrotomy with gentle manual anterior-to-posterior directed pressure using one's index finger on the metaphysis, which reduces the acute component of the SCFE. This technique was described and reported on in 67 consecutive patients with an SCFE; 58 cases involved the traditional unstable SCFE for patients who could not weight bear, and 9 patients were deemed unstable based on a hip effusion diagnosed on ultrasound. In all, 3 (4.7%) patients developed AVN: 2 had moderate SCFE, and in 1 patient the disorder was severe.

Prophylactic Treatment of the Contralateral Hip

The incidence of developing a contralateral SCFE is between 20% and 25%, with younger patients at greatest risk.[78,79] When one sees a unilateral slip in a very young patient, the thought to perform a contralateral prophylactic pinning is warranted. Arguments against prophylactic pinning are that it is unnecessary in 65% of patients, and that the danger of placing a screw into the hip joint is present during prophylactic pinning. Arguments in favor of pinning the contralateral side include (1) that bilateral slips occur up to 25% of the time, (2) that some patients may be unstable, which carries a higher risk for AVN, and (3) that it is a fairly straightforward surgical technique to perform. Little controversy has arisen over whether contralateral pinning should be performed in patients who have a significant endocrinopathy, including patients who have renal disease.[8,80] More controversial discussion focuses on patients who are skeletally immature. Stasikelis utilized the Oxford bone age as a method to predict contralateral slip development. The Oxford bone age analyzes the maturity of the ilium, the triradiate cartilage, the femoral head, the greater trochanter, and the lesser trochanter and sums the scores; higher scores are indicative of skeletal maturity (range, 16 to 26). Contralateral SCFE develops in 85% of patients with a score of 16 and in 11% with a score of 21; no patient with a score of 22 or more developed slip.[81] Later authors have utilized only the triradiate cartilage and have demonstrated little risk for contralateral slip when the triradiate cartilage is closed.[82] Various authors have utilized statistical analyses with many assumptions in an attempt to determine whether prophylactic pinning is appropriate. Although these studies were well done with the use of sophisticated statistics, it has been difficult for investigators to come to a consensus.

The author's practice is to perform a contralateral pinning in all patients who have an open triradiate cartilage that is easily visible (Fig. 42-13). For patients who have a triradiate cartilage that is beginning to close or is closed, in general, the author will not perform a contralateral pinning.

Valgus Slips

As was defined earlier, SCFE most commonly refers to posterior migration of the epiphysis on the metaphysis accompanied by inferior displacement of the epiphysis (Fig. 42-14). Occasionally, however, superior and posterior migration of the epiphysis occurs; this is termed *valgus SCFE*.[51,83,84] An even less likely scenario is one in which the epiphysis slips anteriorly.[85,86] Anteversion of the femur is often seen in hips that develop a valgus SCFE.[83-85]

The clinical presentation is similar to that of the typical SCFE with respect to pain in the hips; patients much more commonly present with a stable SCFE along with the ability to ambulate. The physical examination does not demonstrate obligate external rotation, but instead demonstrates limited adduction due to the anatomic position of the epiphysis. Evaluation of the patient

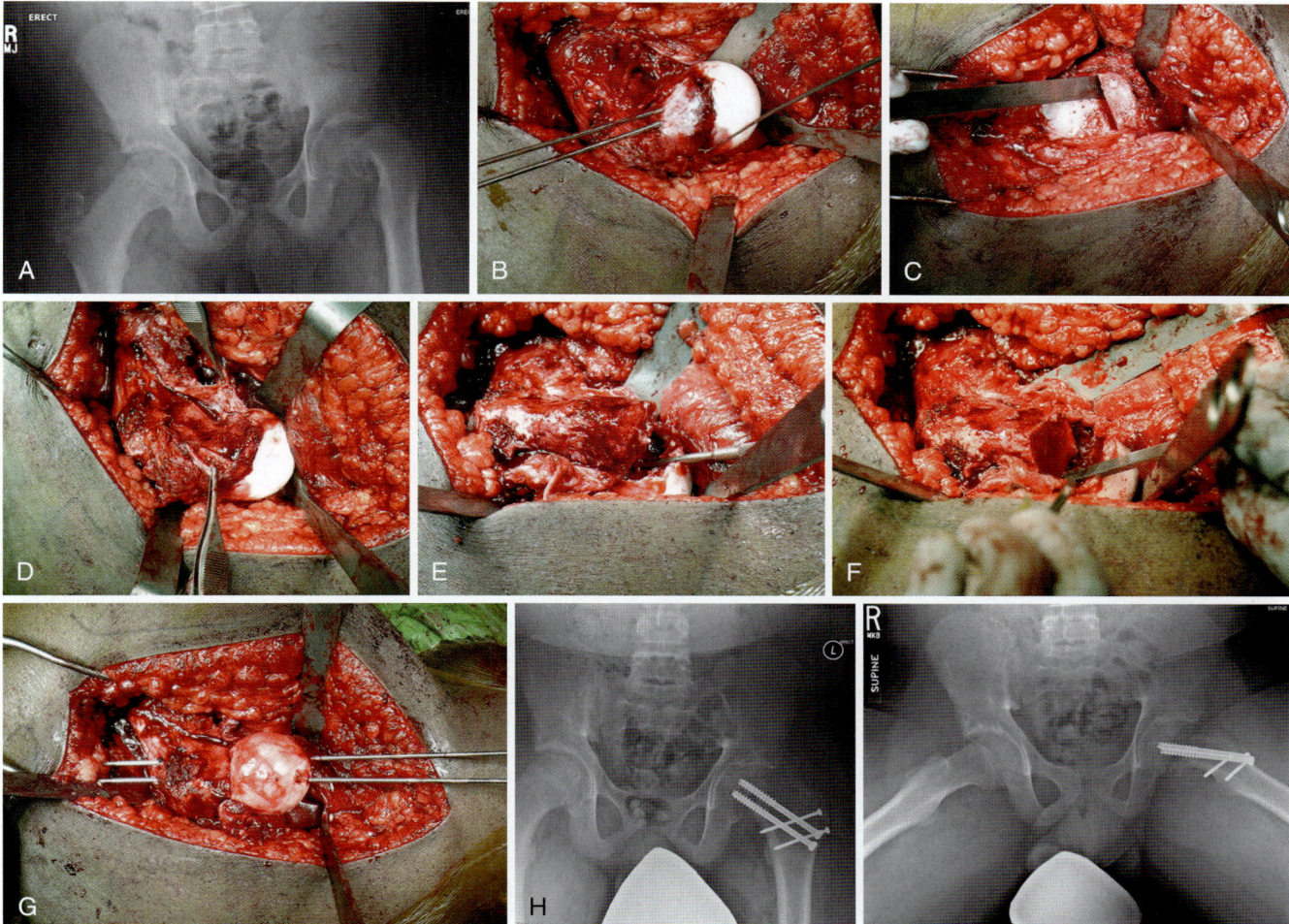

Figure 42-12. Open reduction of slipped capital femoral epiphysis (SCFE). **A,** A left unstable acute-on-chronic SCFE. **B,** The standard surgical dislocation approach as described by Ganz is used to approach the hip, and following the Z-capsulotomy, the epiphysis and the metaphysis are pinned in situ and are dislocated from the acetabulum. A nerve hook is next to the retinacular soft tissue sleeve, which contains the blood vessels to the epiphysis. **C,** The proximal portion of the trochanter is removed using an osteotome, and the soft tissues are carefully dissected off the medial edge. **D,** The medial periosteum and the entire lateral soft tissue sleeve are dissected subperiosteally to gain full access to **(E)** the femoral neck with posterior displacement of the epiphysis. **F,** The femoral neck has been shortened to remove the remodeled bone, and a curved osteotome is used to remove the very hard posterior callus that has developed over time. **G,** Retrograde pinning of the epiphysis onto the metaphysis to allow cannulated screws to be properly placed to secure the epiphysis to the metaphysis. The guide pins are pulled back out of the lateral cortex, so they are just below the femoral head chondral surface. This allows reduction of the epiphysis into the acetabulum and overdrilling in preparation for screw placement. **H,** One year after surgery, no evidence of avascular necrosis (AVN) or chondrolysis is noted.

should include AP and frog-leg lateral pelvic radiographs that demonstrate posterior slip on the frog-leg lateral but a more valgus position or lateralization of the epiphysis on the AP view. In situ pinning is generally performed with good results; however, one needs to be careful because the starting position for the screw is more medial than the traditional slip, and the neurovascular bundle must be protected.[87]

Complications

SCFE can result in several challenging complications, including chondrolysis, avascular necrosis, and femoroacetabular impingement.

Chondrolysis

Chondrolysis is defined as a decreased joint space to 3 mm or less, or a 50% reduction in the joint space relative to the contralateral side. Patients present with decreased range of motion with hip held in a position of external rotation, flexion, and abduction. Mobility of the hip is limited, and pain ensues when movement of the hip is attempted.

The incidence of chondrolysis is wide-ranging from 1.5% to 50% (Fig. 42-15). [88,89] It is more prevalent among females and African Americans, especially in early reports.[90-93] The causes of chondrolysis are

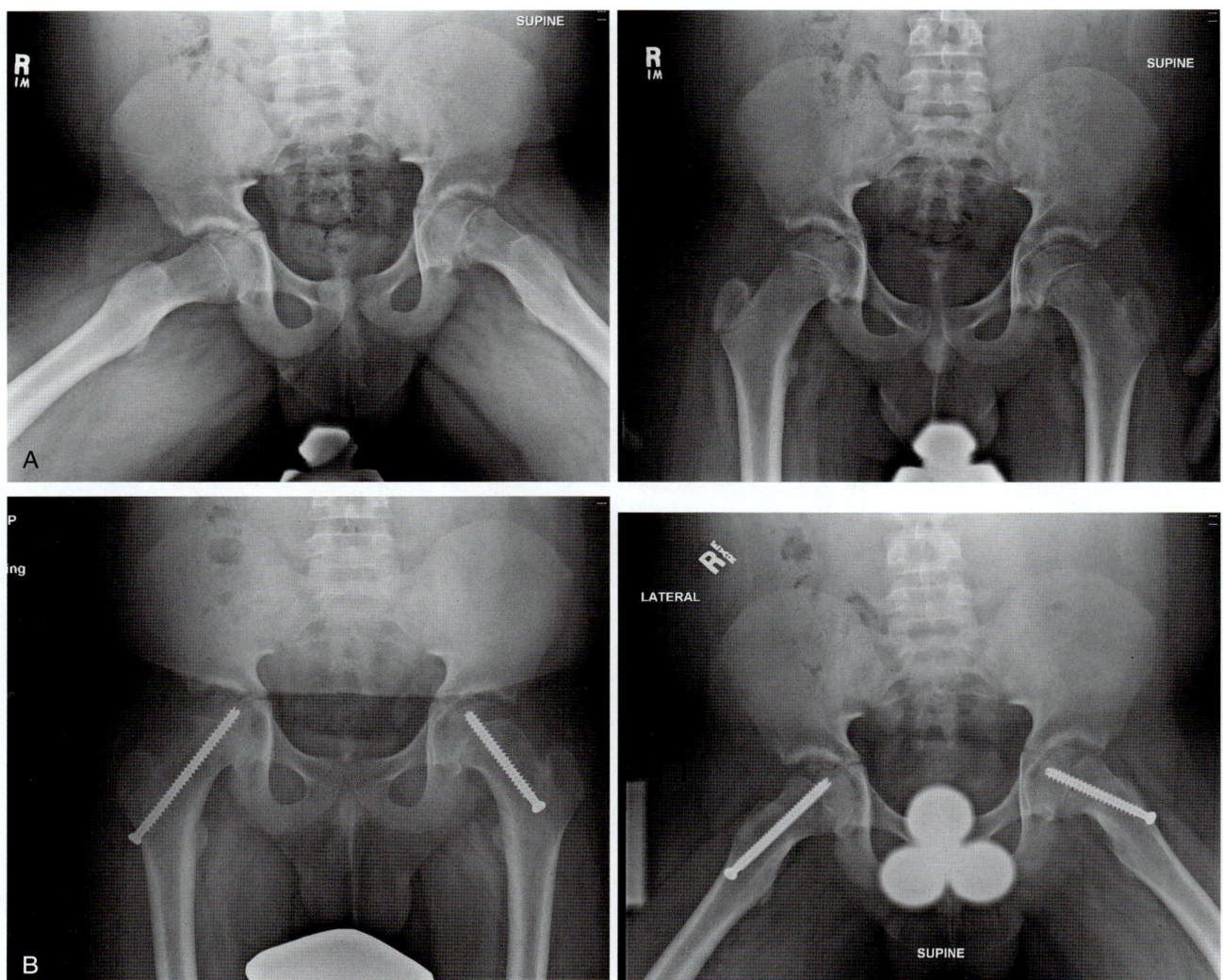

Figure 42-13. Prophylactic pinning of slipped capital femoral epiphysis (SCFE). **A,** Preoperative anteroposterior (AP) and frog-leg lateral radiographs of a 12-year-old boy with open triradiate cartilage demonstrating an obvious left stable SCFE. The AP of the right hip is questionable for an SCFE; however, the lateral does not demonstrate posterior displacement. The patient was asymptomatic, and no pain or obligate external rotation was evident on physical examination. **B,** AP and frog-leg pelvis radiographs following in situ pinning of the left hip and prophylactic pinning of the right.

largely unknown, but it has been associated with pin penetration into the joint.[44,46] This leads to an autoimmune response, confirmed in some studies by an increase in immunoglobulin molecules,[94,95] although other studies demonstrate no association between pin penetration and chondrolysis.[96,97] It is most likely that mechanical injury to the cartilage may stimulate this immune response; whether this occurs with metal implants or with residual deformity with femoroacetabular impingement (FAI), as described by Ganz, is controversial.[98-101]

Treatment for chondrolysis presents many challenges. Attempts to improve symptoms of pain and limited motion have been marginally successful. Treatment is begun by confirming the diagnosis and ruling out an infectious cause of pain; hip aspiration with a septic hip workup may be appropriate. Once the diagnosis has been confirmed, treatment options include offloading of the hip with crutch walking, range-of-motion exercises, and nonsteroidal anti-inflammatory medications. Various surgical treatments have been somewhat unsuccessful; however, procedures such as distraction with an external fixator, subtotal capsulotomy with aggressive continuous passive motion (CPM), and others have been tried.

Avascular Necrosis

The most feared complication associated with SCFE is AVN of the epiphysis. This is not seen when a stable SCFE is present and in situ pin fixation yields a nearly 0% incidence of AVN. It is important that the screw is not placed into the superolateral region of the epiphysis to avoid compromising blood flow to this area.

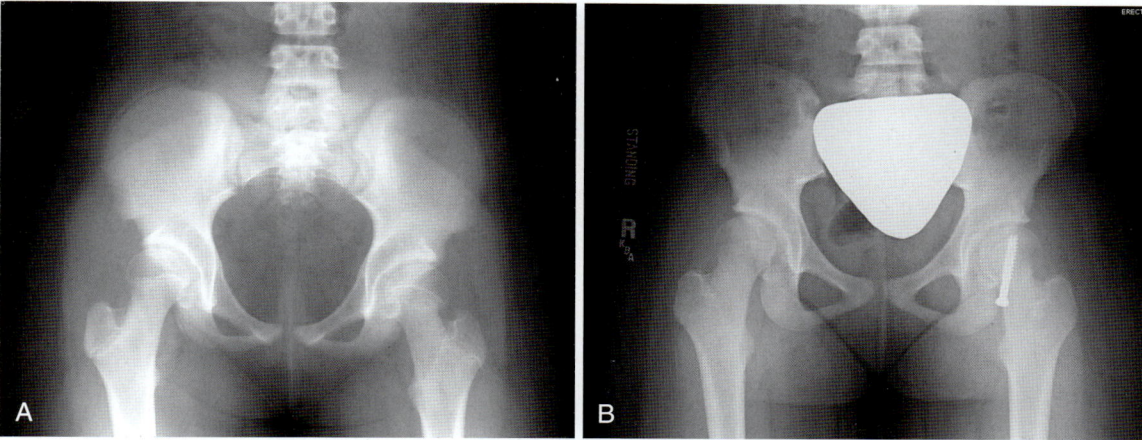

Figure 42-14. Valgus slipped capital femoral epiphysis (SCFE). **A,** Anteroposterior (AP) pelvis radiograph demonstrating a valgus SCFE. Note the superolateral displacement of the epiphysis relative to the metaphysis. **B,** Following in situ pinning, good placement of the screw into the epiphysis is seen. Note the medial starting position of the screw.

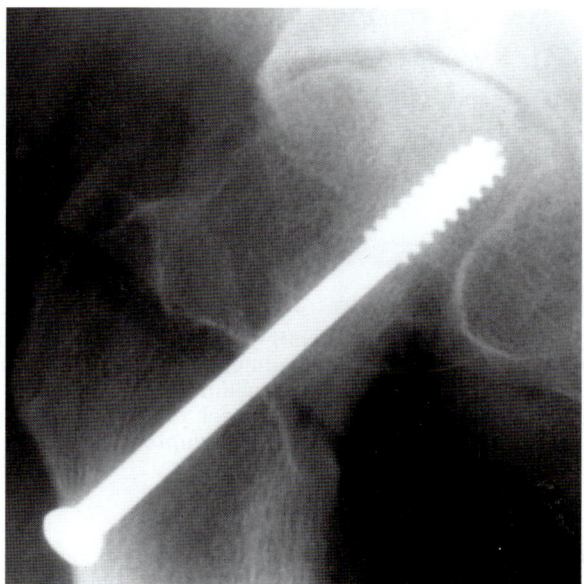

Figure 42-15. Chondrolysis following in situ pinning for a stable slipped capital femoral epiphysis (SCFE). Note the significant joint space narrowing.

In contrast to the stable SCFE, the unstable SCFE is associated with a high incidence of AVN—up to 47%.[63] This AVN may involve partial or total head involvement and has a wide range of symptom presentations from very mild pain, to incapacitating pain with a stiff, almost autofused joint.

The blood supply to the epiphysis has been well studied. Injury to the blood vessels most likely is not due to the initial slip but more likely is due to treatment, along with possible causes of kinking or stretching of the blood vessels during treatment with in situ pin fixation. Intra-articular pressure secondary to hemarthrosis may contribute to this AVN.

Additional radiographic features include lack of osteopenia because bone resorption is prevented by

lack of blood flow. Within 1 year, collapse and destruction of the epiphysis is seen.[10,102] In general, we have not routinely utilized more advanced imaging such as MRI or bone scan in the early period because in large part, this outcome may be the result of ineffective treatment for AVN in the face of slipped capital femoral epiphysis. However, tools are needed to fully assess the epiphysis and to limit the amount of collapse noted with other methods, both surgical and nonsurgical. Treatment for avascular necrosis presents many challenges and includes many options, which may be effective for partial head involvement but not for full head involvement. Osteotomies performed to place the viable femoral head into the weight-bearing zone are appropriate. When total head involvement and total femoral head collapse are seen with incapacitating pain, hip fusion is a viable option with overall good results.[103,104]

Femoroacetabular Impingement Following Slipped Capital Femoral Epiphysis

Femoroacetabular impingement (FAI) can develop following in situ pinning of SCFE; it results in pain, especially with flexion and attempted internal rotation of the hip, and can lead to early osteoarthritis (Fig. 42-16).[105] Because the femoral epiphysis is displaced posteriorly, the metaphysis can cause cam impingement, but retroversion of the acetabulum, which is seen often in SCFE, results in pincer impingement. This impingement can lead to a significant incidence of pathology of the labrum and the articular cartilage and most likely to early osteoarthritis.[106-109]

When a patient presents with FAI secondary to SCFE, the evaluation should include a good physical examination to assess the rotational profile of the patient's hip and the amount of flexion that causes symptoms. Advanced imaging that includes an MRI/arthrogram is important for identifying intra-articular pathology. The author's preference is to perform flexion osteotomy

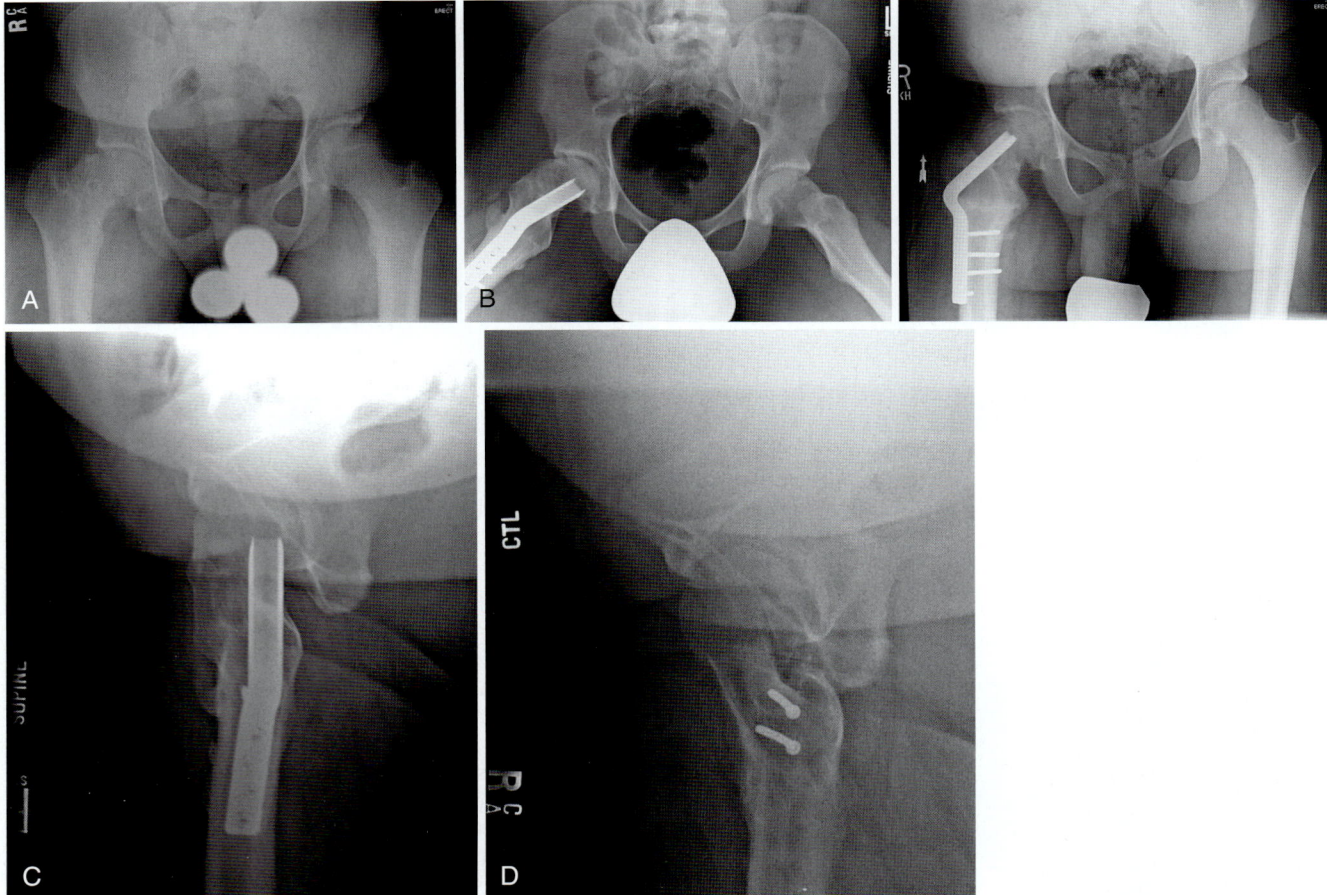

Figure 42-16. Femoroacetabular impingement (FAI) following slipped capital femoral epiphysis (SCFE). **A,** Anteroposterior (AP) pelvis radiograph demonstrates residual deformity from an SCFE that had in situ pinning. **B,** Following a flexion valgus–type (Southwick) osteotomy, a nice restoration of the femoral head acetabular relationship occurs. Note the 60 degrees of flexion on the lateral. **C,** Lateral radiograph demonstrates obvious lack of femoral neck offset. **D,** Following surgical hip dislocation, restoration of the femoral head-neck offset is performed with complete symptom relief. Repair of the labrum was performed at the same procedure.

with some internal rotation if necessary when the amount of deformity is fairly large, but to perform only an osteochondroplasty when the deformity is small. Hip arthroscopy or surgical dislocation is almost always necessary to identify and treat significant intra-articular pathology. Occasionally, osteotomy and surgical dislocation are performed in a staged fashion, when the proximal femoral osteotomy fails to achieve symptom relief.

REFERENCES

1. Kelsey JL: The incidence and distribution of slipped capital femoral epiphysis in Connecticut. J Chronic Dis 23:567–578, 1971.
2. Hagglund G, Hansson LI, Ordeberg G: Epidemiology of slipped capital femoral epiphysis in southern Sweden. Clin Orthop Relat Res 191:82–94, 1984.
3. Loder RT: The demographics of slipped capital femoral epiphysis: an international multicenter study. Clin Orthop Relat Res 322:8–27, 1996.
4. Loder RT, Aronson DD, Bollinger RO: Seasonal variation of slipped capital femoral epiphysis. J Bone Joint Surg Am 72:378–381, 1990.
5. Loder RT: A worldwide study on the seasonal variation of slipped capital femoral epiphysis. Clin Orthop Relat Res 322:28–36, 1996.
6. Loder RT, Aronson DD, Greenfield ML: The epidemiology of bilateral slipped capital femoral epiphysis: a study of children in Michigan. J Bone Joint Surg Am 75:1141–1147, 1993.
7. Alexander C: The etiology of femoral epiphysial slipping. J Bone Joint Surg Br 48:299–311, 1966.
8. Loder RT, Wittenberg B, DeSilva G: Slipped capital femoral epiphysis associated with endocrine disorders. J Pediatr Orthop 15:349–356, 1995.
9. Hansson G, Jerre R, Sanders SM, Wallin J: Radiographic assessment of coxarthrosis following slipped capital femoral epiphysis: a 32-year follow-up study of 151 hips. Acta Radiol 34:117–123, 1993.
10. Loder RT, Richards BS, Shapiro PS, et al: Acute slipped capital femoral epiphysis: the importance of physeal stability. J Bone Joint Surg Am 75:1134–1140, 1993.
11. Kallio PE, Mah ET, Foster BK, et al: Slipped capital femoral epiphysis: incidence and clinical assessment of physeal instability. J Bone Joint Surg Br 77:752–755, 1995.
12. Lubicky JP: Chondrolysis and avascular necrosis: complications of slipped capital femoral epiphysis. J Pediatr Orthop B 5:162–167, 1996.
13. Peterson MD, Weiner DS, Green NE, Terry CL: Acute slipped capital femoral epiphysis: the value and safety of

urgent manipulative reduction. J Pediatr Orthop 17:648–654, 1997.

14. Stevens DB, Short BA, Burch JM: In situ fixation of the slipped capital femoral epiphysis with a single screw. J Pediatr Orthop B 5:85–89, 1996.

15. Muller E: On the deflection of the femoral neck in childhood. Clin Orthop Relat Res 48:7, 1966.

16. Ziebarth K, Zilkens C, Spencer S, et al: Capital realignment for moderate and severe SCFE using a modified Dunn procedure. Clin Orthop Relat Res 467:704–716, 2009.

17. Southwick WO: Osteotomy through the lesser trochanter for slipped capital femoral epiphysis. J Bone Joint Surg Am 49:807–835, 1967.

18. Guzzanti V, Falciglia F: Slipped capital femoral epiphysis: comparison of a roentgenographic method and computed tomography in determining slip severity. J Pediatr Orthop 11:6–12, 1991.

19. Chung SM, Batterman SC, Brighton CT: Shear strength of the human femoral capital epiphyseal plate. J Bone Joint Surg Am 58:94–103, 1976.

20. Litchman HM, Duffy J: Slipped capital femoral epiphysis: factors affecting shear forces on the epiphyseal plate. J Pediatr Orthop 4:745–748, 1984.

21. Gelberman RH, Cohen MS, Shaw BA, et al: The association of femoral retroversion with slipped capital femoral epiphysis. J Bone Joint Surg Am 68:1000–1007, 1986.

22. Stanitski CL, Woo R, Stanitski DF: Femoral version in acute slipped capital femoral epiphysis. J Pediatr Orthop B 5:74–76, 1996.

23. Mirkopulos N, Weiner DS, Askew M: The evolving slope of the proximal femoral growth plate relationship to slipped capital femoral epiphysis. J Pediatr Orthop 8:268–273, 1988.

24. Pritchett J, Perdue KD: Mechanical factors in slipped capital femoral epiphysis. J Pediatr Orthop 8:385–388, 1988.

25. Hennessy MJ, Jones KL: Slipped capital femoral epiphysis in a hypothyroid adult male. Clin Orthop Relat Res 165:204–208, 1982.

26. Heyerman W, Weiner D: Slipped epiphysis associated with hypothyroidism. J Pediatr Orthop 4:569–573, 1984.

27. Moorefield WG, Jr, Urbaniak JR, Ogden WS, Frank JL: Acquired hypothyroidism and slipped capital femoral epiphysis: report of three cases. J Bone Joint Surg Am 58:705–708, 1976.

28. Blethen SL, Rundle AC: Slipped capital femoral epiphysis in children treated with growth hormone: a summary of the National Cooperative Growth Study experience. Horm Res 46:113–116, 1996.

29. Fidler MW, Brook CG: Slipped upper femoral epiphysis following treatment with human growth hormone. J Bone Joint Surg Am 56:1719–1722, 1974.

30. Razzano CD, Nelson C, Eversman J: Growth hormone levels in slipped capital femoral epiphysis. J Bone Joint Surg Am 54:1224–1226, 1972.

31. Sakano S, Yoshihashi Y, Miura T: Slipped capital femoral epiphysis during treatment with recombinant human growth hormone for Turner syndrome. Arch Orthop Trauma Surg 114:237–238, 1995.

32. Nixon JR, Douglas JF: Bilateral slipping of the upper femoral epiphysis in end-stage renal failure: a report of two cases. J Bone Joint Surg Br 62:18–21, 1980.

33. Switzer P, Bell HM: Slipping of the capital femoral epiphysis with renal rickets: a case report. Can J Surg 16:330–332, 1973.

34. Jingushi S, Hara T, Sugioka Y: Deficiency of a parathyroid hormone fragment containing the midportion and 1,25-dihydroxyvitamin D in serum of patients with slipped capital femoral epiphysis. J Pediatr Orthop 17:216–219, 1997.

35. Loder RT, Starnes T, Dikos G, Aronsson DD: Demographic predictors of severity of stable slipped capital femoral epiphyses. J Bone Joint Surg Am 88:97–105, 2006.

36. Ledwith CA, Fleisher GR: Slipped capital femoral epiphysis without hip pain leads to missed diagnosis. Pediatrics 89:660–662, 1992.

37. Matava MJ, Patton CM, Luhmann S, et al: Knee pain as the initial symptom of slipped capital femoral epiphysis: an analysis of initial presentation and treatment. J Pediatr Orthop 19:455–460, 1999.

38. Klein A, Joplin RJ, Reidy JA, Hanelin J: Roentgenographic features of slipped capital femoral epiphysis. Am J Roentgenol Radium Ther Nucl Med 66:361–374, 1951.

39. Maussen JP, Rozing PM, Obermann WR: Intertrochanteric corrective osteotomy in slipped capital femoral epiphysis: a long-term follow-up study of 26 patients. Clin Orthop Relat Res 259:100–110, 1990.

40. Mayer L: The importance of early diagnosis in the treatment of slipping femoral epiphysis. J Bone Joint Surg Am 19:1046, 1937.

41. Steel HH: The metaphyseal blanch sign of slipped capital femoral epiphysis. J Bone Joint Surg Am 68:920–922, 1986.

42. Parsch K, Weller S, Parsch D: Open reduction and smooth Kirschner wire fixation for unstable slipped capital femoral epiphysis. J Pediatr Orthop 29:1–8, 2009.

43. Lindaman LM, Canale ST, Beaty JH, Warner WC: A fluoroscopic technique for determining the incision site for percutaneous fixation of slipped capital femoral epiphysis. J Pediatr Orthop 11:397–401, 1991.

44. Walters R: Joint destruction: a sequel of unrecognized pin penetration in patients with slipped capital femoral epiphysis. In The hip, St Louis, 1980, CV Mosby, pp 145.

45. Ward WT, Stefko J, Wood KB, Stanitski CL: Fixation with a single screw for slipped capital femoral epiphysis [published erratum appears in J Bone Joint Surg Am 75:1255, 1993]. J Bone Joint Surg Am 74:799–809, 1992.

46. Stambough JL, Davidson RS, Ellis RD, Gregg JR: Slipped capital femoral epiphysis: an analysis of 80 patients as to pin placement and number. J Pediatr Orthop 6:265–273, 1986.

47. Blanco JS, Taylor B, Johnston CE 2nd: Comparison of single pin versus multiple pin fixation in treatment of slipped capital femoral epiphysis. J Pediatr Orthop 12:384–389, 1992.

48. Aronsson DD, Loder RT: Treatment of the unstable (acute) slipped capital femoral epiphysis. Clin Orthop Relat Res 322:99–110, 1996.

49. Aronson DD, Carlson WE: Slipped capital femoral epiphysis: a prospective study of fixation with a single screw [published erratum appears in J Bone Joint Surg Am 74:1274, 1992]. J Bone Joint Surg Am 74:810–819, 1992.

50. de Sanctis N, Di Gennaro G, Pempinello C, et al: Is gentle manipulative reduction and percutaneous fixation with a single screw the best management of acute and acute-on-chronic slipped capital femoral epiphysis? A report of 70 patients. J Pediatr Orthop B 5:90–95, 1996.

51. Howorth M: Slipping of the upper femoral epiphysis. J Bone Joint Surg Am 331:734, 1949.

52. Lehman WB, Grant A, Rose D, et al: A method of evaluating possible pin penetration in slipped capital femoral epiphysis using a cannulated internal fixation device. Clin Orthop Relat Res 186:65–70, 1984.

53. Bassett GS: Bone endoscopy: direct visual confirmation of cannulated screw placement in slipped capital femoral epiphysis. J Pediatr Orthop 13:159–163, 1993.

54. Baynham GC, Lucie RS, Cummings RJ: Femoral neck fracture secondary to in situ pinning of slipped capital femoral epiphysis: a previously unreported complication. J Pediatr Orthop 11:187–190, 1991.

55. Canale ST, Casillas M, Banta JV: Displaced femoral neck fractures at the bone-screw interface after in situ fixation of slipped capital femoral epiphysis. J Pediatr Orthop 17:212–215, 1997.

56. Riley PM, Weiner DS, Gillespie R, Weiner SD: Hazards of internal fixation in the treatment of slipped capital femoral epiphysis. J Bone Joint Surg Am 72:1500–1509, 1990.

57. Goodwin RC, Mahar AT, Oswald TS, Wenger DR: Screw head impingement after in situ fixation in moderate and severe slipped capital femoral epiphysis. J Pediatr Orthop 27:319–325, 2007.

58. Heyman CH, Herndon CH: Epiphysiodesis for early slipping of the upper femoral epiphysis. J Bone Joint Surg Am 36:539–555, 1954.

59. Weiner DS, Weiner S, Melby A, Hoyt WA Jr: A 30-year experience with bone graft epiphysiodesis in the treatment of slipped capital femoral epiphysis. J Pediatr Orthop 4:145–152, 1984.

60. Adamczyk MJ, Weiner DS, Hawk D: A 50-year experience with bone graft epiphysiodesis in the treatment of slipped capital femoral epiphysis. J Pediatr Orthop 23:578–583, 2003.

61. Ward WT, Wood K: Open bone graft epiphysiodesis for slipped capital femoral epiphysis. J Pediatr Orthop 10:14–20, 1990.

62. Aadalen RJ, Weiner DS, Hoyt W, Herndon CH: Acute slipped capital femoral epiphysis. J Bone Joint Surg Am 56:1473–1487, 1974.

63. Loder RT, Richards BS, Shapiro PS, et al: Acute slipped capital femoral epiphysis: the importance of physeal stability. J Bone Joint Surg Am 75:1134–1140, 1993.

64. Maeda S, Kita A, Funayama K, Kokubun S: Vascular supply to slipped capital femoral epiphysis. J Pediatr Orthop 21:664–667, 2001.

65. Herrera-Soto JA, Duffy MF, Birnbaum MA, Vander Have KL: Increased intracapsular pressures after unstable slipped capital femoral epiphysis. J Pediatr Orthop 28:723–728, 2008.

66. Chen RC, Schoenecker PL, Dobbs MB, et al: Urgent reduction, fixation, and arthrotomy for unstable slipped capital femoral epiphysis. J Pediatr Orthop 29:687–694, 2009.

67. Dunn DM: The treatment of adolescent slipping of the upper femoral epiphysis. J Bone Joint Surg Br 46:621–629, 1964.

68. Dunn DM, Angel JC: Replacement of the femoral head by open operation in severe adolescent slipping of the upper femoral epiphysis. J Bone Joint Surg Br 60:394–403, 1978.

69. Fish J: Cuneiform osteotomy in slipped capital femoral epiphysis. J Bone Joint Surg Am 56:1301, 1974.

70. Fish JB: Cuneiform osteotomy of the femoral neck in the treatment of slipped capital femoral epiphysis. J Bone Joint Surg Am 66:1153–1168, 1984.

71. Fish JB: Cuneiform osteotomy of the femoral neck in the treatment of slipped capital femoral epiphysis: a follow-up note. J Bone Joint Surg Am 76:46–59, 1994.

72. Velasco R, Schai PA, Exner GU: Slipped capital femoral epiphysis: a long-term follow-up study after open reduction of the femoral head combined with subcapital wedge resection. J Pediatr Orthop B 7:43–52, 1998.

73. DeRosa GP, Mullins RC, Kling TF Jr: Cuneiform osteotomy of the femoral neck in severe slipped capital femoral epiphysis. Clin Orthop Relat Res 322:48–60, 1996.

74. Hauge MF: Wedge osteotomy in slipped femoral epiphysis; with special reference to technique. Acta Orthop Scand 28:51–65, 1958.

75. Wagner L, Donovan M: Wedge osteotomy of neck of femur in advanced cases of displaced upper femoral epiphysis: 10 year study. Am J Surg 78:281, 1949.

76. Ganz R, Gill TJ, Gautier E, et al: Surgical dislocation of the adult hip a technique with full access to the femoral head and acetabulum without the risk of avascular necrosis. J Bone Joint Surg Br 83:1119–1124, 2001.

77. Parsch K, Zehender H, Buhl T, Weller S: Intertrochanteric corrective osteotomy for moderate and severe chronic slipped capital femoral epiphysis. J Pediatr Orthop B 8:223–230, 1999.

78. Jerre R, Billing L, Hansson G, et al: Bilaterality in slipped capital femoral epiphysis: importance of a reliable radiographic method. J Pediatr Orthop B 5:80–84, 1996.

79. Jerre R, Billing L, Hansson G, Wallin J: The contralateral hip in patients primarily treated for unilateral slipped upper femoral epiphysis: long-term follow-up of 61 hips. J Bone Joint Surg Br 76:563–567, 1994.

80. Loder RT, Hensinger RN: Slipped capital femoral epiphysis associated with renal failure osteodystrophy. J Pediatr Orthop 17:205–211, 1997.

81. Acheson R: The Oxford method of assessing skeletal maturity. Clin Orthop Relat Res 10:19–39, 1957.

82. Trueta J: The normal vascular anatomy of the human femoral head during growth. J Bone Joint Surg Br 39:358–394, 1957.

83. Fahey JJ, O'Brien ET: Acute slipped capital femoral epiphysis: review of the literature and report of ten cases. J Bone Joint Surg Am 47:1105–1127, 1965.

84. Segal LS, Weitzel PP, Davidson RS: Valgus slipped capital femoral epiphysis: fact or fiction? Clin Orthop Relat Res 322:91–98, 1996.

85. Duncan JW, Lovell WW: Anterior slip of the capital femoral epiphysis: report of a case and discussion. Clin Orthop Relat Res 110:171–173, 1975.

86. Kampner SL, Wissinger HA: Anterior slipping of the capital femoral epiphysis: report of a case. J Bone Joint Surg Am 54:1531–1536, 1972.

87. Shank CF, Thiel EJ, Klingele KE: Valgus slipped capital femoral epiphysis: prevalence, presentation, and treatment options. J Pediatr Orthop 30:140–146, 2010.

88. Kennedy JP, Weiner DS: Results of slipped capital femoral epiphysis in the black population. J Pediatr Orthop 10:224–227, 1990.

89. Meier MC, Meyer LC, Ferguson RL: Treatment of slipped capital femoral epiphysis with a spica cast [see comments]. J Bone Joint Surg Am 74:1522–1529, 1992.

90. Bennet GC, Koreska J, Rang M: Pin placement in slipped capital femoral epiphysis. J Pediatr Orthop 4:574–578, 1984.

91. Cruess RL: The pathology of acute necrosis of cartilage in slipping of the capital femoral epiphysis: a report of two cases with pathological sections. J Bone Joint Surg Am 45:1013–1024, 1963.

92. Ingram AJ, Clarke MS, Clarke CS Jr, Marshall WR: Chondrolysis complicating slipped capital femoral epiphysis. Clin Orthop Relat Res 165:99–109, 1982.

93. Orofino C, Innis J, Lowrey C: Slipped capital femoral epiphysis in Negroes. J Bone Joint Surg Am 42:1079, 1960.

94. Eisenstein A, Rothschild S: Biochemical abnormalities in patients with slipped capital femoral epiphysis and chondrolysis. J Bone Joint Surg Am 58:459–467, 1976.

95. Mankin H, Sledge C, Rothschild S, et al: Chondrolysis of the hip. In Third open scientific meeting of the Hip Society, St Louis, 1975, CV Mosby.

96. Greenough CG, Bromage JD, Jackson AM: Pinning of the slipped upper femoral epiphysis—a trouble-free procedure? J Pediatr Orthop 5:657–660, 1985.

97. Hale D, Barrett IR: Chondrolysis following slipped capital femoral epiphysis. J Bone Joint Surg Br 71:882, 1989.

98. Ganz R, Gill TJ, Gautier E, et al: Surgical dislocation of the adult hip: a technique with full access to the femoral head and acetabulum without the risk of avascular necrosis. J Bone Joint Surg Br 83:1119–1124, 2001.

99. Ganz R, Parvizi J, Beck M, et al: Femoroacetabular impingement: a cause for osteoarthritis of the hip. Clin Orthop Relat Res 417:112–120, 2003.

100. Leunig M, Casillas MM, Hamlet M, et al: Slipped capital femoral epiphysis: early mechanical damage to the acetabular cartilage by a prominent femoral metaphysis. Acta Orthop Scand 71:370–375, 2000.

101. Spencer S, Millis MB, Kim YJ: Early results of treatment of hip impingement syndrome in slipped capital femoral epiphysis and pistol grip deformity of the femoral head-neck junction using the surgical dislocation technique. J Pediatr Orthop 26:281–285, 2006.

102. Krahn TH, Canale ST, Beaty JH, et al: Long-term follow-up of patients with avascular necrosis after treatment of slipped capital femoral epiphysis. J Pediatr Orthop 13:154–158, 1993.

103. Callaghan JJ, Brand RA, Pedersen DR: Hip arthrodesis: a long-term follow-up. J Bone Joint Surg Am 67:1328–1335, 1985.

104. Sponseller PD, McBeath AA, Perpich M: Hip arthrodesis in young patients: a long-term follow-up study. J Bone Joint Surg Am 66:853–859, 1984.

105. Ganz R, Parvizi J, Beck M, et al: Femoroacetabular impingement: a cause for osteoarthritis of the hip. Clin Orthop Relat Res 417:112–120, 2003.

106. Leunig M, Casillas MM, Hamlet M, et al: Slipped capital femoral epiphysis: early mechanical damage to the acetabular cartilage by a prominent femoral metaphysis. Acta Orthop Scand 71:370–375, 2000.

107. Sink EL, Zaltz I, Heare T, Dayton M: Acetabular cartilage and labral damage observed during surgical hip dislocation for stable slipped capital femoral epiphysis. J Pediatr Orthop 30:26–30, 2009.

108. Abraham E, Gonzalez MH, Pratap S, et al: Clinical implications of anatomical wear characteristics in slipped capital femoral epiphysis and primary osteoarthritis. J Pediatr Orthop 27:788–795, 2007.

109. Mamisch TC, Kim YJ, Richolt JA, et al: Femoral morphology due to impingement influences the range of motion in slipped capital femoral epiphysis. Clin Orthop Relat Res 467:692–698, 2009.

CHAPTER 43

Inflammatory Arthritis in the Child and Adolescent

Anthony A. Stans and Thomas G. Mason

INTRODUCTION

Inflammatory arthritis (IA) in children and adolescents represents a collection of medical conditions that may affect the axial and appendicular joints of the musculoskeletal system of children and teenagers. These conditions are not uncommon and can have substantial impact on functional status and quality of life. Hip involvement in these conditions is frequently associated with worse outcomes.[1]

IA in children and adolescents encompasses two diagnostic groups: juvenile rheumatoid arthritis (JRA) and the spondyloarthropathies. Many pediatric rheumatologists prefer the term *juvenile idiopathic arthritis (JIA)* to describe the IA of children and adolescents. Many similarities and some subtle differences in the definitions of JRA[2] and JIA[3] and their criteria and their subtypes are highlighted in Boxes 43-1 and 43-2. The primary difference between these definitions is the inclusion of many of the spondyloarthropathies in JIA. Uniting features of these conditions include age of onset and their chronic nature. For the purposes of this chapter, JRA terminology will be used, and the spondyloarthropathies will be discussed separately.

The term *spondyloarthropathies* (spondy) refers to a group of inflammatory conditions in which the spine and/or peripheral joints are affected in a characteristic pattern that is clinically different from JRA. Conditions that compose the group of spondy are listed in Box 43-3. Because the arthropathy of these conditions may be its initial manifestation, criteria for the early diagnosis of spondyloarthropathies have been developed and are shown in Box 43-4.[4] Although the clinical definitions of psoriasis and forms of inflammatory bowel disease are beyond the scope of this chapter, criteria[5] for the diagnosis of ankylosing spondylitis (AS) are shown in Box 43-5.

EPIDEMIOLOGY AND RISK FACTORS

The incidence and prevalence of JRA vary with the population studied, but an incidence of about 1 new case per 10,000 children per year and a prevalence of about 1 in 1000 children were found in a population-based cohort.[6] Of this cohort, about two thirds were pauciarticular onset, 10% were systemic onset, and the rest were polyarticular onset. Girls are more likely to develop JRA than boys, except for the systemic-onset subtype, which seems to have no apparent gender predilection. Studies from other centers show a higher prevalence of polyarticular-onset JRA, likely a reflection of the referral nature of those centers studied.

The epidemiology of spondy in children and adolescents is less straightforward, primarily because of lack of uniform terminology and precise definitions of these conditions. Anywhere from 1% to 20% of children seen at pediatric rheumatology centers may have spondy.[7] The prevalence of ankylosing spondylitis (AS) ranged from around 70 to 210 cases per 100,000 adults, and AS has an incidence of between 7 and 9 cases per 100,000 person-years, depending on the population studied.[8] Of patients diagnosed with AS, about 10% to 20% will be diagnosed before 17 years of age—juvenile ankylosing spondylitis (JAS)—although there are populations with higher juvenile prevalence in Mexico and Korea.[9] Boys generally are more likely to develop spondyloarthropathies.

BOX 43-1. CRITERIA FOR THE DIAGNOSIS OF JUVENILE RHEUMATOID ARTHRITIS (JRA)[2]

Clinical Features
- Onset before 16 years of age
- Swelling or two of the following: joint tenderness, decreased range of motion (ROM), painful ROM, or joint warmth
- At least 6 weeks of symptoms
- No other cause

Subtypes
- Pauciarticular: four or fewer joints, fever not prominent
- Polyarticular: five or more joints, fever not prominent
- Systemic onset: prominent fever; rash, polyarticular or pauciarticular

BOX 43-2. CRITERIA FOR THE DIAGNOSIS OF JUVENILE IDIOPATHIC ARTHRITIS (JIA)[3]

Clinical Features
- Onset before 16 years of age
- Swelling or two of the following: joint tenderness, decreased range of motion (ROM), painful ROM, or joint warmth
- At least 6 weeks of symptoms
- No other cause

Subtypes
- Oligoarticular: four or fewer joints, fever not prominent
- Polyarticular: five or more joints, fever not prominent
- Systemic onset: prominent fever; rash, polyarticular or pauciarticular
- Includes arthritis related to inflammatory bowel disease (IBD), psoriasis (PsA), ankylosing spondylitis (AS), and enthesitis-related arthropathy (ERA)

BOX 43-3. SPONDYLOARTHROPATHIES

Psoriatic arthropathy (PsA)
Arthritis associated with inflammatory bowel disease (IBD)
Ankylosing spondylitis (AS)
Reactive arthritis (ReA)
Undifferentiated spondyloarthropathy (Usp)

BOX 43-4. CRITERIA FOR THE DIAGNOSIS OF EARLY SPONDYLOARTHROPATHIES[4]

Synovitis, usually in lower extremity, asymmetrical
Inflammatory back pain, and at least one of the following:
- Family history of a spondyloarthropathy
- Psoriasis
- Inflammatory bowel disease
- Recent acute diarrhea or nongonococcal urethritis
- Enthesitis
- Sacroiliac (SI) pain or x-ray changes

Note: The presence of *A* and/or *B* plus at least one of the other findings is required to make this diagnosis.

BOX 43-5. CRITERIA FOR THE DIAGNOSIS OF ANKYLOSIS SPONDYLITIS (AS)[5]

Moderate bilateral sacroiliac radiographic changes
Severe unilateral sacroiliac radiographic changes
Reduced range of motion (ROM) in lumbar spine
Decreased chest expansion
Inflammatory back pain
- Chronic
- Morning stiffness
- Improved with activity

Note: The presence of at least one radiographic criterion and one clinical criterion is required to make the diagnosis of AS. Features of inflammatory back pain (IBP) are shown.

PATHOPHYSIOLOGY

JRA and spondy are chronic inflammatory conditions that affect the axial and appendicular musculoskeletal system. In general, these conditions are believed to be autoimmune, suggesting that established immune mechanisms somehow become "misguided" and initiate and propagate damage to these structures. This is an area of intense and evolving research. Components of innate immune system, adaptive immune system, cytokines, autoantibodies, and molecular genetics are examples of aspects of the immune system being studied for these conditions.

Of these areas, the association of spondy with HLA B-27 (see earlier) and the development of autoantibodies clearly have the greatest clinical relevance. Autoantibodies are antibodies that have affinity for self and are a hallmark of "autoimmune" conditions. Autoantibodies add prognostic information about forms of IA, but are not required for diagnosis of IA.

Although many types of autoantibodies are known, for children with IA, two are most useful for clinical management. The first of these is rheumatoid factor (RF). An RF is an antibody that has affinity to another antibody; several types of RF have been identified.

Genetic associations for JRA have been described but do not presently have prominent clinical applications. For spondy, however, the association with the class I HLA B-27 molecule is clinically important. The presence of B-27 is correlated with axial involvement in these conditions, and it may be found in almost 90% of teenagers with AS.[10]

Usually, serum RF is measured by enzyme-linked immunosorbent assay (ELISA)—a sensitive, inexpensive technique. The presence of RF in the serum of children with polyarticular JRA increases the likelihood of damage and progressive disease, but most children with polyarticular JRA are RF(−).

The other important autoantibody in children with IA is antinuclear antibody (ANA). Similar to RF, most children with IA are ANA negative, but in children with pauciarticular JRA, the likelihood of uveitis is increased if ANA is found in the serum. Because knowledge of levels of these autoantibodies does not generally help in the longitudinal management of children who have IA, they are not generally sequentially assessed.

CLINICAL FEATURES AND DIAGNOSIS

The key to diagnosing JRA and spondy in children is recognizing the patterns of clinical manifestations of these conditions. Criteria for JRA include at least 6 weeks of symptoms. Similarly, spondyloarthropathies are chronic conditions. Although acute joint inflammation could be associated with the initial presentation of one of these conditions, other causes of joint inflammation such as infection must be strongly considered in this setting. Septic arthritis is a medical emergency that cannot be overlooked. JRA and spondy are chronic, inflammatory conditions. Clinical features of inflammation are highlighted in Box 43-6.

The most common form of JRA, based on population studies, is pauciarticular JRA (pauciJRA). It is defined as arthritis in four or fewer joints, not associated with fever and other extra-articular features such as rash, adenopathy, and so forth[2] (Box 43-7). *Arthritis* of JRA is defined as swelling or two of the following: joint tenderness, pain with range of motion (ROM), decreased ROM, or joint warmth in a diarthrodial joint.[2]

The "typical" case of pauciJRA presents in a preschool-aged girl with a painless limp and synovitis of a knee or ankle. Joint pain often is not the primary reason for evaluation of children with pauciJRA. Often, someone may notice that the child "walks funny" or seems to have a swollen joint, but that it does not seem particularly tender. This paradox may be contributed to by an insidious onset of disease, limited communication capacity of the child, the developing capacity for ambulation in this age group, or other factors. A knee effusion in a 10-year-old boy with pauciJRA is shown in Figure 43-1*A* and *B*. Most of these children do well, but a subset may develop involvement in other joints. Additional joint involvement in children with pauciJRA occurring more than 6 months after diagnosis is known as *extended pauciarticular JRA*. Estimates vary, but as many as one third of children with pauciJRA could become "extended," with a higher likelihood in those with symmetrical and upper extremity presentation.[11]

One of the most important features of pauciJRA is the increased incidence of uveitis, which is found in about 15% of patients.[12] The development of uveitis is associated with the presence of ANA in the serum. The uveitis is usually asymptomatic but, if untreated, can have devastating visual consequences. It is mandatory for all children who have pauciJRA, especially if they are ANA positive, to undergo an ophthalmologic screening program for this potential complication. Girls who are diagnosed before the age of 7, and who have a positive ANA, are at highest risk and may need to be seen as often as every 3 months for screening.

Polyarticular JRA (polyJRA), defined as five or more joints with arthritis at the time of diagnosis, has many clinical features that are similar to those of rheumatoid

---

BOX 43-6.   INFLAMMATORY FEATURES OF RHEUMATIC DISEASE

History
- Morning stiffness
- Fever, constitutional symptoms
- Response to previous anti-inflammatory Rx

Physical examination
- Red, warm, swollen, tender (Celsius criteria) joints
- Restricted range of motion (ROM)
- Associated findings: rash, uveitis, etc.
- Adenopathy, hepatosplenomegaly

Laboratory studies
- Increased erythrocyte sedimentation rate (ESR)
- Increased C-reactive protein (CRP)
- Anemia, leukocytosis, thrombocytosis
- Autoantibodies
- Radiographic changes

BOX 43-7.   APPROACH TO THE CHILD WITH INFLAMMATORY ARTHRITIS (IA)*

Acute Arthritis
- Trauma
- Infection

Chronic Arthritis
- Fever, rash
  - sJRA
- No fever, rash
  - >4 joints
    - polyJRA
  - ≤4 joints
    - pauciJRA
- Spine involvement, SI involvement, enthesitis, psoriasis, IBD, anterior uveitis
  - Spondyloarthropathy
- Chronic arthritis with other features (renal, CNS, etc.)
  - CTD
  - Vasculitis

CNS, Central nervous system; *CTD,* connective tissue disease; *IBD,* inflammatory bowel disease; *pauciJRA,* pauciarticular juvenile rheumatoid arthritis; *polyJRA,* polyarticular juvenile rheumatoid arthritis; *sJRA,* systemic-onset juvenile rheumatoid arthritis.
*Shown are prominent clinical features of the subtypes of IA.

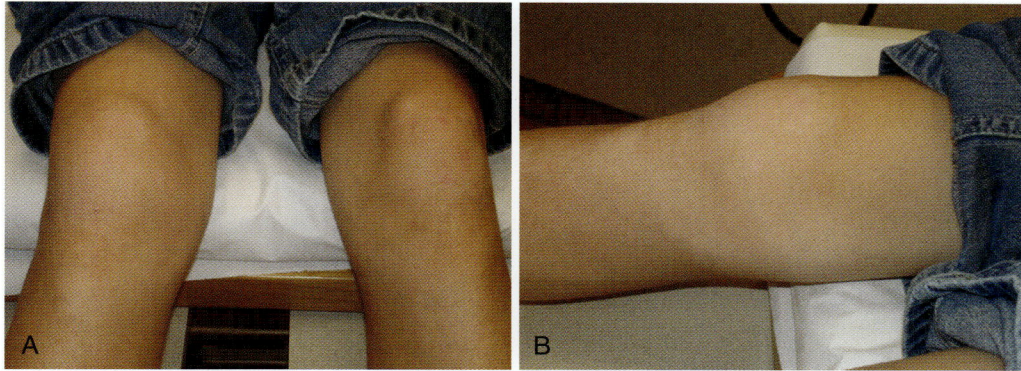

Figure 43-1. A and **B,** This 11-year-old boy has an effusion in his right knee. Note the soft tissue enlargement medial to the patella along the medial joint line. He had diminished flexion but no pain with range of motion (ROM).

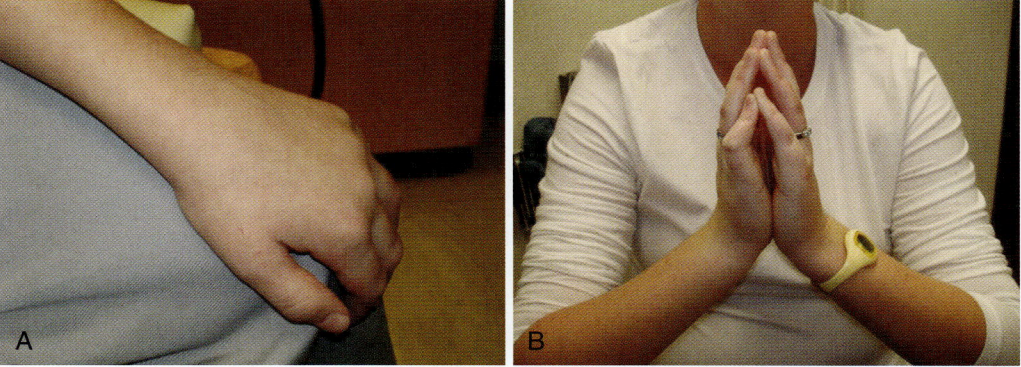

Figure 43-2. A, Left wrist of a 13-year-old girl with chronic polyarticular juvenile rheumatoid arthritis (JRA). Note the prominent synovial tissue on the dorsum of the wrist. **B,** Note decreased passive extension of the wrists and the boutonnière deformity of the right fifth finger in this same patient.

arthritis in the adult. Similar to pauciJRA, polyJRA does not have fever as a major clinical feature. Frequently, symmetrical small joint synovitis with pain, loss of function, and morning stiffness is the pattern at presentation. Soft tissue swelling, restricted ROM, and small joint changes in a 13-year-old girl with polyJRA are shown in Figure 43-2A and B. Large joints, including the hips, may also be involved at the time of diagnosis, or they may become involved in the course of polyJRA. Subcutaneous nodules, typically over extensor surfaces, may be seen in some cases. Also, a few cases of polyJRA will have an associated RF in the serum. The presence of nodules and RF increases the likelihood of joint destruction and worse clinical outcomes.

In addition to the large number of joints affected, subcutaneous nodules, and RF, radiographic changes such as joint space narrowing (JSN) and cortical erosions increase the likelihood of a worse clinical outcome for children with polyJRA. An example of erosive radiographic changes in a teenager with polyJRA is shown in Figure 43-3A and B.

The least common form of JRA is systemic-onset JRA (sJRA). Unlike pauciJRA and polyJRA, sJRA seems to have no age or gender predilection. These children appear ill and have undergone extensive evaluation for occult infection, malignancy, and so forth. Fevers and

the accompanying irritability are prominent. The fever pattern shown in Figure 43-4 is typical for sJRA in that the temperature is usually normal (or even subnormal) in the morning, but is markedly increased in the afternoon and evening. A faint, pink, macular evanescent rash may also be seen, typically with fever spikes. An example of this rash is shown in Figure 43-5.

Joint involvement in sJRA is frequently pauciarticular, but can be polyarticular. Involvement of the wrists is characteristic of sJRA. Extra-articular features, in addition to fever and rash, include prominent adenopathy, hepatosplenomegaly, and serositis. These extra-articular features may be seen in up to half of children with sJRA in the course of their illness.[13]

When spondy occurs in children or adolescents, an asymmetrical oligoarthritis is often the clinical pattern at presentation. This is frequently seen in a lower extremity joint, similar to the ankle shown in Figure 43-6. About 10% to 15% of patients with psoriasis (Fig. 43-7) or inflammatory bowel disease (IBD) will develop an associated spondyloarthropathy, which may precede the rash or enteritis. Boys may be a little more likely to develop these conditions than girls. In an older child with an asymmetrical oligoarthritis, a family history of psoriasis increases the chances of developing psoriatic arthritis—one form of spondyloarthropathy. Also, the

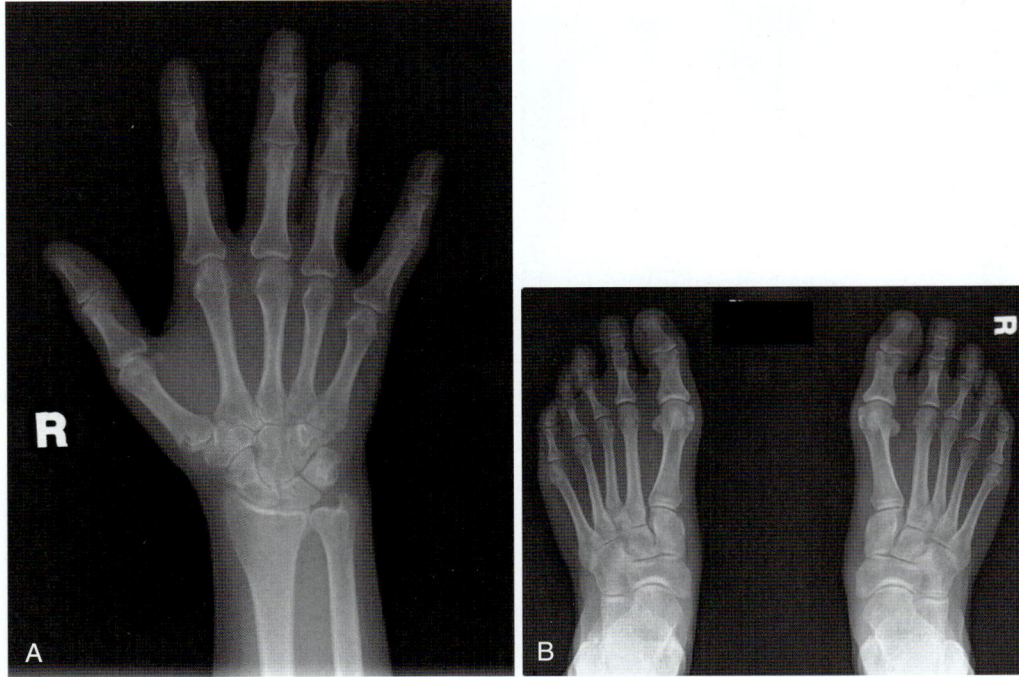

Figure 43-3. A, X-rays of the hands and wrists of a 16-year-old girl with seropositive polyarticular juvenile rheumatoid arthritis (JRA) after 18 months of disease. In spite of weekly methotrexate, these erosive changes developed over the previous year. **B,** X-rays of the feet of the same girl. Her erosive changes in the metatarsophalangeal (MTP) joints are unchanged from the previous study done 1 year ago.

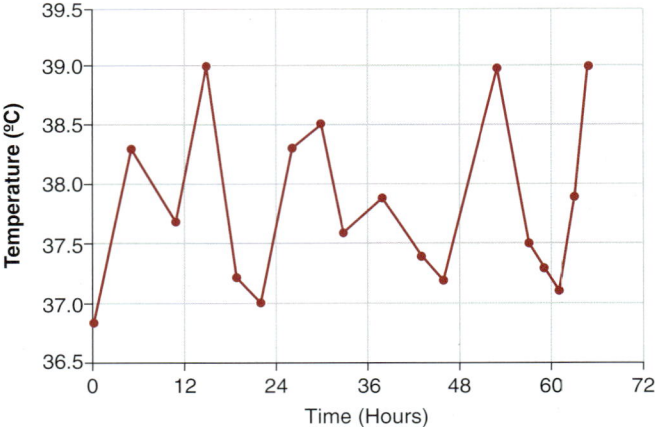

Figure 43-4. Fever curve in a child with systemic-onset juvenile rheumatoid arthritis (sJRA). Early morning temperatures are normal (or occasionally subnormal) but dramatically increase in the afternoon and evening. *(Courtesy E. Rabinovich, M.D., M.P.H.)*

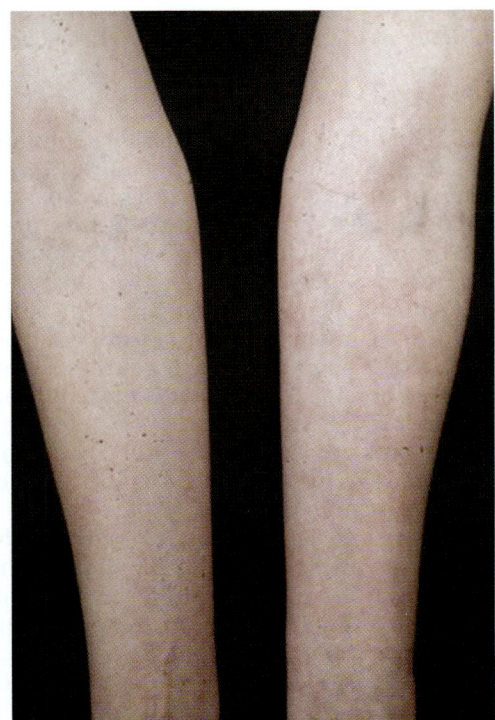

Figure 43-5. This nonspecific macular erythema, typically seen on the trunk (especially during periods of fever), is an example of the rash seen in children with systemic-onset juvenile rheumatoid arthritis (sJRA). *(Courtesy E. Rabinovich, M.D., M.P.H.)*

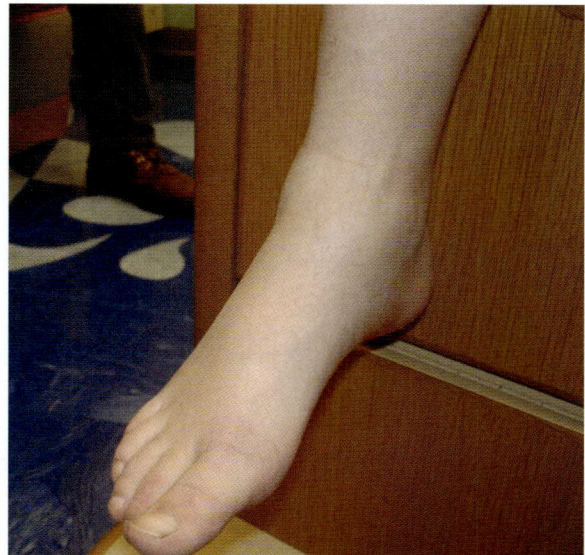

Figure 43-6. This 9-year-old boy has right ankle synovitis with soft tissue swelling just medial to the medial malleolus.

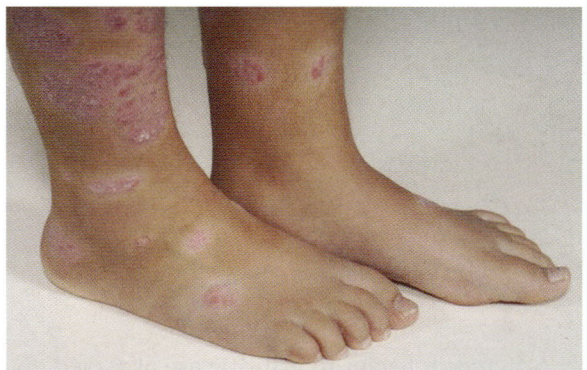

Figure 43-7. Raised, scaly plaques from psoriasis. *(Courtesy D. Davis, M.D.)*

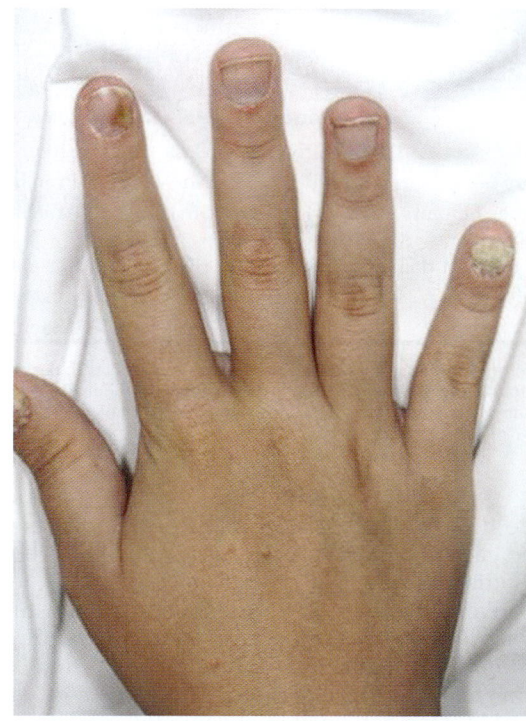

Figure 43-8. Nail changes with psoriasis. Marked onycholysis and nail pitting of the fifth finger are shown, along with some early nail changes in the second finger. *(Courtesy D. Davis, M.D.)*

presence of nail changes, shown in Figure 43-8, increases the odds of developing psoriatic arthritis.

The other common presentation of spondy in children and adolescents is inflammatory back pain (IBP). Features of IBP include stiffness, pain improved by activity, location in the buttocks, and chronicity. These symptoms often reflect sacroiliitis. Radiographic confirmation of sacroiliitis is often a late clinical finding, although magnetic resonance imaging (MRI) appears to hold promise for detecting early changes that may precede standard radiographic changes by many years in patients who eventually develop AS.[14]

Spondy shares other clinical features besides an inflammatory arthritis and spondylitis. One of these is enthesitis, which refers to inflammation at the insertions of ligaments such as the patellar tendon or the Achilles tendon. Another feature is oral mucositis, which is painful but does not scar. Finally, children and teenagers with spondyloarthropathies frequently

develop anterior uveitis, which usually presents with red, painful eyes (can be unilateral too). This uveitis is different from the posterior uveitis of pauciJRA, which is almost always asymptomatic.

Hip involvement in JRA is uncommon at diagnosis but can develop in up to 50% of cases over the first 6 years of disease.[1] Most JRA-related hip disease develops in children with polyJRA. The child may have groin pain or pain referred to the greater trochanter or the distal femur. A limp may be noted, and pain with ROM and decreased ROM of hip are found on examination. Loss of internal rotation is often an early finding. Hip involvement in spondy is very uncommon at presentation but may develop later, particularly in adolescents and young adults with AS.

DIFFERENTIAL DIAGNOSIS

Acute presentation of hip pain in a child or teenager requires strong consideration of a septic process such as septic arthritis or osteomyelitis, particularly if the child is febrile, cannot ambulate or bear weight, appears toxic, or has risk factors. Sterile, postinfectious hip synovitis (also known as *toxic synovitis*) can be painful, but by definition is self-limiting.

A child or adolescent presenting with chronic isolated hip pain or evidence of hip dysfunction without the features listed previously is not likely to have IA. The differential diagnosis in these children would

Table 43-1. Key Clinical Features of the Three Forms of Juvenile Rheumatoid Arthritis (JRA)

	PauciJRA	PolyJRA	sJRA
Gender	Girls	Girls	Either
Fevers	No	No	Prominent
Number of joints involved	0-4	>5	At least 1
Risk for joint damage	Low	High	Variable
ANA	Common	Rare	Absent
RF	Rare	Occasional	Absent

ANA, Serum antinuclear antibodies; *pauciJRA,* pauciarticular juvenile rheumatoid arthritis; *polyJRA,* polyarticular juvenile rheumatoid arthritis; *RF,* serum rheumatoid factor; *sJRA,* systemic-onset juvenile rheumatoid arthritis.

include hip dysplasia, Legg-Calvé-Perthes disease, and slipped capital femoral epiphysis, all of which were previously discussed.

Hip involvement in IA is uncommon at the time of diagnosis but can develop over the course of these conditions. Involvement of other joints and extra-articular features are clues to the diagnosis of various forms of IA. One category of chronic inflammatory conditions that may have an inflammatory arthropathy consists of systemic connective tissue disorders (CTDs) including inflammatory muscle diseases such as juvenile dermatomyositis (JDMS), systemic lupus erythematosus (SLE), and scleroderma. The other category of chronic inflammatory conditions that may include features of an inflammatory arthropathy is the vasculitides. The vasculitides and CTDs are uncommon systemic illnesses that often can adversely affect internal organs and may require systemic immunosuppressive treatment to control symptoms and prevent damage. An approach to the differential diagnosis of JRA and spondy is shown in Table 43-1.

TREATMENT

Once the diagnosis of one of these forms of IA is made in a child or adolescent, the next step is assessment of key variables that influence choices about therapy. In general, decisions for treating these conditions are based on assessments of pain, disability, or dysfunction, and risk for progression and damage. Utilization of both medication-based therapy and physical and occupational therapy is based on these variables. Surgical intervention usually is indicated when these therapies have failed.

The pain from IA can be assessed in several ways, but asking the parent or child to indicate on a 0 to 10 scale, with 10 being the worst pain ever, is a straightforward, frequently used method. Similarly, several validated tools are available to assess the functional status of children with JRA; the most frequently used of these is the Childhood Health Assessment Questionnaire (CHAQ).[15] As with its adult counterpart, the Health Assessment Questionnaire (HAQ), eight domains of

---

BOX 43-8.   FUNDAMENTALS OF THE MANAGEMENT OF CHRONIC DISEASE IN CHILDREN

Ensure effective communication between providers and family.
Provide a clear understanding of diagnosis and significance.
Maintain social and physical activities as much as possible.
Facilitate continued academic development.
Provide high-quality primary care.

BOX 43-9.   SELECT NONSURGICAL THERAPIES FOR CHILDREN AND ADOLESCENTS WITH INFLAMMATORY ARTHRITIS (IA)

Level 1
• PT: stretching, increased ROM
• PT: splint
• PT: strengthening exercises
Level 2
• NSAIDs: ibuprofen, naproxen
• Intra-articular corticosteroids
Level 3
• Methotrexate
• Other DMARDs
• Biologics
• Systemic corticosteroids

DMARDs, Disease-modifying antirheumatic drugs; *NSAIDs,* nonsteroidal anti-inflammatory drugs; *PT,* physical therapy; *ROM,* range of motion.

---

daily activities relevant to arthritis are assessed on a 0 to 3 scale, with 3 representing complete inability to do that activity. Then a composite score is developed. Although the values from these scales are somewhat arbitrary, the relative change in their value can be an adjunct to clinical assessments of joint tenderness, swelling, and acute-phase reactants.

Once an assessment of pain and functional status has been completed, consideration of the natural history of the type of IA along with an assessment of markers of prognosis is the next step. As was noted previously, this is done primarily by checking for serum autoantibodies (RF) and radiographs of the affected joint. Radiographic changes such as JSN and erosion are markers for a worse outcome in children with JRA.[16]

Nonsurgical Therapies

Children with chronic health issues and their families have many health care–related needs. These are summarized in Box 43-8. An overview of potential nonsurgical therapies for IA is shown in Box 43-9. Most children with pauciJRA will need level 1 and level 2 therapies for their articular disease. They will need careful ophthalmologic follow-up as well. Children with refractory disease and those who develop "extended pauci-JRA" will likely progress to level 3 medications.

Children with polyJRA are at high risk of damage and are likely to need level 3 therapies. Level 1 and level 2 therapies may be useful but generally have not been shown to retard disease progression, similar to level 3 medications. The child with polyJRA who has a positive RF and x-ray changes is at highest risk for poor outcome. Because of this, such children are started with level 3 medications, usually methotrexate, along with level 1 and 2 therapies.

Children with sJRA present the clinician with basically two "diseases": arthritis and associated extra-articular features. The proportions of these two components can vary widely from a primarily febrile illness to a primary inflammatory arthritis that is potentially destructive. Therapy for the febrile portion primarily consists of nonsteroidal anti-inflammatory drugs (NSAIDs) and systemic corticosteroids. Management of the arthritis of sJRA is similar to that of pauciJRA and polyJRA and is based on the number of joints involved. Children with sJRA do not have positive RF but can have a destructive arthritis, similar to children with polyJRA.

Children with spondyloarthropathies are frequently managed similarly to children and adolescents with pauciJRA with level 1 and level 2 therapies. If an associated condition (such as psoriasis or IBD) is present, appropriate management of it is indicated as well. Because spine involvement often is not present at the outset, monitoring for spine or sacroiliac (SI) pain and assessment of spinal ROM are important steps in follow-up for children.

Surgical Therapies

Improved medical management and the development of joint arthroplasty have dramatically changed surgical treatment of JRA over the past 40 years. Surgical synovectomy resulted in inconsistent pain relief, and intermediate and long-term follow-up showed no change in the natural history of the disease.[17,18] Osteotomy of the proximal femur was used in the past with poor success to improve the position of the femur relative to the pelvis in the painful, contracted hip and has the harmful consequence of distorting proximal femoral anatomy, compromising the results of later total hip arthroplasty (THA). Hip involvement is often bilateral; therefore arthrodesis is contraindicated. For most JRA patients with hip involvement, level 1, 2, and 3 medical treatment is able to control the disease until patients reach adolescence, when arthroplasty becomes an acceptable option for those with severe pain and functional disability. For the uncommon patient with joint space preservation and significant joint contracture, soft tissue release may be beneficial.[19]

Surgical Indications

Before any surgical treatment is provided, medical management must be optimized and all viable nonoperative treatment options exhausted. Level 2 and 3 medical management by a rheumatologist is essential. Physical therapy is used to maximize joint range of motion and muscle strength. Hip abduction and extension are the two planes of motion most often limited by JRA. Use of a knee immobilizer or a hip abduction pillow at night may be useful for improving hip extension and abduction. The indication for soft tissue hip contracture release is found in the rare patient with joint preservation and significant functional limitation caused by restricted range of motion. Pain, marked contracture, and joint destruction are indications for THA.

Severe hip arthritis caused by JRA most commonly occurs in patients with polyJRA. Multiple joint involvement limits the patient activity level, reduces demands placed on prosthetic joints, and improves arthroplasty longevity when compared with patients of similar age without JRA undergoing THA. Severe contracture with destruction of multiple joints requires a thoughtful surgical strategy, which often necessitates multiple joint arthroplasty. Hip arthroplasty is typically recommended before knee arthroplasty in the same limb; good hip range of motion is necessary for effective knee arthroplasty rehabilitation. Hip disease is often bilateral in polyJRA, and the surgeon should be prepared to consider bilateral THA under the same anesthetic or staged arthroplasties with a short time interval between procedures to allow rapid mobilization and rehabilitation.

Young patients with severe JRA are at risk of having their adolescence stolen from them by their disease as they sit immobile in a wheelchair. Although good judgment should cause the surgeon to pause (and pause again) before performing THA in an adolescent, when severe pain, contracture, and joint destruction exist, total joint arthroplasty can dramatically improve patient function and quality of life.

Preoperative Planning

Preoperative evaluation should include the following radiographs:

1. Anteroposterior (AP) pelvis
2. AP femur
3. True lateral of the hip and proximal femur

Templating of THA components is essential to ensure that components are available to fit the small size and distorted anatomy frequently encountered in JRA patients.

Description of Technique(s)

Soft tissue release is occasionally indicated in the young patient with hip contracture. Hip abduction and extension are the two planes of motion most often limited by JRA. A 2 to 5 cm transverse or longitudinal incision, centered over the adductor longus tendon, is used for adduction contracture release. The adductor longus is always released, the adductor magnus is never released, and the adductor brevis as well as gracilis release are titrated to achieve the desired result of 30 degrees abduction with the hip extended. Test for gracilis contracture by assessing hip abduction with the knee flexed and then in extension. If the adductor brevis and gracilis are completely released and persistent adduction is present, the cause is likely contracture of the medial hip capsule. With the adductor longus and brevis released and retracted, dissection proceeds along the anterior surface of the adductor magnus, deep to the pectineus, to the medial femoral neck. Hohmann or Chandler retractors can be placed anterior and posterior to the femoral neck, exposing the medial hip capsule for release.

Hip flexion contracture is released through an oblique, anterior "bikini" incision centered 2 to 3 cm distal to the anterior superior ileac spine (ASIS) (Fig. 43-9). Dissection proceeds in the interval between the tensor fascia lata and the sartorius muscles, exposing the iliopsoas and the rectus femoris origin at the anterior inferior iliac spine (AIIS). Fractional lengthening of the iliopsoas at the pelvic brim should be performed first. Flexion of the hip relaxes the iliopsoas, allowing it to be retracted anteriorly and permitting dissection along the deep surface of the muscle. Here the tendinous portion of the iliopsoas is released under direct vision, leaving the muscle fibers intact. Now the rectus femoris origin is assessed. If significant contracture of the rectus femoris prevents hip extension to neutral, especially if the contracture is made worse by knee flexion, then the rectus femoris origin may be released. Finally, assess the hip capsule, and if the hip still cannot be extended to neutral, then the anterior capsule may be released. Our preference is to release in a "Z" fashion (Fig. 43-10A and B), which in theory may reduce the likelihood of creating hip instability. Patients undergoing anterior capsular release are placed in a hip abduction pillow

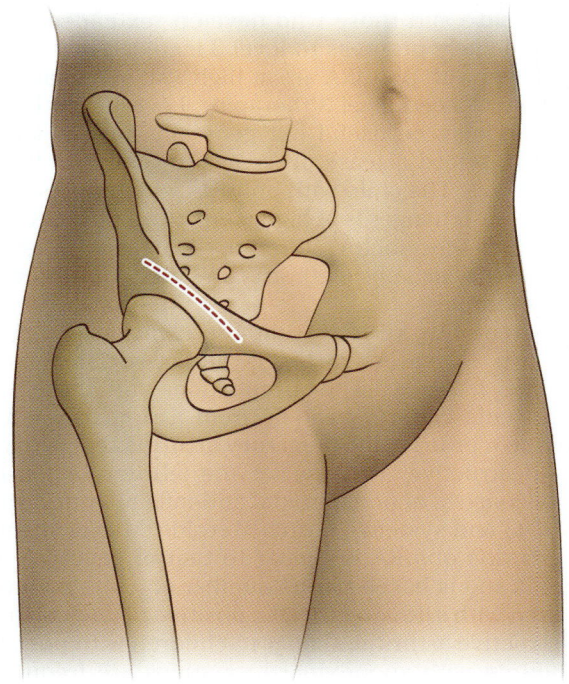

Figure 43-9. Hip flexion contracture release is performed through an oblique anterior "bikini" incision centered approximately 3 cm distal to the anterior superior iliac spine (ASIS).

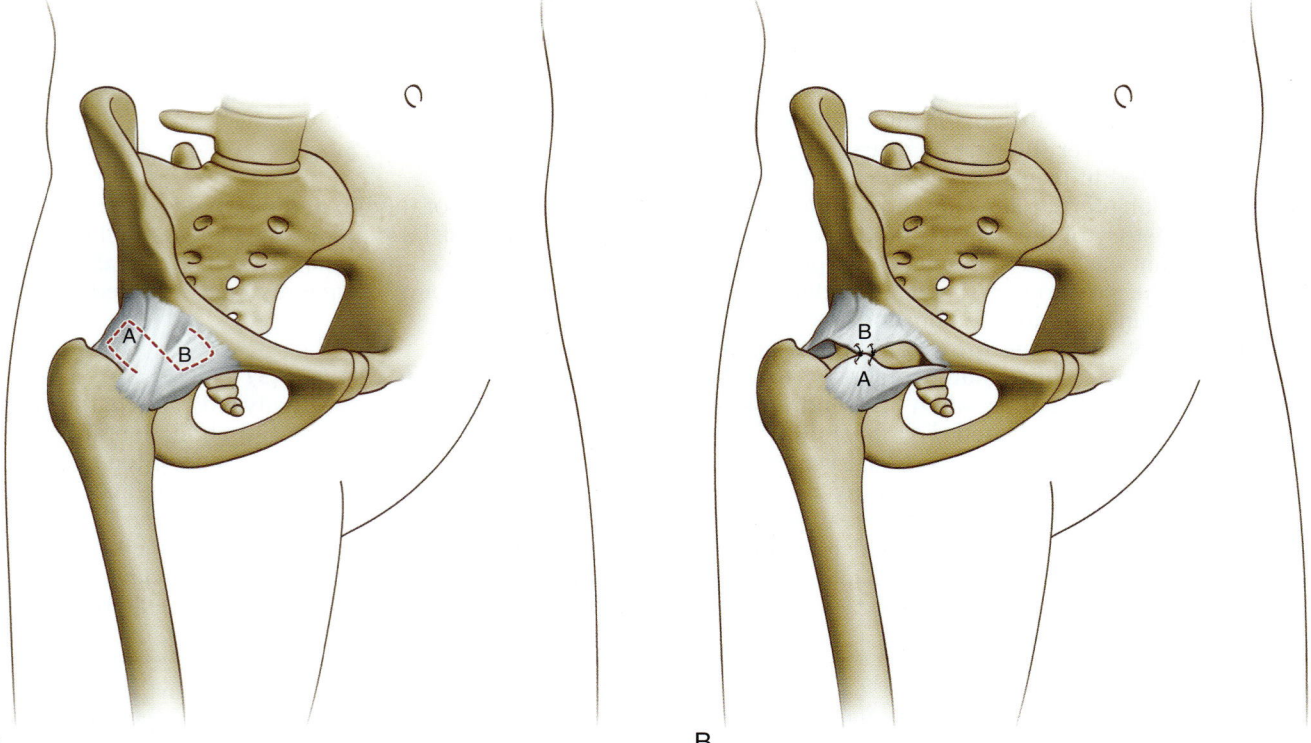

A   B

Figure 43-10. When necessary, anterior capsulotomy is performed in a "Z" fashion, **(A)** which allows lengthening and partial closure **(B)** of the capsule to prevent instability.

postoperatively; this further reduces the risk of hip instability and has the added benefit of holding the hip in an extended position.

Detailed THA technique is described in Section IX, "Primary Hip Arthroplasty." Special considerations that must be kept in mind when THA is performed in JRA patients include diminutive anatomy, distorted anatomy, and poor bone quality. Diminutive anatomy is a result of young patient age, preponderance of female over male patients, and effects of severe systemic disease and its treatment on growth. Anatomy is distorted by bone destruction, femoral head protrusion in osteoporotic bone, and soft tissue contracture. Hastings and colleagues described a group of JRA patients with a unique pathologic anatomic variation characterized by small femoral head size in a capacious acetabulum, which he proposed was caused by destruction of femoral head cartilage and associated enchondral ossification needed for circumferential femoral head growth.[20]

Whether to use cemented or uncemented components in JRA patients continues to be a source of discussion among arthroplasty surgeons. Because revision surgery is a certainty, bone-preserving, uncemented components are appealing. Relatively poor survival of cemented acetabular components in young patients has resulted in most surgeons choosing uncemented acetabular components with good results. Acetabular protrusion is common in JRA. The resultant absence of bone on the acetabular side may be managed with a morselized autologous femoral head bone graft placed behind a press-fit acetabular component.

Uncemented femoral components have not fared as well because abnormal anatomy and poor bone quality compromise uncemented femoral fixation. Such patients may benefit from cemented technique, while uncemented femoral components are reserved for those with excellent bone quality and near normal anatomy. A common compromise is to use a hybrid combination of a cemented femoral component and an uncemented acetabular component. To improve longevity, alternative bearing surfaces may be employed, but no long-term studies in JRA patients are available to demonstrate superiority over metal and polyethylene bearing surfaces. Ceramic-on-ceramic bearing surfaces have the potential to last decades with minimal wear debris, and the brittle material properties of ceramic are less likely to result in implant fracture when used in lightweight, low-demand JRA patients (Fig. 43-11A and B). To avoid polyethylene failure and particulate debris formation with resultant osteolysis, every effort should be made to maximize polyethylene thickness.

Variations/Unusual Situations

Severe hip arthritis is often bilateral in polyJRA patients, occasionally causing patients to become wheelchair bound; this contributes to the development of bilateral hip flexion contractures. The surgeon must choose an approach that allows ample anterior soft tissue contracture release at the time of arthroplasty. In patients with severe bilateral disease, bilateral THA under the same anesthetic, or staged bilateral arthroplasty with a short time interval between hips, is essential to get patients up walking and rehabilitated. A comprehensive strategy that considers all joints involved by JRA is essential. Frequently, total knee replacement (arthroplasty) (TKA) is also indicated in JRA patients who are candidates for THA. In a patient needing THA and TKA, THA is typically performed first, to provide the hip motion necessary for successful TKA rehabilitation.

Postoperative Care

Rapid rehabilitation is a primary concern following THA in JRA patients. Even when uncemented components are used, weight bearing as tolerated is encouraged. Standard dislocation precautions are employed. Adolescent patients are much less likely to experience deep venous thrombosis. Mechanical compression devices

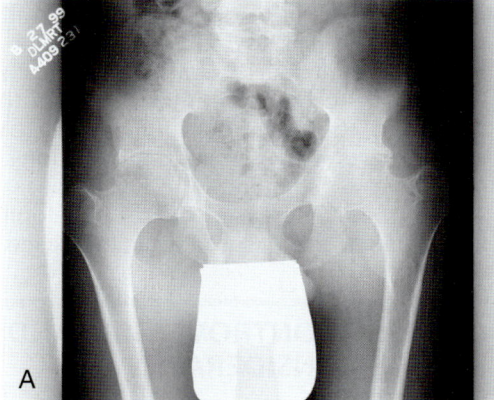
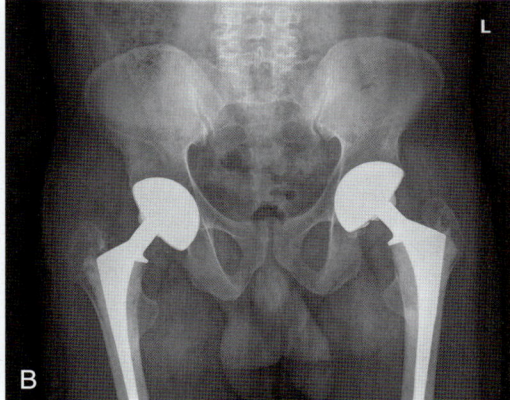

Figure 43-11. Despite optimal medical management, this 14-year-old young man with polyarticular juvenile rheumatoid arthritis (polyJRA) experienced progressive bilateral hip arthritis and was limited to painful household ambulation, requiring a wheelchair for all community mobility. **A,** The anteroposterior (AP) pelvis radiograph demonstrates mild protrusion of the femoral heads, the suggestion of adduction contracture, and marked joint space narrowing. **B,** Nine years following bilateral hybrid total hip arthroplasty using ceramic-on-ceramic bearing surfaces, the patient is fully ambulatory in the community without pain and without the need for a wheelchair or ambulatory aids.

and baby aspirin provide reasonable deep vein thrombosis (DVT) prophylaxis, unless patients have additional risk factors.

Results

Patient series have been published that describe THA results in young patients in which JRA is combined with other diagnoses,[21] but few available reports specifically report THA results in a series of patients including only JRA patients. Chmell reported long-term results of cemented THA in JRA patients demonstrating 85% survival of the femoral component and 70% survival for the acetabular component at an average follow-up of 15 years.[22] Wroblewski published a report on 292 Charnley cemented arthroplasties performed in young rheumatoid and JRA patients with a mean follow-up of 15 years.[23] With revision for any indication as an end point, survival was 74% at 25 years' follow-up. The main indication for revision was acetabular loosening. Lehtimaki and colleagues published the results of Charnley cemented THA performed in JRA patients reporting femoral component survival of 92% and acetabular component survival of 88% at 15 years.[24] In summary, one can expect femoral component survival of 85% to 90% and acetabular component survival of 70% to 85% at 15 to 20 years' follow-up after cemented THA.

Because uncemented THA is a newer technology, published results following uncemented THA in JRA patients are not available with the same length of follow-up as with cemented THA. At mean follow-up of 11 years, McCullough reported the results of 42 hydroxyapatite-coated femoral components inserted in JRA patients, noting that 4 (9.5%) components had failed.[25] All four failures occurred in patients younger than 16 years at the time of surgery. Odent and colleagues reported the results of 62 uncemented total hip arthroplasties implanted in 34 JRA patients with average follow-up of 6 years.[26] Survivorship analysis indicates survival rates of 100% for the femoral component and 90% for the acetabular component at 13 years. As longer follow-up becomes available, there will be greater clarity as to whether uncemented THA in JRA patients provides better bone preservation with the same durability as cemented THA.

Complications

Because of relatively low patient numbers in the JRA THA series, little statistical information is available regarding complication rates, but review of the series referenced in this chapter demonstrated several descriptive trends. Despite the use of immunosuppressive medication by most JRA patients undergoing THA, the infection rate appears to be low. Appropriate use of perioperative antibiotics and meticulous use of aseptic technique appear sufficient to maintain a low infection rate. Children and adolescents have a low incidence of deep vein thrombosis compared with adults, and the young age of JRA patients at the time of arthroplasty may be protective. Routine DVT prophylaxis trending toward conservative prophylaxis is appropriate for this age group. Polyethylene wear and aseptic loosening appear to be the primary problems encountered with THA in JRA patients. Improvements in uncemented component design and alternative bearing surfaces hold the potential to reduce these complications.

PROGNOSIS

Prognosis is different for various forms of IA in children and adolescents. For children with pauciJRA, the long-term outlook is very good, as long as the disease does not progress to an extended status. In population-based studies with long-term follow-up, articular outcomes are good,[27] although other non–population-based studies[28,29] demonstrate more long-term disability from juvenile arthritis.

As was previously noted, children with polyJRA are at higher risk for damage and disability. Risk factors for poorer outcomes include younger age at diagnosis, positive RF, poorer functional status, higher numbers of joints involved, and radiographic changes. Significant advances in medical therapies have improved clinical outcomes in children with poly JRA. Earlier recognition and earlier initiation of appropriate therapy are also likely contributors to improved clinical outcomes.

Children with sJRA generally have the worst outcomes, but multiple reasons may explain this. Some of these are related to the disease process; others are related to the medications often used to treat sJRA. These children frequently are treated with systemic corticosteroids, increasing the risk of growth issues, infection, osteoporosis, and so forth. Arthritis can be as destructive as it is in children with polyJRA. On the other hand, more than one third of children with sJRA will have a "monophasic" illness[12] that seems to remit after treatment without recurrence. It is not clear how those who will have this more benign course at the time of diagnosis can be identified.

Prognosis for most children with spondyloarthropathies is similar to that for pauciJRA. Most will present with a clinical picture with some similarities to pauciJRA such as oligoarthritis, lower extremity involvement, and so forth. Risk of damage from the arthritis related to the spondyloarthropathies is generally lower than with polyJRA or sJRA. The prognosis for axial involvement in spondyloarthropathies is not clear, given the low prevalence of spine involvement in this age group. Because of the longer duration of disease than for adult counterparts with AS, children and adolescents with AS may have worse spine function.[30] These patients with AS may be at increased risk of developing severe hip involvement, as measured by an increased rate of THA.[10]

CURRENT CONTROVERSIES AND FUTURE CONSIDERATIONS

One of the challenges in managing children and adolescents with various forms of IA is deciding how "aggressive" to be with medical management. As outlined earlier, accurate clinical assessment and an understanding of the natural history of the type of IA are mandatory for making informed decisions about treatment.

Fortunately, many children will do well with relatively "low-risk" interventions. Still, when powerful immuno-suppressive medications are administered to children, each treatment decision requires a careful risk/benefit ratio assessment with both short- and long-term perspectives.

REFERENCES

1. Spencer CH, Bernstein BH: Hip disease in juvenile rheumatoid arthritis. Curr Opin Rheumatol 14:536–541, 2002.
2. Cassidy JT, Levinson JE, Bass JC, et al: A study of classification of criteria for a diagnosis of juvenile rheumatoid arthritis. Arthritis Rheum 29:274–281, 1986.
3. Petty RE, Southwood TE, Baum J, et al: Revision of the proposed classification criteria for juvenile idiopathic arthritis: Durban 1997. J Rheumatol 25:1991–1994, 1997.
4. Dougados M, Van Der Linden S, Juhlin R, et al: The European spondyloarthropathy study group preliminary criteria for the classification of spondyloarthropathy. Arthritis Rheum 34:1218–1227, 1991.
5. van der Linden SM, Valkenburg HA, Cats A: Evaluation of diagnostic criteria for ankylosing spondylitis: a proposal for modification of the New York criteria. Arthritis Rheum 27:361–368, 1984.
6. Peterson LS, Mason T, Nelson AM, et al: Juvenile rheumatoid arthritis in Rochester, Minnesota, 1960-1993. Is the epidemiology changing? Arthritis Rheum 39:1385–1390, 1996.
7. Rosenberg AM: Juvenile onset spondyloarthropathies. Curr Opin Rheumatol 12:425–429, 2000.
8. van der Linden SM, van der Heijde D, Maksymowych WP: Ankylosing spondylitis. In Firestein GS, Budd RC, Harris ED (eds): Kelley's textbook of rheumatology, ed 8, Philadelphia, 2008, WB Saunders.
9. Burgos-Vargas R, Vazquez-Mellado J, Cassis N, et al: Genuine ankylosing spondylitis in children: a case-control study of patients with early definitive disease according to adult onset criteria. J Rheumatol 23:2140–2147, 1996.
10. Gensler LS, Ward MM, Reveille JD, et al: Clinical, radiographic and functional differences between juvenile-onset and adult-onset ankylosing spondylitis: results from the PSOAS cohort. Ann Rheum Dis 67:233–237, 2008.
11. Al-Matar MJ, Petty RE, Tucker LB, et al: The early pattern of joint involvement predicts progression in children with oligo-articular onset (pauciarticular) juvenile rheumatoid arthritis. Arthritis Rheum 46:2708–2715, 2002.
12. Saurenmann RK, Levin AV, Feldman BM, et al: Prevalence, risk factors, and outcome of uveitis in juvenile idiopathic arthritis. Arthritis Rheum 56:647–657, 2007.
13. Singh-Grewal D, Schneider R, Bayer N, Feldman BM: Predictors of disease course and remission in systemic juvenile idiopathic arthritis: significance of early clinical and laboratory features. Arthritis Rheum 54:1595–1601, 2006.
14. Bennett AN, McGonagle D, O'Connor P, et al: Severity of baseline magnetic resonance imaging-evident sacroiliitis and HLA-B27 status in early inflammatory back pain predict radiographically evident ankylosing spondylitis at eight years. Arthritis Rheum 58:3413–3418, 2008.
15. Singh G, Athreya BH, Fries JF, Goldsmith DP: Measurement of health status in children with juvenile rheumatoid arthritis. Arthritis Rheum 37:1761–1769, 1994.
16. Magni-Manzoni S, Rossi F, Pistorio A, et al: Prognostic factors for radiographic progression, radiographic damage, and disability in juvenile idiopathic arthritis. Arthritis Rheum 48:3509–3517, 2003.
17. Mogesen B, Brattstrom H, Ekelund L, et al: Synovectomy of the hip in juvenile chronic arthritis. J Bone Joint Surg Br 64:295–299, 1982.
18. Moreno Alvarez MJ, Espada G, Maldonado-Cocco JA, Gagliardi SA: Long-term followup of hip and knee soft tissue release in juvenile chronic arthritis. J Rheum 19:1608–1610, 1992.
19. Witt JD, McCullough CJ: Anterior soft-tissue release of the hip in juvenile chronic arthritis. J Bone Joint Surg Br 76:267–270, 1994.
20. Hastings DE, Orsini E, Myers P, Sullivan J: An unusual pattern of growth disturbance of the hip in juvenile rheumatoid arthritis. J Rheum 21:744–747, 1994.
21. Torchia ME, Klassen RA, Bianco AJ: Total hip arthroplasty with cement in patients less than twenty years old: long-term results. J Bone Joint Surg Am 78:995–1003, 1996.
22. Chmell MJ, Scott RD, Thomas WH, Sledge CB: Total hip arthroplasty with cement for juvenile rheumatoid arthritis: results at a minimum of ten years in patients less than thirty years old. J Bone Joint Surg Am 79:44–52, 1997.
23. Wroblewski BM, Siney PD, Fleming PA: Charnley low-frictional torque arthroplasty in young rheumatoid and juvenile rheumatoid arthritis: 292 hips followed for an average of 15 years. Acta Orthop 78:206–210, 2007.
24. Lehtimaki MY, Lehto MU, Kautiainen H, et al: Survivorship of the Charnley total hip arthroplasty in juvenile chronic arthritis: a follow-up of 186 cases for 22 years. J Bone Joint Surg Br 79:792–795, 1997.
25. McCullough CJ, Remedios D, Tytherleigh-Strong G, et al: The use of hydroxyapatite-coated CAD-CAM femoral components in adolescents and young adults with inflammatory polyarthropathy: ten-year results. J Bone Joint Surg Br 88:860–864, 2006.
26. Odent T, Journeau P, Prieur AM, et al: Cementless hip arthroplasty in juvenile idiopathic arthritis. J Pediatric Orthop 25:465–470, 2005.
27. Peterson LS, Mason T, Nelson AM, et al: Psychosocial outcomes and health status of adults who have had juvenile rheumatoid arthritis: a population-based study. Arthritis Rheum 40:2235–2240, 1997.
28. Foster HE, Marshall N, Myers A, et al: Outcomes in adults with juvenile idiopathic arthritis: a quality of life study. Arthritis Rheum 48:767–775, 2003.
29. Minder K, Nierwerth M, Listing J, et al: Long-term outcome in patients with juvenile idiopathic arthritis. Arthritis Rheum 46:2392–2401, 2002.
30. Stone M, Warren RW, Bruckel J, et al: Juvenile-onset ankylosing spondylitis is associated with worse functional outcomes than adult-onset ankylosing spondylitis. Arthritis Care Res 53:445–451, 2005.

Section VI

TRAUMATIC DISORDERS OF THE HIP

CHAPTER 44

Femoral Neck Fracture

Thuan V. Ly and Marc F. Swiontkowski

INTRODUCTION

Intracapsular femoral neck fractures are common in the elderly population after a simple fall.[1] However, femoral neck fractures in physiologically young adults are less common and represent approximately 5% of the total.[2-4] These younger patients are active, have minimal medical problems, and have good bone quality. Femoral neck fracture in these young patients generally occurs after a motor vehicle accident or other high-energy mechanism. It is important to understand the osseous and vascular anatomy, the mechanism of injury, associated injuries, the fracture pattern, and the goals of treatment. Although achieving anatomic reduction and stable internal fixation is imperative, other treatment variables, such as time to surgery, the role of capsulotomy, and fixation methods, are debated. Knowledge of treatment options and potential complications is beneficial in understanding and managing femoral neck fracture in young adults.

Anatomy

Femoral head blood supply comes from three main sources: the medial femoral circumflex artery (MFCA), the lateral femoral circumflex artery (LFCA), and the obturator artery.[5-8] The largest contributor to the femoral head, especially the superolateral aspect of the femoral head, is the MFCA.[8] The lateral epiphyseal artery complex originates from the MFCA and courses along the posterosuperior aspect of the femoral neck before supplying the femoral head. Terminal branches supplying the femoral head are intracapsular; thus disruption or distortion of these terminal branches likely plays a significant role in the development of osteonecrosis.[9-12] Variables that have been hypothesized as contributing to femoral head osteonecrosis include vascular damage from the initial femoral neck fracture,[4,12-15] the quality of reduction or fixation of the fracture (restoring flow to the distorted arteries),[4,16-20] elevated intracapsular pressure (tamponade from blood),[12,21-26] and the position of the implants.[27]

INDICATIONS/CONTRAINDICATIONS

Poor bone density, multiple medical problems, and propensity to fall are major risk factors for a femoral neck fracture in elderly patients. In the physiologically young adult, a substantial axial load with the hip in an abducted position is the mechanism that will produce a displaced femoral neck fracture.[4,16] Clinical evaluation of these patients should include a thorough trauma workup, as they frequently have other injuries.[16,28-30] Diagnosis and treatment of femoral neck fractures in young adults should be done immediately after other life- and limb-threatening injuries are managed. Patients with displaced femoral neck fracture will have a shortened, flexed, and externally rotated lower extremity. For incomplete or nondisplaced fracture of the femoral neck, internal rotation of the limb and heel-strike usually will produce pain in the hip and groin region.

PREOPERATIVE PLANNING

Radiographic evaluation should include anteroposterior (AP) and lateral plain radiographs of the entire femur, as well as an AP radiograph of the pelvis. The

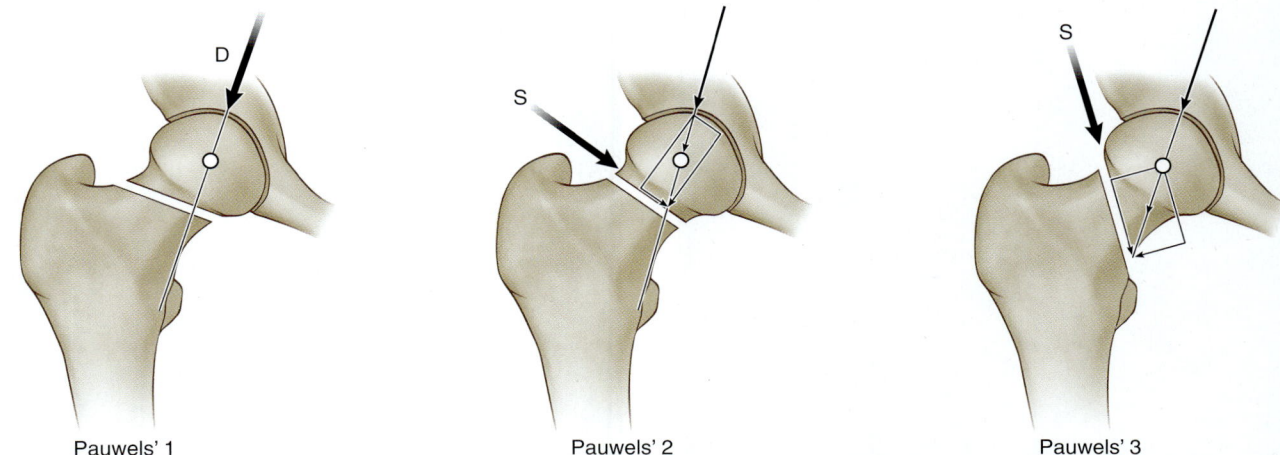

Pauwels' 1   Pauwels' 2   Pauwels' 3

Figure 44-1. Pauwels' classification. (Modified with permission from Bartonicek J: Pauwels' classification of femoral neck fractures: correct interpretation of the original. J Orthop Trauma 15:358–360, 2001.)

fracture pattern seen in young adults is different than that of elderly patients. Elderly patients with poor bone quality or a low-energy injury usually sustain an intertrochanteric hip fracture or a subcapital femoral neck fracture. A transverse fracture pattern with impaction at the fracture site is common. In young adults with better bone quality, higher-energy mechanisms of injury usually cause a basicervical or more distal neck fracture. This occurs from an axially loaded, high-energy force onto an abducted hip. The fracture pattern has a tendency to be more vertically oriented and biomechanically more unstable.[31-35] These characteristics have important implications for obtaining and maintaining stable fixation, both of which are necessary for healing to occur.

Despite known limitations, femoral neck fractures in elderly patients are frequently described using the Garden classification.[36,37] In this age group, treatment is often based on whether the fracture is nondisplaced or impacted (grades I and II) or displaced (grades III and IV). The Garden classification is not as useful for describing femoral neck fractures in young adults. Pauwels' classification[31] (Fig. 44-1) is more descriptive for young adults with femoral neck fractures. The fracture pattern can indicate the relative stability of the fracture and can predict the difficulty of obtaining stable fixation. A femoral neck fracture line less than 30 degrees from the horizontal plane is a Pauwels' type I, one that has an angle with the horizontal between 30 and 50 degrees is a Pauwels' type II, and one that has an angle greater than 50 degrees is a Pauwels' type III. The type I femoral neck fracture has greater intrinsic stability. Type III femoral neck fractures, the least stable, are seen in young adults more frequently than in the elderly. Type III fracture patterns are more difficult to treat and are associated with increased risks of fixation failure, malunion, nonunion, and osteonecrosis, probably because of greater shear at the fracture site related to the vertical nature of the fracture line.[31-35]

PRINCIPLES OF MANAGEMENT AND TREATMENT ALGORITHM

The authors generally consider patients younger than 65 years old as "young" and those over 75 years old as "elderly." Patients between 65 and 75 years of age are judged to be young or elderly based on their "physiologic" age. Those who are active and have high functional demands, have good bone quality, and have minimal medical problems are considered "young"; those who have low functional demands (use assistive device for ambulation), chronic illness, or poor bone quality are considered "elderly."

For the elderly patient, goals include restoring mobility with weight bearing as tolerated and minimizing complications associated with prolonged bed rest. The patient's age and functional demand make preserving the femoral head less important. A hemiarthroplasty or a total hip replacement often accomplishes this best.[38-41]

In the physiologically young and active adult, the goals are to preserve the femoral head, avoid osteonecrosis, and achieve union. Avoiding an arthroplasty is highly desirable. It is generally agreed that anatomic reduction with stable internal fixation is paramount for a good outcome. Nevertheless, other issues such as closed versus open reduction, the role of capsulotomy, and time to surgery remain controversial. Method of fixation is also a variable, but it is less controversial.

Fracture pattern alone determines the treatment of nondisplaced fractures. These include both valgus impacted (Garden grade I) and complete but nondisplaced (Garden grade II) femoral neck fractures. They should be treated with internal fixation.[42,43] Nonoperative management of nondisplaced femoral neck fractures is associated with higher complication rates and increased risk for displacement.[42] Patients should be transferred carefully over to the fracture table to avoid

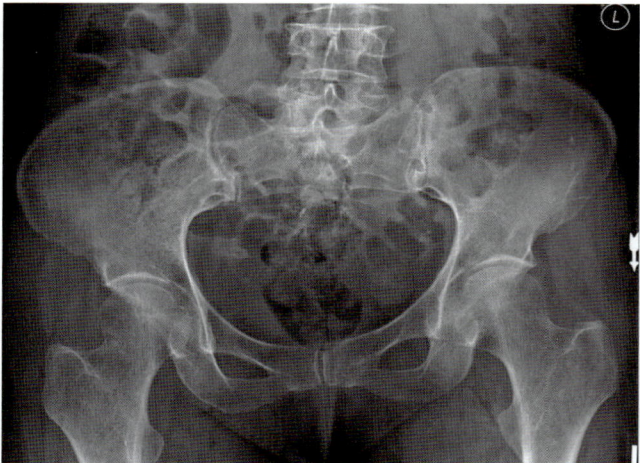

Figure 44-2. Anteroposterior radiograph of pelvis, demonstrating displaced right femoral neck fracture.

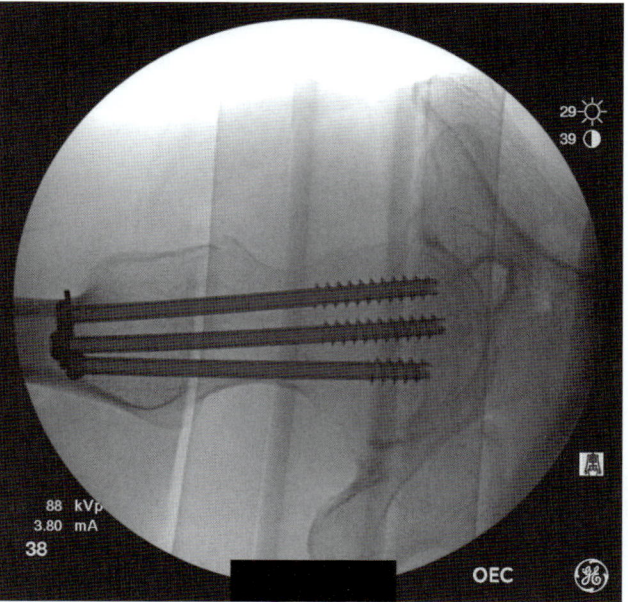

Figure 44-4. Intraoperative C-arm images. A lateral view emphasizes the spread of the three cancellous screws for optimal fixation.

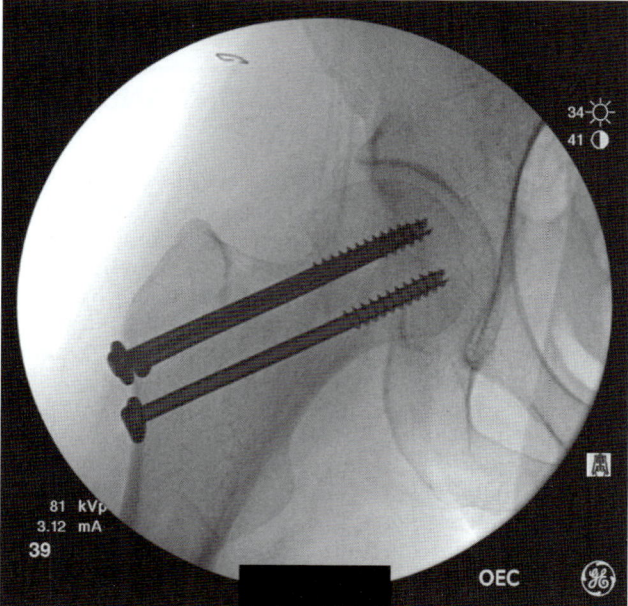

Figure 44-3. Intraoperative C-arm images. Anteroposterior view shows internal fixation with three cancellous screws in an inverted triangle configuration.

further displacement of the femoral neck fracture. Internal fixation in situ with three cannulated cancellous screws is recommended (Figs. 44-2, 44-3, and 44-4).

Patient selection for internal fixation can be more difficult with displaced fracture variants.[44] Factors to consider when deciding whether to proceed with open reduction and internal fixation of displaced femoral neck fractures include the patient's chronological and physiologic age, level of activity, bone quality, associated comorbidities, and fracture pattern and characteristics. Although multiple treatment algorithms have been used and published, the best protocol remains debatable.[44-49] It is generally recommended that displaced femoral neck fractures in patients who are

physiologically younger than age 65 years should have an open reduction and internal fixation. Patients over the age of 75 years with low-energy injuries, poor bone quality, and displaced subcapital fracture patterns should be considered candidates for hemiarthroplasty or total hip arthroplasty (THA) to avoid the higher rate of secondary operations.[50] As for patients between the ages of 65 and 75 years, the trend in the treatment algorithm is to perform a THA, especially if they are active and have high functional demands.[51-53]

Arthroplasty has been reported to have less revision surgery, more rapid mobilization, and better function.[39,50,52] Bhandari and associates[50] published a meta-analysis comparing internal fixation with arthroplasty (hemiarthroplasty, bipolar arthroplasty, and total hip arthroplasty) for treatment of displaced femoral neck fractures. They reviewed 14 studies with a total of 1933 patients. They concluded that performing arthroplasty for displaced femoral neck fracture reduced the risk of secondary operation. Secondary operation after internal fixation was often a result of nonunion and avascular necrosis. However, infection rate, blood loss, and operative time were increased in the arthroplasty group. More recent randomized controlled trials by Blomfeldt and colleagues[39] and Keating and coworkers[52] also reported a decrease in reoperation rate with arthroplasty. Blomfeldt and associates[39] evaluated outcomes at 4 years of mentally competent, relatively healthy elderly patients who underwent internal fixation or THA for displaced femoral neck fracture. The rate of reoperation was 47% for internal fixation and 4% for THA. Using the Charnley score and the EuroQol-5D (EQ-5D) index to assess hip function and health-related quality of life, respectively, investigators concluded that THA performed better. Keating and colleagues[52] randomized 207 patients and compared reduction and fixation, bipolar hemiarthroplasty, and THA. They reported reoperation rates of 39% for the fixation group, 9% for the THA group, and 5% for the hemiarthroplasty group. Arthroplasty was found to have better functional outcomes as measured by a hip rating questionnaire and the EQ-5D index.

Hemiarthroplasty is the preferred treatment for low-functioning community or nursing home ambulatory patients. Performing hemiarthroplasty in more active, mobile, and independent living older patients raises concerns for acetabular erosion, as well as poor functional and pain ratings. Baker and coworkers[38] randomized 81 active individuals to THA or hemiarthroplasty for displaced femoral neck fracture. At a mean follow-up of 3 years, fewer complications, improved walking distances, and a higher Oxford Hip Score were noted for the THA group. More than 60% of living patients in the hemiarthroplasty group showed acetabular erosion on radiograph. In another randomized controlled trial, Blomfeldt and associates[52a] compared bipolar hemiarthroplasty with THA for displaced femoral neck fracture in active and lucid patients. They showed that THA resulted in better hip function (Harris Hip Score) but no significant difference in the health quality-of-life measure between the two groups. In summary, evidence suggests that THA is the better treatment for displaced femoral neck fracture in the right patients. These include patients >65 years of age who are competent, active, and community ambulatory, with preexisting hip disease (osteoarthritis, rheumatoid arthritis).[53,53a]

The author's preferred treatment algorithm is to perform arthroplasty for patients age >65 years with poor bone quality and a high degree of comminution. THA is preferred for patients who are community ambulators who are lucid, independent, and have a life expectancy >5 years. Hemiarthroplasty is ideal for patients who are low-demand, minimal ambulators who have cognitive impairment and a short life expectancy. No evidence indicates superior function or durability of bipolar as compared with unipolar, and unipolar is more cost-effective. Cemented stems are recommended for patients with poor bone quality or low demand. The authors reserve uncemented stems for patients with good bone stock who have higher functional demands and are younger.

DESCRIPTION OF TECHNIQUE(S)

Surgical Approach

After the patient is medically optimized, surgical fixation of the femoral neck should proceed expeditiously. The injured limb should be left shortened and externally rotated while surgery is awaited. Several authors have shown that intracapsular pressure changes vary with hip position in femoral neck fracture.[22,26,54] Intracapsular pressure is greatest when the hip is in extension with internal rotation, and decreases significantly when the hip is in flexion with external rotation.

Preoperative skin traction is ineffective in reducing pain and avoiding complications.[55-58]

Closed reduction is attempted by flexing the hip to 45 degrees with the hip slightly abducted, then extending and internally rotating the leg while applying longitudinal traction. The quality of the reduction is judged on the basis of the fluoroscopic image before percutaneous fixation is performed. Only an anatomic reduction should be accepted; otherwise proceed with an open reduction and internal fixation.[45,59,60] The authors' preference is to have the patient in the supine position, on a radiolucent table, with the leg draped free, but some prefer to have the patient in traction on a fracture table. The supine position provides optimal visualization for fracture reduction and ease of fluoroscopic imaging; in addition, other orthopedic or surgical teams can address associated injuries with the patient supine.

If open reduction is required, then a Watson-Jones approach is used[61,62] (Fig. 44-5). A straight lateral incision is made over the lateral proximal femur. Proximally, the incision is curved anteriorly toward the gluteal pillar of the ilium. The tensor fascia is retracted anteriorly while the gluteus medius is retracted posteriorly.

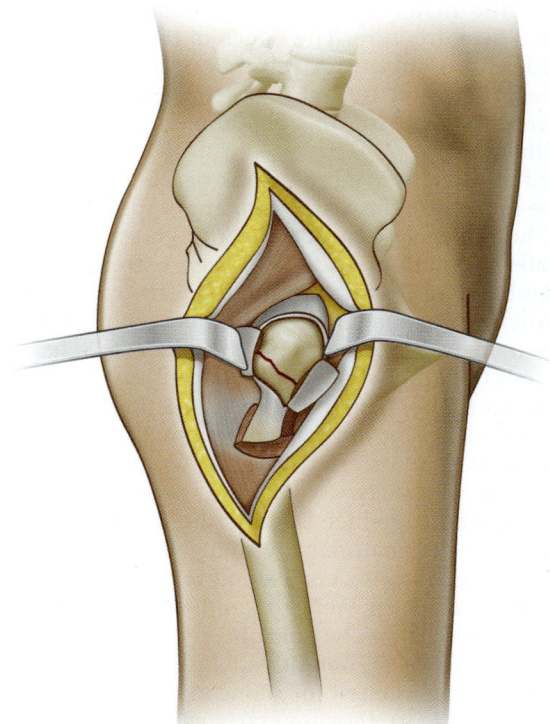

Figure 44-5. Watson-Jones anterolateral exposure to the hip for open reduction of femoral neck fracture. The interval between the tensor fascia and the gluteus medius is exposed. T-capsulotomy with visualization of the femoral neck fracture. (Redrawn from Swiontkowski MF: Intracapsular hip fractures. In Browner BD, Jupiter JB, Levine AM, Trafton PG [eds]: Skeletal trauma, basic science, management, and reconstruction, ed 3, Philadelphia, 2003, Saunders, p 1735.)

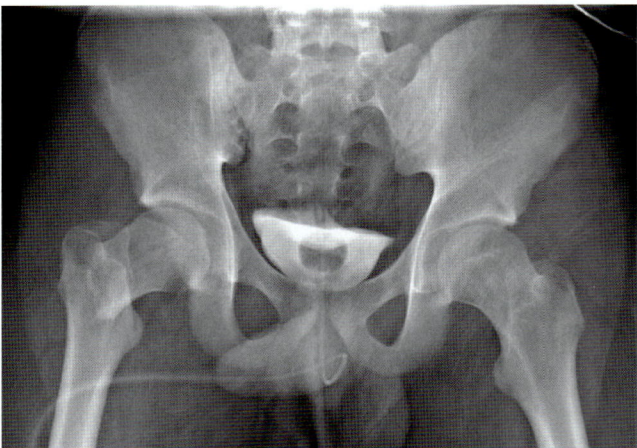

Figure 44-6. Anteroposterior radiograph of pelvis, displaced right femoral neck fracture from motor vehicle accident.

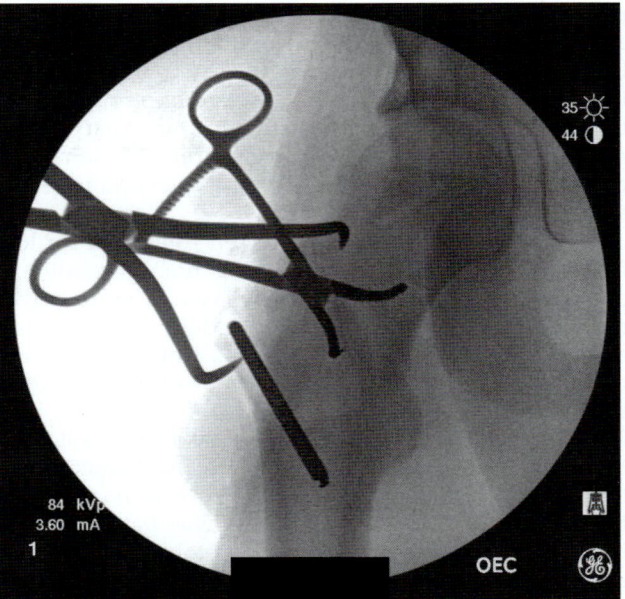

Figure 44-7. Intraoperative C-arm images. Anteroposterior view demonstrating utilization of 5-mm Schanz pin and Weber clamps to reduce the femoral neck fracture.

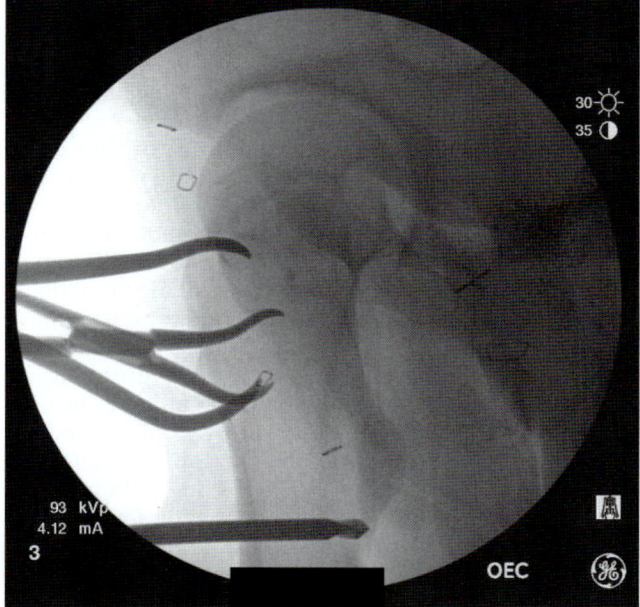

Figure 44-8. Intraoperative C-arm images. Lateral view demonstrating utilization of 5-mm Schanz pin and Weber clamps to reduce the femoral neck fracture.

The pericapsular fat is then swept off to allow visualization of the anterior hip capsule. The vastus lateralis can be slightly elevated off the greater trochanteric ridge for further visualization. A T-capsulotomy, with release of the capsule of the intertrochanteric ridge, is performed in line with the femoral neck. This allows decompression of the hematoma and direct visualization of the femoral neck fracture. The edges of the capsule can be tagged with a suture for retraction. Inserting a small, pointed Hohmann retractor outside the capsule onto the anterior part of the acetabular rim can aid in visualization.

For the reduction, a bone hook or a 5-mm Schanz pin can be applied to the distal segment of the fracture. The bone hook can be placed onto the greater trochanter for lateral traction, and the lower extremity can be manipulated and externally rotated. This will disimpact the fracture and facilitate reduction with an internal rotation maneuver. Alternatively, place a Schanz pin from anterior to posterior several centimeters distal to the fracture site. This can aid in manipulation of the distal fragment. For the proximal segment, 2-mm Kirschner wires can be inserted into the femoral head, functioning as joysticks to lift the proximal fragment anteriorly and to reduce the fracture. Once the femoral neck fracture is anatomically reduced by direct visualization of the anterior cortex and is confirmed by fluoroscopic imaging, a Weber clamp or 2-mm Kirschner wires can provisionally hold the reduction (Figs. 44-6, 44-7, 44-8, and 44-9). Definitive fixation can be attained with three cannulated or noncannulated cancellous screws (Fig. 44-10). Closure starts with loose reapproximation of the capsule with nonabsorbable sutures. The fascia and subcutaneous tissue are closed over a drain with absorbable sutures, followed by dermal sutures or staples for the skin. Another approach using a modified Smith-Peterson surgical exposure has been described.[63] This allows direct access to and visualization of the femoral neck fracture, especially the subcapital region. However, a separate incision is required for implant insertion.

VARIATIONS/UNUSUAL SITUATIONS

Ipsilateral femoral neck fracture can occur in 2% to 6% of all femoral shaft fractures.[64-71] These concomitant ipsilateral injuries can be challenging to reduce, and the best methods of fixation are debatable.[64,66,71] The femoral neck fracture is often a Pauwels' type III and

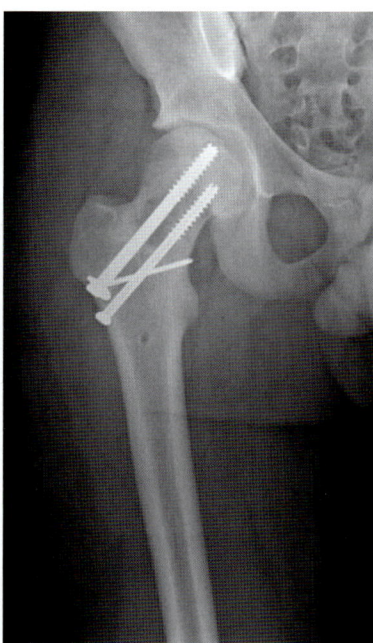

Figure 44-9. Anteroposterior radiograph showing a healed femoral neck.

nondisplaced. Treatment of the femoral neck should be a priority in the sequence of managing this combination. Methods of fixation include sliding hip screw (SHS) and a long side plate, cancellous screws or an SHS and a retrograde intramedullary nail or plate fixation of the shaft fracture, cephalomedullary (second-generation) nails, and a proximal femoral locked plate. A recent retrospective review of 40 patients with ipsilateral femoral neck and shaft fractures suggested that the preferred method is open reduction and internal fixation of the femoral neck with cancellous screws or SHS and retrograde nailing of the shaft fracture. This method resulted in greater accuracy of reduction and improved healing of fractures.[65]

POSTOPERATIVE CARE

The postoperative regimen used by the authors includes antibiotics for 24 hours, deep venous thrombosis prophylaxis with low-molecular-weight heparin or Coumadin for 4 to 6 weeks, depending on the patient's ambulatory status and comorbid medical conditions, and physical therapy consultation. Patients are mobilized and are instructed to be toe touch weight bearing (TTWB) with crutches or a walker for 12 weeks. Patients can progress to full weight bearing when they have the strength and balance to do so. They are instructed to wean off of crutch support when able to ambulate without a significant limp. Monthly radiographs are taken to assess for healing and any evidence of femoral head osteonecrosis. A reasonable clinical indicator that the femoral head is still viable is relative femoral head

osteopenia on the injured side as compared with the normal side on an AP pelvis radiograph. Single photon emission computed tomography (SPECT) can be performed to evaluate the chance of developing femoral head osteonecrosis, preferably within the first 3 postoperative weeks. If uptake is less than 90%, the chance of developing osteonecrosis is increased.[72] Magnetic resonance imaging (MRI) is not a good predictor of posttraumatic osteonecrosis.[73,74] The authors have found that patients who develop femoral head osteonecrosis usually have persistent groin and trochanteric pain that does not resolve with time. If a patient does not have pain and has a normal radiograph at 24 months, he or she is unlikely to develop osteonecrosis. A femoral neck fracture is healing when the patient is asymptomatic and the fracture line is fading radiographically. It is completely healed when the patient is asymptomatic and the fracture is no longer visible. If any question remains (persistent pain) about healing at 4 to 6 months postoperatively, a computed tomography (CT) scan may be obtained to assess fracture union.

RESULTS

In younger and more active patients with femoral neck fracture, preserving the femoral head with internal fixation is desirable. A healed femoral neck fracture, without the development of osteonecrosis, leads to a good functional outcome.[18,27,32,49,75-78] The ability to achieve a good outcome by decreasing fixation failure and the rate of nonunion depends on several factors that the surgeon can control, namely, the quality of reduction and obtaining a stable fixation.[76,79-81] Jain and associates[82] compared early and delayed fixation of subcapital hip fractures in patients 60 years of age and younger. Functional outcomes were assessed with the Short-Form-36 (SF-36) and Western Ontario and McMaster University (WOMAC) Osteoarthritis Index instruments. With a minimum of 2 years' follow-up, investigators found a significant difference (P = .03) in rates of avascular necrosis (six patients in the delayed fixation group, and no patient in the early fixation group). They found no significant difference between early and delayed fixation groups with regard to functional outcomes. No significant difference in outcome was observed between displaced and nondisplaced fractures. However, a larger number of patients and longer follow-up would be needed to determine whether there is a difference between the two groups. El-Abed and colleagues[83] reported the outcomes of hemiarthroplasty and dynamic hip screw fixation for treatment of displaced subcapital hip fractures. Function was measured by physicians using the Matta Functional Hip Score and by the patient using the SF-36. When the Matta scoring systems were used, 70% of patients in the internal fixation group were found to have good to excellent results compared with 42% in the hemiarthroplasty group. Significant agreement (r = 0.64) was noted between patients' perceptions (SF-36) and physicians' perceptions (Matta Functional Hip Score) of outcomes.

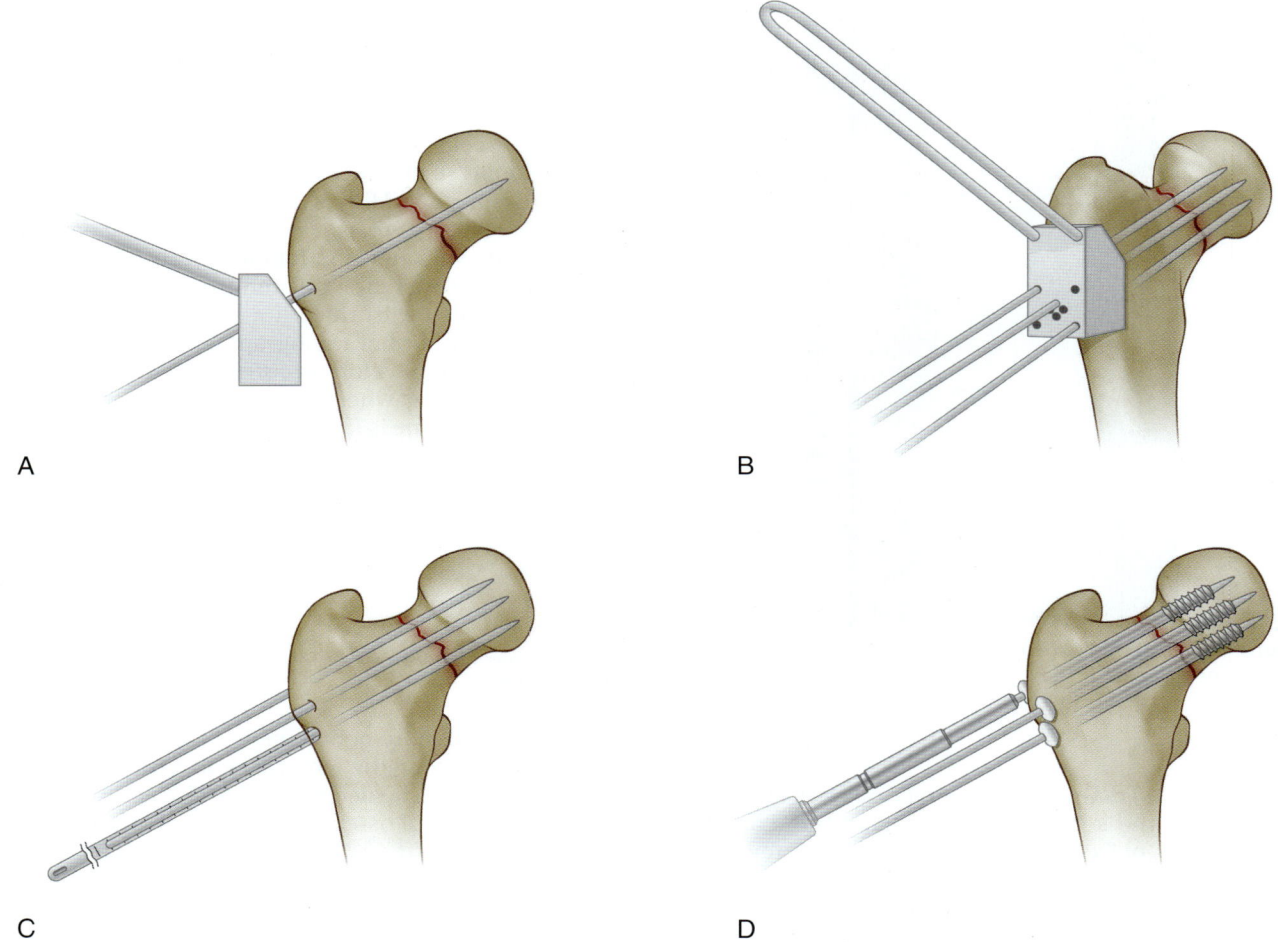

A

B

C

D

Figure 44-10. Internal fixation of a femoral neck fracture with a cannulated screw system. **A** and **B,** Reduction is confirmed and three parallel guide wires are placed using the guide and fluoroscopic control. **C,** Lengths of the wires are measured. **D,** Screws are inserted over the guide wires to a preselected depth. (Redrawn from Swiontkowski MF: Intracapsular hip fractures. In Browner BD, Jupiter JB, Levine AM, Trafton PG [eds]: Skeletal trauma, basic science, management, and reconstruction, ed 3, Philadelphia, 2003, Saunders, p 1737.)

COMPLICATIONS

The two most challenging complications of femoral neck fracture in the young adult are femoral head osteonecrosis and nonunion. Osteonecrosis in a young patient is a devastating complication because of the limited treatment options as compared with elderly patients with osteonecrosis of the femoral head. Osteonecrosis in the elderly is less likely to be symptomatic because of lower functional demands and reduced levels of activity. Fortunately, total hip replacement is a good option that provides consistently good results for elderly patients with symptomatic osteonecrosis. However, no good alternative treatment is available for the young patient with symptomatic osteonecrosis. Younger age and higher function demands make prosthetic replacement more likely to be associated with complications and durability problems, and this approach should be a last resort. Reconstructive options to preserve the hip include osteotomy to unload the segmental area of femoral head collapse, femoral head core decompression, free vascularized bone grafting, hemi-resurfacing of the femoral head, and hip arthrodesis.[84,85] The best method for addressing this difficult complication is prevention, which entails the surgeon doing everything possible under his or her control to minimize further vascular injury to the femoral head, including prompt reduction, intracapsular decompression, anatomic reduction, stable fixation, and close postoperative monitoring for osteonecrosis.

Nonunion is another challenging complication of femoral neck fracture. The rate of nonunion is between 10% and 30%.[4,28,86,87] Fortunately, a valgus-producing osteotomy is a good surgical management option for this problem.[82-92] The goal of treatment is to create an environment that allows for healing. This means converting shear force to compressive force at the fracture site. A valgus-producing intertrochanteric osteotomy accomplishes this by changing the vertical femoral fracture line to a horizontal one, thus allowing for compression.

Marti and coworkers[88] published the largest series of 50 patients treated with Pauwels' abduction osteotomy for femoral neck nonunion. Average age was 53 years, and average follow-up was 7.1 years. Forty-three of 50 femoral necks with nonunion healed, and all osteotomies healed. The average hip score for 37 of these 43 healed fractures was 91. The seven femoral neck fractures that did not heal underwent prosthetic replacement. More recently, Anglen[92] reported his own series of 13 patients treated with a valgus intertrochanteric osteotomy for failed fixation of the femoral neck. All were younger than 60 years of age, and average follow-up time was 25 months. All osteotomies healed. Eleven of 13 had good to excellent functional outcomes. The two poor outcomes had segmental osteonecrosis and went on to have joint replacement.

CURRENT CONTROVERSIES AND FUTURE CONSIDERATIONS

- Fixation methods
- Role of capsulotomy
- Timing of surgery

Fixation Methods

Multiple clinical and biomechanical studies have evaluated the type and number of cancellous screws necessary for treatment of femoral neck fracture.[32-35,79,93,94] A major limitation of these studies is that their conclusions are all based on osteoporotic bone models. However, the basic biomechanical principles should still apply to young adults with good bone density. For most femoral neck fractures, fixation with multiple cancellous lag screws is recommended. Three cancellous lag screws parallel to one another and perpendicular to the fracture line obtain optimal compression at the fracture.[79] Pauwels' type I and II fracture variants are most amenable to this type of fixation. These three cancellous lag screws should be in an inverted triangle configuration (two proximal screws and one distal screw) because this apex-distal screw orientation has less risk of producing a subtrochanteric fracture when compared with the apex-proximal orientation.[95,96] The most inferior screw should rest on the medial femoral neck of the distal fragment to resist varus displacement. A fourth screw does not increase mechanical strength enough in most femoral neck fractures to justify its use, but if posterior comminution occurs, a fourth screw is recommended.[49,97] Two cannulated screws provide inadequate fixation for a displaced femoral neck fracture.[98,99] Care should be taken to not enter the femoral shaft too distally because a subtrochanteric fracture can occur, especially with multiple perforations of the lateral femoral cortex.

Basicervical femoral neck fracture with comminution is a fracture variant for which an SHS will provide more stable fixation than three cancellous screws.[33,34] Blair and coworkers[93] recommend SHS fixation based on their biomechanical cadaver study evaluating three different fixation techniques for treatment of basicervical femoral

neck fracture. They found that a derotation screw located superior to the SHS did not provide increased fixation after the SHS was placed. However, the authors still use a derotational screw to prevent rotation of the femoral head during insertion of the compression screw.

Pauwels' type III fracture remains a difficult challenge. The dominant shear force with this high-angle fracture pattern lends itself to higher rates of failure and nonunion.[31-35,99,100] The authors' preference for treating Pauwels' type III fracture is open reduction and internal fixation with three cannulated screws. Attaining anatomic reduction and adequate fixation remains the key to successful treatment of femoral neck fracture in young adults, as with any other fracture. Failure is often a result of not adequately achieving these goals. The procedure is best accomplished through an open approach to visualize the fracture, anatomic reduction of the fracture, and fracture compression with three screws, optimally placed in parallel. The first screw should be placed inferiorly along the calcar, the second should be placed posteriorly along the neck, and the third should be placed superiorly at the tensile surface of the fracture. It is important to have good spread if not divergent placement of the three screws on the lateral view (see Fig. 44-4). This helps to maintain the reduction and decreases the risk of nonunion.[101]

Others use an SHS for more vertically oriented femoral neck fractures (Pauwels' type III) (Figs. 44-11, 44-12, and 44-13). Baitner and associates found that fixation with an SHS resulted in less inferior femoral head displacement, less shearing displacement, and a greater load to failure when compared with fixation with three cannulated cancellous screws.[33] Bonnaire and Weber[34] looked at four different methods of fixation for Pauwels' type III cadaveric femoral neck fractures, including an SHS with a derotational screw, an SHS without a derotational screw, cancellous screws, and a 130-degree angled blade plate. They concluded that the SHS with the derotational screw is the best implant for this fracture pattern. However, routinely using these large compression hip

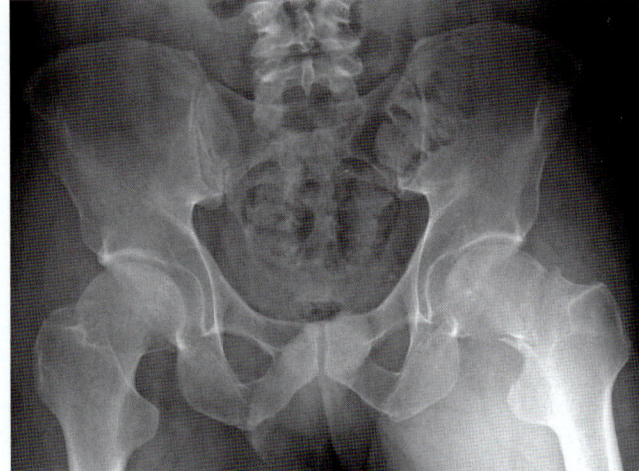

Figure 44-11. Anteroposterior radiograph of pelvis of a 49-year-old male with displaced (Pauwels' type III) left femoral neck fracture.

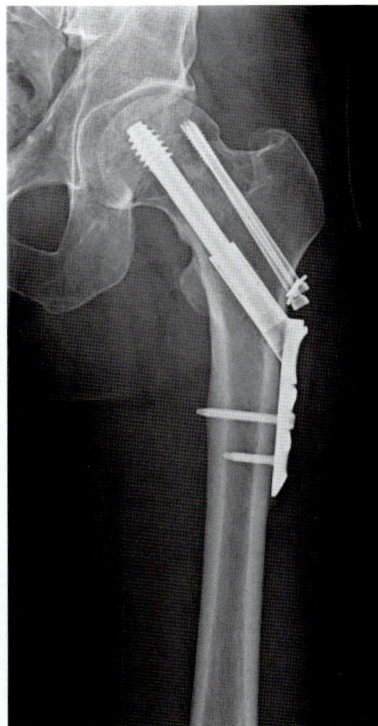

Figure 44-12. Anteroposterior radiograph after open reduction and internal fixation with a sliding hip screw and two cancellous screws.

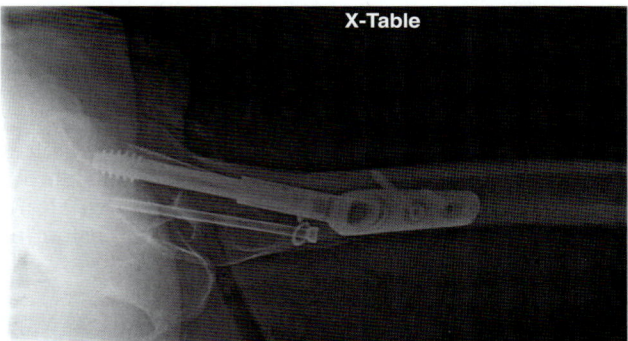

Figure 44-13. Lateral hip radiographs after open reduction and internal fixation with a sliding hip screw and two cancellous screws.

screws raises several concerns, including the amount of bone removed if subsequent reconstruction is required for nonunion, the risk of disrupting the blood supply to the femoral head if imperfectly placed, and the inability to adequately control rotation without insertion of an additional derotational screw.[27,45]

Aminian and associates[102] compared the biomechanical stability of the fixed-angle proximal femoral locking plate (PFLP), 7.3-mm cannulated screws, 135-degree dynamic hip screws (DHSs), and the 95-degree dynamic condylar screw (DCS) for fixation of Pauwels' type III femoral neck fractures. Using cadaveric femurs, they found that the strongest construct was the PFLP,

followed by DCS, DHS, and last, the three cannulated screw model. PFLP allows for multiple fixed-angle points of fixation into the femoral head. However, proper anatomic reduction and compression of the fracture is necessary before fixation, as the PFLP does not allow for fracture compression. Clinical experience with the PFLP is insufficient to recommend its routine use.

Role of Capsulotomy

Capsulotomy in femoral neck fracture remains controversial, and the practice varies by trauma surgeon, region, and country. Both animal and clinical studies suggest a theoretical advantage to performing a capsulotomy. Animal studies[12,21] have shown that increased hip intracapsular pressure results in a tamponade effect and may reduce blood flow to the femoral head. Multiple clinical studies[22-26] have looked at intracapsular pressure measurement in impacted or nondisplaced femoral neck fractures. Intracapsular pressure in nondisplaced femoral neck fractures can exceed normal hip pressure. Investigators found that decompressing the intracapsular hematoma via a capsulotomy or aspiration reduces intracapsular pressure. This decrease in intracapsular pressure results in improved blood flow to the femoral head and may reduce femoral head ischemia.[12,21,23,24,26] This tamponade effect is a possible cause of avascular necrosis, because avascular necrosis has been observed even in some nondisplaced fractures.[18,43,87,103]

Other variables hypothesized to be related to osteonecrosis include the amount of initial fracture displacement,[4,16,18] disruption of the blood supply at the time of fracture,[15,19] the quality of fracture reduction or postreduction malalignment,[4,16-18,20] the time between fracture and reduction,[4,16,17,104,105] postoperative time to full weight-bearing status,[20,82] fracture nonunion,[4,14,18] loss of fracture reduction,[17] and associated ipsilateral femoral neck and shaft fractures.[16,66-70] No solid evidence has been presented as to which factor or combination of factors places the patient at greater risk for femoral head osteonecrosis.

Too few femoral neck fractures occur in the young population to allow a randomized controlled trial with a sufficient sample size to evaluate the role of capsulotomy. Table 44-1 shows a summary of the available literature on femoral neck fractures in young adults with the rate of femoral head osteonecrosis and its relationship to capsulotomy. Until conclusive data are gathered through prospective, controlled trials, the authors recommend doing a capsulotomy. It is easy to perform and adds minimal time and risk to the procedure. Most important, it may help a small subset of patients that otherwise would develop osteonecrosis of the femoral head. The authors believe the pooled evidence indicates that intracapsular pressure plays a role in approximately 15% of patients. No evidence suggests that complications are related to performing an open anterior capsulotomy (directly visualizing the capsule and performing a capsulotomy). However, the authors have seen the scalpel blade detach from the knife handle during a percutaneous capsulotomy (Fig. 44-14). The

Table 44-1. Summary of Literature on Femoral Neck Fractures in Young Adults*

Author	Year	No. of Patients	Osteonecrosis	Capsulotomy
Protzman	1976	22	19	Not reported
Kofoed	1982	17	7	0
Swiontkowski	1984	27	5	17
Tooke	1985	32	6	Not reported
Visuri	1988	12	5	2
Shih	1989	121	32	Not reported
Gerber	1993	54	5	47
Robinson	1995	46	8	0
Gautam	1998	25	3	25
Jain	2002	38	6	1 (aspiration)
Lee	2003	42	10	3
Upadhyay	2004	48 (CRIF)	7 (CRIF)	0
		44 (CRIF)	8 (ORIF)	44
Haidukewych	2004	73	17	22
Total		601	138 (23%)	

CRIF, Closed reduction internal fixation; *ORIF*, open reduction internal fixation.
*Numbers of osteonecrosis cases were reported, along with whether capsulotomy was performed.

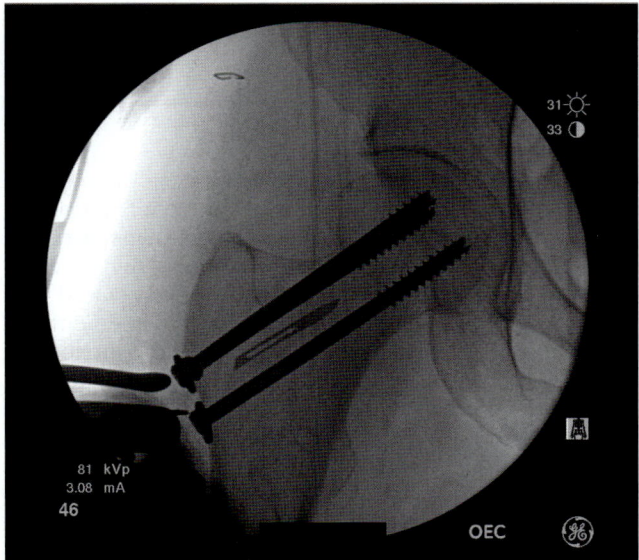

Figure 44-14. Intraoperative C-arm images. A no. 10 blade detached from the knife handle during a percutaneous capsulotomy.

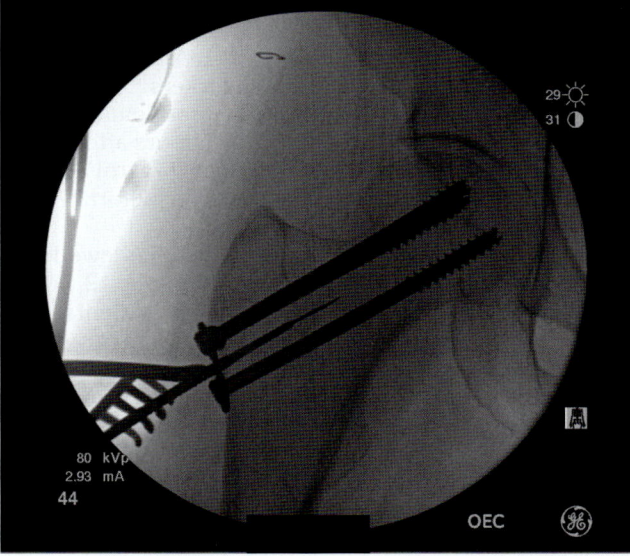

Figure 44-15. Intraoperative C-arm images. Anteroposterior view of percutaneous capsulotomy with a no. 10 blade.

blade was easily retrieved. For femoral neck fractures that are successfully closed, reduced, and percutaneously pinned, we recommend performing a percutaneous capsulotomy with a no. 10 blade (Figs. 44-15 and 44-16). The surgeon should make sure that the blade is fully seated on the knife handle and should slide the blade over the anterior trochanter in line with the center of the femoral neck on AP C-arm images; then the capsulotomy should be performed in the lateral view (make sure you are right on top of the femoral neck bone by feeling on fluoroscopic images). If a small

incision (5 cm) is made and the iliotibial band is split for pinning, a flash of hematoma should be seen to ooze out when the capsulotomy is complete.

Timing of Surgery

The timing of surgery for femoral neck fracture remains controversial, and available data remain inconclusive. Advocates of early surgery suggest that the main advantages of prompt reduction of displaced femoral neck fractures include unkinking the vessels and performing

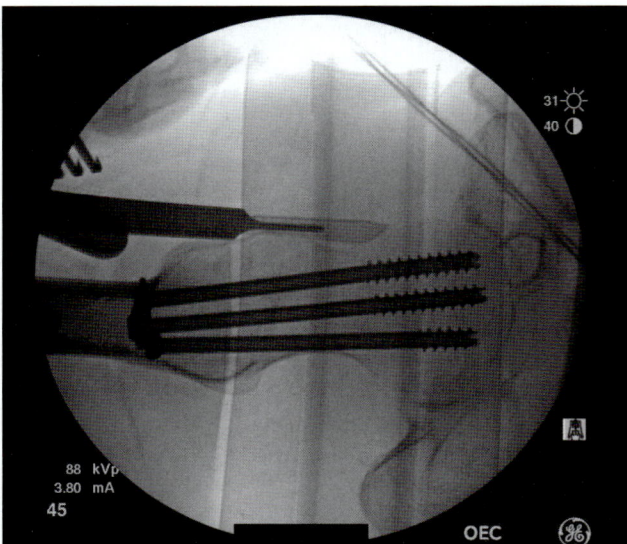

Figure 44-16. Intraoperative C-arm images. Lateral view of percutaneous capsulotomy with a no. 10 blade.

intracapsular decompression to remove the offending agent of increased intracapsular pressure.[5,16,106] This improves and restores blood flow to the femoral head, minimizing the risk of femoral head osteonecrosis.[7,21,23,24,26] Swiontkowski and coworkers[16] had previously recommended that treatment of femoral neck fracture should be performed within 8 hours after injury. Other studies suggest that early surgery (within 6 to 12 hours) can decrease the rate of femoral head osteonecrosis.[17,104,106-108]

Jain and associates[82] retrospectively reviewed and compared early (<12 hours) and delayed (>12 hours) fixation of subcapital hip fracture in 38 patients. Subjects were 60 years of age or younger, and average age was 46.4 years. Radiographic evidence of osteonecrosis developed in 16% of patients, all of whom were in the delayed fixation group. Only 1 of 38 patients had aspiration of the intracapsular hematoma. Age, fracture displacement, and method of fracture fixation did not influence the development of osteonecrosis. Using SF-36 and WOMAC, investigators found no difference in functional results between patients who developed osteonecrosis and those who did not have osteonecrosis. They concluded that delayed treatment led to an increased rate of osteonecrosis but did not affect functional outcomes.

Several studies reported no differences in the rate of osteonecrosis with surgery delayed longer than 24 hours. Haidukewych and colleagues[18] retrospectively reviewed 83 femoral neck fractures in patients between the ages of 15 and 50 years. Osteonecrosis occurred in 23%. Investigators reported that 13 of 53 (25%) patients with femoral neck fractures who were treated within 24 hours after diagnosis developed osteonecrosis. Four of 20 (20%) patients who were treated longer than 24 hours after diagnosis developed osteonecrosis. Given the small sample size, the difference was not significant. Upadhyay and coworkers[87] performed a prospective,

randomized study comparing open reduction internal fixation (ORIF) and closed reduction internal fixation (CRIF) in young adults with Garden grades III and IV femoral neck fractures. A total of 102 patients were randomized, with 44 in ORIF (a Watson-Jones approach with a T-shaped incision in the capsules) and 48 in CRIF (closed reduction and percutaneous pinning). No significant difference in osteonecrosis was noted between the two groups (14.6% for CRIF and 18.2% for ORIF) at 2 years' follow-up. Risk factors such as age, gender, time to surgery (<48 hours or >48 hours), and posterior comminution did not affect the development of osteonecrosis. Most patients in this series were treated longer than 48 hours after injury.

The multiple factors mentioned here make it difficult to come to a final conclusion regarding the timing of surgery. Many articles have specifically evaluated the influence of time to reduction and fixation on outcome. Until conclusive data are available, the authors recommend that surgery should be done on an urgent basis. This implies that ORIF of the femoral neck should be performed as soon as the patient is considered medically stable and is cleared to undergo anesthesia. Urgent operation allows early reduction, capsular decompression, restoration of anatomy, and potential restoration of femoral head vascularity achieved by unkinking the vessels.

CONCLUSION

Femoral neck fractures in young adults are uncommon. They usually occur as a result of high-energy trauma, and patients often have associated injuries. Osteonecrosis of the femoral head and nonunion are the two most common and challenging complications associated with femoral neck fractures. Initial fracture displacement and disruption of femoral head blood flow are contributing factors that are outside of the surgeon's control. However, numerous factors within the surgeon's control can help to minimize and prevent these complications. Key factors in the treatment of femoral neck fractures include early diagnosis, early surgery, anatomic reduction, capsular decompression, and stable internal fixation.

REFERENCES

1. Christodoulou NA, Dretakis EK: Significance of muscular disturbances in the localization of fractures of the proximal femur. Clin Orthop Relat Res 187:215–217, 1984.
2. Robinson CM, Court-Brown CM, McQueen MM, Christie J: Hip fractures in adults younger than 50 years of age. epidemiology and results. Clin Orthop Relat Res 312:238–246, 1995.
3. Askin SR, Bryan RS: Femoral neck fractures in young adults. Clin Orthop Relat Res 114:259–264, 1976.
4. Protzman RR, Burkhalter WE: Femoral-neck fractures in young adults. J Bone Joint Surg Am 58:689–695, 1976.
5. Claffey TJ: Avascular necrosis of the femoral head: an anatomical study. J Bone Joint Surg Br 42:802–809, 1960.
6. Howe WW Jr, Lacey T, Schwartz RP: A study of the gross anatomy of the arteries supplying the proximal portion of the femur and the acetabulum. J Bone Joint Surg Am 32:856–866, 1950.

7. Sevitt S: Avascular necrosis and revascularisation of the femoral head after intracapsular fractures: a combined arteriographic and histological necropsy study. J Bone Joint Surg Br 46:270–296, 1964.

8. Trueta J, Harrison MH: The normal vascular anatomy of the femoral head in adult man. J Bone Joint Surg Br 35:442–461, 1953.

9. Arnoldi CC, Lemperg RK: Fracture of the femoral neck. II. Relative importance of primary vascular damage and surgical procedure for the development of necrosis of the femoral head. Clin Orthop Relat Res 129:217–222, 1977.

10. Arnoldi CC, Linderholm H: Fracture of the femoral neck. I. Vascular disturbances in different types of fractures, assessed by measurements of intraosseous pressures. Clin Orthop Relat Res 84:116–127, 1972.

11. Stromqvist B: Femoral head vitality after intracapsular hip fracture: 490 cases studied by intravital tetracycline labeling and tc-MDP radionuclide imaging. Acta Orthop Scand Suppl 200:1–71, 1983.

12. Swiontkowski MF, Tepic S, Perren SM, et al: Laser doppler flowmetry for bone blood flow measurement: correlation with microsphere estimates and evaluation of the effect of intracapsular pressure on femoral head blood flow. J Orthop Res 4:362–371, 1986.

13. Zetterberg CH, Irstam L, Andersson GB: Femoral neck fractures in young adults. Acta Orthop Scand 53:427–435, 1982.

14. Visuri T, Vara A, Meurman KO: Displaced stress fractures of the femoral neck in young male adults: a report of twelve operative cases. J Trauma 28:1562–1569, 1988.

15. Kregor PJ: The effect of femoral neck fractures on femoral head blood flow. Orthopedics 19:1031–1036; quiz 1037–1038, 1996.

16. Swiontkowski MF, Winquist RA, Hansen ST Jr: Fractures of the femoral neck in patients between the ages of twelve and forty-nine years. J Bone Joint Surg Am 66:837–846, 1984.

17. Lee CH, Huang GS, Chao KH, et al: Surgical treatment of displaced stress fractures of the femoral neck in military recruits: a report of 42 cases. Arch Orthop Trauma Surg 123:527–533, 2003.

18. Haidukewych GJ, Rothwell WS, Jacofsky DJ, et al: Operative treatment of femoral neck fractures in patients between the ages of fifteen and fifty years. J Bone Joint Surg Am 86:1711–1716, 2004.

19. Barnes R, Brown JT, Garden RS, Nicoll EA: Subcapital fractures of the femur: a prospective review. J Bone Joint Surg Br 58:2–24, 1976.

20. Maruenda JI, Barrios C, Gomar-Sancho F: Intracapsular hip pressure after femoral neck fracture. Clin Orthop Relat Res 340:172–180, 1997.

21. Woodhouse CF: Dynamic influences of vascular occlusion affecting the development of avascular necrosis of the femoral head. Clin Orthop Relat Res 32:119–129, 1964.

22. Bonnaire F, Schaefer DJ, Kuner EH: Hemarthrosis and hip joint pressure in femoral neck fractures. Clin Orthop Relat Res 353:148–155, 1998.

23. Harper WM, Barnes MR, Gregg PJ: Femoral head blood flow in femoral neck fractures: an analysis using intra-osseous pressure measurement. J Bone Joint Surg Br 73:73–75, 1991.

24. Holmberg S, Dalen N: Intracapsular pressure and caput circulation in nondisplaced femoral neck fractures. Clin Orthop Relat Res 219:124–126, 1987.

25. Crawfurd EJ, Emery RJ, Hansell DM, et al: Capsular distension and intracapsular pressure in subcapital fractures of the femur. J Bone Joint Surg Br 70:195–198, 1988.

26. Stromqvist B, Nilsson LT, Egund N, et al: Intracapsular pressures in undisplaced femoral neck fractures. J Bone Joint Surg Br 70:192–194, 1988.

27. Brodetti A: The blood supply of the femoral neck and head in relation to the damaging effects of nails and screws. J Bone Joint Surg Br 42:794, 1960.

28. Dedrick DK, Mackenzie JR, Burney RE: Complications of femoral neck fracture in young adults. J Trauma 26:932–937, 1986.

29. Tooke SM, Favero KJ: Femoral neck fractures in skeletally mature patients, fifty years old or less. J Bone Joint Surg Am 67:1255–1260, 1985.

30. Sadat-Ali M, Ahlberg A: Fractured neck of the femur in young adults. Injury 23:311–313, 1992.

31. Bartonicek J: Pauwels' classification of femoral neck fractures: correct interpretation of the original. J Orthop Trauma 15:358–360, 2001.

32. Broos PL, Vercruysse R, Fourneau I, et al: Unstable femoral neck fractures in young adults: treatment with the AO 130-degree blade plate. J Orthop Trauma 12:235–239; discussion 240, 1998.

33. Baitner AC, Maurer SG, Hickey DG, et al: Vertical shear fractures of the femoral neck: a biomechanical study. Clin Orthop Relat Res 367:300–305, 1999.

34. Bonnaire FA, Weber AT: Analysis of fracture gap changes, dynamic and static stability of different osteosynthetic procedures in the femoral neck. Injury 33(Suppl 3):C24–C32, 2002.

35. Stankewich CJ, Chapman J, Muthusamy R, et al: Relationship of mechanical factors to the strength of proximal femur fractures fixed with cancellous screws. J Orthop Trauma 10:248–257, 1996.

36. Garden RS: Low-angle fixation in fractures of the femoral neck. J Bone Joint Surg Br 43:647, 1961.

37. Garden RS: Malreduction and avascular necrosis in subcapital fractures of the femur. J Bone Joint Surg Br 53:183–197, 1971.

38. Baker RP, Squires B, Gargan MF, Bannister GC: Total hip arthroplasty and hemiarthroplasty in mobile, independent patients with a displaced intracapsular fracture of the femoral neck: a randomized, controlled trial. J Bone Joint Surg Am 88:2583–2589, 2006.

39. Blomfeldt R, Tornkvist H, Ponzer S, et al: Comparison of internal fixation with total hip replacement for displaced femoral neck fractures. randomized, controlled trial performed at four years. J Bone Joint Surg Am 87:1680–1688, 2005.

40. Blomfeldt R, Tornkvist H, Ponzer S, et al: Internal fixation versus hemiarthroplasty for displaced fractures of the femoral neck in elderly patients with severe cognitive impairment. J Bone Joint Surg Br 87:523–529, 2005.

41. Tidermark J, Ponzer S, Svensson O, et al: Internal fixation compared with total hip replacement for displaced femoral neck fractures in the elderly: a randomised, controlled trial. J Bone Joint Surg Br 85:380–388, 2003.

42. Cserhati P, Kazar G, Manninger J, et al: Non-operative or operative treatment for undisplaced femoral neck fractures: a comparative study of 122 non-operative and 125 operatively treated cases. Injury 27:583–588, 1996.

43. Chen WC, Yu SW, Tseng IC, et al: Treatment of undisplaced femoral neck fractures in the elderly. J Trauma 58:1035–1039; discussion 1039, 2005.

44. Bhandari M, Devereaux PJ, Tornetta P 3rd, et al: Operative management of displaced femoral neck fractures in elderly patients: an international survey. J Bone Joint Surg Am 87:2122–2130, 2005.

45. Swiontkowski MF: Intracapsular fractures of the hip. J Bone Joint Surg Am 76:129–138, 1994.

46. Macaulay W, Yoon RS, Parsley B, et al; DFACTO Consortium: Displaced femoral neck fractures: is there a standard of care? Orthopedics 30:748–749, 2007.

47. Probe R, Ward R: Internal fixation of femoral neck fractures. J Am Acad Orthop Surg 14:565–571, 2006.

48. Shah AK, Eissler J, Radomisli T: Algorithms for the treatment of femoral neck fractures. Clin Orthop Relat Res 399:28–34, 2002.

49. Bosch U, Schreiber T, Krettek C: Reduction and fixation of displaced intracapsular fractures of the proximal femur. Clin Orthop Relat Res 399:59–71, 2002.

50. Bhandari M, Devereaux PJ, Swiontkowski MF, et al: Internal fixation compared with arthroplasty for displaced fractures of the femoral neck: a meta-analysis. J Bone Joint Surg Am 85:1673–1681, 2003.

51. Rogmark C, Carlsson A, Johnell O, Sernbo I: A prospective randomised trial of internal fixation versus arthroplasty for displaced fractures of the neck of the femur: functional outcome for 450 patients at two years. J Bone Joint Surg Br 84:183–188, 2002.

52. Keating JF, Grant A, Masson M, et al: Randomized comparison of reduction and fixation, bipolar hemiarthroplasty, and total hip arthroplasty: treatment of displaced intracapsular hip fractures in healthy older patients. J Bone Joint Surg Am 88:249–260, 2006.

52a. Blomfeldt R, Tornkvist H, Eriksson K, et al: A randomized controlled trial comparing bipolar hemiarthroplasty with total hip replacement for displaced intracapsular fractures of the femoral neck in elderly patients. J Bone Joint Surg Br 89:160–165, 2007.

53. Heetveld MJ, Rogmark C, Frihagen F, Keating J: Internal fixation versus arthroplasty for displaced femoral neck fractures: what is the evidence? J Orthop Trauma 23:395–402, 2009.

53a. Schmidt AH, Leighton R, Parvizi J, et al: Optimal arthroplasty for femoral neck fractures: is total hip arthroplasty the answer? J Orthop Trauma 23:428–433, 2009.

54. Soto-Hall R, Johnson LH, Johnson RA: Variations in the intra-articular pressure of the hip joint in injury and disease: a probable factor in avascular necrosis. J Bone Joint Surg Am 46:509–516, 1964.

55. Jerre R, Doshe A, Karlsson J: Preoperative skin traction in patients with hip fractures is not useful. Clin Orthop Relat Res 378:169–173, 2000.

56. Anderson GH, Harper WM, Connolly CD, et al: Preoperative skin traction for fractures of the proximal femur: a randomised prospective trial. J Bone Joint Surg Br 75:794–796, 1993.

57. Finsen V, Borset M, Buvik GE, Hauke I: Preoperative traction in patients with hip fractures. Injury 23:242–244, 1992.

58. Needoff M, Radford P, Langstaff R: Preoperative traction for hip fractures in the elderly: a clinical trial. Injury 24:317–318, 1993.

59. Keller CS, Laros GS: Indications for open reduction of femoral neck fractures. Clin Orthop Relat Res 152:131–137, 1980.

60. Chua D, Jaglal SB, Schatzker J: Predictors of early failure of fixation in the treatment of displaced subcapital hip fractures. J Orthop Trauma 12:230–234, 1998.

61. Swiontkowski MF: Femoral neck fractures: open reduction internal fixation. In Wiss DA (ed): Master techniques in orthopaedic surgery, fractures, Philadelphia, 1998, Lippincott Williams & Wilkins, p 213.

62. Watson-Jones R: Fractures of the neck of the femur. Br J Surg 23:787, 1936.

63. Molnar RB, Routt ML Jr: Open reduction of intracapsular hip fractures using a modified Smith-Petersen surgical exposure. J Orthop Trauma 21:490–494, 2007.

64. Bhandari M: Ipsilateral femoral neck and shaft fractures. J Orthop Trauma 17:138–140, 2003.

65. Bedi A, Karunakar MA, Caron T, et al: Accuracy of reduction of ipsilateral femoral neck and shaft fractures—an analysis of various internal fixation strategies. J Orthop Trauma 23:249–253, 1990.

66. Alho A: Concurrent ipsilateral fractures of the hip and femoral shaft: a meta-analysis of 659 cases. Acta Orthop Scand 67:19–28, 1996.

67. Wolinsky PR, Johnson KD: Ipsilateral femoral neck and shaft fractures. Clin Orthop Relat Res 318:81–90, 1995.

68. Swiontkowski MF: Ipsilateral femoral shaft and hip fractures. Orthop Clin North Am 18:73–84, 1987.

69. Peljovich AE, Patterson BM: Ipsilateral femoral neck and shaft fractures. J Am Acad Orthop Surg 6:106–113, 1998.

70. Plancher KD, Donshik JD: Femoral neck and ipsilateral neck and shaft fractures in the young adult. Orthop Clin North Am 28:447–459, 1997.

71. Cannada LK, Viehe T, Cates CA, et al: A retrospective review of high-energy femoral neck-shaft fractures. J Orthop Trauma 23:254–260, 2009.

72. Stromqvist B, Brismar J, Hansson LI, Palmer J: Technetium-99m-methylenediphosphonate scintimetry after femoral neck fracture: a three-year follow-up study. Clin Orthop Relat Res 182:177–189, 1984.

73. Speer KP, Spritzer CE, Harrelson JM, Nunley JA: Magnetic resonance imaging of the femoral head after acute intracapsular fracture of the femoral neck. J Bone Joint Surg Am 72:98–103, 1990.

74. Asnis SE, Gould ES, Bansal M, et al: Magnetic resonance imaging of the hip after displaced femoral neck fractures. Clin Orthop Relat Res 298:191–198, 1994.

75. Gautam VK, Anand S, Dhaon BK: Management of displaced femoral neck fractures in young adults (a group at risk). Injury 29:215–218, 1998.

76. Krischak G, Beck A, Wachter N, et al: Relevance of primary reduction for the clinical outcome of femoral neck fractures treated with cancellous screws. Arch Orthop Trauma Surg 123:404–409, 2003.

77. Bout CA, Cannegieter DM, Juttmann JW: Percutaneous cannulated screw fixation of femoral neck fractures: the three point principle. Injury 28:135–139, 1997.

78. Partanen J, Saarenpaa I, Heikkinen T, et al: Functional outcome after displaced femoral neck fractures treated with osteosynthesis or hemiarthroplasty: a matched-pair study of 714 patients. Acta Orthop Scand 73:496–501, 2002.

79. Szita J, Cserhati P, Bosch U, et al: Intracapsular femoral neck fractures: the importance of early reduction and stable osteosynthesis. Injury 33(Suppl 3):C41–C46, 2002.

80. Heetveld MJ, Raaymakers EL, Luitse JS, Gouma DJ: Rating of internal fixation and clinical outcome in displaced femoral neck fractures: a prospective multicenter study. Clin Orthop Relat Res 454:207–213, 2007.

81. Estrada LS, Volgas DA, Stannard JP, Alonso JE: Fixation failure in femoral neck fractures. Clin Orthop Relat Res 399:110–118, 2002.

82. Jain R, Koo M, Kreder HJ, et al: Comparison of early and delayed fixation of subcapital hip fractures in patients sixty years of age or less. J Bone Joint Surg Am 84:1605–1612, 2002.

83. El-Abed K, McGuinness A, Brunner J, et al: Comparison of outcomes following uncemented hemiarthroplasty and dynamic hip screw in the treatment of displaced subcapital hip fractures in patients aged greater than 70 years. Acta Orthop Belg 71:48–54, 2005.

84. Beris AE, Payatakes AH, Kostopoulos VK, et al: Non-union of femoral neck fractures with osteonecrosis of the femoral head: treatment with combined free vascularized fibular grafting and subtrochanteric valgus osteotomy. Orthop Clin North Am 35:335–343, ix, 2004.

85. Gomez-Castresana F, Perez Caballer A, Ferrandez Portal L: Avascular necrosis of the femoral head after femoral neck fracture. Clin Orthop Relat Res 399:87, 2002.

86. Kofoed H: Femoral neck fractures in young adults. Injury 14:146–150, 1982.

87. Upadhyay A, Jain P, Mishra P, et al: Delayed internal fixation of fractures of the neck of the femur in young adults: a prospective, randomised study comparing closed and open reduction. J Bone Joint Surg Br 86:1035–1040, 2004.

88. Marti RK, Schuller HM, Raaymakers EL: Intertrochanteric osteotomy for non-union of the femoral neck. J Bone Joint Surg Br 71:782–787, 1989.

89. Schoenfeld AJ, Vrabec GA: Valgus osteotomy of the proximal femur with sliding hip screw for the treatment of femoral neck nonunions: the technique, a case series, and literature review. J Orthop Trauma 20:485–491, 2006.

90. Hartford JM, Patel A, Powell J: Intertrochanteric osteotomy using a dynamic hip screw for femoral neck nonunion. J Orthop Trauma 19:329–333, 2005.

91. Kalra M, Anand S: Valgus intertrochanteric osteotomy for neglected femoral neck fractures in young adults. Int Orthop 25:363–366, 2001.

92. Anglen JO: Intertrochanteric osteotomy for failed internal fixation of femoral neck fracture. Clin Orthop Relat Res 341:175–182, 1997.

93. Blair B, Koval KJ, Kummer F, Zuckerman JD: Basicervical fractures of the proximal femur: a biomechanical study of 3 internal fixation techniques. Clin Orthop Relat Res 306:256–263, 1994.

94. Kauffman JI, Simon JA, Kummer FJ, et al: Internal fixation of femoral neck fractures with posterior comminution: a biomechanical study. J Orthop Trauma 13:155–159, 1999.

95. Oakey JW, Stover MD, Summers HD, et al: Does screw configuration affect subtrochanteric fracture after femoral neck fixation? Clin Orthop Relat Res 443:302–306, 2006.

96. Bjorgul K, Reikeras O: Outcome of undisplaced and moderately displaced femoral neck fractures. Acta Orthop 78:498–504, 2007.

97. Holmes CA, Edwards WT, Myers ER, et al: Biomechanics of pin and screw fixation of femoral neck fractures. J Orthop Trauma 7:242–247, 1993.

98. Krastman P, van den Bent RP, Krijnen P, Schipper IB: Two cannulated hip screws for femoral neck fractures: treatment of choice or asking for trouble? Arch Orthop Trauma Surg 126:297–303, 2006.

99. Weinrobe M, Stankewich CJ, Mueller B, Tencer AF: Predicting the mechanical outcome of femoral neck fractures fixed with cancellous screws: an in vivo study. J Orthop Trauma 12:27–36; discussion 36–37, 1998.

100. Liporace F, Gaines R, Collinge C, Haidukewych GJ: Results of internal fixation of Pauwels type-3 vertical femoral neck fractures. J Bone Joint Surg Am 90:1654–1659, 2008.

101. Gurusamy K, Parker MJ, Rowlands TK: The complications of displaced intracapsular fractures of the hip: the effect of screw positioning and angulation on fracture healing. J Bone Joint Surg Br 87:632–634, 2005.

102. Aminian A, Gao F, Fedoriw WW, et al: Vertically oriented femoral neck fractures: mechanical analysis of four fixation techniques. J Orthop Trauma 21:544–548, 2007.

103. Asnis SE, Wanek-Sgaglione L: Intracapsular fractures of the femoral neck: results of cannulated screw fixation. J Bone Joint Surg Am 76:1793–1803, 1994.

104. Manninger J, Kazar G, Fekete G, et al: Avoidance of avascular necrosis of the femoral head, following fractures of the femoral neck, by early reduction and internal fixation. Injury 16:437–448, 1985.

105. Manninger J, Kazar G, Fekete G, et al: Significance of urgent (within 6h) internal fixation in the management of fractures of the neck of the femur. Injury 20:101–105, 1989.

106. Swiontkowski MF, Tepic S, Rahn BA, et al: The effect of fracture on femoral head blood flow: osteonecrosis and revascularization studied in miniature swine. Acta Orthop Scand 64:196–202, 1993.

107. Zetterberg C, Elmerson S, Andersson GB: Epidemiology of hip fractures in Goteborg, Sweden, 1940-1983. Clin Orthop Relat Res 191:43–52, 1984.

108. Gerber C, Strehle J, Ganz R: The treatment of fractures of the femoral neck. Clin Orthop Relat Res 292:77–86, 1993.

CHAPTER 45

Intertrochanteric Fractures

Andrew H. Schmidt and Richard F. Kyle

KEY POINTS

- The treatment of intertrochanteric femur fractures is nearly always operative.
- Compression hip screws are best used in stable fracture patterns and are associated with low rates of complications when properly positioned within the center of the femoral head.
- Cephalomedullary nails are the implant of choice for fractures without a stable lateral cortex and for reverse-oblique fractures, which have increased complications of loss of fixation and poorer functional outcomes when compression hip screws are used.
- Historically, cephalomedullary nails have been associated with higher rates of revision surgery than compression hip screws, largely because of the increased risk of postoperative femur fracture. However, this complication seems to be decreasing with current nail designs, and more recent series have found no increased risk of femoral fracture in patients treated with cephalomedullary nails compared with compression hip screws.[1]

INTRODUCTION

Intertrochanteric fractures of the upper femur occur in the region of the femur bounded by the femoral neck and lesser trochanter medially and the greater trochanter laterally. These fractures occur in two circumstances: with high-energy trauma in the younger patient, and following a simple fall in the older patient. The latter type of fracture is typically associated with senile osteoporosis. Intertrochanteric fractures present in a wide variety of patterns that range from simple to complex and may be minimally displaced or widely displaced. Similar to the proximal humerus, the proximal femur often fractures into typical fragments, which in the femur include the femoral neck and head, the greater and lesser trochanters, and the femoral shaft (Fig. 45-1). Extension of the fracture may occur distally along the femoral shaft, confusing the distinction between intertrochanteric fractures and subtrochanteric fractures.

These fractures are easily diagnosed in the patient with a known or suspected fall on the basis of pain and deformity of the limb, which typically is shortened and externally rotated. Plain radiographs confirm the diagnosis in most cases. Occasionally, a patient with hip pain has normal radiographs; in this case, magnetic resonance imaging should be done. Bone marrow edema or a cortical break in the trochanteric region can be considered evidence of a nondisplaced fracture.

The standard of care for these injuries is surgical stabilization. Nonoperative care of displaced fractures almost always results in varus malunion of the proximal femur with limb shortening and rotational deformity, unless some sort of skeletal traction can be maintained. Even more important, nonoperative care of displaced and/or unstable fractures requires prolonged recumbency of the patient, whereas patients usually can be mobilized in some manner immediately after surgery.

INDICATIONS/CONTRAINDICATIONS

Nonoperative Care

Nonoperative treatment of intertrochanteric fractures is appropriate for those patients with radiographically occult fractures who can be mobilized without too much pain. If this approach is chosen, patients (and their families) need to be warned about the possibility of later displacement, and frequent radiographic follow-up is necessary. Rarely, patients with displaced fractures are not viewed as candidates for surgery or anesthesia because of severe medical comorbidities. When nonoperative management is chosen, such patients need careful medical management and attentive nursing care to prevent thromboembolism, malnutrition, decubitus ulcers, or other complications of prolonged recumbency. Large series reported in the literature indicate that results comparable with those reported after surgery can be obtained with skeletal traction.[2]

Operative Management

Historical Background

Intertrochanteric femur fractures have been managed traditionally with compression (also referred to as *sliding*) hip screws that allow collapse of the facture along the axis of the lag screw, thereby creating bone-to-bone contact that in turn increases stability and leads to reliable healing. The widespread adoption of the compression hip screw that occurred during the

1980s dramatically reduced the incidence of nonunion and loss of fixation that occurred with earlier fixed-angle devices. In the 1990s, cephalomedullary nails were introduced for use in intertrochanteric fractures, yet their role in the management of these fractures is still somewhat controversial. Intramedullary devices offer a potentially less invasive approach to fixation of intertrochanteric fractures compared with plate fixation with a compression hip screw. Recent investigations of

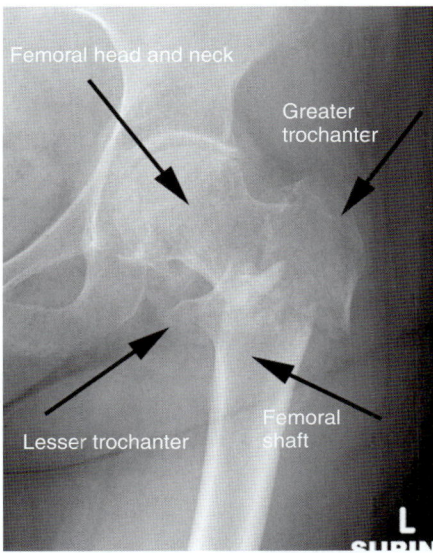

Figure 45-1. Anteroposterior radiograph of a comminuted intertrochanteric fracture, demonstrating classic fracture fragments and displacement. This particular fracture is an example of the newly described Kyle type V fracture, in which an associated fracture occurs at the base of the femoral neck.

the functional outcomes of elderly patients with unstable fracture patterns have highlighted problems associated with loss of reduction due to collapse, which in turn causes limb shortening and loss of the abductor moment arm with potential pain, limp, and poor functional outcomes (Fig. 45-2).[3-5] Fracture collapse after initial reduction and fixation is less common when intramedullary devices are used, so that cephalomedullary nails are now commonly used in patients with unstable fracture patterns, such as those with loss of integrity of the lateral wall of the greater trochanter and reverse-obliquity fractures.[5,6] However, large series of patients comparing compression hip screws with intramedullary nails demonstrate that patients treated with intramedullary nails have a higher overall rate of revision surgery during the first year.[7] For these reasons, the compression hip screw remains the implant of choice at many centers for the treatment of intertrochanteric fractures.[8]

Current Surgical Practice

Surgery is the standard of care for intertrochanteric fractures. Surgical options include external fixation, internal fixation with a compression hip screw, and internal fixation with an intramedullary device, typically a so-called *cephalomedullary nail* (sometimes referred to as an *intramedullary hip screw*). Any of these options can be considered for almost any fracture, and the optimum implant for a given fracture type is a matter of considerable debate.

External fixation is not commonly done, despite reports of success.[9] Very few orthopedic surgeons have experience in the management of intertrochanteric fractures with external fixation, and the need for prolonged care of external fixation pins, as well as complications of pin infection and later fracture through pin sites, makes this technique unpopular.

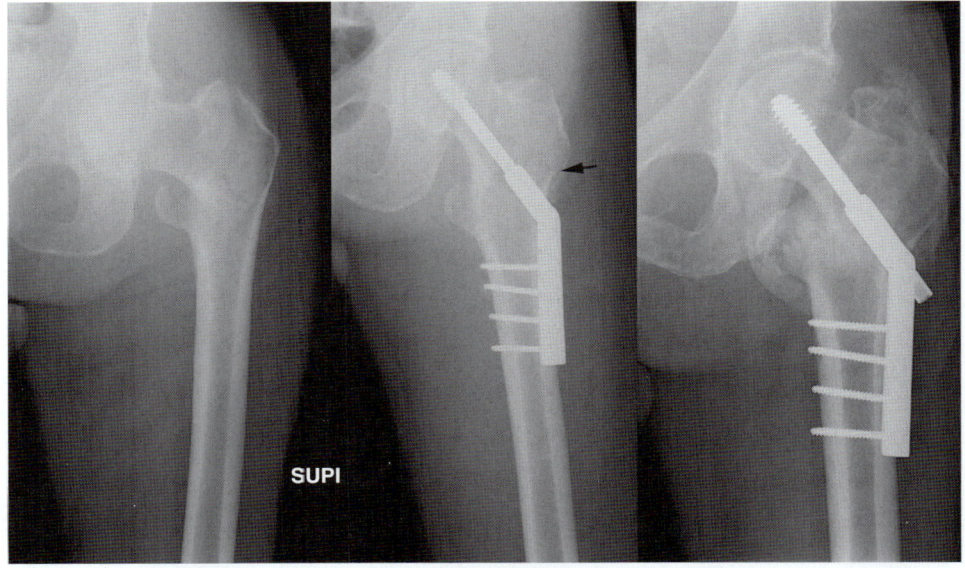

Figure 45-2. Serial anteroposterior radiographs of a patient showing progressive collapse of a compression hip screw comparing the immediate postoperative image *(middle panel)* with another image 5 months later *(right panel)*. The *arrow* in the middle panel shows loss of integrity of the lateral wall of the greater trochanter, which is associated with excessive collapse when sliding hip screws are used.

Compression hip screws represent the traditional standard for operative care of intertrochanteric femur fractures. Loss of fixation is rare when the lag screw is placed within the center of the femoral head, as noted by Kyle and associates[10] and more recently quantified by Baumgaertner and colleagues[11] as the so-called *tip-apex distance* (TAD). Although compression hip screws can be used successfully with any fracture of the proximal femur,[8] recent evidence suggests that use of these devices in specific unstable fracture patterns may lead to increased collapse and/or loss of fixation. Traditionally, loss of the posteromedial buttress of the proximal femur, including the posterior aspect of the femoral neck and the lesser trochanter, has been considered the hallmark of instability (Fig. 45-3). Kyle and coworkers documented that collapse, cutout, and nonunion occurred in 25% of patients with a combined intertrochanteric-femoral neck fracture, which they newly described in their paper.[3] This particular type of fracture, which they described as the Kyle type V fracture, has severe comminution of the greater trochanter and associated femoral neck fracture (see Fig. 45-1), which led to complete collapse of the sliding hip screw in nearly half of the cases in their series, and in 100% of failed cases.[3] Other authors have highlighted loss of the integrity of the lateral wall of the greater trochanter as a risk factor for loss of reduction with compression hip screws (see Fig. 45-2, *middle panel*).[6,12,13] Another fracture pattern that is widely considered to be a contraindication for the use of a compression hip screw is the reverse-oblique fracture (Fig. 45-4). The general consensus, supported by the literature, is that use of a compression hip screw in reverse-oblique fractures leads to frequent complications (Fig. 45-5).[14,15] These unstable fracture patterns must be recognized because recent literature has documented shortening of the femoral neck, loss of the abductor moment arm, limb length discrepancy, and, most important, poorer functional outcomes in patients with unstable fractures treated

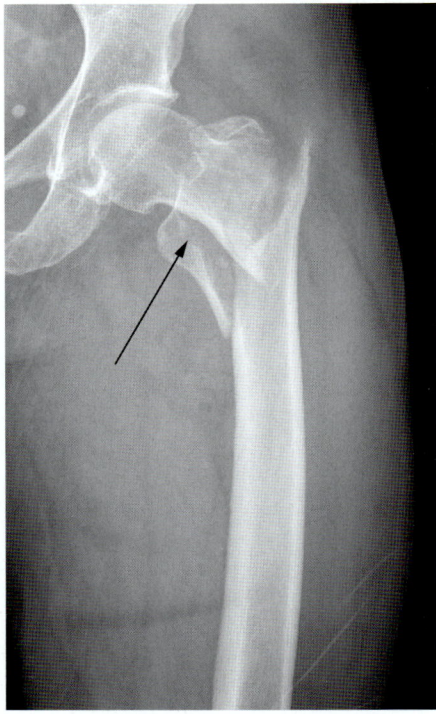

Figure 45-3. Example of an intertrochanteric femur fracture with a large posteromedial fragment *(arrow)*.

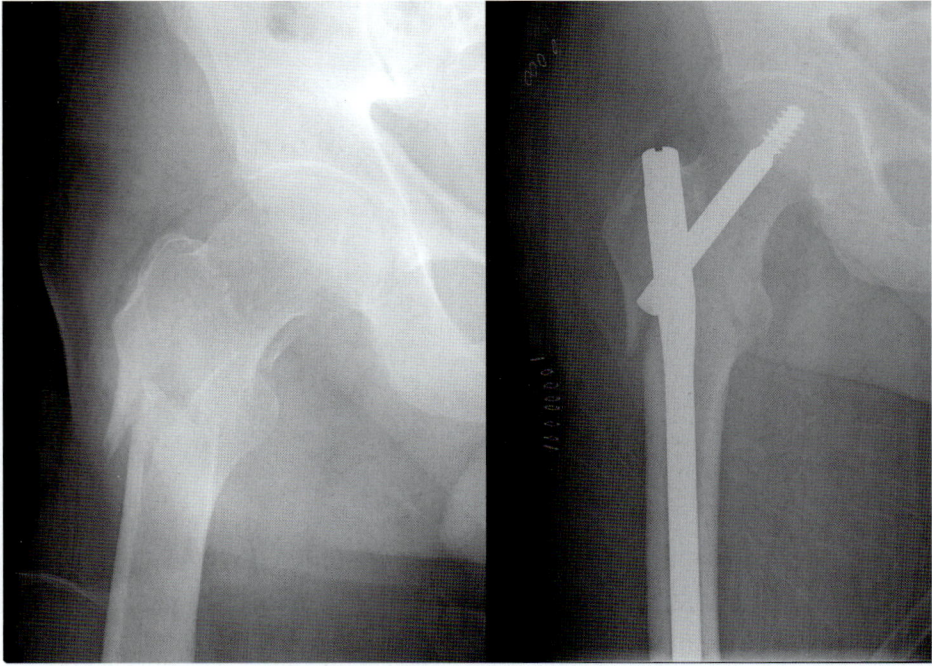

Figure 45-4. Preoperative *(left panel)* and postoperative *(right panel)* anteroposterior radiographs of a reverse-obliquity fracture of the proximal femur, reduced and stabilized with a cephalomedullary nail.

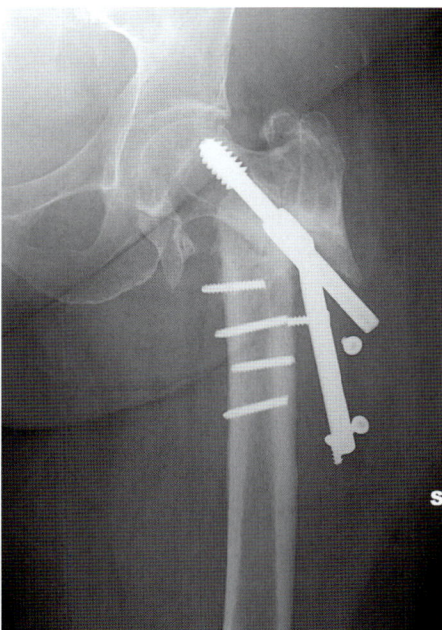

Figure 45-5. Example of catastrophic loss of fixation of a reverse-obliquity fracture treated with a sliding hip screw. Note the evidence of toggling of the lag screw within the femoral head, which occurred after the sliding screw collapsed maximally, and before ultimate failure by pulling out of the screws from the femoral shaft.

with compression hip screws.[16,17] Thus, routine use of compression hip screws in unstable fracture patterns, such as those with loss of the lateral buttress, is now discouraged.

Intramedullary implants, such as the cephalomedullary nail, are being used increasingly for intertrochanteric fractures (Fig. 45-6). Cephalomedullary nails are available in both short and long versions. Short intramedullary devices have been plagued by intraoperative and postoperative fractures.[17-24] In contrast, long cephalomedullary nails have been associated with anterior femoral cortical perforation due to mismatch between the radius of curvature of these nails and the femur.[25,26] This is more of an issue when most of the femoral canal is intact, as is the case when nails are used for very proximal femoral fractures.[26] Intramedullary nails have theoretical benefits. First, their intramedullary position buttresses the proximal femur, thereby preventing excessive collapse of the femoral neck and preventing shortening. Second, by virtue of the more medial position, they experience less loading because of a shorter moment arm. However, as was pointed out by Zlowodzki and associates, this is true only for 135-degree compression hip screws; a high-angle (150-degree) hip screw actually has a shorter moment arm than a 135-degree intramedullary hip screw.[27] In addition, neck shaft angles of intramedullary nails are usually limited to a few angles (typically 125 or 130 degrees) that are "built in," and the position of the guide pin is determined by the position of the nail in the femur, so that achieving ideal center-center position of the lag screw within the

femoral head is potentially more difficult to attain with these devices.[28] This is especially true in patients with a neck shaft angle less than 125 degrees, in whom a sliding hip screw would allow better implant placement within the femoral head.[28]

Another important difference between compression hip screws and cephalomedullary nails is their relative cost. Nails may cost three to four times more than a standard compression hip screw. This fact must be considered in light of evidence that overall outcomes remain good in patients treated with the less expensive compression hip screws,[8] and that overall revision surgery rates at 1 year may be higher in patients treated with nails.[7]

Evidence-Based Approach to Choice of Fixation

The decision regarding choice of a compression hip screw or a cephalomedullary nail for a given patient is complex and depends on many factors related to the patient, the fracture, the surgeon, and the environment in which care is provided. Therefore, it is worthwhile to develop an evidence-based approach to the care of these injuries.

A number of level I and II prospective clinical trials have been published that compare compression hip screws with intramedullary devices.* Although a detailed analysis of all of these studies is beyond the scope of this chapter, they can be summarized as follows (Table 45-1). In general, no consistent, statistically significant, and clinically relevant differences have been found among any perioperative factors between groups of patients treated with a compression hip screw or a cephalomedullary nail. In contrast, functional differences, when present, seem to be of a larger magnitude and favor intramedullary devices, especially in unstable fracture patterns.[4,5,16,17,24] Finally, distinct differences in complications are evident, with femoral shaft fracture complicating many reported series of cephalomedullary nails,[18,19,24,29] whereas loss of reduction and implant cut-out are more common following use of a compression hip screw, especially in unstable fractures characterized by loss of integrity of the lateral wall of the greater trochanter, associated femoral neck fracture, or extension in the subtrochanteric region of the femur.[3,6,12,13,18]

PREOPERATIVE PLANNING

Radiographic Evaluation

Imaging

First, an anteroposterior (AP) radiograph of the pelvis and both AP and lateral radiographs of the injured hip and femur are obtained. It is important that an AP view be done with both traction and internal rotation of the injured leg. Koval and associates found that the addition of the traction–internal rotation AP radiograph to a

---

*References 4, 5, 16-20, 22, 23, and 29-33.

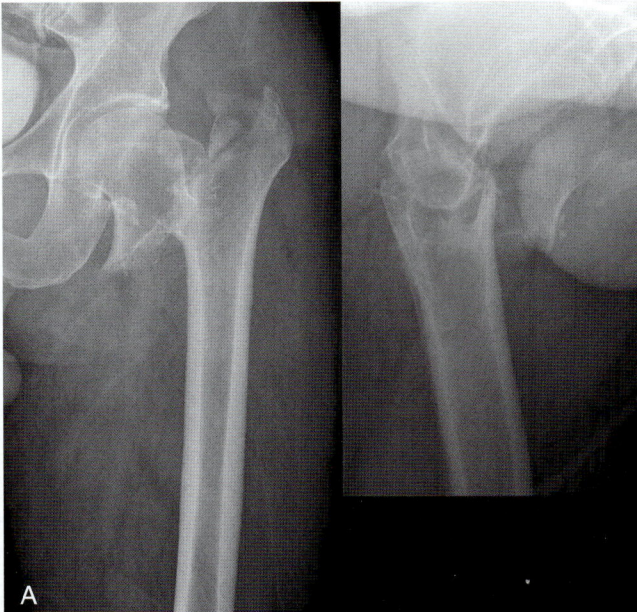

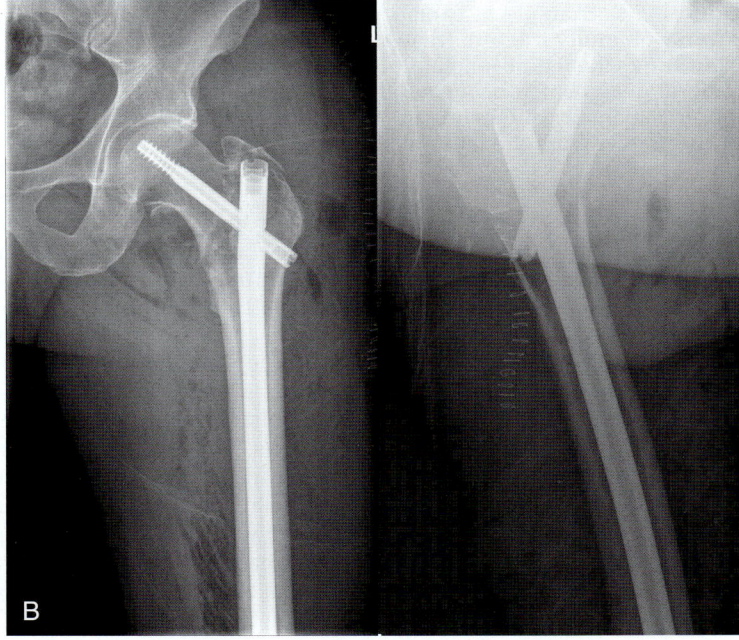

Figure 45-6. Example of an intertrochanteric fracture of the femur treated with a cephalomedullary nail. **A,** Preoperative anteroposterior and lateral radiographs. **B,** Postoperative radiographs following reduction and cephalomedullary nailing.

series of standard hip x-rays led to a change in classification in nearly 10% of cases, and that half of these changes would have affected the choice of treatment.[34] The entire femur should be visualized in case a long nailing procedure is done and might provide evidence of something that could complicate nailing, such as malunion of a previous distal femur fracture, unexpected hardware, or another bone abnormality. Computed tomography usually is not necessary but may be considered if further information about the fracture is desired, or if concern is raised about associated injury to the pelvis. From the imaging studies, one can assess the fracture pattern and the degree of comminution, and can begin to assess fracture stability as discussed here.

Assessment of Stability

Palm and associates and Gotfried identified the integrity of the lateral wall of the greater trochanter as an important predictor of complications; thus special attention should be paid to this area during preoperative planning.[6,12,13] In addition, comminution of the greater trochanter, especially when associated with a fracture of the femoral neck, is an indicator of instability and a high likelihood of failure if a compression hip screw is used.[3]

Table 45-1. Summary of Level I and II Studies Comparing Intramedullary Fixation Versus Compression Hip Screws for Intertrochanteric Fractures

Series	Comparison	Perioperative Parameters	Functional Outcomes	Complications
Adams et al	IM nail vs. DHS, n = 400		No difference in early outcomes or at 1 year	DHS: statistically insignificant lower cut-out, femur fracture, need for revision
Ahrengart et al	Gamma nail vs. CHS, n = 426	CHS: less OR time in whole series, but equal in unstable fractures; less blood loss		Nail: problems with distal interlocking, higher malposition, cut-out, and femoral fracture
Baumgaertner et al	IMHS vs. SHS, n = 135	Nail: less OR time; less blood loss	No difference	
Bridle et al	Gamma nail vs. DHS, n = 100	No difference	No differences at 6 months	Loss of reduction equal Nail: 4% femoral fractures
Hardy et al	IMHS vs. CHS, n = 100	CHS: less OR time IMHS: less blood loss	IMHS: better mobility at 1, 3, 6, 12 months	CHS: 2% loss of fixation IMHS: 6% intraoperative fractures, less sliding and shortening
Leung et al	Gamma nail vs. DHS	Nail: smaller incision; less blood loss	Nail: earlier full weight bearing	Nail: postop femoral shaft fracture
Little et al	Long Holland nail vs. DHS, n = 190	DHS: less OR time; less radiation time Nail: less blood loss; less transfusion	Better in nail group	DHS: 2.1% cut-out Nail: no cut-out
O'Brien et al	Gamma nail vs. CHS, n = 101	No difference	No difference	No difference
Pajarinen et al	PFN vs. DHS, n = 108		Nail: faster return to preoperative gait function	No difference
Radford et al	IM nail vs. SHS, n = 200	No difference	Equal	No difference
Saudan et al	IM nail vs. SHS, n = 206	No difference	Equal	No difference
Utrilla et al	Gamma nail vs. CHS, n = 210	No difference in surgical time Nail: lower transfusion	Nail: improved gait in patients with unstable fractures	No difference

CHS, Compression hip screw; *DHS,* dynamic hip screw; *IM,* intramedullary; *IMHS,* intramedullary hip screw; *OR,* operating room; *PFN,* proximal femoral nail; *SHS,* sliding hip screw.

DESCRIPTION OF TECHNIQUE(S)

General Issues

The strength of fixation of an intertrochanteric hip fracture following surgery is determined by five distinct variables: bone quality, fragment geometry, fracture reduction, implant design, and implant placement.[35] The first two variables—bone quality and fragment geometry—are not under the surgeon's control. However, the remaining three factors—fracture reduction, implant design, and placement of the implant—are directly controlled by the surgeon and have an impact on the results of treatment.

Surgical Technique

Reduction

As stated already, optimum reduction of an intertrochanteric femur fracture is an important determinant of a successful outcome. In treating a displaced fracture, use of a fracture table can greatly facilitate imaging, fracture reduction, and implant placement.

To reduce the fracture, gentle traction is applied to the leg, and any external rotation of the distal fragment is corrected. Once a provisional reduction of the fracture is obtained with acceptable rotation and length on the AP view of the hip, one should obtain lateral views using the image intensifier. Using the lateral view of the hip, one may correct flexion or extension of the distal fragment by elevating or lowering the foot while maintaining all previous reduction maneuvers. One must also beware of posterior sag of the distal fragment at the fracture site, which if present can be corrected with a table extension or a well-placed crutch.

Occasionally, acceptable reduction will not be attainable by closed means, even with the fracture table. In such cases, fracture fragments may need to be disimpacted or directly manipulated before they can be reduced. In these cases, one first can attain provisional correction of alignment, rotation, and length with the fracture table and then can use more traditional reduction clamps and/or pins to attain and maintain fracture reduction during fixation (Fig. 45-7). A very important point about the surgical technique is that reduction of the fracture must be attained before any fixation is inserted, and the reduction achieved must be maintained during fixation.

Surgical Fixation

Compression Hip Screw

With the patient appropriately positioned on the fracture table, an acceptable reduction is obtained as described previously. A surgical incision is made along the lateral aspect of the thigh beginning about 5 cm below the tip of the greater trochanter and extending distally for 5 to 15 cm, depending on the preferences of the surgeon (Fig. 45-8). Many surgeons prefer to begin with a small incision used for initial guide wire placement, with the incision extended distally as needed. Distal fixation of the side plate to the femoral shaft can be done percutaneously if a less invasive surgical approach is desired. The iliotibial band is exposed and is incised in line with the skin incision. The vastus lateralis muscle may be split bluntly in line with the proximal femur to gain direct access to the fracture, or it may be elevated off of the lateral intramuscular septum. Either way, the origin of the vastus lateralis may need to be elevated off of the flare of the distal greater trochanter, so that soft tissues do not impede later placement of surgical instruments or the hip screw itself.

The starting point for the femoral head guide pin is determined using fluoroscopy. The location of the correct starting point will vary depending on the neck shaft angle of the implant to be used. A higher-angle (more valgus) implant will require a starting point that

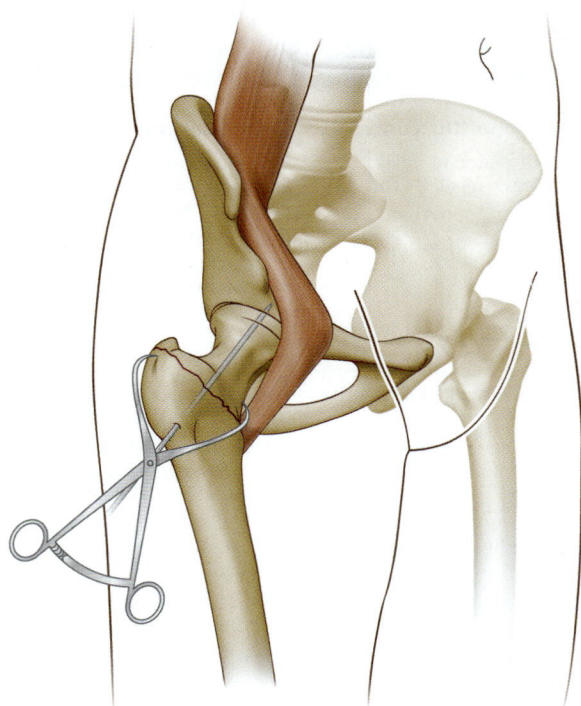

Figure 45-7. Artist's drawing showing how a pointed reduction clamp can be placed around a pertrochanteric fracture to maintain provisional reduction before insertion of internal fixation (whether an intramedullary nail or a compression hip screw).

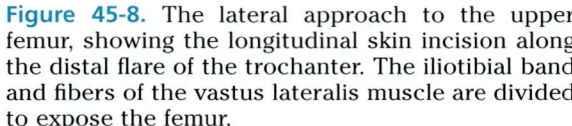

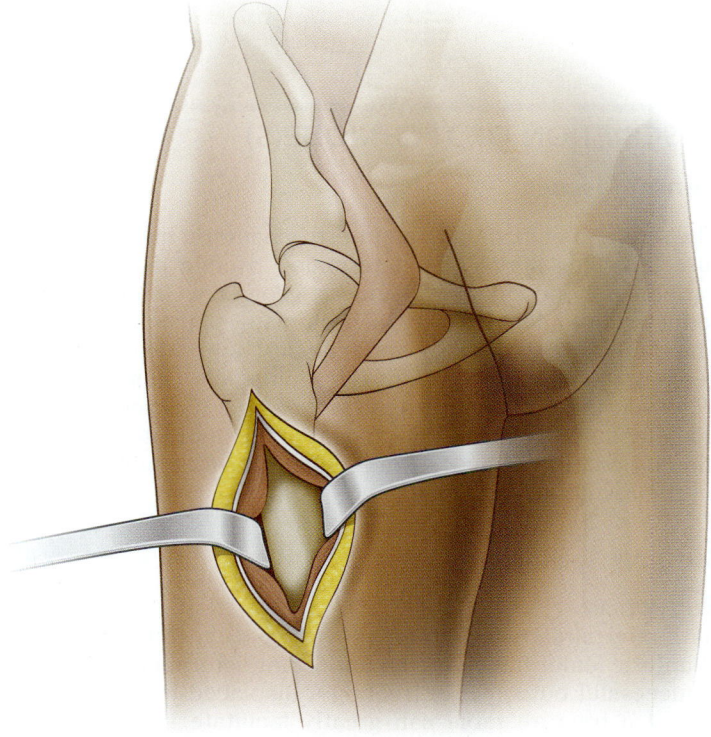

Figure 45-8. The lateral approach to the upper femur, showing the longitudinal skin incision along the distal flare of the trochanter. The iliotibial band and fibers of the vastus lateralis muscle are divided to expose the femur.

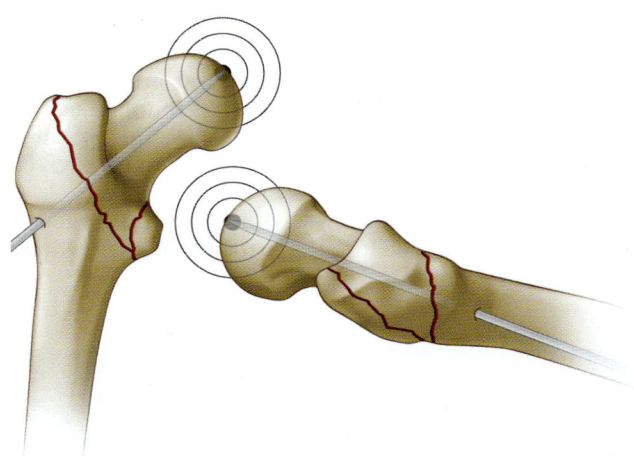

Figure 45-9. Depiction of correct placement of a guide pin in the center of the femoral neck and head, as shown in these drawings of the proximal femur from posterior *(left)* and lateral *(right)* perspectives.

is placed more distally on the femur. Using the desired implant angle targeting guide, a guide pin is drilled from the posterolateral femoral cortex into the center of the femoral neck, aiming slightly anteriorly to take into account the anteversion of the femoral neck. When the correct position of the guide pin has been determined using AP fluoroscopic views, correct central positioning of the guide pin in the lateral view has to be confirmed as well (Fig. 45-9). Central placement of the guide pin in the femoral head is the most important step in avoiding complications when a compression hip screw is used. The guide pin must be properly centered in the femoral neck and head on both AP and lateral views.[10] Once the guide pin is appropriately positioned, it is advanced to the subchondral bone at the apex of the femoral head. Kyle and associates were the first to demonstrate that a marked reduction in complications was associated with the center-center position of the compression hip screw within the subchondral bone of the femoral head.[10]

A useful intraoperative assessment of the position of the guide pin in the femoral head is the so-called *tip-apex distance* (TAD) described by Baumgaertner and colleagues.[11,36] The TAD is the sum of the distance (in millimeters) from the apex of the femoral head to the tip of the inserted guide pin as measured on both AP and lateral radiographic views. The risk of cut-out increases dramatically when the TAD exceeds 25 mm.[11] Rotation of the leg can affect the measurement of TAD.[37]

With the central guide pin in place, the length of the lag screw is measured and the reaming depth determined. When the guide pin is placed just beneath subchondral bone, many surgeons subtract 5 to 10 mm of length from the guide pin measurement when choosing the length of the femoral head lag screw. The cortical reamer is preset for the desired reaming depth and is slowly advanced over the guide pin. One should monitor the progression of the reamer during insertion using intermittent fluoroscopy, because serious

complications can occur if the guide pin penetrates the pelvis. In general, it is not necessary to ream to the end of the guide pin. If desired, a tap is placed over the guide pin and is advanced by hand to the reaming depth. This step is not necessary in patients with poor bone density. The cannulated lag screw, equal in length to the final reaming depth, is then advanced by hand over the guide pin until it is seated in subchondral bone.

The side plate barrel is advanced over the femoral head lag screw and is impacted down to the femur, aligning it with the femoral shaft. Some systems are "keyed," requiring proper rotational orientation of the lag screw during its insertion to align the plate with the bone. Other systems are keyless and can be inserted as a single unit. According to surgeon preference, the plate can be placed submuscularly or in an "open" fashion. Once impacted, the plate is affixed to the femoral shaft with two to six bicortical screws. Two screws are sufficient for most stable fractures, but more screws may be needed in cases of severe osteoporosis to prevent screw pull-out from the femoral shaft.

Cephalomedullary Nail

Cephalomedullary nails used for fixation of pertrochanteric fractures usually are inserted through a trochanteric starting point. Many variations of trochanteric nails are available commercially; some have one larger femoral neck screw, while others use two smaller-diameter screws. Most are available in both short and long versions. Use of these devices requires the same reduction strategies already described for the compression hip screw. Nails usually are inserted using a percutaneous technique, although fracture clamps may be needed for more displaced fractures. Cephalomedullary nails have proved to be predictable devices for both simple and complex intertrochanteric fractures, including the reverse-oblique pattern. Intramedullary nails have more mechanical advantages than compression hip screws because their location is closer to the center of the femoral head, resulting in a shorter lever arm from the femoral head to the load-bearing axis of the implant. Unlike nails used for femoral shaft fractures, distal fixation of the nail does not depend solely on interlocking screw fixation because the nail is surrounded by intact cortical bone.

Patient positioning and initial fracture reduction are performed as described previously. The skin incision for nail insertion is made 3 to 5 cm above the tip of the greater trochanter and is generally 2 to 4 cm in length. The gluteus medius fascia is exposed and is split sharply toward the greater trochanter. Finally, an awl or guide pin is advanced to the tip of the greater trochanter. For a cephalomedullary nail, the ideal starting point is in the anterior third of the trochanter on the lateral view and at the medial aspect of the apex of the trochanter on the AP view (Fig. 45-10).

After reduction of the fracture is ensured, the starting pin or awl is advanced from the starting point into the intertrochanteric region of the femur approximately 3 cm. The pin should aim at the center of the medullary canal. Once the pin is properly placed, it is over-reamed to create an opening sufficient for guide wire and nail placement. A ball-tipped guide wire is placed in the starting portal and is advanced into the distal femur while acceptable reduction of the fracture is ensured. The position of the guide wire should be checked fluoroscopically on both AP and lateral radiographic projections before reaming.

After the guide wire is placed and its position confirmed, the femur is prepared for nail insertion. Typically, the proximal nail diameter does not vary among nails of a given manufacturer; therefore, the proximal femur is reamed to a specific size, while the distal femur is reamed 1 mm larger than the intended nail diameter. Once the desired distal reaming diameter has been achieved, the surgeon reams the proximal opening according to the specific technique for a given nail.

The nail is assembled with its proximal targeting device and is advanced into the proximal femur by hand

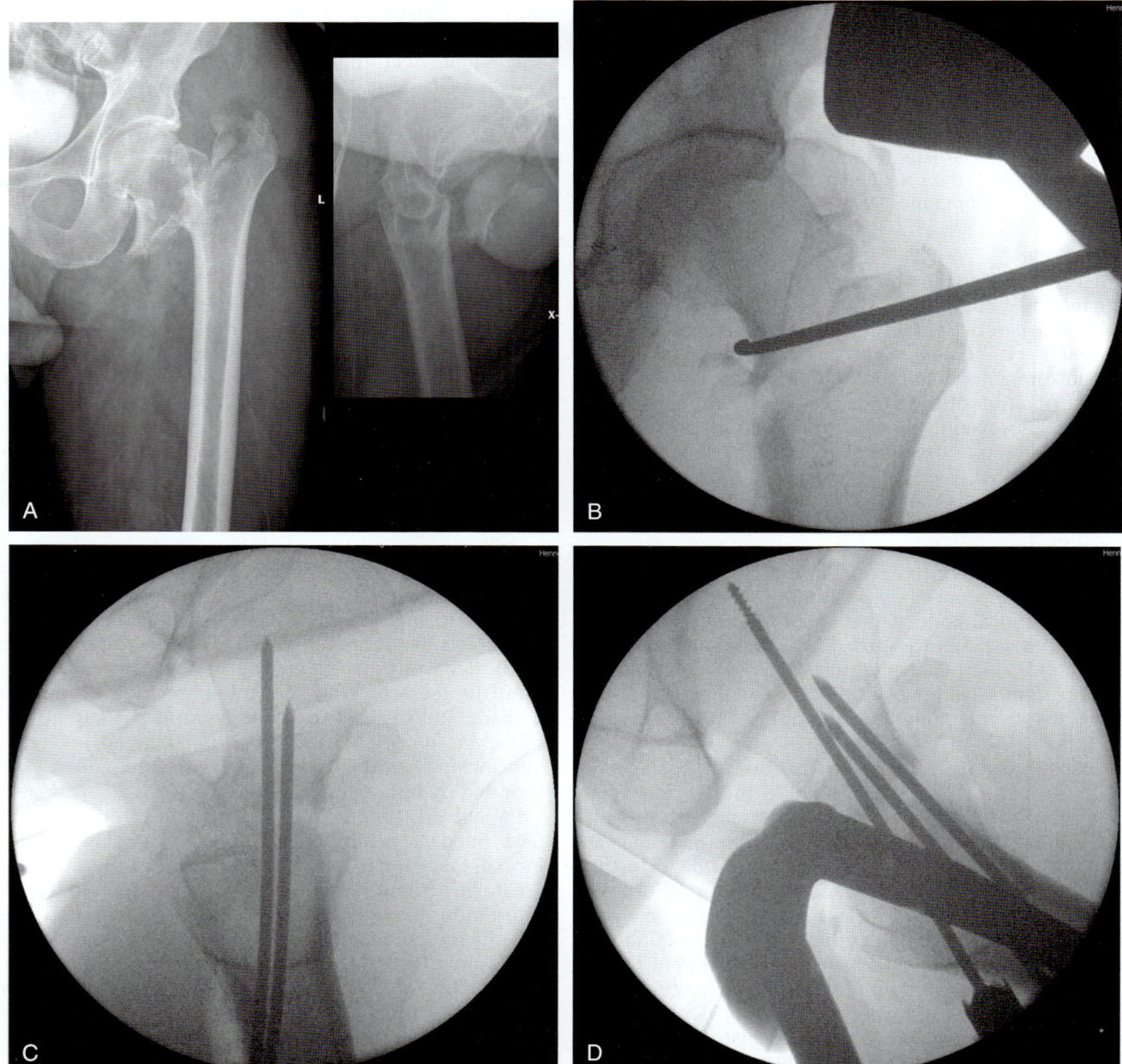

Figure 45-10. Steps in cephalomedullary nailing. **A,** Anteroposterior and lateral images of the upper femur, showing a completely displaced peritrochanteric fracture. **B,** Intraoperative fluoroscopy image showing reduction of the fracture with a bone hook applied over the anterior femoral neck to engage the medial neck and apply a lateral-proximal vector to the femoral head-neck fragment. **C,** After reduction, two K-wires were placed anteriorly to stabilize the fracture in a reduced position. **D,** The nail is inserted and the guide pin for the proximal screw targeted in the center of the femoral head.

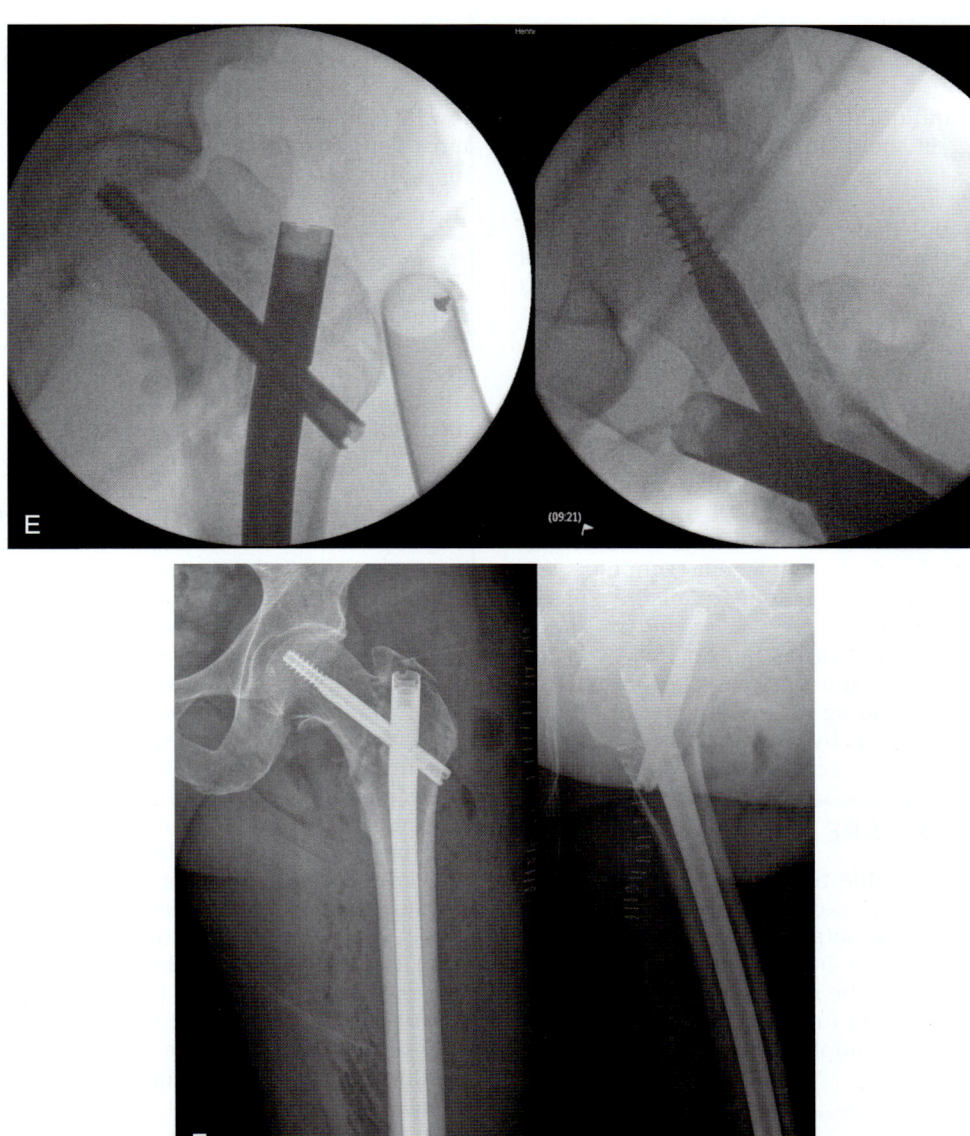

Figure 45-10, cont'd E, Intraoperative fluoroscopic views of the final lag screw and proximal nail. **F,** Final radiographic images.

over the guide wire. Final nail depth and orientation are checked radiographically on the AP view, and once the nail has been inserted to the desired depth, the ball-tipped guide wire should be removed and the targeting jig rotated to approximately 20 degrees of anteversion to target the femoral neck and head. The nail is appropriately seated when the lag screw drill targets the center of the femoral neck and head, or is slightly inferior to the center on the AP radiographic view.

Correct placement of the femoral head lag screw depends on correct initial guide pin placement using AP and lateral views. Moving the plane of the C-arm 20 degrees toward the patient's head while viewing the lateral image will effectively lengthen the femoral neck on the image and will allow better determination of guide pin position with the femoral neck. Typically, the

surgeon inserts the guide pin first while using the AP view and advances the guide pin roughly halfway into the femoral neck. If the guide pin is too high or low within the femoral neck, the wire should be removed and the nail depth should be gently adjusted. Once the guide pin is centered in the femoral neck on the AP view, the correct anteversion must be obtained and checked using the lateral view. The guide pin should be as close to the apex of the femoral head as possible; use of the same TAD criteria described for the compression hip screw is appropriate. Once the correct guide pin position within the femoral head has been achieved, the length of the corresponding lag screw is measured. Finally, distal locking of the nail is recommended for unstable patterns where rotational control is indicated.

TIPS AND PEARLS

- The AP radiograph of the injured leg should be taken while the leg is held in traction and internal rotation.[34]
- Measurement of the tip-apex distance[11] can be affected by rotation of the limb.[37] Correct interpretation of measurements therefore depends on knowledge of the position of the leg with regard to adduction/abduction, as well as internal or external rotation.
- Reduction of the fracture must be obtained prior to fixation, because the implants will not correct malreduction themselves and will not allow for fragment manipulation after insertion. In particular, beware of posterior sag when performing surgery with the patient supine, and maintain manual correction of this throughout the procedure.
- To avoid femoral shaft fracture, always insert a trochanteric nail by hand after sufficient reaming.
- In general, the authors prefer longer nails because of the reduced risk of later fracture at the tip of the implant and less risk of fixation failure. However, one must beware of mismatch between the bow of the femur and the nail, leading to possible perforation of the anterior distal femur by the tip of the nail.

POSTOPERATIVE CARE

At present, it is impossible to provide evidence-based guidelines regarding best practices in the postoperative or subacute period in patients convalescing from repair of a hip fracture.[38] After intramedullary fixation, it appears that patients can be mobilized within 24 hours of surgery with immediate full weight bearing without mechanical failure of the implants or loss of fixation.[39]

RESULTS

The results of treatment of intertrochanteric fractures are not perfectly defined. Advanced age, with related preexisting medical comorbidities as well as functional compromise, makes outcome assessment difficult. Patients may demonstrate measurable deficits after fracture healing compared with "normal," but yet fully return to their own baseline. Thus, it is important to somehow use a given patient's preinjury level of function as the comparison, but this may be very difficult to do.

A fairly detailed description of the outcomes of intertrochanteric fractures was recently provided by Chirodian and associates, who studied 1024 consecutive cases managed with a sliding hip screw.[8] Mean patient age was 82 years, and 78% were female. Seventy-five percent of the fractures were judged to be unstable. At 1-year follow-up, 69% of patients were alive. The vast majority (95%) had minimal or no pain, 85% returned to their prefracture living arrangement, and 50% regained their level of mobility. Complications of surgical fixation occurred in 4% of cases, and just less than 3% required

further surgery as a result. These data confirm that overall fixation failure and reoperation rates for trochanteric fractures fixed with a sliding hip screw are low. The final outcome in surviving patients is good, and most patients return to their prefracture level of accommodation and mobility.[8]

COMPLICATIONS

Complications can be broadly divided into three categories: (1) perioperative complications, including mortality, blood loss, medical complications such as thromboembolism, and wound healing problems; (2) mechanical problems, including loss of fixation, refracture, or implant failure; and (3) fracture healing problems, such as malunion or nonunion.

Overall, medical complications are common in these fragile patients. The choice of fracture fixation has some impact on surgical time and blood loss, but differences between implants are fairly small. Overall, published case series do indicate some differences in complications of cut-out, hardware failure, or femoral fracture depending on the choice of implant.

Aros and colleagues reported a large sample of 43,659 patients who underwent surgical repair of an intertrochanteric fracture between 1999 and 2001, representing a 20% sample of Medicare beneficiaries.[7] Mortality was 15% at 30 days and 31% at 1 year, without significant differences depending on the type of stabilization (compression hip screw vs. intramedullary nail). However, revision surgery was needed more commonly in the nail group, with an odds ratio of 1.35 (95% confidence interval, 1.16 to 1.57). Despite the increased need for revision surgery in the nail group, length of index hospital stay, inpatient days during the first 6 months, and costs were only slightly greater in the nail group.[7]

Failure of fixation is influenced by poor bone density and inappropriate patient activity, both of which are beyond the surgeon's direct control. Fracture reduction, implant choice, and implant position are also significant contributors to loss of fixation. The importance of implant position within the center of the femoral head and close to subchondral bone was described by Kyle and coworkers in 1979.[10] In 1995, Baumgaertner and associates defined the TAD as a key variable influencing the risk of implant cut-out from the femoral head.[11] In a later series, Baumgaertner and colleagues showed that awareness of the TAD led to decreased failure.[36] Pervez and coworkers reviewed 23 cases of cut-out and compared them with 77 successfully treated cases. The TAD (corrected for magnification) was the most significant difference between groups, followed by lag screw position on the lateral radiograph, reduction of the fracture in the anteroposterior radiograph, and uncorrected TAD.[40]

Nonunion without implant cut-out of the femoral head rarely occurs. When it does happen, and when the proximal femoral bone and the acetabulum remain healthy, revision open reduction and internal fixation with a blade plate and bone grafting can be successful in more than 90% of cases.[41]

It is clear that complications after intramedullary nailing are different than after use of a compression hip screw. The predominant problem after nailing is fracture, especially when short nails are used. The frequency of this complication has led some authors to recommend that short trochanteric nails should not be used for intertrochanteric fractures.[38] The incidence of fracture collapse appears to be lower when nails are used compared with compression hip screws, especially in unstable fracture patterns.[22] Loss of fixation and cut-out can be minimized by valgus reduction when a compression hip screw is used. A rare complication of intramedullary nails used in intertrochanteric fractures is the so-called *Z effect*, which occurs in nail designs that use two screws for femoral head fixation.[42] The overall incidence of this complication is unknown. With repetitive loading, the inferior screw sometimes backs out of the femoral head while the superior screw migrates farther medially. The reasons for this phenomenon are not understood, although differences in bone density between the femoral head and neck may contribute.[42]

CURRENT CONTROVERSIES AND FUTURE CONSIDERATIONS

- What is the role of minimally invasive plating and/or computer navigation in the treatment of intertrochanteric fractures? Although such techniques are now being reported,[43] long-term studies must be done to document improved outcomes and/or fewer complications before these techniques should be routinely adopted.
- Implant cost should be considered given our current socioeconomic climate. No evidence suggests that the higher cost of cephalomedullary implants is justified on the basis of superior outcomes or fewer complications for routine intertrochanteric femur fractures.

REFERENCES

1. Bhandari M, Schemitsch E, Jönsson A, et al: Gamma nails revisited: gamma nails versus compression hip screws in the management of intertrochanteric fractures of the hip: a meta-analysis. J Orthop Trauma 23:460–464, 2009.
2. Bong SC, Lau HK, Leong JC, et al: The treatment of unstable intertrochanteric fractures of the hip: a prospective trial of 150 cases. Injury 13:139–146, 1981.
3. Kyle RF, Ellis TJ, Templeman DC: Surgical treatment of intertrochanteric hip fractures with associated femoral neck fractures using a sliding hip screw. J Orthop Trauma 19:1–4, 2005.
4. Little NJ, Verma V, Fernando C, et al: A prospective trial comparing the Holland nail with the dynamic hip screw in the treatment of intertrochanteric fractures of the hip. J Bone Joint Surg Br 90:1073–1078, 2008.
5. Platzer P, Thalhammer G, Wozasek GE, Vécsei V: Femoral shortening after surgical treatment of trochanteric fractures in nongeriatric patients. J Trauma 64:982–989, 2008.
6. Im GI, Shin YW, Song Y-J: Potentially unstable intertrochanteric fractures. J Orthop Trauma 19:5–9, 2005.
7. Aros B, Tosteson ANA, Gottlieb DJ, Koval KJ: Is a sliding hip screw or IM nail the preferred implant for intertrochanteric fracture fixation? Clin Orthop Relat Res 466:2827–2832, 2008.
8. Chirodian N, Arch B, Parker MJ: Sliding hip screw fixation of trochanteric hip fractures: outcome of 1024 procedures. Injury 36:793–800, 2005.
9. Kazakos K, Lyras DN, Verettas D, et al: External fixation of intertrochanteric fractures in elderly high-risk patients. Acta Orthop Belg 73:44–48, 2007.
10. Kyle RF, Gustilo RB, Premer RF: Analysis of six hundred and twenty-two intertrochanteric hip fractures: a retrospective and prospective study. J Bone Joint Surg Am 61:216, 1979.
11. Baumgaertner M, Curtin S, Lindskog D, Keggi J: The value of the tip-apex distance in predicting failure of fixation of peritrochanteric fractures of the hip. J Bone Joint Surg Am 77:1058–1064, 1995.
12. Gotfried Y: The lateral trochanteric wall: a key element in the reconstruction of unstable pertrochanteric hip fractures. Clin Orthop Relat Res 425:82–86, 2004.
13. Palm H, Jacobsen S, Sonne-Holm S, et al: Integrity of the lateral femoral wall in intertrochanteric hip fractures: an important predictor of a reoperation. J Bone Joint Surg Am 89:470–475, 2007.
14. Brammer TJ, Kendrew J, Khan RJK, Parker MJ: Reverse obliquity and transverse fractures of the trochanteric region of the femur: a review of 101 cases. Injury 36:851–857, 2005.
15. Haidukewych GJ, Israel TA, Berry DJ: Reverse oblique fractures of the intertrochanteric region of the femur. J Bone Joint Surg Am 83:643–650, 2001.
16. Pajarinen J, Lindahl J, Michelsson O, et al: Pertrochanteric femoral fractures treated with a dynamic hip screw or a proximal femoral nail: a randomised study comparing post-operative rehabilitation. J Bone Joint Surg Br 87:76–81, 2005.
17. Utrilla AL, Reig JS, Muñoz FM, Tufanisco CB: Trochanteric gamma nail and compression hip screw for trochanteric fractures: a randomized, prospective, comparative study in 210 elderly patients with a new design of the gamma nail. J Orthop Trauma 19:229–233, 2005.
18. Adams CI, Robinson CM, Court-Brown CM, McQueen MM: Prospective randomized controlled trial of an intramedullary nail versus dynamic screw and plate for intertrochanteric fractures of the femur. J Orthop Trauma 15:394–400, 2001.
19. Ahrengart L, Törnkvist H, Fornander P, et al: A randomized study of the compression hip screw and gamma nail in 426 fractures. Clin Orthop Relat Res 401:209–222, 2002.
20. Baumgaertner MR, Curtin SL, Lindskog DM: Intramedullary versus extramedullary fixation for the treatment of intertrochanteric hip fractures. Clin Orthop Relat Res 348:87–94, 1998.
21. Crawford CH, Malkani AL, Cordray S, et al: The trochanteric nail versus the sliding hip screw for intertrochanteric hip fractures: a review of 93 cases. J Trauma 60:325–329, 2006.
22. Hardy DC, Descamps PY, Krallis P, et al: Use of an intramedullary hip-screw compared with a compression hip screw with a plate for intertrochanteric femoral fractures: a prospective, randomized study of one hundred patients. J Bone Joint Surg Am 80:618–630, 1998.
23. Harrington P, Nihal A, Singhania AK, Howell FR: Intramedullary hip screw versus sliding hip screw for unstable intertrochanteric femoral fractures in the elderly. Injury 33:23–28, 2002.
24. Leung KS, So WS, Shen WY, Hui PW: Gamma nails and dynamic hip screws for peritrochanteric fractures: a randomized prospective study in elderly patients. J Bone Joint Surg Br 74:345–351, 1992.
25. Egol KA, Chang EY, Cvitkovic J, et al: Mismatch of current intramedullary nails with the anterior bow of the femur. J Orthop Trauma 18:410–415, 2004.
26. Hwang JH, Oh JK, Han SH, et al: Mismatch between PFNa and medullary canal causing difficulty in nailing of the pertrochanteric fractures. Arch Orthop Trauma Surg 28:1443–1446, 2008.
27. Zlowodzki M, Bhandari M, Brown GA: Misconceptions about the mechanical advantages of intramedullary devices for treatment of proximal femur fractures. Acta Orthop 77:169–170, 2006.
28. Walton NP, Wynn-Jones H, Ward MS, Wimhurst JA: Femoral neck-shaft angle in extra-capsular proximal femoral fracture fixation; does it make a TAD of difference? Injury 36:1361–1364, 2005.
29. Bridle SH, Patel AD, Bircher M, Calvert PT: Fixation of intertrochanteric fractures of the femur: a randomized prospective

comparison of the gamma nail and the dynamic hip screw. J Bone Joint Surg Br 73:330–334, 1991.

30. O'Brien PJ, Meek RN, Blachut PA, et al: Fixation of intertrochanteric hip fractures: gamma nail versus dynamic hip screw. A randomized, prospective study. Can J Surg 38:516–520, 1995.

31. Papasimos S, Koutsojannis CM, Panagopoulos A, et al: A randomised comparison of AMBI, TGN and PFN for treatment of unstable trochanteric fractures. Arch Orthop Trauma Surg 125:462–468, 2005.

32. Radford PJ, Needoff M, Webb JK: A prospective randomised comparison of the dynamic hip screw and the gamma locking nail. J Bone Joint Surg Br 75:789–793, 1993.

33. Saudan M, Lübbeke A, Sadowski C, et al: Pertrochanteric fractures: is there an advantage to an intramedullary nail? A randomized, prospective study of 206 patients comparing the dynamic hip screw and proximal femoral nail. J Orthop Trauma 16:386–393, 2002.

34. Koval KJ, Oh CK, Egol KA: Does a traction-internal rotation radiograph help to better evaluate fractures of the proximal femur? Bull Hosp Jt Dis 66:102–106, 2008.

35. Kaufer H: Mechanics of the treatment of hip injuries. Clin Orthop Relat Res 146:53–61, 1980.

36. Baumgaertner MR, Solberg BD: Awareness of tip-apex distance reduces failure of fixation of trochanteric fractures of the hip. J Bone Joint Surg Br 79:969–971, 1997.

37. Kumar AJS, Parmar VN, Kolpattil S, et al: Significance of hip rotation on measurement of 'Tip Apex Distance' during fixation of extracapsular proximal femoral fractures. Injury 38:792–796, 2007.

38. Beaupre LA, Jones CA, Saunders LD, et al: Best practices for elderly hip fracture patients: a systematic overview of the evidence. J Gen Intern Med 20:1019–1025, 2005.

39. Efstathopoulos NE, Nikolaou VS, Lazarettos JT: Intramedullary fixation of intertrochanteric hip fractures: a comparison of two implant designs. Int Orthop 31:71–76, 2007.

40. Pervez H, Parker MJ, Vowler S: Prediction of fixation failure after sliding hip screw fixation. Injury 35:994–998, 2004.

41. Haidukewych GJ, Berry DJ: Salvage of failed internal fixation of intertrochanteric hip fractures. Clin Orthop Relat Res 412:184–188, 2003.

42. Strauss EJ, Kummer FJ, Koval KJ, Egol KA: The "Z-Effect" phenomenon defined: a laboratory study. J Orthop Res 25:1568–1573, 2007.

43. Chong KW, Wong MK, Rikhraj IS, Howe TS: The use of computer navigation in performing minimally invasive surgery for intertrochanteric hip fractures: the experience in Singapore. Injury 37:755–762, 2006.

CHAPTER 46

Subtrochanteric Fractures

George Haidukewych

- The subtrochanteric region experiences extremely high forces that challenge fixation constructs.
- Muscular deforming forces flex, abduct, and externally rotate short proximal fragments, making reduction and fixation difficult.
- Intramedullary fixation is biomechanically favorable and should be considered the treatment of choice for these injuries.
- Accurate starting point placement and reduction during reaming and nail passage are important to avoid malreduction (typically varus, flexion, and external rotation).
- Clamp-assisted reduction and judicious use of cerclage cables can be effective in improving reductions and construct stability. Biologically friendly techniques are important to avoid further fracture devitalization.

INTRODUCTION

Subtrochanteric fractures occur in the proximal femur between the inferior aspect of the lesser trochanter and a distance extending about 5 cm distally. These fractures generally occur in two patient age distributions: the young, polytraumatized population from a high-energy injury, and the osteopenic older population, usually following a low-energy fall from a standing height.[1,2] The subtrochanteric region of the femur is one of the most highly stressed zones in the human skeleton, and tensile or compressive stresses can exceed several multiples of body weight. The frequently short proximal fragments are deformed by the hip flexors and abductors, which may make accurate reduction and fixation challenging. Internal fixation strategies for managing these fractures fall into one of two categories: intramedullary fixation or some form of plating. Many specific challenges must be overcome to ensure stable proximal fragment fixation performed in a biologically friendly manner while accurate alignment and implant position are attained.

INDICATIONS/CONTRAINDICATIONS

Surgical stabilization is the treatment of choice for subtrochanteric fractures in adults. Internal fixation and early patient mobilization to avoid the negative impact of prolonged recumbency are preferred. Although plates such as the angled blade plate or proximal femoral locking plates can be useful for unusually "short" proximal fragments, intramedullary techniques should be considered the preferred stabilization strategy because of their mechanical superiority and biologically friendly implantation methods. Several studies have demonstrated clinical superiority of nails versus plates. Although a detailed analysis of each of these studies is beyond the scope of this chapter, the reader is referred to extensive references on this subject at the end of this chapter for further reading.

PREOPERATIVE PLANNING

For young patients, attention should be focused on prioritization of treating life-threatening injuries using standard Advanced Trauma Life Support (ATLS) protocols. The fractured limb is examined with careful circumferential examination of the skin to rule out an open fracture. The neurovascular status of the limb should be documented. Elderly patients are medically optimized preoperatively.

Radiographic Evaluation

Quality anteroposterior and lateral radiographs provide enough information to guide treatment of the vast majority of subtrochanteric fractures. The length of the proximal fragment and the diameter of the diaphysis distally should be evaluated. A traction view may be helpful in defining fracture geometry and location, if the initial views are unclear. Any proximal fracture extension into the piriformis fossa or greater trochanter, or involvement of the lesser trochanter, can influence the choice of implant. If any concern is raised about fracture extension into the piriformis fossa or the greater trochanter, a computed tomographic scan can be obtained; however, the author finds these rarely necessary. Several classifications exist for subtrochanteric fractures; however, the author finds the Russell-Taylor method the most useful. The Russell-Taylor classification[3] (Fig. 46-1) may guide the surgeon in determining the integrity of the proximal fragment, which historically has facilitated decision making regarding nail or plating choices. The classification is divided based on whether the piriformis fossa is involved and whether the lesser trochanter is involved.

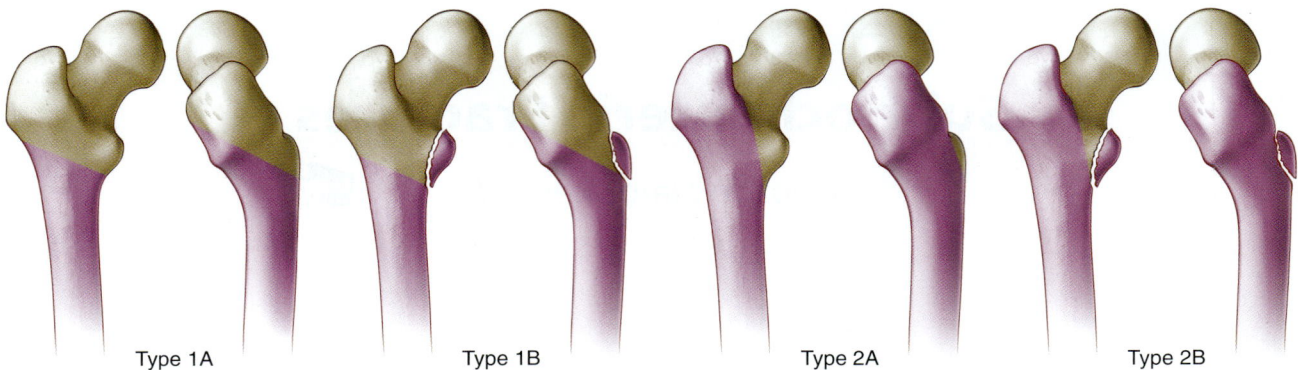

Type 1A   Type 1B   Type 2A   Type 2B

Figure 46-1. Russell-Taylor classification of subtrochanteric fractures of the femur. (Redrawn from Russell TA, Taylor JC: Subtrochanteric fractures of the femur. In Browner BD, Jupiter JB, Levine AM, Trafton PG [eds]: Skeletal trauma, vol 2, Philadelphia, 1992, Saunders, pp 1490–1492.)

Previously, this information would guide decision making regarding standard locking of an intramedullary nail from greater to lesser trochanter or the need for so-called *reconstruction nailing* with cephalomedullary-type fixation. In the past, piriformis fossa extension proximally required plating techniques because surgeons were concerned about losing capture of the proximal fragment during a nailing using a piriformis fossa starting point; the nail could "fall out the back" of the proximal fragment.[1,4] With more contemporary nailing techniques that enter the tip of the greater trochanter, these issues have become less problematic. The common theme for all the various classification schemes proposed is that fractures are classified based on the integrity of the proximal fragment. With modern nailing techniques, however, these classifications no longer influence a "nail versus plate" decision, but may influence the locking configuration. Typically, a standard greater to lesser trochanter locking screw configuration can be used for one-piece proximal fragments, and cephalomedullary locking is used for more complex proximal fragment involvement (Figs. 46-2 through 46-4).

DESCRIPTION OF TECHNIQUE OF INTRAMEDULLARY NAILING OF A SUBTROCHANTERIC FRACTURE

The author prefers to position the patient supine on a fracture table with the involved leg in a traction boot and the other leg placed in the lithotomy position. The use of a fracture table greatly facilitates obtaining a clear proximal-lateral fluoroscopic radiograph, especially in heavy patients, and allows the surgeon to fine-tune the reduction, leg length, and alignment and hold the leg in place during the nailing procedure. Some have advocated the lateral position to facilitate starting point location and reduction by flexing the distal fragment to align with the proximal fragment deformity. This may be of benefit in heavier patients. The lateral position, however, may not be practical in polytraumatized patients. In general, a percutaneous approach is used

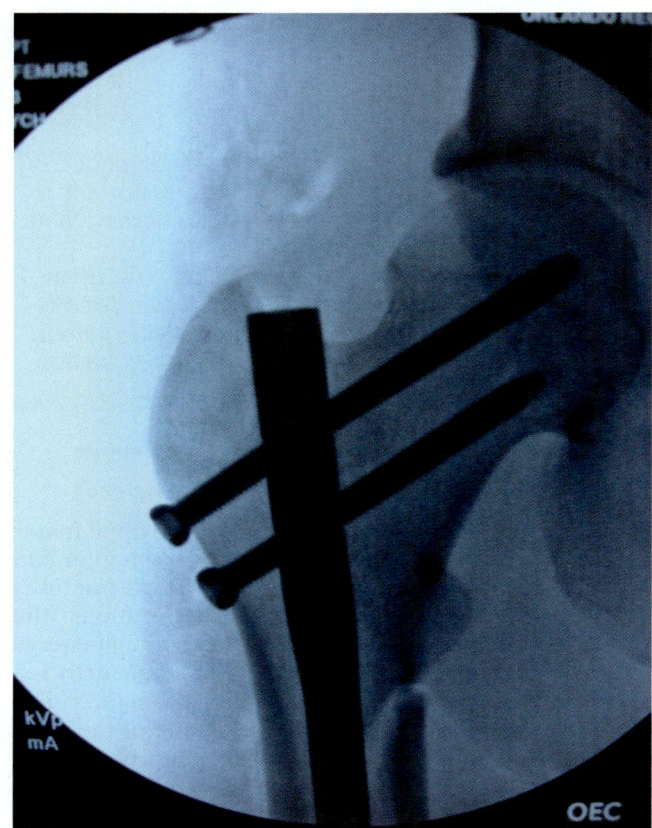

Figure 46-2. Postoperative radiograph of proximal fragment fixation with an intramedullary nail.

for nailing. The author prefers to take a guide pin and place this along the skin laterally, proximal to the greater trochanter, to determine the appropriate nail trajectory and skin entry site to obtain entry into the tip of the greater trochanter. Once this trajectory is known, a stab incision is made in the proximal gluteal area. The incisions required to get the appropriate trajectory can be deceptively proximal. An incision is made in the proximal gluteal area, and a guide pin is placed down to the tip of the trochanter. The author prefers to treat these

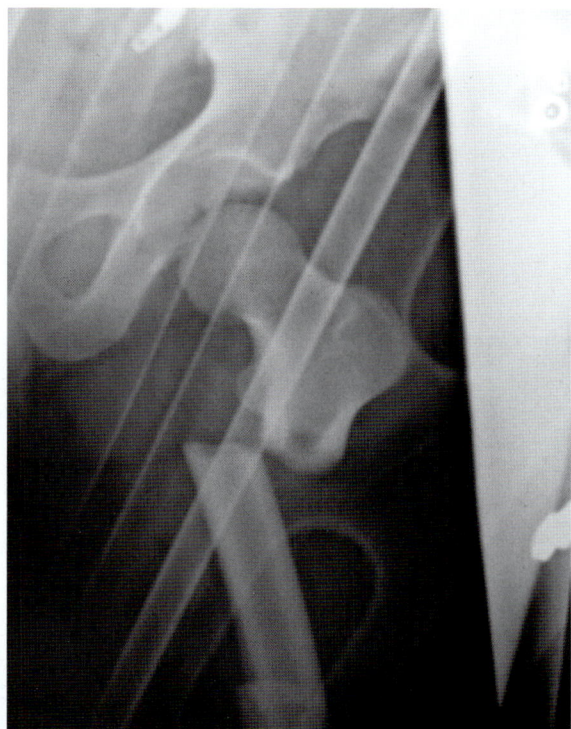

Figure 46-3. Segmental subtrochanteric fracture in a young polytraumatized male.

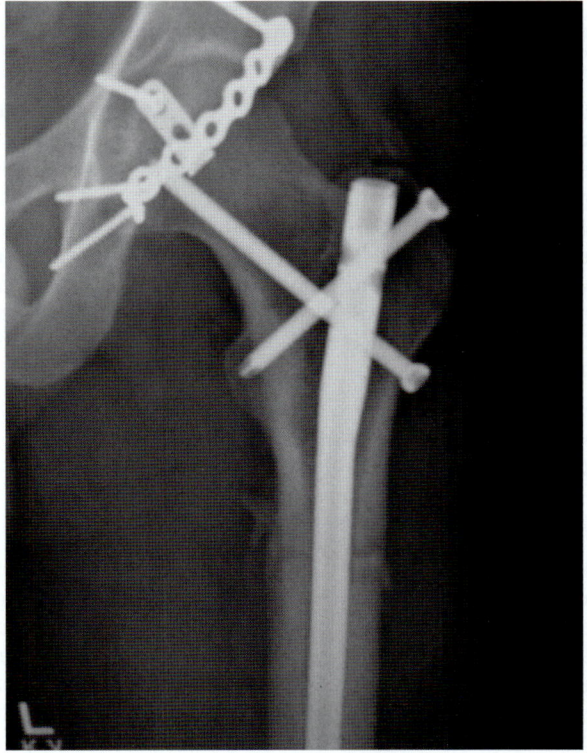

Figure 46-4. Postoperative radiograph after reduction and intramedullary fixation.

fractures with a starting point in the tip of the greater trochanter. The guide pin is placed into the tip of the trochanter or just a few millimeters medially.[5] It is very important not to start even a little lateral to the tip of the trochanter, because this will tend to move the starting point farther laterally with canal preparation and may result in excessive varus of the proximal fragment. The guide pin is placed in the proximal fragment, and the appropriate starter reamer is passed using soft tissue protection sleeves. The guide pin is placed across the fracture.

For "low" (more distal) subtrochanteric fractures that have some intact diaphysis, reduction tools can be used to assist with guide wire placement. These maneuvers are useless if the proximal fragments are short and have large, capacious, osteopenic canals. Appropriate measurements are taken. It is important to avoid running the reamers until the reamer head is well inside the proximal fragment. This will avoid excessive reaming of the starting hole, which can lateralize the entry angle (the starting hole can become an oval). Reaming is performed, and the nail is inserted in the usual fashion. The author selects a nail 1 to 2 mm smaller than the reamer that provided first "chatter" in the diaphysis. Nail length is chosen based on surgeon preference. The author routinely uses long nails and locks them statically distally. Locking screw fixation is placed into the femoral head or neck or into the lesser trochanter based on the indications already discussed. True lateral fluoroscopic projections are used to guide center-center placement of cephalomedullary fixation. In reality, the author typically chooses some form of cephalomedullary fixation for these fractures, because it is difficult to rule out any proximal fracture extensions, and fixation of the femoral head and neck essentially avoids any potential problems with nail containment. Most modern nailing systems allow standard ("greater to lesser trochanteric") or cephalomedullary locking with the same implant.

A "high" subtrochanteric fracture should never be reamed in an unreduced position. If the patient is positioned on the fracture table and significant deformity is still noted in the proximal fragment after gentle traction is applied, then the author typically will attempt some simple percutaneous technique to try to reduce the proximal fragment. This can involve a ball spike pusher placed from anterior to posterior, some form of joystick such as a Schanz pin placed in the lateral cortex, or, more commonly, a percutaneous clamp placed through a very small incision over the lateral femur. The proximal fragment is then reduced, moving it into an extended position, an adducted position, and an internally rotated position relative to its unreduced position. This "reversal" of deforming forces essentially moves the tip of the greater trochanter (or piriformis fossa) into an ideal position to gain access for a starting point, and a starting point can be made in an accurate fashion (Fig. 46-5*A* and *B*). Many different instruments can achieve the reduction; however, the author prefers a percutaneous clamp because it can be repositioned easily (unlike a Schanz pin) and typically will not slip easily (as a ball pike pusher will do). Additionally, a clamp typically

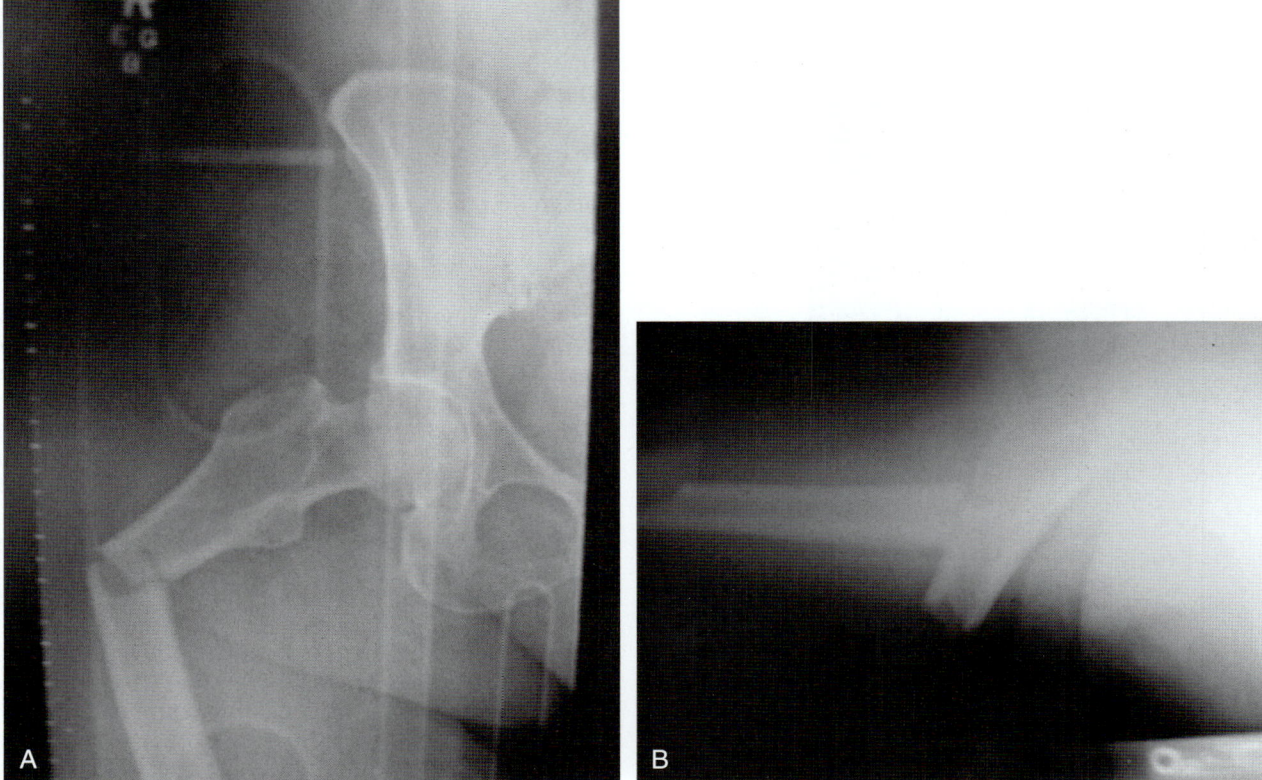

Figure 46-5. A and **B,** Typical flexion, abduction, and external rotation deformity of the proximal fragment.

does not require an assistant to constantly hold it in a reduced position. If one reams the fracture in an unreduced position, it will remain unreduced after the nail is passed because there is no reduction effect of passing the nail, unlike the situation when a diaphyseal femoral fracture is reamed. This typically results in a proximal fragment that is left in varus, external rotation, and flexion—a difficult deformity to manage. It is also important to note that small incisions to improve reduction should not be equated with large incisions with excessive stripping, evacuation of the fracture hematoma, and broad blunt retractors used to reduce the fracture under direct vision. This is not recommended because it will devitalize the tissues and may contribute to nonunion. Cerclage cables generally should be discouraged; however, they occasionally can be useful for supplemental fixation of long spiral or long oblique patterns because nailing these patterns can often leave them distracted. The entire construct is checked fluoroscopically under biplanar evaluation to ensure that excellent fixation and appropriate implant position and length are achieved. The distal femur is evaluated fluoroscopically, especially in the lateral view, in elderly patients with osteopenia and bowed femoral shafts to make sure no distal nail penetration of the cortex occurs anteriorly. The wounds are then irrigated and closed in layers in the usual fashion.

POSTOPERATIVE CARE

The patient is given prophylactic intravenous antibiotics and thromboembolic prophylaxis per surgeon preference. Patients are mobilized on the first postoperative day and are allowed to bear weight as tolerated with gait aids. The author recommends two-arm support (crutches or a walker) for 6 to 12 weeks, depending on fracture geometry and bone quality. Radiographs are obtained at the 6- and 12-week mark, and patients are followed until union, which should be noted by the 4-month mark.

VARIATIONS/UNUSUAL SITUATIONS

Operative Treatment—Plates

Although intramedullary techniques have become the preferred treatment for subtrochanteric fractures, plating is an attractive alternative in some situations. Plating techniques can be useful for subtrochanteric fractures with very short proximal fragments that can be extremely difficult to nail. Several categories of plates can be useful, ranging from a traditional sliding hip screw, a dynamic condylar screw, a 95-degree condylar blade plate, and various locking proximal femoral plates. The obliquity of the fracture should be evaluated carefully if a plating strategy is chosen. For so-called *reverse-obliquity* and *transverse patterns*, sliding hip screws should not be used, as proximal fragment lateralization is uncontrolled and fixation failure has been reported. A 95-degree angled blade plate or a locking plate is a better choice because it resists these proximal lateralizing forces. More recently, anatomically precontoured proximal femoral locking plates were developed to facilitate fixation of such short fractures; however, limited data have documented their efficacy to date. Common features of any plating technique include the need for a relatively large dissection and the fact that plating must be done in a biologically friendly manner (discussed later) to allow relatively rapid healing.[1,6-13] Plates are inherently biomechanically inferior to nails because of their more lateral position (longer lever arm on the proximal fixation) and their non–load-sharing characteristics; therefore, it is critical that a biologically friendly (indirect reduction) technique be chosen for their implantation.

The author generally reserves plating techniques for nonunions and malunions.

PEARLS AND PITFALLS

The most common pitfall of treating any subtrochanteric fracture is malreduction: typically varus, flexion, and external rotation of the proximal fragment with some distraction at the fracture site. Nails are often inserted too laterally in the greater trochanter as well. To avoid this, the author does not hesitate to perform a clamp-assisted nailing, because recent series have shown that this has no detrimental effect on union rates and improves clinical alignment. When plating techniques are used, it is critical to perform these in a biologically friendly fashion, so that only the lateral aspect of the femur is visualized by the surgical dissection. Plating techniques are biomechanically inferior, and although they can be used effectively, they are very dependent on indirect reduction (and bony contact to allow load sharing) to allow rapid healing and avoid hardware failure.

RESULTS

Published data regarding intramedullary fixation of subtrochanteric fractures have generally been good with a high rate of clinical union and a low rate of reoperation. Malalignments are common, and these surgeries can be difficult, with long operative times and significant blood loss. Multiple studies support the superiority of nailing techniques over plating techniques.[1,14-31] Plating techniques can also be effective; however, the best outcomes have been reported with fixed-angle devices implanted with the use of technically demanding indirect reduction techniques. Published data on the management of nonunions have generally demonstrated

Table 46-1. Recent Data on Results of Fixation of Subtrochanteric Femur Fractures

Author, Year	No. of Patients	Treatment	Outcomes
Starr, 2006[36]	34	CMN	100% union, no difference between gamma and recon nailing configuration
Afsari et al, 2009[37]	44	Clamp-assisted CMN	98% union rate
Neogi, 2009[38]	40	IRB plating	100% union
Celebi, 2006[6]	33	IRB plating	100% union
Rahme, 2007[39]	58	RCT nail vs. plate	Plate 28% failure, nails 0% failure
Shukla, 2007[26]	57	CMN	95% union, varus associated with poor results
Cheng, 2005[40]	64	CMN	100% union
Miedel, 2005[41]	16	Nail vs. plate	Plate 17% failure, nail 0% failure

CMN, Cephalomedullary nailing; *IRB,* indirect reduction biologic; *RCT,* randomized controlled trial.

good outcomes if stable proximal fragment fixation can be obtained (Table 46-1).

COMPLICATIONS

Malunion

Malunion can result in varus alignment to the proximal femur, which decreases abductor efficiency by a more proximal position of the greater trochanter. This can also affect limb length and rotation.[32] The amount of deformity that is problematic remains undefined, so the surgeon will have to individualize treatment decisions based on patient complaints and physical examination. No large published series on the management of proximal subtrochanteric malunion are available; however, corrective osteotomy may be indicated if the deformity is severe. The author prefers to use a 95-degree angled blade plate in this situation, because the plate can be placed in the proximal fragment and corrective osteotomy performed at the apex of the deformity, and when the plate is reduced to the femoral shaft, correct alignment is usually obtained—similar to the technique used for indirect reduction of acute fractures. The blade typically can be placed in the inferior femoral head—an area unlikely to be violated by previous internal fixation devices.

Nonunion

Nonunion is a rare but problematic complication of subtrochanteric fracture. Treatment of nonunion will vary; however, the surgeon must determine whether the fracture is aligned in a suitable fashion and can be treated with an exchange nailing, or whether there is concomitant malalignment that will require realignment via a full nonunion takedown. In general, if the nonunion is well aligned and was previously nailed, the author prefers to perform an exchange nailing with a larger-diameter nail in a closed fashion. A nail with a different locking screw configuration into the proximal fragment may provide better fixation if bony defects from prior fixation are present. If hardware failure has occurred, if the proximal fragment is short, or if malalignment is problematic, the author prefers an open plating technique with a 95-degree blade plate. Usually a full nonunion takedown—removing all fibrous tissue from the nonunion site—will be required, and compression must be achieved. Several studies have demonstrated that successful union can be attained as long as stable proximal fragment fixation can be attained.[33-35] Arthroplasty may play a role in multiply operated nonunion in the elderly patient, especially if the proximal fragment has massive bone defects from prior fixation attempts or articular damage from screw cut-out.

Infection

Infection remains one of the most challenging complications to manage and is often associated with nonunion. Early postoperative infection is managed with débridement, retention of stable hardware, and a period of intravenous organism-specific antibiotics. Chronic infection or infection with loose or broken hardware is managed by removal of all hardware, irrigation and débridement, and a period of intravenous organism-specific antibiotics. Intramedullary antibiotic spacers can be useful as well to provisionally stabilize the subtrochanteric region. Definitive fixation with or without bone grafting is performed after eradication of infection. For extremely unstable fractures, temporary external fixation can be useful until definitive fixation can occur.

CONTROVERSIES AND FUTURE DIRECTIONS

- Navigated or robotized reduction of complex proximal fragment deformities may minimize malunion.
- Percutaneous, jig-targeted proximal femoral locking plates may address some of the reduction, alignment, and biological challenges of fixation in this region.
- Nails with innovative locking configurations may be applicable to a wide variety of subtrochanteric fracture patterns.

REFERENCES

1. Bedi A, Toanle T: Subtrochanteric femur fractures. Orthop Clin N Am 35:473–483, 2004. Review.
2. Fielding JW, Magliato HJ: Subtrochanteric fractures. Surg Gynecol Obstet 122:555–569, 1966.
3. Russell TA, Taylor JC: Subtrochanteric fractures of the femur. In Browner BD, Jupiter JB, Levine AM, Trafton PG (eds): Skeletal trauma, vol 2, Philadelphia, 1992, Saunders, pp 1490–1492.
4. Garnavos C, Peterman A, Howard PW: The treatment of difficult proximal femoral fractures with the Russell-Taylor reconstruction nail. Injury 30:407–415, 1999.
5. Ostrum RF, Marcantonio A, Margurger R: A critical analysis of the eccentric starting point for trochanteric intramedullary femoral nailing. J Orthop Trauma 19:681–686, 2005.
6. Celebi L, Cam M, Muratli HH, et al: Indirect reduction and biological internal fixation of comminuted subtrochanteric fractures of the femur. Injury 37:740–750, 2006.
7. Hasenboehler EA, Agudelo JF, Morgan SJ, et al: Treatment of complex proximal femoral fractures with the proximal femur locking compression plate. Orthopedics 30:618–623, 2007.
8. Kinast C, Bolhofner BR, Mast JW, et al: Subtrochanteric fractures of the femur: results of treatment with the 95 condylar blade-plate. Clin Orthop Relat Res 28:122–130, 1989.
9. Krettek C, Muller M, Miclau T: Evolution of minimally invasive plate osteosynthesis (MIPO) in the femur. Injury 32(Suppl 3):SC14–SC23, 2001.
10. Krettek C, Schandelmaier P, Miclau T, Tscherne H: Minimally invasive percutaneous plate osteosynthesis (MIPPO) using the DCS in proximal and distal femoral fractures. Injury 28(Suppl 1):A20–A30, 1997.
11. Neher C, Ostrum RF: Treatment of subtrochanteric femur fractures using a submuscular fixed low-angle plate. Am J Orthop 32(9 Suppl):29–33, 2003.
12. Perren SM: Evolution of the internal fixation of long bone fractures: the scientific basis of biological internal fixation: choosing a new balance between stability and biology. J Bone Joint Surg Br 84:1093–1110, 2002.
13. Sanders R, Regazzoni P: Treatment of subtrochanteric femur fractures using the dynamic condylar screw. J Orthop Trauma 3:206–213, 1989.
14. Brien WW, Wiss DA, Becker V Jr, Lehman T: Subtrochanteric femur fractures: a comparison of the Zickel nail, 95 degrees blade plate, and interlocking nail. J Orthop Trauma 5:458–464, 1991.
15. Broos PL, Reynders P: The use of the unreamed AO femoral intramedullary nail with spiral blade in nonpathologic fractures of the femur: experiences with eighty consecutive cases. J Orthop Trauma 16:150–154, 2002.
16. French BG, Tornetta P: Use of an interlocked cephalomedullary nail for subtrochanteric fracture stabilization. Clin Orthop Relat Res 348:95–100, 1998.
17. Kraemer WJ, Hearn TC, Powell JN, et al: Fixation of segmental subtrochanteric fractures: a biomechanical study. Clin Orthop Relat Res 332:71–79, 1996.
18. Kummer FJ, Olsson O, Pearlman CA, et al: Intramedullary versus extramedullary fixation of subtrochanteric fractures: a biomechanical study. Acta Orthop Scand 69:580–584, 1998.
19. Lee PC, Hsieh PH, Yu SW, et al: Biologic plating versus intramedullary nailing for comminuted subtrochanteric fractures in young adults: a prospective, randomized study of 66 cases. J Trauma 63:1283–1291, 2007.
20. Leung KS, Tang N, Yue W: Early clinical experience of gamma nail: AP nailing with fluoro-navigation. Osteosynthesis and Trauma Care 13:46–49, 2005.
21. Mahonmed MN, Harrington IJ, Hearn TC: Biomechanical analysis of the Medoff sliding plate. J Trauma 48:93–100, 2000.
22. Pai CH: Dynamic condylar screw for subtrochanteric femur fractures with greater trochanteric extension. J Orthop Trauma 10:317–322, 1996.
23. Pugh KJ, Morgan RA, Gorczyca JT, et al: A mechanical comparison of subtrochanteric femur fracture fixation. J Orthop Trauma 12:324–429, 1998.
24. Rantanen J, Aro HT: Intramedullary fixation of high subtrochanteric femoral fractures: a study comparing two implant designs, the gamma nail and the intramedullary hip screw. J Orthop Trauma 12:249–252, 1998.
25. Robinson CM, Houslian S, Khan LA: Trochanteric entry long cephalomedullary nailing of subtrochanteric fractures caused

by low-energy trauma. J Bone Joint Surg Am 87:2217–2226, 2005.

26. Shukla S, Johnston P, Ahmad MA, et al: Outcome of traumatic subtrochanteric femoral fractures fixed using cephalomedullary nails. Injury 38:1286–1293, 2007.

27. Trafton PG: Subtrochanteric-intertrochanteric femoral fractures. Orthop Clin North Am 18:59–71, 1987.

28. Van Doorn R, Stapert JW: The long gamma nail in the treatment of 329 subtrochanteric fractures with major extension into the femoral shaft. Eur J Surg 166:240–246, 2000.

29. Waddell JP: Subtrochanteric fractures of the femur: a review of 130 patients. J Trauma 19:585–592, 1979.

30. Wiss DA, Brien WW: Subtrochanteric fractures of the femur: results of treatment by interlocking nailing. Clin Orthop Relat Res 283:231–236, 1992.

31. Wu CC, Shin CH, Lee ZL: Subtrochanteric fractures treated with interlocking nailing. J Trauma 31:326–333, 1991.

32. Guggenheim JJ, Probe RA, Brinker MR: The effects of femoral shaft malrotation on lower extremity anatomy. J Orthop Trauma 18:658–664, 2004.

33. Barquet A: The treatment of subtrochanteric nonunions with the long gamma nail: twenty-six patients with a minimum 2-year follow-up. J Orthop Trauma 19:294, 2005.

34. deVries JS, Kloen P, Boren SO, et al: Treatment of subtrochanteric nonunions. Injury 37:203–211, 2006.

35. Haidukewych GJ, Berry DJ: Non-union of fractures of the subtrochanteric region of the femur. Clin Orthop Relat Res 419:185–188, 2004.

36. Starr AJ, Hay MT, Reinert CM, et al: Cephalomedullary nails in the treatment of high-energy proximal femur fractures in young patients: a prospective, randomized comparison of trochanteric versus piriformis fossa entry portal. J Orthop Trauma 20:240–246, 2006.

37. Afsari A, Liporace F, Lindvall E, et al: Clamp-assisted reduction of high subtrochanteric fractures of the femur. J Bone Joint Surg Am 91:1913–1918, 2009.

38. Neogi DS, Trikha V, Mishra KK, et al: Biological plate fixation of comminuted subtrochanteric fractures with the dynamic condylar screw: a clinical study. Acta Orthop Belg 75:497–503, 2009.

39. Rahme DM, Harris IA: Intramedullary nailing versus fixed angle blade plating for subtrochanteric femoral fractures: a prospective randomized controlled trial. J Orthop Surg 15:278–281, 2007.

40. Cheng MT, Chiu FY, Chuang TY, et al: Treatment of complex subtrochanteric fracture with the long gamma AP locking nail: a prospective evaluation of 64 cases. J Trauma 58:304–311, 2005.

41. Miedel R, Ponzer S, Törnkvist H, et al: The standard gamma nail or the Medoff sliding plate for unstable trochanteric and subtrochanteric fractures: a randomized, controlled trial. J Bone Joint Surg Br 87:68–75, 2005.

Acetabular Fracture

Brett Bolhofner

INTRODUCTION

The acetabulum is a socket-like structure contained within the innominate bone (Fig. 47-1). It consists of two basic components: the anterior and posterior columns.[1] It is a complex three-dimensional structure, which, in contrast to long bones, is more difficult to visualize and understand from standard planar radiographs. Fractures of the acetabulum provide unique challenges in diagnosis and treatment. Although many surgeons may be comfortable with even difficult fractures on the femoral side of the hip, the same cannot be said for the pelvic side. Reasons for this include the difficulty of (1) understanding the complex three-dimensional geometry of the innominate bone of which the acetabulum is a part, (2) safely accessing the fracture fragments, which may lie deep within the pelvic anatomy, and then (3) accurately reducing and fixing the fractures themselves. Surgical treatment of these injuries depends on knowledge and skill regarding the intrapelvic structures, which often are not part of the acumen of the orthopedic surgeon. Although complications and surgical misadventures in long bone surgery may contribute to morbidity confined to the musculoskeletal system and the particular extremity involved, complications in this type of surgery may also involve multiple unfamiliar organ systems to which the orthopedist often is not exposed.

In contrast to other "articular" reductions, surgical treatment of acetabular fracture is frequently an indirect reduction of the joint, because the actual articular surface is rarely directly visualized. Essentially, bony landmarks are reduced and reconstructed, and the articular reduction is assessed radiographically.

Entire volumes and fellowships have been dedicated to this complex subject, so the purpose of this chapter is to provide an overview and/or review for the unfamiliar reader who may encounter these injuries.

The basic problems are as follows:
1. Assessment of fracture pattern.
2. Decision for surgery: Will outcome be improved by surgical intervention? Is surgery indicated, feasible, or advisable?
3. Difficult and complex surgical approaches.
4. Difficulty accessing, reducing, and fixing fracture fragments.

INCIDENCE AND ETIOLOGY

The incidence of acetabular fracture is believed to be approximately 3 in 100,000 patients; primary causes include motor vehicle accidents and falls from a height.[2] Although many are high-energy injuries, low-energy fractures may occur in situations of bony insufficiency. The primary mechanism is a blow to the femur at the level of the knee or trochanter. Because of the infinite positions of the femur related to the pelvis at the time of injury, as well as the infinite directions and amounts of force, fracture pattern variability is high. Acetabular fractures frequently may be associated with other life-threatening injuries.

CLASSIFICATION

The classification of Leournal and Judet,[1] which has been shown to have high interobserver and intraobserver reliability, remains the standard.[3] Classification consists of the following five elementary patterns (Fig. 47-2):
1. Anterior wall fracture
2. Anterior column fracture
3. Posterior wall fracture
4. Posterior column fracture
5. Transverse fracture

Five associated fracture patterns include the following (Fig. 47-3):
1. Anterior column plus posterior hemitransverse
2. Posterior column plus posterior wall

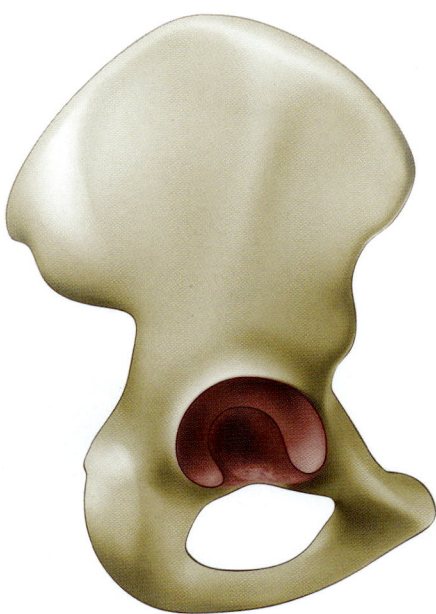

Figure 47-1. Innominate bone with acetabulum.

3. Transverse plus posterior wall
4. T-shaped fractures
5. Both-column fractures

Infinite variations in fracture geometry may exist in nature. The purpose of this classification was not just merely to categorize fracture patterns but to define which surgical approach would best fit the particular fracture pattern, because no single approach is ideal for all of these injuries.

INDICATIONS

Main considerations for deciding on nonoperative versus operative treatment include the following:
1. Displacement
2. Location
3. Stability
4. Patient-related factors

The goal of surgical intervention is to restore the articular surface to anatomicity when and if possible, so that hip joint function may be preserved and ensuing arthrosis may be prevented. Incongruity is poorly tolerated in this load-bearing joint[4,5] and likely will lead to poor outcomes.

Nonoperative Treatment

Less than 3 mm of articular incongruity is probably the threshold that would be accepted for nonoperative treatment, but of course, other factors such as patient age, comorbidities, and the location of the displacement matter as well.[1] An intact roof arc or weight-bearing dome has been shown to be the most critical area to assess and relates most closely to the prognosis for the secondary development of arthrosis[4,6-8] (Fig. 47-4). Roof arc measurements may not be helpful, however, in both column fractures, where relative congruence of the acetabular fragments to the head may exist, even though the hip is not in its proper location in space relative to the axial skeleton. Furthermore, roof arc measurements are not useful for all fracture patterns: for example, they would not be helpful at all for determining the need for surgical intervention for posterior wall fractures. Close clinical and radiographic follow-up is necessary in nonoperative treatment to evaluate the patient for any secondary displacement during early healing. Stress views may be helpful in predicting secondary displacement for fractures where the stability of the hip is uncertain from radiographs alone.[9]

Operative Treatment

Patient-related factors including age, medical comorbidities, survivability, activity, and functional level, and whether or not the fracture can actually be reconstructed, must be considered in the decision for surgical intervention or nonoperative treatment.

Summary of Surgical Indications

1. Loss of congruency between the femoral head and the acetabulum
2. Greater than 2 mm displacement of the weight-bearing dome
3. Instability or 25% or more of wall involvement in posterior wall fractures
4. Significant intra-articular loose fragments (not small foveal fragments)

When surgical intervention is contemplated, the timing is important, because better results have been reported when surgery is undertaken within 3 weeks of injury. In general, adequate time for assessment of the fracture pattern and the patient as a whole should be taken; however, there are a few indications for immediate intervention; these include irreducible fracture dislocation of the hip, open fracture, and fractures with progressive neurologic or vascular compromise. Local tissue conditions, including the presence of a Morelle-Lavalle injury, abrasions, etc., must be considered.

PREOPERATIVE PLANNING AND ASSESSMENT

Assessment of the patient as a whole is paramount because associated injuries, some of which may be life threatening, may be present.

Specific evaluation of the fracture itself includes initial plain radiographs followed by Judet views,[1] which are 45 degree oblique radiographs. This involves turning the patient 45 degrees, which may require sedation in the acute setting. Judet views, as initially described, are necessary to define fracture patterns in a bone of complex shape within the limitation of single-plane imaging. Computed tomography (CT) scanning is necessary to evaluate specific intra-articular fractures, including especially marginal impaction. Three-dimensional CT scanning has not yet replaced Judet views but may

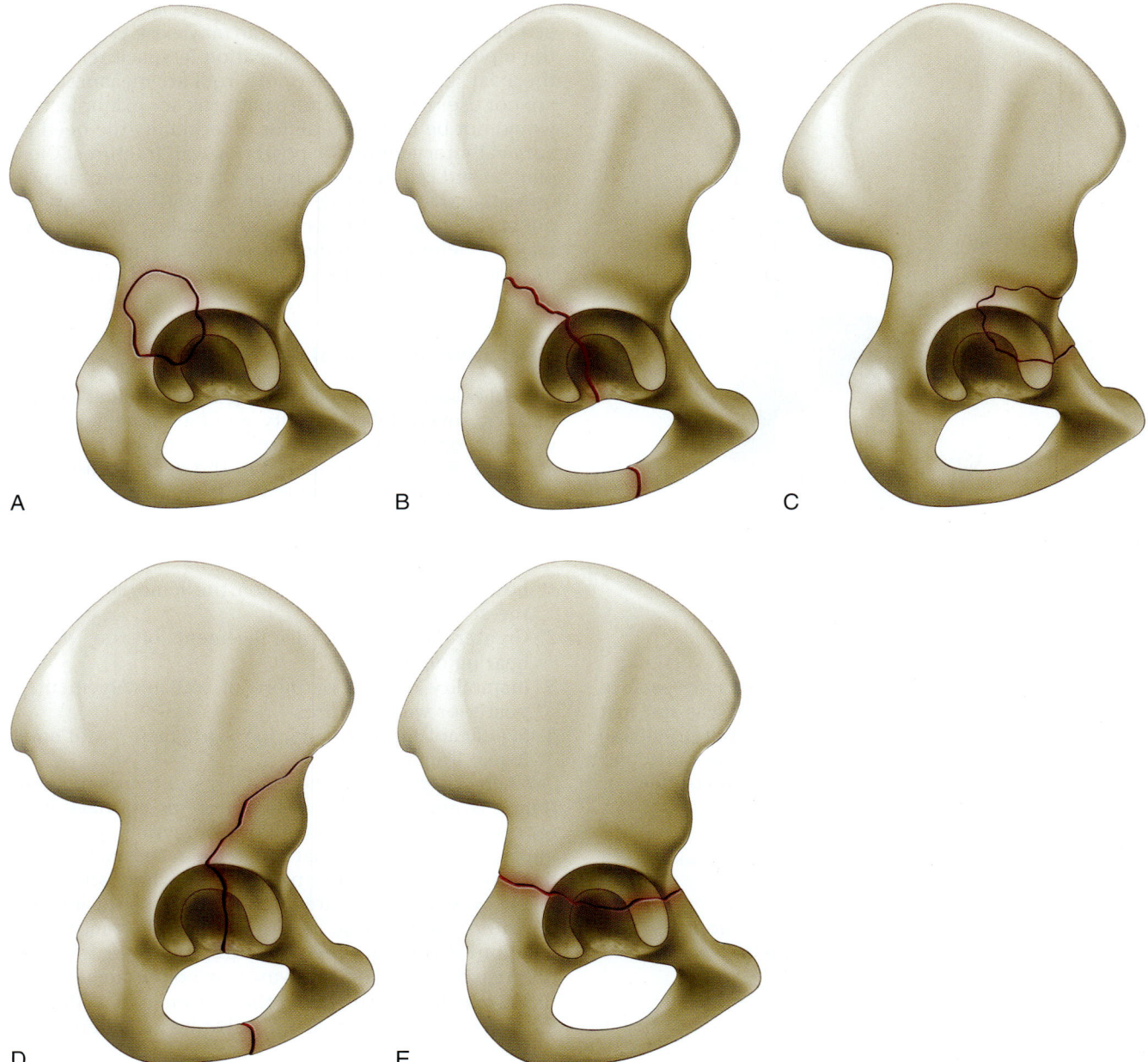

Figure 47-2. Elementary fracture patterns according to Letournel and Judet. **A,** Posterior wall. **B,** Posterior column. **C,** Anterior wall. **D,** Anterior column. **E,** Transverse.

provide the surgeon with a clearer picture of the fracture lines and their displacements and does not require turning the acutely injured patient.

Once the decision for surgery has been made, the following basic requirements must be present:

1. Experienced surgeon
2. Good operating room team with adequate assistance
3. A surgical table that facilitates reduction and imaging (Fig. 47-5)
4. Adequate intraoperative imaging
5. A large volume of specialized reduction clamps and instruments (Fig. 47-6)
6. Specialized implants, including extra-long screws and plates that can be contoured readily (reconstruction plates)

SURGICAL TECHNIQUE AND APPROACHES

Surgical approaches are selected according to the fracture pattern. They may be divided into two basic categories:

1. *Extrapelvic or posterior approaches:* These include the Kocher-Langenbeck, extended iliofemoral, and

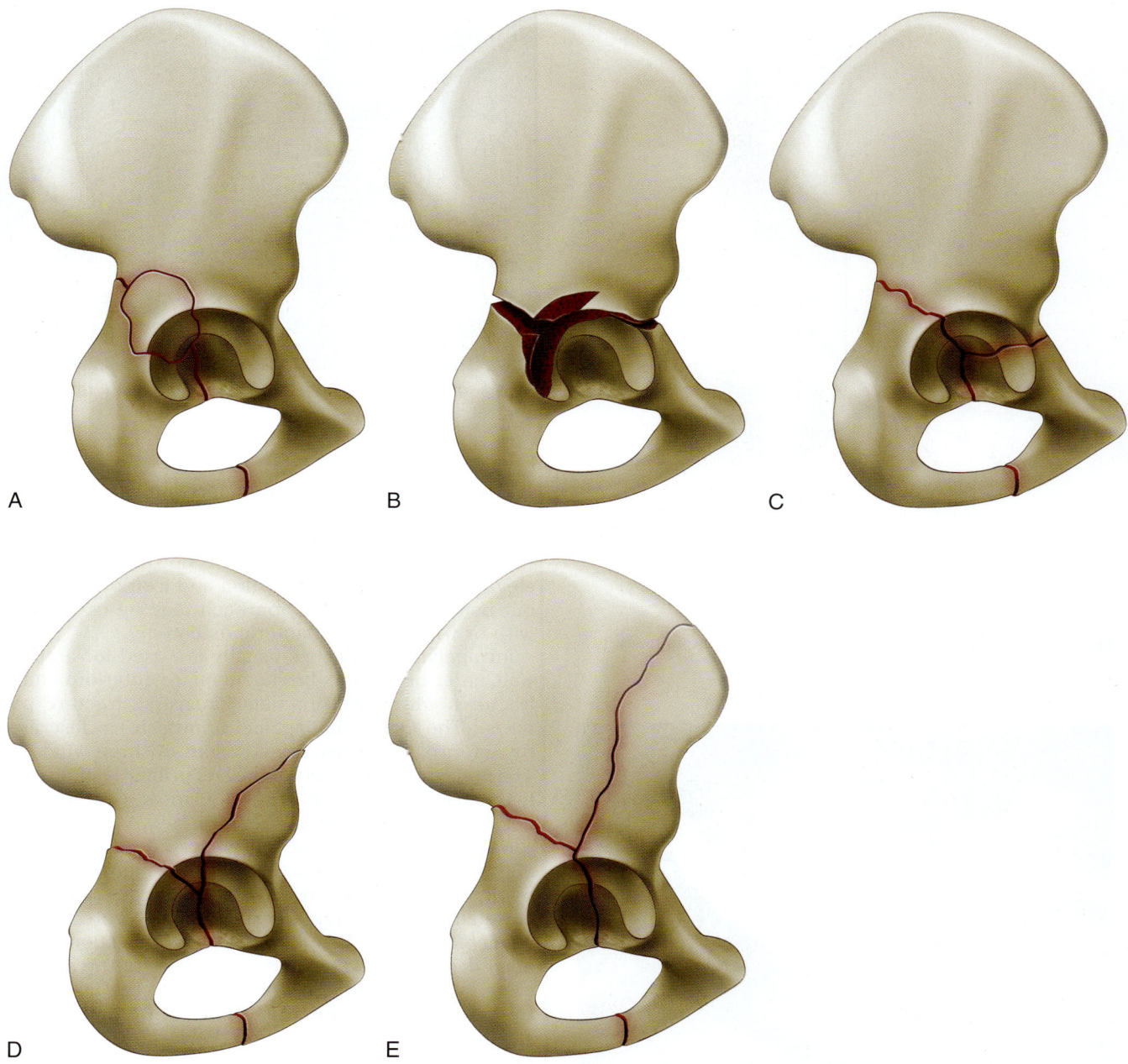

A

B

C

D

E

Figure 47-3. Associated fracture patterns according to Letournel and Judet. **A,** Posterior column posterior wall. **B,** Transverse posterior wall. **C,** T-shaped fractures. **D,** Anterior column posterior hemitransverse. **E,** Both columns.

Gibson straight lateral approaches with or without trochanteric osteotomy or surgical dislocation[10] (Fig. 47-7).

2. *Intrapelvic or anterior approaches:* These include the ilioinguinal and modified Stoppa approaches. Multiple miscellaneous combined surgical approaches also have been described (Fig. 47-8).

The Kocher-Langenbeck surgical approach is most suitable for posterior fracture pathology, including posterior wall fractures, posterior column fractures, and some transverse fractures. This approach involves a posterolateral curvilinear incision, splitting the gluteus maximus, and may be carried out in the prone or lateral

position. The external rotators are transected for access to the retroacetabular surface. Transection should be carried out at least a centimeter from the femoral insertion of the short rotators—very different from the way they are detached during a posterior approach for a total hip arthroplasty, because of vascular concerns regarding the blood supply to the femoral head. The approach is limited distally by the quadratus femoris and proximally by the superior gluteal neurovascular bundle.

The extended iliofemoral approach[1] exposes the entire external aspect of the ileum essentially by elevating the musculature as a large posteriorly based flap or

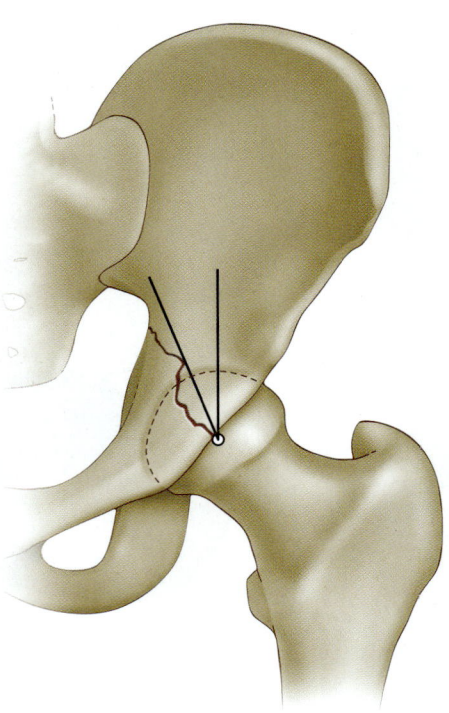

Figure 47-4. Anteroposterior (AP) roof arc measurement.

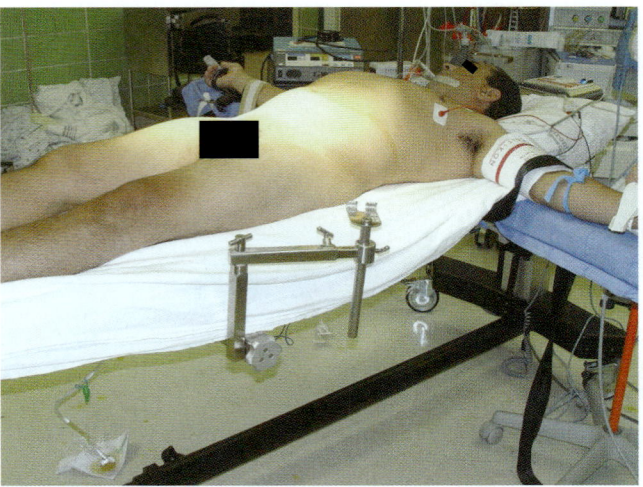

Figure 47-5. Patient supine on a radiolucent table equipped with a lateral traction apparatus. One of various options for an anterior or intrapelvic approach.

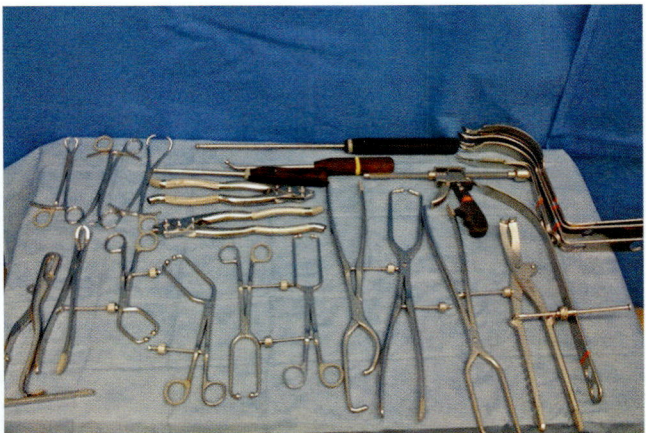

Figure 47-6. Various specialized clamps, reduction tools, and retractors.

The Gibson or straight lateral incision may be carried out in the prone or lateral position. The gluteus maximus is not split but is retracted as a whole posteriorly. Further, the external rotators are not divided but are elevated, and fracture reduction and fixation is carried out beneath them. This approach may be carried out with or without a trochanteric osteotomy.

Intrapelvic approaches usually are used for anterior wall, anterior column, both-column, or anterior column fractures with posterior hemitransverse fracture patterns.[1] The classic ilioinguinal approach as described by Letournal involves development of three windows. The first or lateral window consists primarily of the iliac fossa. The second or middle window is developed between the iliopsoas and femoral nerve laterally and the iliac vessels medially. This window requires incision of the iliopectineal fascia. The medial window is formed by dividing the rectus transversely to access the space of Retzius. Neurovascular structures are protected and retracted during this approach. Modifications have been described allowing greater access to the ilium by more lateral positioning and extending the incision to the posterior superior iliac spine.[14] Alternatively, the sartorius–tensor fascia lata interval has been described as a modification to allow access to the hip joint anteriorly.[15]

The modified Stoppa anterior surgical approach[16] involves a transverse suprapubic incision and division of the rectus in the midline without transection. The ipsilateral hip is flexed, and the surgeon works from the contralateral side of the table. The rectus, neurovascular structures, and iliopsoas are retracted anteriorly, allowing access to the true pelvis and portions of the pelvic rim. This approach is frequently combined with application of lateral traction and also with the lateral (first) window of the ilioinguinal approach via a Smith Peterson approach (two incisions) (Fig. 47-9A-D).

A combination of approaches may be necessary for specific fractures and acetabular fractures associated with pelvic ring and proximal femur lesions. The choice of procedure will depend on accurate preoperative fracture assessment.

pedicle with or without a trochanteric osteotomy. It is usually reserved for certain T-shaped fractures, certain both-column fractures, and some transverse fractures with associated posterior wall pathology. It is most often indicated in complex fractures older than 3 weeks. Various modifications of the iliofemoral approach have been described.[10,11] Heterotopic ossification and devitalization of muscle and bone are primary concerns with this approach.[12,13]

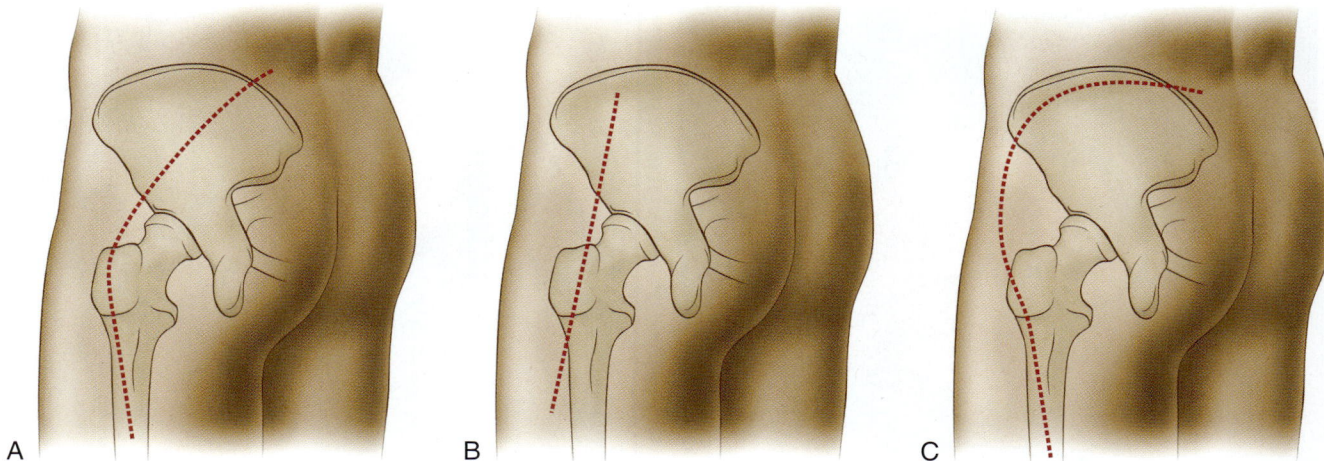

Figure 47-7. Extrapelvic or posterior incisions. **A,** Kocher-Langenbeck. **B,** Gibson. **C,** Extended iliofemoral.

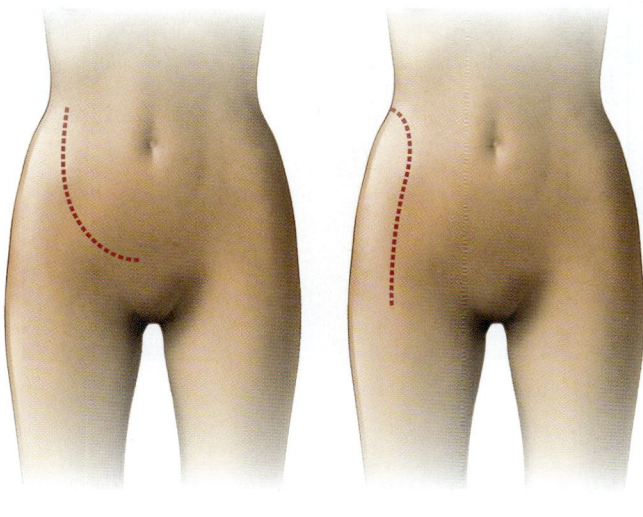

Figure 47-8. Intrapelvic or anterior incisions. **A,** Ilioinguinal. **B,** Stoppa (optional Smith Peterson or lateral window—dotted line).

SURGICAL APPROACH BY FRACTURE PATTERN

Following are general guidelines:

1. *Posterior wall:* extrapelvic or posterior approach
2. *Posterior column:* extrapelvic or posterior approach
3. *Posterior column with posterior wall:* extrapelvic or posterior approach
4. *Anterior wall:* intrapelvic or Smith Peterson approach
5. *Both-column fracture:* intrapelvic and extrapelvic surgical approaches, depending on fracture pattern and displacements. Possible combined intrapelvic and extrapelvic approaches (Fig. 47-10*A-J*)
6. *Transverse fracture:* extrapelvic and/or intrapelvic, depending on the level of the transverse fracture and displacement

7. *Transverse fracture plus posterior wall:* extrapelvic approach or combined intrapelvic and extrapelvic approaches, depending on the transverse pattern
8. *T-shaped fracture:* extrapelvic or combined approaches
9. *Anterior plus posterior hemitransverse:* intrapelvic
10. *Posterior column plus posterior wall:* extrapelvic or posterior approach

THE SPECIAL CASE OF THE POSTERIOR WALL

Because fractures of the posterior wall are the most common type of acetabular fracture, and because they are the type of acetabular fracture most likely to be treated by the orthopedic surgeon, they are deserving of special discussion. This is especially true because although they may appear relatively simple, fractures of the posterior wall have disproportionately poor results compared with other fracture types.[4,17]

As many as one third of acetabular fractures may be posterior wall injuries. Poorer results have been attributed to (1) delays in reduction, (2) intra-articular comminution and marginal impaction, (3) avascular necrosis, and (4) age greater than 50 years.[17] These situations, along with residual postoperative displacement, give the poorest prognosis for arthritis.[18]

Patient assessment includes evaluating the patient for the presence of a dislocation and reducing it promptly. Sciatic nerve function needs to be evaluated and documented. Once a posterior wall fracture has been diagnosed, and the hip, when dislocated, has been reduced, the size of the posterior fragment and the stability of the hip should be assessed clinically and radiographically. This may involve examination or stress views under anesthesia.[9] Assessment of the need for operative treatment focuses on the amount of the posterior wall involved and the stability of the hip. Unstable fractures need immediate reduction, along with the application of skeletal traction to maintain the hip in a

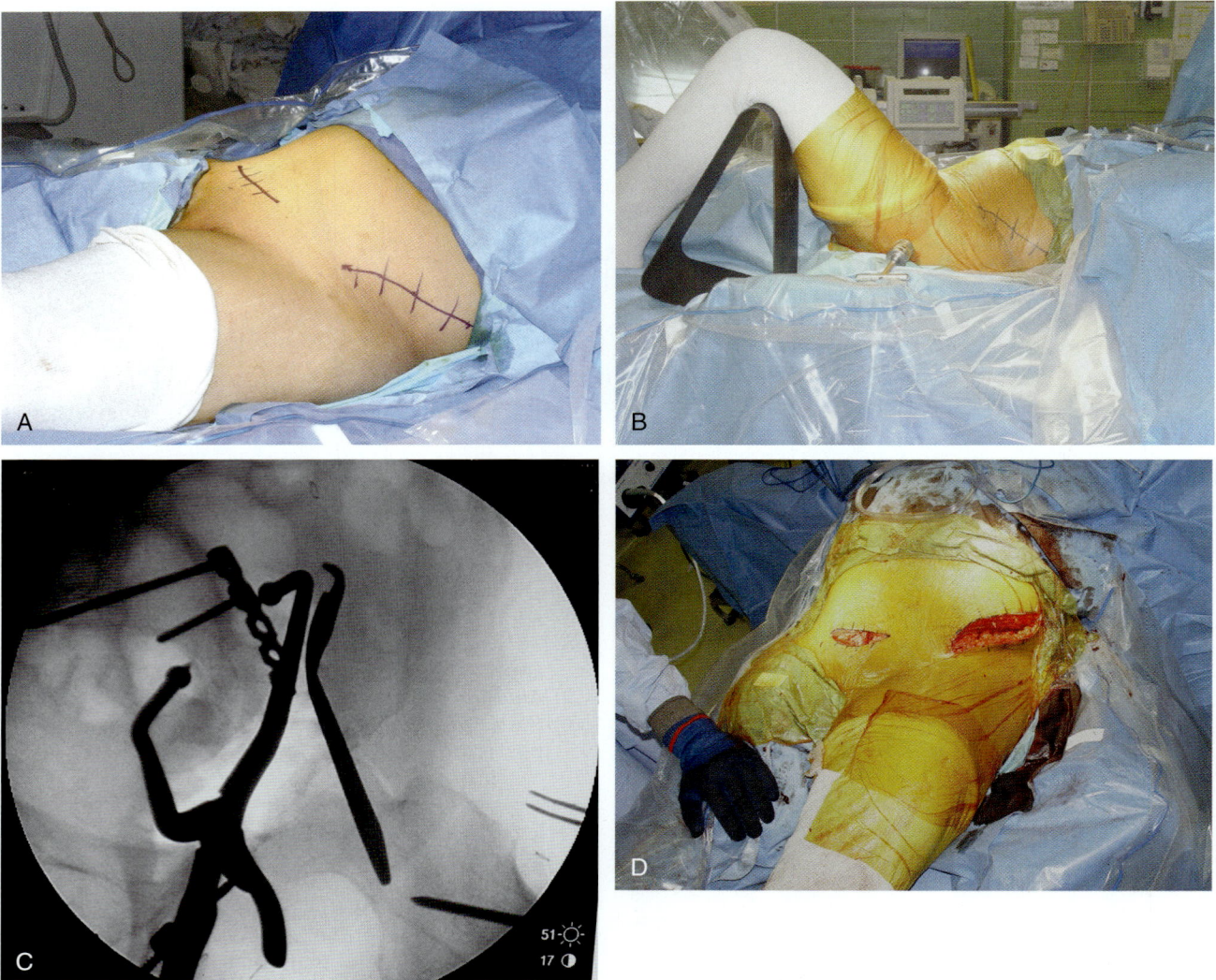

Figure 47-9. Modified Stoppa with lateral window. **A,** Planned incisions with draping. **B,** Operative side leg flexed to relax iliopsoas. Lateral traction apparatus attached to seven-handle Chuck and Schantz screw. **C,** Intraoperative fluoro view with clamp, plate, retractor, and Schantz screw. **D,** Incisions at time of closure.

reduced position until internal fixation can be carried out. Even small posterior wall defects may have significant biomechanical implications.[19]

Fixation is carried out via the use of plates and screws, along with bone grafting for marginal articular impaction. The role of bioabsorbable fixation for small marginal impaction or comminuted fragments is not clearly defined. Labral and rim lesions may require the addition of a spring plate and/or suture anchors. It is imperative as fixation approaches the rim that plates or screws do not come into contact with the femoral head. The viability of the femoral head may be assessed at the time of surgery by drilling a 2 mm drill hole and observing whether or not the head bleeds.

In general, the femoral head is used as a template[1] for reduction of posterior wall fractures. Surgical hip dislocation has been advocated[10]; this allows direct visualization of the articular reconstruction but circumvents using the head as a template. However, for the overwhelming majority of fractures, this maneuver is not necessary and a routine Kocher-Langenbeck approach will suffice.

Improved results have been reported with contemporary open reduction internal fixation (ORIF) techniques.[17] Even with improved hip scores, however, the Musculoskeletal Function Assessment (MFA) demonstrates incomplete recovery with respect to activities of daily living.[18,20]

The goals of surgery are to remove loose bodies (Fig. 47-11), repair marginal impaction and comminution, and restore hip stability. Removal of intra-articular loose bodies requires the hip to be dislocated or subluxated. Marginal articular impaction, which may be present in about one third of posterior wall lesions,[21] should be disimpacted, grafted, and secured with independent fixation or by closing down the posterior wall over the fragments (Fig. 47-12A-D). The quality of reduction is best evaluated by CT scan rather than plain films.[22]

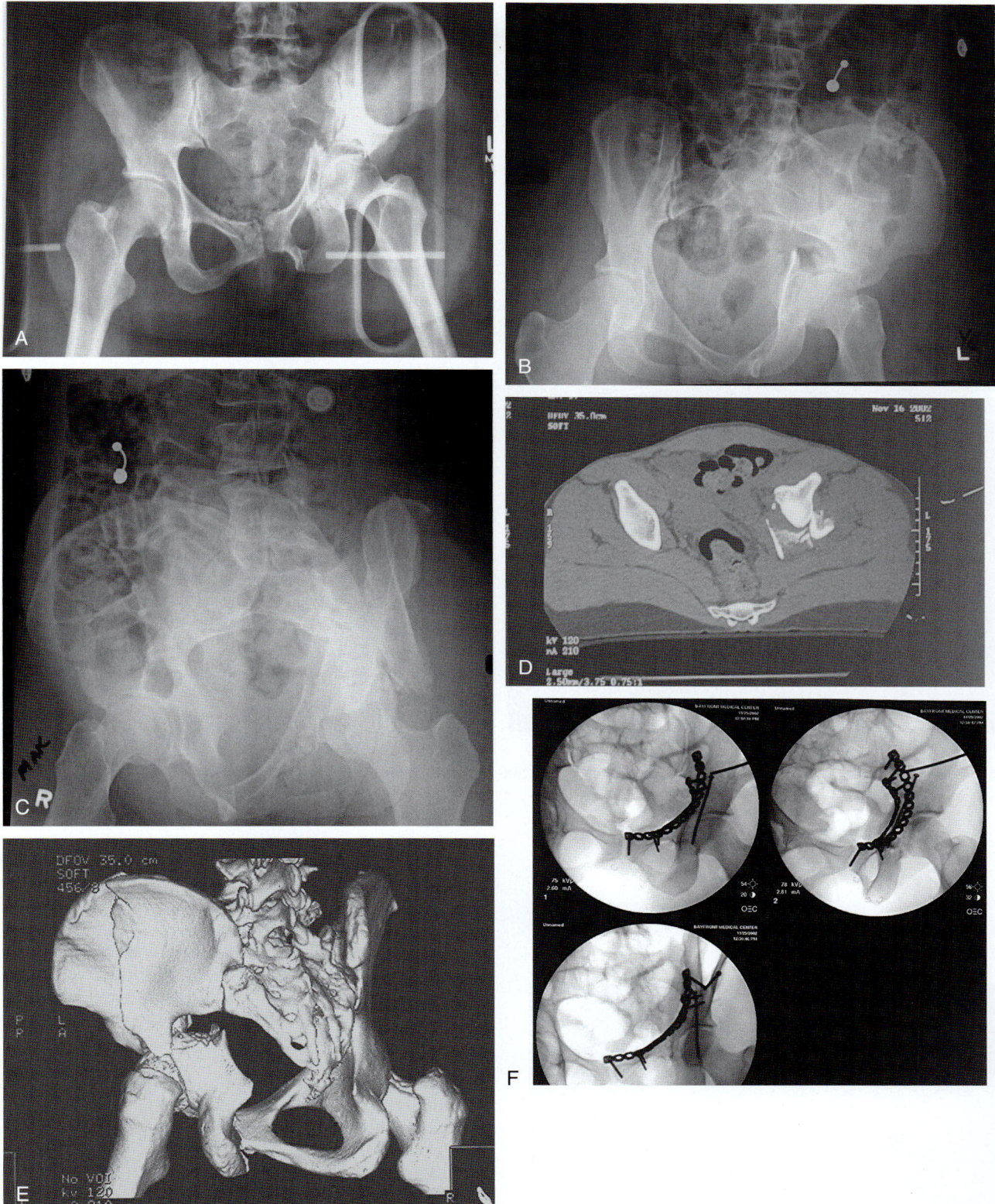

Figure 47-10. Both-column fracture in a 28-year-old woman. **A,** Anteroposterior (AP) emergency department radiograph. **B,** Ilial oblique Judet view. **C,** Obturator oblique Judet view. Spur sign laterally. **D,** Axial computed tomography (CT) cut. **E,** Three-dimensional (3D) CT view. No articular surface remains attached to the iliac wing. **F,** Intraoperative fluoroscopic views after reduction and fixation via anterior (modified Stoppa) approach.

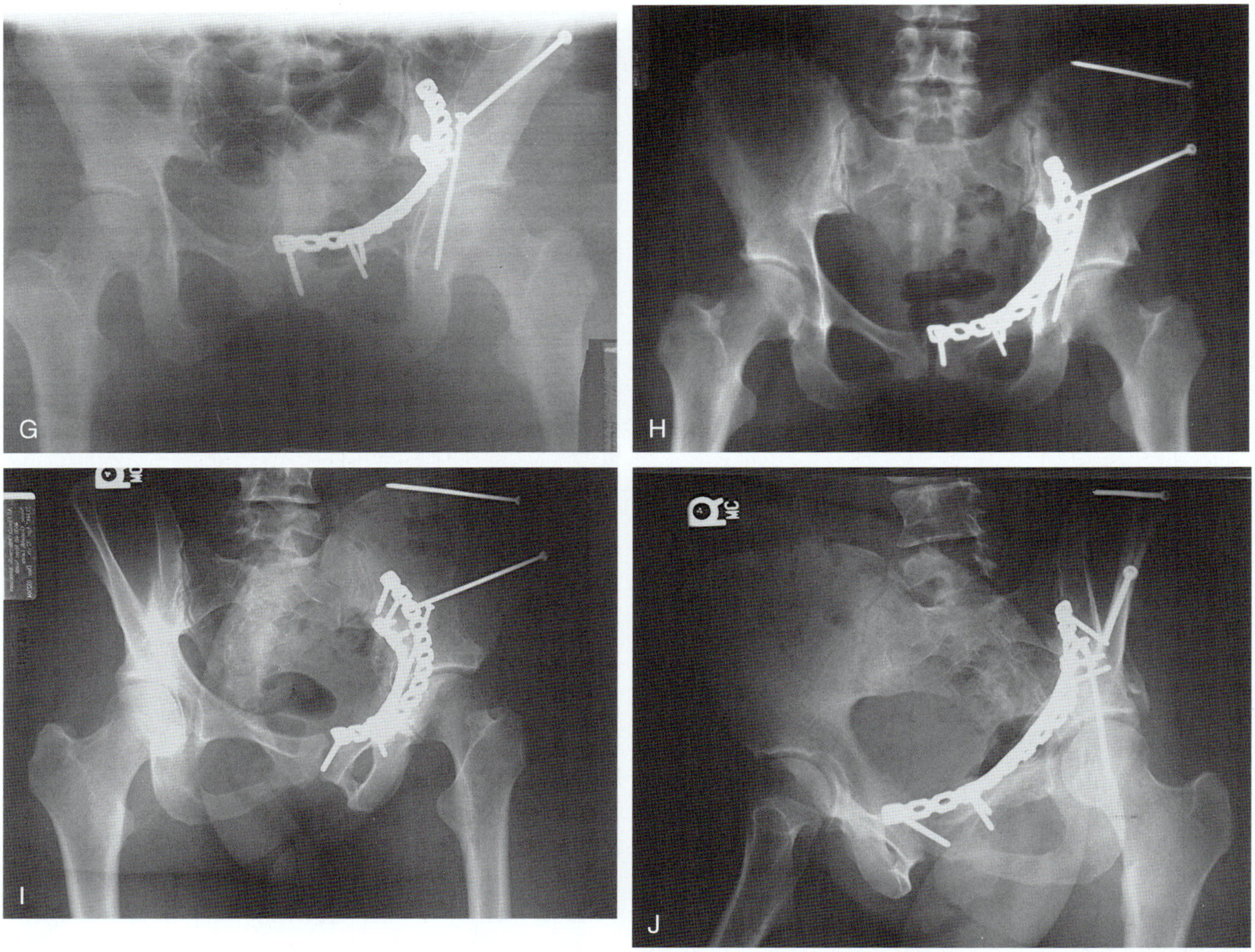

Figure 47-10. cont'd G, Immediate postop AP view. **H,** Six-year follow-up AP view. **I,** Six-year follow-up iliac oblique. **J,** Six-year follow-up obturator oblique.

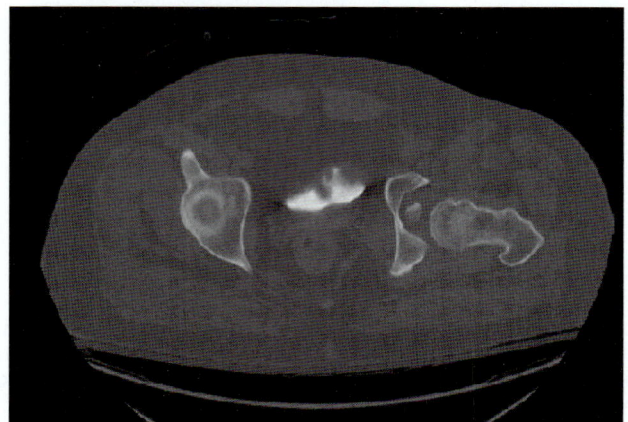

Figure 47-11. Axial computed tomography (CT) cut showing intra-articular loose fragment.

POSTOPERATIVE CARE

Patients are mobilized as with other articular injuries with no or minimal weight bearing and early range of motion. Appropriate deep vein thrombosis (DVT)/pulmonary embolus (PE) and heterotopic ossification prophylaxis measures are taken.

Follow-up radiographs are then taken at monthly intervals for the first 3 to 6 months, and weight bearing is usually progressed after 3 months. Patients receive annual follow-up for a time after recovery for assessment of possible onset of arthrosis.

It is rarely necessary or desirable to remove appropriately placed hardware.

RESULTS/OUTCOMES

For all fracture patterns as a whole, approximately 80% good to excellent results[1,4] have been reported for those fractures operated on within 3 weeks and accurately

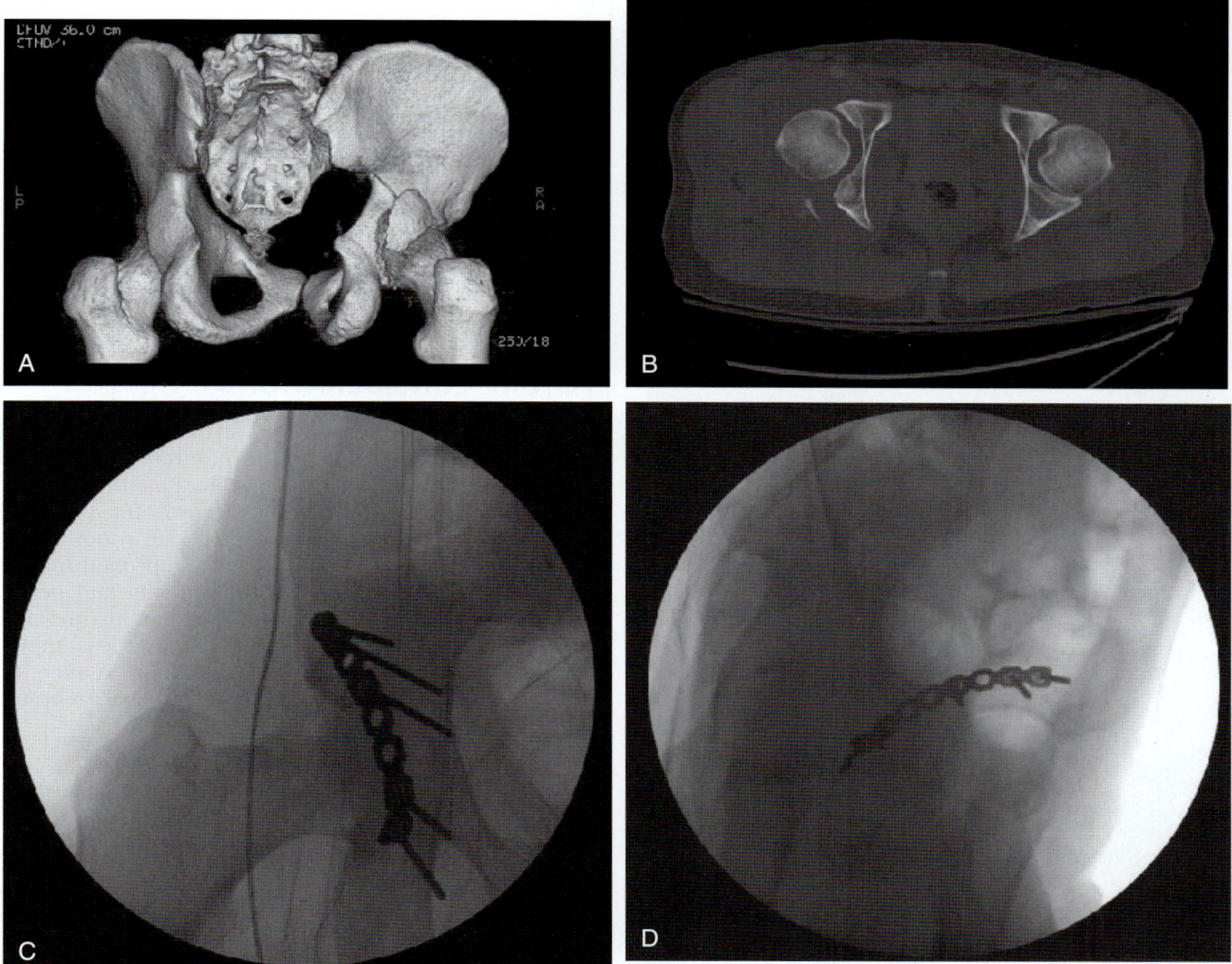

Figure 47-12. Displaced posterior wall fracture and nondisplaced posterior column. **A,** Three-dimensional (3D) computed tomography (CT) image of a displaced posterior wall fracture and a nondisplaced posterior column. **B,** Axial CT cut of same fracture showing posterior marginal impaction. **C,** Intraoperative anteroposterior (AP) with plate. **D,** Intraoperative oblique showing posterior wall reconstruction and fixation. No intra-articular hardware.

reduced. After 3 weeks, good to excellent results drop off to approximately 65% because of surgical and biological complications.[23] Outcome may be further dependent on the surgeon's experience. Poor results may be encountered early in the learning curve.[24]

Meta-analysis of 3670 fractures reported in 2005 shows that the most common long-term complication was arthritis, which occurred in approximately 20% of patients. Late complications such as heterotopic ossification and avascular necrosis occurred in about 10%. Only 8% of patients required a secondary operation. The overall infection rate was 4.4%. Noncontrollable factors affecting functional outcome included the type of fracture, femoral head damage, and associated injuries and comorbidities. Controllable factors included timing of surgery, choosing the correct surgical approach, and the quality of the reduction. Poorest results were noted in anterior wall fractures.[25]

Although good results have been described in elderly patients,[26] patients with difficult fracture patterns and poor bone quality may be treated by combined open reduction internal fixation and total hip arthroplasty, for which good results have been reported[27,28] (Fig. 47-13A and B).

COMPLICATIONS

Complications are a major concern in acetabular fractures, particularly when surgical treatment is selected for these challenging injuries. Complications may be injury related or treatment related or both, and include nerve palsy, heterotopic ossification, and infection.

Iatrogenic nerve injury may be minimized by vigilance during retraction and leg positioning. In the prone or lateral position, this involves placing the hip in

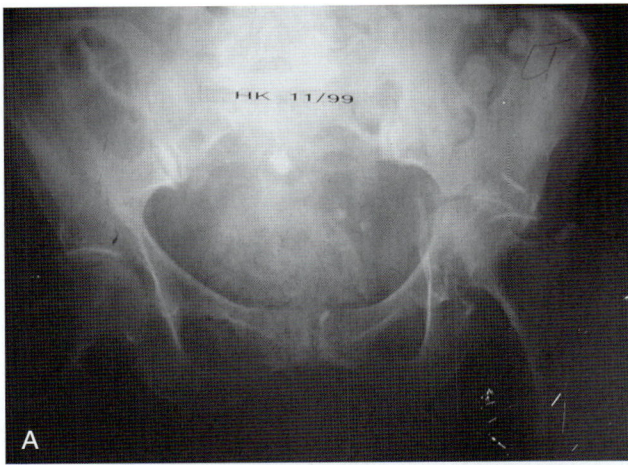

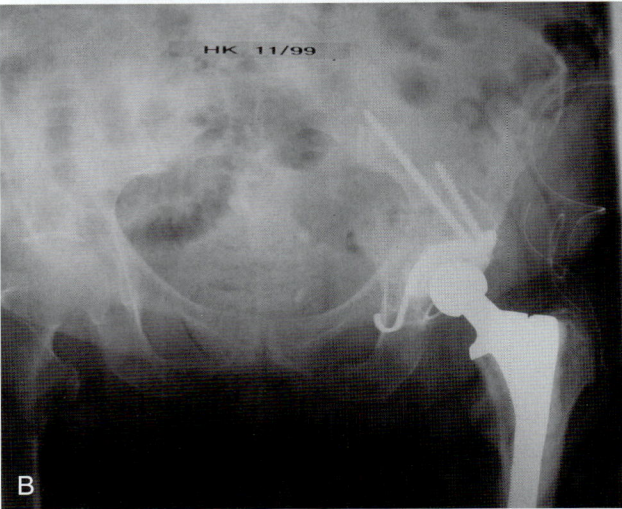

Figure 47-13. A, Elderly patient with porotic bone and displaced acetabular fracture. Note gull-wing appearance of superior articular surface. **B,** 14-month postop antero-posterior (AP) view after primary total hip with Ganz ring. The femoral head was used as bone graft behind the ring.

extension with the knee in flexion to minimize tension on the sciatic nerve in extrapelvic approaches. Nerve monitoring, which has been advocated by some,[29] may or may not be available or helpful.[30] Femoral, obturator, and sciatic nerve injuries are possible with anterior or intrapelvic approaches.

Problematic heterotopic ossification, which is worse with extrapelvic approaches, may be reduced by the use of indomethacin and/or radiation.[31-33] Problems with heterotopic ossification may be further prevented by selection of an intrapelvic approach whenever possible, removal of devitalized muscle and tissue, and avoidance of extensive muscle retraction or unnecessary dissection intraoperatively.

Deep vein thrombosis and pulmonary embolism, which are always considerations in fractures of the pelvis and acetabulum, have been shown by systematic review to have no definitive clinically superior protocol for prevention.[34] The diagnosis of DVT in the presence of a pelvic or acetabular fracture may be difficult, and

it has been shown that magnetic resonance (MR) and CT venography, although once advocated,[35] may not be reliable.[36]

Low-molecular-weight heparin started within 24 hours of injury has been recommended and can be associated with a low incidence of DVT and PE[37]; however, it is clear from the literature that additional clinical trials are needed.

Morbidly obese patients are more likely to have increased blood loss at the time of surgery, an increased incidence of DVT perioperatively, and as much as a five times greater likelihood of wound infection.[38]

FUTURE CONSIDERATIONS

Because operatively achieved articular reduction is paramount for good outcome, any future development toward better achieving and evaluating these reductions will have a reasonable chance for enhanced results. This might include mechanical, robotized, or navigated reduction combined with improved imaging (direct or indirect), both intraoperatively and perioperatively. Although such innovations may further facilitate less invasive surgical approaches with less implied morbidity, they probably will not soon reduce the degree of difficulty associated with surgical treatment of these injuries.

REFERENCES

1. Letournal E: Fractures of the acetabulum, Paris, France, 1993, Springer-Verlag.
2. Laird A, Keating JF: Acetabular fractures: a 16 year prospective epidemiological study. J Bone Joint Surg Br 87:969–973, 2005.
3. Beaule PE, Dorey FJ, Matta JM: Letournel classification for acetabular fractures: assessment of interobserver and intraobserver reliability. J Bone Joint Surg Am 85:1704–1709, 2003.
4. Matta JM, Anderson LM, Epstein HC, Hendrivk P: Fractures of the acetabulum: a retrospective analysis. Clin Orthop Relat Res 205:230–240, 1986.
5. Olson SA, Bay BK, Hamel A: Biomechanics of the hip joint and the effects of fracture of the acetabulum. Clin Orthop Relat Res 339:92–104, 1997.
6. Matta JM, Mehne DK, Roff R: Fractures of the acetabulum: early results of a prospective study. Clin Orthop Relat Res 205:241–250, 1986.
7. Matta JM, Meritt PO: Displaced acetabular fractures. Clin Orthop Relat Res 230:893–897, 1988.
8. Olson SA, Matta JM: The computerized tomography subchondral arc: a new method of assessing acetabular articular continuity after fracture. J Orthop Trauma 7:402–413, 1993.
9. Tornetta P III: Displaced acetabular fractures: indications for operative and non-operative management. J Am Acad Orthop Surg 9:18–28, 2001.
10. Siebenrock KA, Gautier E, Woo AK, Ganz R: Surgical dislocation of the femoral head for joint débridement and accurate reduction of fractures of the acetabulum. J Orthop Trauma 16:543–552, 2002.
11. Reinert CM, Bosse MJ, Poka JA, et al: A modified extensile exposure for the treatment of complex or malunited acetabular fractures. J Bone Joint Surg Am 70:329–337, 1988.
12. Starr AJ, Watson JT, Reinert CM, et al: Complications following the T extensile approach for acetabular fracture surgery: report of forty-three patients. J Orthop Trauma 16:535–542, 2002.
13. Griffin DB, Beaule PE, Matta JM: Safety and efficacy of the extended iliofemoral approach in the treatment of complex

fractures of the acetabulum. J Bone Joint Surg Br 87:1391–1396, 2005.

14. Weber TG, Mast JW: The extended ilioinguinal approach for specific both column fractures. Clin Orthop Relat Res 305:106–111, 1994.

15. Kloen P, Siebenrock KA, Ganz R: Modification of the ilioinguinal approach. J Orthop Trauma 16:586–593, 2002.

16. Cole JD, Bolhofner BR: Acetabular fracture fixation via a modified Stoppa limited intrapelvic approach: description of operative technique and preliminary treatment results. Clin Orthop Relat Res 305:112–123, 1994.

17. Moed BR, Willson Carr SE, Watson JT: Results of operative treatment of fractures of the posterior wall of the acetabulum. J Bone Joint Surg Am 84:752–758, 2002.

18. Kredor HJ, Rozen N, Berchoff CM, et al: Determinants of functional outcome after simple and complex acetabular fractures involving the posterior wall. J Bone Joint Surg Br 88:776–782, 2006.

19. Olson SA, Bay BK, Chapman MW, Sharkey NA: Biomechanical consequences of fractures and repair wall of the acetabulum. J Bone Joint Surg Am 77:1184–1192, 1995.

20. Moed BR, McMichael JC: Outcomes of posterior wall fractures of the acetabulum. J Bone Joint Surg Am 87:1170–1176, 2007.

21. Brumback RJ, Holt ES, McBride MS, et al: Acetabular depression fracture accompanying posterior fracture dislocation of the hip. J Orthop Trauma 4:42–48, 1990.

22. Moed BR, Carr SE, Gruson KI, et al: Computed tomographic assessment of fractures of the posterior wall of the acetabulum after operative treatment. J Bone Joint Surg Am 85:512–522, 2003.

23. Johnson EE, Matta JM, Mast JW, Letournel E: Delayed reconstruction of acetabular fractures 21-120 days following injury. Clin Orthop Relat Res 305:138-151, 1994.

24. Wright R, Barrett K, Christie MJ, Johnson KD: Acetabular fractures: long-term follow up of open reduction and internal fixation. J Orthop Trauma 8:397–403, 1994.

25. Giannoudis PV, Grutz MRW, Papakostidis C, Dinopoulos H: Operative treatment of displaced fractures of the acetabulum: a meta-analysis. J Bone Joint Surg Br 87:2–9, 2005.

26. Helfet DL, Borelli J, DiPasquale T: Fractures in elderly patients. J Bone Joint Surg Am 74:753–765, 1992.

27. Boraiah S, Ragsdale M, Achor T, et al: Open reduction internal fixation and primary total hip arthroplasty of selected acetabular fractures. J Orthop Trauma 23:243–248, 2009.

28. Mears DC, Velyuis JH: Acute total hip arthroplasty for selected displaced acetabular fractures: two to twelve year results. J Bone Joint Surg Am 84:1–9, 2002.

29. Helfet DL, Schmeling GJ: Somatosensory evoked potential monitoring in the surgical treatment of acute displaced acetabular fractures: results of a prospective study. Clin Orthop Relat Res 301:213–220, 1994.

30. Haidukewych GJ, Scaduto J, Herscovici D Jr, et al: Iatrogenic nerve injury in acetabular fracture surgery: a comparison of monitored and unmonitored procedures. J Orthop Trauma 16:297–301, 2002.

31. Bosse MJ, Poka A, Reinert CM, et al: Heterotopic ossification as a complication of acetabular fracture: prophylaxis with low-dose irradiation. J Bone Joint Surg Am 70:1231–1237, 1988.

32. Burd TA, Lowry KJ, Anglen JO: Indomethacin compared with localized irradiation for the prevention of heterotopic ossification following surgical treatment of acetabular fractures. J Bone Joint Surg Am 83:1783–1788, 2001.

33. Matta JM, Siebenrock KA: Does indomethacin reduce heterotopic bone formation after operations for acetabular fractures? A prospective randomized study. J Bone Joint Surg Br 79:959–963, 1997.

34. Slobogean GP, Lefaivre KA, Nicolaov S, O'Brien PJ: A systemic review of thromboprophylaxis for pelvic and acetabulum fractures. J Orthop Trauma 23:379–384, 2009.

35. Montgomery KD, Potter HG, Helfet DL: Magnetic resonance venography to evaluate the deep venous system of the pelvis in patients who have an acetabular fracture. J Bone Joint Surg Am 77:1639–1649, 1995.

36. Stover MD, Morgan SJ, Bosse MJ, et al: Prospective comparison of contrast enhanced computed tomography versus magnetic resonance venography in the detection of occult deep pelvic vein thrombosis in patients with pelvic and acetabular fractures. J Orthop Trauma 16:613–621, 2002.

37. Steele N, Doclenhoff RM, Ward HJ, Morse MH: Thromboprophylaxis in pelvic and acetabular trauma surgery: the role of early treatment with low-molecular weight heparin. J Bone Joint Surg Br 87:209–212, 2005.

38. Karunakar MA, Shah SN, Jerabek S: Body mass as a predictor of complications after operative treatment of acetabular fractures. J Bone Joint Surg Am 87:1498–1502, 2005.

CHAPTER 48

Hip Dislocation and Femoral Head Fractures

Kenneth J. Koval and Philip J. Kregor

KEY POINTS

- Hip dislocations and femoral head fractures are the result of high-energy trauma and usually are associated with other injuries.
- Posterior hip dislocations are much more common than anterior dislocations.
- Patients who have sustained a posterior hip dislocation usually present with the hip in a position of flexion, internal rotation, and adduction; those with an anterior dislocation present with the hip in marked external rotation with mild flexion and abduction.
- A dislocated hip is considered an orthopedic urgency and should be addressed as soon other life-threatening injuries have been addressed. The hip should be reduced on an urgent basis (i.e., within 6 hours) to minimize the risk of femoral head osteonecrosis.
- Indications for open reduction of a dislocated hip include (1) an inability to reduce the hip by closed means, (2) a nonconcentric reduction, and (3) an associated acetabular fracture causing hip instability.
- Femoral head fractures occur in the frontal plane of the femoral head. Therefore fixation of the fracture is addressed most easily via an anterior approach.
- Indications for open reduction of a femoral head fracture include (1) 1 to 2 mm displacement of the articular surface of the femoral head, particularly if it is at or above the foveal area; (2) intra-articular fragments, which cause hip incongruity; (3) a significantly displaced infrafoveal femoral head fragment, which may limit hip motion; and (4) an associated posterior wall fracture causing hip instability.

INTRODUCTION

Hip dislocations and femoral head fractures are usually the result of high-energy trauma.[1-3] Associated injuries are common and include chest, abdominal, craniofacial, and other musculoskeletal trauma.[1-7] Hip dislocations can be divided into anterior and posterior types, and femoral head fractures are classified according to the fracture location in the femoral head, as well as the

presence of an associated fracture (e.g., femoral neck or acetabular fracture).

Treatment principles for patients with either injury include (1) careful clinical evaluation to detect associated injuries; (2) emergent gentle closed or, if necessary, open reduction, followed by assessment of hip stability; (3) radiographic evaluation (including computed tomography [CT] scan) for congruency of reduction and any associated fractures; and (4) treatment of residual joint incongruity, removal of clinically significant intra-articular fragments, and establishment of hip stability.

EPIDEMIOLOGY AND RISK FACTORS

Posterior hip dislocations are much more common than anterior dislocations; anterior dislocations constitute 10% to 15% of traumatic dislocations of the hip,[1-3,7] and posterior dislocations account for the remainder. True shear-type fractures in the frontal plane of the femoral head occur in 10% of posterior dislocations.[7] Indentation lesions of the femoral head occur in 25% to 75% of anterior dislocations.[7]

Hip dislocations and femoral head fractures are usually associated with other injuries, either systemic or musculoskeletal. Suraci reported that 95% of patients who sustained a hip dislocation after a motor vehicle accident had an associated injury requiring inpatient management.[5] Ipsilateral knee injuries are particularly common. In a series of 187 patients who sustained a dislocation or a fracture dislocation of the hip, Tabuenca and Truan reported that 25% sustained a major knee injury.[8] In another series, 89% of patients who sustained a hip dislocation had visible evidence of soft tissue injury about the ipsilateral knee[9]; magnetic resonance imaging (MRI) revealed acute meniscal tear in 22% of patients, bone bruise in 33%, effusion in 37%, cruciate ligament injury in 25%, collateral ligament injury in 21%, and periarticular knee fracture in 15%.

Sciatic nerve injury occurs in 10% to 15% of hip dislocations.[10-12] The peroneal division is affected more frequently than the tibial branch because it is tethered at the pelvis and at the fibular neck. Additionally, the fascicles of the peroneal division are fewer in number, larger, and less protected by connective tissue. Partial return of function in sciatic nerve palsy can be expected in more than 50% of affected patients.

ANATOMY AND PATHOPHYSIOLOGY

The hip joint is inherently stable; more than 400 N of force is required to distract the hip.[13] Hip stability is conferred by both osseous and ligamentous restraints, as well as by femoral head congruity with the acetabulum. The labrum deepens the acetabulum and enhances joint stability.[14] The hip joint capsule is formed by thick longitudinal fibers supplemented by much stronger ligamentous condensations (iliofemoral, pubofemoral, and ischiofemoral ligaments) that run in a spiral fashion, preventing excessive hip extension. Seventy percent of the femoral head articular surface is involved in load transfer; therefore damage to this surface may lead to the development of post-traumatic arthritis.[7]

The main vascular supply to the femoral head originates from the medial and lateral femoral circumflex arteries—branches of the profunda femoral artery.[1-3,7] An extracapsular vascular ring is formed at the base of the femoral neck with ascending cervical branches that pierce the hip joint at the level of the capsular insertion. These branches ascend along the femoral neck and enter the bone just inferior to the cartilage of the femoral head. The artery of the ligamentum teres, a branch of the obturator artery, may contribute blood supply to the epiphyseal region of the femoral head.

The sciatic nerve exits the pelvis at the greater sciatic notch. A certain degree of variability exists in the relationship of the nerve to the piriformis muscle and short external rotators of the hip. Most frequently, the sciatic nerve exits the pelvis deep to the muscle belly of the piriformis.

Force transmission resulting in hip dislocation or femoral head fracture arises from one of three common sources[7,15-20]: (1) the anterior surface of the flexed knee striking an object (e.g., dashboard injury); (2) the sole of the foot, with the ipsilateral knee extended (e.g., foot on brake pedal); or (3) the greater trochanter (e.g., lateral impact). Less frequently, the force resulting in hip dislocation may be applied to the posterior pelvis with the ipsilateral foot or knee acting as the counterforce. The direction of dislocation (anterior or posterior) is ultimately determined by the position of the lower extremity at injury and the direction of the pathologic force.

Anterior dislocations result from hip abduction and external rotation.[7,21] The amount of hip flexion determines whether one sustains a superior or inferior (obturator) type of anterior hip dislocation. Inferior dislocations are the result of simultaneous abduction, external rotation, and hip flexion; superior (iliac or pubic) dislocations are the result of abduction, external rotation, and hip extension. In anterior dislocations, one may also sustain a femoral head impaction fracture secondary to the femoral head impacting the acetabular margin.

Posterior dislocations usually result from direct impact to the flexed knee with the hip in varying degrees of flexion.[7,22] If the position of the hip is neutral or slightly adducted at the time of impact, a simple dislocation (no acetabular fracture) will likely occur. However, a femoral head fracture may occur as a result of avulsion by the ligamentum teres or impaction by the posterior acetabular rim. If the hip is in abduction, a posterior-superior rim of the acetabulum fracture usually results.

For the hip to dislocate, the ligamentum teres and a portion of the hip capsule must be disrupted.[3] Tears of the acetabular labrum and associated muscle commonly occur.[23] The capsule of the hip may be stripped off of the acetabulum or femur as a cuff secondary to rotational forces or may be split by direct pressure.[21] In anterior dislocations, the hip capsule is usually disrupted anteriorly and inferiorly. In posterior dislocations, the capsule may be disrupted inferoposteriorly or directly posteriorly, depending on the position of the hip at impact.

CLINICAL FEATURES AND DIAGNOSIS

Clinical Examination

A full trauma survey is essential because of the high-energy mechanism of injury and the likelihood of associated injuries. The patient may be obtunded or unconscious at the time of hospital presentation and unable to give a clear history of the accident or to complain of other areas of potential injury. Patients presenting with hip dislocations typically are unable to move the injured lower extremity and report severe hip pain.

Patients who have sustained a posterior hip dislocation usually present with the hip in a position of flexion, internal rotation, and adduction; those with an anterior dislocation present with the hip in marked external rotation with mild flexion and abduction. The appearance and alignment of the extremity, however, are dependent on the presence or absence of associated ipsilateral extremity injuries.

One must perform a careful neurovascular examination because injury to the sciatic nerve or to femoral neurovascular structures may have occurred at dislocation. Sciatic nerve injury may result from stretching of the nerve over the posteriorly dislocated femoral head. Posterior wall fragments from the acetabulum may have pierced or partially lacerated the nerve. Usually the peroneal portion of the sciatic nerve is affected, with little if any dysfunction of the tibial nerve. Injury to femoral artery, vein, or nerve is rare but may occur as a result of an anterior dislocation.

Radiographic Evaluation

A dislocated hip is usually apparent on an anteroposterior (AP) radiograph of the pelvis (Fig. 48-1); femoral head fracture may be subtler and more difficult to diagnose. On the AP view of the pelvis, the two femoral heads should appear similar in size, and the hip joints symmetrical. In posterior dislocations, the affected femoral head should appear smaller than the

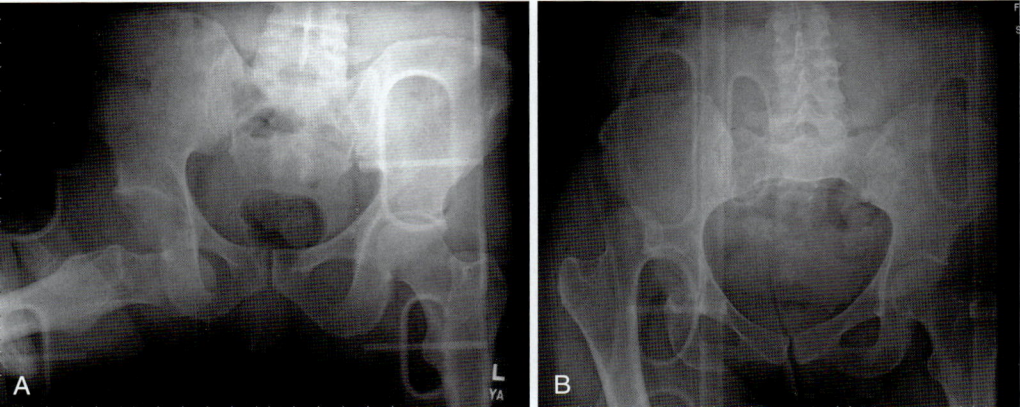

Figure 48-1. A dislocated hip is usually apparent on the anteroposterior (AP) pelvis radiograph. **A,** An anterior dislocation. **B,** A posterior dislocation.

contralateral side because of the closer distance of the femoral head to the radiographic cassette; in anterior dislocation, the femoral head should appear slightly larger than the normal hip.[7] The position of the femoral shaft should be noted (adducted or abducted), as well as the relative appearance of the greater and lesser trochanters, because they may indicate pathologic internal or external hip rotation. One must carefully evaluate the femoral neck to rule out the presence of a femoral neck fracture before any manipulative reduction is performed. Although it is usually not necessary for diagnosis of hip dislocation or fracture dislocation, a cross-table lateral view of the injured hip may help to distinguish a posterior from an anterior dislocation.

Full radiographic evaluation of a dislocated hip can usually wait until after an attempt is made at hip reduction and should include a repeat AP pelvis, cross-table lateral of the hip, and 45 degree oblique (Judet) views of the pelvis. The repeat AP pelvis is necessary to assess hip congruency after reduction; the cross-table lateral is used to evaluate the integrity of the femoral neck. Forty-five degree oblique (Judet) views of the hip are helpful in ascertaining the presence of associated femoral head fracture, osteochondral fragments, the integrity of the acetabulum, and joint congruence. The obturator oblique Judet view is particularly helpful in diagnosing femoral head and neck fractures, posterior wall fractures, and joint incongruity.

In general, CT scan is not needed before hip reduction unless a high level of suspicion for a nondisplaced femoral neck fracture is present. A 2 mm cut CT scan is usually obtained after closed hip reduction to assess the adequacy of reduction and to rule out associated acetabular and femoral head fractures[3] (Fig. 48-2). Frontal plane CT reconstructions are helpful in characterizing associated femoral head fractures. If hip reduction cannot be attained through closed means, a CT scan should be obtained before open reduction to help identify offending structures, such as incarcerated bone fragments from the femoral head or a posterior wall fracture, or soft tissue interposition.

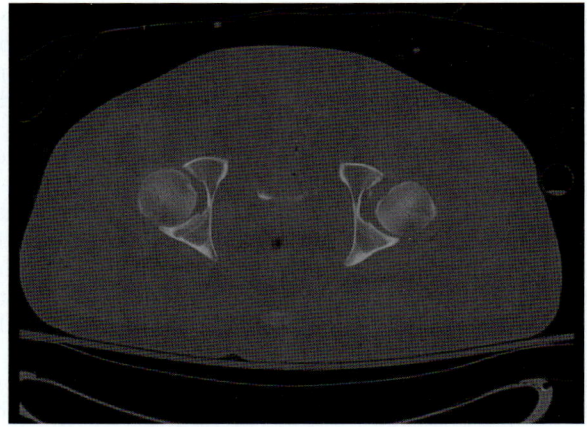

Figure 48-2. Computed tomography (CT) scan after closed reduction of the hip showing asymmetrical joint spaces with widening of the left hip joint.

The role of MRI in the evaluation of hip dislocation is controversial.[7,23] MRI may prove useful in the evaluation of hip labrum integrity and femoral head vascularity; however, the usefulness of MRI in predicting femoral head osteonecrosis after dislocation has not been established.

CLASSIFICATION

Several classifications have been described for hip dislocations and femoral head fractures (Boxes 48-1 through 48-5). In general, hip dislocations are classified on the basis of (1) the relationship of the femoral head to the acetabulum, and (2) the presence or absence of associated fractures. The Stewart and Milford classification for posterior hip dislocations also addresses the question of hip stability after reduction.[24] The Brumback classification of femoral head fractures takes into account the size of the femoral head fragment, the

BOX 48-1. THOMPSON AND EPSTEIN CLASSIFICATION FOR POSTERIOR HIP DISLOCATION (FIG. 48-3)

Type I   Simple dislocation with or without an insignificant posterior wall fragment
Type II   Dislocation associated with a single large posterior wall fragment
Type III   Dislocation with a comminuted posterior wall fragment
Type IV   Dislocation with fracture of the acetabular floor
Type V   Dislocation with fracture of the femoral head

From Thompson VP, Epstein HC: Traumatic dislocation of the hip: a survey of two hundred and four cases covering a period of twenty-one years. J Bone Joint Surg Am 33:746–778, 1951.

BOX 48-2. STEWART AND MILFORD CLASSIFICATION FOR POSTERIOR HIP DISLOCATIONS

Type I   Simple dislocation without fracture
Type II   Dislocation with one or more acetabular rim fractures but sufficient remaining acetabular socket such that the hip is clinically stable after hip reduction
Type III   Dislocation with acetabular rim fracture producing clinical instability after hip reduction
Type IV   Dislocation with associated femoral head or neck fracture

From Stewart MJ, Milford MW: Fracture-dislocation of the hip: an end-result study. J Bone Joint Surg Am 36:315–342, 1954.

BOX 48-3. EPSTEIN CLASSIFICATION FOR ANTERIOR HIP DISLOCATIONS (FIG. 48-3.)

Type I   Superior dislocations, including both pubic and subspinous locations
IA   No associated fracture
IB   Associated fracture or impaction of the femoral head
IC   Associated fracture of the acetabulum
Type II   Inferior dislocations, including both obturator and perineal locations
IIA   No associated fracture
IIB   Associated fracture or impaction of the femoral head
IIC   Associated fracture of the acetabulum

From Epstein HC: Traumatic dislocations of the hip. Clin Orthop Relat Res 92:116–142, 1973; Epstein HC, Wiss DA: Traumatic anterior dislocation of the hip. Orthopedics 8:130, 132–134, 1985.

BOX 48-4. PIPKIN CLASSIFICATION FOR FEMORAL HEAD FRACTURES (FIG. 48-4)

Type I   Hip dislocation with fracture of the femoral head inferior to the fovea
Type II   Hip dislocation with fracture of the femoral head superior to the fovea
Type III   Type I or II injury associated with fracture of the femoral neck
Type IV   Type I or II injury associated with fracture of the acetabular rim

From Pipkin G: Treatment of grade IV fracture-dislocation of the hip. J Bone Joint Surg Am 39:1027–1042, 1957.

BOX 48-5. BRUMBACK CLASSIFICATION FOR FEMORAL HEAD FRACTURES (FIG. 48-5)

Type 1A   Posterior hip dislocation with femoral head fracture involving the inferomedial (non–weight-bearing) portion of the head, minimal or no fracture of the acetabular rim, and a stable hip after reduction
1B   Type 1A with significant acetabular fracture and hip instability after reduction
Type 2A   Posterior hip dislocation with femoral head fracture involving the superomedial (weight-bearing) portion of the head, minimal or no fracture of the acetabular rim, and a stable hip after reduction
2B   Type 2A with significant acetabular fracture and hip instability after reduction
Type 3A   Any hip dislocation with an associated femoral neck fracture
3B   Any hip dislocation with an associated femoral neck and head fracture
Type 4A   Anterior hip dislocation with indentation of the superolateral weight-bearing surface of the femoral head
4B   Anterior hip dislocation with transchondral shear fracture of the weight-bearing surface of the femoral head
Type 5   Central fracture-dislocations of the hip with fracture of the femoral head

From Brumback RJ, Kenzora JE, Levitt L, et al: Fractures of the femoral head. Hip 181–206, 1987.

TREATMENT

Hip Dislocations

A dislocated hip is considered an orthopedic urgency; the hip should be reduced on an emergent basis to minimize the risk of femoral head osteonecrosis.[1-3] Timely hip reduction may assist in restoring normal hip vascularity, thus reducing the duration of femoral head ischemia. Studies have shown that the long-term prognosis worsens if reduction (closed or open) is delayed

direction of hip dislocation, and hip stability.[25] The Orthopaedic Trauma Association (OTA) classification of hip dislocations and femoral head fractures is part of a universal classification system and is used primarily for research purposes.[26]

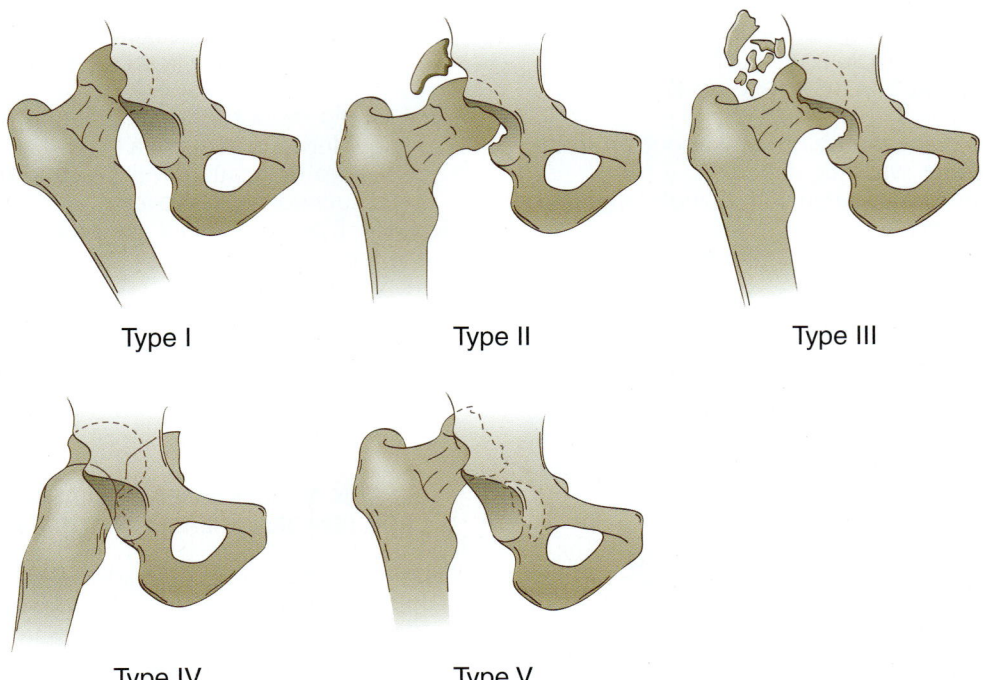

Type I   Type II   Type III

Type IV   Type V

Figure 48-3. Thompson and Epstein classification for posterior hip dislocations. *(Redrawn from Browner B, Jupiter J, Levine A, Trafton P [eds]: Skeletal trauma: fractures, dislocations, ligamentous injuries, ed 3, Philadelphia, 2002, Saunders, Chapter 46.)*

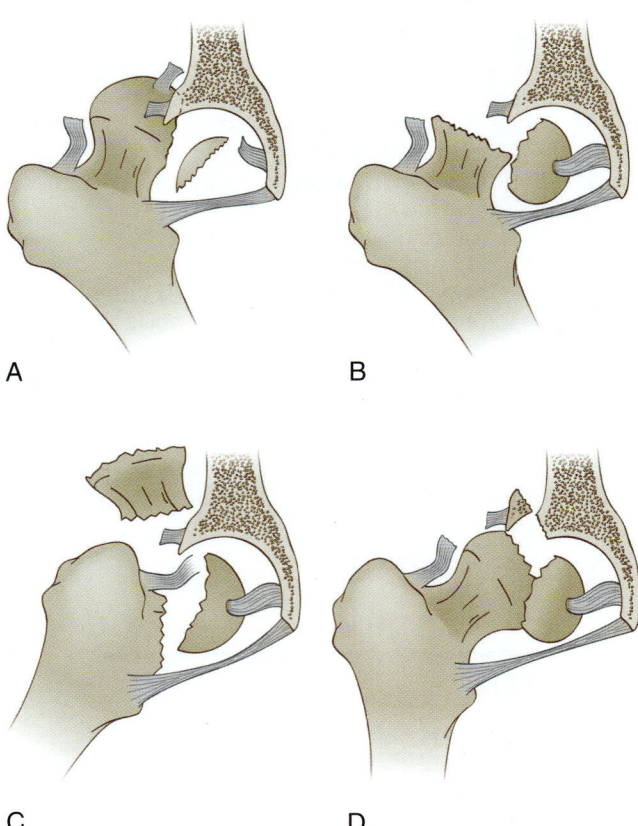

A   B

C   D

Figure 48-4. Pipkin classification for femoral head fractures. *(Redrawn from Bucholz RW, Heckman JD, Court-Brown CM, Tornetta P [eds]: Rockwood and Green's fractures in adults, ed 7, Philadelphia, 2009, Lippincott Williams & Wilkins, Chapter 46.)*

by more than 12 hours.[24,30] However, before either closed or open reduction is performed, adequate radiographic imaging should be obtained to rule out the presence of an associated femoral neck fracture; an associated nondisplaced femoral neck fracture is a contraindication to attempted closed reduction. In such cases, screw fixation of the femoral neck should be performed before closed reduction or during open reduction.

Ideally, closed reduction should be attempted with the patient under general anesthesia to minimize the risk of further damage to the articular cartilage. However, closed reduction is often performed in the emergency department with the patient under conscious sedation with good muscle relaxation. Either way, it is important to attempt hip reduction in as gentle a manner as possible to avoid further damage to the articular cartilage or displacement of an associated fracture. If adequate personnel are available and good conscious sedation is achieved, only one or two good attempts at closed reduction should be made. Repeated reduction attempts by inexperienced personnel should not be allowed; after one or two unsuccessful attempts at closed reduction are made by an experienced individual, the patient should be taken to the operating room for closed or open reduction under general anesthesia.

Closed Reduction

Regardless of the hip dislocation direction, closed reduction should be attempted with in-line traction. One should use continuous traction rather than repeated jerky motions to help overcome contracted muscle forces and to minimize the risk of additional iatrogenic osseous and soft tissue injury. After

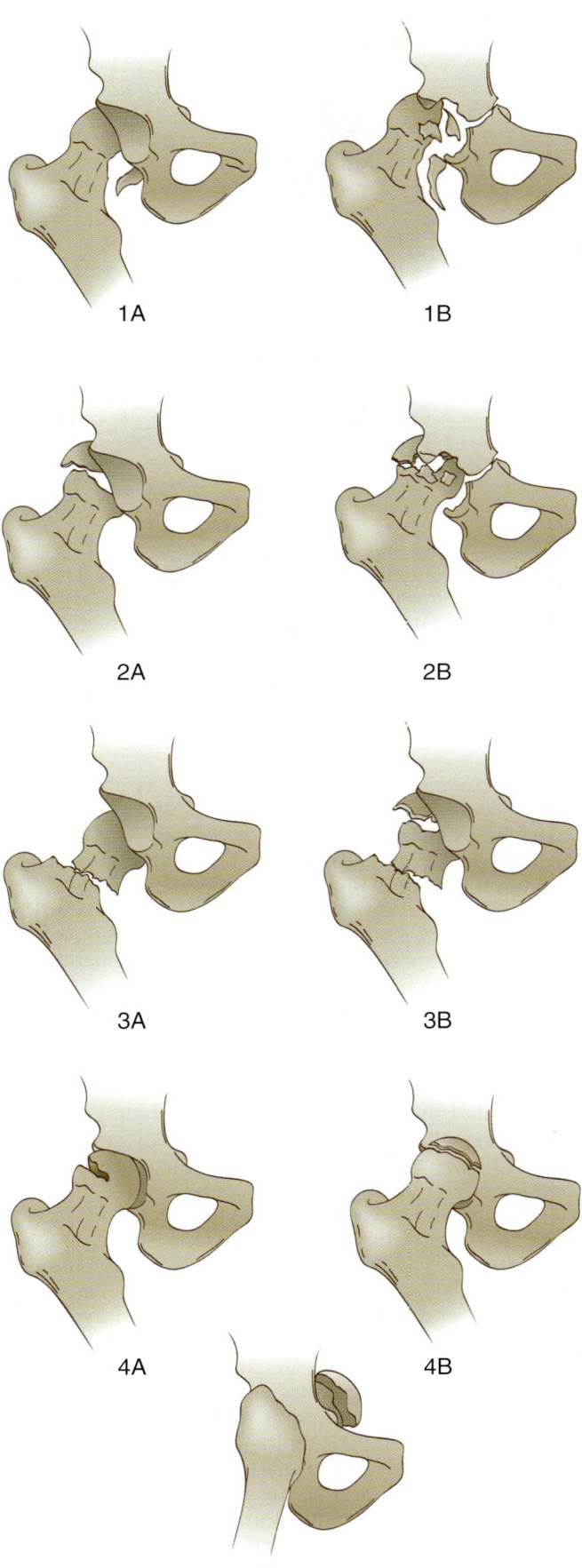

1A   1B

2A   2B

3A   3B

4A   4B

5

Figure 48-5. Brumback classification for femoral head fractures. *(Redrawn from Bucholz RW, Heckman JD, Court-Brown CM, Tornetta P [eds]: Rockwood and Green's fractures in adults, ed 7, Philadelphia, 2009, Lippincott Williams & Wilkins, Chapter 46.)*

reduction of a posterior hip dislocation, one should place a knee immobilizer to minimize the risk of repeat dislocation while additional radiographic studies are obtained. Several methods may be used to achieve closed reduction of a posterior hip dislocation:

- Allis method[3,7,31] (Fig. 48-6): The patient is placed supine with the surgeon standing above the patient. In-line traction is applied while the assistant stabilizes the patient's pelvis through countertraction. The surgeon slowly increases the traction force while flexing the hip to approximately 70 to 90 degrees. Gentle hip rotation and slight adduction may help the femoral head clear the acetabular lip. A lateral force to the proximal thigh may assist in hip reduction, provided by a sheet wrapped around the inner thigh on the side of the involved hip.
- Stimson gravity technique[3,7,32] (Fig. 48-7): The patient is placed prone with the affected leg hanging off the side of a stretcher or bed. This places the extremity in 90 degree hip flexion. The knee is flexed 90 degrees, and the assistant stabilizes the pelvis while the surgeon applies an anteriorly directed force on the posterior aspect of the proximal calf. Gentle rotation of the limb may assist in reduction.
- Bigelow and reverse Bigelow maneuvers[2,7,33]: These maneuvers have been associated with iatrogenic femoral neck fracture and are infrequently used as reduction techniques. With the Bigelow maneuver, the patient is positioned supine and the surgeon applies longitudinal limb traction. The adducted and internally rotated thigh is then flexed to a minimum of 90 degrees. The femoral head is levered into the acetabulum through hip abduction, external rotation, and extension. In the reverse Bigelow maneuver, used for anterior dislocations, traction is applied in the line of the deformity. The hip then is adducted, sharply internally rotated, and extended.

An anterior-inferior hip dislocation can be reduced with modification of the Allis technique. In-line femoral traction is applied with the hip mildly flexed.[34] The hip is gently internally rotated and adducted while a laterally directed force is applied to the inner thigh with the use of a sheet. For an anterior-superior hip dislocation, in-line traction is applied until the femoral head is at the level of the acetabulum; the hip then is gently internally rotated.

Once the hip has been reduced and verified radiographically, hip stability is assessed by gently moving the hip through a range of motion.[1-3,7] In the presence of an associated posterior wall fracture, one can fluoroscopically assess hip stability by placing the hip in 90 degrees of flexion, 20 degrees of adduction, with slight internal rotation, while applying a posteriorly directed

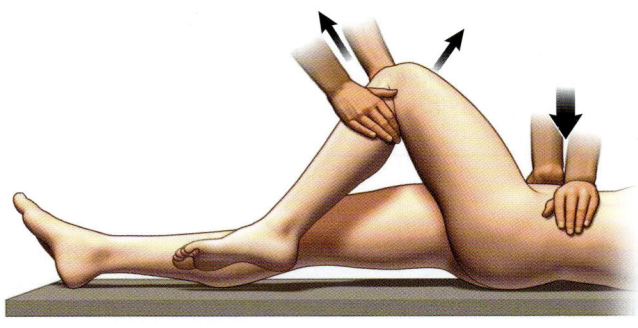

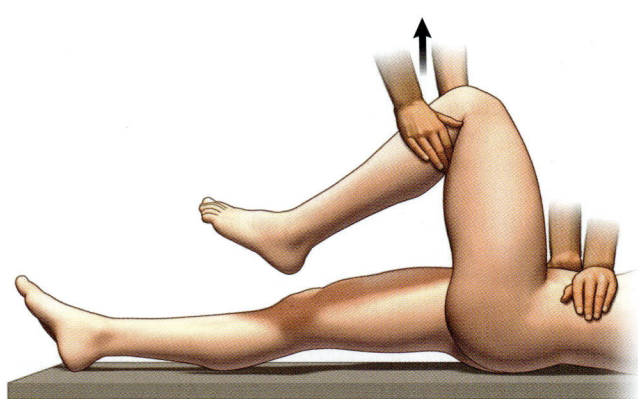

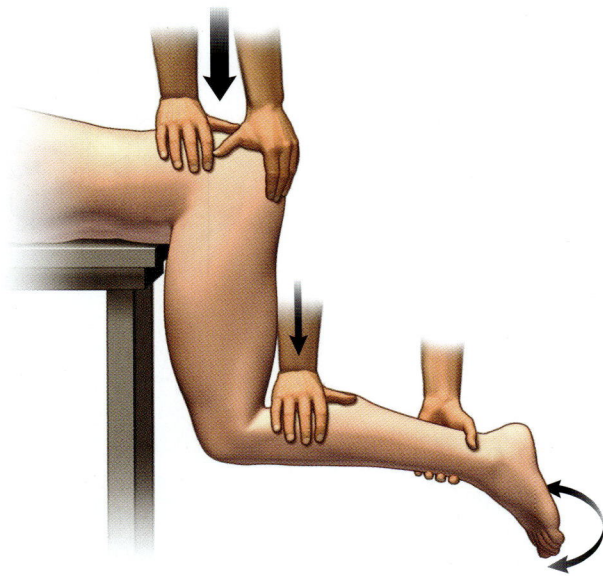

Figure 48-7. The Stimson gravity technique for hip reduction. *(Redrawn from Egol K, Koval KJ, Zuckerman JD [eds]: Handbook of fractures, ed 3, Philadelphia, 2009, Lippincott Williams & Wilkins.)*

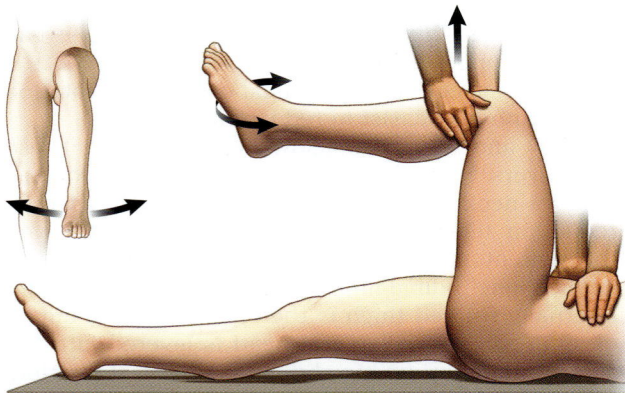

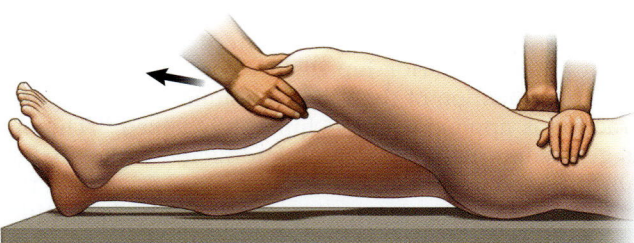

Figure 48-6. The Allis reduction technique for hip reduction. *(Redrawn from Egol K, Koval KJ, Zuckerman JD [eds]: Handbook of fractures, ed 3, Philadelphia, 2009, Lippincott Williams & Wilkins.)*

force.[1-3] Any evidence of hip incongruity during the stress examination indicates hip instability.

If the radiographs show no evidence of subluxation or incongruity and no evidence of instability to range-of-motion testing is found, the hip is determined to be stable. However, the hip should still be evaluated by 2 mm cut CT to confirm that the hip is concentric and to rule out the presence of intra-articular fragments and injury to the femoral head and/or acetabulum.[3] If the hip is concentric on CT scan, closed treatment should serve as definitive management. Retained osseous fragments in the fovea of the hip joint in the presence of a concentric reduction are not an indication for open treatment.[3] However, any incongruity on radiographs or CT scans could signify the presence of bony or chondral fragments or soft tissue interposition and is an indication for open reduction.

Although it is generally accepted that one should obtain a CT after hip reduction, controversy continues over the predictive value of a negative CT to rule out intra-articular pathology.[35,36] Mullis and Dahners[35] and Yamamoto and associates[36] reported a high incidence of intra-articular loose bodies despite negative plain radiographs and thin-cut CT scans. Because of these findings, some investigators advocate open reduction or hip arthroscopy after hip dislocation to evaluate and remove particulate debris.[35,36] In the future, MRI studies may be useful in diagnosing the presence of chondral injury or soft tissue interposition. However, MRI is rarely used in clinical practice and may not be as sensitive as CT in evaluating for retained bony fragments.

Open Reduction

Indications for open reduction of a dislocated hip include (1) an inability to close reduce the hip, (2) a nonconcentric reduction, and (3) an associated acetabular fracture causing hip instability. In the presence of an ipsilateral femoral neck fracture, closed reduction of the hip should not be attempted. The hip fracture should first be provisionally or definitively stabilized; this should be followed by gentle closed or open reduction of the dislocated hip.

Up to 15% of hip dislocations are irreducible.[1-3] In anterior dislocations, buttonholing of the femoral head through the hip capsule or soft tissue interposition (e.g., rectus, capsule, labrum, psoas) may prevent closed reduction.[1-3] In posterior dislocations, buttonholing of the femoral head through the short external rotators, soft tissue interposition (piriformis, gluteus maximus, capsule, ligamentum teres, or labrum), or an interposed osseous fragment may prevent hip reduction.[1-3]

In the setting of an irreducible dislocation, one should perform an urgent open reduction in an effort to restore femoral head blood flow.[1-3] Before open reduction, a CT should be obtained to help identify incarcerated bone fragments from the femoral head or the posterior wall or from soft tissue interposition. However, if obtaining the CT would substantially delay the timing of hip reduction, one should proceed with open reduction and then obtain the CT.

The timing for open reduction after nonconcentric reduction is less crucial than for irreducible dislocation because the femoral head is contained within the acetabulum, and theoretically, blood flow should have been restored to the femoral head. One should obtain a preoperative CT scan to help determine the cause of incongruity; surgery should be performed in a timely manner when a well-rested and qualified surgical team is available. Before surgery, sufficient traction should be placed on the limb to distract the hip and prevent grinding of any incarcerated fragments on the remaining femoral head and acetabular cartilage.

Assessment of hip joint congruence after hip reduction can be difficult. Any widening of the hip may indicate a block to reduction (Fig. 48-8). On plain radiographs, the joint space and measurement from the femoral head to the ilioischial line should be equal for both hips. In a reduced hip, all of the CT sections should demonstrate a congruent relationship between the head and the anterior and posterior articular surfaces.

Open reduction should be performed from the direction of the hip dislocation.[1-3,7] Posterior dislocations are reduced via a Kocher-Langenbach approach. The sciatic nerve should be protected with the hip and knee flexed throughout the case. The acetabulum is examined for potential loose bodies, and the femoral head evaluated for chondral damage before hip reduction. Use of a femoral distractor can help to distract the hip and remove loose fragments within the joint. One should be sure that all fragments that were visualized in preoperative imaging studies are removed during surgery. After the hip has been cleared of loose bodies and soft tissue, the hip is reduced. If there exists an associated

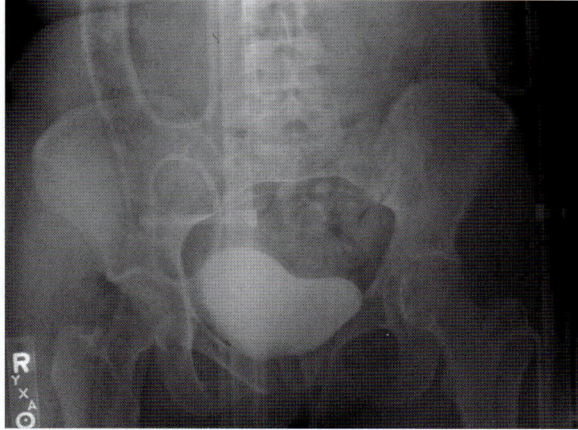

Figure 48-8. Widening of the right hip joint after closed reduction with evidence of a retained fragment in the superior joint space.

posterior wall fracture that is less than 20% of the entire acetabular rim, one should perform stability testing, with fixation of these fragments as needed.[1-3,7] However, some surgeons advocate for fixation a posterior wall fragment of any size because the surgical approach has already been performed. After confirmation of femoral head reduction, one should repair the capsule and the soft tissue. Suture anchors in the periphery of the acetabular wall are helpful for labral repair.

Anterior dislocations can be reduced via an anterior (Smith-Petersen) or an anterolateral (Watson-Jones) approach. The Smith-Petersen approach affords better visualization of the anterior aspect of the hip and femoral head.[1-3,7] This approach also facilitates femoral head reduction and stabilization. Given the frontal plane nature of the femoral head fracture, the screws should be oriented from anteromedial to posterolateral. The anterolateral approach allows access to anterior and posterior aspects of the hip through the same skin incision, if needed; it also enables treatment of combined fractures of the femoral head and neck. The direct lateral (Hardinge) approach affords exposure to anterior and posterior aspects of the hip through a single incision.

Regardless of the approach used, the hip joint should be cleared of all debris and thoroughly irrigated before reduction. A femoral distractor can help to distract the hip; alternatively, one can place an external fixator pin in the femoral neck to help manipulate the proximal femur. The cartilage of the femoral head and acetabulum should be inspected before hip reduction; one should also attempt to repair avulsed soft tissue and labral tears.

Traditionally, fragments of bone within the fovea have not been believed to require removal. In the absence of other surgical indications (e.g., large posterior wall fragment, femoral head fracture), no clear indication for surgical intervention was evident. Typically, these fragments represent chondral or osteochondral fragments pulled off by the ligamentum teres, and they are not thought to be prone to migration into the articular surface of the joint. However, some authors advocate removal of these fragments through open or arthroscopically assisted means.[1-3,38,39] Fragments that are incarcerated between the articular surfaces of the femoral head and the acetabulum mandate removal to minimize the possibility of chondral injury and subsequent osteoarthritis.

Open arthrotomy is the standard method of removal of incarcerated fragments. Reports have described arthroscopic lavage and removal of small fragments of incarcerated bone after hip dislocation.[35,36,38,39] Mullis and Dahners reported the results of arthroscopy on 39 hips after posterior dislocation or fracture/dislocation and found loose bodies in 92% of cases.[35] Yamamoto and colleagues reported similar findings in 11 cases of hip dislocation.[36] In eight hips, they found loose bodies that had not been visualized on preoperative radiographs or CT scans. Philippon and coworkers reported a retrospective review of 14 professional athletes who sustained a simple hip dislocation during active competition and underwent arthroscopic evaluation.[38] All 14 patients had evidence of labral tears and chondral injuries; 11 had loose osteochondral lesions. None of these studies reported whether loose body removal improved patient outcome with a lower incidence of later osteoarthritis.

Femoral Head Fractures

Treatment of femoral head fractures is dependent on fracture location and any associated injuries.[3,7] For Pipkin type I fractures (femoral head inferior to the fovea), closed treatment is recommended if the fracture is nondisplaced or minimally displaced (<1 to 2 mm step-off) and the hip is stable.[3,7] With further fracture displacement, open reduction and internal fixation with countersunk small fragment screws, subarticular headless screws, or absorbable pins using an anterior approach is recommended[3,7,40] (Fig. 48-9). One can excise small fragments if they do not sacrifice stability; however, it is unknown what size fragment influences dynamic hip stability. Therefore if surgical reduction is performed, all reasonable attempts should be made to reconstruct the normal femoral head.

Only nondisplaced Pipkin type II fractures (femoral head superior to the fovea) should be treated without surgery. This situation is relatively rare; careful scrutiny of the obturator oblique Judet view or of frontal plane CT reconstructions will often reveal significant (>1 to 2 mm) fracture displacement. The Smith-Petersen approach is the workhorse for Pipkin II fractures with fracture stabilization involving the use of countersunk small fragment screws, subarticular headless screws, or absorbable pins (Fig. 48-10).

The prognosis for Pipkin type III fractures (femoral head fracture with associated fracture of the femoral neck) is poor and depends on the displacement of the femoral neck fracture.[3,7] In younger individuals, urgent open reduction and internal fixation of the femoral neck should be performed, followed by reduction and internal fixation of the femoral head. Fortunately, these injuries are very rare. One can use an anterior (Smith-Petersen) or anterolateral (Watson-Jones) approach. In older individuals with a displaced femoral neck fracture, prosthetic replacement is usually performed.

Pipkin type IV fractures (femoral head fracture with associated fracture of the acetabulum) are treated in conjunction with the acetabular fracture. Multiple options are available for treatment of a Pipkin type IV injury. The surgical approach is dictated by the size, displacement, and stability of the femoral head and the posterior wall fracture. Options include (1) nonoperative treatment of both the femoral head and the posterior wall fracture; (2) treatment of the femoral head fracture via a Smith-Petersen approach, examination under anesthesia of hip stability, and fixation of the posterior wall fracture, if required, via a Kocher-Langenbeck approach; and (3) treatment of both injuries simultaneously via a Ganz trochanteric flip osteotomy with surgical dislocation of the femoral head[41] (the advantage of this approach is that it allows for total and simultaneous control of both fractures)

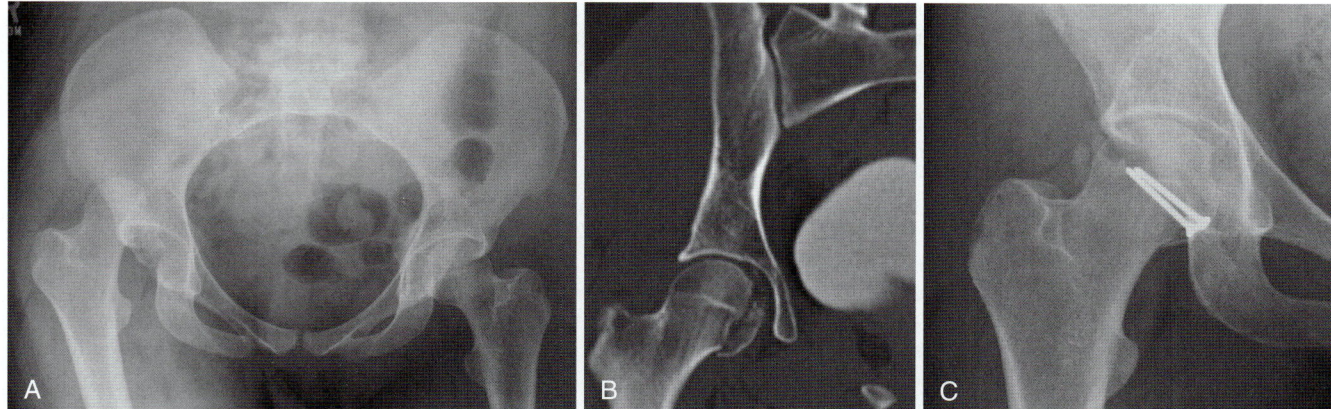

Figure 48-9. Pipkin I femoral head fracture reduced and stabilized through an anterior approach using multiple countersunk screws. **A,** Initial radiograph showing the posterior hip dislocation. **B,** Computed tomography (CT) showing the Pipkin I fracture. **C,** Postoperative radiograph.

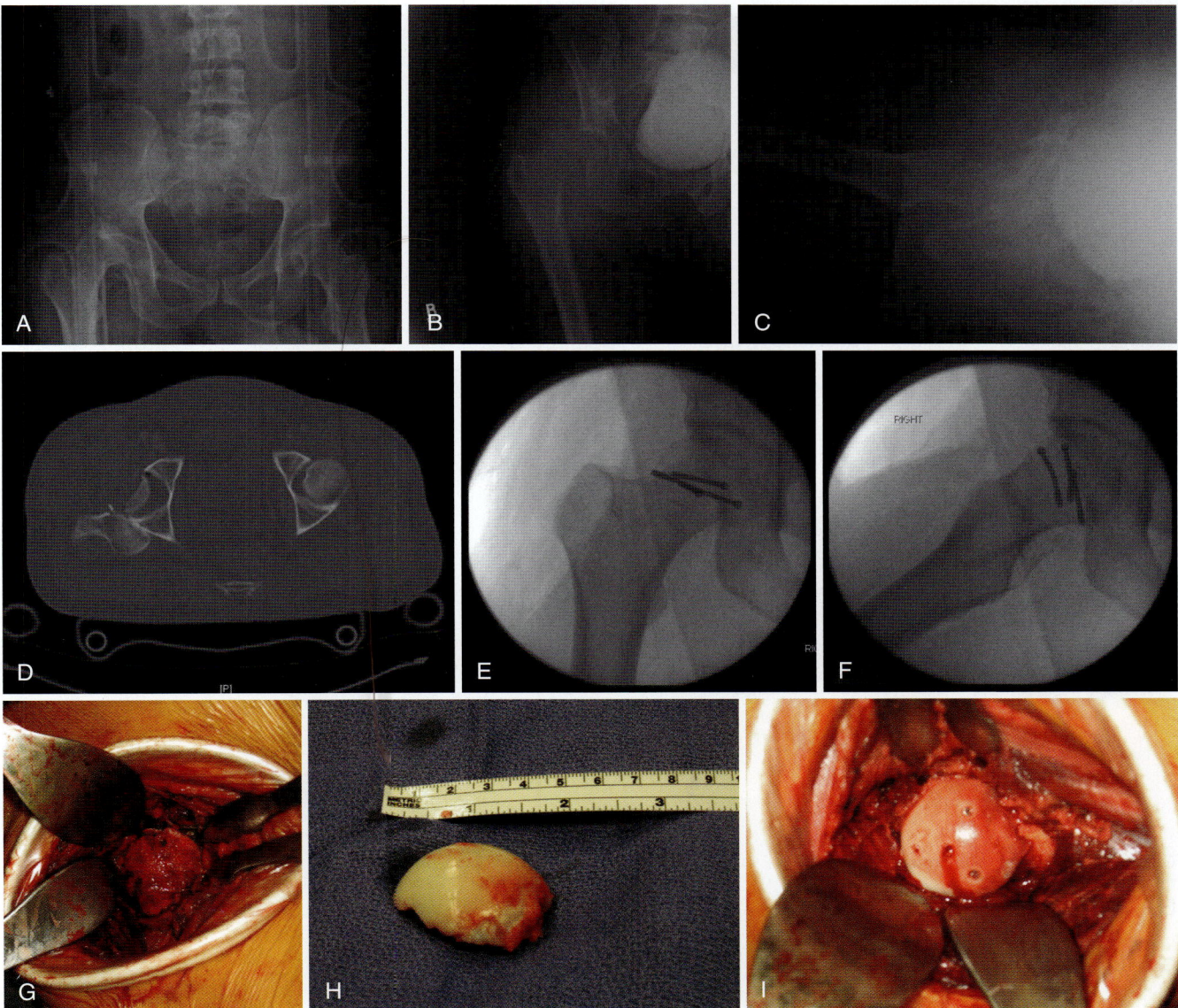

Figure 48-10. Pipkin II fracture reduced and stabilized through an anterior approach. **A** through **D,** Anteroposterior (AP) pelvis, AP hip, cross-table lateral of hip, and computed tomography (CT) scan demonstrating a Pipkin II femoral head fracture. **E** and **F,** Final AP and lateral radiographs after reduction and fixation. **G** through **I,** Intraoperative photographs showing the size and location of the fracture fragment before and after fixation. *(Case courtesy Mark Munro, MD.)*

(Fig. 48-11). In a Pipkin type IV injury, the "posterior" wall fracture is often more *superior,* and the trochanteric flip allows easy access to this location without traction on the superior gluteal neurovascular complex or the gluteus medius musculature. With dislocation of the femoral head, the femoral head fracture is easily addressed. In a foveal/suprafoveal fracture, the ligamentum teres will need to be transected to reduce the femoral head fragment. The labrum and the capsule are repaired as well as possible. If the posterior wall fracture is located superiorly, even a relatively small fragment can cause hip instability and should be repaired. In this case, the plate should be positioned peripherally along the acetabular rim and directed toward the anterior inferior iliac spine.

Femoral head fractures associated with anterior dislocations are more difficult to manage. Small impaction fractures, typically located on the superior aspect of the femoral head, require no specific treatment, but the fracture size and location have prognostic implications.[7] Impaction fractures, which involve a large portion of the femoral head, should be surgically treated with fracture disimpaction, elevation, and bone grafting[3]; biomechanical studies have demonstrated that a 2 cm^2 area of impaction in the weight-bearing portion of the femoral head significantly affects the contact force distribution of the hip.[42] Displaced transchondral fractures that result in nonconcentric hip reduction require open reduction and excision or internal fixation, depending on the fragment size and location.

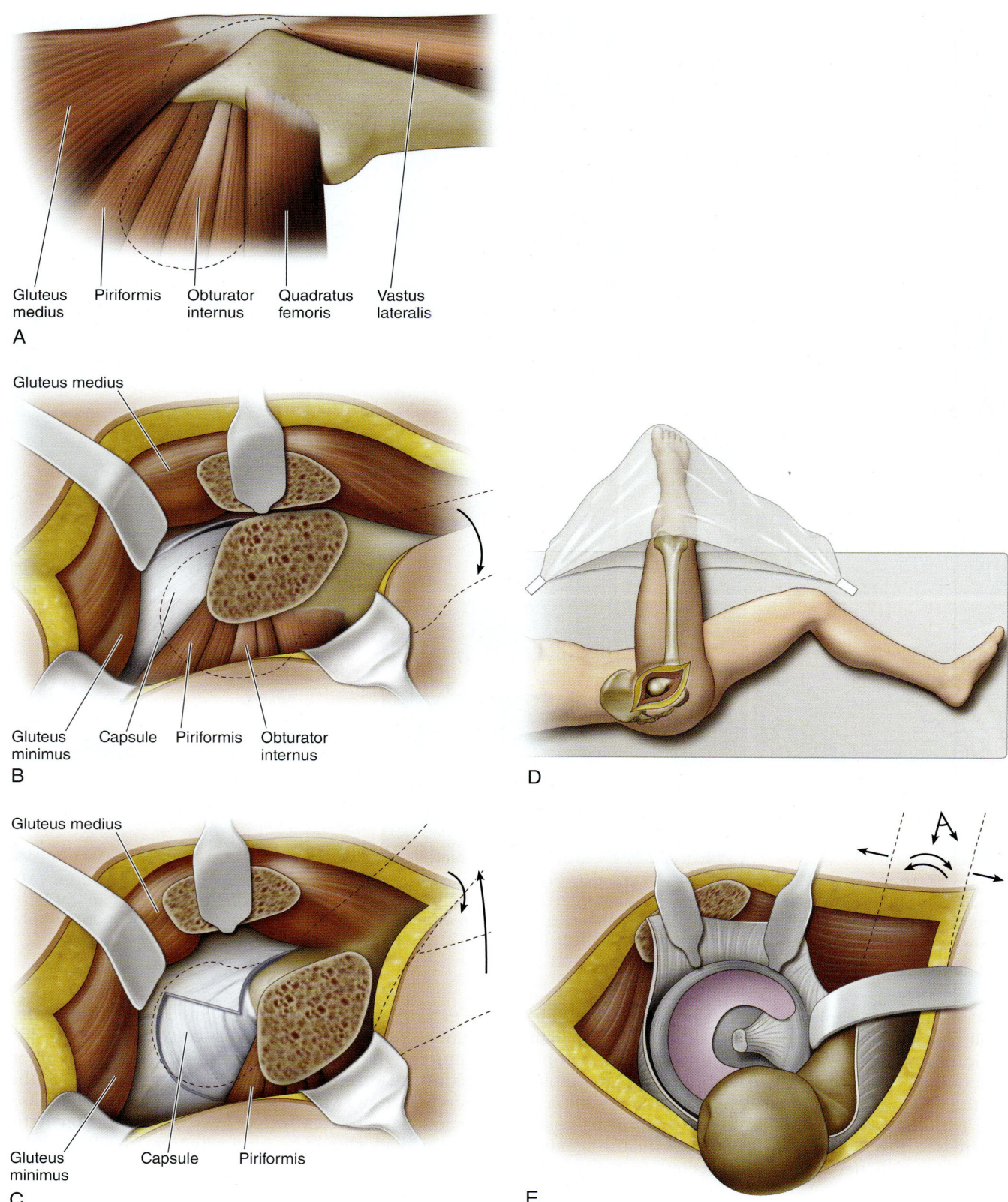

Gluteus
medius

Piriformis

Obturator
internus

Quadratus
femoris

Vastus
lateralis

A

Gluteus medius

Gluteus
minimus

Capsule

Piriformis

Obturator
internus

B

D

Gluteus medius

Gluteus
minimus

Capsule

Piriformis

C

E

Figure 48-11. The Ganz trochanteric flip. (*Redrawn from Ganz R, Gill TJ, Gautier E, et al: Surgical dislocation of the adult hip. J Bone Joint Surg Br 83:1119–1124, 2001.*)

Rehabilitation

Early controlled motion is the goal after any joint injury; joint immobilization can result in intra-articular adhesions and arthritis and therefore should be avoided. Although some investigators have recommended a temporary period of traction or balanced suspension after hip dislocation and reduction until the patient's initial pain has subsided,[7] this protocol has not proved beneficial. In general, controlled passive range-of-hip motion exercises and early mobilization are thought to benefit the patient's overall condition and should be initiated on the basis of clinical range of hip stability. Extremes of motion should be avoided for 4 to 6 weeks to allow capsular and soft tissue healing, dependent on the direction of dislocation. For posterior dislocations, one should avoid the extremes of hip flexion, adduction, and internal rotation. A knee immobilizer may be utilized in the acute setting after posterior hip dislocation to avoid these "at risk" positions. For anterior dislocations, one should avoid extension, abduction, and external rotation.

For a simple hip dislocation that is clinically stable on range-of-motion testing, the patient is mobilized once comfortable. Although early weight bearing has not been shown to add to the initial ischemic insult, the usual recommendation is for protected weight bearing for 4 to 6 weeks after hip dislocation.[3,7] Rehabilitation should include strengthening exercises for the musculature about the hip. Return to high-demand activities and sports should be delayed 6 to 12 weeks or until hip strength is near normal.

For dislocations with associated fractures, patient mobilization, hip range of motion, and weight bearing status are generally dictated by the associated injury. For an associated posterior wall fracture, full weight bearing is generally delayed for 8 to 12 weeks. A similar protocol is usually recommended after fixation of an associated femoral head or neck fracture; progression to weight bearing is based on the radiographic appearance of the associated fracture.

PROGNOSIS

In general, anterior dislocations without femoral head injury have a better long-term prognosis than posterior dislocations.[43] Dreinhofer and associates reported a 75% acceptable result rate after anterior dislocation compared with 48% after posterior dislocation.[44] The prognosis after simple hip dislocation has been reported to be good to excellent in 48% to 95% of patients.[3,44,45] This range of good results may be related to differing patient age, time to reduction, method of reduction, postreduction management, associated injuries, and duration of follow-up.[7] The outcome for individual patients depends mostly on the development of osteonecrosis or post-traumatic arthritis. In the absence of these potential complications, the prognosis after hip dislocation is generally good.

Vecsei and colleagues reported a series of 82 patients who sustained a hip dislocation.[46] Treatment consisted of hip reduction within 6 hours of the injury under general anesthesia followed by full weight bearing as tolerated after 14 days. Forty-three patients were available for follow-up, which ranged from 6 months to 19 years. Radiologic signs of arthritis were seen in 17 (40%) patients, but osteonecrosis was noted in only one hip.

The most important prognostic factor is probably the time from injury to hip reduction.[1-3,7] The longer the interval between injury and hip reduction, the worse the result. Stewart and Milford reported 88% good results if the hip was reduced within 12 hours.[12] Likewise, Brav found that hip reduction after 12 hours increased the percentage of unsatisfactory results from 22% to 52%.[30] Morton reported excellent results only in patients whose hips were reduced within 12 hours.[47] Reigstad found no instances of osteonecrosis or post-traumatic arthritis when simple dislocations were reduced within 6 hours.[48] Furthermore, higher rates of osteonecrosis and arthritis were found by Hougaard and Thomsen if the time to relocation was longer than 6 hours.[49]

Associated injuries have a negative prognostic effect on the clinical result. Dreinhofer and coworkers[44] and Yang and associates[50] reported poorer results in patients who had sustained multiple severe injuries. Pape and colleagues reported a series of 29 consecutive patients who had sustained 31 traumatic hip dislocations and had an Injury Severity Score (ISS) exceeding 18 points.[51] Thirteen patients were available for follow-up at a mean of 8 years after injury. The clinical results at latest follow-up were excellent in three, good in seven, and fair in four hips. Five patients had radiographic evidence of early hip degeneration, and seven patients had osteonecrosis of the femoral head.

Patients who sustain associated femoral head fractures have similar poor outcomes.

Pipkin types I and II are reported to have the same prognosis as a simple dislocation if hip reduction occurs within 6 hours.[3,7,44] Pipkin type IV injuries seem to have roughly the same prognosis as acetabular fractures without a femoral head fracture.[3,7] Pipkin type III injuries have a very poor prognosis. Anterior hip dislocations have been reported to have a higher incidence of associated femoral head injuries (transchondral or indentation type) when compared with posterior dislocations.[3,7] The only patients with excellent results in most authors' series after anterior dislocation are those without an associated femoral head injury.[3,7,44,52]

Yoon and associates reported a series of 30 femoral head fractures.[53] Smaller fragments were excised while larger fragments were internally stabilized. The femoral head was replaced in all Pipkin type IV fractures. After a mean follow-up of 3 to 10 years, the clinical outcome was excellent in 7, good in 15, fair in 4, and poor in 1, and the radiographic outcome was excellent in 15, good in 7, fair in 4, and poor in 1. On the basis of their findings, these investigators concluded that (1) excision of the small fragment is a good choice of treatment in Pipkin type I fractures, (2) early reduction with stable internal fixation is appropriate in type II and III fractures, and (3) arthroplasty is indicated in type IV fractures. Given the ability to address posterior wall fractures, this view might be considered extreme.

Marchetti and colleagues reported a series of 33 patients who sustained a Pipkin fracture and were followed for a mean of 49 months.[54] The overall results were 67% good, 18% fair, and 15% poor; no excellent results were reported. The Pipkin classification scheme was a useful predictor of outcome; patients with Pipkin type I or II had statistically significant better outcomes than did those who sustained Pipkin type III or IV. No statistically significant differences in outcomes or complication rates were noted when time to hip reduction was compared with the operative approach.

Giannoudis and coworkers recently reported the results of a systematic literature review for femoral head fractures, focusing on management, complications, and clinical results.[55] Mean patient age was 38.9 years, with a mean follow-up of 55.6 months. For Pipkin type I fractures, fragment excision seemed to give better results than internal fixation. For Pipkin type II fractures, anatomic reduction and stable fixation yielded the best results. The overall wound infection rate was 3.2%, and the rate of sciatic nerve palsy was 3.95%. Late complications included post-traumatic arthritis (20%), heterotopic ossification (16.8%), and osteonecrosis (11.9%).

COMPLICATIONS

Osteonecrosis has been reported in 5% to 40% of hip dislocations,* and increased risk has been associated with longer time from injury to hip reduction (>6 to 24 hours).[3,7] However, some authors suggest that osteonecrosis may result from the initial injury and not from prolonged dislocation.[7] Osteonecrosis may become clinically apparent up to 5 years after injury. Repeated reduction attempts may increase the risk of osteonecrosis. Post-traumatic osteoarthritis is the most frequent long-term complication of hip dislocation[3,7,27]; its incidence is dramatically higher when associated with acetabular fractures or transchondral fractures of the femoral head. Recurrent dislocation is rare (<2%), although patients with decreased femoral anteversion are at risk for recurrent posterior dislocation, and those with increased femoral anteversion may be prone to recurrent anterior dislocation.[7]

Sciatic nerve injury occurs in 10% to 15% of hip dislocations.[10-12] Sciatic nerve injury is usually caused by stretching of the nerve from a posteriorly dislocated head or from a displaced fracture fragment. The prognosis is unpredictable, but most authors report 40% to 50% full recovery.[7] Electromyographic (EMG) studies are indicated at 3 to 4 weeks for baseline and prognostic information and guidance. If no clinical or electrical improvement is seen by 1 year, surgical intervention may be considered. If sciatic nerve injury occurs after a closed reduction, then entrapment of the nerve is likely and surgical exploration is indicated. Injury to the

femoral nerve and femoral vascular structures has been reported after anterior dislocation.[7]

Heterotopic ossification is common after posterior fracture dislocation and may be related to the initial muscular damage and hematoma formation.[3,7] Surgical intervention increases the incidence of heterotopic ossification. Prophylaxis against heterotopic ossification includes indomethacin for 6 weeks or use of radiation. Thromboembolism may occur after hip dislocation owing to traction-induced intimal injury to the vasculature. Patients should be given adequate prophylaxis consisting of compression stockings, sequential compression devices, and chemoprophylaxis, particularly if placed in traction for any length of time.

CURRENT CONTROVERSIES AND FUTURE CONSIDERATIONS

- *The role of MRI in the evaluation of hip dislocation:* MRI is superior to CT in evaluating soft tissue status; however, CT gives better osseous details. Furthermore, CT scan is easier to obtain in an emergent setting. Although MRI may prove useful in evaluating the vascularity of the femoral head, the usefulness of MRI in predicting osteonecrosis of the femoral head after injury has not been established.
- *The role of hip arthroscopy after hip dislocation:* Arthroscopy can be used to lavage and remove small fragments from the hip joint. However, the size of the fragments that can be removed arthroscopically is limited; in addition, only certain areas of the hip can be accessed arthroscopically. Finally, no study has proved whether loose body removal improves patient outcome by lowering the incidence of resultant osteoarthritis.
- *Open versus closed hip reduction:* Although most authors recommend urgent closed hip reduction, some advocate open reduction for all dislocations and fracture-dislocations to remove fragments from the joint and to reconstruct associated fractures. No studies have documented whether outcomes are improved with open or closed reduction as long as the hip joint is congruous and clinically stable to range-of-motion testing.

REFERENCES

1. Tornetta P, Mostafavi H: Hip dislocation: current treatment regimens. J Am Acad Orthop Surg 5:27–36, 1997.
2. Foulk DM, Mullis BH: Hip dislocation: evaluation and management. J Am Acad Orthop Surg 18:199–209, 2010.
3. Tornetta P III: Hip dislocations and fractures of the femoral head. In Bucholz RW, Heckman JD, Court-Brown C (eds): Fractures in adults, vol 2, ed 6, Philadelphia, 2006, Lippincott Williams & Wilkins, pp 1715–1752.
4. Gillespie WJ: The incidence and pattern of knee injury associated with dislocation of the hip. J Bone Joint Surg Br 57:376–378, 1975.
5. Suraci AL: Distribution and severity of injuries associated with hip dislocations secondary to motor vehicle accidents. J Trauma 26:458–460, 1986.
6. Wu CC, Shih CH, Chen LH: Femoral shaft fractures complicated by fracture-dislocations of the ipsilateral hip. J Trauma 34:70–75, 1993.

---

*References 3, 7, 24, 27, 30, 43, and 56 to 60.

7. Hip dislocations and femoral head fractures. In Egol KA, Koval KJ, Zuckerman JD (eds): Handbook of fractures, ed 4, Philadelphia, 2010, Lippincott Williams & Wilkins, pp 360–377.
8. Tabuenca J, Truan JR: Knee injuries in traumatic hip dislocation. Clin Orthop Relat Res 377:78–83, 2000.
9. Schmidt GL, Sciulli R, Altman GT: Knee injury in patients experiencing a high-energy traumatic ipsilateral hip dislocation. J Bone Joint Surg Am 87:1200–1204, 2005.
10. Upadhyay SS, Moulton A: The long-term results of traumatic posterior dislocation of the hip. J Bone Joint Surg Br 63:548–551, 1981.
11. Epstein HC: Traumatic dislocations of the hip. Clin Orthop Relat Res 92:116–142, 1973.
12. Stewart MJ, Milford LW: Fracture-dislocation of the hip: an end-result study. J Bone Joint Surg Am 36:315–342, 1954.
13. Fairbairn KJ, Mulligan ME, Murphey MD, Resnik CS: Gas bubbles in the hip joint on CT: an indication of recent dislocation. AJR Am J Roentgenol 164:931–934, 1995.
14. Crawford MJ, Dy CJ, Alexander JW, et al: The 2007 Frank Stinchfield Award. The biomechanics of the hip labrum and the stability of the hip. Clin Orthop Relat Res 465:16–22, 2007.
15. Kundu ZS, Mittal R, Sangwan SS, Sharma A: Simultaneous asymmetric bilateral hip dislocation with unilateral fracture of the femur-peculiar mode of trauma in a case. Eur J Orthop Surg Traumatol 13:255–257, 2003.
16. Martinez AA, Gracia F, Rodrigo J: Asymmetrical bilateral traumatic hip dislocation with ipsilateral acetabular fracture. J Orthop Sci 5:307–309, 2000.
17. Dudkiewicz I, Salai M, Horowitz S, Chechik A: Bilateral asymmetric traumatic dislocation of the hip joints. J Trauma 49:336–338, 2000.
18. Kaleli T, Alyuz N: Bilateral traumatic dislocation of the hip: simultaneously one hip anterior and the other posterior. Arch Orthop Trauma Surg 117:479–480, 1998.
19. Lam F, Walczak J, Franklin A: Traumatic asymmetrical bilateral hip dislocation in an adult. Emerg Med J 18:506–507, 2001.
20. Maqsood M, Walker AP: Asymmetrical bilateral traumatic hip dislocation with ipsilateral fracture of the femoral shaft. Injury 27:521–522, 1996.
21. Pringle JH, Edwards AH: Traumatic dislocation at the hip joint: an experimental study on the cadaver. Glasgow Med J 139:25–40, 1943.
22. Upadhyay SS, Moulton A, Burwell RG: Biological factors predisposing to traumatic posterior dislocation of the hip: a selection process in the mechanism of injury. J Bone Joint Surg Br 67:232–236, 1985.
23. Laorr A, Greenspan A, Anderson MW, et al: Traumatic hip dislocation: early MRI findings. Skeletal Radiol 24:239–245, 1995.
24. Stewart MJ, Milford MW: Fracture-dislocation of the hip: an end-result study. J Bone Joint Surg Am 36:315–342, 1954.
25. Brumback RJ, Kenzora JE, Levitt L, et al: Fractures of the femoral head. Hip 181–206, 1987.
26. Orthopaedic Trauma Association: Fracture and dislocation compendium. J Orthop Trauma 10:112, 1996.
27. Thompson VP, Epstein HC: Traumatic dislocation of the hip: a survey of two hundred and four cases covering a period of twenty-one years. J Bone Joint Surg Am 33:746–778, 1951.
28. Epstein HC, Wiss DA: Traumatic anterior dislocation of the hip. Orthopedics 8:130, 132–134, 1985.
29. Pipkin G: Treatment of grade IV fracture-dislocation of the hip. J Bone Joint Surg Am 39:1027–1042, 1957.
30. Brav EA: Traumatic dislocation of the hip: Army experience and results over a twelve-year period. J Bone Joint Surg Am 44:1115–1134, 1952.
31. Allis OH: The hip, Philadelphia, 1895, Dornan.
32. Stimson LA: Five cases of dislocation of the hip. NY Med J 50:118–121, 1889.
33. Sahin V, Karakas ES, Aksu S, et al: Traumatic dislocation and fracture-dislocation of the hip: a long-term follow-up study. J Trauma 54:520–529, 2003.
34. Walker WA: Traumatic dislocations of the hip joint. Am J Surg 50:545–549, 1940.
35. Mullis BH, Dahners LE: Hip arthroscopy to remove loose bodies after traumatic dislocation. J Orthop Trauma 20:22–26, 2006.
36. Yamamoto Y, Ide T, Ono T, Hamada Y: Usefulness of arthroscopic surgery in hip trauma cases. Arthroscopy 19:269–273, 2003.
37. Epstein HC: Posterior fracture-dislocations of the hip: long-term follow-up. J Bone Joint Surg Am 56:1103–1127, 1974.
38. Philippon MJ, Kuppersmith DA, Wolff AB, Briggs KK: Arthroscopic findings following traumatic hip dislocation in 14 professional athletes. Arthroscopy 25:169–174, 2009.
39. Svoboda SJ, Williams DM, Murphy KP: Hip arthroscopy for osteochondral loose body removal after a posterior hip dislocation. Arthroscopy 19:777–781, 2003.
40. Swiontkowski MF, Thorpe M, Seiler JG, Hansen ST: Operative management of displaced femoral head fractures: case-matched comparison of anterior versus posterior approaches for Pipkin I and Pipkin II fractures. J Orthop Trauma 6:437–442, 1992.
41. Ganz R, Gill TJ, Gautier E, et al: Surgical dislocation of the adult hip. J Bone Joint Surg Br 83:1119–1124, 2001.
42. Konrath GA, Hamel AJ, Guerin J, et al: Biomechanical evaluation of impaction fractures of the femoral head. J Orthop Trauma 13:407–413, 1999.
43. Sanders S, Tejwani N, Egol KA: Traumatic hip dislocation—a review. Bull NYU Hosp Jt Dis 68:91–96, 2010.
44. Dreinhöfer KE, Schwarzkopf SR, Haas NP, Tscherne H: Isolated traumatic dislocation of the hip: long-term results in 50 patients. J Bone Joint Surg Br 76:6–12, 1994.
45. Hunter GA: Posterior dislocation and fracture-dislocation of the hip: a review of fifty-seven patients. J Bone Joint Surg Br 51:38–44, 1969.
46. Vécsei V, Schwendenwein E, Berger G: Hip dislocation without bone injuries. Orthopade 26:317–326, 1997.
47. Morton KS: Traumatic dislocation of the hip: a follow-up study. Can J Surg 3:67–74, 1959.
48. Reigstad A: Traumatic dislocation of the hip. J Trauma 20:603–606, 1980.
49. Hougaard K, Thompson PB: Traumatic posterior dislocation of the hip—prognostic factors influencing the incidence of avascular necrosis of the femoral head. Arch Orthop Trauma Surg 106:32–35, 1986.
50. Yang RS, Tsuang YH, Hang YS, Liu TK: Traumatic dislocation of the hip. Clin Orthop Relat Res 265:218–227, 1991.
51. Pape HC, Rice J, Wolfram K, et al: Hip dislocation in patients with multiple injuries: a followup investigation. Clin Orthop Relat Res 377:99–105, 2000.
52. Amihood S: Anterior dislocation of the hip. Injury 7:107–110, 1975.
53. Yoon TR, Rowe SM, Chung JY, et al: Clinical and radiographic outcome of femoral head fractures: 30 patients followed for 3-10 years. Acta Orthop Scand 72:348–353, 2001.
54. Marchetti ME, Steinberg GG, Coumas JM: Intermediate-term experience of Pipkin fracture-dislocations of the hip. J Orthop Trauma 10:455–461, 1996.
55. Giannoudis PV, Kontakis G, Christoforakis Z, et al: Management, complications and clinical results of femoral head fractures. Injury 40:1245–1251, 2009.
56. Armstrong JR: Traumatic dislocation of the hip joint: review of 101 dislocations. J Bone Joint Surg Br 30:430–445, 1948.
57. Paus B: Traumatic dislocations of the hip: late results in 76 cases. Acta Orthop Scand 21:99–112, 1951.
58. Hougaard K, Thomsen PB: Coxarthrosis following traumatic posterior dislocation of the hip. J Bone Joint Surg Am 69:679–683, 1987.
59. Upadhyay SS, Moulton A, Srikrishnamurthy K: An analysis of the late effects of traumatic posterior dislocation of the hip without fractures. J Bone Joint Surg Br 65:150–152, 1983.
60. Reigstad A: Traumatic dislocation of the hip. J Trauma 20:603–606, 1980.

SECTION VII

TUMORS OF THE HIP

CHAPTER 49

Evaluation of Bone Lesions Around the Hip

Eric A. Silverstein

INTRODUCTION

The hip is a common location for many soft tissue and osseous neoplasms in addition to tumor simulators. It is the role of the orthopaedic surgeon to recognize and be aware of these lesions in order to treat them appropriately or refer these patients in a timely fashion. The spectrum of disease varies from latent benign to overly aggressive malignancies.

This chapter will focus on the epidemiology and clinical evaluation of neoplasms arising around the hip. An overview of common lesions and their treatment is presented. Chapter 50 will cover specific treatment techniques for benign tumors. Chapter 51 will cover malignant tumors, and Ch. 52 will discuss the treatment of metastatic disease in detail.

EPIDEMIOLOGY OF HIP LESIONS

A variety of lesions are found in and around the hip. The age range is by no means absolute; however, certain neoplasms, such as Ewing's sarcoma, are rarely seen beyond the age of 25. Most bone tumors have a predilection for males, with few exceptions. The plethora of hip lesions include broad categories such as tumor simulators (infection, congenital and endocrine disorders,

genetic sequelae, and those unexplained), benign and malignant primary bone tumors, synovial-based disease, and metastatic/bone marrow–based disease. Table 49-1 summarizes most of the lesions found around the hip.[1-8]

Clinical Evaluation

The history is key in approaching a patient with a suspected tumor about the hip. The patient's presenting age is an important factor in narrowing down the differential diagnosis. Although any tumor can theoretically occur at any age, there are characteristic age distributions to benign and malignant tumors which will focus the attention of the clinician toward the most likely candidates. These are outlined in Table 49-1.

Obviously, a personal or family history of malignancy or other tumorous condition of bone is relevant. A genetic basis is understood for a number of bone tumors and suspected for many for which it has not yet been ascertained. Particularly in any patient with a history of prior malignancy, the presence of a new tumor about the hip must prompt suspicion for metastatic disease.

The patient's presenting pain is an essential aspect of the evaluation. Lesions may be diagnosed incidentally, they may present with mechanical pain, or they may present with true night pain. The last is pain which is present characteristically at night such that it will actually awaken patients from a sound sleep. Lesions which are found incidentally are most likely be to benign; those which present with mechanical pain are concerning for impending pathologic fracture. Patients presenting with true night pain will raise a high suspicion for malignancy.

The presence of a mass is also an important aspect of the history. The hip and pelvis region are deep-seated structures, so any mass which is detected is usually large and advanced by the time it is clinically apparent. Soft tissue tumors will often present with a painless mass even when malignant and quite large. Fortunately, only a tiny fraction of soft tissues masses presenting in adults represent malignancy.

Clinical Examination

The standard orthopedic examination of the hip joint is performed in any patient presenting with a suspected tumor. Examination is best expressed in degrees of motion as well as percentage comparison of the

Table 49-1. Most Common Lesions Around the Hip

Bone Lesion	Age Range, yr (approximate)	Male-to-Female (ratio)	Category
Fibrous dysplasia (FD) McCune-Albright syndrome	Lifetime	1:1	Tumor simulator
Brown tumor (hyperparathyroidism)	>30	1:3	Tumor simulator
Paget's disease	>50	M>F	Tumor simulator
Osteomyelitis	Any age	1:1	Tumor simulator
Avascular necrosis (AVN)/bone infarct	Any age		Tumor simulator
Hip dysplasia	Congenital	M<F	Tumor simulator
Gorham's disease	Any age Usually <40	1:1	Tumor simulator
Intraosseous cyst	20-60	2:1	Tumor simulator
Unicameral bone cyst (UBC)	5-15	2:1	Tumor simulator
Aneurysmal bone cyst (ABC) Primary vs. secondary	5-30	1:1 (>♀)	Tumor simulator

Nonossifying fibroma (NOF)
  Jaffe-Campanacci syndrome
  Neurofibromatosis
	5-20	1.5:1	Benign bone neoplasms

Desmoplastic fibroma	<30	1:1	Benign bone neoplasms
Liposclerosing myxoid fibrous tumor (LSMFT)	20-60	1:1	Benign bone neoplasms
Exostosis (osteochondroma) Multiple hereditary exostosis (MHE)	5-20	2:1 2:1	Benign bone neoplasms

Langerhans' cell histiocytosis (LCH)
  Eosinophilic granuloma
  Hand-Schüller-Christian disease
  Letterer-Siwe disease
	5-20	2:1	Benign bone neoplasms

Giant cell tumor (GCT)	20-40	1:1 (>♀)	Benign bone neoplasms
Chondroblastoma	10-25	3:1	Benign bone neoplasms
Osteoid osteoma (OO)	5-30	2.5:1	Benign bone neoplasms
Osteoblastoma	10-30	2:1	Benign bone neoplasms
Chondroma Enchondroma	Any age	1:1	Benign bone neoplasms
Intraosseous hemangioma/lymphangioma Cystic angiomatosis	Any age	1.5:1	Benign bone neoplasms
ΔPigmented villonodular synovitis (PVNS)	20-50	1:1 (>♀)	Benign synovial disease
ΔSynovial osteochondromatosis	20-50	1.5:1	Benign synovial disease

Chondrosarcoma
  Central
  Clear cell
	
	40-70
	20-50
		
		1.4:1
		1.4:1
			Primary bone malignancy

Ewing's sarcoma	5-25	1.5:1	Primary bone malignancy
Osteosarcoma (high grade)	10-30 >50 (Paget's or post radiation)	1.5:1	Primary bone malignancy
Malignant fibrous histiocytosis of bone	Any age (except children)	1:1 (>♂)	Primary bone malignancy
Hemangioendothelioma	Any age	2:1	Primary bone malignancy
Chordoma	30-70 (sacral)	2:1	Primary malignancy
Metastatic disease • Five most common primary sites: breast, lung, thyroid, kidney, and prostate	>40	Dependent on tumor type	Bone malignancy
Multiple myeloma Plasmacytoma	>40	1.4:1	Bone malignancy
Lymphoma Primary lymphoma of bone	 15-70	 1.5:1	Bone malignancy

Δ, Synovial-based disease (not bone).

opposite side. Any maneuvers which elicit pain during the examination should be noted for further evaluation. In addition to a standard orthopedic joint evaluation, a full oncologic examination should be performed. This includes an assessment of any masses, evaluation for lymphadenopathy, and any skin changes which may be present in the region of the tumor. Masses should be investigated for the presence of any Tinel's sign, mobility, tenderness, or pulsation. The presence of hepatosplenomegaly or other findings suggestive of disseminated disease are noted. As well, skin manifestations of any systemic disease or genetic syndrome (for example: café au lait spots suggestive of neurofibromatosis) are noted.

Patients with a large mass or destructive lesion will often have compromise of neurologic function in the limb. Careful testing of sciatic nerve function is critical. Although pulses may be palpable, in the setting of a large mass, the ankle brachial index may be decreased due to compression of vascular structures. Deep venous thromboses are common in patients presenting with large malignant masses around the hip and the limb should be assessed for swelling or other stigmata of this. It is helpful to measure the circumference of the limb compared to the uninvolved side at defined points.

Imaging

Characteristics that make an osseous lesion aggressive and concerning include an associated soft tissue mass, periosteal elevation, permeative appearance, large size and rapid growth. Plain film radiographs provide the first assessment of any patients presenting with a potential tumor about the hip. Radiographs have the advantage of defining any bony lesions as lytic, blastic, or having a mixed characteristic. They help determine whether a mass is producing osteoid or has matrix calcification. Additionally, even in patients with soft tissues masses alone, radiographs can define soft tissue calcifications which can be helpful in the evaluation process.

Radiographs provide a rapid assessment of present or impending fracture. However, it is important to remember that up to a third of bony mineral must be lost before a lesion is apparent of plain film radiographs. In imaging lesions around the pelvis, inlet and outlet as well as Judet views are helpful in evaluating periacetabular or iliac wing lesions. Proximal femoral lesions are adequately evaluated by AP and lateral radiographs of the hip. It is important to obtain full length radiographs of the entire femur to evaluate for the presence of any skip or distal lesions which are not immediately apparent on plain films of the hip itself.

Magnetic resonance imaging provides the most sensitive evaluation of tumoral processes in the bone marrow and the greatest definition of soft tissues masses. In obtaining an MRI scan, images before and after administration of gadolinium contrast are always obtained in evaluating potential tumors about the hip. At least one T1 weighted sequence which evaluates the entire extent of the bone is used to evaluate for skip lesions. Most commonly this is a coronal T1 weighted sequence of the femur. T1 weighted sequences provide a sensitive

evaluation for marrow replacing processes to fully define the extent of lesions. Contrast enhancement patterns help separate cystic from solid masses in the evaluation of these patients.

Computed tomography is the most sensitive method to define bony architecture around the hip and provides a rapid assessment of whether any matrix or osteoid production is present. CT can be combined with angiography to define any vascular encasement by tumor. It also provides an efficient mechanism to evaluate for an impending pathologic fracture when plain film radiographs may not clearly demonstrate loss of bony trabeculae or cortical compromise.

In addition to its role for local imaging of the tumor, CT of the chest, abdomen, and pelvis is most commonly utilized as a part of staging studies for patients with suspected or proven malignancy. Although CT of the chest is the most defined study for staging of sarcomas, our practice is to obtain CT images of the abdomen and pelvis for any patient who has a malignancy extending at or above the level of the inguinal ligament to identify any regional metastases which may be missed by CT of the chest alone.

Technetium bone scan is used to define whether a process is active or latent and is a component of staging of most bony malignancies. Although false negatives can be seen (such as in the case of multiple myeloma or in very aggressive lytic tumors), the bone scan is a reliable method for evaluation of most bony processes around the hip and pelvis. In those cases in which it proves unreliable, a bone survey can be used.

The role of positron emission tomography (PET) scanning is evolving at this time. PET is established for the evaluation of patients with aggressive carcinomas among several other malignancies. As it relies upon metabolic uptake by tumor cells, it is less reliable in evaluation of patients with low or intermediate grade malignancies. The role of PET in evaluating patients with high-grade sarcomas is currently under study. PET scans are usually combined with a low resolution CT scan for co-registration of anatomic abnormalities.

Not all imaging modalities are necessary in all patients. Many benign lesions have characteristic appearances on plain radiographs and no further local imaging is necessary. The most common imaging protocol to define suspected lesions around the hip combines plain film radiographs with contrast enhanced MR scans. This combination of imaging is usually adequate to form a differential diagnosis, evaluate the likelihood of malignancy and plan an appropriate oncologic biopsy. Further imaging will be described in the other chapters in this section pursuant to individual lesions.

Biopsy

Biopsy confirmation of suspected histology is usually required. The hazards of a poorly planned biopsy have been well established by Dr. Mankin in a series of studies.[9-10] Poorly planned biopsies will frequently alter the surgical options available for patients and may preclude limb salvage in the setting of a sarcoma diagnosis. Additionally, in adults presenting with suspected metastatic disease, proper staging studies will usually yield the diagnosis without the need for biopsy or may identify a safer alternative site to sample. Dr. Rougraff and colleagues established a protocol of history, routine laboratory studies, bone scan, and CT of the chest, abdomen, and pelvis as identifying the site of primary disease in 85 percent of patients.[11]

The key principle to musculoskeletal biopsy is that the biopsy tract must be able to be excised with the definitive resection if the tumor proves to be a primary sarcoma.[12] For this reason there is the strong recommendation that a musculoskeletal biopsy either be performed or directed by a surgeon who is prepared carry out the definitive resection should a sarcoma be diagnosed. Most biopsies around the hip and pelvis can be performed either through a direct lateral approach for lesions of the proximal femur or along the line of the iliac crest for lesions of the pelvis. This follows the utilitarian incision to the hip as described by Enneking. Biopsies performed along this line are readily excised at the time of surgery.

A tension always exists between performing an open versus a closed biopsy. Open biopsies have the advantage of obtaining a large volume of tissue for histopathologic analysis, particularly if advanced cytogenic or other tests are necessary. They are generally considered the gold standard for diagnosis. However, open biopsies are not without risk; when compared to percutaneous biopsy they expose a larger area of tissue to contamination which will require ultimate excision should a malignancy be proven.

Percutaneous biopsy varies from fine needles (which yield very limited samples) to large bore core needles which can provide samples with preserved architecture. Large bore core needle biopsies directed by CT or magnetic resonance imaging can be used to access areas of the tumor which are likely to be most representative while minimizing areas of soft tissue contamination.[13-14] Percutaneous core needle biopsies must be carefully planned with the performing radiologist as well as pathologist to ensure that representative tissue is obtained in a sufficient quantity to allow a diagnosis while maintaining a safe trajectory. We will often tattoo the site of the biopsy with a small drop of methylene blue to allow it to be identified later for subsequent surgical resection. The ultimate decision for closed versus open biopsy is tailored to the clinical situation and influenced by institutional practice patterns and resources. Cultures are sent in addition to histology studies.

Should an open biopsy be necessary, it is critical that the most direct route to the tumor be used for sampling. Classic anatomic planes are deliberately avoided during these procedures to minimize contamination of multiple compartments. Rather, the approach usually goes directly to the tumor through the edge of an anatomic compartment which can be excised en bloc with the tumor as a more classic plane of approach is used. Major neurovascular structures are deliberately avoided during the course of the biopsy so that they will not be subject to contamination when the tumor is sampled. Very careful hemostasis is practiced and a drain is almost always left during an open biopsy of the proximal femur or pelvis to minimize the resulting hematoma and potential zone of contamination. Nonabsorbable Ethibond sutures are used at closing the fascia following the biopsy so that they can be identified at the time of surgery to be certain that the area is excised fully.

PATHOPHYSIOLOGY, CLINICAL FEATURES, RADIOGRAPHIC APPEARANCE, DIFFERENTIAL DIAGNOSIS, TREATMENT, AND PROGNOSIS

Tumor Simulators

This category encompasses tumor-like lesions ("pseudotumors") that generally are reactive or hyperplastic tissue responses. This definition does carry some ambiguity, and semantics may play a role. Therefore, certain lesions, such as aneurysmal bone cyst (ABC) and unicameral bone cyst (UBC), may be considered a tumor simulator or a benign bone tumor.

Fibrous Dysplasia (FD)

Fibrous dysplasia is a benign intramedullary fibro-osseous dysplastic lesion first described by Lichtenstein in 1938 with an origin linked to an activating mutation in the gene that encodes the α-subunit of stimulatory G protein ($G_s\alpha$). This results in developmental failure in the remodeling of primitive bone to mature lamellar bone. The consequence is biomechanically inferior bone that is non–stress oriented and prone to fracture. The process can be monostotic or polyostotic, and the most extreme presentation is McCune-Albright syndrome, which consists of polyostotic disease with café au lait spots and hyperfunction of multiple endocrine glands. Monostotic disease is fairly common and is not hereditary. Most lesions are asymptomatic and are found incidentally. However, a fairly common clinical presentation consists of bone pain, deformity, and fatigue/pathologic fracture. Wide variability in radiographic features is seen on plain radiographs. The classic pattern is a "ground-glass" appearance. However, cortical thinning, expansile remodeling, endosteal scalloping, and mixed radiolucency and radiodensity are common. Other findings may include coxa vara, shepherd's crook deformity, and protrusio acetabuli (Fig. 49-1). A computed tomography (CT) scan is the best imaging modality, but magnetic resonance imaging (MRI) is often helpful, especially in cases of cystic formation. A radionuclide bone scan will frequently be hot. Histopathology normally demonstrates a bland-spindle cell stroma with embedded trabeculae of woven (immature) bone with no osteoblastic rimming. This is often referred to as an "alphabet soup" appearance.

The diagnosis of fibrous dysplasia is often made on clinical and imaging presentation only. However, with atypical lesions, a biopsy is prudent. The differential diagnosis includes simple bone cysts, osteofibrous dysplasia, nonossifying fibroma, chondroma, low-grade

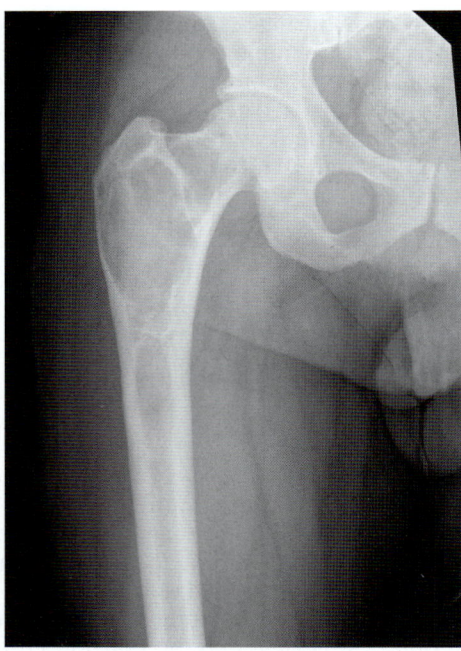

Figure 49-1. Anterior-posterior (AP) radiograph of the hip demonstrating a "ground glass" appearance with mild varus remodeling characteristic of fibrous dysplasia.

intramedullary osteosarcoma, and rarely Paget's disease. The clinical course is variable. Adults are often more symptomatic than children. There is no cure. Surgery is performed to prevent pathologic fracture, to correct limb alignment, and to decrease pain likely to result from fatigue fractures. The best options include the use of hardware or cortical allografts because the process (particularly if still active) can rapidly resorb most bone grafts. Bisphosphonates have shown efficacy in decreasing bone pain in patients with active symptomatic polyostotic disease. Cases of sarcoma developing within areas of fibrous dysplasia have been reported rarely.[1-3,5-8,15-17]

"Brown Tumor"

These pseudotumors are rare sequelae of primary hyperparathyroidism that has a delay in diagnosis or remains untreated. Primary hyperparathyroidism is caused by an adenoma of a single parathyroid gland in approximately 80% of cases, less likely both glands, hyperplasia, or cancer. Uncontrolled increased secretion of parathyroid hormone (PTH) causes an increase in gastrointestinal tract calcium absorption, renal tubular reabsorption of calcium in the kidney, and osteoclastic destruction of bone. This normally results in hypercalcemia and can present with symptoms such as lethargy, confusion, impaired mentation, depression, muscular weakness, loss of appetite, anorexia, nausea and vomiting, constipation, polydypsia/polyuria, nephrolithiasis, peptic ulcer, pancreatitis, and heart problems. This process can also cause profound bone changes. A "brown tumor" is one such consequence that is evident on x-ray as lytic areas, sometimes with

expansile remodeling of the cortex and pathologic fractures. These may simulate metastatic bone disease. The diagnosis usually can be established by blood tests showing hypercalcemia, hypophosphatemia, and an elevated PTH, assuming normal renal function. A biopsy of these lesions shows variable results, including hyperplastic tissue that is fibrous, fibro-osteoid, and giant cell rich; however, lesions can mimic a giant cell tumor, a reparative giant cell granuloma, or an aneurysmal bone cyst. Treatment consists of surgical excision of the parathyroid adenoma. Bone tumors will normally resolve; however, in cases of pathologic fracture or impending fracture, they generally are treated with internal fixation.[2-6,18]

Unicameral Bone Cyst (UBC) (Simple Bone Cyst)

These lesions are common in skeletally immature patients, particularly males. They represent a centrally located cystic lesion of bone that originates in the metaphysis and normally migrates toward the diaphysis with skeletal growth. They are filled with fluid similar to serum. Most are asymptomatic until presentation with a pathologic fracture. X-rays typically demonstrate a central radiolucency in the metadiaphyseal region with significant attenuation and possible mild expansile remodeling. Bone scans normally show little to no uptake unless a fracture is present. CT and MRI show fluid content within the lesion, but a fluid-fluid level characteristic of an aneurysmal bone cyst will not be seen. Bone septation is often seen in varying amounts from ridges along the inner surface of the cortex. The characteristic "fallen leaf" sign may be seen in the presence of a pathologic fracture, which represents a fragment of cortex that sinks into the fluid of the cyst. Histopathology shows a thin membrane walling the cyst that is made of loose fibrous tissue with cells that may resemble endothelial or synovial cells. Hemosiderin, giant cells, and woven bone intermixed are not uncommon. Biopsies usually are not indicated unless atypical. The differential diagnosis includes aneurysmal bone cyst and fibrous dysplasia. Treatment is provided for those at risk of fracture, particularly those with active cysts (adjacent to physis, single cavity with a very thin cortex), one or more recent fractures, and weight-bearing bones. Observation is reasonable for inactive cysts and those at low risk of fracture. Surgical treatment options are still debatable. Many use an aspiration and injection technique with corticosteroids or a combination of autogenous bone marrow and demineralized bone matrix. However, open curettage and bone grafting with or without internal fixation still has utility, especially in lesions around the hip, where structural stability is critical.[2-4,17,19-23]

Aneurysmal Bone Cyst (ABC)

These lesions are considered hyperplastic pseudotumors, which normally are seen in patients younger than 30 years of age. They are thought to be the result of a reactive reparative process that is hemorrhagic. They can be primary or secondary (to a large number of tumors). ABC generally presents as an enlarging, occasionally painful mass. Growth can vary greatly and at times it can be explosive. Malignant transformation has not been documented, and rarely spontaneous involution is seen. Radiographically, lesions are radiolucent with expansile remodeling or a "blow-out" appearance within the metaphysis. They can propagate to the epiphysis and diaphysis and often are eccentric with an "eggshell-thin" outer cortex. Occasionally, they are subperiosteal and can appear septated. Bone scans show predominantly peripheral uptake. CT and MRI often show the characteristic fluid-fluid level representing the separation of blood components. MRI with or without intravenous gadolinium demonstrates rim enhancement consistent with cystic properties. Grossly, an ABC often has a paper-thin reactive shell of bone that has a bluish tinge from old blood in the cavity. Histopathology is consistent with bland stromal cells lining the cavity of bone with multinucleated giant cells. Giant cells often cluster around the edges of the vascular lakes ("blood lakes"). Hemosiderin is usually present. Principal lesions in the differential diagnosis include simple bone cyst, giant cell tumor, and telangiectatic osteosarcoma. Treatment consists of extensive curettage with local adjuvant and reconstruction in most cases. However, with severe bone loss, en bloc resection may be needed. Recurrence rates vary from 20% to 40% without adjuvant, but can exceed 50% in the most aggressive form. External beam radiation can be used for difficult or dangerous surgical regions (e.g., sacrum or spine) and is fairly effective at low doses. Embolization is rarely used in cases not amenable to surgery or radiation and has unpredictable results.*

Benign Bone Neoplasms

This category consists of bony lesions with variably aggressive tendencies that are benign. Details are abridged and are mostly focused on the hip region.

Nonossifying Fibroma (NOF) (Fibrous Cortical Defect, Fibrous Xanthoma...)

This is the most common benign bone tumor. It is normally seen in childhood and rarely beyond the age of 20. Although it is a common bone lesion, nonossifying fibroma is uncommon around the hip. These tumors localize to the metaphysis, and most cases are asymptomatic. Radiographically, they are distinct with a small osteolytic defect located eccentrically in the metaphysis, but they can grow to a moderate size. A scalloped appearance is typical. The major axis is oriented parallel to the length of the bone. The lesion is mentioned here because the differential diagnosis can include fibrous dysplasia, chondromyxoid fibroma, unicameral and aneurysmal bone cysts, benign fibrous histiocytoma (histopathology identical but clinically more aggressive), giant cell tumor, and, rarely, malignant fibrous histiocytoma. Almost all lesions are treated conservatively unless the diagnosis is uncertain or the lesion atypical.[1-4,7,16]

Exostosis (Osteochondroma)

This neoplasm is a common developmental dysplasia of the peripheral growth plate that presents as a hamartomatous outgrowth of cartilage undergoing enchondral ossification. It can be solitary or multiple. These are usually apparent by the age of 5, or earlier in the setting of multiple hereditary exostoses. They often present as a painless, slow-growing, hard, fixed mass. Symptoms are often linked to mechanical irritation of surrounding soft tissues and bursal inflammation. Multiple hereditary exostoses present with multiple lesions, short stature, bony deformity, and commonly coxa valga with excessive anteversion. Radiographs may show a sessile or pedunculated (stalklike) lesion located in the metaphysis, which will be seen further from the growth plate as the child matures. Often the exostosis is pointing away from the physis. The radiographic hallmark is continuity of the medullary canals between the lesion and the host bone. This is easily seen on x-rays and CT scan (Fig. 49-2). Grossly, the tumor is composed of a bony base and a cartilaginous cap that is "cauliflower-like." Rarely, malignant transformation of a solitary osteochondroma into a chondrosarcoma may occur; this risk is generally believed to be less than 1%. However, in hereditary syndromes such as multiple hereditary exostosis (MHE), the risk of malignant transformation somewhere in the body may be as high as 25%. Evidence of transformation in adults includes (1) rapid growth and new onset of pain, (2) cartilaginous cap greater than 2 cm thick on MRI, (3) sudden or marked increase in radioisotope uptake on bone scan, and (4) presence of a soft tissue mass confirmed by CT or MRI. The

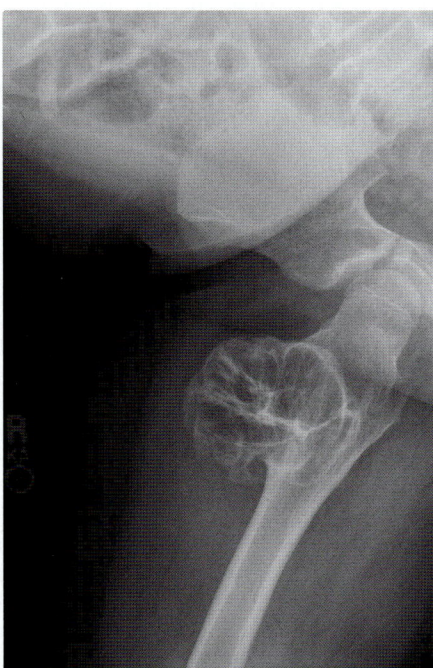

Figure 49-2. Frog-leg lateral radiograph of the hip showing a large osteochondroma (exostosis) in a skeletally immature patient with multiple hereditary exostosis (MHE).

---

*References 2-4, 7, 8, 17, 24, and 25.

differential diagnosis includes periosteal chondroma and parosteal osteosarcoma.

Indications for surgical treatment of osteochondroma include cosmesis, mechanical irritation and dysfunction, and deformity correction. Prophylactic removal to prevent sarcomatous transformation generally is not indicated. Treatment involves marginal excision including removal of the entire cartilaginous cap and the overlying perichondrium to minimize local recurrence. In MHE, neglected hip deformity can become severe and require a fairly extensive operation for removal. If malignant transformation occurs, it generally produces a low-grade chondrosarcoma, which requires a wide surgical excision.[1-4,26,27]

Langerhans' Cell Histiocytosis (eosinophilic granuloma)

Often described as the "great imitator," eosinophilic granuloma may present with monostotic or polyostotic disease. The origin is unknown, but it is considered a granulomatous inflammatory process. With rare exceptions, this is a pediatric disease. Most lesions present with pain and/or swelling. Vertebral plana and back pain constitute a classic presentation, but the proximal femur and the pelvis are common regions of disease involvement. Blood tests may show a slight increase in the erythrocyte sedimentation rate and rarely mild peripheral eosinophilia. Radiographic features vary greatly from well-contained radiolucencies surrounded by reactive bone to permeative lytic lesions with cortical destruction and even a soft tissue mass. Bone scans may show increased uptake, but skeletal surveys are more reliable in that one third of lesions are "cold." Lesions are hypervascular and thus are enhanced with intravenous (IV) contrast. MRI shows increased signals on T1 and T2. Microscopically, the tissue is composed of loose sheets of histiocyte-like cells (Langerhans' cells) infiltrated by eosinophils. Under electron microscopy, Langerhans' cells show numerous inclusion bodies in the cytoplasm called *Bierbeck granules,* which have a "tennis racket" appearance. Occasionally, the differential diagnosis can be difficult because of the variable presentation. This includes osteomyelitis, Ewing's sarcoma, Hodgkin's lymphoma, and non-Hodgkin's lymphoma, in addition to others. Solitary eosinophilic granuloma spontaneously heals in most cases. Therefore, surgery is rarely indicated, except for a biopsy or a lesion at risk for pathologic fracture. The recurrence rate is low. Radiation and chemotherapy are sometimes used for polyostotic disease presentations, especially when extraskeletal disease is present.*

Giant Cell Tumor (GCT)

This active and often aggressive benign tumor is found in young adults and has a predilection for epiphyses of bone. It is rare in patients with open growth plates. More than 50% of cases are located at the knee; however, the hip is not an uncommon site. The lesion is considered to have a fibrohistiocytic origin. Pulmonary

metastases are possible in 1% to 5% of cases, despite the benign designation. Multicentric disease is even less common (<1%). The most common clinical presentation is pain; pathologic fracture occurs in approximately 10% of cases. On radiographs, a latent lesion (uncommon) appears as a subtle, radiolucent defect that is well marginated in the epiphysis. In most cases, lesions are aggressive and present as geographic radiolucent lesions with a thin rim of reactive bone, or more poorly defined lesions with destruction of the cortex and a soft tissue mass. These lesions frequently extend from the epiphysis to the metaphysis with associated subchondral plate destruction. Bone scans show increased uptake, and CT scans are helpful in staging to identify cortical breakthrough and lung involvement. MRI typically shows low signal intensity on T1 and high signal intensity on T2 but is the most sensitive modality for finding a soft tissue mass and intra-articular involvement. The classic histopathology demonstrates bland stromal cells with uniform large, vesiculated nuclei mixed with many multinucleated giant cells, generous vascularity, and areas of necrosis. Giant cell nuclei appear nearly identical in size and shape to stromal cell nuclei, making them difficult to discern.

The differential diagnosis includes conventional chondrosarcoma, clear cell chondrosarcoma, malignant fibrous histiocytoma, osteolytic forms of osteosarcoma (i.e., telangiectatic), metastatic cancer, multiple myeloma, chondroblastoma, aneurysmal bone cyst, giant cell reparative granuloma, histiocytic fibroma, and "brown tumor." Treatment in most cases comprises extended curettage, local adjuvant (e.g., argon beam coagulation, liquid nitrogen, phenol), high-speed burring, and reconstruction with allograft or methylmethacrylate. Wide excision is used for multiply recurrent disease, intra-articular involvement, wide bone destruction, and some cases of pathologic fracture. Radiation or embolization is used for rare cases not amenable to surgery. The use of radiation has been associated with risk of malignant degeneration into a high-grade sarcoma.[1-4,8,30-32]

Chondroblastoma

Chondroblastoma accounts for 1% of primary bone tumors. Similar to GCTs, they originate in the epiphyses or apophyses of bones and spread toward the metaphysis. They often present with moderate pain for a long duration with occasional mild functional impairment (mimicking internal derangement). Lesions are often active and may simulate malignancy. Distant metastasis to the lungs is rarely seen, and sarcomatous transformation has been reported. Radiographically, most lesions are small (between 2 and 4 cm) and radiolucent and may include small areas of mineralization. They usually are well marginated and located within the metaepiphyseal region of bone. Bone scans are hot, and CT scans better delineate punctate mineralization and proximity to the physis. MRI is helpful in the search for a soft tissue mass with aggressive tumors. Histopathology shows large, polygonal cells (chondroblasts) that form a "paving stone" arrangement or mosaic-like pattern. Frequently, giant cells are seen. Approximately one

---

*References 2-4, 6, 7, 17, 28, and 29.

third of the time, "chicken wire" calcification is noted; this represents an area of confluent mineralization between chondroblasts, forming a lacelike appearance. The differential diagnosis includes GCT, clear cell chondrosarcoma, enchondroma, ABC, Brodie's abscess, and, rarely, chondromyxoid fibroma. Most chondroblastomas can be treated successfully with aggressive curettage with local adjuvant. Rarely, cases with extensive bony destruction or recurrent lesions may require wide excision and reconstruction.[2-4,7,8,33-35]

Osteoid Osteoma

An osteoid osteoma is an interesting benign bone tumor commonly known for its proclivity of causing night pain and non–activity-related pain dramatically relieved by nonsteroidal anti-inflammatories. It is normally seen in patients younger than 30 years of age, and its most common location is the proximal femur. In addition to pain, which can be exacerbated by alcohol or direct pressure, some have a palpable hard mass from reactive bone. On x-ray, the lesion normally presents as a small, round intracortical radiolucency ("nidus") surrounded by abundant reactive bone. However, an intramedullary lesion often is difficult to see and has little reactive change. The nidus rarely is beyond 1 to 2 cm in greatest dimension. Secondary radiographic changes are possible, especially in long-standing lesions. Bone scans are hot ("double-density sign" may be present from partial nidus ossification), and CT scan, the study of choice, normally delineates the nidus, which is radiolucent but may ossify over time (Fig. 49-3). MRI is not particularly helpful or useful in most cases. Microscopically, the center of the nidus consists of non–stress-oriented bars of osteoid bounded by osteoblasts, which are surrounded by a peripheral rim of fibrovascular proliferations. The differential diagnosis includes osteosarcoma, osteoblastoma, Brodie's abscess, stress fracture, and sclerosing osteoperiostitis. The typical clinical course

is spontaneous resolution, but this often takes an average of 3 to 5 years. However, most patients are symptomatic, and a trial of anti-inflammatories is prudent. This is rarely tolerated for long after the diagnosis is made. Most patients prefer surgical intervention, and the technique of choice is CT-guided radiofrequency ablation. The success rate is approximately 85% to 90%. This is true for local recurrent disease, as well as with a second attempt. Rarely, if the disease is multiply recurrent, open biopsy and curettage are required to verify the diagnosis and eliminate the lesion.[2-4,7,17]

Enchondroma

Often considered an intramedullary hamartoma rather than a benign bone tumor, enchondroma is commonly seen in almost all ages. It is rarely symptomatic and most often is found incidentally. Many describe the lesions as remnants of hyaline cartilage derived from the physis that remain within the medullary canal. After skeletal maturity, these normally heavily calcify. Malignant transformation of solitary enchondroma is very rare (<1%) but is difficult to quantify because most cases are asymptomatic and are not diagnosed. Rarely, polyostotic forms of the lesion (e.g., Ollier's disease, Maffucci's syndrome) may cause deformity, fracture, and malignant transformation into chondrosarcoma. On x-ray and CT scan, these radiolucent lesions are usually geographic with stippled calcifications ("popcorn" or "ring-like"). However, in adulthood, lesions often become increasingly radiodense. They are often centrally based and may cause intracortical scalloping. Scalloping by itself is not indicative of malignant transformation, but the addition of aggressive radiolucencies, periosteal elevation, and a soft tissue mass does indicate this. Bone scans often show uptake at varying levels, depending on the activity of the lesion. MRI shows low signal intensity on a T1 sequence and mostly high signal intensity on a T2, with areas of low signal intensity from any mineralization present. Microscopically, these appear as lobules of actively proliferating cartilage with no atypia. Most enchondromas are easily recognized on x-ray, unless they are minimally calcified, and can be followed on serial x-rays without biopsy. Differential diagnosis when not calcified includes fibrous dysplasia, simple bone cyst, and chondroblastoma (if epiphyseal). However, mineralized lesions can simulate a bone infarct or, more important, low-grade chondrosarcoma. In cases of symptomatic lesions or atypical characteristics, a biopsy and curettage is standard practice. The risk of local recurrence in adults is low.[1-4,7,33,36,37] Note that all intraosseous cartilaginous lesions in the pelvis are considered malignant (e.g., pelvic enchondromas are not recognized but rather represent [usually low-grade] chondrosarcomas).

Malignant Bone Neoplasms

This section focuses on primary and metastatic lesions, which are most common in the pelvis and proximal femur. It highlights common clinical presentations and key areas to identify for diagnosis.

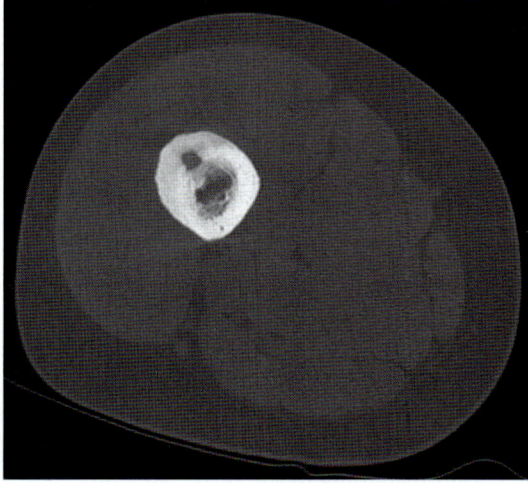

Figure 49-3. Axial computed tomography (CT) scan of the femur demonstrating an osteoid osteoma with a radiolucent "nidus."

Chondrosarcoma

(This section briefly details central and clear cell variants only.)

Central Chondrosarcoma. This primary malignant tumor of bone produces neoplastic cartilage. It is found most frequently in the pelvis and proximal femur. Chondrosarcoma most commonly presents in patients older than 40 years of age as a centrally located lesion. The typical clinical presentation is a painful, slow-growing mass, which is usually firm. Tumor grade dramatically affects the prognosis. Stage I (low-grade) lesions have an excellent 5-year survival of approximately 85%, whereas stage II lesions (high-grade) have a fair prognosis with survival rates of about 60%, and less for dedifferentiated forms. Radiographically, low-grade chondrosarcomas can look similar to enchondromas. However, most chondrosarcomas (particularly higher-grade lesions) demonstrate permeative destruction, fluffy calcification and radiodensities, aggressive endosteal scalloping, periosteal elevation, and often a soft tissue mass. Bone scan routinely shows increased uptake with extension often beyond the radiographic features. CT scans show properties similar to those shown on x-ray, with more pronounced calcifications, radiolucencies, and permeative changes, and a poorly circumscribed edge (Fig. 49-4). MRI, is low signal intensity on T1 and very high on T2, is very helpful in showing bone marrow involvement and the presence of a soft tissue mass. Key imaging features used to distinguish chondrosarcoma from enchondroma include (1) large size and increasing size, (2) periosteal reaction, (3) deep broad endosteal scalloping, (4) permeative changes, (5) cortical thickening, and (6) soft tissue mass. As mentioned earlier, pelvic lesions are by definition considered chondrosarcomas rather than enchondromas. Histopathology can be difficult to differentiate between low-grade lesions versus enchondromas; however, high-grade lesions often show increasing hyperplasia, anaplasia, and pleomorphism with larger and multiple nuclei per lacunae. Highest-grade lesions often do not resemble cartilage. With careful investigation, low-grade lesions may show invasion of Haversian canals with cartilaginous tissue, encircling of bone fragments by cartilage, and "bands of fibrosis." Differential diagnosis includes chondroma, synovial osteochondromatosis, chondromyxoid fibroma, and chondroblastic osteosarcoma. Biopsies of chondrosarcomas are carefully correlated with imaging findings to arrive at the final diagnosis.

Treatment for most chondrosarcomas consists of wide surgical excision (Fig. 49-5), but some espouse the use of intralesional curettage with adjuvant in low-grade lesions that are not axially based; intralesional therapy is never recommended for pelvic lesions but may be used in experienced hands for select femoral lesions. Advanced tumors may require radical resection. Chemotherapy and radiation have no significant role in central chondrosarcoma.[2-4,7,8,33,36-43]

Clear Cell Chondrosarcoma. Clear cell chondrosarcoma is an interesting variant of chondrosarcoma that has a predilection for the epiphyses of bones, particularly the femoral head. It is found in younger patients than central chondrosarcoma. It often presents as a slow-growing lesion with indolent pain for several years before diagnosis. X-rays show an expansile, radiolucent lesion in the metaepiphyseal region, which resembles the differential diagnosis of chondroblastoma and GCT. A thin sclerotic margin is common. The lesion may lack

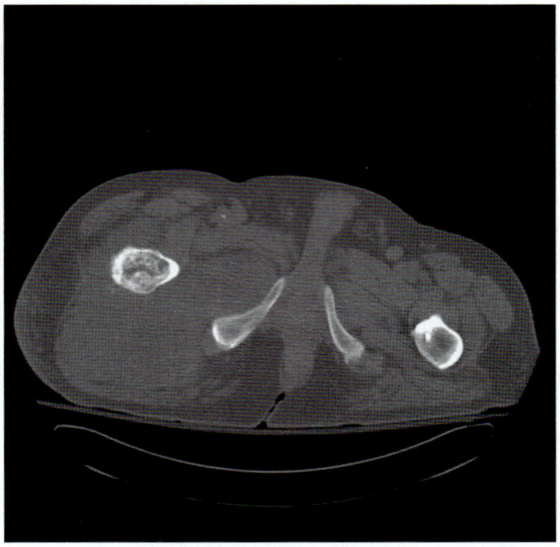

Figure 49-4. Axial computed tomography (CT) scan of the proximal femur and pelvis in a patient with a high-grade central chondrosarcoma. A large soft tissue mass is seen with small regions of calcification.

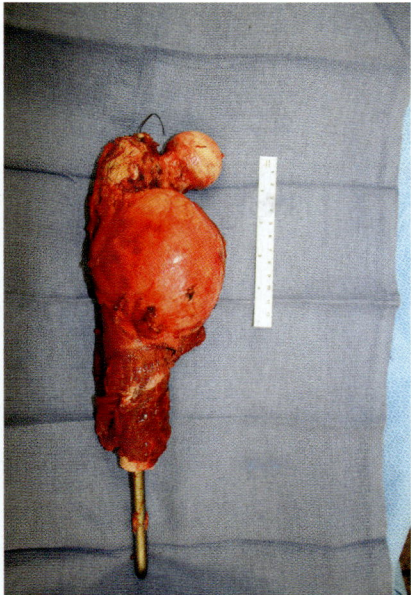

Figure 49-5. Gross pathoanatomy of an intermediate-grade central chondrosarcoma of the proximal femur. The lesion was originally low grade and presented with a pathologic fracture that was mistakenly fixated with an intramedullary nail without prior biopsy.

mineralization. CT scan may be helpful in eliciting faint calcifications, and MRI typically shows high signal intensity on T2-weighted sequences, along with lack of a soft tissue mass and intramedullary extension. Most patients present as stage IA (low grade and intracompartmental). Treatment consists of wide, en bloc excision with reconstruction. Chemotherapy and radiotherapy have no role.[2-4,40,44-46]

Ewing's Sarcoma

Ewing's sarcoma is a primary malignant neoplasm of uncertain origin that is composed of small round cells. It is found in the pelvis and femur (among other bones) of young patients, frequently between the ages of 5 and 25. Unlike other sarcomas, which predominantly present with pain and/or a mass, Ewing's sarcoma may resemble an infection with clinical symptoms such as fever, malaise, and weight loss. Consistent with the clinical picture, blood tests may reveal elevated lactic dehydrogenase (LDH), increased erythrocyte sedimentation rate (ESR), leukocytosis, and anemia. Radiographic presentation is variable, with early disease showing a permeative, ill-defined radiolucent process with a wide zone of transition and poorly visible margins. As the disease progresses, periosteal elevation ("onion skin"), Codman's triangles, enlargement of the bony diaphysis, and a disproportionately large soft tissue mass usually are noted. CT scan helps further define the amount of bony destruction, the extraosseous extent, risk for pathologic fracture, and regional lymph node involvement (Fig. 49-6). MRI is normally of low signal intensity on T1 and high on T2, and is helpful in defining bone marrow extension, soft tissue involvement, and sites of skip lesions. Bone scan is useful in showing metastatic bone disease.

Generous large-bore needle or careful open biopsy is important for diagnosis because adequate tissue is needed for cytogenetic studies used in the diagnosis of Ewing's sarcoma. Histopathology shows uniform sheets of small round blue cells; however, large areas of necrosis and hemorrhage are common. Occasionally, "pseudorosettes" are seen; these represent six to eight cells in a circle about an unstained or slightly eosinophilic clear center. Differential diagnosis includes osteomyelitis, lymphoma, mesenchymal chondrosarcoma, small cell osteosarcoma, metastatic neuroblastoma, metastatic small cell carcinoma, eosinophilic granuloma, and embryonal rhabdomyosarcoma. These tumors in general are very aggressive and, like all sarcomas, metastasize to the lungs first. However, more advanced cases may show metastatic bone and visceral disease. The definitive diagnosis can be determined by the presence of a CD99 cell marker and defined translocation of chromosomes 11 and 22 in most cases. The translocation forms a fusion protein called *EWS-FL1*.

Ewing's sarcoma is treated with neoadjuvant chemotherapy, local control, and further adjuvant chemotherapy. Local control may be accomplished by radiation, surgery, or both. The decision to use surgery and/or radiation in local control of Ewing's sarcoma is highly individualized. Five-year survival for nonmetastatic patients is about 65%.[2-4,7,38,43,47-51]

Metastatic Bone Disease

Metastatic bone disease accounts for the vast majority of malignant skeletal lesions, far more than primary lesions. The pelvis and the proximal femur are frequently involved. The skeleton is the third most common target of metastatic cancer after lung and liver, respectively. Most metastatic disease is seen after the age of 40. Carcinoma of the breast, lung, thyroid, kidney, or prostate is the source of a great majority of metastatic bone lesions. It is important for an orthopedic surgeon to first recognize a lesion of potential concern. Aggressive features include a large tumor (>5 cm), permeative changes, periosteal reaction, a soft tissue mass, and pathologic fracture (e.g., atraumatic avulsion of the lesser trochanter) (Fig. 49-7). Clinically, most patients present with pain that increases in severity over time, is not relieved by rest, and often persists at night, even preventing sleep. However, many skeletal metastatic lesions are asymptomatic and are found through screening and staging. The workup in a patient with suspected metastatic bone disease includes

1. Thorough medical history and physical examination
2. Routine laboratory tests
   a. Complete blood count (CBC), chemistry panel (chem-10), serum protein electrophoresis (SPEP), urine protein electrophoresis (UPEP), prostate-specific antigen (PSA), LDH, thyroid-stimulating hormone (TSH), free triiodothyronine (T_3), alkaline phosphatase, liver function tests (LFTs), ESR, C-reactive protein (CRP), nutrition panel, and others per patient history
3. Plain radiography of involved region
4. Whole-body bone scan (technetium-99)
5. CT scan of the chest, abdomen, and pelvis with and without oral and intravenous contrast

This protocol will identify the primary site of disease in more than 85% of patients. Often a biopsy is not necessary, and if one is necessary, studies often reveal a safer site to biopsy (biopsy of lesions around the hip may increase the risk of pathologic fracture).

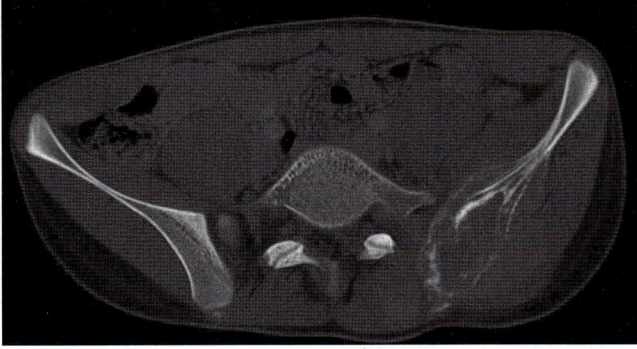

Figure 49-6. Computed tomography (CT) scan of the pelvis in a patient with Ewing's sarcoma shows an aggressive pattern with a soft tissue mass, permeative bone changes, and an abundant layered periosteal reaction ("onion skin").

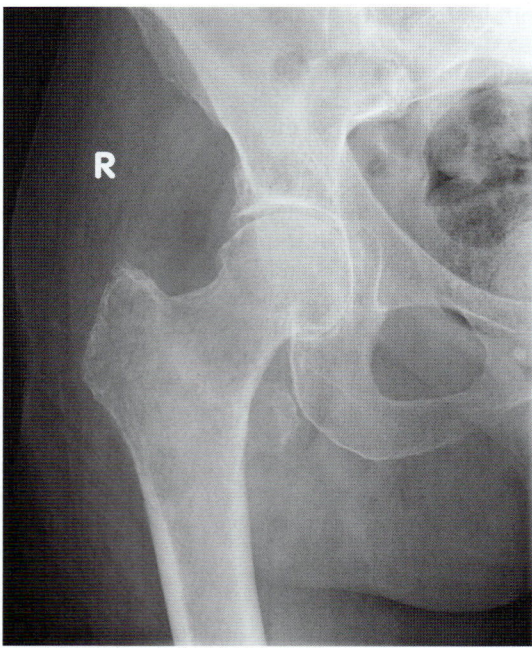

Figure 49-7. Anterior-posterior (AP) radiograph of the hip with early permeative changes and an atraumatic avulsion of the lesser trochanter in a patient with metastatic adenocarcinoma.

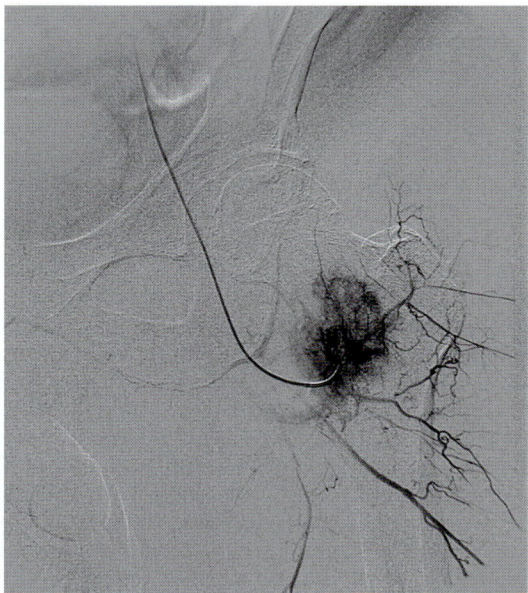

Figure 49-8. Angiogram and embolization of a suspected renal cell carcinoma performed preoperatively, showing a large vascular blush consistent with its hypervascularity.

Some metastatic lesions have well-defined characteristics. For example, most prostatic lesions are radiodense, whereas those from the thyroid, kidney, and lung are radiolucent. The breast often demonstrates both properties. Lesions found in the hand and/or feet are more likely the result of a primary lung lesion. However, a pulsatile mass with a bruit is likely associated with renal cell carcinoma, and its bleeding tendency may require preoperative embolization (Fig. 49-8). After a complete staging workup has been performed, the next step is biopsy. This should be carefully planned and executed with future surgery in mind. The patient should be referred promptly if the surgeon is not comfortable with the definitive procedure or has suspicion of a primary lesion. Extreme caution should be used when it is assumed that a lesion is metastatic, especially in a patient with a cancer history. If a pathologic fracture is present without a known diagnosis, biopsy with frozen section is recommended. These steps will help avoid the pitfalls of misdiagnosis (e.g., sarcoma) and morbidity to the patient. Once the diagnosis has been established, the goal of treatment is to provide a better quality of life through pain relief, improved functional status, and possibly prolonged survival. Surgical management will be addressed in detail in a subsequent chapter. However, other options exist beyond surgery, including chemotherapy, radiotherapy, and radiofrequency ablation. The use of these is patient and disease specific. The current standard of care includes intravenous infusions of bisphosphonates (i.e., zoledronic acid or pamidronate), which have been shown to decrease bone pain and reduce the number of

pathologic fractures. Unfortunately, this can cause avascular necrosis of the jaw, a rare but serious complication. Overall, patients require a multidisciplinary approach, and because average survival of patients with metastatic bone disease has improved, more aggressive treatment may be considered in select cases (particularly prostate and breast cancer). Among the most common sources of metastatic bone cancer, adenocarcinoma of the lung has the worst prognosis.[2,3,52-72]

Multiple Myeloma
Multiple myeloma is a systemic malignant tumor of the bone marrow that usually involves multiple sites and arises from plasma cells. It is second to metastatic disease in frequency of malignant bone lesions found in patients older than 40 years of age. The initial clinical presentation often consists of mild to moderate bone pain that usually is relieved by rest. However, fatigue secondary to anemia and vague nonspecific symptoms are common. With advancing disease, more pronounced systemic signs and symptoms are seen; these may include fever and infection, weight loss, severe anemia, bleeding, hypercalcemia, renal insufficiency, amyloidosis, jaundice, and pathologic fracture. Most clinical sequelae are secondary to excessive and abnormal production of monoclonal immunoglobulins. Early blood tests may be normal, but most patients with myeloma have positive SPEP or UPEP. UPEP is more sensitive and often detects light chain proteins that may not be detected by a standard SPEP (Bence-Jones protein). In cases of more severe disease, several blood tests may be abnormal, such as (1) elevated ESR, (2) low hematocrit and less likely pancytopenia, (3) elevated serum blood urea nitrogen (BUN) and creatinine, (4) hypercalcemia,

(5) elevated alkaline phosphatase, (6) hyperuricemia, and (7) abnormal liver function tests.

Radiographically, initial x-rays may show only diffuse osteopenia. However, as the disease progresses, radiolucent lesions are seen with little to no reactive bone around them. Although the lesions may become large and may appear aggressive, periosteal reaction is rare. Because these lesions do not incite a significant osteoblastic response, bone scans may show little to no uptake. As a result, a whole-body skeletal survey is a more effective staging modality. MRI can help demonstrate the extent of bone marrow and soft tissue involvement if needed (usually for evaluation of spinal lesions). CT is helpful in determining the risk of pathologic fracture and often shows the characteristic "punched out" lesions (Fig. 49-9). It is important to note that lesions composed of myeloma are hypervascular and will enhance with contrast. Histopathology is consistent with that of other small round blue cell tumors. However, in some cases, plasma cells may have a "clock-faced" or "wagon-wheel" appearance. Differential diagnosis includes small round blue cell tumors (lymphoma, Hodgkin's disease, Ewing's sarcoma) and metastatic carcinoma.

Patients may present with elevated serum protein studies and bone marrow findings that confirm the diagnosis; in this setting, a patient with multiple characteristic lytic lesions does not require biopsy. However, in cases in which the diagnosis is uncertain, biopsy provides definitive confirmation. A needle biopsy is preferred because of the significant bleeding tendency. In addition, the bone marrow needs to be biopsied for evaluation of systemic disease. Fortunately, multiple myeloma is sensitive to radiation and chemotherapy; the expanding role of stem cell transplant is increasing

the likelihood of durable disease remission. Average survival after diagnosis is approximately 3 years, but many patients survive much longer.

Surgical management in multiple myeloma is used to address present and impending fractures caused by mechanical destruction of bone. Bisphosphonates are recommended to prevent pathologic fracture and to reduce bone pain. It is interesting to note that patients can have a solitary lesion of plasma cells called a *plasmacytoma* with no systemic involvement, but nearly all patients progress to multiple myeloma.[2-4,61,73,74]

CURRENT CONTROVERSIES AND FUTURE CONSIDERATIONS

- Debate continues regarding treatment of low-grade malignancies with extensive curettage and adjuvant versus wide surgical excision.
- It is recommended that a biopsy be performed (or at least directed) by the surgeon, who is comfortable in performing the definitive procedure.
- It will become more of a challenge to provide long-lasting stable reconstruction after tumor excision because patients are living longer.
- It is hoped that targeted therapy will provide better outcomes in the future for patients with sarcoma and other malignancies that spread to the bone.

REFERENCES

1. Enneking WF, Conrad EU 3rd: Common bone tumors. Clin Symp 41:1–32, 1989.
2. Enneking WF: Clinical musculoskeletal pathology seminar, Gainesville, Fla, 1998, University of Florida.
3. Campanacci M: Bone and soft tissue tumors: clinical features, imaging, pathology, and treatment, ed 2 (completely rev ed), Wein, Austria, 1999, Springer.
4. Dorfman HD, Czerniak B: Bone tumors, St Louis, Mosby, 1998, p ix.
5. Gould CF, Ly JQ, Lattin GE Jr, et al: Bone tumor mimics: avoiding misdiagnosis. Curr Probl Diagn Radiol 36:124–141, 2007.
6. Mankin HJ: Pathophysiology of orthopaedic diseases: great educators, Rosemont, Ill, 2006, American Academy of Orthopaedic Surgeons.
7. Vigorita VJ, Ghelman B, Mintz D: Orthopaedic pathology, ed 2, Philadelphia, 2008, Wolters Kluwer Lippincott Williams and Wilkins.
8. Simon MA, Springfield DS: Surgery for bone and soft-tissue tumors, Philadelphia, 1998, Lippincott-Raven Publishers.
9. Mankin HJ, Lange TA, Spanier SS: The hazards of biopsy in patients with malignant primary bone and soft-tissue tumors. J Bone Joint Surg Am 64:1121–1127, 1982.
10. Mankin HJ, Mankin CJ, Simon MA: The hazards of biopsy revisited: Members of the Musculoskeletal Tumor Society. J Bone Joint Surg Am 78:656–663, 1996.
11. Rougraff BT, Kneisl JS, Simon MA: Skeletal metastases of unknown origin: a prospective diagnostic strategy. J Bone Joint Surg Am 75:1276–1281, 1993.
12. Scarborough MT: The biopsy. Instr Course Lect 53:639–644, 2004.
13. Carrino JA, Khurana B, Ready JE, et al: Magnetic resonance imaging-guided percutaneous biopsy of musculoskeletal lesions. J Bone Joint Surg Am 89:2179–2187, 2007.
14. Ng CS, Salisbury JR, Darby AJ, et al: Radiologically guided bone biopsy: results of 502 biopsies. Cardiovasc Intervent Radiol 21:122–128, 1998.

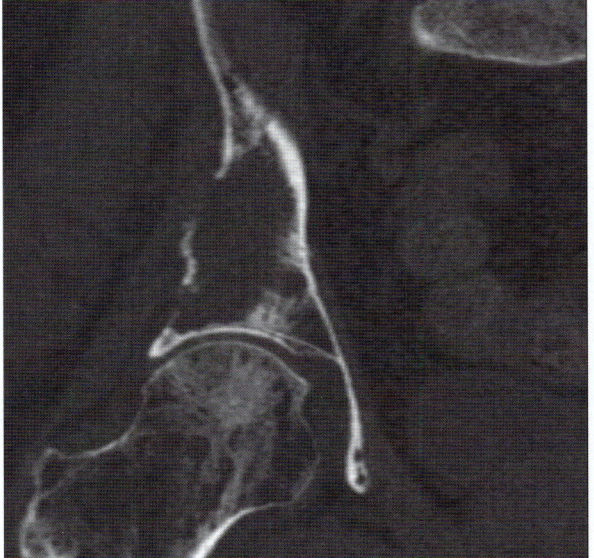

Figure 49-9. Coronal computed tomography (CT) reformat of the hip in a patient with multiple myeloma, showing the classic "punched out" lesions in the proximal femur and more aggressive changes in the periacetabular region.

15. DiCaprio MR, Enneking WF: Fibrous dysplasia: pathophysiology, evaluation, and treatment. J Bone Joint Surg Am 87:1848–1864, 2005.
16. Marks KE, Bauer TW: Fibrous tumors of bone. Orthop Clin North Am 20:377–393, 1989.
17. Ruggieri P, Angelini A, Montalti M, et al: Tumours and tumour-like lesions of the hip in the paediatric age: a review of the Rizzoli experience. Hip Int 19(Suppl 6):S35–S45, 2009.
18. Diamanti-Kandarakis E, Livadas S, Tseleni-Balafouta S, et al: Brown tumor of the fibula: unusual presentation of an uncommon manifestation. Report of a case and review of the literature. Endocrine 32:345–349, 2007.
19. Baig R, Eady JL: Unicameral (simple) bone cysts. South Med J 99:966–976, 2006.
20. Lokiec F, Ezra E, Khermosh O, Wientroub S: Simple bone cysts treated by percutaneous autologous marrow grafting: a preliminary report. J Bone Joint Surg Br 78:934–937, 1996.
21. Lokiec F, Wientroub S: Simple bone cyst: etiology, classification, pathology, and treatment modalities. J Pediatr Orthop B 7:262–273, 1998.
22. Parman LM, Murphey MD: Alphabet soup: cystic lesions of bone. Semin Musculoskelet Radiol 4:89–101, 2000.
23. Wilkins RM: Unicameral bone cysts. J Am Acad Orthop Surg 8:217–224, 2000.
24. Gibbs CP Jr, Hefele MC, Peabody TD, et al: Aneurysmal bone cyst of the extremities: factors related to local recurrence after curettage with a high-speed burr. J Bone Joint Surg Am 81:1671–1678, 1999.
25. Mendenhall WM, Zlotecki RA, Gibbs CP, et al: Aneurysmal bone cyst. Am J Clin Oncol 29:311–315, 2006.
26. Weiner DS, Hoyt WA Jr: The development of the upper end of the femur in multiple hereditary exostosis. Clin Orthop Relat Res 137:187–190, 1978.
27. Porter DE, Benson MK, Hosney GA: The hip in hereditary multiple exostoses. J Bone Joint Surg Br 83:988–995, 2001.
28. Azouz EM, Saigal G, Rodriguez MM, Podda A: Langerhans' cell histiocytosis: pathology, imaging and treatment of skeletal involvement. Pediatr Radiol 35:103–115, 2005.
29. Kilpatrick SE, Wenger DE, Gilchrist GS, et al: Langerhans' cell histiocytosis (histiocytosis X) of bone: a clinicopathologic analysis of 263 pediatric and adult cases. Cancer 76:2471–2484, 1995.
30. Thomas DM, Skubitz KM: Giant cell tumour of bone. Curr Opin Oncol 21:338–344, 2009.
31. Werner M: Giant cell tumour of bone: morphological, biological and histogenetical aspects. Int Orthop 30:484–489, 2006.
32. Yasko AW: Giant cell tumor of bone. Curr Oncol Rep 4:520–526, 2002.
33. Giudici MA, Moser RP Jr, Kransdorf MJ: Cartilaginous bone tumors. Radiol Clin North Am 31:237–259, 1993.
34. Rajaram A, Tamurian RM, Reith JD, Bush CH: Hip pain in an 18-year-old man. Clin Orthop Relat Res 466:248–254, 2008.
35. Springfield DS, Capanna R, Gherlinzoni F, et al: Chondroblastoma: a review of seventy cases. J Bone Joint Surg Am 67:748–755, 1985.
36. Marco RA, Gitelis S, Brebach GT, Healey JH: Cartilage tumors: evaluation and treatment. J Am Acad Orthop Surg 8:292–304, 2000.
37. Weiner SD: Enchondroma and chondrosarcoma of bone: clinical, radiologic, and histologic differentiation. Instr Course Lect 53:645–649, 2004.
38. Damron TA, Ward WG, Stewart A: Osteosarcoma, chondrosarcoma, and Ewing's sarcoma: National Cancer Data Base report. Clin Orthop Relat Res 459:40–47, 2007.
39. Eriksson AI, Schiller A, Mankin HJ: The management of chondrosarcoma of bone. Clin Orthop Relat Res 153:44–66, 1980.
40. Gelderblom H, Hogendoorn PC, Dijkstra SD, et al: The clinical approach towards chondrosarcoma. Oncologist 13:320–329, 2008.
41. Lee FY, Mankin HJ, Fondren G, et al: Chondrosarcoma of bone: an assessment of outcome. J Bone Joint Surg Am 81:326–338, 1999.
42. Pring ME, Weber KL, Unni KK, Sim FH: Chondrosarcoma of the pelvis: a review of sixty-four cases. J Bone Joint Surg Am 83:1630–1642, 2001.
43. Weber K, Damron TA, Frassica FJ, Sim FH: Malignant bone tumors. Instr Course Lect 57:673–688, 2008.
44. Bjornsson J, Unni KK, Dahlin DC, et al: Clear cell chondrosarcoma of bone: observations in 47 cases. Am J Surg Pathol 8:223–230, 1984.
45. Donati D, Yin JQ, Colangeli M, et al: Clear cell chondrosarcoma of bone: long time follow-up of 18 cases. Arch Orthop Trauma Surg 128:137–142, 2008.
46. Unni KK, Dahlin DC, Beabout JW, Sim FH: Chondrosarcoma: clear-cell variant. A report of sixteen cases. J Bone Joint Surg Am 58:676–683, 1976.
47. Bernstein M, Kovar H, Paulussen M, et al: Ewing's sarcoma family of tumors: current management. Oncologist 11:503–519, 2006.
48. Grier HE: The Ewing family of tumors: Ewing's sarcoma and primitive neuroectodermal tumors. Pediatr Clin North Am 44:991–1004, 1997.
49. Ludwig JA: Ewing sarcoma: historical perspectives, current state-of-the-art, and opportunities for targeted therapy in the future. Curr Opin Oncol 20:412–418, 2008.
50. Subbiah V, Anderson P, Lazar AJ, et al: Ewing's sarcoma: standard and experimental treatment options. Curr Treat Options Oncol 10:126–140, 2009.
51. Weber KL, Sim FH: Ewing's sarcoma: presentation and management. J Orthop Sci 6:366–371, 2001.
52. Aaron AD: Treatment of metastatic adenocarcinoma of the pelvis and the extremities. J Bone Joint Surg Am 79:917–932, 1997.
53. Bertin KC, Horstman J, Coleman SS: Isolated fracture of the lesser trochanter in adults: an initial manifestation of metastatic malignant disease. J Bone Joint Surg Am 66:770–773, 1984.
54. Bickels J, Dadia S, Lidar Z: Surgical management of metastatic bone disease. J Bone Joint Surg Am 91:1503–1516, 2009.
55. Biermann JS, Holt GE, Lewis VO, et al: Metastatic bone disease: diagnosis, evaluation, and treatment. J Bone Joint Surg Am 91:1518–1530, 2009.
56. Damron TA, Sim FH: Surgical treatment for metastatic disease of the pelvis and the proximal end of the femur. Instr Course Lect 49:461–470, 2000.
57. Frassica FJ, Gitelis S, Sim FH: Metastatic bone disease: general principles, pathophysiology, evaluation, and biopsy. Instr Course Lect 41:293–300, 1992.
58. Harrington KD: Orthopaedic management of extremity and pelvic lesions. Clin Orthop Relat Res 312:136–147, 1995.
59. Jacofsky DJ, Haidukewych GJ: Management of pathologic fractures of the proximal femur: state of the art. J Orthop Trauma 18:459–469, 2004.
60. Jacofsky DJ, Haidukewych GJ, Zhang H, Sim FH: Complications and results of arthroplasty for salvage of failed treatment of malignant pathologic fractures of the hip. Clin Orthop Relat Res 427:52–56, 2004.
61. Lin JT, Lane JM: Bisphosphonates. J Am Acad Orthop Surg 11:1–4, 2003.
62. Manoso MW, Frassica DA, Lietman ES, Frassica FJ: Proximal femoral replacement for metastatic bone disease. Orthopedics 30:384–388, 2007.
63. Marco RA, Sheth DS, Boland PJ, et al: Functional and oncological outcome of acetabular reconstruction for the treatment of metastatic disease. J Bone Joint Surg Am 82:642–651, 2000.
64. Mehrotra B, Ruggiero S: Bisphosphonate complications including osteonecrosis of the jaw. Hematology Am Soc Hematol Educ Program 356–360, 515, 2006.
65. Papagelopoulos PJ, Mavrogenis AF, Soucacos PN: Evaluation and treatment of pelvic metastases. Injury 38:509–520, 2007.
66. Quinn RH, Drenga J: Perioperative morbidity and mortality after reconstruction for metastatic tumors of the proximal femur and acetabulum. J Arthroplasty 21:227–232, 2006.
67. Schneiderbauer MM, von Knoch M, Schleck CD, et al: Patient survival after hip arthroplasty for metastatic disease of the hip. J Bone Joint Surg Am 86:1684–1689, 2004.
68. Selek H, Başarir K, Yildiz Y, Sağlik Y: Cemented endoprosthetic replacement for metastatic bone disease in the proximal femur. J Arthroplasty 23:112–117, 2008.
69. Sim FH: Metastatic bone disease: philosophy of treatment. Orthopedics 15:541–544, 1992.

70. Sim FH: Metastatic bone disease of the pelvis and femur. Instr Course Lect 41:317–327, 1992.

71. Swanson KC, Pritchard DJ, Sim FH: Surgical treatment of metastatic disease of the femur. J Am Acad Orthop Surg 8:56–65, 2000.

72. Varadhachary GR, Abbruzzese JL, Lenzi R: Diagnostic strategies for unknown primary cancer. Cancer 100:1776–1785, 2004.

73. Dagan R, Morris CG, Kirwan J, Mendenhall WM: Solitary plasmacytoma. Am J Clin Oncol 32:612–617, 2009.

74. Harousseau JL, Shaughnessy J Jr, Richardson P: Multiple myeloma. Hematology Am Soc Hematol Educ Program 237–256, 2004.

CHAPTER 50

Benign Bone Tumors

Bruno Fuchs and Peter S. Rose

KEY POINTS

- Many benign tumors about the hip require only observation and reassurance.
- The aggressiveness of treatment is matched to the aggressiveness of the tumor.
- Surgical treatment for benign tumors most commonly consists of curettage or marginal excision.

INTRODUCTION

Benign bone tumors about the hip and pelvis represent a varied group of rare lesions. As benign entities, they are characterized by autonomous growth but lack the ability to metastasize. Therefore benign tumors may be thought of as a local but not a systemic problem. Benign tumors around the hip are most common in young patients and on average affect males more frequently than females, although they may occur at any age.

Dr. Silverstein in Chapter 49 reviewed the evaluation and common features of tumorous conditions presenting about the hip. This chapter will review treatment modalities for patients presenting with benign tumors with specific recommendations for commonly encountered benign tumors. In contrast to patients presenting with malignancies, those with benign tumors in general require less aggressive/less radical treatment. Additionally, the role of adjuvant chemotherapy or radiotherapy is rare in the treatment of benign conditions.

EVALUATION

Patients are evaluated as outlined by Dr. Silverstein in Chapter 49. Many benign conditions have characteristic imaging features and do not require biopsy. For example, nonossifying fibroma and enchondroma are conditions that are diagnosed generally by imaging modalities alone. Occasionally, biopsy will be necessary and should be carried out in keeping with the principles outlined in Chapter 49. The key feature of biopsy requires that minimal tissue be contaminated, and that the biopsy tract be excisable by a limb salvage procedure should a primary sarcoma requiring en bloc resection be diagnosed.

Occasionally, benign conditions will present in a multifocal manner. For example, patients with hereditary multiple exostoses or Ollier's syndrome will present with disseminated benign tumors. These patients usually are detected on physical examination and by history to clue the clinician into the presence of multifocal lesions. Additionally, standard radiographs of the pelvis and femur would usually alert the clinician to the presence of more than one lesion. If a multifocal process is suspected, it is appropriate to obtain a baseline skeletal survey or bone scan to obtain an initial characterization of the extent of the process. Although benign, these processes often have a predisposition to malignancy.

Most benign conditions that arise about the hip are unifocal. Once the diagnosis of a benign tumor about the hip has been established, a careful treatment plan is tailored to the patient. This plan considers the anatomic location and extent of the lesion, its histology and accordant predicted biological behavior, the patient's expectations and needs, and available surgical and other treatment options. Many benign conditions do not require surgery and can be observed or treated by lesser means. It is rare for benign conditions to require major reconstructive techniques, which would compromise patient function.

TREATMENT OPTIONS

A variety of treatment options are available for patients with benign conditions. They may be summarized as follows:

1. Watchful waiting
2. Medical therapy
3. Injection/percutaneous treatment
4. Radiofrequency or cryoablation
5. Curettage with or without adjuvant treatment
6. Internal fixation
7. Marginal excision
8. Surgical resection

These treatment techniques are tailored to the individual patient's condition. We will discuss each option and will provide clinical examples of how these treatments may be used in individual patients. Treatment protocols for common benign lesions will follow.

Watchful Waiting

A large number of benign conditions around the hip can be identified and characterized as benign on the basis of their imaging characteristics. Many do not require surgical treatment. For example, a nonossifying fibroma/

fibrous cortical defect diagnosed about the hip joint is typically found asymptomatically and requires no specific treatment. Another example of this would be an enchondroma. These conditions rarely if ever require surgical treatment; however, they should often be observed through serial imaging to ensure stability of the process. For example, as outlined in Chapter 49 by Dr. Silverstein, low risk is often present for a lesion that initially appears to be an enchondroma to develop into a low-grade chondrosarcoma. Patients who present with imaging studies that implicate an enchondroma are recommended to undergo serial radiograph examinations to ensure stability of the lesion. Experience shows that the risk of pathologic fracture through incidentally detected lesions of this nature is quite low.[1] Other benign lesions that are commonly observed include small osteochondromas that are not causing mechanical problems.

Medical Therapy

Many benign conditions may not require interventional management but may benefit from drug therapy. For example, bisphosphonates may be used in the treatment of patients with fibrous dysplasia.[2] The classic medical management of osteoid osteoma involves the use of aspirin, nonsteroidal anti-inflammatory drugs, or cyclooxygenase (COX)-2 inhibitors. Medical therapy may be used in patients who have benign conditions that can have both active and latent phases. Medical therapy thus is used to alleviate symptoms until the condition "burns itself out." Drug therapy provided in this manner allows alleviation of symptoms without the morbidity and risk associated with an interventional procedure.

Injection Therapy

Various benign conditions may be treated with percutaneous injection therapy. For example, unicameral bone cysts are thought to respond to a variety of injection techniques.[3,4] Methylprednisolone injection is commonly administered and in a randomized trial was superior to injection of bone marrow aspirate for unicameral bone cysts.[5]

Injection therapy is generally provided under computed tomography (CT) or fluoroscopic guidance. These treatments offer the benefit of low risk for any individual procedure; however, multiple procedures are often necessary. Technical considerations around providing injection therapy include the use of radiopaque injectate to ensure that intravenous injection is not occurring within the bone. As well, patients may require a period of non–weight bearing to allow healing of the lesion as the treatment takes effect. Therefore these treatments are used more commonly in pediatric patients than in adults.

Selective embolization may be categorized under injection therapy. Embolization can be used as an adjunct in the treatment of benign lesions around the hip and pelvis. For example, data are available to support the role of serial embolization of patients with giant cell tumors that are found in surgically inaccessible areas.[6]

Radiofrequency Ablation/Cryoablation

Benign lesions may be ablated with the use of thermal techniques (heat via radiofrequency ablation or cold via cryoablation). The classic lesion amenable to this is an osteoid osteoma. Previously, osteoid osteomas were treated by open surgical means to excise the nidus. Experience has demonstrated that ablation of the nidus via percutaneous radiofrequency ablation provides excellent and immediate pain relief for patients.[7,8] Percutaneous ablation procedures are generally performed under CT guidance using a minimally invasive approach. A guide wire is placed in the desired location on the skeleton, and then a cannulated drill is used to bridge the cortex and advance the ablation probe (Fig. 50-1).

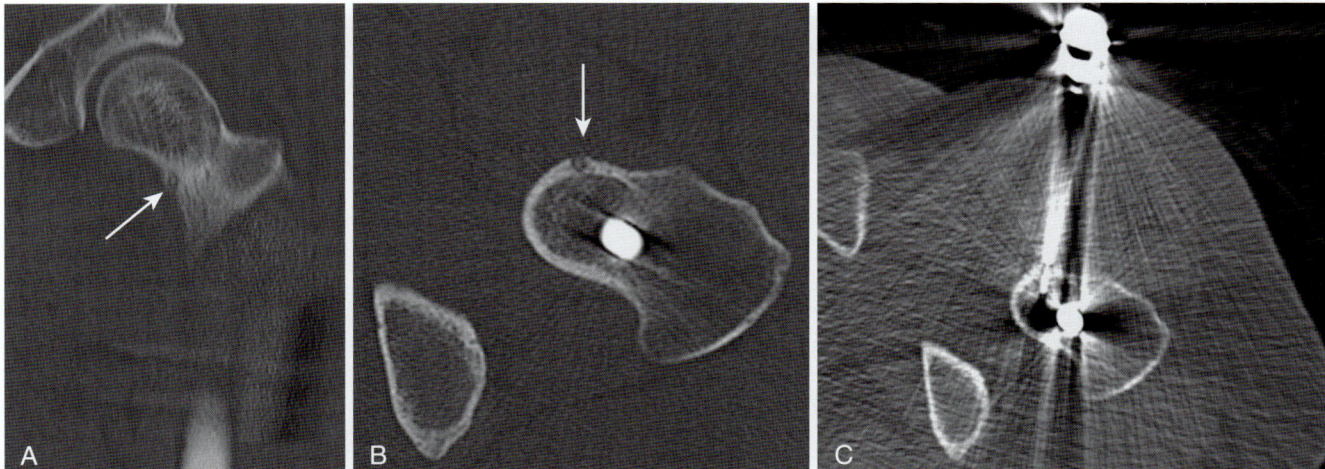

Figure 50-1. Radiofrequency (RF) ablation of an osteoid osteoma of the femoral neck. The patient had been treated erroneously with a sliding hip screw for a presumed stress fracture. **A,** Coronal computed tomography (CT) and **(B)** axial CT demonstrate a characteristic nidus. **C,** RF ablation resulted in immediate pain relief.

This procedure is safe and well tolerated; it is usually performed under sedation or light general anesthesia on an outpatient basis. Careful shielding is necessary to minimize necrosis of the surrounding skin.

Recurrence rates following percutaneous ablation may approach 15%; however, these recurrences generally are readily handled with repeat ablation procedures and are usually due to suboptimal placement of the initial ablation catheter. Note that in lesions that are juxta-articular to the hip joint, a transient hemarthrosis may occur post procedure. This usually causes only temporary discomfort for the patient.[7,8]

Curettage

Curettage of benign bone lesions is usually coupled with grafting of the curettage cavity and has high efficacy in reducing painful symptoms.[9] Curettage is the most common open surgical treatment for benign bone tumors. It is usually performed for active tumors such as giant cell tumors or chondroblastomas or for select

eosinophil granulomas that are causing significant symptoms. The surgical approach for curettage is determined by the anatomic location of the lesion. In general, the most direct access point is chosen; this results in minimal damage to surrounding tissues. A direct lateral approach is used most commonly for lesions about the trochanteric region; surgical hip dislocation may be entertained for careful access to juxta-articular lesions.

Curettage is most commonly performed open with wide exteriorization of the lesion to provide good visualization and access to the lesion. Surrounding soft tissues are draped away to minimize contamination and implanting of tumor seeds (Fig. 50-2). Alternatively, less invasive techniques may be applied with curettage performed under fluoroscopic guidance and arthroscopy equipment used subsequently to evaluate the cavity, which is formed to detect residual tumor (Fig. 50-3).

A variety of grafts may be used to fill the curettage defect; those chosen usually vary with surgeon preference and patient wishes.[10] Autogenous graft is clearly the gold standard for these purposes; however, it is of

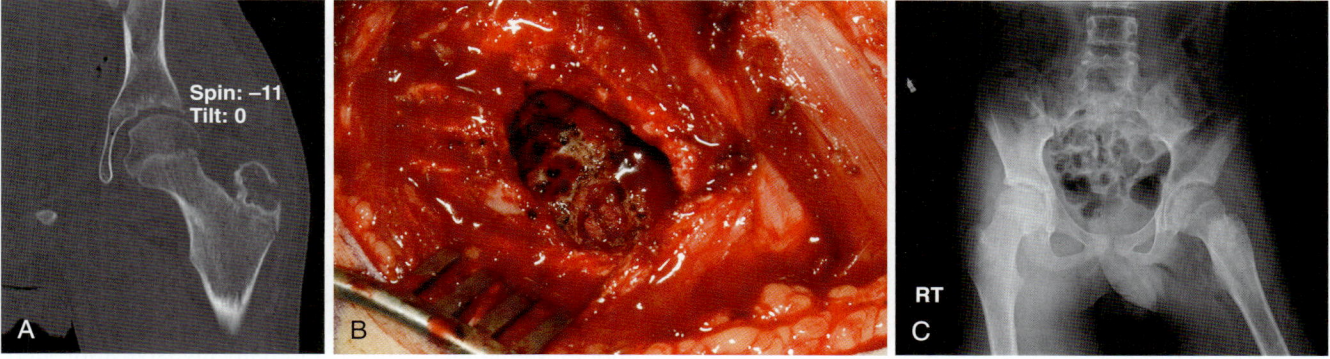

Figure 50-2. Open curettage of a chondroblastoma of the trochanteric apophysis. **A,** Coronal computed tomography (CT) demonstrates a lesion. **B,** Wide exteriorization of the lesion is performed. **C,** Radiograph demonstrating allograft incorporation.

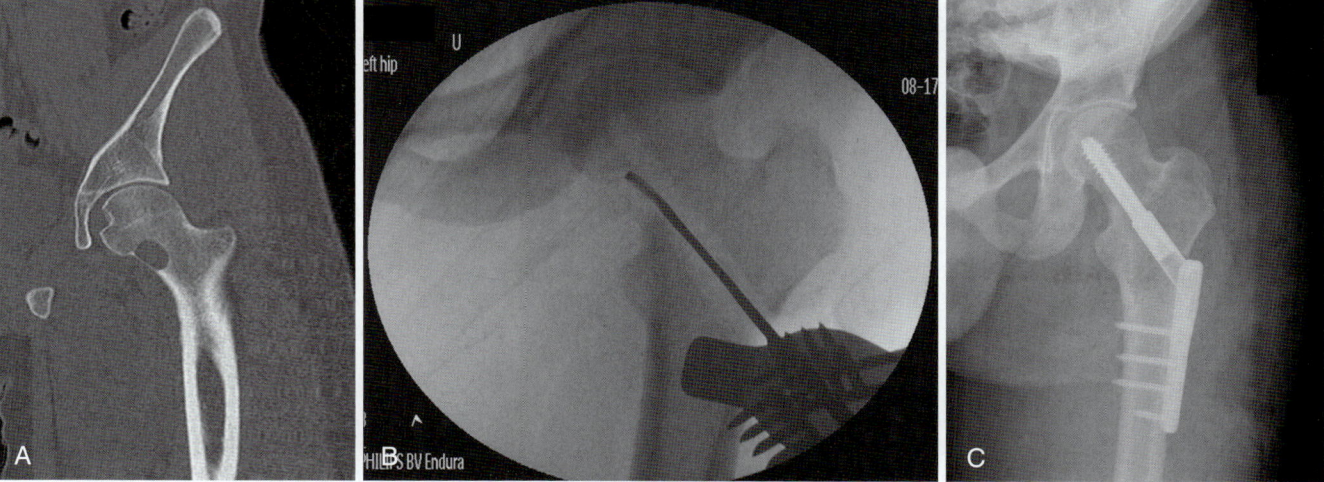

Figure 50-3. Fluoroscopically guided curettage of cystic fibrous dysplasia of the hip with grafting and internal fixation. **A,** Preoperative computed tomography (CT) image. **B,** Fluoroscopically guided curettage. **C,** Postoperative image.

potentially limited supply and is associated with harvest morbidity. Additionally, if autograft is used in the treatment of benign bone tumors, the surgeon should carefully segregate the instruments and the operative field of the bone graft harvest from the bone graft of the lesion itself to minimize the theoretical risk of transplantation of benign tumors from one area to another.

In addition to autograft, cancellous and corticocancellous allografts, as well as calcium sulfate and other bone graft substitutes, are successfully employed in the treatment of these lesions[4,11,12] (Fig. 50-4). Although potentially attractive, the role of recombinant bone morphogenetic protein (BMP) has not been established in the treatment of benign bone lesions. Because BMP acts as a transcription factor and can potentially activate residual tumor cells, its use is relatively contraindicated in the treatment of benign bone tumors.

Methylmethacrylate bone cement may also be used to fill voids after curettage and to provide immediate structural stability. Bone cement is most commonly used in the treatment of giant cell tumor of bone. Although conflicting results are seen in the literature, bone cement appears to reduce the likelihood of tumor recurrence. Whether this is due to chemical or thermal ablation of microscopic residual tumor cells or whether it occurs merely because a more thorough curettage is performed when cement (with its immediate stability) is used is unclear.[13-16]

Curettage may be divided into three primary categories. Simple curettage involves mechanical removal of tumor from a cavity. This minimizes damage to healthy bone and other structures in the area but poses the risk of leaving residual microscopic tumor behind. Simple curettage may be augmented with mechanical curettage. Most commonly this includes the use of a high-speed burr to treat the walls of the curettage cavity once simple curettage has been completed. This allows extension of the apparent "margin" of tumor removal. More aggressive curettage may be accomplished by the use of chemical and/or thermal adjuvants, as is discussed later. In the treatment of aggressive benign conditions such as giant cell tumor or chondroblastoma, more aggressive adjuvant treatment is seen to increase the likelihood of cure/lesion eradication.

Adjuvant Treatments

Chemical and thermal adjuvants enhance the efficacy of curettage. They are used to achieve chemical or thermal ablation of the cavity rim to eradicate microscopic residual tumor cells, which are believed to be a cause of lesion recurrence.

Chemical curettage may be provided by a variety of chemical adjuvants, which vary in their risk and effectiveness in an inverse pattern. The simplest chemical adjuvant is distilled water, which is used to provide osmotic lysis of surrounding cells. This is a very safe treatment that has a minimal impact on surrounding healthy tissue. Distilled water, however, has limited effectiveness in comparison with more aggressive techniques. Similarly, hydrogen peroxide diluted 50% or in pure strength can be instilled directly into the cavity. Hydrogen peroxide is believed to have relatively increased effectiveness compared with distilled water but causes modestly increased damage to surrounding tissues.[17] Hydrogen peroxide may be used in juxta-articular lesions for which an attempt is being made to save the native articulation. Ethanol is effective in a similar manner but does pose a fire hazard.[18]

Phenol, the most common chemical adjuvant, is used in the treatment of aggressive benign bone tumors. Phenol provides a caustic burn to surrounding tissues in an attempt to ablate residual tumor cells.[19] It will burn native cells similarly. Reports conflict as to the efficacy of phenol as an adjuvant in treating benign bone tumors.[14,20,21] Once phenol is applied, it is subsequently neutralized with an alcohol solution. Phenol requires special handling and should be avoided by pregnant caregivers in the operating room. As well, the alcohol used to neutralize phenol is flammable. Thus if electrical/ heat ablation techniques as described here are applied,

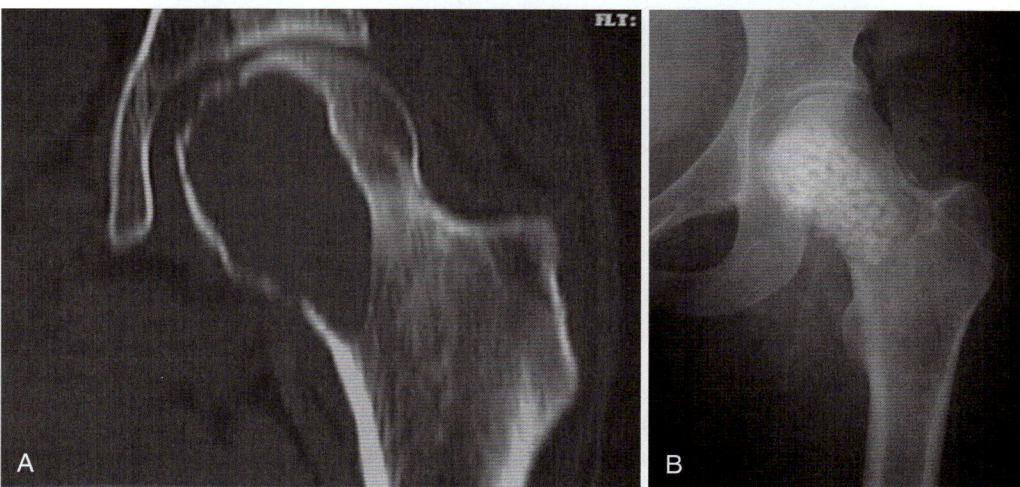

Figure 50-4. Calcium sulfate pellets used to treat a benign bone cyst. **A,** Preoperative computed tomography (CT). **B,** Postoperative radiograph.

they should likely be performed before instillation of phenol and subsequent alcohol treatment to minimize the risk of fire caused by the neutralizing alcohol solution.

Thermal adjuvants extend the efficacy of curettage in the treatment of benign bone lesions. Thermal adjuvants may be grouped into those that provide heat and those that provide cooling as their source of thermal ablation. The prototypical thermal adjuvant is cryotherapy. This was pioneered by Dr. Marcove in the 1960s and 1970s for the treatment of benign bone tumors. Cryotherapy involves the direct instillation of liquid nitrogen into a tumor cavity (by a direct pour technique or by a spray technique). Commercially available cryoprobes can provide point cryotherapy at the end of an instrument.[22]

Cryotherapy has excellent efficacy in the treatment of aggressive benign bone tumors such as giant cell tumor.[23] However, cryotherapy presents real risks for complications; skin necrosis, subsequent pathologic

fracture, and even intraoperative nitrogen embolism have been noted with the use of cryotherapy. The last complication is potentially fatal in rare circumstances. The clinician must carefully weigh the risks and benefits associated with this powerful adjuvant therapy in the treatment of individual patients. That said, cryotherapy serves as an excellent modality to help achieve local control in the treatment of aggressive benign conditions.

Thermal burning of the cavity may be used to provide adjuvant treatment for benign bone tumors. The argon beam coagulator can provide a thermal burn to a tumor cavity (Fig. 50-5). This instrument allows direct control of the surfaces being coagulated. In contrast to chemical adjuvants and the methods used most commonly to deliver cryotherapy, the argon beam coagulator likely provides more controlled delivery around critical structures such as adjacent joints and physes. If the argon beam coagulator is used in conjunction with a flammable chemical adjuvant such as phenol or alcohol, it is

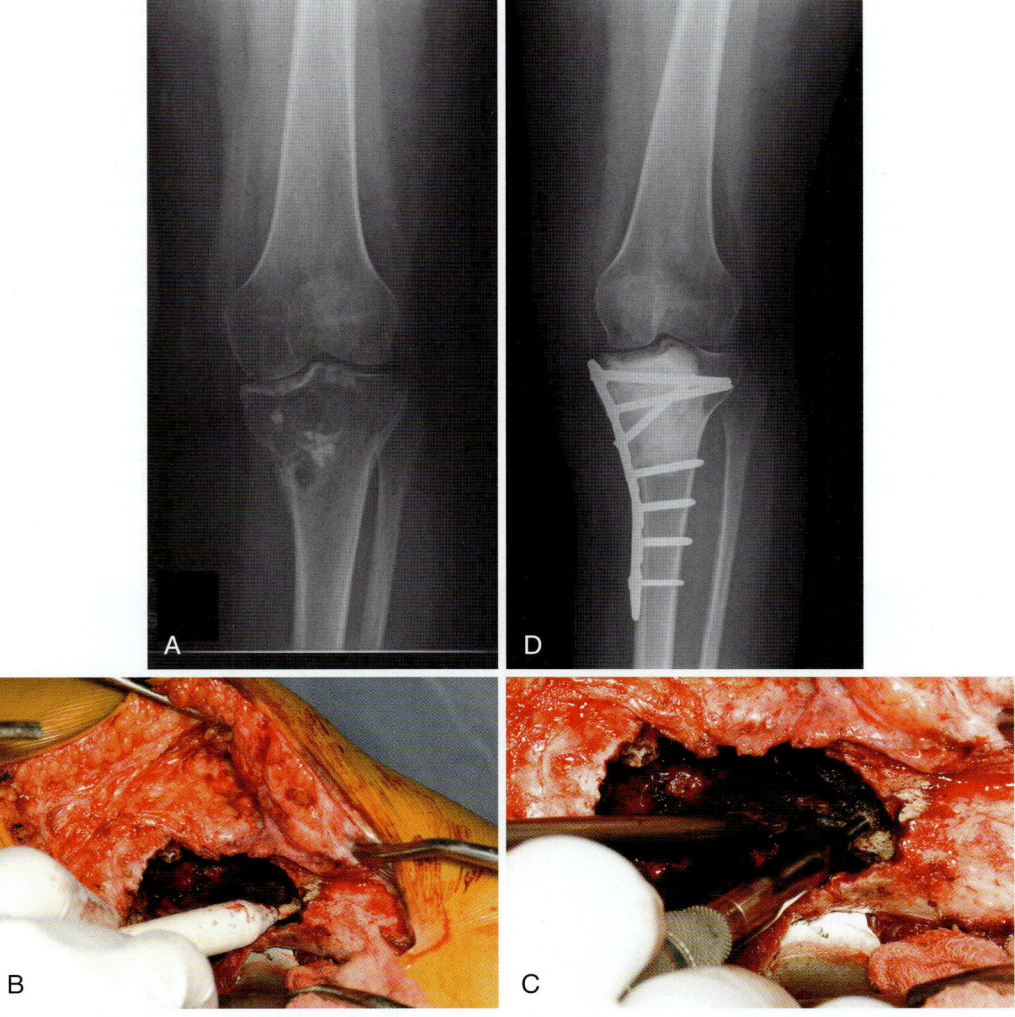

Figure 50-5. Use of the argon beam coagulator and a high-speed burr in the treatment of a recurrent giant cell tumor of bone (this example is in the proximal tibia). **A,** Preoperative radiograph. **B,** Use of the argon beam coagulator and (**C**) high-speed burr as thermal and mechanical adjuvants for tumor removal. **D,** Radiograph after internal fixation and cementation of the defect.

recommended that it be employed first to minimize the risk of intraoperative fire, as was described earlier. Good initial results have been obtained with this technique in the treatment of giant cell tumors and aneurysmal bone cysts.[24,25]

Use of these aggressive adjuvants is generally reserved for experienced surgeons, who develop and refine the technique by their applications. Comparative studies of their relative efficacies are lacking at this time. The decision to use specific chemical or thermal adjuvants in the treatment of aggressive benign bone tumors is heavily influenced by surgeon preference and institutional practice patterns.

Internal Fixation

A variety of benign bone tumors may progress to the point that there is risk of impending pathologic fracture or pain caused by relative mechanical insufficiency of the bone but not requiring discrete treatment of the lesion. The classic example of this is fibrous dysplasia, which commonly affects a long segment of the bone. It is classically refractory to bone grafting procedures. Best results in the treatment of fibrous dysplasia that does not respond to bisphosphonates are seen with internal fixation, usually with intramedullary devices to maintain mechanical alignment of the bone.[26] Also, supplementary fixation is commonly used after curettage procedures for this and other tumors, to augment mechanical stability and to minimize the risk of pathologic fracture after the curettage procedure has taken place.

If fibrous dysplasia affects the entire bone or a large segment of it, intramedullary fixation is indicated. With internal fixation of bone tumors that have a more defined and limited extent, care should be taken to minimize contamination of other areas of the bone. For example, internal fixation after curettage of a giant cell tumor around the hip joint probably would best utilize a plate and screw or perhaps a short intramedullary device. The use of a long intramedullary device would be relatively contraindicated because it could transfer residual cells throughout the bone, potentially leading to multifocal giant cell tumor disease throughout the femur.

Marginal Excision

Select benign tumors may best be treated by marginal surgical excision if they are causing difficulty. For example, an osteochondroma around the hip joint that is causing mechanical symptoms owing to its impingement on other structures is best treated by marginal excision of the lesion itself, with an osteotomy through its stalk. Marginal excision of this nature does not require that a wide margin be achieved with the sacrifice of a cuff of surrounding normal tissue. Rather, the marginal excision proceeds in the plane around the tumor itself to effect complete removal. This is appropriate in the treatment of benign tumors, which have a low propensity for recurrence or are most efficiently treated by complete excision. Another example would

involve treatment of a deep intramuscular lipoma about the hip. Marginal excision of these benign lesions is appropriate if they are causing symptoms. However, the benign nature of the tumor does not justify the sacrifice of normal tissue.

Surgical Resection

Rarely, very aggressive benign tumors may require true resection in a manner similar to malignant lesions. Examples include a very aggressive giant cell tumor, particularly in the presence of minimal remaining bone stock and pathologic fracture. Such treatment is provided reluctantly because of the functional loss inherent in such aggressive treatments. Resection techniques are discussed by Dr. Rose in Chapter 51.

SPECIFIC TREATMENT RECOMMENDATIONS

The treatment options described previously are used solely or in combination to treat benign tumors about the hip. Specific treatment recommendations for commonly encountered bone tumors follow.

Fibrous Dysplasia

The key aspect of the treatment of fibrous dysplasia around the hip is a clinical assessment of the fracture risk involved. Fibrous dysplasia often presents in the femoral neck with an impending or even incomplete or present pathologic fracture (Fig. 50-6A). When symptomatic in the femoral neck, fibrous dysplasia is nearly always treated surgically to minimize the risk of a femoral neck fracture. Fibrous dysplasia may also present in the diaphysis of the femur. In this setting, fracture risk may not be so high, although the lesion may still be symptomatic. The framework of Mirel's criteria is used to evaluate the overall risk of fracture.[27] Patients with significant and immediate weight-bearing pain are judged to be at higher risk of fracture.

Patients who are not believed to be at high risk of fracture from fibrous dysplasia are usually treated initially with bisphosphonates.[2] This treatment provides very low morbidity and reasonable efficacy in the treatment of these lesions. Patients who are judged to be at greater risk of fracture are treated with internal fixation. If any clinical deformity is present, it is important to maintain or reestablish the appropriate mechanical axis of the femur during treatment.[26] Isolated femoral neck lesions may be treated with a side plate and screw construct; lesions that extend into the diaphysis are usually treated with a cephalomedullary rod.

It is attractive and usually customary to curet and graft the lesions of fibrous dysplasia at the time of surgery. This allows for pathologic confirmation of the lesion; however, bone grafting should be performed with the knowledge that the lesion usually heals with additional areas of fibrous dysplasia.[26] Thus the surgeon should design the internal fixation in such a way that it

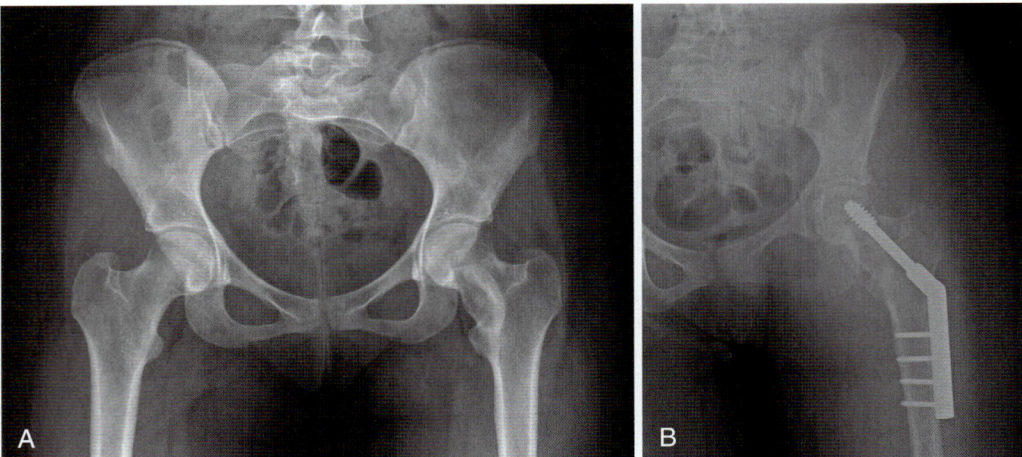

Figure 50-6. Fibrous dysplasia of the femoral neck. **A,** Lesion with developing stress fracture in the femoral neck of an 18-year-old woman. **B,** Patient had immediate relief of symptoms with side plate and screw fixation. Note that the screw is placed in the center of the remaining bone rather than in the center of the femoral neck.

will be appropriate for stabilizing the lesion that is being treated.

Giant Cell Tumor

Giant cell tumors about the hip most commonly arise in the proximal femur around the epiphysis or around the trochanteric apophysis. When possible, they are treated intralesionally to preserve the native hip joint. Wide resection is used for other, more expendable locations (e.g., fibula head) or for tumors with extensive soft tissue extensions and/or pathologic fractures.[28] Although wide resection presents a lower risk of recurrence, it is associated with higher risks of complications and increased functional impairment.

Intralesional treatment with allograft filling has reported recurrence rates between 12% and 65%. Use of polymethylmethacrylate (PMMA) may decrease recurrence rates, although results of studies that have explored this topic are conflicting. Conflicting efficacy reports have been obtained for chemical adjuvants as well.[13-25,29] In nearly all cases of giant cell tumor about the hip, supplementary internal fixation is added to decrease the risk of postprocedure fracture.

Our general practice is to perform joint-preserving surgery when possible for patients with giant cell tumor of the proximal femur. Lesions in this area are treated by extended curettage as outlined earlier, coupled with a combination of mechanical, chemical, and/or thermal adjuvant. The resulting cavity may be filled with bone graft or methylmethacrylate at the surgeon's discretion. PMMA is favored for immediate stability, easy detection of recurrence, and its potential tumorilytic effects (Fig. 50-7).

With recurrent tumors, extensive lesions with significant extraosseous mass, and displaced pathologic fractures, preservation of the native joint may not be practical. In these cases, arthroplasty is preferred. A careful decision is made by the treating surgeon regarding whether to perform a hemiarthroplasty or a total

hip arthroplasty in this setting. Expanding the procedure to include an acetabular component violates the natural anatomic barrier to tumor extension into the pelvis and potentially places the patient at risk for recurrent tumor in this area. Giant cell tumors can metastasize to the lungs, so chest imaging of these patients is indicated.

Enchondroma

Enchondromas are commonly seen around the proximal femur. They are usually discovered incidentally and do not require specific treatment. However, the clinician must always be alert for the potential of aggressive behavior or even malignancy. These lesions are generally observed through "watchful waiting." Serial radiographs are obtained to ensure stability of the lesion. In the rare case that an enchondroma is believed to be symptomatic, surgical treatment involves careful curettage and surgical fixation.

Osteochondroma

Osteochondromas usually cause mechanical symptoms around the hip with impingement upon musculotendinous or visceral structures (Fig. 50-8). When they are present, treatment consists of simple excision by transection of the lesion at its stalk or base. The recurrence rate is negligible with this treatment. Clinicians must be careful about the stress riser, which results from transection of the tumor at its stalk. Patients are usually placed on activity restrictions and occasionally benefit from prophylactic fixation (e.g., sliding hip screw) if a large cortical defect is created as part of the excision.

Osteoid Osteoma

Osteoid osteoma may be an occult cause of hip pain in young adults. Particularly when eccentric, lesions may be difficult to visualize other than with CT (see Fig.

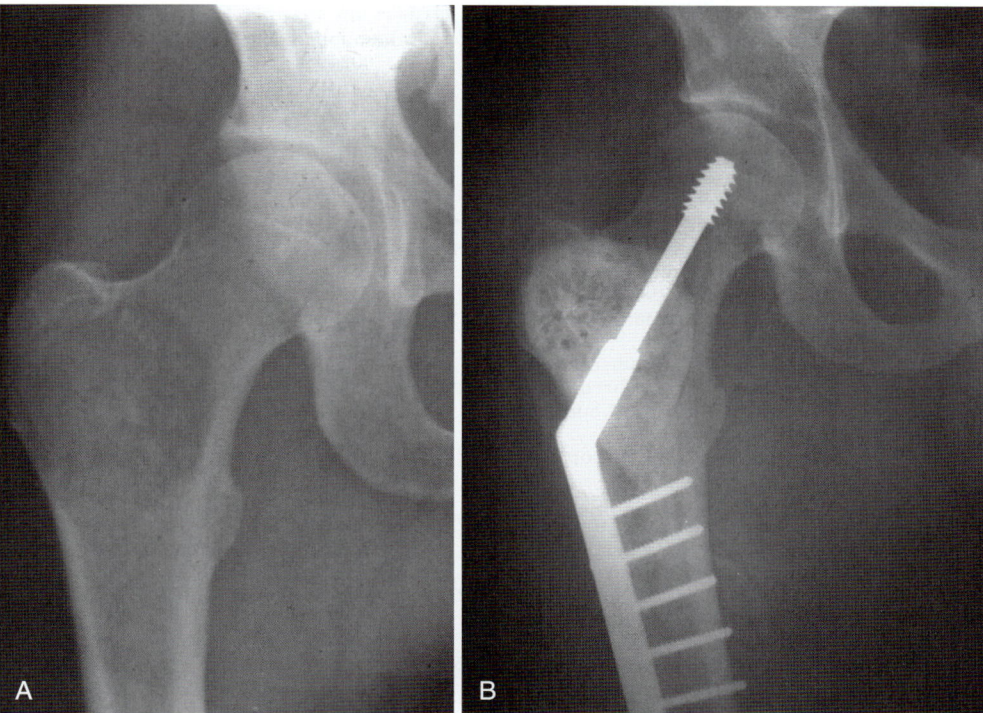

Figure 50-7. Giant cell tumor of the trochanteric apophysis. **A,** Presenting imaging. **B,** Resolution of pain after curettage, cementation, and internal fixation.

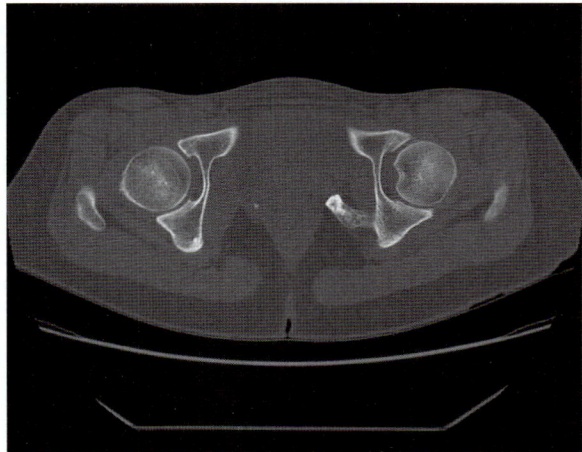

Figure 50-8. Periacetabular osteochondroma presented with dyspareunia. Tumor underwent simple excision.

50-1). The first line of treatment for osteoid osteoma is percutaneous radiofrequency or cryoablation.[7,8] The selection of one modality over the other is based on surgeon preference and institutional practice patterns. A small increased risk of fracture is probably noted in the weeks following an ablation, and patients are advised to maintain activity restrictions during this time. However, it is usually not necessary to provide any supplementing or internal fixation in this setting.

Chondroblastoma

Chondroblastomas arise in epiphyseal or apophyseal regions of the skeleton. They are commonly seen in the

proximal femur, particularly in children with open physes.[30] Chondroblastoma is treated similarly to giant cell tumor of bone, through joint-preserving intra-lesional procedures (see Fig. 50-2). Recurrence rates as high as 32% have been recorded, and proximal femur lesions appear to be at high risk for recurrence.[30,31] Like giant cell tumors, chondroblastomas occasionally metastasize to the lungs, and chest imaging is indicated.

CONCLUSIONS

Most benign lesions about the hip require no treatment or are well treated with minimal morbidity for the patient. To achieve a diagnosis and exclude malignancy, evaluation proceeds as outlined in Chapter 49 by Dr. Silverstein. A variety of techniques can be adapted to the treatment of benign bone lesions about the hip; they are tailored to the needs of the individual patient and the presenting histology.

The initial treatment of benign lesions about the hip is always conservative in an attempt to maximize patient function and outcome (nonoperatively or with lesser surgical procedures). In select aggressive lesions, this does pose a risk of recurrence; however, a conservative approach is supported by the benign nature of the lesion and the high likelihood that less aggressive treatment will be successful. In patients in whom more limited approaches fail, aggressive resection as outlined in Chapter 51 for the treatment of malignant tumors may be performed to salvage recurrent benign conditions. For example, giant cell tumors are usually treated initially by an attempt at curettage with the use of adjuvants to preserve the native hip joint and maximize patient function. If recurrence precludes salvage of the limb, the techniques of resection and reconstruction outlined by Dr. Rose in Chapter 51 can maintain patient function.

REFERENCES

1. Arata MA, Peterson HA, Dahlin DC: Pathological fractures through non-ossifying fibromas: review of the Mayo Clinic experience. J Bone Joint Surg Am 63:980–988, 1981.
2. DiMeglio LA: Bisphosphonate therapy for fibrous dysplasia. Pediatr Endocrinol Rev 4(Suppl 4):440–445, 2007.
3. Rougraff BT, Kling TJ: Treatment of active unicameral bone cysts with percutaneous injection of demineralized bone matrix and autogenous bone marrow. J Bone Joint Surg Am 84:921–929, 2002.
4. Wilkins RM: Unicameral bone cysts. J Am Acad Orthop Surg 8:217–224, 2000.
5. Wright JG, Yandow S, Donaldson S, Marley L, on Behalf of The Simple Bone Cyst Trial Group: A randomized clinical trial comparing intralesional bone marrow and steroid injections for simple bone cysts. J Bone Joint Surg Am 90:722–730, 2008.
6. Hosalkar HS, Jones KJ, King JJ, Lackman RD: Serial arterial embolization for large sacral giant-cell tumors: mid-to long-term results. Spine 32:1107–1115, 2007.
7. Cribb GL, Goude WH, Cool P, et al: Percutaneous radiofrequency thermocoagulation of osteoid osteomas: factors affecting therapeutic outcome. Skeletal Radiol 34:702–706, 2005.
8. Donkol RH, Al-Nammi A, Moghazi K: Efficacy of percutaneous radiofrequency ablation of osteoid osteoma in children. Pediatr Radiol 38:180–185, 2008.
9. Moretti VM, Slotcavage RL, Crawford EA, et al: Curettage and graft alleviates athletic-limiting pain in benign lytic bone lesions. Clin Orthop Relat Res 469:283–288, 2011.
10. Hak DJ: The use of osteoconductive bone graft substitutes in orthopaedic trauma. J Am Acad Orthop Surg 15:525–536, 2007.
11. Hou HY, Wu K, Wang CT, et al: Treatment of unicameral bone cyst: a comparative study of selected techniques. J Bone Joint Surg Am 92:855–862, 2010.
12. Shih HN, Su Jy, Hsu KY, Hsu RW: Allogeneic cortical strut for benign lesions of the humerus in adolescents. J Pediatr Orthop 17:433–436, 1997.
13. Balke M, Schremper L, Gebert C, et al: Giant cell tumor of bone: treatment and outcome of 214 cases. J Cancer Res Clin Oncol 134:969–978, 2008.
14. Arbeitsgemeinschaft K, Becker WT, Dohle J, et al: Local recurrence of giant cell tumor of bone after intralesional treatment with and without adjuvant therapy. J Bone Joint Surg Am 90:1060–1067, 2008.
15. Ghert MA, Rizzo M, Harrelson JM, Scully SP: Giant-cell tumor of the appendicular skeleton. Clin Orthop Relat Res 400:201–210, 2002.
16. Kivioja AH, Blomqvist C, Hietaniemi K, et al: Cement is recommended in intralesional surgery of giant cell tumors: a Scandinavian Sarcoma Group study of 294 patients followed for a median time of 5 years, Acta Orthop 79:86–93, 2008.
17. Nicholson NC, Ramp WK, Kneisl JS, Kaysinger KK: Hydrogen peroxide inhibits giant cell tumor and osteoblast metabolism in vitro. Clin Orthop Relat Res 347:250–260, 1998.
18. Jones KB, DeYoung BR, Morcuende JA, Buckwalter JA: Ethanol as a local adjuvant for giant cell tumor of bone. Iowa Orthop J 26:69–76, 2006.
19. Quint U, Vanhofer U, Harstrick A, Muller RT: Cytotoxicity of phenol to musculoskeletal tumour. J Bone Joint Surg Br 78:984–985, 1996.
20. Durr HR, Maier M, Jansson V, et al: Phenol as an adjuvant for local control in the treatment of giant cell tumour of the bone. Eur J Surg Oncol 25:610–618, 1999.
21. Trieb K, Bitzan P, Lang S, et al: Recurrence of curetted and bone-grafted giant-cell tumours with and without adjuvant phenol therapy. Eur J Surg Oncol 27:200–202, 2001.
22. Robinson D, Yassin M, Nevo Z: Cryotherapy of musculoskeletal tumors—from basic science to clinical results. Technol Cancer Res Treat 3:371–375, 2004.
23. Malawer MM, Bickels J, Meller I, et al: Cryosurgery in the treatment of giant cell tumor: a long-term followup study. Clin Orthop Relat Res 359:176–188, 1999.
24. Cummings JE, Smith RA, Heck RK Jr: Argon beam coagulation as adjuvant treatment after curettage of aneurysmal bone cysts: a preliminary study. Clin Orthop Relat Res 468:231–237, 2010.
25. Lewis VO, Wei A, Mendoza T, et al: Argon beam coagulation as an adjuvant for local control of giant cell tumor. Clin Orthop Relat Res 454:192–197, 2007.
26. Guille JT, Kumar SJ, Macewen GD: Fibrous dysplasia of the proximal part of the femur: long-term results of curettage and bone-grafting and mechanical realignment. J Bone Joint Surg Am 80:648–658, 1998.
27. Mirels H: Metastatic disease in long bones: a proposed scoring system for diagnosing impending pathologic fractures. Clin Orthop Relat Res 249:256–264, 1989.
28. McDonald DJ, Sim FH, McLeod RA, Dahlin DC: Giant cell tumor of bone. J Bone Joint Surg Am 68:235–242, 1986.
29. Klenke FM, Wenger DE, Inwards CY, et al: Giant cell tumor of bone: risk factors for recurrence. Clin Orthop Relat Res 469:591–599, 2011.
30. Sailhan F, Chotel F, Parot R: Chondroblastoma of bone in a pediatric population. J Bone Joint Surg Am 91:2159–2168, 2009.
31. Ramappa AJ, Lee FY, Tang P, et al: Chondroblastoma of bone. J Bone Joint Surg Am 82:1140–1145, 2000.

CHAPTER 51

Primary Malignant Bone Tumors

Peter S. Rose

KEY POINTS

- Primary malignant tumors about the hip are rare.
- Early recognition is critical in curative treatment.
- Chemotherapy or radiation may be indicated, depending on histology. Durable limb salvage techniques are applicable to most patients.

INTRODUCTION

Primary malignant processes frequently present in the hip region. Prompt recognition of these patients is critical, as a window for cure often exists. These lesions are treated with resection with or without adjuvant therapies, depending on histology. With few exceptions, wide surgical resection of all disease is required for long-term survival. Limb salvage procedures are possible in 85% to 90% of cases, and modern techniques give durable prosthetic reconstructions. This chapter will address the treatment of primary bone and soft tissue sarcomas about the hip.

EPIDEMIOLOGY

Although sarcomas can present in any age group, classic patterns have been observed and documented. Osteosarcoma is the most common bone sarcoma with the best characterized epidemiology. Approximately 500 cases per year arise in the United States. Although mutations in the retinoblastoma gene can lead to osteosarcoma, most cases arise sporadically.[1]

Data from more than 2000 cases of osteosarcoma treated over a 100 year period highlight the presentation of this tumor (Fig. 51-1). Males account for a modest majority of cases, and most patients are in the second or third decade of life. The hip region (including proximal femur and pelvis) is the second most common site of disease after the knee. The skeletal distribution of osteosarcoma roughly parallels the amount of skeletal growth at various sites.

Other sarcomas have similar distributions. Chondrosarcoma and Ewing's sarcoma are the next most common primary bone tumors about the hip. Chondrosarcoma arises in an older patient population than osteosarcoma and most commonly involves the pelvis or proximal femur region. Ewing's sarcoma shows a similar age distribution to osteosarcoma but has more tumors in the hip and pelvis region. Extra-abdominal soft tissue sarcomas present in middle-aged to older adult patients, with the thigh and buttock regions being the most frequent sites of disease. Although true bony invasion is rare, these tumors may encase the sciatic nerve or femoral artery and often abut the bone directly.

GENERAL CONSIDERATIONS

Staging and Biopsy

Patients presenting with a primary malignant tumor about the hip joint require accurate diagnosis and staging for proper management. Staging involves defining the local and systemic extent of disease. Local imaging begins with plain radiographs of the affected area (even for patients with soft tissue sarcomas). Patients with bony tumors should undergo imaging of the entire femur and pelvis to identify any discontiguous sites of disease (skip lesions). Magnetic resonance imaging is used to characterize marrow involvement and soft tissue masses or extensions. Select tumors may require computed tomography (CT) angiography to define vascular invasion or encasement.

The systemic extent of disease is evaluated with computed tomography of the chest and bone scintigraphy (for bony tumors) to complete oncologic staging. Although CT of the abdomen and pelvis is not part of routine oncologic staging for sarcomas, we employ this approach in any patient whose primary tumor involves the pelvis or extends above the inguinal ligament, to detect any regional metastases that might be missed with imaging of the chest and tumor site alone. The role of positron emission tomography (PET) is currently evolving in the staging evaluation of primary tumors. Select histologies (e.g., myxoid liposarcoma) may have specific additional staging protocols.[2]

Although many lesions have a characteristic appearance on imaging studies, biopsy is generally needed to establish diagnosis before malignant conditions are treated. We generally use image-guided (fluoroscopic, CT, or ultrasound) biopsy as the first-line invasive sampling method for tumors. High diagnostic accuracy is seen in the hands of experienced pathologists.[3] Open biopsy is reserved for unsuccessful core needle biopsy. The biopsy approach, whether open or percutaneous, should be carefully planned to target high-yield

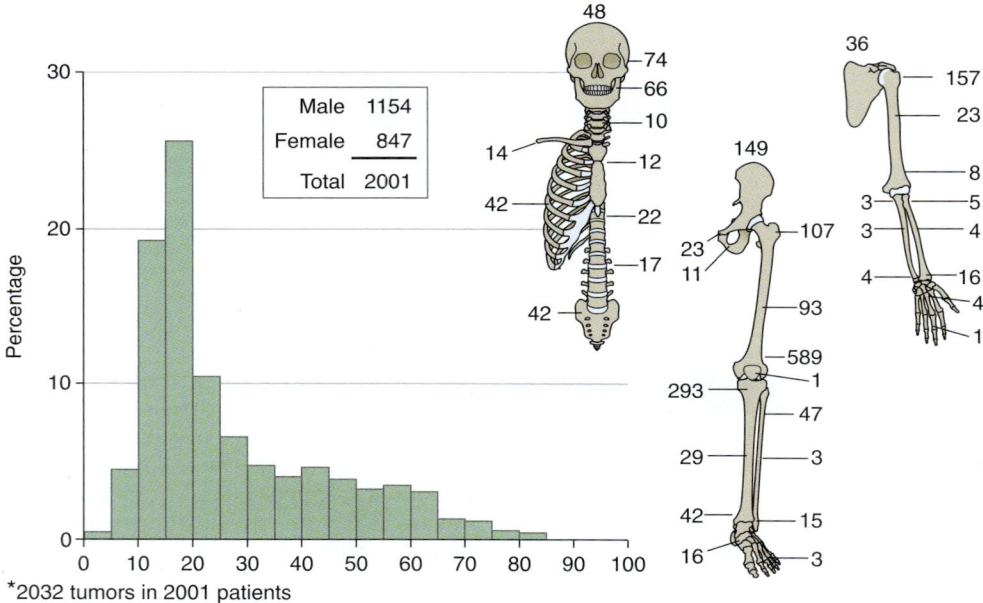

Figure 51-1. Age, sex, and skeletal distribution of osteosarcoma in 2001 patients.

areas of the lesion and to allow excision of the biopsy tract and any contaminated tissues at the time of definitive resection. Poorly planned biopsy can severely compromise ultimate patient outcomes.[4] In the case of open biopsy, transverse incisions are never used, and care is taken to split individual muscles rather than open classic planes to minimize the zone of biopsy site contamination.

Adjuvant Therapy

Adjuvant chemotherapy and/or radiation therapy is the standard of care in high-grade primary bony malignancies. Chemotherapy improves the survival of patients with localized Ewing's sarcoma and osteosarcoma from approximately 15% to approaching 70% or greater. Additionally, long-term disease-free survival is seen even in patients with limited metastatic disease treated with aggressive surgery and chemotherapy. Essentially all standard regimens for these tumors employ two to four cycles of chemotherapy preoperatively. Surgical resection is accomplished with a minimal delay in therapy, followed by multiple postoperative cycles.[1,5]

The critical nature of chemotherapy in these diseases highlights the importance of an accurate initial diagnosis before therapy commences. The chemotherapy response as assessed by the necrosis seen in the resected tumor specimen is predictive of overall survival. That said, up-front surgery followed by an equivalent total number of postoperative chemotherapy cycles yielded identical clinical outcomes in the only study that directly examined this.[6]

Radiotherapy may be used in the treatment of Ewing's sarcoma and is commonly used in the treatment of soft tissue sarcoma. High-dose radiation can be used in place of surgery for local control in Ewing's sarcoma, when resection is not possible or practical. Although no prospective randomized studies have compared surgery versus radiotherapy for local control in Ewing's sarcoma, available data appear to indicate that surgery or surgery combined with radiation may be superior to radiation alone.[7,8] Additionally, long-term complications are seen following radiation for Ewing's sarcoma.[9]

Local control of soft tissue sarcomas is improved with the use of radiotherapy. Radiation for soft tissue sarcomas may be administered preoperatively or postoperatively and has been examined in a prospective randomized study. Preoperative therapy engenders a higher wound complication rate but allows a lower dose to be administered to a smaller volume of tissue.[10] Although initial wound complications are more frequent with preoperative therapy, long-term limb function appears better as the result of less ultimate edema and fibrosis.[11] The use of preoperative versus postoperative radiotherapy is often influenced by institutional practice patterns and specific patient situations.

Use of chemotherapy for soft tissue tumors is best considered investigational. Multiple studies (most retrospective) have found conflicting results, and a high-quality meta-analysis revealed modest survival benefits in patients with high-grade tumors.[12] Relatively few studies of chemotherapy in soft tissue sarcoma are "clean." Most mix patients with different histologies and use varying treatment regimens. Just as the results of chemotherapy for bone sarcoma would be difficult to interpret if osteosarcoma, chondrosarcoma, and Ewing's sarcoma were lumped together, interpretation of chemotherapy results for soft tissue sarcoma is nuanced and complex. Adjuvant chemotherapy for these conditions is best given under the advice and management of an experienced sarcoma oncologist in a clinical trial until further data are available.[13]

Patients in whom soft tissue tumors are excised with a periosteal margin following radiation have a high risk of subsequent femur fracture and may benefit from prophylactic fixation.[14] This usually is not done at the time of tumor resection to avoid increasing the magnitude of an already complex procedure. Patients can be allowed to recover from the initial surgery with final margin status assessed and flap healing accomplished before prophylactic nailing is done.

MEDICAL CONSIDERATIONS

Patients requiring hip surgery for oncologic indications are at elevated risk of postoperative complications compared with general orthopedic patients. Preoperative chemotherapy can leave patients malnourished and immunosuppressed. Patients treated with doxorubicin (Adriamycin)-containing regimens (which are commonly used for sarcoma chemotherapy) are at risk for cardiomyopathy and arrhythmia. Patients are at risk for colonization with resistant bacteria from their frequent interaction with the health care system.

It is invaluable to meet with the patient and his/her medical/pediatric oncologist immediately before planned resection for patients on chemotherapy to assess fitness for surgery. One primary consideration is that the patient should not be neutropenic when entering a large surgery. As well, inferior survival is seen in patients with a delay to chemotherapy resumption longer than 21 days postoperatively in high-grade bone sarcoma (Fig. 51-2).[15] Meeting with the medical/pediatric oncology team immediately preoperatively allows for planned resumption of chemotherapy following surgical resection.

Thromboembolic disease is seen more frequently in patients with sarcoma resection than metastatic disease or standard joint arthroplasty.[16] Patients with soft tissue sarcoma may present with venous thrombosis from vascular compression. Surgical site infection is seen in ≈10% of patients.[17] The use of radiotherapy increases this risk further, particularly if an endoprosthesis is placed.[18] These frequent complications highlight the complexity of medical care in an oncologic population.

Surgical Approach

The first critical assessment in approaching patients with primary malignancies around the hip is suitability for limb salvage. The two central tenets of limb salvage surgery are that (1) oncologic outcome should be the same as amputation, and (2) function should be equal to or better than amputation. Close scrutiny is given to involvement of the acetabulum, external iliac/femoral vessels, and sciatic nerve by tumor. These areas are often the places where critical margins can occur in primary tumors about the hip.

Surgical resection of the acetabulum, external iliac vessels, or sciatic nerve can be accomplished with good functional outcomes. However, if two or three of these structures require resection, patient function significantly falls while complication rates increase. Resection of the sciatic nerve, acetabulum, and external iliac vessels implies such a large tumor and engenders such a high likelihood of complications that patients generally will have better oncologic and functional outcomes with an amputation. Decisions when two of these three

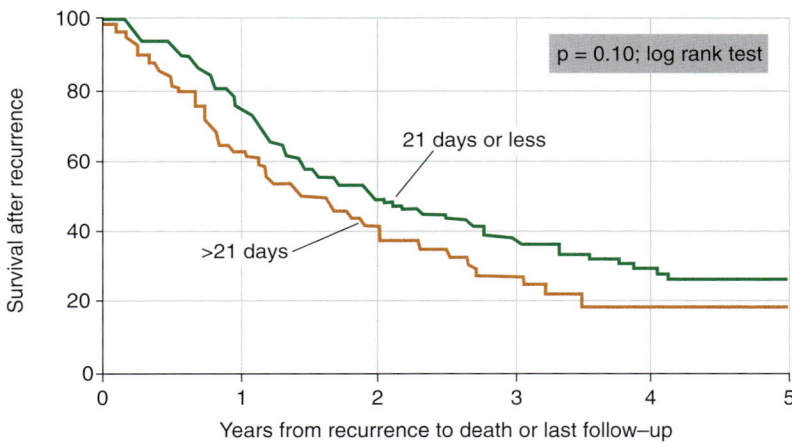

Suvival after recurrence	Number (%) still at risk				
	Year 1	Year 2	Year 3	Year 4	Year 5
21 days or less (N = 157)	103 (65.6)	59 (37.6)	34 (21.7)	20 (2.7)	12 (7.6)
>21 days (N = 62)	34 (54.8)	19 (30.6)	10 (61.1)	34 (9.1)	3 (4.8)
	95% confidence interval				
21 days or less (N = 157)	68.0-82.3	41.3-58.3	29.4-47.0	21.8-39.8	18.6-36.9
>21 days (N = 62)	51.3-76.8	30.2-57.2	17.1-43.6	9.3-35.4	9.3-35.4

Figure 51-2. Kaplan-Meier curves comparing survival after recurrence according to whether the delay in the resumption of chemotherapy after definitive surgery was longer than 21 days as opposed to within 21 days. (Redrawn from Imran H, Enders F, Krailo M, et al: Effect of time to resumption of chemotherapy after definitive surgery on prognosis for non-metastatic osteosarcoma. J Bone Joint Surg Am 91:604–612, 2009.)

structures are involved are individualized, but very strong consideration should be given to amputation in such cases as a way to likely provide better ultimate functional and oncologic outcomes. When amputation is contemplated, preoperative meetings between the patient and a prosthetist are valuable.

When limb salvage is appropriate, the location and extent of the primary tumor dictate the ultimate surgical approach. Our most common approach to tumors about the hip is a direct lateral approach. All bony and nearly all relevant soft tissue structures can be accessed through this method, and the approach can be extended to access the entire femur if needed. The incision can be extended up around the iliac crest to access the pelvis and "T'd" to provide extension into an ilioinguinal approach. A poorly placed biopsy site may require alteration of this approach or a separate incision to resect the biopsy tract in continuity with the tumor.

Large oncologic resections around the hip and pelvis may be associated with significant hemorrhage. Use of autologous blood salvage ("cell-saver") is contraindicated in the setting of malignancy. We administer prophylactic antibiotics around the time of surgery only and are liberal in our use of drains; these are often left for low wall suction for the first 2 to 3 days after surgery to minimize any fluid collections. A 12 French pediatric chest tube can be used in this manner and connected to a pleurovac to maintain a sterile circuit. When drains are near implants, we try to remove them by day 3. Given the amount of dissection and the often large areas of tissue "dead space" following resection, we often use vacuum-assisted wound therapy to provide negative pressure across an incision after primary closure. It has been our experience that we avoid the persistent weeping surgical wound at hip or hemipelvectomy incisions by using this technique.[19]

Oncologic resection may lead to extensive soft tissue defects. Similarly, radiated wounds present significant healing challenges. Healthy muscle and fascia should be used to cover implants whenever possible. This hip region often lends itself to local soft tissue transfer (e.g., gracilis flap) or regional flap coverage (vertical rectus abdominis turndown flap). If free flap coverage is needed, the femoral or profundus system provides ready sites of anastomosis.

When vascular structures are encased by tumor, resection and reconstruction of involved blood vessels can be performed (Fig. 51-3). The complication rate from these procedures is formidable, however.[20] Direct vascular invasion often heralds metastatic disease.

RECONSTRUCTIVE OPTIONS

Soft Tissue Tumors

Reconstructive options are individualized to the needs of the patient. Many soft tissue resections require little formal reconstruction. In the event that significant skin is excised, split-thickness skin grafting may be needed. Local muscle transfer may serve to cover vascular or nervous structures or to recentralize the extensor mechanism if an asymmetrical portion of the quadriceps is resected.

Resection of the sciatic nerve is often required with soft tissue sarcomas of the buttock region. Ultimate function for these patients is surprisingly good, although they require bracing and physical therapy to achieve these goals.[21]

If tumor extends to but does not infiltrate bone, resection may be accomplished with a periosteal margin. Our practice is to treat these patients with preoperative radiation and surgical resection using the periosteum as a margin, and then to provide a boost dose with intraoperative radiotherapy. Postoperatively, patients are at risk for insufficiency fractures that are difficult to heal.[14] We maintain them in a protected weight-bearing stance until all wounds heal, and then proceed with prophylactic intramedullary fixation 8 to 12 weeks postoperatively. This delay allows an initial magnetic resonance (MR) scan to be obtained after postoperative changes have regressed and before susceptibility artifact from an implant is present.

Malignant Bone Tumors

Multiple reconstructive options following wide bony resections about the hip are available, depending on which combination of acetabulum, proximal femur, and femoral diaphysis is resected. Reconstructions use some combination of vascularized autograft, allograft, and prosthetics.

Resection of the femoral diaphysis alone is generally treated with intercalary allografts to preserve the native hip joint (Fig. 51-4). Grafts may be fixed with plates or intramedullary devices. Although union rates are similar with the two approaches, fracture rates may be lower with the use of intramedullary fixation.[22] Vascularized free fibula or periosteal graft transfer can be used to augment healing of the host-allograft junction.[23]

Resection that includes sacrifice of the proximal femur may be reconstructed by iliofemoral or ischiofemoral arthrodesis, pseudarthrosis, osteoarticular allograft, endoprosthesis, or alloprosthetic composite. Arthrodesis and pseudarthrosis techniques are less frequently employed, as techniques of more anatomic reconstruction of the hip joint have advanced. Similarly, osteoarticular allografts are less frequently employed about the hip than the knee. These techniques suffer from high rates of fracture and infection.[24,25] The line of force transmission through the femoral neck (as opposed to along the long axis of the allograft) places osteoarticular allografts of the hip at a mechanical disadvantage and predisposes them to fracture.

Modular endoprosthetic reconstruction is the most common reconstruction following resection of the proximal femur (Fig. 51-5). Modular systems allow tremendous flexibility and intraoperative adaptation of reconstructions. These implants probably have the most reproducible initial and intermediate-term functional results. Long-term results suffer from mechanical and septic failure, as would be expected from such large procedures.[26-28] The largest series with minimum 10 year follow-up for megaprostheses demonstrated 10 year

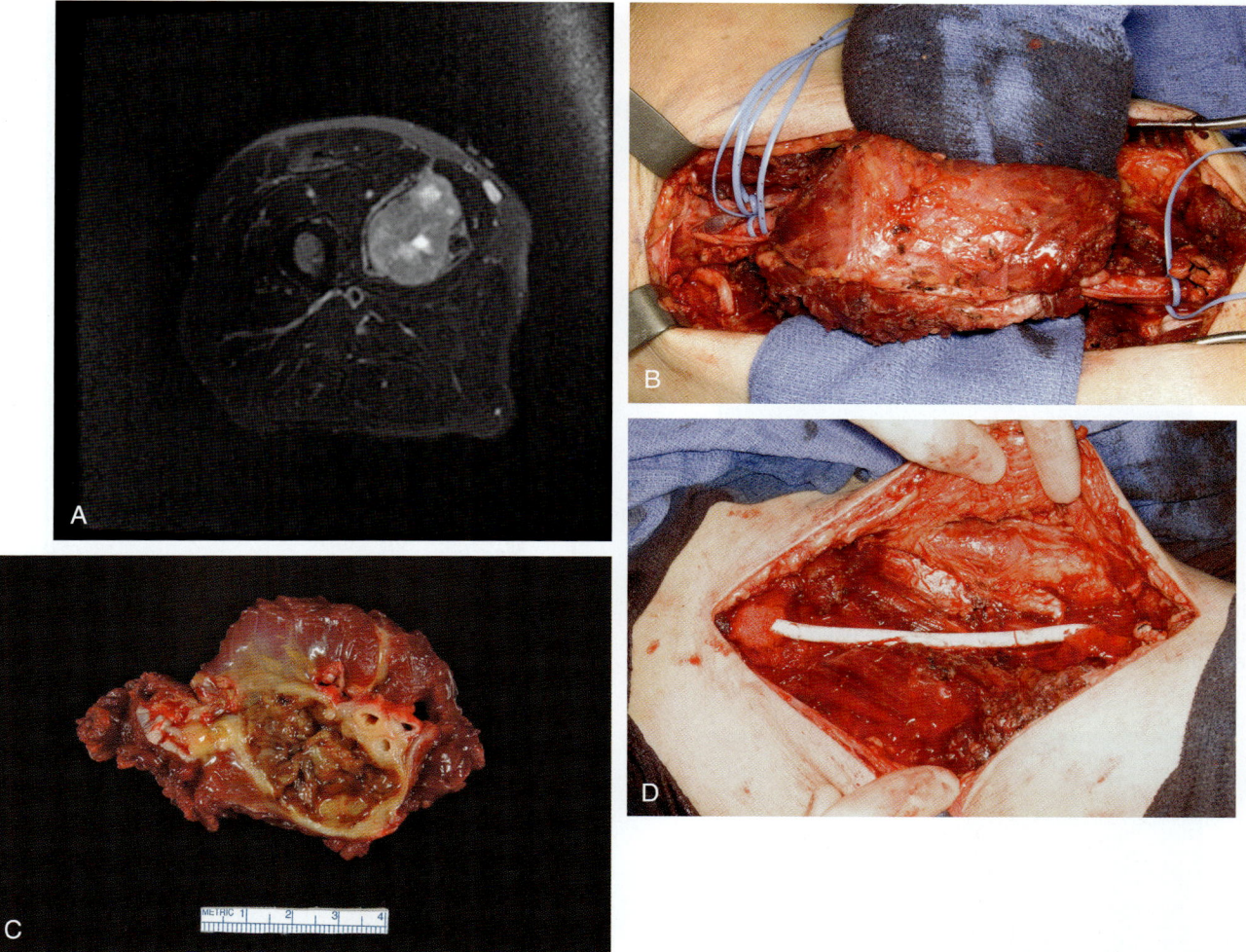

Figure 51-3. Wide excision of high-grade soft tissue sarcoma of the thigh. **A,** Magnetic resonance (MR) demonstrating tumor encasement of femoral vessels. **B,** Specimen immediately before removal, with vessels entering and exiting the lesion. **C,** Cut tumor demonstrating vessel encasement. **D,** Vascular reconstruction.

survival from mechanical failure of 78%, and survival from any failure of 64%.[26] Equivalent outcomes are reported after cemented or cementless fixation. Although these prostheses have holes for soft tissue attachments, experience shows that this is not a predictable way to ensure function. Our preferred method is to suture remaining abductor muscles to the vastus lateralis and fascia lata and to purse-string the remaining capsule around the neck of the implant to maximize function and stability. Stability can possibly be enhanced by lengthening the limb to tension the remaining soft tissue envelope. Additionally, we routinely place the prosthesis with exaggerated anteversion to combat the common tendency of posterior dislocation after extensive oncologic resection.

Allograft prosthetic composite reconstructions offer the potential of prosthetic durability with the functional benefits of soft tissue reconstruction (Fig. 51-6). Improved abductor strength and function have been shown in some series, and clinical experience has shown a lower rate of dislocation caused by an enhanced

ability to repair the capsular tissue of the graft to the host over standard megaprostheses. Even when the native capsule has to be excised, suture anchors may be used to attach the allograft capsule to the acetabular rim. The reoperation rate is greater than 50% for patients surviving longer than 2 years, however.[29] We favor a technique with a transverse osteotomy, although many surgeons prefer the increased allograft-host junction surface area and rotational stability that a step cut affords. The prosthesis is cemented into the allograft and is cemented or press-fit into host bone at the surgeon's preference.[28,30] Alloprosthetic composite reconstructions are more complicated and lengthier procedures compared with endoprosthetic reconstructions. A lead time is needed to obtain a size-matched allograft. Finally, these reconstructions may be best suited to patients not requiring adjuvant chemotherapy or radiotherapy that would impair union across the allograft-host junction.

When the native acetabulum can be spared, we favor the use of a monopolar or bipolar femoral head. Unless

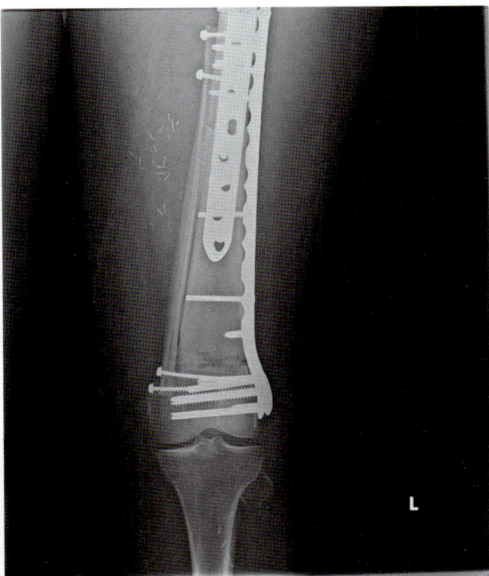

Figure 51-4. Intercalary allograft reconstruction augmented with vascularized fibula following resection of a diaphyseal osteosarcoma (similar techniques are used for more proximal tumors).

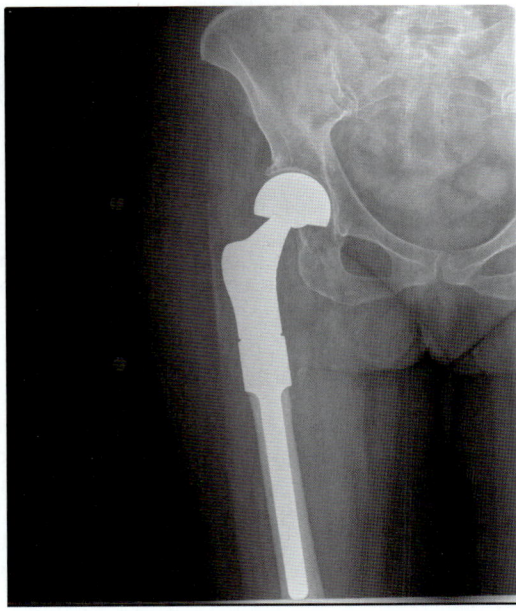

Figure 51-5. Endoprosthetic reconstruction following proximal femur replacement.

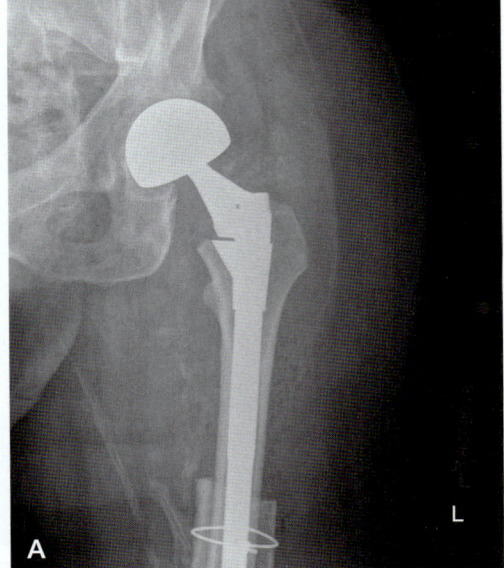

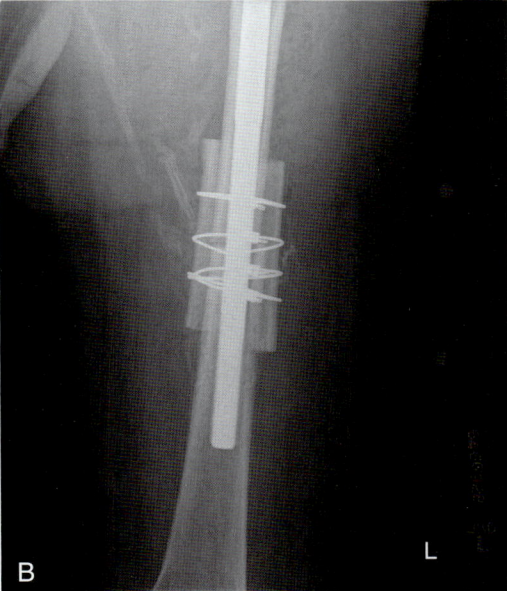

Figure 51-6. Allograft-prosthetic composite reconstruction **(A)** proximal and **(B)** distal.

severe arthritis is present, we do not routinely perform a total hip arthroplasty for several reasons. First, this potentially contaminates the ilium in case an unanticipated positive margin or tumor spillage occurs. Second, this increases the risk of dislocation. We do not favor the use of constrained liners because of their high loosening and failure rates even in conventional arthroplasty situations. Finally, expansion of the procedure beyond its oncologic goals increases the complexity of an already large surgery. All patients undergoing

reconstruction are treated with an abduction brace and protected weight bearing for a period of 6 to 8 weeks to promote healing of the soft tissue envelope and stability of the implant.

Tumors necessitating resection of the acetabulum provide significantly greater reconstructive challenges. These procedures become type II internal hemipelvectomies (periacetabular resections) that may be combined with iliac wing resections (type I internal hemipelvectomy) and pubic excisions (type III internal hemipelvectomy), along with femoral resection. Reconstructive options include arthrodesis, pseudarthrosis, structural pelvic allografts, the saddle prosthesis and its variations, custom pelvic prostheses, and novel pelvic implants (Fig. 51-7). The best functional results

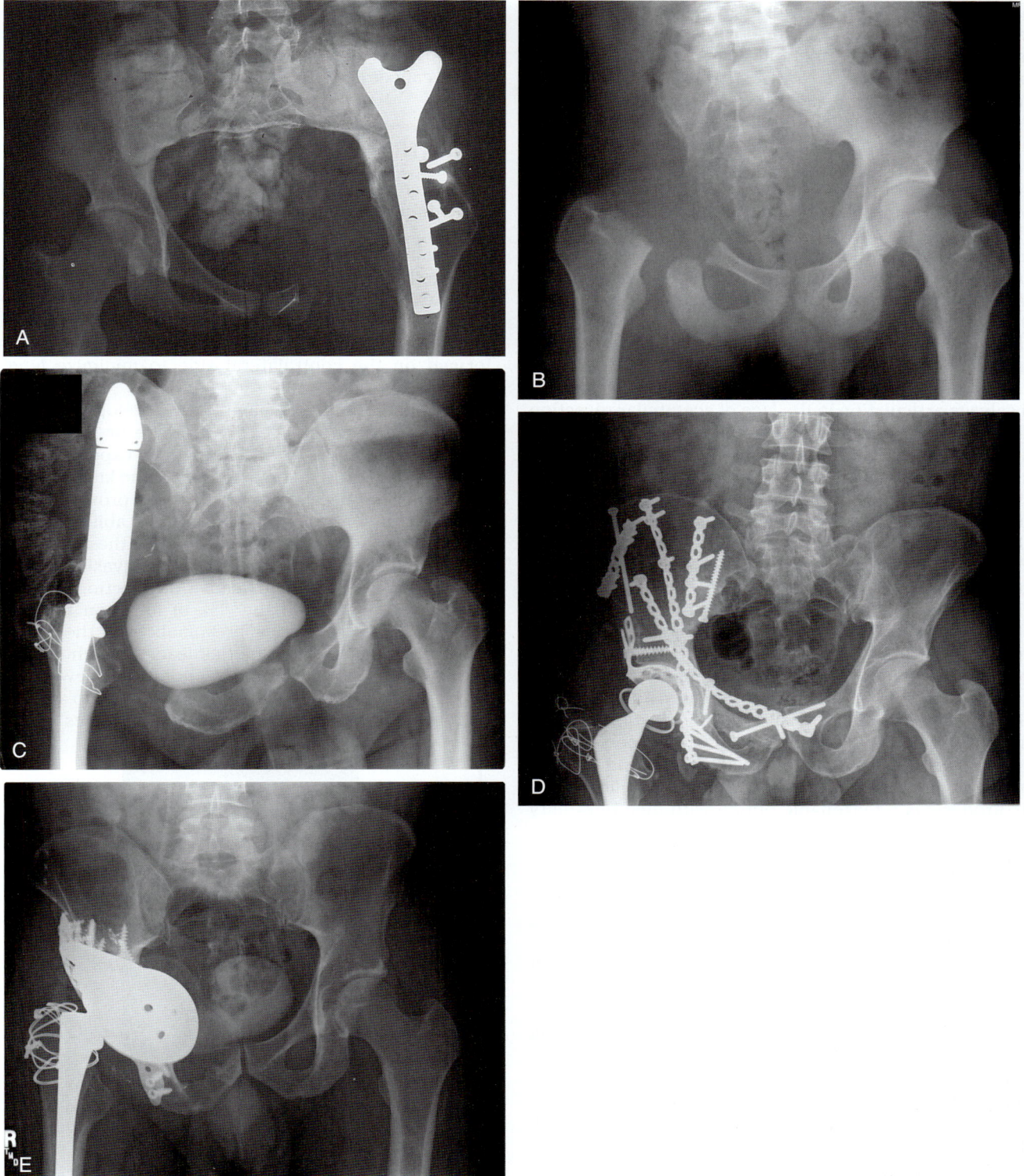

Figure 51-7. Reconstructive options following periacetabular resections. **A,** Iliofemoral arthrodesis. **B,** Pseudarthrosis (Friedman-Eilber resection arthroplasty). **C,** Saddle prosthesis. **D,** Structural pelvic allograft reconstruction. **E,** Tantalum trabecular metal reconstruction.

are seen in these patients when femorosacral continuity is achieved.[31] Enthusiasm for complex reconstructions in these patients is tempered by the recognition of perioperative complication rates well in excess of 50%, particularly for infection.

Because of the magnitude of the oncologic resection and the high complication rate of periacetabular tumor reconstructions, pseudarthrosis (Friedman-Eilber resection arthroplasty) is a common reconstruction technique following type II internal hemipelvectomy (Fig. 51-7B). Surprisingly good function is achieved by many patients, although the results for any individual patient are difficult to predict.[32] This option is attractive in patients requiring immediate resumption of postoperative chemotherapy, in whom a deep allograft or prosthetic infection that delayed adjuvant therapy could negatively impact ultimate survival.

The saddle prosthesis has been developed to provide a salvage articulation in the face of acetabular resection (Fig. 51-7C). It offers the advantage of a simple reconstruction that can be efficiently performed. Results suffer from frequent dislocation, nerve palsy, and infection. Even with high morbidity, the functional results of this construct probably confer a benefit compared with the disadvantages of external hemipelvectomy.[33] Whether this reconstruction provides any benefit over pseudarthrosis is controversial.

Large pelvic allografts have been mated to hip prostheses in an attempt to perform a biological reconstruction (Fig. 51-7D). Although select patients achieve remarkable function, the results are heavily influenced by a deep infection rate of 50% or greater. Rates of infection are influenced by the size of the resection and the ultimate graft, which is necessary.[34] We reserve these reconstructions for highly selected patients. When minimal iliac wing requires resection, iliofemoral arthrodesis is a reasonable option with high durability and modest risk of late infection.

New experience is being gained with the use of trabecular metal implants in the reconstruction of pelvic defects (Fig. 51-7E). These implants have shown favorable results in the treatment of radiation osteonecrosis of the pelvis and in reconstruction of cavitary defects caused by metastatic disease.[35] Early experience with these reconstructions in patients with primary tumor resections is promising.[36]

Infection is an unfortunately common complication following large oncologic surgeries. Infection complicates more than 10% of extremity reconstructive procedures and a much higher percentage of pelvic procedures.[34,37] More than one third of patients with infected prostheses ultimately require amputation.[37] Radiotherapy significantly increases this risk as well.[18] Infection is treated with aggressive two-stage exchange protocols and culture-directed antibiotics in the hope of salvaging these situations.

Several different implants are available from various manufacturers. The superiority of any one implant over another has never been demonstrated (and probably never will be). The rarity of primary tumor cases and the heterogeneity of oncologic resections and adjuvant therapies preclude any well-matched comparisons.

Literature reports on these topics are limited to modest case series of contemporary implants, or large series that span decades of evolution of clinical practice at major cancer centers.

PEDIATRIC PATIENTS

Special considerations are needed in treating pediatric patients. Resections commonly require sacrifice of the proximal femoral physis and/or the triradiate cartilage. The resulting leg length discrepancy may be accepted, managed by shoe lift, or treated surgically. In growing patients, the operative limb usually can be lengthened by 1 to 2 cm at the time of resection to decrease the ultimate leg length discrepancy. Epiphysiodesis is performed on the contralateral side to minimize length discrepancy.

Expandable implants have been developed to allow lengthening of prostheses by invasive or noninvasive mechanisms (Fig. 51-8).[38,39] The greatest experience with these implants has taken place about the knee, and this experience has been extrapolated to the proximal femur. Although they are very useful in their ability to minimize ultimate leg length discrepancy, these implants suffer from high ultimate failure rates. Invasive expandable implants are a major cause of infection in megaprostheses.[37] Although the risk of infection from any single expansion episode if presumably low, the cumulative effect of multiple surgeries leads to high ultimate septic failure. These implants should be viewed as a "bridge" to adulthood with later conversion to a permanent fixed prosthesis if the patient survives his/her

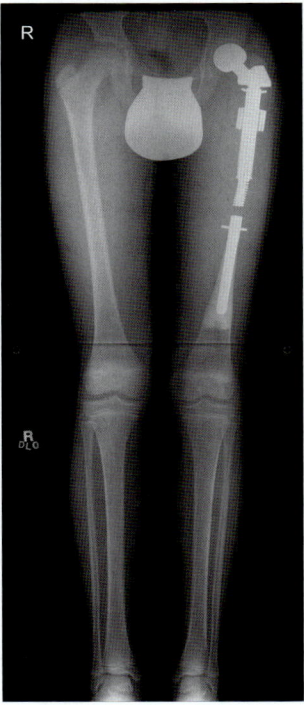

Figure 51-8. Expandable implant in a child: 3.5 years with four expansions following tumor resection; leg length discrepancy is less than 3 mm.

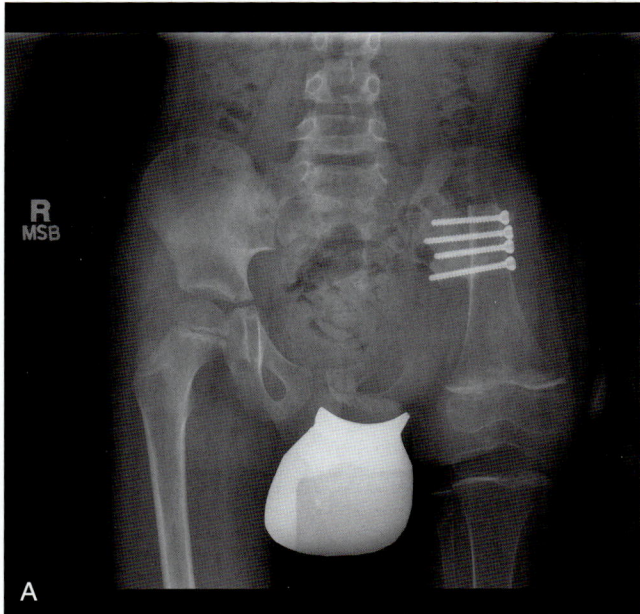

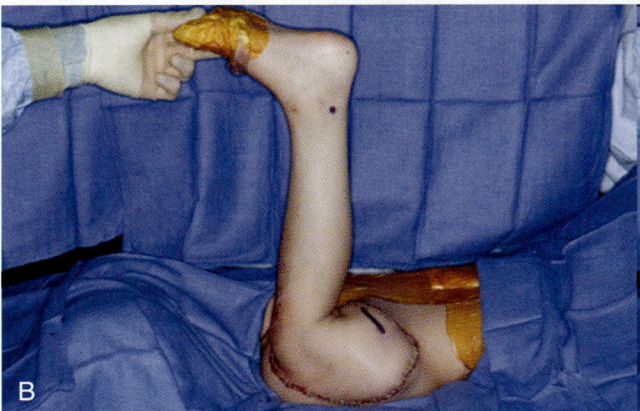

Figure 51-9. Hip rotationplasty in a 7-year-old child following resection of proximal femur osteosarcoma. **A,** Radiograph. **B,** Clinical photograph at surgery.

Table 51-1. Interval for Postoperative Surveillance Based on Tumor Grade

Time Since Diagnosis	Low Grade	High Grade
0-2 years	4-6 months	3-4 months
3-5 years	8-12 months	6 months
6-10 years	24 months	12 months
>10 years	2-5 years	24 months

of the local site as well as the chest and other bones (for bony sarcomas via technetium bone scan). As mentioned earlier, tumors extending into the pelvis are suitable for abdomen and pelvis imaging as well.

COMMENTS ON SPECIFIC TUMOR HISTOLOGIES

Osteosarcoma

Osteosarcoma (also osteogenic sarcoma) is the most common primary bone sarcoma. The 100 year Mayo Clinic Rochester experience (1905-2005) totals 2032 tumors in 2001 patients. Of these, 107 were located in the proximal femur, 183 in the pelvis, and 93 in the femoral diaphysis. Pain is the most common presenting symptom. The hallmark of the tumor, neoplastic osteoid production, is usually visible on radiographs (Fig. 51-10).

Most patients are children or young adults; rarely the tumor will arise in older patients, often as a secondary lesion in pagetic or radiated bone. Treatment of osteosarcoma patients has been revolutionized by the development of adjuvant chemotherapy over the past four decades. Long-term survival has improved from ≈15% to nearly 70% for patients presenting with clinically localized disease (Fig. 51-11).[41,42] Patients with pelvic tumors have a poorer prognosis, likely as the result of larger tumor size at presentation and difficulty in achieving tumor-free margins. Whether proximal femoral lesions have a poorer prognosis is not clear.

Standard treatment protocols call for two to four cycles of preoperative (neoadjuvant) chemotherapy, wide surgical resection, and additional chemotherapy.[1] Agents include doxorubicin, cisplatin, methotrexate, and ifosfamide. The practice of neoadjuvant chemotherapy for osteosarcoma developed in the 1970s to allow treatment to commence while custom limb salvage implants were being fabricated. With the advent of modern modular reconstruction systems, immediate limb salvage surgery is usually possible. A single prospective randomized trial analyzing the benefit of immediate surgery versus neoadjuvant chemotherapy found no significant difference in patient survival or limb salvage rates with either approach.[6] Most surgeons favor preoperative chemotherapy to shrink tumor masses and facilitate resection. Additionally, analysis of tumor necrosis in the resected specimen gives valuable prognostic information.[43]

cancer. Very young patients are candidates for hip rotationplasty (Fig. 51-9). Young patients treated with hemiarthroplasty reconstructions predictably develop acetabular dysplasia.[40] The long-term implications of this are not yet known.

POSTOPERATIVE SURVEILLANCE

Patients treated for primary malignancies about the hip require long-term surveillance for local or distant recurrence of disease. Exact protocols are not standardized, and clinicians recognize that the highest risk of recurrence occurs in the first 2 years after treatment. Late recurrence of sarcoma (even beyond 10 years) is well recognized.

Surveillance protocols for patients on clinical trials are predefined. For other patients, a reasonable strategy is outlined in Table 51-1. Surveillance includes imaging

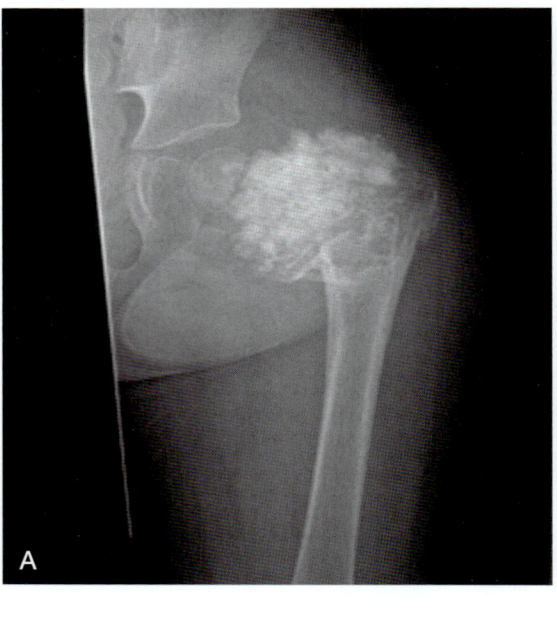

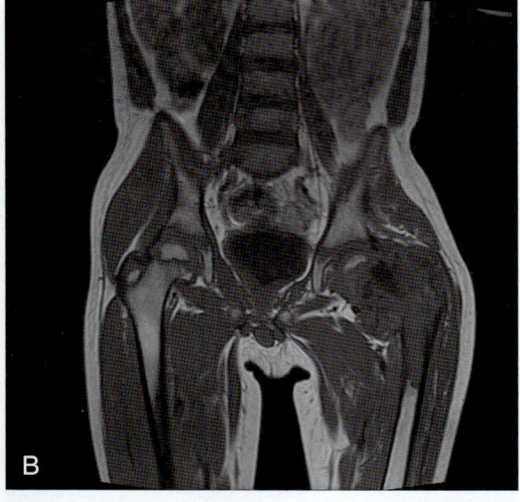

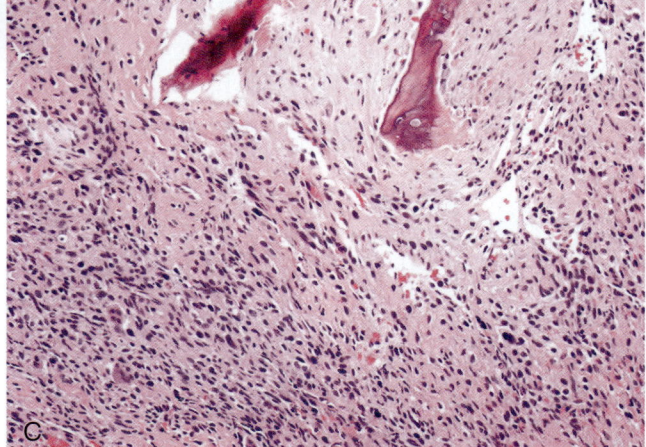

Figure 51-10. Presentation of osteoblastic osteosarcoma. **A,** Radiographs demonstrate a permeative, aggressive lesion with neoplastic osteoid formation. **B,** Magnetic resonance (MR) scan demonstrates extent of tumor and extraosseous mass. **C,** Histology shows high-grade spindle cell malignancy with neoplastic osteoid formation.

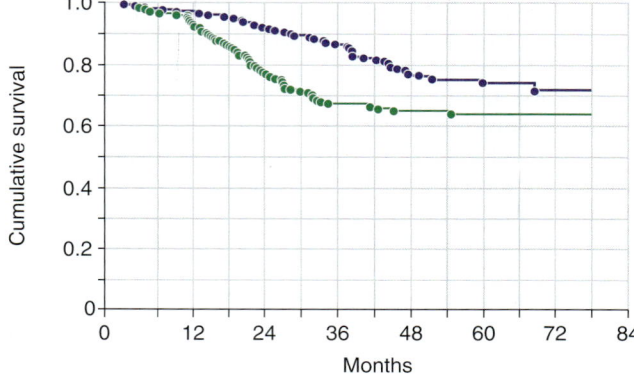

Figure 51-11. Overall and event-free survival in extremity osteosarcoma treated with aggressive chemotherapy. (With permission, Figure 1, Ferrari S, Smeland S, Mercuri M, et al: Neoadjuvant chemotherapy with high-dose ifosfamide, high-dose methotrexate, cisplatin, and doxorubicin for patients with localized osteosarcoma of the extremity: a joint study by the Italian and Scandinavian Sarcoma Groups. J Clin Oncol 23:8845–8852, 2005.)

Reconstructive options for patients with osteosarcoma are as outlined earlier. Large extraosseous soft tissue masses frequently require extensive muscle and bony resection to achieve a wide margin. Margin and tumor necrosis closely correlate with risk of recurrence (which in turn correlates with survival), emphasizing the need to aggressively resect these malignancies.[44] After curative treatment, the risk of developing a second malignancy is greater than 3% at 10 years.[45]

Chondrosarcoma

Chondrosarcoma, the second most common primary bone sarcoma, is frequently seen in the hip and pelvis region. Of 895 chondrosarcomas reported by Dahlin and Unni, 99 arose in the proximal femur and 191 in the adjacent pelvis.[46,47] Chondrosarcomas arise in middle-aged patients as compared with osteogenic or Ewing's sarcoma. Most tumors are slow growing and present with a long history of local or referred pain. Radiographic interpretation can be hampered by overlying bowel gas for pelvic lesions. However, cortical thickening, scalloping, and matrix mineralization are common findings in chondrosarcoma. Axial imaging is often needed to adequately visualize these lesions, particularly in the pelvis/acetabulum. Images should be carefully scrutinized for any areas of dedifferentiation, where a high-grade neoplasm develops within a lower-grade chondrosarcoma.

No effective treatments for chondrosarcoma other than surgery are known. The role of chemotherapy for the rare dedifferentiated lesion is controversial.[48] Select low-grade femoral lesions can be treated with intralesional removal and use of local adjuvants (Fig. 51-12).[49] This should not be performed in the pelvis, as local recurrence is universal following intralesional procedures here.[50] Additionally, chondrosarcomas (particularly higher-grade lesions) are very implantable tumors; careful planning from biopsy to resection and reconstruction is required for oncologic cure. Biopsy tracts should be excised at the time of treatment. If intralesional resection is done for low-grade extremity lesions, towels or drapes should protect adjacent soft tissue from contamination during tumor removal. A

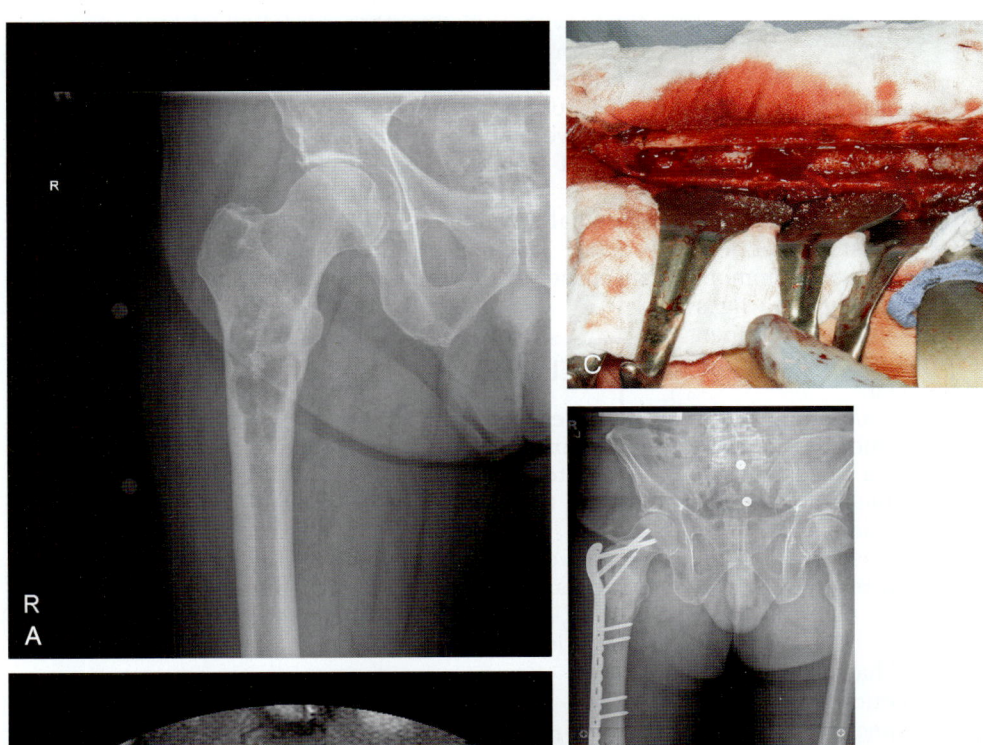

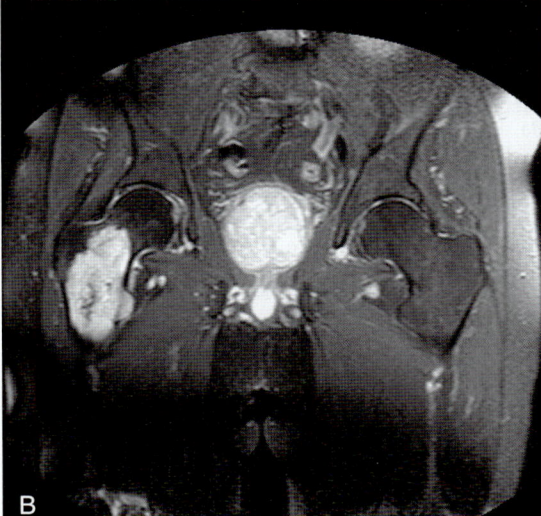

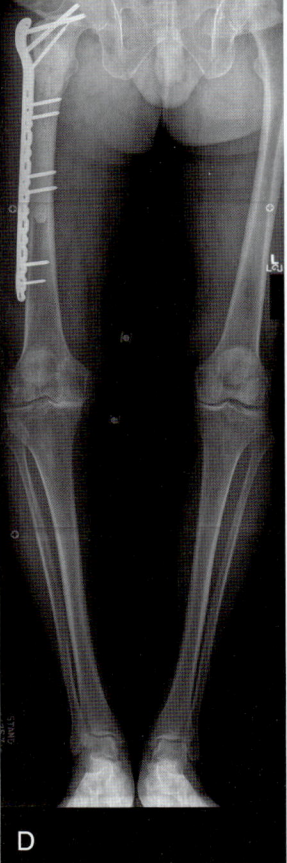

Figure 51-12. Intralesional treatment of a low-grade chondrosarcoma. **A,** Presenting radiograph of a grade I chondrosarcoma. **B,** T2-weighted magnetic resonance imaging (MRI). **C,** Tumor is curettaged, burred, and treated with phenol. Note protection of soft tissues from contamination. **D,** Methylmethacrylate and plate reconstruction provide immediate stability and facilitate detection of any future tumor recurrence.

separate setup is used for tumor removal and reconstruction instruments to prevent contamination.

Intermediate- or higher-grade femoral lesions and all pelvic lesions should be treated with wide resection. Our group treats all pelvic cartilaginous tumors as malignant (e.g., we do not recognize the existence of pelvic enchondromas). Local recurrence and survival correlate with margin status in these patients.[51-53] Overall survival is heavily influenced by grade and pelvic location; survival over 90% is seen with low-grade lesions, but survival falls to ≈25% for high-grade tumors.[54] Extensive soft tissue masses may be present but are not as common as those seen in osteogenic or Ewing's sarcoma.

Ewing's Sarcoma

Ewing's sarcoma is an aggressive tumor of children and young adults. Approximately 25% of Ewing's tumors arise in the vicinity of the hip joint. Patients may present with constitutional symptoms including fever and elevated erythrocyte sedimentation rate that mimic infection. Radiographs show extensive periosteal reaction, and large extraosseous soft tissue masses are common. Bone marrow biopsy is used in the staging of Ewing's sarcoma, so if this diagnosis is suspected and an open biopsy is being performed, the surgeon should be prepared to perform this procedure as well.

Standard treatment for Ewing's sarcoma consists of neoadjuvant chemotherapy, surgery and/or radiation therapy to achieve local control, and then further chemotherapy. Agents include doxorubicin, ifosfamide, etoposide, vincristine, actinomycin D, and cyclophosphamide. Survival is similar to osteosarcoma with modern treatments. Tumor necrosis in resected specimens is predictive of outcome, as it is in osteosarcoma patients.[44]

No prospective randomized trials have compared radiation therapy versus surgical resection in the management of Ewing's sarcoma. Retrospective comparisons of the two modalities usually are poorly matched and underpowered. However, the clinical experience at Mayo Clinic Rochester favors resection whenever possible. Local recurrence appears to be less in patients treated surgically.[7,8] As well, radiation therapy is associated with significant long-term morbidity.[9] Radiation may be used as an adjunct to surgical resection in cases of close margins at critical structures. If it is anticipated that radiation may be employed, reconstruction is best performed with a cemented endoprosthesis. Very young patients may be treated initially with radiation in the knowledge that if they survive, they will ultimately require some form of orthopedic intervention for the limb.

Malignant Soft Tissue Tumors

A large number of histologies are incorporated in the category of malignant soft tissue tumors. Common examples include liposarcoma, synovial sarcoma, leiomyosarcoma, malignant peripheral nerve sheath tumor, and pleomorphic spindle cell sarcoma. Malignant fibrous histiocytoma (MFH) used to be the most frequently diagnosed soft tissue sarcoma. However, recent advances in tumor subtyping have caused this diagnosis to be abandoned as a discrete entity. Most tumors previously termed *MFH* now fall under the category of undifferentiated pleomorphic spindle cell sarcoma.

From a practical surgical standpoint, malignant soft tissue tumors are treated similarly, with wide excision (see Fig. 51-3). Adjuvant radiation therapy is employed to decrease the risk of local recurrence. As discussed earlier, radiation may be given preoperatively or postoperatively with benefits derived from each approach. Our practice is to treat soft tissue sarcoma preoperatively with radiation therapy followed by wide resection. An intraoperative boost dose can be used to help sterilize close margins.

The use of chemotherapy in soft tissue sarcoma is controversial with current protocols under study. Current evidence and experience suggest that benefit may be derived from chemotherapy in patients with synovial sarcoma and potentially large high-grade sarcomas. The use of such therapy should be carefully discussed with an experienced sarcoma oncologist.[12,13]

CONCLUSIONS

Treatment of primary sarcomas about the hip is a complex but rewarding aspect of orthopedic surgery. Accurate diagnosis and staging are required before proper treatment can be initiated. Wide resection of tumors is necessary for cure, and a variety of reconstructive options can be individualized for particular patients. A close partnership and teamwork between patient, surgeon, and radiation and medical oncologists are critical for success.

REFERENCES

1. Messerschmidt PJ, Garcia RM, Abdul-Karim FW, et al: Osteosarcoma. J Am Acad Orthop Surg 17:515–527, 2009.
2. Schwabb JH, Boland PJ, Antonescu C, et al: Spinal metastases from myxoid liposarcoma warrant screening with magnetic resonance imaging. Cancer 110:1815–1822, 2007.
3. Mitsuyoshi G, Naito N, Kawai A, et al: Accurate diagnosis of musculoskeletal lesions by core needle biopsy. J Surg Oncol 94:21–27, 2006.
4. Mankin HJ, Mankin CJ, Simon MA: The hazards of biopsy revisited: members of the Musculoskeletal Tumor Society. J Bone Joint Surg Am 78:656–663, 1996.
5. Bernstein M, Kovar H, Paulussen M, et al: Ewing's sarcoma family of tumors: current management. Oncologist 11:503–519, 2006.
6. Goorin AM, Schwartzentruber DJ, Devidas M, et al: Presurgical chemotherapy compared with immediate surgery and adjuvant chemotherapy for nonmetastatic osteosarcoma: Pediatric Oncology Group Study POG-8651. J Clin Oncol 15:1574–1580, 2003.
7. Donati D, Yin J, Di Bella C, et al: Local and distant control in non-metastatic pelvic Ewing's sarcoma patients. J Surg Oncol 96:19–25, 2007.
8. Toni A, Neff JR, Sudanese A, et al: The role of surgical therapy in patients with nonmetastatic Ewing's sarcoma of the limbs. Clin Orthop Relat Res 286:225–240, 1993.
9. Fuchs B, Valenzuela RG, Inwards C, et al: Complications in long term survivors of Ewing sarcoma. Cancer 98:2687–2692, 2003.

10. O'Sullivan B, Davis AM, Turvotte R, et al: Preoperative versus postoperative radiotherapy in soft-tissue sarcoma of the limbs: a randomized trial. Lancet 359:2235–2241, 2002.

11. Davis AM, O'Sullivan B, Turcotte R, et al: Late radiation morbidity following randomization to preoperative versus postoperative radiotherapy in extremity soft tissue sarcoma. Radiother Oncol 75:48–53, 2005.

12. Sarcoma Meta-analysis Collaboration: Adjuvant chemotherapy for localized resectable soft-tissue sarcoma of adults: meta-analysis of individual data. Lancet 350:1647–1654, 1997.

13. Schlieman M, Smith R, Kraybill WG: Adjuvant therapy for extremity sarcomas. Curr Treat Options Oncol 7:456–463, 2006.

14. Holt GE, Griffin AM, Pintilie M, et al: Fractures following radiotherapy and limb salvage surgery for lower extremity soft-tissue sarcomas: a comparison of high-dose and low-dose radiotherapy. J Bone Joint Surg Am 87:315–319, 2005.

15. Imran H, Enders F, Krailo M, et al: Effect of time to resumption of chemotherapy after definitive surgery on prognosis for non-metastatic osteosarcoma. J Bone Joint Surg Am 91:604–612, 2009.

16. Nathan SS, Simmons KA, Lin PP, et al: Proximal deep vein thrombosis after hip replacement for oncologic indications. J Bone Joint Surg Am 88:1066–1070, 2006.

17. Morris CD, Sepkowitz K, Fonshell C, et al: Prospective identification of risk factors for wound infection after lower extremity oncologic surgery. Ann Surg Oncol 10:778–782, 2003.

18. Jeys L, Luscombe JS, Grimer RJ, et al: The risks and benefits of radiotherapy with massive endoprosthetic replacement. J Bone Joint Surg Br 89:1352–1355, 2007.

19. Webb LA: New techniques in wound management: vacuum assisted wound closure. J Am Acad Orthop Surg 10:303–311, 2002.

20. Ghert MA, Davis AM, Griffin AM, et al: The surgical and functional outcome of limb-salvage surgery with vascular reconstruction for soft tissue sarcoma of the extremity. Ann Surg Oncol 12:1102–1110, 2005.

21. Fuchs B, Davis AM, Wunder JS, et al: Sciatic nerve resection in the thigh: a functional evaluation. Clin Orthop Relat Res 382:34–41, 2001.

22. Vander Griend RA: The effect of internal fixation on the healing of large allografts. J Bone Joint Surg Am 76:657–663, 1994.

23. Friedrich JB, Moral SL, Bishop AT, et al: Free vascularized fibula graft salvage of complications of long-bone allograft after tumor reconstruction. J Bone Joint Surg Am 90:93–100, 2008.

24. Mankin HJ, Hornicek FJ, Raskin KA: Infection in massive bone allografts. Clin Orthop Relat Res 432:210–216, 2005.

25. Sorger JI, Hornicek FJ, Zavatta M, et al: Allograft fractures revisited. Clin Orthop Relat Res 382:66–74, 2001.

26. Jeys LM, Kulkarni A, Grimer RJ, et al: Endoprosthetic reconstruction for treatment of musculoskeletal tumors of the appendicular skeleton and pelvis. J Bone Joint Surg Am 90:1265–1271, 2008.

27. Potter BK, Chow VE, Adams SC, et al: Endoprosthetic proximal femur replacement: metastatic versus primary tumors. Surg Oncol 18:343–349, 2009.

28. Zehr RJ, Enneking WF, Scarborough MT: Allograft prosthesis composite versus megaprosthesis in proximal femoral reconstruction. Clin Orthop Relat Res 322:207–223, 1996.

29. Langlais F, Lambiotte JC, Collin P, Thomazeau H: Long-term results of allograft composite total hip prostheses for tumors. Clin Orthop Relat Res 414:197–211, 2003.

30. Donati D, Giacomini S Gozzi E, Mercuri M: Proximal femur reconstruction by an allograft prosthesis composite. Clin Orthop Relat Res 394:192–200, 2002.

31. O'Connor MI, Sim FH: Salvage of the limb in the treatment of malignant pelvic tumors. J Bone Joint Surg Am 71:481–494, 1989.

32. Schwartz AJ, Kiatisevi P, Eilber FC, et al: The Friedman-Eilber resection arthroplasty of the pelvis. Clin Orthop Relat Res 467:2825–2830, 2009.

33. Aljassir F, Deadel GP, Turcotte RE, et al: Outcome after pelvic resection reconstructed with saddle prosthesis. Clin Orthop Relat Res 438:36–41, 2005.

34. Beadel GP, McLaughlin CE, Wunder JS, et al: Outcome of two groups of patients with allograft-prosthetic reconstruction of pelvic tumor defects. Clin Orthop Relat Res 438:30–35, 2005.

35. Rose PS, Halasy M, Trousdale RT, et al: Preliminary results of tantalum acetabular components for THA after pelvic radiation. Clin Orthop Relat Res 453:195–198, 2006.

36. Khan FA, Rose PS, Sim FH, Lewallen DG: Acetabular reconstruction with porous tantalum implants in patients with periacetabular bone tumors. Paper presented at the International Society of Limb Salvage/Musculoskeletal Tumor Society Combined Meeting, Boston, Mass, September 2009.

37. Jeys LM, Grimer RJ, Carter SR, Tillman RM: Periprosthetic infection in patients treated for an orthopaedic oncological condition. J Bone Joint Surg Am 87:842–849, 2005.

38. Arkader A, Viola DC, Morris CD, et al: Coaxial extendible knee equalizes limb length in children with osteogenic sarcoma. Clin Orthop Relat Res 459:60–65, 2007.

39. Neel MD, Wilkins RM, Rao BN, Kelly CM: Early experience with a noninvasive expandable prosthesis. Clin Orthop Relat Res 415:42–81, 2003.

40. Manoso MW, Boland PJ, Healey JH, et al: Acetabular development after bipolar hemiarthroplasty for osteosarcoma in children. J Bone Joint Surg Br 87:1658–1662, 2005.

41. Bacci G, Longhi A, Versari M, et al: Prognostic factors for osteosarcoma of the extremity treated with neoadjuvant chemotherapy: 15 year experience in 789 patients treated at a single institution. Cancer 106:1154–1161, 2006.

42. Ferrari S, Smeland S, Mercuri M, et al: Neoadjuvant chemotherapy with high-dose ifosfamide, high-dose methotrexate, cisplatin, and doxorubicin for patients with localized osteosarcoma of the extremity: a joint study by the Italian and Scandinavian Sarcoma Groups. J Clin Oncol 23:8845–8852, 2005.

43. Meyers PA, Heller G, Healey J, et al: Chemotherapy for non-metastatic osteosarcoma: the Memorial Sloan-Kettering experience. J Clin Oncol 10:5–15, 1992.

44. Picci P, Rougraff B, Bacci G, et al: Prognostic significance of histopathologic response to chemotherapy in nonmetastatic Ewing's sarcoma of the extremities. J Clin Oncol 11:1763–1769, 1993.

45. Aung L, Gorlick RG, Shi W, et al: Second malignant neoplasms in long-term survivors of osteosarcoma: the Memorial Sloan-Kettering Cancer Center experience. Cancer 95:1728–1734, 2002.

46. Pritchard DJ, Lunke RJ, Taylor WF, et al: Chondrosarcoma: a clinicopathologic and statistical analysis. Cancer 45:149, 1980.

47. Unni KK: Dahlin's bone tumors: general aspects and data on 11,087 cases, Springfield, Ill, 1996, Charles C Thomas, p 227.

48. Dickey ID, Rose PS, Fuchs B, et al: Dedifferentiated chondrosarcoma: the role of chemotherapy with updated outcomes. J Bone Joint Surg Am 86:2412–2418, 2004.

49. Leerapun T, Hugate RR, Inwards CY, et al: Surgical management of conventional grade I chondrosarcoma of long bones. Clin Orthop Relat Res 463:166–172, 2007.

50. Streitburger A, Ahrens H, Balke M, et al: Grade I chondrosarcoma : the Munster experience. J Cancer Res Clin Oncol 135:543–550, 2009.

51. Pring ME, Weber KL, Unni KK, Sim FH: Chondrosarcoma of the pelvis: a review of 64 cases. J Bone Joint Surg Am 83:1630–1642, 2001.

52. Schwab J, Wenger D, Unni K, Sim F: Does local recurrence impact survival in low-grade chondrosarcoma of the long bones? Clin Orthop Relat Res 462:175–180, 2007.

53. Weber KL, Pring ME, Sim FH: Treatment and outcome of recurrent pelvic chondrosarcoma. Clin Orthop Relat Res 397:19–28, 2002.

54. Lee FY, Mankin HJ, Fondren G, et al: Chondrosarcoma of bone: an assessment of outcome. J Bone Joint Surg Am 81:326–338, 1999.

CHAPTER 52

Metastatic Disease Around the Hip

Joseph H. Schwab and Francis J. Hornicek

KEY POINTS

- Metastatic bone disease is a relatively common problem that will become more common as the population ages.
- Pain and loss of mobility as a result of bone metastasis can severely impair a patient's quality of life.
- The treatment of bone metastasis is a multidisciplinary endeavor, and treatment decisions should be made collectively.
- Surgery is often an integral part of the palliation of metastatic bone disease.
- The goal of surgery should be to allow immediate weight bearing.
- The scope of bone metastasis dwarfs that of primary bone tumors, of which fewer than 2000 are diagnosed each year.

INTRODUCTION

More than 1.5 million new cases of cancer will be diagnosed this year in the United States. It is estimated that 562,340 people will die from cancer in the United States in 2009.[1] Lung, breast, and prostate cancers are the three most common forms of cancer; all three commonly spread to bone. Renal and thyroid carcinomas are also known to be osteophilic. Jaffe reported a 90% incidence of bone metastasis during autopsy of patients who succumbed to osteophilic tumor.[2] Furthermore, the incidence of bone metastasis is expected to increase as the population ages. Although management of primary bone tumors is generally reserved for those specifically trained in orthopedic oncology, the sheer volume of bone metastasis mandates that all orthopedic surgeons should be aware of the principles of management. The purpose of this chapter is to introduce the reader to current concepts in the management of patients with metastasis about the hip joint. The management of bone metastasis is a multidisciplinary endeavor; therefore, nonsurgical management will also be discussed.

EPIDEMIOLOGY AND RISK FACTORS

It is estimated that more than 14 million people worldwide are suffering from cancer, and that 70% to 90% of those with late-stage disease have significant pain.[3]

Bone metastasis contributes significantly to the prevalence of pain in this patient population. The axial and appendicular skeletons are the most common sites of metastatic disease. A report on more than 300 cases of bone metastasis stated that bones in and around the hip joint are involved in 66% of cases.[4] Similarly, Galasko and associates found the pelvis to be involved in 66% of cases and the femur in more than half of cases of metastatic breast carcinoma.[5]

Paget was the first to popularize the concept that some tumors have a predilection for spreading to bone. At the time, competing views were put forth on how and where secondary cancers occurred. One popular theory of the time was that cells spread to other organs via the blood and became trapped in their parenchyma vis à vis an embolism. This theory was supported by Virchow, who believed that embolism was a critical means by which secondary cancers occurred. Paget disagreed with this view and mentioned the work of Langenbech, who thought that each embolic cell should be considered as a separate living entity. Further, he credited Fuchs, who noted that some organs were "predisposed" to secondary cancer. Paget stated, "When a plant goes to seed, its seeds are carried in all directions; but they can only live and grow if they fall on congenial soil." He noted that breast and thyroid cancers have a predilection to spread to bone that cannot be explained by embolic theory alone.[6]

Subsequent studies have confirmed that some cancers spread to bone more frequently than others. Abrams and associates described their autopsy findings in 167 cases of breast cancer in which 73% of cases had bony involvement.[7] The same report found that 32% of lung and 24% of renal cell patients had bony metastases at autopsy.[7] Prostate cancer is well known to spread to the skeleton. When one is considering risk factors for metastatic disease to bone, the most likely tissues of origin include lung, breast, prostate, thyroid, and renal cell. Patients with a history of these malignancies are at higher risk for developing bony disease. Multiple myeloma should also be considered, because it is the most primary tumor in bone.

PATHOPHYSIOLOGY

Although the location and speed with which tumors metastasize to other sites vary considerably, all tumor cells generally must clear five hurdles before they can grow in a different organ: cancer initiation, local invasion, circulation, infiltration, and colonization. Some cancers pass through these stages rapidly (such as non–small cell lung cancer, in which metastasis has often occurred by the time the primary tumor is detected).[8] Others, such as breast and prostate, pass through these stages more slowly. Indeed distant spread may not be detected for years after the primary tumor has been detected and treated.[9] In addition to the speed with which cancers spread, the location to which they spread is unique. Although breast commonly spreads to bone, it also commonly spreads to the liver and lungs. Prostate cancer, in contrast, generally spreads to the bones only late in the course of dissemination.[10]

Cancer initiation requires the cancer cells to grow in a heterogeneous way.[11] For cancer cells to grow, they must be able to circumvent normal anatomic constraints that ordinarily would keep order. For instance, they must be able to break through the basement membrane and grow locally. This exposes cells to selective pressures that each cell must overcome. For instance, if a tumor is growing locally, it may outgrow its blood supply and then is exposed to a hypoxic environment. Some cells will not be able to grow in these conditions, and other cells adapt to the conditions by producing hypoxia-inducible factor. This triggers a series of events that allow the cell to grow and even thrive in this new hypoxic environment. This is an example of how cells might be "selected" to grow in an otherwise hostile environment. A key component of this concept is that cells within a colony are heterogeneous. Cells must display genomic instability for the heterogeneity to persist. So the progeny of the original aberrant cell may look very different genetically from that of its sister cells from the same original cell. If all cells in a colony were similar, then "selection" could not occur, because survival would be an all or none phenomenon.[11]

After cancer begins, cells must be able to break through their local basement membrane and grow into their local extracellular matrix. As mentioned, hypoxia is one environmental stress to which cancer cells may be exposed. Hypoxia stimulates, among other things, cancer cells to develop their own vascular supply. Some genes are known to be important in this stage of cancer development, including *VEGF, MMP-9,* and *MMP-1*.[11] Another important component of this stage of cancer development is known as *epithelial-to-mesenchymal transition*.[12,13] Epithelial cells generally respect the basement membrane as a boundary, and they have polarity that reflects their orientation to the membrane. Mesenchymal cells do not have the same polarity, nor do they respect the basement membrane as a barrier. One can see how this sort of transition would be favorable for the growth and spread of carcinoma.[12,13]

Once cancer cells have mastered their local environment, they must be able to enter the circulatory system and survive. At this point, it may seem only a matter of semantics whether metastasis has occurred or not. However, simply entering the circulation is no guarantee that metastasis will follow. Animal models have shown that less than 0.01% of circulation tumor cells form metastasis.[14] The circulatory system exposes cells to new stresses that they must overcome, including turbulent flow and circulation immune cells. If cells survive here, they must still be able to traverse the endothelium of a new organ site. Once there, they must be able to grow into and through a new organ with distinct extracellular conditions. One can imagine that the extracellular environment in the breast is very different from that found in bone.

Why then do some tumors spread to bone, whereas others do not? This question and the concepts leading up to it are areas of active research. The spine is the most common site of osseous metastasis; Batson proposed that the valveless venous system surrounding the spine was the primary reason for the higher number of bone metastases in the spine.[15] This is akin to the embolic theory of metastasis, which Paget had argued was an insufficient explanation for the predilection of some cancers to certain organs.[6] Although most researchers agree that embolism and anatomy are secondary to genetic components of metastasis, important anatomic considerations should be kept in mind. Bone marrow sinusoids (capillaries) contain fenestrations that allow the ingress and egress of hematopoietic cells.[16] This may contribute to how cancer cells enter the bone.

Entering the bone marrow is not sufficient for macrometastasis to occur. Tumor cells must be able to live and grow within the extracellular matrix of bone. This necessarily requires the breakdown of bone, which is a task that only osteoclasts can accomplish. Some cancer cells produce factors that directly activate osteoclasts (parathyroid-related peptide [PTHrP], interleukin [IL]-11, IL-6), granulocyte macrophage colony-stimulating factor (GM-CSF), and tumor necrosis factor-alpha (TNF-α).[17-20] GM-CSF directly stimulates osteoclastogenesis. PTHrP, IL-11, IL-6, and TNF-α all stimulate osteoblasts to produce receptor activator of nuclear factor-κB ligand (RANKL), which stimulates osteoclast formation. Expression of cytokines that stimulate osteoclasts may not be unique to cancers that enter the bone marrow sinusoids; however, their production may offer a survival advantage only in areas rich in osteoclasts. Therefore, these cells are selected to grow in bone, rather than other cells that may accompany them into the marrow. These same cells may not thrive in the liver or lung, where other cytokines offer a survival advantage.

The contribution of the molecular mechanisms behind metastasis is clear. However, the vascular contribution to metastasis still has merit. The valveless venous system surrounding the axial skeleton and parts of the pelvis are subject to stagnation, particularly during episodes of increased intra-abdominal pressure, such as during Valsalva.[15] Additionally, larger bones have more area in which metastatic cells can accumulate and a corresponding larger blood supply, delivering more cells.

When one considers the pathophysiology of metastatic bone disease, the gross biomechanical properties of metastatic lesions must be considered. When a lesion is seen on plain radiographs, the biomechanical properties of the affected bone are not equivalent to those of normal pre-metastatic bone. This is clear, but how much does the lesion affect the structural quality of the bone? Hipp and colleagues determined that both lytic and blastic metastases weaken bone, but lytic lesions weaken bone to a greater extent. Lytic lesions have a greater impact on the strength and stiffness of bone through their disruption of mineral, organic, and structural components of bone. Blastic lesions disrupt the trabecular framework of bone; this is detrimental to overall stiffness and fatigue properties, while sparing bone strength.[21] Lytic lesions in the cortex force an accumulation of stress in the bone surrounding the lesion. This so-called *stress riser* can lead to a fracture. A lesion that measures 20% of the overall bone diameter decreases the bending strength of bone by 40%.[22] However, even small cortical disruptions can significantly decrease the structural integrity of bone. One biomechanical study evaluated the energy-absorbing capacity of bone after drill holes were made in the femoral shaft. The holes measured between 2.8 mm and 3.6 mm, which is roughly ⅛ of an inch. Such lesions reduced the energy-absorbing capacity of bone by 55%, leading to torsion-type fractures.[23] An "open section" defect describes the situation in which the size of a lesion is greater than the diameter of the bone. This defect reduces bending strength by 90%. However, the femur is most likely to break when a torsional load is applied, as when a patient pivots when rising from a chair.[22]

CLINICAL FEATURES AND DIAGNOSIS

Pain is the most important and most common symptom of bony metastasis. It is the most feared complication of cancer in general, and most people perceive that death from cancer will be painful. Nearly 70% of cancer patients report that severe pain may lead them to consider suicide.[24-26] In spite of this, cancer pain was reported to be undertreated by 86% of cancer physicians.[27] The orthopedic surgeon has a vital role to play in the management of cancer pain.

Prostaglandins and osteoclast-activating factors sensitize nociceptors and produce hyperalgesia and pain during osteolysis.[28] This can produce pain even when the structural integrity of bone remains relatively intact. Patients often complain of a deep aching pain that often prevents them from sleeping. A key part of the history with regard to this pain is that it troubles them even when they are lying down. This is different from pain that occurs only when the patient is ambulating or bearing weight. Pain that is relieved by rest is more likely related to a structural problem and is termed *functional* or *mechanical pain.* It is very important to distinguish these two presentations. The first may respond to systemic therapy or radiation therapy, whereas the second will not likely respond to either.

Pain about the hip may be referred from the spine. An L1 compression fracture may compress the exiting nerve roots, causing referred pain to the hip/groin area (Fig. 52-1). Alternatively, knee pain can be the only

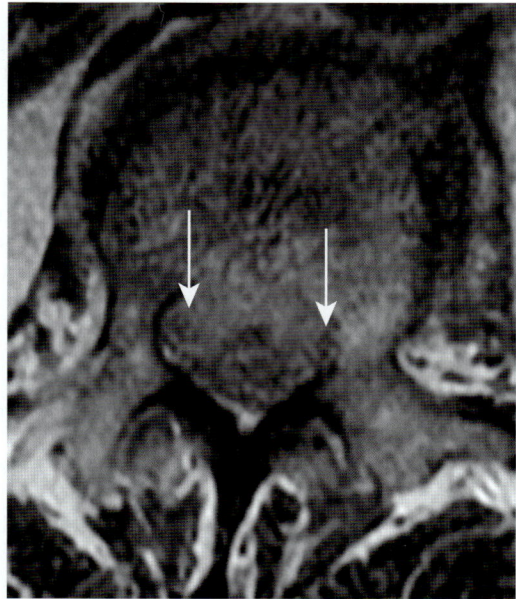

Figure 52-1. This sagittal, T2-weighted magnetic resonance image (MRI) was taken from a patient who described bilateral groin pain. Images of her hips were negative. This pathologic fracture at L1 was causing compression of her exiting nerve roots. Subsequent biopsy revealed metastatic carcinoma.

manifestation of hip pathology. In general, acetabular, femoral head, and neck and pubic rami pathology will manifest as groin pain. Gentle rotation of the femoral head may help distinguish intracapsular pathology from pubic rami pathology. Tenderness over the pubic ramus can also help distinguish these areas. As with other types of hip pain, patients may demonstrate a Trendelenburg gait as they try to unload their hip joint. Groin pain with straight-leg raise or pain with passive rotation of the hip may indicate hip pathology.

It is important to assess the patient's ability to ambulate. It is one of the key features that determine prognosis and treatment options. The inability to ambulate may prevent patients from being considered for systemic therapy or clinical trials. Ambulation is used as a surrogate for overall function. It is important for the orthopedist to help determine whether the patient's functional capacity is the problem, or whether his/her inability to ambulate is amenable to surgery.

Hypercalcemia of malignancy is the most common paraneoplastic condition in patients with cancer.[29] It has been reported to occur in nearly half of patients with metastatic breast carcinoma to bone.[30,31] Dehydration is a common problem in patients treated with chemotherapy for metastatic disease. This can exacerbate an underlying hypercalcemia. Increased serum levels of calcium can occur from robust osteoclastic resorption, which is seen with widely metastatic bone disease. Some carcinomas express PTHrP, which causes hypercalcemia as a result of secondary hyperparathyroidism. Patients with hypercalcemia can become lethargic, fatigued, and anorexic. Patients may become comatose and/or may develop cardiac arrhythmia if left untreated.[32]

Initial management of such patients consists of fluid resuscitation with normal saline. Thiazide diuretics should be stopped because they foster calcium retention. Once the patient has been adequately hydrated, a loop diuretic may be given because it helps clear calcium via the urine.[33] In addition, bisphosphonates have been approved for the treatment of hypercalcemia.

Plain radiographs are an important part of the assessment of any bony pain. This is particularly true in patients suspected of having metastatic disease. Lytic or sclerotic lesions are often detected with plain radiographs. However, a normal x-ray does not completely rule out a metastatic focus in that 30% to 50% of bone must be destroyed before it is detected on plain radiographs. Judet views of the pelvis should also be included in the workup of hip pain in patients suspected of metastatic disease, because they provide useful information regarding the anterior and posterior column. If surgery of the hip is planned, then full-length femur x-rays are mandated. It is important to not miss a subclinical lesion in the femur. If such a lesion is not sought, then a short-stemmed prosthesis may be inadvertently placed just above it. If this lesion later fractures, reconstruction becomes more complex owing to the previously placed prosthesis.

When a lesion is detected, the treating physician should ask two questions. Is this lesion primary or metastatic? If this lesion is metastatic, are other lesions present? Bone scintigraphy is the imaging modality best suited to answer this second question.[34] Bone scans allow the activity of osteoblasts to be tracked. The radiolabeled diphosphate is taken up by osteoblasts and deposited into hydroxyapatite. Those areas of the skeleton in which osteoblasts are more active will lay down more radioactive tracer, which will be detected in the displayed images. A positive bone scan must be followed by plain radiography because a positive scan is not specific. In addition, a negative bone scan does not necessarily rule out metastasis. Myeloma is notorious for being negative on bone scans owing to its failure to elicit an osteoblastic response. This is likely related to the ability of myeloma to stimulate the expression of RANKL by cells other than osteoblasts.[35,36]

Radiographs serve as the mainstay for surgical evaluation of metastatic bone disease. However, if radiographs are equivocal, computed tomography is the best modality to further characterize the structural integrity of the bone. It is particularly useful about the hip because it provides useful information about the dome of the acetabulum and the quality of the anterior and posterior column.[37] It will also allow better visualization of subtle fractures.

Magnetic resonance imaging (MRI) is another modality that has a place in the analysis of metastatic disease. MRI is most commonly employed for spinal lesions, in which the ability to view marrow infiltration and nervous structures is useful. MRI may be used to detect tumor infiltration of bone marrow (and avoid a biopsy) in a patient with a positive bone scan but normal radiographic and/or computed tomography (CT) imaging. It is also useful in cases of occult fracture when a CT is

negative.[38] However, in cases of known metastatic disease, plain radiographs and CT are often better tests, in that they provide actionable information in a cost-effective and time-efficient manner. For example, if a patient has known metastasis to the bones and has pain in the femur, it is best to order plain radiographs first. CT scan will provide further information about the structural quality of the bone if the situation remains unclear, and the additional information will influence the decision for surgery. MRI may show marrow disease that is not detected on plain x-ray or CT, but the presence of marrow disease is not particularly helpful in a patient with known metastasis.

When surgery is planned for patients with particularly vascular tumors such as thyroid, renal, and hepatocellular carcinoma, arteriography and embolization is considered to prevent excessive blood loss if the lesion is to be entered at the time of surgery. If wide resection is planned (e.g., a proximal femur metastatic renal cell lesion), embolization may not be necessary.

The decision to proceed with surgery is predicated on the need to treat a fracture or prevent an impending fracture. Predicting which lesions will lead to a fracture is not always easy. Several studies provide useful parameters that one can use as a guide. Lytic disease involving more than 2.5 cm of the femoral cortex has been identified as a means to predict impending fracture in the femur.[39] Subsequent studies have used painful lesions eroding more than 50% of the femoral diameter as a benchmark for surgery.[40] This criterion was later changed to include painful lesions involving more than 30% of the femoral diameter that have failed radiation treatment.[41] Another study added painful lesions involving the subtrochanteric region as at high risk for fracture.[42] However, one of the largest studies evaluating more than 516 lesions in 203 patients with metastatic breast cancer could not correlate pain or lesion size with fracture risk.[43] In addition, a biomechanical study failed to demonstrate a strong correlation between prediction of fracture risk based on interpretation of plain radiography and CT with actual mechanical strength of bone.[44] A follow-up study from the same group found that bone mineral content as assessed by dual energy x-ray absorptiometry (DEXA) could be useful in predicting failure in patients with lytic lesions.[45] Subsequent studies have demonstrated that quantitative computed tomography may be useful in predicting fractures.[46]

In 1989 Mirel proposed a scoring system to predict impending fracture based on four criteria, including lesion location, size (relative to the diameter of the shaft), pain, and radiographic appearance[47] (Table 52-1). Mirel's criteria have since become the most common framework for evaluation of patients with metastatic skeletal disease. Scores can range from 4 to 12. Higher scores predicting fracture were given to lesions about the hip (peritrochanteric), lesions involving more than $\frac{2}{3}$ the diameter of the bone, lytic lesions, and painful lesions. Two groups emerged from this study. One group, which did not have a fracture, had a mean score of 7; the other group, which did have a fracture, had a mean score of 10. Significant overlap was noted between the two groups. One third of patients who developed a

Table 52-1. The Mirel Scoring System

Variable	1	2	3
Site	Upper limb	Lower limb	Peritrochanteric
Pain	Mild	Moderate	Severe
Lesion	Blastic	Mixed	Lytic
Size	< ⅓	⅓ - ⅔	> ⅔

Adapted from Mirels H: Metastatic disease in long bones: a proposed scoring system for diagnosing impending pathologic fractures. Clin Orthop Relat Res 249:256, 1989.

fracture had a score below 10. The criteria proposed in this study serve as a useful starting point when one is considering a metastatic lesion; however, there are no fully validated criteria on which one can completely base one's decision. Although means of quantifying fracture risk are improving, a pragmatic approach balancing anticipated load on the hip relative to its load-bearing capacity must be kept in mind. Each patient must be evaluated with this concept in mind, and quantitative assessments must be used as an adjuvant to one's clinical acumen.

DIFFERENTIAL DIAGNOSIS

It is important to keep in mind that noncancerous causes of hip pain may be at hand, and they should be considered. Many patients are immunocompromised and are prone to joint sepsis and zoster infection. Many chemotherapeutic regimens include dexamethasone. The use of steroids is associated with osteonecrosis, and osteonecrosis should be on the differential as well. Osteoporosis is a major problem in cancer patients, and insufficiency fractures should be kept in mind. Although bisphosphonates are used to help prevent insufficiency fractures, they have been associated with subtrochanteric fractures as well.[48,49]

TREATMENT

Radiation

Radiation therapy is standard treatment for bony metastasis. The goals of radiation are pain relief and local tumor control. It should be the considered as first-line treatment in bony metastasis without impending fracture. Adjuvant radiation is also standard after surgical reconstruction to help minimize the risk of local tumor recurrence and construct failure.

Radiation therapy achieves partial pain relief in 80% to 90% of patients, and it achieves complete pain relief in 50% to 85%.[50,51] Breast and prostate seem to have a better response than other histologic subtypes. Doses greater than 4000 cGy delivered in multiple fractions seem to be most efficacious.[52,53]

Once a fracture has occurred about the hip, radiation is most commonly used as an adjuvant following surgical stabilization. A study of pathologic fracture in rats demonstrated that fractures treated with 2000 cGy of radiation would not heal unless they were rigidly immobilized.[54] Rigid internal fixation demonstrates higher union rates than external immobilization. Primary bone healing seems to be less sensitive to the detrimental effects of radiation than is secondary bone healing. One explanation for this is that secondary bony healing must go through a phase of hyaline cartilage formation. Cartilage growth is stymied by radiation.[55] In clinical practice, bone healing is dependent on tumor histology, adjuvant treatments, local tumor burden, and other factors that make it unreliable. Except in rare circumstances, surgical treatment of pathologic fractures should be carried out in a manner that provides predictable function without the need for osseous union. This leads to frequent arthroplasty procedures and liberal use of bone cement to augment rod (or more rarely plate) stabilization of fractures.

When osseous metastases are widespread, bone-seeking isotopes are useful means of delivering systemic radiation to bone. Examples of such agents include strontium-89 and samarium-153, which are incorporated into the bony matrix by active osteoblasts.

Systemic Therapy

An explosion of new cancer therapies has been seen in the last decade. However, few agents have been accepted as widely as bisphosphonates. Numerous prospective randomized trials have demonstrated improvement in patient-reported pain, improved quality of life, and delay in onset of skeletal-related events in patients with metastatic bone disease treated with bisphosphonates. The newest generation of nitrogen-containing agents seems to be most effective.[56-63] These agents directly inhibit osteoclast function, thereby preventing bone resorption.[56] Reports of osteonecrosis of the jaw and low-energy, subtrochanteric femur fractures are causes for vigilance.[49,64]

More recently, anti-RANKL antibodies have been shown to be effective in preventing osteoporosis-related skeletal events in men receiving androgen deprivation for prostate cancer.[65] This is likely only the beginning of additional agents that modulate the balance between RANKL and osteoprotegerin.[66]

Surgical Management

General Considerations

Pathologic fractures about the hip generally are treated surgically. The caveat to this occurs when patients are asymptomatic (e.g., anterior iliac spine avulsion fractures, pubic ramus fractures), or when they have a life expectancy less than 1 month. Goals of surgery should be to allow immediate and durable weight bearing on the limb. The surgeon must be cognizant that other lesions may exist, and the entire femur must be well visualized before a definitive plan is determined. Solitary lesions should be biopsied before a final surgical plan is made, to confirm metastatic disease rather than the presence of a second primary lesion. Rare (and controversial) indications for resection of solitary metastatic lesions are known. Barring rare cases of wide resection of disease, patients treated for metastases are treated with postoperative radiotherapy.

In most cases, a pathologic fracture or an impending fracture secondary to metastatic disease will not be a solitary lesion. In these cases, wide resection of the metastasis is not indicated. However, removing bulky disease may have some merit. This will improve the effectiveness of postop radiation and may help reduce pain. Surgical adjuvants such as liquid nitrogen may also be considered when one is treating a tumor that is poorly responsive to chemotherapy and radiation. Recurrent lesions can lead to failure of fixation. This is particularly true when plates and screws are utilized. Methylmethacrylate can be used to help fill defects left after bulky tumor removal. Methylmethacrylate is strongest in compression and can be useful as a medial buttress to help support prosthetic reconstruction.

The overall health of patients with metastatic disease is often quite different from that of patients without cancer. Cancer patients are often in a catabolic state before undergoing surgery. Their nutrition is often further compromised by poor intake secondary to chemotherapy side effects. Therefore, careful consideration of the caloric needs of each patient is important. Malnourished patients are more likely to have trouble with wound healing. One may consider checking a prealbumin in the perioperative setting to get an idea of the nutritional status of the patient. Dehydration is commonly seen in cancer patients; this may exacerbate hypercalcemia and other metabolic abnormalities. Careful assessment of fluids and electrolytes is mandatory.

Osteoporosis often accompanies metastatic disease to bone and adjuvant treatments employed in cancer therapy. This has an obvious impact on surgical fixation; however it may also come into play in patient positioning. One must be extra-vigilant to avoid iatrogenic fractures.

Pulmonary metastases may also be present; these can decrease the pulmonary reserve of patients. When the patient is placed in the lateral position, a ventilation/perfusion mismatch occurs, which may be problematic if pulmonary disease is particularly severe.

Liver metastasis may adversely impact liver function. This may come into play during surgery, as clotting factors may not be optimized. In addition, platelet function may be adversely impacted. This could lead to significant problems with hemostasis. Furthermore, postoperative anticoagulation with vitamin K inhibitors may be influenced by altered liver function.

Brain metastasis may impact decisions regarding postoperative anticoagulation. One must be wary of cerebrovascular accidents secondary to hemorrhage from a metastatic focus in the brain.

Finally, patients with metastatic disease and often recent adjuvant therapies are at increased risk for infection and thromboembolic disease. Postoperative care is carefully coordinated around adjuvant therapies; this may impair wound healing, suppress the immune system, or alter thrombotic risk. Because patients on chemotherapy and with other metastases may have unpredictable responses to warfarin therapy, low-molecular-weight heparin is more commonly used for thromboembolic prophylaxis in this patient population.

Percutaneous Treatment of Pelvic Metastasis

A trend toward percutaneous procedures has been noted in radiation recalcitrant pelvic lesions. Percutaneous methylmethacrylate injection, radiofrequency ablation, microwave ablation, and cryoablation have been described. Percutaneous injection of methylmethacrylate has been used as a means of treating pathologic fractures in the pelvis. Proponents argue that the approach is minimally invasive and allows immediate weight bearing. Furthermore, adequate pain relief and improved quality of life have been reported following percutaneous acetabuloplasty.[67,68] Careful assessment of periacetabular bone is a must, to avoid intrapelvic or intra-articular polymethylmethacrylate (PMMA) extravasation. The technique is not appropriate when the weight-bearing subchondral bone has been destroyed.

Similarly, radiofrequency ablation and cryoablation have been used in a palliative manner.[69,70] One prospective trial reported a clinically significant drop in pain after radiofrequency ablation in 59 of 62 (95%) patients.[71] These modalities are useful alternatives to open procedures; however, the decision to proceed with a percutaneous procedure rather than an open procedure should be made in collaboration with an orthopedic surgeon experienced in pelvic reconstruction.

Femoral Neck and Head Fractures

Metastatic lesions in the epiphysis of the femoral head are best treated with hemiarthroplasty (Fig. 52- 2). The length of the stem used is dependent on the present or anticipated tumor load in the rest of the femur. Full-length femoral x-rays must be obtained before a fully informed decision is made. Cemented (rather an ingrowth) components are favored because of the need for chemotherapy and radiotherapy, which would make ingrowth components unreliable in this setting. The goal of surgery is to provide full weight bearing in the immediate postoperative period for patients in whom general deconditioning or other skeletal lesions may impair their ability to safely mobilize in a limited weight-bearing capacity. Transcervical fractures of the femoral neck secondary to metastatic disease are best treated with hemiarthroplasty. Nonprosthetic fixation methods have led to high rates of nonunion. One study reported 24 nonunions out of 24 transcervical fractures after attempted fixation without prosthetic reconstruction.[5]

Intertrochanteric Fractures

Pathologic intertrochanteric fractures are most commonly treated with calcar replacing hemiarthroplasty; an alternative for carefully selected patients is treatment with curettage followed by reconstruction with a plate and screws coupled with methylmethacrylate (Fig. 52-3). A cemented, long-stemmed hemiarthroplasty

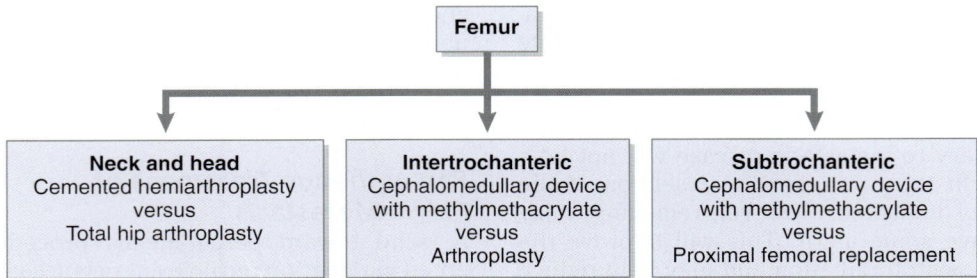

```
Femur
├── Neck and head
│   Cemented hemiarthroplasty
│   versus
│   Total hip arthroplasty
├── Intertrochanteric
│   Cephalomedullary device
│   with methylmethacrylate
│   versus
│   Arthroplasty
└── Subtrochanteric
    Cephalomedullary device
    with methylmethacrylate
    versus
    Proximal femoral replacement
```

Figure 52-2. This algorithm helps organize the surgical approach to pathologic fracture or impending fracture of the proximal femur.

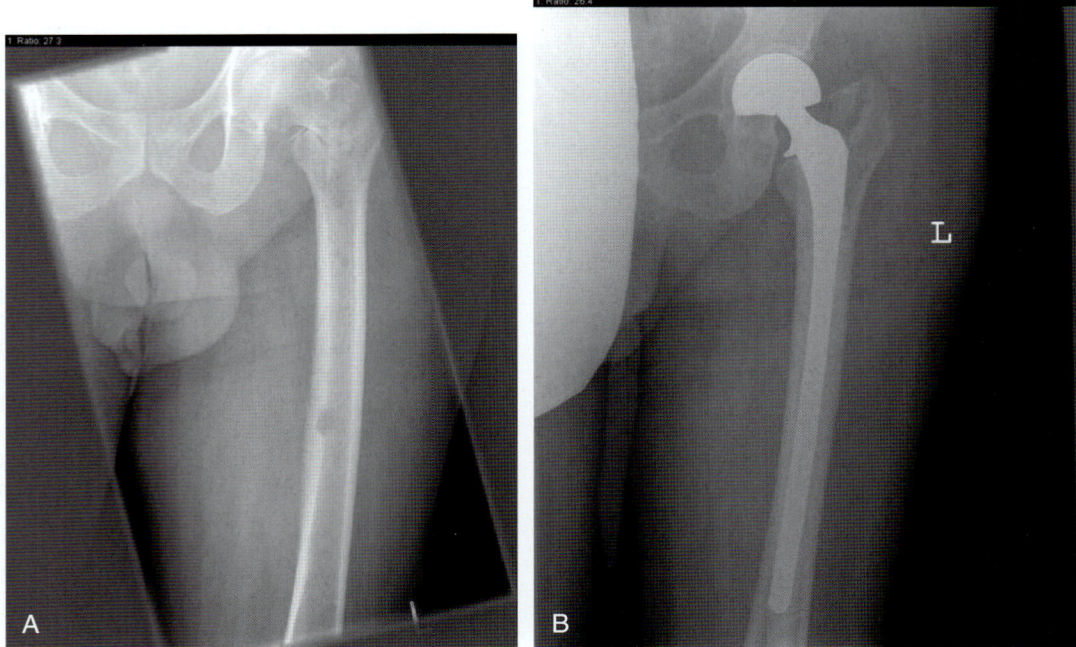

Figure 52-3. A, This preoperative plain radiograph demonstrates the pathologic intertrochanteric fracture as well as a lytic lesion farther down the femoral shaft. **B,** The fracture was treated with a cemented hemiarthroplasty with a long stem spanning the lytic lesion.

eliminates concern for disease progression in the femoral head or neck, which may necessitate reoperation.[72] In addition, it allows impending lesions to be treated with one operation. This follows the "one bone, one operation" mantra espoused by some. One may consider venting the femur with a quarter inch drill bit before reaming. The vent decreases embolic load by reducing intraosseous pressures encountered during reaming. The advantage of curettage and cementation is that it retains the native hip joint and decreases the patient's exposure to embolic material, which occurs with reaming. Care must be taken when plate and screws are used for these fractures because the medial calcar may be disrupted. Methylmethacrylate can be used as a buttress in this setting to help avoid varus collapse and failure of fixation. The disadvantage of plate and screw reconstruction is that is relies on local radiation and/or chemotherapy to prevent further compromise of adjacent bone. In addition, it does not address other areas of the femur that may be involved in the disease,

and as such is reserved for carefully selected patients with favorable (chemosensitive and radiosensitive) pathology.

Subtrochanteric Fractures

Subtrochanteric fractures secondary to metastatic disease can be particularly challenging to treat. Intramedullary rod fixation is the most common treatment option in this setting.[4,42] For proximal lesions, many surgeons favor a cemented, long-stemmed hemiarthroplasty versus a cemented, proximal femoral replacement in cases with severe bone destruction, to help avoid hardware failure associated with tumor progression.[73] In either case, we generally curettage bulky disease before stabilizing the fracture. Methylmethacrylate can be used to fill cavitary lesions. A transverse subtrochanteric fracture is recognized as a complication of long-term bisphosphonate usage.[49] It is important to distinguish between a bisphosphonate-related fracture and a fracture secondary to metastatic disease. In the former case, we generally would use an intramedullary rod to stabilize the fracture. In addition, radiation would not be needed and in fact would be contraindicated.

Acetabular Fractures

Pathologic fractures about the acetabulum may be treated with protective weight bearing and radiation therapy if they are nondisplaced and no impending fractures exist on the femoral side. This treatment may be augmented by percutaneous cement injection, as described earlier. Surgery may become necessary if pain persists in spite of radiation and a period of protective weight bearing. Cheng reported a series of such fractures treated successfully without surgery.[74]

In cases with more severe bone destruction, or with femoral-sided lesions requiring surgery, multiple options are available to help reconstruct the hip. Bone loss can be severe, and methylmethacrylate alone may be insufficient to reconstruct the destroyed bone. The general principle is that the load being transmitted through damaged bone must be transferred to normal healthy bone. This is accomplished by using flanged cups, cages, metal wedges, and/or metal pins, in addition to methylmethacrylate.[75-77] The goal should be to allow the acetabular cup to sit in its anatomic position with the aid of the modalities mentioned earlier.

Harrington classified periacetabular lesions on the basis of whether lateral, superior, or medial cortices were intact.[78] Class 1 lesions involve trabecular bone about the acetabular, but cortical bone remains intact. A cemented acetabular cup coupled with an appropriate femoral-sided prosthesis is sufficient treatment in these cases. Methylmethacrylate can be placed into the destroyed periacetabular bone via a cortical window, or by placing a trocar into the cavity and injecting the cement—similar to a percutaneous approach (Fig. 52-4).

The medial cortex is destroyed in Harrington class 2 lesions. Reconstruction of the hip involves a cemented cup, but an acetabular cage can be utilized to transfer loads to adjacent healthier bone. These lesions can be viewed as one would view a protrusio acetabulum. Available reconstructive options for protrusio acetabulum can be used for Harrington type 2 lesions, with the caveat that methylmethacrylate ought to be strongly considered.

Harrington type 3 lesions pose a significant challenge. In this scenario, lateral cortices of the acetabulum and the dome are destroyed (Fig. 52-5). This scenario does not lend itself to cage or protrusio cup reconstruction because of lack of supportive local bone. Transferring loads to normal bone means spanning cavitary defects in multiple plains. Harrington described placing pins in a retrograde fashion from the cavitary defect into healthy bone posteriorly and superiorly. The cavitary defect is then filled with methylmethacrylate. Modifications of this technique have been described, in which pins are placed in an antegrade fashion from the iliac wing into the cavitary defect.[37,79] Although satisfactory clinical results are possible with this technique, lack of normal bone stock exposes pelvic viscera and vascular structures not normally encountered during hip reconstruction.

PROGNOSIS

When one considers prognosis with regard to patients with metastatic bone disease, it is important to keep in mind that survival is often difficult to predict. Clearly, histology, extent of disease, and adjuvant therapy options impact prognosis. One study from Sloan Kettering pointed out that even experienced oncologists are correct only about a third of the time when predicting survival.[80] In addition, cancer treatments are evolving. Newer agents are extending the lives of patients with metastatic disease by as much as 6 months.[81] Still it is useful to consider general guidelines for survival when one is considering surgery. For instance, patients with breast and prostate metastases generally will live longer than 1 year, whereas those with non–small cell lung cancer are more likely to live about 8 to 9 months. Decisions about surgery should be made with the consultation of the patient and medical oncology and radiation oncology staff.[82]

CURRENT CONTROVERSIES AND FUTURE CONSIDERATIONS

Use of percutaneous ablative procedures with or without methylmethacrylate reconstruction is gaining popularity secondary to their minimally invasive nature. These procedures are performed by surgeons and interventional radiologists. Indications for these procedures are

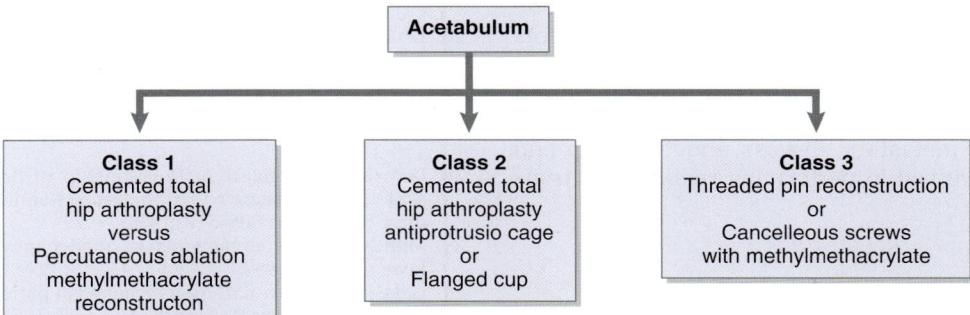

Figure 52-4. This algorithm uses the Harrington classification to organize the approach to destructive lesions about the acetabulum.

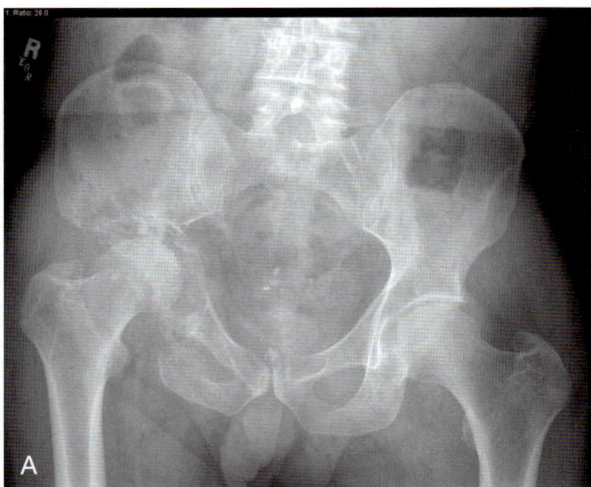

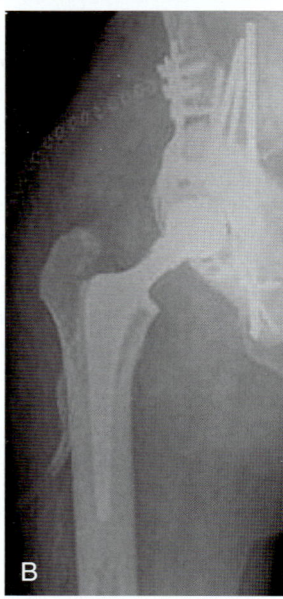

Figure 52-5. A, This anteroposterior pelvic plain radiograph shows a destructive lesion compromising the dome, lateral walls, and medial wall of the acetabulum. **B,** Harrington recommended augmenting the acetabulum with screws or wires into normal bone, with polymethylmethacrylate (PMMA) used to fill the defect.

in flux, and the decision to perform a particular surgical procedure or to use radiation alone ought to be made by committee rather than by a single individual. Consensus does not exist as to when to proceed with open surgery versus percutaneous surgery. Investigation of this subject is hampered by the heterogeneity of patients presenting with metastatic disease about the hip and the difficulty involved in performing randomized trials in this setting.

REFERENCES

1. Jemal A, Siegel R, Ward E, et al: Cancer statistics, 2009. CA Cancer J Clin 59:225–249, 2009.
2. Jaffe H: Tumors and tumorous conditions of bones and joints, Philadelphia, 1958, Lea and Febiger.
3. World Health Organization (WHO): Report of the WHO Expert Committee on Cancer Pain Relief and Active Supportive Care: cancer pain relief with a guide to opioid availability, Geneva, Switzerland, 1996, WHO.
4. Habermann ET, Sachs R, Stern RE, et al: The pathology and treatment of metastatic disease of the femur. Clin Orthop Relat Res 169:70–82, 1982.
5. Galasko CS: Skeletal metastases and mammary cancer. Ann R Coll Surg Engl 50:3–28, 1972.
6. Paget S: The distribution of secondary growths in cancer of the breast. Lancet 1:571–573, 1889.
7. Abrams HL, Spiro R, Goldstein N: Metastases in carcinoma: analysis of 1000 autopsied cases. Cancer 3:74–85, 1950.
8. Hoffman PC, Mauer AM, Vokes EE: Lung cancer. Lancet 355:479–485, 2000.
9. Karrison TG, Ferguson DJ, Meier P: Dormancy of mammary carcinoma after mastectomy. J Natl Cancer Inst 91:80–85, 1999.
10. Edlund M, Sung SY, Chung LW: Modulation of prostate cancer growth in bone microenvironments. J Cell Biochem 91:686–705, 2004.
11. Chiang AC, Massague J: Molecular basis of metastasis. N Engl J Med 359:2814–2823, 2008.
12. Mani SA, Guo W, Liao MJ, et al: The epithelial-mesenchymal transition generates cells with properties of stem cells. Cell 133:704–715, 2008.
13. Yang J, Weinberg RA: Epithelial-mesenchymal transition: at the crossroads of development and tumor metastasis. Dev Cell 14:818–829, 2008.
14. Chambers AF, Groom AC, MacDonald IC: Dissemination and growth of cancer cells in metastatic sites. Nat Rev Cancer 2:563–572, 2002.
15. Batson O: The role of the vertebral veins in the spread of metastasis. Ann Intern Med 16:38–45, 1942.
16. Kopp HG, Avecilla ST, Hooper AT, Rafii S: The bone marrow vascular niche: home of HSC differentiation and mobilization. Physiology (Bethesda) 20:349–356, 2005.
17. Yin JJ, Selander K, Chirgwin JM, et al: TGF-beta signaling blockade inhibits PTHrP secretion by breast cancer cells and bone metastases development. J Clin Invest 103:197–206, 1999.
18. Mundy GR: Metastasis to bone: causes, consequences and therapeutic opportunities. Nat Rev Cancer 2:584–593, 2002.
19. Kang Y, Siegel PM, Shu W, et al: A multigenic program mediating breast cancer metastasis to bone. Cancer Cell 3:537–549, 2003.
20. Park BK, Zhang H, Zeng Q, et al: NF-kappaB in breast cancer cells promotes osteolytic bone metastasis by inducing osteoclastogenesis via GM-CSF. Nat Med 13:62–69, 2007.
21. Hipp J RA, Hayes W: Mechanical properties of trabecular bone within and adjacent to osseous metastasis. J Bone Miner Res 7:1165, 1992.
22. McBroom RC, Hayes W: Strength reductions from metastatic cortical defects in long bones. J Orthop Res 6:369, 1988.
23. Brooks DB, Burstein AH, Frankel VH: The biomechanics of torsional fractures: the stress concentration effect of a drill hole. J Bone Joint Surg Am 52:507–514, 1970.
24. Cleeland CS, Gonin R, Hatfield AK, et al: Pain and its treatment in outpatients with metastatic cancer. N Engl J Med 330:592–596, 1994.
25. Cleeland CS: The impact of pain on the patient with cancer. Cancer 54(suppl 11):2635–2641, 1984.
26. Levin DN, Cleeland CS, Dar R: Public attitudes toward cancer pain. Cancer 56:2337–2339, 1985.
27. Von Roenn JH, Cleeland CS, Gonin R, et al: Physician attitudes and practice in cancer pain management: a survey from the Eastern Cooperative Oncology Group. Ann Intern Med 119:121–126, 1993.
28. Galasko CS, Bennett A: Relationship of bone destruction in skeletal metastases to osteoclast activation and prostaglandins. Nature 263:508–510, 1976.
29. Mundy GR: Hypercalcemia of malignancy revisited. J Clin Invest 82:1–6, 1988.
30. Galasko CS, Burn JI: Hypercalcaemia in patients with advanced mammary cancer. Br Med J 3:573–577, 1971.
31. Plunkett TA, Smith P, Rubens RD: Risk of complications from bone metastases in breast cancer: implications for management. Eur J Cancer 36:476–482, 2000.

32. Ralston SH, Gallacher SJ, Patel U, et al: Cancer-associated hypercalcemia: morbidity and mortality. Clinical experience in 126 treated patients. Ann Intern Med 112:499–504, 1990.
33. Stewart AF: Clinical practice: hypercalcemia associated with cancer. N Engl J Med 352:373–379, 2005.
34. Hamaoka T, Madewell JE, Podoloff DA, et al: Bone imaging in metastatic breast cancer. J Clin Oncol 22:2942–2953, 2004.
35. Giuliani N, Bataille R, Mancini C, et al: Myeloma cells induce imbalance in the osteoprotegerin/osteoprotegerin ligand system in the human bone marrow environment. Blood 98:3527–3533, 2001.
36. Giuliani N, Colla S, Sala R, et al: Human myeloma cells stimulate the receptor activator of nuclear factor-kappa B ligand (RANKL) in T lymphocytes: a potential role in multiple myeloma bone disease. Blood 100:4615–4621, 2002.
37. Marco RA, Sheth DS, Boland PJ, et al: Functional and oncological outcome of acetabular reconstruction for the treatment of metastatic disease. J Bone Joint Surg Am 82:642–651, 2001.
38. Rizzo PF, Gould ES, Lyden JP, Asnis SE: Diagnosis of occult fractures about the hip: magnetic resonance imaging compared with bone-scanning. J Bone Joint Surg Am 75:395–401, 1993.
39. Snell W, Beals RK: Femoral metastases and fractures from breast cancer. Surg Gynecol Obstet 119:22–24, 1964.
40. Parrish FF, Murray JA: Surgical treatment for secondary neoplastic fractures: a retrospective study of ninety-six patients. J Bone Joint Surg Am 52:665–686, 1970.
41. Murray JA, Bruels MC, Lindberg RD: Irradiation of polymethylmethacrylate: in vitro gamma radiation effect. J Bone Joint Surg Am 56:311–312, 1974.
42. Zickel RE, Mouradian WH: Intramedullary fixation of pathologic fractures and lesions of the subtrochanteric region of the femur. J Bone Joint Surg Am 58:1061–1066, 1976.
43. Keene JS, Sellinger DS, McBeath AA, Engber WD: Metastatic breast cancer in the femur: a search for the lesion at risk of fracture. Clin Orthop Relat Res 203:282–288, 1986.
44. Hipp J: Predicting pathologic fracture risk in the management of metastatic bone defects. Clin Orthop Relat Res 312:120–135, 1995.
45. Michaeli DA, Inoue K, Hayes WC, Hipp JA: Density predicts the activity-dependent failure load of proximal femora with defects. Skeletal Radiol 28:90–95, 1999.
46. Snyder BD, Hauser-Kara DA, Hipp JA, et al: Predicting fracture through benign skeletal lesions with quantitative computed tomography. J Bone Joint Surg Am 88:55–70, 2006.
47. Mirels H: Metastatic disease in long bones: a proposed scoring system for diagnosing impending pathologic fractures. Clin Orthop Relat Res 249:256–264, 1989.
48. Lenart BA, Lorich DG, Lane JM: Atypical fractures of the femoral diaphysis in postmenopausal women taking alendronate. N Engl J Med 358:1304–1306, 2008.
49. Neviaser AS, Lane JM, Lenart BA, et al: Low-energy femoral shaft fractures associated with alendronate use. J Orthop Trauma 22:346–350, 2008.
50. Tong D, Gillick L, Hendrickson F: The palliation of symptomatic osseous metastases: final results of the study by the Radiation Therapy Oncology Group. Cancer 50:893–899, 1982.
51. Vargha ZO, Glicksman AS, Boland J: Single-dose radiation therapy in the palliation of metastatic disease. Radiology 93:1181–1184, 1969.
52. Arcangeli G, Giovinazzo G, Saracino B, et al: Radiation therapy in the management of symptomatic bone metastases: the effect of total dose and histology on pain relief and response duration. Int J Radiat Oncol Biol Phys 42:1119–1126, 1998.
53. Blitzer P: Reanalysis of the RTOG study of the palliation of symptomatic osseous metastasis. Cancer 55:1468, 1985.
54. Bonarigo BC, Rubin P: Nonunion of pathologic fractures after radiation therapy. Radiology 88:889–898, 1967.
55. Gainor BJ, Buchert P: Fracture healing in metastatic bone disease. Clin Orthop Relat Res 178:297–302, 1983.
56. Costa L, Major PP: Effect of bisphosphonates on pain and quality of life in patients with bone metastases. Nat Clin Pract 6:163–174, 2009.
57. Rosen LS: Efficacy and safety of zoledronic acid in the treatment of bone metastases associated with lung cancer and

other solid tumors. Semin Oncol 29(6 Suppl 21):28–32, 2002.
58. Rosen LS: New generation of bisphosphonates: broad clinical utility in breast and prostate cancer. Oncology 18(5 Suppl 3):26–32, 2004.
59. Rosen LS, Gordon D, Kaminski M, et al: Long-term efficacy and safety of zoledronic acid compared with pamidronate disodium in the treatment of skeletal complications in patients with advanced multiple myeloma or breast carcinoma: a randomized, double-blind, multicenter, comparative trial. Cancer 98:1735–1744, 2003.
60. Rosen LS, Gordon D, Tchekmedyian NS, et al: Long-term efficacy and safety of zoledronic acid in the treatment of skeletal metastases in patients with nonsmall cell lung carcinoma and other solid tumors: a randomized, Phase III, double-blind, placebo-controlled trial. Cancer 100:2613–2621, 2004.
61. Rosen LS, Gordon D, Tchekmedyian S, et al: Zoledronic acid versus placebo in the treatment of skeletal metastases in patients with lung cancer and other solid tumors: a phase III, double-blind, randomized trial—the Zoledronic Acid Lung Cancer and Other Solid Tumors Study Group. J Clin Oncol 21:3150–3157, 2003.
62. Rosen LS, Gordon DH, Dugan W Jr, et al: Zoledronic acid is superior to pamidronate for the treatment of bone metastases in breast carcinoma patients with at least one osteolytic lesion. Cancer 100:36–43, 2004.
63. Wardley A, Davidson N, Barrett-Lee P, et al: Zoledronic acid significantly improves pain scores and quality of life in breast cancer patients with bone metastases: a randomised, crossover study of community vs hospital bisphosphonate administration. Brit J Cancer 92:1869–1876, 2005.
64. Vahtsevanos K, Kyrgidis A, Verrou E, et al: Longitudinal cohort study of risk factors in cancer patients of bisphosphonate-related osteonecrosis of the jaw. J Clin Oncol 27:5356–5362, 2009.
65. Smith MR, Egerdie B, Hernandez Toriz N, et al: Denosumab in men receiving androgen-deprivation therapy for prostate cancer. N Engl J Med 361:745–755, 2009.
66. Roodman GD: Mechanisms of bone metastasis. N Engl J Med 350:1655–1664, 2004.
67. Scaramuzzo L, Maccauro G, Rossi B, et al: Quality of life in patients following percutaneous PMMA acetabuloplasty for acetabular metastasis due to carcinoma. Acta Orthop Belg 75:484–489, 2009.
68. Maccauro G, Liuzza F, Scaramuzzo L, et al: Percutaneous acetabuloplasty for metastatic acetabular lesions. BMC Musculoskel Disord 9:66, 2008.
69. Callstrom MR, Atwell TD, Charboneau JW, et al: Painful metastases involving bone: percutaneous image-guided cryoablation—prospective trial interim analysis. Radiology 241:572–580, 2006.
70. Callstrom MR, Charboneau JW, Goetz MP, et al: Painful metastases involving bone: feasibility of percutaneous CT- and US-guided radio-frequency ablation. Radiology 224:87–97, 2002.
71. Goetz MP, Callstrom MR, Charboneau JW, et al: Percutaneous image-guided radiofrequency ablation of painful metastases involving bone: a multicenter study. J Clin Oncol 22:300–306, 2004.
72. Wedin R, Bauer HC: Surgical treatment of skeletal metastatic lesions of the proximal femur: endoprosthesis or reconstruction nail? J Bone Joint Surg 87:1653–1657, 2004.
73. Weber KL, Randall RL, Grossman S, Parvizi J: Management of lower-extremity bone metastasis. J Bone Joint Surg Am 88(Suppl 4):11–19, 2006.
74. Cheng DS, Seitz CB, Eyre HJ: Nonoperative management of femoral, humeral, and acetabular metastases in patients with breast carcinoma. Cancer 45:1533–1537, 1980.
75. Stark A, Bauer HC: Reconstruction in metastatic destruction of the acetabulum: support rings and arthroplasty in 12 patients. Acta Orthop Scand 67:435–438, 1996.
76. Benevenia J, Cyran FP, Biermann JS, et al: Treatment of advanced metastatic lesions of the acetabulum using the saddle prosthesis. Clin Orthop Relat Res 426:23–31, 2004.

77. Allan DG, Bell RS, Davis A, Langer F: Complex acetabular reconstruction for metastatic tumor. J Arthroplasty 10:301–306, 1995.

78. Harrington K: The management of acetabular insufficiency secondary to metastatic malignant disease. J Bone Joint Surg Am 63:653–664, 1981.

79. Tillman RM, Myers GJ, Abudu AT, et al: The three-pin modified "Harrington" procedure for advanced metastatic destruction of the acetabulum. J Bone Joint Surg 90:84–87, 2008.

80. Nathan SS, Healey JH, Mellano D, et al: Survival in patients operated on for pathologic fracture: implications for end-of-life orthopedic care. J Clin Oncol 23:6072–6082, 2005.

81. Motzer RJ, Hutson TE, Tomczak P, et al: Sunitinib versus interferon alfa in metastatic renal-cell carcinoma. N Engl J Med 356:115–124, 2007.

82. Biermann WA, Cantor RI, Fellin FM, et al: An evaluation of the potential cost reductions resulting from the use of clodronate in the treatment of metastatic carcinoma of the breast to bone. Bone 12(Suppl 1):S37–S42, 1991.

NONARTHROPLASTY TREATMENT OF HIP PATHOLOGY

CHAPTER 53

Hip Arthroscopy for Nonstructural Hip Problems

J.W. Thomas Byrd

INTRODUCTION

Femoroacetabular impingement (FAI) and dysplasia are the two most common structural problems implicated in hip pathology. However, numerous nonstructural problems are associated with disorders of the hip joint and hip region. These include macrotrauma, repetitive overuse microtrauma, consequences of kinetic and kinematic disorders, and intrinsic tissue disease. Hip problems manifested by painful symptoms are often the culmination of multifactorial causes. Underlying disease may render some joints more susceptible to acute injury. For example, acute subluxations and dislocations encountered among contact sports, which are relatively low-velocity injuries compared with those resulting from vehicular trauma, often have underlying findings of impingement.[1] It is likely that owing to the underlying morphology, the hip is rendered more susceptible to luxation by the levering effect.

Numerous soft tissue disorders around the hip can cause problems and may be amenable to endoscopic intervention. The collective group of coxa saltans, which includes snapping of the iliopsoas tendon and iliotibial band and possibly other less evident entities, can be corrected endoscopically.[2-4] Bursectomy can be performed, and many cases of recalcitrant trochanteric bursitis may actually represent painful abductor tendinopathies.[5-7] Keep in mind that some of these disorders may be incidental, normally occurring observations, and others can occur as a normal consequence of aging or of subtle gait abnormalities. It is a challenge to the clinician to distinguish pathologic processes from normal variations. It is also important to keep in mind that several disorders may coexist, and one must differentiate which are the principal problems and how they should best be managed. Recommendations may range from simple activity modifications, to structured conservative treatment, to surgical intervention.

INDICATIONS/CONTRAINDICATIONS

For nonstructural problems, the most common indication for arthroscopy is pain caused by some type of pathologic condition that can be corrected by arthroscopic techniques. Rarely is arthroscopy considered in the presence of a painless disorder. Often, patients may present for assessment with modest symptoms that are not sufficient to create a functional problem. Under these circumstances, thoughtful observation and other nonoperative treatments may be appropriate. If symptoms are worsening in the presence of recognized pathology, it may be prudent to be proactive in considering surgical intervention. Keep in mind that various disorders may coexist, which can include pathologic conditions and anomalies that are not responsible for the patient's symptoms. For example, hip joint pathology may occur in conjunction with a snapping iliopsoas tendon, which may or may not be a contributing cause of pain warranting correction.

Contraindications to hip arthroscopy are few. Most important is simply ensuring that the patient's condition is amenable to and appropriate for arthroscopic intervention. Another important consideration is ensuring that the patient's expectations can be practically met by the procedure. Surgery in the presence of unreasonable expectations will be a failure regardless of the skill with which the procedure is performed. Advanced disease states such as severe degenerative arthritis are contraindications simply because arthroscopy cannot reasonably be of any benefit. Some severe deformities, wound problems, and medical conditions may contraindicate arthroscopy or possibly even any type of surgery.

PREOPERATIVE PLANNING

Imaging studies are an important part of the diagnostic workup and surgical planning. Radiographs reveal joint morphology and underlying structural disorders, as well as the presence of degenerative disease. It is important to keep in mind that damage within the joint is typically substantial before radiographic changes become evident. Thus reasonable joint space preservation may not preclude the existence of considerable degenerative disease. Also, subtle radiographic changes should be taken as serious evidence of advanced pathology.

Conventional magnetic resonance imaging (MRI) is an important component of most preoperative planning for hip surgery. Its reliability for detecting intra-articular pathology may be variable, but it is often helpful to rule out disorders that will not benefit from arthroscopy, such as avascular necrosis, transient regional osteoporosis, and many others. Gadolinium arthrography with MRI (MRA) is better but is not completely reliable for detecting all intra-articular pathology. Injecting anesthetic along with contrast is a valuable tool in substantiating that the hip joint is the source of symptoms. In cases of multiple pain generators, intra-articular injection helps to distinguish how much the hip is contributing.[8] Assessing the patient's response to the injection can be important in making the decision for surgery. In general, imaging studies are good for assessing labral pathology but may be less reliable in detecting associated articular damage. This is important when one is counseling patients because the uncertain extent of articular damage is often a limiting factor in the success of arthroscopy. Computed tomography has a significant role in assessing bony architecture and the three-dimensional morphology of the joint but is less often enlightening for soft tissue problems about the hip.

Problematic snapping of the iliopsoas tendon and the iliotibial band is mostly identified from the history and examination findings. This snapping is usually a dynamic phenomenon, not predictably reproduced with examination under anesthesia, and the arthroscopic findings do little to substantiate the diagnosis. Abductor tendinopathies can be a normal consequence of aging but can also be a source of relevant clinical pathology. Thus the clinical findings dictate how aggressive one should be with lesions encountered in the peritrochanteric space.

DESCRIPTION OF TECHNIQUE

The technique illustrated is being performed with the patient in supine position.[9,10] The important principles for performing safe, effective, reproducible arthroscopy are the same whether the patient is in the lateral decubitus or supine orientation. Portal placements, relationships of extra-articular structures, and arthroscopic anatomy are all the same regardless of positioning.

EQUIPMENT

A standard fracture table or custom distraction device is needed to achieve effective joint space separation. The C-arm is important for precise placement of instrumentation within the joint. Extra-length arthroscopy

instruments are also available to accommodate the dense surrounding soft tissue.

ANESTHESIA

The procedure is commonly performed with the patient under general anesthesia. It can be performed under epidural but requires an adequate motor block to ensure optimal distractibility of the joint.

INTRA-ARTICULAR (CENTRAL) COMPARTMENT

Setup

The perineal post is heavily padded and lateralized against the medial thigh of the operative hip (Fig. 53-1). This aids in achieving the optimal traction vector (Fig. 53-2) and reduces pressure directly on the perineum, lessening the risk of neuropraxia of the pudendal nerve. Neutral rotation achieves a constant relationship between the topographic landmarks and the joint. Slight flexion may relax the capsule, but excessive flexion should be avoided because this places undue tension on the sciatic nerve and may block access to the anterior portal. Typically, about 50 pounds of force is needed to distract the joint. In general, the goal is to use the minimum force necessary to achieve adequate distraction while keeping traction time as brief as possible. Two hours is usually recognized as a reasonable limit for traction.

Portals

Three standard portals provide optimal access for the central compartment (Figs. 53-3 and 53-4). Two of these (anterolateral and posterolateral) are placed laterally over the superior margin of the greater trochanter at its anterior and posterior borders. The anterior portal is

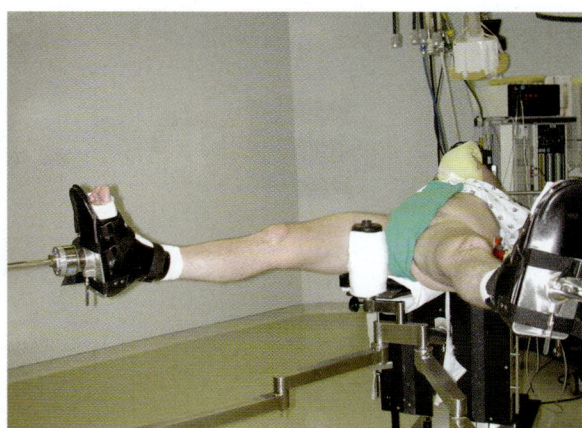

Figure 53-1. The patient is positioned on the fracture table so that the perineal post is placed as far laterally as possible toward the operative hip resting against the medial thigh. *(Courtesy J. W. Thomas Byrd, MD, Nashville, Tenn.)*

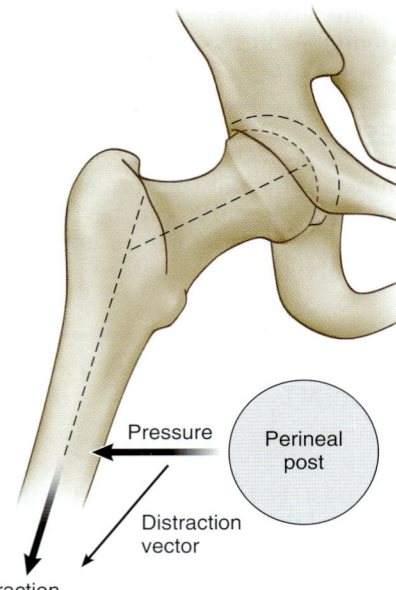

Figure 53-2. The optimal vector for distraction is oblique relative to the axis of the body and more closely coincides with the axis of the femoral neck than the femoral shaft. This oblique vector is partially created by abduction of the hip and is partially accentuated by a small transverse component to the vector created by lateralizing the perineal post. *(Courtesy J. W. Thomas Byrd, MD, Nashville, Tenn.)*

placed at the site of intersection of a sagittal line drawn distally from the anterior superior iliac spine and a transverse line across the tip of the greater trochanter. With careful orientation to the landmarks in relation to the joint, these portals are a safe distance from the surrounding major neurovascular structures.[11] Additional portals may be needed occasionally Most common is a more distal mid-anterior portal for placing anchors in conjunction with labral repair. The more distal position is necessary to ensure that the anchor diverges at the rim to avoid perforating the acetabular surface.

Diagnostic Procedure

After traction is applied, a spinal needle is placed from the anterolateral position and the joint is distended with fluid. The anterolateral portal is then established under fluoroscopic control for introduction of the arthroscope (Fig. 53-5). Careful attention is necessary to avoid perforating the labrum or scuffing the articular surface.[12] Using the 70 degree scope, the anterior and posterolateral portals are placed under direct arthroscopic view as well as under fluoroscopy for precise entry into the joint. Diagnostic and operative arthroscopy is then achieved by interchanging the arthroscope with instruments between the three established portals. Use of both 70 degree and 30 degree scopes provides optimal viewing despite limitations of

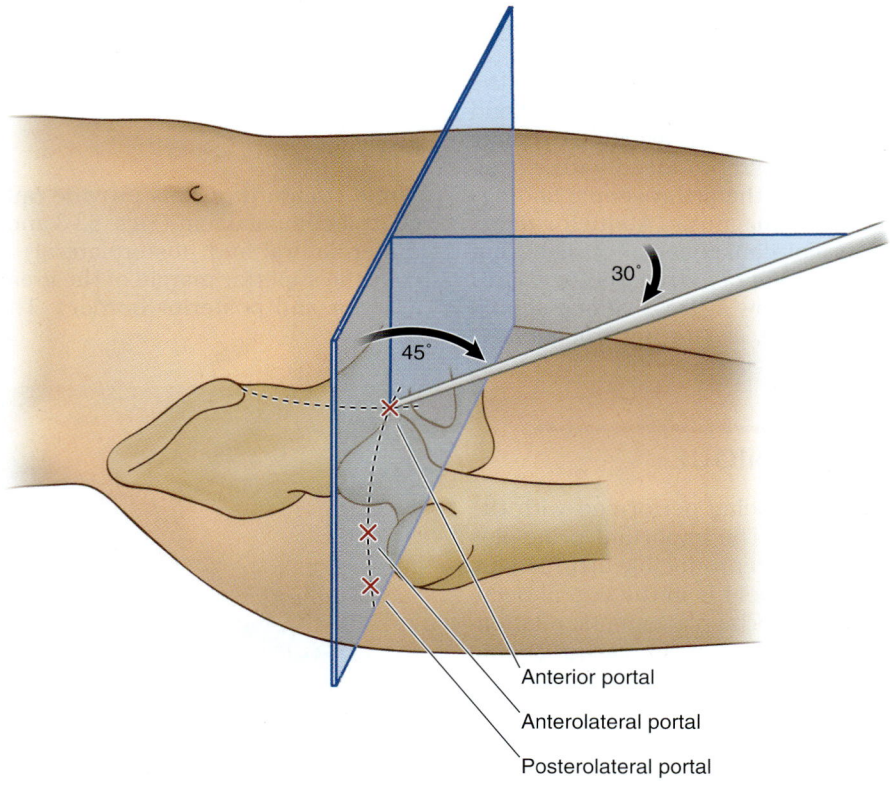

Figure 53-3. The site of the anterior portal coincides with the intersection of a sagittal line drawn distally from the anterior superior iliac spine and a transverse line across the superior margin of the greater trochanter. The direction of this portal courses approximately 45 degrees cephalad and 30 degrees toward the midline. The anterolateral and posterolateral portals are positioned directly over the superior aspect of the trochanter at its anterior and posterior borders. *(Redrawn from Byrd JWT: Hip arthroscopy utilizing the supine position. Arthroscopy 10:275–280, 1994.)*

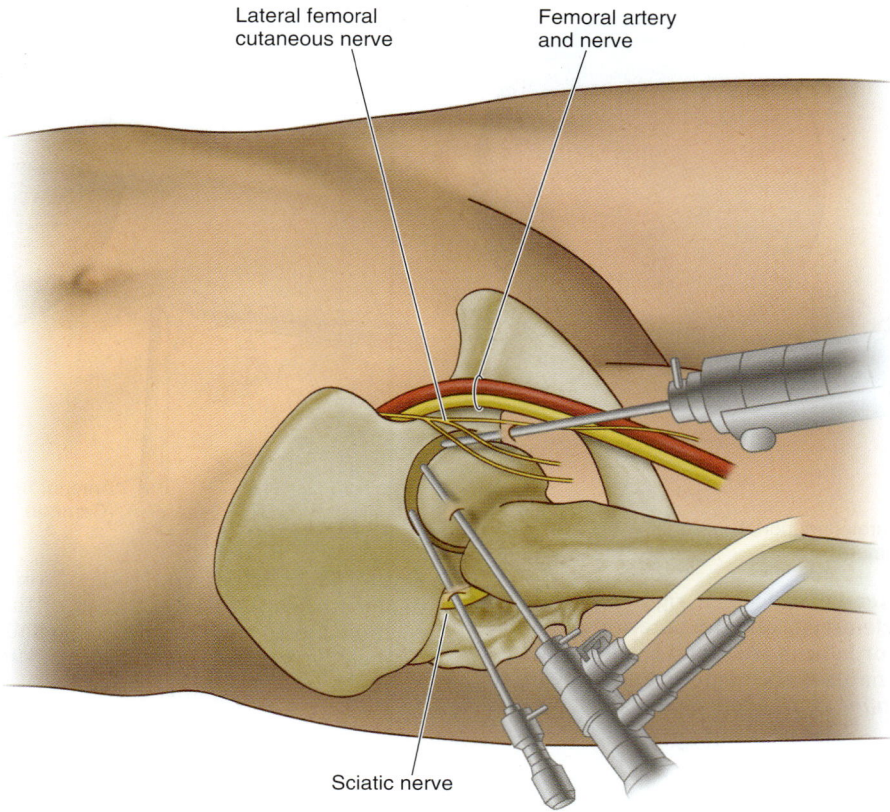

Figure 53-4. The relationship of major neurovascular structures to the three standard portals is demonstrated. The femoral artery and nerve lie well medial to the anterior portal. The sciatic nerve lies posterior to the posterolateral portal. Small branches of the lateral femoral cutaneous nerve lie close to the anterior portal. Injury to these is avoided by utilizing proper technique in portal placement. The anterolateral portal is established first because it lies most centrally in the safe zone for arthroscopy. *(Courtesy J. W. Thomas Byrd, MD, Nashville, Tenn.)*

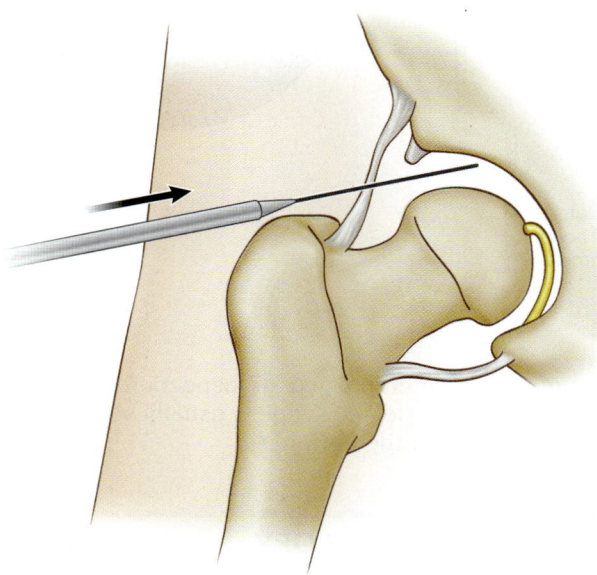

Figure 53-5. The arthroscope cannula is passed over a guide wire that was inserted through a prepositioned spinal needle. Fluoroscopy aids in avoiding contact with the femoral head or perforating the acetabular labrum.

maneuverability within the joint (Figs. 53-6 through 53-9). If needed, supplemental portals can be placed under similar arthroscopic control.

PERIPHERAL COMPARTMENT

Positioning

Routine arthroscopy of the peripheral compartment is performed after arthroscopy of the intra-articular compartment has been completed. The instruments are removed, the traction released, and the hip flexed approximately 45 degrees (Fig. 53-10). This relaxes the capsule, providing access to the peripheral compartment. Note that when correction of impingement is performed, a capsulotomy is needed for exposure and facilitates movement between the central and peripheral compartments without the need to remove the instruments. This technique is described in Chapter 54.

Portal Placement

At least two portals are used routinely to access the peripheral compartment. These include the

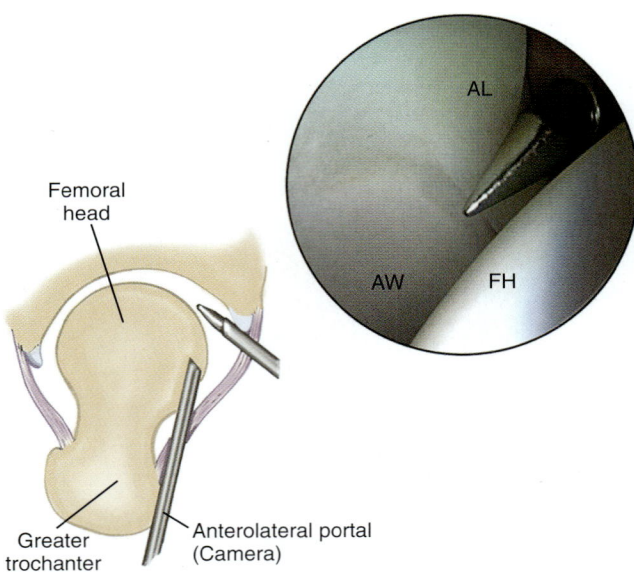

Femoral head

Greater trochanter

Anterolateral portal (Camera)

Figure 53-6. Arthroscopic view of a right hip from the anterolateral portal demonstrates the anterior acetabular wall (AW), the anterior labrum (AL), and the femoral head (FH). The anterior cannula is seen entering underneath the labrum. *(Courtesy Smith & Nephew Endoscopy, Andover, Mass [artwork].)*

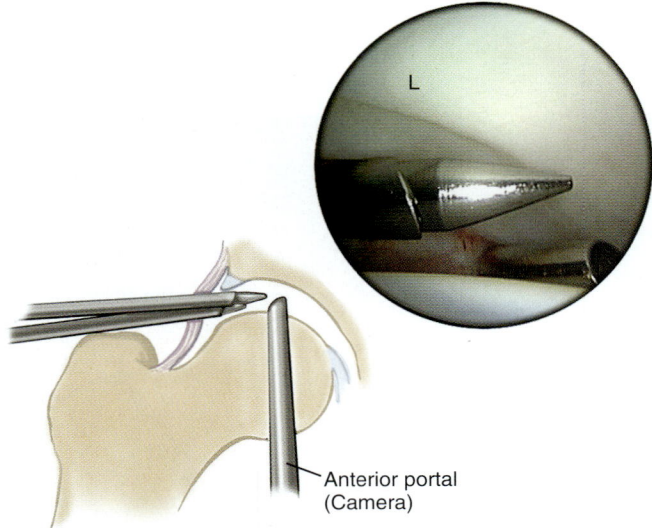

Anterior portal (Camera)

Figure 53-7. Arthroscopic view from the anterior portal demonstrates the lateral aspect of the labrum (L) and its relationship to the lateral two portals. *(Courtesy Smith & Nephew Endoscopy, Andover, Mass [artwork].)*

Figure 53-8. Arthroscopic view from the posterolateral portal demonstrates the posterior acetabular wall (PW), the posterior labrum (PL), and the femoral head (FH). *(Courtesy Smith & Nephew Endoscopy, Andover, Mass [artwork].)*

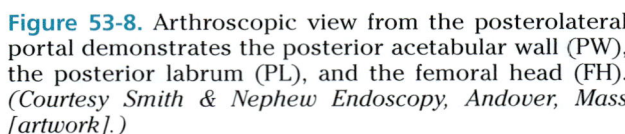
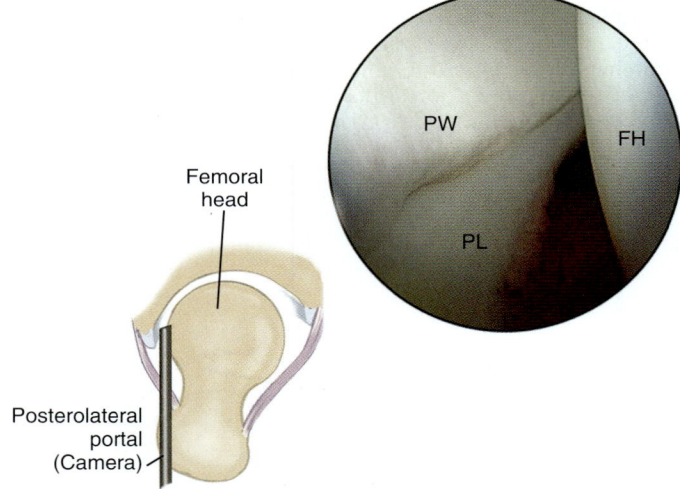

Femoral head

Posterolateral portal (Camera)

anterolateral portal and an ancillary portal established 4 to 5 cm distally. A broad safe zone in which to work is present, and numerous variations on portal placement are available. It is simply important to be consistent in portal choices for reproducibility of placement and for orientation to the anatomy of the periphery.

Diagnostic Procedure

The anterolateral portal is redirected onto the anterior neck of the femur (Fig. 53-11). The ancillary portal is then established distally under direct arthroscopic and fluoroscopic guidance (Fig. 53-12). The arthroscope and

instruments are interchanged for inspection (Figs. 53-13 and 53-14). The 30 degree scope is usually sufficient for most work done in the periphery.

ILIOPSOAS BURSOSCOPY

Positioning

Flexion is slightly less (15 to 20 degrees) than that used to view the peripheral compartment. The hip is externally rotated; this moves the lesser trochanter to a position that is more anterior and accessible to the portals.

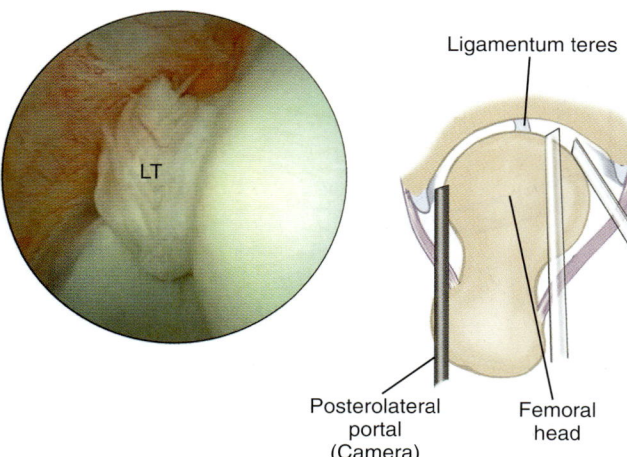

Ligamentum teres

LT

Posterolateral
portal
(Camera)

Femoral
head

Figure 53-9. The acetabular fossa can be inspected from all three portals to view the ligamentum teres (LT) with its accompanying vessels traversing in a serpentine fashion from its more posteriorly placed acetabular attachment. *(Courtesy Smith & Nephew Endoscopy, Andover, Mass [artwork]. Reprinted with permission. Byrd JWT: The supine position. In Byrd JWT, editor: Operative hip arthroscopy, New York, 1998, Thieme Medical Publishers [arthroscopic image].)*

Portals

Two portals are needed for viewing and using instrumentation within the bursa (Fig. 53-15). These portals are distal to those used for the peripheral compartment and require fluoroscopy for precise positioning. They may be slightly more anterior for complete access to the area of the lesser trochanter.

Diagnostic Procedure

The spinal needle is placed directly on the lesser trochanter under fluoroscopy. With the arthroscope introduced, a second portal is established. Adhesions or fibrinous debris within the bursa may have to be débrided to achieve clear visualization (see Fig. 53-15). Staying next to bone avoids straying into the medial soft tissues.

TROCHANTERIC BURSOSCOPY (PERITROCHANTERIC SPACE)

Positioning

Positioning is the same as for arthroscopy of the central compartment, but no traction is needed.

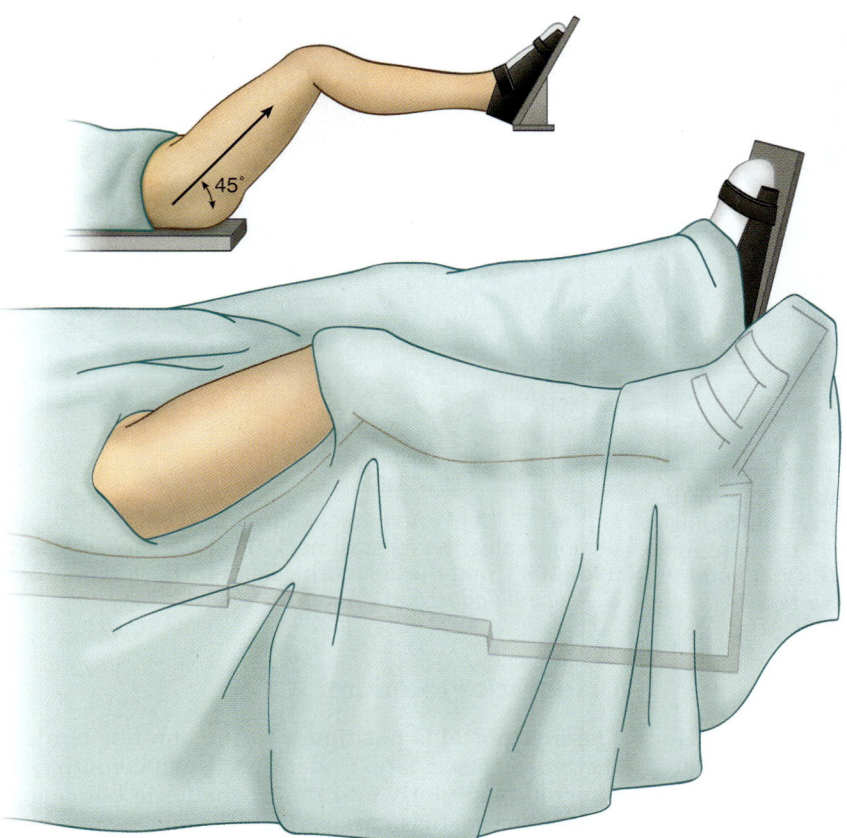

45°

Figure 53-10. The operative area remains covered in sterile drapes while traction is released and the hip is flexed 45 degrees. *Inset,* Illustrates the position of the hip without the overlying drape.

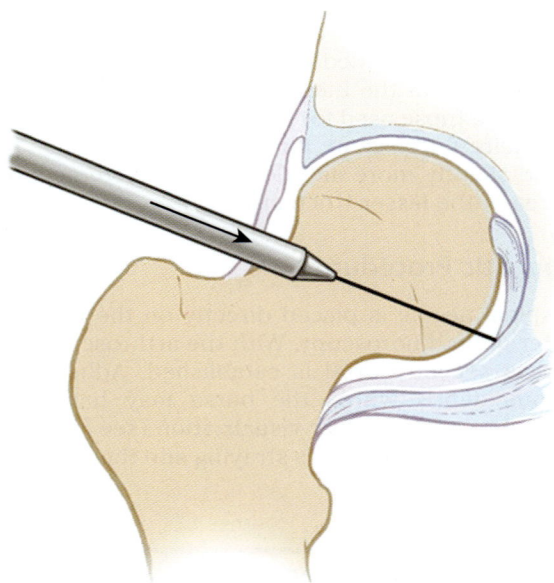

Figure 53-11. From the anterolateral entry site, the arthroscope cannula is redirected over the guide wire through the anterior capsule onto the neck of the femur. *(Courtesy Smith & Nephew Endoscopy, Andover, Mass.)*

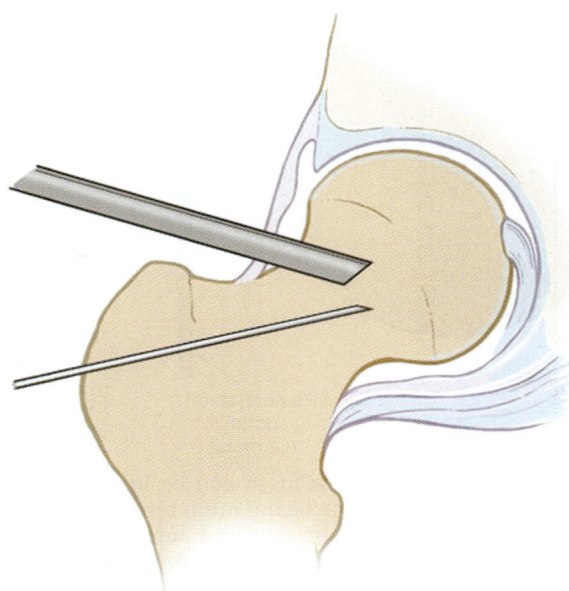

Figure 53-12. With the arthroscope in place, prepositioning is performed with a spinal needle for placement of an ancillary portal distally. *(Courtesy Smith & Nephew Endoscopy, Andover, Mass.)*

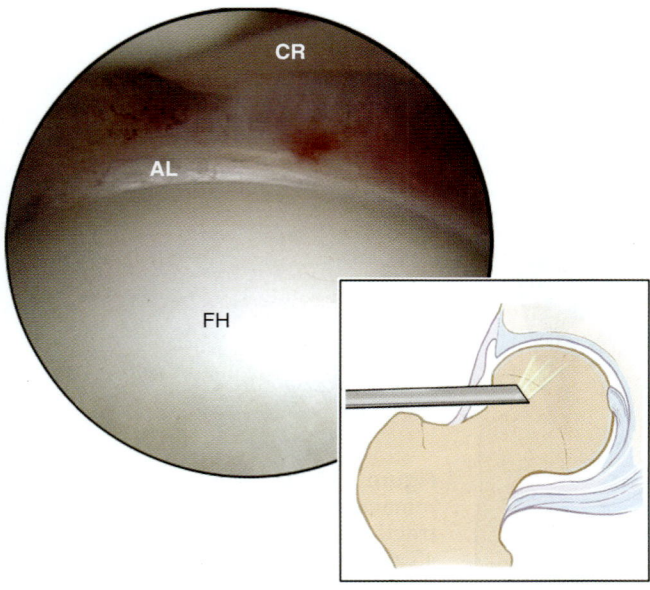

Figure 53-13. Peripheral compartment viewed superiorly demonstrates the anterior portion of the joint, including the articular surface of the femoral head (FH), the anterior labrum (AL), and the capsular reflection (CR). *(Courtesy Smith & Nephew Endoscopy, Andover, Mass [artwork].)*

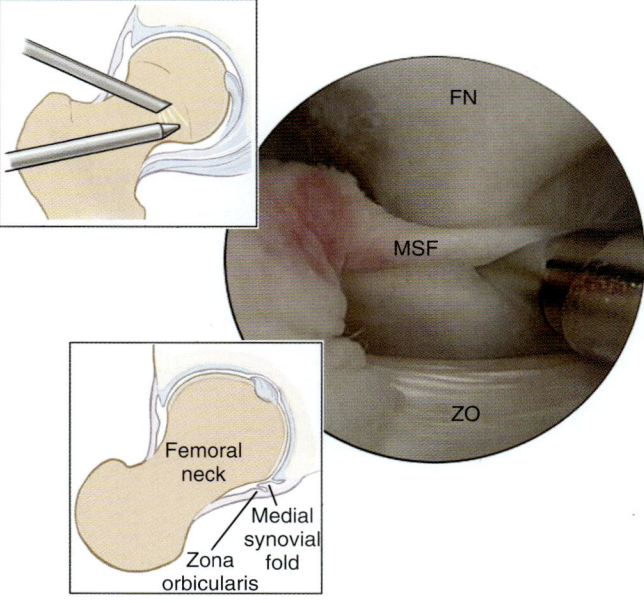

Figure 53-14. Peripheral compartment viewed medially demonstrates the femoral neck (FN), the medial synovial fold (MSF), and the zona orbicularis (ZO). *(Courtesy Smith & Nephew Endoscopy, Andover, Mass [artwork].)*

Portals

At least two portals are needed for routine endoscopy. These are best placed from the anterior for initial development of the space within the trochanteric bursal region (Fig. 53-16). Supplementary portals may be needed for various operative procedures.

Diagnostic Procedure

The first portal is positioned at the anterior border of the tensor fascia lata. Under fluoroscopic control, it is directed posteriorly into the trochanteric bursa at the level of the vastus lateralis ridge. Placing the portal just lateral to this ridge aids in having the cannula pass

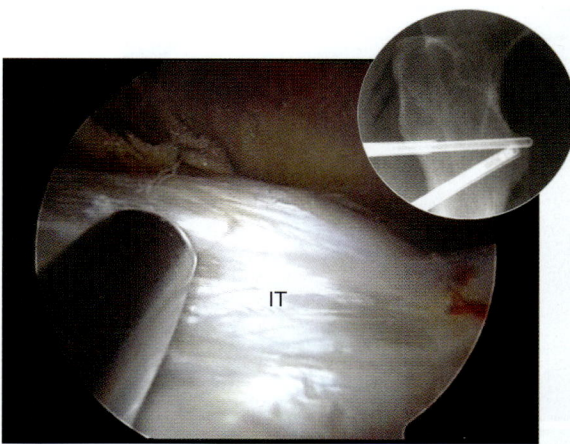

Figure 53-15. The arthroscope and the shaver are positioned within the iliopsoas bursa directly over the lesser trochanter, allowing identification of the fibers of the iliopsoas tendon (IT) at its insertion site.

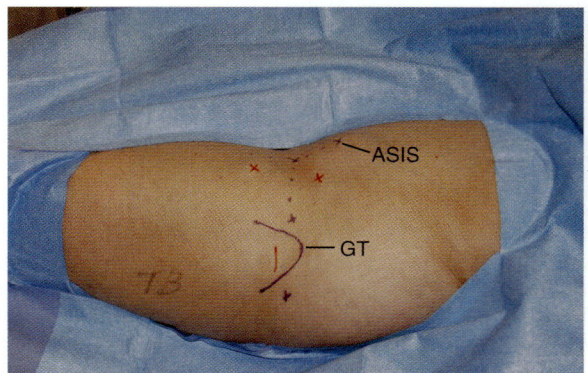

Figure 53-16. Viewed from this left hip, two portals (red x's) provide access to the peritrochanteric space from the anterior position. These are positioned proximal and distal to the vastus lateralis ridge, which is marked on the surface by a red line. The greater trochanter (GT) and the anterior superior iliac spine (ASIS) are marked, as are standard arthroscopy portals for the central compartment (purple x's). *(Courtesy J. W. Thomas Byrd, MD, Nashville, Tenn.)*

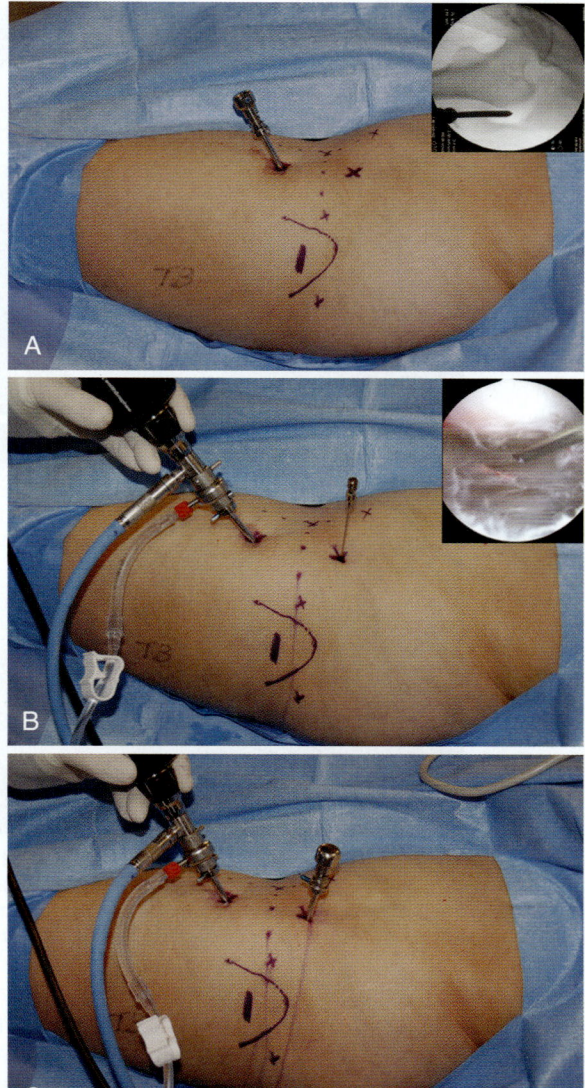

Figure 53-17. A, The distal portal is placed into the peritrochanteric space. The fluoroscopic image illustrates positioning of the portal underneath the iliotibial band at the vastus lateralis ridge, which is the lateral-most prominence of the greater trochanter. This location avoids penetration of the gluteus medius or the vastus lateralis. **B,** The second portal is then placed under direct arthroscopic visualization. Prepositioning is performed with a 17 gauge spinal needle. **C,** A working portal has been established, and arthroscopy is facilitated by switching the arthroscope and instruments between the two portals. *(Courtesy J. W. Thomas Byrd, MD, Nashville, Tenn.)*

underneath the iliotibial band without perforating the muscular portion of the gluteus medius insertion or the vastus lateralis origin immediately above and below the vastus ridge (Fig. 53-17). Under direct arthroscopic visualization, a second portal is then placed above the initial portal for removal of debris and development of the trochanteric space.

SPECIFIC SITUATIONS AND RESULTS

Labral Débridement

Labral débridement can be performed effectively via the three standard portals. Small capsulotomies at the portal sites improve maneuverability to allow access to the damaged tissue. The focus is selective débridement with removal of damaged tissue while healthy tissue is

preserved and a stable transition zone created (Fig. 53-18). Excessive labral excision has deleterious effects.[13] Most damaged tissue can be débrided with a mechanical shaver. Conservative thermal treatment with a radiofrequency device can aid in creating a smooth transition to healthy tissue, preserving more of the labral substance. Because cellular water content is increased in diseased tissue, it preferentially responds to thermal application. The response of healthy labrum

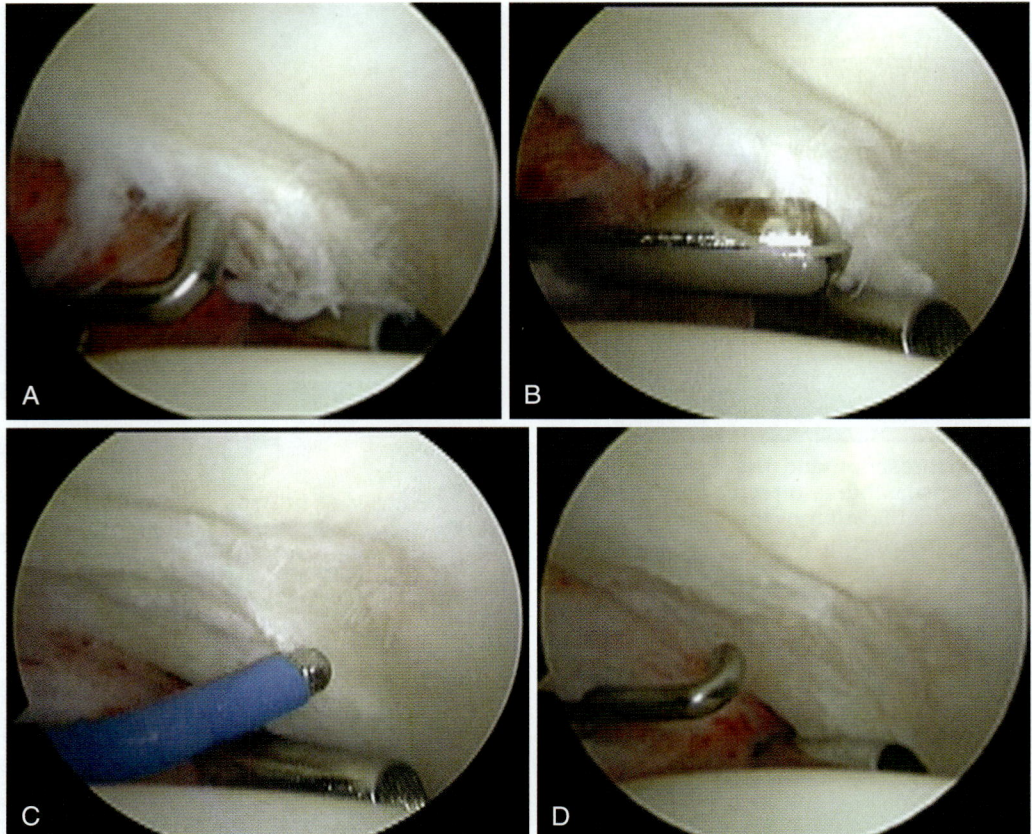

Figure 53-18. Arthroscopic view of the right hip from the anterior portal. **A,** A fragmented labral tear with degeneration within its substance is identified. **B,** Débridement is initiated with the power shaver. **C,** A portion of the comminuted labral tear is conservatively stabilized with a radiofrequency probe. **D,** The damaged portion has been removed, preserving the healthy substance of the labrum. *(Courtesy J. W. Thomas Byrd, MD, Nashville, Tenn.)*

is less brisk and provides a visual indication of a healthy transition zone. After simple débridement procedures have been performed, crutches are used for only a few days to normalize gait, and normal activities may be cautiously resumed within 1 to 2 months.

The labrum is the most frequently damaged structure in the hip, and tears are the most predictably recognized pathology observed with imaging technology. Numerous reports on labral débridement in the hip have been put forth describing moderately favorable results.[14-16] Excessive labrectomy leads to more quickly progressive degenerative disease.[13] Byrd and Jones reported 83% successful outcomes at 10 years' follow-up among patients without arthritis.[17] Similar to the findings of other studies, patients with evidence of arthritis did poorly. Most of these studies predate some of our current understanding of the causes of labral tears, especially femoroacetabular impingement.

Labral Repair

Simple labral repair can be performed by coapting the tear to the articular edge of the acetabular rim (Fig. 53-19). The greatest damage is typically noted on the articular surface of the labrum, while the capsular side is patent and is not violated with this technique. More commonly, labral mobilization and refixation are performed in conjunction with acetabular rim trimming for pincer impingement; these are addressed from the capsular side (see Chapter 54).

With simple repair, suture anchors are placed adjacent to the articular surface on the articular side of the labrum. A more distally based portal is usually necessary to ensure that the anchor diverges from the surface of the acetabulum, thus avoiding perforating the subchondral bone (Fig. 53-20). The articular surface is visualized while the anchor hole is drilled. Subtle rippling of the articular cartilage may be the only indication that the hole violates the subchondral bone. If this occurs, the position must be changed. Placing the anchor onto the face of the articular surface is not necessary to reapproximate the labrum to the acetabular rim. Unlike the shoulder, the goal is not to create a bolster, but simply to re-create the labral seal. Placing the anchor too far away from the articular surface does not allow the labral seal to be reconstituted and is thus ineffective in re-creating any of the protective labral function.

Because most tears extend from the anterolateral rim of the acetabulum, accessory portals for anchor placement are typically found between the anterolateral and anterior portals. A large-diameter disposable cannula is

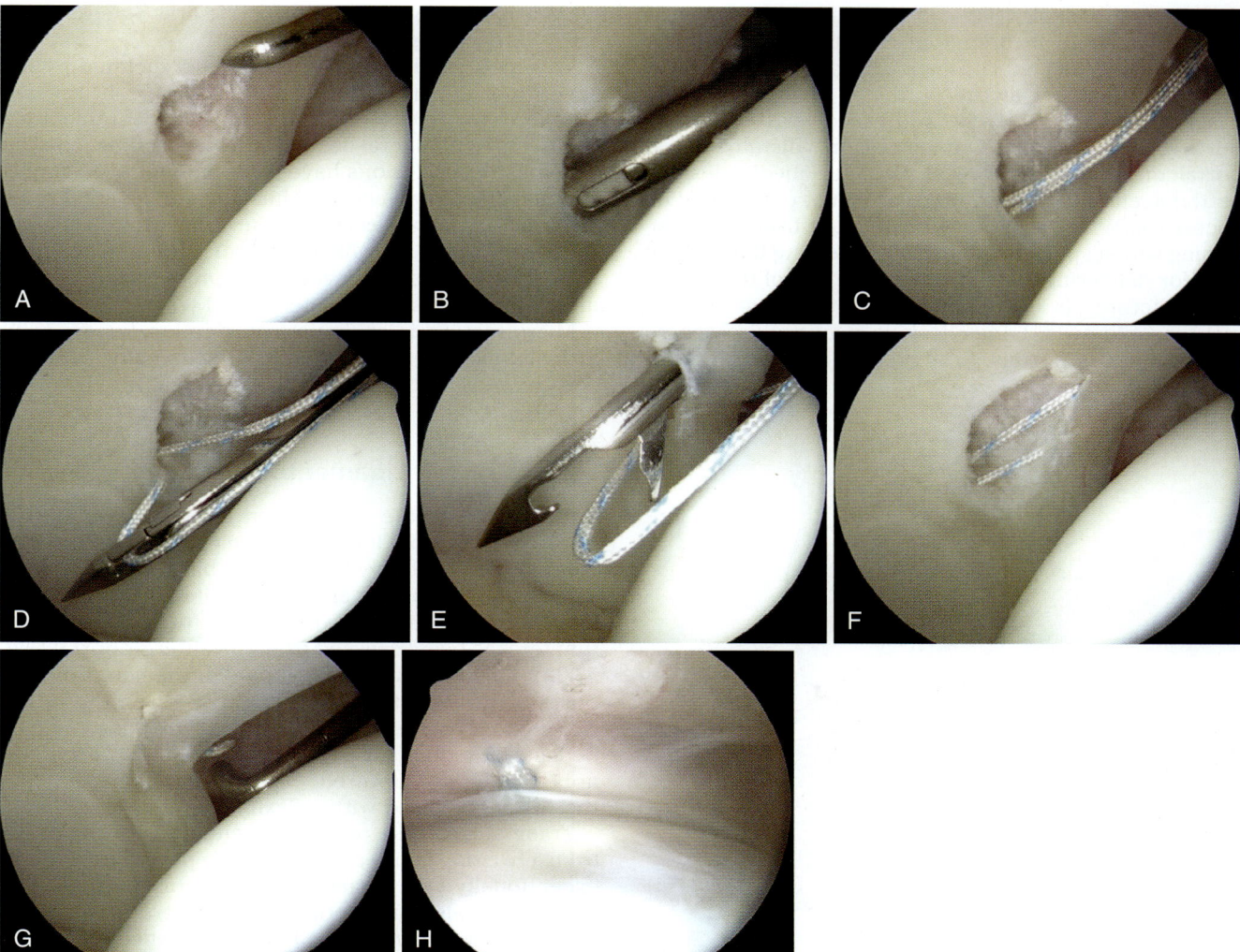

Figure 53-19. A right hip is viewed from the anterolateral portal. **A,** A tear of the anteromedial labrum is probed. **B,** A suture anchor is being seated at the acetabular rim. **C,** Both suture limbs lie anterior to the labrum. **D,** One suture limb is being passed deep into the hip. **E,** The penetrating device has been passed through the labrum to grasp this limb of the suture. **F,** Both suture limbs have been passed through the labrum in a mattress fashion. **G,** The suture has been tied, securing the labrum back to the acetabular rim. **H,** Viewed from the peripheral compartment, the repair suture is away from the articular surface of the femoral head. *(Courtesy J. W. Thomas Byrd, MD, Nashville, Tenn.)*

needed in the anterior or anterolateral portal for suture management. The suture limbs are passed through the substance of the labrum with soft tissue penetrator devices or suture shuttle technique. If the quality of the tissue is sufficient, it is preferable to place the sutures in a mattress fashion to avoid suture interposition of material being between the labrum and the articular surface of the femoral head. Sometimes, looping the suture may be necessary (but less desirable) to ensure approximation of tissue of reasonable quality. After repair, crutches are used for 1 month; during this time, external rotation and maximal flexion, which might stress the repair site, are avoided. Full healing is anticipated at about 3 months.

Early data on labral repairs have been reported with modest results.[18,19] These results will undoubtedly improve with refinement of repair techniques and enhanced understanding of appropriately selected lesions. Greater experience is being gained in labral refixation performed in conjunction with correction of pincer impingement.

Chondroplasty/Microfracture

Chondroplasty is performed with hand instruments and mechanical shavers via the three standard portals with maneuverability facilitated by small capsulotomies. Like the labrum, judicious use of a radiofrequency (RF) device may aid in creating a stable transition zone, allowing preservation of a greater amount of healthy cartilage. Indiscriminate use can be detrimental, resulting in greater chondrocyte cell death. Crutches are used only for comfort, and recovery can be variable depending on the severity of the damage.

Microfracture is appropriately indicated for grade IV lesions with healthy surrounding cartilage, especially in younger individuals (Fig. 53-21). Specially designed curettes may aid in preparing the subchondral bone, removing the calcified layer, and sharply creating stable articular shoulders at the border of the lesion. Most cases can be effectively addressed with standard portals, but sometimes an accessory distally based portal may improve access. Also, for medial lesions on the acetabular side, a more proximal portal may be necessary. When accessory portals are used, prepositioning with a spinal needle aids in selecting the optimal spot for delivering instruments to the site of the lesion. Microfracture is performed with various angled arthroscopic awls. Larger lesions may require access from numerous portals. Protected weight bearing with

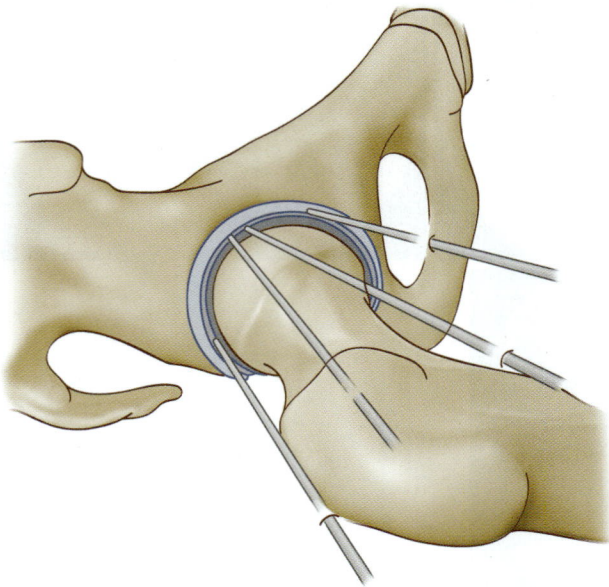

Figure 53-20. Viewed from the right hip, a more distally based entry site is used for anchor placement *(arrow)* to ensure that it diverges from the articular surface of the acetabulum. *(Courtesy J. W. Thomas Byrd, MD, Nashville, Tenn.)*

emphasis on range of motion for the first 8 weeks facilitates fibrocartilaginous healing.

Results of chondroplasty are usually dictated by the severity of the global degenerative disease. In general, chondral treatment tends to be less favorable than treatment with labral lesions. However, data confirm that most labral lesions have some amount of accompanying articular damage, and imaging studies tend to be less reliable for assessing the severity of the articular problem. Thus, the likelihood of chondral damage should be anticipated, even when preoperative assessment may suggest an isolated labral tear.

Microfracture is an imperfect solution for grade IV articular lesions, but the results are generally favorable and the morbidity is minimal, other than the inconvenience of a more protracted rehabilitation strategy.[20-22]

Lesions of the Ligamentum Teres

The function of the ligamentum teres in adulthood is poorly understood. Indiscriminate resection of the ligament should probably be avoided, but ruptures can be a source of symptoms and can be effectively débrided. Like most contents of the acetabular fossa, the ligamentum teres is best accessed from the anterior portal (Fig. 53-22). This is complemented by débridement from the posterolateral portal, which can best reach the posterior contents of the fossa. Curved shaver blades may be beneficial. Redundant portions of the ligament that are not completely ruptured can be decompressed and thermally stabilized with a flexible RF device.

Traumatic rupture of the ligamentum teres can occur from a twisting injury and has been reported to respond exceptionally well to arthroscopic débridement.[23] The ligament is also susceptible to degenerative rupture, especially a hypertrophic form often encountered in conjunction with dysplasia.[24] Lesions of the ligamentum teres can be quite painful; although they may respond to arthroscopic débridement, sometimes other associated pathology may be more of a determinant of the outcomes of treatment.

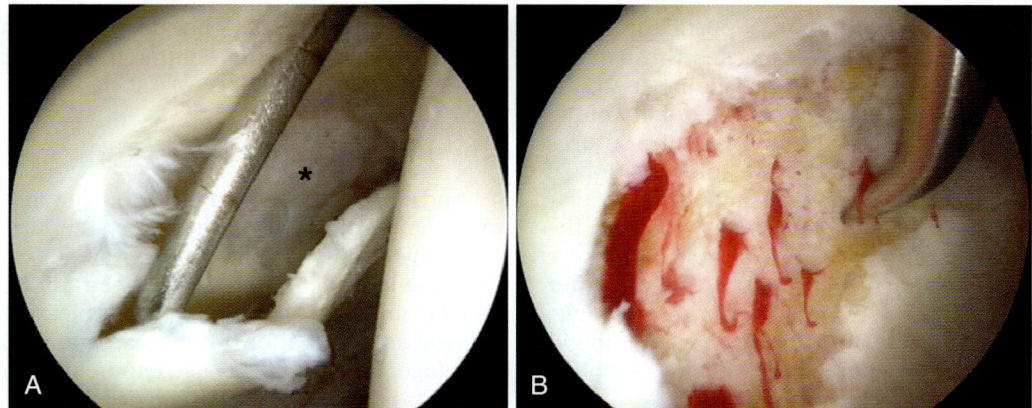

Figure 53-21. Right hip viewed from the anterolateral portal. **A,** Grade IV articular delamination of the anterolateral acetabulum is being unroofed with a probe, revealing the underlying subchondral bone *(asterisk).* **B,** An arthroscopic awl is being used to create multiple perforations into the subchondral bone, resulting in vascular return. *(Courtesy J. W. Thomas Byrd, MD, Nashville, Tenn.)*

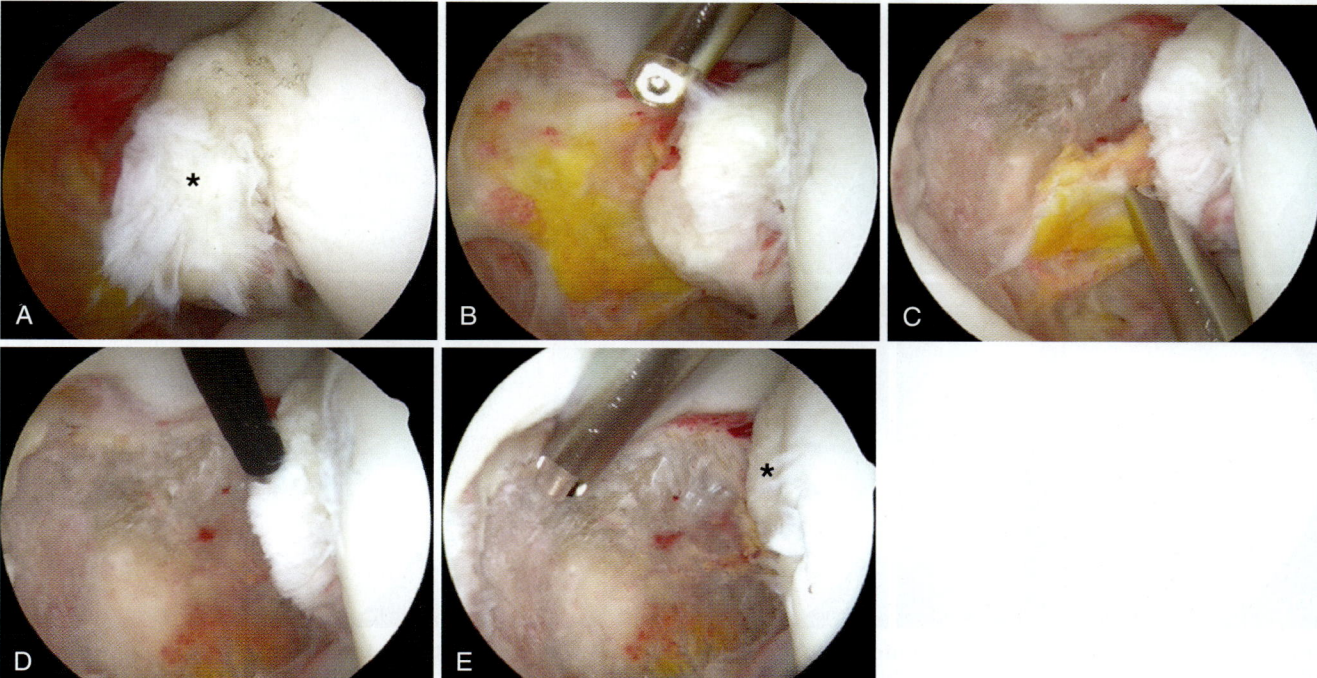

Figure 53-22. The right hip is viewed from the anterolateral portal. **A,** A ruptured ligamentum teres is identified *(asterisk).* **B,** Initial débridement is begun with a shaver from the anterior portal. **C,** Débridement is continued with the shaver from the posterolateral portal. **D,** Decompression of some of the redundant fibers is completed with a flexible radiofrequency (RF) device. **E,** Débridement of the ruptured portion is complete, preserving some of the intact inferior fibers *(asterisk).* *(Courtesy J. W. Thomas Byrd, MD, Nashville, Tenn.)*

Synovectomy

Although a total synovectomy cannot be performed, an extensive arthroscopic synovectomy can be accomplished (Fig. 53-23). Synovial disease may emanate from the acetabular fossa and can be excised from the anterior and posterolateral portals with straight and curved shaver blades aided by RF ablation. However, more diffuse disease necessitates access from the peripheral compartment. Standard arthroscopy portals, as well as numerous adjunct portals, may be necessary to complete the synovectomy.

Although few reports have described arthroscopic synovectomy in the hip, the indications are comparable to those established for other joints. Synovectomy for inflammatory arthritides is infrequently necessary because of improved pharmacologic management. The most common synovial disorder reported in the literature is synovial chondromatosis.[25,26] When the lesions are ossified, the diagnosis is usually evident, but when they are nonossified, the diagnosis may be elusive on preoperative studies and may become evident only at the time of arthroscopy.[25] In this author's experience, the second most common synovial disease encountered in the hip is pigmented villonodular synovitis (PVNS). This may present in a nodular or diffuse pattern. Arthroscopic synovectomy seems to be an appropriate first line of surgical management, especially because secondary joint damage is often advanced at the time of initial presentation and may contraindicate an extensive open procedure. Regardless of the technique used, close follow-up for residual or recurrent disease is important.

Loose Bodies

Retrieval of symptomatic loose bodies represents the clearest indication for hip arthroscopy (Fig. 53-24). The diagnosis is often evident, the importance of loose body removal has been well substantiated, and arthroscopy offers a much less invasive alternative to traditional open techniques.[27,28] Retrieval can be difficult. Graspers of various sizes with various angles and some with teeth may be needed for retrieval. If soft tissue attachments are present, leaving a small tag makes it easier to grasp the fragment rather than chasing it as it floats free in the joint. Small loose bodies can be retrieved through conventional cannulas, and slotted cannulas aid in retrieval of larger ones. It is important to dilate the soft tissues before attempting to retrieve sizable loose bodies. They are most likely to dislodge at the capsule, fascia, and skin. Thus deeply incising these areas can be important for clearing the retrieved fragments. In the peripheral compartment, various supplementary portals can be used as needed to access free fragments.

The origin of loose bodies is variable and includes synovial chondromatosis, trauma, and sequelae of osteochondritis dissecans with Perthes disease. The prognosis is variable, depending on associated pathology, but retrieval of symptomatic fragments is often

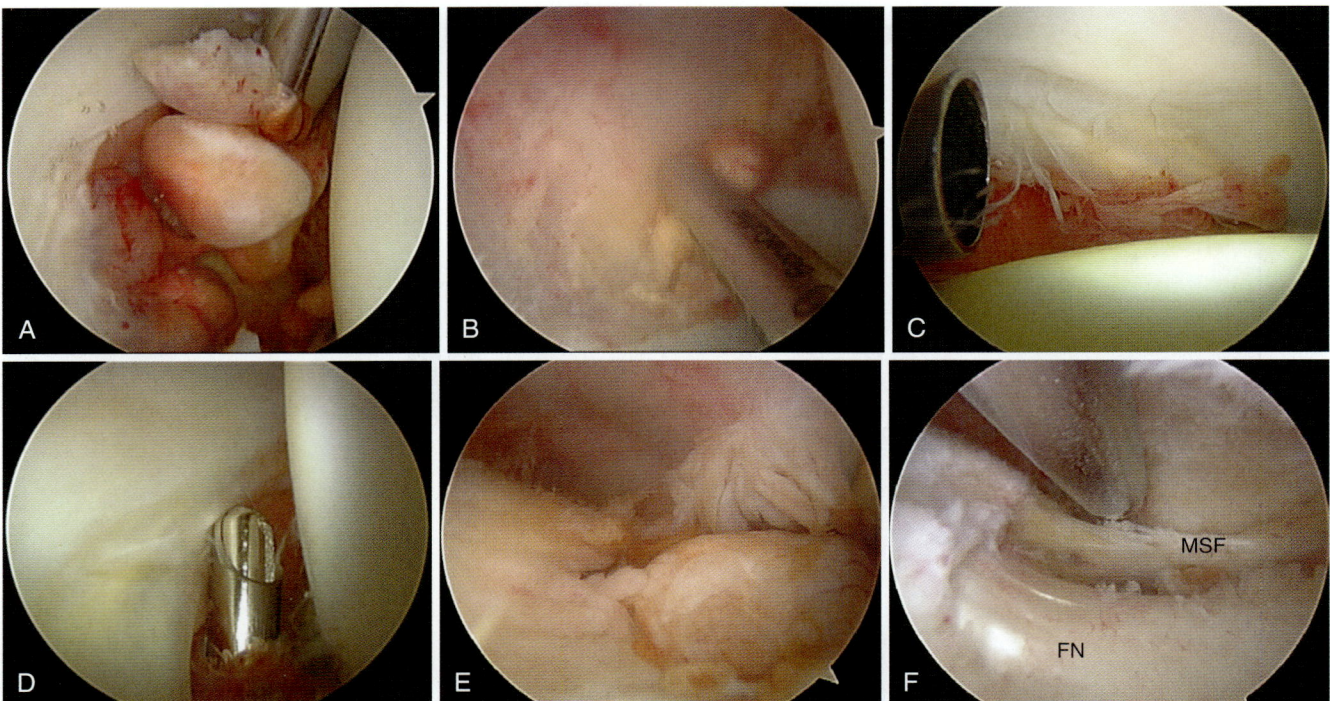

Figure 53-23. The right hip with pigmented villonodular synovitis is viewed from the anterolateral portal. **A,** Viewed medially, synovial disease within the acetabular fossa is débrided from the anterior portal. **B,** Synovectomy of the fossa is completed with the shaver from the posterolateral portal. **C,** Viewed posteriorly, further synovial disease is evident behind the labrum. **D,** Synovectomy of the posterior capsule is accomplished from the posterolateral portal. **E,** Viewed in the periphery, the normal anatomy is obscured by synovial disease. **F,** The same view after synovectomy reveals the anterior neck of the femur (FN) and the medial synovial fold (MSF). *(Courtesy J. W. Thomas Byrd, MD, Nashville, Tenn.)*

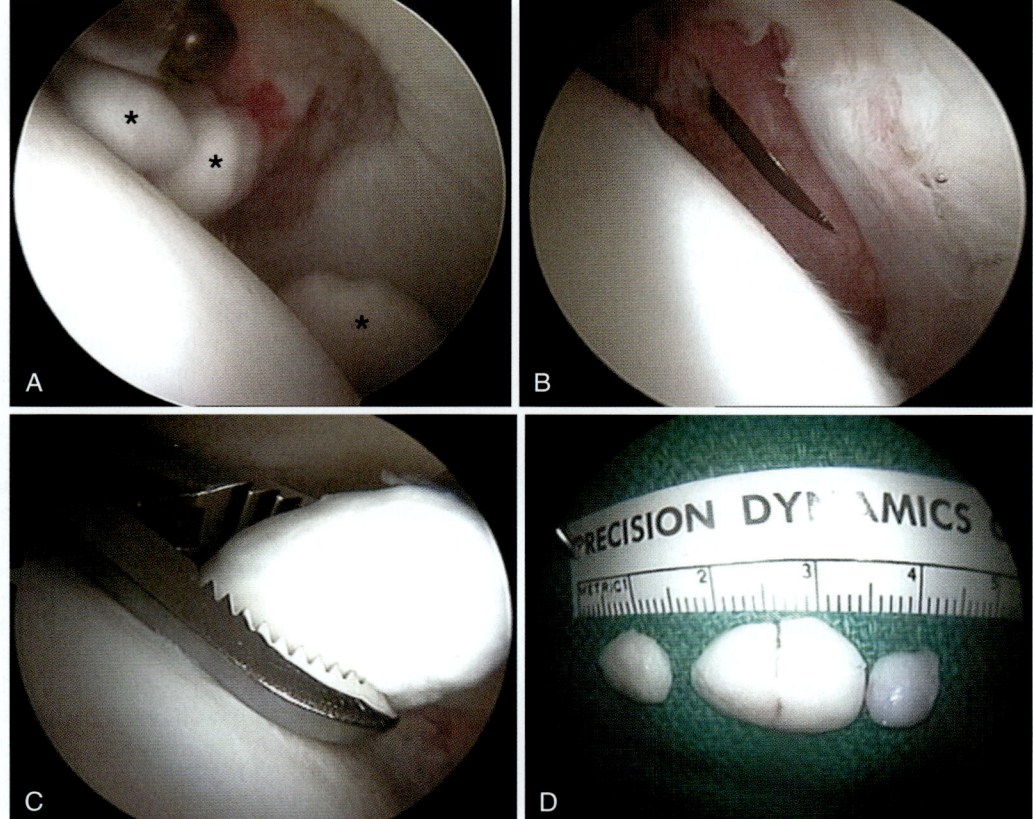

Figure 53-24. Arthroscopic view of the right hip from the anterolateral portal. **A,** Viewed medially, loose bodies are identified *(asterisks).* **B,** Viewed anteriorly, the anterior capsular incision is enlarged with an arthroscopic knife to facilitate removal of the fragments. **C,** One of the fragments is being retrieved. **D,** Loose bodies can be removed whole. *(Reprinted with permission from Byrd JWT: Hip arthroscopy in athletes. In Byrd JWT, editor: Operative hip arthroscopy, ed 2, New York, 2005, Springer, pp 195–203.)*

gratifying and avoids further secondary damage due to third body wear. With synovial chondromatosis, it is difficult to ensure a complete synovectomy, and residual disease can lead to recurrence of loose bodies, necessitating repeat arthroscopy.

Iliopsoas Tendon

Three methods are available for transecting the tendinous portion of the iliopsoas. One, which is not formally described in the literature, is performed from the central compartment while the hip is under traction. The tendon is exposed by incising the capsule medially from the anterior portal. The tendinous portion is then transected (Fig. 53-25).

A more popular technique is performed via the peripheral compartment (Fig. 53-26).[29] A window is made in the thin medial capsule above the zona orbicularis at the level of the medial synovial fold. Opening the capsule will expose the tendinous portion of the

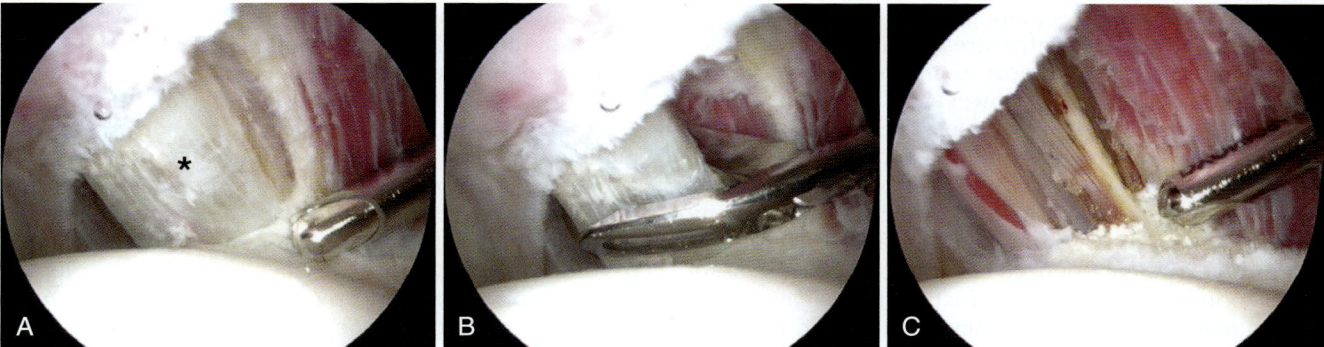

Figure 53-25. A, Viewed anteriorly from the anterolateral portal in the central compartment of this right hip, the iliopsoas tendon has been exposed *(asterisk)*. B, The tendon is released with a cutting hand instrument. C, The tendon is then released, revealing the muscular portion, which is preserved. *(Courtesy J. W. Thomas Byrd, MD, Nashville, Tenn.)*

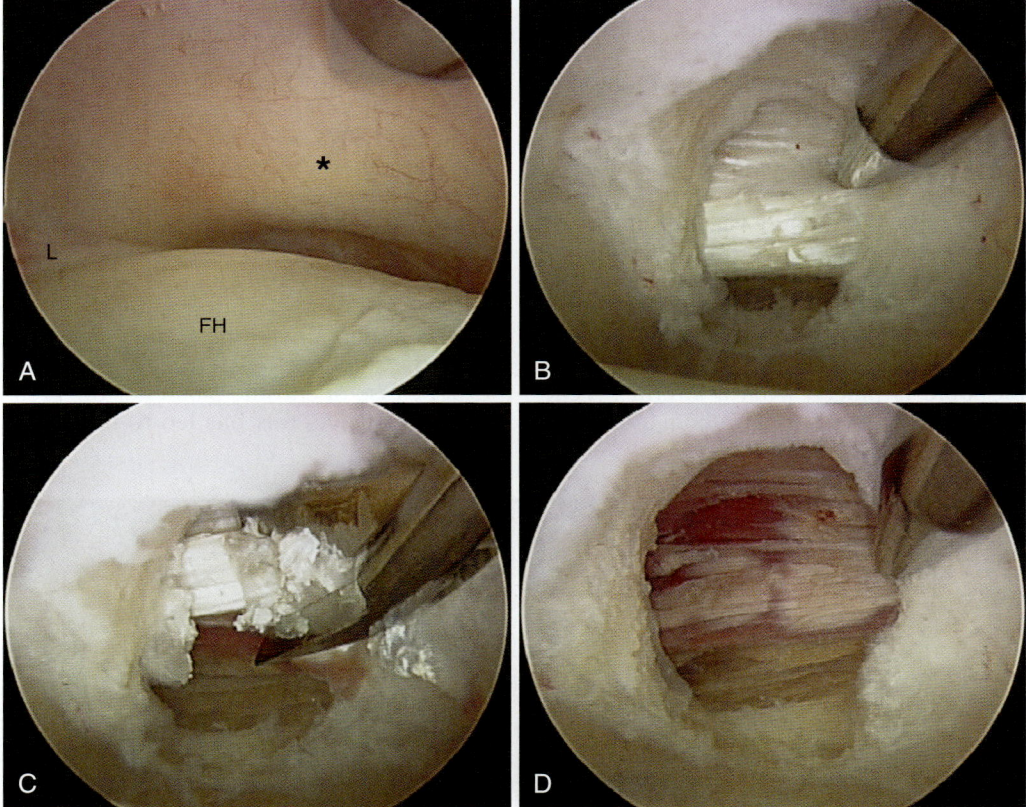

Figure 53-26. The right hip is viewed from the peripheral compartment. A, Fibers of the iliopsoas tendon *(asterisk)* are visible through the thin medial capsule anterior to the femoral head (FH) and labrum (L). This is located directly above the zona orbicularis at the level of the medial synovial fold. B, A small capsular window is created, exposing the iliopsoas tendon. C, A cutting hand instrument is used to release the tendinous portion of the iliopsoas. D, The tendon has been released, revealing the muscular portion of the iliopsoas, which is preserved. *(Courtesy J. W. Thomas Byrd, MD, Nashville, Tenn.)*

iliopsoas, which is then transected with combinations of hand cutters, shavers, and RF. The femoral neurovascular structures lie anterior and is separated from the operative field by the psoas muscle.

A third technique is performed within the iliopsoas bursa, releasing the tendon from its insertion on the lesser trochanter. The small muscular portion of the iliacus, which attaches directly to bone, is preserved (Fig. 53-27).[2,3]

Snapping of the iliopsoas tendon often occurs as an incidental asymptomatic finding. Surgery is indicated only if symptomatic snapping is intolerable to the patient despite conservative treatment. With a correct diagnosis, surgery is almost uniformly successful in eliminating the snapping. However, in a few cases, the source of the snapping may be less well defined, resulting in a small failure rate. Several reports have documented that most cases have associated intra-articular pathology, emphasizing the importance of arthroscopy of the joint in conjunction with release of the tendon.[2,3] In a prospective randomized study, Ilizaliturri and associates obtained comparable results by releasing the tendon from the peripheral compartment and from the lesser trochanter.[30] Residual hip flexor weakness is one potential concern of this procedure, but it is rarely a symptomatic problem. Heterotopic ossification has been reported as a complication of surgical release of the iliopsoas; thus this operation warrants prophylaxis with a nonsteroidal anti-inflammatory medication.[31] Crutches are used for 2 to 4 weeks to regain a normal gait pattern with return to full activities anticipated at 3 months.

Snapping Iliotibial Band

Snapping of the iliotibial (IT) band can be effectively corrected with a simple incisional tendoplasty.[4] A modified cruciate method originally reported as an open procedure has been adapted to an endoscopic technique performed from within the peritrochanteric space (Fig. 53-28).[32] Viewing takes place from within the space, and an arthroscopic knife is placed from a lateral percutaneous approach. An 8 to 10 cm longitudinal incision is made in the IT band directly over the greater trochanter with two small pairs of 1 to 1.5 cm transverse cuts. The loose edges may be débrided, but further resection is not necessary. The length of the incisions is dictated by the size of the patient and the amount of tightness. A diamond-shaped incision has also been described, performed from the superficial surface (Fig. 53-29). This is exposed by developing a space within the overlying subcutaneous tissues. With either technique, immediate weight bearing is allowed with crutches as necessary for 1 to 2 weeks. Aggressive activities are avoided for the first 2 months to allow adequate return of muscle strength and hip girdle function.

Snapping of the IT band is a common asymptomatic condition that rarely requires surgical intervention. Incisional tendoplasties have proved effective with minimal morbidity and ease of recovery, and are amenable to endoscopic adaptation. Extensive z-plasty techniques have been described but represent much more complex procedures for a relatively simply problem, offering no advantage with the burden of greater morbidity.[33,34] Correction of a snapping IT band is a simple procedure that requires thoughtful attention to the details. Inadequate release may fail to resolve the disorder, but excessive release can compromise the abductor mechanism, resulting in a virtually unsalvageable problem.

Trochanteric Bursectomy

Endoscopic trochanteric bursectomy is easily performed with standard portals for the peritrochanteric space (see Figs. 53-16 and 53-17). Removal of adhesions and bursal tissue is facilitated by switching between two anteriorly based portals. This is sometimes used simply as a preliminary step in developing the peritrochanteric space.

Trochanteric bursectomy is reserved for recalcitrant painful trochanteric bursitis that has failed conservative treatment, including activity modification, physical therapy, and corticosteroid injections. However, the exact cause of chronic pain over the greater trochanter is often elusive; this has led to use of the term *greater*

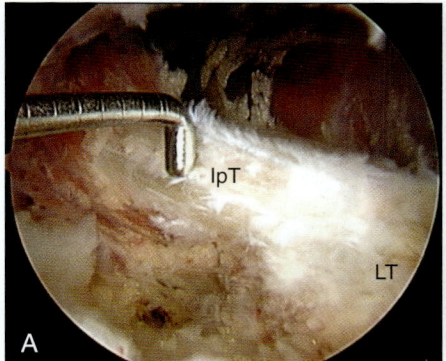 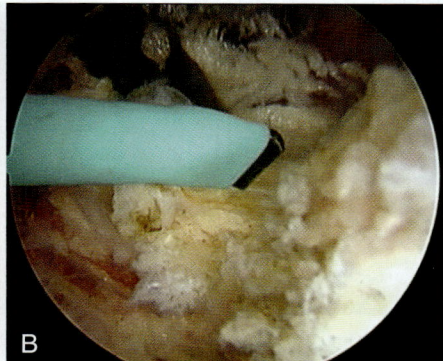 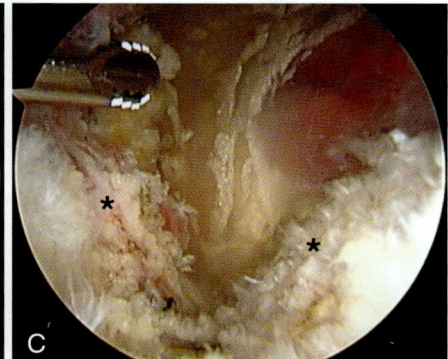

Figure 53-27. View from the iliopsoas bursa of the right hip. **A,** The iliopsoas tendon (IpT) is being probed adjacent to its insertion on the lesser trochanter (LT). **B,** A flexible radiofrequency (RF) device is being used to divide the tendon. **C,** Completing the division, the tendon edges *(asterisks)* are noted to separate. *(Courtesy J. W. Thomas Byrd, MD, Nashville, Tenn.)*

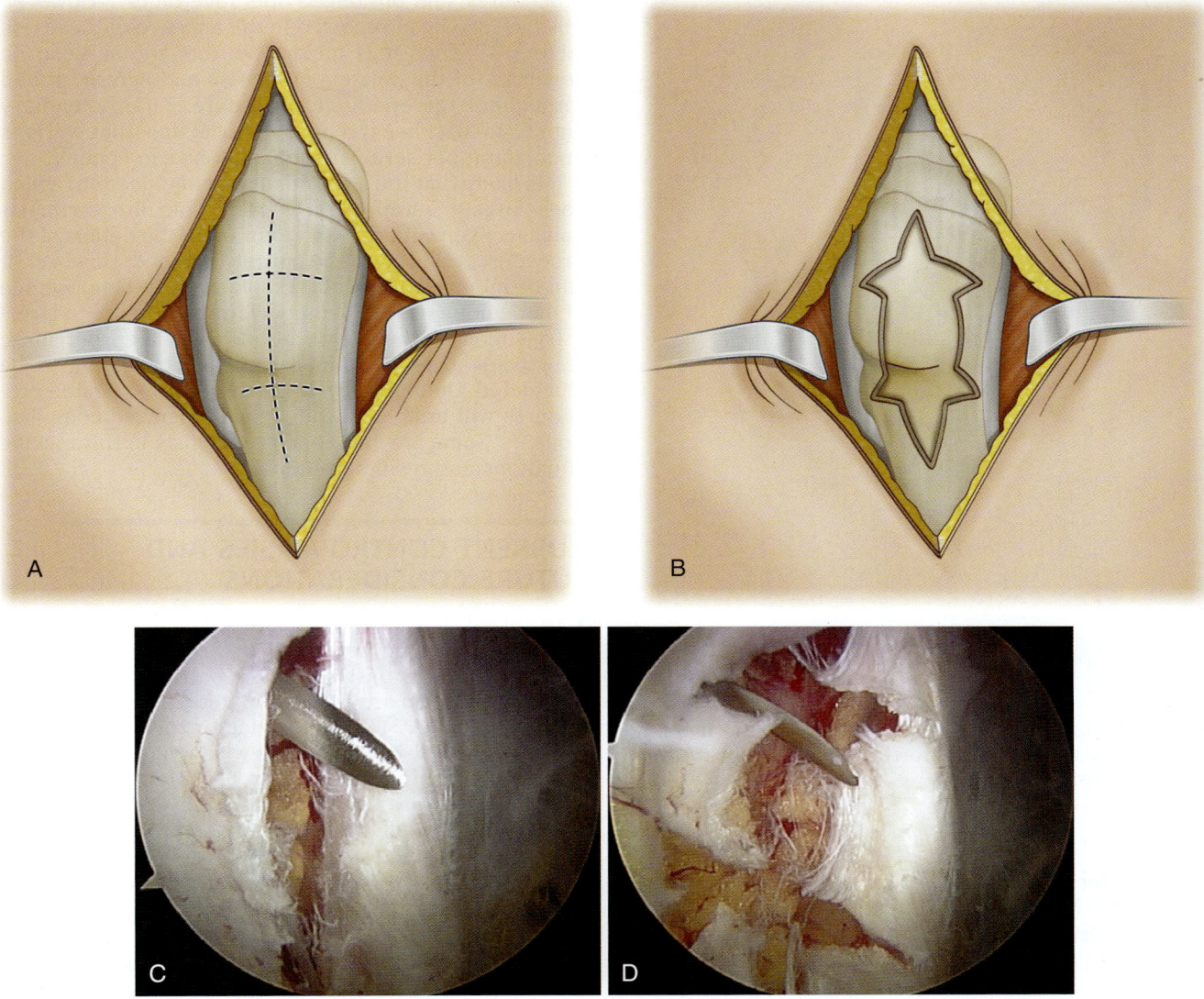

Figure 53-28. A, Illustration depicts the modified cruciate incision. **B,** A relaxing effect on the iliotibial band is illustrated. **C,** As viewed from the peritrochanteric space of a right hip from the anterior portal, the longitudinal limb of the modified cruciate incision is being created with an arthroscopic knife. **D,** The modified cruciate incision is being completed with relaxation of the iliotibial band. *(Courtesy J. W. Thomas Byrd, MD, Nashville, Tenn.)*

trochanteric pain syndrome, which is less specific but perhaps more accurate in encompassing other causes of lateral pain besides simple bursitis.[7] Because of the sometimes elusive nature of the diagnosis, the results of bursectomy, although often favorable, can be variable.[5,6]

Abductor Tendinopathies

Débridement of partial tears of the gluteus medius or minimus can be performed. However, partial tears often exist on the deep surface, covered by intact tendon, and may be less evident without unroofing the intact portion. Repair can be performed by using techniques comparable with rotator cuff repair in the shoulder (Fig. 53-30). The insertion site is prepared by light decortication,

developing a bleeding bony bed to stimulate healing of the repair. Anchors with high pull-out strength are necessary for secure fixation. The tendon edges are lightly débrided to ensure reapproximation of quality tissue. Sutures can be passed using a variety of retrograde and antegrade techniques. Crutches are necessary for 6 weeks, and an abduction brace may help to protect the repair site. Precautions are necessary for up to 4 months.

Management of abductor tendinopathies is in a state of evolution. Tendinopathies are often diagnosed on magnetic resonance imaging (MRI). However, this type of tendon degeneration may occur as a normal consequence of aging; thus it is important that the patient's clinical findings correlate with the documented pathology. Endoscopic management may be appropriately

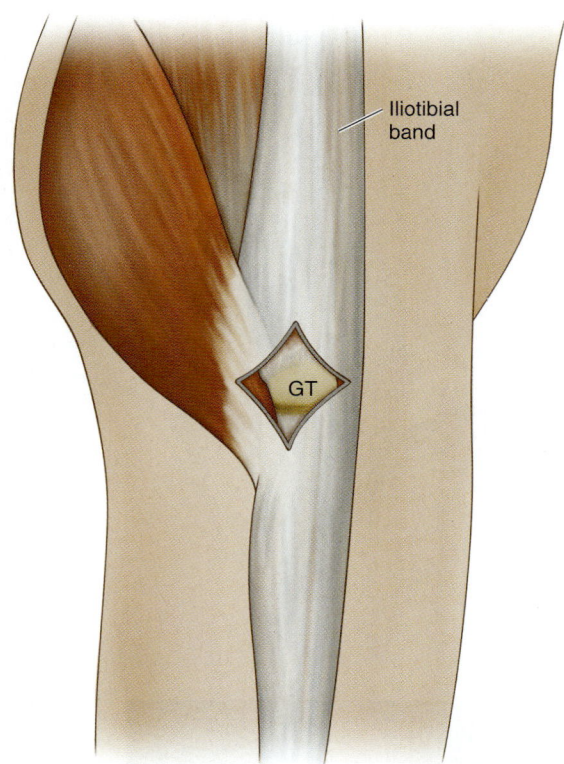

Figure 53-29. A diamond-shaped release of the iliotibial band as described by Ilizaliturri. *(Courtesy J. W. Thomas Byrd, MD, Nashville, Tenn.)*

indicated for recalcitrant cases that fail conservative treatment.[35] More favorable results may be expected with traumatic lesions with good quality tissue.

COMPLICATIONS

Reported complication rates associated with large hip arthroscopy series range from 1.3% to 6.4%.[36-38] Most of these complications are minor or transient, but a few major complications have been reported. Traction neuropraxia is usually associated with prolonged procedures and excessive traction but can occur even within established guidelines. With normal precautions, it is expected that the condition should be transient and recovery complete. Direct trauma to the major neurovascular structures should be avoidable with thoughtful orientation to the landmarks and careful technique in portal placement. The consequences of these types of injuries are generally devastating. Small branches of the lateral femoral cutaneous nerve invariably lie around the anterior portal. Even with careful technique, there is a 0.5% chance of incurring a small patch of reduced sensation in the lateral thigh with the use of instrumentation around one of these branches.

Potentially life-threatening intra-abdominal extravasation of fluid has been reported.[39] This is generally attributed to fresh acetabular fractures, extra-articular procedures, and prolonged operative times.[37] However, this has also been reported in the absence of these risk factors.[40,41] Thus it is imperative that the surgeon be cognizant of the balance of ingress and egress of fluid throughout the operative procedure. Fatal pulmonary embolism has been reported, reflecting that various uncommon but serious complications can occur.[42]

It is likely that the most common complication, which goes largely unreported, is iatrogenic intra-articular damage. Even with careful attention to the details of the procedure, this cannot be entirely avoided. However, it can be minimized, and this emphasizes the importance of meticulous technique in performing the procedure.

Last, many of the complications associated with more recent advanced techniques are just beginning to be elucidated. Undoubtedly, these more sophisticated procedures will bring a new array of recognized complications.[43,44] Some are mentioned previously in the specific situations and results sections.

CURRENT CONTROVERSIES AND FUTURE CONSIDERATIONS

- Dysplasia is not a contraindication to arthroscopy, but it cannot be corrected by arthroscopic means. Arthroscopy is best suited for patients with painful symptoms who are not candidates for periacetabular osteotomy (PAO) because of factors of age and severity of damage, but who otherwise still are not candidates for total hip arthroplasty. The role of arthroscopy in patients who are candidates for PAO is limited. Caution is needed because an arthroscopic procedure may provide transient relief, delaying a PAO and ultimately resulting in further avoidable secondary damage. Occasionally, arthroscopy may be beneficial as a staging procedure and in assessing the severity of damage and helping to determine the value of PAO.
- Many cases of FAI are amenable to arthroscopic intervention, but some are better served by open techniques. Another question remains regarding how clearly arthroscopic correction of FAI is superior to simpler arthroscopic procedures that address only secondary damage. More morbidity and protracted recovery are associated with these more extensive procedures. Time will tell whether these results are better than those described with some historically reported simpler techniques.
- Labral preservation makes sense, and the purpose of an intact labrum has been well defined. However, it is unclear how this equates to management of a damaged labrum. Unique technical and rehabilitation challenges associated with labral repair do not exist with simple débridement procedures. The hope is that labral repair restores labral function, providing better long-term results.
- Abductor tendinopathies may be clinically relevant but sometimes exist as coincidental findings on MRI. Defining who can benefit from technical abilities to repair the tendon remains a work in progress.
- Reconstructive procedures are being developed. Autologous tissue has been used to restore a deficient

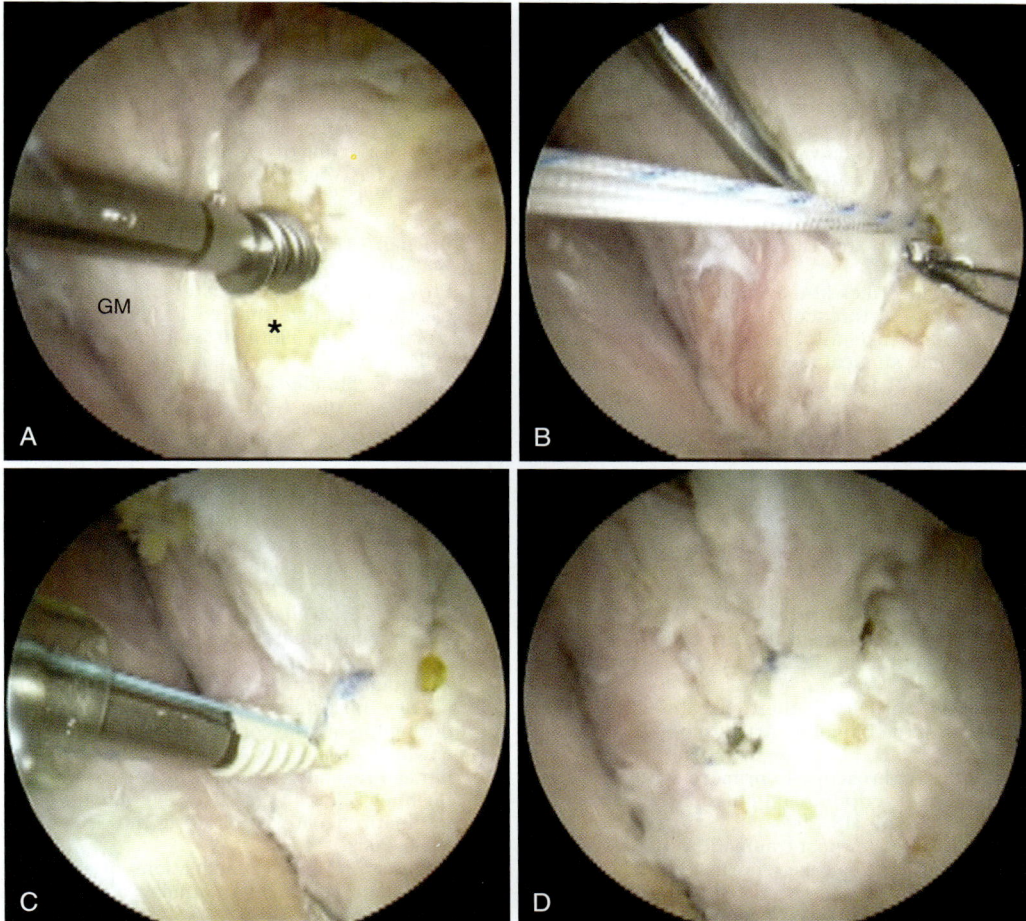

Figure 53-30. The peritrochanteric space of the right hip is viewed from an anterior portal. **A,** A suture anchor is being inserted into the bony bed of the footprint *(asterisk)* of the gluteus medius tendon. The tendon (GM) has been retracted posteriorly. **B,** A penetrating device has been passed through the anterior fiber of the gluteus medius to shuttle the sutures through the tendon. **C,** The tendon has been reapproximated to the footprint with the suture limbs passed through a knotless anchor for further distal fixation. **D,** The final fixation construct is viewed with the tendon restored to the greater trochanter. *(Courtesy J. W. Thomas Byrd, MD, Nashville, Tenn.)*

labrum, but its current clinical application is not defined. The role of the ligamentum teres in adulthood is not understood, but preliminary methods for ligament reconstruction have already been developed. Similar to other joints, restoration of lost articular cartilage is an unsolved problem. Microfracture has some efficacy with minimal morbidity, but better restorative methods are clearly needed.

• The distinction between arthroscopic and open methods will become less clear as open methods become less invasive, and as the arthroscope finds a role in arthroscopically assisted open techniques.

REFERENCES

1. Philippon MJ, Kuppersmith DA, Wolff AB, Briggs KK: Arthroscopic findings following traumatic hip dislocation in 14 professional athletes. Arthroscopy 25:169–174, 2009.
2. Byrd JWT: Evaluation and management of the snapping iliopsoas tendon. Instr Course Lect 55:347–355, 2006.
3. Ilizaliturri VM, Villalobos FE, Chaidez PA, et al: Internal snapping hip syndrome: treatment by endoscopic release of the iliopsoas tendon. Arthroscopy 21:1375–1380, 2005.
4. Ilizaliturri VM, Jr, Martinez-Escalante FA, Chaidez PA, Camacho-Galindo J: Endoscopic iliotibial band release for external snapping hip syndrome. Arthroscopy 22:505–510, 2006.
5. Fox JL: The role of arthroscopic bursectomy in the treatment of trochanteric bursitis. Arthroscopy 18:E34, 2002.
6. Baker CL, Jr, Massie RV, Hurt WG, Savory CG: Arthroscopic bursectomy for recalcitrant trochanteric bursitis. Arthroscopy 23:827–832, 2007.
7. Kingzett-Taylor A, Tirman PF, Feller J, et al: Tendinosis and tears of gluteus medius and minimus muscles as a cause of hip pain: MR imaging findings. AJR Am J Roentgenol 173:1123–1126, 1999.
8. Byrd JWT, Jones KS: Diagnostic accuracy of clinical assessment, MRI, gadolinium MRI, and intraarticular injection in hip arthroscopy patients. Am J Sports Med 32:1668–1674, 2004.
9. Byrd JWT: The supine approach. In Byrd JWT, editor: Operative hip arthroscopy, ed 2, New York, 2005, Springer, pp 145–169.
10. Byrd JWT: Hip arthroscopy by the supine approach. Instr Course Lect 55:325–336, 2006.
11. Byrd JWT, Pappas JN, Pedley MJ: Hip arthroscopy: an anatomic study of portal placement and relationship to the extraarticular structures. Arthroscopy 11:418–423, 1995.
12. Byrd JWT: Avoiding the labrum in hip arthroscopy. Arthroscopy 16:770–773, 2000.
13. Espinosa N, Beck M, Rothenfluh DA, et al: Treatment of femoroacetabular impingement: preliminary results of labral

refixation. Surgical technique. J Bone Joint Surg Am 89(Suppl 2):36–53, 2007.

14. Farjo LA, Glick JM, Sampson TG: Hip arthroscopy for acetabular labrum tears. Arthroscopy 13:409, 1997.

15. Santori N, Villar RN: Acetabular labral tears: result of arthroscopic partial limbectomy. Arthroscopy 16:11–15, 2000.

16. Kamath AF, Componova R, Baldwin K, et al: Hip arthroscopy for labral tears: review of clinical outcomes with 4.8-year mean followup. Am J Sports Med 37:1721–1727, 2009.

17. Byrd JWT, Jones KS: Hip arthroscopy for labral pathology: prospective analysis with 10-year follow-up. Arthroscopy 25:365–368, 2009.

18. Murphy KP, Ross AE, Javernick MA, Lehman RA: Repair of the adult acetabular labrum. Arthroscopy 22:567.e1–567.e3, 2006.

19. Kelly BT, Weiland DE, Schenker ML, Philippon MJ: Arthroscopic labral repair in the hip: surgical technique and review of the literature. Arthroscopy 21:1496–1504, 2005.

20. Byrd JWT, Jones KS: Microfracture for grade IV chondral lesions of the hip. Arthroscopy 20:SS–89,41, 2004.

21. Philippon MJ, Schenker ML, Briggs KK, Maxwell RB: Can microfracture produce repair tissue in acetabular chondral defects? Arthroscopy 24:46–50, 2008.

22. Byrd JWT, Jones KS: Arthroscopic "femoroplasty" in the management of cam-type femoroacetabular impingement. Clin Orthop Relat Res 467:739–746, 2009.

23. Byrd JWT, Jones KS: Traumatic rupture of the ligamentum teres as a source of hip pain. Arthroscopy 20:385–391, 2004.

24. Gray AJR, Villar RN: The ligamentum teres of the hip: an arthroscopic classification of its pathology. Arthroscopy 13:575–578, 1997.

25. McCarthy JC, Bono JV, Wardell S: Is there a treatment for synovial chondromatosis of the hip joint? Arthroscopy 13:409–410, 1997.

26. Boyer T, Dorfmann H: Arthroscopy in primary synovial chondromatosis of the hip: description and outcome of treatment. J Bone Joint Surg Br 90:314–318, 2008.

27. Byrd JWT: Hip arthroscopy for post-traumatic loose fragments in the young active adult: three case reports. Clin J Sport Med 6:129–134, 1996.

28. Epstein H: Posterior fracture-dislocations of the hip: comparison of open and closed methods of treatment in certain types. J Bone Joint Surg Am 43:1079–1098, 1961.

29. Wettstein M, Jung J, Dienst M: Arthroscopic psoas tenotomy. Arthroscopy 22:907.e1–907.e4, 2006.

30. Ilizaliturri VM, Chaidez C, Villegas P, et al: Prospective randomized study of 2 different techniques for endoscopic iliopsoas tendon release in the treatment of internal snapping hip syndrome. Arthroscopy 25:159–163, 2009.

31. Byrd JWT, Polkowski GG, Jones KS: Endoscopic management of the snapping iliopsoas tendon. In Proceedings of the 2009 Annual Meeting of the American Academy of Orthopaedic Surgeons, Las Vegas, February 25–28, 2009, p 787.

32. Byrd JWT: Snapping hip. Oper Techn Sports Med 13:46–54, 2005.

33. Brignall CG, Stainsby GD: The snapping hip: treatment by Z-plasty. J Bone Joint Surg Br 73:253–254, 1991.

34. Provencher MT, Hofmeister EP, Muldoon MP: The surgical treatment of external coxa saltans (the snapping hip) by Z-plasty of the iliotibial band. Am J Sports Med 32:470–476, 2004.

35. Voos JE, Shindle MK, Pruett A, et al: Endoscopic repair of gluteus medius tendon tears of the hip. Am J Sports Med 37:743–747, 2009.

36. Clarke MT, Arora A, Villar RN: Hip arthroscopy: complications in 1054 cases. Clin Orthop Relat Res 406:84–88, 2003.

37. Sampson TG: Complications of hip arthroscopy. Clin Sports Med 20:831–835, 2001.

38. Byrd JWT: Complications associated with hip arthroscopy. In Byrd JWT, editor: Operative hip arthroscopy, New York, 1998, Thieme, pp 171–176.

39. Bartlett CS, DiFelice GS, Buly RL, et al: Cardiac arrest as a result of intraabdominal extravasation of fluid during arthroscopic removal of a loose body from the hip joint of a patient with an acetabular fracture. J Orthop Trauma 12:294–300, 1998.

40. Ladner B, Nester K, Cascio B: Abdominal fluid extravasation during hip arthroscopy. Arthroscopy 26:131–135, 2010.

41. Fowler J, Owens BD: Abdominal compartment syndrome after hip arthroscopy. Arthroscopy 26:128–130, 2010.

42. Bushnell BD, Dahners LE: Fatal pulmonary embolism in a polytraumatized patient following hip arthroscopy. Orthopedics 32:56, 2009.

43. Ilizaliturri VM, Jr: Complications of arthroscopic femoroacetabular impingement treatment: a review. Clin Orthop Relat Res 467:760–768, 2009.

44. Souza BGS, Polesello G, Ono NK, et al: Complications in hip arthroscopy. In Proceedings of the 2009 Annual Meeting of the American Academy of Orthopaedic Surgeons, Las Vegas, February 25–28, 2009, p 787.

CHAPTER 54

Hip Arthroscopy for Structural Hip Problems

Marc Philippon, Bruno G. Schroder e Souza, and Karen K. Briggs

KEY POINTS

- Structural abnormalities are the main causes of labral pathology in the hip.
- Femoroacetabular impingement and developmental hip dysplasia are causes of osteoarthritis in the hip.
- Arthroscopy is an effective, reproducible, and less invasive method of treating intra-articular problems in the hip.
- Morphologic alterations that accompany most of these lesions should be treated at the time of hip arthroscopy.
- Patient selection, correct surgical indication, and observation of the technical aspects of surgery are paramount for the success of the procedure.

INTRODUCTION

Arthroscopy has been used successfully to address intra-articular hip pathology due to functional or morphologic alterations of the hip. Historically, trauma was believed to be the cause of most labral tears in the hip; however, improved understanding of physiopathology has revealed that up to 80% of such lesions are related to subtle structural problems.[1] For many years, this led surgeons to classify most hip osteoarthritis cases as primary or idiopathic.[2,3] However, both the femur and the acetabulum can present with abnormal shapes that predispose to impingement, instability, or both, which ultimately induce degenerative changes of osteoarthritis.[2,4,5] Hip arthroscopy aims to treat intra-articular damage and its causes, preferably in the early stages of the disease. It has been shown to improve symptoms and is expected to improve joint biomechanics to prevent or delay the natural progression of joint degeneration.[5]

A common structural problem is developmental dysplasia of the hip (DDH), in which the acetabulum is shallow, is inclined laterally, and insufficiently covers the femoral head.[6-8] In this situation, the labrum is known to function as a key factor in joint stability and is usually hypertrophic.[6] Higher stress loads on the lateral margin of the acetabulum and labrum were found to occur in an inverse relation to acetabular coverage, as shown by the center edge angle.[9] The lesser the coverage, the greater the stresses that are found, and the earlier joint degeneration is observed.[8,10] Whenever the labrum fails to manage those stresses, it presents with a tear or detachment. Subluxation, joint incongruence, and rapid progression to joint degeneration have been documented.[10,11]

On the other hand, the acetabulum can present with excessive coverage leading to joint impingement at the extremes of range of motion.[12,13] Examples of such morphologic alterations include coxa profunda and protrusio acetabuli, in which the center of rotation of the femoral head lies too medially in an abnormally deep socket.[14] Another condition is general acetabular retroversion, in which the whole acetabulum is oriented posteriorly, producing anterior overcoverage, predisposing to impingement against the femoral neck during hip flexion, and relative undercoverage posteriorly. Focal acetabular retroversion is seen more commonly, and the superior hemisphere of the acetabulum is posteriorly oriented, provoking localized impingement on the anterior superior aspect of the acetabular rim, proximal to the psoas valley or U, in between the origins of the heads of the rectus femoris muscle.[14]

In many instances, the femur is the site of the deformity. A posterior tilt of the femoral head relative to the axis of the femoral neck is often observed after slipped femoral capitis (clinical or subclinical).[2,3,5] The decreased femoral head-neck offset is responsible for a cam effect, in which that region is forced into the acetabulum, especially on hip flexion, adduction, and internal rotation.[12,15] This effect can also be elicited in maximum abduction, when the bump is more laterally based. In many cases, the center of rotation of the femoral head is in line with the femoral neck axis, but insufficient offset is present. Cam deformities seem to be deleterious to the hip joint because they can predispose to impingement at earlier degrees of range of motion, inducing cartilage and labral damage.[9,12,16] Other variations on proximal femur morphology, such as excessive anteversion and coxa valga, can be components of DDH and can worsen joint function.

To restore normal interaction between femur and acetabulum, hip arthroscopy can be used to modify the shape of the femoral head-neck junction and the acetabular rim.[17,18] When correctly indicated, the arthroscopic approach provides the great advantages of effective treatment, low morbidity, reproducibility,[19,20] and excellent results.[21-23]

INDICATIONS/CONTRAINDICATIONS

Hip arthroscopy is indicated to correct intra-articular conditions, specifically, labral tears, chondral lesions, loose bodies, ligament teres pathology, and capsular disease, which often are observed in the presence of trauma or functional or structural alterations in the hip.[24-26] Femoroacetabular impingement (FAI) is probably the most common indication. The presence of symptoms, along with radiographic evidence of impingement and chondral and/or labral lesions, is a clear indication for surgical treatment.[17,23,24,26-28] No conservative measure has been shown to be effective when intra-articular lesions are already present. Operative treatment focuses on improving clearance of hip motion and alleviating femoral abutment against the acetabular rim to relieve pathologic stresses in the labrum and the articular cartilage.[9] This is achieved by acetabular osteoplasty (or rim trimming) and femoral osteochondroplasty (cam resection).[17,18] Localized acetabular retroversion and the presence of an anterior-superior bump in the femoral head-neck junction are optimal indications. A completely deepened socket, as in coxa profunda or protrusio acetabuli cases, is treatable arthroscopically; however, the procedure may be technically demanding. Besides correcting morphologic factors leading to impingement, treatment of concurrent intra-articular lesions is paramount.

Mild hip dysplasia can be treated with arthroscopy.[29] Great functional and pain improvement was reported when intra-articular loose bodies and ligamentum teres tears were present in the dysplastic joint.[29] Although labral repair may reestablish joint physiology in mildly dysplastic joints, no arthroscopic treatment has been developed to date for the treatment of acetabular bone undercoverage. In the presence of hip dysplasia, complete resection of the labrum is contraindicated because the condition worsens joint instability, and this has been related to faster development of joint degenerative disease.[5] More severe hip dysplasia is often better treated with open approaches in young patients.[30] However, even in these patients, hip arthroscopy can be performed before or after reorientating osteotomies to mend intra-articular pathology.[31]

Advanced joint degenerative disease, with massive chondral loss and radiographic joint space of less than 2 mm, has been related to worse outcomes[23] and is a relative contraindication for hip arthroscopy. In such patients, mechanical causes of symptoms such as loose bodies or an entrapped labrum may be possible indications for surgery. Previous hip surgery[32,33] or a history of joint infection[34] is not a contraindication. However, effective revision hip arthroscopy is a demanding procedure because scar tissue is often present, as is altered anatomy in some cases. Extra-articular infection without joint extension should be treated completely before any arthroscopic procedure can be considered because of the risk of development of pioarthrosis. Obesity poses extra difficulty for the procedure, in that joint distraction may be challenging and the instruments can become hard to maneuver or may not reach the necessary depth.[35] Other conditions that impede adequate join distraction such as severe protrusio acetabuli, dense heterotopic bone formation, and joint ankylosis are also contraindications.[35]

PREOPERATIVE PLANNING

Preoperative assessment begins with an adequate history and physical examination.[36,37] The physician should be able to distinguish between intra-articular and extra-articular sources of pain based on symptoms and signs elicited by the evaluation.[6,36,38,39]

Radiographic assessment is paramount in defining the cause of the condition.[18,36,37] Almost all morphologic causes of hip problems can be evident on a series of radiographs (Tables 54-1 and 54-2). The anteroposterior (AP) pelvis in the supine position, a lateral view of the proximal femur (cross-table, Dunn, or its modifications), and a false profile of the pelvis are often enough to disclose both impingement and dysplasia. An AP pelvis roentgenogram should be obtained in all patients. Pelvic positioning must be considered when radiographic signs associated with pincer impingement are interpreted. With the coccyx and the symphysis pubis aligned, the pelvis should be in neutral flexion-extension.[40] Pincer-type impingement can be diagnosed on this view when the patient has acetabular retroversion and coxa profunda.[13] Dysplasia and proximal femur deformities can also be seen on this view.[40,41] Signs of acetabular dysplasia are presented in Table 54-2. The center edge angle is of special interest for surgical planning. Bone resection for correction of pincer deformity should not decrease that angle to below 25 degrees because of the risk of creating instability.[42,43] Intraoperative fluoroscopic methods to quantify the amount of actual resection have been described.[44,45] Another study correlated the amount of resection in millimeters with the reduction in the center edge (CE) angle. The formula derived from that study (CE angle reduction = 1.8 + [0.64 × rim reduction in millimeters]) also provides an estimate for maximal resection.[46]

A lateral view of the proximal femur is essential for the diagnosis of cam impingement. Because the abnormality is typically seen in the anterolateral portion of the head-neck junction, it may not be evident on an AP pelvic radiograph. A cross-table lateral view (with the hip in 10 degrees of internal rotation) is the authors' preferred view. Correlation between radiographs and surgical findings is paramount in guiding resection of the correct amount of bone in the femoral neck. Remnants of the physeal scar can be used to guide the surgeon as to where to begin the femoral osteoplasty. Although insufficient resection can cause persistent impingement, over-resection can lead to risk of femoral neck fracture[47] and may impair an adequate sealing effect in the labrum.[44]

In some cases, signs of dysplasia can be disclosed only in the false profile view of the pelvis, as described by Lequesne.[48] The anterior center edge angle (vertical-center-anterior [VCA]) is calculated in this radiologic view. The patient stands at an angle 65 degrees oblique

Table 54-1. Radiographic Signs of FAI

Type	Measurement	Sign of Impingement	Definition
Pincer	Acetabular retroversion	Crossover sign positive[13]	The anterior acetabular rim line lies lateral to the posterior rim in the cranial part of the acetabulum and crosses the latter in the distal part of the acetabulum, forming a figure-of-eight configuration. This is a sign of focal overcoverage of the anterosuperior acetabulum.
	Acetabular depth	Profunda/protrusio[70]	Coxa profunda is identified when the medial wall of the acetabulum lies on or medial to the ilioischial line. Protrusio acetabuli, which represents the more severe form of coxa profunda, is diagnosed when the femoral head crosses the ilioischial line.
	CE angle	>39 degrees[10]	Angle subtended by a vertical line (in relation to the pelvis) and a line connecting the femoral head center with the lateral edge of the acetabulum.
	Ischial spine sign	Positive[71]	Consists of a preeminent projection of that structure to the pelvis in AP radiograph. It denotes not only global acetabular retroversion, but also the involvement of the whole hemipelvis in the deformity.
	Posterior wall sign	Positive[13]	Indicates the presence of a prominent posterior wall. The posterior line lies lateral to the femoral center; this can cause posterior impingement with reproducible pain in hip extension and external rotation. In a normal hip, the visible outline of the posterior rim descends approximately through the center point of the femoral head. Conversely, a deficient posterior wall has the posterior rim line medial to the femoral head center. A deficient posterior wall is often correlated with acetabular retroversion or dysplasia; an excessive posterior wall can often be seen in hips with coxa profunda or protrusio acetabuli but can also occur as an isolated entity.
	Acetabular inclination	Tonnis angle <0 degrees[72]	Angle is subtended by the horizontal line of the pelvis and the line connecting the most lateral and most medial parts of the sclerotic bone in the acetabular weight-bearing sourcil.
	Congruency	Incongruence (convergent)[41,73]	Incongruence is defined as nonparallel contours of the femoral head and acetabulum. It is considered convergent if the articular distance is increased medially and decreased laterally.
Cam	Alpha angle	>42 to 50 degrees[41,74]	Angle is subtended by the axis of the femoral neck and the line between the center of the femoral head and the point when the head first loses its sphericity.
	Pistol grip deformity	Present[75]	Classic deformity of the femoral head-neck junction in which the offset is lost, resembling the shape of the grip of an old pistol.
	Head-neck offset ratio	<0.17[41,76]	Three parallel lines are drawn, with line 1 drawn through the center of the long axis of the femoral neck, line 2 drawn through the anterior-most aspect of the femoral neck, and line 3 drawn through the anterior-most aspect of the femoral head. The head-neck offset ratio is calculated by measuring the distance between lines 2 and 3 and dividing by the diameter of the femoral head.
	Triangular index	R > r + 2 mm[77]	The radius (r) of the femoral head is measured. Then $\frac{1}{2}$ r and the corresponding perpendicular height (H) to the cortex are measured. The pathologically increased radius (R) is found by applying the Pythagorean law for triangular figures $$(r^2 + H^2 = R^2).$$
	Head-neck offset	<9 mm[78]	Three parallel lines are drawn, with line 1 drawn through the center of the long axis of the femoral neck, line 2 drawn through the anterior-most aspect of the femoral neck, and line 3 drawn through the anterior-most aspect of the femoral head. The head-neck offset is the perpendicular distance between lines 2 and 3.

AP, Anteroposterior; *CE,* center edge; *FAI,* femoroacetabular impingement.

Table 54-2. Radiographic Signs of Hip Dysplasia

Measurement	Sign of Dysplasia	Definition
Acetabular inclination	Tonnis angle >10 degrees[79]	Angle subtended by the horizontal line of the pelvis and the line connecting the most lateral and most medial parts of the sclerotic bone in the acetabular weight-bearing sourcil.
CE angle	<25 degrees[10]	Angle is subtended by a vertical line (in relation to the pelvis) and a line connecting the femoral head center.
Extrusion index[79]	>20%[80]	The femoral head is measured horizontally. The index is calculated by dividing the size of the uncovered portion of the femoral head by the size of the head.
Congruency	Incongruence (convergent)[41,73]	Incongruence is defined as nonparallel contours of femoral head and acetabulum. It is considered divergent if the articular distance is increased laterally and decreased medially.
Shenton's line	Superior migration of the femur[41]	Line formed by the inferior margin of the femoral neck and the superior border of the obturator foramen.
Lateralization of the femoral head	Lateralized (>10 mm)[41]	The hip center is considered lateralized if the medial aspect of the femoral head is greater than 10 mm from the ilioischial line.
Sharps' acetabular angle	>42 degrees[81]	Angle subtended by the horizontal line of the pelvis connecting both teardrop signs and the line of the teardrop to the most lateral point of the acetabular articular surface.
Anterior center edge angle (VCA)	<20 degrees[48]	Angle subtended by the line connecting the center of both femoral heads and the one between the center of the femoral head and the anterior-most edge of the acetabulum articular surface.

CE, Center edge; *VCA*, vertical-center-anterior.

to the x-ray beam, with the foot on the affected side parallel to the x-ray cassette. The focal distance is 1 meter. The beam is centered by using the tip of the greater trochanter as the horizontal center. The vertical center is located midway between the symphysis pubis and the anterior superior iliac spine.[40,41,48] A VCA angle of 25 degrees is regarded as normal, 20 to 25 degrees as borderline, and less than 20 degrees as pathologic. The threshold of abnormality of the VCA angle may be even lower. Some studies suggest that the normal value is equal to or greater than 17 degrees.[49] The presence of hip dysplasia should preclude further bone resection and alerts the surgeon to be more conservative with the labrum. Yet on this view, joint space narrowing on the anterior superior or on the posterior inferior aspect of the acetabulum can be evidence of more advanced joint degeneration than might be expected by isolated analysis of the AP radiograph.[41]

DESCRIPTION OF TECHNIQUES

Arthroscopic Treatment of Femoroacetabular Impingement

After thorough inspection, a capsulotomy is performed about 1 cm distal and parallel to the labral margin. Leaving a cuff of intact capsule next to the labrum will ease visualization of the peripheral compartment and may help to prevent postoperative adhesions. Although preserving the iliofemoral ligament by avoiding excessive anterior extension of the capsulotomy anteriorly is desired, this should not impede adequate exposition and instrumentation. The ligament can be repaired afterward. At all stages, the capsulotomy should be performed under direct visualization. The lateral retinacular vessels, which are an important source of blood supply to the femoral head, lie on the lateral synovial fold and should be at risk if blind manipulation is performed too laterally.[47]

Acetabular Rim Trimming With Labral Takedown

When the labrum is detached at its base, it should be separated in the watershed zone, so that the underlying bone deformity (pincer) can be corrected. The labrum is reattached with suture anchors. First, the chondrolabral junction is delineated by controlled application of a monopolar radiofrequency (RF) chisel to better define the tear to prevent sacrificing healthy labral tissue. Chondral flaps are removed after demarcation with the aid of the same RF device. The area between the labrum and the capsule is then dissected with a shaver, and the labrum is completely detached from the acetabular rim. The acetabular bone overhang, responsible for the pincer deformity, is removed, before or after complete labral detachment, with a motorized burr blade. The amount of rim resection should be estimated preoperatively by analysis of the image examinations. The lateral portal is used to perform most of the resection, although switching of portals is essential for assessment of complete work. The current labral repair technique will be detailed in a separate item.

PEARL

- Use of a radiofrequency device to delineate the limit of the chondro-labral junction prevents the sacrifice of healthy labral tissue and helps to stabilize adjacent acetabular cartilage.

Acetabular Rim Trimming Without Labral Takedown

In cases without labral tear and in which a minimum amount of acetabular bone resection is required, rim trimming can be performed without labral takedown. To obtain adequate space to work between the capsule and the labrum, articular traction is released, the capsulotomy is extended, and the peripheral compartment is usually treated first. With a shaver in the space between the capsule and the labrum, the resection is then performed as planned (Fig. 54-1). Articular traction is introduced again, and inspection of the labrum is performed. The stability of the labrum should be thoroughly inspected to ensure adequate support from the remaining acetabular rim. If inadequate bone remains, failure of the watershed zone is expected (Fig. 54-2). On revision surgery, in cases with no additional fixation of labrum to bone, intraoperative findings showed a labral tear at the transition (watershed) zone and adherence of the labrum to the adjacent capsule, despite no history of new trauma. Anchor placement with suture fixation of the labrum to the acetabulum is recommended despite not taking down the labrum (Fig. 54-3). Besides preventing failure of the watershed zone, this practice allows a more active rehabilitation process, which is believed to help prevent adhesions and to allow early return to most activities.

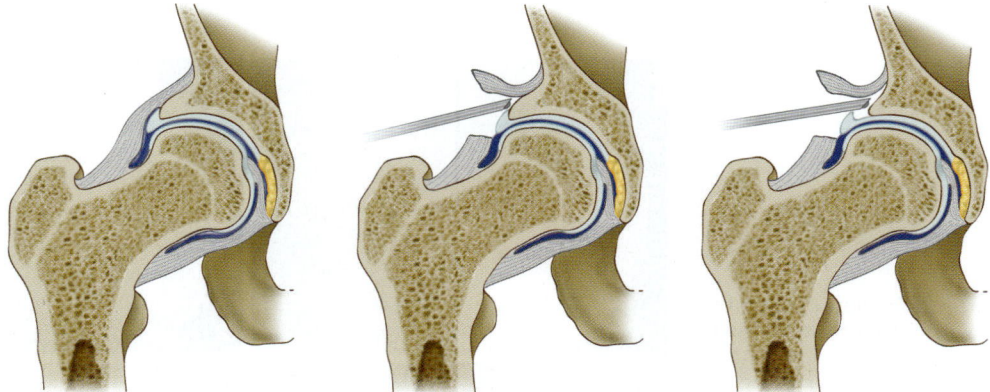

Figure 54-1. Illustration demonstrating rim trimming of the acetabular rim for pincer impingement without takedown of the labrum.

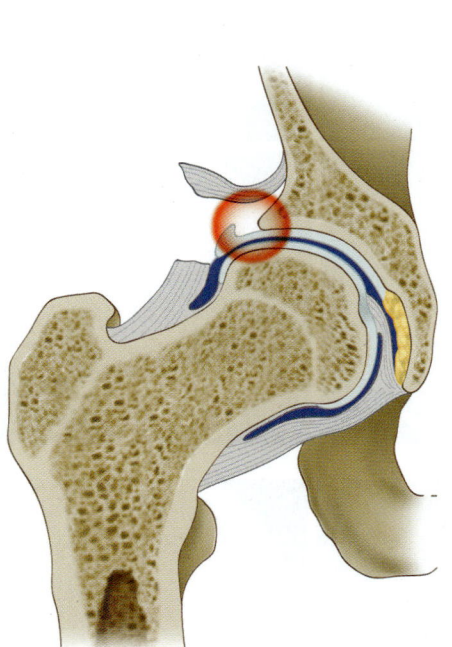

Figure 54-2. If the labrum is not repaired, after rim trimming without labral takedown, the abnormal mobility of the labrum causes the thin chondro-labral junction to fail. Labral tear and capsule-labral adhesions have been documented in this situation.

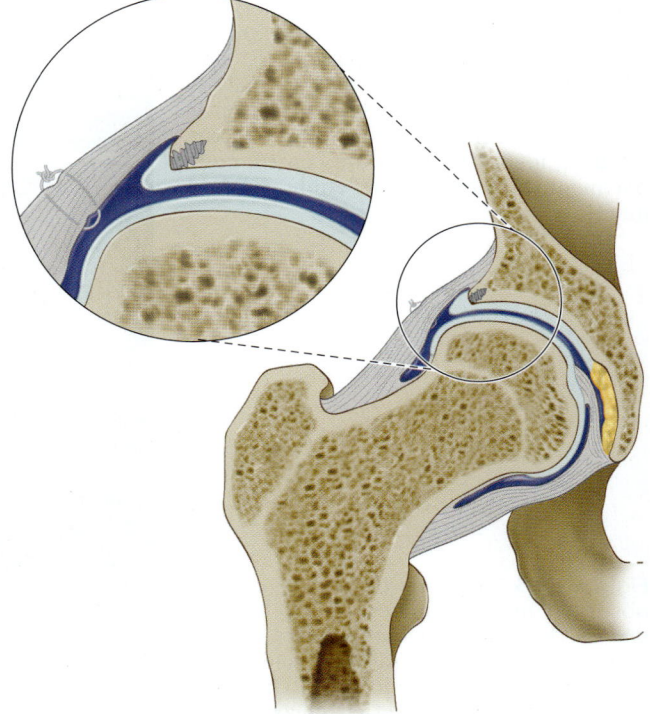

Figure 54-3. Illustration of no labral detachment, but repair of the labrum with anchors. This is advised to allow early rehabilitation.

The technique for anchor placement without labral detachment is similar to that described for labral repair (Figs. 54-4 and 54-5). It may be slightly more difficult to inspect constantly the entry point and the articular surface during anchor insertion. Suture fixation follows the same technique, but with the need to pierce the chondro-labral junction to pass one of the suture limbs between the labrum and the acetabulum.

PITFALL

- After rim trimming without labral takedown, repair with anchors is often necessary to prevent abnormal labral mobility and consequent failure at the watershed zone.

Femoral Osteoplasty (Cam Resection)

It is important to note that isolated pincer lesions occur in only about 10% of cases.[16] In most cases, femoral deformities coexist and should be addressed; not doing so risks treatment failure. To approach the peripheral compartment, traction is released. As the hip is flexed, the capsulotomy is inspected from outside and is enlarged distally to allow better visualization. In some cases, the zona orbicularis may be very tight, and an additional incision starting at the medial aspect of the capsulotomy running distally in the direction of the femoral neck may be necessary. After inspection of the femoral deformity, the femoral head-neck junction is reshaped. Some authors recommended first contouring the bump with the motorized burr, then resecting the

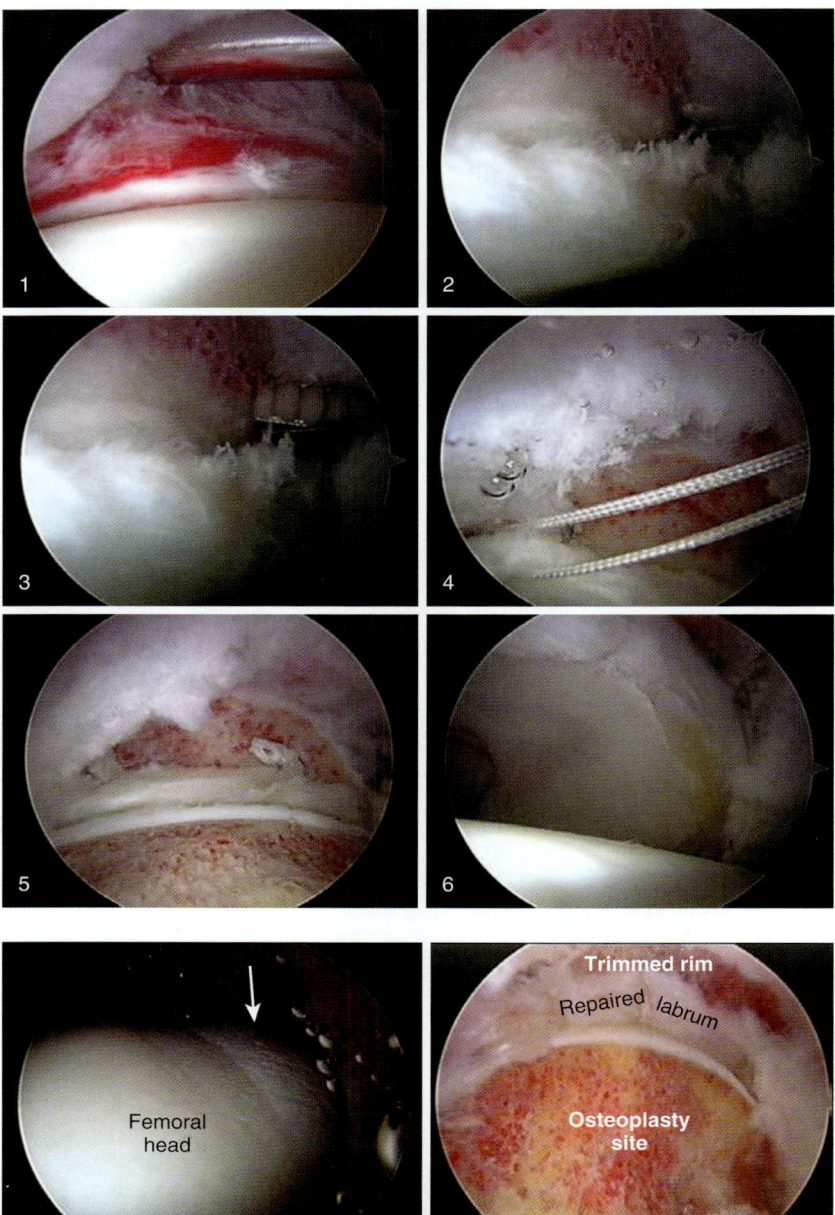

Figure 54-4. Arthroscopic view of acetabular rim trimming without labral takedown. (1) Dissection between the capsule and the labrum is seen (note bruising of the labrum caused by the impingement); (2) after rim trimming, the labrum is attached only to the articular cartilage and a guide is placed to drill the anchor hole; (3) a bioabsorbable anchor is placed on the rim; (4) the suture is looped around the labrum for adequate fixation; (5) with traction released, the labral seal is re-established and good labral fixation is confirmed; and (6) under traction, the repair is inspected from the central compartment showing an intact chondro-labral junction.

Figure 54-5. A, Cam deformity can be observed as a prominent bump (*yellow arrow*). **B,** After the osteoplasty, normal concavity of the femoral head-neck junction is re-established, and the hip is tested dynamically under direct visualization.

bone within the contours. Another approach is to resect the most prominent part of the deformity and progress until visual appraisal of sufficient resection is obtained. In some cases, a thin osteotome may be necessary to remove a medial osteophyte in the femoral head. A preoperative idea of the amount of resection needed can be derived from evaluation of radiographs. The adequacy of the osteoplasty is then confirmed by dynamic evaluation of the joint under direct arthroscopic vision (Fig. 54-6). Any sign of impingement should elicit further bone reshaping or labral contouring. The need for additional labral fixations is commonly noted at this time in the surgery, and suture anchors are used to provide better attachment to the labrum. In athletes, the sports gesture is reproduced to disclose any potential conflict between the femur and the labrum. Further resection is performed as deemed necessary. The objective is to obtain maximum range of motion without impingement. Dynamic fluoroscopy may aid in determining the adequacy of bone resection,[44,45] but it does not substitute for direct arthroscopic inspection.[23] After this, the capsule is closed so that faster healing is obtained and iatrogenic instability can be prevented.[42] The skin is closed in usual fashion, and compressive dressings are applied.

Labral Treatment

Once labral pathology has been evidenced during surgery, correction is necessary. The most common cause of labral lesions is structural alterations.[1] This association must be recognized previously because it demands specific treatment under risk of failure of the surgical repair or suboptimal outcome.[50-52] The strategy used to manage the labrum will depend on the underlying bone morphology, the quality of the labral tissue, and the type of lesion.[50] A causative classification of labral tears can be used to delineate the treatment[36,50,53] (Table 54-3). In the category of labral tears secondary to morphologic alterations (category 1), a large labrum (width ≥7 mm) with a simple tear or detachment usually can be repaired.

In the presence of femoroacetabular impingement (category 1a), acetabular rim trimming, femoral osteoplasty, or both are advised. In this condition, whenever the tissue quality allows, labral repair is preferred to labral débridement.[18,23,52] In cases of severe labral insufficiency, labral reconstruction with iliotibial band autograft may be an option in very active or young patients.[54,55] In cases of isolated fraying and flapping lesions, simple débridement can be considered if the

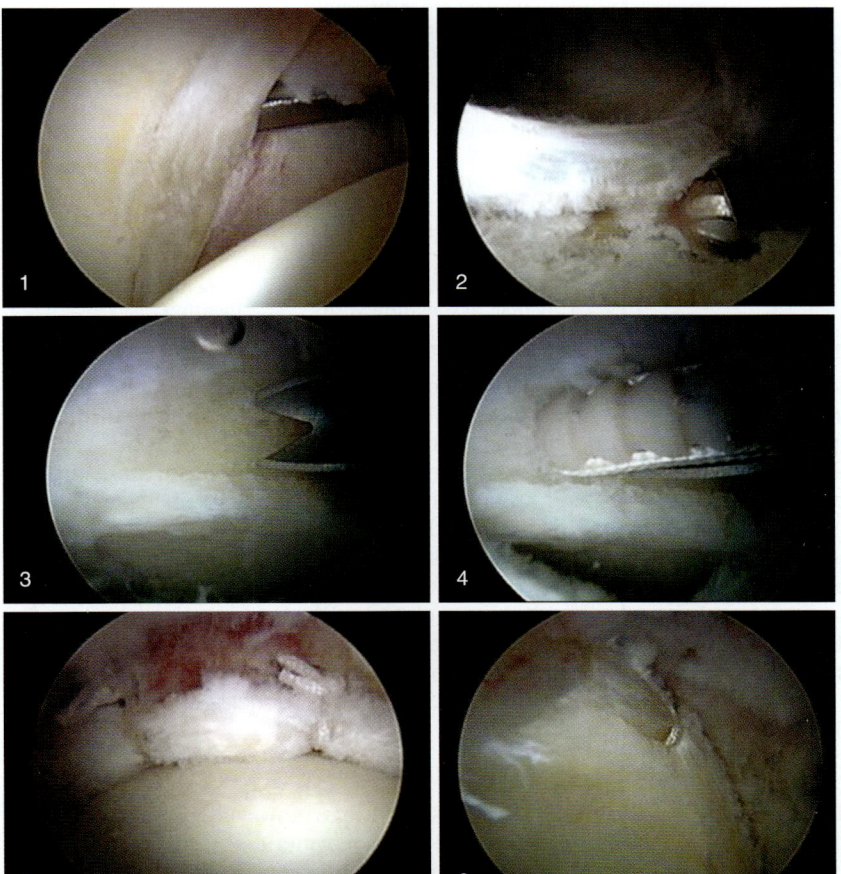

Figure 54-6. Arthroscopic view of acetabular rim trimming with labral takedown. (1) An arthroscopic blade is used to complete the labral detachment; (2) rim trimming is performed with an arthroscopic burr blade; (3) adequate position of the guide is about 2 mm away from the cartilage surface; (4) a bioabsorbable anchor is driven into the hole; (5) labral repair is inspected from the peripheral compartment with traction released; and (6) inspection from the central compartment shows excellent labral apposition.

Table 54-3. Causes of Labral Pathology

Type	Base Condition	Typical Labral Morphology	Typical Labral Lesion	Common Location*
1. Morphologic alterations	A. Femoroacetabular impingement			
	Cam	Normal	Labral tear (usually base detachment in the watershed zone associated with chondral lesion)	Anterior-superior
	Pincer	Hypotrophic	Labral degeneration (bruising, fraying with eventual cysts and ossification)	Anterior and posterior-superior
	Mixed-type	Normal/hypotrophic areas	Labral tear associated with degeneration signs	Same as pincer
	B. Dysplasia	Hypertrophic	Myxoid degeneration and/or detachment from the osseous rim	Antero-superior
2. Functional alterations	A. Instability	Normal	Labral tear (usually base detachment in the watershed zone)	Anterior
	B. Iliopsoas impingement	Normal	Inflammation, labral tear or mucoid degeneration. Scarring to the anterior capsule	3 o'clock
3. Trauma	A. Subluxation	Normal	Variable	Posterior/Anterior
	B. Dislocation	Normal	Variable	Posterior/Anterior
	C. Fractures	Normal	Variable	Posterior/Anterior
	D. Iatrogenic	Normal	Labral perforation or detachment	12 o'clock
4. "DIRT"	A. Degenerative hip disease	Hypotrophic	Labral degeneration (yellow color, bruising, fraying with eventual cysts and ossification)	Global
	B. Infectious disease	Variable	Intense synovitis, capsule-labral adhesions, association with loose bodies	Global
	C. Rheumatologic conditions	Variable	Synovitis, pannus, adhesion, labral degeneration, calcium deposits	Global
	D. Tumors	Variable	Labral invasion, labral tear, association with loose bodies	Depend on tumor location

remaining labrum is large enough and the underlying condition was corrected (e.g., isolated cam).[56]

On the other hand, patients with developmental dysplasia of the hip (category 1b) usually rely mostly on the hypertrophic labrum to maintain joint homeostasis.[6,8,10,11] In those cases, extensive labral débridement should be avoided to minimize the risk of creating an unstable joint.* Labral repair may be performed in cases of mild dysplasia, or after more severe deformities have been corrected by a periacetabular osteotomy.[30,31] In the presence of structural causes, however, labral repair has shown to be the treatment of choice.[23,52]

For the degenerative labrum (category 4), mechanical débridement of nonviable tissue is performed using a 4.5 mm full radius shaver. Preserving as much of the viable acetabular labrum as possible is important to optimize joint congruence, evenly distribute force contact loads, and prevent further joint degeneration. Tear size does not preclude arthroscopic fixation, and even with large tears, labral repair can be a viable option.[58] Preserving viable tissue is important, but recognizing an unstable construct is also necessary. Some cases present with extremely degenerative labra, and repair is not possible. Irreparable labra are usually those with complex tears, segmental deficiencies, and small widths associated with degenerative changes.[54,55] In these cases, labral reconstruction has emerged as a new option to improve biomechanics and symptoms in young active patients and those with signs of hip instability.[54,55]

Labral Repair

Most labral lesions are due to femoroacetabular impingement; if it is present, treatment should address that condition under risk of premature failure of the repair. Mechanical débridement of nonviable tissue is

*References 8, 42, 43, 50, 53, and 57.

performed using a shaver. Often a previously unrecognized flap or area of gross delamination becomes more apparent. The quality of the tissue and the nature of the tear are evaluated at this point. A bleeding cancellous bone bed is desired for labral re-fixation because of the relatively avascular nature of the labrum. Experimental studies have demonstrated that it is able to heal directly to the bone, as well as to the surrounding capsule.[59] The acetabular rim provides solid fixation to the anchors and a stable base to allow the labral repair. One bioabsorbable 2.9 mm anchor is used for every 1 cm on average of labral detachment. Smaller anchors might be required in smaller patients and in cases in which the acetabular wall is thinner (3 and 9 o'clock). Additional anchors should be placed as needed to provide good stability and shape to the labrum, so that it can exert its physiologic functions. Bioabsorbable anchors are preferred for many reasons. The difficulty involved in removing metallic anchors in revision surgery is probably the most important.

PEARL

- Although a 2.9 mm anchor usually provides the best purchase, smaller anchors may be necessary, especially at thinner portions of the acetabular wall (3 and 9 o'clock).

Anchors are placed about 2 mm off the acetabular rim in the area of the rim trimming under direct visualization of the entry point and the adjacent articular surface. In general, the anterolateral portal allows insertion of anchors into the anterolateral aspect of the acetabulum, where most lesions are found. As the guide sleeve is directed toward the trimmed acetabular margin, in a divergent direction to avoid intra-articular penetration, a cranial angle of about 30 to 45 degrees is often observed in the coronal plane. As more anterior placements are necessary, a forward inclination of the guide is performed. This can be limited at the 2 o'clock position (considering the right acetabulum), where the insertion angle may be too acute. For insertion of anterior-most anchors, therefore, the mid-anterior portal may be used. Fluoroscopy can be used during the procedure to ensure optimal placement.[44,45]

While drilling the path of the anchor, it is critical to visualize the articular surface of the acetabulum to ensure that the articular surface is not being compromised. If bulging of the articular surface is noticed, the angle of the anchor must be redirected. Only then should the anchor be placed.

PITFALLS

- In patients with coxa vara, the anterolateral portal usually remains relatively more proximal to the acetabular rim. Failure to incline the guide proximally will lead to intra-articular penetration of the anchor.
- Inappropriate entry point and guide angulation may lead to intra-articular penetration of the anchor, chondral damage, or inadequate fixation.

A clear 8.25 mm cannula is introduced through the working portal, and the suture wires are drawn back through it. It can be inserted before the guiding stick for the anchor; however, in more extreme positions, it may hinder the mobility of the guide. The next step is to deliver a limb of suture between the labrum and the acetabular rim with a suture passer. The suture is then retrieved over the labrum. The loop suture is tied down using standard arthroscopic knot-tying techniques.

A trans-labral suture stitch may be performed in thick labra when less labral eversion is desired. In this case, one limb of the suture is delivered intra-articularly between the labrum and the acetabular rim. Then the labrum is pierced with the suture passer in its midsubstance in an outside-in direction, and a loop of the intra-articular limb of the suture is pulled through. The arthropierce is removed from the labrum and is used to pull the free end of the same suture limb completely through the loop, retrieving it through the cannula. At this point, as both limbs of the suture are tensioned simultaneously, the labrum gets closer to the acetabular rim, allowing a suture-free margin of it to be in contact with the femoral head. The suture is then tied down using standard arthroscopic knot-tying techniques.

PEARL

- Trans-labral sutures may be used in thicker portions of the labrum when the objective is to minimize labral eversion.

Labral Reconstruction

In very active young patients and in those with signs of hip instability with irreparable labral lesions, labral reconstruction might be considered. Severely hypotrophic labra, with complex tears or segmental deficiency, are usually impossible to repair. A technique for labral reconstruction using autologous fascia lata grafts has been developed to treat patients with these conditions.[54,55] After the original labrum is considered unviable and a decision for reconstruction has been made, débridement of the remaining labrum is performed in the area in which it was considered unhealthy. The objective is to obtain a regular and stable rim for re-fixation of the new labrum. The need for a bleeding cancellous bed cannot be overemphasized in this condition, because vascular ingrowth to the free graft must occur from this site. As soon as adequate margins for the labrum anastomosis are achieved and the acetabular rim is prepared, measurement of the gap without labrum is taken. We often use the tip of the 5.5 mm motorized burr as a parameter to perform this measurement. At this point, the arthroscope is retrieved from the joint and traction is released.

With the leg straight and internally rotated, a longitudinal incision comprising the skin and subcutaneous tissue is performed over the great trochanter. The iliotibial tract is exposed, and a rectangle of tissue is retrieved. The longitudinal axis of the graft should correspond to 130% to 140% of the intra-articular distance measured, and the transverse axis should be about 1 inch. After the graft is cleared from all muscular and fatty tissue, it is tubulized with the use of absorbable sutures. Strong suture is placed at each end of the graft to tension it. Additionally, a loop of suture is left in the proximal end of the graft. The graft is then bathed in platelet-rich plasma. It should provide a tubular structure with about 7 mm width and enough length to substitute the missing labrum.

After the leg is put back into traction, a suture anchor is placed at the anterior-most part of the labrum defect on the acetabular rim. The limbs of the suture should be inside an 8.25 mm transparent cannula placed on the mid-anterior portal. The graft is then transfixed at its distal portion with one of the suture limbs. An arthroscopic sliding knot is performed, and the labrum is pushed within the joint through the cannula. After good fixation of the distal portion is obtained, the portals are switched and an anchor is placed at the lateral-most part of the defect in the acetabular rim. One of the limbs of the suture is passed through the suture loop in the proximal (posterior) end of the graft. The graft is then pushed into position by a sliding knot, and an additional loop suture around the labrum is performed to grant its attachment. Another anchor should be placed in the mid-portion of the defect to provide adequate fixation and anatomic contour to the labrum, as in the technique for labral re-fixation. Attention must be paid to the anastomosis so that no redundant tissue causes conflict with the joint.

VARIATIONS/UNUSUAL SITUATIONS

Some morphologic conditions require special consideration and some modifications of the technique. In patients with coxa vara, the anterolateral portal usually remains relatively more proximal to the acetabular rim. In these patients, failure to incline the guide proximally when the anchor is placed will lead to intra-articular penetration. In such conditions, attentive placement of the portal and an adequate entry point are paramount to avoid complications.

Some patients with cam deformity and a normal center edge angle may present with an abnormally increased Tonnis angle. This exaggerated lateral inclination of the weight-bearing surface should raise attention for a potentially unstable joint. When necessary, bone resection of a pincer deformity should be extremely cautious, because the resection can create a dysplastic conformation, increasing joint stresses and the risk of subluxation. Simple labral débridement is not acceptable in this condition because of the underlying potential instability.

In patients with hip dysplasia, the joint capsule may be stretched through repetitive stresses, worsening the instability. In these patients, besides labral repair, capsular plication or thermal capsulorrhaphy is often necessary to restore joint homeostasis.

No age restriction is applied in arthroscopic treatment of the hip. However, patients with an open physis should not be treated with femoroplasty because of the risk of halting growth and eliciting deformity.[60] In cases

of symptomatic femoroacetabular impingement, a possible approach is to treat the acetabular rim and the labrum while restricting impingement-related movement. Later treatment of the cam deformity may be warranted in cases of persistent symptoms at or close to the expected date of physeal closure.

POSTOPERATIVE CARE

The rehabilitation protocol for labral reconstruction does not differ from the one we use for labral repair.[61,62] We instruct patients to walk with 20 pounds of foot-flat weight bearing and to engage in 4 hours per day of continuous passive motion (CPM) for 2 weeks. This period of time is increased to 6 to 8 hours per day for 8 weeks if microfracture is performed to treat associated chondral lesions. We recommend that the patient lie prone for 2 hours per day to prevent hip flexion contracture while using the CPM machine. An antirotation bolster to prevent hip external rotation when supine is used for 14 to 21 days after surgery. A hip brace is used to restrict extension and external rotation during gait for 14 to 21 days. Physical therapy is used to restore first passive and then active motion followed by strength. Passive hip circumduction motions are recommended to prevent adhesions. Endurance strengthening should be commenced after motion is maximized and good stability in gait and movement can be demonstrated.

Before being cleared for sports-specific training, the asymptomatic patient should be able to succeed in the Hip Sports Test. This test is administered by a physical therapist or a certified athletic trainer and consists of four components designed to assess muscle endurance, patients' ability to maintain adequate form during exercise without compensatory movements, and the absence of pain even in highly demanding situations such as deep hip flexion and pivoting movements. Once the athlete scores 17 or more points out of 20, he/she is allowed to return to sports-specific practice with decreased risk for reinjury, new injury, or recurrence of symptoms.[63]

RESULTS

Arthroscopic surgery results compare favorably with most outcomes reported with open surgical dislocation to treat femoroacetabular impingement. When studies with similar populations of professional athletes were compared, hip arthroscopy was shown to have a shorter recovery time and an earlier return to sports time.[64,65] The rate of return to sports in patients with FAI treated with arthroscopy has been reported. Philippon and colleagues[66] reported on 45 professional athletes who underwent arthroscopic treatment for FAI and associated pathologies; 93% returned to the professional level and 78% remained active at this level at a mean of 1.6 years' follow-up.

Labral repair using suture anchors to reattach the labrum to the acetabular rim has been shown to be an effective treatment option for patients with a detached or torn labrum. Several authors have published early clinical results of labral repair showing that patients experience significant improvement in function at least 6 months postoperatively and continue to experience improvement in clinical outcome measurements after that.[23,27,52] In a retrospective comparative study, Larson[52] analyzed the outcomes of arthroscopic labral débridement and re-fixation. In this series, good to excellent results were noted in 66.7% of patients with labral débridement, and 89.7% of hips in the labral re-fixation group had those results in the last follow-up ($P = .01$). The authors concluded that labral re-fixation resulted in better modified Harris Hip Scores and a greater percentage of good to excellent results compared with labral débridement in a minimum 1 year follow-up. In another study, Philippon[23] reported on FAI patients with chondro-labral dysfunction treated arthroscopically, with a minimum 2 years' follow-up. A significant improvement in the modified Harris Hip Score (HHS) of 24 points on average (from 58 to 84) was noted, with a median patient satisfaction of 9 (scale, 1 to 10) and 8.9% conversions to total hip replacement. Multivariable analysis revealed that labral repair rather than débridement was a statistically significant independent predictor of better functional outcome.[23] Additional predictors of a better outcome were the preoperative modified HHS ($P = .018$) and a joint space ≥2 mm ($P = .005$).

Results of labral reconstruction in 37 patients with a minimum 1 year follow-up were recently published.[54,55] Average age was 37 years (range, 18 to 55 years), and the time from initial injury to labral reconstruction was 36 months (range, 1 month to 12 years). Average time to follow-up was 18 months (range, 12 to 32 months). Indications for the procedure included irreparable labral tears or insufficient labral tissue in young patients or those with potential hip instability. Average preoperative modified Harris Hip Score improved from 62 (range, 35 to 92) to an average of 85 (range, 53 to 100) ($P = .001$). Median patient satisfaction was 8 out of 10 (range, 1 to 10). Patients who were treated within a year of injury had higher functional scores. Four (8%) patients needed subsequent total hip arthroplasty. The independent predictor of patient satisfaction with outcome following labral reconstruction was age younger than 30 years.

COMPLICATIONS

The surgeon beginning to perform hip arthroscopies should not be confronted with all the original complications experienced by pioneers of hip arthroscopy because surgical protocols for a safe procedure have been created, and specific instruments are readily available for both lateral and supine positions. Most recent studies report complication rates ranging from 0.5% to 6.4%.[47,67] Nonetheless, hip arthroscopy is a challenging procedure with a steep learning curve and should be attempted only after specific training.[35]

Complications have been categorized as musculoskeletal, neurologic, and vascular-ischemic.[67] The possible mechanism of each complication provided the subdivisions for this classification (Table 54-4). Attempts have also been made to classify complications according to severity. Major complications cause definitive consequences to the patient or may require another surgery

Table 54-4. Reported and Potential Complications of Hip Arthroscopy

Complication Type		Examples
Musculoskeletal	Instrument breakage	Guide wire breakage Forceps breakage
	Intra-articular structural damage	Articular cartilage scuff Iatrogenic labral lesion
	Extra-articular structural damage	Iatrogenic muscle lesion Iatrogenic tendon lesion* Myositis ossificans HO of the iliopsoas tendon Pericapsular HO Trochanteric bursitis
	Adhesions	Adhesion
	Fracture	Femoral neck stress fracture
	Joint instability	Hip dislocation (macroinstability) Hip instability (microinstability)
	Infection	Superficial wound infection Pioarthrosis
Neurologic	Related to portal placement	Meralgia paresthetica Neuropraxia of LFCN Femoral nerve injury*
	Related to articular distraction	Sciatic nerve palsy Femoral nerve palsy Sympathetic reflex
	Related to compression	Pudendal nerve palsy Loss of erection
	Related to manipulation	Direct injury of the femoral nerve* Direct injury of the sciatic nerve* Direct injury of the gluteus superior nerve*
Vascular and Ischemic	Related to venous stasis	Deep venous thrombosis Vulvae edema
	Related to ischemia	Skin necrosis of the perineum Osteonecrosis of the femoral head
	Related to fluid extravasation	Cardiac arrest Abdominal compartment syndrome Edema
	Related to bleeding	Wound bleeding Perineal lacerations Hematomas Great vessel injuries*

HO, Heterotopic ossification; *LFCN*, lateral femoral cutaneous nerve.
*Potential complications, not yet reported in the literature.

for their solution. Intermediate complications can be healed with medical treatment or may resolve spontaneously after some time. Minor complications may occur intraoperatively and can be managed during the procedure.

Specifically with regard to FAI surgery, some complications have been reported. Femoral neck fractures,[67,68] hip dislocations,[69] hip instability, and postoperative adhesions are the most serious and should be avoided by correct surgical indication, attentive surgical technique, and appropriate patient education.

CURRENT CONTROVERSIES AND FUTURE CONSIDERATIONS

- The effects of open and arthroscopic treatment of FAI on the natural history of the disease remain to be evaluated.
- Validated algorithms are required to determine the best indications for open surgery over an arthroscopic approach in patients with abnormal hip structure.
- Specially designed studies are required to further validate the advantages of acetabular labrum repair over simple débridement.
- Indications for labral reconstruction need to be further elucidated.
- Alternative biomaterials for labral reconstruction and chondral treatment are expected to be developed. The objective is to improve the condition of patients with more extensive joint damage while preventing or delaying the need for total joint replacement.
- Some new complications have been observed with the development of arthroscopic treatment of FAI. Identification of risk factors for those complications and validation of effective preventive measures are needed.

REFERENCES

1. Wenger DE, Kendell KR, Miner MR, Trousdale RT: Acetabular labral tears rarely occur in the absence of bony abnormalities. Clin Orthop Relat Res 426:145–150, 2004.
2. Ganz R, Leunig M, Leunig-Ganz K, Harris WH: The etiology of osteoarthritis of the hip: an integrated mechanical concept. Clin Orthop Relat Res 466:264–272, 2008.
3. Murray RO: The aetiology of primary osteoarthritis of the hip. Br J Radiol 38:810–824, 1965.
4. Clohisy JC, Nunley RM, Carlisle JC, Schoenecker PL: Incidence and characteristics of femoral deformities in the dysplastic hip. Clin Orthop Relat Res 467:128–134, 2009.
5. Millis MB, Kim YJ: Rationale of osteotomy and related procedures for hip preservation: a review. Clin Orthop Relat Res 405:108–121, 2002.
6. Klaue K, Durnin CW, Ganz R: The acetabular rim syndrome: a clinical presentation of dysplasia of the hip. J Bone Joint Surg Br 73:423–429, 1991.
7. Li PLS, Ganz R: Morphologic features of congenital acetabular dysplasia. Clin Orthop Relat Res 416:245–253, 2003.
8. Weinstein SL: Natural history of congenital hip dislocation (CDH) and hip dysplasia. Clin Orthop Relat Res 225:62–76, 1987.
9. Chegini S, Beck M, Ferguson SJ: The effects of impingement and dysplasia on stress distributions in the hip joint during sitting and walking: a finite element analysis. J Orthop Res 27:195–201, 2009.
10. Wiberg G: Studies on dysplastic acetabula and congenital subluxation of the hip joint: with special reference to the complication of osteoarthritis. Acta Chir Scand 83(Suppl 58):28–38, 1939.
11. Cooperman DR, Wallensten R, Stulberg SD: Acetabular dysplasia in the adult. Clin Orthop 75:79–85, 1983.
12. Ganz R, Parvizi J, Beck M, et al: Femoroacetabular impingement: a cause for osteoarthritis of the hip. Clin Orthop Relat Res 417:112–120, 2003.
13. Reynolds D, Lucac J, Klaue K: Retroversion of the acetabulum: a cause of hip pain. J Bone Joint Surg Br 81:281–288, 1999.
14. Vandenbussche E, Saffarini M, Taillieu F, Mutschler C: The asymmetric profile of the acetabulum. Clin Orthop Relat Res 466:417–423, 2008.
15. Leunig M, Casillas MM, Hamlet M, et al: Slipped capital femoral epiphysis: early mechanical damage to the acetabular cartilage by a prominent femoral metaphysis. Acta Orthop Scand 71:370–375, 2000.
16. Beck M, Kalhor M, Leunig M, Ganz R: Hip morphology influences the pattern of damage to the acetabular cartilage: femoroacetabular impingement as a cause of early osteoarthritis of the hip. J Bone Joint Surg Br 87:1012–1018, 2005.
17. Philippon MJ, Schenker ML: A new method for acetabular rim trimming and labral repair. Clin Sports Med 25:293–297, 2006.
18. Philippon MJ, Stubbs AJ, Schenker ML, et al: Arthroscopic management of femoroacetabular impingement: osteoplasty technique and literature review. Am J Sports Med 35:1571–1580, 2007.
19. Mardones R, Lara J, Donndorff A, et al: Surgical correction of "cam-type" femoroacetabular impingement: a cadaveric comparison of open versus arthroscopic débridement. Arthroscopy 25:175–182, 2009.
20. Zumstein M, Hahn F, Sukthankar A, et al: How accurately can the acetabular rim be trimmed in hip arthroscopy for pincer-type femoral acetabular impingement: a cadaveric investigation. Arthroscopy 25:164–168, 2009.
21. Byrd JW, Jones KS: Arthroscopic femoroplasty in the management of cam-type femoroacetabular impingement. Clin Orthop Relat Res 467:739–746, 2009.
22. Ilizaliturri VM, Jr, Orozco-Rodriguez L, Acosta-Rodríguez E, Camacho-Galindo J: Arthroscopic treatment of cam-type femoroacetabular impingement: preliminary report at 2 years minimum follow-up. J Arthroplasty 23:226–234, 2008.
23. Philippon MJ, Briggs KK, Yen YM, Kuppersmith DA: Outcomes following hip arthroscopy for femoroacetabular impingement with associated chondrolabral dysfunction: minimum two-year follow-up. J Bone Joint Surg Br 91:16–23, 2009.
24. Kelly BT, Williams RJ, 3rd, Philippon MJ: Hip arthroscopy: current indications, treatment options, and management issues. Am J Sports Med 31:1020–1037, 2003.
25. Philippon MJ, Schenker ML: Arthroscopy for the treatment of femoroacetabular impingement in the athlete. Clin Sports Med 25:299–308, 2006.
26. Byrd JW: Hip arthroscopy: surgical indications. Arthroscopy 22:1260–1262, 2006.
27. Espinosa N, Rothenfluh DA, Beck M, et al: Treatment of femoroacetabular impingement: preliminary results of labral refixation. J Bone Joint Surg Am 88:925–935, 2006.
28. Maheshwari AV, Malik A, Dorr LD: Impingement of the native hip joint. J Bone Joint Surg Am 89:2508–2518, 2007.
29. Byrd JW, Jones KS: Hip arthroscopy in the presence of dysplasia. Arthroscopy 19:1055–1060, 2003.
30. Steppacher SD, Tannast M, Ganz R, Siebenrock KA: Mean 20-year followup of Bernese periacetabular osteotomy. Clin Orthop Relat Res 466:1633–1644, 2008.
31. Ilizaliturri VM, Jr, Chaidez PA, Valero FS, Aguilera JM: Hip arthroscopy after previous acetabular osteotomy for developmental dysplasia of the hip. Arthroscopy 21:176–181, 2005.
32. Krueger A, Leunig M, Siebenrock KA, Beck M: Hip arthroscopy after previous surgical hip dislocation for femoroacetabular impingement. Arthroscopy 23:1285–1289, 2007.
33. Philippon MJ, Schenker ML, Briggs KK, et al: Revision hip arthroscopy. Am J Sports Med 35:1918–1921, 2007.
34. Nusem I, Jabur MK, Playford EG: Arthroscopic treatment of septic arthritis of the hip. Arthroscopy 22:902.e1–e3, 2006.

35. McCarthy JC, Lee JA: Arthroscopic intervention in early hip disease. Clin Orthop Relat Res 429:157–162, 2004.

36. Philippon MJ, Souza BGS: Identifying labral tears in daily practice. Sports Med Update 2:3–6, 2009.

37. Philippon MJ, Maxwell RB, Johnston TL, et al: Clinical presentation of femoroacetabular impingement. Knee Surg Sports Traumatol Arthrosc 15:1041–1047, 2007.

38. Burnett RS, Della Rocca GJ, Prather H, et al: Clinical presentation of patients with tears of the acetabular labrum. J Bone Joint Surg Am 88:1448–1457, 2006.

39. Wyss TF, Clark JM, Weishaupt D, Notzli HP: Correlation between internal rotation and bony anatomy in the hip. Clin Orthop Relat Res 460:152–158,2007.

40. Tannast M, Goricki D, Beck M, et al: Hip damage occurs at the zone of femoroacetabular impingement. Clin Orthop Relat Res 466:273–280, 2008.

41. Clohisy JC, Carlisle JC, Beaulé PE, et al: A systematic approach to the plain radiographic evaluation of the young adult hip. J Bone Joint Surg Am 90(Suppl 4):47–66, 2008.

42. Matsuda DK: Acute iatrogenic dislocation following hip impingement arthroscopic surgery. Arthroscopy 25:400–404, 2009.

43. Maeyama A, Naito M, Moriyama S, Yoshimura I: Evaluation of dynamic instability of the dysplastic hip with use of triaxial accelerometry. J Bone Joint Surg Am 90:85–92, 2008.

44. Larson CM, Wulf CA: Intraoperative fluoroscopy for evaluation of bony resection during arthroscopic management of femoroacetabular impingement in the supine position. Arthroscopy 25:1183–1192, 2009.

45. Matsuda DK: Fluoroscopic templating technique for precision arthroscopic rim trimming. Arthroscopy 25:1175–1182, 2009.

46. Philippon MJ, Wolff AB, Briggs KK, et al: Acetabular rim reduction for the treatment of femoroacetabular impingement correlates with preoperative and postoperative center-edge angle. Arthroscopy 26(6):757–761, 2010.

47. Ilizaturri VM, Jr: Complications of arthroscopic femoroacetabular impingement treatment: a review. Clin Orthop Relat Res 467:760–768, 2009.

48. Lequesne M, de Seze S: Le faux profil du bassin: nouvelle incidence radiographique pour l'étude de la hanche: son utilité dans les dysplasies et les differentes coxopathies. Rev Rhum 28:643–652, 1961.

49. Crockarell JR, Jr, Trousdale RT, Guyton JL: The anterior centre-edge angle: a cadaver study. J Bone Joint Surg Br 82:532–534, 2000.

50. Philippon MJ, Souza BGS, Briggs KK: Hip arthroscopy and labral treatment in patients with femoroacetabular impingement. Minerva Ortop Traumatol 60:293–302, 2009.

51. Bardakos NV, Vasconcelos JC, Villar RN: Early outcome of hip arthroscopy for femoroacetabular impingement: the role of femoral osteoplasty in symptomatic improvement. J Bone Joint Surg Br 90:1570–1575, 2008.

52. Larson CM, Giveans MR: Arthroscopic débridement versus refixation of the acetabular labrum associated with femoroacetabular impingement. Arthroscopy 25:369–376, 2009.

53. Philippon MJ, Schroder E, Souza BG, et al: Labrum: resection, repair and reconstruction sports medicine and arthroscopy review. Sports Med Arthrosc 18(2):76–82, 2010.

54. Philippon MJ, Briggs KK, Hay C, et al: Arthroscopic labral reconstruction in the hip using iliotibial band autograft: technique and early outcomes. Arthroscopy 26:750–756, 2010.

55. Philippon MJ, Souza BGS, Briggs KK: Rekonstruktion des Labrum acetabulare mit autologem Fascia lata-Transplantat. Arthroskopie 22:306–311, 2009.

56. Byrd JW, Jones KS: Hip arthroscopy in athletes: 10-year follow-up. Am J Sports Med 37:2140–2143, 2009.

57. Parvizi J, Bican O, Bender B, et al: Arthroscopy for labral tears in patients with developmental dysplasia of the hip: a cautionary note. J Arthroplasty 24(Suppl 6):110–113, 2009.

58. Philippon MJ: New frontiers in hip arthroscopy: the role of arthroscopic hip labral repair and capsulorrhaphy in the treatment of hip disorders. Instr Course Lect 55:309–316, 2006.

59. Philippon MJ, Arnoczky SP, Torrie A: Arthroscopic repair of the acetabular labrum: a histologic assessment of healing in an ovine model. Arthroscopy 23:376–380, 2007.

60. Philippon MJ, Yen YM, Briggs KK, et al: Early outcomes after hip arthroscopy for femoroacetabular impingement in the athletic adolescent patient: a preliminary report. J Pediatr Orthop 28:705–710, 2008.

61. Enseki KR, Martin RL, Draovitch P, et al: The hip joint: arthroscopic procedures and postoperative rehabilitation. J Orthop Sports Phys Ther 36:516–525, 2006.

62. Philippon MJ, Christensen JC, Wahoff MS: Rehabilitation after arthroscopic repair of intra-articular disorders of the hip in a professional football athlete. J Sport Rehabil 18:118–134, 2009.

63. Souza BGS, Philippon MJ, Briggs KK, Wahof M: Sports test: an objective method to assess the ability to return to sports after hip arthroscopy. Paper presented at the 1st Annual Scientific Meeting of the International Society for Hip Arthroscopy, New York, NY, 2009.

64. Bizzini M, Notzli HP, Maffiuletti NA: Femoroacetabular impingement in professional ice hockey players: a case series of 5 athletes after open surgical decompression of the hip. Am J Sports Med 35:1955–1959, 2007.

65. Philippon MJ, Weiss DR, Kuppersmith DA, et al: Arthroscopic labral repair and treatment of femoroacetabular impingement in professional hockey players. Am J Sports Med 38:99–104, 2010.

66. Philippon M, Schenker M, Briggs K, Kuppersmith D: Femoroacetabular impingement in 45 professional athletes: associated pathologies and return to sport following arthroscopic decompression. Knee Surg Sports Traumatol Arthrosc 15:908–914, 2007.

67. Souza BGS, Polesello GC, Honda EK, et al: Complications in hip arthroscopy. In Proceedings of the 2009 Annual Meeting of the American Academy of Orthopaedic Surgeons, Las Vegas, 2009.

68. Sampson TG: Arthroscopic treatment of femoroacetabular impingement. Am J Orthop 37:608–612, 2008.

69. Benali Y, Katthagen BD: Hip subluxation as a complication of arthroscopic débridement. Arthroscopy 25:405–407, 2009.

70. Barjhoux P, Francois B, Vignon G: [Acetabular protrusion, coxa profunda, deepened acetabulum]. Sem Hop 32:3955–3962, 1956.

71. Kalberer F, Sierra RJ, Madan SS, et al: Ischial spine projection into the pelvis: a new sign for acetabular retroversion. Clin Orthop Relat Res 466:677–683, 2008.

72. Tönnis D, Heinecke A: Acetabular and femoral anteversion: relationship with osteoarthritis of the hip. J Bone Joint Surg Am 81:1747–1770, 1999.

73. Yasunaga Y, Ikuta Y, Kanazawa T, et al: The state of the articular cartilage at the time of surgery as an indication for rotational acetabular osteotomy. J Bone Joint Surg Br 83:1001–1004, 2001.

74. Nötzli HP, Wyss TF, Stöcklin CH, et al: The contour of the femoral head-neck junction as a predictor for the risk of anterior impingement. J Bone Joint Surg Br 84:556–560, 2002.

75. Stulberg SD: Unrecognized childhood hip disease: a major cause of idiopathic osteoarthritis of the hip. In Cordell LD, Harris WH, Ramsey PL, MacEwen GD, editors: The hip: proceedings of the Third Open Scientific Meeting of the Hip Society, St Louis, 1975, CV Mosby, pp 212–228.

76. Peelle MW, Della Rocca GJ, Maloney WJ, et al: Acetabular and femoral radiographic abnormalities associated with labral tears. Clin Orthop Relat Res 441:327–333, 2005.

77. Gosvig KK, Jacobsen S, Palm H, et al: A new radiological index for assessing asphericity of the femoral head in cam impingement. J Bone Joint Surg Br 89:1309–1316, 2007.

78. Eijer H, Leunig M, Mahomed MN, Ganz R: Cross-table lateral radiographs for screening of anterior femoral head-neck offset in patients with femoro-acetabular impingement. Hip Int 11:37–41, 2001.

79. Reimers J: The stability of the hip in children: a radiological study of the results of muscle surgery in cerebral palsy. Acta Orthop Scand Suppl 184:1–100, 1980.

80. Murphy SB, Ganz R, Müller ME: The prognosis in untreated dysplasia of the hip. J Bone Joint Surg Am 77:985–989, 1995.

81. Sharp IK: Acetabular dysplasia: the acetabular angle. J Bone Joint Surg Br 43:268–272, 1961.

CHAPTER 55

Open Surgical Débridement for Femoroacetabular Impingement

Rafael J. Sierra and Robert T. Trousdale

KEY POINTS

- Trochanteric slide osteotomy with anterior capsulotomy and anterior dislocation of the hip provides
  - A 360-degree view of the acetabulum for acetabular rim trimming and/or labral repair and reconstruction
  - Complete access to the femoral head and neck junction with a direct view of retinacular vessels that allows safe débridement of cam lesions
- Intraoperative ROM testing is important in evaluating the adequacy of a corrective surgical procedure.
- Supervised rehabilitation is valuable in enhancing recovery.

INTRODUCTION

Femoroacetabular impingement (FAI) occurs when the proximal femur repeatedly contacts the native acetabular rim during normal or abnormal hip range of motion (ROM).[1-5] It most commonly occurs with flexion and internal rotation but may also occur with extension and external rotation. It is well recognized now that FAI is a mechanism that leads to osteoarthritis (OA),[1-4] and its role as a prearthritic hip condition has been studied extensively. Treatment of FAI is aimed at restoration of normal structural anatomy about the hip.[5,6] Open surgical hip dislocation has been the gold standard for management of the patient with FAI.[6-8] The aim of this chapter is to discuss the indications, contraindications, technique, and postoperative care associated with surgical hip dislocation for treatment of FAI.

INDICATIONS

A good candidate for femoroacetabular impingement (FAI) surgery through surgical hip dislocation is a patient who (1) has reasonably preserved articular cartilage, (2) has a correctable structural abnormality that involves both femoral and acetabular sides with or without labral chondral pathology, and (3) understands limitations and outcomes of the procedure. Relative contraindications include (1) patients into the fourth and fifth decades of life or greater, (2) patients with Tonnis grade II osteoarthritis (OA) unless extremely young, (3) patients with a retroverted acetabulum with poor posterior coverage (a reverse periacetabular osteotomy [PAO] would be a better option), and (4) patients with anterior translation of the femoral head into an anterior acetabular cartilage defect, as seen radiographically or on magnetic resonance imaging (MRI). Absolute contraindications include (1) patients with Tonnis grade III or higher OA, (2) patients with hip pain with an uncorrectable structural deformity, (3) infection, and (4) the older patient with advanced degenerative joint disease for whom total hip arthroplasty (THA) would be a better option.

PREOPERATIVE PLANNING

The anteroposterior pelvic radiograph provides useful information for planning a surgical hip dislocation. Interpretation of this x-ray, however, is very sensitive to the position of the pelvis at the time of exposure. It is commonly accepted now that a well-centered anteroposterior pelvic view is obtained when there is symmetry of the iliac wings and of the obturator foramina, and when the coccyx is at a point in the midline at a distance 0 to 2 cm above the symphysis pubis.[9] A well-centered radiograph is very important in assessing structural anomalies about the pelvis and the proximal femur. Plain radiographs are used to assess retroversion of the acetabulum or whether coxa profunda or protrusion is present[10-13] and to study the shape of the proximal femur. The shape of the femoral head is classified as "pistol grip" if the lateral contour of the femoral head extends in a convex shape to the base of the neck, and is classified as *aspherical* if the epiphysis of the head protrudes laterally out of a circle drawn around the contour of the head.[6,14,15]

An MRI arthrogram also helps with preoperative planning. The protocol for obtaining magnetic resonance arthrography (MRA) has been described previously.[16] In brief, axial, coronal, oblique, sagittal oblique, and radial sequences are obtained. This last sequence is useful for evaluating the proximal femur and for calculating the alpha angle, and it has been useful in evaluating the localization of labral tears (see Chapter 31).[17] Acetabular cartilage degeneration is less reliably seen on MRI.[18-21] Assessment of the status of the cartilage is very important when surgical intervention is planned. In

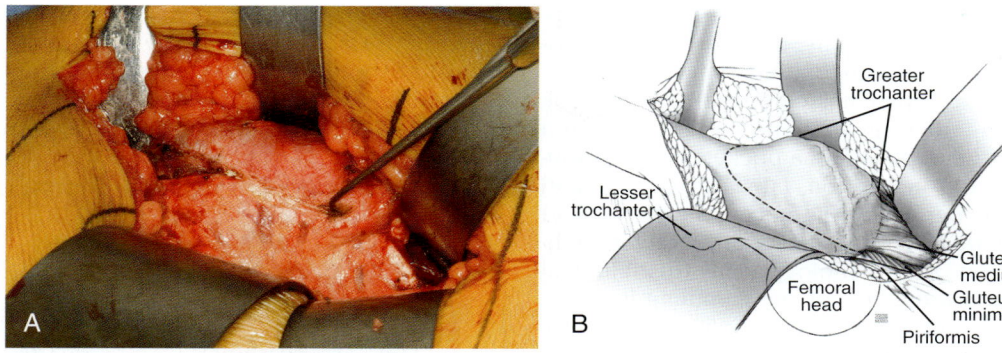

Figure 55-1. Surgical photograph and illustration depicting the posterior aspect of the trochanter with external rotators. Osteotomy should be performed 5 mm anterior to the posterior overhang of the trochanter. Posterior dissection should be carried out between the piriformis and the gluteus minimus.

patients with FAI, the cartilage lesion is often anterosuperior, and in patients with advanced cam-type FAI, this may be seen as extensive chondral lesions as a result of the outside-to-in shearing mechanism. Superior and lateral acetabular cyst formation can also be seen on MRI and is indicative of more advanced disease.

For patients with symptomatic coxa profunda or protrusio, surgical hip dislocation for acetabular rim trimming would be the treatment of choice for management of their global overcoverage; however, they may benefit from a PAO or intertrochanteric osteotomy. Patients with large retroverted acetabulae with labral pathology who require rim trimming are also good candidates for surgical hip dislocation. Patients with isolated cam impingement with a normal acetabular contour and minimal labral pathology may be treated with less invasive procedures such as hip arthroscopy[22-37] or the anterior Hueter or Smith-Petersen approach.[38-40] Indications for less invasive procedures are continually evolving, and there is certainly a trend toward less invasive techniques for management of patients with FAI. Only time will tell whether the results of arthroscopic treatment are comparable with those of open treatment.

DESCRIPTION OF TECHNIQUE

The patient is placed in the lateral decubitus position. A straight incision distal to the iliac crest crossing anterior to the greater trochanter and over the proximal femur is made. For the fascial incision, a Gibson approach, which preserves the anterior aspect of the gluteus maximus, or a Kocher-Langenbech split of the gluteus maximus can be performed. We prefer the Kocher-Langenbech because the length of the skin incision is smaller, allowing access to the posterior aspect of the hip. The trochanteric bursa is incised longitudinally with the incision. Then a trigastric trochanteric osteotomy is performed. The osteotomy should not be performed under, but should end within, the trochanter proximally to protect the medial femoral circumflex artery as it courses superiorly behind the greater trochanter, and to ensure that most of the tendon fibers of the piriformis remain on the stable portion of the

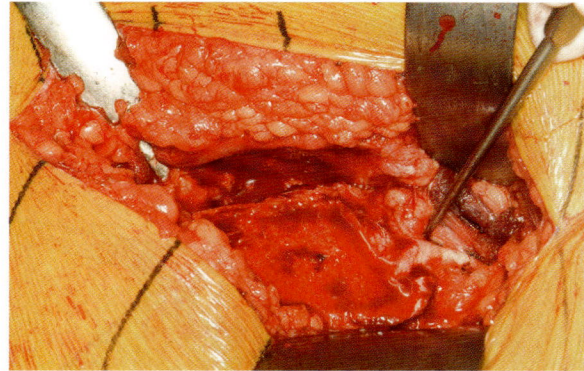

Figure 55-2. Surgical photograph depicting preservation of the piriformis and its attachment to the stable part of the trochanter.

trochanter (Figs. 55-1A and B). A safe distance is 5 mm anterior to the trochanteric overhang. The stable trochanter is preserved with most or almost all the piriformis and all the other external rotators (Fig. 55-2). A capsular exposure is performed posteriorly in between the interval of the piriformis and the gluteus minimus. Staying proximal to the piriformis tendon diminishes the risk of damage to the anastomosis between the deep branch of the medial femoral circumflex and the inferior gluteal artery that runs inferior to the piriformis. Elevate the gluteus minimus off the superior and posterior capsule down to the sciatic notch. The superior dissection can be carried anteriorly to the reflected head of the rectus, which becomes visible over the acetabular rim. Anteriorly and inferiorly, the insertions of the short head of the minimus onto the capsule should be released. The trochanteric fragment is retracted anteriorly throughout this exposure, facilitated by increasing flexion and abduction. A Z-shaped capsulotomy is started by carrying the capsulotomy along the long axis of the neck from distal to proximal, starting at the anterosuperior edge of the stable trochanter and coursing toward the acetabular rim (Fig. 55-3). The capsulotomy should be carried out with a knife from inside-out, so that the labrum is not damaged as the rim is approached

(Fig. 55-4*A* and *B*). The distal limb of the Z-shaped capsulotomy is made longitudinally, anteriorly, and inferiorly at the level of the psoas tendon.

The femoral head is then dislocated with a bone hook by cutting the round ligament. The leg is flexed and externally rotated and placed in a pocket. The acetabulum is exposed, and inspection, labral takedown, and rim trimming are performed as necessary (Fig. 55-5*A* and *B*). Where to do the rim trimming or labral reattachment depends on the pathology, but this surgical approach allows 360 degrees of rim trimming if necessary. Refixing the labrum is achieved with nonabsorbable suture anchors into the acetabular rim (Fig. 55-6). The knot should be tied over the rim outside the joint, taking care to pass this suture through the undersurface of the labrum, so it is not reattached in an inverted manner.

The femoral head and neck osteochondroplasty is then performed. We routinely use spherical templates to gauge the shape of the femoral head at the beginning of the osteochondroplasty and again at the end (Fig. 55-7*A* and *B*). It is important to always visualize the

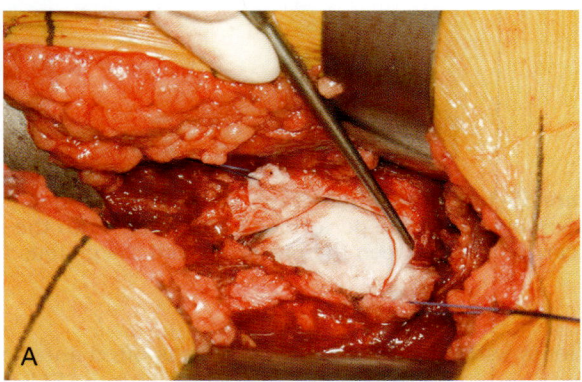

A

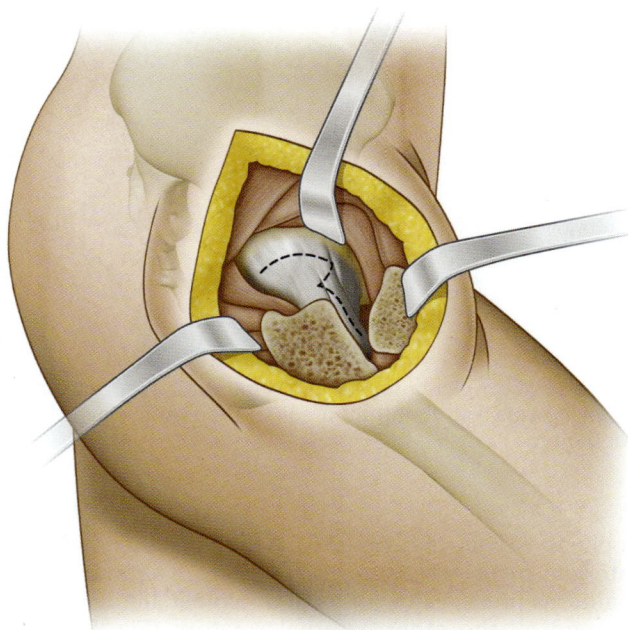

Figure 55-3. Z-shaped capsulotomy performed on the right hip. The capsulotomy is carried along the long axis of the neck from distal to proximal, starting at the anterior superior edge of the stable trochanter and moving toward the acetabular rim.

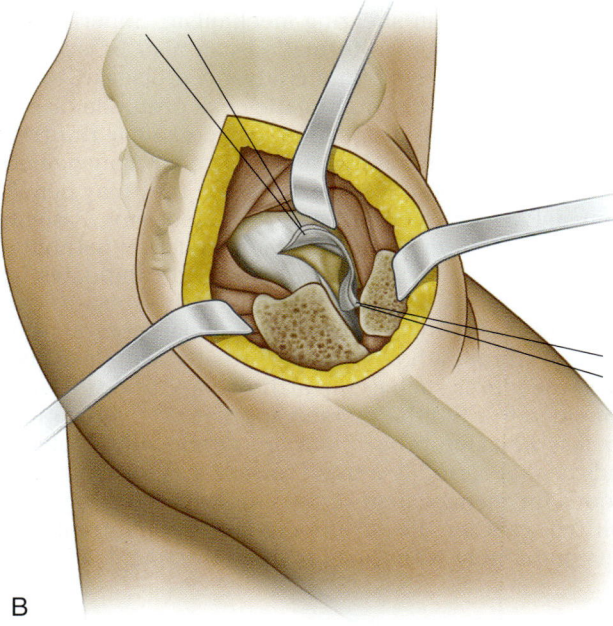

B

Figure 55-4. The capsulotomy should be carried out with a knife from inside-out, always with visualization of the labrum to prevent iatrogenic injury.

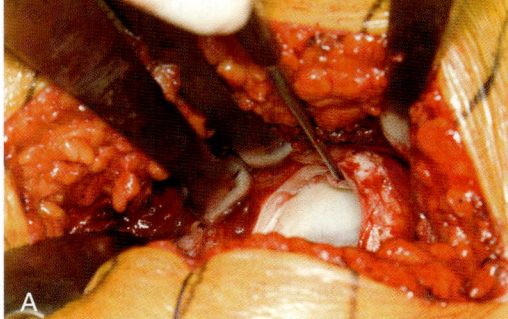

A

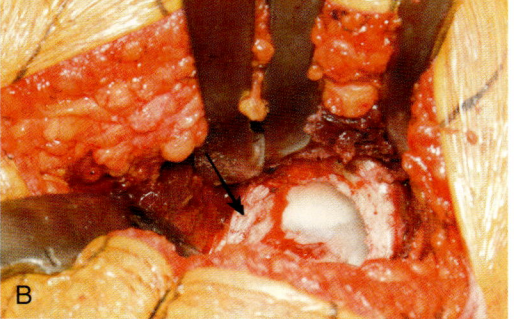

B

Figure 55-5. A, A 33-year-old female with combined pincer and cam impingement shows a cleavage lesion of the acetabular cartilage located in the anterior superior rim. **B,** Intraoperative photo depicting takedown of the labrum and 5 mm of rim trimming. The labrum is then reattached to the rim with suture anchors.

retinaculum, especially in cases of large cam lesions in which the cam lesion includes the top of the retinacular vessels. If a cam problem is present above or around the retinacular vessels, it is safer to bring the osteotome proximal to distal, not too deep, because it may damage the intraosseous vessels. Reduce the hip and check ROM for impingement. Internal rotation free from impingement should be obtained, and the surgeon should aim for 45 degrees of internal rotation at 90 degrees of flexion. Commonly, bone wax is placed into the cancellous bone of the head-neck junction to prevent capsular adhesions.

A loose capsular closure is performed, and finally the trochanteric reattachment is made with two or three 4.5-mm screws. These screws should be placed deep into the trochanter to prevent screw irritation, although routine removal of screws may be a better practice.

VARIATIONS/UNUSUAL SITUATIONS

Relative neck lengthening with relief of superior and posterior trochanteric impingement can be a therapeutic step, as in patients with high-riding trochanters or

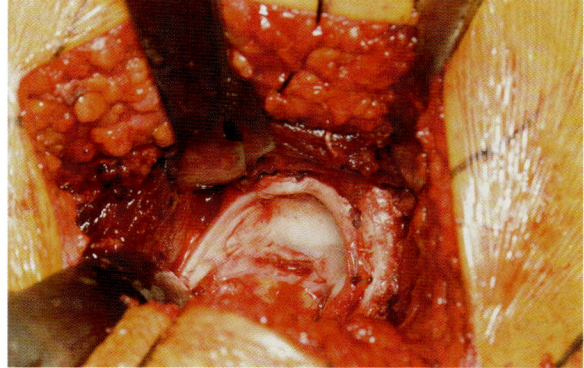

Figure 55-6. Reattachment of the labrum to the acetabular rim has been performed with suture anchors. Knots are tied on the outside part of the acetabular rim. The labrum is not looped, but the outermost part of the labrum is traversed with a suture to prevent inversion of the labrum at the time of reattachment.

as an extension of the approach if a femoral neck osteotomy is intended. This procedure implies removal of the posterior stable part of the trochanter until it is flush with the posterior femoral neck and the axilla of the trochanteric femoral neck junction is exposed in its entirety. This exposure is the workhorse for all other procedures that are performed around the neck (osteotomy or head reductions for slipped capital femoral epiphyses).

Surgical hip dislocation is more difficult to perform when the patient has undergone previous surgery to the hip because there may be notable scarring of the anterior capsule, making the plane between the capsule and the muscle difficult to create. In cases of Perthes disease, it is important to avoid bringing the osteotomy too far anteriorly; this may risk injury to the large femoral head. The anterior capsule in Perthes disease is thin and is difficult to repair consistently. The surgeon should be aware of the large redundant labrum in patients with Perthes hip because iatrogenic injury of the labrum may occur. In large male patients, muscle relaxation is commonly used to expose the hip adequately for the acetabular work.

Care should be taken at the time of trochanteric reattachment. Stable fixation of the trochanter should be achieved at the time of surgery. In most cases, screws alone can be used without the use of washers. In patients who have soft bone, the use of washers may be an adjuvant to fixation but should not be relied on as the sole fixation.

The Deficient Labrum

In patients with a deficient labrum caused by severe degeneration or tearing or previous resection, reconstruction of the labrum with autogenous soft tissue has been described.[41] We have described use of the round ligament for reconstruction of the deficient labrum with good results (Fig. 55-8). If the round ligament is deficient or of small size and the labral defect is large, then autogenous fascia lata also can be used to reconstruct the labrum. It is unclear at this time whether the labral graft may restore the negative intraarticular pressures that may prevent continued cartilage damage.

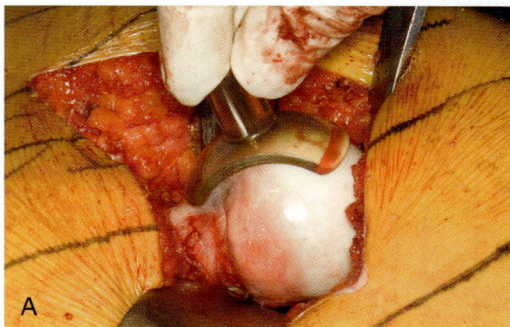
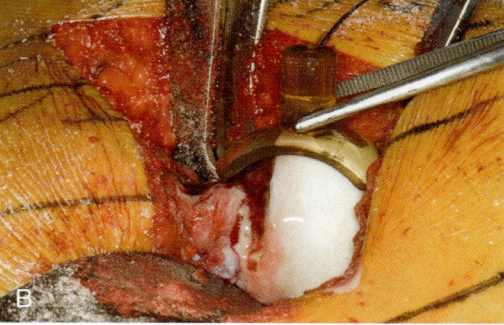

Figure 55-7. A, Picture depicting the acetabular offset gauge before femoral osteochondroplasty. **B,** Picture showing the acetabular gauge after femoral osteochondroplasty has been performed. Femoral osteochondroplasty has been performed over the superior and lateral aspects of the retinacular vessels, which are shown in this picture.

POSTOPERATIVE CARE

Supervised stepwise progressive hip rehabilitation is indicated after surgical dislocation. Patients undergoing surgery for FAI are mobilized on the day after surgery. Weight bearing is limited to toe touch weight bearing for 4 weeks and then is progressed to partial weight bearing at 6 weeks, and full weight bearing by week 8, unless trochanteric healing is delayed. Flexion of the hip is limited to 90 degrees in patients in whom labral repair or reconstruction has been performed. Most patients at 8 weeks show good trochanteric healing. After 6 weeks, abductor strengthening exercises are begun. Continuous passive motion machines are used for 8 hours a day for 6 weeks because this may prevent anterior capsular adhesions. The patient should be able to ambulate without assistive devices at 8 weeks from surgery, and limp should disappear around 3 months with this therapy protocol.

RESULTS

Published results of surgical hip dislocation for management of FAI are shown in Table 55-1.[42-46] Early experience

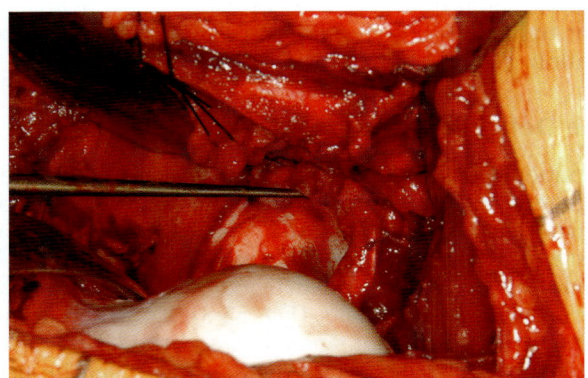

Figure 55-8. The probe shows the reconstructed labrum with autogenous ligamentum teres.

with the surgical technique was reported by Beck and colleagues.[42] Average age at the time of surgery was 36. Nineteen patients with no previous hip surgery who underwent surgical hip dislocation were reviewed at a minimum of 4 years and a mean of 4.7 years. Thirteen hips showed substantial improvement, 2 hips remained unchanged, and 4 hips had worsening symptoms. Five hips required a THA at an average of 3.1 years. Poor outcomes were seen in patients with Tonnis grade 2 OA and in those with intraoperative evidence of extensive cartilage damage with cleavage lesions that involved one third to one half of the cartilage width or deep fissuring of cartilage in the weight-bearing zone. No significant complications were associated with the procedure. Espinosa and associates[43] reported the results of surgical hip dislocation in patients with FAI with special emphasis on the results of labral refixation. At 2 years, 94% of patients who had labral refixation had good or excellent results compared with 76% of patients who had labral resection. This study underscores the importance of trying to preserve the labrum at the time of surgical hip dislocation. Peters and Erickson[46] reported the results in a group of patients with higher grades of arthritis. Thirty hips in 29 patients with a mean age of 31 years were followed for an average of 32 months. Both femoral and acetabular sides were addressed in most patients. The average Harris Hip Score improved from 70 to 87 points at the time of last follow-up. Four of the 30 hips, all in female patients, were considered failures because of pain or progressive arthrosis. Three hips were converted to THA. This study showed that adequate patient selection is imperative for good surgical results. More recently, Graves and Mast[44] reported their good results in a select group of patients with minimal OA at short-term follow-up.

COMPLICATIONS

Poor results are commonly seen in patients who are poor candidates for the procedure; therefore adequate patient selection is imperative for good surgical results. First and foremost, the patient with a severe arthritic

Table 55-1.	Surgical Hip Dislocation and Femoroacetabular Impingement					
Study	**No. of Hips (Patients)**	**Mean Age in Years (range)**	**Mean Follow-up in Years (range)**	**No. of Patients With ≥Tonnis Grade 2 OA Preoperative (%)**	**Average Preoperative Score**	**Postoperative Score**
Beck et al[42]	19 (19)	36 (21–52)	4.7 (4.2–5.2)	2 (10.5)	14.1	16.5
Murphy et al[45]	23 (23)	35.4 (17–54)	5.2 (2–12)	4 (17)	13.2	16.9
Espinosa et al[43]	Group 1 (labral resection), 25 (20) Group 2 (labral reattachment), 35 (32)	30 (20–40)	NR	0	12 12	15 17
Peters and Erickson[46]	30 (29)	31 (16–51)	2.6 (?)	2	NA	NA
Graves and Mast[44]	48 (46)	33 (18–51)	38 (6–67)	1	13	16.8

NA, Not applicable; *NR,* not reported.

hip is not a good candidate for the procedure. Patients with extensive acetabular cartilage cleavage lesions and femoral cam lesions initially may show improvement in their pain and function, but extensive damage will preclude patients from obtaining a good result, and hip symptoms may continue to deteriorate over time. Another poor candidate for the procedure is the patient with minor structural changes, normal MRI, good ROM, and severe hip pain. These patients' symptoms often do not improve with surgical hip dislocation or with any other form of hip surgery (e.g., arthroscopy, anterior mini open procedures) because there is little to correct.

Complications of the surgical procedure have been well described. The first published article on the surgical technique reported on 213 patients who underwent the procedure.[8] Most important, no instances of osteonecrosis of the femoral head occurred. Two patients had partial neuropraxia of the sciatic nerve, which resolved spontaneously. Three patients had failure of the trochanteric fixation. Heterotopic ossification occurred in 37% of hips. Brooker grade 1 heterotopic bone occurred in 68 hips, grade 2 in 9 hips, and grade 3 in 2 hips. Two patients required surgical intervention to improve ROM for symptomatic heterotopic ossification. In addition, 7 patients (6 women) developed a saddle-backed deformity around the buttock after the Kocher-Langenbeck incision. The patient who is at high risk of developing problems with trochanteric fixation usually is an active smoker who does not comply with weight-bearing restrictions after surgery, although careful surgical technique and trochanteric fixation are prerequisites for adequate healing of the trochanter.

CURRENT CONTROVERSIES AND FUTURE CONSIDERATIONS

As more information is obtained on the natural history of FAI, prophylactic treatment in the absence of notable symptoms may be warranted in the future. However, currently such treatment is not recommended. Prophylactic treatment would have to be combined with universal implementation of early detection of hip disease and less invasive procedures for management of FAI. Hip arthroscopy and less invasive procedures that can manage the structural deformity about the hip have become popular for management of FAI. As hip arthroscopy techniques become more sophisticated, an increasing number of hips will be treated with this technique, and only difficult hips with complex pathomorphology will remain as an indication for surgical dislocation. A diligent study of radiographs, MRI, and patient ROM could guide the choice of treatment for patients with FAI, and less invasive surgical procedures could potentially accelerate the recovery of patients undergoing these procedures.

REFERENCES

1. Ganz R, Parvizi J, Beck M, et al: Femoroacetabular impingement: a cause for osteoarthritis of the hip. Clin Orthop Relat Res 417:112–120, 2003.
2. Tannast M, Goricki D, Beck M, et al: Hip damage occurs at the zone of femoroacetabular impingement. Clin Orthop Relat Res 466:273–280, 2008.
3. Ganz R, Leunig M, Leunig-Ganz K, Harris WH: The etiology of osteoarthritis of the hip: an integrated mechanical concept. Clin Orthop Relat Res 466:264–272, 2008.
4. Beck M, Kalhor M, Leunig M, Ganz R: Hip morphology influences the pattern of damage to the acetabular cartilage: femoroacetabular impingement as a cause of early osteoarthritis of the hip. J Bone Joint Surg Br 87:1012–1018, 2005.
5. Sierra RJ, Trousdale RT, Ganz R, Leunig M: Hip disease in the young, active patient: evaluation and nonarthroplasty surgical options. J Am Acad Orthop Surg 16:689–703, 2008.
6. Lavigne M, Parvizi J, Beck M, et al: Anterior femoroacetabular impingement: part I. Techniques of joint preserving surgery. Clin Orthop Relat Res 418:61–66, 2004.
7. Leunig M, Beck M, Dora C, Ganz R: Femoroacetabular impingement: etiology and surgical concepts. Oper Tech Orthop 15:247–255, 2005.
8. Ganz R, Gill TJ, Gautier E, et al: Surgical dislocation of the adult hip: a technique with full access to femoral head and acetabulum without the risk of avascular necrosis. J Bone Joint Surg Br 83:1119–1124, 2001.
9. Siebenrock KA, Karlbertmatten DF, Ganz R: Effect of pelvic tilt on acetabular retroversion: a study of pelves from cadavers. Clin Orthop Relat Res 407:241–248, 2003.
10. Ezoe M, Naito M, Inoue T: The prevalence of acetabular retroversion among various disorders of the hip. J Bone Joint Surg Am 88:372–379, 2006.
11. Giori NJ, Trousdale RT: Acetabular retroversion is associated with osteoarthritis of the hip. Clin Orthop Relat Res 417:263–269, 2003.
12. Reynolds D, Lucas J, Klaue K: Retroversion of the acetabulum: a cause of hip pain. J Bone Joint Surg Br 81:281–288, 1999.
13. Li PL, Ganz R: Morphologic features of congenital acetabular dysplasia: one in six is retroverted. Clin Orthop Relat Res 416:245–253, 2003.
14. Harris WH: Etiology of osteoarthritis of the hip. J Bone Joint Surg Am 213:20–33, 1986.
15. Tanzer M, Noiseux N: Osseous abnormalities and early osteoarthritis: the role of hip impingement. Clin Orthop Relat Res 429:170–171, 2004.
16. Locher S, Werlen S, Leunig M, Ganz R: [MR-arthrography with radial sequences for visualization of early hip pathology not visible on plain radiographs]. Z Orthop Ihre Grenzgeb 140:52–57, 2002.
17. Notzli HP, Wyss TF, Stoecklin CH, et al: The contour of the femoral head-neck junction as a predictor for the risk of anterior impingement. J Bone Joint Surg Br 84:556–560, 2002.
18. Kassarjian A, Yoon LS, Belzile E, et al: Triad of MR arthrographic findings in patients with cam-type femoroacetabular impingement. Radiology 236:588–592, 2005.
19. Leunig M, Podesywa D, Beck M, et al: Magnetic resonance arthrography of labral disorders in hips with dysplasia and impingement. Clin Orthop Relat Res 418:74–80, 2004.
20. Leunig M, Werlen S, Ungersböck A, et al: Evaluation of the acetabular labrum by MR arthrography. J Bone Joint Surg Br 79:230–234, 1997.
21. Toomayan GA, Holman WR, Major NM, et al: Sensitivity of MR arthrography in the evaluation of acetabular labral tears. Am J Roentgenol 186:449–453, 2006.
22. Byrd JW: Hip arthroscopy: evolving frontiers. Oper Tech Orthop 14:58–67, 2004.
23. Byrd JW, Jones KS: Arthroscopic femoroplasty in the management of cam-type femoroacetabular impingement. Clin Orthop Relat Res 467:739–746, 2009.
24. Byrd JW, Jones KS: Hip arthroscopy in the presence of dysplasia. Arthroscopy 19:1055–1060, 2003.
25. Costa ML, Villar RN: Labrum acetabulare: arthroskipische diagnose unde Behandlung degenerativer und traumatischer Läsionen. Orthopäde 35:54–58, 2006.
26. Dienst M, Godde S, Seil R, et al: Hip arthroscopy without traction: in vivo anatomy of the peripheral hip joint cavity. Arthroscopy 17:924–931, 2001.
27. Dorrell JH, Catterall A: The torn acetabular labrum. J Bone Joint Surg Br 68:400–403, 1986.

28. Guanche CA, Bare AA: Arthroscopic treatment of femoroacetabular impingement. Arthroscopy 22:95–106, 2006.

29. Ilizaliturri VM, Jr, Orozco-Rodriguez L, Acosta-Rodriguez E, Camacho-Galindo J: Arthroscopic treatment of cam-type femoroacetabular impingement: preliminary report at 2 years minimum follow-up. J Arthroplasty 23:226–234, 2008.

30. Kelly B, Weiland DE, Schenker MS, Philippon MJ: Arthroscopic labral repair in the hip: surgical technique and review of the literature. Arthroscopy 21:1496–1504, 2005.

31. McCarthy JC, Lee J: Hip arthroscopy: indications and technical pearls. Clin Orthop Relat Res 441:180–187, 2005.

32. McCarthy JC, Mason JB, Wardell SR: Hip arthroscopy for acetabular dysplasia: a pipe dream? Orthopedics 21:977–979, 1998.

33. Philippon MJ, Briggs KK, Yen YM, Kuppersmith DA: Outcomes following hip arthroscopy for femoroacetabular impingement with associated chondrolabral dysfunction: minimum two-year follow-up. J Bone Joint Surg Br 91:16–23, 2009.

34. Phillipon MJ, Schenker ML: A new method for acetabular rim trimming and labral repair. Clin Sports Med 25:293–297, 2006.

35. Sampson TG: Hip morphology and its relationship to pathology: dysplasia to impingement. Oper Tech Sports Med 13:37–45, 2005.

36. Stähelin L, Stähelin T, Jolles BM, Herzog RF: Arthroscopic offset restoration in femoroacetabular cam impingement: accuracy and early clinical outcome. Arthroscopy 24:51–57, 2008.

37. Wettstein M, Dienst M: [Hip arthroscopy for femoroacetabular impingement]. Orthopäde 35:85–93, 2006.

38. Clohisy JC, McClure JT: Treatment of anterior femoroacetabular impingement with combined hip arthroscopy and limited anterior decompression. Iowa Orthop J 25:164–171, 2005.

39. Laude F, Sariali E, Nogier A: Femoroacetabular impingement treatment using arthroscopy and anterior approach. Clin Orthop Relat Res 467:747–752, 2009.

40. Ribas M, Marin-Pena OR, Regenbrecht B, et al: Hip osteoplasty by an anterior minimally invasive approach for active patients with femoroacetabular impingement. Hip Int 17:91–98, 2007.

41. Sierra RJ, Trousdale RT: Labral reconstruction using the ligamentum teres capitis: report of a new technique. Clin Orthop Relat Res 467:753–759, 2009.

42. Beck M, Leunig M, Parvizi J, et al: Anterior femoroacetabular impingement: part II. Mid-term results of surgical treatment. Clin Orthop Relat Res 418:67–73, 2004.

43. Espinosa N, Rothefluh DA, Beck M, et al: Treatment of femoroacetabular impingement: preliminary results of labral refixation. J Bone Joint Surg Am 88:925–935, 2006.

44. Graves ML, Mast JW: Femoroacetabular impingement: do outcomes reliably improve with surgical dislocations? Clin Orthop Relat Res 467:717–723, 2009.

45. Murphy S, Tannast M, Kim YJ, et al: Débridement of the adult hip for femoroacetabular impingement: indications and preliminary clinical results. Clin Orthop Relat Res 429:178–181, 2004.

46. Peters CL, Erickson JA: Treatment of femoroacetabular impingement with surgical dislocation and débridement in young adults. J Bone Joint Surg Am 88:1735–1741, 2006.

CHAPTER 56

Pelvic Osteotomies for Hip Dysplasia

Robert T. Trousdale

KEY POINTS

- Pelvic osteotomy is the treatment of choice for young patients with symptomatic hip dysplasia in the absence of marked secondary degenerative disease.
- Pelvic osteotomy allows medialization of the hip center, correction of version abnormalities, and creation of a more normal horizontal weight-bearing surface.
- The Bernese periacetabular osteotomy has many advantages over other types of pelvic osteotomies and is the procedure of choice in many centers.

INTRODUCTION

Reorientation pelvic osteotomy is the treatment of choice for young patients with symptomatic structural disorders of the acetabulum in the absence of severe secondary changes.[1] These structural problems can be grouped into three categories: classic developmental dysplasia, retrotorsional abnormalities of the acetabulum, and post-traumatic problems. During the past 20 years, various techniques of acetabular reorientation have evolved, making the procedure relatively reliable, reproducible, and durable. Many patients who present with hip pain are not good candidates for arthroplasty because of their young age and limited activity level; some often have reasonable articular cartilage present.

Patients with classic developmental hip dysplasia typically have varying degrees of anatomic abnormalities.[2] On the acetabular side, the joint socket usually is shallow, anteverted, and lateralized, and femoral head coverage is deficient anteriorly and superiorly. The versional status of the acetabulum may be retrotorted in up to 25% of the acetabula. On the femoral side, the head can be small, the neck shaft angle is typically increased, and the femoral canal is narrow. These structural abnormalities lead to decreased contact between the femoral head and the acetabulum and an increased body weight lever arm from excessive lateralization of the hip center of rotation. Relatively high forces transmitted through this decreased surface area can lead to secondary degenerative joint disease over time.

In young patients with symptomatic hip dysplasia with viable articular cartilage, reorientation of the acetabulum is the procedure of choice. Pelvic osteotomy increases the hip contact area and allows for medialization of the hip center of rotation, which decreases the body weight lever arm. These improvements in the mechanics about the hip joint are expected to reduce pain and protect the articular cartilage from further degenerative changes.

Many types of pelvic osteotomies have been described.[1] Single, double, triple, and various periacetabular osteotomies improve mechanics about the hip joint. Each technique has advantages and disadvantages. The Bernese periacetabular osteotomy developed by Ganz and others[3] in the early 1980s is currently the acetabular procedure of choice in many centers (Table 56-1). It has many advantages: It can be done through one incision through a series of straight, reproducible, extra-articular osteotomies. It allows for large corrections in all necessary directions. The osteotomy is inherently stable because the posterior column of the hemipelvis remains intact, and the orthogonal cuts render some stability to the fragment once it has been mobilized. In addition, minimal internal fixation is required. No casting or bracing is needed, and early ambulation is possible. The vascularity of the acetabular fragment via the inferior gluteal artery is preserved, and an arthrotomy can be done without further risk of devascularization of the osteotomized fragment. The shape of the true pelvis is not markedly changed, allowing women who become pregnant after the procedure to have a vaginal delivery. Furthermore, the procedure can be done without taking down the abductors, which facilitates a relatively rapid recovery (Fig. 56-1).[4-11]

INDICATIONS/CONTRAINDICATIONS

Reorientation pelvic osteotomy may be offered to young patients with symptomatic hip dysplasia without excessive proximal migration of the hip center of rotation and with no more than mild to moderate degenerative changes of the articular surface. Because most of the structural abnormality is located on the acetabular side of the joint, correction is best attained with a pelvic osteotomy.[12,18] Joint congruity also is important. Having a relatively round acetabulum that matches a relatively round femoral head probably produces a more reliable and durable outcome. Examination of the hip under fluoroscopy and functional radiographs can be helpful in ensuring that reasonable joint congruity is present.

Table 56-1. Results of Periacetabular Osteotomy for Dysplastic Hips

Study	No. of Osteotomies (patients)	Mean Age (range), yr	Mean Follow-up (range if available), yr	No. (%) of Patients With Tonnis Grade ≥2 OA Preop	Progression Tonnis Grade ≥1 Without Subsequent Surgery	No. (%) of Conversions to THR or Fusion	Clinical Results: Type of Score: Preop (Postop)	Negative Prognostic Factors	Comments
Kralj et al[7]	26 (26)	34 (18-50)	12 (7-15)	5 (19.2)	18 (69)	4 (15)	WOMAC: 66 (63)	Grade of OA, high peak contact stresses	Possible selection bias
Siebenrock et al[10]	71 (60)	29.3 (13-56)	11.3 (10.0-13.8)	13 (18)	14 (25)	12 (17)	73% G/E d'Aubigné: 14.6 (16.3)	Patient age, grade of OA; labral lesion, poor correction	Not specific to classic dysplasia
Trumble et al[11]	123 (115)	32.9 (14-54)	4.3 (2-10)	38 (30)	6 of 56 with grade ≥1 preop	7 (6)	83% G/E	Grade of OA; poor correction	Not specific to classic dysplasia
Clohisy et al[4]	16 (13)	17.6 (13-32)	4.2	0	5 (31)	0	87% G/E Harris: 73 (91)*	False acetabulum	
Matta et al[17]	66 (58)	33.6 (19-51)	4 (2-10)	28 (39)	4 (6) 18 <1 grade	5 (8)	76% G/E 60% improved clinically	Grade of OA	Not specific to classic dysplasia; difficulty with ideal fragment position
Trousdale et al[18]	42 (42)	37 (11-56)	4 (2-8)	9 (21)	4 (9)	6 (14)	Harris: 62 (86)	Grade 3 OA	All patients had OA preop; decreased postop ROM
Crockarell et al[5]	21 (19)	21 (17-43)	3.2 (2.0-4.3)	3 (14)	2 (9)	1 (5)	Harris: 62 (86)	NR	Decreased postop ROM; fragment position difficult

*Excludes two dissatisfied hips.
G/E, Good/excellent; NR, not reported; OA, osteoarthritis; postop, postoperatively; preop, preoperatively; ROM, range of motion; THR, total hip replacement; WOMAC, Western Ontario and McMaster University Osteoarthritis Index.

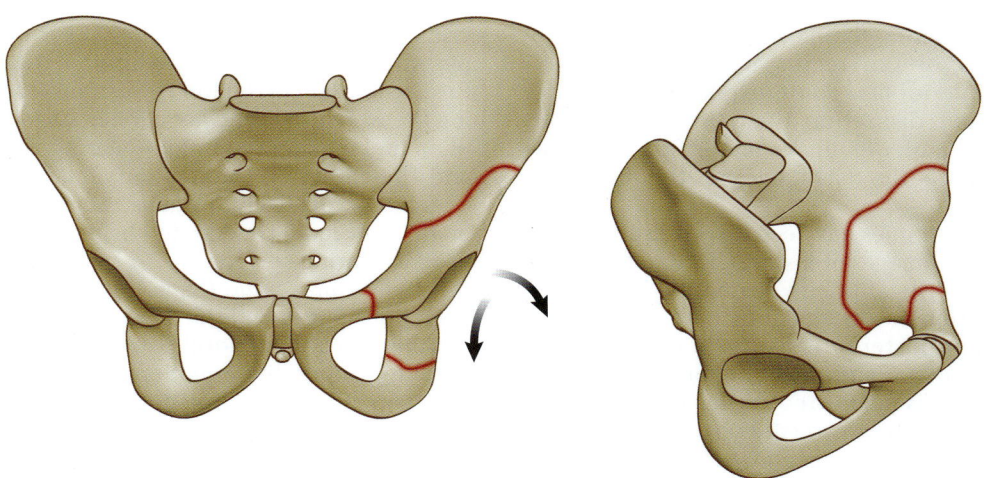

Figure 56-1. The location of bone cuts for a Bernese periacetabular osteotomy.

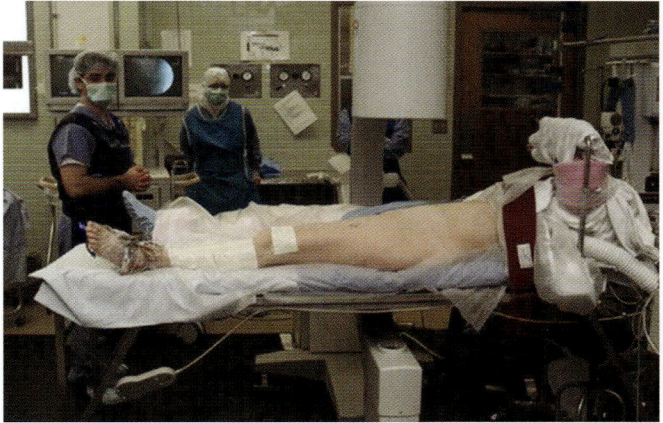

Figure 56-2. Intraoperative photograph showing preparation with fluoroscopy and electromyographic (EMG) monitoring.

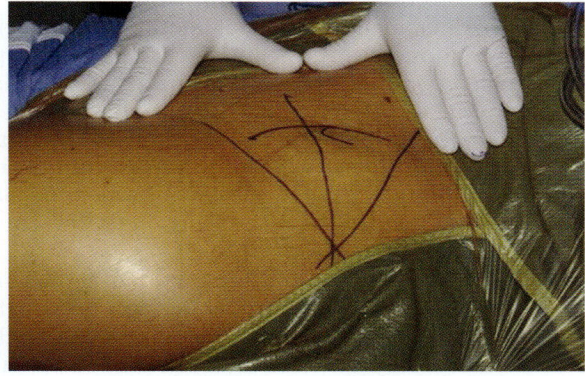

Figure 56-3. Intraoperative photograph showing the location of a skin incision on the patient's left hip.

The extent of acceptable secondary arthrosis or incongruity depends in part on the patient's age and expectations, and on potential future demands that will be placed on the hip joint.[13] A Chiari osteotomy, a shelf osteotomy, and arthroplasty are reasonable options when congruity or arthrosis makes the success of a reconstructive osteotomy unlikely.

SURGICAL TECHNIQUE

Regional epidural anesthesia is used in most patients. We have abandoned the use of preoperative autologous blood donation because intraoperative cell saver appears quite helpful in minimizing the need for allogeneic blood. Presently, the allogeneic transfusion rate at our institution is less than one in four patients.

The patient is placed on an image table, and an indwelling urinary catheter is inserted. The sciatic and femoral nerves are monitored with intraoperative electromyography to minimize the chance of neurologic injury[14,15] (Fig. 56-2). Beginning in 1992, we used an anterior incision, which provided exposure by the inner and outer tables of the pelvis. Four years later, we began to use the same skin incision to perform the osteotomy while exposing only the inner aspect of the pelvis, leaving the abductors intact on the outer aspect of the ilium.[16,17] This approach has dramatically improved the rate of healing, time to weight bearing, and resolution of the postoperative limp.

The incision typically begins along the border of the iliac crest, proceeds along the anterosuperior iliac spine, and continues distally, ending approximately 3 cm distal and anterior to the greater trochanter[19] (Fig. 56-3). The plane between the tensor fascia lata and the sartorius is then developed, and the deep fascia over the tensor fascia lata is incised to avoid direct injury to the lateral femoral cutaneous nerve. The sartorius origin is reflected from the anterosuperior iliac spine. The hip is then flexed and adducted, and the inner table of the pelvis is exposed to the sciatic notch. The pubis is exposed by retracting the iliopsoas tendon medially. The direct head of the rectus is reflected distally from the anteroinferior iliac spine, exposing the anterior hip capsule. Blunt dissection then proceeds distally and medially, and under an image intensifier, a scissors is used to palpate the ischium and the obturator foramen.

Performing osteotomies has become relatively routine with the help of an image intensifier. We use the image intensifier at four critical points during the osteotomy: first during initiation of the ischial osteotomy, and then to obtain an anteroposterior (AP) image to ensure that the osteotomy is distal and medial enough and is oriented properly. The ischial osteotome is left in place as a guide for the final osteotomy (the posterior iliac osteotomy). Often, this osteotome can be palpated medially and distally over the quadrilateral surface. The pubic bone is exposed using a Hohmann retractor, and the image is checked to ensure that one is medial enough, which prevents entry of the osteotomy into the joint. The pubic osteotomy is then performed in an oblique fashion, proximal-medial to distal-lateral, which facilitates mobilization of the fragment. The iliac cut typically is made at or just distal to the anterosuperior iliac spine. An AP image is obtained to ensure that the cut is high enough above the joint to allow satisfactory fixation of the distal fragment. It is often helpful to orient the iliac cut slightly distally to ensure that when the iliac cut is turned to connect with the ischial cut, the cut is distal to the top of the sciatic notch.

The image intensifier is quite helpful with the final osteotomy. A 45-degree oblique radiograph shows the posterior column of the acetabulum, ensuring that the posterior osteotomy is extra-articular and does not violate the posterior column. Once the cuts are made, the fragment is mobilized. Occasionally, the "corners" of the cuts can impinge or catch, limiting mobilization. Care must be taken to avoid hinging the fragment with correction. This error is easily detected, both on palpation and radiographically. The acetabular teardrop should be seen to flip radiographically to confirm that the fragment is not hinging. If a fragment is hinging posteriorly and inferiorly, the corner can be trimmed with an osteotome or a rongeur, facilitating mobility. When all three osteotomies are completed in the proper location, the posterior column should be left intact, and the acetabular fragment should be free and mobile.

The most difficult part of the operation is obtaining proper correction. One should think of the proper correction in four different planes: proper medialization of the hip center of rotation, proper acetabular version, proper lateral coverage, and proper AP coverage of the femoral head. In reality, there is only one perfect correction for each dysplastic hip, and errors in correction in any of these planes can lead to suboptimal coverage. When assessing correction, a true AP radiograph of the pelvis should be obtained. Ensuring that the pelvis is not tilted in any direction facilitates proper assessment of acetabular version and medialization. A true AP radiograph should have symmetrical obturator foramina, with the coccyx ending approximately 1 cm proximal to the symphysis pubis. In patients with bilateral dysplasia, the medial aspect of the femoral head is placed just lateral (0 to 5 mm) to the ilioischial line. Proper lateral correction is best assessed by normalizing the weight-bearing acetabular surface of the acetabulum and making the weight-bearing surface between 0 and 10 degrees off the horizontal. It is important not to overcorrect laterally because this can lead to impingement and may potentially bring the fovea into the weight-bearing surface.

If the Tonnis angle (angle of acetabular sourcil) has been normalized and the Wieberg angle is still less than optimal, a varus femoral osteotomy should be considered. Intraoperative functional views with fluoroscopy can help in that decision-making process. Anterior correction and anteversion are critical; it is very easy to overcorrect the fragment anteriorly, leading to anterior impingement of the femoral head-neck junction on the anterior rim of the acetabulum with secondary limitation of hip flexion. In extreme cases, anterior overcorrection can lead to posterior subluxation of the femoral head. On a true AP radiograph of the pelvis, the relationship of the anterior and posterior acetabular rims relative to the lateral edge of the weight-bearing surface indicates the amount of anteversion. The anterior wall should cover approximately one third of the femoral head, and the posterior wall should cover about half of the femoral head; both walls should meet at the lateral aspect of the acetabular sourcil. If the anterior wall covers less of the femoral head than the posterior wall, and if they meet at the lateral aspect of the sourcil on a true AP radiograph of the pelvis, then the socket is adequately anteverted. If the posterior wall meets the sourcil medial to the anterior wall, then the socket has been retroverted. Once correction in all planes is deemed satisfactory, temporary smooth pins are removed and replaced with three 4.5-mm , fully threaded cortical screws (Fig. 56-4). The hip capsule is then opened for assessment of the labrum. If the labrum is detached from the rim and is repairable, it is fixed with sutures. If it is frayed and irreparable, an elliptical excision is performed. One should verify that the hip can be flexed up to 110 to 115 degrees without impingement of the femoral head-neck junction on the acetabular rim. If impingement is noted, the socket must be checked to ensure that it is not retroverted. If socket anteversion is believed to be appropriate, an osteochondroplasty is performed at the anterior head-neck junction to improve the femoral head-neck junction.

POSTOPERATIVE MANAGEMENT AND REHABILITATION

On the first postoperative day, drains are removed and the patient is mobilized with ambulatory aids. Intravenous antibiotics are used for 24 hours. Epidural and urinary catheters are left in place for 24 to 48 hours. Aspirin is used for 6 weeks for deep vein thrombosis prophylaxis. Weight bearing as tolerated, abduction exercises, aquatherapy, and stationary bike exercises begin at 4 weeks.

Acetabular Retrotorsion

Retroversion of the acetabulum has been increasingly recognized over the past 10 years as a potential source of hip discomfort. It is defined as a posteriorly oriented acetabular opening (reference to the sagittal plane) and can be seen as an isolated entity or associated with classic hip dysplasia. It also is seen after injury to the triradiate cartilage in a child or in association with bladder exstrophy or Legg-Calvé-Perthes disease.

Patients with a retroverted acetabulum typically present with groin pain that can be reproduced with flexion and internal rotation of the hip. This pain is most likely secondary to impingement of the head-neck junction against the prominent retroverted anterolateral edge of the acetabulum. The diagnosis of acetabular retroversion can be made by computed tomography (CT) with horizontal acetabular cross-sections or on the basis of a crossover sign on the true AP radiograph. Radiographically, on a true AP radiograph of the pelvis in neutral inclination, the anterior wall of a normal acetabulum covers about one third of the femoral head, and the posterior wall covers about half of the femoral head; they meet at the lateral edge of the sourcil. In a retroverted acetabulum, the posterior wall is across from the anterior wall and meets the sourcil medial to the anterior wall; this is called the *crossover sign.*

A posterior wall sign is present when the outline of the posterior wall is more medial than the center of the femoral head, indicating relatively less posterior femoral head coverage. Magnetic resonance imaging (MRI) with intra-articular gadolinium commonly shows changes in the acetabular rim and the anterior head-neck junction.

Labral abnormalities, and later articular cartilage delamination, can be seen at the anterior-lateral acetabular rim. Retroversion of the acetabulum has been implicated in the development of secondary arthritis as a result of recurrent impingement. When nonsurgical treatment fails, surgical intervention is considered. Because anterior rim lesions are secondary to the structural bony problems, arthroscopic débridement alone does not solve the primary pathology and is not likely a permanent solution.

Acetabular reorientation, which increases anteversion, has been reported to improve all of the following: clinical hip scores; hip internal rotation, flexion, and adduction; and radiographic coverage of the hip (Fig. 56-5).[10]

An alternative treatment for a retroverted socket is trimming of the anterior aspect of the acetabular rim. This is indicated when the socket is in retrotorsion in the presence of satisfactory posterior coverage. Trimming also can be considered in patients with severely compromised anterior articular cartilage as noted on MRI.

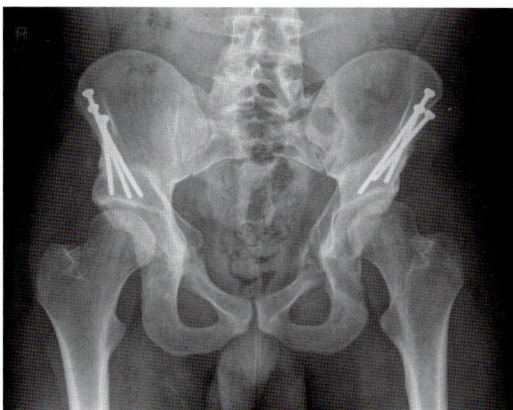

Figure 56-4. Postoperative anteroposterior (AP) radiographs of bilateral classic hip dysplasia before and after correction.

RESULTS

Over the past 10 to 15 years, many published clinical studies have reported results of periacetabular osteotomy. Most of these studies showed major radiographic improvement in biomechanics about the hip joint, and all studies showed significant improvement in hip pain and function scores. A 20-year experience with this operation has been described, and at long-term

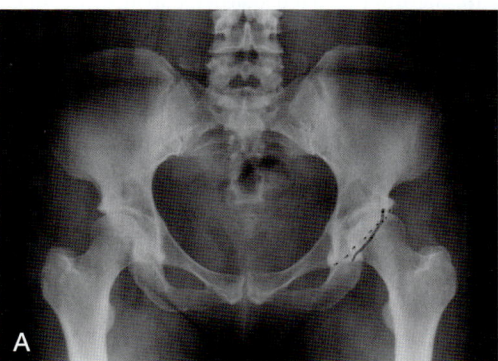
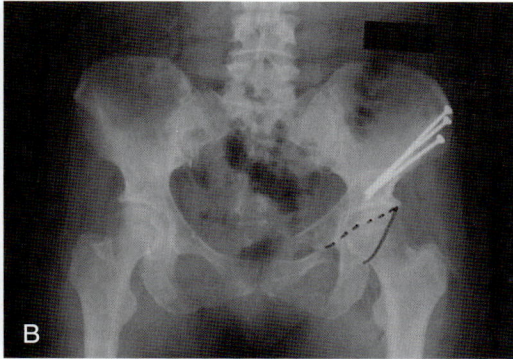

Figure 56-5. Preoperative **(A)** and postoperative **(B)** anteroposterior (AP) radiographs of a retroverted left socket and an anteverted socket after correction. The dotted line is drawn at the anterior wall.

follow-up, the group from Bern revealed hip joint survivorship of 82% at an average follow-up of more than 11 years. In all, 73% of patients had good to excellent results clinically; factors associated with failure have included advanced arthrosis at the time of surgery, older patient age, inadequate correction, and labral pathology. These results have been repeated at multiple centers throughout the world. Data from Rochester, Minnesota, Boston, and many other hip centers have shown significant improvement both clinically and radiographically in most patients who undergo this operation.

COMPLICATIONS

Periacetabular osteotomy is a complex operation. Nerve injury, including damage to the lateral femoral cutaneous nerve and the sciatic, femoral and obturator nerves, can occur. Some centers have used intraoperative electromyographic (EMG) monitoring in an attempt to decrease the risk of damage to the sciatic and femoral nerves during the procedure; however, it remains unproven whether this technology decreases neuropraxia rates. Intra-articular fracture is a rare occurrence seen in less than 1% of patients. The use of intraoperative fluoroscopy minimizes the risk of this serious complication. Nonunion can occur. Iliac nonunion is extremely rare, but depending on the osteotomy displacement, superior pubic ramus nonunion can occur in up to 7% to 10% of patients. Most patients who have pubic nonunion are asymptomatic. Ischial nonunion can occur rarely and is associated with ligamentous laxity or iatrogenic extension of the ischial osteotomy in the lesser sciatic foramen. Vascular injury is extremely uncommon. Osteonecrosis of the acetabulum can occur if the osteotomy is done too close to the joint. The most common complication after this osteotomy is poor positioning of the fragment.

CONCLUSION

Acetabular osteotomy is the treatment of choice for young active patients with symptomatic structural abnormalities of the acetabulum in the absence of severe secondary degenerative changes. Reorientation pelvic osteotomy can provide pain relief, improve acetabular coverage, and decrease joint surface contact forces in patients with classic dysplasia, retrotorted orientation of the acetabulum, or, rarely, post-traumatic problems.

REFERENCES

1. Tonnis D: Congenital dysplasia and dislocation of the hip, Berlin, 1987, Springer-Verlag.
2. Murphy SB, Kijewski PK, Millis MB, Harless A: Acetabular dysplasia in the adolescent and young adult. Clin Orthop Relat Res 261:213–223, 1990.
3. Ganz R, Klaue K, Vinh TS, Mast JW: A new periacetabular osteotomy for the treatment of hip dysplasias: technique and preliminary results. Clin Orthop Relat Res 232:26–36, 1988.
4. Clohisy JC, Barrett SE, Gordon JE, et al: Periacetabular osteotomy for the treatment of severe acetabular dysplasia. J Bone Joint Surg Am 87:254–259, 2005.
5. Crockarell J, Trousdale RT, Cabanela ME, Berry DJ: Early experience and results with the periacetabular osteotomy: the Mayo Clinic experience. Clin Orthop Relat Res 363:45–53, 1999.
6. Davey JP, Santore RF: Complications of periacetabular osteotomy. Clin Orthop Relat Res 353:33–37, 1999.
7. Kralj M, Mavcic B, Antolic V, et al: The Bernese periacetabular osteotomy: clinical, radiographic and mechanical 7-15-year follow-up of 26 hips. Acta Orthop 76:833–840, 2005.
8. Mayo KA, Trumble SJ, Mast JW: Results of periacetabular osteotomy in patients with previous surgery for hip dysplasia. Clin Orthop Relat Res 363:73–80, 1999.
9. Myers SR, Eijer H, Ganz R: Anterior femoroacetabular impingement after periacetabular osteotomy. Clin Orthop Relat Res 363:93–99, 1999.
10. Siebenrock KA, Schöll E, Lottenbach M, Ganz R: Bernese periacetabular osteotomy. Clin Orthop Relat Res 363:9–20, 1999.
11. Trumble SJ, Mayo KA, Mast JW: The periacetabular osteotomy: minimum 2 year followup in more than 100 hips. Clin Orthop Relat Res 363:54–63, 1999.
12. Murphy SB, Millis MB, Hall JE: Surgical correction of acetabular dysplasia in the adult. A Boston experience. Clin Orthop Relat Res 1999;363:38–44.
13. Trousdale RT, Ekkernkamp A, Ganz R: Periacetabular osteotomy for the dysplastic hip with osteoarthritis. J Bone Joint Surg 1995;77-A:73–85.
14. McGrory BJ, Trousdale RT: Tips of the trade: Sterile EMG monitoring during hip and pelvis surgery. Orthop Rev 1994;23:274.
15. Pring ME, Trousdale RT, Cabanela ME, Harper CM: Intraoperative electromyographic monitoring during periacetabular osteotomy. Clin Orthop Relat Res 400:158–164, 2002.
16. Hussell JG, Mast JW, Mayo KA, et al: A comparison of different surgical approaches for the periacetabular osteotomy. Clin Orthop Relat Res 363:64–72, 1999.
17. Matta JM, Stover MD, Siebenrock K: Periacetabular osteotomy through the Smith-Peterson approach. Clin Orthop Relat Res 363:21–32, 1999.
18. Trousdale RT: Recurrent anterior hip instability after a simple hip dislocation. Clin Orthop Relat Res 408:189–192, 2003.
19. McGrory BJ, Trousdale RT, Cabanela ME, Ganz R: Bernese periacetabular osteotomy: surgical techniques. J Orthop Tech 1247:179–191, 1993.

CHAPTER 57

Femoral Osteotomy

Miguel E. Cabanela

INTRODUCTION

It is now well established that degenerative arthritis of the hip is generally the consequence of sometimes subtle, sometimes obvious morphologic abnormalities of the joint that produce articular cartilage loads in excess of what the cartilage can tolerate. These abnormalities often become mildly symptomatic early in life. However, although they can be very limiting in the life of a young active adult, they often are not symptomatic enough to justify joint replacement. Furthermore, the longevity of joint replacement in young patients is limited by problems of polyethylene wear and resulting osteolysis, and new bearing surfaces have shown their own set of problems.

Consequently, there has been a resurgence of interest in *joint preservation surgery*. If a symptomatic joint deformity that reduces the cartilage surface area and results in excessive loads on the articular cartilage above what the cartilage can tolerate for proper viability and function can be corrected by a *geometric* operation that would increase the area of cartilage available for load and therefore decrease the load per unit area, this would potentially obviate the need for a joint replacement or may delay such surgery. The objectives of the osteotomy most often are to correct the anatomic abnormality, optimize hip congruity, decrease cartilage load/unit area to a level compatible with good function, and improve joint biomechanics. In addition, osteotomy can make the range of motion more functional and can help eliminate fixed deformities.

From a clinical perspective, osteotomy should reduce patient symptoms, help delay the development or progression of osteoarthritis, and therefore delay the need for joint replacement. Thus by its nature, osteotomy often is a temporizing operation, and its results, which

are somewhat unpredictable and temporary, are correlated with the fact that the biological capacity of the cartilage to regenerate is not fully predictable or understood. Perhaps the results of osteotomy should not be judged by the same parameters used to judge replacement surgery.

Osteotomy about the hip can be performed on both sides of the joint, that is, the pelvis and the proximal femur. Currently, pelvic osteotomy is far more popular because as techniques have reached significant maturity, the corrective power of the procedure is greater, and the number of patients who can benefit from the procedure is larger. Furthermore, in most patients with hip dysplasia, the anatomic abnormality is more severe on the pelvic side of the joint. In this chapter, we will discuss the remaining few indications for an osteotomy of the proximal femur, an operation that is older than pelvic osteotomy but is more limited in scope of applications and usefulness.

Historically, the operation is almost 200 years old. Barton,[1] in 1827, reported on an intertrochanteric osteotomy performed on a sailor with a post-traumatic deformity of the proximal femur. Kirmisson,[2] in 1984, described an osteotomy through the proximal femur to treat developmental dysplasia. Surgeons from Germany and Austria introduced modifications to the Kirmisson osteotomy in the first part of the 20th century. Names such as VonBaeyer,[3] Lorenz,[4] and Schanz[5] are associated with developmental dysplasia of the hip (DDH). The first report of a proximal femoral osteotomy to treat osteoarthritis was that of McMurray[6] in 1935. He attempted to change the line of load by a large medial displacement of the distal fragment, thereby unloading the articular cartilage. He also introduced the concept of the *vascular effect* of the osteotomy, whereby increased vascularity brought about by osteotomy healing would have a beneficial effect on the articular cartilage.

It was Pauwels[7-9] in 1950 who clearly revolutionized the concept of femoral osteotomy by introducing the concept of valgus and varus osteotomies to increase the weight-bearing surface area of the hip joint. Bombelli,[10] in the 1970s, further expanded the Pauwels doctrine by introducing the concept of correction in the sagittal plane by adding flexion or extension to the varus or valgus angulation in an effort to further increase the weight-bearing surface area of the hip joint. Modern day femoral osteotomies are based on the ideas of Pauwels and Bombelli.

CURRENT INDICATIONS OF FEMORAL OSTEOTOMIES

Patients considered good candidates for femoral osteotomies are those with morphologic hip joint abnormalities in which realignment of the proximal femur would increase the joint contact area. The prime indication is developmental dysplasia with coxa valga. Patients with avascular necrosis and small lesions occasionally can be helped by femoral osteotomy. Those with posttraumatic deformities such as femoral neck nonunion or proximal femoral malunion also may be good candidates for the procedure. Patients with other conditions such as the residua of slipped capital femoral epiphysis (SCFE) or Perthes, or leg length inequality, may be treated occasionally by proximal femoral osteotomy.

Inflammatory arthritis, severe stiffness, and active infection contraindicate the procedure.

Factors that should be considered in decisions regarding an osteotomy are patient age, weight, and occupation (manual laborer vs. sedentary), the condition of the lumbar spine and ipsilateral knee, and leg lengths.

Developmental Dysplasia

The most common anatomic abnormality in dysplasia is found in the acetabulum. Its abnormal slope and deficiency causes the center of rotation of the hip to displace laterally and the femoral head to be poorly covered laterally, anteriorly, and superiorly. This problem is helped by pelvic osteotomy. Sometimes however, associated excessive anteversion and valgus of the proximal femur is the dominant deformity. In this instance—coxa valga luxans of Bombelli—a femoral osteotomy can improve head coverage, medialize the center of rotation, improve function, and, by decreasing the load per unit area of cartilage, decrease pain.[11]

Prerequisites for a varus intertrochanteric osteotomy include the presence of a spherical femoral head, an increased neck shaft angle, relatively minor acetabular involvement, and good to excellent range of motion. The patient should have no pain with the hip in an abducted position. Radiologically, improvement of femoral head coverage in abduction is a favorable sign, as is satisfactory anterior head coverage in the false profile view. Mild deficiency of anterior coverage can be helped by adding a little extension to the abduction or varus osteotomy.

Varus osteotomy potentially produces marked limb shortening, but this can be minimized by a straight osteotomy made transversely across the proximal femur at the level of the lesser trochanter, followed by repair of the proximal fragment after it is abducted, without removal of a wedge of bone. The resultant gap reliably fills with bone over time. Because of shortening of abductor muscles that occurs with this surgery, abductor weakness persists for a long time, even up to a year, and it is advisable to place patients on a prolonged abductor strengthening exercise program. Finally, it is important to recognize that the osteotomy is unlikely to be the final operation; therefore, it is advisable to avoid producing significant deformities of the proximal femur, which may make the subsequent arthroplasty very difficult. Thus, extending the proximal fragment more than 20 degrees and/or abducting it more than 20 to 25 degrees is not recommended. If greater abduction is necessary, simultaneous greater trochanteric osteotomy and advancement is necessary. Otherwise, the trochanter would overlie the femoral canal, and it would be necessary to osteotomize it at the time of arthroplasty to avoid abductor muscle injury (Fig. 57-1).

When a varus osteotomy of the proximal femur is performed, medial displacement of the distal fragment is necessary to preserve the mechanical axis of the extremity and avoid eccentric knee loads.

It could be said that the results of varus femoral osteotomies correlate with the severity of the pathology treated. If the operation is performed in patients with no or minimal degenerative disease, good to excellent results have been reported in 70% to 90% of patients with follow-up longer than 10 years.[12-16] As occurs with osteotomies about the knee, results deteriorate with the passage of time.

Adduction or valgus intertrochanteric osteotomy for dysplasia is done very rarely today in North America. The classical indication is the "out-of-round" femoral head with a large medial osteophyte (Bombelli called this the *capital drop osteophyte*), an increased neck shaft angle, poor acetabular coverage, and a proximally

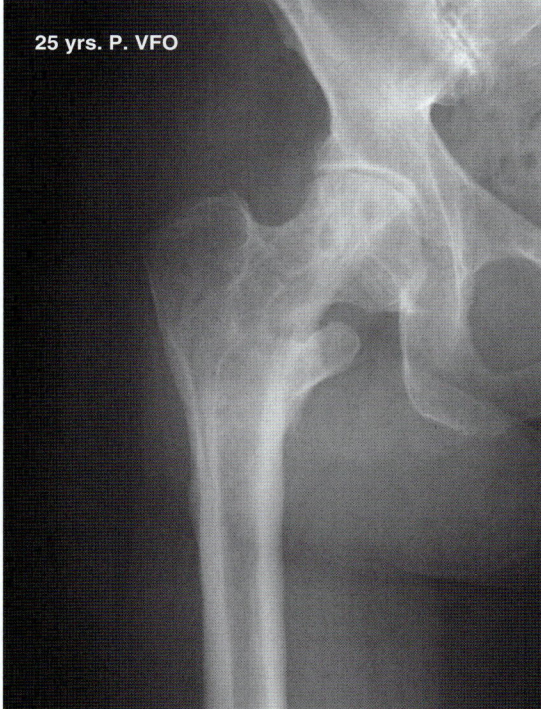

25 yrs. P. VFO

Figure 57-1. Anteroposterior radiograph of the hip of a 72-year-old woman 25 years after a varus intertrochanteric osteotomy. She has become symptomatic enough to undergo joint arthroplasty. Note the position of the trochanter overlying the femoral canal. A trochanteric osteotomy may be advisable for arthroplasty.

migrated greater trochanter. An adduction (valgus) and extension osteotomy in this situation would improve joint congruity, unload the superior lateral joint space, and improve joint mechanics by loading the medial osteophyte. Bombelli thought that adduction of the proximal fragment would increase tension on the lateral capsule, and that this might stimulate cartilage metaplasia on the acetabular rim with the passage of time.

Candidates for this osteotomy should have adequate range of hip motion and particularly should be comfortable or should experience reduced pain with the legs crossed in extension (hip adducted). Radiologically, the preoperative x-ray in adduction should show improved joint congruity.

Because valgus osteotomies are done in patients who already have degenerative joint disease, they fall into the category of salvage procedures. Results therefore are less predictable than those of varus osteotomies and typically of lesser quality. Survivorship of the procedure before conversion to arthroplasty at 5 years has been reported in the realm of 50% to 70%.[17,18] Patients therefore should be carefully selected, and realistic expectations should be emphasized before this operation is begun.

In truth, these surgeries are performed far less frequently today, when it appears that the results and longevity of arthroplasty in young patients have become more predictable.

Sequelae of SCFE and Perthes

Both conditions are causes of early degenerative joint disease in young adults. SCFE results in posterior and medial displacement of the epiphysis, and the typical complaint is limited hip flexion combined with external rotation deformity of the limb and symptoms of femoroacetabular impingement.

Because this problem occurs early in life, surgical correction may be advisable, even if symptoms are relatively mild (not in an asymptomatic patients, however). The risk of avascular necrosis potentially is high if correction is attempted at the site of deformity in the femoral neck, although special methods and exposures to avoid this problem are under development. Therefore, some believe that the most logical site of correction would be at the intertrochanteric level, and that the procedure of choice is a flexion osteotomy combined at times with internal rotation of the shaft fragment. It is advisable to add an anterior capsulotomy of the hip to facilitate extension. Sometimes, adduction (valgus) of the proximal fragment can be added to move the lateral "bump" (which occurs near the head-neck junction and causes impingement) away from the acetabular rim to improve abduction. Capsulotomy, direct inspection of the femoral head after the osteotomy, and removal of the offending bump are often added to the procedure today.

When performing these procedures, one should think of the future and should strive to avoid severe distortion of the proximal femoral anatomy, so that arthroplasty is not made exceedingly difficult when, not if, it becomes necessary.

Avascular Necrosis

Intertrochanteric femoral osteotomy is seldom used today in the management of avascular necrosis of the femoral head. The objective of osteotomy in avascular necrosis would be to rotate the femoral head so that weight bearing is performed by good bone supporting noncollapsed articular cartilage, thus moving necrotic bone away from weight bearing. Logically then, the necrotic process should be limited to small portions of the femoral head, so that rotation away from load bearing can be executed. Because most avascular necroses are fairly extensive, the number of patients for whom this procedure is applicable is very limited.

With this in mind, it is obvious that osteotomy is not indicated before collapse of the articular cartilage has occurred; thus in Ficat stages I and II, osteotomy is not indicated. Osteotomy is not indicated when joint damage is present (stage IV). Thus there is only a narrow range of osteotomy indications, specifically when collapse is beginning, and only if the necrotic segment is small. The size of the lesion can be assessed with plain radiographs in two planes, or more accurately with computed tomography (CT) scans. One can draw the necrotic arc angles (Kerboull angles) on radiographs by tracing the segment of the head involved by the necrotic process on an anteroposterior and a lateral radiograph, and then summing the angles. If the sum is less than 200 degrees, osteotomy may be considered. The origin of the necrotic process probably plays a role in the osteotomy indication. Patients with avascular necrosis secondary to steroids or to alcohol intake usually have very large lesions and seldom are candidates for osteotomy; on the contrary, post-traumatic necrosis can be more segmental, and patients with this diagnosis more often are candidates.

Osteotomies can be rotational or angular. The transtrochanteric rotational osteotomy of Sugioka enjoyed a brief period of popularity in North America because of its theoretical advantages: the ability to rotate even a large lesion away from weight bearing, and the early satisfactory results reported. For success, however, this procedure requires preservation of the posterior column artery on which the femoral head blood supply is based. Sugioka has reported good to excellent results in a large number of patients with up to 11 years of follow-up.[19,20] These results could not be duplicated by others in Japan,[21] Europe, or the United States. Our own results show progressive collapse or very symptomatic degenerative joint disease in 83% of patients with 5 years of follow-up.[22] The technique is technically demanding and has been virtually abandoned in North America today.

Valgus and varus with flexion or extension added have been advocated and may be indicated in exceptional cases with segmental necrosis small enough to be moved away from weight bearing without significant disruption of joint mechanics. Typical reports show improvement in around 70% of cases.[23-25]

As long-term results of joint replacement in the young patient and in those with avascular necrosis improve, and as indications of joint replacement are extended, femoral osteotomy is used less frequently in treating these patients.

Nonunion of Femoral Neck Fracture

Femoral neck nonunion remains a very good indication for osteotomy in the young patient if the head appears mostly viable. Femoral head viability can be assessed by scintigraphy or preferably by magnetic resonance imaging (MRI). The presence of small areas of avascular necrosis is not a contraindication for osteotomy.[26]

The femoral neck fractures most likely to evolve toward nonunion are those with a vertical fracture line (Pauwels type 3). The rationale of treatment by osteotomy is to horizontalize the fracture line so that shearing forces at the fracture site are converted into compressive forces, thus enhancing fracture union. To

do this, a valgus osteotomy is carried out, and the ideal fixation device is an offset angle blade plate with an angle of 110 degrees, 120 degrees, or, uncommonly, 130 degrees. This requires careful preoperative templating and very careful execution[27]; the plate has to be anchored in remaining good bone in the head, and an adequate bridge between the point of entry of the blade into the side of the proximal femur and the osteotomy site must exist, so that fixation is not compromised.

In a small series of 15 patients with femoral neck nonunion treated by valgus osteotomy, we showed that the union rate was 80% and femoral head salvage was 67% (Figs. 57-2 through 57-4).[26] In our experience, however, the presence of a postoperative limp was common. We believe this is related to the mechanical effect of decreased offset and the abductor lever arm caused by femoral neck shortening and valgus

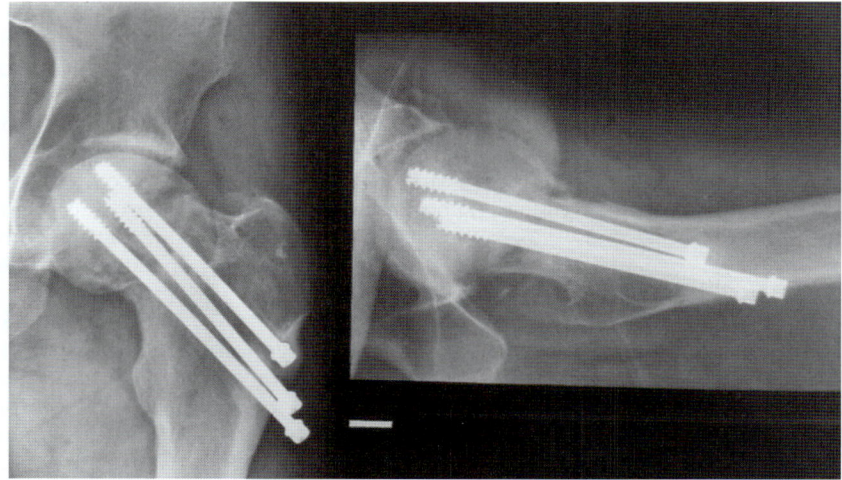

Figure 57-2. Anteroposterior and lateral hip radiographs of a 20-year-old man 12 months after a femoral neck fracture. The patient has severe hip pain.

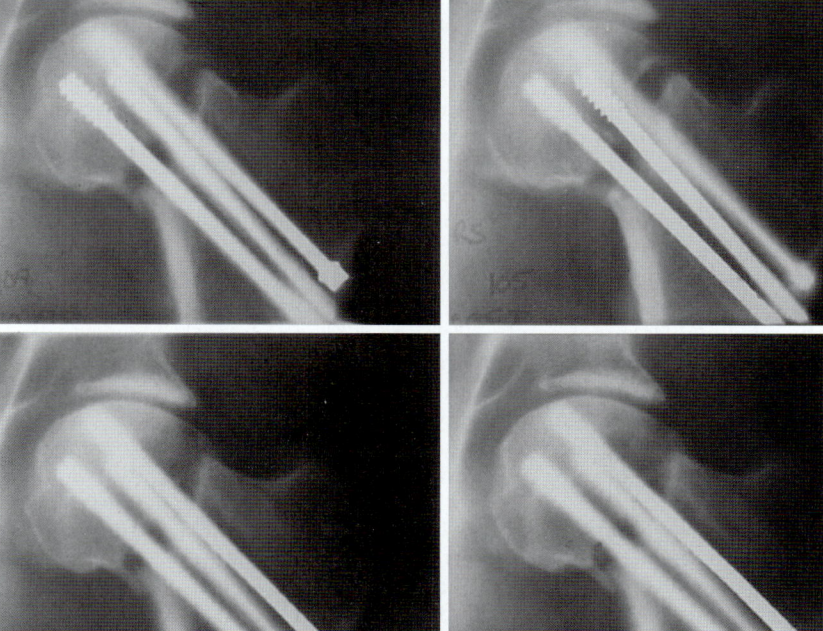

Figure 57-3. Anteroposterior tomograms of the same hip, confirming the presence of a nonunion.

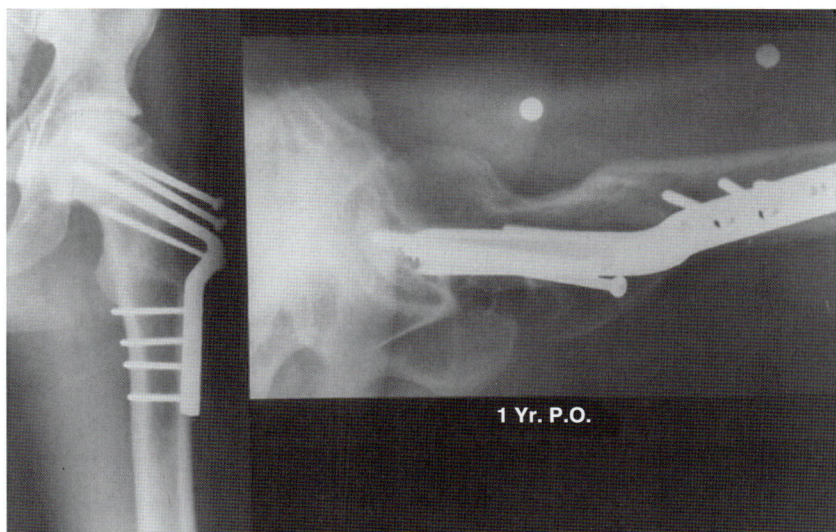

Figure 57-4. Anteroposterior and lateral hip radiographs of the same patient 1 year after valgus osteotomy. Note that both the osteotomy and the fracture have healed.

1 Yr. P.O.

osteotomy. It was our impression, after examining these patients, that excessive valgus and horizontalization of the fracture site should be avoided to minimize undesirable effects on gait.

Contraindications for this valgus osteotomy include advanced age (joint replacement is clearly preferred for such patients), significant femoroacetabular incongruity, and severe bone loss. As mentioned, evidence of small areas of avascular necrosis is not a contraindication to osteotomy. The presence of avascular necrosis may decrease the quality of the clinical result, although it does not interfere with fracture union.

TECHNIQUE AND COMPLICATIONS

By and large, the techniques proposed by Müller[28] using a blade plate for osteotomy fixation are the most commonly used methods today. These techniques are described in detail elsewhere.

Essential elements of a technically successful osteotomy include the following:

- Proper preoperative templating with accurate planning of the angle of correction in both anteroposterior and lateral planes. Particularly important are the point of entry of the chisel and subsequent blade in the lateral cortex of the femur, the length of penetration of the blade into the proximal femur and therefore the length of the blade, the inclination of the plate in relation to the longitudinal axis of the femur, which will determine the amount of flexion or extension of the osteotomy, and the choice of offset on the blade plate, which will determine the medial or lateral translation of the distal femur (this is important for preserving proper limb alignment and avoiding improper loading of the ipsilateral knee).
- Careful execution of the technique. This demands fluoroscopic monitoring of chisel insertion in the predetermined position. The path for the blade is made by the chisel; driving the chisel in and out several times with small blows of the hammer facilitates

creating a good path for the blade and minimizes the risk of creating a different path when the blade is inserted.
- Planning should include identifying the presence of an adequate bridge of bone between the osteotomy and the point of entry of the blade (at least 1.5 cm) to avoid fracture of this bony bridge, which would place in peril the fixation of the osteotomy.
- If adequate fixation is obtained, there is no need for external immobilization. However, partial weight bearing with crutch support for 8 weeks is necessary before full unrestricted weight bearing is allowed.
- Abduction strengthening exercises are advisable because abductor weakness after intertrochanteric osteotomy is the rule. It is not uncommon to have an abductor limp for up to a year after a varus osteotomy.

Complications of osteotomy include failure of fixation, which most commonly is related to technical execution of the procedure. Fixation problems can lead to nonunion, in which case reoperation may be necessary to refix the osteotomy or, depending on the circumstances, to convert to joint replacement. Hemorrhage, nerve palsy, or infection can occur; these events are not specific to this procedure, and they are uncommon.

TOTAL HIP ARTHROPLASTY AFTER INTERTROCHANTERIC OSTEOTOMY

Almost by definition, all osteotomies have a finite life, and eventually the wear and tear process in the joint requires a joint arthroplasty. Over the past two decades, femoral osteotomy has been performed with less and less frequency. Thus conversion of osteotomy to hip replacement is not a common procedure today. Most osteotomy conversions occurred in the first two decades of hip joint replacement; therefore, experience with conversion is by and large based on cemented replacement.

Early experience with cemented hip replacement after osteotomy showed that the procedure was technically difficult, intraoperative and postoperative complications were common, and, perhaps because of this, the infection rate was high.[29-32] Among the technical difficulties, hardware removal and the need for a trochanteric osteotomy to gain access to the hip were cited. Deformity of the proximal femur by the previous osteotomy made conversion for total hip arthroplasty (THA) more difficult. All these challenges prolonged operative time in these cases. In addition, and perhaps in part because of all these reasons, prosthesis survival after this procedure appears to be slightly worse in some publications than after cemented primary hip replacement for osteoarthritis.

These experiences have taught us several lessons. First, when an intertrochanteric osteotomy is done, the proximal femoral anatomy should be distorted as little as possible, so that execution of a subsequent THA is not hampered (see Fig. 57-1). It is better to avoid the wedge osteotomy technique, especially at the subtrochanteric level; this would make a re-osteotomy mandatory at the time of arthroplasty. Second, routine hardware removal after the osteotomy has healed is a minor procedure with small risks; it can help avoid technical problems and can shorten operative time at the time of arthroplasty.

Published experience on cementless hip arthroplasty after proximal femoral osteotomy is limited. The author's tendency is to use diaphyseal fixation when doing this procedure today, because metaphyseal fixation may be hampered by the altered anatomy of the proximal femur.

FINAL CONSIDERATIONS

Given the enormous popularity of hip replacement over the past three decades, it is unfortunate that both patients and surgeons in North America appear to have lost interest in alternative procedures. As a result of this, the expertise needed to perform an osteotomy has become more and more restricted to a few specialized hip surgery centers.

Yet there is no question that in selected young patients, femoral osteotomy can provide many years of good pain relief and satisfactory hip function. Certain patients with developmental dysplasia, slipped capital femoral epiphysis, and femoral neck nonunion may be excellent candidates for proximal femoral osteotomy. Less frequently, the procedure may be indicated for other diagnoses. Patients who are potential candidates for this procedure should be educated about its advantages and disadvantages, as well as the potential problems of the alternative, namely, having hip joint replacement at a young age.

REFERENCES

1. Barton JR: On the treatment of ankylosis by the formation of artificial joints. North Am Med J 3:269–310, 1827.

2. Kirmisson E: De l'osteotomie sous-trochanterienne applique a certains cas de la luxation congenitale de la hanche. Rev Orthop 5:137–146, 1984.

3. Von-Baeyer H: Behandlung von nicht-reparier-baren Angeborenen Huftuerre-Kungen. Munch Med Wochenschr 65:1216, 1918.

4. Lorenz A: Uber die Behandling der irreponiblen argeborenen Huftluxation und der Schenkel halspeudarthrose mittels babelung. Wien Klin Wochenscher 32:997, 1919.

5. Schanz A: Fur Behandling der veralteten angeborenen Hufturrenkung. Munch Med Wochenschr 69:930k, 1922.

6. McMurray TP: Osteoarthritis of the hip joint. Br J Surg 22:716–727, 1935.

7. Pauwels F: Biomechanics of the normal and diseased hip: theoretical foundation, technique and results of treatment. An atlas, New York, 1976, Springer.

8. Pauwels F: Der Schenkelhalsbruch ein mechanisches Problem: Grundlagen des heilungsvorganges Prognose and kausale Therapie, Stuttgart, 1935, Ferdinand Enke Verlag.

9. Pauwels F: Uber eine kausale Behandlung der coxa valga luxans. Zeitschr Orthop 79:305–315, 1950.

10. Bombelli R: Osteoarthritis of the hip: pathogenesis and consequent therapy, Berlin, 1976, Springer.

11. Sanchez-Sotelo J, Trousdale RT, Berry DJ, et al: Surgical treatment of developmental dysplasia of the hip in adults. I. Nonarthroplasty options. J Am Acad Orthop Surg 10:321–333, 2002.

12. Iwase T, Hasegawa Y, Kawamoto K, et al: Twenty years' follow-up of intertrochanteric osteotomy for treatment of the dysplastic hip. Clin Orthop Relat Res 331:245–255, 1996.

13. Marti RK, Schuller HM, Raaymakers EL: Intertrochanteric osteotomy for non-union of the femoral neck. J Bone Joint Surg Br 71:782–787, 1989.

14. Miegel RE, Harris WH: Medial-displacement intertrochanteric osteotomy in the treatment of osteoarthritis of the hip: a long-term follow-up study. J Bone Joint Surg Am 66:878–887, 1984.

15. Pellicci PM, Hu S, Garvin KL, et al: Varus rotational femoral osteotomies in adults with hip dysplasia. Clin Orthop Relat Res 272:162–166, 1991.

16. Weisl H: Intertrochanteric osteotomy for osteoarthritis: a long-term follow-up. J Bone Joint Surg Br 62:37–42, 1980.

17. Gotoh E, Inao S, Okamoto T, et al: Valgus-extension osteotomy for advanced osteoarthritis in dysplastic hips: results at 12 to 18 years. J Bone Joint Surg Br 79:609–615, 1997.

18. Maistrelli GL, Gerundini M, Fusco U, et al: Valgus-extension osteotomy for osteoarthritis of the hip: indications and long-term results. J Bone Joint Surg Br 72:653–657, 1990.

19. Sugioka Y, Hotokebuchi T, Tsutsui H: Transtrochanteric anterior rotational osteotomy for idiopathic and steroid-induced necrosis of the femoral head: indications and long-term results. Clin Orthop Relat Res 277:111–120, 1992.

20. Sugioka Y, Katsuki I, Hotokebuchi T: Transtrochanteric rotational osteotomy of the femoral head for the treatment of osteonecrosis: follow-up statistics. Clin Orthop Relat Res 169:115–125, 1982.

21. Sugano N, Takaoka K, Ohzono K, et al: Rotational osteotomy for nontraumatic avascular necrosis of the femoral head. J Bone Joint Surg Br 74:734–739, 1992.

22. Dean MT, Cabanela ME: Transtrochanteric anterior rotational osteotomy for avascular necrosis of the femoral head: long term results. J Bone Joint Surg Br 75:597–601, 1993.

23. Mont MA, Fairbank AC, Jinnah RH, et al: Varus osteotomy for avascular necrosis of the femoral head: results of long-term follow-up. Paper presented at the Annual Meeting of the American Academy of Orthopaedic Surgeons, New Orleans, Louisiana, February 26, 1994.

24. Mont MA, Fairbank AC, Krackow KA, et al: Corrective osteotomy for osteonecrosis of the femoral head. J Bone Joint Surg Am 78:1032–1038, 1996.

25. Scher MA, Jakim I: Intertrochanteric osteotomy and autogenous bone grafting for avascular necrosis of the femoral head. J Bone Joint Surg Am 75:1119–1133, 1993.

26. Mathews V, Cabanela ME: Femoral neck nonunion treatment. Clin Orthop Relat Res 419:57–64, 2004.

27. Mast JW, May KA: The intertrochanteric osteotomy for non-union or malunion of fractures of the proximal femur. Semin Arthroplasty 8:51–68, 1997.
28. Müller ME: Intertrochanteric osteotomy: indication, preoperative planning, technique. In Schatzker J, editor: The intertrochanteric osteotomy, Berlin, 1984, Springer-Verlag, pp 26–66.
29. Benke GI, Baker AS, Dounis E: Total hip replacement after upper femoral osteotomy: a clinical review. J Bone Joint Surg Br 64:570–571, 1982.
30. Boos N, Krushell R, Ganz R, et al: Total hip arthroplasty after previous proximal femoral osteotomy. J Bone Joint Surg Br 79:247–253, 1997.
31. Ferguson GM, Cabanela ME, Ilstrup DM: Total hip arthroplasty after failed intertrochanteric osteotomy. J Bone Joint Surg Br 76:252–257, 1994.
32. Soballe K, Boll KL, Kofod S, et al: Total hip replacement after medial-displacement osteotomy of the proximal part of the femur. J Bone Joint Surg Am 71:692–697, 1989.

CHAPTER 58

Femoral Head Sparing Procedures for Osteonecrosis of the Hip

Michael A. Mont, Michael G. Zywiel, and Edward H. Becker

KEY POINTS

- Early diagnosis is critical in maximizing success with femoral head-sparing surgical procedures for osteonecrosis.
- One should select the least invasive procedure possible for a given stage of osteonecrosis.
- Use of core decompression or percutaneous drilling procedures is appropriate only in precollapse disease.
- Success rates with femoral head-sparing procedures are much lower if more than 2 mm of femoral head collapse is present, or if the necrotic lesion is large.
- Certain nonarthroplasty procedures (e.g., vascularized fibular grafting) are technically complex and should not be attempted without appropriate training.
- Many patients will eventually progress to femoral collapse, although nonarthroplasty procedures may delay this by a decade or longer. Nevertheless, it may be preferable to avoid procedures that could complicate future arthroplasty options.

INTRODUCTION

Multiple treatment options are available for osteonecrosis of the femoral head. If the disease has progressed to severe femoral head collapse and/or acetabular damage, only a hip arthroplasty will markedly relieve pain and improve function. However, for lesions that are not as advanced, multiple joint-preserving treatments have been successfully utilized to improve symptoms and delay or prevent arthroplasty.

Early diagnosis and accurate staging of the disease are important for selecting the optimal treatment. Different treatment modalities are indicated for different stages of the disease, and overall success rates are higher at earlier disease stages. Therefore, it is important to understand how to make the earliest possible diagnosis based on history and physical examination and how to plan treatment based mostly on radiographic indices.

To make an early diagnosis, the clinician should understand that osteonecrosis is frequently associated with one or more risk factors such as corticosteroid or excessive alcohol use (Box 58-1), which, if present in combination with symptoms, should trigger a low threshold for radiographic evaluation. The most common clinical symptoms of osteonecrosis include deep, throbbing groin pain and limited range of motion, especially of internal rotation.[1] Pain may be localized to the buttock, thigh, or knee. It often occurs with hip movement or weight-bearing activities, although rest pain is noted in more advanced disease. Pain usually has a gradual onset, although acute onset of symptoms may occur. Some patients have minimal pain; others are asymptomatic, irrespective of radiographic appearance.

Radiographically, osteonecrosis has a wide range of findings, and many different classification systems have been used to characterize this disease and to help stage it for diagnosis, treatment, and prognosis. For example, in one recent report, more than 23 classification systems were cited. Fortunately, most publications have described one of five commonly used systems (Table 58-1).[2-6] However, the present authors have found it more useful to understand four primary radiographic factors in staging and planning the most appropriate head-sparing procedure for these patients. These radiographic features include (1) precollapse or postcollapse (presence of crescent sign) femoral heads, with precollapse lesions having the best prognosis, (2) size of the lesion, with larger lesions having a worse prognosis than small or medium-sized lesions, (3) amount of femoral head depression, with greater than 2 mm appearing to be the cutoff for not using head-preserving procedures, and (4) acetabular involvement with disease, in which head-preserving procedures should not be used. Some authors have characterized the location of the lesion as important in determining prognosis and a treatment plan, as outlined by the Japanese Orthopaedic Association. For example, lateral lesions have a worse prognosis than medial lesions, and central lesions are more intermediate. The present authors have found that location sometimes adds little prognostic information to the size evaluation because most lateral lesions are large, and medially located lesions are usually small.

In the following description of various head-preserving procedures, we will discuss where different procedures are used based on these four radiographic features. In addition, if the clinician is reviewing the literature, one can easily convert these features into different classification systems.

BOX 58-1. RISK FACTORS FOR OSTEONECROSIS OF THE FEMORAL HEAD

Direct Risk Factors
- Traumatic fracture and/or dislocation
- Sickle cell disease
- Radiation
- Chemotherapy
- Myeloproliferative disorders
- Thalassemia
- Caisson disease

Associated Risk Factors
- Corticosteroid use
- Alcohol abuse
- Tobacco abuse
- Systemic lupus erythematosus
- Organ transplant
- Gastrointestinal disorder
- Pregnancy
- Genetic inheritance
- Coagulation deficiency

To analyze these radiographic features, it is necessary only to get good quality anteroposterior and frog-leg lateral radiographs, as well as magnetic resonance imaging (MRI) scans. When the disease is obvious (e.g., postcollapse disease with a crescent sign), it may not even be necessary to obtain an MRI evaluation. However, MRI examinations are more than 99% sensitive and specific for the disease, and rapid low-cost screening protocols have been developed that take approximately 15 minutes to perform. Other screening tests such as bone scans, computed tomography scans, and bone biopsies, although of historical importance, are not necessary for the diagnosis of osteonecrosis. For example, in one recent study, bone scanning missed 44% of symptomatic osteonecrotic lesions in 48 patients who were otherwise diagnosed with MRI.[7] Computed tomography scanning is not recommended because it exposes patients to unnecessary radiation risks.

Once osteonecrosis has been diagnosed and characterized radiographically, a treatment plan can be proposed. The radiographic evaluation, in the authors' opinion, is of paramount importance over other demographic factors in formulating this strategy. However,

Table 58-1. Overview of Various Staging Systems for Osteonecrosis of the Femoral Head

Ficat and Arlet[2] Stage	Description	University Of Pennsylvania[6]* Stage	Description	Association Research Circulation Osseous[3] Stage	Description	Japanese Orthopaedic Association (Ohzono)[5]† Stage	Description	Marcus, Enneking, and Massam[4] Stage	Description
I	Normal radiographic appearance	0	Normal	0	None	1	Demarcation line	1	Mottled areas of increased density on plain radiographs
II	Diffuse sclerotic or cystic lesions	I	Positive findings on bone scan or magnetic resonance imaging	1	Normal findings on radiography or computed tomography; positive findings with at least one other technique	2	Early flattening without demarcation line around necrotic area	2	Demarcation zone of increased radiodensity surrounding lesion
III	Subchondral fracture	II	Diffuse sclerotic or cystic lesions	2	Sclerosis, osteolysis, focal porosis	3	Cystic lesions	3	Subchondral lucency (crescent sign)
IV	Femoral head collapse, osteoarthritis, acetabular changes	III	Stop-off in contour of subchondral bone	3	Crescent sign and/or flattening of articular surface			4	Flattening of femoral head
		IV	Flattening of femoral head	4	Osteoarthritis, acetabular changes			5	Flattening and compression of necrotic zone; narrowing of joint space
		V	Joint narrowing or acetabular changes					6	Progressive erosion of femoral head; degenerative arthritis
		VI	Advanced degenerative changes						

*Further stratified as A,B, or C, depending on severity.
†Stratified by medial to lateral weight-bearing area involvement.

one may occasionally consider various demographic factors such as patient age or morbidity in deciding on a procedure. For example, one would be more likely to try a head-preserving procedure in an 18-year-old patient versus a 62-year-old patient who might be served better with a hip arthroplasty procedure. In addition, patients who have many comorbidities may not want to risk a procedure with a higher risk of failure necessitating reoperation, and may opt for a more definitive procedure. With these considerations in mind, the various nonarthroplasty procedures that have been used to treat osteonecrosis of the femoral head will be discussed, including indications and contraindications for each procedure, the surgical technique and relevant variations, postoperative care, results, and complications.

CORE DECOMPRESSION AND PERCUTANEOUS DRILLING

Core decompression is a surgical technique that involves removing a cylindrical core of bone from the proximal femur, creating a tract that extends from the subchondral region of the femoral head to the extraosseous space adjacent to the lateral proximal femur. This technique was originally described by Ficat and Arlet[8] and by Hungerford[9] as a method of diagnosis by histologic examination of removed bone and as a method of pain reduction. This procedure is no longer necessary for the diagnosis of osteonecrosis because magnetic resonance imaging is currently the preferred modality.[10,11] Core decompression continues to be used for pain reduction and to slow the progression of disease, although some controversy continues regarding the degree to which the procedure influences the natural course of this disease. It is believed that bone removal may reduce intramedullary pressure caused by various factors such as increased adipocyte density or venous congestion within the bone, which are associated with osteonecrosis.[12] Multiple animal and human studies have reported neovascularization and improved osseous blood flow following core decompression.[13,14] This has been described as a simple, low-morbidity method of treating osteonecrosis, although some studies have reported complication rates of 10% or higher.

Indications and Contraindications

Core decompression can be used in patients who have precollapse osteonecrosis of the femoral head. Success rates are highest in patients who have Ficat and Arlet stage I disease (changes visible on magnetic resonance imaging only) and in those who have smaller lesions encompassing less than 25% of the volume of the femoral head. However, the procedure has been demonstrated to slow or arrest progression in Ficat and Arlet stage II and III disease, albeit less frequently. Because of the minimally invasive nature of the procedure and the low associated morbidity, especially when percutaneous drilling techniques are used, core decompression

may be an excellent first choice of surgical treatment for osteonecrosis in many patients with precollapse disease. It should not be used for patients with advanced postcollapse disease or very large stage II and III lesions that have a high risk of progression or have already collapsed.

Preoperative Planning

Little preoperative planning is necessary for this procedure. A recent magnetic resonance study of both hips should be obtained and examined to determine the size and location of the osteonecrotic lesion and to evaluate for lesions in the contralateral hip. Bilateral osteonecrosis of the hips occurs in up to 85% of patients, and most asymptomatic hips progress to symptomatic disease and/or femoral head collapse. Given the low morbidity of core decompression, surgeons may consider decompressing both hips if asymptomatic disease of the contralateral joint is identified on magnetic resonance imaging. In addition to the necessary instruments, surgeons should ensure that intraoperative fluoroscopy and a radiolucent table are available for the procedure.

Description of Techniques

Core decompression has traditionally been performed with trephines or cannulated drill bits that have diameters of between 5 and 10 mm. These instruments are driven through the femoral neck into the head under fluoroscopic guidance. Various materials, such as bone graft and osteogenic proteins, may be placed into the tracts, or the channels may be left open. Complications can occur if the drill hole is started too distally relative to the femoral metaphysis, which may result in a subtrochanteric fracture. Additionally, the drill hole may be extended too far, damaging the articular cartilage and leading to loose bodies within the joint capsule.

Technique: Modified Hungerford
- Position the patient supine on a fracture table.
- Using fluoroscopy as a guide, make a 2 to 3 cm longitudinal incision in the midlateral thigh at the level of the lesser trochanter, and split the fascia lata in the direction of its fibers.
- Using a cannulated drill or cortical reamer, create a 10 mm window in the lateral cortex of the femur at the level of the superior margin of the lesser trochanter.
- Introduce an 8 to 10 mm trephine through the cortical window over a K wire, and use image guidance to drive the trephine medially and proximally up the femoral neck toward the center of the lesion, with prior magnetic resonance imaging or plain film radiographs as a guide to determine optimal positioning.
- Use image intensification to track progress of the trephine in both anteroposterior and frog-leg lateral projections, ensuring that the cortices are not breached, and that the tip does not penetrate the articular cortex of the femoral head (Fig. 58-1).

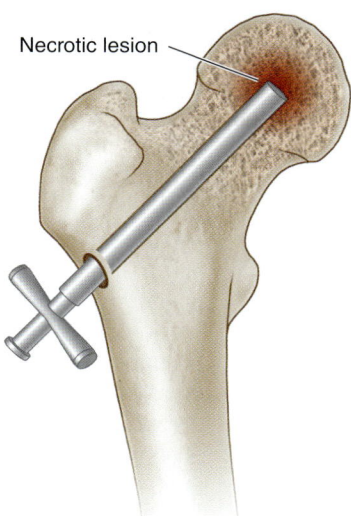

Figure 58-1. Introduction of an 8 to 10 mm trephine through a cortical window in the metaphysis of the proximal femur, advancing up the femoral neck into the necrotic lesion *(indicated by the arrow).*

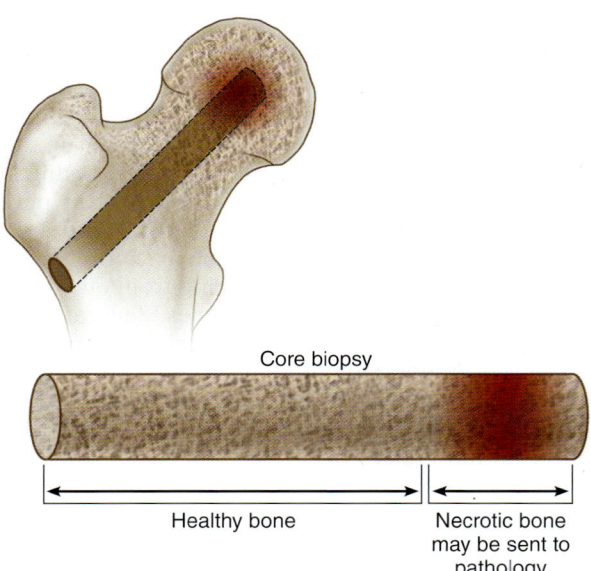

Figure 58-2. The trephine is withdrawn along with a core of both necrotic and viable cancellous bone. The necrotic material can be sent for histopathologic analysis.

- Once the lesion has been reached, the trephine is withdrawn along with the K wire and a core of trabecular bone (Fig. 58-2).
- Once the procedure is complete, the wound is closed in layers, with one or two sutures used to close the skin incision.

A newer modified core decompression technique, which is really a percutaneous drilling procedure, has been described by Song and associates[15] and Mont and colleagues[16] and involves using a smaller-diameter drill bit or a Steinman pin (2 to 3 mm) inserted percutaneously to create the core tracts. Multiple drillings are created in an attempt to sufficiently decompress the diseased region. In addition, bone matrix or growth factors can be placed into the tracts. Potential advantages of this technique include percutaneous insertion rather than a surgical incision, shorter surgical time, and less tissue damage. In addition, this technique may be associated with a lower risk of fracture or collapse.

Technique as Described by Mont

- Position the patient supine on the fracture table.
- Under fluoroscopic guidance, insert a 3.2 to 3.4 mm Steinman pin percutaneously into the lateral thigh at the level of the superior margin of the lesser trochanter.
- Keeping the Steinman pin perpendicular to the femoral shaft, penetrate the lateral cortex and enter the intramedullary canal.
- Angle the Steinman pin proximally and medially parallel to the neck of the femur, and advance the pin through the medullary canal toward the lesion in the femoral head, checking progress using fluoroscopy in both anteroposterior and lateral views to ensure that the cortex is not breached.
- Extend the tract to the subchondral bone, taking care to not breach the articular surface.
- For small and medium-sized lesions, two passes are made into the diseased area (previously identified using magnetic resonance imaging or plain film radiographs), using a single common entry point in the lateral cortex. The pin should not be withdrawn from the wound between passes. The authors make three passes for large lesions.
- The Steinman pin is withdrawn, and the entry point into the skin is covered with an adhesive bandage.

Variations and Unusual Situations

Core decompression is a relatively simple and safe procedure that can be used in virtually all patients with the appropriate indications. Use of intraoperative fluoroscopy to guide the path of the intraosseous channel allows accommodation of virtually any anatomic variations of the proximal femur, such as hip dysplasia, slipped capital femoral epiphysis, post-traumatic anatomic changes, or a pistol grip deformity of the proximal femur. Regardless of the femoral anatomy, surgeons should ensure that the femoral cortex is not penetrated, and that the decompression tract reaches the lesion in the subchondral space.

Steinberg and coworkers described a variation of the modified Hungerford technique.[17] After the initial core tract is made, two additional passes are made into other areas of the necrotic lesion through the same cortical entry point, using 5 or 6 mm trephines. Then, the large-diameter trephine is reintroduced with the aid of a trocar and is used as a guide to loosely place morselized cancellous bone and/or bone growth–stimulating substances into the decompressed lesion. The rationale for this procedure as described by the authors was to stimulate revascularization and bone growth.

Table 58-2. Recent Studies Reporting Outcomes of Core Decompression and Percutaneous Drilling

Author/Year	Technique	Number of Hips	Months Follow-up (Range)	Additional Surgery, n (%)	Radiographic Failure, n (%)
Chen et al/2000[105]	Core	27	28 (12-128)	—	10 (37)
Lavernia and Sierra/2000[23]	Core	67	41	16 (24)	—
Maniwa et al/2000[25]	Core	26	94 (53-164)	8 (31)	—
Specchiulli et al/2000[28]	Core	20	67	4 (20)	4 (20)
Piperkovski/2001[106]	Core	39	48	4 (8)	—
Yoon et al/2001[30]	Core	39	61 (24-118)	19 (49)	—
Aigner et al/2002[18]	Core	45	69 (31-120)	7 (16)	12 (27)
Hernigou et al/2003[22]	Core	189	84 (60-132)	34 (18)	39 (21)
Wirtz et al/2003[107]	Core	51	(36-132)	18 (35)	—
Gangji et al/2004[20]	Core	8	24	2 (25)	5 (63)
Lieberman et al/2004[24]	Core	17	53 (26-94)	3 (18)	3 (18)
Bellot et al/2005[19]	Core	31	(1-176)	19 (61)	19 (61)
Ha et al/2006[21]	Core	18	(50-96)	—	14 (78)
Neumayr et al/2006[27]	Core	17	36	3 (18)	—
Marker et al/2008[26]	Percutaneous	79	24 (20-39)	27 (34)	27 (34)
Song et al/2007[15]	Percutaneous	163	87 (60-134)	50 (31)	—
Wang et al/2009[58]	Percutaneous	59	28 (12-40)	7 (12)	14 (24)

Postoperative Care

Recommended postoperative care has been similar regardless of the decompression technique used. Patients are typically discharged home on the same day of the procedure or on the following morning. They are mobilized before discharge, using a single crutch or cane in the contralateral hand. In cases of bilateral hip decompressions, two crutches or canes are used. Patients are advised to maintain partial weight bearing until a follow-up visit at approximately 6 weeks after the procedure. Patients are then allowed to progress to full weight bearing as tolerated but are counseled to avoid high-impact activities for 12 months and are encouraged to perform regular home-based abductor-strengthening exercises. One year after the core decompression procedure is performed, patients are evaluated clinically and radiographically for disease progression and/or femoral head collapse. If no evidence of disease progression is found, all restrictions are lifted, although patients are encouraged to return for regular annual follow-up examinations to monitor for radiographic signs of delayed disease progression.

Results

Over the past several decades, considerable variability has been noted in reported results of various decompression techniques for osteonecrosis of the femoral head. The literature includes a paucity of well-designed comparative studies and considerable heterogeneity in study populations in terms of lesion size, location, and radiographic stage. Reporting of results is further complicated by differences in the definition of successful and/or failed treatment, with different authors alternately measuring success as preservation of the native joint, no radiographic progression of disease, or no symptomatic progression.

Overall results of core decompression reported over the last decade as measured by the avoidance of further surgery range from 42% to 86% at mean follow-up times from 24 to 94 months, with most studies reporting survival rates in the range of 70% to 85% over this period (Table 58-2).[15,18-31] Success rates as measured by an absence of radiographic progression are more variable and somewhat more modest, ranging from 30% to 86% over a similar range of follow-up times. Several studies have consistently reported that superior survival rates are seen in earlier radiographic stages of the disease (stages I and II) and with smaller, more medially located lesions.[15,16,23,30,32-34]

Some authors raise concerns about the degree, if any, to which core decompression affects the natural course of the disease,[27,35-37] noting that many small early-stage lesions do not progress, even without surgical treatment. One well-controlled study did not confirm an effect with core decompression.[27] However, several comparative studies and literature reviews have demonstrated consistently poorer survival rates for hips treated nonoperatively and overall failure rates approximately double those seen with core decompression.[38-40]

In summary, although a number of patients treated with core decompression eventually do progress to further surgical treatment, this procedure is minimally invasive (especially when performed using the percutaneous small-diameter technique), can be performed quickly with minimal technical requirements, has very low morbidity, provides immediate symptomatic relief in the large majority of patients, and may successfully delay further surgical treatment for many years in many patients who otherwise are offered much larger procedures, if not joint arthroplasty. For these reasons, the

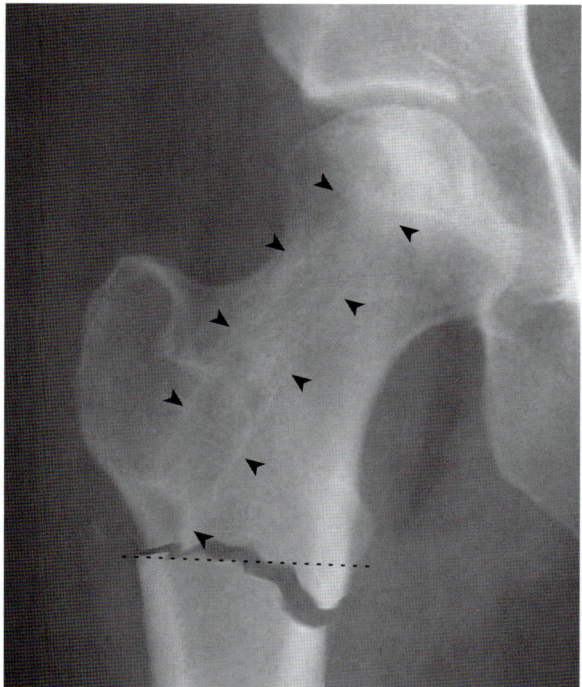

Figure 58-3. Subtrochanteric fracture involving the lateral cortical entry point of a recent core decompression tract *(arrowheads)*. Note that the entry point is below the level of the proximal lesser trochanter *(dashed line)*, which increases the risk of postoperative fracture. *(Copyright Mount Sinai Hospital Inc., Baltimore, Md.)*

authors advocate the use of percutaneous core decompression for the treatment of symptomatic precollapse small to medium-sized lesions.

Complications

The principal risks of core decompression are related to the anesthesia of the surgery because the procedure itself has few complications. Authors experienced in core decompression typically report complication rates well below 1%. Patients treated with large-diameter trephine core decompression are at risk for proximal femur fracture should a fall occur in the early postoperative period, when the proximal femur is structurally weakened and the bone has not yet fully healed (Fig. 58-3). Improper placement of the trephine in the diaphysis of the femur can account for most fractures. However, the rate of these complications is low and can be further minimized by ensuring that an appropriate entry point is used in the metaphysis opposite to the proximal margin of the lesser trochanter, and that a period of postoperative protected weight bearing is strictly followed.

STRUCTURAL BONE GRAFTING

Structural bone grafting is a more invasive procedure than core decompression, so it is typically utilized for patients who have failed core decompression, or who

would not be appropriate candidates for core decompression owing to large lesions or more advanced stages of disease. The general procedure for bone grafting involves soft tissue dissection to access the femur, removal of a window of cortical bone to access the intramedullary space, débridement of the necrotic bone, placement of the bone graft material, replacement of the bone window, and wound closure. Various types of bone grafting material can be used, including nonvascularized iliac crest, fibula, or tibia autograft or allograft; synthetic bone graft material such as demineralized bone matrix and corticocancellous bone chips; or vascularized fibular or muscle-pedicle autograft. In addition, growth factors such as bone marrow and bone morphogenetic proteins 2 and 7 have been added to the graft material in an attempt to stimulate new bone growth. Although a number of procedures have been described, they can be broadly divided into two categories: nonvascularized and vascularized bone grafting. Additionally, a few recent reports have described implantation of nonbiological porous tantalum metal rods, which may act like a structural bone graft. The rationale for bone grafting is multifold: (1) The technique provides a mechanism to decompress the femoral head, reducing intramedullary pressure; (2) it removes some or all of the necrotic bone, eliminates a source of inflammation, and provides a more suitable environment for the growth of viable bone; (3) it provides structural support with bone graft for the articular surface to prevent further collapse; and (4) it provides a mechanism for the placement of bone growth factors to stimulate healing. An additional rationale for the use of vascularized bone grafting is to introduce healthy viable bone into the lesion as a replacement for necrotic tissue.

Nonvascularized Bone Grafting

Indications and Contraindications

Indications for nonvascularized bone grafting include a Ficat stage II or III lesion with less than 2 mm of femoral head collapse. Failure of core decompression to adequately address the symptoms of osteonecrosis might also be an indication. It should not be used in patients who have articular cartilage defects that are greater than 1 cm in diameter, delaminated cartilage, acetabular changes, or very large areas of necrosis (>30% of the head) because they will not have high success rates with this procedure.

Preoperative Planning

Preoperative planning should include magnetic resonance imaging and/or plain film radiographs of the affected hip to accurately define the size and location of the necrotic area. This is important so that the necrotic lesion can be approached most directly with any type of nonvascularized bone grafting. The surgeon should additionally ensure that sufficient graft material is available if bone allograft is being used.

Description of Techniques

Three different techniques have been described for nonvascularized grafting of the femoral head: (1)

Phemister, (2) trapdoor, and (3) lightbulb techniques. The Phemister technique, the first one reported, was used originally for the treatment of post-traumatic osteonecrosis.[41] It consisted of creating two core decompression tracts with 8 to 10 millimeter trephines and placing a core of graft material into the tracts. Modifications of this technique were reported by a number of authors for nontraumatic osteonecrosis,[42-45] including the use of a single core decompression tract and the use of various graft sources such as tibial, fibular, or iliac crest autografts and fibular allograft.

Modified Phemister Technique

- Position the patient supine on a fracture table; make a 2 to 3 cm lateral incision centered at the level of the lesser trochanter and deepen the incision, splitting the fascia lata along the direction of its fibers.
- Introduce a K wire under fluoroscopic guidance through the lateral cortex of the proximal femoral metaphysis, and drill it up the femoral neck into the center of the necrotic lesion.
- Drill into the necrotic lesion using a 9 mm cannulated drill bit over the K wire, extending the tract to the subchondral bone within 5 mm of the articular surface.
- Prepare a graft of similar length to the decompression tract, rounding the proximal end and tapering slightly toward a larger distal diameter to allow for a press fit. Autologous corticocancellous tibial or iliac crest bone can be used as the graft material, or intact fibular autograft or allograft may be used.
- Press-fit the graft into the decompression tract, using fluoroscopy to confirm placement and ensuring that the rounded proximal end is in the subchondral space (Fig. 58-4).

To improve visualization and débridement of the necrotic lesion, Meyers and associates proposed introducing iliac cancellous autograft through a cortical window in the articular surface of the femoral head, directly above the necrotic lesion.[46,47] This approach was later modified by Mont and colleagues, who described the use of iliac cancellous and cortical graft through an articular trapdoor.[48]

Trapdoor Procedure

- With the patient in a true lateral position, arthrotomy is performed through the anterolateral or posterolateral approach. Perform a capsulotomy and dislocate the hip.
- Using a marking pen, outline a 1.5 cm square on the articular surface that will be removed to access the intramedullary space.
- The window is cut by using an oscillating saw and angling the blade toward the center of the trapdoor while cutting to create a beveled edge. Once all four sides have been cut, the osteochondral trapdoor is removed and retained (Fig. 58-5).
- Using a high-speed burr and curettes, all necrotic bone is removed until bleeding cancellous bone is visualized throughout the base of the lesion (Fig. 58-6A and B). A penlight can be periodically inserted into the cavity to improve visualization and ensure that all necrotic bone has been removed.
- Two or three cortical struts are impacted into the base of the intraosseous cavity (in the technique reported by Meyers, only cancellous bone was used). Fill the remaining void with cancellous bone, with added demineralized bone matrix if desired, and replace the osteochondral trapdoor; fix it in place using three absorbable pins (Fig. 58-7).
- Reduce the hip joint and close the wound in layers over a drain.

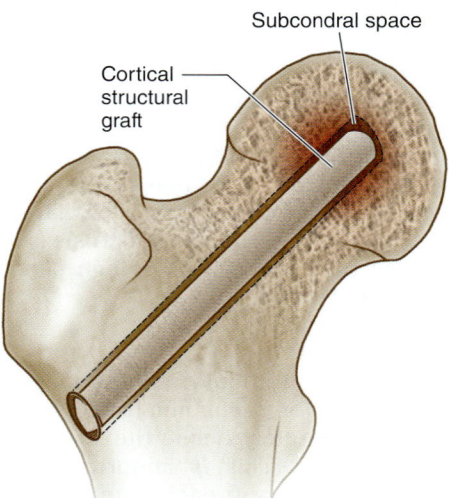

Figure 58-4. The Phemister technique for bone grafting involves placing a cortical structural graft into a core decompression tract, ensuring that the rounded end of the graft lies in the subchondral space of the decompressed lesion *(indicated by the arrow)*.

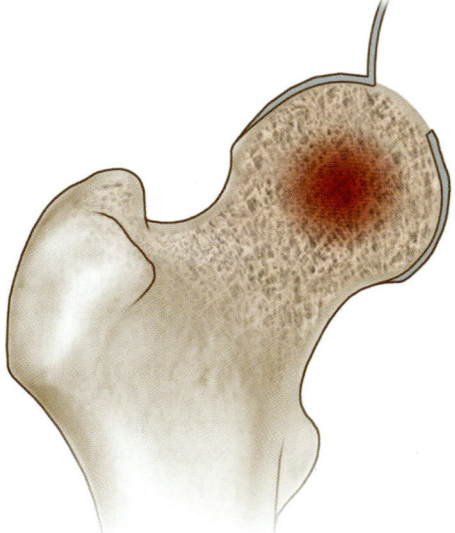

Figure 58-5. A trapdoor is created in the articular surface of the femoral head and the subsequent flap is lifted utilizing either scalpel dissection (pictured) or a small oscillating saw (instrument not pictured).

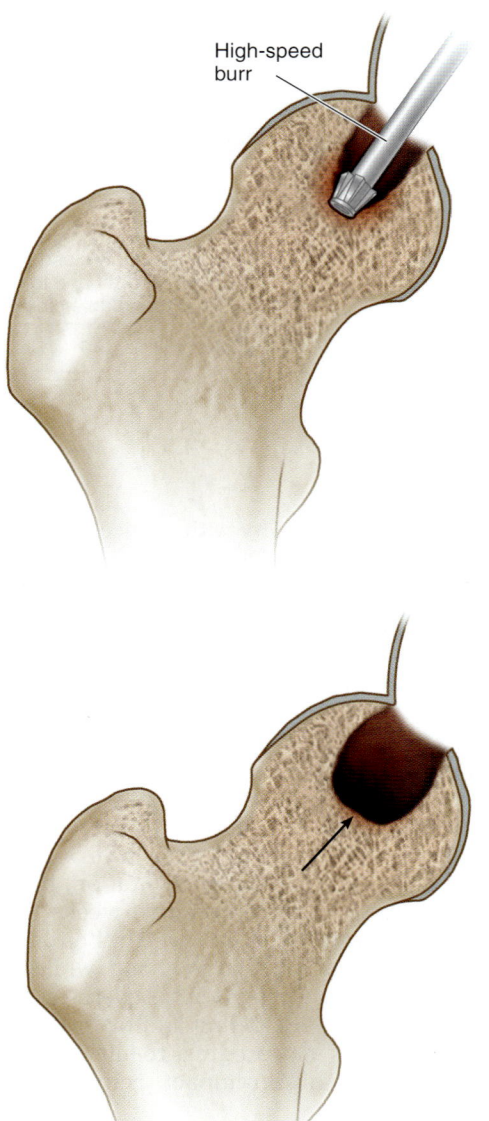

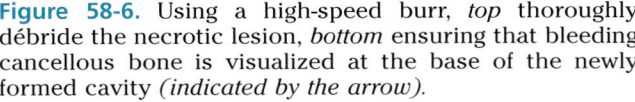

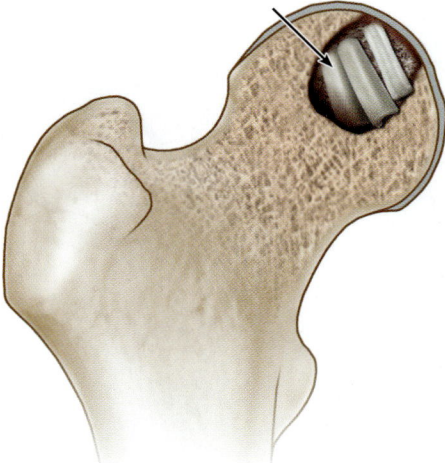

Figure 58-7. Impact cortical struts into the base of the cavity *(indicated by the arrow),* fill the remaining void with morselized bone graft, and replace the trapdoor, fixing it with absorbable pins.

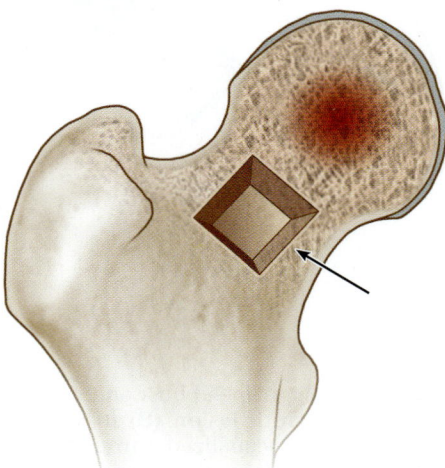

Figure 58-6. Using a high-speed burr, *top* thoroughly débride the necrotic lesion, *bottom* ensuring that bleeding cancellous bone is visualized at the base of the newly formed cavity *(indicated by the arrow).*

Figure 58-8. Using a small oscillating saw, create a trapdoor in the anterior femoral neck, just distal to the articular surface of the head *(as indicated by the arrow). (Modified from Seyler TM, Marker DR, Ulrich SD, et al: Nonvascularized bone grafting defers joint arthroplasty in hip osteonecrosis. Clin Orthop Relat Res 466:1125–1132, 2008. Used with permission.)*

Rosenwasser and associates reported a modification of the trapdoor technique known as the *lightbulb procedure,* which allows access to the necrotic lesion in the femoral head for débridement and bone grafting without the need for dislocation of the hip joint.[49]

Lightbulb Procedure
- Expose the anterior capsule using an anterior or anterolateral approach, positioning the patient as appropriate.
- The hip capsule is opened from the base of the femoral neck to the acetabulum, and the incision is extended 180 degrees around the circumference of the neck.

- Create a trapdoor in the anterior femoral neck, just distal to the articular surface of the femoral head, making beveled cuts using a small oscillating saw, as described for the trapdoor technique (Fig. 58-8).
- Using a high-speed burr and curettes, thoroughly débride the necrotic lesion all the way to the subchondral bone of the femoral head (Fig. 58-9A), using a penlight to enhance visualization and ensure that bleeding cancellous bone is present at the base of the cavity (Fig. 58-9B).

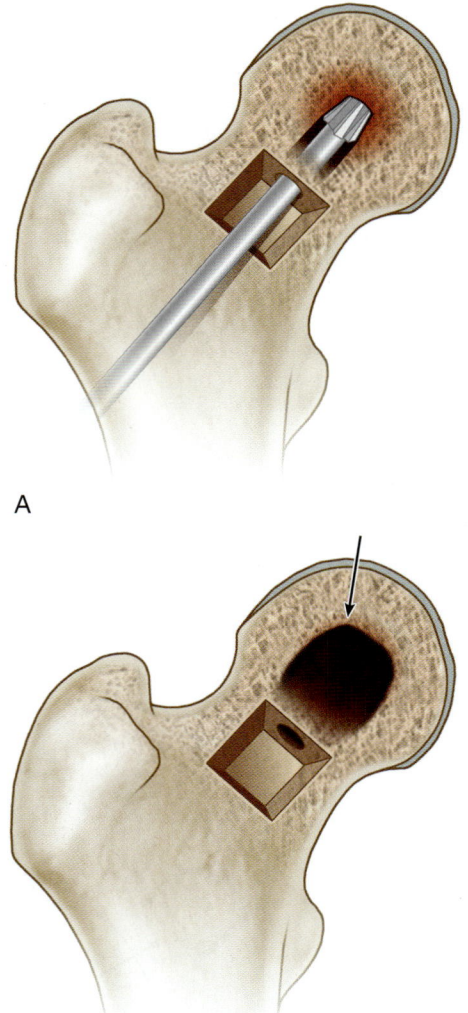

A

B

Figure 58-9. A, Use a high-speed burr and curettes to thoroughly débride the necrotic lesion, **(B)** ensuring that bleeding cancellous bone is visualized throughout the newly formed cavity *(indicated by the arrow). (Modified from Seyler TM, Marker DR, Ulrich SD, et al: Nonvascularized bone grafting defers joint arthroplasty in hip osteonecrosis. Clin Orthop Relat Res 466:1125–1132, 2008. Used with permission.)*

- Pack the cavity with cortical and/or cancellous iliac bone graft, mixed with demineralized bone matrix if desired.
- Replace the cortical trapdoor, fixing it in place with three absorbable pins (Fig. 58-10).
- Close the wound in layers over a drain.

Postoperative Care

Regardless of the specific bone grafting technique used, a considerable period of protected weight bearing should be followed to protect the weakened proximal femoral bone and allow osseous regeneration to occur. Patients can be discharged from the hospital as soon as they are able to mobilize, typically on postoperative day

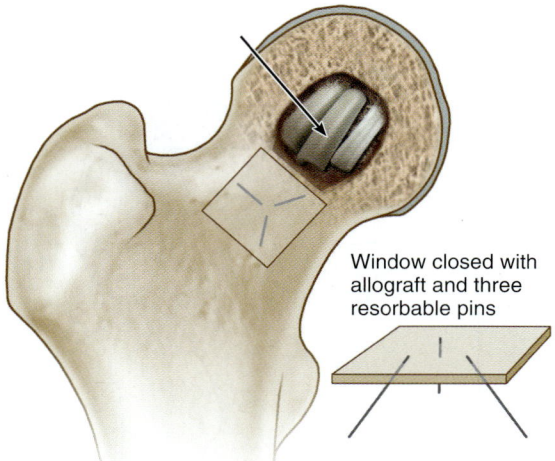

Window closed with allograft and three resorbable pins

Figure 58-10. Pack the cavity with cortical and/or cancellous bone graft *(indicated by the arrow)*, and replace the cortical window, fixing it in place with three absorbable pins. *(Modified from Seyler TM, Marker DR, Ulrich SD, et al: Nonvascularized bone grafting defers joint arthroplasty in hip osteonecrosis. Clin Orthop Relat Res 466:1125–1132, 2008. Used with permission.)*

one or two. A 6 week period of toe touch weight bearing is recommended, accompanied by daily gentle range-of-motion exercises. Patients should be advised to avoid hip flexion beyond 90 degrees, as well as excessive abduction, adduction, or external rotation. If no radiographic disease progression is seen at 6 weeks' follow-up, the patient may progress to 50% weight bearing using a crutch or cane in the contralateral hand, while performing abductor muscle strengthening exercises and gait training. If adequate remodeling and/or healing is seen at 3 months, patients may progress to full weight bearing with avoidance of higher-impact activities until 12 months.

Results

Initial results with the Phemister technique were favorable, but longer-term follow-up revealed less positive outcomes. Nelson and colleagues reported that 13 of 17 patients with stage II disease at the time of bone grafting showed radiographic progression of at least one stage within 2 years.[50] Similar rates of progression were seen in stage III and IV hips, with many patients progressing to hip arthroplasty, especially in stage IV disease. Results with the modified technique reported by Buckley and coworkers were more positive, with 18 of 20 patients with stage II disease having no radiographic or symptomatic progression at a mean follow-up of 8 years (range, 2 to 19 years).[44] Some authors have compared this technique with vascularized bone grafting and have found that the vascularized technique had superior results. For example, Kim and associates compared 23 hips with large precollapse and postcollapse lesions treated with vascularized fibular grafting versus 23 hips matched by lesion stage and size treated with nonvascularized fibular bone grafting and found collapse in

35% of vascularized grafts and in 70% of nonvascularized grafts at a mean follow-up of 4 years.[51] Similar results were reported by Plakseychuk and associates.[52] However, advantages of the modified Phemister technique were that it was the least invasive and had the lowest morbidity. Nevertheless, it was more difficult to visualize and remove necrotic bone with this technique, and reported success rates varied widely.[53-56] Possibly because of the combination of these factors and the doubtful increased success of bone grafting over core decompression alone, this technique has largely fallen out of favor.

More consistent results were reported for bone grafting using the trapdoor technique (Table 58-3), which provided the advantage of excellent visualization of the necrotic lesion and allowed thorough débridement of diseased bone without compromising the structural integrity of the femoral neck or trochanteric region. Clinical success rates ranged from 71% to 89% for stage III and early stage IV disease, and radiographic success rates ranged from 70% to 73% at follow-up times of 3 to 5 years.[48] Although no major complications have been reported with this technique, concern has been expressed about possible lasting damage to the articular cartilage with this procedure and the potential for future medium and long-term arthritic complications.

The most recently described technique, the lightbulb technique, was used by Rosenwasser and colleagues to treat 15 hips in 13 patients, with 12 of 14 hips (86%) available for review at a mean follow-up of 12 years (range, 10 to 15 years) remaining pain free.[49] Mont and coworkers reported outcomes of the lightbulb technique in 21 hips in 19 patients at a mean follow-up of 48 months (range, 36 to 55 months), with successful preservation of the native joint in 18 patients (86%).[57] Wang

and associates described 90% survival of 138 hips at a mean follow-up of 25 months (range, 7 to 45 months),[58] and Chang and colleagues reported 73% survival of 11 hips at a mean follow-up of 61 months (range, 30 to 103 months).[59] Both authors noted considerably higher survival in hips that had not collapsed at the time of the grafting procedure (100% and 93%, respectively).

Complications

Early results with the Phemister technique were complicated by occasional catastrophic failure as a result of subtrochanteric or femoral neck fracture. Although infrequent, these complications necessitated immediate revision to a total hip arthroplasty, which was particularly complex in cases of subtrochanteric fracture. This complication has not been reported with the trapdoor or the lightbulb technique, both of which were well tolerated in most patients without major complications in the early postoperative period. Ultimately, although these procedures delayed the need for total hip arthroplasty by several years in most patients, and over a decade in some, the primary complication experienced by most patients was radiographic and symptomatic progression of disease, with eventual need for hip arthroplasty.

Variations and Unusual Situations

A recent variation on the Phemister technique involves the implantation of a porous trabecular metal rod into the core decompression tract in place of the traditional structural bone graft. The procedure is initially performed as described earlier for the Phemister technique but with use of a 10 mm drill bit, following by introduction and fixation of a distally threaded rod that spans from the subchondral bone of the femoral head to the

Table 58-3. Results of the Use of Bone Grafting for Treatment of Osteonecrosis of the Femoral Head

Author/Year	Technique	Number of Hips	Months Follow-up, n (range)	Clinical Failure Rate, %
Ko et al/1995[108]	Trapdoor technique and/or osteotomies	14	53 (24-108)	15
Mont et al/1998[48]	Trapdoor technique	30	56 (30-60)	27
Steinberg et al/2001[17]	Phemister technique	312	63 (23-146)	36
Plakseychuk et al/2003[52]	Phemister technique	50	60 (36-96)	64
Rijnen et al/2003[45]	Phemister technique	28	50 (24-119)	29
Lieberman et al/2004[24]	Phemister technique	17	53 (26-94)	18
Kim et al/2005[51]	Phemister technique	30	50 (36-67)	65
Israelite et al/2005[109]	Phemister technique	276	NA (24-145)	38
Wang et al/2005[110]	Phemister technique	28	26 (24-39)	35
Keizer et al/2006[55]	Phemister technique	80	84 (36-NA)	69
Saito et al/1988[111]	Lightbulb technique	18	48 (24-168)	28
Scher and Jakim/1999[98]	Lightbulb technique	50	96 (36-168)	14
Rosenwasser et al/1994[49]	Lightbulb technique	15	138 (108-180)	13
Seyler et al/2008[112]	Lightbulb technique	47	28 (12-50)	32
Wang et al/2009[58]	Lightbulb technique	138	25 (7-42)	10
Chang et al/2009[59]	Lightbulb technique plus wire coil	11	61 (30-103)	27

NA, Not available.

entrance point in the lateral cortex. This rod is made of a porous trabeculated tantalum metal that has a similar elasticity to native bone. The rationale for this procedure is to provide structural support to the subchondral bone while providing a scaffold to promote ingrowth of healthy native bone after the decompression procedure is performed. Initial indications for this procedure included symptomatic Ficat and Arlet stage II disease without previous surgical or electrical stimulation treatment. However, this technique has been used in patients with disease stage presentation ranging from symptomatic stage I disease to stage III disease with minimal collapse of the articular surface.

Although the initial results were promising, survivorship at 4 years has been reported at approximately 70% in three separate studies (Table 58-4)[29,60,61] with failure most commonly occurring as a result of collapse of the femoral head around a stable implant.[62] At best, these outcomes are similar to those reported in more recent studies of core decompression alone for similar radiographic stages of osteonecrosis of the femoral head, raising concerns about whether the use of tantalum rods provides any advantages. Of additional concern are some reports of catastrophic early failures, specifically femoral neck and shaft fractures requiring revision to total hip arthroplasty.[63,64] Whether revision is performed after proximal femoral fracture or after disease progression, the surgery is frequently more complex because of the need to remove the typically well-fixed implant.

Although a better understanding of the mechanisms of failure of tantalum rods and potential modifications to the surgical indications and techniques may improve future outcomes with this technique, at the present time it does not appear that they provide any benefit; in fact, they may potentially complicate future revisions to total hip arthroplasty.

Vascularized Bone Grafting

Vascularized bone grafting is an alternative to nonvascularized grafting that utilizes bone tissue that has direct vascularity in an attempt to improve the viability of the graft. Two different methods of vascularized bone grafting have been utilized: free vascularized fibula transplantation and muscle-pedicle bone grafting. These procedures require considerable technical expertise, especially in the case of free vascularized fibular grafting.

Indications and Contraindications

Indications for vascularized bone grafting are similar to those for nonvascularized grafting, namely, stage II to stage III disease. Because these procedures are quite invasive and, in the case of free vascularized grafting, depend partially on healing of a microvascular anastomosis, they are indicated primarily in younger patients 20 to 40 years of age with good healing potential. Some authors have recommended that these procedures not be used in stage III disease, with large lesions involving more than 50% of the femoral head, or with a Kerboul angle of 300 degrees or more because of the high incidence of disease progression.[65-67] These grafting procedures similarly are not recommended for patients with considerable head flattening or with more than 2 mm collapse of the femoral head.

Patients should be assessed for their potential for compliance with postoperative rehabilitation and avoidance of lifestyle factors that may interfere with healing, such as ongoing excessive alcohol consumption or tobacco smoking. Poor compliance with these factors and vascular compromise of the lower extremity are considered contraindications for the procedure, although ongoing corticosteroid therapy is not.

Table 58-4. Recent Studies Evaluating the Outcome of Trabecular Metal Rod Implantation

Authors/Year	Implant Used	Number of Hips (Number of Patients)	Follow-up Duration in Months (Range)	Survival/ Survivorship
Varitimidis et al/2009[61]	Tantalum (9 stage II, 7 stage III, 10 stage IV)	31 (26)	38 (15-71)	100% at 12 months 96% at 24 months 76% at 36 months 68% at 48 months
Tanzer et al/2008[62]	Tantalum (stage II)	15	13 (3-36)	N/A—failure analysis
Shuler et al/2007[113]	Tantalum vs. fibular graft	24 rod; 21 fibular	39 (27-59)	86%
Nadeau et al/2007[114]	Tantalum (3 stage III; 15 stage IV)	18 (15)	23 (12-48)	44% at 24 months 44% survival at FFU
Aldegheri et al/2007[63]	Tantalum (6 stage I; 9 stage II)	15 (10)	15 (8-24)	80% survival at FFU
Veillette et al/2006[29]	Tantalum (1 stage I, 49 stage II, 8 stage III)	58 (52)	24 (6-52)	92% at 12 months 82% at 24 months 68% at 48 months
Tsao et al/2005[60]	Tantalum (1 stage I, 93 stage II; 7 stage III, 12 stage IV)	113 (98)	2 years for each	For stage II hips: 85% at 12 months 79% at 24 months 73% at 36 months 73% at 48 months

Preoperative Planning

Careful preoperative planning is recommended to maximize the chances of success. Accurate staging of the disease and assessment of lesion size and location should be performed using recent radiographs and magnetic resonance imaging to ensure that the patient is an appropriate candidate for the procedure, and to note where graft placement is necessary. The participation of two experienced surgeons greatly shortens the required operative time because this allows fibular harvesting to be performed concurrently with preparation and grafting of the proximal femur.

Description of Techniques

Free Fibular Grafting As Described by Urbaniak.[68]

Because free vascularized fibular grafting is a complex procedure, it is best performed with two experienced surgeons operating concurrently on the fibula and the proximal femur. Although a single surgeon may require up to 7 hours to complete this operation, two experienced surgeons may be able to complete the procedure in approximately 3 hours.

The patient is placed in the lateral decubitus position, and the whole lower extremity is prepped up to the level of the iliac crest. A stocking is placed over the leg up to the level of the midthigh, and a sterile tourniquet is placed just proximal to the knee to provide hemostasis of the leg during fibular harvest.

Approach to and Preparation of Donor Vessels

- Approach the hip using a curved anterolateral skin incision over the proximal femur. Carry the dissection down through the subcutaneous tissue. Identify and split the interval between the tensor fascia lata and the gluteus medius muscles, and place a self-retaining retractor.
- Identify the donor vessels, the ascending branch of the lateral femoral circumflex artery, and two accompanying veins between the vastus intermedius and rectus femoris muscles. Cut the origin of the vastus lateralis from the vastus ridge, and reflect it distally at the posterior attachment to expose the lateral femur.
- Detach the origin of the vastus intermedius muscle using a right angle dissector and a knife, taking care to transect all fibers to provide a more proximal trough to accommodate anastomosed vessels without tension. Do not extend the dissection medial to the encountered fat layer to avoid damaging the femoral nerve and vessels.
- Retract the reflected vastus intermedius and vastus lateralis muscles anteriorly, exposing the aponeurosis between the anterolateral femur and the rectus femoris muscle. Sweep away the adjacent fat pad, exposing the ascending branch of the lateral femoral circumflex vessel and its two accompanying veins. These branches are consistently found 8 to 10 cm distal to the anterior superior iliac spine and can be distinguished by their ascending course; the other branches of the lateral circumflex artery have a transverse and descending course.
- Under loupe magnification, dissect the vessels individually down to their origin, starting from the first

major division of the artery and veins. Place small vascular clips just distal to the first bifurcation; this will ensure optimal vessel size match and sufficient length for a tension-free anastomosis. Use small clips on any small branches encountered along the dissection to ensure hemostasis.
- Once a 4 cm length of each vessel has been freed, the vessels can be clipped and transected, and retractors can be removed to proceed with preparation of the femoral head (Fig. 58-11).

Preparation of the Femoral Head

- Position the C-arm over the hip in such a way that both anteroposterior and frog-leg lateral views can be obtained without repositioning the arm. Beginning at the junction of the posterior and middle thirds of the lateral femur, approximately 2 cm distal to the vastus ridge, introduce a 3 mm guide pin up the femoral neck and into the center of the necrotic lesion in the femoral head. Check progress using fluoroscopy in anteroposterior and lateral projections to ensure optimal placement and to confirm that sufficient space remains between the guide pin and the cortices to accommodate subsequent reaming.
- Starting with a 10 mm reamer, create a channel over the guide pin, reaming to within 3 to 5 mm of the articular surface of the femoral head. Proceed with progressively larger reamers until the diameter of the donor fibula is reached, typically 16 mm for women and 19 mm for men. As the reamers are withdrawn, clean the flutes, disposing of any necrotic bone but retaining viable cancellous bone for subsequent grafting. Use a filtered suction tip to capture viable cancellous bone from the slurry expressed during the reaming process for subsequent grafting.
- For larger lesions or in patients with remaining necrotic bone visible on fluoroscopy after reaming is complete, use a ball reamer to remove the remaining diseased bone. Renografin can be introduced into the reamed canal for better visualization of any remaining necrotic lesion on fluoroscopy. Continue reaming until all diseased bone has been removed, taking care not to compromise the subchondral plate of the articular surface (Fig. 58-12).
- Using a curette, remove cancellous bone from the greater trochanter for use as additional graft material. Once all necrotic bone has been removed from the lesion, place the collected cancellous bone into the cavity within the femoral head. Start with the harvested trochanteric bone followed by the fragments collected during reaming, impacting them into place with a customized impaction device with depth markings on the shaft, taking care to provide sufficient tunnel depth to accommodate the harvested fibular graft.
- Confirm adequate grafting by introducing water-soluble contrast into the tunnel to allow visualization of the obliteration of the reamed cavity on both anteroposterior and lateral fluoroscopic projections.

Fibular Harvest

- After the leg is exsanguinated and the tourniquet is inflated, a straight lateral incision is made in line with the sulcus between the posterior and lateral

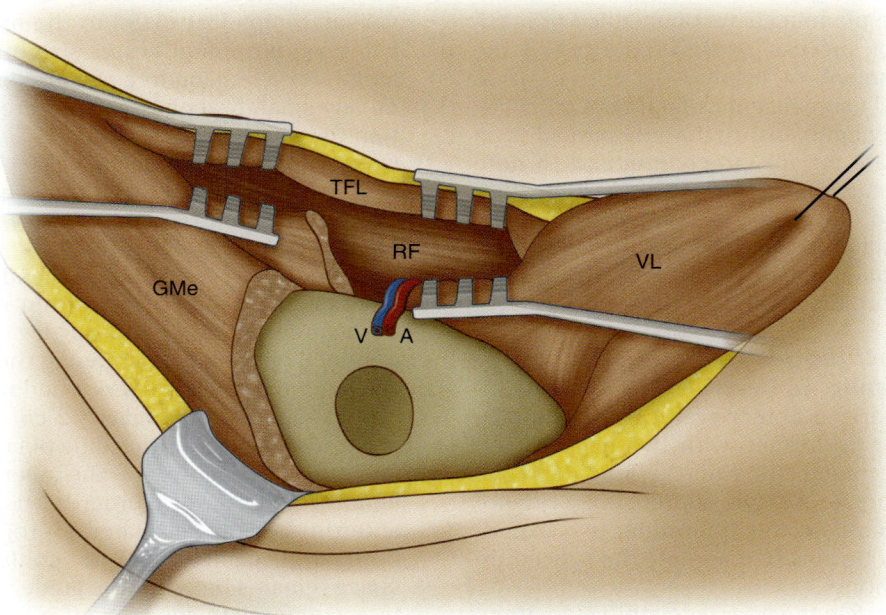

Figure 58-11. The origin of the vastus intermedius muscle is released to facilitate a tension-free anastomosis between the ascending lateral circumflex artery (a) and vein (v). The tensor fascia lata (TFL) and rectus femoris (RF) muscles are retracted anteriorly, and the vastus lateralis (VL) muscle is retracted distally to improve visualization for preparation of the femoral head. *GMe,* Gluteus medius muscle. (*Redrawn from Urbaniak JR, Coogan P, Gunneson E, Nunley J: Treatment of osteonecrosis of the femoral head with free vacularized fibular grafting: a long-term follow-up study of one hundred and three hips. J Bone Joint Surg Am 77:681–694, 1995. Used with permission.*)

compartments of the leg, starting 10 cm distal to the fibular head and terminating 10 cm proximal to the lateral malleolus.

- The lateral compartment is incised, and the peroneal muscles are bluntly elevated off the posterior intermuscular septum in an anterior direction and are held with self-retaining retractors, exposing the fibula.
- Sharp dissection is used to separate the peroneal muscles from the fibula, stopping when the anterior intermuscular septum is seen along the whole length of the exposed fibular fragment. A thin, 1 to 2 mm cuff of muscle should be retained on the fibula to preserve the periosteum.
- The exposed anterior intermuscular septum is divided, and the musculature of the anterior compartment is elevated off the fibula, preserving the periosteum and a thin cuff of muscle and exposing the interosseous membrane.
- The anterior musculature is gently retracted anteromedially along with the deep peroneal nerve and the anterior tibial artery, and the interosseous membrane is divided using a right angle blade.
- The posterior intermuscular septum is incised, exposing the musculature of the posterior compartment.
- The distal pedicle of the peroneal vessels is identified at the level of the distal flexor hallucis longus muscle. After a right angle clamp is placed between the pedicle and the fibula, two malleable retractors are passed between the clamp and the bone to protect the vessels during the osteotomy. After it has been

confirmed that at least 10 cm of fibula will remain distal to the osteotomy site, an oscillating saw is used to transect the bone with copious irrigation to prevent thermal necrosis. A hemoclip is used to fix the distal pedicle to the fibula to prevent avulsion during the remainder of the harvest.

- After the proximal peroneal pedicle deep to the soleus muscle is identified and the superficial peroneal nerve exposed on the surface of the peroneus longus muscle is protected, the proximal osteotomy is performed in a manner similar to that already described. Ensure that an appropriate length of fibula is harvested to fit the length of the femoral canal measured using the graduated impactor. A bone clamp is placed around the fibula to control motion during the subsequent pedicle dissection.
- Dissect the vascular pedicle from distal to proximal after using hemostatic clamps and a microsurgical knife to isolate and transect the distal vessels. Release the fibula and the vascular pedicle from adjoining muscles in a systematic fashion. Use hemostatic clips to manage any perforating vessels while dissecting at least 4 cm of free proximal vascular pedicle. Once this has been established, use hemostatic clips to ligate the vessels and divide them just distal to their origin from the posterior tibial vessels.
- Pass the freed fibular graft (Fig. 58-13) to the back table for preparation, and let down the tourniquet while irrigating the wound and addressing any continuing bleeding.

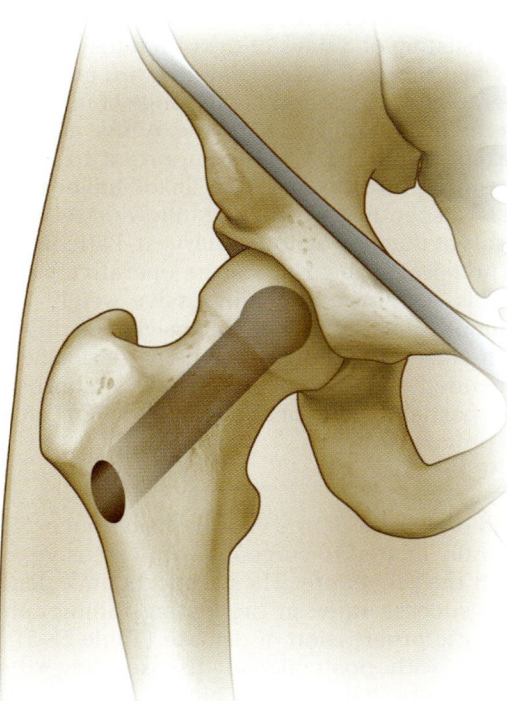

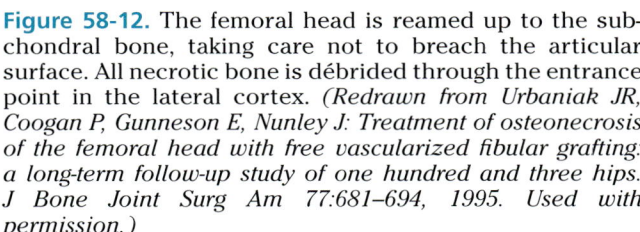

Figure 58-12. The femoral head is reamed up to the subchondral bone, taking care not to breach the articular surface. All necrotic bone is débrided through the entrance point in the lateral cortex. *(Redrawn from Urbaniak JR, Coogan P, Gunneson E, Nunley J: Treatment of osteonecrosis of the femoral head with free vascularized fibular grafting: a long-term follow-up study of one hundred and three hips. J Bone Joint Surg Am 77:681–694, 1995. Used with permission.)*

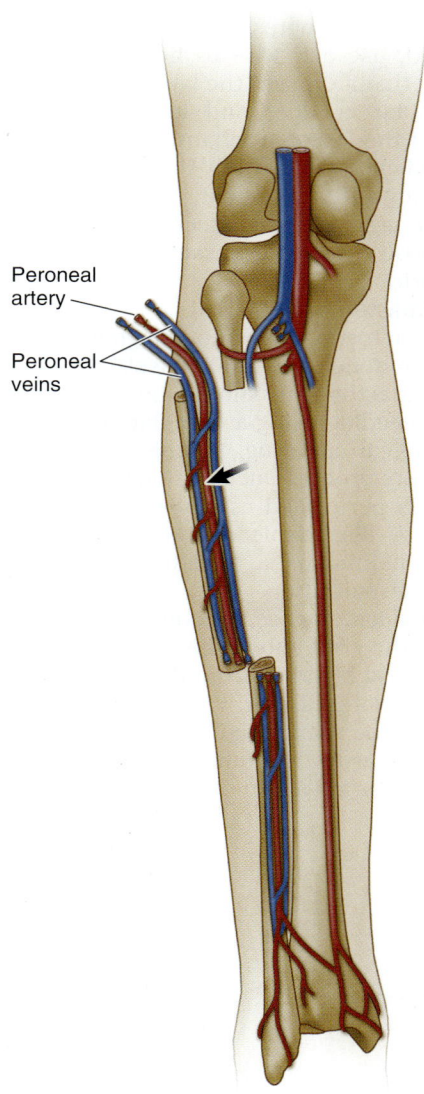

Figure 58-13. The femoral graft is harvested from the ipsilateral leg, ensuring that at least 10 cm of fibula remains proximal to the lateral malleolus, and that the vascular pedicle is well protected throughout the harvesting procedure, so as not to avulse any feeder vessels. *(Redrawn from Urbaniak JR, Coogan P, Gunneson E, Nunley J: Treatment of osteonecrosis of the femoral head with free vacularized fibular grafting: a long-term follow-up study of one hundred and three hips. J Bone Joint Surg Am 77:681–694, 1995. Used with permission.)*

Fibular Preparation

- Place the graft on a saline-soaked sponge, and separate the individual vessels of the pedicle. Inject heparinized lactated Ringer's solution into each of the three vessels, inspecting for any vascular leaks. If found, these should be repaired with microvascular techniques.
- Select one vein for grafting and ligate the other with a hemostatic clip. Measure the diameter of the fibular graft, and use this to guide the final reaming size for the proximal femoral canal.
- The vascular pedicle is reflected from the proximal fibula until a large feeder vessel is seen, and with copious irrigation, an oscillating saw is use to transect the graft at this level. Once the final required graft length is known from the measurement made with the graduated impactor, this dimension is marked on the distal femur, and a 1 cm distal periosteal cuff is created and reflected proximal to the distal osteotomy mark. An oscillating saw is then used to make the distal cut, and the reflected periosteum and distal pedicle are secured to the fibula with a 4-0

absorbable suture to prevent avulsion during graft insertion.

Placement of the Fibular Graft Into the Femoral Head

- After all contrast material has been removed from the reamed canal, the fibular graft is inserted with the vascular pedicle positioned superiorly and anteriorly and recessed in the natural fibular sulcus. The graft should be inserted along the posterior wall of the canal to minimize pressure on the pedicle.

- Using a bone tamp, gently impact the graft into place while checking progress using fluoroscopy. Once fully advanced, use a K wire to hold the graft in place, ensuring that it crosses the lateral femoral cortex and both fibular cortices and inserts into the medial cortex of the lesser trochanter. Ensure that the vascular pedicle is adequately protected from compression during wire placement.
- Once the graft has been secured, remove the C-arm and expose the donor vessels using a self-retaining four-quadrant retractor.

Vessel Anastomosis

- Using a microscope or loupe magnification as appropriate, the donor and graft vessels are anastomosed. Venous anastomosis should be performed first to control bleeding using a vascular coupling device or microsurgical suturing techniques, depending on surgeon preference. Once complete, the arterial anastomosis is performed using 8-0 or 9-0 monofilament sutures. A disposable suction mat of contrasting color is helpful as a backdrop while suturing to enhance visualization.
- Once the anastomoses are complete (Fig. 58-14), perfusion of the graft should be confirmed by observing for endosteal bleeding from the implanted fibula.
- The vastus lateralis and vastus intermedius muscles should not be reattached to prevent compromise of the blood flow to the graft. The wound is then closed in layers over a suction drain.

Postoperative Care

Patients should receive thromboprophylaxis postoperatively, consisting of 3 days of dextran infusion followed by daily aspirin for 6 weeks. Patients are mobilized on postoperative day one and begin range-of-motion exercises of the ipsilateral ankle and toe. Active and passive dorsiflexion of the great toe is important to prevent a flexion contracture because the flexor hallucis longus muscle is susceptible to scarring following reflection of the muscle at the time of fibular harvest. Patients should remain non–weight bearing on the operative side for 6 weeks; this is followed by progressive weight bearing until 6 months, at which time full weight bearing is permitted. If staged procedures are being performed, it is recommended that they be performed 3 months apart to allow partial weight bearing on one limb after the second procedure.

Results

Reported outcomes of free vascularized fibular grafting are generally limited to surgeons with extensive experience with the procedure. These reports have generally excellent success rates in preventing radiographic or symptomatic progression of disease (Table 58-5), even in patients with postcollapse disease. Nevertheless, several authors have found higher survivorship in patients with precollapse disease. Using the modified Marcus staging system, Urbaniak and associates reported 5 year survivorship in stage II hips of 91%,

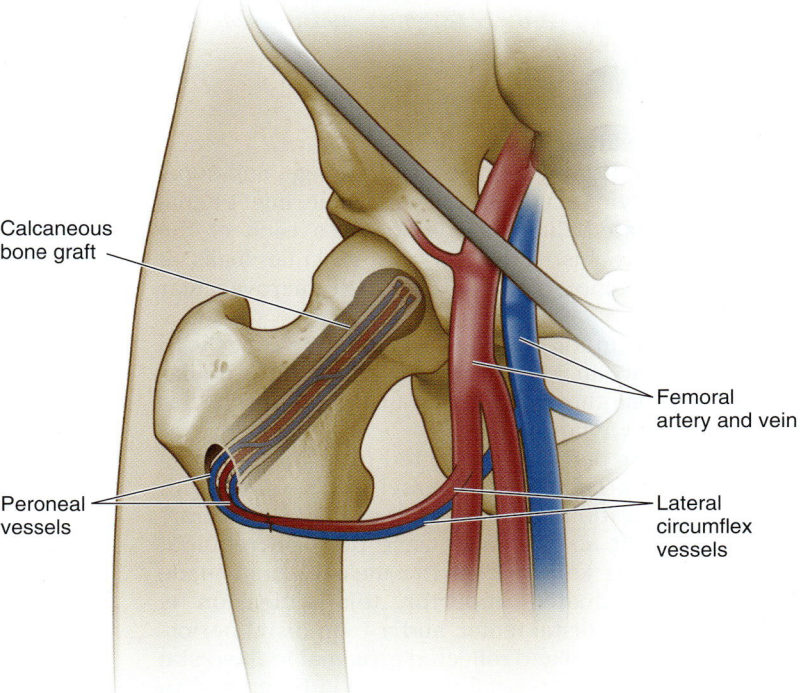

Figure 58-14. The cavity in the femoral head is filled with cancellous bone graft to minimize any intraosseous voids after fibular implantation. The peroneal vessels are anastomosed to the previously prepared ascending branches of the lateral femoral circumflex vessels, which arise from the femoral artery and vein. *(Redrawn from Urbaniak JR, Coogan P, Gunneson E, Nunley J: Treatment of osteonecrosis of the femoral head with free vacularized fibular grafting: a long-term follow-up study of one hundred and three hips. J Bone Joint Surg Am 77:681–694, 1995. Used with permission.)*

Calcaneous bone graft

Femoral artery and vein

Peroneal vessels

Lateral circumflex vessels

Table 58-5. Recently Reported Results of the Use of Vascularized Bone Grafting

Author/Year	Graft	Age (Range) in Years	Months Follow-up (Range)	Additional Surgery, n (%)	Radiographic Failure, n (%)
Dean et al/2001[115]	Fibula	15 (9-18)	52 (24-120)	8 (15)	18 (33)
Judet and Gilbert/2001[116]	Fibula	35 (20-64)	216 (180-264)	18 (25)	33 (48)
Soucacos et al/2001[70]	Fibula	32 (16-54)	56 (12-120)	14 (8)	83 (45)
Plakseychuk et al/2003[52]	Fibula	44 (23-52)	60 (36-96)	NA	21 (42)
Berend et al/2003[71]	Fibula	34 (9-57)	52 (24-144)	73 (33)	73 (33)
Rizzo et al/2004[117]	Fibula	NA	NA	2 (6)	NA
Le Nen et al/2004[118]	Fibula	39	42 (minimum 15)	NA	13 (81)
Garberina et al/2004[119]	Fibula	34	58 (minimum 24)	8 (24)	8 (24)
Zhang et al/2004[120]	Fibula	NA	12 (6-18)	NA	1 (4)
Kim et al/2005[51]	Fibula	43 (24-52)	50 (36-66)	3 (13)	13 (57)
Marciniak et al/2005[121]	Fibula	34 (16-61)	96 (60-180)	57 (56)	59 (58)
Stubbs et al/2005[122]	Fibula	13 (9-20)	47 (36-75)	0 (0)	0 (0)
Yen et al/2006[123]	Fibula	38 (28-52)	(minimum 36)	2 (9)	4 (18)
Roush et al/2006[124]	Fibula	34 (15-48)	90 (79-100)	48 (24)	62 (31)
Kawate et al/2007[66]	Fibula	39 (15-61)	84 (36-144)	13 (18)	35 (49)
Yoo et al/2008[72]	Fibula	36 (13-63)	167 (120-284)	13 (10)	48 (39)
Eisenschenk et al/2001[125]	Ilium	NA	60 (6-120)	8 (9)	44 (54)
Noguchi et al/2001[126]	Ilium	40 (21-55)	52 (18-81)	2 (11)	5 (28)
Zhang et al/2003[127]	Ilium	36 (16-57)	NA	NA	2 (1)
Fuchs et al/2003[128]	Ilium	34 (16-51)	162 (60-240)	15 (34)	35 (8)
Nagoya et al/2004[129]	Ilium	35 (17-62)	103 (36-204)	NA	19 (54)
Matsusaki et al/2005[130]	Ilium	38 (21-51)	51 (18-133)	3 (18)	5 (29)
Nakamura et al/2005[131]	Ilium	28 (16-45)	81 (36-180)	1 (8)	2 (17)
Yen et al/2006[123]	Ilium	40 (26-63)	(minimum 48)	4 (10)	17 (44)
Baksi et al/2009[80]	Ilium	36 (16-62)	198 (120-258)	NA	43 (24)

NA, Not available.

compared with 77% in stage III disease, 71% in stage IV, and 73% in stage V disease in a review of 103 consecutive hips treated with free vascularized fibular grafting.[69] At a mean follow-up of 5 years (range, 1 to 10 years), Soucacos and colleagues reported radiographic progression in 5% of stage II hips with none progressing to total hip arthroplasty,[70] while 48% of stage IV hips progressed radiographically and 12% underwent eventual total hip arthroplasty. In a review of 121 procedures performed in hips with stage IV disease with a mean follow-up of 5.7 years (range, 5 to 12 years), Berend and coworkers reported 65% native joint survival at final follow-up,[71] with larger lesions trending toward a higher failure rate. In contrast, Yoon and associates reviewed outcomes of 124 hips in 110 patients with stage II and III disease at the time of vascularized fibular grafting, at a mean follow-up of 14 years (range, 10 to 24 years).[72] The authors reported native joint survivorship of 93% at 10 years and 83% at 20 years, with higher rates of radiographic progression in larger and more laterally location lesions, although no difference in radiographic stage was seen. Yoon and colleagues additionally found significantly lower success rates in patients older than 35 years of age at the time of fibular grafting,[72] and Urbaniak and coworkers reported a trend toward higher failure rates in patients older than 30 years of age.[69] In general, when performed by experienced surgeons, this procedure has good success rates in preventing disease progression and delaying total hip arthroplasty in both precollapse and early postcollapse disease.

Complications

A measurable incidence of a number of different graft and donor site complications has been reported, with most found at the donor site. In a review of 1270 procedures performed over a 17 year period, Gaskill and associates reported a 17% complication rate, with 12% of cases occurring at the donor site.[73] The most common findings included great toe flexion contractures (37% of all donor site complications), ankle pain or tenderness (36%), and sensory deficits (14%). Motor weakness was identified in 8 of 1270 cases. The most common graft site complications included pin migration (43% of graft site complications), heterotopic ossification (26%), and femoral fracture (13%). The overall complication rate was considerably lower than in an earlier report by the same senior author, which reviewed 247 procedures performed over the 12 year period preceding the most recent report. At that time, Vail and Urbaniak reported a 24% incidence of donor site complications,[74] including an overall 10% incidence of transient motor weakness months postoperatively, decreasing to 2% at a minimum of 5 years' follow-up, a 12% incidence of sensory deficits, and persistent ankle pain in 12% of patients at 5 years postoperatively. Yoo and associates reported an overall incidence of great toe flexion contractures of 11% in 151 cases, as well as two peroneal nerve palsies that resolved within 18 months and two subtrochanteric fractures.[72] Lee and colleagues assessed the incidence of subtrochanteric fracture following fibular grafting, finding an overall incidence of 4%, which increased to 14% in bilateral procedures.[75] In contrast, Soucacos and coworkers reported lower complication rates, with four flexion contractures of the great toe and no peroneal nerve deficits in 228 hips.[70] Davis and colleagues additionally reported that patients who underwent total hip arthroplasty after a failed free vascularized fibular graft had worse clinical outcomes as compared with matched patients who did not undergo the grafting procedure before hip arthroplasty.[76] Although some authors have had very low complication rates with this procedure, it appears that a considerable incidence of a wide range of postoperative complications may exist with this vascularized fibular grafting, which may have a long learning curve.

Variations and Unique Situations

An alternate technique for vascularized bone implantation is the muscle-pedicle graft with several reported variations. This technique was first reported by Meyers and associates for the treatment of post-traumatic osteonecrosis.[77] After a posterior approach to the hip, a segment of cortical bone with the attached insertion of the quadratus femoris muscle is elevated off the proximal femur. A cortical window is made in the posterior neck of the femur, and after the necrotic lesion is débrided, the cortical bone graft is inserted through the bony window into the bony channel extending up into the femoral head. Other authors have reported the use of various muscle pedicles with bone taken from the ilium.[78,79] Although one author has reported survivorship of 91% at 15 years in 82 patients with stage II disease at the time of surgery,[80] very few reports have described the use of these techniques, and they are not currently in general use.

OSTEOTOMIES

A variety of osteotomies of the proximal femur have been utilized for the treatment of osteonecrosis of the femoral head. In all cases, the rationale behind their use is to shift the diseased section of the femoral head to a non–weight-bearing portion of the joint, unloading the necrotic lesion while allowing the loaded articulation to take place on a healthy section of the articular surface. Two categories of osteotomies are commonly used for the treatment of osteonecrosis: the proximal femoral rotational osteotomy (anterior or posterior) and the intertrochanteric angular osteotomy (flexion, extension, valgus, varus, and various combinations). These are technically demanding procedures with variable reported success rates. Regarding rotational

osteotomies, excellent success rates have been reported from the Far East, specifically from Japan and South Korea, and results in North America and Europe have been less than optimal. This has led some authors to speculate that anatomic variations between different populations may contribute to success or failure with these procedures. For example, Dean and Cabanela speculated that the posterior capsule may be more lax in East Asian populations, improving the outcomes of proximal femoral rotational osteotomy.[81]

Indications and Contraindications

The principal indication for treatment with an osteotomy is limited precollapse disease with preservation of the acetabular articular cartilage, as well as sufficient femoral bone and articular cartilage to provide a healthy load-bearing region following the osteotomy. For a rotational osteotomy, it is recommended that sufficient unaffected bone be available to occupy at least one third of the load-bearing portion of the acetabulum.[82,83]

Concerning angular osteotomies, the valgus osteotomy is indicated when the osteonecrotic segment is limited to the anterosuperior portion of the femoral head with minimal posterior involvement, and the varus osteotomy is indicated when an arc of at least 20 degrees of unaffected bone is present on the lateral aspect of the femoral head.

Contraindications for the use of osteotomy are patients older than 45 years of age, whole femoral head necrosis, and poor general health or other factors that might adversely affect bone healing.

Preoperative Planning

Careful preoperative evaluation of the size, location, and extent of the lesion, preferably with magnetic resonance imaging to appreciate the relationship between the necrotic area and surrounding bony anatomy in three dimensions, is required. This will allow selection of the most appropriate osteotomy for shifting load bearing to an area of healthy bone and cartilage.

Description of Procedures

A full description of surgical techniques and postoperative care for various osteotomies can be found in Chapter 57.

Results

The transtrochanteric rotational osteotomy has been largely successful in Asian countries (Table 58-6). Sugioka and associates reported that all 51 consecutive hips with stage III and IV disease treated with a posterior rotational femoral osteotomy had avoided total hip arthroplasty at a mean follow-up of 12 years (range, 1.2 to 21 years).[84] The senior author had reported earlier that 143 of 154 hips (93%) treated with an anterior femoral rotational osteotomy had more than one third of the femoral articular surface intact immediately after

Table 58-6. Overview of Recent Studies Investigating the Use of Proximal Femoral Osteotomies

Author/Year	Type of Osteotomy	Number of Hips	Months Follow-up, n (Range)	Success Rate, %
Hisatome et al/2004[132]	Anterior rotational	25	77 (41-149)	60
Matsusaki et al/2005[130]	Anterior rotational plus vascularized bone graft	17	51 (18-133)	71
Sakano et al/2004[133]	Curved intertrochanteric varus	20	48 (8-149)	90
Mont et al/1996[93]	Intertrochanteric	37	138 (60-216)	76
Simank et al/2001[134]	Intertrochanteric	75	72 (18-228)	75
Pavlovcic and Dolinar/2002[97]	Intertrochanteric plus cancellous bone graft	32	204 (108-312)	72
Gallinaro and Masse/2001[135]	Intertrochanteric flexion	24	122 (48-144)	63
Schneider et al/2002[94]	Intertrochanteric flexion	63	50 (31-161)	7
Schneider et al/2002[94]	Rotational	29	97 (79-295)	43
Drescher et al/2003[95]	Intertrochanteric flexion	70	125 (36-244)	73
Fuchs et al/2003[128]	Intertrochanteric flexion plus vascularized bone graft	44	162 (60-240)	66
Koo et al/2001[136]	Rotational	17	54 (42-78)	100
Hasegawa et al/2003[137]	Rotational	77	84 (60-132)	78
Zhang et al/2004[138]	Rotational	23	54	73
Chen et al/2004[139]	Rotational	20	23 (5-46)	63
Onodera et al/2005[140]	Rotational	38	48 (25-84)	58
Rijnen et al/2005[90]	Rotational	26	104 (79-120)	35
Nakamura et al/2005[131]	Rotational plus vascularized bone graft	12	81 (36-180)	83
Ikemura et al/2007[141]	Anterior rotational	44	34 (17-55)	100
Yoon et al/2008[88]	Modified rotational	43	37 (24-52)	93
Sugioka and Yamamoto/2008[84]	Posterior rotational	46	144 (14-252)	65
Biswal et al/2009[87]	Rotational	60	84 (18-156)	73

the procedure and had avoided total hip arthroplasty at follow-up times ranging from 3 to 16 years (range not reported).[82] Other authors from Asian countries have reported more modest but still generally excellent results, with survival rates between 56% and 93% reported in adult patients at follow-up times between 2 and 13 years.[85-88] However, European and North American surgeons have consistently reported poor results with this procedure, with many authors reporting survival rates of less than 50% and as low as 17%, at follow-up times ranging from 2 to 14 years.[81,89-92] Many of these authors have claimed to abandon the procedure.

Success rates in Europe and North America have been higher with the intertrochanteric angular osteotomy. Mont and colleagues reported the outcomes of 37 corrective varus osteotomies in 34 patients at a mean follow-up of 12 years (range, 5 to 18 years), finding that 26 hips (76%) were doing well at final follow-up.[93] Schneider and coworkers reviewed the outcomes of 69 hips treated with a flexion osteotomy, finding 70% survivorship at 5 years and 50% at 10 years. However, the authors noted that hips with smaller necrotic lesions had better outcomes, with 5 and 10 year survivorship of 90% and 61%, respectively, in hips with a Kerboul angle of less than 180 degrees.[94] Other authors have reported generally excellent results,[95-98] with 5 year

survivorship between 70% and 90% reported, along with 15 year survivorship between 40% and 86%.

Complications

Complications are common because the procedure is technically demanding. Rijnen and associates reported two cases of broken fixation screws, one case of screw migration, two trochanteric nonunions, and one femoral fracture below the healed osteotomy in 26 hips that underwent femoral rotational osteotomy, as well as an overall rate of complications requiring reoperation of 31%.[90] Iwasada and colleagues reported 8 complications in 48 hips (13%), including 4 hips with varus deformity and 2 subtrochanteric fractures.[85] Several authors have reported high rates of intraoperative and postoperative complications for total hip arthroplasty after a previous proximal femoral osteotomy, although it is not clear whether previous osteotomy results in significantly decreased survival when compared with hip arthroplasty without a previous history of proximal femoral osteotomy.[99-103] Although excellent success rates have been reported in specific patient groups, the present authors no longer utilize osteotomies to treat osteonecrosis because of considerable failure rates with such an invasive procedure and potential difficulties with future revision to a total hip arthroplasty.

CURRENT CONTROVERSIES AND FUTURE CONSIDERATIONS

- Should core decompression be used to treat asymptomatic lesions, given that most are likely to progress to symptomatic disease and/or collapse?
- Is it worth treating patients with early collapse disease utilizing head-preserving procedures when the results of modern total hip arthroplasty are excellent?
- What are the most optimal bone growth factors, angiogenic stimulating factors, and other peptides that can be used to enhance healing?
- Can cartilage lesions be treated separately to salvage hips in the future as various chondroprotective techniques become more successful?
- Can we further evaluate various patient demographic factors such as genomic screening as predictors of outcome of these procedures?
- Do pharmacologic agents (e.g., bisphosphonates, statins, vasodilators) have a place in enhancing these joint-preserving procedures?
- Are mechanical perturbing agents (e.g., electrical stimulation, ultrasound, shock waves) available that can enhance these procedures in the future?

DISCUSSION

A survey of members of the American Association of Hip and Knee Surgeons found that most of its members utilize core decompression to treat osteonecrosis, although fewer utilize nonoperative modalities or other techniques to treat the disease.[104] The conclusion was that insufficient prospective studies have compared the relative success of these treatments. Additionally, available reports have examined different patient populations, procedures, evaluation techniques, and follow-up times, so it is difficult to compare these studies or to combine them in a meta-analysis. Nevertheless, it is clear that all of these techniques have shown success in improving symptoms and/or delaying total hip arthroplasty, and all of these techniques have greater success rates when performed for patients who have Ficat stage I or II lesions.

Various patient-specific factors must be considered when a treatment plan for osteonecrosis is selected, including age/life expectancy, health, comorbidities, and activity level of the patient. Young or active patients who undergo a total hip arthroplasty are likely to require a revision at some point in their lives. These patients should be considered as candidates for procedures that delay total joint arthroplasty such as core decompression or bone grafting. If procedures are performed at a sufficiently early stage, they may substantially improve a patient's function and reduce pain, while delaying joint arthroplasty.

REFERENCES

1. Mont MA, Jones LC, Hungerford DS: Nontraumatic osteonecrosis of the femoral head: ten years later. J Bone Joint Surg Am 88:1117–1132, 2006.
2. Ficat RP: Idiopathic bone necrosis of the femoral head: early diagnosis and treatment. J Bone Joint Surg Br 67:3–9, 1985.
3. Gardeniers JW; ARCO Committee on Terminology and Staging: Report on the committee meeting at Santiago de Compostela. ARCO Newsletter 5:79–82, 1993.
4. Marcus ND, Enneking WF, Massam RA: The silent hip in idiopathic aseptic necrosis: treatment by bone-grafting. J Bone Joint Surg Am 55:1351–1366, 1973.
5. Ohzono K, Saito M, Sugano N, et al: The fate of nontraumatic avascular necrosis of the femoral head: a radiologic classification to formulate prognosis. Clin Orthop Relat Res 277:73–78, 1992.
6. Steinberg ME, Hayken GD, Steinberg DR: A quantitative system for staging avascular necrosis. J Bone Joint Surg Br 77:34–41, 1995.
7. Mont MA, Ulrich SD, Seyler TM, et al: Bone scanning of limited value for diagnosis of symptomatic oligofocal and multifocal osteonecrosis. J Rheumatol 35:1629–1634, 2008.
8. Ficat RP, Arlet J: Functional investigation of bone under normal conditions. In Ficat RP, Arlet J, Hungerford DS, editors: Ischemia and necrosis of bone, Baltimore, 1980, Williams & Wilkins, pp 29–52.
9. Hungerford DS: Treatment of ischemic necrosis of the femoral head. In Evarts CM, editor: Surgery of the musculoskeletal system, New York, 1983, Churchill Livingstone, pp 5–29.
10. Hauzeur JP, Pasteels JL, Schoutens A, et al: The diagnostic value of magnetic resonance imaging in non-traumatic osteonecrosis of the femoral head. J Bone Joint Surg Am 71:641–649, 1989.
11. Bassett LW, Gold RH, Reicher M, et al: Magnetic resonance imaging in the early diagnosis of ischemic necrosis of the femoral head: preliminary results. Clin Orthop Relat Res 214:237–248, 1987.
12. Hungerford DS, Zizic TM: Pathogenesis of ischemic necrosis of the femoral head. Hip 249–262, 1983.
13. Wang GJ, Dughman SS, Reger SI, Stamp WG: The effect of core decompression on femoral head blood flow in steroid-induced avascular necrosis of the femoral head. J Bone Joint Surg Am 67:121–124, 1985.
14. Simank HG, Graf J, Kerber A, Wiedmaier S: Long-term effects of core decompression by drilling: demonstration of bone healing and vessel ingrowth in an animal study. Acta Anat (Basel) 158:185–191, 1997.
15. Song WS, Yoo JJ, Kim YM, Kim HJ: Results of multiple drilling compared with those of conventional methods of core decompression. Clin Orthop Relat Res 454:139–146, 2007.
16. Mont MA, Ragland PS, Etienne G: Core decompression of the femoral head for osteonecrosis using percutaneous multiple small-diameter drilling. Clin Orthop Relat Res 429:131–138, 2004.
17. Steinberg ME, Larcom PG, Strafford B, et al: Core decompression with bone grafting for osteonecrosis of the femoral head. Clin Orthop Relat Res 386:71–78, 2001.
18. Aigner N, Schneider W, Eberl V, Knahr K: Core decompression in early stages of femoral head osteonecrosis—an MRI-controlled study. Int Orthop 26:31–35, 2002.
19. Bellot F, Havet E, Gabrion A, et al: [Core decompression of the femoral head for avascular necrosis]. Rev Chir Orthop Reparatrice Appar Mot 91:114–123, 2005.
20. Gangji V, Hauzeur JP, Matos C, et al: Treatment of osteonecrosis of the femoral head with implantation of autologous bone-marrow cells: a pilot study. J Bone Joint Surg Am 86:1153–1160, 2004.
21. Ha YC, Jung WH, Kim JR, et al: Prediction of collapse in femoral head osteonecrosis: a modified Kerboul method with use of magnetic resonance images. J Bone Joint Surg Am 88(Suppl 3):35–40, 2006.
22. Hernigou P, Bachir D, Galacteros F: The natural history of symptomatic osteonecrosis in adults with sickle-cell disease. J Bone Joint Surg Am 85:500–504, 2003.
23. Lavernia CJ, Sierra RJ: Core decompression in atraumatic osteonecrosis of the hip. J Arthroplasty 15:171–178, 2000.
24. Lieberman JR, Conduah A, Urist MR: Treatment of osteonecrosis of the femoral head with core decompression and human bone morphogenetic protein. Clin Orthop Relat Res 429:139–145, 2004.

25. Maniwa S, Nishikori T, Furukawa S, et al: Evaluation of core decompression for early osteonecrosis of the femoral head. Arch Orthop Trauma Surg 120:241–244, 2000.
26. Marker DR, Seyler TM, Ulrich SD, et al: Do modern techniques improve core decompression outcomes for hip osteonecrosis? Clin Orthop Relat Res 466:1093–1103, 2008.
27. Neumayr LD, Aguilar C, Earles AN, et al: Physical therapy alone compared with core decompression and physical therapy for femoral head osteonecrosis in sickle cell disease: results of a multicenter study at a mean of three years after treatment. J Bone Joint Surg Am 88:2573–2582, 2006.
28. Specchiulli F: Core decompression in the treatment of necrosis of the femoral head: long-term results. Chir Organi Mov 85:395–402, 2000.
29. Veillette CJ, Mehdian H, Schemitsch EH, McKee MD: Survivorship analysis and radiographic outcome following tantalum rod insertion for osteonecrosis of the femoral head. J Bone Joint Surg Am 88(Suppl 3):48–55, 2006.
30. Yoon TR, Song EK, Rowe SM, Park CH: Failure after core decompression in osteonecrosis of the femoral head. Int Orthop 24:316–318, 2001.
31. Lee MS, Hsieh PH, Chang YH, et al: Elevated intraosseous pressure in the intertrochanteric region is associated with poorer results in osteonecrosis of the femoral head treated by multiple drilling. J Bone Joint Surg Br 90:852–857, 2008.
32. Fairbank AC, Bhatia D, Jinnah RH, Hungerford DS: Long-term results of core decompression for ischaemic necrosis of the femoral head. J Bone Joint Surg Br 77:42–49, 1995.
33. Mazieres B, Marin F, Chiron P, et al: Influence of the volume of osteonecrosis on the outcome of core decompression of the femoral head. Ann Rheum Dis 56:747–750, 1997.
34. Mont MA, Jones LC, Pacheco I, Hungerford DS: Radiographic predictors of outcome of core decompression for hips with osteonecrosis stage III. Clin Orthop Relat Res 354:159–168, 1998.
35. Markel DC, Miskovsky C, Sculco TP, et al: Core decompression for osteonecrosis of the femoral head. Clin Orthop Relat Res 323:226–233, 1996.
36. Lafforgue P, Dahan E, Chagnaud C, et al: Early-stage avascular necrosis of the femoral head: MR imaging for prognosis in 31 cases with at least 2 years of follow-up. Radiology 187:199–204, 1993.
37. Koo KH, Kim R, Ko GH, et al: Preventing collapse in early osteonecrosis of the femoral head: a randomised clinical trial of core decompression. J Bone Joint Surg Br 77:870–874, 1995.
38. Mont MA, Carbone JJ, Fairbank AC: Core decompression versus nonoperative management for osteonecrosis of the hip. Clin Orthop Relat Res 324:169–178, 1996.
39. Stulberg BN, Davis AW, Bauer TW, et al: Osteonecrosis of the femoral head: a prospective randomized treatment protocol. Clin Orthop Relat Res 268:140–151, 1991.
40. Steinberg ME: Core decompression of the femoral head for avascular necrosis: indications and results. Can J Surg 38(Suppl 1):S18–S24, 1995.
41. Phemister DB: Treatment of the necrotic head of the femur in adults. J Bone Joint Surg Am 31:55–66, 1949.
42. Boettcher WG, Bonfiglio M, Smith K: Non-traumatic necrosis of the femoral head. II. Experiences in treatment. J Bone Joint Surg Am 52:322–329, 1970.
43. Bonfiglio M, Bardenstein MB: Treatment by bone-grafting of aseptic necrosis of the femoral head and non-union of the femoral neck (Phemister technique). J Bone Joint Surg Am 40:1329–1346, 1958.
44. Buckley PD, Gearen PF, Petty RW: Structural bone-grafting for early atraumatic avascular necrosis of the femoral head. J Bone Joint Surg Am 73:1357–1364, 1991.
45. Rijnen WH, Gardeniers JW, Buma P, et al: Treatment of femoral head osteonecrosis using bone impaction grafting. Clin Orthop Relat Res 417:74–83, 2003.
46. Meyers MH: The treatment of osteonecrosis of the hip with fresh osteochondral allografts and with the muscle pedicle graft technique. Clin Orthop Relat Res 130:202–209, 1978.
47. Meyers MH, Convery FR: Grafting procedure in osteonecrosis of the hip. Semin Arthroplasty 3:189–197, 1991.
48. Mont MA, Einhorn TA, Sponseller PD, Hungerford DS: The trapdoor procedure using autogenous cortical and cancellous bone grafts for osteonecrosis of the femoral head. J Bone Joint Surg Br 80:56–62, 1998.
49. Rosenwasser MP, Garino JP, Kiernan HA, Michelsen CB: Long term followup of thorough débridement and cancellous bone grafting of the femoral head for avascular necrosis. Clin Orthop Relat Res 306:17–27, 1994.
50. Nelson LM, Clark CR: Efficacy of Phemister bone grafting in nontraumatic aseptic necrosis of the femoral head. J Arthroplasty 8:253–258, 1993.
51. Kim SY, Kim YG, Kim PT, et al: Vascularized compared with nonvascularized fibular grafts for large osteonecrotic lesions of the femoral head. J Bone Joint Surg Am 87:2012–2018, 2005.
52. Plakseychuk AY, Kim SY, Park BC, et al: Vascularized compared with nonvascularized fibular grafting for the treatment of osteonecrosis of the femoral head. J Bone Joint Surg Am 85:589–596, 2003.
53. Dunn AW, Grow T: Aseptic necrosis of the femoral head: treatment with bone grafts of doubtful value. Clin Orthop Relat Res 122:249–254, 1977.
54. Smith KR, Bonfiglio M, Montgomery WJ: Non-traumatic necrosis of the femoral head treated with tibial bone-grafting: a follow-up note. J Bone Joint Surg Am 62:845–847, 1980.
55. Keizer SB, Kock NB, Dijkstra PD, et al: Treatment of avascular necrosis of the hip by a non-vascularised cortical graft. J Bone Joint Surg Br 88:460–466, 2006.
56. Mont MA, Jones LC, Sotereanos DG, et al: Understanding and treating osteonecrosis of the femoral head. Instr Course Lect 49:169–185, 2000.
57. Mont MA, Etienne G, Ragland PS: Outcome of nonvascularized bone grafting for osteonecrosis of the femoral head. Clin Orthop Relat Res 417:84–92, 2003.
58. Wang BL, Sun W, Shi ZC, et al: Treatment of nontraumatic osteonecrosis of the femoral head using bone impaction grafting through a femoral neck window. Int Orthop 34:635–639, 2010.
59. Chang Y, Hu CC, Chen DW, et al: Local cancellous bone grafting for osteonecrosis of the femoral head. Surg Innov 16:63–67, 2009.
60. Tsao AK, Roberson JR, Christie MJ, et al: Biomechanical and clinical evaluations of a porous tantalum implant for the treatment of early-stage osteonecrosis. J Bone Joint Surg Am 87(Suppl 2):22–27, 2005.
61. Varitimidis SE, Dimitroulias AP, Karachalios TS, et al: Outcome after tantalum rod implantation for treatment of femoral head osteonecrosis: 26 hips followed for an average of 3 years. Acta Orthop 80:20–25, 2009.
62. Tanzer M, Bobyn JD, Krygier JJ, Karabasz D: Histopathologic retrieval analysis of clinically failed porous tantalum osteonecrosis implants. J Bone Joint Surg Am 90:1282–1289, 2008.
63. Aldegheri R, Taglialavoro G, Berizzi A: The tantalum screw for treating femoral head necrosis: rationale and results. Strategies Trauma Limb Reconstr 2:63–68, 2007.
64. Fung DA, Frey S, Menkowitz M, Mark A: Subtrochanteric fracture in a patient with trabecular metal osteonecrosis intervention implant. Orthopedics 31:614, 2008.
65. Urbaniak JR, Harvey EJ: Revascularization of the femoral head in osteonecrosis. J Am Acad Orthop Surg 6:44–54, 1998.
66. Kawate K, Yajima H, Sugimoto K, et al: Indications for free vascularized fibular grafting for the treatment of osteonecrosis of the femoral head. BMC Musculoskelet Disord 8:78, 2007.
67. Kerboul M, Thomine J, Postel M, Merle d'Aubigné R: The conservative surgical treatment of idiopathic aseptic necrosis of the femoral head. J Bone Joint Surg Br 56:291–296, 1974.
68. Aldridge JM, 3rd, Berend KR, Gunneson EE, Urbaniak JR: Free vascularized fibular grafting for the treatment of postcollapse osteonecrosis of the femoral head: surgical technique. J Bone Joint Surg Am 86(Suppl 1):87–101, 2004.
69. Urbaniak JR, Coogan PG, Gunneson EB, Nunley JA: Treatment of osteonecrosis of the femoral head with free vascularized fibular grafting: a long-term follow-up study of one hundred and three hips. J Bone Joint Surg Am 77:681–694, 1995.
70. Soucacos PN, Beris AE, Malizos K, et al: Treatment of avascular necrosis of the femoral head with vascularized fibular transplant. Clin Orthop Relat Res 386:120–130, 2001.
71. Berend KR, Gunneson EE, Urbaniak JR: Free vascularized fibular grafting for the treatment of postcollapse

osteonecrosis of the femoral head. J Bone Joint Surg Am 85:987–993, 2003.

72. Yoo MC, Kim KI, Hahn CS, Parvizi J: Long-term followup of vascularized fibular grafting for femoral head necrosis. Clin Orthop Relat Res 466:1133–1140, 2009.

73. Gaskill TR, Urbaniak JR, Aldridge JM 3rd: Free vascularized fibular transfer for femoral head osteonecrosis: donor and graft site morbidity. J Bone Joint Surg Am 91:1861–1867, 2009.

74. Vail TP, Urbaniak JR: Donor-site morbidity with use of vascularized autogenous fibular grafts. J Bone Joint Surg Am 78:204–211, 1996.

75. Lee KH, Kim HM, Kim YS, et al: Subtrochanteric fracture after free vascularised fibular grafting for osteonecrosis of the femoral head. Injury 39:1182–1187, 2008.

76. Davis ET, McKee MD, Waddell JP, et al: Total hip arthroplasty following failure of free vascularized fibular graft. J Bone Joint Surg Am 88(Suppl 3):110–115, 2006.

77. Meyers MH, Harvey JP, Jr, Moore TM: Treatment of displaced subcapital and transcervical fractures of the femoral neck by muscle-pedicle-bone graft and internal fixation: a preliminary report on one hundred and fifty cases. J Bone Joint Surg Am 55:257–274, 1973.

78. Baksi DP: Treatment of osteonecrosis of the femoral head by drilling and muscle-pedicle bone grafting. J Bone Joint Surg Br 73:241–245, 1991.

79. Zhao D, Xu D, Wang W, Cui X: Iliac graft vascularization for femoral head osteonecrosis. Clin Orthop Relat Res 442:171–179, 2006.

80. Baksi DP, Pal AK, Baksi DD: Long-term results of decompression and muscle-pedicle bone grafting for osteonecrosis of the femoral head. Int Orthop 33:41–47, 2009.

81. Dean MT, Cabanela ME: Transtrochanteric anterior rotational osteotomy for avascular necrosis of the femoral head: long-term results. J Bone Joint Surg Br 75:597–601, 1993.

82. Sugioka Y, Hotokebuchi T, Tsutsui H: Transtrochanteric anterior rotational osteotomy for idiopathic and steroid-induced necrosis of the femoral head: indications and long-term results. Clin Orthop Relat Res 277:111–120, 1992.

83. Miyanishi K, Noguchi Y, Yamamoto T, et al: Prediction of the outcome of transtrochanteric rotational osteotomy for osteonecrosis of the femoral head. J Bone Joint Surg Br 82:512–516, 2000.

84. Sugioka Y, Yamamoto T: Transtrochanteric posterior rotational osteotomy for osteonecrosis. Clin Orthop Relat Res 466:1104–1109, 2008.

85. Iwasada S, Hasegawa Y, Iwase T, Kitamura S, Iwata H: Transtrochanteric rotational osteotomy for osteonecrosis of the femoral head. 43 patients followed for at least 3 years. Arch Orthop Trauma Surg 116:447–453, 1997.

86. Sugano N, Takaoka K, Ohzono K, et al: Rotational osteotomy for non-traumatic avascular necrosis of the femoral head. J Bone Joint Surg Br 74:734–739, 1992.

87. Biswal S, Hazra S, Yun HH, et al: Transtrochanteric rotational osteotomy for nontraumatic osteonecrosis of the femoral head in young adults. Clin Orthop Relat Res 467:1529–1537, 2009.

88. Yoon TR, Abbas AA, Hur CI, et al: Modified transtrochanteric rotational osteotomy for femoral head osteonecrosis. Clin Orthop Relat Res 466:1110–1116, 2008.

89. Tooke SM, Amstutz HC, Hedley AK: Results of transtrochanteric rotational osteotomy for femoral head osteonecrosis. Clin Orthop Relat Res 224:150–157, 1987.

90. Rijnen WH, Gardeniers JW, Westrek BL, et al: Sugioka's osteotomy for femoral-head necrosis in young Caucasians. Int Orthop 29:140–144, 2005.

91. Belal MA, Reichelt A: Clinical results of rotational osteotomy for treatment of avascular necrosis of the femoral head. Arch Orthop Trauma Surg 115:80–84, 1996.

92. Grigoris P, Safran M, Brown I, Amstutz HC: Long-term results of transtrochanteric rotational osteotomy for femoral head osteonecrosis. Arch Orthop Trauma Surg 115:127–130, 1996.

93. Mont MA, Fairbank AC, Krackow KA, Hungerford DS: Corrective osteotomy for osteonecrosis of the femoral head. J Bone Joint Surg Am 78:1032–1038, 1996.

94. Schneider W, Aigner N, Pinggera O, Knahr K: Intertrochanteric osteotomy for avascular necrosis of the head of the femur: survival probability of two different methods. J Bone Joint Surg Br 84:817–824, 2002.

95. Drescher W, Furst M, Hahne HJ, et al: Survival analysis of hips treated with flexion osteotomy for femoral head necrosis. J Bone Joint Surg Br 85:969–974, 2003.

96. Maistrelli G, Fusco U, Avai A, Bombelli R: Osteonecrosis of the hip treated by intertrochanteric osteotomy: a four- to 15-year follow-up. J Bone Joint Surg Br 70:761–766, 1988.

97. Pavlovcic V, Dolinar D: Intertrochanteric osteotomy for osteonecrosis of the femoral head. Int Orthop 26:238–242, 2002.

98. Scher MA, Jakim I: Late follow-up of femoral head avascular necrosis managed by intertrochanteric osteotomy and bone grafting. Acta Orthop Belg 65(Suppl 1):73–77, 1999.

99. Ferguson GM, Cabanela ME, Ilstrup DM: Total hip arthroplasty after failed intertrochanteric osteotomy. J Bone Joint Surg Br 76:252–257, 1994.

100. Kawasaki M, Hasegawa Y, Sakano S, et al: Total hip arthroplasty after failed transtrochanteric rotational osteotomy for avascular necrosis of the femoral head. J Arthroplasty 20:574–579, 2005.

101. Shinar AA, Harris WH: Cemented total hip arthroplasty following previous femoral osteotomy: an average 16-year follow-up study. J Arthroplasty 13:243–253, 1998.

102. Rijnen WH, Lameijn N, Schreurs BW, Gardeniers JW: Total hip arthroplasty after failed treatment for osteonecrosis of the femoral head. Orthop Clin North Am 40:291–298, 2009.

103. Hungerford DS: Treatment of osteonecrosis of the femoral head: everything's new. J Arthroplasty 22:91–94, 2007.

104. McGrory BJ, York SC, Iorio R, et al: Current practices of AAHKS members in the treatment of adult osteonecrosis of the femoral head. J Bone Joint Surg Am 89:1194–1204, 2007.

105. Chen CH, Chang JK, Huang KY, et al: Core decompression for osteonecrosis of the femoral head at pre-collapse stage. Kaohsiung J Med Sci 16:76–82, 2000.

106. Piperkovski T: Results of treatment in patients with nontraumatic avascular necrosis of the femoral head by monitor assisted core decompression. Roentgenol Radiol 40:281–284, 2001.

107. Wirtz DC, Rohrig H, Neuss M: Core decompression for avascular necrosis of the femoral head. Oper Orthop Traumatol 15:288–303, 2003.

108. Ko JY, Meyers MH, Wenger DR: "Trapdoor" procedure for osteonecrosis with segmental collapse of the femoral head in teenagers. J Pediatr Orthop 15:7–15, 1995.

109. Israelite C, Nelson CL, Ziarani CF, et al: Bilateral core decompression for osteonecrosis of the femoral head. Clin Orthop Relat Res 441:285–290, 2005.

110. Wang CJ, Wang FS, Huang CC, et al: Treatment for osteonecrosis of the femoral head: comparison of extracorporeal shock waves with core decompression and bone-grafting. J Bone Joint Surg 87:2380–2387, 2005.

111. Saito S, Ohzono K, Ono K: Joint-preserving operations for idiopathic avascular necrosis of the femoral head: results of core decompression, grafting and osteotomy. J Bone Joint Surg Br 70:78–84, 1988.

112. Seyler TM, Marker DR, Ulrich SD, et al: Nonvascularized bone grafting defers joint arthroplasty in hip osteonecrosis. Clin Orthop Relat Res 466:1125–1132, 2008.

113. Shuler MS, Rooks MD, Roberson JR: Porous tantalum implant in early osteonecrosis of the hip: preliminary report on operative, survival, and outcomes results. J Arthroplasty 22:26–31, 2007.

114. Nadeau M, Seguin C, Theodoropoulos JS, Harvey EJ: Short term clinical outcome of a porous tantalum implant for the treatment of advanced osteonecrosis of the femoral head. McGill J Med 10:4–10, 2007.

115. Dean GS, Kime RC, Fitch RD, et al: Treatment of osteonecrosis in the hip of pediatric patients by free vascularized fibular graft. Clin Orthop Relat Res 386:106–113, 2001.

116. Judet H, Gilbert A: Long-term results of free vascularized fibular grafting for femoral head necrosis. Clin Orthop Relat Res 386:114–119, 2001.

117. Rizzo M, Clifford PE, Gunneson EE, Urbaniak JR: Physicians and health professionals with osteonecrosis of the femoral head: results of management with free vascularized fibular grafting. J Surg Orthop Adv 13:30–37, 2004.

118. Le Nen D, Genestet M, Dubrana F, et al: [Vascularized fibular transplant for avascular necrosis of the femoral head: 16 cases]. Rev Chir Orthop Reparatrice Appar Mot 90:722–731, 2004.

119. Garberina MJ, Berend KR, Gunneson EE, Urbaniak JR: Results of free vascularized fibular grafting for femoral head osteonecrosis in patients with systemic lupus erythematosus. Orthop Clin North Am 35:353–357, x, 2004.

120. Zhang C, Zeng B, Xu Z, et al: [Treatment of osteonecrosis of femoral head with free vascularized fibula grafting]. Zhongguo Xiu Fu Chong Jian Wai Ke Za Zhi 18:367–369, 2004.

121. Marciniak D, Furey C, Shaffer JW: Osteonecrosis of the femoral head: a study of 101 hips treated with vascularized fibular grafting. J Bone Joint Surg Am 87:742–747, 2005.

122. Stubbs AJ, Gunneson EB, Urbaniak JR: Pediatric femoral avascular necrosis after pyarthrosis: use of free vascularized fibular grafting. Clin Orthop Relat Res 439:193–200, 2005.

123. Yen CY, Tu YK, Ma CH, et al: Osteonecrosis of the femoral head: comparison of clinical results for vascularized iliac and fibula bone grafting. J Reconstr Microsurg 22:21–24, 2006.

124. Roush TF, Olson SA, Pietrobon R, et al: Influence of acetabular coverage on hip survival after free vascularized fibular grafting for femoral head osteonecrosis. J Bone Joint Surg Am 88:2152–2158, 2006.

125. Eisenschenk A, Lautenbach M, Schwetlick G, Weber U: Treatment of femoral head necrosis with vascularized iliac crest transplants. Clin Orthop Relat Res 386:100–105, 2001.

126. Noguchi M, Kawakami T, Yamamoto H: Use of vascularized pedicle iliac bone graft in the treatment of avascular necrosis of the femoral head. Arch Orthop Trauma Surg 121:437–442, 2001.

127. Zhang NF, Li ZR, Zhang XZ, Wang W: [Vascularized iliac bone grafting for avascular necrosis of the femoral head]. Zhonghua Wai Ke Za Zhi 41:125–129, 2003.

128. Fuchs B, Knothe U, Hertel R, Ganz R: Femoral osteotomy and iliac graft vascularization for femoral head osteonecrosis. Clin Orthop Relat Res 412:84–93, 2003.

129. Nagoya S, Nagao M, Takada J, et al: Predictive factors for vascularized iliac bone graft for nontraumatic osteonecrosis of the femoral head. J Orthop Sci 9:566–570, 2004.

130. Matsusaki H, Noguchi M, Kawakami T, Tani T: Use of vascularized pedicle iliac bone graft combined with transtrochanteric rotational osteotomy in the treatment of avascular necrosis of the femoral head. Arch Orthop Trauma Surg 125:95–101, 2005.

131. Nakamura Y, Kumazawa Y, Mitsui H, et al: Combined rotational osteotomy and vascularized iliac bone graft for advanced osteonecrosis of the femoral head. J Reconstr Microsurg 21:101–105, 2005.

132. Hisatome T, Yasunaga Y, Takahashi K, Ochi M: Progressive collapse of transposed necrotic area after transtrochanteric rotational osteotomy for osteonecrosis of the femoral head induces osteoarthritic change: mid-term results of transtrochanteric rotational osteotomy for osteonecrosis of the femoral head. Arch Orthop Trauma Surg 124:77–81, 2004.

133. Sakano S, Hasegawa Y, Torii Y, et al: Curved intertrochanteric varus osteotomy for osteonecrosis of the femoral head. J Bone Joint Surg Br 86:359–365, 2004.

134. Simank HG, Brocai DR, Brill C, Lukoschek M: Comparison of results of core decompression and intertrochanteric osteotomy for nontraumatic osteonecrosis of the femoral head using Cox regression and survivorship analysis. J Arthroplasty 16:790–794, 2001.

135. Gallinaro P, Masse A: Flexion osteotomy in the treatment of avascular necrosis of the hip. Clin Orthop Relat Res 386:79–84, 2001.

136. Koo KH, Song HR, Yang JW, et al: Trochanteric rotational osteotomy for osteonecrosis of the femoral head. J Bone Joint Surg Br 83:83–89, 2001.

137. Hasegawa Y, Sakano S, Iwase T, et al: Pedicle bone grafting versus transtrochanteric rotational osteotomy for avascular necrosis of the femoral head. J Bone Joint Surg Br 85:191–198, 2003.

138. Zhang NF, Li ZR, Yang LF, et al: [Transtrochanteric rotational osteotomy for osteonecrosis of the femoral head]. Zhonghua Wai Ke Za Zhi 42:1477–1480, 2004.

139. Chen WP, Tai CL, Shih CH, et al: Selection of fixation devices in proximal femur rotational osteotomy: clinical complications and finite element analysis. Clin Biomech 19:255–262, 2004.

140. Onodera S, Majima T, Abe Y, et al: Transtrochanteric rotational osteotomy for osteonecrosis of the femoral head: relation between radiographic features and secondary collapse. J Orthop Sci 10:367–373, 2005.

141. Ikemura S, Yamamoto T, Jingushi S, et al: Use of a screw and plate system for a transtrochanteric anterior rotational osteotomy for osteonecrosis of the femoral head. J Orthop Sci 12:260–264, 2007.

CHAPTER 59

Arthrodesis and Resection Arthroplasty of the Hip

Michael J. Taunton and Robert T. Trousdale

Arthrodesis

KEY POINTS

- Indications for arthrodesis of the hip include young active patients with arthritis, in whom other forms of reconstruction will likely fail at an unacceptably high rate.
- Surgical technique greatly influences outcome; sparing of the abductor mechanism is key for later reconstruction.
- The optimal position for hip fusion is 20 to 30 degrees of flexion, 5 to 7 degrees of adduction, and 5 to 10 degrees of external rotation, with shortening kept to a minimum.
- Modern techniques quote a 78% to 83% fusion rate.
- Conversion to total hip arthroplasty can have a favorable outcome, but rates of aseptic loosening, heterotopic ossification, and limp are higher than for primary total hip arthroplasty.

INTRODUCTION

Operative arthrodesis of the hip is defined by any method that effectively fuses the ilium and the proximal femur, eliminating the hip joint and its motion. Thus, arthrosis of the hip joint and accompanying pain are eliminated.

Hip arthrodesis was a commonly performed procedure in the United States up until other forms of motion-sparing, pain-relieving reconstruction became available. However, with the advent of hip arthroplasty, each decade the number of hip arthrodeses decreases. Unfortunately for the young patient, the durability of current components of total hip arthroplasty cannot compete with patients' lifestyle, and this often leads to revision. The success of total hip arthroplasty has improved in recent decades with quoted success of modern components in patients younger than 50 years of age to be 87% at 10 years for uncemented Harris Galante acetabular components,[1] 95% at 7 years for Exeter cemented femoral components, and 90% for an uncemented grit-blasted straight tapered titanium femoral stem at 20 years.[2] Even with exceedingly favorable results, many patients younger than 50 will need at least one revision of total hip arthroplasty in their lifetime.

Preoperative discussion in patients with end-stage arthrosis of the hip younger than 40 years of age must include discussions of the pros and cons of salvage procedures such as arthrodesis. Although surgeons' enthusiasm for the procedure and patients' acceptance of fusion may be low, hip arthrodesis may be an important consideration in a select patient population with end-stage arthrosis of the hip. A properly positioned, fused hip joint can offer long-term pain relief and good function.[3-6] However, as the results of total hip arthroplasty improve with further development of implants, bearing surfaces, and techniques, hip fusion may become even more limited. Discussions between patient and physician with the patient's best interest in mind, combined with quality data, will continue to direct decision making.

HISTORICAL PERSPECTIVE

In the United States in 1908, F. H. Ablee first discussed arthrodesis of the hip for advanced arthrosis in five patients.[7] Indications for most early reports included tuberculous hips in younger patients and unilateral osteoarthritis in older patients. Arthrodesis was first used for old congenital dislocation by Heusner, by Lampugnani, and by Albert as early as 1885, according to Nové-Josserand.[8] In the early 1900s, many methods of extra-articular arthrodesis were described.[9-11] Ghormley, in 1931, and Henderson, in 1933, described their techniques of arthrodesis, used chiefly in tuberculous hips.[12,13] Ghormley advocated a combined intra-articular and extra-articular arthrodesis and pointed out that the risk of spreading tuberculosis by opening the superior surface of the capsule was minimal. Henderson recommended clean removal of tuberculous tissue and combined intra-articular and extra-articular fusion for tuberculosis of the hip.

Trumble, in 1932,[14] and Brittain, in 1941,[15,16] described techniques for ischiofemoral arthrodesis. Brittain's method of arthrodesis involved making a subtrochanteric osteotomy with special chisels and placing a tibial autograph strut from the subtrochanteric osteotomy into the ischium. Patients were kept in plaster cast immobilization for 4 months postoperatively.

In 1938, Watson-Jones advocated internal fixation of the femoral head to the pelvis by a long Smith-Petersen nail.[17] This was later refined and described in combination with iliac grafting. Watson-Jones reported in 1956 an incidence of 94% sound bone fusion in 120 patients who had arthrodesis of the hip for osteoarthritis who had been observed for a minimum of 5 years.[18,19] Immobilization in a double hip spica for at least 4 months was considered essential by these authors. Lange reported the largest series (500 patients) of the technique with 85% perfect results.[20]

Thompson and Cholmeley, both in 1956, advocated routine subtrochanteric osteotomy for all patients having arthrodesis of the hip.[21,22] Both Thompson and Cholmeley concluded that success occurred more frequently when the grafting operation was combined with or followed by osteotomy. Thompson noted a 90% rate of union in those patients having combined hip fusion and osteotomy against a prior 26% rate of union in patients in whom fusion was attempted without osteotomy for osteoarthritis.[22]

Charnley, in 1953, advocated central dislocation of the femoral head in surgical arthrodesis of the hip and subsequently reported excellent or good results in 88% of 105 patients treated by this method. Even though many of his patients did not obtain fusion, they were included in the 88% good results.[23] Medialization of the hip center lowered joint reaction forces across the hip by shortening the lever arm from the center of gravity. Schneider applied the concepts of Charnley's arthrodesis and added the Cobra-headed plate arthrodesis.[24]

These reports and others had relatively short follow-up and focused on fusion rates with different intra-articular and extra-articular techniques with and without internal fixation. Many reports required prolonged immobilization in plaster cast for 6 weeks to 4 months to achieve fusion.

Callaghan and Sponseller were some of the first to report the long-term outcomes of patients with arthrodesis of the hip. Sponseller cited that 78% of patients were satisfied with the arthrodesis, and all were able to work; 57% had some low back pain, and 45% had knee discomfort. Only 13% had undergone total hip arthroplasty on the arthrodesed hip.[6] Callaghan retrospectively reviewed 28 patients with an average follow-up of 38 years after arthrodesis through various techniques. About 60% of patients had pain in the ipsilateral knee, with onset on average 23 years after arthrodesis. Back pain was similar, with an average onset of 25 years after arthrodesis. Seventy percent of patients could walk farther than 1 mile. Based on their results, investigators believed that the optimal position for fusion was in approximately 5 degrees of adduction and 35 to 40 degrees of flexion. The authors concluded that a patient with an arthrodesis of the hip could function at a high level for many years and would be able to work at most occupations. Pain in the back and knee was a common sequela, especially at long-term follow-up. However, symptoms usually are not incapacitating and generally had their onset many years after the arthrodesis.[4]

INDICATIONS/CONTRAINDICATIONS

Indications

- Monoarticular hip osteoarthritis, especially in a young, high-demand patient
- Hip arthrosis after fracture
- Unilateral end-stage avascular necrosis of the femoral head
- History of unilateral septic arthritis of the hip with end-stage arthritis
- Salvage of prior surgery (e.g., osteotomy)
- Unilateral hip dysplasia with end-stage arthritis
- Patients with contraindications to total hip arthroplasty (THA) with end-stage disease
- Muscular or neurologic deficiencies about the hip in the setting of end-stage arthrosis

Contraindications

- Polyarticular arthritis
- Rheumatoid arthritis
- Active infection
- Bilateral hip disease or dysplasia
- Spondylosis
- Radiographic knee arthritis
- Knee instability

Only after appropriate exhaustion of nonsurgical modalities, such as activity modification, anti-inflammatories, and the use of assistive devices, can an operative salvage procedure such as fusion be entertained. A strong indication for arthrodesis of the hip is a young patient (generally defined as 1 less than 40 years of age) who is healthy with high demands (such as a heavy laborer) and end-stage monoarticular osteoarthritis of the hip. Patients with neurologic or muscular abnormalities that would compromise the function of the abductor musculature after total hip arthroplasty may also be better suited for arthrodesis. Other relative indications include hip arthrosis after fracture, end-stage unilateral avascular necrosis of the femoral head, a history of unilateral septic arthritis of the hip with end-stage arthritis, salvage of prior surgery (e.g., osteotomy), unilateral hip dysplasia with end-stage arthritis, and other patients with contraindications to THA with end-stage hip disease.

Strong contraindications for arthrodesis of the hip include active infection, inflammatory arthritis such as rheumatoid arthritis or systemic lupus erythematosus, older patients with osteoarthritis that can be managed with total hip arthroplasty, and those with bilateral hip disease. Radiographs of the patient's lumbar spine, contralateral hip, and bilateral knees should be obtained. Although early changes in back and knee arthritis are not an absolute contraindication, various authors have reported poorer results with spondylosis, gonarthrosis, and knee instability.[4,25]

Other relative contraindications include patients who are not able to comply with postoperative rehabilitation and limited weight bearing, especially the obese. The patient's lifestyle must be taken into consideration.

Those with a job or a desire for activity such as climbing, sitting for long periods of time, and repetitive stooping or squatting may not be best served by arthrodesis. The patient's overall psychological condition should be assessed for tolerance of the procedure and rehabilitation.

PREOPERATIVE PLANNING

An important component of the preoperative plan is a precise and careful discussion of the options and expected functional outcome of the arthrodesis. The physician-patient relationship is very important in this situation for a positive outcome. Patients should be counseled that although the motion of the hip joint will be obliterated, they will be allowed to resume all activities. The reality of the salvage situation must be conveyed to enable the patient to have realistic and appropriate expectations after the procedure.

To help define the bony anatomy and any bony deformities that may be encountered at arthrodesis, enhanced radiographic evaluation is indicated. Routine standing anteroposterior (AP) pelvis, Judet, and AP and cross-table lateral views of the femur should be obtained. These films will allow the surgeon to assess leg length discrepancy, offset, rotation, and angular deformity. Additionally, the acetabular bone stock and points of fixation can be more readily assessed with Judet films. If the pelvic anatomy or bone deficiency is more complex, preoperative three-dimensional computed tomography (CT) reconstructions of the pelvis and proximal femur may assist the surgeon in proper positioning and fixation of the arthrodesis.

Routine preoperative laboratory tests should be obtained. However, in addition, erythrocyte sedimentation rate, C-reactive protein, and complete blood count with differential are advised in patients with a history of infection. If any of these tests are abnormal, preoperative hip joint aspiration with cell count and culture will help rule out chronic infection. Patients with remote histories of inflammatory disease may have to be evaluated by a rheumatologist and may need to be reconsidered for fusion if active inflammatory disease is present. Preoperative blood donation or intraoperative blood salvage may be indicated because blood loss may necessitate transfusion.

DESCRIPTION OF TECHNIQUE(S)

Positioning of the Hip Arthrodesis

Positioning of the arthrodesis has been developed as a position of the limb that best accommodates normal activities of daily living. Patients with unilateral hip fusion walk with a gait that is somewhat slow, asymmetrical, and arrhythmic. Compensation for absent hip motion is accomplished by increased transverse and sagittal rotation of the pelvis, increased motion in the sound hip, and increased flexion of the knee throughout the stance phase on the fused side.[26-28] Positioning can

have a large effect on the durability of the fusion and the joints adjacent to it.[4] The optimal position of hip fusion is 5 to 7 degrees of adduction, 20 to 30 degrees of hip flexion, and 5 to 10 degrees of external rotation. Limb shortening is kept to a minimum. Gore and associates stated, "Relationships between the fusion position, certain physical traits, and walking performance suggest that the best gait can be expected in young patients who have free motion of the lumbar spine, the sound hip, and the knee on the side of fusion, and who have equal limb lengths and a hip fused in a position that includes excessive adduction."[27] It is important to note that Fulkerson found that in children with long-term follow-up, the fused hip can drift into excessive adduction over time. In these patients, it is advisable to fuse in neutral adduction.[29,30] Activities that require hip flexion are most difficult for patients, who find that sitting in tight spaces such as airplanes is difficult. Additionally, simple activities of daily living such as donning and doffing socks and bending are troublesome. Some women may have difficulty with sexual activity. The patient and the surgeon must accept the limitations of the procedure and must position the fusion in the most functional and durable position.

Techniques

Anterior Plating Technique. The modern anterior approach to arthrodesis described by Beaule and associates is done through an extended Smith-Petersen approach with the patient supine on a radiolucent table. Depending on the type of table used, the leg may be prepped free and supported intraoperatively for optimal positioning, or the leg may be held by the table in the proper position if a traction table is used. An incision is made from just superior-lateral to the anterior superior iliac spine to below the greater trochanter, lateral to the course of the lateral cutaneous femoral nerve. The fascia over the tensor fascia lata is incised and elevated off of the muscle medially. Tensor, sartorius, and rectus muscles are released from their insertions, and a complete anterior capsulectomy is performed. After the extended Smith-Petersen approach, the internal aspects of the ilium, hip, and proximal femur are well seen. The traction table can facilitate distraction and/or dislocation of the hip for preparation of the bony surfaces. The acetabulum is curetted and reamed, and a bleeding cancellous surface is obtained, if possible. The surface of the femoral head is likewise denuded and is shaped with female reamers, if available. A conforming fit of the femoral head and acetabulum is important for successful fusion. At this point, proper positioning of the hip joint is obtained, or it is re-evaluated for fusion. Flexion is checked and measured relative to the angle of the femoral shaft and the floor. The foot and the patella are used to judge rotation. Fluoroscopy is helpful to identify the horizontal axis, defined as a line between the anterior superior iliac spines. The mechanical axis of the femur can also be identified by fluoroscopy by a line subtended between the center of the femoral head and the center of the knee or the center of the weight-bearing dome of the talus. When the position is correct, a long 6.5 mm cancellous lag screw is placed from the lateral aspect of the greater trochanter to the femoral head into the ilium to obtain medialization and compression of the femoral head. A 12 or 14 hole 4.5 mm low-contact dynamic compression (LCDC) plate is then modeled to the anterior contour of the femur, pelvic brim, and proximal femur. The released vastus lateralis, rectus femoris, and sartorius muscles are reattached. The abductors are spared and pelvic deformity is minimized, making later conversion to THA less technically challenging. Bone graft may be added from the ilium or from allograft sources and placed around the site of fusion. Deep drains are placed, and the wound is closed in standard fashion.[31]

Screw Technique. The procedure may also be carried out in a lateral position through an anterolateral approach. The patient is positioned in the lateral position on the traction table. An incision is made over the lateral aspect of the greater trochanter. The fascia over the greater trochanter is incised in line with its fibers. The anterior one third of the gluteus medius is elevated from the greater trochanter. The anterior capsule is excised. The leg is externally rotated, and the hip is dislocated anteriorly. The rectus is released, and the capsule is released to assist with retracting the femur for acetabular exposure. The acetabulum is curetted and reamed. The femoral head is prepared likewise. The hip is then relocated and is placed in proper position for arthrodesis. A guide pin for a fixed angle hip screw is inserted from the greater trochanter through the femoral head into the supra-acetabular bone. The path is drilled, and a hip screw of appropriate length is placed. The lateral side plate is placed in standard fashion, and the surfaces are compressed. Then three 6.5 mm cancellous screws are placed along the axis of the hip screw for added compression. Cancellous bone chips can be added around the rim of the femur and acetabulum for added osteoconductive potential. The abductors are reattached in standard fashion, and the wound is closed in layers. A double hip spica cast is placed and kept for 3 months. The fusion is re-evaluated at that time and is converted to a single leg spica for an additional 4 to 6 weeks.

POSTOPERATIVE CARE

Standard postoperative antibiotics are maintained for 24 hours. Drains are removed when output has declined to less than 50 mL over 8 hours. Deep venous thrombosis prophylaxis should be maintained with a comprehensive protocol as with total hip arthroplasty, including but not limited to mechanical and dynamic compression garments and chemical thromboprophylaxis. Whether casting has been chosen or not (based on the rigidity of internal fixation and surgeon preference), weight bearing should be limited to no more than 30 lb for the first 6 to 8 weeks. If not treated with a cast, the patient should not sit at any angle greater than 60 degrees so as not to stress the fixation of the fusion. AP and lateral radiographs of the pelvis are obtained at 3 months to assess the fusion, and every 6 weeks thereafter until fusion is obtained. Activity and weight bearing are progressed when bony fusion has been achieved and pain has subsided.

RESULTS

In Callaghan's review of 28 Iowa patients who had been fused from 1923 to 1966 with a variety of techniques, and with an average follow-up of 35 years, 22 of the 28 remained fused; in 6, the arthrodesed hip had been converted to total hip replacement. Average age at fusion was 25 years. Low back pain was present in 61%, and knee pain was present in 57%. Arthrodesis reliably relieved patients' pain but limited lifestyle to some degree. Patients fused in abduction had more back pain than those fused in neutral or adduction (78% vs. 50% to 60%). Additionally, those fused in adduction had a lower rate of knee pain and radiographic changes in the knee than those fused in abduction (43% vs. 78%). Patients fused in a more flexed position (average 33 degrees) tended not to have back pain compared with those fused in a less flexed position, who had back pain (average 29 degrees). Most patients were unsure whether in hindsight they would have preferred a total hip arthroplasty or an arthrodesis (Table 59-1).

With more modern fusion techniques and with a group of primary fusion and re-fusion patients, Brien reviewed 16 patients who had undergone hip arthrodesis utilizing an anteriorly placed compression plate an average of 4.5 years after surgery. The rationale for the anteriorly based plate is that future conversion to total hip arthroplasty should be considered at the time of planning for hip fusion. Rates of conversion to THA range from 13% to 21%.[4,6] In this study, 63% of patients failed to unite, and 100% of those were re-fusions. Half of those with pseudarthroses were accepted by patients, and few significant restrictions in functional activities were reported.[25] However, in a retrospective review by Matta, at an average follow-up of 25 months, 83% achieved solid fusion by clinical and radiographic

Table 59-1. Long-Term Results of Hip Arthrodesis				
Author	Number of Hips	Mean Follow-up, yr	Mean Patient Age, yr	Results
Sponseller (1984)	53	38	14	17% contralateral hip pain 45% ipsilateral knee pain 57% back pain
Callaghan (1985)	28	37	25	28% contralateral hip pain 57% ipsilateral knee pain 61% back pain

criteria. Seventy-five percent of patients in that study had no or minor restrictions when participating in their former sports activities, and half regained the ability to work at their former jobs or in new occupations.[32]

COMPLICATIONS

Today, the major complication of arthrodesis may be patient dissatisfaction. Most patients know or have seen someone with a total hip arthroplasty and desire that level of function and hip motion. An open conversation about the procedure is very important. Proper patient education, combined with excellent surgical technique, may decrease this concern. Fusion position adjustment, based on the patient's daily activity and interests, may enhance acceptance of an arthrodesis. Some authors have suggested a trial of spica casting before arthrodesis to "test out" the position and make modifications to the position preoperatively.

Malunion is the major complication of hip arthrodesis. Modern reports cite a high rate ($\approx$80% to 90%) of union with modern techniques.[31,32] However, Brien found that patients with previous failed fusion or bone loss have a high risk of nonunion.[25] A single plate may not be adequate to neutralize forces across the hip joint, particularly in cases such as multiply operated hips, re-fusion, or avascular necrosis, when the contact surface area between the femoral head and the acetabulum is reduced. In these cases, supplemental fixation with lateral plates and additional bone graft may be indicated.[25]

CURRENT CONTROVERSIES AND FUTURE CONSIDERATIONS

- A properly positioned, fused hip joint can offer long-term pain relief and good function.
- Most authors believe that an optimal position can maximize outcome.
- A superior method of fixation, approach, and postoperative immobilization has not been clearly defined by any prospective study and is unlikely to be performed in the future.
- As the results of total hip arthroplasty improve with further development of implants, bearing surfaces, and techniques, hip fusion may be even less frequently performed.
- Discussions between patient and physician with the patient's best interest in mind, combined with quality data, will continue to direct decision making.

REFERENCES

1. Duffy GP, Prpa B, Rowland CM, Berry DJ: Primary uncemented Harris-Galante acetabular components in patients 50 years old or younger: results at 10 to 12 years. Clin Orthop Relat Res 427:157–161, 2004.
2. Aldinger PR, Jung AW, Pritsch M, et al: Uncemented grit-blasted straight tapered titanium stems in patients younger than fifty-five years of age: fifteen to twenty-year results. J Bone Joint Surg Am 91:1432–1439, 2009.
3. Beaulé PE, Matta JM, Mast JW: Hip arthrodesis: current indications and techniques. J Am Acad Orthop Surg 10:249–258, 2002.
4. Callaghan JJ, Brand RA, Pedersen DR: Hip arthrodesis: a long-term follow-up. J Bone Joint Surg Am 67:1328–1335, 1985.
5. Karol LA, Halliday SE, Gourineni P: Gait and function after intra-articular arthrodesis of the hip in adolescents. J Bone Joint Surg Am 82:561–569, 2000.
6. Sponseller PD, McBeath AA, Perpich M: Hip arthrodesis in young patients: a long-term follow-up study. J Bone Joint Surg Am 66:853–859, 1984.
7. Albee FH: Arthritis deformans of the hip: report of a new operation. JAMA 50:1553–1554, 1908.
8. Nové-Josserand G: Les nouvelles application de l'arthrodèse de la hanche. Paris Méd 45:63–68, 1922.
9. Rogers MHP: Operative treatment of old hip disease. J Orthop Surg II:589, 1920.
10. Spiers HW: An end-result study of arthrodesis for non-tubercular affections of the hip joint. J Orthop Surg II:515, 1920.
11. Wilson JC: Extra-articular fusion of the tuberculous hip joint. Calif West Med XXVII:774, 1927.
12. Ghormley R: Use of the anterior superior spine and crest of the ilium in surgery of the hip joint. J Bone Joint Surg Am 13:784–798, 1931.
13. Henderson MS: Combined intra-articular and extra-articular arthrodesis for tuberculosis of the hip joint. J Bone Joint Surg Am 15:51–57, 1933.
14. Trumble HC: A method of fixation of the hip joint by means of extra-articular bone graft. Austral N Z J Surg 1:413–420, 1932.
15. Brittain HA: Ischiofemoral arthrodesis. Br J Surg 29:93, 1941.
16. Brittain HA: Ischio-femoral arthrodesis. J Bone Joint Surg Br 30:642–650, 1948.
17. Watson-Jones R: Arthrodesis of the osteoarthritic hip. JAMA 110:278, 1938.
18. Watson-Jones R: Arthrodesis of the osteoarthritic hip joint. J Bone Joint Surg Br 38:353–377, 1956.
19. Watson-Jones R: Discussion on treatment of unilateral osteoarthritis of the hip joint. Proc R Soc Med XXXVIII:363–368, 1945.
20. Lange M: Arthrodesis of the hip: review of a series of more than five hundred cases. J Int Coll Surg 29:638–643, 1958.
21. Cholmeley JA: Femoral osteotomy in extra-articular arthrodesis of the tuberculous hip. J Bone Joint Surg Br 38:342–352, 1956.
22. Thompson FR: Combined hip fusion and subtrochanteric osteotomy allowing early ambulation. J Bone Joint Surg Am 38:13–22, 1956.
23. Charnley J: Treatment of mono-articular arthritis of the hip by the central dislocation operation. J Bone Joint Surg Br 38:592–593, 1956.
24. Schneider R: Hip arthrodesis with the cobra head plate and pelvic osteotomy. Reconstr Surg Traumatol 14:1–37, 1974.
25. Brien WW, Golz RJ, Kuschner SH, et al: Hip joint arthrodesis utilizing anterior compression plate fixation [see comment]. J Arthroplasty 9:171–176, 1994.
26. Ahlback SO, Lindahl O: Hip arthrodesis: the connection between function and position. Acta Orthop Scand 37:77–87, 1966.
27. Gore DR, Murray MP, Sepic SB, Gardner GM: Walking patterns of men with unilateral surgical hip fusion. J Bone Joint Surg Am 57:759–765, 1975.
28. Hauge MF: The knee in patients with hip joint ankylosis: clinical survey and bio-mechanical aspects. Acta Orthop Scand 44:485–495, 1973.
29. Fulkerson JP: Arthrodesis for disabling hip pain in children and adolescents. Clin Orthop Relat Res 128:296–302, 1977.
30. Fulkerson JP: Hip arthrodesis. Clin Orthop Relat Res 182:309–310, 1984.
31. Stover MD, Beaulé PE, Matta JM, Mast JW: Hip arthrodesis: a procedure for the new millennium? Clin Orthop Relat Res 418:126–133, 2004.
32. Matta JM, Siebenrock KA, Gautier E, et al: Hip fusion through an anterior approach with the use of a ventral plate. Clin Orthop Relat Res 337:129–178, 1997.

Resection Arthroplasty

KEY POINTS

- Although rarely a primary indication, resection arthroplasty maintains its importance.
- Modern resection preserves the femoral neck to preserve length for possible future reconstruction.
- Addition of osteotomies or soft tissue reconstructions to resection arthroplasty remains controversial.
- Resection is a powerful treatment for infection about the hip joint.
- Main goals are to relieve pain, restore some function, and eradicate infection.

INTRODUCTION

Resection arthroplasty of the hip consists of removal of the femoral head and a variable amount of femoral neck, proximal femur, and/or acetabulum. Additions of osteotomies and soft tissue reconstructions have been described.

HISTORICAL PERSPECTIVE

Resection arthroplasty of the hip joint was originally described in the 1800s as a primary procedure for treatment of destructive conditions of the hip joint, chiefly tuberculosis. In present day, it is usually employed as a salvage procedure for failed arthroplasty. However, the relevance of the procedure is maintained in a variety of special situations.

One of the first descriptions of resection arthroplasty can be found in the obituary of Mr. Anthony White, a surgeon at Westminster Hospital, who began practice in 1816. The account describes his treatment of a 9-year-old boy with post-traumatic septic arthritis about the hip joint. "Mr. White removed the head and neck of the femur, with a portion just below the trochanter minor, from the dorsum of the ilium."[1,2] The boy made a dramatic recovery after 1 year of rehabilitation.

J. R. Barton, of Philadelphia, Pennsylvania, described in 1827 the creation of a pseudarthrosis of the hip joint by dividing the femur between the trochanters in a patient with post-traumatic arthrosis.[3]

Tuberculous disease of the hip was maintained as a major indication for resection of the hip in the 1800s. In 1928, Mr. G. R. Girdlestone, an orthopedic surgeon at Wingfield Orthopaedic Hospital, Headington, Oxford, described a wide excision of the upper end of the femur, including the head, neck, and trochanters, for severe septic infection of a tuberculous hip in an adult in whom ankylosis was not taking place. This was done through a transverse incision, with removal of a wide sector of tissue, including the greater trochanter and the lower half of the gluteus medius and minimus, leaving a broad trough leading straight down to the hip. The wound was left open and was allowed to heal from the bottom up. Girdlestone also described an extra-articular pseudarthrosis, first performed in 1923,[4] which had the purpose of "relieving strain on a grumbling hip," to correct deformity and to restore movement below the hip. Active infection was seen as a contraindication. A transverse incision was made, and the greater trochanter was chiseled off with the abductors attached. A section of bone consisting of the femoral neck from the subcapital region to the lesser trochanter was removed, diagonally. The greater trochanter was then applied to the shaft "rather than to the neck as originally described by Sir Robert Jones."[5] This was done to prevent a bony bridge between the shaft and the head. The aim was a free false joint.[6]

In 1943, Girdlestone described an application of the wide excision technique to pyogenic infections of the hip joint.[7,8] In 1945, he described the use of extra-articular pseudarthrosis for the treatment of unilateral hip osteoarthritis.[9]

In 1950, R. G. Taylor, from the same institution as Mr. Girdlestone, described the results of a modified Girdlestone resection in 93 patients. Instead of the transverse incision, a Smith-Petersen approach[10] was employed. A broad gouge was used to remove the anterior and upper rims of the acetabulum. The neck was osteotomized at the intertrochanteric line, and the head and the neck were removed. Indications included unilateral arthritis in 59, bilateral in 14, ankylosing spondylitis in 11, infection in 2, and fractures in the remaining. Results were classed as good in 83 cases and poor in 7 cases. Three patients died as a result of the operation. This case review of the cases of Mr. G. R. Girdlestone, Mr. W. B. Foley, Mr. J. C. Scott, and Professor J. Trueta outlines what we now know as *Girdlestone resection arthroplasty.*[4]

Instability, weakness, and shortening of the extremity were noted by many authors, and a variety of different techniques to improve function of the resected hip were described. In 1950, Gruca discussed a technique of resection and "dynamic" osteotomy of the proximal femur. He recognized the optimal biomechanics of the hip joint and discussed three important points: (1) If the trochanter is elevated above the axis, the abductors become less effective; (2) the lever arm of the abductors is a function of the distance from the abductor attachment to the center of rotation; and (3) a greater distance from the center of rotation to the center of gravity increases the force needed by the abductors. This was accomplished by resection of the hip joint followed by a step-cut osteotomy through the intertrochanteric area, bringing the medial fragment medially into the acetabulum, and the greater trochanter laterally to increase tension on the abductors. They reviewed 224 cases with 90% satisfactory outcomes in patients with quiescent tuberculosis. These patients had a painless stable joint and a range of movement varying from 40% to 100% of normal.[11]

Milch[12,13] popularized a one-stage resection-angulation osteotomy, recognizing that "experience quickly demonstrated that the primary resection of the femoral head necessitated a prolonged period of traction to prevent upward dislocation of the shaft." His paper in 1955 described a primary resection of the head and neck and a subtrochanteric osteotomy that was fixed in a valgus position, was congruent with the lateral pelvic wall (205 to 210 degrees), and was fixed with a Moore-Blount blade plate. Evaluation of 64 procedures revealed 69% with "good" pain relief and 53% with "good" motion.[12] This description, unlike Gruca's,[11] pertained to a more heterogeneous population consisting of many arthritic conditions, and only 3% had tuberculosis. Osteoarthritis was the primary diagnosis in 27%.

The addition of osteotomies about resections brought about comparison studies. Shepard, in a study comparing cup arthroplasty, Judet arthroplasty, osteotomy, and resection arthroplasty with or without osteotomy, reviewed 70 patients with resections. Over a period greater than 5 years, results in patients who had simple excision of the head and neck were rather better than those for Batchelor's operation.[14] In fact, this operation provided relief of pain more consistently than any other operation whose results were reviewed. However, results of the Trendelenburg test and stability were improved in the group that underwent Batchelor's operations; this may be due to increased pelvic support or to enhancement of the mechanical advantage of the abductor muscles.[14,15]

In 1965, Lipscomb from the Mayo Clinic reviewed 349 patients who underwent bilateral operations on the hips for chronic disease.[16] These operations consisted of resection arthroplasties, cup arthroplasties, osteotomies, and arthrodesis. He emphasized that for some patients with severe bilateral disease, such as those with rheumatoid arthritis, relief of pain, a useful range of motion, and instability are preferable to a long rehabilitation, as would be needed after arthrodesis, osteotomies, or cup arthroplasties.

Even as the use of hip replacement arthroplasty became more mainstream, the importance of resection arthroplasty was noted for patients who for reason of infection, age, or another disability were not candidates for hip replacement surgery. Parr[2] reviewed 44 patients with resection arthroplasties, 5 of whom had abduction osteotomies at 30 degrees of abduction. Eighty percent were relieved of preoperative pain. Although a small number, the authors believed that the range of motion in the angulation osteotomy group was superior, and that the angulation osteotomy increased stability and was a worthwhile adjunct. Results of 32 patients followed for longer than 2 years after simple Girdlestone resection arthroplasty were reported by Murray[17,18] in 1964, and 30 had no pain.

The advent of a reliable solution for most hip pathology using a femoral endoprosthesis or total hip arthroplasty has in effect moved resection arthroplasty to a salvage procedure. The preceding historical discussion outlines the development of and concepts behind resection arthroplasty and the rationale for its employment. However, even today, patients who are unsuitable for advanced reconstruction may benefit from resection. The focus of this section will be on resection

arthroplasty as a procedure, not as salvage of resection of a total hip arthroplasty.

INDICATIONS/CONTRAINDICATIONS

Indications

Primary Indications
- Nonunions about the hip joint
- Pyogenic arthritis
- Tuberculous arthritis
- Ankylosing spondylitis
- Severe rheumatoid arthritis
- Neurologic disorders—spastic
- Acetabuli protrusio
- Charcot arthropathy
- Tumors about the proximal femur and/or acetabulum
- Osteoarthritis in noncompliant patients
- Prior hip arthrodesis

Secondary Indications
- Failed total hip arthroplasty, especially failed constrained cups
- Failed fixation of femoral neck fractures
- Failed THA in nonambulator; ethanol or substance abuse with other problems
- Failed THA in the poorly compliant

Secondary to the development of total hip arthroplasty, improved fracture fixation, and advanced chemotherapy for infectious and inflammatory disease, resection arthroplasty has declined as a first-line option for the treatment of hip joint pathology. However, in certain situations, resection is a viable option as a primary or a salvage procedure. From the 1800s through the mid 20th century, resection arthroplasty was an effective treatment to relieve pain, increase range of motion, eradicate infection, and enhance overall function. It was first applied to tuberculous and pyogenic infections of the hip, but because of its success, it was expanded to treat osteoarthritis, rheumatoid arthritis, failed fixation of fractures about the hip, ankylosing spondylitis, congenital hip dislocation, and severe femoral and acetabular deformity.* Resection arthroplasty in the medically unstable patient with septic arthritis may be a life-preserving procedure. Pressure sores that are refractory to treatment, septic arthritis in nonambulatory patients, and paraplegia with hip fusion may be effectively treated with resection arthroplasty.[29-31]

Patient populations with poor bone stock, frail medical conditions, or infection recalcitrant to treatment may not be safely treated by one- or two-stage revision total hip arthroplasty. It is in these patients that resection arthroplasty remains an acceptable salvage procedure. In this chapter, we will focus on nonsalvage indications for the procedure and techniques to maximize the benefits of treatment.

---

*References 1, 3, 4, 7, 11, 14, and 18 to 28.

Contraindications

Relative contraindications for resection arthroplasty include patients who could be more effectively managed with hemiarthroplasty or total hip arthroplasty. Other contraindications include patients who are ambulatory but morbidly obese and those who lack the necessary upper extremity strength for use of upper extremity supports such as a walker or crutches, because these are invariably needed over the long term or in the recovery period.

PREOPERATIVE PLANNING

The approach to planning a resection arthroplasty parallels the workup for consideration of total hip arthroplasty. A complete history and physical examination with special attention to comorbidities and social situations is important.

Special attention to comorbid conditions such as neurologic disease, ethanol (EtOH) or other substance abuse, other infections, autoimmune disease, or history of diabetes mellitus or cancer can allow the practitioner to have these diseases fully evaluated before making a final decision regarding resection arthroplasty.

If infection is part of the preoperative concerns, blood cultures, complete blood count, erythrocyte sedimentation rate, C-reactive protein, hip joint aspiration (with culture and cell count of the synovial fluid), and possibly bone scan should be considered before the procedure is performed.

Radiographic evaluation includes AP pelvis and lateral films in most nonemergent situations. CT can be of assistance in cases of arthrodesis take-down for identification of the femoral neck.[32] Judet films can be of assistance for identification of pelvic ring fractures and pelvic discontinuity. Ultrasound, magnetic resonance imaging (MRI), and other advanced imaging may assist in identification of the extent of disease in an infection and in identification of abscesses that may be managed at the same time as resection arthroplasty.

DESCRIPTION OF TECHNIQUE(S)

In the original description of the procedure,[1] White treated a 9-year-old boy with post-traumatic pyogenic arthritis of the hip with resection by "removing the head and neck of the femur with a portion just below the trochanter minor, from the dorsum of the ilium." In Girdlestone's first description of an extra-articular pseudarthrosis, first performed in 1923[4] for quiescent tuberculous hip pathology, a transverse incision was made; the greater trochanter was chiseled off with the abductors attached. A section of bone consisting of the femoral neck from the subcapital region to the lesser trochanter was removed, diagonally. The greater trochanter was then applied to the shaft "rather than to the neck as originally described by Sir Robert Jones."[5] This was done to prevent a bony bridge between the shaft and the head. This procedure is distinctly different from his historical wide resection initially used in active tuberculous infection of the hip, as described earlier.

As indications for resection arthroplasty increased from tuberculous arthritis of the hip, so did modifications of the procedure. Girdlestone later reported the use of resection in unilateral osteoarthritis of the hip, and results of the procedure were reported by Taylor in 1950.[4] They described using a broad gouge to remove the anterior and upper rim of the acetabulum to assist with dislocation of the hip, then dividing the femoral neck at the base with a hand-saw or a Gigli saw. All sharp edges were rounded.

Modern approaches for the procedure are varied. Often, one may need to consider the approach used for a prior procedure and incorporate the incision when reasonable. The Smith-Petersen,[10] anterolateral, direct lateral,[33] and posterolateral approaches are often cited, but any standard longitudinal approach may be implemented. The Smith-Petersen[10] approach has the advantage of preserving the gluteus medius and the tensor fascia lata and their nerve supply. The incision can be made from the anterior one third of the greater trochanter to just anterior to the anterior superior iliac spine. This incision may be extended proximally around the crest of the ilium if a more extensile approach is desired. The fascia overlying the tensor fascia lata is incised and is elevated off of the muscle anteriorly, leading to a fatty plane on the anterior aspect of the femoral neck. Vessels in this fatty layer can be clamped and cauterized. The capsule may be divided with an H-shaped or L-shaped capsulotomy. If a more extensile approach for acetabular exposure is necessary, extension of the capsulotomy may extend to the superior acetabular rim, and the tensor fascia lata may be carefully detached from its origin from the ilium, taking care to watch for perforators. It is important to not remove the origin of the gluteus medius to preserve abductor strength and stability in gait.

The femoral neck is osteotomized at the level of the intertrochanteric line or proximal to it. The femoral head and neck are then removed, along with a variable amount of capsule. Often, underlying pathology dictates the level of the neck resection, especially in fracture cases. If infection or tumor is present, one must remove affected bone to most effectively cure the disease. Grauer reviewed the results of 48 resection arthroplasties for various conditions and developed four types of femoral neck resection that correlated with clinical outcomes of walking, function, and level of activity. Type I resection left a remnant of the femoral neck that measured more than 1.5 cm. Type II resection left a smaller remnant ($\leq$1.5 cm). Type III resection was performed through the intertrochanteric line, and type IV resection was performed distal to the intertrochanteric line, after which only a narrow spike of the proximal part of the femur remained. A positive correlation was noted between shortening and the level of the resection ($P < .01$). The authors believed that use of a more proximal level of resection may have improved stability, allowing patients to remain relatively active. The finding of increased sclerosis on the acetabular rim indicated that stress was being transferred to the acetabulum.[22]

A consideration that must be made for each resection is the possibility that the patient may become in the future a candidate for total hip arthroplasty. In these cases, preservation of femoral bone stock is also of importance.

On the acetabular side, most surgeons recommend excision of soft tissues around the acetabular margin limited to removal of debris, grossly infected tissues, and any projecting bone.[2,25,27] If total hip arthroplasty is a possibility in the future, conservative removal of acetabular bone stock is indicated. Girdlestone and Taylor described using a broad gouge to remove the anterior and upper rim of the acetabulum. The gouge enters the bone half an inch above the upper margin of the acetabulum. They believed that creating a rim of the acetabulum parallel to the intertrochanteric resection of the femur would decrease bony contact and pain.

The capsule is divided on entry to the joint and may be interposed to prevent bone-on-bone contact, especially when the acetabular rim is left intact.[25] Others have closed the capsule without interposition with good results.[18]

In cases of infection, a complete synovectomy, complete débridement of all involved bone and soft tissues, decompression of any abscesses, and reaming of the acetabular cartilage are important for eradication of disease.

After capsular closure, deep drains are inserted and the wound is closed in layers, taking care to restore muscular anatomy during closure for stability and control of the extremity.

VARIATIONS/UNUSUAL SITUATIONS

As with the historical nature of the pseudarthrosis, numerous descriptions and variations on the procedure have been provided. However, a few notable variations deserve mention, including angulation osteotomies and reconstructions combined with the resection procedure.

The angled osteotomy was popularized by Milch and Batchelor separately[12,13,19,34-36] as treatments for arthrosis of the hip. Milch described approaching the hip though a lateral iliofemoral incision, which extends from the anterior superior iliac spine to the base of the trochanter and downward along the lateral aspect of the femur. The intermuscular space between the tensor fascia lata and the gluteus medius is bluntly opened. The capsule is incised along the acetabular margin and is turned down as a flap. The hip is dislocated, and resection of the femoral head and neck is completed along the intertrochanteric line. The capsular flap is sutured over the cut surface at the base of the neck. The upper end of the femur is exposed, and a Moore-Blount blade plate is inserted, so that the apex of the angle of the plate, which is determined before the procedure is performed (angle is from 205 to 210 degrees), lies at a predetermined level of osteotomy. The femoral osteotomy is then made, and the distal fragment is abducted to match the angle of the plate and is internally rotated 20 to 30 degrees. The plate is then fixed to the distal fragment with screws.[12]

According to Batchelor, the procedure can be performed by a two-stage or one-stage approach. In the two-stage approach, the resection is performed through a direct anterior Smith-Petersen approach by resecting the femoral head and neck at the intertrochanteric line. The surgeon then returns a few days later through a posterolateral approach for the second-stage osteotomy. In the one-stage procedure, the anterolateral approach allows resection of the head and neck and exposure of the upper end of the femur for osteotomy. Resection of the head and neck is carried out through the intertrochanteric line, making a smooth interface. The acetabular osteophytes are removed, and all surfaces are made smooth for a nonpainful interface. The osteotomy is carried out 12 to 18 mm below the lesser trochanter. A wedge of bone is removed to create a 40 degree angulation deformity of the proximal femur. The osteotomy is then internally fixed with a plate. Full weight bearing is allowed when the osteotomy has healed.[37]

Coventry reported in 1964 that 57 patients at the Mayo Clinic had a Colonna reconstruction after resection, with more than 90% attaining improvement.[21,38] He recommended this technique over Girdlestone resection or Batchelor's osteotomy. The Colonna reconstruction is performed through a lateral approach. The fascia is divided, and all muscles attached to the greater trochanter are carefully divided near their insertions. The upper end of the femur is left covered by a thin layer of muscle and fibrous tissue. The capsule is opened longitudinally and afterward is divided transversely, close to the greater trochanter, with as much of the capsule preserved as possible. The limb is adducted and rotated outward; the upper end of the femur is freed by cutting the piriformis, gemelli, quadratus femoris, and obturator muscles close to their insertions. Resection is completed at the intertrochanteric line, and the greater trochanter is sunk deeply inside the acetabulum. The thickened capsule and abductor muscles are then pulled down while the limb is held in about 20 degrees of abduction. Fibers of the vastus lateralis are identified and separated subperiosteally to expose the shaft of the femur. A bony trough is made on the lateral aspect as far down as the abductor muscles will reach when the limb is in about 20 degrees of abduction. Two small drill holes are made in the shaft of the femur in an anteroposterior plane, and the muscles are sutured into place. The vastus lateralis is then carefully reefed over the new insertions of the gluteus medius and gluteus minimus muscles; the wound is closed in layers. A long plaster spica is applied from the metatarsal heads to the axilla with the limb in about 20 degrees of abduction and in full extension. Patients were kept in plaster for 4 weeks; range of motion was begun and walking was allowed at 8 weeks.[39] This historical procedure most likely would not be tolerated by today's patient and carries considerable risk for venous thrombosis and other stasis complications.

POSTOPERATIVE CARE

After modern Girdlestone resection arthroplasty, patients, depending on overall ambulatory and functional status, may be kept in light skin traction for comfort while in bed. Shortening of the extremity is inevitable, and prolonged immobilization with bed rest and traction is fraught with complications. To prevent deep venous thrombosis and respiratory complications, patients may be mobilized to the chair on postoperative day one and may be mobilized non–weight bearing with a walker or crutches. After 3 months, the patient may begin to bear weight as tolerated. At this time, accommodative shoe wear may be fabricated to equalize leg lengths.

RESULTS

Results of resection arthroplasty are variable. Patient variables such as infection, bone loss, bilateral disease, age, and comorbid conditions are all factors (Fig. 59-1A and B). Other variables, such as surgeon technique, primary versus secondary procedures, and combined procedures, are also factors. Salvage procedures produce much poorer results than primary procedures, even for the same indications.[40] However, the goals of the procedure are the same: good pain relief, restoration of function, and, in infection situations, eradication of infection. Negative results of the procedures are predictable; loss of strength, limb shortening, and limp are noted in most patients postoperatively.[23,25]

Results of primary resection arthroplasty include reliable relief of pain, reasonable restoration of function, and overall patient satisfaction[4,11-13,19,23,37] (Table 59-2).

Control of infection is excellent in primary situations with success greater than 90%. Grauer reviewed 48 patients with resection arthroplasties, 5 of which were primary procedures for infection. All primary procedures eradicated infection. Three recurrences (out of 43) were reported in patients with resection of prior arthroplasty with retained cement. All were treated successfully with repeat débridement.[22] Tuli was able to cure 27 of 30 patients with tuberculous and pyogenic infection with primary resection.[27] Parr attained healing in 26 of 28 patients.[2]

In Shepard's comprehensive review of the results of 314 patients with arthroplasty of the hip, including Judet arthroplasty, cup arthroplasty, displacement osteotomy, Batchelor's procedure, and resection arthroplasty, "a fair result is more likely than an excellent one, but late poor results are few. Relief of pain is better after excision of the head and neck than after any other operation reviewed." In one of the more modern papers, Parr in 1971 reviewed 41 patients with Girdlestone resection "who, because of age, infection, or other disability, were not considered to be candidates for the more sophisticated hip reconstruction operations." Eighty percent were relieved of their preoperative pain. Eighty-four percent continued to have good pain relief. Six patients who were initially relieved of preoperative pain began to have pain on weight bearing several months after the operation. The authors attributed this to the femur abutting against the lateral portion of the acetabulum. Virtually all patients had intermittent aching pain when fatigued. Although pain was sufficient to limit activities to some degree, no patient was dissatisfied with the result because of it.[2]

Comparison of functional outcomes of resection arthroplasties between authors is difficult. Outcome measures and endpoints vary. Twenty-one percent are unlimited walkers according to Ballard.[40] Some variation in functional outcome has been noted based on unilateral and bilateral resections. In a study by Grauer, among patients who had a unilateral procedure, 38% had a good score and 62% had a poor score for walking; 41% had a good score and 60% had a poor score for function. Of 6 patients who had a bilateral procedure, only 1 had a good score for walking and none had a good functional result.[22]

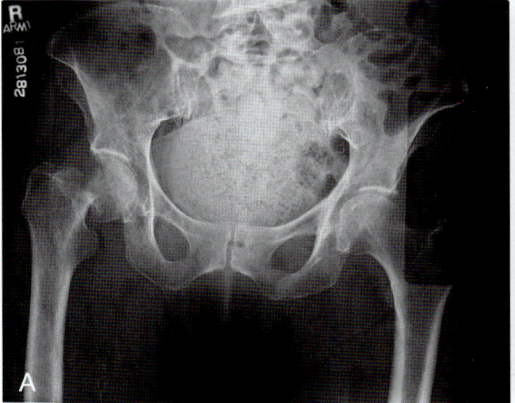
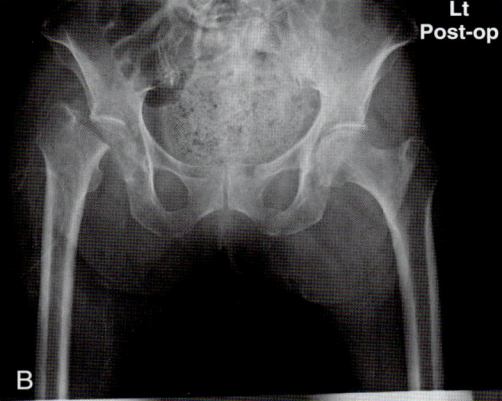

Figure 59-1. Case example. **A,** Preoperative anteroposterior (AP) pelvis radiograph of an 89-year-old female with dementia and severe memory loss, renal insufficiency, and atrial fibrillation admitted with an acute femoral neck fracture. **B,** Postoperative AP pelvis radiograph after primary Girdlestone resection arthroplasty.

Table 59-2. Primary Resection Arthroplasty of the Hip: Review of the Literature

Author	# Resections	Follow-up, yrs	Diagnosis	Pain	Eradication of Infection	Function/Walking	Patient Satisfaction
Ballard	46	8.0	Multiple	29.6% no pain 51.2% fatigue pain	96% eradicated	21% unlimited walking Average Iowa HS 76.0	72%
Milch	64	NA	Multiple (most arthritis)	93% marked improvement	NA	Satisfactory motion in 53%	NA
Grauer	48	3.8	Multiple	35% good relief	94% eradicated	Activity only slightly improved	NA
Haw	40	10	Multiple	47% pain-free 25% satisfactory	100% eradicated	NA	77%
Murray	32	3.5	Multiple	94% pain free 6% slight pain	NA	31/32 ambulatory, all had increased function	NA
Parr	38	3.5	Multiple	80% relieved of preoperative pain	83% eradicated	32/38 became ambulatory Average Iowa HS 70	NA
Shepard	70		Multiple	78%			Unilateral: 70% Bilateral: 26%
Taylor	93		Multiple			83/93 good 7/93 poor 3/93 died in surgery	
Tuli	30		Tuberculous	80%	90%	90% sit.	53% good 30% fair 17% poor

HS, Hip score; *NA,* not applicable.
Modified from Ballard WT, Lowry DA, Brand RA: Resection arthroplasty of the hip. J Arthroplasty 10:772–779, 1995.

Satisfaction in patients with resection arthroplasty as a primary procedure is around 70% to 80%. Function and pain relief tend to hold steady or improve with time. Virtually all patients require ambulatory aids at long-term follow-up. Average shortening of the leg is 1 to 2.5 inches.[18,22,27,40] A Trendelenburg gait is common. Most studies did not consider a Trendelenburg gait, leg length discrepancy, or instability of the joint as failure. The goals of the procedure—pain relief, eradication of infection, and functional motion—were achieved in most patients.*

COMPLICATIONS

Recurrence of infection is uncommon in most series, but Grauer noted recurrence of infection in 3 of 48 resections done for infection in primary septic arthritis or infected arthroplasty.[22] Patients with resistant organisms or with retained cement or foreign material are seen as at higher risk for recurrent infection. For the resection-angulation procedure, Milch noted 6 deaths postoperatively, wound infection in 3 of 64 patients, 3% transient peroneal nerve palsy, loss of fixation in 11%, and excessive formation of callus in 6%.[12] Patients with the need for bilateral resections universally do worse than those treated with a unilateral procedure.[2,12,14]

CURRENT CONTROVERSIES AND FUTURE CONSIDERATIONS

Current indications for resection include relief of pain and control of infection in patients in whom, for many reasons, a more sophisticated arthroplasty is not indicated or is not safe, or in patients who are unable to tolerate advanced procedures or rehabilitation. Resection of the head and neck has become primarily a salvage procedure for failed total hip arthroplasty, but its use as a primary procedure yields reliable results in properly selected and emotionally prepared patients. In the future, the indications may become even narrower, but the procedure remains a cost-effective and important procedure in the management of arthrosis of the hip joint.

REFERENCES

1. Obituary of Mr. Anthony White. Lancet 53:324, 1849.
2. Parr PL, Croft C, Enneking WF: Resection of the head and neck of the femur with and without angulation osteotomy: a follow-up study of thirty-eight patients. J Bone Joint Surg Am 53:935–944, 1971.
3. Barton JR: On the treatment of ankylosis by the formation of artificial joints. North Am Med Surg J 3:279–400, 1827.
4. Taylor RG: Pseudarthrosis of the hip joint. J Bone Joint Surg Br 32:161–165, 1950.
5. Jones SR: Orthopedic surgery of injuries, London, 1921, Oxford University Press, Humphrey Milford, p 450.

*References 2-4, 7, 18, 22, 23, 26, 27, 39, and 41.

6. Girdlestone GR: Arthrodesis and other operations for tuberculosis of the hip. In The Robert Jones birthday volume: a collection of surgical essays, London, 1928, Oxford University Press, p 347.
7. Girdlestone GR: Acute pyogenic arthritis of the hip: an operation giving free access and effective drainage. Lancet 241:419–421, 1943.
8. Girdlestone GR: Acute pyogenic arthritis of the hip: an operation giving free access and effective drainage, 1943. Clin Orthop Relat Res 466:258–263, 2008.
9. Girdlestone GR: Discussion on treatment of unilateral osteoarthritis of the hip-joint. In Proceedinqs of the Royal Society of Medicine XXXVIII:363–368, 1945.
10. Smith-Petersen MN: Treatment of malum coxae senilis, old slipped upper femoral epiphysis, intrapelvic protrusion of the acetabulum, and coxa plana by means of acetabuloplasty. J Bone Joint Surg Am 18:869, 1936.
11. Gruca A: The treatment of quiescent tuberculosis of the hip joint by excision and "dynamic" osteotomy. J Bone Joint Surg Br 32:174–182, 1950.
12. Milch H: The resection-angulation operation for hip-joint disabilities. J Bone Joint Surg Am 37:699–717, 1955.
13. Milch H: Surgical treatment of the stiff, painful hip—the resection-angulation operation. Clin Orthop Relat Res 31:48–57, 1963.
14. Shepherd MM: A further review of the results of operations on the hip joint. J Bone Joint Surg Br 42:177–204, 1960.
15. Muller KH: Resection or the femoral head and neck and resection angulation osteotomy. In Tronzo R, editor: Surgery of the hip joint, Philadelphia, 1973, Lea & Febiger, pp 644–656.
16. Lipscomb PR: Reconstructive surgery for bilateral hip-joint disease in the adult. J Bone Joint Surg Am 47:1–30, 1965.
17. Murray MP, Gore DR, Clarkson BH: Walking patterns of patients with unilateral hip pain due to osteo-arthritis and avascular necrosis. J Bone Joint Surg Am 53:259–274, 1971.
18. Murray WR, Lucas DB, Inman VT: Femoral head and neck resection. J Bone Joint Surg Am 46:1184–1197, 1964.
19. Batchelor JS: Excision of the femoral head and neck for ankylosis and arthritis of the hip. Postgrad Med J 24:241–248, 1948.
20. Belzunegui J, Maíz O, López L, et al: Hydatid disease of bone with adjacent joint involvement: a radiological follow-up of 12 years. Br J Rheumatol 36:133–135, 1997.
21. Coventry MB: Salvage of the painful hip prosthesis. J Bone Joint Surg Am 46:200–212, 1964.
22. Grauer JD, Amstutz HC, O'Carroll PF, Dorey FJ: Resection arthroplasty of the hip. J Bone Joint Surg Am 71:669–678, 1989.
23. Haw CS, Gray DH: Excision arthroplasty of the hip. J Bone Joint Surg Br 58:44–47, 1976.
24. Klein N, Moore T, Capen D, Green S: Sepsis of the hip in paraplegic patients. J Bone Joint Surg Am 70:839–843, 1988.
25. Scott JC: Pseudarthrosis of the hip. Clin Orthop Relat Res 31:31–38, 1963.
26. Sharma H, De Leeuw J, Rowley DI: Girdlestone resection arthroplasty following failed surgical procedures. Int Orthop 29:92–95, 2005.
27. Tuli SM, Mukherjee SK: Excision arthroplasty for tuberculous and pyogenic arthritis of the hip. J Bone Joint Surg Br 63:29–32, 1981.
28. Vatopoulos PK, Diacomopoulos GJ, Demiris CS, et al: Girdlestone's operation: a follow-up study. Acta Orthop Scand 47:324–328, 1976.
29. Klein NE, Luster S, Green S, et al: Closure of defects from pressure sores requiring proximal femoral resection. Ann Plast Surg 21:246–250, 1988.
30. Ryan MD, Henderson JJ: The management of an old fused hip after the occurrence of paraplegia. Paraplegia 30:220–222, 1992.
31. Evans GR, Lewis VL, Jr, Manson PN, et al: Hip joint communication with pressure sore: the refractory wound and the role of Girdlestone arthroplasty. Plast Reconstr Surg 91:288–294, 1993.
32. Akiyama H: Computed tomography-based navigation to determine the femoral neck osteotomy and location of the acetabular socket of an arthrodesed hip. J Arthroplasty 24:1292.e1–1292.e4, 2009.
33. Hardinge K: The direct lateral approach to the hip. J Bone Joint Surg Br 64:17–19, 1982.
34. Batchelor JS: Excision of the femoral head and neck for ankylosis and arthritis of the hip. Overseas Post-Graduate Medical Journal 2:448–456, 1948.
35. Batchelor JS: Pseudarthrosis for ankylosis and arthritis of the hip: Proceedings of the British Orthopaedic Association. J Bone and Joint Surg Br 31:1, 1949.
36. Pirtle RT: The Whitman abduction method in the treatment of hip fracture. Am J Surg 122–123, 1921.
37. Batchelor JS: The surgery of the hip. Proceedings of the Royal Society of Medicine 52:355–360, 1959.
38. Lewis RC, Jr, Ghormley RK: Colonna reconstruction of the hip: results in 57 cases. Proceedings of the Staff Meetings of the Mayo Clinic 29:605–613, 1954.
39. Colonna PC: The trochanteric reconstruction operation for ununited fractures of the upper end of the femur. J Bone Joint Surg Br 42:5–10, 1960.
40. Ballard WT, Lowry DA, Brand RA: Resection arthroplasty of the hip. J Arthroplasty 10:772–779, 1995.
41. Bohler M, Salzer M: Girdlestone's modified resection arthroplasty. Orthopedics 14:661–666, 1991.

PRIMARY HIP ARTHROPLASTY

CHAPTER 60

Long-Term Results of Total Hip Arthroplasty

William N. Capello and James A. D'Antonio

INTRODUCTION

Total hip arthroplasty over the past five decades has evolved to become a remarkable reconstructive procedure that relieves pain, restores function, and returns patients to independent activities of daily living. This chapter will discuss the long-term results of primary total hip replacement, both cemented and cementless. We have elected to discuss acetabular and femoral component results separately, and we have included a discussion of bearings and their influence on long-term fixation. When possible, articles quoted will have at least a 10-year follow-up.

FEMORAL COMPONENTS IN PRIMARY TOTAL HIP REPLACEMENT

Femoral component fixation, once the major reason for revision in primary total hips, has improved to the point where we can expect the component to survive for decades. Advances in prosthetic design, implant finishes, instrumentation, and cementing technique have led to improved fixation of both cementless and cemented femoral components.

CEMENTED FIXATION

Since Sir John Charnley popularized the use of polymethylmethacrylate as a fixative for femoral implants, the use of cement and the results of that form of fixation have served as the standard by which all other methods of fixation have been gauged. The Norwegian Arthroplasty Register for the year 2007 shows that more than 70% of primary total hips done that year had cemented femoral fixation.[1] However, if one separates out those patients who are younger than 60, the same registry for the same year shows only 35% of patients in that subset having cement fixation. Without a registry, it is difficult to determine accurately the usage of cement in femoral fixation in the United States; however, it appears that cementless fixation is becoming increasingly popular among U.S. surgeons. Long-term studies of cemented components show excellent durability. Lewthwaite and colleagues from Exeter in a challenging group of patients 50 years of age and younger followed for 10 to 17 years reported no femoral component revisions due to aseptic loosening over that time interval.[2] Buckwalter, Callaghan, and others in Iowa looked at the Charnley hip at a minimum of 25 years of follow-up and found some deterioration as the result of fixation over time; even at 25 years, 90% of femoral components in those patients still alive remained in place and were functioning well. A similar paper by the same group from Iowa looked at 25-year results of patients younger than 50 at the time of their index surgery; this was a follow-up of a previous report of a 20-year follow-up.[3] Over that intervening time interval, no deterioration of fixation of the femoral component was noted.

The Australian Orthopaedic Association National Joint Replacement Registry looks at survivorship in the form of revision per 100 observed component-years. Figure 60-1 shows that the durability of cemented stems, whether with cemented sockets or in hybrid form, is fairly consistent over various age groups; in fact, better survival than their cementless counterparts is evident at each interval presented.[4] Over the past 20 years, improvements in prosthetic design, a better understanding of surface finish as it relates to implant survival, and better cement handling techniques have contributed to improve the durability of cemented femoral components.

In our own experience, two studies have looked at cemented femoral components.[5,6] One group of 131 cemented total hips, followed between 5 and 12 years,

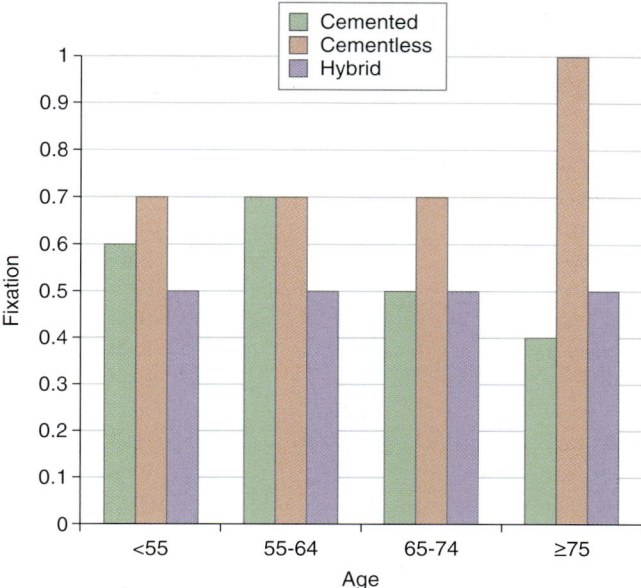

Figure 60-1. Primary conventional total hip replacements requiring revision by fixation and age. *(Data from the Australian Orthopaedic Association: National Joint Replacement Registry, 2007.)*

underwent revision for aseptic loosening at 2.3%. An additional patient was noted radiographically at 11-year follow-up to have a loose stem, yielding a total mechanical failure rate of 3.1% for cemented stems. The second study, which focused on hybrid hips with an average of 9 years of follow-up (range, 5 to 12 years), involved 102 hips and had a mechanical failure rate of 2%. In both instances, the canal had been vigorously reamed at the time of the index total hip. In both series, a second-generation cement technique was used; this consisted of plugging of the canal, brushing, cleaning of the canal, retrograde loading with a cement gun, and proximal pressurization. At that time, no attempt was made to reduce cement porosity through centrifugation or vacuum mixing. In both studies, we were able to achieve femoral component fixation of 97% out to 11 years of follow-up.

CEMENTLESS FIXATION

This section will describe cementless fixation of femoral components as it relates only to total hip arthroplasty. It will not include hemiarthroplasties or press-fit arthroplasties that are never expected to achieve biological fixation. Over the past 15 years, a variety of means of securing the femoral component in a cementless fashion have evolved. All share one common characteristic, that is, the need for stable initial fixation followed by biological fixation in the form of bone ingrowth or ongrowth onto the prosthetic surface. Various surface treatments have been shown to be very effective in establishing the long-term durability of cementless femoral components. These include porous coated surfaces—both those confined to the proximal part of

the implant and those extensively covering the implant. Roughened surfaces such as arc deposit or plasma spray applications, and in some cases simply roughing the titanium substrate through grit blasting, have provided an excellent milieu for bone ongrowth. In addition, ceramic coatings such as hydroxylapatite have been applied to finely roughen substrates of titanium or grossly roughened surfaces and have proved successful.

Two basic stem designs have evolved over the years for use in primary hip replacement. One is the use of diaphyseal fixation with a cylindrical stem that is slightly oversized to the preparation and achieves excellent interference when press-fit through this mechanism. The best example of this type of fixation is the anatomic medullary locking (AML) prosthesis. Engh and coworkers,[7] who popularized the use of this implant, followed a series of patients for a minimum of 10 years. The average age of patients in that group at the time of surgery was 55 years. Among 174 patients remaining from that group, only 3 were noted to have clinical aseptic loosening. An additional 2 stems were judged to be radiographically loose but were unrevised over the same period. All of these 5 stems were judged to be undersized at the time of initial implantation.

A second type of stem is a proximally fixed implant. Almost all of these have a wedge shape with taper built into them. A number of articles have reported excellent results with these implants. Lombardi and associates looked at 191 Mallory-Head implants (Biomet, Warsaw, Ind) followed for 14.5 years. Of these 191 implants, 61 had an additional hydroxylapatite coating over the plasma spray. The remaining 131 did not contain hydroxylapatite, only plasma spray. At follow-up, survivorship of those stems with just the plasma spray was 99.2%, and of those with hydroxylapatite plus the plasma spray, 100%.[7] Archibeck and colleagues, using a proximally fitted implant with fiber mesh placed circumferentially, had excellent results in a young group of patients followed a minimum of 9 years. Thus far, no femoral revisions have been reported in this group, and none were radiographically loose.[8] Teloken reported on a cobalt chrome proximally fixed implant, the TriLock (Medartis, Basel, Switzerland), with 10 to 15 years of follow-up. No femoral loosenings were noted, and two components showed evidence of radiographic instability. This was out of a total of 49 hips followed during that time.[9]

Cementless femoral fixation seems to be the most popular choice among surgeons for patients who are relatively young. Even the Norwegian Registry for the year 2007 showed that among this subset of patients, more than 60% received cementless component fixation (Fig. 60-2). The Australian Registry shows that 60% of all patients undergoing primary total hips received cementless femoral fixation in the year 2007 (Fig. 60-3).

Our own experience with hydroxylapatite-coated stems spans 21 years (Table 60-1). This prospective study began in 1987 and involves patients from four centers. The implant has a tapered, double-wedged configuration made of titanium alloy; it has a roughened surface attained through grit blasting, and a 50-micron

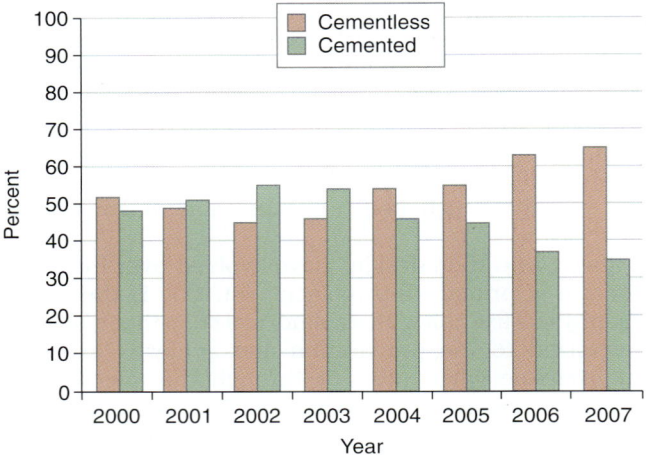

Figure 60-2. Cementless femoral components in patients younger than 60 years. *(Data from the Norwegian Arthroplasty Registry, 2007.)*

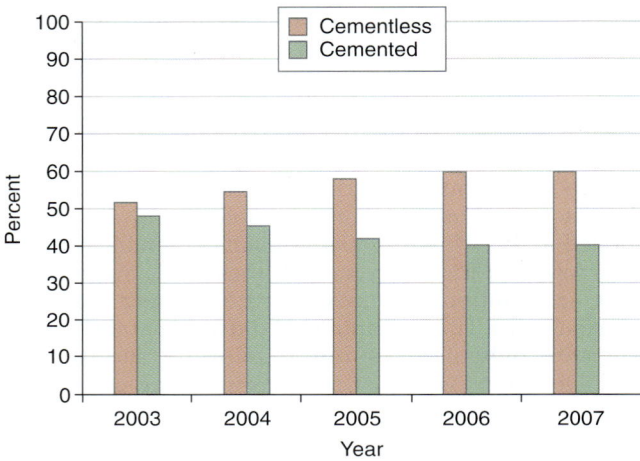

Figure 60-3. Percentage of femoral components used in primary conventional total hip replacements, 2003 to 2007. *(Data from the Australian Orthopaedic Association: National Joint Replacement Registry, 2007.)*

Table 60-1. Stem Survivorship of Omnifit Hydroxylapatite (HA) (N = 262)

Survivorship	HA Stem Revision for Any Reason (N = 262)	HA Stem Revision Due to Aseptic Failure (N = 262)
1 year	99.24%	100%
2 years	98.84%	100%
3 years	98.84%	100%
4 years	98.94%	100%
5 years	98.44%	100%
6 years	98.03%	100%
7 years	97.62%	100%
8 years	97.21%	100%
9 years	97.21%	100%
10 years	96.79%	100%
11 years	95.92%	99.55%
12 years	95.47%	99.55%
13 years	95.01%	99.55%
14 years	95.01%	99.55%
15 years	95.01%	99.55%
16 years	94.43%	99.55%
17 years	94.43%	99.55%
18 years	94.43%	99.55%
19 years	94.43%	99.55%
20 years	94.43%	99.55%
21 years	94.43%	99.55%

layer of hydroxylapatite has been plasma sprayed to the upper third of the implant. The average age of patients at the time of implantation was 51.8 years, half are males, and 67% carried the diagnosis of osteoarthritis. At 21 years, 94.43% of the stems remain in place, and survivorship with aseptic loosening as the end point is 99.5%. Only one has been revised for aseptic loosening. This stem has shown remarkable durability in this young group of patients followed now for two decades. We have also documented the remodeling changes that occurred around this implant.[10] It appears that remodeling changes continue for many years post implantation. We have noted that even between 15 and 20 years of follow-up, fairly significant changes occurred. A second study, involving the same stem, is also prospective and multicentered but has a control group relative to the bearing surface. This study involved ceramic-on-ceramic bearings compared with a metal and polyethylene bearing. Of a total of 475 hips, 65.5% were male, and

average age at the time of surgery was 53 years. Four stems (0.84%) have been revised since the study began, none for aseptic loosening. By combining these two studies, we have 737 patients followed between 13 and 21 years with only one known case of aseptic loosening that occurred at 9.5 years post implantation.

The popularity of cementless fixation in the United States is related to the ease of implantation when contrasted with the technical skills needed to create a perfect bone-cement interface in cemented fixation. In addition, decreased operative time and recent reports of good results among all age groups have combined to make cementless fixation a very popular method of securing femoral components in the United States.[11,12]

THE ACETABULAR COMPONENT

Introduction

Total hip arthroplasty has become a highly successful treatment for disabling arthritis of the hip; however, reconstruction on the acetabular side remains a challenge. Many factors including age, sex, bone quality, diagnosis, component positioning, surgical technique, and implant design can have a significant influence on both short- and long-term survivorship of the reconstruction. Although cement fixation for the socket remains dominant in many countries, its use in North America has sharply declined because of reports of high aseptic loosening rates over time.[14-17] These experiences gave rise to the development and use of cementless components. Although the design of cementless components has evolved toward improved survivorship for aseptic loosening, reports of revision for any reason over the past 20 years remain similar for cemented and cementless acetabular components and remain higher than comparable rates of failure on the femoral side.[2,15-17]

The Cemented Cup

Cementing an acetabular implant is highly technically dependent, and long-term fixation is directly influenced by the initial bone and cement preparation. It would also appear that fixation results can be influenced by poor bone quality, and some surgeons are reluctant to use cement in the face of significant cardiopulmonary disease. Major advantages of a cemented all-polyethylene acetabular component include less wear and lower prosthetic cost. However, these components do not provide intraoperative flexibility to change cup position or the modularity provided by cementless sockets.

Cemented acetabular fixation can be durable, and reports in the literature describe excellent survivorship. Ranawat reported 81% survivorship at 15 years in his group of patients. If only those with osteoarthritis were assessed, survivorship improved to 98% at that time interval.[13] Weber had similar good results, with 99% survivorship at 10 years and 85% at 20 years.[14] Even in a very challenging group of patients, those younger than 50 years, the Exeter group reported 97.6% survivorship at 10 years. However, when radiographic criteria were included, the overall failure rate jumped to 18.7%.[2] Additional reports with 10- to 25-year follow-up have shown increasing acetabular loosening rates over time, even with the use of second-generation cement techniques. Buckwalter reported for patients with more than 25 years of follow-up a revision rate for aseptic loosening of 28%; 16% had additional radiographic loosening.[3] Likewise, Mulroy at minimum 14 years and Ballard at 10 to 15 years found revisions for aseptic loosening of 10% and 24% and radiographic loosening in an additional 42% and 17%.[14,17] Our own experience with a contemporary cementing technique in 114 primary acetabular components yielded a mechanical failure rate of 18.4%. Those patients with primary osteoarthritis had a lower rate of failure (14.0%) than those with rheumatoid arthritis (38.9%). Fifty-seven of the acetabular components were metal-backed, and 57 were non–metal-backed. The incidence of revision of metal-backed components was 5.3% compared with 14% for non–metal-backed components. However, no difference was noted in total mechanical failure rates for these two groups of 15.8% for metal-backed versus 21% for non–metal-backed.[6]

It is interesting to look at national registries to see to what extent cemented acetabular components are still being used. The Norwegian Registry for the year 2007 shows that in primary total hips, cemented acetabular components are being used in 85% of cases (Fig. 60-4). However, among patients younger than 60 years

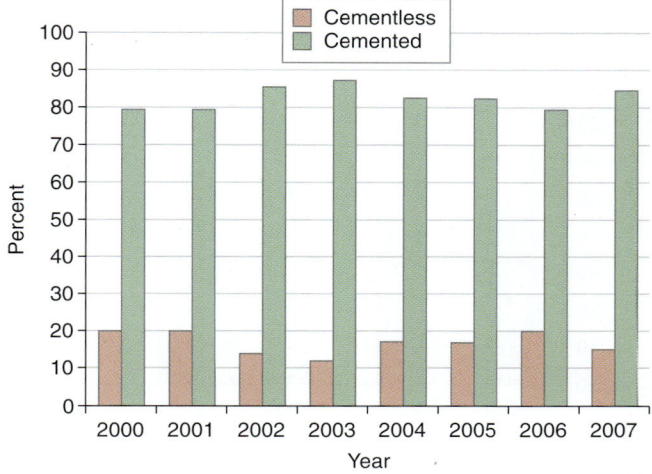

Figure 60-4. Cementless acetabular components, all patients. *(Data from the Norwegian Arthroplasty Registry, 2007.)*

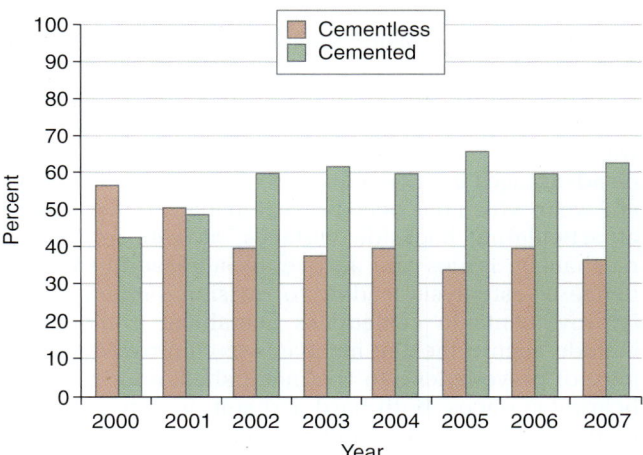

Figure 60-5. Cementless acetabular components in patients younger than 60 years. *(Data from the Norwegian Arthroplasty Registry, 2007.)*

undergoing primary hip replacement, the number decreases to 63% (Fig. 60-5). The Australian Registry, also for the year 2007, shows that only 40% of acetabular components used were cemented (Fig. 60-6).

In general terms, the use of cemented acetabular components in North America is much less than in Europe or even Australia at this time.

Cementless Fixation

Cementless fixation of the acetabular component has evolved over the past three decades and now includes devices with mechanical interlock such as threaded components, devices that have a two-dimensional roughened surface for tissue ongrowth, and finally surfaces that provide three-dimensional interlock with porous coatings. In addition, hydroxylapatite (HA) components are available, with the HA coating applied to

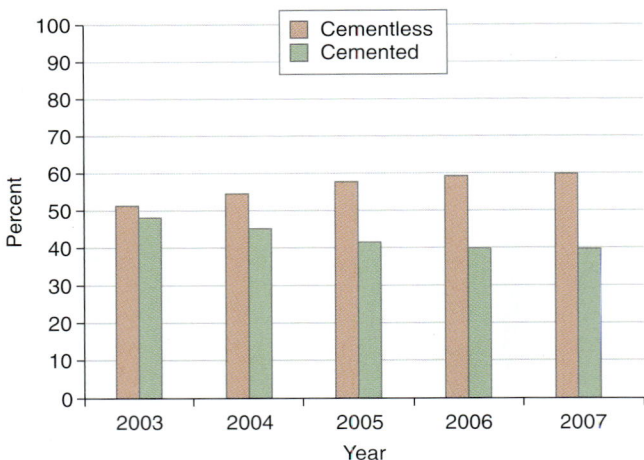

Figure 60-6. Percentage of acetabular components used in primary conventional total hip replacements, 2003 to 2007. *(Data from the Australian Orthopaedic Association: National Joint Replacement Registry, 2007.)*

roughened two-dimensional or three-dimensional ingrowth surfaces. Major advantages of cementless fixation include the ability to exchange the liner and make adjustments to the component position intraoperatively; also, current experience indicates that fixation with interlock of bone is not as time sensitive. Major disadvantages include a history of increased polyethylene wear, which has been present in many designs, both at articulating backside surfaces, as well as locking mechanism issues and an overall increase in the incidence of osteolysis leading to revision surgery. Major improvements in cementless acetabular components include secure locking mechanisms, improved conformity of polyethylene to the metal shell, and improved bearing surfaces, both hard and soft, inserted into the modular component, yielding far less wear than conventional polyethylene.

Plasma-sprayed surfaces without hydroxylapatite and smooth press-fit hydroxylapatite-coated implants have had mixed results.[15,16] Porous ingrowth preparations (cobalt chrome and titanium) and titanium fiber mesh have been used long term with great success from a fixation standpoint.[17,18] In recent years, tantalum and titanium cancellous structured materials have been developed that provide not only a three-dimensional interlock of bone, but also greater flexibility to minimize stress shielding in the acetabulum.

One of the more successful ingrowth surfaces for fixation has been that of titanium fiber mesh.[9,22,26,27] Several articles have described outstanding clinical results out to 20 years of follow-up. Utting, in patients younger than 50 years, reported survivorship of the acetabular component alone of 94% at a mean of 13.6 years. However, survivorship for component plus liner declined to 84%, and adding impending acetabular revisions reduced survivorship on the acetabular side to 78.7% at a mean of 13.6 years.[24] Curry reported no aseptic loosening of the Harris-Galante (HG)-II titanium fiber mesh component (Zimmer, Indianapolis, Ind) at 10 years; very high failure rates related to osteolysis and liner dissociation

were documented with this particular implant.[19] Archibeck, in a series of 100 patients (91 hips) younger than 50 years, using the same cup design, recorded survivorship revision for aseptic loosening of 98% and for revision for any reason of 87.5%.[9] Gaffey, reporting on cementless fixation at 15 years, described survivorship of 81% for revision for any reason, but revision for clinical failure showed survivorship at 94%.[22] In terms of fixation, the HG-I cementless socket performed better than the cemented acetabular component, but the wear rate associated with the cementless component and the incidence of osteolysis were greater. An article by Della Valle reporting on 124 hips treated with the HG cup followed for a minimum of 20 years shows excellent results; survivorship of 96% is reported with endpoints of aseptic loosening and radiographic loosening.[30]

Engh looked at a group of acetabular components, all followed for at least 15 years, that consisted of cobalt chrome and titanium. Some had ancillary spike fixation, others rim screw fixation, and a third subset just press-fit fixation. All had a three-dimensional ingrowth surface of beads or titanium fiber mesh. Survivorship range at 15 years for aseptic loosening was 94.7% to 100%, but for revision for any reason it was 71.6% to 82.9%. The press-fit group had better survivorship for aseptic loosening than the group with ancillary spike fixation or the group rim screw fixation.[25] Hamilton, after 15 years of experience with three cementless socket designs, reported survivorship revision for aseptic loosening of 95.3% (range, 95.3% to 99.6%) and a survivorship revision rate for any reason of 74.9% (range, 70.1% to 89.3%).[23]

Two reports on threaded hydroxylapatite-coated cups have shown high survivorship and excellent clinical results at minimum 10-year follow-up. Tindall reported 99% survivorship at 13 years for revision for any reason and survivorship of 100% for aseptic loosening.[20] Epinette reported a survivorship of 98.2% for revision for any reason and for aseptic loosening a survivorship of 99.4%.[21]

Our own experience with a variety of cup designs involved in prospective studies began in 1987. Results, comparing survivorship over time for acetabular revision due to aseptic loosening versus acetabular revision for any reason as endpoints, are outlined in Tables 60-2 and 60-3. Four different acetabular surface designs were used and followed prospectively: a titanium microstructured press-fit design, a relatively smooth grit-blasted HA-coated socket, an HA-coated grit-blasted threaded component, and a Ti Arc deposited press-fit. The smooth titanium HA-coated implant had no failures in the first 3 years but then began to show a progressive failure rate over time. Survivorship at 21 years for revision for aseptic loosening as an endpoint was 45%, and survivorship for revision for any reason was 35%. This contrasted with findings for the porous press-fit component, which, at 21 years, shows survivorship for revision for aseptic loosening of 97.37% and survivorship for revision for any reason of 83.88%. The threaded HA cup had survivorship for revision for aseptic loosening of 85.54% and survivorship for revision for any reason of 72.07%. Redesign of the press-fit cup provided for a layer of arc

Table 60-2. Comparison of Survivorship Over Time With Acetabular Revision as End Point

Survivorship	Porous DG (from HA Study) (N = 44)	HA PF (N = 72)	HA TH (N = 143)	Sys I (MS ABC) (n = 95)	Sys II (HA ABC) (N = 99)	Control (MS PSL) (N = 95)	Trident (ABC) (N = 186)
1 year	100%	100%	99.30%	100%	98.95%	100%	100%
2 years	100%	98.57%	99.30%	100%	98.95%	98.92%	100%
3 years	100%	98.57%	99.30%	100%	98.95%	98.92%	100%
4 years	100%	97.14%	99.30%	100%	98.95%	98.92%	100%
5 years	100%	91.26%	98.56%	98.89%	98.95%	98.92%	100%
6 years	100%	89.76%	96.34%	98.89%	98.95%	98.92%	100%
7 years	100%	85.27%	96.34%	98.89%	98.95%	98.92%	100%
8 years	94.87%	79.29%	95.59%	98.89%	98.95%	98.92%	100%
9 years	94.87%	76.24%	94.83%	98.89%	98.95%	98.92%	100%
10 years	94.87%	71.60%	93.31%	98.89%	98.95%	98.92%	
11 years	94.87%	70.04%	91.02%	98.89%	98.95%	91.86%	
12 years	94.87%	68.34%	89.46%		98.95%		
13 years	94.87%	68.34%	87.00%				
14 years	91.60%	62.24%	85.33%				
15 years	88.08%	57.78%	84.46%				
16 years	88.08%	55.16%	78.47%				
17 years	88.08%	52.40%	78.47%				
18 years	83.88%	46.88%	78.47%				
19 years	83.88%	41.02%	72.07%				
20 years	83.88%	35.16%	72.07%				
21 years	83.88%	35.16%	72.07%				

Table 60-3. Comparison of Survivorship Over Time With Acetabular Revision Due to Aseptic Loosening of Acetabular Component as End Point

Survivorship	Porous DG (from HA Study) (N = 44)	HA PF (N = 72)	HA TH (N = 143)	Sys I (MS ABC) (n = 95)	Sys II (HA ABC) (N = 99)	Control (MS PSL) (N = 95)	Trident (ABC) (N = 186)
1 year	100%	100%	100%	100%	100%	100%	100%
2 years	100%	100%	100%	100%	100%	100%	100%
3 years	100%	100%	100%	100%	100%	100%	100%
4 years	100%	98.53%	100%	100%	100%	100%	100%
5 years	100%	93.98%	100%	100%	100%	100%	100%
6 years	100%	92.44%	100%	100%	100%	100%	100%
7 years	100%	87.82%	100%	100%	100%	100%	100%
8 years	97.37%	83.20%	100%	100%	100%	100%	100%
9 years	97.37%	80.06%	100%	100%	100%	100%	100%
10 years	97.37%	75.28%	98.45%	100%	100%	100%	
11 years	97.37%	75.28%	97.67%	100%	100%	100%	
12 years	97.37%	71.89%	96.87%		100%		
13 years	97.37%	71.89%	95.18%				
14 years	97.37%	67.59%	94.33%				
15 years	97.37%	65.34%	93.45%				
16 years	97.37%	62.62%	89.43%				
17 years	97.37%	62.62%	89.43%				
18 years	97.37%	56.92%	89.43%				
19 years	97.37%	51.23%	85.54%				
20 years	97.37%	45.54%	85.54%				
21 years	97.37%	45.54%	85.54%				

deposited titanium that created a significantly roughened outer surface of the implant to which hydroxylapatite was then applied. This socket was used in a prospective, randomized, ceramic-on-ceramic bearing study that also featured a microstructured titanium cup with ceramic-on-ceramic bearings and a microstructured titanium cup that received a control conventional polyethylene. Survivorship (see Tables 60-2 and 60-3) for aseptic loosening as an endpoint for porous microstructured cups with and without ceramic bearings was 100% at 11 years, and for the arc deposited HA socket, 100% at 12 years. Survivorship revision for any reason as an endpoint was as follows: microstructured component with ceramic bearings, 98.89%; arc deposited HA cup with ceramic bearings, 98.95%; and microstructured socket with conventional polyethylene used as a control, 91.6%.

As mentioned previously, cementless acetabular fixation has not enjoyed the same popularity in Europe as it has in North America. Again, the Norwegian Registry, for the year 2007, showed that only 15% of acetabular components used were cementless, although in patients younger than 60 years, that number increased to 37%. In Australia, for the same year, 60% of acetabular components used in primary total hip arthroplasty were cementless. Cementless acetabular fixation allows a surgeon several options. The surgeon can change the orientation of the component at the time of surgery without compromising fixation. The modularity that is available allows the surgeon to choose varying bearing surfaces, as well as a variety of liner options, as necessary. Finally, revision of the component for sepsis, aseptic loosening, or even well-fixed acetabular components has been made much easier with the use of instruments such as the Explant System (Zimmer).

In the past decade, newer surface configurations to enhance fixation and perhaps decrease overall cup stiffness have been designed utilizing a foamed cancellous structure of titanium and/or tantalum. An 8- to 10-year radiographic follow-up study using porous tantalum acetabular components for total hip arthroplasty reported no revisions for aseptic loosening.[22]

The Influence of Bearings

Major reasons for revision of cementless sockets over the past 15 years have been wear and osteolysis. The combination of poor locking mechanisms, lack of congruity of polyethylene to shell, and increased wear at the bearing surface, as well as in some cases at the backside of the polyethylene liner, has led to accelerated wear, increased wear debris, osteolysis, and the need for reoperation. Over the past 15 years, new bearing surfaces have become available in North America, including the hard-on-hard (ceramic-on-ceramic and cobalt chrome metal-on-metal) surface and the newly introduced highly cross-linked polyethylenes. These bearings show significantly less wear than metal or ceramic bearings on conventional polyethylene, and over the past 10 years, they have clinically demonstrated a very low incidence of osteolysis.

Current cementless acetabular designs promise excellent biological fixation and resistance to aseptic loosening over time. However, it remains to be seen whether survivorship using revision for any reason as an endpoint will show improvement over known long-term results of cemented acetabular components. Because of new implant designs and bearings, revisions for osteolysis and failure of the modular bearing surface may be markedly decreased, thereby promising to increase the overall longevity of total hip arthroplasty.

CURRENT CONTROVERSIES/FUTURE CONSIDERATIONS

One of the current concerns with cemented femoral fixation is this: How durable is the fixation, given the seemingly increasing demand for increased activities among younger patients? Another worry, at least in the United States is this: Is cemented femoral fixation becoming a lost art, given the current popularity of cementless fixation?

Debate continues to surround cementless femoral fixation relative to stress shielding and extent of coating. Included in this concern is whether shortening the femoral stem will promote more proximal load transfer, or whether it will simply lead to increased implant loosening and/or pain. Debate also surrounds the extent of coating needed for long-term cementless femoral fixation. Although both proximally fixed implants and extensively coated ones have excellent results at 15 to 20 years, some question whether continuing the coating to the proximal part of the implants will lead to extended durability out to 20 to 30 years.

Acetabular fixation concerns are similar:
- What are the long-term consequences of stress shielding?
- Will improvement in bearing surfaces actually translate into added longevity and durability?
- Will surface designs providing for two- or three-dimensional interlock be superior for long-term fixation?

We believe that future implant systems will attempt to address these concerns. More flexible acetabular components, minimizing stress shielding, may demand entirely different bearing surfaces. Femoral stem material and geometry may change as well to promote better proximal stress transfer.

These are just a few of the current concerns and future challenges that await the implant surgeons of tomorrow.

REFERENCES

1. The Norwegian Arthroplasty Register Group: The Norwegian Arthroplasty Register, 2007.
2. Lewthwaite SC, Squires B, Gie GA, Timperley AJ, Ling RS: The Exeter universal hip in patients 50 years or younger at 10 to 17 years follow up. Clin Orthop Relat Res 466:324–331, 2008.
3. Buckwalter AE, Callaghan JJ, Liu SS, et al: Results of Charnley total hip arthroplasty with use of improved femoral cementing techniques. J Bone Joint Surg Am 88:1481–1485, 2006.
4. Australian Orthopaedic Association: National Joint Replacement Registry, 2007.
5. Meneghini ME, Feinberg JR, Capello WN: Primary hybrid total hip arthroplasty with a roughened femoral stem: integrity of the stem cement interface. J Arthroplasty 18:299–307, 2003.

6. Hirose I, Capello WN, Feinberg JR, Shirer RM: Primary cemented total hip arthroplasty: five to twelve year clinical and radiographic follow up. Iowa Orthop J 15:43–47, 1995.

7. Lombardi AV, Berend KR, Mallory TH: Hydroxylapatite coated titanium porous plasma spray tapered stem. Clin Orthop Relat Res 453:81–85, 2006.

8. Archibeck MJ, Surdam JW, Schultz SC, et al: Cementless total hip arthroplasty in patients 50 years or younger. J Arthroplasty 21:476–483, 2006.

9. Teloken MA, Bissett G, Hozack WJ, et al: Ten to fifteen year follow up after total hip arthroplasty with a tapered cobalt chromium femoral component (Tri-Lock) inserted without cement. J Bone Joint Surg Am 84:2140–2144, 2002.

10. Capello WN, D'Antonio JA, Geesink RG, et al: Late remodeling around a proximally HA coated tapered titanium femoral component. Clin Orthop Relat Res 467:155–165, 2009.

11. Capello WN, D'Antonio JA, Feinberg JR, Manley MT: Hydroxylapatite coated total hip femoral components in patients less than fifty years old: clinical and radiographic results after five to eight years of follow up. J Bone Joint Surg Am 79:1023, 1997.

12. Keisu KS, Orozco F, Sharkey PF, et al: Primary cementless total hip arthroplasty in octogenarians: two to eleven year follow-up. J Bone Joint Surg Am 83:359, 2001.

13. Ranawat AS, Ranawat CS: The cemented acetabulum: rationale and technique. In The adult hip, vol 2, 2nd ed, Baltimore, 2004, Lippincott Wilkins, pp 940–945.

14. De Jong PT, de Man FHR, Haverkamp D, Marti RK: The long-term outcome of the cemented Weber acetabular component in total hip replacement using a second-generation cementing technique. J Bone Joint Surg Br 91:31–36, 2009.

15. Jiranek WA, Whidden DR, Johnston WT: Late loosening of press fit cementless acetabular components. Clin Orthop Relat Res 418:172–178, 2004.

16. Manley MT, Capello WN, D'Antonio JA, et al: Fixation of acetabular cups without cement in total hip arthroplasty: a comparison of three different implant surfaces at a minimum duration of follow up of five years. J Bone Joint Surg Am 80:1175–1185, 1998.

17. Gaffey JL, Callaghan JJ, Pedersen DR, et al: Cementless acetabular fixation at fifteen years: a comparison with the same surgeon's results following acetabular fixation with cement. J Bone Joint Surg Am 86:257–261, 2004.

18. Hamilton WG, Calendine CL, Buikirch SE, et al: Acetabular fixation options: first generation modular cup curtain calls and caveats. J Arthroplasty 22(Suppl 1):75–81, 2007.

19. Curry HG, Lynskey TG: Harris Galante II acetabular cup: a survival analysis. J Orthop Surg 16:201–205, 2008.

20. Tindall A, James KD, Slack R, et al: Long-term follow up of a hydroxylapatite ceramic coated threaded cup: an analysis of survival and fixation at up to fifteen years. J Arthroplasty 22:1079–1082, 2007.

21. Epinette JA, Manley MT, D'Antonio JA, et al: A 10 year minimum follow up of hydroxylapatite coated threaded cups. J Arthroplasty 18:140–148, 2003.

22. Macheras G, Konstantinos K, Athanassios K, et al: Eight to ten year clinical and radiographic outcome of a porous tantalum monoblock acetabular component. J Arthroplasty 24:705–709, 2009.

30. Della Valle CJ, Mesko NW, Quigley L, et al: Primary total hip arthroplasty with a porous coated acetabular component: concise follow up at minimum of 20 years. A previous report. J Bone Joint Surg Am 91:1130–1135, 2009.

SUGGESTED READINGS

Capello WN, D'Antonio JA, Geesink RG, et al: Late remodeling around a proximally HA coated tapered titanium femoral component. Clin Orthop Relat Res 467:155–165, 2009.
Details of long-term remodeling around titanium/hydroxylapatite (Ti/HA) stems.

Engh CA, Hopper RH, Engh CA, Jr: Long term porous coated cup survivorship using spikes, screws, and press-fitting for initial fixation. J Arthroplasty 19:54–60, 2004.
Long-term experience with fully coated cementless implants.

Lewthwaite SC, Squires B, Gie GA, et al: The Exeter universal hip in patients 50 years or younger at 10 to 17 years follow up. Clin Orthop Relat Res 466:324–331, 2008.
Impressive results with cemented implants in young population.

Lombardi AV, Berend KR, Mallory TH: Hydroxylapatite coated titanium porous plasma spray tapered stem. Clin Orthop Relat Res 453:81–85, 2006.
Intermediate- to long-term follow-up of tapered stems with and without hydroxylapatite (HA).

The Norwegian Arthroplasty Register, 2007, and the Australian Orthopaedic Association: National Joint Replacement Registry, 2007.
Comprehensive detailed look at trends and outcomes of large numbers of patients treated with various implants and techniques.

CHAPTER 61

Rating Systems and Outcomes of Total Hip Arthroplasty

Conor J. Hurson and Michael J. Dunbar

KEY POINTS

- The outcome of THA is generally excellent, yielding a large standard effect size.
- The large standard effect size associated with THA introduces a paradox of outcomes assessment, in that patients find it subjectively difficult to interpret subtle differences in outcomes associated with the introduction of new THA technology in the face of overall improvement post surgery.
- The gold standard for assessment of outcomes after hip arthroplasty is prosthesis survivorship. It is limited by the fact that revision status is a relatively blunt metric and generally is nonrepresentative of function, degree of pain relief, and overall patient satisfaction after hip arthroplasty.
- Higher-precision metrics and scoring systems are necessary to help introduce the next phase of surgical innovation.
- Survivorship for THA is generally improving over time.
- All rating systems are a construct for the "true" outcome. As such, all rating systems are subject to variable bias.

INTRODUCTION

The Oxford English Dictionary defines outcome as the result or effect of treatment.[1] Rating systems are tools or metrics used to assess an outcome. Numerous types of rating systems have been proposed for assessment of the outcome of total hip arthroplasty (THA). These include objective metrics, usually completed by the surgeon or allied health care professional, and subjective metrics, usually completed by the patient. Traditionally, and early in the development of THA, outcomes have concentrated on objective outcomes to record the success of the THA in terms of survivorship or reduction in complications. This was a necessary first step in the introduction, evolution, and refinement of THA as a viable and highly successful procedure. However, because the World Health Organization (WHO) has defined health as "...not only the absence of infirmity and disease but also a state of physical, mental and social well-being,"[2] subjective outcomes have become more prevalent to augment some of the blunter objective outcome metrics.

Hip arthroplasty has been shown to have a major impact on health-related quality of life when preoperative status and postoperative status are compared.[3-7] Such profound results make preoperative and postoperative comparisons of different prosthetic designs, surgical techniques, and so forth, using a given questionnaire, difficult to interpret and potentially irrelevant because assumed subtle differences in questionnaire results would be lost in the large signal. Paradoxically, the signal for preoperative and postoperative comparisons after hip arthroplasty is so loud (large) that in effect it functions as noise and obscures the subtler signal of interest. Additionally, hip arthroplasty innovation has made it inherently difficult to distinguish between subtle changes in treatments (Fig. 61-1). Therefore, a surgeon should carefully consider the various outcome metrics available before deciding which is most effective and appropriate for the desired application.

Although some consensus has been reached regarding which categories of outcome metrics should be applied to arthroplasty patients, no agreement is known as to which specific metrics are most appropriate. Instead, multitudes of metrics have been put forward in the literature, and new metrics continue to be introduced. Researchers are subsequently forced to choose a metric based on its published psychometric properties, or based on precedence and extraneous political factors. This practice has led to significant variation in the reporting of outcomes post arthroplasty. Although general trends in outcomes can be contrasted with various outcome metrics, subtler differences in outcomes are lost in the psychometric variability between outcome tools. Consequently, the need for consensus on the most appropriate outcome metrics for wide-scale employment was alluded to by Lord Kelvin when he said, "I often say that when you can measure what you are speaking about, and express it in numbers, you know something about it; but when you cannot measure it, when you cannot express it in numbers, your knowledge is of a meagre and unsatisfactory kind."[8]

Outcome metrics have been criticized because of the perception that they yield "soft" data, at least in comparison with more standardized technological laboratory tests that permeate the medical field, such as serum potassium or hemoglobin. Such tests are believed to yield "hard" data because the method for such tests is well described, the precisions are high, and the reproducibility is excellent. Still, the perception that questionnaires yield only soft data must not prevent clinically

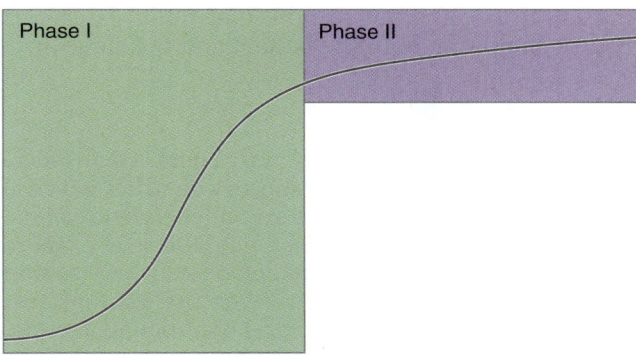

Phase I

Phase II

Figure 61-1. Asymptote of surgical innovation for total hip arthroplasty. Phase 1 innovation involved radical changes in technology from innovation to innovation (largely historic). Phase 2 represents modern, substantially more subtle innovative changes.

relevant questionnaire data from being utilized, because these data, perhaps more than any other, speak to the humanistic side, or art, of medicine.

BACKGROUND

Objective Outcome Metrics

One of the earliest assessments of hip mobility was devised in 1931 by Fergusson and Howarth to assess patients with slipped upper femoral epiphysis.[9] In this purely objective assessment, points were allocated for hip flexion and abduction, as well as for adduction and hyperextension. In 1954, Merle d'Aubigné and Postel further developed the evaluation tool into a hip scoring system by including a subjective component that scored pain.[10]

The hip scoring system of Merle d'Aubigné and Postel was modified by Charnley in 1972, and has since become one of the most widely used hip assessment tools by orthopedic surgeons. The Charnley modification of the Merle d'Aubigné and Postel hip score assesses hip movements, pain, and walking. It is important to note that these categories require input from both the patient and the surgeon (or subjective and objective information), and the scores from each section are not combined for a total score.

The Harris Hip Score, developed in 1969, is one of the most widely used scoring systems to report outcomes following THA. It is a clinician-completed scoring system used to evaluate pain, function, range of motion, and absence of deformity. The function of a patient is decided by walking habits and the ability to do specified activities.

Surgeon-derived outcome measures can differ significantly from patient satisfaction after THA.[11] Discrepancies between patient and surgeon perspectives are particularly large when patients are dissatisfied with replacement surgery. Thus, appraising the success of a THA using objective information exclusively will account for only a portion of the complete picture; therefore, subjective metrics are an important component of a hip scoring system.

Inclusion of Subjective Metrics

Subjective components in scoring systems became increasingly prevalent after the WHO altered its definition of health. Objective measures are unable to capture the mental and social well-being of patients. Unfortunately, subjectivity can make it difficult to make comparisons between different scoring systems; even the same scoring system reproduced in different languages can produce inconsistent results.[12]

Reporting of total scores can have the effect of blurring results. Individual section scores may not be proportional and cannot be meaningfully added together. Proportionality is particularly difficult to achieve when objective (e.g., radiologic measurements) and subjective (e.g., patient pain assessments) composite scores are combined.

Four types of questionnaires include at least subjective components: General Health, Disease Specific, Joint Specific, and Patient Specific. Each of these will be discussed in the "Basic Science" section of this chapter (Box 61-1).

Precision Objective Metrics

Over the past decade, high-precision metrics such as radiostereometric analysis (RSA) and gait analysis have become increasingly available. Currently, these techniques are used mainly as research tools, but as they evolve and less expensive surrogates are validated, their use will become more pervasive and essential to assessment of arthroplasty outcomes.

Survivorship

The gold standard for assessment of outcomes after THA is prosthesis survivorship. This survival analysis has been a powerful tool in the long-term assessment of replacement arthroplasty and allows comparison among types or series of joint replacements. Survivorship analysis was first used in orthopedics by Dobbs in 1980[13] and remains popular today.

Survival analysis provides very useful information; for this reason, many countries have developed joint replacement registries. These are national databases that monitor the survival of implants based on many variables, such as material, fixation technique, and size.

Although survival analysis is an essential tool for measuring THA outcomes, it is a crude one.

Survivorship is based on an endpoint (e.g., revision, death) and often fails to account for the complexity of the variables involved. An implant can be revised (or not revised) for a variety of reasons; therefore large sample sizes can be required to allow conclusions about a particular procedure. Hence, survival analysis has no predictive power, and its applications are limited to post hoc and trend analyses.

Chaotic Innovation

Unfortunately, the introduction of new technology usually does not follow a stepwise algorithm and could be considered chaotic. The initial step, preclinical testing, is robust in North America. However, instead of being incorporated into prospective randomized studies before general release, new technologies are often made immediately available to a wide surgical community. Little emphasis is placed on formal study of clinical outcomes. Only a few specialized academic centers conduct prospective randomized studies; this again introduces a reporting bias into the literature. Finally, most published studies on new technology are retrospective in nature, often published after the technology has already changed. See Figure 61-2 for an illustration that demonstrates chaotic innovation.

BASIC SCIENCE

Outcome Metrics

With the advent of prosthetic components that demonstrate predictably good results, it became evident that more formalized outcome metrics were necessary. The initial response was that surgeons assessed the results of their interventions. Purely surgeon-derived outcome assessments were quickly shown to be inadequate without subjective data. Sir John Charnley, in 1972, modified the Merle d'Aubigné and Postel hip score to assess the outcome of his prosthesis; this system has become one of the most widely used hip scoring systems. This score assesses hip movement, pain, and

walking. It is important to note that these categories require input from both the patient and the surgeon.

Survival Analysis

The Kaplan-Meier[14] method is most commonly used to estimate prosthesis survival and to construct survival plots. It provides results that are independent of time intervals, in that survival is estimated at every failure time. Statistically significant differences can be assessed by using the log rank test. However, the log rank test does not allow adjustment for confounding factors. Relative risks for revision can be assessed and adjustments made for differences between compared groups (e.g., age, gender, diagnosis, other confounding factors) by using the Cox multiple regression model.

A 95% confidence interval should be given when survival results are presented. These can be presented in tables or on curves (Fig. 61-3). Murray and associates[15] recommended the inclusion of a "worst case" curve—in which all patients lost to follow-up are considered failures—to provide a statistically accurate statement of survival. In addition, Lettin and colleagues[16] recommended that at least 40 surviving subjects are required to produce reliable results.

Revision is a definite and easily reproducible endpoint that can be influenced by extraneous factors such as a patient's fitness for surgery and severity of pain. Other endpoints, such as the presence of severe pain, low functional scores, and radiographic failure, should also be included.

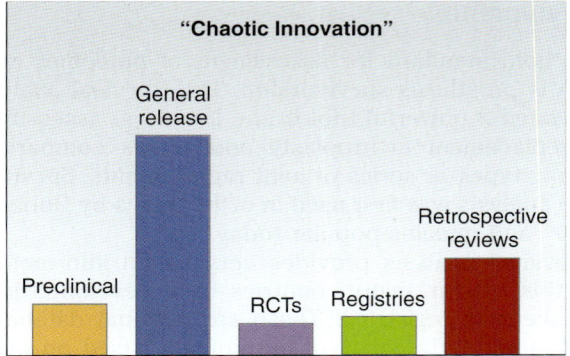

Figure 61-2. Unfortunately, the introduction of new technology usually does not follow a stepwise algorithm and could be considered chaotic.

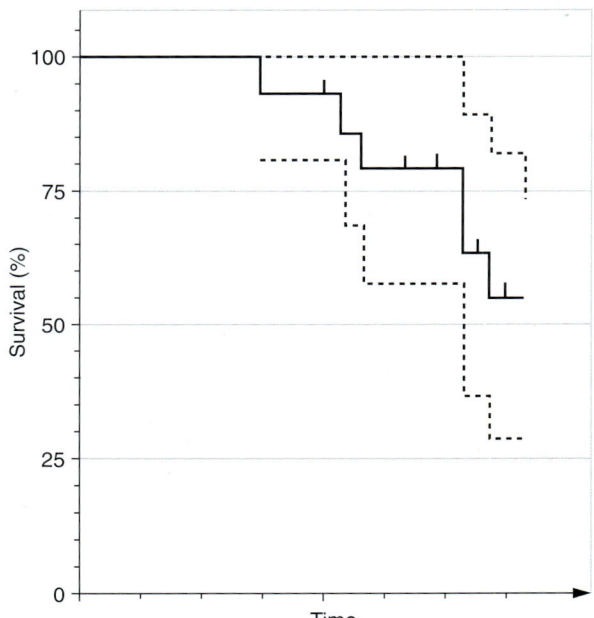

Figure 61-3. An example of a survival curve with a 95% confidence interval. The survival curve is represented by the solid line, for the sample of subjects. Confidence intervals, represented by the dotted line, become wider as the sample size decreases over time.

Arthroplasty Registries

Arthroplasty registries use prosthesis survival as the primary outcome. Survival analysis is a definitive metric that facilitates comparison of outcomes between nations. Currently, 15 national arthroplasty registries have the potential to compare and contrast survivorship outcomes.[17-20] However, such comparisons are limited with respect to variations in demographics, including age at time of operation, diagnostic groupings, body mass index, gender, and activity levels. Research efforts are directed at defining the demographics of each nation/center in detail so that the denominator of the comparative data can be determined. Without this level of research, comparison of outcomes in survivorship between nations/centers is prone to misinterpretation. Furthermore, the specific method of defining survivorship should be standardized.[15] For example, Cox's regression is a particularly useful method because it accounts for other factors such as age and gender, which are known to have an effect on outcomes. If such factors are not considered in outcome analyses, reported differences in survival curves between various prostheses are difficult to interpret, particularly on an international basis.

Arthroplasty registries function best as a surveillance tool for implant failure. As such, favorable and unfavorable trends in the outcomes of certain prostheses can be easily determined and disseminated back to the orthopedic community in a quality improvement feedback cycle. However, because arthroplasty registries are surveillance tools, there is an inherent lag in the reporting of outcomes; this creates a potential for suboptimal implants or techniques to penetrate into and become part of the clinical norm before detection by the registry. A more accurate and predictive form of survivorship analysis would have the advantage of limiting new technology and techniques to fewer patients than is necessary to see trends with arthroplasty registries.

The gold standard for assessment of outcomes after hip arthroplasty is prosthesis survivorship. However, modern advances in prosthetic design and technique are such that the threshold for joint arthroplasty has moved from salvage operations performed in extreme cases to an intervention designed to improve the quality of life in patients who otherwise might cope without surgery. Hence, judging the success of the surgery may relate more to subtler improvements in quality of life, including relief of pain and improvement in function. Furthermore, technological innovation has improved the design of prostheses, ensuring survival in situ, barring infection, for at least a decade with relative certainty.[18,21,22] Consequently, the homogeneity of current prostheses (with respect to stable and lasting designs) has produced an emerging emphasis on quantifying subtler outcomes after arthroplasty.

Limitation of Survivorship Analysis

Arthroplasty registries rely on revision status as the sole endpoint for defining outcomes after arthroplasty. Revision status is a useful measure because it is relatively easy to define and the incidence of revision is definite. Although definitive, revision status is a relatively blunt metric and is generally nonrepresentative of function, degree of pain relief, and overall patient satisfaction after knee arthroplasty. Furthermore, different surgeons have different thresholds for performing revisions, and not all patients who require revision surgery undergo the procedure because of coexisting medical problems, personal wishes, and so forth.[23] Revision status yields data only on the small minority of operations that fail.[24] The same set of arguments generally holds true for the outcome of continuous migration, as defined by RSA, which essentially acts as a surrogate for revision status. Although some evidence suggests that subjective outcomes may be correlated with RSA-defined migration patterns, this phenomenon is not widely reported in the literature.[25]

Subjective Outcomes

Pythagoras mused that "man is a measure of all things."[26] The implication of this statement speaks to the conceptualization that the distinction between mind and body is blurred, or indeed that there is no distinction at all. Although the Western philosophical distinction between mind and body has its origins with the ancient Greeks, it was the works of Renés Descartes that formalized the modern distinction between mind and body.[27] According to Descartes, the rational soul is an entity distinct from the body that may or may not be aware of signals passing through the body via interfibrillar spaces. The interfibrillar spaces (i.e., the sensory nervous system) were "extended" into the physical world, while the rational soul (i.e., consciousness) was not. This distinction between mind and body has persisted into modern Western medical thought.

In 1947, the WHO defined health as follows: "Health is not only the absence of infirmity and disease but also a state of physical, mental and social well-being." This definition reintroduced the concept that mind and body are in fact one and the "well-being" of the mind and body combined represents health. Subsequently, the measurement of health moved from simply defining the success of a procedure by determining its effect on infirmity and disease, to the more ambitious approach of defining what effect the intervention had on physical, mental, and social well-being. By this definition, it was no longer adequate to define the outcome of a hip arthroplasty, for example, simply by stating what the range of motion was or what the impact was on mobility. Instead, a more comprehensive metric was needed.

The definition of health put forth by the WHO was perhaps the impetus for the modern movement to measure physical, mental, and social well-being. The first attempts at quantifying general health involved single-item global ratings that were designed to augment organ-specific or more physiologic outcomes. Over time, a large number of questionnaires were developed that asked more questions around various aspects of health, such that separate scores for each of these health domains were generated. Domains that attempted to account for physical, mental, and social well-being included Emotional Reaction, Sleep, Social Isolation, Body Pain, and Social Functioning, for example. Advanced study and refinement of these tools continue today. The introduction and evolution of generic (or general) health measurements have been well documented.[28] Measurements of this sort are often referred to as "subjective" and are difficult to quantify. Still, some form of logical metric was imperative for further research. This dilemma was eloquently alluded to by Lord Kelvin when he said, "I often say that when you can measure what you are speaking about, and express it in numbers, you know something about it; but when you cannot measure it, when you cannot express it in numbers, your knowledge is of a meager and unsatisfactory kind."[8] The WHO continues to be interested in this area of outcomes research. At a workshop in January of 2000 under the umbrella of the Bone and Joint Decade 2000-2010, the need to standardize outcome metrics for musculoskeletal research was discussed.[29]

Although the WHO definition of health may be largely responsible for the emergence of general health outcome questionnaires, the first aspect of the definition, that is, "…the absence of infirmary or disease…," has not been lost on researchers. Similar evolution of health outcome questionnaires focused on the organ (or site) or physiologic process (disease) that has come about.

SUBJECTIVE HEALTH OUTCOME QUESTIONNAIRES

Psychometric Considerations: What Makes a Good Questionnaire?

Definition of Psychometrics

Psychometrics can be defined as "the scientific measurement of mental capacities and processes and of personality."[30] In other words, psychometrics is the process that allows researchers to apply scientific methods to the measurement of subjective outcomes. In practical terms, the published psychometric properties of a questionnaire pertain mostly to validation of the questionnaire, or to defining how well the questionnaire measures what it is supposed to measure, in a global sense. The validation process usually involves three specific aspects of questionnaire testing: validity, reliability, and responsiveness.

Validity

Validity refers more specifically (as opposed to validation) to how well the questionnaire measures the question of interest. Validity can take many forms, and numerous synonyms have been utilized in conjunction with it. These include criterion, construct, convergent, divergent, and content validity. Before one can comment on the validity of a questionnaire, the results of the questionnaire must be compared with something.

Criterion Validity. Criterion validity refers to comparison of the metric versus a "gold standard." For example, a thermometer is the gold standard for measuring body temperature. If a questionnaire was designed to measure body temperature, the items within may inquire about how warm the patient felt, whether the patient had chills, and so forth. Results of this questionnaire could be directly correlated with the gold standard (criterion). Unfortunately, there is no gold standard for knee arthroplasty.[31,32] Consequently, questionnaires for knee arthroplasty usually are validated against a postulated effect that should result from the intervention. Such a postulation is referred to as a construct.

Construct Validity. Construct validity may be determined against another previously validated questionnaire or a consensus statement, for example. Divergent and convergent validity can be used as a check for the construct in that items within a questionnaire that relate to knee function, for example, should improve after knee arthroplasty (convergent), while items that are not related to the knee, such as eating, should not change (divergent).

A note of caution is warranted when construct validity is considered. Construct validity in the absence of a gold standard, as is the case with knee arthroplasty, is problematic. Often, questionnaires are validated against another questionnaire that has been validated previously. Further investigation may reveal that the previously validated questionnaire has been validated against a construct. Hence, a circuitous logical argument can be associated with outcome questionnaires with potential sophistic implications. There is no "cogito ergo sum" on which to base construct validity in the absence of a gold standard.

Content Validity. Content validity addresses whether a questionnaire has a sufficient number of items and adequately covers the domain of interest.[33] For example, if a questionnaire is designed to measure how much mobility a patient has gained from a knee arthroplasty intervention, then by inference, a patient who scores well on the questionnaire could be assumed to have good mobility. However, if the items within the questionnaire do not ask specifically about mobility, then the inference (not necessarily the questionnaire) is invalid. Questionnaires with good content validity cover the target behavior well and subsequently provide for valid inferences. Content validity can be tested by investigating the frequency distribution of scores produced by a questionnaire or the domains within. In particular, floor and ceiling effects are important when content validity is assessed. A floor effect occurs when a respondent scores the lowest (i.e., the best) possible score on a questionnaire. Thus, if a patient were to clinically become better, the questionnaire would be unable to reflect that change. The content of the behavior would not be covered, and inferences would be invalid. The same argument holds true for the ceiling effect, which occurs in an opposite direction.

Reliability

Reliability refers to the ability of an outcome metric to remain unchanged when applied on two separate occasions when no clinical change has occurred. Essentially, in its most basic sense, reliability is the measure of the noise within a metric and can be conceptualized by the following equation:

$$\text{Reliability} = \frac{\text{Subject Variability}}{\text{Subject Variability} + \text{Measurement Variability}}$$

For an outcome metric to have acceptable reliability, it must, by the definition proposed here, have limited measurement variability.

Outcome metrics have been criticized because of the perception that they yield "soft" data, at least in comparison with more standardized technological laboratory tests that permeate the medical field, such as serum potassium or hemoglobin. Such tests are believed to yield "hard" data because the method used for such tests is well described, the precisions are high, and the reproducibility is excellent. Still, the perception that questionnaires yield only soft data must not prevent clinically relevant questionnaire data from being utilized, because these data, perhaps more than any other, speak to the humanistic side, or art, of medicine. Such an argument was well described by Feinstein when he said the following: "If we say that cardiac size became smaller, that cardiac rhythm became normal, and that certain enzyme levels became normal, the description could pertain to a rat, a dog, or a person. But if we say that chest pain disappeared, that the patient was able to return to work, and [that] the family was pleased, we have given a human account of human feelings and observations."

Classically, the test-retest reliability of an outcome metric is investigated by determining the intraclass correlation coefficient (ICC).[34] The ICC is advantageous over other correlation coefficients, such as Spearman or Pearson, because it is not biased by the order in which pairs of data are compared. Subsequently, learning effects that may occur when a questionnaire is applied on two separate occasions will not influence the ICC. An ICC value between 0.60 and 0.79 can be considered fair, 0.80 to 0.89 good, and 0.90 and above excellent. Test-retest reliability values greater than 0.90 are required if consideration is being given to employing a questionnaire in a discriminative application on a patient-to-patient basis, as opposed to discriminating between groups.[35]

Test-retest reliability is related to the number of items within a questionnaire because the true variance will increase as the square of the number of items, while the error variance will increase linearly with the number of items.[33] Generally then, the greater the number of items within a questionnaire, the higher the test-retest value will be. This may have implications for questionnaire selection when good test-retest reliability is required, given the large variation in the number of items per questionnaire. Item reduction comes at the expense of test-retest reliability.

Reliability can also be investigated using Cronbach's alpha statistic.[36,37] Cronbach's alpha addresses the homogeneity of items (questions) within an outcome questionnaire domain or total score and is complementary to the ICC as a metric of reliability. Cronbach's alpha is used primarily in the development of a questionnaire as a means of reducing the number of items within a scale because the statistic determines the inter-item correlation for each item within a domain. A value from 0 to 1 is produced, and a value of 0.60 to 0.79 is indicative of fair internal consistency, 0.80 to 0.89 good internal consistency, and greater than or equal to 0.90 excellent internal consistency.[38] Cronbach's alpha is calculated n times for a scale (n = number of items within the scale) with one item omitted each time. If the value for Cronbach's alpha increases with the omission of an item, then that item can be argued to be deviating from the area of interest inquired about within the scale and can therefore be omitted from the finalized scale. Cronbach's alpha is used when the items within a scale are polychotomous. Dichotomous items, such as those in the Nottingham Health Profile (NHP), require a variation of Cronbach's alpha known as the *Kuder Richardson formula*.[25]

As alluded to previously, health outcome questionnaires have been criticized for yielding soft data, and the softness or hardness of data generally refers to the reliability of the questionnaire (both ICC and Cronbach's alpha). However, when relevant health outcome questionnaires are evaluated in a target population, questionnaires have been shown to demonstrate fair to excellent reliability and therefore can be considered relatively hard. Generally, disease/site-specific questionnaires produce harder data than general health questionnaires. Some "hard" and "objective" data yield distinctly poor ICC values, making them actually rather "soft."[39]

Responsiveness

Responsiveness is the measure of the ability of a questionnaire to detect change when it is applied on separate occasions and a clinically significant change has occurred between applications. By definition, responsiveness is related to longitudinal application of a questionnaire; however, as outlined earlier, the purpose of this study was to define appropriate questionnaires for cross-sectional discriminative application. Nevertheless, determining the responsiveness of a questionnaire is integral to the validation process. Although responsiveness may have been defined previously for a questionnaire, investigations have often been performed on dissimilar populations; therefore investigating responsiveness among the target population is necessary. Questionnaire validation is a dynamic unending process.[40]

Several methods of determining responsiveness are known, including the standardized effect size.[32,41-44] *Standardized effect size* is calculated by subtracting the results of a questionnaire at time 2 from the results of the same questionnaire at time 1 and dividing the difference by the standard deviation of the test results from time 1. Time 1 and time 2 together represent a period over which a clinically significant change should have occurred, such as before and after a therapeutic intervention, whether drug therapy or surgery, for example. A standardized effect size of 0.2 is considered small, 0.5 moderate, and greater than 0.8 large.[45]

Knee and hip arthroplasties have been shown to have a major impact on health-related quality of life when preoperative status is compared with postoperative status.[3-7] In fact, Dawson and associates showed a standardized effect size greater than 2.0 for hip arthroplasty when the Oxford-12 Item Knee Score was applied preoperatively and postoperatively.[6] Such a standardized effect size can be considered profound, especially when a standardized effect size of 0.8 is considered large. Such profound results make preoperative and postoperative comparisons of different prosthetic designs, surgical techniques, and so forth, using a given questionnaire, difficult to interpret and potentially irrelevant, because assumed subtle differences in questionnaire results would be lost in the large signal. Paradoxically, the signal for preoperative and postoperative comparisons after knee arthroplasty is so loud (large) that in effect, it functions as noise and obscures the subtler signal of interest. Therefore, it may be more relevant to calculate responsiveness using an alternative method and/or to follow arthroplasty patients longitudinally between time 2 (a defined postoperative period) and time 3. In this case, the large signal of the operative intervention would not obscure the subtler signal of interest.

The Receiver Operating Characteristic Curve (ROC Curve)

The receiver operating characteristic curve (ROC curve) has been shown to be of value as a surrogate to classic responsiveness measures when longitudinal data are not available.[41,43,46,47] This is particularly relevant for the reasons listed earlier, and because the Swedish Knee Arthroplasty Registry (SKAR) to date has not applied questionnaires in a longitudinal fashion. The ROC curve method originated from the operation of radar equipment during the Second World War. At that time, radar operators and others were interested in optimizing the signal-to-noise ratio of their receivers. Initially, as the gain on equipment was increased, the signal correspondingly increased rapidly. However, at some point, the gain in noise was greater than the gain in signal. This represents the "cut-point" of interest, and essentially the cut-point represents the dichotomization of continuous data. To construct an ROC curve, the true-positive rate (sensitivity) of a test is plotted on the Y-axis and the false-positive rate (1-specificity) on the X-axis. These two values are determined for each possible cut-point, and a curve is subsequently generated. The area under the ROC curve is used as a gauge of the discriminative ability of the test, with an area of 1.0 representative of a perfectly discriminative test and an area of 0.5 a nondiscriminative test. An example of an ROC curve is shown in Figure 61-4. In this case, Questionnaire A has better discriminative ability than Questionnaire B.

Sources of Bias When Outcomes Are Assessed

Health outcome questionnaires are subject to bias from several sources. First, patient demographics may influence the results of questionnaire scores. Advanced age (>85 years) has been shown to have an adverse effect on subjective assessment after knee arthroplasty, as has low socioeconomic status, at least in North America.[48,49] Gender has also been found to affect the results of health outcome questionnaires, particularly when used in association with hip or knee arthroplasty; women tend to report greater pain and physical function limitation after hip or knee arthroplasty.[50] Comorbidity has been shown to adversely affect the results of knee arthroplasty, as assessed by questionnaire, for both joint-related and medical problems.[49,51] Charnley was aware of the potential biasing effect of comorbidity; this was largely the impetus for the Charnley comorbidity classification proposed for hip arthroplasty.[52] Gender, age, and comorbidity should be factored when outcomes after hip or knee arthroplasty are compared. Socioeconomic status probably does not have as significant an impact in a homogeneous country such as Sweden.

Mode of Administration of Questionnaires

The mode of administration also significantly biases the results of health outcomes questionnaires. When a questionnaire is self-completed by the patient after knee surgery, as opposed to being administered by the investigator, resulting questionnaire scores have been shown to be significantly worse.[53] Also, nonresponders to a self-administered postal survey on quality of life tend to report worse quality of life than responders on a follow-up telephone survey.[54] Therefore, assessment of the status of nonresponders is probably warranted when a low response rate occurs with administration of a questionnaire.

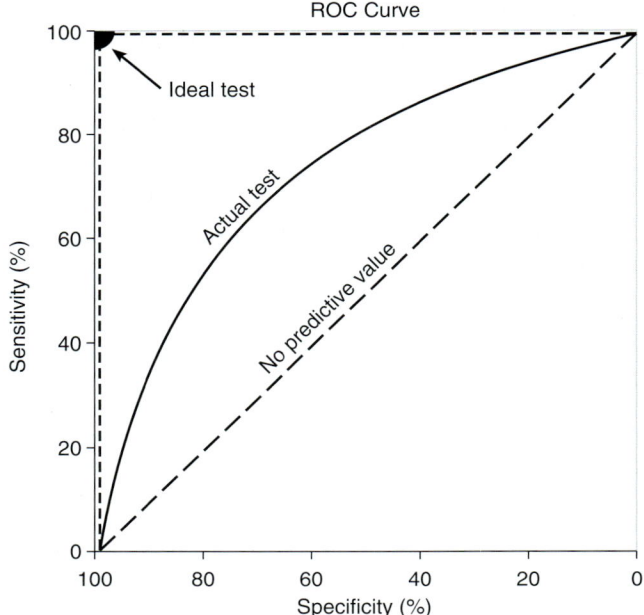

Figure 61-4. Typical receiver operating characteristic (ROC) curve.

Types of Outcome Questionnaires

General Health Outcomes

Since the WHO modified the definition of health to include "…a state of physical, mental and social well-being," measurement of health has moved from simply defining the success of a procedure by its effect on infirmity and disease, to defining what effect the intervention had on physical, mental, and social well-being.[23] By this definition, it was no longer adequate to define the outcome of an arthroplasty, for example, by simply stating the prosthesis survival rate. This change in philosophy led to the development of general health outcome questionnaires; examples that have been used in arthroplasty research include the 36-Item Short-Form Health Survey (SF-36),[55] the 12-Item Short-Form Health Survey (SF-12),[56] the Nottingham Health Profile (NHP),[57] the Sickness Impact Profile (SIP),[58] and the EuroQual questionnaires.[59] General health questionnaires focus on patients' perceptions of their own health, including such diverse domains as ability to sleep, energy level, mood, and perception of body pain. These questionnaires are limited neither to specific disease nor to patient cohort.

Disease-Specific Outcomes

In an effort to avoid the surgeon bias associated with objective outcomes, additional disease-specific questionnaires were introduced to arthroplasty patients. Disease-specific questionnaires attempt to isolate the signal of interest by focusing questions around a particular disease state. In the 1980s, the Lequesne Index of Severity for the Knee (ISK)[60,61] and the Western Ontario and MacMaster Universities Osteoarthritis Index (WOMAC)[62,63] were introduced.

Joint-Specific Outcomes

Site-specific questionnaires attempt to isolate the signal in a similar fashion by focusing questions on a specific region of the body. The Oxford-12 Item Knee and Hip Scores (Oxford-12) were later developed and released in 1998 for use with knee and hip arthroplasty patients as site-specific questionnaires.[6,7]

Patient-Specific Outcomes

Patient-specific questionnaires, such as the Patient-Specific Index,[64] use a novel approach to limit the noise within a questionnaire by asking patients to choose their own goals or objectives before an intervention and by requesting that they subsequently rate or score how well those objectives have been accomplished.

Single-Item Questionnaires

Global or single-item questionnaires, such as those regarding patient satisfaction, are the most aggressive in their effort to limit noise by asking a single direct question regarding the state or condition of interest.[65,66]

Interest is increasing in the use of patient reports of the outcomes of their surgical operations as an accurate indication of the results. Bream and Black reviewed 62 studies of health status and found that patients' views of their level of disability reflect clinicians' views and can be relied upon to provide an accurate indication of the outcome of elective surgery.[67] Gandhi[68] reported a low to moderate relationship between self-reported (WOMAC and SF-36) and performance-based tools (timed-up-and-go). He stated that both tests are needed to assess the true level of patient disability.

Several authors have suggested that the simultaneous use of general health and disease/site-specific questionnaires yields complementary data.[69-71]

Frequently Used Outcome Questionnaires

General Health Questionnaires

36-Item Short-Form Health Survey (SF-36). This widely used general health questionnaire allows comparison across many conditions and interventions. It consists of 36 questions with Likert-box response keys. Item scaling is both dichotomous and polychotomous. Eight domain scores ranging from 0 to 100 are generated. These include Body Pain, Physical Functioning, Vitality, General Health, Social Functioning, Role-Physical, Role-Emotion, and Mental Health. A score of 100 represents the best possible health state. Two summary scales of physical and mental health are generated for the SF-36: the Physical Component Summary (PCS), and the Mental Component Summary (MCS). Their scoring is similar to that used for summary scores of the SF-12.

12-Item Short-Form Health Survey (SF-12). The SF-12 contains 12 items from the SF-36 Health Survey. It was originally developed in 1994 as a shorter alternative to the SF-36 for studies for which a 36-item form was too long. The SF-12 contains one or two items that measure each of the eight concepts included in the SF-36. The SF-12 consists of 12 questions with a Likert-box response key. Item scaling is both dichotomous and polychotomous. Scores are transformed into two weighted summary scores called the *Physical Component Summary* (PCS) and the *Mental Component Summary* (MCS). Weights are calculated via z- and t-transformation so that an average population sample will record a score of 50 for each summary, and a score change of 10 points represents one standard deviation. A score above 50 represents a perception of better health than the average population.

EuroQual Questionnaire. EuroQual-5D is an example of a general health questionnaire. The EuroQual-5D is a system that evaluates five dimensions of a patient's health (mobility, self-care, usual activities, pain/discomfort, and anxiety/depression). Each dimension includes three levels (no problems, some/moderate problems, extreme problems). The patient's health state is defined by combining one level from each of the five dimensions, with +1 as the best and −0.594 as the worst possible outcome.

Disease-Specific Questionnaire

Western Ontario and McMaster Universities Osteoarthritis Index (WOMAC). The disease-specific WOMAC questionnaire inquires about pain with activity and the

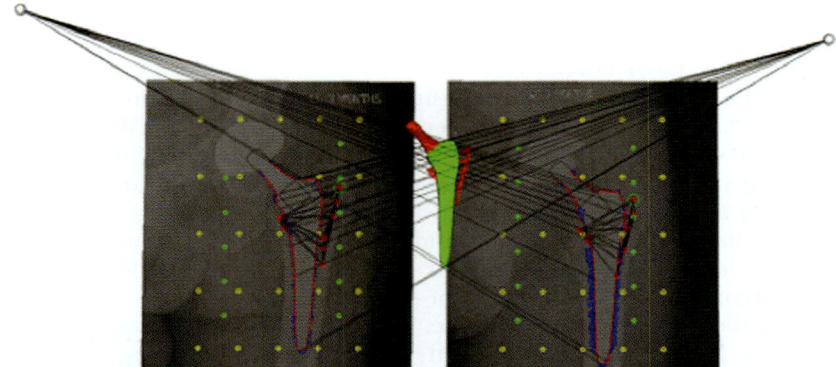

Figure 61-5. Example of a radiostereometric analysis (RSA) examination analysis using RSA software to find the position of the total hip replacement. The femur is represented by the tantalum beads inserted during surgery.

ability to perform activities such as stair climbing, putting on shoes and socks, and so forth. It consists of 24 Likert-box questions broken down into three domains: Pain (five questions), Stiffness (two questions), and Physical Function (17 questions). Scores range from 0 to 20 for Pain, from 0 to 8 for Stiffness, and from 0 to 68 for Physical Function. A score of 0 represents the best possible health state. Items are scaled with five boxes for each question ranging from 0 to 4.

Joint-Specific Questionnaire

Oxford-12 Item Knee Score (Oxford-12). The Oxford-12 Item Knee Score is a relatively new and well-validated outcome questionnaire designed specifically for use with knee arthroplasty patients. Twelve questions are posed that relate specifically to the knee. Each question has a Likert-box response key from 1 to 5. A single score is produced ranging from 12 to 60, with 12 indicating the best possible health state.

PRECISION OBJECTIVE METRICS

Radiosteroemetric Analysis

Radiostereometric analysis (RSA) is a precise outcome tool that has accurate and reliable predictive ability with regard to implant aseptic loosening and thus survivorship.[72,73] At the time of surgery, radiodense tantalum markers are placed into the host bone, and these beads are used to mark the implant. Postoperatively, biplanar simultaneous stereo x-rays of the joint are taken through a calibration cage with known fiducial points (Fig. 61-5). The generated images are then imported into an RSA software analysis package, and micromotion at the interface of the implant and the host bone is calculated in three dimensions. These three vectors are combined into a metric of overall motion—maximum total point motion (MTPM). At 6-month intervals, MTPM is plotted on the Y-axis against serial x-ray measures (on the X-axis) (Fig. 61-6). RSA curves follow a typical pattern: The implanted prosthesis stabilizes with respect to MTPM over time, or it continues to migrate. If the prosthesis stabilizes, revision for aseptic loosening is unlikely. Conversely, if the prosthesis

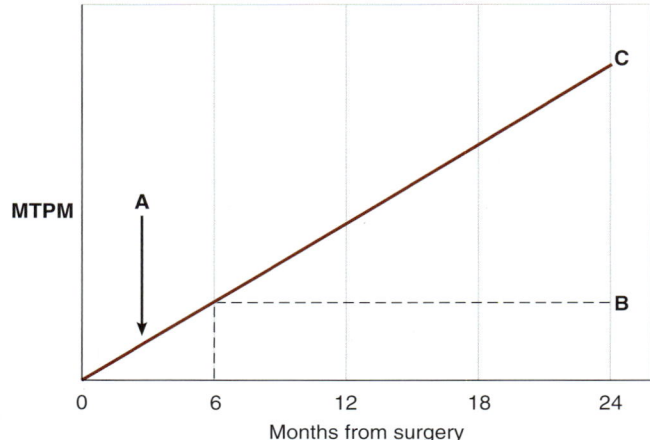

Figure 61-6. Typical radiostereometric analysis (RSA) curve. Maximum total point motion (MTPM) is on the Y-axis. *A,* All prostheses initially migrate. *B,* Some components stabilize and are unlikely to be revised for aseptic loosening. *C,* Some components continue to migrate and are likely to be revised for aseptic loosening. The two curves differentiate early.

continues to migrate, revision for aseptic loosening is significantly more likely. The power of RSA is such that variation in MTPM patterns can be differentiated accurately as early as 1 year postoperatively, and as few as 30 to 40 patients need to be exposed to the experimental technology.

It is the author's opinion that RSA is a critical technology for the rational development of new techniques and implants. As new techniques and implants are introduced, earlier concerns over health quality improvement and cost savings can be effectively addressed. National registries, although useful in overseeing the introduction of new technology, offer outcomes on a near real-time basis and hence are not predictive. RSA has the potential to predict the long-term survivorship of new implants and technologies.

Gait and EMG

Interest is increasing in using quality of gait as an adjunct to standard outcome measures to assess patient outcomes following hip arthroplasty. In investigating the correlation between objective and subjective evaluation of patients with total hip replacement, Lindemann[74] suggests that the WOMAC questionnaire might not reflect walking performance, and that gait analysis is recommended to gain objective information about the quality of gait.

Limitations of Precision Objective Metrics

RSA, gait analysis, and electromyography (EMG) studies are limited by their cost and lack of availability. RSA suites and gait laboratories generally are available only in specialized centers. The costs involved make these additional studies available only for research purposes. The future of these outcome metrics lies in the use of inexpensive surrogate measures, which are validated to replace their expensive alternatives.

FUTURE DIRECTIONS

The future direction of hip outcomes involves standardizing international agreement on outcomes and combining data from national registries. Continued implementation of precise metrics secondary to reduced costs will allow early detection of poor implants and techniques.

Future Directions: Registries

National registries are well established in the Nordic countries and are becoming established in other nations, including Canada. It is logically predictable that the current and future proliferation of information technology will motivate and facilitate linking of national registries. Meaningful comparisons between nations using health outcome questionnaires are possible but will be problematic unless several prerequisites are fulfilled. The first prerequisite involves standardizing the questionnaires employed. A consensus between nations is necessary regarding which questionnaires should be used. Obviously, agreed upon questionnaires should be available in translated and subsequently validated versions for the respective nations. Several types of questionnaires should be agreed upon to optimize for specific applications, as outlined earlier. The second prerequisite involves the establishment of demographic norms for each nation. Such norms would provide the "denominator" required to compare outcome results. The final prerequisite involves more detailed subjective descriptions of the natural history of hip arthroplasty, including the effects of complications. Currently, the natural history is not well described, hence making the creation of hypothetical constructs difficult. Because the natural subjective history of revised and unrevised hip arthroplasty patients is not well defined, neither is the construct. This weakens test results. The work of national registries will be instrumental in this capacity.

Future Directions: Questionnaires

Validation of outcome questionnaires is a dynamic process, and continued investigation of the performance of a questionnaire across multiple types of applications on various cohorts is required. Also, repeat surveying of existing subjects may allow identification of subtler variations in outcome between types of techniques and prostheses. This would also serve to test the evaluative ability of the questionnaire.

Current scoring systems are based largely on traditional outcomes of pain relief and limited return to functional activities. However, patients' expectations have increased; most are no longer satisfied with just pain relief but demand to be able to return to significant physical activities, including recreational activities.

It is almost impossible to distinguish even significant functional differences, such as the ability to walk over uneven ground, run, or participate in vigorous recreational activities, using current outcome measures. This limitation has led to the introduction of new, higher-precision scoring systems such as the High-Activity Arthroplasty Score (HAAS), which was specifically developed to assess subtle variations in functional ability after lower limb arthroplasty with particular regard to highly functioning individuals.[75]

This scoring system includes four categories of activities: walking, running, stair climbing, and activity level. The aim was to produce a measure that would remove any ceiling effect by including high-demand activities. For example, a maximum score would mean that a patient has the ability to walk over rough ground longer than 1 hour, run more than 5 kilometers, climb stairs two at a time, and play competitive sports.

This higher-precision scoring system should improve our ability to discern subtle outcome differences in highly functioning individuals.

Future Directions: RSA

Future exciting developments in RSA technology include model-based RSA, image-based RSA, and inducible displacement. Model-based RSA and image-based RSA enable assessment of micromotion in total joint replacement without the use of marker beads. Inducible displacement is the reversible motion generated in response to an applied external load. Its measurement should allow accurate assessment of fixation of an implant at any point after surgery, thus predicting the likelihood of early failure.[76,77]

RSA technology is becoming increasingly available and easier to implement, with custom RSA suites, improved instruments, and centralized secure data analysis available to any institution interested in using high-precision metrics to assess arthroplasty outcomes.

Future Directions: Gait

The use of novel portable gait analysis systems (e.g., the Walkabout Portable Gait Monitor, INNOMED Expert Systems Inc., Hammonds Plains, Nova Scotia, Canada) that use triaxial accelerometers to measure the three-dimensional motion of the center of mass has been shown to be effective in quantifying the quality of gait. These portable gait analysis systems have taken basic gait analysis out of the gait laboratory and into the outpatient clinic, allowing easy assessment during preoperative and postoperative clinic visits.

REFERENCES

1. The Oxford English dictionary, definition of "health," New York, 2010, Oxford University Press.
2. McHorney CA: Generic health measurement: past accomplishments and a measurement paradigm for the 21st century. Ann Intern Med 127(8 Pt 2):743–750, 1997.
3. Laupacis A, Bourne R, Rorabeck C, et al: The effect of elective total hip replacement on health-related quality of life. J Bone Joint Surg Am 75:1619–1626, 1993.
4. Rissanen P, Aro S, Slatis P, et al: Health and quality of life before and after hip or knee arthroplasty. J Arthroplasty 10:169–175, 1995.
5. Ritter MA, Albohm MJ, Keating EM, et al: Comparative outcomes of total joint arthroplasty. J Arthroplasty 10:737–741, 1995.
6. Dawson J, Fitzpatrick R, Carr A, Murray D: Questionnaire on the perceptions of patients about total hip replacement. J Bone Joint Surg Br 78:185–190, 1996.
7. Dawson J, Fitzpatrick R, Murray D, Carr A: Questionnaire on the perceptions of patients about total knee replacement. J Bone Joint Surg Br 80:63–69, 1998.
8. Thompson SP: Life of Lord Kelvin, Chelsea, NY, 1976, Chelsea Publishing.
9. Fergusson AB, Howarth MB: Slipping of the upper femoral epiphysis. JAMA 97:1867–1872, 1931.
10. d'Aubigné RM, Postel M: The classic: functional results of hip arthroplasty with acrylic prosthesis, 1954. Clin Orthop Relat Res 467:7–27, 2009.
11. Lieberman JR, Dorey F, Shekelle P, et al: Differences between patients' and physicians' evaluations of outcome after total hip arthroplasty. J Bone Joint Surg Am 78:835–838, 1996.
12. Su CT, Parham LD: Generating a valid questionnaire translation for cross-cultural use. Am J Occup Ther 56:581–585, 2002.
13. Dobbs HS: Survivorship of total hip replacements. J Bone Joint Surg Br 62:168–173, 1980.
14. Kaplan EL, Meier P: Nonparametric estimation from incomplete observations. J Am Stat Assoc 53:457–481, 1958.
15. Murray DW, Carr AJ, Bulstrode C: Survival analysis of joint replacements. J Bone Joint Surg Br 75:697–704, 1993.
16. Lettin AW, Ware HS, Morris RW: Survivorship analysis and confidence intervals: an assessment with reference to the Stanmore total knee replacement. J Bone Joint Surg Br 73:729–731, 1991.
17. Espehaug B, Havelin LI, Engesaeter LB, et al: Early revision among 12,179 hip prostheses: a comparison of 10 different brands reported to the Norwegian Arthroplasty Register, 1987-1993. Acta Orthop Scand 66:487–493, 1995.
18. Herberts P, Malchau H: Long-term registration has improved the quality of hip replacement: a review of the Swedish THR Register comparing 160,000 cases. Acta Orthop Scand 71:111–121, 2000.
19. Puolakka TJ, Pajamaki KJ, Halonen PJ, et al: The Finnish Arthroplasty Register: report of the hip register. Acta Orthop Scand 72:433–441, 2001.
20. Robertsson O, Dunbar MJ, Knutson K, et al: The Swedish Knee Arthroplasty Register: 25 years experience. Bull Hosp Jt Dis 58:133–138, 1999.
21. Knutson K, Lewold S, Robertsson O, Lidgren L: The Swedish Knee Arthroplasty Register: a nation-wide study of 30,003 knees 1976-1992. Acta Orthop Scand 65:375–386, 1994.
22. Robertsson O, Knutson K, Lewold S, Lidgren L: Knee arthroplasty for osteoarthrosis and rheumatoid arthritis 1986-1996. Presented at the Scientific Exhibit SE028, AAOS Annual Meeting, Anaheim, Calif, February 4-8, 1999.
23. Dunbar MJ: Subjective outcomes after knee arthroplasty. Acta Orthop Scand Suppl 72:1–63, 2001.
24. Apley AG: An assessment of assessment. J Bone Joint Surg Br 72:957–958, 1990.
25. Hilding MB, Backbro B, Ryd L: Quality of life after knee arthroplasty: a randomized study of 3 designs in 42 patients, compared after 4 years. Acta Orthop Scand 68:156–160, 1997.
26. Strohmeier J, Westbrook P: Divine harmony: the life and teachings of Pythagoras, Berkeley, Calif, 1999, Berkeley Hill Books.
27. Descartes R: A discourse on method: meditations and principles, Vale, Guernsey, 1986, Guernsey Press Company Limited.
28. McHorney CA: Generic health measurement: past accomplishments and a measurement paradigm for the 21st century, Ann Intern Med 127(8 Pt 2):743–750, 1997.
29. Bone and joint decade, Workshop. Available at: http://www.bonejointdecade.org. Accessed July 23, 2010.
30. Brown L: The new shorter Oxford English dictionary, New York, NY, 1993, Oxford University Press.
31. Kirshner B, Guyatt G: A methodological framework for assessing health indices. J Chronic Dis 38:27–36, 1985.
32. Kreibich DN, Vaz M, Bourne RB, et al: What is the best way of assessing outcome after total knee replacement? Clin Orthop Relat Res 331:221–225, 1996.
33. Streiner DL, Norman GR: Health measurement scales: a practical guide to their development and use, New York, NY, 1998, Oxford University Press.
34. Bland JM, Altman DG: Measurement error and correlation coefficients. BMJ 313:41–42, 1996.
35. Ware JE, Jr, Sherbourne CD: The MOS 36-item Short-Form Health Survey (SF-36). I. Conceptual framework and item selection. Med Care 30:473–483, 1992.
36. Cronbach LJ, Meehl PE: Construct validity in psychological tests. Psychol Bull 52:281–302, 1955.
37. Bland JM, Altman DG: Cronbach's alpha. BMJ 314:572, 1997.
38. Feinstein AR: Clinimetrics, New Haven, Conn, 1987, Yale University Press.
39. Ryd L, Karrholm J, Ahlvin P: Knee scoring systems in gonarthrosis: evaluation of interobserver variability and the envelope of bias. Score Assessment Group. Acta Orthop Scand 68:41–45, 1997.
40. Nunnally JC, Bernstein IH: Psychometric theory, New York, NY, 1994, McGraw-Hill.
41. Deyo RA, Centor RM: Assessing the responsiveness of functional scales to clinical change: an analogy to diagnostic test performance. J Chronic Dis 39:897–906, 1986.
42. Guyatt G, Walter S, Norman G: Measuring change over time: assessing the usefulness of evaluative instruments. J Chronic Dis 40:171–178, 1987.
43. Essink-Bot ML, Krabbe PF, Bonsel GJ, Aaronson NK: An empirical comparison of four generic health status measures: the Nottingham Health Profile, the Medical Outcomes Study 36-item Short-Form Health Survey, the COOP/WONCA charts, and the EuroQol instrument. Med Care 35:522–537, 1997.
44. Wright JG, Young NL: A comparison of different indices of responsiveness. J Clin Epidemiol 50:239–246, 1997.
45. Meenan RF, Kazis LE, Anthony JM, Wallin BA: The clinical and health status of patients with recent-onset rheumatoid arthritis. Arthritis Rheum 34:761–765, 1991.
46. Hanley JA, McNeil BJ: The meaning and use of the area under a receiver operating characteristic (ROC) curve. Radiology 143:29–36, 1982.
47. Centor RM: Signal detectability: the use of ROC curves and their analyses. Med Decis Making 11:102–106, 1991.
48. Callahan CM, Drake BG, Heck DA, Dittus RS: Patient outcomes following tricompartmental total knee replacement: a meta-analysis. JAMA 271:1349–1357, 1994.
49. Brinker MR, Lund PJ, Barrack RL: Demographic biases of scoring instruments for the results of total knee arthroplasty. J Bone Joint Surg Am 79:858–865, 1997.
50. Katz JN, Wright EA, Guadagnoli E, et al: Differences between men and women undergoing major orthopedic surgery for degenerative arthritis. Arthritis Rheum 37:687–694, 1994.
51. Hawker G, Wright J, Coyte P, et al: Health-related quality of life after knee replacement. J Bone Joint Surg Am 80:163–173, 1998.

52. Charnley J: Low friction arthroplasty of the hip, Berlin, 1979, Springer-Verlag.
53. Hoher J, Bach T, Munster A, et al: Does the mode of data collection change results in a subjective knee score? Self-administration versus interview. Am J Sports Med 25:642–647, 1997.
54. Hill A, Roberts J, Ewings P, Gunnell D: Non-response bias in a lifestyle survey. J Public Health Med 19:203–207, 1997.
55. Brazier JE, Harper R, Jones NM, et al: Validating the SF-36 health survey questionnaire: new outcome measure for primary care. BMJ 305:160–164, 1992.
56. Ware J Jr, Kosinski M, Keller SD: A 12-item Short-Form Health Survey: construction of scales and preliminary tests of reliability and validity. Med Care 34:220–233, 1996.
57. Hunt SM, McKenna SP, McEwen J, et al: A quantitative approach to perceived health status: a validation study. J Epidemiol Community Health 34:281–286, 1980.
58. Pollard WE, Bobbitt RA, Bergner M, et al: The Sickness Impact Profile: reliability of a health status measure. Med Care 14:146–155, 1976.
59. EuroQol: a new facility for the measurement of health-related quality of life. The EuroQol Group. Health Policy 16:199–208, 1990.
60. Lequesne M: Informational indices: validation of criteria and tests. Scand J Rheumatol Suppl 80:17–28, 1989.
61. Lequesne MG, Mery C, Samson M, Gerard P: Indexes of severity for osteoarthritis of the hip and knee: validation—value in comparison with other assessment tests. Scand J Rheumatol Suppl 65:85–89, 1987.
62. Bellamy N, Buchanan WW: Outcome measurement in osteoarthritis clinical trials: the case for standardisation. Clin Rheumatol 3:293–303, 1984.
63. Bellamy N, Buchanan WW, Goldsmith CH, et al: Validation study of WOMAC: a health status instrument for measuring clinically important patient relevant outcomes to antirheumatic drug therapy in patients with osteoarthritis of the hip or knee. J Rheumatol 15:1833–1840, 1988.
64. Wright JG, Young NL: The patient-specific index: asking patients what they want. J Bone Joint Surg Am 79:974–983, 1997.
65. Robertsson O, Dunbar M, Pehrsson T, et al: Patient satisfaction after knee arthroplasty: a report on 27,372 knees operated on between 1981 and 1995 in Sweden. Acta Orthop Scand 71:262–267, 2000.
66. Robertsson O, Dunbar MJ: Patient satisfaction compared with general health and disease-specific questionnaires in knee arthroplasty patients. J Arthroplasty 16:476–482, 2001.
67. Bream E, Black N: What is the relationship between patients' and clinicians' reports of the outcomes of elective surgery? J Health Serv Res Policy 14:174–182, 2009.
68. Gandhi R, Tsvetkov D, Davey JR, et al: Relationship between self-reported and performance-based tests in a hip and knee joint replacement population. Clin Rheumatol 28:253–257, 2009.
69. Hawker G, Melfi C, Paul J, et al: Comparison of a generic (SF-36) and a disease specific (WOMAC) (Western Ontario and McMaster Universities Osteoarthritis Index) instrument in the measurement of outcomes after knee replacement surgery. J Rheumatol 22:1193–1196, 1995.
70. Lieberman JR, Dorey F, Shekelle P, et al: Outcome after total hip arthroplasty: comparison of a traditional disease-specific and a quality-of-life measurement of outcome. J Arthroplasty 12:639–645, 1997.
71. Patrick DL, Deyo RA: Generic and disease-specific measures in assessing health status and quality of life. Med Care 27(3 Suppl):S217–S232, 1989.
72. Karrholm J, Herberts P, Hultmark P, et al: Radiostereometry of hip prostheses: review of methodology and clinical results. Clin Orthop Relat Res 344:94–110, 1997.
73. Ryd L: Micromotion in knee arthroplasty: a roentgen stereophotogrammetric analysis of tibial component fixation. Acta Orthop Scand Suppl 220:1–80, 1986.
74. Lindemann U, Becker C, Unnewehr I, et al: Gait analysis and WOMAC are complementary in assessing functional outcome in total hip replacement. Clin Rehabil 20:413–420, 2006.
75. Talbot S, Hooper G, Stokes A, Zordan R: Use of a new high-activity arthroplasty score to assess function of young patients with total hip or knee arthroplasty. J Arthroplasty 25:268–273, 2010.
76. Fukuoka S, Yoshida K, Yamano Y: Estimation of the migration of tibial components in total knee arthroplasty: a roentgen stereophotogrammetric analysis. J Bone Joint Surg Br 82:222–227, 2000.
77. Wilson DA, Astephen JL, Hennigar AW, Dunbar MJ: Inducible displacement of a trabecular metal tibial monoblock component. J Arthroplasty 25:893–900, 2010.

CHAPTER 62

Preoperative Planning and Templating for Primary Hip Arthroplasty

Tad M. Mabry

INTRODUCTION

Pain relief and restoration of function remain the two primary goals of total hip arthroplasty (THA). The critical first step in achieving these goals is preoperative planning, which must begin as soon as a patient is determined to be a candidate for THA.[1] The purpose of this chapter is to describe a method of comprehensive surgical planning that will serve to maximize patient outcomes both in the perioperative period and over the lifetime of the hip reconstruction.

INDICATIONS/CONTRAINDICATIONS

Comprehensive surgical planning should be performed in advance of all hip reconstructive procedures. The scope of this planning stage must encompass more than simple templating for implant sizes.[2] Failure to precisely plan all aspects of the hip reconstruction could result in a number of potentially preventable complications, such as loosening, fracture, instability, and leg length inequality.[2-8]

TECHNIQUE: PREOPERATIVE PLANNING

Patient Selection

Great care must be exercised in selecting arthroplasty as the treatment for derangements about the hip. In general, total hip arthroplasty (THA) should be reserved for patients with severe hip pathology who have failed a comprehensive nonoperative treatment program, and who are capable, both physically and cognitively, of recovering from the surgery. In addition to assessment of the patient's overall health status, several key historical features should be ascertained, including the quality, severity, and location of pain; impact on activities; prior treatments; need for gait aids; and patient perception of limb length.[2] Extra-articular pain generators, such as spinal pathology (stenosis, radiculopathy), vascular pathology (vascular claudication), trochanteric bursitis, or stress fracture (pelvis, proximal femur), should be considered during the history-taking process.

Many patients presenting for possible conversion to a primary THA have undergone prior hip surgery, such as osteotomy or internal fixation of fractures. Details of these procedures should be elucidated, including indications for surgery and the presence or absence of postoperative complications such as infection. Whenever possible, it is best to obtain and review old operative notes to better understand any potential alterations to the local anatomy.

Details of the physical examination are found elsewhere in this text; however, this portion of the patient selection process should focus on four main features: confirmation of intra-articular pathology as the pain generator, exclusion of extra-articular pain generators, detailed evaluation of the neurovascular status of the entire limb, and assessment of true and apparent leg length.

Assessment of leg length bears special mention because leg length discrepancy is one of the major causes of patient dissatisfaction following THA.[9-11] The surgeon must consider the combination of patient perception and objective measurements when planning the reconstruction to provide appropriate preoperative patient counseling and to best manage leg length discrepancy during surgery.

Radiographic Evaluation

High-quality radiographs of known magnification are essential for both patient selection and templating for THA.[6,12-15] Many surgeons utilize a three-view radiographic evaluation, including anteroposterior (AP) views of the pelvis and proximal femur, as well as a true lateral view of the affected hip(s). The AP pelvis allows side-to-side comparison of the hips and radiographic leg length measurement. The AP proximal femur provides complete visualization of the upper femur, which allows more accurate templating of the femoral reconstruction. Where possible, these AP views should be obtained with the hips internally rotated 10 to 15 degrees. This will compensate for femoral neck anteversion and will bring the neck into full profile, thus avoiding underestimation of the patient's femoral offset. The true lateral view allows visualization of overhanging osteophytes near the anterior or posterior acetabular walls. This view also allows femoral templating in the sagittal plane. A "frog-leg" lateral view of the proximal femur may be used in place of, or as a supplement to, the true lateral view with respect to femoral templating.

Optimization

As was previously noted, preoperative planning should begin as soon as the patient is deemed to be a candidate for THA. The surgeon should consider four separate issues related to medical optimization of the patient before surgery: medical clearance, blood management, infection prevention strategy, and venous thromboembolic (VTE) prophylaxis.

The need for preoperative medical clearance certainly depends on the overall health of the patient. At the time of the original surgical consultation, the patient's past medical history should be specifically examined for risk factors that would necessitate further preoperative workup, such as cardiovascular disease, pulmonary disease, immunodeficiency, rheumatologic conditions, corticosteroid dependence, bleeding diathesis, hypercoagulability, diabetes mellitus, tobacco dependence, alcohol abuse, or other chronic conditions. Patients should be questioned regarding the

details of any prior invasive surgeries and any complications encountered following these procedures. Patients identified as having significant medical risks should be referred to an internal medicine physician for further evaluation and preoperative medical optimization before elective surgical intervention is provided. Aside from benefits to the patient in the preoperative and intraoperative time periods, the results of this medical evaluation will be put to use later in formulating the postoperative care plan.

Blood management is another part of the comprehensive surgical plan and must be considered for each patient individually.[16] Blood management is further explored elsewhere in this text. In general terms, there are three areas in which the surgeon may intervene to decrease the need for allogeneic blood transfusion. These areas include increasing the starting hemoglobin, minimizing intraoperative blood loss, and lowering the transfusion trigger to a lower level of hemoglobin/hematocrit.

The first step in this process is evaluation of the patient's preoperative blood counts. Patients with chronic anemia may benefit from stimulated erythropoiesis to elevate starting hemoglobin during the preoperative period if identified in a timely fashion. Preoperative autologous donation is another method of blood management that must be instituted at the appropriate time. Furthermore, the surgeon must decide in the preoperative period whether to utilize antifibrinolytic medications or blood salvage devices intraoperatively to minimize loss of blood.

Issues related to the mitigation of infection risk must be considered during the preoperative planning stage.[17] Areas of active infection remote to the affected joint must be identified and completely treated before elective THA is performed. If there is a possibility of sepsis in the affected joint, this must be identified before conversion to arthroplasty. Antibiotic allergies must be identified so that the appropriate intravenous antibiotic prophylaxis is available in the operating room. Allergies also must be considered if the surgeon intends to utilize prophylactic antibiotics in any cement that may be used as part of the joint reconstruction. Patients taking immunosuppressive drugs (e.g., post transplant, rheumatoid arthritis) may need to have these regimens adjusted in the perioperative period to promote wound healing and minimize the risk of infection.[18,19]

Interest has arisen in preoperative decolonization regimens aimed at individuals colonized with *Staphylococcus aureus*.[20,21] Patients must be screened for the presence of *S. aureus* 2 to 4 weeks preoperatively. Colonized patients typically receive 5 days of twice-daily mupirocin ointment applied to the anterior nares. Patients may also be given chlorhexidine skin scrubs during this time period. Patients colonized with methicillin-resistant *S. aureus* (MRSA) are given intravenous vancomycin rather than a cephalosporin as antibiotic prophylaxis. These regimens have proved very effective in lowering the rate of surgical site infection due to *S. aureus*.

Finally, the strategy for VTE prophylaxis should be determined preoperatively. All patients are at high risk for VTE following hip arthroplasty.[22] There are many postoperative VTE prophylaxis regimens from which to choose, and the particular method should be selected after the risks of bleeding versus the risks of clotting are considered for each individual patient.[23,24] Risk factors that may further elevate the postoperative clotting risk must be ascertained before surgery. Some of the more common diagnoses that could add to the risk of postoperative VTE in the hip arthroplasty population include malignancy (active or occult), prior VTE, estrogen-containing medications, obesity, and thrombophilia (inherited or acquired).[22]

Each of these issues related to medical optimization (medical clearance, blood management, infection mitigation, and VTE prophylaxis) must be taken into account during the preoperative planning stage to maximize patient outcomes.

Templating

Templating the hip reconstruction serves multiple important purposes in the preoperative planning stage of total hip arthroplasty. First, careful templating will improve the surgeon's ability to restore favorable biomechanics to the joint, including leg length and offset. Second, templating will allow the surgeon to determine which implants will be required to carry out the reconstruction. Implant selection on both sides of the joint is determined by local anatomy, periarticular bone quality, and surgeon experience. In some cases, special devices may have to be made available that are not standard at the surgeon's hospital. Third, templating allows the surgeon to take note of osseous deformity and local landmarks that will facilitate appropriate component placement. Proper implant placement will benefit the patient in both the short term (e.g., decreased dislocation risk) and the long term (e.g., wear of the bearing surface) following THA. Finally, the templating process allows the surgeon to think in three dimensions and becomes a rehearsal of the reconstruction to be performed. Following is a stepwise approach to templating for primary THA.

Step 1: Determine the Magnification

It is critical to first determine the magnification of the radiographs to be templated, because all subsequent steps are based on measurements that have been appropriately corrected.[12] This is most often done by utilizing some type of external magnification marker at the time of radiographic exposure.[12,13]

Step 2: Identify Radiographic Landmarks

Several landmarks will be referenced during the templating process and should now be identified.[25] Three landmarks on the pelvis will be particularly useful for templating the acetabular component (Fig. 62-1): (1) The first landmark, the base of the radiographic teardrop, represents the inferomedial acetabulum. The inferior edge of the cup is typically placed at this level in the absence of significant deformity. (2) The ilioischial line should be identified and marked, because the

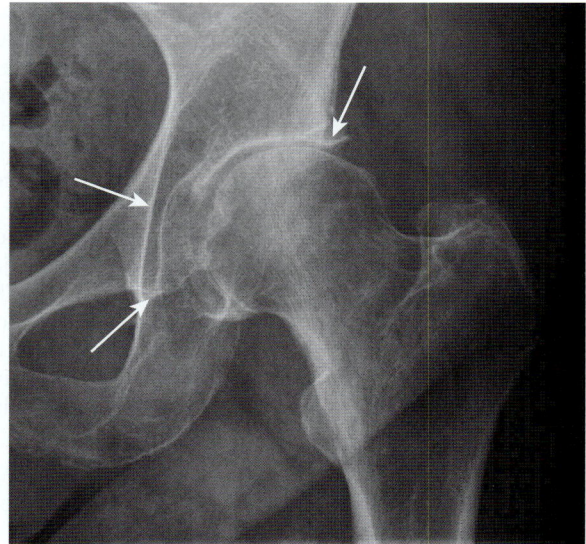

Figure 62-1. The three primary pelvic landmarks *(clockwise from the bottom)* include the base of the radiographic teardrop, the ilioischial line, and the superolateral margin of the acetabulum.

acetabular component is typically medialized no further than this point. (3) The location of the superolateral edge of the acetabulum is also noted at this stage. Coverage of the cup with respect to this point will be assessed during the templating process, and again intraoperatively.

Step 3: Assess Leg Length

Assessment of leg length involves synthesis of information gathered from the history, physical examination, and radiographs. The goal of the hip reconstruction is to restore equal leg length while maintaining appropriate joint stability. Typically, this involves maintaining existing leg length or lengthening a shortened limb. Occasionally, it is necessary to lengthen the limb to optimize hip stability, because avoidance of postoperative dislocation is a higher priority than avoidance of leg length inequality.[26]

To assess radiographic leg length at the hip, one first must create a pelvic reference line. This is most commonly identified as an inter-teardrop line.[25] However, one may also utilize a line connecting the most distal aspects of the sacroiliac joints and the most inferior aspects of the ischia, or a line connecting symmetric portions of the obturator foramina. The surgeon may then measure from the pelvic reference line to a fixed point on each femur, such as the lesser trochanter, the greater trochanter, or the center of rotation. Any difference from side to side represents radiographic leg length difference at the hip (Fig. 62-2). It is important to consider that leg length difference may be present at a site distal to the hip (e.g., healed tibia fracture, ankle fusion), and final decisions regarding intraoperative correction are made after all these data points are considered.

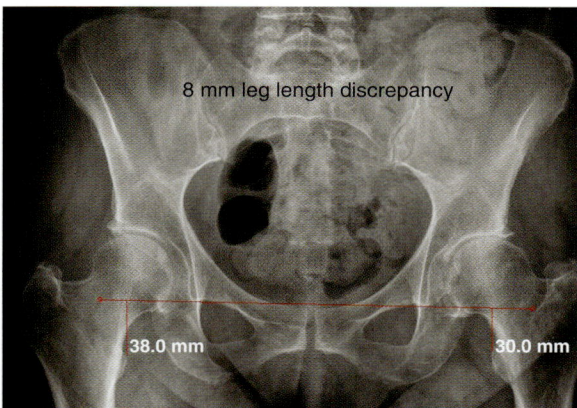

Figure 62-2. An inter-teardrop line has been drawn on this anteroposterior (AP) pelvis radiograph to serve as a reference line. The distance from this line to the lesser trochanter is 8 mm less on the patient's left than on the right, indicating that the left leg is approximately 8 mm shorter.

Step 4: Identify Areas of Deformity

Before templating for the component size and position, the surgeon must identify any areas of deformity around the acetabulum or the femur. On the acetabular side, sites of deformity could include excessive version, osteophytes, dysplasia, retained hardware, or post-traumatic/postsurgical changes related to previous fracture or osteotomy about the acetabulum. Areas of concern on the femoral side may include trochanteric overhang, coxa vara, coxa valga, excessive anteversion, retained hardware, or post-traumatic/postsurgical changes related to previous fracture or osteotomy about the proximal femur. When significant deformity exists on either side of the joint, it might be helpful to template both the normal (unaffected) hip and the diseased hip. Planning reconstruction in the setting of significant deformity is discussed in detail elsewhere in the text.

Step 5: Template the Acetabulum

The acetabulum should always be templated before the femur is templated, because this will establish the center of rotation (COR) for the hip reconstruction. In general terms, the medial edge of the socket should be placed near the ilioischial line to medialize the hip center of rotation. A medialized COR is advantageous because it decreases the joint reactive forces by way of a decrease in the body weight lever arm. The lateral border of the radiographic teardrop may also be used as the intended level of cup medialization, and may even represent a more constant landmark.[27,28] The goal abduction angle is approximately 45 degrees from the pelvic reference line. The size may then be determined as a "best fit" that avoids excessive removal of bone. The amount of lateral coverage is assessed with respect to the previously identified superolateral margin of the native acetabular bone stock (Fig. 62-3). This evaluation will be put to use intraoperatively. For example, if the acetabular component was templated to a position

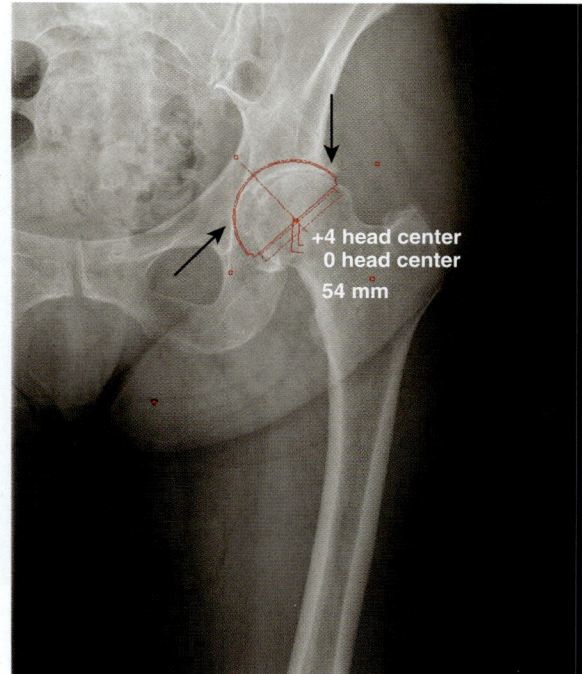

Figure 62-3. In this anteroposterior (AP) radiograph of a left hip, note the position of the templated acetabular component. The medial edge of the socket is immediately adjacent to the ilioischial line (medial arrow). Very good coverage of the socket is seen at the superolateral margin of the acetabulum (superior arrow). As in this case, many acetabular component systems offer both standard and lateralized offset liner options.

flush with the superolateral edge of the native acetabulum, this position should be confirmed under direct visualization in the operating room. If the new socket is recessed inside of this position at the time of surgery, this should alert the surgeon to the possibility of component malposition, such as overmedialization or vertical cup placement (Fig. 62-4A and B).

Once these steps have been performed, the new center of rotation can be marked. It is important to make a notation of the standard hip center, as well as any offset hip center options that may be available with the given acetabular device.

In addition to identifying the implant size and position, the surgeon must now decide whether to proceed with cemented or uncemented acetabular fixation. This decision typically is influenced by surgeon preference and experience, host bone quality, and host activity level.

Finally, once the size and type of acetabular component have been selected, the surgeon will have an idea of the bearing surface options and head sizes available. This information may play a role in decision making regarding the surgical approach to the hip. Patients deemed at higher risk for postoperative instability (e.g., Parkinson's disease, dementia, spasticity, alcoholism, hip fracture) are often treated with large-diameter bearings when possible. If such bearings are not available or

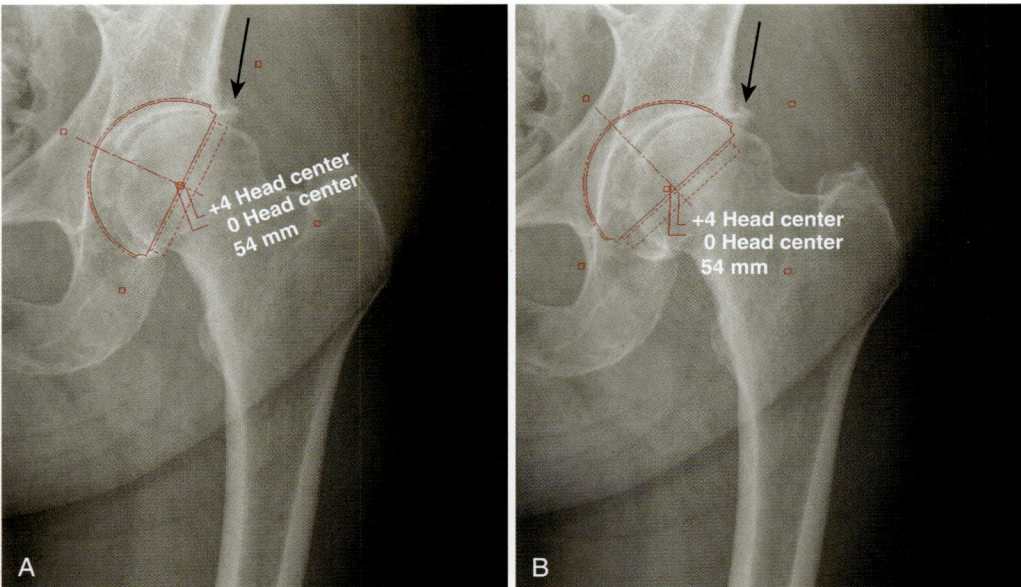

Figure 62-4. Anteroposterior (AP) radiograph of the same patient's left hip. These images simulate what may be noted intraoperatively if the acetabular component **(A)** is placed too far vertically or **(B)** is over-medialized. In both cases, the edge of the component is recessed medial to the previously templated cup position flush with the superolateral margin of the acetabulum *(see arrow)*.

are not desirable within a given acetabular component size range, the surgeon may choose to utilize a surgical approach that is intended to maximize postoperative stability.[29-33]

Step 6: Template the Femur

If the key feature of acetabular templating is establishment of the new hip center of rotation, then key features of femoral templating include establishment of the new hip offset and correction of any leg length discrepancy. The surgeon must determine the goals for leg length correction and hip offset, and then must choose the correct stem that will fulfill these goals.[34] In general terms, the surgeon will first select the intended mode of stem fixation. Most modern cemented stems are available in a variety of sizes and offsets that will allow accurate reconstruction of proper hip biomechanics. The same is true for most modern uncemented stems, including tapered stems, extensively porous-coated stems, and modular stems. The choice of stem fixation type is influenced by surgeon preference and experience, host bone quality, and host activity level.

Once the method of stem fixation is chosen, stem templates are analyzed with respect to size and position within the host bone that will properly restore predetermined biomechanical needs. The stem *size* required is a function of the local anatomy and the nature of each stem's individual design characteristics. The stem *position* within the bone will determine the length and offset.

In the absence of a preoperative leg length discrepancy, the femur is templated in such a way as to place the stem with a standard (+0) head at the same level as the templated hip COR. If a preoperative leg length discrepancy is to be corrected at surgery, the femur is templated with a standard head at a level superior to

the templated COR. For example, to correct 1 cm of shortening, the femur is templated 1 cm superior to the planned COR (Fig. 62-5A and B). Once the femur is templated, the surgeon may make a note of the desired position of the femoral neck osteotomy. This is most often determined with respect to a fixed point on the femur, such as the lesser trochanter, the greater trochanter, or the femoral head.[2,25]

Offset is assessed in a similar fashion. The goal at surgery is typically to maintain, or to slightly increase, the offset of the affected hip with respect to the normal hip.[2,25] A reduction in hip offset may lead to inadequate soft tissue tension and to increased risk of postoperative instability. Occasionally, the surgeon must lengthen the limb to provide the necessary soft tissue tension if the offset cannot be re-established. During femoral templating, the position of a standard (+0) prosthetic femoral head should be assessed with respect to the new acetabular COR. If the templated prosthetic femoral head lies *medial* to the planned COR, an increased offset will result; however, if it lies *lateral* to the planned COR, a decrease in the offset will be produced (Fig. 62-6A and B).

If significant loss of femoral offset is noted during templating, the surgeon should assess whether the offset could be restored with any of the following: a high offset stem, an offset liner, or a different stem design with greater offset. If the templating process reveals a significant gain of femoral offset, it must be determined whether the amount of increased offset is desirable, or if it should be lessened with the use of a more medialized acetabular position or a change in stem design. Bear in mind that the true offset of the native proximal femur may be underestimated if radiographs are obtained with the hips externally rotated.[2]

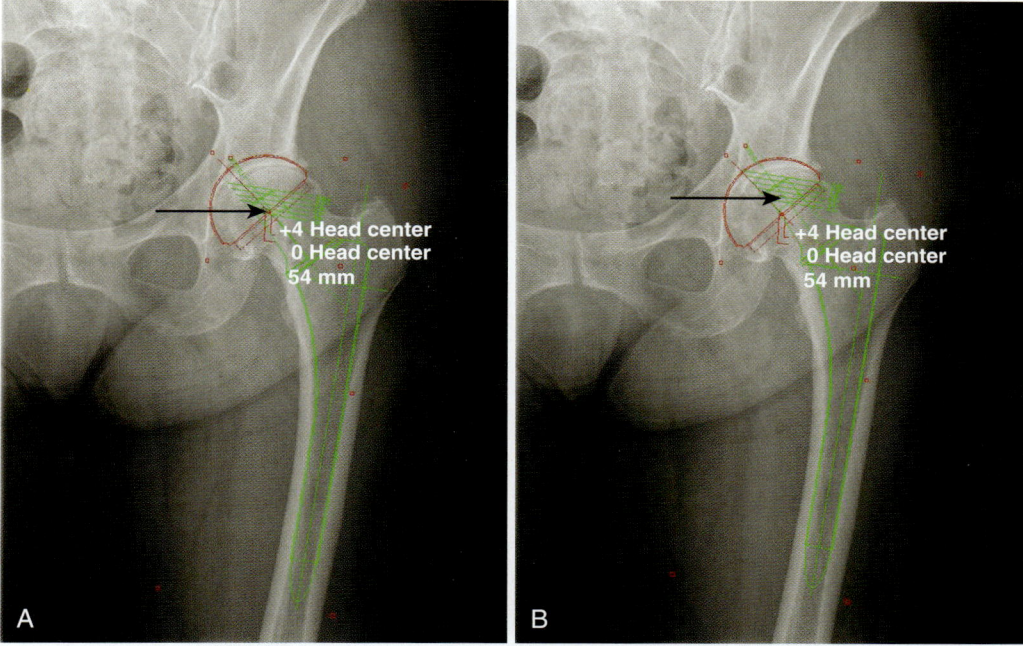

Figure 62-5. Femoral templating is performed on the left hip to correct for approximately 1 cm of shortening of the affected hip. **A,** No change in leg length is effected when the femoral head is templated at the level of the new center of rotation (COR). **B,** The femoral component must be templated in a position 1 cm proximal to this level to effect the intended leg length correction.

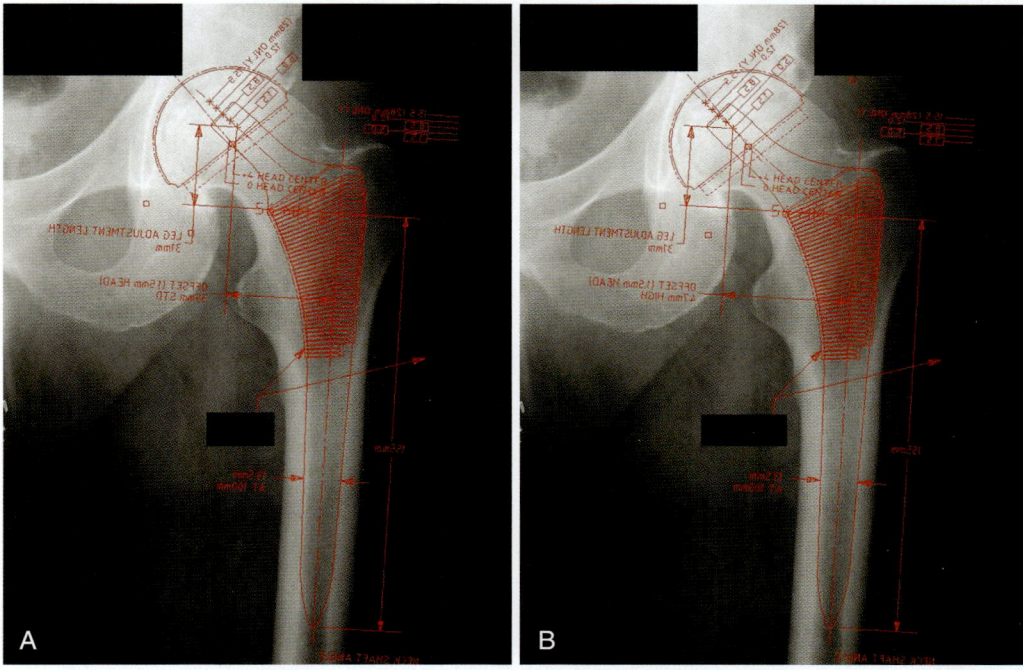

Figure 62-6. This left hip is being templated with both standard and high-offset uncemented stems with the intention of correcting a small leg length inequality, as noted by the position of the templated prosthetic head slightly proximal to the templated center of rotation (COR). **A,** The offset will be maintained when the femoral head lies at the same level in the mediolateral direction as the templated COR. **B,** The high-offset stem moves the femoral head position medial to the templated COR, which will increase the femoral offset.

It is also critical to assess the position of the greater trochanter with respect to the femoral diaphysis. In some cases, significant trochanteric overhang may necessitate special consideration. Preoperative identification of trochanteric overhang might allow the surgeon

to minimize the risk of fracture through alteration of the surgical approach or stem design.

Occasionally, the stem choice will change during this process. For example, the surgeon may begin this process having chosen to utilize an uncemented, tapered stem. During templating, it may become clear that a mismatch exists between metaphyseal size and diaphyseal diameter. If a significant amount of diaphyseal bone would have to be removed for placement of an appropriately sized tapered stem, the surgeon may choose instead to utilize a modular stem or an extensively porous-coated stem that would necessitate less bone removal (Fig. 62-7A through C). Another possibility might be seen in the patient with a wide metaphysis and a wide diaphysis. If the surgeon began templating with an extensively porous-coated stem, it could become clear that this stem would be large and stiff, and the

decision might be made to utilize cemented stem fixation (Fig. 62-8A and B).

Postoperative Needs Assessment

The final phase of preoperative planning involves consideration of each individual patient's postoperative needs. Patients with certain medical needs may require postoperative intensive care unit (ICU) monitoring or the availability of other specialized personnel; this must be arranged preoperatively whenever possible. Needed postoperative bracing or special orthoses should be

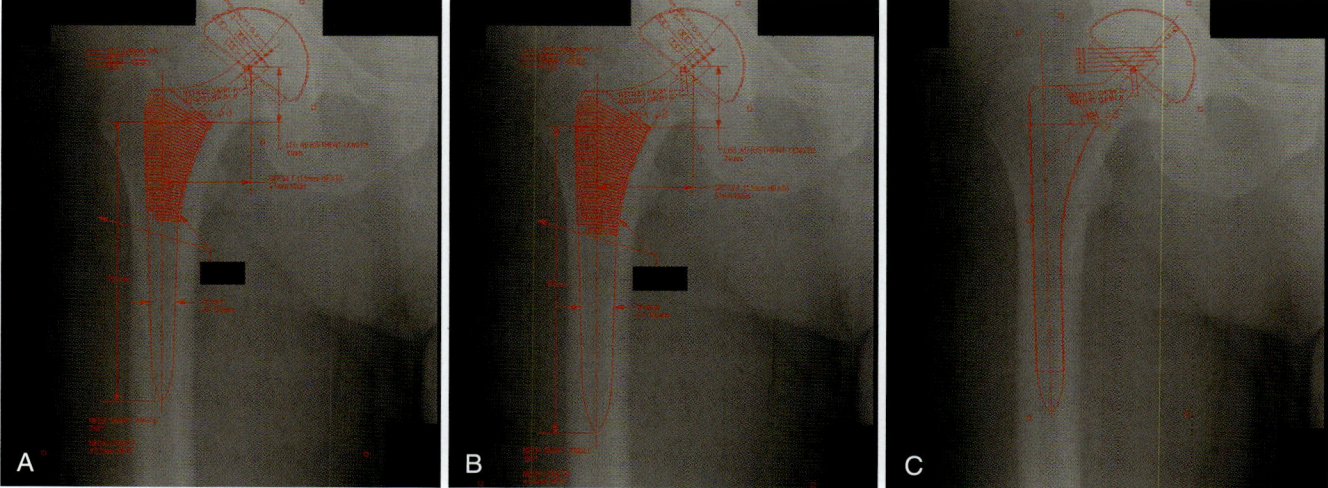

Figure 62-7. In this large patient, a relative mismatch is seen between the metaphysis and the diaphysis. **A,** In templating for a tapered stem, it is noted that diaphyseal contact is achieved before the metaphysis is appropriately filled. **B,** When a larger tapered stem is chosen, a need for substantial diaphyseal reaming is noted. **C,** In this case, an extensively porous-coated, diaphyseal engaging stem is chosen to minimize the bone loss required for stem preparation.

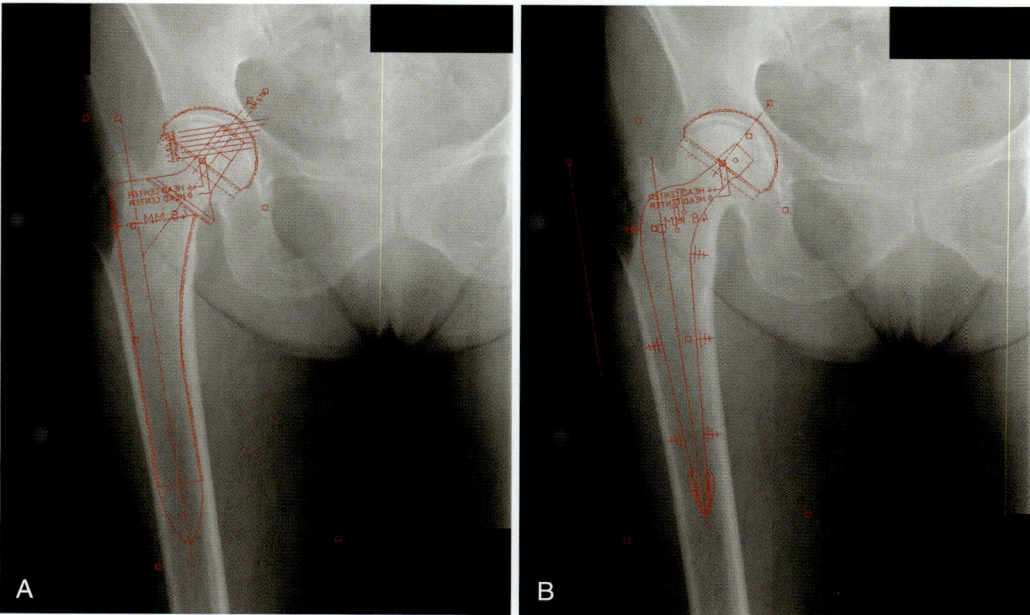

Figure 62-8. This patient presents with both a wide metaphysis and a wide diaphysis. **A,** The extensively porous-coated stem is quite large and would be very stiff. **B,** In this case, a cemented stem is chosen.

planned in advance of surgery to allow timely fitting in the postoperative period. Finally, patients should be counseled preoperatively with respect to post–hospital discharge planning. A realistic assessment of the patient's ability to discharge directly to home should be made preoperatively. Patients who require skilled care in the post-hospital phase of recovery should work on the discharge plan ahead of the surgery to avoid a prolonged hospital stay.

VARIATIONS/UNUSUAL SITUATIONS

The technique described embodies the planning process for most routine hip arthroplasties. Variations in this technique typically apply only to the templating process and are related to areas of deformity or previous surgery. All patients will benefit from the outlined approach to patient selection, radiographic evaluation, host optimization, and postoperative needs assessment. Specific diagnoses that might impart enough deformity to change the templating process include hip dysplasia, prior hip arthrodesis, and previous fracture. Planning for primary total hip arthroplasty for such specific conditions is covered in detail elsewhere in the text.

CURRENT CONTROVERSIES AND FUTURE CONSIDERATIONS

Templating for primary total hip arthroplasty began with direct marking on printed radiographs using acetate implant templates. Over time, digital imaging and digital templating have become more common. Several studies have compared the results of digital versus analogue templating.[6,14,15] Digital templating has been found to be both safe and effective.

CONCLUSION

This chapter has described one method of comprehensive preoperative surgical planning. Key features of this process include patient selection, radiographic evaluation, host optimization, templating, and postoperative needs assessment. Surgeons utilizing such an approach can expect to improve their own efficiency as well as patient outcomes following primary total hip arthroplasty.

REFERENCES

1. Muller ME: Lessons of 30 years of total hip arthroplasty. Clin Orthop Relat Res 274:12–21, 1992.
2. Della Valle AG, Padgett DE, Salvati EA: Preoperative planning for primary total hip arthroplasty. J Am Acad Orthop Surg 13:455–462, 2005.
3. Eggli S, Pisan M, Muller ME: The value of preoperative planning for total hip arthroplasty. J Bone Joint Surg Br 80:382–390, 1998.
4. Bourne RB, Rorabeck CH: Soft tissue balancing: the hip. J Arthroplasty 17(4 Suppl 1):17–22, 2002.
5. Carter LW, Stovall DO, Young TR: Determination of accuracy of preoperative templating of noncemented femoral prostheses. J Arthroplasty 10:507–513, 1995.
6. Iorio R, Siegel J, Specht LM, et al: A comparison of acetate vs digital templating for preoperative planning of total hip arthroplasty: is digital templating accurate and safe? J Arthroplasty 24:175–179, 2009.
7. McAuley JP, Ridgeway SR: Preoperative planning to prevent dislocation of the hip. Orthop Clin North Am 32:579–586, 2001.
8. Schmalzried TP: Preoperative templating and biomechanics in total hip arthroplasty. Orthopedics 28(8 Suppl):s849–s851, 2005.
9. Maloney WJ, Keeney JA: Leg length discrepancy after total hip arthroplasty. J Arthroplasty 19(4 Suppl 1):108–110, 2004.
10. Ranawat CS, Rao RR, Rodriguez JA, et al: Correction of limb-length inequality during total hip arthroplasty. J Arthroplasty 16:715–720, 2001.
11. Ranawat CS, Rodriguez J: Functional leg-length inequality following total hip arthroplasty. J Arthroplasty 12:359–364, 1997.
12. Bono JV: Digital templating in total hip arthroplasty. J Bone Joint Surg Am 86(Suppl 2):118–122, 2004.
13. Crooijmans HJ, Laumen AM, van Pul C, et al: A new digital preoperative planning method for total hip arthroplasties. Clin Orthop Relat Res 467:909–916, 2009.
14. Kosashvili Y, Shasha N, Olschewski E, et al: Digital versus conventional templating techniques in preoperative planning for total hip arthroplasty. Can J Surg 52:6–11, 2009.
15. The B, Verdonschot N, van Horn JR, et al: Digital versus analogue preoperative planning of total hip arthroplasties: a randomized clinical trial of 210 total hip arthroplasties. J Arthroplasty 22:866–870, 2007.
16. Clark CR: Perioperative blood management in total hip arthroplasty. Instr Course Lect 58:167–172, 2009.
17. Marculescu CE, Osmon DR: Antibiotic prophylaxis in orthopedic prosthetic surgery. Infect Dis Clin North Am 19:931–946, 2005.
18. Howe CR, Gardner GC, Kadel NJ: Perioperative medication management for the patient with rheumatoid arthritis. J Am Acad Orthop Surg 14:544–551, 2006.
19. Nowicki P, Chaudhary H: Total hip replacement in renal transplant patients. J Bone Joint Surg Br 89:1561–1566, 2007.
20. Hacek DM, Robb WJ, Paule SM, et al: Staphylococcus aureus nasal decolonization in joint replacement surgery reduces infection. Clin Orthop Relat Res 466:1349–1355, 2008.
21. Rao N, Cannella B, Crossett SS, et al: A preoperative decolonization protocol for Staphylococcus aureus prevents orthopaedic infections. Clin Orthop Relat Res 466:1343–1348, 2008.
22. Geerts WH, Bergqvist D, Pineo GF, et al: Prevention of venous thromboembolism: American College of Chest Physicians evidence-based clinical practice guidelines (8th edition). Chest 133(6 Suppl):381S–453S, 2008.
23. Haas SB, Barrack RL, Westrich G: Venous thromboembolic disease after total hip and knee arthroplasty. Instr Course Lect 58:781–793, 2009.
24. Johanson NA, Lachiewicz PF, Lieberman JR, et al: American Academy of Orthopaedic Surgeons clinical practice guideline on prevention of symptomatic pulmonary embolism in patients undergoing total hip or knee arthroplasty. J Bone Joint Surg Am 91:1756–1757, 2009.
25. Gonzalez AD, Slullitel G, Piccaluga F, et al: The precision and usefulness of preoperative planning for cemented and hybrid primary total hip arthroplasty. J Arthroplasty 20:51–58, 2005.
26. Austin MS, Hozack WJ, Sharkey PF, et al: Stability and leg length equality in total hip arthroplasty. J Arthroplasty 18(3 Pt 2):88–90, 2003.
27. Goodman SB, Adler SJ, Fyhrie DP, et al: The acetabular teardrop and its relevance to acetabular migration. Clin Orthop Relat Res 236:199–204, 1988.
28. Unnanuntana A, Wagner D, Goodman SB: The accuracy of preoperative templating in cementless total hip arthroplasty. J Arthroplasty 24:180–186, 2009.
29. Engh CA Sr: Optimizing stability and leg length. In Lieberman JR, Berry DJ, editors: Advanced reconstruction hip, Rosemont, Ill, 2005, American Academy of Orthopaedic Surgeons, pp 105–112.
30. Lewallen DG: Primary total hip arthroplasty: anterolateral and direct lateral approaches. In Lieberman JR, Berry DJ, editors: Advanced reconstruction hip, Rosemont, Ill, 2005, American Academy of Orthopaedic Surgeons, pp 11–15.

31. Parvizi J, Picinic E, Sharkey PF: Revision total hip arthroplasty for instability: surgical techniques and principles. J Bone Joint Surg Am 90:1134–1142, 2008.

32. Soong M, Rubash HE, Macaulay W: Dislocation after total hip arthroplasty. J Am Acad Orthop Surg 12:314–321, 2004.

33. Woo RY, Morrey BF: Dislocations after total hip arthroplasty. J Bone Joint Surg Am 64:1295–1306, 1982.

34. Garvin KL: Primary total hip arthroplasty: preoperative planning and templating. In Lieberman JR, Berry DJ, editors: Advanced reconstruction hip, Rosemont, Ill, 2005, American Academy of Orthopedic Surgeons, pp 41–46.

SUGGESTED READINGS

Bono JV: Digital templating in total hip arthroplasty. J Bone Joint Surg Am 86(Suppl 2):118–122, 2004.

This article reviews the digital approach to preoperative templating and demonstrates a stepwise approach to the templating process.

Della Valle AG, Padgett DE, Salvati EA: Preoperative planning for primary total hip arthroplasty. J Am Acad Orthop Surg 13:455–462, 2005.

This recent review article discusses the rationale and importance of preoperative planning. The reader will also find a step-by-step guide to proper templating, including cases involving significant deformity (e.g., dysplasia, protrusio, lateralized acetabulum, leg length discrepancy).

Maloney WJ, Keeney JA: Leg length discrepancy after total hip arthroplasty. J Arthroplasty 19(4 Suppl 1):108–110, 2004.

This article reviews the preoperative clinical and radiographic examination of the patient with leg length discrepancy. Intraoperative techniques of leg length assessment are also discussed in detail.

Ranawat CS, Rao RR, Rodriguez JA, et al: Correction of limb-length inequality during total hip arthroplasty. J Arthroplasty 16:715–720, 2001.

This article reviews in detail a comprehensive approach to the correction of leg length discrepancy during total hip arthroplasty (THA). The authors describe preoperative evaluation, templating, and surgical execution of the appropriate plan.

CHAPTER 63

Resurfacing Hip Arthroplasty: Evolution, Design, Indications, and Results

Michael L. Caravelli and Thomas Parker Vail

KEY POINTS

- The success of the first generation of resurfacing implants was limited by inferior manufacturing processes and materials that were the best available at the time.
- Improvements in the understanding of tribology; improvements in materials, design, and surgical technique; and the insight of clinicians have led to the evolution of contemporary resurfacing designs, which in many cases have limited the early failure mechanisms previously seen.
- Successful RHA does have its limitations. The technique is challenging, results are not consistent, the number of patients ideally indicated for the procedure is limited, and the consequences of unanticipated wear mechanisms and the local effects of metal ions remain unresolved.
- Clinical reports of success with hip resurfacing in the most demanding cohort of joint arthroplasty patients support its continued use and development.

INTRODUCTION

Modern total hip arthroplasty is considered one of the most successful surgical treatments ever developed. Its current form resulted from an evolution of ideas starting in the late 19th century. Resurfacing hip arthroplasty (RHA) is one adaptation along the course of this evolution. RHA was conceptualized and then championed as a technique that better replicated the normal anatomy of the hip and conserved host bone. In its early clinical application, RHA was met with unanticipated complications including femoral fracture, osteonecrosis, materials failure, and implant loosening. Today, with the advent of bearing material improvements and better understanding of tribology as related to large-diameter hip bearings, RHA remains a viable option for hip reconstruction in properly indicated patients. Issues and concerns associated with patient selection, risks associated with metal bearings, and exacting surgical techniques continue to limit wide adoption of the technology.

HISTORY AND EVOLUTION

Before 1900, treatment for osteoarthritis of the hip was dominated by joint excision and amputation. Toward the end of the 19th century, interest developed in interpositional materials that were founded on the successes of Heinrich Helferich, who used interpositional tissue successfully to treat temporomandibular joint arthritis.[1] The lack of reliable results of interposition forced the development of other techniques. Marius Smith-Petersen, in Boston, Massachusetts, is credited with the development in 1923 of the concept of mould arthroplasty, a technique that may be considered the grandparent to resurfacing hip arthroplasty (RHA). Smith-Petersen conceptualized mould arthroplasty as the introduction of a biologically inert material that would be removed after it successfully served to "guide nature's repair so that defects would be eliminated."[2] Unfortunately, because of the formation of fibrocartilage beneath the mould, the material was not mechanically stable; thus this procedure did not become the expected panacea. In most cases, the mould was left in place, serving as a permanent rather than a temporary interpositional graft. From these origins, the procedure, which was initially conceived as a temporary interposition, evolved into a more permanent femoral hemiresurfacing. The *mould arthroplasty* concept came to be referred to in the literature as *cup arthroplasty*. The cup substrate material evolved over time, starting with the original glass and transitioning through viscaloid, pyrex, and vitallium. Outcomes for these devices did show some early benefit in terms of pain control, but gait, motion, material performance, and consequently implant survival were unpredictable.[3-9]

Parallel to the development of cup arthroplasty was the introduction of a femoral endoprosthesis. The Judet brothers, in 1950, garnered popularity for their published *resection-reconstruction technique,* which involved implantation of a femoral component made from an acrylic resin. Their favorable early results set the stage for further development of resurfacing implants, but limited ability to withstand stresses at the hip joint and acetabular erosion caused by the articulation with acrylic material posed significant problems.[10]

Sir John Charnley was given credit for developing the first total resurfacing arthroplasty. He had developed a two-piece low-friction resurfacing device made of Teflon (polytetrafluoroethylene) that unfortunately failed rapidly as the result of wear. Although Teflon had very favorable low-friction characteristics, it proved vulnerable to shear loading and abrasive wear. After Charnley's attempt to resurface the proximal femur, a number of devices came to the foreground. In 1960, Townley introduced the total articular resurfacing arthroplasty (TARA), a metal-on-polyurethane bearing with a stemmed resurfacing femoral component. Townley changed the socket to polyethylene, but his rate of failure from aseptic loosening due to frictional torque or osteolysis from the large-diameter head still was unacceptably high.[11,12] In 1967, Maurice Muller created a metal-on-metal (MOM) surface replacement. Reportedly, he abandoned the MOM device in favor of the low-friction metal-on-polyethylene (MOP) total hip arthroplasty in 1968, also because of problems of loosening attributed to high frictional torque through the bearing, which caused untimely disruption of the bone-cement interface.[13] Gerard, in 1970, took a different approach, unifying the concepts of hemiresurfacing of the femur and "mould arthroplasty." He resurfaced the femur with a Luck cup and inserted it into an Aufranc cup that approximated the diameter of the host acetabulum. Treatment of pain over the short term was acceptable, but after 2 years, complications due to resorption of femoral bone, femoral fracture, and acetabular medialization were seen.[14] RHA implant systems, also referred to in the literature as *socket-cup devices,* out of Japan with MOP bearings were reported over short-term to mid-term time periods. Furuya, in 1971, created a socket-cup arthroplasty that, despite alterations in bearing materials, required revision to total hip arthroplasty in 7 out of 12 cases.[15] Nishio, in 1972, designed an uncemented socket and cup replacement of the hip. He reported that 86% of patients had pain relief and only 3 of 67 hips required revision.[16] Tanaka's hybrid arthroplasty with a cemented polyethylene acetabulum and uncemented femoral component yielded pain relief in 97% of patients, and no component revisions were required at the time of publication.[17] In Italy, the Paltrinieri-Trentani surface arthroplasty was implanted, with 12% of cases failing as the result of neck fracture or component loosening.[18] The efforts of Freeman, Wagner, Eicher and Capello, Amstutz, and Buechel and Pappas were comparable.[19-23]

Cumulative review of the results of first-generation resurfacing devices revealed two main complications. First, the interaction of the large bearing surfaces caused high frictional torque, presumably causing loosening of the socket, and the hard-on-soft articulation led to higher levels of volumetric wear and acetabular osteolysis. Second, there was a high incidence of femoral neck fracture presumably due to notching of the superior neck—a practice that was accepted because of the contemporary teaching that the femoral component should be in 140 degrees of valgus for proper stress transfer through the components. With the guarded results of RHA and the international success that Charnley enjoyed with his low-friction arthroplasty concept, the orthopedic community weighted the effort of innovation toward optimizing the MOP total hip arthroplasty (THA). Although these first-generation resurfacing

devices differed in form, the consistent rationale in this era was the belief that these procedures were bone conserving and were indicated for patients younger than 60 years, in whom a Charnley low-friction THA was relatively contraindicated because of the greater difficulty and likelihood of future revision. Charnley's low-friction THA had become the preferred procedure for patients older than 60 years; however, a predictable solution for treating the young patient with hip osteoarthritis still was not clear. Experience gained during these years did help build an appreciation for the meticulous technique and sound design required for successful use of RHA.

Metal-on-metal (MOM) bearings were introduced during the early development of hip arthroplasty as a low-wear, low-friction, durable, and biologically stable bearing combination. The Muller, McKee-Farrar, Ring, Wiles, Stanmore, and Sivash total hip systems and various hemiarthroplasty combinations were being used at the time. Results with MOM bearings in these first-generation implants were not satisfactory.[13] A high rate of component loosening due to frictional torque, equatorial seizing of matched bearings, fatigue fracture of the acetabulum, and infection; concern about systemic effects of metal ions; and the early success of the Charnley THA played a role in sidelining the MOM bearing. A rejuvenation of interest in MOM bearings emerged in the late 1980s. Published comparative studies between the McKee-Farrar and Charnley implants demonstrated comparable mid- to long-term survival of MOM bearings, stimulating discussion and further development of the technology.[24,25] From 1983 to 1988, Bernard Weber and Sulzer Orthopaedics manufactured the Metasul bearing. The design consisted of a CoCrMo alloy bearing with a 28-mm or 32-mm metal head articulating with a metal socket as an inlay in polyethylene. RHA components were designed by Heinz Wagner and Derek McMinn. The Wagner RHA, introduced between 1990 and 1992, had an inlay-forged CoCrMo articulating surface with a grit-blasted titanium surface coating at the bone interfaces. The McMinn prosthesis, introduced between 1991 and 1993, had a cast CoCrMo design with an acetabular component with hydroxyapatite (HA) coating and peripheral fins for rotational stability. Both designs led to improved results in terms of loosening, and neither was associated with femoral fracture.[23,26]

Concurrently, efforts were being made to improve acetabular component fixation in total hip arthroplasty. Aseptic loosening of cemented acetabular components was a considerable problem at mid-term follow-up.[27,28] Jones and Hungerford and Jasty and associates published early works on the pathophysiology of this problem.[29,30] Porous-coated acetabular components that would achieve biological fixation were developed. The Harris-Galante cup and the porous-coated monatomic (PCA) cup were two of the early prototypes. By the mid-1990s, sufficient evidence and positive survivorship data supported the durability of porous-coated acetabular components.[28,31-33]

With advanced knowledge of large bearing function and the possibility of a durable biological cementless

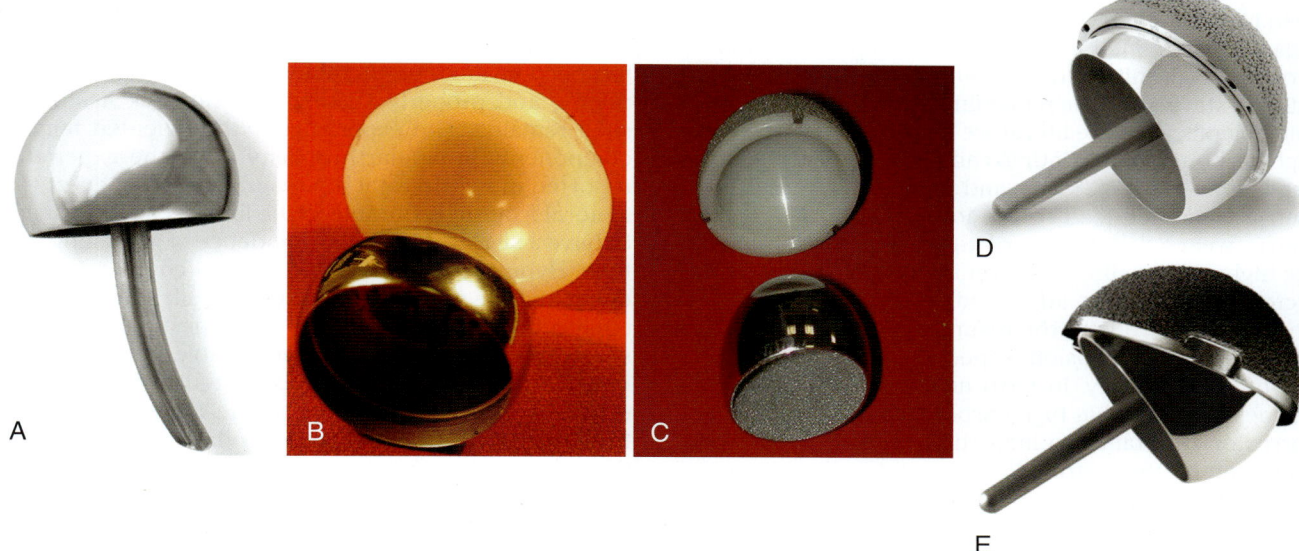

Figure 63-1. A, Total articular resurfacing arthroplasty (TARA) hemiresurfacing component. **B,** Total hip articular replacement by internal eccentric shells (THARIES) resurfacing components. **C,** Porous surface replacement (PSR). **D,** Birmingham resurfacing components. **E,** Conserve Plus (Wright Medical Technology, Arlington, TN) resurfacing components.

acetabular fixation, the stage was now set for development of the RHA systems that are currently in use. An evolution over four decades resulted in improvements in materials, acetabular fixation, bearing function, and implant technique. Figure 63-1 illustrates an evolution from femoral hemiresurfacing to MOP bearings to the current MOM bearings.

The Wagner prosthesis was manufactured by Protek AG (Bern, Switzerland), a company founded by Maurice Muller. The McMinn prosthesis underwent a series of evolutions through Corin Medical to become the Cormet 2000 (Corin Medical, Cirencester, Glos, United Kingdom) and subsequently the Birmingham Hip (Smith and Nephew, London, United Kingdom). Harlan Amstutz after his initial work with the THARIES (total hip articular replacement by internal eccentric shells) resurfacing components developed the Conserve Plus system with Orthomet (Minneapolis, Minn), a company that was purchased by Wright Medical (Clarion, Iowa). Biomet (Warsaw, Ind) designed the ReCap system. DePuy (Warsaw, Ind) designed the articular surface replacement (ASR) system. Zimmer (Warsaw, Ind) designed the Durom system. The final common system was a hybrid design with a cementless acetabular component and a cemented femoral component. This is the current standard.

DESIGN

Tribology is the study of interacting surfaces in tangential motion. The main principles that define this interaction are friction, lubrication, and wear. Its study, therefore, includes material properties of the bearing surfaces, bearing geometry, joint kinematics, and load patterns. These properties are then modified by the dynamic interaction between surfaces manifested by joint lubrication, joint kinematics, and contact area. A brief review of these material properties facilitates understanding of the evolution of design of RHA components.

Friction is an extrinsic force that develops from the interaction of two moving solid objects. Its magnitude is a result of the physical and chemical microstructure of the contacting surfaces. Early MOM components were believed to have failed early as the result of high frictional torque that disrupted the skeletal fixation, clinically manifested by early acetabular loosening.[34,35] In an acetabular bearing, frictional torque (Q) is determined by the formula $Q = \mu R r$, where μ is the friction coefficient, R is the vertical component of the load in the plane of measurement, and r is the radius of the femoral head.[36] In simplistic terms, the frictional torque is proportional to the coefficient of friction between articulating surfaces, the load, and the radius of the femoral head. A catastrophic example of excessive frictional torque would be instantaneous cup displacement or fracture of the cement mantle or host bone, but frictional torque in an MOM implant has been shown to be an order of magnitude less than would be required for this to occur in a metal-on-polyethylene bearing.[37,38] Lower levels of frictional torque over time, however, can be quantified by progressive component loosening and wear, defined as erosion of material from a solid surface due to its interaction with another surface.

The measurement of wear is of much greater importance in evaluating these articulating materials because of the clinical implications of osteolysis and subsequent aseptic loosening. The dominant wear modes seen in hip arthroplasty are adhesive, abrasive, and corrosive. Specifically, with MOM implants, adhesive wear, because of the self-polishing ability of CoCrMo alloys and matched bearing hardness, is less prominent than that seen in unmatched bearing couples. Wear in MOM bearings, as determined in hip simulator studies, is characterized by an initial "running-in" period followed by a "steady-state" over the remaining lifetime of the implant. Conclusions from the literature have demonstrated that high carbon content CoCrMo alloys (>0.20% C), femoral heads greater than 28 mm, and the lowest practical diametric clearance lead to the lowest quantitative volumetric wear.[39-41] With regard to carbon distribution in the high-carbon alloy, however, there have been contradictory results that still need to be worked out.[42,43] Another concern with the resurgence of MOM bearings is the effect of corrosion, especially with higher levels of Co^{2+} systemically. In vitro analysis by Yan and colleagues suggests that high-carbon alloys have sufficient corrosion resistance to limit the total volumetric wear produced by the bearing.[44]

Lubrication conditions seen in MOM bearings exert a significant influence on volumetric wear. Lubrication regimens include boundary lubrication, mixed lubrication, and fluid film lubrication. Boundary lubrication relies on physicochemical interactions between lubricating fluid, any additives, and contacting solid surfaces. Fluid film lubrication occurs with entrainment of lubricant between interacting solid surfaces, preventing their contact. Mixed lubrication demonstrates characteristics of both. Theoretical predictions of the predominant lubrication regimen are made with the lambda ratio: Λ = Theoretical minimum film thickness/Composite surface roughness. A $\Lambda \leq 1$ leads to boundary lubrication, $1 \leq \Lambda \leq 3$ leads to mixed lubrication, and $\Lambda \geq 3$ leads to fluid film lubrication.[36] Modern manufacturing techniques have succeeded in producing accurate bearing geometry and highly polished bearing surfaces that optimize the potential for articulation in the fluid film lubrication regimen. Fluid film thickness is influenced by diametric clearance of the bearing, defined as the distance between the outer diameter of the convex surface and the inner diameter of the concave surface. Recommended diametric clearances typically are based on in vitro data, but the smallest practical clearance that will not lead to equatorial seizing, along with a femoral articulating surface that deviates less than 10 μm from sphericity and surface roughness less than 0.05 μm, maximizes the potential for the articulation to operate in the fluid film lubrication regimen. It is also important to point out the need for a durable acetabular component that undergoes minimal deformation with implantation, as this can alter the expected clearance.[45,46]

Aside from the tribologic requirements for a successful RHA bearing are biological considerations including the potential for biological fixation. As was discussed earlier, first-generation RHA components and MOM bearings with large-diameter heads experienced short-term failure from acetabular component loosening. The cause of these early failures likely was multifactorial and included inferior component fixation with early-generation cement techniques, high levels of wear particles caused by a large-diameter metal head articulating with conventional polyethylene, and higher frictional

torque than was seen with the 22-mm articulation used by Charnley. With the evolution of porous-coated sockets, biological fixation of the acetabular component has become more predictable. Yet the challenge of positioning and properly seating a monoblock acetabular shell remains. The experience with cemented femoral components in hemiarthroplasty[47] and the experience reported in hybrid total hip resurfacing[26,48] suggest that femoral fixation is durable in the first decade but seems to have a slightly increasing incidence of loosening over time. Hypothesized causes of femoral component loosening include selection of cases with structurally inadequate host bone, osteolysis from particulate debris, stress shielding causing undesirable femoral neck remodeling, host bone necrosis related to thermal properties of cement or damage to the blood supply, and fracture. If local bone necrosis is related to the cement, there may be some theoretical advantage of using a cementless femoral component, provided that biological fixation could be achieved. Several groups have published their early results on cementless femoral resurfacing prostheses, but no consensus has been reached on their clinical application or durability at this time.[49-51]

INDICATIONS

RHA is indicated as an alternative to total hip replacement in a select group of patients with good proximal femoral bone quality for whom a metal-on-metal bearing is an acceptable risk. The key to defining proper indications for RHA is to identify when the risk-to-benefit ratio for RHA is more favorable than the risk-to-benefit ratio for THA. Current indications include the patient for whom the benefits of bone conservation are maximal. Thus, the ideal candidate is generally younger and consequently has a higher likelihood of ipsilateral revision, desires a high-activity lifestyle, and possesses good proximal femoral bone quality. Registry data suggest that smaller size, female gender, and age over 70 years may predispose to greater risk of complications or reoperation, and younger, larger male patients may be the better candidates.[52,53]

The most difficult challenge associated with THA performance has traditionally been associated with the young and active male patient. Lower component survivorship rates in this population due to wear and osteolysis have been hypothesized to be a result of insufficient ability of the bearing material and implants to tolerate increased activity levels and an extended life span.[54] The young patient after any arthroplasty, therefore, has a significantly greater probability of requiring revision hip reconstruction in the future, although low risk in the first decade, periprosthetic fracture, bone loss due to stress shielding, infection, and substrate failure remain long-term concerns with total hip replacement. The typical patient for whom RHA is considered has symptomatic hip osteoarthritis, is between 30 and 60 years of age (average age 49, compared with 67 for THA),[55] and is still employed and physically active. Current data from the Central Intelligence Agency estimate average life expectancy in the United States to be 78.11 years.[56] This would require many of these young patients to get well more than 20 years from the time of receiving their implants—an achievement that cannot be reliably expected based on current survivorship results. Unfortunately, results of revision hip reconstruction are inferior to those of primary reconstruction. Higher rates of dislocation, perioperative and postoperative complications, lower functional scores, and decreased implant survivorship have been demonstrated after revision hip reconstruction.[57-60] RHA offers a potential alternative to the failed total hip scenario in that the femoral resurfacing component can be revised to a stemmed femoral component—a procedure that is less demanding, technically, than a standard femoral component revision. Conversion of resurfacing to a total hip has been shown in small series to be a stable, durable alternative to THA over the short and mid-term that does not appear to limit the effectiveness of THA.[61,62] Nevertheless, it must be recognized that the complexity of revising a hip resurfacing device is related to the diagnosis at the time of revision. Patients with uncomplicated fracture or aseptic loosening can be more easily revised with higher functional expectations than patients revised because of an adverse soft tissue reaction that causes local tissue destruction with muscle necrosis.

Not all of the proposed advantages of hip resurfacing have been proved. Proposed advantages of RHA include femoral bone preservation, uncomplicated revision in most cases, a low dislocation rate, durability of the metal-bearing couple, and a more physiologic reconstruction as measured by an improved gait pattern and fewer activity limitations. Risks associated with RHA, on the other hand, are not theoretical and have been well described in the literature. Some complications of hip resurfacing have been related to early experience and a "learning curve."[63-65] Higher rates of component loosening, primarily on the femoral side, may be due to patient selection and technical issues such as cement technique and component malposition. Causes of aseptic loosening of the acetabular component differ little from those of THA and include failure to achieve primary fixation, full component seating, and impingement. Progressive femoral neck narrowing, femoral neck fracture, femoral head-neck necrosis, acetabular and femoral component loosening, and sequelae from metal particles are the most frequent complications associated with RHA. Acetabular malposition in RHA such as a high lateral opening angle or increased anteversion may predispose to edge loading, which has been shown to elevate wear rates and both systemic and local ion levels.[66] The consequences of metal particles and ions have yet to be fully and conclusively elucidated. However, it is clear that a spectrum of local tissue reactions from benign to severe is associated with exposure to metal ions. These reactions have been described as having features of hypersensitivity, as demonstrated by perivascular lymphocytic infiltration. More dramatic clinical presentations with pain and local fluid accumulation, fibrosis, and muscle and tendon necrosis have been described in association with high local levels of chromium and cobalt ions. This potential led to a medical device alert in April and May of 2010 from the Medicines and Healthcare Products Regulatory Agency, an agency of the Department of Health in the United Kingdom.[67-70]

RHA is an acceptable option when there does not exist a major biomechanical problem such as leg length discrepancy, coxa vara, or a severe sequela of a childhood hip disorder such as developmental dysplasia (DDH) or Perthes disease. Although it is possible to make some minor changes in the location of the hip center when placing the acetabular component during hip resurfacing, it is not possible to lengthen the leg or increase the offset substantially. Success rates with resurfacing have been lower with DDH, Perthes, and osteonecrosis of the femoral head than with osteoarthritis, in part because of the biomechanical limitations of a resurfacing construct. Abnormal femoral morphology described as a head-to-neck ratio less than 1.2, short neck length, femoral head cysts larger than 1 cm, and decreased bone density increases the risk of femoral neck fracture.[71,72]

Absolute contraindications to RHA, similar to THA, include active infection of the hip joint and the presence of systemic infection. Patients with known metal hypersensitivity should be avoided, although presently no test is predictive of clinical problems for a joint implant related to metal sensitivity. Patients with renal insufficiency are not good candidates for resurfacing because ions released from the bearing surface are cleared through the kidneys. Women of childbearing age should be approached with caution or eliminated from consideration for hip resurfacing because of known potential for fetal exposure by metal ions and lack of complete understanding of potential adverse effects to a fetus of ion exposure.

RESULTS

Validation for the use of RHA even in properly indicated patients requires evidence supporting its benefit versus contemporary total hip arthroplasty. Failures in early-generation RHA were due to component loosening, femoral neck fracture, and osteolysis. Although all of these failure mechanisms are reported with today's devices, tribologic and design advances have decreased the incidence of these complications substantially. Current published revision rates are 2% to 7% over 2 to 5 years of follow-up.[67,73-81] RHA and conventional stemmed implants with cobalt chrome on highly cross-linked polyethylene (HXPE) bearing can be compared on the basis of cost-effectiveness, implant survival, stability, overall complication rates, and functional results. Potential failure mechanisms unique to RHA with an MOM bearing include femoral neck fracture, failure of the femoral component, local ion effects on soft tissue, and systemic release of metal ions.

In 2009, a utilization analysis on the use of metal bearings was published by Bozic and coworkers.[82] Bearing surface use was compared with demographic data, and the frequency of MOM bearing use was found to be related to the following: (1) patient age younger than 65 years, (2) patient age greater than 65 years with private insurance, (3) patient sex, with males more likely to have received an MOM bearing, and (4) surgery performed in the Midwest, South, or West.[82] Previously published data by McKenzie and associates were not able to demonstrate the cost-effectiveness of MOM RHA until revision rates were less than those seen in primary THA. Their study, however, was limited in the quantity of data available at the time of publication related to RHA outcomes.[83] Current published data from our institution, based on demographics and utilization data, suggest that MOM RHA may be clinically effective and cost-effective for men younger than 60 years and for women younger than 50 years.[52]

Cumulative survival data in RHA are limited to 5 to 10 years. Current analyses demonstrate contemporary RHA implant design survival rates ranging from 95% to 99.8%.[48,64,67,73-80,84-87] Although these optimistic rates have been seen in the short and early mid-term, other studies of first-generation RHA devices show dramatic decreases in survival at 4 years—a finding that promotes healthy concerns about the long-term viability of contemporary systems.[88] Survival rates of primary cementless THA in all comers are comparable at similar duration of follow-up with current RHA. Comparative data from the Australian Joint Registry support these findings.[75] Also remarkable and somewhat a matter of concern is the variability in revision rates by hospital, surgeon, and implant. Rates of survival in younger patients are often questioned, but McAuley and associates showed that survivorship for all THA components at 5 years in patients younger than 50 years nears 97%.[54] Femoral component survival alone was no different. McAuley's review of other series shows component survival of cementless stems to be 93% to 100%. The nearest direct comparison in the literature comes from Pollard and colleagues,[89] who studied RHA versus hybrid THA in age-matched patients (average 50 years old) followed for a mean of 80 months. Eight percent of hybrid THAs required revision—three patients for osteolysis and one for instability. Six percent of RHA patients required revision. All four required revision for femoral component failure.[89] Subsets of larger male patients undergoing RHA have demonstrated superior survival when compared with cementless total hip arthroplasty in large registry comparisons.[90] No comparative data exist to distinguish hybrid versus cementless RHA.

Advocates of RHA since its inception have focused on bone preservation as a primary benefit of the procedure relative to THA. This is related primarily to the femoral side. It is on the femoral side that most complications, including component loosening and fracture, have been seen. On the other hand, contemporary cementless acetabular components used for RHA or THA vary little in the amount of host bone required for insertion. A theoretical benefit of femoral bone preservation is the ease of revision in the setting of femoral component failure. Clinical support of this observation has been illustrated by Ball and colleagues and McGrath and coworkers.[61,62] Investigators performed direct

comparisons of femoral failures of RHA converted to THA. Functional outcomes were similar between groups in both studies. Intraoperative variables, including operative blood loss and duration of hospitalization, were not significantly different. Operative time was significantly longer in the conversion group in McGrath's study, but was statistically similar in the trial of Ball and associates. Radiographic evaluation demonstrated equivalent achievement of biological fixation in the two groups. One femoral stem became loose 1 year after conversion in the McGrath's cohort. Complications in the Ball study included the following: in the conversion group: a femoral nerve palsy, intraoperative femur fracture, and postoperative myocardial infarction; in the primary THA group, two femur fractures (one intraoperative and one postoperative periprosthetic), three femoral nerve palsies, and one deep infection. In the McGrath cohort, reported complications included peroneal nerve palsy and a dislocation in the conversion group with no reported complications in the primary THA group. In summary, conversion of RHA to THA in the setting of femoral failure is comparable in terms of safety, clinical outcomes, and technical execution.[61,62] Direct comparisons, to our knowledge, between RHA conversions and THA revisions have not been done.

As was mentioned earlier, complications of greater concern with contemporary RHA include femoral component loosening and fracture and local and systemic effects of metal ion release. Other complications shared between RHA and primary THA include perioperative medical complications, venous thromboembolism, nerve injury, dislocation, and formation of heterotopic ossification. These complications are reviewed in detail elsewhere in this text.

Retention of femoral head and neck bone introduces the potential for unique complications related to RHA. Stress distribution in a resurfaced femoral head is intended to pass through the primary compressive trabeculae. Preparation of the femur or notching of the neck, theoretically, can lead to stress risers in the retained femoral bone. The varus and external rotation moment created with weight bearing can then lead to fracture. One can understand how sensitive the complication of femoral neck fracture, in the setting of RHA, is in terms of surgical technique and bone quality. Reported series have published femoral neck fracture rates of 1.5%,[91] 1.7%,[92] 1%,[48] and 2.8% (0.4% after the first 70 cases).[63] Another potential cause contributing to femoral loosening consequent to femoral preparation is interruption of the femoral head and neck blood supply with subsequent osteonecrosis. Beaulé and coworkers[93] showed decreased blood flow signal after cylindrical reaming of the femur. The clinical consequences of injury to the blood supply from femoral preparation manifesting as osteonecrosis and loosening are not clearly defined.

Local and systemic effects of metal ions have been frequently discussed but clinically less often encountered in the setting of RHA and MOM THA. Benefits of MOM articulations include stability due to large-diameter heads (LDHs), durability, and lower volumetric wear rates, decreasing the potential for osteolysis that causes aseptic loosening. MOM articulations, however, produce low levels of local and systemic cobalt and chromium ions, about whose long-term effects and target tissues we currently have limited understanding. Pain, joint effusions, aseptic loosening, and osteolysis have been reported as potential complications of delayed-type metal hypersensitivity reaction and/or release of metal ions.[69,94,95] Increased acetabular anteversion and inclination have been demonstrated to increase the volume of metal ion release, perhaps as the result of a less favorable lubrication regimen or impingement.[96] The effect of bearing size in the literature is equivocal.[97,98] The osteolytic potential of these particles is not completely understood.

RHA was envisioned as a more physiologic alternative to a total hip in that it more accurately restored the native hip center and offset. Dislocation rates in the literature range from 0 to 1.5% in RHA[26,64,99] and from 2% to 5% in THA.[100,101] RHA, employing LDHs and MOM bearings, limits intrinsic instability, but the consequences of bearing wear are not yet clear. Use of larger-diameter heads has decreased the incidence of dislocation by increasing the jump distance.[102-104] The in vivo wear rate and the capacity to generate clinically significant osteolysis in MOM bearings, however, are still awaiting long-term follow-up.[105] HXPE, over the short term and mid-term, appears to have decreased rates of osteolysis and aseptic loosening, but clinical experience is insufficient to predict survivorship at 20 to 30 years. Current data suggest that femoral head penetration rates on HXPE are consistently lower than rates seen in conventional ultrahigh-molecular-weight polyethylene.[106-111] Only Geerdink and associates, with a mean 8-year follow-up, have shown significantly lower rates of osteolysis radiographically with HXPE.[108]

Range-of-motion (ROM) and activity differences in the literature have shown favorable results. Vail and colleagues in a comparison study of primary THA versus RHA showed statistically significant increases in overall ROM and hip flexion.[81] The cohort reported by Back and coworkers had hip flexion of 110.41 degrees.[74] Lavigne and associates,[112] on the other hand, in attempting to control for the potential bias of larger femoral heads and patient selection in RHA, showed no significant difference when comparing LDH THA versus RHA. Gait pattern study has yielded equivocal results, but Mont and colleagues, with better-matched patient groups than were seen in previous studies, demonstrated improved speed and kinetic measurements that neared normal values.[113] Evidence of return to athletic activity has been demonstrated.[114] Limited published data have concluded demonstrably superior clinical function versus similar patients treated with THA, but Lavigne and coworkers in 2008 showed a significant increase in the level of athletic participation using validated functional outcome measurements.[115] Functional outcomes of a well-functioning total hip and a well-functioning hip resurfacing seem to be comparable with patients demonstrating the capability to participate in high activity with either type of implant.

FUTURE DIRECTIONS AND CURRENT CONTROVERSIES

RHA was introduced originally to provide a solution for young patients whose activity level and longevity would exceed the functional limits of Charnley's low-friction arthroplasty. The future of resurfacing lies with the same clinical dilemma that was apparent in Charnley's early days. Because the lower limit of age for patients undergoing arthroplasty now dips often into the third and fourth decades, we cannot be certain that any option available today will last a lifetime.

Current controversies regarding resurfacing center upon whether the technology should be reserved for only the most ideal candidates; whether the risk of femoral neck fracture, component loosening, and exposure to metal ions is balanced by the value of bone conservation; and whether the procedure is so technically challenging that it should be limited to certain surgeons or centers. Given these concerns, future directions must address metal ion issues through changes or improvements in materials that minimize or eliminate metal ion exposure. Implants must be designed for the most extreme loading conditions, which might include complete subluxation of the articulation onto the rim of the acetabular component during the course of physical activity. Retrievals must be analyzed to extract the secrets associated with well-functioning bearings and the problems that lead to failure. Finally, instrumentation, education, and training must be optimized to eliminate the variability in results that is reflected in today's registries.

REFERENCES

1. Grigoris P, Roberts P, Panousis K, Bosch H: The evolution of hip resurfacing arthroplasty. Orthop Clin North Am 36:125–134, vii, 2005.
2. Smith-Petersen MN: Evolution of mould arthroplasty of the hip joint. J Bone Joint Surg Am 30:59–75, 1948.
3. Bickel WH, Babb FS: Cup arthroplasty of the hip. J Bone Joint Surg Am 30:647–656, 1948.
4. Law WA: Post-operative study of vitallium mould arthroplasty of the hip joint. J Bone Joint Surg Am 30:76–83, 1948.
5. Law WA: Hip joint reconstruction by vitallium mould arthroplasty. Rheumatism 3:157–161, 1948.
6. Gibson A: Vitallium-cup arthroplasty of the hip joint: review of approximately 100 cases. J Bone Joint Surg Am 31:861–868, 1949.
7. Stinchfield FE, Carroll RE: Vitallium-cup arthroplasty of the hip joint: an end-result study. J Bone Joint Surg Am 31:628–638, 1949.
8. Adams JC: A reconsideration of cup arthroplasty of the hip, with a precise method of concentric arthroplasty. J Bone Joint Surg Br 35:199–208, 1953.
9. Aufranc OE: Constructive hip surgery with the vitallium mold; a report on 1,000 cases of arthroplasty of the hip over a fifteen-year period. J Bone Joint Surg Am 39:237–248; passim, 1957.
10. Judet J, Judet R: The use of an artificial femoral head for arthroplasty of the hip joint. J Bone Joint Surg Br 32:166–173, 1950.
11. Head WC: Total articular resurfacing arthroplasty: analysis of component failure in sixty-seven hips. J Bone Joint Surg Am 66:28–34, 1984.

12. Mesko JW, Goodman FG, Stanescu S: Total articular replacement arthroplasty: a three- to ten-year case-controlled study. Clin Orthop Relat Res 300:168–177, 1994.

13. Muller ME: The benefits of metal-on-metal total hip replacements. Clin Orthop Relat Res 311:54–59, 1995.

14. Gerard Y: Hip arthroplasty by matching cups. Clin Orthop Relat Res 134:25–35, 1978.

15. Furuya K, Tsuchiya M, Kawachi S: Socket-cup arthroplasty. Clin Orthop Relat Res 134:41–44, 1978.

16. Nishio A, Eguchi M, Kaibara N: Socket and cup surface replacement of the hip. Clin Orthop Relat Res 134:53–58, 1978.

17. Tanaka S: Surface replacement of the hip joint. Clin Orthop Relat Res 134:75–79, 1978.

18. Trentani C, Vaccarino F: The Paltrinieri-Trentani hip joint resurface arthroplasty. Clin Orthop Relat Res 134:36–40, 1978.

19. Amstutz HC, Kim WC, Thomas BJ, Mai ŁL: THARIES: two-year to six and one half-year results. Hip 185–197, 1982.

20. Buechel FF, Drucker D, Jasty M, et al: Osteolysis around uncemented acetabular components of cobalt-chrome surface replacement hip arthroplasty. Clin Orthop Relat Res 298:202–211, 1994.

21. Capello WN, Ireland PH, Trammell TR, Eicher P: Conservative total hip arthroplasty: a procedure to conserve bone stock. Part I. Analysis of sixty-six patients. Part II. Analysis of failures. Clin Orthop Relat Res 134:59–74, 1978.

22. Freeman MA, Cameron HU, Brown GC: Cemented double cup arthroplasty of the hip: a 5 year experience with the ICLH prosthesis. Clin Orthop Relat Res 134:45–52, 1978.

23. Wagner M, Wagner H: Preliminary results of uncemented metal on metal stemmed and resurfacing hip replacement arthroplasty. Clin Orthop Relat Res 329(Suppl):S78–S88, 1996.

24. August AC, Aldam CH, Pynsent PB: The McKee-Farrar hip arthroplasty: a long-term study. J Bone Joint Surg Br 68:520–527, 1986.

25. Jacobsson SA, Djerf K, Wahlstrom O: A comparative study between McKee-Farrar and Charnley arthroplasty with long-term follow-up periods. J Arthroplasty 5:9–14, 1990.

26. McMinn D, Treacy R, Lin K, Pynsent P: Metal on metal surface replacement of the hip: experience of the McMinn prothesis. Clin Orthop Relat Res 329(Suppl):S89–S98, 1996.

27. Clohisy JC, Harris WH: Matched-pair analysis of cemented and cementless acetabular reconstruction in primary total hip arthroplasty. J Arthroplasty 16:697–705, 2001.

28. Schulte KR, Callaghan JJ, Kelley SS, Johnston RC: The outcome of Charnley total hip arthroplasty with cement after a minimum twenty-year follow-up: the results of one surgeon. J Bone Joint Surg Am 75:961–975, 1993.

29. Jasty MJ, Floyd WE 3rd, Schiller AL, et al: Localized osteolysis in stable, non-septic total hip replacement. J Bone Joint Surg Am 68:912–919, 1986.

30. Jones LC, Hungerford DS: Cement disease. Clin Orthop Relat Res 225:192–206, 1987.

31. Schmalzried TP, Wessinger SJ, Hill GE, Harris WH: The Harris-Galante porous acetabular component press-fit without screw fixation: five-year radiographic analysis of primary cases. J Arthroplasty 9:235–242, 1994.

32. Smith SE, Estok DM 2nd, Harris WH: Average 12-year outcome of a chrome-cobalt, beaded, bony ingrowth acetabular component. J Arthroplasty 13:50–60, 1998.

33. Tompkins GS, Jacobs JJ, Kull LR, et al: Primary total hip arthroplasty with a porous-coated acetabular component: seven-to-ten-year results. J Bone Joint Surg Am 79:169–176, 1997.

34. McKee GK, Chen SC: The statistics of the McKee-Farrar method of total hip replacement. Clin Orthop Relat Res 95:26–33, 1973.

35. Wilson PD Jr, Amstutz HC, Czerniecki A, et al: Total hip replacement with fixation by acrylic cement: a preliminary study of 100 consecutive McKee-Farrar prosthetic replacements. J Bone Joint Surg Am 54:207–236, 1972.

36. Dumbleton JH: Tribology of natural and artificial joints, New York, NY, 1981, Elsevier Scientific Publishing.

37. Lu Z, McKellop H: Frictional heating of bearing materials tested in a hip joint wear simulator. Proc Inst Mech Eng H 211:101–108, 1997.

38. Wagner M, Wagner H: Medium-term results of a modern metal-on-metal system in total hip replacement. Clin Orthop Relat Res 379:123–133, 2000.

39. Dowson D, Hardaker C, Flett M, Isaac GH: A hip joint simulator study of the performance of metal-on-metal joints. Part II. Design. J Arthroplasty 19:124–130, 2004.

40. Dowson D, Hardaker C, Flett M, Isaac GH: A hip joint simulator study of the performance of metal-on-metal joints. Part I. The role of materials. J Arthroplasty 19:118–123, 2004.

41. Dowson D, Jin ZM: Metal-on-metal hip joint tribology. Proc Inst Mech Eng H 220:107–118, 2006.

42. Chan FW, Bobyn JD, Medley JB, et al: Engineering issues and wear performance of metal on metal hip implants. Clin Orthop Relat Res 333:96–107, 1996.

43. Streicher RM, Semlitsch M, Schon R, et al: Metal-on-metal articulation for artificial hip joints: laboratory study and clinical results. Proc Inst Mech Eng H 210:223–232, 1996.

44. Yan Y, Neville A, Dowson D: Understanding the role of corrosion in the degradation of metal-on-metal implants. Proc Inst Mech Eng H 220:173–181, 2006.

45. Lin ZM, Meakins S, Morlock MM, et al: Deformation of press-fitted metallic resurfacing cups. Part 1. Experimental simulation. Proc Inst Mech Eng H 220:299–309, 2006.

46. Yew A, Udofia I, Jagatia M, Jin ZM: Analysis of elastohydrodynamic lubrication in McKee-Farrar metal-on-metal hip joint replacement. Proc Inst Mech Eng H 218:27–34, 2004.

47. Bezwada HP, Shah AR, Harding SH, et al: Cementless bipolar hemiarthroplasty for displaced femoral neck fractures in the elderly. J Arthroplasty 19:73–77, 2004.

48. Amstutz HC: Hip resurfacing: principles, indications, technique, and results, Philadelphia, Pa, 2008, Saunders/Elsevier.

49. Amstutz HC, Le Duff MJ: Cementing the metaphyseal stem in metal-on-metal resurfacing: when and why. Clin Orthop Relat Res 467:79–83, 2009.

50. Beaule PE: Removal of acetabular bone in resurfacing arthroplasty of the hip. J Bone Joint Surg Br 88:838, 2006.

51. Gross TP, Liu F: Metal-on-metal hip resurfacing with an uncemented femoral component: a seven-year follow-up study. J Bone Joint Surg Am 90(Suppl 3):32–37, 2008.

52. Bozic KJ, Pui CM, Ludeman MJ, et al: Do the potential benefits of metal-on-metal hip resurfacing justify the increased cost and risk of complications? Clin Orthop Relat Res 468:2301–2312, 2010.

53. Graves S: 2009 annual report: hip and knee replacement. Presented at the Australian Orthopaedic Association Meeting, Brisbane, Australia, August 5–7, 2009.

54. McAuley JP, Szuszczewicz ES, Young A, Engh CA Sr: Total hip arthroplasty in patients 50 years and younger. Clin Orthop Relat Res 418:119–125, 2004.

55. Lingard EA, Muthumayandi K, Holland JP: Comparison of patient-reported outcomes between hip resurfacing and total hip replacement patients. J Bone Joint Surg Br 91:1550–1554, 2009.

56. U.S. Central Intelligence Agency: The CIA world factbook, New York, 2009, Skyhorse Publishing.

57. Engh CA, Glassman AH, Griffin WL, Mayer JG: Results of cementless revision for failed cemented total hip arthroplasty. Clin Orthop Relat Res 235:91–110, 1988.

58. Hunter GA, Welsh RP, Cameron HU, Bailey WH: The results of revision of total hip arthroplasty. J Bone Joint Surg Br 61:419–421, 1979.

59. Kavanagh BF, Ilstrup DM, Fitzgerald RH Jr: Revision total hip arthroplasty. J Bone Joint Surg Am 67:517–526, 1985.

60. Pellicci PM, Wilson PD Jr, Sledge CB, et al: Revision total hip arthroplasty. Clin Orthop Relat Res 170:34–41, 1982.

61. McGrath MS, Marker DR, Seyler TM, et al: Surface replacement is comparable to primary total hip arthroplasty. Clin Orthop Relat Res 467:94–100, 2009.

62. Ball ST, Le Duff MJ, Amstutz HC: Early results of conversion of a failed femoral component in hip resurfacing arthroplasty. J Bone Joint Surg Am 89:735–741, 2007.

63. Marker DR, Seyler TM, Jinnah RH, et al: Femoral neck fractures after metal-on-metal total hip resurfacing: a prospective cohort study. J Arthroplasty 22:66–71, 2007.

64. Mont MA, Schmalzried TP: Modern metal-on-metal hip resurfacing: important observations from the first ten years. J Bone Joint Surg Am 90(Suppl 3):3–11, 2008.

65. Nunley RM, Della Valle CJ, Barrack RL: Is patient selection important for hip resurfacing? Clin Orthop Relat Res 467:56–65, 2009.

66. Williams S, Leslie I, Isaac G, et al: Tribology and wear of metal-on-metal hip prostheses: influence of cup angle and head position. J Bone Joint Surg Am 90(Suppl 3):111–117, 2008.

67. Daniel J, Pynsent PB, McMinn DJ: Metal-on-metal resurfacing of the hip in patients under the age of 55 years with osteoarthritis. J Bone Joint Surg Br 86:177–184, 2004.

68. Hallab NJ, Jacobs JJ: Biologic effects of implant debris. Bull NYU Hosp Jt Dis 67:182–188, 2009.

69. Willert HG, Buchhorn GH, Fayyazi A, et al: Metal-on-metal bearings and hypersensitivity in patients with artificial hip joints: a clinical and histomorphological study. J Bone Joint Surg Am 87:28–36, 2005.

70. Medical Device Alert: All metal-on-metal (MoM) hip replacements, Victoria, London, United Kingdom, 2010, Medicines and Healthcare Products Regulatory Agency.

71. Beaule PE, Dorey FJ, LeDuff M, et al: Risk factors affecting outcome of metal-on-metal surface arthroplasty of the hip. Clin Orthop Relat Res 418:87–93, 2004.

72. Schmalzried TP, Silva M, de la Rosa MA, et al: Optimizing patient selection and outcomes with total hip resurfacing. Clin Orthop Relat Res 441:200–204, 2005.

73. Amstutz HC, Le Duff MJ: Eleven years of experience with metal-on-metal hybrid hip resurfacing: a review of 1000 conserve plus. J Arthroplasty 23:36–43, 2008.

74. Back DL, Dalziel R, Young D, Shimmin A: Early results of primary Birmingham hip resurfacings: an independent prospective study of the first 230 hips. J Bone Joint Surg Br 87:324–329, 2005.

75. Buergi ML, Walter WL: Hip resurfacing arthroplasty: the Australian experience. J Arthroplasty 22:61–65, 2007.

76. De Smet KA: Belgium experience with metal-on-metal surface arthroplasty. Orthop Clin North Am 36:203–213, ix, 2005.

77. Heilpern GN, Shah NN, Fordyce MJ: Birmingham hip resurfacing arthroplasty: a series of 110 consecutive hips with a minimum five-year clinical and radiological follow-up. J Bone Joint Surg Br 90:1137–1142, 2008.

78. Hing CB, Back DL, Bailey M, et al: The results of primary Birmingham hip resurfacings at a mean of five years: an independent prospective review of the first 230 hips. J Bone Joint Surg Br 89:1431–1438, 2007.

79. Steffen RT, Pandit HP, Palan J, et al: The five-year results of the Birmingham hip resurfacing arthroplasty: an independent series. J Bone Joint Surg Br 90:436–441, 2008.

80. Treacy RB, McBryde CW, Pynsent PB: Birmingham hip resurfacing arthroplasty: a minimum follow-up of five years. J Bone Joint Surg Br 87:167–170, 2005.

81. Vail TP, Mina CA, Yergler JD, Pietrobon R: Metal-on-metal hip resurfacing compares favorably with THA at 2 years followup. Clin Orthop Relat Res 453:123–131, 2006.

82. Bozic KJ, Kurtz S, Lau E, et al: The epidemiology of bearing surface usage in total hip arthroplasty in the United States. J Bone Joint Surg Am 91:1614–1620, 2009.

83. McKenzie L, Vale L, Stearns S, McCormack K: Metal on metal hip resurfacing arthroplasty: an economic analysis. Eur J Health Econ 4:122–129, 2003.

84. Mont MA, Seyler TM, Ulrich SD, et al: Effect of changing indications and techniques on total hip resurfacing. Clin Orthop Relat Res 465:63–70, 2007.

85. Stulberg BN, Trier KK, Naughton M, Zadzilka JD: Results and lessons learned from a United States hip resurfacing investigational device exemption trial. J Bone Joint Surg Am 90(Suppl 3):21–26, 2008.

86. Della Valle CJ, Nunley RM, Raterman SJ, Barrack RL: Initial American experience with hip resurfacing following FDA approval. Clin Orthop Relat Res 467:72–78, 2009.

87. Schachter AK, Lamont JG: Surface replacement arthroplasty of the hip. Bull NYU Hosp Jt Dis 67:75–82, 2009.

88. Yue EJ, Cabanela ME, Duffy GP, et al: Hip resurfacing arthroplasty: risk factors for failure over 25 years. Clin Orthop Relat Res 467:992–999, 2009.

89. Pollard TC, Baker RP, Eastaugh-Waring SJ, Bannister GC: Treatment of the young active patient with osteoarthritis of the hip: a five- to seven-year comparison of hybrid total hip arthroplasty and metal-on-metal resurfacing. J Bone Joint Surg Br 88:592–600, 2006.

90. American Orthopaedic Association (AOA): National Joint Replacement Registry annual report 2007, Rosemont, Ill, 2007, AOA.

91. Shimmin AJ, Back D: Femoral neck fractures following Birmingham hip resurfacing: a national review of 50 cases. J Bone Joint Surg Br 87:463–464, 2005.

92. Cossey AJ, Back DL, Shimmin A, et al: The nonoperative management of periprosthetic fractures associated with the Birmingham hip resurfacing procedure. J Arthroplasty 20:358–361, 2005.

93. Beaulé PE, Campbell P, Shim P: Femoral head blood flow during hip resurfacing. Clin Orthop Relat Res 456:148–152, 2007.

94. Davies AP, Willert HG, Campbell PA, et al: An unusual lymphocytic perivascular infiltration in tissues around contemporary metal-on-metal joint replacements. J Bone Joint Surg Am 87:18–27, 2005.

95. Park YS, Moon YW, Lim SJ, et al: Early osteolysis following second-generation metal-on-metal hip replacement. J Bone Joint Surg Am 87:1515–1521, 2005.

96. Langton DJ, Jameson SS, Joyce TJ, et al: The effect of component size and orientation on the concentrations of metal ions after resurfacing arthroplasty of the hip. J Bone Joint Surg Br 90:1143–1151, 2008.

97. Daniel J, Ziaee H, Salama A, et al: The effect of the diameter of metal-on-metal bearings on systemic exposure to cobalt and chromium. J Bone Joint Surg Br 88:443–448, 2006.

98. Vendittoli PA, Mottard S, Roy AG, et al: Chromium and cobalt ion release following the Durom high carbon content, forged metal-on-metal surface replacement of the hip. J Bone Joint Surg Br 89:441–448, 2007.

99. Amstutz HC, Grigoris P, Dorey FJ: Evolution and future of surface replacement of the hip. J Orthop Sci 3:169–186, 1998.

100. Quesada MJ, Marker DR, Mont MA: Metal-on-metal hip resurfacing: advantages and disadvantages. J Arthroplasty 23:69–73, 2008.

101. Shimmin A, Beaule PE, Campbell P: Metal-on-metal hip resurfacing arthroplasty. J Bone Joint Surg Am 90:637–654, 2008.

102. Beaule PE, Schmalzried TP, Udomkiat P, Amstutz HC: Jumbo femoral head for the treatment of recurrent dislocation following total hip replacement. J Bone Joint Surg Am 84:256–263, 2002.

103. Crowninshield RD, Maloney WJ, Wentz DH, et al: Biomechanics of large femoral heads: what they do and don't do. Clin Orthop Relat Res 429:102–107, 2004.

104. Stuchin SA: Anatomic diameter femoral heads in total hip arthroplasty: a preliminary report. J Bone Joint Surg Am 90(Suppl 3):52–56, 2008.

105. Jacobs JJ, Hallab NJ: Loosening and osteolysis associated with metal-on-metal bearings: a local effect of metal hypersensitivity? J Bone Joint Surg Am 88:1171–1172, 2006.

106. Bragdon CR, Kwon YM, Geller JA, et al: Minimum 6-year followup of highly cross-linked polyethylene in THA. Clin Orthop Relat Res 465:122–127, 2007.

107. Dumbleton JH, D'Antonio JA, Manley MT, et al: The basis for a second-generation highly cross-linked UHMWPE. Clin Orthop Relat Res 453:265–271, 2006.

108. Geerdink CH, Grimm B, Vencken W, et al: Cross-linked compared with historical polyethylene in THA: an 8-year clinical study. Clin Orthop Relat Res 467:979–984, 2009.

109. Glyn-Jones S, Isaac S, Hauptfleisch J, et al: Does highly cross-linked polyethylene wear less than conventional polyethylene in total hip arthroplasty? A double-blind, randomized, and controlled trial using roentgen stereophotogrammetric analysis. J Arthroplasty 23:337–343, 2008.

110. Gomez-Barrena E, Puertolas JA, Munuera L, Konttinen YT: Update on UHMWPE research: from the bench to the bedside. Acta Orthop 79:832–840, 2008.

111. McCalden RW, MacDonald SJ, Rorabeck CH, et al: Wear rate of highly cross-linked polyethylene in total hip arthroplasty: a randomized controlled trial. J Bone Joint Surg Am 91:773–782, 2009.

112. Lavigne M, Therrien M, Nantel J, et al: The John Charnley Award. The functional outcome of hip resurfacing and large-head THA is the same: a randomized, double-blind study. Clin Orthop Relat Res 468:326–336, 2010.

113. Mont MA, Seyler TM, Ragland PS, et al: Gait analysis of patients with resurfacing hip arthroplasty compared with hip osteoarthritis and standard total hip arthroplasty. J Arthroplasty 22:100–108, 2007.

114. Naal FD, Maffiuletti NA, Munzinger U, Hersche O: Sports after hip resurfacing arthroplasty. Am J Sports Med 35:705–711, 2007.

115. Lavigne M, Masse V, Girard J, et al: [Return to sport after hip resurfacing or total hip arthroplasty: a randomized study]. Rev Chir Orthop Reparatrice Appar Mot 94:361–367, 2008.

FURTHER READING

Bozic KJ, Pui CM, Ludeman MJ, et al: Do the potential benefits of metal-on-metal hip resurfacing justify the increased cost and risk of complications? Clin Orthop Relat Res 468:2301–2312, 2010.

A detailed analysis of the use of metal-on-metal (MOM) bearings in hip arthroplasty related to the value added to the patient from use of the technology.

Dowson D: Tribologic principles in metal-on-metal hip joint design. Proc Inst Mech Eng H 220:161–171, 2006.

Application of tribologic principles to current implant designs.

Dowson D, Jin ZM: Metal-on-metal hip joint tribology. Proc Inst Mech Eng H 220:107–118, 2006.

A technical review of tribology of metal-on-metal (MOM) bearing surfaces.

Grigoris P, Roberts P, Panousis K, Bosch H: The evolution of hip resurfacing arthroplasty. Orthop Clin North Am 36:125–134, vii, 2005.

A comprehensive review of the evolution of hip resurfacing arthroplasty.

Jacobs JJ, Urban RM, Hallab NJ, et al: Metal-on-metal bearing surfaces. J Am Acad Orthop Surg 17:69–76, 2009.

A comprehensive review of the biological effects related to the use of metal-on-metal (MOM) bearings.

Shimmin A, Beaule PE, Campbell P: Metal-on-metal hip resurfacing arthroplasty. J Bone Joint Surg Am 90:637–654, 2008.

A Current Concepts review that discusses pertinent concepts, literature, and controversies.

CHAPTER 64

Resurfacing Hip Arthroplasty: Techniques

Thomas P. Schmalzried

KEY POINTS

- Obtaining adequate femoral and acetabular exposure is the key to accurate component insertion.
- Neck notching and vigorous component impaction predispose to femoral neck fracture.
- The recommended femoral pin orientation is neutral to slight valgus and neutral version relative to the native neck.
- Properly press-fitting a monoblock resurfacing acetabular component can be more challenging than with a modular total hip.
- The role of proper acetabular component placement cannot be overemphasized.

INTRODUCTION

More than 10 years of experience with metal-metal resurfacing utilizing hybrid fixation (cemented femur and cementless socket) has been documented. Although implant technology and instrumentation will evolve, several technical principles have been established. Femoral neck fracture is the most common cause of early resurfacing failure. Neck notching and vigorous component impaction predispose to femoral neck fracture. Cobalt-chromium alloy monoblock resurfacing acetabular components osseointegrate somewhat less reliably than modular titanium alloy components.[1] Acetabular lateral opening angles greater than 50 degrees, retroversion, or high combined anteversion is associated with increased wear, higher ion levels, and increased risk of revision.[2-4]

PREOPERATIVE PLANNING

Quality radiographs in multiple planes are helpful in assessing hip deformity and planning the resurfacing procedure. An anteroposterior (AP) pelvis with the beam centered on the pubis, a "frog" lateral, and Johnson's or "shoot-through" lateral are recommended. It is helpful to appreciate the *deformity pattern*. At one end of the spectrum is the patient with anterior femoral acetabular impingement (FAI). These hips tend to be found in males (larger stature) and to have normal or reduced femoral valgus (higher femoral offset); the

head tends to be relatively posterior and inferior on the neck, and low combined anteversion is seen frequently. At the other end of the spectrum is the dysplastic hip. These hips usually are seen in females (smaller stature) and have increased femoral valgus (reduced femoral offset); the head tends to be relatively centered on the neck, and combined anteversion (femoral plus acetabular anteversion) is increased. The deformity pattern has implications for both femoral and acetabular component positioning. Johnson's lateral is useful for assessing anterior and posterior aspects of the hip and the potential for postoperative FAI (Fig. 64-1).

The goals of templating are to get an estimate of component size and to visualize the orientation of the components relative to the patient's bony anatomy. The diameter of the femoral neck determines the smallest component size that can be used; the acetabulum determines the largest size possible. The outer diameter of the resurfacing acetabular component should be within 2 mm of what would be used for a total hip in that acetabulum.[5] Acetabular component positioning goals are not different from those of total hip replacement. Some medialization is desirable with a lateral opening angle in the 40- to 45-degree range. On the femoral side, relative varus component positioning should be avoided. The longitudinal position of the femoral component can be adjusted for limb length. Because the socket is medialized and the femoral offset is unchanged by resurfacing, the offset of the hip tends to be decreased by resurfacing[5] (Fig. 64-2).

EXPOSURE

Resurfacing can be performed through several approaches. Regardless of the surgical approach, the principles of exposure for resurfacing are similar. Goals include a circumferential view of the femoral head/neck during femoral preparation and a circumferential view of the acetabulum during acetabular preparation (Fig. 64-3). The major difference in exposure compared with total hip replacement is the capsular release (resection). Capsular release is needed to mobilize the proximal femur to (1) elevate the head out of the wound for femoral preparation and (2) translate the proximal femur for acetabular exposure. The extent of the release can be variable, depending on the degree of stiffness. Care must be taken in retractor placement and in performance of the capsular release not to stray from the

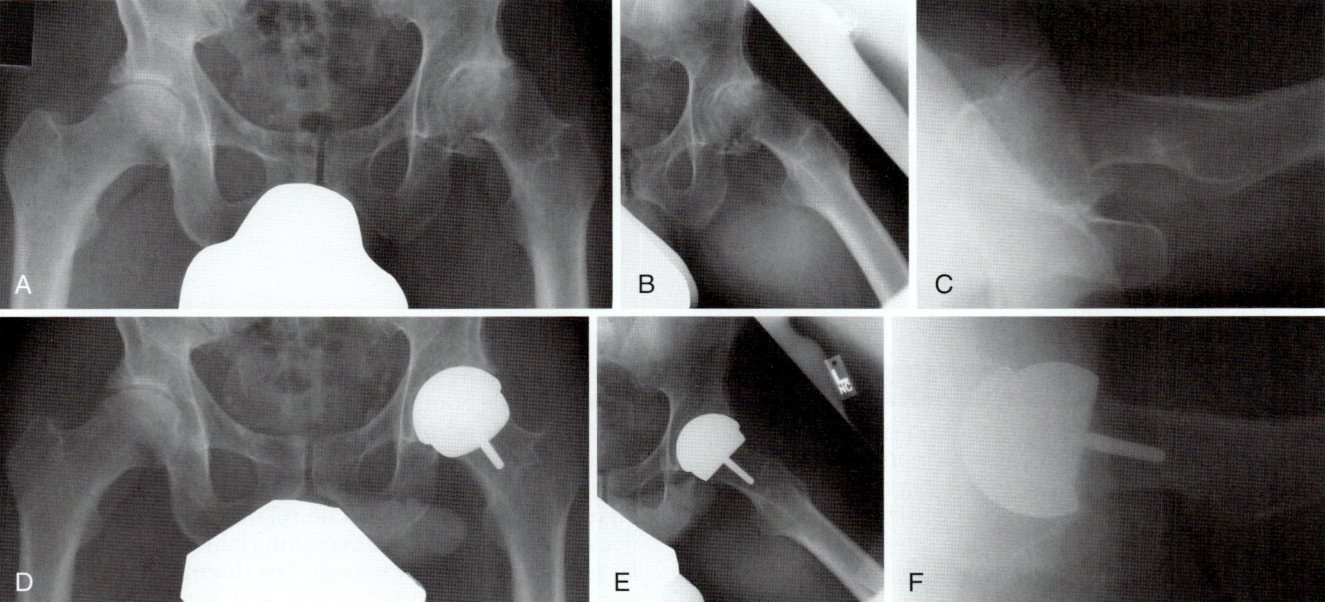

Figure 64-1. Radiographic evaluation. This patient has more of a dysplastic deformity pattern. **A,** Low anteroposterior (AP) pelvis centered on the pubis. Note that an external rotation position of the femur results in an apparent increase in neck valgus. **B,** Modified frog lateral. **C,** Johnson's shoot-through lateral. Note the calcified anterior labrum/osteophyte. **D,** Postoperative AP pelvis. Note the low lateral opening angle of the socket and the valgus orientation of the femoral component. **E,** Postoperative modified frog lateral. The femoral component is slightly anteverted. **F,** Postoperative shoot-through lateral demonstrating socket anteversion and removal of the calcified anterior labrum/osteophyte flush with the anterior rim of the socket.

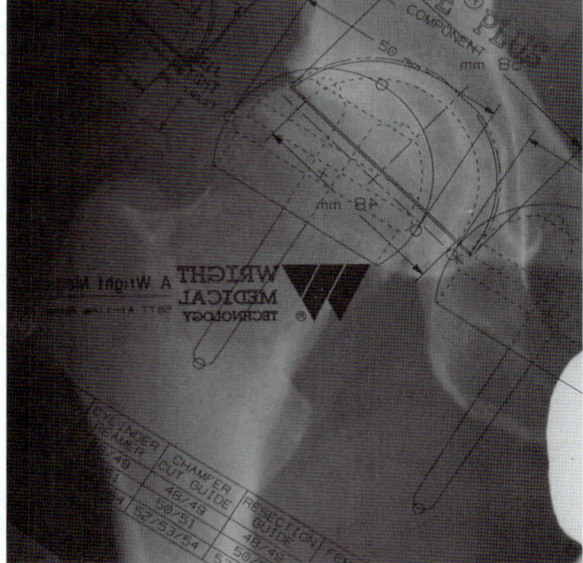

Figure 64-2. Templating. The acetabular component template is positioned first using the teardrop as a medial reference. The lateral opening angle target is 40 to 45 degrees. The femoral component template is aligned with the neck axis. The neck diameter determines the smallest possible femoral component size.

joint and risk injury to adjacent nerves and vessels and the iliopsoas tendon. Partial excision of a hypertrophic capsule can facilitate acetabular exposure. The author tries not to disrupt any soft tissue (e.g., capsule, synovium) on the femoral neck.

FEMORAL PREPARATION

The author prefers to prepare the femoral head first, but this is not necessary. Reducing the bulk of the proximal femur can facilitate acetabular exposure. The concern is that the reamed femoral bone may be damaged during acetabular exposure and preparation.

Conceptually, the operation is more a resurfacing around the neck than a resurfacing of the head per se. Several femoral pin guidance systems (e.g., mechanical, computer-assisted, shape matching) are available, but the goal of pin placement is the same. Although there are many degrees of freedom, major considerations include (1) native neck shaft orientation and (2) the position of the head center relative to the neck center. These factors influence the intended orientation of the femoral component (valgus and version) and the entry point of the guide pin on the femoral head. In patients with a "pistol-grip" or "slip-type" deformity, the entry point is superior and anterior on the head to translate the femoral component to increase the anterior head offset relative to the neck. In patients with dysplasia and increased combined anteversion, the entry point is closer to the head center, and care should be taken to maintain posterior femoral offset. The recommended pin orientation is neutral to slight valgus and neutral version relative to the native neck. The author uses a large goniometer to check the pin-shaft axis and ensure that it is within a couple of degrees of the preoperative plan and will reposition the pin if needed.

Essentially all available systems have a stylus to check "clearance" around the femoral neck from the

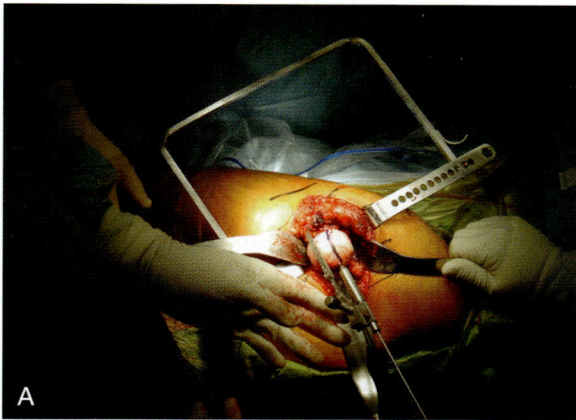

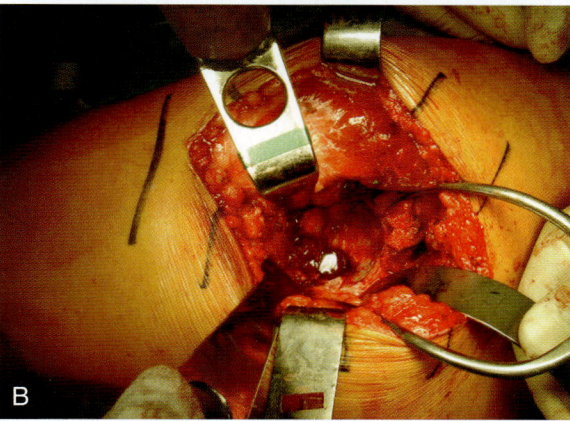

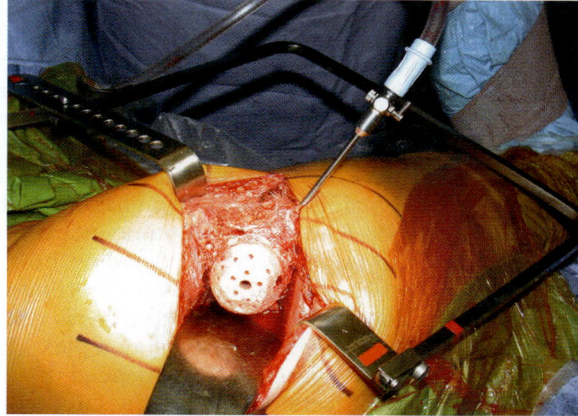

Figure 64-4. Proximal femoral suction. Wall suction drawn through a small-diameter cannula inserted into the greater or lesser trochanter can stop bleeding from the reamed femoral head bone. The cannula is in the lesser trochanter in this example.

Figure 64-3. A, Femoral exposure and guide pin placement. For this posterior approach on a left hip, the patient's leg is to the left. The ipsilateral knee is flexed to about 90 degrees, and the foot is pointed toward the ceiling (hip internally rotated). A flat retractor under the femoral neck elevates the head and protects the posterior tissues. Anterior and posterior cobra retractors facilitate a 360-degree view around the head and neck. A guide pin has been placed along the neck axis, and the orientation/clearance is being checked with a stylus. **B,** Acetabular exposure. Same patient, left hip, posterior approach, the leg is to the left. The femoral head has been prepared and retracted anterior beneath the abductor. The surgeon has a 360-degree view of the socket.

femoral guide pin (see Fig. 64-3A). The tip should not touch bone anywhere around the neck. Special attention should be given to the anterior-superior region. Tension stresses are greatest in this region of the neck, and a cortical violation here (so-called *notch*) increases the risk of a postoperative fracture.

CEMENTING

Cemented fixation of femoral knee components is highly consistent and durable. This is due to the accessibility of cut bone surfaces and elimination of back-bleeding (use of a tourniquet). The same conditions can be achieved for femoral resurfacing if proximal femoral suction is utilized. Wall suction drawn through a small-diameter cannula inserted into the greater or lesser

trochanter can stop bleeding from the reamed femoral head bone (Fig. 64-4).

The cementing technique has been implicated in femoral failures of current-generation resurfacing arthroplasties. Debate continues regarding the relative merits of "cup filling" techniques with low-viscosity cement compared with manual application of moderate-viscosity cement. Regardless, the goals of femoral component resurfacing are the same: uniform cement penetration of 2 to 5 mm over the available fixation surface and full seating of the component (no polar cement cap) without the use of high-impact forces that can fracture trabecular bone. Variables influencing cement penetration, distribution into the prepared femoral head, and the force required to seat the component include (1) density of the bone, (2) viscosity of the cement, (3) the amount of cement used, (4) how the cement is applied, and (5) the space or clearance between the prepared bone and the inside of the component.[6,7]

ACETABULAR PREPARATION AND COMPONENT POSITIONING

Acetabular reaming for resurfacing is no different than for total hip replacement. Differences have been noted between the various acetabular resurfacing systems regarding the recommended difference in nominal diameter of the last reamer and in nominal diameter of the component. Properly press-fitting a monoblock resurfacing acetabular component can be more challenging than with a modular total hip. Cobalt-chromium alloy resurfacing components are stiffer than titanium alloy modular components. No holes are seen through the resurfacing component, so it is more difficult to tell whether the component is fully seated.

The role of proper acetabular component placement cannot be overemphasized.[8] It is even more important in resurfacing than in total hip replacement because of the generally lower head-to-neck ratio and the inability to adjust femoral version. An unsatisfactory acetabular component position has been associated with instability, pain, increased wear, and adverse local tissue reactions (ALTRs) and revision. Pelvic, acetabular, and femoral anatomy is variable, so it is illogical to have the same fixed target position for all patients. The hip arthroplasty surgeon actually faces two challenges: (1) determining the desired acetabular component position for *that patient* (the target), and (2) deciding how to reasonably attain that position in surgery (hitting the target). An abduction angle of 40 ± 10 degrees is generally satisfactory. Anteversion is more complex. The desired amount of anteversion is influenced by the amount of femoral anteversion and by the cup abduction angle. *Combined anteversion* of greater than 25 degrees is generally satisfactory, and more than 40 degrees may be too much.

Templating can be used to approximate the relationship between bony landmarks and the intended position of the implant. Most constant is the medial wall of the acetabulum (AP view). The anterior rim of the native acetabulum generally can be visualized on the shoot-through lateral, and this can serve as a reference for anteversion (see Fig. 64-1C). These internal landmarks can be used in conjunction with external landmarks (e.g., orientation of the acetabular component insertion handle relative to the plane of the patient, the operating room [OR] table, the OR). As an additional check, it is common that the posterior-superior portion of the properly positioned component is uncovered, indicating a reduction in cup abduction relative to the native anatomy. The amount of anteversion relative to the native anatomy can be assessed by comparing the location of the anterior edge of the component with that of the native acetabulum. For example, if bone extends beyond the anterior rim of the component (and the component is seated near the medial wall), it is likely that anteversion has been increased. The transverse acetabular ligament (TAL) serves as an internal reference for the version of the native acetabulum.

If the deformity pattern indicates low combined native anteversion, the anteversion of the resurfacing socket can be increased. Overhanging calcified anterior labrum, osteophyte, and/or anterior wall should be excised flush to the rim of the component. Conversely, if the deformity pattern indicates increased combined native anteversion, the anteversion of the resurfacing socket can be reduced. Such cases often have a more valgus femoral neck, and it is especially important to keep the socket lateral opening angle near 40 degrees. With its deformity pattern, less cup anteversion and a low lateral opening angle will increase femoral head coverage and will keep the anterior-inferior edge of the cup away from the psoas tendon.

The intraoperative range of motion should be evaluated with consideration for the limits of flexion; at 90 degrees of flexion, it is desirable to have at least 45 degrees of internal rotation before anterior impingement and full extension, with at least 30 degrees of external rotation before posterior impingement. If in doubt about component positions, an intraoperative

radiograph or FluoroSpot (MABTECH AB, Strand, Sweden) is recommended.

CURRENT CONTROVERSIES AND FUTURE DIRECTIONS

Controversy is ongoing regarding the cementing technique, especially with regard to how much cement (if any) should be applied directly to the femoral head and how much cement (if any) should be poured into the femoral resurfacing shell. Regardless of technique, the goal is complete seating of the component with intrusion of cement into all of the available fixation area. To address issues related to cement fixation, cementless femoral components may be used. Clinical experience with cementless femoral components is relatively limited, and only time will tell which method of fixation is preferable.

The greatest challenges for future resurfacing technology include determining the optimal component positions for individual patients, and consistently implanting components in the desired position. Better mechanical guides, intraoperative imaging, computer-assisted surgery, so-called *shape-matching* (patient-specific) guides, and robotics should prove helpful.

REFERENCES

1. Morlock MM, Bishop N, Zustin J, et al: Modes of implant failure after hip resurfacing: morphological and wear analysis of 267 retrieval specimens. J Bone Joint Surg Am 90(Suppl 3):89–95, 2008.
2. De Haan R, Campbell PA, Su EP, De Smet KA: Revision of metal-on-metal resurfacing arthroplasty of the hip: the influence of malpositioning of the components. J Bone Joint Surg Br 90:1158–1163, 2008.
3. De Haan R, Pattyn C, Gill HS, et al: Correlation between inclination of the acetabular component and metal ion levels in metal-on-metal hip resurfacing replacement. J Bone Joint Surg Br 90:1291–1297, 2008.
4. Langton DJ, Jameson SS, Joyce TJ, et al: The effect of component size and orientation on the concentrations of metal ions after resurfacing arthroplasty of the hip. J Bone Joint Surg Br 90:1143–1151, 2008.
5. Silva M, Lee KH, Heisel C, et al: The biomechanical results of total hip resurfacing arthroplasty. J Bone Joint Surg Am 86:40–46, 2004.
6. Bitsch RG, Heisel C, Silva M, Schmalzried TP: Femoral cementing technique for hip resurfacing arthroplasty. J Orthop Res 25:423–431, 2007.
7. Bitsch RG, Loidolt T, Heisel C, Schmalzried TP: Cementing techniques for hip resurfacing arthroplasty: development of a laboratory model. J Bone Joint Surg Am 90(Suppl 3):102–110, 2008.
8. Schmalzried TP: The importance of proper acetabular component positioning and the challenges to achieving it. Oper Tech Orthop 19:132–136, 2009.

FURTHER READINGS

Mont MA, Schmalzried TP: Modern metal-on-metal hip resurfacing: important observations from the first ten years. J Bone Joint Surg Am 90(Suppl 3):3–11, 2008.
    As the title suggests, this review summarizes the lessons learned from a decade of metal-metal hip resurfacing. It also includes some speculation regarding future directions for the technology.

Schmalzried TP: The importance of proper acetabular component positioning and the challenges to achieving it. Oper Tech Orthop 19:132–136, 2009.

This technical monograph summarizes the clinical importance of acetabular component position, regardless of the bearing, and describes methods to improve preoperative planning, acetabular component positioning, and postoperative assessment.

Schmalzried TP, Silva M, de la Rosa M, et al: Optimizing patient selection and outcomes with total hip resurfacing. Clin Orthop Relat Res 441:200–204, 2005.

Patient demographics have been consistently correlated with clinical outcomes with hip resurfacing. This study describes a simple grading system that can be used to identify the best hips for resurfacing.

CHAPTER 65

Cemented Acetabular Components

Fares S. Haddad and Adam M.M. Cohen

KEY POINTS
• Although cemented THR continues to be the most commonly performed of all THR types, the cemented acetabular component is often the "weak link" in the longevity of a fully cemented total hip replacement.
• Each patient must undergo plain radiographic examination to allow accurate templating and planning of the operation.
• Best practice in performing the technique of cementing the component is described.
• Limitations of the procedure are explained.
• Results of the procedure are discussed.

INTRODUCTION

Total hip replacement (THR) has been performed for osteoarthritis for nearly 50 years. The start of the revolution that has been total hip replacement began when John Charnley developed *low-friction arthroplasty*.[1] Charnley used a stainless steel femoral head 22 mm in diameter articulating with a high-density polyethylene following initial use of Teflon for the acetabulum, which failed badly. The components were cemented in originally with dental cement[2] and subsequently with specifically designed bone cements.[3]

A cemented acetabular replacement is a composite of materials with different moduli of elasticity compared with bone. The cement, which acts as a grout between the articulating component and the bone, allows torque forces produced at the articulation to be transmitted to the bone to minimize the shear stress effect on the bone (Fig. 65-1).

Cemented acetabular components have been shown to work well in patients over the age of 65, but their survival in young patients and in those with rheumatoid arthritis, dysplasia, or revision surgery is not as good.[4]

INDICATIONS/CONTRAINDICATIONS

Indications for using a cemented acetabular component when performing a total hip replacement (THR) are often debated. Cemented components have been used since the dawn of total hip arthroplasty and therefore have a long track record.[5-7] Cemented THR continues to be the most commonly performed procedure of all THR types.[4] However, it is commonly pointed out that the cemented acetabular component is the "weak link" in the longevity of a fully cemented total hip replacement.[4,5]

The age of the patient is an important consideration in deciding the most appropriate implant. Patients over the age of 65 constitute a significant proportion of patients undergoing THR.[4] Factors that affect component choice in this age group include underlying pathology, medical comorbidities, osteopenia, and the surgeon's skills/preferences. Evidence suggests that cemented total hip replacement in this age group is an acceptable technique, given that with modern cementing methods the replacement can be expected to last 20 years in 90% of patients.[4] In the younger patient (<65 years), the argument to use a cemented acetabular component is more difficult to make,[8] although each case should be considered on its merits.

Patients with osteopenia who require hip replacement are poor candidates for uncemented components because of the risk of pelvic fracture and the difficulty in attaining adequate primary stability. The more logical choice is a cemented acetabulum. In the United States, cemented acetabular components have been replaced by cementless fixation in many centers. Reasons for this include observed poor results of cemented "metal-backed" components[9] and perceived difficulties of using bone cement in an effective manner. Therefore, many surgeons may struggle when faced with an irradiated acetabulum, severe osteopenia, or metabolic bone disease, all of which are good indications for cementation.

Cemented fixation of the acetabulum remains the most commonly used method in certain parts of Europe.[4,10,11] Most other countries performing total hip arthroplasty have been using uncemented acetabular implants more commonly. The cemented all-polyethylene component is much cheaper to insert, and its use in experienced hands produces excellent long-term results. The Ranawat Orthopaedic Center uses an all-polyethylene component in patients over the age of 60 years who have osteoarthritis of the hip. Exclusions for the cemented method include the following:

- Excessive bleeding following reaming
- Extensive cyst formation
- Inflammatory arthropathies
- Dysplasia

Table 65-1. Results of Cemented Acetabular Components

Author/Date	Prosthesis	No. of Hips	Minimum F/U, yr	Revision Rate, %
Delee/1977	Charnley	141	10	NR
Stauffer/1982	Charnley	231	10	3
Poss/1988	Mixed	267	11	3.1
Ritter/1992	Charnley	238	10	4.6
Wroblewski/1993	Charnley	193	18	3
Kavanagh/1994	Charnley	112	20	16
Callaghan/2004	Charnley	27	30	12
Della Valle/2004	Charnley	40	20	23

F/U, Follow-up; *NR*, not reported.

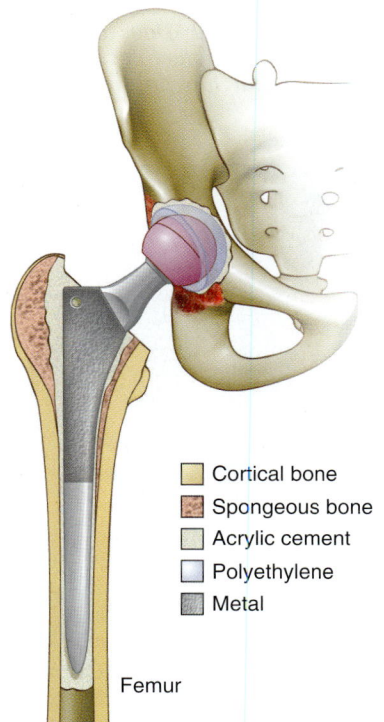

Cortical bone
Spongeous bone
Acrylic cement
Polyethylene
Metal

Femur

Figure 65-1. Line drawing of cemented total hip arthroplasty (THA).

- Protrusio deformities
- Significant cardiopulmonary disease

These indications/exclusions are by no means exclusive. Such criteria can produce excellent results.[12] Various studies of cemented acetabular components are summarized in Table 65-1.

PREOPERATIVE PLANNING

Preoperative planning is an essential part of hip replacement surgery. It serves many functions including the following:

- Ensuring that appropriate implants are obtained prior to surgery
- Ensuring that correct sizes are available

- Providing knowledge of the anatomic challenges of each individual hip
- Restoring appropriate biomechanics
- Avoiding leg length inequalities
- Reducing intraoperative complications

Each patient must undergo plain radiographic examination for accurate planning of the operation. An anteroposterior pelvic view with the extremities internally rotated 15 degrees that includes the proximal third of the femora and a lateral view of the affected hip should be routine. The basic principle is to restore normal hip anatomy and therefore biomechanics. Modern templating is often performed on digital radiographs using commercially available templating programs. Therefore, it is imperative to obtain accurate scaling of the radiographic view. This requires the use of a templating ball of known dimension with every radiograph taken for arthroplasty surgery.

Accurate templating improves with experience; however, certain conventions, when followed, enhance the accuracy of acetabular templating.[13] Positioning of the acetabular component predicts the center of rotation of the replaced joint and therefore is an essential step in the process. One of the main objectives is to provide sufficient support for the acetabular component within the native socket. The "teardrop" is an important reference point, indicating the acetabular floor. The lateral lip of the teardrop corresponds to the outer acetabular floor, and the medial lip corresponds to the inner floor. The template should not be placed medial to this anatomically consistent point. The abduction angle should be 40 to 45 degrees. A 2-mm allowance for the bone cement should be taken into consideration when the size and position of the acetabular component are assessed (Fig. 65-2).

If complex anatomic deformities are noted, or if the socket is very deficient, a computed tomography (CT) scan is often helpful.

Among the potential advantages of cemented acetabular components, avoidance of acetabular fracture is important. Patients with relative osteoporotic bone, which may not be appreciated on preoperative radiographs, are at increased risk of this complication with uncemented cups. Similarly, iliopsoas irritation from retroverted or overhanging uncemented cups is a problem avoided with the cemented option.[14] Finally,

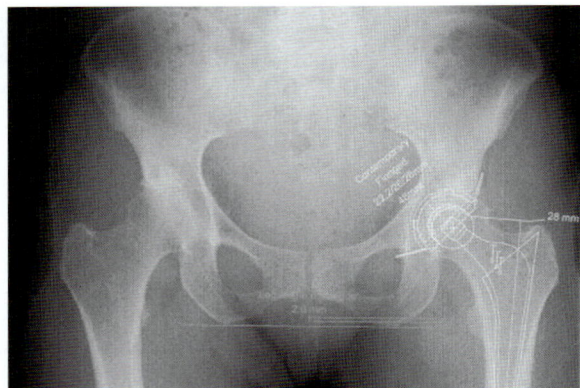

Figure 65-2. Templating for cemented total hip arthroplasty (THA).

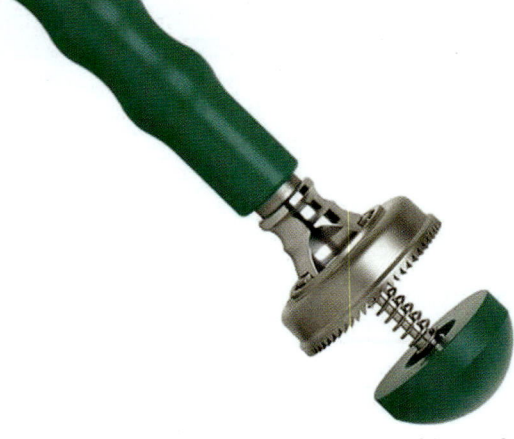

Figure 65-3. Acetabular rim cutter. *(From Conroy JL, Chawda M, Kaushal R, et al: Does use of a "rim cutter" improve quality of cementation of the acetabular component of cemented Exeter total hip arthroplasty? J Arthroplasty 24:71–75, 2009.)*

the stress-shielding phenomenon has been described in association with uncemented implants. This problem seems to be avoided with cemented cups because stresses are distributed over a wider area compared with the very stiff implants used in uncemented cups, which concentrate the stresses.[15]

However, the use of cemented cups limits the clinician to the use of polyethylene and does not allow for the use of modern bearing surfaces. Despite this, improvements in polyethylene manufacture have produced ultrahigh-molecular-weight polyethylene, which has very favorable wear characteristics, especially when used in conjunction with harder bearings such as ceramic heads.

DESCRIPTION OF TECHNIQUE

Exposure

A cemented acetabular component may be inserted by a variety of different approaches. It is not the purpose of this chapter to recommend a particular method. However, the approach used must provide 360-degree exposure of the acetabulum. The transverse acetabular ligament (TAL) is an important anatomic landmark across the floor of the acetabulum.[16] It is imperative to expose the TAL as an indicator of true anteversion of the acetabulum. Osteophytes may grow over the TAL, obscuring its position. These osteophytes must be removed before reaming. The labrum and extraneous soft tissue should be removed to expose the edge of the acetabulum. Obvious peripheral osteophytes may be removed at this stage.

Reaming

The process of reaming is designed to expose sufficient cancellous bone to allow effective interdigitation of cement with bone.[17] Initial reamer selection should facilitate reaming of the acetabular floor. The direction of reaming must represent the position in which the definitive component is expected to lie. Therefore, an abduction angle of 35 to 40 degrees and an anteversion angle of 20 to 30 degrees are appropriate. Successive reamers

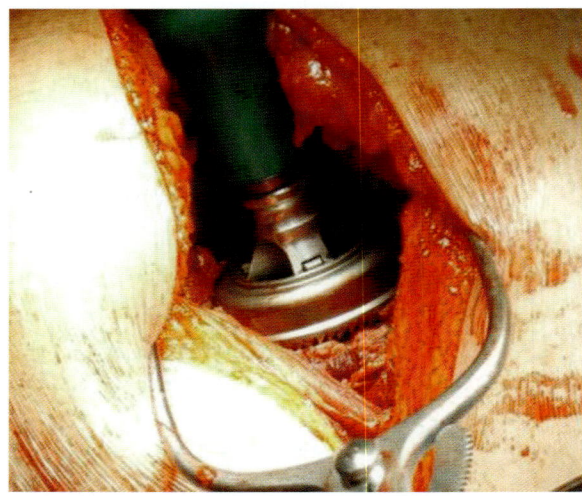

Figure 65-4. Rim cutter in use. *(From Conroy JL, Chawda M, Kaushal R, et al: Does use of a "rim cutter" improve quality of cementation of the acetabular component of cemented Exeter total hip arthroplasty? J Arthroplasty 24:71–75, 2009.)*

are chosen to remove remaining cartilage. Reamers must be sharp, and excessive pressure should not be necessary. The presence of bleeding cancellous bone indicates that sufficient reaming has been performed. Unlike the technique of reaming required for cementless cups, it is beneficial to ream through the subchondral bone to improve the potential for interdigitation of the cement mantle.[18,19] Any residual cartilage in the periphery of the acetabulum should be removed with a sharp curette. This avoids the subsequent use of a larger-diameter reamer, which otherwise might remove more peripheral bone than is absolutely necessary.

As reaming progresses, there is a tendency to ream excessively into the posterior column. Gentle pressure with the hand nearest to the acetabulum in an anterior direction helps to prevent potentially uneven reaming.

The recently introduced rim cutter (Figs. 65-3 and 65-4) has been claimed to help with pressurization and therefore with the quality of the cement mantle in cemented hip arthroplasty.[20] This device is designed for use with flanged polyethylene cups. Its use produces a flat rim at the periphery of the acetabulum to aid seating of the flange of the polyethylene cup (Fig. 65-5). This provides a seal, which improves pressurization of the cement as the cup is being inserted.[21]

Drill Holes

The use of drill holes with cemented cups is essential in providing torsional resistance at the bone-cement interface (Fig. 65-6). Between five and eight drill holes measuring 5 to 10 mm in diameter should be placed into the roof of the acetabulum, as well as in the ischium and pubis.[22] These holes should be made with a step drill to prevent penetration into the pelvis. The drill holes should be made at 90 degrees to the acetabular bone and chamfered to reduce edge stresses.[23] Any cysts that are curetted may also be used as cement fixation holes.

Cementing Technique

The priority in using cement is to obtain a good bone-cement interface. Bleeding from the bony bed hinders

a good bone-cement interface; therefore reducing bleeding through hypotensive anesthesia[18] may improve the long-term outcome. Pulsatile lavage is essential in cleaning the cancellous bed of any loose bone fragments and blood, which otherwise would affect cement interdigitation. Cleaning drill holes through pulsed lavage and removing any soft tissue that may have become stuck in the cancellous bone also have proved helpful.

Maintaining a dry acetabular bed before the introduction of cement may be facilitated by the use of an iliac wing aspirator.[20] This device, designed by John Timperley (Fig. 65-7), is placed into the iliac wing before cement is introduced into the acetabulum. The effect is to remove blood from the cancellous bone to improve the cement-bone interface. Use of an iliac wing aspirator has been shown to improve cement intrusion into the bone.[24]

Preferences for the type of cement to be used vary, but primarily, the cement must be easy to handle for the purposes of introducing cement into the acetabulum. Two mixes of cement is sufficient for most acetabula. Once the cement can be taken into the hand without sticking to the glove, it should be placed into the dry acetabulum and pressurized. Pressurization may be achieved with a proprietary device such as the Exeter (Stryker, Kalamazoo, Mich) acetabular pressurizer. Pressure should be maintained for an additional 2 to 3 minutes, depending on the type of cement used.

Insertion of Component

All polyethylene acetabular components are the most commonly used for cemented acetabula.[4] Components should be introduced into the cement on an introducer, with the inferior lip advanced into its position in relation to the TAL. Pressure applied to the introducer will sink the component into the cement to the predetermined position of abduction angle. Once the prosthesis is in the correct position, constant pressure should be applied to the introducer to force cement into the

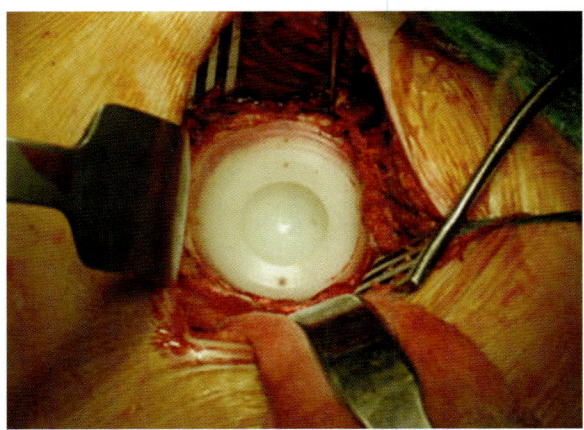

Figure 65-5. Rim-seated flanged polyethylene cup. *(Courtesy Exeter Total Hip, Exeter, United Kingdom.)*

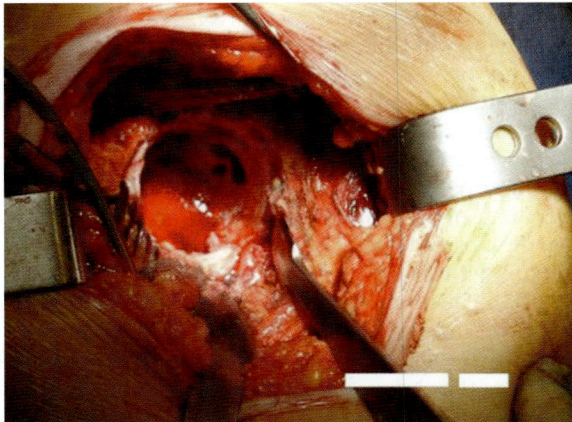

Figure 65-6. Acetabular drill holes.

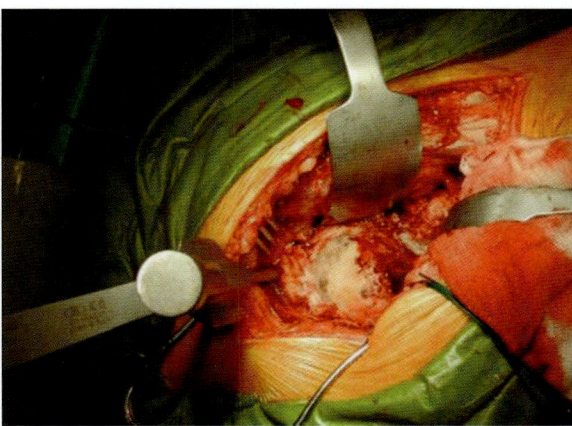

Figure 65-7. Iliac wing aspirator. *(From Sierra RJ, Timperley JA, Gie GA: Contemporary cementing technique and mortality during and after Exeter Total Hip arthroplasty. J Arthroplasty 24:325–332, 2009.)*

cancellous bone. The Exeter cup is a contemporary ultrahigh-molecular-weight polyethylene cup with a flange that is cut to fit the reamed and rim-cut acetabulum. As the flange comes to rest on the rim-cut edge, trapped cement is pressurized further, thus improving penetration.[20,21] The introducer should be removed and exchanged for a ball-pusher to retrieve any extruded cement before it cures. Pressure should be maintained until the cement has fully polymerized.

Any residual osteophytes that might cause impingement and levering should be trimmed away once the cement has hardened (Fig. 65-8).

Unusual Situations/Variations

Situations in which the acetabulum is significantly deformed as a result of dysplasia or previous fracture present special problems. In these scenarios, techniques that provide additional support for the cemented component may be necessary.

Dysplastic hips may be reconstructed with a cemented technique, but the use of block allografts, frozen or an autograft taken from the femoral head or from the iliac wing, and peripheral cages may be necessary, depending on the area of bony deficiency. Results in this situation depend on the experience of the surgeon. Also, dysplasia may present as a relatively straightforward shallow acetabulum or as a more problematic low dislocation or high dislocation. Long-term results for cemented acetabula worsen according to the increasing severity of dysplasia.[25]

Protrusio acetabuli may be a primary pathology or may occur secondary to osteoarthritis, inflammatory arthritis, and septic arthritis, or as a result of trauma (central fracture dislocation). Reconstruction of these acetabular deformities using a cemented technique requires the use of impaction grafting to the acetabular floor. A wire mesh or an acetabular reconstruction cage is fixed over the impacted graft, and a cup is cemented into the construct.

Following acetabular trauma, grafting may be necessary for uncontained defects that require an anchored graft or a morselized graft for contained defects.

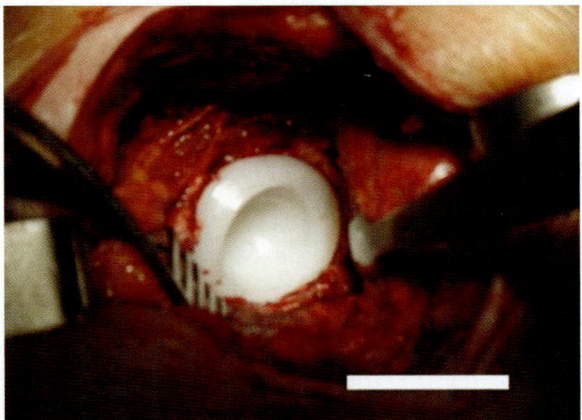

Figure 65-8. Implanted polyethylene cup.

Postoperative Care

Patients who have had cemented acetabula require no special postoperative regimens. Suction drains are a matter of a surgeon's personal preference. Typically, three doses of intravenous broad-spectrum antibiotic and appropriate antithrombotic prophylaxis are necessary.

The mobilization regimen following cemented acetabular reconstruction depends very much on the indication for the reconstruction and therefore on the technical difficulties encountered. A primary cemented acetabulum should allow immediate full weight-bearing mobilization, and in keeping with most postoperative regimens, flexion beyond 90 degrees particularly with internal rotation should be discouraged. In cases where the procedure has been a complex primary, especially in cases where structural grafting has been necessary, it may be appropriate for the patient to remain partially weight bearing for 6 to 12 weeks.

A physiotherapist should be involved in preoperative and postoperative management of patients undergoing total hip arthroplasty. Following surgery, patients should be educated regarding isometric quadriceps and gluteus exercises, transfers, and good gait pattern, and they should be advised about inappropriate movements that may lead to dislocation.

Outcomes

Traditional cemented total hip replacements now have extremely long follow-up.[4,5,7,26] Charnley and Exeter cemented hip replacements have been followed worldwide.

The Charnley hip replacement[1] has published results of 30-year survivorship.[7,27] It is clear that this cemented hip replacement lasts. However in terms of survivorship of the acetabular component, results are inferior in comparison with the femoral component. The original series of Charnley replacements were inserted via trochanteric osteotomy with the use of unsophisticated cementing methods.[28,29] The use of high-density polyethylene acetabula began in 1962. Nine- to 10-year results for these components were reported in 1973 by Charnley and Cupic.[28] Cup wear in this group of patients was measured by the relatively simple method of measuring linear wear on an anteroposterior (AP) view of the pelvis. Results of this analysis showed an average wear of 1.1 mm on 170 radiographs in 1973. Among 409 patients in this study, three cases of radiographic acetabular loosening occurred, of which one had been revised 7 years postoperatively and one was revised 9 years postoperatively; another had not been operated on because of lack of symptoms. In an additional two cases, reoperation was performed to address suspected problems with the acetabular component. Subsequent analysis of these cases until 1976 revealed three more cases of acetabular failure.

From 1976 until 1978, 357 Charnley THRs were performed at the Iowa Methodist Medical Center with so-called *second-generation cementing techniques*.[30] Revised cementing techniques have helped with respect to femoral component longevity but have made little impact on the acetabular side. Madey and associates were able to follow 356 of their patients.[30] The acetabular component was revised because of aseptic loosening in 17 (5%) of the entire series and in 14 (10%) of the 142 hips that survived for at least 15 years. By comparison, only 4 cases of aseptic loosening were reported in the entire series of 356 for the femoral component, and among survivors to 15 years, 3 cases of femoral component loosening were reported.

In 1993, Hodgkinson and colleagues reported their results with Charnley's "flanged" acetabular component[31] following experimental evidence that a flanged socket exerts much greater pressure on setting bone cement.[32] Their results showed that at 10 years, flanged cups had improved radiologic demarcation in comparison with unflanged cups.

In 1979, when the technique of acetabular component insertion was modified to include pulsed lavage, preservation of subchondral bone, and multiple fixation holes and components to improve pressurization, Cornell and Ranawat showed enhanced durability of acetabular fixation.[33] In a subsequent paper, Ranawat postulated that long-term fixation of the component could be assessed by the initial postoperative radiograph if radiolucent lines were present or absent in zone 1.[34]

Crites reviewed the results of Ritter in 2000.[18] He compared acetabular introduction techniques of the 1970s, 1980s, and 1990s. Metal-backed polyethylene cups failed at a significantly greater rate than their predecessors. During the 1990s however, it became clear that compression-molded all-polyethylene cups performed well. Authors concluded that five factors were essential for the long-term success of acetabular components:

1. Good cancellous acetabular bed with particular attention to zone 1
2. Complete coverage of the component within the bony acetabulum
3. Pulsed lavage irrigation of the cancellous bone
4. Drying of the acetabulum with thrombin or a vasoconstricting agent
5. Pressurization of the entire acetabulum at the same time

Mullins and coworkers reviewed their long-term (30-year) outcomes with Charnley THR through a posterior approach.[27] A total of 228 Charnley LFA procedures were performed between 1972 and 1976. Only five cases of aseptic loosening occurred in the acetabular components inserted in this series. In this series, a Charnley cup with a long posterior wall was implanted using first-generation cementing techniques.

The Exeter experience with cemented components is also well documented in the orthopedic literature. Although much of this work refers to survivorship of the Exeter femoral stem, the outcome with the cup is known in most cases. In 2002, the Exeter group reported on 325 Exeter Universal hip replacements.[35] These cemented, polished, double-tapered, modular stems were implanted with cemented polyethylene cups, which in 94% of cases were metal-backed. Survivorship of the cups after 12 years (with revision of the acetabular component for aseptic loosening as the endpoint) was 96.86%. By comparison, survivorship of the femoral component was 100%. A radiographic view was possible in 201 hips at the time of review and was obtained as anteroposterior and lateral images. Migration of the socket was noted in 4% of hips. Radiolucent lines affected all three zones[36] in 17% of cases. No evidence of pelvic osteolysis was found. Four sockets had been revised at the time of the review in 1998; an additional three, which were radiologically loose at the time of review, were subsequently revised. All sockets were metal-backed. Metal-backed sockets were discontinued in 1990, when it became apparent that the metal back was responsible for the generation of polyethylene and cement debris as a result of fretting against the polyethylene and cement.[37] Further investigation has yielded indifferent results with metal-backed polyethylene cups.[38]

In a patient population younger than 50, results with cemented cups are inferior to those in older patients. Lewthwaite and colleagues[39] reported in 2008 on 130 cemented hip replacements performed in patients at an average age of 42 years. Mean follow-up was 12.5 years. On the acetabular side, 97% of the cups were the cemented type. Including revisions, 23 (18.7%) of the acetabular components were judged to have failed clinically or radiographically at the time of final review.

The rim cutter is a device that was developed to try to improve cement mantle quality. Thus far, its use has improved the "quality" of cementation through improved cement penetration and mantle thickness.[21] Conroy and colleagues performed a randomized controlled trial in 40 patients to assess the effects of the rim cutter on cement mantles using a flanged acetabular component.[21] Statistically significant improvement in cement penetration in zone 1 and in cement mantle thickness in zones 2 and 3 was noted.

The iliac wing aspirator is another device designed to improve the penetration of cement into acetabular bone during insertion of the cemented component (see Fig. 65-3). Assessment of this device was performed in 2005 by Hogan and associates[40] to look at penetration of the cement into the iliac wing. Their findings were that penetration was significantly greater in the group in which the device was used. Subsequently, in 2009, John Timperley published results of a radiographic and radiostereometric study in 38 patients randomly allocated to one of two groups.[24] All operations were performed in an identical manner, other than that the iliac wing aspirator was used in one of the groups. Results showed no difference in proximal migration between the two groups. No improvement in fixation was proved from measured translations and rotations of the socket in the suction group. Investigators found no difference in the number or extent of radiolucent lines or in the depth of cement penetration when the iliac suction device was used in conjunction with contemporary cementing techniques. Although no differences were reported in this publication, the authors stated that longer-term outcomes will show differences, because they believe that the iliac wing aspirator is likely to improve the longevity of cemented fixation.

Complications

Complications specific to a cemented acetabular component may be classified according to events occurring because of exposure for the operation and those occurring as a result of the use of polymethylmethacrylate.

Retractors are essential in exposure of the acetabulum in preparation for a cemented component. Insufficient exposure results in failure to prepare the acetabular rim adequately, which often leads to a poor cement technique with consequences for long-term outcomes of the procedure. Homan-type retractors are often used anteriorly and inferiorly. A posterior approach to the hip exposes the sciatic nerve to potential damage, particularly with placement of an inferior retractor. If the inferior retractor is placed too far posteriorly, its tip may injure the sciatic nerve as it passes through the greater sciatic notch. Similarly, if this "inferior" retractor is positioned too far anteriorly, the obturator artery is placed at risk. A retractor placed anteriorly, which is necessary to move the femoral neck away from the acetabulum, could cause damage to the iliac/femoral artery. However, if this anterior retractor is placed more proximally, the psoas is more muscular in this region and therefore provides a greater degree of protection to the artery. Branches of the obturator artery may be divided, causing profuse bleeding from the inferior aspect of the acetabulum during instrumentation or dissection of the anteroinferior part of the acetabulum. Arterial injury during THR is rare. Most of the literature refers to case reports. Bergqvist and colleagues[41] reported on four cases of vascular injury during total hip arthroplasty (THA) and reviewed the literature. Calligaro and coworkers[42] reviewed all their THAs between 1989 and 2002. Acute arterial complications were noted in 8 (0.08%) of their series. The incidence of sciatic and/or femoral nerve palsy following THA is 1% to 3% that of primary THA, with the incidence increasing following revision arthroplasty, particularly in patients with congenitally dislocated hips. Most nerve injuries are partial and temporary, and they occur more frequently in female patients.[43] Often the cause of sciatic nerve palsy is unknown, but a hematoma is occasionally found in cases where re-exploration has been performed. The obturator nerve is also at risk from retractor injury or dissection around the anteroinferior acetabulum. The use of cement during acetabular component insertion may place this nerve at additional risk if the cement that extrudes is not controlled or retrieved from the inferior aspect of the acetabulum. The effect of the exothermic reaction or the presence of a bolus of hardened cement theoretically may cause damage to local nerves. Cement can pass beneath the transverse acetabular ligament into the superolateral aspect of the obturator foramen.

The use of polymethylmethacrylate bone cement often raises concerns about the production of microemboli during pressurization and the consequences of this. Although publications have proved the effect of cement pressurization on the production of microemboli in the cemented femoral stem,[44] no studies show that microemboli occur during insertion of a cemented acetabular component of a primary THA.

High-Risk Patient

Older patients tend to be regarded as at higher risk in terms of the potential for complications following THA.[45,46] The potential embolic effect of bone cement on the cardiovascular system of older patients provides sufficient reason for surgeons to be cautious when using bone cement in these patients. However, it is older patients who benefit most from the cemented form of THA in that the act of inserting the prosthesis is much less mechanically traumatic for the bones.

Patients who are 50 years old or younger are poor candidates for cemented acetabular components given the inferior results reported in this group of patients.[4] Also, patients with coexisting or comorbid disease require special attention before, during, and after cemented total hip arthroplasty. The presence of coexisting disease predicts whether older patients will develop postoperative complications.[36] Obesity and smoking present significant risks for patients undergoing cemented hip arthroplasty, given their association with cardiac and respiratory diseases.

Ultimately, one wants to use an implant that will last for the rest of the patient's life. This is not always possible, and the difficulty of the resulting revision will depend on the component used at the first operation. Cemented cups often fail between the cement and the bone, resulting in loosening in this plane, which makes removal of the component relatively easy. By contrast, uncemented cups may be difficult to remove in cases where localized osteolysis has occurred, and removal of the cup is necessary to graft the resulting defect.[47] Other reasons for having to remove a well-fixed cup, such as liner wear, recurrent dislocation, and infection, pose similar problems—problems that are potentially easier to overcome with a cemented cup.

Issues such as the post irradiation pelvis are also better served with a cemented cup, given the inferior results described in this situation.[48]

CURRENT CONTROVERSIES

Cemented acetabular components are a very good and cost-effective choice for certain patients. Cemented arthroplasty has the longest clinical follow-up data—a fact that cannot be disputed—which show that this form of hip arthroplasty works well. Primary problems with the use of cemented components are the technical nature of the operation and the risk of late loosening; it is the desire to avoid these problems that has prompted the search for alternative fixation methods. Cemented components must be inserted with good technique to obtain good, consistent results; unless a surgeon is well trained in the use of cement, results will be inferior. Surgeons training in the modern era must not ignore the results of traditional methods and should at every opportunity consider which implant fixation is going to work for each specific patient.

Current research in cemented hip replacement is striving for improved longevity of fixation. The successful use of flanged cups with rim fitting has yet to be proved clinically. Iliac wing aspiration certainly improves the penetration of cement into bone but has yet to be shown to improve survival of the implant.

Other issues that require clarification through future research efforts include the following:

- The best cement consistency/working characteristic to improve fixation
- The use of highly cross-linked polyethylene, which appears very promising for cemented acetabular components
- The best counter face—metal, ceramic, or oxinium
- Ongoing technological advances in improving the quality of cementation

REFERENCES

1. Charnley J: Low friction arthroplasty of the hip: theory and practice, New York, 1979, Springer-Verlag.
2. Haboush E: A new operation for arthroplasty of the hip based on biomechanics, photoelasticity, fast-setting dental acrylic, and other considerations. Bull Hosp Jt Dis 14:242–277, 1953.
3. Charnley J: Acrylic cement in orthopaedic surgery, Baltimore, 1970, Williams & Wilkins.
4. Swedish Hip Arthroplasty Register: Annual report 2007, Lund, Sweden, 2007, Swedish Hip Arthroplasty Register.
5. Wroblewski BM, Siney BA: Charnley low friction arthroplasty of the hip: long term results. Clin Orthop Relat Res 292:191–201, 1993.
6. Older J: Charnley low friction arthroplasty: a worldwide retrospective review at 15 to 20 years. J Arthroplasty 17:675–680, 2002.
7. Callaghan JJ, Templeton JE, Liu SS, et al: Results of Charnley total hip arthroplasty at a minimum of thirty years: a concise follow-up of a previous report. J Bone Joint Surg Am 86:690–695, 2004.
8. Lewthwaite SC, Squires B, Gie GA, et al: The Exeter Universal hip in patients 50 years or younger at 10-17 years' followup. Clin Orthop Relat Res 466:324–331, 2008.
9. Dalstra M, Huiskes R: The influence of metal-backing in cemented cups. Orthop Trans 15:459, 1991.
10. National Joint Registry for England and Wales: 6th annual report 2009, Hempstead, United Kingdom, 2009, NJR.
11. The Norwegian Arthroplasty Register: 2007 report, Bergen, Norway, 2007, NAR.
12. Levy B, Berry D, Pagnano M: Long-term survivorship of cemented all-polyethylene acetabular components in patients >75 years of age. J Arthroplasty 15:461–467, 2000.
13. Della Valle AG, Padgett DE, Salvati EA: Preoperative planning for primary total hip arthroplasty. J Am Acad Orthop Surg 13:455–462, 2005.
14. Ala Eddine T, Rémy F, Chantelot C, et al: Iliopsoas conflict with the total hip arthroplasty cup: diagnostic approach and therapeutic modalities in nine cases. J Bone Joint Surg Br 84(Suppl I):51–52, 2002.
15. Pitto RP, Bhargava A, Pandit S, et al: Retroacetabular stress-shielding in THA. Clin Orthop Relat Res 466:353–358, 2008.
16. Archbold HAP, Mockford B, Molloy D, et al: The transverse acetabular ligament: an aid to orientation of the acetabular component during primary total hip replacement. J Bone Joint Surg Br 88:883–886, 2006.
17. Ranawat CS, Rawlins BA, Harju VT: Effect of modern cement technique on acetabular fixation total hip arthroplasty: a retrospective study in matched pairs. Orthop Clin North Am 19:599–603, 1988.
18. Crites BM, Berend ME, Ritter MA: Technical considerations of cemented acetabular components: a 30-year evaluation. Clin Orthop Relat Res 381:114–119, 2000.
19. Flivik G, Kristiansson I, Kesteris U, Ryd L: Is removal of subchondral bone plate advantageous in cemented cup fixation? A randomized RSA study. Clin Orthop Relat Res 448:164–172, 2006.
20. Sierra RJ, Timperley JA, Gie GA: Contemporary cementing technique and mortality during and after Exeter total hip arthroplasty. J Arthroplasty 24:325–332, 2009.
21. Conroy JL, Chawda M, Kaushal R, et al: Does use of a "rim cutter" improve quality of cementation of the acetabular component of cemented Exeter total hip arthroplasty? J Arthroplasty 24:71–75, 2009.
22. Mburu G, Aspden RM, Hutchison JD: Optimizing the configuration of cement keyholes for acetabular fixation in total hip replacement using Taguchi experimental design. Proc Inst Mech Eng 213:485–492, 1999.
23. Mootanah R, Jarrett P, Ingle P, et al: Configuration of anchorage holes affects cemented fixation of the acetabular component in total hip replacement: an in vitro study. Technol Health Care 16:19–30, 2008.
24. Timperley AJ, Whitehouse SL, Hourigan PG: The influence of a suction device on fixation of a cemented cup using RSA. Clin Orthop Relat Res 467:792–798, 2009.
25. Chougle A, Hemmady MV, Hodgkinson JP: Severity of hip dysplasia and loosening of the socket in cemented total hip replacement: a long-term follow-up. J Bone Joint Surg Br 87:16–20, 2005.
26. Callaghan JJ, Templeton JE, Liu SS, et al: Results of Charnley total hip arthroplasty at a minimum of thirty years. J Bone Joint Surg Am 86:690–695, 2004.
27. Mullins MM, Norbury W, Dowell JK, Heywood-Waddington M: Thirty-year results of a prospective study of Charnley total hip arthroplasty by the posterior approach. J Arthroplasty 22:833–839, 2007.
28. Charnley J, Cupic Z: The nine and ten year results of low friction arthroplasty of the hip. Clin Orthop Relat Res 95:9–25, 1973.
29. Stauffer RN: Ten-year follow-up study of total hip replacement. J Bone Joint Surg Am 64:983–990, 1982.
30. Madey SM, Callaghan JJ, Olejniczak JP, et al: Charnley total hip arthroplasty with use of improved techniques of cementing. J Bone Joint Surg Am 79:53–64, 1997.
31. Hodgkinson JP, Maskell AP, Ashok PB, Wroblewski M: Flanged acetabular components in cemented Charnley hip arthroplasty: ten year follow-up of 350 patients. J Bone Joint Surg Br 75:464–467, 1993.
32. Shelley P, Wroblewski BM: Socket design and cement pressurisation in the Charnley low-friction arthroplasty. J Bone Joint Surg Br 70:358–363, 1988.
33. Comell CN, Ranawat CS: The impact of modern cement techniques on acetabular fixation in cemented total hip replacement. J Arthroplasty 1:197–202, 1986.
34. Ranawat C, Deshmukh R, Peters L, Umlas M: Prediction of the long-term durability of all-polyethylene cemented sockets. Clin Orthop Relat Res 317:89–105, 1995.
35. Williams HDW, Browne G, Gie GA, et al: The Exeter Universal cemented femoral component at 8 to 12 years. J Bone Joint Surg Br 84:324–334, 2002.
36. Delee JG, Charnley J: Radiological demarcation of cemented sockets in total hip replacement. Clin Orthop Relat Res 121:20–32, 1976.
37. Dalstra M, Huiskes R: The influence of metal-backing in cemented cups. Orthop Trans 15:459, 1991.
38. Ritter MA, Keating EM, Faris PM, Brugo G: Metal-backed acetabular cups in total hip arthroplasty. J Bone Joint Surg Am 72:672–677, 1990.
39. Lewthwaite SC, Squires B, Gie GA, et al: The Exeter Universal hip in patients 50 years or younger at 10-17 years' followup. Clin Orthop Relat Res 466:324–331, 2008.
40. Hogan N, Azhar A, Brady O: An improved acetabular cementing technique in total hip arthroplasty: aspiration of the iliac wing. J Bone Joint Surg Br 87:1216–1219, 2005.
41. Bergqvist D, Carlsson AS, Ericsson BF: Vascular complications after total hip arthroplasty. Acta Orthop Scand 54:157–163, 1983.
42. Calligaro KD, Dougherty MJ, Ryan S, Booth RE: Acute arterial complications associated with total hip and knee arthroplasty. J Vasc Surg 38:1170–1175, 2003.
43. Edwards BN, Tullos HS, Noble PC: Contributory factors and etiology of sciatic nerve palsy in total hip arthroplasty. Clin Orthop Relat Res 218:136–141, 1987.

44. Patterson BM, Healey JH, Cornell CN, Sharrock NE: Cardiac arrest during hip arthroplasty with a cemented long-stem component: a report of seven cases. J Bone Joint Surg Am 73:271–277, 1991.
45. Wurtz LD, Feinberg JR, Capello WN, et al: Elective primary total hip arthroplasty in octogenarians. J Gerontol Series A Biol Sci Med Sci 58:M468–M471, 2003.
46. Brander VA, Malhotra S, Jet J, et al: Outcome of hip and knee arthroplasty in persons aged 80 years and older. Clin Orthop Relat Res 345:67–78, 1997.
47. Maloney WJ, Herzwurm P, Paprosky W, et al: Treatment of pelvic osteolysis associated with a stable acetabular component inserted without cement as part of a total hip replacement. J Bone J Surg Am 79:1628–1634, 1997.
48. Jacobs JJ, Kull LR, Frey GA, et al: Early failure of acetabular components inserted without cement after previous pelvic irradiation. J Bone Joint Surg Am 77:1829–1835, 1995.

FURTHER READING

Callaghan JJ, Templeton JE, Liu SS, et al: Results of Charnley total hip arthroplasty at a minimum of thirty years: a concise follow-up of a previous report. J Bone Joint Surg Am 86:690–695, 2004.
An article proving that the Charnley prosthesis has stood the test of time even after 30 years. This article shows that 88% of original prostheses were intact at final follow-up.

Crites BM, Berend ME, Ritter MA: Technical considerations of cemented acetabular components: a 30-year evaluation. Clin Orthop Relat Res 381:114–119, 2000.
This article shows, in a very scientific way, how improvements in cementing technique over a number of years have improved the fixation that can be attained with a cemented acetabular component.

Ranawat CS, Peters LE, Umlas ME: Fixation of the acetabular component: the case for cement. Clin Orthop Relat Res 344:207–215, 1997.
Dr. Ranawat summarizes why the cemented acetabulum is durable, reproducible, and financially viable in a well-selected population of patients.

CHAPTER 66

Uncemented Acetabular Components

Neil P. Sheth and Craig J. Della Valle

INTRODUCTION

Cemented acetabular component fixation in total hip arthroplasty (THA) was introduced in the early 1960s by Sir John Charnley. Early results demonstrated favorable clinical outcomes with radiographic loosening rates of less than 5%.[1] The use of cement remained the major mode of acetabular component fixation until longer-term (>10-year follow-up) results demonstrated rates of radiographic loosening as high as 60%.[1-9] Improvements in cement technique throughout the 1970s and 1980s led to improved femoral component durability, but similar benefits were not recognized on the acetabular side.[6,10,11] In addition, the surgical technique for cemented acetabular fixation is technically demanding, and even in expert hands, radiographic outcomes were not always found to be ideal. Furthermore, the lack of liner modularity rendered few options for optimizing intraoperative

stability. Based on these factors, interest mounted in a new approach to acetabular component fixation. Specifically, biological fixation of acetabular components through insertion of a cementless device developed as an alternative method of reconstruction in the hope that a biological bond between implant and host bone would provide greater long-term durability, along with a simpler, more reproducible surgical technique and greater intraoperative flexibility.

Cementless acetabular fixation brought about the advent of novel designs and cup geometries and the use of different implant materials in conjunction with various surface coatings that would lead to initial implant stability and long-term biological fixation. Factors critical to obtaining adequate stability and biological fixation were identified, and methods of cup insertion were developed. Radiographic and clinical evaluation at more than 20 years postoperatively has shown favorable results[12] that have made hemispherical, porous-coated, cementless acetabular devices with or without adjunctive screw fixation the implant of choice in most North American centers for primary total hip arthroplasty.

GENERAL CONSIDERATIONS

Requirements for bone ingrowth include biocompatibility of the surface material, an appropriate pore size, adequate surface contact with host bone, and initial stability during the incorporation process.[13-16] Pilliar and associates demonstrated that excessive micromotion greater than 150 μm at the bone-implant interface resulted in fibrous tissue infiltration behind the acetabular component as opposed to bone ingrowth.[17] Bobyn and colleagues determined that the optimal pore size for bone ingrowth to occur was between 100 μm and 400 μm.[18] As a result of these findings, in the early 1980s, porous-coated hemispherical cups were introduced, including porous-coated anatomic (PCA, Howmedica, Rutherford, NJ), Harris-Galante (Zimmer, Warsaw, Ind) (Fig. 66-1), and anatomic medullary locking cups (AML, DePuy, Warsaw, Ind).

Implant Materials

Titanium and Cobalt-Chromium Alloys

Various materials were initially used in the manufacture of cementless acetabular components, including

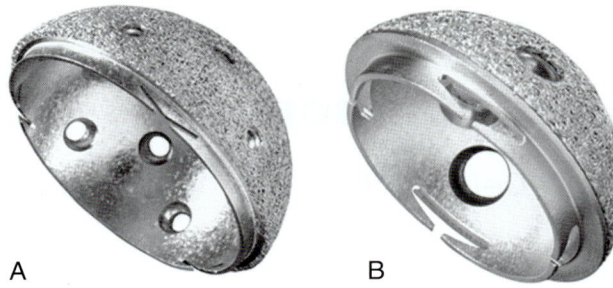

Figure 66-1. Harris-Galante (HG)-1 and HG-2 cups.

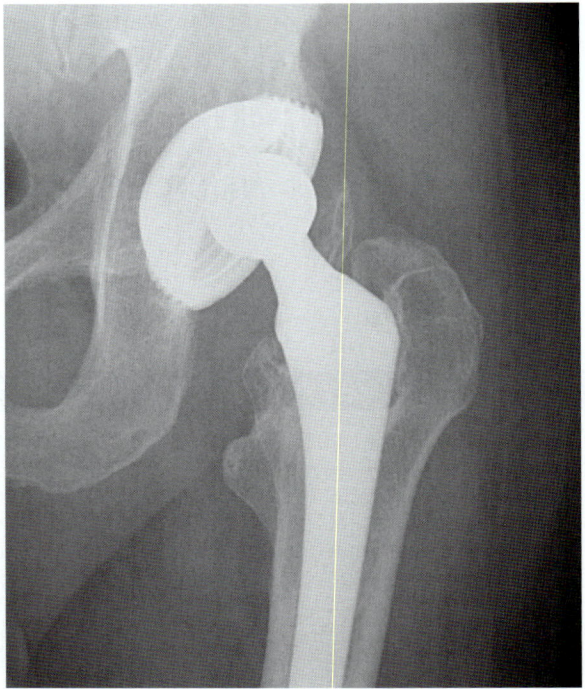

Figure 66-2. Anteroposterior (AP) radiograph of a threaded acetabular cup. *(Courtesy Dr. William L. Jaffe, MD.)*

nonmetallic materials (such as all-polyethylene or all-ceramic components, which met with high failure rates as there was no surface by which ingrowth could support long-term stability) and, more commonly, titanium[19] or cobalt-chromium alloys. Both metal-based materials are biocompatible and are capable of supporting bone ingrowth; however, quantitatively, titanium has shown increased bone density, deeper penetration, and a greater degree of mean bone ingrowth as compared with cobalt-chromium components.[20]

Additional benefits are associated with titanium as an implant material. Titanium has a lower modulus of elasticity, closer to that of cancellous bone, theoretically yielding a lesser degree of stress remodeling of the host pelvic bone. In addition, it is a more flexible material, lending itself to easier insertion, especially if a press-fit technique is used, and is associated with potentially lower insertional acetabular fracture risk.[21] From a manufacturing perspective, titanium is easier to handle than cobalt-chromium, and, in the arena of health care cost containment, titanium is less expensive.[21]

Implant Shape

The concept of "cement disease" became popular as a reason for loss of fixation of cemented acetabular implants. By eliminating cement, the hope was that acetabular fixation would be more durable. The first generation of cementless acetabular components were designed with several different geometries and were classified by Morscher and associates[22] into five different types: (1) cylindrical, (2) square, (3) cone type, (4) ellipsoid or oblong, and (5) hemispherical. Of these design types, the most popular designs used are presented in the following paragraphs.

Among the more common early "cementless" designs were threaded acetabular components, designed in the early 1970s. Most of these designs did not possess a surface coating and therefore relied upon a mechanical interlock between the device and the host bone, rather than biological fixation, to achieve stable implant fixation. Some specific designs included the Lord cup, along with Mittelmeier, Mecring, T-Tap, and S-ROM Anderson implants. Several studies reported initial satisfactory results, but longer-term follow-up revealed loosening rates of nearly 60% and early revision rates for aseptic loosening as high as 31% at 10 years.[23-28]

Several theories regarding the reasons for unacceptable rates of migratory failure with first-generation threaded implants became prevalent. It was thought that screwing in a cementless implant led to increased stresses at the implant-bone (thread) interface, resulting in subsequent pressure necrosis, bone resorption, and fibrous tissue interposition.[23,29] Retrieval studies supported the postulation that fibrous tissue filled in between the threaded surfaces, yielding inadequate host-bone contact to support long-term fixation.[30,31]

As compared with hemispherical cup designs, threaded components were more difficult to reproducibly insert in the proper position. Acetabular bed preparation for threaded components was challenging and often led to poorer mechanical stability compared with hemispherical cups because of a lesser degree of surface area contact with host bone. In addition, many systems used an awkward insertional handle, which predisposed to vertical cup positioning, especially in obese patients.[21]

The failure of first-generation cementless devices brought about so-called *second-generation threaded cementless implants* that incorporated a porous or grit-blasted surface to enhance biological fixation via bone ingrowth or ongrowth, respectively. Despite the shortcomings of threaded designs, these devices relied upon the threads for initial mechanical stability and the surface coating for long-term biological fixation. Cups with this design included the Zweymüller (grit-blasted titanium; Zimmer), the S-ROM Super Cup (titanium-sintered beads; DePuy), and the Arc-2f (hydroxyapatite-coated; Osteonics, Stryker Orthopaedics, Mahway, NJ) (Fig. 66-2). Medium-term results demonstrated extremely low rates of radiographic failure; however, these devices had numerous problems that resulted in a move toward alternative designs, including difficulty with insertion and high rates of polyethylene wear.[28,32,33] Incorporation of a surface coating with the early threaded design feature supported the importance of initial mechanical stability in conjunction with biological fixation for long-term implant stability.

Hemispherical cups are classified as having single or dual geometry design. Dual geometry components exhibit an enlarged radius at the rim of the component and were designed to maximize the surface area of contact for biological ingrowth. The dual geometry design gained enthusiasm in attempts to avoid adjunctive fixation to enhance the initial mechanical stability of the implanted acetabular component. Concern has arisen that design features may decrease total contact between the component and the surrounding host bone, specifically at the dome portion of the implant, leading to decreased bone ingrowth. Bauer and coworkers[34] evaluated two dual geometry cup designs at the time of postmortem retrieval and found evidence of increased bone ingrowth at the peripheral rim as compared with the dome. The authors compared this design to threaded cups and determined that a greater degree of bone apposition was seen with the dual geometry design, but bone ingrowth was less than was suggested by radiographs.[34] Most cementless acetabular devices in use today are single geometry in design, mostly because of the ease of acetabular bed preparation and reproducible insertion.[21]

The final shape to be considered is the hemi-ellipsoid shape of the Zimmer trabecular metal component. This device exhibits a gradual transition in interference from the peripheral rim (2 mm) to the dome (0 mm). The rationale behind this design is that it maximizes peripheral interference stability, minimizes the potential for early bottoming out, and eliminates the discontinuity associated with dual geometry designs. This interference fit plays an important role in monoblock-type implants, into which screws cannot be inserted for supplemental fixation (Fig. 66-3).

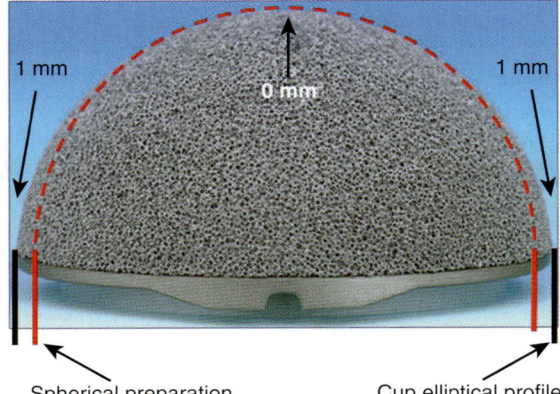

Figure 66-3. Hemi-ellipsoid shape of a trabecular metal acetabular monoblock shell. (*Courtesy Zimmer, Warsaw, Ind.*)

Surface Coatings

With the understanding that surface coatings were of critical importance in achieving clinical success with an uncemented acetabular component, several different surface preparations were developed. Hydroxyapatite (HA) coatings gained popularity as osteoconductive surface coatings for acetabular components, secondary to good early and intermediate results when applied to cementless femoral components.[35,36] Unfortunately, when applied to the back of a cementless acetabular component without an underlying porous surface, when the HA resorbed over time, a high rate of failure ensued, because no ingrowth or ongrowth surface could provide long-term fixation.[37] Hydroxyapatite is still popular, however, and improved results have been associated with the use of HA in conjunction with porous-coated or grit-blasted surfaces.[38-40]

Calcicoat

The basic requirements for bone ingrowth became evident and included factors such as material biocompatibility, optimal pore size, initial implant stability, and intimate contact at the interface between the component and the host bone. Adjuvant techniques, specifically the use of a calcium phosphate ceramic (Calcicoat, Zimmer), were devised to further enhance bony ingrowth into porous materials.[41] Ducheyne and associates[42] demonstrated increased strength and skeletal fixation and volume of bone formation with the use of porous implants impregnated with a calcium phosphate slurry. Other authors attempted to replicate the study; although they were unsuccessful in reproducing the results,[43] the concept of a bioreactive coating on an inert porous metal to enhance biological fixation became attractive.

Rivero and colleagues[41] used an in vivo animal model to evaluate porous titanium fiber implants for cementless skeletal fixation treated with a calcium phosphate coating applied with a plasma flame-spray as compared with matched-pair controls. Implants were inserted into the humeri and olecranons of 36 adult dogs and were harvested and biomechanically tested over a 6-week period at 2-week intervals. Calcicoat-treated implants demonstrated 24% greater shear strength ($P < .01$) than matched-pair controls at 4 weeks. The osteoconductive properties of Calcicoat were thought to allow for bone formation in direct contact with the coating on the titanium fibers. The authors concluded that although the volume of bone growth was not different between groups, Calcicoat as a ceramic coating may serve to enhance the skeletal fixation of porous metal implants.

Other studies have clinically evaluated various coating surfaces such as Calcicoat. Laursen and coworkers[44] assessed the 3-year results of porous-coated Trilogy acetabular components as compared with Trilogy acetabular cups coated with HA and tricalcium phosphate (TCP). All cups were inserted using a press-fit technique and were evaluated by dual-emission x-ray absorptiometry (DEXA) scan to determine periprosthetic bone density. At the time of final follow-up, no difference was noted between the two cohorts in terms

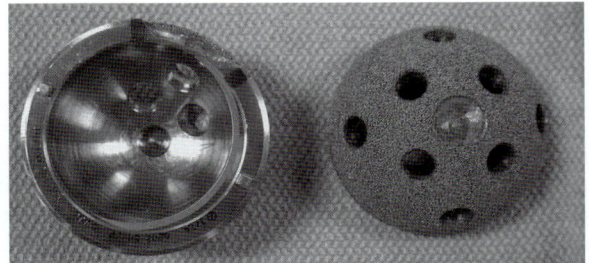

Figure 66-4. Modular tantalum cementless acetabular cup.

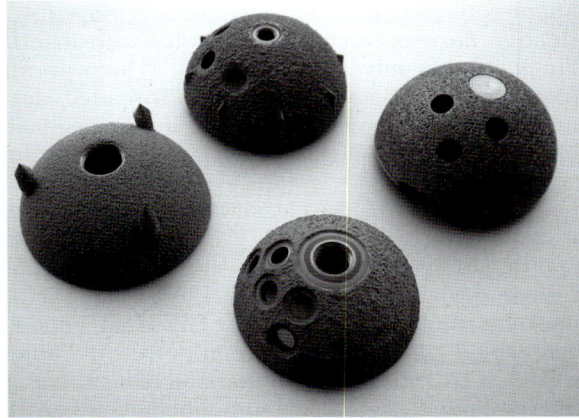

Figure 66-5. Cementless acetabular components with different fixation options, including spikes, pegs, or screws.

of periprosthetic bone density. However, the authors concluded that heavier patients regained more bone mineral; this supports the assumption that load is beneficial for bone remodeling.[44]

Porous Metals

Significant enthusiasm has surrounded the use of recently introduced so-called *porous metals* that have biomechanical properties similar to those of cancellous bone. Metals such as tantalum possess a volume porosity of 70% to 80%, a modulus of elasticity of 3 GPa (same order of magnitude as cancellous bone), and frictional characteristics that encourage bone ingrowth[45] (Fig. 66-4).

Several early clinical and radiographic evaluations were conducted using tantalum acetabular components for primary total hip arthroplasty (THA). These studies described acceptable results comparable with those of conventional cementless components; however, no direct comparative studies suggest a clear advantage over components manufactured from standard materials such as titanium.[46-48] In addition, in the single component that has been studied most widely, a high rate of dislocation was observed; this was hypothesized to be secondary to femoral neck impingement against the rim of the polyethylene liner.

In one recent study, Gruen and colleagues[48] evaluated 574 patients at 2 to 5 years after the index THA. At final follow-up, only 412 of the original patient cohort were available for radiographic analysis, although 100% demonstrated evidence of osseointegration. A total of 10 hips (1.7%) required revision: six (1%) for recurrent dislocation, one (0.2%) for traumatic cup loosening, and three (0.5%) for infection. Although short-term results seem favorable, longer-term clinical studies are required to determine the efficacy of porous tantalum and other porous metals.

METHODS OF UNCEMENTED ACETABULAR CUP FIXATION

Immediate implant stability is critical for achieving osseointegration. Although line-to-line insertion and fixation with supplemental screws for fixation were popular in the past, most surgeons currently use a press-fit technique wherein the acetabulum is reamed to 1 to 2 mm below the size of the component inserted

with or without the use of supplemental screws, pegs, or spikes for adjunctive fixation.

Supplemental Fixation

Although supplemental fixation with screws has been associated with high rates of osseointegration,[31,49] concerns have been raised regarding screws and associated screw holes as pathways for wear particles that lead to osteolysis.[50] Further, fretting corrosion between the screws and the metal shell is an additional concern with the use of screws for adjunctive fixation.

Cook and coworkers conducted a histologic study comparing the degree of bone ingrowth attained with the use of components with spikes, pegs, or screws (Fig. 66-5). The authors were able to demonstrate that the distribution of bone ingrowth surrounded the pegs or spikes, but was greater surrounding cups secured with adjunctive screws, because this design allowed visualization of bone-implant contact upon insertion—a factor that has been shown to influence bone ingrowth. They concluded that the use of peripheral spikes or pegs may prevent adequate seating of the cementless device, thereby reducing the surface area of contact between the porous surface and the host bone. Concerns surfaced regarding difficulty in repositioning a malpositioned cup with peripheral fins or spikes. In addition, several retrieval studies have shown increased bone ingrowth adjacent to screws compared with other regions of the cup.[31,51]

Biomechanical analyses of these modes of adjunctive fixation further demonstrated that the use of screws may convert torsional forces to compressive forces, thereby preloading the bone-prosthesis interface and increasing the contact area, further promoting bone ingrowth.[52] Using in vitro models, Lachiewicz and associates[53] showed that significantly greater torque was required for screw failure as compared with spikes and pegs, and Stiehl and colleagues[54] revealed less micromotion with the use of screw fixation compared with pegs.

Although ample literature supports the use of screws, other studies have demonstrated excellent clinical success of components when dome spikes or peripheral pegs and fins were used. Engh and colleagues[55] reported 15-year survivorship of 95% for tri-spiked cementless acetabular components with revision for aseptic loosening as an endpoint.

With improved, low wear–bearing surfaces, concerns regarding screw holes as access channels for wear particles may no longer be relevant, because the particle load with alternative bearings and highly cross-linked polyethylene may be below the level required to induce osteolysis. Long-term studies are required to make a definitive conclusion, because this concept pertains to implant longevity.

An additional important consideration to be addressed regarding supplemental screw fixation is the risk of neurovascular injury associated with errant screw placement. Through the combination of defined acetabular quadrants, improved understanding of pelvic anatomy, and increased surgeon experience in placing acetabular screws, the risk for neurovascular injury has been dramatically reduced by placement of screws in the posterosuperior quadrant with careful measurement of screw length.[56]

Press-Fit Technique

The concept of a pure *press-fit technique* without the use of screws for component insertion was developed to avoid the use of screws for the reasons previously described. The acetabulum is under-reamed by 1 mm to 2 mm, and then the component is impacted into place. This method of cup insertion is dependent upon the viscoelastic or time-dependent properties of bone to allow deformation and recoil to obtain initial implant stability.[52]

On initial evaluation of the press-fit technique, it was evident that radiolucencies at the periphery of the acetabular shell were less prevalent; however, gaps at the dome were more common. By 2 years, dome gaps were no longer visible, suggesting bone formation at the pole of the component.[57] In vitro analysis, however, showed that gaps greater than 2 mm are not compatible with bone formation and subsequently increase the effective joint space for synovial fluid and wear with debris access to trabecular bone behind the component.[58]

Both Won and associates and Steihl and colleagues demonstrated in a cadaveric model that press-fit insertion with under-reaming by 1 mm resulted in better component mechanical stability than line-to-line insertion with the use of supplemental screw fixation.[54,59] Based on this and other studies, it seems that the depth and accuracy of acetabular reaming may be more important than the presence of supplemental fixation modalities (e.g., spikes, pegs, screws) for attaining mechanical stability.

Finite element models have been used to evaluate loading conditions at the periphery of cementless devices. Acetabular strains registered at the periphery of hemispherical cups inserted using a press-fit technique were the highest, resulting in greater compressive bone forces, thus enhancing cup stability.[60,61] Component oversizing of 2 mm rather than 1 mm was needed to augment this; however, greater amounts of under-reaming increase the risk for acetabular fracture. This may be dependent on acetabular component size; in general, larger amounts of under-reaming are acceptable for larger components.

Comparisons were made between hemispherical and dual geometry cup designs that possess a wider radius at the mouth of the implant compared with the dome; this is intended to increase press-fit at the rim of the acetabulum. Dual geometry designs when tested biomechanically produced higher strain rates at the periphery than were produced by hemispherical cups but resulted in less deformation of the acetabular bone stock. Theoretically, such dual geometry designs would require less force for proper implant seating and would potentially decrease the risk of acetabular fracture upon insertion. However, although higher strains were recorded at the periphery with dual geometry designs, hemispherical cups exhibited better overall implant stability; thus the dual geometry design concept, for the most part, has fallen out of favor.[60,61]

The risk of creating a periprosthetic acetabular fracture is a concern that surfaced when the press-fit technique of insertion was introduced. This technique of insertion relies upon hoop stresses generated within the acetabulum to help maintain component stability. The tenet that is inherent to this technique is that the host bone is able to tolerate the hoop stresses that are generated. Insertion of significantly oversized components may result in inadequate acetabular component seating and possible fracture of acetabular walls or columns. Kim and associates[62] showed that 18 of 30 (60%) acetabular fractures occurred during insertion of cementless devices using a press-fit technique. Acetabular fractures were more likely with components that were oversized by 4 mm than 2 mm. Sharkey and colleagues reported 13 periprosthetic acetabular fractures, of which 9 were recognized intraoperatively, during implantation of a hemispherical cup using a press-fit technique and under reaming by 1 mm to 3 mm. Of the 13 patients, 6 had osteoarthritis, 3 had osteonecrosis of the femoral head, 2 had rheumatoid arthritis, and the remaining patients were treated for developmental dysplasia or a hip fracture nonunion. Fractures identified intraoperatively were addressed by a variety of methods including screw augmentation in and around the cup, use of autologous bone graft at the fracture site, and/or protected weight bearing and immobilization postoperatively. Two cases identified postoperatively required acetabular component revision because of radiographic evidence of component migration. As a result, the authors identified two additional predisposing clinical risk factors for periprosthetic acetabular fracture—osteoporosis and rheumatoid arthritis.[63]

POLYETHYLENE LINERS AND MODULARITY

The introduction of modular polyethylene liners in the 1980s addressed concerns over intraoperative flexibility to maximize stability and allow for modular exchange of the bearing surface in cases of wear. Although this design advancement provided potential benefits, it also introduced unanticipated problems such as backside wear (wear associated with an additional interface between the polyethylene liner and the metal shell) and the potential for liner dissociation.[64]

Wear of the polyethylene liner seemed to be a greater problem than with cemented, all-polyethylene components. Wear rates exhibited by cementless acetabular cups were in the range of 0.10 mm/yr to 0.25 mm/yr[11,50,65-73] compared with 0.07 mm/yr to 0.15 mm/yr[2,7,9,10,74] with cemented, all-polyethylene cups. First-generation cementless devices in some instances utilized a liner of inadequate thickness often combined with larger, 32-mm heads that caused increased volumetric wear and wear-related complications. Further, suboptimal locking mechanisms and rough inner surfaces in some cases led to substantial backside wear of the liner, which exacerbated the particle load. Another factor that contributed to increased wear rates was the use of gamma-irradiation in air for polyethylene sterilization during this time.

The effect of liner thickness on polyethylene wear rates has been evaluated by several authors. Contact stresses between the femoral head and the acetabular liner increase as the thickness of the liner decreases. With thin polyethylene liners, the liner behaves like the stiffer underlying metal shell, leading to increased failure rates due to early fatigue failure.[32,67] Bartel and associates[75] demonstrated via finite element analysis that contact stresses dramatically increased when the liner thickness was less than 6 mm. Berry and colleagues[76] reported an increased risk of polyethylene wear and liner fracture when the thickness was less than 5 mm.

Congruency between the liner and the inner surface of the shell is another important component of wear generation in cementless acetabular fixation. Irregularities in the surface from design features such as screw holes or fenestrations may result in areas of unsupported polyethylene, leading to cold flow of the polyethylene and further backside wear. Nonuniform congruency between the two surfaces can result in micromotion between the shell and the liner; this is hypothesized to increase retroacetabular osteolysis.[14,50,67,68]

Early cementless acetabular components were plagued by poor liner locking mechanisms. The first-generation PCA locking mechanism failed secondary to cracks in the liner and resulting deformation of the anti-rotation notch in the polyethylene rim.[66] The Mallory-Head prosthesis utilized a hexagonal liner locking mechanism, which resulted in excessive motion between the shell and the liner and subsequent increased wear and acetabular lysis.[77] Harris-Galante 1 and 2 utilized tines for locking the liner into place. These tines were reported to break, creating the potential for liner dissociation.

In an effort to expand the armamentarium to restore offset and address intraoperative instability in primary THA, different design features such as elevated rims and lateral or extended offset were incorporated into polyethylene liners. One study by Archibeck and coworkers[78] evaluated the use of extended offset and its effect on cementless acetabular component fixation. The authors retrospectively reviewed more than 1900 primary THA procedures, among which a 7-mm extended offset polyethylene liner was used in 120 cases. The aseptic acetabular loosening rate was 0.12% for the standard offset liner group compared with 4.0% for the offset liner group at a minimum of 2 years' follow-up (mean, 3.6 years; range, 2 to 9 years). Acetabular component survivorship was significantly less ($P < .01$) for the offset liner group compared with the standard liner group at 6 years. The authors concluded that even though offset liners are useful for restoring hip mechanics and may assist in addressing THA instability, the increased loosening rate may be attributed to the transfer of increased torsional loads to the prosthesis.[78]

It is evident that although benefits are provided by the introduction of modularity in cementless acetabular implants, this approach has been associated with problems. In response to these problems, newer designs have incorporated more secure locking mechanisms often combined with a polished inner cup surface to decrease backside wear. Although newer, more wear-resistant bearing surfaces may decrease the prevalence of some of these issues, the presence of a secure locking mechanism is required for optimal results.

RADIOGRAPHIC EVALUATION OF CEMENTLESS ACETABULAR COMPONENT FIXATION

The presence of progressive radiolucencies (particularly if >2 mm in width), a change in the acetabular component opening angle of greater than 5 degrees, broken screws, and component migration of 2 to 3 mm are the most universally agreed upon findings of a loose component. Serial radiographs are often the best way to identify these abnormalities and to define and monitor osteolysis.[74,79-82]

The implant-bone interface is most commonly described using the zones of Delee and Charnley. They divided the retroacetabular region into three equivalent zones: zone I was most lateral, zone III was most medial, and zone II was intervening[83] (Fig. 66-6A and B). Martell and associates[84] modified this classification by subcategorizing zone II into two additional zones, for a total of five zones. Although radiolucencies are common at the bone-implant interface, they should not be progressive and should not be greater than 2 mm in width.

In an effort to further delineate the radiographic criteria for cementless acetabular component stability, Udomkiat and associates[85] compared preoperative radiographs versus intraoperative findings. The presence of specific preoperative radiographic findings (Box 66-1) was associated with a sensitivity of 94%, a specificity of 100%, and a negative predictive value of 97% for component loosening. The authors also showed that the presence of gaps less than 2 mm on immediate postoperative radiographs was not associated with the subsequent development of radiolucent lines, progressive radiolucency, or component loosening.

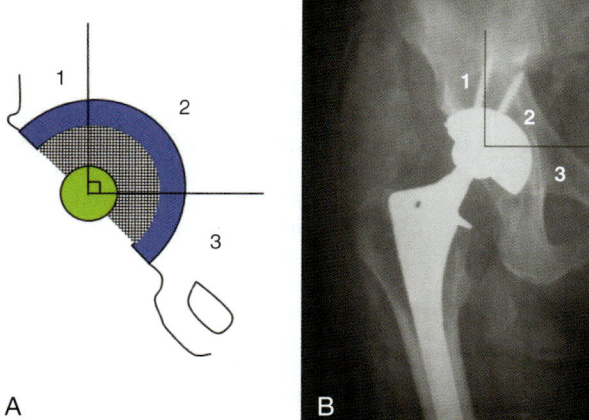

A

B

Figure 66-6. **A,** Cartoon illustration, and **(B)** anteroposterior (AP) hip radiograph demonstrating Delee and Charnley zones of acetabular osteolysis.

BOX 66-1. RADIOGRAPHIC SIGNS OF CEMENTLESS COMPONENT LOOSENING

- Radiolucent lines that appear after 2 years
- Progression of radiolucent lines after 2 years
- Radiolucent lines in all three zones
- Radiolucent lines 2 mm or wider in any zone
- Component migration

CEMENTLESS ACETABULAR COMPONENT RETRIEVAL DATA

Retrieval studies have helped to demonstrate the in vivo behavior of an implant, which in turn can be correlated with its radiographic appearance and clinical performance. Although initial retrievals were performed at the time of revision, better data can be obtained from the study of components retrieved at the time of death. Such studies have provided an understanding of (1) the implant-bone interface with regard to the host tissue's response and biological fixation, (2) the histologic correlation with the radiographic appearance of biological fixation and the patient's clinical outcome, and (3) the geographic distribution of wear debris and resulting osteolysis.[86]

Engh and associates[79] assessed nine porous-coated acetabular implants retrieved at death and found that the mean amount of bone ingrowth was 32%, and the average area density was 48%. The authors further correlated this histologic finding with radiographic analysis of the same patients for evidence of loosening or signs of bone ingrowth. They concluded that there was no correlation between the histologic and radiographic appearance of the implants. Radiographs consistently underestimated the degree of gap formation between the implant and the host bone and overestimated the degree of bone ingrowth. Gaps at the implant-bone interface were uniformly filled with fibrous tissue without evidence of particulate debris–related osteolysis.

Pidhorz and colleagues[31] evaluated 11 Harris-Galante porous cups inserted with the use of supplemental screw fixation at a mean of 41 months. The percent bone ingrowth histologically was near 30%, and evidence revealed significantly increased bone mass surrounding screw holes with, as opposed to those without, screws. Polyethylene debris was present in both filled and empty holes. The fraction of bone ingrowth was higher, nearing 50%. Particulate debris was found to track along the screws at the screw-bone interface, although no evidence of radiolucency was seen on radiographs. In both studies, Harris-Galante porous acetabular components demonstrated a relationship between the absence of radiographic radiolucency and the amount of bone present at the interface. The authors speculated that the presence of particulate wear debris along the screws may indicate that screws serve as a conduit for wear debris to gain access to the retroacetabular bone; the region surrounding the screws may extend the effective joint space.

Bloebaum and coworkers[87] retrieved seven porous acetabular components that were functioning well radiographically as well as clinically at the time of death. Six of the seven components were inserted by adjunctive fixation using screws. Approximately 84% of the porous coating surface was in contact with host bone, but an average of 12% of the space available in the porous coating was occupied by bone ingrowth. This was comparable with the 12.1% calculated by Pidhorz and associates.[88]

A more recent study by Urban and colleagues[89] evaluated the performance of Harris-Galante (HG) porous-coated hemispherical acetabular devices at the time of postmortem retrieval with regard to particle-induced granuloma formation and backside liner wear. A total of 36 cups (19 HG-1 and 17 HG-2) implanted with two to five screws were retrieved at a mean of 8 years (range, 2 to 21 years). Each acetabular implant was evaluated for overall fraction of bone ingrowth; extent of bone, marrow, fibrous tissue, and particle-induced granuloma surrounding the porous coating surface; and quantitative degree of backside and polyethylene bearing surface wear. The overall fraction of bone ingrowth was calculated to be $12.1 \pm 6.6\%$. The interface between the porous coating and the surrounding host bone was composed of $37.5 \pm 16.9\%$ bone, $30.8 \pm 22.9\%$ fibrous tissue, and $3.0 \pm 7.1\%$ granuloma, with the remainder being a mixture of fibrocartilage, marrow elements, and screw holes. Damage scores used to evaluate backside wear correlated with the extent of polyethylene-induced granuloma formation and increased with increasing duration of implantation. The mean polyethylene-bearing surface volumetric wear was 44 mm^3/yr and increased with time but did not correlate with the extent of granuloma formation in tissue present at the interface. The authors concluded excellent durability of biological fixation of porous-coated acetabular components at over two decades. The phenomenon of granuloma formation at the interface correlated with backside liner wear and not with bearing surface wear. The long-term success of these devices still requires close monitoring for osteolysis as time from implantation increases.

Third-generation hemispherical porous-coated acetabular devices (Trilogy Cup, Zimmer) addressed issues associated with a poor locking mechanism and an unpolished surface finish leading to increased backside wear. Urban and associates[90] conducted a study at the time of postmortem retrieval of 14 Trilogy acetabular components at a mean of 7.4 years (range, 1 to 12 years) post implantation. This study was designed similarly to the study mentioned previously by the same group, and these data were compared with retrieval data observed in the Harris-Galante components. Investigators reported that third-generation components exhibited significantly reduced liner backside wear with complete absence of particle-induced granuloma formation at the interface surface up to 12 years following implantation. The authors concluded that the improved locking mechanism and better stability between the liner and the metal shell were effective design features in limiting backside wear and migration of polyethylene particles from the joint, both of which contribute to pelvic osteolysis.

Retrieval studies have allowed a few general conclusions to be derived regarding uncemented acetabular component fixation. At the time of autopsy, porous acetabular implants appear to be well fixed, with approximately 30% of the surface bone ingrown to the underlying host bone, irrespective of the type of porous cementless device used. The use of screws is associated with increased bone density, but concern has been raised regarding wear debris gaining access to the retroacetabular space via screws and screw holes.

CLINICAL RESULTS OF CURRENT CEMENTLESS ACETABULAR COMPONENTS

Cementless acetabular implants have demonstrated excellent clinical results in the short to intermediate term (less than 10-year follow-up) with a range of aseptic

loosening from 0% to as high as 18% (e.g., PCA cup); the revision rate has ranged from 0% to 3.3%[69-73,91-96] (Table 66-1). However, cemented acetabular cup fixation has also exhibited excellent results in the short and intermediate term.[1] It was not until longer-term follow-up was evaluated that high rates of aseptic loosening and revision were recognized.[1-9] Longer-term follow-up—longer than 10 years—is available for the most commonly used cementless acetabular devices, including Harris-Galante 1 and 2 porous cups, the PCA cup, the AML cup, and some other devices.

An initial comparison analysis between cemented and cementless devices was conducted in patients undergoing bilateral single-stage primary total hip arthroplasty. Twenty-one patients were treated with a Harris-Galante-1 acetabular component on one side and a cemented all-polyethylene Charnley cup on the contralateral side. At 27-month follow-up, no difference was reported between the two sides with respect to radiographic loosening or clinical outcome.[97] This study supported the fact that both types of acetabular fixation were acceptable in the short term, but that longer-term studies were required for definitive answers to the question of whether cementless fixation is preferable over the use of cement.

Harris-Galante (HG-1 and HG-2) (Zimmer) porous acetabular components are the most studied of all cementless acetabular components. The cup consists of a titanium shell with a titanium fiber metal mesh diffusion bonded to the shell for bone ingrowth, with capability for 4.5-mm (HG-1) or 5.1-mm cancellous screw placement for fixation performed using a line-to-line technique. Several studies have demonstrated excellent long-term (>10 years) results with a range of aseptic loosening from 0% to 4.4%, and a revision rate ranging from 0% to 3.3%[12,14,65,98-104] (Table 66-2).

A recently published study by Della Valle and associates evaluated 20-year follow-up of patients with the HG-1 porous acetabular component.[12] A total of 114 patients of the original cohort of 204 patients were

Table 66-1. Intermediate-term Follow-up of Porous Acetabular Cups

Type of Cup	Author	Mean Length of Follow-up, yr	Number of Cups	Radiographically Loose, n (%)	Revised for Loosening, n
HG-1	Berger	8.6	91	2 (2)	0
HG-1	Bohm	7.9	264	0 (0)	0
HG	Callaghan	8.5	131	0 (0)	0
HG-1	Dunkley	7	55	0 (0)	0
HG-1	Goldberg	8.6	123	0 (0)	0
HG-1	Latimer	7	136	0 (0)	0
HG-1	Ricci	7	123	0 (0)	0
HG-1/2	Soto	7.3	93	1 (1)	1
HG-1/2	Tompkins	8.3	173	0 (0)	0
Trilogy	Amenábar	11.2	127	1 (.1)	1
PCA	Malchau	7	539	96 (18)	18
AML	Piston	7.5	35	0 (0)	0
AML	Zicat	8.5	74	3 (4)	1

AML, Anatomic medullary locking; *HG,* Harris-Galante; *PCA,* porous-coated anatomic.

Table 66-2. Long-term Follow-up of the Harris-Galante Porous Acetabular Cup

Type of Cup	Author	Mean Length of Follow-up, yr	Number of Cups	Radiographically Loose, n (%)	Revised for Loosening, n
HG-2	Archibeck	10	74	2 (3)	1
HG-1	Callaghan	14	72	0 (0)	0
HG-1/2	Clohisy	10	196	0 (0)	0
HG-1	Crowther	11	56	0 (0)	0
HG-1	Maloney	10	168	1 (0.6)	0
HG-1	Parvizi	14.9	90	0 (0)	0
HG-1/2	Rasquinha	13.5	204	0 (0)	0
HG-1	Della Valle	20	114	5 (4)	5

HG, Harris-Galante.

Table 66-3. Long-term Follow-up of the Porous-Coated Anatomic Acetabular Component

Type of Cup	Author	Mean Length of Follow-up, yr	Number of Cups	Radiographically Loose, n (%)	Revised for Loosening, n
PCA	Bojescul	15.6	64	19 (30)	17
PCA	Hastings	10.3	73	13 (18)	7
PCA	Healy	12.3	53	6 (11)	6
PCA	Kawamura	12	187	12 (6)	8
PCA	Kim	11.2	116	8 (7)	8
PCA	Tsao	10	91	3 (3)	3

PCA, Porous-coated anatomic.

available for review. Kaplan-Meier survivorship of the acetabular component was 96% in terms of revision for aseptic loosening or radiographic evidence of loosening as an endpoint. Fourteen hips (12.3%) with well-fixed acetabular shells underwent revision for a modular liner exchange. The authors concluded that wear-related complications continue to be the major mode of failure.

Ihle and colleagues[105] recently reported on 20-year follow-up using a different titanium acetabular device, the titanium-coated RM cementless acetabular cup. This specific prosthesis was manufactured from ultrahigh-molecular-weight polyethylene, sterilized in gamma irradiation and air, and coated with a thin layer of titanium particles. Initial fixation was achieved with two anchoring pegs and supplemental screw fixation. Mean time to follow-up was 19.3 years with a range from 17.4 to 20.9 years, and no patients were lost at time of final follow-up. Ninety-three primary THAs were performed in 80 patients with a survivorship of 94% when revision for aseptic loosening was used as an endpoint. This study demonstrates reliable long-term fixation with another titanium-coated acetabular device, with revisions done primarily for osteolysis and polyethylene wear. The authors concluded that reduction in wear-induced osteolysis continues to be the major future challenge for implant longevity in primary THA.

The Morscher acetabular prosthesis is another titanium device that has been reported to demonstrate excellent long-term survivorship. The prosthesis is a nonmodular, monoblock, flexible cup with the polyethylene liner directly compression-molded into a titanium mesh shell. Lack of modularity does not allow for supplemental screw fixation at the time of implantation. Gwynne-Jones and associates[106] reviewed 113 patients who underwent primary THA with the Morscher prosthesis. A total of 125 implants were inserted, and mean time to follow-up was 11 years (range, 9 to 13 years). At the time of final follow-up, no revisions were done for aseptic loosening. Kaplan-Meier analysis at 13 years demonstrated survivorship of 96.8% with THA revision for any reason used as an endpoint, and 95.7% with acetabular reoperation for any cause used as an endpoint. Results paralleled those of the original designer of the prosthesis, whose study demonstrated 97.5% survivorship when revision for aseptic loosening was used at 15-year follow-up.[107] Clinical results with the Morscher prosthesis further support the use of titanium-backed metal shell for cementless acetabular reconstruction in primary THA in attempts to achieve long-term biological fixation.

The PCA acetabular component is composed of a cobalt-chromium shell with a cobalt-chromium–sintered bead surface. Initial mechanical stability was achieved with the use of pegs at the periphery; this cup design did not accommodate supplemental screw fixation. Long-term follow-up has demonstrated high failure rates secondary to wear and osteolysis. These components were typically implanted with concomitant use of a 32-mm head; this resulted in the use of a thin polyethylene liner that was predisposed to catastrophic wear. The range of aseptic loosening was 3.3% to 30%, with an associated revision rate ranging from 3.3% to 26.5%[108-113] (Table 66-3).

The AML cementless device is a beaded cobalt-chromium alloy component. Fewer long-term studies are available in which the AML acetabular prosthesis was evaluated. One study published by Belmont and colleagues[114] evaluated the AML cementless acetabular device at a minimum of 20 years' follow-up. A total of 119 THAs from the original cohort of 223 THAs were available for follow-up at a mean of 22 years; the survival rate was 85.8 ± 5.2%.

In general, clinical results of the AML cementless cup parallel those of the PCA acetabular component.[112,115] The rate of aseptic loosening ranged from 3.8% to 4%, with an associated range of revision for loosening from 2.3% to 3.8%. The AML device, similar to the PCA, often was implanted with larger-diameter (32-mm) femoral heads that resulted in suboptimal polyethylene thickness in many cases.

Review of long-term data reveals that stable, long-term biological fixation can be achieved. Wear of the polyethylene liner and osetolysis constitute a common mode of failure that may be improved with the use of more wear-resistant bearing surfaces.

INDICATIONS/CONTRAINDICATIONS

Most patients have adequate acetabular bone stock to support a cementless acetabular component, and this method of reconstruction accounts for the vast majority of primary total hip arthroplasties performed in North America. Cemented components, however, may be more appropriate for patients with severe osteopenia and inadequate bone strength to support a cementless component, as can be seen in some patients with severe inflammatory arthritis of the hip (Fig. 66-7A and B). At some centers, cemented all-polyethylene acetabular components are still used for low-demand patients.

Radiation necrosis of the pelvis is a relative contraindication to the use of a cementless acetabular component.[116] Unfortunately, equally bad results have been reported for cemented all-polyethylene components in this clinical scenario, with rates of acetabular component loosening as high as 52%.[117] If true radiation necrosis of the pelvis is present, consideration should be given to the use of a reconstruction cage that spans from the ilium to the ischium with multiple screws for fixation to create a biomechanically strong construct. Intraoperatively, lack of bleeding cancellous bone in the acetabular bed is an indicator that bone ingrowth is unlikely to occur.

It is important to recognize, however, that true radiation necrosis of the pelvis is rare with more modern techniques of radiation delivery for the treatment of pelvic tumors. Kim and associates[118] retrospectively reviewed 58 patients (66 hips) who underwent primary cementless THA following radiation therapy for prostate cancer. At the time of final follow-up, 51 patients (58 hips) were available for evaluation. Mean time to follow-up was 4.8 years, and minimal follow-up occurred at 2 years. None of the patients underwent revision of the acetabular component for aseptic loosening. Two femoral components were revised: one for periprosthetic fracture, and another for stem subsidence (Fig. 66-8A and B).

TECHNIQUE OF CEMENTLESS ACETABULAR COMPONENT INSERTION

Preoperative Planning

Preoperative planning is an essential part of performing a total hip arthroplasty. Clear overlay templates are utilized (Fig. 66-9) to estimate acetabular component size; if, intraoperatively, size varies by more than 4 mm from the planned size, intraoperative radiographs are recommended to ensure that a component of

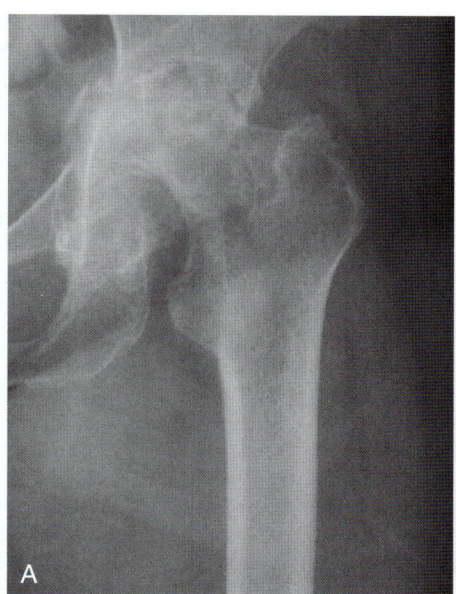
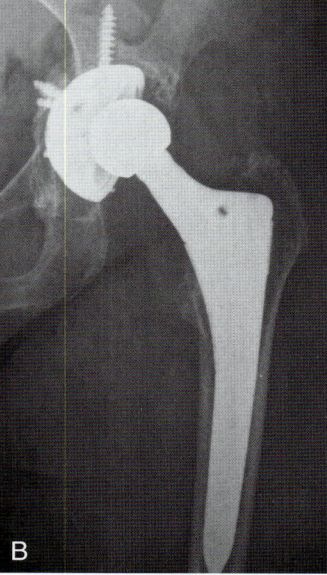

Figure 66-7. A, Preoperative anteroposterior (AP) hip radiograph of a patient with severe rheumatoid arthritis. **B,** Thirteen-month postoperative hip radiograph demonstrating failure of the cementless acetabular device with migration of the cup into a vertical position. Cemented acetabular fixation may have been an alternative option for this patient.

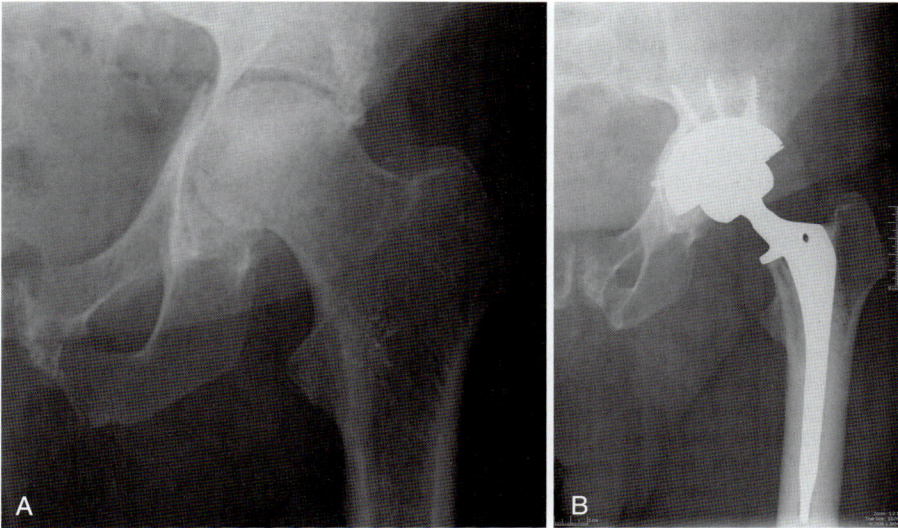

Figure 66-8. A, Preoperative anteroposterior (AP) hip radiograph with radiation necrosis of the left hip and associated medial wall fracture. **B,** Postoperative radiograph of the left hip following cementless acetabular reconstruction with several screws used for supplemental fixation.

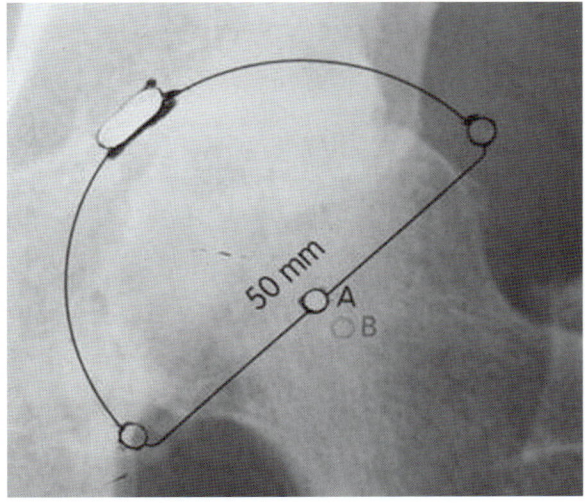

Figure 66-9. Acetabular template used preoperatively to determine the size of the acetabular component. The template is positioned so that subchondral bone is being engaged by the component throughout the entire region of contact.

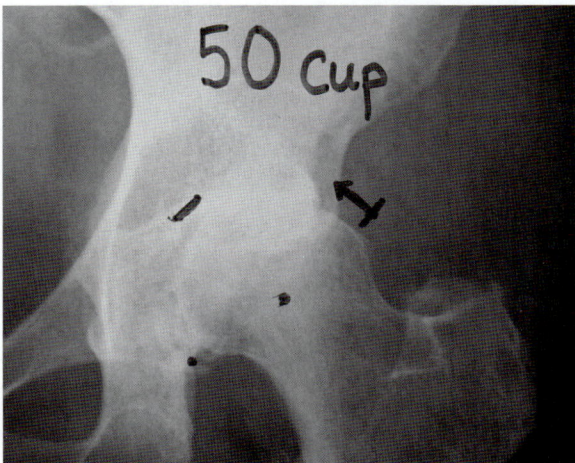

Figure 66-10. Final template cup size with an arrow situated laterally to demonstrate the amount of uncovered cup.

appropriate size is being inserted. Templating will also allow the surgeon to identify patients with smaller components, which may necessitate the use of smaller-diameter femoral heads to maintain adequate polyethylene thickness. These may not be routinely available unless arrangements are made ahead of time.

Templating also assists in determining appropriate component orientation and position to accurately re-create offset and optimize both stability and wear characteristics. Specifically, in patients with large amounts of femoral offset, over-medialization of the component can lead to altered biomechanics and the potential for instability or abductor weakness. Finally, templating the desired abduction angle preoperatively

(ideally, approximately 40 degrees) assists the surgeon intraoperatively in ensuring appropriate component position. Specifically, measuring the amount of the acetabular component that should be uncovered laterally is a good approach to ensure that the cup is not placed in a position that is too vertical (Fig. 66-10). Femoral component templating goes hand in hand with acetabular templating to ensure that leg length and offset are restored, in addition to estimating appropriate femoral component size.

Description of Surgical Technique

A press-fit technique, with or without adjunctive screw fixation, is most commonly used in North America. Excellent exposure can be attained by using a number of different surgical approaches. Following hip dislocation, femoral neck osteotomy is performed at the templated level and the acetabulum exposed. If a posterior approach to the hip is selected, adequate anterior release is required to allow for retraction of the femur anteriorly and direct access to the acetabulum; inadequate release risks reaming and component insertion in retroversion. Once an anterior acetabular retractor is placed, the anterior wall should be easily visualized; if not, additional anterior capsular release is required. A posterior retractor is then placed between the posterior capsule and the posterior wall to complete the exposure. A third retractor may be required superiorly for full visualization of the acetabulum (Fig. 66-11). Remaining labral tissue is resected circumferentially with a long-handled scalpel or by electrocautery.

The transverse acetabular ligament is identified next, and the cotyloid fossa is carefully cleared of soft tissue with the use of electrocautery; care must be exercised because branches of the obturator vessels can be lacerated, possibly leading to bleeding that is difficult to control (Fig. 66-12). The transverse acetabular ligament

will serve as a guide to acetabular component version, and the floor of the cotyloid fossa represents the outer table of the medial wall; this is used to guide the depth of acetabular reaming.

Based on the preoperative template, a reamer that is 4 mm smaller than the templated size is used as the first reamer (e.g., if templating to a cup size of 52 mm, start with a 48-mm reamer). The reamer is started superficially in the acetabulum to ensure that peripheral osteophytes are removed during the reaming process (Fig. 66-13). At first, the reamer is gently advanced in line with the transverse acetabular ligament and the desired angle of acetabular component insertion. While reaming, it is important to apply slight anterior and medial pressure to ensure that the posterior wall is not sacrificed during reaming, as is the tendency with a posterior approach to the hip. The reamer is advanced until the appropriate amount of medialization is attained, as again judged by the floor of the true acetabulum as visualized in the cotyloid fossa (Fig. 66-14).

The next reamer of even size is used in a similar fashion, and reaming progresses until contact is

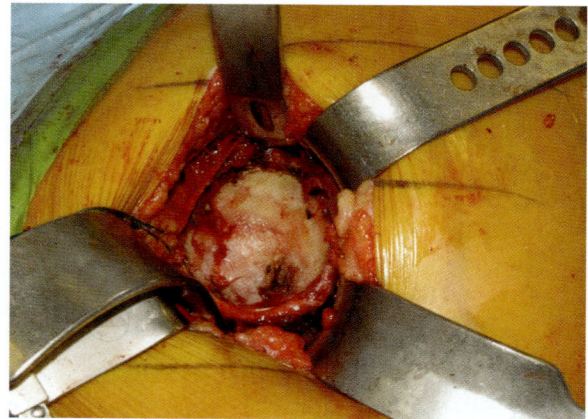

Figure 66-11. Acetabular exposure with retractors in place.

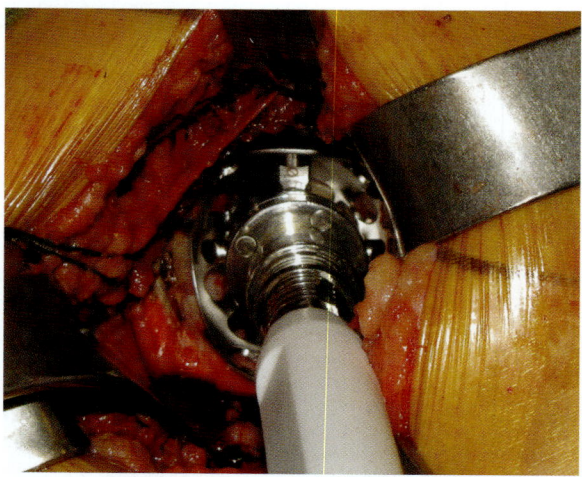

Figure 66-13. Reaming of the acetabulum with a 50-mm reamer.

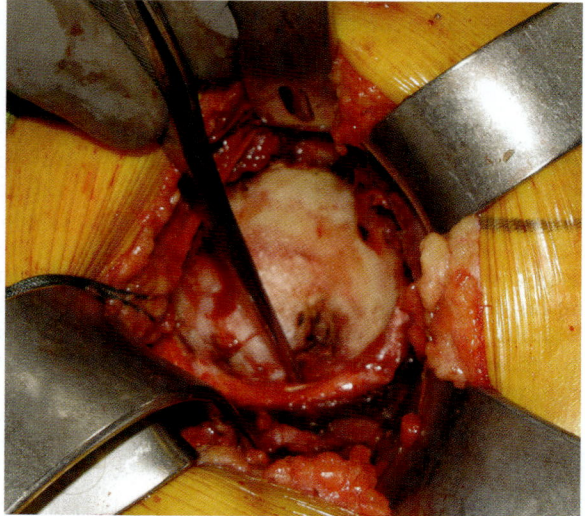

Figure 66-12. Image depicting the transverse acetabular ligament. This structure can be used as a landmark to determine the appropriate acetabular component version.

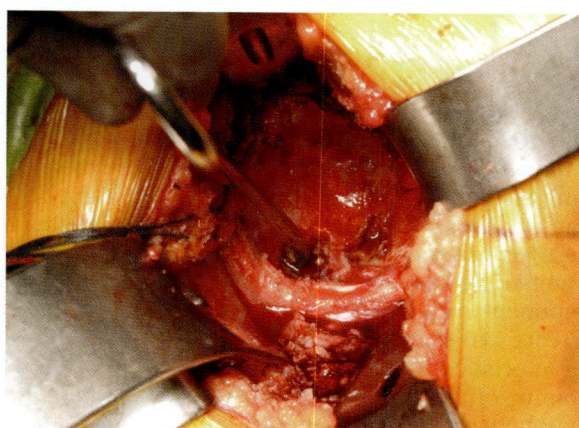

Figure 66-14. Image depicting the cotyloid fossa after acetabular reaming.

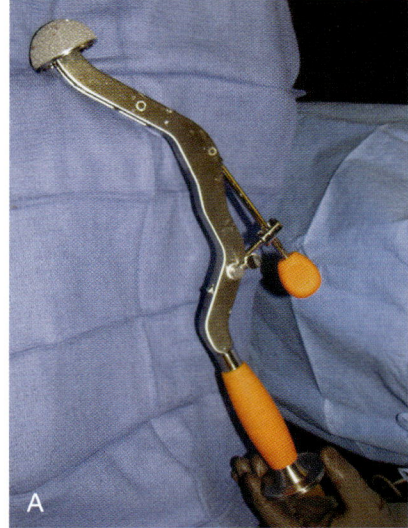
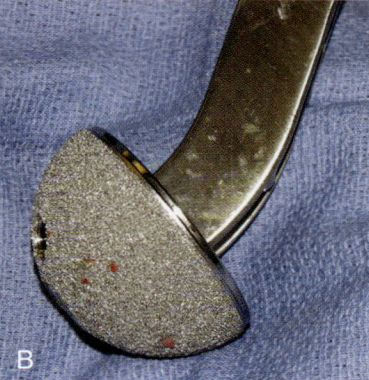

Figure 66-15. A, Offset acetabular inserter with **(B)** a porous, cementless, hemispherical acetabular component attached to the end.

achieved circumferentially with the reamer and the appropriate depth of reaming has been achieved. Depending on the implant system being used, under-reaming by 1 or 2 mm is performed. Depending on surgeon preference, a trial can now be inserted to check implant stability.

Although an offset cup inserter is the author's preference, a straight insert is often easier to use because forces are transmitted more directly (Fig. 66-15A and B). With the transverse acetabular ligament used as a guide, the component is inserted at approximately 20 degrees of anteversion and 40 degrees of cup abduction. A variable but typically small amount of the component should be uncovered laterally to ensure that the cup is not too vertical, as determined by preoperative templating; similarly, from a posterior approach, the component should lie behind the anterior wall of the acetabulum to ensure appropriate anteversion (Fig. 66-16).

A cup with three screw holes is typically used, and the component is inserted in such a way that the screw holes are situated in the posterosuperior quadrant of the acetabulum (the so-called *safe-zone*). The desired component is then impacted into place until tactile and auditory cues indicate that it is fully seated; if a cup with screw holes is used, visual confirmation can be performed via the screw holes themselves. Two screws of adequate length to engage the far cortex (but not so long so as to risk neurovascular injury) are inserted into the posterosuperior quadrant (Fig. 66-17A and B). Once the screws have been inserted and stability confirmed, a trial or final liner can be placed, based on surgeon preference. Osteophytes can then be trimmed around the acetabular component, but care should be taken to ensure that the component lies fully behind the anterior wall of the acetabulum because an exposed acetabular component anteriorly may predispose to iliopsoas tendinitis and groin pain (Fig. 66-18A and B). Following preparation of the proximal femur, with the trial broach in place, the hip is carefully trialed to ensure restoration of leg length and offset and a stable reconstruction. In

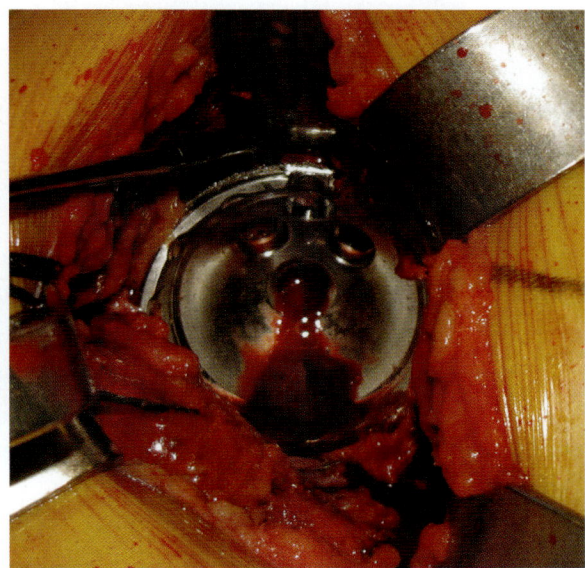

Figure 66-16. Acetabular cup implanted with a small degree of uncoverage of the cup laterally.

some cases, reorientation of the newly implanted component may be required to achieve these goals, and the surgeon should not hesitate to change component position if necessary (Fig. 66-19).

Summary of Complications

When using these devices, one must be cognizant that several complications are potentially associated with cementless acetabular cup insertion. As was previously discussed, fracture of the acetabular walls or the pelvis itself can occur. First and foremost, appropriate exposure of the acetabulum is required, and meticulous removal of the labrum and any overhanging capsule eases component insertion. Forceful impaction of the cup is to be avoided, particularly in patients with poor

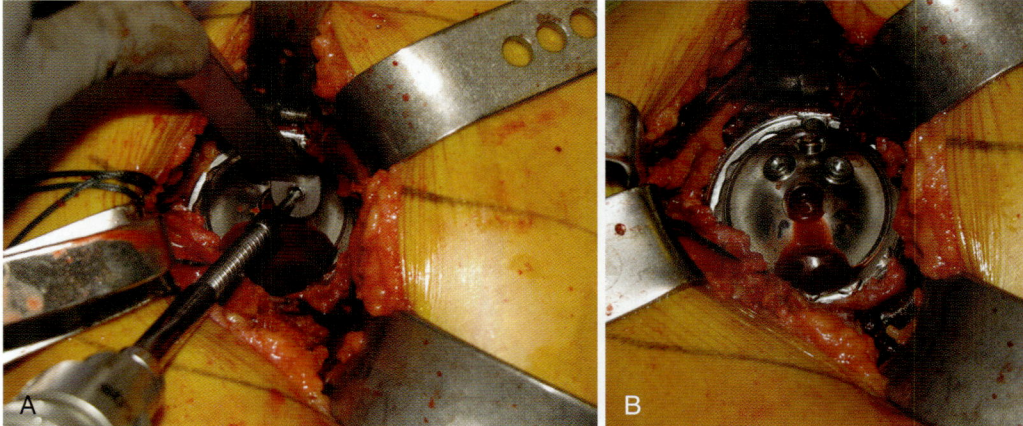

Figure 66-17. A, A drill is used to create a track for proper screw insertion. It is important to make sure that the drill guide is seated perpendicularly to the screw hole to ensure that the screws sit flush with the metal shell. **B,** An image of an implanted acetabular cup with two screws through the acetabular metal shell into the acetabular host bone.

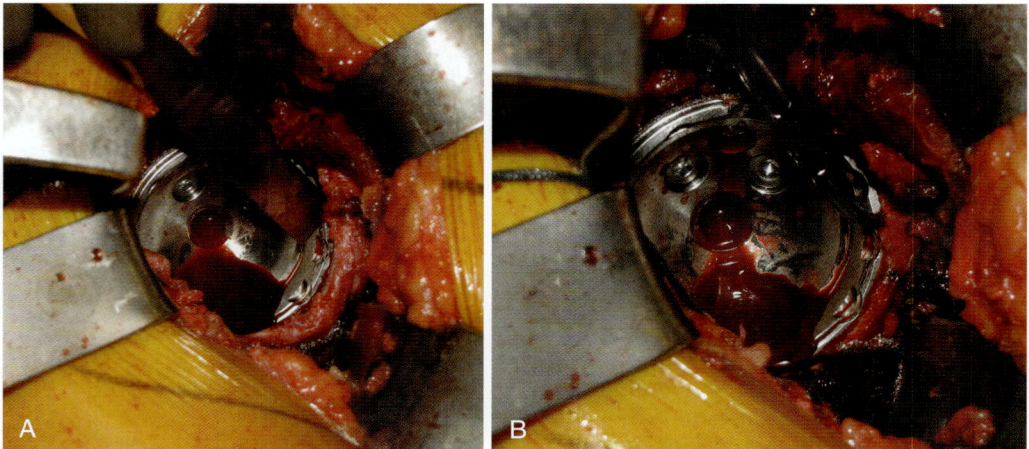

Figure 66-18. A, Resection of osteophytes once the acetabular component has been implanted. **B,** Post resection of the osteophyte.

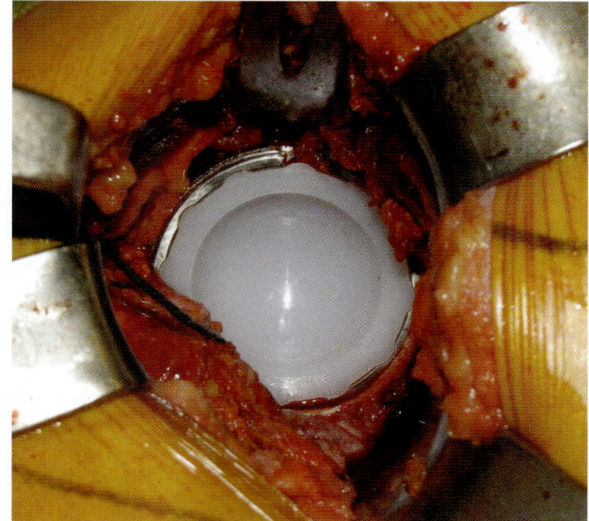

Figure 66-19. Final acetabular component in position with polyethylene liner locked into the metal shell.

bone stock. If a press-fit is not initially obtained, the component should be removed, appropriate exposure ensured, and an attempt made at reinsertion once the edges of the acetabulum are found to be free of soft tissue. In some cases, additional reaming may be required; if difficulty is encountered, a trial component may be helpful before repeated attempts are made at insertion (Fig. 66-20*A* and *B*).

The possibility for neurovascular injury is associated with the use of adjunctive screw fixation, as was previously described. The likelihood of this type of injury was decreased after specific acetabular quadrants were defined and surgeons had gained more experience with cementless devices.[56] Quadrants are defined from anterior to posterior by a line that connects the anterior superior iliac spine and the ischium. This line is bisected across the acetabulum to define superior to inferior. The risk to neurovascular structures traversing the pelvis is minimized when screws are placed in the posterosuperior quadrant of the acetabulum.

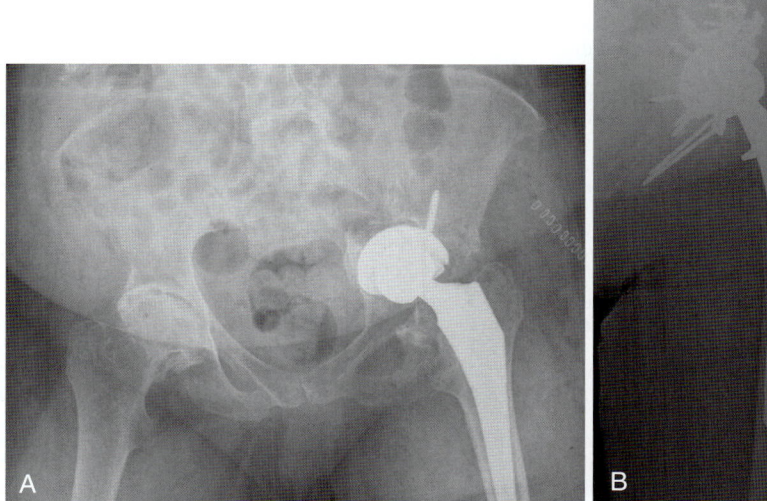

Figure 66-20. A, Patient transferred with a periprosthetic acetabular fracture caused by forceful impaction during cementless acetabular component insertion and poor underlying bone stock; fracture was identified on a radiograph taken in the recovery room immediately postoperatively. **B,** Postoperative anteroposterior (AP) hip radiograph following open reduction internal fixation (ORIF) and cementless acetabular reconstruction.

Appropriate component positioning is of critical importance in achieving clinical success and in avoiding instability and wear-related problems. The ideal position of an acetabular component should be at 35 to 45 degrees of abduction or inclination and 15 to 20 degrees of anteversion.[77] Although newer-generation bearing surfaces offer the promise of reduced wear and decreased risk of longer-term wear-related sequelae, they seem to be very sensitive to component malposition.

CURRENT CONTROVERSIES AND FUTURE DIRECTIONS

Approximately 25 years of experience with cementless acetabular devices has shown that long-term biological fixation can be achieved with durability that is improved over that of acetabular components inserted with cement. However, further improvement can be achieved in some areas.

Although long-term fixation with most cementless designs has been adequate, use of surface coatings that may enhance bone ingrowth may further improve results, particularly in the revision setting. Several "porous metals" have been introduced in an attempt to increase the extent of biological fixation. Although early results as outlined previously are encouraging, long-term results are unknown.

Additional developments in bearing surface technology are needed because wear-related complications continue to be a major mode of failure. Similarly, the risk of revision secondary to instability remains, and better bearing surfaces that allow for more physiologically sized femoral heads and improved surgical techniques may decrease this risk. Failures related to infection continue to occur; implants that resist

infection would greatly decrease the risk of this common mode of failure.

Acknowledgment

The authors would like to acknowledge Dr. Jorge O. Galante, MD, for his historical perspective and experience in the design and development of cementless acetabular devices. His guidance was helpful in the completion of this work.

REFERENCES

 1. Charnley J: Low friction arthroplasty of the hip: theory and practice, Berlin, 1979, Springer-Verlag.
 2. Clohisy JC, Harris WH: Matched-pair analysis of cemented and cementless acetabular reconstruction in primary total hip arthroplasty. J Arthroplasty 16:697–705, 2001.
 3. Garcia-Cimbrelo E, Munuera L: Early and late loosening of the acetabular cup after low-friction arthroplasty. J Bone Joint Surg Am 74:1119–1129, 1992.
 4. Kavanagh BF, Wallrichs S, Dewitz M, et al: Charnley low-friction arthroplasty of the hip: twenty-year results with cement. J Arthroplasty 9:229–234, 1994.
 5. Madey SM, Callaghan JJ, Olejniczak JP, et al: Charnley total hip arthroplasty with use of improved techniques of cementing: the results after a minimum of fifteen years of follow-up. J Bone Joint Surg Am 79:53–64, 1997.
 6. Mulroy WF, Estok DM, Harris WH: Total hip arthroplasty with use of so-called second-generation cementing techniques: a fifteen-year-average follow-up study. J Bone Joint Surg Am 77:1845–1852, 1995.
 7. Schulte KR, Callaghan JJ, Kelley SS, Johnston RC: The outcome of Charnley total hip arthroplasty with cement after a minimum twenty-year follow-up: the results of one surgeon. J Bone Joint Surg Am 75:961–975, 1993.
 8. Stauffer RN: Ten-year follow-up study of total hip replacement. J Bone Joint Surg Am 64:983–990, 1982.
 9. Wroblewski BM: 15-21-year results of the Charnley low-friction arthroplasty. Clin Orthop Relat Res 211:30–35, 1986.
10. Ballard WT, Callaghan JJ, Sullivan PM, Johnston RC: The results of improved cementing techniques for total hip

arthroplasty in patients less than fifty years old: a ten-year follow-up study. J Bone Joint Surg Am 76:959–964, 1994.

11. Smith SE, Estok DM, 2nd, Harris WH: Average 12-year outcome of a chrome-cobalt, beaded, bony ingrowth acetabular component. J Arthroplasty 13:50–60, 1998.

12. Della Valle CJ, Mesko NW, Quigley L, et al: Primary total hip arthroplasty with a porous-coated acetabular component: a concise follow-up, at a minimum of twenty years, of previous reports. J Bone Joint Surg Am 91:1130–1135, 2009.

13. Jones LC, Hungerford DS: Cement disease. Clin Orthop Relat Res 225:192–206, 1987.

14. Maloney WJ, Galante JO, Anderson M, et al: Fixation, polyethylene wear, and pelvic osteolysis in primary total hip replacement. Clin Orthop Relat Res 369:157–164, 1999.

15. Morscher E, Berli B, Jockers W, Schenk R: Rationale of a flexible press fit cup in total hip replacement: 5-year followup in 280 procedures. Clin Orthop Relat Res 341:42–50, 1997.

16. Morscher EW: Current status of acetabular fixation in primary total hip arthroplasty. Clin Orthop Relat Res 274:172–193, 1992.

17. Pilliar RM, Lee JM, Maniatopoulos C: Observations on the effect of movement on bone ingrowth into porous-surfaced implants. Clin Orthop Relat Res 208:108–113, 1986.

18. Bobyn JD, Pilliar RM, Cameron HU, Weatherly GC: The optimum pore size for the fixation of porous-surfaced metal implants by the ingrowth of bone. Clin Orthop Relat Res 150:263–270, 1980.

19. Galante J, Rostoker W, Lueck R, Ray RD: Sintered fiber metal composites as a basis for attachment of implants to bone. J Bone Joint Surg Am 53:101–114, 1971.

20. Jasty M, Bragdon CR, Haire T, et al: Comparison of bone ingrowth into cobalt chrome sphere and titanium fiber mesh porous coated cementless canine acetabular components. J Biomed Mater Res 27:639–644, 1993.

21. Savory C, Hamilton W, Engh CS, et al: Hip designs. In American Academy of Orthopaedic Surgeons, editors: Orthopaedic knowledge update 3, Rosemont, Ill, 2006, AAOS, pp 345–368.

22. Morscher EW: Cementless total hip arthroplasty. Clin Orthop Relat Res 181:76–91, 1983.

23. Bruijn JD, Seelen JL, Feenstra RM, et al: Failure of the Mecring screw-ring acetabular component in total hip arthroplasty: a three- to seven-year follow-up study. J Bone Joint Surg Am 77:760–766, 1995.

24. Engh CA, Griffin WL, Marx CL: Cementless acetabular components. J Bone Joint Surg Br 72:53–59, 1990.

25. Fox GM, McBeath AA, Heiner JP: Hip replacement with a threaded acetabular cup: a follow-up study. J Bone Joint Surg Am 76:195–201, 1994.

26. Lord G, Bancel P: The madreporic cementless total hip arthroplasty: new experimental data and a seven-year clinical follow-up study. Clin Orthop Relat Res 176:67–76, 1983.

27. Malchau H, Herberts P, Wang YX, et al: Long-term clinical and radiological results of the Lord total hip prosthesis: a prospective study. J Bone Joint Surg Br 78:884–891, 1996.

28. Pupparo F, Engh CA: Comparison of porous-threaded and smooth-threaded acetabular components of identical design: two- to four-year results. Clin Orthop Relat Res 271:201–206, 1991.

29. Huiskes R: Finite element analysis of acetabular reconstruction: noncemented threaded cups. Acta Orthop Scand 58:620–625, 1987.

30. Bobyn JD, Engh CA, Glassman AH: Radiography and histology of a threaded acetabular implant: one case studied at two years. J Bone Joint Surg Br 70:302–304, 1988.

31. Pidhorz LE, Urban RM, Jacobs JJ, et al: A quantitative study of bone and soft tissues in cementless porous-coated acetabular components retrieved at autopsy. J Arthroplasty 8:213–225, 1993.

32. Delaunay CP, Kapandji AI: Survivorship of rough-surfaced threaded acetabular cups: 382 consecutive primary Zweymuller cups followed for 0.2-12 years. Acta Orthop Scand 69:379–383, 1998.

33. Epinette JA, Manley MT, D'Antonio JA, et al: A 10-year minimum follow-up of hydroxyapatite-coated threaded cups: clinical, radiographic and survivorship analyses with comparison to the literature. J Arthroplasty 18:140–148, 2003.

34. Bauer TW, Stulberg BN, Ming J, Geesink RG: Uncemented acetabular components: histologic analysis of retrieved hydroxyapatite-coated and porous implants. J Arthroplasty 8:167–177, 1993.

35. Capello WN, D'Antonio JA, Manley MT, Feinberg JR: Hydroxyapatite in total hip arthroplasty: clinical results and critical issues. Clin Orthop Relat Res 355:200–211, 1998.

36. Geesink RG, Hoefnagels NH: Six-year results of hydroxyapatite-coated total hip replacement. J Bone Joint Surg Br 77:534–547, 1995.

37. Manley MT, Capello WN, D'Antonio JA, et al: Fixation of acetabular cups without cement in total hip arthroplasty: a comparison of three different implant surfaces at a minimum duration of follow-up of five years. J Bone Joint Surg Am 80:1175–1185, 1998.

38. Chung YY, Kim J, Lim CH, et al: Measurement of extent of bone ongrowth and hydroxyapatite absorption in retrieved acetabular cups. J Orthop Sci 13:198–201, 2008.

39. Gabbar OA, Rajan RA, Londhe S, Hyde ID: Ten- to twelve-year follow-up of the furlong hydroxyapatite-coated femoral stem and threaded acetabular cup in patients younger than 65 years. J Arthroplasty 23:413–417, 2008.

40. Jaffe WL, Morris HB, Nessler JP, et al: Hydroxylapatite-coated acetabular shells with arc deposited titanium surface roughening and dual radius design. Bull NYU Hosp Jt Dis 65:257–262, 2007.

41. Rivero DP, Fox J, Skipor AK, et al: Calcium phosphate-coated porous titanium implants for enhanced skeletal fixation. J Biomed Mater Res 22:191–201, 1988.

42. Ducheyne P, Hench LL, Kagan A, 2nd, et al: Effect of hydroxyapatite impregnation on skeletal bonding of porous coated implants. J Biomed Mater Res 14:225–237, 1980.

43. Eschenroeder HC, Jr, McLaughlin RE, Reger SI: Enhanced stabilization of porous-coated metal implants with tricalcium phosphate granules. Clin Orthop Relat Res 216:234–246, 1987.

44. Laursen MB, Nielsen PT, Soballe K: Bone remodelling around HA-coated acetabular cups: a DEXA study with a 3-year follow-up in a randomised trial. Int Orthop 31:199–204, 2007.

45. Levine B, Della Valle CJ, Jacobs JJ: Applications of porous tantalum in total hip arthroplasty. J Am Acad Orthop Surg 14:646–655, 2006.

46. Bargiotas K, Maziloas K, Karachalios T, et al: Total hip arthroplasty using trabecular metal acetabular component: middle-term results. In American Academy of Orthopaedic Surgeons, Rosemont, Ill, 2005, pp 368–369.

47. Bobyn JD, Poggie RA, Krygier JJ, et al: Clinical validation of a structural porous tantalum biomaterial for adult reconstruction. J Bone Joint Surg Am 86(Suppl 2):123–129, 2004.

48. Gruen TA, Poggie RA, Lewallen DG, et al: Radiographic evaluation of a monoblock acetabular component: a multicenter study with 2- to 5-year results. J Arthroplasty 20:369–378, 2005.

49. Sumner DR, Jasty M, Jacobs JJ, et al: Histology of porous-coated acetabular components: 25 cementless cups retrieved after arthroplasty. Acta Orthop Scand 64:619–626, 1993.

50. Callaghan JJ, Kim YS, Brown TD, et al: Concerns and improvements with cementless metal-backed acetabular components. Clin Orthop Relat Res 311:76–84, 1995.

51. Cook SD, Barrack RL, Thomas KA, Haddad RJ, Jr: Quantitative analysis of tissue growth into human porous total hip components. J Arthroplasty 3:249–262, 1988.

52. Curtis MJ, Jinnah RH, Wilson VD, Hungerford DS: The initial stability of uncemented acetabular components. J Bone Joint Surg Br 74:372–376, 1992.

53. Lachiewicz PF, Suh PB, Gilbert JA: In vitro initial fixation of porous-coated acetabular total hip components: a biomechanical comparative study. J Arthroplasty 4:201–205, 1989.

54. Stiehl JB, MacMillan E, Skrade DA: Mechanical stability of porous-coated acetabular components in total hip arthroplasty. J Arthroplasty 6:295–300, 1991.

55. Engh C: Long-term porous-coated survivorship using spikes, screws and using press-fitting for initial fixation. In American Association of Hip and Knee Surgeons, Dallas, 2003, AAHKS.

56. Wasielewski RC, Cooperstein LA, Kruger MP, Rubash HE: Acetabular anatomy and the transacetabular fixation of

screws in total hip arthroplasty. J Bone Joint Surg Am 72:501–508, 1990.

57. Schmalzried TP, Wessinger SJ, Hill GE, Harris WH: The Harris-Galante porous acetabular component press-fit without screw fixation: five-year radiographic analysis of primary cases. J Arthroplasty 9:235–242, 1994.

58. Sandborn PM, Cook SD, Spires WP, Kester MA: Tissue response to porous-coated implants lacking initial bone apposition. J Arthroplasty 3:337–346, 1988.

59. Won CH, Hearn TC, Tile M: Micromotion of cementless hemispherical acetabular components: does press-fit need adjunctive screw fixation? J Bone Joint Surg Am 77:484–489, 1995.

60. Ries MD, Harbaugh M: Acetabular strains produced by oversized press fit cups. Clin Orthop Relat Res 334:276–281, 1997.

61. Ries MD, Harbaugh M, Shea J, Lambert R: Effect of cementless acetabular cup geometry on strain distribution and press-fit stability. J Arthroplasty 12:207–212, 1997.

62. Kim YS, Callaghan JJ, Ahn PB, Brown TD: Fracture of the acetabulum during insertion of an oversized hemispherical component. J Bone Joint Surg Am 77:111–117, 1995.

63. Sharkey PF, Hozack WJ, Callaghan JJ, et al: Acetabular fracture associated with cementless acetabular component insertion: a report of 13 cases. J Arthroplasty 14:426–431, 1999.

64. Gonzalez Della Valle A, Ruzo PS, Li S, et al: Dislodgment of polyethylene liners in first- and second-generation Harris-Galante acetabular components: a report of eighteen cases. J Bone Joint Surg Am 83:553–559, 2001.

65. Archibeck MJ, Berger RA, Jacobs JJ, et al: Second-generation cementless total hip arthroplasty: eight to eleven-year results. J Bone Joint Surg Am 83:1666–1673, 2001.

66. Astion DJ, Saluan P, Stulberg BN, et al: The porous-coated anatomic total hip prosthesis: failure of the metal-backed acetabular component. J Bone Joint Surg Am 78:755–766, 1996.

67. Barrack RL: Concerns with cementless modular acetabular components. Orthopedics 19:741–743, 1996.

68. Barrack RL, Folgueras A, Munn B, et al: Pelvic lysis and polyethylene wear at 5-8 years in an uncemented total hip. Clin Orthop Relat Res 335:211–217, 1997.

69. Berger RA, Kull LR, Rosenberg AG, Galante JO: Hybrid total hip arthroplasty: 7- to 10-year results. Clin Orthop Relat Res 333:134–146, 1996.

70. Callaghan JJ, Tooma GS, Olejniczak JP, et al: Primary hybrid total hip arthroplasty: an interim followup. Clin Orthop Relat Res 333:118–125, 1996.

71. Dunkley AB, Eldridge JD, Lee MB, et al: Cementless acetabular replacement in the young: a 5- to 10-year prospective study. Clin Orthop Relat Res 376:149–155, 2000.

72. Latimer HA, Lachiewicz PF: Porous-coated acetabular components with screw fixation: five- to ten-year results. J Bone Joint Surg Am 78:975–981, 1996.

73. Tompkins GS, Jacobs JJ, Kull LR, et al: Primary total hip arthroplasty with a porous-coated acetabular component: seven-to-ten-year results. J Bone Joint Surg Am 79:169–176, 1997.

74. Nayak NK, Mulliken B, Rorabeck CH, et al: Osteolysis in cemented versus cementless acetabular components. J Arthroplasty 11:135–140, 1996.

75. Bartel DL, Bicknell VL, Wright TM: The effect of conformity, thickness, and material on stresses in ultra-high molecular weight components for total joint replacement. J Bone Joint Surg Am 68:1041–1051, 1986.

76. Berry DJ, Barnes CL, Scott RD, et al: Catastrophic failure of the polyethylene liner of uncemented acetabular components. J Bone Joint Surg Br 76:575–578, 1994.

77. Illgen R, 2nd, Rubash HE: The optimal fixation of the cementless acetabular component in primary total hip arthroplasty. J Am Acad Orthop Surg 10:43–56, 2002.

78. Archibeck MJ, Cummins T, Junick DW, White RE, Jr: Acetabular loosening using an extended offset polyethylene liner. Clin Orthop Relat Res 467:188–193, 2009.

79. Engh CA, Zettl-Schaffer KF, Kukita Y, et al: Histological and radiographic assessment of well functioning porous-coated acetabular components: a human postmortem retrieval study. J Bone Joint Surg Am 75:814–824, 1993.

80. Maloney WJ, Peters P, Engh CA, Chandler H: Severe osteolysis of the pelvic in association with acetabular replacement without cement. J Bone Joint Surg Am 75:1627–1635, 1993.

81. Massin P, Schmidt L, Engh CA: Evaluation of cementless acetabular component migration: an experimental study. J Arthroplasty 4:245–251, 1989.

82. Schmalzried TP, Harris WH: The Harris-Galante porous-coated acetabular component with screw fixation: radiographic analysis of eighty-three primary hip replacements at a minimum of five years. J Bone Joint Surg Am 74:1130–1139, 1992.

83. DeLee JG, Charnley J: Radiological demarcation of cemented sockets in total hip replacement. Clin Orthop Relat Res 121:20–32, 1976.

84. Martell JM, Pierson RH, 3rd, Jacobs JJ, et al: Primary total hip reconstruction with a titanium fiber-coated prosthesis inserted without cement. J Bone Joint Surg Am 75:554–571, 1993.

85. Udomkiat P, Wan Z, Dorr LD: Comparison of preoperative radiographs and intraoperative findings of fixation of hemispheric porous-coated sockets. J Bone Joint Surg Am 83:1865–1870, 2001.

86. Peters CL: The cementless acetabular component. In Callaghan JJ, Rosenberg AG, Rubash HE, editors: The adult hip, Philadelphia, 2007, Lippincott Wilkins & Wilkins, pp 946–968.

87. Bloebaum RD, Mihalopoulus NL, Jensen JW, Dorr LD: Postmortem analysis of bone growth into porous-coated acetabular components. J Bone Joint Surg Am 79:1013–1022, 1997.

88. Pidhorz LE, Urban RM, Jacobs JJ, et al: [Histological study of the porous coating of the uncemented acetabulum: apropos of 11 implants removed at autopsy]. Chirurgie 119:334–339, 1993.

89. Urban R, Hall DJ, Jacobs JJ, et al: Long-term fixation and potential failure mechanisms in cementless acetabular components retrieved post-mortem. In Transaction of the Orthopaedic Research Society, Rosemont, Ill, 2007, ORS.

90. Urban R, Hall DJ, Dahlmeier EL, et al: Reduced backside wear, particle migration, and osteolysis in third generation cementless acetabular components retrieved postmortem. In ORS, Las Vegas, 2009, ORS.

91. Bohm P, Bosche R: Survival analysis of the Harris-Galante I acetabular cup. J Bone Joint Surg Br 80:396–403, 1998.

92. Goldberg VM, Ninomiya J, Kelly G, Kraay M: Hybrid total hip arthroplasty: a 7- to 11-year followup. Clin Orthop Relat Res 333:147–154, 1996.

93. Piston RW, Engh CA, De Carvalho PI, Suthers K: Osteonecrosis of the femoral head treated with total hip arthroplasty without cement. J Bone Joint Surg Am 76:202–214, 1994.

94. Ricci WM, Westrich GH, Lorei M, et al: Primary total hip replacement with a noncemented acetabular component: minimum 5-year clinical follow-up. J Arthroplasty 15:146–152, 2000.

95. Soto MO, Rodriguez JA, Ranawat CS: Clinical and radiographic evaluation of the Harris-Galante cup: incidence of wear and osteolysis at 7 to 9 years follow-up. J Arthroplasty 15:139–145, 2000.

96. Zicat B, Engh CA, Gokcen E: Patterns of osteolysis around total hip components inserted with and without cement. J Bone Joint Surg Am 77:432–439, 1995.

97. Onsten I, Carlsson AS, Sanzen L, Besjakov J: Migration and wear of a hydroxyapatite-coated hip prosthesis: a controlled roentgen stereophotogrammetric study. J Bone Joint Surg Br 78:85–91, 1996.

98. Amenábar P, Della Valle CJ, Royce B, et al: Third generation cementless acetabular components: clinical and radiographic results at a minimum of 10 years. In American Academy of Orthopaedic Surgeons, Las Vegas, 2008, AAOS.

99. Callaghan JJ, Gaffey JL, Goetz DD: Cementless acetabular fixation at 15 years with the HG1 cup: comparison to the gold standard Charnley. In American Association of Hip and Knee Surgeons, Dallas, 2002, AAHKS.

100. Clohisy JC, Harris WH: The Harris-Galante porous-coated acetabular component with screw fixation: an average ten-year follow-up study. J Bone Joint Surg Am 81:66–73, 1999.

101. Crowther JD, Lachiewicz PF: Survival and polyethylene wear of porous-coated acetabular components in patients less than fifty years old: results at nine to fourteen years. J Bone Joint Surg Am 84:729–735, 2002.

102. Gaffey JL, Callaghan JJ, Pedersen DR, et al: Cementless acetabular fixation at fifteen years: a comparison with the same surgeon's results following acetabular fixation with cement. J Bone Joint Surg Am 86:257–261, 2004.

103. Parvizi J, Sullivan T, Duffy G, Cabanela ME: Fifteen-year clinical survivorship of Harris-Galante total hip arthroplasty. J Arthroplasty 19:672–677, 2004.

104. Rasquinha VJ, Dua V, Rodriguez JA, Ranawat CS: Fifteen-year survivorship of a collarless, cemented, normalized femoral stem in primary hybrid total hip arthroplasty with a modified third-generation cement technique. J Arthroplasty 18(7 Suppl 1):86–94, 2003.

105. Ihle M, Mai S, Pfluger D, Siebert W: The results of the titanium-coated RM acetabular component at 20 years: a long-term follow-up of an uncemented primary total hip replacement. J Bone Joint Surg Br 90:1284–1290, 2008.

106. Gwynne-Jones DP, Garneti N, Wainwright C, et al: The Morscher press fit acetabular component: a nine- to 13-year review. J Bone Joint Surg Br 91:859–864, 2009.

107. Berli BJ, Ping G, Dick W, Morscher EW: Nonmodular flexible press-fit cup in primary total hip arthroplasty: 15-year followup. Clin Orthop Relat Res 461:114–121, 2007.

108. Bojescul JA, Xenos JS, Callaghan JJ, Savory CG: Results of porous-coated anatomic total hip arthroplasty without cement at fifteen years: a concise follow-up of a previous report. J Bone Joint Surg Am 85:1079–1083, 2003.

109. Hastings DE, Tobin H, Sellenkowitsch M: Review of 10-year results of PCA hip arthroplasty. Can J Surg 41:48–52, 1998.

110. Healy WL, Casey DJ, Iorio R, Appleby D: Evaluation of the porous-coated anatomic hip at 12 years. J Arthroplasty 17:856–863, 2002.

111. Kawamura H, Dunbar MJ, Murray P, et al: The porous coated anatomic total hip replacement: a ten- to fourteen-year follow-up study of a cementless total hip arthroplasty. J Bone Joint Surg Am 83:1333–1338, 2001.

112. Kim YH, Kim JS, Cho SH: Primary total hip arthroplasty with the AML total hip prosthesis. Clin Orthop Relat Res 360:147–158, 1999.

113. Tsao AK, Lavernia CJ, Drakeford M: Porous coated anatomic hip replacement: the first 100: an eight to ten year review. Orthop Trans 18:1190, 1995.

114. Belmont PJ, Jr, Powers CC, Beykirch SE, et al: Results of the anatomic medullary locking total hip arthroplasty at a minimum of twenty years: a concise follow-up of previous reports. J Bone Joint Surg Am 90:1524–1530, 2008.

115. Engh CA, Jr, Culpepper WJ, 2nd, Engh CA: Long-term results of use of the anatomic medullary locking prosthesis in total hip arthroplasty. J Bone Joint Surg Am 79:177–184, 1997.

116. Jacobs JJ, Kull LR, Frey GA, et al: Early failure of acetabular components inserted without cement after previous pelvic irradiation. J Bone Joint Surg Am 77:1829–1835, 1995.

117. Massin P, Duparc J: Total hip replacement in irradiated hips: a retrospective study of 71 cases. J Bone Joint Surg Br 77:847–852, 1995.

118. Kim KI, Klein GR, Sleeper J, et al: Uncemented total hip arthroplasty in patients with a history of pelvic irradiation for prostate cancer. J Bone Joint Surg Am 89:798–805, 2007.

FURTHER READING

Clohisy JC, Harris WH: The Harris-Galante porous-coated acetabular component with screw fixation: an average ten-year follow-up study. J Bone Joint Surg Am 81:66–73, 1999.
This study demonstrates mid-term results with titanium, hemispherical, cementless acetabular components inserted with screws.

Della Valle CJ, Mesko NW, Quigley L, et al: Primary total hip arthroplasty with a porous-coated acetabular component: a concise follow-up, at a minimum of twenty years, of previous reports. J Bone Joint Surg Am 91:1130–1135, 2009.
This publication demonstrates at 20-year follow-up durable long-term fixation with titanium, hemispherical, cementless acetabular components inserted with screws.

Levine B, Della Valle CJ, Jacobs JJ: Applications of porous tantalum in total hip arthroplasty. J Am Acad Orthop Surg 14:646–655, 2006.
This review article explains the use of porous tantalum, the next generation of porous ingrowth surfaces, as it pertains to total joint arthroplasty.

Maloney WJ, Galante JO, Anderson M, et al: Fixation, polyethylene wear, and pelvic osteolysis in primary total hip replacement. Clin Orthop Relat Res 369:157–164, 1999.
In the absence of infection, implant longevity is associated with minimizing polyethylene wear and avoiding subsequent osteolysis and bone loss. Maloney and associates describe methods by which to define osteolysis and bone loss while defining risk factors for increased polyethylene wear.

Zicat B, Engh CA, Gokcen E: Patterns of osteolysis around total hip components inserted with and without cement. J Bone Joint Surg Am 77:432–439, 1995.
Zicat and colleagues describe predictable patterns of osteolysis associated with cementless and cemented acetabular components.

CHAPTER 67

Cemented Femoral Components

Andrew J. Timperley, Jonathan R. Howell, Matthew J.W. Hubble, Graham A. Gie, and Sarah L. Whitehouse

KEY POINTS

- Cemented stems (Fig. 67-1) are indicated in patients in *all* age groups who require a hip arthroplasty for *any* pathology (Fig. 67-2).
- Results from national joint registries confirm that cemented taper-slip femoral components yield predictable excellent results in the hands of surgeons of all levels of experience.
- The use of collarless polished tapered stems confers significant advantages in the restoration of hip biomechanics in that *stem size, stem offset, leg length,* and *version* are all independently variable.
- If an additional operation is ever required on the hip to correct problems unconnected with femoral fixation, the implant is, in practical terms, modular at the stem-cement interface. The stem can be knocked out of a well-fixed cement mantle and the same, or a smaller, stem recemented into the existing cement mantle at the end of the operation. This technique allows for correction of leg length, offset, and version, even in the revision situation.

INTRODUCTION

Although Philip Wiles[1] of the Middlesex Hospital in London must be credited with the introduction of the first *total* hip replacement in 1958, it was Charnley who was the first to use acrylic cement to anchor the stem of an intramedullary femoral prosthesis,[2] and McKee and Watson-Farrar[3] of Norwich who were the first to use cement for fixation of the acetabular cup. It can be argued that acrylic bone cement is probably the most abused biomaterial, literally and figuratively, in use in orthopedic surgery. A cursory review of the literature shows that the surgical techniques employed when cement is chosen as the method of fixation are of great importance, but surgeons have blamed failure of cemented hip arthroplasty on fundamental failings of cement as a biomaterial,[4] rather than on failure of the surgeon to appreciate the surgical steps necessary to use the material appropriately. Polymethylmethacrylate bone cement (PMMA) has no adhesive properties, and fixation using this material mandates that the surgeon establish a strong mechanical interlock with cement against host bone.[5] Lars Linder[6] pointed out that osseointegration "should be regarded not as an exclusive reaction to a specific implant material, but as the expression of a non-specific and basic healing potential in bone." Malcolm[7] demonstrated, in man, that acrylic bone cement can remain osseointegrated over the long term, thereby maintaining sound mechanical fixation of the implant. The cement-bone interface is thereby protected from intrusion of fluid under pressure containing particulate debris.

Detractors of the use of cement ignore the other beneficial attributes that are a corollary of its use. As it is used today, acrylic cement subserves several functions: Not only is it the means by which the implant is fixed to the bone, it is also an integral part of the mechanism of load transmission into the femur and is fundamentally just as much a part of the "implant" as the metallic component. Moreover, the viscoelastic properties of PMMA allow it to act as a load spreader, a shock absorber, and a decoupler of differential movements of structures of different modulus and structural rigidity.[8]

GENERAL CONSIDERATIONS

Shen,[9] an engineer, suggested that cemented femoral components can be divided into two basic types (Fig. 67-3). *Taper-slip* or *force-closed* stems are exemplified by the original polished flatback Charnley (Zimmer, Warsaw, Indiana) and the polished Exeter (Stryker Inc., Newbury, United Kingdom) stems that routinely subside within the cement mantle without fracturing it. With these stems, stability is maintained by a balance of forces across the stem-cement interface with no form of bond between the two. *Composite-beam* or *shape-closed* stems cannot, by definition, subside within the cement, and stability is maintained by the bond that arises when the surface contours of the stem are matched and cement is applied to it.[10] Kärrholm showed in a radiostereometric assay (RSA) study[11] that subsidence of the stem at the stem-cement interface regularly occurred not only with taper-slip stems, but also with composite-beam stems, thus calling into question the whole concept of the composite-beam stem.

Good results can be obtained using composite-beam stems, but they are less forgiving in terms of surgical technique.[12,13] The basic surgical techniques described here for contemporary femoral cementing are valid for both types of stem. If a composite-beam stem is to be used, it is essential that a complete cement mantle of adequate thickness is established, as well as solid

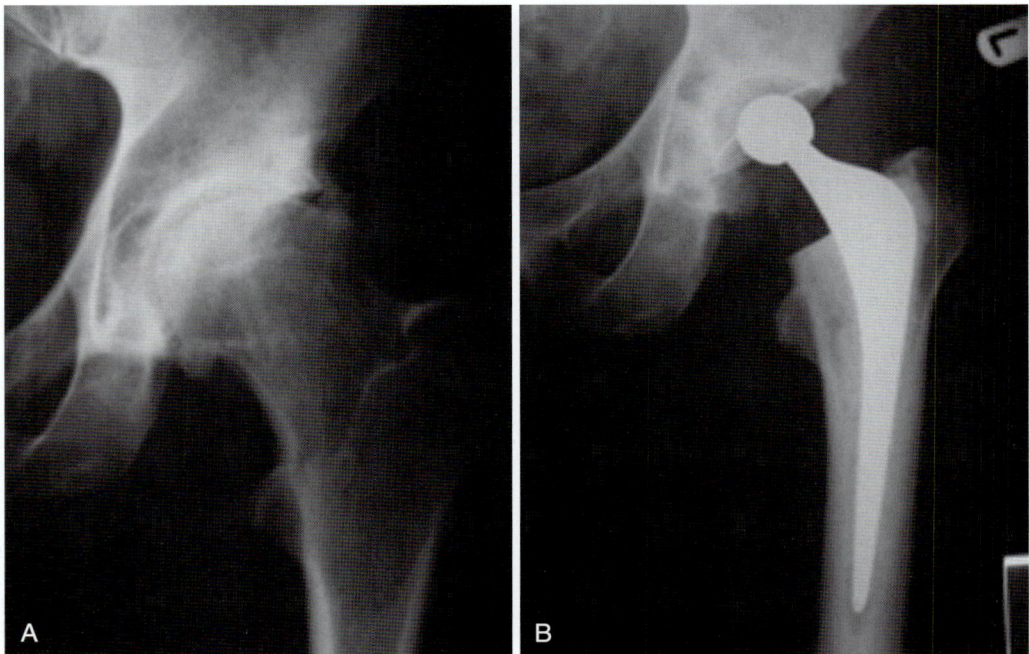

Figure 67-1. A cemented femoral component can reliably reproduce the biomechanics of the hip because femoral offset, leg length, and version all are independently variable.

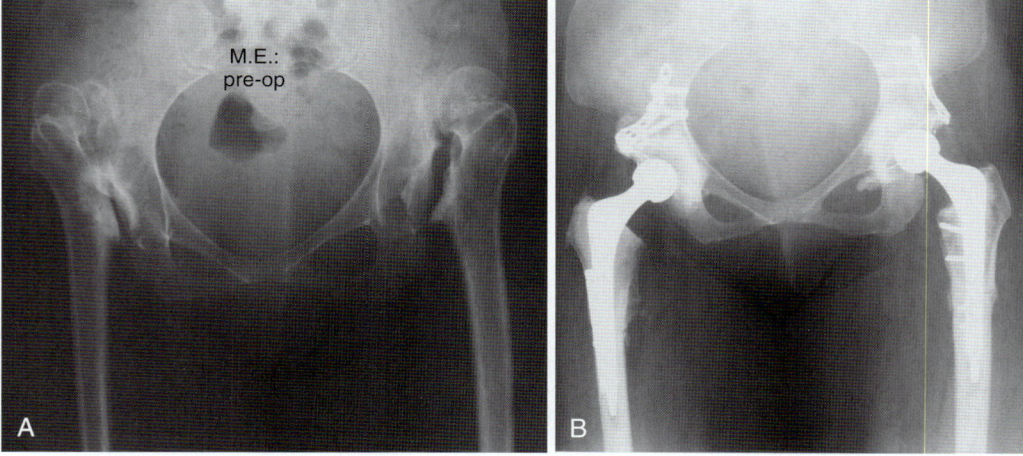

Figure 67-2. Cemented femoral components can be used for any pathology. In the case illustrated, subtrochanteric femoral osteotomies have been necessary in the treatment of bilateral Crowe IV developmental dysplasia of the hip (DDH).

fixation at both the stem-cement interface and the cement-bone interface. Scheerlinck[12] points out that although in vivo both concepts of stem fixation have proved effective, they cannot work together, and it is important to understand on which principle a particular stem relies.

In contrast to the variable results of composite-beam components, taper-slip stems have been demonstrated to yield excellent results in all existing national joint registries,[14-16] as well as in individual publications from multiple centers. In engineering practice, the taper is one of the strongest and most reliable methods of transmitting not only axial but also torsional forces between one component and another. In the context of the

cemented stem, subsidence of the tapered stem is analogous to engagement of the taper; if the stem is to function effectively as a taper, it *must not* in any way be fixed to the cement or end-bearing. Shen[9] and Howie[17] point out that the taper-slip system is more forgiving in terms of surgical technique, and the success of the concept is demonstrated by the fact that all major manufacturers of hip implants now have such stems in their portfolio. In contemporary practice, they are by far the most widely used cemented stems throughout the world.

To function by the taper-slip principle, a stem must be tapered in shape and must have a polished surface; also, there must be no feature on the device, such as a collar, that could prevent the stem from subsiding

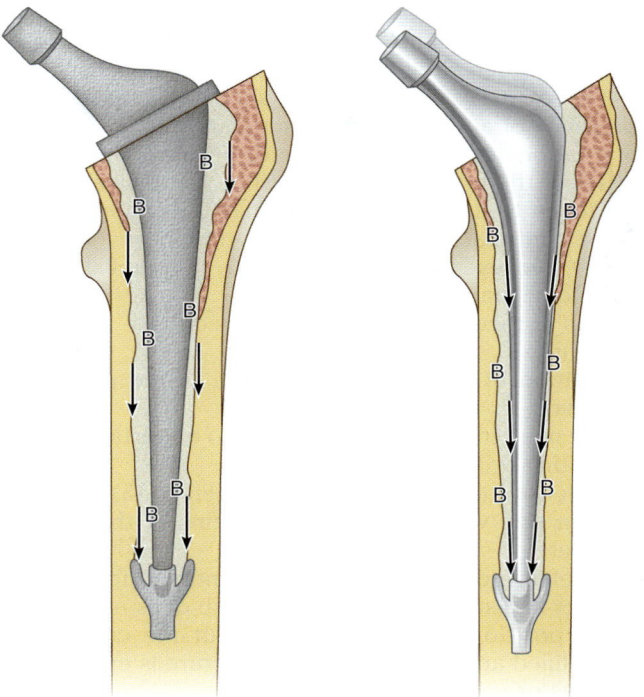

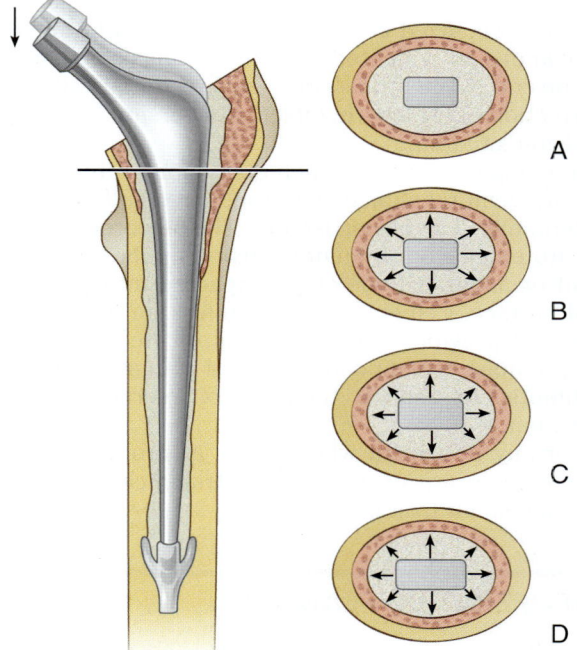

Figure 67-3. A composite beam stem is demonstrated on the left. The stem is bonded to cement *(B)*, and shear forces are transmitted directly to the cement-bone interface *(arrows)*. A taper-slip stem is demonstrated on the right. Shear forces are transmitted to the stem-cement interface, where subsidence occurs *(arrows)* and the cement-bone interface is protected *(B)*.

Figure 67-4. Transverse sections at the level of the line on the femur are shown. **A,** The unloaded situation. **B,** On loading, radial compressive stresses are induced in the cement. **C,** As the stem has subsided, a larger cross-section is accommodated by the cement, generating hoop tensile stresses within the cement mantle. **D,** On resting, residual hoop strain persists, and stress relaxation occurs within the cement of these tensile forces. The loading regimen is now dominated by compression at the stem-cement interface, within the cement, and across the cement-bone interface.

within the cement mantle. A stem with these characteristics can take advantage of the viscoelastic behavior of acrylic bone cement in that movement is allowed at the stem-cement interface without damage to the internal surface of the cement mantle. This subsidence has three important effects:

- Because a force on the stem produces subsidence at the stem-cement interface, it does not induce damaging shear forces at the biological interface, that is, the bone-cement interface. This is in contradistinction to a composite-beam stem in which shear forces exerted on the cement by the stem are transmitted directly to the biological interface.
- As the stem subsides, it generates hoop tensile forces and radial compression within the cement (Fig. 67-4). Radial compressive forces serve to protect the cement-bone interface from any shear forces; they also load the bone. During periods of rest, tensile strain persists and stress relaxation of cement occurs, dissipating hoop tensile stresses.[18] This mechanism protects the cement against fatigue fracture, and the whole loading regimen is dominated by compressive forces. Crowninshield and associates[19] noted, "Load transmission by compression across the stem-cement boundary may be the only reliable mechanism of loading in vivo."
- Subsidence of the polished taper within the cement increases the torsional stability of the stem.[20]

With contemporary cementing, observed subsidence of the stem within the cement is approximately 1.3 mm at 17 years' follow-up.[21] It continues very slowly throughout the life of the implant, but with contemporary cementing, this is not of clinical importance with regard to leg length.[22]

INDICATIONS/CONTRAINDICATIONS OF CEMENTED FEMORAL COMPONENTS

Cemented femoral stems can be considered for any patient who requires a hip arthroplasty. Cemented, taper-slip devices are recognized as delivering the gold standard in terms of long-term fixation.[21-23] Use of a collarless, polished, tapered, cemented stem confers significant advantages over cementless designs in that stem size, stem offset, leg length, and version all are independently variable, allowing faithful re-creation of hip biomechanics no matter what the original deformity. Over the longer term, use of a taper-slip stem also confers an advantage if an additional operation is required to address problems with the hip other than femoral fixation. The device is, in effect, modular at the stem-cement interface, and the stem can be knocked out of a well-fixed cement mantle and another stem of similar design cemented into the existing cement mantle at the end of the procedure.[24] This technique allows for correction of leg length, offset, and version, even in the revision situation.

In complex cases in which distortion of the anatomy occurs, femoral shortening procedures and de-rotation osteotomies can be carried out. The osteotomy site can be protected from cement intrusion by the use of autograft or allograft bone chips impacted into the endosteal surface. Cement fixation confers an advantage in cases of previous septic arthritis of the hip, because acrylic bone cement can be loaded with an appropriate antibiotic to reduce the risk of recrudescence of infection.

For any patient in whom a hip arthroplasty is indicated, there are no specific contraindications for the use of cement fixation.

PREOPERATIVE PLANNING

The aim of preoperative planning is to determine the correct position of the components to allow restoration of the anatomic center of rotation of the joint, and to re-create the correct leg length and offset. Preoperative planning also helps the surgeon predict, before the start of the procedure, the need for appropriate instrumentation, prostheses, and, occasionally, bone graft. A major advantage of scaled *digital* templating is that implant templates can be imported at the correct size rather than at the assumed 120% magnification, as is the case with acetates. The image taken for templating must be taken with a scale on the image. An ideal scale for hip replacement is a total hip replacement (THR) on the contralateral side, where the size of the femoral head is known. The next best system is for a marker of known size to be placed in the plane of the femoral head. We have established a convention to position a HipScaler (www.hipscaler.com) on all anteroposterior (AP) x-rays of the pelvis taken at our institution, thereby reducing the need to take additional films for this purpose.

Clinical examination of the patient is an essential part of the preoperative assessment, so that the surgeon is aware of any true or apparent leg length discrepancy or fixed contracture of the hip, or the presence of fixed pelvic obliquity. In the absence of a navigation system, it is the responsibility of the operating surgeon personally to position the patient on the operating table so that he or she is aware of the relative position of the pelvis to the horizontal and vertical planes.

Radiologic Assessment

X-rays ideally should be taken with the hip internally rotated by 15 degrees. If the film is not taken in this position, with the x-ray beam perpendicular to the femoral neck, the x-ray will suggest a more valgus femoral neck with reduced offset and a higher center of rotation in relation to the femur than is actually the case. In addition to the clinical assessment, the x-ray

profile of the lesser trochanter will give the surgeon a clue to any rotational deformity of the femur.

The surgeon should determine whether there is deficiency or excess of bone and should identify (1) the presence of any leg length discrepancy, (2) the center of rotation of the acetabulum and the femur, and (3) the offset of the hip (the distance from the neutral axis of the femur to the center of rotation of the femoral head). If the contralateral hip is normal, this makes planning easier, because the goal is usually to re-establish native hip biomechanics.

This process allows the surgeon to plan the following:
- Position of the center of rotation of the prosthetic socket
- The need to remove any bone or to undertake a bone grafting procedure
- Offset of the stem to be inserted (Fig. 67-5)
- Stem size within the range of stems of the desired offset
- Level of neck resection (this is not critical with a taper-slip stem because neck length does not control the position of the prosthesis, but the cut can be modified appropriately if the structure is excessively varus or valgus)
- Depth of the stem insertion in relation to the tip of the greater trochanter
- The need for any unusual procedures such as subtrochanteric femoral osteotomy and shortening, with or without de-rotation of the proximal fragment, primary impaction grafting, etc.

RESULTS

Survivorship data with the longest follow-up when a double-tapered, collarless, polished cemented stem has been used have been published by the Exeter team (from the Exeter stem). At the 33rd year of follow-up, stem survivorship with the endpoint of revision for aseptic loosening was 93.5% (95% confidence interval [CI], 90.0% to 97.0%).[22] In the "worst case scenario,"[25,26] in which all cases lost to follow-up are regarded as failures from aseptic stem loosening, survivorship was 85.8% with a 95% CI of 81.3% to 90.3%. Of 433 hips in the series, 14 have been revised for aseptic stem loosening (3.46%). Two of these were re-revisions, and two had previously undergone intertrochanteric osteotomy. None have been revised for aseptic loosening since the 20th year of the survivorship study, and none have been lost to follow-up since that time. These results were achieved with first-generation cementing techniques and with surgeons of widely differing experience, illustrating that excellent results can be attained with a stem functioning by the taper-slip principle, despite relatively poor quality cementing by today's standards. The Exeter Universal stem, which had an identical surface finish and a very slight difference in stem geometry but functions in exactly the same way, was introduced in 1988. The 17-year survivorship with the endpoint of revision for aseptic stem loosening was 100% in the series published by the design center.[21] In a separate

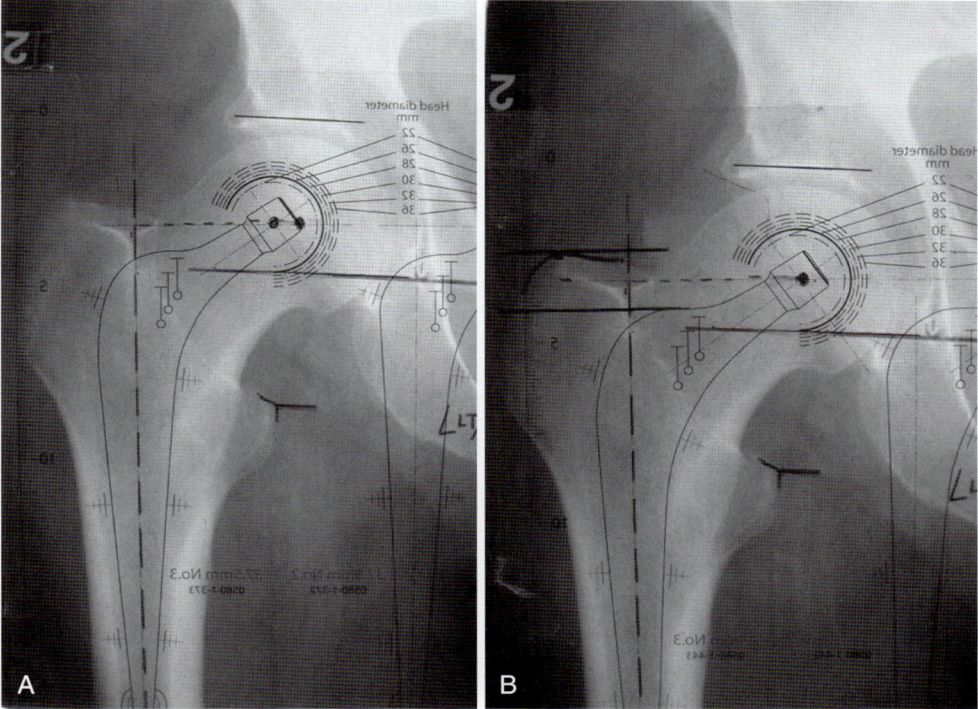

Figure 67-5. **A,** A template of a femoral component of insufficient offset has been laid on the x-ray. **B,** A femoral component with a greater offset is chosen, and it now can be seen that the center of rotation of the prosthesis coincides with that of the native hip. Leg length is unchanged.

study of results in patients younger than 50 years[27] at the time of surgery (average age at surgery, 42 years), with no case lost to follow-up, stem survivorship was 100% with revision for aseptic stem loosening as the endpoint, and 99% for all causes of stem revision, including periprosthetic fracture. This occurred at 10 to 17 years' (average, 12.5 years') follow-up. No case showed focal femoral osteolysis.

Many reports from other centers have described results with stems that function by the taper-slip principle.[28-49] Burston[50] reported results in patients younger than 50 and concluded, "… the performance of polished tapered stems in patients younger than 50 years is excellent, with stem survival and subsidence equivalent to the older, standard hip arthroplasty population. They compare very favorably with other stem designs that have been reported among the younger patients. With ease of insertion and such predictable behavior, this type of stem has to be the benchmark for comparison to other stem designs, including uncemented stems and resurfacing implants, in this young age group." All papers cited reported a consistent pattern of behavior with regard to femoral components, irrespective of the experience of the operating surgeon, and demonstrated similar results to those obtained in Exeter with benign radiologic appearances, a small degree of subsidence within the cement mantle, and satisfactory clinical outcomes.

Survivorship analysis, as used in hip registries, is a powerful tool in the long-term assessment of arthroplasty because it gives a more realistic presentation of longevity than is provided by simple examination of

failure rates. The behavior of the polished Exeter Universal stem in the Swedish and Norwegian Hip Registries is, in general, in line with results from elsewhere.[15,51-55] Furnes and associates[55] reported that the Exeter had the lowest percentage revision rate at 15 years (3.0%) and the smallest increment in revision rate between 10 and 15 years (from 2.2% to 3.0%) among the 10 most commonly used cements in Norway. A study from Finland[56] of patients aged 55 years or older undergoing surgery for osteoarthritis found that the only femoral and acetabular component combination to have a survivorship greater than 90% at 15 years was the Exeter Universal/Exeter All-Polyethylene couple. The most recent study from the Swedish Registry[15] includes a detailed analysis of implant survival for all diagnoses and all reasons for revision from 1992 to 2007, and allows separation of the results of different cups with the same variety of stem. The combination of the Cenator flanged cemented cup with the Exeter polished Universal stem (660 hips) shows survivorship at 5 and 10 years of 99.5% and 98.8%, respectively.

TECHNIQUES

Overview of Technique

The aim of contemporary cementing techniques is to establish direct contact between cement and living bone without an intervening cellular layer. To this end, it is important to leave strong trabecular bone in the proximal femur[57] and to prepare the surface adequately

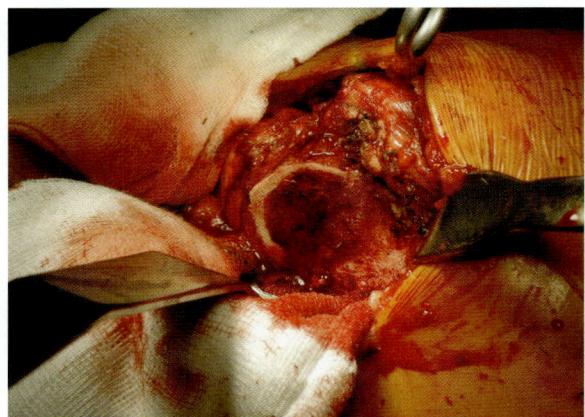

Figure 67-6. Exposure of the top end of the femur through a posterior approach after neck section.

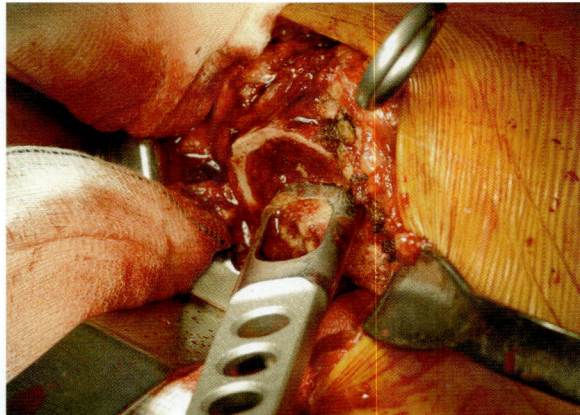

Figure 67-7. A box chisel is used to open the proximal femur, with particular attention to opening the canal lateral to the mid axis of the femur.

for application and pressurization of polymethylmethacrylate into the interstices of the bone. The femur must be prepared with the use of a pressurized lavage system, following which the surface is dried with hydrogen peroxide–soaked ribbon gauze. The plugged canal is then filled with cement in retrograde fashion with the use of a gun, and more cement is injected through a proximal femoral seal, thereby forcing the material into the bone and, by maintaining pressure within the canal, protecting the interface from the deleterious effects of bleeding.[58,59]

A stem of the correct offset is inserted to a prerehearsed depth in an appropriate degree of version. This technique is described in detail in the following section.

Exposure and Bone Preparation

Any of the routine approaches can be used to prepare the femur for cementing, although at our institution, a posterior approach, which is described here, is favored.

In routine cases, the obturator internus, the gemelli, and a portion of the quadratus femoris are divided, but usually it is not necessary to divide the anterior capsule, the iliopsoas, the femoral insertion of the gluteus maximus, or the piriformis. A femoral elevator is used to deliver the femur into the wound, and a gluteus medius retractor serves to adequately expose the proximal femur (Fig. 67-6).

The level of the neck cut is not important when a polished, tapered, collarless stem is used. Preoperative templating will have established whether abnormal preexisting varus or valgus angulation of the femoral neck is present. With coxa vara, the neck cut can be made in a low position and the stem will need to be inserted further into the femoral canal than is normal. In cases of coxa valga, the neck cut is slightly longer than normal, so that a stem will be well supported within the canal.

It is very important to open up the proximal end of the femur 1 cm lateral to the axis of the shaft so that the instruments can be introduced down the midline of the femoral medullary canal. This can be accomplished

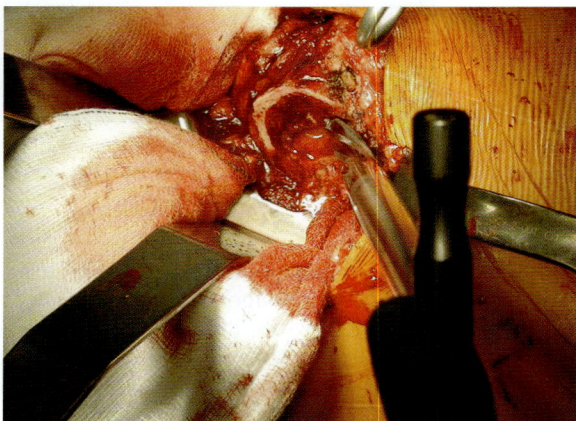

Figure 67-8. If the lateral canal has been opened adequately, the taper pin reamer will point toward the middle of the popliteal fossa.

by using a box chisel (Fig. 67-7). Taper pin reamers point directly to the middle of the popliteal fossa if the lateral canal has been opened adequately (Fig. 67-8). The canal is lavaged and aspirated before any instrument is introduced. The size of the canal at a level immediately distal to the stem tip is established with the use of sizers, and a PMMA plug of this diameter can be opened, ready for later implantation.

Rasping and First Trial Reduction

Rasps of appropriate offset, as determined by templating, are used sequentially, usually starting one size smaller than the predicted stem size (Fig. 67-9). Rasps allow for an adequate cement mantle, and the lateral edge is useful in further opening the posterolateral aspect of the trochanter. By looking at the distance between the tip of the greater trochanter and the shoulder of the rasp, the depth of insertion is compared with that predicted at templating. It is important not to use an oversized rasp, but to preserve 2 to 3 mm of strong cancellous bone within the proximal femur. The

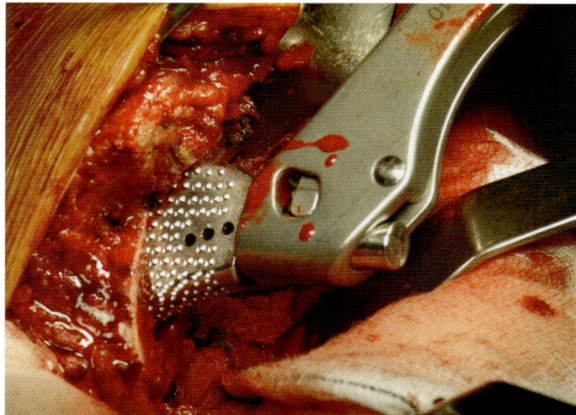

Figure 67-9. The appropriate rasp is introduced into the canal. The lateral edge of the rasp is useful in opening the lateral canal. Care is taken to leave strong cancellous bone within the proximal femur.

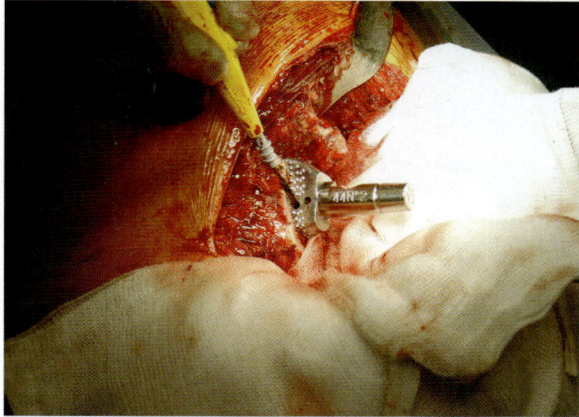

Figure 67-10. After trial reduction, a mark is made on the femur opposite one of the markers on the rasp to illustrate the correct depth of stem insertion.

thickness of the cement mantle is not critical with this type of implant because cement fracture is not a mode of failure of the device.

The leg length is determined by how far the implant is introduced down the canal. If, on trial reduction of the rasp, the leg is found to be long, then the rasp can be introduced further into the canal until the correct leg length is established. Conversely, if the leg is too short, a further trial reduction can be carried out with a locating pin in the rasp holding it out to the correct level, or, if sufficient strong bone is present in the proximal femur, a larger rasp can be introduced to the correct level.

Range of motion, soft tissue tension, and the stability of the hip are checked in all positions of the joint. A careful assessment is made for impingement of hard or soft tissues because this must be addressed if it is found to compromise stability. Inappropriate leg length is dealt with by changing the depth of insertion of the rasp; fine adjustment to offset may be made with a +4 mm or a −4 mm head, with corresponding fine adjustment to the change in length. Very occasionally, a stem of different offset may be deemed appropriate. It is never necessary to use a greater range of neck lengths with this system; thus problems that occur when skirted devices are implanted are avoided. All extended or reduced neck options affect leg length and offset. It is one of the great advantages of this type of cemented hip system that these two parameters can be independently varied.

A mark is made on the femoral neck adjacent to one of the marks on the rasp (Fig. 67-10). This indicates the depth of insertion of the definitive stem. The order can be given to start mixing the cement while final preparation of the femur is carried out.

Final Preparation of the Femur and Cementing

The cement restrictor is introduced, and a pressurized lavage system is employed to wash the canal aggressively (Fig. 67-11). A 2-inch ribbon gauze soaked in

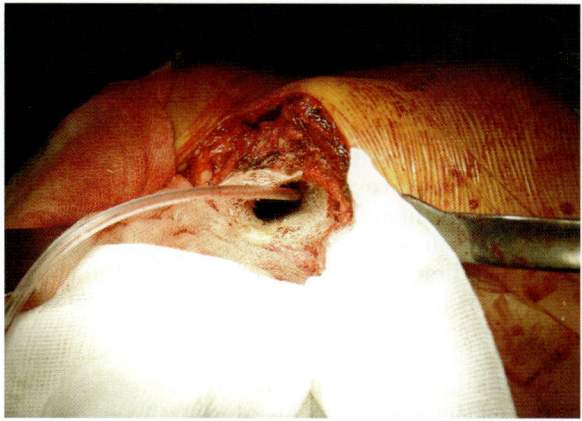

Figure 67-11. While the cement is being mixed, the femoral canal is thoroughly lavaged. The bone in the proximal end of the femur should appear pearly white after lavage of blood and marrow contents.

hydrogen peroxide is introduced over a suction catheter, the end of which is left at the level of the distal plug; this serves to promote stasis and further cleans the trabecular bone.[58] As an alternative, adrenaline-soaked ribbon gauze or ice-cold rolls may be used.[60] The canal is now ready for the introduction of cement.

At our institution, bone cement containing antibiotics is used routinely. Mixing is carried out in a low vacuum; we do not use full vacuum mixing to reduce porosity because it has not been found to confer any advantage in the medium term, especially if a force-closed design of stem is used.[61,62] Two 40-g mixes of cement are used routinely.

The femoral canal is cleared except for the suction catheter, which is left in place on top of the plug until it blocks as the cement is introduced. Simplex at 21° C is ready for injection into the canal about 2 minutes after mixing commences. The canal is filled in retrograde fashion, the nozzle of the gun is cut level with the distal femoral seal, and more cement is injected through

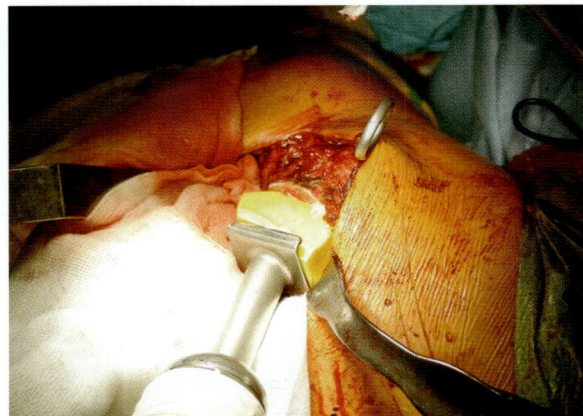

Figure 67-12. Cement is introduced in retrograde fashion over the top of a distal plug. When the canal is full, further cement is injected into the closed cavity through a proximal femoral seal, and pressure is maintained until the cement viscosity is high enough for stem introduction.

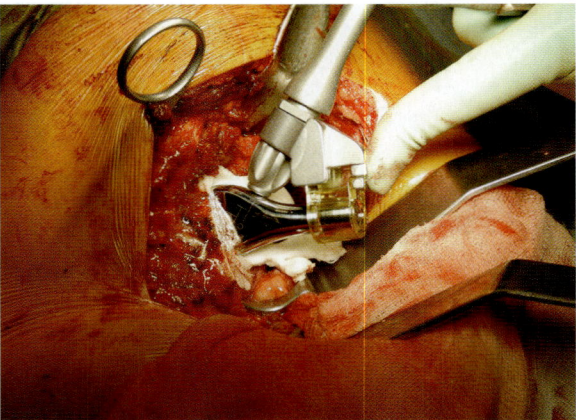

Figure 67-13. The stem is inserted to the depth previously rehearsed and is marked for correct leg length.

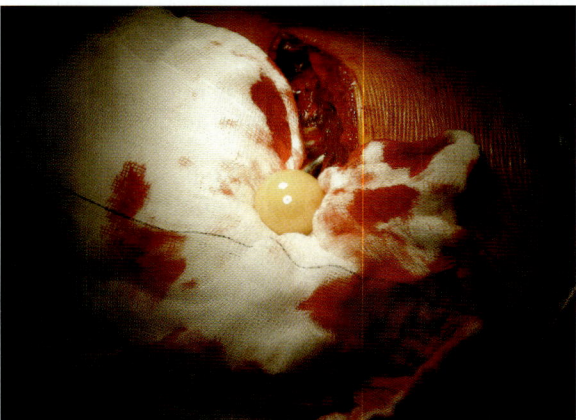

Figure 67-14. A further trial reduction is carried out before the definitive head is applied to the stem, in this case a ceramic head.

the seal to force cement into the interstices of the trabecular bone (Fig. 67-12). There should be steady extrusion of fat and marrow through the proximal femoral cortex. Pressure is maintained until the cement is doughy enough for the stem to be introduced. This usually occurs approximately 5 minutes from the start of mixing if the theater temperature is 21° C. A bolus of cement is retained in the surgeon's hand as another indicator of the correct moment to insert the stem.

The stem is preheated in a bath of saline at 60° C, with the aim of accelerating polymerization of the cement once it is introduced into the femoral canal. A secondary benefit of this technique is that porosities are reduced at the stem-cement interface,[63] although this may not be clinically relevant. The implant should be thoroughly dried before insertion.

Stem Introduction and Final Trial Reduction

The stem should be introduced with the point of entry close to the post area margin of the cut surface of the femoral neck. This point of entry reduces the possibility of a cement mantle deficiency in the lower part of zone 8 and the upper part of zone 9.[64] Particular attention should be paid to the entry point if a direct lateral approach to the hip has been used, because there is a tendency for the stem to be inserted from front to back, and for the tip to be adjacent to the posterior cortex. As the stem is inserted, the opening of the canal medial to the stem is occluded by the surgeon's thumb with the aim of maximizing cement-bone interface pressure in the proximal femur. Version and alignment of the stem are checked as the stem is introduced. The implant is inserted until the appropriate mark corresponding to that on the rasp is adjacent to the mark on the femur (Fig. 67-13).

Once the stem has been inserted, it should not be moved within the cement mantle during the polymerization process. Pressure is applied through a sorbothane "horse-collar," which is positioned around the implant

on top of the cement mantle. The effect of this is to slow the rate of fall of pressure within the femur, so that the interface is protected until polymerization is complete.[8]

After polymerization is complete, cement is removed from the cut surface of the femoral neck, a head is applied to the implant, and a further trial reduction is performed. Further fine tuning can be carried out with a different neck length. It is essential that the hip is stable, and that all impingement issues have been addressed by the end of the procedure.

Once the definitive head has been applied (Fig. 67-14), the hip is reduced and the capsule and short rotators are reattached through drill holes in the greater trochanter.

Practical Tips

1. Sufficient time should be spent on templating. This will give an indication not only of the size and offset, but also of the depth of insertion of the prosthesis.
2. If the predetermined size of broach is too tight, check the entry point. It is probably not lateral and posterior enough.

3. It is important to preserve the strong cancellous bone along the calcar. At least 2 to 3 mm of cancellous bone should be available for cement interlock.
4. Use of a powered lavage system is mandatory to clean the bone surface.
5. Pressurization of the cemented canal should be maintained before, during, and after insertion of the stem until the cement has completely cured.

COMPLICATIONS

Death following elective total hip arthroplasty is a relatively rare event and, according to several sources, is less in this relatively healthy surgical cohort of patients than in the general population of the same age group.[65-67] The latest National Joint Registry (NJR) of England and Wales[16] report indicates a significantly reduced mortality rate (less than half) at 1 year following primary total hip replacement (1.9%; 95% CI, 1.8% to 2.0%) than is seen in the general population of England and Wales, using age- and gender-adjusted standardized mortality ratios (SMRs). Indeed, this SMR is slightly less for cemented hips (0.46; 95% CI, 0.42 to 0.50) than for cementless hips (0.49; 95% CI, 0.42 to 0.57). These figures are mirrored in the Australian Orthopaedic Association (AOA) National Joint Replacement Registry (NJRR),[14] with a standardized mortality of 2.4% for primary total hip replacement.

One cause of sudden intraoperative death during arthroplasty is venous embolization of marrow contents. This phenomenon occurs during instrumentation of any long bone.[68] At the time of arthroplasty, it can occur when cement is used,[69-71] but it has also been reported with cementless implants.[70,71] Improvements in operative technique designed to minimize these intramedullary pressures were associated with a reduction greater than threefold in overall intraoperative mortality rate.[72] A randomized prospective study comparing cemented with uncemented stems in total hip arthroplasty reported no difference in the prevalence of fat or bone marrow embolism.[73] In Exeter[68] and elsewhere,[74] recommendations have been made for the prevention of these cardiovascular aberrations. In his review of mortality and contemporary cementing techniques during a cemented THR with the Exeter stem, Sierra[75] reported one operative death in a series of 9082 total hips over a 17-year period—a 0.01% prevalence of sudden death. With current contemporary cementing techniques and a specialized anesthetic protocol, he suggested that the incidence of sudden death during cemented THR should be "near zero."

The NJR report[16] includes revision rates at 3 months of 0.2% for cemented and 0.5% for cementless procedures, with the difference increasing by 1 year to 0.3% for cemented and 1.0% for cementless total hips. This trend continues to 3 years (0.9% cemented, 1.9% cementless). The AOA NJRR[14] also reports a significantly higher risk of revision for cementless compared with cemented (Adj HR = 1.46; 95% CI, 1.27 to 1.68; $P < .001$) and hybrid conventional total hip replacements (Adj HR = 1.43; 95% CI, 1.30 to 1.58; $P < .001$), which were adjusted for age

and gender. At 7 years, the cumulative percent revision is 3.0% for both hybrid and cemented total hip replacements and 3.9% for cementless total hip replacement ($P < .001$). Between 1998 and 2007, the Swedish Registry[15] reports a significantly increased revision risk for uncemented implants, with a relative risk (RR) of 1.37 (95% CI, 1.13 to 1.67) after adjustment for age, gender, diagnosis, bilaterality, and approach. It is interesting to note that the risk of early revision (within 2 years) for uncemented implants is almost double that for cemented implants—RR, 1.86 (95% CI, 1.55 to 2.23)—where infection is excluded.

It has been shown that mortality following revision THR is more than double the rate after primary surgery—0.33 to 0.84[76] and 0.4 to 0.9[77] for primary and revision surgeries, respectively. The increased risk of revision with cementless implants, coupled with the significantly increased mortality rate at revision surgery,[76-78] indicates that the balanced risk of mortality is significantly reduced if a cemented prosthesis is used at primary operation.

Reducing Risk During Hip Arthroplasty

Every effort should be made intraoperatively to reduce the possibility of embolization of fat and marrow contents, whether the hip is to be cemented[72] or cementless.[70,71,79]

Pressurized Lavage
Thorough lavage of the medullary cavity with a pressurized system is mandatory to reduce the embolic load[74,80-82] and has been shown to improve fixation of the femoral component.[54] Lavage should be carried out before any instrumentation of the medullary cavity is performed.[83]

Cement Restrictor/Plug
Evidence supports the use of a cement restrictor to reduce physiologic disturbance.[84,85]

Suction Catheter
The safest way to introduce cement is in retrograde fashion from a gun. A suction catheter placed distally above the plug must be used to reduce pressure at the cement/marrow-vessel interface during cement insertion.[72] A reduction in intramedullary pressure has been reported to lead to a threefold reduction in intraoperative mortality.[72] If the canal is adequately cleaned, and if the patient is adequately prepared and monitored during the procedure, then cement pressurization appears to confer no disadvantage with regard to risk and improves fixation of the femoral component.[15,16,75]

SUMMARY AND FUTURE CONSIDERATIONS

In the history of hip arthroplasty, there has never been more evidence than there is now to support the routine use of cemented femoral components that function by the taper-slip principle. Multiple publications, including those of national joint registries, are testament to the longevity of these implants in terms of mechanical loosening. In addition, these implants confer practical advantages for the surgeon to accurately re-create the native hip biomechanics, because stem size, femoral offset, leg length, and version all are independently variable. The implants preserve bone stock in the femur over the long term compared with uncemented devices, and if a revision procedure is required on the hip for a reason other than femoral loosening, a cement-in-cement procedure can be carried out. Even in the revision situation, the same flexibility remains to vary offset, leg length, and version separately to deliver an optimal result. Because it is not necessary to disturb the biological interface, the risk to the patient in terms of morbidity and mortality is reduced, and the revision procedure is faster and less expensive. If more evidence is required to support the case for cemented components, multiple publications support the health care economic argument for their routine use.

REFERENCES

1. Wiles P: The surgery of the osteoarthritic hip. Br J Surg 45:488–497, 1958.
2. Charnley J: Surgery of the hip-joint: present and future developments. Br Med J 1:821–826, 1960.
3. McKee GK, Watson-Farrar J: Replacement of arthritic hips by the McKee-Farrar prosthesis. J Bone Joint Surg Br 48:245–259, 1966.
4. Jones LC, Hungerford DS: Cement disease. Clin Orthop Relat Res 225:192–206, 1987.
5. Benjamin JB, Gie GA, Lee AJ, et al: Cementing technique and the effects of bleeding. J Bone Joint Surg Br 69:620–624, 1987.
6. Linder L: Osseointegration of metallic implants. I. Light microscopy in the rabbit. Acta Orthop Scand 60:129–134, 1989.
7. Malcolm AJ: Cemented and hydroxyapatite-coated hip implants: an autopsy retrieval study. In Morrey B, editor: Biological, material, and mechanical considerations of joint replacement, New York, 1993, Raven Press, pp 39–50.
8. Lee AJ, Ling RS, Gheduzzi S, et al: Factors affecting the mechanical and viscoelastic properties of acrylic bone cement. J Mater Sci Mater Med 13:723–733, 2002.
9. Shen G: Femoral stem fixation: an engineering interpretation of the long-term outcome of Charnley and Exeter stems. J Bone Joint Surg Br 80:754–756, 1998.
10. Huiskes R, Verdonschot N, Nivbrant B: Migration, stem shape, and surface finish in cemented total hip arthroplasty. Clin Orthop Relat Res 355:103–112, 1998.
11. Kärrholm J, Nivbrant B, Thanner J, et al: Radiostereometric evaluation of hip implant design and surface finish: micromotion of cemented femoral stems. Presented at the 67th Annual Meeting of the American Academy of Orthopaedic Surgeons, Orlando, March 15–19, 2000.
12. Scheerlinck T, Casteleyn PP: The design features of cemented femoral hip implants. J Bone Joint Surg Br 88:1409–1418, 2006.
13. Lachiewicz PF, Kelley SS, Soileau ES: Survival of polished compared with precoated roughened cemented femoral components: a prospective, randomized study. J Bone Joint Surg Am 90:1457–1463, 2008.
14. Australian Orthopaedic Association: National Joint Replacement Registry annual report, Adelaide, Australia, 2008, AOA.
15. Kärrholm J, Garellick G, Rogmark C, Herberts P: Swedish Hip Arthroplasty Register annual report 2007, Lund, Sweden, 2008, Swedish Hip Arthroplasty Register.
16. National Joint Registry for England and Wales: 5th annual report, Hempstead, United Kingdom, 2009, NJR.
17. Howie CR. In Callaghan JJ, Rosenberg AG, Rubash HE, editors: The adult hip, vol 2, Philadelphia, 2007, Lippincott, Williams and Wilkins, p 186.
18. Lee AJC: The time dependent properties of polymethylmethacrylate bone cement: the interaction of shape of femoral stems, surface finish and bone cement. In Learmonth ID, editor: Interfaces in total hip arthroplasty, New York, 1999, Springer, pp 11–19.
19. Crowninshield RD, Brand RA, Johnston RC, Milroy JC: The effect of femoral stem cross-sectional geometry on cement stresses in total hip reconstruction. Clin Orthop Relat Res 146:71–77, 1980.
20. Lee AJC, Thomson A: Torsional stability of a polished, collarless, tapered total replacement hip joint stem under vertical load: an in vitro investigation. Proc Inst Mech Eng H 225:77–85, 2011.
21. Carrington NC, Sierra RJ, Gie GA, et al: The Exeter Universal cemented femoral component at 15 to 17 years: an update on the first 325 hips. J Bone Joint Surg Br 91:730–737, 2009.
22. Ling RS, Charity J, Lee AJ, et al: The long-term results of the original Exeter polished cemented femoral component: a follow-up report. J Arthroplasty 24:511–517, 2009.
23. Wroblewski BM, Siney PD, Fleming PA: Charnley low-frictional torque arthroplasty: follow-up for 30 to 40 years. J Bone Joint Surg Br 91:447–450, 2009.
24. Duncan WW, Hubble MJ, Howell JR, et al: Revision of the cemented femoral stem using a cement-in-cement technique: a five- to 15-year review. J Bone Joint Surg Br 91:577–582, 2009.
25. Murray DW, Britton AR, Bulstrode CJ: Loss to follow-up matters. J Bone Joint Surg Br 79:254–257, 1997.
26. Murray DW, Carr AJ, Bulstrode C: Survival analysis of joint replacements. J Bone Joint Surg Br 75:697–704, 1993.
27. Lewthwaite SC, Squires B, Gie GA, et al: The Exeter Universal hip in patients 50 years or younger at 10-17 years' followup. Clin Orthop Relat Res 466:324–331, 2008.
28. Rockborn P, Olsson SS: Loosening and migration of Exeter THR. J Bone Joint Surg Br 76:507–511, 1994.
29. Weidenhielm LR, Mikhail WE, Nelissen RG, Bauer TW: Cemented collarless (Exeter-CPT) versus cementless collarless (PCA) femoral components: a 2- to 14-year follow-up evaluation. J Arthroplasty 10:592–597, 1995.
30. Chiu KH, Shen WY, Tsui HF, Chan KM: Experience with primary Exeter Total Hip arthroplasty in patients with small femurs: review at average follow-up period of 6 years. J Arthroplasty 12:267–272, 1997.
31. Fitzpatrick R, Shortall E, Sculpher M, et al: Primary total hip replacement surgery: a systematic review of outcomes and modelling of cost-effectiveness associated with different prostheses. Health Technol Assess 2:1–64, 1998.
32. Howie DW, Middleton RG, Costi K: Loosening of matt and polished cemented femoral stems. J Bone Joint Surg Br 80:573–576, 1998.
33. Middleton RG, Howie DW, Costi K, Sharpe P: Effects of design changes on cemented tapered femoral stem fixation. Clin Orthop Relat Res 355:47–56, 1998.
34. Sherfey JJ, McCalden RW: Mid-term results of Exeter vs Endurance cemented stems. J Arthroplasty 21:1118–1123, 2006.
35. Wroblewski BM, Siney PD, Fleming PA: Triple taper polished cemented stem in total hip arthroplasty: rationale for the design, surgical technique, and 7 years of clinical experience. J Arthroplasty 16(Suppl 3):37–41, 2001.
36. Franklin J, Robertsson O, Gestsson J, et al: Revision and complication rates in 654 Exeter Total Hip replacements, with a maximum follow-up of 20 years. BMC Musculoskelet Disord 4:6, 2003.
37. Howie DW, Costi K, McGee MA: Results of cemented collarless double taper femoral stems at primary THR. Presented at the 11th Meeting of the Combined Orthopaedic Associations—Science Art and Humanity in Orthopaedics, Sydney, Australia, 2004, Australian Orthopaedic Association.
38. McCombe P, Williams SA: A comparison of polyethylene wear rates between cemented and cementless cups: a prospective, randomised trial. J Bone Joint Surg Br 86:344–349, 2004.
39. Ek ET, Choong PF: Comparison between triple-tapered and double-tapered cemented femoral stems in total hip arthroplasty: a prospective study comparing the C-Stem versus the Exeter Universal early results after 5 years of clinical experience. J Arthroplasty 20:94–100, 2005.
40. Sundberg M, Besjakov J, Carlsson A, et al: Movement patterns of the C-stem femoral component: an RSA study of 33 primary total hip arthroplasties followed for two years. J Bone Joint Surg Br 87:1352–1356, 2005.

41. Field RE, Singh PJ, Latif AM, et al: Five-year prospective clinical and radiological results of a new cannulated cemented polished Tri-Taper femoral stem. J Bone Joint Surg Br 88:315–320, 2006.
42. Hook S, Moulder E, Yates PJ, et al: The Exeter Universal stem: a minimum ten-year review from an independent centre. J Bone Joint Surg Br 88:1584–1590, 2006.
43. McCombe P: Initial results of the Exeter Universal femoral component: a 7 year review. J Bone Joint Surg Br 81(Suppl 1):8, 1999.
44. Yates PJ, Quraishi NA, Kop A, et al: Fractures of modern high nitrogen stainless steel cemented stems: cause, mechanism, and avoidance in 14 cases. J Arthroplasty 23:188–196, 2008.
45. de Kam DC, Klarenbeek RL, Gardeniers JW, et al: The medium-term results of the cemented Exeter femoral component in patients under 40 years of age. J Bone Joint Surg Br 90:1417–1421, 2008.
46. Makela K, Eskelinen A, Pulkkinen P, et al: Cemented total hip replacement for primary osteoarthritis in patients aged 55 years or older: results of the 12 most common cemented implants followed for 25 years in the Finnish Arthroplasty Register. J Bone Joint Surg Br 90:1562–1569, 2008.
47. Miller D, Choksey A, Jones P, Perkins R: Medium to long term results of the Exeter bipolar hemiarthroplasty for femoral neck fractures in active, independent patients: 5-13 year follow-up. Hip Int 18:301–306, 2008.
48. Myers GJ, Morgan D, O'Dwyer K: Exeter-Ogee total hip replacement using the Hardinge approach; the ten to twelve year results. Hip Int 18:35–39, 2008.
49. Young L, Duckett S, Dunn A: The use of the cemented Exeter Universal femoral stem in a District General Hospital: a minimum ten-year follow-up. J Bone Joint Surg Br 91:170–175, 2009.
50. Burston BJ, Yates PJ, Hook S, et al: Cemented polished tapered stems in patients less than 50 years of age: a minimum 10-year follow-up. J Arthroplasty 25:692–699, 2010.
51. Malchau H, Herberts P, Eisler T, et al: The Swedish Total Hip Replacement Register. J Bone Joint Surg Am 84(Suppl):22–20, 2002.
52. Malchau H, Herberts P, Ahnfelt L: Prognosis of total hip replacement in Sweden: follow-up of 92,675 operations performed 1978-1990. Acta Orthop Scand 64:497–506, 1993.
53. Iwase T, Wingstrand I, Persson BM, et al: The ScanHip total hip arthroplasty: radiographic assessment of 72 hips after 10 years. Acta Orthop Scand 73:54–59, 2002.
54. Malchau H, Herberts P, Soderman P, Oden A: Prognosis of total hip replacements: update and validation of results from the Swedish National Hip Arthroplasty Registry 1979-1998, 2000. Presented at the 67th Annual Meeting of the American Academy of Orthopaedic Surgeons, Orlando, FL, March 15-19, 2000.
55. Furnes O, Havelin LI, Espehaug B: Femoral components: cemented stems for everybody? In Breusch SJ, Malchau H, editors: The well-cemented total hip arthroplasty, Heidelberg, Germany, 2005, Springer Verlag, pp 216–220.
56. Makela KT, Eskelinen A, Pulkkinen P, et al: Total hip arthroplasty for primary osteoarthritis in patients fifty-five years of age or older: an analysis of the Finnish arthroplasty registry. J Bone Joint Surg Am 90:2160–2170, 2008.
57. Halawa M, Lee AJ, Ling RS, Vangala SS: The shear strength of trabecular bone from the femur, and some factors affecting the shear strength of the cement-bone interface. Arch Orthop Trauma Surg 92:19–30, 1978.
58. Majkowski RS, Bannister GC, Miles AW: The effect of bleeding on the cement-bone interface: an experimental study. Clin Orthop Relat Res 299:293–297, 1994.
59. Heyse-Moore GH, Ling RSM: Current cement techniques. In Marti RK, editor: Progress in cemented total hip surgery and revision, Amsterdam, 1983, Excerpta Medica, pp 71–86.
60. Bannister GC, Young SK, Baker AS, et al: Control of bleeding in cemented arthroplasty. J Bone Joint Surg Br 72:444–446, 1990.
61. Malchau H, Herberts P, Garellick G, et al: Prognosis of total hip replacement: update of results and risk-ratio analysis. Presented at the 69th Annual Meeting of the American Academy of Orthopaedic Surgeons, Dallas, February 13–17, 2002.
62. Ling RS, Lee AJ: Porosity reduction in acrylic cement is clinically irrelevant. Clin Orthop Relat Res 355:249–253, 1998.
63. Dall DM, Miles AW, Juby G: Accelerated polymerization of acrylic bone cement using preheated implants. Clin Orthop Relat Res 211:148–150, 1986.
64. Gruen TA, McNeice GM, Amstutz HC: "Modes of failure" of cemented stem-type femoral components: a radiographic analysis of loosening. Clin Orthop Relat Res 141:17–27, 1979.
65. Nunley RM, Lachiewicz PF: Mortality after total hip and knee arthroplasty in a medium-volume university practice. J Arthroplasty 18:278–285, 2003.
66. Sharrock NE, Cazan MG, Hargett MJ, et al: Changes in mortality after total hip and knee arthroplasty over a ten-year period. Anesth Analg 80:242–248, 1995.
67. Barrett J, Losina E, Baron JA, et al: Survival following total hip replacement. J Bone Joint Surg Am 87:1965–1971, 2005.
68. Ling RSM: Complications of total hip replacement, Edinburgh, 1984, Churchill Livingstone.
69. Dearborn JT, Harris WH: Postoperative mortality after total hip arthroplasty: an analysis of deaths after two thousand seven hundred and thirty-six procedures. J Bone Joint Surg Am 80:1291–1294, 1998.
70. Gelinas JJ, Cherry R, MacDonald SJ: Fat embolism syndrome after cementless total hip arthroplasty. J Arthroplasty 15:809–813, 2000.
71. Arroyo JS, Garvin KL, McGuire MH: Fatal marrow embolization following a porous-coated bipolar hip endoprosthesis. J Arthroplasty 9:449–452, 1994.
72. Parvizi J, Holiday AD, Ereth MH, Lewallen DG: The Frank Stinchfield Award. Sudden death during primary hip arthroplasty. Clin Orthop Relat Res 369:39–48, 1999.
73. Kim YH, Oh SW, Kim JS: Prevalence of fat embolism following bilateral simultaneous and unilateral total hip arthroplasty performed with or without cement: a prospective, randomized clinical study. J Bone Joint Surg Am 84:1372–1379, 2002.
74. Byrick RJ, Bell RS, Kay JC, et al: High-volume, high-pressure pulsatile lavage during cemented arthroplasty. J Bone Joint Surg Am 71:1331–1336, 1989.
75. Sierra RJ, Timperley JA, Gie GA: Contemporary cementing technique and mortality during and after Exeter Total Hip arthroplasty. J Arthroplasty 24:325–332, 2008.
76. Zhan C, Kaczmarek R, Loyo-Berrios N, et al: Incidence and short-term outcomes of primary and revision hip replacement in the United States. J Bone Joint Surg Am 89:526–533, 2007.
77. Sharkey PF, Shastri S, Teloken MA, et al: Relationship between surgical volume and early outcomes of total hip arthroplasty: do results continue to get better? J Arthroplasty 19:694–699, 2004.
78. Doro C, Dimick J, Wainess R, et al: Hospital volume and inpatient mortality outcomes of total hip arthroplasty in the United States. J Arthroplasty 21(6 Suppl 2):10–16, 2006.
79. Pitto RP, Koessler M, Draenert K: The John Charnley Award. Prophylaxis of fat and bone marrow embolism in cemented total hip arthroplasty. Clin Orthop Relat Res 355:23–34, 1998.
80. Christie J, Robinson CM, Singer B, Ray DC: Medullary lavage reduces embolic phenomena and cardiopulmonary changes during cemented hemiarthroplasty. J Bone Joint Surg Br 77:456–459, 1995.
81. Breusch SJ, Reitzel T, Schneider U, et al: [Cemented hip prosthesis implantation—decreasing the rate of fat embolism with pulsed pressure lavage]. Orthopade 29:578–586, 2000.
82. Pitto RP, Koessler M, Kuehle JW: Comparison of fixation of the femoral component without cement and fixation with use of a bone-vacuum cementing technique for the prevention of fat embolism during total hip arthroplasty: a prospective, randomized clinical trial. J Bone Joint Surg Am 81:831–843, 1999.
83. Clarius M, Heisel C, Breusch SJ: Pulmonary embolism in cemented total hip arthroplasty. In Breusch SJ, Malchau H, editors: The well-cemented total hip arthroplasty, Heidelberg, Germany, 2005, Springer Verlag, pp 320–331.
84. Heisel C, Norman T, Rupp R, et al: In vitro performance of intramedullary cement restrictors in total hip arthroplasty. J Biomech 36:835–843, 2003.
85. McCaskie AW, Barnes MR, Lin E, et al: Cement pressurisation during hip replacement. J Bone Joint Surg Br 79:379–384, 1997.

CHAPTER 68

Uncemented Extensively Porous-Coated Femoral Components

C. Anderson Engh, Jr., Christi J. Sychterz Terefenko, and Charles A. Engh, Sr.

KEY POINTS

- 98% stem survivorship at 20 years
- The implant can be used for all diagnoses and in all qualities of bone.
- Defining characteristics of the stem include its non-tapered cylindrical distal geometry with extensive porous coating.
- The surgical technique is a reamed technique.
- The goal of the surgical technique is to obtain 5 cm of diaphyseal scratch fit.

INTRODUCTION

In response to early failures of some cemented femoral components, porous-coated femoral stem technology was developed in the 1970s. The concept behind the design was that live bone in contact with a three-dimensional metal implant surface would grow into and interdigitate with the porous surface to provide a means of stable implant fixation[1-3] (Fig. 68-1).

In 1983, the Food and Drug Administration approved the first porous-coated femoral implant for use without cement. This implant, the anatomic medullary locking stem (AML, DePuy, Warsaw, Ind), was characterized by a circumferentially porous-coated, straight, nontapered distal cylindrical rod coupled with a circumferentially porous-coated proximal metaphyseal triangular shape. Current studies of the AML have documented 98% femoral component survivorship at 20 years.[4] Excellent results with this stem have been reported in scenarios historically not deemed appropriate for porous-coated fixation, as in patients with avascular necrosis or rheumatoid arthritis, and in the elderly with osteoporosis.[5-7]

Today, extensively porous-coated femoral implants are available from many manufacturers. Hallmarks of these implants include the presence of a three-dimensional beaded circumferential porous coating on two thirds or more of the femoral stem. Because application of the porous surface requires reheating, which weakens the metal substrate, these stems are typically made of cobalt-chrome rather than titanium. The shape of the typical extensively porous-coated stem is a cylinder distally for fixation in the femoral diaphysis, and a triangle proximally to fit the patient's femoral metaphysis. Diaphyseal diameters range from 10.5 mm to 22.5 mm, usually in 1- to 1.5-mm increments. Each diaphyseal diameter is accompanied by two to three metaphyseal sizes, which allow for different femoral offsets (Fig. 68-2).

Surgical implantation of an extensively porous-coated stem is a reamed technique wherein the femur is machined to fit the implant. The cylindrical parallel sides of the implant contact the diaphyseal femoral cortex. Initial fixation is attained with a "scratch fit" of the porous coating, which contacts at least 5 cm of diaphyseal bone. The initial rigid fixation obtained with this technique allows subsequent ingrowth of bone or osseointegration of the stem. This osseointegration accounts for the extremely durable implant fixation.

Through analyses of well-functioning implants retrieved postmortem,[8-15] extensively porous-coated femoral implants have been studied more thoroughly than many other designs of cementless stems. The extent and quality of bone ingrowth, the amount of implant micromotion, and the bone remodeling process have been well documented through such studies[8-15] and serve to complement an ever growing clinical experience.[4,16-20] Clinical experience has further addressed design concerns such as thigh pain and periprosthetic bone loss secondary to stress shielding.[21,22] Both thigh pain and stress shielding are thought to result from the mismatch of modulus between the host bone and the much stiffer cobalt-chrome stem. To date, however, the proximal bone loss that occurs to some extent with all uncemented implant systems has not demonstrated negative long-term clinical consequences.[22] Clinical experience has not shown practical complications such as failure of fixation, implant fracture, or femoral fracture from bone remodeling.

INDICATIONS AND CONTRAINDICATIONS

Indications, contraindications, and alternative treatment options for the use of extensively porous-coated femoral components are the same as they are for any other form of hip arthroplasty. The patient should be skeletally mature with clinical and radiographic evidence of hip joint deterioration. The patient should have had an adequate trial of nonoperative care and should not have active infection at the surgical site. Patients with a femoral diaphysis smaller than 10.5 mm are not candidates for this type of implant. For those with a femoral diaphysis larger than 22.5 mm, although

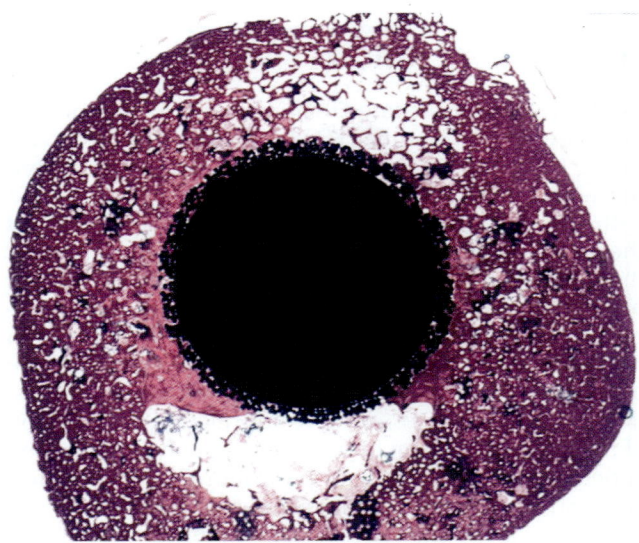

Figure 68-1. Histologic slide showing cross-section of a femoral porous-coated total hip prosthesis with bone ingrowth into the beaded implant surface.

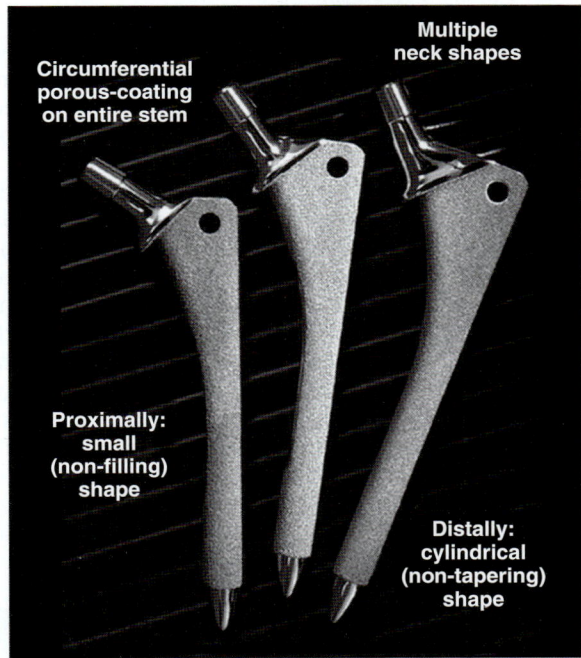

Figure 68-2. The shape of the typical extensively porous-coated stem is a cylinder distally for fixation in the femoral diaphysis, and a triangle proximally to fit the patient's femoral metaphysis. Pictured here are extensively porous-coated anatomic medullary locking (AML) femoral components.

standard implant sizes are not available, custom implants can be used. Femoral angular and rotational deformities can be addressed with the use of a femoral osteotomy.

PREOPERATIVE PLANNING

Surgical planning of a total hip replacement with an extensively porous-coated femoral component is similar

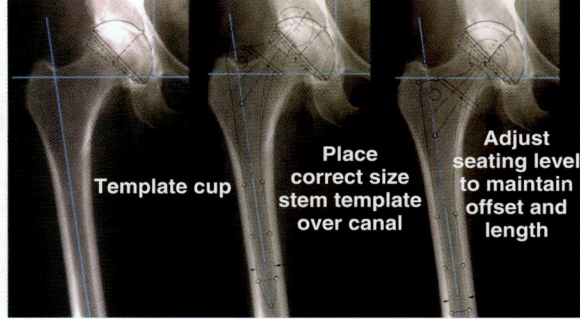

Figure 68-3. Radiographs demonstrating the templating process. First, the acetabular template is placed on the anteroposterior pelvic film to determine the rotational center of the hip joint. Next, a femoral implant template that appears to contact the medial and lateral diaphyseal bone for a length of 5 cm is chosen. Finally, the template is raised and lowered along the femoral axis until the center of the implant coincides with the previously determined acetabular center.

to planning for other implants. A preoperative physical examination is needed to confirm adequate abductor strength and must include an assessment of leg length. Radiographic evaluation should include a low anteroposterior (AP) pelvic film and a true lateral of the proximal one half of the femur. The AP pelvic film should be centered at or below the level of the lesser trochanter and should include approximately 2 cm of pelvic bone above the acetabulum, as well as the femoral diaphysis distally. For this radiograph, the patient ideally internally rotates the femur approximately 15 degrees, so that the femur is imaged in the same plane in which the implant template is created. Signs of a properly rotated femur include overlapping of the anterior and posterior portions of the greater trochanter and a reduced lesser trochanteric profile. With the femur properly rotated, the patient's offset and the shape of the femoral metaphysis are most accurately displayed for templating. Although offset and metaphyseal dimensions are visible on a unilateral AP femoral view, it is not possible to determine the radiographic hip length relative to the patient's contralateral side. Before surgical planning with templates is begun, the surgeon must reconcile any differences that exist between the leg length determined by physical examination and the length determined with an AP pelvic radiograph. With those two measurements, the surgeon can determine the targeted surgical leg length correction and can begin the templating process.

The templating process begins by placing the acetabular template on the AP pelvic film to determine the rotational center of the hip joint (Fig. 68-3). Attention then is turned to the femur. The femoral diaphysis dictates stem diameter and stem alignment. A template that appears to contact the medial and lateral diaphyseal bone for a length of 5 cm is chosen (see Fig. 68-3). The template is raised and lowered along the femoral axis until the center of the implant coincides with the previously determined acetabular center. If the target leg length correction includes lengthening of the leg, then the femoral implant center will sit above the acetabular center by the planned correction amount. A metaphyseal size is chosen to re-create or slightly increase femoral offset. On the radiograph, relative horizontal locations between the femoral head and the acetabular center represent femoral offset.

With the femoral template positioned, the distance from the tip of the greater trochanter to the lateral aspect of the femoral template and the distance from the lesser trochanter to the calcar aspect of the femoral template are recorded, so that these measurements can be checked and duplicated at surgery (Fig. 68-4). Additionally, the extent to which the greater trochanter overhangs the axis of the femur is noted. This is helpful in determining how lateral the surgeon needs to be to avoid varus alignment of the stem. Last, with a straight 6-inch-long template on the lateral radiograph, the surgeon must confirm that the femoral component will not create a notch in the distal anterior femoral cortex.

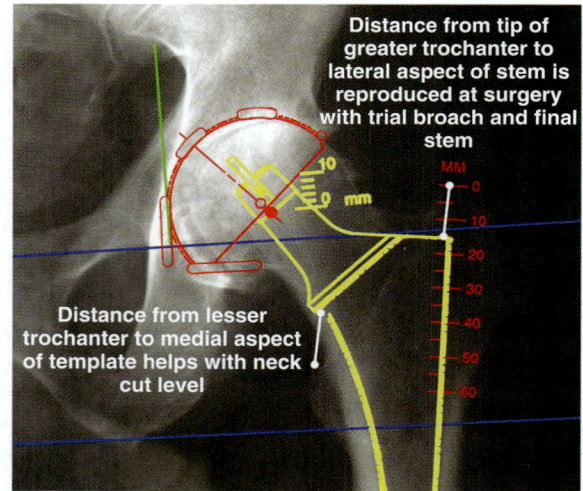

Figure 68-4. With the femoral template positioned correctly, radiographic measurements are recorded for later use during surgery.

SURGICAL TECHNIQUE

Extensively porous-coated femoral stems are well suited for posterior and modified Hardinge surgical approaches to the hip joint. Because the stem is straight, oriented to the diaphysis, and 6 inches long, it is not easily used with anterior approaches that emphasize protection of the gluteus medius. After dislocation of the hip joint, the level of the femoral neck osteotomy is determined by the templating process. When visible, the lesser trochanter is a good reference, but the exact distance from the lesser trochanter can be difficult to measure because of its rounded contours. With today's smaller incisions, the greater trochanter, or more specifically, the junction of the anterior portion of the greater trochanter and the superior femoral neck, can be a more accurate reference. Some patients with a valgus neck shaft angle will have a neck cut that is high and simply transects the femoral neck (Fig. 68-5). Other patients with some degree of coxa vara will have a neck cut that requires an osteotomy below the superior aspect of the femoral neck and likely will require a second more vertical cut to complete the full osteotomy (see Fig. 68-5). It is acceptable to be conservative with a high femoral neck cut and leave bone to be milled away at a later time. However, a high femoral neck cut that leaves too much femoral neck may make acetabular exposure more difficult.

Next, a chisel or a high-speed bur is used to create the pilot hole at the piriformis fossa. For the pilot hole, most if not all of any remaining posterior and lateral femoral neck typically is removed. An initial 8-mm reamer finds the femoral canal and is passed by hand. As the femoral diaphysis guides the initial reamer, the surgeon notes whether the location of the pilot hole needs to be changed. At all times, the surgeon must ensure that reamers are directed by the distal endosteal cortices, and that the direction of reaming is not influenced by an overhanging greater trochanter or a portion of the femoral neck. Reaming is continued in 0.5-mm increments until the surgeon encounters distal cutting

Figure 68-5. Radiograph demonstrating the level of femoral neck resection for different femoral geometries. Patients with a valgus neck shaft angle will have a neck cut that is high and simply transects the femoral neck. Patients with some degree of coxa vara will have a neck cut that requires an osteotomy below the superior aspect of the femoral neck and will likely require a second more vertical cut to complete the full osteotomy.

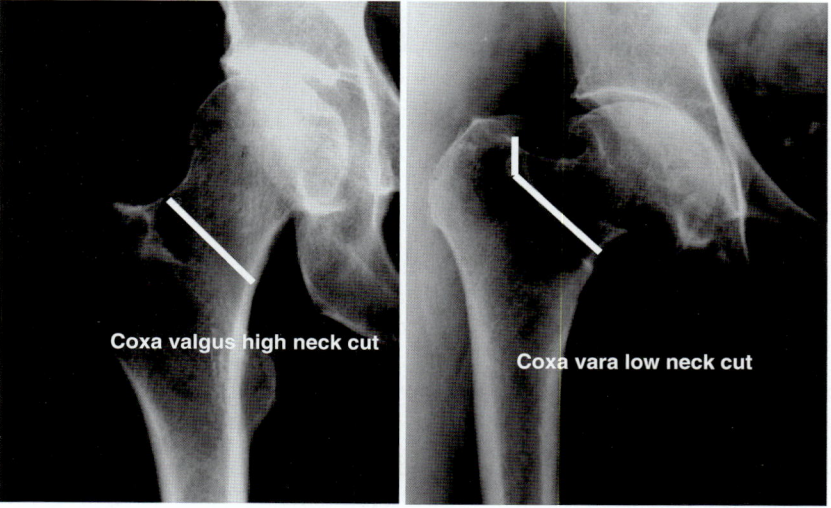

resistance over at least 5 cm of the femoral isthmus. Typically, the final reamer diameter will be 0.5 mm smaller than the size of the actual stem to be implanted to obtain a tight "scratch fit" and ensure adequate stem-femur contact. Markings on the reamer that correspond to the level of the femoral calcar or the tip of the greater trochanter help the surgeon determine the depth of reaming. When combined with the templated positions of the stem, these reamer marks are helpful for preventing distal over-reaming, which could weaken the anterior cortex by endosteal notching. These reamer markings are also helpful for determining the length of scratch fit that will be attained.

Proponents of extensively porous-coated stems agree that diaphyseal fixation requires precise cylindrical reaming. However, an equally precise proximal metaphyseal preparation is also important. The last step in femoral preparation is preparing the proximal femur to accept the proximal triangular geometry of the stem. This can be done by using broaches or a milling-type reamer. When possible, a larger proximal triangle should be used to increase femoral offset, thus enhancing rotational stability and increasing the amount of porous surface available for bone ingrowth. Precise proximal preparation will prevent gaps between the bone and the implant, protecting against the ingress of joint fluid, which could result in a pathway for late-onset femoral osteolysis.

When the broach can be inserted to the templated location and the neck is flush with the broach, the hip is reduced with the use of a trial neck segment. Hip joint stability, leg length, and femoral offset are then checked. If the leg is too long, the broach is lowered in the femur with care not to fracture the proximal femur. Occasionally, a milling device or a high-speed bur is needed to remove proximal cortical bone, allowing the stem to be lowered further. If leg length is good but additional femoral offset is required for hip stability, there are two options. First, if the femoral metaphysis can accommodate it, offset can be increased without lowering the stem by simply using a larger proximal triangular shape. Alternatively, the stem can be lowered and combined with the use of a longer ball, resulting in more offset without lengthening the leg. With currently available larger-diameter heads, the latter option is viable because femoral head skirts that limit range of motion are not as common with larger heads as they were with smaller head sizes. A final technique tip is to perform the trial reduction with a ball of mid length. This allows the use of a ball of shorter or longer length once the femoral implant is inserted.

The stem is inserted by hand until cortical contact requires the use of a hammer. If the stem is 10 cm or more proud of its final seating level, if it does not advance easily at first, or if the patient has strong bone, the surgeon can decide to further ream the femoral canal to the diameter of the implant rather than keeping it under-reamed by 0.5 mm. This decision, like that of how hard to hit the stem without fracturing the femur, is a matter of experience. As a guideline, the initial femoral impaction blows should seat the stem about 5 mm at a time. As the stem advances, the same hammer blows will move the stem only 0.5 to 1.0 mm. This amount of advancement over the final 2 cm of seating is appropriate. Stems being implanted into patients with hard bone may advance only every other hammer blow. Often the force of each hammer blow will have to be increased slightly for the final 5 mm of femoral seating. The force required to implant an extensively porous-coated femoral component is considerably greater than that needed for a tapered stem. A tapered stem inserted with the same force will likely split the proximal femur. The parallel sides and cylindrical shape of an extensively porous-coated stem make this stem less prone to insertional femoral fracture than a triangular or wedge-shaped stem.

VARIATIONS AND UNUSUAL SITUATIONS

Extensively porous-coated femoral components can be used in patients who require some form of femoral osteotomy at the time of arthroplasty, because the stem bypasses the osteotomy and is fixed to the diaphysis—not to the proximal bone weakened by the osteotomy. Cases of high-riding developmental dysplasia that need shortening, angular, or rotational osteotomy are well suited to this implant design (Fig. 68-6). Distal rotational control is excellent with the rough cylindrical scratch fit, and the proximal fragment of the osteotomy is well controlled by the triangular metaphyseal segment of the implant. Although a step-cut osteotomy can be used, it is not required. This technique can also be used in patients who have a deformity secondary to a previous varus or valgus reconstructive osteotomy. Distal fixation with an extensively porous-coated femoral component is also helpful in cases that require a greater trochanteric osteotomy. A trochanteric osteotomy weakens the proximal femur and might prohibit the use of a proximally coated or wedge-shaped stem. An example would be conversion of a hip fusion to a total hip in which a greater trochanteric osteotomy facilitates exposure of the hip joint. The distal fixation bypasses the osteotomy that was required for exposure.

POSTOPERATIVE CARE

Postoperative care of patients implanted with extensively porous-coated femoral components is similar to that of patients with other types of total hip arthroplasty. Historically, weight bearing has been limited for a 6-week period. Current protocols, however, allow immediate weight bearing as tolerated.[23] Although full weight bearing may be acceptable for most patients, in some, a 3- to 6-week period of 50% or less weight bearing is beneficial. The decision to limit weight bearing typically is based on the length of scratch fit, the ease of stem insertion, and the appearance of the postoperative radiograph. Those patients with a good scratch fit intraoperatively and a normal x-ray postoperatively are routinely allowed to bear weight as tolerated. However,

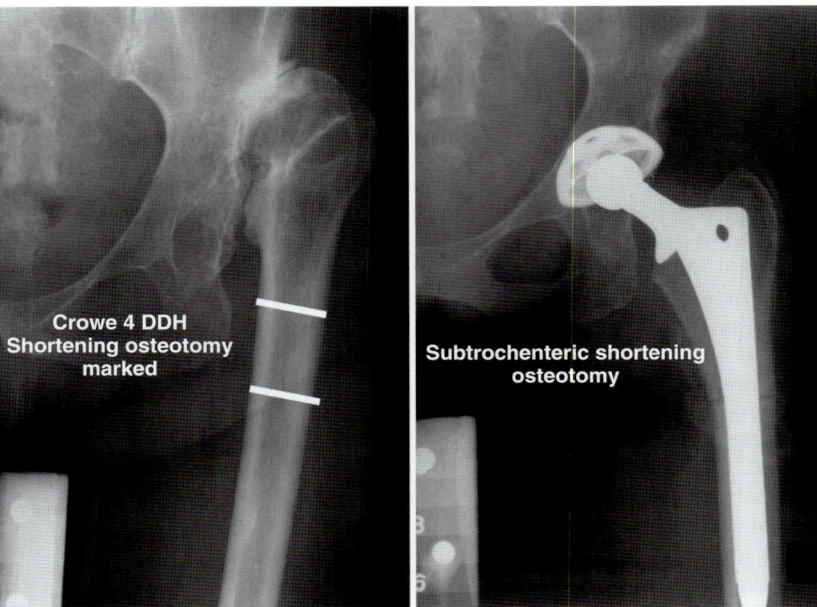

Figure 68-6. Extensively porous-coated femoral components can be used in patients who require some form of femoral osteotomy at the time of arthroplasty, because the stem bypasses the osteotomy and is fixed to the diaphysis—not to the proximal bone weakened by the osteotomy. Cases of high-riding developmental dysplasia that need shortening, angular, or rotational osteotomy are particularly well suited to this implant design.

patients in whom stems are inserted easily or are undersized on the postoperative radiograph, or in whom a diaphyseal hairline fracture exists, should limit weight bearing for 3 to 6 weeks postoperatively.

RESULTS

Extensively porous-coated femoral components have been studied more extensively than perhaps any other type of cementless implant. Although the 20-year survivorship data alone present a compelling statistic, these data have only recently become available. Early studies were performed on radiographs and on specimens retrieved postmortem. Postmortem analysis of retrieved extensively porous-coated stems has (1) confirmed the occurrence of bone ingrowth into the stem's surface, (2) described the resulting mechanical stability, (3) evaluated the effect of bone ingrowth on femoral remodeling, and (4) confirmed that circumferential ingrowth seals the effective joint space.[9-15,24] These studies were followed by clinical publications that addressed concerns such as stress shielding and thigh pain, as well as by studies that supported the use of extensively porous-coated stems in patients with altered bone physiology.[5-7,21,22,28,29] This section summarizes this body of work.

The first autopsy study on extensively coated stems confirmed the occurrence of bone ingrowth into the stem's surface.[9] It revealed that, on average, bone grew into 35% of the available porous implant surface (range, 25% to 43%). Moreover, it showed that the pattern of ingrowth was predictable, with the most consistent growth occurring at the termination of the porous coating.[9] Following confirmation of osseointegration, the stability of ingrown stems was tested. Mechanical testing of autopsy-retrieved specimens demonstrated that the relative motion between bone and implant was

less than 20 μm and was completely elastic.[10] Subsequent research documented the effect of this ingrowth on how the femur was remodeled. Dual-emission x-ray absorptiometry (DEXA) and videodensitometric analysis revealed that implantation of an extensively porous-coated stem resulted in an average loss of 23% of the bone mineral content of the femur (range, 5% to 47%) post implantation.[11-14] This bone loss occurred on a gradient and typically was greatest adjacent to the proximal one third of the implant. Moreover, studies showed that the magnitude of the loss was highly correlated with the patient's initial quality of bone.[14,15] Patients with low bone mineral content preoperatively (osteopenia or osteoporosis) had more pronounced proximal bone loss after arthroplasty than those with high initial bone mineral content (Fig. 68-7). Bone loss secondary to implantation of an extensively porous-coated stem was not found to be correlated with stem size, patient weight, duration of implantation, or patient age.[14,15]

Specimens retrieved postmortem were also used to examine the effect of circumferential porous coating on the migration of wear debris adjacent to uncemented femoral components.[24] As has been previously documented, access of wear particles to the endosteum of the femur can lead to osteolysis, which can compromise implant stability and femoral structural integrity. One study analyzed five femoral specimens with bone-ingrown and fibrous-encapsulated femoral implants retrieved at autopsy after a mean 95 months in situ (range, 53 to 132 months).[24] Histologic examination of the bone revealed small areas of granulation tissue and polyethylene particles at the level of the lesser trochanter in two cases but no evidence of polyethylene particles or granuloma at the mid or distal portion of any implant. These findings implied that circumferential porous coating of cementless femoral components could prevent distal migration of polyethylene wear

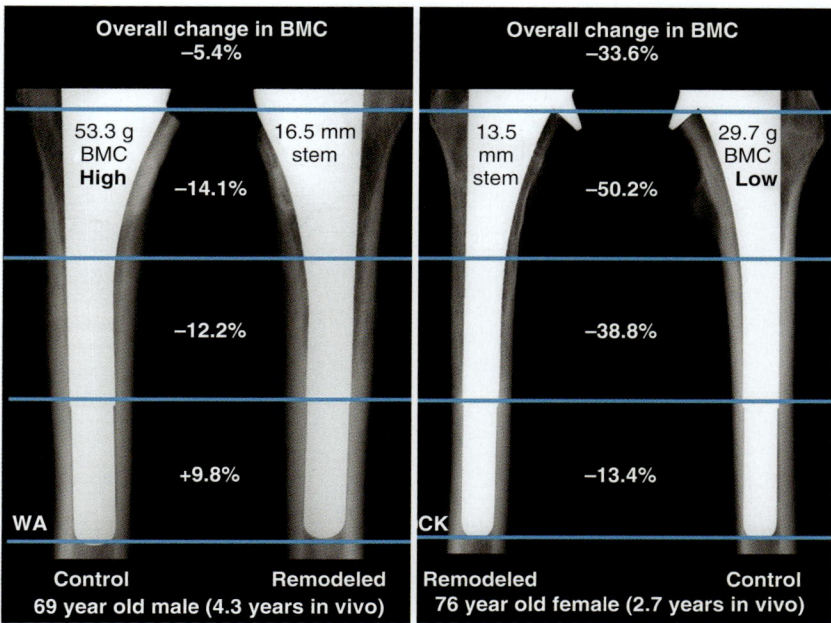

Figure 68-7. Radiographs demonstrating the overall change in bone mineral content (BMC) for two patients following total hip arthroplasty (THA). Typically, a gradient of bone loss follows hip arthroplasty, with the greatest loss occurring proximally and the least occurring distally. Further, the amount of overall bone loss has been found to correlate with the patient's preoperative bone mineral content. Patients with high preoperative BMC *(left)* lose less bone after THA than those with low preoperative BMC *(right)*.

debris along the bone-implant interface in both bone-ingrown and fibrous-encapsulated femoral implants.

Because postmortem retrieval specimens are difficult to obtain, early clinical studies of extensively porous-coated stems focused on defining the radiographic appearance of bone-ingrown, fibrous-stable, and loose cementless femoral components. In a study of 97 hips implanted with AML stems and 51 hips implanted with other cementless stems, the authors devised a means of grading fixation that could be applied to any cementless femoral implant.[17] Implant stability was assessed through review of serial radiographs noting the presence or absence of the following indicators: spot welds, implant migration, radiolucent lines, calcar modeling, femoral distal pedestal formation, and/or particle shedding. Signs that a stem was well fixed by bone ingrowth included the presence of spot welds to endosteal bone at the termination of the porous coating, calcar atrophy, and the absence of migration (Fig. 68-8). In contrast, signs of failed ingrowth included the presence of extensive radiolucent lines adjacent to the porous coating, stem migration, and the presence of a distal pedestal (see Fig. 68-8).

With direct confirmation of osseointegration through autopsy analysis and a clear radiographic definition of an ingrown stem, it became easier for clinical researchers to document the survivorship of extensively porous-coated stems.[4,16,18-20] Although most publications referenced herein originate from the institute that developed extensively porous-coated stems, other centers have duplicated these clinical results, and some have similarly confirmed better than 95% survivorship of porous-coated stems.[25-27] Studies have also documented high porous-coated stem survivorship in patients with altered bone quality. One study of 203 patients who were 65 years or older at the time of hip replacement surgery reported 97% femoral survivorship at 12 years

post arthroplasty.[7] Another study of 64 patients with rheumatoid arthritis implanted with extensively porous-coated stems demonstrated 98% femoral stem survivorship at 10 years.[6] Even a study of 45 young patients (mean age at surgery, 31 years) with avascular necrosis thought to have altered femoral physiology reported no failures at a mean of 9 years' follow-up.[5]

Despite excellent femoral survivorship spanning 20 years and multiple diagnoses, concerns remained about stress shielding and thigh pain. To address concerns about bone loss secondary to stress shielding, clinical and radiographic results of 48 total hip arthroplasties (THAs) in patients with easily visible proximal bone loss were compared with results from 160 THAs without proximal bone loss.[22] At a mean 14-year follow-up, the study showed that patients with radiographically evident proximal bone loss secondary to stress shielding were no more likely to be revised, to have particle-induced osteolysis, or to have thigh pain than patients without proximal bone loss. Similarly, although thigh pain has been reported in 8% to 14% of patients implanted with extensively porous-coated stems,[1,16,18,28] it rarely limits a patient's activity or satisfaction with the hip replacement.[21,28,29] McAuley and associates, while addressing concerns about extensively porous-coated stems, reported a 12% incidence of thigh pain, but noted that the pain limited activity in only 3% of patients.[28] Likewise, a study of 1415 extensively porous-coated femoral components assessed outcomes as a function of stem diameter.[21] Activity-limiting thigh pain was present in 3.6% of patients with the smallest-diameter stems and in 2.5% of patients with the largest-diameter stems (range, 18 to 21 mm). The study concluded that patients with large-diameter extensively porous-coated femoral components were no more likely to be revised, to loosen, or to have thigh- or activity-limiting pain than those with smaller-diameter stems.

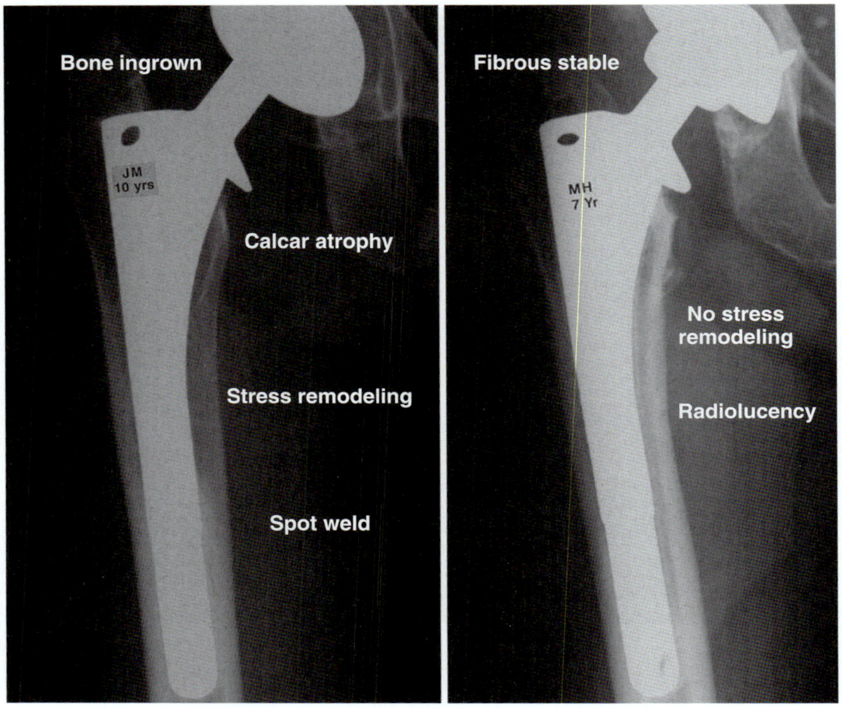

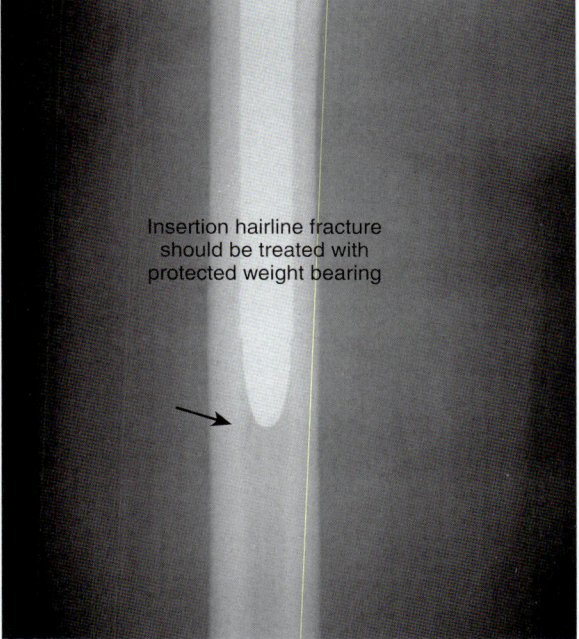

Figure 68-8. Examples of bone-ingrown and fibrous-stable stems. Signs that a stem is well fixed by bone ingrowth include the presence of spot welds to endosteal bone at the termination of the porous coating, calcar atrophy, and the absence of migration. Signs of failed ingrowth include the presence of extensive radiolucent lines adjacent to the porous coating, stem migration, and the presence of a distal pedestal.

COMPLICATIONS

Insertion of extensively porous-coated stems, like other press-fit cementless stems, can be associated with femoral fractures that must be addressed. In choosing a stem size, surgeons must balance between undersizing the stem, which can result in a loose prosthesis, and oversizing the stem to obtain more rigid fixation, which can result in an insertional femoral fracture.

A study in 1989 reviewed the type and treatment of femoral fractures that occurred with insertion of an extensively porous-coated stem.[30] In 1318 hip arthroplasties performed between 1977 and 1986, 39 insertional fractures (3%) were reported.[30] The study found that fractures were more common in women, and that their occurrence decreased over time as surgical technique and instruments were refined. Only half of the fractures were diagnosed intraoperatively. Proximal fractures were less common than distal fractures and were more likely to be diagnosed intraoperatively. When an insertional fracture was diagnosed intraoperatively, the stability of the implant was tested with additional impaction and torque testing consisting of reduction and dislocation of the hip and a thorough examination with range of motion. With a stable implant, incomplete proximal fractures were treated simply with protective weight bearing, and displaced proximal fractures were treated with cerclage wires. Proximal fractures with a resultant unstable stem were treated with a longer and slightly larger-diameter extensively porous-coated stem to ensure secure distal fixation.

The most common type of distal fracture, a nondisplaced cortical fissure, was typically discovered on postoperative radiographs, was visible only on a single

Figure 68-9. The most common type of distal fracture, a nondisplaced cortical fissure, is typically discovered on postoperative radiographs.

view, and did not involve the posterior femoral cortex (Fig. 68-9). Surgeons should suspect this type of fracture intraoperatively if the stem that advanced 0.5 mm to 1 mm with each impaction suddenly advances 2 mm or more. It can be treated with protective weight bearing without compromising long-term fixation. Displaced distal fractures are treated with open reduction and internal fixation using a cable screw plate, while retaining the femoral component if the stem is stable. If the fracture is displaced and the stem is unstable, the fracture should be bypassed with a longer, extensively porous-coated stem.

Occasionally, extensively porous-coated stems will need to be removed for pain, stem breakage, or infection. The technique for removal was described in 1992.[31] Emphasis was placed on obtaining serial radiographs to determine whether the stem to be removed was stable or loose. Loose stems that demonstrate migration are easily removed. Stable stems are removed by sectioning the stem between the proximal triangular portion and the distal cylindrical portion with a metal cutting bur through a cortical window or by performing an extended trochanteric slide osteotomy (Fig. 68-10). If an extended trochanteric slide osteotomy is not used, the interface between implant and bone in the proximal metaphysis is divided with thin osteotomes. Because proximal medial ingrowth is common with this implant design, it is necessary to remove the collar of the implant with a high-speed bur to gain access to this area. This difficulty can be overcome with the extended trochanteric osteotomy and the use of a gigli saw to separate the medial bone-implant interface. The cylindrical distal portion of the stem is removed using trephines designed to match the implant diameter. The trephines must be irrigated frequently to prevent heat necrosis of the bone. In addition, the trephines become dull with use, and several trephines of the same diameter are typically necessary for a single case. In cases in which a new stem will be inserted, surgeons should consider bypassing the trephined area to avoid fractures resulting from femoral notching or heat necrosis that may have occurred during removal of the stem.

CURRENT CONTROVERSIES AND FUTURE CONSIDERATIONS

- After 20 years of clinical use,
  - Will proximal bone resorption contribute to stem or trochanteric fracture?
  - Will porous coating delaminate, leading to loosening?
- How often do proximally coated stems become distally fixed?
  - When they do, will they cause thigh pain or trochanteric fracture?
  - How difficult is it to remove a tapered distally fixed stem?

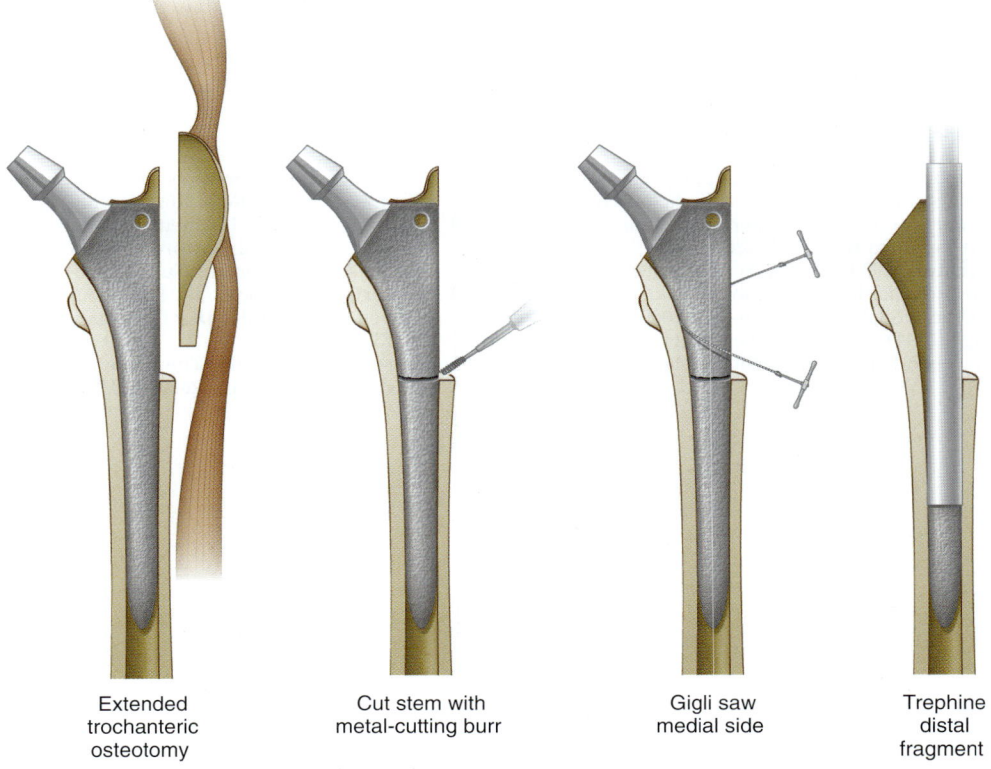

Extended	Cut stem with	Gigli saw	Trephine
trochanteric	metal-cutting burr	medial side	distal
osteotomy			fragment

Figure 68-10. Removal of a bone-ingrown stem is a multistep process. First, a cortical window or an extended trochanteric slide osteotomy is created. Next, the stem is sectioned with a metal cutting bur between the proximal triangle and the distal cylindrical portion of the stem. Because proximal medial ingrowth is common with this implant design, it is necessary to remove the collar of the implant with a high-speed bur to gain access to this area. A gigli saw can be used to separate the medial bone-implant interface. Finally, the cylindrical distal portion of the stem is removed using trephines designed to match the implant diameter.

REFERENCES

1. Engh CA, Bobyn JD, Glassman AH: Porous-coated hip replacement: the factors governing bone ingrowth, stress shielding, and clinical results. J Bone Joint Surg Br 69:45–55, 1987.
2. Bobyn JD, Pilliar RM, Cameron HU, et al: The optimum pore size for the fixation of porous-surfaced metal implants by the ingrowth of bone. Clin Orthop Relat Res 150:263–269, 1980.
3. Collier JP, Mayor MB, Chae JC, et al: Macroscopic and microscopic evidence of prosthetic fixation with porous-coated materials. Clin Orthop Relat Res 235:173–180, 1988.
4. Belmont PJ, Jr, Powers CC, Beykirch SE, et al: Results of the anatomic medullary locking total hip arthroplasty at a minimum of twenty years: a concise follow-up of previous reports. J Bone Joint Surg Am 90:1524–1530, 2008.
5. Hartley WT, McAuley JP, Culpepper WJ, et al: Osteonecrosis of the femoral head treated with cementless total hip arthroplasty. J Bone Joint Surg Am 82:1408–1413, 2000.
6. Jana AK, Engh CA, Jr, Lewandowski PJ, Hopper RH, Jr, Engh CA: Total hip arthroplasty using porous-coated femoral components in patients with rheumatoid arthritis. J Bone Joint Surg Br 83:686–690, 2001.
7. McAuley JP, Moore KD, Culpepper WJ, 2nd, Engh CA: Total hip arthroplasty with porous-coated prostheses fixed without cement in patients who are sixty-five years of age or older. J Bone Joint Surg Am 80:1648–1655, 1998.
8. Sychterz CJ, Claus AM, Engh CA: What we have learned about long-term cementless fixation from autopsy retrievals. Clin Orthop Relat Res 405:79–91, 2002.
9. Engh CA, Hooten JP, Jr, Zettl-Schaffer KF, et al: Evaluation of bone ingrowth in proximally and extensively porous-coated anatomic medullary locking prostheses retrieved at autopsy. J Bone Joint Surg Am 77:903–910, 1995.
10. Engh CA, O'Connor D, Jasty M, et al: Quantification of implant micromotion, strain shielding, and bone resorption with porous-coated anatomic medullary locking femoral prostheses. Clin Orthop Relat Res 285:13–29, 1992.
11. Engh CA, McGovern TF, Bobyn JD, Harris WH: A quantitative evaluation of periprosthetic bone-remodeling after cementless total hip arthroplasty. J Bone Joint Surg Am 74:1009–1020, 1992.
12. Maloney WJ, Sychterz C, Bragdon C, et al: Femoral bone remodeling after total hip arthroplasty: the skeletal response to well fixed femoral components inserted with and without cement. Clin Orthop Relat Res 333:15–26, 1996.
13. McAuley JP, Sychterz CJ, Engh CA Sr: Influence of porous coating level on proximal femoral remodeling: a postmortem analysis. Clin Orthop Relat Res 371:146–153, 2000.
14. Sychterz CJ, Engh CA: The influence of clinical factors on periprosthetic bone remodeling. Clin Orthop Relat Res 322:285–292, 1996.
15. Sychterz CJ, Topoleski LD, Sacco M, Engh CA Sr: Effect of femoral stiffness on bone remodeling after uncemented arthroplasty. Clin Orthop Relat Res 389:218–227, 2001.
16. Engh CA, Massin P: Cementless total hip arthroplasty using the anatomic medullary locking stem: results using a survivorship analysis. Clin Orthop Relat Res 249:141–158, 1989.
17. Engh CA, Massin P, Suthers KE: Roentgenographic assessment of the biologic fixation of porous-surfaced femoral components. Clin Orthop Relat Res 257:107–128, 1990. Erratum in Clin Orthop Relat Res 284:310–312, 1992.
18. Engh CA, Jr, Culpepper WJ, 2nd, Engh CA: Long-term results of use of the anatomic medullary locking prosthesis in total hip arthroplasty. J Bone Joint Surg Am 79:177–184, 1997.
19. Engh CA, Jr, Claus AM, Hopper RH, Jr, Engh CA: Long-term results using the anatomic medullary locking hip prosthesis. Clin Orthop Relat Res 393:137–146, 2001.
20. Chen CJ, Xenos JS, McAuley JP, et al: Second-generation porous-coated cementless total hip arthroplasties have high survival. Clin Orthop Relat Res 451:121–127, 2006.
21. Engh CA, Jr, Mohan V, Nagowski JP, et al: Influence of stem size on clinical outcome of primary total hip arthroplasty with cementless extensively porous-coated femoral components. J Arthroplasty 24:554–559, 2009.
22. Engh CA, Jr, Young AM, Engh CA, Sr, Hopper RH, Jr: Clinical consequences of stress shielding after porous-coated total hip arthroplasty. Clin Orthop Relat Res 417:157–163, 2003.
23. Woolson ST, Adler NS: The effect of partial or full weight bearing ambulation after cementless total hip arthroplasty. J Arthroplasty 17:820–825, 2002.
24. Von Knoch M, Engh CA, Sr, Sychterz CJ, et al: Migration of polyethylene wear debris in one type of uncemented femoral component with circumferential porous coating: an autopsy study of 5 femurs. J Arthroplasty 15:72–78, 2000.
25. Nercessian OA, Wu WH, Sarkissian H: Clinical and radiographic results of cementless AML total hip arthroplasty in young patients. J Arthroplasty 16:312–316, 2001.
26. Chiu KY, Tang WM, Ng TP, et al: Cementless total hip arthroplasty in young Chinese patients: a comparison of 2 different prostheses. J Arthroplasty 16:863–870, 2001.
27. Kronick JL, Barba ML, Paprosky WG: Extensively coated femoral components in young patients. Clin Orthop Relat Res 344:263–274, 1997.
28. McAuley JP, Culpepper WJ, Engh CA: Total hip arthroplasty: concerns with extensively porous coated femoral components. Clin Orthop Relat Res 355:182–188, 1998.
29. Brown TE, Larson B, Shen F, Moskal JT: Thigh pain after cementless total hip arthroplasty: evaluation and management. J Am Acad Orthop Surg 10:385–392, 2002.
30. Schwartz JT, Jr, Mayer JG, Engh CA: Femoral fracture during non-cemented total hip arthroplasty. J Bone Joint Surg Am 71:1135–1142, 1989.
31. Glassman AH, Engh CA: The removal of porous-coated femoral hip stems. Clin Orthop Relat Res 285:164–180, 1992.

CHAPTER 69

Uncemented Tapered Femoral Components

Kristoff Corten and Robert B. Bourne

INTRODUCTION

During the early 1980s, with total hip arthroplasty (THA) becoming a much more established procedure, concerns surrounding the use of cement fixation started to surface. The longevity of first-generation cementing techniques was being questioned, especially in young, active patients.[1-5] The more frequent occurrence of osteolysis, which in retrospect was erroneously attributed to "cement disease," promoted renewed interest in both improved cementing techniques and cementless fixation with ingrowth or ongrowth of bone to stem. The first generation of cementless femoral stems produced mixed results, with problems related to fixation failure, thigh pain, wear, and osteolysis.[6-10] Subsequent generations of uncemented femoral stems have been developed to address these complications and have achieved longevity after 10 years that is at least comparable with that of their cemented counterparts[11-20] (Table 69-1).

Various cementless THA designs are currently available, and good long-term results are now reported most often. In general, uncemented stems can be grouped into three design categories: anatomic, cylindrical, and tapered. The main differences among these choices include component shape, metallurgy, and head/neck design. Furthermore, the coating surface can vary in extent (proximally vs. fully coated) and in surface properties (e.g., hydroxyapatite, porous, fiber/metal coated). These design features result in different fixation modes, which may influence clinical results.

Anatomic designed femoral stems such as porous coated anatomic (PCA, Howmedica, Rutherford, NJ) are manufactured from a cobalt-chrome (Co-Cr) alloy and achieve fixation by proximal ingrowth. Modular mismatch, endosteal irritation, and lack of ingrowth all were implicated in the high prevalence of symptomatic thigh pain with this implant. At our institution, we prospectively reviewed 311 PCA hip replacements in 279 patients.[21] The mean follow-up was 12 years (range, 10 to 14 years) in 168 patients with 187 PCA replacements. The overall survival rate at 14 years with revision for any reason as the endpoint was 90 ± 5.4%, whereas the survival rate of the femoral component was 95 ± 3.6%.[21] This was similar to the 4% revision rate for aseptic loosening of the stem at 15 years that was reported by Bojescul.[22] Reported prevalence of thigh pain was 36%[21] and 13%,[22] respectively. Osteolysis and wear of the polyethylene liner were the two most important indications for revision at long term.[21,22]

Fully porous-coated cylindrical stems such as anatomic medullary locking (AML) stems (DePuy, Warsaw, Ind) achieve primarily distal diaphyseal fixation. This Co-Cr stem has a sintered-bead porous surface. Several reviews have reported on an unselected, consecutive series of 223 patients with an AML stem,[13,15,23,24] and results of 119 hips in 113 patients with a minimum follow-up of 20 years (mean, 22 years) have been reported.[13] A vast majority of revisions were directed toward the acetabular component (TriSpike, DePuy), and 77 patients (65%) continued to retain all components. Six stems (3%) were radiographically loose, of which four cases had undergone revision. Ninety-six percent of stems achieved bone ingrowth, and none of them subsequently loosened. At the time of the most recent follow-up, 18 hips (16%) were associated with moderate and 9 (8%) with severe functional limitations. Survivorship upon analysis of the stem, with revision for aseptic loosening as the endpoint, was 99 ± 1.5% at 15 years[23] and 98.3 ± 1.9% at 20 years.[13] Femoral osteolytic lesions were present in 25 of 68 hips (37%) with minimum 20-year radiographic follow-up.[13] Although thigh pain was not reported in this series, an earlier publication reported an incidence of 8%.[24] Osteolysis and polyethylene wear were the most frequent complications associated with this total hip system.[13,15,23,24]

Uncemented, tapered femoral components were designed to allow for stable initial three-point fixation and a graduated load transfer to the proximal femur, which reduces excessive proximal stress shielding and

Table 69-1. Uncemented, Tapered Femoral Components With Minimum 10-Year Follow-up Have Been Reported With Survivorships from 94% to 100%*

	Patient Number	Stem Type	Mean Follow-up, yr	Survivorship of Stem at Max Follow-up	Incidence of Thigh Pain, %
Cylindrical Extensively Coated Stems					
Engh 2001[7]	129	AML	13.9	98.9	8
Belmont 2008[13]	119	AML	22	98.3	NA
Anatomic Stems					
Kawamura 2001[21]	187	PCA	12	94.9	36
Bojescul 2003[22]	64	PCA	15.6	92	12.5
Tapered Stems					
Schramm 2000[75]	89	CLS	10.3	100	17
Aldinger 2003[7]	262	CLS	12	95	0
Aldinger 2009[7]	257	CLS	17	94	0
Sakalkale 1999[42]	71	Tri-Lock	11.5	100	1.4
Purtill 2001[41]	49	Tri-Lock	15	100	2
Teloken 2002[43]	49	Tri-Lock	15	100	2
Capello 2003[40]	111	Omnifit HA	11.3	98.9	2.6
Bourne 2001[14]	307	MH	10-13	99	3
Mallory 2001[18]	120	MH	12.2	97.5	3.4
Au 2009[26]	126	MH	20	99	NA
Grubl 2001[7]	133	Zweymuller	10.7	99	3
Garcia-Cimbrelo 2003[16]	104	Zweymuller	11.3	95.4	13.5
Suckel 2009[79]	314	Zweymuller	15	98	NA
Parvizi 2004[60]	104	Taperloc	10	100	NA
McLaughlin 2008[19]	145	Taperloc	20	99	4

*The prevalence of thigh pain with tapered stems varies between stem designs but also between studies focusing on a particular design. Cylindrical extensively coated stems and anatomic stems have reported survivorships of 98% to 99% and 92% to 95%, respectively; both designs are associated with a high prevalence of thigh pain.
AML, Anatomic medullary locking; *PCA*, porous-coated anatomic; *CLS*, cementless locking stem; *MH*, Mallory-Head; *NA*, not applicable.

Table 69-2. Overview of the Metallurgy, Coating, and Geometric Features of the Most Common Uncemented, Tapered Stem Designs

Stem	Company	Metallurgy	Taper	Collar	Surface	Extent of Coating
Zweymuller	AlloPro AG, Baar, Switzerland	Ti	Wedged	No	Corundum blasting	Full
Mallory-Head	Biomet, Warsaw, Ind	Ti	3D	No	Plasma-sprayed proximal third, grit-blasted middle third, and matte-finished distal third	Proximal and middle thirds
Taperloc	Biomet Warsaw, Ind	Ti	2D	No	Plasma-spray	
Tri-Lock	DePuy, Warsaw, Ind	Co-Cr	2D	No	Sintered beads	60% proximal
CLS	Centerpulse, Zurich, Switzerland	Ti	2D (rectangular, flutes)	No	Corundum blasting	Full
Synergy	Smith and Nephew, Memphis, Tenn	Ti	3D	No	Porous or HA	Proximal
Summit	DePuy, Warsaw, Ind	Ti	3D	No	Porous or HA	Proximal

2D, Two-dimensional; *3D*, three-dimensional; *CLS*, cementless locking stem; *Co-Cr*, cobalt-chrome; *HA*, hydroxyapatite; *Ti*, titanium.

decreases the risk for thigh pain (Table 69-2). We reported on the 10- to 13-year performance of a nonconsecutive series of 307 Mallory-Head THAs (Biomet, Warsaw, Ind) in 283 patients.[25] Overall 10-year Kaplan-Meier survivorship was 90% for hip replacement and 99% for the stem. Mild stress shielding limited to Gruen zones 1 and 7 was seen in 50% of patients, and activity-related thigh pain was present in only 3%.[25] In addition, 20-year results of a randomized controlled trial (RCT) conducted at our institution to compare the results of cementless and cemented fixation of Mallory-Head THA showed that the survival rate of the stem was 99%, with only 1 stem out of 126 revised for periprosthetic fracture. The 20-year survival rate of the cementless system (76%) was significantly higher than that of cemented THA (63%) (*P* = .018).[26]

In general, not the stem but the acetabular component has been shown to be the weakest link in early-generation cementless THA systems, and long-term survivorship of anatomic, cylindrical, and some tapered designed stems can be considered good to excellent.[11-20] However, concerns regarding subsidence with some designs,[11,12,27] thigh pain,[7,13,15,21,28-30] and stress shielding[31,32] have been raised. Uncemented three-dimensional (3D)-tapered femoral components rely on initial three-point fixation followed by proximal porous ingrowth for continued stability. Subsidence does not seem to be a problem with proximally coated tapered-stem designs.[25,26,33] When osseointegration has occurred at approximately 12 weeks, a graduated load transfer is induced by the tapered design; this reduces excessive proximal stress shielding, as we have shown in a multicenter, randomized, controlled trial in which proximal coated stems were compared with cylindrical extensively coated stems.[34] In addition, the elastic modularity of the titanium alloy approaches the modularity of the femoral bone; this could reduce the prevalence of thigh pain.[25] Our experience has been that in terms of fixation, avoidance of thigh pain and stress shielding, with a cementless, proximally coated, tapered femoral component, based on a Titanium alloy (Ti), indeed seems to be a promising option. In this chapter, we will review the design rationale and the surgical technique of tapered cementless stems, as well as currently available outcomes studies.

DESIGN RATIONALE FOR TAPERED FEMORAL COMPONENTS

Cementless tapered femoral components require good initial fixation by means of proper femoral size selection and the design features (i.e., oversized porous coating, antirotation fins) of tapered (usually 3D-taper) stems. There is little doubt that the principle of obtaining good initial femoral fixation is of importance in promoting good long-term fixation between the component and the host bone. Excessive initial micromotion greater than 40 to 75 μm will lead to the formation of fibrous connective tissue at the bone-stem interface.[35,36] Tapered femoral components gain initial three-point, self-locking fixation, which also provides rotational stability (Fig. 69-1).

Popular cementless tapered stems may feature a two-dimensional (2D) coronal or sagittal femoral taper or a 3D-tapered design; the most important difference is that 3D-tapered stems have a transverse taper, in addition to coronal and sagittal tapers. When a tapered component is forced into the cylindrical medullary canal of the femur, hoop stresses are set up. The femoral bone is viscoelastic; this implies that when a tapered stem is introduced into the slightly smaller medullary canal, creep and stress relaxation will occur. Initially, three-point fixation and press-fit will be noted, which implies that when an equilibrium is set up, the axially loaded tapered stem will not advance any farther.[37] Over time, viscoelastic relaxation of the bone can occur and the press-fit will lessen. Further advancement of the implant within the bone is prevented by three-point fixation, the

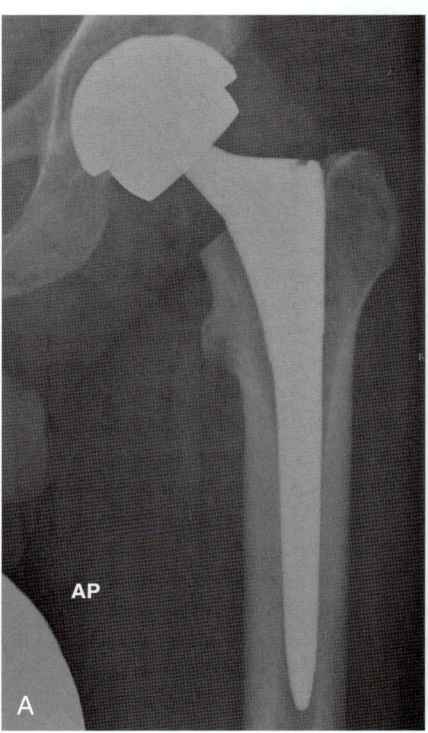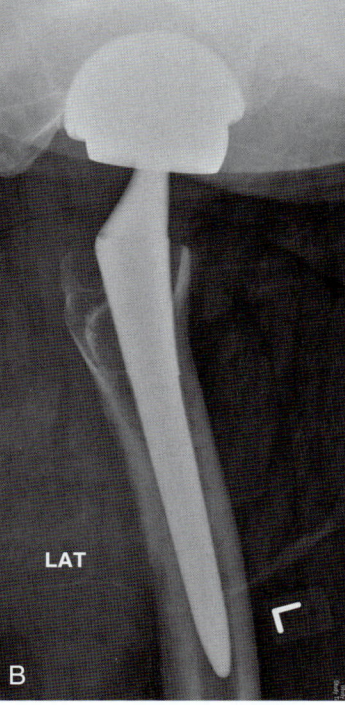

Figure 69-1. Anteroposterior (AP) and lateral (LAT) radiographs of a total hip replacement using a cementless tapered femoral component (Synergy, Smith and Nephew, Memphis, Tenn). On the lateral view, note the three-point fixation of the femoral component with posterior cortical contact proximally, anterior contact at the metaphyseal/isthmic junction, and posterior distal contact.

high roughness and friction of the porous or hydroxy-apatite surface, and the 3-degree tapered design. The initial and intermediate stability of the component within the bone will allow for appositional bone formation on the component surface. This appositional bone in turn will connect to the endosteal bone at approximately 12 weeks.[38] In other words, the design of the tapered component allows for stable initial mechanical fixation, which in turn allows for biological fixation over a period of approximately 3 months in the metaphyseal region. As a consequence, the proximal femur is subjected to a more favorable gradual loading profile, which may be responsible for reduced stress shielding and the relatively low prevalence of thigh pain observed with the use of tapered femoral components.[7,17,18,39-43] The use of a collar in cementless tapered stems would interfere with initial implant impaction and the secondary small amount of "settling" of the component. Therefore, tapered stems are usually collarless.

Achieving initial rotational stability is of paramount importance for long-term fixation. The Zweymuller stem is a 2D-tapered stem that achieves its rotational stability through its rectangular cross-section and the lock achieved by sharp corners of the stem with cortical bone. Most contemporary cementless tapered stems are round in cross-section, feature a 3-degree three-dimensional longitudinal taper, and obtain additional rotational stability through the use of longitudinal fins. Newer-generation tapered stems such as the Synergy stem (Smith and Nephew, Memphis, Tenn) are 3D tapered at the proximal, porous-coated part of the stem by the addition of a 3-degree taper in the transverse

plane. This configuration more closely mimics the proximal geometry of the femur, which is narrower medially (calcar and medial neck) than laterally (greater trochanter) (Fig. 69-1 through 69-3). Tapered stems with circular cross-sections and longitudinal flutes that provide rotational stability also exist. Wagner[44] promoted such stems in patients with dysplastic hips, in whom the proximal femur is not morphologically suited to an oval or rectangular stem. The circular shape allows for correction of anteversion and reduces the risk for intraoperative fracture. Highly satisfactory successful outcomes with no thigh pain were reported in a 9-year follow-up study of 635 implants.[44]

A modular mismatch between stem and surrounding bone might lead to an increased incidence of endosteal irritation and thigh pain.[7,28] Most tapered cementless stems are made of a titanium (Ti) alloy with aluminum and vanadium (Ti-6Al-4V). This alloy has the greatest fatigue resistance of all Ti alloys and is 50% less stiff than Co-Cr alloys used in earlier cementless designs that were associated with a high incidence of thigh pain.[21,22,25] In addition, Ti has been histologically demonstrated to be very biocompatible, with ongrowth (e.g., plasma-sprayed surface) or ingrowth (e.g., porous surface) of the bone to the stem surface.[38] This property of Ti alloys enabled Albrektsson to coin the term "osseointegration."[38] More recently, the application of bioactive coatings such as hydroxyapatite (HA), to which Ti specifically lends itself, has been shown to enhance the process of osseointegration.[45] However, this has not resulted in improved long-term survivorship in comparison with porous-coated designs without HA

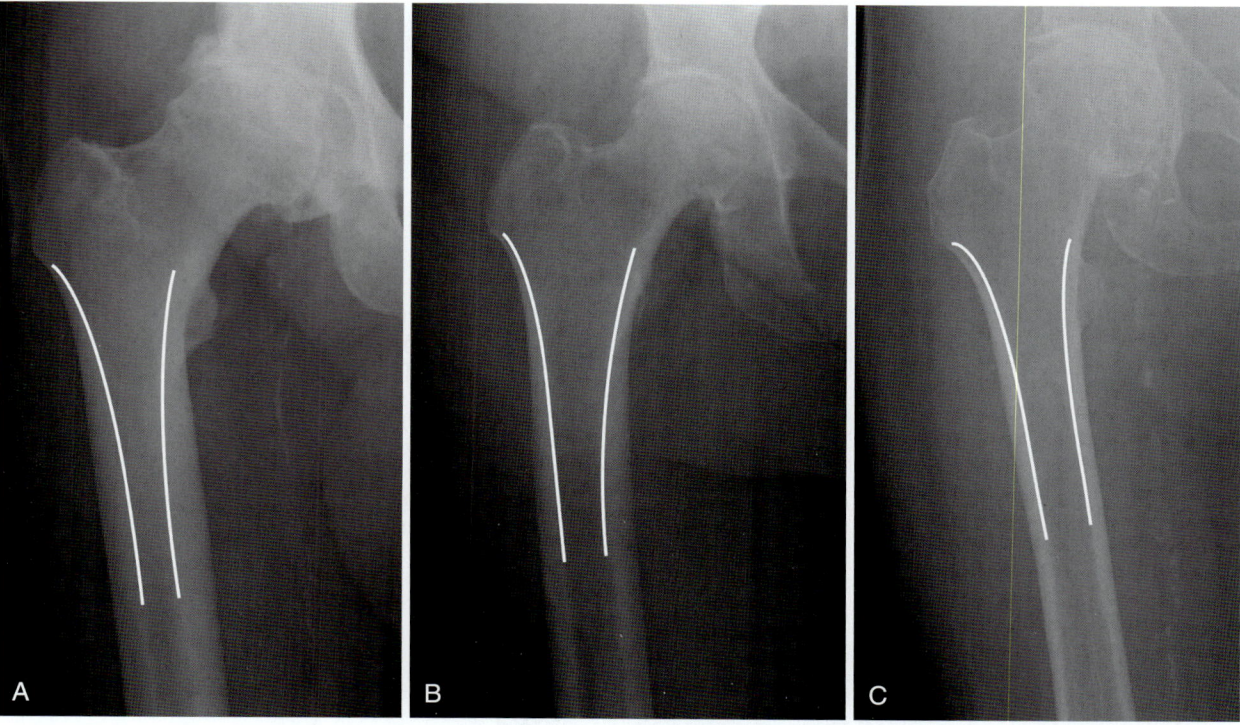

Figure 69-2. Anteroposterior hip radiographs demonstrating the three varying proximal femoral morphologies using the Dorr classification: type **A** (champagne flute), type **B** (funnel-shaped), and type **C** (cylindrical).

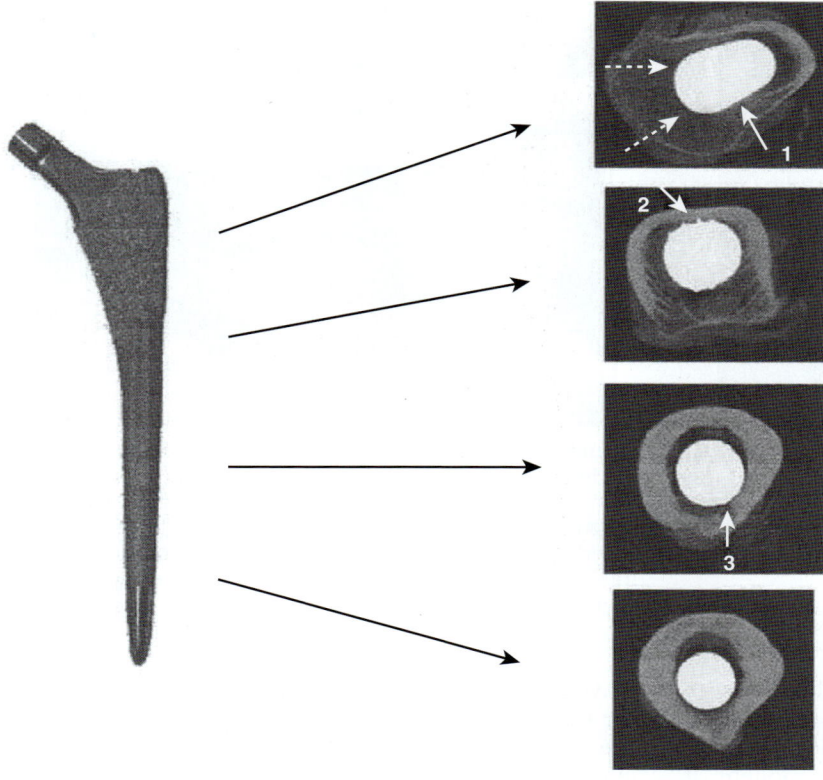

Figure 69-3. Computed tomograms demonstrating where a cementless tapered femoral component (Synergy, Memphis, Tenn) contacts the cortical bone proximally, mid stem, and distally.

coating.[20] Furthermore, circumferential proximal coated surfaces seem protective in preventing femoral osteolysis distal to the level of the lesser trochanter.[26]

The mechanical properties of tapered stems imply that they, theoretically, work best in proximal femoral morphologies with tapered medullary shapes, because the congruency between the 3-degree taper of the implant and the morphology of the proximal femur allows maximal implant-to-bone contact. According to the Dorr classification,[46] Dorr type A or B femurs would be ideally suited for tapered stems. However, in our clinical practice, we sometimes use these stems in Dorr type C femurs with good clinical results (see Fig. 69-2).

SURGICAL TECHNIQUE

Preoperative Planning

Preoperative planning is a very important step of any THA procedure. A low-centered anteroposterior (AP) radiograph of the pelvis and a true lateral radiograph of the affected hip are needed to assess leg length, the anatomic femoral configuration, the level of the femoral neck cut, offset, and stem size.

Pelvic obliquity, pelvic symmetry, and other leg abnormalities (i.e., malunion, growth arrest, deformity) must be considered when leg length discrepancies are assessed. In most cases, a horizontal line can be drawn through the teardrops (inferior aspects of the pelvic quadrilateral plates). A vertical line drawn through the center of the femoral heads or the tip of the greater or

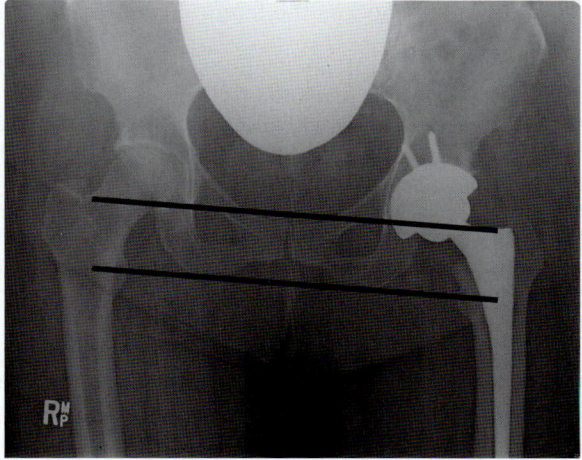

Figure 69-4. Two options for assessing leg length on an anteroposterior pelvic radiograph using lines joining the teardrops (superior line) or the transischial line (inferior line). When the patient has a fixed flexion contracture of the hip, the line joining the teardrops is preferred.

lesser trochanter will detect any leg length that has to be made up. Some surgeons prefer to use a horizontal line to join the ischial tuberosities instead of the inter-teardrop line, but occasionally a fixed flexion contracture of the hip can render these landmarks erroneous (Fig. 69-4).

It is important to preoperatively estimate the anatomic relationship of the tip of the greater trochanter to the medullary canal of the femur. This will allow the

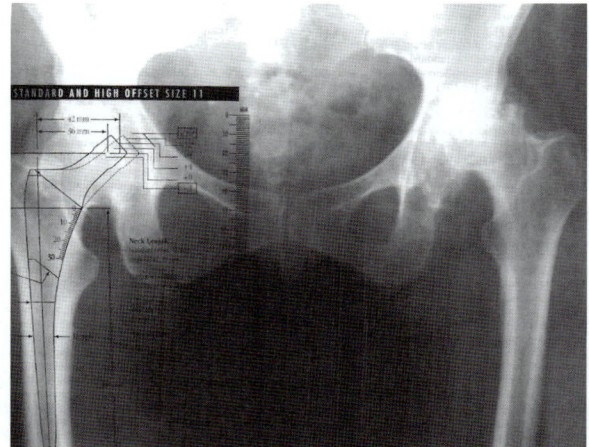

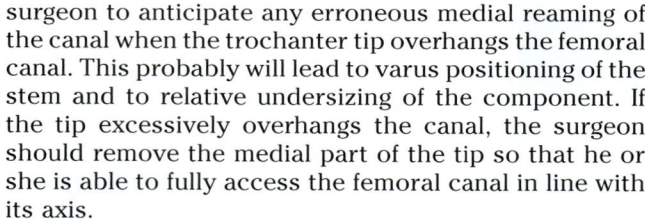

Figure 69-5. Templating of ipsilateral and contralateral hips is recommended on an anteroposterior radiograph where magnification has been determined, because the ipsilateral hip often has an external rotation contracture, making it difficult to determine the size of the component and offset required.

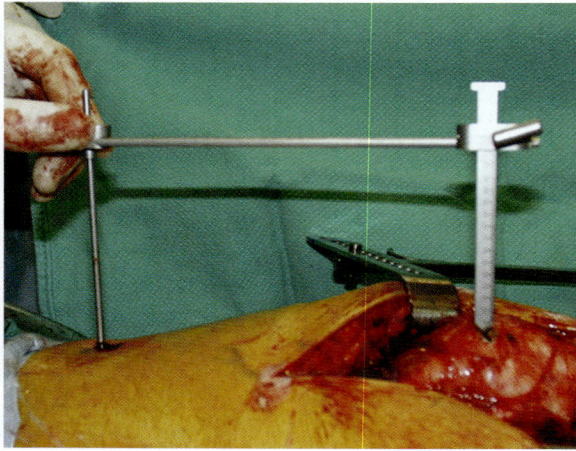

Figure 69-6. The authors' preferred method of determining leg length and offset restoration, using a pin placed in the iliac crest and a detachable leg length/offset guide. Leg length and offset are determined before the hip is dislocated, then are reassessed with the trial components and final components in place to verify that the required corrections have been made.

surgeon to anticipate any erroneous medial reaming of the canal when the trochanter tip overhangs the femoral canal. This probably will lead to varus positioning of the stem and to relative undersizing of the component. If the tip excessively overhangs the canal, the surgeon should remove the medial part of the tip so that he or she is able to fully access the femoral canal in line with its axis.

Usually, the femoral neck cut is one fingerbreadth (approximately 1 cm) proximal to the lesser trochanter. Preoperative templating will allow the surgeon to adjust the level of the neck cut. A lower neck cut will allow for deeper engagement of the stem in the femoral canal and may be necessary to avoid leg lengthening in a patient with a short—often varus—femoral neck or to avoid excessive femoral stem anteversion in dysplastic femurs with excessive anteversion. A higher femoral neck cut will allow for a relatively higher press-fit of the stem in the proximal femur, which may be necessary to lengthen a short leg or to compensate for a higher valgus neck shaft angle.

Offset restoration is a particularly important aspect of soft tissue balancing that will in turn determine implant stability and long-term survival.[47-50] Soft tissue balancing is important to avoid dislocation by tensioning soft tissues, preventing impingement, and improving abductor function and resultant hip joint reaction forces by restoring normal abductor resting length. For offset estimation, the surgeon needs radiographs in which the lower extremities are in neutral rotation. This is sometimes a problem in arthritic hips with external rotation contractures that lead to an underestimation of the true offset. Oblique radiographs sometimes may be beneficial,[51] but more important, templating of the contralateral and ipsilateral hip is recommended (Fig. 69-5). Multiple operative factors such as the level of the femoral neck osteotomy, the varus/valgus positioning of the stem, and the position of the acetabular component

may have an influence on restoration of normal abductor resting length of the replaced hip. Intraoperatively, the use of a special caliper may help in assessing the amount of leg lengthening that has occurred during surgery and may indicate the degree of restoration of the femoral offset. The jig we use (Smith and Nephew) consists of a pin placed in the iliac crest. It also has an adjustable side arm that is fixed to the pin and allows measurement of both leg length and offset to a point indicated on the greater trochanter. This is done before dislocation of the hip and following trial reduction (see also "Surgical Technique"). This allows the surgeon to anticipate any measured length and offset discrepancies (Fig. 69-6). The geometry of the femoral component also plays an important role in restoring the femoral offset. We compared the original Mallory-Head stem design with a 135-degree neck shaft angle versus the newer Synergy stem, with a 131-degree neck shaft angle and two offset options in terms of restoring femoral head offset.[52] Patients with unilateral osteoarthritis were included, and AP radiographs were taken with the leg 15 to 20 degrees internally rotated. In keeping with the criterion that successful restoration of the offset was within 4 mm of the nonoperated side, femoral offset was restored in 99 of 109 patients (91%) in the Synergy group, and in 38 of 93 patients (41%) in the Mallory-Head group.[52]

Finally, the stem size will be determined by the diameter of the femoral canal, but most important, it also will be determined by the anatomic and biomechanical requirements of the proximal femur such as the femoral offset.

Surgical Technique

The surgical procedure using a tapered uncemented femoral component is simple and straightforward. Cementless tapered stems can be inserted using any of the traditional surgical approaches (anterolateral, posterior, transtrochanteric, and minimally invasive). In our institution, we prefer to use a direct lateral Hardinge or posterolateral surgical approach. Before dislocating the femoral head, we fix a pin to the iliac crest and use the cautery and a marking pen to identify a landmark on the greater trochanter. The leg length/offset jig is then fixed to the pin and set at the level of the trochanter landmark, with the leg in a position that can be reproduced later on with the trial components in place. Following the femoral neck osteotomy, the acetabulum is reconstructed using the surgical technique pertinent to use of the intended acetabular component. We usually first insert a trial liner. The leg is externally rotated and the lower limb is placed in a leg bag placed on the side opposite to the surgeon. The femoral canal is opened with the use of a box osteotome. It is important to stay as lateral and posterior as possible. The use of a blunt Hohman retractor behind the greater trochanter and a Hohman retractor behind the posterior cortex to elevate the proximal femur into the wound is recommended. Sequential tapered reamers are used to enlarge the femoral canal. Care is taken to prevent damage to the gluteus medius muscle. During reaming it is important to stay as lateral as possible. Failure to do so may result in ultimate varus placement of the component. If

necessary, and as assessed on preoperative templating, it might be helpful to remove some medial bone of the tip of the greater trochanter with a broach or a rongeur. Reaming is stopped when the templated size reamer reaches the osteotomy level. If reaming is held up at a smaller size than templated, varus malpositioning is the usual cause. Next, the broaches are used to further prepare the femoral canal. The first broach used should be at least two sizes smaller than the templated size. If progression of the broach is slow, the surgeon should consider two steps: (1) rasping of the lateral aspect of the femoral canal to correct for any varus malpositioning, and (2) careful partial extraction and reintroduction of the broach to clear its teeth to overcome resistance to further introduction of the broach. Full seating of the broach is established when the level of the femoral neck osteotomy is reached. The broach handle is toggled using the antirotation side bar on the handle to observe the potential for rotatory movement between the broach and the bone. If any rotation of the stem still occurs, upsizing of the stem is probably required. With the broach seated, a calcar reamer may be used to remove some prominent bone, which bears a potential for impingement. At this stage, a trial reduction can be done with the final broach in place to assess for stability of the hip (Fig. 69-7). Changes to stem offset, neck

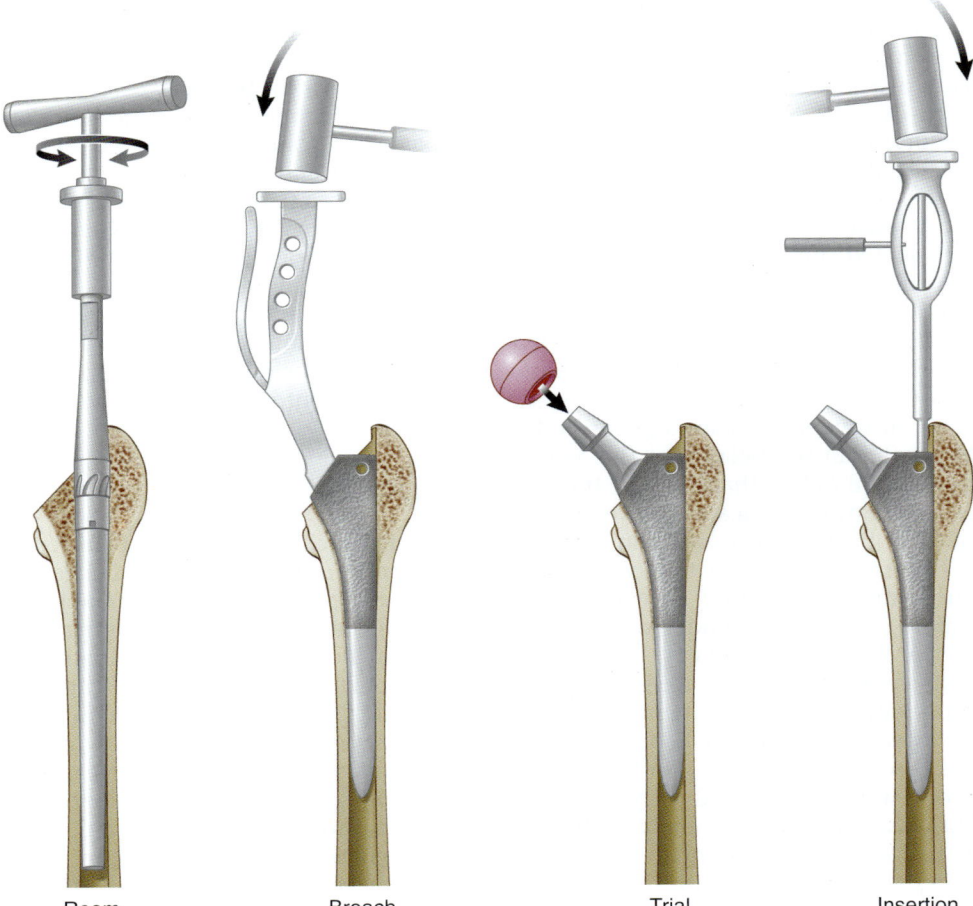

Ream	Broach	Trial	Insertion

Figure 69-7. A pictorial representation demonstrating the four easy steps of inserting a cementless tapered femoral component (i.e., ream, broach, trial, and insert).

length, femoral neck cut, and acetabular liner can still be made. With the trial components in place, the leg length/offset jig can be reapplied to the pin. Assessment of the position of the previously set jig relative to the previously identified trochanter landmark will allow evaluation of whether any adjustments to the stem or the liner (with or without offset) would improve hip biomechanics. The hip is taken through a full range of movement, and soft tissue tension is assessed. External rotational stability of the hip should be tested in extension, and stability in maximal internal rotation in 90 degrees of flexion should be evaluated. Also, any potential for impingement is investigated and offending osteophytes are removed. If this is satisfactory, the definitive stem and liner can be inserted.

A cementless, tapered stem should be engaged in the femoral canal by first gently toggling so that the distance of the proximal border of the coating is within 1 cm of the femoral osteotomy. If this cannot be achieved, one should not attempt to tap the stem down, because this might lead to excessive hoop stresses, which in turn may lead to a calcar fracture. Instead, one should re-evaluate the position of the stem in the canal (often the stem is in varus alignment) or even re-broach if deemed necessary. Again the stem is toggled down to the required 1 cm from its final position. The stem then is gently tapped into place using a light mallet. The stem is seated when no further advancement of the stem occurs on gently striking the introducer. Often this is accompanied by a change in sound and feel. A gentle rotational torque is also used to assess for rotational stability (see Fig. 69-7).

A final trial reduction with the jig assessment is performed using a trial femoral head. After cleaning and drying of the femoral taper, the definitive femoral head is applied. A washout is performed, and the acetabulum is inspected for the presence of any particulate debris. The hip is then reduced under direct vision.

We allow our patients to bear weight as tolerated when using cementless tapered femoral components, recognizing that postoperative management with regard to weight bearing is controversial. Some surgeons prefer protected weight bearing in the belief that this would minimize the micromotion to less than 150 μm, thereby optimizing the osseointegration. Pacanti showed that it is more important to observe the manner in which a patient carries out a particular activity than which specific activities the patient is allowed to carry out.[53] Woolson looked at 46 patients who underwent 50 consecutive primary AML replacements.[54] Twenty-four patients (25 hips) were allowed full weight bearing immediately postoperatively, and 24 patients (25 hips) were instructed to bear weight of 50 lb or less for 6 weeks. The Harris Hip Score at 2 years for the partial weight-bearing group was 95 compared with 97 for the full weight-bearing group. Radiographic analysis showed that both groups had evidence of adequate osseointegration. The authors concluded that with this prosthesis and with good initial intraoperative stem stability, immediate postoperative full weight bearing did not cause any problems.[54]

Table 69-3. Algorithm for Femoral Component Selection

	Cementless	Cemented
Age, yr	<75	>75
Medullary shape	Funnel shaped	Cylindrical
Bone disease	Osteoarthritis Avascular necrosis	Irradiated Paget
Demand	High	Low

Based on our assessment of a number of studies, we have developed a "typical algorithm" for selection of the femoral component. This selection is based on the patient's age, the shape of the proximal femoral medullary canal, the type of arthritis, and patient demand. With this algorithm, at least 85% to 90% of patients at our unit undergoing a primary THA do receive a cementless tapered stem (Table 69-3).

AVOIDING AND DEALING WITH COMPLICATIONS

Intraoperative Femoral Fracture

The procedure of impacting a broach or a cementless tapered component carries with it some risk of creating an intraoperative fracture, particularly in patients with poor bone stock. Berry reviewed 23,980 primary hip replacements and found an overall intraoperative periprosthetic fracture rate of 1%.[55] The intraoperative fracture rate was 0.3% (68/20,859) for cemented and 5.4% (170/3121) for uncemented stems of all types.[55] We reviewed a series of 442 Mallory-Head stems and found an intraoperative fracture rate of 5% (21/442 stems). Fractures were treated successfully with no adverse events by backing out the stem and cerclage-wiring the proximal femur. The same component was reinserted, and the patient was restricted to touch weight bearing for 6 weeks.[14]

Thigh Pain

The high incidence of thigh pain reported with earlier cementless stem designs challenged the popularity of the uncemented femoral component. It is important for the surgeon to understand which factors influence thigh pain, so he or she can anticipate any problems that might occur postoperatively. Thigh pain is multifactorial and is associated with several features of an uncemented stem, but other causes of thigh pain must be excluded, such as infection, stress fracture, and spinal pathology. Review of our experience with the PCA implant showed that thigh pain was correlated with subsidence, cortical hypertrophy, and sclerosis at the tip of the stem.[21] However, we also found cortical hypertrophy around the distal one third of the Mallory-Head stem in nearly 50% of cases, but we were unable to correlate this with a high incidence of thigh pain (6%).[25] In other words, the surgeon should evaluate thigh pain in light of the specific features of each implant and the radiographic findings in each case.

Thigh pain occurs in association with several features of an uncemented stem. The modular mismatch between stem and bone, the diaphyseal fit of the stem, and the time interval following surgery are probably the most important factors. The metallurgy and design of the implant influence the incidence of thigh pain, and an increased modular mismatch between stem and bone, as can be found in Co-Cr stems, may cause endosteal irritation and has been associated with thigh pain.[7,13,28-30] Stems with a cylindrical diaphyseal press-fit[9,17,18,24,39-43] have been associated with a higher incidence of thigh pain than those with a proximal press-fit.[9,11,12,27] The extent of the coating and the size of the stem may also influence the incidence of thigh pain,[32,34,56] which seems to be associated with the time interval following surgery.[29,34,56] The incidence and intensity of thigh pain seem to decrease over time, and only 50% of patients with thigh pain report pain on consecutive time intervals following surgery.[56] Factors that have not been associated with thigh pain include age, gender, diagnosis, and stem alignment in the coronal plane.[24,27]

In most cases, thigh pain symptoms are tolerable and the patient is able to live with the symptoms. Explanation about the cause of the pain and expected improvement over time might help the patient to comprehend what is going on; conservative treatment should be sufficient. In some cases, however, the discomfort is disabling, leading to an unsatisfied patient. Revision of the femoral component or augmentation of the femur at the tip of the stem with cortical strut grafting has been suggested as a salvage procedure.[57]

Stress Shielding

Stress shielding can be found in all total hip replacements—both cemented and uncemented implants—with the most important difference being that bone loss around cemented implants seems to be progressive after 3 years, whereas with uncemented stems, it has been reported to cease at 1 to 2 years.[9,31,58-61] Similar to thigh pain, stress shielding is influenced by several features of the uncemented stem, such as metallurgy and the extent of coating (see later). The clinical relevance of stress shielding of the proximal femur following cementless implants remains uncertain and in our practice is certainly no indication for revision surgery in the asymptomatic patient. In addition, patients with a greater baseline bone mineral density (BMD) (≥80th percentile) can be expected to have a greater percentage of bone loss over time with no adverse effects in the intermediate follow-up.[34]

Stem Subsidence

The tapered design allows for some initial minimal subsidence of the stem. Few long-term studies have reported any subsidence, and none of the subsided stems had to be revised.[11,12,25,27] Aldinger[12] reported on a 15- to 20-year follow-up series of 127 THAs with a cementless locking stem (CLS) in a group of patients younger than 55 years. Among 101 hips available for radiographic analysis, 1 stem (1%) had subsided for greater than 5 mm.[12] One stem had subsided in another series in which 186 of 250 CLS stems were followed radiographically for 15 to 20 years by Aldinger.[11] In a consecutive series of 98 CLS stems followed by Min, 7 stems (7%) had more than 5 mm nonprogressive subsidence and 24 stems (26%) had radiolucent lines, but none of the stems had been revised or were considered to be loose at an average follow-up of 7.7 years.[27] Mulliken[25] reported on the radiographic stability of 416 Mallory-Head stems. Forty-four stems had measurable subsidence, which was greater than 5 mm in 5 stems (1%). This subsidence stabilized at 6 months in all but 2 stems and continued after 1 year in 1 stem. The patient was pain free, and the stem had not been revised.[25] Several authors concluded that initial limited subsidence of a tapered femoral component does not demonstrate component loosening and in fact may be desirable to achieve optimal mechanical fixation.[19,25,43,62]

Dislocation

Dislocation is the leading early complication of THA.[63] Recurrent hip dislocation occurs in 60% of patients after a first-time dislocation, and 15% to 40% of patients may require reoperation.[33,64,65] The causes of dislocation are multifactorial and include patient-related factors (e.g., neuromuscular disorders, substance abuse, female gender, advancing age), surgical parameters (e.g., posterior approach, poor soft tissue balancing), and implant features (e.g., poor restoration of offset, poor head-to-neck ratio). The surgical approach bears a major contribution to preventing hip instability. We performed an extensive literature review involving 13,203 primary THAs meeting the criteria based on variables previously shown to affect stability.[66] The dislocation rate was 0.55% for the direct lateral approach, 2.2% for the anterolateral approach, and 3.2% for the posterior approach (4% without posterior repair and 2% with posterior repair).[66] We reviewed 1515 primary THAs in 1333 patients performed at our center.[67,68] The direct lateral approach was used, and follow-up occurred at 2 to 10 years. We observed only 6 hip dislocations (0.4%). All occurred within the first year following surgery. Four of the 6 patients had an acetabular inclination and anteversion outside the safe zone as described by Lewinnek[69] (40 ± 10 degrees of inclination and 15 ± 10 degrees of anteversion). Twelve percent of patients had a limp; this was comparable with the 18% to 26% incidence reported in the literature.[69,70]

Achieving an adequate soft tissue balance in primary THA is very important. Preoperative templating on standardized radiographs assists with selection of an implant of appropriate size and the location of the appropriate neck cut. Intraoperative use of a leg length/offset caliper helps to reproduce the leg length and offset (see earlier, "Surgical Technique"). In addition, offset restoration is aided by the availability of a femoral stem with different offsets[52] and acetabular sockets with the option of a lateralized acetabular liner.

Stability can be determined intraoperatively by performing special maneuvers such as the "shuck test," in which the surgeon tries to distract the THA in an inferior direction to assess soft tissue tension. Another test is the "drop kick" test, where the hip is held in extension and the knee is flexed to 90 degrees. If the limb is over-lengthened, there is a tendency for the knee to spring back into extension. Finally, impingement of the stem on the acetabular component is looked for during surgery, and periacetabular osteophytes are routinely excised. Whenever possible, skirted femoral necks on modular femoral heads are avoided because they may lead to impingement and dislocation. The use of femoral heads smaller than 28 mm is avoided if possible, because they are associated with increased dislocation potential.[71]

CLINICAL RESULTS

With regard to the clinical results of tapered, uncemented stems, three specific clinical parameters should be discussed and compared with other designs: (1) thigh pain, (2) stress shielding, and (3) survivorship. Five different types of tapered uncemented stems have been reported with a minimum 10-year follow-up (see Table 69-1). These stems include the Zweymuller Alloclassic (Alloclassic-SL, AlloPro AG, Baar, Switzerland), the Cementless Locking Stem (CLS, Sulzer Medica, Baar, Switzerland), the Mallory-Head stem (Biomet, Warsaw, Ind), the Taperloc (Biomet, Warsaw, Ind), and the Tri-Lock stem (DePuy).

Thigh Pain

Thigh pain occurs in association with distal canal reaming,[9] Co-Cr implants,[13,30] and tight fit.[9] Thigh pain does not seem to be associated with alignment of tapered stems into the femoral bone.[27] The incidence of thigh pain at the tip of a Ti-tapered stem, without radiographic signs of loosening, is comparable with (3%)[27,28] or even lower[11,12] than that seen in patients with cemented stems and is lower than that observed in anatomic Co-Cr stem designs[7,72,28,29] or some cylindrical distal fixation designs.*

In an RCT carried out at our center, 126 cemented and 124 cementless Mallory-Head THAs were compared.[28] The incidence of mild thigh pain was 3% in both groups.[28] Other Ti-based, tapered stems such as the CLS stem have been reported, with incidences of thigh pain comparable with or even less than those of cemented stems.[11,12,27] Aldinger[12] reported on the 15- to 20-year results of 154 CLS stems in patients younger than 55 years. These CLS stems have an ongrowth surface and are specifically designed so that they do not obtain a press-fit in the upper diaphysis. None of the 127 hips available for follow-up as reported by Aldinger[12] had any thigh pain, but 12 stems (8%) had been revised, including 5 for aseptic loosening and 5 for periprosthetic

fracture. No patient reported any thigh pain in another series of 250 CLS stems followed for 15 to 20 years by Aldinger.[11] Twelve stems (3%) had been revised for aseptic loosening and 9 (2.5%) for a periprosthetic fracture. In a consecutive series of 98 CLS stems followed by Min, 5% of patients had slight thigh pain that did not affect functional outcome scores.[27] Seven stems (7%) had more than 5 mm nonprogressive subsidence and 24 stems (26%) had radiolucent lines, but no stems had been revised or were considered to be loose at an average follow-up of 7.7 years.[27]

Numerous studies looking at the use of a tapered uncemented stem confirm the lower incidence of thigh pain compared with that reported in some anatomic and cylindrical cementless implants.*

We compared the 2-year incidence of thigh pain in the first 94 patients receiving a Mallory-Head prosthesis, with 110 patients receiving a PCA component.[7] For the Mallory-Head group, the incidence of thigh pain was 7% and 3% at 1 year and 2 years, respectively. For the PCA components, this was 13% and 23%, respectively. Less modular mismatch and less endosteal irritation were believed to be responsible for these improved results in the tapered stem design.[7] In another study,[29] rates of slight to mild thigh pain with the PCA stem were in excess of 20% at 3 to 4 years, but the incidence decreased over time to 12% at a minimum of 10 years of follow-up.

Early, minimum 2-year results of 307 AML stems showed high incidences of pain (14%) and limp (21%). In most cases, the pain was occasional, was felt in the thigh at the level of the tip of the stem, and was delayed in onset (usually after walking several blocks). In most patients, this delayed onset "end-of-stem" pain was associated with a limp.[9] A minimum 10-year follow-up study of 174 AML stems showed that 2 (1%) hips had been revised specifically for thigh pain.[24] In 13 of 154 hips (8%) that did not undergo revision surgery, pain in the thigh was reported. In 7 patients, the pain was mild or did not limit their activity. The remaining 6 patients believed that the pain limited their activity, but only 2 (1%) were dissatisfied with the result of the operation. The authors were unable to establish any relationship between pain that limited the patient's activity and the size of the stem or the patient's diagnosis, age, or gender.[24] The Prodigy stem (DePuy) was developed to overcome the problems with thigh pain and stress shielding noted with the AML stem. This Co-Cr cylindrical component was fully porous coated, which is more than the 4/5 coating of the AML stem, except for the distal bullet. In addition, a medial diaphyseal cutout was incorporated to decrease the flexural rigidity of the stem. Hennessy reported on the minimum 10-year results (range, 10 to 12 years) of 100 Prodigy stems in 86 patients, and only 2 patients (2%) reported thigh pain at last follow-up.[32]

The incidence of thigh pain between studies should be compared cautiously because the incidence of thigh pain associated with a particular implant can fluctuate dramatically when studies are compared.† Several

---

*See References 9, 17, 18, 24, and 39-43.

---

*See References 7, 9, 17, 18, 24, 28, 29, 39-43, and 73.
†See References 11-13, 16, 17, 27, 29, and 74.

explanations can be put forth. The incidence and intensity of thigh pain are multifactorial and seem to be related to the follow-up period, the stem size, the way the patient is questioned about it, and whether the results are retrospectively or prospectively evaluated.[29,34,56] A multicenter RCT compared the minimum 2-year results of 198 proximally coated, Ti alloy, tapered Synergy stems (Smith and Nephew) versus 190 Prodigy stems.[34] No differences in functional scores were reported. All patients at each time interval were asked specifically about the presence of thigh pain. A high incidence of preoperative thigh pain (70%) was related to the underlying diagnosis of osteoarthritis, but no differences were noted between groups. At 6 months, there were no differences between groups, with 11% of the Synergy group and 15% of the Prodigy group reporting thigh pain. Also, the incidences of thigh pain at 1 year (11% Synergy and 14% Prodigy) and at 2 years (9% Synergy and 6% Prodigy) were not different between groups. It must be emphasized that in this study, data were prospectively collected and patients were asked repeatedly and directly about the presence of thigh pain, which explains the slightly higher incidences than were previously reported.[75,76] The incidence of thigh pain was retrospectively compared between 118 Co-Cr and 123 Ti-alloy Tri-Lock stems.[56] A slightly lower percentage of patients reported thigh pain at year 2 (8.7%) than at year 1 (9.5%). However, among 192 patients with 1- and 2-year follow-up information, only 9 patients (4.7%) reported thigh pain at both assessments. Average visual analog scale (VAS) pain intensity levels at 1 and 2 years were 1.30 and 1.37, respectively. Comparable rates of thigh pain (7.5% to 9.5%) were reported at 1- and 2-year follow-up among patients receiving Co-Cr and Ti stems. Stem size appeared to be an important determinant of thigh pain at 1 year, with smaller sizes (<10 cm in length) reporting a significantly lower incidence of thigh pain than larger sizes (3% and 15%, respectively). The significance level disappeared after 2 years (6% and 11%, respectively). VAS intensity appeared to be higher in the larger stem size groups. The authors concluded that not the elastic modulus of the stem but the moment of inertia, which is changed by the stem size, was the determining factor for the development of postoperative thigh pain.[56] In another minimum 2-year follow-up study (mean, 4.7 years) comparing 199 Co-Cr and 191 Ti-based Tri-Lock stems, the incidence of thigh pain was 5% for the whole group, but 7% of Co-Cr stems and 3% of Ti stems were associated with thigh pain. It is interesting to note that Dorr C-type femurs were associated with the lowest prevalence of thigh pain (1.8%). No correlation between stem size and thigh pain was found in this study.[73]

Stress Shielding

Stress shielding can be found in all total hip replacements, both cemented and uncemented.[59] Dual-energy x-ray absorptiometry (DEXA) of femurs containing cemented prostheses has demonstrated marked loss of BMD of greater than 40% as early as 1 to 3 years postoperatively.[61] This loss of BMD is equal to, if not greater than, that seen in cementless stems.[60] Moreover, unlike the situation around stems inserted without cement, bone loss around cemented implants seems to be progressive after 3 years of follow-up.[60,61]

The long-term fixation of any uncemented stem depends on how the region of femoral bone around the stem adapts to the prevailing stress distribution. Several features of uncemented stems might influence the extent of proximal stress shielding. Ample evidence indicates that proximal stress shielding around first-generation, well-fixed, Co-Cr, extensively coated implants such as the AML stem is considerable (18%).[31] This stress shielding may be related to the extent of the surface coating, but it also may be a direct result of the stiffness of the Co-Cr stem, which may cause a modular mismatch between the stem and the bone. However, Hennessy[32] reported that radiographic stress shielding at 10 years with the Prodigy stem, which is a modification of the AML stem, was found to be mild in 54% (41 hips), moderate in 26% (20 hips), and severe in 1% (1 hip) of cases. In other words, the incidence of stress shielding noted with a fully coated stem and an improved modulus of elasticity in comparison with the stiffer AML stem remained high. This indicates that the extent of coating might be a very important parameter for stress shielding. In an RCT, MacDonald[34] compared femoral BMD changes with DEXA scanning in 72 patients following the Synergy and Prodigy stem at a minimum of 2 years' follow-up (mean, 6.4 years). No differences were found except for the BMD change in Gruen zone 7, which was 24% with the fully coated stem and 15% with the proximally coated stem. At 2 years' follow-up, the Synergy stem demonstrated substantial bone loss in Gruen zones 1, 6, and 7, and the Prodigy stem revealed an almost identical pattern, with substantial bone loss in Gruen zones 1, 2, 6, and 7. It is interesting to note that the authors found that patients with a greater baseline BMD (≥80th percentile) were at greater risk of having a greater percentage of bone loss over time. The effect of stem size on bone loss was also evaluated. The Prodigy stem showed no differences in percentage of bone loss associated with stem size. However, larger stem sizes within the Synergy group were associated with a greater percentage of bone loss in Gruen zone 7.[34]

The configuration of the press-fit of the stem may also play an important role. Gibbons compared the change in BMD of the AML stem with that of the CLS stem.[78] These stems have a comparable extent of coating but differ in terms of metallurgy and initial press-fit. Investigators used DEXA scanning at a mean of 40 months for the AML stem and 52 months for the CLS stem. They found that the greatest loss of BMD was located in Gruen zone 7 and the least loss in Gruen zone 5. Loss of BMD was greater in all zones with the AML stem compared with the CLS stem, but only to a statistically significant level in Gruen zones 6 and 7. The press-fit principle of the CLS stem is that it allows a more gradual distribution of stress from proximal to distal because there is only a proximal press-fit and no press-fit in the upper diaphysis. This creates a more physiologic loading situation with less proximal stress shielding than occurs with the AML stem, which has a diaphyseal fit. Aldinger reported on a prospective longitudinal study of the CLS stem with a median follow-up of 84 months including 26 patients and a separate cross-sectional study with a median follow up of 156 months involving 35 patients.[58] Results showed that after the initial remodeling process, which lasted a year, no further bone loss occurred up to 84 months.[58] In addition, the minimum 15-year follow-up study of Aldinger in patients 55 years of age or younger treated with the CLS stem showed that no patients had radiographic stress shielding according to the criteria of Engh.[9] These findings were confirmed in another study by Aldinger involving 257 CLS stems followed for at least 17 years.[11]

Long-Term Results

Delauney[73] assessed 133 THAs using the Zweymuller Alloclassic stem and subdivided patients into two subgroups. One group was younger than 65 years and was deemed to have "an excellent bone stock." The second group included patients of all ages. One hundred eighteen replacements were reviewed with a mean follow-up of 7 years, and overall survivorship at 10 years was 95.4%. No difference in survivorship was noted between groups, but an early reoperation rate and proximal stress shielding were more common in the group of patients of all ages. Proximal stress shielding was observed in 7.6% of patients, and the incidence of thigh pain was 2.5%.[73] Grubl[17] reported on the 10-year results of 133 hips with the Zweymuller prosthesis from a consecutive series of 200 patients. Three stems were revised—none for aseptic loosening. The probability of survival of the stem was 99%, and the incidence of thigh pain was 3%.[17] Garcia-Cimbrelo[16] followed 104 hips with a Zweymuller implant in a consecutive series of 124 implants for a minimum of 10 years (mean, 11 years). At maximum follow-up, no stems were revised. The worst case scenario survivorship at 12 years was 85.3%; this was due mainly to failure of the acetabular components. The cumulative probability of having femoral osteolysis was 17% at 12 years. The prevalence of thigh pain was 13.5%.[16] Finally, Suckel[79] presented the minimum 15-year results of 320 Zweymuller THAs, of which 150 were available for follow-up. The survival rate of the stem was 98% after 17 years. Radiographic stress shielding was found in Gruen zones 1 (12%) and 7 (18%).[79]

The CLS component was introduced by Spotorno during the mid-1980s. Aldinger reported on a consecutive series of 354 THAs with the CLS stem.[39] Mean follow-up was 12 years (range, 10 to 15 years), and overall survivorship with aseptic loosening as the endpoint was 95% at 12 years. However, taking into account 8 revisions of the stem for infection and 3 for periprosthetic fracture, overall survival was 92% at 12 years. Radiolucent lines less than 2 mm were noted in Gruen zones 1 and 7 in 16% and 14% of cases, respectively. The high rate of acetabular loosening was a concern in this study. Schramm reported a series of 107 hips (94 patients) with the CLS stem that were followed for a mean of 10.3 years (range, 10 to 12 years).[75] Grade 3 osteolysis was seen in 35% of patients. Mild, occasional

thigh pain noted in 17% of patients did not interfere with work or activities. A consecutive report on 257 hips with a mean 17-year follow-up (range, 15 to 20 years) was published by Aldinger.[11] The femoral component was revised in 35 hips: 8 for infection, 9 for periprosthetic fracture with stem loosening, 1 for traumatic loosening, and 17 for aseptic loosening. Survival of the stem was 88% at 17 years, and survival of the stem with revision for aseptic loosening as the endpoint was 94% at 17 and 20 years. No thigh pain was reported. No distal femoral osteolysis was found. No instance of distal cortical hypertrophy was seen, and no obvious stress shielding was reported. Pedestal formation at the tip of the prosthesis was seen in 31 hips (17%). In another study, Aldinger[12] reported on the 15- to 20-year results of 154 CLS stems in patients younger than 55 years. Twelve stems (8%) had been revised, including 5 for aseptic loosening and 5 for periprosthetic fracture.

Mallory[18] reported the 10-year minimum follow-up of 120 primary Mallory-Head THAs. Three stems (2.5%) had to be revised because of aseptic loosening, yielding 97.5% survivorship. He reported the incidence of mild or absent thigh pain as 96.6%. Distal femoral osteolysis was observed in less than 2% of cases.[18] We reported on the 10- to 13-year performance of a nonconsecutive series of 307 Mallory-Head THAs in 283 patients.[14] Overall 10-year Kaplan-Meier survivorship was 90% for the hip replacement and 99% for the stem. Again, a vast majority of revisions were directed toward the acetabular component, and none of the stems was revised for aseptic loosening. No stems were radiographically loose. Mild stress shielding limited to Gruen zones 1 and 7 was seen in 153 (50%) patients. It is interesting to note that some distal cortical hypertrophy was noted in about 50% of patients, but this was not correlated with an increased incidence of thigh pain because activity-related thigh pain was present in only 10 (3%) patients.[14] Similarly, 20-year results of an RCT conducted at our institution to compare the results of cementless and cemented fixation of the Mallory-Head THA showed that the survival rate of the stem was 99%, with only 1 stem of 126 being revised for aseptic loosening. The 20-year survival rate of the cementless THA (76%) was still significantly higher than that of the cemented THA (63%) (P = .018).[26]

McLaughlin[19] reported on the 20-year results (range, 18 to 22 years) of 145 Taperloc stems. Sixty-five hips in 58 patients were still available for follow-up, and 80 patients had died. Including those who had died, 1 patient had undergone revision of the stem for aseptic loosening, and a total of 13 stems (9%) had been revised for any reason. In 8 hips (6%), the femoral component was revised during acetabular revision, but in all 8 of these revisions, the femoral component was well fixed to the bone. The 22-year Kaplan-Meier survivorship, with revision of the femoral component for any reason as the endpoint, was 87%, and the prevalence of revision for aseptic loosening of the femoral component was less than 1%. In addition, Parvizi[20] has shown that adding hydroxyapatite to the coating of the stem does not influence the survival of this stem at 10 years.

Teloken[43] published 10- to 15-year follow-up results of the Tri-Lock stem in 67 hips (58 patients). Forty-nine hips (45 patients) were available for review. No revisions were needed for aseptic loosening of the stem. The prevalence of thigh pain was 2%. Sakalkale[42] reported on 71 THAs with a minimum 10-year follow-up (mean, 11.5 years) in 60 patients using the Tri-Lock. The overall mechanical failure rate was 5%, and the incidence of thigh pain (1.4%) was very low.[42] Purtill and coauthors[41] reported their 15-year experience with the Tri-Lock and the Taperloc used in patients with osteoarthritis or rheumatoid arthritis, and in octogenarians. The overall incidence of thigh pain was 2% with the Tri-Lock system and 4% with the Taperloc system. Thigh pain was noted in 4% of octogenarians and in 2% of patients with rheumatoid arthritis. Twelve percent of the Tri-Lock stems had to be revised, but this was caused by lack of modularity during acetabular revision.[41]

Osseointegration has been questioned in patients in whom the bone stock is not deemed of appropriate morphology to accept a tapered femoral component. Typically this corresponds to the Dorr type C femur. Keisu,[80] however, reported on a 2- to 11-year follow-up series of 123 Taperloc stems in 114 patients ranging from 80 to 89 years old. Twenty-three patients (26%) had Dorr type C femurs. For the 92 hips that were available for review, Harris Hip Scores improved from a mean of 42 to a mean of 82 at last follow-up. No femoral components had to be revised, and all components showed stable bone ingrowth. The authors concluded that cementless fixation in octogenarians was safe, effective, and durable.[80] This conclusion is supported by our clinical experience with the Synergy stem.

CONCLUSIONS

Tapered, anatomic, and cylindrical cementless stems with distal fixation all demonstrate durable fixation with good long-term survivorship. Tapered stems manufactured from titanium alloy induce a graduated load transfer to the proximal femur, which reduces excessive proximal stress shielding. In addition, the elastic modularity of the titanium alloy approaches the modularity of the femoral bone; as a consequence, a low incidence of thigh pain has been found. Appropriate morphology of the proximal femoral anatomy such as a Dorr type A or B femur together with a femur of suitable surface finish will increase the chance of osseointegration, although few problems have been found with Dorr type C femurs. In addition, a number of improvements have accompanied the evolution of cementless tapered femoral components. These have included a better femoral neck design to enhance the range of motion without impingement and options to restore leg length and femoral offset.

REFERENCES

1. Collis DK: Cemented total hip replacement in patients who are less than fifty years old. J Bone Joint Surg Am 66:353–359, 1984.
2. Dorr LD, Takei GK, Conaty JP: Total hip arthroplasties in patients less than forty-five years old. J Bone Joint Surg Am 65:474–479, 1983.
3. Ranawat CS, Atkinson RE, Salvati EA, Wilson PD Jr: Conventional total hip arthroplasty for degenerative joint disease in patients between the ages of forty and sixty years. J Bone Joint Surg Am 66:745–752, 1984.
4. Stauffer RN: Ten-year follow-up study of total hip replacement. J Bone Joint Surg Am 64:983–990, 1982.
5. Sutherland CJ, Wilde AH, Borden LS, Marks KE: A ten-year follow-up of one hundred consecutive Muller curved-stem total hip-replacement arthroplasties. J Bone Joint Surg Am 64:970–982, 1982.
6. Callaghan JJ, Dysart SH, Savory CG: The uncemented porous-coated anatomic total hip prosthesis: two-year results of a prospective consecutive series. J Bone Joint Surg Am 70:337–346, 1988.
7. Campbell AC, Rorabeck CH, Bourne RB, et al: Thigh pain after cementless hip arthroplasty: annoyance or ill omen. J Bone Joint Surg Br 74:63–66, 1992.
8. Dodge BM, Fitzrandolph R, Collins DN: Noncemented porous-coated anatomic total hip arthroplasty. Clin Orthop Relat Res 269:16–24, 1991.
9. Engh CA, Bobyn JD, Glassman AH: Porous-coated hip replacement: the factors governing bone ingrowth, stress shielding, and clinical results. J Bone Joint Surg Br 69:45–55, 1987.
10. Ritter MA, Keating EM, Faris PM: A porous polyethylene-coated femoral component of a total hip arthroplasty. J Arthroplasty 5:83–88, 1990.
11. Aldinger PR, Jung AW, Breusch SJ, et al: Survival of the cementless Spotorno stem in the second decade. Clin Orthop Relat Res 467:2297–2304, 2009.
12. Aldinger PR, Jung AW, Pritsch M, et al: Uncemented grit blasted straight tapered titanium stems in patients younger than 55 years of age: fifteen to twenty year results. J Bone Joint Surg (Am) 91:1432–1439, 2009.
13. Belmont PJ Jr, Powers CC, Beykirch SE, et al: Results of the anatomic medullary locking total hip arthroplasty at a minimum of twenty years: a concise followup of previous reports. J Bone Joint Surg (Am) 90:1524–1530, 2008.
14. Bourne RB, Rorabeck CH, Patterson JJ, Guerin J: Tapered titanium cementless total hip replacements: a 10- to 13-year followup study. Clin Orthop Relat Res 393:112–120, 2001.
15. Engh CA, McGovern TF, Engh CA, Jr, Macalino GE: Clinical experience with the anatomic medullary locking (AML) prosthesis for total hip replacement. In Morrey BF, editor: Biological, material, and mechanical considerations of joint replacement, New York, 1993, Raven Press, pp 167–184.
16. Garcia-Cimbrelo E, Cruz-Pardos A, Madero R, Ortega-Andreu M: Total hip arthroplasty with use of the cementless Zweymuller Alloclassic system: a ten- to thirteen-year follow-up study. J Bone Joint Surg Am 85:296–303, 2003.
17. Grubl A, Chiari C, Gruber M, et al: Cementless total hip arthroplasty with a tapered, rectangular titanium stem and a threaded cup: a minimum ten-year follow-up. J Bone Joint Surg Am 84:425–431, 2002.
18. Mallory TH, Lombardi AV Jr, Leith JR, et al: Minimal 10-year results of a tapered cementless femoral component in total hip arthroplasty. J Arthroplasty 16(Suppl 1):49–54, 2001.
19. McLaughlin JR, Lee KR: Total hip arthroplasty with an uncemented tapered component. J Bone Joint Surg 90:1290–1296, 2008.
20. Parvizi J, Sharkey PF, Hozack WJ, et al: Prospective matched-pair analysis of hydroxy-apatite coated and uncoated femoral stems in total hip arthroplasty: a concise follow-up of a previous report. J Bone Joint Surg Am 86:783–786, 2004.
21. Kawamura H, Dunbar MJ, Murray P, et al: The porous coated anatomic total hip replacement: a ten- to fourteen-year follow-up study of a cementless total hip arthroplasty. J Bone Joint Surg Am 83:333–338, 2001.
22. Bojescul JA, Xenos JS, Callaghan JJ, Savory CG: Results of the porous coated anatomic total hip arthroplasty without cement at fifteen years. J Bone Joint Surg (Am) 85:1079–1083, 2003.
23. Engh CA Jr, Claus AM, Hopper RH, Jr, Engh CA: Long-term results using the anatomic medullary locking hip prosthesis. Clin Orthop Relat Res 393:137–146, 2001.

24. Engh CA Jr, Culpepper WJ, 2nd, Engh CA: Long-term results of use of the anatomic medullary locking prosthesis in total hip arthroplasty. J Bone Joint Surg Am 79:177–184, 1997.

25. Mulliken BD, Bourne RB, Rorabeck CH, Nayak N: A tapered titanium femoral stem inserted without cement in a total hip arthroplasty: radiographic evaluation and stability. J Bone Joint Surg Am 78:1214–1225, 1996.

26. Au K, Corten K, Bourne RB, et al: Cemented and cementless total hip arthroplasty: a randomized controlled trial at 17 to 21 years of follow-up. Presented at Canadian Orthopaedic Association Meeting, Whistler, British Columbia, July 3–6, 2009.

27. Min BW, Song KS, Bae KC, et al: The effect of stem alignment on the results of total hip arthroplasty with a cementless tapered-wedge femoral component. J Arthroplasty 23:418–423, 2008.

28. Rorabeck CH, Bourne RB, Laupacis A, et al: A double-blind study of 250 cases comparing cemented with cementless total hip arthroplasty: cost-effectiveness and its impact on health-related quality of life. Clin Orthop Relat Res 298:156–164, 1994.

29. Xenos JS, Callaghan JJ, Heekin RD, et al: The porous-coated anatomic total hip prosthesis, inserted without cement: a prospective study with a minimum of ten years of follow-up. J Bone Joint Surg Am 81:74–82, 1999.

30. Yoon TR, Rowe SM, Kim MS, et al: Fifteen- to 20- year results of uncemented tapered fully porous-coated cobalt chrome stems. Int Orthop 32:317–323, 2008.

31. Engh CA, Bobyn JD: The influence of stem size and extent of porous coating on femoral bone resorption after primary cementless hip arthroplasty. Clin Orthop Relat Res 231:7–28, 1988.

32. Hennessy DW, Callaghan JJ, Liu SS: Second-generation extensively porous-coated THA stems at minimum 10 year follow-up. Clin Orthop Relat Res 467:2290–2296, 2009.

33. Li E, Meding JB, Ritter MA, et al: The natural history of a posteriorly dislocated total hip replacement. J Arthroplasty 14:964–968, 1999.

34. MacDonald SJ, Rosenzweig S, Guerin JS, et al: Proximally versus fully porous coated femoral stems: a multicenter randomized trial. Clin Orthop Relat Res 468:424–431, 2010.

35. Burke DW, Bragdon CR, O'Connor DO, et al: Dynamic measurement of interface mechanics in vivo and the effect of micromotion on bone ingrowth into a porous surface device under controlled loads in vivo. Trans Orthop Res Soc 16:103, 1991.

36. Jasty M, Bragdon C, Burke D, et al: In vivo skeletal responses to porous-surfaced subjected to small induced motions. J Bone Joint Surg 79:707–714, 1997.

37. Mallory TH, Head WC, Lombardi AV, Jr: Tapered design for the cementless total hip arthroplasty femoral component. Clin Orthop Relat Res 344:172–178, 1997.

38. Albrektsson T, Branemark PI, Hansson HA, Lindstrom J: Osseointegrated titanium implants: requirements for ensuring a long-lasting, direct bone-to-implant anchorage in man. Acta Orthop Scand 52:155–170, 1981.

39. Aldinger PR, Breusch SJ, Lukoschek M, et al: A ten- to 15-year follow-up of the cementless Spotorno stem. J Bone Joint Surg Br 85:209–214, 2003.

40. Capello WN, D'Antonio JA, Feinberg JR, Manley MT: Ten-year results with hydroxyapatite-coated total hip femoral components in patients less than fifty years old: a concise follow-up of a previous report. J Bone Joint Surg Am 85:885–889, 2003.

41. Purtill JJ, Rothman RH, Hozack WJ, Sharkey PF: Total hip arthroplasty using two different cementless tapered stems. Clin Orthop Relat Res 393:121–127, 2001.

42. Sakalkale DP, Eng K, Hozack WJ, Rothman RH: Minimum 10-year results of a tapered cementless hip replacement. Clin Orthop Relat Res 362:138–144, 1999.

43. Teloken MA, Bissett G, Hozack WJ, et al: Ten to fifteen-year follow-up after total hip arthroplasty with a tapered cobalt-chromium femoral component (tri-lock) inserted without cement. J Bone Joint Surg Am 84:2140–2144, 2002.

44. Wagner H, Wagner M: Cone prosthesis for the hip joint. Arch Orthop Trauma Surg 120:88–95, 2000.

45. Oonishi H, Yamamoto M, Ishimaru H, et al: The effect of hydroxyapatite coating on bone growth into porous titanium alloy implants. J Bone Joint Surg Br 71:213–216, 1989.

46. Dorr LD, Faugere MC, Mackel AM, et al: Structural and cellular assessment of bone quality of proximal femur. Bone 14:231–242, 1993.

47. Devane PA, Horne JG: Assessment of polyethylene wear in total hip replacement. Clin Orthop Relat Res 369:59–72, 1999.

48. McGrory BJ, Morrey BF, Cahalan TD, et al: Effect of femoral offset on range of motion and abductor muscle strength after total hip arthroplasty. J Bone Joint Surg Br 77:865–869, 1995.

49. Sakalkale DP, Sharkey PF, Eng K, et al: Effect of femoral component offset on polyethylene wear in total hip arthroplasty. Clin Orthop Relat Res 388:125–134, 2001.

50. Schmalzried TP, Shepherd EF, Dorey FJ, et al: The John Charnley Award. Wear is a function of use, not time. Clin Orthop Relat Res 381:36–46, 2000.

51. Claus AM, Engh CA Jr, Sychterz CJ, et al: Radiographic definition of pelvic osteolysis following total hip arthroplasty. J Bone Joint Surg (Am) 85:1519–1526, 2003.

52. Dolhain P, Tsigaras H, Bourne RB, et al: The effectiveness of dual offset stems in restoring offset during total hip replacement. Acta Orthop Belg 68:490–499, 2002.

53. Pancanti A, Bernakiewicz M, Viceconti M: The primary stability of a cementless stem varies between subjects as much as between activities. J Biomech 36:777–785, 2003.

54. Woolson ST, Adler NS: The effect of partial or full weight bearing ambulation after cementless total hip arthroplasty. J Arthroplasty 17:820–825, 2002.

55. Berry DJ: Epidemiology: hip and knee. Orthop Clin North Am 30:183–190, 1999.

56. Lavernia C, D'Appuzo M, Hernandez V, Lee D: Thigh pain in primary total hip arthroplasty: the effects of elastic moduli. J Arthroplasty 19(Suppl 2):10–16, 2004.

57. Brown TE, Larson B, Shen F, Moskal JT: Thigh pain after cementless total hip arthroplasty: evaluation and management. J Am Acad Orthop Surg 10:385–392, 2002.

58. Aldinger PR, Sabo D, Pritsch M, et al: Pattern of periprosthetic bone remodeling around stable uncemented tapered hip stems: a prospective 84-month follow-up study and a median 156-month cross-sectional study with DXA. Calcif Tissue Int 73:115–121, 2003.

59. Deleted in proof.

60. Bobyn JD, Mortimer ES, Glassman AH, et al: Producing and avoiding stress shielding: laboratory and clinical observations of noncemented total hip arthroplasty. Clin Orthop Relat Res 274:79–96, 1992.

61. Hughes SS, Furia JP, Smith P, Pellegrini VD: Atrophy of the proximal part of the femur after total hip arthroplasty without cement: a quantitative comparison of cobalt-chromium and titanium femoral stems with use of dual x-ray absorptiometry. J Bone Joint Surg Am 77:231–239, 1995.

62. McCarthy CK, Steinberg CC, Agren M, et al: Quantifying bone loss from the proximal femur after total hip arthroplasty. J Bone Joint Surg Am 73:774–778, 1991.

63. Parvizi J, Keisu KS, Hozack WJ, et al: Primary total hip arthroplasty with an uncemented femoral component: a long-term study of the Taperloc stem. J Arthroplasty 19:151–156, 2004.

64. Johnsen SP, Sørensen HT, Lucht U, et al: Patient-related predictors of implant failure after primary total hip replacement in the initial, short- and long-terms. J Bone Joint Surg Br 88:1303–1308, 2006.

65. Woo RY, Morrey BF: Dislocations after total hip arthroplasty. J Bone Joint Surg Am 64:1295–1306, 1982.

66. Yuan L, Shih C: Dislocation after total hip arthroplasty. Arch Orthop Trauma Surg 119:263–266, 1999.

67. Masonis JL, Bourne RB: Surgical approach, abductor function, and total hip arthroplasty dislocation. Clin Orthop Relat Res 405:46–53, 2002.

68. Demos HA, Rorabeck CH, Bourne RB, et al: Instability in primary total hip arthroplasty with the direct lateral approach. Clin Orthop Relat Res 393:168–180, 2001.

69. Lewinnek GE, Lewis JL, Tarr R, et al: Dislocations after total hip-replacement arthroplasties. J Bone Joint Surg Am 60:217–220, 1978.

70. Moskal JT, Mann JW 3rd: A modified direct lateral approach for primary and revision total hip arthroplasty: a prospective analysis of 453 cases. J Arthroplasty 11:255–266, 1996.

71. Stephenson PK, Freeman MA: Exposure of the hip using a modified anterolateral approach. J Arthroplasty 6:137–145, 1991.

72. Kelley SS, Lachiewicz PF, Hickman JM, Paterno SM: Relationship of femoral head and acetabular size to the prevalence of dislocation. Clin Orthop Relat Res 355:163–170, 1998.

73. Healy WL, Tilzey JF, Iorio R, et al: Prospective, randomized comparison of cobalt-chrome and titanium Trilock femoral stems. J Arthroplasty 24:831–836, 2009.

74. Delaunay C, Bonnomet F, North J, et al: Grit-blasted titanium femoral stem in cementless primary total hip arthroplasty: a 5- to 10-year multicenter study. J Arthroplasty 16:47–54, 2001.

75. Schramm M, Keck F, Hohmann D, Pitto RP: Total hip arthroplasty using an uncemented femoral component with taper design: outcome at 10-year follow-up. Arch Orthop Trauma Surg 120:407–412, 2000.

76. Callaghan JJ, Templeton JE, Liu SS, et al: Improved results using extensively coated THA stems at minimum 5-year followup. Clin Orthop Relat Res 453:91–96, 2006.

77. Danesh-Clough T, Bourne RB, Rorabeck CH, McCalden R: The mid-term results of a dual offset uncemented stem for total hip arthroplasty. J Arthroplasty 22:195–203, 2007.

78. Gibbons CE, Davies AJ, Amis AA, et al: Periprosthetic bone mineral density changes with femoral components of differing design philosophy. Int Orthop 25:89–92, 2001.

79. Suckel A, Geiger F, Kinzl L, et al: Long-term results for the uncemented Zweymuller/Alloclassic hip endoprosthesis. J Arthroplasty 24:846–853, 2009.

80. Keisu KS, Orozco F, Sharkey PF, et al: Primary cementless total hip arthroplasty in octogenarians: two- to eleven-year follow-up. J Bone Joint Surg Am 83:359–363, 2001.

FURTHER READING

Belmont PJ Jr, Powers CC, Beykirch SE, et al: Results of the anatomic medullary locking total hip arthroplasty at a minimum of twenty years: a concise followup of previous reports. J Bone Joint Surg Am 90:1524–1530, 2008.

Bobyn JD, Mortimer ES, Glassman AH, et al: Producing and avoiding stress shielding: laboratory and clinical observations of noncemented total hip arthroplasty. Clin Orthop Relat Res 274:79–96, 1992.

Bojescul JA, Xenos JS, Callaghan JJ, Savory CG: Results of the porous coated anatomic total hip arthroplasty without cement at fifteen years. J Bone Joint Surg Am 85:1079–1083, 2003.

Campbell AC, Rorabeck CH, Bourne RB, et al: Thigh pain after cementless hip arthroplasty: annoyance or ill omen. J Bone Joint Surg Br 74:63–66, 1992.

Engh CA Jr, Culpepper WJ, 2nd, Engh CA: Long-term results of use of the anatomic medullary locking prosthesis in total hip arthroplasty. J Bone Joint Surg Am 79:177–184, 1997.

McLaughlin JR, Lee KR: Total hip arthroplasty with an uncemented tapered component. J Bone Joint Surg Am 90:1290–1296, 2008.

Oonishi H, Yamamoto M, Ishimaru H, et al: The effect of hydroxy-apatite coating on bone growth into porous titanium alloy implants. J Bone Joint Surg Br 71:213–216, 1989.

Rorabeck CH, Bourne RB, Laupacis A, et al: A double-blind study of 250 cases comparing cemented with cementless total hip arthroplasty: cost-effectiveness and its impact on health-related quality of life. Clin Orthop Relat Res 298:156–164, 1994.

CHAPTER 70

Uncemented Short Metaphyseal Femoral Components

S. David Stulberg and Ronak M. Patel

KEY POINTS

- Metaphyseal fit and ingrowth can provide rotational and axial stability without distal diaphyseal support.
- Bone remodeling after insertion of metaphyseal engaging short stems shows endosteal condensation and cortical hypertrophy in the proximal metaphyseal region of the femur.
- Functional Harris hip scores and Western Ontario and McMaster University (WOMAC) Osteoarthritis Index pain scores are equivalent in patients with metaphyseal engaging short stems and uncemented stems of conventional length.
- The surgical technique used for accurately, reproducibly inserting metaphyseal short stems is virtually identical to the technique used for inserting cementless stems of conventional length.
- Short stems reduce the incidence of periprosthetic fracture associated with metaphyseal-diaphyseal mismatch.

INTRODUCTION

Total hip arthroplasty (THA) is a highly successful, safe, and cost-effective intervention for the treatment of patients with moderate and severe degenerative arthritis. Porous-coated, uncemented femoral stems were introduced in the 1980s for use in total hip arthroplasty. Uncemented stems, which achieve their fixation by porous diaphyseal fixation or by porous metaphyseal fixation–nonporous diaphyseal contact, produce dependable long-term fixation and pain-free function in patients of all ages and bone quality and in those with a wide range of clinical function.[1-59] Uncemented, porous femoral implants are now used routinely in virtually all patients undergoing primary THA in North America. Despite the documented success of these implants, uncemented stems are currently being used in patients whose size, age, level of physical activity, and bone quality present particular challenges for uncemented fixation technologies. These challenges include (1) the need for very long-term fixation; (2) the preservation of proximal femoral bone stock; (3) the potential need for effective femoral component revision; (4) the desire to reproduce a wide range of proximal femoral extra-articular anatomic variations with the provision of multiple offset options; (6) the elimination of thigh pain in extremely active patients of all ages and bone quality;

and (7) the ability to insert implants safely, securely, and reproducibly via specific surgical approaches (e.g., direct anterior) that are currently being evaluated and promoted. The success that has been achieved with uncemented femoral stems of a wide range of designs is now encouraging investigators to consider uncemented femoral implant concepts that address these challenges without compromising the high level of success attainable with current uncemented femoral components.

In particular, clinicians have expressed an interest in short uncemented stem designs that rely for their stability on femoral metaphyseal fixation. The purposes of this chapter are to (1) review the principles underlying these types of femoral components, (2) describe the various design characteristics of these stems, (3) summarize initial clinical results with these stems, and (4) suggest the direction that these design concepts may take in the near future.

FUNCTIONS OF THE DIAPHYSEAL AND METAPHYSEAL PORTIONS OF UNCEMENTED FEMORAL STEMS

To understand the design rationale that is currently being applied to short, metaphyseal engaging femoral stems, it is important to consider the function of each portion of a femoral implant. The section of the femoral component that engages the diaphysis contributes to the initial stability of the device. This portion of the component may be cylindrical or tapered (Fig. 70-1*a* through *c*). Tapered stems may be two-dimensional (a coronal taper and a nontapered rectangular lateral border) or three-dimensional (tapered in both coronal and sagittal planes). The diaphyseal engaging stem may be made of cobalt-chrome alloy or titanium alloy. It may be fully coated with a three-dimensional porous surface, a thin layer of hydroxyapatite, a grit-blasted finish of varying degrees of roughness, or a combination of some or all of these surfaces. The diaphyseal portion of the stem may be polished. The femoral stem may have flutes to resist rotation and/or slots to reduce stiffness. The intended function of the diaphyseal portion of a femoral stem is reflected in its shape, metallurgy, and surface treatment.

Cylindrical, cobalt-chromium, extensively porous coated stems (e.g., anatomic medullary locking [AML])

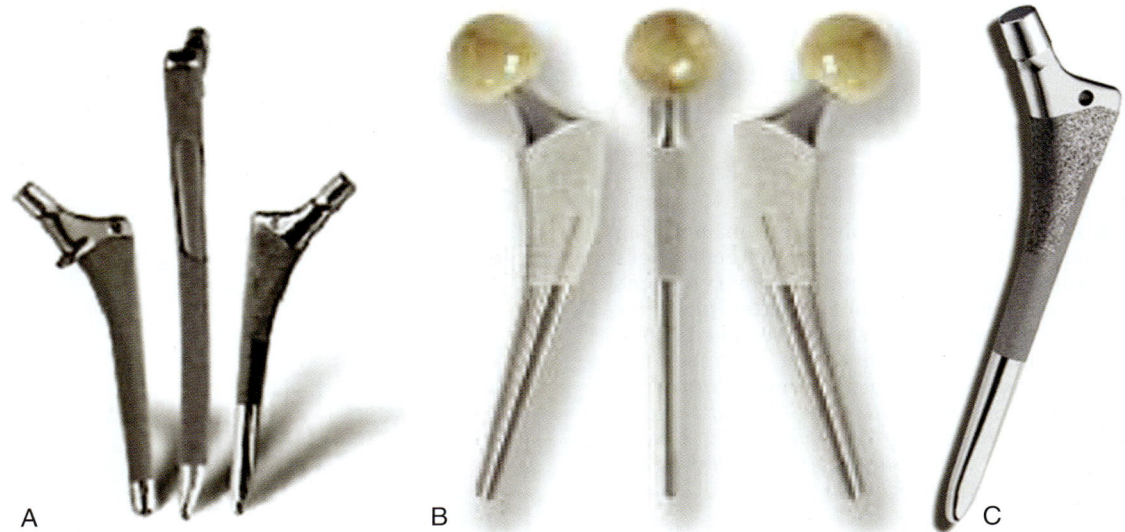

A   B   C

Figure 70-1. A through **C,** The section of the femoral component that engages the diaphysis contributes to the initial stability of the device. This portion of the component may be cylindrical or tapered and may be porous coated, hydroxyapatite coated, grit-blasted, smooth, or a combination. **A,** Cylindrical with various coating lengths. **B,** Narrow tapered stem. **C,** Anatomic tapered stem.

are designed to provide rigid initial **and** long-term fixation in the diaphysis. Initial axial fixation is achieved by tightly engaging a significant segment of the endosteal diaphyseal cortex. Although this engagement with the diaphysis may provide initial rotational stability, the porous coating also provides some resistance to rotational stresses. Long-term fixation is achieved by bone ingrowth into the porous coating. The long-term clinical and radiographic results of cylindrical, extensively coated stems have been extensively documented.[21,22,60-72] The long-term stability of stems of this design is excellent in patients of all ages and bone quality. Consistent concerns associated with these stems have included stress shielding and thigh pain[11,66,67,72-83] (Fig. 70-2). Cylindrical stems without porous coating may be made of cobalt-chromium or titanium alloys. The surfaces may be grit-blasted to varying degrees or polished. Cylindrical stems with a titanium alloy core and a flexible polymer coating are also available.[27,46,84] These stems are designed to provide a degree of initial axial and rotational fixation by coming in contact with the diaphysis, but they avoid the stress shielding and thigh pain that might be associated with large, long, metal cylindrical stems.

Cylindrical femoral components with absence of a diaphyseal porous coating rely on metaphyseal bone contact to enhance their initial axial and, especially, rotational stability. Moreover, these stems seek long-term fixation through bone ingrowth or ongrowth at the metaphysis. These stems achieve metaphyseal stability by attempting to optimize resistance to rotation with rectangular shapes, lateral antirotation ridges, or wedge shapes. Some implants with uncoated cylindrical stems seek to achieve rotational stability and optimized proximal bone restoration by maximizing the fit and fill of the metaphysis (e.g., the PCA implant). All current metaphyseal engaging implants with nonporous coated

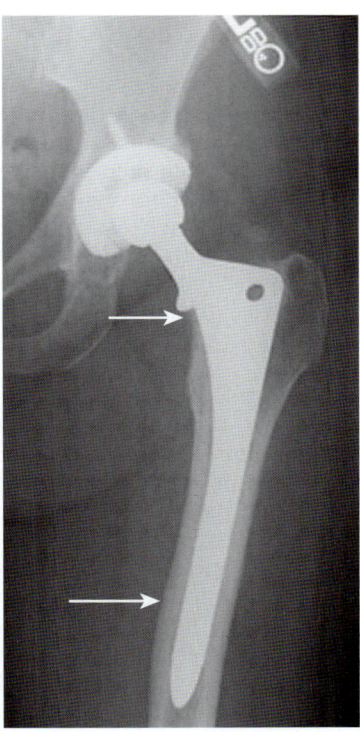

Figure 70-2. Consistent concern associated with extensively porous-coated, cylindrical stems has been stress shielding. Poor bone remodeling in a well-fixed, extensively porous-coated femoral stem.

diaphyseal stems seek to increase rotational stability and positive bone remodeling with metaphyseal circumferential porous coatings or ongrowth surfaces. Numerous reports of follow-up longer than 10 years indicate that femoral components with cylindrical stems without ingrowth or ongrowth coating are associated with

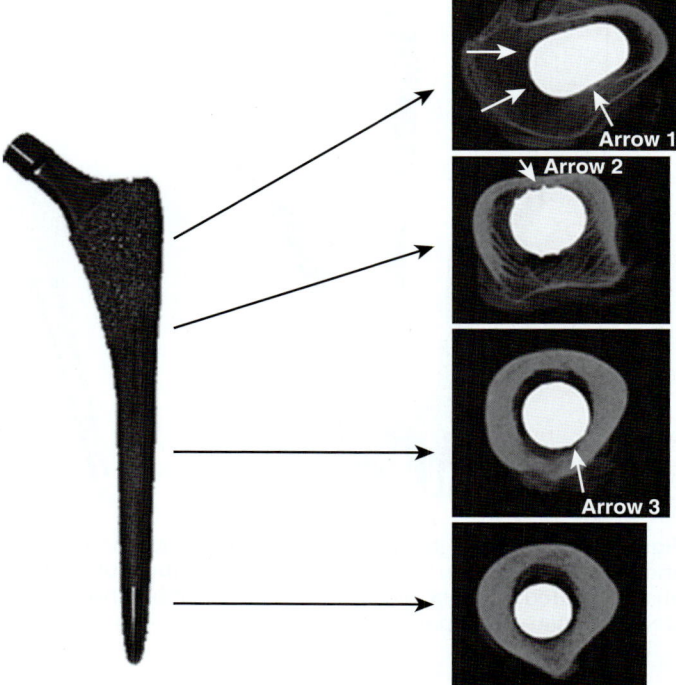

Figure 70-3. Computed tomography scan images from four regions along the length of a tapered cementless femoral implant (Synergy). Proximally, primary cancellous contact occurs. In the proximal quarter, posterior cortical contact is noted *(arrow 1)*. In the second quarter, anterior cortical contact is evident *(arrow 2)*. In the third quarter, cortical contact is seen posteriorly *(arrow 3)*. *(Courtesy Busch CA, Bourne RB: The tapered femoral stem. In Callahan JJ, Rosenberg AG, Rubash HE, editors: The adult hip, ed 2, Philadelphia, 2007, Lippincott Williams & Wilkins, pp 1025–1035.)*

durable fixation and very satisfactory and reliable clinical results.* The goals of stems of this design are to reduce the incidence of thigh pain and stress shielding associated with extensively porous-coated, cylindrical stems while retaining, through osseointegration in the metaphysis, durable fixation. In general, stems of this design appear to be associated with a lower incidence of thigh pain and less proximal stress shielding than extensively coated, cobalt-chromium, cylindrical stems.[†]

Tapered uncemented femoral components seek to achieve fixation in two phases.[100] Initial rigid fixation is achieved by three-point self-locking fixation (Fig. 70-3). When the tapered stem is securely inserted into the cylindrical femur, hoop stresses are generated. When stress relaxation of the femur has occurred, equilibrium is set up between bone and stem, and the axially loaded tapered component will not advance. In principle, this mechanism of initial axial fixation works best in proximal femoral morphologies with tapered medullary shapes. Therefore stems of this design are best applied to Dorr type A (champagne fluted) and type B (funnel shaped) and are less well suited to type C (cylindrical shape) femurs.[90,100] The proximal component taper seeks to maximize implant-bone contact with the intramedullary proximal femoral shaft taper and to provide a gradual loading profile to the proximal femur.

Establishment of rotational stability of tapered stems is critical for achieving initial rigid fixation of tapered stems. Some tapered stem designs (e.g., Zweymuller [Zimmer Inc., Swindon, United Kingdom] and

cementless locking stem [CLS]) are rectangular. Some (e.g., Taperloc, Biomet, Warsaw, Ind) have antirotation lateral ridges. Other stems (e.g., the Synergy stem, Smith & Nephew, Fort Washington, Pa) have wedge-shaped proximal geometries. Still others (e.g., the ABG stem, Stryker Corporation, Berkshire, United Kingdom) have anatomically shaped metaphyseal designs that seek to achieve rotational stability by maximizing fit and fill in the proximal femur (Fig. 70-4).

The second stage of fixation sought by tapered stems occurs in the metaphysis and depends on the presence of a circumferential ingrowth or ongrowth surface.[100] It is believed that the more extensive the area of contact between implant and metaphyseal bone contact, the more secure will be the secondary fixation, and the more positive will be the proximal bone restoration and remodeling. The goals of tapered stems are to achieve rigid durable fixation, to eliminate thigh pain, and to minimize stress shielding. A substantial number of studies have established the clinical and radiographic reliability and durability of tapered stems of many designs.* In general, the use of femoral components with tapered diaphyseal stems is associated with less thigh pain than implants with cylindrical stems.[9,74,77,83,100]

In summary, the diaphyseal portions of femoral stems, both cylindrical and tapered, are designed to provide primary axial stability to the component and varying degrees of rotational stability. These portions of the implant are particularly critical for achievement of rigid initial fixation. The metaphyseal portion of femoral implants provides initial rotational stability. Provision

---

*References 4, 5, 7, 12-14, 16, 20, 24, 25, 29, 31, 34, 43, 51, and 85-99.
[†]References 4, 14, 16, 25, 31, 43, 60, 76, 77, 83, 85, 89, 90, and 96.

*References 2, 3, 6, 7, 9, 10, 15, 17, 18, 26, 28, 32, 36, 37, 39-43, 45, 48-50, 53-59, 95, and 100-111.

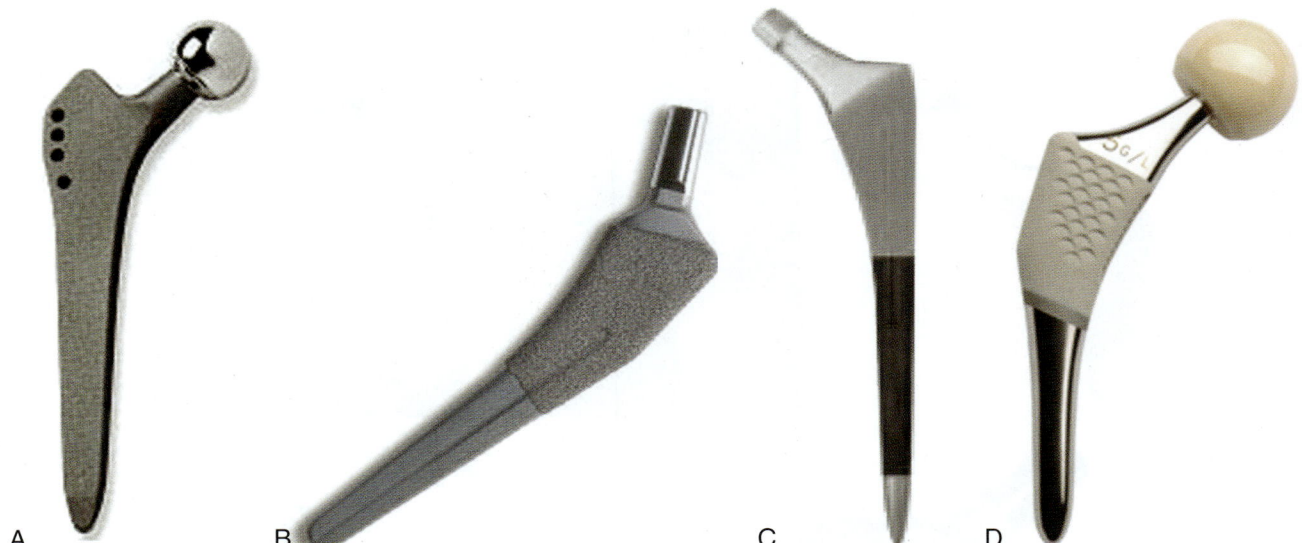

A   B   C   D

Figure 70-4. Tapered stem designs may achieve proximal stability with **(A)** rectangular shapes (Zweymuller); **(B)** antirotation lateral wedges (Taperloc); **(C)** wedge-shaped proximal geometries (Synergy); and **(D)** anatomic-fit/fill-metaphyseal designs (ABG). **A,** Tapered stem with antirotational rectangular shape (Zweymuller). **B,** Tapered stem with antirotation ridges (Taperloc). **C,** Tapered stem with wedge metaphyseal design (Synergy). **D,** Tapered stem with anatomic metaphyseal design (ABG).

of this stability may be particularly important in stems of tapered designs or polished cylindrical designs, in which localized bone contact and absence of porous coating reduce that resistance to rotation provided by the diaphyseal portion of these implants.

DESIGN RATIONALE AND REQUIREMENTS FOR UNCEMENTED, SHORT, METAPHYSEAL ENGAGING STEMS

Short, uncemented, metaphyseal engaging stems seek to address the following issues: (1) the need for very long-term fixation in young patients; (2) the preservation of proximal femoral bone stock, particularly in young patients and patients with poor proximal femoral bone quality; (3) the potential need for effective, bone-preserving femoral component revision; (4) the elimination of thigh pain in extremely active patients of all ages and bone quality; and (5) the ability to insert implants safely, securely, and reproducibly using specific surgical approaches, in particular, the direct anterior approach.[112] Developers of these stems believe that these goals can be best attained by femoral components that achieve secure enough initial fixation in the metaphysis that the axial and rotational stability provided by the diaphyseal portion of the femoral implant is not important or perhaps even necessary. Long-term fixation of these short components is achieved, it is hoped, in the same manner as that achieved by tapered implants (i.e., metaphyseal ingrowth or ongrowth).

A wide variety of short stem designs have been introduced over the past few years (Fig. 70-5). Although some of these stems incorporate unique design characteristics, many are simply shortened versions of currently available cementless stems. A classification of these short, metaphyseal engaging stems has not yet been developed; however, currently available implants fall into one of two categories: (1) standard neck resection and (2) femoral neck sparing. The former implants are frequently shortened versions of currently available uncemented stems of standard length; the latter often incorporate new, unique design features. Although no accepted definition of "short stem" has been identified, most implants seeking this designation are 110 mm or less from the level of the top of the prosthesis neck to the tip of the stem.

Experience with stems that are shortened versions of cementless stems of standard length and that are inserted using a standard level of neck resection has been gradually accumulating over the past 4 years.[106,112-115] Stems included in this category may have shortened tapered or cylindrical diaphyseal-reaching stems and metaphyseal shapes that range from currently available two- or three-dimensional taper shapes that achieve 2-point wedge fixation in the metaphysis[113] to anatomic shapes that seek to fit and fill the metaphysis.[112] Investigators of these shortened versions of cementless implants of standard length (e.g., the Taperloc Microplasty stem, Biomet; the Citation Short, Stryker) anticipate that the proximal, metaphyseal fixation provided by stems of standard length will be adequate to achieve initial and long-term stability of the shorter versions.

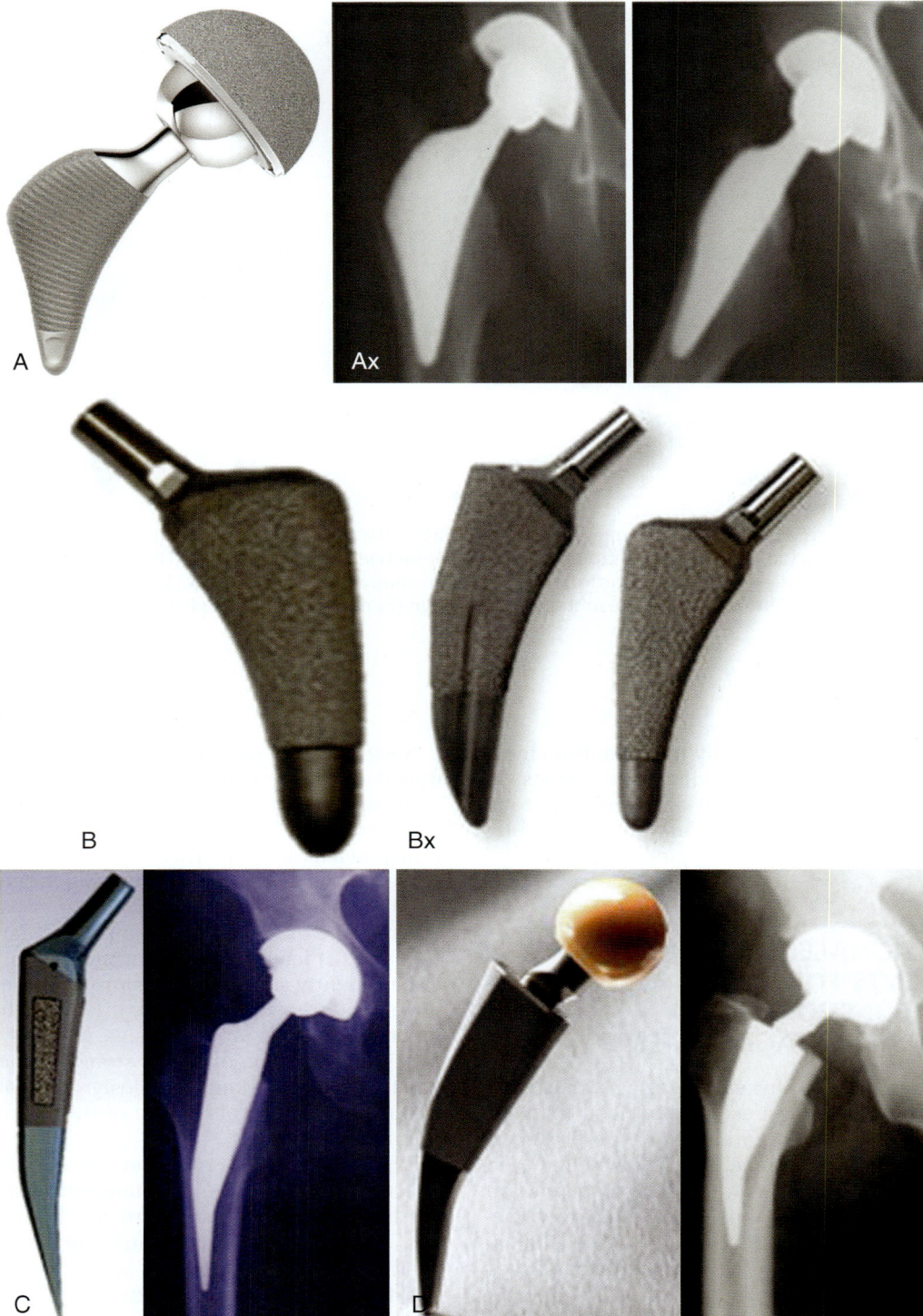

Figure 70-5. A wide variety of short stem designs have been introduced in the past few years. **A,** Proxima stem. **B,** Microplasty Balance and Taperloc stems. **C,** Mayo stem. **D,** Metha stem.

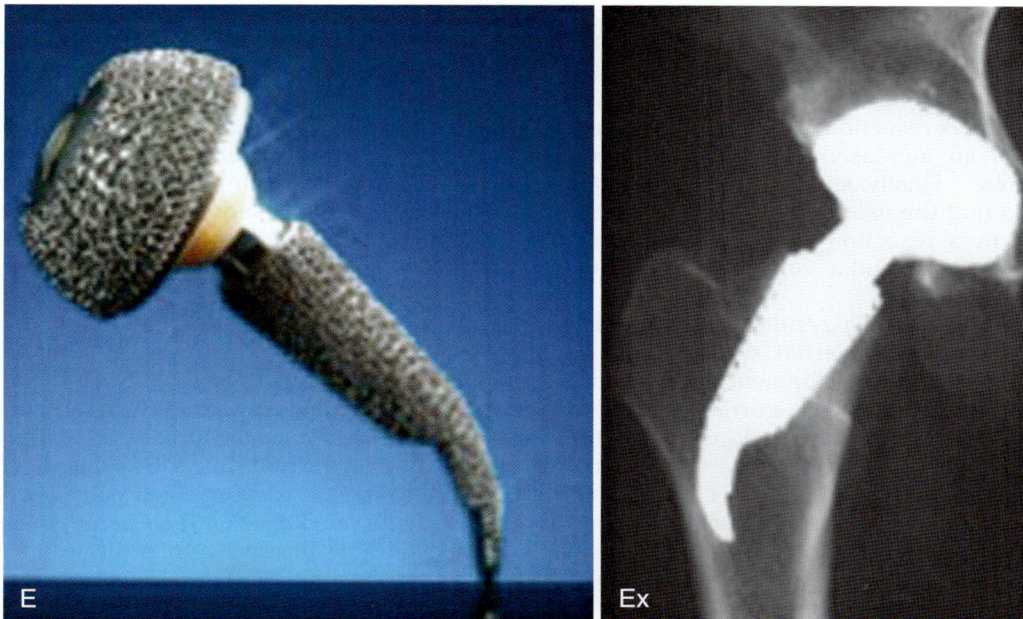

Figure 70-5, cont'd E, Eska stem.

Although extensive laboratory work examining the characteristics of femoral stems, including stem length, has been done for cemented femoral implants, little research has focused on the impact of stem length on the performance of uncemented femoral components.[71,116-118] Therefore, virtually no laboratory evidence underlies the current clinical use of short stems. Early adopters of these types of devices hope that the extremely reliable midterm clinical and radiographic results with stems of standard length will be replicated by the shortened implants. In this early evaluation phase of these short stems, investigators have tended to restrict the use of these devices to patients with good bone quality, those who are younger, and patients who are not excessively large. Moreover, investigators tend to follow a somewhat less aggressive return to full activity and weight bearing than normal.[119,120] These stems are being inserted using all of the surgical approaches and current surgical techniques employed for their standard length counterparts. Initial clinical and radiographic results with these shortened stems of standard metaphyseal design have been encouraging. No reports have described an increased incidence of early stem subsidence or loosening, of unsatisfactory or atypical clinical and functional results, or of inadequate bone ingrowth or remodeling. However, reports on the use of these stems at this time are sparse and describe short-term results from centers responsible for the development of these stems or from centers very familiar with the use of devices of standard length. Nevertheless, it is noteworthy that, unlike the experience with surface replacement arthroplasties, these favorable initial results appear to have been achieved with little if any learning curve. If results in the hands of these initial users are sustained and replicated by the general orthopedic surgical community, it is conceivable that surgeons familiar with the use of devices of standard length can relatively easily adopt the shorter versions. What must be established, however, is whether implants of varying metaphyseal design will produce equally satisfactory clinical and radiographic results when their stems are shortened.

The concept of high femoral neck resection in association with the use of cementless stems has been discussed and evaluated since the earliest days of uncemented total hip arthroplasty.[121-128] The rationale for this concept has been based on the belief that additional initial implant stability and optimal proximal femoral neck preservation can be achieved with this design. Proponents of this concept have suggested that important bone and soft "tissue sparing" occurs with the use of these implants. This tissue preservation is believed to enhance implant fixation, reduce symptoms associated with surgical trauma, improve abductor muscle function, and provide additional bone stock if future procedures are necessary. Both conventional-length (Freeman, Whiteside, Pipino) and short (Mayo) stems have been combined with the concept of high femoral neck resection.

Although results reported by the developers of uncemented femoral components inserted with high femoral neck resection have been encouraging,[116,123,125,129-132] widespread use of these devices has not yet occurred. A number of reasons have been proposed for the slow adoption of this concept. The surgical technique for inserting stems of this design is more difficult than more standard neck resection approaches. The long retained femoral neck can make exposure of the acetabulum difficult. Accurate, reproducible alignment of the femoral stem within the diaphysis may be difficult to accomplish. Restoration of accurate leg length and avoidance of lengthening of the extremity may be difficult to achieve. Moreover, the high neck resection limits exposure of the metaphysis and may reduce the extent and reliability with which metaphyseal fit and contact can be achieved. Concerns have been raised that the combination of high neck resection and short stems may be associated with an increased incidence of proximal femoral fractures.[117] Finally, surgeons and investigators have suggested that the use of implants inserted using a high femoral neck resection may result in increased bone-bone impingement and a consequent reduction in range of motion.

Nevertheless, encouraging results with the original short-stemmed implants inserted with a high neck resection have led to the development of a substantial number of new designs that are currently in various phases of clinical evaluation. Development of these devices is being spurred by a renewed interest in the use of the direct anterior approach for THA, the desire for surgical and implant approaches that minimize soft tissue and bone trauma, and a concern about proximal bone preservation and positive bone remodeling. Increasing concerns regarding the use of metal-on-metal surface replacement arthroplasties are also stimulating interest in the development of reliable, safe, tissue-preserving short-stemmed femoral implants as a possible alternative to surface replacements.

EVOLUTION OF AND EXPERIENCE WITH METAPHYSEAL-ENGAGING SHORT STEMS

For many years, our center has had an interest in the development and application of metaphyseal-engaging short-stemmed femoral components. This interest focused on four issues related to cementless femoral fixation: (1) optimizing load transfer to the proximal femur and preserving femoral bone stock[80,133]; (2) eliminating the potential for proximal metaphyseal and distal diaphyseal mismatch (Fig. 70-6a and b); (3) facilitating the use of potentially less invasive surgical exposures, especially the direct anterior approach; and (4) making possible a bone-conserving revision of the well-fixed, ingrown femoral component, if this was ultimately required. We believed that these issues could and should be addressed without compromising the results that are achievable with current cementless femoral components of standard length. Specifically, the goal was to identify design characteristics of metaphyseal-engaging short-stemmed femoral components that (1) could be inserted reproducibly with a surgical technique that was associated with a minimal learning curve; (2) provided secure enough initial fixation to allow immediate, full weight bearing; (3) allowed a high level of function without thigh pain; (4) could be used in patients of all ages with all bone types; and (5) provided durable fixation with positive proximal femoral bone remodeling.

A pilot clinical study was initiated in 2002 using custom-made short-stem implants.[112] We had had extensive experience with primary custom-made primary femoral components with a conventional stem length. We had accumulated clinical and radiographic data over 10 years that indicated that these stems allowed a high level of function and were associated with extremely reliable uniform, proximal bone ingrowth and dexa-study established proximal load transfer[133] (Fig. 70-7). The customization process allowed us to define and optimize the metaphyseal contact of the device with bone. This extensive and predictable metaphyseal contact would, we hypothesized, reduce the importance of a diaphyseal-engaging stem (Fig. 70-8).

The stems were titanium alloy implants circumferentially coated in the proximal one third to one half with hydroxyapatite on a porous plasma spray surface. The

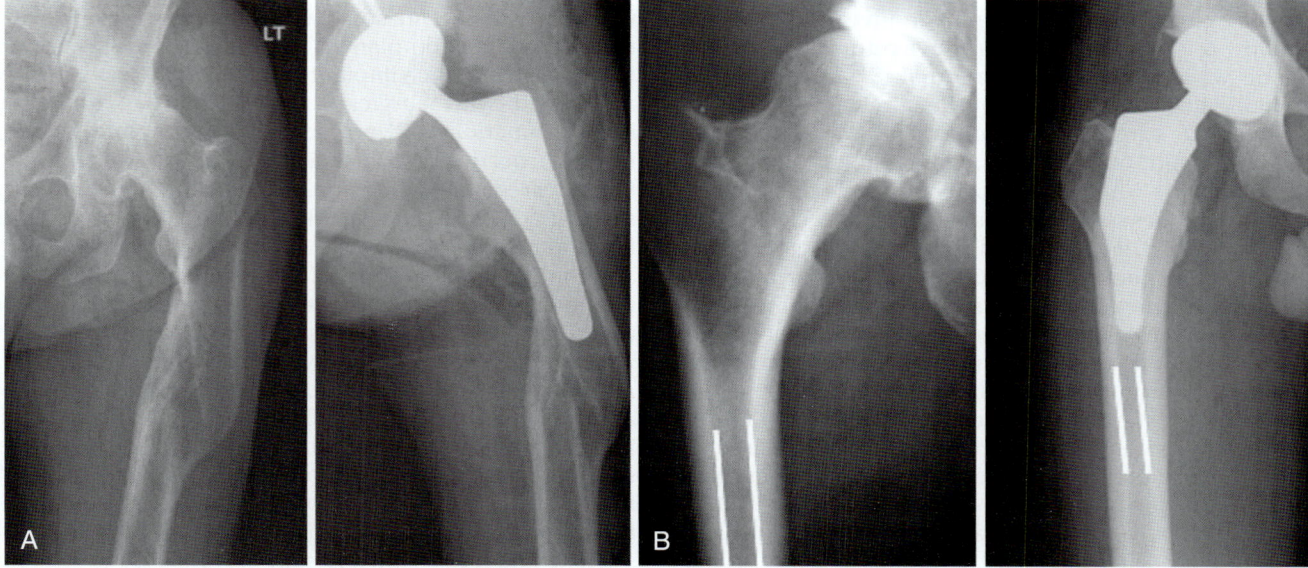

Figure 70-6. Two types of proximal-distal mismatch treated with metaphyseal-engaging, short-stem devices. **A,** Proximal femoral fracture. **B,** Wide metaphysis, narrow diaphysis in a young, robust male patient.

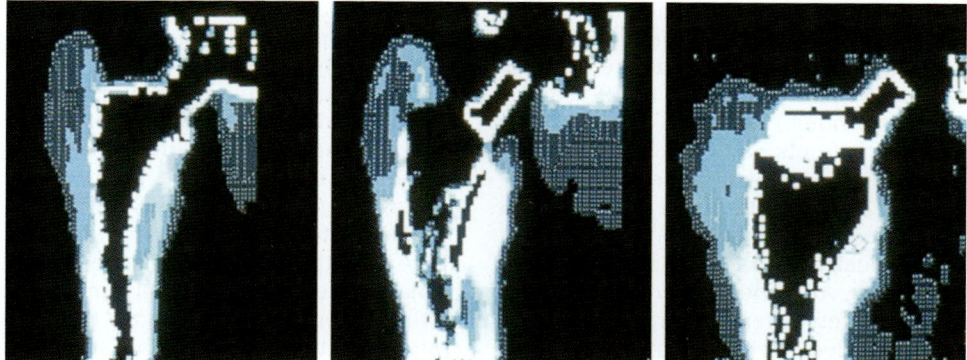

Figure 70-7. Positive bone remodeling over 3 years in a patient with a custom-made femoral stem of coventional length. *(From Wixson RL, Stulberg SD, Van Flandern GJ, Puri L: Maintenance of proximal bone mass with an uncemented femoral stem analysis with dual-energy x-ray absorptiometry. J Arthroplasty 12:365–372, 1997.)*

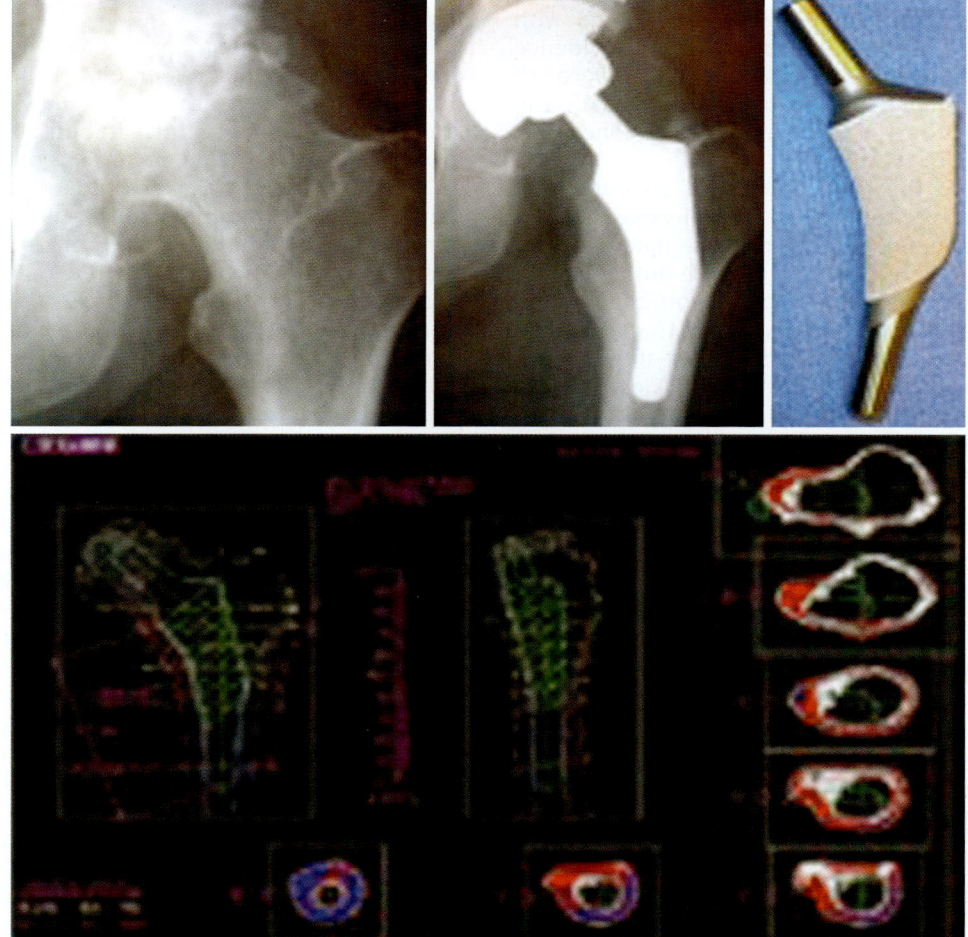

Figure 70-8. A short-stem custom implant was designed from computed tomography (CT) reconstructions using design rules that maximized proximal fit and fill and extended the stem to just beyond the metaphyseal-diaphyseal junction.

remainder of the stem was polished. Average stem length, measured from the base of the femoral neck to the tip of the stem, was 90.4 mm (range, 70 to 105 mm). Stem length was established on computed tomography (CT) scan. Stems were designed to reach the point at which the femoral metaphyseal cortices became parallel and merged with the diaphysis (see Fig. 70-8). The

stems were cylindrical. The implants were inserted using a less invasive, posterolateral exposure that was identical to the surgical technique that had been used to insert custom implants of conventional length.

Sixty-five stems were inserted into 60 consecutive patients undergoing cementless primary total hip arthroplasty (37 men, 23 women). At the time the study was performed, the senior author's indication for cementless total hip arthroplasty was patients younger than age 70. The average age of patients at the time of implant insertion was 56 years (range, 16 to 69 years). The average body mass index (BMI) was 29.1 (range, 26.3 to 54.6). Fifty-seven patients had osteoarthritis and three had avascular necrosis. Twenty-one hips (32%) had Dorr type A bone, 39 hips (60%) had Dorr type B bone, and 5 hips (8%) had Dorr type C bone. Patients have been followed clinically and radiographically for 7 years (minimum, 4 years). All patients were allowed to bear full weight immediately after surgery. Crutch or cane support was continued until the patient walked without a limp.

The average Harris hip score rose from 49 preoperatively to 93 postoperatively. No occurrence of thigh pain has been reported. Two dislocations occurred, one of which required an acetabular revision. No perioperative fractures and no complications were associated with the femoral stem. All stems have radiographic evidence of bone ingrowth. The radiographic pattern of ingrowth included bone bridging and endosteal condensation in the proximal one third of the femur (Gruen zones 1, 2, 6, and 7) (Fig. 70-9).

The purpose of the pilot study was to determine whether extensive, predictable metaphyseal contact with a press-fit, circumferentially porous-coated implant with a short stem could provide reliable initial fixation and durable bone ingrowth. Encouraging clinical and radiographic results of this study led us to carry out a clinical evaluation of an off-the-shelf short-stem device. A variety of commercially available metaphyseal-engaging porous-coated femoral implants of conventional length were evaluated with CT scans. The implant whose metaphyseal femoral shape most closely matched that of the custom-made implants was the Stryker

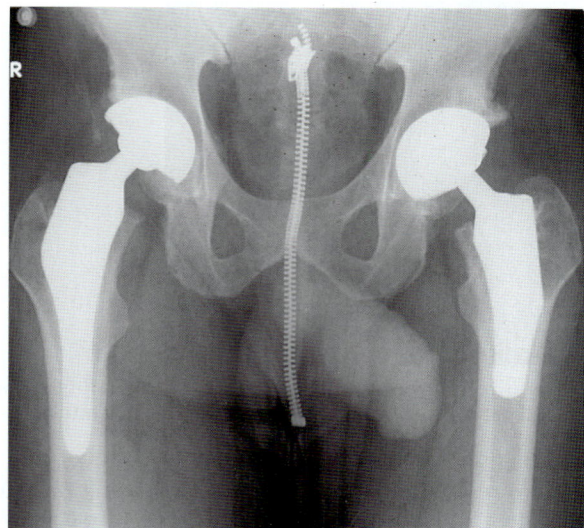

Figure 70-9. Bone remodeling of the proximal femur 4 years after implantation of a short-stem custom-made implant *(left hip)* is similar to bone remodeling observed 10 years after implantation of a custom-made implant of conventional length *(right hip).*

Citation Anatomic Stem. The stem of this device was then shortened to match the length of the short custom implants (Fig. 70-10).

The stems are made of titanium alloy implants circumferentially coated in the proximal one third with hydroxyapatite on a porous plasma spray surface. A transition portion of the stem distal to the porous coating is grit-blasted. The remainder of the stem is polished. Stem length and diameter vary proportionately with the size of the metaphyseal portion of the implant. Average stem length measured from the base of the femoral neck to the tip of the stem was 97 mm (range, 90 to 110 mm). The stem is cylindrical. The metaphyseal portion of the stem is designed to maximize fit and fill and therefore is anatomic in shape. Implants were inserted using a less invasive, posterolateral exposure that was identical to the surgical technique that had been used to insert the short custom implants.

One hundred ninety-four stems were inserted into consecutive patients undergoing primary cementless total hip arthroplasty. Unlike clinically evaluated short-stem custom implants, the Citation Short implant was inserted into all patients, regardless of age, sex, diagnosis, or bone type. One hundred thirty-four hips had clinical and radiographic follow-up information at a minimum of 24 months (range, 24 to 33 months). The average age of patients at the time of implant insertion was 70 years (range, 32 to 95 years). Average BMI was 28 (range, 19 to 63). One hundred eight hips (58%) had Dorr type A bone, 65 hips (35%) had Dorr type B bone, and 14 hips (7%) had Dorr type C bone. All patients were allowed to bear full weight immediately after the surgery. Crutch or cane support was continued until the patient walked without a limp.

The average Harris hip score rose from 52 preoperatively to 92 postoperatively. The clinical results are not significantly different from those achieved with the short custom implant. No occurrence of thigh pain has been reported. Two dislocations occurred, both of which required a polyethylene liner revision. One intraoperative undisplaced periprosthetic fracture was treated with cerclage wiring, and one postoperative minimally displaced fracture with slight component subsidence has not required surgical treatment. All of the stems have radiographic evidence of bone ingrowth. The radiographic pattern of ingrowth included bone bridging and endosteal condensation in the proximal one third of the femur (Gruen zones 1, 2, 6, and 7). The pattern of bone condensation is somewhat more localized than that seen with custom implants and may reflect the somewhat less predictable metaphyseal contact of the off-the-shelf device. Eight stems were placed in varus. This positioning did not adversely affect Harris hip scores or bone ingrowth (Fig. 70-11). The Harris hip scores of patients with Dorr C bone were similar (HHS-100) to those of all other patients.[92] Varus positioning of the implant tended to occur in younger males with Dorr A bone and high offset femoral necks. The robust lateral shoulder of the implant tended to force the device into varus in these patients. Forty-seven patients were older than 70 years at the time of

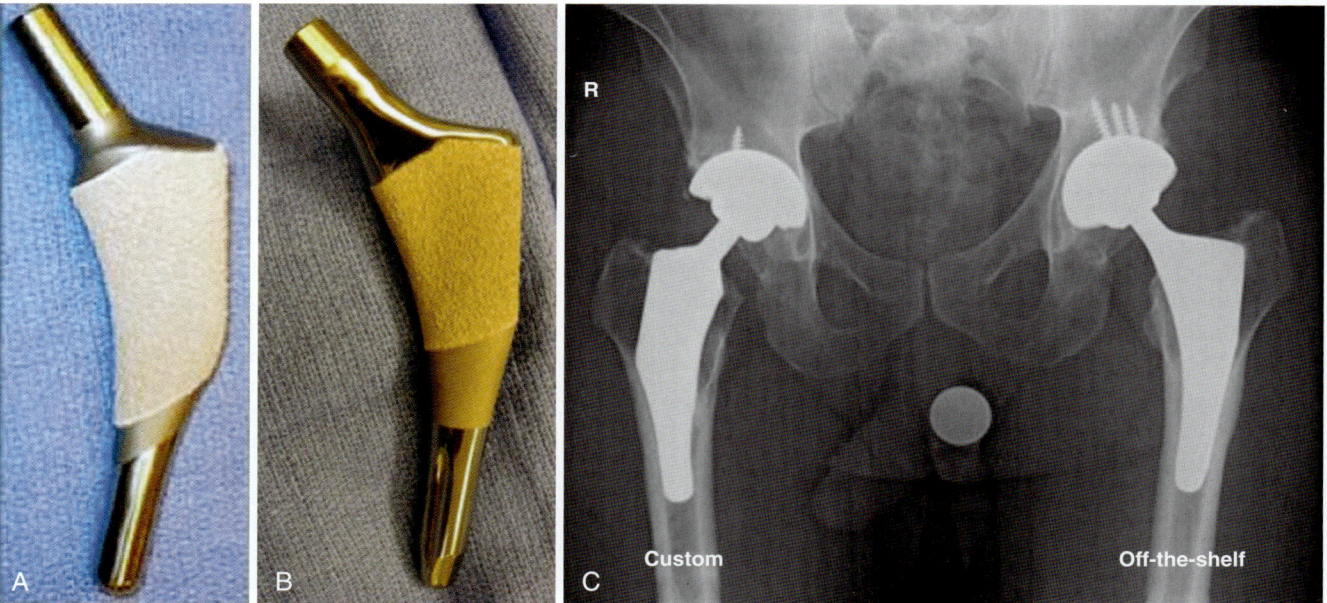

Figure 70-10. The off-the-shelf metaphyseal-engaging short stem had a proximal metaphyseal geometry that was very similar to that of the custom-made short stem.

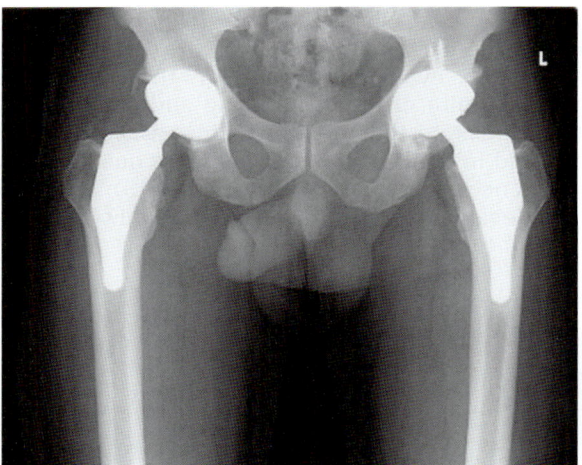

Figure 70-11. Varus position of a short metaphyseal-engaging stem *(left hip)* does not alter clinical or radiographic results 4 years after surgery.

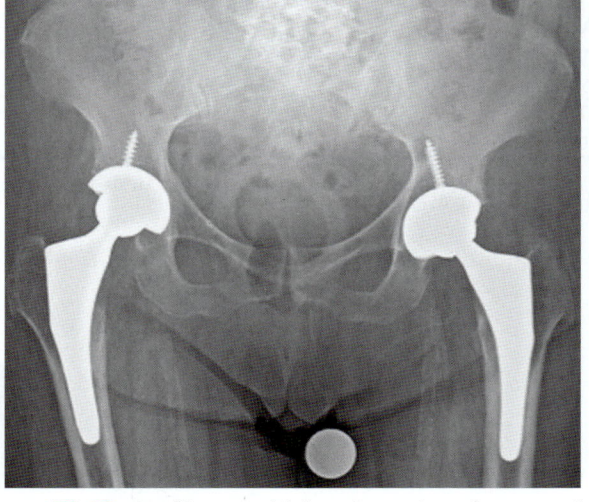

Figure 70-12. An 88-year-old female patient 2 years after insertion of bilateral off-the-shelf short-stem implants.

component implantation (Fig. 70-12). The Harris hip scores of these patients (HHS-88) did not differ from those of all other patients (HHS-92) (Table 70-1).

Results of these evaluations suggest to us that short-stemmed, uncemented, circumferentially proximally porous-coated femoral implants that fill and engage the proximal metaphysis provide reliable, secure fixation to at least 7 years. Use of stems of this design appears to be associated with clinical results that are identical to those of implants of conventional length and with radiographic results that indicate reliable bone ingrowth and positive bone remodeling of the proximal femur. Although varus positioning of these implants did not appear to adversely impact clinical or radiographic

outcomes, the reliable elimination of thigh pain and the avoidance of cortical hypertrophy may require accurate placement of short implants with stems that are designed to avoid significant cortical contact. Our experience with the Citation Short implant suggests that accurate placement of the stem may be influenced by the proximal-lateral geometry of the implant, and that a cylindrical stem is likely to impinge upon the lateral cortex if the device is placed in varus. Therefore, we are currently evaluating a metaphyseal-engaging stem whose proximal geometry is similar to that of the stems that we have previously studied, but whose lateral shoulder has been eliminated and whose distal portion has been tapered. Although initial results with these stems are encouraging, follow-up is too short to determine whether issues related to stem positioning and stem cortical abutment have been addressed successfully.

SUMMARY

Uncemented stems of conventional length produce dependable long-term fixation and pain-free function in patients of all ages and bone quality and in those with a wide range of clinical function. Surgeons with a wide

Table 70-1. Results: Short Custom Stem vs. Short Off-the-Shelf Stem		
Results	**Custom**	**Off-the-Shelf**
Harris hip score (preop)	49	52
Harris hip score (postop)	93	92
Harris hip score (patients >70 years)	NA	88
Harris hip score (Dorr type C)	NA	92
Harris hip score (varus position)	NA	100
WOMAC (preop)	NA	50
WOMAC (postop)	NA	5
WOMAC (postop; patients >70 years)	NA	6
Thigh pain	0	0
Complications		

NA, Not applicable; *WOMAC*, Western Ontario and McMaster University Osteoarthritis Index.

range of experience can insert them safely, reproducibly, and successfully. Uncemented, porous femoral implants are now used routinely in virtually all patients undergoing primary THA. Interest in short, uncemented, metaphyseal-engaging femoral components is being stimulated by the rapidly increasing frequency with which orthopedic surgeons perform total hip surgery in patients whose size, age, level of physical activity, and bone quality present particular challenges for current uncemented femoral fixation technologies. These challenges include (1) the need for very long-term fixation; (2) the preservation of proximal femoral bone stock; (3) the potential need for femoral component revision; (4) the desire to reproduce a wide range of proximal femoral extra-articular anatomic variations with provision of multiple offset options; (5) the elimination of thigh pain in extremely active patients of all ages and bone quality; and (6) the ability to insert implants safely, securely, and reproducibly through specific surgical approaches (e.g., direct anterior) that are currently being evaluated and promoted. Increasing concerns regarding the use of metal-on-metal surface replacement arthroplasties are also stimulating interest in the development of reliable, safe, tissue-preserving, short-stemmed femoral implants as a possible alternative to surface replacements.

Relatively little basic science is available to guide surgeons in the selection of emerging short-stem designs. There is a need to develop preclinical and post-implantation evaluation tools for these short-stem implants. Finite element modeling and simulated and actual stress testing of implants of various designs implanted in femurs with varying bone quality characteristics need to be carried out (Fig. 70-13), as do post-implant evaluations of initial implant stability. Roentgen

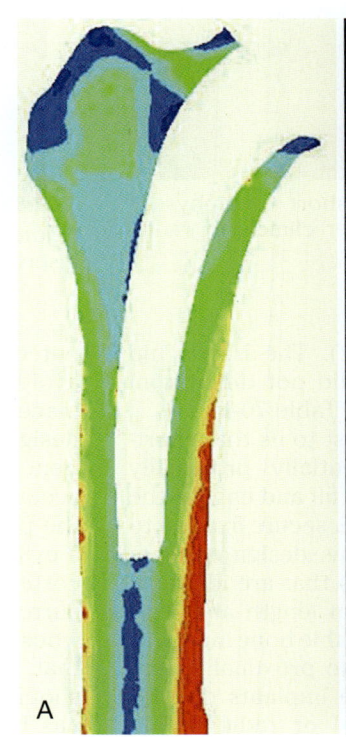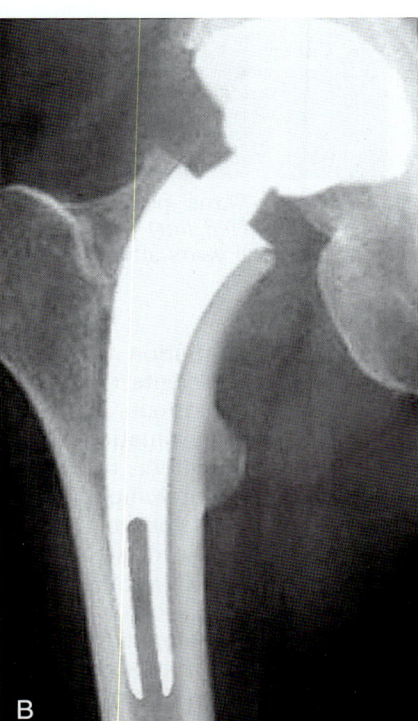

Figure 70-13. A finite element analysis of the ARC high neck resection femoral short stem demonstrating load transfer to the proximal femur performed in premarket evaluation. **A,** Finite element analysis. **B,** Two years post implantation of the ARC stem, appearing to corroborate proximal load transfer predicted by finite element modeling. *(Courtesy Tim McTighe.)*

A   B

stereophotogrammetric analysis (RSA) is a sensitive tool for measuring implant stability, and its use should be encouraged, especially for uniquely shaped short stems and stems designed to be inserted using a high femoral neck resection technique. Postimplantation evaluations should be initiated to assess bone remodeling. Bone remodeling around short-stemmed devices may vary significantly from design to design and is likely to reflect many factors, including bone-implant contact, implant-coating technology, component metallurgy, and implant geometry. The nature and quality of this remodeling may have as important an impact on implant durability as the quality of initial implant fixation. Issues related to long-term bone remodeling might differ, as they do with stems of conventional length, from those that are important for initial implant fixation.

Although lessons learned during the evolution to current uncemented femoral stems of conventional length may be helpful, they provide no assurance that short stems that retain many of the design characteristics of their longer counterparts will match the success of these devices. Moreover, surgeons are now being confronted with a number of intriguing short stem designs that have relatively short clinical follow-up and still unclear indications. Thus, surgeons would be wise to proceed cautiously and thoughtfully with the incorporation of short-stem femoral stem technology into their surgical armamentarium.

Nevertheless, early experiences with uncemented, metaphyseal-engaging short femoral stems do provide guidelines for surgeons interested in this technology. It is apparent that if the design of these stems is similar to that of their longer counterparts, then the learning curve for inserting these implants will probably be short. It should be possible for surgeons to incorporate these short stems into their hip replacement practice without significantly altering their current surgical technique. It also is clear that initial rigid fixation, particularly in rotation, will require extensive metaphyseal contact. Such contact is most likely to be associated with the most optimum proximal bone remodeling. Circumferential porous coatings, with or without hydroxapatite, in the metaphyseal regions of these devices are likely to enhance initial fixation and probably are preferable to grit-blasted finishes. However, it is not known how far down the implant such coatings should extend. This may vary with stem design and may have a significant impact on both initial fixation and long-term bone remodeling. Although it may be wise to proceed more cautiously than usual with resumption of vigorous activity when short-stemmed devices are used, the author's initial experience with devices that extensively engage the metaphysis suggests that it will be possible and safe to allow patients with short-stemmed implants to resume activities in the same way as with components of conventional length. It may also be wise to proceed cautiously with the use of short-stemmed devices in patients with poorer bone quality (Dorr type C). This is particularly true with the use of short tapered stems, which were originally designed to engage the taper of the proximal femur that is present in Dorr type A and B bone. However, our experience with devices that extensively engage the metaphysis suggests that it should be possible and safe to insert these implants in all patients regardless of bone quality. Finally, it remains to be seen whether revision of well-fixed, cementless, metaphyseal-engaging short stems is more bone conserving than revision of cementless implants of conventional length. Virtually no information on this issue is available. If, as developers hope, these short implants are able to achieve the clinical and radiographic results associated with cementless components of conventional length, and if it is possible to revise these implants with minimal bone loss, then the role of cementless, short, metaphyseal-engaging implants will be compelling.

REFERENCES

1. Albrektsson T, Brånemark PI, Hansson HA, Lindström J: Osseointegrated titanium implants: requirements for ensuring a long-lasting, direct bone-to-implant anchorage in man. Acta Orthop Scand 52:155–170, 1981.
2. Aldinger PR, Breusch SJ, Lukoschek M, et al: A ten- to 15-year follow-up of the cementless spotorno stem. J Bone Joint Surg Br 85:209–214, 2003.
3. Aldinger PR, Jung AW, Pritsch M, et al: Uncemented grit-blasted straight tapered titanium stems in patients younger than fifty-five years of age: fifteen to twenty-year results. J Bone Joint Surg Am 91:1432–1439, 2009.
4. Archibeck MJ, Berger RA, Jacobs JJ, et al: Second-generation cementless total hip arthroplasty: eight to eleven-year results. J Bone Joint Surg Am 83:1666–1673, 2001.
5. Berry DJ, Harmsen WS, Ilstrup D, et al: Survivorship of uncemented proximally porous-coated femoral components. Clin Orthop Relat Res 319:168–177, 1995.
6. Bidar R, Kouyoumdjian P, Munini E, Asencio G: Long-term results of the ABG-1 hydroxyapatite coated total hip arthroplasty: analysis of 111 cases with a minimum follow-up of 10 years. Rev Chir Orthop Traumatol 95:579–587, 2009.
7. Bodén H, Salemyr M, Sköldenberg O, et al: Total hip arthroplasty with an uncemented hydroxyapatite-coated tapered titanium stem: results at a minimum of 10 years' follow-up in 104 hips. J Orthop Sci 11:175–179, 2006.
8. Bojescul JA, Xenos JS, Callaghan JJ, Savory CJ: Results of porous-coated anatomic total hip arthroplasty without cement at fifteen years: a concise follow-up of a previous report. J Bone Joint Surg Am 85:1079–1083, 2003.
9. Bourne RB, Rorabeck CH: A critical look at cementless stems: taper designs and when to use alternatives. Clin Orthop Relat Res 355:212–223, 1998.
10. Bourne RB, Rorabeck CH, Patterson JJ, Guerin J: Tapered titanium cementless total hip replacements: a 10- to 13-year followup study. Clin Orthop Relat Res 393:112–120, 2001.
11. Bugbee WD, Culpepper WJ, 2nd, Engh CA Jr, Engh CA Sr: Long-term clinical consequences of stress-shielding after total hip arthroplasty without cement. J Bone Joint Surg Am 79:1007–1012, 1997.
12. Burt CF, Garvin KL, Otterberg ET, Jardon OM: A femoral component inserted without cement in total hip arthroplasty: a study of the Tri-Lock component with an average ten-year duration of follow-up. J Bone Joint Surg Am 80:952–960, 1998.
13. Callaghan JJ: The clinical results and basic science of total hip arthroplasty with porous-coated prostheses. J Bone Joint Surg Am 75:299–310, 1993.
14. Capello WN, D'Antonio JA, Jaffe WL, et al: Hydroxyapatite-coated femoral components: 15-year minimum followup. Clin Orthop Relat Res 453:75–80, 2006.
15. Carl HD, Ploetzner J, Swoboda B, et al: Cementless total hip arthroplasty in patients with rheumatoid arthritis using a tapered designed titanium hip stem minimum: 10-year results. Rheumatol Int 31:353–359, 2011.

16. Clohisy JC, Harris WH: The Harris-Galante uncemented femoral component in primary total hip replacement at 10 years. J Arthroplasty 14:915–917, 1999.

17. Delaunay C, Bonnomet F, North J, et al: Grit-blasted titanium femoral stem in cementless primary total hip arthroplasty: a 5- to 10-year multicenter study. J Arthroplasty 16:47–54, 2001.

18. Delaunay C, Kapandji AI: Survival analysis of cementless grit-blasted titanium total hip arthroplasties. J Bone Joint Surg Br 83:408–413, 2001.

19. Dodge BM, Fitzrandolph R, Collins DN: Noncemented porous-coated anatomic total hip arthroplasty. Clin Orthop Relat Res 269:16–24, 1991.

20. Dorr LD, Takei GK, Conaty JP: Total hip arthroplasties in patients less than forty-five years old. J Bone Joint Surg Am 65:474–479, 1983.

21. Engh CA: Porous-coated fixation forever. Orthopedics 17:775–776, 1994.

22. Engh CA Jr, Culpepper WJ 2nd, Engh CA: Long-term results of use of the anatomic medullary locking prosthesis in total hip arthroplasty. J Bone Joint Surg Am 79:177–184, 1997.

23. Epinette JA, Manley MT: Uncemented stems in hip replacement—hydroxyapatite or plain porous: does it matter? Based on a prospective study of HA Omnifit stems at 15-years minimum follow-up. Hip Int 18:69–74, 2008.

24. Eskelinen A, Remes V, Helenius I, et al: Uncemented total hip arthroplasty for primary osteoarthritis in young patients: a mid- to long-term follow-up study from the Finnish Arthroplasty Register. Acta Orthop 77:57–70, 2006.

25. Gabbar OA, Rajan RA, Londhe S, Hyde ID: Ten- to twelve-year follow-up of the furlong hydroxyapatite-coated femoral stem and threaded acetabular cup in patients younger than 65 years. J Arthroplasty 23:413–417, 2008.

26. Garcia-Cimbrelo E, Cruz-Pardos A, Madero R, Ortega-Andreu M: Total hip arthroplasty with use of the cementless Zwey-muller Alloclassic system: a ten- to thirteen-year follow-up study. J Bone Joint Surg Am 85:296–303, 2003.

27. Goosen JH, Castelein RM, Runne WC, et al: Long-term results of a soft interface- (Proplast-) coated femoral stem. Acta Orthop 77:585–590, 2006.

28. Grübl A, Chiari C, Gruber M, et al: Cementless total hip arthroplasty with a tapered, rectangular titanium stem and a threaded cup: a minimum ten-year follow-up. J Bone Joint Surg Am 84:425–431, 2002.

29. Hallan G, Lie SA, Furnes O, et al: Medium- and long-term performance of 11,516 uncemented primary femoral stems from the Norwegian arthroplasty register. J Bone Joint Surg Br 89:1574–1580, 2007.

30. Healy WL, Casey DJ, Iorio R, Appleby D: Evaluation of the porous-coated anatomic hip at 12 years. J Arthroplasty 17:856–863, 2002.

31. Hellman EJ, Capello WN, Feinberg JR: Omnifit cementless total hip arthroplasty: a 10-year average followup. Clin Orthop Relat Res 364:164–174, 1999.

32. Hofmann AA, Feign ME, Klauser W, et al: Cementless primary total hip arthroplasty with a tapered, proximally porous-coated titanium prosthesis: a 4- to 8-year retrospective review. J Arthroplasty 15:833–839, 2000.

33. Kim YH, Kim JS, Oh SH, Kim JM: Comparison of porous-coated titanium femoral stems with and without hydroxyapatite coating. J Bone Joint Surg Am 85:1682–1688, 2003.

34. Kim YH, Oh SH, Kim JS: Primary total hip arthroplasty with a second-generation cementless total hip prosthesis in patients younger than fifty years of age. J Bone Joint Surg Am 85:109–114, 2003.

35. Landor I, Vavrik P, Sosna A, et al: Hydroxyapatite porous coating and the osteointegration of the total hip replacement. Arch Orthop Trauma Surg 127:81–89, 2007.

36. Leali A, Fetto J: Promising mid-term results of total hip arthroplasties using an uncemented lateral-flare hip prosthesis: a clinical and radiographic study. Int Orthop 31:845–849, 2007.

37. Mallory TH, Lombardi AV Jr, Leith JR, et al: Minimal 10-year results of a tapered cementless femoral component in total hip arthroplasty. J Arthroplasty 16(8 Suppl 1):49–54, 2001.

38. Manning DW, Rubash HE: The proximally ingrown stem. In Barrack RL editor: The hip, Philadelphia, 2006, Lippincott Williams & Wilkins.

39. Marshall AD, Mokris JG, Reitman RD, et al: Cementless titanium tapered-wedge femoral stem: 10- to 15-year follow-up. J Arthroplasty 19:546–552, 2004.

40. McLaughlin JR, Lee KR: The outcome of total hip replacement in obese and non-obese patients at 10- to 18-years. J Bone Joint Surg Br 88:1286–1292, 2006.

41. McLaughlin JR, Lee KR: Total hip arthroplasty with an uncemented tapered femoral component. J Bone Joint Surg Am 90:1290–1296, 2008.

42. McLaughlin JR, Lee KR: Total hip arthroplasty with an uncemented tapered femoral component in patients younger than 50 years. J Arthroplasty 26:9–15, 2011.

43. Meding JB, Galley MR, Ritter MA: High survival of uncemented proximally porous-coated titanium alloy femoral stems in osteoporotic bone. Clin Orthop Relat Res 468:441–447, 2010.

44. Moyer JA, Metz CM, Callaghan JJ, et al: Durability of second-generation extensively porous-coated stems in patients age 50 and younger. Clin Orthop Relat Res 468:448–453, 2010.

45. Müller LA, Wenger N, Schramm M, et al: Seventeen-year survival of the cementless CLS Spotorno stem. Arch Orthop Trauma Surg 130:269–275, 2010.

46. Nagi ON, Kumar S, Aggarwal S: The uncemented isoelastic/isotitan total hip arthroplasty: a 10-15 years follow-up with bone mineral density evaluation. Acta Orthop Belg 72:55–64, 2006.

47. Ostbyhaug PO, Klaksvik J, Romundstad P, Aamodt A: Primary stability of custom and anatomical uncemented femoral stems: a method for three-dimensional in vitro measurement of implant stability. Clin Biomech 25:318–324, 2010.

48. Parvizi J, Keisu KS, Hozack WJ, et al: Primary total hip arthroplasty with an uncemented femoral component: a long-term study of the Taperloc stem. J Arthroplasty 19:151–156, 2004.

49. Parvizi J, Sharkey PF, Hozack WJ, et al: Prospective matched-pair analysis of hydroxyapatite-coated and uncoated femoral stems in total hip arthroplasty: a concise follow-up of a previous report. J Bone Joint Surg Am 86:783–786, 2004.

50. Purtill JJ, Rothman RH, Hozack WJ, Sharkey PF: Total hip arthroplasty using two different cementless tapered stems. Clin Orthop Relat Res 393:121–127, 2001.

51. Reigstad O, Siewers P, Røkkum M, Espehaug B: Excellent long-term survival of an uncemented press-fit stem and screw cup in young patients: follow-up of 75 hips for 15-18 years. Acta Orthop 79:194–202, 2008.

52. Rosenberg AG: Fixation for the millennium: the hip. J Arthroplasty 17(4 Suppl 1):3–5, 2002.

53. Sakalkale DP, Eng K, Hozack WJ, Rothman RH: Minimum 10-year results of a tapered cementless hip replacement. Clin Orthop Relat Res 362:138–144, 1999.

54. Schramm M, Keck F, Hohmann D, Pitto RP: Total hip arthroplasty using an uncemented femoral component with taper design: outcome at 10-year follow-up. Arch Orthop Trauma Surg 120:407–412, 2000.

55. Suckel A, Geiger F, Kinzl L, et al: Long-term results for the uncemented Zweymuller/Alloclassic hip endoprosthesis: a 15-year minimum follow-up of 320 hip operations. J Arthroplasty 24:846–853, 2009.

56. Swanson TV: The tapered press fit total hip arthroplasty: a European alternative. J Arthroplasty 20(4 Suppl 2):63–67, 2005.

57. Teloken MA, Bissett G, Hozack WJ, et al: Ten to fifteen-year follow-up after total hip arthroplasty with a tapered cobalt-chromium femoral component (tri-lock) inserted without cement. J Bone Joint Surg Am 84:2140–2144, 2002.

58. Yoon TR, Rowe SM, Kim MS, et al: Fifteen- to 20-year results of uncemented tapered fully porous-coated cobalt-chrome stems. Int Orthop 32:317–323, 2008.

59. Zweymuller K: A cementless titanium hip endoprosthesis system based on press-fit fixation: basic research and clinical results. Instr Course Lect 35:203–225, 1986.

60. Engh CA, Bobyn JD: The influence of stem size and extent of porous coating on femoral bone resorption after primary cementless hip arthroplasty. Clin Orthop Relat Res 231:7–28, 1988.

61. Engh CA, Bobyn JD, Glassman AH: Porous-coated hip replacement: the factors governing bone ingrowth, stress shielding, and clinical results. J Bone Joint Surg Br 69:45–55, 1987.

62. Engh CA, Jr, Claus AM, Hopper RH Jr, Engh CA: Long-term results using the anatomic medullary locking hip prosthesis. Clin Orthop Relat Res 393:137–146, 2001.

63. Engh CA, Hooten JP, Jr, Zettl-Schaffer KF, et al: Porous-coated total hip replacement. Clin Orthop Relat Res 298:89–96, 1994.

64. Engh CA, Hopper RH, Jr: The odyssey of porous-coated fixation. J Arthroplasty 17(4 Suppl 1):102–107, 2002.

65. Engh CA, Massin P: Cementless total hip arthroplasty using the anatomic medullary locking stem: results using a survivorship analysis. Clin Orthop Relat Res 249:141–158, 1989.

66. Engh CA, et al: A quantitative evaluation of periprosthetic bone-remodeling after cementless total hip arthroplasty. J Bone Joint Surg Am 74:1009–1020, 1992.

67. Gibbons CE, Davies AJ, Amis AA, et al: Periprosthetic bone mineral density changes with femoral components of differing design philosophy. Int Orthop 25:89–92, 2001.

68. Kawamura H, Dunbar MJ, Murray P, et al: The porous coated anatomic total hip replacement: a ten to fourteen-year follow-up study of a cementless total hip arthroplasty. J Bone Joint Surg Am 83:1333–1338, 2001.

69. Kim YH, Kim JS, Cho SH: Primary total hip arthroplasty with the AML total hip prosthesis. Clin Orthop Relat Res 360:147–158, 1999.

70. Kim YH, Kim VE: Cementless porous-coated anatomic medullary locking total hip prostheses. J Arthroplasty 9:243–252, 1994.

71. Kirk KL, Potter BK, Lehman RA, Jr, Xenos JS: Effect of distal stem geometry on interface motion in uncemented revision total hip prostheses. Am J Orthop 36:545–549, 2007.

72. McAuley JP, Culpepper WJ, Engh CA: Total hip arthroplasty: concerns with extensively porous coated femoral components. Clin Orthop Relat Res 355:182–188, 1998.

73. Bobyn JD, Mortimer ES, Glassman AH, et al: Producing and avoiding stress shielding: laboratory and clinical observations of noncemented total hip arthroplasty. Clin Orthop Relat Res 274:79–96, 1992.

74. Bourne RB, Rorabeck CH, Ghazal ME, Lee MH: Pain in the thigh following total hip replacement with a porous-coated anatomic prosthesis for osteoarthrosis: a five-year follow-up study. J Bone Joint Surg Am 76:1464–1470, 1994.

75. Bragdon CR, Burke D, Lowenstein JD, et al: Differences in stiffness of the interface between a cementless porous implant and cancellous bone in vivo in dogs due to varying amounts of implant motion. J Arthroplasty 11:945–951, 1996.

76. Brown TE, Larson B, Shen F, Moskal JT: Thigh pain after cementless total hip arthroplasty: evaluation and management. J Am Acad Orthop Surg 10:385–392, 2002.

77. Campbell AC, Rorabeck CH, Bourne RB, et al: Thigh pain after cementless hip arthroplasty: annoyance or ill omen. J Bone Joint Surg Br 74:63–66, 1992.

78. Dan D, Germann D, Burki H, et al: Bone loss after total hip arthroplasty. Rheumatol Int 26:792–798, 2006.

79. Harvey EJ, Bobyn JD, Tanzer M, et al: Effect of flexibility of the femoral stem on bone-remodeling and fixation of the stem in a canine total hip arthroplasty model without cement. J Bone Joint Surg Am 81:93–107, 1999.

80. Herrera A, Panisello JJ, Ibarz E, et al: Comparison between DEXA and finite element studies in the long-term bone remodeling of an anatomical femoral stem. J Biomech Eng 131:041013, 2009.

81. Mueller LA, Nowak TE, Haeberle L, et al: Progressive femoral cortical and cancellous bone density loss after uncemented tapered-design stem fixation. Acta Orthop 81:171–177, 2010.

82. Pitto RP, Hayward A, Walker C, Shim FB: Femoral bone density changes after total hip arthroplasty with uncemented taper-design stem: a five year follow-up study. Int Orthop 34:783–787, 2010.

83. Saito J, Aslam N, Tokunaga K, et al: Bone remodeling is different in metaphyseal and diaphyseal-fit uncemented hip stems. Clin Orthop Relat Res 451:128–133, 2006.

84. Ritter MA, Keating EM, Faris PM: A porous polyethylene-coated femoral component of a total hip arthroplasty. J Arthroplasty 5:83–88, 1990.

85. Baltopoulos P, Tsintzos C, Papadakou E, et al: Hydroxyapatite-coated total hip arthroplasty: the impact on thigh pain and arthroplasty survival. Acta Orthop Belg 74:323–331, 2008.

86. Bauer TW, Geesink RC, Zimmerman R, McMahon JT: Hydroxyapatite-coated femoral stems: histological analysis of components retrieved at autopsy. J Bone Joint Surg Am 73:1439–1452, 1991.

87. Capello WN, D'Antonio JA, Feinberg JR, Manley MT: Ten-year results with hydroxyapatite-coated total hip femoral components in patients less than fifty years old: a concise follow-up of a previous report. J Bone Joint Surg Am 85:885–889, 2003.

88. Dalton JE, Cook SD, Thomas KA, Kay JF: The effect of operative fit and hydroxyapatite coating on the mechanical and biological response to porous implants. J Bone Joint Surg Am 77:97–110, 1995.

89. Dorr LD, Absatz M, Gruen TA, et al: Anatomic porous replacement hip arthroplasty: first 100 consecutive cases. Semin Arthroplasty 1:77–86, 1990.

90. Dorr LD, Faugere MC, Mackel AM, et al: Structural and cellular assessment of bone quality of proximal femur. Bone 14:231–242, 1993.

91. Dorr LD, Lewonowski K, Lucero M, et al: Failure mechanisms of anatomic porous replacement I cementless total hip replacement. Clin Orthop Relat Res 334:157–167, 1997.

92. Dorr LD, Wan Z, Song M, Ranawat A: Bilateral total hip arthroplasty comparing hydroxyapatite coating to porous-coated fixation. J Arthroplasty 13:729–736, 1998.

93. Haddad RJ Jr, Cook SD, Thomas KA: Biological fixation of porous-coated implants. J Bone Joint Surg Am 69:1459–1466, 1987.

94. Meding JB, Ritter MA, Keating EM, Faris PM: Comparison of collared and collarless femoral components in primary uncemented total hip arthroplasty. J Arthroplasty 12:273–280, 1997.

95. Meding JB, Ritter MA, Keating EM, et al: A comparison of collared and collarless femoral components in primary cemented total hip arthroplasty: a randomized clinical trial. J Arthroplasty 14:123–130, 1999.

96. Mont MA, Yoon TR, Krackow KA, Hungerford DS: Clinical experience with a proximally porous-coated second-generation cementless total hip prosthesis: minimum 5-year follow-up. J Arthroplasty 14:930–939, 1999.

97. Noble PC, Alexander JW, Lindahl LJ, et al: The anatomic basis of femoral component design. Clin Orthop Relat Res 235:148–165, 1988.

98. Oonishi H, Yamamoto M, Ishimaru H, et al: The effect of hydroxyapatite coating on bone growth into porous titanium alloy implants. J Bone Joint Surg Br 71:213–216, 1989.

99. Pancanti A, Bernakiewicz M, Viceconti M: The primary stability of a cementless stem varies between subjects as much as between activities. J Biomech 36:777–785, 2003.

100. Busch CA, Bourne RB: The tapered femoral stem. In Callahan JJ, Rosenberg AG, Rubash HE editors: The adult hip, ed 2, Philadelphia, 2007, Lippincott Williams & Wilkins, pp 1025–1035.

101. Bodén HS, Sköldenberg OG, Salemyr MO, et al: Continuous bone loss around a tapered uncemented femoral stem: a long-term evaluation with DEXA. Acta Orthop 77:877–885, 2006.

102. Keisu KS, Orozco F, Sharkey PF, et al: Primary cementless total hip arthroplasty in octogenarians: two to eleven-year follow-up. J Bone Joint Surg Am 83:359–363, 2001.

103. Mallory TH, Head WC, Lombardi AV Jr: Tapered design for the cementless total hip arthroplasty femoral component. Clin Orthop Relat Res 344:172–178, 1997.

104. Mallory TH, Lombardi AV Jr, Leith JR, et al: Why a taper? J Bone Joint Surg Am 84(Suppl 2):81–89, 2002.

105. Martell JM, Pierson RH, 3rd, Jacobs JJ, et al: Primary total hip reconstruction with a titanium fiber-coated prosthesis inserted without cement. J Bone Joint Surg Am 75:554–571, 1993.

106. Mazoochian F, Schrimpf FM, Kircher J, et al: Proximal loading of the femur leads to low subsidence rates: first clinical

results of the CR-stem. Arch Orthop Trauma Surg 127:397–401, 2007.

107. McLaughlin JR, Lee KR: Total hip arthroplasty with an uncemented femoral component: excellent results at ten-year follow-up. J Bone Joint Surg Br 79:900–907, 1997.

108. Mulliken BD, Bourne RB, Rorabeck CH, et al: A tapered titanium femoral stem inserted without cement in a total hip arthroplasty: radiographic evaluation and stability. J Bone Joint Surg Am 78:1214–1225, 1996.

109. Ragab AA, Kraay MJ, Goldberg VM: Clinical and radiographic outcomes of total hip arthroplasty with insertion of an anatomically designed femoral component without cement for the treatment of primary osteoarthritis: a study with a minimum of six years of follow-up. J Bone Joint Surg Am 81:210–218, 1999.

110. Rothman RH, Hozack WJ, Ranawat A, Moriarty L: Hydroxyapatite-coated femoral stems: a matched-pair analysis of coated and uncoated implants. J Bone Joint Surg Am 78:319–324, 1996.

111. Sinha RK, Dungy DS, Yeon HB: Primary total hip arthroplasty with a proximally porous-coated femoral stem. J Bone Joint Surg Am 86:1254–1261, 2004.

112. Stulberg SD, Dolan M: The short stem: a thinking man's alternative to surface replacement. Orthopedics 31:885–886, 2008.

113. Emerson RH, et al: Short term clinical outcomes of the Taperloc® Microplasty™ stem [internal document], Warsaw, Ind, 2009, Biomet Inc.

114. Chen HH, Morrey BF, An KN, Luo ZP: Bone remodeling characteristics of a short-stemmed total hip replacement. J Arthroplasty 24:945–950, 1995.

115. Renkawitz T, Santori FS, Grifka J, et al: A new short uncemented, proximally fixed anatomic femoral implant with a prominent lateral flare: design rationals and study design of an international clinical trial. BMC Musculoskelet Disord 9:147, 2008.

116. Falez F, Casella F, Panegrossi G, et al: Perspectives on metaphyseal conservative stems. J Orthop Traumatol 9:49–54, 2008.

117. Jakubowitz E, Seeger JB, Lee C, et al: Do short-stemmed prostheses induce periprosthetic fractures earlier than standard hip stems? A biomechanical ex-vivo study of two different stem designs. Arch Orthop Trauma Surg 129:849–855, 2009.

118. Carlson L, Albrektsson B, Freeman MA: Femoral neck retention in hip arthroplasty: a cadaver study of mechanical effects. Acta Orthop Scand 59:6–8, 1988.

119. Hol AM, van Grinsven S, Lucas C, et al: Partial versus unrestricted weight bearing after an uncemented femoral stem in total hip arthroplasty: recommendation of a concise rehabilitation protocol from a systematic review of the literature. Arch Orthop Trauma Surg 130:547–555, 2010.

120. Thien TM, Ahnfelt L, Eriksson M, et al: Immediate weight bearing after uncemented total hip arthroplasty with an anteverted stem: a prospective randomized comparison using radiostereometry. Acta Orthop 78:730–738, 2007.

121. Freeman MA: Why resect the neck? J Bone Joint Surg Br 68:346–349, 1986.

122. Freeman MA, McLeod HC, Levai JP: Cementless fixation of prosthetic components in total arthroplasty of the knee and hip. Clin Orthop Relat Res 176:88–94, 1983.

123. Mannan K, Freeman MA, Scott G: The Freeman femoral component with hydroxyapatite coating and retention of the neck: an update with a minimum follow-up of 17 years. J Bone Joint Surg Br 92:480–485, 2010.

124. Pipino F, Molfetta L: Femoral neck preservation in total hip replacement. Ital J Orthop Traumatol 19:5–12, 1993.

125. Whiteside LA, Amador D, Russell K: The effects of the collar on total hip femoral component subsidence. Clin Orthop Relat Res 231:120–126, 1988.

126. Whiteside LA, Easley JC: The effect of collar and distal stem fixation on micromotion of the femoral stem in uncemented total hip arthroplasty. Clin Orthop Relat Res 239:145–153, 1989.

127. Whiteside LA, McCarthy DS, White SE: Rotational stability of noncemented total hip femoral components. Am J Orthop 25:276–280, 1996.

128. Whiteside LA, White SE, McCarthy DS: Effect of neck resection on torsional stability of cementless total hip replacement. Am J Orthop 24:766–770, 1995.

129. Gagala J, Mazurkiewicz T: [Early experiences in the use of Mayo stem in hip arthroplasty]. Chir Narzadow Ruchu Ortop Pol 74:152–156, 2009.

130. Goebel D, Schultz W: The Mayo cementless femoral component in active patients with osteoarthritis. Hip Int 19:206–210, 2009.

131. Hagel A, Hein W, Wohlrab D: Experience with the Mayo conservative hip system. Acta Chir Orthop Traumatol Cech 75:288–292, 2008.

132. Tadeusz N, Adam N, Lukasz N: [Total hip replacement in young patients with use of Mayo prosthesis—early result of treatment]. Chir Narzadow Ruchu Ortop Pol 72:319–321, 2007.

133. Wixson RL, Stulberg SD, Van Flandern GJ, Puri L: Maintenance of proximal bone mass with an uncemented femoral stem analysis with dual-energy x-ray absorptiometry. J Arthroplasty 12:365–372, 1997.

CHAPTER 71

Highly Cross-Linked Polyethylene Bearings

*J. Benjamin Jackson III, John L. Masonis,
and Thomas Fehring*

KEY POINTS

- Highly cross-linked polyethylene has demonstrated wear rate reduction of between 40% and 95% over conventional polyethylene.
- Current evidence in the literature does not reveal significant rates of osteolysis or autoimmune reaction to highly cross-linked polyethylene.
- Medium-term studies have not demonstrated significant adverse events with highly cross-linked polyethylene and would support its continued use.
- Questions still remain about the long-term significance of reactive oxygen species formation during the cross-linking process.

BACKGROUND

The success of total hip arthroplasty (THA) has been well documented. Since its inception in the 1960s, the major obstacles to success in THA have been component fixation and articular bearing wear. With documented improvements in durable component fixation over the past four decades, wear remains the most troublesome issue in THA. Materials utilized for the acetabular articular bearing in THA have included Teflon, polyurethanes, metal alloys, ceramics, and polyethylenes. Over the past four decades, modifications to the structure and production of polyethylene have shown both positive and negative effects. Polyethylene remains the most widely utilized acetabular bearing surface in the world. Our knowledge of its structure and performance will strongly influence the future of total hip arthroplasty.

POLYETHYLENE MANUFACTURING

Commercial production of ultra-high-molecular-weight polyethylene (UHMWPE) began in the early 1950s. The largest current manufacturer of UHMWPE resin is Ticona (Florence, Ky). All Ticona resins are labeled "GUR." Current medical/orthopedic grade resins include GUR 1020, 1120, 1050, and 1150. The numeric label following GUR explains the details of the resin. The first digit (1) indicates that the resin is for orthopedic usage. The second digit represents the presence (1) or absence (0) of calcium stearate. The third digit indicates the

molecular weight of the resin. The final digit is used for manufacturing corporate coding (1). Although other resins (1900 series produced by Hercules Powder, Wilmington, Del) have been utilized for orthopedic purposes and clinically studied, they are no longer in production. The remainder of this chapter will focus on the current GUR resins in clinical usage (GUR 1020 and GUR 1050).[1]

Polyethylene is composed of repeating ethylene monomers, each of which contains two carbon atoms. Polyethylene molecules contain a crystalline region and an amorphous region. The polyethylene chains can be described as low or high density based on their molecular weight and chain length. Polyethylene begins as a resin or powder and is fabricated into bulk form for orthopedic implant designs. Resins are developed into bulk material by direct compression molding or are machined from ram-extruded bars or large molded sheets.

The mechanical properties of any given polyethylene implant are affected by the resin, the molecular weight, and preparation of the material. The temperature, pressure, and cooling rate during the manufacture of polyethylene will influence its ultimate properties. Final component preparation is completed by direct compression molding (the polyethylene is melted and then is solidified in its desired shape) or by machining the material into its desired shape.

STERILIZATION

Sterilization of polyethylene has become an area of expanded interest. The three current methods of sterilization include ethylene oxide gas, gas plasma, and radiation. A combination of these techniques is utilized in the production of highly cross-linked polyethylene (HCLPE). Ethylene oxide sterilization is completed in an enclosed chamber because of the toxicity of the gas. Following diffusion of ethylene oxide into polyethylene and adequate time for clearance, the polyethylene is biologically sterile. The mechanical properties of polyethylene are unchanged following ethylene oxide sterilization. Gamma radiation sterilization of polyethylene has been utilized for many years. The radiation dosage has varied by manufacturer, but a minimum dose of 2.5 rads is required for adequate sterilization. Radiation sterilization does affect the mechanical properties of polyethylene. Although initially believed to be benign, radiation sterilization can have both positive and negative effects on polyethylene mechanical properties and wear characteristics.

CROSS-LINKING

Cross-linking of polyethylene involves the formation of a complex structure containing multiple polyethylene molecules. Initially, polyethylene cross-linking was an unintentional by-product of radiation sterilization. However, further research found that cross-linked polyethylene is a more mechanically stable material that is more resistant to wear. Manufacturers now use gamma or electron beam radiation to cross-link polyethylene. When polyethylene is irradiated, the polyethylene chains are broken and the molecules are able to re-form with increased cross-linking to adjacent polyethylene molecules, or they become free radicals that are capable of bonding to other molecules present in the material. If oxygen is present at the time of irradiation, the free radical polyethylene molecule can bond to oxygen, thus incorporating oxygen into the polymer structure. Oxygen free radical deposition has been shown to negatively affect the long-term mechanical properties of polyethylene through oxidation.[2]

Once oxidation was recognized as a major contributor to polyethylene wear, multiple strategies were employed to prevent oxygen bonding to free radicals. These strategies include gamma radiation in an oxygen-depleted environment (e.g., nitrogen vacuum) and the addition of other molecules (e.g., vitamin E) to "scavenge" free radicals and prevent oxygen bonding. Although cross-linking improves the wear characteristics of polyethylene, there is a downside to gamma radiation—it impairs the mechanical strength of polyethylene. The tensile strength and fatigue strength of polyethylene are inversely proportional to the amount of radiation applied to the material. Therefore, the dosage of gamma radiation and cross-linking must be regulated to maximize wear resistance while minimizing the risk of material fatigue failure (fracture). Table 71-1

summarizes the current production techniques used in first- and second-generation HCLPE.

CLINICAL RESULTS

Radiographic Analysis of Polyethylene Wear Rates

Numerous authors have attempted to systematically evaluate the wear rates of first- and second-generation HCLPE components. These studies have used radiostereometric analysis and computer-assisted edge detection techniques (Martell method)[4] for analysis of wear, creep, and penetration rates. Both short- and, more recently, intermediate-term clinical studies have been reported with a maximum follow-up of 7.6 years (Table 71-2).

Six studies have documented radiographic wear rates with more than 6 years of follow-up[6-10] (Table 71-3). Three of these studies used retrospective comparison designs that evaluated first-generation HCLPE versus conventional polyethylene (CPE). McCalden and associates[10] evaluated the wear rate of Longevity versus Trilogy liners using Martell methods and documented a 50% relative wear rate reduction in the HCLPE cohort at a mean of 6.8 years. Rajadhyaksha and colleagues[12] evaluated the wear rate of Crossfire (HCLPE) versus Nitrogen Vac (CPE), using Martell methods, and documented a 74% relative wear reduction in the HCLPE cohort at a mean of 6.1 years. Rohr and coworkers[34] evaluated the wear rate of Crossfire (HCLPE) versus Exeter (CPE) using radiostereometric analysis and documented a 74% relative wear reduction in the HCLPE cohort at a mean of 6 years.

Two additional retrospective studies have evaluated HCLPE wear rates at more than 6 years post implantation. Bragdon and associates evaluated the wear of two distinct HCLPE liners (Longevity and Durasul) at a mean of 6.9 years. Using Martell methods, both cohorts documented extremely low linear wear rates at less than

Table 71-1. Highly Cross-Linked Polyethylene Production Methods

Polyethylene Manufacturing Process

First Generation	GUR	Temp, ° Celsius	Radiation, mrad	Radiation	Thermal Treatment	Sterilization Method	Free Radicals
Longevity (Zimmer)	1020	40	10	Electron beam	Melted	Gas plasma	No
Marathon (DePuy)	1020	21	5	Gamma	Melted	Gas plasma	No
XLPE (Smith and Nephew)	1020	21	10	Gamma	Melted	Ethylene oxide	No
Durasul (Zimmer)	1020	125	9.5	Electron beam	Melted	Ethylene oxide	No
Crossfire (Stryker)	1020	21	7.5	Gamma	Annealed	Gamma in nitrogen	Yes
Second Generation							
Acrom-XL (Biomet)	1020	21	5	Gamma	Annealing and mechanical	Gas plasma	Yes
Crossfire X3 (Stryker)	1050	21	9.9 (3 × 3.3)	Gamma	Annealing	Gas plasma	Yes
E-poly (Biomet)	1020	21	10	Electron beam	Treated with Vitamin E	Gamma in nitrogen	Yes

Table 71-2. Clinical Wear Studies of HCLPE

Author	Design	Participants Analyzed	Implant	Mean Follow-up, yr	Detection Method	Rate
Bragdon et al	Retrospective	72 = HCLPE Group 1	Longevity	6.9	Martell method	−.001 mm/yr
		128 = HCLPE Group 2	Durasul			−.001 mm/yr
Bragdon et al	Retrospective comparative	53 = HCLPE 58 = CPE	Durasul Unclear	3.7	Martell method	.018 mm/yr .144 mm/yr
Bitsch et al		32 = HCLPE 24 = CPE	Marathon Enduron	5.8	Martell method	.031 mm/yr .178 m/yr
Calvert et al	RCT	59 = HCLPE 60 = CPE	Marathon Enduron	4	PolyWare auto	.0239 mm/yr .1276 mm/yr
D'Antonio et al	Retrospective comparative	56 = HCLPE 53 = CPE	Crossfire N_2/Vac	4.9 5.3	Modified Livermore Method	.055 mm/yr .138 mm/yr
Digas et al	Two RCTs combined data	28 = HCLPE 19 = HCLPE	Durasul Longevity	5	RSA	0 mm/yr 0 mm/yr
Dorr et al	Prospective comparative	31 = HCLPE 35 = CPE	Durasul Unclear	5	Martell method	.029 mm/yr .065 mm/yr
Engh et al	RCT	76 = HCLPE 72 = CPE	Marathon Enduron	4.3	Martell method	.01 mm/yr .20 mm/yr
Garvin et al	Retrospective	56 = HCLPE	Longevity	2	Martell method	.041 mm/yr
García-Rey et al	RCT	45 = HCLPE 45 = CPE	Durasul Sulene	5.5	AutoCAD	.006 mm/year .038 mm/yr
Geller et al	Prospective	45 = HCLPE	Longevity	3.3	Martell method	0 mm/yr
Glyn-Jones et al	RCT	26 = HCLPE 25 = CPE	Longevity CPE	3	RSA	.003 mm/yr .007 mm/yr
Heisel et al	Prospective cohort	34 = HCLPE 24 = CPE	Marathon Enduron	2.75 2.2	Martell method	.02 mm/yr .13 mm/yr
Hopper et al	Retrospective comparative	48 = HCLPE 50 = CPE	Marathon Enduron	2.8 2.9	Martell method	.08 mm/yr .18 mm/yr
Krushell et al	Case control	40 = HCLPE 40 = CPE	Crossfire Standard Series II	4 4.1	Ramakrishnan method	.05 mm/yr .12 mm/yr
Lachiewicz et al	Retrospective	90 = HCLPE	Longevity	5.7	Martell method	.004 mm/yr
Manning et al	Case control	30 = HCLPE Group 1	Longevity	2.6	Martell method	.007 mm/yr
		108 = HCLPE Group 2	Durasul			.007 mm/yr
		214 = CPE	Unclear	4		.174 mm/yr
Martell et al	RCT	24 = HCLPE 22 = CPE	Crossfire N_2/Vac	2.3	Martell method	.12 mm/yr .20 mm/yr
McCalden et al	RCT	42 = HCLPE 47 = CPE	Longevity Trilogy	6.8	Martell method	−.029 mm/yr .057 mm/yr
Nakahara et al	Retrospective	94 = HCLPE	Longevity	6.7	PolyWare auto	−.014 mm/yr
Rajadhyaksha et al	Retrospective comparative	27 = HCLPE 27 = CPE	Crossfire N_2/Vac	5.9 6.3	Martell method	.022 mm/yr .085 mm/yr
Rohrl et al		10 = HCLPE 20 = CPE	Crossfire Exeter	6 5	RSA	.006 mm/year .072 mm/yr
Shia et al	Retrospective	70 = HCLPE	Longevity	4	Martell method	.003 mm/yr
Triclot et al	RCT	33 = HCLPE 34 = CPE	Durasul Sulene	4.9		.025 mm/yr .106 mm/yr
Whittaker et al	Retrospective	47 = HCLPE Group 1	Reflection XLPE	6.42	Martell method	.026 mm/yr
		36 = HCLPE Group 2	Longevity	7.64		.025 mm/yr

CPE, Conventional polyethylene; *HCLPE*, highly cross-linked polyethylene; *RCT*, randomized controlled trial; *RSA*, radiostereometric analysis.

Table 71-3. Six-Year Clinical Study Results

Study	Design	Material	Implant	Follow-up, yr	Detection Method	Wear Rate
Bragdon et al	Retrospective	72 = HCLPE 128 = HCLPE	Longevity Durasul	6.9	Martell	.001 mm/yr .001 mm/yr
McCalden et al	RCT	42 = HCLPE 47 = CPE	Longevity Trilogy	6.8	Martell	.029 mm/yr .057 mm/yr
Nakahara et al	Retrospective	94 = HCLPE	Longevity	6.7	PolyWare	.014 mm/yr
Rajadhyaksha et al	Retrospective comparative	27 = HCLPE 27 = CPE	Crossfire N$_2$/Vac	5.9 6.3	Martell	.022 mm/yr .085 mm/yr
Rohrl et al	Prospective Comparative	10 = HCLPE 20 = CPE	Crossfire Exeter	6 5	RSA	.006 mm/yr .072 mm/yr
Whittaker et al	Retrospective	47 = HCLPE 36 = HCLPE	Reflection XLPE Longevity	6.42 7.64	Martell	.026 mm/yr .025 mm/yr

CPE, Conventional polyethylene; *HCLPE*, highly cross-linked polyethylene; *RCT*, randomized controlled trial; *RSA*, radiostereometric analysis.

0.001 mm/yr, with 0.01 mm total penetration. Nakahara and colleagues reviewed Longevity (HCLPE) liners at a mean of 6.7 years post implantation using computer Polywear methods and documented a total penetration of 0.03 mm.

It is interesting to note that every published clinical study evaluating first-generation HCLPE versus CPE has shown a decreased wear rate in the HCLPE cohort between 2 and 6 years post implantation versus the CPE cohort. Relative wear reduction has ranged from 31% to 95%. No published studies have explored second-generation HCLPE wear rates with follow-up greater than 5 years. Recent data have reported an increase in the wear rate of HCLPE between 5 and 8 years post implantation after very low wear rates during the initial 5 years of clinical evaluation.[11] The cause of this increase in wear rate is not clear, and further follow-up is needed to determine whether this trend will continue.

Radiographic Osteolysis Evaluation

HCLPE has demonstrated lower volumetric wear rates in hip simulator evaluations. However, concern has been raised regarding the smaller size of particles produced during the wear of HCLPE and the potential immunologic reaction to these particles. The main reason for this concern is the potential for osteolysis. A total of 26 clinical studies listed in Table 71-2 evaluated the clinical and radiographic performance of HCLPE at follow-up of 2.2 to 7.6 years. Ten of these studies commented on the presence or absence of osteolysis. Within the 10 studies, no cases of radiographic osteolysis surrounding the involved HCLPE hip arthroplasty were reported. In contrast, Rajadhyksha and coworkers reported a 26% osteolysis rate in the CPE (N$_2$/Vac) cohort at 6.3 years' follow-up, and Bitsch and associates reported a 33% osteolysis rate in the CPE (Enduron) cohort at 5 years' follow-up.[5,12]

HCLPE Liner Failures and Retrieval Data

Several studies have looked at the short-term clinical characteristics of highly cross-linked polyethylene. Retrieved liners were examined for surface wear, oxidation, mechanical properties, penetration, and wear rates. Both penetration and wear rates for HCLPE are decreased compared with CPE retrieved liners.[13-15] Kurtz and associates found that the penetration rate was .04 mm/yr and was comparable with that of clinical wear studies. Knahr and colleagues reported that the linear wear rates of their two retrieval liners at intermediate-term follow-up were .01 mm/yr and .015 mm/yr. Salineros and coworkers described 46 retrieved HCLPE liners that were implanted for 12 to 96 months and reported an 80% reduction of wear and a 90% reduction of creep with HCLPE liners as compared with CPE liners in their comparative retrieval study.

Several authors have reported an increase in surface damage, including scratching and cracking, with HCLPE as compared with conventional polyethylenes.[16-18] These observations have raised questions about the long-term wear characteristics of HCLPE and whether it differs from CPE. Muratoglu and associates found that surface scratching, in particular, was able to be reversed when HCLPE retrieved liners were re-melted. Surface scratches were not changed when the CPE liners were re-melted. This finding suggests that the HCLPE liner deformation was plastic in nature and did not reflect true liner volume loss. Despite the surface scratching, HCLPE liner retrievals were not revised for osteolysis or wear.

One distinct trade-off that occurs with higher levels of cross-linking is the drop in mechanical strength of the polyethylene with regard to fracture risk. Cole and colleagues reported on the effects of gamma radiation and its relationship to fatigue crack behavior and fracture toughness.[19] Clinical reports of HCLPE liner fatigue fracture have been put forth. Tower and coworkers reported on four Longevity (HCLPE) liner fractures that were retrieved and evaluated.[18] All four liners demonstrated fatigue fracture at the superior rim adjacent to the locking mechanism groove. Based on these and other retrievals, we can conclude that HCLPE designs should avoid (1) decreased polyethylene thickness at the rim of the locking mechanism, (2) unsupported polyethylene rims, and (3) cup implantation at high abduction angles (>50 degrees) due to stress on the superior rim of the liner (Fig. 71-1).

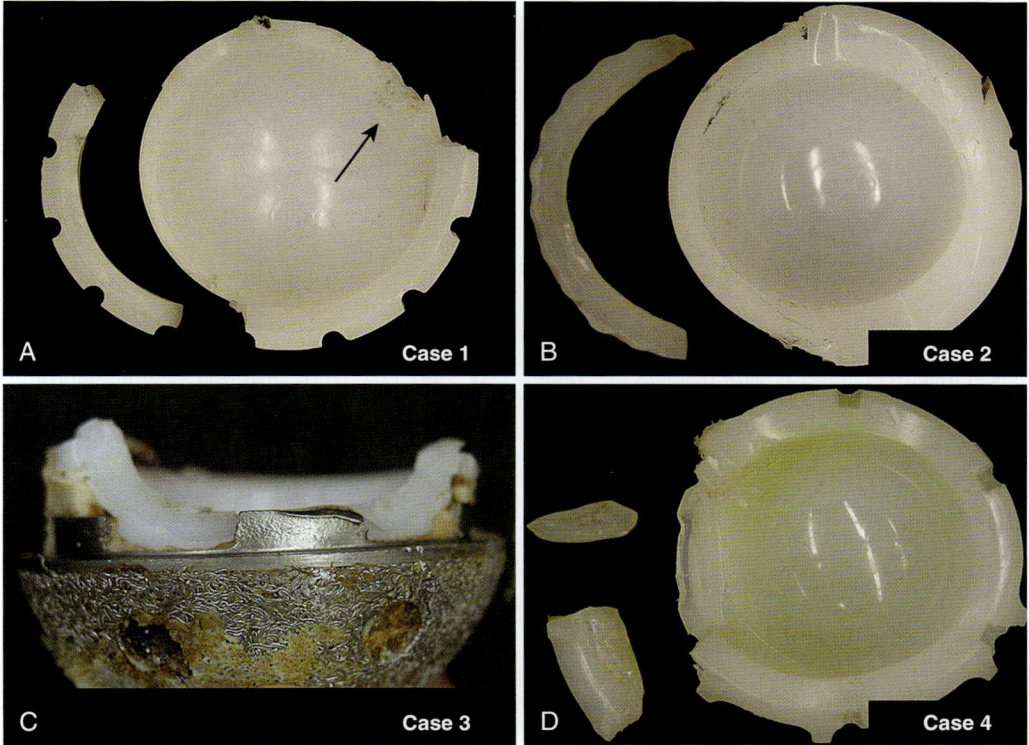

Figure 71-1. Photographs of acetabular liner rim fractures of Longevity, XLPE, Durasul, and Marathon liners, respectively. *(From Furmanski J, Anderson M, Bal S, et al: Clinical fracture of cross-linked UHMWPE acetabular liners. Biomaterials 30:5572–5582, 2009.)*

Free radical formation remains a topic of controversy in HCLPE liner development. Oxidation from free radical formation has been linked to prior CPE failure.[20] Two questions remain with regard to free radicals and HCLPE. First, what method of preparation can limit the number of free radicals in the HCLPE? Second, does long term oxidation occur in vivo? Wannomae and coworkers suggested that the production process influences the amount of oxidation. In their review of 26 HCLPE liners, liners produced via annealing had a tenfold higher level of oxidation and crystallinity when compared with melted liners.[2] Investigators suggested that melting may be a more effective way to achieve increased quenched free radicals, rather than by annealing. Despite this finding, annealed HCLPE liners have yielded excellent in vivo clinical data with no evidence of osteolysis at 6-year follow-up.[21,22]

Evidence is now available to support the concept that in vivo oxidation may occur in both CPE and HCLPE liners. Retrieved liners have been examined by using the Fourier transform infrared spectroscopy method for oxidation analysis. Results reveal that the greatest areas of oxidation typically occur in regions of the liner that experience minimal wear (such as the rim of the liner). Studies have demonstrated that the rim oxidation of HCLPE is more significant and shows a near exponential increase with increased time in vivo.[2,21,22] The significance of oxidation with long-term wear in HCLPE is currently unknown. In the absence of rim impingement,

10-year retrieval data suggest that rim oxidation has no effect on the clinical performance of these liners.[21]

SUMMARY

Polyethylene is the most commonly used bearing surface in total hip arthroplasty. The past decade has shown an explosion in the modification and development of HCLPE materials. Laboratory and short-term clinical data have predicted and documented a significant reduction in wear of between 40% and 95%. More important, radiographic and clinical studies to date have demonstrated no cases of osteolysis or increased immunologic reaction to the particulate debris of HCLPE.

The fatigue strength of HCLPE is reduced when compared with that of CPE; this should be recognized in acetabular component design and implantation to avoid liner fracture. Unsupported HCLPE and thin HCLPE at the point of peripheral locking mechanisms should be avoided. Similarly, acetabular component position should avoid abduction angles greater than 50 degrees as well as neck impingement, both of which place the peripheral HCLPE at risk for fracture. It is this same region of the polyethylene that has been shown to be most susceptible to in vivo oxidation.

Despite some recent evidence that suggests increased HCLPE wear rates between 5 and 8 years post implantation, the clinical performance of first-generation HCLPE has been excellent, and its continued use is justified on the basis of available clinical data. Longer follow-up is mandatory to determine which production method is superior and to delineate future failure mechanisms.

REFERENCES

1. Gordon A, D'Lima D, Colwell C: Highly cross linked polyethylene in total hip arthroplasty. J Am Acad Orthop Surg 14:511–523, 2006.
2. Wannomae KK, Bhattacharyya S, Freiberg A, et al: In vivo oxidation of retrieved cross-linked ultra-high-molecular-weight polyethylene acetabular components with residual free radicals. J Arthroplasty 21:1005–1011, 2006.
3. Chiesa R, Tanzi MC, Alfonsi S, et al: Enhanced wear performance of highly crosslinked UHMWPE for artificial joints. J Biomed Mater Res 50:381–387, 2000.
4. Martell JM, Verner JJ, Incavo SJ: Clinical performance of a highly cross-linked polyethylene at two years in total hip arthroplasty: a randomized prospective trial. J Arthroplasty 18(7 Suppl 1):55–59, 2003.
5. Bitsch RG, Loidolt T, Heisel C, et al: Reduction of osteolysis with use of Marathon cross-linked polyethylene: a concise follow-up, at a minimum of five years, of a previous report. J Bone Joint Surg Am 90:1487–1491, 2008.
6. Bragdon CR, Kwon YM, Geller JA, et al: Minimum 6-year follow-up of highly cross-linked polyethylene in THA. Clin Orthop Relat Res 465:122–127, 2007.
7. D'Antonio JA, Manley MT, Capello WN, et al: Five-year experience with Crossfire highly cross-linked polyethylene. Clin Orthop Relat Res 441:143–150, 2005.
8. Digas G, Karrholm J, Thanner J, Herberts P: 5-year experience of highly cross-linked polyethylene in cemented and uncemented socket: two randomized studies using radiostereometric analysis. Acta Orthop 78:746–754, 2007.
9. Lachiewicz PF, Heckman DS, Soileau ES, et al: Femoral head size and wear of highly cross-linked polyethylene at 5 to 8 years. Clin Orthop Relat Res 467:3290–3296, 2009.
10. McCalden RW, MacDonald SJ, Roraback CH, et al: Wear rate of highly cross-linked polyethylene in total hip arthroplasty: a randomized controlled trial. J Bone Joint Surg Am 91:773–782, 2009.
11. Malcheau 5-8 yr HCLPE data
12. Rajadhyaksha AD, Brotea C, Cheung Y, et al: Five-year comparative study of highly cross-linked (Crossfire) and traditional polyethylene. J Arthroplasty 24:161–167, 2009.
13. Kurtz SM, Austin MS, Azzam K, et al: Mechanical properties of retrieved highly cross-linked Crossfire liners after short-term implantation. J Arthroplasty 20:840–849, 2005.
14. Knahr K, Pospischill M, Kottig P, et al: Retrieval analyses of highly cross-linked polyethylene acetabular liners four and five years after implantation. J Bone Joint Surg Br 89:1036–1041, 2007.
15. Salineros MJ, Crowninshield RD, Laurent M, et al: Analysis of retrieved acetabular components of three polyethylene types. Clin Orthop Relat Res 465:140–149, 2007.
16. Muratoglu OK, Greenbaum ES, Bragdon CR, et al: Surface analysis of early retrieved acetabular polyethylene liners: a comparison of conventional and highly cross-linked polyethylenes. J Arthroplasty 19:68–77, 2004.
17. Tower SS, Currier JH, Currier BH, et al: Rim cracking of the cross-linked Longevity polyethylene acetabular liner after total hip arthroplasty. J Bone Joint Surg Am 89:2212–2217, 2007.
18. Cole JC, Lemons JE, Eberhardt AW: Gamma irradiation alters fatigue crack behavior and fracture toughness in 1900H and GUR 1050 UHMWPE. J Biomed Mater Res 63:559–566, 2002.
19. Kurtz SM, Hozack WJ, Purtill JJ, et al: 2006 Otto Aufranc Award Paper: significance of in vivo degradation for polyethylene in total hip arthroplasty. Clin Orthop Relat Res 453:47–57, 2006.
20. Currier BH, Currier JH, Mayor MB, et al: Evaluation of oxidation and fatigue damage of retrieved Crossfire polyethylene acetabular cups. J Bone Joint Surg Am 89:2023–2029, 2007.
21. Crowninshield RD: Murtoglu OK, on behalf of the Implant Wear Symposium 2007 Engineering Work Group: How have new sterilization techniques and new forms of polyethylene influenced wear in total joint replacement? J Am Acad Orthop Surg 16(Suppl 1):S80, 2008.
22. Calvert GT, Devane PA, Felden J, et al: A double-blind, prospective, randomized controlled trial comparing highly cross-linked and conventional polyethylene in primary total hip arthroplasty. J Arthroplasty 24:505–510, 2009.
23. Dorr LD, Wan Z, Shahrdar C, et al: Clinical performance of a Durasul highly cross-linked polyethylene acetabular liner for total hip arthroplasty at five years. J Bone Joint Surg Am 20:1816–1821, 2005.
24. Engh CA, Stepniewski AS, Ginn SD, et al: A randomized prospective evaluation of outcomes after total hip arthroplasty using cross-linked Marathon and non-cross-linked Enduron polyethylene liners: Dorr Award. J Arthroplasty 21(Suppl 2):17–25, 2006.
25. García-Rey E, Garcia-Cimrelo E, Cruz-Pardos A, Ortega-Chamarro J: New polyethylenes in total hip replacement: a prospective, comparative clinical study of two types of liner. J Bone Joint Surg Br 90:149–153, 2008.
26. Garvin KL, Hartman CW, Mangla J, et al: Wear analysis in THA utilizing oxidized zirconium and cross-linked polyethylene. Clin Orthop Relat Res 467:141–145, 2009.
27. Geller JA, Malchau H, Bragdon C, et al: Large diameter femoral heads on highly cross-linked polyethylene: minimum 3-year results. Clin Orthop Relat Res 447:53–59, 2006.
28. Glyn-Jones S, McLardy-Smith P, Gill HS, Murray DW: The creep and wear of highly cross-linked polyethylene: a three-year randomized, controlled trial using radiostereometric analysis. J Bone Joint Surg Am 90:556–561, 2008.
29. Heisel C, Silva M, Dela Rosa MA, Schmalzried TP: Short-term in vivo wear of cross-linked polyethylene. J Bone Joint Surg Am 86:748–751, 2004.
30. Hopper RH, Young AM, Orishima KF, McAuley JP: Correlation between early and late wear rates in total hip arthroplasty with application to the performance of Marathon cross-linked polyethylene liners. J Arthroplasty 18(Suppl 1):60–67, 2003.
31. Krushell RJ, Fingeroth RJ, Cushing MC: Early femoral head penetration of a highly cross-linked polyethylene liner vs a conventional polyethylene liner: a case controlled study. J Arthroplasty 20(Suppl 3):73–76, 2005.
32. Manning DW, Chiang PP, Martell JM, et al: In vivo comparative wear study of traditional and highly cross-linked polyethylene in total hip arthroplasty. J Arthroplasty 20:880–886, 2005.
33. Nakahara I, Nakamura N, Nishii T, et al: Minimum five-year follow-up wear measurement of Longevity highly cross-linked polyethylene cup against cobalt-chromium or zirconia heads. J Arthroplasty 25:1182–1187, 2010.
34. Rohrl SM, Li MG, Nilsson KG, Nivbrant B: Very low wear of non-remelted highly cross-linked polyethylene cups: an RSA study lasting up to 6 years. Acta Orthop 78:739–745, 2007.
35. Shia DS, Clohisy JC, Schinsky MF, et al: THA with highly cross-linked polyethylene in patients 50 years or younger. Clin Orthop Relat Res 467:2059–2065, 2009.
36. Triclot P, Grosjea G, El Masri F, et al: A comparison of the penetration rate of two polyethylene acetabular liners of different levels of cross-linking: a prospective randomized trial. J Bone Joint Surg Br 89:1439–1445, 2007.
37. Whittaker JP, Charron KD, McCalden RW, et al: Comparison of steady state femoral head penetration rates between 2 highly cross-linked polyethylenes in total hip arthroplasty. J Arthroplasty 680–686, 2010.

CHAPTER 72

Metal-on-Metal Bearings

Philip A. O'Connor, Brent A. Lanting, and Steven J. MacDonald

---

KEY POINTS

Advantages of Metal-on-Metal Bearings
- Exhibit extremely low wear rates (40 to 100 times less than conventional metal-on-polyethylene in vitro)
- Allow the use of thinner acetabular cups and larger femoral heads
- Osteolysis is rare

Disadvantages of Metal-on-Metal Bearings
- Production of metal ions (cobalt and chromium)
- Hypersensitivity reactions and pseudotumors
- High revisions of some prosthesis leading to implant recall
- Contraindicated in patients with renal failure
- Theoretical carcinogenic concerns

INTRODUCTION

Metal-on-metal (MOM) articulations evolved simultaneously with Charnley's low-friction arthroplasty (LFA). Inadequate clearances, poor manufacturing tolerances, and poor implantation technique all lead to early failure and the demise of first-generation MOM implants. The resurgence of interest in alternatives to the LFA followed observations of failure secondary to polyethylene wear and osteolysis, particularly in younger, more active patients. After 2 decades, newer manufacturing capabilities and greater understanding of tribology allowed the development of second-generation MOM total hip arthroplasty (THA). In MOM bearings, wear volume has been shown to decrease as femoral head size increases, hence the development of modern resurfacing-type implants, using thinner acetabular components and large-diameter femoral heads. Modular, large MOM bearings offer the potential for low wear rates, greater stability, and less impingement with increased head-to-neck ratios. In 2005, metal-on-metal bearings accounted for 35% of all hip arthroplasties performed in the United States.[1] However, recent reports of lymphocytic aggregates, elevated metal ion concentrations, and hypersensitivity reactions[2] have raised concerns regarding the safety of MOM bearings. Furthermore, registry data have indicated a revision rate of greater than 10% for some implants within 10 years.[3] Implant and radiographic features that contribute to early failure are not completely understood, and only limited short to midterm results are available. Concerns for local and systemic toxicity and elevated revision rates are present in spite of improved wear performance.

DEVELOPMENT OF METAL-ON-METAL BEARINGS

The wear properties of metal for arthroplasty were recognized as far back as 1938 by Smith-Peterson. It was on the recommendation of his dentist that he turned to Vitallium, a cobalt-chrome alloy, after earlier failures of his "mold arthroplasty." Several long-term reports on these implants have been put forth, and the longest implant is known to have survived 56 years.[4] Philip Wiles of Middlesex implanted the first metallic THA, which was made of stainless steel. The components were ground to fit together accurately. He used his design in 1938 on six patients with Still's disease but reported very limited success.[5] Little evidence remains of his efforts because nearly all radiographs were lost during World War II. Further modifications were made, and in 1957, his new implant was inserted into eight patients—again with limited success. Kenneth McKee had worked as a registrar to Wiles and in Norwich went on to develop his own THA. After a visit to America in 1953, he came across the Thompson prosthesis, which he would then mate with his cast cobalt-chromium cloverleaf socket, which was fixed by screws. Charnley's use of acrylic cement provided the breakthrough for vastly improved femoral fixation. McKee would later modify the femoral stem, initially by burring down the undersurface of the neck.

Eventually a new design was developed. John Watson-Farrar was registrar to McKee, and it was his suggestion that a larger femoral component should be used. The final version of the McKee-Farrar was produced in 1965. The 38-mm femoral head articulated with a thin cobalt-chromium cup. Several long-term reports highlight the success of this MOM construct, with the longest series reporting nearly 30 years' follow-up.[6] Clinical success was limited, and early component loosening was attributed to poor manufacturing quality, variable tolerance, and failure of fixation.[7] Early loosening of the acetabular component, due to equatorial contact, was one of the reasons why this design was abandoned. In Surrey, Peter Ring designed an acetabular component that he mated with a 40-mm Moore prosthesis, and the components were wrapped together. His design was inserted without the use of acrylic cement because the acetabular component had a long thread that was screwed into the ilium. Ring reported one series with survivorship of 85% at 6 to 11 years.[8] Varying modification of the implants took place, with an eventual move to polyethylene cups that proved to be inferior.

Weber observed that several Müller-McKee replacements were still functioning after 25 years.[9] Implants that did produce long-term survivorship were noted to have little or no wear or incidence of osteolysis.[10,11] As a result, he was motivated to re-explore MOM bearing couples, reasoning that low wear and low friction were contributing factors to the longevity of the implants he observed. Failure of the McKee-Farrar implant was due to design deficiencies rather than to accelerated wear, and the low wear rates seen might limit the production of wear particles and the development of osteolysis. At the end of the 1970s, Weber approached Sulzer Brothers Limited (Sulzer Inc., Winterthur, Switzerland) to ask for help in developing a modern MOM couple with better manufacturing precision and tolerances. It was already thought that high carbon content of the cobalt-chromium-molybdenum (Co-Cr-Mo) alloy could provide improved lower wear.[9] The Metasul THA (Zimmer, Inc., Warsaw, Ind) produced by Sulzer consisted of a 28-mm or 32-mm modular metal Co-Cr-Mo femoral head and an acetabular metal inlay embedded in the polyethylene cup, with a four-layer sintered stainless steel mesh surface for enhanced cement fixation. In 1988, Weber started to implant the Metasul bearings, commencing the era of second-generation MOM bearings. Although the initial second-generation MOM bearings measured 28 or 32 mm, MOM designs quickly evolved. In a desire to maximize the benefits of increased stability and range of motion, head sizes increased to reach the 40- to 50-mm range. Cup designs included metal inlay liner in a polyethylene cup, hemispherical cups with modular liners, and monoblock, sub-hemispherical acetabular components. Several cup design features resulted in a sub-hemispherical articulation. To increase cup stiffness, the dome was thickened. To allow fluid ingress, the cup edges were rounded. Some cups had specialized insertional tools that locked within the cup. A sub-hemispherical cup also decreased impingement potential. Griffin and associates investigated 33 cups of different sizes from six companies. Notably, the mean articular arc was 160.5 degrees; with the smallest articular arc being 151.8 degrees.[12]

WEAR

Standard THA with a metal head articulating against a polyethylene couple has yielded highly predictable and reproducible good results. The search for alternative bearings has occurred in part because of observed osteolysis and component failure. In addition, younger patients are now presenting for arthroplasty who will have increased tribiological demands placed on their implants compared with those reported in currently available historic long-term outcome data. Data from the Swedish Hip Arthroplasty Register reveal 21-year survivorship with Charnley's prosthesis of 81.7% in primary hip osteoarthritis.[13] Metal bearings have evolved in hip arthroplasty to meet the challenge of reducing wear-related failure for a more active, younger population with an increased life expectancy. One million cycles in a hip joint simulator has been compared with 1-year prosthetic use by the patient. However, Schmalzried and associates[14] reported on a group of 33 patients with well-functioning THAs and noted that the average patient's walking activity approached 2 million cycles per year, and up to 3.5 million cycles per year in highly active people.[15]

The most significant advantage of the use of a MOM bearing couple in THA is the clearly documented reduction in wear of the bearing surface.[16] Wear portends bearing failure, and rates for MOM articulations have been estimated to be up to 100 times lower than those of metal-on-polyethylene (MOP) couples.[16] Polyethylene wear particles induce osteolysis through a well-understood inflammatory cascade.[17] Schulte and coworkers measured wear rates of Charnley's MOP prostheses on radiographs. At 20 years, they reported an average wear rate of 0.074 mm/yr.[18] A vast majority of PE wear particles are between 0.1 and 0.5 μm, and particles smaller than 0.5 μm are of the critical size for macrophage activation. Metal ion production can occur with a conventional MOP bearing from the femoral component through corrosion and/or fretting at the head-neck coupling.[19] Estimates of wear rates from MOM McKee-Farrar implants retrieved at 20 years were 0.0042 mm/yr, that is, 25 times lower than MOP rates.

Metal bearings exhibit a complex tribology. Wear is dependent on metallurgy, design, geometry, radial clearance, lubrication, loading regimen, kinematics, and component position.[20] Cobalt-chromium-molybdenum is the most commonly used alloy for MOM bearings; however, it should be emphasized that metal bearings represent a large heterogeneous group. The wear pattern of MOM bearings exhibits two distinct phases, as demonstrated in laboratory simulator experiments.[16,21,22] An initial "bedding-in" period is seen for the first million cycles, or the first year in vivo, during which self-polishing of the bearing takes place. The subsequent "steady-state" phase exhibits a lower continuous wear rate. The mean linear wear rate of a MOM hip has been shown to be about 5 μm/yr, and this corresponds to a volumetric wear of 1 mm^3/yr.[23] This is approximately 40 times lower in linear wear as compared with MOP articulations. Retrieval studies[24] of 118 Metasul MOM bearings documented a linear rate of wear of 5 μm/yr, which is at least 20 times less than that of MOP. The volumetric rate of wear of 0.3 mm^3/yr is at least 60 times less than that of MOP (17.9 mm^3/yr). Langton looked at 15 Articular Surface Replacement (ASR) hips (Depuy Orthopaedics, Inc., Warsaw, Ind) explanted at a mean of 18 months, and demonstrated a mean linear wear rate of 2.9 μm.[25] Increased variation was reported by Schmidt and coworkers on 11 McKee-Farrar hips explanted at a mean of 16.3 years, with linear wear rates ranging from 0.1 to 300 μm/yr.[26] Witzleb et al reported higher levels of volumetric wear rates in

10 Birmingham Hip Resurfacing (BHR) hips (Smith & Nephew Orthopaedics, Memphis, Tenn) explanted at a mean of 13 months, with volumetric wear rates of up to 27 mm³/yr.[27] Component type and size and position all play important clinical roles that are not been fully described in a laboratory setting, which may result in in vivo differences in wear rates.

Wear rate has been implicated in the development of pseudotumours. Higher wear rates and greater prevalence of edge wear have been demonstrated in a group of 18 patients with resurfacings revised for pseudotumor compared with 18 patients revised for other reasons.[28] Volumetric wear (3.3 ± 5.7 mm3/yr) was six times greater and the linear wear rate (8.4 ± 8.7 µm/yr) was three times greater for the pseudotumor group than for the control group. The argument that cup position is correlated to higher wear due to edge loading as measured by ion levels was re-enforced by a recent paper that examined MOM revisions for pseudotumors, with revisions for other reasons as a control group.[29] In this article, thirty resurfacing hips were retrieved—8 for pseudotumor formation—and were assessed with a roundness machine. Those hips that had a pseudotumor were found to have a higher rate of wear of the femoral component (8.1 µm/yr [range, 2.75 to 25.4 µm/yr]) than those that did not have a pseudotumour (1.8 µm/yr [range, 0.82 to 4.14 µm/yr]). Acetabular component pseudotumour revisions also showed increased wear, at 7.36 µm/yr (range, 1.61 to 24.9 µm/yr), versus 1.28 µm/yr (range, 0.81 to 3.33 µm/yr). Wear patterns were consistent with edge loading.

METALLURGY

Carbon carbides are produced when carbon reacts with metal at high temperatures. Heat treatment (annealing) of high-carbon (0.266 wt %) Co-Cr-Mo alters the size and percentage of carbides on the bearing surface, allowing the hard carbides to diffuse into the softer matrix material. Single-treatment annealing leads to smaller carbides in the material, whereas double-treatment annealing leads to almost no visible carbides under scanning electron microscpy (SEM). Kinburn examined the effects of carbides on wear in three different as cast high-carbon components.[30] Their results indicate that "heat treatment by solution annealing of a Co-Cr-Mo material significantly increased the wear rates." Dowson performed a hip simulator study to compare various combinations of 36-mm, high- and low-carbon, wrought and cast Co-Cr-Mo femoral heads.[31] The low-carbon material exhibited higher wear than the high-carbon wrought material. No significant difference was noted between wrought and cast high-carbon materials. High-carbon/high-carbon pairings show the lowest wear rates in hip joint simulator tests.[32]

The ability to establish fluid-film lubrication is a major factor in the very low wear rates seen in MOM hips. Head diameter and diametrical clearance are central to this concept. The wear rate of MOM is reduced with a larger head size in combination with lower clearances; this is in contradistinction to MOP bearings. In Charnley's LFA, wear was shown to be proportional to the sliding distance. By reducing the femoral head diameter, he aimed to reduce wear volume. Charnley chose a femoral head diameter that was half the diameter of the polyethylene socket. In contrast, lubrication analysis of metal bearings reveals that as the head size increased, the potential to achieve fluid-film lubrication also increased, resulting in reduced wear.[33] Dowson has shown that as diametrical clearance increased, both bedding-in wear and steady-state wear increased significantly.[31] So the most advantageous design of an MOM bearing includes low clearance and a larger diameter. The challenge with lower clearances, in particular with a monoblock design, is that cups can deflect on insertion, which can potentially lead to equatorial binding.[34] Additionally, manufacturing tolerances are a factor in the ability to effectively reduce clearances, once again because of the concern of too small a clearance, leading to equatorial binding.

METAL PARTICLES

Metallic debris particles are in the order of 10 to 50 nm in size.[35] However, the volume of metallic particles produced is much greater. Corrosion of particles, on exposure to periprosthetic fluids, releases metal ions into the surrounding tissue. Subsequent dissemination of chromium (Cr) and cobalt (Co) ions throughout the body has raised concerns about elevated serum, urinary, and tissue levels. Doorn and colleagues[36] were able to estimate the total number of particles produced per year in vivo because wear volumes of the prostheses and the particle size had been determined. They estimated that from 6.7×10^{12} to 2.5×10^{14} metal particles were produced per year in three different patients with MOM THAs. This figure is 13 to 500 times greater than that of the 5×10^{11} ultra-high-molecular-weight polyethylene (UHMWPE) particles produced in a typical MOP prosthesis. Production of metallic debris has raised concerns regarding metal ion levels and tissue hypersenstivity reactions, the biological effects of which remain uncertain.

Metal Ion Analysis

MOM THA wear, with production of metal particles, has led to concern for systemic exposure to metal ions. In 1973, Coleman[37] reported analytical techniques for the measurement of cobalt and chromium in blood and urine in a series of 12 patients undergoing THA, 9 of whom had MOM bearings and 3 of whom had MOP bearings. Study results showed an almost threefold elevation of chromium in whole blood, an 11-fold increase in cobalt, a 15-fold increase in chromium in urine, and a 48-fold cobalt increase in urine in patients with MOM components. Elevated systemic ion levels has been used as a marker for localized pathology, with Bosker and associates reporting that patients with elevated serum ion levels were at a four times higher risk of developing pseudotumor.[38] Also, systemic toxicity has been reported secondary to elevated ion levels.[39,40] This has led to increasing interest in the measurement and monitoring of ion levels of patients with MOM hips.

Lazennec and coworkers analyzed the metal ion concentration of patients in their cohort. Sampling was performed at 3 months, 6 months, 1 year, and every year postoperatively until the last endpoint was reached. Chromium and cobalt levels were assayed in plasma using inductively coupled optical emission spectrometry (ICP-OES).[41] Median serum cobalt levels at 9 years were 1.55 µg/L with little variation observed over time. Serum chromium levels at 9 years were 1.49 µg/L and showed a slight decrease over time. In eight patients who underwent revision for aseptic loosening, the median cobalt was almost 17 times higher at 26 µg/L. Investigators report one revision case for persistent and unexplained pain with well-fixed implants. Grossly elevated serum cobalt levels were detected, and at operation, massive and macroscopic metallosis was observed in the joint. The patient's symptoms settled after exchange of bearing surfaces with ceramic-on-ceramic. In an additional study, it has been seen that after revision, metal ions significantly decrease.[42] Pre-revision cobalt was 307.1 nM/L (range, 25 to 2300 nM/L), and chrome was 204.5 nM/L (range, 25 to 850 nM/L). After revision, cobalt levels decreased to 6.6 nM/L (range, 1.7 to 23.8 nM/L), and chrome levels to 67.3 nM/L (range, 19 to 885 nM/L). In this study, one patient with persistently elevated ion levels after revision was awaiting revision for a contralateral MOM THA.

Several published series of second-generation MOM total hip systems have shown elevated cobalt and chromium levels in blood and/or urine. These show a fivefold to 10-fold increase from preoperative to postoperative blood cobalt values (average preoperative blood cobalt level, 0.15 µg/L; postoperative level, 1.0 µg/L).[43] MacDonald and coworkers[44] performed a prospective, randomized, blinded clinical trial in 41 patients to evaluate MOM versus MOP THAs. Patients were assessed preoperatively and postoperatively using erythrocyte metal ion analysis of cobalt, chromium, and titanium (Co, Cr, Ti), as well as urine metal ion analysis (Co, Cr, Ti). Patients were followed for a minimum of 2 years. Those who had MOM inserts had on average a 7.9-fold increase in erythrocyte cobalt, a 2.3-fold increase in erythrocyte chromium, a 1.7-fold increase in erythrocyte titanium, a 35.1-fold increase in urine cobalt, a 17.4-fold increase in urine chromium, and a 2.6-fold increase in urine titanium at 2 years' follow-up. Patients receiving a polyethylene insert had no change in erythrocyte titanium, urine cobalt, or urine chromium and a 1.5-fold increase in erythrocyte cobalt, a 2.2-fold increase in erythrocyte chromium, and a 4.2-fold increase in urine titanium. Forty-one percent of patients receiving metal-on-metal articulations had increasing metal ion levels at the latest follow-up.

Although it is known that ion levels rise after MOM THAs compared to those in control patients, and that elevated ion levels may be indicative of pathologic wear, challenges to the interpretation of serum ion levels are known. Results from patients that have had bilateral MOM articulations are more difficult to interpret because ion levels are greater than, but not double, that of unilateral cases.[45] Also, serum ion levels increase with increased activity of the patient.[46] Finally, differences between MOM THAs and resurfacings have been identified, limiting the ability to extrapolate knowledge. A meta-analysis was conducted that reviewed comparative studies of MOM total versus resurfacing hip arthroplasties.[47] This study was limited by the relatively small number of subjects, and of large head MOM THA cases. Only metal cobalt levels only were found to be lower in the resurfacing group, and it was found that chrome levels were not affected.

Problems with comparison of published data on metal ion concentrations are due to lack of uniformity. Specimens analyzed in publications include whole blood, serum, erythrocytes, urine, synovial fluid, periprosthetic tissue, and remote tissue. Blood and urine are the most commonly assayed samples. Guidelines on standardized methods for sampling, storing, processing, analyzing, and reporting have been established.[48] Retrieval analysis[24] has provided important data on wear in MOM bearings, but surrogate markers of wear in MOM hip arthroplasties are needed, because it is not possible to measure wear radiographically.[49] Serum metal levels can provide some comparative information on the performance of MOM hip arthroplasty systems as long as patient demographics, activity level, and renal function, as well as analytical technique used are comparable.[49] Finally, the effect of time of exposure is not understood. Griffin and colleagues found that ion levels did not correlate with extent of soft tissue damage, but the time in situ did have statistical significance.[50] However, significance is lost once ion levels and time in situ are combined. Bernstein and coworkers reported on 163 Metasul 28-mm MOM hips at 8.9 years (range, 7-13 years) and noted that cobalt levels peaked at 4 years at 2.87 µg/L, subsequently decreased to 2.0 µg/L after 9 years.[51] Chrome levels increased to five years to 0.75 µg/L and then decreased after 7 years to 0.56 µg/L. Griffin and associates describe an increase in soft tissue damage with increased time in situ with a time to revision of less than 5 years; therefore, it is unknown whether soft tissue damage is due to time in situ or to steadily climbing ion levels.[50] However, the potential for increased soft tissue damage with increased time in-situ needs to be considered.

Healthcare regulatory bodies such as the MHRA recommend following serum ion levels in patients with MOM articulations. However, the impact of elevated ions levels is not well understood. A safe level of metal ion concentration has yet to be defined for patients with MOM hip arthroplasties, and to date, only a fraction of the estimated 600,000 MOM hip arthroplasties implanted have undergone metal ion analysis. Although serum ions levels may provide clinical information about the wear rate of the MOM articulation and potential for sub-optimal function,[45] absolute values do not provide information on the extent of soft tissue destruction found intra-operatively.[50] This finding was corroborated in another recent paper, which recommended MRI cross-sectional imaging for MOM follow-up.[52]

Component Position

Higher wear rates have been reported with acetabular components inserted with a cup inclination greater than 50 degrees in MOP bearings.[53] Brodner examined three patients with cup inclinations of 58 degrees, 61 degrees, and 63 degrees who had serum chromium levels of 10.4 µg/L, 33.6 µg/L, and 12.1 µg/L, and serum cobalt levels of 4.9 µg/L, 26.8 µg/L, and 12.9 µg/L. The overall study group had a median chromium concentration of 1.1 µg/L and a median cobalt level of 0.5 µg/L. Although Brodner and associates reported that no statistical difference in correlation could be detected between three groups of varying cup inclination, multiple other authors did find this difference.[54] Angadji and colleagues[55] examined the effect of cup inclination on MOM bearings in vitro using six MoM bearings with a head diameter of 40 mm. Three different angles of cup inclination were examined: 35 degrees, 50 degrees, and 60 degrees. Higher wear rates were seen with steeper inclination during steady-state wear. As cup inclination increased, the observed wear pattern progressed from polar to the cup rim. Williams and colleagues[56] performed a hip joint simulator study to examine the role of increased cup inclination and wear in MOM bearings. Cups placed at 55 degrees showed a fivefold increase in steady-state wear over cups placed at an angle of 45 degrees. The wear pattern at a higher inclination was noted to move toward the superior edge of the cup. DeHaan and associates[57] reported a statistically significant increase in blood chromium and cobalt levels with steeply inclined cup position. Mean values for cobalt were 9.8 µg/L (range, 0.6 to 111.3 µg/L; 95% confidence interval [CI], 4.4 to 15.1) for components at greater than 55 degrees, and 2.4 µg/L (range, 0.4 to 31.5 µg/L; 95% CI, 1.8 to 2.9) for components at less than 55 degrees. Mean values for chromium were 9.7 µg/L (range, 0.6 to 94.6 µg/L; 95% CI, 5.3 to 14.1) for components at greater than 55 degrees, and 3.6 µg/L (range, 0.2 to 32.2 µg/L; 95% CI, 2.8 to 4.3) for components at less than 55 degrees of abduction.

Similarly, work by Langton and colleagues[58] confirmed a positive correlation between the inclination of the acetabular component and concentrations of cobalt ($r = 0.439$; $P < .001$) and chromium ($r = 0.372$; $P = .011$). This finding was supported by Hart and colleagues, who found an increase in ion levels with cup inclination of greater than 50 degrees; albeit in a small patient number.[59] An additional study revealed similar findings, using direct measurement of wear in 45 retrieved resurfacings.[60] Using 5 µm as the cutoff between low and high wear resurfacings, it was demonstrated that low-wearing hips were within 30 to 50 degrees of abduction twice as often as the higher-wear hips. Acetabular and combined version was only weakly correlated with increased wear. However, the impact of patient-specific biomechanics cannot be disregarded. In a group of four subjects, motion pathway, computed tomography (CT) imaging and finite element analysis (FEA) were analyzed by Mellon and associates.[61] Based on gait cycle and stair descent motion analysis, cup position as measured by CT, and published hip contact forces, FEA was conducted for 1-degree intervals of cup inclination. This group demonstrated that cup position should not be considered in isolation, and that patient motion patterns do influence the potential for edge loading.

Optimal cup position is a combination of coronal and sagittal plane positioning. It can be seen that a frontal plane cup position of greater than 50 degrees should be avoided. In hip resurfacing components, the recommended lateral opening angle should be between 40 degrees and 45 degrees, and combined anteversion (acetabular and femoral) should be 20 degrees to 30 degrees.[62]

CLINICAL OUTCOME (Table 72-1)

A 10-year outcome of the Metasul MOM bearing was published by Eswaramoorthy.[63] A cemented Stuehmer-Weber polyethylene acetabular component with a Metasul bearing was used in 52 hips, and an Allofit uncemented component with a Metasul insert was used in the other 52 hips. The cohort consisted of 100 patients undergoing 104 hip arthroplasties. In all, 15 patients had died before their 10-year review, and all deaths were reported to be unrelated to their well-functioning THAs. Three patients were lost to follow-up; this left 82 patients (85 hips) as the study group. Six revisions were performed, only one of which was done for confirmed infection. One revision was performed in another jurisdiction, and no details were available. Three preocedures were performed for pain, of which two had histologic changes typical of aseptic lymphocytic vasculitis–associated lesion (ALVAL). The reason for revision in the sixth case was presumed infection, although no organism was cultured. Survivorship of the Metasul MOM bearing in this series was 94% at 10 years.

A cohort followed for a minimum of 5 years was reported by Sharma and associates.[64] They performed a retrospective review of 222 patients who had undergone THA with Metasul articular bearings, with a mean age at surgery of 70 years (range, 47 to 86 years) and with mean follow-up of 7.33 years (range, 5 to 11.4 years). Two types of acetabular components were utilized: the cemented Weber Metasul cup and the cementless Armor cup with a Metasul insert. Loosening of the acetabular component occurred in two patients at 3.7 years and 6 years, respectively. Both underwent revision to cementless Armor cups. One dislocation of a cup occurred at 1 year but was believed to be due to technical fault at implantation with failure to graft an uncontained superior acetabular defect. A liner dissociation subsequently occurred. For the cohort as a whole, the survivorship rate was 95.5% at 12 years.

Saito and colleagues[65] presented their 5-year clinical and metal ion analysis of patients undergoing hip arthroplasty with the Metasul hip system. The study group consisted of 90 patients undergoing 106 hip arthroplasties. None of this group was lost to follow-up, and mean age at surgery was 57.8 years (range, 42 to 79 years). Only one patient required revision because of a liner

Table 72-1. Clinical Results of Second-Generation Metal-on-Metal Total Hip Arthroplasties

Study	Prosthesis	Number of Hips	Mean Age (range), yr	Disease	Mean Follow-up (range), yr	Outcome
Weber[9]	Metasul	105	59 (21.6-77.6)	OA 48 DDH 23 RA 7 AVN 4 Other 18	3.5 (2-7)	Early loosening of three stems and one acetabular component; one late stem loosening at 6 years
Dorr et al[114]	Metasul	56	70 (35-85)		5.2 (4-6.8)	98.2% acetabular survival, 100% femoral survival at 7 years
Wagner et al[115]	Metasul	75	48.8 (18-75)	OA 25 DDH 33 AVN 5 Other 12 OA 52	5 (3.66-7.33)	Three revisions (one late infection and two HO)
Lombardi et al[116]	M²a	78	49.3 (26-73)	OA 52 AVN 13 Other 7	3.29 (1.64-5.4)	100% survival
MacDonald et al[44]	M²a	22	60.9 (44.4-75.2)	OA 22	3.2 (2.2-3.9)	100% survival
Eswaramoorthy et al[63]	Metasul	100	61.6 (44-84)	OA 97 DDH 3 AVN 1 Other 3	10.8 (10.2-12.2)	94% survivorship at 10 years; 1 aseptic loosening; 2 ALVAL; 2 sepsis
Sharma et al[64]	Metasul	209 (187 patients)	70 (47-86)	OA 147 DDH 1 AVN 2 RA 12 Other 25	7.33 (5-11.4)	Femoral 100% Acetabulum 95.5% 3 revisions (2 osteolysis, 1 instability)
Long et al[117]	Metasul	161 (154 patients)	55.5 (27-83)	OA 112 DDH 4 AVN 39 RA 3 Other 3	6.5 (2-9)	Revision rate 3.7% Acetabulum 100% Femoral 99.4% Other 1.2%
Saito et al[65]	Metasul	106	57.8 (42-19)	OA 83 AVN 12 RA 11	6.4 (5-8)	99% (1 revision for liner dissociation at 6 years)
Dorr et al[118]	Metasul	127	72 (20-84)	OA 96 AVN 12 DDH 3 RA 1 Other 5	7-11	96.8% 4 revisions (1 osteolysis, 3 instability)
Lazennec et al[41]	Metasul	134	54 (30-60)	OA 121 AVN 13	9 (7-11)	91% acetabulum 99% femoral stem
Engh et al[119]	Ultramet 36 mm	131	53 (25-78)	OA 101 DDH 10 AVN 9 RA 4 Other 7	5 (5-7)	98%
Grübl et al[64]	Metasul	105 (98 patients)	56 (22-79)	OA 59 DDH 19 AVN 16 RA 4 Other 7	10	98.6% 4 revisions No aseptic loosening
Kindsfater et al[76]	Pinnacle	95 (95 patients)	53.5 (34-70)	OA 87 AVN 4 RA 2 DDH 1 Other 1	6 (5-8)	97.8% at 7 years 1 revision for fracture 1 revision for instability
Hug et al[68]	ASR	190 (172 patients)	50 (17-78)		3 (1-5)	87% at 40 months Metallosis (9 patients), Aseptic cup loosening (8), fracture (2), Infection (2), Other (3)

ALVAL, Aseptic lymphocytic vasculitis–associated lesion; *AVN,* avascular necrosis; *DDH,* developmental dysplasia of the hip; *HO,* heterotopic ossification; *OA,* osteoarthritis; *RA,* rheumatoid arthritis.
Modified with permission from MacDonald SJ, Mehin R: Metal on metal: clinical results with modern implants. Semin Arthroplasty 14:123–130. Copyright © 2003, with permission from Elsevier.

dissociation. Serum chromium concentrations were determined only at last follow-up and showed elevated levels in cases of bilateral MOM bearings (twofold) and unilateral MOM bearings (twofold) as compared with the MOP bearing group. This is remarkably lower than levels described in other reports.

Lazennec and coworkers[41] reported on a consecutive series of 113 patients who underwent primary hip arthroplasty using the 28-mm Metasul hip system with cemented acetabular and femoral components. The mean age of the group was 54 years (range, 30 to 60 years). Four patients were lost to follow-up, with the remaining 109 patients (138 hips) available for complete follow-up 7 to 11 years postoperatively. Interim serum cobalt, chromium, and titanium levels were obtained and analyzed using ICP-OES. Eight revisions were performed for loose Metasul cemented cups with radiolucencies greater than 2 mm, axial migration, and osteolysis. Investigators report a case with persistent unexplained pain and a serum cobalt level greater than 20-fold higher than the detection limit. At the time of revision, no abnormality was observed, apart from massive and microscopic metallosis in the joint. The bearing surfaces were changed to ceramic-on-ceramic implants, and the symptoms disappeared. The median serum cobalt level was relatively constant over the study period at fivefold to more than sixfold greater than the 0.3-µg/L detection limit. This differs from the findings of other researchers. In addition, median chromium and titanium levels were relatively constant. Because of the high rate of acetabular loosening, the authors no longer use MOM bearings. Overall, a disappointing survivorship of 91% was reported at a mean of 9 years, along with concerns over the durability of another 26% of cups.

Grübl and coworkers[66] conducted a retrospective review of a series of 98 patients (105 hips) undergoing cementless primary THA using an MOM bearing. Average patient age was 56 years (range, 22 to 79 years), and the follow-up period was a minimum of 10 years. Fifteen patients died, eight were lost to follow-up, and two could perform only telephone contact. In all, 73 patients were available for follow-up. Clinical, radiographic, and metal ion assays were performed at 10-year follow-up. A total of 22 patients underwent serum analysis for cobalt and chromium. The median serum concentration for cobalt was 0.75 µg/L (range, 0.3 to 5.0 µg/L) and for chromium 0.95 µg/L (range, 0.3 to 58.6 µg/L). Two patients had markedly high values; the first was a 90-year-old patient with documented renal impairment, and no cause was identified in the second, who subsequently underwent revision, after which her levels returned to the median for the overall group. Five patients were diagnosed with a primary tumor during the study period; this is consistent with the expected incidence rate. Ten-year survivorship was 98.6% (95% CI, 96 to 100).

Garbuz and colleagues[67] conducted a randomized clinical trial to examine the clinical outcomes of a large-head MOM versus a resurfacing hip arthroplasty. A total of 73 patients were randomly assigned to receive a Durom (Zimmer Inc., Winterthur, Switzerland)

resurfacing femoral and acetabular component or a Durom acetabular component and an M/L Taper (Zimmer) stem with a 28-mm Metasul (Zimmer) head via a Cr-Co alloy sleeve adapter. A total of 26 patients underwent metal serum–metal ion measurement at baseline and 1 year postoperatively. Results analyzed at 1 year postoperatively of an intragroup comparison of patients who received the large-head MOM THA showed a 46-fold increase in serum Co from preoperative median values of 0.11 µg/L (interquartile range, 0.1 to 0.2 µg/L) to the postoperative median of 5.09 µg/L (interquartile range, 3.0 to 7.5 µg/L). The resurfacing group showed only a 3.9-fold increase. Intergroup median serum levels for cobalt at 1 year postoperatively were 10-fold higher in the large-head MOM group than in the resurfacing group. Elevations in serum chromium ion levels were also seen to be statisically significant, with a 10.7-fold increase observed in the intragroup comparison of the large-head MOM group. Because the bearing surface was identical in the two groups, investigators attributed the markedly elevated serum cobalt and chromium levels to the modular connections of the large-head MOM group. They no longer recommend this particular design but acknowledge that further work is warranted to verify that their results are not solely implant dependent.

MacDonald and coworkers reported on the results of a prospective randomized blinded clinical trial performed to evaluate polyethylene versus metal bearing surfaces in THA while addressing specifically metal ions in both blood and urine. Results of the ion analysis have been described previously. Twenty-three patients received the M²a MOM liner, and 18 patients received the polyethylene insert. The acetabular component was titanium, and the metal liner was modular and was inserted into the titanium shell. All femoral heads were 28 mm in diameter. A standard Mallory Head (Biomet Inc., Warsaw, Ind) titanium femoral component was used in all patients. Although the primary outcome in this series involved metal ions, secondary outcome measures included Western Ontario and McMaster University (WOMAC) Osteoarthritis Index scores, Harris hip scores, and Short-Form 12 scores. No differences were noted in either group at an average of 3.2 years follow-up (range, 2.2 to 3.9 years). No clinical complications and no radiographic concerns were reported at latest follow-up.[44]

However, recent reports for large head MOM hips have caused concern among clinicians. A recent report with 12- to 74-month follow-up of the ASR described a 13% revision rate based on 190 hips.[68] A report based on 1167 procedures in the Australian registry data demonstrated a cumulative revision rate of the ASR XL acetabular system at 5 years to be 9.3%.[3] When adjusted for age, and sex the revision rate was four times it was for all other conventional THAs, irrespective of the surgical volume of the center. This hip system had a much higher 5-year revision rate for metal sensitivity, loosening and infection compared with MOP. In comparison to other MOM hips, the revision rate was 2.5 times greater. Revision rates for the ASR resurfacing system at 5 years post-operatively were almost 11%—much higher than the 4% reported for all other resurfacings. When adjusted for age and sex, this revision rate was twice that of other resurfacings. Head size did impact revision rates, with head sizes less than 44 mm having five times the revision rate of ASR resurfacing head sizes greater than 55 mm. Revision rates for the ASR resurfacing system did appear to be impacted by the volume of the surgical center.

Because of worrisome early reports and registry data, authors have tried to provide a higher level of evidence by analyzing current literature via systematic review or meta-analysis. A meta-analysis of eight randomized controlled trials (RCTs) comparing MOM to MOP THAs in 974 hips.[69] Although Titanium levels increased for both groups compared to pre-operatively, no differences in erythrocyte or urine Titanium levels were noted between groups. Cobalt and chrome levels increased compared to pre-operatively for the MoM, with continued increase in value in serum and erythrocyte levels at 6, 12, and 24 months. No increase in cobalt or chrome levels was observed in the MOP group. In comparison to MOP, the MOM cobalt and chrome levels were increased for both blood and urine levels at 12 and 24 months. Revision rates were not different between groups. However, this meta-analysis had significant limitations. MOM hips used featured 28 mm heads with a follow-up of less than 4 years in most of the papers examined. More limiting to the study's usefulness was that only 6 studies provided reoperation rates. A second group conducted a systematic review of 18 studies that compared all bearing surfaces in 3404 hips.[70] MOM hips were found to have worse Harris hip scores than MOP hips. Of the two papers comparing MOM with MOP, no difference in revision rates were reported. However, this systematic review also was limited by the short follow-up of included papers, with only one article following to 5 years. There also was a relatively low number of patients in each paper; with no papers featuring over 200 patients.

Turning to registry data, data from England and Wales, based on more than 31,000 implants, produced some concerning findings. The resultant conclusion was that MOM THA should not be implanted.[71] Because the ASR has an elevated revision rate compared to other MOM THAs, it was excluded in an attempt to prevent data skew. The overall revision rate at 5 years was 6.2%—higher than for any other articular surface combination. With increased time in situ, an increased rate of revision was reported. Head size was an independent predictor of revision, with a 2% increase in the hazard of revision for each increase in head diameter. Revision rates were higher for women, and younger women were at higher risk of revision when compared with older women. For 60-year-old women, the revision rate for 46 mm MOM THA at 5 years was 6.1%—much higher than the 1.6% revision rate for a cemented 28-mm MOP.

Registry data from Australia revealed that the number of MOM hips at risk at 7 years is 1446, whereas 11,539 MOP hips are at risk.[72] The cumulative revision rate for MOM with heads larger than 28 mm is 7.7%. However, the cumulative revision rate of MOM with heads smaller than 28 mm is 4.4% at 7 years. This is identical to the rate of revision for MOP with the same head size. The rate of revision for MOP hips with head sizes greater than 28 mm was 3.2% at 7 years. With 32 mm used as the cutoff, revision rates of MOM hips smaller than this were 4.5% at 7 years; and 8.4% if greater than 32 mm. The increased rate of revision for heads larger than 32 mm is seen in both genders. The revision rate in heads larger than 32 mm varies according to the implant, with the highest rate of revision at 5 years seen with the ASR at 7.8%, and the lowest with the Articul/Eze head and Ultamet acetabulum combination (DePuy Orthopaedics) at 3.5%. Age was also a factor; revision rates for hip resurfacing at 7 years were 5.6% in patients younger than 55 but 7.3% for those older than 65. The revision rate at 7 years was higher for females (9.3%) than males (4.5%). For MOM THAs at five years, revision rates were proportional to head size: 3.6% if smaller than 28 mm, 4.2% if 30 to 32mm, 6.0% if 36 to 40mm, and 6.4% if larger than 40 mm. As opposed to MOM THA, in hip resurfacings, head size was inversely proportional to revision rates at 7 years, with 13.8% of heads smaller than 44 mm being revised, as well as 8.8% of heads between 45 and 49 mm, 3.7% of heads between 50 and 54 mm, and 2.2% of heads bigger than 55 mm. No gender difference was apparent. Revision rates at 7 years were approximately 10.3% for both males and females for heads smaller than 50 mm, and 3.4% for heads greater than 50 mm. The BHR had the lowest revision rate at 5 years of 3.5%; the ASR had the highest at 5 years at 10.9%.

Graves and associates published the results of the International Consortium of Orthopaedic Registries, looking primarily to combine the outcomes of the Australian, England and Wales, and New Zealand registries.[73] This consortium concluded that MOM THA with heads greater than 32 mm were more than twice as likely to require revision than those with heads smaller than 32 mm, at a rate of 9.4% at 7 years for heads larger than 32 mm, and 4.5% for heads smaller than 32 mm. Implant-specific outcomes at 5 years showed revision rates ranging from 3.5 to 7.8%. The highest listed revision rate was for the Bionik—8% at 3 years. Larger heads had increased rates of loosening, infection, and metal sensitivity when compared with smaller heads as the indication for revision. The consortium also reviewed results for hip resurfacings. The subgroup with the best performance was the males less than 65 years old, with large metal heads. However, this group had a revision rate that was similar to conventional total hip replacements.

Specific patient subgroups tend to respond differently to specific MOM hips. For example, the outcomes to the Birmingham Hip Resurfacing implant was examined in 646 hips at an average of 8 years (1 to 12 years) (554 patients) in one study.[74] In females, the 10-year survivorship was 74%. However, in males younger than 50 years treated for osteoarthritis, survivorship was 99% at 1 years. Pseudotumor formation and revision rates were higher in smaller cups. Overall, the revision rate for pseudotumour was 7.5%, but the incidence of pseudotumour was sensitive to component size and gender. The incidence was 18.8% in females and 28.8% in components smaller than 46 mm. In components greater than 50 mm, the incidence was 0%. These worrisome findings were not concluded in a publication from Birmingham, which looked at the influence of head size and gender on BHRs.[75] The study was based on 2123 BHRs— 799 female, with an average follow-up of 3.5 years (0 to 10.9 yrs). A total of 655 patients had follow-up beyond 5 years. Incremental decreases of head size by 4 mm showed a hazard rate of 4.9 in this study. The hazard rate for gender was not statistically significant. However, this study reported 95.5% survivorship at 10 years based on 20 patients with that length of follow-up.

Obscuring our ability to clearly differentiate outcomes with MOM hips is the variety of implants available. Although it is clear that some systems have a high failure rate, others do not. It has been shown that sub-hemispherical, monoblock shells do have a higher failure rate and should be approached with caution. However, modular acetabular MOM components may not have a high failure rate. For example, 85 Pinnacle MOM hips (DePuy Orthopaedics) with modular acetabular components with minimum follow-up of 5 years have been shown to have 97.8% survivorship at a mean of 7 years.[76]

In summary, significant concern has arisen regarding MOM THAs. The elevated revision rate has led some analysts to alarming conclusions because of the number of implants used. In patients older than 65, Medicare data alone indicates there are 49,646 MOM THAs implanted between 2005 and 2009 in the United States.[77] Although the number of hips involved is not known, 93,000 ASRs were manufactured, which is a matter of concern given the high revision rates seen so far.[3] These concerns have caused some regulatory bodies to recommend cessation of clinical use for all MOM. However,

this recommendation may be premature. Although monoblock, sub-hemispherical cups with large-diameter heads have a higher rate of revision, reports on survivorship for modular, hemispherical shells with smaller heads are much less worrisome. Long-term outcomes for correctly positioned, hemispherical modular acetabula articulating with head sizes around 28-32 mm need to be analyzed. Also, for younger males, large diameter resurfacings have been reported to have very good medium-term outcomes. Therefore, further follow-up is needed for these specific subgroups to gain a better understanding on the risks and benefits associated with MOM THAs.

IMMUNE RESPONSE (Table 72-2)

Metal sensitivity as a cause of aseptic loosening was proposed as far back as 1974.[78] In that study of McKee-Farrar arthroplasties, tissue adjacent to the bearings showed elevated chromium and cobalt levels compared with controls. Histologic examination showed macrophage and lymphocyte aggregates. All metals in contact with biological systems can corrode and generate metal ions that may stay bound to local tissues, or they may bond to protein moieties that are transported in the bloodstream and to lymphatics, hence to remote organs.[79] These metalloproteins can activate the immune system. Activation of T lymphocytes results in cytokine production (interferon-γ, tumor necrosis factor-α, receptor activator of nuclear factor κB ligand [RANKL], interleukin-1, and interleukin-2) and increased activation of macrophages.[80] Metal ions implicated in sensitivity reactions include nickel (Ni), cobalt (Co), chromium (Cr), titanium (Ti), vanadium (V), and tantalum (Ta).[50]

Table 72-2. Cobalt and Chromium Levels of Metal-on-Metal Implants

Study	Implant	Analytical Technique	Sample	No. of Implants	Time in Vivo, yr	Cobalt Levels, parts per billion	Chromium Levels, parts per billion
Brodner et al[54]	Metasul*	AAS	Serum	27	1	1.1	—
Brodner et al[120]	Metasul	AAS	Serum	36	5	0.7	—
Savarino et al[121]	Metasul	AAS	Serum	15	2	0.88	—
Savarino et al[121]	Metasul	AAS	Serum	15	4.3	0.81	—
Witzleb et al[122]	Metasul	AAS	Serum	60	2	1.70	4.28
Savarino et al[123]	Metasul	AAS	Serum	42	4	1.57	2.10
Grüb et al[66]	Metasul	AAS	Serum	22	10	0.75	0.95
Lazennac et al[41]	Metasul	ICP-MS	Serum	56	9	1.55	1.49
Saito et al[65]	Metasul	AAS	Serum	50	6.4	—	0.85
Dahlstrand et al[124]	Metasul	ICP-MS	Serum	54	2	1.01	1.15
	Metasul Average					**1.1**	**1.8**
MacDonald et al[44]	M²a†	ICP-MS	Erythrocytes	22	2	1.10	2.50
Rasquinha et al[125]	M²a	AAS	Serum	10	6	1.55	0.84
	M²a Average					**1.33**	**1.67**
Garbuz et al[67]	Durom‡	ICP-MS	Serum	26	2	5.38	2.88

AAS, Atomic absorption spectrophotometry; *ICP-MS*, inductively coupled plasma mass spectrometry.
*Zimmer Inc., Winterthur, Switzerland.
†Biomet Inc., Warsaw, Ind.
‡Zimmer Inc., Winterthur, Switzerland.

The dermal sensitivity most commonly seen is Ni, followed by Co and then Cr. The level of Ni sensitivity in the general population may be as high as 17%.[81] Dermal patch testing is commonly used to assess hypersensitivity to metal; however, it is unclear what relationship this has for prosthetic implants. The cascade involved differs in that it is a delayed cell-mediated response. Langerhans cells contained in the dermis are specific antigen-presenting cells (APCs) that are absent in deep periprosthetic tissues.[82] No dominant APC has been identified in the periprosthetic milieu. The incidence of metal sensitivity in well-functioning THAs has been estimated to be as low as less than 1% to as high as 25%.[80] Malfunctioning MOM implants produce high wear and are associated with effusions, pain, and osteolysis. No gold standard test is available for diagnosis of hypersensitivity to metal implants. The diagnosis is typically suspected on the basis of clinical criteria. Patients with metallic implants may be sensitized to metal debris because peripheral blood monocytes have been shown to produce elevated cytokine levels.[83] Hallab and colleagues[84] hypothesize that lymphocyte metal-induced reactivity increases with metal exposure. They describe a triple assay technique of lymphocyte activation (lymphocyte transformation testing [LTT], lymphocyte migration inhibition, and cytokine profiling).[85] Another observed feature of MOM bearings is the reduction in lymphocyte subsets,[86] the clinical significance of which currently remains unknown.

Histologic Examination

Aseptic lymphocytic vasculitis–associated lesion (ALVAL) is a term that was first used by Wilert and associates in 2005.[87] This newly described phenomenon has been documented only with second-generation MOM prostheses. Patients typically have persisting unexplained pain, effusions, and periprosthetic osteolysis and present on average 2 years postoperatively. Changes are seen histologically and are characterized by a prominent perivascular and/or diffuse lymphocytic infiltration. At revision surgery, areas of necrosis have been observed but typically without notable wear debris.[88,89] Pandit and colleagues[90] described a series of "pseudotumors" occurring in 17 patients (3 bilateral) who had undergone MOM resurfacing arthroplasties. All patients were female and presented postoperatively at a mean of 17 months (range, 0 to 60 months). The most common presenting symptom was discomfort in the groin, on the lateral aspect of the hip, or in the buttock. Other findings included dislocation, instability symptoms, and the presence of a lump, rash, or femoral nerve palsy. Erythrocyte sedimentation rate (ESR) and C-reactive protein (CRP) were normal in 15 of the 17 patients. Plain radiographs showed no lucency around either component. Cup inclination angles varied between 22 degrees and 75 degrees, with seven cases having angles between 40 degrees and 45 degrees. Ultrasonography, MRI, CT, and hip arthrography were used to image the joints further. The most common finding was a cystic mass lying posterolateral to the joint. Histologically, lesions were characterized by the presence of metal wear particles, extensive necrosis, and macrophage and lymphocytic infiltrates. Twelve patients underwent revision surgery; all symptoms improved in eight patients and settled completely in four. In a follow-up report,[91] the outcome after revision for pseudotumor was noted to be poor, with low functional outcome scores and a major complication rate of 50%. Recurrent dislocations, nerve palsies, further component loosening, and recurrence of pseudotumors were observed. Hart and associates further characterized MRI findings by classifying them.[92] A pseudotumour type 1 is thin walled and fluid filled, type 2a is thick walled and fluid filled, type 2b is thick walled with variable signal on T2 imaging, and type 3 is solid, with a mixed signal on MRI.

Chromosomal Anomalies

Potential mutagenic damage in peripheral blood lymphocytes undergoing revision arthroplasty for predominantly MOP THAs was examined by Doherty and associates.[93] An increase in both aneuploidy and chromosomal translocations was noted when compared with controls. Genetic changes can be normal as a result of aging and environmental factors. The authors propose that monitoring of genetic damage coupled with measurement of metal ion levels may aid in the monitoring of long-term effects of different bearings in joint arthroplasty. A subsequent report[94] has shown chromosomal abnormalities to be increased in patients with well-functioning Metasul MOM hip replacements. Whole blood analysis confirmed an expected rise in peripheral whole blood Cr and Co levels after 2 years, but no statistical correlation was noted between metal ion levels in whole blood and chromosomal translocations and aneuploidy, except for molybdenum.

Dunstan and coworkers[95] examined the level of chromosomal abnormalities in peripheral blood in a cohort of nine patients with MOM prostheses who previously had been treated for varying primary bone tumors. They were analyzed along with a control group of six patients who had no implant. Of the nine patients with an original MOM prosthesis, four had undergone later revision to MOP bearings and were considered as a separate subgroup. Original diagnoses included giant cell tumor of bone (two), Ewing's sarcoma, chondrosarcoma, and synovial chondromatosis. Original diagnoses in the revised group included giant cell tumor of bone (two) and chondrosarcoma (two). A statistically significant elevation of chromosomal abnormalities—both aneuploidy gain and structural aberrations—was observed in patients with an MOM hip bearing compared with age- and sex-matched controls; this was absent in the group revised to an MOP bearing.

In addition to observations of chromosomal abnormalities in peripheral blood of patients with MOM prostheses, synovial fluid containing metallic debris has been shown to cause an elevation in DNA damage to in vitro cultures of fibroblasts.[96] No documented result indicates that any increase in observed DNA damage or chromosomal abnormalities results in the occurrence of de novo malignancy. In conclusion, the clinical significance of these studies remains uncertain.

CARCINOGENICITY

Metal ion elevation in blood and urine samples of patients with well-functioning MOM THAs has been well documented. Concerns have arisen regarding the long-term effects of raised metal ion exposure, particularly in the younger patient population suitable for MOM bearings, who may have exposure over several decades. A consistent metal ion production level is seen in the well-functioning prosthesis, even during steady-state wear. In vitro studies have shown metal ions to be toxic to macrophages and hepatocyes,[97-99] and some animal studies have reported an elevated carcinoma rate when exposed to elevated levels of chromium, cobalt, and nickel.[100-102] Because of their small size, metal particles can spread to distant organ sites, especially to regional lymph nodes, liver, and spleen.[103-105] Campbell[106] has reported on the autopsy findings of a patient with a McKee-Farrar prosthesis in place for 29 years. Particle size identified was on average 77 nm; approximately half of the findings were consistent with Co-Cr, and the remainder were consistent with Cr oxides. The greatest numbers of particles were found in the abdominal lymph nodes but particles were also seen in the liver, spleen, and other lymph nodes. No evidence of end-organ damage was identified in any of the tissues.

Visuri[107] examined the incidence of cancer after MOM THA and conventional MOP arthroplasty in comparison with the general population in Finland. The series consisted of 579 patients who had a McKee-Farrar MOM and 1585 who had MOP. During the follow-up period, 113 malignant cancers were diagnosed in the MOM group. Total cancer incidence in both groups was less than that expected in the general population. The standardized incidence ratio for all cancers in the MOM arthroplasty group was 0.95 (95% CI, 0.79 to 1.13). This was not statistically greater than the standardized ratio for patients having MOP THAs (0.76; 95% CI, 0.68 to 0.86). The combined standardized incidence ratio for lymphoma and leukemia in patients who had MOM total hip arthroplasty was 1.59 (95% CI, 0.82 to 2.77) and 0.59 in those who had MOP THA (95% CI, 0.29 to 1.05). A linkage study involving the National Joint Registry of England and Wales and hospital statistics was conducted with similar results.[108] Stemmed MOM hips had lower rates of cancer than expected (1.15% in men vs. an expected 1.45%, 0.84% vs. 1.22% in women). Resurfacings showed even lower rates (0.48% in men vs. an expected rate of 0.77%, 0.56% in women vs. an expected 0.73%). Resurfacings were found to have lower rates of prostate cancer, haematologic cancers or any cancer when compared with other bearings. Gillespie[109] initially reported an increase in incidence of tumors of the lymphatic and hematopoietic system, but this was refuted in a later publication.[110]

As was previously discussed by MacDonald,[111] all these studies are significantly underpowered to detect clinically relevant differences. After 40 years of clinical use, no epidemiologic evidence suggests increased risk of malignancy in patients with MOM bearings. Conflicting data have been obtained regarding the ability of metal ions to cross the placenta[112,113]; however, most surgeons avoid implanting MOM prostheses into women of childbearing age.

FUTURE DIRECTIONS

Currently, only medium-term clinical results are available for MOM bearings. Evidence suggests that subhemispherical acetabula placed in excessive inclination with large head articulation have a significant predisposition to early failure, as do small-diameter heads, in hip resurfacings. However, long-term outcomes of modular, hemispherical cups in good position with smaller articular heads remain unclear. Also unclear are the long-term outcomes of resurfacing arthroplasties in young males with large heads who appear to have the best subgroup results. Close follow-up of patients with MOM hips is needed and may require the use of serum ion levels or cross-sectional imaging, as well as local and systemic examination for toxicity. Although the elevated revision rate in registry data has caused some countries to recommend cessation of utilization, this recommendation may be premature. At this time, caution is recommended before implantation of stemmed MOM THAs, as is careful consideration of the type of prosthesis when large head resurfacing is considered in specific patients.

REFERENCES

1. Bozic KJ, Kurtz S, Lau E, et al: The epidemiology of bearing surface usage in total hip arthroplasty in the United States. J Bone Joint Surg Am 91(7):1614–1620, 2009.
2. Neumann DR, Thaler C, Hitzl W, Huber M, Hofstadter T, Dorn U: Long-term results of a contemporary metal-on-metal total hip arthroplasty: A 10-year follow-up study. J Arthroplasty 25(5):700–708, 2010.
3. de Steiger RN, Hang JR, Miller LN, Graves SE, Davidson DC: Five-year results of the ASR XL acetabular system and the ASR hip resurfacing system: An analysis from the Australian orthopaedic association national joint replacement registry. J Bone Joint Surg Am 93(24):2287–2293, 2011.
4. Wright DM, Alonso A, Rathinam M, Sochart DH: Smith-petersen mould arthroplasty: An ultra-long-term follow-up. J Arthroplasty 21(6):916–917, 2006.
5. Wiles P: The surgery of the osteo-arthritic hip. Clin Orthop Relat Res 417:3–16, 2003.
6. Brown SR, Davies WA, DeHeer DH, Swanson AB: Long-term survival of McKee-farrar total hip prostheses. Clin Orthop Relat Res 402:157–163, 2002.
7. Dandy DJ, Theodorou BC: The management of local complications of total hip replacement by the McKee-Farrar technique. J Bone Joint Surg Br 57(1):30–35, 1975.
8. Ring PA: Five to fourteen year interim results of uncemented total hip arthroplasty. Clin Orthop Relat Res (137):87–95, 1978.
9. Weber BG: Experience with the metasul total hip bearing system. Clin Orthop Relat Res (329 Suppl):S69–77, 1996.
10. Jantsch S, Schwagerl W, Zenz P, Semlitsch M, Fertschak W: Long-term results after implantation of McKee-farrar total hip prostheses. Arch Orthop Trauma Surg 110(5):230–237, 1991.
11. Higuchi F, Inoue A, Semlitsch M: Metal-on-metal CoCrMo McKee-farrar total hip arthroplasty: Characteristics from a long-term follow-up study. Arch Orthop Trauma Surg 116(3):121–124, 1997.
12. Griffin WL, Nanson CJ, Springer BD, Davies MA, Fehring TK: Reduced articular surface of one-piece cups: A cause of runaway wear and early failure. Clin Orthop Relat Res 468(9):2328–2332, 2010.

13. Malchau H, Herberts P, Eisler T, Garellick G, Soderman P: The swedish total hip replacement register. J Bone Joint Surg Am 84-A(Suppl 2):2–20, 2002.

14. Silva M, Shepherd EF, Jackson WO, Dorey FJ, Schmalzried TP: Average patient walking activity approaches 2 million cycles per year: Pedometers under-record walking activity. J Arthroplasty 17(6):693–697, 2002.

15. Schmalzried TP, Szuszczewicz ES, Northfield MR, et al: Quantitative assessment of walking activity after total hip or knee replacement. J Bone Joint Surg Am 80(1):54–59, 1998.

16. Clarke IC, Good V, Williams P, et al: Ultra-low wear rates for rigid-on-rigid bearings in total hip replacements. Proc Inst Mech Eng H 214(4):331–347, 2000.

17. Holt G, Murnaghan C, Reilly J, Meek RM: The biology of aseptic osteolysis. Clin Orthop Relat Res 460:240–252, 2007.

18. Schulte KR, Callaghan JJ, Kelley SS, Johnston RC: The outcome of charnley total hip arthroplasty with cement after a minimum twenty-year follow-up. the results of one surgeon. J Bone Joint Surg Am 75(7):961–975, 1993.

19. Jacobs JJ, Skipor AK, Patterson LM, et al: Metal release in patients who have had a primary total hip arthroplasty. A prospective, controlled, longitudinal study. J Bone Joint Surg Am 80(10):1447–1458, 1998.

20. Fisher J, Jin Z, Tipper J, Stone M, Ingham E: Tribology of alternative bearings. Clin Orthop Relat Res 453:25–34, 2006.

21. Lee R, Essner A, Wang A: Tribological considerations in primary and revision metal-on-metal arthroplasty. J Bone Joint Surg Am 90(Suppl 3):118–124, 2008.

22. Firkins PJ, Tipper JL, Saadatzadeh MR, et al: Quantitative analysis of wear and wear debris from metal-on-metal hip prostheses tested in a physiological hip joint simulator. Biomed Mater Eng 11(2):143–157, 2001.

23. Rieker C, Shen M, Kottig P: In-vivo tribological performance of 177 metal-on-metal hip articulations. In Eiker C, Oberholzer S, Wyss U, editors: World tribology forum in arthroplasty, Bern, Switzerland, 2001, Hans Huber, p 137.

24. Sieber HP, Rieker CB, Kottig P: Analysis of 118 second-generation metal-on-metal retrieved hip implants. J Bone Joint Surg Br 81(1):46–50, 1999.

25. Langton DJ, Jameson SS, Joyce TJ, Hallab NJ, Natu S, Nargol AV: Early failure of metal-on-metal bearings in hip resurfacing and large-diameter total hip replacement: A consequence of excess wear. J Bone Joint Surg Br 92(1):38–46, 2010.

26. Schmidt M, Weber H, Schon R: Cobalt chromium molybdenum metal combination for modular hip prostheses. Clin Orthop Relat Res (329 Suppl):S35–47, 1996.

27. Witzleb WC, Hanisch U, Ziegler J, Guenther KP: In vivo wear rate of the birmingham hip resurfacing arthroplasty. A review of 10 retrieved components. J Arthroplasty 24(6):951–956, 2009.

28. Glyn-Jones S, Roques A, Taylor A, et al: The in vivo linear and volumetric wear of hip resurfacing implants revised for pseudotumor. J Bone Joint Surg Am 93(23):2180–2188, 2011.

29. Kwon YM, Glyn-Jones S, Simpson DJ, et al: Analysis of wear of retrieved metal-on-metal hip resurfacing implants revised due to pseudotumours. J Bone Joint Surg Br 92(3):356–361, 2010.

30. Kinbrum A, Unsworth A: The wear of high-carbon metal-on-metal bearings after different heat treatments. Proc Inst Mech Eng H 222(6):887–895, 2008.

31. Dowson D, Hardaker C, Flett M, Isaac GH: A hip joint simulator study of the performance of metal-on-metal joints: Part I: The role of materials. J Arthroplasty 19(8 Suppl 3):118–123, 2004.

32. Firkins PJ, Tipper JL, Ingham E, Stone MH, Farrar R, Fisher J: Influence of simulator kinematics on the wear of metal-on-metal hip prostheses. Proc Inst Mech Eng H 215(1):119–121, 2001.

33. Chan FW, Bobyn JD, Medley JB, Krygier JJ, Tanzer M: The otto aufranc award. wear and lubrication of metal-on-metal hip implants. Clin Orthop Relat Res 369:10–24, 1999.

34. Squire M, Griffin WL, Mason JB, Peindl RD, Odum S: Acetabular component deformation with press-fit fixation. J Arthroplasty 21(6 Suppl 2):72–77, 2006.

35. Lee JM, Salvati EA, Betts F, DiCarlo EF, Doty SB, Bullough PG: Size of metallic and polyethylene debris particles in failed cemented total hip replacements. J Bone Joint Surg Br 74(3):380–384, 1992.

36. Doorn PF, Campbell PA, Worrall J, Benya PD, McKellop HA, Amstutz HC: Metal wear particle characterization from metal on metal total hip replacements: Transmission electron microscopy study of periprosthetic tissues and isolated particles. J Biomed Mater Res 42(1):103–111, 1998.

37. Coleman RF, Herrington J, Scales JT: Concentration of wear products in hair, blood, and urine after total hip replacement. Br Med J 1(5852):527–529, 1973.

38. Bosker BH, Ettema HB, Boomsma MF, Kollen BJ, Maas M, Verheyen CC: High incidence of pseudotumour formation after large-diameter metal-on-metal total hip replacement: A prospective cohort study. J Bone Joint Surg Br 94(6):755–761, 2012.

39. Mao X, Wong AA, Crawford RW: Cobalt toxicity–an emerging clinical problem in patients with metal-on-metal hip prostheses? Med J Aust 194(12):649–651, 2011.

40. Tower SS: Arthroprosthetic cobaltism: Neurological and cardiac manifestations in two patients with metal-on-metal arthroplasty: A case report. J Bone Joint Surg Am 92(17):2847–2851, 2010.

41. Lazennec JY, Boyer P, Poupon J, et al: Outcome and serum ion determination up to 11 years after implantation of a cemented metal-on-metal hip prosthesis. Acta Orthop 80(2):168–173, 2009.

42. Ebreo D, Khan A, El-Meligy M, Armstrong C, Peter V: Metal ion levels decrease after revision for metallosis arising from large-diameter metal-on-metal hip arthroplasty. Acta Orthop Belg 77(6):777–781, 2011.

43. MacDonald SJ: Can a safe level for metal ions in patients with metal-on-metal total hip arthroplasties be determined? J Arthroplasty 19(8 Suppl 3):71–77, 2004.

44. MacDonald SJ, McCalden RW, Chess DG, et al: Metal-on-metal versus polyethylene in hip arthroplasty: A randomized clinical trial. Clin Orthop Relat Res 406:282–296, 2003.

45. Van Der Straeten C, Grammatopoulos G, Gill HS, Calistri A, Campbell P, De Smet KA: The 2012 otto aufranc award: The interpretation of metal ion levels in unilateral and bilateral hip resurfacing. Clin Orthop Relat Res 2012.

46. Khan M, Takahashi T, Kuiper JH, Sieniawska CE, Takagi K, Richardson JB: Current in vivo wear of metal-on-metal bearings assessed by exercise-related rise in plasma cobalt level. J Orthop Res 24(11):2029–2035, 2006.

47. Kuzyk PR, Sellan M, Olsen M, Schemitsch EH: Hip resurfacing versus metal-on-metal total hip arthroplasty—are metal ion levels different? Bull NYU Hosp Jt Dis 69(Suppl 1):S5–11, 2011.

48. MacDonald SJ, Brodner W, Jacobs JJ: A consensus paper on metal ions in metal-on-metal hip arthroplasties. J Arthroplasty 19(8 Suppl 3):12–16, 2004.

49. Jacobs JJ, Skipor AK, Campbell PA, Hallab NJ, Urban RM, Amstutz HC: Can metal levels be used to monitor metal-on-metal hip arthroplasties? J Arthroplasty 19(8 Suppl 3):59–65, 2004.

50. Griffin WL, Fehring TK, Kudrna JC, et al: Are metal ion levels a useful trigger for surgical intervention? J Arthroplasty 27(8 Suppl):32–36, 2012.

51. Bernstein M, Desy NM, Petit A, Zukor DJ, Huk OL, Antoniou J: Long-term follow-up and metal ion trend of patients with metal-on-metal total hip arthroplasty. Int Orthop 36(9):1807–1812, 2012.

52. Macnair RD, Wynn-Jones H, Wimhurst JA, Toms A, Cahir J: Metal ion levels not sufficient as a screening measure for adverse reactions in metal-on-metal hip arthroplasties. J Arthroplasty 2012.

53. Kennedy JG, Rogers WB, Soffe KE, Sullivan RJ, Griffen DG, Sheehan LJ: Effect of acetabular component orientation on recurrent dislocation, pelvic osteolysis, polyethylene wear, and component migration. J Arthroplasty 13(5):530–534, 1998.

54. Brodner W, Bitzan P, Meisinger V, Kaider A, Gottsauner-Wolf F, Kotz R: Elevated serum cobalt with metal-on-metal articulating surfaces. J Bone Joint Surg Br 79(2):316–321, 1997.

55. Angadji A, Royle M, Collins SN, Shelton JC: Influence of cup orientation on the wear performance of metal-on-metal hip replacements. Proc Inst Mech Eng H 223(4):449–457, 2009.

56. Williams S, Leslie I, Isaac G, Jin Z, Ingham E, Fisher J: Tribology and wear of metal-on-metal hip prostheses: Influence of cup angle and head position. J Bone Joint Surg Am 90(Suppl 3):111–117, 2008.

57. De Haan R, Pattyn C, Gill HS, Murray DW, Campbell PA, De Smet K: Correlation between inclination of the acetabular component and metal ion levels in metal-on-metal hip resurfacing replacement. J Bone Joint Surg Br 90(10):1291–1297, 2008.

58. Langton DJ, Jameson SS, Joyce TJ, Webb J, Nargol AV: The effect of component size and orientation on the concentrations of metal ions after resurfacing arthroplasty of the hip. J Bone Joint Surg Br 90(9):1143–1151, 2008.

59. Hart AJ, Buddhdev P, Winship P, Faria N, Powell JJ, Skinner JA: Cup inclination angle of greater than 50 degrees increases whole blood concentrations of cobalt and chromium ions after metal-on-metal hip resurfacing. Hip Int 18(3):212–219, 2008.

60. Hart AJ, Ilo K, Underwood R, et al: The relationship between the angle of version and rate of wear of retrieved metal-on-metal resurfacings: A prospective, CT-based study. J Bone Joint Surg Br 93(3):315–320, 2011.

61. Mellon SJ, Kwon YM, Glyn-Jones S, Murray DW, Gill HS: The effect of motion patterns on edge-loading of metal-on-metal hip resurfacing. Med Eng Phys 33(10):1212–1220, 2011.

62. Schmalzried TP: Metal-metal bearing surfaces in hip arthroplasty. Orthopedics 32(9):10, 2009.3928/01477447-20090728-06.

63. Eswaramoorthy V, Moonot P, Kalairajah Y, Biant LC, Field RE: The metasul metal-on-metal articulation in primary total hip replacement: Clinical and radiological results at ten years. J Bone Joint Surg Br 90(10):1278–1283, 2008.

64. Sharma S, Vassan U, Bhamra MS: Metal-on-metal total hip joint replacement: A minimum follow-up of five years. Hip Int 17(2):70–77, 2007.

65. Saito S, Ryu J, Watanabe M, Ishii T, Saigo K: Midterm results of metasul metal-on-metal total hip arthroplasty. J Arthroplasty 21(8):1105–1110, 2006.

66. Grubl A, Marker M, Brodner W, et al: Long-term follow-up of metal-on-metal total hip replacement. J Orthop Res 25(7):841–848, 2007.

67. Garbuz DS, Tanzer M, Greidanus NV, Masri BA, Duncan CP: The john charnley award: Metal-on-metal hip resurfacing versus large-diameter head metal-on-metal total hip arthroplasty: A randomized clinical trial. Clin Orthop Relat Res 468(2):318–325, 2010.

68. Hug KT, Watters TS, Vail TP, Bolognesi MP: The withdrawn ASR THA and hip resurfacing systems: How have our patients fared over 1 to 6 years? Clin Orthop Relat Res 2012.

69. Qu X, Huang X, Dai K: Metal-on-metal or metal-on-polyethylene for total hip arthroplasty: A meta-analysis of prospective randomized studies. Arch Orthop Trauma Surg 131(11):1573–1583, 2011.

70. Sedrakyan A, Normand SL, Dabic S, Jacobs S, Graves S, Marinac-Dabic D: Comparative assessment of implantable hip devices with different bearing surfaces: Systematic appraisal of evidence. BMJ 343:d7434, 2011.

71. Smith AJ, Dieppe P, Vernon K, Porter M, Blom AW: National Joint Registry of England and Wales. Failure rates of stemmed metal-on-metal hip replacements: Analysis of data from the national joint registry of england and wales. Lancet 379(9822):1199–1204, 2012.

72. Australian Orthopaedic Association National Joint Replacement Registry: Annual report. 2010.

73. Graves SE, Rothwell A, Tucker K, Jacobs JJ, Sedrakyan A: A multinational assessment of metal-on-metal bearings in hip replacement. J Bone Joint Surg Am 93(Suppl 3):43–47, 2011.

74. Murray DW, Grammatopoulos G, Pandit H, Gundle R, Gill HS, McLardy-Smith P: The ten-year survival of the birmingham hip resurfacing: An independent series. J Bone Joint Surg Br 94(9):1180–1186, 2012.

75. McBryde CW, Theivendran K, Thomas AM, Treacy RB, Pynsent PB: The influence of head size and sex on the outcome of birmingham hip resurfacing. J Bone Joint Surg Am 92(1):105–112, 2010.

76. Kindsfater KA, Sychterz Terefenko CJ, Gruen TA, Sherman CM: Minimum 5-year results of modular metal-on-metal total hip arthroplasty. J Arthroplasty 27(4):545–550, 2012.

77. Bozic KJ, Lau EC, Ong KL, Vail TP, Rubash HE, Berry DJ: Comparative effectiveness of metal-on-metal and metal-on-polyethylene bearings in medicare total hip arthroplasty patients. J Arthroplasty 27(8 Suppl):37–40, 2012.

78. Evans EM, Freeman MA, Miller AJ, Vernon-Roberts B: Metal sensitivity as a cause of bone necrosis and loosening of the prosthesis in total joint replacement. J Bone Joint Surg Br 56-B(4):626–642, 1974.

79. Jacobs JJ, Gilbert JL, Urban RM: Corrosion of metal orthopaedic implants. J Bone Joint Surg Am 80(2):268–282, 1998.

80. Hallab N, Merritt K, Jacobs JJ: Metal sensitivity in patients with orthopaedic implants. J Bone Joint Surg Am 83-A(3):428–436, 2001.

81. Dotterud LK, Smith-Sivertsen T: Allergic contact sensitization in the general adult population: A population-based study from northern norway. Contact Dermatitis 56(1):10–15, 2007.

82. Jacobs JJ, Campbell PA, T Konttinen Y, Implant Wear Symposium 2007 Biologic Work Group: How has the biologic reaction to wear particles changed with newer bearing surfaces? J Am Acad Orthop Surg 16(Suppl 1):S49–S55, 2008.

83. Lee SH, Brennan FR, Jacobs JJ, Urban RM, Ragasa DR, Glant TT: Human monocyte/macrophage response to cobalt-chromium corrosion products and titanium particles in patients with total joint replacements. J Orthop Res 15(1):40–49, 1997.

84. Hallab NJ, Anderson S, Caicedo M, Skipor A, Campbell P, Jacobs JJ: Immune responses correlate with serum-metal in metal-on-metal hip arthroplasty. J Arthroplasty 19(8 Suppl 3):88–93, 2004.

85. Hallab NJ, Mikecz K, Jacobs JJ: A triple assay technique for the evaluation of metal-induced, delayed-type hypersensitivity responses in patients with or receiving total joint arthroplasty. J Biomed Mater Res 53(5):480–489, 2000.

86. Hart AJ, Skinner JA, Winship P, et al: Circulating levels of cobalt and chromium from metal-on-metal hip replacement are associated with CD8+ T-cell lymphopenia. J Bone Joint Surg Br 91(6):835–842, 2009.

87. Willert HG, Buchhorn GH, Fayyazi A, et al: Metal-on-metal bearings and hypersensitivity in patients with artificial hip joints. A clinical and histomorphological study. J Bone Joint Surg Am 87(1):28–36, 2005.

88. Shimmin A, Beaule PE, Campbell P: Metal-on-metal hip resurfacing arthroplasty. J Bone Joint Surg Am 90(3):637–654, 2008.

89. Ollivere B, Darrah C, Barker T, Nolan J, Porteous MJ: Early clinical failure of the birmingham metal-on-metal hip resurfacing is associated with metallosis and soft-tissue necrosis. J Bone Joint Surg Br 91(8):1025–1030, 2009.

90. Pandit H, Glyn-Jones S, McLardy-Smith P, et al: Pseudotumours associated with metal-on-metal hip resurfacings. J Bone Joint Surg Br 90(7):847–851, 2008.

91. Grammatopolous G, Pandit H, Kwon YM, et al: Hip resurfacings revised for inflammatory pseudotumour have a poor outcome. J Bone Joint Surg Br 91(8):1019–1024, 2009.

92. Hart AJ, Satchithananda K, Liddle AD, et al: Pseudotumors in association with well-functioning metal-on-metal hip prostheses: A case-control study using three-dimensional computed tomography and magnetic resonance imaging. J Bone Joint Surg Am 94(4):317–325, 2012.

93. Doherty AT, Howell RT, Ellis LA, et al: Increased chromosome translocations and aneuploidy in peripheral blood lymphocytes of patients having revision arthroplasty of the hip. J Bone Joint Surg Br 83(7):1075–1081, 2001.

94. Ladon D, Doherty A, Newson R, Turner J, Bhamra M, Case CP: Changes in metal levels and chromosome aberrations in the peripheral blood of patients after metal-on-metal hip arthroplasty. J Arthroplasty 19(8 Suppl 3):78–83, 2004.

95. Dunstan E, Ladon D, Whittingham-Jones P, Carrington R, Briggs TW: Chromosomal aberrations in the peripheral blood of patients with metal-on-metal hip bearings. J Bone Joint Surg Am 90(3):517–522, 2008.

96. Davies AP, Sood A, Lewis AC, Newson R, Learmonth ID, Case CP: Metal-specific differences in levels of DNA damage caused by synovial fluid recovered at revision arthroplasty. J Bone Joint Surg Br 87(10):1439–1444, 2005.

97. Catelas I, Petit A, Vali H, et al: Quantitative analysis of macrophage apoptosis vs. necrosis induced by cobalt and chromium ions in vitro. Biomaterials 26(15):2441–2453, 2005.

98. Gunaratnam M, Grant MH: The interaction of the orthopaedic metals, chromium VI and nickel, with hepatocytes. J Mater Sci Mater Med 12(10-12):945–948, 2001.

99. Huk OL, Catelas I, Mwale F, Antoniou J, Zukor DJ, Petit A: Induction of apoptosis and necrosis by metal ions in vitro. J Arthroplasty 19(8 Suppl 3):84–87, 2004.

100. Heath JC, Freeman MA, Swanson SA: Carcinogenic properties of wear particles from prostheses made in cobalt-chromium alloy. Lancet 1(7699):564–566, 1971.

101. Lewis CG, Sunderman FW, Jr: Metal carcinogenesis in total joint arthroplasty. animal models. Clin Orthop Relat Res (329 Suppl):S264–8, 1996.

102. Memoli VA, Urban RM, Alroy J, Galante JO: Malignant neoplasms associated with orthopedic implant materials in rats. J Orthop Res 4(3):346–355, 1986.

103. Shea KG, Lundeen GA, Bloebaum RD, Bachus KN, Zou L: Lymphoreticular dissemination of metal particles after primary joint replacements. Clin Orthop Relat Res 338:219–226, 1997.

104. Urban RM, Jacobs JJ, Tomlinson MJ, Gavrilovic J, Black J, Peoc'h M: Dissemination of wear particles to the liver, spleen, and abdominal lymph nodes of patients with hip or knee replacement. J Bone Joint Surg Am 82(4):457–476, 2000.

105. Urban RM, Tomlinson MJ, Hall DJ, Jacobs JJ: Accumulation in liver and spleen of metal particles generated at nonbearing surfaces in hip arthroplasty. J Arthroplasty 19(8 Suppl 3):94–101, 2004.

106. Campbell P, Urban RM, Catelas I, Skipor AK, Schmalzried TP: Autopsy analysis thirty years after metal-on-metal total hip replacement. A case report. J Bone Joint Surg Am 85-A(11):2218–2222, 2003.

107. Visuri T, Pukkala E, Paavolainen P, Pulkkinen P, Riska EB: Cancer risk after metal on metal and polyethylene on metal total hip arthroplasty. Clin Orthop Relat Res (329 Suppl):S280–9, 1996.

108. Smith AJ, Dieppe P, Porter M, Blom AW: National Joint Registry of England and Wales. Risk of cancer in first seven years after metal-on-metal hip replacement compared with other bearings and general population: Linkage study between the national joint registry of England and Wales and hospital episode statistics. BMJ 344:e2383, 2012.

109. Gillespie WJ, Frampton CM, Henderson RJ, Ryan PM: The incidence of cancer following total hip replacement. J Bone Joint Surg Br 70(4):539–542, 1988.

110. Gillespie WJ, Henry DA, O'Connell DL, et al: Development of hematopoietic cancers after implantation of total joint replacement. Clin Orthop Relat Res (329 Suppl):S290–6, 1996.

111. MacDonald SJ: Metal-on-metal total hip arthroplasty: The concerns. Clin Orthop Relat Res 429:86–93, 2004.

112. Ziaee H, Daniel J, Datta AK, Blunt S, McMinn DJ: Transplacental transfer of cobalt and chromium in patients with metal-on-metal hip arthroplasty: A controlled study. J Bone Joint Surg Br 89(3):301–305, 2007.

113. Brodner W, Grohs JG, Bancher-Todesca D, et al: Does the placenta inhibit the passage of chromium and cobalt after metal-on-metal total hip arthroplasty? J Arthroplasty 19(8 Suppl 3):102–106, 2004.

114. Dorr LD, Wan Z, Longjohn DB, Dubois B, Murken R: Total hip arthroplasty with use of the metasul metal-on-metal articulation. four to seven-year results. J Bone Joint Surg Am 82(6):789–798, 2000.

115. Wagner M, Wagner H: Medium-term results of a modern metal-on-metal system in total hip replacement. Clin Orthop Relat Res 379:123–133, 2000.

116. Lombardi A, Mallory T, Alexiades M: Short-term results of the M2a-taper metal-on-metal articulation. J Arthroplasty 16:122–128, 2001.

117. Long WT, Dorr LD, Gendelman V: An american experience with metal-on-metal total hip arthroplasties: A 7-year follow-up study. J Arthroplasty 19(8 Suppl 3):29–34, 2004.

118. Dorr LD, Wan Z, Sirianni LE, Boutary M, Chandran S: Fixation and osteolysis with metasul metal-on-metal articulation. J Arthroplasty 19(8):951–955, 2004.

119. Engh CA, Jr, MacDonald SJ, Sritulanondha S, Thompson A, Naudie D, Engh CA: 2008 John Charnley award: Metal ion levels after metal-on-metal total hip arthroplasty: A randomized trial. Clin Orthop Relat Res 467(1):101–111, 2009.

120. Brodner W, Bitzan P, Meisinger V, Kaider A, Gottsauner-Wolf F, Kotz R: Serum cobalt levels after metal-on-metal total hip arthroplasty. J Bone Joint Surg Am 85-A(11):2168–2173, 2003.

121. Savarino L, Granchi D, Ciapetti G, et al: Ion release in stable hip arthroplasties using metal-on-metal articulating surfaces: A comparison between short- and medium-term results. J Biomed Mater Res A 66(3):450–456, 2003.

122. Witzleb WC, Ziegler J, Krummenauer F, Neumeister V, Guenther KP: Exposure to chromium, cobalt and molybdenum from metal-on-metal total hip replacement and hip resurfacing arthroplasty. Acta Orthop 77(5):697–705, 2006.

123. Savarino L, Greco M, Cenni E, et al: Differences in ion release after ceramic-on-ceramic and metal-on-metal total hip replacement. Medium-term follow-up. J Bone Joint Surg Br 88(4):472–476, 2006.

124. Dahlstrand H, Stark A, Anissian L, Hailer NP: Elevated serum concentrations of cobalt, chromium, nickel, and manganese after metal-on-metal alloarthroplasty of the hip: A prospective randomized study. J Arthroplasty 24(6):837–845, 2009.

125. Rasquinha VJ, Ranawat CS, Weiskopf J, Rodriguez JA, Skipor AK, Jacobs JJ: Serum metal levels and bearing surfaces in total hip arthroplasty. J Arthroplasty 21(6 Suppl 2):47–52, 2006.

CHAPTER 73

Ceramic-on-Ceramic Bearings

Aaron Carter and Peter F. Sharkey

KEY POINTS

- Ceramic-on-ceramic bearings in total hip arthroplasty were first implemented as a solution to wear debris and subsequent osteolysis seen in traditional bearing surfaces.
- Ceramics are hard, scratch-resistant, wear-resistant, low-friction, thermodynamically stable, chemically inert, biocompatible, and resistant to corrosion.
- Concerns about ceramics include risk of fracture, the phenomenon of stripe wear, motion-related noise, impingement, and limitations in component options available to the surgeon.
- Early ceramics experienced a high fracture rate; however, owing to manufacturing and design advances, modern ceramics have shown promising clinical results.
- Ceramics are best used in a young active population in whom wear and osteolysis are concerns.

INTRODUCTION

The most frequently used bearing surface in total hip arthroplasty (THA) is the metal head articulating with an ultra-high-molecular-weight polyethylene socket. It is considered the standard bearing surface for THA in the United States. As the indications for THA are extending to a younger and more active population, the focus has been moving toward increasing the longevity of these implants. Wear debris from polyethylene leading to periprosthetic osteolysis is considered the major long-term complication resulting in the need for revision.[1-3] The extent of osteolysis is of major importance not only in terms of the likelihood of failure, but also in terms of the complexities of obtaining fixation of new components during revision surgery and the long-term success of the revision surgery itself.[1] The need for improved bearing surfaces has led to cross-linking of polyethylene via a variety of methods. These advancements have greatly improved the wear characteristics of polyethylene.[4,5] Studies have shown that cross-linking polyethylene in an articulation with a metal or a ceramic head can reduce wear by more than 50%.[6-8] However, cross-linking polyethylene may weaken the polyethylene, causing catastrophic failure with cracking of the liner.[9-11]

Ceramics were originally introduced as a solution to the problems of friction and wear seen in metal-on-polyethylene and metal-on-metal configurations. The intended goal of the ceramic-on-ceramic bearing is to reduce biologically active wear debris, thereby minimizing the occurrence of osteolysis and aseptic loosening.[12] The standard ceramic-on-ceramic articulation is the alumina-on-alumina bearing. Both in vitro and clinical retrieval studies have demonstrated a significant reduction in wear and particle production when compared with metal on polyethylene articulations.[13-17] Osteolysis in these bearings appears to be minimal or nonexistent.[18,19] Although osteolysis has only rarely been identified with the ceramic-on-ceramic articulation, potential disadvantages have been identified. Ceramics are hard, brittle materials that lack fracture toughness. Improvements in processing and machining of ceramics have reduced fracture risk; however, this complication has not yet been eliminated.[15,20-24] Other disadvantages of ceramic-on-ceramic articulations include stripe wear, motion-related noise, impingement, and limited head and liner options.

This chapter will review the basic science of ceramic-on-ceramic bearings, including mechanical properties, advantages, and disadvantages of this articulation. Clinical studies related to ceramic-on-ceramic bearings will be summarized, and future directions will be discussed.

BASIC SCIENCE

History

The ceramic-on-ceramic articulation was first introduced by Pierre Boutin and associates in 1970 as an alternative to the conventional metal-on-polyethylene total hip.[25] Early results for this first prosthesis showed promise; however, ceramic fracture was a matter of concern.[26] High fracture rates were attributable to the large grain sizes, low density, and impurity of the alumina.[27] Prior fixation methods involved gluing the head to the stem with a resin or screwing it in place.[26] As the production of surgical-grade dense alumina ceramic evolved, strong fixation of the ceramic head to the metal stem was achieved with the introduction of the Morse taper in 1977, significantly reducing the risk of fracture to 2%.[26,28] Current alumina production techniques have brought the fracture rate to 0.004%.[29] With the reduction in the risk of fracture, acetabular component fixation leading to loosening and subsequent revision became the major long-term problem for these devices. Various methods of fixation were explored, finally leading to the use of porous-coated titanium shells with modular acetabular inserts press-fit into bone.[26] Despite their use in Europe, alumina femoral heads only became available in the early 1980s in the United States, with ceramic-on-ceramic alumina bearing surfaces available by the early 2000s.[30] Alumina has been a standardized material since 1984 (International Standard Organization [ISO] 6474).[26]

GENERAL STATEMENTS ABOUT CERAMICS

The two ceramic materials currently in clinical use as bearing surfaces are aluminum oxide (alumina) and zirconium oxide (zirconia). The ceramic-on-ceramic bearing surface is an alumina-on-alumina bearing surface because zirconia produces high wear when articulating against itself.[31] These materials exist in their highest oxidation state, allowing excellent biocompatibility, thermodynamic stability, chemical inertness, and resistance to corrosion.[31] Ceramics are water insoluble and have excellent compression strength but poor bending strength.[28,31] Because of their mechanical properties, ceramics are considered hard and brittle in nature.

Use of proprietary ceramic processing methods by each manufacturer reflects the fact that all ceramics are not alike and subtle differences exist between ceramics manufactured by each company.

MANUFACTURING PROCESS

Alumina ceramics are manufactured under a complex process involving multiple steps under intense and optimal quality control. The mechanical properties of the final product rely heavily on proper performance of these manufacturing steps.[26]

The current third generation of ceramic processing consists of mixing aluminum oxide powder with organic bonding agents, water, and lubricants.[27] The mixture is isostatically pressed into a mold that will give it its final shape. The formed piece is then dried, while the water is evaporated, and a thermal process removes the organic binder. The product is then sintered at a very high temperature (between 1600° C and 1800° C) under high pressure. The quality and purity of the initial powder and control of precision over the thermal process applied affect the final microstructure of the ceramic.[26,28] Mechanical strength and tribological characteristics are determined by the purity, porosity, and grain size through the ceramic. When ceramics were first produced, longer sintering times were necessary to achieve full or nearly full density; however, larger grain size resulted, thus reducing overall strength and contributing to early failures.[27,31] The addition of materials such as CaO or MgO prevented grain growth, allowing manufacturers to achieve smaller grain sizes and thus higher strength and reliability.[31] These additions in the

late 1980s and early 1990s would be considered second-generation ceramics, which would later give rise to the third-generation ceramics in use today.[27] The third-generation ceramics were developed in 1994 and constitute ceramics that employ hot isostatic pressing, further resulting in smaller grain size, minimal grain boundaries and inclusions, and increased burst strength and wear resistance.[29] Currently, four major companies in the world meet the technologically demanding and complex process requirements needed to produce medical grade ceramics, including Ceraver Osteal (Roissy, France), Ceramtec AG (Stuttgart, Germany), Morgan Advanced Ceramics (Rugby, UK), and Kyocera (Kyoto, Japan).[26] Since 2003, several companies have released ceramics for use in the United States (Wright Medical Technology, Arlington, Tenn; Stryker-Howmedica-Osteonics, Allendale, NJ; Encore Medical, Austin, Tex; Smith & Nephew, Memphis, Tenn; Biomet, Warsaw, Ind; DePuy Orthopaedics, Warsaw, Ind; Zimmer, Warsaw, Ind; Stelkast, McMurray, Pa; and Exactech, Gainesville, Fla).[26,32]

Flaws in the manufacturing process can lead to catastrophic ceramic fracture. Crack propagation and subsequent fracture can result from flaws as small as the size of a few alumina grains.[31] Improvements in the manufacturing process such as diminishing the size of grains used for fabricating components have reduced the risk of fracture. When ceramics were first introduced, the average grain size was 50 μm. The alumina used today has an average grain size of 2 μm, contributing to the substantial decrease in risk of catastrophic fracture.[33]

ALUMINA CERAMICS MECHANICAL PROPERTIES

Alumina ceramic is a highly oxidized, hard, stable monophasic polycrystalline form of industrial sapphire.[34] Because of its high oxidation state, alumina exists in a low state of energy and exhibits a high state of thermodynamic stability. It has a high thermal conductivity coefficient and exhibits excellent resistance to corrosion. Alumina is also biologically inert and is resistant to further oxidation because of its fully oxidized state.[31] The ionic structure of alumina creates a hydrophilic state, resulting in fluid film lubrication and leading to higher wettability compared with orthopedic polymers and metals.[26,35] This increases lubrication of the joint. The intrinsic hardness of alumina makes it highly abrasion and wear resistant.[26,36] The hardness of alumina increases resistance to scratching, making it much less likely to scratch than titanium or cobalt chrome alloys. The only material that is capable of scratching alumina is diamond. Scratch resistance makes alumina resistant to third-body wear.[37]

Alumina has strong compression strength despite poor bending characteristics. Alumina also lacks the ability to deform under high stress owing to its stiffness. This has limited ceramic use to only the femoral head and the cup liner. Polyethylene has the capability to mold around the femoral head if any inconsistency is present between articular surfaces. Ceramics lack this capability and are subject to high wear rates if any articulation mismatch occurs.[13,38] Clearance between the ceramic femoral head and the socket must be over 50 μm to prevent grain detachment and third-body wear.[39] Lack of ceramic deformation makes the points of contact between articulation surfaces smaller than with metal-on-polyethylene articulations. Advances in manufacturing techniques since 1993 have made it unnecessary to factory-match components.

Mechanical and biological factors have been linked to cement fragmentation and eventual loosening.[35] The stiffness of alumina ceramics is roughly 300 times higher than that of cancellous bone and is 190 times higher than that of polymethylmethacrylate (PMMA).[26] This modulus mismatch alters the stress distribution across the ceramic-cement-bone interface. This in combination with stress shielding makes microfracture of cement likely.[35] In addition, the low damping capacity of alumina may increase the risk of cement or bone microfracture due to excess transmission of impact loading.[35] These properties prevent the use of ceramics in the manufacture of stem or socket components.

Alumina ceramics are brittle because of excellent compression strength and low bending strength. Ceramics exhibit a linear elastic behavior and low fracture toughness, causing them to break without warning.[26] The risk of ceramic fracture is determined by the initial flaws of the ceramic. The incidence of fracture has substantially decreased over time owing to smaller grain size, fewer impurities, laser etching, and proof testing. The burst strength of alumina has improved over time from 38 kilonewtons (1977) to 98 kilonewtons (1998), far exceeding the U.S. Food and Drug Administration (FDA) limit of 46 kilonewtons.[26]

TRIBOLOGICAL PROPERTIES

Tribology is the science of the mechanisms of friction, lubrication, and wear of interacting surfaces that are in relative motion. In vitro studies and retrieval analysis have provided useful information on the function and behavior of ceramic-on-ceramic prostheses.

Numerous in vitro wear studies have documented the low friction and wear of alumina on alumina.[40,41] Low surface roughness secondary to small grain size, hardness contributing to scratch resistance, and enhanced wettability and fluid film lubrication result in the excellent tribological properties of the alumina articulation. In vitro testing has demonstrated that two phases of wear are present.[42] The first million cycles constitute the "run-in" phase, and wear rates for alumina on alumina range between 0.1 and 0.3 mm³ per million cycles.[42,43] The second phase is termed the *steady-state* phase, and volumetric wear rates decrease to less than 0.01 mm³.[42,43] This wear is considerably less when compared with the traditional metal-on-polyethylene bearing, and in some studies is up to 5000 times less.[26,37,42,44]

Accelerated wear can occur in alumina-on-alumina couples in certain clinical situations. A unique phenomenon of stripe wear occurs from microseparation during the swing phase of gait, or when the ball is levered out of the socket by impingement, resulting in edge loading and accelerated wear over a discreet area. Conditions associated with ceramic wear include vertical cup position, femoral neck impingement, and femoral head separation.[45] In vitro testing that simulates microseparation has been able to reproduce wear rates and patterns comparable with those seen clinically.[21] Wear as high as 1.24 mm³ per million cycles can occur with separation and stripe wear. Particles produced from wear also exhibit a bimodal distribution that is speculated to be generated by two separate mechanisms in vivo. Nanometer-size particles (5 to 90 nm) are produced from polishing under normal articulating conditions. Micrometer-size particles (0.05 to 3.2 μm) are produced by stripe wear and transgranular fracture of the ceramic.[21,46]

Numerous retrieval studies have been performed to analyze the performance of ceramic-on-ceramic bearings. One study examined alumina component retrieval associated with aseptic loosening of the socket at a mean of 11 years after implantation.[13] Components were classified into three groups: (1) low wear with no visible sign of wear; (2) stripe wear with a visible oblong worn area on the femoral heads and penetration less than 10 μm/yr; and (3) severe wear with visible loss of material on both components, and maximum penetrations greater than 150 μm. Examination of the 11 components revealed massive wear on two devices, and the remaining nine components demonstrated linear wear rates less than 15 μm/yr. The authors concluded that one type of wear has a negligible effect on the long-term life of the implant, and a second type of wear leads to catastrophic destruction of the bearing surface. Clinical wear rates of the bearing surface vary, ranging from 0.3 μm/yr to 5.0 mm/yr.[37,44,47] Improvement in alumina quality, in addition to factors responsible for a load increase (weight, young age, and male gender) or for impairment in the load distribution over the component surfaces (large grain size, nonoptimal initial cup inclination, and cup migration and/or tilting), can account for these variations.[13] It is important to note, however, that most catastrophic wear has been reported in products produced before 1990.[13,27,29] Recent wear rates have been consistently below 15 μm/yr.[13,47]

WEAR DEBRIS AND TISSUE RESPONSE

In vitro and in vivo studies have shown that alumina debris is biologically inert and well tolerated. The small size and the low volume of alumina wear particles generated result in a low level of bioactivity.[12,18,48-50] In contrast with polyethylene or metallic particles, giant cells have not been observed in contact with alumina wear particles. One study compared 12 periprosthetic membranes collected during revision surgery for aseptic component loosening in an alumina-on-alumina articulation, and compared them with membranes collected from metal-on-polyethylene bearings.[35] In the alumina-on-alumina group, the mild cellular reaction was in fact due to the use of zirconia ceramic particles in the cement as an opacifying agent. The zirconia ceramic was present in large enough amounts to illicit a small macrophage response, which subsequently contributed to component loosening. No cellular reaction to the alumina particles was noted, which contrasted with the polyethylene debris generated from the metal-on-polyethylene group.

Osteolysis associated with alumina-on-alumina bearings has been reported rarely. One study demonstrated a high revision rate (27%) due to aseptic loosening in a cohort of 69 hips when the bearing was made with ceramics consisting of large grain size and high porosity.[38] These factors resulted in a large production of debris and osteolysis. Another observation found periprosthetic tissue from alumina-on-alumina couples retrieved at revision surgery to have lower prostaglandin E_2 levels than tissue obtained from hips with metal on polyethylene.[38]

A separate study demonstrated that alumina and polyethylene debris stimulate release of tumor necrosis factor (TNF).[51] Cell mortality and the amount of TNF released increase with the size and concentration of alumina particles. This same study also showed that polyethylene particles cause greater release of TNF, stimulating up to 8 to 10 times the quantity of ceramic particles.[51] Alumina particles have been shown to induce macrophage apoptosis, which provides a mechanism to explain the lower levels of TNF. This could also explain the differences seen in osteolysis patterns of ceramic-on-ceramic when compared with metal-on-polyethylene articulations.[50]

CERAMIC ADVANTAGES

The primary advantage of using a ceramic-on-ceramic articulation is decreased wear and osteolysis.[7,18,26,41,43] Osteolysis is considered the major phenomenon preventing development of a longer-lasting hip replacement. As the indications for total hip arthroplasty have been extended to younger, healthier, and more active patients, the need to eliminate wear and osteolysis has become more apparent.

The tribological properties of alumina make ceramics ideal for the articular surfaces of total hip arthroplasty. The surface roughness of alumina has been greatly reduced with reduced grain size and improved polishing technology resulting from advances in material processing. The inherent hard characteristics of alumina make the material resistant to scratches, minimizing third-body wear from bone, cement, or metal debris. Alumina ceramic is also considered to have high compression strength and low bioreactivity. One advantage of ceramics over metal-on-metal bearings is that they do not increase serum or cellular ion content.[52,53] The ionic properties of alumina in combination with body fluids make the ceramic surface wettable, creating a fluid film that decreases friction. Low wear rates in combination with minimal bioreactivity decrease the likelihood of osteolysis. With current implant design and advanced ceramic processing, osteolysis has not been reported in follow-up as long as 18.5 years.[19]

CURRENT CONTROVERSIES AND FUTURE DIRECTIONS

Major Ceramic Concerns

Fracture

Ceramic fracture is caused by the propagation of nanometric cracks when an unexpected high load pressure is applied to the material.[28] Cracks are created when the stress-intensity factor is higher than the fatigue limit ($K1_0$) of the ceramic. When the stress-intensity factor (K1) exceeds the fracture toughness ($K1_c$), the ceramic will fracture abruptly without warning.[28] In normal physiologic conditions, the stress intensity should not reach the fatigue limit.[54] Imperfections in the materials can initiate cracks. These initial cracks will grow at different velocities, depending on the size of the initial flaw, the quality of the alumina material, and the load applied.[26]

The poor quality of the initial ceramics resulted in a high incidence of component fracture. Over time, decreased grain size, higher density, fewer impurities, improvements in ceramic processing, laser etching, and proof testing have decreased the risk of catastrophic fracture. The incidence of fracture in the 1990s was 0.8%, and today it is between 0.004% and 0.010% —a 200-fold decrease.[20,29] However, fractures still occur.[22-24,55,56] Owing to the more demanding nature of ceramic production compared with metal and polyethylene components, the incidence of catastrophic failure will likely always be higher.

Proof testing involves subjecting ceramic components to stresses greater than those expected to break the weak components and thus remove flawed products that are likely to fail. The tests are designed to be non-destructive but stringent enough to remove weak parts. Proof testing, however, is not 100% effective because components likely to fail are not always eliminated. In 1998, a manufacturing change resulted in a 1 in 3 clinical failure rate of zirconia femoral heads despite proof testing.[30]

Proper surgical technique is extremely important in that malpositioning can lead to component fracture. Ceramics are less resistant to nonuniform loading owing to their high modulus of elasticity, making initial component positioning vital to the longevity of the implant. During implantation, generation of any stress intensity factors should be avoided.[28] Any foreign body between the trunion and the head, or strong impaction of the head on the trunion with a mallet, should be avoided.[28] Only after the ceramic head is concentrically placed on the metal trunion should the head be impacted.[23,28] Rotation of the femoral head during insertion ensures concentricity, and failure to do so can lead to malalignment, point contact stresses, and increased risk of failure.[20] Uniformity of the manufacturer between head and stem is important in that taper angles differ between companies.[33] It is also theoretically possible to nonconcentrically place the ceramic liner into the metal acetabular shell; however, the long-term consequences of this have not yet been reported.[20,57]

Ceramic component fracture is a medical emergency that requires immediate revision surgery. Revision surgery due to ceramic fracture involves a thorough synovectomy and débridement to remove as much ceramic debris as possible.[58] This is important because ceramic debris embedded in the soft tissue can lend itself to third-body wear or accelerated wear if a metal-on-polyethylene bearing surface is used. Ceramic replacement heads are usually not an option because the trunion is commonly damaged in fracture. Even with immediate intervention and proper surgical technique, revision for fracture still carries a greater risk of less than optimal outcome. One study found that revision for fracture carried a 63% survival rate at 5 years (Figs. 73-1 and 73-2).[58]

Stripe Wear

Retrieval studies have reported that the most commonly observed pattern of wear was a stripe scar on the femoral head and the rim of the socket.[15] Originally thought to be associated with the poor quality of first-generation alumina, the stripe wear phenomenon has also been shown in modern alumina bearings.[15] Stripe

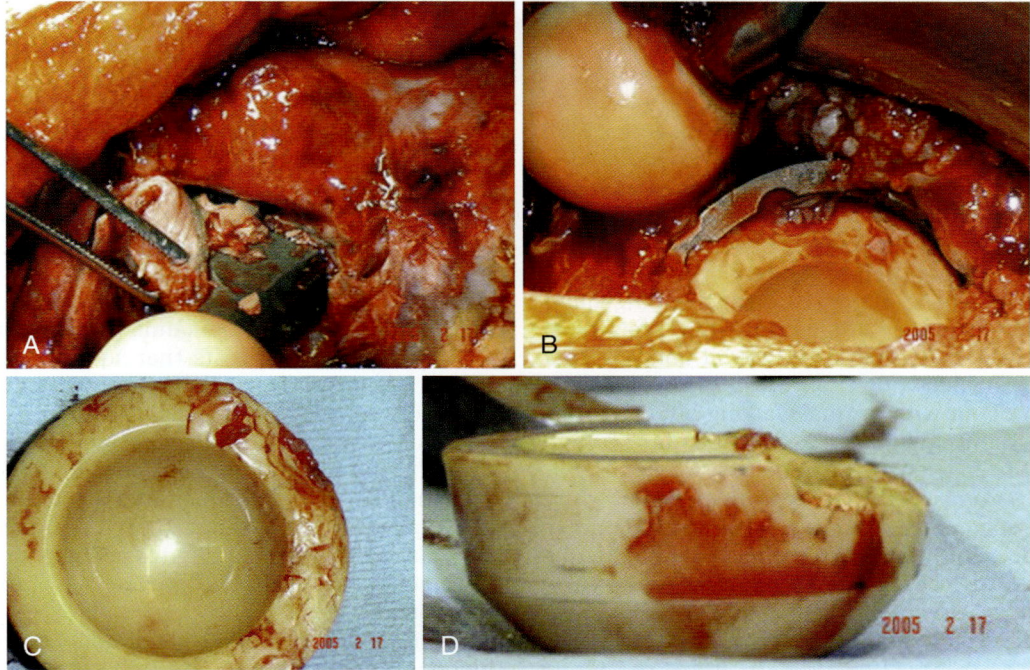

Figure 73-1. Ceramic liner fragmentation and anterior margin damage. **A,** Debris seen around the femoral stem. **B,** Liner fractured at the anterior margin in situ and after removal (**C** and **D**). *(From McCarthy MJ, Halawa M: Case report: lining up the liner: 2 case reports of early ceramic liner fragmentation. J Arthroplasty 22:1217–1222, 2007.)*

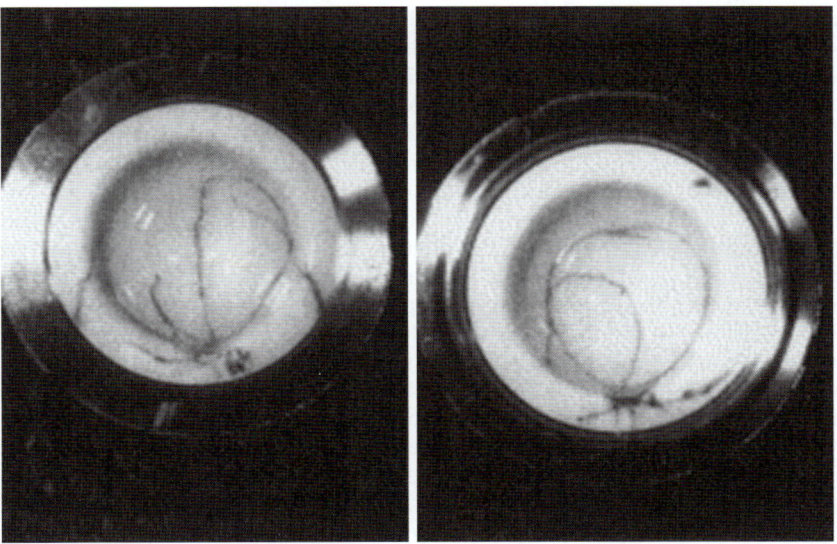

Figure 73-2. Examples of fractured liners. Cracks were stained to aid in visualization. *(From Maher SA, Lipman JD, Curley LJ, et al: Mechanical performance of ceramic acetabular liners under impact conditions. J Arthroplasty 18:936–941, 2003.)*

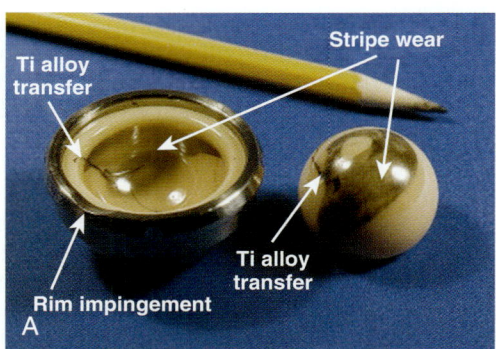
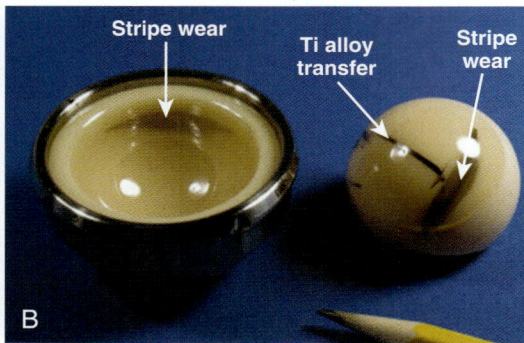

Figure 73-3. A, An acetabular component retrieved from a patient with squeaking hip shows evidence of impingement. Note the indentation of the metal rim generated by the femoral neck. **B,** Components retrieved from a patient with squeaking hip show stripe wear on the femoral head and the acetabular component. *(From Restrepo C, Parvizi J, Kurtz SM, et al: The noisy ceramic hip: is component malpositioning the cause? J Arthroplasty 23:643–649, 2008.)*

wear is of concern because of its association with a high rate of volumetric wear, averaging 1.24 mm^3 per million cycles in one study.[21] A bimodal distribution of nanometer- and micrometer-sized particles is also produced, which increases tissue response. Stripe wear is said to result from microseparation of the ball from the socket during the swing phase of gait or during impingement of the trunion on the acetabular rim, which has been replicated in vitro.[21] A separate retrieval analysis that mapped wear stripes, however, suggested that most stripes do not occur with normal walking but with edge loading when the hip is flexed, as with climbing a high step or rising from a chair.[59] A recent study by Taylor and associates concluded that wear stripes caused by edge loading may be associated with bearing noise during edge loading alone or during normal articulation.[60] When stripe wear occurs, surface roughness increases greatly, along with the coefficient of friction of the bearing surface (Fig. 73-3).

The Squeaking Hip

Motion-related noise is a phenomenon that is unique to hard-on-hard bearing surfaces in total hip arthroplasty. The noise can be so disconcerting that revision surgery is requested by the patient. Patients with alumina-on-alumina bearings have described this motion-related noise as squeaking. The incidence of squeaking in North America following ceramic-on-ceramic total hip arthroplasty has ranged from 0% to 3%.[61] Direct questioning of patients, however, has suggested that the incidence of squeaking is higher than was previously reported. Jarrett and colleagues reported that 14 (10.7%) of 131 patients with ceramic-on-ceramic bearings had audible squeak when directly questioned through administration of a questionnaire.[61] Of these 14 patients, one patient (<1%) reported squeaking before administration of the questionnaire. Four patients (3%) were able to reproduce the squeak through the combination of weight bearing and movement from 60 degrees of flexion to 0 degrees or full extension. One study in the Netherlands reported a 21% incidence of reproducible squeaking with the use of direct questioning, supporting the argument that this phenomenon is underreported.[62]

Numerous mechanisms have been proposed to determine the cause of the squeaking hip; however, the exact cause is still being debated. Technical factors such as mismatch in bearing surface and shorter neck length, as well as patient factors including younger age, taller height, and heavier weight, have been associated with squeaking.[62-64] Demographic factors may indicate the increased mechanical demands placed on the bearings. One in vitro test suggests that squeaking is a problem of lubrication, and that this noise occurs when the film fluid between two surfaces is disrupted.[64] Other studies have suggested that squeaking is related to cup position.[65,66] A study by Restrepo and coworkers reviewed the incidence of 999 ceramic-on-ceramic total hip arthroplasties and found that 28 patients reported squeaking.[67] When matched against a control group, however, no significant difference in acetabular position was found.

Retrieval analysis of noisy ceramic bearings has been inconclusive because interpretation of findings is limited by lack of a control group. Stripe wear and metallic staining have been noticed on noisy retrieved bearings.[60] This could be associated with the ceramic head subluxing and making contact with the protective metal rim around the ceramic or the acetabular shell. Squeaking most likely occurs when stripe wear develops and the bearing surface coefficient of friction increases greatly. Motion then can create enormous system energy, which vibrates the metal components. The measured frequency of squeaking is consistent with the vibration of titanium.

Management of squeaking begins with informing the patient that the occurrence of noise may be possible in an otherwise well-functioning arthroplasty. Patient perception that the prosthesis is malfunctioning may prompt litigation. Reassurance is appropriate because currently, there is no association between noise and a deteriorating articular surface. For most patients, squeaking is not problematic, and noise can be avoided by activity modification.[65] In some patients, the noise may be persistent enough that the patient is emotionally distraught and revision surgery is indicated. Intraoperatively, the cup and stem need to be carefully inspected to ensure appropriate position and fixation. Revision to a metal-on-polyethylene articulation will avoid the possibility of further squeaking because metal-on-metal articulations have been reported to make noise also.

Other Ceramic Concerns

Ceramic articulations are limited in the number of femoral head size and neck length options available to the surgeon. Traditional metal-on-polyethylene articulations have increased head sizes, modular head lengths, and liner options. Most ceramic-on-ceramic systems, however, have only two size liner diameters and paired head girths available for a given acetabular component. Offset and lipped acetabular liners are not produced because of concerns of impingement and chipping. In addition, collared heads are not manufactured, and this reduces the neck length options available. Because two crucial goals of THA are to equalize limb length and maximize stability, loss of head and liner options may be the most substantial disadvantage of ceramic-on-ceramic systems.[20] Clinically, the incidence of hip instability is low, however, after ceramic-on-ceramic THA.[7,57,68-70]

Impingement of the femoral component trunion on the ceramic liner edge can lead to chipping of the ceramic liner or notching of the femoral component.[7,20] To prevent this, one manufacturer (Stryker Orthopaedics, Kalamazoo, Mich) has added a protective metal rim to the ceramic shell liner. Even with this protective rim in place, impingement still may occur, leading to femoral neck notching and debris generation.

CLINICAL STUDIES

Since its introduction in the early 1970s, the ceramic-on-ceramic couple has been used in more than 150,000 total hip arthroplasties, primarily in Europe and Japan.[26] Poor quality alumina and less sophisticated technology initially resulted in a high failure rate, mostly caused by fracture. Component fixation also proved problematic in that cementing an all-acetabular component led to high aseptic loosening rates.[19,71] More modern implants have resulted in favorable clinical outcomes in terms of pain relief, durability, and decreased risk of fracture.

Hamadouche and associates reported on a consecutive series of 118 ceramic-on-ceramic arthroplasties (106 patients) performed between 1979 and 1980. Alumina heads measuring 32 mm with an all-alumina socket were used.[19] At 18.5 to 20 years' follow-up, 45 patients (51 hips) were alive and had not had a revision, 25 patients (25 hips) had undergone revision of one or both components, 27 patients (30 hips) had died, and 9 patients (12 hips) had been lost to follow-up. The mean Merle d'Aubigné functional hip score increased from 10.3 ± 2.2 points before surgery to 16.2 ± 1.8 points at the time of the most recent follow-up. No component fractures were noted, wear was not radiographically detectable, and only 3 of 118 hips had evidence of osteolysis. This study showed that minimal wear rates combined with limited osteolysis can be expected up to 20 years postoperatively, provided that sound acetabular component fixation is obtained.

Studies have also been published regarding the clinical outcome of younger patients receiving ceramic-on-ceramic arthroplasty. The same group of surgeons that conducted the previously mentioned study examined the results of ceramic-on-ceramic bearings in patients younger than age 55.[72] A total of 62 consecutive patients (71 hips) received hybrid alumina-on-alumina prostheses with a cemented titanium alloy stem, a 32-mm alumina head, and a press-fit metal-backed socket with an alumina insert. The component survival rate at 9 years' minimum follow-up was 93.7% with revision for any cause. In this series, no component fractures occurred, no radiographically measured wear was noted, and only two cases revealed minimal osteolysis.

Another study by Ha and colleagues reported encouraging data from intermediate-term results.[55] In all, 67 patients (78 hips) younger than age 50 underwent primary total hip arthroplasty utilizing a single cementless prosthesis design with an alumina-on-alumina articulation. At minimum 5 years' follow-up, one patient died and two were lost to follow-up. Of the remaining 64 patients (74 hips), good component fixation and no signs of osteolysis or wear were noted. The mean preoperative Harris hip score of 51 points improved to 94 points at the time of final follow-up. Two patients dislocated and were successfully treated with closed reduction. Other studies have been published supporting this data and demonstrating that alumina-on-alumina bearing surfaces seem to be a valuable alternative to the standard metal-on-polyethylene system for young patients.[73,74]

As interest in ceramic-on-ceramic articulations increased in the late 1990s, several U.S. device manufacturers began Investigational Device Exemption studies with ceramic articulations. Stryker Orthopaedics and Wright Medical Technology have published minimum 5-year results of total hip arthroplasties using ceramic bearings. These bearings were made by Ceramtec AG.

The Stryker Orthopaedics study examined 316 patients (328 hips) with ceramic-on-ceramic bearings implanted and matched them to a control group with metal-on-polyethylene bearings.[7] The patients in the study were fairly young, with an average age of 54 years at the time of index arthroplasty. At an average 5-year follow-up, equivalent Harris hip scores were reported in both groups (mean, 97). Proximal femoral osteolysis was noted in 0.6% of the ceramic group compared with 22.1% radiographically identifiable osteolysis in the metal-on-polyethylene group. Also of note, only 1.8% of patients in the ceramic group underwent revision, whereas 7.4% in the metal-on-polyethylene group required revision surgery. No catastrophic failures of the ceramics occurred; however, nine insertional ceramic chip fractures did occur. Stryker has since added a titanium sleeve to the ceramic acetabular insert, reducing the risk of chip fracture. However, this modification in design has raised concern over impingement on the metal sleeve, resultant metallosis, and increased risk of squeaking.[75]

In the Wright Medical Technology study, 1484 patients (1709 hips) underwent total hip arthroplasty with ceramic-on-ceramic bearings.[70] The mean age of patients studied was 52.1 years. The 8-year survival rate for any implant-related complication was 97%. The 8-year survival rate of the acetabular component was 99.9%, the femoral component 98.0%, and the bearing surface 99.0%. The catastrophic fracture rate was 0.2% (three liners, one femoral head), and three reoperations were required for dislocation (two early, one recurrent). One flaw in this study was that follow-up at greater than 5 years was available for only 633 of the 1709 patients.

Numerous studies have been published in the 3- to 8-year range that also indicate that ceramic-on-ceramic arthroplasty provides a promising bearing surface.[7,45,70,76-79] Additional studies with long-term follow-up data are warranted to determine the true potential of this articulation.

FUTURE DIRECTIONS

Alumina Matrix Composite (AMC)

Composite materials were first discovered when industrial manufacturers began investigating the method of transformation toughening as a means to strengthen alumina. Alumina matrix composite (AMC) is composed of small zirconia grains incorporated into the alumina matrix. These new mixed-oxide ceramics seem to provide a better ceramic in terms of fracture toughness without decreasing the sliding properties.[26] Composite ceramics also have the luxury of providing more component options (the offer of few component options is a limitation of alumina-on-alumina bearings).[80,81] Benchtop testing in one study demonstrated that AMC on alumina and AMC on AMC produce significantly lower wear rates than hot isostatically pressed (HIPed) alumina.[81] The same study also noted that AMC showed similar wear mechanisms and wear debris in previous alumina retrieval studies. AMC was first clinically used in the United States in June 2000 as a ceramic-on-polyethylene bearing. Currently, data showing the clinical performance of AMC-on-AMC bearings are just starting to be produced.[80,82]

SUMMARY

The ceramic-on-ceramic articulation was originally implemented to solve the long-term complication of wear and associated osteolysis found with more traditional bearing surfaces. Ceramics have the desired characteristics of hardness, wettability, significantly diminished wear, and biocompatibility. Early to mid-term results with the ceramic-on-ceramic articulation have shown promise in that patients have relief of pain and restoration of function equivalent to those seen with conventional total hip arthroplasties. However, ceramics do have several drawbacks. Although rare, catastrophic fracture of the head or liner is a medical emergency requiring immediate revision surgery.

Motion-related noise such as squeaking can be so bothersome to the patient that revision surgery will be required with an otherwise well-functioning implant. These complications may even prompt litigation for the surgeon. Another disadvantage is the limitation in head and liner options available to the surgeon, which can make the surgery more technically demanding. The long-term consequences of stripe wear and impingement have yet to be determined. Ceramic-on-ceramic bearings should be implanted only in young, highly active patients who are likely to have implant failure caused by wear and osteolysis. These factors should be taken into consideration when a ceramic-on-ceramic system is utilized. Only after informed consent has been obtained and the patient has acknowledged understanding of the potential risks associated with ceramic-on-ceramic bearings should surgery be performed.

REFERENCES

1. Harris WH: Wear and periprosthetic osteolysis: the problem. Clin Orthop Relat Res 393:66–70, 2001.
2. Soto MO, Rodriguez JA, Ranawat CS: Clinical and radiographic evaluation of the Harris-Galante cup: incidence of wear and osteolysis at 7 to 9 years follow-up. J Arthroplasty 15:139–145, 2000.
3. Kurtz S, Mowat F, Ong K, et al: Prevalence of primary and revision total hip and knee arthroplasty in the United States from 1990 through 2002. J Bone Joint Surg Am 87:1487–1497, 2005.
4. Geller JA, Malchau H, Bragdon C, et al: Large diameter femoral heads on highly cross-linked polyethylene: minimum 3-year results. Clin Orthop Relat Res 447:53–59, 2006.
5. Harris WH: Cross-linked polyethylene: why the enthusiasm? Instr Course Lect 50:181–184, 2001.
6. Harris WH, Muratoglu OK: A review of current cross-linked polyethylenes used in total joint arthroplasty. Clin Orthop Relat Res 430:46–52, 2005.
7. D'Antonio J, Capello W, Manley M, et al: Alumina ceramic bearings for total hip arthroplasty: five-year results of a prospective randomized study. Clin Orthop Relat Res 436:164–171, 2005.
8. Dorlot JM, Christel P, Meunier A: Wear analysis of retrieved alumina heads and sockets of hip prostheses. J Biomed Mater Res 23(A3 Suppl):299–310, 1989.
9. Bradford L, Baker D, Ries MD, Pruitt LA: Fatigue crack propagation resistance of highly crosslinked polyethylene. Clin Orthop Relat Res 429:68–72, 2004.
10. Bradford L, Kurland R, Sankaran M, et al: Early failure due to osteolysis associated with contemporary highly cross-linked ultra-high molecular weight polyethylene: a case report. J Bone Joint Surg Am 86:1051–1506, 2004.
11. Birman MV, Noble PC, Conditt MA, et al: Cracking and impingement in ultra-high-molecular-weight polyethylene acetabular liners. J Arthroplasty 20(7 Suppl 3):87–92, 2005.
12. Archibeck MJ, Jacobs JJ, Black J: Alternate bearing surfaces in total joint arthroplasty: biologic considerations. Clin Orthop Relat Res 379:12–21, 2000.
13. Prudhommeaux F, Hamadouche M, Nevelos J, et al: Wear of alumina-on-alumina total hip arthroplasties at a mean 11-year followup. Clin Orthop Relat Res 379:113–122, 2000.
14. Isaac GH, Wroblewski BM, Atkinson JR, Dowson D: A tribological study of retrieved hip prostheses. Clin Orthop Relat Res 276:115–125, 1992.
15. Yamamoto T, Saito M, Ueno M, et al: Wear analysis of retrieved ceramic-on-ceramic articulations in total hip arthroplasty: femoral head makes contact with the rim of the socket outside of the bearing surface. J Biomed Mater Res B Appl Biomater 73:301–307, 2005.
16. Fruh HJ, Willmann G: Tribological investigations of the wear couple alumina-CFRP for total hip replacement. Biomaterials 19:1145–1150, 1998.

17. Mochida Y, Boehler M, Salzer M, Bauer TW: Debris from failed ceramic-on-ceramic and ceramic-on-polyethylene hip prostheses. Clin Orthop Relat Res 389:113–125, 2001.
18. Bizot P, Nizard R, Hamadouche M, et al: Prevention of wear and osteolysis: alumina-on-alumina bearing. Clin Orthop Relat Res 393:85–93, 2001.
19. Hamadouche M, Boutin P, Daussange J, et al: Alumina-on-alumina total hip arthroplasty: a minimum 18.5-year follow-up study. J Bone Joint Surg Am 84:69–77, 2002.
20. Barrack RL, Burak C, Skinner HB: Concerns about ceramics in THA. Clin Orthop Relat Res 429:73–79, 2004.
21. Nevelos J, Ingham E, Doyle C, et al: Microseparation of the centers of alumina-alumina artificial hip joints during simulator testing produces clinically relevant wear rates and patterns. J Arthroplasty 15:793–795, 2000.
22. McLean CR, Dabis H, Mok D: Delayed fracture of the ceramic femoral head after trauma. J Arthroplasty 17:503–504, 2002.
23. Michaud RJ, Rashad SY: Spontaneous fracture of the ceramic ball in a ceramic-polyethylene total hip arthroplasty. J Arthroplasty 10:863–867, 1995.
24. Rhoads DP, Baker KC, Israel R, Greene PW: Fracture of an alumina femoral head used in ceramic-on-ceramic total hip arthroplasty. J Arthroplasty 23:1239e25–e30, 2008.
25. Boutin P: Total hip arthroplasty using a ceramic prosthesis: Pierre Boutin (1924-1989). Clin Orthop Relat Res 379:3–11, 2000.
26. Hannouche D, Hamadouche M, Nizard R, et al: Ceramics in total hip replacement. Clin Orthop Relat Res 430:62–71, 2005.
27. Capello WN, Dantonio JA, Feinberg JR, Manley MT: Alternative bearing surfaces: alumina ceramic bearings for total hip arthroplasty. Instr Course Lect 54:171–176, 2005.
28. Hannouche D, Nich C, Bizot P, et al: Fractures of ceramic bearings: history and present status. Clin Orthop Relat Res 417:19–26, 2003.
29. Willmann G: Ceramic femoral head retrieval data. Clin Orthop Relat Res 379:22–28, 2000.
30. Masonis JL, Bourne RB, Ries MD, et al: Zirconia femoral head fractures: a clinical and retrieval analysis. J Arthroplasty 19:898–905, 2004.
31. Skinner HB: Ceramic bearing surfaces. Clin Orthop Relat Res 369:83–91, 1999.
32. FDA premarket approvals database, Silver Spring, Md, 2009, Food and Drug Administration Center for Devices and Radiological Health.
33. Sedel L: Evolution of alumina-on-alumina implants: a review. Clin Orthop Relat Res 379:48–54, 2000.
34. Hamadouche M, Sedel L: Ceramics in orthopaedics. J Bone Joint Surg Br 82:1095–1099, 2000.
35. Lerouge S, Huk O, Yahia L, et al: Ceramic-ceramic and metal-polyethylene total hip replacements: comparison of pseudo-membranes after loosening. J Bone Joint Surg Br 79:135–139, 1997.
36. Endo MM, Barbour PS, Barton DC, et al: Comparative wear and wear debris under three different counterface conditions of crosslinked and non-crosslinked ultra high molecular weight polyethylene. Biomed Mater Eng 11:23–35, 2001.
37. Cooper JR, Dowson D, Fisher J, Jobbins B: Ceramic bearing surfaces in total artificial joints: resistance to third body wear damage from bone cement particles. J Med Eng Technol 15:63–67, 1991.
38. O'Leary JF, Mallory TH, Kraus TJ, et al: Mittelmeier ceramic total hip arthroplasty: a retrospective study. J Arthroplasty 3:87–96, 1988.
39. Sedel L: The tribology of hip replacement: European Instructional Course Lectures. EFORT 3:25–33, 1997.
40. Boutin P, Christel P, Dorlot JM, et al: The use of dense alumina-alumina ceramic combination in total hip replacement. J Biomed Mater Res 22:1203–1232, 1988.
41. Clarke IC: Role of ceramic implants: design and clinical success with total hip prosthetic ceramic-to-ceramic bearings. Clin Orthop Relat Res 282:19–30, 1992.
42. Oonishi H, Clarke IC, Good V, et al: Alumina hip joints characterized by run-in wear and steady-state wear to 14 million cycles in hip-simulator model. J Biomed Mater Res A 70:523–532, 2004.
43. Clarke IC, Good V, Williams P, et al: Ultra-low wear rates for rigid-on-rigid bearings in total hip replacements. Proc Inst Mech Eng H 214:331–347, 2000.
44. Davidson JA, Poggie RA, Mishra AK: Abrasive wear of ceramic, metal, and UHMWPE bearing surfaces from third-body bone, PMMA bone cement, and titanium debris. Biomed Mater Eng 4:213–229, 1994.
45. Greene JW, Malkani AL, Kolisek FR, et al: Ceramic-on-ceramic total hip arthroplasty. J Arthroplasty 24(6 Suppl):15–18, 2009.
46. Tipper JL, Hatton A, Nevelos JE, et al: Alumina-alumina artificial hip joints. Part II. Characterisation of the wear debris from in vitro hip joint simulations. Biomaterials 23:3441–3448, 2002.
47. Jazrawi LM, Bogner E, Della Valle CJ, et al: Wear rates of ceramic-on-ceramic bearing surfaces in total hip implants: a 12-year follow-up study. J Arthroplasty 14:781–787, 1999.
48. Sedel L: Ceramic hips. J Bone Joint Surg Br 74:331–332, 1992.
49. Catelas I, Petit A, Zukor DJ, et al: Induction of macrophage apoptosis by ceramic and polyethylene particles in vitro. Biomaterials 20:625–630, 1999.
50. Petit A, Catelas I, Antoniou J, et al: Differential apoptotic response of J774 macrophages to alumina and ultra-high-molecular-weight polyethylene particles. J Orthop Res 20:9–15, 2002.
51. Catelas I, Petit A, Marchand R, et al: Cytotoxicity and macrophage cytokine release induced by ceramic and polyethylene particles in vitro. J Bone Joint Surg Br 81:516–521, 1999.
52. Savarino L, Padovani G, Ferretti M, et al: Serum ion levels after ceramic-on-ceramic and metal-on-metal total hip arthroplasty: 8-year minimum follow-up. J Orthop Res 26:1569–1576, 2008.
53. Grübl A, Weissinger M, Brodner W, et al: Serum aluminium and cobalt levels after ceramic-on-ceramic and metal-on-metal total hip replacement. J Bone Joint Surg Br 88:1003–1005, 2006.
54. Willmann G: Ceramics for total hip replacement—what a surgeon should know. Orthopedics 21:173–177, 1998.
55. Ha YC, Koo KH, Jeong ST, et al: Cementless alumina-on-alumina total hip arthroplasty in patients younger than 50 years: a 5-year minimum follow-up study. J Arthroplasty 22:184–188, 2007.
56. Min BW, Song KS, Kang CH, et al: Delayed fracture of a ceramic insert with modern ceramic total hip replacement. J Arthroplasty 22:136–139, 2007.
57. Garino JP: Modern ceramic-on-ceramic total hip systems in the United States: early results. Clin Orthop Relat Res 379:41–47, 2000.
58. Allain J, Roudot-Thoraval F, Delecrin J, et al: Revision total hip arthroplasty performed after fracture of a ceramic femoral head: a multicenter survivorship study. J Bone Joint Surg Am 85:825–830, 2003.
59. Walter WL, Insley GM, Walter WK, Tuke MA: Edge loading in third generation alumina ceramic-on-ceramic bearings: stripe wear. J Arthroplasty 19:402–413, 2004.
60. Taylor S, Manley MT, Sutton K: The role of stripe wear in causing acoustic emissions from alumina ceramic-on-ceramic bearings. J Arthroplasty 22(7 Suppl 3):47–51, 2007.
61. Jarrett CA, Ranawat AS, Bruzzone M, et al: The squeaking hip: a phenomenon of ceramic-on-ceramic total hip arthroplasty. J Bone Joint Surg Am 91:1344–1349, 2009.
62. Keurentjes JC, Kuipers RM, Wever DJ, Schreurs BW: High incidence of squeaking in THAs with alumina ceramic-on-ceramic bearings. Clin Orthop Relat Res 466:1438–1443, 2008.
63. Morlock M, Nassutt R, Janssen R, et al: Mismatched wear couple zirconium oxide and aluminum oxide in total hip arthroplasty. J Arthroplasty 16:1071–1074, 2001.
64. Chevillotte C, Trousdale RT, Chen Q, et al: The 2009 Frank Stinchfield Award. "Hip squeaking": a biomechanical study of ceramic-on-ceramic bearing surfaces. Clin Orthop Relat Res 468:345–350, 2010.
65. Walter WL, O'Toole GC, Walter WK, et al: Squeaking in ceramic-on-ceramic hips: the importance of acetabular component orientation. J Arthroplasty 22:496–503, 2007.
66. Affatato S, Traina F, Mazzega-Fabbro C, et al: Is ceramic-on-ceramic squeaking phenomenon reproducible in vitro? A long-term simulator study under severe conditions. J Biomed Mater Res B Appl Biomater 91:264–271, 2009.

67. Restrepo C, Parvizi J, Kurtz SM, et al: The noisy ceramic hip: is component malpositioning the cause? J Arthroplasty 23:643–649, 2008.

68. Murphy SB, Ecker TM, Tannast M: Two- to 9-year clinical results of alumina ceramic-on-ceramic THA. Clin Orthop Relat Res 453:97–102, 2006.

69. Mai K, Hardwick ME, Walker RH, et al: Early dislocation rate in ceramic-on-ceramic total hip arthroplasty. HSS J 4:10–13, 2008.

70. Murphy S, Ecker T, Tannast M, et al: Experience in the United States with alumina ceramic-ceramic total hip arthroplasty. Semin Arthroplasty 17:120–124, 2006.

71. Nizard RS, Sedel L, Christel P, et al: Ten-year survivorship of cemented ceramic-ceramic total hip prosthesis. Clin Orthop Relat Res 282:53–63, 1992.

72. Bizot P, Hannouche D, Nizard R, et al: Hybrid alumina total hip arthroplasty using a press-fit metal-backed socket in patients younger than 55 years: a six- to 11-year evaluation. J Bone Joint Surg Br 86:190–194, 2004.

73. Yoo JJ, Kim YM, Yoon KS, et al: Contemporary alumina-on-alumina total hip arthroplasty performed in patients younger than forty years: a 5-year minimum follow-up study. J Biomed Mater Res B Appl Biomater 78:70–75, 2006.

74. Bizot P, Banallec L, Sedel L, Nizard R: Alumina-on-alumina total hip prostheses in patients 40 years of age or younger. Clin Orthop Relat Res 379:68–76, 2000.

75. Murali R, Bonar SF, Kirsh G, et al: Osteolysis in third-generation alumina ceramic-on-ceramic hip bearings with severe impingement and titanium metallosis. J Arthroplasty 23:1240e13–e19, 2008.

76. Lusty PJ, Tai CC, Sew-Hoy RP, et al: Third-generation alumina-on-alumina ceramic bearings in cementless total hip arthroplasty. J Bone Joint Surg Am 89:2676–2683, 2007.

77. Garcia-Cimbrelo E, Garcia-Rey E, Murcia-Mazon A, et al: Alumina-on-alumina in THA: a multicenter prospective study. Clin Orthop Relat Res 466:309–316, 2008.

78. Bierbaum BE, Nairus J, Kuesis D, et al: Ceramic-on-ceramic bearings in total hip arthroplasty. Clin Orthop Relat Res 405:158–163, 2002.

79. Capello WN, D'Antonio JA, Feinberg JR, et al: Ceramic-on-ceramic total hip arthroplasty: update. J Arthroplasty 23(7 Suppl):39–43, 2008.

80. Masson B: Emergence of the alumina matrix composite in total hip arthroplasty. Int Orthop 33:359–363, 2009.

81. Stewart TD, Tipper JL, Insley G, et al: Long-term wear of ceramic matrix composite materials for hip prostheses under severe swing phase microseparation. J Biomed Mater Res B Appl Biomater 66:567–573, 2003.

82. Lombardi AV Jr, Berend KR, Seng BE, et al: Delta ceramic-on-alumina ceramic articulation in primary THA: prospective, randomized FDA-IDE study and retrieval analysis. Clin Orthop Relat Res 468:367–374, 2010.

FURTHER READING

Barrack RL, Burak C, Skinner HB: Concerns about ceramics in THA. Clin Orthop Relat Res 429:73–79, 2004.
Addresses concerns with the ceramic-on-ceramic articulation, as well as with conditions associated with ceramic wear.

Hannouche D, Hamadouche M, Nizard R, et al: Ceramics in total hip replacement. Clin Orthop Relat Res 430:62–71, 2005.
A summary of the ceramic-on-ceramic articulation regarding in vitro and in vivo wear rates, focusing primarily on wear debris and histologic tissue examination.

Hannouche D, Nich C, Bizot P, et al: Fractures of ceramic bearings: history and present status. Clin Orthop Relat Res 417:19–26, 2003.
A retrospective review that focuses on the complication of ceramic fracture in patients receiving the ceramic-on-ceramic articulation.

Jarrett CA, Ranawat AS, Bruzzone M, et al: The squeaking hip: a phenomenon of ceramic-on-ceramic total hip arthroplasty. J Bone Joint Surg Am 91:1344–1349, 2009.
A study that focuses on the incidence of the squeaking hip phenomenon in hard-on-hard bearing articulating surfaces.

Lombardi AV, Jr, Berend KR, Seng BE, et al: Delta ceramic-on-alumina ceramic articulation in primary THA: prospective, randomized FDA-IDE study and retrieval analysis. Clin Orthop Relat Res 468:367–374, 2010.
A study and retrieval analysis of patients who received a delta ceramic femoral head articulating with an alumina liner compared with an alumina-on-alumina bearing surface and zirconia-on-polyethylene articulations.

Masson B: Emergence of the alumina matrix composite in total hip arthroplasty. Int Orthop 33:359–363, 2009.
The properties of the alumina matrix composites and their role in total hip arthroplasties are addressed in this article.

Restrepo C, Parvizi J, Kurtz SM, et al: The noisy ceramic hip: is component malpositioning the cause? J Arthroplasty 23:643–649, 2008.
This study examines component malpositioning as a contributing factor in the origin of a squeaking hip in ceramic-on-ceramic bearing surfaces.

Skinner HB: Ceramic bearing surfaces. Clin Orthop Relat Res 369:83–91, 1999.
A general overview of ceramic-on-ceramic articulations, including properties, wear rates, and concerns.

CHAPTER 74

Computer Navigation in Hip Arthroplasty and Hip Resurfacing

Rupesh Tarwala and Lawrence D. Dorr

KEY POINTS

- Successful total hip arthroplasty (THA) depends on proper positioning of components.
- Computer navigation helps in accurate cup position and reduces chances of human error.
- Navigation is a very useful tool in avoiding malposition of the cup in minimal incision surgery.
- Restoration of leg length and offset is most accurate with navigation.
- Center of rotation (COR) can be achieved within 2 to 3 mm and increases the longevity of the arthroplasty.

RATIONALE AND INDICATIONS

Since Smith-Petersen designed a successful hip arthroplasty operation in the 1930s, hip surgery has been the glory operation for orthopedics. Each decade has brought improvement. Austin-Moore replaced the femoral head with a monoblock stemmed prosthesis in the 1940s. The 1950s saw metal-on-metal articulations for the first time. The revolution occurred in the 1960s, when Charnley used acrylic cement to fix the acetabular and femoral components, which resulted in much greater patient satisfaction than the press-fit stems with monoblock heads of the 40s and 50s. Charnley's results with all-polyethylene cups bettered those achieved with McKee-Farrar metal-on-metal designs, so the Charnley hip replacement became the gold standard around the world.

Innovation did not stop with Charnley. Charles Engh led the move to bone ingrowth fixation with the anatomic medullary locking (AML) design in the late 1970s. The 1980s saw an explosion of implant designs and companies. Total hip replacement and, subsequently, total knee replacement made orthopedics a commercial bonanza, and every new small company had its own implants. The advantage for surgeons was that the best designs were soon revealed, and bone ingrowth fixation gradually became dominant. The focus in the decade of the 1990s was the articulation surface, and metal-on-metal, ceramic-on-ceramic, and highly crossed linked polyethylene significantly increased the longevity of operations. By the decade of the 2000s, fixation was a certainty with confidence in the durability of the articulation.

Failures in the decade of the 2000s can be attributed to failure of performance of the operation by the surgeon. Surgeons operate using their experience, instinct, and intuition to create a result. This is effective for most patients. However, all surgeons have outliers, and with hip replacement, these outliers occur when the surgeon does not implant the components in the correct position. The version of both the femoral component[1-3] and the acetabular component[4-7] is misjudged, even by experienced surgeons.

With predictability of fixation and articulation surfaces, it is incumbent on arthroplasty surgeons to make the predictability of component position secure. The only method to do this requires the use of machines in the operating room to overcome human errors of judgment. Judgment errors are most common with the acetabulum because it is attached to the pelvis, which is further influenced by the spine and the longitudinal axis of the body. The surgeon's judgment of cup position is confounded by the pelvis being buried under skin, fat, and muscle. Estimation of pelvic position is worse when the operation is performed in the lateral position because pelvic landmarks are more hidden than when the supine position is used.

Femoral component anteversion can be estimated by the surgeon more easily than acetabular position because more bony landmarks are evident. The femoral neck proximally can be sighted, as can the epicondyles distally, to judge the axis of the femur. With cemented stems, because the stem is smaller than the canal and can be manipulated inside the canal, the anteversion can be more precisely controlled by the surgeon. Errors are still made, as was evidenced in two reports.[1,3] Surgeons have much less control with cementless stems, which are rigidly press-fit in a fixed bony structure. The bony structure itself varies from retroversion to high degrees of anteversion.[8] Insertion of a stem is controlled by femoral bony neck anteversion, the anterior-posterior isthmus at the level of the lesser trochanter, and diaphyseal bone by both external radius and internal thickness of the posterior cortex (type A, B, C bone[9]). In fact, estimates by the same experienced surgeon have the same precision for stem anteversion (11.3 degrees)[2] and cup anteversion (12.3 degrees).[4] This precision means that the estimate can be wrong by these many degrees. By contrast, the precision of computer navigation in the same studies was less than 5 degrees for both stem and cup. For surface replacement, computer navigation is used to center the stem and cup; this nearly eliminates the risk of neck notching.

Whether the arthroplasty is conventional or surface, the principles of cup position are the same. The most important technical factor in cup position is COR, which should be within 2 mm of anatomic for greatest durability of the arthroplasty.[10] The COR has the most influence on impingement: if it is lateralized, the metal neck can impact the edge of the metal shell (risk increases with poor combined anteversion); if it is superior or medialized, the risk of bone-on-bone impingement increases unless femoral offset, or hip length, is increased (by the use of an offset stem or by lengthening of the hip/leg).

Inclination and anteversion of the cup also have rigid criteria for success. Inclination cannot exceed 45 degrees for optimal wear[11]; when it exceeds 50 degrees, it causes runaway wear with metal-on-metal[12,13] and increases the risk of breakage of ceramic[14] or highly cross-linked polyethylene.[15] Cup anteversion can be targeted to a mean of 20 degrees with a cemented stem. With cementless stem anteversion, the anteversion of the cup must be adjusted to the stem anteversion to position the arthroplasty within the safe zone of combined anteversion of 25 to 50 degrees (37 ± 12 degrees), with men usually 25 to 35 degrees and women 30 to 50 degrees (the more flexible the patient's hip, the bigger the combined anteversion).[16] With a cementless stem, the femoral preparation should be done first to determine the stem anteversion; the cup anteversion should then be created to provide the desired combined anteversion.

Quantitative knowledge in the operating room is required to reproduce COR and to correct inclination and anteversion of the cup in 100% of patients. Tilt of the pelvis must be known to align the cup inclination and anteversion on the coronal plane of the body, which is the functional plane for the patient.[17,18] Stem anteversion should be quantitatively known also. Quantitative knowledge is not possible without a machine in the operating room, that is, computer navigation or robotic guidance. This chapter will outline the principles of technique in using computer guidance in the operating room and the results reported when this is done.

TECHNICAL CONSIDERATIONS

Pelvic Registration

The tools needed for computer navigation in the operating room need to be calibrated. This calibration is done by the scrub person while the patient is prepared for anesthesia. The pelvic registration is done with the patient supine on the operating table. The pelvic skin is prepped with a sterilization chemical and is draped so the registration device is attached to the iliac crest under sterile conditions. Three threaded pins are inserted obliquely at the thickest portion of the crest (where a bone graft usually is taken). The pointer guide must contact bone for most accurate registration, so to minimize skin damage, puncture wounds are made with a no. 15 scalpel. The anterior posterior plane (APP) of

the pelvis is registered by touching the two anterior superior iliac spines and the pubis near the pubic tubercles. At the completion of registration of the APP, the drapes are removed and the array is removed from the attachment device to the pelvis; the patient is then prepared for the operation.

If the operation is to be done with the patient in the lateral position, the patient is now turned to the lateral position and is fixed securely with two anterior and two posterior posts (Fig. 74-1). The patient's skin is prepared with a sterile chemical, and when draped the pelvic array must be draped into the field. The longitudinal axis of the body is measured by touching the posterior pelvic and chest supports, creating a triangle between them (see Fig. 74-1). This axis allows the software to determine the pelvic tilt (APP angle to the body axis). Knowledge of the degrees of pelvic tilt allows the acetabular component inclination and anteversion to be positioned on the coronal plane.

After the incision has exposed the greater trochanter, a small unicortical screw is inserted for measurement of leg length and offset, with the legs aligned on top of each other by the tibial tubercles and heels. This measurement is repeated after reconstruction of the hip is completed and reduction of the hip is done. Both legs are kept in the same position, as for the measurement before reconstruction. The computer will report the change in hip length and offset (Fig. 74-2A and B). It is critical that the same assistant align the leg position for measurements before and after reconstruction.

Femoral Preparation

No matter the approach used, the femoral neck is cut at the level determined by the surgeon. The femur is prepared first; this represents a paradigm change in conventional hip replacement.[16] Preparing the femur first allows the surgeon to estimate femoral anteversion and position the cup to provide a correct combined anteversion of mean 37 ± 12 degrees. The femoral component anteversion can be more accurately measured by computer navigation, as we have done,[2,16] but this requires pins in the femoral diaphysis, and we have learned that these pins cause residual pain for 6 to 8 weeks for many patients. Because the femoral anteversion can be estimated within 5 degrees with experience, we have stopped measuring femoral anteversion with navigation.

Acetabular Preparation

The acetabulum is exposed by retraction of the femur anteriorly or posteriorly, depending on the approach. We use the posterior approach, and this will provide the basis of our description. If difficulty is encountered with anterior retraction of the femur, the surgeon should release the anterior-superior capsule and the reflected head of the rectus muscle; this will facilitate the maneuver. With the acetabulum in full view, the labrum is excised, as is the pulvinar from the cotyloid notch. Removal of the pulvinar from the cotyloid notch allows registration of the cortical bone of the notch, and this

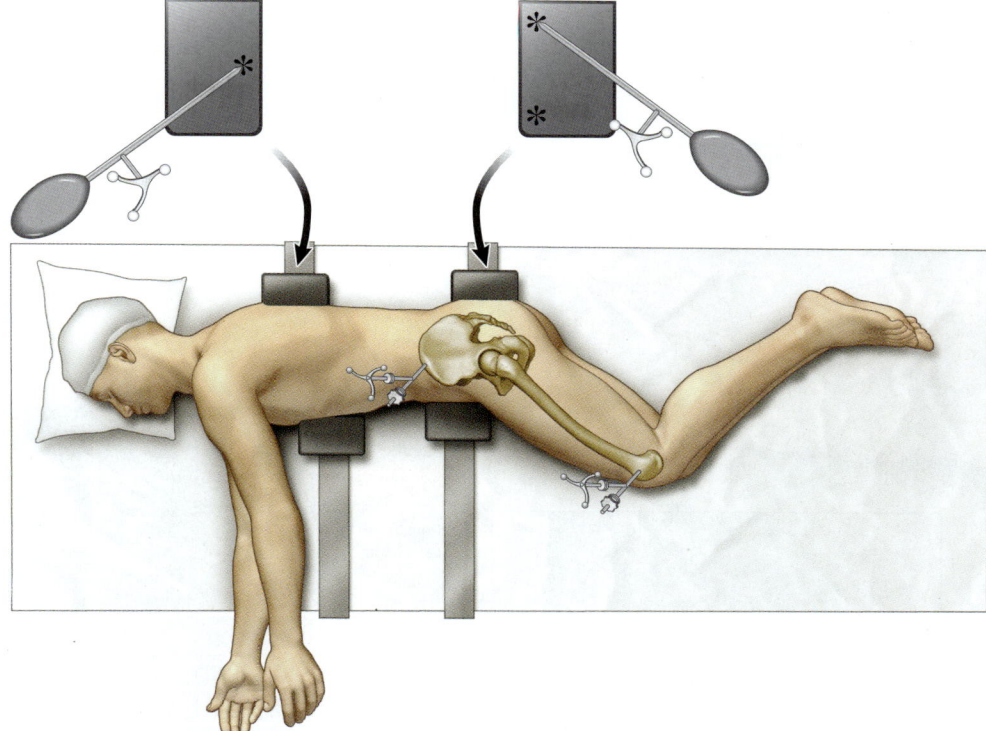

Figure 74-1. Patient properly secured with two padded posts supporting the chest and two padded pelvic supports. The pointer guide (your spoon-shaped instrument) is used to register the longitudinal axis of the body by touching the posterior posts in a triangular shape *(asterisks)* with two points on the pelvic support and one on the chest support.

enables the software to calculate the medial wall of the anatomic acetabulum by combining these points with those on the acetabular wall. Sixteen points are taken on the walls, while osteophytes are avoided (Fig. 74-3A). Four additional points are taken in the cotyloid notch. These 20 points allow the software to compute the anatomic center of rotation and the acetabular bony position relative to the pelvis (Fig. 74-3B). Measurement of the longitudinal axis of the body and computer determination of pelvic tilt, which was done by touching the posterior supports, allow the cup to be positioned in the combined anteversion safe zone according to the axis of the body (functional position), rather than just in relationship to the pelvis (anatomic plane).

The bony anatomic inclination and anteversion of the natural acetabulum can be measured with computer navigation. This gives the surgeon information for superior cup coverage. It educates the surgeon as to the necessity of medialization of the acetabulum to provide coverage of the acetabular cup at an inclination less than 45 degrees, because anatomic inclination of the bony acetabulum occurs at a mean of 55 degrees.[19] Forty percent of bony acetabula have inclination even greater than 55 degrees. Anatomic anteversion in arthritic acetabula is measured at a mean of 11 to 13 degrees, so the cup anteversion most often exceeds that which would be obtained by an "anatomic cup position," using the bony walls or the transverse acetabular ligament. The vertical native inclination is the reason

why the posterior-superior edge of the acetabular cup is commonly uncovered by bone, with up to 3 mm of metal left exposed. If the metal cup were entirely covered by the native acetabulum, the inclination would be too great or the cup would have been reamed superiorly and medially (i.e., the center of rotation elevated 5 mm or more).

Additional information obtained by registration of the acetabulum includes the approximate acetabular diameter. We have found that the precision of this measurement is 2 to 3 mm, but it does give good information regarding the starting size of the reamer to be used in the acetabulum.

The surgeon should control the depth of reaming (Fig. 74-4A and B) so that the COR of the cup is 2 mm superior and 4 to 5 mm medial. Each surgeon needs to know the depth required for the cup system that is in use. We need to ream 3 to 5 mm superior for cup COR to be 2 mm superior because of cup and polyethylene thickness. Control of COR is the most valuable technical feature of navigation. It is the singular technical accomplishment that can prevent impingement. The goal of hip arthroplasty is to replace the COR of the femur into the COR of the acetabulum (i.e., restore the anatomic COR). Attaining this COR means that the cup coverage is correct, so neck-on-cup component impingement will be avoided when combined with correct inclination and anteversion. Reconstruction of acetabular COR means that the offset will be correct if the correct level of bone

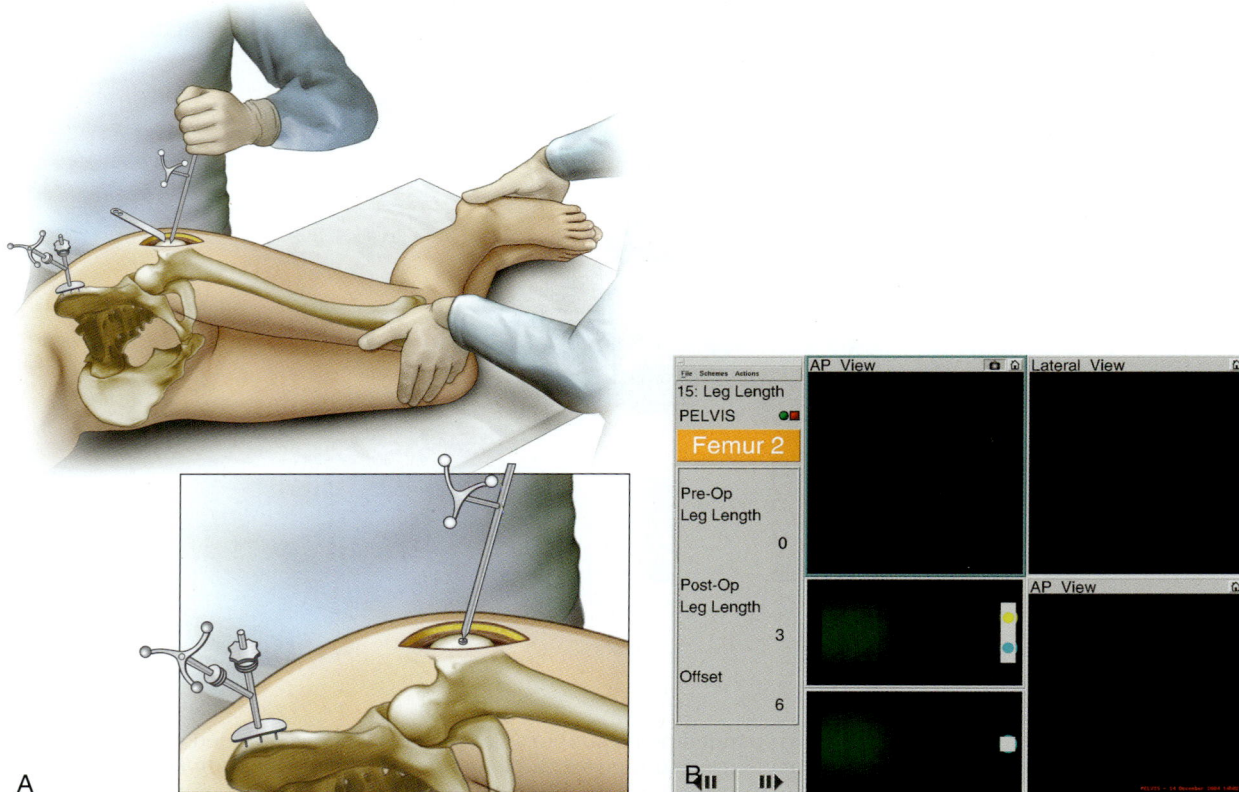

Figure 74-2. A, A pelvic array is fixed to the iliac crest by three pins. A 3.2-mm screw is inserted into the prominence of the greater trochanter as a reference site for measuring leg length and offset. The pointer guide touches the screw head to register preoperative values into the computer and is touched again after reconstruction to obtain the change in length and offset. **B,** The legs are overlaid by aligning the patellae and the heels during length and offset measurements. This ensures that the leg is in the same position. The pelvic array is seen on the iliac crest. A retractor exposes the screw, which the pointer guide touches.

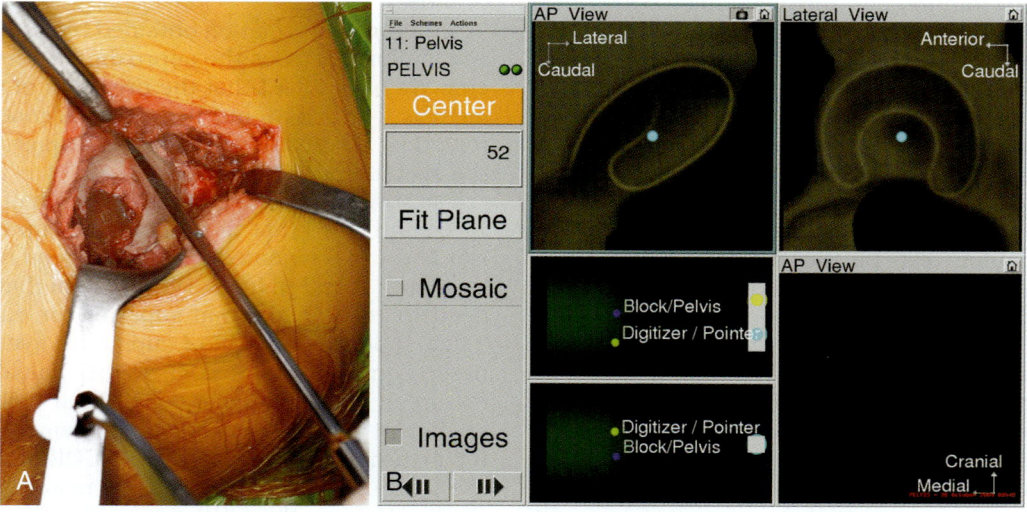

Figure 74-3. A, Intraoperative view of the pointer guide touching the periphery of the acetabulum. The central cotyloid notch is avoided for this measurement, as are osteophytes. **B,** After 16-point registration of the acetabulum, the computer screen shows the acetabular center of rotation in the two planes. Four additional points in the cotyloid notch show the medial wall. On the left side of the screen, in the box under the word "center," the diameter of the acetabulum is given (52 mm in this patient).

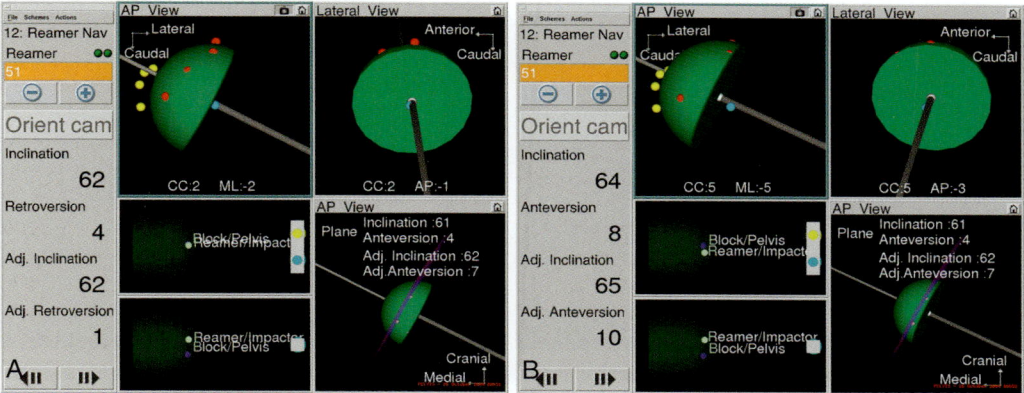

Figure 74-4. A, Computer screen showing the information available during reaming. In the left column, the angles of the reamer are given. Because this reaming is done transversely, the inclination is steep. The reamer can be adjusted into anteversion as desired. Relatively little anteversion occurs in the reamer during transverse removal of the ridge. The upper two quadrants show the reamer and its position in the acetabulum. The CC number (2) means that the reamer is 2 mm superior to the center of rotation of the osseous acetabulum. The ML number (−2) means that the reamer is 2 mm medial to the osseous center (COR). In the upper right quadrant, the CC number (2) means that the reamer is 2 mm superior, and the AP number (−1) means that the reamer is 1 mm posterior from the center. This gives the surgeon complete information with regard to the change in acetabular COR induced by reaming. **B,** The reamer has been advanced to the level of the medial wall, as can be seen as it touches the yellow dots. In the upper right quadrant, the AP number indicates that the center has been moved 3 mm posteriorly. The upper left quadrant shows that the center of rotation has been elevated 5 mm and medialized 5 mm. The lower right quadrant provides a graphic illustration of coverage of the cup with the reamer in its current position compared with values of the native acetabulum.

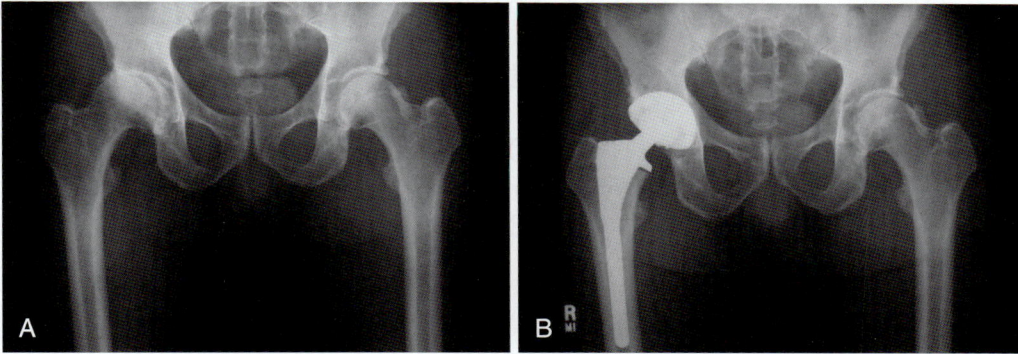

Figure 74-5. A, Preoperative x-ray with superior lateral migration of the femoral head means that the offset should be reduced if the correct hip center of rotation (COR) of the cup and stem is restored. **B,** COR is restored, as is the offset and the length (which means that leg lengths are equal).

cut is made on the femur (Fig. 74-5). The level of the neck cut can be determined easily by preoperative templating, which determines the level of cut necessary to restore the femoral head COR. If the COR is not restored, the offset must be increased to avoid bone-on-bone impingement (Fig. 74-6).

The second advantage of navigation is seen as quantitative and precise control of the inclination and anteversion of the cup. Inclination must be below 45 degrees to optimize wear, and because the computer has 4 to 5 degrees of precision, we place inclination at 38 to 40 ± 2 degrees,[4] which means that the superior-posterior edge of the cup is usually uncovered by 3 ± 2 mm. Anteversion of the cup is determined by femoral component anteversion. With men, the least combined anteversion is 25 degrees, and rarely do they require 40 degrees. Thirty to thirty-five degrees is common because men

who get osteoarthritis commonly have a cam impingement deformity, which is associated with low combined anteversion of the anatomic hip. So the cementless femoral component anteversion often is less than 10 degrees, even 0 to 5 degrees, which means that the cup anteversion may need to be near 30 degrees. It is difficult to antevert the cup more than 30 degrees because the metal shell will protrude above the posterior bony wall, and this ensures component impingement in extension and external rotation of gait.

Cup Placement

A trial cup is placed using a cup holder with an attached array, which allows the surgeon to receive real-time information on medialization, center of rotation, and anterior-posterior positioning of the cup. The computer

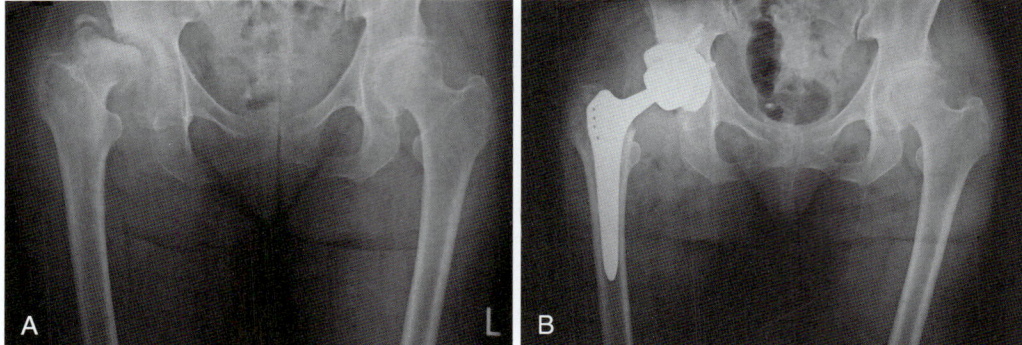

Figure 74-6. A, Preoperative x-ray with severe superior lateral migration of the femur; this results in an inability to restore the center of rotation (COR) of the acetabulum. **B,** Reconstruction requires increased offset of the hip to prevent bone-on-bone impingement and to keep the gluteus medius muscle length correct. The hip length is correct.

Figure 74-7. Computer screen showing seating of the acetabular cup with the position of the center of rotation (COR) 2 mm superior, 4 mm medial, and 2 mm posterior. (Cup COR differs from reaming COR.) The adjusted inclination is 40 degrees and the adjusted anteversion 28 degrees. The numbers in the lower right are those of the osseous acetabulum.

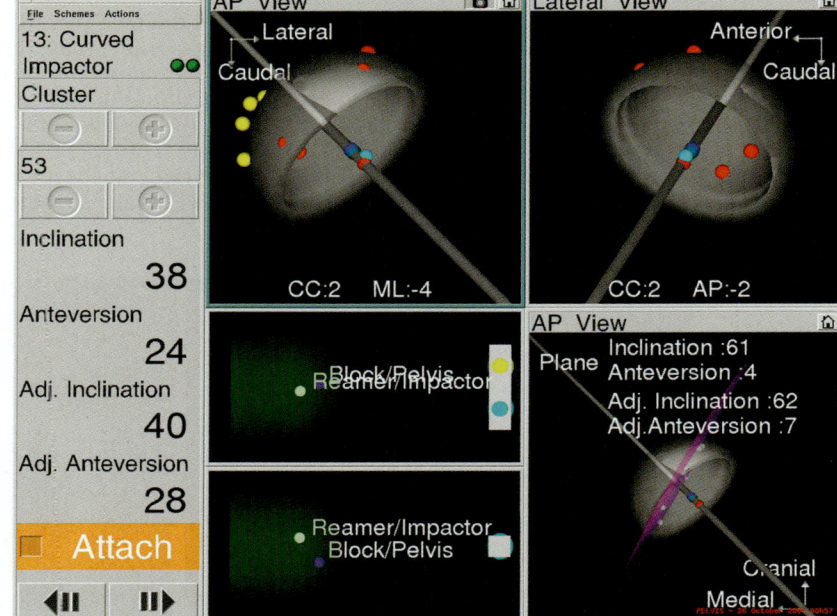

screen displays the inclination, adjusted inclination, anteversion, and adjusted anteversion. Adjusted values should be selected because they are adjusted for the patient's pelvic tilt and therefore are in the functional position of the coronal plane. If the cup has a COR that is lateralized, the acetabular bone should be reamed deeper. If the COR is 5 mm or more superior, the depth must be visually and manually assessed. If the anterior-superior edge of the cup is below the anterior-superior bony acetabulum, bone-on-bone impingement of the greater trochanter on the pelvis (anterior-inferior ischial spine) can occur with resultant dislocation. The periphery of the acetabulum should be reamed for the next larger cup without increasing the depth, so that the COR is displaced more laterally.

Once these are ascertained, the trial component is removed and the acetabular component is implanted using a cup holder with an attached array (Fig. 74-7). After cup implantation, if screws are added, inclination and anteversion may change. These measurements can

be confirmed by touching the edge of the metal shell six times. The numbers are displayed in the lower right quadrant of the screen. This same maneuver can be repeated after the liner has been placed (Fig. 74-7A and B). The periphery of the liner is touched six times, and if the inclination or anteversion changes by 5 degrees or more after impaction of the liner, the cup is not rigidly fixed, and the surgeon will need to correct this.

Leg Length and Offset

After the stem has been inserted and the trial head attached, the hip is relocated. The legs are overlaid, and the pointer guide touches the greater trochanter screw. The software computes changes in leg length and offset. If these changes are consistent with preoperative determination of desired changes, the real head is attached. If the offset or the hip length is not what is desired, adjustments will have to be made to the neck length of the femur or the position of the stem relative to the neck cut. For instance, with a neutral head, if the offset were increased by 3 mm but the leg length was increased and unacceptable at 6 mm, a short head should be used to decrease hip length. If a short head corrected leg length but caused impingement by decreasing the offset, an offset stem should be selected or an additional neck cut performed, so that length decreases while offset would again increase. These are decision problems that occur when the COR is not correctly restored. With correct restoration of the acetabular COR and the femoral COR, leg length and offset changes will occur as expected.

Quantitative knowledge of leg length and offset is of tremendous benefit in confirming the manual measurements of the surgeon.

RESULTS

In THA, the anterior or posterior tilt of the pelvis changes the position of the acetabular component on the coronal plane of the body as compared with its anatomic position in the pelvic bone. Lembeck and associates[20] found that pelvic tilt ranges from −27 to +3 degrees, and that pelvic reclination of 1 degree will lead to functional anteversion of the cup of approximately 0.7 degree. In our study of 477 hips, we found that the distribution of tilt had a range of 25 degrees posterior to 20 degrees anterior and confirmed Lembeck's conversion factor (we had 0.8 degree).[21] Ten-degree pelvic tilt creates an absolute error of 8 degrees in judging the cup on the coronal plane; this is additive to measurement errors of the surgeon's estimate. We proved that measurement of pelvic tilt during the performance of THA will improve the accuracy of cup position as measured on the coronal plane.[21]

Evidence that computer navigation enhances precision and reduces the number of outliers in THA has been found in several studies.[4,7,22,23] In our study of 101 hips, the surgeon's estimate for cup position was compared with computer navigation values.[4] We found that

even the experienced surgeon had precision of 11.5 degrees for inclination and of 12.3 degrees for anteversion, while the computer had precision of 4.4 degrees for inclination (bias of 0.03 degree) and 4.1 degrees for anteversion (bias of 0.73 degree).[4] In our study of 109 consecutive cementless stem positions, we found that only 45% were between 10 and 20 degrees of anteversion.[2] This means that the surgeon must judge the cementless stem anteversion. The surgeon can be consistent in this judgment over time, but precision in the first 50 hips is 11.3 degrees.[2] These findings of an experienced surgeon's precision suggest that all surgeons need the help of computer navigation to obtain quantitative knowledge in the operating room for correct component position in 100% of hips.

Reconstruction of the hip with hip arthroplasty requires correction of the hip joint. The femur has been taken for granted, and most studies focus on reconstruction of the acetabulum. Therefore a safe zone of the acetabulum is frequently discussed without reference to the femur. With cementless total hip replacement (THR), the surgeon must be aware of the anteversion of both femur and cup.[16] This is termed *combined anteversion* and has been recognized since 1970.[24] In a study of 200 adult cadavers, combined anteversion for men was a mean 29.6° and for women 33.5°, with femoral anteversion a mean 11.6 degrees (men were 11.1 degrees and women 12.2 degrees).[25] A finite element study of THR found that optimal combined anteversion to avoid impingement was 37.3 degrees.[26] It is interesting to note that this is the same mean found in our clinical study.[16] Mathematical models have confirmed combined anteversion to be the measurement that must be considered to avoid impingement.[27] Clinical use of combined anteversion found men to be between 25 and 35 degrees and women up to 45 degrees,[28] which is consistent with our data of 25 to 40 degrees for men and 30 to 50 degrees for women.[16] Our studies prove that computer navigation is more precise than surgeon's judgment for femoral or acetabular

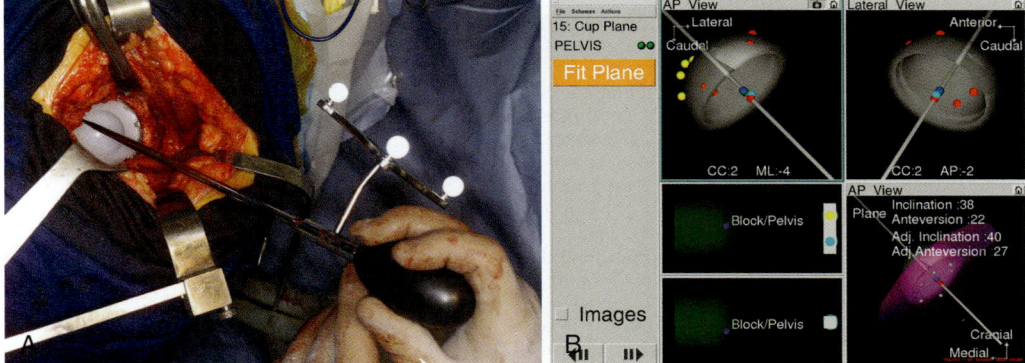

Figure 74-8. The final measurement can be repeated once the plastic liner has been inserted into the metal shell by touching the periphery of the liner at six points. In our experience, insertion of the liner changes the inclination/anteversion numbers by up to 3 degrees, but this is of no clinical significance, especially with a margin of measurement error of 2 degrees. **B,** The final values are seen in the lower right, with confirmed inclination of 40 degrees and anteversion of 27 degrees.

anteversion, with precision for both of 5 degrees as confirmed by postoperative computed tomography (CT) scans.[2,4] With computer navigation, 96% of hips were in a safe zone of combined anteversion of 25 to 50 degrees.[16] In this study, we accepted stems that were retroverted, which today, outside of the study, we would not do. Therefore, 100% of hips should be able to be in the safe zone with computer navigation. We have experienced dislocations with retroverted stems. A retroverted Zweymuller (Zimmer, Warsaw, Ind) is converted by us to an Anatomic APR (Zimmer), which will provide satisfactory anteversion of the stem. For retroverted cementless stems, conversion to a cemented stem corrects the version. Modular necks are an option but offer limited anteversion modification of 5 to 7 degrees, which is of little help with a 5-degree retroverted stem.

Perhaps the two perplexing intraoperative decisions for the surgeon are ensuring correct cup position and deciding leg length. Quantitative knowledge in the operating room simplifies these decisions, no matter whether the arthroplasty is conventional or surface. The combination of surgeon experience and intuition with absolute numbers makes these decisions completely predictable. Our data on leg length and offset reconstruction using computer navigation confirm this statement. Eighty-two hips in patients with unilateral arthritis (contralateral normal hip) had leg length restored within 6 mm in 99%, with one outlier, who had a Crowe III dysplastic hip. Seventy-eight of 82 hips had offset within 6 mm; four outliers had valgus hips, which required an increase in offset greater than 6 mm. We found that the key to optimal length and offset is restoration of the center of rotation of the hip within 5 mm (see Figs. 74-7 and 74-8). We strive to keep the COR at 2 to 3 mm superior for longevity of the arthroplasty.[10] Medialization is, on average, less than 5 mm to permit correct coverage of the cup with abduction less than 45 degrees.

REFERENCES

1. Wines AP, McNicol D: Computed tomography measurement of the accuracy of component version in total hip arthroplasty. J Arthroplasty 21:696–701, 2006.
2. Dorr LD: Femoral anteversion of cementless stems for total hip arthroplasty. J Bone Joint Surg Am In press.
3. Pierchon F, Pasquier G, Cotten A, et al: Causes of dislocation of total hip arthroplasty: CT study of component alignment. J Bone Joint Surg Br 76:45–48, 1994.
4. Dorr LD, Malik A, Wan Z, et al: Precision and bias of imageless computer navigation and surgeon estimates for acetabular component position. Clin Orthop Relat Res 465:92–99, 2007.
5. Digioia AM, 3rd, Jaramaz B, Plakseychuk AY, et al: Comparison of a mechanical acetabular alignment guide with computer placement of the socket. J Arthroplasty 17:359–364, 2002.
6. Babisch JW, Layher F, Amiot LP: The rationale for tilt-adjusted acetabular cup navigation. J Bone Joint Surg Am 90:357–365, 2008.
7. Parratte S, Argenson JN: Validation and usefulness of a computer-assisted cup-positioning system in total hip arthroplasty: a prospective, randomized, controlled study. J Bone Joint Surg Am 89:494–499, 2007.
8. Husmann O, Rubin PJ, Leyvraz PF, et al: Three-dimensional morphology of the proximal femur. J Arthroplasty 12:444–450, 1997.
9. Dorr LD, Faugere MC, Mackel AM, et al: Structural and cellular assessment of bone quality of proximal femur. Bone 14:231–242, 1993.
10. Karachalios T, Hartofilakidis G, Zacharakis N, et al: A 12- to 18-year radiographic follow-up study of Charnley low-friction arthroplasty: the role of the center of rotation. Clin Orthop Relat Res 296:140–147, 1993.
11. Patil S, Bergula A, Chen PC, et al: Polyethylene wear and acetabular component orientation. J Bone Joint Surg Am 85(Suppl 4):56–63, 2003.
12. De Haan R, Pattyn C, Gill HS, et al: Correlation between inclination of the acetabular component and metal ion levels in metal-on-metal hip resurfacing replacement. J Bone Joint Surg Br 90:1291–1297, 2008.
13. Hart AJ, Buddhdev P, Winship P, et al: Cup inclination angle of greater than 50 degrees increases whole blood concentrations of cobalt and chromium ions after metal-on-metal hip resurfacing. Hip Int 18:212–219, 2008.
14. Nizard RS, Sedel L, Christel P, et al: Ten-year survivorship of cemented ceramic-ceramic total hip prosthesis. Clin Orthop Relat Res 282:53–63, 1992.
15. Ries MD: Complications in primary total hip arthroplasty: avoidance and management: wear. Instr Course Lect 52:257–265, 2003.
16. Dorr LD, Malik A, Dastane M, et al: Combined anteversion technique for total hip arthroplasty. Clin Orthop Relat Res 467:119–127, 2009.
17. DiGioia AM, Jaramaz B, Blackwell M, et al: The Otto Aufranc Award. Image guided navigation system to measure intraoperatively acetabular implant alignment. Clin Orthop Relat Res 355:8–22, 1998.
18. DiGioia AM, Hafez MA, Jaramaz B, et al: Functional pelvic orientation measured from lateral standing and sitting radiographs. Clin Orthop Relat Res 453:272–276, 2006.
19. Dorr LD: Hip arthroplasty: minimally invasive techniques and computer navigation, Philadelphia, 2005, WB Saunders Elsevier.
20. Lembeck B, Mueller O, Reize P, et al: Pelvic tilt makes acetabular cup navigation inaccurate. Acta Orthop 76:517–523, 2005.
21. Zhu J, Wan Z, Dorr LD: Quantification of pelvic tilt in total hip arthroplasty. Clin Orthop Relat Res 468:571–575, 2010.
22. Jolles BM, Genoud P, Hoffmeyer P: Computer-assisted cup placement techniques in total hip arthroplasty improve accuracy of placement. Clin Orthop Relat Res 426:174–179, 2004.
23. Kalteis T, Handel M, Herold T, et al: Greater accuracy in positioning of the acetabular cup by using an image-free navigation system. Int Orthop 29:272–276, 2005.
24. McKibbin B: Anatomical factors in the stability of the hip joint in the newborn. J Bone Joint Surg Br 52:148–159, 1970.
25. Maruyama M, Feinberg JR, Capello WN, et al: The Frank Stinchfield Award. Morphologic features of the acetabulum and femur: anteversion angle and implant positioning. Clin Orthop Relat Res 393:52–65, 2001.
26. Widmer KH, Zurfluh B: Compliant positioning of total hip components for optimal range of motion. J Orthop Res 22:815–821, 2004.
27. Yoshimine F: The safe-zones for combined cup and neck anteversions that fulfill the essential range of motion and their optimum combination in total hip replacements. J Biomech 39:1315–1323, 2006.
28. Ranawat CS: Modern techniques of cemented total hip arthroplasty. Tech Orthop 6:17–25, 1991.

FURTHER READING

DiGioia AM, Jaramaz B, Blackwell M, et al: The Otto Aufranc Award. Image guided navigation system to measure intraoperatively acetabular implant alignment. Clin Orthop Relat Res 355:8–22, 1998.
Image guided system introduced to provide intraoperative feedback to surgeon regarding pelvic location on operating table with a goal of improving cup position.

Dorr LD: Hip arthroplasty: minimally invasive techniques and computer navigation, Philadelphia, 2005, WB Saunders Elsevier.

Computer navigation is very important for proper positioning of component in minimally invasive total hip arthroplasty.

Dorr LD, Malik A, Dastane M, et al: Combined anteversion technique for total hip arthroplasty. Clin Orthop Relat Res 467:119–127, 2009.

Combined anteversion can be achieved within safe zone with computer navigation which is very important in avoiding impingement, dislocation, accelerated wear and pain after total hip arthroplasty.

Dorr LD, Malik A, Wan Z, et al: Precision and bias of imageless computer navigation and surgeon estimates for acetabular component position. Clin Orthop Relat Res 465:92–99, 2007.

Precision of computer navigation is better than surgeon estimation and is within 5 degrees for inclination and anteversion of cup.

Parratte S, Argenson JN: Validation and usefulness of a computer-assisted cup-positioning system in total hip arthroplasty. A prospective, randomized, controlled study. J Bone Joint Surg Am 89:494–499, 2007.

The computer navigation system significantly reduces the number of outliers as compared to free hand in cup positioning during THA.

Zhu J, Wan Z, Dorr LD: Quantification of Pelvic Tilt in Total Hip Arthroplasty. Clin Orthop Relat Res 468:571, 2010.

The computer navigation system compensates for interindividual variability of pelvic tilt and improves accuracy of cup position in total hip arthroplasty.

PRIMARY TOTAL HIP ARTHROPLASTY IN SPECIFIC CONDITIONS

CHAPTER 75

Hip Dysplasia

Ryan Cordry and Richard Santore

KEY POINTS

- Congenital dislocation of the hip (CDH) and developmental dysplasia of the hip (DDH) are diagnoses that often lead to secondary osteoarthritis at a relatively young age; total hip arthroplasty (THA) has become a safe, effective, and durable treatment for these patients.
- Compared with THA for nondysplastic arthritic hips, these cases pose a higher degree of technical difficulty and include greater perioperative risks, which are increased in proportion to the severity of the dysplasia.
- Special anatomic features include decreased acetabular diameter and volume, increased femoral anteversion, insufficient femoral offset, proximal femoral valgus or varus deformities, and small and straight proximal femoral dimensions.
- Careful preoperative planning, as well as anticipation of contingencies, is critical for the procedure to be performed successfully.
- Use of smaller components and head diameters, modular components, acetabular medialization, bone grafts, intraoperative x-rays, cages, femoral osteotomy in high-grade (Crowe IV) cases, and vigilance in protection of major nerves should be anticipated.
- Recognizing the need for special surgical considerations and techniques, even in the setting of mild dysplasia, is important.
- In deference to the high complication rate, long-term nonoperative management of Crowe IV hips should always be considered in patients who present with painless limp.

INTRODUCTION

The most common underlying cause of secondary osteoarthritis of the hip is congenital hip disease.[1-4] The spectrum of deformities can be quite large. This range represents a continuum from subtle acetabular dysplasia to progressively increasing degrees of subluxation, culminating with complete dislocation. When this process is recognized early, and before significant secondary arthritis, joint preservation surgeries may be possible to delay or prevent the need for hip replacement. In general, joint-preserving surgery is not

appropriate once Tonnis II changes are present. However, even Tonnis I arthritis is sometimes best managed nonoperatively until natural progression dictates total hip arthroplasty (THA). When significant articular destruction has resulted in arthritis, THA is the most reliable and appropriate procedure to relieve pain and restore function.

Total hip arthroplasty can be performed in the presence of mild dysplasia, much as in primary osteoarthritis. However, even in mild dysplasia, it is important to anticipate the possible need for special surgical considerations and techniques. Reconstructing the arthritic hip in the setting of severe dysplasia can be one of the most challenging circumstances facing hip surgeons. This chapter covers the indications, surgical approaches, component selection, complications, and techniques used to prepare the hip surgeon for the challenges associated with reconstructing the dysplastic hip.

CLASSIFICATION

Several classification systems have been developed to characterize dysplastic hips in the adult population. The two most frequently used systems are those of Crowe[5] and Hartofilakidis.[6,7] Both of these systems are relatively easy to use and require only a plain anteroposterior (AP) radiograph of the pelvis. These systems are useful for guiding treatment and providing prognostic information. The system devised by Mendes[8] is more complex and is focused on surgical planning.

The Crowe system[5] is based on the ratio of the distance the upper femur has migrated proximally relative to the femoral head diameter. A reference line that connects the teardrops of both hips is drawn. Despite the presence of dysplasia, the inferomedial femoral head-neck junction is generally readily recognizable. A point is marked at this position, and the distance from the reference line is carefully measured. The height of the pelvis and the superior-to-inferior diameter of the femoral head should be measured; in practice, however, only one of these two measurements is required. Occasionally, obtaining an accurate measurement of the diameter of the femoral head may be difficult owing to severe bilateral deformity or suboptimal radiographic technique. Because the femoral head diameter is typically 20% of the height of the pelvis, pelvic height may be substituted in calculating the ratio of migration. In normal hips, the inferomedial head-neck junction will sit within a few millimeters of the reference line drawn to connect the teardrops. In class I dysplasia, this point will sit cephalad to the reference line at a distance that is less than 50% of the diameter of the femoral head (<10% of the height of the pelvis). Class II dysplasia is present when this point has migrated 50% to 75% of the diameter of the femoral head (or 10% to 15% of the height of the pelvis). Class III dysplasia is identified with a migration distance of 75% to 100% of the femoral head diameter (or 15% to 20% of the pelvic height). When the proximal femur has migrated more than 100% of the diameter of the femoral head (or 20% of the height of the pelvis), the dysplasia is defined as class IV (Fig. 75-1).

The classification system proposed by Hartofilakidis segregates adult dysplastic hips into one of three categories: dysplastic, low dislocation, or high dislocation.[6,7] Dysplastic hips may be subluxated; however, the femoral head is still contained within the true acetabulum. When the femoral head articulates with a false acetabulum, which overlaps the true acetabulum, a low dislocation is identified. This is noted when the inferior lip of the false acetabulum overlaps the superolateral lip of the true acetabulum. When no overlap is encountered and the femoral head is articulating with a false acetabulum located proximal and posterior to the true acetabulum, a high dislocation is identified. This classification system is intuitive and easy to use (Figs. 75-2 through 75-4).

Mendes[8] proposed a classification system that is more focused on surgical planning of the hip arthroplasty and involves concepts beyond radiographic features alone. Its clinical application has not been validated for reproducibility/reliability or for its prognostic information. Nevertheless, it is a useful tool when preparing and templating the reconstructive procedure. There are two general categories of dysplastic hips according to this system: subluxated and high. For each type of hip, priorities are established to guide the procedure. Primary consideration is given to bone stock and acetabular inclination. Bone stock may be considered adequate or deficient. Acetabular inclination is characterized as normal or superior. Characterizing soft tissue abnormalities, based on the presence of weakness or contracture, constitutes the secondary consideration. Tertiary considerations evaluate such factors as leg length inequality, pelvic obliquity, knee valgus, or lumbar curvature. Clearly, taking into consideration all of the unique clinical aspects of dysplasia makes intuitive sense.

A recent study[9] showed excellent intraobserver and interobserver reproducibility and reliability for the Crowe and Hartofilakidis classification systems. This confirms the utility of these systems in comparing results among treating surgeons and centers. The manner in which these systems guide treatment for the surgeon is discussed throughout the chapter. Several other studies have reported the prognostic implication of these two classification schemes[10-12]; one found an increased rate of revision and loosening of the acetabular component in Crowe IV hips compared with Crowe I through III.[12] Cameron and associates[10] showed that Crowe I hips undergoing THA had equal Harris Hip scores and limp after THA as patients undergoing THA for nondysplastic osteoarthritis. Patients after THA for Crowe II through IV showed progressively lower Harris Hip scores. High complication rates were noted in Crowe III (25%) and IV hips (50%), with no increase in rate of complications in the Crowe I or II group.

ANATOMY

Understanding the pathologic anatomy of the dysplastic hip is important when considering its reconstruction. Anatomic changes are present on both the acetabular and femoral sides of the joint and are proportional to the severity of dysplasia.[5,13,14] Both bony and soft tissue alterations are common. Computed tomography (CT) scans, although not essential for the diagnosis or treatment of dysplasia, afford a more detailed appreciation of the bony changes present in these hips. These morphologic differences from typical hips form the basis of the potential pitfalls of this operation.

Dysplastic hips are smaller and architecturally abnormal as compared with normal adult hips. The femoral head is small and can become flattened.[15] The femoral neck is generally shorter and the upper femur more anteverted compared with age-matched controls.[14] Even mildly dysplastic joints have increased femoral anteversion compared with normal adult controls.[14,16,17] This anteversion is a rotational deformity localized to the proximal femoral diaphysis rather than the neck itself and is not related to coxa valga.[14,16,17] The proximal femoral canal is straighter and narrower, particularly in the coronal plane.[5,13-16] The greater trochanter is found more posteriorly[5,13] and is soft and underdeveloped.[15] Proximal femoral bone is also smaller and weaker than in nondysplastic hips and is more prone to intraoperative fracture.

Structural changes to the acetabulum of adults with congenital hip disease are also common. Volumetric insufficiency describes the appearance of the dysplastic acetabulum with or without dislocation. Dunn and Hess[15] described the pathologic anatomy associated with 22 congenitally dislocated hips of 16 patients undergoing THA. The acetabula in their series appeared small, shallow, and poorly developed. In cases of late dislocation after years of subluxation, investigators noted erosion of the superior aspect of the acetabulum. This significantly worsened already shallow sockets and complicated attainment of coverage of the acetabular component. They reported extremely soft bone directly superior to the true acetabulum due to chronic lack of weight bearing in this area.

Hartofilakidis and colleagues[7] analyzed 431 hips and described their morphology based on the severity of dysplasia. They classified these hips as dysplasia, low dislocation, or high dislocation. Of these, all 325 dysplastic hips had a deficiency of the superior segment of the acetabulum. In each of the low dislocations, a deficiency of the anterior and posterior segments was evident, and all high dislocations had a deficiency of the entire rim. All low and high dislocations had a narrow

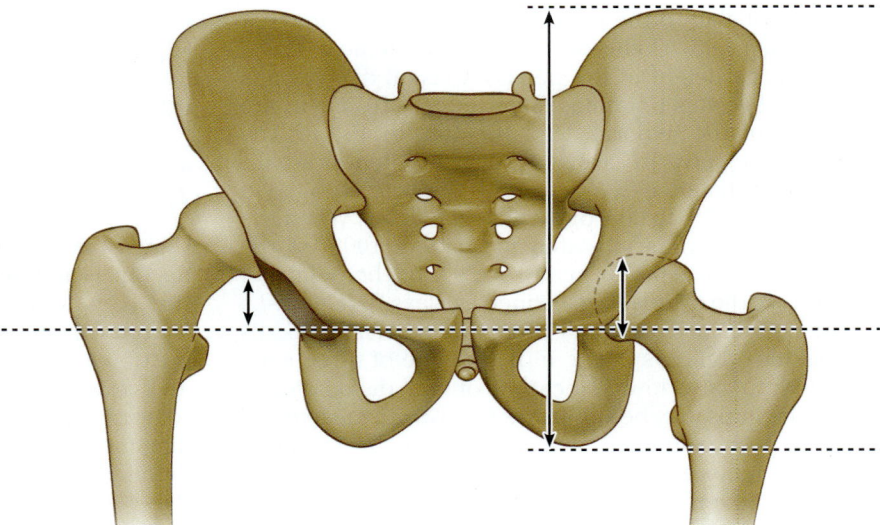

Figure 75-1. Measurements used in the Crowe grading system. *(Redrawn from Sanchez-Sotelo J, Berry DJ, Trousdale RT, Cabanela ME: Surgical treatment of developmental dysplasia of the hip in adults: II. Arthroplasty options. J Am Acad Orthop Surg 10:334–344, 2002.)*

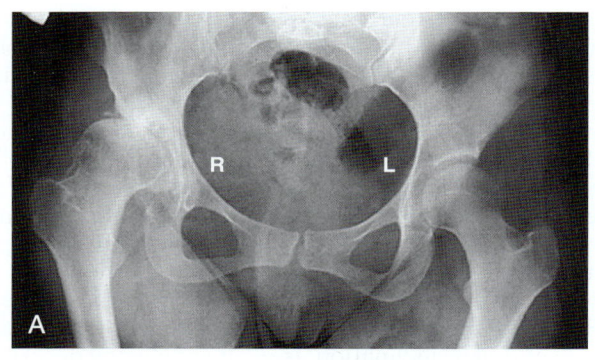

Figure 75-2. The Hartofilakidis dysplastic hip. Radiograph **(A)** and line drawing **(B)** of a 28-year-old woman who had a dysplastic hip on the right. *(From Hartofilakidis G, Stamos K, Karachalios T, et al: Congenital hip disease in adults: classification of acetabular deficiencies and operative treatment with acetabuloplasty combined with total hip arthroplasty. J Bone Joint Surg Am 78:683–692, 1996. Part **B** redrawn.)*

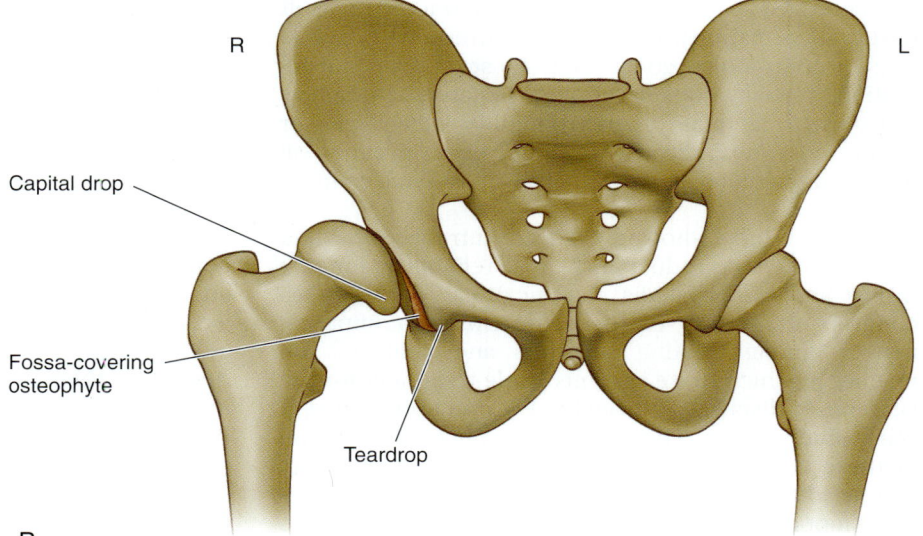

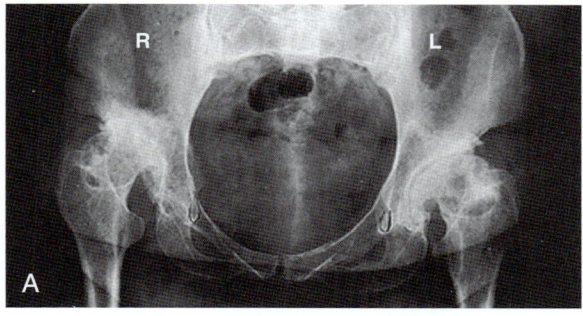

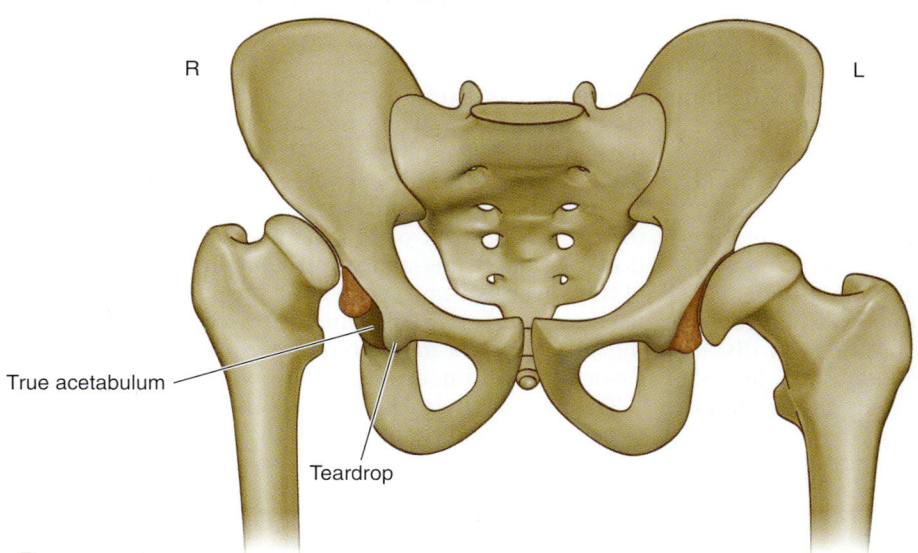

True acetabulum

Teardrop

B

Figure 75-3. The Hartofilakidis low dislocation *(right hip)* and dysplastic *(left hip)* hip. **A,** A 44-year-old woman who had bilateral congenital hip disease. **B,** Line drawing of the same hips showing the differences between a low dislocation and a dysplastic hip with approximately the same degree of subluxation. *(From Hartofilakidis G, Stamos K, Karachalios T, et al: Congenital hip disease in adults: classification of acetabular deficiencies and operative treatment with acetabuloplasty combined with total hip arthroplasty. J Bone Joint Surg Am 78:683–692, 1996. Part **B** redrawn.)*

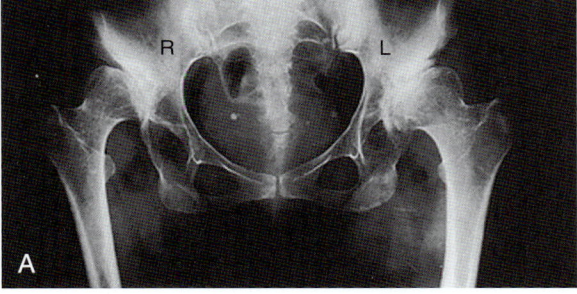

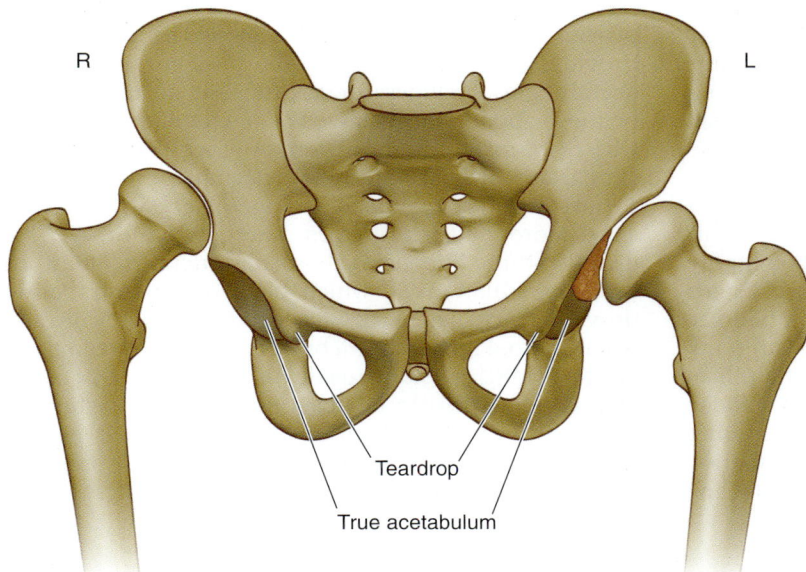

Teardrop

True acetabulum

B

Figure 75-4. The Hartofilakidis high dislocation. Radiograph **(A)** and line drawing **(B)** of a 42-year-old woman who had a high dislocation of the hip on the right and a low dislocation on the left. *(From Hartofilakidis G, Stamos K, Karachalios T, et al: Congenital hip disease in adults: classification of acetabular deficiencies and operative treatment with acetabuloplasty combined with total hip arthroplasty. J Bone Joint Surg Am 78:683–692, 1996. Part **B** redrawn.)*

opening of the acetabulum and inadequate depth. Posterosuperior bone stock was decreased in 32 of 43 (74%) low dislocations and in 56 of 63 (89%) high dislocations.

Soft tissues are also abnormal. Neurovascular structures are shortened and are no more likely to stretch than in normal hips. Hamstring, quadriceps, and adductor muscles are shortened. As the femoral head migrates proximally, the abductors shorten and insert on the proximal femur from a more horizontal direction. This variance in the orientation of muscles needs to be anticipated during the surgical approach to the hip to avoid unintended damage to the abductors. Harris and coworkers[18] in a report of their early experience with 22 patients in the setting of developmental dysplasia of the hip (DDH) described the anatomic alterations present in 27 hips. They noted proximal displacement of the femoral nerve and profunda femoris artery. The femoral nerve was vulnerable to injury as the proximal femur was retracted anteriorly for exposure of the acetabulum. Additionally, the profunda femoris artery passed closer to the inferior pole of the acetabulum, which may predispose it to injury. They also found an elongated hip capsule, which had a proximal rather than distal orientation. The hip capsule was frequently thickened and was described as having an hourglass shape. Dunn and Hess[15] found the superior portion of the capsule to firmly adhere to the abductors, while the inferior portion frequently obscured the true acetabulum.

PREOPERATIVE EVALUATION

The importance of a detailed history and physical examination cannot be overemphasized. It is important to understand what limitations patients are experiencing, as well as their desired level of activity. Patients with Crowe grade II or III disease frequently present at younger ages than those with grade I or IV. These younger patients may have expectations of resuming high levels of activity.

Many patients with DDH will present before advanced osteoarthritic changes are present. Prearthritic patients with definite structural abnormalities about the hip may be candidates for acetabular and/or femoral osteotomy. These joint-preserving procedures may delay the need for arthroplasty and may diminish some of the challenges for the arthroplasty surgeon. However, these procedures are not the subject of this chapter.

As in typical primary osteoarthritis of the hip, patients may experience groin or buttock pain as a direct result of their diseased hip. Ipsilateral knee pain is commonly reported in patients with dysplastic hips. Leg length discrepancy, muscle weakness, and pelvic obliquity may cause a limp and secondary lumbosacral symptoms and problems. Pelvic obliquity and leg length differences can be clinically assessed by placing blocks under the short leg until the pelvis is leveled, by measuring the distance from the umbilicus and the anterosuperior iliac spine (ASIS) to the tip of the medial malleolus, or

by performing a scanogram. These assessments should assist the surgeon in determining how much lengthening is desired during the reconstructive procedure.

Stiffness about the hip joint should be assessed so the clinician can further understand any soft tissue releases that may be required. Hip flexion contracture functionally shortens the lower extremity, thereby adversely affecting the patient's gait. The contracture is most readily observed in the supine position and during gait. The supine patient should be able to place the affected thigh flat on the examination table without accentuating lumbar lordosis. Full extension of the knee should be confirmed to ensure that the restricted motion is isolated to the hip. Observation of a patient during gait is likely to reveal an obvious limp with a short stride, toe-walking, and increased lumbar lordosis during the stance phase. Treatment of the flexion contracture with anterior capsule and/or iliopsoas tendon release will improve hip extension, alleviate compensatory hyperlordosis of the lumbar spine, reduce functional leg length inequality, and facilitate true lengthening of the lower extremity. The need for this adjunctive soft tissue surgery is determined on a case-by-case basis; the procedure is more frequently appropriate in DDH associated with neuromuscular conditions.

The patient should be closely observed while walking to assess the gait pattern. Leg length discrepancy, pain, and muscle weakness are the three contributing factors to the limp in DDH patients. Any real leg length inequality can be normalized with a lift placed on or in the shoe of the short extremity. If the limp persists in spite of the lift, other causes should be considered. Pain causing an antalgic gait may be assessed by injecting a local anesthetic into the hip joint. Documentation of the Trendelenburg sign as well as the patient's abductor strength against gravity and manual resistance in the side-lying position is helpful in describing the degree of weakness present. Poor abductor function may result from proximal femoral migration or reduced femoral offset. Optimizing abductor function is a critical component of the successful hip reconstruction.

Radiographic evaluation should include a standard anteroposterior (AP) view of the pelvis, including both hips, an AP of the involved hip, and a true lateral of the proximal femur. A false profile view of the involved hip provides additional valuable information regarding the acetabulum. It allows for assessment of anterior and posterior bone stock, as well as acetabular version. As was previously noted, full-length standing orthoroentgenograms of bilateral lower extremities may be used to further quantify leg length inequality when necessary. More detailed images, such as CT scans that include three-dimensional reconstructions, may be used for situations in which plain radiographs fail to provide clarity, in cases of high-grade deformity, or when custom implants will be used. Magnetic resonance imaging (MRI) is seldom useful in the presence of established osteoarthritic changes about a dysplastic hip, although its utility when joint preservation is considered is significant. Imaging results should be correlated with history and physical examination findings.

INDICATIONS

Hip pain due to osteoarthritis, which limits activities of daily living, is the most common indication for arthroplasty. Most patients presenting with secondary osteoarthritis caused by developmental dysplasia of the hip will describe pain in the involved groin, hip, or buttock. Other reports may include limp, weakness, leg length inequality, or ipsilateral knee pain due to ambulating with the dislocated hip. Leg length inequality causing pelvic obliquity and compensatory lumbar lordosis may provoke low back pain.

Patients with grade II or III dysplasia according to Crowe[5] tend to develop osteoarthritis earlier in life. Counter to intuition, some patients with bilateral grade IV disease may function relatively well despite significant radiographic abnormalities. These patients ambulate with a "waddling" gait bilaterally, with similar leg lengths and relatively limited pain. They frequently respond favorably to oral analgesic medication and a brief period of activity modification. A short course of ambulating with an assistive device such as a crutch or a cane is frequently a powerful tool that may postpone the need for arthroplasty. A course of physical therapy for muscle strengthening exercises may provide relief of symptoms. Delaying surgical intervention in these patients until symptoms worsen is prudent. This subset of patients carries the greatest risk of surgical complications and reduced survivorship. When symptoms are well tolerated, life-long nonoperative management is not inappropriate for these patients.

SURGICAL EXPOSURE/APPROACH

Several approaches have been described in the treatment of congenital hip disease by total hip arthroplasty. In the setting of mild dysplasia or low dislocation, relatively standard approaches should suffice. However, it is important to anticipate the need to use small acetabular components inserted with deliberate medialization and the need to use relatively smaller femoral heads. Higher offset in the femoral stem can compensate for the decrease in abductor muscle tension that occurs with deliberate acetabular medialization. On the femoral side, precautions to avoid intraoperative fracture and strategies to deal with increased anteversion are needed even in mild dysplasia. Moderate dysplasia may require additional visualization at the time of arthroplasty, and extensile approaches should be favored. When a high dislocation is present, even more exposure is necessary owing to the need to control leg length, balance soft tissue tension, perform osteotomy of the proximal femur, and assess/treat acetabular bone deficiency. Preoperative evaluations, both clinical and radiographic, as well as careful preoperative planning of the selected procedure, are crucial for guiding the necessary approach (Fig. 75-5A-C).

Greater trochanteric osteotomy[19] or a trochanteric slide[20] is a useful approach. This approach allows for excellent exposure of the acetabulum and is useful for Crowe II through IV dysplasia. The trochanteric slide provides less control of abductor tensioning but in milder cases allows the treating surgeon to adjust the

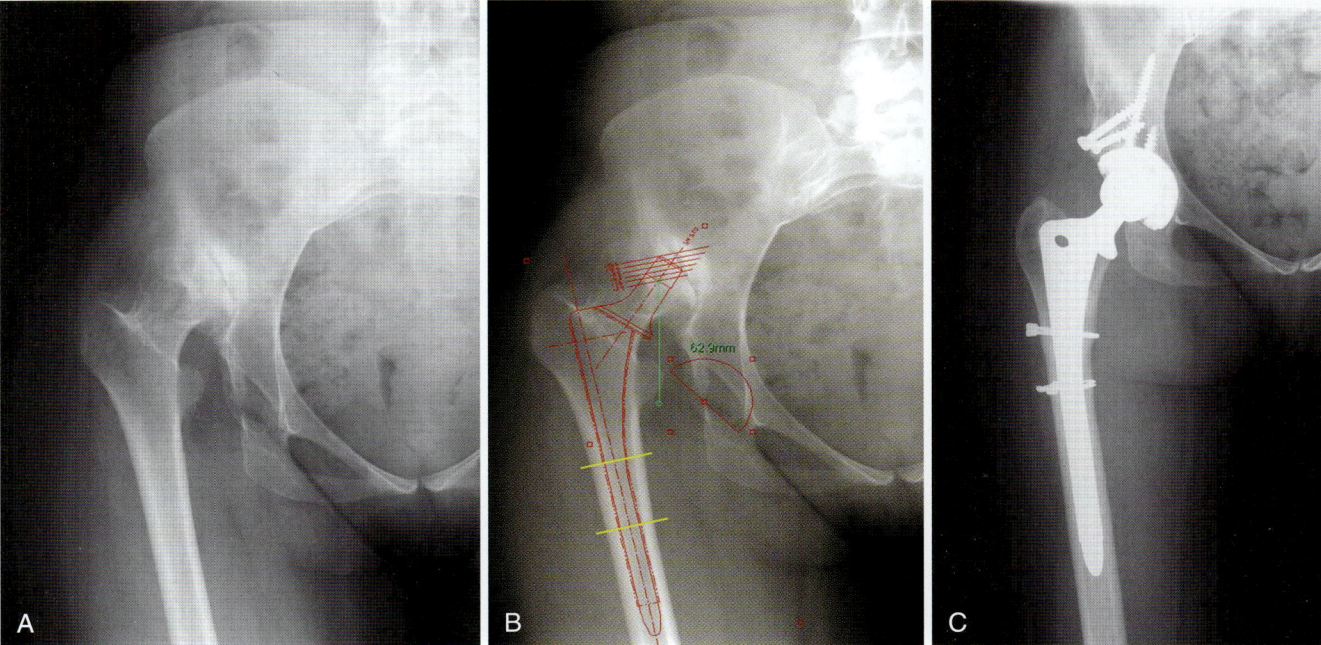

Figure 75-5. **A,** A 30-year-old woman with severe pain in the right hip and no previous surgery on the right hip. **B,** Radiograph demonstrating the preoperative templating process. **C,** Anteroposterior radiograph made 2 years postoperatively. *(From Krych AJ, Howard JL, Trousdale RT, et al: Total hip arthroplasty with shortening subtrochanteric osteotomy in Crowe type-IV developmental dysplasia. J Bone Joint Surg Am 91:2213–2221, 2009.)*

abductor tension as the lower extremity is lengthened during the hip reconstruction. A nonunion rate of approximately 10% should be anticipated even in the hands of very experienced surgeons. However, several authors have noted an acceptably low complication rate.

Another option for the dislocated hip is a subtrochanteric osteotomy.[21] This osteotomy is helpful in management of leg length, tension on major nerves, and rotation of the proximal femur. This approach allows the femur to be shortened to avoid excessive lengthening as the hip center of rotation is restored to the more distal true acetabulum. When the lower extremity is lengthened by more than 2 cm, the need for shortening osteotomy should be anticipated. By retracting the proximal portion of the osteotomized femur anteriorly or superiorly, excellent exposure of the acetabulum is possible. Once the true hip center is re-established and the hip is reduced, measured resection of the proximal femoral shaft can be performed (Fig. 75-6). One recent series of 28 Crowe IV hips had a 7% osteotomy nonunion rate but reported acceptable overall results at an average of 4.8 years' follow-up using this approach.[22]

Several other approaches have been described. Lai and associates[23] used pre-arthroplasty external fixation with distraction for patients with more than 4 cm limb length discrepancy to equalize leg lengths. Total hip arthroplasty was then performed without the need for

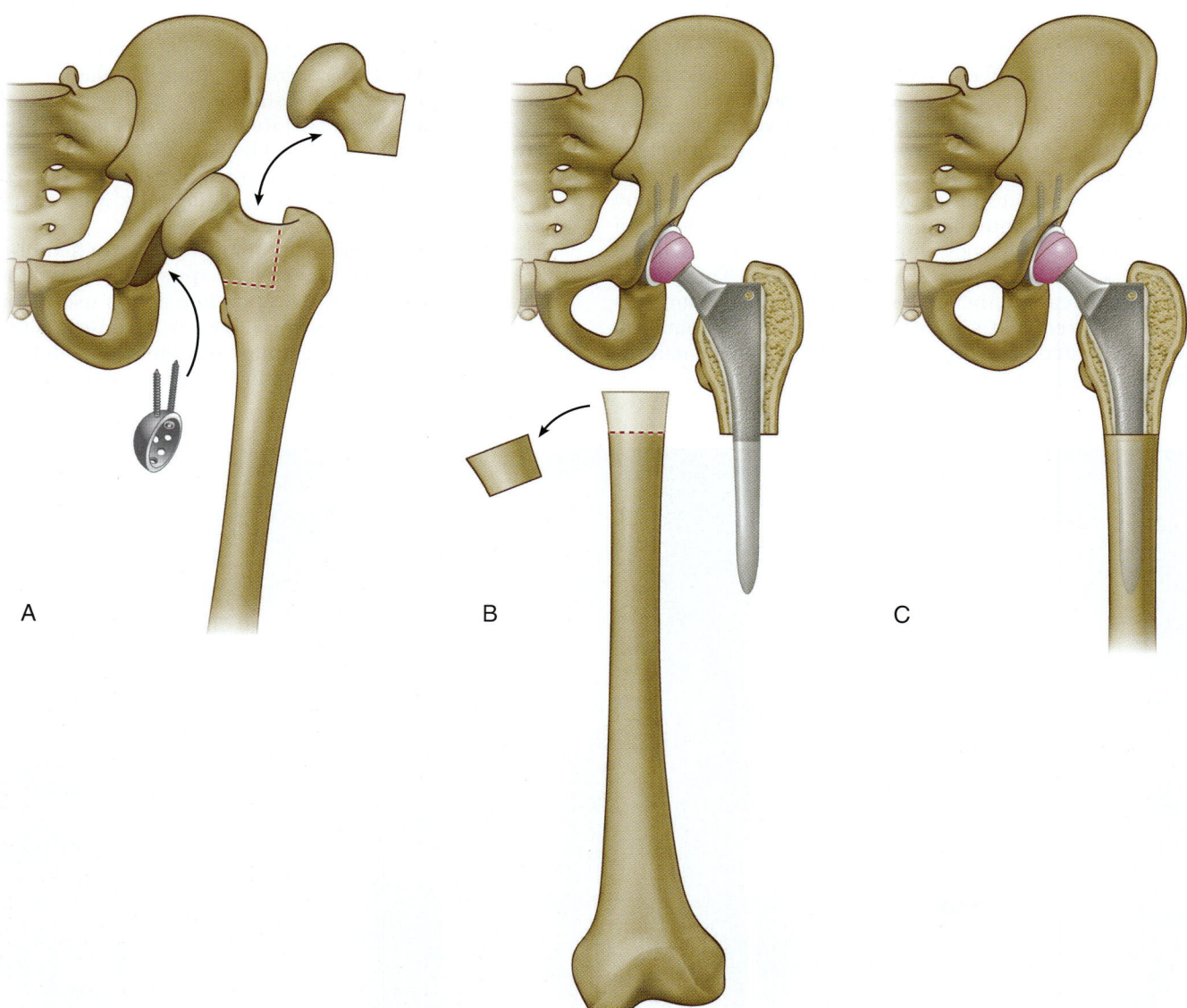

A   B   C

Figure 75-6. A, Femoral head osteotomy is followed by acetabular resurfacing. **B,** Femoral preparation, subtrochanteric osteotomy, and reduction of the proximal hip segment allow assessment of the femoral bone overlap, which defines the amount of shortening required. **C,** The osteotomy is transfixed by the long stem implant, and the hip is reduced. *(Redrawn from Bernasek TL, Haidukewych GJ, Gustke KA, et al: Total hip arthroplasty requiring subtrochanteric osteotomy for developmental hip dysplasia: 5- to 14-year results. J Arthroplasty 22[6 Suppl 2]:145–150, 2007.)*

shortening osteotomy. Their follow-up averaged over 10 years in a series of 48 patients and included no infections, nerve palsies, or dislocations. Cameron and colleagues[10] used the Smith-Peterson approach in all of their Crowe IV and in 30% of their Crowe III hips, along with a modified Watson-Jones approach in lower Crowe grades. Their study reported a significantly higher rate of complications and poorer outcomes in the more severely dysplastic hips, but the surgical approach was not controlled in this study.

Acetabular Reconstruction

Reconstruction of the acetabulum requires specific considerations in the adult with congenital hip disease, and it is critical to perform this stage of the procedure with precision.[24] The acetabular reconstruction (level, depth, size, and orientation) determines to a large degree the type of femoral reconstruction that will be performed and therefore influences the optimal surgical approach. Difficulties experienced in acetabular reconstruction are related to dealing with the lack of bone stock and poor bone quality and re-creating the true hip center of rotation. Placement of a sufficiently small acetabular component helps to achieve adequate coverage of the implant without violating anterior or posterior walls. Additional techniques to augment acetabular component coverage when needed in more severe dysplasia are individually discussed in the next section. One important principle in acetabular reconstruction is that the linear distance between anterior and posterior acetabular walls is the principal determinant of the appropriate outer diameter of the component. A common mistake is to plan the size of the acetabular component based on perceived medial-to-lateral distance of the socket on an AP radiograph of the pelvis. In most cases, a component judged to "fit" on the AP view is also of sufficient diameter to damage (or destroy entirely) the anterior or posterior walls, or both. Acetabular cages serve as a valuable backup in such cases.

Several strategies are useful for successfully placing the acetabular component at the level of the true hip center in mild to moderate dysplasia. Exposure of the most inferior aspect of the acetabulum allows a Homan, Cobra, or other retractor to be placed at the margin for confirmation of the level. Intraoperative radiographs, whether taken routinely or only as needed, are useful for confirming the position of the acetabulum. A small drill bit may be passed through the fovea to the medial wall of the acetabulum. Usually, 10 to 15 mm of depth will be encountered at the correct level, which will facilitate appropriate medialization of the component. Beware of cases of coxa profunda, however, as there may be only 1 to 3 mm of bone between the visible floor of the fovea and the true inner floor of the pelvis. Reaming should begin in the center of the acetabulum based on the anterior and posterior walls, not based on the perceived medial to lateral distance. The first reamer should have an outer diameter equal to the measured diameter of the femoral head. As reaming continues, deepening of the acetabulum should be performed carefully to avoid reaming eccentrically into the anterior or posterior walls. Necessary corrections must be made to continue reaming centrally. Because of the generally smaller size of the acetabulum after the first few sizes, further increases in acetabular reamer diameter should be performed in 1-mm increments. Trial components should be liberally used to assess for a snug fit as soon as it becomes possible; it is important to avoid the concept of using "the largest component possible." Rather, the correct philosophy is to use the smallest component that gives an excellent press-fit, and the determining variable is the anterior-to-posterior diameter of the acetabulum. The femoral head size is then adjusted as needed to provide adequate liner thickness. Despite the advent of highly cross-linked polyethylene, 22-mm femoral heads are still appropriate for acetabular components with outside diameters of 48 mm or less.

Methods for Improving Coverage

Because of the poor bone stock present in the acetabular region of patients with dysplasia, several modifications to the procedure have been developed. Mild uncovering of the component because of anterolateral acetabular deficiency is acceptable in cementless acetabular reconstruction. The exact amount of the component that may remain unsupported has not been scientifically established; however, there is some consensus that two thirds of the component should be supported by host bone. Whenever some of the component is uncovered, screws should be used for adjunctive fixation. In more severe cases of subluxation or dislocation, when adequate coverage is not present or the component is unstable, alternative means of gaining support must be undertaken. The most commonly used modifications include the addition of an autogenous bone graft, controlled fracture of the medial wall, or use of an acetabular cage. Each of these methods is employed to avoid displacement of the hip center proximally and/or laterally in the region of the false acetabulum. All of these approaches should be performed using small acetabular components to further increase coverage and compensate for the hypoplastic anatomy. It is useful to have small cages available as backup in cases of high-grade dysplasia. Some European surgeons use cages on a routine basis for dysplasia; however, publications describing this approach are very few.

Autogenous Bone Grafting. Autogenous bone grafting with the patient's resected femoral head, as first described by Harris and Crothers,[18] has many advantages. It is autogenous, is readily available during the procedure, and has sufficient size and strength to lend support to the acetabular component (Fig. 75-7A-C). It can be used to augment coverage of the acetabular component and provide additional bone stock if a revision is required. However, it is technically demanding and has been associated with loosening of cemented acetabular components, although one study by Chougle[25] did not show this association. Investigators reviewed 206 patients who underwent cemented THA in 292 hips, 48 of whom underwent structural bone grafting. Risk of aseptic loosening was not increased in their patients treated with femoral head autografting as

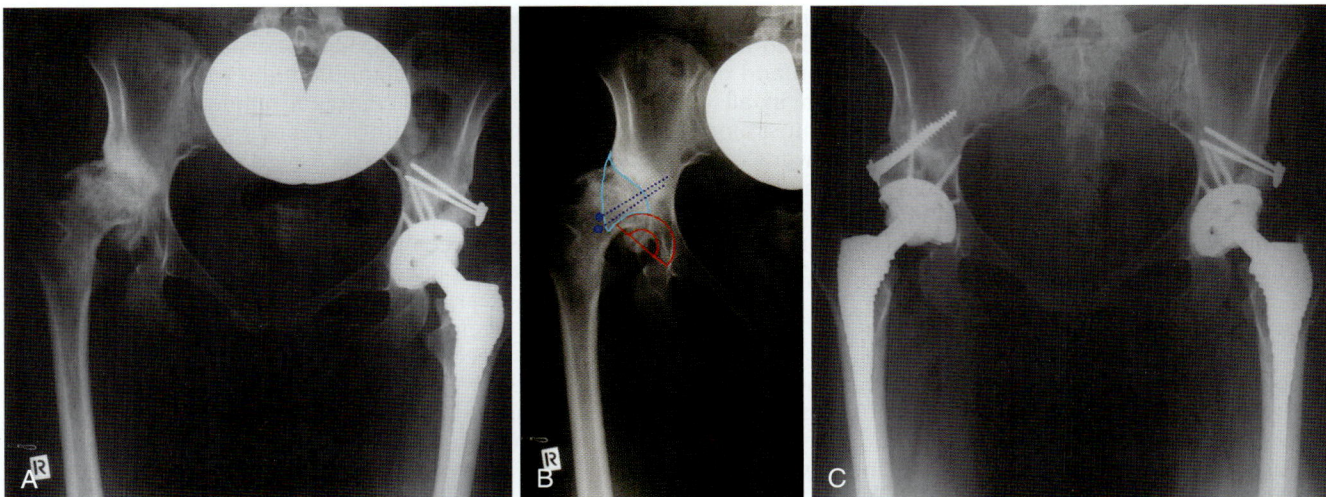

Figure 75-7. A, Preoperative radiograph of a patient with developmental dysplasia of the hip and severe degenerative arthritis. **B,** Preoperative sketch of the planned arthroplasty. **C,** Postoperative result. *(From Hendrich C, Engelmaier F, Mehling I, et al: Cementless acetabular reconstruction and structural bone-grafting in dysplastic hips: surgical technique. J Bone Joint Surg Am 89:54–67, 2007.)*

compared with those without. Their autografts covered at least 25% of the component, but no mention was made of the upper limit. Fixation strength of the autograft may be increased with the use of bolts; however, large fragment screws are generally sufficient.[26] Many studies have shown exceptional rates of radiographic union of the autograft, whether cemented or cementless acetabular reconstruction is performed.[27-35]

Medial Protrusio Technique. The "cotyloplasty" technique is a useful means of improving acetabular component coverage while maintaining the hip center of rotation at the intended level.[15] This procedure involves controlled penetration or fracture of the medial wall of the acetabulum in the region of the cotyloid fossa, which provides improved lateral coverage of the implant. Before insertion of the component, the medial wall can be bone grafted with morselized autograft from the femoral head and/or acetabular reamings.

Early reports[15] were based on use of a wire mesh to contain the graft and a cemented technique. More recently, proponents have used a cementless technique and no wire mesh.[36] Biomechanically medializing the hip center of rotation decreases joint reaction forces and was a principle of the classic Charnley low-friction arthroplasty. However, this does not appear to decrease the rate of wear as significantly as other variables.[37] Opponents of this approach note the risks of protrusio and dissociation of the component from the pelvis. Excellent results and no problems with healing of the medial acetabular wall have been reported.[7,36] As was noted previously, it is important to factor in the effect on femoral offset when a medialization technique is used on the acetabular side of the reconstruction.

Using an Elevated or Lateral Hip Center of Rotation. Appropriate placement of the hip center of rotation has been a topic of debate.[33,38-42] Proximal[39,41,42] and lateral[33] placement of the hip center (as in the region of the false acetabulum) has been shown to increase the

rate of failure of cemented acetabular components. Linde and associates[41] compared outcomes at average follow-up of 9 years in hips reconstructed with a center of rotation above the acetabular roof with those performed at or below that level. They found that cemented acetabular components in hips with an elevated center of rotation had a 42% rate of loosening compared with 13% in those reconstructed at a more normal level. Stans and colleagues[42] showed a similar correlation.

Re-establishing the true hip center of rotation in patients with a high dislocation requires substantial lengthening of the lower extremity. Although this may serve to improve a leg length discrepancy in unilateral disease, it also may contribute to complications such as nerve palsy. Simultaneous femoral shortening should be done to prevent overlengthening and thereby prevent such complications. The ilium in the region of the false acetabulum is generally thin and provides little lateral coverage. Previously discussed techniques significantly improve lateral coverage of the acetabular component when reconstruction is performed at the anatomic position; however, these approaches may be insufficient when performed at the false acetabulum. For these reasons, most authors advocate placement of the hip center at the level of the true acetabulum.[39,41,42] This approach results in less force transmitted across the joint, lower rates of aseptic loosening, and less leg length inequality. Rarely, in Crowe II and III hips, the true acetabulum is so poorly developed that the surgeon may be left with no viable alternative to a high hip center placement.

Cemented Acetabular Reconstruction

Early in the history of THA, acetabular reconstruction was routinely performed with cement. Initially, Harris and Crothers[18] showed promising results in severely dysplastic or dislocated hips with cemented acetabular components using femoral head autografting. Midterm results at an average of 7.1 years proved less encouraging.[30] Further follow-up of these patients at an average 16.6 years revealed much higher rates of revision (29%) and radiographic loosening (additional 31%).[43] This series showed an increased risk of failure associated with younger age and increased coverage provided by the bone graft. More recent series have shown acceptable mid- to long-term results with cemented components when the amount of structural support provided by the graft is limited to 40% to 50% or less.[32-35] Some surgeons routinely reconstruct dysplastic acetabula with acetabular cages and cemented liners. Clinical, peer-reviewed reports of this option are sparse in the literature, however. Except in the context of a cemented cup within a cage, cemented acetabular reconstruction is largely a historical technique in North America, given the superior results with cementless fixation.

Cementless Acetabular Reconstruction

As THA evolved to more biological means of fixation, more information became available on the mid- to long-term survival of cementless acetabular reconstruction in dysplastic and dislocated hips.[44-46] Cementless acetabular fixation provides the surgeon some flexibility when choosing the appropriate position for placement of the acetabular component. In contrast to cemented acetabular reconstruction, cementless fixation has shown durability with placement of an acetabular component at a more proximal position, a so-called *high hip center*. This may be beneficial in cases of severe soft tissue contracture, when leg lengthening is not desirable, or when significant periacetabular bone loss has taken place. This technique typically requires smaller acetabular components but may reduce the need for structural bone grafting. Restoring the true hip center of rotation by placing the component as medially and distally as possible is generally favored, however, for several reasons, including improved biomechanics. In this position, contact with host bone is maximized to provide optimal stability of the component. Compared with proximal positioning, a larger component may be used, which improves polyethylene thickness and/or femoral head diameter. Improving containment of the component reduces the need for structural autograft, thereby limiting early implant migration and/or rotation associated with early graft resorption. Placing the acetabular component more distally may reduce leg length inequality.

Hampton and Harris published their series of cementless acetabular reconstruction at an average 16 years.[46] They noted survival of 92% of their 21 hips using radiographic loosening or revision as the endpoint. Several other series also indicate favorable results at mid- to long-term follow-up when employing cementless techniques.[26,29,31,44,45] Ito and associates[45] had no revisions of cementless acetabular components due to aseptic loosening at more than 10 years of follow-up. Hendrich and colleagues published their results in 47 patients with 56 THAs.[26] They reported 11-year survival rates of 91.6% and 88.9% with endpoints of revision and loosening,

respectively. Cementless acetabular reconstruction has become the preferred method in North America.[47]

FEMORAL COMPONENT

Anatomic abnormalities present in the femur depend on the severity of dysplasia. As stated previously, the proximal aspect of the femur is typically smaller, narrower, straighter, weaker, and more anteverted (occasionally severely anteverted) than in normal hips. These factors must be considered when addressing the femur during arthroplasty. Additionally, disuse osteoporosis results in thin cortices and increases the risk of intraoperative fracture. Smaller standard components may suffice in cases of mild dysplasia. In more severe cases with or without osteotomy, however, modular or custom implants may be very useful, if not absolutely necessary.

Further accommodations may need to be made based on the type of acetabular reconstruction performed. As was stated previously, when a high hip center of rotation is restored to the normal anatomic position, a femoral shortening osteotomy may be required. Additionally, when smaller acetabular components are implanted, a smaller femoral head may be necessary to ensure adequate polyethylene thickness. Stem designs that offer options in femoral offset and anteversion are desirable. Occasionally, components from different companies may be paired together to optimize the beneficial characteristics of different designs. Caution must be taken when employing this technique for "22-mm" femoral head diameters, however. Femoral heads and corresponding acetabular liners from the era of Sir John Charnley were actually $\frac{7}{8}$ inch (roughly 22.22 mm) in diameter. Although some manufacturers still use $\frac{7}{8}$-inch bearing surfaces, most contemporary manufacturers use small heads that measure the exact metric 22 mm. Accordingly, whenever use of a 22-mm-diameter femoral head is contemplated, it is a good principle to use femoral and acetabular components from the same manufacturer.

Biant and coworkers[48] followed 21 patients with 28 Crowe III or IV hips after THA using a cementless cylindrical modular femoral component. This component features a smaller-diameter cylindrical design with less severe proximal flare to accommodate the straighter, narrower femoral canals in this population. Investigators performed femoral shortening in 21% of their patients. Modularity allowed the surgeon to determine the anteversion of the component independently from the proximal femoral diaphysis. After 10 years of follow-up, no loose stems were found and no femoral revisions were performed.

COMPLICATIONS

The risk of complications from surgery in dysplastic hips is higher than in typical osteoarthritis (OA). In fact, early complications and technical difficulties led Charnley and Feagin[13] to recommend against replacement of congenitally dislocated hips. Most commonly, leg length discrepancy, aseptic loosening, nerve palsy, instability, intraoperative fracture, and migration compromised the success of the procedure. Our understanding of pathologic anatomy and our experience in addressing these issues have improved. Despite improving clinical results, however, complication rates associated with reconstruction of the dysplastic hip remain higher than in THA performed for DJD. Cameron and associates[10] showed that the rate of complication is related to the severity of disease as classified by the Crowe system. Group I and II hips were shown to have no more complications than nondysplastic hips, and group III and IV hips had overall 25% and 50% complication rates, respectively. Hartofilakidis and associates[6] noted 14 complications in 42 total hip arthroplasties (33%) performed for neglected DDH. Nine of these patients presented with "low" dislocations, and 33 presented with "high" dislocations. Their series included two femoral nerve palsies, three fixed abduction contractures, one femoral fracture requiring fixation, three femoral cortex perforations not requiring fixation, three greater trochanter nonunions, and three cases of heterotopic ossification. They had no infections in their series and reported overall satisfactory clinical results. Both Crowe[5] and Eskelinen[49] reported an overall rate of complication of 19%. Several studies have shown high rates of dislocation ranging from 10% to 16%.[22,30,50]

Farrell[51] studied patients undergoing total hip arthroplasty who sustained motor nerve palsies. Investigators reviewed 27,004 THAs and identified 47 patients who sustained motor nerve palsies; a diagnosis of DDH and lengthening of the lower extremity were independent risk factors for postoperative nerve palsy. Farrell and colleagues described an average lengthening of 1.7 cm in their patients with motor nerve palsies on clinical examination compared with an average of 1.1 cm in a matched cohort without motor nerve palsies.[51] Although a maximum threshold of 4 cm of lengthening has been discussed,[52] Schmalzried and coworkers[53] and Eggli and associates[54] found no correlation between the amount of leg lengthening and the development of postoperative nerve palsy; rather, both found the preoperative diagnosis of DDH alone to be an independent risk factor. Schmalzried and colleagues[53] reviewed 3126 THA procedures and noted that more than 80% of lesions were localized to the sciatic nerve or one of its branches. Less than 20% of the lesions were encountered in the femoral nerve. Investigators reported a 5.3% incidence in DDH cases compared with 1.3% in uncomplicated primary THAs and 3.2% in revision THAs. Eggli and coworkers[54] correlated the development of motor nerve palsy with the difficulty of the procedure. Investigators advocated for exposure of the sciatic nerve to monitor position and tension throughout the procedure. If significant lengthening is anticipated, compensatory shortening must be considered to prevent postoperative nerve dysfunction. Intraoperative monitoring of evoked potentials of major nerves, although not established as a standard technique, has obvious intuitive attractiveness in high-grade cases.

Previous Operations

Several recent studies have focused on the results of total hip arthroplasty following previous osteotomy. Although these joint-sparing procedures were commonly presumed to improve eventual outcomes of total hip arthroplasty, few studies were available to support this claim. Chiari osteotomies are somewhat difficult to convert to total hip arthroplasty. Conversion from prior periacetabular osteotomy appears to be less troublesome, unless iatrogenic retroversion is significant.

Minoda[55] compared 10 THAs in which prior Chiari osteotomy was performed with 20 dysplastic or dislocated hips in which no previous surgery had been performed. They found that the prior osteotomy group had longer operative times, increased blood loss, and altered biomechanics (decreased abductor force and verticalized joint forces), which may compromise results. However, this study did not clearly show a difference in clinically relevant outcomes.

Baque[56] retrospectively reviewed eight hips that underwent periacetabular osteotomy (PAO) and later THA. Both procedures were performed through anterior Smith-Peterson approaches. Investigators discovered no complications and did not require bone grafting for acetabular coverage in any of the hips. Parvizi and associates[57] showed that prior PAO did not compromise results of eventual THA and reported their results with 41 THAs at average 7-year follow-up. Investigators noted an acceptable number of complications; however, 23 of the 41 hips had acetabular retroversion, which complicated proper positioning of the acetabular component. They recommended careful observation of acetabular component position.

CONCLUSION

Although replacement of arthritic hips due to degenerative dysplasia of the hip is challenging, it remains the most reproducible and reliable procedure in alleviating the symptoms of advanced arthritis in this setting. Careful planning and specialized surgical considerations are needed throughout the spectrum of DDH cases, from mild to most severe. Current techniques are capable of producing acceptable to excellent long-term results. Placement of the acetabular component near the true hip center and with satisfactory coverage is important. Use of small modular components that accommodate the pathologic anatomy is recommended. Modular femoral components can play a useful role. Complications can be minimized by achieving adequate exposure, avoiding overlengthening of the limb, and implanting the components in appropriate position. It is important to note that the high rate of revision is due not only to the cause of the arthritis, but also to the relatively young age and higher levels of activity of this patient population.

CURRENT CONTROVERSIES/ FUTURE DIRECTIONS

Many of the current controversies facing total hip arthroplasty in the congenitally dislocated or dysplastic hip are the same as those facing total hip arthroplasty in general. Repeated studies confirming the true, long-term clinical results of total hip arthroplasty using highly cross-linked ultra-high-molecular-weight polyethylene in these patients are needed. The relatively younger age of patients in this population may make alternative bearing surfaces seem more attractive. Improved wear of highly cross-linked polyethylene and recent concerns regarding some alternative bearing surfaces leave this an area that warrants further investigation. Additionally, the durability and long-term clinical success of newer "mini" and "micro" implants have not been clearly established in dysplastic and dislocated hips.

REFERENCES

1. Stulberg D, Harris WH: Acetabular dysplasia and development of osteoarthritis of hip. In Harris WH, editor: The hip, proceedings of the Second Open Scientific Meeting of The Hip Society, St Louis, 1974, CV Mosby, p 82.
2. Aronson J: Osteoarthritis of the young adult hip: etiology and treatment. Instr Course Lect 35:119–128, 1986.
3. Harris WH: Etiology of osteoarthritis of the hip. Clin Orthop Relat Res 213:20–33, 1986.
4. Hartofilakidis G, Karachalios T, Stamos KG, et al: Epidemiology, demographics, and natural history of congenital hip disease in adults. Orthopedics 23:823–827, 2000.
5. Crowe JF, Mani VJ, Ranawat CS: Total hip replacement in congenital dislocation and dysplasia of the hip. J Bone Joint Surg Am 61:15–23, 1979.
6. Hartofilakidis G, Stamos K, Ioannidis TT: Low friction arthroplasty for old untreated congenital dislocation of the hip. J Bone Joint Surg Br 70:182–186, 1988.
7. Hartofilakidis G, Stamos K, Karachalios T, et al: Congenital hip disease in adults: classification of acetabular deficiencies and operative treatment with acetabuloplasty combined with total hip arthroplasty. J Bone Joint Surg Am 78:683–692, 1996.
8. Mendes DG, Said MS, Aslan K: Classification of adult congenital hip dysplasia for total hip arthroplasty. Orthopedics 19:881–887; quiz 888–889, 1996.
9. Yiannakopoulos CK, Chougle A, Eskelinen A, et al: Inter- and intra-observer variability of the Crowe and Hartofilakidis classification systems for congenital hip disease in adults. J Bone Joint Surg Br 90:579–583, 2008.
10. Cameron HU, Botsford DJ, Park YS: Influence of the Crowe rating on the outcome of total hip arthroplasty in congenital hip dysplasia. J Arthroplasty 11:582–587, 1996.
11. Linde F, Jensen J: Socket loosening in arthroplasty for congenital dislocation of the hip. Acta Orthop Scand 59:254–257, 1988.
12. Numair J, Joshi AB, Murphy JC, et al: Total hip arthroplasty for congenital dysplasia or dislocation of the hip: survivorship analysis and long-term results. J Bone Joint Surg Am 79:1352–1360, 1997.
13. Charnley J, Feagin JA: Low-friction arthroplasty in congenital subluxation of the hip. Clin Orthop Relat Res 91:98–113, 1973.
14. Noble PC, Kamaric E, Sugano N, et al: Three-dimensional shape of the dysplastic femur: implications for THR. Clin Orthop Relat Res 417:27–40, 2003.
15. Dunn HK, Hess WE: Total hip reconstruction in chronically dislocated hips. J Bone Joint Surg Am 58:838–845, 1976.
16. Sugano N, Noble PC, Kamaric E, et al: The morphology of the femur in developmental dysplasia of the hip. J Bone Joint Surg Br 80:711–719, 1998.
17. Argenson JN, Ryembault E, Flecher X, et al: Three-dimensional anatomy of the hip in osteoarthritis after developmental dysplasia. J Bone Joint Surg Br 87:1192–1196, 2005.
18. Harris WH, Crothers O, Oh I: Total hip replacement and femoral-head bone-grafting for severe acetabular deficiency in adults. J Bone Joint Surg Am 59:752–759, 1977.
19. English TA: The trochanteric approach to the hip for prosthetic replacement. J Bone Joint Surg Am 57:1128–1133, 1975.
20. Glassman AH, Engh CA, Bobyn JD: Proximal femoral osteotomy as an adjunct in cementless revision total hip arthroplasty. J Arthroplasty 2:47–63, 1987.
21. Symeonides PP, Pournaras J, Petsatodes G, et al: Total hip arthroplasty in neglected congenital dislocation of the hip. Clin Orthop Relat Res 341:55–61, 1997.
22. Krych AJ, Howard JL, Trousdale RT, et al: Total hip arthroplasty with shortening subtrochanteric osteotomy in Crowe type-IV developmental dysplasia. J Bone Joint Surg Am 91:2213–2221, 2009.
23. Lai KA, Shen WJ, Huang LW, Chen MY: Cementless total hip arthroplasty and limb-length equalization in patients with unilateral Crowe type-IV hip dislocation. J Bone Joint Surg Am 87:339–345, 2005.
24. Haddad FS, Masri BA, Garbuz DS, Duncan CP: Primary total replacement of the dysplastic hip. Instr Course Lect 49:23–39, 2000.
25. Chougle A, Hemmady MV, Hodgkinson JP: Long-term survival of the acetabular component after total hip arthroplasty with cement in patients with developmental dysplasia of the hip. J Bone Joint Surg Am 88:71–79, 2006.
26. Hendrich C, Mehling I, Sauer U, et al: Cementless acetabular reconstruction and structural bone-grafting in dysplastic hips. J Bone Joint Surg Am 88:387–394, 2006.
27. Rodriguez JA, Huk OL, Pellicci PM, Wilson PD Jr: Autogenous bone grafts from the femoral head for the treatment of acetabular deficiency in primary total hip arthroplasty with cement: long-term results. J Bone Joint Surg Am 77:1227–1233, 1995.
28. Lee BP, Cabanela ME, Wallrichs SL, Ilstrup DM: Bone-graft augmentation for acetabular deficiencies in total hip arthroplasty: results of long-term follow-up evaluation. J Arthroplasty 12:503–510, 1997.
29. Spangehl MJ, Berry DJ, Trousdale RT, Cabanela ME: Uncemented acetabular components with bulk femoral head autograft for acetabular reconstruction in developmental dysplasia of the hip: results at five to twelve years. J Bone Joint Surg Am 83:1484–1489, 2001.
30. Gerber SD, Harris WH: Femoral head autografting to augment acetabular deficiency in patients requiring total hip replacement: a minimum five-year and an average seven-year follow-up study. J Bone Joint Surg Am 68:1241–1248, 1986.
31. Silber DA, Engh CA: Cementless total hip arthroplasty with femoral head bone grafting for hip dysplasia. J Arthroplasty 5:231–240, 1990.
32. Kobayashi S, Saito N, Nawata M, et al: Total hip arthroplasty with bulk femoral head autograft for acetabular reconstruction in developmental dysplasia of the hip. J Bone Joint Surg Am 85:615–621, 2003.
33. Iida H, Matsusue Y, Kawanabe K, et al: Cemented total hip arthroplasty with acetabular bone graft for developmental dysplasia: long-term results and survivorship analysis. J Bone Joint Surg Br 82:176–184, 2000.
34. Bobak P, Wroblewski BM, Siney PD, et al: Charnley low-friction arthroplasty with an autograft of the femoral head for developmental dysplasia of the hip: the 10- to 15-year results. J Bone Joint Surg Br 82:508–511, 2000.
35. Inao S, Matsuno T: Cemented total hip arthroplasty with autogenous acetabular bone grafting for hips with developmental dysplasia in adults: the results at a minimum of ten years. J Bone Joint Surg Br 82:375–377, 2000.
36. Dorr LD, Tawakkol S, Moorthy M, et al: Medial protrusio technique for placement of a porous-coated, hemispherical acetabular component without cement in a total hip arthroplasty in

patients who have acetabular dysplasia. J Bone Joint Surg Am 81:83–92, 1999.

37. Wan Z, Boutary M, Dorr LD: The influence of acetabular component position on wear in total hip arthroplasty. J Arthroplasty 23:51–56, 2008.

38. Russotti GM, Harris WH: Proximal placement of the acetabular component in total hip arthroplasty: a long-term follow-up study. J Bone Joint Surg Am 73:587–592, 1991.

39. Pagnano W, Hanssen AD, Lewallen DG, Shaughnessy WJ: The effect of superior placement of the acetabular component on the rate of loosening after total hip arthroplasty. J Bone Joint Surg Am 78:1004–1014, 1996.

40. Kaneuji A, Sugimori T, Ichiseki T, et al: Minimum ten-year results of a porous acetabular component for Crowe I to III hip dysplasia using an elevated hip center. J Arthroplasty 24:187–194, 2009.

41. Linde F, Jensen J, Pilgaard S: Charnley arthroplasty in osteoarthritis secondary to congenital dislocation or subluxation of the hip. Clin Orthop Relat Res 227:164–171, 1988.

42. Stans AA, Pagnano MW, Shaughnessy WJ, Hanssen AD: Results of total hip arthroplasty for Crowe Type III developmental hip dysplasia. Clin Orthop Relat Res 348:149–157, 1998.

43. Shinar AA, Harris WH: Bulk structural autogenous grafts and allografts for reconstruction of the acetabulum in total hip arthroplasty: sixteen-year-average follow-up. J Bone Joint Surg Am 79:159–168, 1997.

44. Anderson MJ, Harris WH: Total hip arthroplasty with insertion of the acetabular component without cement in hips with total congenital dislocation or marked congenital dysplasia. J Bone Joint Surg Am 81:347–354, 1999.

45. Ito H, Matsuno T, Minami A, Aoki Y: Intermediate-term results after hybrid total hip arthroplasty for the treatment of dysplastic hips. J Bone Joint Surg Am 85:1725–1732, 2003.

46. Hampton BJ, Harris WH: Primary cementless acetabular components in hips with severe developmental dysplasia or total dislocation: a concise follow-up, at an average of sixteen years, of a previous report. J Bone Joint Surg Am 88:1549–1552, 2006.

47. Cabanella M: Total hip arthroplasty: degenerative dysplasia of the hip. In Lieberman J, Berry D, editors: Advanced reconstruction, hip, Rosemont, Ill, 2005, American Academy of Orthopaedic Surgeons, p 116.

48. Biant LC, Bruce WJ, Assini JB, et al: Primary total hip arthroplasty in severe developmental dysplasia of the hip: ten-year results using a cementless modular stem. J Arthroplasty 24:27–32, 2009.

49. Eskelinen A, Helenius I, Remes V, et al: Cementless total hip arthroplasty in patients with high congenital hip dislocation. J Bone Joint Surg Am 88:80–91, 2006.

50. Woolson ST, Harris WH: Complex total hip replacement for dysplastic or hypoplastic hips using miniature or microminiature components. J Bone Joint Surg Am 65:1099–1108, 1983.

51. Farrell CM, Springer BD, Haidukewich GJ, Morrey BF: Motor nerve palsy following primary total hip arthroplasty. J Bone Joint Surg Am 87:2619–2625, 2005.

52. Edwards BN, Tullos HS, Noble PC: Contributory factors and etiology of sciatic nerve palsy in total hip arthroplasty. Clin Orthop Relat Res 218:136–141, 1987.

53. Schmalzried TP, Amstutz HC, Dorey FJ: Nerve palsy associated with total hip replacement: risk factors and prognosis. J Bone Joint Surg Am 73:1074–1080, 1991.

54. Eggli S, Hankemayer S, Müller ME: Nerve palsy after leg lengthening in total replacement arthroplasty for developmental dysplasia of the hip. J Bone Joint Surg Br 81:843–845, 1999.

55. Minoda Y, Kadowaki T, Kim M: Total hip arthroplasty of dysplastic hip after previous Chiari pelvic osteotomy. Arch Orthop Trauma Surg 126:394–400, 2006.

56. Baque F, Brown A, Matta J: Total hip arthroplasty after periacetabular osteotomy. Orthopedics 32:399, 2009.

57. Parvizi J, Burmeister H, Ganz R: Previous Bernese periacetabular osteotomy does not compromise the results of total hip arthroplasty. Clin Orthop Relat Res 423:118–122, 2004.

Previous Acetabular Fracture

Michael D. Ries

INTRODUCTION

Total hip arthroplasty (THA) is an effective treatment for post-traumatic arthritis. However, results of THA after previous acetabular fracture are generally less favorable than results of primary THA for osteoarthritis or inflammatory arthritis.[1-9] After prior acetabular fracture, a number of issues may increase the complexity of THA; these include protrusio deformity, cavitary bone defects, segmental peripheral bone loss, prior infection, retained hardware, limb shortening, sciatic nerve palsy, abductor deficiency, and heterotopic bone formation.

Patients with post-traumatic arthritis after prior acetabular fracture can present to the reconstructive surgeon with a wide spectrum of challenges. However, favorable results can generally be achieved with careful preoperative planning and use of surgical techniques, including removal of hardware when necessary, identification of the sciatic nerve, bone grafting or modular augmentation of acetabular defects, use of a large cementless cup or cage with screw fixation, and perioperative radiation therapy or nonsteroidal anti-inflammatory drugs (NSAIDs), to minimize the risk of recurrent heterotopic bone formation.

INDICATIONS/CONTRAINDICATIONS

Indications for THA after prior acetabular fracture include pain unresponsive to conservative therapy resulting from post-traumatic arthritis or avascular necrosis, and functional impairment caused by limited hip range of motion or limb shortening. Active infection is a contraindication to THA. Factors that may increase the risk of failure or complications after THA include prior infection, high patient activity level, and abductor deficiency.

PREOPERATIVE PLANNING

Radiographic Evaluation

Radiographic evaluation includes an anteroposterior (AP) view of the pelvis, as well as AP and lateral views of the affected hip. Additional Judet views can be helpful to delineate bony deformity in the anterior and posterior columns, the presence of discontinuity, and the location of retained hardware. Acetabular fractures that involve the anterior or posterior columns disrupt the anatomy of the medial acetabular wall (Fig. 76-1). Medialization of the cup to the acetabular floor will result in cup placement medial to the anatomic position of the acetabulum. Prior fracture of the posterior wall without fracture of either column does not disrupt the floor or medial wall of the acetabulum so the cup can be medialized to the anatomic acetabular floor (Fig. 76-2).

Prior acetabular trauma, which included a fracture of the anterior or posterior column or a transverse fracture, typically results in a deformity in which the inferior hemipelvis is displaced medially. Figure 76-3*A* illustrates a healed transverse acetabular facture with retained screws in the anterior and posterior columns. Kohler's line *(yellow line)* on the *(left)* noninvolved acetabulum is illustrated from the medial border of the sciatic notch to the lateral border of the obturator foramen. However, the hemipelvis inferior to the sciatic notch *(white arrow)* of the right post-traumatic hip has been displaced medially. Figure 76-3*B* illustrates the templated position of an acetabular cup, which has been medialized to the acetabular floor. However, because the acetabular floor and teardrop *(purple*

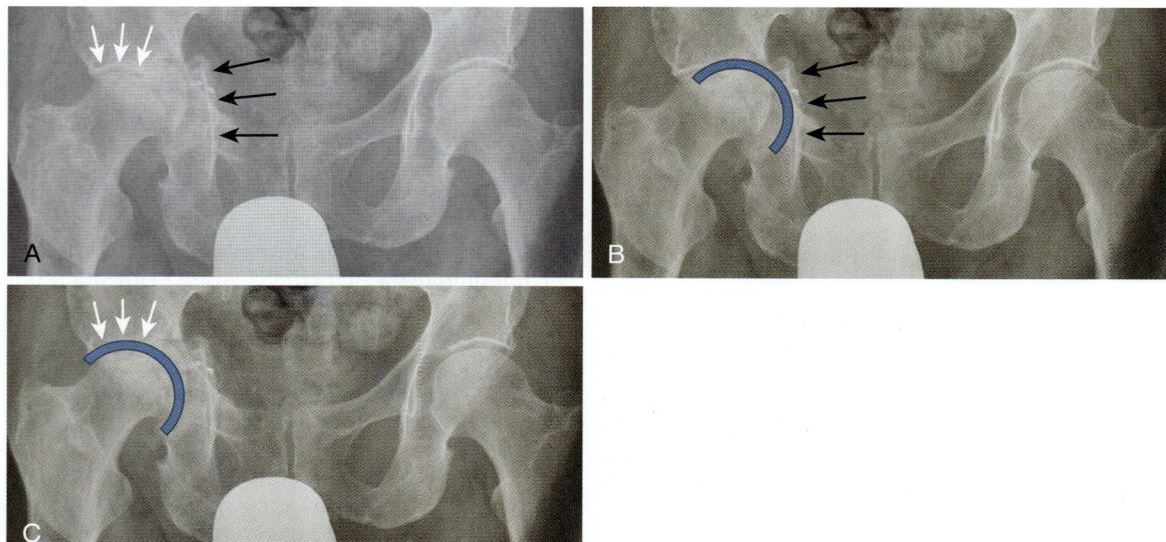

Figure 76-1. A, An anteroposterior (AP) pelvic radiograph demonstrates a healed acetabular fracture with medial displacement of the acetabular floor *(black arrows)*. The superior acetabular dome *(white arrows)* was not involved in the fracture and remains in its anatomic position. **B,** If the acetabular cup is medialized to the acetabular floor, the center of the hip will be displaced medially relative to its native anatomic position. **C,** If the cup is positioned along the superior dome and lateral to the acetabular floor, the cup center will be restored to its prefracture anatomic location.

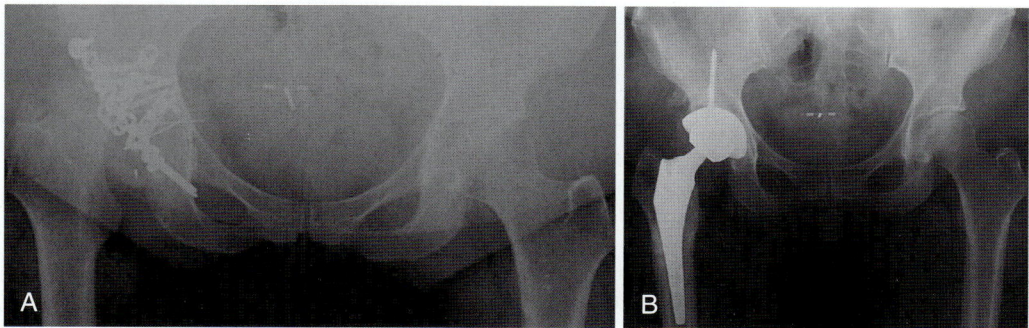

Figure 76-2. A, An anteroposterior (AP) radiograph illustrates a fracture of the posterior wall that has been plated. However, the columns were not fractured, so the acetabular floor is not displaced. **B,** A postoperative radiograph illustrates that the cup has been medialized to the acetabular floor and the hardware removed. Because the acetabular floor was not displaced, the hip center remains in its anatomic position.

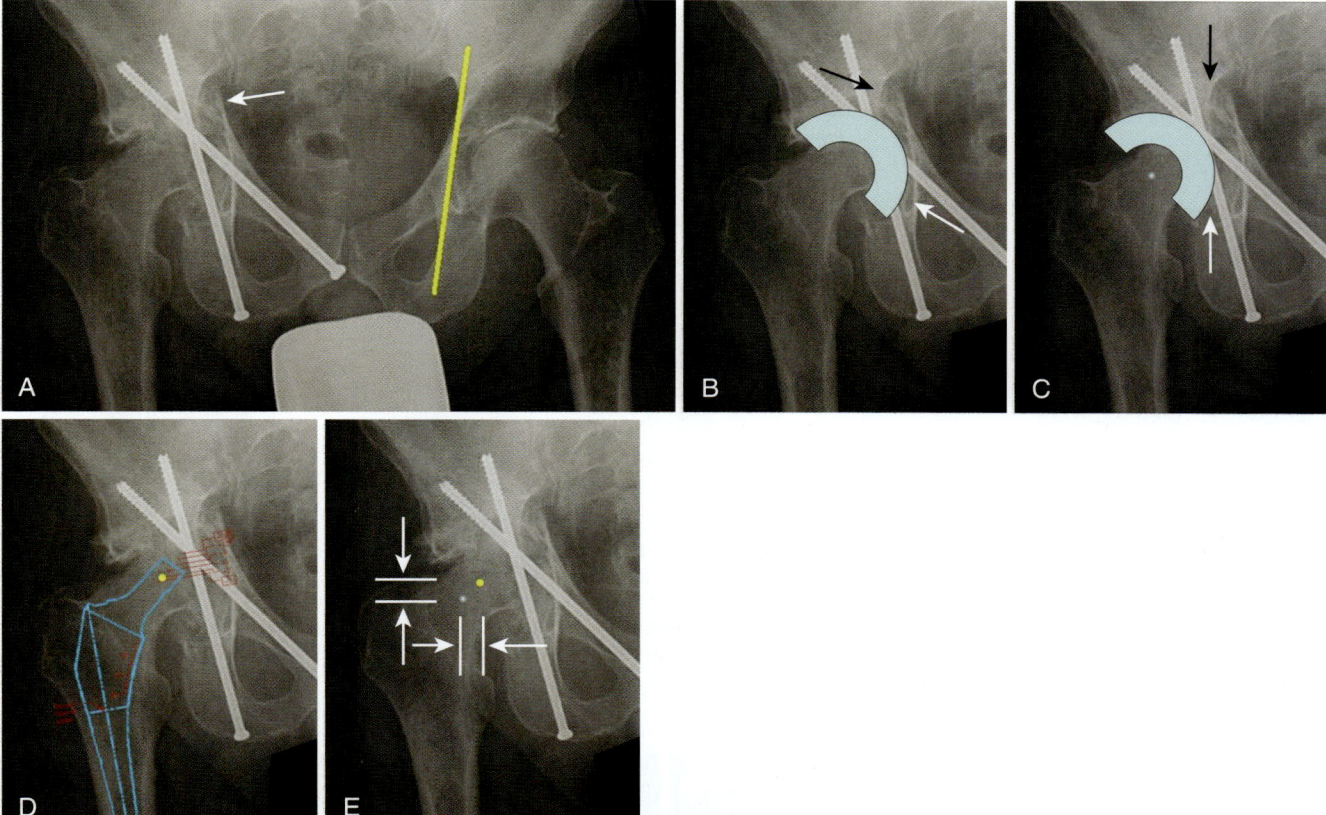

Figure 76-3. A, An anteroposterior (AP) pelvic radiograph illustrates a healed transverse acetabular fracture with post-traumatic arthritis. Kohler's line *(yellow line)* on the *(left)* noninvolved acetabulum extends from the medial border of the sciatic notch to the lateral border of the obturator foramen. The acetabular floor inferior to the sciatic notch *(white arrow)* of the right post-traumatic hip has been displaced medially. **B,** The templated position of an acetabular cup that has been medialized to the acetabular floor will result in excessive medialization of the hip relative to the normal anatomic hip center. Because the acetabular floor and teardrop *(white arrow)* are displaced medially, the cup is medial to the anatomic position of the sciatic notch *(black arrow).* This will result in medialization of the hip relative to the upper hemipelvis. **C,** A more favorable cup position is illustrated. The cup is lateralized relative to the existing acetabular floor. The inferior cup *(white arrow)* is now lateral to the teardrop but is no longer displaced medially relative to the anatomic position of the sciatic notch (black arrow). The templated hip center is illustrated at the center of the cup. **D,** After the acetabular component position has been templated, the femoral component should be templated. The center of the templated femoral head is illustrated as a yellow dot. **E,** The center of the templated acetabular cup *(shown in Fig. 76-3C)* and the center of the templated femoral head *(black dot in Fig. 76-3D)* are illustrated. The expected change in leg length (distance between vertical arrows) and lateral offset (distance between horizontal arrows) can be determined by the difference in position of the center of the acetabular cup and the center of the femoral head.

arrow) are displaced medially, the cup is medial to the anatomic position of the sciatic notch *(black arrow).* This will result in medialization of the hip relative to the upper hemipelvis.

Figure 76-3C illustrates a more favorable cup position. The cup is lateralized relative to the acetabular floor. The inferior cup *(white arrow)* is now lateral to the teardrop but is no longer displaced medially relative to the anatomic position of the sciatic notch *(black arrow).* The templated hip *(center)* is illustrated at the center of the cup.

After the acetabular component position has been templated, the femoral component position should be templated (Fig. 76-3D). The center of the femoral head is illustrated as a yellow dot. Figure 76-3E illustrates the expected change in leg length (distance between

vertical arrows) and lateral offset (distance between horizontal arrows).

DESCRIPTION OF TECHNIQUE

Prior skin incisions should be used when possible. The hip can be exposed through any standard approach. However, if prior posterior hardware is present, a posterior approach allows exposure of the hardware for removal.

Reaming should start with a relatively large-diameter reamer to enlarge the acetabular rim and permit support of the cup primarily on the remaining intact peripheral bony rim. If a small reamer is used, excessive medialization may result (Fig. 76-4A), but a larger reamer will

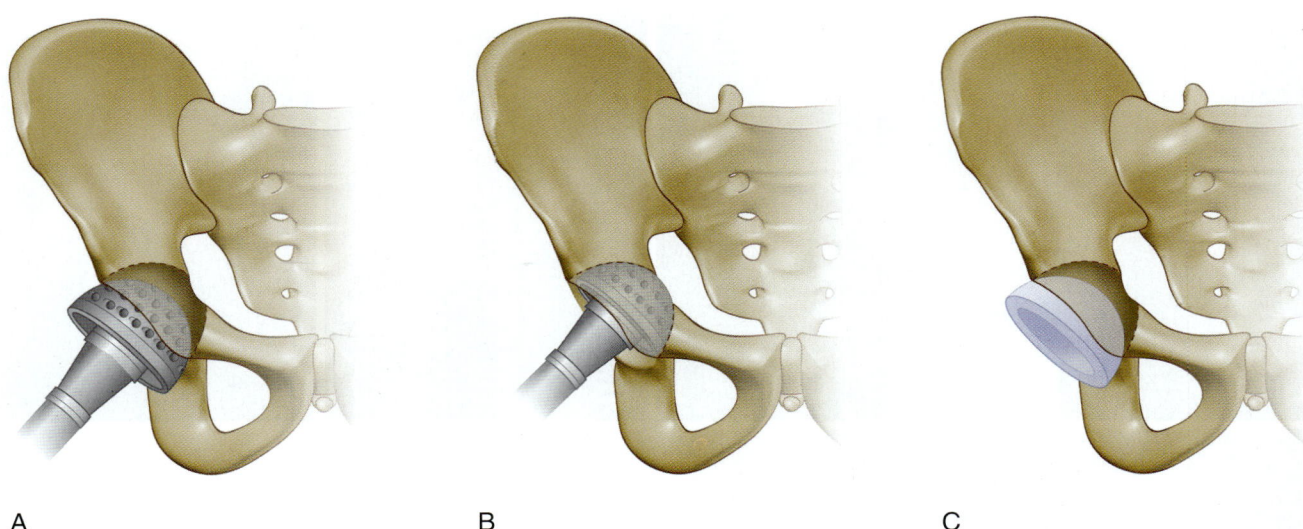

A   B   C

Figure 76-4. A, Reaming should start with a large-diameter reamer, which contacts the remaining acetabular rim. The reamer should be held in a relatively lateralized position to expand the rim and allow the cup to be supported on the peripheral bony rim. **B,** If a small reamer is used and reamed to the acetabular floor, the cup may be positioned medial to the anatomic hip center. **C,** A slightly oversized rim fit cup is supported on the remaining peripheral host bone. Morselized bone graft *(dark area)* from the acetabular reamings or the femoral head can be used to fill the cavitary medial defect.

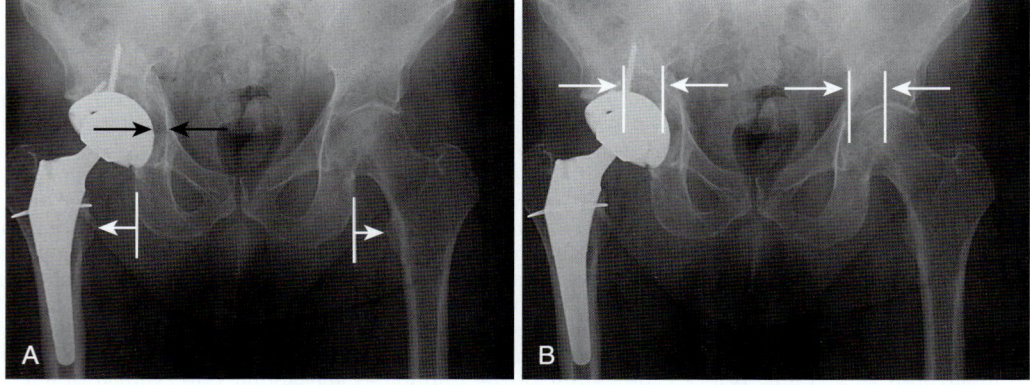

Figure 76-5. A illustrates a postoperative radiograph of the hip after placement of the hip in the position templated in Figure 76-3. The acetabular cup is lateralized relative to the teardrop *(black arrows)*. The femoral offset measured from the lateral border of the ischium to the lesser trochanter *(distance between white arrows)* is greater on the right compared with the normal left hip. **B** illustrates that the lateral distances from the sciatic notch to the center of the femoral head for left and right hips are equal. This re-establishes the normal prefracture position of the center of the hip.

engage the acetabular rim and prevent further medialization of the hip center (Fig. 76-4B).

Medial cavitary bone defects are filled with morselized bone autograft obtained from the femoral head or acetabular reamings. Figure 76-4C illustrates the medial bone graft and cup, which are supported on the acetabular rim.

Figure 76-5A illustrates a postoperative radiograph of the hip templated in Figure 76-3. The acetabular cup is lateralized relative to the teardrop *(black arrows)*. The femoral offset measured from the lateral border of the ischium to the lesser trochanter *(distance between white arrows)* is greater on the right compared with the normal left hip.

Figure 76-5B illustrates that the lateral distance from the sciatic notch to the center of the femoral head for the left and right hips is equal. This re-establishes the normal prefracture position of the center of the hip.

VARIATIONS/UNUSUAL SITUATIONS

Posterior plates and screws will frequently protrude into the acetabulum, requiring removal, but hardware from anterior column plating typically does not require removal. Figure 76-6A illustrates retained anterior column and posterior column plates. If prior posterior hardware is present, a posterior approach provides

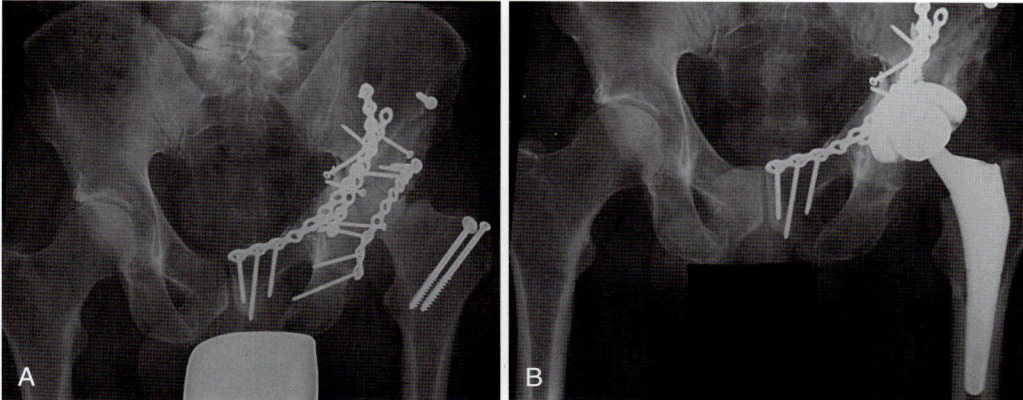

Figure 76-6. A, An anteroposterior (AP) pelvic radiograph illustrates retained anterior and posterior plates from prior open reduction internal fixation (ORIF). Judet views can also be helpful to visualize the location of hardware and to provide the exposure needed for hardware removal. Removal of the anterior plate would require an ilioinguinal approach. However, anterior column hardware rarely protrudes into the acetabulum and requires removal for total hip arthroplasty (THA). The posterior plate can be removed through a conventional posterior approach during THA. **B,** A postoperative AP radiograph illustrates THA after removal of the posterior hardware.

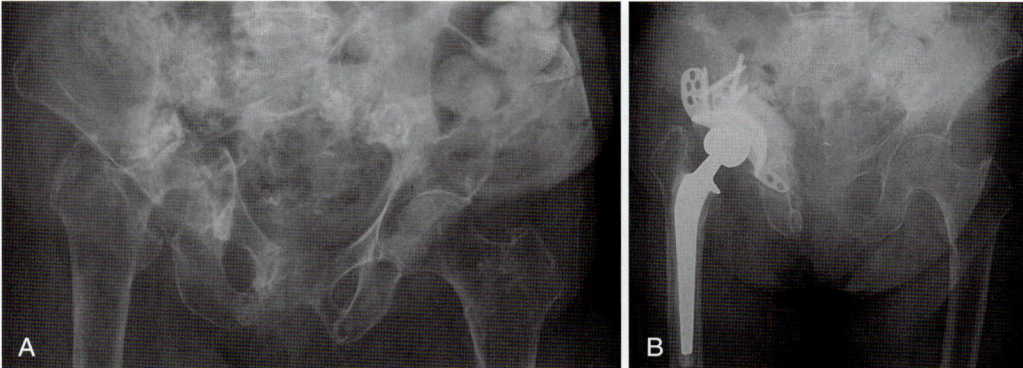

Figure 76-7. A, An 88-year-old woman with severe osteoporosis presented with an untreated displaced acetabular fracture. **B,** The acetabular rim was nonsupportive, so a reconstruction cage was implanted. Morselized bone graft was packed into the medial defect.

exposure to mobilize the sciatic nerve and remove posterior plates and screws. Figure 76-6*B* illustrates the implant position after posterior hardware removal.

Patients with severe osteoporosis or segmental bone loss may not have adequate peripheral bone to support a cementless cup. If rim fixation is not feasible, then a reconstruction cage should be used (Fig. 76-7).

If significant HO is present after prior acetabular fracture and requires removal, recurrent HO may be seen after THA. Patients who have HO removed during THA should be treated with perioperative radiation therapy or postoperative NSAIDs to minimize the risk of recurrent HO formation (Fig. 76-8).

POSTOPERATIVE CARE

Weight bearing should be restricted after THA for post-traumatic arthritis if bone grafting is required, or if

implant stability relies substantially on screw fixation to allow optimal bone healing and ingrowth to occur.

RESULTS

Excellent results can be achieved with THA after prior acetabular fracture. However, reported outcomes are quite variable. Berry and Halasey observed a relatively high rate of failure at 10 years' follow-up in 33 patients (34 hips) treated with uncemented acetabular components.[5] Nine patients had acetabular revisions, including four who had the shell revised (one for loosening, one for loosening and dislocation, and two for osteolysis) and five for liner exchanges (three for polyethylene wear and two for dislocation). The authors concluded that uncemented sockets had a low rate of loosening, but polyethylene wear and osteolysis were problematic. Several other authors have observed failure rates higher

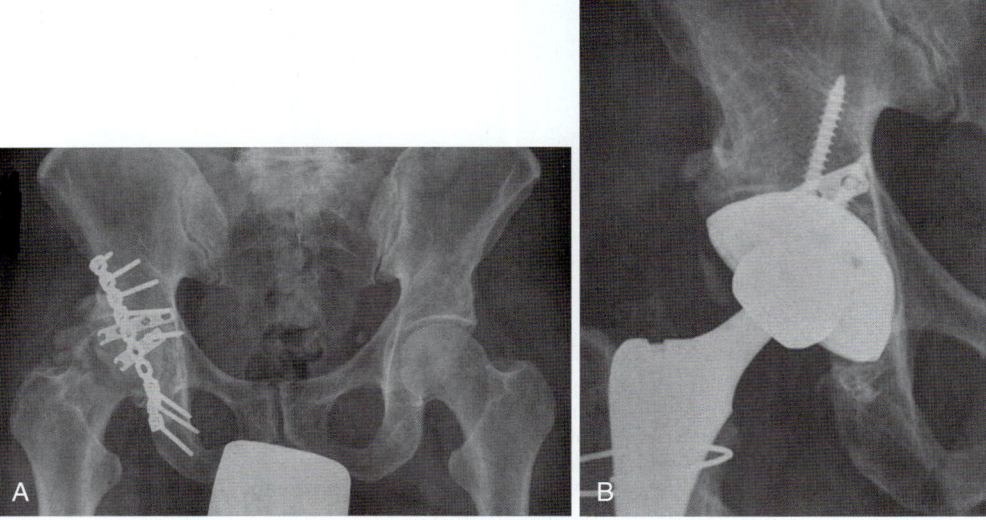

Figure 76-8. A, An anteroposterior (AP) radiograph illustrates heterotopic ossification that developed after prior open reduction internal fixation (ORIF) of an acetabular fracture. **B,** During total hip arthroplasty (THA), the heterotopic ossification (HO) was removed, then postoperative radiation therapy was administered. Two years after THA, the HO has not re-formed.

than THA for nontraumatic arthritis. Sermon and colleagues reported a 22% revision rate in 57 hips treated with THA after prior acetabular fracture at 30.7 months' follow-up.[7] Ranawat and associates reported on 32 patients treated with THA for post-traumatic arthritis after previous acetabular fracture, 24 of whom had prior ORIF.[3] Five-year survivorship was only 79% with revision, loosening, dislocation, or infection as an end point, but survivorship for aseptic loosening was 97%. Earlier failure was associated with nonanatomic restoration of the hip center and prior infection. Weber and coworkers reported on 66 patients who underwent THA for post-traumatic arthritis after prior acetabular fracture.[6] The mean age at the time of THA was 52 years. At 9.6 years' follow-up, 17 patients had a revision, and 10-year survivorship for the acetabular component was 87%. Age younger than 50 years, weight of 80 kilograms or more, and large acetabular bony deficiencies were significant risk factors for aseptic loosening. However, Bellabarbara and associates reported on 30 patients who had excellent results with THA after prior acetabular fracture.[10] Ten-year survivorship was 97%, and the authors concluded that intermediate-term clinical results of THA with cementless acetabular reconstruction for post-traumatic arthritis after acetabular fracture were similar to those after THA for nontraumatic arthritis, regardless of whether the acetabular fracture had been internally fixed initially. Results of these studies demonstrate a range of outcomes and indicate that the relative success of the arthroplasty is dependent on a number of factors, including the severity of the original fracture and the presence or absence of prior infection, bony deformity, HO, and sciatic nerve palsy, as well as the surgical technique and implant fixation method used.

COMPLICATIONS

Patients with previous infection have a higher risk of developing postoperative infection. Poorly vascularized tissue from prior trauma and surgery may increase the risks of nonunion and infection. In an immunocompromised patient with chronic infection and pelvic bone loss after THA for post-traumatic arthritis, salvage of a functioning THA may not be possible (Fig. 76-9).

Abductor weakness can occur from prior surgery and trauma, resulting in increased risk of dislocation after THA. However, dislocation risk can be reduced with the use of a large-diameter femoral head.

Patients with prior acetabular fracture and HO who require removal of HO during THA have increased risk of recurrent HO formation. This risk can be minimized with the use of perioperative radiation therapy or postoperative NSAIDs.

Prior acetabular fracture may be associated with limb shortening and scarring around the sciatic nerve. Dissection required for THA and restoration of leg length can contribute to sciatic nerve palsy. Sciatic nerve function should be carefully assessed preoperatively and the sciatic nerve identified and protected during surgery, especially if it is anticipated that lengthening of the limb is required to achieve a more normal position.

Many patients who have acetabular fractures are young active males; this situation is associated with higher risk of failure due to wear and loosening after THA. However, newer bearing surfaces with greater durability and wear resistance than conventional ultra-high-molecular-weight polyethylene (UHMWPE) may improve the longevity of THA in this patient population.

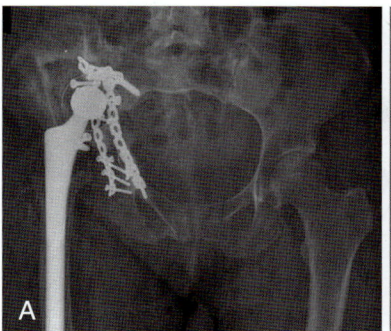 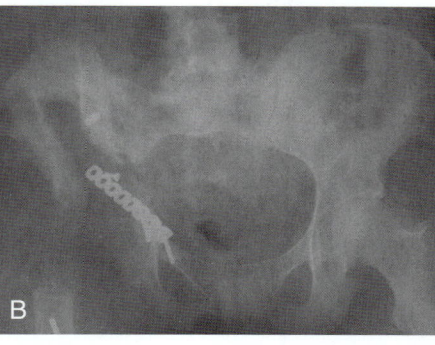 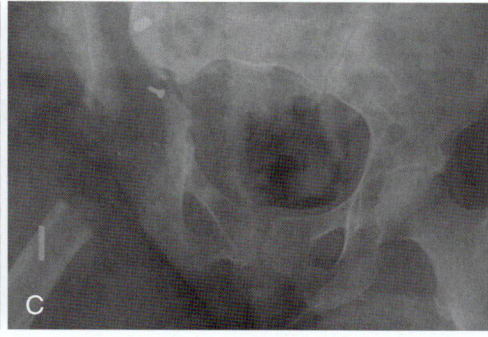

Figure 76-9. A, A 56-year-old woman with a history of intravenous drug abuse had undergone total hip arthroplasty (THA) 10 years previously for post-traumatic arthritis after anterior and posterior plating of an acetabular fracture. She had been treated with multiple I and D's and suppressive antibiotic therapy. She was unable to ambulate and presented with both anterior and posterior draining hip sinuses, sciatic nerve palsy, chronic pain, and limb shortening. **B,** Staged excision arthroplasty was performed. The THA and the posterior plate were removed through a posterior approach. An antero-posterior (AP) pelvic radiograph illustrates the extent of bone loss and the retained anterior column plate. **C,** Anterior débridement and removal of the anterior plate were performed through a separate ilioinguinal approach. Although the hip function remains unchanged from the preoperative condition, clinical signs of infection have resolved, and the patient's level of pain is improved.

CURRENT CONTROVERSIES AND FUTURE CONSIDERATIONS

- Areas of segmental bone loss requiring structural support can be augmented with femoral head autograft, allograft, or metal augmentation. Early results with trabecular metal augmentation of acetabular defects have been favorable.[11] However, metal augmentation does not restore bone stock, which may be necessary in young patients who could require future revision surgery.
- Newer techniques in acetabular fracture trauma management include less invasive surgical exposures and computer navigation. This may result in better preservation of soft tissue vascularity and bone stock for future THA.

REFERENCES

1. Mears DC, Velyvis JH: Primary total hip arthroplasty after acetabular fracture. J Bone Joint Surg 82:1328–1353, 2000.
2. Jimenez ML, Tile M, Schenk RS: Total hip replacement after acetabular fracture. Orthop Clin N Am 28:435–446, 1997.
3. Ranawat A, Zelken J, Helfet D, Buly R: Total hip arthroplasty for posttraumatic arthritis after acetabular fracture. J Arthroplasty 42:759–767, 2009.
4. Berry D: Total hip arthroplasty following acetabular fracture. Orthopaedics 22:837–839, 1999.
5. Berry DJ, Halasy M: Uncemented acetabular components for arthritis after acetabular fracture. Clin Orthop Relat Res 405:164–167, 2002.
6. Weber M, Berry D, Harmsen WS: Total hip arthroplasty after operative treatment of an acetabular fracture. J Bone Joint Surg Am 80:1295–1305, 1998.
7. Sermon A, Broos P, Vandersch P: Total hip replacement for acetabular fractures: results in 121 patients operated between 1983 and 2003. Injury 39:914–921, 2008.
8. Swanson MA, Huo MH: Total hip arthroplasty for post-traumatic arthritis after previous acetabular fracture. Semin Arthroplasty 19:303–306, 2008.
9. Glas PY, Béjui-Hugues J, Carret JP: Total hip arthroplasty after treatment of acetabular fracture. Rev Chir Orthop Repar Appereil Moteurpril 91:124–131, 2005.
10. Bellabara C, Berger RA, Bentley CD, et al: Cementless acetabular reconstruction after acetabular fracture. J Bone Joint Surg Am 83:868–876, 2001.
11. Kosashvili Y, Backstein D, Safir O, et al: Acetabular revision using an anti-protrusion (ilio-ischial) cage and trabecular metal acetabular component for severe acetabular bone loss associated with pelvic discontinuity. J Bone Joint Surg Br 91:870–876, 2009.

CHAPTER 77

Previous Proximal Femoral Fracture and Proximal Femoral Deformity

John F. Tilzey and Richard Iorio

INTRODUCTION

The presence of proximal femoral deformities secondary to previous fracture or orthopedic disease may make femoral reconstruction during total hip arthroplasty difficult, or impossible, with routine femoral implants and techniques.

INDICATIONS

During total hip arthroplasty (THA), most variations in anatomy of the proximal femur can be treated with standard femoral components, cemented and cementless. The proximal femur may be considered deformed when the anatomy precludes the use of standard total hip implants and requires complex techniques and atypical components more often associated with revision THA. This variation in anatomy may be due to developmental dysplasia of the hip or other developmental abnormalities, trauma with previous surgical intervention, or metabolic bone disease.

Berry[1] devised a method of classifying femoral deformity principally determined by anatomic site with subclassification of deformity secondary to geometry: A = torsional anteversion or retroversion; B = angular such as varus and valgus, or flexion and extension; C = translational; and D = size alterations (larger or smaller bone than usual) and cause of the deformity (i.e., developmental, metabolic, previous osteotomy, or previous fracture) (Box 77-1). The anatomic site and the type of deformity will affect choice of implant, implant size, and need for possible osteotomy. The Paprosky classification of femoral deficiency[2] is useful in preoperative planning with regard to choice of implant and surgical technique (Box 77-2).

Deformities of the femoral neck include excessive anteversion, as is most commonly seen in developmental dysplasia of the hip (DDH). Operative options for excessive anteversion include a low neck osteotomy and diaphyseal fixation with a fully porous-coated stem or a proximal modular stem with optimum stem version obtained by final placement of the stem within the proximal sleeve.

Deformity involving the greater trochanter can present as trochanteric overhang or proximal femoral varus malalignment. Therefore, straight access to the proximal femoral canal can be compromised, causing varus malalignment of the implant. A greater trochanteric osteotomy (see Case 3) trochanteric slide or a subtrochanteric osteotomy can be used to facilitate straight access to the femoral diaphysis. The proximal femur and the greater trochanter are repaired to the construct and lateralized; this can improve abductor muscle tension and lever arm moment.

With deformities of the metaphysis and the proximal femoral diaphysis caused by fracture malunion or previous corrective osteotomy, an osteotomy at the level of the deformity may be required to allow distal fixation and proximal reconstruction. In these cases, a proximal modular stem or an extensively porous-coated stem may be useful.

Metal-on-metal total hip resurfacing arthroplasty has become a popular procedure for patients with hip arthrosis, especially younger male patients, with a reasonably predictable intermediate outcome and a low complication rate.[3] Mont and colleagues[4] suggested that another potential advantage of total hip resurfacing arthroplasty is preservation of proximal native femoral bone, which may make hip resurfacing an option for those patients with a proximal femoral deformity, intramedullary sclerosis as in Paget's disease, or retained hardware, which may make reconstruction with a stemmed femoral component more difficult.

CONTRAINDICATIONS

Contraindications to arthroplasty in these complex cases are similar to those for primary THA. Patients with Paget's disease in the active, lytic phase of bone resorption may have vascular proliferation and associated bone pain. THA performed during this phase may be associated with increased intraoperative blood loss, increased bone pain, perioperative systemic hypercalcemia and accelerated bone resorption, and increased risk of local bone resorption around the hip implants. This active, lytic phase of Paget's disease may present a relative contraindication to total hip arthroplasty. Pagetoid lytic activity can be assessed with a technetium bone scan. Serum alkaline phosphatase is an indicator of bone formation, and urinary hydroxyproline excretion is an indicator of bone resorption. These levels may be used as markers, in conjunction with the bone scan, to correlate the extent and activity level of the disease. Preoperative medical management of the active lytic phase of Paget's disease with systemic antiresorptive agents may decrease the risk of complications. Sarcomatous degeneration of pagetoid bone occurs in less than 1% of patients. If pagetoid changes become rapidly destructive and increasingly painful with associated cortical erosions, with or without a soft tissue mass, sarcomatous degeneration must be considered.

PREOPERATIVE PLANNING

Careful preoperative planning is mandatory in these complex cases and cannot be overemphasized. Deformity of the proximal femur, retained hardware, and sclerosis of the femoral canal can all be determined with the use of conventional radiographs. Occasionally, a CT scan may be useful in assessing possible fracture or nonunion. Magnetic resonance imaging is rarely useful unless sarcomatous degeneration is suspected. Obtaining previous operative reports and identifying which implants are in place can aid in extraction and may provide information that is useful for future planned reconstruction.

Magnification markers make templating of components more predictable. In cases where nonunion and retained hardware exist, preoperative workup routinely includes serum C-reactive protein (CRP) and erythrocyte sedimentation rate (ESR) as sensitive screening markers for occult infection.[5] If these markers are elevated, then aspiration of the hip joint or biopsy of the nonunion site for culture is necessary. At the time of surgery, frozen section analysis of local tissue is performed on intraoperative tissue specimens from areas of retained hardware; this tissue is also sent for culture in the setting of conversion arthroplasty.

Templating of components on the anteroposterior (AP) and lateral radiograph will determine whether an osteotomy, either of the trochanter or at the apex of the deformity, will be required (Figs. 77-1 and 77-2). The lateral radiograph is useful to determine any apex anterior or posterior deformity because perforation of the femur can occur with a straight stem. For all complex cases, intraoperative fluoroscopy is used with the patient on a radiolucent operating table.

Choice of femoral stem is determined preoperatively, usually with an alternative reconstruction option as a backup (i.e., proximal modular stem with a fully porous-coated diaphyseal fitting stem as a backup).

Digital imaging has proved useful in preoperative planning for these complex cases. Specifically, digital

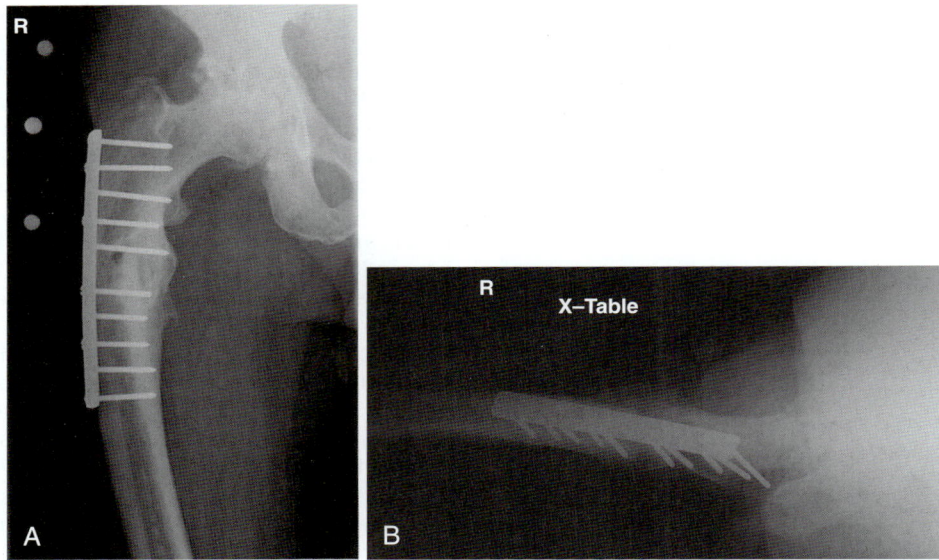

Figure 77-1. A, Preoperative anteroposterior x-ray and **(B)** lateral x-ray. Patient had previous open reduction and internal fixation of a subtrochanteric femur fracture with subsequent proximal femoral varus malunion.

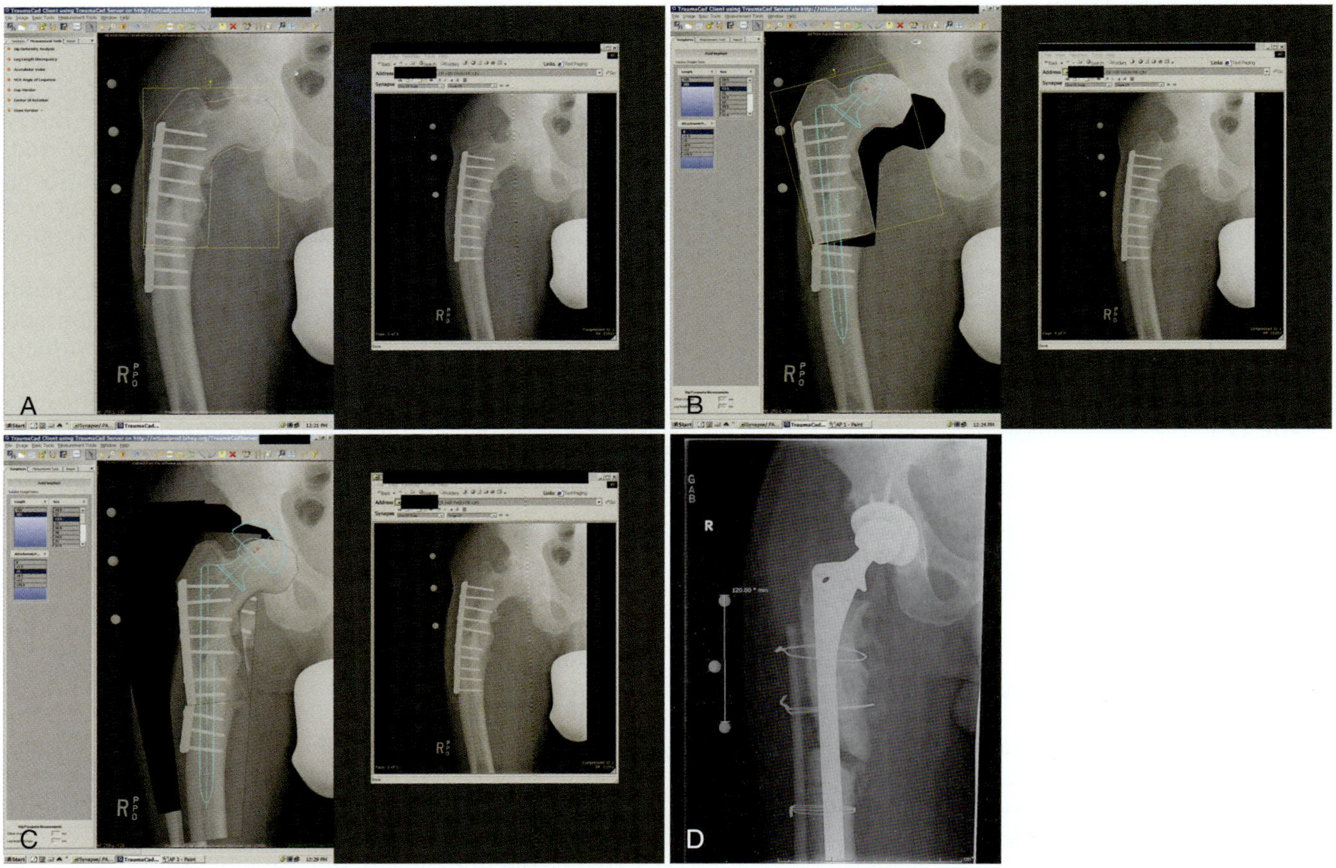

Figure 77-2. Sequence of images using a digital templating system to correct deformity and to determine the appropriate femoral implant for reconstruction. **A,** Proximal femoral segment is outlined. **B,** Appropriate deformity is corrected. **C,** Fully porous-coated femoral implant is selected and sized. **D,** Postoperative anteroposterior radiograph.

templating can be a useful adjunct for correction of deformity in the setting of arthroplasty for proximal femoral deformity.

DESCRIPTION OF TECHNIQUES

The surgical approach and the choice of femoral reconstructive implant are determined on a case-by-case basis. Deformity of the femur or retained hardware is recognized by careful preoperative planning.

Retained Hardware

In all cases where retained hardware is removed, the femoral stem should span the distal screw hole by two diameters of the femoral canal to reduce the risk of fracture through a stress riser postoperatively. Choice of femoral component in these cases is predominantly cementless, and fixation can be obtained with a wedge-tapered design with a proximal modular or anatomic cylindrical design.

Exposure

Surgical approaches are similar to primary THA and usually reflect the surgeon's preference. Previous surgical incisions are marked and can be incorporated if they do not compromise exposure. If exposure will be compromised, a new incision is made. Often a distal extensile incision is made in-line with the lateral femur if an osteotomy is planned or lateral proximal hardware is to be removed. A distal extensile approach is preferred; the aponeurosis of the vastus lateralis is incised approximately 1 to 2 cm anterior to the linea aspera, and the muscle fibers are reflected anteriorly over the femur.

Prosthetic Choice

An uncemented femoral component is chosen in most cases. However, in elderly patients, when hardware is removed from the proximal femur and a cemented stem is chosen, previous screw holes need to be plugged with unicortical screws or bone graft to prevent extrusion of cement.

Proximally coated modular stems can be used in Paprosky type 1 femurs with an intact femoral metaphysis. Typical examples include THA following failed internal fixation for femoral neck fracture or noncomplex intertrochanteric femur fracture with arthrosis, which requires hardware removal. Typically, the hip is dislocated before hardware removal to avoid fracture through stress risers created by removed hardware. Cerclage wiring of the proximal femur can reduce the risk of fracture during broaching. Lateral screw holes need to be bypassed by at least two cortical diameters with the stem.

Deformities of the greater trochanter may include trochanteric overhang in a varus femur or overgrowth. An overhanging greater trochanter makes straight access to the lateral endosteal cortex difficult with potential varus positioning of a straight implant. Use of the "cookie-cutter" osteotome to remove medial overhanging bone followed by placement of the straight reamer in slight valgus can provide straight access to the canal. Alternatively, a high-speed power tool can be used to lateralize the site of proximal trochanteric entry.

A high-riding, overgrown trochanter may cause impingement on the pelvis with flexion and rotation, as well as decreased abductor moment arm function. An osteotomy can be performed with advancement to a more suitable distal and lateral position (Fig. 77-3).

In most cases of developmental hip dysplasia, the stem of choice has a proximal modular design. However, those femurs with metaphyseal bone loss such as in Paprosky type II deformities make this stem design unsuitable. The metaphyseal sleeve is impacted into the milled bone and gives proximal and rotational stability with bone in-growth. Prophylactic cerclage wiring should be considered in cases with thin cortices. The stem is fluted with distal slots, which, following reaming

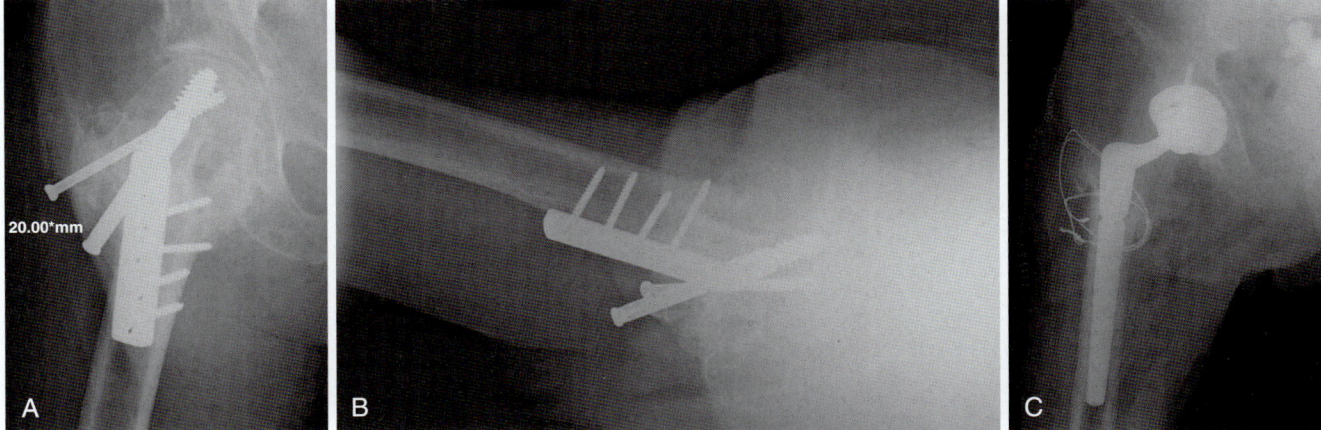

Figure 77-3. A, Anteroposterior radiograph shows failed internal fixation of an intertrochanteric femur fracture with severe deformity and nonunion. **B,** Lateral radiograph. **C,** Postoperative radiograph following total hip arthroplasty with a mid-modular femoral component and a trochanteric osteotomy, bypassing screw-hole stress risers.

of the femoral diaphysis, gives the stem distal rotational stability. The version of the stem is determined by its position in the femoral diaphysis when the orientation of the proximal femur is abnormally positioned.

Extensively porous-coated stems are designed to obtain rigid axial and rotational stability in diaphyseal femoral bone. They are suitable for Paprosky type II and III deformities and require a rigid diaphyseal fit as determined with straight reaming. If a straight stem is used, this will result in three-point fixation when placed into a bowed femur. Use of a preoperative lateral femoral radiograph will help the clinician determine whether to select a straight or a bowed stem, or perhaps an apical osteotomy in severe deformities. Intraoperative fluoroscopy is frequently used to ensure that straight rigid reamers are not compromising the anterior cortex of the femur.

Mid-modular stems generally are used in Paprosky type III and IV femurs, enabling independent metaphyseal and diaphyseal sizing. The distal stem fixation provides rotational and axial stability. The proximal body can provide options for length and rotational freedom for version orientation when a metaphyseal/diaphyseal size mismatch occurs.

Distal stem options include conical, porous-coated, and fluted designs. The conical distal stem provides immediate diaphyseal rotational control and axial stability. The stem is heavy grit-blasted and is available in straight and bowed designs. The proximal cone body can be independent of the distal stem, and cone-shaped reamers machine the proximal femoral bone.

Osteotomy

The use of straight stems in cases involving angular deformity may compromise the greater trochanter or the femoral diaphysis with perforation or fracture. In these cases, femoral osteotomy is indicated. Usually the osteotomy is performed at the apex of the deformity, and preoperative planning will determine whether a bi-planar osteotomy is required. A transverse, subtrochanteric osteotomy is simplest and leads to predictable results for stability and healing.

UNUSUAL SITUATIONS

Case 1

50-year-old male. Traumatic arthritis right hip, with deformity of the femoral neck, Paprosky type I femur. Underwent right THA with a proximal modular stem (Fig. 77-4).

Case 2

82-year-old male with failed internal fixation of a right femoral neck fracture. Underwent right THA with a proximal coated tapered stem with prophylactic cerclage wiring (Fig. 77-5).

Case 3

53-year-old male with history of Legg-Calvé-Perthes disease with deformity of the greater trochanter and proximal femur. Underwent osteotomy of the greater trochanter and advancement (Fig. 77-6).

Case 4

47-year-old male with malunion and failure of fixation following an intertrochanteric proximal femur fracture.

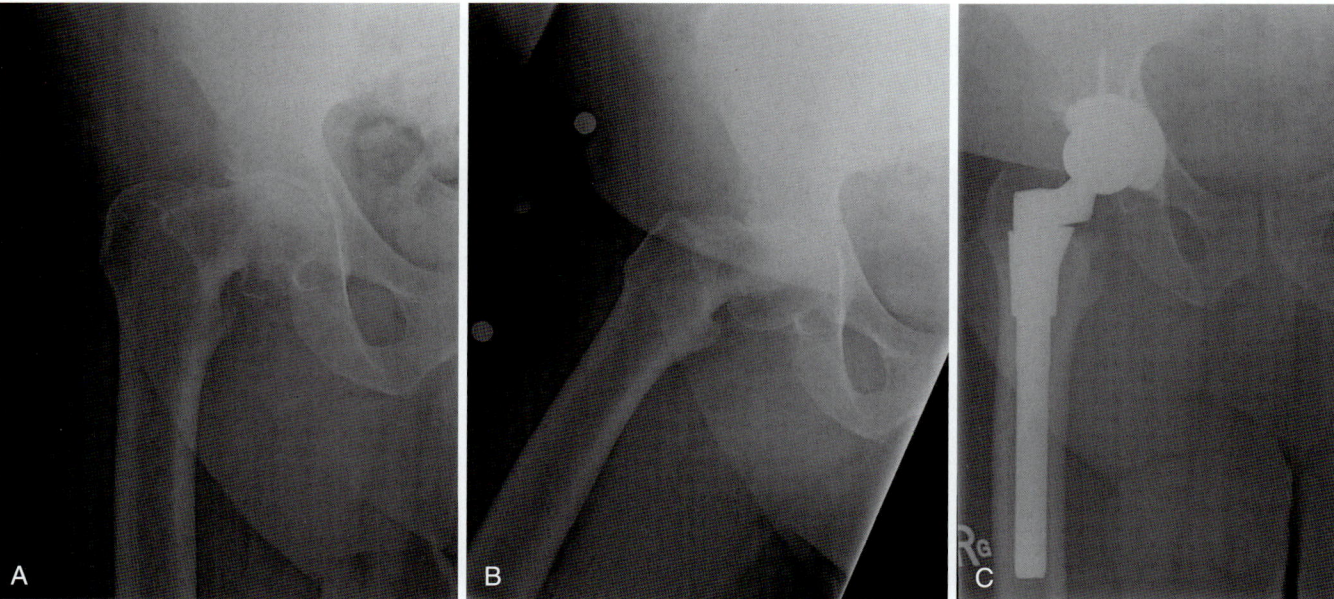

Figure 77-4. Case 1. A, Anteroposterior radiograph showing significant coxa vara with hip arthrosis. **B,** Lateral radiograph demonstrates retroversion deformity of the femoral neck. **C,** Postoperative anteroposterior radiograph following total hip arthroplasty (THA) with a proximal modular stem.

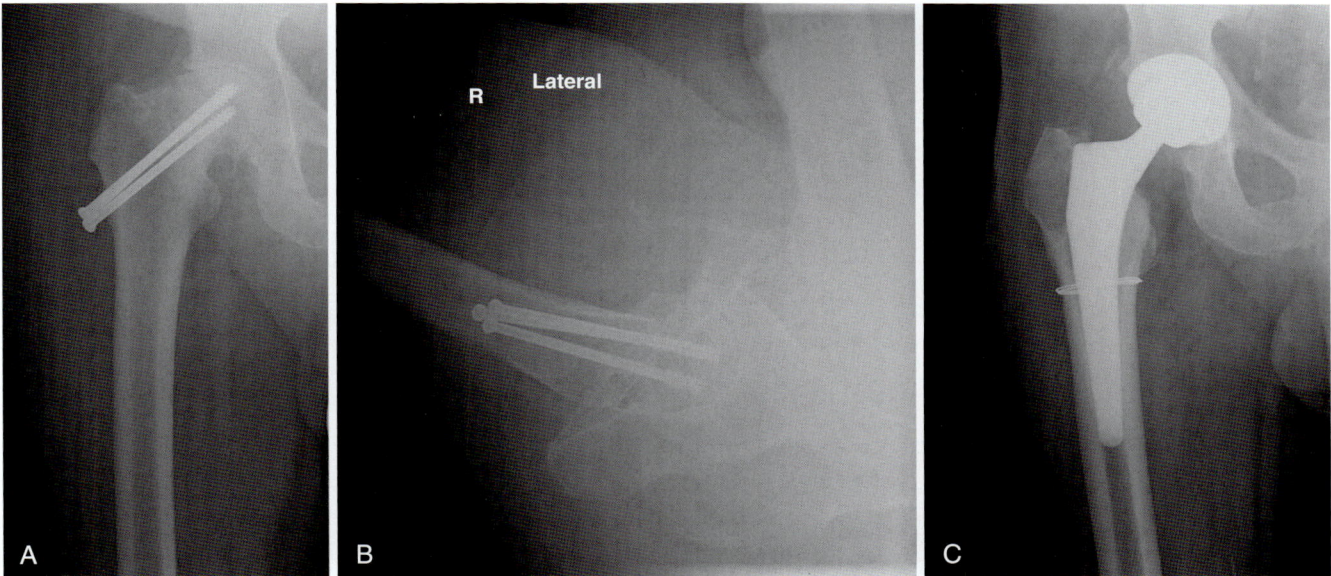

Figure 77-5. Case 2. A, Anteroposterior radiograph demonstrates failure of internal fixation and arthrosis. **B,** Lateral radiograph shows no significant deformity of the distal femoral neck. **C,** Postoperative anteroposterior radiograph following total hip arthroplasty (THA). Femoral reconstruction was done with a proximally coated tapered wedge stem. Prophylactic cerclage wires were placed before broaching of the endosteal canal to reduce the risk of perioperative fracture.

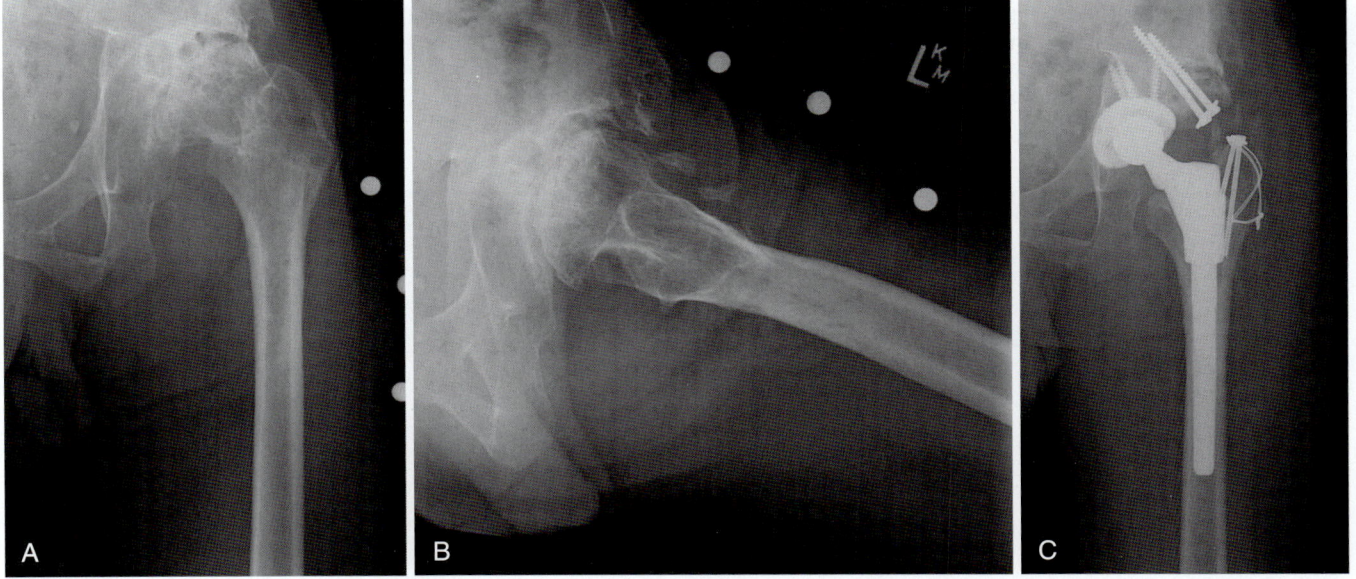

Figure 77-6. Case 3. A, Anteroposterior radiograph shows severe arthrosis of the hip with trochanteric deformity. **B,** Lateral radiograph shows that the greater trochanteric deformity is anterior. **C,** Postoperative radiograph following total hip arthroplasty (THA) with a proximal modular stem and trochanteric osteotomy and advancement.

Underwent left THA with a proximal modular stem (Fig. 77-7).

Case 5

44-year-old female with left proximal femoral varus deformity. Underwent left THA with proximal modular stem and trochanteric osteotomy and advancement. Note slight varus position of the stem, which was

believed to be acceptable and preferable to performing a subtrochanteric osteotomy (Fig. 77-8).

Case 6

52-year-old female with history of fibrous dysplasia and failed hybrid right THA 3 years before presentation. Underwent revision right THA with proximal femoral osteotomy; reconstruction was done with a mid-modular stem (Fig. 77-9).

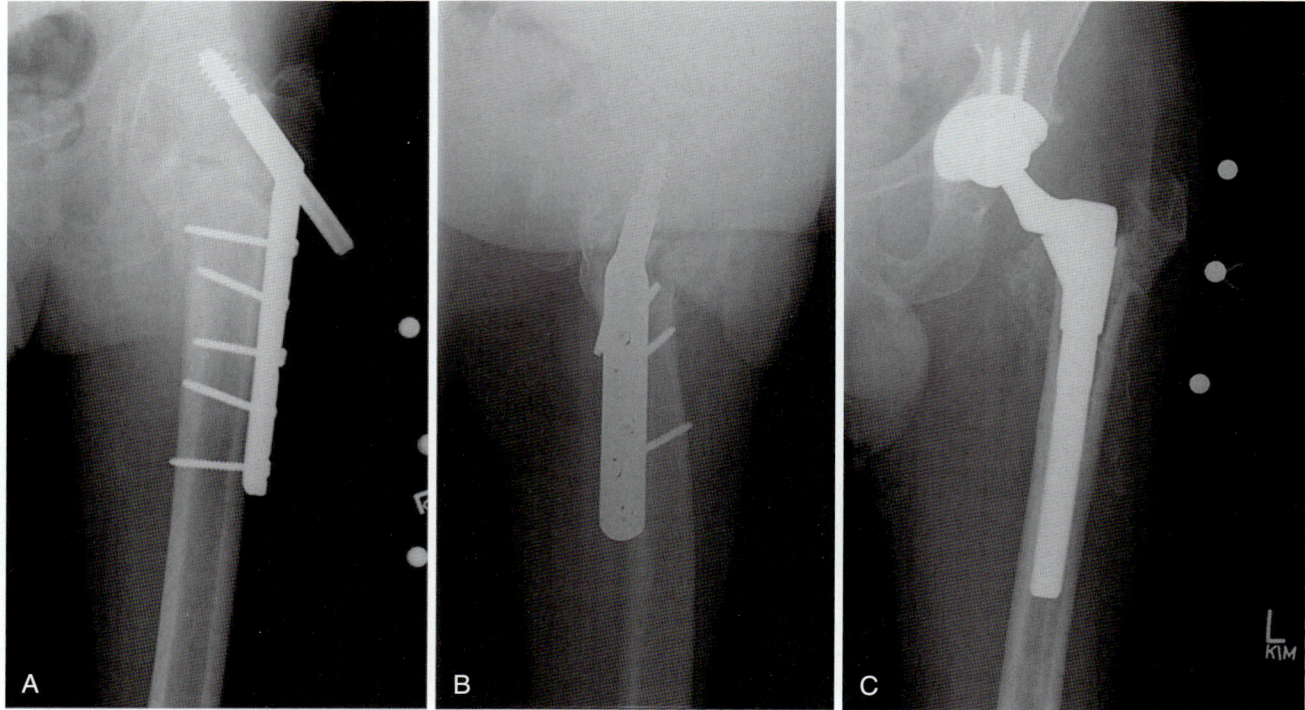

Figure 77-7. **Case 4. A,** Anteroposterior radiograph: failed internal fixation of an intertrochanteric femur fracture. **B,** Lateral radiograph: proximal femoral metaphysis is intact. **C,** Postoperative radiograph following total hip arthroplasty (THA) with a proximal modular femoral stem. The greater trochanter did not require osteotomy, but overhang was reduced to enable lateral endosteal canal entry. The femoral stem bypasses distal cortical stress risers by more than two canal cortices; supplemental plating was not necessary.

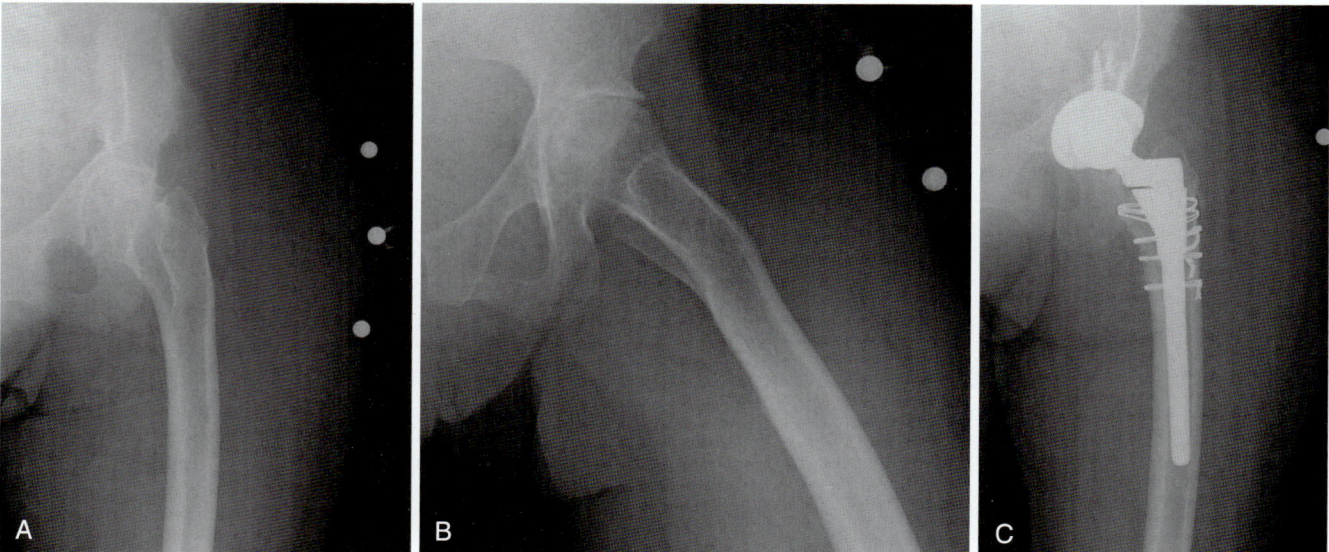

Figure 77-8. **Case 5. A,** Anteroposterior radiograph shows proximal femoral varus and deformity of the greater trochanter. **B,** Lateral radiograph demonstrates significant anteversion of the proximal femur. **C,** Postoperative radiograph following total hip arthroplasty (THA) with a proximal modular femoral stem and greater trochanteric osteotomy and advancement. Note the slight varus position of the stem, which was determined to be acceptable intraoperatively, rather than performing a subtrochanteric osteotomy.

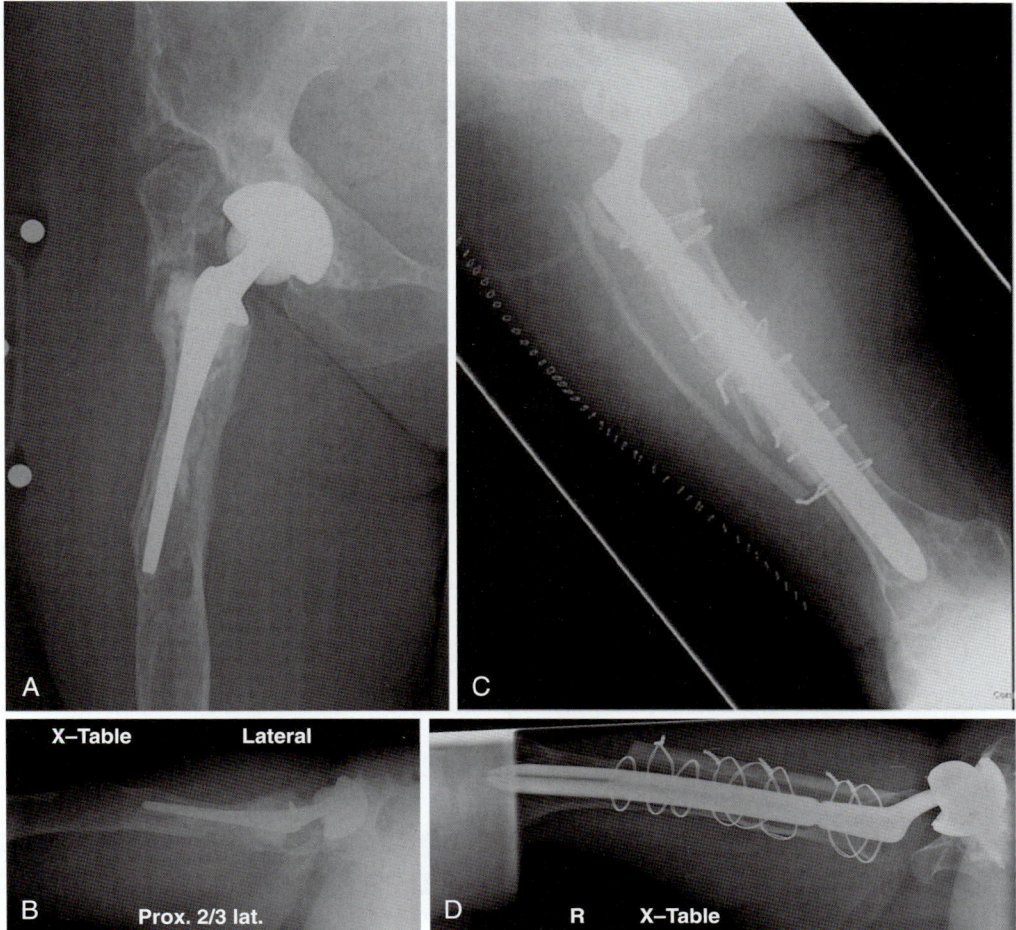

Figure 77-9. Case 6. A, Anteroposterior radiograph shows failed cemented femoral reconstruction, greater trochanteric deformity, and nonunion. **B,** Lateral radiograph demonstrates a severely deformed proximal femur. **C** and **D,** Postoperative anteroposterior and lateral radiographs following revision total hip arthroplasty (THA) with proximal femoral osteotomy and femoral reconstruction with a mid-modular conical proximal body to restore offset and length, and a fluted distal stem that provided distal axial and rotational stability.

POSTOPERATIVE CARE

Immediate partial weight bearing is allowed in cases with a transverse subtrochanteric osteotomy, as this allows effective dynamization of the osteotomy. Otherwise, weight bearing is decided on a case-by-case basis. Radiographs are obtained at 6 weeks if there is no change in the position of the osteotomy; with a change in implant position, the patient can begin weight bearing as tolerated.

RESULTS

THA With Proximal Femoral Deformity

Very little information can be found in the literature analyzing THA in those patients with a deformed proximal femur (Table 77-1). These are small series of patients in case studies without controls and with intermediate follow-up.

Holtgreve and Hungerford (1989)[6] reported on a small series of 9 hips (see Table 77-1) in which a proximal femoral osteotomy was used with a cementless femoral component. For primary hip patients (3 hips: 2 with DDH), the mean Harris hip score (HHS) was 94; for those patients with revision THA (6 hips), the mean HHS was 84. In primary cases, the osteotomy healed in an average of 15 weeks compared with 27 weeks in revision cases. The HHS for primary THA in this series was therefore comparable with that in routine THA and was less in revision THA.

Papagelopoulos and associates[7] reported on their series of 31 hips with proximal femoral osteotomy (20 primary and 11 revision) with a mean follow-up of 4.6 years. The HHS was 77 and 73 for primary and revision hips, respectively, with an average time to union of the osteotomy of 35 weeks. Fifty-five percent of the primary cases had undergone previous hip surgery. Ten reoperations (32%) were performed in 8 patients; 4 hips in the primary group and 2 in the revision cohort required femoral revision. The overall nonunion rate at the osteotomy site was 13%.

Table 77-1. Results of THA for Proximal Femoral Deformities

	Number of Hips	Level of Evidence	Cemented vs. Cementless	Mean Follow-up	Outcome	Complications
Holtgreve and Hungerford (1989)	9 hips (6 revisions, 3 primary)	IV	Cementless	47 months	HHS 94 primary and 84 revisions; osteotomy healed at 15 weeks and 27 weeks for primary and revision hips, respectively	1 plate removal 1 peroneal nerve palsy 1 delayed union 1 intraoperative fracture
Papagelopoulos et al (1996)	31 hips (11 revisions, 20 primary)	IV	Cementless	4.6 years	HHS 77 primary and 73 revisions; average time to union, 35 weeks	7 intraoperative femur fractures 4 nonunion 4 instability 4 aseptic loosening 1 osteolysis 1 deep infection 32% reoperation rate
Onodera et al (2006)	14 hips (primary)	IV	Cementless	61 months	HHS 82	6 intraoperative fractures 1 nonunion 1 dislocation 1 stem subsidence 1 revision
Mont et al (2008)	17 total hips (resurfacing arthroplasties)	IV	Hip resurfacing	3 years	HHS 92	2 revisions (same patient)

HHS, Harris hip score.

Table 77-2. Results of THA After Conversion from Failed Fracture Fixation

	Number of Hips	Cemented vs. Cementless	Mean Follow-up	Survivorship
Mehlhoff et al (1991)	27 hips (14 femoral neck, 13 intertrochanteric)	Both	34 months	
Haidvkewych and Berry (2003)	60 hips (failed intertrochanteric)	57 cemented stems 3 uncemented	65 months	100% at 7 years 87.5% at 10 years
Mabry et al (2004)	84 hips (femoral neck nonunion)	Cemented Charnley	12.2 years	93% at 10 years 76% at 20 years

Onodera and colleagues (2006)[8] reported on their series of 14 primary hips with mean follow-up of 61 months. Postsurgery HHS was 82, and all but one osteotomy healed. These authors used a proximal modular stem, which provided rotational stability for both proximal and distal segments of the transverse osteotomy.

Mont and coworkers (2008)[4] reported on a case series of total hip resurfacing arthroplasty in patients with a proximal deformity of less than 20^0 or retained hardware that would complicate placement of conventional femoral components. At intermediate (3 years) follow-up, 16 hips had an HHS of 92. One patient had undergone two revisions (one for femoral neck fracture and the other for cup loosening). The authors concluded that hip resurfacing arthroplasty can be associated with excellent results at early follow-up in patients with proximal femoral deformity.

THA After Conversion from Failed Fracture Fixation

Mabry and associates (2004)[9] reported on the long-term follow-up of THA conversion in 84 hips for femoral fracture nonunion using a Charnley cemented THA. At 10 and 20 years' follow-up, survivorship was 93% and 76%, respectively. Among those patients younger than 65 years, 20-year survivorship was 65% compared with 95% in patients older than 65. When their data were compared with the general population for THA, results were slightly inferior,[10] with 84% survivorship at 20 years (Table 77-2).

Haidukewych and Berry (2003)[11] followed 60 hips with failed intertrochanteric fracture treatment: 57 cases used cemented stems and 3 utilized uncemented stems. Twenty-eight patients underwent hemiarthroplasty. Mean follow-up was 65 months with 44 surviving

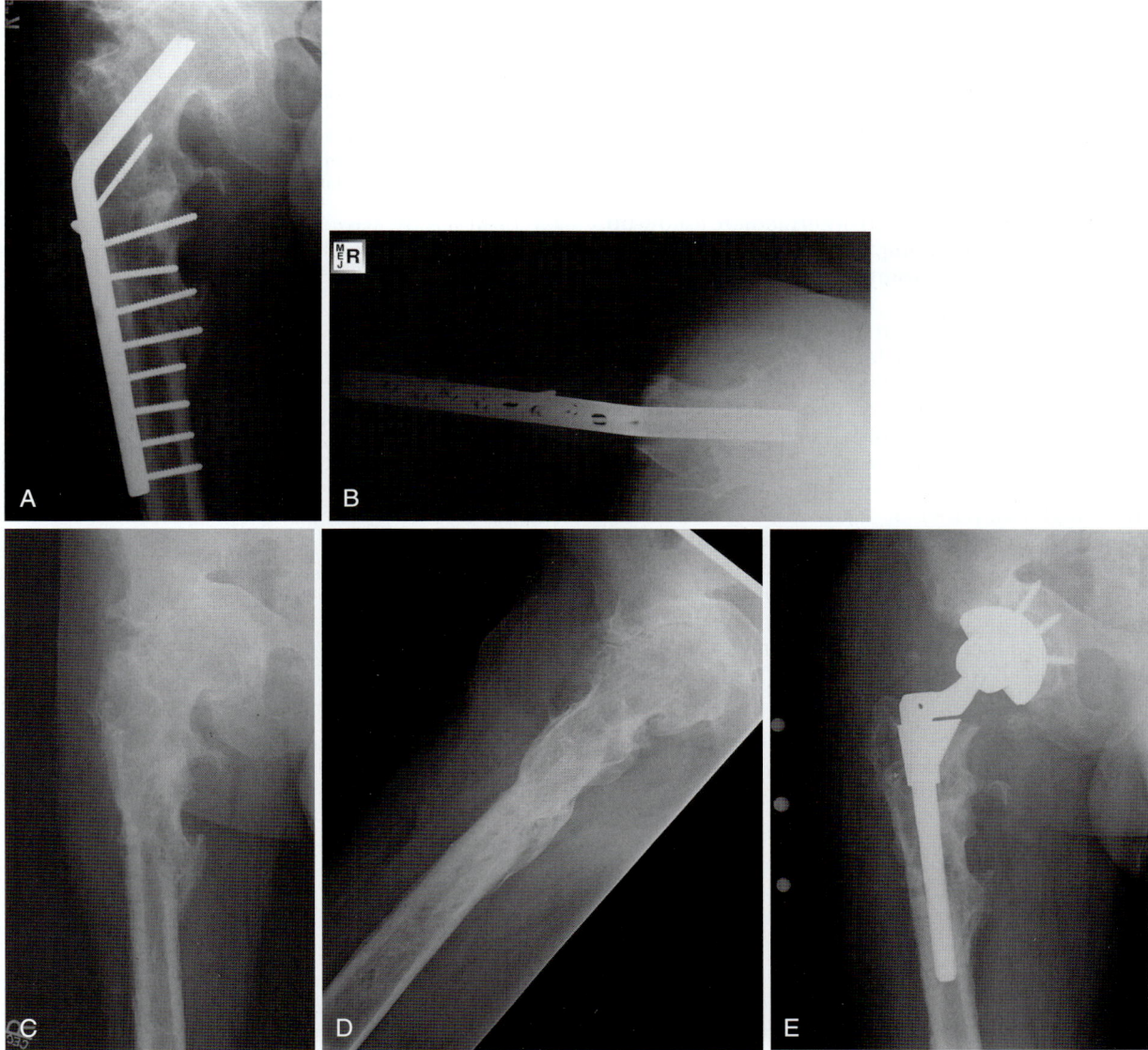

Figure 77-10. A, Preoperative anteroposterior radiograph showing traumatic arthrosis of the right hip. **B,** Lateral radiograph. Staged removal of internal fixation device, anteroposterior **(C)** and lateral **(D)** radiographs. **E,** Anteroposterior radiograph following staged total hip arthroplasty (THA) with a proximal modular femoral component.

hips. Five patients (8%) underwent reoperation, and only two of those patients underwent revision arthroplasty—one patient for aseptic loosening of both components at 8 years, and one patient for severe osteolysis at 10 years. The other three reoperations were performed for trochanteric nonunion, painful trochanteric hardware, and hematoma evacuation. Survivorship was 100% at 7 years and 87.5% at 10 years.

COMPLICATIONS

Total hip arthroplasty in these patients is associated with a greater number of intraoperative and postoperative complications compared with routine primary THA

patients. Careful preoperative planning can help reduce these risks. In cases of failed fracture fixation, waiting at least 3 months post surgery before revision is indicated because of the risk of infection and the benefits of fracture consolidation and bone healing, unless the patient is substantially incapacitated with pain. High-risk patients include those elderly patients in the early postsurgery period who are at risk of increased mortality associated with fractures around the hip. Infection risk is always increased when arthroplasty is performed after previous surgical intervention.

In all cases of complex THA, use of intraoperative fluoroscopy reduces the risk of intraoperative complications, particularly in those patients with poor bone quality. This technique is useful when reaming the endosteum to avoid perforating the anterior cortex with straight rigid reamers. Prophylactic cerclage wires can also reduce the risk of intraoperative fracture.

CURRENT CONTROVERSIES AND FUTURE CONSIDERATIONS

- Long-term outcome in these patients is unknown; most studies are reported with intermediate follow-up, so the use of current implant systems with intra-operative femoral osteotomy is not yet validated with long-term data.
- Poorer outcome has been demonstrated in those patients undergoing THA for femoral neck fracture following internal fixation; the reasons for this remain unclear but may be related to poorer bone quality.
- The recent increased use of larger femoral heads in conjunction with highly cross-linked polyethylene acetabular liners may decrease the risk of dislocation in these high-risk patients.
- Staging of procedures (hardware removal and/or osteotomy) in these complex cases of previous fracture surgery may be an option to decrease peri-operative complications; however, little evidence is available to support better outcomes with this approach (Fig. 77-10).

REFERENCES

1. Berry DJ: Total hip arthroplasty in patients with proximal femoral deformity. Clin Orthop Relat Res 369:262–272, 1999.
2. Park JH, Paprosky WG, Jablonsky WS, Lawrence JM: Femoral strut allografts in cementless revision total hip arthroplasty. Clin Orthop Relat Res 295:172–178, 1993.
3. Treacy RB, McBryde CW, Pynsent PB: Birmingham hip resurfacing arthroplasty: a minimum follow-up of five years. J Bone Joint Surg Br 87:167–170, 2005.
4. Mont MA, McGrath MS, Ulrich SD, et al: Metal-on-metal total hip resurfacing arthroplasty in the presence of extra-articular deformities or implants. J Bone Joint Surg Am 90(Suppl 3): 45–51, 2008.
5. Greidanus NV, Masri BA, Garbuz DS, et al: Use of erythrocyte sedimentation rate and C-reactive protein level to diagnose infection before revision total knee arthroplasty: a prospective evaluation. J Bone Joint Surg Am 89:1409–1416, 2007.
6. Holtgrewe JL, Hungerford DS: Primary and revision total hip replacement without cement and with associated femoral osteotomy. J Bone Joint Surg Am 71:1487–1495, 1989.
7. Papagelopoulos PJ, Trousdale RT, Lewallen DG: Total hip arthroplasty with femoral osteotomy for proximal femoral deformity. Clin Orthop Relat Res 332:151–162, 1996.
8. Onodera S, Majima T, Ito H, et al: Cementless total hip arthroplasty using the modular S-ROM prosthesis combined with corrective proximal femoral osteotomy. J Arthroplasty 21:664–669, 2006.
9. Mabry TM, Prpa B, Haidukewych GJ, et al: Long-term results of total hip arthroplasty for femoral neck fracture nonunion. J Bone Joint Surg Am 86:2263–2267, 2004.
10. Kavanagh BF, Wallrichs S, Dewitz M, et al: Charnley low-friction arthroplasty of the hip: twenty-year results with cement. J Arthroplasty 9:229–234, 1994.
11. Haidukewych GJ, Berry DJ: Hip arthroplasty for salvage of failed treatment of intertrochanteric hip fractures. J Bone Joint Surg Am 85:899–904, 2003.
12. Mehlhoff T, Landon GC, Tullos US: Total hip arthroplasty following failed internal fixation of hip fractures. Clin Orthop Relat Res 269:32–37, 1991.

CHAPTER 78

Metabolic Bone Disease

Steven J. Fitzgerald and David G. Lewallen

PAGET'S DISEASE

Introduction

Paget's disease affects 1% of the U.S. population over the age of 40.[1] It is a chronic localized disorder of bone marked by increased bone turnover, specifically, resorption, formation, and remodeling resulting in the replacement of normal matrix with a weakened and enlarged bone. Both monostotic and polyostotic forms are possible as defined by the number of involved skeletal sites. Paget's can affect any bone but is most common in the pelvis and femur, and is polyostotic in 76% of cases.[2-5] Overall prevalence, including both forms, increases with age, with a 1.2:1 male-to-female ratio in the United States.[1] Prevalence varies geographically; Paget's is most common in Europe among those of Anglo-Saxon ancestry and is rare in Africa and Asia.[6,7] Population studies from both Europe and New Zealand have suggested that the severity of Paget's disease has decreased over the past 40 years, and an increase in the monostotic form of the disease has been noted, especially among women.[8,9]

Pathoanatomy

Paget's disease is often diagnosed incidentally but can present with generalized bone pain. With proximal femoral and hip involvement, it can be difficult to differentiate generalized bone pain from active disease, stress fracture, or radiculopathy from intra-articular pathology. Intra-articular injection in this situation may aid in differentiating the source of pain.[10] Malignant transformation and Paget's sarcoma occur in less than 1% of patients but carry a poor prognosis and should be included in the differential when symptomatic patients with Paget's disease of the hip are evaluated.[11] Destructive bone changes and a soft tissue mass superimposed on typical pagetoid bone patterns with recently increased pain may suggest possible sarcomatous change.

Bone pain generally correlates with disease activity. Disease activity can be followed by monitoring of serum alkaline phosphatase and urinary pyridinium crosslinks. Increased bone turnover results in increased excretion of type I collagen breakdown products, and the compensatory osteoblastic activity results in increased alkaline phosphatase activity.

The exact cause of Paget's remains unknown; however, a viral origin was first proposed in 1974, after the discovery of virus-like inclusion bodies in the osteoclasts of affected bone.[12] A viral cause continues to be a focus of current research, with implications for the paramyxovirus family.[13] Multiple molecular markers have also been implicated in the disease process, including interleukin-6, a resorptive cytokine found in the bone marrow of affected patients.[14] Additional work has been undertaken to investigate increased expression of genes that inhibit apoptosis, which leads to a relative increase in the number of osteoclasts.[15] It is more common among relatives of those with Paget's disease, with first-degree relatives having a seven-fold increased chance of developing Paget's disease.[16] Genetic studies and linkage analysis have implicated the sequestrosome 1 gene and multiple other genetic loci as candidate regions for Paget's disease.[15,17] Extensive osteolysis, large numbers of osteoclasts and osteoblasts, and rapid formation of disorganized woven bone remain the histologic hallmarks of pagetoid bone.[18]

A frequent association with disabling hip disease leading to hip arthroplasty has been well established, but it remains unclear whether osteoarthritis is more common in patients with Paget's disease than in age-matched controls.[4,19,20] It has been postulated that the pagetic process and deformity predispose patients to develop degenerative arthritis at an accelerated rate secondary to juxta-articular bony enlargement,

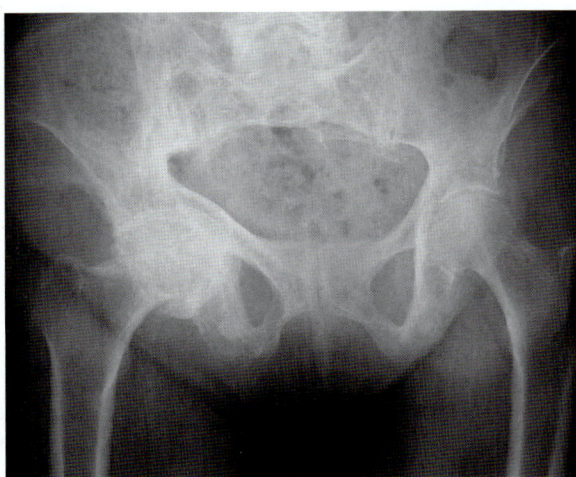

Figure 78-1. Typical acetabular wear pattern seen in Paget's disease.

Table 78-1. Antiresorptive Agents for Paget's Disease of Bone

Agent	Trade Name	Dosage
Risedronate	Actonel	30 mg by mouth daily for 2 months
Alendronate	Fosamax	40 mg by mouth daily for 6 months
Zoledronate	Reclast	5 mg IV once every 12 months
Salmon calcitonin	Miacalcin	50-100 U subcutaneous injection daily for 6-18 months

From References 25 and 26.

resulting in incongruity, altered biomechanics secondary to bowing, and altered subchondral support.[21-23]

In the region of the hip, characteristic varus bowing of the femur, coxa vara, and acetabular protrusio are commonly seen in patients with Paget's. Subcapital fracture, nonunion of the proximal femur, and a distorted and sclerotic canal can complicate treatment. Both medial and concentric wear patterns of the hip joint are common[23,24] (Fig. 78-1). Hypervascularity characteristic of the active lytic phase of the disease may be associated with increased intraoperative blood loss. Appropriate medical management, including consultation with an endocrinologist, can help mitigate the risk of intraoperative bleeding, as well as postoperative periimplant bone resorption.

Alternative Treatment

Analgesics and nonsteroidal anti-inflammatory drugs (NSAIDs) can be used to reduce bone pain in patients with active disease; however, antiresorptive medications have become the mainstay of modern medical treatment of Paget's disease of bone. Antiresorptive medications act by decreasing the osteoclast-mediated bone resorption characteristic of Paget's disease, both by decreasing active symptoms and reducing future complications. Two main classes of antiresorptive medications are available in the United States: (1) calcitonin and (2) bisphosphonates. Salmon calcitonin is less effective than nitrogen-containing bisphosphonates and requires daily subcutaneous injection.[25] The nitrogen-containing bisphosphonates alendronate, risedronate, and zoledronate acid have all shown varying degrees of effectiveness and potency when serum alkaline phosphatase levels are used as measurement of active disease.[25,26] Zoledronate has proved particularly effective in arresting active disease and provides the convenience of one-time intravenous dosing over 15 minutes.[26] A summary of commonly used bisphosphosphonates and dosing regimens is provided in Table 78-1. Antiresorptive therapy can be used to treat pain caused by

Paget's disease and to prevent or slow the development of osteoarthritis and advancing deformity. Antiresorptive therapy is also thought to be effective before surgery for reducing intraoperative bleeding due to hypervascularity in active disease, as well as the potential for postoperative bone resorption.[25-29] No consensus is seen in the literature regarding the timing of perioperative bisphosphonate therapy. The timing and dosing of antiresorptive therapy should be prescribed in consultation with and monitored by an endocrinologist secondary to potential side effects.[21] Nonsurgical treatment of degenerative arthritis associated with Paget's disease is the same as that provided for idiopathic osteoarthritis and includes anti-inflammatory agents, activity modification, and gait aids.

Surgical Treatment

Both cemented and uncemented total hip arthroplasty have been used successfully to treat degenerative hip disease secondary to Paget's disease, and good to excellent results have been reported for both. Nevertheless, no consensus has been reached regarding choice of implant or fixation technique. Direct comparison of available studies is difficult owing to confounding variables, results spanning two decades, small numbers of patients, differing implant designs, and evolving techniques. The degree of deformity, the amount of bone loss, and the need for osteotomy require implant selection and technique adjustment based on individual patient pathology. However, reported revision rates appear to be higher with the use of cemented implants. Results of available studies using cemented and uncemented implants are summarized in Tables 78-2 and 78-3. The use of hybrid THA in a Paget's patient with severe proximal femoral involvement is demonstrated in Figures 78-2 and 78-3.

Technique

Preoperative Planning. All patients should have full-length radiographs of the femur, in addition to standard hip films, before surgery. This allows assessment of femoral deformity and extent of bony involvement. Additionally, full-length standing radiographs of the entire extremity may help in assessment of lower leg involvement and may facilitate preoperative planning and decision making on the need for an associated osteotomy. Additional axial imaging, including magnetic

Table 78-2. Cemented Total Hip Arthroplasty for Paget's Disease of the Hip

Authors	Number of Hips	Mean Age, yr	Mean follow-up, yr, n (range)	Results
Merkow et al (1984)	21	68.6	5 (2-11)	18 of 21 good to excellent; 2 revisions
McDonald and Sim (1987)	52	69.9	8.8 (3-15)	39 of 52 good to excellent; 9 revisions
Ludkowski and Wilson-McDonald (1988)	37	71.5	7.8 (1-18.4)	26 of 37 good to excellent; 0 revisions
Sochart and Porter (2000)	98	67.4	10.4 (5.5-20)	81 of 98 good to excellent; 8 revisions

From References 24, 36, 47, and 48.

Table 78-3. Uncemented Total Hip Arthroplasty for Paget's Disease of the Hip

Authors	Number of Hips	Mean Age, yr	Mean follow-up, yr, n (range)	Results
Hozack et al (1999)	5	68	5.8 (4.8-8.8)	5 of 5 good to excellent
Kirsch et al (2001)	20	72	6 (4.8)	18 of 20 good to excellent; 0 revisions
Parvizi et al (2002)	19	71.3	7 (2-15)	16 of 19 good to excellent; 0 revisions
Lusty et al (2007)	23	75	6.7 (3-14.6)	22 of 23 good to excellent
Wegrzyn et al (2010)	37	74.2	6.6 (2-16.2)	27 of 37 good to excellent

From References 31 and 49 through 52.

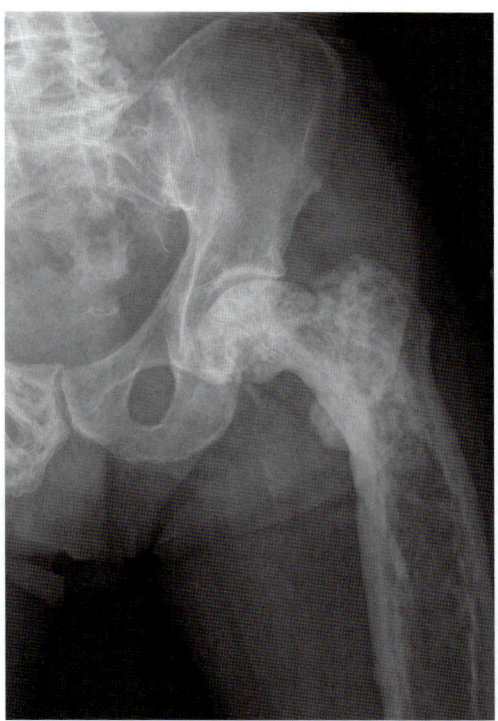

Figure 78-2. Paget's disease with severe proximal femoral involvement.

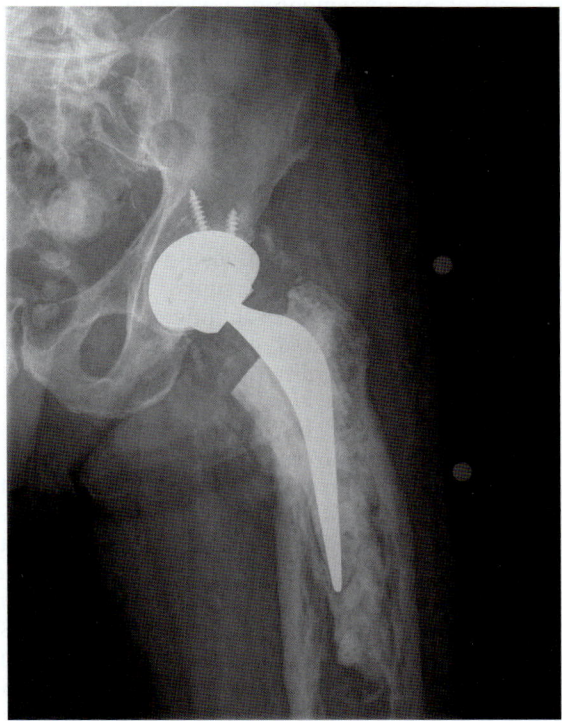

Figure 78-3. Paget's disease with severe proximal femoral involvement after hybrid total hip arthroplasty (THA).

resonance imaging (MRI) or computed tomography (CT), may be warranted in the setting of cortical erosion or soft tissue mass and concern for sarcomatous degeneration. Hypervascularity may lead to increased intraoperative blood loss, greater than usual fluid and blood replacement requirements, and decreased intraoperative visualization. An associated risk of cardiac enlargement and altered ventricular function in polyostotic disease involving more than 15% of the skeleton is present. Some patients may develop high-output cardiac failure.[30] An adequate anesthesia plan regarding resuscitation and use of an intraoperative blood salvage system is recommended. Preoperative medical management of active disease can help to minimize the risk of bleeding and can aid in intraoperative evaluation of the bone-implant interface, as well as achievement of a dry surgical field, if cemented techniques are used.

Exposure. Paget's disease of the hip without deformity can be approached as any other total hip arthroplasty using an anterolateral, posterior, or trochanteric approach, depending on surgeon experience and preference. Coxa vara and femoral bowing can complicate entry into the femoral canal, making it difficult to avoid varus stem positioning, encroachment on the trochanter, and trochanteric fracture. Trochanteric or femoral osteotomy may be necessary to facilitate dislocation, prevent fracture, and achieve optimum implant positioning.

Bony Preparation. Protrusio deformity is common in Paget's disease and may produce technical challenges related to the severity of bone loss. Reaming to expand the periphery without deepening the socket is advised to prevent worsening of the protrusio deformity. Cystic lesions can be curetted and bone grafted with autologous reamings.

Femoral preparation involves the elimination of fibrous pagetoid tissue and shaping of the often sclerotic canal. It is helpful to have high-speed burrs available as well as flexible reamers for preparation of the canal, in case hard sclerotic bone is encountered, precluding the use of standard rasps and instrumentation. Intraoperative fluoroscopy or plain x-ray is advisable to confirm reamer position within the canal and to correct broach or trial position.

Prosthesis Implantation. On the acetabular side, inability to produce a dry acetabular bed may compromise cement interdigitation with bone, preventing successful fixation of a cemented cup; this may necessitate use of an uncemented acetabular component. Intermediate-term follow-up from the Mayo Clinic with the use of an uncemented cup in pagetoid bone appears promising.[31] With use of an uncemented cup, peripheral fit against an intact rim and the use of multiple screws are required to prevent cup migration and allow for bony ingrowth. Medial acetabular bone grafting or use of an oversized hemispherical cup may be helpful in restoring the anatomic hip center, as well as the availability of offset liners to compensate for a medialized cup position in a protrusio deformity.[32] Cement fixation in combination with a cage, or an uncemented cup-cage construct with a cemented liner, may be required if extremely poor bone quality or significant bone loss is encountered.

Bowing of the femur may necessitate femoral osteotomy to allow stem placement. Femoral osteotomy for coxa vara in Paget's disease has been well described with the use of both cemented and uncemented stems.[33,34] Use of a long cemented implant, an extensively coated implant, or a modular tapered stem may be required to bypass mechanically insufficient proximal bone and achieve diaphyseal fixation (Fig. 78-4). Osteotomy may be complicated by delayed union in Paget's disease, especially in a diaphyseal location.[34] Therefore a one-stage approach to limit the total period of disability is preferred. If cemented femoral fixation is used in combination with corrective osteotomy, care must be taken to avoid cement extravasation into the osteotomy site, inhibiting union. Strut grafts spanning the area of the osteotomy may be useful to facilitate union and stability; however, invasion of strut allografts with pagetoid bone has been reported.[35] Regardless of

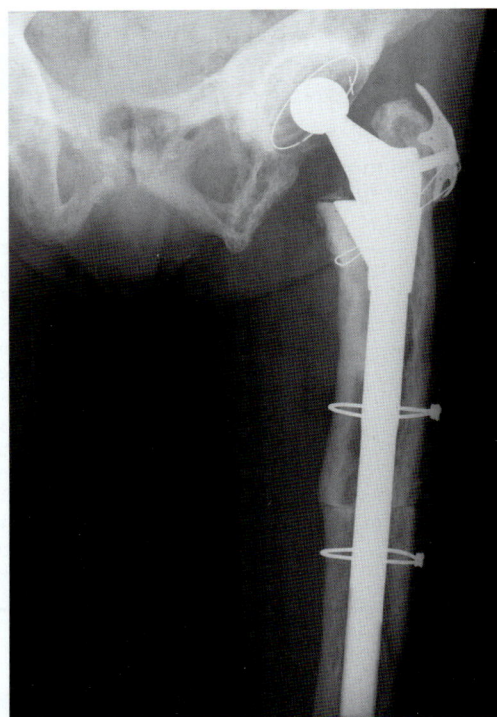

Figure 78-4. Paget's disease treated with femoral osteotomy and total hip arthroplasty (THA) with a modular uncemented stem.

the method of fixation, stem length should ensure that the stem tip is not placed in a region of diseased bone to prevent further varus remodeling and stress fracture at the stem tip.

Wound Closure. Wound closure is performed in a routine manner in this patient population, according to the preference of the surgeon. Adequate hemostasis and use of drains are recommended to help prevent hematoma formation, wound breakdown, and infection.

Postoperative Regimen. When an osteotomy is performed, we routinely limit weight bearing until radiographic union is evident. Patients with Paget's disease undergoing THA are at increased risk of developing heterotopic ossification, with rates ranging from 28% to 52%.[31,36,37] Patients should be treated with prophylactic postoperative radiation or placed on a prophylactic drug regimen for prevention.[38,39] Potential postoperative bone loss secondary to hypervascular metabolic effects as well as immobility should be anticipated; therefore, early mobilization should be advised. Early postoperative follow-up is recommended to monitor for bone loss and to monitor osteotomy union. Postoperative treatment with antiresorptive therapy may be beneficial in reducing bone loss. Any sudden change in status heralded by increasing pain should be investigated for a developing stress fracture or for rapidly increasing bone resorption.

TOTAL HIP ARTHROPLASTY: RENAL OSTEODYSTROPHY, RENAL TRANSPLANT, AND DIALYSIS

Renal osteodystrophy describes the skeletal complications of end-stage renal disease secondary to a range of disorders, including secondary hyperparathyroidism, hypocalcemia, hyperphosphatemia, impaired production of 1,25-dihydroxycholecalciferol, altered skeletal response to parathyroid hormone (PTH), and abnormal PTH gene transcription. It is also found in patients with end-stage renal disease who have been overtreated with calcium and vitamin D or have aluminum intoxication from dialysis.[40] Total hip arthroplasty in patients with end-stage renal disease, either on dialysis or after renal transplant, can be complicated by systemic medical conditions, poor bone quality, and increased risk of complications.

The adult patient with osteodystrophy requiring THA after renal transplant usually presents with osteonecrosis or osteoarthritis secondary to long-term steroid use; indeed, osteonecrosis was the most frequent diagnosis requiring THA in this population.[41] However, since the early 1980s with the advent of cyclosporine for immunosuppression, decreasing the need for steroid use after transplant, fewer cases of transplant-associated osteonecrosis have been seen.[42,43]

Results

Total hip arthroplasty has been reported in patients on dialysis, with 76% good to excellent clinical results in a small series, but it carries a high rate of perioperative complications, increased rates of infection, and associated increased short-term mortality.[43-46] Deep infection rates as high as 19% have been reported in patients undergoing THA while on dialysis, and rates of perioperative and short-term postoperative mortality have been reported to be as high as 58%.[45,46] No consensus has been reached regarding cemented versus cementless fixation in the treatment of patients on dialysis with osteoarthritis or osteonecrosis with THA; mixed results have been reported using both techniques. It is clear, however, that results are inferior to those in patients undergoing THA with primary osteoarthritis; increased risk of infection, higher rates of perioperative complications, and increased risk of mortality have all been observed.

The overall outcome of THA in patients with chronic renal failure who underwent renal transplant is reported to be better than results in patients undergoing THA while on dialysis.[45] However, a retrospective direct comparison study from the Mayo Clinic of 28 patients (36 hips) after renal transplant and 9 patients (9 hips) undergoing renal dialysis found a higher incidence of complications (61%) in the transplant group than in the dialysis group (33%).[43] However, this almost twofold difference in complications was not reported as significant. Investigators also found a higher rate of reoperation (33%) in the transplant group compared with the

dialysis (22%) group. However, these results have been attributed to longer follow-up time for transplant patients in the Mayo Clinic study and to a higher mortality rate in the dialysis group, creating an artificially lower rate of complications.

Efforts to optimize implant fixation should be pursued, employing techniques similar to those used in osteoporotic elderly patients with poor bone quality due to underlying metabolic bone disease. Although THA in patients with chronic renal failure on dialysis and after renal transplant can be successful in reducing pain and improving function, surgeons should approach this population with objective analysis of risks and benefits, and should counsel patients regarding the associated risk of complications.

REFERENCES

1. Altman RD, Bloch DA, Hochberg MC, Murphy WA: Prevalence of pelvic Paget's disease of bone in the United States. J Bone Miner Res 15:461–465, 2000.
2. Cameron HU: Total knee replacement in Paget's disease. Orthop Rev 18:206–208, 1989.
3. Guyer PB, Chamberlain AT, Ackery DM, Rolfe EB: The anatomic distribution of osteitis deformans. Clin Orthop Relat Res 156:141–144, 1981.
4. McDonald D, Sim F: Hip arthroplasty in Paget's disease. In Morrey BF, editor: Reconstructive surgery of the joints, ed 2, New York, 1996, Churchill Livingstone, pp 115–121.
5. Ziegler R, Holz G, Rotzler B, Minne H: Paget's disease of bone in West Germany: prevalence and distribution. Clin Orthop Relat Res 194:199–204, 1985.
6. Mirra JM: Pathogenesis of Paget's disease based on viral etiology. Clin Orthop Relat Res 217:162–170, 1987.
7. Yip KM, Lee YL, Kumta SM, Lin J: The second case of Paget's disease (osteitis deformans) in a Chinese lady. Singapore Med J 37:665–667, 1996.
8. Poor G, Donath J, Fornet B, Cooper C: Epidemiology of Paget's disease in Europe: the prevalence is decreasing. J Bone Miner Res 21:1545–1549, 2006.
9. Cundy HR, Gamble G, Wattie D, et al: Paget's disease of bone in New Zealand: continued decline in disease severity. Calcif Tissue Int 75:358–364, 2004.
10. Crawford RW, Gie GA, Ling RS, Murray DW: Diagnostic value of intra-articular anaesthetic in primary osteoarthritis of the hip. J Bone Joint Surg Br 80:279–281, 1998.
11. Klippel JH: Primer on the rheumatic diseases, ed 13, New York, 2008, Springer.
12. Rebel A, Malkani K, Basle M, Bregeon C: Osteoclast ultrastructure in Paget's disease. Calcif Tissue Res 20:187–199, 1976.
13. Basle MF, Russell WC, Goswami KK, et al: Paramyxovirus antigens in osteoclasts from Paget's bone tissue detected by monoclonal antibodies. J Gen Virol 66(Pt 10):2103–2110, 1985.
14. Roodman GD, Kurihara N, Ohsaki Y, et al: Interleukin 6: a potential autocrine/paracrine factor in Paget's disease of bone. J Clin Invest 89:46–52, 1992.
15. Haslam SI, Van Hul W, Morales-Piga A, et al: Paget's disease of bone: evidence for a susceptibility locus on chromosome 18q and for genetic heterogeneity. J Bone Miner Res 13:911–917, 1998.
16. Siris ES, Ottman R, Flaster E, Kelsey JL: Familial aggregation of Paget's disease of bone. J Bone Miner Res 6:495–500, 1991.
17. Laurin N, Brown JP, Morissette J, Raymond V: Recurrent mutation of the gene encoding sequestosome 1 (SQSTM1/p62) in Paget disease of bone. Am J Hum Genet 70:1582–1588, 2002.
18. Seitz S, Priemel M, Zustin J, et al: Paget's disease of bone: histologic analysis of 754 patients. J Bone Miner Res 24:62–69, 2009.
19. Graham J, Harris WH: Paget's disease involving the hip joint. J Bone Joint Surg Br 53:650–659, 1971.

20. Renier JC, Fanello S, Bos C, Audran M: An etiologic study of Paget's disease. Rev Rhum Engl Ed 63:606–611, 1996.
21. Altman RD: Arthritis in Paget's disease of bone. J Bone Miner Res 14(Suppl 2):85–87, 1999.
22. Helliwell PS: Osteoarthritis and Paget's disease. Br J Rheumatol 34:1061–1063, 1995.
23. Altman RD: Musculoskeletal manifestations of Paget's disease of bone. Arthritis Rheum 23:1121–1127, 1980.
24. Ludkowski P, Wilson-MacDonald J: Total arthroplasty in Paget's disease of the hip: a clinical review and review of the literature. Clin Orthop Relat Res 255:160–167, 1990.
25. Siris ES, Lyles KW, Singer FR, Meunier PJ: Medical management of Paget's disease of bone: indications for treatment and review of current therapies. J Bone Miner Res 21(Suppl 2):P94–P98, 2006.
26. Reid IR, Hosking DJ: Bisphosphonates in Paget's disease. Bone 49:89–94, 2011.
27. Oakley AP, Matheson JA: Rapid osteolysis after revision hip arthroplasty in Paget's disease. J Arthroplasty 18:204–207, 2003.
28. Avioli LV: Paget's disease: state of the art. Clin Ther 9:567–576, 1987.
29. Merkow RL, Lane JM: Paget's disease of bone. Orthop Clin North Am 21:171–189, 1990.
30. Arnalich F, Plaza I, Sobrino JA, et al: Cardiac size and function in Paget's disease of bone. Int J Cardiol 5:491–505, 1984.
31. Parvizi J, Schall DM, Lewallen DG, Sim FH: Outcome of uncemented hip arthroplasty components in patients with Paget's disease. Clin Orthop Relat Res 127–134, 2002.
32. Lewallen DG: Hip arthroplasty in patients with Paget's disease. Clin Orthop Relat Res 369:243–250, 1999.
33. Namba RS, Brick GW, Murray WR: Revision total hip arthroplasty with correctional femoral osteotomy in Paget's disease. J Arthroplasty 12:591–595, 1997.
34. Parvizi J, Frankle MA, Tiegs RD, Sim FH: Corrective osteotomy for deformity in Paget disease. J Bone Joint Surg Am 85:697–702, 2003.
35. Cameron HU, Fornasier VL, Van Zyl DV: Strut allograft invasion by Paget's disease of bone: a case report. Can J Surg 43:140–141, 2000.
36. McDonald DJ, Sim FH: Total hip arthroplasty in Paget's disease: a follow-up note. J Bone Joint Surg Am 69:766–772, 1987.
37. Stauffer RN, Sim FH: Total hip arthroplasty in Paget's disease of the hip. J Bone Joint Surg Am 58:476–478, 1976.
38. Ferguson DJ, Itonaga I, Maki M, et al: Heterotopic bone formation following hip arthroplasty in Paget's disease. Bone 34:1078–1083, 2004.
39. Iorio R, Healy WL: Heterotopic ossification after hip and knee arthroplasty: risk factors, prevention, and treatment. J Am Acad Orthop Surg 10:409–416, 2002.
40. Tejwani NC, Schachter AK, Immerman I, Achan P: Renal osteodystrophy. J Am Acad Orthop Surg 14:303–311, 2006.
41. Bucci JR, Oglesby RJ, Agodoa LY, Abbott KC: Hospitalizations for total hip arthroplasty after renal transplantation in the United States. Am J Transplant 2:999–1004, 2002.
42. Landmann J, Renner N, Gachter A, et al: Cyclosporin A and osteonecrosis of the femoral head. J Bone Joint Surg Am 69:1226–1228, 1987.
43. Shrader MW, Schall D, Parvizi J, et al: Total hip arthroplasty in patients with renal failure: a comparison between transplant and dialysis patients. J Arthroplasty 21:324–329, 2006.
44. Gualtieri G, Vellani G, Dallari D, et al: Total hip arthroplasty in patients dialyzed or with renal transplants. Chir Organi Mov 80:139–145, 1995.
45. Lieberman JR, Fuchs MD, Haas SB, et al: Hip arthroplasty in patients with chronic renal failure. J Arthroplasty 10:191–195, 1995.
46. Sakalkale DP, Hozack WJ, Rothman RH: Total hip arthroplasty in patients on long-term renal dialysis. J Arthroplasty 14:571–575, 1999.
47. Merkow RL, Pellicci PM, Hely DP, Salvati EA: Total hip replacement for Paget's disease of the hip. J Bone Joint Surg Am 66:752–758, 1984.
48. Sochart DH, Porter ML: Charnley low-friction arthroplasty for Paget's disease of the hip. J Arthroplasty 15:210–219, 2000.
49. Hozack WJ, Rushton SA, Carey C, et al: Uncemented total hip arthroplasty in Paget's disease of the hip: a report of 5 cases with 5-year follow-up. J Arthroplasty 14:872–876, 1999.
50. Kirsh G, Kligman M, Roffman M: Hydroxyapatite-coated total hip replacement in Paget's disease: 20 patients followed for 4-8 years. Acta Orthop Scand 72:127–132, 2001.
51. Lusty PJ, Walter WL, Walter WK, Zicat B: Cementless hip arthroplasty in Paget's disease at medium-term follow-up (average of 6.7 years). J Arthroplasty 22:692–696, 2007.
52. Wegrzyn J, Pibarot V, Chapurlat R, et al: Cementless total hip arthroplasty in Paget's disease of bone: a retrospective review. Int Orthop 34:1103–1109, 2010.

CHAPTER 79

Osteonecrosis of the Hip

Kevin L. Garvin

KEY POINTS

- Patients with avascular necrosis of the hip are likely to
  - Have abnormal bone quality of the hip and femur
  - Be younger than patients with osteoarthritis of the hip
  - Have a systemic disease associated with the osteonecrosis
  - Suffer from complications that are unique to their associated systemic disease and abnormal bone
  - Pose unique technical challenges during their total hip arthroplasty surgery
- The acetabular bone in patients with osteonecrosis is often of poor quality, and the surgeon must be careful in reaming the acetabulum. Aggressive reaming of the acetabulum can lead to loss of bone stock and proximal placement of the acetabular component.

INTRODUCTION

Total hip arthroplasty (THA) for osteonecrosis of the hip poses several unique challenges when compared with hip replacement for osteoarthritis[1-10]; these include abnormal bone quality of osteonecrosis, the young age of the patient who typically develops osteonecrosis, and underlying diseases associated with osteonecrosis.[2,3,7,11-13] Surgical challenges may also be present because of previous hip surgery performed to help prevent femoral head collapse. Surgery to preserve the femoral head via core decompression with or without adjunct bone graft or an osteotomy to rotate the osteonecrotic segment from the weight-bearing area of the femoral head is commonly performed. The purpose of this chapter is to provide essential information to assist in the management of patients with osteonecrosis. Defining features and teaching points relevant to THA for patients with osteonecrosis are discussed as well.[14-16]

The quality of acetabular and proximal femoral bone in patients with osteonecrosis is far from normal. Arlot and associates evaluated bone histomorphometry in 77 patients with osteonecrosis of the femoral head.[2] All patients were ambulatory, and none was confined to a bed or wheelchair. Among these patients, factors associated with osteonecrosis included steroids (15 patients) and alcoholism (33 patients) and were unknown in the remaining patients (29). Bone biopsy and histomorphometric analysis were performed on horizontal transiliac crest bone. Trabecular bone volume, trabecular osteoid volume, trabecular osteoid surface, thickness index of osteoid seams, total resorption surfaces, calcification rate, tetracycline-labeled surfaces, and bone formation rates at the basic multicellular unit level and at the tissue level were determined. Results suggested a marked decrease in osteoblastic appositional rate and in bone formation rate at cell and tissue levels. The extent of disease has also been studied. Calder[3] examined 16 patients with advanced osteonecrosis of the hip (Ficat III and IV)[11] and compared them with 19 patients with osteoarthritis who had undergone THA. Histologic specimens from the hip and the proximal femur were examined. Extensive osteonecrosis extending to 4 cm below the lesser trochanter was identified. Overall, a statistically significant difference in extent of disease was noted between the two groups ($P < .001$). This report may explain why patients with osteonecrosis are more likely to develop early aseptic loosening of the femoral prosthesis.[3,17-19]

The second challenging factor that affects the results of surgery for this patient population is age. In general, patients with osteonecrosis are younger than those undergoing total hip replacement for osteoarthritis. Results of THA in younger patients have not been as good as in an older population.[19-21] By definition, this group is more active than their elderly counterparts; this may account for the difference in results.[9,18,19,22-27]

Systemic diseases associated with osteonecrosis are a third factor contributing to the poor results of THA. Steroids, alcoholism, connective tissue disease, sickle cell disease, end-stage renal failure, human immunodeficiency virus (HIV), and trauma all possess characteristics that may compromise early and long-term results of total hip arthroplasty.[7,12,13,26] Furthermore, the complications associated with total hip arthroplasty in these patients are unique and occur more frequently than complications of THA in patients with osteoarthritis.

Surgery to correct the problem of osteonecrosis is not always successful, thereby leading to total hip arthroplasty. Alterations to the surgical site caused by previous surgery may pose a substantial challenge to the surgeon at the time of joint replacement and therefore are another factor contributing to the poor results of total hip replacement in this population. Core decompression with placement of a fibular strut graft, tantalum construct, or dowel poses unique challenges. Intertrochanteric osteotomy may result in abnormal and scarred anatomy.[28-32] Finally, because of abnormalities related to age, bone quality, and previous surgery, thorough preoperative planning, meticulous surgery, and selection of the correct implant are imperative for achieving a good result in this patient population.

INDICATIONS AND CONTRAINDICATIONS

Indications for total hip arthroplasty in patients with osteonecrosis include disabling pain and loss of function and are present in this population of patients at an average age that is younger than patients with osteoarthritis. The heavy demand over a longer time requires that the prosthesis is durable, thus minimizing the risk of early revision. Modest expectations and a lower level of activity may increase implant durability and longevity. Unfortunately, it is unlikely that this population will become less active after surgery because one of their main goals is to obtain relief from pain so they can be more active.

Relative and absolute contraindications to hip replacement also exist for patients with osteonecrosis of the hip. Many of these patients are at increased risk for complications after hip replacement, but the operation itself is not contraindicated. However, because many of these patients at baseline are at increased risk for infection, the presence of active infection before elective hip replacement must be ruled out and is an absolute contraindication to surgery. One example of this problem is the patient on dialysis who is especially prone to infection. It is incumbent on the treating surgeon to make certain that infection is not present before elective hip replacement is performed. The same is true for patients on steroids and for those who are immunocompromised because of medications used to treat their underlying disease process.

Peripheral vascular disease is also common in patients with end-stage renal disease. Evaluation of peripheral arterial blood flow should be performed preoperatively to assess the presence of peripheral vascular disease. In addition to systemic and diffuse disease processes that require preoperative evaluation, local problems challenge the surgical reconstruction or may be a contraindication to hip replacement.

Retained hardware after osteotomy or fracture fixation increases the risk for infection. Low-grade or active infection may be present in these patients as well. If an infection is suspected, staged surgical removal of the retained hardware, débridement, and antibiotics are necessary before total hip replacement is performed.

PREOPERATIVE PLANNING

Preoperative planning for total hip arthroplasty focuses on optimization of underlying medical conditions in these patients and on their orthopedic evaluation. In addition, it is important that appropriate preoperative planning for the hip surgery is performed. This process of preoperative planning and templating helps to identify technical factors that may require special attention.

DESCRIPTION OF TECHNIQUE

Surgical reconstruction and total hip replacement for patients with avascular necrosis can pose unique challenges. Overall, the quality of bone in this patient population is less robust than that in their osteoarthritis counterparts. Fracture of the bone at the time of surgical implantation of the total hip components caused by osteoporotic bone is possible, and the surgeon must take caution while reaming and broaching the bone. Because of the osteoporotic bone, it may be prudent to place a prophylactic wire around the femur to prevent a fracture.

A unique group of patients with avascular necrosis is the sickle cell patient population, whose repeated sickle cell crises may result in deformity of the femur and a narrow sclerotic femoral canal. Preparation of the femur for femoral component placement requires careful surgical technique and possible use of high-speed reaming tools with radiographic assistance to avoid fracture or component malposition.

Finally, techniques like hip resurfacing arthroplasty are not indicated for this population of patients with femoral head osteotomy and osteoporosis.

TECHNICAL VARIATIONS/ UNUSUAL SITUATIONS

Specifically, total hip arthroplasty after osteotomy or after core decompression with a fibular bone graft or tantalum placement requires careful planning for surgery. Total hip arthroplasty after previous osteotomy is a technically difficult operation. Kawasaki and associates[15] studied 15 hips converted to total hip arthroplasty after a failed transtrochanteric rotational osteotomy. The authors compared these hips with those of a control group of 16 with avascular necrosis who had not had prior osteotomy and were treated with total hip arthroplasty. In the study group of osteotomy patients, surgery was significantly longer than in the primary total hip arthroplasty group ($P = .003$), and perioperative blood loss was greater ($P = .036$). The authors attributed these difficulties to rotational changes in the geometry of the proximal femur after anterior or posterior rotational osteotomy. The authors did not report more frequent complications during surgery for the osteotomy group, but this is not the experience of other surgeons. At least two previous studies[28] reported a greater risk of complications in a group of patients with osteotomy before total hip arthroplasty. In only one patient in the two studies did the complication result in revision surgery.[15]

Core decompression followed by the use of a fibula bone graft or a tantalum implant is not always a successful treatment for patients with avascular necrosis of the hip. If the hip is converted to a total hip arthroplasty, the retained fibular bone or the tantalum implant must be adequately removed to allow for proper placement of the femoral component. Tanzer and colleagues[33] performed a total hip replacement for 17 hips in which a porous tantalum implant had been used for the treatment of Steinberg stage II osteonecrosis of the hip. During the hip replacement surgery in 13 of the 15 hips, large quantities of metallic debris from the implant were present at the femoral neck base after the implant had been transected. The long-term effect of the tantalum particles is unknown, but they could potentially accelerate wear of the prosthetic bearing. The authors reported that less debris could possibly be generated if the implant was cored out or transected with an osteotome rather than with a high-speed oscillating saw. Shuler and coworkers[34] reported on 24 patients treated with a tantalum implant for avascular necrosis; 3 of these patients had their hip converted to a total hip arthroplasty. None had complications, but the authors reported concern about third-particle wear.

POSTOPERATIVE CARE

Postoperative care of patients with avascular necrosis who have received a total hip replacement is similar to that of other patients with the same procedure. Any deviation in the care of these patients is individualized and is based on unique characteristics of the patient and specific surgical nuances.

RESULTS

Results of total hip replacement for patients with avascular necrosis have improved greatly over the past two decades. The results of total hip replacement using cemented components were not as good in patients with osteonecrosis as in patients with osteoarthritis. Patients' young age, increased activity, and poor bone quality were all thought to play a role in the poor results.[30] The advent of cementless hip replacement brought better midterm results in patients with osteonecrosis, as reported in nine studies totaling 489 patients (Table 79-1).[6,23,24,35-41] At an average follow-up of 6 years 9 months, the failure rate on average was 16.3%. Risks of dislocation and infection were 2% and 1.9%, respectively. Recent results with the use of alternative bearings are also improved when compared with previous reports. Four studies (Table 79-2)[17,25,42-44] totaling 252 hips in 212 patients followed for an average of 7 years and 7 months had a failure rate of less than 13%. Three of these studies had failure rates of 0, 3.89%, and 4%, and one study with cemented acetabular components had a failure rate of 31%. Risks of dislocation and infection were still significant (1.78%, 1.45%) in this challenging population. It is likely that additional studies using highly cross-linked polyethylene and cobalt chrome articulations will show improved results as well.

COMPLICATIONS

Total hip replacement for the treatment of avascular necrosis is associated with a higher risk of complications when compared with the same procedure performed for osteoarthritis.[18,29,36,45,46] Ortiguera and associates[18] studied a matched-pair analysis of 188 hips with long-term follow-up. Results of revision were comparable except in patients younger than 50 years. In the younger than 50 years population, revision ($P < .005$) and mechanical failure ($P > .05$) rates for the osteonecrosis group were significantly greater. Dislocations also occurred more frequently in the osteonecrosis group than in the osteoarthritis group.[18] The underlying disease process associated with osteonecrosis is challenging for the patient and the surgeon. Perhaps the group at greatest risk of complications is the sickle cell disease population. Sickle cell disease patients possess unique medical problems as well as bony problems.[12] Dense sclerotic bone with a narrow canal increases the risk of fracture and canal perforation during preparation of the femur for component placement. Clarke and colleagues[7] reported on 27 hips in patients with sickle cell disease. In nine of the hips, hard sclerotic bone obliterated the femoral canal, leading to perforation and femoral fracture in four hips.[7]

Lieberman and coworkers[10] reported on 16 patients with chronic renal failure who underwent hip replacement for avascular necrosis. In this multicenter study, the frequency of infection was 19% and the mortality rate was 45% at an average follow-up of 55 years. Naito and associates[47] reported a 12% infection rate in 15 patients. Sakalkale and colleagues[48] and Sunday and coworkers[49] reported alarmingly high mortality rates of 58% at short-term follow-up averaging 31 months (1 month to 11 years) and 29%, respectively. More recently, Nagoya and associates[50] retrospectively reviewed 11 total hip arthroplasties in just seven patients receiving long-term dialysis for chronic renal failure. At an average follow-up of longer than 8 years, only two of the components showed central migration of the bipolar heads. The authors did report two deaths (at 3 years and 4 years after surgery).

Systemic lupus erythematosus, human immunodeficiency virus, and other serious medical diseases are also associated with osteonecrosis of the hip. Larger studies on these topics will ultimately help us determine whether these patient populations are also at risk for more frequent perioperative complications and early failure of their replaced hips.[26,51,52]

CURRENT CONTROVERSIES AND FUTURE CONSIDERATIONS

- Patients with avascular necrosis of the hip are some of the most difficult to manage because of their associated medical conditions and challenging surgical reconstruction procedures.

Table 79-1. Uncemented Total Hip Arthroplasty for Osteonecrosis Without Alternative Bearings*†

Study	# Hips	Age, yr	Gender	Follow-up Average	Preop HHS	Postop HHS	Failure	Revision	Loose	Infected	Dislocated
Katz et al, Clin Orthop Relat Res (1992)						84					
Lins et al, Clin Orthop Relat Res (1993)	34/33	43	25 M 14 F	60 mo	42	86	2 inf (5.4%)	No rev	1 cup (2.7%)	2	1
Brinker et al, J Arthroplasty (1994)	84/64	39.9 (40)	37 M 27 F	68 mo	52.9	87.9	10 fem 5 acetab 15 of 81 (18%)	11.10%	18%	0	0
Phillips et al, Clin Orthop Relat Res (1994)	20/15	45	62 mo	NR	88	20	4 (20%)	0	4 (20%)	1 (5%)	NR
Piston et al, J Bone Joint Surg Am (1994)	38/33	32	19 M 11 F	90 mo	2.7/6*	5.7/6*	3 (9%) loose	2/6	3(9%)	1 (3%)	2 (6%)
Kim et al, Clin Orthop Relat Res (1995)	78/61	48	45 M 16 F	86 mo	45.6	90.3	20.50%	11.50%	NR	NR	NR
D'Antonio et al, Clin Orthop Relat Res (1997)	53/44	41	29 M 24 F	82 mo	45	90	?	30%	1 infected (1.9%)		2 disl (3.7%)
Stulberg et al, Clin Orthop Relat Res (1997)	98/64	41	42 M 22 F	88 mo	NR	NR	22 (4 osteolysis) 25%	21%		NR	NR
Chiu et al, J Arthroplasty 1997	36/29	47	20 M 9 F	70 mo	37	84	0	0	NR	0	NR
Hartley et al, J Bone Joint Surg Am (2000)	48/39	31	30 M 15 F	125 mo	NR	NR			1 (2%)	1 (2%)	3 (6%)
Total	489/382	41	247 M 138 F	81 mo	45	87	16.30%	10.70%	11%	1.90%	2.00%

HHS, Harris hip score; NR, not rated.
*Merle d'Aubigné score.
†Results of total hip arthroplasty for osteonecrosis using uncemented components. Alternative bearings were not used in any of the studies.

Table 79-2. Uncemented Total Hip Arthroplasty for Osteonecrosis With Alternative Bearings*

Study	Hips/Patients	Age, yr	Gender	Follow-up Average	Preop HHS	Postop HHS	Failure	Revision	Loose	Infected	Dislocated
Nich et al, Clin Orthop Relat Res (2003)†	52/41	40	25 M 16 F	16 yr			16 (31%)	16 (31%)		2 (3.8%)	2 (3.8%)
Alumina-alumina											
Mont et al, J Bone Joint Surg Am (2006)	52/41	38	30 M 11 F	3 yr	30	92	2 (4%)	2 (4%)	0%	1 (2%)	1 (2%)
Uncemented THA											
Seyler et al, J Bone Joint Surg Am (2006)	79/70	45.2	54 M 16 F	4.2 yr	48.8	96	3 (3.8%)	3 (3.8%)	0	0	1 (1.3%)
Alumina-alumina											
Baek et al, J Bone Joint Surg Am (2008)	71/60	39.1	53 M 7 F	7.1 yr	56.8	97	0	0	0	0	0
Alumina-alumina											
Fenollosa et al, J Bone Joint Surg (2006)	25/23										
Alumina-alumina											
Total	254/212	40.6	162 M 50 F	7.6 yr	44.2	95	12.96%	12.96%	0	1.45%	1.78%

HHS, Harris hip score.
*Results of total hip arthroplasty for osteonecrosis using uncemented components and alternative bearing materials.
†Cemented acetabular components.

- Surface arthroplasty and femoral head resurfacing arthroplasty are controversial treatments for these patients at this time.
- Future considerations will focus on improving the host and in turn the bone of the host.
- Providing this young population with a durable hip is an ongoing goal.
- In conclusion, results of total hip replacement in this challenging population of patients with osteonecrosis have improved since early reports of cemented total hip arthroplasty.
- Improved understanding of disease processes and better medical management have resulted in fewer perioperative complications.
- Results of total hip arthroplasty are better with modern designs using porous implants and modern bearing materials.

REFERENCES

1. Marker DR, Seyler TM, McGrath MS, et al: Treatment of early stage osteonecrosis of the femoral head. J Bone Joint Surg Am 90(Suppl 4):175–187, 2008.
2. Arlot ME, Bonjean M, Chavassieux PM, Meunier PJ: Bone histology in adults with aseptic necrosis: histomorphometric evaluation of iliac biopsies in seventy-seven patients. J Bone Joint Surg Am 65:1319–1327, 1983.
3. Calder JD, Pearse MF, Revell PA: The extent of osteocyte death in the proximal femur of patients with osteonecrosis of the femoral head. J Bone Joint Surg Br 83:419–422, 2001.
4. Archibeck MJ, Berger RA, Jacobs JJ, et al: Second-generation cementless total hip arthroplasty. eight to eleven-year results. J Bone Joint Surg Am 83:1666–1673, 2001.
5. Buckwalter AE, Callaghan JJ, Liu SS, et al: Results of Charnley total hip arthroplasty with use of improved femoral cementing techniques. a concise follow-up, at a minimum of twenty-five years, of a previous report. J Bone Joint Surg Am 88:1481–1485, 2006.
6. Chiu KH, Shen WY, Ko CK, Chan KM: Osteonecrosis of the femoral head treated with cementless total hip arthroplasty: a comparison with other diagnoses. J Arthroplasty 12:683–688, 1997.
7. Clarke HJ, Jinnah RH, Brooker AF, Michaelson JD: Total replacement of the hip for avascular necrosis in sickle cell disease. J Bone Joint Surg Br 71:465–470, 1989.
8. Issack PS, Botero HG, Hiebert RN, et al: Sixteen-year follow-up of the cemented spectron femoral stem for hip arthroplasty. J Arthroplasty 18:925–930, 2003.
9. Kantor SG, Huo MH, Huk OL, Salvati EA: Cemented total hip arthroplasty in patients with osteonecrosis: a 6-year minimum follow-up study of second-generation cement techniques. J Arthroplasty 11:267–271, 1996.
10. Lieberman JR, Fuchs MD, Haas SB, et al: Hip arthroplasty in patients with chronic renal failure. J Arthroplasty 10:191–195, 1995.
11. Ficat RP: Idiopathic bone necrosis of the femoral head: early diagnosis and treatment. J Bone Joint Surg Br 67:3–9, 1985.
12. Huo MH, Salvati EA, Browne MG, et al: Primary total hip arthroplasty in systemic lupus erythematosus. J Arthroplasty 7:51–56, 1992.
13. Jacobs B: Epidemiology of traumatic and nontraumatic osteonecrosis. Clin Orthop Relat Res 130:51–67, 1978.
14. Squire M, Fehring TK, Odum S, et al: Failure of femoral surface replacement for femoral head avascular necrosis. J Arthroplasty 20:108–114, 2005.
15. Kawasaki M, Hasegawa Y, Sakano S, et al: Total hip arthroplasty after failed transtrochanteric rotational osteotomy for avascular necrosis of the femoral head. J Arthroplasty 20:574–579, 2005.
16. Dean MT, Cabanela ME: Transtrochanteric anterior rotational osteotomy for avascular necrosis of the femoral head: long-term results. J Bone Joint Surg Br 75:597–601, 1993.
17. Baek SH, Kim SY: Cementless total hip arthroplasty with alumina bearings in patients younger than fifty with femoral head osteonecrosis. J Bone Joint Surg Am 90:1314–1320, 2008.
18. Ortiguera CJ, Pulliam IT, Cabanela ME: Total hip arthroplasty for osteonecrosis: matched-pair analysis of 188 hips with long-term follow-up. J Arthroplasty 14:21–28, 1999.
19. Wroblewski BM, Siney PD, Fleming PA: Charnley low-frictional torque arthroplasty for avascular necrosis of the femoral head. J Arthroplasty 20:870–873, 2005.
20. Grecula MJ, Grigoris P, Schmalzried TP, et al: Endoprostheses for osteonecrosis of the femoral head: a comparison of four models in young patients. Int Orthop 19:137–143, 1995.
21. Kobayashi S, Eftekhar NS, Terayama K, Joshi RP: Comparative study of total hip arthroplasty between younger and older patients. Clin Orthop Relat Res 339:140–151, 1997.
22. Garino JP, Steinberg ME: Total hip arthroplasty in patients with avascular necrosis of the femoral head: a 2- to 10-year follow-up. Clin Orthop Relat Res 334:108–115, 1997.
23. Hartley WT, McAuley JP, Culpepper WJ, et al: Osteonecrosis of the femoral head treated with cementless total hip arthroplasty. J Bone Joint Surg Am 82:1408–1413, 2000.
24. Kim YH, Oh JH, Oh SH: Cementless total hip arthroplasty in patients with osteonecrosis of the femoral head. Clin Orthop Relat Res 320:73–84, 1995.
25. Mont MA, Seyler TM, Plate JF, et al: Uncemented total hip arthroplasty in young adults with osteonecrosis of the femoral head: a comparative study. J Bone Joint Surg Am 88(Suppl 3):104–109, 2006.
26. Mont MA, Jones LC, Hungerford DS: Nontraumatic osteonecrosis of the femoral head: ten years later. J Bone Joint Surg Am 88:1117–1132, 2006.
27. Saito S, Saito M, Nishina T, et al: Long-term results of total hip arthroplasty for osteonecrosis of the femoral head: a comparison with osteoarthritis. Clin Orthop Relat Res 244:198–207, 1989.
28. Boos N, Krushell R, Ganz R, Muller ME: Total hip arthroplasty after previous proximal femoral osteotomy. J Bone Joint Surg Br 79:247–253, 1997.
29. Dorr LD, Takei GK, Conaty JP: Total hip arthroplasties in patients less than forty-five years old. J Bone Joint Surg Am 65:474–479, 1983.
30. Dorr LD, Luckett M, Conaty JP: Total hip arthroplasties in patients younger than 45 years: a nine- to ten-year follow-up study. Clin Orthop Relat Res 260:215–219, 1990.
31. Ferguson GM, Cabanela ME, Ilstrup DM: Total hip arthroplasty after failed intertrochanteric osteotomy. J Bone Joint Surg Br 76:252–257, 1994.
32. Soballe K, Boll KL, Kofod S, et al: Total hip replacement after medial-displacement osteotomy of the proximal part of the femur. J Bone Joint Surg Am 71:692–697, 1989.
33. Tanzer M, Bobyn JD, Krygier JJ, Karabasz D: Histopathologic retrieval analysis of clinically failed porous tantalum osteonecrosis implants. J Bone Joint Surg Am 90:1282–1289, 2008.
34. Shuler MS, Rooks MD, Roberson JR: Porous tantalum implant in early osteonecrosis of the hip: preliminary report on operative, survival, and outcomes results. J Arthroplasty 22:26–31, 2007.
35. Katz RL, Bourne RB, Rorabeck CH, McGee H: Total hip arthroplasty in patients with avascular necrosis of the hip. follow-up observations on cementless and cemented operations. Clin Orthop Relat Res 281:145–151, 1992.
36. Lins RE, Barnes BC, Callaghan JJ, et al: Evaluation of uncemented total hip arthroplasty in patients with avascular necrosis of the femoral head. Clin Orthop Relat Res 297:168–173, 1993.
37. Brinker MR, Rosenberg AG, Kull L, Galante JO: Primary total hip arthroplasty using noncemented porous-coated femoral components in patients with osteonecrosis of the femoral head. J Arthroplasty 9:457–468, 1994.
38. Phillips FM, Pottenger LA, Finn HA, Vandermolen J: Cementless total hip arthroplasty in patients with steroid-induced

avascular necrosis of the hip: a 62-month follow-up study. Clin Orthop Relat Res 303:147–154, 1994.

39. Piston RW, Engh CA, De Carvalho PI, Suthers K: Osteonecrosis of the femoral head treated with total hip arthroplasty without cement. J Bone Joint Surg Am 76:202–214, 1994.

40. D'Antonio JA, Capello WN, Manley MT, Feinberg J: Hydroxyapatite coated implants: total hip arthroplasty in the young patient and patients with avascular necrosis. Clin Orthop Relat Res 344:124–138, 1997.

41. Stulberg BN, Singer R, Goldner J, Stulberg J: Uncemented total hip arthroplasty in osteonecrosis: a 2- to 10-year evaluation. Clin Orthop Relat Res 334:116–123, 1997.

42. Nich C, Sariali E, Hannouche D, et al: Long-term results of alumina-on-alumina hip arthroplasty for osteonecrosis. Clin Orthop Relat Res 417:102–111, 2003.

43. Yoo JJ, Kim YM, Yoon KS, et al: Alumina-on-alumina total hip arthroplasty: a five-year minimum follow-up study. J Bone Joint Surg Am 87:530–535, 2005.

44. Seyler TM, Bonutti PM, Shen J, et al: Use of an alumina-on-alumina bearing system in total hip arthroplasty for osteonecrosis of the hip. J Bone Joint Surg Am 88(Suppl 3):116–125, 2006.

45. Del Savio GC, Zelicof SB, Wexler LM, et al: Preoperative nutritional status and outcome of elective total hip replacement. Clin Orthop Relat Res 326:153–161, 1996.

46. Mont MA, Hungerford DS: Non-traumatic avascular necrosis of the femoral head. J Bone Joint Surg Am 77:459–474, 1995.

47. Naito M, Ogata K, Shiota E, et al: Hip arthroplasty in haemodialysis patients. J Bone Joint Surg Br 76:428–431, 1994.

48. Sakalkale DP, Hozack WJ, Rothman RH: Total hip arthroplasty in patients on long-term renal dialysis. J Arthroplasty 14:571–575, 1999.

49. Sunday JM, Guille JT, Torg JS: Complications of joint arthroplasty in patients with end-stage renal disease on hemodialysis. Clin Orthop Relat Res 397:350–355, 2002.

50. Nagoya S, Nagao M, Takada J, et al: Efficacy of cementless total hip arthroplasty in patients on long-term hemodialysis. J Arthroplasty 20:66–71, 2005.

51. Petsatodis GE, Antonarakos PD, Christodoulou AG, et al: Cementless total hip arthroplasty for osteonecrosis of the femoral head after allogenic bone marrow transplantation. J Arthroplasty 24:414–420, 2009.

52. Ries MD, Barcohana B, Davidson A, et al: Association between human immunodeficiency virus and osteonecrosis of the femoral head. J Arthroplasty 17:135–139, 2002.

CHAPTER 80

The Neuromuscular Hip

Mathias P.G. Bostrom and Michael B. Cross

KEY POINT

- Neuromuscular hip disorders can be classified as intrinsic or extrinsic. Both types may be spastic or flaccid.
- Patients with intrinsic neuromuscular disorders (e.g., cerebral palsy, myelomeningocele), or in whom a neuromuscular affliction occurs while the hip is still in early development (e.g., poliomyelitis, encephalitis, cerebrovascular accident, childhood spinal cord injury, brain trauma), are at increased risk for hip subluxation-dislocation.
- Treatment options for the adult with painful dislocated hip include (1) head-neck resection with or without interposition arthroplasty, (2) hip arthrodesis, and (3) total hip replacement.
- In extrinsic movement disorders (e.g., dyskinesis, athetosis, Parkinson's disease, multiple sclerosis) hip subluxation-dislocation is rare but is frequently associated with contractures about the hip; these patients often develop painful degenerative arthritis.
- Goals of treatment in adult spastic neuromuscular hip are (1) to prevent contractures, and (2) if the dysplastic hip becomes painful or the sitting position and perineal care become difficult because of contractures, to perform salvage procedures to improve function and eliminate pain.

INTRODUCTION

Although relatively rare, adult patients with hip pathology secondary to neuromuscular disorders remain a unique and varied group of patients who require different approaches to the care of their hip disease. The goal of this chapter is to describe the unique nature of these pathologies while presenting appropriate treatment algorithms for the care of these special patients and their hip pathology.

Although the definition varies among clinicians, in this chapter we will define a *neuromuscular disorder* as any disease that involves any part of the muscle or nerve. This includes myopathies, muscular dystrophies, upper and lower motor neuron diseases/injuries, neurodegenerative disorders, movement disorders, and diseases of the neuromuscular junction. Similarly, we will

define *adult neuromuscular hip disorders* as pathology of the hip directly or indirectly caused by neuromuscular disease states. These disorders can be categorized further into intrinsic and extrinsic disorders.

In the literature, it has been shown repeatedly that muscle imbalance about the hip caused by an underlying neuromuscular disease can result in subluxation and dislocation of the hip in growing children and may predispose adult patients to degenerative joint disease of the hip. Specifically, the muscle imbalance that directly causes acquired hip instability and dysfunction is due to the presence of strong hip flexors and adductors that overpower weaker or absent hip extensors and abductors. Although the direct cause of the instability is this muscle imbalance, the underlying cause of the hip dysfunction may involve intrinsic or extrinsic factors. Intrinsic muscle imbalance about the hip manifests during childhood and plays the primary role in subsequent hip problems. Extrinsic causes of neuromuscular imbalance occur in stable hips and play a secondary role in the development of osteoarthritis and contractures in later life.

The two basic types of paralysis or paresis are flaccid paralysis, which is caused by injury to the lower motor neurons or peripheral nerves, and spastic paralysis, which is caused by injury to the upper motor neurons or the cortex of the brain. In approaching the neuromuscular hip, certain differences between flaccid and spastic paralysis must be delineated. The spastic muscle has increased tone and often functions in both phases of gait (i.e., in phase and out of phase). The flaccid muscle has decreased tone but always functions according to its normal role. Both spastic and flaccid types of pareses are found in both intrinsic and extrinsic disorders.

Extrinsic movement disorders, such as dyskinesis, athetosis, Parkinson's disease, and multiple sclerosis (which may be more specifically classified as a demyelinating disorder), may have elements of spasticity, but hip subluxation-dislocation is rare in this group of patients because the onset of disease usually occurs after growth is complete. However, movement disorders are frequently associated with contractures about the hip, and these patients often develop painful degenerative arthritis.

On the other hand, children who are born with intrinsic neuromuscular disorders (e.g., cerebral palsy, myelomeningocele), or in whom a neuromuscular affliction occurs while the hip is still in early development (e.g., poliomyelitis, encephalitis, cerebrovascular accident, childhood spinal cord injury, brain trauma), are at increased risk for hip subluxation-dislocation. In these children, frequent examinations and hip x-rays can detect and even predict those hips at risk. If detected, botulinum toxin A injections, early muscle releases or transfers, and appropriate varus rotation femoral osteotomies can improve hip stability. Still, in spite of treatment, a number of hips remain subluxated or dislocated and thus can be a source of pain and disability in the adult.

Although diminished sensation itself plays no role in hip instability, the lack thereof is an important consideration in planning surgery, as well as in the prognosis of the joint. For example, intact sensation is usually present in cerebral palsy but may be diminished in adult patients who have had a cerebrovascular accident. Additionally, myelomeningocele patients have significant loss of sensation, but polio patients have intact sensation.

Sensation in general does not play a role in hip instability; however, compromised proprioception may play a role. Clearly diminished or absent proprioception, whether it existed preoperatively or was compromised as the result of surgery about the hip, may cause instability after total hip arthroplasty. Unfortunately, assessing proprioception about the hip is challenging clinically, and therefore truly assessing its role is difficult.

INTRINSIC DISORDERS

Spasticity

Among intrinsic neuromuscular hip disorders, major causes of spasticity include cerebral palsy, cerebrovascular accident, and spinal cord injury in the young child. Despite differing origins, the hip pathology seen in these patients is similar; thus their treatment may be approached in a like manner. Among the more severely neurologically affected children with any one of these disorders, hip subluxation or dislocation often occurs. As was noted earlier, the direct cause of hip instability is muscle imbalance resulting from strong hip adductors and flexors overpowering weaker hip abductors and extensors. Coxa valga, increased femoral anteversion, and pelvic obliquity also contribute to the problem of hip instability. However, scoliosis plays less of a role, except for its relationship to pelvic obliquity. In the subluxated or dislocated hip, the uncovered femoral capital epiphysis becomes deformed and often becomes associated with painful arthritic changes later in life. Early treatment during childhood consists of nonoperative measures such as physical therapy, bracing, wheelchair modifications, botulinum toxin A injections, and operative treatment, including muscle releases and transfers to obtain muscle balance and early varus rotation femoral osteotomies to better stabilize the hip(s). When the acetabulum is deficient, acetabuloplasty should also be considered as operative treatment. Although these procedures may be suitable for the growing child, salvage operations are usually necessary in the treatment of adult patients.

In the adult patient, regardless of the cause and ambulatory status, the goal of treatment is to preserve or restore a functional range of painless hip motion in all patients. In the cerebral palsy population, the most severely involved patients (e.g., spastic quadriplegics) have the greatest frequency of mental retardation and seizure disorder, and often suffer from malnutrition, especially if they reside in large institutions. They are also the most likely patients to develop subluxation or dislocation of the hip. In fact, the incidence in this group is reported to be as high as 50% to 60%. Further, among hips that dislocate, approximately 50% will become painful. In addition to causing pain, subluxation-dislocation of the hip is often accompanied by contractures (e.g., adduction and/or flexion), which prevent standing, limit or prohibit sitting, and make perineal care difficult.

Therefore, the goals of treatment of the adult spastic neuromuscular hip are twofold: (1) prevent contractures, and (2) if the dysplastic hip becomes painful or the sitting position and perineal care become difficult because of contractures, perform salvage procedures to improve function and eliminate pain.

The uncovered, unprotected, growing femoral capital epiphysis is subjected to deforming forces from overlying spastic hip abductors and the tight superior capsule, and to the pressure of the elongated and hypertrophied ligamentum teres. The former two produce the pathognomonic flattening of the superolateral portion of the spastic subluxated-dislocated femoral head, and the latter, that is, the ligamentum teres, produces medial notching. The combination creates the typical "triangulation" effect (Fig. 80-1).

In young children who still have significant growth, a deformed femoral head can remodel after reduction. In early adult years, if the femoral head is not deformed, femoral and pelvic osteotomies may achieve adequate femoral head coverage with functional range of motion. On the other hand, in the adult, if the femoral head is deformed, repositioning it in the acetabulum will result in an incongruous and painful joint. Valgus or Schantz pelvic support osteotomies may relieve hip pain, but the abducted position of the hip may prevent wheelchair sitting, which is essential for the severely involved patient. As outlined by the treatment algorithm in Figure 80-2, the three traditional treatments of the painful, dislocated hip in the adult are (1) head-neck resection with or without interposition arthroplasty, (2) hip arthrodesis, and (3) total hip replacement.

Head-Neck Resection and Interposition Arthroplasty

Resection arthroplasty, as described by Girdlestone,[30] has not been traditionally recommended for spastic cerebral palsy patients, given its high incidence of stiffness, seating difficulty, heterotopic ossification, and proximal migration of the femur.[31] Castle and Schneider in 1978 were the first to describe an extensive proximal femoral resection with interposition arthroplasty. In this operation, the proximal femur is resected below the

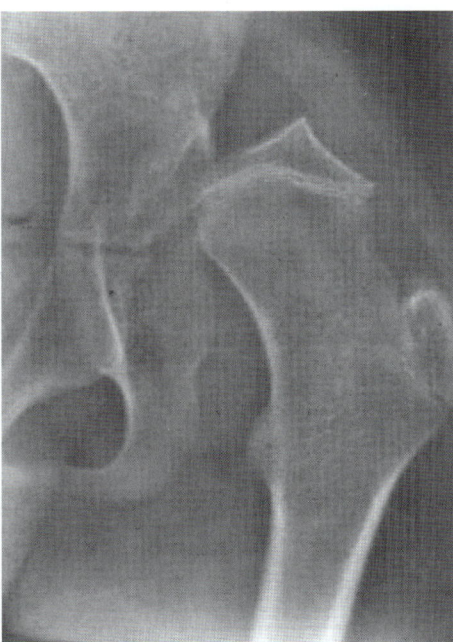

Figure 80-1. Radiograph of a hip demonstrating the "triangulation" effect with flattening of the superolateral femoral head caused by spastic hip abductors and a tight superior capsule, and medial notching of the head caused by the ligamentum teres.

level of the lesser trochanter, the capsule is closed over the acetabulum with the detached end of the iliopsoas tendon, and the vastus lateralis is sutured over the stump of the proximal femur. Then, the abductor muscle mass is interposed between the two (Fig. 80-3). In their series, they reported good long-term pain relief, improved sitting, and ease of perineal care in 12 patients (Table 80-1).[7]

This technique was further modified by McCarthy and associates, who published the largest series to date in 1988 by combining the results of groups of severely neurologically involved, institutionalized patients from Massachusetts and Arkansas. In their procedure, using extraperiosteal dissection, they resected the proximal femur to 3 cm below the level of the lesser trochanter (at a line drawn from the distal ischium); they performed this procedure on 58 proximal femurs in 34 patients, with ages ranging from 15 to 60 years. Pain was relieved and sitting was improved in 33 of the 34 patients. Still, ectopic bone was noted in 53 hips: 32 with just capping of the proximal femur, 12 hips with a lateral spike of the proximal femur, and 9 with bone interposed between the acetabulum and the femur. However, only 3 hips required revision because of heterotopic bone formation.

McHale and colleagues described a procedure that included adductor release, resection of the femoral head and neck, valgus proximal femoral osteotomy to achieve 45 degrees of abduction, suturing of the psoas tendon to the ligamentum teres, and capsulorrhaphy, followed by postoperative spica casting for 3 weeks. In all 5 patients, investigators noted improved sitting,

pain, and range of motion with no cases of proximal femoral migration and less heterotopic ossification.

In 1999, Widmann and coworkers reported on outcomes at The Hospital for Special Surgery (HSS). In all, 13 patients (18 hips) with an average age of 26.6 years underwent proximal femoral resection–interposition arthroplasty. Postoperatively, 6 hips were treated with skeletal traction and 9 hips were treated with skin traction. Five hips in the study had postoperative localized radiation at 700 cGy. Investigators reported statistically significant improvements in pain, perineal care, and sitting ability. In addition, range of motion improved with respect to flexion, extension, and especially abduction, where motion improved from 10.6 degrees preoperatively to 43.6 degrees postoperatively. In addition, a significant difference in postoperative heterotopic ossification was noted among patients treated with postoperative radiation. No difference in proximal femoral migration occurred in patients treated with skin traction, as opposed to skeletal traction.

Still, although Bleck was an early proponent of head-neck resection, the incidence of recurring pain and heterotopic bone formation has altered his advocacy.[4] Because of poor results, several authors have abandoned this procedure. In 2008, to combat the problem of proximal femoral migration and to allow for immediate upright sitting, Lampropulos and associates published results in a series of 4 hips in 3 patients who had undergone proximal femoral resection–interpositional arthroplasty as described by Castle and Schneider, with the addition of an external fixator for articulated hip distraction. All patients showed improvement in pain, perineal care, and sitting tolerance. One patient had proximal femoral migration above the level of the acetabulum with associated pain requiring a revision resection, and all patients had some degree of heterotopic ossification that did not interfere with outcomes. Complications associated with the external fixator were not seen.[32]

Although most authors have achieved favorable results with this procedure, it is important for the clinician to understand the limitations and contraindications of the procedure. Proximal femoral resection is contraindicated in walking patients because the restored limb cannot bear weight. It should not be performed in young, growing children because of upward migration and heterotopic bone formation in this group, which usually occur by the third to the fifteenth week. Furthermore, notwithstanding the complexity of attempted reconstruction, in the young child the potential for achieving satisfactory hip function with reduction and appropriate osteotomies makes this far preferable to proximal femoral resection. Finally, in all patients following proximal femoral resection, pain may be present for several months.

Hip Arthrodesis

Arthrodesis of a painful hip joint has been a time-honored orthopedic solution for treatment of the painful arthritic hip in the young adult; however, its use in neuromuscular disorders about the hip is less well documented. Indications for arthrodesis include disabling

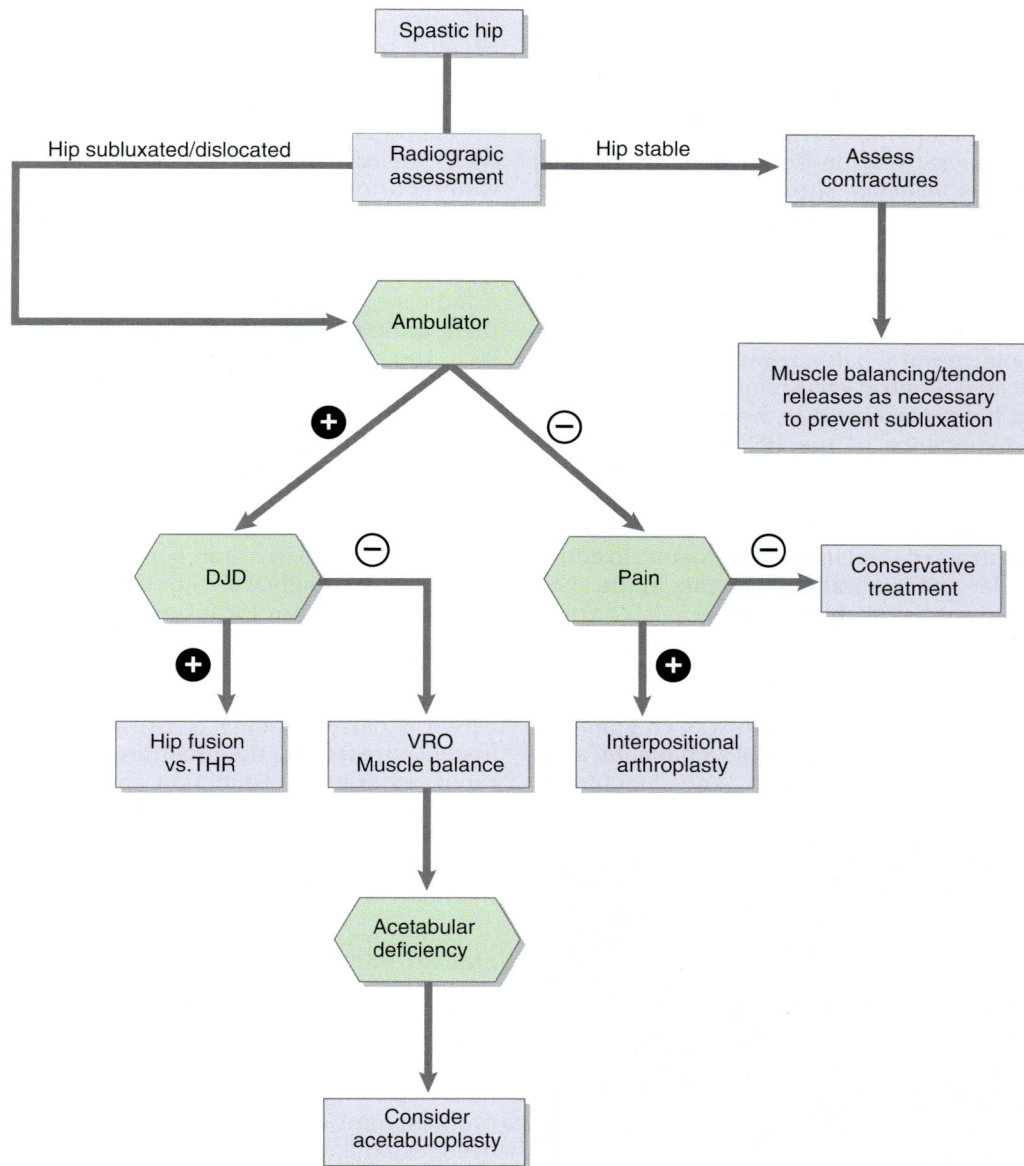

Figure 80-2. Treatment algorithm for the spastic hip.

hip pain, a normal contralateral hip, and no evidence of spinal deformity. Thus, because most painful, subluxated, or dislocated hips occur in severely neurologically involved patients who have contralateral hip dysplasia, as well as spinal deformity, hip arthrodesis as a surgical option in this population is relatively limited. Advantages of a successfully arthrodesed hip include elimination of pain, improved ability to sit and stand, and long-term durability. Disadvantages include the high incidence of failure and the need for prolonged postoperative immobilization. The latter may be reduced or eliminated with the use of larger and stronger internal fixation devices such as an AO-Cobra plate or the use of an external fixator. Although these stronger internal devices may improve fusion rates, they should be used with caution because a possible future total hip arthroplasty may be compromised if the abductor muscles are excessively weakened.

In 1986, Root and colleagues reported on 8 cerebral palsy patients with ages ranging from 13 to 34 years who had unilateral hip arthrodeses.[22] All patients had painful arthrosis of the hip associated with subluxation or dislocation. Of the original 8 patients, 6 fused successfully and 2 required revisions. One of the revisions was ultimately converted to a total hip replacement. Fucs and coworkers published the largest series in 2003, when they analyzed 14 patients with spastic cerebral palsy and painful chronic hip dislocations or subluxations that were treated with hip arthrodesis.[51] Six hips were stabilized with an AO-DCP 4.5-mm plate, 4 hips with an AO-Cobra plate, and 3 hips with 6.5-mm cancellous screws. One hip was initially stabilized with Kirschner wires and went on to develop a nonunion, which was eventually revised with a Cobra plate. A hip spica was used on 8 patients, and 1 of the patients who was not casted developed a nonunion. Among the 14 hips,

11 hips fused without a nonunion. Three patients developed a pseudarthrosis with aseptic loosening of the hardware requiring reoperation, and all 3 cases eventually fused. All patients noted relief of pain, and of the 3 sitting patients preoperatively, 2 became household ambulators postoperatively. In addition, most of the bedridden patients became sitters, and ambulatory patients maintained or improved their ambulatory status.

Total Hip Arthroplasty

Total hip replacement is a successful treatment option for painful hips in cerebral palsy, regardless of whether the hip is dislocated. Contrary to Koffman's poor experience with total hip replacement in 5 patients reported in 1981,[13] the experience of the HSS of 19 total hip replacements in 18 patients with an average follow-up of 10 years was remarkably good.[6] Whereas Koffman used various constrained prostheses, the HSS series reported no constrained total hip replacements. In addition, all acetabular and femoral components in the HSS series were fixed with polymethylmethacrylate. Four hips had bone graft augmentation for a deficient acetabulum. Notably, a postoperative hip spica cast was used in 16 of 18 patients to prevent dislocation and promote healing of the greater trochanter. Pain was completely resolved at long-term follow-up in 16 of 18 patients, and 12 patients improved by at least one functional

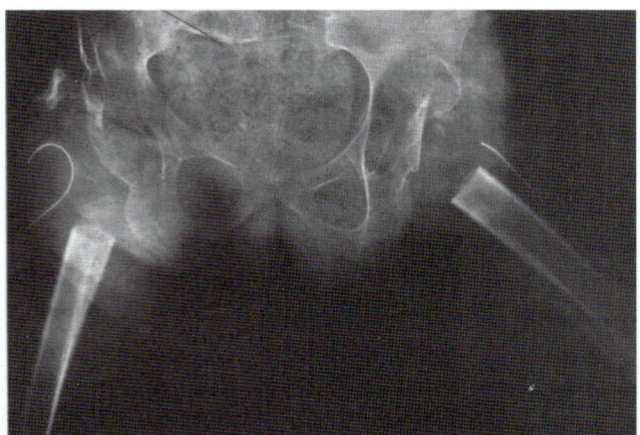

Figure 80-3. Anteroposterior radiograph of a pelvis demonstrating bilateral proximal femoral resections.

category. Two patients had recurrent dislocation because of component malposition, and both had successful revisions. Thus, survivorship was 95% at 10 years when the endpoint was loosening, and 86% when the endpoint was revision for any reason. Similar results were published in 2009 by Schroeder and associates, who reported on 18 total hip replacements in 16 ambulatory cerebral palsy patients. However, their series had slightly higher dislocation and acetabular loosening rates.[33]

Indications for performing a total hip replacement in the spastic patient include the following:

1. Hip pain refractory to medication.
2. Decreased function in standing, limited sitting, and difficulty with perineal hygiene.
3. Potential standing or walking, transfer ability, or upright sitting in a wheelchair.

Mental retardation is not an absolute contraindication, but patients who are severely retarded and essentially bedridden are not good candidates. Although adolescents initially were not believed to be candidates because of concern for future revision, adolescence is no longer considered a major contraindication, and recent reports have demonstrated good outcomes in this age group,[34] in part because the activity level of cerebral palsy patients is usually decreased so that loading stresses on the prosthesis are less. In addition, rapid restoration of function and pain-free movement after surgery makes this procedure very desirable. Still, it is important to realize that patients with cerebral palsy do have a higher frequency of complications than the uninvolved population.

Flaccid Paralysis

The intrinsic neuromuscular disorders associated with flaccid paralysis include poliomyelitis, myelomeningocele, and Charcot-Marie-Tooth disease. Fortunately, with worldwide polio vaccination, this disorder and its problems are seen less frequently today than in past decades. Still, past experience with polio provides the basis for understanding and treating this group of neuromuscular disorders. Study of the effects of muscle paralysis on bone growth and the development of deformity not only provides the rationale for treatment, but also has enhanced our knowledge and concepts of normal joint function and gait.

Table 80-1. Interpositional Arthroplasty in Cerebral Palsy

Authors (ref)	Hips, *N*	Patients, *N*	Outcome	Heterotopic Ossification
Castle and Schneider (7)	14	12	All improved	—
Koffman (13)	16	10	All improved	100%
Baxter and D'Astous (2)	5	4	Good	—
McCarthy et al (16)	58	34	33 patients with pain relief	98%
Widmann et al (31)	18	13	All improved	89% (less with postop XRT)
Lampropulos (32)	4	3	All improved	100%

XRT, Radiotherapy.

Poliomyelitis

Poliomyelitis is caused by a virus that mainly affects the anterior horn cells of the spinal cord and certain motor nuclei of the brainstem; thus, sensation is intact and intelligence is not altered. As a result, the patient can cooperate, and the success of restoration of muscle balance by release or transfer can be measured. As in the spastic patient, hip subluxation-dislocation in polio patients is generally caused by flexors and adductors overpowering weaker abductors and extensors, often in association with pelvic obliquity. In most cases, the hip on the "high" side is adducted, and the hip on the "low" side may have an abduction contracture. A classification system has been developed for the fixed pelvic obliquity seen in poliomyelitis; it is based on a combination of the level of the pelvis in relation to the short limb, and the direction and severity of scolioisis.[37] In the young child, coxa valga and excessive femoral anteversion also contribute to the development of hip instability. The "flail" polio hip, on the other hand, rarely dislocates, and if seen, it is usually the result of marked pelvic obliquity and abduction contracture of the contralateral limb. In this situation, release of the abductors as recommended by Eberle may result in reduction just by leveling the pelvis.[8]

To obtain a stable hip, muscle balancing is always necessary and often must be combined with femoral and pelvic osteotomies. For the most part, the young child with hip subluxation is treated by a combination of procedures to improve muscle balance with adductor transfers to the ischium or with iliopsoas transfers laterally to the greater trochanter (Fig. 80-4).[18,19] When the contralateral hip has been in abduction, the contracture must be released as well, or secondary pelvic obliquity can lead to recurrence of subluxation even after surgical reduction. If coxa valga and femoral anteversion are associated with the subluxation-dislocation, varus rotation osteotomy is indicated. Acetabulum insufficiency can be corrected by pelvic osteotomies such as Pemberton or shelf-type procedures, the innominate osteotomy of Salter, the sliding osteotomy of Chiari, or the triple osteotomy of Steel. Lau and colleagues reported on 39 patients with an average age at surgery of 13.4 years and average follow-up of 9.3 years, who had undergone muscle transfers, femoral osteotomies, and/or pelvic osteotomies, and published good results in 46% and satisfactory results in 24%.[36] Although these procedures are generally reserved for children, one can achieve a successful, painless reduction using the same procedures

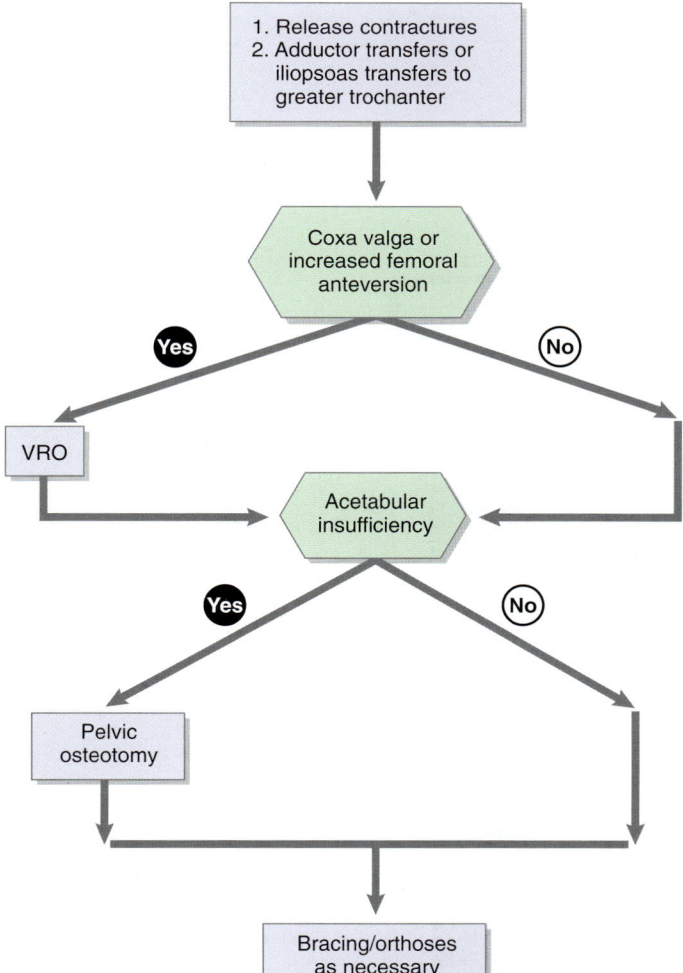

Figure 80-4. Treatment algorithm for the unstable hip in adult patients with poliomyelitis.

in a young adult with similar dysplasia and without arthritic changes.

The completely dislocated hip is rarely painful; however, older polio patients with subluxation of the hips are prone to develop painful arthritis. The femoral head deformity seen in spastic subluxation-dislocation does not occur in poliomyelitis. The uncovered femoral head may demonstrate medial flattening caused by pressure from the hypertrophied ligamentum teres, but not the superolateral flattening associated with the spastic subluxated-dislocated hip.

Regardless, in the ambulating adult polio patient, the arthritic painful hip can be very disabling. A Chiari or varus rotational osteotomy may provide pain relief if the arthritis is not advanced. However, the presence of advanced arthritic changes and decreased range of motion precludes pelvic or femoral osteotomy (Fig. 80-5). At this stage, the only alternatives are hip arthrodesis and total hip arthroplasty. In today's world, most patients would strongly prefer a total hip replacement to an arthrodesis. As was noted earlier, the advantages of an arthrodesis are that it relieves pain and it allows sitting and walking. More important for the patient with

flaccid paralysis, it does not rely upon muscle strength or balance for stability and function. A total hip arthroplasty also provides a functional painless range of motion and permits sitting and walking. However, when loss of muscle power is significant, especially if hip abductors are absent, hip stability is jeopardized. A constrained prosthesis may help to relieve this problem, but an arthrodesis should be considered if significant muscle weakness is present. Given the low prevalence of polio in today's society, the literature on outcomes of total hip replacement or arthrodesis is minimal.

Myelomeningocele

The number of new cases of myelomeningocele has decreased in recent years with advances in obstetrics and folate supplementation. However, the survival rate of these patients has increased significantly over the past two decades because of emphasis on early closure of the spinal defect and on insertion of a ventriculoperitoneal shunt to treat hydrocephalus. Thus, the prevalence of adult hip pathology in this patient population is still noteworthy. Also, treatment of these hip deformities in children is complicated by associated sensory

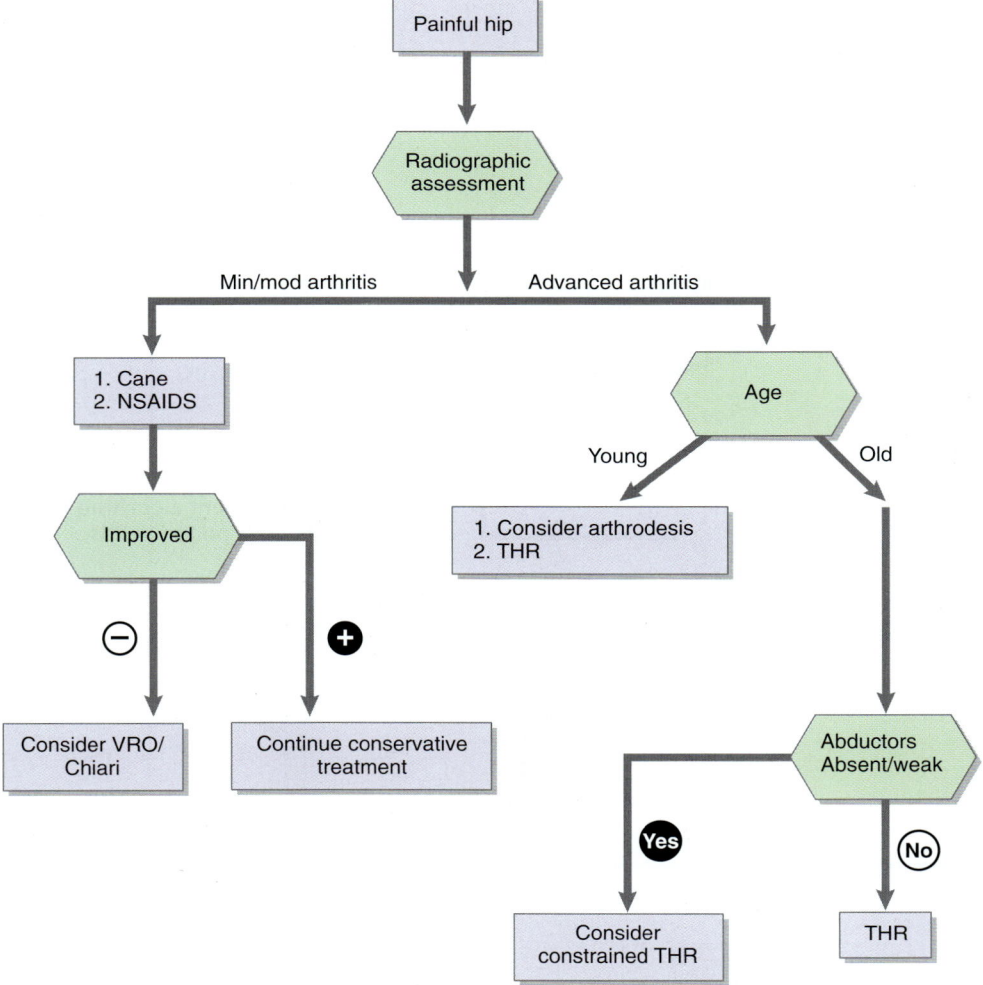

Figure 80-5. Treatment algorithm for the stable arthritic hip in adult patients with poliomyelitis.

deficits in the lower extremities, as well as by frequent pelvic obliquity.

The level of the lesion, defined as the lowest active functioning nerve root, determines not only the patient's ability to walk but also the patient's risk of developing hip instability (Fig. 80-6). High-level involvement as seen with high thoracic or lumbar levels rarely leads to hip instability. Patients with muscle power to L2 will walk only with braces and crutches and generally become wheelchair bound by their adolescent years. Patients with intact L3 and L4 nerve roots have good quadriceps and the potential to be community ambulators, although they may require orthotics. Their prognosis improves if hamstring activity is present as well. The incidence of hip subluxation is greatest in patients with these levels because hip flexors and adductors remain intact, and hip extensors and abductors are absent or weak. According to Sharrard, 60% of these children will develop hip subluxation by age 3 if left untreated.[24] The L5 level with strong quadriceps, active hamstrings, and the presence of some abductor or extensor activity rarely develops hip instability. Likewise, in general, patients with the S1 level or below do not develop hip instability.

General agreement is evident in the literature that no attempt should be made to reduce hips if quadriceps function is not present. Contractures should be treated with releases or osteotomies to facilitate the use of braces for standing and sitting. Dislocation in this group, whether unilateral or bilateral, does not become painful in adult life, and sufficient range of motion remains for functioning in a wheelchair. Because dislocation is rare at L5 and is never seen at S1, these hips do not present future problems.

Controversy exists regarding whether one should aggressively treat the dislocated hip of a patient with

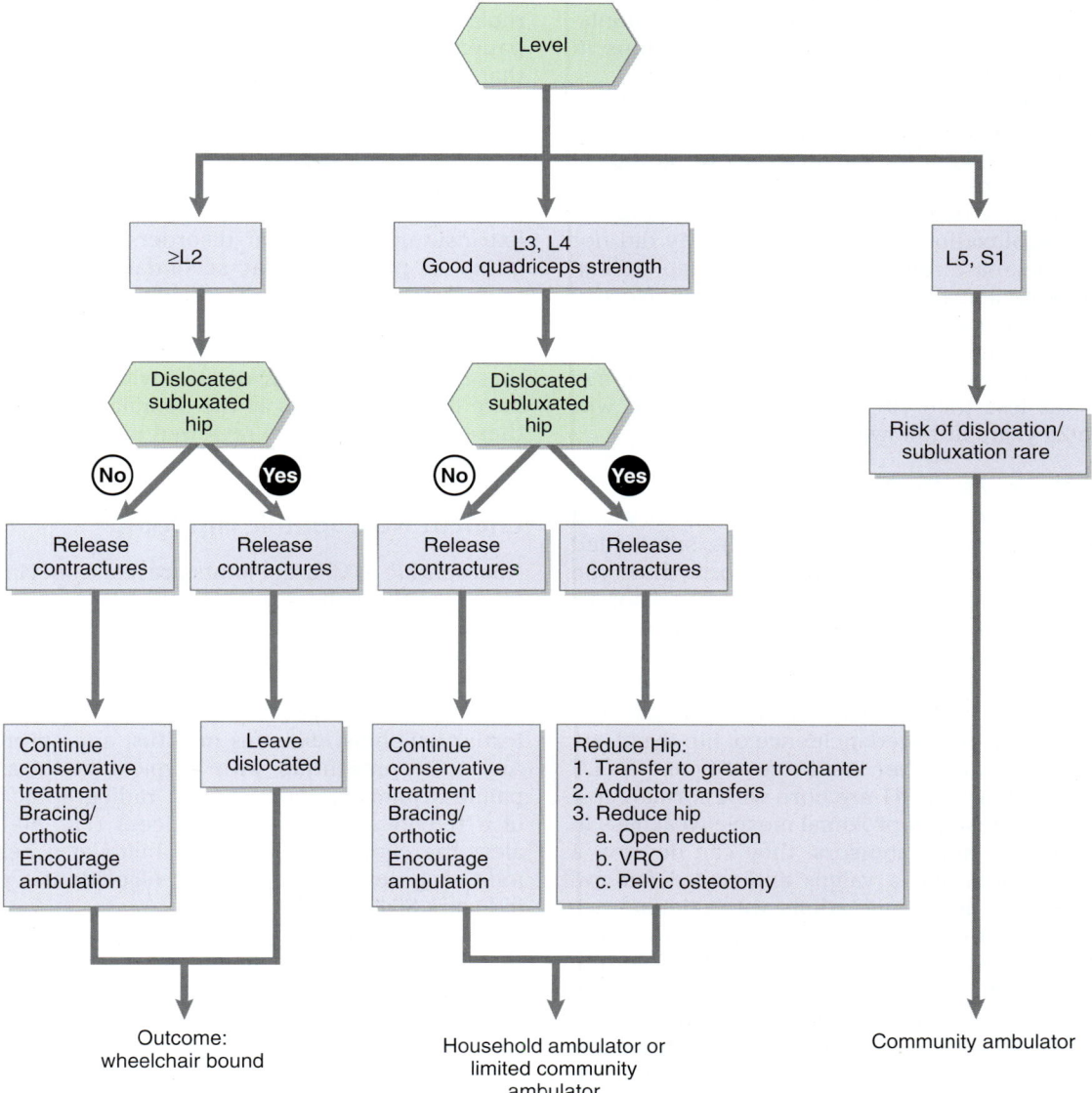

Figure 80-6. Treatment algorithm for the hip in patients with myelomeningocele with expected ambulatory outcomes.

L3 or L4 level involvement. Some authors recommend no treatment except for the correction of contractures, and others recommend reducing all subluxated or dislocated hips. Open reduction, varus rotational osteotomy, pelvic osteotomy, and any combination of these procedures are often necessary to reduce hips. Some authors recommend iliopsoas transfer to the greater trochanter or an external oblique transfer to the greater trochanter.[18,23,29,38] The goal of these operations is to locate the hip and improve abductor strength. In addition, the adductors are often transferred to the ischium to remove a deforming force and reinforce hip extension.

The question of the importance of hip stability for ambulation remains unanswered. Root and coworkers reviewed more than 100 myelomeningocele patients.[3] Surgical reduction of the hip above an L2 level uniformly failed. Of the hips with an L5 and S1 level, all were stable. Of 30 hips with an L3 and L4 level, 60% had persistent instability, including those in which reduction and maintenance of reduction were achieved. Ambulation improved with increased stability of the hips in patients with good quadriceps function.

Feiwell and associates reported in 1979 on 76 patients with myelomeningocele over the age of 5 who failed to achieve hip stability.[10] In the mid-lumbar group of patients, stability did not influence ambulation. No hip was painful if there had been no prior surgery, and the presence of subluxation-dislocation instability did not significantly decrease range of motion. For hip subluxation in these patients, investigators recommended surgical intervention, including adductor tenotomy, medial capsulotomy of the hip, or iliopsoas release if these structures were contracted. However, the average follow-up was less than 10 years, and no patient was older than 29 years at follow-up.

Charcot-Marie-Tooth Disease

Charcot-Marie-Tooth (CMT) disease is a sensory and motor peripheral neuropathy that can be subdivided into type I, which is the demyelinating form, and type II, which is the axonal form. Patients with this disorder often present with symmetrical distal muscle weakness, decreased reflexes in the lower extremity, and less involvement of the proximal muscles. Walker and associates reported in 1994, in their review of 100 patients with CMT, that the estimated incidence of hip dysplasia is 6% to 8.1%, with a higher incidence of type I CMT.[28] Although patients with CMT are born with normal hips, over time, as the result of proximal muscle weakness in the hip abductors and extensors, they can develop a shallow acetabulum and a valgus anteverted femoral neck.[40] In children and young adults with minimal evidence of hip arthritis, pelvic and varus femoral osteotomies can be performed to provide a more stable hip. However, it is best to address the acetabular deficiency before treating the proximal femur, and then to make an intraoperative decision to treat the femur if both abnormalities are present.[40] Although patients with Charcot-Marie-Tooth rarely develop symptomatic hip instability as children, they may develop painful osteoarthritis in later years, leading to the need for total hip

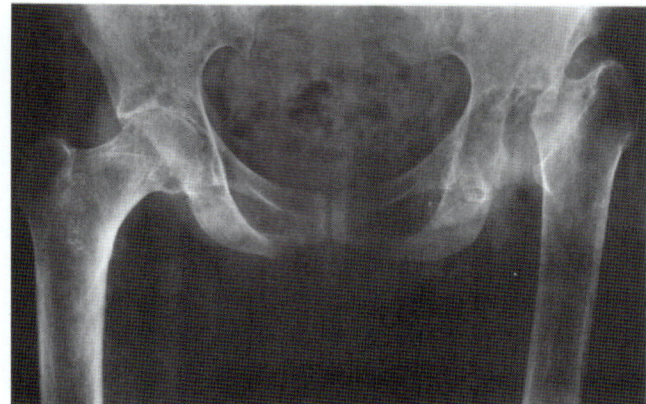

Figure 80-7. Anteroposterior radiograph of a pelvis with a painless left neuropathic hip joint.

arthroplasty.[14,28] The issue of instability with total hip replacement in these patients is the same as in the patient with polio. If muscle weakness is so profound that the arthroplasty is unstable, a constrained device may be necessary to provide stability.

EXTRINSIC DISORDERS

Extrinsic neuromuscular disorders make up a diverse group of problems that secondarily involve the hip joint. In these disorders, muscle imbalance with hip subluxation-dislocation plays a secondary role, but contractures about the hip frequently develop. Some of these disorders are associated with spasticity; others have flaccid paralysis as the dominant feature. Each of these disorders will be reviewed individually, although the treatment algorithms may be similar.

Charcot Neuropathic Hip Joint

Neuropathic or Charcot joints present a special problem for the orthopedic surgeon, regardless of the specific joint involved. The critical element in treating a patient with a neuropathic hip joint is to establish the diagnosis.* Charcot joints can be caused by a variety of diseases and disease processes. The most common include tertiary syphilis, diabetes mellitus, and syringomyelia. Any joint presenting with atypical findings such as painless joint dysfunction and radiographic evidence of a relentless destructive process (Fig. 80-7) should alert the clinician to the possibility of a neuropathic joint. A generalized diagnostic algorithm is presented in Figure 80-8.

If the joint remains painless and functional, no treatment is recommended. If pain is present and function is impaired, conservative treatment with protected weight bearing should be extended as long as possible before any type of surgical procedure is considered. If nonoperative treatment fails, available surgical options include arthrodesis, total hip replacement, and resection

---

*References 1, 5, 11, 17, 20, 21, and 25.

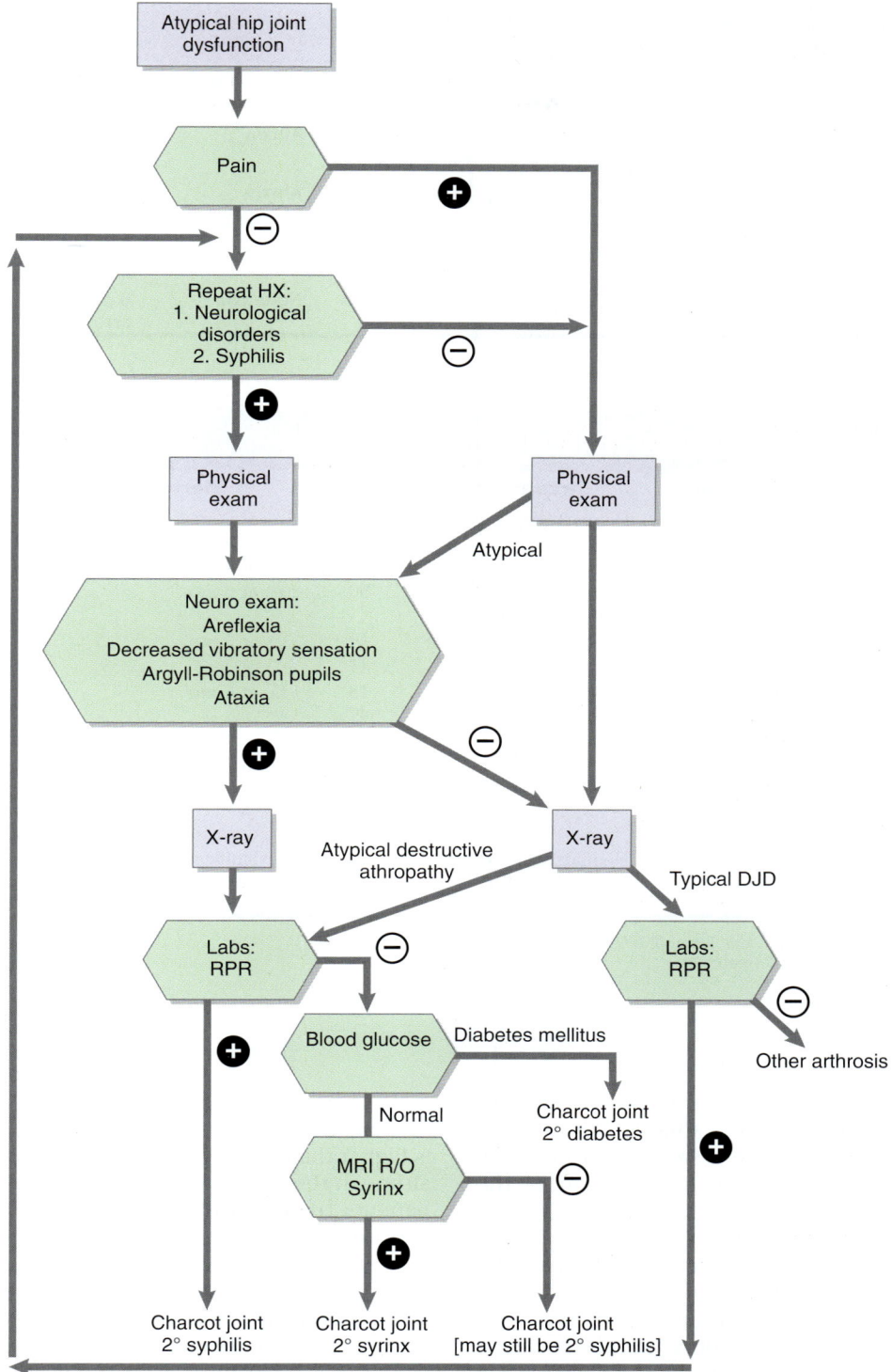

Figure 80-8. Diagnostic algorithm of a suspected Charcot hip joint.

arthroplasty. Treatment with hip arthrodesis has been associated with an unacceptable rate of nonunion that, historically, has been reported to be as high as 100%.[11] Total hip arthroplasty also has a high failure rate, especially in patients with significant neurologic findings or ataxia. Although the number of patients treated with total hip arthroplasty reported in the literature is small, most likely reflecting the low incidence of neuropathic hips, nearly all of them have done poorly (Table 80-2). In fact, of the dozen or so cases reported in the literature, only one patient was stated to have done well with a total hip arthroplasty, which the authors attributed to the fact that the patient was not ataxic.[25] The remainder did poorly even when treated with a broad range of total

Table 80-2. Total Hip Arthroplasty and Charcot Hips

Authors (ref)	Cases, N	Prosthesis Type	Diagnosis	Neurologic Involvement	Outcome
Ritter and DeRosa (20)	1	McKee/Farrar	Tabes dorsalis	Ataxia	Multiple dislocations
McKee (17)	1	McKee/Farrar	Tabes dorsalis		Femoral/acetabular loosening
Buchholz (5)	1	St. George	Tabes dorsalis	Ataxia	Failed
Sprenger and Foley (25)	1	St. George	Tabes dorsalis	No ataxia	Good at 7 years
Baldini et al (1)	4	Multiple	Tabes dorsalis	Ataxia	Recurrent dislocations and/or loosening
Robb et al (21)	1	Charnley	Tabes dorsalis	No ataxia	6 dislocations → resection arthroplasty

Table 80-3. Hip Fracture in Parkinson's Disease

Authors (ref)	Fracture Type	Treatment	Hips, N	Mortality	D
Couglin et al	Fem neck Intertrochanteric	Hemiarthroplasty CRIF	27 22	60% at 6 mo* 27% at 6 mo* 47% at 6 mo†	35% dislocation rate*
Staeheli et al (26)	Displaced fem neck	Hemiarthroplasty	50	20% at 6 mo	UTI, 20%; pneumonia, 10%
Eventov et al (9)	Fem neck Intertrochanteric	Hemiarthroplasty CRIF	34 11	31% at 3 mo†	
Turcotte et al (27)	Nondisplaced fem neck Displaced fem neck Intertrochanteric	In situ pinning Hemiarthroplasty CRIF	13 47 34	14% at 6 mo†	5 dislocations*
Londos et al (15)	Nondisplaced fem neck Displaced fem neck	In situ pinning CRIF	8 24	28% at 2 yr†	33% healing complications† 6 nonunions, 3 segmental collapses*
Idjadi et al (42)	Fem neck Intertrochanteric	Hemiarthroplasty Internal fixation Internal fixation	8 5 18	No significant differences from general population	Not specifically reported

CRIF, Closed reduction internal fixation; *fem*, femoral; *UTI*, urinary tract infection.
*Data reflect specific fracture type and treatment.
†Data reflect entire study.

hip designs. This limited evidence strongly indicates that prosthetic replacement of a Charcot hip joint is contraindicated. Resorting to a resection arthroplasty may be the only viable solution in treatment of the painful hip in these patients.

Treatment of hip fractures in a Charcot hip joint is also problematic. Internal fixation has been documented to do as poorly as prosthetic replacement. Thus treatment with restricted weight bearing may be the most prudent option. A delayed resection arthroplasty can be performed at a later date if the joint subsequently becomes painful.

Parkinson's Disease

Degenerative arthritis of the hip in patients with Parkinson's disease may occur through natural processes or following hip fracture, but the overall incidence is unknown. On the other hand, given the high incidences of vitamin D and calcium deficiency and osteoporosis,

and the high fall rate, among patients with Parkinson's disease, the incidence of hip fracture in these patients is higher than in the general elderly population.[43,44] Thus although the literature is sparse regarding outcomes in patients treated with total hip arthroplasty, extensive literature describes the treatment of hip fracture in patients with Parkinson's disease (Table 80-3).[9,15,26,27,42] In fact, to our knowledge, the only recent paper reporting on outcomes following total hip replacement in patients with Parkinson's disease was authored by Weber and colleagues, who reported on 107 total hip arthroplasties in 98 patients. A total of 58 hip arthroplasties were performed for osteoarthrosis, and concurrent tendon release for contracture was performed in 8 patients. Investigators reported only 6 dislocations and no dislocation in any primary total hip replacement. At 7-year follow-up on 75 hips, 51 patients had died, and function was directly related to the stage of Parkinson's disease.[41]

With regard to femoral neck fractures in these patients, controversy exists as to whether the most appropriate surgical option is pinning or primary hip arthroplasty. Eventov and his associates in 1983 reported on 62 Parkinson's patients with hip fracture.[9] Among these patients, 39 were subcapital and 23 were intertrochanteric in location. A total of 34 patients with subcapital fracture had undergone primary hemiarthroplasty, 11 patients with intracapsular fracture had had nail plate insertion, and 12 had refused surgery. Five patients were too medically unstable for surgery. Regardless of fracture type, these patients had high mortality and morbidity rates, and bronchial pneumonia was the most frequent complication. Patients treated with surgery had better functional results and a better quality of life. Staeheli and colleagues in 1981 reported on 49 patients with 50 femoral neck fractures of the Garden III or Garden IV type treated with endoprosthetic replacement of the femoral head (hemiarthroplasty).[26] In all, 10 patients died within 6 months of surgery. This rate is higher than the mortality rate in the first year postoperatively in a general hip fracture population.[12] Complications included urinary tract infection and pneumonia. Investigators reported only 1 postoperative dislocation, and 80% of the survivors could walk. The authors attribute the good results to rapid mobilization of patients postoperatively and to the release of contracted adductor muscles at the time of surgery.

Turcotte and colleagues in 1988 in their series reported that hemiarthroplasty was not as good as simple internal fixation of the fracture.[27] Their study group consisted of 87 patients with 94 fractures. Group A consisted of 13 patients with Garden I or II fractures treated with in situ pinning. Group B consisted of 47 hips in 41 patients with Garden III or IV fractures, all of whom had undergone hemiarthroplasty. Group C consisted of 34 hips in 33 patients with extracapsular femoral neck fracture requiring closed reduction and internal fixation. The authors found that the incidence of complications was twice as high in the hemiarthroplasty group as in the internal fixation group, with 4 wound infections and 5 dislocations occurring in this series.

Londos, Nielsen, and Strongvist in 1989 recommended internal fixation over primary hip arthroplasty for Parkinson's patients.[15] They treated 32 patients with femoral neck fracture with internal fixation. A total of 24 displaced fractures were complicated by 6 nonunions and 3 segmental femoral head collapses. Among 8 nondisplaced fractures, 1 case of segmental collapse was diagnosed. Healing complications occurred in 33% of patients. Three patients with complications required total hip replacement. Investigators compared healing complications with those of a nonambulatory population of 547 patients. Among 151 uncomplicated fractures, healing complications occurred in 8%. Among 196 patients with displaced fractures, healing complications occurred in 40% of survivors. Although these authors recommended internal fixation over primary arthroplasty in Parkinson's patients with femoral neck fracture, it would seem logical that primary arthroplasty should be performed in both patient populations for displaced fractures.

Idjadi and associates performed a prospective study in 2005 to examine 920 community-dwelling patients treated for a hip fracture and compared the subgroup of patients who had Parkinson's disease (31 patients) against remaining patients.[42] They found that patients with Parkinson's disease were hospitalized significantly longer and were more likely to be sent to a skilled nursing facility on discharge. Further, after surgery, patients with Parkinson's disease declined in their ability to perform activities of daily living (ADLs) independently. However, investigators found no difference in ambulatory ability and mortality within the first year postoperatively.

Treatment of these fractures remains problematic with a high rate of complications, including frequent dislocation of hips treated with hemiarthroplasty. However, the literature is contradictory with respect to an increased mortality rate among patients with Parkinson's disease who have hip fractures. Whether these higher complication rates can be extrapolated to those patients with Parkinson's disease undergoing total hip arthroplasty is not known, given the limited literature available on this topic. Given the findings of Weber and colleagues, with aggressive pharmacologic treatment it is possible that patients with degenerative hip disease undergoing total hip arthroplasty may behave differently from more debilitated Parkinson's disease patients suffering from hip fracture. Further, use of supplemental calcium, vitamin D, and bisphosphonates may be an important pharmacologic intervention to help prevent hip fracture in this population.[45]

Multiple Sclerosis

Painful hip flexion adduction contractures in patients with advanced multiple sclerosis are very difficult to treat. What further complicates treatment is that by the time these develop, patients are in an end stage of their disease and often have knee flexion contractures and contracted upper extremities as well. At this stage, patients usually become aphasic but remain mentally alert. Early release of contracted hip adductors, flexors, and iliopsoas muscles, as well as hamstrings, is essential to prevent painful fixed joint deformities. These contractures may recur, but with peripheral nerve blockade such as phenol, alcohol, or botulinum toxin A, the relentless progression of the deformity can be substantially delayed. Unfortunately, the progressive nature of multiple sclerosis often leads to a nihilistic surgical approach.

Once contractures are fixed and severe, patients develop painful decubiti or pelvic obliquity and often are unable to sit or even lie comfortably. Despite the fact that these patients are essentially terminal, multiple extensive soft tissue procedures may provide pain relief and some improvement in sitting. Occasionally, a proximal femoral resection is warranted for pain relief. Because of prolonged steroid use and diminished function and strength, fractures about the hip, particularly of the femoral neck and trochanter, are matters of concern.[46]

Adult-Onset Cerebrovascular Accident (Stroke), Upper Motor Neuron Spinal Cord Injury, and Head Injury

As noted earlier, hip subluxation-dislocation rarely occurs in adult-onset spasticity due to brain or upper spinal cord injury. On the other hand, hip joint contractures are frequent. Thus early, intensive physical therapy is important for maintenance of hip range of motion. This is especially true in the patient who is comatose for an extended period. Unless regularly manipulated through a normal range of motion, these hips will develop significant contractures.

If the patient survives the initial insult, whether it is due to a traumatic event or a cerebrovascular accident, efforts should be directed toward regaining functional ambulation. That being said, patients left with greater neurologic impairment most likely will end up wheelchair bound. Regardless, at least a 90-degree range of hip flexion/extension is necessary for sitting or standing, and this should be the treatment goal. Among these patients, usually the hip flexors and adductors are less impaired than the hip extensors and abductors. As a result, simple tenotomies of the involved muscles may be helpful in restoring balance. One major reason why balance is so important in this population is the higher rate of falls; bone loss on the paretic side results in an increased rate of hip/femur fracture in these patients.[47,50] Still, functional recovery after surgical treatment of hip fracture is similar to that of patients who have not had a prior cerebrovascular accident.[49]

Another problem in these patients, especially those with traumatic brain injury, is the propensity for heterotopic ossification, which can also limit joint motion. This excessive bone must be allowed to fully mature before resection is attempted; otherwise more extensive heterotopic bone formation may occur post resection. One good indicator of bone maturation is serum alkaline phosphatase levels, which should return to normal before an attempt is made at resection. After surgical resection, multimodal prophylaxis to prevent recurrence must be instituted, including low-dose radiation, nonsteroidal anti-inflammatory agents, and early mobilization.

Older stroke patients are more prone to degenerative joint disease of the hip and should be treated according to the same guidelines as the general population. However, they may require release of contracted adductor or hip flexor muscles at the time of the total hip arthroplasty. The adductor tenotomy can be performed percutaneously just before the patient is positioned for hip arthroplasty, and the iliopsoas can be released from its insertion on the lesser trochanter during exposure of the joint. Further, current literature suggests an increased risk of heterotopic ossification following total hip replacement in this population, with a reported incidence of 36%; thus prophylaxis may be warranted in these patients.[48]

Total hip replacement is also recommended for younger patients who, in addition to sustaining head injuries, develop painful post-traumatic arthritis or even avascular necrosis. Because their spasticity is usually profound, these patients should be immobilized postoperatively in a hip spica cast or a hip abduction brace for 3 to 4 weeks to prevent dislocation or contracture.

Spinal Cord Injury

Just as in juvenile patients, spinal cord injuries in adults can result in significant spasticity of the muscles around the hip. Although subluxation and dislocation usually are not problems in the adult patient, as they are in children, spasticity can lead to contractures that require appropriate early releases. If degenerative arthritis does develop, total hip arthroplasty may be indicated for pain relief. On the other hand, if the patient is a nonambulator with severe contractures and skin problems, resection arthroplasty may be a more viable option. Although not as prevalent as in traumatic brain injury patients, heterotopic ossification does occur with some frequency and should be approached as in patients with traumatic brain injury.

CONCLUSION

As with any disease process, prevention of hip pathology in patients with intrinsic neuromuscular disease is much more rewarding and results in better outcomes than treatment provided once the hip becomes unstable. Thus early treatment in childhood to preserve hip stability is essential. Treatment for hip problems in patients with extrinsic neuromuscular disease is much more problematic and depends on the progressive nature of the disease, the functional level of the patient, and the degree of pain suffered.

REFERENCES

1. Baldini N, Sudanese A, Toni A: Total prosthetic replacement in tabetic arthropathy of the hip joint. Ital J Orthop Traumatol 11:193, 1985.
2. Baxter MP, D'Astous JL: Proximal femoral resection-interposition arthroplasty: salvage hip surgery for the severely disabled child with cerebral palsy. J Pediatr Orthop 6:681, 1986.
3. Benton LJ, Salvati EA, Root L: Reconstructive surgery in the myelomeningocele hip. Clin Orthop Relat Res 110:261, 1975.
4. Bleck EE: The hip in cerebral palsy. Orthop Clin North Am 11:79, 1980.
5. Buchholz H: Personal communication, 1981.
6. Buly RL, Huo M, Root L, et al: Total hip arthroplasty in cerebral palsy: long-term follow-up results. Clin Orthop Relat Res 296:148, 1993.
7. Castle ME, Schneider C: Proximal femoral resection-interposition arthroplasty. J Bone Joint Surg Am 60:1051, 1978.
8. Eberle C: Pelvic obliquity and the unstable hip after poliomyelitis. J Bone Joint Surg Br 64:300, 1982.
9. Eventov I, Moreno M, Geller E, et al: Hip fractures in patients with Parkinson's syndrome. J Orthop Trauma 23:98, 1983.
10. Feiwell E, Sakai D, Blatt T: The effect of hip reduction on function in patients with myelomeningocele: potential gains and hazards of surgical treatment. J Bone Joint Surg Am 60:169, 1978.
11. Johnson J: Neuropathic fractures and joint injuries. J Bone Joint Surg Am 49:1, 1967.
12. Kenzura JE, McCarthy RE, Lowell JD, et al: Hip fracture mortality: relation to age, treatment, preoperative illness, time of

surgery, and complications. Clin Orthop Relat Res 186:45, 1984.

13. Koffman M: Proximal femoral resection or total hip replacement in severely disabled cerebral-spastic patients. Orthop Clin North Am 12:91, 1981.

14. Kumar SJ, Marks HG, Bowen JR, et al: Hip dysplasia associated with Charcot-Marie-Tooth disease in the older child and adolescent. J Pediatr Orthop 5:511, 1985.

15. Londos E, Nilsson LT, Stromqvist B: Internal fixation of femoral neck fractures in Parkinson's disease: 32 patients followed for 2 years. Acta Orthop Scand 60:682, 1989.

16. McCarthy RE, Simon S, Douglas B, et al: Proximal femoral resection to allow adults who have severe cerebral palsy to sit. J Bone Joint Surg Am 70:1011, 1988.

17. McKee G: Personal communication, 1981.

18. Mustard WT: Iliopsoas transfer for weakness of the hip abductors. J Bone Joint Surg Am 24:647, 1952.

19. Nickel VL, Perry J, Garret A, et al: Paralytic dislocation of the hip. J Bone Joint Surg Am 48:1021, 1966.

20. Ritter M, DeRosa G: Total hip arthroplasty in a Charcot joint: a case report with six year follow-up. Orthop Rev 6:51, 1977.

21. Robb JE, Rymaszewski LA, Reeves BF, et al: Total hip replacement in a Charcot joint: brief report. J Bone Joint Surg Br 70:489, 1988.

22. Root L, Goss JR, Mendes J: The treatment of the painful hip in cerebral palsy by total hip replacement or hip arthrodesis. J Bone Joint Surg Am 68:590, 1986.

23. Sharrard WJ: Posterior iliopsoas transplantation and the treatment of paralytic dislocation of the hip. J Bone Joint Surg Br 46:426, 1964.

24. Sharrard WJ: Management of paralytic subluxation and dislocation of the hip in myelomeningocele. Dev Med Child Neurol 25:374, 1983.

25. Sprenger TR, Foley CJ: Hip replacement in a Charcot joint: a case report and historical review. Clin Orthop Relat Res 165:191, 1982.

26. Staeheli JW, Frassica FJ, Sim FH: Prosthetic replacement of the femoral head for fracture of the femoral neck in patients who have Parkinson disease. J Bone Joint Surg Am 70:565, 1988.

27. Turcotte R, Godin C, Duchesne R, et al: Hip fractures and Parkinson's disease: a clinical review of 94 fractures treated surgically [see comments]. Clin Orthop Relat Res 256:132, 1990.

28. Walker JL, Nelson KR, Heavilon JA, et al: A. Hip abnormalities in children with Charcot-Marie-Tooth disease. J Pediatr Orthop 14:54, 1994.

29. Yngve DA, Lindseth RE: Effectiveness of muscle transfers in myelomeningocele hips measured by radiographic indices. J Pediatr Orthop 2:121, 1982.

30. Girdlestone G: Acute pyogenic arthritis of the hip: an operation giving free access and effective drainage. Lancet 1:419, 1943.

31. Widmann RF, Do TT, Doyle SM, et al: Resection arthroplasty of the hip for patients with cerebral palsy: an outcome study. J Pediatr Orthop 19:805, 1999.

32. Lampropulos M, Puigdevall M, Zapazko D, et al: Proximal femoral resection and articulated hip distraction with an external fixator for the treatment of painful spastic hip

33. dislocation in pediatric patients with spastic quadriplegia. J Pediatr Orthop B 17:27, 2008.

33. Schroeder K, Hauck C, Wiedenhofer B, et al: Long-term results of hip arthroplasty in ambulatory patients with cerebral palsy. Int Orthop 34:335, 2010.

34. Blake SM, Kitson J, Howell JR, et al: Constrained total hip arthroplasty in a pediatric patient with cerebral palsy and painful dislocation of the hip: a case report. J Bone Joint Surg Br 88:655, 2006.

35. Laguna R, Barrientos J: Total hip arthroplasty in paralytic dislocation from poliomyelitis. Orthopedics 31:179, 2008.

36. Lau JH, Parker JC, Hsu LC, Leong JC: Paralytic hip instability in poliomyelitis. J Bone Joint Surg Br 68:528, 1986.

37. Lee DY, Choi IH, Chung CY, et al: Fixed pelvic obliquity after poliomyelitis: classification and management. J Bone Joint Surg Br 79:190, 1997.

38. Lorente Molto FJ, Martinez Garrido I: Retrospective review of L3 myelomeningocele in three age groups: should posterolateral iliopsoas transfer still be indicated to stabilize the hip? J Pediatr Orthop B 14:177, 2005.

39. Walker JL, Nelson KR, Heavilon JA, et al: Hip abnormalities in children with Charcot-Marie-Tooth disease. J Pediatr Orthop 14:54, 1994.

40. Chan G, Bowen JR, Kumar SJ: Evaluation and treatment of hip dysplasia in Charcot-Marie-Tooth disease. Orthop Clin North Am 37:203, 2006.

41. Weber M, Cabanela ME, Sim FH, et al: Total hip replacement in patients with Parkinson's disease. Int Orthop 26:66, 2002.

42. Idjadi JA, Aharonoff GB, Su H, et al: Hip fracture outcomes in patients with Parkinson's disease. Am J Orthop 34:341, 2005.

43. Bezza A, Ouzzif Z, Naji H, et al: Prevalence and risk factors of osteoporosis in patients with Parkinson's disease. Rheumatol Int 28:1205, 2008.

44. Fink HA, Kuskowski MA, Taylor BC, et al: Association of Parkinson's disease with accelerated bone loss, fractures and mortality in older men: the Osteoporotic Fractures in Men (MrOS). Osteoporos Int 19:1277, 2008.

45. Sato Y, Honda Y, Iwamoto J: Risedronate and ergocalciferol prevent hip fracture in elderly men with Parkinson disease. Neurology 68:911, 2007.

46. Stenager E, Jensen K: Fractures in multiple sclerosis. Acta Neurol Belg 91:296, 1991.

47. Pouwels S, Lamohamed A, Leufkens B, et al: Risk of hip/femur fracture after stroke: a population-based case-control study. Stroke 40:3281, 2009.

48. DiCaprio MR, Huo MH, Zatorski LE, Keggi K: Incidence of heterotopic ossification following total hip arthroplasty in patients with prior stroke. Orthopedics 27:41, 2004.

49. Youm T, Aharonoff G, Zuckerman JD, Koval KJ: Effect of previous cerebrovascular accident on outcome after hip fracture. J Orthop Trauma 14:329, 2000.

50. Ramnemark A, Nilsson M, Borssen B, Gustafson Y: Stroke, a major and increasing risk factor for femoral neck fracture. Stroke 31:1572, 2000.

51. de Moraes Barros Fucs PM, Svartman C, de Assumpcao RM, Kertzman PF: Treatment of the painful chronically dislocated and subluxated hip in cerebral palsy with hip arthrodesis. J Pediatr Orthop 23:529, 2003.

CHAPTER 81

Previous Hip Arthrodesis

Mark J. Spangehl

KEY POINTS

- Conversion of a previously arthrodesed hip to total hip replacement is indicated for pain relief in surrounding joints, and less often for pain relief in the fused hip. However, patients may also seek conversion because of disability related to the immobile hip, or before undergoing ipsilateral total knee replacement.[11-13]
- Surgical exposure is dependent upon the type of arthrodesis and the presence and location of hardware, but it typically requires a more extensile approach (standard or extended trochanteric osteotomy or trochanteric slide). The inferior aspect of the acetabulum is the most important landmark to help with preparation and placement of the socket.
- Abductor strength may continue to improve for 2 to 3 years after conversion.[14,15]
- Range of motion remains restricted compared with conventional primary total hip replacements.
- Full function, without pain or the use of walking aids, and a negative Trendelenburg sign can be obtained in only a minority of cases, yet a large majority of patients are satisfied with the result of their conversion.

INTRODUCTION

Changing patient expectations and improved results with hip replacement have led to a decreased demand for hip arthrodesis. Fusion of the hip is now rarely performed for end-stage degenerative hip disease. Nevertheless, hip fusion allows for long-term pain relief and provides adequate function for individuals who may not be candidates for total hip replacement. However, the disability resulting from an arthrodesed hip may, over time, result in the need for conversion of the fused hip to a total hip replacement.

Total hip replacement after previous hip arthrodesis is a challenging procedure. It may be considered in patients who have developed pain and disability in surrounding joints as a result of increased stress placed on these joints by the stiff hip. Long-term sequelae of hip arthrodesis include an increased incidence of pain and degenerative changes in the lumbar spine, ipsilateral knee, and contralateral hip.[1-10]

INDICATIONS/CONTRAINDICATIONS

Indications for conversion of an arthrodesed hip to a total hip replacement most commonly include disabling low back pain, ipsilateral knee pain, and contralateral hip pain.[1-10] Increased degenerative changes occur in these joints owing to increased stress placed through the joints juxtaposed to the fused hip. Poor range of motion after knee replacement in patients with ipsilateral hip arthrodesis has been documented, and conversion of the fused hip to a mobile hip before knee replacement has been advocated by some authors.[11-13]

Although pain in the fused hip typically is not an indication for surgery, increasing pain from a pseudarthrosis and functional disability from a malpositioned arthrodesis are additional indications for conversion.

Last, even in the absence of the previous indications, patients may seek conversion of an arthrodesed hip to a mobile hip replacement as they become less willing to accept the inconvenience and increased energy expenditure during gait that an arthrodesed hip places on activities of daily living.[16,17]

Alternatives to conversion of an arthrodesed hip relate to treatment of the symptomatic joint or joints around the fused hip. Generally, conversion of the fused hip is undertaken after nonoperative treatment of these joints has failed. Failed nonoperative management of low back pain is the most common reason for conversion. Surgical treatment of mechanical low back pain should not be considered until after conversion of a fused hip is performed. Surgical management of mechanical low back pain before conversion of a fused hip is much less likely to be successful because of ongoing stress placed through the lumbar spine as a result of the fused hip. Pain relief in the ipsilateral knee or the contralateral hip is less predictable after conversion of a fused hip (see "Results"), and surgical treatment may be required before or after conversion of the fused hip depending on the severity of symptoms and degenerative changes in these joints.

Absolute contraindications to conversion of an arthrodesed hip are similar to those for primary or revision hip replacement surgery. Active or suspected infection and poor medical health are contraindications to this surgery. Relative contraindications include young age in a patient in whom the hip is fused in an acceptable position (20 degrees flexion, 5 degrees external rotation, neutral abduction/adduction),[3] particularly if returning to heavy labor; severely distorted anatomy that would preclude restoration of near-normal biomechanics or would place the hip replacement at high risk of failure; and poor or absent abductor musculature.

Patients who expect complete or near-complete relief of symptoms in surrounding joints or a normally functioning hip replacement must be counseled as to the outcome of conversion of an arthrodesed hip to a hip replacement (see "Results"). Results typically are not comparable with those of primary hip replacement, and although improvement is noted in the symptoms of surrounding joints, particularly low back pain, complete relief of symptoms is unlikely.

PREOPERATIVE PLANNING

Routine preoperative radiographs (anteroposterior [AP] pelvis, AP hip, and true lateral hip) are usually the only imaging studies required preoperatively, provided that no significant distortion of anatomy or usual placement of hardware is noted (Fig. 81-1A through C). If distorted anatomy is present (e.g., extra-articular arthrodesis, large amount of heterotopic bone), a preoperative computed tomography (CT) scan is helpful for defining anatomy and identifying anterior or inferomedial bone bridges or hardware.

Electromyography need not be used routinely in the preoperative workup for evaluation of abductor function. The use of electromyography to assess gluteal muscle function is of limited value and does not correlate well with postoperative abductor function.[12] Postoperative abductor muscle function can be best predicted by preoperative palpation of contracting abductor musculature and, more important, by intraoperative assessment of muscles.[15,18] The intraoperative assessment has been shown to correlate well with return of postoperative abductor function.[7,14,15] Even

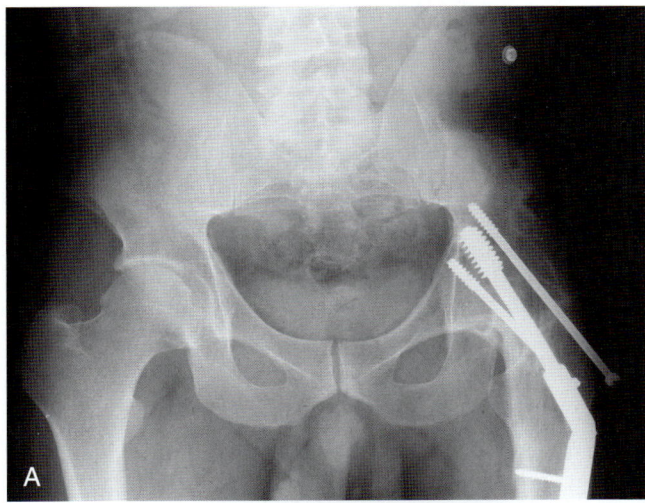

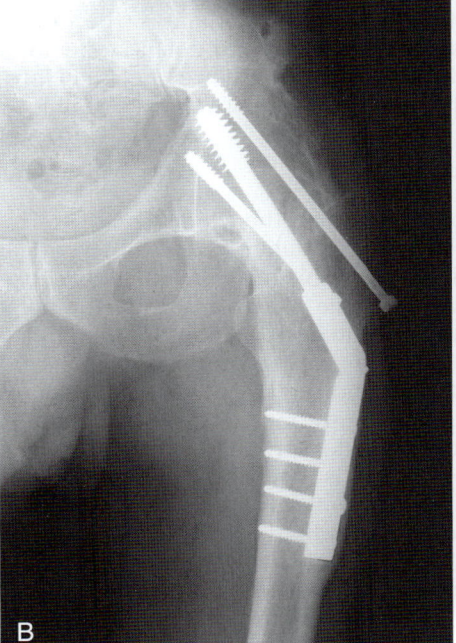

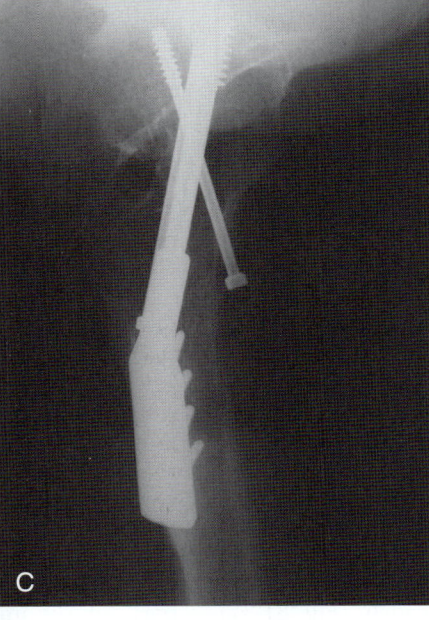

Figure 81-1. **A** through **C,** Routine preoperative radiographs before takedown of a left hip fusion. **A,** Anteroposterior (AP) pelvis radiograph of a 46 y/o male who underwent left hip arthrodesis at the age of 32 for post-traumatic arthritis. He was a laborer working on a pipeline. **B,** AP left hip radiograph. **C,** True lateral left hip radiograph. Note that the trochanter is present and is not damaged. (*Radiographs courtesy Dr. M. Cabanela, Mayo Clinic Rochester.*)

severely atrophied muscle can recover acceptable function if it otherwise appears intact and healthy (bleeding and red in appearance).

Additional equipment, apart from that required for insertion of the implants, should be available. Metal cutting burrs, broken screw extractors, and fluoroscopy may be required to remove hardware or to identify bony landmarks. Additionally, the surgeon should be familiar with the technique that was used for the index arthrodesis of the hip because this may influence the exposure and the need for bone removal, particularly with an extra-articular arthrodesis.

DESCRIPTION OF TECHNIQUE

Technique

Conversion of a hip arthrodesis to total hip replacement is a technically demanding procedure. Important technical considerations include adequate exposure with maintenance or restoration of abductor function, removal of hardware, if present, and careful identification of bony landmarks to ensure proper implant orientation.

Exposure

Positioning is done by surgeon preference, but typically the patient is placed in a lateral decubitus position because this allows for a more extensile acetabular exposure if required. The skin incision is dictated by the previous incisions and the need for hardware removal. If no incision is present, a lateral incision is used, centered over the trochanter and curving posteriorly at the proximal end. Any hardware overlying the trochanter and the proximal femur is removed. If a previous trochanteric osteotomy was performed at the time of fusion, and if the hardware is beneath the trochanter and the outer table of the pelvis (e.g., Cobra plate), then a classic trochanteric osteotomy is required (Fig. 81-2). Otherwise, a trochanteric slide with retraction of the trochanteric fragment anteriorly generally provides sufficient exposure and reduces additional trauma to the abductors. A short extended osteotomy, with soft tissue attachments maintained, may be preferred to facilitate closure and healing of the osteotomy. A more formal or a longer extended osteotomy may be required if a proximal femoral deformity that requires correction is present. If a trochanteric fragment is absent because of previous surgery, a posterior approach with anterior elevation of the remaining abductors, along with the anterior portion of the vastus lateralis, can be used. Soft tissues are then further cleared from the arthrodesis and the proximal femur for identification of the femoral neck. If a bony bridge exists between the femur and the ischium, the bridge is osteotomized and resected before or after osteotomy of the femoral neck. Care should be taken to protect the sciatic nerve in this region. The femoral neck is then identified and retractors placed around the neck anteriorly and posteriorly (Fig. 81-3). An initial femoral neck osteotomy is made somewhat

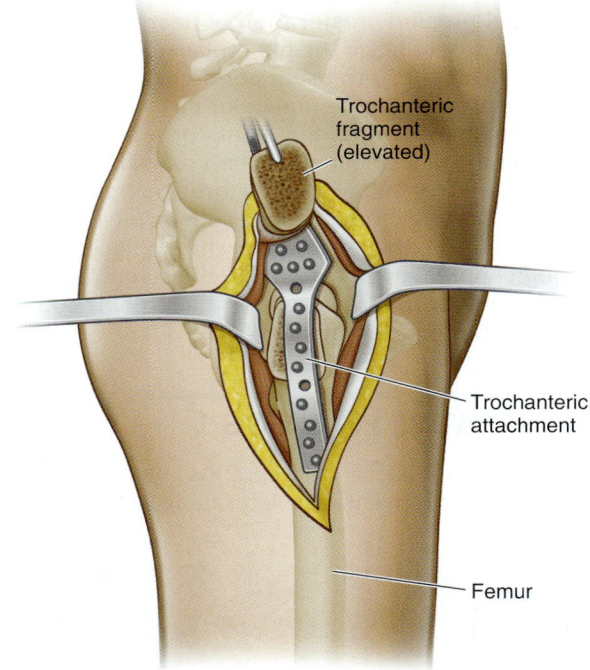

Femur labels:
- Trochanteric fragment (elevated)
- Trochanteric attachment
- Femur

Figure 81-2. Illustration of a hip exposure using a classic trochanteric osteotomy elevating the trochanter off of a Cobra plate. The trochanter is reflected superiorly to the left and is held with a clamp, exposing the Cobra plate laying on the lower ilium above the acetabulum. The trochanteric bed is also seen over the Cobra plate because the trochanter had been fixed over the plate at the time of fusion.

more proximally than the anticipated final cut, and further release of soft tissues around the proximal femur improves exposure. Based on preoperative templating and identification of bony landmarks (the greater or lesser trochanter), a revised and definitive femoral neck cut is performed. A slightly lower neck cut provides additional exposure to prepare the acetabulum.

Bone Preparation

Bony preparation is begun on the acetabular side. The inferior aspect of the acetabulum is the most critical landmark to be identified. This may be difficult because of the bone overlying the floor of the acetabulum; however, this landmark may be located by identifying the superior aspect of the obturator foramen and placing a retractor around the most inferior portion of the acetabulum. The anterior and posterior walls must also be identified for proper placement of the reamer before reaming is begun. A blunt retractor carefully placed over the anterior wall is helpful in maintaining exposure and orienting oneself to the anterior wall. Once this is accomplished, the acetabulum is carefully deepened and widened with reamers. Often, particularly in cases of spontaneous fusion, as the acetabulum is deepened, soft tissues (transverse

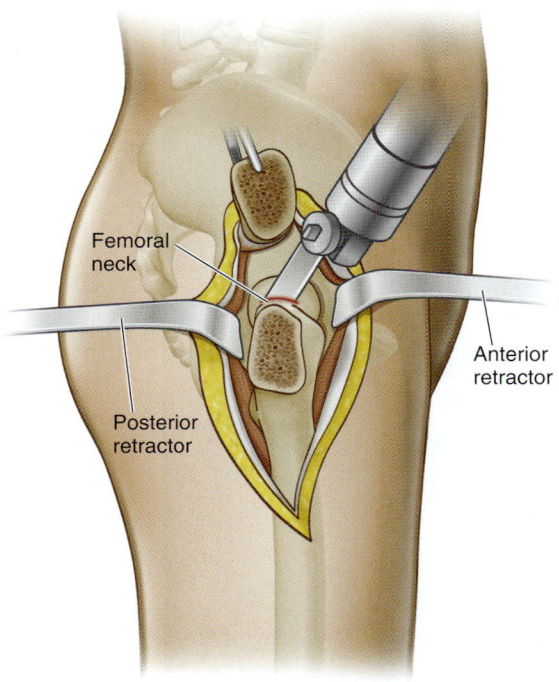

Figure 81-3. Illustration of the hip exposed with retractors placed anteriorly *(top)* and posteriorly *(bottom)* around the femoral neck. A femoral neck osteotomy is then made. An initial cut can be made more proximally, and once the femur is mobilized, a second definitive cut can be made more distally.

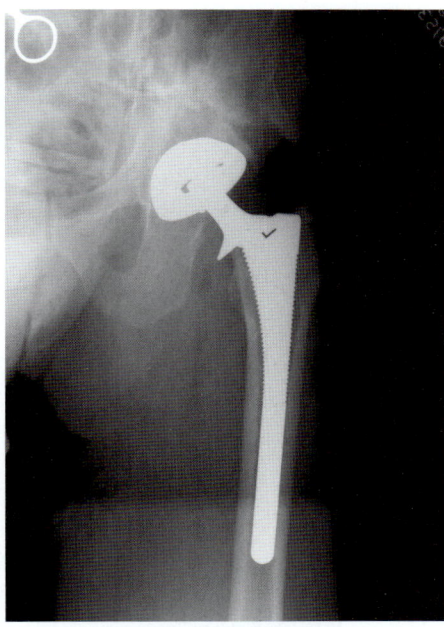

Figure 81-4. Intraoperative radiographs *(same patient as Fig. 81-6)* with trial implants in place ensuring proper positioning of both acetabular and femoral components. *(Radiographs courtesy Dr. M. Cabanela, Mayo Clinic Rochester.)*

acetabular ligament or remnants of the ligamentum teres) are recognized in the floor of the acetabulum. Careful attention to the thickness of the anterior and posterior walls is necessary during preparation of the socket. An intraoperative radiograph may be helpful early in preparation of the socket to ensure proper positioning of the reamer in the superior-inferior direction (Fig. 81-4). Additionally, if severe distortion of the anatomy is noted, placement of a K-wire as a marker before a radiograph is obtained will assist in orientation. Once the acetabulum is prepared, a trial socket is inserted. Femoral preparation is then performed according to the type of femoral implant used.

Prosthesis Implantation

Femoral prosthetic selection depends on the patient's bone quality, the presence of any cortical defects or stress risers related to hardware removal, and the amount of deformity in the proximal femur, as well as the plan for its correction. The patient's age and activity level, and the surgeon's general preference regarding implant fixation, are also factors considered in selection of the prosthesis.

On the acetabular side, uncemented fixation can be used. In cases of distorted anatomy or defects in bone, autogenous bone graft from the femoral head and supplemental screw fixation may be required. On the femoral side, an uncemented implant is generally favored because most patients undergoing conversion would be in a relatively younger age group (younger than 70 years) and would have bone of sufficient quality to support stable fixation with an uncemented implant. Proximal fixation may be used if the proximal metaphyseal bone is of good quality (Fig. 81-5A and B). Distal fixation typically is used if the proximal metaphyseal bone is distorted or is significantly compromised by prior hardware or deformity; if an extended trochanteric osteotomy is required for exposure or correction of deformity; or if a long plate was removed from the proximal femur, because the presence of multiple stress risers and stress-shielded bone under the plate would make proximal fixation less appropriate because of risk of fracture (Fig. 81-6A and B). Rarely, the femur may have considerable disuse osteopenia, making stable fixation with an uncemented implant difficult. The use of a cemented stem may be more appropriate in this situation with care taken to avoid cement at the trochanteric osteotomy interface.

A large femoral head and liner (36 mm or larger) is preferred, particularly if the abductors are deficient, or if the patient is at high risk for postoperative instability.

Before final component implantation, a trial reduction is performed to decide the appropriate neck length for soft tissue tension and leg lengths. Palpation of the sciatic nerve should be performed to ensure that it is mobile with the hip slightly flexed and the knee extended. If excess tension on the nerve is noted, the neck length or the femoral component position may need to be adjusted. The risk of stretching the sciatic

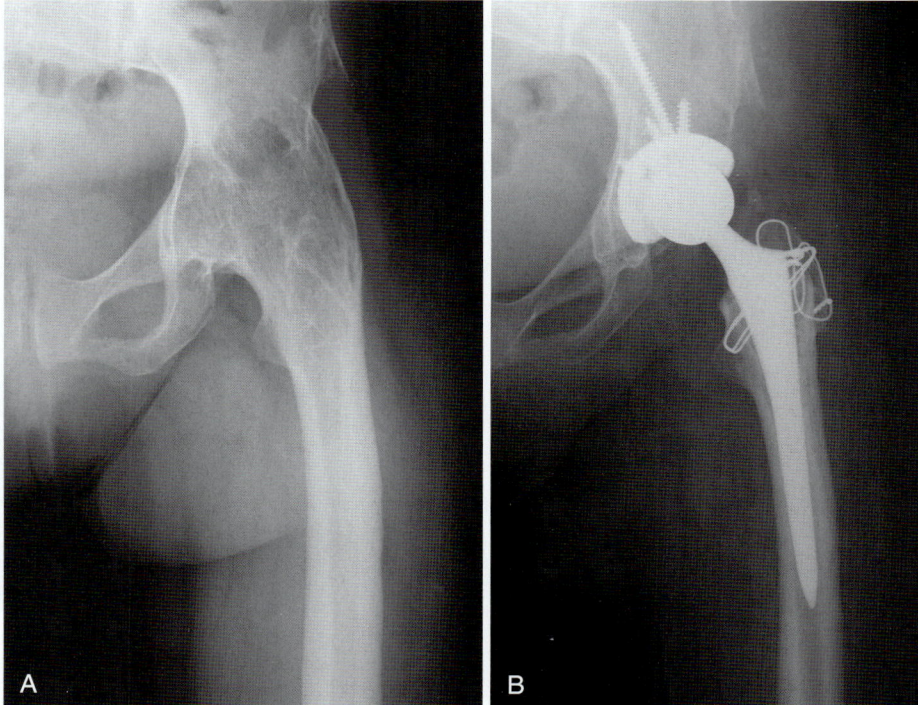

Figure 81-5. Preoperative and postoperative radiographs of a 34-year-old female who injured her hip at age 13, resulting in an arthrodesis. **A,** Preoperative anteroposterior (AP) hip. Note the varus deformity involving the proximal femur. The metaphyseal bone is of good quality. **B,** Postoperative AP radiograph of the hip. A proximal porous-coated implant was used, avoiding the need to osteotomize and correct the deformity. A fully porous-coated implant relying on distal fixation would have required a corrective osteotomy. *(Radiographs courtesy Dr. R. Trousdale, Mayo Clinic Rochester.)*

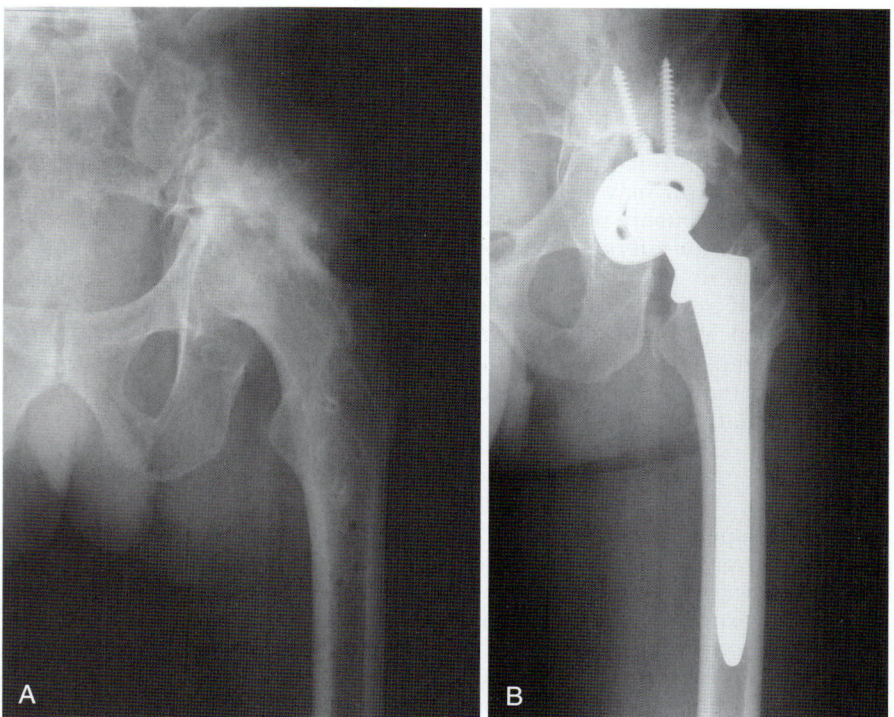

Figure 81-6. **A** and **B,** Preoperative and postoperative radiographs of conversion of a hip fusion to total hip replacement. **A,** AP left hip showing hip fusion for post-traumatic arthritis in a 39-year-old male. He had sustained multiple injuries from a motor vehicle accident. Arthrodesis had been achieved with an anterior plate, which was subsequently removed. Note the screw holes in the proximal femur. **B,** AP radiograph of the left hip postconversion. A fully porous-coated implant was used for the femoral reconstruction. *(Radiographs courtesy Dr. M. Cabanela, Mayo Clinic Rochester.)*

nerve likely depends on the age of the patient and the amount of shortening that is noted at the time of arthrodesis. In most cases, the lower extremity will be short relative to the opposite side before conversion is performed. Excessive lengthening (>3 to 4 cm) should be avoided because of concerns about injury to the sciatic or femoral nerves, and because of difficulties associated with trochanteric reattachment.

Before closure, the hip should be placed through a range of motion to assess positions of risk for dislocation and to carefully inspect for bony impingement. Even if no direct bony contact occurs, areas of potential impingement should be removed. The converted hip will lack the motion of a primary hip replacement immediately after conversion; however, over time this may improve. Increased motion over time may result in bony impingement, potentially causing pain or instability, hence the need to remove possible areas of impingement at the time of conversion.

Wound Closure

The trochanteric osteotomy is closed with wires or cables. A claw or grip device can be avoided if a short extended osteotomy is used. If the trochanter is absent, the abductors or lateral scar tissue may be sutured to the proximal femur and closed to the posterior soft tissue sleeve. Alternatively, the tensor fascia lata may be sutured to the trochanter or the proximal femur to improve abductor function. An adductor tenotomy or psoas tendon release may be required if hip abduction is limited.

Tips and Pearls

Additional trauma to the abductors should be minimized as much as possible, and, if the location of the hardware or the prior incision allows, a more abductor-sparing approach is preferred (trochanteric osteotomy or posterior approach).

A slightly lower femoral neck cut will provide for additional exposure and working room while the acetabulum is prepared.

The inferior aspect of the acetabulum is an important landmark to assist in proper cup placement.

If the acetabular anatomy is markedly distorted, placement of a K-wire and an intraoperative x-ray taken early during socket preparation will assist in proper placement of the acetabular component.

An adductor tenotomy will help hip abduction if the adductors are excessively tight.

Remove areas of potential bony impingement (even if direct bony impingement is not seen at the time of conversion) because range of motion will likely improve over time, causing possible bony impingement and pain or instability.

VARIATIONS/UNUSUAL SITUATIONS

Some older techniques of hip arthrodesis result in intrapelvic hardware (washers and nuts used for screw fixation across the joint). The hardware can remain against the inner table of the pelvis, deep to the iliacus muscle; a separate retroperitoneal exposure is not required to remove the hardware.

Patients whose hip fusions were secondary to tuberculosis infection represent a unique group because of the concern of reactivation of quiescent tuberculosis. In a large series of 208 converted hips, patients who had a history of prior septic tuberculosis infection received a combination of rifampicin, isoniazid, and ethambutol for 6 weeks preoperatively and 3 months postoperatively.[19] However, these authors did not state how many patients in their series received this treatment.

POSTOPERATIVE CARE

Weight bearing after conversion depends on the adequacy of trochanteric fixation, the type of implants used, and the surgeon's philosophy regarding weight bearing after primary or revision total hip replacement. Patients with good trochanteric fixation may be allowed to partially bear weight; however, if the quality of fixation is at all in doubt, touch weight bearing should be maintained for 6 to 8 weeks after surgery. Active abduction is delayed for 8 weeks after surgery to allow for adequate trochanteric or abductor healing. Once the trochanteric osteotomy or abductors are well healed, active abduction exercises are started and are continued for at least a year. Improvement in abductor function has been noted to occur for 2 years or longer after surgery.[14,15]

Most conversions of an arthrodesed hip to a mobile hip replacement will remain stiff compared with the usual motion seen after primary hip replacement.[7,14,15] Patients with severely deficient or absent abductors may be at increased risk for dislocation, particularly if good motion is noted at the time of surgery. These patients should be braced in a hip abduction orthosis, restricting flexion and adduction for 6 to 12 weeks. Patients who are noted to remain stiff at the time of conversion can begin appropriate stretching exercises, avoiding extreme positions of risk for instability.

Routine antibiotics and thromboembolic prophylaxis should be given. Prophylaxis against heterotopic ossification is not routinely required. However, if the arthrodesis occurred spontaneously, or if the patient has risk factors for the development of heterotopic bone, then prophylaxis, preferably with radiation therapy, should be used. Extensive use of anti-inflammatories should be avoided because this may delay or prevent trochanteric union, particularly if the bone and surrounding soft tissues are compromised.

RESULTS

Conversion of a previous hip arthrodesis to a total hip replacement is usually undertaken to relieve pain in surrounding joints, pain from a pseudarthrosis, or pain attributed to muscle fatigue in the fused hip, and to improve function and gait efficiency by converting a fused joint to a mobile joint. Therefore, results can be separated into (1) relief of symptoms in surrounding joints, (2) function and pain of the converted hip, (3) survival of the converted hip replacement, and (4) general patient satisfaction.

Pain Relief

Lower back pain is the most common complaint after long-standing hip fusion and thus is the most common indication for surgery. Most patients (between 61% and 94%) demonstrate significant improvement in lower back symptoms.[5,7,14,18,20] However, patients need to be counseled that up to one third may experience no improvement in lower back symptoms because of advanced degenerative changes. In a study of 45 patients undergoing conversion, 22 reported that their symptoms improved, and in 14 patients, symptoms were unchanged.[14] The authors noted that back pain is always improved in patients who have mild degenerative changes. Pain relief in other surrounding joints is less predictable and depends mostly on the degree of degenerative change of the affected joint. Patients with more advanced degenerative change eventually may require surgical treatment of those joints. Ipsilateral knee pain was improved in only one third of patients in one series.[15] However, other authors have reported somewhat more favorable results, with decreased knee pain in 10 of 15 patients in whom knee pain was present before the time of conversion.[14] Four patients in this series required total knee replacement soon after conversion. Similarly, relief of contralateral hip pain depends on the extent of degenerative change present within the hip.

Function and Pain of the Converted Hip

Patients generally are pleased with the function of the converted hip, accepting inferior results compared with routine primary hip replacement in exchange for increased mobility of the converted hip. Despite good patient satisfaction, outcomes consisting of decreased muscle strength, a greater need for walking aids, and poorer range of motion are more frequently seen in converted hips when compared with primary hip replacements.* Abductor muscle strength can continue to improve for years after surgery, with some authors noting improvement for up to 3 years, or longer, after conversion.[14,15] However, a substantial number of patients require walking aids and continue to limp after conversion. In several studies, the need for a walking aid ranged from 33% to 61%.[5-7,21] Some authors have shown that between 14% (5 of 36) and 74% (34 of 46) required greater walking aid support (e.g., from requiring nothing to using a cane, or from a cane to a walker) postoperatively.[15,22] Reduced range of motion, compared with routine primary hip replacement, is more commonly noted after conversion, with average flexion arcs

of between 74 and 88 degrees reported.[7,14,15] Approximately half of converted hips fail to achieve motion greater than 90 degrees.[7,14,15] Leg length discrepancy is usually improved after conversion. Generally the side of fusion is the shorter limb, and conversion decreases the discrepancy. The ability to equalize leg lengths depends on the magnitude of the discrepancy preoperatively, and the amount of scarring and the ability to release soft tissues without excessively lengthening the limb. A number of series have reported an improvement in leg length inequality, with average lengthening of the limb ranging from 2.2 to 2.9 cm without complications.[12,15,18] Improvement in leg length inequality can also be expected on the basis of correction of deformity. Correction of severe flexion or abduction deformity will reduce leg length inequality even in the absence of a change in true leg lengths. Residual pain in the converted hip is generally modest, but again is somewhat more common than after routine primary hip replacement. In a large series of 208 conversions, 79% were pain free or had minimal pain.[19] In another series of 45 conversions, 96% of patients were pain free postoperatively in the converted hip.[14]

Survival of the Converted Total Hip Replacement

Survival of the converted hip replacement shows variable results depending on the series reported. Most series have combined various types of hip replacements, including cemented and uncemented implants, with results that often span decades. This variable use of implants and prolonged duration of reporting make interpretation and comparison between series, or extrapolation to contemporary implants, impossible. Nevertheless, some authors have reported excellent survival results. A large series of 208 conversions reported 96% survival at 10 years and 90% at 15 years with revision for any reason as an endpoint.[19] Another recent study of 45 consecutive conversions demonstrated 10-year survival of 91%.[14] Other reports have been less encouraging; one series of previously surgically fused patients reported mechanical failure in 11 of 60 hips at 9 to 15 years' follow-up, and another reported a 15% (7 of 46) failure rate with similar follow-up.[10,22] The authors of the latter study relate most of the failures to the use of inferior prostheses.[22] In some series, implant survival has been related to spontaneous versus surgical fusion. Some series have reported higher failure rates in patients who had surgical fusions[5,15]; others have noted no difference.[14,19,21]

Overall Patient Satisfaction

Despite a less predictable outcome compared with primary total hip arthroplasty, the common occurrence of a limp, and the need for a walking aid in many patients, overall patient satisfaction is high. Functional outcomes are more similar to those of revision hip replacement than primary hip replacement, yet patients generally are happy with the restored mobility and improved function that the converted hip usually provides.

---

*See References 5, 7, 14, 15, 21, and 22.

Table 81-1. Results of Various Studies on Conversion of Hip Arthrodesis to Total Hip Replacement*†

Author/Year	No. of Hips	Average Age at Conversion, yr (range)	Follow-up, yr (range)	Age at Fusion	Age at Conversion	Duration of Fusion	Spontaneous vs. Surgical Fusion	Other Results
Peterson et al/2009	30	52.5 (27-70)	10.4 (2-20.5)	Not reported	<50 years: higher failure rate, but better function	<30 years: higher failure rate, but better function	Surgical fusion: higher failure	86% 5-year and 75% 10-year survival: 10 unsuccessful (3 for pain, 7 for failure); 2 dislocations
Joshi et al/2002	208	51 (20-80)	9.2 (2-26)	≤Age 15: poorer outcome ? Related to underdeveloped abductors; >15 better functional scores	Not reported	Not reported	Spontaneous fusion: slightly higher functional result	96% 10-year and 90% 15-year survival: 5 dislocations (4 in patients fused at age <15); 15 nerve palsies; 79% min pain or pain free; 83% good/excellent function
Hamadouche et al/2001	45	55.8 (28-80)	8.5 (5-21)	No impact	No impact	Trend for higher functional scores with shorter duration of fusion	No impact	91% 10-year survival: walking ability was associated with quality of gluteal muscles intraoperatively; walking improved for 2-3 years; 50% used cane
Reikeras et al/1995	46	58 (33-75)	8 (5-13)	Younger age at fusion: more satisfied	Not reported	Shorter duration: more satisfied	Not reported	76% good/ excellent; 85% satisfied; 74% walking aid: 15.2 revisions
Kilgus et al/1990	41	53 (24-75)	7 (2-16.5)	Not reported	<50: higher failure rate	Not reported	Surgical fusion: higher failure rate	4 deep infections; 5 mechanical failures; decreased Trendelenburg sign in patients whose abductor moment arm was restored; 74% required walking aid
Strathy and Fitzgerald/1988	80	50 (21-70)	10.4 (9-15)	Not reported	<50: higher failure rate	No impact	Surgical fusion: higher failure rate	9 deep infections; 1 failure in 20 spontaneous fused vs. 20 failures in surgically fused; 30 of 80 had poor results

*Highlighting variables affecting outcome.
†Only studies with a minimum of 30 hips are included in the table.

Various reports have shown that patient satisfaction ranged from 72% to 100%.[6,14,15,18,20]

Some authors have noted that longer duration of fusion, younger age at conversion (<50 years of age), multiple surgeries, and surgical arthrodesis were all risk factors for poorer clinical outcome.[5,10,14,15] Better results are generally reported in patients who were older at the time of conversion, who had had a spontaneous fusion, and whose abductors were in relatively good condition[5,10,15] (Table 81-1).

COMPLICATIONS

The types of complications that occur after conversion of an arthrodesed hip to a total hip replacement are similar to those seen with primary total hip replacement performed for degenerative joint disease; however, the incidence of complications is generally greater. The incidence of infection is usually higher, with reported rates in series that included 40 or more patients ranging from 0% to 11.3%.[10,15,19,21-23] Nerve palsy is more commonly seen after conversion; one large series reported an incidence of 7% (15 of 208 hips), another series 5% (4 of 86), with almost equal numbers of femoral and sciatic nerve palsies, and a third series 13% (15 of 112), with 11 having sciatic nerve involvement.[19-21] Dislocation does not seem to be substantially greater after takedown of arthrodesis; this may be related to the fact that the average range of motion is less than that of primary total hip replacement. Many authors have reported zero dislocations in reasonably large series of patients (45 to 112 patients).[7,14,20] However, patients with very deficient or absent abductors may be at increased risk of dislocation. In one large series of 208 conversions, 4 of 5 dislocations occurred in patients who were younger than 15 years of age at the time of hip fusion.[19] The authors concluded that underdeveloped abductors increase the risk of dislocation. Trochanteric nonunion reportedly has been as high as 14%, although other series report a lower incidence of approximately 5%.[7,19] The use of a trochanteric slide with maintenance of the vastus lateralis attachment or a short extended trochanteric osteotomy allowing wire or cable fixation of the proximal lateral cortex, while also maintaining the soft tissue attachments, may reduce the occurrence of trochanteric nonunion. Heterotopic bone (HO) formation was reported to occur in 13% of a large series of 208 patients.[19] No prophylaxis against heterotopic bone formation was used in any of these patients. Only 3 of 28 hips had Brooker class III heterotopic bone; the remaining patients had lesser-grade ossification. No patient had any functional limitation as a result of HO.

CURRENT CONTROVERSIES AND FUTURE CONSIDERATIONS

- The optimal patient population in which conversion of a previous hip arthrodesis can be expected to produce the best outcome is a matter of ongoing debate. Literature accounts conflict regarding how variables of age at time of fusion, duration of fusion, surgical versus spontaneous fusion, and age at time of conversion affect outcome (see Table 81-1).
- Relief of pain in surrounding joints, particularly back pain, is the main indication for conversion, yet patients need to be counseled that up to one third will experience no improvement in back symptoms. Despite this, most patients are satisfied and happy that they underwent the conversion procedure.
- It is very likely that the need for conversion of hip arthrodesis to hip replacement will continue to decrease as indications for hip arthrodesis also decrease in the industrialized world. This may not hold true for other areas of the world, where hip arthrodesis may still be an appropriate procedure for younger patients with hip disease.

REFERENCES

1. Beaule PE, Matta JM, Mast JW: Hip arthrodesis: current indications and techniques. J Am Assoc Orthop Surg 10:249–258, 2002.
2. Callaghan JJ, Brand RA, Pedersen DR: Hip arthrodesis: a long-term follow-up. J Bone Joint Surg Am 67:1328–1335, 1985.
3. Duncan CP, Spangehl MJ, Beauchamp CP, McGraw R: Hip arthrodesis: an important option for advanced disease in the young adult. Can J Surg 38(Suppl 1):S39–S45, 1995.
4. Panagiotopoulos KP, Robbins GM, Masri BA, Duncan CP: Conversion of hip arthrodesis to total hip arthroplasty. Instr Course Lect 50:297–305, 2001.
5. Peterson ED, Nemanich JP, Altenburg A, Cabanela ME: Hip arthroplasty after previous arthrodesis. Clin Orthop Relat Res 467:2880–2885, 2009.
6. Safer D, Dick W, Morscher E: Total hip arthroplasty after arthrodesis of the hip joint. Arch Orthop Trauma Surg 120:176–178, 2000.
7. Sirikonda SP, Beardmore SP, Hodgkinson JP: Role of hip arthrodesis in current practice: long term results following conversion to total hip arthroplasty. Hip Int 18:263–271, 2008.
8. Sponseller PD, McBeath AA, Perpich M: Hip arthrodesis in young patients: a long-term follow-up study. J Bone Joint Surg Am 66:853–859, 1984.
9. Stover MD, Beaule PE, Matta JM, Mast JW: Hip arthrodesis: a procedure for the new millennium? Clin Orthop Relat Res 418:126–133, 2004.
10. Strathy GM, Fitzgerald RH: Total hip arthroplasty in the ankylosed hip: a ten year follow-up. J Bone Joint Surg Am 70:963–966, 1988.
11. Garvin KL, Pellicci PM, Windsor RE, et al: Contralateral total hip arthroplasty or ipsilateral total knee arthroplasty in patients who have a long-standing fusion of the hip. J Bone Joint Surg Am 71:1355–1362, 1989.
12. Rittmeister M, Starker M, Zichner L: Hip and knee replacement after longstanding hip arthrodesis. Clin Orthop Relat Res 371:136–145, 2000.
13. Romness DW, Morrey BF: Total knee arthroplasty in patients with prior ipsilateral hip fusion. J Arthroplasty 7:63–70, 1992.
14. Hamadouche M, Kerboull L, Meunier A, et al: Total hip arthroplasty for the treatment of ankylosed hips: a five- to twenty-one-year follow-up study. J Bone Joint Surg Am 83:992–998, 2001.
15. Kilgus DJ, Amstutz HC, Wolgin MA, Dorey FJ: Joint replacement for ankylosed hips. J Bone Joint Surg Am 72:45–54, 1990.
16. Gore DR, Murray MP, Sepic SB, Gardner GM: Walking patterns of men with unilateral surgical hip fusion. J Bone Joint Surg Am 57:759–765, 1975.
17. Waters RL, Barnes G, Husserl T, et al: Comparable energy expenditure after arthrodesis of the hip and ankle. J Bone Joint Surg Am 70:1032–1037, 1988.
18. Brewster RC, Coventry MB, Johnson EW Jr: Conversion of the arthrodesed hip to a total hip arthroplasty. J Bone Joint Surg Am 57:27–30, 1975.

19. Joshi AB, Markovic L, Hardinge K, Murphy JC: Conversion of a fused hip to total hip arthroplasty. J Bone Joint Surg Am 84:1335–1341, 2002.

20. Hardinge K, Murphy JC, Frenyo S: Conversion of hip fusion to Charnley low-friction arthroplasty. Clin Orthop Relat Res 211:173–179, 1986.

21. Kim YH, Oh SH, Kim JS, Lee SH: Total hip arthroplasty for the treatment of osseous ankylosed hips. Clin Orthop Relat Res 414:136–148, 2003.

22. Reikeras O, Bjerkreim I, Gundersson R: Total hip arthroplasty for arthrodesed hips: 5- to 13-year results. J Arthroplasty 10:529–531, 1995.

23. Kreder HJ, Williams JI, Jaglal S, et al: A population study in the Province of Ontario of the complications after conversion of hip or knee arthrodesis to total joint replacement. Can J Surg 42:433–439, 1999.

CHAPTER 82

Protrusio Acetabuli

Douglas E. Padgett

KEY POINTS

- Clinical signs of protrusio acetabuli include groin pain, limited hip abduction, and often, a hip flexion contracture. Radiographic findings of the femoral head medial to the ilioischial line confirm the diagnosis of protrusio acetabuli.
- Preoperative planning for THR in protrusio should focus on restoration of offset on both acetabular and femoral sides. The key is to recognize that the anticipated socket will not lie in contact with the acetabular fossa but should be lateral, resulting in a gap medially between implant and bone.
- In exposing the hip with protrusio acetabuli, remember that forceful attempts at dislocation can result in fracture or significant soft tissue injury. Wide capsular exposure should help identify the proximal aspect of the femur: the neck and the trochanter. To facilitate dislocation, it is recommended to use bone hooks to provide lateral traction to the femur. If dislocation is not possible, in situ femoral neck osteotomy is indicated.
- Most complications that occur during exposure can be prevented by avoiding forceful manipulation of the femur. Anticipated use of in situ neck osteotomy or trochanteric osteotomy is much safer and is more predictable.
- The primary bone defect encountered in protrusio is a medial acetabular defect. This can be successfully managed by using the resected femoral head as autograft. The autograft bone should be denuded of cartilage remnants and morselized into 3- to 5-mm bits of graft, which can be compacted into the medial defect using a circular impactor or reamers in the reverse mode.

INTRODUCTION

Total hip arthroplasty has clearly been demonstrated to be a successful intervention for alleviation of pain and improvement in overall function.[1] Much of the functional improvement that occurs after total hip replacement (THR) can be attributed to increased range of motion.[2,3] Determinants of range of motion are dependent upon many factors, including implant position, intrinsic properties of the patient's soft tissues, and bony anatomy.[4] Prior chapters in this section have dealt with total hip arthroplasty in the setting of insufficient bone coverage as encountered in developmental dysplasia, as well as after fracture. The purpose of this chapter will be to discuss the evaluation and treatment of patients with protrusio acetabuli, in whom bony overcoverage is the prime problem.

Protrusio acetabuli—protrusion of the floor of the acetabulum into the true pelvis—was originally described by Otto, whose writing was later excerpted by Pomeranz.[5] As the acetabulum migrates medially, so does the femoral head. Radiographic features of **protrusio** are several, but most authors agree that (1) the floor of the acetabulum lies medial to the ilioischial line; (2) the femoral head is at or medial to the ilioischial line; (3) the center edge angle is greater than 40 degrees; and (4) the acetabular roof angle is negative[6,7] (Fig. 82-1). It has been suggested that the pattern of joint loading as a consequence of acetabular protrusion differs from that of the "normal" native hip. Specifically, larger joint reaction forces are found across the medial aspect of the femoral head, and over time, medial osteoarthritis ensues.[8] In some instances, the acetabular fossa lies medial to the ilioischial line, but the femoral head remains lateral to the ilioischial line, and the roof angle is normal. This condition, known as ***coxa profunda,*** is associated with intact articular cartilage and may be treated by joint preservation surgery such as acetabular rim trimming[9] (Fig. 82-1*A* through *C*).

The cause of protrusio acetabuli is not entirely clear. Two main categories of the condition have been identified: primary and secondary. Primary protrusio acetabuli is considered by some to be an acquired condition caused by incomplete or delayed fusion of the triradiate cartilage. The resulting chondrodystrophy leads to abnormal development of the medial wall of the acetabulum, resulting in protrusion.[10] McBride and associates nicely described the secondary causes of protrusio acetabuli, which include infectious, neoplastic, inflammatory, metabolic, traumatic, and genetic causes.[11] In addition, iatrogenic protrusio resulting from primary total hip arthroplasty has been observed (Fig. 82-2).

INDICATIONS/CONTRAINDICATIONS

The indication for total hip arthroplasty in the patient with protrusio acetabuli is similar to that in most other degenerative conditions about the hip: notably pain and loss of function. The clinical presentation of the patient

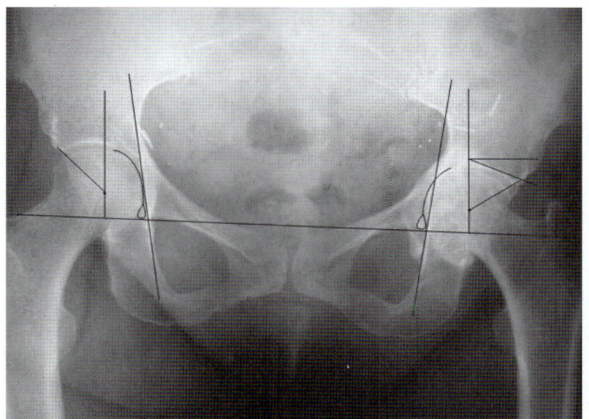

Figure 82-1. Radiograph of pelvis demonstrating the features of protrusio acetabuli.

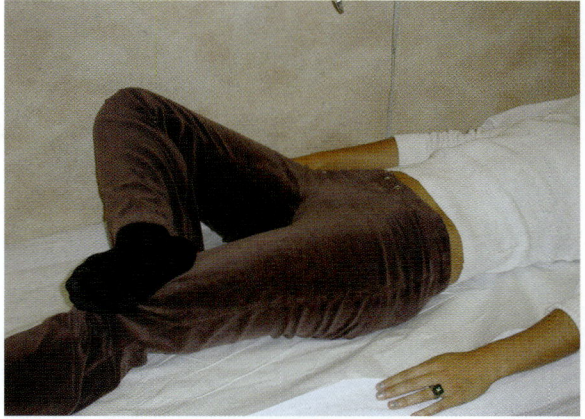

Figure 82-3. External rotation of the hip.

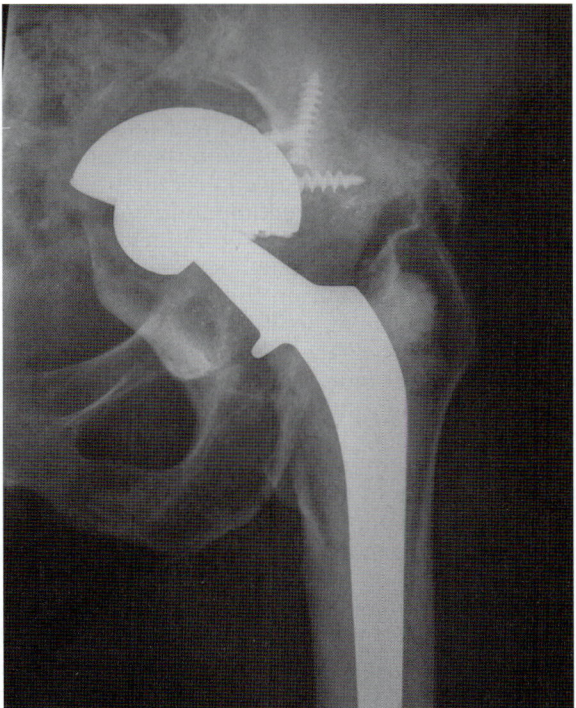

Figure 82-2. Iatrogenic protrusio resulting in catastrophic pelvic migration of the implant.

with protrusio acetabuli consists of groin pain as well as restriction in mobility. Often, the symptoms have been long-standing, and as stiffness ensues, pain is a less predominant feature. However, functional impairment is very noticeable. Given the higher prevalence of this condition in females, the diagnosis of hip pathology is often brought to the attention of the patient during annual pelvic examination, whereupon leg abduction is markedly diminished. In addition, as loss of hip extension (flexion contracture) progresses, patients develop a hyperlordotic posture and, not uncommonly, report having mechanical low back pain. Any of these symptoms should alert the clinician to the possibility of hip pathology and protrusion.

Physical examination of the patient with protrusio acetabuli commences with observation of gait. As stated, hyperlordosis of the lumbar spine and a shortened stance phase are hallmark features, especially in instances of bilateral disease. Given the high association of this condition with a variety of metabolic and rheumatologic conditions,[11] a general skeletal survey may be indicated. This includes cervical spine, upper extremities, thoracolumbar spine, hips, and knees, as well as foot and ankle.

Hip-specific features often include the presence of significant hip flexion contractures, as evidenced by the Thomas test. Frontal plane flexion often is not compromised, and the patient can continue with activities such as bike riding. However, the major obstacle is getting onto and off of the bicycle. Hip abduction is significantly compromised, as is rotation, especially external rotation (Fig. 82-3). Documentation of limb length equality is extremely important, especially when performance of a unilateral arthroplasty is contemplated.

Radiographic features of protrusio acetabuli have already been described. It cannot be emphasized enough that a feature often missed by clinicians is significant loss of medial joint space, as well as migration. Commonly, the presence of an "intact" superolateral joint space is interpreted as a "normal hip," and other sources of pain are investigated. This is often the case in the patient with stiffness, flexion contracture, and hyperlordosis of the lumbar spine who will be worked up for lumbosacral pathology. Educating colleagues who deal with spinal conditions about this common presentation has been successful in guiding patients to the appropriate treating physician.

Because of the frequent association of this condition with metabolic and rheumatic conditions, laboratory investigation is routinely suggested. Baseline complete blood counts and rheumatologic screening can be ordered, although direct referral to a rheumatologist for independent evaluation of these patients is preferable.

The primary indication for total hip arthroplasty in these patients consists of pain and loss of function as a result of motion loss in the presence of joint space obliteration. Although anti-inflammatory medications

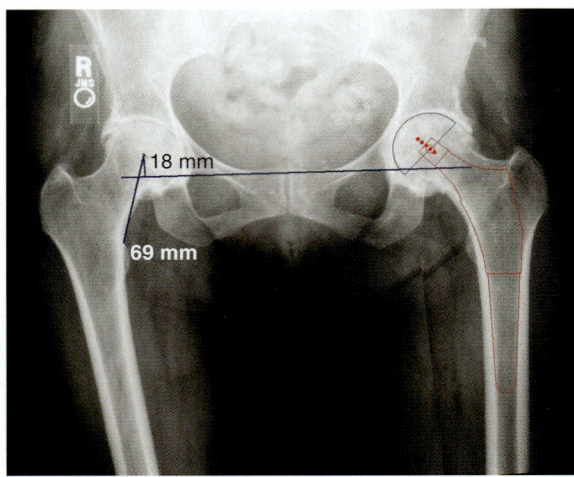

Figure 82-4. Anteroposterior (AP) radiograph of a preoperative plan for total hip arthroplasty in a patient with protrusio acetabuli. Preoperative templating is intended to facilitate restoration of the anatomical hip center and normal offset.

may alleviate some of the symptoms, function rarely improves. The role of physical therapy for the stiff, contracted patient is somewhat limited, and this intervention may be of marginal benefit in strengthening the patient in anticipation of surgery.

Contraindications for total hip arthroplasty in the patient with protrusio acetabuli are much the same as in other conditions:

1. Active infection
2. Neuromuscular conditions affecting abductor function
3. Cognitive dysfunction
4. Pain and stiffness in the presence of intact articular cartilage.

Joint preservation in the form of osteotomy (femur or acetabulum), acetabuloplasty, or a combination of any of these[12] should be considered for this condition.

PREOPERATIVE PLANNING

Preoperative planning for total hip arthroplasty in the setting of protrusio acetabuli should represent a synthesis of physical examination findings and thorough assessment by radiography. As has been stated, the four features of importance noted on examination include the following:

1. Leg length discrepancy (actual or functional)
2. Extent of contractures (flexion/adduction)
3. Degree of stiffness (rotation)
4. Unilateral disease/bilateral disease

These features may determine how effectively one can restore limb lengths. In cases of bilateral disease where reconstruction of only one hip is intended, discussion with the patient regarding the likelihood of the operative leg feeling, and probably actually being, longer is essential to minimize patient dissatisfaction postoperatively. The degree of stiffness of the affected hip is an early indication of how difficult exposure/

dislocation may be and of the potential need for alternative techniques for joint mobilization.

The goal of preoperative planning is restoration of the biomechanics of the hip to optimize range of motion, maximize efficiency of hip musculature, and minimize adverse loading conditions across the articulation.[13] The preoperative plan is a stepwise approach that is based on standardized radiographs. The key radiograph is the anteroposterior pelvic radiograph (Fig. 82-4). Most standard anteroposterior (AP) radiographs are approximately 20% magnified, as are standard templates from manufacturers. This should be confirmed by verification of magnification. The technique is as follows:

1. Draw in the inter-teardrop line. This line has been demonstrated to be the most reliable and reproducible landmark on the AP radiograph and the least affected by pelvic rotation.[14]
2. A perpendicular line is drawn from the inter-teardrop line to the lesser trochanter on each side. These distances are measured and compared. In typical superolateral osteoarthritis of the hip, the affected side will be shorter than the "nonaffected" side. This difference represents the limb length discrepancy attributable to hip pathology (and only hip pathology). It should be compared with the clinical assessment of limb length. Flexion contractures and coronal plane contractures (abduction/adduction) will affect clinical limb lengths. This will be further discussed in the chapter on limb length inequality.
3. The center of rotation on the "nonaffected" side is identified. The use of hemispherical acetabular templates can assist. Place the hemispherical template on the circumference of the femoral head, adjusting the size to match the sphericity. Mark the center of rotation. Note that this measurement does not take into account the articular cartilage layer and can vary by 1 to 2 mm.
4. Measure the distance from the lesser trochanter to the center of rotation on the "nonaffected" side (LT-COR).
5. The acetabular templates are now used on the symptomatic side. Two key issues are involved in templating the socket in protrusio acetabuli: **size and location.** The **size** of the acetabular socket is determined by the hemisphere that can be placed at the base of the teardrop and is angled 40 degrees superolateral. Both edges of the hemispherical template should fit at these points. The template will go beyond some of the subchondral bone in the dome: This is expected and represents the amount of bone to be reamed. The **location** of this cup should be on the periphery of the acetabular rim. In protrusio acetabuli, the templated socket will not contact the acetabular fossa. This is to be expected. The gap between the template and the medial extent of the fossa represents the area where bone graft is expected to be placed. This should be noted! The COR of the templated cup is then marked and recorded.
6. Note whether any difference between the two templated CORs is evident. If no difference between the CORs is noted, femoral reconstruction should match

the opposite side by mimicking the lesser trochanter–to–center of rotation measurement (LT-COR). If the reconstructed side has a COR greater than the "non-affected" side, the difference between the two numbers must be ADDED to the LT-COR measurement. If the COR on the reconstructed side is less than that on the "nonaffected" side, the difference between the two numbers is SUBTRACTED from the LT-COR measurement.

7. Femoral templating is then performed. Factors to consider include type of fixation and the ability to restore the mechanics of the hip, including offset. Pay particular attention to **femoral offset** when templating. Socket lateralization and bone grafting will increase lateralization of the femur from the patient's preoperative condition. This additional lateralization may cause excessive tension on the iliotibial band/abductors, resulting in an abduction contracture and significant functional leg lengthening, which can take months to rehabilitate. Regardless of the method of femoral fixation, mimicking the LT-COR and accounting for changes in acetabular effect upon COR will aid in minimizing limb length discrepancy.

8. Femoral measurements for planning include the level of the neck osteotomy, the size of the reamers and the implant to be inserted, and the final LT-COR measurement.

SURGICAL TECHNIQUE

The surgical technique of total hip arthroplasty in the hip with protrusio acetabuli can be broken down into three distinct aspects:
1. Surgical approach and exposure
2. Acetabular preparation and bone graft and cup insertion
3. Femoral preparation and component insertion

Surgical exposure of the hip with protrusio acetabuli should never be taken for granted. Regardless of the intended surgical approach, mobilization of the femur may be difficult owing to inward migration of the femoral head, as well as stiffness of the joint. The usual landmarks encountered in the arthritic hip, such as the greater trochanter and the femoral neck, may be difficult to assess owing to distortion. In using the posterolateral approach, a straight lateral incision is centered over the trochanter, extending from 1.5 cm above the trochanter distally for a distance of 6 to 8 cm. After the deep fascial layer is incised, a self-retaining retractor is inserted, and an attempt is made to identify the posterolateral trochanter, external hip rotators, and posterior neck.

Caveat: If the protrusio is severe, distinguishing between the greater trochanter and the posterior wall of the acetabulum may be difficult. Peeling back the external rotators and the posterior capsule and rotating the hip can provide clues as to the exact location (Fig. 82-5).

At this stage, mobilization of the femur is required. Three options are available for complete exposure:
1. Controlled dislocation with a bone hook
2. In situ neck osteotomy

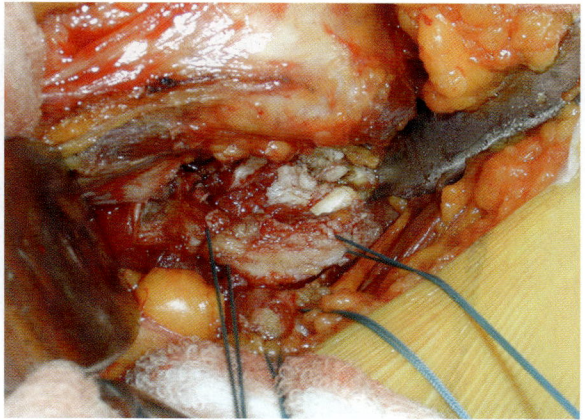

Figure 82-5. Tagged external rotators and posterior capsule revealing underlying posterior neck.

3. Trochanteric osteotomy followed by neck osteotomy

For most hips with protrusio acetabuli, **controlled dislocation** using a bone hook is possible; the key is to perform as complete a capsular incision as possible. In the case of a posterolateral approach, the capsule is incised from the level of the insertion of the reflected head of the rectus tendon all the way posteroinferiorly to the lesser trochanter. During this capsular release, a periodic check to ensure that the incision remains on the femur (not the posterior acetabulum) is performed by rotating the femur internally and externally and palpating landmarks. At this point, a pointed bone hook is placed beneath the inferior femoral neck, and as the assistant flexes and internally rotates the hip, lateral traction is applied, and the proximal femur is lifted out of the acetabulum (Fig. 82-6). If the femur is not sliding easily out of the acetabulum, then the soft tissue release is extended, or an alternative option is considered. **DO NOT FORCEFULLY ATTEMPT TO DISLOCATE THE HIP!** Forceful attempts at dislocation may result in fracture of the posterior wall of the acetabulum (Fig. 82-7), fracture of the proximal femur, or major ligamentous injury to the knee.

For the hip with more extensive protrusion and/or stiffness, such that controlled dislocation is not possible, **in situ neck osteotomy** is the preferred method used for exposure. The key to performing in situ neck osteotomy is identification of anatomic landmarks for localization. As in the controlled dislocation, capsular reflection and soft tissue release are crucial. In addition, frequent checks of anatomic landmarks using femoral rotation are advised. If possible, identify the lesser trochanter to approximate the level of the neck osteotomy. Alternatively, if the head-neck junction is visible or palpable, this is an excellent landmark. The key is to cut as high on the neck as possible: a secondary re-cut at the preoperatively planned level can be performed later. The goal at this juncture is extensive femoral mobilization. The hip is placed in a full extension position, and the leg is internally rotated 30 degrees. The osteotomy is performed just distal to the acetabular wall, ensuring a "high" neck cut (Fig. 82-8). Following the neck

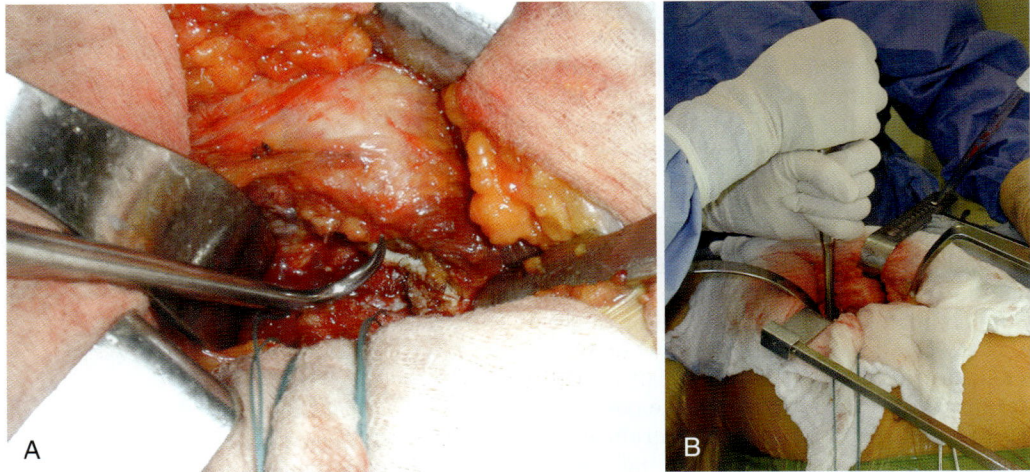

Figure 82-6. A and **B,** Pointed bone hook for controlled dislocation.

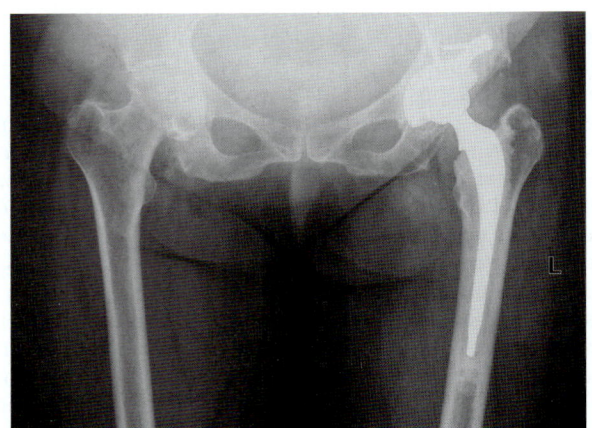

Figure 82-7. Fracture of the posterior wall of the acetabulum resulting from forceful hip dislocation requiring posterior pelvic plating.

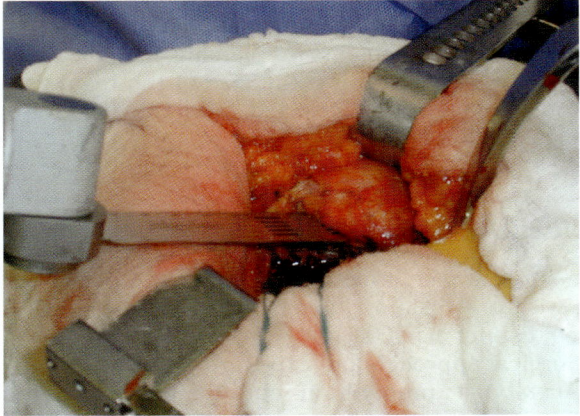

Figure 82-8. In situ neck cut with the saw blade entering just distal to the posterior wall. This ensures a "high" neck cut.

osteotomy, the hip can now be fully rotated, and a second neck resection is fashioned at a more precise and appropriate level. The proximal neck and head section is removed using a skid or a periosteal elevator.

In instances of severe protrusio with no discernible interval between the trochanter and the posterior wall of the acetabulum, a **trochanteric osteotomy** is recommended (Fig. 82-9). The extent of the trochanteric osteotomy is dependent upon the extent of mobilization of the trochanter required for visualization of the neck. This can vary from a trochanteric "flip"–sized fragment to a more extensive extended trochanteric osteotomy. Preoperative assessment of the radiographs will aid in determining the location and extent of the osteotomy.

Following femoral mobilization and neck osteotomy, **acetabular preparation** is performed. As in all aspects of orthopedic surgery, surgical exposure is critical; therefore, placement of acetabular retractors to optimize visualization is required. When a posterior

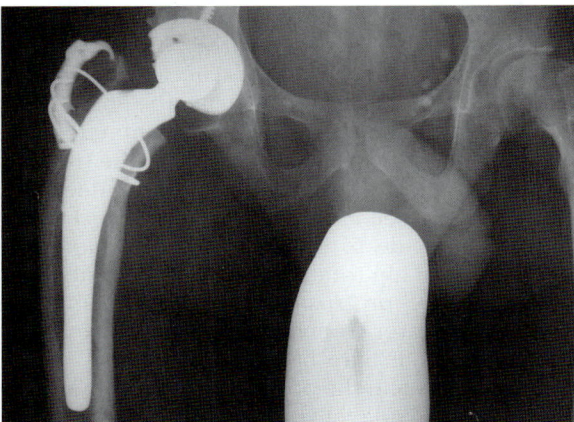

Figure 82-9. Trochanteric osteotomy performed for exposure and mobilization in this complex primary total hip arthroplasty.

approach is used, four regions require retraction. Initially, a curved Hohmann-type retractor moves the femur anteriorly. At the apex of the incision, a large Steinman pin is used to reflect the gluteus medius and minimus away from the acetabular vault. An angled Hohmann-type retractor is then placed posteriorly; it is preferably driven into the ischial tuberosity. Finally, a blunt retractor can be placed beneath the transverse acetabular ligament to complete the 360-degree exposure of the acetabulum. Removal of labral remnants is performed, although in many cases the labrum is calcified/ossified, requiring removal with a heavy knife or a rongeur. Unlike the typical osteoarthritic hip with superolateral cartilage loss and migration, the protrusio acetabuli will not have any discernible pulvinar or medial osteophyte. It is important to remember that the medial wall is thin and medialized. Commence at this point with a small-diameter reamer (preferably sharp); the goal is to gently remove any remaining articular cartilage while sparing the underlying bone. A small amount of bleeding bone is ideal. The concern at this juncture is less about acetabular shape and more about simply removing remaining cartilage. Any cartilage interface may compromise the ability of bone graft to adequately heal to underlying host bone, or may inhibit osseous integration if placed directly against a porous substrate.

Once the acetabular vault has been denuded of articular cartilage, the periphery of the acetabulum is sized by manually placing reamers into the socket mouth; the goal is peripheral fit/fixation. At this point, proceed with this size reamer, and insert on power until the reamer is 1 to 2 mm below the rim of the acetabulum. This is the desired depth of insertion. Remember: **Do not bottom out the reamer!** The goal is to lateralize the socket. Sequentially enlarge the reamers until a good solid rim fit is obtained. This width of rim contact can range anywhere from 5 to 7 mm to as much as 20 mm, depending on the unique anatomy of the protrusio encountered. Maximizing bone contact in conjunction with implant stability is essential to ensure biological fixation. This should correspond to the templated socket size, and a gap should remain between the bottom of the reamer and the host bone; this is the region to be bone grafted.

Acetabular bone graft is often required in cases of protrusio acetabuli. Whether socket fixation is achieved by cement, is cemented with a reinforcement ring, or is cementless, the goal for reconstruction is to bring the socket center out laterally from its medial position to a more anatomic location. Options for the medial defect may include autograft, allograft, or bone synthetics. [15,16] Because it is readily available, femoral head autograft is most frequently used. Although excellent results have been reported using solid femoral head autograft in conjunction with medial mesh,[17] the use of particulate graft has increased in popularity. Observation of the predictable pattern of medial particulate graft consolidation and formation of dense sclerotic bone has been shown in revision total hip arthroplasty.[18] The technique initially involves graft harvesting; a useful method is to take small-diameter acetabular reamers and ream directly into the femoral head remnant. This will have to be done several times with periodic stops for removal of the cancellous bone graft from inside the reamer. Once all of the cancellous bone graft is obtained, the graft is then delivered into the mouth of the acetabulum. The final reamer used for acetabular preparation is introduced and is placed in a "reverse" mode. The graft should then be compressed with the reverse reamer in such a manner as to fill the defect (Fig. 82-10). The grafted area should feel "solid." If this is not the case, more graft is added. Once grafting is completed, socket insertion is performed. The type of acetabular fixation to be used is based upon surgeon preference. Cement, cement reinforcement rings, and noncemented porous-coated implants have all produced satisfactory results, but the current trend is to use cementless fixation. The acetabular shell is impacted into position. The shell to be inserted is the same size as, or is 1 to 2 mm larger in diameter than, the last reamer, depending on shell design. Because of the presence of the bone graft and the peripheral rim contact, the shell will have an excellent fit and is quite stable. However, with extensive medial bone graft, the use of adjuvant screw fixation is suggested for added stability (Fig. 82-11 & 82-12). At this point, it is important to confirm that the acetabular shell is at the socket rim and has not migrated medially. The acetabular liner is not inserted at this time; it should be noted that usually there is no need for any type of offset liner when this technique is used.

Femoral preparation is now performed. The type of femoral reconstruction is based upon preoperative assessment of bone morphology, bone quality, and

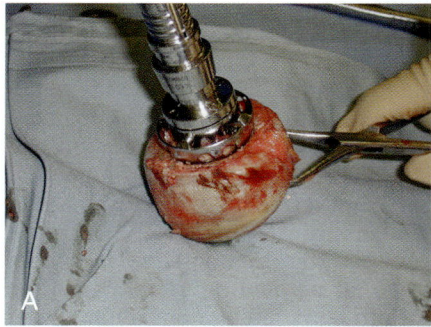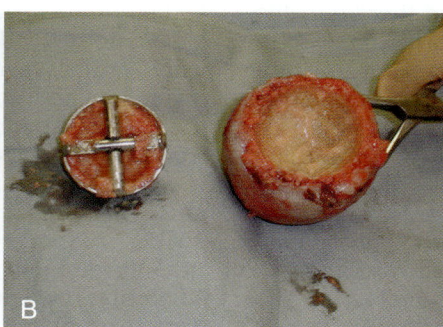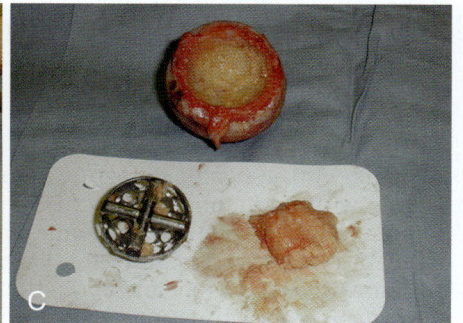

Figure 82-10. A through **C,** Autologous femoral head bone graft preparation using the technique of morselized bone and a reamer on reverse.

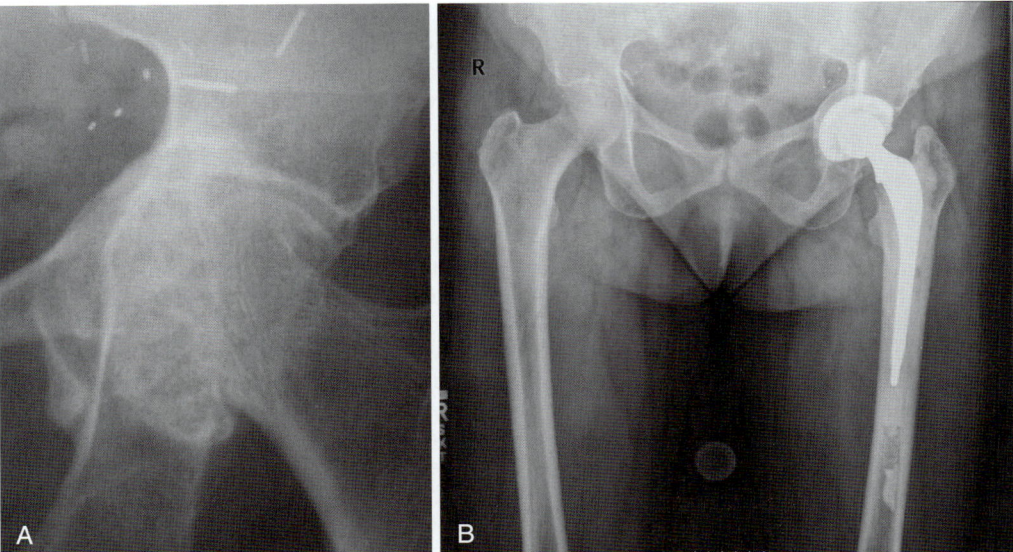

Figure 82-11. A Preoperative and 5-year postoperative radiographs demonstrating protrusio acetabuli reconstructed with the technique of medial bone graft, noncemented socket, and supplemental screw fixation. **B,** Five-year follow-up x-ray.

surgeon preference. As stated previously, the goal is to restore normal hip mechanics. The key task following femoral preparation and trial insertion is to check for impingement during range of motion. Impingement can be seen in the form of

1. A prosthetic femoral neck against the socket liner construct
2. A prosthetic neck against the acetabular rim
3. Bone-to-bone impingement (i.e., trochanter against pelvis)

Any of these can occur as a consequence of failure to restore adequate lateral offset of the femur. This must be checked both in flexion/internal rotation (posterior stability check) and in extension/abduction/external rotation (anterior stability check). If leg lengths and stability are satisfactory, final femoral component insertion is performed.

Closure is performed in the usual manner. Note that in the case of moderate to severe protrusio acetabuli, because of the lateral translation of the femur, it is common that the posterior soft tissue envelope of capsule and short rotators will not "reach" the posterolateral trochanter for repair. Unfortunately, mobilization of the capsule often is not sufficient, and there remains a soft tissue defect. This lack of soft tissue check rein serves as a reminder of how critical implant position and avoidance of impingement are in determining overall stability of the hip.

Often the patient with moderate to severe protrusio presents with a significant hip flexion contracture, as well as with adduction contractures. For many years, percutaneous adductor tenotomy had been recommended at the conclusion of total hip arthroplasty in the patient with significant abduction limitation. The performance of tenotomy has generally declined and is considered optional. Most patients, given appropriate improvement in lateral offset and relief of pain, can

recover this mobility simply by following an appropriate physiotherapy regimen.

VARIATIONS AND CAVEATS

The principal features of the technique have been highlighted throughout this chapter. The main variation consists of the extent of protrusio and how its severity influences all aspects of the procedure. In summary, the pertinent points are as follows:

1. Surgical exposure
2. Controlled dislocation or in situ neck resection
3. Acetabular inspection and cartilage removal
4. Socket preparation and bone grafting
5. Socket insertion ensuring rim fixation
6. Femoral insertion and check for stability

POSTOPERATIVE CARE

Postoperative features mandatory for any reconstruction involve two main questions: weight-bearing status and motion restrictions or precautions.

Despite the wide range of bone defects encountered when protrusio acetabuli is reconstructed, with adequate bone grafting and solid peripheral rim support of the socket supplemented with adjuvant screw fixation, **weight bearing as tolerated** is permitted (assuming satisfactory femoral fixation). The rationale is the need to immediately start loading the medially grafted bone to further compress the construct.

As mentioned, preoperative flexion deformity and adduction contracture are common. Patients often describe "apparent" limb lengthening due to hip center lateralization, which results in tightness along the iliotibial band (ITB)/tensor fascia lata. **Avoid** prescription of a shoe/heel lift; rather, it is better to start working at ITB stretching to encourage the pelvis to level out. The one exception is the patient in whom severe lumbar pain occurs. In that situation, short-term use of an orthotic may be appropriate. In addition to ITB stretching, patients must be instructed in how to perform anterior capsular stretching exercises by performing a modified Thomas stretch. This should be done daily and frequently. Progress in overcoming the hip flexion contracture can be gauged by gradual correction of the lumbar lordosis.

RESULTS

Excellent results of total hip arthroplasty in the setting of protrusio acetabuli have been reported since the days of Charnley.[19] In their original description, the authors documented the excellent outcome using cemented all-polyethylene acetabular components, with the medial defect filled with either bone cement or bone graft and no need for acetabular reinforcement mesh. The case for solid bone graft to fill the medial bone defect was made by Heywood.[20] In his series of nine procedures in which the technique of bulk medial autograft was used, all grafts were found to be incorporated, and all patients functioned well clinically. It was several years later that Crowninshield and colleagues performed finite element analysis, supporting the basic concept of restoring the more "normal" location of the acetabular center by lateralizing the cup. Their work suggested that sockets in a protruded location produced greater stresses along the medial pelvic wall. These stresses could affect the quality of the bone-cement interface and might lead to early failure of the interface.[21] The concept of restoration of the "anatomic" center of rotation was further supported by the clinical experience of Ranawat and associates.[22] In a select series of 35 total hip arthroplasties performed in patients with protrusio acetabuli, these authors were able to correlate radiographic evidence of implant loosening with suboptimal component position. Implants placed 1 cm or farther outside (superior or medial) of the anatomic triangle, representing an ideal position for the socket center of rotation, demonstrated a substantially higher incidence of progressive radiolucent lines suggestive of loosening.

Over time, several centers have validated the concept of medial grafting with or without the use of reinforcement rings and a cemented acetabular socket. McCollum and colleagues reported their early success in 32 patients using bulk medial graft. In 7 of these patients, a completely absent medial wall was compensated for with the use of a protrusio acetabular ring. Between 2 and 8 years' follow-up (mean, 4.7 years), all grafts had healed and no cases of socket loosening were reported.[23] An excellent subsequent follow-up of this cohort was provided by Gates and coworkers, who reported that at a mean of 12.8 years' follow-up, 20% of this group had acetabular loosening manifest by superior migration or, less commonly, recurrence of medial protrusio. These results were similar to the results of longer-term cemented socket fixation for nonprotrusio hips.[24] The predictable incorporation of femoral head graft was nicely shown by Ebert and associates, who reported 4-year results of the Heywood technique with bulk autograft. In their series of 35 hips, all grafts demonstrated consolidation, and no socket demarcations were identified on any radiographs.[25]

Although these results were outstanding, attempts at simply grafting the medial defect and avoiding the need for a fixed acetabular component appealed to some. Wilson and colleagues, using a technique of ground cancellous bone graft in conjunction with bipolar arthroplasty, showed graft incorporation in 17 of 22 hips reconstructed using this technique.[26] However, Brien and others reported on 18 patients who underwent acetabular reconstruction using the morselized grafting technique with a bipolar implant and noted that only 4 of the 18 (22%) demonstrated graft incorporation. These authors concluded that bone graft subjected to motion was prone to resorption, and that a fixed socket appeared warranted in these cases.[27]

Despite the success of medial bone graft and cemented socket fixation, by the late 1980s, socket fixation had clearly evolved to the use of press-fit porous-coated implants. Uncemented fixation in primary and revision total hip arthroplasty had by this time become the primary mode of socket fixation.[28,29] However, several reports have described the use of cementless acetabular fixation in the treatment of protrusio acetabuli. Mullaji and Marawar,[30] in a consecutive series of 30 hips using impacted morselized autogenous bone and a cementless socket, reported 100% graft incorporation and no instances of socket loosening at a mean of 4.2 years' follow-up. Krushell and colleagues employed a similar morselized bone grafting technique but used a dual geometry cementless socket for acetabular fixation. In their series of 29 hips evaluated at a mean of 4 years, these authors noted complete radiographic incorporation of bone graft in 93% and no instances of socket loosening, although in 17% of cases, some radiolucent lines were noted.[31] Because of these excellent results, the technique of morselized cancellous bone graft and cementless socket fixation appears to remain the recommended method of reconstruction at this time.

COMPLICATIONS OF PROTRUSIO ACETABULI

Complications associated with treatment of the patient with protrusio acetabuli are almost always technical in nature. Failure to lateralize the socket, leaving it in a more protruded position, is more of a technical flaw than a complication. However, overly vigorous graft insertion resulting in an inadvertent medial "blowout" is clearly a complication to be avoided. As seen in Figure 82-2, iatrogenic fracture in both primary and revision surgery is a real possibility. Steady graft compression using the reamer in reverse mode rather than bold impaction with a heavy mallet is the favored approach. Patients at greatest risk for this complication tend to be females with osteopenia/osteoporosis. GO SLOWLY!

FUTURE CONSIDERATIONS

Protrusio acetabuli is becoming a more frequently recognized entity. As our understanding of the pathoanatomy of both coxa profunda and protrusio increases, earlier recognition of the entity may allow sooner intervention, before global cartilage loss has occurred. The role of joint salvage procedures continues to evolve, and we eagerly await the results of studies evaluating the success of treatments such as acetabular rim trimming and osteotomy. However, techniques for reconstruction of the degenerative hip affected by protrusio acetabuli are well grounded at this time, and improvement in function and relief of pain are predictable following total joint arthroplasty.

REFERENCES

1. Charnley J: The long term results of low-friction arthroplasty of the hip performed as a primary intervention. J Bone Joint Surg Br 54:61–71, 1973.
2. Harris WH: Traumatic arthritis of the hip after dislocation and acetabular fractures: treatment by mold arthroplasty: an end-result study using a new method of result evaluation. J Bone Joint Surg Am 51:737–755, 1969.
3. Davis KE, Ritter MA, Berend ME, Meding JB: The importance of range of motion after total hip arthroplasty. Clin Orthop Relat Res 465:180–184, 2007.
4. Padgett DE, Lipman J, Robie B, Nestor BJ: Influence of total hip design on dislocation: a computer model and clinical analysis. Clin Orthop Relat Res 447:48–52, 2006.
5. Pomeranz MM: Intrapelvic protrusion of the acetabulum (Otto pelvis). J Bone Joint Surg Am 14:663–686, 1932.
6. Hooper JC, Jones EW: Primary protrusion of the acetabulum. J Bone Joint Surg Br 53:23–29, 1971.
7. Gates HS, III, Poletti SC, Callaghan JJ, McCollum DE: Radiographic measurements in protrusio acetabuli. J Arthroplasty 4:347–351, 1989.
8. Pawels F, Furlong RJ, Maquet P (trans): Biomechanics of the normal and diseased hip: theoretical foundation, technique and results of treatment—an atlas, Berlin, 1976, Springer-Verlag, pp 129–169.
9. Leunig M, Huff TW, Ganz R: Femoroacetabular impingement: treatment of the acetabular side. Instr Course Lect 58:223–229, 2009.
10. Alexander C: The aetiology of primary protrusio acetabuli. Br J Radiol 38:567–580, 1965.
11. Mcbride MT, Muldoon MP, Santore RF, et al: Protrusio acetabuli: diagnosis and treatment. J Am Acad Orthop Surg 9:79–88, 2001.
12. Leunig M, Nho SJ, Turchetto L, Ganz R: Protrusio acetabuli: new insights and experience with joint preservation. Clin Orthop Relat Res 467:2241–2250, 2009.
13. Della Valle AG, Padgett DE, Salvati EA: Preoperative planning for primary total hip arthroplasty. J Am Acad Orthop Surg 13:455–462, 2005.
14. Massin P, Schmidt L, Engh CA: Evaluation of cementless acetabular component migration: an experimental study. J Arthroplasty 4:245–251, 1989.
15. Rosenberg WW, Schreurs BW, de Waal Malefijt MC, et al: Impacted morsellized bone grafting and cemented primary total arthroplasty for acetabular protrusio in patients with rheumatoid arthritis: an 8-11 year follow-up study of 36 hips. Acta Orthop Scand 71:143–146, 2000.
16. Matsuno H, Yasuda T, Yudoh K, et al: Cementless cup supporter for protrusio acetabuli in patients with rheumatoid arthritis. Int Orthop 24:15–18, 2000.
17. Heywood AW: Hip replacement arthroplasty in rheumatoid arthritis. Ann Chir Gynaecol Suppl 198:76–80, 1985.
18. Padgett DE, Kull L, Rosenberg A, et al: Revision of the acetabular component without cement after total hip arthroplasty: three to six year followup. J Bone Joint Surg Am 75:663–673, 1993.
19. Sotelo-Garza A, Charnley J: The results of Charnley arthroplasty of hip performed for protrusio acetabuli. Clin Orthop Relat Res 132:12–18, 1978.
20. Heywood AW: Arthroplasty with solid bone graft for protrusio acetabuli. J Bone Joint Surg Br 62:332–326, 1980.
21. Crowinshield RD, Brand RA, Pedersen DR: A stress analysis of acetabular reconstruction in protrusio acetabuli. J Bone Joint Surg Am 65:495–499, 1983.
22. Ranawat CS, Zahn MG: Role of bone grafting in correction of protrusio acetabuli by total hip arthroplasty. J Arthroplasty 1:131–137, 1986.
23. McCollum DE, Nunley JA, Harrelson JM: Bone grafting in total hip replacement for acetabular protrusio. J Bone Joint Surg Am 62:1065–1073, 1980.
24. Gates HS III, McCollum DE, Poletti SC, Nunley JA: Bone-grafting in total hip arthroplasty for protrusio acetabuli: a follow-up note. J Bone Joint Surg Am 72:248–251, 1990.
25. Ebert FR, Hussain S, Krackow KA: Total hip arthroplasty for protrusio acetabuli: a 3- to 9- year follow up of the Heywood technique. Orthopedics 15:17–20, 1992.
26. Wilson MG, Nikpoor N, Aliabadi P, et al: The fate of acetabular allografts after bipolar revision arthroplasty of the hip: a radiographic review. J Bone Joint Surg Am 71:1469–1479, 1989.
27. Brien WW, Bruce WJ, Salvati EA, et al: Acetabular reconstruction with a bipolar prosthesis and morselized bone grafts. J Bone Joint Surg Am 72:1230–1235, 1990.
28. Schmalzried TP, Harris WH: The Harris-Galante porous-coated acetabular component with screw fixation: radiographic analysis of eighty-three primary hip replacements at a minimum of five years. J Bone Joint Surg Am 74:1130–1139, 1992.
29. Tanzer M, Drucker D, Jasty M, Harris WH: Revision of the acetabular component with an uncemented Harris-Galante porous coated prosthesis. J Bone Joint Surg Am 74:987–994, 1992.
30. Mullaji AB, Marawar SV: Primary total hip arthroplasty in protrusio acetabuli using impacted morsellised bone grafting and cementless cups: a medium-term radiographic review. J Arthroplasty 22:1143–1149, 2007.
31. Krushell RJ, Fingeroth RJ, Gelling B: Primary total hip arthroplasty using a dual-geometry cup to treat protrusio acetabuli. J Arthroplasty 23:1128–1131, 2008.

CHAPTER 83

Sickle Cell Disease

Megan A. Swanson and Michael H. Huo

KEY POINTS

- This is a systemic disease; consider obtaining magnetic resonance imaging (MRI) of the asymptomatic contralateral hip. MRI can identify early-stage femoral head osteonecrosis that may be amenable to nonarthroplasty and nonsurgical treatments. Patients are immunodeficient (owing to functional asplenia) and have a high rate of pyogenic infection. Additionally, a multidisciplinary care plan must be instituted to coordinate all of the involved disciplines, including hematology, infectious disease, cardiology, pain management, rehabilitation medicine, and anesthesiology.
- Characteristic changes in the osseous architecture of the symptomatic hip have been observed. The proximal femur may have areas of sclerosis and even complete canal obliteration secondary to osseous infarction. Marrow hyperplasia may lead to widening of the metaphyseal medullary canal and thinning of the trabeculae and cortices. The femoral head is usually flattened with significant subchondral collapse. Acetabular protrusio is also common. All of these may necessitate special considerations for implant selection and alteration in surgical technique to optimize fixation and biomechanics, and to avoid complications during surgery.
- The perioperative management plan is modified in four core areas: (1) Monitor fluid resuscitation and oxygenation to prevent a sickling crisis, cardiac fluid overload, and acute chest syndrome; (2) consider extended administration of antibiotics, and assess sources of infection such as ipsilateral extremity venous stasis ulcers. It is recommended to obtain intraoperative cultures and histopathology to rule out hip joint infection; (3) optimize hemostasis to minimize wound drainage, hematoma formation, and other bleeding complications that may increase the need for blood transfusion in a patient population at risk for alloimmunization and blood transfusion reaction; and (4) provide pain management with consideration for epidural analgesia and regional nerve blocks because almost all of these patients have a narcotic tolerance owing to long-term narcotic use to manage painful sickle crises. On occasion, consideration should be given to prevention of sickling and subsequent crises with a trial of temporary sympathectomy.
- Discuss potential technical challenges, higher risks of complications, and reduced prosthesis survivorship with these patients. Likewise, the potential for articular surface wear is increased because most of these patients are young and active.

INTRODUCTION

Sickle cell disease is a hematological disorder characterized by deformation of red blood cells into an abnormal, rigid, and sickled shape (Fig. 83-1). Sickling decreases erythrocyte flexibility, leading to a variety of complications; it occurs because of a mutation in the hemoglobin gene. Sickle cell disease is relatively common in populations inhabiting tropical and subtropical regions of the world. One third of all indigenous inhabitants of sub-Saharan Africa carry the gene. An interesting clinical relationship has been noted between sickle cell disease and malaria; those with only one of the two gene alleles for sickle cell disease are more resistant to malaria because affected red cells are more resistant to infestation by the malaria *Plasmodium*.

Sickle cell syndrome encompasses a wide spectrum of clinical manifestations depending on the number and type of gene mutations. Sickle cell anemia represents a specific form of sickle cell disease. Patients are homozygous for the gene mutation resulting in hemoglobin S, hence sickle cell anemia is also referred to in the medical literature as *HbSS*, *SS disease*, or *hemoglobin S*. Patients with a heterozygous gene pattern (one sickle gene and one normal gene) are referred to as *HbAS* or *sickle cell trait*. Other less common forms of sickle cell syndrome include sickle–hemoglobin C disease (HbSC), sickle beta-plus-thalassemia (HbS/β+), and sickle beta-zero-thalassemia (HbS/β0). These other forms of sickle cell disease are compound heterozygous patterns in which the patient has only one copy of the mutation that causes HbS and one copy of another abnormal hemoglobin allele.

Heterozygous patients are often asymptomatic. Homozygous patients have severe anemia, recurrent painful crises, pyogenic infections, and chronic end-organ necrosis and infarction (e.g., splenic, osseous). A wide range in the prevalence of osteonecrosis of the femoral head has been reported in the literature, and it is dependent upon the sickle cell genotype: The

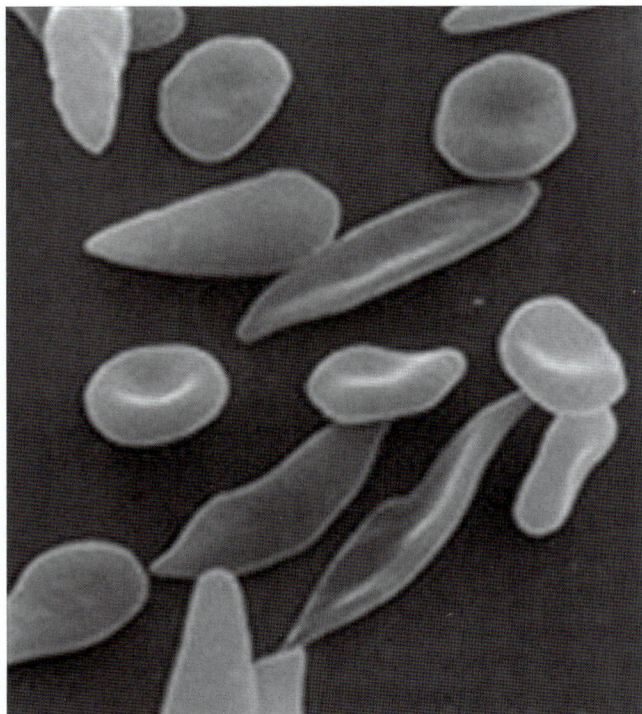

Figure 83-1. Sickling of the red blood cell.

Table 83-1. Ficat and Arlet Classification System

Stage	Radiographic Finding
I	None (evident only on magnetic resonance imaging [MRI])
II	Diffuse sclerosis, cysts (visualized on radiographs)
III	Subchondral fracture (crescent sign with or without head collapse)
IV	Femoral head collapse, acetabular involvement, and joint destruction (osteoarthritis)

Table 83-2. University of Pennsylvania (Steinberg) Classification System

Stage	Criteria
0	Normal radiograph, bone scan, and magnetic resonance imaging (MRI)
I	Normal radiograph, abnormal bone scan and/or MRI A: Mild (<15% of femoral head affected) B: Moderate (15% to 30% of femoral head affected) C: Severe (>30% of femoral head affected)
II	Cystic and sclerotic changes in femoral head A: Mild (<15% of femoral head affected) B: Moderate (15% to 30% of femoral head affected) C: Severe (>30% of femoral head affected)
III	Subchondral collapse without flattening (crescent sign) A: Mild (<15% of articular surface) B: Moderate (15% to 30% of articular surface) C: Severe (>30% of articular surface)
IV	Flattening of the femoral head A: Mild (<15% of surface and <2 mm of depression) B: Moderate (15% to 30% of surface and 2 mm to 4 mm of depression) C: Severe (>30% of surface and >4 mm of depression)
V	Joint narrowing or acetabular changes A: Mild B: Moderate C: Severe
VI	Advanced degenerative changes

prevalence of osteonecrosis was greatest in the group with in Sβ0 genotype (13.1 percent), followed by those with the hemoglobin SS genotype (10.2 percent), those with the hemoglobin SC genotype (8.8 percent), and patients with the Sβ+ genotype (5.8 percent).[1-3] Femoral head osteonecrosis develops before the age of 35 years in nearly half of all patients with HbSS.[4,5] Bilateral hip involvement is seen in 40% to 91% of patients.[6-9] Historically, life expectancy was often shortened[10] because of the many complications; however, advances in medical therapy have improved life expectancy. This has led to an increasing number of patients in need of medical and surgical management of femoral head osteonecrosis. Primary total hip arthroplasty (THA) in patients with sickle cell disease requires an understanding of the musculoskeletal manifestations associated with sickle cell disease, as well as the variety of medical problems that may complicate the perioperative and postoperative periods and compromise the clinical outcome.

INDICATIONS/CONTRAINDICATIONS

Treatment of precollapse femoral head osteonecrosis includes physical therapy, statins, bisphosphonates, core decompression, and bone grafting with or without growth factors.[11] Some surgeons have performed total hip resurfacing in appropriate patients.[12,13] Patients with sickle cell disease and end-stage femoral head osteonecrosis are indicated for THA when other treatments are no longer effective. Absolute contraindications include active infection and severe medical problems that are not optimized. Primary resection arthroplasty and hip fusion generally are not desirable in this patient population owing to young age, bilaterality of hip disease, and difficulty in achieving fusion in necrotic bone. Femoral osteotomy is associated with a poor outcome because it does not alter disease progression.[14] Hemiarthroplasty is not indicated because of abnormal acetabular bone stock and/or the presence of protrusio.

The decision of what surgical option to undertake is based upon the stage of femoral head osteonecrosis. Multiple staging systems have been proposed to describe the changes and evolution of osteonecrosis of the hip.[15] The three most commonly used are the Ficat and Arlet,[16] University of Pennsylvania (Steinberg),[17] and Association Research Circulation Osseous (ARCO)[18] classification systems (Tables 83-1 through 83-3). Regardless of the classification system used, evaluation of the radiograph and of MRI images should be based on the size of the lesion and the presence of sclerosis or cysts, crescent sign, head depression, and/or

Table 83-3. Association Research Circulation Osseous (ARCO) Classification System

Stage	Findings	Techniques	Subclassification	Quantitation
0	None	Radiography, CT, scintigraphy, MRI	No	No
I	Radiography and CT normal At least ONE other technique is positive	Scintigraphy, MRI	Location of lesion Medial Central Lateral	Area of involvement (percentage) A: Minimal (<15%) B: Moderate (15% to 30%) C: Extensive Length of crescent A:<15% B: 15% to 30% C: >30% Surface collapse and dome depression A: <15% and <2 mm B: 15% to 30% and 2 mm to 4 mm C: >30% and >4 mm
II	Sclerosis, osteolysis, focal porosis	Radiography, CT, scintigraphy, MRI	Same as stage I	Same as stage I
III	Crescent sign and/or flattening of articular surface	Radiography and CT	Same as stage I	Same as stage I
IV	Osteoarthritis, acetabular changes, joint destruction	Radiography only	No	No

CT, Computed tomography; MRI, magnetic resonance imaging.
Reproduced from Mont et al: Systematic analysis of classification systems for osteonecrosis of the femoral head. JBJS 99:16–26, 2006.

collapse, as well as acetabular changes. McGrory and associates[19] recently reported on current practices of members of the American Association of Hip and Knee Surgeons (AAHKS) in treating adults with femoral head osteonecrosis. Total hip arthroplasty was reported to be the most frequent intervention for treatment of post-collapse (Steinberg stage III, IV, V, and VI) osteonecrosis. Core decompression was reported to be the most commonly offered intervention for symptomatic precollapse (Steinberg stages I and II) osteonecrosis. Less common treatments included nonoperative management, osteotomy, vascularized and nonvascularized bone grafting, hemiarthroplasty, and arthrodesis.

Efforts are being made to evaluate surgical treatment options with the specific goal of preventing progression of femoral head collapse in hips with moderate disease (stage II). Multiple studies have provided evidence supporting the use of core decompression for stages I and II.[20-22] However, Moran[23] has suggested that core decompression will not work as well in sickle cell patients because it does not address the primary underlying pathology of vaso-occlusion. In addition, many of these patients already have advanced head collapse upon initial presentation for evaluation. Marker and colleagues[24] reviewed the literature for early-stage femoral head osteonecrosis. They recommended following the treatment algorithm proposed by Seyler and coworkers[25] (Fig. 83-2).

PREOPERATIVE PLANNING

The clinical assessment should include level of pain, functional limitation, history of nonsurgical management, prior infections, prior surgeries, and overall medical status. The clinical examination should include range of motion of the hip, specifically noting contractures, the presence/location of prior incisions and wounds, measurement of limb lengths, and checking for vascular insufficiency and ulcerations of the legs. Attention must be paid to the contralateral hip because many patients have bilateral hip disease.

A high likelihood of rapid progression of symptoms and head collapse is reported in sickle cell patients with asymptomatic femoral head osteonecrosis.[26] Hernigou and associates[26] studied the natural history of 121 asymptomatic hips opposite symptomatic hips in 121 sickle cell disease patients. The mean length of follow-up was 14 years. At the time of initial evaluation, 56 asymptomatic hips were classified as Steinberg stage 0, 42 hips as stage I, and 23 hips as stage II. At the time of final follow-up, pain had developed in 110 previously asymptomatic hips (91%), and head collapse had occurred in 93 hips (77%). Symptoms always preceded collapse. Of the 56 hips that were classified as Steinberg stage 0, 47 hips (84%) had developed symptoms, and 34 (61%) had experienced head collapse at final follow-up. Of the 42 asymptomatic stage I hips, 40 (95%) became symptomatic within 3 years, and 36 (86%) had head collapse. Of the 23 asymptomatic stage II hips, all became symptomatic (100%) within 2 years, and all (100%) had head collapse. The average interval between onset of pain and head collapse was 11 months. At the time of final follow-up, 91 hips (75%) had required surgical treatment. These findings validated the same authors' previously published results demonstrating that sickle cell disease patients with symptomatic femoral head osteonecrosis deteriorate rapidly,[27] and sharply contrasted with the natural history of the contralateral hip in patients with osteonecrosis as observed in other

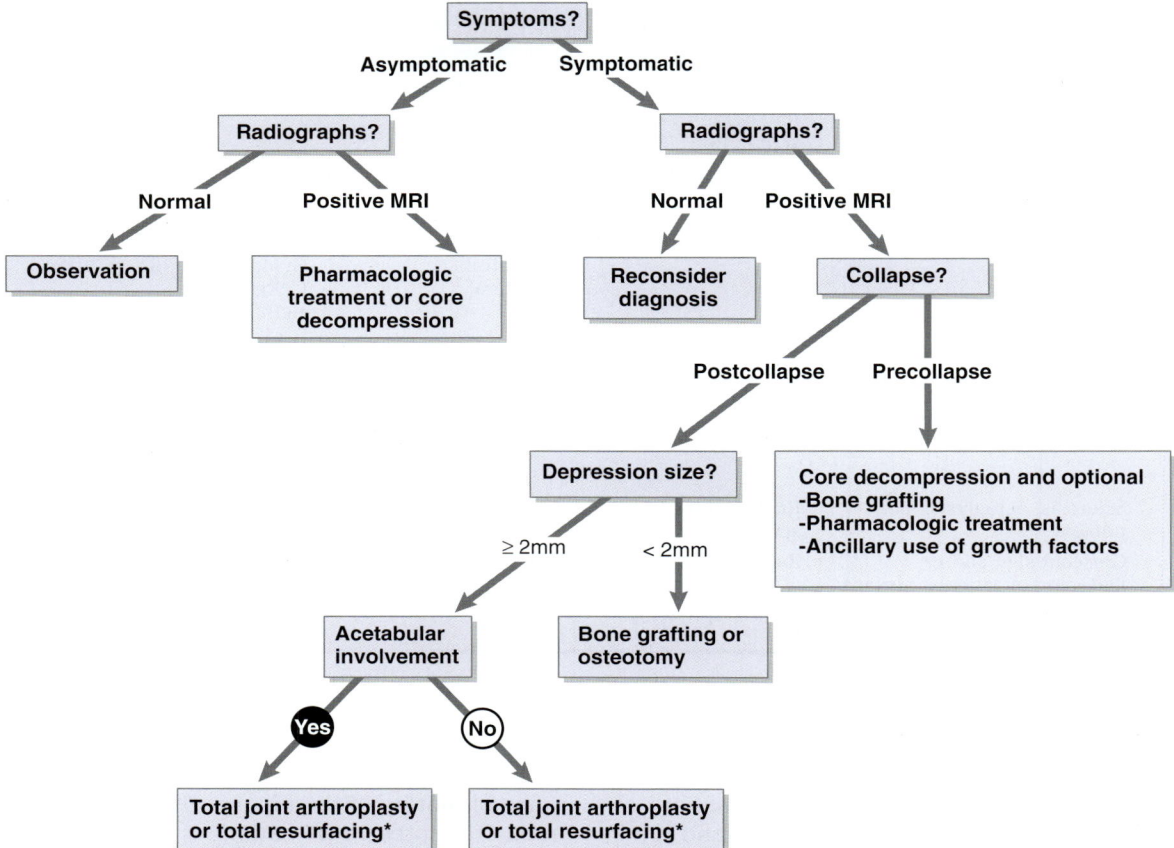

Figure 83-2. Treatment for osteonecrosis of the hip should be determined on the basis of both clinical and radiographic assessments. *Hip resurfacing remains an option in selected patients, in particular those with extra-articular deformity of the upper femur. However, many patients with hemoglobinopathy also have renal dysfunction, which would preclude the use of metal-on-metal articulation. Moreover, metal-on-metal articulation such as that seen in hip resurfacing is contraindicated in women of childbearing age. *MRI,* Magnetic resonance imaging. *(Redrawn from Seyler TM, Marker D, Mont MA: Osteonecrosis. In Klippel JH, Stone JH, Crofford LJ, White PH [eds]: Primer on the rheumatic diseases, ed 13, New York, 2008, Springer, p 571.)*

conditions. Additionally, Davidson and colleagues[28] noted only a 5% progression rate in contralateral asymptomatic hips at the time of initial presentation.

Radiographic assessment should include evaluation of acetabular protrusion and coverage of the femoral head, canal sclerosis, previous core decompression tract (with or without bone grafting), canal geometry, and any pelvic obliquity. Hernigou and coworkers[8] have outlined the radiographic features of 52 patients (95 hips) with sickle cell disease. They noted that pathologic changes differed from those observed in patients with femoral head osteonecrosis secondary to other causes. Using standard radiographic images of the hip (Fig. 83-3), the authors noted that osteochondritis dissecans was less common than in non–sickle cell disease patients. Coxa plana was more common, with premature growth plate closure resulting in a short femoral neck without significant alteration in the neck shaft angle. However, if premature closure of only the medial portion of the physis occurred, this would lead to widening of the femoral neck and varus deformity. Protrusio acetabuli[29] was also more common in sickle cell disease patients. It is important to note that the proximal femur may have areas of sclerosis and frank canal obliteration secondary to repeated bone infarctions. Conversely, marrow hyperplasia may lead to widening of the metaphyseal medullary canal and thinning of the trabeculae and cortices, which may predispose to fracture during surgical preparation and insertion of the implant.

A multidisciplinary program for preoperative evaluation that includes hematology, infectious disease, cardiology, pain management, physiotherapy, rehabilitation, and anesthesiology should be instituted. Sickle cell patients are anemic; Jeong and associates[30] recommend preoperative transfusion or plasmapheresis to achieve a hemoglobin level greater than 11 g/dL and a hematocrit level greater than 30%. Moreover, it is important to achieve circulating levels of hemoglobin A (HgbA) greater than 30% and hemoglobin S (HgbS) levels less than 30%. The rate of HgbS polymer formation is dependent upon the HgbS concentration; thus reduction in HgbS levels will reduce complications. However, this aggressive transfusion regimen may be associated with more transfusion-related complications in association with a 20% to 30% rate of alloimmunization in

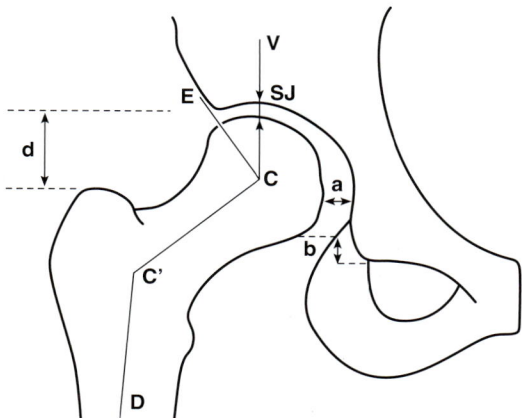

Figure 83-3. Drawing showing the radiographic indices of the hip. Lateral subluxation **(a)** was considered to be present when the distance **(a)** was greater than 10 mm. Superior subluxation **(b)** was measured by the step-off in the Shenton line, by projecting the inferior surface of the femoral neck and relating it to the obturator foramen. Because femoral rotation may alter this measurement, only a break greater than 5 mm was considered abnormal. The center angle of Wiberg (formed by VCE) was considered insufficient when it measured less than 20 degrees. The articulotrochanteric distance **(d)** was determined by measurement of the distance between the proximal pole of the femoral head and the top of the trochanter. The superior joint space (SJ) was measured on a vertical line at 90 degrees from the horizontal line drawn between the inferior aspects of the teardrops of both hips. The neck shaft angle is formed by CC'D. The average value is 123 degrees, and the standard deviation is 7 degrees. *(Redrawn from Hernigou P, Galacteros F, Bachir D, Goutallier D: Deformities of the hip in adults who have sickle cell disease and had avascular necrosis in childhood. J Bone Joint Surg Am 73:81–92, 1991.)*

these patients.[31,32] Preoperative administration of folic acid and recombinant erythropoietin may also be beneficial.

Sickle cell disease (SCD) patients are often immunodeficient owing to functional asplenia and are susceptible to bacteremia and hematogenous seeding of multiple joints by polysaccharide-encapsulated microorganisms. *Staphylococcus aureus* is the most common cause of osteomyelitis and periprosthetic THA infection in these patients.[33] In addition to obtaining a thorough infectious disease history, both legs should be checked for venous stasis ulcers, and extended-duration postoperative antibiotics should be instituted.[34]

Acute chest syndrome (ACS) is the second most common cause of hospitalization in SCD; it accounts for more than 25% of premature deaths in sickle cell disease. It is estimated that half of all patients with SCD will develop ACS at least once in their lives.[35] ACS is a noninfectious vaso-occlusive crisis of the pulmonary vasculature. It can come on suddenly and can range from being very mild to fatal. Its main signs and symptoms include dyspnea, chest pain, fever, cough, and new pulmonary infiltrates on chest x-ray. It is a form of lung injury that can progress to adult respiratory distress syndrome. Recent sickle cell crises, including ACS,

should be completely resolved before any elective surgery is undertaken.

DESCRIPTION OF TECHNIQUE

The principal technical challenges are present on the femoral side. The surgical approach should be decided at the surgeon's discretion. Hip dislocation may be challenging owing to ankylosis and acetabular protrusio; accordingly, femoral neck osteotomy in situ may be desirable to avoid fracture from excessive manipulation of the leg. Femoral canal preparation is complicated by areas of sclerosis and thinned cortices. Rates of intraoperative fracture and perforation are higher than in routine osteoarthritis patients; they have been reported to range from 4.9% to 18.2%.[34,36] Technique modifications include using a high-speed drill to locate the femoral canal under fluoroscopic guidance and using flexible reamers before using rigid reamers.[9,37] Intraoperative radiographs may assist in confirming proper femoral canal preparation and stem insertion and in excluding any fracture or perforation. Marrow hyperplasia may lead to a widened metaphyseal region, challenging optimal fit and fixation of the stem. Durable cementless fixation is difficult to achieve in sclerotic necrotic bone. In contrast, cement fixation has been documented to be associated with high rates of infection and mechanical loosening.[33,38,39]

Many patients may have coxa breva, femoral head flattening, and acetabular protrusio. These changes alter hip biomechanics with regard to offset, leg length, and abductor tension. Careful preoperative planning, implant selection, and surgical technique are required to minimize complications such as dislocation and Trendelenburg gait after the operation. If acetabular protrusio is present, bone grafting may be necessary. The acetabulum may have areas of irregular sclerosis and thinning, leading to increased risk of eccentric reaming and even column fractures. Adjunct screw fixation and surface modification (such as hydroxyapatite coating) of the cup are recommended to optimize cup stability and bone ingrowth.

TIPS AND PEARLS

- Place drill bit/high-speed drill, guide wire, and flexible reamers under direct fluoroscopic guidance to initiate femoral canal preparation.
- Use a high-speed burr to improve alignment of the femoral component by removing residual bone graft from previous procedures.[40]
- Perform in situ osteotomy of the femoral neck to facilitate safe hip dislocation.
- Have bone allograft or substitutes available for acetabular protrusio.
- Consider intraoperative bone cultures and histopathology analysis to rule out occult infection before prosthesis implantation.[39]
- Employ strict hemostasis to minimize wound drainage, hematoma formation, and other bleeding

complications that may increase the need for blood transfusion in a patient population at risk for alloimmunization and transfusion reaction.

- Monitor fluid resuscitation and oxygenation to prevent a sickling crisis, cardiac fluid overload, and acute chest syndrome.
- Use epidural analgesia and regional nerve blocks to treat patients who may have developed a narcotic tolerance. Consider sympathectomy to prevent sickling and subsequent crises.[9]

POSTOPERATIVE CARE

The patient's fluid status and pulmonary function and pain management should be monitored closely. Jeong and associates[30] noted that patients should be monitored postoperatively for sickle cell–related events such as vaso-occlusive crises and acute chest syndrome (a new pulmonary infiltrate involving at least one full lung segment, excluding atelectasis). Currently recommended indications for postoperative transfusion in sickle cell patients consist of (1) Hgb level below 10 mg/dL, (2) signs and symptoms of anemia (including tachycardia, syncope, angina, and high output failure), (3) acute central nervous system complications from hypoxia or anemia, (4) sequestration crisis, (5) acute chest syndrome with hypoxia, and (6) acute hemorrhage.[41] The rate of late prosthetic infection has been reported to range from 17% to 72%.[38,42,43] Given the increased risk of late hematogenous seeding of the prosthesis, lifelong antibiotic prophylaxis for dental, gastrointestinal, and urological procedures is advisable. Standard perioperative venous thromboprophylaxis should be administered.

RESULTS

Reported results of primary THA in sickle cell disease are mixed. Most studies report high patient satisfaction reflected by a standardized hip outcome scale, pain reduction, and functional improvement. However, much of the literature reports high rates of infection, fixation loosening, and revision (Table 83-4). Advances in new bearing surfaces and improved surgical technique may offer some promise. We will specifically focus on three recent citations on THA outcome in sickle cell disease, femoral head osteonecrosis, and very young patients.

Hernigou and colleagues[44] retrospectively reviewed 312 THAs performed in 244 patients with sickle cell disease. A total of 126 women and 118 men were included. Mean patient age at the time of surgery was 32 years, and minimum follow-up was 5 years (mean, 13 years; range, 5 to 25 years). The overall revision rate for all causes was 16% (48 hips). Revision was done in 10 hips (3%) for infection at a mean of 11 years (range, 7 to 15 years). Additional revisions were done in 21 cups (8%) and 17 stems (5%) for aseptic loosening at a mean of 14 years. Medical complications occurred after 85 operations (27%), and orthopedic complications were reported in 42 cases (13%). These rates of revisions and

complications are higher than those seen in primary THAs performed for osteoarthritis.

Dastane and coworkers[45] reviewed outcomes of THA using a metal-on-metal coupling in a selected group of 107 patients with 112 hips. These patients were all younger than 60 years of age at the time of the THA. In all, 27 patients had femoral head osteonecrosis (30 hips), and 80 patients had osteoarthritis (82 hips). Cement fixation was used in 14 stems, and cementless fixation in 98 stems. Overall, five mechanical complications were due to impingement—two with unexplained pain, two dislocations, and one liner disassociation. At a minimum follow-up of 2.2 years (mean, 5.5 years; range, 2.2 to 11.7 years), no periarticular osteolysis was observed in either group. No stem was loose. No cup loosening or revision was necessary in the femoral head osteonecrosis group. One cup revision for aseptic loosening was necessary in the osteoarthritis group. No difference in clinical outcome measures was noted. However, these data reflect only very short-term follow-up. Longer follow-up is necessary to determine whether metal-on-metal coupling will remain durable and without complications from metal ion release or wear debris, specifically in sickle cell disease patients.

In summary, primary THA in sickle cell disease patients can predictably offer pain relief and functional improvement. Complications are more numerous than after routine THA performed for other reasons and in other patient populations. Major limitations continue to involve fixation durability. Further improvements in fixation durability and reduction of articulation wear are needed.

COMPLICATIONS

Medical complications can be minimized by using a multidisciplinary approach, as was previously outlined. Hemostasis, infection prevention, and optimal pain management are critical in reducing overall complications and enhancing patient rehabilitation.[9,30]

The principal complications associated with THA are infection, fixation loosening, and dislocation. Average rates of early and late postoperative wound infection have been reported to be nearly 20% in multiple studies (see Table 83-4). The most common microorganism is *Staphylococcus aureus*.[46,47] Moran and coworkers[33] stated that there is no need to administer any specific prophylaxis against *Salmonella* because no such infection has been reported around a THA in a sickle cell patient. Investigators indicated that the most common reason for THA failure was aseptic loosening of cemented acetabular cups. Other studies have reported decreased rates of aseptic loosening and infection when cementless fixation has been used.[38,39,48] Additionally, Hickman and associates[48] reported a dislocation rate of 26%. We previously cited the need for careful preoperative planning, implant selection, and surgical technique to address deformed anatomy and to optimize hip biomechanics to minimize the risk of dislocation. The risk of dislocation may be improved by soft tissue repair, selection of high-offset stem designs, and use of

Table 83-4. Studies of Primary Total Hip Arthroplasty in Sickle Cell Disease

Authors	Year	Primary THAs	Mean Follow-up in Years (range)	Results
Hernigou et al	2008	312 THAs (244 pts)	13 (5-25)	27% medical complications immediately postop 13% orthopedic complications immediately postop 8% cups revised for aseptic loosening at mean of 14 years 5% stems revised for aseptic loosening at mean of 14 years 3% revised for infection at mean of 11 years (range, 7-15)
Dastane et al	2008	132 THAs (101 pts) Ceramic	6.9 (1-26.5)	10-year survivorship: 82.1% 9% cups revised for aseptic loosening 1.5% stems revised for aseptic loosening 2% both stem and cup revised for aseptic loosening
Nizard et al	2008	30 THAs (27 hips) Metal-on-metal Any origin of osteonecrosis	5.5 (2.2-11.7)	No osteolysis or aseptic loosening observed No revisions
Ilyas and Moreau	2002	36 THAs 18 patients: bilateral and simultaneous Cementless	5.7 (2-10)	11% wound infection No stems revised for loosening 6% revision rate 50% complication rate
Al-Mousawi	2002	35 THAs Cemented	9.5 (5-15)	20% revision rate—6 revised for aseptic loosening and 1 revised for deep infection HHS: 36->86
Hickman and Lachiewicz	1997	15 THAs Cementless	6	No evidence of acetabular loosening 5/15 (33%) had >2000 mL intraoperative blood loss HHS: 36->94
Moran et al	1993	22 THAs	4.8	HHS: 47->88
Acurio and Friedman	1992	35 THAs 17 cemented 18 cementless	7.5	59% of cemented THAs revised 22% of cementless THAs revised
Clarke et al	1989	27 THAs 13 cemented 14 cementless	5.5	15% femoral fracture/perforation Average EBL 1390 mL in cemented arthroplasties
Bishop et al	1988	17 THAs 15 cemented 2 cementless	8.9	24% revision rate 29% complication rate
Hanker and Amstutz	1988	9 THAs	6.5	63% revision rate

EBL, Estimated blood loss; *HHS*, Harris hip score; *pts*, patients; *THA*, total hip arthroplasty.

larger-diameter articulations with alternative bearing surfaces.

CURRENT CONTROVERSIES AND FUTURE CONSIDERATIONS

- Cemented versus cementless fixation
  - Cement provides immediate, rigid fixation and decreased risk of fractures and perforations. It may also be associated with less blood loss. Cementless fixation reportedly is associated with lower rates of aseptic loosening and infection. The most favorable fixation method has yet to be determined.
- Ceramic-on-ceramic and metal-on-metal bearing couplings
  - Ceramic-on-ceramic bearing couplings show promise in early studies in young patients and require linger term follow-up. Metal-on-metal bearing couplings should be used very cautiously

given recent reports regarding metal ion debris and associated side effects.
- Use of total hip resurfacing for the treatment of femoral head osteonecrosis has had promising short-term results in some recent studies.[12,13] However, few of the patients in these studies had sickle cell disease. Therefore, clinical data are insufficient to support the efficacy and durability of hip resurfacing in sickle cell disease patients at this time.
- Functional outcomes of THAs following previous vascularized fibular graft
  - Davis and associates[40] compared 12 THAs done following previous vascularized fibular grafting with 36 THAs done for femoral head osteonecrosis treated without previous bone grafting. No difference in migration of the cup or the stem was noted between control and study groups at comparable follow-up intervals. However, clinical hip scores were substantially worse in patients who had undergone previous vascularized fibular grafting.

This could be due to morbidity at the graft donor site rather than to differences in THA performance.

- Role of nonvascularized bone grafting to defer THA
  - Seyler and colleagues[49] reviewed 33 patients (39 hips) with osteonecrosis of the hip who had undergone nonvascularized bone grafting procedures with supplemental osteogenic protein 1 (OP-1) using a trapdoor at the head-neck junction. The authors reported that 18 of 22 Ficat stage II patients did not require further hip surgery over a minimum 24-month follow-up period.
- Physical therapy and core decompression used as treatment modalities for symptomatic stage I, II, and III osteonecrosis in sickle cell disease patients
  - In a prospective multicenter study, Neumayr and coworkers[50] evaluated the safety of core decompression and compared the results of decompression and physical therapy with those of physical therapy alone for the treatment of femoral head osteonecrosis in sickle cell disease patients. Forty-six patients (46 hips) with Steinberg stage I, II, or III femoral head osteonecrosis were randomized to one of two treatment arms: (1) core decompression followed by a physical therapy program, or (2) a physical therapy program alone. After a mean of 3 years, the hip survival rate was 82% in the group treated with core decompression and physical therapy, and 86% in the group treated with physical therapy alone. According to a modification of the Harris hip score, the mean clinical improvement was 18.1 points for patients treated with core decompression and physical therapy compared with 15.7 points for those treated with physical therapy alone.

REFERENCES

1. Chung SM, Ralston EL: Necrosis of the femoral head associated with sickle-cell anemia and its genetic variants: a review of the literature and study of thirteen cases. J Bone Joint Surg Am 51:33–58, 1969.
2. Chung SM, Alavi A, Russell MO: Management of osteonecrosis in sickle-cell anemia and its genetic variants. Clin Orthop Relat Res 130:158–174, 1978.
3. Milner PF, Kraus AP, Sebes JI, et al: Sickle cell disease as a cause of osteonecrosis of the femoral head. N Engl J Med 325:1476–1481, 1991.
4. Ware HE, Brooks AP, Toye R, Berney SI: Sickle cell disease and silent avascular necrosis of the hip. J Bone Joint Surg Br 73:947–949, 1991.
5. Marouf R, Gupta R, Haider MZ, et al: Avascular necrosis of the femoral head in adult Kuwaiti sickle cell disease patients. Acta Haematol 110:11–15, 2003.
6. Athanassiou-Metaxa M, Kirkos J, Koussi A, et al: Avascular necrosis of the femoral head among children and adolescents with sickle cell disease in Greece. Haematologica 87:771–772, 2002.
7. Lavernia CJ, Sierra RJ: Core decompression in atraumatic osteonecrosis of the hip. J Arthroplasty 15:171–178, 2000.
8. Hernigou P, Galacteros F, Bachir D, Goutallier D: Deformities of the hip in adults who have sickle cell disease and had avascular necrosis in childhood. J Bone Joint Surg Am 73:81–92, 1991.
9. Clarke HJ, Jinnah RH, Brooker AF, Michaelson JD: Total replacement of the hip for avascular necrosis in sickle cell disease. J Bone Joint Surg Br 71:465–470, 1989.
10. Platt OS, Brambilla DJ, Rosse WF, et al: Mortality in sickle cell disease: life expectancy and risk factors for early death. N Engl J Med 330:1639–1644, 1994.
11. Marker DR, Seyler TM, McGrath MS, et al: Treatment of early stage osteonecrosis of the femoral head. J Bone Joint Surg Am 90(Suppl 4):175–187, 1998.
12. Revell MP, McBryde CW, Bhatnagar S, et al: Metal-on-metal hip resurfacing in osteonecrosis of the femoral head. J Bone Joint Surg Am 88(Suppl 3):98–103, 2006.
13. Mont MA, Seyler TM, Marker DR, et al: Use of metal-on-metal total hip resurfacing for the treatment of osteonecrosis of the femoral head. J Bone Joint Surg Am 88(Suppl 3):90–97, 2006.
14. Schneider W, Aigner N, Pinggera O, Knahr K: Intertrochanteric osteotomy for avascular necrosis of the head of the femur: survival survival probability of two different methods. J Bone Joint Surg Br 84:817–824, 2002.
15. Mont MA, Maralunda GA, Jones LC, et al: Systematic analysis of classification systems for osteonecrosis of the femoral head. J Bone Joint Surg Am 88(Suppl 3):16–25, 2006.
16. Ficat RP, Arlet J. In Hungerford D, editor: Ischemia and necrosis of bone, Baltimore, 1980, Williams & Wilkins.
17. Steinberg ME, Hayken GD, Steinberg DR: A quantitative system for staging avascular necrosis. J Bone Joint Surg Br 77:34–41, 1995.
18. Gardeniers JWM: Report of the committee of staging and nomenclature. ARCO News Letter 5:79–82, 1993.
19. McGrory BJ, York SC, Iorio R, et al: Current practices of AAHKS members in the treatment of adult osteonecrosis of the femoral head. J Bone Joint Surg Am 89:1194–1204, 2007.
20. Steinberg ME, Larcom PG, Strafford B, et al: Core decompression with bone grafting for osteonecrosis of the femoral head. Clin Orthop Relat Res 386:71–78, 2001.
21. Castro FP, Barrack RL: Core decompression and conservative treatment for avascular necrosis of the femoral head: a meta-analysis. Am J Orthop 29:187–194, 2000.
22. Smith SW, Fehring TK, Griffin WL, Beaver WB: Core decompression of the osteonecrotic femoral head. J Bone Joint Surg Am 77:674–680, 1995.
23. Moran MC: Osteonecrosis of the hip in sickle cell hemoglobinopathy. Am J Orthop 24:18–24, 1995.
24. Marker DR, Seyler TM, McGrath MS, et al: Treatment of early stage osteonecrosis of the femoral head. J Bone Joint Surg Am 90(Suppl 4):175–187, 2008.
25. Seyler TM, Marker D, Mont MA: Osteonecrosis. In Klippel JH, Stone JH, Crofford LJ, White PH, editors: Primer on the rheumatic diseases, ed 13, New York, 2008, Springer, p 571.
26. Hernigou P, Habibi A, Bachir D, Galacteros F: The natural history of asymptomatic osteonecrosis of the femoral head in adults with sickle cell disease. J Bone Joint Surg Am 88:2565–2589, 2006.
27. Hernigou P, Bachir D, Galacteros F: The natural history of symptomatic osteonecrosis in adults with sickle-cell disease. J Bone Joint Surg Am 85:500–504, 2003.
28. Davidson JL, Coogan PG, Gunneson EE, Urbaniak JR: The asymptomatic contralateral hip in osteonecrosis of the femoral head. In Urbaniak JR, Jones JP, editors: Osteonecrosis: etiology, diagnosis, and treatment, Rosemont, Ill, 1997, American Academy of Orthopaedic Surgeons, pp 231–240.
29. Armbuster TG, Guerra J, Jr, Resnick D, et al: The adult hip: an anatomic study. Part I. The bony landmarks. Radiology 128:1–10, 1978.
30. Jeong GK, Ruchelsman DE, Jazrawi LM, Jaffe WL: Total hip arthroplasty in sickle cell hemoglobinopathies. J Am Acad Orthop Surg 13:208–217, 2005.
31. Vichinsky EP, Neumayr LD, Haberkern C, et al: The perioperative complication rate of orthopedic surgery in sickle cell disease: report of the National Sickle Cell Surgery Study Group. Am J Hematol 62:129–138, 1999.
32. Vichinsky EP, Haberkern CM, Neumayr L, et al: A comparison of conservative and aggressive transfusion regimens in the perioperative management of sickle cell disease. The Preoperative Transfusion in Sickle Cell Disease Study Group. N Engl J Med 333:206–213, 1995.
33. Moran MC, Huo MH, Garvin KL, et al: Total hip arthroplasty in sickle cell hemoglobinopathy. Clin Orthop Relat Res 294:140–148, 1995.
34. Gunderson C, D'Ambrosia RD, Shoji H: Total hip replacement in patients with sickle-cell disease. J Bone Joint Surg Am 59:760–762, 1997.

35. Castro O, Brambilla DJ, Thorington B, et al: The acute chest syndrome in sickle cell disease: incidence and risk factors. Blood 84:643–649, 1994.

36. Epps C, Castro O: Complications of total hip replacement in sickle cell disease. Orthop Trans 2:236–237, 1978.

37. Al-Mousawi F, Malki A, Al-Aradi A, et al: Total hip replacement in sickle cell disease. Int Orthop 26:157–161, 2002.

38. Acurio MT, Friedman RJ: Hip arthroplasty in patients with sickle-cell haemoglobinopathy. J Bone Joint Surg Br 74:367–371, 1992.

39. Ilyas I, Moreau P: Simultaneous bilateral total hip arthroplasty in sickle cell disease. J Arthroplasty 17:441–445, 2002.

40. Davis ET, McKee MD, Waddell JP, et al: Total hip arthroplasty following failure of free vascularized fibular graft. J Bone Joint Surg Am 88(Suppl 3):110–115, 2006.

41. Garden MS, Grant RE, Jebraili S: Perioperative complications in patients with sickle cell disease: an orthopedic perspective. Am J Orthop 25:353–356, 1996.

42. Bishop AR, Roberson JR, Eckman JR, Fleming LL: Total hip arthroplasty in patients who have sickle-cell hemoglobinopathy. J Bone Joint Surg Am 70:853–855, 1988.

43. Hanker GJ, Amstutz HC: Osteonecrosis of the hip in the sickle-cell diseases: treatment and complications. J Bone Joint Surg Am 70:499–506, 1988.

44. Hernigou P, Zilber S, Filippini P, et al: Total hip arthroplasty in adult osteonecrosis related to sickle cell disease. Clin Orthop Relat Res 466:300–308, 2008.

45. Dastane MR, Long WT, Wan Z, et al: Metal-on-metal hip arthroplasty does equally well in osteonecrosis and osteoarthritis. Clin Orthop Relat Res 466:1148–1153, 2008.

46. Epps CH, Jr, Bryant DD, III, Coles MJ, Castro O: Osteomyelitis in patients who have sickle-cell disease: diagnosis and management. J Bone Joint Surg Am 73:1281–1294, 1991.

47. D'Ambrosia RD, Shoji H, Heater R: Secondarily infected total joint replacements by hematogenous spread. J Bone Joint Surg Am 58:450–453, 1976.

48. Hickman JM, Lachiewicz PF: Results and complications of total hip arthroplasties in patients with sickle-cell hemoglobinopathies: role of cementless components. J Arthroplasty 12:420–425, 1997.

49. Seyler TM, Marker DR, Ulrich SD, et al: Nonvascularized bone grafting defers joint arthroplasty in hip osteonecrosis. Clin Orthop Relat Res 466:1125–1132, 2008.

50. Neumayr LD, Aguilar C, Earles AN, et al, and the National Osteonecrosis Trial in Sickle Cell Anemia Study Group: Physical therapy alone compared with core decompression and physical therapy for femoral head osteonecrosis in sickle cell disease. J Bone Joint Surg Am 88:2573–2582, 2006.

FURTHER READING

Firth PG, Head CA: Sickle cell disease and anesthesia. Anesthesiology 101:766–785, 2004.

Huo MH, Friedlaender GE, Marsh JS: Orthopaedic manifestations of sickle-cell disease. Yale J Biol Med 63:195–207, 1990.

McCarthy I: The physiology of bone blood flow: a review. J Bone Joint Surg Am 88(Suppl 3):4–8, 2006.

Mont MA, Jones LC, Hungerford DS: Nontraumatic osteonecrosis of the femoral head: ten years later. J Bone Joint Surg Am 88:1117–1132, 2006.

Steinberg MH: Management of sickle cell disease. N Engl J Med 340:1021–1030, 1999.

CHAPTER 84

High Body Mass Index

C. Lowry Barnes

KEY POINTS

- Careful preoperative planning, along with pharmacologic consultation, is essential for optimal results in obese patients undergoing THA.
- Early postoperative mobilization, although possibly more difficult for obese patients, is critical to avoid decline in function, as well as thromboembolic and respiratory complications.
- Intraoperative radiographic evaluation is important in obese patients to assist the surgeon in attaining proper acetabular cup placement and leg length equality.
- Prolonged wound drainage and higher infection rates are known risks for obese patients undergoing THA.
- Higher complication rates among obese patients undergoing THA may be reduced if bariatric surgery is performed before THA.

INTRODUCTION

The most recent data (2005) from the World Health Organization (WHO) estimate that approximately 1.6 billion people age 15 and older are overweight (i.e., body mass index [BMI] ≥25) (Table 84-1), and that at least 400 million people worldwide are obese (i.e., BMI ≥30).[1] WHO data predict that by 2015, approximately 2.3 billion adults will be overweight, and more than 700 million will be obese. In 2008, six states had an obesity prevalence of greater than 30%, and Colorado was the only state with an obesity prevalence of less than 20%. Between 1991 and 2000, the number of people in the United States in the obese category grew by 60%.[2] In the United States, obesity trails only cancer and coronary heart disease as the third most costly diet- and inactivity-related disease, at $117 billion annually.[3] Total hip arthroplasty (THA) in obese patients presents the surgeon with challenges associated with the surgical procedure itself, the increased risk of perioperative complications, and postoperative recovery and performance of the implant. This chapter will focus on those aspects of THA performed in patients with high BMI (Table 84-2).

INDICATIONS/CONTRAINDICATIONS

The most common indication for THA is osteoarthritis. Several studies have shown that obesity is likely to play a role in the development of osteoarthritis of the hip.[4-8] Clinicians have postulated that "obese" (BMI, 30 to 39.9 kg/m^2) and "morbidly obese" (i.e., BMI ≥40 kg/m^2) patients undergoing THA pose greater technical difficulty for the surgeon, have more postoperative complications, and have poorer short- and long-term outcomes than "ideal weight" (BMI, 20 to 24.9 kg/m^2) or "overweight" (BMI, 25 to 29.9 kg/m^2) patients. In 1982, Sir John Charnley stated that obesity should be a contraindication to performing THA.[9] Some surgeons advise obese patients to lose weight before undergoing THA, believing that THA in an obese patient would be technically demanding and would likely lead to increased postoperative morbidity.[10] Possible concerns have included increased risk of infection, thromboembolism, and early implant failure (e.g., fatigue fracture).

Implant manufacturers today include some patient selection caveats in their precautionary statements to surgeons and include warnings in their product inserts, for example, "patients should be able to control their weight"; "excessive weight may adversely affect the implant"; "heavy patients can place high loads on the prosthesis which may lead to failure"; and "complications or failure may be more likely in heavy patients."

PREOPERATIVE PLANNING

Preoperative planning for obese patients does not differ, in general, from planning for nonobese patients. Standard radiographic imaging should be performed. A radiographic marker may be more important for sizing because of increased distance between the hip and the radiographic plate. To facilitate postoperative evaluation and long-term follow-up, additional preoperative assessments can be valuable (e.g., Harris hip scores, Short Form [SF]-12 or SF-36).

It is advisable to encourage obese patients to attempt to increase upper body strength preoperatively because they must utilize an overhead frame on the hospital bed to assist in achieving early mobilization. As with all THA procedures, early mobilization is important to avoid an overall decline in function, venous thromboembolism, and respiratory complications. In addition,

Table 84-1. International Classification of Adult Underweight, Overweight, and Obesity According to BMI

Classification	BMI, kg/m²	
	Principal Cutoff Points	Additional Cutoff Points
Underweight	<18.50	<18.50
Severe thinness	<16.00	<16.00
Moderate thinness	16.00-16.99	16.00-16.99
Mild thinness	17.00-18.49	17.00-18.49
Normal range	18.50-24.99	18.50-22.99
		23.00-24.99
Overweight	≥25.00	≥25.00
Pre-obese	25.00-29.99	25.00-27.49
		27.50-29.99
Obese	≥30.00	≥30.00
• Obese class I	30.00-34.99	30.00-32.49
		32.50-34.99
• Obese class II	35.00-39.99	35.00-37.49
		37.50-39.99
• Obese class III	≥40.00	≥40.00

Data from World Health Organization (WHO): Physical status: the use and interpretation of anthropometry, report of a WHO Expert Committee, WHO Technical Report Series 854, Geneva, 1995, WHO; World Health Organization: Obesity: preventing and managing the global epidemic, report of a WHO Consultation, WHO Technical Report Series 894, Geneva, 2000, WHO; and World Health Organization (WHO)/International Association for the Study of Obesity (ASO)/International Obesity Taskforce (IOTF): The Asia-Pacific perspective: redefining obesity and its treatment, Melbourne, Australia, 2000, Health Communications.

preoperative plans for other accommodative equipment should be made, such as a wide bedside commode and a wide walker. Preoperative planning should also include pharmacologic consultation to ensure careful administration of narcotic pain medications because obese patients often cannot tolerate as much narcotic as simple calculations based on an increased BMI might suggest. Finally, consideration should be given to bariatric surgery before elective primary THA for selected patients.

DESCRIPTION OF SURGICAL TECHNIQUE: VARIATIONS IN OBESE PATIENTS

Few differences in operative technique have been described for obese patients undergoing THA. In general, a minimally invasive approach should be avoided in obese patients; however, any approach and incision that can achieve easy and adequate exposure while protecting the soft tissues is appropriate (Fig. 84-1). The author prefers a straight lateral position on the operating table, which allows fat/excess skin to "fall away" (Figs. 84-2 through 84-5), combined with an anterolateral approach and a cementless socket and stem. When a modular neck prosthesis is used, it is preferable to use a short straight neck to avoid increasing the risk of fatigue fracture of the femoral neck. For obese patients, low wear with large heads is preferred in the absence of other contraindications.

Intraoperative radiographic evaluation allows the surgeon to determine proper cup placement. With obese patients, a tendency to place the cup in a more abducted position in the acetabulum should be avoided, especially with hard-on-hard bearings, because this may result in increased wear. Intraoperative radiographs allow the surgeon to assess the equality of leg length, which can be more difficult to determine in obese patients. At the conclusion of the operation, two drains are placed: one deep to the fascia and the other in the subcutaneous space; then, a waterproof, compliant dressing is applied (Fig. 84-6).

POSTOPERATIVE CARE

Studies have shown that obesity is associated with a number of operative and postoperative complications, making careful medical and pharmacologic management a priority. Obesity is an independent risk factor for type 2 diabetes mellitus, which is known to be associated with postoperative morbidity.[11] Specifically, because of the strong association between diabetes and obesity, as well as the predictive value of diabetic glucose control and the risk of infectious complications, preoperative screening of obese patients for hemoglobin A1c (Hgb_{A1c}) levels may be advisable. Obesity is also associated with postoperative deep vein thrombosis (DVT) and pulmonary embolism after joint replacement surgery.[12,13] Prolonged wound drainage and higher rates of wound infection are other well-known morbidities in the obese THA population.[14,15] Prophylaxis against DVT is a must, and patients must be monitored closely after discharge as well. They are especially at risk for wound problems because of the need for DVT prophylaxis with low-molecular-weight heparin, fondaparinux, or warfarin and associated large "dead space" areas for hematoma development.[16] Postoperative mobilization and activity are to be encouraged.

EFFECTS OF OBESITY ON THA: RESULTS/COMPLICATIONS

It has been shown in a European study that orthopedic surgeons and their referring physicians have differing opinions about what patient factors affect long-term outcome after primary THA. Sturmer and associates[17] used a standard questionnaire to conduct a multicenter, cross-sectional survey of 304 orthopedic surgeons and 314 referring physicians at 22 centers from 12 European countries. The questionnaire asked about seven patient characteristics and their effects on long-term outcome after THA. Participants were asked, "How would each of the following patient characteristics in your view affect the chances of a favorable long-term outcome of hip replacement (pain and function)?" Participant physicians were asked to make one choice to answer each question: (1) increases the chances of favorable outcome, (2) does not affect outcome, or (3) decreases the chances of favorable outcome. The seven patient characteristics were male gender, old age (>80 years),

Table 84-2. Summary of Representative Studies

Study/Date	Design	Comparison (# Hips)	Outcomes/ Variables	Authors' Conclusions	Authors' Limitations
Malinzak/2009	Retrospective	Deep infection (13)/ noninfected (2775)	BMI, diabetes, osteoarthritis, rheumatoid	Obesity, diabetes, younger age risk factors for joint arthroplasty infection	Retrospective, nonidentical perioperative management
Andrew/2008	Prospective, multicenter	Nonobese (1069)/ obese (332)/morbidly obese (18)	Oxford hip score (OHS), rate of dislocation, blood transfusion, deep infection, DVT, PE, revision	No significant difference between groups for mean change in OHS at 5 years, rate of dislocation, or rate of revision	Only 18 morbidly obese patients
Walsh/2009	Retrospective	PE (30)/no PE (5755)	Age, BMI, gender, ASA grade, physical activity level, DVT prophylaxis	Increasing age, increased BMI, female gender associated with increased risk of PE	Multicenter study may allow acquisition of more PE cases, which should allow for study of various DVT prophylaxis regimens and other risk factors
Fehring/2007	Retrospective	Increases in BMI 1990-2005 (# cases not given)	BMI increase, Medicare reimbursement	BMI of total joint arthroplasty patients has increased significantly over time; reimbursement has not kept pace	As a tertiary referral center, may receive more obese patients from referral
Lübbeke/2007	Prospective cohort study	Nonobese (1906)/ obese (589)/men vs. women	Main complications, HHS, WOMAC	Obesity increased infection rate in women (not in men); functional outcome and satisfaction slightly lower in obese women; no difference among men	Lack of information about patients' activity level, small number of revisions, short follow-up time
Patel/2007	Retrospective	Nonobese/obese (total, 1211)	BMI, blood loss, operative time, prophylaxis against DVT, length of stay, duration of wound drainage	Morbid obesity, low-molecular-weight heparin, greater wound drainage were associated with prolonged wound drainage; prolonged drainage was associated with a higher rate of infection	None stated
McLaughlin/2006	Retrospective	Nonobese (100)/ obese (109)	BMI, revisions, perioperative complications, HHS	No difference between groups in clinical and radiologic outcomes, complications, or revisions	None stated
Sadr Azodi/2006	Retrospective	Nonobese (1167)/ overweight and obese (2142); tobacco use vs. no tobacco use	Length of stay, complications	Smoking and obesity substantially increase risk of complications; high BMI was statistically significantly correlated with longer hospital stay.	Data obtained from registry; data may be missing or incomplete
Moran/2005	Prospective	BMI (800)	HHS, SF-36; reoperation, death, dislocation, deep/ superficial infection	No relationship between BMI and any complications found; BMI predicted slightly lower HHS at 6 and 18 months	Power of the study may be too low.

Table 84-2. Summary of Representative Studies—cont'd

Study/Date	Design	Comparison (# Hips)	Outcomes/ Variables	Authors' Conclusions	Authors' Limitations
Ibrahim/2005	Retrospective	Nonobese (179)/obese (164)	Complications/ reoperation/self-administered questionnaire for satisfaction	No difference in satisfaction between nonobese and obese; no significant difference in complications or revision surgery; at minimum 1-year follow-up, BMI >30 is not associated with an increase in complications or reoperation	Short follow-up period; complications assessed subjectively by patient questionnaire
Mantilla/2003	Case control	PE (116)/no PE (116)	BMI, ASA grade, prophylaxis against thromboembolic events	In patients undergoing lower extremity arthroplasty, obesity, poor ASA grade, lack of thromboprophylaxis are independent risk factors for thromboembolic events.	Findings show relative risk is greater than absolute risk.
Sturm/2002	Retrospective	Smoking, drinking, obesity (10,000)	17 common chronic health conditions; SF-12; spending on inpatient and ambulatory care; medication use	Obesity has significantly greater effects on chronic conditions and causes a greater increase in patient care costs than are seen with smoking.	None stated
Stickles/2001	Retrospective	BMI <25 (131); 25-30 (223); 30-35 (119); 35-40 (51); >40 (27)	Patient satisfaction, complications; WOMAC and SF-36	No difference between obese and nonobese patients in satisfaction, decision to undergo THA again; slightly increased risk for complications among obese	Only ≈24% of preoperative data are usable because patients were excluded if no 1-year follow-up data were available.
White/2000	Retrospective	Rehospitalization for thromboembolism after THA (297)/ unmatched controls (592)	Demographic, surgical, medical; BMI	BMI ≥25 associated with rehospitalization for thromboembolism	Diagnostic bias and selection bias
Chan/1996	Prospective	Nonobese (85)/obese (81)	Preoperative and postoperative quality of life; modified HHS and Rosser Index Matrix	No significant difference in quality of life scores at 1 and 3 years; relative body weight alone does not influence the benefits of THA	None stated
Jiganti/1993	Retrospective	Nonobese (270)/obese (41)	Complications	No significant differences between nonobese and obese patients	More rheumatoid patients in nonobese group (steroids could affect wound healing and infection rates, thus increasing complications)

ASA, American Society of Anesthesiologists; *BMI,* body mass index; *DVT,* deep vein thrombosis; *HHS,* Harris hip score; *PE,* pulmonary embolism; *SF,* short form; *THA,* total hip arthroplasty; *WOMAC,* Western Ontario and McMaster University Osteoarthritis Index.

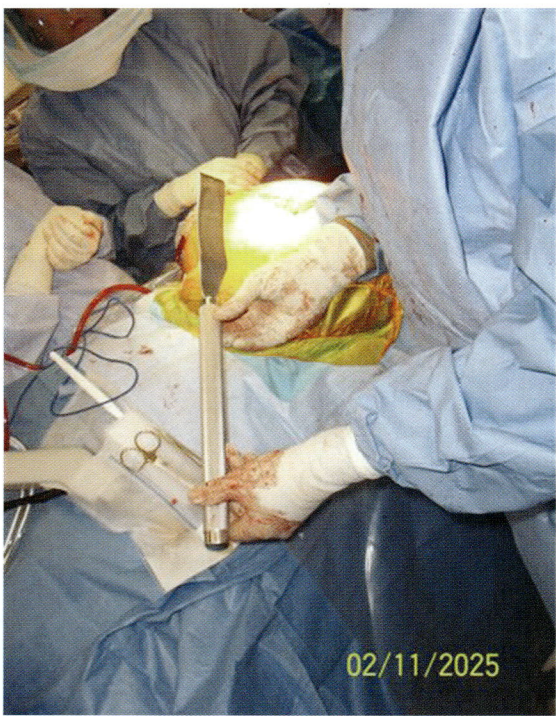

Figure 84-1. Long femoral elevating retractors are used in obese patients.

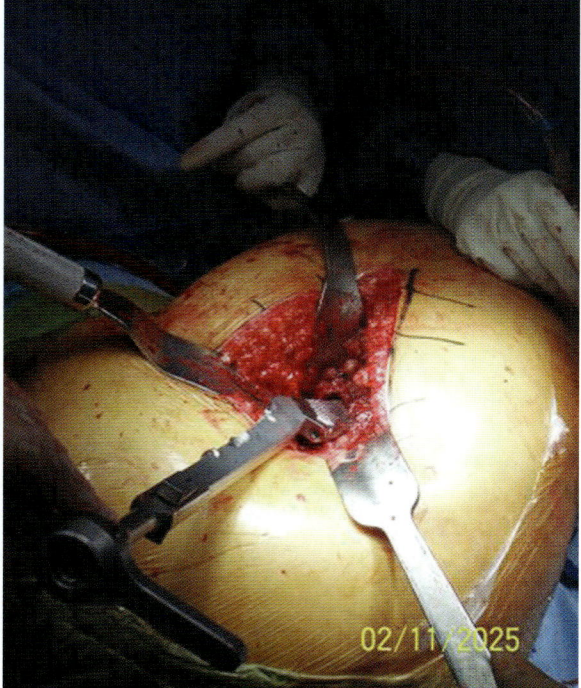

Figure 84-2. With appropriate use of retractors, excellent proximal femoral visualization can be attained.

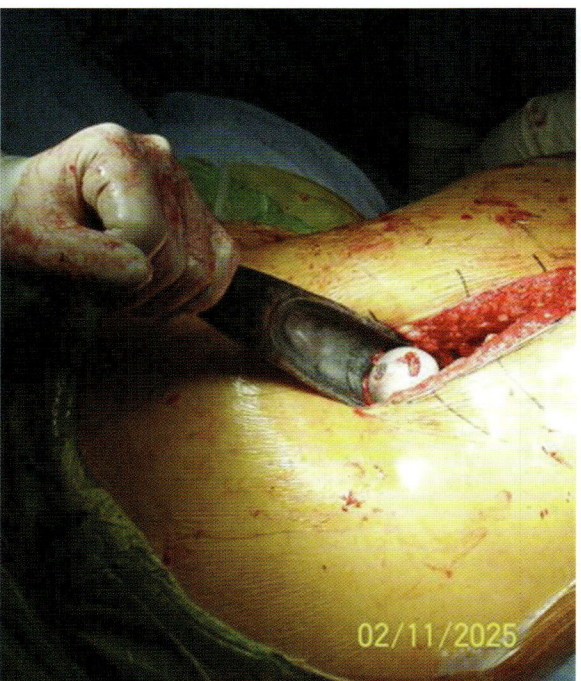

Figure 84-3. A hip slide functions as a shoehorn to allow a clear pathway for hip reduction.

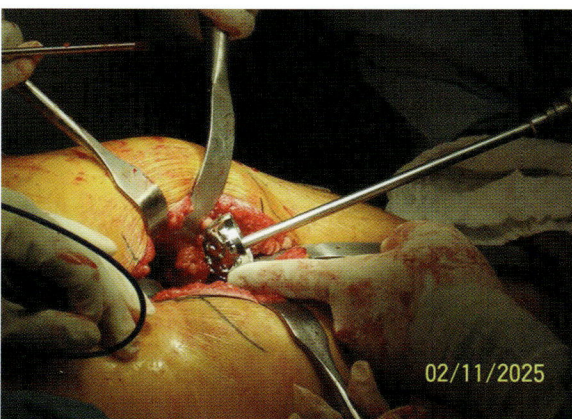

Figure 84-4. Visualization during reaming is increased when a thinner reamer driveshaft is used. Easily removable reamer baskets allow for placement of the reamer basket into the acetabulum and subsequent attachment of the reamer driveshaft.

young age (<50 years), obesity, medical comorbidity, rheumatoid arthritis, and poor bone quality. Responses were analyzed using the Cochran-Mantel-Haenszel statistic.

A majority of participants in both groups of physicians believed that patient gender did not affect the chances of a favorable outcome. For old age patients, 56.2% of referring physicians believed that chances of a favorable outcome would be decreased, as did 40.5% of orthopedic surgeons, yet 23.3% of surgeons thought that old age increased the chance of success. For young age patients, 39.7% of surgeons thought chances of a favorable outcome would be decreased, and 37.1% of them thought young age increased the chances of success. Among referring physicians, a greater percentage (46.6%) thought that young age increased the chances of success. When considering obesity, 80.9% of orthopedic surgeons thought that this factor would decrease the chances of success, as did 89.1% of

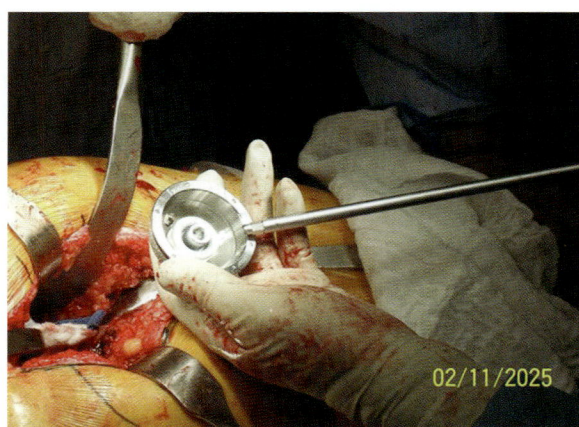

Figure 84-5. A two-piece inserter for the acetabulum allows easy isolated placement of acetabular components into the reamed acetabulum before engagement with the impactor, which is narrow in diameter to allow for better visualization.

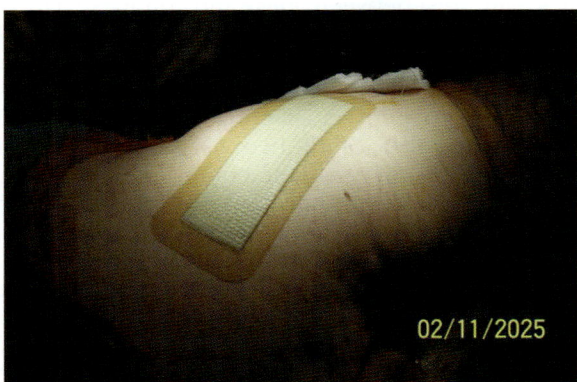

Figure 84-6. A waterproof, compliant dressing helps prevent blistering and allows sealing of the wound dressing.

referring physicians. Statistical analysis of these responses revealed that differences in mean scores between orthopedic surgeons and referring physicians were statistically significant for old age ($P < .0001$), young age ($P < .006$), and obesity ($P < .006$). No major differences in mean response scores between physician groups were noted for significant comorbidities, rheumatoid arthritis, and poor bone quality, although a majority of participants in both groups agreed that these conditions would decrease the chance of a favorable long-term result.[17] In many European countries, referral by a physician to an orthopedic surgeon is required for the patient to undergo THA. Results of this study showed that referring physicians believe that patients who are old or overweight, or who have comorbidities, might not benefit from THA; thus, they may not refer patients who would actually benefit from this procedure. Although orthopedic surgeons could not agree on the influence of "old age" on THA outcome, it may be concluded that referring physicians are even less well informed about the results of studies evaluating the success of total joint replacement in patients with

variable physical and medical characteristics and conditions.

Studies of factors affecting long-term outcome of THA have reported variable results. For example, although it is generally agreed that patient gender does not independently affect the success or failure of the procedure, studies have shown that men can have better outcomes with regard to activities of daily living.[18,19] Using age as a predictor of outcome after THA has also been inconsistent, with some studies associating advanced age with poorer outcomes[20-29] and others finding no adverse effect related to advanced age.[30,31] Along with age in years as a predictor of long-term outcome after THA, patient functional status and quality of life should be considered.[31]

With specific regard to obesity, Chan and Villar[32] prospectively studied quality of life in obese patients after THA using Harris hip scores and the Rosser Index Matrix. Of 166 patients with adequate follow-up data, 85 were nonobese (BMI <25), 56 were grade I (mildly obese; BMI, 25 to 29.9), 25 were grade II and above (moderately obese; BMI, 30 to 39.9), and 1 patient had a BMI greater than 40 and was included in the grade II and above group. Average weights of patients in the different groups were not statistically significantly different. Quality of life scores for the nonobese group improved significantly at 1 year post THA ($P < .001$) and remained similar at the 3-year post-THA time point. For the grade I obese group, average scores improved significantly at both 1- and 3-year follow-up ($P < .001$ for both time periods). The grade II and above obese group showed improvements of similar magnitude in their quality of life scores, but because of the smaller number of patients in this group, improvements were not statistically significant. These results indicate that quality of life improvement for nonobese, mildly obese, and moderately obese showed no differences between groups, leading the authors to conclude that patients should not be excluded from undergoing THA based on obesity alone.[32]

Sadr Azodi and colleagues[33] retrospectively studied the impact of obesity on postoperative complications and length of hospital stay after THA. They categorized patients as "highly obese" if BMI was greater than 35. Of the 3309 male patients studied, 2142 (64.8%) were considered overweight or obese. They found that BMI was significantly associated with increased length of hospital stay ($P < .001$); the mean length of stay for overweight patients was 4.7% (95% confidence interval [CI], 2.0 to 7.3) longer, and for obese patients was 7.09% (95% CI, 2.9 to 11.1) longer, than for patients of normal weight. Patients with increased BMI spent up to 7% longer in the hospital than normal weight patients. The authors found a trend for increased risk of postoperative complications with increasing BMI ($P = .082$); obese patients had a 58% increased risk (odds ratio [OR], 1.58; 95% CI 1.06 to 2.35) compared with patients of normal weight; study authors defined systemic complications as venous thromboembolism, acute cardiac or cerebrovascular events, postoperative anemia, blood transfusion or gastrointestinal bleeding, urinary tract infection, and pneumonia.[33]

Namba and coworkers[15] prospectively evaluated 1071 THA patients to review the effects of obesity on perioperative morbidity. Their study categorized obesity as BMI greater than 30, high obesity as BMI greater than 35, and morbid obesity as BMI greater than 40. Patient data were obtained using a prospective joint replacement registry, and postoperative complications (superficial and deep space infections) were recorded up to 1 year post THA. Researchers defined superficial infection as wound drainage or erythema requiring intravenous antibiotics and prolonged hospital stay, or readmission, and deep infection as any infection treated operatively or with a positive culture.

Reviewers found that the mean BMI of highly obese patients was significantly greater than the mean BMI of non–highly obese patients (39.5 vs. 27; $P < .001$). Highly obese patients had significantly higher rates of two comorbid conditions compared with non–highly obese patients: diabetes mellitus, 14% vs. 9% ($P < .04$) and hypertension, 53% vs. 36% ($P < .001$). A trend for increased infection rate was observed among highly obese patients (1.3% vs. 0.3%; $P = .09$); the odds ratio yielded a 4.3 times higher risk for infection in highly obese patients.[15]

Andrew and associates[34] conducted a prospective study of 1356 THA patients (1421 hips) from seven centers to determine whether clinical outcomes for obese versus nonobese patients differed. Patients were grouped according to BMI: nonobese (BMI < 30), obese (BMI 30 to < 40), and morbidly obese (BMI ≥ 40). Change in the Oxford hip score (OHS) was the primary outcome measure, and dislocation, hemorrhage requiring transfusion, deep infection, perioperative DVT requiring anticoagulation therapy, pulmonary embolism, and revision surgery were secondary outcomes. At 5 years post THA, 795 nonobese, 249 obese, and 15 morbidly obese hips were available for follow-up. Mean absolute OHS values (although improved greatly for each BMI group) of the obese and morbidly obese groups were significantly worse than that of the nonobese group ($P = .005$). However, all OHS results improved from preoperative values, thus illustrating the clinical benefit of THA for patients with an excessive BMI.[34]

A 2005 prospective study conducted in the United Kingdom consisted of 759 patients (800 hips) undergoing THA who were evaluated preoperatively and at 6 and 18 months postoperatively using SF-36 and Harris hip scores.[35] Researchers recorded length of stay, death, dislocation, reoperation, superficial and deep wound infections, blood loss and need for transfusion, and concomitant medical problems (e.g., smoking, cancer, atherosclerosis, cardiac disease, diabetes mellitus, osteoporosis, thromboembolism). All patients completed the preoperative HHS and SF-36, and 774 were assessed at 6 months and 687 at 18 months post THA. The mean BMI was 27.8 kg/m² (range, 17 to 49 kg/m²). A statistically significant improvement in HHS scores as compared with preoperative scores was noted at 6 and 18 months ($P < .0001$). A total of 7 deep and 56 superficial wound infections were reported; univariate analysis indicated that BMI might be associated with higher rates of superficial infection and lower HHS at the two postoperative time points ($P < .05$). However, additional statistical evaluation of postoperative HHS using multiple regression analysis showed that BMI was *not* a significant independent predictor of superficial wound infection. Multiple regression analysis further noted that a postoperative increase in BMI was inversely related to a change in Harris hip score at 6-month ($P = .02$) and 18-month ($P < .001$) evaluations; for every 1-point increase in BMI, the HHS decreased by 0.25 at 6 months and by 0.35 points at 18 months. Body mass index did not have an effect on early THA failure. The authors added that although higher patient body weight places a greater load on the arthroplasty, obese patients tend to be less active, which may temper the effect of greater BMI on the durability of the implant.[35]

One recent study evaluated the effects of obesity on complications, functional outcome, and satisfaction after THA with emphasis on identifying differences between men and women.[36] This prospective study evaluated 2495 THAs (2186 patients), comparing outcomes of interest between obese and nonobese patients. The primary outcome was the prevalence of "main" complications (deep infection, dislocation, and revision); secondary outcomes included disease-specific quality of life, patient satisfaction, and general health, assessed using HHS, SF-12, two visual analogue scales measuring pain relief and function, and the Western Ontario and McMaster University Osteoarthritis Index (WOMAC). Obesity was more prevalent in male patients (26.7% vs. 20.5%). With a follow-up period ranging from 3 to 72 months, 91 hips with main complications were reported: Infection was more prevalent in the hips of obese patients (1.7% vs. 0.4%). Obesity in women was associated with infection (prevalence ratio of obese vs. nonobese women was 16.1; 95% CI, 3.4 to 75.7), but obesity among male patients did not appear to be associated with an increased infection rate (rate ratio, 1.0; 95% CI, 0.2 to 5.3). For dislocation, the adjusted rate ratio was 2.4 (95% CI, 1.4 to 4.2) among obese patients, and the prevalence of dislocation was approximately twice as high among men, but the relative rate increase due to obesity was higher in women (rate ratio, 3.0 vs. 1.8). Revision THA was performed in 13 nonobese and 8 obese patients (adjusted rate ratio, 2.0; 95% CI, 0.9 to 4.8). Among hips available for 5-year follow-up, 81% of hips in the nonobese group and 70% in the obese group had good to excellent results as measured by the HHS. Investigators found that obesity was related to increased infection and dislocation rates, as well as an increased need for revision due to septic loosening. Further, obese women had higher rates of infection than obese men, as well as lower functional outcome and less satisfaction with THA than obese men.[36]

Patel and colleagues[14] studied the factors possibly related to prolonged wound drainage and their effects on rate of wound infection and longer hospital stay. They retrospectively reviewed the records of 1211 primary THAs, 15 of which developed acute infection postoperatively. Their analysis revealed that morbid obesity and prolonged wound drainage were statistically associated ($P = .001$), and that prolonged wound drainage led to significantly prolonged length of hospital stay ($P < .001$). Their analysis also revealed that for each day of prolonged wound drainage, the risk of wound infection increased by 42% following THA.[14]

Stickles and coworkers[37] reviewed the relationship between obesity and patient subjective assessments of outcome after THA using the SF-36 instrument and the WOMAC questionnaire. They found no difference between obese and nonobese patients in terms of self-reported patient satisfaction, whether they would undergo total joint arthroplasty again, a physical component summary, a mental component summary, and WOMAC (all $P > .05$). The only difference between obese and nonobese patients was that obese patients reported difficulty in negotiating stairs at the 1-year postarthroplasty time point (odds ratio, 1.2 to 1.3). This observation, however, may apply to obese individuals in general, not just those who are post THA. [37]

Jiganti and associates[38] in 1993 reported on the safety of total joint arthroplasty performed in an obese population and noted that losing weight before total joint arthroplasty may have little effect on the patient's postoperative course. Through a retrospective review of 51 nonobese and 103 obese THA patients, they found that intravenous fluid administration and total blood loss were slightly higher for obese patients, and that operative time was significantly longer for obese THA patients ($P < .001$). Investigators reported 0.29 minor complications per nonobese patient and 0.22 per obese patient. A total of 0.22 major complications occurred per nonobese patient and 0.10 per obese patient.[38]

A 2005 report by Ibrahim and colleagues[39] assessed the effects of obesity on complications and reoperations after THA with a minimum of 1-year follow-up via a self-administered validated questionnaire. Patient satisfaction with the procedure was high, and no difference between obese and nonobese patient groups was noted. Similarly, no difference in length of hospital stay, American Society of Anesthesiologists (ASA) grade, or proportion of intraoperative complications, total complications, or revision procedures was observed. However, because of the short follow-up period in this study, the authors note that long-term studies are still necessary to determine further effects of obesity on outcomes of THA.[39]

A Mayo Clinic study found that preemptive bariatric surgery is beneficial for morbidly obese patients undergoing total joint arthroplasty. Parvizi and coworkers[40] reported the results of THA in seven patients who underwent bariatric surgery before their total joint procedure. Average time from bariatric surgery to joint replacement was 23 months (range, 7 to 65 months). One staged bilateral THA and six unilateral THAs were reported. The follow-up period averaged 3.7 years (range, 2 to 11 years), and no patients were lost to follow-up. No radiographic evidence of loosening or wear of components was noted at the latest follow-up evaluation. Postoperatively, two cases of DVT were treated successfully with intravenous heparin and oral warfarin for 3 months. In two hips, superficial infection was treated with oral antibiotics. One revision was performed in a patient who underwent primary THA at age 25. After the bariatric surgery, the patient lost more than 40% of her weight and became very physically active, which may have contributed to early failure. In this series, patients who first underwent bariatric surgery had very acceptable results after total joint arthroplasty with few complications.[40]

Super-Obese Patients

Although the studies reviewed have shown, in general, acceptable and even equal results for obese and morbidly obese patients undergoing THA, one report focused on studying "super-obese" patients with BMI greater than 50. Polga and associates[41] retrospectively reviewed the outcomes of 41 patients (43 hips) who underwent THA between 1996 and 2006, all with BMI greater than 50 (range, 50 to 77). The mean age of patients at surgery was 56.8 years, and the mean follow-up period was 36.8 months. In all, 17 surgical complications (39.5%) and 7 (17%) medical complications occurred; 5 patients died between 3 and 28 months postoperatively. Ten hips had prolonged wound drainage. The major complication rate was 12.2%, which included 15 reoperations (5 patients): 1 for irrigation and débridement with component retention, 3 for recurrent dislocation (2 of which became chronically infected requiring resection), 1 for periprosthetic fracture that also became infected and required resection, and 1 fractured stem that required revision 4 years after the index THA. Two intraoperative complications (1 acetabular fracture and 1 femur fracture) were treated at the time of primary THA. These high rates of complications should alert surgeons to counsel super-obese patients about the importance of weight loss before THA and suggest the advantages of preoperative referral to a bariatric surgeon.[41]

Infection

In multiple studies, infection risk has been shown to be higher following THA in obese patients. Peersman[42] reported that prior open surgical procedures, immunosuppression, poor nutrition, hypokalemia, diabetes mellitus, obesity, and tobacco use increased the chance of developing surgical site infection. Malinzak and colleagues[43] retrospectively compared cases of deep infection with noninfected cases of both total knee arthroplasty (TKA) and THA with the goal of determining infection rates and risk factors. The infection rate for THA was 0.47% (13 of 2775). Patients with BMI greater than 50 (both knee and hip arthroplasties) were 18.3 times more likely to develop infection than were patients with BMI less than 50 ($P < .0001$). Additionally, patients with diabetes were 3 times as likely as nondiabetic patients to experience an infection ($P < .0027$). When data for the 13 infected THAs were examined, no variables were found to be significantly different from those of noninfected THAs (e.g., age, BMI, simultaneous or single hip procedures). This study showed that obesity, diabetes, and younger age are all risk factors for developing infection after total joint replacement procedures are performed.[43]

Thromboembolic Complications

A recent large study reviewed the records of 5832 total hip or knee patients to determine the preoperative, intraoperative, and postoperative risk factors for an increased incidence of pulmonary embolism.[44] Overall, 30 pulmonary emboli were reported. Statistical analysis determined that increased age (OR, 1.07; $P = .004$), increased BMI (OR, 1.11; $P < .001$), and female gender (OR, 7.54; $P = .05$) were associated with increased risk of developing pulmonary embolism (PE) after total joint arthroplasty.[43] An earlier study compared patients who underwent primary hip or knee arthroplasty and experienced PE or DVT within 30 days of surgery versus patients who underwent the same operation by the same surgeon and did not have a thromboembolic event.[45] Their review found that increased BMI ($P = .031$; OR, 1.5 for each 5-kg/m^2 BMI increase) and an ASA physical status score of 3 or greater ($P = .005$; OR, 2.6) were independent risk factors for increasing the likelihood of PE or DVT. White and colleagues[46] examined California Medicare records from 1993 through 1996 and found 297 patients 65 years of age or older who had been rehospitalized for thromboembolism within 3 months post THA. Comparison with 592 unmatched controls revealed that BMI of 25 or greater was associated with embolism and rehospitalization (OR, 2.5; 95% CI, 1.8 to 3.4). Investigators also reported that use of pneumatic compression in patients with BMI less than 25 and administration of prophylactic warfarin after discharge were independently protective against thromboembolic events.[45]

CURRENT CONTROVERSIES AND FUTURE CONSIDERATIONS

- As the population ages and as obesity becomes more prevalent, orthopedic surgeons will encounter more patients who are older and heavier who desire total joint arthroplasty.
- Most published studies of THA in obese patients are relatively recent; studies with longer-term follow-up will be necessary to evaluate the effect of obesity on the durability of the implanted devices.
- Longer-term follow-up studies may also identify implant designs that are more appropriate for obese patients and the increased demand they place on the joints.

CONCLUSIONS

Variable results regarding the effects of obesity on THA have been reported in multiple studies in which complications and outcomes were reviewed. Patient satisfaction and absolute functional outcome may be lower for obese versus nonobese patients, yet obese patients enjoy functional improvement comparable with that of their nonobese counterparts when compared according to preoperative status. Total hip arthroplasty should not be reserved for patients with lower BMI (and denied to obese patients on the basis of perceived increases in

complications, failures, revisions, operative time, blood loss, and surgical difficulty). However, it does appear that some differences exist for obese men and obese women in terms of postoperative complications; this should be discussed with patients as part of their preoperative evaluation and counseling. Many studies acknowledge limitations, such as short-term follow-up, small numbers of patients due to missing data, patients lost to follow-up, and low statistical power; it should be recognized that variations in stated results and conclusions can be attributed to different statistical methods. Even when the variable results of studies of THA in obese patients are considered, collectively virtually all studies report restoration of patient function, pain relief, and acceptable levels of patient satisfaction, which are the primary goals of THA, with increased risk of some perioperative complications.

REFERENCES

1. World Health Organization: Available at: http://www.who.int/mediacentre/factsheets/fs311/en/. Accessed September 2, 2009.
2. Mokdad AH, Bowman BA, Ford ES, et al: The continuing epidemics of obesity and diabetes in the United States. JAMA 286:1195–1200, 2001.
3. Centers for Disease Control: Available at: http://www.cdc.org/task_forces/prevention/WebPhyAct_Medical_Costs.htm. Accessed September 2, 2009.
4. Marks R, Allegrante JP: Body mass indices in patients with disabling hip osteoarthritis. Arthritis Res 4:112–116, 2002.
5. Wendelboe AM, Hegmann KT, Biggs JJ, et al: Relationships between body mass indices and surgical replacements of knees and hip joints. Am J Prev Med 25:290–295, 2003.
6. Karlson EW, Mandl LA, Aweh GN: Total hip replacement due to osteoarthritis: the importance of age, obesity, and other modifiable risk factors. Am J Med 114:93–98, 2003.
7. Stürmer T, Gunther KP, Brenner H: Obesity, overweight and patterns of osteoarthritis: the Ulm osteoarthritis study. J Clin Epidemiol 53:307–313, 2000.
8. Harms S, Larson R, Sahmoun AE, Beal JR: Obesity increases the likelihood of total joint replacement surgery among younger adults. Int Orthop 31:23–26, 2007.
9. Charnley J: Long-term results of low-friction arthroplasty. Hip 42–49, 1982.
10. Horan F: Obesity and joint replacement. J Bone Joint Surg Br 88:1269–1271, 2006.
11. Adams JP, Murphy PG: Obesity in anaesthesia and intensive care. Br J Anaesth 85:91–108, 2000.
12. Lowe GD, Haverkate F, Thompson SG: Prediction of deep vein thrombosis after elective hip replacement surgery by preoperative clinical and haemostatic variables: the ECAT DVT Study. European Concerted Action on Thrombosis. Thromb Haemost 81:879–886, 1999.
13. Abdollahi M, Cushman, Rosendaal FR: Obesity: risk of venous thrombosis and the interaction with coagulation factor levels and oral contraceptive use. Thromb Haemost 89:493–498, 2003.
14. Patel VP, Walsh M, Sehgal B, et al: Factors associated with prolonged wound drainage after primary total hip and knee arthroplasty. J Bone Joint Surg Am 89:33–38, 2007.
15. Namba RS, Paxton L, Fithian DC, Stone ML: Obesity and perioperative morbidity in total hip and total knee arthroplasty patients. J Arthroplasty 20(Suppl 3):46–50, 2005.
16. Burnett RSJ, Clohisy JJC, Wright RW, et al: Failure of the American College of Chest Physicians-1A protocol for Lovenox in clinical outcomes for thromboembolic prophylaxis. J Arthroplasty 22:317–324, 2007.
17. Stürmer T, Dreinhöfer K, Gröber-Grätz D, et al: Differences in the views of orthopaedic surgeons and referring practitioners on the determinants of outcome after total hip replacement. J Bone Joint Surg Br 87:16–19, 2005.

18. Young NL, Cheah D, Waddell JP, Wright JG: Patient characteristics that affect the outcome of total hip arthroplasty: a review. Can J Surg 41:188–195, 1998.

19. Holtzman J, Saleh K, Kane R: Gender differences in functional status and pain in a Medicare population undergoing elective total hip arthroplasty. Med Care 40:461–470, 2002.

20. Nilsdotter AK, Petersson IF, Roos EM, Lohmander LS: Predictors of patient relevant outcome after total hip replacement for osteoarthritis: a prospective study. Ann Rheum Dis 62:923–930, 2003.

21. Pettine HA, Aamlid BC, Cabanela ME: Elective total hip arthroplasty in patients older than 80 years of age. Clin Orthop Relat Res 266:127–132, 1991.

22. Boettcher WG: Total hip arthroplasties in the elderly: morbidity, mortality, and cost effectiveness. Clin Orthop Relat Res 274:30–34, 1992.

23. Levy RN, Levy CM, Snyder J, Digiovanni J: Outcome and long-term results following total hip replacement in elderly patients. Clin Orthop Relat Res 316:25–30, 1995.

24. Towheed TE, Hochberg MC: Health-related quality of life after total hip replacement. Semin Arthritis Rheum 26:483–491, 1996.

25. Braeken AM, Lochhaas-Gerlach JA, Gollish JD, et al: Determinants of 6-12 month postoperative functional status and pain after elective total hip replacement. Int J Qual Health Care 9:413–418, 1997.

26. Brander VA, Malhotra S, Jet J, et al: Outcome of hip and knee arthroplasty in persons aged 80 years and older. Clin Orthop Relat Res 345:67–78, 1997.

27. Espehaug B, Havelin LI, Angesaeter LB, et al: Patient satisfaction and function after primary and revision total hip replacement. Clin Orthop Relat Res 351:135–148, 1998.

28. Garellick G, Malchau H, Herberts P, et al: Life expectancy and cost utility after total hip replacement. Clin Orthop Relat Res 346:1414–1451, 1998.

29. Nilsdotter AK, Lohmander LS: Age and waiting time as predictors of outcome after total hip replacement for osteoarthritis. Rheumatology 41:1261–1267, 2002.

30. Jones CA, Voaklander DC, Johnston DW, Suarez-Almazor ME: The effect of age on pain, function, and quality of life after total hip and knee arthroplasty. Arch Intern Med 161:454–460, 2001.

31. March LM, Cross MJ, Lapsley H, et al: Outcomes after hip or knee replacement surgery for osteoarthritis: a prospective cohort study comparing patients' quality of life before and after surgery with age-related population norms. Med J Aust 171:235–238, 1999.

32. Chan CLH, Villar RN: Obesity and quality of life after primary hip arthroplasty. J Bone Joint Surg Br 78:78–81, 1996.

33. Sadr Azodi O, Bellocco R, Eriksson K, Adami J: The impact of tobacco use and body mass index on the length of stay in hospital and the risk of post-operative complications among patients undergoing total hip replacement. J Bone Joint Surg Br 88:1316–1320, 2006.

34. Andrew JG, Palan J, Kurup HV, et al: Obesity in total hip replacement. J Bone Joint Surg Br 90:424–429, 2008.

35. Moran M, Walmsley P, Gray A, Brenkel IJ: Does body mass index affect the early outcome of primary total hip arthroplasty? J Arthroplasty 20:866–869, 2005.

36. Lübbeke A, Stern R, Garavaglia G, et al: Differences in outcomes of obese women and men undergoing primary total hip arthroplasty. Arthritis Rheum 57:327–334, 2007.

37. Stickles B, Phillips L, Brox WT, et al: Defining the relationship between obesity and total joint arthroplasty. Obes Res 9:219–223, 2001.

38. Jiganti JJ, Goldstein WM, Williams CS: A comparison of the perioperative morbidity in total joint arthroplasty in the obese and nonobese patient. Clin Orthop Relat Res 289:175–179, 1993.

39. Ibrahim T, Hobson S, Beiri A, Esler CN: No influence on body mass index on early outcome following total hip arthroplasty. Int Orthop 29:359–361, 2005.

40. Parvizi J, Trousdale RT, Sarr MG: Total joint arthroplasty in patients surgically treated for obesity. J Arthroplasty 15:1003–1008, 2000.

41. Polga DJ, Altenburg A, Trousdale RT, Lewallen DG: Complications following total hip arthroplasty in the superobese, BMI >50. Presented at the Annual Meeting of the American Academy of Orthopaedic Surgeons, Las Vegas, February 26, 2009.

42. Peersman G: Infection in total knee replacement. Clin Orthop Relat Res 392:15–23, 2001.

43. Malinzak RA, Ritter MA, Berend ME, et al: Morbidly obese, diabetic, younger, and unilateral joint arthroplasty patients have elevated total joint arthroplasty infection rates. J Arthroplasty 24(Suppl 1):84–88, 2009.

44. Walsh MG, Preston C, Patel V, DiCesare PE: Risk factors for acute pulmonary embolism following total hip and knee arthroplasty. J Orthop 5:10, 2008. Available at: http://www.jortho.org/2008/5/2/310/index.htm. Accessed September 3, 2009.

45. Mantilla CB, Horlocker TT, Schroeder DR, et al: Risk factors for clinically relevant pulmonary embolism and deep venous thrombosis in patients undergoing primary hip or knee arthroplasty. Anesthesiology 99:552–560, 2003.

46. White RH, Gettner S, Newman JM, et al: Predictors of rehospitalization for symptomatic venous thromboembolism after total hip arthroplasty. N Engl J Med 343:1758–1764, 2000.

REVISION TOTAL HIP ARTHROPLASTY

CHAPTER 85

Evaluation of the Failed Total Hip Arthroplasty

*Randy Rizek, Rajiv Gandhi, Khalid Syed,
and Nizar Mahomed*

INTRODUCTION

Total hip arthroplasty (THA) continues to be one of the most successful orthopedic procedures, improving function and providing significant pain relief among the majority of patients. However, complications do arise postoperatively that can threaten the longevity of the prosthesis. The most common modes of failure following THA include aseptic loosening, infection, dislocation, and periprosthetic fracture. A systematic approach beginning with a thorough history and physical examination aids in determining an accurate diagnosis and the need for a revision procedure.

CLINICAL EVALUATION

Pain is the most common presentation of a patient with a failed total hip arthroplasty (THA). Characterizing the temporal onset, duration, severity, location, and quality of the pain is essential in determining whether the symptoms are due to intrinsic hip pathology or extrinsic causes (Table 85-1). If the patient's preoperative pain remains unresolved postoperatively in the absence of a pain-free interval, the original diagnosis prior to surgery should be questioned. If the pain differs and is worse postoperatively, the underlying cause is most likely the surgery itself, as in cases of infection, hematoma, component instability, loosening, impingement, or fracture. A delay in the onset of pain postoperatively suggests that the inciting problem may be the implant itself, as can be seen in loosening, chronic infection, or osteolysis.

Determining the location of painful symptoms aids in narrowing the differential diagnosis. Pain localized over the lateral aspect of the hip/thigh may result from trochanteric bursitis, suture/wire irritation, osteolysis, muscle strain, or a fracture. Groin or buttocks pain is typical of vascular or neurogenic claudication, acetabular loosening, or osteolysis. Other causes include iliopsoas impingement and tendinitis due to acetabular retroversion or a prominent acetabular implant.[1] Hematoma, various types of hernias, and gynecologic/genitourinary problems are less frequent. Buttocks pain that is associated with radiation distal to the knee is suggestive of spine pathology such as degenerative disk disease or spinal stenosis. Patients with iliopsoas tendinitis describe pain with movements that involve active hip flexion and rotation, such as getting up from a seated position. Thigh pain can be attributable to a loose femoral component, whereby micromotion occurs between the bone and the prosthesis owing to a mismatch in their modulus of elasticity.[2,3] However, patients could still have pain despite the presence of a well-fixed cemented or cementless femoral component.

It is important to note circumstances that aggravate and alleviate symptoms. Night pain or pain at rest is suggestive of an underlying infection or malignancy. Painful symptoms associated with activity that are relieved with rest could be due to a loose component, a subtle fracture, or vascular or neurogenic claudication. Pain that is severe with initiating movements, such as getting out of a chair, but resolves once active is associated with early component loosening, spondyloarthrosis, or iliopsoas tendinitis.[4] Any history of a traumatic event, such as a sudden slip or fall, preceding the onset of painful symptoms raises the suspicion of traumatic loosening or fracture. Patients with a history of hip and spine pathology may experience increasing pain postoperatively as a result of an increase in their activity levels.

One of the main goals of obtaining a history from a patient with a potentially failed THA is to rule out infection. An infected THA is classified into one of three categories based on onset of symptoms and the underlying cause of the infection.[5] Stage I infections occur in the immediate postoperative period, and patients can

Table 85-1. Differential Diagnosis of Pain Following Hip Replacement

Intrinsic Causes	Extrinsic Causes
Infection: acute, delayed, late, hematogenous	Lumbar spine disease: stenosis, disk herniation, spondylolysis/ spondylolisthesis
Aseptic loosening	Malignant tumor: primary, secondary
Pain at stem tip (modulus mismatch)	Peripheral vascular disease
Greater trochanter nonunion	Metabolic disease
Wear debris synovitis	Stress and insufficiency fracture
Periprosthetic fracture	Nerve injury: sciatic, femoral, lateral cutaneous
Osteolysis	Iliopsoas tendinitis
Occult instability	Hernia: femoral, inguinal, obturator
	Complex regional pain syndrome
	Other gastrointestinal, genitourinary, or gynecologic disease

From Duffy P, Masri BA, Garbuz D, Duncan CP: Evaluation of patients with pain following total hip replacement. Instr Course Lect 55:223–232, 2006.

present with systemic signs of infection such as fever, chills, sweating, and constant pain, along with a red, swollen wound that is draining purulent material. However, this classic presentation of a septic THA is rare.[5] Most patients with acute infection of a THA present within the first 12 weeks of surgery with a history of pain and serous wound drainage. The challenge is differentiating whether the infection is superficial or has penetrated the deep fascia to the periprosthetic space.

Stage II infections originate from the index procedure but may involve an acute or delayed low-grade, indolent process. They occur between 6 and 24 months after surgery with increasing pain and a gradually declining level of activity. Pain usually occurs at rest and during weight bearing but is not as severe as with an acutely infected THA. There may be a history of previous infection from another source that preceded the hip symptoms. The patient must be questioned regarding whether there was a delay in the discharge, prolonged use of antibiotics, night pain, or a history of persistent wound drainage.

Stage III infections are the least common and the easiest to diagnose. The clinical presentation consists of sudden onset of hip pain without a history of perioperative sepsis. Pain on weight bearing or any movement of the hip along with rest pain is characteristic of a late deep infection after the patient has been asymptomatic for 2 years or longer after surgery. It occurs as the result of hematogenous spread from another remote source. Patients usually can recall a previous dental procedure, respiratory infection, genitourinary procedure or infection, or open skin lesion before the onset of symptoms. However, medications such as antibiotics or steroids can mask these symptoms. Immunocompromised patients, intravenous (IV) drug users, and patients who

require frequent urinary catheterizations are at high risk for stage III infection.

Clinical assessment of a patient with a problem following THA includes determining the presence of subluxation or dislocation. Patients will describe a sensation of popping or clicking, suggesting that the hip is coming into and out of the joint. They can also present with an acute dislocation precipitated by a traumatic event. Most dislocations occur within the first year of surgery.[6] Patient factors such as gender, body habitus, a history of neuromuscular or cognitive disorders, and alcohol use are shown to increase the rate of dislocation.[7] Any previous history of hip surgery and the surgical approach utilized should be determined. In the setting of acute dislocation, information surrounding the episode, including any history of previous dislocations, is crucial in elucidating the cause of instability.

Identifying the patient's functional status requires a thorough evaluation to assess the impact that the problematic THA is having on daily activities. Several standardized scales are available to assist in quantifying a patient's level of disability and pain; these include the Western Ontario and McMaster University (WOMAC) Osteoarthritis Index and Short Form (SF)-36.[8] These scales can also be useful in assessing postoperative improvement.

The patient's medical history and a review of systems should be obtained. Most often, THA is performed on members of the elderly population, who are likely to have comorbidities that predispose them to postoperative complications. Risk factors for infection as discussed previously should be ruled out. Any history of venous ulcers or vascular insufficiency may necessitate a vascular surgery consultation. If the patient has been immobilized postoperatively, the risk of developing a pulmonary embolism and deep vein thrombosis is high, requiring appropriate workup. A positive cardiac history will require preoperative assessment to ensure medical optimization and to determine whether surgical intervention is a viable treatment option. Patients who have received previous pelvis irradiation treatment with radiation osteonecrosis are not suitable for porous-coated implants if revision hip surgery is required.[9] Previous hip operations should be documented. The presence of constitutional symptoms should not be overlooked, thereby avoiding the danger of missing an underlying infection or malignant process.

Finally, an attempt should be made to obtain all operative records from the primary surgery along with the implant labels. These provide insight into any technical challenges that may have arisen. They also describe the type and size of implant that was used, providing information that is invaluable in preoperative planning and assessment of compatibility if revision surgery is indicated.

PHYSICAL EXAMINATION

A complete musculoskeletal examination must be performed when a patient presents with a problem following THA. The contralateral hip, both knees, and the lumbar spine are incorporated into the routine examination to rule out pathology from referred sources. The examination should begin with an assessment of the patient's gait, which can help identify a leg length discrepancy, antalgia, or abductor weakness. A leg length discrepancy (LLD) of 2.5 cm or greater can cause a limp with a vaulting-type gait pattern, but its effect on mechanical failure or correlation with the onset of low back pain is inconclusive.[10] Although its functional implications are not well defined, a substantial LLD is dissatisfying to the patient and is a common reason for litigation. It must be determined whether it is a true or apparent LLD. True leg length can be measured from the anterior superior iliac spines to the medial malleoli of the ankles. A true bony inequality exists if the two measurements are unequal. The LLD should be compared with measurements taken postoperatively because increasing discrepancy would suggest gradual subsidence of the components.[11] An apparent leg length discrepancy is identified by measuring the distance from the umbilicus to the medial malleoli. In the absence of a true LLD, an apparent LLD can occur owing to pelvic obliquity, adduction, or flexure contracture.

A Trendelenburg gait can be observed when the abductor muscles are weak or nonfunctional, whereby the unsupported hip drops during the midstance phase of the gait cycle, and the patient exhibits a characteristic lurch to compensate for the instability. The abductors can be tested against gravity by having the patient abduct his leg while in the lateral decubitus position.

The skin should be carefully examined with particular attention to the condition of the primary incision and its usefulness for revision surgery. Inspection for signs of inflammation, persistent drainage, or healed sinus tracks should be documented. Palpation can aid in localizing the source of symptoms in that tenderness along the scar suggests a possible neuroma. The greater trochanter, femur, and pubic rami should be palpated to rule out a possible trochanteric bursitis, occult fracture, or metastatic deposit. The iliac fossa and inguinal region should be examined for fullness or masses that may suggest the presence of hernias.

The hip and adjacent joints should be taken through full active and passive ranges of motion. Pain at the extremes suggests component loosening, and pain with any form of movement may indicate an infection or an inflammatory process. Impingement or instability will cause pain in a particular position or movement. Pain caused by trochanteric bursitis, gluteal calcific tendinitis, and heterotopic ossification can be exacerbated by resisted abduction. Pain with resisted hip flexion or passive hip extension may suggest iliopsoas tendinitis,[1] and pain with passive straight-leg raise is indicative of a lumbar spine radiculopathy.

A detailed neurovascular examination is essential in ruling out neurogenic or vascular causes of symptoms. Patients with a history of spine pathology are at increased risk for nerve palsy.[12] Preoperative documentation of any motor or sensory deficits should be obtained. Direct nerve injury can result from surgical trauma, traction, retractors, limb lengthening, positioning, or thermal or pressure injury from cement.[10] The peroneal division of the sciatic nerve is the most commonly injured nerve, as is demonstrated by weakness in ankle dorsiflexion and decreased/loss of sensation to the dorsum of the foot.[13] This should be carefully assessed in the setting of limb lengthening. Injury to the tibial division is rare but is seen with weakness of the knee flexors and ankle plantarflexors.[14]

The vascular integrity of the limb should be closely scrutinized. Any sign of vascular compromise or insufficiency should warrant further investigation. A swollen, tender calf should raise suspicion of a deep venous thrombosis, and incisions from a previous vascular bypass surgery may necessitate a vascular consultation.

Further abdominal, pelvic, and rectal examinations may be warranted in an effort to rule out causes of referred pain.

IMAGING OF THE FAILED TOTAL HIP REPLACEMENT

Evaluation of the failed total hip replacement (THR) requires knowledge of diagnostic imaging options. These imaging tools have evolved in diagnostic accuracy, and the choice of test ordered by the evaluating physician must reflect some understanding of the sensitivity and specificity of these tests. As a reminder for the reader, the sensitivity of a test represents its true positive rate; specificity refers to the true negative rate.

Standard evaluation of the failed THR should include an anteroposterior (AP) view of the pelvis centered on the pubic symphysis, an AP view of the affected hip, and a shoot-through lateral of the affected hip. Radiographs should cover the full extent of the prosthesis, including the entire column of cement if a cemented femoral component exists. In addition to alignment and positioning of the components, areas of osteolysis, femoral bowing, cement mantle fractures, and cortical thinning can be seen. Positioning the limb in 15 to 20 degrees of internal rotation allows for an accurate assessment of the femoral neck shaft angle and offset. Measurement of the femoral canal diameter can be difficult with magnification errors; however, standardization with marker films can be helpful.

Patients with pelvic and acetabular osteolysis or post-traumatic deformities may be assessed with Judet views to evaluate the integrity of the anterior and posterior columns. These radiographs should be reviewed for heterotopic ossification, and those with Brooker grade 3 or 4 disease should be considered for prophylaxis following revision surgery. This prophylaxis may consist of postoperative radiation or oral indomethacin.

Clinical examination and imaging of a painful metal-on-metal bearing hip replacement must consider the possibility of an inflammatory "pseudotumor." This pseudotumor signifies a high-grade inflammatory reaction in the soft tissues, and although the exact cause is unclear, it is believed to be mediated by a lymphocytic reaction to local cobalt and chromium ions. Patients with these reactions may present with regional hip pain, a palpable soft tissue mass, spontaneous dislocation, or associated nerve palsies.[15,16]

Ultrasound is likely the best imaging modality of choice if a pseudotumor is first suspected. Magnetic resonance imaging findings can include a soft tissue mass with muscle necrosis and cystic fluid collections. X-ray findings may show an elevated acetabular cup abduction angle because this is believed to be associated with elevated ion levels. The best reported treatments are pseudotumor excision and a change in the bearing surface.[15,16]

Osteolysis and Wear

Osteolysis is a major reason for failure following THA. It is a biological process caused by particle debris that leads to bone loss around the prosthesis. The cause is multifactorial and is influenced by patient, implant, and surgical factors. The terms *osteolysis* and *aseptic loosening* have been used interchangeably in the literature, but they refer to the same biological process occurring at the metal-bone or cement-bone interface. Clinical manifestations of osteolysis can range from slowly progressive radiolucencies around a previously well-fixed component that can result in mechanical loosening to rapidly expansile radiolucent lesions that may or may not result in mechanical loosening. Therefore, it is essential for orthopedic surgeons who perform THA to be aware of the clinical and radiographic patterns of osteolysis.

Causes

The osteolytic process is initiated by particulate debris generated from wear sources, most of which come from the bearing surfaces of the implant. Wear debris can consist of polyethylene, polymethylmethacrylate, metals, or ceramics. The size, shape, and concentration of these particles influence the extent of osteolysis that occurs. Wear has been shown to consist mostly of submicron polyethylene particles generated from a cobalt-chromium-polyethylene articulation.[17] These particles are known to illicit an enhanced host immune response, whereby macrophages ingest particle debris, leading to activation of an inflammatory cascade. These inflammatory markers initiate osteoclast activity and inhibit osteoblast activity, which leads to the resorption of bone. Because this process compromises the metal-bone or cement-bone interface, micromotion of the implant occurs; this can lead to the production of additional wear debris and eventual mechanical loosening.

The extent of osteolysis and loosening is influenced by particle access to the prosthesis interface. Particles can travel within the new prosthetic joint and in the potential space around the prosthesis-bone interface, which is referred to as the *effective joint space*.[18] Access to the effective joint space is influenced by implant factors such as shape, size, and extent of porous coating.

Risk Factors

Specific factors that place a patient at increased risk of osteolysis include age, male gender, and high levels of activity. Young patients have been specifically shown to have higher rates of acetabular loosening and osteolysis, but age does not influence the rate of femoral loosening.[19] The generation of wear debris is generally higher among more active individuals and is not associated with a patient's weight.[20,21] It is thought that aerobic activity is well tolerated as opposed to high-impact activities such as running or repetitive heavy lifting.[20]

Implant-related factors are known to effect the generation of wear debris. Polyethylene sterilized by gamma irradiation in a vacuum rather than in air demonstrates increased fatigue strength and wear resistance. Oxidation of polyethylene in an inert atmosphere leads to cross-linking between polymer chains.[22] Highly cross-linked polyethylene has been shown to generate lower rates of wear debris.[23] Polyethylene thickness less than 6 mm is associated with higher rates of osteolysis.[24] Alternate bearing surfaces have been introduced to increase the longevity of THA and have demonstrated improved wear characteristics. Hard surfaces such as ceramic articulating with cross-linked polyethylene or ceramic demonstrate minimal amounts of osteolysis.[17,25] Modern metal-on-metal bearings generate a lower volume of wear and smaller particulate debris, but the long-term effects of metallosis remain unknown. Other surgical factors associated with increased wear rate include malalignment of the acetabular component and failure to restore femoral offset.[26]

Diagnosis

Osteolysis can exist in the absence of clinical symptoms, making the diagnosis challenging. The patient may remain asymptomatic despite evidence of periprosthetic radiolucencies or enlarging focal defects on plain radiographs. It is recommended that serial radiographs be performed during the first 5 to 7 years of follow-up to screen for evidence of ingrowth and the presence of radiolucencies or loosening. Computed tomography (CT) scans should be utilized to screen young, active patients following THA for evidence of osteolysis.

Patients typically begin to present with pain when bone loss leads to implant loosening or a periprosthetic fracture. Pain localized to the thigh is usually associated with femoral loosening, and groin or buttock pain is associated with acetabular loosening. Pain occurs with activity and can be present at night. The presence of a periprosthetic infection should always be considered in cases of failed THA, because the signs and symptoms mimic those of aseptic failure. Other less common causes of femoral osteolysis should also be considered, such as metastatic carcinoma, multiple myeloma, lymphoma, stress shielding, and premature cement mantle fracture.[22]

Radiology and Classification

Femoral Component

To evaluate for aseptic loosening of cemented femoral components, the categories of definitely loose, probably loose, and possibly loose should be used. *Definitely loose* is defined as migration of the femoral stem, a new continuous lucent line at the stem-cement interface, a stem fracture, or fracture of the cement mantle.[27] *Probably loose* is defined as a continuous lucent line at the cement-bone junction. *Possibly loose* is defined by a radiolucent line between 50% and 100% of the cement-bone interface. It should be noted that cement-bone lucencies are commonly seen, and although they may represent aseptic loosening, they also may be due to nonfilling of the canal with cement, remodeling, and neocortex formation. Aseptic loosening demonstrates progressive and localized endosteal scalloping on subsequent films; neocortex formation with remodeling appears as a nonprogressive linear radiolucency. The four modes of failure of cemented femoral stems were described by Gruen as pistoning, medial midstem pivot, calcar pivot, and bending cantilever fatigue.[28] Gruen divided the femoral component into seven radiographic zones where radiolucency can develop in cemented or uncemented stems (Fig. 85-1). Progressive radiolucency within these zones is indicative of femoral loosening.

Uncemented femoral stems that are well fixed are characterized by the absence of radiolucent lines adjacent to the porous coating and the presence of spot welds. Cortical atrophy and stress shielding may be seen just proximal to these spot welds.[3] Any subsidence of an uncemented implant as seen by an increase in vertical distance between the top of the greater trochanter and the shoulder of the prosthesis is generally considered a sign of instability. A bony pedestal is an endosteal condensation of bone that may or may not extend across the intramedullary canal. It is considered evidence of lack of bony ingrowth as the stem attempts to obtain vertical stability. A bony pedestal at the distal

tip would likely not occur in a bony ingrown stem because with a stable stem, stress transfer to bone occurs at the level of the proximal porous coating.

Temmerman and associates examined the utility of plain radiography, subtraction arthrography, nuclear arthrography, and bone scintigraphy in diagnosing aseptic loosening of the femoral component. They concluded that both bone scintigraphy and nuclear arthrography made a significant contribution to the diagnosis beyond that made by plain radiography alone.[29]

Use of magnetic resonance imaging (MRI) in the diagnosis of aseptic loosening of uncemented femoral stems has been evaluated in a few studies. One group found that high signal on T1 and short tau inversion recovery (STIR) MRI was associated with radiographic signs surgical and pathologic findings of loosening.[30] MRI with metal artifact reduction techniques has been demonstrated to be a valuable tool in diagnosing abductor tendon avulsion injury following hip arthroplasty.[31]

Radiographic evaluation of a second-generation metal-on-metal bearing surface total hip replacement warrants special consideration here. Particle-induced osteolysis is considered a major cause of aseptic loosening in cemented and uncemented metal-on-polyethylene total hips; however, this disease may also occur in metal hips. Beaule and colleagues reported on a case of progressive osteolysis at the distal tip of the femoral stem in an uncemented second-generation metal-on-metal total hip that required revision surgery.[32] Similarly, other authors reported on 10 hips with evidence of osteolysis around a metal-on-metal bearing total hip replacement.[33] These authors suggest that the cause was an immunology response to metal ions in the periprosthetic soft tissue. Specifically, they point to antigen-specific sensitization of T cells as a mediator of this process.[33] Most reported cases of osteolysis around these implants occur on the femoral side.

Acetabular Component

The diagnostic evaluation of a loose acetabular component is generally considered more difficult than evaluation of the femoral component.[34] Reported imaging techniques include plain radiographs, subtraction arthrography, bone scintigraphy, and CT.

Plain radiographs can be used to assess acetabular cups for aseptic loosening based on the zones defined by DeLee and Charnley.[35] Loosening of cemented acetabular components usually begins at the cement-bone interface. Cups with greater than 2 mm lucency in all three zones or in zones 1 and 2 are likely to be loose. Any cups that demonstrate signs of migration are considered definitely loose. Radiolucent lines around cementless acetabular cups are less reliable for loosening than those around cemented acetabular cups. Definite signs of loosening include migration of the cup, screw breakage, fracture of the shell, and shedding of the porous surface.

When an osteolytic defect is evaluated, plain radiographs have the limitation of trying to evaluate a three-dimensional defect with two-dimensional imaging. The AP view of the hip provides good information about the dome and floor of the acetabulum; however, it can be

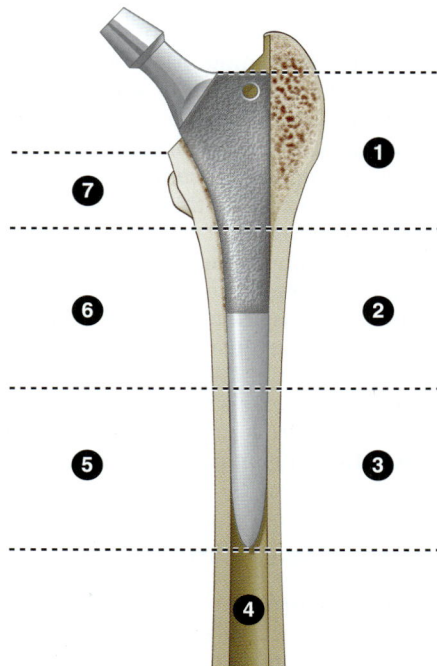

Figure 85-1. Division of the femoral prosthesis into the seven Gruen zones.

difficult to distinguish between osteolysis of the anterior and posterior columns.[36] Judet views may be helpful for better evaluating the acetabular columns. Many studies have shown that plain radiographs alone underestimate the size and number of acetabular defects.[37,38] A systematic review and meta-analysis of this topic concluded that the sensitivity and specificity of plain radiographs alone in detecting aseptic loosening of acetabular cups were 70% and 80%, respectively.[39] Three commonly used classifications for acetabular bone defects are the American Academy of Orthopedic Surgeons (AAOS) classification, the Paprosky classification, and gross classifications (Boxes 85-1 through 85-3). When these classifications were reviewed with the use of plain radiographs, intraobserver and interobserver reliability was found to be low.[40]

Many patients with early osteolysis are asymptomatic[41,42]; however, the extent of osteolysis has been shown to predict the outcome of revision surgery.[43,44] Therefore, early and accurate detection of acetabular osteolysis is essential. A study comparing the diagnostic accuracy of plain radiography, subtraction arthrography, and nuclear arthrography in the diagnosis of aseptic loosening of uncemented acetabular cups determined that the combination of plain radiographs and one other imaging modality provided the most information.[39] However, the utility of these imaging techniques is limited by the expertise of the interpreters.[39] CT scans employing a metal artifact minimization protocol have been shown to be more accurate than plain radiographs in identifying sites of, and quantifying the extent of, acetabular osteolysis.[45-47]

MRI performed to detect acetabular lysis has been shown to be useful in cadaveric studies; however, future work in vivo is still needed.[36] The benefit of MRI versus CT scans is the absence of any ionizing radiation and superior soft tissue contrast. Moreover, some authors have shown an ability to image synovitis secondary to particle disease, which may precede osteoclastic bone resorption and osteolysis.[48]

BOX 85-1. AAOS CLASSIFICATION

Type I.   Segmental deficiency
          IA. Peripheral
          IB. Central (medial wall absent)
Type II. Cavitary
Type III. Combined deficiency
Type IV. Pelvic discontinuity
Type V.   Arthrodesis

AAOS, American Academy of Orthopedic Surgeons.

BOX 85-2. PAPROSKY CLASSIFICATION

Type I.   Supportive rim with no bone lysis or migration
Type II. Distorted hemisphere with intact supportive columns and <2 cm superomedial or superolateral migration
          A. Superomedial
          B. Superolateral (no superior dome)
          C. Medial only
Type III. Superior migration >2 cm and severe ischial and medial osteolysis
          A. Kohler's line intact, 30%-60% of component supported by graft (bone loss 10 o'clock to 2 o'clock)
          B. Kohler's line not intact, >60% of component supported by graft (bone loss 9 o'clock to 5 o'clock)

BOX 85-3. GROSS CLASSIFICATION

Type I.   Contained defect with intact rim and columns
Type II. Noncontained
          A. Shelf/minor column:
              Loss of <50% of host acetabulum in contact with cup
          B. Major column:
              >50% loss of acetabulum that is in contact with the cup
              Loss of one or both columns

PERIPROSTHETIC INFECTION

Incidence and Epidemiology

A significant decrease in the rate of infection following THA, which ranged from 7% to 10%, has been noted since its introduction by Charnley in the 1960s.[49] Modern infection rates of 0.3% to 1.7%[50,51] have been attributed to the use of prophylactic antibiotics, body exhaust systems, laminar flow, and other surgical precautions. Despite the low rate of periprosthetic joint infection, it remains the second most common complication of THA,[52] and prevalence is expected to rise with the increasing number of THAs being performed.[53] The consequences of periprosthetic infection are associated with a substantial socioeconomic burden.[54] They involve multiple revision surgeries, prolonged periods of patient disability, and inferior functional outcomes. It is crucial to differentiate periprosthetic infection from other mechanisms of prosthetic failure because treatment options vary widely.

Risk Factors

Unfortunately, no definitive test is known to diagnose an infection following THA with absolute certainty. The surgeon must rely on a combination of clinical findings and interpretation of preoperative and intraoperative investigations. Several patient-related risk factors for developing a periprosthetic infection have been identified: higher American Society of Anesthesiologists (ASA) score, morbid obesity, previous revision arthroplasty, previous infection of a prosthetic joint, smoking history, rheumatoid arthritis, neoplasm, immunosuppression, and diabetes mellitus. Identified surgical risk factors include long operative time (>2.5 hours), allogenic transfusion, postoperative atrial fibrillation, myocardial infarction, urinary tract infection, prolonged hospitalization, and *Staphylococcus aureus* bacteremia.[55]

Pathophysiology

The most commonly identified organisms among periprosthetic infections are clustered gram-positive cocci (*S. aureus* and *Staphylococcus epidermidis*).[51] They interact with the implant by producing a biofilm glycocalyx, which protects it from being eradicated by the host's immune system and conventional antimicrobial agents. Concern is growing regarding the increasing isolation of resistant strains, such as methicillin-resistant *S. aureus* and *S. epidermidis*.[56]

Periprosthetic infections are commonly classified according to the timing and mechanism of their presentation. Acute infection results from an organism's direct inoculation during the procedure from the skin or a draining wound, and the patient becomes symptomatic within the initial postoperative period. Delayed infection occurs as the result of contamination from the air, from surgical equipment, or from the prosthesis itself; this delay in presentation is due to the time required for the organisms to proliferate. Late infection is the result of hematogenous seeding of the implant by organisms in the bloodstream due to recent surgical treatment, dental manipulation, or remote infection. Recent studies have indicated that late infections represent most infections—a finding that reveals a shift from early reports suggesting that acute infection was more common.[57] This change may reflect improved surgical practices and techniques.[58]

Clinical Features and Diagnosis

Performing a history and physical examination aids in diagnosing with a high degree of certainty most cases of acute infection (stage I) or chronic infection (stage III) in the presence of draining sinus. Any additional investigations would be used to confirm the high suspicion of infection. Identifying the presence of a subacute infection (stage II) is more problematic owing to an overlap of symptoms and signs with aseptic failure. Therefore, additional radiographic and serologic investigations are needed to differentiate between the various mechanisms of failure.

Radiographs have low sensitivity and specificity in diagnosing periprosthetic infection. Radiographic features such as loosening, osteolysis, and endosteal scalloping are also seen in the setting of aseptic failure.[59] CT and MRI studies are not widely used owing to artifact interference from the prosthesis. Radionuclide studies are helpful in excluding the diagnosis of infection. Technetium-99 m (Tc-99 m) bone scanning when combined with indium-111 has higher specificity than when the tests are performed alone.[60] The technetium scan identifies areas of high metabolic activity, and the indium-111 scan identifies areas of inflammation; this differentiates sites of infection from fracture or bone remodeling. Studies examining the role of fluorodeoxyglucose positron-emission tomography (FDG-PET) as a screening modality have reported sensitivity of 90% and specificity of 89% for diagnosing infection around THA.[61] However, this modality is not widely available and remains under investigation.

Initial laboratory workup consists of measuring erythrocyte sedimentation rate (ESR) and C-reactive protein (CRP) level, which are nonspecific markers of inflammation. Both ESR and CRP normally increase following THA, reaching peak levels within 3 to 5 days postoperatively. CRP reaches its peak value earlier than ESR and subsequently normalizes by about 3 weeks postoperatively.[62] ESR returns to normal levels at a slower rate (6 to 12 months) and may stay elevated for 6 weeks.[63] Elevated ESR and CRP levels 3 months after THA are highly suggestive of infection in the absence of inflammatory arthropathies, heterotopic ossification, systemic illness, or recent surgery. An ESR greater than 30 to 35 mm/hr is considered abnormal, with sensitivity and specificity of 82% and 85%, respectively.[64] CRP was a more useful screening tool for infection because a level greater than 10 mg/L was found to have sensitivity of 86% and specificity of 92%.[65] Although these markers are not diagnostic, the combined use of these tests is necessary when evaluating a possible infected THA. Another serologic test for detecting infection that is currently being investigated is measurement of the serum level of interleukin-6 (IL)-6.[66] IL-6 is a product of monocytes and macrophages and is found to be elevated in the presence of periprosthetic infection. It is elevated postoperatively but normalizes within 48 hours and is not elevated in patients with aseptic failure.

Preoperative aspiration of the hip joint for cell count and culture is an important tool when evaluating possible infection following THA. It should not be used as a screening tool but should be used selectively to help confirm the diagnosis of infection.[65] The sensitivity and specificity of aspirated cultures are higher in patients with positive ESR and CRP tests. Repeating the aspiration when there is a high clinical suspicion of infection despite an initial negative aspiration increases culture sensitivity.[67] The procedure should be performed under image guidance and not through areas that are potentially cellulolytic. Antibiotics should be discontinued 2 weeks before aspiration to achieve optimal sensitivity and specificity.[67] Fluid aspirations also allow for preoperative isolation of the infecting organism and its antibiotic sensitivities, which is useful in determining the types of antibiotics used preoperatively or combined with cement during revision surgery. With respect to the aspirated cell count, a leukocyte count greater than 50.0×10^9 per liter and a neutrophil count greater than 80% are consistent with a prosthetic hip infection.[65] A gram stain may be performed on the aspirated joint fluid, but its low sensitivity and specificity have rendered it an ineffective test.[68,69]

Intraoperative studies are utilized to help confirm the diagnosis when there is clinical suspicion of a periprosthetic infection but preoperative tests including joint aspiration are negative and an organism cannot be isolated. Frozen sections of tissue obtained from the joint capsule or periprosthetic material is examined to identify histologic evidence of acute inflammation. Studies have demonstrated that a frozen section is suggestive of infection if it contains at least five neutrophils in each of three 400× high-power microscopic fields found beneath the surface of the membrane.[58] To increase its sensitivity, tissue samples should be obtained from areas that are most inflamed, and antibiotics should be discontinued before the time of collection.

Most studies have used the results of intraoperative cultures as the "gold standard" to define the presence or absence of a periprosthetic infection. However, the test is not 100% reliable, with recent studies reporting negative predictive values between 84% and 88%.[70] In an effort to improve its accuracy, it is recommended that five or six specimens be retrieved, and that two or three positive tests be considered diagnostic for infection.[69] Culture swabs of sinus tracts should be avoided. Clean instruments must be used when retrieving the sample, which must be transferred directly to the culture bottle without additional handling and sent directly to the laboratory for processing. Preoperative antibiotics are discontinued 2 weeks before surgery, and intraoperative antibiotics should be withheld until the tissue samples are retrieved by sharp dissection without excessive cauterization.[58] Ultrasonification of the removed prosthesis to isolate adherent organisms from the biofilm has been suggested as a useful diagnostic tool.[71-73] This technique demonstrated improved sensitivity when antibiotics were administered within 2 weeks of surgery. Collaboration between the surgeon and the pathologist is essential when rare organisms are isolated and the clinical relevance of the pathology is determined.

Future Directions

New molecular techniques have been developed to aid in the diagnosis of periprosthetic infection. Polymerase chain reaction (PCR) assays have the ability to detect bacterial DNA and RNA from small quantities of starting material. Forward and reverse primers designed to match specific bacterial DNA sequences are used, such as the 16S rRNA, which is commonly found on all bacterial species. PCR possesses the advantage of providing a rapid diagnosis while detecting bacterial DNA in culture-negative samples due to antimicrobial therapy. The major limitation of this technique is its susceptibility to contamination, which has led to a high prevalence of false-positives.[74-76] Combining specific PCR assays to detect targeted organisms instead of using broad-spectrum PCR assays is a strategy currently under investigation.[77,78] Other techniques include the use of microarray and proteomics technologies, which involve detecting organism-specific bacterial RNA genes and proteins.[79] The challenge remains to provide a diagnostic test with a high degree of accuracy that can direct clinical management.

DISLOCATION

Dislocation following total hip arthroplasty continues to be a troubling complication despite advances in surgical techniques and component design. Risk factors have been identified among patients, surgical techniques, and components. It is the second most common reason for revision surgery following aseptic loosening. Determining the underlying cause of instability is critical in determining appropriate management.

Epidemiology

The incidence of dislocation following primary THA among large case studies is less than 5%.[80,81] A comprehensive review performed by Morrey of 35,000 procedures revealed an average dislocation rate of 2.24%, whereby individual rates varied from 0.7% to 7%.[82] Variability among reports can be attributed to different surgical approaches, prosthesis designs, and postoperative regimens. The prevalence of instability is likely underestimated because studies measure only dislocation events, not the presence of instability. The use of newer implants and improved techniques has aimed to decrease the dislocation rate. However, increased use of THA among populations with significant comorbidities, along with modularity that causes impingement, has likely neutralized those advantages. The longer patients are followed after the first dislocation, the higher is the prevalence of dislocation. Most dislocations occur within the first few months after surgery and according to most studies are unlikely to be followed by recurrent dislocations.[83] However, dislocations that occur after 3 months have a higher rate of redislocation.

Patient Factors

Patient-related factors have been identified that predispose individuals to dislocation following THA. The female gender is a significant risk factor for instability; women dislocate three to four times more frequently than men 5 years after the index THA.[84,85] Possible explanations include soft tissue laxity and decreased muscle tone and bone density. Women have been shown to have more frequent late dislocations as well. Late dislocations have also been correlated with younger age, history of trauma, previous episodes of subluxation, and the presence of cognitive or motor neurologic impairment.[83,86]

Any history of previous surgery of the hip such as previous THA, osteotomy, open reduction internal fixation (ORIF), and arthrodesis is a significant risk factor for postoperative dislocation following THA.[6] This event can be attributed to soft tissue trauma including damage to external rotators and abductors, which would compromise hip stability. Dislocation rates are lower when more complete soft tissue repair is performed.

The presence of comorbidities such as neuromuscular disorders, psychosis, or alcoholism is associated with a higher incidence of dislocation.[87,88] These factors impair the patient's ability to control hip position and comply with hip precautions, thus increasing the frequency of falls.

A significant association between preoperative diagnosis and rate of dislocation has not been shown. Although the dislocation rate is higher among patients undergoing THA for developmental dysplasia, no statistical difference in dislocation rates has been noted between patients with osteoarthritis, rheumatoid arthritis, and osteonecrosis.[6]

Elderly patients (>75 years) were found to have higher dislocation rates, but statistical significance is lacking. Increased fracture risk, poor soft tissues, increased cognitive impairment, and noncompliance with hip precautions likely confound this association. Despite the belief that obese or tall patients would have increased rates of dislocation owing to soft tissue impingement or increased lever arms, weight and height are not statistically significant factors influencing instability.

Surgical Factors

Surgical factors that influence dislocation rates include surgical approach, surgeon's experience level, component orientation, and restoration of soft tissue tension.

Multiple studies have demonstrated a higher dislocation rate with THA utilizing the posterior approach compared with the anterolateral or direct lateral approach.[6,89,90] This is attributed to loss of restraint and stability when the posterior capsule and the short external rotators are compromised. There is also a tendency to position the acetabular component in retroversion with the posterior approach owing to inadequate visualization of the cup and anterior interference by the femur. However, a dramatic decrease in dislocations with the posterior approach was shown if the posterior capsule and the short external rotators are specifically repaired to their insertion on the greater trochanter.[91]

Surgeon experience has been shown to influence dislocation rates.[92,93] Surgeons who perform two or fewer THAs per year have significantly higher complications. A study examining a series of THAs performed using the posterior approach found that surgeons who performed 15 or fewer THAs have twice as many dislocations when compared with surgeons who perform a greater number of THAs.[92] The dislocation rate becomes consistent among surgeons when 30 or more THAs are performed per year.

Component positioning is considered one of the key variables that predispose to dislocation. It is recommended based on computer modeling that the acetabular component be placed in a safe zone of 45 ± 10 degrees of abduction and 20 ± 10 degrees of anteversion.[94] Dislocation rates increase from 1.5% to 6.1% when the acetabular component is placed outside of 40 degrees of adduction and 15 degrees of anteversion.[95] Excessive anteversion of the femoral component should be avoided; the recommended position is 10 to 20 degrees of anteversion. Interaction between the cup and the femoral stem position offers the opportunity to compensate for cup malpositioning by adjusting the femoral

stem position. It is recommended that a combined position of 40 degrees of anteversion is optimal. In addition, excessive medial or superior placement of the cup can compromise THA stability.

Soft tissue structures around the hip should be reestablished in an effort to minimize dislocation rates. These structures provide a passive resistant force at the hip, preventing femoral head separation from the acetabulum. A popular way to reestablish soft tissue tension consists of matching preoperative and postoperative limb lengths.

Implant Factors

Implant factors should be considered when evaluating an unstable THA. These include femoral head size, femoral offset, femoral head-to-acetabulum ratio, and liner profile. However, it is difficult to attribute instability to any factor in isolation because it is a multifactorial problem with many confounding factors.

Larger femoral head sizes have long been theorized to decrease the rate of dislocation owing to a greater primary arc of motion and increased femoral head displacement necessary to cause dislocation. However, clinical correlation between larger femoral head sizes and dislocation rates is lacking. Clinical studies in the setting of revision surgery have demonstrated improved hip stability using 28- and 32-mm heads when compared with 22-mm heads.[86] The use of highly cross-linked polyethylene and alternate bearings has allowed increased use of larger femoral heads.[96] A larger femoral head size while avoiding the use of a skirt on the neck increases the femoral head-to-neck ratio, which increases the arc of motion to impingement, thus decreasing the chance of dislocation.[97]

Restoring femoral offset is critical to properly tension the abductors and enhance hip stability. Low femoral offset has been linked with higher rates of dislocation. The ability to increase femoral offset is a design advantage that increases soft tissue tensioning without excessive leg lengthening.

Use of elevated liners affects hip stability by increasing the amount of contact with the femoral head in the area that is likely to dislocate. However, the elevated rim can create prosthetic impingement leading to dislocation. One study showed that elevated liners decreased the dislocation rate of primary THA using a posterior approach, but longer follow-up showed no difference owing to smaller numbers, hence elevated liners were not recommended for routine use.[98] Newer versions of liners are available that are intended to change the arc of motion without decreasing it.

Clinical Features and Diagnosis

Evaluation of an unstable THA involves performing a complete history and physical with careful review of imaging studies, as outlined in the preceding section. The history will reveal the position of the leg before and after the dislocation and the mechanism of the inciting event. Posterior dislocations tend to occur with hyperflexion and internal rotation of the hip; anterior dislocations occur with hyperextension and external rotation. If there is a history of recurrent dislocations, one must rule out the presence of multidirectional instability, which occurs when different mechanisms lead to dislocation. Unidirectional versus multidirectional instability can be distinguished under fluoroscopic examination. The chance of recurrence is higher if the dislocation occurred by means of a low-energy mechanism.

Determining the chronology of the dislocation is essential in elucidating the underlying cause and the chance of recurrence. Most dislocations occur within the first 3 months after surgery and are typically caused by incomplete scar formation and relaxed soft tissues. These dislocations are less likely to be recurrent. Dislocations that occur between 3 months and 5 years are typically caused by component malposition or dysfunction of the trochanter/abductor complex. When dislocations occur 5 years or later from the index procedure, they are considered late dislocations. Late dislocations make up less than 1% of dislocations and frequently require revision surgery. A recurrence rate of 60% has been reported.[6,83,95,99] This subset of patients has a greater range of motion, especially in flexion, caused by stretching of the pseudocapsule, which leads to dislocation. Another theory for the instability among late dislocators is that the presence of polyethylene wear debris synovitis causes the head to sit deeper in the cup, leading to earlier impingement.[100] Predictors of late dislocation include female gender, younger age at index THA (63 years), history subluxation without dislocation, an episode of trauma, marked weight loss, and a recent decline in cognitive or neurologic function.[81] Radiographic predictors of instability among this group consist of acetabular component malposition, polyethylene wear greater than 2 mm, and a loose implant with migration.

PERIPROSTHETIC FRACTURES

Periprosthetic fractures are a devastating complication that is increasing in frequency owing to the increasing numbers of THAs and revision procedures performed, the increasing number of elderly patients with osteoporosis, surgeon preference for cementless implants, and utilization of minimally invasive techniques that compromise exposure. They are associated with significant morbidity and mortality. Therefore, an in-depth understanding of risk factors and classification systems is necessary to guide management.

Epidemiology

Periprosthetic fractures can occur intraoperatively and postoperatively around the femur and/or the acetabulum. Periprosthetic fractures are the third most common reason for revision surgery after aseptic loosening and dislocation. Fractures about the femur are reported to occur more frequently, which is likely a result of the difficulty involved in recognizing acetabular fractures. The Mayo Clinic Joint Registry reported intraoperative

periprosthetic fracture rates of 0.3% and 5.4% for cemented and uncemented primary THAs, respectively.[101] The incidence among revision THAs was 3.6% for cemented prostheses and 20.9% for uncemented prostheses, respectively. The prevalence of postoperative femoral fractures was reported in the same study to be 1% after primary THA and 4% after revision surgery.

Risk Factors

Risk factors for femoral periprosthetic fracture in patients undergoing primary THA include bone fragility and osteopenia, rheumatoid arthritis, female gender, and the presence of bony deformity. In the setting of revision surgery, risk factors consist of decreased bone stock, altered bone morphology or defects, the presence of hardware, and cortical perforations with extruded cement. The use of cementless implants is a risk factor in primary and revision settings owing to the technique of press-fitting the prostheses. Impaction bone grafting is also associated with risk of periprosthetic fracture, and prophylactic measures are advised. Postoperative periprosthetic fractures usually occur spontaneously or as the result of minor trauma. The presence of a bony lesion or deficiency predisposes the prosthesis to fracture. More than 70% of postoperative periprosthetic fractures are reported to be associated with femoral loosening.[102] Therefore, careful screening for any evidence of prosthetic loosening can prevent the occurrence of postoperative periprosthetic fracture.

Classification

The Vancouver classification system is used to help guide management of intraoperative and postoperative periprosthetic femur fractures. Intraoperative fractures are grouped as proximal metaphyseal, diaphyseal, or distal diaphyseal (including distal metaphysis). These three groups are further divided on the basis of the presence of a cortical perforation, a nondisplaced linear crack, or a displaced unstable fracture. For postoperative periprosthetic fractures, classification takes into account the site of the fracture, the stability of the implant, and the quality of surrounding bone. Type A fractures occur within the trochanteric region (AG at the greater trochanter, AL at the lesser trochanter), type B fractures are noted in proximal areas of the preexisting stem or just distal to it, and type C fractures arise far below the femoral stem. Type B fractures are subdivided into three groups according to the stability of the implant and the quality of bone stock. Type B1 fractures have a well-fixed implant, type B2 fractures have loose but adequate bone stock, and type B3 fracture implants are loose with poor bone stock.

Diagnosis

Patients commonly present with pain localized to the thigh or groin after a minor fall or activity. A history of start-up pain may be suggestive of a loose femoral component. A sudden inability to bear weight during the postoperative period and the presence of a deformity are suggestive of a periprosthetic fracture. AP and lateral radiographs of the pelvis and the full length of the femur are required to rule out the presence of periprosthetic fracture or osteolysis. Specialized radiographs such as Judet views of the acetabulum or a CT scan may be necessary to delineate nondisplaced fractures.

A high index of suspicion and identification of risk factors are critical for recognition of intraoperative fractures. Periprosthetic acetabular fractures can occur spontaneously, traumatically, owing to pelvic discontinuity, or during removal of well-fixed components. The columns need to be assessed intraoperatively for stability, and the amount of host bone coverage must be scrutinized to determine its ability to provide mechanical support. During insertion of the cementless stem, sudden loss of resistance may suggest an iatrogenic fracture. Clinical and radiographic assessments performed intraoperatively are required to ensure stability of the component before leaving the operative room if a periprosthetic fracture is suspected.

REFERENCES

1. Lachiewicz PF, Kauk JR: Anterior iliopsoas impingement and tendinitis after total hip arthroplasty. J Am Acad Orthop Surg 17:337–344, 2009.
2. McAuley JP, Culpepper WJ, Engh CA: Total hip arthroplasty: concerns with extensively porous coated femoral components. Clin Orthop Relat Res 355:182–188, 1998.
3. Engh CA, Massin P, Suthers KE: Roentgenographic assessment of the biologic fixation of porous-surfaced femoral components. Clin Orthop Relat Res 257:107–128, 1990.
4. Duffy P, Masri BA, Garbuz D, Duncan CP: Evaluation of patients with pain following total hip replacement. Instr Course Lect 55:223–232, 2006.
5. Fitzgerald RH, Jr: Infected total hip arthroplasty: diagnosis and treatment. J Am Acad Orthop Surg 3:249–262, 1995.
6. Woo RY, Morrey BF: Dislocations after total hip arthroplasty. J Bone Joint Surg Am 64:1295–1306, 1982.
7. Soong M, Rubash HE, Macaulay W: Dislocation after total hip arthroplasty. J Am Acad Orthop Surg 12:314–321, 2004.
8. Pollard B, Johnston M, Dixon D: Theoretical framework and methodological development of common subjective health outcome measures in osteoarthritis: a critical review. Health Qual Life Outcomes 5:14, 2007.
9. Jacobs JJ, Kull LR, Frey GA, et al: Early failure of acetabular components inserted without cement after previous pelvic irradiation. J Bone Joint Surg Am 77:1829–1835, 1995.
10. Canale ST, Campbell WC: Campbell's operative orthopaedics, ed 10, St Louis, 2003, Mosby, p 4283.
11. Cuckler JM, Star AM, Alavi A, Noto RB: Diagnosis and management of the infected total joint arthroplasty. Orthop Clin North Am 22:523–530, 1991.
12. Pritchett JW: Lumbar decompression to treat foot drop after hip arthroplasty. Clin Orthop Relat Res 303:173–177, 1994.
13. Barrack RL, Burnett RS: Preoperative planning for revision total hip arthroplasty. Instr Course Lect 55:233–244, 2006.
14. DeHart MM, Riley LH, Jr: Nerve injuries in total hip arthroplasty. J Am Acad Orthop Surg 7:101–111, 1999.
15. Clayton RA, Beggs I, Salter DM, et al: Inflammatory pseudotumor associated with femoral nerve palsy following metal-on-metal resurfacing of the hip: a case report. J Bone Joint Surg Am 90:1988–1993, 2008.
16. Pandit H, Glyn-Jones S, McLardy-Smith P, et al: Pseudotumours associated with metal-on-metal hip resurfacings. J Bone Joint Surg Br 90:847–851, 2008.
17. Sinha RK, Shanbhag AS, Maloney WJ, et al: Osteolysis: cause and effect. Instr Course Lect 47:307–320, 1998.
18. Schmalzried TP, Jasty M, Harris WH: Periprosthetic bone loss in total hip arthroplasty: polyethylene wear debris and the concept of the effective joint space. J Bone Joint Surg Am 74:849–863, 1992.
19. Neumann L, Freund KG, Sorensen KH: Total hip arthroplasty with the Charnley prosthesis in patients fifty-five years old and less: fifteen to twenty-one-year results. J Bone Joint Surg Am 78:73–79, 1996.
20. Mont MA, LaPorte DM, Mullick T, et al: Tennis after total hip arthroplasty. Am J Sports Med 27:60–64, 1999.
21. Schmalzried TP, Shepherd EF, Dorey FJ, et al: The John Charnley Award. Wear is a function of use, not time. Clin Orthop Relat Res 381:36–46, 2000.
22. Dunbar MJ, Blackley HR, Bourne RB: Osteolysis of the femur: principles of management. Instr Course Lect 50:197–209, 2001.
23. Hermida JC, Bergula A, Chen P, et al: Comparison of the wear rates of twenty-eight and thirty-two-millimeter femoral heads on cross-linked polyethylene acetabular cups in a wear simulator. J Bone Joint Surg Am 85:2325–2331, 2003.
24. Ries MD: Complications in primary total hip arthroplasty: avoidance and management: wear. Instr Course Lect 52:257–265, 2003.
25. Urban JA, Garvin KL, Boese CK, et al: Ceramic-on-polyethylene bearing surfaces in total hip arthroplasty: seventeen to twenty-one-year results. J Bone Joint Surg Am 83:1688–1694, 2001.
26. Patil S, Bergula A, Chen PC, et al: Polyethylene wear and acetabular component orientation. J Bone Joint Surg Am 85(Suppl 4):56–63, 2003.
27. Harris WH, McCarthy JC, Jr, O'Neill DA: Femoral component loosening using contemporary techniques of femoral cement fixation. J Bone Joint Surg Am 64:1063–1067, 1982.
28. Gruen TA, McNeice GM, Amstutz HC: "Modes of failure" of cemented stem-type femoral components: a radiographic analysis of loosening. Clin Orthop Relat Res 141:17–27, 1979.
29. Temmerman OP, Raijmakers PG, Berkhof J, et al: Diagnostic accuracy and interobserver variability of plain radiography, subtraction arthrography, nuclear arthrography, and bone scintigraphy in the assessment of aseptic femoral component loosening. Arch Orthop Trauma Surg 126:316–323, 2006.
30. Sugimoto H, Hirose I, Miyaoka E, et al: Low-field-strength MR imaging of failed hip arthroplasty: association of femoral periprosthetic signal intensity with radiographic, surgical, and pathologic findings. Radiology 229:718–723, 2003.
31. Twair A, Ryan M, O'Connell M, et al: MRI of failed total hip replacement caused by abductor muscle avulsion. AJR Am J Roentgenol 181:1547–1550, 2003.
32. Beaulé PE, Campbell P, Mirra J, et al: Osteolysis in a cementless, second generation metal-on-metal hip replacement. Clin Orthop Relat Res 386:159–165, 2001.
33. Park YS, Moon YW, Lim SJ, et al: Early osteolysis following second-generation metal-on-metal hip replacement. J Bone Joint Surg Am 87:1515–1521, 2005.
34. Li DJ, Miles KA, Wraight EP: Bone scintigraphy of hip prostheses: can analysis of patterns of abnormality improve accuracy? Clin Nucl Med 19:112–115, 1994.
35. DeLee JG, Charnley J: Radiological demarcation of cemented sockets in total hip replacement. Clin Orthop Relat Res 121:20–32, 1976.
36. Weiland DE, Walde TA, Leung SB, et al: Magnetic resonance imaging in the evaluation of periprosthetic acetabular osteolysis: a cadaveric study. J Orthop Res 23:713–719, 2005.
37. Claus AM, Engh CA, Jr, Sychterz CJ, et al: Radiographic definition of pelvic osteolysis following total hip arthroplasty. J Bone Joint Surg Am 85:1519–1526, 2003.
38. Saleh KJ, Holtzman J, Gafni A, et al: Reliability and intraoperative validity of preoperative assessment of standardized plain radiographs in predicting bone loss at revision hip surgery. J Bone Joint Surg Am 83:1040–1046, 2001.
39. Temmerman OP, Raijmakers PG, David EF, et al: A comparison of radiographic and scintigraphic techniques to assess aseptic loosening of the acetabular component in a total hip replacement. J Bone Joint Surg Am 86:2456–2463, 2004.

40. Campbell DG, Garbuz DS, Masri BA, Duncan CP: Reliability of acetabular bone defect classification systems in revision total hip arthroplasty. J Arthroplasty 16:83–86, 2001.

41. Hozack WJ, Mesa JJ, Carey C, Rothman RH: Relationship between polyethylene wear, pelvic osteolysis, and clinical symptomatology in patients with cementless acetabular components: a framework for decision making. J Arthroplasty 11:769–772, 1996.

42. Johnston RC, Fitzgerald RH, Jr, Harris WH, et al: Clinical and radiographic evaluation of total hip replacement: a standard system of terminology for reporting results. J Bone Joint Surg Am 72:161–168, 1991.

43. Engelbrecht DJ, Weber FA, Sweet MB, Jakim I: Long-term results of revision total hip arthroplasty. J Bone Joint Surg Br 72:41–45, 1990.

44. Maloney WJ, Peters P, Engh CA, Chandler H: Severe osteolysis of the pelvis in association with acetabular replacement without cement. J Bone Joint Surg Am 75:1627–1635, 1993.

45. Puri L, Wixson RL, Stern SH, et al: Use of helical computed tomography for the assessment of acetabular osteolysis after total hip arthroplasty. J Bone Joint Surg Am 84:609–614, 2002.

46. Robertson DD, Magid D, Poss R, et al: Enhanced computed tomographic techniques for the evaluation of total hip arthroplasty. J Arthroplasty 4:271–276, 1989.

47. Stulberg SD, Wixson RL, Adams AD, et al: Monitoring pelvic osteolysis following total hip replacement surgery: an algorithm for surveillance. J Bone Joint Surg Am 84(Suppl 2):116–122, 2002.

48. Potter HG, Nestor BJ, Sofka CM, et al: Magnetic resonance imaging after total hip arthroplasty: evaluation of periprosthetic soft tissue. J Bone Joint Surg Am 86:1947–1954, 2004.

49. Charnley J, Eftekhar N: Postoperative infection in total prosthetic replacement arthroplasty of the hip-joint: with special reference to the bacterial content of the air of the operating room. Br J Surg 56:641–649, 1969.

50. Phillips JE, Crane TP, Noy M, et al: The incidence of deep prosthetic infections in a specialist orthopaedic hospital: a 15-year prospective survey. J Bone Joint Surg Br 88:943–948, 2006.

51. Pulido L, Ghanem E, Joshi A, et al: Periprosthetic joint infection: the incidence, timing, and predisposing factors. Clin Orthop Relat Res 466:1710–1715, 2008.

52. Herberts P, Malchau H: Long-term registration has improved the quality of hip replacement: a review of the Swedish THR Register comparing 160,000 cases. Acta Orthop Scand 71:111–121, 2000.

53. National Hospital Discharge Survey: Survey results and products, Atlanta, 2009, Centers for Disease Control and Prevention.

54. Sculco TP: The economic impact of infected total joint arthroplasty. In Instructional course lectures, American Academy of Orthopaedic Surgeons, Rosemont, Ill, 1993, American Academy of Orthopaedic Surgeons, pp 349–351.

55. Choong PF, Dowsey MM, Carr D, et al: Risk factors associated with acute hip prosthetic joint infections and outcome of treatment with a rifampinbased regimen. Acta Orthop 78:755–765, 2007.

56. Parvizi J, Azzam K, Ghanem E, et al: Periprosthetic infection due to resistant staphylococci: serious problems on the horizon. Clin Orthop Relat Res 467:1732–1739, 2009.

57. Schmalzried TP, Amstutz HC, Au MK, Dorey FJ: Etiology of deep sepsis in total hip arthroplasty: the significance of hematogenous and recurrent infections. Clin Orthop Relat Res 280:200–207, 1992.

58. Bauer TW, Parvizi J, Kobayashi N, Krebs V: Diagnosis of periprosthetic infection. J Bone Joint Surg Am 88:869–882, 2006.

59. Tigges S, Stiles RG, Roberson JR: Appearance of septic hip prostheses on plain radiographs. Am J Roentgenol 163:377–380, 1994.

60. Palestro CJ, Swyer AJ, Kim CK, Goldsmith SJ: Infected knee prosthesis: diagnosis with In-111 leukocyte, Tc-99 m sulfur colloid, and Tc-99 m MDP imaging. Radiology 179:645–648, 1991.

61. Zhuang H, Duarte PS, Pourdehnad M, et al: The promising role of 18F-FDG PET in detecting infected lower limb prosthesis implants. J Nucl Med 42:44–48, 2001.

62. Larsson S, Thelander U, Friberg S: C-reactive protein (CRP) levels after elective orthopedic surgery. Clin Orthop Relat Res 275:237–242, 1992.

63. Carlsson AS: Erythrocyte sedimentation rate in infected and non-infected total-hip arthroplasties. Acta Orthop Scand 49:287–290, 1978.

64. Lachiewicz PF, Rogers GD, Thomason HC: Aspiration of the hip joint before revision total hip arthroplasty: clinical and laboratory factors influencing attainment of a positive culture. J Bone Joint Surg Am 78:749–754, 1996.

65. Spangehl MJ, Masri BA, O'Connell JX, Duncan CP: Prospective analysis of preoperative and intraoperative investigations for the diagnosis of infection at the sites of two hundred and two revision total hip arthroplasties. J Bone Joint Surg Am 81:672–683, 1999.

66. Di Cesare PE, Chang E, Preston CF, Liu CJ: Serum interleukin-6 as a marker of periprosthetic infection following total hip and knee arthroplasty. J Bone Joint Surg Am 87:1921–1927, 2005.

67. Barrack RL, Harris WH: The value of aspiration of the hip joint before revision total hip arthroplasty. J Bone Joint Surg Am 75:66–76, 1993.

68. Della Valle CJ, Scher DM, Kim YH, et al: The role of intraoperative Gram stain in revision total joint arthroplasty. J Arthroplasty 14:500–504, 1999.

69. Atkins BL, Athanasou N, Deeks JJ, et al: Prospective evaluation of criteria for microbiological diagnosis of prosthetic-joint infection at revision arthroplasty. J Clin Microbiol 36:2932–2939, 1998.

70. Parvizi J, Ghanem E, Menashe S, et al: Periprosthetic infection: what are the diagnostic challenges? J Bone Joint Surg Am 88(Suppl 4):138–147, 2006.

71. Dobbins JJ, Seligson D, Raff MJ: Bacterial colonization of orthopedic fixation devices in the absence of clinical infection. J Infect Dis 158:203–205, 1998.

72. Neut D, van Horn JR, van Kooten TG, et al: Detection of biomaterial-associated infections in orthopaedic joint implants. Clin Orthop Relat Res 413:261–268, 2003.

73. Tunney MM, Patrick S, Curran MD, et al: Detection of prosthetic joint biofilm infection using immunological and molecular techniques. Methods Enzymol 310:566–576, 1999.

74. Corless CE, Guiver M, Borrow R, et al: Contamination and sensitivity issues with a real-time universal 16S rRNA PCR. J Clin Microbiol 38:1747–1752, 2000.

75. Meier A, Persing DH, Finken M, Böttger EC: Elimination of contaminating DNA within polymerase chain reaction reagents: implications for a general approach to detection of uncultured pathogens. J Clin Microbiol 31:646–652, 1993.

76. Newsome T, Li BJ, Zou N, Lo SC: Presence of bacterial phage-like DNA sequences in commercial Taq DNA polymerase reagents. J Clin Microbiol 42:2264–2267, 2004.

77. Kobayashi N, Bauer TW, Togawa D, et al: A molecular gram stain using broad range PCR and pyrosequencing technology: a potentially useful tool for diagnosing orthopaedic infections. Diagn Mol Pathol 14:83–89, 2005.

78. Sakai H, Procop GW, Kobayashi N, et al: Simultaneous detection of Staphylococcus aureus and coagulase-negative staphylococci in positive blood cultures by real-time PCR with two fluorescence resonance energy transfer probe sets. J Clin Microbiol 42:5739–5744, 2004.

79. Deirmengian C, Lonner JH, Booth RE: The Mark Coventry Award. White blood cell gene expression: a new approach toward the study and diagnosis of infection. Clin Orthop Relat Res 440:38–44, 2005.

80. Berry DJ, von Knoch M, Schleck CD, Harmsen WS: The cumulative long-term risk of dislocation after primary Charnley total hip arthroplasty. J Bone Joint Surg Am 86:9–14, 2004.

81. von Knoch M, Berry DJ, Harmsen WS, Morrey BF: Late dislocation after total hip arthroplasty. J Bone Joint Surg Am 84:1949–1953, 2002.

82. Mahoney CR, Pellicci PM: Complications in primary total hip arthroplasty: avoidance and management of dislocations. Instr Course Lect 52:247–255, 2003.

83. Ali Khan MA, Brakenbury PH, Reynolds IS: Dislocation following total hip replacement. J Bone Joint Surg Br 63:214–218, 1981.

84. Coventry MB: The treatment of fracture-dislocation of the hip by total hip arthroplasty. J Bone Joint Surg Am 56:1128–1134, 1974.

85. Hedlundh U, Fredin H: Patient characteristics in dislocations after primary total hip arthroplasty: 60 patients compared with a control group. Acta Orthop Scand 66:225–228, 1995.

86. Alberton GM, High WA, Morrey BF: Dislocation after revision total hip arthroplasty: an analysis of risk factors and treatment options. J Bone Joint Surg Am 84:1788–1792, 2002.

87. Woolson ST, Rahimtoola ZO: Risk factors for dislocation during the first 3 months after primary total hip replacement. J Arthroplasty 14:662–668, 1999.

88. Paterno SA, Lachiewicz PF, Kelley SS: The influence of patient-related factors and the position of the acetabular component on the rate of dislocation after total hip replacement. J Bone Joint Surg Am 79:1202–1210, 1997.

89. Morrey BF: Difficult complications after hip joint replacement: dislocation. Clin Orthop Relat Res 344:179–187, 1997.

90. Roberts JM, Fu FH, McClain EJ, Ferguson AB, Jr: A comparison of the posterolateral and anterolateral approaches to total hip arthroplasty. Clin Orthop Relat Res 187:205–210, 1984.

91. Pellicci PM, Bostrom M, Poss R: Posterior approach to total hip replacement using enhanced posterior soft tissue repair. Clin Orthop Relat Res 355:224–228, 1998.

92. Hedlundh U, Ahnfelt L, Hybbinette CH, et al: Surgical experience related to dislocations after total hip arthroplasty. J Bone Joint Surg Br 78:206–209, 1996.

93. Kreder HJ, Deyo RA, Koepsell T, et al: Relationship between the volume of total hip replacements performed by providers and the rates of postoperative complications in the state of Washington. J Bone Joint Surg Am 79:485–494, 1997.

94. D'Lima DD, Urquhart AG, Buehler KO, et al: The effect of the orientation of the acetabular and femoral components on the range of motion of the hip at different head-neck ratios. J Bone Joint Surg Am 82:315–321, 2000.

95. Lewinnek GE, Lewis JL, Tarr R, et al: Dislocations after total hip-replacement arthroplasties. J Bone Joint Surg Am 60:217–220, 1978.

96. Cuckler JM, Moore KD, Lombardi AV Jr, et al: Large versus small femoral heads in metal-on-metal total hip arthroplasty. J Arthroplasty 19(8 Suppl 3):41–44, 2004.

97. Lawton RL, Morrey BF: Dislocation after long-necked total hip arthroplasty. Clin Orthop Relat Res 422:164–166, 2004.

98. Sultan PG, Tan V, Lai M, Garino JP: Independent contribution of elevated-rim acetabular liner and femoral head size to the stability of total hip implants. J Arthroplasty 17:289–292, 2002.

99. Fackler CD, Poss R: Dislocation in total hip arthroplasties. Clin Orthop Relat Res 151:169–178, 1980.

100. Hamilton WG, McAuley JP: Evaluation of the unstable total hip arthroplasty. Instr Course Lect 53:87–92, 2004.

101. Berry DJ: Epidemiology: hip and knee. Orthop Clin North Am 30:183–190, 1999.

102. Lindahl H, Malchau H, Herberts P, Garellick G: Periprosthetic femoral fractures classification and demographics of 1049 periprosthetic femoral fractures from the Swedish National Hip Arthroplasty Register. J Arthroplasty 20:857–865, 2005.

FURTHER READING

Pandit H, Glyn-Jones S, McLardy-Smith P, et al: Pseudotumors associated with metal-on-metal hip resurfacings. J Bone Joint Surg Br 90:847–851, 2008.

The authors reported on female patients who presented with symptoms following metal-on-metal hip resurfacings. They estimate that approximately 1% of patients who have a metal-on-metal resurfacing develop a pseudotumor within 5 years. The cause is unknown and is probably multifactorial. A toxic reaction to an excess of particulate metal wear debris or a hypersensitivity reaction to a normal amount of metal debris may be causative.

Park YS, Moon YW, Lim SJ, et al: Early osteolysis following second-generation metal-on-metal hip replacement. J Bone Joint Surg Am 87:1515–1521, 2005.

The authors performed a retrospective study investigating the association of metal hypersensitivity and early osteolysis of total hip arthroplasty with the use of metal-on-metal bearings. They found that patients with early osteolysis had a significantly higher rate of hypersensitivity reactions to cobalt compared with controls. Retrieved periprosthetic tissues showed no evidence of metallic staining, but histologic analysis revealed a perivascular accumulation of CD3-positive T cells and CD68-positive macrophages and absence of both particle-laden macrophages and polymorphonuclear cells. Immunohistochemical analysis revealed that bone-resorbing cytokines such as interleukin (IL)-1beta and tumor necrosis factor (TNF) were produced mainly by infiltrating lymphocytes and activated macrophages. These findings raise the possibility that early osteolysis in patients with this second-generation metal-on-metal hip replacement is associated with abnormalities consistent with delayed-type hypersensitivity to metal.

Parvizi J, Azzam K, Ghanem E, et al: Periprosthetic infection due to resistant staphylococci: serious problems on the horizon. Clin Orthop Relat Res 467:1732–1739, 2009.

The authors examined the effectiveness of surgical treatment in treating infection of total hip or knee arthroplasty caused by methicillin-resistant staphylococcal strains and variables influencing treatment success. They found that débridement and retention of prosthesis were not as successful in eradicating infection compared with a two-stage exchange arthroplasty, and that preexisting cardiac disease was associated with a higher failure rate in treating infection.

Pill SG, Parvizi J, Tang PH, et al: Comparison of fluorodeoxyglucose positron emission tomography and (111)indium-white blood cell imaging in the diagnosis of periprosthetic infection of the hip. J Arthroplasty 21(6 Suppl 2):91–97, 2006.

The authors compared the accuracy of fluorodeoxyglucose positron emission tomography (FDG-PET) with that of technetium-99 m sulfur colloid indium-111–labeled white blood cell scintigraphy (TcSC-Ind BM/WBC) in the diagnosis of periprosthetic infection. FDG-PET correctly diagnosed 20 of 21 infected cases (sensitivity, 95.2%) and ruled out infection in 66 of 71 aseptic hips (specificity, 93%) corresponding to a positive predictive value of 80% (20/25) and a negative predictive value of 98.5% (66/67). They concluded that FDG-PET is a promising diagnostic tool for distinguishing septic from aseptic painful hip prostheses.

Temmerman OP, Raijmakers PG, Berkhof J, et al: Diagnostic accuracy and interobserver variability of plain radiography, subtraction arthrography, nuclear arthrography, and bone scintigraphy in the assessment of aseptic femoral component loosening. Arch Orthop Trauma Surg 126:316–323, 2006.

The authors evaluated the diagnostic accuracy and interobserver reliability of the four techniques in patients referred for evaluation of their femoral hip prostheses. They found considerable interobserver variability with all four techniques. A multivariate regression analysis revealed that bone scintigraphy and nuclear arthrography together made a significant contribution to the diagnosis when used in combination with plain radiography, and are, when plain radiography is inconclusive, useful additional diagnostic techniques for the detection of femoral component loosening.

CHAPTER 86

Preoperative Planning and Templating for Revision Hip Arthroplasty

Jay Patel and Kevin Bozic

KEY POINTS

- Preoperative planning begins with a thorough history and physical examination to determine the cause and location of hip pain, the general medical condition of the patient, and the functional goals of the patient.
- Radiographic evaluation is helpful in determining the cause of hip arthroplasty failure and in assessing component type, component alignment, bone stock, and infectious or osteolytic processes.
- Infection is a source of primary hip arthroplasty failure that should not be missed; evaluation requires familiarity with diagnostic algorithms.
- Using appropriate techniques and tools during component removal allows bone stock preservation at the time of revision.
- Templating allows the surgeon to anticipate the need for specific surgical instruments, components, and bone grafts intraoperatively.

INTRODUCTION

Revision total hip arthroplasty (THA) is a complex procedure associated with inferior patient outcomes, higher rates of complications, and greater hospital resource utilization compared with primary THA.[1-4] Furthermore, the number of revision THA procedures is expected to increase in proportion to the substantial increase in primary THA procedures.[5] Much effort has historically been placed on improving implant design, materials, and surgical techniques to improve outcomes of revision surgery. Although these efforts have generated many benefits, preoperative planning is an imperative, but often overlooked, step in anticipating the added challenges of revision surgery and minimizing complications. The process of preoperative planning for revision THA surgery is not algorithmic but includes three consistent steps.

First, the surgeon must diagnose the specific mode and cause of failure. Patient complaints can often be vague, and a thorough history, physical examination, and diagnostic evaluation are required to determine why revision surgery is indicated. Second, the surgeon must identify the goals of surgery. This entails identifying the technical goals of surgery, such as improving abductor tension or improving alignment of the acetabulum, and determining the patient-oriented goals of surgery, such as reducing hip pain or preventing hip dislocation. The patient must actively contribute to the goals of surgery and be made aware of the risks of surgery. Third, the surgeon must create a surgical plan that involves templating, anticipating alternative surgical methods, and ensuring that all necessary implants, instruments, and bone grafts are readily available on the day of surgery. The entire preoperative planning process is critical to the success of the surgery.

PREOPERATIVE DIAGNOSIS

The preoperative planning process begins during the patient's first office visit. The surgeon should listen carefully to the patient's complaint and begin to establish the surgeon-patient relationship. The history and physical examination should be thorough and should include significant detail about the hip, as well as general medical conditions. Hospital records, previous radiographs, and all previous operative reports, with implant labels, should be brought to the visit.

Patients often present with reports of pain or instability of the hip (Fig. 86-1). The pain should be defined in terms of its quality, severity, onset, progression, and location, as well as alleviating and exacerbating factors. The type of pain can be suggestive of a diagnosis. Aseptic loosening commonly presents with pain, which is worse with activity and is improved with rest. Pain in the groin or the gluteal region can be suggestive of a loose acetabular component, whereas pain in the thigh is suggestive of problems of the femoral component.[6,7] Groin pain occasionally can be due to hernias, lymphadenopathy, psoas abscess, or various gynecologic or genitourinary causes.[6-8] Start-up pain or pain with walking a few steps is also a hallmark of a loose femoral component.[6,7] If the patient had a pain-free interval after surgery, existing pain may be due to late infection, aseptic loosening, stress fracture, or osteolysis.[6,7,9] Persistent pain after surgery without a pain-free interval is suggestive of early infection, failure to obtain initial implant stability, periprosthetic fracture, or misdiagnosis of the original problem.[6,7,9] Constant pain, pain at rest, or night pain may be due to infection or malignancy.[9] Pain associated with a decreased range of motion (ROM) is a sign of infection, heterotopic ossification, subsidence, or acetabular protrusio. Acute pain

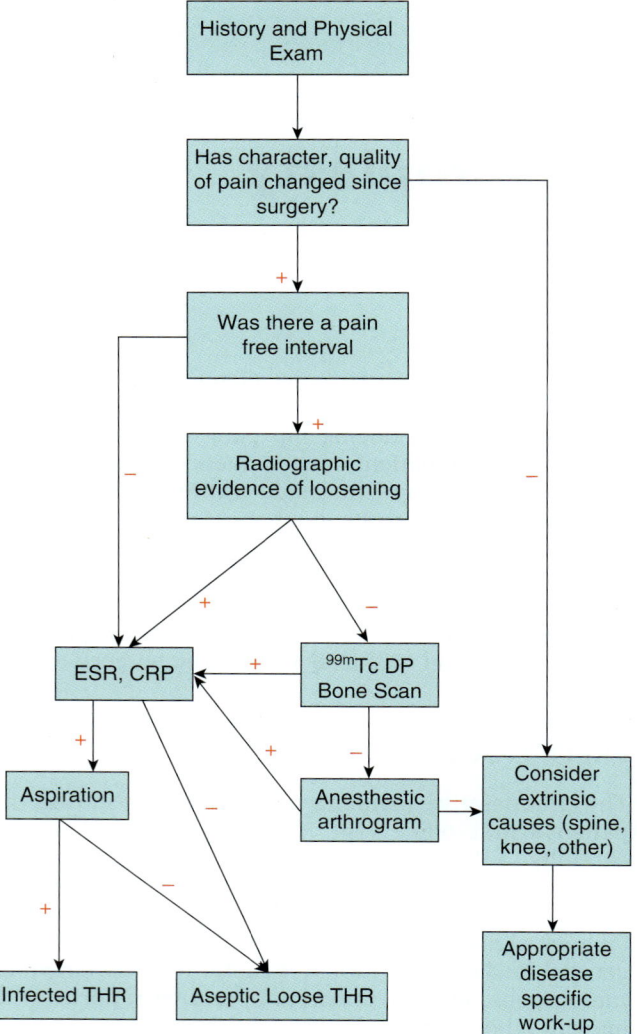

Figure 86-1. Algorithm to evaluate painful total hip arthroplasty (THA).

BOX 86-1. DIFFERENTIAL DIAGNOSIS FOR PAINFUL TOTAL HIP ARTHROPLASTY

Intrinsic Causes
- Infection
- Mechanical loosening
- Cemented
- Cementless
- Tip of stem pain (modulus mismatch)
- Stress fracture
- Periprosthetic fracture
- Nonunion
- Osteolysis
- Occult instability
- Inflammatory bursitis, tendinitis (trochanteric, iliopsoas)

Extrinsic Causes
- Lumbar spine disease
- Stenosis
- Disk herniation
- Spondylolysis or spondylolisthesis
- Peripheral vascular disease
- Nerve injury or irritation (sciatic, femoral, meralgia paresthetica)
- Causalgia or complex regional pain syndrome
- Metabolic disease (Paget's disease, osteomalacia)
- Malignancy or metastases
- Hernia (femoral, inguinal, obturator)
- Referred pain

From Bozic KJ, Rubash HE: The painful total hip replacement. Clin Orthop Relat Res 420:18, 2004.

---

is associated with hip dislocation and periprosthetic fracture. Patients with lumbar spine disease may be more active after hip arthroplasty, causing exacerbation of their neurogenic claudication.[10]

Thigh pain, although sometimes associated with a loose femoral component, is more commonly associated with well-fixed porous ingrowth or press-fit femoral components. Persistent thigh pain with no radiographic evidence of loosening has been described in 12% to 41% of patients with cementless implants,[11,12] although with modern implants and techniques, it is probably less common now. Some patients with persistent thigh pain have also been found to have well-fixed femoral components at the time of surgery.[13,14] Femoral component revision can be indicated for continued thigh pain despite well-fixed components. Tip of stem pain may be caused by modulus mismatch between a stiff cementless femoral stem and the less stiff surrounding bone.[9]

Hip instability is another common chief complaint. For these patients, a history of dislocation, including the number of dislocations, the timing of dislocation relative to the date of surgery, the position of the leg at the time of dislocation, the surgical approach used for the index procedure, and the method of reduction of the hip should be elicited. For patients who have symptoms of instability without dislocation, identifying the position of the leg when instability arises is important. Preoperative live fluoroscopy may be obtained to demonstrate the positions of impingement and instability. Causes of instability include inadequate soft tissue tension, component malposition, and bony impingement.

Intrinsic hip pain after hip arthroplasty must be distinguished from pain from extrinsic causes (Box 86-1). Intrinsic causes of pain include mechanical loosening, sepsis, stress fracture, implant failure, modulus mismatch, and subluxation or impingement.[9] Extrinsic causes of pain include lumbar spine disease, neurogenic or vascular claudication, trochanteric pain syndrome related to bursitis, abductor avulsion, tendinitis or abductor deficiency, peripheral nerve dysfunction, abductor or iliopsoas tendinitis, femoral or inguinal hernia, and malignancy.[9] A snapping hip may be confused with hip subluxation. Nonunion of the greater trochanter or painful hardware at the trochanter, from cerclage wires or a trochanter fixation plate, produces pain over the trochanter. Spinal stenosis can create radicular pain in the hip, thigh, and gluteal region. Vascular claudication from aortoiliac artery stenosis or in the gluteal branches can cause pain that is worse with activity, better with rest, and also present in the calf if distal run-off is poor. Although vascular claudication is typically due to atherosclerotic disease, it may also be caused by vascular injury during the primary surgery or by malpositioned acetabular screws.

Periprosthetic joint infection should be considered in all patients with a painful THA (see Fig. 86-1). Important elements of the history should include whether the patient is experiencing fevers, chills, or drainage from the wound. Patients who have a history of infection, postoperative hematoma, prolonged wound drainage, previous revision surgery, night pain, or pain with rest have a higher probability of developing infection. A history of other systemic infections, diabetes, nutritional deficiency, or immunocompromised status must also be elicited. Procedures that may cause transient bacteremia such as dental work, colonoscopy, or cystoscopy put the patient at risk for bacteria seeding the hip.

Identifying the patient's functional status, both before the index arthroplasty procedure and at the current time, is important when determining the goals of surgery. The surgeon should document whether the patient is household or community ambulatory, what distances the patient can walk without taking a rest, whether walking aids such as canes or walkers are used, whether the patient has caretaker assistance, and what activities of daily living the patient is able to perform. Because younger, more active patients are now undergoing primary hip arthroplasty procedures, the surgeon should also understand what types of sports and fitness activities the patient wishes to be able to do. Quantitative functional outcome measures, including the Harris hip score, can be helpful in assessing a patient's functional status both before and after THA.

A comprehensive medical evaluation is necessary to ensure that the patient's overall health is optimized before surgery is begun. Poor dentition can increase the risk of infection; therefore patients should undergo dental cleaning or obtain dentures well in advance of the date of surgery. Poor nutrition is also a risk factor for infection; the nutritional status of patients can be assessed at the preoperative planning stage by measuring serum albumin, prealbumin, and total protein in high-risk patients.[15-18] Patients with low prealbumin are at risk of poor wound healing and may need nutritional supplementation before the time of surgery. Peripheral vascular disease can increase the chance of infection, venous stasis ulcers, and deep venous thrombosis (DVT). If the patient has had a previous recent DVT, a lower extremity ultrasound is indicated to confirm resolution. In some cases, as in periprosthetic fracture or dislocation, surgery must be done immediately. In those cases, if a DVT is present, surgery should be delayed, or an inferior vena cava filter should be placed to prevent symptomatic pulmonary embolus. Similarly, if the patient is at risk of stasis because of poor ambulatory status from severe disability, recurrent dislocation, or periprosthetic fracture, a preoperative ultrasound may be considered to rule out DVT. Revascularization procedures for arterial insufficiency should be done in advance of revision hip arthroplasty procedures when in the opinion of a vascular surgeon the circulation is too poor to allow proper wound healing. This is a rare occurrence.

Urologic disorders such as benign prostate hyperplasia, urinary retention, and urinary tract infection should be addressed by a urologist. Urinary tract infections are common in the revision hip arthroplasty population and may put the hip at risk of being seeded as well. Hematologic disorders are also important to know about and are rarely identified. Difficulty with clotting or prolonged wound drainage during previous hip surgery may put the patient at risk for hematoma formation and wound infection. Preoperative hemoglobin levels should be measured to assess for anemia. The use of erythropoietin preoperatively to raise hemoglobin levels and reduce the amount of postoperative blood transfused may be considered.[19] Patients with body mass index greater than 35 are at increased risk of dislocation and would benefit from weight reduction,[20] although this is often futile. Cardiac and pulmonary comorbidities should be optimized before surgery to reduce anesthetic and surgical risks. Patients with a history of coronary bypass surgery, coronary stents, or congestive heart failure may need a preoperative pharmacologic stress test or cardiac catheterization if indicated. Diabetic patients should have their blood sugar control improved before undergoing surgery. Poor glycemic control has been shown to be associated with increased risk of stroke, urinary tract infection, ileus, postoperative hemorrhage, blood transfusion, wound infection, and death.[21]

PHYSICAL EXAMINATION

The physical examination of a patient with a painful THA should involve a comprehensive evaluation of both lower extremities and the spine, along with a full motor, sensory, and neurovascular examination.

Patients with a failed THA can have a number of gait patterns. Trendelenburg gait is a sign of hip abductor dysfunction and is more common after the direct lateral approach.[9] Causes of hip abductor dysfunction can include poor strength, poor abductor tension, superior gluteal nerve injury, trochanteric nonunion, and a failed repair. In addition to causing a limp, poor abductor strength can put the patient at risk of dislocation. If a trochanteric fracture or a nonunion occurs, this may be repaired at the time of surgery, although such repairs are not very predictable when done late. If abductor function is absent, a constrained liner may have to be available at the time of surgery. An extensor lurch occurs when the back hyperextends during the stance phase to compensate for a weak gluteus maximus. Drop foot gait, a sign of peroneal nerve injury, is manifested by the patient using high degrees of hip and knee flexion to clear the foot during the swing phase. During antalgic gait, the patient may use short steps to minimize motion at the hip. Finally, during short leg gait, a sign of limb length discrepancy, the pelvis will be noted to tilt downward, and the shoulder will be tilted upward on the short leg side.

Examination of previous incisions can guide both diagnosis and treatment planning. Existing scars and previous operative reports should be reviewed to determine which surgical approach has been used in the past. Previous wounds should be inspected for signs of infection, including warmth, erythema, fluctuance, wound drainage, and sinus tracts. In rare cases of chronic wounds with exposed prosthesis, bone, or hardware, muscle flap coverage by a plastic surgeon may be required. Local wound care is possible for small superficial wounds.[22] The surgical approach for revision surgery is guided by both the anatomic exposure that is required and the familiarity of the surgeon with particular approaches. Skin bridges between old and new incisions, or in cases where two incisions are required at the time of revision surgery, should be maximized to preserve skin blood supply. Commonly, extensile approaches are required to safely remove existing prostheses, treat bone deficiency, and implant revision components. The posterior approach is frequently used because it can be easily extended both proximally and distally.

Limb length discrepancy is common after failed primary hip arthroplasty and should be corrected as much as possible at the time of revision surgery. In many cases, however, full correction is not feasible, and patients should be counseled accordingly. Multiple methods may be used to measure limb length discrepancy. True limb length discrepancy is the distance from the anterior superior iliac spine to the medial malleolus with no pelvic tilt. The apparent limb length discrepancy is the distance from the umbilicus to the medial malleolus. Preferably true and apparent leg lengths should be measured with graduated blocks because patients with lumbar spine disease and fixed pelvic obliquity or both may present with notable differences between their true and apparent limb length discrepancies.[9] When significant deformity, scoliosis, flexion contractures, or obesity is present, a scanogram radiographic series or a computed tomography scan may be necessary. Progressive limb shortening after the primary procedures is suggestive of mechanical failure of fixation.[9]

Range of motion should be carefully measured to determine which positions re-created the patient's pain and/or instability symptoms. Pain with active ROM or extremes of motion can be indicative of loosening, whereas pain with passive ROM is suggestive of sepsis. Pain with a positive straight-leg raise suggests sciatic nerve irritation. Apprehension in certain positions is indicative of instability or impingement. Patients with instability may have a palpable or audible click during ROM. Pain with resisted hip flexion and passive extension is associated with iliopsoas tendinitis.[9] Limited ROM may occur secondary to ankylosis of the hip or acetabular protrusio. The Thomas test, a test for hip flexion deformity, is positive when flexion of the unaffected hip causes the affected leg to lift off the examination table and lumbar lordosis is maintained.

A detailed neurovascular examination, including motor, sensory, and peripheral vascular examinations, should be performed to assess for neurogenic or vascular causes of pain and dysfunction. Patients with spinal stenosis are at risk for peripheral nerve injury from the "double crush" phenomenon as a result of retraction or excessive limb lengthening.[6]

RADIOGRAPHIC EVALUATION

Preoperative planning for revision hip arthroplasty requires evaluation of serial plain radiographs. Multiple radiographic views can be used to obtain information about bone stock, migration, and osteolysis. Care must be taken to ensure that proper radiographic technique is used, including orientation, penetration, and rotation.

The anteroposterior (AP) pelvis view provides information about limb lengths by comparing the distance from the lesser trochanter to the interischial line. Although Kohler's line, or the ilioischial line, is used to assess for medial position of the cup, the acetabular teardrop has been found to be a more reliable landmark for detection of medial and superior migration.[23] The AP hip view is best obtained with 15 degrees of internal rotation of the lower limbs to best approximate the femoral neck shaft angle. Patients with contractures can be positioned semiprone to allow a perpendicular view of the femoral neck.[6] Adequate lateral film of the hip should include the entire prosthesis, cement column, and bow of the femur.[6] The shoot-through lateral technique, obtained with a 45-degree angled beam with the affected hip extended and the contralateral side flexed, is used to assess acetabular version. For patients with hip flexion contracture, a Lowenstein lateral, or a "table down lateral," can be obtained with the affected hip and knee flexed and the patient positioned in a lateral decubitus. The advantage of a Lowenstein lateral is that it demonstrates the femoral bow. In particular, if a femoral prosthesis longer than 15 cm is anticipated, it is helpful to evaluate the femoral bow preoperatively. A full-length AP and lateral view of the femur is indicated in cases of periprosthetic fracture, anticipated osteotomy, and ipsilateral hardware or total knee arthroplasty with stemmed implants. Judet views assist in evaluating bone stock and the integrity of the anterior and posterior columns.

Identifying which components may have to be removed is an important part of the radiographic evaluation. In an epidemiologic study of revision total hip arthroplasty, 41.1% of operations involved all component revision, 13.2% involved femoral component revision, 12.7% involved acetabular components, and 12.6% involved femoral head and liner exchange.[3] Loosening of a cemented femoral component can be classified radiographically.[24] Possible loosening is present when a radiolucent line spans 50% to 100% of the bone-cement interface. Probable loosening is characterized by a continuous or 2-mm-wide line at the bone-cement interface. Definite loosening is present when the following are noted: stem migration, a new continuous radiolucent line at the prosthesis-cement interface, prosthesis fracture, or cement fracture. Porous ingrowth stems can have signs of osseointegration, which include endosteal spot welds and radiodense lines around the coated part of the stem, calcar atrophy, a stable distal stem, and absence of a pedestal.[11] Failed osseointegration, on the other hand, is demonstrated by reactive lines around the porous stem and by the lack of endosteal spot welds, as well as implant migration distally or into varus.[11] In cemented acetabular cups, loosening can be estimated by the number of 2-mm demarcation zones identified on radiographs.[25] Migration of the cup and cement mantle together is defined as socket break-in, and migration of the cup relative to the cement is defined as socket break-out.[6] Findings have been mixed regarding the use of radiographs to determine whether porous ingrowth acetabular components are well fixed.[26,27] Migration, screw breakage, and component fracture, however, are definite signs of failure of cementless cups. Continuous radiolucent lines and evidence of bead shedding suggest probable loosening.

The degree and location of bone loss must be determined during the planning stage. Kitamura and associates demonstrated that the AP radiograph has 67% sensitivity and 72% specificity for detecting acetabular osteolysis.[28] Sensitivity improved to 90% when the osteolysis lesion volume was greater than 10 cm[3]. Thomas and colleagues demonstrated the value of Judet oblique radiographs in identifying osteolysis lesions. In a retrospective review of patients undergoing revision hip arthroplasty, the mean osteolytic area on AP radiograph was 384 mm[2], whereas the area on obturator oblique and iliac oblique radiographs was 790 mm[2] and 512 mm[2], respectively. Claus and coworkers reported that although multiple radiographic views allow for better approximation of osteolysis size and location, radiographs still have limitations. In their study, the sensitivity of detecting an osteolysis lesion on a single radiograph was 41.5%, but sensitivity increased to only 73.6% when four views were obtained. Saleh and associates have described a classification system based on standardized plain radiographs that is reliable for predicting bone loss at the time of revision surgery.[29]

Computed tomography (CT) imaging has been found to better demonstrate osteolytic lesions than plain radiographs[30] (Fig. 86-2). Kitamura and associates demonstrated how CT imaging can be used to differentiate osteolysis from preexisting bone defects by the

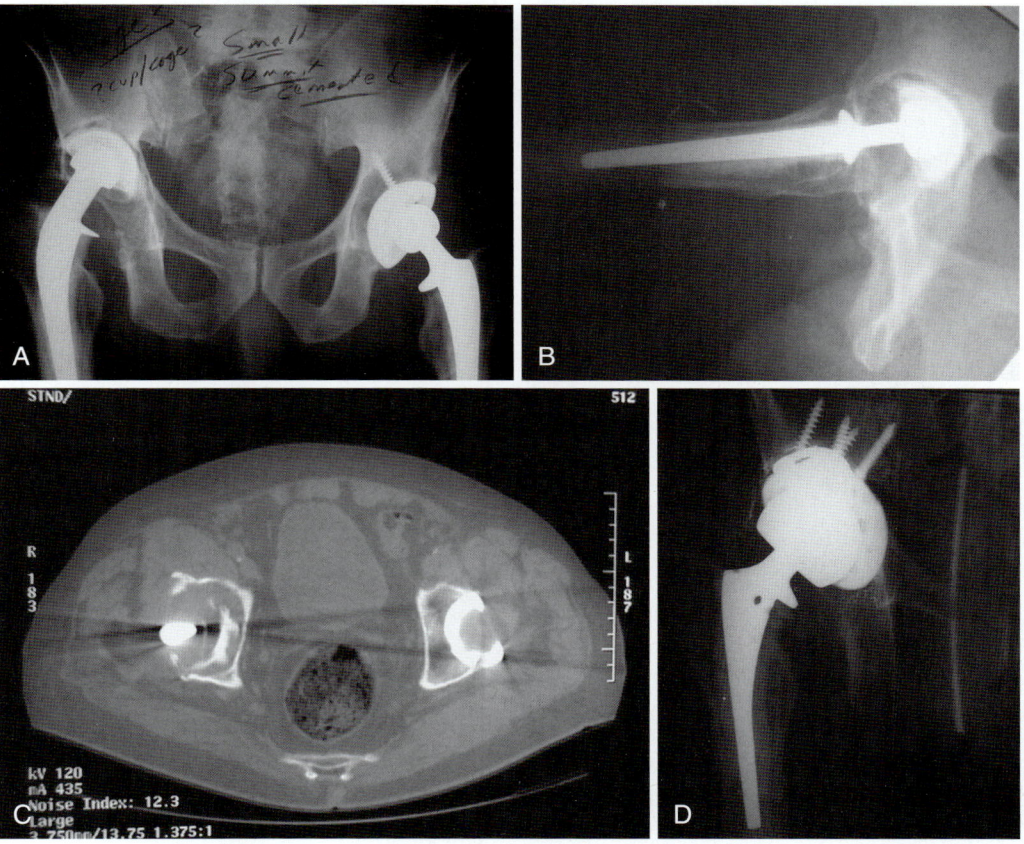

Figure 86-2. Imaging of acetabular osteolysis. **A** and **B,** Anteroposterior (AP) and lateral views demonstrating acetabular osteolysis with superior migration of the acetabular component. **C,** Computed tomography (CT) scan better demonstrating location and volume of acetabular bone loss. **D,** Revision of acetabular component with tantalum cup with augment. *(Courtesy Robert Gorab, MD.)*

identification of communication pathways. Lesions without communication pathways were smaller and not associated with cortical erosions, whereas lesions with pathways were larger with erosions. In their study, cortical erosions were a hallmark of osteolysis lesions.[31] To avoid radiation exposure, some have used new magnetic resonance imaging (MRI) protocols to assess for acetabular osteolysis. Weiland and colleagues reported that MRI has a sensitivity of 95% for osteolysis detection.[32] Walde and coworkers found that the sensitivity of detecting osteolytic lesions was 51% for radiographs, 74% for CT, and 95% for MRI. Although MRI was found to have higher sensitivity than CT, CT was found to be more accurate in detecting lesion volume.[33]

Multiple classification systems for bone deficiency have been devised,[34-38] and the reader is referred to

Chapter 89 for details. The American Academy of Orthopaedic Surgeons (AAOS) Committee on the Hip has described classification systems for the acetabulum and the femur that differentiate between segmental and cavitary deficiencies[34,35] (Boxes 86-2 and 86-3). The Paprosky classification of acetabular and femoral defects has also been widely adopted[36,38] (Boxes 86-4 and 86-5). Paprosky type I and II acetabular defects can

---

BOX 86-2. AAOS CLASSIFICATION OF BONE DEFICIENCIES: ACETABULUM

I. Segmental deficiency
  Peripheral
  Superior
  Anterior
  Posterior
  Central
II. Cavitary deficiency
  Peripheral
  Superior
  Anterior
  Posterior
  Central
III. Combined deficiency
IV. Pelvic discontinuity
V. Arthrodesis

AAOS, American Academy of Orthopaedic Surgeons.

BOX 86-3. AAOS CLASSIFICATION OF BONE DEFICIENCIES: FEMUR

I. Segmental deficiency
  Proximal
  Partial
  Complete
  Intercalary
  Greater trochanter
II. Cavitary deficiency
  Cancellous
  Cortical
  Ectasia
III. Combined deficiency
IV. Malalignment
  Rotational
  Angular
V. Femoral stenosis
VI. Femoral discontinuity

AAOS, American Academy of Orthopaedic Surgeons.

BOX 86-4. PAPROSKY CLASSIFICATION OF BONE DEFICIENCIES: ACETABULUM

Type I
- Acetabular rim intact and undistorted
- Acetabulum hemispherical in shape with supportive dome

Type II
- Acetabular rim distorted or has minor deficiencies but fully supportive of hemispherical shell
- At least 50% of hemispherical component in contact with host bone
- Hip center migration less than 3 cm superior to superior obturator line
- Minimal ischial bone loss

Type IIIa
- Marked superolateral acetabular bone loss with greater than one third of acetabular rim circumference deficient
- Hemispherical cup does not have inherent stability on host bone

Type IIIb
- Marked superomedial acetabular bone loss
- Failed implant migration medial to Kohler's line
- Migration greater than 3 cm superior to superior obturator line
- Extensive ischial osteolysis

BOX 86-5. PAPROSKY CLASSIFICATION OF BONE DEFECTS: FEMUR

Type I
- Minimal loss of metaphyseal cancellous bone with an intact diaphysis

Type II
- Extensive loss of metaphyseal bone with a completely intact diaphysis

Type IIIa
- Metaphysis is damaged severely and nonsupportive
- Minimum of 4 cm of intact cortical bone present in the femoral isthmus

Type IIIb
- Severely damaged metaphysis
- Some intact cortical bone present distal to the isthmus (<4 cm)

Type IV
- Extensive metadiaphyseal damage in conjunction with a widened femoral canal

often be managed with hemispherical cementless cups fixed with screws and limited bone grafting. Type IIIa deficiencies may require structural allografts or modular porous metal augments used in combination with cementless cups, bilobed cups, or antiprotrusio cages. Type IIIb deficiencies by definition have an insufficient peripheral rim of bone to support a hemispheric cup and therefore frequently require other reconstructive techniques, such as antiprotrusio cages or custom triflange components.[38] It should be noted that increased use of highly porous metal shells may expand the indications for hemispheric acetabular components in the management of Paprosky IIIa and IIIb defects.[39]

Paprosky type I femoral defects can be treated with cemented stems, proximally coated cementless stems, or 6-inch extensively porous-coated cementless stems. Type II defects can be treated with 6-inch extensively porous-coated cementless stems, cemented long stems, or modular tapered cementless stems. Type IIIa defects, in which more than 4 cm of isthmus is remaining for bony ingrowth, can be managed with 8- or 10-inch extensively porous-coated stems (straight or bowed), impaction grafting, or modular tapered cementless stems. Type IIIb deficiencies, in which less than 4 m of isthmus is remaining, can be treated with 10-inch extensively coated stems, impaction grafting, or modular tapered cementless stems. Finally, type IV defects can be addressed with allograft prosthetic composites, femoral replacing endoprostheses, or modular tapered cementless stems.[36]

Heterotopic ossification can be graded according to the classification described by Brooker.[40] For patients with previous heterotopic ossification or at high risk for developing new heterotopic ossification, low-dose radiation (700 cGray) should be administered 24 hours preoperatively or no more than 48 hours postoperatively.[41,42] Rumi and associates demonstrated that preoperative radiation administered 24 hours preoperatively is more effective than when administered 4 hours, 72 hours, or 3 weeks preoperatively. Porous ingrowth and potential osteotomy sites should be shielded from radiation to prevent nonunion or lack of ingrowth.[43]

INFECTION EVALUATION

Infection must be on the differential diagnosis of all patients undergoing revision THA (see Fig. 86-1). Guidelines regarding the use of laboratory assays, aspiration, intraoperative gram stain, cultures, and nuclear medicine tests are continually being developed. The white blood cell count has been found to be an unreliable indicator of infection.[44,45] Spangehl and colleagues demonstrated that an elevated white blood cell count has only 20% sensitivity, 96% specificity, 54% positive predictive value, and 85% negative predictive value for infection. In their prospective study, the erythrocyte sedimentation rate (ESR) and C-reactive protein (CRP) were found to be more useful preoperative infection

indicators. An ESR was considered elevated if it was greater than 30 mm/hr, and a CRP was elevated if greater than 10 mg/mL. Alone, the ESR has 82% sensitivity, 85% specificity, 58% positive predictive value, and 95% negative predictive value. The CRP was found to be more useful than the ESR, having 96% sensitivity, 92% specificity, 74% positive predictive value, and 99% negative predictive value. CRP may be a more accurate indicator than ESR because in uninfected cases, it normalizes by 3 weeks after surgery, whereas the ESR may remain slightly elevated up to 1 year after surgery.[46] The Spangehl study found that the combination of a normal CRP and a normal ESR is reliable in predicting the absence of infection.[45]

Aspiration has been used to augment the diagnosis of infection. Whereas some surgeons routinely perform preoperative aspirations on all patients undergoing revision THA, others do aspirations only when other laboratory, radiographic, or clinical parameters suggest infection. Aspiration has been demonstrated to have 86% sensitivity, 94% specificity, 67% positive predictive value, and 98% negative predictive value in diagnosing periprosthetic joint infection.[45] Multiple studies have demonstrated that routine preoperative aspiration is not indicated unless other clinical signs or symptoms of infection are noted.[47,48] However, algorithms for using white blood cell count in the setting of elevated CRP and ESR are proving to have greater utility. Schinsky and coworkers recommend using a cutoff of 4200 white blood cells/mL and 80% polymorphonuclear cells.[49] In the setting of an elevated CRP and ESR, the cutoff is reduced to 3000 white blood cells/mL. These cutoffs are much lower than historic cutoffs of 25,000 to 80,000 white blood cells/mL.[49]

Nuclear imaging studies can assist in differentiating loosening from infection. Technetium-99 methylene diphosphonate (^{99}Tc-MDP) bone scintigraphy can identify areas of increased metabolic activity, but when used alone has low sensitivity and specificity for detecting loosening or infection.[50] Technetium-99 colloid sulfur imaging combined with 111-indium–labeled leukocyte scans improves the sensitivity and specificity of the diagnosis of infection.[51,52] Delank and coworkers completed a prospective study of 18F-fluorodeoxyglucose positron emission tomography (18F-FDG-PET) as a new technique to identify infection and loosening in the setting of joint arthroplasty. The technique has 100% sensitivity for septic cases, but differentiation of infection from loosening is not reliable.[53]

Use of intraoperative frozen section analysis and cultures must be coordinated with laboratory and pathology services. A plan of action based on the results of these findings must be established preoperatively. For intraoperative frozen section analysis, Lonner and associates showed that more than 10 polymorphonuclear cells per high-power field is suggestive of infection.[54] Although intraoperative cultures are considered the gold standard for identifying infection, problems of sampling error and a false-positive rate of 8% make their use difficult.[49]

TEMPLATING

The principles of templating for a revision hip arthroplasty begin as many of the same principles for templating a primary procedure. Preoperative templating is based primarily on an AP pelvis radiograph. Both conventional and digital templating techniques are commonly used. With digital radiography becoming more common, surgeons are increasingly using electronic overlays and measurements. Initial studies of digital templating for primary hip arthroplasty have showed promise in predicting actual implant size.[55-61] The benefit of digital techniques for revision arthroplasty, where the potential implant and bone graft needs are broader and less predictable, has yet to be determined.

The first step is to measure the limb length discrepancy. This is done by comparing the distance between the lesser trochanter and the interischial line. The acetabular component is typically templated first. The acetabulum template is positioned with the inferomedial aspect of the component adjacent to the teardrop. The position of the cup must maximize contact with host bone. If there is superior bony deficiency or acetabular distortion, the cup may have to be positioned superiorly to maximize contact. The use of a larger cup, often required for revision arthroplasty, may counter this effect because of the inherent lower center of rotation[7] (Fig. 86-3). Use of a high hip center is sometimes warranted to improve bony ingrowth and reduce the

need for structural allograft (Fig. 86-4). Whereas superolateral positioning of the acetabulum has been associated with increased loosening secondary to greater forces across the joint, superior only positioning does not share the same problem.[62]

The size of the cup is determined by the similar principles of (1) maximizing host bone contact, (2) restoring the native center of rotation, and (3) maximizing hip joint stability. The acetabular template should iteratively be placed against the AP and lateral radiographs of the hip to ensure that the component is sized appropriately. Often, the lateral view can be used to determine whether enough bone in the anterior and posterior columns is available for the given size of the component.

The optimal position of the acetabular component is 45 degrees abducted and 20 degrees anteverted. The range for acceptable abduction is 30 to 50 degrees. Ideally, when the acetabulum is positioned in 45 degrees abduction, it should extend from the teardrop to the superolateral acetabular margin.[6]

The medial extent of the acetabular component should be a few millimeters lateral to the lateral aspect of the teardrop or, less reliably, lateral to the ilioischial line.[23] Components that are medial to the teardrop indicate a medial wall deficit or protrusio acetabuli (Fig. 86-5). The medial position of the acetabulum decreases abductor tension and allows for potential impingement. When there is concern for a thin or deficient medial wall, a pelvic angiogram may assist in

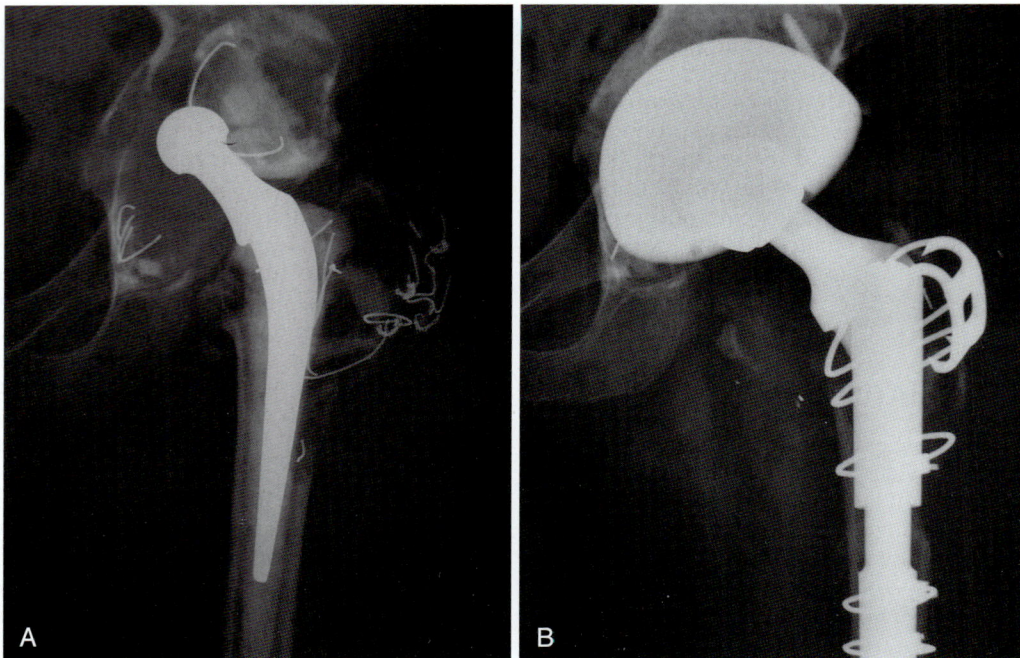

Figure 86-3. Jumbo cup for massive acetabular osteolysis. **A,** Preoperative radiograph demonstrates significant acetabular osteolysis with superolateral migration and rotation. This defect represents a Paprosky IIIb defect. **B,** Postoperative radiograph demonstrates revision with 80-mm jumbo cup restoring hip center. In this case, a hemispherical cup augmented with screw fixation and bone grafting was possible. If a peripheral rim fit was not possible, the acetabulum could be revised with a structural allograft and an antiprotrusio cage or a custom triflange porous-coated cup. *(Courtesy Robert Gorab, MD.)*

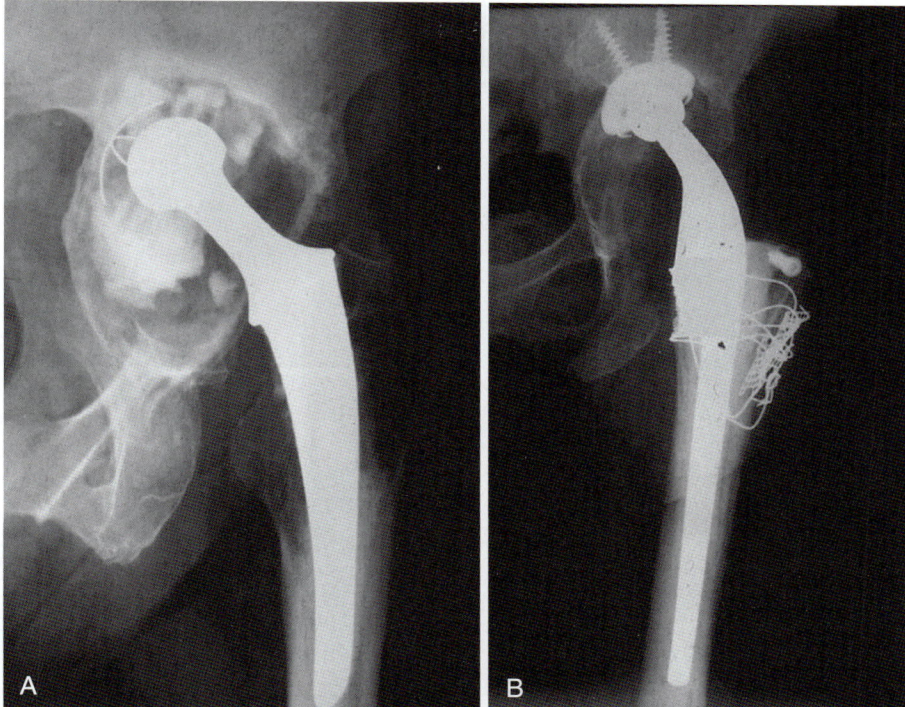

Figure 86-4. High hip center technique for massive acetabular osteolysis. **A,** Preoperative radiograph showing significant acetabular osteolysis. **B,** Postoperative radiograph showing revision using high hip center technique. *(From Bozic KJ, Freiberg AA, Harris WH: The high hip center. Clin Orthop Relat Res 420:101, 2004.)*

determining the relative position of the intrapelvic vessels. Intrapelvic cement or components may lead to vascular injury; therefore a retroperitoneal approach may be warranted to protect the vessels (Fig. 86-6).[63] If there is concern for medial migration of the revision acetabular component, a large-diameter cup or antiprotrusio cage should be available. Lateral component positioning, on the other hand, increases joint reaction forces.

The choice of acetabular component and bone graft depends highly on the degree of bone loss and the quality of the remaining host bone. A vast majority of acetabular revisions can be performed with a hemispheric cementless acetabular component. Generally speaking, if a hemispheric acetabular component is uncovered less than 20%, no bone grafting is required. When the component is uncovered 20% to 40%, a structural graft such as a femoral allograft or metal augments may be needed. If more than 50% to 60% of the cup is uncovered, an antiprotrusio cage with structural bone grafting is usually recommended.[6,7] In cases of contained bony defects, large hemispherical porous-coated components can be placed with impaction grafting of the cavity. A review of 4762 revision total hip arthroplasty procedures from the Norwegian Arthroplasty Register revealed that uncemented acetabular components, both with and without allograft, had lower rates of re-revision compared with cemented acetabular components.[64] Uncontained defects can be addressed with large components, high hip centers, and structural bone grafting.[6] Jumbo, or extra-large, cups allow for greater

host bone contact, minimize elevation of the hip center, distribute the forces of body weight over a greater surface area, and reduce the need for structural bone grafting. A recent review of 89 hip revisions using a jumbo cup demonstrated survival of 93% at 8 years.[65] Bilobed, oblong, and modular cups have been used to treat patients with particular patterns of segmental bone deficiency but with mixed results.[66,67] Antiprotrusio rings are useful in the case of uncontained defects when there is less than 50% contact between the acetabular component and the host bone. The ring protects morselized graft and provides support from the ilium to the inferomedial acetabulum. Rings can also be used with structural grafts that support less than 50% of the cup. Acetabular cages, on the other hand, are useful for large uncontained defects when significant amounts of morselized graft or structural grafts that support more than 50% of the cup are used. Cages provide support from the ilium to the ischium.[68] Pelvic discontinuity can be addressed with a protrusio cage, posterior column reconstruction followed by cementless hemispherical component, a custom triflange implant, or a cup-cage construct.[69]

Bone grafting is a useful adjunct to cementless acetabular reconstruction in revision THA. Structural allografts, although often used in the setting of large, uncontained defects, are characterized by high union rates, but they do have a significant rate of failure secondary to resorption.[70] Typically, such bulk bone grafts are used for superolateral acetabular defects or for posterior wall and column deficiencies. Impaction grafting,

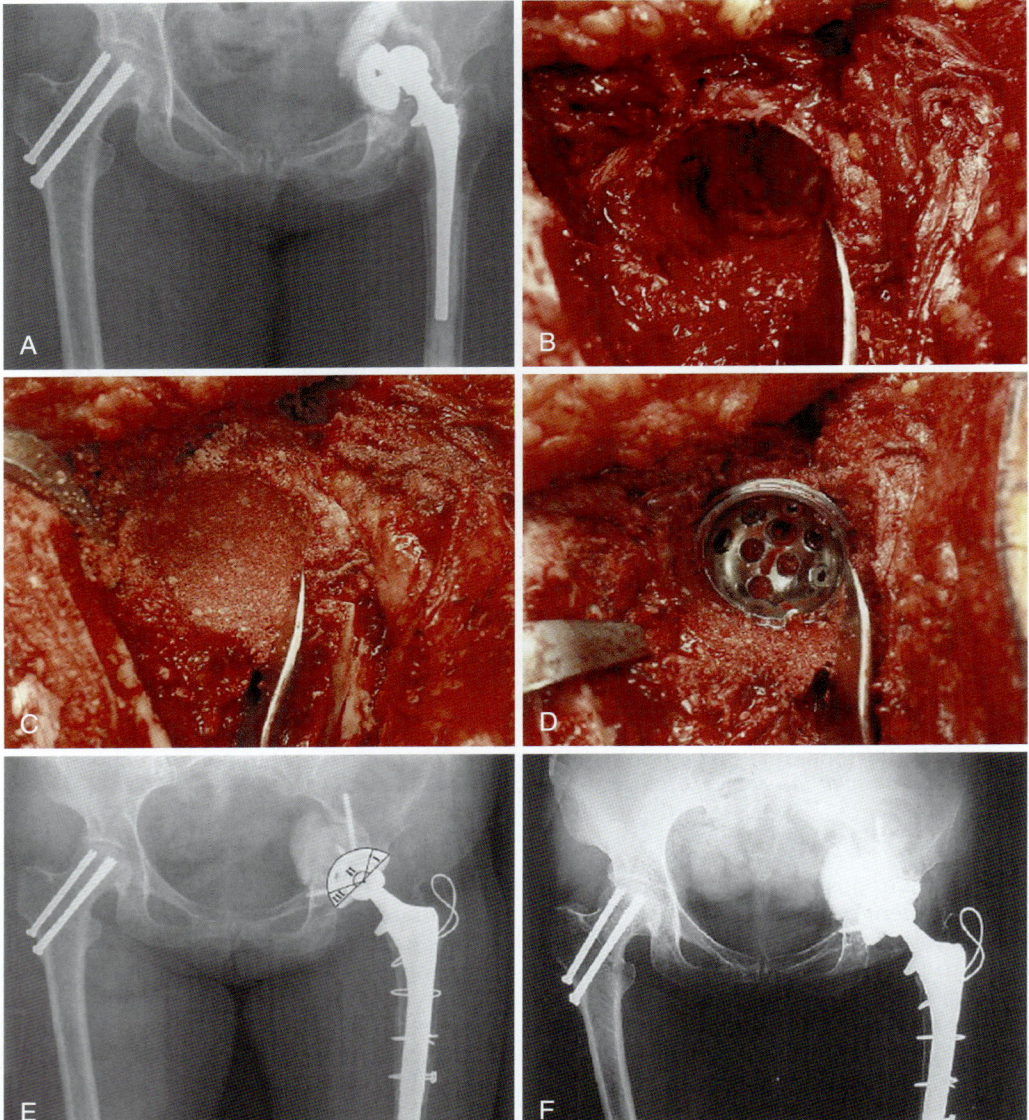

Figure 86-5. Treatment of medial uncontained acetabular defect. **A,** Preoperative radiograph of medial acetabular defect. **B,** Intraoperative view showing medial defect with rim intact. **C,** Morselized allograft packed into medial defect. **D,** Cementless rim fit cup with screws. **E,** Six-week follow-up radiograph. **F,** Eighteen-week follow-up radiograph. *(From Hansen E, Ries M: Revision total hip arthroplasty for large medial [protrusion] defects with a rim-fit cementless acetabular component. J Arthroplasty 21:72, 2006.)*

through the use of morselized allograft, is useful for contained defects.

Well-fixed acetabulum components with nearby adjacent osteolytic lesions can be treated with bone grafting through holes in the acetabular component or through peripheral communication pathways. The acetabular component should be assessed for stability to ensure that it is in fact well fixed. To replace the liner, a new liner may be fixed using a functioning locking mechanism or cemented in place after being scored on the backside to improve cement interdigitation.

Templating of the femoral component begins with obtaining AP and lateral radiographs of the affected hip (Fig. 86-7). The radiograph should include the entire

femoral component and enough distal femoral diaphysis to plan for a long stem. Restoration of stability, limb length, and offset is the goal of femoral reconstruction. Limb length discrepancies can be corrected by relative positioning of the center of rotation of femoral and acetabular components. Soft tissue and neurovascular structures may limit the amount of lengthening that is possible. When acetabular components that alter the center of rotation are used, specialized femoral components that can correct for length and offset should be available. These may include components that are calcar replacing or have increased offset.[7] Offset is best measured on radiographs in which the hip is internally rotated 15 degrees to better demonstrate the femoral

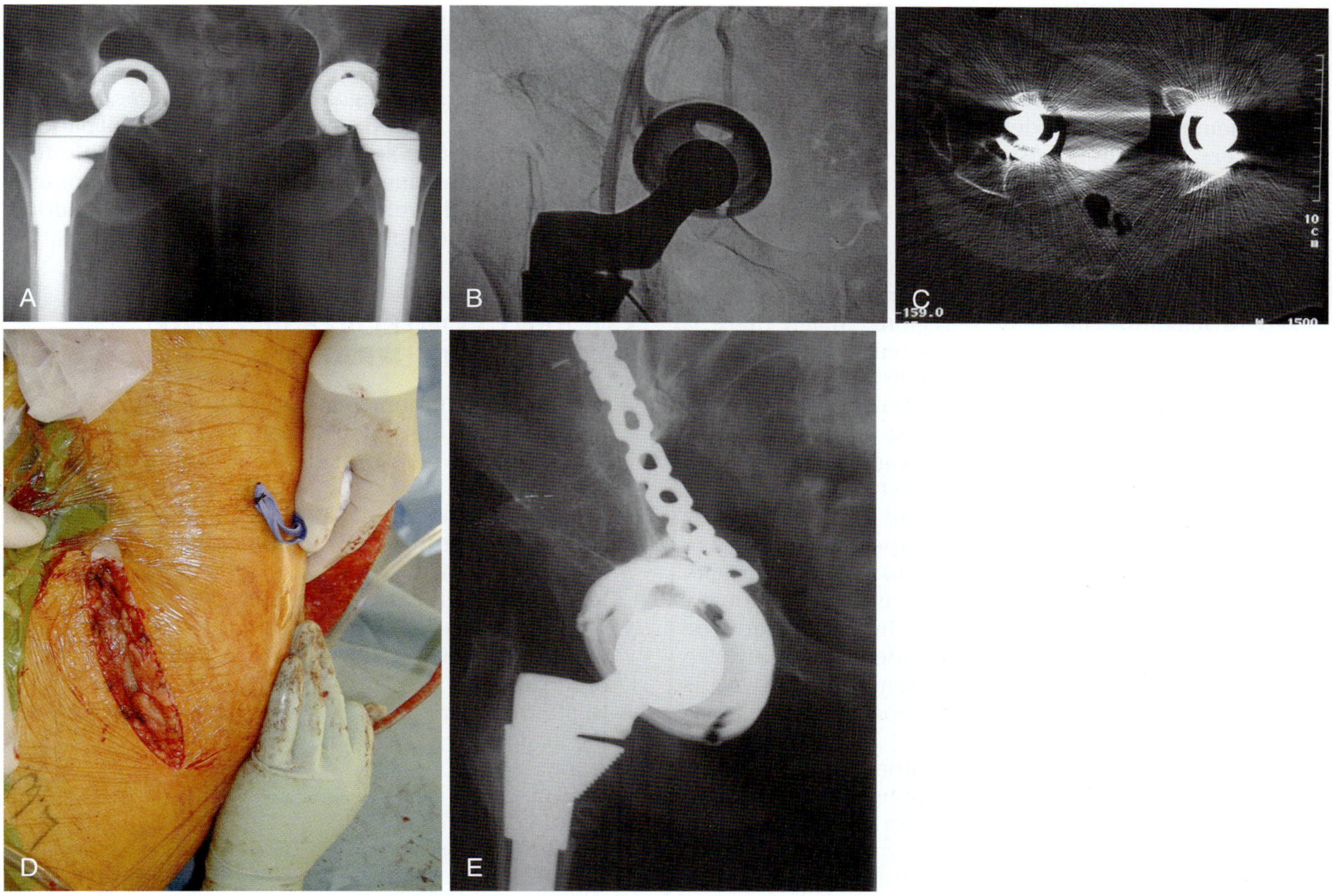

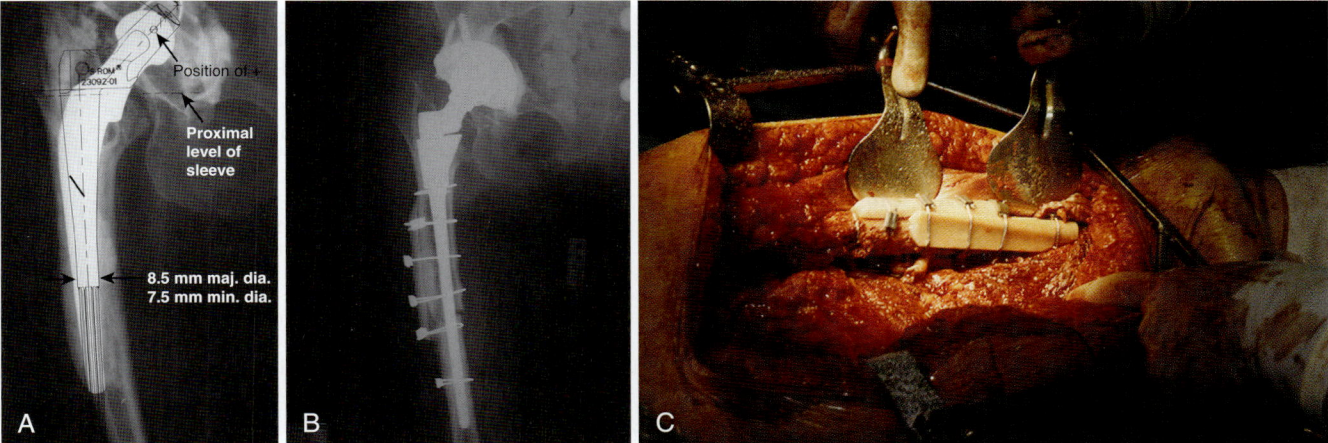

Figure 86-6. Evaluation and treatment of severe acetabuli protrusio. **A,** Preoperative radiograph showing severe protrusio defect. **B,** Preoperative angiogram showing proximity to iliac vessels. **C,** Preoperative computed tomography (CT) scan showing bladder compression. **D,** Intraoperative view of retroperitoneal approach. **E,** Postoperative radiograph of acetabulum revision with internal fixation. *(Courtesy Robert Gorab, MD.)*

Figure 86-7. Femoral component templating. **A,** Preoperative radiograph with template of long-stem prosthesis that demonstrates the need for femoral osteotomy. This defect represents a Paprosky IIIa defect given the unsupportive metaphysis and 4 cm of diaphysis available for scratch fit. **B,** Postoperative radiograph demonstrates revision with long-stem prosthesis with proximal sleeve, allograft, and cerclage fixation. An extended trochanteric osteotomy was done to allow for cement removal and deformity correction. A modular stem was used to correct for torsional remodeling of the proximal femur. **C,** Intraoperative view demonstrates use of strut allografts and cerclage fixation. *(Courtesy Robert Gorab, MD.)*

neck profile. If there is difficulty in determining the offset of the affected side, templating of the contralateral hip may provide the true offset.

The length of the stem should be chosen to bypass distal femoral cortical defects by two to three canal diameters.[71] When extensively coated stems are used, 6 cm of scratch fit in the isthmic region of the diaphysis is recommended for stability.[6] After the length of stem is chosen, the degree of proximal fill is assessed. Because the degree of bone loss in the metaphysis and in the diaphysis may be different, modular implants may be used to maximize fill in both regions. When there is calcar bone loss, calcar replacing stems can replace 15 to 30 mm of length.[7] For more than 30 mm loss from the lesser trochanter, a proximal femoral replacement or an allograft composite prosthesis can be used. Extensively coated stems allow for stability through the presence of a scratch fit, as well as bone ingrowth.[6] Implants with distally fixed stems may be used but can cause stress shielding of the proximal femur. Impaction grafting to improve bone stock within the proximal femur and onlay cortical strut grafts to bypass cavitary or locally segmental bony defects may be required and should be available. Long, tapered stems provide an alternative to impaction grafting in cases where femoral diaphysis is insufficient to attain adequate fixation with a cylindrical, fully porous-coated stem.[72]

The extended trochanteric osteotomy is an excellent tool to safely remove femoral components and to insert long-stemmed prostheses. Whether or not the extended trochanteric osteotomy is planned, familiarity with the technique before any revision hip arthroplasty will allow the surgeon to deal with unanticipated situations. The rate of union of the extended trochanteric osteotomy has been reported to be between 96% and 100%.[73] If proximal femoral varus remodeling has occurred, this osteotomy facilitates placement of a long-stemmed prosthesis while minimizing the risk of cortical perforation.

Cemented femoral prostheses have historically been less reliable for revision arthroplasty. Lack of cancellous bone for cement interdigitation at the time of revision is thought to cause a decrease in shear resistance. Cementation of a femoral component that passes the isthmus is problematic because of difficulty removing the cement at time of re-revision and pressurizing the cement.[7] If a cemented femoral prosthesis is anticipated, allowances for a 2-mm cement mantle should be made. Some surgeons avoid stems longer than 160 to 180 mm because of abutment on the femoral cortex.[7]

An additional challenge associated with templating a revision hip arthroplasty is anticipating how to remove existing implants. Often a large armamentarium of surgical instruments must be available because component extraction can be difficult. Selection of tools and technique must ensure that bone stock will be preserved. Techniques are covered in detail in Chapter 87.

CONCLUSIONS

Thorough preoperative planning is mandatory for successful revision hip arthroplasty. The challenge begins with identifying the exact cause of hip pain and understanding the patient's overall health status. Radiographic analysis provides a wealth of information about the mode of failure and goals of surgery. Infection must be considered at the top of the differential for all patients undergoing revision surgery. Finally, radiographic templating allows the surgeon to anticipate all equipment, component, and grafting material needs for multiple alternative surgical plans.

CURRENT CONTROVERSIES AND FUTURE CONSIDERATIONS

- Economic limitations pose an additional challenge in planning revision hip arthroplasty because resource utilization for revision surgery is higher and is continually rising.
- Improving infection evaluation for THA patients will involve algorithms that combine existing tests with the development of new diagnostic assays with increased sensitivity and specificity.
- The role of computer navigation in improving outcomes of revision hip arthroplasty has yet to be determined.
- Digital templating will likely replace manual templating as digital radiographs become standard.

REFERENCES

1. Bozic KJ, Durbhakula S, Berry DJ, et al: Differences in patient and procedure characteristics and hospital resource use in primary and revision total joint arthroplasty: a multicenter study. J Arthroplasty 20(7 Suppl 3):17, 2005.
2. Bozic KJ, Katz P, Cisternas M, et al: Hospital resource utilization for primary and revision total hip arthroplasty. J Bone Joint Surg Am 87:570, 2005.
3. Bozic KJ, Kurtz SM, Lau E, et al: The epidemiology of revision total hip arthroplasty in the United States. J Bone Joint Surg Am 91:128, 2009.
4. Bozic KJ, Ries MD: The impact of infection after total hip arthroplasty on hospital and surgeon resource utilization. J Bone Joint Surg Am 87:1746, 2005.
5. Iorio R, Robb WJ, Healy WL, et al: Orthopaedic surgeon workforce and volume assessment for total hip and knee replacement in the United States: preparing for an epidemic. J Bone Joint Surg Am 90:1598, 2008.
6. Agarwal S, Freiberg A, Rubash H: Preoperative planning for revision hip arthroplasty. In Callaghan J, Rosenberg A, Rubash H, editors: The adult hip, Philadelphia, 2007, Lippincott Williams & Wilkins, p 1313.
7. Barrack RL, Burnett RS: Preoperative planning for revision total hip arthroplasty. Instr Course Lect 55:233, 2006
8. Gaunt ME, Tan SG, Dias J: Strangulated obturator hernia masquerading as pain from a total hip replacement. J Bone Joint Surg Br 74:782, 1992.
9. Bozic KJ, Rubash HE: The painful total hip replacement. Clin Orthop Relat Res 420:18, 2004.
10. Bohl WR, Steffee AD: Lumbar spinal stenosis: a cause of continued pain and disability in patients after total hip arthroplasty. Spine 4:168, 1979.
11. Engh CA, Massin P, Suthers KE: Roentgenographic assessment of the biologic fixation of porous-surfaced femoral components. Clin Orthop Relat Res 257:107, 1990.
12. Haddad RJ, Jr, Skalley TC, Cook SD, et al: Clinical and roentgenographic evaluation of noncemented porous-coated anatomic medullary locking (AML) and porous-coated anatomic (PCA) total hip arthroplasties. Clin Orthop Relat Res 258:176, 1990.

13. Cook SD, Barrack RL, Thomas KA, Haddad RJ Jr: Tissue growth into porous primary and revision femoral stems. J Arthroplasty 6(Suppl):S37, 1991.
14. Engh CA, Jr, Culpepper WJ, 2nd, Engh CA: Long-term results of use of the anatomic medullary locking prosthesis in total hip arthroplasty. J Bone Joint Surg Am 79:177, 1997.
15. Del Savio GC, Zelicof SB, Wexler LM, et al: Preoperative nutritional status and outcome of elective total hip replacement. Clin Orthop Relat Res 326:153, 1996.
16. Gherini S, Vaughn BK, Lombardi AV, Jr, Mallory TH: Delayed wound healing and nutritional deficiencies after total hip arthroplasty. Clin Orthop Relat Res 293:188, 1993.
17. Greene KA, Wilde AH, Stulberg BN: Preoperative nutritional status of total joint patients: relationship to postoperative wound complications. J Arthroplasty 6:321, 1991.
18. Marin LA, Salido JA, Lopez A, Silva A: Preoperative nutritional evaluation as a prognostic tool for wound healing. Acta Orthop Scand 73:2, 2002.
19. Moonen AF, Thomassen BJ, Knoors NT, et al: Pre-operative injections of epoetin-alpha versus post-operative retransfusion of autologous shed blood in total hip and knee replacement: a prospective randomised clinical trial. J Bone Joint Surg Br 90:1079, 2008.
20. Kim Y, Morshed S, Joseph T, et al: Clinical impact of obesity on stability following revision total hip arthroplasty. Clin Orthop Relat Res 453:142, 2006.
21. Marchant MH, Jr, Viens NA, Cook C, et al: The impact of glycemic control and diabetes mellitus on perioperative outcomes after total joint arthroplasty. J Bone Joint Surg Am 91:1621, 2009.
22. Gusenoff JA, Hungerford DS, Orlando JC, Nahabedian MY: Outcome and management of infected wounds after total hip arthroplasty. Ann Plast Surg 49:587, 2002.
23. Goodman SB, Adler SJ, Fyhrie DP, Schurman DJ: The acetabular teardrop and its relevance to acetabular migration. Clin Orthop Relat Res 236:199, 1988.
24. Harris WH, McCarthy JC, Jr, O'Neill DA: Loosening of the femoral component of total hip replacement after plugging the femoral canal. Hip 228, 1982.
25. DeLee JG, Charnley J: Radiological demarcation of cemented sockets in total hip replacement. Clin Orthop Relat Res 121:20, 1976.
26. Cook SD, Barrack RL, Thomas KA, Haddad RJ, Jr: Quantitative analysis of tissue growth into human porous total hip components. J Arthroplasty 3:249, 1988.
27. Udomkiat P, Wan Z, Dorr LD: Comparison of preoperative radiographs and intraoperative findings of fixation of hemispheric porous-coated sockets. J Bone Joint Surg Am 83:1865, 2001.
28. Kitamura N, Pappedemos PC, Duffy PR, 3rd, et al: The value of anteroposterior pelvic radiographs for evaluating pelvic osteolysis. Clin Orthop Relat Res 453:239, 2006.
29. Saleh KJ, Holtzman J, Gafni A, et al: Reliability and intraoperative validity of preoperative assessment of standardized plain radiographs in predicting bone loss at revision hip surgery. J Bone Joint Surg Am 83:1040, 2001.
30. Puri L, Wixson RL, Stern SH, et al: Use of helical computed tomography for the assessment of acetabular osteolysis after total hip arthroplasty. J Bone Joint Surg Am 84:609, 2002.
31. Kitamura N, Naudie DD, Leung SB, et al: Diagnostic features of pelvic osteolysis on computed tomography: the importance of communication pathways. J Bone Joint Surg Am 87:1542, 2005.
32. Weiland DE, Walde TA, Leung SB, et al: Magnetic resonance imaging in the evaluation of periprosthetic acetabular osteolysis: a cadaveric study. J Orthop Res 23:713, 2005.
33. Walde TA, Weiland DE, Leung SB, et al: Comparison of CT, MRI, and radiographs in assessing pelvic osteolysis: a cadaveric study. Clin Orthop Relat Res 437:138, 2005.
34. D'Antonio J, McCarthy JC, Bargar WL, et al: Classification of femoral abnormalities in total hip arthroplasty. Clin Orthop Relat Res 296:133, 1993.
35. D'Antonio JA, Capello WN, Borden LS, et al: Classification and management of acetabular abnormalities in total hip arthroplasty. Clin Orthop Relat Res 243:126, 1989.
36. Della Valle CJ, Paprosky WG: The femur in revision total hip arthroplasty evaluation and classification. Clin Orthop Relat Res 420:55, 2004.
37. Mallory TH: Preparation of the proximal femur in cementless total hip revision. Clin Orthop Relat Res 235:47, 1988.
38. Paprosky WG, Perona PG, Lawrence JM: Acetabular defect classification and surgical reconstruction in revision arthroplasty: a 6-year follow-up evaluation. J Arthroplasty 9:33, 1994.
39. Meneghini RM, Meyer C, Buckley CA, et al: Mechanical stability of novel highly porous metal acetabular components in revision total hip arthroplasty. J Arthroplasty 25:337, 2010.
40. Brooker AF, Bowerman JW, Robinson RA, Riley LH, Jr: Ectopic ossification following total hip replacement: incidence and a method of classification. J Bone Joint Surg Am 55:1629, 1973.
41. Pellegrini VD, Jr, Gregoritch SJ: Preoperative irradiation for prevention of heterotopic ossification following total hip arthroplasty. J Bone Joint Surg Am 78:870, 1996.
42. Rumi MN, Deol GS, Bergandi JA, et al: Optimal timing of preoperative radiation for prophylaxis against heterotopic ossification: a rabbit hip model. J Bone Joint Surg Am 87:366, 2005.
43. Jasty M, Schutzer S, Tepper J, et al: Radiation-blocking shields to localize periarticular radiation precisely for prevention of heterotopic bone formation around uncemented total hip arthroplasties. Clin Orthop Relat Res 257:138, 1990.
44. Canner GC, Steinberg ME, Heppenstall RB, Balderston R: The infected hip after total hip arthroplasty. J Bone Joint Surg Am 66:1393, 1984.
45. Spangehl MJ, Masri BA, O'Connell JX, Duncan CP: Prospective analysis of preoperative and intraoperative investigations for the diagnosis of infection at the sites of two hundred and two revision total hip arthroplasties. J Bone Joint Surg Am 81:672, 1999.
46. Aalto K, Osterman K, Peltola H, Rasanen J: Changes in erythrocyte sedimentation rate and C-reactive protein after total hip arthroplasty. Clin Orthop Relat Res 184:118, 1984.
47. Fehring TK, Cohen B: Aspiration as a guide to sepsis in revision total hip arthroplasty. J Arthroplasty 11:543, 1996.
48. Lachiewicz PF, Rogers GD, Thomason HC: Aspiration of the hip joint before revision total hip arthroplasty: clinical and laboratory factors influencing attainment of a positive culture. J Bone Joint Surg Am 78:749, 1996.
49. Schinsky MF, Della Valle CJ, Sporer SM, Paprosky WG: Perioperative testing for joint infection in patients undergoing revision total hip arthroplasty. J Bone Joint Surg Am 90:1869, 2008.
50. Lieberman JR, Huo MH, Schneider R, et al: Evaluation of painful hip arthroplasties: are technetium bone scans necessary? J Bone Joint Surg Br 75:475, 1993.
51. Oswald SG, Van Nostrand D, Savory CG, Callaghan JJ: Three-phase bone scan and indium white blood cell scintigraphy following porous coated hip arthroplasty: a prospective study of the prosthetic tip. J Nucl Med 30:1321, 1989.
52. Palestro CJ, Kim CK, Swyer AJ, et al: Total-hip arthroplasty: periprosthetic indium-111-labeled leukocyte activity and complementary technetium-99 m-sulfur colloid imaging in suspected infection. J Nucl Med 31:1950, 1990.
53. Delank KS, Schmidt M, Michael JW, et al: The implications of 18F-FDG PET for the diagnosis of endoprosthetic loosening and infection in hip and knee arthroplasty: results from a prospective, blinded study. BMC Musculoskelet Disord 7:20, 2006.
54. Lonner JH, Desai P, Dicesare PE, et al: The reliability of analysis of intraoperative frozen sections for identifying active infection during revision hip or knee arthroplasty. J Bone Joint Surg Am 78:1553, 1996.
55. Iorio R, Siegel J, Specht LM, et al: A comparison of acetate vs digital templating for preoperative planning of total hip arthroplasty: is digital templating accurate and safe? J Arthroplasty 24:175, 2009.
56. Oddy MJ, Jones MJ, Pendegrass CJ, et al: Assessment of reproducibility and accuracy in templating hybrid total hip arthroplasty using digital radiographs. J Bone Joint Surg Br 88:581, 2006.
57. Specht LM, Levitz S, Iorio R, et al: A comparison of acetate and digital templating for total knee arthroplasty. Clin Orthop Relat Res 464:179, 2007.

58. Kosashvili Y, Shasha N, Olschewski E, et al: Digital versus conventional templating techniques in preoperative planning for total hip arthroplasty. Can J Surg 52:6, 2009.

59. Gonzalez Della Valle A, Comba F, Taveras N, Salvati EA: The utility and precision of analogue and digital preoperative planning for total hip arthroplasty. Int Orthop 32:289, 2008.

60. Gamble P, de Beer J, Petruccelli D, Winemaker M: The accuracy of digital templating in uncemented total hip arthroplasty. J Arthroplasty 25:529, 2010.

61. The B, Verdonschot N, van Horn JR, et al: Digital versus analogue preoperative planning of total hip arthroplasties: a randomized clinical trial of 210 total hip arthroplasties. J Arthroplasty 22:866, 2007.

62. Bozic KJ, Freiberg AA, Harris WH: The high hip center. Clin Orthop Relat Res 420:101, 2004.

63. Petrera P, Trakru S, Mehta S, et al: Revision total hip arthroplasty with a retroperitoneal approach to the iliac vessels. J Arthroplasty 11:704, 1996.

64. Lie SA, Havelin LI, Furnes ON, et al: Failure rates for 4762 revision total hip arthroplasties in the Norwegian Arthroplasty Register. J Bone Joint Surg Br 86:504, 2004.

65. Whaley AL, Berry DJ, Harmsen WS: Extra-large uncemented hemispherical acetabular components for revision total hip arthroplasty. J Bone Joint Surg Am 83:1352, 2001.

66. Berry DJ, Sutherland CJ, Trousdale RT, et al: Bilobed oblong porous coated acetabular components in revision total hip arthroplasty. Clin Orthop Relat Res 371:154, 2000.

67. Chen WM, Engh CA, Jr, Hopper RH, Jr, et al: Acetabular revision with use of a bilobed component inserted without cement in patients who have acetabular bone-stock deficiency. J Bone Joint Surg Am 82:197, 2000.

68. Gross AE, Wong P, Saleh KJ: Don't throw away the ring: indications and use. J Arthroplasty 17(4 Suppl 1):162, 2002.

69. Berry DJ, Lewallen DG, Hanssen AD, Cabanela ME: Pelvic discontinuity in revision total hip arthroplasty. J Bone Joint Surg Am 81:1692, 1999.

70. Shinar AA, Harris WH: Bulk structural autogenous grafts and allografts for reconstruction of the acetabulum in total hip arthroplasty: sixteen-year-average follow-up. J Bone Joint Surg Am 79:159, 1997.

71. Maurer SG, Baitner AC, Di Cesare PE: Reconstruction of the failed femoral component and proximal femoral bone loss in revision hip surgery. J Am Acad Orthop Surg 8:354, 2000.

72. Gutierrez Del Alamo J, Garcia-Cimbrelo E, Castellanos V, Gil-Garay E: Radiographic bone regeneration and clinical outcome with the Wagner SL revision stem: a 5-year to 12-year follow-up study. J Arthroplasty 22:515, 2007.

73. Jando VT, Greidanus NV, Masri BA, et al: Trochanteric osteotomies in revision total hip arthroplasty: contemporary techniques and results. Instr Course Lect 54:143, 2005.

CHAPTER 87

Implant Removal in Revision Hip Arthroplasty

Daniel H. Williams, Donald S. Garbuz, Clive P. Duncan, and Bassam A. Masri

KEY POINTS

- Ensuring maximum possible intact host bone following implant removal provides an optimum platform on which to build a successful hip reconstruction.
- Successful implant removal depends upon careful preoperative planning, which cannot be separated from planning for subsequent hip reconstruction.
- Choice of surgical approach is determined by the design of the implant to be removed, implant fixation, and the cause of implant failure.
- Planned extensile exposure with osteotomy and stable repair is preferable to an unplanned iatrogenic cortical breach or periprosthetic fracture.
- Specific techniques utilizing specific instruments are available to facilitate removal of both loose and solidly fixed cemented and uncemented acetabular and femoral components.

INTRODUCTION

The key aims of revision total hip arthroplasty are (1) to extract failing components, ensuring minimal damage to host bone and soft tissue, (2) to implant new components to provide long-term stable fixation, and (3) to manage bone loss by augmenting deficient bone stock. Preserving the maximum possible intact host bone during implant removal provides an optimum platform on which to build a successful reconstruction. The ease of implant removal depends on the implant design and the method of fixation employed at the primary procedure, how well the primary procedure was performed, the host response to the implant, and the cause of implant failure. Thus the removal of cemented components presents challenges unique to the removal of components fixed without cement. Loose implants may be "tapped" out, whereas solidly fixed components can be technically challenging to remove. This chapter will discuss the principles and techniques applied to different etiologic settings for the removal of failing acetabular and femoral components. Emphasis will be placed on preoperative planning and the surgical approach in the revision setting; discussion will focus on the management of difficult scenarios, such as the distally fixed broken stem.

INDICATIONS/CONTRAINDICATIONS

Once the decision has been made to proceed with revision surgery, general principles dictate that failed or failing implants should be removed and replaced. Certain indications for implant removal are clearer than others. Broken components clearly need to be removed, but the indications for changing implants in cases of instability can be more subtle.

Despite recent improvements in bearing surface material properties, aseptic loosening usually secondary to osteolysis (attributed to the macrophage response to accumulated wear debris) remains one of the main causes of failed hip arthroplasty. Removal of loose implants is clearly indicated, but the paired primary component may be left in situ if solid fixation, component compatibility, and adequate soft tissue balancing can be ensured in combination with the new revision implant. Changing a loose acetabular component may require the replacement of a modular femoral head to achieve these goals. A monoblock stem that is not compatible with the new socket or that provides inadequate soft tissue tension may have to be removed despite being well fixed. Removal might also be necessary during an intended isolated single-component revision when the component to be left in situ is inadvertently damaged (e.g., trunnion damage, scratching of the head on a monoblock stem).

If detected early enough, osteolytic defects around solidly fixed implants with satisfactory position and an intact locking mechanism can be managed without component removal. Bearing surface exchange, with or without bone grafting of the osteolytic defect, may allow satisfactory treatment (see Chapter 88). Cementing a new liner into a well-fixed acetabular shell is a good option in suitable patients[1] if the available liner is not compatible with the in situ socket. This technique can also be considered when a liner of increased constraint, obliquity, or posterior wall height is required for the treatment of instability. This technique necessitates the sole removal of the liner without removing a well-fixed acetabular component—typically an easy task that does not require any specialized techniques.

Cement-in-cement revision of the femur is appropriate when the cause of revision is not on the femoral side and the cement-bone interface remains pristine. Bonding of the new cement to the old mantle is good and allows implantation of a smaller cemented stem. Specific cemented revision stems have recently come to market for this purpose, and the technique has good reported medium-term results.[2-5] The technique is suitable when treating the failed acetabular component where the stem requires removal only to grant access to the acetabulum. Substantial correction of femoral version may not be possible with this technique, although minor correction is possible as long as the cement mantle is not fractured in the process.

Traumatic periprosthetic fractures usually affect the femur. The femoral component may be retained in the treatment of Vancouver classification type A and C fractures, which do not violate the bony interface with the stem or the cement mantle. Type B1 fractures are identified by the presence of a well-fixed stem, which can be retained. Type B2 fractures (with a loose component) and B3 fractures (with inadequate bone) require stem and any cement mantle to be removed before reconstruction is begun.[6]

Two or more episodes of recurrent dislocation indicate the need to proceed to revision in medically fit patients. Well-fixed components may be retained:

- If subtle malalignment of the socket can be treated by retention of the acetabular shell and exchange of the liner to an oblique liner or a liner with an elevated rim
- If exchange to a liner with an increased internal diameter accommodating a larger femoral head is sufficient to prevent dislocation of well-aligned components. Increased femoral head diameter–to–neck diameter ratio increases range of motion to impingement (of the neck upon the acetabular component) and increases the "jump distance" to dislocation once impingement occurs
- If exchange of the femoral head to provide a longer neck length addresses inadequate soft tissue tension
- If exchange to a constrained liner (compatible with a well-fixed and well-aligned acetabular shell) or cementing of a constrained liner into a noncompatible well-fixed shell of adequate diameter is suitable

If these conditions are not met, one or, less commonly, both components may have to be removed.

Recommended treatment of chronic periprosthetic infection requires removal of all foreign implant material, followed usually by a two-stage reconstruction.[7,8]

Other causes of revision specific to the use of alternative bearing surfaces include "squeaking" or rarely fracture of a ceramic-on-ceramic bearing couple, which generally requires implant removal. Management of raised serum metal ions in association with a metal-on-metal bearing couple is controversial.[9] In the symptomatic patient, with or without the presence of so-called *pseudotumor*, removal of components becomes necessary to allow revision to an alternative bearing surface. The same treatment may be recommended in the asymptomatic patient with an overly abducted or anteverted acetabular component. Failure of hip resurfacing secondary to femoral neck fracture clearly requires the removal of at least the femoral component, if not both components, to convert to a non–metal-on-metal bearing surface.

PREOPERATIVE PLANNING

Preoperative planning for implant removal in hip revision surgery cannot be divorced from preoperative planning for hip reconstruction (see Chapter 86). Planning for implant removal focuses on selection of the appropriate approach to the hip, including the requirement for an extensile exposure or osteotomy, and choice of the appropriate instruments required to remove failed components. Planning must therefore consider decisions made at the primary procedure regarding the choice of implant design and the method of fixation employed, how the primary procedure was approached and how well it was performed, the host response to the primary implant, and the cause of implant failure.

Thus relevant documentation and background information from the primary procedure, including implant labels showing the manufacturer, brand, size, and catalogue number of the components, need to be available. The function of the liner locking mechanism of an uncemented component should be understood and specialized tools for removal of the liner made available. The correct screwdriver for screw removal and other specialized tools for implant removal should also be available. On the femoral side, if a cemented stem was precoated with methacrylate, removal may be significantly more challenging, and femoral osteotomy may be required. The distal extent of any porous coating and the point at which any metaphyseal taper meets the cylindrical distal part of the stem should also be known ahead of time.

Up-to-date and previous serial plain radiographs of the hip (if available) should include an anteroposterior (AP) pelvis, a centered AP of the hip and femur, and a lateral radiograph of the involved hip of sufficient length. Forty-five–degree Judet views allow assessment of the integrity of the anterior and posterior columns and the extent of any osteolytic lesions.[10] Vascular contrast studies may be indicated if there is concern that the iliac vessels may be damaged during removal of the acetabular component. If the vessels lie between the implant and the bone, a retroperitoneal approach to the socket would be favored. An adequate picture of the distal extent and distribution of any femoral cement mantle guides the direction of osteotomes, chisels, and other cement removal instruments at the time of revision surgery. A good quality lateral is particularly useful in this regard. Computed tomography (CT) or magnetic resonance imaging (MRI) can demonstrate cement that does not contain radiopaque barium, and a CT scan can provide a more accurate picture of bone loss.[11] The criteria for loosening of cemented[12,13] and uncemented[14] components have been published elsewhere and are beyond the scope of this chapter.

Preparation for an extensile exposure, osteotomy,[15-17] or cortical window[18-22] should be done preoperatively and all suitable instruments made available. The templated length of an extended trochanteric osteotomy (ETO)[15-17] measured on the AP radiograph should ensure that any broken stem, femoral stem porous coating, or retained cement can be readily accessed. Preoperative planning for implant removal cannot be separated from planning for femoral reconstruction, and the templated femoral stem length should bypass the distal extent of any osteotomy by a suitable distance, usually said to be approximately two diaphyseal diameters.

Occasionally, a specific extractor may be required for a particular stem or for part of a stem (in the case of modular stems or a modular centralizer attached distally to an uncemented stem). If unfamiliar with a particular stem design, the surgeon should contact the manufacturer to obtain any specific extraction instructions and to make sure that any required instruments are made available at the time of surgery.

DESCRIPTION OF TECHNIQUES

With a clear understanding of the indications, and after a preoperative plan has been formulated, the surgical approach, acetabular implant removal, and femoral implant removal can be considered.

Surgical Approach

The objectives while approaching the hip during a revision procedure are to adequately expose the hip, preserve bone, preserve soft tissue, and preserve blood supply. The approach should provide sufficient exposure of the components to be removed, any associated bone defects, and any neurovascular structures that require visualization. This allows preservation of the maximum possible intact host bone during implant removal. Planned extensile incisions of sufficient length or osteotomies that can be adequately repaired are preferable to an unplanned iatrogenic cortical breach or periprosthetic fracture.[23] Utilization of previously healed incisions without compromising surgical exposure minimizes additional scar tissue. Finally, avoiding unnecessary devascularization of bone is of paramount importance, particularly in cases of sepsis, where dead bone can act as a nidus for ongoing infection.

The choice of approach depends on the implant design and its method of fixation, how the primary procedure was approached, the degree of bone loss, and the indication for revision. Good circumferential exposure is required to assess whether cemented or uncemented acetabular components require removal. A more extensile exposure to the outer table of the ilium is required if a reconstruction cage or a metal augment is to be removed (or inserted), or if a superolateral or posterior column defect requires assessment (or reconstruction). If removal of a well-fixed femoral cement mantle is indicated, an ETO[15-17] or a cortical window[18-22] will significantly improve visualization, particularly of a long column of distal cement. An ETO also is often deemed necessary for removal of a cemented stem that has been precoated with methacrylate. The rigid implant-mantle bond is strong and makes removal of the stem from above impossible. Osteointegrated uncemented stems present a similar problem, and familiarity with design specifications remains important.

Knowledge of the extent and location of porous coating, the modularity of the prosthesis, the presence of a collar, and the level at which the metaphyseal flare joins the more tubular distal part of the stem will ensure the correct choice of approach. Varus remodeling of the proximal femur (Fig. 87-1), which is more common when the femoral component is loose, may add considerable difficulty to removal of a straight stem from the intact femur and may indicate the need for an osteotomy. A broken stem, cemented or not, also presents a unique problem that also often requires an ETO[15-17] or a cortical window.[18-22]

The incision, superficial and deep dissection used to approach the primary, and any previous revision operation should be taken into account. As much of the previous incision as possible should be used at revision to avoid unnecessary railroad-track incisions and attendant risks of wound-edge necrosis. Skin laxity may allow utilization of an incision that is not optimally positioned so long as the correct fascial incision can be made. Deep dissection through a previous exposure is often best employed. A nonunited greater trochanter may provide an obvious route to the hip joint, and a poorly healed transgluteal approach may be reused. Some controversy continues as to whether a gluteal tear should be incorporated into a transgluteal approach[24] and repaired during closure of the revision, or whether a posterior approach[25,26] should be employed and the gluteal tear ignored. The preferred compromise is reuse of the old gluteal tear, if it affords adequate exposure, and subsequent transosseous repair at the end of the procedure.

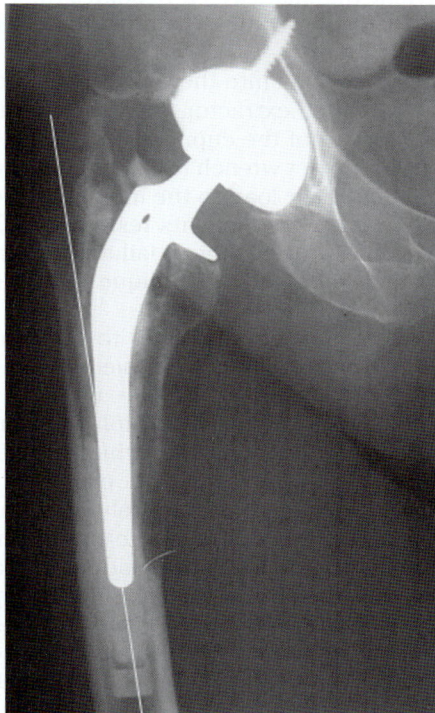

Figure 87-1. Anteroposterior (AP) radiograph showing varus remodeling in response to a stem that has failed with severe osteolysis.

Otherwise, use of a posterior approach is preferred.[25,26] In cases of chronic sepsis, an infected sinus tract, often along the route of the primary approach, is ideally completely excised.

Each of these factors contributing to the choice of approach needs to be balanced with the primary goal of preserving bone during implant removal. The revision arthroplasty surgeon therefore needs to be comfortable not only with the standard anterolateral (see Chapter 18),[24,27-32] posterior (see Chapter 19),[25,26] and transtrochanteric (see Chapter 20)[33,34] approaches to the hip but also with the more extensile approaches, osteotomies, and other specialized exposures (see Chapter 21)[15-22,35-37] required to gain adequate access to the acetabular and femoral components.

The Acetabulum

Good circumferential exposure is required to remove a cemented or an uncemented acetabular component while ensuring optimal preservation of intact host bone.

Removal of the Cemented Acetabular Component

The aim is to loosen the solidly fixed cemented acetabular cup from the underlying polymethylmethacrylate (PMMA) cement by one of five methods:

- The cup-cement bond is disrupted by carefully introducing curved osteotomes at the interface and tapping medially along the interface until the cup can be lifted out.
- The all-polyethylene component can be thinned with sequential acetabular reamers.[38] The rigidity of the polyethylene diminishes as it becomes thinner, and it is lifted out of the cement mantle when sufficiently flexible.
- A hole can be drilled into the polyethylene to accommodate a threaded extractor, which allows disimpaction and removal of the cup.
- A pneumatic impact wrench is used to deliver a repetitive torsional shear load to the implant-cement-bone interface. In eight components tested with this technique, however, one technical failure and one pelvic fracture occurred.[39] This technique is therefore not favored.
- A high-speed burr can be used to section the all-polyethylene cup and remove it piecemeal.

Cement-splitting osteotomes are used to remove the cement in a piecemeal fashion. Cement plugs in large and small holes used to achieve a macro-lock at the primary procedure can be carefully curetted out or burred away. Large intrapelvic extensions of cement require removal only in cases of infection, cases of dysuria secondary to bladder irritation by the cement, and cases of dyspareunia in female patients. In most cases, intrapelvic cement may be left undisturbed because it is outside the surgical field, and its presence will not affect the final reconstruction. If removal is planned, preoperative assessment with intrapelvic contrast studies is required and a retroperitoneal approach employed with the assistance of a general surgery colleague.[40-44] Thus with adequate preoperative planning and operative exposure, the acetabular implant and the cement may be removed safely, under direct vision, with optimal preservation of intact host bone.

Removal of the Solidly Fixed Uncemented Acetabular Component

Achieving optimal bone preservation can be more challenging when the solidly fixed uncemented acetabular shell is removed. The modular liner requires removal to gain access to shell fixation screws or, depending on design, to clearly visualize the bone-implant interface. It can be left in situ if screws were not previously used, or if they have broken. One of five methods can be used to remove the liner:

- A specific manufacturer-designed technique may require specialized tools to undo the locking mechanism.
- It may be possible to insert a lever between the protruding rim of the liner and the circumference of the shell. Any leverage must avoid pivoting against host bone, or an iatrogenic fracture may result.
- A hole may be drilled into the polyethylene liner to accommodate a 6.5-mm screw, which when advanced against the metal shell should extrude the liner.
- The liner may be thinned with sequential acetabular reamers and the flexible remainder easily extracted.
- The liner may be segmented into triangles with a high-speed burr and removed piecemeal. This may allow access to the locking ring for its division or extraction.

Considerable caution must be exercised during removal of the solidly fixed shell. The preferred technique uses short and long blades to loosen the shell's interface with the bone. A curved blade specific to the outside diameter of the shell is attached to a rotating handle device (e.g., Explant Acetabular Removal System, Zimmer, Warsaw, Ind) that is centered in the polyethylene liner by a head component of appropriate size (Fig. 87-2). If the shell is secured with screws, the liner and screws are removed and the liner is replaced. If the liner is severely worn in an eccentric manner, it can be rotated 180 degrees within the shell to place the worn segment inferiorly, or a trial liner of appropriate size is inserted to center the device.[45] Two blades are used sequentially. The first is a truncated blade used to open the interface between the implant and the host bone (Fig. 87-2A). The second—a thin, full-radius blade—is used to completely release the implant from the host bone, minimizing acetabular bone loss (Fig. 87-2B). During 31 procedures using this technique, the time for removal of the shell did not exceed 5 minutes, and the median difference between the diameter of the implant removed and that of the final reamer in the reconstruction was 4 mm. This reflects no more bone loss than the thickness of the blades. The uniform finding in all cases was removal of the acetabular shell devoid of host bone, except the bone that had ingrown within the component.[46,47]

Several other techniques have recently fallen out of favor:

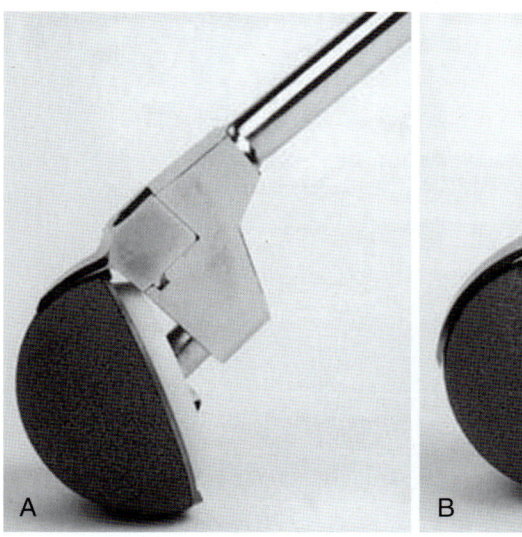
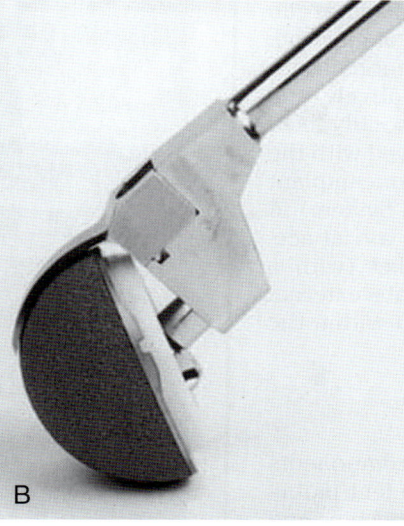

A   B

Figure 87-2. Thin, stiff, size-specific curved blades that match the outside diameter of the acetabular component to be removed. **A,** The shorter blade is used to open the interface at the periphery of the cup. **B,** The longer blade is used to extract the cup with minimal bone loss. *(From Mitchell PA, Masri BA, Garbuz DS, et al: Removal of well-fixed, cementless, acetabular components in revision hip arthroplasty. J Bone Joint Surg Br 85:949–952, 2003.)*

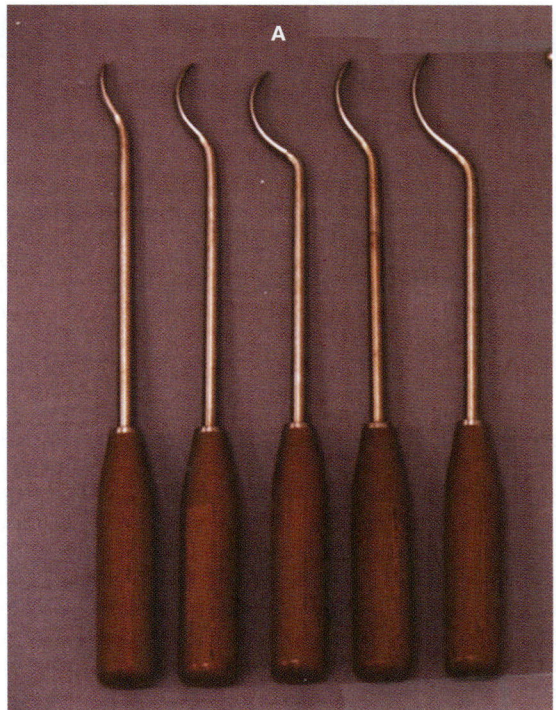

A

Figure 87-3. Curved osteotomes traditionally used for the removal of an uncemented acetabular component.

keyhole made in the superior acetabulum. The punch applies tensile forces to the bone-implant interface, thus loosening the implant. Although no complications were encountered in the initial series of 35 cases, host bone is removed as part of the technique.[48]

- A reciprocating saw blade can be bent and used with power to loosen the shell without loss of medial wall support. Excessive bone destruction can occur, however, if used too aggressively.[49]
- A drill can be introduced through a separate stab incision over the high point of the ilium and advanced through the anterosuperior aspect of the acetabulum. A punch is used to "pop out" the acetabular component with a few blows. In a series of 20 patients, acetabular component removal was accomplished within 10 minutes with one intraoperative fracture.[50]
- The acetabular shell can be sectioned with a metal cutting burr and removed piecemeal.[51] This is time-consuming and risks introducing metal filings into the revised hip joint with the potential for increased polyethylene wear.
- Uncommonly, the shell has a conical screw-home macro-interlock design, once popular in Europe. The rim locking torque insertion wrenches designed for insertion are also useful for extraction and may be available through the manufacturer. If not, then one or more of the techniques outlined earlier will be required.

- The traditional technique loosens the shell using curved osteotomes (Fig. 87-3) with the potential for additional bone loss.
- A pneumatic impact wrench can be used to deliver repetitive torsional shear loads to the implant-bone interface. Among eight components tested with this technique, however, one technical failure and one pelvic fracture occurred.[39] As already stated, this technique is not used for these reasons.
- An angled punch can be impacted against the acetabular component superiorly through a 3- to 4-mm

Removal of the Metal-on-Metal Uncemented Acetabular Component

Following renewed interest in and increased use of the metal-on-metal bearing at primary arthroplasty, more nonmodular metal acetabular components have been encountered at revision surgery. The cause of symptomatic failure of this bearing surface is not yet always fully understood.[9] When the need for revision of this stiff acetabular component is determined, fixation may sometimes be found to be fibrous. A single blow delivered by a punch directed vertically to the inferior edge of the socket circumference at the 6 o'clock position can sometimes "pop" out the cup and is worthy of mention. This is effective in certain implant designs that have not achieved sufficient bone ingrowth. Alternatively, the preferred technique, as for removal of the solidly fixed uncemented acetabular shell, can be employed with the use of short and long blades to loosen the bone-implant interface (e.g., Explant Acetabular Removal System). A trial large bipolar hemiarthroplasty head,[52] a trial acetabular liner,[45] or an all-polyethylene socket (with a smooth congruent backside)[53] of appropriate external diameter may be used to center the system within the socket and facilitate removal.

The Femur

Successful removal of solidly fixed femoral components depends on wide exposure to achieve sufficient mobility of the proximal femur, dislocation of the hip, and component removal while avoiding intraoperative fracture. An extensile posterior approach is often preferred, with preoperative plans made for an ETO if required. If the greater trochanter overhangs the medullary canal, a predisposition to trochanteric fracture exists during implant removal, and the shoulder of the femoral stem must be completely cleared of bone, soft tissue, and any cement before removal is attempted. This will allow a straight line exit of the femoral stem from the canal during attempted removal.

Removal of the Solidly Fixed Cemented Femoral Component

Cemented stems can be smooth, rough, or precoated with methracrylate with a respective increase in bonding to the cement mantle.[54] Once the shoulder of the stem is cleared of cement, a stem extractor can easily remove smooth stems or stems with only light texture. However, very rough or precoated stems may be impossible to remove with only an extractor. Basic principles apply in either situation: initial stem removal followed by cement mantle extraction.

If the cemented stem cannot be removed with a well-fitting extraction device,[55] a combination of thin, flexible osteotomes, cement-removing instruments, and very narrow high-speed burrs is used to loosen the stem from the cement. As discussed, an ETO allows safe exposure of the stem-cement interface,[15] and its planned length depends on knowledge of the area of the stem that is roughened or precoated with methacrylate. If only the metaphyseal portion of the stem is precoated or roughened, the osteotomy needs only to extend to a point just below the metaphysis. Cement can be removed from the stem-cement interface with a narrow pencil-tip burr to loosen the stem. A punch or stem extractor will remove the stem from the remaining mantle. However, if there is precoating or roughening down to the tip of the stem, the ETO must be lengthened to just below the tip, so that the same procedure can be taken more distally to free the whole of the stem.

After stem removal, well-bonded cement may be removed using a combination of long, thin osteotomes, reverse cutting hooks, drills, taps, high-speed burrs

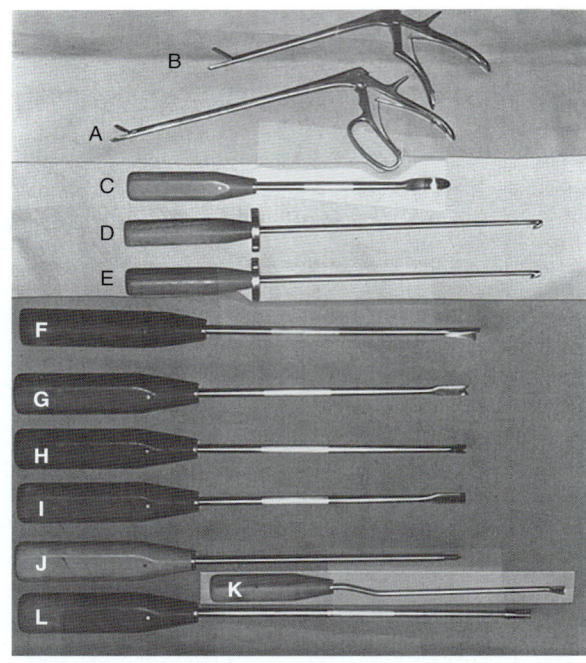

Figure 87-4. Cement removal tools. **A** and **B,** Long and short cement graspers. **C,** Acetabular gouge for removing a polyethylene cup from its cement mantle. **D** and **E,** Reverse cutting hooks. **F,** T-osteotome for loosening, fragmenting, and removing cement piecemeal. **G** and **L,** Cement splitters. **H** and **I,** Cement scoops for separating loosened cement. **J,** Carbide punch for extracting stems from within their cement mantle. **K,** Angled T-osteotome. *(From Masri BA, Mitchell PA, Duncan CP: Removal of solidly fixed implants during revision hip and knee arthroplasty. J Am Acad Orthop Surg 13:18–27, 2005.)*

designed specifically for cement removal, and ultrasonic cement removal tools. PMMA bone cement is generally weaker than cortical bone and is weaker in tension than in compression—properties that are exploited in the design of cement removal instruments (Fig. 87-4). All cement can usually be removed from the intact femur with these instruments, causing minimal damage to the host bone. However, this is the most time-consuming part of any revision procedure and contributes significantly to operative blood loss, operative time, and perioperative morbidity. Careful technique is therefore required to avoid unplanned cortical perforation, which may complicate up to 4.4% of cases,[56] and femoral fracture, which most commonly occurs during cement removal.[57] Once the more proximal cement has been removed, a drill guide is connected to centralizers that match the diameter of the femoral canal.[58] Drills are then used to drill the cement plug, and a variety of taps can be used to engage the plug and tap it out in a retrograde manner (Fig. 87-5). If there is a long column of cement proximal to the plug, it is best to repeat this process several times rather than risk uncontrolled perforation. Any remnants of cement or cement restrictor can then be removed with reverse hooks, and an olive-tipped guide wire can be used as a feeler to ensure that the cortex has not been breached.

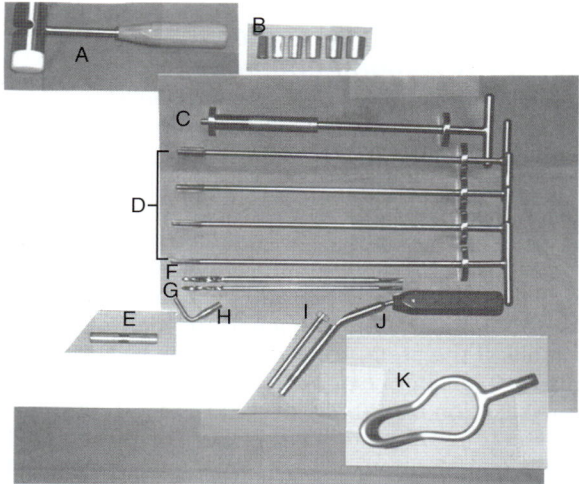

Figure 87-5. Instruments used to remove the femoral stem and the cement plug. The stem extractor system is used to remove a well-fixed stem: **A,** Slap hammer. Following removal of the proximal cement, the plug is extracted retrograde. **B,** Drill guide centralizers (equal to the diameter of the femoral canal). **C,** Handle. **D,** Cement plug taps to engage and extract the plug retrograde. **E,** Assembly tools. **F** and **G,** Cement plug drills. **H,** Assembly tools. **I** and **J,** Drill guides. **K,** Extractor (for a monoblock stem). *(From Masri BA, Mitchell PA, Duncan CP: Removal of solidly fixed implants during revision hip and knee arthroplasty. J Am Acad Orthop Surg 13:18–27, 2005.)*

Alternatively, if the tap fails to engage the cement, the plug can be completely drilled through and a guide wire passed. Intramedullary position can be confirmed with intraoperative fluoroscopy and the plug sequentially reamed over the guide wire. When wide enough, the reverse hooks can be passed and used to extract the remaining cement. A modification of this technique, described by Gray,[59] employs modular manual tools and cannulated reaming instruments again to maximize the safety and efficiency of cement removal. A cement column that is distal to the narrower isthmus of the femur cannot be extracted safely with retrograde plug extraction techniques. This cement can be intentionally displaced distally (if not dealing with infection), extracted via a carefully planned and executed cortical window, or extracted via a very extended trochanteric osteotomy.

If an ETO has not been necessary to remove proximal cement, then a femoral cortical window[18-22] or a controlled cortical perforation technique[60] may improve visualization to remove the distal cement. A headlamp, a handheld light, or endoscopic instrumentation may be used to improve visibility.[61,62] As was previously mentioned, intraoperative fluoroscopy may also be helpful.

Instrumentation is available that delivers high-energy ultrasound, at frequencies greater than 16 kHz, directly to the cement mantle, resulting in heating and melting of the PMMA.[63,64] Damage to adjacent bone is minimized because bone cement maintains a steep temperature gradient of 200° C over 1 mm. Heat is still released, however, and this has been shown to result in bone

necrosis to a depth of 50 μm with the use of ultrasonic instruments over a 10-second period. Irrigation during use is recommended, but this shallow 50-μm depth compares with the 500-μm depth of necrosis seen following exothermic polymerization of the cement.[63-68] The ultrasonic probe is designed to emit an audible high-pitched sound when contact is made with cortical bone. Modular probes designed for use with the ultrasound device include probes for cement perforation, cement grooving, and cement scraping; an L-shaped probe to section cement circumferentially; and a helical-tipped device that allows insertion into the distal cement plug, followed by controlled extraction with retrograde tapping.

In a study of the use of high-energy ultrasound in 90 femoral revision cases, superficial bone burns were seen in 8 (9%) cases, with only 1 femoral shaft perforation (1%).[63] In vitro work has determined that perforation does not occur when the femoral cortical thickness measures 3 mm. When the cortex measures 2 mm, perforation is possible, but loads three to six times greater than those normally used to remove cement are required to do this.[69] Fletcher and associates[70] found that ultrasonic cement removal facilitated a shorter ETO (and subsequent implantation of shorter revision prostheses), and that its use may decrease the requirement for a cortical window.[64] High-frequency ultrasound is considered a safe and efficacious method of cement removal.

Another, now largely historical, technique involves the insertion of fresh PMMA cement into the carefully prepared existing cement mantle inside the femur. Before the cement has cured, an extraction rod with nuts (placed at 1-cm intervals) is inserted into the new cement. Using a series of additional extraction rods, the cement is then segmentally extracted based on the assumption that the PMMA-PMMA bond is stronger than the bone-cement interface. Lithotripsy and laser have also been used to weaken the bone-cement interface, allowing straightforward cement removal, but neither technique is currently in common use.

Removal of the Proximally Coated Cementless Femoral Component
Proximally coated cementless stems achieve primary stability by press-fit that facilitates metaphyseal bone ingrowth through or ongrowth onto a porous or hydroxyapatite proximal coating. These stems are not designed to ingrow in the diaphysis, but any roughened distal portion of the stem may lead to bone ongrowth. If distal ongrowth has occurred, removal may require similar techniques to those used to remove extensively porous-coated stems.

Proximally coated cementless stems can become incredibly well fixed, and the challenge presented in their removal should not be underestimated. The preferred method of removal involves the use of very sharp, flexible osteotomes (Fig. 87-6) or thin, high-speed burrs to break down the metaphyseal bone growth. Repeated attempts are made to remove the stem using a stem extractor[55] by providing a shear stress across the stem-bone interface, thus avoiding unnecessary damage to the femur caused by prolonged use of osteotomes and burrs. A good fit of the stem extractor on the specific type of stem ensures good purchase and maximizes the chance of success. In some cases, a short ETO can facilitate access to the ingrown areas. A Gigli saw can then be placed medially and used to debond the prosthesis, provided there is no medial collar, or when the collar has been completely removed using a metal-cutting burr (see later).

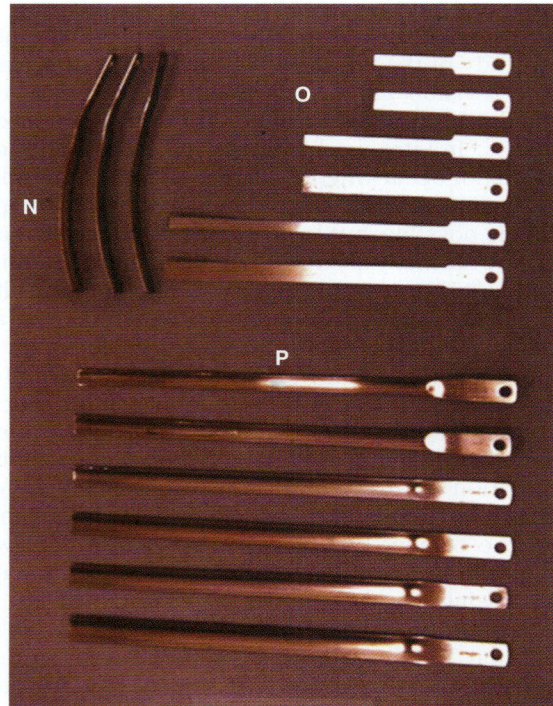

Figure 87-6. Thin flexible osteotomes used to disrupt the bony interface at the metaphyseal portion of a proximally coated cementless stem. The geometry of these osteotomes matches that of the femoral stem. **O** and **P,** Straight osteotomes for the anterior and posterior surfaces. **N,** Curved osteotomes for the medial border and shoulder of the stem. *(From Masri BA, Mitchell PA, Duncan CP: Removal of solidly fixed implants during revision hip and knee arthroplasty. J Am Acad Orthop Surg 13:18–27, 2005.)*

Removal of the Fully Coated Cementless Femoral Component

Removal of a solidly fixed, fully coated stem is time-consuming and may lead to extensive femoral damage. Multiple instruments should be available for this procedure, including broad osteotomes, flexible osteotomes, Gigli saws, high-speed metal-cutting burrs, and multiple trephines with diameters 0.5 mm larger than the stem to be removed. An ETO is performed with the stem in situ. The level of the osteotomy depends on the length of the stem in situ and the length of the revision stem available. If the stem to be removed is relatively short and a revision stem can be used that will provide satisfactory fixation below the level of the existing stem tip, the osteotomy is made at the level of the stem tip.[71] Using a combination of Gigli saws and flexible osteotomes, the osteotomy fragment is lifted off the stem and mobilized in the standard manner. Using the same instruments, the stem is then loosened from the underlying femur and lifted out.

When a long primary or revision stem is removed, the ETO cannot be made at the level of the stem tip because doing so may seriously compromise the fixation of the subsequent revision implant. In this situation, the osteotomy is made at a level that is planned to facilitate satisfactory reconstruction after implant removal. The osteotomy fragment is then mobilized as described to expose the underlying stem, and the stem is sectioned using high-speed metal-cutting burrs. This can be time-consuming, requiring several new burr tips, particularly when sectioning a cobalt-chrome stem. Once the stem is sectioned, the proximal fragment is loosened from the femur and lifted out. The distal segment is loosened using trephines (Fig. 87-7A). As discussed, the exact dimensions of the stem should be known at the planning stage of the procedure. If the stem is not cylindrical, the osteotomy and subsequent sectioning should be made at the point where the broad proximal portion transits to the cylindrical distal section (Fig. 87-7B). It has to be kept in mind that one trephine is never enough, and most sets designed to remove these stems have only one sterile trephine. It is highly recommended that the surgeon determine the size required and order at least five or six sterile trephines ahead of time. Similarly, it is

Figure 87-7. A, Trephines used to extract the cylindrical portion of a fully porous-coated stem. **B,** An extended trochanteric osteotomy (ETO) allows exposure, sectioning of the stem, and removal of the metaphyseal portion. A trephine 0.5 mm larger than the existing stem is used to remove the well-fixed distal portion. *(From Masri BA, Mitchell PA, Duncan CP: Removal of solidly fixed implants during revision hip and knee arthroplasty. J Am Acad Orthop Surg 13:18–27, 2005.)*

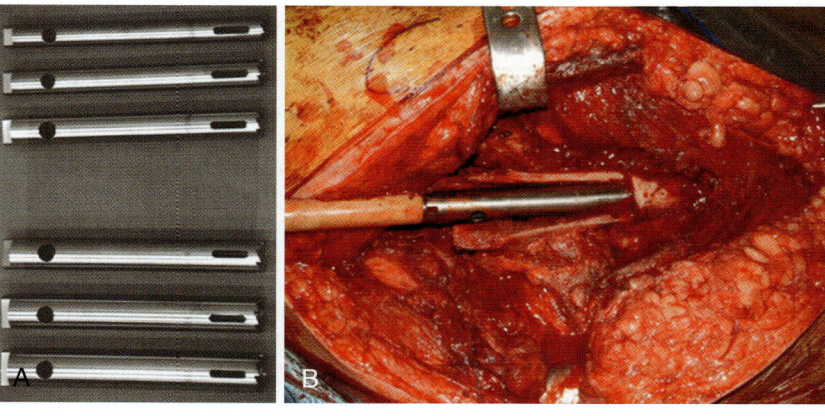

wise to have at least three Gigli saws available because they seize and shred easily against porous-coated stems.

A curved microsagittal saw technique applied via a long cortical window has also been described for removal of a well-fixed stem.[72] A long straight microsagittal saw blade or a thin osteotome is first used to loosen the proximal stem-bone interface. A longitudinal cortical window is fashioned from the level of the saw blade or osteotome to reach the distal end of the porous coat. The window is made as wide as the stem at the corresponding level. The distal portion of the saw blade is then bent with a heavy tissue clamp to make it a quarter circle and is gradually advanced between the stem and the surrounding bone in a circular fashion. The extractor is used to remove the stem when sufficiently loose.

Removal of a Broken Femoral Stem

The broken cementless femoral stem is invariably solidly fixed distally. Removal of this implant is achieved with the same technique described for the long, fully coated stem. Fortunately, these stems usually fracture at the transition zone between broad proximal and cylindrical distal segments. The ETO is made at the level of the stem fracture, and the well-fixed distal portion is removed using trephines[73] (see Fig. 87-7B). A broken cemented stem may be removed using a similar technique, but the osteotomy may have to extend distal to the fracture so that the cement may be removed once the broken stem is removed. The cement around the stem is removed using a high-speed pencil-tip burr. A small divot is then made in the stem using a metal-cutting burr, and a carbide punch is used to tap the broken stem out of the femur. A similar technique may be applied without an ETO using the cortical window[74] or a controlled perforation technique.[60] The divot in the stem can be made through a small anterior perforation in the femur and a carbide punch used to tap out the stem. Multiple divots are often required, and this technique is more technically challenging.

POSTOPERATIVE CARE

In the same way that planning for implant removal cannot be divorced from hip reconstruction planning, so postoperative care relevant to the techniques employed for implant removal cannot be considered in isolation. Suffice it to say that patients who have undergone femoral ETO, cortical window, or a controlled perforation technique are generally instructed to partially bear weight for at least 6 to 12 weeks during the immediate postoperative period.

FUTURE CONSIDERATIONS

- Incremental improvements in implant engineering, design, and material science continue to improve bearing surface tribology and implant fixation. Although it is hoped that these factors will lead to improved longevity of both primary and revision

implants, they inevitably will challenge the techniques of implant removal when removal becomes necessary.
- The best chance of optimizing remaining intact host bone following implant removal is by carefully adhering to the general principles laid down in the recent orthopedic literature and summarized in this chapter.
- Successful preoperative planning considers the design of the implant to be removed and its method of fixation, the host response to the primary implant, and the cause of implant failure. This allows choice and planning of the appropriate approach to the hip, which may include an extensile exposure or osteotomy, and ensures the availability of appropriate instruments to employ the most suitable technique for implant removal.
- The planning and techniques of implant removal are intimately related to the planning and techniques of hip reconstruction.
- Optimal intact host bone following implant removal will provide an optimum platform on which to build a successful hip reconstruction.

REFERENCES

1. Mountney JF, Garbuz DS, Greidanus NV, et al: Cementing constrained acetabular liners in revision hip replacement: clinical and laboratory observations. Instr Course Lect 53:131–140, 2004.
2. Goto KF, Kawanabe KF, Akiyama HF, et al: Clinical and radiological evaluation of revision hip arthroplasty using the cement-in-cement technique. J Bone Joint Surg Br 90:1013–1018, 2008.
3. Quinlan JF, O'Shea KF, Doyle FF, Brady OH: In-cement technique for revision hip arthroplasty. J Bone Joint Surg Br 88:730–733, 2006.
4. Lieberman J, Moeckel BH, Evans BG, et al: Cement-within-cement revision hip arthroplasty. J Bone Joint Surg Br 75:869–871, 1993.
5. Duncan WW, Hubble MJ, Howell JR, et al: Revision of the cemented femoral stem using a cement-in-cement technique: a five- to 15-year review. J Bone Joint Surg Br 91:577–582, 2009.
6. Duncan CP, Masri BA: Fractures of the femur after hip replacement. Instr Course Lect 44:293–304, 1995.
7. Toms AD, Davidson D, Masri BA, Duncan CP: The management of peri-prosthetic infection in total joint arthroplasty. J Bone Joint Surg Br 88:149–155, 2006.
8. Masri BA, Panagiotopoulos KP, Greidanus NV, et al: Cementless two-stage exchange arthroplasty for infection after total hip arthroplasty. J Arthroplasty 22:72–78, 2007.
9. Pandit H, Glyn-Jones S, McLardy-Smith P, et al: Pseudotumours associated with metal-on-metal hip resurfacings. J Bone Joint Surg Br 90:847–851, 2008.
10. Judet RF, Judet JF, Letournel E: Fractures of the acetabulum: classification and surgical approaches for open reduction. J Bone Joint Surg Am 46:1615–1646, 1964.
11. Fehrman DF, McBeath AA, DeSmet AA, Tuite MJ: Imaging barium-free bone cement. Am J Orthop 25:172–174, 1996.
12. Harris WH, McCarthy JC Jr, O'Neill DA: Femoral component loosening using contemporary techniques of femoral cement fixation. J Bone Joint Surg Am 64:1063–1067, 1982.
13. Johnston RC, Fitzgerald RH, Jr, Harris WH, et al: Clinical and radiographic evaluation of total hip replacement: a standard system of terminology for reporting results. J Bone Joint Surg Am 72:161–168, 1990.
14. Engh CA: Technique for revision surgery: biological fixation in total hip arthroplasty, Thorofare, NJ, 1985, Slack, pp 89–107.
15. Younger TI, Bradford MS, Magnus RE, Paprosky WG: Extended proximal femoral osteotomy: a new technique for femoral revision arthroplasty. J Arthroplasty 10:329–338, 1995.

16. Cameron HU: Use of a distal trochanteric osteotomy in hip revision. Contemp Orthop 23:235–238, 1991.

17. Neider E: Revision total hip arthroplasty. In Bauer R, editor: Atlas of hip surgery, New York, 1996, Thieme Medical Publishers Inc., pp 270.

18. Buehler KO, Walker RH: Polymethylmethacrylate removal from the femur using a crescentic window technique. Orthopedics 21:697–700, 1998.

19. Cameron HU: Tips of the trade #29: femoral windows for easy cement removal in hip revision surgery. Orthop Rev 19:909–910, 1990.

20. Klein AH, Rubash HE: Femoral windows in revision total hip arthroplasty. Clin Orthop Relat Res 291:164–170, 1993.

21. Nelson CL, Weber MJ: Technique of windowing the femoral shaft for removal of bone cement. Clin Orthop Relat Res 154:336–337, 1981.

22. Nelson CL, Barnes CL: Removal of bone cement from the femoral shaft using a femoral windowing device. J Arthroplasty 5:67–69, 1990.

23. Jando VT, Greidanus NV, Masri BA, et al: Trochanteric osteotomies in revision total hip arthroplasty: contemporary techniques and results. Instr Course Lect 54:143–155, 2005.

24. Hardinge K: The direct lateral approach to the hip. J Bone Joint Surg Br 64:17–19, 1982.

25. Moore AT: The Moore self-locking Vitallium prosthesis in fresh femoral neck fractures: a new low posterior approach (the Southern exposure). Instr Course Lect 16:309–321, 1959.

26. Marcy GH, Fletcher RS: Modification of the posterolateral approach to the hip for insertion of femoral-head prosthesis. J Bone Joint Surg Am 36:142–143, 1954.

27. McFarland B, Osborne G: Approach to the hip: a suggested improvement on Kocher's method. J Bone Joint Surg Br 36:364–367, 1954.

28. Dall D: Exposure of the hip by anterior osteotomy of the greater trochanter: a modified anterolateral approach. J Bone Joint Surg Br 68:382–386, 1986.

29. Frndak PA, Mallory TH, Lombardi AV, Jr: Translateral surgical approach to the hip: the abductor muscle "split." Clin Orthop Relat Res 295:135–141, 1993.

30. Head WC, Mallory TH, Berklacich FM, et al: Extensile exposure of the hip for revision arthroplasty. J Arthroplasty 2:265–273, 1987.

31. Learmonth ID, Allen PE: The omega lateral approach to the hip. J Bone Joint Surg Br 78:559–561, 1996.

32. Stephenson PK, Freeman MA: Exposure of the hip using a modified anterolateral approach. J Arthroplasty 6:137–145, 1991.

33. Mercati E, Guary AF, Myquel CF, Bourgeon A: A postero-external approach to the hip joint: value of the formation of a digastric muscle. J Chir 103:499–504, 1973.

34. Glassman AH, Engh CA, Bobyn JD: A technique of extensile exposure for total hip arthroplasty. J Arthroplasty 2:11–21, 1987.

35. Masri BA, Campbell DG, Garbuz DS, Duncan CP: Seven specialized exposures for revision hip and knee replacement. Orthop Clin North Am 29:229–240, 1998.

36. Masterson EL, Masri BA, Duncan CP: Surgical approaches in revision hip replacement. J Am Acad Orthop Surg 6:84–92, 1998.

37. Neil MJ, Solomon MI: A technique of revision of failed acetabular components leaving the femoral component in situ. J Arthroplasty 11:482–483, 1996.

38. de Thomasson E, Mazel CF, Gagna GF, Guingand O: A simple technique to remove well-fixed, all-polyethylene cemented acetabular component in revision hip arthroplasty. J Arthroplasty 16:538–540, 2001.

39. Anspach WE III, Lachiewicz PF: A new technique for removal of the total hip arthroplasty acetabular component. Clin Orthop Relat Res 268:152–156, 1991.

40. Roberts JA, Loudon JR: Vesico-acetabular fistula. J Bone Joint Surg Br 69:150–151, 1987.

41. Slater RN, Edge AJ, Salman A: Delayed arterial injury after hip replacement. J Bone Joint Surg Br 71:699, 1989.

42. Head WC: Prevention of intraoperative vascular complications in revision total hip-replacement arthroplasty: a case report. J Bone Joint Surg Am 66:458–459, 1984.

43. Eftekhar NS, Nercessian O: Intrapelvic migration of total hip prostheses: operative treatment. J Bone Joint Surg Am 71:1480–1486, 1989.

44. Grigoris PF, Roberts PF, McMinn DJ, Villar RN: A technique for removing an intrapelvic acetabular cup. J Bone Joint Surg Br 75:25–27, 1993.

45. Taylor PR, Stoffel KK, Dunlop DG, Yates PJ: Removal of the well-fixed hip resurfacing acetabular component: a simple, bone preserving technique. J Arthroplasty 24:484–486, 2009.

46. The Australian National Joint Replacement Registry Annual Report 2008 www.dmac.adelaide.edu.au/aoanjrr.

47. Mitchell PA, Masri BA, Garbuz DS, et al: Removal of well-fixed, cementless, acetabular components in revision hip arthroplasty. J Bone Joint Surg Br 85:949–952, 2003.

48. Daum WJ, Calhoun JH: Removal of the acetabular component minimizing destruction of the bone bed. J Arthroplasty 3:379–380, 1988.

49. Pierson JL, Jasty MF, Harris WH: Techniques of extraction of well-fixed cemented and cementless implants in revision total hip arthroplasty. Orthop Rev 22:904–916, 1993.

50. Markovich GD, Banks SA, Hodge WA: A new technique for removing noncemented acetabular components in revision total hip arthroplasty. Am J Orthop 28:35–37, 1999.

51. Paprosky WG, Weeden SH, Bowling JW, Jr: Component removal in revision total hip arthroplasty. Clin Orthop Relat Res 393:181–193, 2001.

52. Blumenfeld TJ: Removing a well-fixed nonmodular large-bearing cementless acetabular component: a simple modification of an existing removal device. J Arthroplasty 25:491.e1–491.e3, 2010.

53. Olyslaegers CF, Wainwright TF, Middleton RG: A novel technique for the removal of well-fixed cementless, large-diameter metal-on-metal acetabular components. J Arthroplasty 23:1071–1073, 2008.

54. Shen G: Femoral stem fixation: an engineering interpretation of the long-term outcome of Charnley and Exeter stems. J Bone Joint Surg Br 80:754–756, 1998.

55. Bohn WW: Modular femoral stem removal during total hip arthroplasty using a universal modular stem extractor. Clin Orthop Relat Res 285:155–157, 1992.

56. Talab YA, States JD, Evarts CM: Femoral shaft perforation: a complication of total hip reconstruction. Clin Orthop Relat Res 141:158–165, 1979.

57. Meek RM, Garbuz DS, Masri BA, et al: Intraoperative fracture of the femur in revision total hip arthroplasty with a diaphyseal fitting stem. J Bone Joint Surg Am 86:480–485, 2004.

58. Jingushi S, Noguchi YF, Shuto TF, et al: A device for removal of femoral distal cement plug during hip revision arthroplasty: a high-powered drill equipped with a centralizer. J Arthroplasty 15:231–233, 2000.

59. Gray FB: Total hip revision arthroplasty: prosthesis and cement removal techniques. Orthop Clin North Am 23:313–319, 1992.

60. Sydney SV, Mallory TH: Controlled perforation: a safe method of cement removal from the femoral canal. Clin Orthop Relat Res 253:168–172, 1990.

61. Koster GF, Willert HF, Buchhorn GH: Endoscopy of the femoral canal in revision arthroplasty of the hip: a new method for improving the operative technique and analysis of implant failure. Arch Orthop Trauma Surg 119:245–252, 1999.

62. Porsch MF, Schmidt J: Cement removal with an endoscopically controlled ballistically driven chiselling system: a new device for cement removal and preliminary clinical results. Arch Orthop Trauma Surg 121:274–277, 2001.

63. Gardiner RF, Hozack WJ, Nelson CF, Keating EM: Revision total hip arthroplasty using ultrasonically driven tools: a clinical evaluation. J Arthroplasty 8:517–521, 1993.

64. Klapper RC, Caillouette JT, Callaghan JJ, Hozack WJ: Ultrasonic technology in revision joint arthroplasty. Clin Orthop Relat Res 285:147–154, 1992.

65. Brooks AT, Nelson CL, Stewart CL, et al: Effect of an ultrasonic device on temperatures generated in bone and on bone-cement structure. J Arthroplasty 8:413–418, 1993.

66. Caillouette JT, Gorab RS, Klapper RC, Anzel SH: Revision arthroplasty facilitated by ultrasonic tool cement removal. Part I. In vitro evaluation. Orthop Rev 20:353–357, 1991.

67. Caillouette JT, Gorab RS, Klapper RC, Anzel SH: Revision arthroplasty facilitated by ultrasonic tool cement removal. Part II. Histologic analysis of endosteal bone after cement removal. Orthop Rev 20:435–440, 1991.
68. Callaghan JJ, Elder SH, Stranne SK, et al: Revision arthroplasty facilitated by ultrasonic tool cement removal: an evaluation of whole bone strength in a canine model. J Arthroplasty 7:495–500, 1992.
69. Brooks AT, Nelson CL, Hofmann OE: Minimal femoral cortical thickness necessary to prevent perforation by ultrasonic tools in joint revision surgery. J Arthroplasty 10:359–362, 1995.
70. Fletcher MF, Jennings GJ, Warren PJ: Ultrasonically driven instruments in the transfemoral approach: an aid to preservation of bone stock and reduction of implant length. Arch Orthop Trauma Surg 120:559–561, 2000.
71. Bhamra MS, Rao GS, Robson MJ: Hydroxyapatite-coated hip prostheses: difficulties with revision in 4 cases. Acta Orthop Scand 67:49–52, 1996.
72. Kim YM, Lim ST, Yoo JJ, Kim HJ: Removal of a well-fixed cementless femoral stem using a microsagittal saw. J Arthroplasty 18:511–512, 2003.
73. Harris WH, White RE, Jr, Mitchell S, Barber F: Removal of broken stems of total joint components by a new method: drilling, undercutting, and extracting without damage to bone. Hip 37–45, 1981.
74. Moreland JR, Marder RF, Anspach WE, Jr: The window technique for the removal of broken femoral stems in total hip replacement. Clin Orthop Relat Res 212:245–249, 1986.

CHAPTER 88

Osteolysis Around Well-Fixed Hip Replacement Parts

James I. Huddleston III and William J. Maloney

KEY POINTS
• Osteolytic lesions of the pelvis that progress over a 3- to 6-month period in patients with osseointegrated cementless sockets are an indication for operative treatment. Severe polyethylene wear may justify a lower threshold for treatment because it is optimal to intervene before the time when the head wears through the liner and engages the shell.
• Key factors in determining whether the well-fixed shell can be retained include exchangeability of the liner, extent of osseointegration, position of the socket, and type of fixation surface (i.e., two-dimensional [ongrowth] vs. three-dimensional [ingrowth]).
• Indications for operative treatment in cases of femoral osteolysis include progressive lesions, diaphyseal osteolysis, impending fracture, and pain.
• Key factors in determining whether the well-fixed femoral component can be retained include extent of osseointegration, location of the lesion, and exchangeability of the femoral head.
• Although it is clear that implant retention and grafting are appropriate in selected cases, surgeons must have a low threshold for revising the implants if the strict criteria, as outlined in this chapter, are not met.

INTRODUCTION

Aseptic loosening from periprosthetic osteolysis is a common cause of late failure after total hip arthroplasty (THA). In the United States in 2006, 24.7% of 51,345 revision hip procedures were performed for mechanical loosening and bearing surface wear.[1] In this chapter, we present a strategy for managing periprosthetic osteolysis in the setting of well-fixed implants.

Osteolysis was first described by Harris and associates in 1976.[2] At the time, it was believed that this was due to "cement disease."[2-4] Initially seen around cemented femoral components, osteolysis was later observed around cemented acetabular components that failed owing to aseptic loosening. Cementless sockets were then designed to mitigate the failures seen with cemented fixation. Over time, osteolysis was seen around cementless implants as well. It was observed that the processes around cemented and cementless

implants were similar histologically.[5,6] It is now widely accepted that the process of osteolysis is most commonly driven by the biological response to particulate interface wear debris.[5-8]

It is important to note that the natural history of osteolysis in cemented and cementless fixation is different. In cemented fixation, osteolysis involving the bone-cement interface typically leads to aseptic loosening.[9-12] Surgical management in this situation will consist of revision of the entire implant, and the timing depends on the severity of bone loss and the patient's symptoms. In cementless fixation, osteolysis more commonly involves periprosthetic bone, and the implants may remain osseointegrated in the setting of even massive bone loss. Revision of the entire implant and bearing exchange with débridement of the osteolytic granuloma and bone grafting are viable options in this setting.

INDICATIONS

Patients who develop osteolysis around cemented acetabular components generally present with pain. The radiographic pattern of osteolysis in these patients is usually linear and progresses to involve the entire bone-cement interface. When the entire bone-cement interface is involved, the cup becomes loose. The linear pattern precludes grafting, thus there is not a prophylactic surgical treatment that is practical. Pain is the indication for operative treatment in these patients. The timing of intervention should be commensurate with symptoms; many patients with loose cemented sockets report only mild pain that does not warrant surgical intervention immediately.

Indications for operative treatment of osteolysis around cementless acetabular components are less well defined. Patients with loose cementless sockets have pain, thus the indication for revision is straightforward. Controversy exists regarding the timing of operative intervention in cases where the socket remains well-fixed. In these cases, patients often are pain free, and the issue becomes operating on asymptomatic patients.[13] A few small areas of osseointegration can keep cups well-fixed; therefore patients can remain pain free despite expansile lesions.[14,15] In general, most experts agree that osteolytic lesions that progress over a 3- to 6-month period are an indication for operative treatment. Severe polyethylene wear may justify a lower threshold for treatment because it is optimal to intervene before the time when the head wears through the liner and engages the shell. Prompt operative treatment is warranted when the head has worn through the liner because this situation will generate metallosis and an intense local inflammatory response from metal and polyethylene debris.

In planning for surgical treatment, it is important to consider that plain radiographs generally underestimate the size of osteolytic lesions.[11,14,16-21] In addition to standard anteroposterior pelvis, anteroposterior hip, and cross-table lateral views, Judet views (45-degree obturator and iliac oblique views) often provide information regarding the extent of involvement of the anterior and posterior columns. Helical computed tomography (spiral CT) with metal artifact suppression generally provides the most accurate representation of the size and anatomy of osteolytic lesions.[19,21-24]

Patients with femoral osteolysis generally remain asymptomatic until an impending fracture or extensive synovitis is present, except when osteolysis is associated with femoral component loosening. As on the acetabular side, the timing for surgical intervention is controversial. Indications for operative treatment in cases of femoral osteolysis include progressive lesions, diaphyseal osteolysis, impending fracture, and pain.

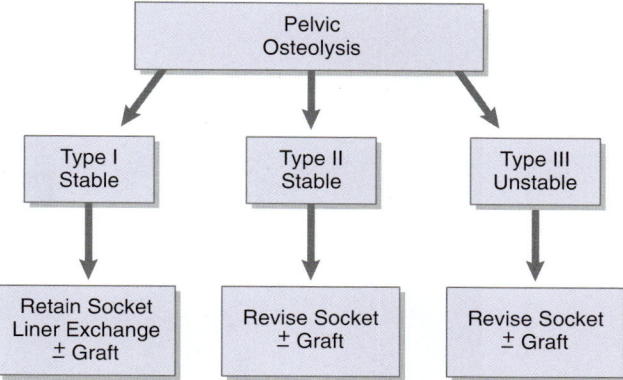

Figure 88-1. This diagram shows the treatment algorithm for management of osteolysis around osseointegrated acetabular components.

ACETABULAR TREATMENT ALGORITHM

The key issue in treating acetabular osteolysis in the setting of a well-fixed shell is whether to retain or remove the cup. Several early reports recommended removing the entire shell to attain adequate access to the lesion.[11,14,15,25] The drawback to this approach is that reconstruction after cup removal is likely to be complex, especially in lesions where the posterior column has been compromised. Key factors in determining whether the shell can be retained include exchangeability of the liner, osseointegration, and type of fixation surface (i.e., two-dimensional [ongrowth] vs. three-dimensional [ingrowth]).

A classification system has been developed to guide surgeons in the treatment of pelvic osteolysis with cementless acetabular components (Fig. 88-1).[10,26-30] A type 1 socket is well positioned, has an ingrowth fixation surface, has a modular liner, and has acceptable survivorship. These cases can be addressed with débridement of the lesion and bone grafting at the surgeon's discretion (Fig. 88-2). Relative contraindications to liner exchange include a damaged shell or locking mechanism and the unavailability of liners with adequate thickness, head size, and/or highly cross-linked polyethylene. An undamaged locking mechanism is only a relative contraindication because it is safe to cement a liner into an appropriate shell.[31,32] Unfortunately, no data are available regarding how much shell damage is permissible. Ongrowth fixation surfaces are a relative contraindication to liner exchange because tensile strength between bone and socket is weaker than the same interface with an ingrowth surface. Hydroxyapatite-coated and macrotextured cups are examples of sockets

that should not be classified as type I.[33-35] Type II sockets are well-fixed but do not meet the criteria for type I sockets. Type II sockets should be removed, and residual bone defects should be managed accordingly. Type III sockets are loose and should be revised.

FEMORAL TREATMENT ALGORITHM

Several key factors must be addressed when treating osteolysis around cementless femoral components. First, stem stability must be determined. Although the surgeon should have an accurate prediction of stability based on interpretation of preoperative radiographs, intraoperative assessment is crucial for corroboration. Second, the extent of osseointegration is an important consideration. The surgeon must be confident that remaining bony apposition to the fixation surface is sufficient to provide long-term implant stability. Third, the location of the lesion is critical. Well-fixed stems with metaphyseal lesions may be retained in many cases. Diaphyseal lesions indicate a connection between the joint space and the distal endosteum.[5] These lesions are difficult to access, and stem revision may be required in the setting of progression of the lesion and/or impending fracture. And fourth, the exchangeability of the femoral head should be considered. If the implant is nonmodular, the head must be in good condition and of sufficient size, and the offset and length must be appropriate, to ensure adequate hip stability.

A classification system has been devised to guide surgeons in the treatment of osteolytic lesions around cementless femoral components (Fig. 88-3).[28] In type I cases, stems are osseointegrated, lesions are predominantly metaphyseal, and the extent of osseointegration is judged sufficient to ensure long-term stability. In this situation, we recommend stem retention, grafting of contained lesions, and exchange of the femoral head (Fig. 88-4). Relative contraindications to stem retention and head exchange include a fixed femoral head that is damaged or insufficient in size or length to provide hip stability, a limited area of osseointegration, diaphyseal osteolysis, appropriate head not available, and a

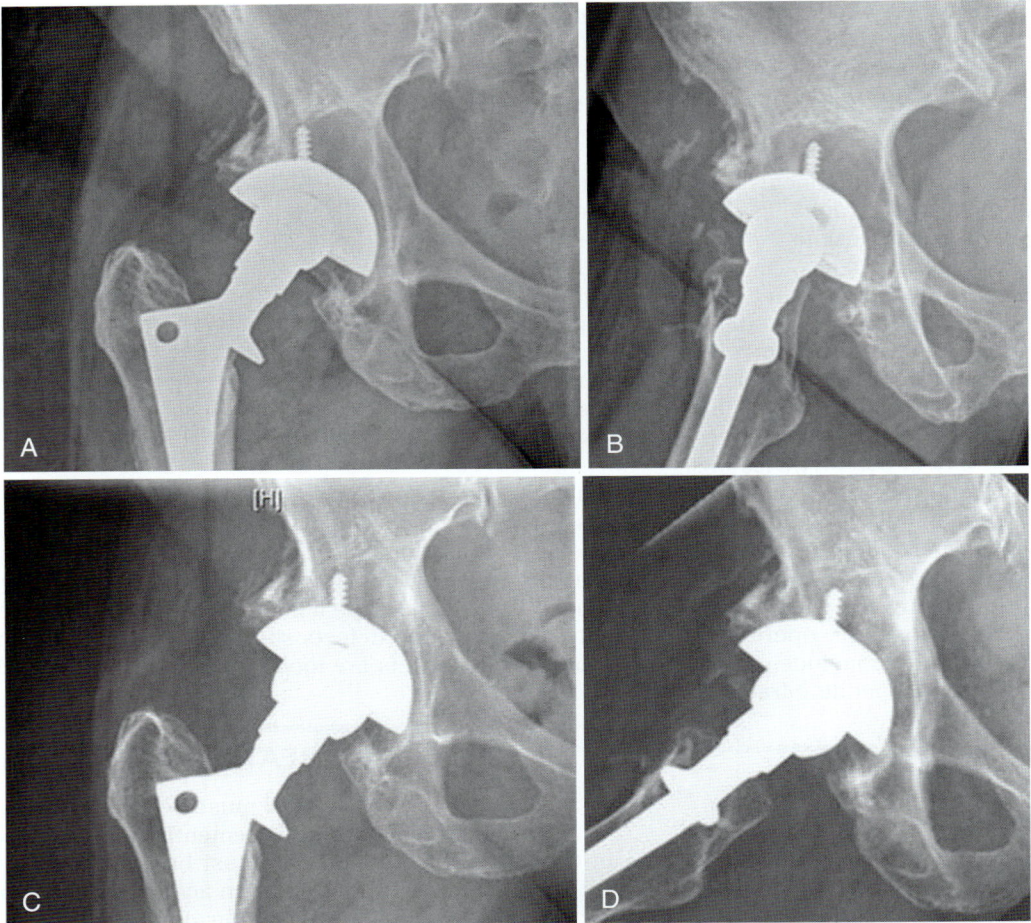

Figure 88-2. These preoperative (**A** and **B**) and 2-year postoperative radiographs (**C** and **D**) show a type I acetabular case treated with socket retention, granuloma débridement, grafting, and liner exchange.

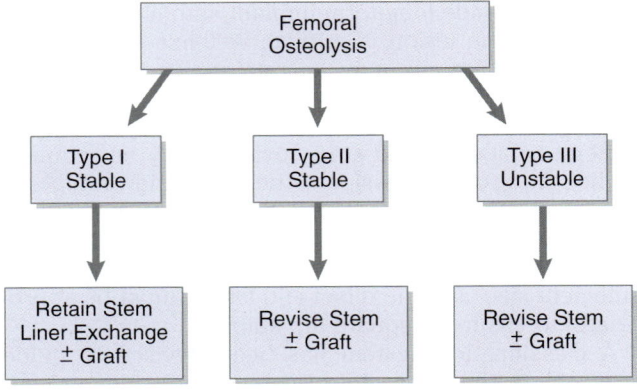

Figure 88-3. This diagram shows the treatment algorithm for management of osteolysis around osseointegrated femoral components.

severely corroded taper. Taper corrosion generates biologically active particulate debris that can lead to third-body wear; it can also weaken the stem and cause implant fracture. In type II cases, the stem is osseointegrated but there is significant diaphyseal osteolysis or insufficient extent of osseointegration, or the femoral head is fixed and damaged. In these cases, we recommend revision of the femoral stem. In type III cases, the stem is loose, thus revision is required.

SURGICAL TECHNIQUE

The surgical approach should allow for wide exposure of the acetabulum, femur, and periprosthetic bone. This will facilitate adequate visualization for testing of socket and stem stability, as well as débridement of the osteolytic granuloma and bone grafting. Prior skin incisions may dictate approach. We recommend that the surgeon ultimately utilize the approach that he/she is most comfortable with. If the femoral component is to be retained, one may consider performing a gluteus maximus tenotomy if the posterior approach is used. This will facilitate retraction of the proximal femur anteriorly. Special care must be taken to protect the trunion once the femoral head has been removed. The finger of a glove can work well for this.

After the fibrous tissue has been removed from the periphery of the socket, the liner can be removed. The surgeon should have knowledge of the manufacturer and type of locking mechanism so that the appropriate

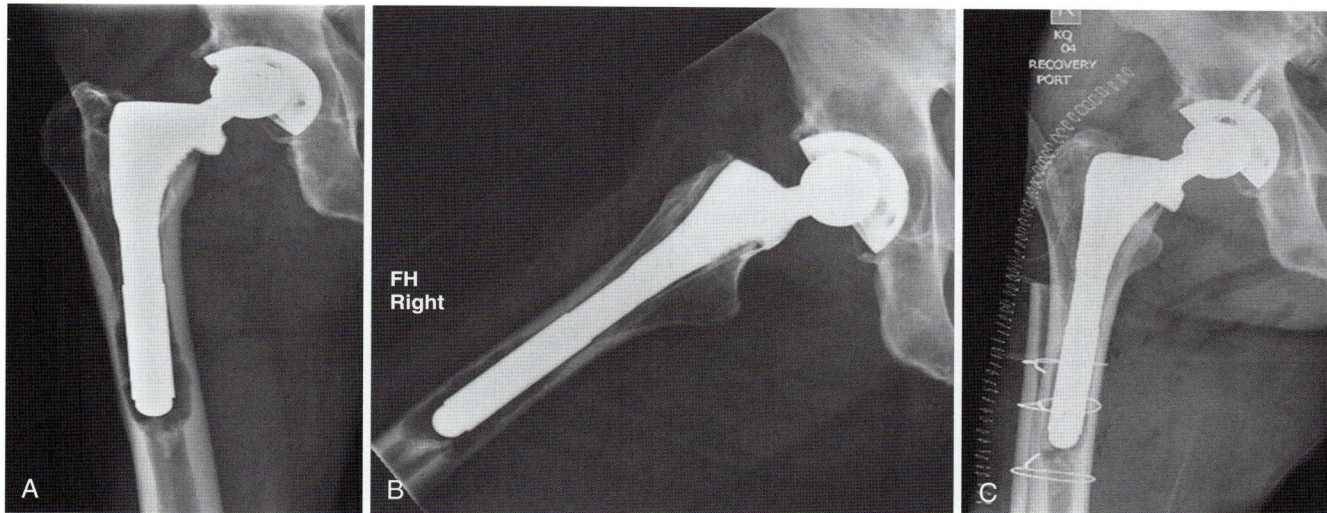

Figure 88-4. These preoperative (**A** and **B**) and early postoperative (**C**) radiographs show a type I femoral case treated with stem retention, head exchange, and grafting through a distal cortical window. A femoral strut allograft was placed prophylactically. The acetabular shell was retained, the acetabular osteolytic defect was débrided and grafted via the screw holes, new screws were placed prophylactically, and the liner was replaced.

extraction tool is available; this will facilitate removal of the liner without damaging the shell and locking mechanism. If an extraction tool does not exist or is unavailable, other methods can be used. Using osteotomes and "screwing" the liner out by drilling a screw through the liner can achieve the same goal with relatively little damage to the lock detail and shell.

Testing for socket stability can occur once any screws are removed. Multiple techniques have been described to test for socket stability.[6,9,10,30] If the cup inserter is available, it will provide a long lever arm. A bone tamp can be used to press on the rim of the cup. If the rim is proud, a heavy needle driver can be used to dislodge the shell from surrounding bone.

Once socket stability has been confirmed, the next step is to gain access to the osteolytic lesions for débridement and bone grafting. Several methods have been described to accomplish this, and the technique used will depend on the location of the lesions. Lesions of the anterior column and symphysis pubis often are not grafted because of difficulty with accessibility. Dome lesions can be grafted through screw holes if present. Because of the difficulty of placing instruments through screw holes, special instruments and bone graft substitutes have been designed to facilitate this process. Specially designed trumpets with a plunger allow effective and efficient placement of up to several cubic centimeters of allograft bone chips.[36] If screw holes are not available, a trap door can be made in the ilium to access the dome. One may consider limiting weight bearing postoperatively if a trap door approach is utilized. Lesions of the posterior column are readily accessible if a posterior approach is utilized. Although a variety of bone void fillers are available, no data are available regarding the efficacy of allograft bone chips or other substitutes in this application.

The technique for grafting of femoral lesions is relatively straightforward. Once the fibrous tissue has been removed from the mouth of the femur, the location and size of the lesion are assessed. The granuloma is then débrided, and contained defects are amenable to bone grafting.

After the osteolytic lesions have been addressed, a trial is performed to assess for hip stability, restoration of offset, and leg length. As with most revisions, we prefer to upsize the femoral head if possible. Patients are allowed to bear weight as tolerated postoperatively. We recommend the use of a hip abduction brace for 6 weeks postoperatively to minimize the risk of dislocation. It has been shown in multiple studies that the risk of dislocation after isolated liner exchange is relatively high.[10,37,38] Timing of the start of abduction exercises will depend on the condition of the greater trochanter.

RESULTS

Follow-up studies on bearing surface exchange for wear and osteolysis have shown that osteolytic lesions may decrease in size or resolve postoperatively. In a study of 35 patients who underwent liner exchange and bone grafting for wear and osteolysis, Maloney and associates reported that one third of the lesions resolved and two thirds of the lesions decreased in size regardless of whether they were grafted or not. Bone graft was used in 74% of the lesions in this series. None of the sockets that were found to be well-fixed intraoperatively loosened at final follow-up.[9] In a similar study with a mean follow-up greater than 6 years, Terfenko and colleagues described that débridement of the osteolytic lesions and bone grafting slowed the progression of osteolysis, and no sockets loosened.[38] Finally, O'Brien and coworkers reported on a series of 23 patients treated with isolated liner exchange and bone grafting of accessible lesions. The authors used computed tomography to quantify lesion size in 18 of the 23 hips. In 17 of 18 hips that were imaged, osteolytic lesions decreased or resolved altogether.[37]

Although it is clear that socket retention with grafting is appropriate in selected cases, the surgeon must have a low threshold to revise the entire shell if the strict criteria, as outlined above, are not met. Hozack and associates recently reported on their results of isolated liner exchange. In their series, 3 of 36 hips treated with socket retention and grafting had failed at 5 years' follow-up. The authors concluded that patients should be warned of an approximate 10% failure rate when the acetabular component is retained.[39] In a study of 1649 revisions, Lie and colleagues hoped to differentiate between the survival of revisions where an uncemented acetabular component was left intact or revised. Using the Norwegian Arthroplasty Register, all cases between 1987 and 2005 with uncemented acetabular components were identified, and 60 different implant styles were included in the analysis. Patients undergoing revision were split into three study groups, in which the liner alone (318 hips), well-fixed shells (398 hips), or loose shells (933 hips) were revised. Subgroups included patients for whom shells were hydroxyapatite-coated and those for whom the femoral component was included in the revision or not. The mean age at revision was 59.2 years, and the most frequent reasons for further revision included dislocation (28%), pain (12%), acetabular loosening (11%), infection (9%), and major wear (8%). Using survival analysis, the authors found that the risk of re-revision was greatest for the group that underwent isolated liner exchange, compared with revision of a well-fixed (relative risk, 0.56) or loose shell (relative risk, 0.56). In addition, re-revisions for pain were less frequent in the group undergoing revision of a well-fixed shell, with a relative risk of 0.20 compared with isolated liner exchange.[40]

Treatment of osteolytic lesions of the proximal femur with osseointegrated femoral components has been successful as well. Bierbaum and coworkers reported on 17 patients who were treated with bone grafting of proximal femoral lesions around stable, cementless femoral implants. At 2 to 6 years' follow-up, 15 of the 17 patients experienced regression of the lesions postoperatively, and no stems loosened.[41] Similar results were reported by Maloney and associates in a series of 15 patients with stems of varying modularity and extent of porous coating. At a minimum of 5 years' follow-up, none of the stems had loosened.[42] The optimal treatment for uncontained lesions is unknown. Min and colleagues reported on 24 hips with a minimum follow-up of 3 years treated with débridement of uncontained femoral osteolytic defects and no femoral grafting during isolated acetabular revision. None of the hips showed progression of any femoral lesions, and all stems remained well-fixed at final follow-up.[43]

FUTURE DIRECTIONS

Although we anticipate that the prevalence of these problems will decrease with increased use of cross-linked polyethylenes and alternative bearing surfaces,

regular monitoring of patients after total hip replacement will still be required. Present efforts to improve implant positioning and to define the optimal bearing surface will likely lead to further reductions in prevalence. Continued investigation of the inflammatory cascade leading to osteolysis may yield targets amenable to nonoperative systemic and local treatment approaches. Finally, genetic testing may afford the opportunity to identify patients who are at high risk for osteolysis.

REFERENCES

1. Bozic KJ, Kurtz SM, Lau E, et al: The epidemiology of revision total hip arthroplasty in the United States. J Bone Joint Surg Am 91:128–133, 2009.
2. Harris WH, Schiller AL, Scholler JM, et al: Extensive localized bone resorption in the femur following total hip replacement. J Bone Joint Surg Am 58:612–618, 1976.
3. Jasty MJ, Floyd WE, 3rd, Schiller AL, et al: Localized osteolysis in stable, non-septic total hip replacement. J Bone Joint Surg Am 68:912–919, 1986.
4. Maloney WJ, Jasty M, Rosenberg A, Harris WH: Bone lysis in well-fixed cemented femoral components. J Bone Joint Surg Br 72:966–970, 1990.
5. Schmalzried TP, Jasty M, Harris WH: Periprosthetic bone loss in total hip arthroplasty: polyethylene wear debris and the concept of the effective joint space. J Bone Joint Surg Am 74:849–863, 1992.
6. Schmalzried TP, Guttmann D, Grecula M, Amstutz HC: The relationship between the design, position, and articular wear of acetabular components inserted without cement and the development of pelvic osteolysis. J Bone Joint Surg Am 76:677–688, 1994.
7. Jacobs JJ, Roebuck KA, Archibeck M, et al: Osteolysis: basic science. Clin Orthop Relat Res 393:71–77, 2001.
8. Harris WH: Wear and periprosthetic osteolysis: the problem. Clin Orthop Relat Res 393:66–70, 2001.
9. Maloney WJ, Herzwurm P, Paprosky W, et al: Treatment of pelvic osteolysis associated with a stable acetabular component inserted without cement as part of a total hip replacement. J Bone Joint Surg Am 79:1628–1634, 1997.
10. Maloney WJ, Paprosky W, Engh CA, Rubash H: Surgical treatment of pelvic osteolysis. Clin Orthop Relat Res 393:78–84, 2001.
11. Maloney WJ, Peters P, Engh CA, Chandler H: Severe osteolysis of the pelvis in association with acetabular replacement without cement. J Bone Joint Surg Am 75:1627–1635, 1993.
12. Zicat B, Engh CA, Gokcen E: Patterns of osteolysis around total hip components inserted with and without cement. J Bone Joint Surg Am 77:432–439, 1995.
13. Schmalzried TP, Fowble VA, Amstutz HC: The fate of pelvic osteolysis after reoperation: no recurrence with lesional treatment. Clin Orthop Relat Res 350:128–137, 1998.
14. Hozack WJ, Mesa JJ, Carey C, Rothman RH: Relationship between polyethylene wear, pelvic osteolysis, and clinical symptomatology in patients with cementless acetabular components: a framework for decision making. J Arthroplasty 11:769–772, 1996.
15. Kavanagh BF, Callaghan JJ, Leggon R, et al: Pelvic osteolysis associated with an uncemented acetabular component in total hip arthroplasty. Orthopedics 19:159–163, 1996.
16. Bobyn JD, Engh CA, Glassman AH: Radiography and histology of a threaded acetabular implant: one case studied at two years. J Bone Joint Surg Br 70:302–304, 1988.
17. Engh CA, Griffin WL, Marx CL: Cementless acetabular components. J Bone Joint Surg Br 72:53–59, 1990.
18. Engh CA, Zettl-Schaffer KF, Kukita Y, et al: Histological and radiographic assessment of well functioning porous-coated acetabular components: a human postmortem retrieval study. J Bone Joint Surg Am 75:814–824, 1993.
19. Puri L, Wixson RL, Stern SH, et al: Use of helical computed tomography for the assessment of acetabular osteolysis

after total hip arthroplasty. J Bone Joint Surg Am 84:609–614, 2002.

20. Southwell DG, Bechtold JE, Lew WD, Schmidt AH: Improving the detection of acetabular osteolysis using oblique radiographs. J Bone Joint Surg Br 81:289–295, 1999.

21. Stulberg SD, Wixson RL, Adams AD, et al: Monitoring pelvic osteolysis following total hip replacement surgery: an algorithm for surveillance. J Bone Joint Surg Am 84(Suppl 2):116–222, 2002.

22. Egawa H, Ho H, Huynh C, et al: A three-dimensional method for evaluating changes in acetabular osteolytic lesions in response to treatment. Clin Orthop Relat Res 468:480–490, 2010.

23. Egawa H, Powers CC, Beykirch SE, et al: Can the volume of pelvic osteolysis be calculated without using computed tomography? Clin Orthop Relat Res 467:181–187, 2009.

24. Egawa H, Ho H, Hopper RH, Jr, et al: Computed tomography assessment of pelvic osteolysis and cup-lesion interface involvement with a press-fit porous-coated acetabular cup. J Arthroplasty 24:233–239, 2009.

25. Mallory TH, Lombardi AV, Jr, Fada RA, et al: Noncemented acetabular component removal in the presence of osteolysis: the affirmative. Clin Orthop Relat Res 381:120–128, 2000.

26. Blaha JD: Well-fixed acetabular component retention or replacement: the whys and the wherefores. J Arthroplasty 17(4 Suppl 1):157–161, 2002.

27. Maloney WJ: Socket retention: staying in place. Orthopedics 23:965–966, 2000.

28. Rubash HE, Sinha RK, Maloney WJ, Paprosky WG: Osteolysis: surgical treatment. Instr Course Lect 47:321–329, 1998.

29. Sinha RK, Shanbhag AS, Maloney WJ, et al: Osteolysis: cause and effect. Instr Course Lect 47:307–320, 1998.

30. Rubash HE, Sinha RK, Paprosky W, et al: A new classification system for the management of acetabular osteolysis after total hip arthroplasty. Instr Course Lect 48:37–42, 1999.

31. Callaghan JJ, Liu SS, Schularick NM: Shell retention with a cemented acetabular liner. Orthopedics 32, 2009.

32. Haft GF, Heiner AD, Callaghan JJ, et al: Polyethylene liner cementation into fixed acetabular shells. J Arthroplasty 17(4 Suppl 1):167–170, 2002.

33. Capello WN, D'Antonio JA, Manley MT, Feinberg JR: Hydroxyapatite in total hip arthroplasty: clinical results and critical issues. Clin Orthop Relat Res 355:200–211, 1998.

34. Manley MT, Capello WN, D'Antonio JA, et al: Fixation of acetabular cups without cement in total hip arthroplasty: a comparison of three different implant surfaces at a minimum duration of follow-up of five years. J Bone Joint Surg Am 80:1175–1185, 1998.

35. Jiranek WA, Whiddon DR, Johnstone WT: Late loosening of press-fit cementless acetabular components. Clin Orthop Relat Res 418:172–178, 2004.

36. Chiang PP, Burke DW, Freiberg AA, Rubash HE: Osteolysis of the pelvis: evaluation and treatment. Clin Orthop Relat Res 417:164–174, 2003.

37. O'Brien JJ, Burnett RS, McCalden RW, et al: Isolated liner exchange in revision total hip arthroplasty: clinical results using the direct lateral surgical approach. J Arthroplasty 19:414–423, 2004.

38. Terefenko KM, Sychterz CJ, Orishimo K, Engh CA, Sr: Polyethylene liner exchange for excessive wear and osteolysis. J Arthroplasty 17:798–804, 2002.

39. Restrepo C, Ghanem E, Houssock C, et al: Isolated polyethylene exchange versus acetabular revision for polyethylene wear. Clin Orthop Relat Res 467:194–198, 2009.

40. Lie SA, Hallan G, Furnes O, et al: Isolated acetabular liner exchange compared with complete acetabular component revision in revision of primary uncemented acetabular components: a study of 1649 revisions from the Norwegian Arthroplasty Register. J Bone Joint Surg Br 89:591–594, 2007.

41. Benson ER, Christensen CP, Monesmith EA, et al: Particulate bone grafting of osteolytic femoral lesions around stable cementless stems. Clin Orthop Relat Res 381:58–67, 2000.

42. Maloney WJ: The surgical management of femoral osteolysis. J Arthroplasty 20(4 Suppl 2):75–78, 2005.

43. Min BW, Song KS, Cho CH, et al: Femoral osteolysis around the unrevised stem during isolated acetabular revision. Clin Orthop Relat Res 467:1501–1506, 2009.

KEY READINGS

Lie SA, Hallan G, Furnes O, et al: Isolated acetabular liner exchange compared with complete acetabular component revision in revision of primary uncemented acetabular components: a study of 1649 revisions from the Norwegian Arthroplasty Register. J Bone Joint Surg Br 89:591–594, 2007.
In a study of 1649 revisions from 1987 to 2005, the authors hoped to differentiate between the survival of revisions where an uncemented acetabular component was left intact or revised. Sixty different implant styles were included in the analysis. Patients undergoing revision were split into three study groups in which the liner alone (318 hips), well-fixed shells (398 hips), or loose shells (933 hips) were revised. Subgroups included patients for whom those shells were hydroxyapatite-coated and those for whom the femoral component was included in the revision or not. The mean age at revision was 59.2 years, and the most frequent reasons for further revision included dislocation (28%), pain (12%), acetabular loosening (11%), infection (9%), and major wear (8%). Using survival analysis, the authors found that the risk of re-revision was greatest for the group that underwent isolated liner exchange compared with revision of a well-fixed (relative risk, 0.56) or loose shell (relative risk, 0.56). In addition, re-revisions for pain were less frequent in the group undergoing revision of a well-fixed shell, with a relative risk of 0.20 compared with isolated liner exchange.

Maloney WJ: The surgical management of femoral osteolysis. J Arthroplasty 20(4 Suppl 2):75–78, 2005.
The author reports the results of 15 patients treated with stem retention and grafting. The stems were of varying modularity and extent of porous coating. At a minimum of 5 years' follow-up, none of the stems had loosened.

Maloney WJ, Herzwurm P, Paprosky W, et al: Treatment of pelvic osteolysis associated with a stable acetabular component inserted without cement as part of a total hip replacement. J Bone Joint Surg Am 79:1628–1634, 1997.
The authors report the results of 35 patients who underwent liner exchange and bone grafting for wear and osteolysis. One third of the lesions resolved, and two thirds of the lesions decreased in size, regardless of whether they were grafted or not. Bone graft was used in 74% of the lesions in this series. None of the sockets that were found to be well-fixed intraoperatively had loosened at final follow-up.

CHAPTER 89

Acetabular Reconstruction: Classification of Bone Defects and Treatment Options

Geoffrey Wright and Wayne G. Paprosky

KEY POINTS

- Successful reconstruction of the acetabulum during revision total hip arthroplasty requires a thorough understanding of host bone defects. In an attempt to better define these defects, classification systems are used. The most commonly used systems are the American Academy of Orthopaedic Surgeons (AAOS) and Paprosky classifications of acetabular defects.
- The Paprosky classification is based on the antero-posterior (AP) pelvis radiograph. It uses four separate criteria to determine the classification: superior migration of the cup, the amount of ischial osteolysis, the amount of teardrop osteolysis, and the position of the cup relative to Kohler's line.
- Several different options are available for reconstruction of the acetabulum, including hemispherical cementless cups, jumbo cups, bilobed cups, high hip center, impaction grafting of the acetabulum, bulk structural allograft, antiprotrusio cages, and highly porous acetabular cups. Each has its own advantages and disadvantages.

INTRODUCTION

Over the past decade, improvements in technology and surgical technique have made acetabular revision more successful and straightforward. The main goals of acetabular revision are (1) to extract failed implants with minimal bone and soft tissue damage, (2) to implant new components that provide long-term pain relief and good function, and (3) to manage bone deficiencies effectively and if possible restore bone stock.

The location and degree of acetabular bone loss can be predicted with the use of preoperative radiographs. New instruments and techniques have made removal of existing components easier. During surgery, stable implant fixation is required to obtain a good long-term clinical result. Restoring the optimal position of the acetabulum is important for providing the highest likelihood of hip stability. These factors must be addressed in the planning process of the reconstruction and can be completed in such a way that the likelihood of success is optimized.

Classification systems are used throughout orthopedics, and reconstructive surgery is no different. The ideal classification system should be simple to use and should have excellent intraobserver and interobserver reliability and validity. It should provide an accurate enough description to facilitate communication between providers, assist with preoperative evaluation, allow for determination of the most appropriate treatment options, and predict outcomes after surgery. Unfortunately, such an ideal classification system rarely exists.

This chapter will discuss the two most popular classification systems used to describe acetabular bone defects. It will review how the type of defect as determined from preoperative radiographs, the author's approach to complicated cases, and the different treatment options available for acetabular reconstruction.

INDICATIONS/CONTRAINDICATIONS

The decision to proceed with revision hip surgery is the endpoint of a complex decision-making process involving the patient and the surgeon. It should consider the severity of the patient's symptoms, along with the patient's function, disability, and general health, as well as the surgeon's experience. However, revision hip arthroplasty usually is not indicated unless a specific problem is identified that can be surgically corrected.

Indications for acetabular revision include symptomatic aseptic loosening, failure of fixation, infection, wear, osteolysis, and instability. Revision may be indicated for an asymptomatic patient who has progressive osteolysis, severe wear, or bone loss that could compromise a future reconstruction. Historically, the most common indication for acetabular revision has been loosening of the acetabular component. However, Bozic and associates, using the Healthcare Cost and Utilization Project Nationwide Inpatient Sample database, recently found that the most common cause of revision hip surgery was instability or dislocation (22.5%).[1] Mechanical loosening and infection were next in frequency at 19.7% and 14.8%, respectively. Instability or dislocation was the most common cause of an isolated acetabular revision (33%), and mechanical loosening was the second most common indication (24%). In this study, 54% of all cases required revision of the acetabulum.

Contraindications for revision of the acetabular component include severe bone loss precluding allograft fixation or implant fixation, uncontrolled infection, and medical comorbidities that preclude surgery. In these patients, nonsurgical treatment such as activity modification, ambulatory aids, and oral analgesics may be appropriate.

CLASSIFICATION SYSTEMS

AAOS Classification

The American Academy of Orthopaedic Surgeons (AAOS) classification of bone defects, as described by D'Antonio and associates, identifies the pattern and location of bone loss but does not quantify the defect (Box 89-1).[2,3] This system, which was developed by evaluating 83 AP and lateral hip radiographs and comparing results intraoperatively, is probably the most commonly used classification in the literature. It is based on two basic categories: segmental and cavitary defects. A segmental defect (type I) is defined as complete loss of bone in the hemisphere of the acetabulum, peripherally or centrally. A central segmental defect involves loss of the medial wall of the acetabulum. A cavitary deficiency (type II) is defined as volumetric bony loss of the acetabulum with an intact rim. These defects can occur peripherally or centrally. Medial cavitary defects involve loss of bone centrally with an intact medial wall, as in most cases of protrusio. The peripheral defects in types I and II are further divided by anatomic position: medial, superior, anterior, or posterior. Combined segmental and cavitary defects (type III) occur frequently. These include defects due to a failed,

migrated endoprosthesis and those defects seen in developmental dysplasia.

Pelvic discontinuity (type IV) is an unusual condition in which the superior pelvis and the inferior pelvis are separated. Typically, this occurs through a transverse acetabular fracture through weak and deficient bone. Identifying features on preoperative radiographs include a visible fracture line through the anterior and posterior columns, a break in Kohler's line such that the superior pelvis and the inferior pelvis are offset relative to one another, and rotation of the inferior aspect of the hemipelvis relative to the superior aspect, which is often seen as asymmetry of the obturator rings.[4]

Arthrodesis is considered the final type of acetabular defect (type V) in this classification. Although this classification does define acetabular defects, its major flaw as a classification system is that it does not address the management of these defects.

Paprosky Classification

The Paprosky classification system is based on the severity of bone loss and on the ability to obtain cementless fixation for a given bone loss pattern.[5-7] It was initially developed by evaluating the AP pelvis radiograph and comparing this information with intraoperative findings. The Paprosky classification system was designed to provide guidance on when cementless components are appropriate and when other techniques should be used. The key to this classification is determining the ability of the remaining host bone to provide initial stability to a hemispherical cementless acetabular component until ingrowth occurs. Intraoperative decisions are based on findings when trial components are used; however, intraoperative findings can often be predicted by the preoperative AP radiograph of the pelvis when this classification system is used.

Careful interpretation of the AP radiograph can predict the type of defect and can allow the surgeon to plan for the acetabular reconstruction. Four criteria are used to assess the preoperative radiograph: (1) superior migration of the hip center, (2) ischial osteolysis, (3) teardrop osteolysis, and (4) position of the implant relative to Kohler's line (Table 89-1).

Superior migration of the hip center represents bone loss in the acetabular dome involving the anterior and posterior columns. Superior and medial migration indicates greater involvement of the anterior column. Superior and lateral migration indicates greater involvement of the posterior column. The amount of superior migration is measured as the distance in millimeters (adjusted for magnification) relative to the superior obturator line, or a line drawn from the top of each obturator foramen.

Ischial osteolysis indicates bone loss from the inferior aspect of the posterior column, including the posterior wall. The amount of ischial osteolysis is quantified by measuring the distance (adjusted for magnification) from the most inferior extent of the lytic area to the superior obturator line. Mild ischial osteolysis is defined as less than 7 mm, and severe ischial osteolysis is defined as greater than 15 mm.

BOX 89-1. AMERICAN ACADEMY OF ORTHOPAEDIC SURGEONS ACETABULAR DEFICIENCY CLASSIFICATION

Type I   Segmental defect
  • Peripheral
  • Central
Type II   Cavitary defect (intact rim)
  • Peripheral
  • Central
Type III Combined defect
Type IV   Pelvic discontinuity
Type V   Arthrodesis

Modified from D'Antonio JA, Capello WN, Borden LS, et al: Classification and management of acetabular abnormalities in total hip arthroplasty. Clin Orthop Relat Res 243:127, 1989.

Table 89-1. Paprosky Classification of Acetabular Defects

Defect	Rim	Walls	Columns	Migration	Teardrop Lysis
Type 1	Intact	Intact	Intact/Supportive	None	None
Type 2	Distorted	Distorted	Intact/Supportive	<2 cm	
Type 2A	Distorted	Intact	Intact/Supportive	Superomedial	Minimal
Type 2B	Missing	Distorted	Intact/Supportive	Superolateral	Minimal
Type 2C	Distorted	Intact	Intact/Supportive	Medial	Severe
Type 3	Missing	Compromised	Nonsupportive	>2 cm	
Type 3A	Missing	Compromised	Nonsupportive	Superolateral	Moderate
Type 3B	Missing	Compromised	Nonsupportive	Superomedial	Severe

Modified from Paprosky WG, Perona PG, Lawrence JM: Acetabular defect classification and surgical reconstruction in revision arthroplasty: a 6-year follow-up evaluation. J Arthroplasty 9:34, 1994.

Teardrop osteolysis indicates bone loss from the inferior and medial aspects of the acetabulum, including the inferior aspect of the anterior column, the lateral aspect of the pubis, and the medial wall. Moderate osteolysis is defined as partial destruction of the teardrop with maintenance of the medial limb of the teardrop. Severe involvement is defined as complete obliteration of the teardrop.

Medial migration of the component relative to Kohler's line represents a deficiency of the anterior column. Kohler's line, or the ilioischial line, is defined as a line connecting the most lateral aspect of the pelvic brim and the most lateral aspect of the obturator foramen on an anteroposterior radiograph of the pelvis. The medial aspect of the implant is lateral to Kohler's line with grade 1 migration and medial to the line with grade 3 migration. With grade 2 migration, migration to Kohler's line or slight remodeling of the iliopubic and ilioischial lines occurs without a break in continuity.

With a Paprosky type 1 defect, minimal bone loss is noted (Fig. 89-1). The acetabular rim and walls are intact and supportive without distortion. The acetabulum is hemispherical, and there may be small focal areas of contained bone loss. The anterior and posterior columns are intact. The preoperative radiograph shows no superior migration of the component, no evidence of osteolysis in the ischium or teardrop, and grade 1 medial migration (Kohler's line has not been violated). A hemispherical cementless implant is almost completely supported by native bone; however, a large cup may be required. Full inherent stability is achieved, and particulate grafting can be used to fill the minor areas of bone loss.

In a type 2 defect, the acetabular rim and walls are distorted, but the host bone is adequate to support a cementless acetabular component. The anterior and posterior columns remain intact and supportive. On the preoperative radiograph of a type 2 defect, superior migration of the hip center is less than 3 cm from the superior obturator line, osteolysis of the ischium is mild (<7 mm distal to the obturator line), and osteolysis of the teardrop is not substantial. At least 50% of the surface area of the component is in contact with host bone for potential ingrowth, and good mechanical support can be provided entirely by host bone. The trial

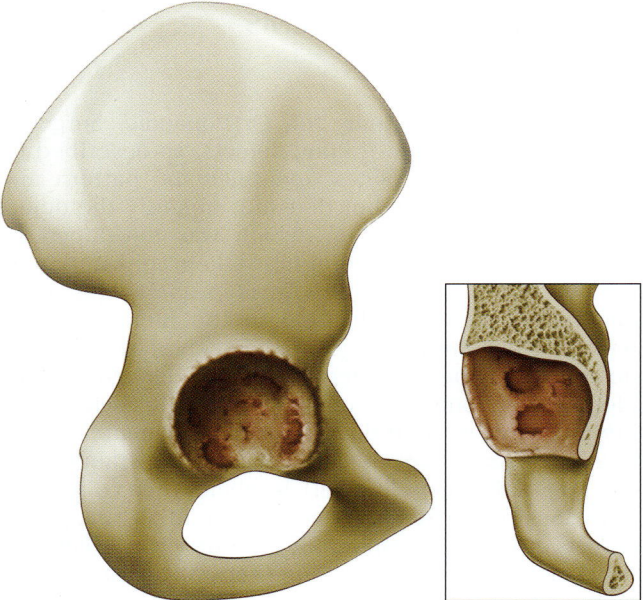

Figure 89-1. Type 1 acetabular defect. The rim is intact and the columns are fully supportive of a hemispherical component. Only localized bone lysis is noted. *(Redrawn from Paprosky WG, Perona PG, Lawrence JM: Acetabular defect classification and surgical reconstruction in revision arthroplasty: a 6-year follow-up evaluation. J Arthroplasty 9:34, 1994.)*

component has full inherent stability; however, the hip center may be elevated as much as 1.5 cm to achieve superior contact and support.

Type 2 defects are subdivided into types A, B, and C, according to the bone loss pattern. Type 2A defects are oval enlargements of the acetabulum caused by superior bone lysis; however, the superior rim of the acetabulum is intact (Fig. 89-2). Migration of the component into a cavitary defect is evident medial to a thinned superior rim and is directed superior or superior medial. This migration is less than 2 cm. In most patients, the defect can be treated with particulate allograft because the remaining superior rim provides a buttress for containment of the allograft.

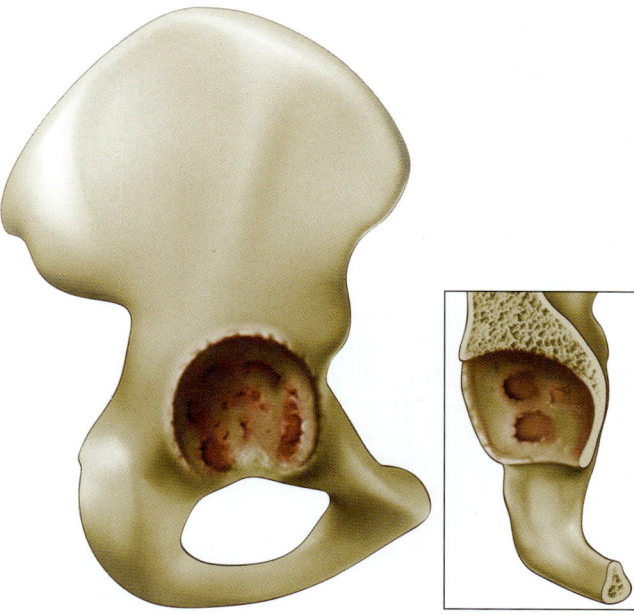

Figure 89-2. Type 2A acetabular defect. The rim remains intact; however, it is enlarged superiorly to create an oval. *(Redrawn from Paprosky WG, Perona PG, Lawrence JM: Acetabular defect classification and surgical reconstruction in revision arthroplasty: a 6-year follow-up evaluation. J Arthroplasty 9:35, 1994.)*

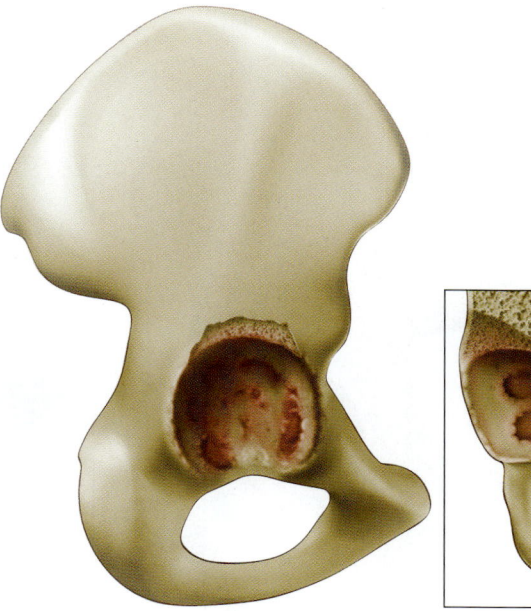

Figure 89-3. Type 2B acetabular defect. The superior rim is absent; however, the column remains fully supportive. *(Redrawn from Paprosky WG, Perona PG, Lawrence JM: Acetabular defect classification and surgical reconstruction in revision arthroplasty: a 6-year follow-up evaluation. J Arthroplasty 9:36, 1994).*

In a type 2B defect, the superior acetabular rim is missing (Fig. 89-3). Usually, less than one third of the circumference of the superior rim is deficient. This defect is not contained. The remaining anterior and posterior rims and columns are supportive of an implant. Migration of the component occurs superior and lateral because the acetabular rim is deficient. Most reconstructions are done without grafting of the segmental defect because stability can be achieved through the remaining columns. Occasionally, an allograft can be used to restore bone stock; however, it is not supportive of the implant.

Type 2C defects (Fig. 89-4*A* and *B*) have a medial wall defect and migration of the acetabular component medial to the Kohler line. The rim of the acetabulum is intact and will support a hemispherical component. Reconstruction of these defects is similar to the treatment of protrusio acetabuli in the setting of a primary arthroplasty. Sequentially larger reamers are used until the acetabular rim is engaged. Particulate bone graft can be placed medially to lateralize the hip center of rotation back to its anatomic position.

In Paprosky type 3 defects, major acetabular bone loss has occurred. The acetabular rim and walls are compromised, and the anterior and posterior columns are nonsupportive. The remaining acetabular rim will not provide adequate initial component stability to achieve reliable biological fixation; therefore the trial implant lacks full intrinsic stability. The acetabular component has migrated proximally more than 2 cm. These defects are subdivided into two types.

Type 3A defects (Fig. 89-5*A* and *B*) involve more than one third but not more than one half of the circumference of the acetabular rim. The rim defect is usually located between the 10 o'clock and 2 o'clock positions. The medial wall of the acetabulum is present; therefore migration of the acetabular component is superolateral. Typically, the acetabular component has migrated more than 2 cm superiorly. Preoperative radiographs show superior and lateral migration of the component greater than 3 cm above the obturator line (with adjustment for magnification). Ischial lysis is mild to moderate, extending less than 15 mm inferior to the obturator line. Partial destruction of the teardrop is seen, but the medial limb usually is still present. The component is even with or lateral to Kohler's line, and the ilioischial and iliopubic lines are intact. Enough host bone is in contact with the ingrowth surface of a hemispherical component to attain durable biological fixation (meaning that more than 50% of the surface area of the cementless cup is in contact with host bone). However, the trial components are only partially stable, and support of the implant with a structural augment or allograft is necessary in the short term to provide initial stability.

Type 3B defects (Fig. 89-6*A* and *B*) involve more than half of the circumference of the acetabular rim, usually extending from the 9 o'clock to the 5 o'clock position. The failed acetabular component migrates superiorly and medially because the medial wall has been destroyed. Patients with a type 3B defect are at high risk for pelvic discontinuity; this possibility must be thoroughly evaluated at the time of reconstruction.

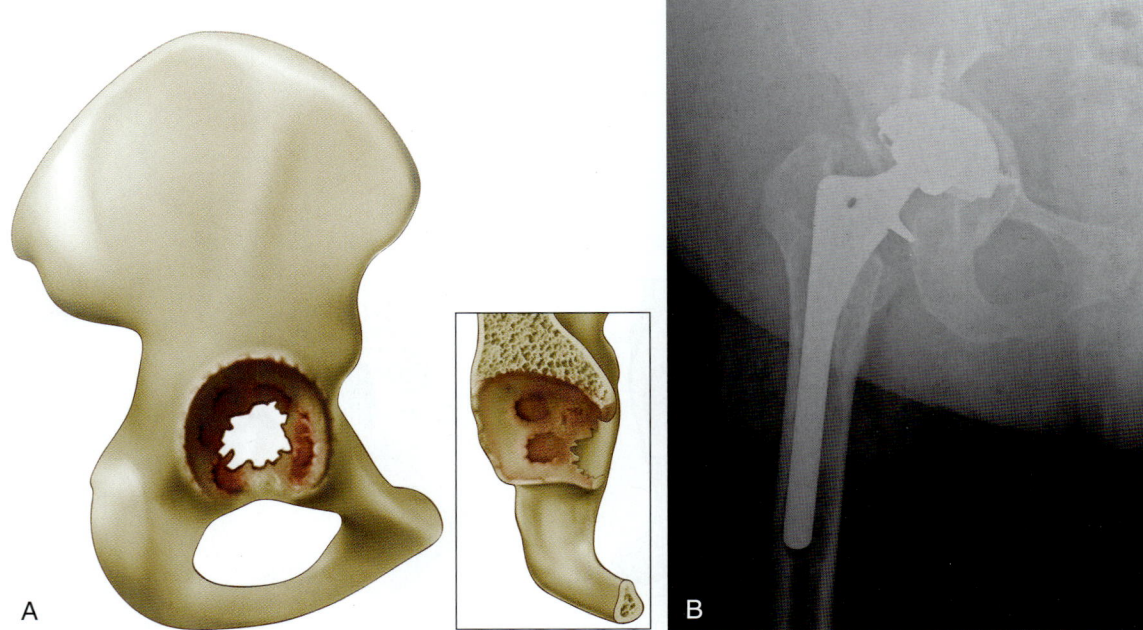

A

B

Figure 89-4. **A**, Type 2C acetabular defect. The rim is enlarged and the medial wall is destroyed. The teardrop may be obliterated as well. *(Redrawn from Paprosky WG, Perona PG, Lawrence JM: Acetabular defect classification and surgical reconstruction in revision arthroplasty: a 6-year follow-up evaluation. J Arthroplasty 9:37, 1994.)* **B,** Radiograph demonstrating a Type 2C acetabular defect. The teardrop is obliterated and the component has migrated medially past Kohler's line.

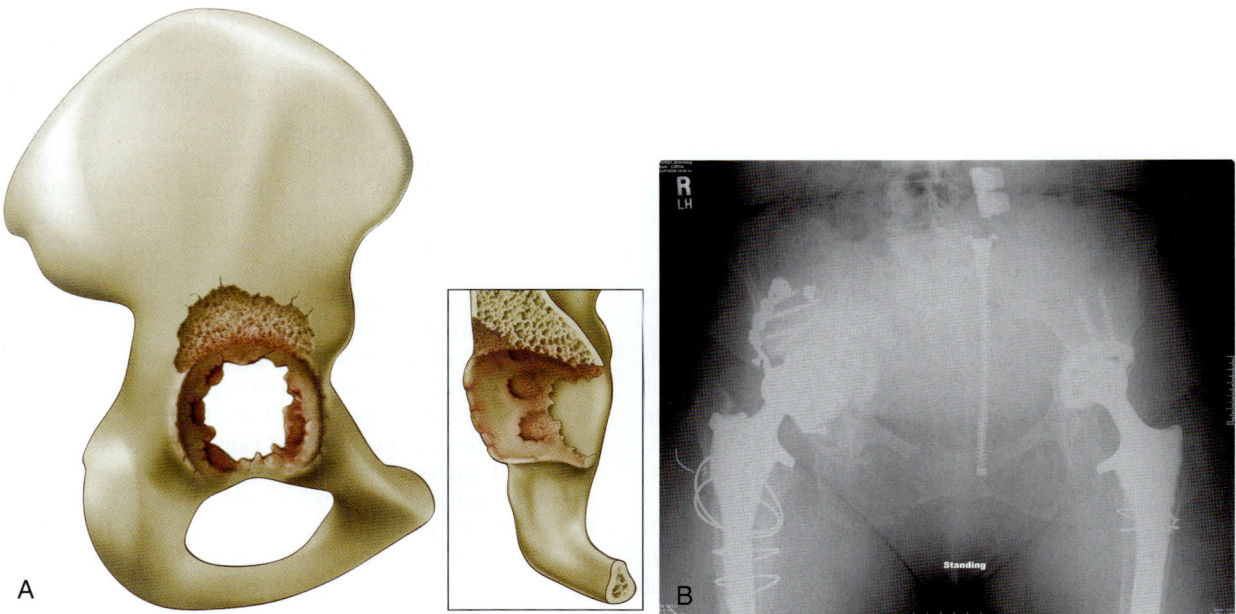

A

B

Figure 89-5. **A,** Type 3A acetabular defect. Bone loss along the superior rim and dome of the acetabulum. The medial teardrop is still present. *(Redrawn from Paprosky WG, Perona PG, Lawrence JM: Acetabular defect classification and surgical reconstruction in revision arthroplasty: a 6-year follow-up evaluation. J Arthroplasty 9:38, 1994.)* **B,** The right hip demonstrates a type 3A defect with superolateral migration of the acetabular component. The acetabular component has eroded superiorly and shifted to a vertical position. The left hip demonstrates placement of the acetabular component with a high hip center.

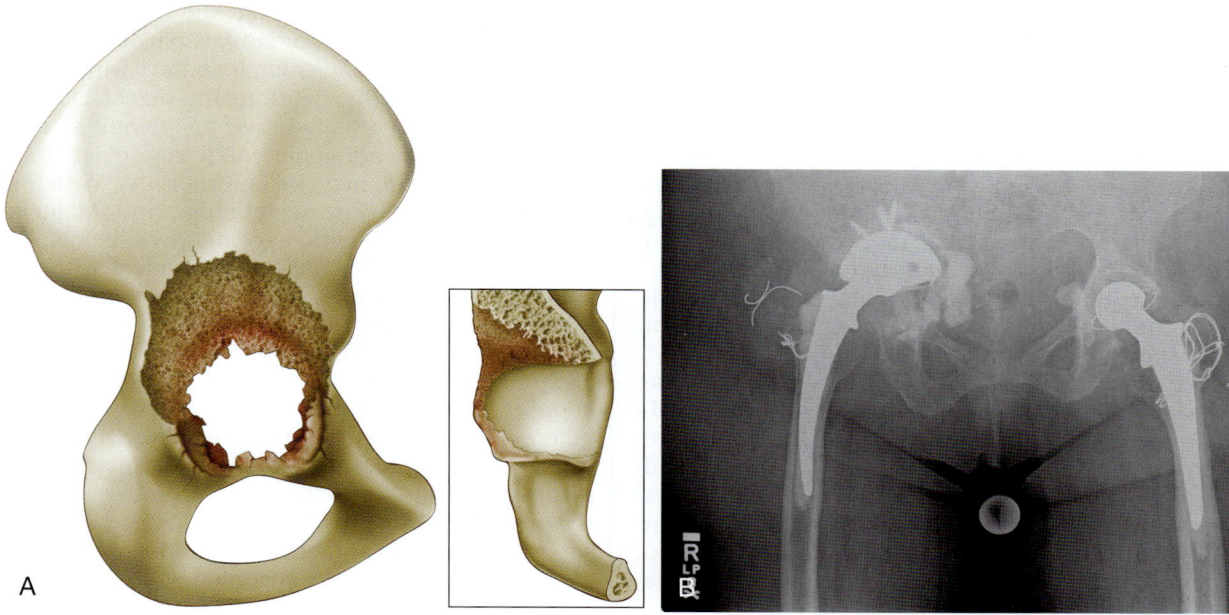

Figure 89-6. A, Type 3B acetabular defect. Complete obliteration of the medial teardrop and severe lysis. Columns are not supportive. *(Redrawn from Paprosky WG, Perona PG, Lawrence JM: Acetabular defect classification and surgical reconstruction in revision arthroplasty: a 6-year follow-up evaluation. J Arthroplasty 9:39, 1994.)* **B,** The right hip shows a type 3B defect with superomedial migration. The medial wall is destroyed with subsequent migration of the cup and cement into the pelvis. Severe bone loss is evident.

Preoperative radiographs often show severe ischial osteolysis, complete destruction of the teardrop, migration medial to Kohler's line, and migration greater than 3 cm superior to the obturator line. Less than 40% of the ingrowth surface of the acetabular component is in contact with host bone. Inherent stability is not achievable with a trial implant. Alternative techniques are often required with these defects.

RELIABILITY AND VALIDITY OF THE CLASSIFICATION SYSTEMS

Any classification system must undergo validity and reliability testing to be universally accepted. In Paprosky's original paper, 92.5% agreement was reported between preoperative and intraoperative assessment or an assessment of the validity of the system.[6] Gozzard and coworkers evaluated both of the discussed classification systems by having two orthopedic consultants and two orthopedic registrars examine 25 radiographs on two separate occasions.[8] The validity of the Paprosky system, or the comparison between preoperative and intraoperative findings, was found to be good. The reliability of a system is defined as its ability to grade a given degree of bone stock loss in a consistent manner. Intraobserver reliability ranged from poor to good, depending on the experience of the observer, with the registrars having higher scores. Interobserver agreement was moderate in both classification systems.

In a separate study evaluating the AAOS and Paprosky systems, Campbell examined interobserver and intraobserver reliability for 33 hips needing revision hip arthroplasty.[9] The originators of each system—three expert orthopedic surgeons and three senior residents—reviewed the films on two separate occasions at a minimum of 2 weeks apart. Overall reliability was poor for both systems. Intraobserver reliability of the originators was moderate for both, with the Paprosky classification being slightly more reliable. However, intraobserver reliability among orthopedic surgeons and residents was poor. Interobserver reliability was poor for both. Although these studies show that neither of these classification systems is perfect, both agree that some form of classification should be used to facilitate communicate between surgeons and to compare outcomes.

PREOPERATIVE PLANNING

Preoperative planning is a critical aspect of any reconstructive hip surgery but is particularly important in revision surgery. The surgeon must anticipate instrument, bone graft, and implant requirements for the surgery, as well as which reconstructive options may be needed, based on what may be found intraoperatively.

A complete history and physical examination should be completed, and medical clearance should be obtained, before revision acetabular surgery is performed. These procedures can take a long time and can result in significant blood loss, especially if the femoral component is being removed; therefore all of the patient's existing medical conditions should be well controlled before surgery is begun. The patient should be aware of potential medical and surgical complications, and realistic goals should be discussed with the patient preoperatively. Discussion should include information on postoperative weight-bearing status and limitations, along with long-term outcome expectations.

Every attempt should be made to identify the cause or causes of the implant failure. The type of pain is important in that patients with start-up pain usually have loose components, and those with continuous unrelenting pain may be more likely to have an ongoing infection. The preoperative status of the muscles and neurovascular structures should be identified, specifically the function of the hip abductors. In patients with deficient abductors, larger femoral heads or constraint in the acetabular construct may be required.

Every patient undergoing revision surgery should be screened for infection with at least an erythrocyte sedimentation rate and C-reactive protein. The erythrocyte sedimentation rate should be less than 30 mm/hr and the C-reactive protein less than 10 mg/L. If these values are elevated or inconclusive, aspiration of the joint should be performed because treatment for an infected prosthesis is different from treatment for other events leading to revision arthroplasty.

Standard preoperative radiographs should include an anteroposterior pelvis film, an anteroposterior hip film, a lateral radiograph of the hip, and a shoot-through lateral radiograph. The shoot-through lateral is particularly helpful for evaluating the posterior column, which is often obscured by the cup on other films. Judet oblique pelvic views can be helpful if pelvic discontinuity is suspected. Although not required, three-dimensional imaging such as computed tomography (CT) scans may be helpful in accurately determining the pattern of the acetabular defect. CT scans are probably most helpful in patients with significant medial migration of the acetabular component when used to evaluate the proximity of neurovascular structures.

Algorithmic Approach

The authors' approach to revision of the acetabulum is shown in the accompanying chart (Fig. 89-7). Although this is not all encompassing, it does provide an excellent guide for approaching these difficult cases. Currently, we use a posterolateral approach to the hip for all acetabular revisions. Other approaches can be used, depending on the severity of the revision and the surgeon's experience. Careful evaluation of the preoperative radiographs is essential in determining how to proceed with the operation.

Our initial decision depends on the superior migration of the hip center before the revision is performed. If the hip center has migrated less than 3 cm above the superior obturator line, the defect is classified as type I or type II. The surgeon must then determine whether full inherent stability can be achieved with a trial component. If this can be done, a hemispherical cementless implant is utilized. If migration is medial to Kohler's line, the defect is classified as type IIC, and the rim will support the hemispherical implant.

If the hip center has migrated more than 3 cm superior to the superior obturator line, or if the surgeon is unable to achieve full inherent stability of the hemispherical trial component, the defect is classified as type III. If a trial component has partial inherent stability, there is generally enough contact with host bone to support ingrowth; therefore the defect is type IIIA. Type IIIA defects usually have an oblong shape, but occasionally they are spherical. If the defect is spherical, a jumbo cup may be appropriate. With oblong remodeling of the host acetabulum, options include a structural allograft with a cementless hemispherical cup, a modular trabecular metal augment with a hemispherical cup, or a high hip center hemispherical cup. The former two options are appropriate when restoration of an anatomic hip center is desired. With both the allograft and the modular augment, the goal is to provide support to a hemispherical implant that has partial inherent stability until supportive ingrowth into the cup is adequate. Advantages of an allograft include positive results that last longer than with other techniques and restoration of bone for future reconstruction if necessary. Potential advantages of a modular cup-and-augment system include less stripping of the ilium and less mobilization of the abductors, which results in a technically easier and faster procedure. Also the augment does not have the potential for resorption. Disadvantages of this method include its unknown long-term durability, the potential for debris generation at the interface, the potential for fatigue failure, and the inability to restore bone stock for future revisions.

When the hemispherical trial component has no inherent stability, the defect is classified as type IIIB. Once a pelvic discontinuity has been ruled out, options for treatment of such defects include (1) nonbiological fixation with an impaction allograft supported with a cage, or with a structural allograft (an acetabular allograft or a distal femoral allograft) supported with a cage, and (2) biological fixation with a modular trabecular metal system or a custom triflanged implant.

In the presence of pelvic discontinuity, we determine intraoperatively whether the discontinuity appears to be acute, with the potential for healing, or chronic, without the potential for healing. If healing is possible, we use a compression plate across the dissociation, as well as one of the reconstructive approaches described previously for a type IIIB defect. When there is no potential for healing, we distract the discontinuity and insert bone graft into the defect. The initial stability of the structural graft or the modular reconstruction is greatly enhanced by distraction (as opposed to compression, with which there is little chance for the host bone to bring about healing of the discontinuity).[10]

TREATMENT OPTIONS FOR ACETABULAR DEFECTS

Several options are available for acetabular revision. These options are divided into two major categories based on the type of fixation. *Biological fixation* refers to any surgical option that requires direct contact with host bone and osteointegration into the acetabular shell

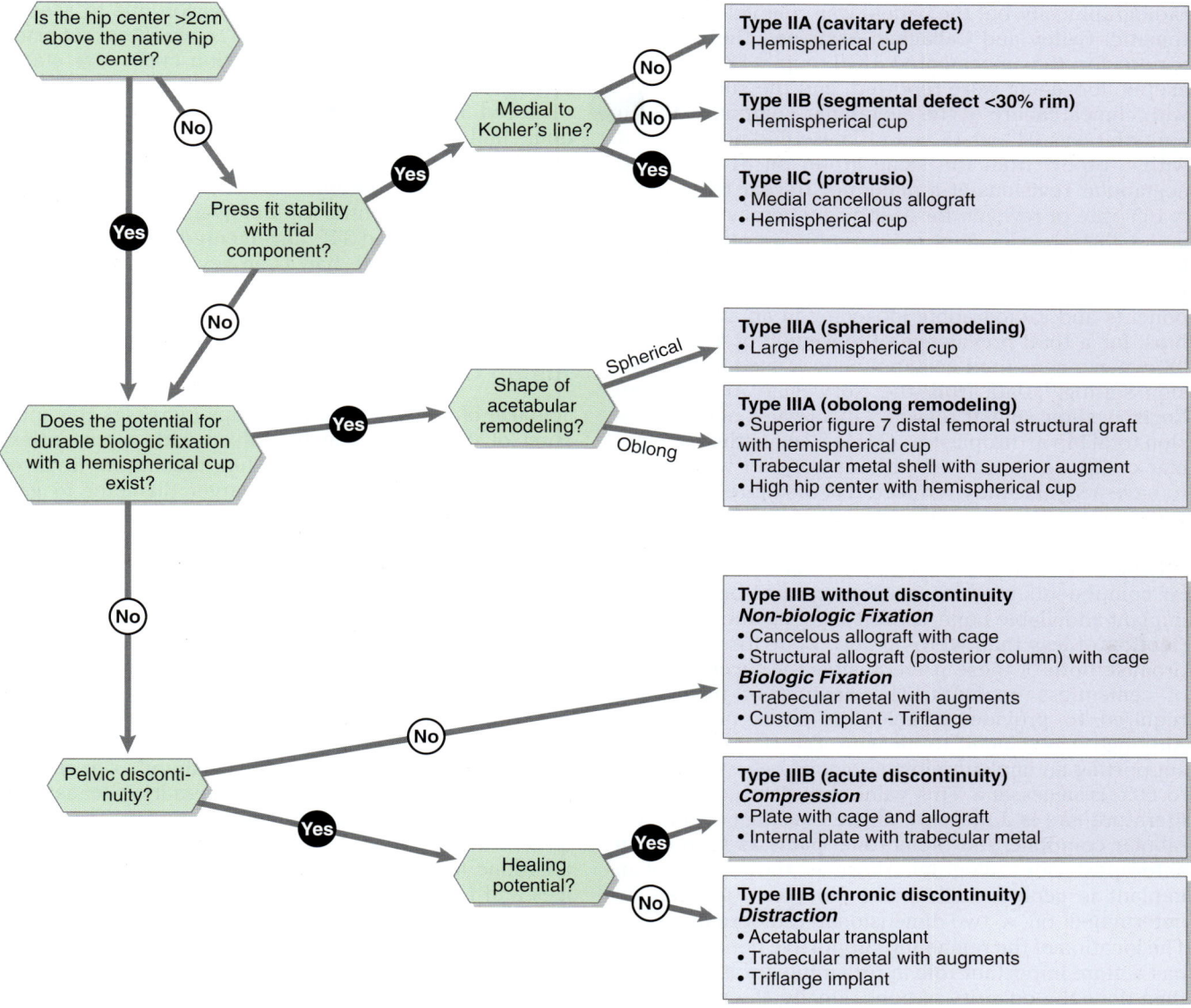

Figure 89-7. Algorithmic approach to acetabular reconstruction. *(Redrawn from Sporer SM, Paprosky WG, O'Rourke MR: Managing bone loss in acetabular revision. Instr Course Lect 55:290, 2006.)*

to provide long-term fixation. Biological fixation techniques include the use of a hemispherical uncemented cup at the anatomic hip center or a high hip center (>2 cm superior to the native hip center), a jumbo cup (66 to 80 mm), a bilobed or oblong cup, an uncemented hemispherical cup supported by structural allograft, and a modular cementless implant system. *Nonbiological fixation* refers to any method of reconstruction that achieves stability of the acetabular component through a mechanical construct without the need for osteointegration between the acetabular shell and the host bone. Nonbiological fixation techniques include cementing of a polyethylene cup, use of a superior structural allograft and a cemented polyethylene cup with or without an antiprotrusio cage, impaction grafting with or without an antiprotrusio cage, and application of a total acetabular allograft.

Hemispherical Porous-Coated Cementless Acetabular Component

Cementless biological fixation has become the preferred method of fixation in acetabular revisions because it provides a combination of good results and a straightforward technique that is applicable to most revisions. Rates of failure for cemented fixation in the revision setting have been higher than for cementless fixation. Templeton and associates reviewed 28 patients (32 hips) at 12.9 years who had undergone revision of a cemented acetabular component to an uncemented Harris-Galante 1 (HG-1) component.[11] No cases of aseptic loosening of the cup were noted. Two cups had migrated from their initial placement; one had stabilized at 3 months and was unchanged at 9.8 years, when the patient died, and the other cup had migrated radiographically, but the patient was completely asymptomatic. Gaffey and Callaghan examined their 15-year results for the uncemented HG-1 cup.[12] No cases of aseptic loosening were reported, and the survival rate with clinical failure of the acetabular component as an endpoint was 94% at 15 years. These findings contrast with a report from the same group on 81 cemented acetabular revisions at a minimum 10-year follow-up.[13] A 16% rate of revision for aseptic acetabular loosening and a 33% prevalence of radiographic aseptic acetabular loosening were noted. Estok and Harris reported re-revision of 7 (22%) of 32 cemented acetabular components and radiographic loosening in an additional 6 hips, for a total prevalence of loosening of 41% (13 of 32) when a cemented acetabulum was used in the revision setting.[14] Data from the Norwegian Arthroplasty Registry show similar results.[15] In a review of 4726 revision total hip arthroplasties (THAs), cementless acetabular components with or without allograft were found to have a significantly reduced risk of failure compared with cemented components (relative risk [RR] = 0.37 and 0.66, respectively).

Reliable and durable fixation of cementless acetabular components requires intimate contact between the implant and viable bone, as well as mechanical stability (motion of less than 40 to 50 μm). Bone loss can compromise both of these prerequisites for successful use of cementless implants. The amount of host bone required to provide durable fixation is not known. Although it is difficult to measure the amount of bone supporting an implant, most surgeons believe that 50% to 60% is necessary. This value was derived from the literature and is a measure of the coverage of the acetabular component in the coronal plane as seen on an anteroposterior radiograph. However, the support of an implant is geometrically more complex than can be determined on a two-dimensional radiograph alone. The location of the remaining supportive bone probably has a more important role in providing durable fixation than does the quantity of bone. Finally, the percentage of bone necessary to support the implant probably decreases as the implant size increases because of the increased surface area.

Cementless porous-coated hemispherical sockets have performed well and have demonstrated a low failure rate in multiple studies. Park and Della Valle have followed 138 hips in 132 patients revised with a HG-1 acetabular component for a mean of 20 years.[16] Twenty-one of the hips underwent repeat acetabular revision with the most common cause being infection (8) and instability (8). A total of 4 acetabular components were radiographically loose, of which only 1 had undergone revision. The other 3 patients died before undergoing revision. Six patients had undergone isolated liner exchanges with retention of the cup; this was recommended in 4 other patients. The 20-year survival of the acetabular component with revision for aseptic loosening or radiographic evidence of definite loosening was 95%. The 20-year survival with revision for any reason was 82%. In a study on the results of 122 cementless revisions with the HG-1 cup at an average of 12 years, Hallstrom and colleagues reported a rate of aseptic loosening of 11% and a rate of revision due to aseptic loosening of 4%.[17] Moskal and coworkers reported that 94% of 32 uncemented revision cups were stable after 3- to 9-year follow-up.[18] Lachiewicz and Poon reviewed 57 uncemented revision cups and found that none had loosened after a mean 7-year follow-up.[19] Tanzer and associates reported that 2 of 140 revision cups had failed because of aseptic loosening after a mean of 41 months of follow-up.[20] Silverton and colleagues reviewed 115 uncemented revision sockets and found that none had been revised for loosening, and 1 was radiographically loose after 7 to 11 years of follow-up.[21]

Jumbo Cups

The use of jumbo cementless cups increases the spectrum of cases that can be solved with a cementless hemispherical component. This technique involves reaming the acetabulum to a larger diameter to gain contact of the large socket against the remaining rim of the acetabulum. It was first used as an alternative to structural allograft in treating cavernous acetabular deficiencies.[22] Although the definition of the jumbo cup varies from at least 60 to 70 mm in the literature, good intermediate- to long-term success has been reported even in cases with severe bone loss.

Large porous-coated cups have several advantages over standard-size implants. The surface contact area between the component and the host bone is maximized, thereby increasing the likelihood of ingrowth. Structural allograft is often unnecessary because the defect is filled by the acetabular component. The center of rotation of the hip is more closely restored to an anatomic location because the large cup often lateralizes and lowers the center of rotation. This results in improved soft tissue tension about the hip and reduces the risk of femoral-pelvic impingement. Theoretically, this should lead to fewer dislocations.

Whatley and colleagues in a series of extra-large cups from the Mayo Clinic reviewed 89 acetabular revisions with HG-1 and HG-2 cups at a mean follow-up of 7.2 years.[23] Only 4 cups were revised: 2 for loosening, 1 for infection, and 1 for recurrent dislocation. Two other hips had radiographic signs of loosening as well. The most common complication reported was dislocation in 11 patients, of whom only 4 required surgery and only 1 required the acetabular component to be changed. The probability of survival of the acetabular component was 93% at 8 years. Patel reviewed 43 acetabular revisions with mean 10-year results treated with jumbo cups.[24] Two components were revised for loosening, and 2 other cases were complicated by dislocation. Investigators calculated a 92% survival rate using Kaplan-Meier.

Disadvantages of this technique include (1) that host bone is not restored and (2) that converting the often oblong defect to a large hemisphere requires removal of bone. However, as long as superior support, a posterior column, and at least 50% host bone contact are present, the results of acetabular revision with jumbo cups have been good.[25]

High Hip Center

An alternative to the jumbo component, which may require the removal of significant anterior and posterior column bone, is to implant a cementless hemispherical component in a superior location. This technique is most useful when the acetabular deficiency is much larger superoinferior than anteroposterior. It avoids the use of structural bone graft and places the component on native bone. Typically, the high hip center is defined as being a minimum of 35 mm proximal to the interteardrop line. Cementless fixation of the cup should be used because cemented fixation has shown failure rates as high as 50%.[26] Dearborn and Harris reported on 46 patients who underwent cementless revision THA with a high hip center at a mean 10-year follow-up.[27] They noted a 6% mechanical loosening rate and an 11% dislocation rate (5 cases, 3 of which were recurrent).

Disadvantages of this technique include the nonanatomic location of the hip center of rotation, lack of soft tissue tension, and risk of femoral-pelvic impingement, which may explain the high dislocation rate experienced by Dearborn. Other studies have shown that dislocation rates with a high hip center may not be significantly higher than with other techniques.[28] Another disadvantage of this method of treating acetabular defects is that significant leg length discrepancy can occur or can remain if the femoral component is not revised at the same time. Several authors have noted high rates of femoral failure in revision THA with a high hip center. With cemented components, Pagnano[29] noted an increased rate at greater than 15 mm superior migration, and Kelly[30] noted a 25% femoral loosening rate.

Bilobed or Oblong Cups

The acetabular defect often seen in revision arthroplasty has an oval shape. Bilobed or oblong cementless implants are an option in these situations. Oblong cups are smaller in the mediolateral and anteroposterior dimensions then hemispherical components of the same superoinferior dimension. This technique avoids removal of host bone when the acetabulum is not hemispherical. Theoretically, it decreases the risk of reaming the anterior and posterior columns and disrupting the medial wall. Advantages of this technique include an increased surface contact area between porous metal and native acetabular bone, avoidance of structural bone grafts, and the potential to normalize the center of hip rotation. Use of these cups requires that the superior aspect of the component be placed against superior host bone, and that the inferior portion of the implant be supported by the intact anterior and posterior columns.[31]

Results have been varied. Chen and Engh reported on 41 acetabular revisions in 38 patients using bilobed components.[32] Of 34 patients (37 hips) with 41 months of follow-up, 9 (24%) bilobed implants were loose or were probably loose. Factors that were predictive of failure included disruption of Kohler's line or medial wall destruction, greater than 2 cm superior migration, and undersizing of the component (defined as the inferior aspect of the component not extending to or distal to the interteardrop line). The Mayo Clinic reported their early results (mean of 5 years) using bilobed components in 38 revisions.[33] Only one revision for loosening was reported, and this patient had greater than 50% of the implant placed on structural allograft from a previous surgery. The mean center of rotation of the hip decreased from 37 mm to 25 mm superior to the interteardrop line. Harris hip scores improved from 54 to a mean of 90. Investigators concluded that in select defects, specifically, large superolateral segmental defects, bilobed implants yielded good early results. However, it was difficult to predict their use on the basis of preoperative radiographs, and the components were often difficult to insert and required special reamers or a double reaming technique. More recently, Moskal and associates used bilobed cups in 11 patients with AAOS type III defects.[34] At 5 years, no revisions or planned revisions had occurred, average leg length discrepancy decreased form 34 mm to 7 mm, and Harris hip scores improved from 36 to 85. Investigators concluded that bilobed components offer a viable option for reconstruction of AAOS type III defects without the use of a structural bone graft or cement while maximizing host bone–implant contact and restoring the native hip center.

Disadvantages of this technique include that no bone is restored for future surgeries, and these implants are difficult to insert. As was stated previously, it is also difficult to predict their use preoperatively. Last, this technique should be not used in cases of pelvic discontinuity.[35]

Impaction Grafting and Cement

Each of the techniques discussed thus far offers no benefit in restoring bone loss for later reconstruction. Impaction grafting was developed in an attempt to restore bone. This technique involves impacting cancellous bone graft into bone deficiencies and cementing an acetabular component into the impacted bone (Fig. 89-8). If peripheral segmental deficiencies are present, wire mesh is used to reconstruct the defect before bone impaction. This technique was popularized by Schreurs and colleagues.[36] In their recent study of 20- to 25-year follow-up on 62 acetabular revisions, the implant survival rate was 85% with revision for loosening as the endpoint. Kaplan-Meier survivorship for the cup with revision for any reason was 75% at 20 years. The same group described their results in rheumatoid arthritis patients undergoing revision arthroplasty with this technique.[37] Kaplan-Meier analysis showed that the probability of survival of the acetabular component at 12 years was 80% with removal of the cup for any reason as the endpoint and 85% with aseptic loosening as the endpoint.

Although the ability to restore bone is encouraging, results have not been universal because this is a technically demanding technique. Knight reported on 74 consecutive cases of primary and revision total hip

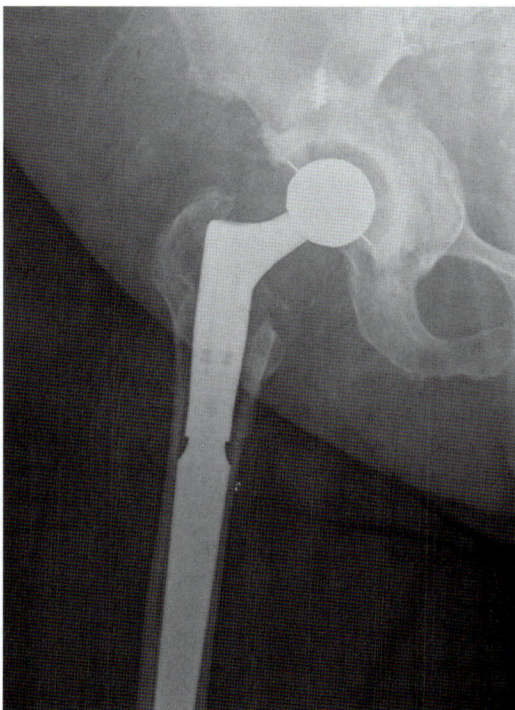

Figure 89-8. Impaction grafting of a Paprosky 2C defect with cancellous bone graft and a cemented polyethylene acetabular component. Preoperative x-rays were shown in Figure 89-4*B*.

arthroplasties.[38] Although all grafts appeared to unite, 20% of the cups were possibly or definitely loose at a mean of 40 months. The authors noted that loosening was associated with AAOS type III defects, use of allograft versus autograft, and initial cup abduction of 50 degrees or more. Kaplan-Meier survivorship analyses found 31% loosening rates and 15% revision rates at 5 years.

Outcomes of this technique seem to deteriorate with increasing bone deficiency. In a study of 71 acetabular revisions with mean follow-up of 7 years, van Haaren and coworkers found that 20 components required revision because of aseptic loosening.[39] Fourteen of the 20 failures had AAOS type III or IV defects. Overall survival of the acetabular component was 72%. Bodt, in a review of 181 cemented revision total hip arthroplasties with 173 acetabular and 79 femoral reconstructions with impaction bone grafting, noted 97% overall survival at 4 years.[40] However, investigators did not recommend this technique in Paprosky type 3 defects.

Structural Bulk Allografts

Bone defects can be filled with metal, bone graft, or bone substitute. Particulate allograft is used most frequently and may have the best potential for restoring bone loss. Structural bulk allografts have also been used with some success. These grafts are generally used for large segmental bone deficiencies, most commonly involving the superolateral acetabulum or the posterior wall and column. They have the potential to restore bone stock and appear to have a high rate of union to the pelvis.

Early results indicated that this technique was successful; however, long-term follow-up has not been as positive. Shinar and Harris, in a series of 70 primary and revision total hip arthroplasties using bulk structural graft and cemented acetabular components, reported a rate of revision or loosening of 60% at 16 years.[41] All of the grafts united; however, only 15 were allografts. Investigators also found that as the amount of the graft covering the acetabular component increased, the rate of failure increased. Twenty-one (78%) of 27 acetabular components that remained rigidly fixed were supported by graft over less than 50% of the contact area. Among components that were revised, only 9 of 25 (36%) had less than 50% coverage. Of 9 acetabular components with 30% or less of the contact area supported by graft, none were revised. Pollack and Whiteside found similar results in a series of 20 acetabular allografts performed for revision total hip arthroplasty.[42] With a minimum of 2 years of follow-up, only 7 of 20 revealed no change in the position of the cup. However, if the expectation was to restore adequate bone stock to allow reconstruction with a cementless cup, all but 3 of the revisions would be considered successes because biopsies taken at the time of revision showed viable bone.

Gross noted that the rate of failure of the cup was higher if it was supported by less than 50% of host bone.[43] Therefore he proposed using a reinforcement ring or cage in situations where the bulk allograft supports more than 50% of the acetabular component. Results show problems with the protective cages in that it does not provide biological fixation, and loosening or breakage of the cage occurs eventually. If the cage fails after 5 years, bone stock has been restored, and a cementless cup without structural grafting can be carried out.

Primary concerns with a bulk allograft include the risks of resorption and collapse over time. In a recent study of 23 hips with Paprosky type IIIA defects treated with cementless hemispherical cups and bulk distal femoral allograft, success was reported in 17 hips at a minimum 10-year follow-up.[44] Allograft resorption was noted in 8 of 23 cups. Jasty and Harris described a high rate of acetabular bone graft collapse and socket loosening when most of a cemented socket is supported by bone grafts.[45]

Antiprotrusio Cages

In patients with severe acetabular bone loss, biological fixation can be extremely difficult, if not impossible, to achieve. In these patients, when a stable uncemented hemispherical component cannot be achieved, acetabular reinforcement rings or antiprotrusio cages have been used. These devices provide a large surface area that distributes the forces of the hip joint over the remaining host bone. This large surface area also helps to resist migration of the component. Cages are able to bridge defects and protect bone graft placed behind them. They are fixed with multiple screws and provide nonbiological fixation. Therefore breakage or mechanical loosening is a large concern. The rate of mechanical failure reported in the literature varies between 0 and 15% in early and midterm follow-up studies.[46] However, decision criteria for the use of cages vary significantly in these studies. When used for larger acetabular defects, Udomkiat and Dorr reported a high failure rate when more than 60% of the superior weight-bearing bone was deficient and was filled with only cement and particulate allograft.[47] Perka and Ludwig in a review of 63 cages showed that antiprotrusio cages have a higher failure rate when used, if a large posterior column deficiency is present.[48]

As stated previously, cages have been used in association with bulk allograft. Saleh and associates reviewed 13 patients treated with structural allograft and acetabular cages.[49] Three patients had failed (1 for graft resorption and 2 for recurrent dislocation) and had undergone resection arthroplasties. At a mean 10-year follow-up, 77% (10 of 13) of acetabular reconstructions with a massive allograft and cage have achieved satisfactory results.

Cages have also been used in cases of chronic pelvic discontinuity. Berry reported on the Mayo Clinic experience with the Burch-Schneider antiprotrusio cage in 13 patients.[4] The socket remained stable in all patients, with probable healing of the discontinuity in 11 patients. Two patients had unsatisfactory results: one for recurrent instability and the other for nonunion of the discontinuity. However, Paprosky in his series of 16 pelvic discontinuities treated with acetabular cages reported a 31% loosening rate at 5 years.[50]

A new use of acetabular cages, the cup cage technique, is now being used in an attempt to restore bone stock in the most severe cases of acetabular bone loss. This technique involves bone-grafting the defect, placing a hemispherical cementless cup for biological fixation, and using a cage on top of it to provide initial mechanical stability (Fig. 89-9A and B). The cage will protect the cementless metal cup while ingrowth and stabilization occur. The cage places the articulating hip center at the correct anatomic level. Only early result are available for this technique; however, they are promising. Kosashvili and colleagues with 44 months of follow-up and with failure defined as migration of a component of greater than 5 mm reported no clinical or radiographic evidence of loosening in 23 of 26 hips treated with this technique for pelvic discontinuity.[51] The mean Harris hip score improved from 46 to 76 points at 2 years.

Highly Porous Acetabular Cups and Augment Systems

Modular highly porous acetabular systems including cups and metal augments are being used with increasing frequency. Trabecular metal (Zimmer, Warsaw, Ind) is the most widely studied of these systems although others are available. It has a high coefficient of friction. Its pore diameter is within the optimal limits for bone and soft tissue ingrowth, and it has a structural stiffness similar to cancellous bone. These properties theoretically provide excellent initial stability, extensive bone ingrowth, and minimal stress shielding. The surgical technique consists of fixing highly porous metal augments to the pelvis with multiple screws, securing the shell to the augment with a small amount of bone cement, and subsequently attaching the shell to the

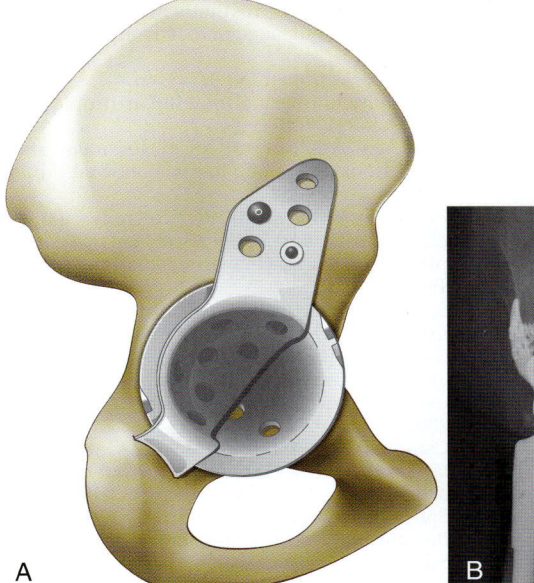
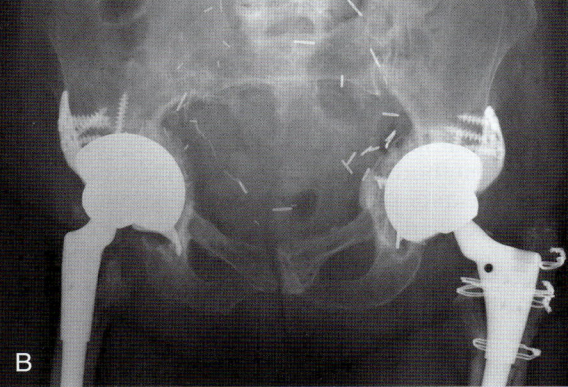

A   B

Figure 89-9. A, Diagram of cup cage technique. *(Redrawn from Kosashvili Y, Backstein D, Safir O, et al: Acetabular revision using an anti-protrusion [ilio-ischial] cage and trabecular metal acetabular component for severe acetabular bone loss associated with pelvic discontinuity. J Bone Joint Surg Br 91:870–876, 2009.)* **B,** Radiograph of cup cage technique used bilaterally for pelvis discontinuity. *(From Kosashvili Y, Backstein D, Safir O, et al: Acetabular revision using an anti-protrusion [ilio-ischial] cage and trabecular metal acetabular component for severe acetabular bone loss associated with pelvic discontinuity. J Bone Joint Surg Br 91:870–876, 2009.)*

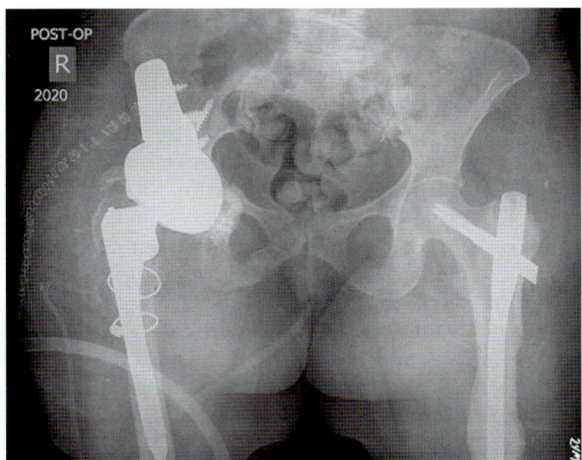

Figure 89-10. Radiograph of an acetabular reconstruction demonstrating the use of trabecular metal augments and an acetabular cup.

pelvis with multiple dome screws (Fig. 89-10). Only early results of this technique have been reported. Unger reviewed 60 patients who underwent revision total hip arthroplasties with a mean follow-up of 42 months.[52] Most cups were able to be implanted without screws. Only one case of aseptic loosening occurred, and Harris hip score improved from 75 to 94 points. Fletcher reported on 23 acetabular revisions of Paprosky type 3 defects, of which 8 had chronic pelvic discontinuity.[53] No additional plating or bone grafting was used. No mechanical failures occurred over a mean of 35 months.

Those highly porous metal acetabular components are challenging the idea that at least 50% of host bone is needed for cementless fixation without a cage. In a recent study by Lakstein on 53 revision acetabular arthroplasties performed with trabecular metal cups with 50% or less contact with native bone, only two cups required revision owing to loosening, and 2 others had radiographic evidence of loosening at 2-year follow-up.[54]

CURRENT CONTROVERSIES/ FUTURE CONSIDERATIONS

Many options are available for the treatment of bone defects in revision total hip arthroplasty. However, to determine the best method of treating these defects, a validated, reliable, and reproducible classification system should be applied. Given the complexity of these deformities, this is a very difficult task, as proven by several recent studies. Further development of an ideal classification system that can be used to better describe the defects and aid in the determination of optimal treatment methods is needed.

The relatively small number of significant or high-grade defects in a given practice makes determining the optimal treatment method difficult. To obtain better information on this, large multicenter studies and utilization of total joint registries are needed to determine longer-term outcomes. Comparison studies are also

needed because many published studies focus on one particular treatment option.

SUMMARY

Successful reconstruction of the acetabulum during revision total hip arthroplasty requires a thorough understanding of host bone defects. Although there may not be an ideal classification system by which to describe these defects, the Paprosky system can accurately predict the defect based on the preoperative AP pelvis radiograph. This system can also assist in the decision-making process of which reconstruction option to use. Currently, many defects are reconstructed using cementless hemispherical components with jumbo cups, high hip centers, or bilobed cups. Alternative techniques, including impaction grafting, bulk structural allograft, and acetabular cages, can be used with more severe acetabular deficiencies. However, as methods of cementless acetabular reconstruction have improved, the use of these alternative techniques has decreased. Modular highly porous acetabular systems are becoming very popular, and early results show tremendous promise. However, long-term results of these systems are not yet known.

REFERENCES

1. Bozic KJ, Kurtz SM, Lau E, et al: The epidemiology of revision total hip arthroplasty in the United States. J Bone Joint Surg Am 91:128–133, 2009.
2. D'Antonio JA, Capello WN, Borden LS, et al: Classification and management of acetabular abnormalities in total hip arthroplasty. Clin Orthop Relat Res 243:126–137, 1989.
3. D'Antonio JA: Periprosthetic bone loss of the acetabulum: classification and management. Orthop Clin North Am 23:279–290, 1992.
4. Berry DJ, Lewallen DG, Hanssen AD, Cabanela ME: Pelvic discontinuity in revision total hip arthroplasty. J Bone Joint Surg Am 81:1692–1702, 1999.
5. Paprosky WG, Burnett RS: Assessment and classification of bone stock deficiency in revision total hip arthroplasty. Am J Orthop 31:459, 2002.
6. Paprosky WG, Perona PG, Lawrence JM: Acetabular defect classification and surgical reconstruction in revision arthroplasty: a 6-year follow-up evaluation. J Arthroplasty 9:33–44, 1994.
7. Sporer SM, Paprosky WG, O'Rourke MR: Managing bone loss in acetabular revision. Instr Course Lect 55:287–297, 2006.
8. Gozzard C, Blom A, Taylor A, et al: A comparison of the reliability and validity of bone stock loss classification systems used for revision hip surgery. J Arthroplasty 18:638–642, 2003.
9. Campbell DG, Garbuz DS, Masri BA, et al: Reliability of acetabular bone defect classification systems in revision total hip arthroplasty. J Arthroplasty 16:83, 2001.
10. Sporer SM, O'Rourke M, Paprosky WG: The treatment of pelvic discontinuity during acetabular revision. J Arthroplasty 20(4 Suppl 2):79, 2005.
11. Templeton JE, Callaghan JJ, Goetz DD, et al: Revision of a cemented acetabular component to a cementless acetabular component: a ten- to fourteen-year follow-up study. J Bone Joint Surg Am 83:1706–1711, 2001.
12. Gaffey JL, Callaghan JJ, Pedersen DR, et al: Cementless acetabular fixation at fifteen years: a comparison with the same surgeon's results following acetabular fixation with cement. J Bone Joint Surg Am 86:257–261, 2004.

13. Katz RP, Callaghan JJ, Sullivan PM, Johnston RC: Long-term results of revision total hip arthroplasty with improved cementing technique. J Bone Joint Surg Br 79:322–326, 1997.

14. Estok DM, 2nd, Harris WH: Long-term results of cemented femoral revision surgery using second-generation techniques: an average 11.7-year follow-up evaluation. Clin Orthop Relat Res 299:190–202, 1994.

15. Lie SA, Havelin LI, Furnes ON, et al: Failure rates for 4762 revision total hip arthroplasties in the Norwegian Arthroplasty Register. J Bone Joint Surg Br 86:504–509, 2004.

16. Park DK, Della Valle CJ, Quigley L, et al: Revision of the acetabular component without cement: a concise follow-up, at twenty to twenty-four years, of a previous report. J Bone Joint Surg Am 91:350–355, 2009.

17. Hallstrom BR, Golladay GJ, Vittetoe DA, Harris WH: Cementless acetabular revision with the Harris-Galante porous prosthesis: results after a minimum of ten years of follow-up. J Bone Joint Surg Am 86:1007–1011, 2004.

18. Moskal JT, Danisa OA, Shaffrey CI: Isolated revision acetabuloplasty using a porous-coated cementless acetabular component without removal of a well-fixed femoral component: a 3- to 9-year follow-up study. J Arthroplasty 12:719–727, 1997.

19. Lachiewicz PF, Poon ED: Revision of a total hip arthroplasty with a Harris-Galante porous-coated acetabular component inserted without cement: a follow-up note on the results at five to twelve years. J Bone Joint Surg Am 80:980–984, 1998.

20. Tanzer M, Drucker D, Jasty M, et al: Revision of the acetabular component with an uncemented Harris-Galante porous-coated prosthesis. J Bone Joint Surg Am 74:987–994, 1992.

21. Silverton CD, Rosenberg AG, Sheinkop MB, et al: Revision of the acetabular component without cement after total hip arthroplasty: a follow-up note regarding results at seven to eleven years. J Bone Joint Surg Am 78:1366–1370, 1996.

22. Emerson RH, Jr, Head WC: Dealing with the deficient acetabulum in revision hip arthroplasty: the importance of implant migration and use of the jumbo cup. Semin Arthroplasty 4:2–8, 1993.

23. Whaley AL, Berry DJ, Harmsen WS: Extra-large uncemented hemispherical acetabular components for revision total hip arthroplasty. J Bone Joint Surg Am 83:1352–1357, 2001.

24. Patel JV, Masonis JL, Bourne RB, Rorabeck CH: The fate of cementless jumbo cups in revision hip arthroplasty. J Arthroplasty 18:129–133, 2003.

25. Jasty M: Jumbo cups and morselized graft. Orthop Clin North Am 29:249–254, 1998.

26. Callaghan JJ, Salvati EA, Pellicci PM, et al: Results of revision for mechanical failure after cemented total hip replacement, 1979 to 1982. J Bone Joint Surg Am 67:1074–1085, 1985.

27. Dearborn JT, Harris WH: High placement of an acetabular component inserted without cement in a revision total hip arthroplasty: results after a mean of ten years. J Bone Joint Surg Am 81:469–480, 1999.

28. Ito H, Matsuno T, Aoki Y, Minami A: Acetabular components without bulk bone graft in revision surgery: a 5- to 13-year follow-up study. J Arthroplasty 18:134–139, 2003.

29. Pagnano W, Hanssen AD, Lewallen DG, Shaughnessy WJ: The effect of superior placement of the acetabular component on the rate of loosening after total hip arthroplasty. J Bone Joint Surg Am 78:1004–1014, 1996.

30. Kelley S: High hip center in revision arthroplasty. J Arthroplasty 9:503–510, 1994.

31. DeBoer DK, Christie MJ: Reconstruction of the deficient acetabulum with an oblong prosthesis: three- to seven-year results. J Arthroplasty 13:674–680, 1998.

32. Chen WM, Engh CA, Jr, Hopper RH, Jr, et al: Acetabular revision with use of a bilobed component inserted without cement in patients who have acetabular bone-stock deficiency. J Bone Joint Surg Am 82:197–206, 2000.

33. Berry DJ, Sutherland CJ, Trousdale RT, et al: Bilobed oblong porous coated acetabular components in revision total hip arthroplasty. Clin Orthop Relat Res 371:154–160, 2000.

34. Moskal JT, Higgins ME, Shen J: Type III acetabular defect revision with bilobed components: five-year results. Clin Orthop Relat Res 466:691–695, 2008.

35. Köster G, Willert HG, Köhler HP, Döpkens K: An oblong revision cup for large acetabular defects: design rationale and two- to seven-year follow-up. J Arthroplasty 13:559–569, 1998.

36. Schreurs BW, Keurentjes JC, Gardeniers JW, et al: Acetabular revision with impacted morsellised cancellous bone grafting and a cemented acetabular component: a 20- to 25-year follow-up. J Bone Joint Surg Br 91:1148–1153, 2009.

37. Schreurs BW, Luttjeboer J, Thien TM, et al: Acetabular revision with impacted morselized cancellous bone graft and a cemented cup in patients with rheumatoid arthritis: a concise follow-up, at eight to nineteen years, of a previous report. J Bone Joint Surg Am 91:646–651, 2009.

38. Knight JL, Fujii K, Atwater R, Grothaus L: Bone-grafting for acetabular deficiency during primary and revision total hip arthroplasty: a radiographic and clinical analysis. J Arthroplasty 8:371–382, 1993.

39. van Haaren EH, Heyligers IC, Alexander FG, Wuisman PI: High rate of failure of impaction grafting in large acetabular defects. J Bone Joint Surg Br 89:296–300, 2007.

40. Boldt JG, Dilawari P, Agarwal S, Drabu KJ: Revision total hip arthroplasty using impaction bone grafting with cemented nonpolished stems and Charnley cups. J Arthroplasty 16:943–952, 2001.

41. Shinar AA, Harris WH: Bulk structural autogenous grafts and allografts for reconstruction of the acetabulum in total hip arthroplasty: sixteen-year-average follow-up. J Bone Joint Surg Am 79:159–168, 1997.

42. Pollock FH, Whiteside LA: The fate of massive allografts in total hip acetabular revision surgery. J Arthroplasty 7:271–276, 1992.

43. Gross AE, Goodman S: The current role of structural grafts and cages in revision arthroplasty of the hip. Clin Orthop Relat Res 429:193–200, 2004.

44. Sporer SM, O'Rourke M, Chong P, et al: The use of structural distal femoral allografts for acetabular reconstruction: average ten-year follow-up. J Bone Joint Surg Am 87:760, 2005.

45. Jasty M, Harris WH: Salvage total hip reconstruction in patients with major acetabular bone deficiency using structural femoral head allografts. J Bone Joint Surg Br 72:63–67, 1990.

46. Berry DJ: Antiprotrusio cages for acetabular revision. Clin Orthop Relat Res 420:106–112, 2004.

47. Udomkiat P, Dorr LD, Won YY, et al: Technical factors for success with metal ring acetabular reconstruction. J Arthroplasty 16:961–969, 2001.

48. Perka C, Ludwig R: Reconstruction of segmental defects during revision procedures of the acetabulum with the Burch-Schneider anti-protrusio cage. J Arthroplasty 16:568–574, 2001.

49. Saleh KJ, Jaroszynski G, Woodgate I, et al: Revision total hip arthroplasty with the use of structural acetabular allograft and reconstruction ring: a case series with a 10-year average followup. J Arthroplasty 15:951–958, 2000.

50. Paprosky W, Sporer S, O'Rourke MR: The treatment of pelvic discontinuity with acetabular cages. Clin Orthop Relat Res 453:183–187, 2006.

51. Kosashvili Y, Backstein D, Safir O, et al: Acetabular revision using an anti-protrusion (ilio-ischial) cage and trabecular metal acetabular component for severe acetabular bone loss associated with pelvic discontinuity. J Bone Joint Surg Br 91:87–876, 2009.

52. Unger AS, Lewis RJ, Gruen T: Evaluation of a porous tantalum uncemented acetabular cup in revision total hip arthroplasty: clinical and radiological results of 60 hips. J Arthroplasty 20:1002–1009, 2005.

53. Flecher X, Sporer S, Paprosky W: Management of severe bone loss in acetabular revision using a trabecular metal shell. J Arthroplasty 23:949–955, 2008.

54. Lakstein D, Backstein D, Safir O, et al: Trabecular metal cups for acetabular defects with 50% or less host bone contact. Clin Orthop Relat Res 467:2318–2324, 2009.

FURTHER READING

D'Antonio JA, Capello WN, Borden LS, et al: Classification and management of acetabular abnormalities in total hip arthroplasty. Clin Orthop Relat Res 243:126–137, 1989.
The original article describing the AAOS classification system.

Johanson NA, Driftmier KR, Cerynik DL, Stehman CC: Grading acetabular defects: the need for a universal and valid system. J Arthroplasty 25:425–431, 2010.

A concise review of the different classification systems and any validity and reliability testing that the systems have undergone.

Paprosky WG, Perona PG, Lawrence JM: Acetabular defect classification and surgical reconstruction in revision arthroplasty: a 6-year follow-up evaluation. J Arthroplasty 9:33–44, 1994.

The original article describing the Paprosky classification system.

Saleh KJ, Holtzman J, Gafni A, et al: Development, test reliability and validation of a classification for revision hip arthroplasty. J Orthop Res 19:50, 2001.

Describes another classification system, which may have the greatest interobserver reliability of any system to date. This system is based on an estimation of anticipated remaining bone stock following removal of a failed implant.

CHAPTER 90

Acetabular Revision:
Uncemented Hemispherical Components

Adolph V. Lombardi, Jr. and Joseph J. Kavolus

KEY POINTS

- A cementless hemispherical acetabular component has become the preferred system to employ for most acetabular revisions.
- Radiographic evidence of polyethylene wear with significant osteolysis warrants acetabular revision even in the absence of clinical or functional symptoms.
- The most critical feature of preoperative planning is careful evaluation of anteroposterior (AP) and lateral radiographs. A computed tomography (CT) scan with three-dimensional (3D) reconstructions can be extremely useful in determining the degree of osteolysis and in assisting with effective preoperative planning.
- Removal of cementless acetabular components has been revolutionized by newer extraction tools. These new devices are size-specific, blade-shaped devices that literally cut the bone at the prosthesis-bone interface.
- In revision total hip arthroplasty, press-fit fixation is compromised, and screws should be placed circumferentially around the acetabulum, where good bone stock is present.

INTRODUCTION

Revision of the acetabular component of a total hip arthroplasty (THA) poses a unique set of challenges for the reconstructive surgeon. A full appreciation of the reason for the revision will assist in preoperative planning and execution of an appropriate acetabular reconstruction. Several reasons are known for revision of the acetabular component; they include polyethylene wear with or without osteolysis, aseptic loosening, mechanical failure, recurrent dislocation, acetabular component malposition, and septic loosening. The challenges of acetabular revision are related to loss of bone stock, alteration of the hip center of rotation, and the need to achieve stability of the prosthesis. The aims of revision are (1) to reconstitute acetabular deficits with the primary goal of re-creating the anatomy and biomechanics of the physiologic joint, and (2) to achieve stable fixation while taking special precautions to preserve bone in the event a repeat revision is required.

Over the past 30 years, a cementless hemispherical component has become the preferred system to employ for most acetabular revisions.[1-3] Paramount to revision success is that the implant has initial stability to promote bone ingrowth and remodeling of the acetabulum to ensure long-term viability of the arthroplasty. Implant stability is directly related to the characteristics of the acetabular bone deficits, which, therefore, determine the specifics of the reconstruction process. A standard porous cementless hemispherical shell secured with multiple screws is the implant of choice but is feasible only with at least 50% host-bone contact. The utility of hemispherical shells is expanded by utilizing a jumbo cup with a slightly high hip center.[4-9] The recent introduction of ultraporous metal surfaces with superior bone ingrowth capability has further increased the capabilities of cementless hemispherical acetabular revision.[2,3,10-20]

INDICATIONS

The driving tenet in the vast majority of arthroplasty procedures is that the physician should operate on the basis of the patient's complaints, not the patient's radiographs. However, in acetabular revision, this is not always the case. Patients presenting with polyethylene wear with or without osteolysis may have varying degrees of symptoms ranging from none to severe incapacitating pain. The physical examination may reveal a range from normal findings to significant limp and instability with recurrent dislocations. Radiographic evidence of polyethylene wear with significant osteolysis warrants acetabular revision even in the absence of clinical or functional symptoms. Some surgeons believe that even a marginal degree of osteolysis warrants revision because radiographs underestimate the degree of osteolysis.[21-27] Computed tomography (CT) scan evaluation of patients has documented a far greater degree of osteolysis than can be evaluated utilizing standard radiographic techniques.[21-27]

Imaging studies can be combined with knowledge of the track record of specific devices. For example, a patient presenting with wear and osteolysis who has a liner of a type of polyethylene known to have a poor track record of wear should be considered for revision because this polyethylene liner is associated with significant wear and osteolysis.[28] The debate in this specific group of patients involves whether a complete component revision is necessary, or whether isolated polyethylene exchange with retention of the acetabular component should be considered. The requisites for isolated polyethylene exchange alone include an acetabular component that is well-fixed, is in satisfactory position, has a satisfactory track record for component fixation, and has a satisfactory locking mechanism or adequate size to allow cementation of appropriate polyethylene into the device. Patients should be cautioned that this liner exchange does not imply that the procedure is simple or low risk. Instability following polyethylene liner exchange has been reported to be as high as 15% in patients who have undergone the surgical procedure via a posterior approach.[29-31] The direct lateral approach has minimized this complication.[32-34] In this specific patient population, complete acetabular revision should be considered and is the required course of action in the setting of damage to the locking mechanism or the actual component itself, which precludes the replacement of a new polyethylene liner or the cementation of an appropriate liner into the component, a malpositioned component, or a migrated or unstable component that fails stability testing during the operative intervention.

Symptomatic patients should undergo a complete history and physical examination. Patients presenting with acetabular component loosening will generally localize pain to the groin, buttock, and anterior medial thigh. Pain is generally associated with weight-bearing activities. Patients frequently describe classic start-up pain, which is severe, with the first few steps, followed by a diminution of the severity of pain as the patient ambulates. On physical examination, the patient will ambulate with a limp, noting pain in the groin. Pain is generally elicited with the patient supine performing a straight-leg raise and again localizing the pain to the groin. Radiographic evaluation generally reveals radiolucent lines at the component-bone interface. These may vary from radiolucencies limited to one or two of the DeLee and Charnley zones to radiolucencies involving all three zones.[35] Radiolucencies in zones I and II are more indicative of loosening than is an isolated radiolucent line in zone III. Serial radiographs are always useful to determine the stability of an acetabular component with respect to cranial and medial migration. Further imaging studies that may prove useful are CT scans, which can critically evaluate the bone-prosthesis interface and can reveal the degree of osteolysis and osteopenia surrounding the acetabular component.

Increased utilization of alternate bearings in recent years has led to the introduction of several new indications for complete acetabular revision. In patients who have a ceramic-on-ceramic bearing, the incidence of squeaking has been reported to be anywhere from 0.2% to 21%.[36-40] A variety of causes have been described. Several reports indicate that squeaking is component specific.[36,41,42] Component malposition with associated impingement has been reported in several studies.[40,43,44] The ensuing metal transfer from the impingement or from corrosion and modular junctions may lead to metal transfer, which appears to be a cause of significant squeaking.[43,45,46] Although squeaking itself has not been shown to have any deleterious effects on the arthroplasty, if secondary to component malposition and impingement, the impingement may cause a stress riser on the femoral neck and ultimately fracture of the femoral neck.[43] Additionally, squeaking has been the sole indication for acetabular component revision in patients whose lifestyle is affected by the squeaking itself.[38,40,47]

The resurgence of metal-on-metal total hip arthroplasty has brought not only the enhanced stability afforded by large-head reconstruction, but also concerns over adverse tissue reaction to metal debris.[48,49] Two components have been withdrawn from the market[50,51]; therefore patients presenting with these components in place with any symptoms should be counseled on the possible need for acetabular revision. Symptomatic patients with metal-on-metal articulation may undergo serum metal ion screening. The Medicines and Healthcare products Regulatory Agency (MHRA) in the United Kingdom has recommended that all patients implanted with metal-on-metal devices should receive follow-up at least annually for 5 years, and more frequently if symptomatic.[52] In addition, thorough investigation of symptomatic or at risk patients should include serum ion testing of cobalt and chromium levels, with a second test performed after a modest time interval in selected patients with elevated metal levels. Cross-sectional imaging studies including ultrasound or magnetic resonance imaging (MRI) should be performed, and revision considered if imaging reveals soft tissue reactions, fluid collections, or tissue masses.[52] In light of a recent case report of cobalt toxicity in two patients who received metal-on-metal hip implants,[53] the American Academy of Orthopaedic Surgeons has warned patients with metal-on-metal devices to inform their doctor or orthopedic surgeon of any new pain or increase in pain 3 months after hip replacement surgery.[54] Patients can also be evaluated with a lymphocytic proliferation assay to determine reactivity to various metals.[49,55]

Patients presenting with acute instability with recurrent dislocation following primary hip arthroplasty should be evaluated carefully for component position. Appropriate anteroposterior (AP) and lateral radiographs maybe sufficient to determine the degree of abduction and anteversion. A CT scan may also be useful in patients with symptomatic metal-on-metal articulations. Late instability in patients who have metal-on-polyethylene articulations may be secondary to severe wear and shortening of the extremity with resultant capsular laxity. Patients may be treated with acetabular liner exchange.[32-34] Leg length can be restored or enhanced with modular head/neck exchange,[56,57] and the option for utilization of a larger head may be considered to enhance stability.[58-60]

It is imperative to rule out sepsis in all patients undergoing total hip revision arthroplasty. A careful history is important and may raise or lower the physician index of suspicion with respect to a septic process. Specifically, did the patient have any wound healing issues following the primary arthroplasty? Was the patient treated with antibiotics for wound erythema or extremity cellulitis? Are there any constitutional symptoms suggestive of infection, such as fever, chills, night sweats, etc.? Have there been any recent septic processes such as a dental abscess, upper respiratory infection, or urinary tract infection? Inflammatory markers consisting of a complete blood count (CBC) with differential, erythrocyte sedimentation rate (ESR), and C-reactive protein (CRP) should be obtained on all patients. If these inflammatory markers are abnormal, hip aspiration should be performed, not only for culture and sensitivity, but also for cell count. Recent literature documents that a synovial fluid white blood cell count (WBC) greater than 2000/mL with more than 60% poly-morphonuclear sites is indicative of infection.[61,62] An indium WBC scan may be helpful in further delineating sepsis as the cause.[63] Finally, at the time of surgical intervention, specimens can be sent for pathology testing, with a look at the number of white cells per high-power field. More than five cells per high-power field is suggestive of infection, and certainly more than 10 WBCs per high-power field is diagnostic of infection.[64]

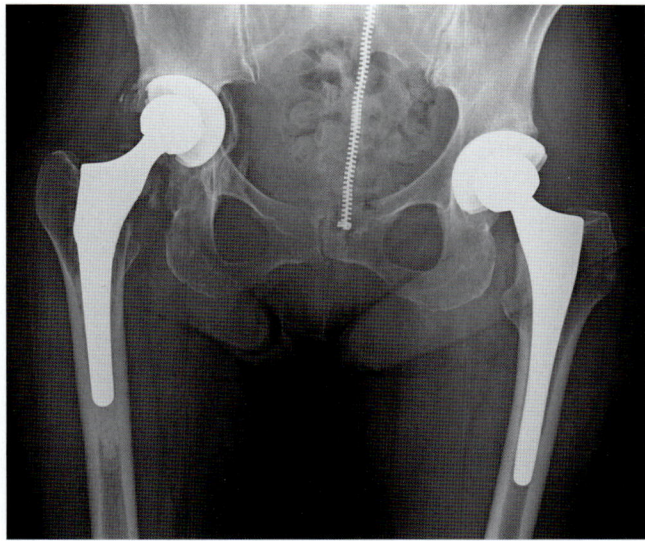

Figure 90-1. Anteroposterior (AP) radiograph of the pelvis of a 69-year-old female patient demonstrates bilateral total hip arthroplasty with acetabular findings of the right hip significant for bone deficiency in zone III, complete radio-lucency, polyethylene wear, and component migration.

PREOPERATIVE PLANNING

Paramount in planning is assessment of the severity and location of acetabular bone deficits. Managing these deficits during the reconstruction is one of the greatest challenges of hip revision. The primary aim of the surgical reconstruction is component stability. Integral to this fundamental requirement is comprehension of the current state of the acetabular bone stock. Preoperative planning starts with the basics: a comprehensive history and physical examination. Does the patient have a history of developmental dysplasia of the hip, Legg-Calvé-Perthes disease, or slipped capital femoral epiphysis? Were any nonarthroplasty surgical procedures performed, and when were they performed? The date of the primary hip arthroplasty and of any required subsequent procedures would be determined. Were there any perioperative complications? Did the primary procedure proceed without difficulty? Were there any concerns regarding the surgical site? Was the patient allowed to fully weight-bear following the procedure? If the patient was limited to protective weight bearing, for how long, and what was offered as an explanation for protected weight bearing? How long did the patient use assistive devices? How quickly did the patient feel that he or she resumed normal gait? Has the patient had any episodes of subluxation or actual dislocation? Has the patient experienced any grinding, clicking, squeaking, or other audible symptoms? The nature, location, and onset of pain should be explored.

Physical examination commences with the assessment of gait. Is the gait normal, antalgic, or Trendelenburg? Is the pelvis level, or is there pelvic obliquity secondary to a leg length discrepancy or spinal deformity? Leg length discrepancy can be assessed with the patient standing, by placing blocks of various thicknesses under the shorter extremity until the pelvis is deemed level. Alternatively, leg length can be evaluated

with the patient in the supine position. A straight-leg raise test with the patient supine may elicit pain in the groin or buttock if the acetabular component is loose. Range of motion should be assessed. Patients who are experiencing anterior dislocation may have apprehension with full extension and external rotation; those who are experiencing posterior subluxation/dislocation may have significant apprehension with flexion, internal rotation, and adduction of the hip.

Radiographic evaluation should commence with a standard AP radiograph (Fig. 90-1). The intersection of the transischial line with the proximal femur is useful in determining leg length. Assessment of the Ranawat triangle is useful in determining whether the center of rotation has been restored.[65,66] Furthermore, an evaluation of the acetabular component with respect to Kohler's line is useful in detecting restoration of the center of the head. The abduction angle can be clearly determined on the AP radiograph. Concentric circles can be used to evaluate the degree of polyethylene wear. The AP pelvis is also carefully evaluated for any evidence of osteolysis, and the presence or absence of radiolucent lines in the zones of DeLee and Charnley is noted. If available, evaluation of serial radiographs is helpful in determining whether any cranial or medial migration of the acetabular component has occurred. A lateral radiograph should be evaluated for appropriate anteversion of the acetabular component (Fig. 90-2). If further detail is required, a CT scan with three-dimensional reconstructions can be acquired to determine component position, as well as degree of osteolysis, which is often underestimated by plain radiographs (Fig. 90-3).[67-69]

The condition of the acetabulum should be graded using a radiographic classification system. The Paprosky classification is outlined in Chapter 89. The degree and

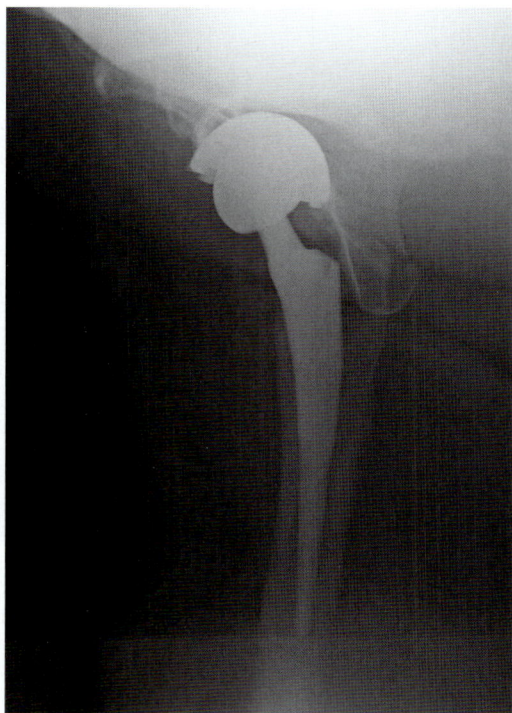

Figure 90-2. A lateral radiograph should be evaluated for appropriate anteversion of the acetabular component. In this case, the acetabular component has migrated into excessive anteversion.

severity of bone loss will determine whether three-point fixation can be attained, which is a requisite for utilization of a cementless hemispherical acetabular component. A review of the previous operative report should reveal the size of the component present and will assist the surgeon in determining the approximate size of the revision acetabular component. This information will be useful in obtaining appropriately sized components, corresponding polyethylene liners, and femoral head options. Furthermore, the need for any special equipment specific to removal of a particular implant can be determined. A treatment plan for the osteolysis should be outlined preoperatively, and appropriate bone graft material should be made available.

DESCRIPTION OF TECHNIQUE

When the decision is made between the surgeon and the patient to proceed with revision arthroplasty, appropriate medical clearance should be obtained. The patient is assessed by anesthesia staff upon arrival on the day of surgery. After successful induction of anesthesia, the patient is evaluated in the supine position to assess leg length. The patient then is placed in a lateral decubitus position with the operative extremity facing the operative field. The extremity is prepped and draped in standard fashion. Previous surgical incisions are outlined. The hip is approached by utilizing as much of the previous skin incision as possible. The actual approach to the hip will vary depending on the surgeon's preference. The most common approaches utilized are the posterior lateral and direct lateral (anterior lateral). In cases of difficult exposure, a trochanteric slide osteotomy or an extended trochanteric osteotomy may be required.[70] The senior author's preference is the direct lateral approach.[71] Upon completion of the skin incision, the fascia is incised along the line of the incision, identifying the lateral aspect of the femur. Commencing 3 to 4 cm distal to the vastus tubercle, the vastus lateralis is split along the lateral aspect of the femur (Fig. 90-4).

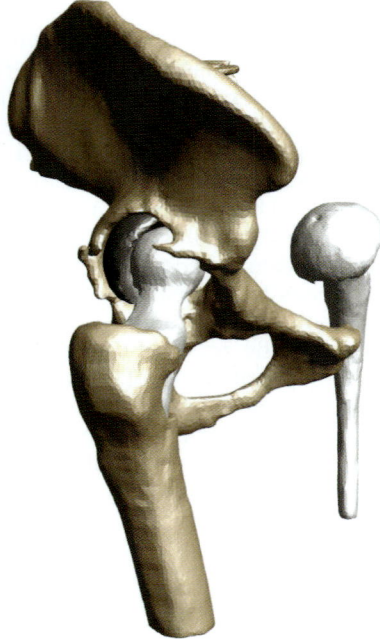

Figure 90-3. A three-dimensional reconstruction from a computed tomography scan further illustrates the extent of acetabular bone loss.

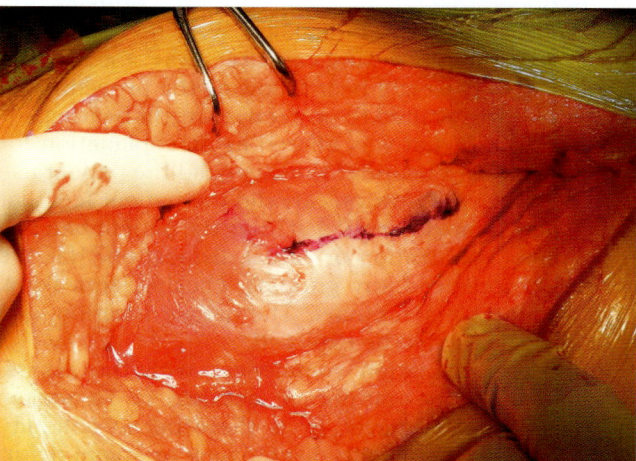

Figure 90-4. Using a direct lateral approach, the vastus lateralis is split along the lateral aspect of the femur, commencing 3 to 4 cm distal to the vastus tubercle, as shown here.

This dissection is carried proximally in continuity with the gluteus medius and minimus, elevating approximately the anterior one third of the abductors. The femoral neck of the femoral component is identified, and the capsule is incised in the direction of the femoral neck, extending superiorly to the rim of the acetabulum. Dislocation occurs with the flexion in external rotation–adduction maneuver (Fig. 90-5). Exposure is facilitated by releasing the iliopsoas tendon from the lesser trochanter, if required. If the femoral component is modular, the head/neck unit can be removed (Fig. 90-6). If the femoral component is to be removed, this procedure should be performed at this time to facilitate exposure of the acetabulum. The acetabulum is exposed by placing an anterior retractor approximately 1 cm above the pubis. A posterior sharp, long Hohmann retractor is now placed into the ischium to displace the femur posteriorly. Finally, a spike is driven in at the 12 o'clock position approximately 1 cm above the acetabular

component. Circumferential exposure of the acetabulum is required, and all scar tissue should be excised.

In the case of a cemented acetabular component, the cement-component interface can be interrupted with curved osteotomes specifically designed to accomplish this task. By separating the component from the cement, initially there is less chance to create an acetabular fracture or to unnecessarily damage the remaining acetabular bone stock. Avoid levering an instrument against the bony acetabulum to prevent acetabular fracture. This is especially critical when working in the posterior-superior portion of the acetabulum because this region of the acetabulum is vital to the subsequent reconstruction. Cement that is extruded beyond the medial wall of the acetabulum usually can be left, thereby avoiding damage to vascular, neurologic, and urologic structures. However, extraneous cement should be removed from the interpelvic region when established that its presence creates a mechanical obstruction, or that it is associated with infection. If one encounters difficulty removing the polyethylene with curved osteotomes, then the acetabulum can be removed with a high-speed burr, while cutting it in the classic pie-shaped method.[70] The remaining cement generally can be removed with osteotomes and rongeurs. Occasionally, a high-speed burr is required.

The removal of cementless acetabular components has been revolutionized by newer extraction tools. These new devices are size-specific blade-shaped devices that literally cut the bone at the prosthesis-bone interface (Fig. 90-7). They are now provided by several manufacturers. The first step requires the use of a shorter cutting blade with an appropriately sized centering ball, which corresponds to the inner diameter of the acetabular component, that is, the size of the removed femoral head. By seating this device and identifying the rim, one can circumferentially clean the rim of the acetabular component (Fig. 90-8). One can then proceed with further dissection at the prosthesis-bone interface if no screws are present. However, if screws

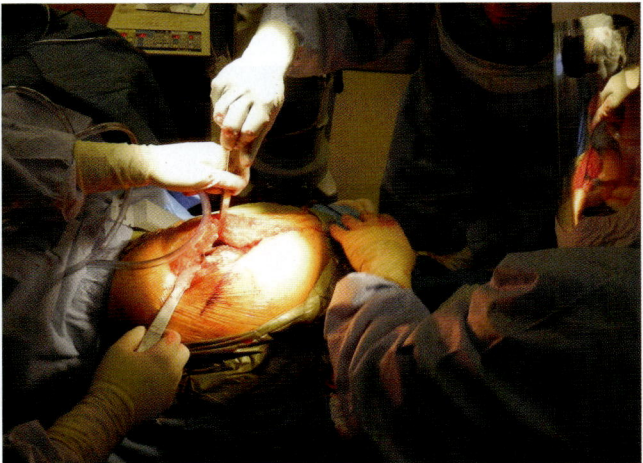

Figure 90-5. Dislocation occurs with the flexion in external rotation–adduction maneuver performed by the assistant.

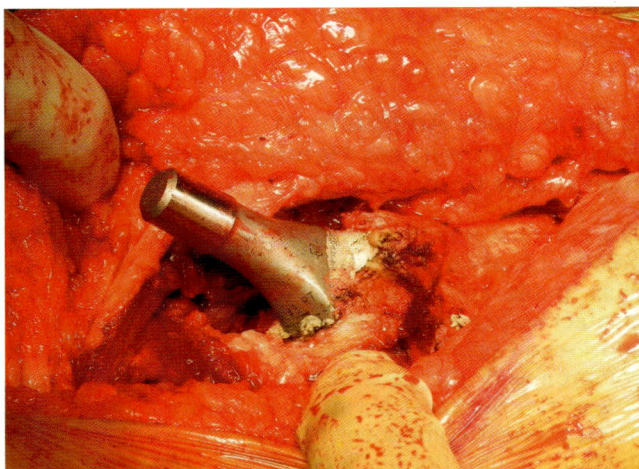

Figure 90-6. The modular head/neck unit of the femoral component is removed to facilitate exposure of the acetabulum.

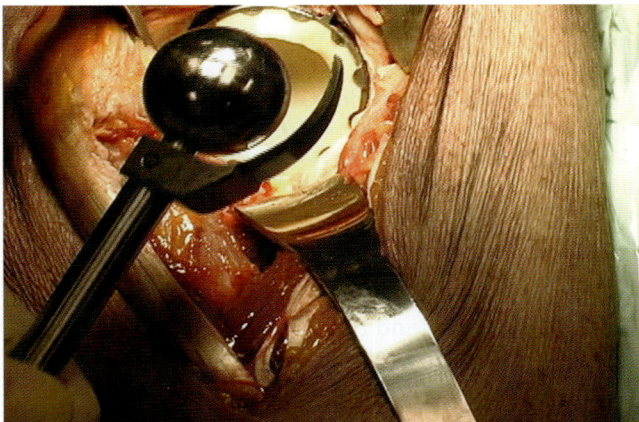

Figure 90-7. Removal of cementless acetabular components has been revolutionized by newer extraction tools. These new devices are size-specific blade-shaped devices that literally cut the bone at the prosthesis-bone interface.

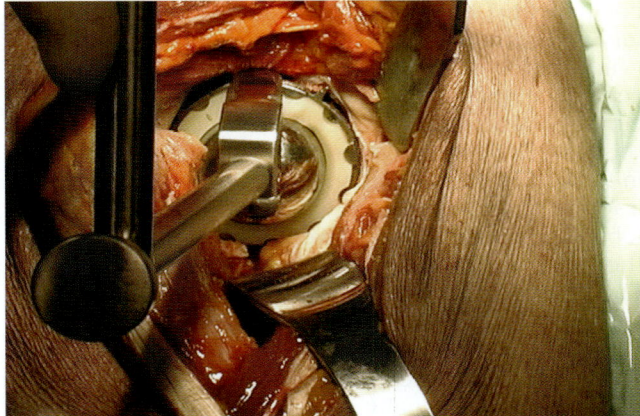

Figure 90-8. The rim of the acetabulum is identified, and the component removal device is seated. The surgeon can then clean the rim of the acetabular component circumferentially.

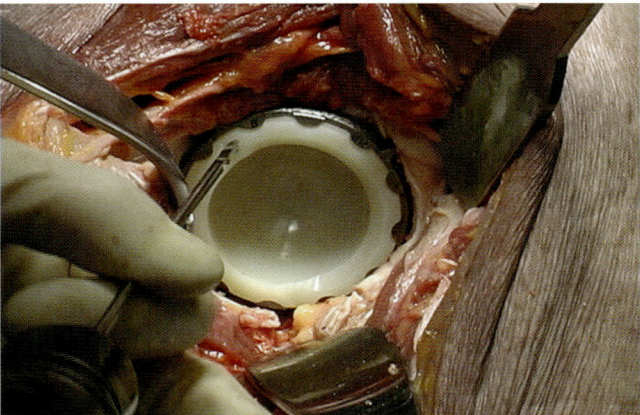

Figure 90-9. The atraumatic tool technique can be used to remove the polyethylene in the absence of a device-specific extraction tool. The first step is to drill a pilot hole with a 3.2-mm drill bit through the polyethylene at the rim to the metal of the acetabular component.

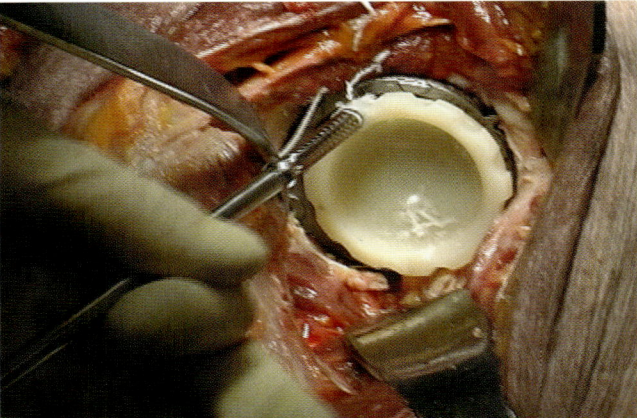

Figure 90-10. The second step of the atraumatic tool technique is to use a 6.5-mm screw on power to engage the polyethylene and, when it hits the metal of the acetabular component, force the polyethylene out. All bone screws are then removed, and the polyethylene is reinserted, to accommodate the size-specific, bladed component removal device.

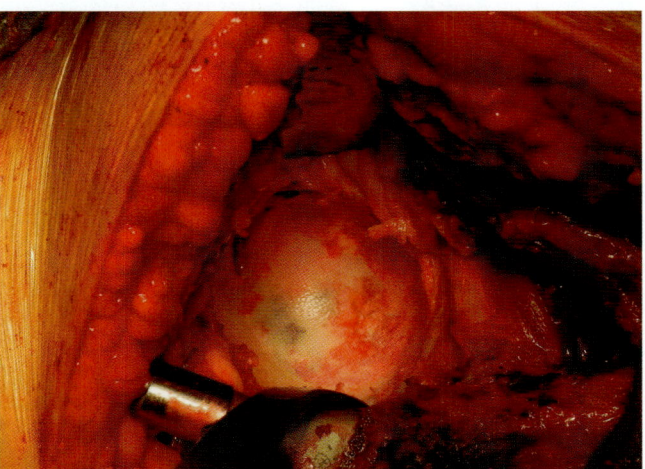

Figure 90-11. With the acetabular component removed, curettes and rongeurs are used to remove any soft tissue debris. The structural integrity of the acetabulum is then evaluated.

are present, then the polyethylene must be removed. If the extraction tool needed to remove the polyethylene is not available, one can use the atraumatic tool technique. This involves drilling a hole with a 3.2-mm drill bit through the polyethylene to the metal of the acetabular component (Fig. 90-9). A 6.5-mm screw is then used on power. The screw will engage the polyethylene, and when it hits the metal, the acetabular component will force the polyethylene out (Fig. 90-10). At this point, the screws can be removed and the polyethylene can be reinserted. One can then complete acetabular removal first with the short and then with the long blade. These devices have allowed essentially atraumatic removal of the acetabular components. More important, little to no bone is lost when these devices are used. When a broken screw is encountered, a trephine is necessary for its removal. With the acetabular component removed, curettes and rongeurs are used to remove any soft tissue debris. At this point, the structural integrity of the acetabulum should be evaluated (Fig. 90-11).

Is Bone Stock Adequate to Secure a Cementless Hemispherical Acetabular Component?

The essential requirement is the ability to obtain three points of fixation. These points include contacts in the ilium, pubis, and ischium. If the rim of the acetabulum is intact and cavitary defects are present, these may be addressed easily with morselized allograft. If the rim is compromised, the general consensus is that at least 50% of the rim must be intact to secure a cementless hemispherical component.[2,3] However, with the introduction of ultraporous components, there are some who believe that stability and ingrowth of these components can be accomplished with less than 50% of the rim.[2,3] Furthermore, the introduction of ultraporous augments has allowed for the strategic reconstruction of the rim of the acetabulum.

Once the acetabular component has been removed, the acetabulum has been assessed, and a determination made that reconstruction will be accomplished with a cementless hemispherical component, the acetabulum is reamed. The size of the initial reamer is usually the size of the acetabular component that was removed. Orientation of the reaming is critical at this juncture to avoid a significantly high hip center. Identify the pubis and ischium and the obturator foramen. By doing so, the reamer can be positioned correctly and superior component placement avoided (Fig. 90-12). A common error is to simply ream in the direction to which the acetabular component has migrated. To avoid excessive medialization of the acetabular component, identify the ilium, pubis, and ischium, and avoid seating the reamer deeper to these structures. Reaming in acetabular revision is not the same as reaming the acetabulum in primary surgery. Unlike in primary arthroplasty, the subchondral bone plate is no longer intact, and the bone is significantly osteopenic. Therefore reaming must be carried out with a gentle hand and is occasionally performed with the reamer in reverse. This allows the surgeon to identify the size of the acetabulum without removing any significant bone stock. To determine the appropriate size, the surgeon should ream until a frictional fit is obtained. However, the degree of frictional fit is somewhat less exact than in primary surgery.

Understanding the specific features of the selected hemispherical shell will assist in size determination. Important in these considerations is the nature of the cementless surface—Is it a beaded surface, a fragmental surface, an aggressive plasma spray surface, or an ultraporous surface? Are there adjunct fixation modalities such as spikes, fins, or a rimmed flare? Ultimately, manufacturing trials are used to determine the appropriate size (Fig. 90-13). In devices that are not rim-flared, the author prefers to use a component that is 2 mm larger than the trial. Once the reaming and sizing process is completed, cavitary defects are treated with morselized allograft. The author prefers to use a corticocancellous mixture obtained in various quantities from a commercial bone bank (Fig. 90-14). The graft is impacted with a combination of bone tamps and the reverse reaming process (Fig. 90-15).

Within the same series of acetabular components, most manufacturers provide solid components, cluster hole components, and multihole components. Because the quality of press-fit in revision cases is generally not as good as in primary cases, the author prefers to utilize adjunctive screw fixation. Therefore a multihole cup is almost always selected (Fig. 90-16). Attention must be paid to seating the acetabular component for optimal

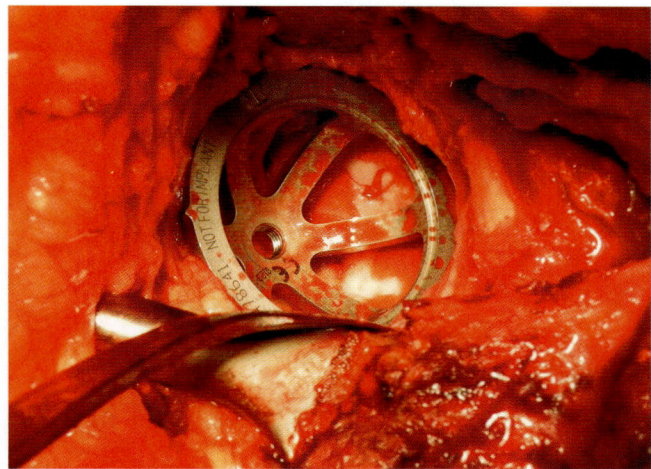

Figure 90-13. The manufacturer's trials are used to determine the appropriate size and, in this case, to assess the deficiency of the bone stock present.

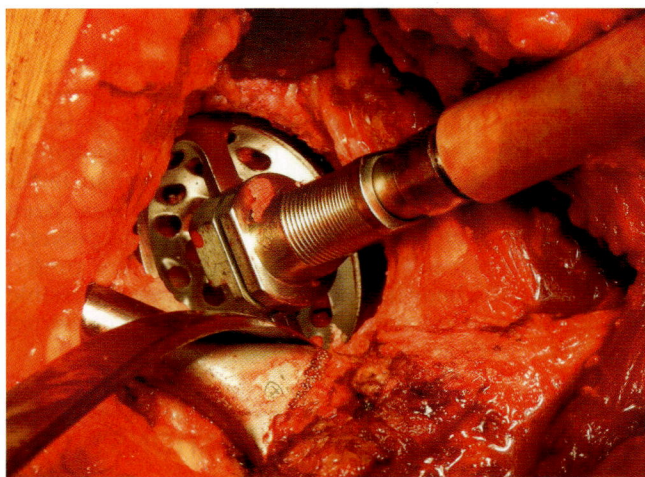

Figure 90-12. Orientation of the reaming is critical to avoid a significantly high hip center. The pubis, ischium, and obturator foramen are identified to position the reamer correctly and avoid superior component placement.

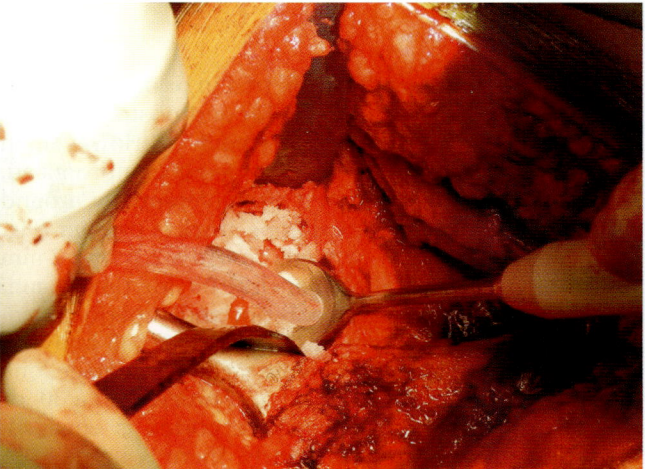

Figure 90-14. Once the reaming and sizing process has been completed, cavitary defects are treated with morselized allograft. Corticocancellous mixture obtained from a commercial bone bank is impacted with a combination of bone tamps and the reverse reaming process.

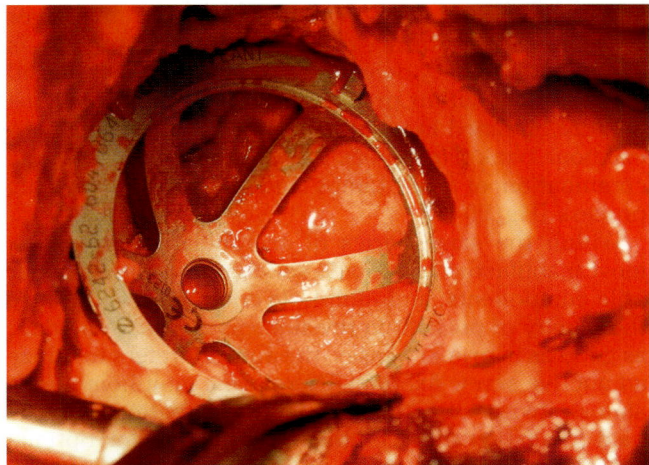

Figure 90-15. The manufacturer's trials are again placed, and reconstitution of bone stock is noted.

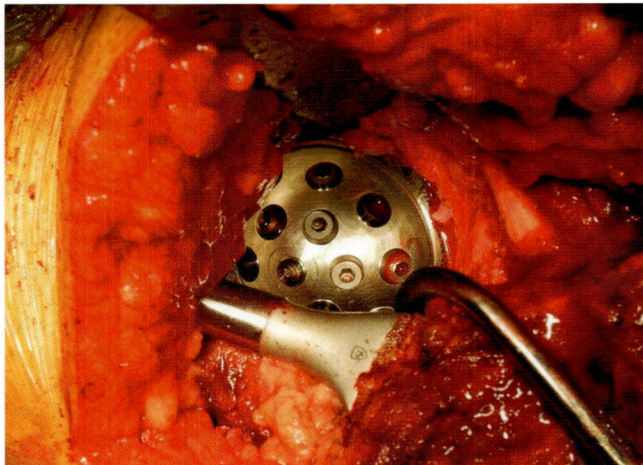

Figure 90-17. Screws are used as adjunct fixation and are placed circumferentially around the acetabulum, where good bone stock is present.

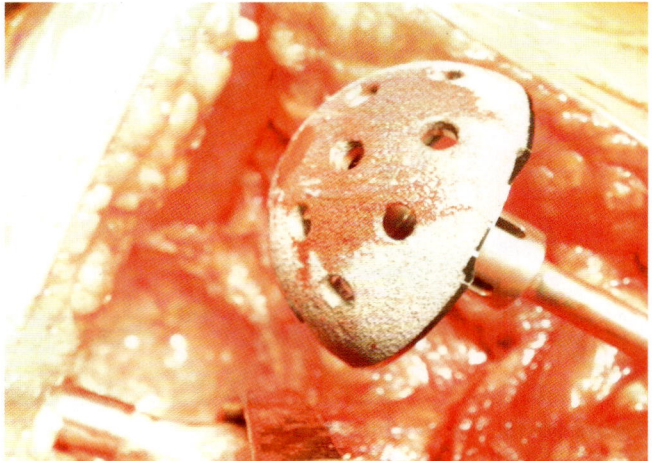

Figure 90-16. A multihole ultraporous cup is utilized in most revision cases.

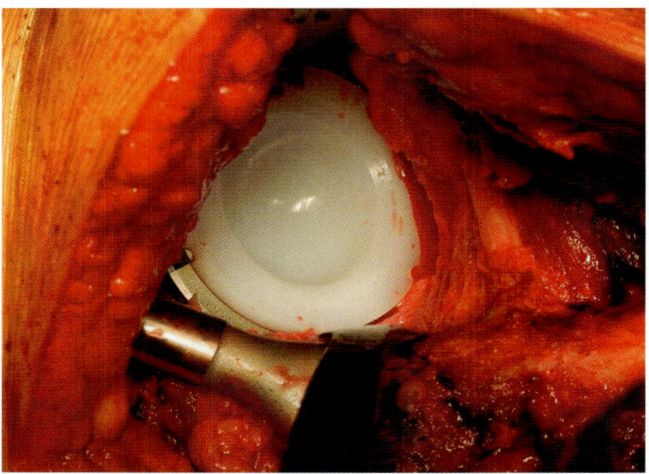

Figure 90-18. Once the acetabular component has been secured with multiple screws, the appropriate polyethylene liner is placed.

screw placement. As per the dictum in primary cementless hip arthroplasty, the superior and posterior quadrants are ideal for screw placement.[72-75] However, in revision arthroplasty, press-fit fixation is compromised, and screws should be placed circumferentially around the acetabulum, where good bone stock is present (Fig. 90-17). The senior author tends to use a 2.7- or 3.2-mm drill bit rather than a 4.5-mm drill bit for the 6.5-mm acetabular screws. In the posterior and superior quadrants, screw lengths can vary from 30 to 40 mm and sometimes even longer. To avoid vascular damage, one can start with a 20-mm drill bit and proceed to a 30- or 40-mm drill bit until the opposite cortex is engaged. Posterior inferiorly and anteriorly, there is no need to use a drill bit longer than 20 mm. In these regions where the bone may be osteopenic, occasionally the depth gauge can be used alone without drilling. In addition to placing screws in the superior and posterior quadrants, the senior author favors placement of screws into the pubis and ischium. The number of screws utilized is dependent on the degree of rim reaming, the degree of press-fit, and the quality of screw purchase. It is the author's impression that when it comes to supplemental screw fixation, more screws are better than fewer screws. Once the acetabular component has been secured with multiple screws, the appropriate polyethylene liner is placed (Fig. 90-18). It is the authors' preference to use the liner that allows for the largest possible femoral head to enhance the stability of the reconstruction (Figs. 90-19 and 90-20).

VARIATIONS/UNUSUAL SITUATIONS

Variations in the utilization of cementless hemispherical acetabular components occur when these devices are used in the presence of significant uncontained deficits. The introduction of ultraporous metal technology has

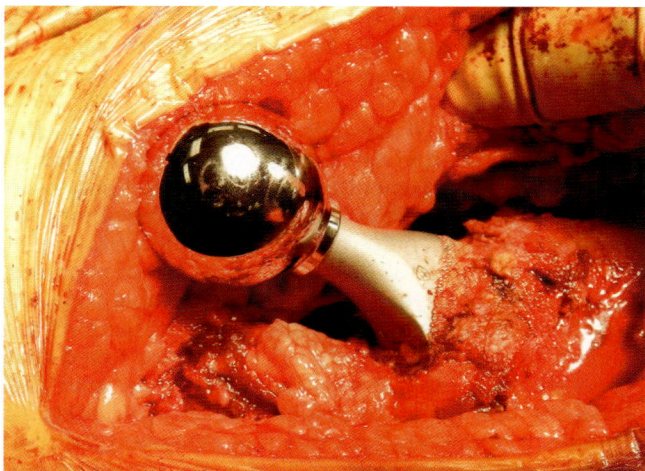

Figure 90-19. The largest possible femoral head is utilized to enhance stability.

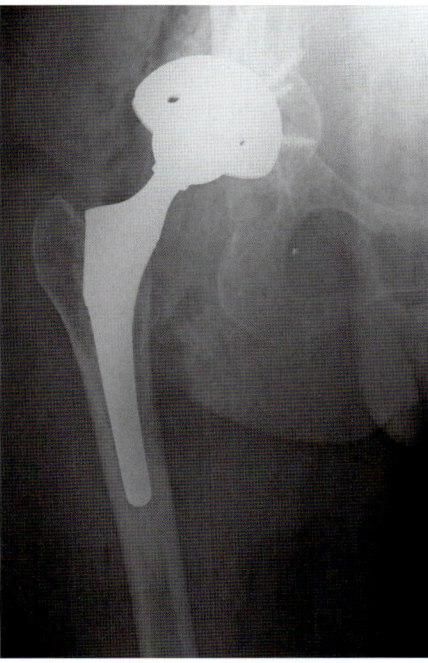

Figure 90-20. Postoperative anteroposterior (AP) radiograph of the pelvis demonstrates revision acetabular components in satisfactory position and alignment.

enhanced the ability to stabilize cementless acetabular components. Augments can be utilized to correct rim deficiencies. These augments are frequently used to reconstruct the dome of the acetabulum, and therefore are placed on the wing of the ilium to reconstruct the posterior superior support of the acetabular component. Additionally, smaller augments can be utilized in the ischium or the pubis to provide support for the acetabular component in zone III. The ultraporous cementless acetabular component with or without the combination of augments has been used to treat pelvic discontinuity.[3,16,17,20,76-80] The technique is described as a distraction technique, wherein a jumbo cup with or without augments is used to distract the discontinuity and therefore promote healing directly to the porous metal in the ilium, pubis, and ischium. The technique involves grafting the discontinuity, distracting it with a large acetabular component, and placing screws into the ilium, pubis, and ischium. Depending on the stability of the acetabular reconstruction and the degree of purchase of the screws, this construct may need to be protected with a cage placed over the cementless device.

Another variation involves complete absence of the medial wall with the rim intact. The medial wall deficit can be converted into a contained deficit with the use of mesh and then filled with a morselized allograft. A structural allograft can be contoured that is larger than the medial deficit such that it is concave on the outer surface and convex on the inner surface to match the size of the acetabular component. Generally, a large femoral head is useful for assisting with containment of a significant medial wall deficit. The final method is to contain the deficit with the use of porous metal augments. These augments can reconstruct the floor of the acetabulum. A layer of cement can be used to unitize the augments to the acetabular component, which then obtains biological fixation on the rim.

POSTOPERATIVE CARE

Postoperative management of the patient who has undergone revision total hip arthroplasty is dictated by the extent of the surgical reconstruction performed. Three main factors dictate the postoperative physical therapy and rehabilitation program: status of the wound, stability of the arthroplasty, and integrity of the prosthetic reconstruction. With respect to the status of the wound, one must be cognizant of the fact that revision arthroplasty requires a significant amount of wound dissection and therefore surgical trauma. A meticulous technique of hemostasis should be considered. The liberal use of hemostatic agents such as topical thrombin and gel foam is appropriate. The introduction of bipolar diathermia has been shown to enhance hemostasis during hip arthroplasty and therefore may be considered in the revision scenario.[81,82]

The stability of the arthroplasty as determined at the time of reduction is a critical factor in the postoperative physical therapy and rehabilitation program. The physical therapist should be apprised of any concerns regarding stability and therefore should admonish the patient with hip precautions and review techniques of transferring into and out of bed, rising from a toilet, ascending and descending stairs, riding in a vehicle, and sitting only in chairs of adequate height. The physical therapist should also be aware of the surgical approach used to perform the operative procedure. If a trochanteric osteotomy was performed, there should be an appropriate delay in the commencement of hip abduction exercises, whereas this may not be necessary if a posterolateral or anterolateral approach was utilized. Because there is ongoing concern about dislocation in revision hip arthroplasty, some surgeons have advocated the utilization of a hip abduction orthosis for the first 6 weeks postoperatively,[83,84] although this is not a universally accepted practice, and it should not be considered the standard of care.

Finally, the integrity of the surgical reconstruction is a critical factor in determining the weight-bearing status of the patient. Most patients will need to use a double limb support—a walker or crutches—for the first 6 to 12 weeks postoperatively. The actual degree of weight bearing generally commences with toe touch or protected partial weight bearing and ultimately progresses to full weight bearing over the first 3-month period at the surgeon's discretion.

RESULTS

Over the past several years, multiple published reports have documented excellent intermediate- to long-term survivorship of cementless acetabular components in revision arthroplasty.[6,7,85-96] For a standard acetabular revision, employing a porous-coated cementless acetabular component in a procedure without complications, Ito and associates reported 93% survival in 66 patients (75 hips) at an average follow-up of 15.6 years.[89] The introduction of ultraporous metal technology has further enhanced the success of acetabular revision with hemispherical devices.[8-14,17,18,20,97-99] In a direct comparison of titanium and tantalum acetabular components, tantalum implants were found to radiographically achieve better fixation and to produce better results at 6 months.[100] These results, augmented by the fact that ultraporous implants have demonstrated success in otherwise difficult revisions and maintain superior mechanical stability, explain why they are considered today's prosthesis of choice for revision arthroplasty.

COMPLICATIONS

Short-term complications of cementless acetabular component revision involve infection, dislocation, and loss of fixation. With respect to infection, it should be noted that these procedures are complex, usually requiring extended surgical times and a large array of instrumentation, which therefore enhances potential for contamination of the operative field. Factors that can minimize the incidence of infection include optimization of the patient's preoperative medical condition, meticulous perioperative planning, procurement of all necessary equipment before commencement of the surgical procedure, immediate availability of all prosthetic components, meticulous surgical technique, and appropriate perioperative antibiotics.

Dislocation remains a concern following primary and revision total hip arthroplasties but has been reported to occur more than three times more frequently in revision hip arthroplasty.[101] Meticulous attention to soft tissue dissection and, more important, repair of all soft tissues at the conclusion of the operative intervention can decrease the potential for dislocation. With the introduction of highly cross-linked polyethylene,

surgeons have opted to utilize larger femoral heads, which promote stability by increasing the range of motion before impingement and by increasing the jump distance.[1,48,102]

Loss of fixation represents failure to adhere to the principles outlined in the surgical technique section of this chapter. For a cementless acetabular component to be successful in the revision scenario, three-point fixation must be augmented with multiple-screw fixation. In a report describing 138 cementless acetabular revisions at a minimum of 15 years of follow-up, the most common complications were infection and recurrent instability.[85] A follow-up of the same study 5 years later found that reoperation for other complications such as wear and osteolysis first began to manifest at approximately 12 years postoperatively.[92] A study that evaluated the clinical and radiographic outcomes of cementless acetabular component revisions with morselized allografts demonstrated that the average time for graft incorporation was 12.5 months.[94] However, at an average follow-up of greater than 8 years, osteolysis was the most consistent complication. As was noted previously, osteolysis is a dreaded and well-accepted complication that is often asymptomatic until substantial bone loss has occurred.[21] Fortunately, in short- to intermediate-term follow-up studies, wear of polyethylene has been reduced by over 50%, and resultant osteolysis has been minimized with the introduction of highly cross-linked polyethylene.[24,102-104]

REFERENCES

1. Harris WH: An integrated solution to acetabular revision surgery. Clin Orthop Relat Res 453:178–182, 2006.
2. Issack PS, Nousiainen M, Beksac B, et al: Acetabular component revision in total hip arthroplasty. Part I. Cementless shells. Am J Orthop 38:509–514, 2009.
3. Issack PS, Nousiainen M, Beksac B, et al: Acetabular component revision in total hip arthroplasty. Part II. Management of major bone loss and pelvic discontinuity. Am J Orthop 38:550–556, 2009.
4. Bozic KJ, Freiberg AA, Harris WH: The high hip center. Clin Orthop Relat Res 420:101–105, 2004.
5. Dearborn JT, Harris WH: High placement of an acetabular component inserted without cement in a revision total hip arthroplasty: results after a mean of ten years. J Bone Joint Surg Am 81:469–480, 1999.
6. Hendricks KJ, Harris WH: High placement of noncemented acetabular components in revision total hip arthroplasty: a concise follow-up, at a minimum of fifteen years, of a previous report. J Bone Joint Surg Am 88:2231–2236, 2006.
7. Hendricks KJ, Harris WH: Revision of failed acetabular components with use of so-called jumbo noncemented components: a concise follow-up of a previous report. J Bone Joint Surg Am 88:559–563, 2006.
8. Gustke KA: Jumbo cup or high hip center: is bigger better? J Arthroplasty 19(4 Suppl 1):120–123, 2004.
9. Whaley AL, Berry DJ, Harmsen WS: Extra-large uncemented hemispherical acetabular components for revision total hip arthroplasty. J Bone Joint Surg Am 83:1352–1357, 2001.
10. Bourne RB, McCalden RW, Naudie D, et al: The next generation of acetabular shell design and bearing surfaces. Orthopedics 31(12 Suppl 2):ii, 2008 (orthosupersite.com/view.asp?rID=37179).
11. Fernández-Fairen M, Murcia A, Blanco A, et al: Revision of failed total hip arthroplasty acetabular cups to porous tantalum components: a 5-year follow-up study. J Arthroplasty 25:865–872, 2010.

12. Flecher X, Paprosky W, Grillo JC, et al: Do tantalum components provide adequate primary fixation in all acetabular revisions? Orthop Traumatol Surg Res 96:235–241, 2010.

13. Flecher X, Sporer S, Paprosky W: Management of severe bone loss in acetabular revision using a trabecular metal shell. J Arthroplasty 23:949–955, 2008.

14. Kim WY, Greidanus NV, Duncan CP, et al: Porous tantalum uncemented acetabular shells in revision total hip replacement: two to four year clinical and radiographic results. Hip Int 18:17–22, 2008.

15. Klika AK, Murray TG, Darwiche H, Barsoum WK: Options for acetabular fixation surfaces. J Long Term Eff Med Implants 17:187–192, 2007.

16. Kosashvili Y, Safir O, Backstein D, et al: Salvage of failed acetabular cages by nonbuttressed trabecular metal cups. Clin Orthop Relat Res 468:466–471, 2010.

17. Kosashvili Y, Backstein D, Safir O, et al: Acetabular revision using an anti-protrusion (ilio-ischial) cage and trabecular metal acetabular component for severe acetabular bone loss associated with pelvic discontinuity. J Bone Joint Surg Br 91:870–876, 2009.

18. Lachiewicz PF, Soileau ES: Tantalum components in difficult acetabular revisions. Clin Orthop Relat Res 468:454–458, 2010.

19. Lakstein D, Backstein D, Safir O, et al: Trabecular metal cups for acetabular defects with 50% or less host bone contact. Clin Orthop Relat Res 467:2318–2324, 2009.

20. Sporer SM, Paprosky WG: Acetabular revision using a trabecular metal acetabular component for severe acetabular bone loss associated with a pelvic discontinuity. J Arthroplasty 21(6 Suppl 2):87–90, 2006.

21. Chiang PP, Burke DW, Freiberg AA, Rubash HE: Osteolysis of the pelvis: evaluation and treatment. Clin Orthop Relat Res 417:164–174, 2003.

22. Claus AM, Engh CA, Jr, Sychterz CJ, et al: Radiographic definition of pelvic osteolysis following total hip arthroplasty. J Bone Joint Surg Am 85:1519–1526, 2003.

23. Claus AM, Walde TA, Leung SB, et al: Management of patients with acetabular socket wear and pelvic osteolysis. J Arthroplasty 18(3 Suppl 1):112–117, 2003.

24. Mall NA, Nunley RM, Zhu JJ, et al: The incidence of acetabular osteolysis in young patients with conventional versus highly crosslinked polyethylene. Clin Orthop Relat Res 469:372–381, 2011.

25. Walde TA, Mohan V, Leung S, Engh CA, Sr: Sensitivity and specificity of plain radiographs for detection of medial-wall perforation secondary to osteolysis. J Arthroplasty 20:20–24, 2005.

26. Walde TA, Weiland DE, Leung SB, et al: Comparison of CT, MRI, and radiographs in assessing pelvic osteolysis: a cadaveric study. Clin Orthop Relat Res 437:138–144, 2005.

27. Noordin S, Masri BA, Duncan CP, Garbuz DS: Acetabular bone loss in revision total hip arthroplasty: principles and techniques. Instr Course Lect 59:27–36, 2010.

28. Huddleston JI, Harris AH, Atienza CA, Woolson ST: Hylamer vs conventional polyethylene in primary total hip arthroplasty: a long-term case-control study of wear rates and osteolysis. J Arthroplasty 25:203–207, 2010.

29. Boucher HR, Lynch C, Young AM, et al: Dislocation after polyethylene liner exchange in total hip arthroplasty. J Arthroplasty 18:654–657, 2003.

30. Griffin WL, Fehring TK, Mason JB, et al: Early morbidity of modular exchange for polyethylene wear and osteolysis. J Arthroplasty 19(7 Suppl 2):61–66, 2004.

31. Lachiewicz PF, Soileau E, Ellis J: Modular revision for recurrent dislocation of primary or revision total hip arthroplasty. J Arthroplasty 19:424–429, 2004.

32. O'Brien JJ, Burnett RS, McCalden RW, et al: Isolated liner exchange in revision total hip arthroplasty: clinical results using the direct lateral surgical approach. J Arthroplasty 19:414–423, 2004.

33. Smith TM, Berend KR, Lombardi AV, Jr, et al: Isolated liner exchange using the anterolateral approach is associated with a low risk of dislocation. Clin Orthop Relat Res 441:221–226, 2005.

34. Wade FA, Rapuri VR, Parvizi J, Hozack WJ: Isolated acetabular polyethylene exchange through the anterolateral approach. J Arthroplasty 19:498–500, 2004.

35. DeLee JG, Charnley J: Radiological demarcation of cemented sockets in total hip replacement. Clin Orthop Relat Res 121:20–32, 1976.

36. Keurentjes JC, Kuipers RM, Wever DJ, Schreurs BW: High incidence of squeaking in THAs with alumina ceramic-on-ceramic bearings. Clin Orthop Relat Res 466:1438–1443, 2008.

37. Mai K, Verioti C, Ezzet KA, et al: Incidence of "squeaking" after ceramic-on-ceramic total hip arthroplasty. Clin Orthop Relat Res 468:413–417, 2010.

38. Restrepo C, Matar WY, Parvizi J, et al: Natural history of squeaking after total hip arthroplasty. Clin Orthop Relat Res 468:2340–2345, 2010.

39. Schroder D, Bornstein L, Bostrom MP, et al: Ceramic-on-ceramic total hip arthroplasty: incidence of instability and noise. Clin Orthop Relat Res 469:437–442, 2011.

40. Walter WL, Yeung E, Esposito C: A review of squeaking hips. J Am Acad Orthop Surg 18:319–326, 2010.

41. Restrepo C, Post ZD, Kai B, Hozack WJ: The effect of stem design on the prevalence of squeaking following ceramic-on-ceramic bearing total hip arthroplasty. J Bone Joint Surg Am 92:550–557, 2010.

42. Swanson TV, Peterson DJ, Seethala R, et al: Influence of prosthetic design on squeaking after ceramic-on-ceramic total hip arthroplasty. J Arthroplasty 25(6 Suppl):36–42, 2010.

43. Affatato S, Traina F, Mazzega-Fabbro C, et al: Is ceramic-on-ceramic squeaking phenomenon reproducible in vitro? A long-term simulator study under severe conditions. J Biomed Mater Res B Appl Biomater 91:264–271, 2009.

44. Walter WL, O'Toole GC, Walter WK, et al: Squeaking in ceramic-on-ceramic hips: the importance of acetabular component orientation. J Arthroplasty 22:496–503, 2007.

45. Chevillotte C, Trousdale RT, Chen Q, et al: The 2009 Frank Stinchfield Award. "Hip squeaking": a biomechanical study of ceramic-on-ceramic bearing surfaces. Clin Orthop Relat Res 468:345–350, 2010.

46. Taylor S, Manley MT, Sutton K: The role of stripe wear in causing acoustic emissions from alumina ceramic-on-ceramic bearings. J Arthroplasty 22(7 Suppl 3):47–51, 2007.

47. Matar WY, Restrepo C, Parvizi J, et al: Revision hip arthroplasty for ceramic-on-ceramic squeaking hips does not compromise the results. J Arthroplasty 25(6 Suppl):81–86, 2010.

48. Lombardi AV, Jr, Skeels MD, Berend KR, et al: Do large heads enhance stability and restore native anatomy in primary total hip arthroplasty? Clin Orthop Relat Res 469:1547–1543, 2011.

49. Jacobs JJ, Urban RM, Hallab NJ, et al: Metal-on-metal bearing surfaces. J Am Acad Orthop Surg 17:69–76, 2009.

50. U.S. Food and Drug Administration (FDA): Class 2 Recall Durom cup, 2008 Sep 26 (http://www.accessdata.fda.gov/scripts/cdrh/cfdocs/cfres/res.cfm?id=72719). Accessed November 8, 2010.

51. U.S. Food and Drug Administration (FDA): Class 2 Recall DePuy ASR acetabular implant, 2010 Jul 17 (http://www.accessdata.fda.gov/scripts/cdrh/cfdocs/cfres/res.cfm?id=91225). Accessed November 8, 2010.

52. Medicines and Healthcare products Regulatory Agency (MHRA): Medical device alert: all metal-on-metal (MoM) hip replacements (MDA/2010/033), 2010 Apr 22 (http://www.mhra.gov.uk/Publications/Safetywarnings/MedicalDeviceAlerts/CON079157). Accessed November 4, 2010.

53. Tower SS: Arthroprosthetic cobaltism: neurological and cardiac manifestations in two patients with metal-on-metal arthroplasty. J Bone Joint Surg Am 89:1–5, 2010.

54. American Association of Orthopaedic Surgeons: Metal-on-metal hip replacementorthopaedic surgeons provide awareness and information to patients, medical community at-large, 2010 Oct 29 (http://www6.aaos.org/news/pemr/releases/release.cfm?releasenum=934). Accessed November 8, 2010.

55. Hallab NJ, Mikecz K, Jacobs JJ: A triple assay technique for the evaluation of metal-induced, delayed-type hypersensitivity responses in patients with or receiving total joint arthroplasty. J Biomed Mater Res 53:480–489, 2000.

56. Jones DL, Vigna F, Barrack RL: The use of modularity in revision total hip replacement. Am J Orthop 30:297–302, 2001.

57. McCarthy JC, Bono JV, O'Donnell PJ: Custom and modular components in primary total hip replacement. Clin Orthop Relat Res 344:162–171, 1997.

58. Amstutz HC, Le Duff MJ, Beaulé PE: Prevention and treatment of dislocation after total hip replacement using large diameter balls. Clin Orthop Relat Res 429:108–116, 2004.

59. Sikes CV, Lai LP, Schreiber M, et al: Instability after total hip arthroplasty: treatment with large femoral heads vs constrained liners. J Arthroplasty 23(7 Suppl):59–63, 2008.

60. Skeels MD, Berend KR, Lombardi AV Jr: The dislocator, early and late: the role of large heads. Orthopedics 32:ii, 2009 (orthosupersite.com/view.asp?rID=42837).

61. Deirmengian C, Hallab N, Tarabishy A, et al: Synovial fluid biomarkers for periprosthetic infection. Clin Orthop Relat Res 468:2017–2023, 2010.

62. Mason JB, Fehring TK, Odum SM, et al: The value of white blood cell counts before revision total knee arthroplasty. J Arthroplasty 18:1038–1043, 2003. (Erratum in: J Arthroplasty 24:1293, 2009.)

63. Love C, Marwin SE, Tomas MB, et al: Diagnosing infection in the failed joint replacement: a comparison of coincidence detection 18F-FDG and 111In-labeled leukocyte/99mTc-sulfur colloid marrow imaging. J Nucl Med 45:1864–1871, 2004.

64. Lonner JH, Desai P, Dicesare PE, et al: The reliability of analysis of intraoperative frozen sections for identifying active infection during revision hip or knee arthroplasty. J Bone Joint Surg Am 78:1553–1558, 1996.

65. Ranawat CS, Dorr LD, Inglis AE: Total hip arthroplasty in protrusio acetabuli of rheumatoid arthritis. J Bone Joint Surg Am 62:1059–1065, 1980.

66. Dorr LD, Tawakkol S, Moorthy M, et al: Medial protrusio technique for placement of a porous-coated, hemispherical acetabular component without cement in a total hip arthroplasty in patients who have acetabular dysplasia. J Bone Joint Surg Am 81:83–92, 1999.

67. Egawa H, Ho H, Hopper RH, Jr, et al: Computed tomography assessment of pelvic osteolysis and cup-lesion interface involvement with a press-fit porous-coated acetabular cup. J Arthroplasty 24:233–239, 2009.

68. Garcia-Cimbrelo E, Tapia M, Martin-Hervas C: Multislice computed tomography for evaluating acetabular defects in revision THA. Clin Orthop Relat Res 463:138–143, 2007.

69. Howie DW, Neale SD, Stamenkov R, et al: Progression of acetabular periprosthetic osteolytic lesions measured with computed tomography. J Bone Joint Surg Am 89:1818–1825, 2007.

70. Lombardi AV, Jr: Cement removal in revision total hip arthroplasty. Semin Arthroplasty 3:264–272, 1992.

71. Lombardi AV, Jr, Berend KR: Surgical approach to the hip: direct lateral. In Hozack WJ, Parvizi J, Bender B, editors: Surgical treatment of hip arthritis: reconstruction, replacement, and revision, Philadelphia, 2009, Saunders Elsevier, pp 272–277.

72. Liu Q, Zhou YX, Xu HJ, et al: Safe zone for transacetabular screw fixation in prosthetic acetabular reconstruction of high developmental dysplasia of the hip. J Bone Joint Surg Am 91:2880–2885, 2009.

73. Meldrum R, Johansen RL: Safe screw placement in acetabular revision surgery. J Arthroplasty 16:953–960, 2001.

74. Wasielewski RC, Cooperstein LA, Kruger MP, Rubash HE: Acetabular anatomy and the transacetabular fixation of screws in total hip arthroplasty. J Bone Joint Surg Am 72:501–508, 1990.

75. Wasielewski RC, Galat DD, Sheridan KC, Rubash HE: Acetabular anatomy and transacetabular screw fixation at the high hip center. Clin Orthop Relat Res 438:171–176, 2005.

76. Ballester Alfaro JJ, Sueiro Fernández J: Trabecular metal buttress augment and the trabecular metal cup-cage construct in revision hip arthroplasty for severe acetabular bone loss and pelvic discontinuity. Hip Int 27(Suppl 7):119–127, 2010.

77. Nehme A, Lewallen DG, Hanssen AD: Modular porous metal augments for treatment of severe acetabular bone loss during revision hip arthroplasty. Clin Orthop Relat Res 429:201–208, 2004.

78. Paprosky WG, O'Rourke M, Sporer SM: The treatment of acetabular bone defects with an associated pelvic discontinuity. Clin Orthop Relat Res 441:216–220, 2005.

79. Siegmeth A, Duncan CP, Masri BA, et al: Modular tantalum augments for acetabular defects in revision hip arthroplasty. Clin Orthop Relat Res 467:199–205, 2009.

80. Van Kleunen JP, Lee GC, Lementowski PW, et al: Acetabular revisions using trabecular metal cups and augments. J Arthroplasty 24(6 Suppl):64–68, 2009.

81. Morris MJ, Berend KR, Lombardi AV Jr: Hemostasis in anterior supine intermuscular total hip arthroplasty: pilot study comparing standard electrocautery and a bipolar sealer. Surg Technol Int 20:352–356, 2010.

82. Ulrich SD, Kyle B, Johnson AJ, et al: Strategies to reduce blood loss in lower extremity total joint arthroplasty. Surg Technol Int 20:341–347, 2010.

83. Mallory TH, Vaughn BK, Lombardi AV, Jr, Kraus TJ: Prophylactic use of a hip cast-brace following primary and revision total hip arthroplasty. Orthop Rev 17:178–183, 1988.

84. Dorr LD: Bracing after revision THA: essential, expedient, and economical. Orthopedics 24:228, 2001.

85. Della Valle CJ, Shuaipaj T, Berger RA, et al: Revision of the acetabular component without cement after total hip arthroplasty: a concise follow-up, at fifteen to nineteen years, of a previous report. J Bone Joint Surg Am 87:1795–1800, 2005.

86. Della Valle CJ, Berger RA, Rosenberg AG, Galante JO: Cementless acetabular reconstruction in revision total hip arthroplasty. Clin Orthop Relat Res 420:96–100, 2004.

87. Fabi D, Gonzalez M, Goldstein W, Ahmed M: Acetabular cup revision with the use of the medial protrusio technique at an average follow-up of 6.6 years. J Arthroplasty 25:197–202, 2010.

88. Ito H, Matsuno T, Aoki Y, Minami A: Acetabular components without bulk bone graft in revision surgery: a 5- to 13-year follow-up study. J Arthroplasty 18:134–139, 2003.

89. Ito H, Tanino H, Yamanaka Y, et al: Porous-coated cementless acetabular components without bulk bone graft in revision surgery. J Arthroplasty 25:1307–1310, 2010.

90. Lakemeier S, Aurand G, Timmesfeld N, et al: Results of the cementless Plasmacup in revision total hip arthroplasty: a retrospective study of 72 cases with an average follow-up of eight years. BMC Musculoskelet Disord 11:101, 2010.

91. Leopold SS, Rosenberg AG, Bhatt RD, et al: Cementless acetabular revision: evaluation at an average of 10.5 years. Clin Orthop Relat Res 369:179–186, 1999.

92. Park DK, Della Valle CJ, Quigley L, et al: Revision of the acetabular component without cement: a concise follow-up, at twenty to twenty-four years, of a previous report. J Bone Joint Surg Am 91:350–355, 2009. (Erratum in: J Bone Joint Surg Am 91:2931, 2009.)

93. Sudo A, Hasegawa M, Fukuda A, et al: Acetabular reconstruction using a cementless cup and hydroxyapatite granules: 3- to 8-year clinical results. J Arthroplasty 22:828–832, 2007.

94. Sun C, Lian YY, Jin YH, et al: Clinical and radiographic assessment of cementless acetabular revision with morsellised allografts. Int Orthop 33:1525–1530, 2009.

95. Templeton JE, Callaghan JJ, Goetz DD, et al: Revision of a cemented acetabular component to a cementless acetabular component: a ten to fourteen-year follow-up study. J Bone Joint Surg Am 83:1706–1711, 2001.

96. Traina F, Giardina F, De Clerico M, Toni A: Structural allograft and primary press-fit cup for severe acetabular deficiency: a minimum 6-year follow-up study. Int Orthop 29:135–139, 2005.

97. Simon JP, Bellemans J: Clinical and radiological evaluation of modular trabecular metal acetabular cups: short-term results in 64 hips. Acta Orthop Belg 75:623–630, 2009.

98. Unger AS, Lewis RJ, Gruen T: Evaluation of a porous tantalum uncemented acetabular cup in revision total hip arthroplasty: clinical and radiological results of 60 hips. J Arthroplasty 20:1002–1009, 2005.

99. Weeden SH, Schmidt RH: The use of tantalum porous metal implants for Paprosky 3A and 3B defects. J Arthroplasty 22(6 Suppl 2):151–155, 2007.

100. Jafari SM, Bender B, Coyle C, et al: Do tantalum and titanium cups show similar results in revision hip arthroplasty? Clin Orthop Relat Res 468:459–465, 2010.

101. Phillips CB, Barrett JA, Losina E, et al: Incidence rates of dislocation, pulmonary embolism, and deep infection during the first six months after elective total hip replacement. J Bone Joint Surg Am 85:20–26, 2003.

102. Kelly NH, Rajadhyaksha AD, Wright TM, et al: High stress conditions do not increase wear of thin highly crosslinked UHMWPE. Clin Orthop Relat Res 468:418–423, 2010.

103. Digas G, Kärrholm J, Thanner J, Herberts P: 5-year experience of highly cross-linked polyethylene in cemented and uncemented sockets: two randomized studies using radiostereometric analysis. Acta Orthop 78:746–754, 2007.

104. Mutimer J, Devane PA, Adams K, Horne JG: Highly crosslinked polyethylene reduces wear in total hip arthroplasty at 5 years. Clin Orthop Relat Res 468:3228–3233, 2010.

CHAPTER 91

Acetabular Revision: Impaction Bone Grafting

Matthew J. Wilson and Jonathan R. Howell

INTRODUCTION

Loss of acetabular bone stock is a major challenge in revision hip surgery, and the facility to restore bone stock and thereby re-create the normal biomechanics of the hip joint is an attractive solution. This can be achieved with impaction grafting of the acetabulum, which is an established technique and should be an essential tool in the armamentarium of the modern revision hip surgeon.

Use of large amounts of cement in isolation for the reconstruction of loose acetabular components has been well described,[1] with Sotelo-Garza concluding that there was no difference in the outcome of hip replacement in protrusio whether or not bone graft was used.[2] However, the results of this technique in the revision setting are generally poor, with Amstutz reporting 83% radiographic loosening at only 2 years postoperatively.[3] Callaghan's review of 146 revisions revealed a 34% rate of radiologic loosening or mechanical failure at 3.6 years.[4] Similar results from the Mayo Clinic review of 166 revisions at a mean of 4.5 years revealed probable or possible acetabular loosening in 37.7% of hips, and complete radiolucent lines in 70.9% of cases.[5] Following removal of loose acetabular components, the acetabular interface is often found to be sclerotic, particularly following removal of a cemented socket. In these circumstances, it is not possible to gain adequate osteointegration[6] of the cement at revision, and early loosening is common; therefore the reconstruction of acetabular defects with cement has largely been abandoned. However, impaction bone grafting provides an ideal surface for cement integration *and* has the ability to incorporate, restoring bone stock and re-creating anatomy.

The use of bone graft has its roots in the early days of modern surgery. In 1859, Ollier was credited with describing the first clinical experiment of bone grafting when he attempted to transplant the radius from a rabbit into a tibial nonunion. Subsequent work by Macewen and Ponset on the use of allograft from amputated limbs led to increased interest in the subject.[7] However, the clinical use of bone grafting was hampered by the limited availability of autograft and the inability to store allograft properly. It was the development of bone banks and of methods of freezing allograft at the Hospital for Special Surgery in New York in the late 1940s that secured the future of bone grafting in reconstructive orthopedic surgery. In the 1970s, the first reports on the use of bone graft to treat acetabular deficiencies began to appear. In 1975, Hastings and Parker suggested the use of medial bone graft with a Vitallium mesh, in combination with a cemented acetabular component, for the treatment of primary acetabular protrusio.[8] Further reports by McCollum, Harris, and Heywood confirmed the success of bone graft in acetabular reconstruction.[1,9,10]

The development of cementless techniques for implant fixation has offered an alternative method of acetabular reconstruction. Good results have been reported, both with and without bone graft,[11-13] and most acetabular revisions are performed using these types of implants, particularly in cases where a defect is uncontained and cannot be contained using reinforcement mesh. In our opinion, the successful use of bone graft in large defects relies on adequate loading of the impacted graft, and this can be achieved reliably only by using a cemented socket. The use of an uncemented shell relies on contact with host bone, and loading will occur preferentially at these points of contact. The use of a cemented socket also allows circumferential use of bone graft, in which the cement is in contact with impacted graft over 100% of its interface. This allows restoration of bone stock in all areas of the acetabulum—something that is precluded by the necessity for host bone contact with cementless shells.

In the field of revision hip surgery, the modern techniques of impacting morselized graft to re-create anatomy and to restore bone in the femur and acetabulum have been popularized by units in Nijmegen and Exeter.[14-16] Essential to the technique is the creation of a contained acetabular defect. This in itself can be technically challenging and may require the use of metal reinforcement mesh. Once the acetabular defect has been contained, morselized autograft or allograft is impacted within the cavity to form a stable base before cementation of a polyethylene acetabular component.

This chapter describes the indications, technique, and limitations of impaction bone grafting, in combination with a cemented acetabular component, in the reconstruction of acetabular defects.

INDICATIONS/CONTRAINDICATIONS

Indications

There are three main reasons for the loss of acetabular bone stock in revision hip arthroplasty:
1. Aseptic loosening due to osteolysis
2. Bone loss due to infection
3. Iatrogenic loss during implant removal

The main indication for revision of the acetabular component is painful socket loosening. There are notable differences in the patterns of bone loss that occur around cemented and uncemented components, specifically in their tendencies to migrate or cause extensive osteolysis.

There is no doubt that the survival of a cemented acetabular component is dependent on the quality of the original operation. Previously well-fixed, cemented acetabular components will loosen because of osteolysis caused by particulate debris or by infection. Loosening of cemented sockets has been defined as the development of lucent lines of between 1 mm[17] and 2 mm[18] at the bone-cement interface, or as progressive migration. Once a cemented socket becomes radiologically loose, it will start to migrate and it will often, although not always, become symptomatic, alerting the surgeon to the need for revision surgery.

Periprosthetic bone loss around uncemented components is often classed as silent.[19] Gross suggests that an uncemented shell with at least 50% coverage requires no additional support.[20] A well-supported socket that loses bony support because of osteolysis may need only 50% bony adherence, possibly even less, to remain well-fixed and therefore asymptomatic—despite significant loss of bone stock. Regular, long-term follow-up of these patients is essential to avoid late presentation with catastrophic bone loss. Hartofilakidis performed a comparison review of cemented and uncemented acetabular shells and concluded that the lysis around cemented sockets was linear. However, the lysis around uncemented shells was more aggressive and expansile.[21]

Acetabular impaction grafting is also indicated in primary procedures where there is loss of host bone, such as protrusio acetabuli, acetabular dysplasia, and trauma.

CONTRAINDICATIONS

The only absolute contraindication to impaction grafting is the inability to contain a segmental defect, medial or peripheral, as defined by D'Antonio.[22] Although large defects can be successfully contained, it is the stability and durability of that containment that are essential to the success of impaction grafting. It can be impossible to contain significant defects of the anterior and posterior columns with enough stability to allow effective impaction grafting, and other techniques for reconstruction should be considered in these circumstances. Similarly, large superolateral defects extending down the anterior and posterior columns are difficult to contain with a mesh, and cementless implants may be required in these cases.

Although infection is thought to be a relative contraindication to the use of impacted graft, Rudelli reported a 6.2% recurrence of infection at 8.6 years in 32 patients who underwent one-stage revision of infected, loose total hip replacements. Of these patients, 25 underwent impaction grafting of *both* the femur and the acetabulum, and half required the use of mesh to contain the graft.[23] These results are similar to those reported using a two-stage procedure.[24-26]

EQUIPMENT

A major part of planning any surgery is predicting which equipment is likely to be required. With particular reference to impaction grafting of the acetabulum, the following items should be available in the operating room:
1. Fresh frozen femoral heads: two to three for an average defect
2. Concave femoral head reamers (see Fig. 91-4)
3. A bone mill capable of producing large bone chips. Alternatively, rongeurs may be used.
4. A selection of rim and medial meshes
5. 3.5-mm small fragment screw set
6. Hemispherical acetabular impactors in a selection of sizes.
7. Small peripheral impactors

DESCRIPTION OF TECHNIQUE

Preoperative Procedure

A lateral position is preferred, ensuring that the pelvis is adequately secured with appropriately placed padded props. It is important to align the anterior superior iliac spines in the vertical plane. This, in combination with an assessment of the transverse ligament, helps with final orientation of the new acetabular component.

Perioperative antibiotics should be administered. Multiple tissue samples are sent for culture and, where infection is suspected, frozen section may be requested. The frozen femoral heads are removed from the freezer and are allowed to defrost in sterile, warmed saline while the exposure continues.

Surgical Exposure

An extensile posterior approach generally gives excellent exposure of the acetabulum and the posterior wall and column should plating be necessary. The proximal femur is mobilized; sufficient soft tissue is released, and thickened capsular tissue is removed to allow dislocation of the hip.

Retention of the femoral component can limit visualization and hamper acetabular reconstruction, but the authors' strategy toward the femoral component depends on its method and state of fixation. Clearly, a loose femoral component should be revised using the surgeons' preferred technique for the femoral conditions that exist at the time of revision. However, well-fixed stems do not necessarily require full revision, be they cemented or cementless, and indeed revision of a well-fixed stem or cement mantle may cause unnecessary damage to the femur. For a soundly fixed cemented stem and cement mantle, it is relatively easy to burr away cement over the shoulder of the prosthesis and tap the femoral component from its intact cement mantle. After acetabular reconstruction is complete, a new femoral component can be recemented into the old mantle—the so-called *cement-in-cement technique*.[27] If a cementless femoral component is to be retained and the anterior acetabular wall is intact, then a pocket can be made in the anterosuperior tissues to accommodate the femoral head or trunnion. However, it is often difficult to create a space large enough for the proximal femur, and it is important to avoid imparting excessive force on the anterior wall during exposure of the socket. An alternative approach for well-fixed uncemented stems is use of the trochanteric slide,[28] through which the abductors are safely separated from the femur, thereby allowing circumferential exposure of the acetabulum. Alternatively, if it is necessary to remove a well-fixed uncemented femoral component, an extended trochanteric osteotomy can be used, which also gives excellent exposure of the whole acetabulum.

Whichever, approach is used, retractors are placed anteriorly and posteroinferiorly, with care taken to protect the thin walls of the acetabulum and the sciatic nerve. It is important to identify the transverse ligament, which helps with orientation of the acetabular component and acts as a guide to the level of socket placement. If it is present, the transverse ligament is retained because, apart from its role as a guide to socket placement, it also helps to constrain the bone graft during the impaction process. If the transverse ligament is absent, the teardrop is identified as a guide to the inferior margin of the acetabulum.

Acetabular Assessment

Curettes are used to remove any acetabular membrane, although some medial membrane may be retained if the medial wall is deficient because its removal may be hazardous to structures within the pelvis. Care is taken to preserve the walls of the acetabulum, and the use of reamers is kept to a minimum to avoid removal of host bone. The rim of the defect is completely cleared of soft tissue, the acetabulum lavaged, and the defect assessed (Fig. 91-1).

Once the integrity of the anterior and posterior columns has been confirmed, the acetabulum is assessed for central and peripheral segmental defects. It is useful to position an appropriately sized trial component or acetabular impactor at the level of the transverse ligament in an anatomic position. With the instrument held in the intended anteversion and inclination of the final component, the surgeon can assess the extent of any peripheral defects and how easily they may be contained (Fig. 91-2).

Acetabular Reconstruction

Cavitary Defects

For pure cavitary defects, no additional reconstruction with mesh is required. It is important to establish a bleeding bed for the bone graft, so areas of sclerotic bone should be reamed gently, burred, or drilled with a 2-mm drill until bleeding points are seen throughout the socket.

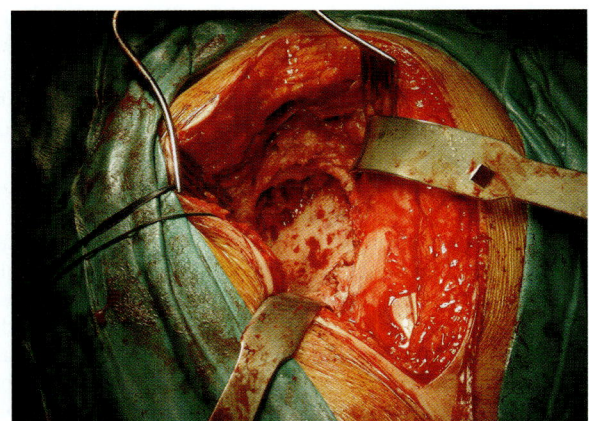

Figure 91-1. The cleared acetabulum prior to assessment of defect.

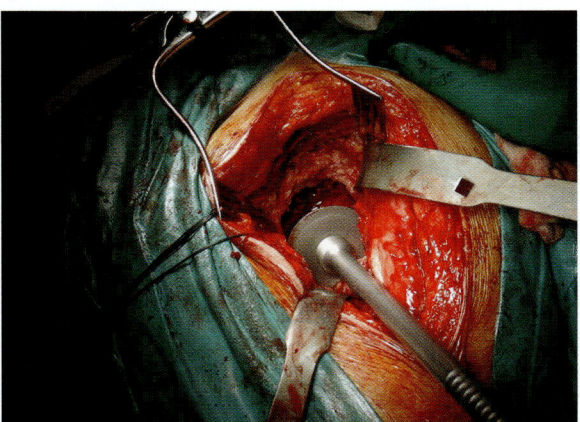

Figure 91-2. Impactor placed in an anatomic position helps to define the defect.

Medial Segmental Defects

Medial segmental defects are common and require reinforcement before impaction grafting is performed. Specific medial meshes or a small rim mesh can be trimmed to size and laid over the defect. A wafer of femoral head or a layer of cancellous graft laid over the defect before insertion of the mesh enhances the stability of the mesh and can improve the reconstruction. If needed, the mesh can be stabilized with two or three small fragment screws. Massive medial segmental defects may require protection with a support ring or cage.

Peripheral Segmental Defects

In the revision of loose cemented sockets, segmental defects are commonly restricted to the superolateral region from approximately 10 o'clock to 2 o'clock. Larger defects involving the anterior and posterior walls may also be seen and can occur after removal of uncemented shells.

Superolateral defects are best closed by applying a rim mesh to the outer aspect of the acetabulum and ilium. Some fibers of the glutei need to be elevated to allow correct placement of the mesh. The mesh should be trimmed to size, ensuring that the sharp edges of cut mesh are not situated along the posterior border, where they risk irritating the sciatic nerve.

When judging the size and orientation of the rim mesh, it is useful to place an appropriately sized impactor within the acetabulum in the orientation intended for the final component. This helps to ensure that the defect is fully contained, and that the mesh is aligned correctly.

The rim mesh is secured to the acetabulum using multiple small fragment screws. Once the rim mesh has been cut to size, the assistant holds it in place with an artery forceps while the surgeon inserts the first screw. This should be placed at the apex of the proximal edge, roughly halfway between its anterior and posterior margins. Having placed this screw, the surgeon reassesses the orientation of the mesh and, if necessary, makes any minor adjustments to its anteversion by rotating the mesh around the apical screw. The next two screws are placed at the anterior and posterior extremities; they are critical to the success of the operation. The screws should be directed into the anterior and posterior columns to establish fixation of the two ends of the mesh. Once they are positioned, the remaining screws are placed at 1-cm intervals around the periphery. All screws should be bicortical, and it does not matter unduly if the screws pass through the cavitary defect, as long as they do not interfere with insertion of the impactor or with cup placement (Fig. 91-3).

Anterior wall defects should be closed with rim mesh; however, for these defects it is usually easier to lay the mesh on the inner surface of the acetabular wall. When they are placed in this fashion, the anterior rim meshes are often stable enough to allow impaction without further stabilization, although screws may be added superiorly and inferiorly with caution to avoid vascular injury (see Fig. 91-3).

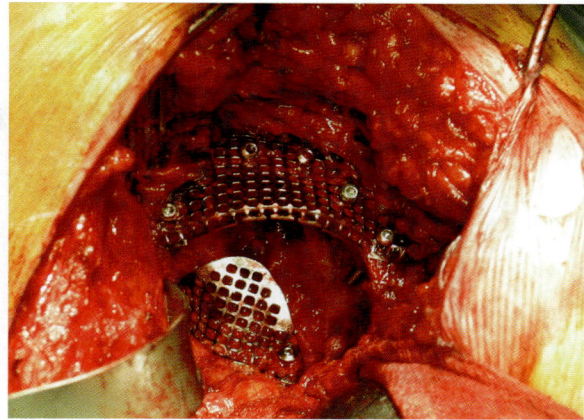

Figure 91-3. Rim mesh held in place with screws. Here an anterior rim mesh has also been inserted.

Graft Preparation

Fresh frozen femoral heads are the preferred source of graft for impaction grafting. It is occasionally possible to plan revision surgery after a contralateral primary hip arthroplasty is performed. In these cases, the femoral head from the primary can be stored for use as autograft, but most defects require more than one femoral head; therefore it is necessary to use a mixture of allograft and autograft.

The preparation of morselized graft can be accomplished by hand, using a saw to section the head, followed by rongeurs, or by using a commercially available bone mill. Surgeons in Nijmegen advocate the use of large chips of approximately 0.5 to 1 cubic centimeter,[27,29] and good evidence suggests that better initial stability is achieved with the use of larger chips.[30] The use of pulse lavage to wash the graft before impaction also improves stability, probably by allowing tighter impaction,[30-32] and it may reduce the risk of disease transmission.[33] Van der Donk showed that graft incorporation was not compromised by washing with pulse lavage.[34] Most commercially available bone mills are not capable of producing chips large enough to meet the demands of impaction grafting in the acetabulum. It has been shown that the average chip size in milled bone is less than 3.5 mm.[35]

The authors recommend that the surgeon remove any remaining cartilage and the cortical bone with concave femoral head reamers (Fig. 91-4). The femoral head is sectioned into quarters with a saw, and then large rongeurs are used to create cancellous bone chips of approximately 0.5 to 1 cm^3. The chips should be washed in a sieve using pulse lavage to remove excess fat and blood. Where there is concern about prior infection or where one-stage revision is performed for infection, 1 g of vancomycin antibiotic powder can be added to each morselized femoral head after lavage and before the time of impaction.

Acetabular Impaction

Bone chips are introduced into the acetabulum and are impacted in layers. Initially, chips are placed into the

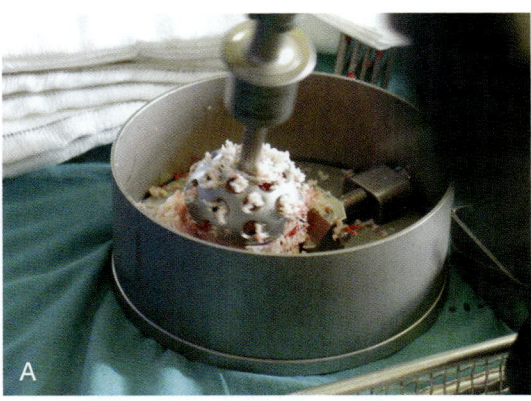
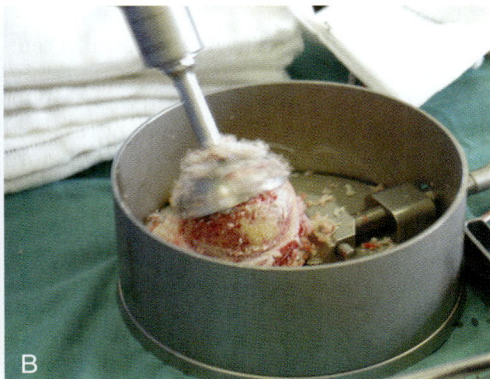

Figure 91-4. Reverse femoral head reamers in use.

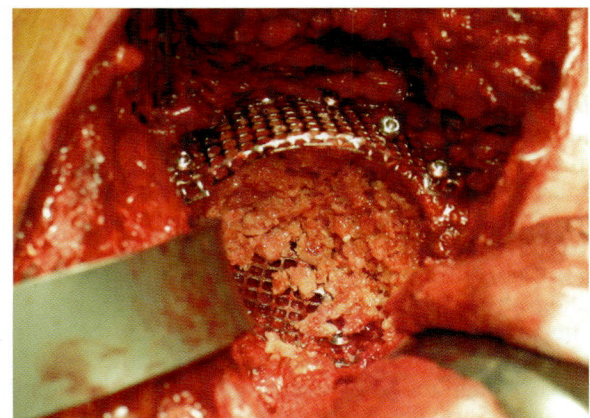

Figure 91-5. Chips are placed into the superior defect.

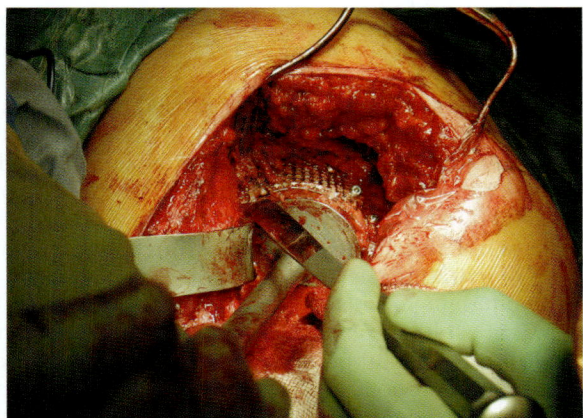

Figure 91-6. Peripheral impaction with the hemispherical impactor held in place.

superior defect (Fig. 91-5) and are impacted around any screws that may be passing across the defect; the surgeon should concentrate on filling the superior cavitary defect. It is a technical mistake to place too much graft medially because this risks lateralizing the socket.

Various impactors are available in commercially available systems. Small impactors and punches should be used to fill small cysts, defects, and gaps around screws. Once these are filled, the graft is impacted using hemispherical impactors of increasing size. Small aliquots of bone are sequentially introduced into the socket defect, and impaction is performed with vigorous hammering using a metal mallet. Impaction needs to be firm enough to create a solid base of bone, but not so hard as to fracture the acetabulum. It is thought that multiple light impactions are superior to fewer, heavy hammer blows. The process of adding bone followed by impaction is repeated until the acetabulum is reconstructed back to the planned anatomic position. The final impactor used should be 4 to 6 mm larger than the true outer diameter of the proposed polyethylene socket to allow for an adequate cement mantle.

Once central impaction is complete, attention should be turned to peripheral impaction, which is a vital step in producing a densely packed bone bed ready for cementing. The assistant maintains pressure on the final impactor, which is left in position, while the surgeon places pieces of graft around the superolateral periphery of the impactor. These bone chips are then impacted using a narrow punch, followed by the addition of more chips around the periphery (Fig. 91-6). This process is repeated until it is no longer possible to impact any further graft under the rim of the socket or mesh.

During peripheral impaction, the hemispherical impactor can be backed off by 1 or 2 mm to allow a better peripheral pack, but care should be taken that peripheral packing does not force the hemispherical impactor out of the socket because this risks lowering the acetabular center of rotation. The final maneuver is to hammer the central impactor back into place. When impaction has been done properly, the packed bone is often so firm that the impactor is gripped by the graft, and some force is required to remove it.

The final impaction should be at least 5 mm thick circumferentially and should have the consistency of cortical bone (Fig. 91-7). At this stage, the trial socket can be offered up and the acetabulum cleaned and dried. A specially designed mesh for washing the graft is available and is used to protect the graft during lavage. Hydrogen peroxide–soaked gauzes are placed in the acetabulum and are pressurized to clean and dry the graft ready for cementing. The authors prefer to use

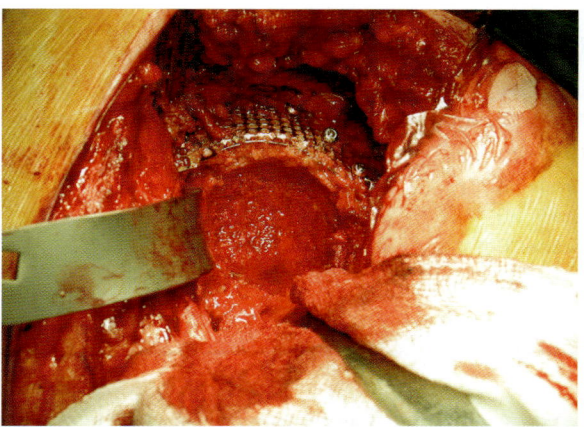

Figure 91-7. Final appearance of impacted socket prior to lavage and drying.

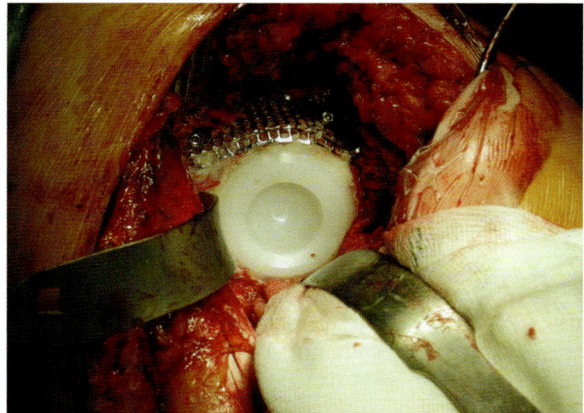

Figure 91-8. Final appearance of cemented socket.

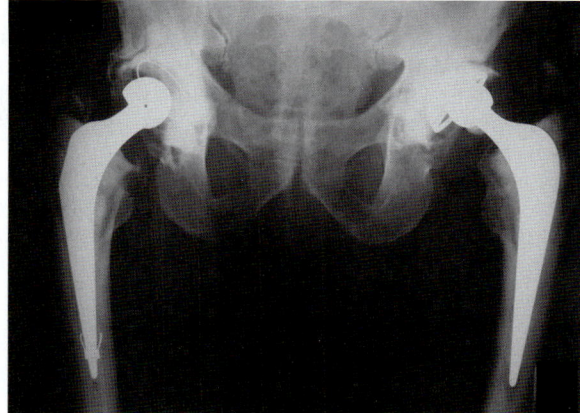

Figure 91-9. Preoperative radiograph with loose cemented sockets.

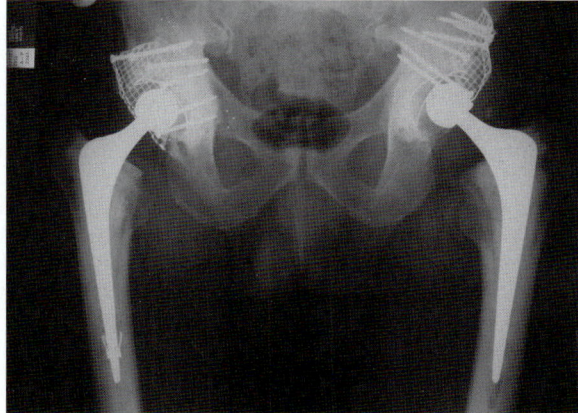

Figure 91-10. Postoperative radiograph with rim mesh and impaction grafting. The well-fixed stems were also revised using the cement-in-cement technique.

a flanged polyethylene component and pressurized cement. The cement is prepared in a closed system with fume extraction and is inserted into the acetabulum once it has reached the correct consistency. This usually happens at least 3 minutes after the addition of monomer. The cement is then pressurized in the acetabulum to force it into the graft for at least an additional minute. As the cement is pressurized, the surgeon may observe fat extruding from the superolateral bone graft surface; this is entirely normal. Cement may leak around the periphery of the graft underneath the pressurizer device, but its extrusion out through the superolateral graft bed indicates inadequate graft packing. The polyethylene socket is inserted at approximately 5 minutes for the cement used by the authors, and considerable force is required to seat the flanged socket. After socket insertion, pressure is maintained on the introducer until the cement has polymerized. The final appearance of the reconstructed socket is shown in Figure 91-8.

Reverse Reaming Versus Impaction Grafting (Figs 91-9 and 91-10)

The technique of "impacting" bone graft by using axial compression through an acetabular reamer in reverse

has been described by some authors.[36,37] Although this technique results in a cosmetically pleasing, hemispherical neo-acetabulum, it should not be used in combination with a cemented component.[38] The compaction achieved is inferior to that obtained using hemispherical impactors and vigorous hammering. Bolder and associates demonstrated significantly greater cup migration using a reverse reaming technique compared with formal impaction grafting. This was particularly true when reverse reaming was combined with slurry graft, in which case migration was three times greater.[35]

POSTOPERATIVE CARE

Patients are routinely mobilized the day after surgery. Fully contained defects should have enough initial stability to allow immediate weight bearing. Studies using radiostereometric analysis (RSA) to assess the effect of weight-bearing status with impaction grafting in the femur have shown no difference between full and partial weight-bearing protocols with respect to migration of a polished, tapered, cemented stem.[39] However, we are not aware of a similar study in the case of acetabular revision. In most cases of impaction grafting, the authors encourage protected weight bearing for a period of 6 weeks, at which time stage check radiographs are taken. Provided there is no change in cup inclination, patients make a gradual return to full weight bearing with the aim of restoring full activities by 3 months postoperatively.

In those cases where a support ring or cage has been used, a similar protocol is followed, but a prolonged period of protected weight bearing may be needed. This will depend on the surgeon's assessment of the stability of the initial construct.

COMPLICATIONS

No studies have reported specific complication rates with particular reference to acetabular impaction bone grafting. High rates of complications have been reported after impaction grafting of the femur, mainly related to femoral fractures.[40] Acetabular fracture during impaction grafting is not frequently reported, despite the need for vigorous, forceful impaction.

Although migration of the acetabular component is commonly noted, RSA studies demonstrate that the rate of migration decreases during the initial postoperative years as the graft incorporates.[41] Further studies are needed to determine any correlation between socket migration and implant failure, but significant migration in defects reconstructed using large meshes may result in fatigue failure of the mesh.

With meticulous attention to surgical technique, the complications of impaction grafting are similar to those of any procedure used in reconstruction of the acetabulum.

RESULTS

The techniques for containing acetabular defects in revision surgery and for their reconstruction with impaction grafting are well established. Results are now being presented from groups other than the originators to suggest that the technique is not only successful but also reproducible.

We have reviewed 339 consecutive hip arthroplasties using impaction bone grafting performed at our institution.[42] Most patients—202—were undergoing their first revision, 46 their second, and 9 their third, and for 4 patients, it was their fourth revision. Forty-four patients were undergoing a primary hip arthroplasty, and 34 second-stage revisions were performed for infection. The average age at surgery was 71 (range, 23 to 96) years, and the average follow-up was 6.1 (range, 4.3 to 8.4) years. No patient was lost to follow-up. The acetabular defects were classified according to Paprosky[43] and are summarized in Table 91-1; the methods of graft containment are summarized in Table 91-2. Complications included 5 nerve injuries (1 femoral and 4 sciatic), 3 of which made a full recovery. In all, 15 deep infections were identified; 8 were new infections (8/305; 2.6%), and 7 were infections of second-stage revisions (7/34; 20.6%). Of 13 dislocations (3.8%), 4 became recurrent, 2 of

which were re-revised. Overall survivorship at 9 to 10 years was 86.5% with reoperation for any reason as the endpoint. Overall survivorship of the socket, with revision for aseptic loosening as the endpoint, was 92.7%.

In 2009, Schreurs published work from Nijmegen on the 20- to 25-year follow-up of 62 revisions using these techniques. The average age at revision surgery was 62 years, and defects were classified as cavitary in 38% of cases and combined in 62%; investigators reported 87% survival with re-revision for aseptic loosening as the endpoint.[44]

A recent follow-up of impaction grafted revisions in patients with rheumatoid arthritis demonstrated 85% survival at 12 years. These results must be considered good in a group of patients who are often young at revision surgery (mean, 57 years in this study), many of whom have marked bone loss.[45]

Azuma and colleagues reported on the fate of 30 hips with a variety of cavitary and segmental defects at 5.8 years. Although no cases were revised, 3 were lost to follow-up, and 2 radiographic failures were reported. In this study, segmental defects were closed with block grafts rather than with wire mesh. Of 2 cases that migrated, 1 socket had been reconstructed using a block graft.[46]

The importance of obtaining adequate stability in segmental reconstruction was highlighted by Comba and coworkers. Thirty-one patients reviewed at 2 to 13.1 years (mean, 51.7 months) revealed 98% survival for aseptic loosening, although 6 were lost to follow-up (worst case survival, 91.3%). Although 48% had segmental defects, a mesh was used in only 11% of cases. In the remainder, the long flange of an Ogee cemented

Table 91-1. Paprosky Classification: Acetabular Defects

Paprosky Classification	No. of Patients
Grade 1	10
Grade 2A	71
Grade 2B	95
Grade 2C	57
Grade 3A	55
Grade 3B	48
Pelvic discontinuity	3

Table 91-2. Methods of Graft Containment in Exeter Series

Method of Graft Containment	No. of Patients
Impaction only	89
Medial mesh	48
Rim mesh	118
Rim and medial mesh	19
Kerboul-Postel plate	53
Reinforcement ring/cage	12

polyethylene component was used to support the lateral graft. All 3 patients with mechanical loosening had segmental defects reconstructed with the socket flange rather than with mesh.[47]

The use of cemented metal-backed components has been proposed.[48] One study reported radiographic survival of 96.4% at 5.8 years, although 5 of 60 hips were not included in the analysis. This type of socket, albeit cemented, primarily loads on the acetabular rim and is secured additionally with screws. In this situation, loading of the graft must be altered; this technique should be considered in isolation and the longer-term results studied.

With impaction grafting, migration of cemented cups can occur as graft is incorporated; long-term follow-up is recommended for this reason. Usually migration is minor and is limited to the first few years after surgery. Once the graft is fully incorporated, migration stops.

Measurement of migration on plain films, using techniques described by Nunn, has an accuracy of 3 mm.[49] However, RSA is considered the gold standard and has been used to measure socket migration in impaction grafting. Of 17 hips reviewed at 5 years, all but 1 had migrated, often by distances that would not have been picked up using plain film measurements. The mean migration was 2.5 mm superiorly, 1.1 mm medially, and 0.9 mm posteriorly. Rates of migration decreased in all directions over 5 years, and 13 of 17 hips had stopped migrating by 4 years.[41] Further follow-up is needed to show if there is any correlation between the degree and the timing of migration, and failure.

Large, peripheral segmental defects can be extremely challenging, and revision surgery is generally associated with poorer results whatever the means of reconstruction. Van Haaren and associates reported only 72% survival in a group of patients of whom 70% had American Association of Orthopaedic Surgeons (AAOS) grade III or IV defects. The authors concluded that failure rates were higher with more severe defects, although they conceded that the cohort did represent their learning curve, and that broadening of indications to include pelvic discontinuity may have affected the results.[41,50] Similar poor results were reported in Buttaro's review of 23 AAOS grade III defects in 2008, demonstrating 90.8% survival at only 36 months. Biopsy specimens demonstrated necrotic graft and fibrous tissue, suggesting that instability was the main cause of failure. Cases presented in the paper suggest that the mesh fixation was not ideal with fewer than the recommended number of screws and poor screw placement. The authors concluded that mesh did not prevent migration, although they noted that despite evidence of migration, patients were largely asymptomatic. Their recommendation was that mesh and graft are good for medium uncontained defects but not for severe defects.[51]

The results for acetabular impaction grafting can be excellent and comparable with those of other reconstructive options. However, the selection of appropriate cases and meticulous surgical technique are critical to a successful outcome.

USE OF SUPPORT RINGS AND CAGES WITH IMPACTION GRAFTING

It has been noted previously that the only contraindication to impaction grafting of the acetabulum is the inability to contain an uncontained defect.

In the case of large medial segmental defects, it may not be possible to provide enough stability to the medial wall with mesh alone, and in these cases, vigorous impaction may lead to prolapse of the graft into the pelvis. Minor medial prolapse of the graft is not usually a concern because it incorporates and remodels well, but a major loss of medial support will inevitably lead to consequent loss of stability of the graft, cement, and acetabular component. Similarly, large peripheral segmental defects may be too large to span using reinforcement mesh, or bone may be insufficient anteriorly and posteriorly to allow solid fixation of the mesh. In these circumstances, it may be necessary to protect the graft with a support ring or cage. Results of revision using these techniques are plentiful but variable in the medium term.[37,45,52-60] Follow-up of more than 10 years is rarely reported, although this may reflect the advanced age of this group of patients.

Results of revision are generally worse in cases with significant acetabular defects. Okano and coworkers reported results at 6.3 years in 31 hips with massive bone loss revised using impacted bone allograft and a Kerboull-type acetabular device. Overall, they recorded a 23% failure rate. However, failure rates were significantly increased when the thickness of the graft was greater than 20 mm as measured on an anteroposterior (AP) radiograph. They recommended the additional use of bulk graft in those cases where more than 2 cm deficiency is anticipated.[53]

Kawanabe and associates, in their 9-year review of 42 hips reconstructed with bone graft and the Kerboull device, reported better results with bulk graft than with morselized chips—82% vs. 53% survival—although ceramic particles were used as a graft expander in the morselized group (see section on alternative to the use of fresh-frozen allograft). As expected, higher rates of failure were seen when the acetabular defects were more severe and uncontained.[59]

Critical to the incorporation of morselized graft is adequate loading according to Wolff's law. The basic purpose of any support ring or cage is to offload and protect the graft, which has inevitable consequences for graft incorporation. Lunn's 5-year review of 35 revision hip replacements using impaction grafting and the Kerboull device demonstrated graft resorption in 7 hips with consequent superior migration of the plate and fracture of the inferior hook.[61]

Antiprotrusio cages such as Birch-Schneider or Contour cages are more rigid and may be more resistant to mechanical failure. Berry and Muller reported 12% failure for aseptic loosening in 42 revised hips, all with combined segmental and peripheral defects, at a mean follow-up of 5 years.[54] Carroll reviewed 63 cases treated with a variety of support rings in combination with impacted graft; all cases were Paprosky grade 3, and 4 with pelvic dissociation were included. Investigators reported relatively good results in this difficult-to-treat group, with 84% survival for aseptic loosening at 8.75 years.[60]

It has been suggested that morselized graft can be compressed and loaded using screws through a Burch-Schneider cage or Muller support ring. Haddad and colleagues reported no aseptic failures and good graft incorporation in 48 hips revised with this technique, although follow-up was limited to 64 months.[37]

HISTOLOGY OF IMPACTED BONE GRAFT

Although autograft is accepted as the ideal material for bony reconstruction,[62,63] a limited supply often necessitates the use of allograft. Despite the proven clinical success of acetabular impaction bone grafting, considerable debate has continued about the ability of allograft to incorporate. A study from Nijmegen reported histologic and mechanical results from impaction grafting of acetabular defects in a goat model. At 6 weeks, investigators showed that two thirds of the interface had become incorporated, and by 24 to 48 weeks, there was complete consolidation and revascularization of the graft. However, of the goats sacrificed at 48 weeks, all were found to have a thick fibrous layer at the bone-cement interface, with a consequent effect on implant stability. The authors suggested that high peak stresses at this interface, which arose because of the relatively thin layers of cement and the inability of the goat to adapt to a reconstructed joint, might have contributed to the formation of this layer. Moreover, they stated that similar interface formation has not been demonstrated in human patients.[64]

Histologic studies in humans have also confirmed incorporation of impacted graft. Buma and coworkers took core biopsies from the grafted acetabula of 8 patients undergoing revision for a variety of reasons, including infection and aseptic loosening. All grafts that had been in place for longer than 8 months showed evidence of incorporation, compared with none of the grafts that were sampled less than 4 months post impaction. Among samples taken more than 15 months postoperatively, graft remnants were extremely scarce, and all samples closely resembled normal trabecular bone.[65]

Allograft is an osteoconductive material that acts as a scaffold for new bone formation. However, histologic studies have demonstrated that new bone is formed within the fibrous stromal tissue,[66] indicating that osteoinduction may also play a role, although the exact mechanism by which this might occur is not clear. In vitro studies have shown the presence of bone morphogenic protein 7 (BMP-7) in specimens of fresh-frozen femoral head and have demonstrated that impaction increases the release of BMP-7.[67] The authors speculated that the strain imparted during impaction results in microfractures, permitting release of BMP-7 from the exposed matrix. This is an area that requires further research before we can conclude that such grafts are osteoinductive.

Studies have also demonstrated that any cartilage fragments left within the graft do not incorporate[66] and risk interfering with the stability of the graft, and hence with long-term survival. Therefore care should be taken to remove cartilage fragments from bone graft before impaction.

Postmortem retrieval studies provide the benefit of removing the bias associated with sampling hips that have failed, but unfortunately such studies are scarce. Heekin and associates studied the grafts from 3 patients who had died after previously undergoing impaction grafting. At 18 months, the graft had vascularized to a depth of 4 mm; by 53 months, the graft had incorporated; and at 85 months, the graft had completely remodeled. Investigators compared the histologic findings with radiographic definitions of graft incorporation in these cases and concluded that although graft incorporates, the rate of incorporation is difficult to assess on postoperative radiographs.[68] Incorporation of graft seems to follow a similar pattern to that of animal experiments, although it occurs at a slower rate. Regardless, the porous nature of morselized trabecular bone allows rapid vascularization and new bone apposition, so that incorporation can occur without structural weakening.

The histologic incorporation of bulk allograft in the acetabulum has not been studied to the same depth. Retrieval and postmortem studies have shown that revascularization and incorporation of bulk allograft are minimal, and that radiographic appearances do not correlate with histologic studies.[69,70] These findings correlate with Enneking's study of massive retrieved allograft, in which he demonstrated that although healing can occur between graft and host, it is limited to the interface between the two.[71] Studies in which both bulk graft and morselized graft from the same patient have been analyzed have demonstrated better incorporation of the morselized graft.[69]

Use of wire mesh to contain graft in the femur has been shown to improve the rate of graft vascularization compared with strut graft. Research has suggested that the holes in the mesh facilitate the passage of bone morphogenic proteins and osteoprogenitor cells into the graft.[72] Similar conclusions were drawn when the incorporation of graft in reconstructed acetabuli was studied using positron emission tomography (PET) scanning. Graft placed in segmental defects took several months to reach the levels of regenerative activity recorded in cavitary defects. Although graft in segmental defects is not in direct contact with host bone, it has been speculated that the vascularized tissue overlying the porous mesh supplies mesenchymal stem cells, which promote graft incorporation.

ALTERNATIVES TO THE USE OF FRESH-FROZEN ALLOGRAFT

Fresh-frozen allograft is the gold standard material for use in impaction grafting.[73] There are two main reasons to research alternatives: increasing demand and the risk of disease transmission.

The growing success of impaction grafting in orthopedic reconstruction will cause the demand for allograft to increase in the future. In the United States, over the next 10 years, an estimated 500,000 operations using bone graft will be performed.[74]

A recent audit of infection related to fresh-frozen allograft reported a 2.5% rate of deep infection and concluded that ongoing use of nonirradiated bone was safe in a regional setting.[75] The potential for disease transmission from fresh allograft is controlled only by donor screening, which has limited ability to adequately screen for viral proteins and prions. Irradiation of bone as secondary sterilization is well proven. However, good evidence indicates that the structural properties are weakened.[76,77] Whether this applies to impacted cancellous bone is not known. Bankes and colleagues compared fresh-frozen and irradiated bone in femoral revision at a mean of 47 months and concluded that there was no difference in outcome.[78] Results of impaction grafting in the acetabulum with irradiated bone have shown 88% survival at a mean of 5 years,[79] compared with the best results using nonirradiated bone of 84% at 16.5 years.[80] Other studies have questioned the ability of irradiated bone to remodel, and long-term follow-up is needed.[81]

The use of xenograft prepared from bovine bone has shown poor results, even in combination with allograft.[82] Hydroxyapatite and tricalcium phosphate (TCP) ceramics have been shown to osteointegrate[83,84] with an optimal pore size of 300 to 400 μm.[85,86] The stability of TCP when used in a 50:50 mix with allograft has been shown to be adequate in experimental studies.[87,88] Integration of TCP particles has been histologically confirmed, and no adverse effect on cement penetration has been noted.[89] Early results with Bonesave, a porous ceramic bone graft substitute used as a graft expander, were reported by Blom and colleagues.[90] No cases of revision were reported at 2 years when Bonesave was used as a 50:50 mix with morselized allograft to reconstruct acetabular defects. The authors reported a high rate of radiolucent lines and concluded that longer follow-up was necessary.

CONCLUSIONS

- The most effective method of preventing socket loosening after total hip replacement in patients with a deficient acetabulum is to reconstruct the acetabulum at the anatomic position using bone graft.[91] Where possible, the same method should be used in cases of acetabular revision.
- Impaction grafting is a technically exacting but reproducible technique.
- Morselized allograft has the ability to incorporate and restore host bone.
- Acceptance of a high hip center has been shown to reduce abductor strength.[92]
- Bone loss from osteolysis, infection, and implant removal and stress shielding can be significant; impaction bone grafting has the ability to restore bone stock and re-create anatomy.

- As the revision burden increases and younger patients undergo hip arthroplasty, the modern revision hip surgeon needs to be familiar with a variety of reconstructive techniques: No single method can be applicable to all scenarios, and appropriate planning is essential.
- Radiographic assessment of acetabular defects is challenging, and often deficiencies are most easily assessed at the time of revision. The ability to adapt the surgical technique to the findings at the time of revision depends on the technical ability of the surgeon and on ensuring that appropriate implants are available.
- Future developments in the form of graft expanders and bioactive materials[93] need careful assessment and long-term follow-up.
- The fate of impaction grafting in large peripheral segmental defects is unclear, and other techniques may prove more appropriate in these situations.
- The use of new technologies such as porous tantalum or similar augments[94] may have a role to play in containing graft, but the long-term fate of these implants is not known.

CURRENT CONTROVERSIES AND FUTURE CONSIDERATIONS

- Further research is needed in bioactive materials and synthetic bone seeded with osteoprogenitor cells.
- The role of porous tantalum in impaction grafting is unclear. The osteoconductive nature of these materials should allow good initial stability and ingrowth potential for bone graft.
- Cages and support rings manufactured from new materials, such as porous tantalum, may allow more ingrowth and provide better long-term outcome in cases of severe acetabular defects.

REFERENCES

1. Harris WH, Jones WN: The use of wire mesh in total hip replacement surgery. Clin Orthop Relat Res 106:117–121, 1975.
2. Sotelo-Garza A, Charnley J: The results of Charnley arthroplasty of hip performed for protrusio acetabuli. Clin Orthop Relat Res 132:12–18, 1978.
3. Amstutz HC, Ma SM, Jinnah RH, Mai L: Revision of aseptic loose total hip arthroplasties. Clin Orthop Relat Res 170:21–33, 1982.
4. Callaghan JJ, Salvati EA, Pellicci PM, et al: Results of revision for mechanical failure after cemented total hip replacement, 1979 to 1982: a two- to five-year follow-up. J Bone Joint Surg Am 67:1074–1085, 1985.
5. Kavanagh BF, Ilstrup DM, Fitzgerald RH, Jr: Revision total hip arthroplasty. J Bone Joint Surg Am 67:517–526, 1985.
6. Malcolm AJ: Cemented and hydroxyapatite-coated hip implants: an autopsy retrieval study. In Morrey BF, editor: Biological, material and mechanical considerations of joint replacement, San Diego, 1993, Raven Press, pp 39–50.
7. Wilson PD: Experiences with the use of refrigerated homogenous bone. J Bone Joint Surg Br 33:301–315, 1951.
8. Hastings DE, Parker SM: Protrusio acetabuli in rheumatoid arthritis. Clin Orthop Relat Res 108:76–83, 1975.
9. Heywood AW: Arthroplasty with a solid bone graft for protrusio acetabuli. J Bone Joint Surg Br 62:332–336, 1980.

10. McCollum DE, Nunley JA, Harrelson JM: Bone-grafting in total hip replacement for acetabular protrusion. J Bone Joint Surg Am 62:1065–1073, 1980.

11. Ito H, Tanino H, Yamanaka Y, et al: Porous-coated cementless acetabular components without bulk bone graft in revision surgery. J Arthroplasty 35:1307–1310, 2010.

12. Jasty M: Jumbo cups and morselized graft. Orthop Clin North Am 29:249–254, 1998.

13. Sporer SM, Paprosky WG, O'Rourke MR: Managing bone loss in acetabular revision. Instr Course Lect 55:287–297, 2006.

14. Slooff TJ, Huiskes R, van Horn J, Lemmens AJ: Bone grafting in total hip replacement for acetabular protrusion. Acta Orthop Scand 55:593–596, 1984.

15. Slooff TJ, Buma P, Schreurs BW, et al: Acetabular and femoral reconstruction with impacted graft and cement. Clin Orthop Relat Res 324:108–115, 1996.

16. Gie GA, Linder L, Ling RS, et al: Impacted cancellous allografts and cement for revision total hip arthroplasty. J Bone Joint Surg Br 75:14–21, 1993.

17. Stauffer RN: Ten-year follow-up study of total hip replacement. J Bone Joint Surg Am 64:983–990, 1982.

18. Tehranzadeh J, Schneider R, Freiberger RH: Radiological evaluation of painful total hip replacement. Radiology 141:355–362, 1981.

19. Lavernia CJ: Cost-effectiveness of early surgical intervention in silent osteolysis. J Arthroplasty 13:277–279, 1998.

20. Gross AE: Restoration of acetabular bone loss 2005. J Arthroplasty 21(4 Suppl 1):117–120, 2006.

21. Hartofilakidis G, Georgiades G, Babis GC: A comparison of the outcome of cemented all-polyethylene and cementless metal-backed acetabular sockets in primary total hip arthroplasty. J Arthroplasty 24:217–225, 2009.

22. D'Antonio JA, Capello WN, Borden LS, et al: Classification and management of acetabular abnormalities in total hip arthroplasty. Clin Orthop Relat Res 243:126–137, 1989.

23. Rudelli S, Uip D, Honda E, Lima AL: One-stage revision of infected total hip arthroplasty with bone graft. J Arthroplasty 23:1165–1177, 2008.

24. Garvin KL, Evans BG, Salvati EA, Brause BD: Palacos gentamicin for the treatment of deep periprosthetic hip infections. Clin Orthop Relat Res 298:97–105, 1994.

25. Garvin KL, Hanssen AD: Infection after total hip arthroplasty: past, present, and future. J Bone Joint Surg Am 77:1576–1588, 1995.

26. Lieberman JR, Callaway GH, Salvati EA, et al: Treatment of the infected total hip arthroplasty with a two-stage reimplantation protocol. Clin Orthop Relat Res 301:205–212, 1994.

27. Duncan WW, Hubble MJ, Howell JR, et al: Revision of the cemented femoral stem using a cement-in-cement technique: a five- to 15-year review. J Bone Joint Surg Br 91:577–582, 2009.

28. Glassman AH, Engh CA, Bobyn CA: A technique of extensile exposure for total hip arthroplasty. J Arthroplasty 2:11–21, 1987.

29. Schreurs BW, Slooff TJ, Buma P, et al: Acetabular reconstruction with impacted morsellised cancellous bone graft and cement: a 10- to 15-year follow-up of 60 revision arthroplasties. J Bone Joint Surg Br 80:391–395, 1998.

30. Arts JJ, Verdonschot N, Buma P, Schreurs BW: Larger bone graft size and washing of bone grafts prior to impaction enhance the initial stability of cemented cups: experiments using a synthetic acetabular model. Acta Orthop 77:227–233, 2006.

31. Dunlop DG, Brewster NT, Madabhushi SP, et al: Techniques to improve the shear strength of impacted bone graft: the effect of particle size and washing of the graft. J Bone Joint Surg Am 85:639–646, 2003.

32. Ullmark G, Nilsson O: Impacted corticocancellous allografts: recoil and strength. J Arthroplasty 14:1019–1023, 1999.

33. Kwong FN, Ibrahim T, Power RA: Incidence of infection with the use of non-irradiated morsellised allograft bone washed at the time of revision arthroplasty of the hip. J Bone Joint Surg Br 87:1524–1526, 2005.

34. van der Donk S, Weernink T, Buma P, et al: Rinsing morselized allografts improves bone and tissue ingrowth. Clin Orthop Relat Res 408:302–310, 2003.

35. Bolder SB, Schreurs BW, Verdonschot N, et al: Particle size of bone graft and method of impaction affect initial stability of cemented cups: human cadaveric and synthetic pelvic specimen studies. Acta Orthop Scand 74:652–657, 2003.

36. Mallory TH, Lombardi AV, Jr, Fada RA, et al: Noncemented acetabular component removal in the presence of osteolysis: the affirmative. Clin Orthop Relat Res 381:120–128, 2000.

37. Haddad FS, Shergill N, Muirhead-Allwood SK: Acetabular reconstruction with morcellized allograft and ring support: a medium-term review. J Arthroplasty 14:788–795, 1999.

38. Bolder SB, Verdonschot N, Schreurs BW: Technical factors affecting cup stability in bone impaction grafting. Proc Inst Mech Eng H 221:81–86, 2007.

39. Ornstein E, Franzen H, Johnsson R, et al: Hip revision with impacted morselized allografts: unrestricted weight-bearing and restricted weight-bearing have similar effect on migration. A radiostereometry analysis. Arch Orthop Trauma Surg 123:261–267, 2003.

40. Pekkarinen J, Alho A, Lepisto J, et al: Impaction bone grafting in revision hip surgery: a high incidence of complications. J Bone Joint Surg Br 82:103–107, 2000.

41. Ornstein E, Franzen H, Johnsson R, et al: Five-year follow-up of socket movements and loosening after revision with impacted morselized allograft bone and cement: a radiostereometric and radiographic analysis. J Arthroplasty 21:975–984, 2006.

42. Rigby MR, Howell JR, Hubble MJ, et al: Acetabular impaction grafting: a consecutive series of 339 total hip arthroplasties. 2009, Unpublished work.

43. Paprosky WG, Magnus RE: Principles of bone grafting in revision total hip arthroplasty: acetabular technique. Clin Orthop Relat Res 298:147–155, 1994.

44. Schreurs BW, Keurentjes JC, Gardeniers JW, et al: Acetabular revision with impacted morsellised cancellous bone grafting and a cemented acetabular component: a 20- to 25-year follow-up. J Bone Joint Surg Br 91:1148–1153, 2009.

45. Schreurs BW, Luttjeboer J, Thien TM, et al: Acetabular revision with impacted morsellised cancellous bone graft and a cemented cup in patients with rheumatoid arthritis: a concise follow-up, at eight to nineteen years, of a previous report. J Bone Joint Surg Am 91:646–651, 2009.

46. Azuma T, Yasuda H, Okagaki K, Sakai K: Compressed allograft chips for acetabular reconstruction in revision hip arthroplasty. J Bone Joint Surg Br 76:740–744, 1994.

47. Comba F, Buttaro M, Pusso R, Piccaluga F: Acetabular reconstruction with impacted bone allografts and cemented acetabular components: a 2- to 13-year follow-up study of 142 aseptic revisions. J Bone Joint Surg Br 88:865–869, 2006.

48. Wang JW, Fong CY, Su YS, Yu HN: Acetabular revision with morsellised allogenic bone graft and a cemented metal-backed component. J Bone Joint Surg Br 88:586–591, 2006.

49. Nunn D, Freeman MA, Hill PF, Evans SJ: The measurement of migration of the acetabular component of hip prostheses. J Bone Joint Surg Br 71:629–631, 1989.

50. van Haaren EH, Heyligers IC, Alexander FG, Wuisman PI: High rate of failure of impaction grafting in large acetabular defects. J Bone Joint Surg Br 89:296–300, 2007.

51. Buttaro MA, Comba F, Pusso R, Piccaluga F: Acetabular revision with metal mesh, impaction bone grafting, and a cemented cup. Clin Orthop Relat Res 466:2482–2490, 2010.

52. Rosson J, Schatzker J: The use of reinforcement rings to reconstruct deficient acetabula. J Bone Joint Surg Br 74:716–720, 1992.

53. Okano K, Miyata N, Enomoto H, et al: Revision with impacted bone allografts and the Kerboull cross plate for massive bone defect of the Acetabulum. J Arthroplasty 25:594–599, 2010.

54. Berry DJ, Muller ME: Revision arthroplasty using an anti-protrusio cage for massive acetabular bone deficiency. J Bone Joint Surg Br 74:711–715, 1992.

55. Kerboull M, Hamadouche M, Kerboull L: The Kerboull acetabular reinforcement device in major acetabular reconstructions. Clin Orthop Relat Res 378:155–168, 2000.

56. Gill TJ, Sledge JB, Muller ME: The management of severe acetabular bone loss using structural allograft and acetabular reinforcement devices. J Arthroplasty 15:1–7, 2000.

57. van der LM, Tonino A: Acetabular revision with impacted grafting and a reinforcement ring: 42 patients followed for a mean of 10 years. Acta Orthop Scand 72:221, 2010.

58. Tanaka C, Shikata J, Ikenaga M, Takahashi M: Acetabular reconstruction using a Kerboull-type acetabular reinforcement device and hydroxyapatite granules: a 3- to 8-year follow-up study. J Arthroplasty 18:719–725, 2010.

59. Kawanabe K, Akiyama H, Onishi E, Nakamura T: Revision total hip replacement using the Kerboull acetabular reinforcement device with morsellised or bulk graft: results at a mean follow-up of 8.7 years. J Bone Joint Surg Br 89:26–31, 2007.

60. Carroll FA, Hoad-Reddick DA, Kerry RM, Stockley I: The survival of support rings in complex acetabular revision surgery. J Bone Joint Surg Br 90:574–578, 2008.

61. Lunn JV, Kearns SS, Quinlan W, et al: Impaction allografting and the Kerboull acetabular reinforcement device: 35 hips followed for 3-7 years. Acta Orthop 76:296–302, 2005.

62. Heiple KG, Chase SW, Herndon CH: A comparative study of the healing process following different types of bone transplantation. J Bone Joint Surg Am 45:1593–1616, 1963.

63. Campbell CJ, Brower T, MacFadden DG, et al: Experimental study of the fate of bone grafts. J Bone Joint Surg Am 35:332–346, 1953.

64. Schimmel JW, Buma P, Versleyen D, et al: Acetabular reconstruction with impacted morselized cancellous allografts in cemented hip arthroplasty: a histological and biomechanical study on the goat. J Arthroplasty 13:438–448, 1998.

65. Buma P, Lamerigts N, Schreurs BW, et al: Impacted graft incorporation after cemented acetabular revision: histological evaluation in 8 patients. Acta Orthop Scand 67:536–540, 1996.

66. van der Donk S, Buma P, Slooff TJ, et al: Incorporation of morselized bone grafts: a study of 24 acetabular biopsy specimens. Clin Orthop Relat Res 396:131–141, 2002.

67. Board TN, Rooney P, Kearney JN, Kay PR: Impaction allografting in revision total hip replacement. J Bone Joint Surg Br 88:852–857, 2006.

68. Heekin RD, Engh CA, Vinh T: Morselized allograft in acetabular reconstruction: a postmortem retrieval analysis. Clin Orthop Relat Res 319:184–190, 1995.

69. Hirose I, Kawauchi K, Kondo S, et al: Histological evaluation of allograft bone after acetabular revision arthroplasty: report of two cases. J Orthop Sci 5:515–519, 2000.

70. Hooten JP, Jr, Engh CA, Heekin RD, Vinh TN: Structural bulk allografts in acetabular reconstruction: analysis of two grafts retrieved at post-mortem. J Bone Joint Surg Br 78:270–275, 1996.

71. Enneking WF, Mindell ER: Observations on massive retrieved human allografts. J Bone Joint Surg Am 73:1123–1142, 1991.

72. Bolder SB, Schreurs BW, Verdonschot N, et al: Wire mesh allows more revascularization than a strut in impaction bone grafting: an animal study in goats. Clin Orthop Relat Res 423:280–286, 2004.

73. Baas J: Adjuvant therapies of bone graft around non-cemented experimental orthopedic implants: stereological methods and experiments in dogs. Acta Orthop Suppl 79:1–43, 2008.

74. Endres S, Kratz M: Gamma irradiation: an effective procedure for bone banks, but does it make sense from an osteobiological perspective? J Musculoskelet Neuronal Interact 9:25–31, 2009.

75. Love D, Pritchard M, Burgess T, et al: Audit of the Douglas Hocking Research Institute bone bank: ten years of non-irradiated bone graft. ANZ J Surg 79:55–61, 2009.

76. Nguyen H, Morgan DA, Forwood MR: Sterilization of allograft bone: effects of gamma irradiation on allograft biology and biomechanics. Cell Tissue Bank 8:93–105, 2007.

77. Vastel L, Meunier A, Siney H, et al: Effect of different sterilization processing methods on the mechanical properties of human cancellous bone allografts. Biomaterials 25:2105–2110, 2004.

78. Bankes MJ, Allen PW, Aldam CH: Results of impaction grafting in revision hip arthroplasty at two to seven years using fresh and irradiated allograft bone. Hip Int 13:1–11, 2009.

79. Buckley SC, Stockley I, Hamer AJ, Kerry RM: Irradiated allograft bone for acetabular revision surgery: results at a mean of five years. J Bone Joint Surg Br 87:310–313, 2005.

80. Schreurs BW, Bolder SB, Gardeniers JW, et al: Acetabular revision with impacted morsellised cancellous bone grafting and a cemented cup: a 15- to 20-year follow-up. J Bone Joint Surg Br 86:492–497, 2004.

81. Mehendale S, Learmonth ID, Smith EJ, et al: Use of irradiated bone graft for impaction grafting in acetabular revision surgery: a review of fifty consecutive cases. Hip Int 19:114–119, 2009.

82. Charalambides C, Beer M, Cobb AG: Poor results after augmenting autograft with xenograft (Surgibone) in hip revision surgery: a report of 27 cases. Acta Orthop 76:544–549, 2005.

83. Itokazu M, Matsunaga T, Ishii M, et al: Use of arthroscopy and interporous hydroxyapatite as a bone graft substitute in tibial plateau fractures. Arch Orthop Trauma Surg 115:45–48, 1996.

84. Ransford AO, Morley T, Edgar MA, et al: Synthetic porous ceramic compared with autograft in scoliosis surgery: a prospective, randomized study of 341 patients. J Bone Joint Surg Br 80:13–18, 1998.

85. Tsuruga E, Takita H, Itoh H, et al: Pore size of porous hydroxyapatite as the cell-substratum controls BMP-induced osteogenesis. J Biochem 121:317–324, 1997.

86. Kuhne JH, Bartl R, Frisch B, et al: Bone formation in coralline hydroxyapatite: effects of pore size studied in rabbits. Acta Orthop Scand 65:246–252, 1994.

87. Bolder SB, Verdonschot N, Schreurs BW, Buma P: Acetabular defect reconstruction with impacted morsellized bone grafts or TCP/HA particles: a study on the mechanical stability of cemented cups in an artificial acetabulum model. Biomaterials 23:659–666, 2002.

88. Bolder SB, Verdonschot N, Schreurs BW, Buma P: The initial stability of cemented acetabular cups can be augmented by mixing morsellized bone grafts with tricalciumphosphate/hydroxyapatite particles in bone impaction grafting. J Arthroplasty 18:1056–1063, 2003.

89. Arts JJ, Gardeniers JW, Welten ML, et al: No negative effects of bone impaction grafting with bone and ceramic mixtures. Clin Orthop Relat Res 438:239–247, 2005.

90. Blom AW, Wylde V, Livesey C, et al: Impaction bone grafting of the acetabulum at hip revision using a mix of bone chips and a biphasic porous ceramic bone graft substitute. Acta Orthop 80:150–154, 2009.

91. Azuma T: [Preparation of the acetabulum to correct severe acetabular deficiency for total hip replacement—with special reference to stress distribution of the periacetabular region after operation]. Nippon Seikeigeka Gakkai Zasshi 59:269–283, 1985.

92. Kiyama T, Naito M, Shinoda T, Maeyama A: Hip abductor strengths after total hip arthroplasty via the lateral and posterolateral approaches. J Arthroplasty 25:76–80, 2010.

93. Mushipe MT, Chen X, Jennings D, Li G: Cells seeded on MBG scaffold survive impaction grafting technique: potential application of cell-seeded biomaterials for revision arthroplasty. J Orthop Res 24:501–507, 2006.

94. Sporer SM, Paprosky WG: The use of a trabecular metal acetabular component and trabecular metal augment for severe acetabular defects. J Arthroplasty 21(6 Suppl 2):83–86, 2006.

FURTHER READING

Comba F, Buttaro M, Pusso R, Piccaluga F: Acetabular reconstruction with impacted bone allografts and cemented acetabular components: a 2- to 13-year follow-up study of 142 aseptic revisions. J Bone Joint Surg Br 88:865–869, 2006.

Hastings DE, Parker SM: Protrusio acetabuli in rheumatoid arthritis. Clin Orthop Relat Res 108:76–83, 1975.

Okano K, Miyata N, Enomoto H, et al: Revision with impacted bone allografts and the Kerboull cross plate for massive bone defect of the acetabulum. J Arthroplasty 25:594–599, 2010.

Schruers BW, Keurentjes JC, Gardeniers JW, et al: Acetabular revision with impacted morsellised cancellous bone grafting and a cemented cup: a 20- to 25-year follow-up. J Bone Joint Surg Br 91:1148–1153, 2009.

Slooff TJ, Huiskes R, van Horn J, Lemmens AJ: Bone grafting in total hip replacement for acetabular protrusion. Acta Orthop Scand 55:593–596, 1984.

van der Donk S, Buma P, Slooff TJ, et al: Incorporation of morselized bone grafts: a study of 24 acetabular biopsy specimens. Clin Orthop Relat Res 396:131–141, 2002.

CHAPTER 92

Acetabular Revision: Rings, Cages, and Custom Implants

Derek R. Johnson, Douglas A. Dennis, and Raymond H. Kim

KEY POINTS

- A thorough radiographic examination, often including computed tomography, is necessary preoperatively to evaluate osseous defects and help identify a pelvic discontinuity.
- The liberal use of a standard or extended trochanteric osteotomy allows for improved visualization and protection of the superior gluteal nerve.
- When the ischium is exposed, careful dissection of the sciatic nerve with the hip in extension and the knee in flexion will minimize the risk of sciatic nerve injury.
- In cases of pelvic discontinuity, posterior column plating will improve construct stability and decrease the likelihood of mechanical failure.
- To minimize the risk of dislocation, use of high-wall, face-changing, or constrained modular polyethylene liners is often necessary.

INTRODUCTION

The goal of acetabular revision surgery is to achieve a stable, pain-free, and functional construct. This can frequently be achieved with the use of larger hemispherical acetabular components. However, in the setting of massive periacetabular bone loss, stable fixation with the use of a standard hemispherical acetabular component may not be possible, and other reconstruction options must be considered.

Numerous treatment methods are available for management of massive acetabular defects in revision total hip arthroplasty (THA). Unfortunately, the clinical results of managing these complex cases are highly variable and are often associated with a high incidence of complications. Treatment methods utilized in an attempt to reconstruct these difficult cases have included implantation of jumbo acetabular components[1] with or without the use of massive structural allografts,[2-5] bipolar hemiarthroplasty,[6] acetabular impaction bone grafting,[7] oblong acetabular components,[8-10] noncustom acetabular reconstruction rings or cages,[11-14] and use of custom triflanged acetabular

components (CTACs).[15-19] This chapter will focus on the treatment of massive periacetabular bone loss in revision THA with use of noncustom rings and cages and custom triflanged acetabular components.

BONE LOSS CLASSIFICATION

The severity of acetabular bone loss in revision total hip arthroplasty (THA) has been classified by Paprosky[5] (Table 92-1) and the American Academy of Orthopedic Surgeons (AAOS; Table 92-2).[20] The bone loss is classified according to the magnitude of bone loss, the amount of acetabular component migration, and the degree of destruction of the anterior and posterior columns.

INDICATIONS

The presence of massive periacetabular bone loss (Paprosky 3B and AAOS III and IV) that precludes the ability to obtain a stable acetabular reconstruction with a traditional hemispherical cup is the primary indication for the use of acetabular cages or a custom triflanged acetabular component (CTAC). The use of bulk allograft and impaction grafting with traditional acetabular components in these cases has failure rates as high as 36% in some series.[2-4,7] The ability of these allografts to incorporate and withstand physiologic loads is questionable and is a likely cause of the unacceptably high failure rates. With the use of cages or a CTAC, however, the ability to bridge the defects and obtain fixation to remaining available host bone is theoretically attained, providing stable fixation and preventing early component migration. An additional advantage of the use of acetabular cages or a CTAC is the ability to place the acetabular component at a correct anatomic level to restore hip biomechanics and stability more accurately.

CONTRAINDICATIONS

The outstanding results and proven long-term success of hemispherical components in revision THA make these devices the components of choice in the presence

Table 92-1. Paprosky Classification of Acetabular Defects

Type	Description
1	• Columns intact • Hemisphere intact • >70% of prosthesis can be in contact with host bone
2A	• Columns intact • Defect below superior dome • Migration of head center <2 cm • No ischial or teardrop lysis • Kohler's line intact
2B	• Columns intact • Superior lateral migration, creating dome defect • Migration of head center <2 cm • Minimal ischial lysis • Kohler's line intact
2C	• Columns intact • Medial wall defect • Medial migration with minimal superior migration of head center
3A	• Columns intact • Severe superior lateral migration, creating >50% dome defect • Migration of head center >2 cm • Kohler's line intact
3B	• Posterior column deficient • Severe superior medial migration • Severe ischial lysis • Kohler's line broken • Possible pelvic discontinuity

Table 92-2. AAOS Classification of Acetabular Defects

Type	Description
I	• No significant bone loss
II	• Columns and rim intact • Contained cavitary loss
III	• Columns may be deficient • Uncontained defect involving <50% of acetabulum
IV	• Columns deficient • Uncontained defect involving >50% of acetabulum • Pelvic discontinuity may be present

AAOS, American Academy of Orthopaedic Surgeons.

of adequate host bone. The cost and complexity of cages and a CTAC limit their indication only to those cases in which adequate host bone for hemispherical cups is not available. In cases in which adequate pelvic bone quality to obtain screw fixation does not exist, or in the setting of persistent infection, cages and CTAC are contraindicated. Finally, use of these devices alone without additional efforts at pelvic stabilization (column plating) is relatively contraindicated in situations with massive bone loss associated with the presence of a pelvic discontinuity.

PREOPERATIVE PLANNING

History and Physical Examination

As with any arthroplasty evaluation, the initial step in management is a thorough history and physical examination. History should include the reason for initial arthroplasty, as well as the reason for any subsequent revision arthroplasty procedures. A detailed investigation for infection is essential, including white blood cell count, erythrocyte sedimentation rate, and C-reactive protein. If these tests are elevated, or if the history indicates infection (previous infection or wound complication, early failure of previous surgery, or constitutional symptoms), hip aspiration and joint fluid analysis are necessary. Previous operative records should be reviewed to note the exposure used and any complications or unusual techniques involved, and to determine the type, size, and fixation method of the currently implanted components. Careful examination should be performed, including inspection of the skin for the presence of fluctuance, warmth, and erythema and for the location and condition of previous skin incisions. The neurovascular status of the limb must be assessed, as well as the symmetry of leg lengths. Also, the motor function of the lower extremities must be evaluated, particularly the function of the abductor musculature, as this can be predictive of future postoperative problems with hip stability.

Radiographic Evaluation

Plain radiographs, including an anteroposterior view of the pelvis and anteroposterior and lateral views of the hip along with the entire prosthesis, should be obtained. If a femoral component revision is planned, anteroposterior and lateral views of the femur undergoing instrumentation are necessary. Iliac and obturator oblique views are helpful in classifying bone loss and in determining whether a pelvic discontinuity is present. Computed tomography (CT) with metal subtraction techniques allows the surgeon to evaluate osseous defects more precisely, including the presence of a pelvic discontinuity, and is essential for the design of a CTAC should this treatment method be selected (Fig. 92-1A and B). Specific CT scan protocols are often required for the production of a CTAC and should be ordered as such to avoid subjecting the patient to multiple CT scans. In cases with significant leg length discrepancy, full-length orthoroentgenograms may be necessary for preoperative leg length assessment.

In scenarios of severe acetabular component protrusio, a CT scan with a concomitant angiogram may be required.[21] This would aid in determining whether intrapelvic vessels or other visceral structures are in close proximity to the failed acetabular component. Anticipation of potential vascular injury would warrant a preoperative vascular surgery consultation and consideration of a retroperitoneal exposure to free vital intrapelvic structures from the acetabular component before it is removed.

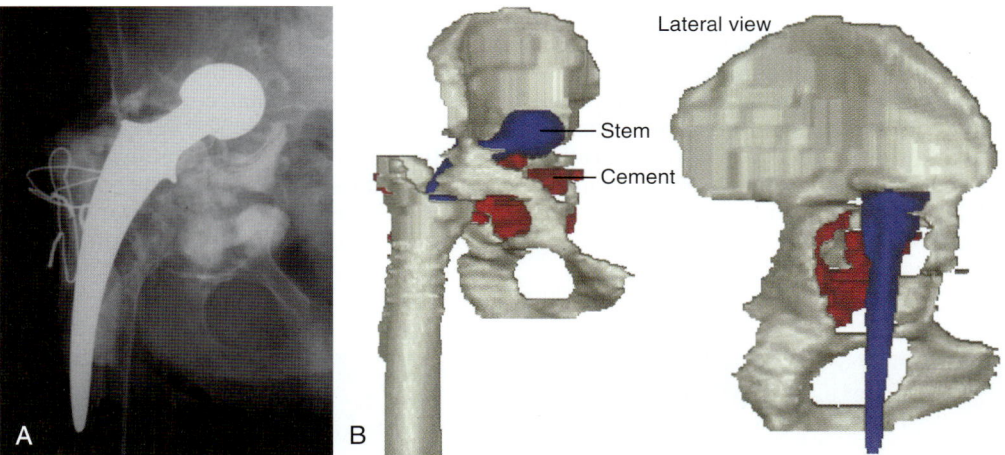

Figure 92-1. A, Anteroposterior radiograph of a failed total hip arthroplasty (THA) with acetabular component loosening and massive periacetabular bone loss. **B,** Three-dimensional images created from a thin cut computed tomography (CT) scan, demonstrating severe acetabular protrusio and a Paprosky 3B acetabular defect.

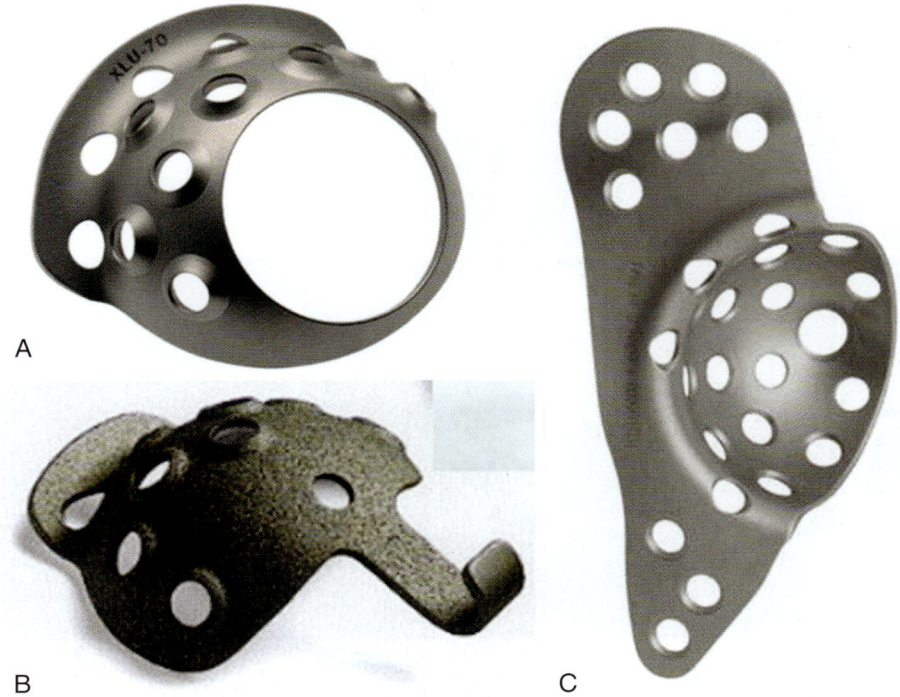

Figure 92-2. Photographs of a Mueller acetabular ring **(A),** a Ganz roof ring **(B),** and an antiprotrusio cage **(C)** utilized for reconstruction of large acetabular bone defects.

Component Design

Numerous designs of noncustom acetabular rings and antiprotrusio cages are available and selected when stable fixation on remaining host bone is not possible (Fig. 92-2). These devices gain stability through fixation to the ischium and ilium, bridge areas of acetabular bone loss, provide support for the acetabular component, and allow for pelvic bone grafting in an environment protected from excessive stress. They are typically designed with some degree of flexibility, allowing the surgeon to manipulate the shape of the cage somewhat intraoperatively to maximize fixation and fit. Polyethylene acetabular components are then cemented into the ring or cage.

The design of a CTAC is finalized preoperatively rather than intraoperatively as with cages. After completion of a thin cut CT with metal subtraction, the manufacturer creates three dimensional (3D) images, as well as a one-to-one computer-aided design (CAD) solid model of the hemipelvis. This 3D model allows for accurate assessment of bone loss and remaining pelvic bone and is utilized to facilitate the design of the CTAC. The surgeon, in conjunction with the design engineer, uses the 3D model to create a clay or acrylic prototype of the CTAC. The surgeon is then able to manipulate the prototype within the 3D hemipelvis and make recommendations to the design engineer regarding cup orientation, the hip center, and the number and position of flange fixation screws. In addition to their use in preoperative planning, these models may be sterilized and used intraoperatively as a trial component to assess position and fit (Fig. 92-3A through G).

Patient-specific considerations, including leg length discrepancy, planned retention or revision of the femoral component, length of the contralateral leg, and size of the current acetabular component, determine the position of the hip center. The vertical head center location can be established by first determining the approximate anatomic position of the head center using the superior aspect of the obturator foramen as a reference point. The remaining bone of the anterior and posterior

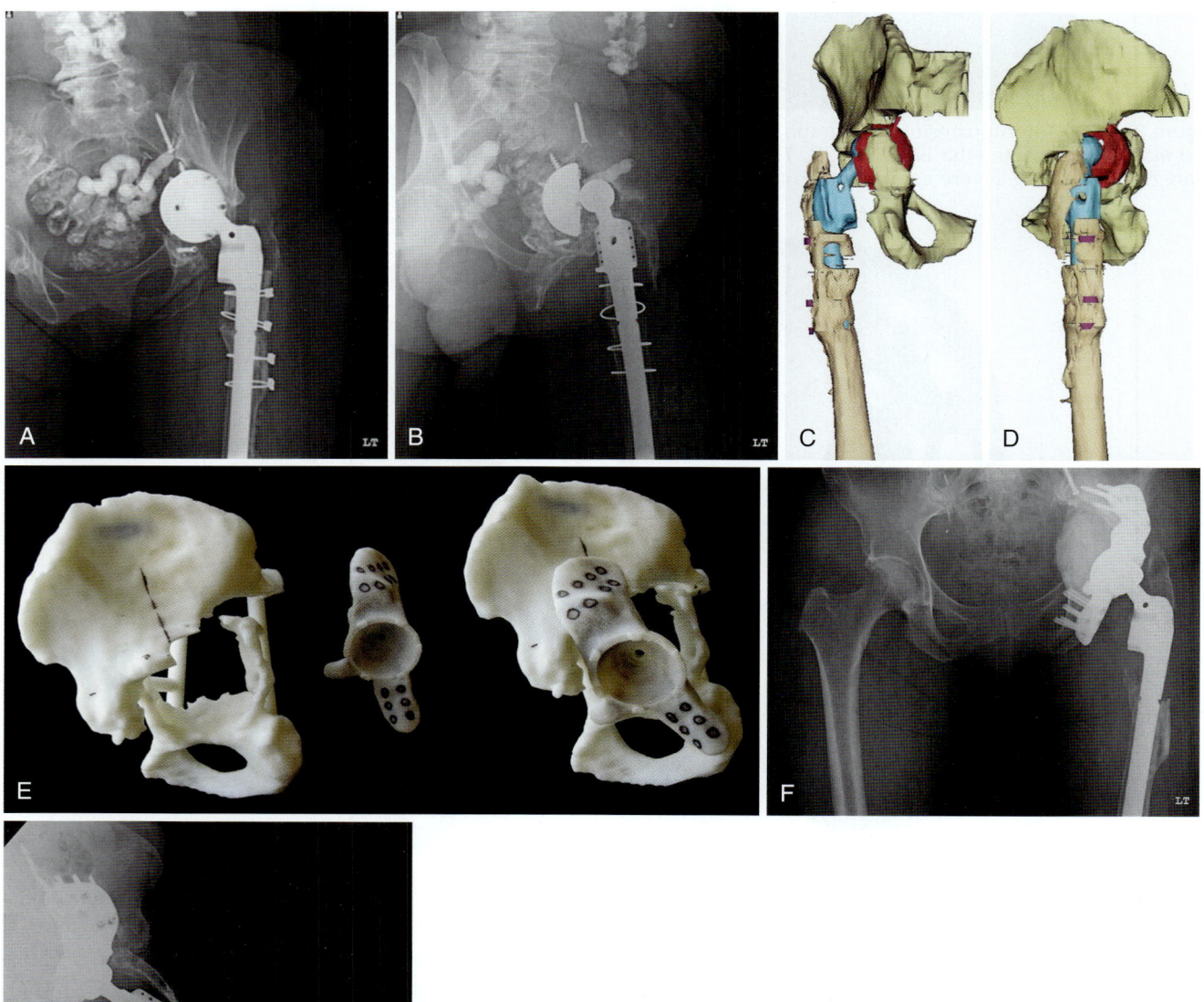

Figure 92-3. Preoperative anteroposterior **(A)** and lateral **(B)** radiographs demonstrating a failed total hip arthroplasty (THA) with acetabular component migration and massive periacetabular bone loss. Three-dimensional anteroposterior **(C)** and lateral **(D)** images demonstrating severe acetabula protrusio and a Paprosky 3B acetabular defect. **E,** Photographs of a one-to-one computer-aided design (CAD) model of a hemipelvis, demonstrating marked periacetabular bone loss, along with the acrylic custom triflanged acetabular component (CTAC) designed for acetabular reconstruction. Postoperative anteroposterior **(F)** and lateral **(G)** radiographs following reconstruction with a CTAC.

columns determines the head center in the coronal plane, whereas flange geometry and component face diameter guide the position of the head center in the sagittal plane. Evaluation of the contralateral hip center, if not distorted by aberrant anatomy or previous joint arthroplasty, can be helpful in determination of the true anatomic hip center. Although it may be desirable to reconstruct the hip center anatomically from a hip biomechanics standpoint, this may not be possible in all cases, particularly if the hip center has been displaced superiorly for an extended period of time and the femoral component is to be maintained. In this situation, a compromise may be needed with some superior positioning of the vertical hip center to reduce the newly reconstructed hip without the risk of neurovascular injury. Obtaining a preoperative anteroposterior radiograph with traction applied to the operative limb may be helpful in assessing laxity of the hip and in subsequently determining where the hip center of the CTAC should be placed.

Establishing anteversion and abduction angles of the cup is necessary to set face orientation. The abduction angle is set 35 to 40 degrees from the horizontal plane, using the plane of the obturator foramen as a reference. The anteversion angle is set at 25 to 30 degrees, using the plane of the iliac wing and the obturator foramen as references.

Upon finalization of implant design, the surfaces of the titanium alloy stock are milled. The iliac and ischial flanges contain multiple rows of screw holes for 6.5-mm screws. Current designs allow the inclusion of threaded holes to accommodate locking screws into some, or all, of the holes. Four to six screw holes in the ischial flange are preferred because they have proved to be the most common site of fixation loss. Two rows of three to four screw holes have proved sufficient for fixation of the iliac flange. The pubic flange is smaller and does not contain screw holes. Dome screw holes may also be placed, depending on the adequacy of the iliac bone stock, to create interlocking-screw fixation with the iliac flange screws. The inner geometry has a modular locking mechanism that can accept any of the modular polyethylene or metal liners typically available for standard acetabular components.

The bone interface of the CTAC, including the flanges, has a porous ingrowth surface to foster osteointegration and may be enhanced by the addition of a hydroxyapatite coating. Although osseous integration has not been proven through histologic retrieval analyses with the use of a CTAC, the ingrowth surface does provide a theoretical fixation advantage not afforded with the use of cages. We suspect that some magnitude of bone ingrowth occurs based on the lack of component migration observed radiographically in most cases now followed out to 10 years. Current CTAC designs allow for easier insertion at the time of operation and provide space behind the implant for additional bone graft. A critical design characteristic involves creating a central dome that has intimate contact with the remaining ilium superiorly to reduce shear stresses on the three fixation flanges. In a hip with massive acetabular bone loss or even pelvic discontinuity, this iliac shelf may be the only

structurally sound bone on which the CTAC may be able to rely.

Throughout the development process of the CTAC, multiple iterations of the prototype are often required, with extensive communication between the surgeon and the design engineer. This is necessary for accurate component preparation, which is critical because the operation is dependent upon the availability of a single component at the time of the operation. Because of the need for careful planning and production of the custom implant, the patient should be made aware that the preoperative process may take up to 2 months to complete. In addition to the extensive planning necessary for using CTAC, the implant is significantly more expensive than cages and "off-the-shelf" implants. For this reason, many hospitals may require prior authorization for its use or may preclude its use altogether.

DESCRIPTION OF TECHNIQUES

Surgical Approach

One can use an extensile anterolateral, posterolateral, or transtrochanteric approach to the hip. The authors' preferred approach is an extensile posterolateral approach with liberal use of a trochanteric slide[22] or a traditional greater trochanteric osteotomy. The addition of a trochanteric osteotomy facilitates exposure and hip dislocation, particularly in cases with severe acetabula protrusio (Fig. 92-4A and B). Additionally, it is helpful to prevent injury to the superior gluteal nerve, which typically is placed under tension during exposure of the ilium as required for implantation of most acetabular cages and custom triflanged acetabular components.

The femoral component should be carefully scrutinized both preoperatively on radiographs and intraoperatively to assess its degree of fixation. Although removal of a well-fixed femur is not encouraged, removal of a marginally fixed stem will improve the acetabular exposure.

If the femoral component is maintained, an anterior capsular release is necessary to create a pocket anteriorly, which allows mobilization of the femur and exposure of the pubis. Extensive release of the anterior and medial femur proximal to the lesser trochanter is often necessary to allow mobilization. Occasionally, release of the iliopsoas and gluteus maximus tendons and an extensive anterior capsulotomy are necessary to mobilize the femur adequately to allow appropriate access to the acetabulum. When the femoral stem is retained, greater dissection is necessary to allow adequate mobilization.

When an antiprotrusio cage is used, subperiosteal exposure of 2 or 3 cm of the ilium above the acetabulum is required. With use of a CTAC, greater exposure of the ilium (3 to 5 cm) is often necessary. Careful dissection to mobilize the gluteus minimus and medius muscles from the iliac wing is required to avoid damage to the superior gluteal neurovascular pedicle. A trochanteric slide or a standard trochanteric osteotomy is performed

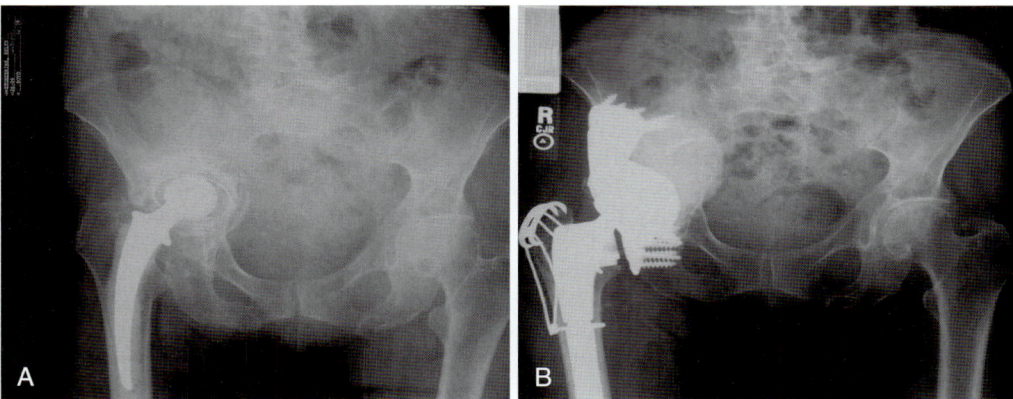

Figure 92-4. A, Preoperative anteroposterior (AP) pelvis radiograph of a failed total hip arthroplasty (THA) with severe periacetabular bone loss and acetabula protrusio. **B,** Postoperative AP pelvis radiograph following revision THA with a custom triflanged acetabular component (CTAC) used with a standard trochanteric osteotomy.

at this point if excessive tension on the neurovascular pedicle is encountered.

It is imperative to identify the sciatic nerve before beginning posterior dissection. Patients with massive periacetabular bone loss have often experienced multiple hip operations, and displacement of the sciatic nerve from its normal anatomic position is possible. The sciatic nerve may be palpated from the level of the greater sciatic notch to below the ischium. If significant scarring of the sciatic nerve is present, meticulous neurolysis is necessary to allow safe mobilization of the nerve posteriorly from the ischium. The sciatic nerve may be further protected by maintaining hip extension and knee flexion while clearing the tissue from the ischium to the level of the hamstring origin. This technique relaxes the tension on the nerve and allows it to fall away from the ischium. The assistant holding the leg should alert the surgeon to foot twitches during exposure of the ischium to create awareness regarding the proximity of the sciatic nerve. Somatosensory evoked potential (SSEP) monitoring may be used to assist in monitoring the sciatic nerve; however, the authors believe that the previously mentioned techniques are sufficient and do not utilize this resource.

After adequate exposure of the acetabulum is attained, the acetabular component, cement, and membrane from the acetabulum may be carefully removed. Unnecessary damage to the remaining acetabular bone should be avoided. After component removal, acetabular bone stock and the adequacy of the exposure for placement of an acetabular cage or CTAC may be assessed.

Acetabular Cage Implantation

When a noncustom antiprotrusio cage is inserted, trial cages should be used to assess appropriate cage size and contour when possible. It is often necessary to customize the cage to fit the deformed anatomy of the patient. Contouring the proximal iliac flange toward the pelvis ensures better contact of the flange with the ilium and the inferior ischial flange to allow for its insertion into the prepared fixation slot in the ischium.

Making a slot in the ischium for the inferior flange allows more horizontal placement of the cup, protects the sciatic nerve from irritation, and provides better fixation than screws into the ischial bone, which is often osteolytic. A high-speed burr may be used to make the slot laterally and to avoid perforation into the obturator foramen. The slot should be oriented in 25 to 30 degrees of anteversion.

Before the cage is inserted, bone grafting should be performed as necessary. Structural allografts can be contoured for superior or posterior column support on the back table and secured into place with screws or a pelvic reconstruction plate. Care is taken when using posterior column screws to avoid placement of screws into the superior dome, where cage screws are necessary. Cancellous allograft can be packed into cavitary defects.

The cage may then be inserted into the pelvis from superior to inferior, with the inferior flange placed into the prepared slot. The dome of the cage should slide into the defect with the superior flange resting against the ilium. The cage should then be secured to the pelvis with multiple 6.5-mm cancellous screws. The first screws should be placed into the dome of the acetabulum to pull the cage firmly up against superior host bone or structural allograft. The number of dome screws into the ilium should be maximized to achieve secure fixation. These screws may be angled up into the posterior column to gain maximum screw length. Any anterior screws are typically much shorter and place the pelvic contents at increased risk. Shorter iliac flange screws may then be placed after secure fixation is attained with the dome screws; this enhances fixation with an interlocking-screw construct[23] (Fig. 92-5A through C).

Currently, biological ongrowth or ingrowth is not typically utilized with noncustom acetabular cages. It is therefore imperative to ensure that the cage is mechanically stable after screw placement. Without rigid mechanical stability, failure of the construct is imminent. Once mechanical stability is obtained with screw fixation, any remaining cavitary defects should be filled with cancellous particulate graft.

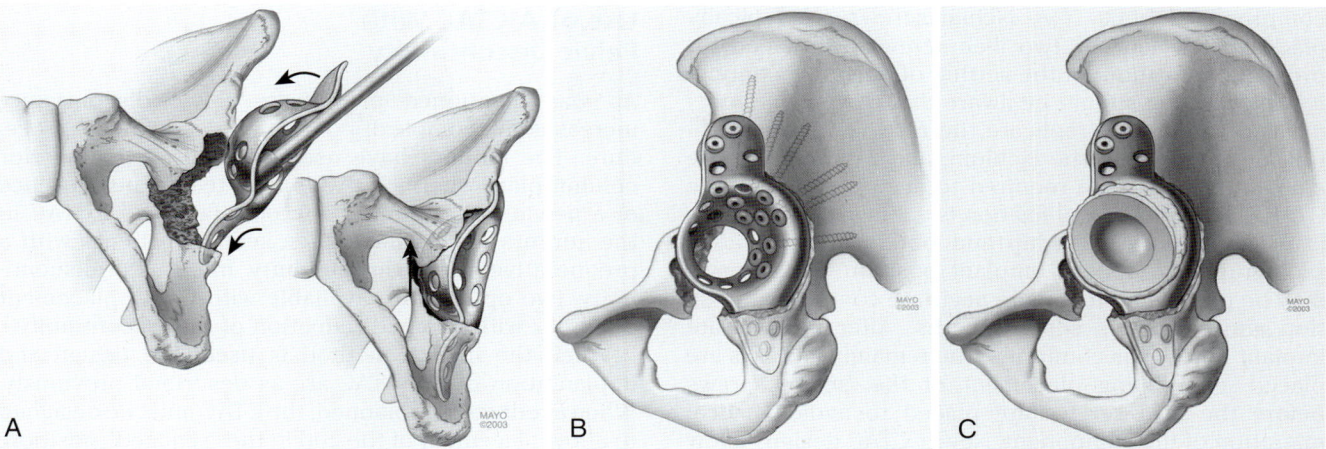

Figure 92-5. A, Diagram of insertion of an antiprotrusio cage into the acetabulum. The cage is inserted superiorly and is impacted into the ischium. *(Copyrighted and used with permission of the Mayo Foundation for Medical Education and Research. All rights reserved.*[23]*)* **B,** Diagram after placement of multiple screws through the dome holes of the cage into the ilium. *(Copyrighted and used with permission of the Mayo Foundation for Medical Education and Research. All rights reserved.*[23]*)* **C,** Diagram demonstrating placement of a cemented polyethylene acetabular component into the antiprotrusio cage. *(Copyrighted and used with permission of the Mayo Foundation for Medical Education and Research. All rights reserved.*[23]*)*

Two liner options are available with the use of a cage: (1) all-polyethylene cemented acetabular components, and (2) modular polyethylene acetabular liners. Regardless of component type, they are cemented into the cage. When a modular polyethylene liner is used, the back side of the component should be roughened with a high-speed burr for better fixation before cementing, taking care to avoid thinning the component too much at the site of burring.

The cement should be mixed into a doughy state and compressed firmly into the cage to allow the cement to interdigitate with cage and underlying bone. Before cementing, the screw heads should be filled with bone wax to allow for removal down the road should that ever become necessary. The liner or porous shell may then be pressed into the cage, taking care to attain the proper cup abduction and anteversion orientation. It is acceptable to alter the orientation of the liner from the cage, but a buttress of cement should cover the entire liner. The liner should be firmly held in place until the cement is fully hardened.

CTAC Implantation

The hemipelvis model created during design of the CTAC is gas-sterilized and referenced during the operative procedure to ensure appropriate implant placement. If the preoperative plan required removal of impeding segments of bone, these are carefully removed to shape the pelvis to accommodate the CTAC. This typically involves a thin rim of bone surrounding a portion of the remaining acetabulum. It is important to avoid removing bone in excess to that which corresponds with the preoperative plans to avoid further destabilizing the pelvis. As with implantation of a non-custom cage, any remaining cement and intervening

fibrous membrane are removed. Cancellous particulate bone graft is then packed into remaining cavitary bone defects.

Initial implantation of the CTAC may be performed via the iliac or ischial flange. However, implanting the iliac flange first is the most common technique because it places less tension on the superior gluteal neurovascular pedicle. Insertion of the acrylic trial first is wise to assess the best final method of insertion and overall fit, as well as the need for additional trimming of bone to maximize fit and position. The initial insertion of the iliac flange can be facilitated by translating the leg proximally with hip flexion and abduction to relax the abductor musculature. The iliac flange can then slide under the hip abductor musculature onto the iliac wing. Care should be taken to avoid undue traction on the superior gluteal nerve and artery via excessive retraction of the gluteus medius and minimus. After implantation of the iliac flange, the knee is flexed and the hip extended to relax the posterior soft tissues. This allows rotation of the pubic and ischial flanges into position. Care must be taken to avoid entrapment of the sciatic nerve underneath the ischial flange during CTAC insertion. The gas-sterilized pelvic model can be referenced again after implantation to ensure that implant position is similar to that described in the preoperative plan. Very little toggle of the implant is possible if the CTAC is in the appropriate position.

Fixation of the CTAC begins with placement of the ischial screws where bone is typically the poorest and severe osteolysis is common. As was previously mentioned, the authors favor placement of four to six screws into the weakened ischial bone. If necessary, cement augmentation of the osteolytic ischium allows for better fixation. The advent of locking screw technology with the CTAC offers improved fixation into this compromised bone. Two ischial screws are typically placed before one or two iliac screws are placed for provisional fixation. In the setting of pelvic discontinuity, the surgeon should be aware that the pelvic model may not accurately replicate the relative in vivo position of the ilium to the ischium, and reduction of the discontinuity may be required to accurately place the CTAC. After provisional fixation is achieved, a trial liner is used to reduce the hip and obtain intraoperative radiographs to confirm implant position. Judet views may be performed to ensure accurate component position and to assess screw lengths. After appropriate implant position is confirmed, the remaining screws are placed, completing placement of the ischial screws before the iliac screws are placed to avoid vertical migration of the component. Newer CTAC designs allow for the placement of dome screws. These may be useful in cases of severe osteolysis to improve iliac fixation via an interlocking-screw construct.

Wound Closure

Wound closure may be performed for either technique in a routine manner. Care should be taken to close any remaining posterior capsule. The trochanteric osteotomy may be repaired with cables or with a trochanteric hooked plate or claw. The authors recommend closing the fascia over a drain to minimize the risk of deep hematoma and possible subsequent infection.

VARIATIONS/UNUSUAL SITUATIONS

Use of A Cage in Pelvic Discontinuity

The presence of a pelvic discontinuity raises the complexity of an already difficult procedure. Although the cage and its flanges offer some stability, additional fixation is often required to provide a stable construct. This can most reliably be accomplished through posterior column plating. Although attaining additional stability of the discontinuity is necessary, it is important to avoid sacrificing fixation of the cage to obtain fixation of the nonunion.

In this situation, exposure should be attained as with cage insertion. Oftentimes, increased posterior column exposure is necessary, and the sciatic nerve may be identified as it courses along the posterior column mobilized away from the direct field of the posterior column. Again, it is important to keep the knee flexed and the hip extended when dissecting posteriorly around the nerve to decrease nerve tension. Bone grafting of the central defect and the nonunion of the posterior column should be performed before acetabular cage insertion.

After secure fixation of the cage is attained, attention may be directed toward securing the posterior column. A 3.5-mm pelvic reconstruction plate can then be contoured to fit the posterior column. The plate should be long enough to allow placement of at least three screws above and below the discontinuity into the ilium and the ischium, respectively.

Use of A CTAC With Pelvic Discontinuity

As was mentioned previously, pelvic discontinuity increases the complexity of this already difficult procedure. The authors have used an additional posterior column plate when a CTAC is inserted in the presence of a pelvic discontinuity. The only failures of CTAC in the authors' hands have been seen in patients with a preoperative pelvic discontinuity. In cases of discontinuity, two options are available with CTAC: placement in situ or with planned reduction of the discontinuity.

When the in situ method is used, the design and implantation of the CTAC are as described previously. When a reduction is planned, the CTAC must be designed to allow placement of the cup in the "reduced" position. With this technique, an intraoperative assessment must be completed to ensure that the relative position of the ischium and ilium will reduce to an anatomic position. Then after the CTAC is placed, the iliac screws should be placed first, before reduction is undertaken. This drives the component into intimate contact with the host bone. The shape of the CTAC, once in contact with host bone, causes the inferior hemipelvis to rotate into position against the component, thus reducing the discontinuity.

Regardless of the technique selected in cases of pelvic discontinuity, the authors have used an additional posterior column plate when inserting a CTAC in the presence of a pelvic discontinuity. Posterior column plating requires additional ischial and iliac exposure, as well as precise planning during the CTAC design, to ensure that there is room for the plate after the CTAC is placed. As with cages, the CTAC should be secured with screw fixation before the posterior column plate is placed, with the hip maintained in extension and the knee flexed during plating, while three or more screws are placed above and below the nonunion. In deficient bone, the use of a locking pelvic reconstruction plate with locking screws may enhance fixation.

The Cup-Cage Construct

A noncustom acetabular cage allows bridging of massive acetabular defects and creation of a stable construct; however, it provides no potential for biological fixation. With this in mind, all cages have the potential for loosening, leading to increased failure rates over time. To overcome this potential weakness of the cage construct, the cup-cage construct has been described, in which a jumbo acetabular revision component is used in conjunction with a noncustom antiprotrusio cage.[24,25] This allows biological fixation with the hemispherical tantalum cup while ensuring temporary fixation with an antiprotrusio cage.

An extensile exposure similar to the one previously described is necessary for this technique. Reaming of the acetabulum is performed to accommodate a jumbo hemispherical cup. Bone grafting is performed as needed. A jumbo trabecular metal (Zimmer, Warsaw, Ind) or other porous metal revision acetabular component is inserted into the large acetabular defect and is secured as well as possible with multiple dome screws. If necessary, a high-speed burr may be used to create holes in the trabecular metal acetabular component that align with available bone and screws to be placed later through holes in the cage. Because of massive bone loss, good stability typically is not achieved with the acetabular component alone. Therefore, an appropriately sized noncustom antiprotrusio cage is inserted directly into the previously implanted acetabular component to enhance fixation of the construct. To place the cage, an ischial slot should be prepared as previously described, and the screw holes of the cage should be aligned with the screw holes of the cup. This is often not possible, but because porous metals are quite soft, it is easy to drill a hole into the porous metal cup through the cage screw hole. Dome screws can then be placed through the cage and the acetabular component into the ilium, followed by screws into the iliac flange of the cage. A polyethylene liner is cemented into the cage, as with a typical cage construct, taking care to interdigitate the cement through the cage and into the tantalum shell (Fig. 92-6A through E). Kosashvili and associates[24] have reported on the use of a cup-cage construct in 26 cases of failed THA with associated pelvic discontinuity. At a mean follow-up duration of 44.6 months, 23 of 26 cases (88.5%) demonstrated a solid construct without clinical or radiographic evidence of loosening, and without posterior column plating.

The authors have favored the use of a CTAC over a cup-cage construct in most cases with severe periacetabular bone loss owing to longer follow-up with the CTAC, as well as the presence of less modularity, which may theoretically result in debris generation or premature failure. However, in cases with a pelvic discontinuity, we have used a cup-cage construct more recently because of the fact that it is easier to add a posterior column plate for further fixation of the discontinuity.

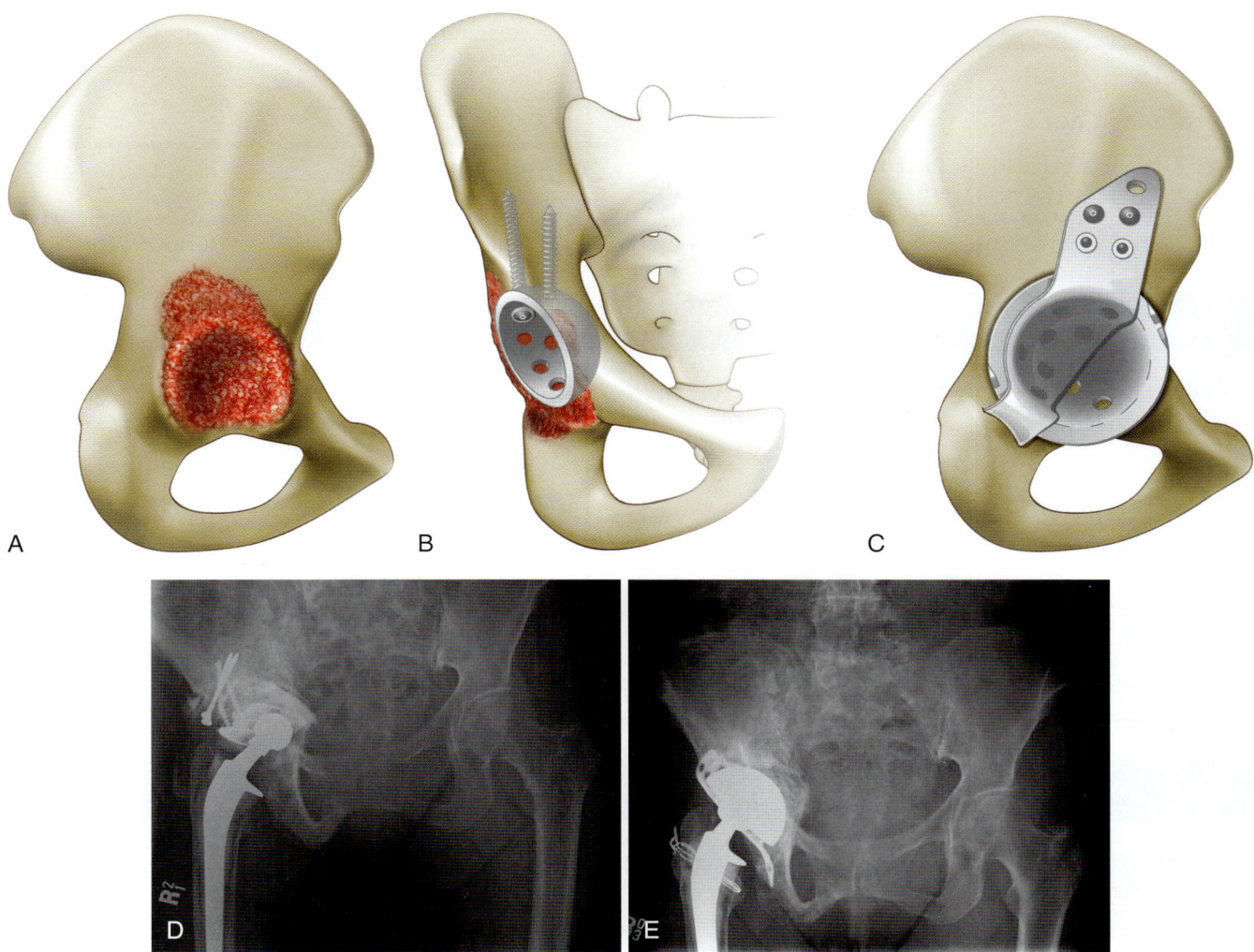

A   B   C

D   E

Figure 92-6. A, Diagram of the technique with use of a cup-cage construct showing the acetabular defect initially packed with particulate bone graft. **B,** Diagram of fixation of a trabecular metal acetabular component with multiple screws. **C,** Diagram following insertion of an acetabular cage into the trabecular metal acetabular component. **D,** Preoperative anteroposterior (AP) pelvis radiograph demonstrating a failed revision total hip arthroplasty (THA) with a 3B acetabular bone defect. *(Courtesy Yona Kosashvili, MD, and Allan Gross, MD.)* **E,** Five-year postoperative AP pelvis radiograph following reconstruction with a cup-cage construct. *(Courtesy Yona Kosashvili, MD, and Allan Gross, MD.)*

With use of a cup-cage construct, the ischial flange is embedded within the ischium, leaving more room for plate placement, whereas with a CTAC, the ischial flange is positioned on the outside of the ischium, and this can preclude plate placement in the desired location.

POSTOPERATIVE CARE

Toe touch weight bearing should be maintained for a period of 1 to 2 months after surgery, followed by partial weight bearing with walking aids for another period of 1 to 2 months. In the setting of a pelvic discontinuity, weight bearing may need to be restricted longer until the surgeon is convinced that the posterior column has reconstituted. Careful monitoring of anticoagulation in the acute period is necessary to avoid hematoma formation. A hip abduction orthosis may aid in preventing dislocation and protecting the trochanteric osteotomy in the acute postoperative period.

RESULTS

Acetabular Cages

Several reports have described the results observed when antiprotrusio cages were used in massive acetabular defects. Most of these studies show 80% to 90% survivorship at midterm (5 to 10 years') follow-up

duration (Table 92-3). It is important to note that a higher failure rate has been reported in the presence of a pelvic discontinuity or severe posterior column deficiency. For this reason, we recommend posterior column plating or use of structural allograft in these cases. It is important to remember that it is impossible to attain biological fixation with noncustom cages; therefore, all are susceptible to mechanical failure over time.

CTAC

Three studies reporting the results of CTAC are available in the literature (Table 92-4). These studies have described very good midterm (2 to 9 years) results with greater than 90% success overall. These series report only one revision for mechanical failure, which was performed in a patient with preoperative pelvic discontinuity. The most common reason for revision was recurrent dislocation requiring conversion to a more constrained liner. An additional study reported use of these devices in 20 cases with a pelvic discontinuity; osseous union of the discontinuity was attained in 18 of the 20 (90%) cases.[17]

COMPLICATIONS

Sciatic nerve injury, although rare, does occur when these complex procedures are performed. This most

Table 92-3. Selected Results With Use of Acetabular Cages

Author	Year	Number of Hips	Mean Age, yr	Mean Follow-up, yr (range)	Results
Peters et al[11]	1995	28	60.7	2.8	• 14% cup migration >3 mm • 7% patients with recurrent dislocation • 18% patients with nonprogressive radiolucent lines • 0 re-revisions
Berry & Muller[12]	1992	42	61 (female) 64 (male)	5 (2-11)	• 12% failure to sepsis • 12% mechanical failure
Gill et al[13]	1998	63	63	8.5 (5-18)	• 5% mechanical failure • 2% failure to sepsis • 2% recurrent dislocation • 5% probable loosening without re-revision
Perka & Ludwig[14]	2001	63	67.4	5.5 (3-10)	• 5% mechanical failure • 5% probable loosening without re-revision

Table 92-4. Selected Results With Use of A CTAC

Author	Year	Number of Hips	Mean Age, yr	Mean Follow-up, yr (range)	Results
Christie et al[15]	2001	67	59	4.5 (2-9)	• 0 mechanical failures • 15% dislocation rate • 8% re-revision for recurrent dislocation
Joshi et al[16]	2002	27	68	5 (4-6)	• 0 mechanical failures • 3% re-revision for dislocation • 3% revision for sciatic nerve palsy
Holt & Dennis[18]	2004	26	68	4.5 (2-7)	• 3% mechanical failures • 6% radiographic loosening without re-revision

CTAC, Custom triflanged acetabular component.

commonly occurs during dissection and is most often observed as traction rather than a direct nerve injury. Caution should be taken to maintain knee flexion and hip extension during dissection and ischial flange placement. Placement of increased tension on posterior retractors, which place tension on the sciatic nerve, must be avoided. Placement of the ischial flange or the posterior column plate in a manner in which it overhangs the ischium will increase the risk of sciatic nerve irritation. In addition, one must be careful to avoid overlengthening of the limb. Often in chronically failed cases, the hip center may be significantly medialized with severe acetabular component protrusio and concomitantly contracted soft tissues. In these cases, once an acetabular cage or CTAC is placed, the limb may be relatively lengthened to the degree that the hip may not be able to be reduced without excessive and potential damage to lower extremity traction. The surgeon should be prepared to revise the femoral component, despite its being well fixed, to achieve an acceptable leg length without excessive nerve tension. This problem is preferably avoided with proper preoperative planning and accurate determination of the desired hip center. After a trial hip reduction, an intraoperative straight-leg raise test should be performed with palpation of the sciatic nerve while slowly flexing the hip and extending the knee to ensure that excessive tension is not present.

Mechanical failure is another common form of failure with these procedures. It occurs most commonly secondary to failure to attain mechanical stability of the cage or CTAC at the initial operative procedure, or failure to stabilize a pelvic discontinuity. If motion of the cage or CTAC is noted at the time of implantation, failure is imminent. Increasing the number of screws or augmenting screw fixation with cement in osteolytic bone may help achieve stability. We recommend posterior column plating and bone graft in all cases of pelvic discontinuity despite the fact that some[17] have achieved success in management of these cases with implantation of a CTAC alone without posterior column plating.

Instability is perhaps the most common complication encountered. This happens for multiple reasons. Weak abductor strength secondary to multiple hip surgeries, capsular insufficiency, trochanteric nonunion, or superior gluteal nerve injury increases the risk of dislocation. Nerve injury may be avoided with the liberal use of a trochanteric osteotomy during the exposure. The surgeon should strive to attain secure fixation of the osteotomy and to protect the abductor mechanism in the acute postoperative phase. Acetabular component malposition is another leading cause of dislocation. Meticulous surgical technique is necessary to ensure appropriate cup position. In some cases, despite excellent surgical technique, stability is difficult to achieve. For this reason, we recommend a low threshold for the use of a high-wall, face-changing, or constrained polyethylene liner, as well as consideration of use of a hip abduction orthosis postoperatively if stability is in question.

REFERENCES

1. Whaley AL, Berry DJ, Harmsen WS: Extra-large uncemented hemispherical acetabular components for revision total hip arthroplasty. J Bone Joint Surg Am 83:1352–1357, 2001.
2. Gross AE: Revision arthroplasty of the acetabulum with restoration of bone stock. Clin Orthop Relat Res 369:198–207, 1999.
3. Saleh KJ, Jaroszynski G, Woodgate I, et al: Revision total hip arthroplasty with the use of structural acetabular allograft and reconstruction ring: a case series with a 10-year average follow-up. J Arthroplasty 15:951–958, 2000.
4. Shinar AA, Harris WS: Bulk structural autogenous grafts and allografts for reconstruction of the acetabulum in total hip arthroplasty: sixteen-year-average follow-up. J Bone Joint Surg Am 79:159–168, 1997.
5. Paprosky WG, Perona PG, Lawrence JM: Acetabular defect classification and surgical reconstruction in revision arthroplasty: a 6-year follow-up evaluation. J Arthroplasty 9:33–44, 1994.
6. Murray WR: Acetabular salvage in revision total hip arthroplasty using the bipolar prosthesis. Clin Orthop Relat Res 251:92–99, 1990.
7. Schreurs BW, Slooff TJ, Gardeniers JW, Buma P: Acetabular reconstruction with bone impaction grafting and a cemented cup: 20 years' experience. Clin Orthop Relat Res 393:202–215, 2001.
8. Sutherland CJ: Early experience with eccentric acetabular components in revision total hip arthroplasty. Am J Orthop 25:284–289, 1996.
9. Berry DJ, Sutherland CJ, Trousdale RT, et al: Bilobed oblong porous coated acetabular components in revision total hip arthroplasty. Clin Orthop Relat Res 371:154–160, 2000.
10. Chen WM, Engh CA, Hopper RH, et al: Acetabular revision with use of a bilobed component inserted without cement in patients who have acetabular bone-stock deficiency. J Bone Joint Surg Am 82:197–206, 2000.
11. Peters CL, Curtain M, Samuleson KM: Acetabular revision with the Burch-Schnieder antiprotrusio cage and cancellous allograft bone. J Arthroplasty 10:307–312, 1995.
12. Berry DJ, Muller ME: Revision arthroplasty using an antiprotrusio cage for massive acetabular bone deficiency. J Bone Joint Surg Br 74:711–715, 1992.
13. Gill TJ, Sledge JB, Muller ME: The Burch-Schneider antiprotrusio cage in revision total hip arthroplasty: indications, principles, and long-term results. J Bone Joint Surg Br 74:716–720, 1998.
14. Perka C, Ludwig R: Reconstruction of segmental defects during revision procedures of the acetabulum with the Burch-Schneider anti-protrusio cage. J Arthroplasty 15:568–574, 2001.
15. Christie MJ, Barrington SA, Brinson MF, et al: Bridging massive acetabular defects with the triflange cup: 2- to 9-year results. Clin Orthop Relat Res 293:216–227, 2001.
16. Joshi AB, Lee J, Christensen C: Results for a custom acetabular component for acetabular deficiency. J Arthroplasty 17:643–648, 2002.
17. Dennis DA: Management of massive acetabular defects in revision total hip arthroplasty. J Arthroplasty 18:121–125, 2003.
18. Holt GE, Dennis DA: Use of custom triflanged acetabular components in revision total hip arthroplasty. Clin Orthop Relat Res 429:209–214, 2004.
19. DeBoer DK, Christie MJ, Brinson MF, Morrison JC: Revision total hip arthroplasty for pelvic discontinuity. J Bone Joint Surg Am 89:835–840, 2007.
20. D'Antonio JA, Capello WN, Borden LS, et al: Classification and management of acetabular abnormalities in total hip arthroplasty. Clin Orthop Relat Res 243:126–137, 1989.
21. Fehring TK, Guilford WB, Baron J: Assessment of intrapelvic cement and screws in revision total hip arthroplasty. J Arthroplasty 7:509–518, 1992.
22. Glassman AH, Engh CA, Bobyn JD: A technique of extensile exposure for total hip arthroplasty. J Arthroplasty 2:11–21, 1987.

23. Berry DJ: Cages. In Barrack RL, editor: Master techniques in orthopedic surgery: the hip, ed 2, Philadelphia, 2005, Lippincott Williams & Wilkins, pp 438–439.

24. Kosashvili Y, Backstein D, Safir O, et al: Acetabular revision using an anti-protrusion (ilio-ischial) cage and trabecular metal acetabular component for severe acetabular bone loss associated with pelvic discontinuity. J Bone Joint Surg Br 91:870–876, 2009.

25. Boscainos PJ, Kellett CF, Maury AC, et al: Management of peri-acetabular bone loss in revision hip arthroplasty. Clin Orthop Relat Res 465:159–165, 2007.

CHAPTER 93

Femoral Revision: Classification of Bone Defects and Treatment Options

Michael Tanzer and Dylan Tanzer

KEY POINTS

- *Revision THA:* Classifying femoral bone defects is a critical part of the preoperative planning required for a successful revision THA.
- *Classification:* Classifying femoral bone defects is a critical part of the preoperative planning required for a successful revision THA. Paprosky, Mallory, the American Academy of Orthopaedic Surgeons, Endo-Klink, Saleh and coworkers, Engh and Glassman, Gustillo and Pasternak, and Chandler and Penenberg have all published classification systems that differ in their complexity and descriptive terms; however, there remains no consensus as to which classification system should be used when bone loss is assessed in the face of revision THA.
- *Femoral bone loss:* Failure of a primary THA typically occurs with varying degrees of femoral bone loss.
- *Treatment options:* Femoral bone loss can be extensive, making it difficult to obtain adequate support of the femoral component at the time of revision surgery. As a result, these bone defects can adversely affect the long-term fixation and survivorship of the revised femoral implant.
- *Reliability:* A useful classification system for femoral bone loss associated with a failed THA should be both reliable and valid. *Reliability* refers to both interobserver reliability, the agreement between different observers, and intraobserver reliability, the agreement of one observer on separate occasions. *Validity* indicates the accuracy with which the classification system describes the true pathology.

INTRODUCTION

Failure of a primary total hip arthroplasty (THA) typically occurs with varying degrees of femoral bone loss. This bone loss can be the result of osteolysis, mechanical loosening, infection, or stress shielding. Regardless of the underlying cause, femoral bone loss can be extensive, making it difficult to obtain adequate support of the femoral component at the time of revision surgery. As a result, these bone defects can adversely affect the long-term fixation and survivorship of the revised femoral implant.

Classifying femoral bone defects is a critical part of the preoperative planning required for a successful revision THA. A classification system that estimates the pattern and degree of bone loss can aid the surgeon in determining the operative plan. The classification system can predict the complexity of the surgery and can provide an algorithmic approach to reconstruction of the femoral deficiency in revision THA. This is necessary to determine which implants, instruments, and bone grafts will be required to be available at the time of revision surgery. Because various reconstructive options are available to revise a failed femoral component, a classification system also allows the uniform comparison of published outcomes of these different reconstructive techniques.

Several classification systems for femoral bone loss associated with a failed THA have been described in the literature. Paprosky, Mallory, Saleh and associates, Engh and Glassman, Gustillo and Pasternak, and Chandler and Penenberg have all published classification systems that differ in their complexity and descriptive terms.[1-6] The emphasis of these different classification systems varies with the objective that each was designed to achieve. Despite their usefulness to the author advocating the classification, none has been universally accepted and used. A comprehensive classification system for femoral deficiencies in revision THA was developed by the American Academy of Orthopaedic Surgeons Committee on the Hip and was reported by D'Antonio and colleagues.[7] Unfortunately, many of the present classification systems are difficult to remember or are inadequate in providing an algorithm for femoral reconstruction. As a result, there remains no consensus as to which classification system should be used when bone loss is assessed in the face of revision THA. The purposes of this chapter are to review the most common classification systems of bone defects associated with femoral revision and, when possible, to link the classification system with treatment options for femoral reconstruction at the time of revision THA.

CLASSIFICATIONS AND TREATMENT OPTIONS

Paprosky Classification

The Paprosky classification for femoral bone loss is commonly used in North America and Europe and attempts to group the revision femur into one of four types based on the integrity of the metaphysis, the remaining isthmic bone and the quality of the host cortices (Table 93-1).[8-10] This classification system is based on the ability of the reconstruction to bypass the compromised proximal femur and attain osteointegration of an extensively coated femoral implant in the femoral diaphysis. In addition to classifying femoral defects, this system provides an algorithmic approach to reconstruction of femoral deficiency in revision total hip arthroplasty (THA).

In a type I defect, there is minimal loss of metaphyseal cancellous bone with an intact femoral diaphysis. This type of bone defect is not common. It is usually seen with a failed cementless, smooth implant such as a failed Austin-Moore prosthesis (Fig. 93-1). Revision THA

is relatively straightforward, and the intact metaphyseal bone allows the use of a cemented or cementless femoral implant. However, inferior results have been reported after revision using a cemented or proximally porous-coated primary hip stem.[11] If a cemented stem is used for the revision, careful canal preparation and removal of the neocortex are mandatory to achieve cement interdigitation and long-term success.[11]

Type II defects are among the more common types of deficiencies. In a type II defect, extensive loss of metaphyseal bone is seen with a completely intact femoral diaphysis. This type of defect is often present after the removal of loose cemented femoral component or in the early stage of loosening of a cementless femoral implant (Fig. 93-2). The deficient metaphyseal cancellous bone precludes revision with a cemented stem. Because the metaphysis remains somewhat supportive, a proximally porous-coated cementless implant with diaphyseal stabilization or an extensively porous-coated implant with distal fixation can be used to revise the failed THA. Type II defects can be associated with varus remodeling of the proximal femur. In these cases, an extended trochanteric osteotomy and a diaphyseal filling implant are required.

Type III defects are subdivided depending on the amount of intact diaphyseal bone available for distal fixation. In type IIIA defects, the femoral metaphysis is severely damaged and nonsupportive, but at least 4 cm of intact cortical bone is present in the femoral diaphysis (Fig. 93-3). At least 4 cm of intact diaphyseal bone is

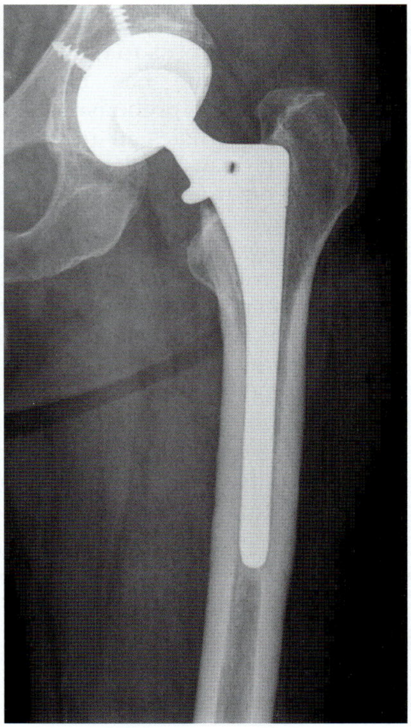

Table 93-1. Paprosky Classification

Type	Femoral Bone Deficiency
1	Minimal loss of metaphyseal cancellous bone with an intact femoral diaphysis
2	Extensive loss of metaphyseal bone with a completely intact femoral diaphysis
3A	Femoral metaphysis severely damaged and nonsupportive, with at least 4 cm of intact cortical bone present in the femoral diaphysis
3B	Nonsupportive severely damaged metaphysis with intact diaphyseal cortical bone less than 4 cm in length
4	Extensive metaphyseal and diaphyseal damage in conjunction with a widened femoral canal

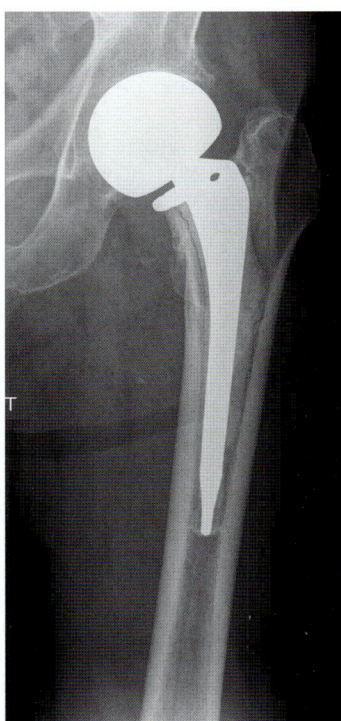

Figure 93-1. An anteroposterior radiograph of a loose cementless femoral component illustrating a type I defect. Minimal loss of the metaphyseal cancellous bone occurs with an intact femoral diaphysis.

Figure 93-2. An anteroposterior radiograph of a loose cemented femoral endoprosthesis illustrating a type II defect. Extensive loss of the metaphyseal bone is noted with a completely intact femoral diaphysis.

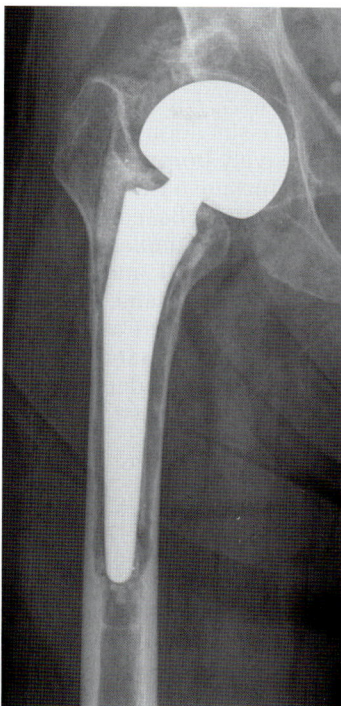

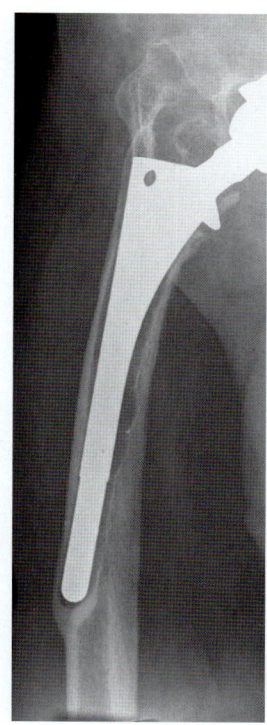

Figure 93-3. An anteroposterior radiograph of a loose cemented femoral endoprosthesis illustrating a type IIIA defect. The femoral metaphysis is severely damaged and nonsupportive, but more than 4 cm of intact cortical bone is present in the femoral diaphysis distal to the failed implant.

Figure 93-4. An anteroposterior radiograph of a loose cementless femoral component that has migrated into varus. The severe varus femoral remodeling associated with this necessitates an extended trochanteric osteotomy at the time of revision surgery to ensure proper implant alignment.

required to have sufficient implant-cortical contact to achieve initial stability and long-term osteointegration.[12] In these cases, revision with an extensively porous-coated femoral implant is used to achieve fixation in the diaphysis. Eight-inch stems are most frequently utilized, but their use can be complicated by perforation of the anterior femoral cortex at the level of the anterior femoral bow. The risk of femoral perforation can be minimized with the use of curved femoral implants. Another reconstructive technique for type IIIA defects is impaction grafting.[8,13-19] Type IIIA defects can be associated with torsional remodeling of the proximal femur into retroversion. In these cases, a modular tapered stem can be used because it allows independent filling of proximal and distal portions of the femur while allowing independent rotation of the two segments to correct the femoral anteversion. Type IIIA defects are frequently associated with varus femoral remodeling that requires an extended trochanteric osteotomy at the time of revision surgery to ensure proper implant alignment and restoration of normal femoral alignment (Fig. 93-4).

Similar to type IIIA defects, type IIIB defects have a severely damaged metaphysis that is nonsupportive. However, in type IIIB defects, the intact diaphyseal cortical bone is less than 4 cm in length (Fig. 93-5). This type of femoral bone deficiency is commonly seen with revision of a failed long cemented stem with a distal plug and a long cement mantle or with cementless stems with substantial distal osteolysis. The short

region of intact cortical bone in type IIIB defects does not tend to provide sufficient initial scratch fit and implant-bone contact to ensure implant stability and ingrowth. As a result, the use of extensively porous-coated stems in these defects has been associated with an unacceptably higher rate of fibrous stable fixation rather than bone ingrowth.[1] Revision with a modular, tapered cementless stem is recommended for these defects.[18,20] The tapered and fluted stem is able to attain excellent initial axial and rotational stability in the face of a very short region of intact isthmus. Modularity allows the impaction of the distal component until it is stable and then provides the ability to build up the proximal segment to restore leg lengths and offset. Impaction grafting also can be used to reconstruct type IIIB defects if the metaphysis is relatively intact with contained defects; if not, it can be reconstructed with mesh, strut grafts, or plates.

In a type IV defect, extensive metaphyseal and diaphyseal damage is noted in conjunction with a widened femoral canal. In these rare cases, the isthmus is nonsupportive, and distal fixation cannot be achieved (Fig. 93-6). Revision with a modular, tapered cementless stem has demonstrated early and promising results for these defects.[8,20] When the proximal femoral cortex is intact, impaction grafting can also be used to reconstruct the femur and restore bone stock. In low-demand elderly patients, a long cemented stem can be used occasionally to revise the loose THA. When the proximal femoral

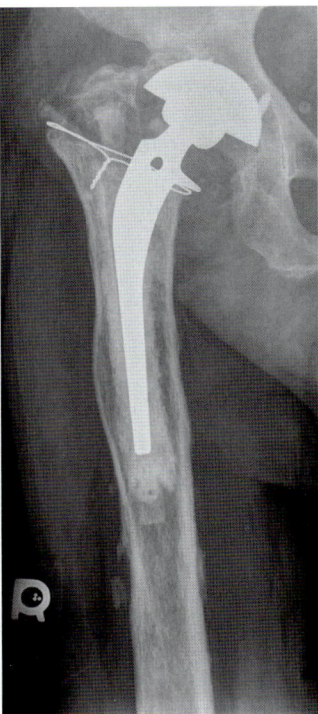

Figure 93-5. An anteroposterior radiograph of a loose cemented femoral component illustrating a type IIIB defect. The metaphysis is severely damaged and nonsupportive. The intact diaphyseal cortical bone distal to the failed stem is less than 4 cm in length.

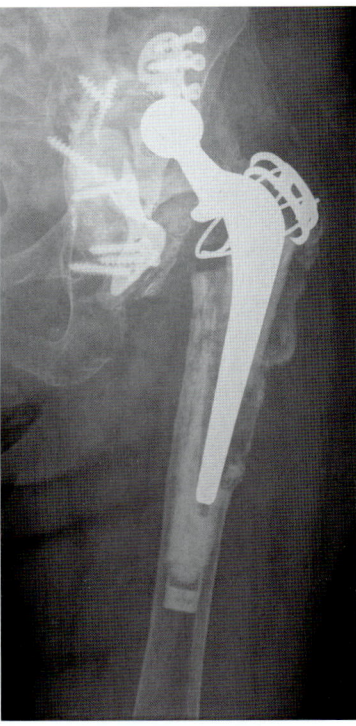

Figure 93-6. An anteroposterior radiograph of a loose cemented femoral component illustrating a type IV defect. Extensive metaphyseal and diaphyseal damage is seen in conjunction with a widened femoral canal.

cortex is deficient, a femoral allograft-prosthesis composite can be used to reconstitute bone stock in younger patients, and a proximal femoral replacement can be used in older patients.[21-24]

The Paprosky classification system is based on the ability of an extensively porous-coated femoral implant to bypass the compromised femur and attain fixation in the femoral diaphysis. Based on this classification, extensively porous-coated implants have demonstrated 96% survivorship in type II and type IIIA defects at 14-year follow-up.[8,12] At the same follow-up, the rate of mechanical failure is reported at 21% for type IIIB or type IV defects.[12] As a result, modular tapered cementless stems are now recommended for reconstruction of the severe femoral defects seen in Paprosky type IIIB and type IV femurs.

Mallory Classification

The Mallory classification is one of the earliest systems that attempts to classify femoral bone loss and provide a guide to treatment.[2] This system describes femoral bone loss as varying degrees of expansive opening of the proximal femur and associated cortical thinning, medullary canal disintegration, and preservation of the femur distal to the failed implant or cement mantle. The classification system divides femoral bone loss into three types based on the integrity of the medullary contents of the femur and the integrity of the cortical bone (Table 93-2). In a type I defect, the cortex and medullary contents remain essentially intact. Loosening occurs only within the medullary canal and does not destroy the medullary canal or the cortical bone. This type of bone loss is frequently seen with a failed cemented THA that was poorly cemented and had a thin cement mantle that did not fill the entire metaphyseal cancellous bone. This type of bone defect can be treated with cemented or cementless femoral components following conventional parameters, similar to a primary THA.

In a type II defect, the medullary contents of the femur are essentially gone, but the cortical tube remains intact. This type of defect occurs after failure of a cemented femoral component in which the cement extended all the way to the metaphyseal cortex, or with femoral loosening and associated endosteal osteolysis that destroys all the cancellous bone. Because the proximal cancellous bone is deficient and the cortical tube

Table 93-2. Mallory Classification	
Type	**Femoral Bone Loss**
I	Intact cortex and medullary contents
II	Intact cortex with deficient medullary contents
III	Deficient cortex and medullary contents
	IIIA Cortical bone loss proximal to the lesser trochanter
	IIIB Cortical bone loss between the lesser trochanter and the isthmus
	IIIC Cortical bone loss to the isthmus and distal

is intact, reconstruction with distal fixation beyond the previous implant is recommended, and cemented implants are avoided in this type of defect.[2]

In type III defects, both the medullary contents and the cortical tube have been destroyed. The destruction of the cortical tube is then graded according to its extent. In type IIIA, cortical bone loss is seen proximal to the lesser trochanter, in type IIIB between the lesser trochanter and the isthmus, and in type IIIC to the isthmus and distal. Mallory recommended a femoral allograft-prosthesis composite to reconstruct and restore the bone stock in type IIIB and IIIC defects.[2]

American Academy of Orthopaedic Surgeons Committee on the Hip Classification

The American Academy of Orthopaedic Surgeons (AAOS) Committee on the Hip Classification introduced a comprehensive classification system to address femoral bony deficiencies in both primary and revision THA (Table 93-3).[7] The goal was to classify bony deficiencies in a uniform manner so as to facilitate both preoperative planning and surgical treatment of these deficiencies. This system is commonly used in North America.

The classification system of femoral abnormalities has two basic categories: segmental and cavitary. Type I defects are segmental femoral defects. A segmental defect is defined as any loss of bone in the supporting cortical shell of the femur (Fig. 93-7). Segmental proximal deficiencies can be further subdivided into partial or complete. Partial proximal segmental bone loss can be located anteriorly, medially, or posteriorly. These defects can be present from proximal through any distal level of the femur. An intercalary defect is a segmental cortical bone defect with intact bone above and below, as is seen with a cortical perforation, with a cortical window, or in the case of severe osteolysis. It is recommended that when intercalary defects are present, the revision implant should bypass the defect by two and one-half canal diameters.[7] Segmental bone loss affecting the greater trochanter is categorized as a separate segmental defect because of the unique and difficult problems that it can present in femoral reconstruction.

Type II defects are cavitary femoral defects. A cavitary defect is a contained lesion and represents an excavation of the cancellous or endosteal cortical bone with no violation of the outer cortical shell of the femur. Three types of cavitary bone loss may occur, according to the degree of bone loss within the femur. Cancellous cavitary defects involve only the cancellous medullary bone. Cortical cavitary defects suggest a more severe type of erosion where, in addition to cancellous loss, the femoral cortex is eroded from within (Fig. 93-8). In the most extreme cases of cavitary defects, the femur becomes ectatic or dilated with complete loss of cancellous bone and severe cortical erosion and thinning.

Type III defects are combined segmental and cavitary femoral defects. Combined deficiencies designate the situation where segmental and cavitary bone losses in the femur coexist. This may result from osteolysis, stem movement, or iatrogenic circumstances. Combined segmental and cavitary defects are the most common defects experienced in revision surgery and are often the result of osteolysis and femoral stem migration (see Fig. 93-6).

Type IV defects are characterized by femoral malalignment. Malalignment is defined as a distortion of the femoral architectural geometry in the rotational or angular plane. This can be seen with varus femoral

Type	Femoral Bone Defect

I	Segmental femoral defects
	    Proximal: partial or complete
	    Intercalary
	    Greater trochanter

II	Cavitary femoral defects
	    Cancellous
	    Cortical
	    Ectatic

III	Combined segmental and cavitary femoral defects

IV	Femoral malalignment
	    Rotational
	    Angular

V	Femoral stenosis
VI	Femoral discontinuity

Table 93-3. AAOS Committee on the Hip Classification

AAOS, American Academy of Orthopaedic Surgeons.

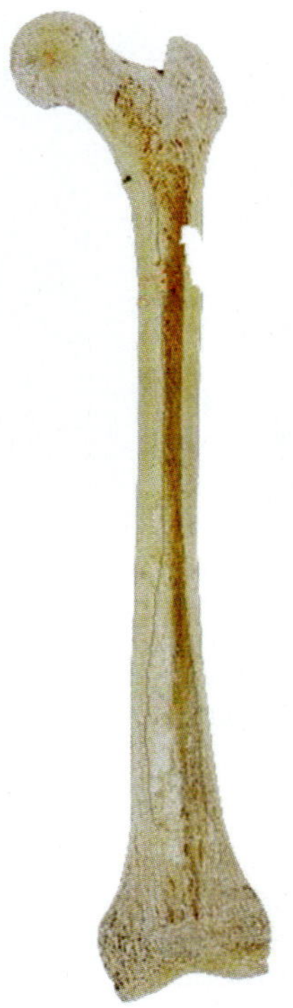

Figure 93-7. Diagrammatic representation of a segmental defect in which loss of the supporting cortical shell of the femur is evident.

remodeling of a loose femoral component (see Fig. 93-4).

A type V deformity occurs when femoral stenosis is present. Femoral stenosis involves the relative or absolute narrowing of the femoral canal, creating partial or complete occlusion of the femoral intramedullary canal. This may result from bony hypertrophy, fracture, or fixation devices.

A type VI defect is observed when there is femoral discontinuity. Femoral discontinuity describes the lack of bony integrity that exists with periprosthetic fracture of the femur or nonunion of a periprosthetic fracture.

To better localize the femoral defects and assist in preoperative planning, the AAOS classification uses levels of involvement (Fig. 93-9). Level I is defined as bone proximal to the inferior portion of the lesser trochanter, level II is from the inferior lesser trochanter to 10 cm distal, and level III involves bone distal to level II. Most defects seen in revision THA occur at levels I and

II. Level III deficiencies most frequently occur with failure of a long-stem prosthesis or with a periprosthetic fracture.

A grading system is used in this classification to grade the reconstructive effort. Grade I is seen when there is complete implant-host bone contact and no bone graft is required. Grade II reconstruction implies that there is incomplete implant-host bone contact but the implant is stable. Bone graft is not necessary but can be used to fill the gaps. In grade III, implant-host bone contact is insufficient to provide stability and structural bone grafting is required.

Overall, this classification system tries to provide a comprehensive description of all types of femoral bone loss, as well as the location of the lost bone. However, it does not fully predict the type of management required for treatment of all these defects. This has been left to other surgeons to develop over time, based on their experience, expertise, and outcomes while using the AAOS classification to communicate their results in the orthopedic literature.

Endo-Klink Classification

The Endo-Klink classification system, which is more commonly used in Europe, classifies femoral bone loss that is commonly seen with a failed cemented femoral component (Table 93-4).[25] In grade 1, the femoral prosthesis is clinically loose and radiolucent lines are noted along the proximal half of the cement mantle. This can be seen with poor cementing, debonding of the femoral prosthesis, or osteolysis. In grade 2, radiolucent lines are present circumferentially around the femoral implant, and the medullary cavity of the proximal part of the femur is expanded by endosteal erosion. In grade 3, bone loss is characterized by expansion of

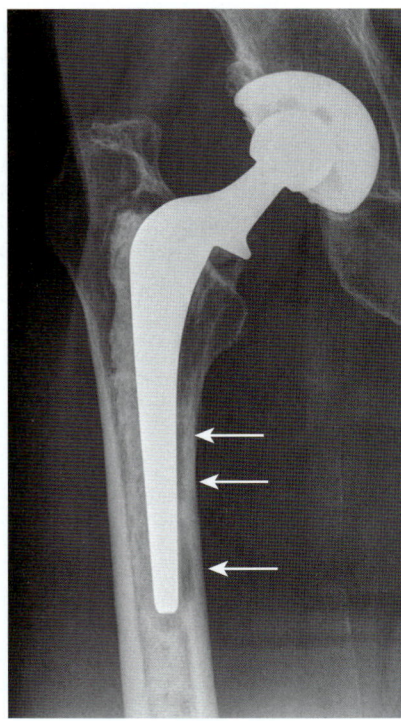

Figure 93-8. An anteroposterior radiograph of a loose cemented femoral component demonstrating cortical cavitary defects along the distal portion of the stem. The arrows denote the region where erosion of the cancellous bone is seen and adjacent cortex from within.

Table 93-4. Endo-Klink Classification	
Grade	**Femoral Bone Loss**
1	Loose implant with radiolucent lines along the proximal half of the cement mantle
2	Circumferential radiolucent lines around the implant; medullary cavity of the proximal part of the femur expanded by endosteal erosion
3	Proximal femoral expansion with widening of the medullary cavity
4	Gross destruction of the proximal third of the femur with involvement of the middle third of the femur

Figure 93-9. Illustration of the level of femoral bone loss according to the American Academy of Orthopaedic Surgeons (AAOS) Committee on the Hip Classification System.

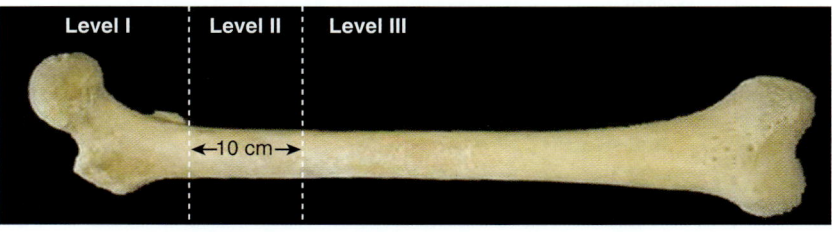

the proximal part of the femur with widening of the medullary cavity. A cortical defect may be present in these cases. In grade 4, gross destruction of the proximal third of the femur occurs with involvement of the middle third of the femur. This precludes the use of a long-stem prosthesis.

Classification of Saleh and Associates

This classification system used a consensus panel of experts to define the dimensions that were important when measuring the severity of a failed THA and then used input from the expert panel to develop a measure of severity (Table 93-5).[3,26] The authors designed the system to extract information from standard radiographs, to be comprehensive and practical, and to provide a guide to specific treatment of each type of bone loss.

In type I femoral defects, there is no notable loss of bone stock. Erosion of the endosteal bone may occur, but there is no involvement of the cortex. This type of bone loss can be dealt with by using a conventional cemented or cementless femoral component.

In type II bone loss, there is a constrained loss of bone stock with cortical thinning. The intramedullary canal is widened, but the cortical sleeve is intact. Reconstructive options include both proximal and distal fixation. Proximal fixation can be achieved with a modular implant, a proximal porous-coated implant, or impaction grafting. Distal fixation can be attained with a long porous-coated implant, a press-fit implant, or a long cemented implant.

In type III bone loss, there is uncontained loss of cortical bone stock involving the calcar and the lesser trochanter. It can be noncircumferential or circumferential, but it must be less than 5 cm in length and proximal to the diaphysis. The noncircumferential defect can be treated with a cortical strut allograft or by bypassing the defect with the femoral stem. If the defect is circumferential, it can be reconstructed by using a calcar replacing femoral implant.

In type IV defects, there is uncontained circumferential loss of bone stock greater than 5 cm in length that extends into the diaphysis. Reconstruction of these defects requires a structural allograft or tumor prosthesis.

Type V defects occur when there is a periprosthetic fracture with circumferential bone loss proximal to the fracture. The bone loss has to be as severe as that described in type IV. Lesser degrees of bone loss in association with a periprosthetic fracture are not classified by this system. Reconstruction requires a tumor prosthesis or a structural femoral allograft with fracture fixation by the femoral stem and osteotomy at the allograft-host junction.

Engh and Glassman Classification

Engh and Glassman observed that a failed THA resulted in three basic patterns of femoral bone stock loss (Table 93-6).[4,27] The classification system is also designed to provide a recommendation as to the implants and the surgical technique required to obtain long-term fixation.

The three types of femoral bone loss in this classification system are mild, moderate, and severe. The progression of bone stock loss usually proceeds from proximal to distal with increasing degrees of damage. In mild or type I bone stock damage, both the metaphysis and the isthmus are intact. After removal of the implant materials, including any cement, the reconstruction is similar to that of a primary THA.

In moderate or type II bone stock damage, there is significant structural damage or absence of portions of the metaphysis with the isthmus remaining intact. With damage or enlargement of the proximal femoral metaphysis, there is only limited potential for bone ingrowth with a proximally porous-coated implant. As a result, the authors recommend the use of a standard fully porous-coated femoral implant that can achieve initial stability and long-term ingrowth in the intact diaphysis.

In severe or type III bone loss, both the metaphysis and the isthmus are damaged. The cortices are commonly thin or even perforated, and there may be an angular deformity of the femur secondary to remodeling around the loose femoral implant. A corrective osteotomy may be required if the deformity prevents insertion of a straight stem. Damage to both the metaphysis and the femoral shaft precludes the possibility of obtaining initial stability with a standard length implant. Reaming the canal to a cylindrical shape for a standard length implant is not possible without risking fracture or thinning the cortices excessively. The best potential for stability and ingrowth lies distally in the diaphysis, farther than the previous implant. As such, the authors

Table 93-5. Saleh Classification

Type	Femoral Bone Loss
I	No notable loss of bone stock
II	Contained loss of bone stock with cortical thinning
III	Uncontained loss of cortical bone stock involving the calcar and the lesser trochanter that is less than 5 cm in length and proximal to the diaphysis
IV	Uncontained circumferential loss of bone stock greater than 5 cm in length that extends into the diaphysis
V	Periprosthetic fracture with circumferential bone loss proximal to the fracture

Table 93-6. Engh and Glassman Classification

Type	Femoral Bone Loss
I or Mild	Intact metaphysis and isthmus
II or Moderate	Significant damage or absence of portions of the metaphysis with the isthmus remaining intact
III or Severe	Damaged metaphysis and isthmus

Table 93-7. Gustilo and Pasternak Classification	
Type	**Femoral Bone Loss**
I	Minimal endosteal or inner cortex bone loss
II	Proximal canal enlargement with 50% or greater cortical thinning
III	Posteromedial wall defect involving the lesser trochanter
IV	Total proximal circumferential loss below the lesser trochanter

Table 93-8. Chandler and Penenberg Classification	
Category	**Femoral Bone Defect**
1	Deficiency of the calcar femorale 1A Intramedullary 1B Total
2	Deficiency of the greater trochanter
3	Cortical thinning
4	Cortical perforation
5	Fracture about or distal to the stem 5A In the host bone 5B In previously used femoral allograft
6	Circumferential deficiency of the metaphysis and the proximal part of the diaphysis 6A Loss of greater trochanter and metaphysis with thin shell of diaphysis remaining 6B Total loss of proximal part of the femur

recommend a long-stem fully porous-coated implant. Morselized bone graft to the proximal deficiencies is not recommended.

Gustilo and Pasternak Classification

This system was devised to classify bone loss that occurred with loosening of a cemented femoral component (Table 93-7).[5] In type I, there is minimal endosteal or inner cortex bone loss. Type II has proximal canal enlargement with cortical thinning of 50% or more. At times, the femur can have a lateral wall defect with an intact circumferential wall. In type III, there is a posteromedial wall defect involving the lesser trochanter, indicating instability, and in type IV, there is total proximal circumferential loss at varying distances below the lesser trochanter. In their series, Gustilo and Pasternak found that 82% of cases were type II or III.[5] They recommended a cemented revision for type I cases in patients older than 65 years of age and cementless femoral revision with bone grafting for all cases.

Chandler and Penenberg Classification

This classification system was described with specific reference to treatment options for femoral bone loss with the use of allografts.[6] In this system, six main categories may exist in isolation or in conjunction with another category (Table 93-8). In category I, there is deficiency of the calcar femorale, where calcar bone loss can be intramedullary (category 1A) or can represent a total deficiency (category 1B). The bone loss in category 2 involves the greater trochanter, category 3 indicates cortical thinning, and category 4 bone loss is seen when there is implant-related or iatrogenic perforation of the femoral cortex. Category 5 denotes that there is a fracture about or distal to the femoral component in the host bone (category 5A) or in a proximal femoral allograft used in a previous revision THA (category 5B). In category 6, there is circumferential deficiency of the metaphysis and the proximal part of the diaphysis. If there is loss of the greater trochanter and metaphysis with a thin shell of diaphysis remaining, this is classified as category 6A, but if there is total loss of the proximal part of the femur, this is classified as category 6B.

CLASSIFICATION RELIABILITY AND VALIDITY

A useful classification system for femoral bone loss associated with a failed THA should be both reliable and valid. *Reliability* refers to both interobserver reliability, the agreement between different observers, and intraobserver reliability, the agreement of one observer on separate occasions. Reliability is measured by the kappa value (κ), which distinguishes true agreement of various observations from agreement due to chance alone.[28] The criteria of Landis and Koch are most commonly used to interpret the kappa value.[29] A kappa value of 0.20 or less implies poor agreement, 0.21 to 0.40 fair agreement, 0.41 to 0.60 moderate agreement, 0.61 to 0.80 good agreement, and 0.80 to 1.00 very good or almost perfect agreement. Because most classification systems are developed for widespread use, reliability must be high among all observers for a system to have clinical utility. If the degree of reliability is low, then the classification system will have limited utility. If the classification system has been shown to be reliable, then testing for validity can be done.

Validity indicates the accuracy with which the classification system describes the true pathology.[30] Validity can be measured by comparison with a gold standard. In the case of femoral bone loss, the gold standard can be the intraoperative assessment of bone loss. Validation of a classification system requires high correlation between preoperative radiographs and intraoperative findings. This comparison of radiographs with the surgeon's intraoperative observations introduces an element of observer bias to the validation process. As a result, validity is much more difficult to measure; therefore it is essential that a classification system has at least a high degree of reliability.

Despite the widespread use of the various classification systems for femoral bone loss, very few studies have looked at the reliability and validity of these femoral bone stock classifications. Gozzard and associates specifically analyzed intraobserver and interobserver reliability of the AAOS, Paprosky, and Endo-Klink classification systems, as well as intraoperative validity of the Paprosky classification.[31] They found that intraobserver agreement varied between individual observers but varied from poor to good (κ range, 0.08 to 0.64). Moderate interobserver agreement was noted for the Endo-Klink (κ = 0.48) and Paprosky (κ = 0.42) classifications, and the AAOS (κ = 0.24) classification had only fair agreement. When the validity of the Paprosky femoral classification was assessed, the authors found moderate agreement between predicted preoperative bone loss identified on radiographs and true intraoperative bone loss as seen at the time of surgery (κ = 0.54).

In another study, Haddad and colleagues assessed intraobserver and interobserver agreement on femoral bone loss using the AAOS, Paprosky, and Mallory classification systems.[32] For both expert and nonexpert evaluators, they found moderate intraobserver agreement (κ range, 0.43 to 0.62) and poor (κ range, 0.12 to 0.29) interobserver agreement for all three classification systems.

Saleh and coworkers assessed their own femoral classification system and found that it was reliable and a valid predictor of bone loss found at the time of surgery.[3] They reported significant agreement in interobserver reliability with a kappa value greater than 0.75. Assessment of the system's validity revealed significant agreement between observers and intraoperative findings with a kappa value greater than 0.75. No independent group has evaluated this classification system to corroborate their findings, and no studies have been done to determine the validity of this classification.

These studies highlight suboptimal interobserver and intraobserver reliability with some of the commonly used classification systems. Furthermore, the validity of any classification system is compromised if the system is not reliable.

CONCLUSIONS

Classification of femoral bone defects in revision THA can help the surgeon characterize the problem, offer guidance in deciding on the ideal treatment, and allow consistent comparisons of surgical outcomes. The ideal classification system should be descriptive to quantify the bone loss, and it should guide treatment options and be both reliable and valid. To date, a number of classifications have been developed and utilized, but none has gained universal acceptance. When critically evaluated, some of the commonly used classification systems in use today have been shown to be unreliable. Thus their use to differentiate treatments and suggest outcomes is not warranted. The comprehensive classification put forward by the AAOS Committee on the Hip may be applicable to all situations, but its complexity diminishes its reliability. More simplistic classifications like the Endo-Klink are more reliable but provide less information and are not extensive enough to address all types of bone loss. The Paprosky classification has

demonstrated moderate reliability and validity. Many other classification systems commonly cited in the literature have not been tested; therefore no evidence indicates whether they are or are not reliable. However, there is no reason to believe that the classification systems that have not been tested would fare any better than those that have.[33] Nonetheless, those classification systems with suboptimal reliability and those that have not been tested are not necessarily without use. They provide a discipline by which to help define pathology and treatment options, and they provide a language to describe that pathology. However, it is necessary to recognize the limitations of existing classification systems and the need to confirm or refine proposed preoperative categories through careful intraoperative observation of actual findings.[33]

CURRENT CONTROVERSIES AND FUTURE DIRECTIONS

- Femoral bone loss classifications characterize the nature of the problem, guide treatment decision making, and allow for uniform reporting of outcomes.
- Various classification systems have been developed and utilized, but none has gained universal acceptance.
- Despite widespread use of various classification systems for femoral bone loss, very few studies have looked at their reliability and validity.
- Some of the commonly used classification systems in use today have been shown to be unreliable.
- Many other classification systems commonly cited in the literature have not been tested; therefore no evidence indicates whether they are or are not reliable.
- It is necessary to recognize the limitations of existing classification systems and the need to confirm their reliability and validity. If required, these classification systems should be refined to meet accepted standards of scientific testing.

REFERENCES

1. Paprosky WG, Aribindi R: Hip replacement: treatment of femoral bone loss using distal bypass fixation. Instr Course Lect 49:119–130, 2000.
2. Mallory TH: Preparation of the proximal femur in cementless total hip revision. Clin Orthop Relat Res 235:47–60, 1988.
3. Saleh KJ, Holtzman J, Gafni A, et al: Reliability and intraoperative validity of preoperative assessment of standardized plain radiographs in predicting bone loss at revision hip surgery. J Bone Joint Surg Am 83:1040–1046, 2001.
4. Engh CA, Glassman AH, Griffin WL, Mayer JG: Results of cementless revision for failed cemented total hip arthroplasty. Clin Orthop Relat Res 235:91–110, 1988.
5. Gustilo RB, Pasternak HS: Revision total hip arthroplasty with titanium ingrowth prosthesis and bone grafting for failed cemented femoral component loosening. Clin Orthop Relat Res 235:111–119, 1988.
6. Chandler HP, Penenberg BL: Bone stock deficiency in total hip replacement: classification and management, Thorofare, NJ, 1989, Slack, pp 19–164.
7. D'Antonio J, McCarthy JC, Bargar WL, et al: Classification of femoral abnormalities in total hip arthroplasty. Clin Orthop Relat Res 296:133–139, 1993.

8. Sporer SM, Paprosky WG: Femoral fixation in the face of considerable bone loss: the use of modular stems. Clin Orthop Relat Res 429:227–231, 2004.

9. Della Valle CJ, Paprosky WG: Classification and an algorithmic approach to the reconstruction of femoral deficiency in revision total hip arthroplasty. J Bone Joint Surg Am 85(Suppl 4):1–6, 2003.

10. Della Valle CJ, Paprosky WG: The femur in revision total hip arthroplasty evaluation and classification. Clin Orthop Relat Res 420:55–62, 2004.

11. Sierra RJ, Cabanela ME: Conversion of failed hip hemiarthroplasties after femoral neck fractures. Clin Orthop Relat Res 399:129–139, 2002.

12. Weeden SH, Paprosky WG: Minimal 11-year follow-up of extensively porous-coated stems in femoral revision total hip arthroplasty. J Arthroplasty 17(4 Suppl 1):134–137, 2002.

13. Elting JJ, Mikhail WE, Zicat BA, et al: Preliminary report of impaction grafting for exchange femoral arthroplasty. Clin Orthop Relat Res 319:159–167, 1995.

13a. Gie GA, Linder L, Ling RS, et al: Impacted cancellous allografts and cement for revision total hip arthroplasty. J Bone Joint Surg Br 75:14–21, 1993.

14. Gie GA, Linder L, Ling RS, et al: Impacted cancellous allografts and cement for revision total hip arthroplasty. J Bone Joint Surg Br 75:14–21, 1993.

15. Schreurs BW, Arts JJ, Verdonschot N, et al: Femoral component revision with use of impaction bone-grafting and a cemented polished stem: surgical technique. J Bone Joint Surg Am 88(Suppl 1 Pt 2):259–274, 2006.

16. Wraighte PJ, Howard PW: Femoral impaction bone allografting with an Exeter cemented collarless, polished, tapered stem in revision hip replacement: a mean follow-up of 10.5 years. J Bone Joint Surg Br 90:1000–1004, 2008.

17. Ornstein E, Linder L, Ranstam J, et al: Femoral impaction bone grafting with the Exeter stem—the Swedish experience: survivorship analysis of 1305 revisions performed between 1989 and 2002. J Bone Joint Surg Br 91:441–446, 2009.

18. Ovesen O, Emmeluth C, Hofbauer C, Overgaard S: Revision total hip arthroplasty using a modular tapered stem with distal fixation: good short-term results in 125 revisions. J Arthroplasty 25:348–354, 2010.

19. Garbuz DS, Toms A, Masri BA, Duncan CP: Improved outcome in femoral revision arthroplasty with tapered fluted modular titanium stems. Clin Orthop Relat Res 453:199–202, 2006.

20. Böhm P, Bischel O: Femoral revision with the Wagner SL revision stem: evaluation of one hundred and twenty-nine revisions followed for a mean of 4.8 years. J Bone Joint Surg Am 83:1023–1031, 2001.

21. Lee SH, Ahn YJ, Chung SJ, et al: The use of allograft prosthesis composite for extensive proximal femoral bone deficiencies: a 2-year to 9.8-year follow-up study. J Arthroplasty 24:1241–1248, 2009.

22. Safir O, Kellett CF, Flint M, et al: Revision of the deficient proximal femur with a proximal femoral allograft. Clin Orthop Relat Res 467:206–212, 2009.

23. Gross AE, Allan DG, Lavoie GJ, Oakeshott RD: Revision arthroplasty of the proximal femur using allograft bone. Orthop Clin North Am 24:705–715, 1993.

24. Friesecke C, Plutat J, Block A: Revision arthroplasty with use of a total femur prosthesis. J Bone Joint Surg Am 87:2693–2701, 2005.

25. Engelbrecht E, Heinert K: Klassifikation und Behandlungsrichtlinien von nochensubstanzverlusten bei Revisionsoperationen am Huftgelenkmittelfristige Ergebnisse: Primare und Revisionsalloarthroplastik Hrsg Endo-Klinik, Berlin, 1987, Springer-Verlag.

26. Saleh KJ, Holtzman J, Gafni A, et al: Development, test reliability and validation of a classification for revision hip arthroplasty. J Orthop Res 19:50–56, 2001.

27. Glassman AH, Engh CA: Cementless revision for femoral failure. Orthopedics 18:851–853, 1995.

28. Cohen J: A coefficient of agreement for nominal scales. Educational and Psychological Measurement 20:37–46, 1960.

29. Landis JR, Koch GG: The measurement of observer agreement for categorical data. Biometrics 33:159–174, 1977.

30. Wright JG, Feinstein AR: Improving the reliability of orthopaedic measurements. J Bone Joint Surg Br 74:287–291, 1992.

31. Gozzard C, Blom A, Taylor A, et al: A comparison of the reliability and validity of bone stock loss classification systems used for revision hip surgery. J Arthroplasty 18:638–642, 2003.

32. Haddad FS, Masri BA, Garbuz DS, Duncan CP: Femoral bone loss in total hip arthroplasty: classification and preoperative planning. Instr Course Lect 49:83–96, 2000.

33. Garbuz DS, Masri BA, Esdaile J, Duncan CP: Classification systems in orthopaedics. J Am Acad Orthop Surg 10:290–297, 2002.

CHAPTER 94

Cemented Femoral Revision in Total Hip Arthroplasty: A View in the 21st Century

Bryan Nestor

KEY POINTS

- The cement-bone interface strength is reduced in revisions owing to loss of cancellous bone and less cement interdigitation with bone.
- The historic rate of cemented femoral component failure was high when cemented revisions were used in all cases owing to mechanical failure of the cement-bone interface.
- Cemented femoral revision now is used mostly in first-time revisions of older, low-demand patients in whom good cancellous bone remains.
- "Cement-within-cement" revision techniques may be used in special circumstances when the cement-bone interface is intact.

INTRODUCTION

Cemented femoral revision has fallen out of popularity as uncemented revision methods have matured. Cemented femoral revision with impaction bone grafting is a special technique that is discussed later. Cemented femoral revision now is used mostly in elderly patients with low activity demands and good remaining cancellous bone, which provides for cement interdigitation with the bone and hence a good mechanical interlock (Fig. 94-1). Cemented revision is also used in special cases in which the old cement mantle is intact and is well bonded to the bone, allowing a "cement-in-cement" technique after removal of the previous prosthesis from the cement.

EARLY EXPERIENCE

Not long after the introduction of cemented total hip arthroplasty, aseptic loosening was recognized as the major cause of failure. Early experience with cemented revisions led most to observe that the results of revision would be less satisfactory than those attained with primary total hip arthroplasty.[1-3] Even by the end of the first decade of total hip arthroplasty in the late 1970s, it was recognized that the best opportunity to attain good long-term fixation was the "first time around," and that most early failures would have been done differently based on recognized technical advances.[3]

In one of the earliest reports of cemented revision total hip arthroplasty by Hunter and associates, only one fourth of patients had a good or excellent result with early follow-up, and results were confounded by the presence of infection. Ultimately, one third of patients were diagnosed with infection, and Girdlestone resection was the final treatment for 31 of 140 revision hip arthroplasties.[2] Amstutz and colleagues reported on 88 patients, of whom 73% underwent cemented femoral revision, and outlined the significant complexity of revision hip arthroplasty with increased blood loss, increased operative time, and increased complications compared with primary hip arthroplasty.[1] Even more disappointing was the 9% incidence of re-revision at short-term follow-up, with an additional 20% showing substantial progressive radiolucencies.[1] Kavanagh and coworkers reviewed 206 hip revisions and reported a mechanical failure rate of 18% and a re-revision rate of 8%.[4] Pellicci and associates reported similar results for 110 hips in 107 patients with a mechanical failure rate of 14% and progressive radiolucencies in 26%.[3] However, with longer follow-up, this same series of patients had a 29% failure rate.[5] Marti and associates reported 85% survival of cemented revisions at 14 years using early techniques from 1974 to 1983.[6]

Numerous studies subsequently documented the high incidence of re-revision, mechanical loosening, and radiographic radiolucencies with early cemented femoral revision techniques and long-term follow-up.[7-11] Correlating with the high rate of radiographic radiolucencies, the use of roentgen stereophotogrammetric analysis confirmed a very high rate and extent of femoral component migration following cemented revision, particularly in cases with severe bone loss.[12,13]

LESSONS LEARNED

As the experience with cemented femoral revision grew, a number of lessons learned from the initial experience contributed to improved clinical results.

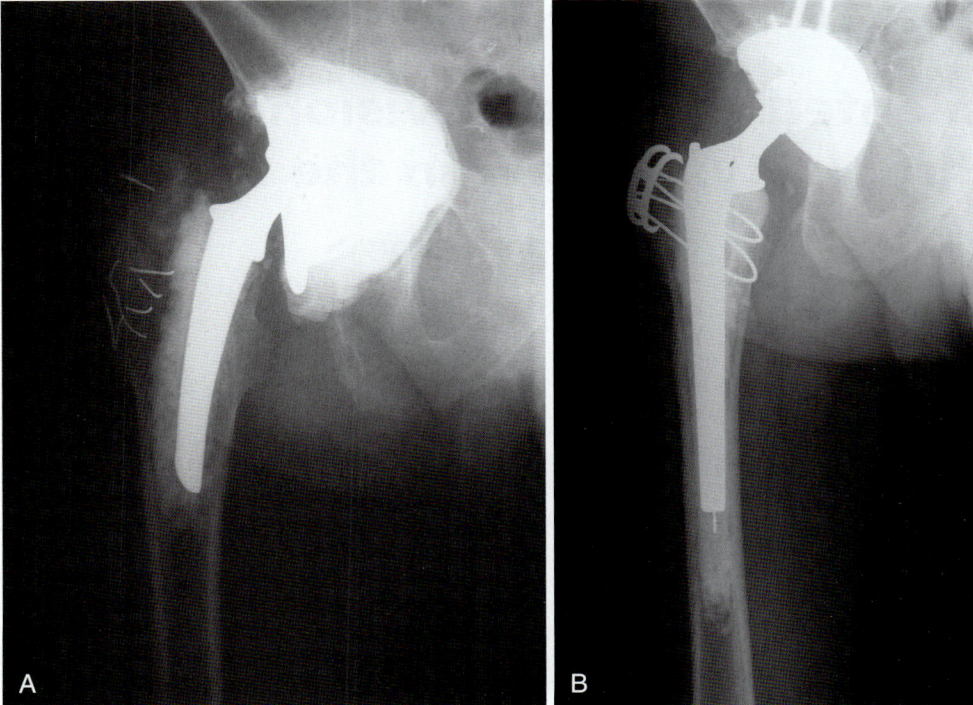

Figure 94-1. A, Hip radiograph of patient with loose femoral stem and good remaining cancellous bone. **B,** Radiograph after revision with cemented calcar replacement femoral component. Note that the good cancellous bone allowed creation of a good bone-cement interface.

Lesson 1: Longer stems can improve cemented femoral fixation

One of the early observations pointed out the advantage of using longer stems that bypassed proximal bone deficiencies and attained fixation in better quality bone distally. Progression of radiolucencies was observed by Callaghan and associates to be significantly less in femoral revisions performed with long-stem prostheses (150 to 230 cm in length).[14] Similarly, using early cement techniques, Turner and colleagues reported decreased progression of femoral radiolucencies and decreased mechanical failure with use of long-stem implants.[15] Crawford and coworkers, using a long stem in a series of 74 femoral revisions performed after 1985, most of which had severe bone loss, found no mechanical failures at a mean follow-up of 5.75 years in 45 hips in which the stem had at least 10 cm of distal fixation.[16] Others using contemporary cement techniques have shown a decreased risk of re-revision when a long-stem femoral component is used.[17,18] Repten and colleagues demonstrated improved survival when the stem extended beyond the most distal extent of bone loss by at least one diameter.[18] Hultmark demonstrated that long-stem fixation had a 93% survival rate free of mechanical loosening compared with a 79% survival rate for standard stems at 10 years.[17] In a biomechanical study using a three-dimensional finite element model, Mann and coworkers showed that a femoral component that bypassed the cancellous bone defect by two femoral diameters was most effective in reducing adverse stresses in the cement mantel and motion and stresses

at the cement-bone interface.[19] Further increases in stem length had only a minor effect.[19]

Lesson 2: Cemented re-revision does poorly

Another early observation was that cemented re-revisions resulted in even less satisfactory clinical and radiographic results than index cemented femoral revisions with a high rate of subsequent mechanical failure.[15,20,21] The poorer results were felt to be secondary to progressive loss of the micro-interlock between cement and cancellous bone. In a biomechanical study, Dohmae and associates demonstrated that bone-cement interface shear strength was reduced to 20.6% of primary strength with the first revision and to 6.8% of primary strength with the second revision.[22]

Lesson 3: Bone loss and time to failure are risk factors for failure

A number of studies have demonstrated a correlation between the prognosis for cemented femoral revision and the degree of bone loss.[17,22,23] This is reflected by the difficulty of obtaining a good cement mantle as defined by Mulroy and Harris.[17,24] Davis and colleagues in a study on 48 cemented femoral revisions for failed uncemented femoral components reported a loosening rate of 29% with minimum 5-year follow-up.[25] The high rate of failure was likely secondary to extensive loss of cancellous bone and to the use of standard length stems in most cases (41/48).[25] Perhaps directly or indirectly related to bone quality, Malchau and coworkers, reporting the results of 16,577 cemented femoral revisions in the Swedish Registry, with and without impaction grafting, noted a 3.3 times increased risk of re-revision when the first revision was performed within 5 years of the index arthroplasty.[26]

Lesson 4: Cement technique matters

As cementing techniques evolved and improved in primary total hip arthroplasty, they were also applied to cemented femoral revision. A number of studies documented increased longevity and lower rates of mechanical failure with the use of improved cementing techniques.[17,24,27-31] Mulroy and associates reported a rate of loosening of 26% at 15.1 years using second-generation techniques (distal cement plug and retrograde canal filling with a cement gun).[24] Hultmark and colleagues found no improvement in outcome with the addition of third-generation techniques (high-pressure canal lavage and tamponade).[17] Although the same authors demonstrated improved femoral component survival with second-generation techniques, linear regression analysis showed that other variables, including age, stem length, radiolucencies, and bone quality, were more important than cement technique in predicting femoral component failure.[17] However, Haydon and associates did report a significant improvement in outcome with third-generation cement techniques.[32]

Lesson 5: Young age increases risk of failure

Young age, generally defined as younger than 55 years of age, has also been associated with increased risk of failure for cemented femoral revision.[17,18,31-33] Increased activity level and physical demands are causative factors frequently cited as leading to higher failure rates.

Lessons Learned: Long-term follow-up

Incorporation of some or all of the lessons learned had a significant impact on long-term survival of cemented femoral revision. Although a number of studies include some patients revised with earlier techniques, most patients represent contemporary techniques and experience. Izquierdo and colleagues in a long-term survival study based on surgery performed from 1982 to 1989 and including infection in one third of patients and a previous revision in 32% reported impressive radiographic 10-year survivorship for the femoral component of 90.5% and 95% survivorship with revision as an endpoint.[34] Iorio, reporting on a more extensive but single surgeon experience from 1971 to 1990 including acetabular revision, revealed clinical survivorship free of revision of 97% at 5 years and 76% at 10 years and radiographic survivorship of 94% at 5 years and 62% at 10 years.[35] In a similar single surgeon study from 1974 to 1990, Raut and coworkers reported 93.9% 10-year femoral survivorship with revision as an endpoint and 91.5% 10-year survivorship with radiographic loosening

as an endpoint, proclaiming the Charnley stem as the gold standard of revision.[36] In another study over the same period—1975 to 1996—but with particular attention to technique, Haydon and associates reported 91% 10-year survivorship for the femoral component free of revision and 71% survivorship with loosening as an endpoint.[32] The authors were able to demonstrate improved survivorship associated with third-generation cement technique and quality of cement mantle.[32] They also reported increased rates of re-revision for patients with poor preoperative bone stock and age greater than 60 years.[32]

Reflecting a more contemporary experience from 1984 to 2003, Howie and colleagues reported 9-year femoral survivorship free of re-revision of 98% with long stems and 93% with standard length stems, prompting the authors to recommend cemented femoral revision in older patients.[37] In a study limited to contemporary technique from 1993 to 1996, Bardou-Jacquet and coworkers reported a 10-year femoral survival rate of 90% and association of survival with number of previous revisions, bone quality, and quality of cementation.[23]

In the only prospective randomized trial comparing cemented femoral revision with uncemented femoral revision with a modular metaphyseal stem (SROM, DePuy, Warsaw, Ind), Iorio and associates reported 92% 5-year survivorship free of re-revision for cemented stems and 94% for the SROM, which was not statistically significant.[35] Most cemented stems used in this study were of standard length (74%), and cement-in-cement technique was used in 23%.[35] Despite their results, the authors reported currently using cemented femoral revision only in older patients with minimal bone loss.[35]

Certainly the success of uncemented femoral revision has tempered enthusiasm for cemented fixation.[38-41] In a recent report on 4762 aseptic revisions in the Norwegian Register from 1987 to 2003, re-cementation of the femoral component was associated with the poorest results.[42]

INDICATIONS

Based on predictable success and ease of use despite severe bone loss,[38-41] the role of cemented femoral revision today is very limited, and utilization should be individualized. When cemented femoral revision is considered, the ideal patient is older, with a life expectancy of fewer than 10 years, with first-time aseptic loosening of a cemented stem, and with minimal bone loss or reasonable bone stock distally. Good remaining cancellous bone improves the likelihood of good cement interdigitation with bone for long-term fixation. The cement-within-cement technique (Fig. 94-2) has limited indications, as is noted in the following sections.

TECHNIQUE

Cemented femoral revision can be accomplished using a variety of surgical approaches. All loose and

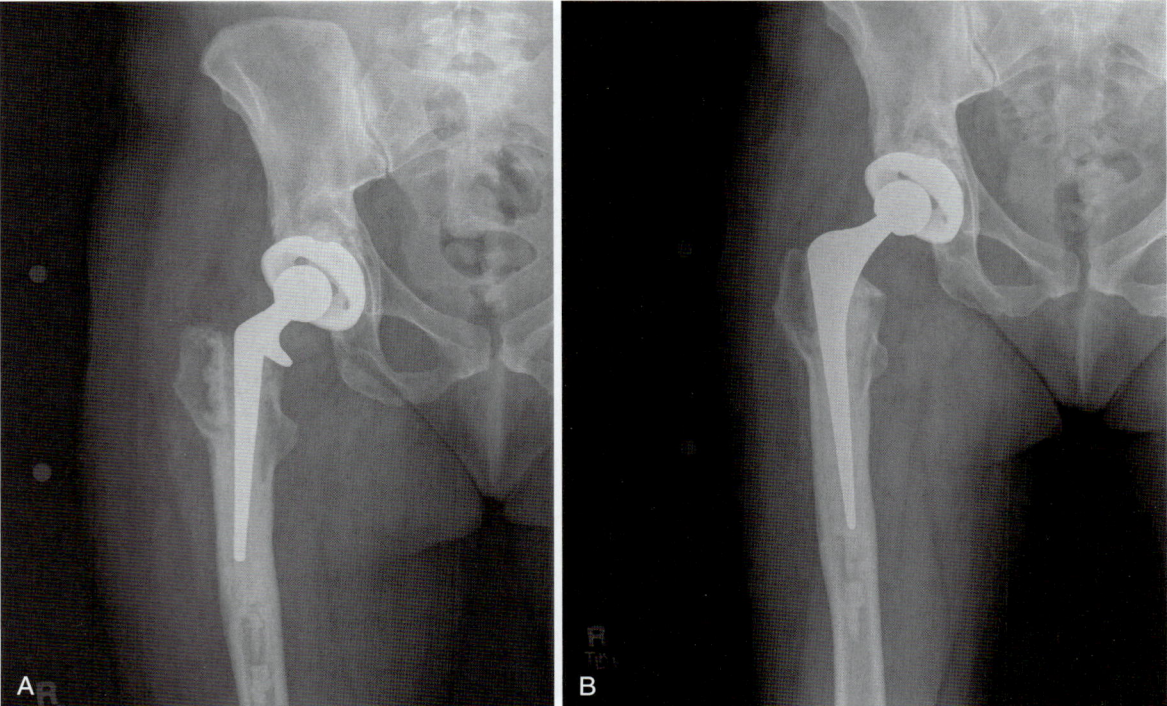

Figure 94-2. A, Hip radiograph of patient with a loose femoral stem that has debonded from a well-fixed cement mantle. **B,** Radiograph after femoral revision using cement-in-cement technique.

fragmented cement, as well as the soft tissue at the bone-cement interface, should be removed. Remaining cancellous bone is preserved, and any areas of hard sclerotic bone are macro-textured with a burr to enhance cement interdigitation. If a "neocortex" is present, it is removed with back biting instruments to expose underlying cancellous bone.

Depending on the extent of bone loss, a longer stem that extends 2 or 3 femoral diameters distal to the plug might be used. If distal bone is insufficient, then an alternative method of fixation must be considered. Cementation technique should include pulsatile lavage after femoral preparation, vacuum mixing of the cement, a distal plug, retrograde filling, and pressurization. When a plastic cement plug fails to attain fixation past the isthmus, a cement plug may be constructed using a small amount of liquid cement, which is injected at a proper position and is allowed to harden (before the main bolus of cement is injected). Stem centralizers may be used but are not always feasible in the revision setting. One of the advantages of cemented revision is the ability to add antibiotics at the surgeon's discretion.

If the cement mantle is intact, then a cement-within-cement technique may be considered. The cement-within-cement technique also may be used when a well-fixed cemented stem needs to be revised for exposure or for mechanical reasons, or when the stem is nonmodular and the head is scratched or otherwise damaged. As long as the stem may be removed without disturbing the cement mantle, a new cemented stem that fits the profile (shape and size) of the cement mantle may be inserted using this technique. Care should be taken to ensure that the implant to be cemented is accommodated in the existing cement mantle, and that sufficient room is available for cementation. The cement mantle is prepared with a burr. Cementation should be performed with the cement in liquid phase.

CONCLUSION

In summary, indications for cemented femoral revision are limited and should be individualized. The most favorable indications involve patients with little bone loss, those with good remaining cancellous bone, and elderly, low-demand patients. For the right indications, reasonable clinical and radiographic outcomes can be expected, at least in the short term to midterm.

REFERENCES

1. Amstutz HC, Ma SM, Jinnah RH, Mai L: Revision of aseptic loose total hip arthroplasties. Clin Orthop Relat Res 170:21–33, 1982.
2. Hunter GA, Welsh RP, Cameron HU, Bailey WH: The results of revision of total hip arthroplasty. J Bone Joint Surg Br 61:419–421, 1979.
3. Pellicci PM, Wilson PD, Jr, Sledge CB, et al: Revision total hip arthroplasty. Clin Orthop Relat Res 170:34–41, 1982.
4. Kavanagh BF, Ilstrup DM, Fitzgerald RH: Revision total hip arthroplasty. J Bone Joint Surg Am 67:517–526, 1985.
5. Pellicci PM, Wilson PD, Jr, Sledge CB, et al: Long-term results of revision total hip replacement: a follow-up report. J Bone Joint Surg Am 67:513–516, 1985.

6. Marti RK, Schuller HM, Besselaar PP, Vanfrank Haasnoot EL: Results of revision of hip arthroplasty with cement: a five- to fourteen-year follow-up study. J Bone Joint Surg Am 72:346–354, 1990.

7. Diekerhof CH, Barnaart LFW, Rozing PM: Long-term clinical results of cemented revision of primary cemented total hip arthroplasties. Acta Orthop Belg 66:376–381, 2000.

8. Engelbrecht DJ, Wever FA, Sweet MBE, Jakim I: Long term results of revision total hip arthroplasty. J Bone Joint Surg Br 72:41–45, 1990.

9. Garcia-Cimbrelo E, Munuera L, Diez-Vazquez V: Long-term results of aseptic cemented Charnley revisions. J Arthroplasty 10:121–131, 1995.

10. Gramkow J, Jensen TH, Varmarken JE, Repten JB: Long-term results after cemented revision of the femoral component in total hip arthroplasty. J Arthroplasty 16:777–783, 2001.

11. Wirta J, Eskola A, Hoikka V, et al: Revision of cemented hip arthroplasties: 101 hips followed for 5 (4-9) years. Acta Orthop Scand 64:263–267, 1993.

12. Franzen H, Mjoberg B, Onnerfalt R: Early loosening of femoral components after cemented revision: a roentgen stereophotogrammetric study. J Bone Joint Surg Br 74:721–724, 1992.

13. Snorrason F, Karrholm J: Early loosening of revision hip arthroplasty: a roentgen stereophotogrammetric analysis. J Arthroplasty 5:217–229, 1990.

14. Callaghan JJ, Salvati EA, Pellicci PM, et al: Results of revision for mechanical failure after cemented total hip replacement, 1979 to 1982: a two- to five-year follow-up. J Bone Joint Surg Am 67:1074–1085, 1985.

15. Turner RH, Mattingly DA, Scheller A: Femoral revision total hip arthroplasty using a long-stem femoral component: clinical and radiographic analysis. J Arthroplasty 2:247–258, 1987.

16. Crawford SA, Siney PD, Wroblewski BM: Revision of failed total hip arthroplasty with a proximal femoral modular cemented stem. J Bone Joint Surg Br 82:684–688, 2000.

17. Hultmark P, Karrholm J, Stromberg C, et al: Cemented first-time revisions of the femoral component. J Arthroplasty 15:551–561, 2000.

18. Repten JB, Jensen S: Risk factors for recurrent aseptic loosening of the femoral component after cemented revision. J Arthroplasty 8:471–478, 1993.

19. Mann KA, Ayers DC, Damron TA: Effects of stem length on mechanics of the femoral hip component after cemented revision. J Orthop Res 15:62–68, 1997.

20. Kavanagh BF, Fitzgerald RH: Multiple revisions for failed total hip arthroplasty not associated with infection. J Bone Joint Surg Am 69:1144–1149, 1987.

21. Repten JB, Varmarken JE, Rock ND, Jensen JS: Unsatisfactory results after repeated revision of hip arthroplasty: 61 cases followed for 5 (1-10) years. Acta Orthop Scand 63:120–127, 1992.

22. Dohmae Y, Bechtold JE, Sherman RE, et al: Reduction in cement-bone interface shear strength between primary and revision arthroplasty. Clin Orthop Relat Res 236:214–220, 1988.

23. Bardou-Jacquet J, Souillac V, Mouton A, Chauveaux D: Primary aseptic revision of the femoral component of a cemented total hip arthroplasty using a cemented technique without bone graft. Orthop Traumatol 95:243–248, 2009.

24. Mulroy WF, Harris WH: Revision total hip arthroplasty with use of so-called second-generation cementing techniques for aseptic loosening of the femoral component: a fifteen year average follow-up study. J Bone Joint Surg Am 78:325–330, 1996.

25. Davis CM 3rd, Berry DJ, Harmsen WS: Cemented revision of failed uncemented femoral components of total hip arthroplasty. J Bone Joint Surg Am 85:1264–1269, 2003.

26. Malchau H, Herberts P, Eisler T, et al: The Swedish total hip replacement register. J Bone Joint Surg Am 84(Suppl):2, 2002.

27. Estok DM, Harris WH: Long-term results of cemented femoral revision surgery using second-generation techniques: an average 11.7-year follow-up evaluation. Clin Orthop Relat Res 299:190–202, 1994.

28. Katz RP, Callaghan JJ, Sullivan PM, Johnston RC: Results of cemented femoral revision total hip arthroplasty using improved cementing techniques. Clin Orthop Relat Res 319:178–183, 1995.

29. Katz RP, Callaghan JJ, Sullivan PM, Johnston RC: Long-term results of revision total hip arthroplasty with improved cementing technique. J Bone Joint Surg Br 79:322–326, 1997.

30. Pierson JL, Harris WH: Effect of improved cementing techniques on the longevity of fixation in revision cemented femoral arthroplasties. J Arthroplasty 10:581–591, 1995.

31. Stromberg CN, Herberts P, Ahnfelt L: Revision total hip arthroplasty in patients younger than 55 years old: clinical and radiologic results after 4 years. J Arthroplasty 3:47–59, 1988.

32. Haydon CM, Mehin R, Burnett S, et al: Revision total hip arthroplasty with use of a cemented femoral component: results at a mean of ten years. J Bone Joint Surg Am 86:1179–1185, 2004.

33. Stromberg CN, Herberts P: Cemented revision total hip arthroplasties in patients younger than 55 years old: a multicenter evaluation of second-generation cementing technique. J Arthoplasty 11:489–499, 1996.

34. Izquierdo RJ, Northmore-Ball MD: Long-term results of revision hip arthroplasty: survival analysis with special reference to the femoral component. J Bone Joint Surg Br 76:34–39, 1994.

35. Iorio R, Healy WL, Presutti AH: A prospective outcomes analysis of femoral component fixation in revision total hip arthroplasty. J Arthroplasty 23:662–669, 2008.

36. Raut VV, Siney PD, Wroblewski BM: Outcome of revision for mechanical stem failure using the cemented Charnley's stem: a study of 399 cases. J Arthroplasty 11:405–410, 1996.

37. Howie DW, Wimhurst JA, McGee MA, et al: Revision total hip replacement using cemented collarless double-taper femoral components. J Bone Joint Surg Br 89:879–886, 2007.

38. Engh CA, Jr, Ellis TJ, Koralewicz LM, et al: Extensively porous-coated femoral revision for severe femoral bone loss: minimum 10-year follow-up. J Arthroplasty 17:955–960, 2002.

39. Head WC, Emerson RH, Higgins LL: A titanium cementless calcar replacement prosthesis in revision surgery of the femur: 13-year experience. J Arthroplasty 16(Suppl):183–187, 2001.

40. Moreland JR, Moreno MA: Cementless femoral revision arthroplasty of the hip: minimum 5 years followup. Clin Orthop Relat Res 393:194–201, 2001.

41. Paprosky WG, Greidanus NV, Antoniou J: Minimum 10-year results of extensively porous-coated stems in revision hip arthroplasty. Clin Orthop Relat Res 369:230–242, 1999.

42. Lie SA, Havelin LI, Furnes ON, et al: Failure rates for 4762 revision total hip arthroplasties in the Norwegian Arthroplasty Register. J Bone Joint Surg Br 86:504–509, 2004.

CHAPTER 95

Femoral Revision: Impaction Bone Grafting

Graham A. Gie

INTRODUCTION

Impaction allografting for reconstruction of bone loss in revision total hip arthroplasty was initially developed for acetabular reconstruction. Experience from Professor Slooff and colleagues from Nijmegen, The Netherlands, who developed impaction bone grafting in the acetabulum in 1979,[1] subsequently contributed toward the application of this technique on the femoral side.

Professor Robin Ling had initially impacted a femoral canal with milled bone (1985) and inserted a femoral component without cement that subsided significantly. To address this shortcoming, this technique was revised by using cemented femoral fixation, and the senior author performed the first case of a contemporary femoral revision with impaction bone grafting in Exeter in 1987. With the goal of achieving a stable reconstruction while restoring proximal femoral bone stock loss, this first case of cemented revision with impaction grafting was carried out using canal sizers as distal impactors and an oversized trial stem as the proximal impactor.

Ling and associates[2] examined the quality of bone from a retrieved specimen 3.5 years post femoral impaction grafting, clearly showing cortical healing and a histologically regenerated cortical zone. As a result, in Exeter, this technique has become the procedure of choice in femoral revision surgery (Fig. 95-1).

INDICATIONS/CONTRAINDICATIONS

Indications

- In situations where avoiding the use of distal fixation long stems is desirable, as in the younger patient
- In revision cemented hip arthroplasty where removal of the preexisting prosthesis and cement mantle leaves behind a smooth and sclerotic endosteal surface; use of this technique provides an interface for mechanical interlocking of cement, with the added benefit of restoring bone stock
- Where the minimum necessary length of scratch fit cannot be attained for the use of fully coated cementless stems
- Where fixation with a conical fluted stem cannot be achieved owing to a reverse cone shape of the femoral canal below the isthmus
- Where the medullary canal is greater than 18 mm, increasing the risk of thigh pain with the use of cementless stems

Contraindications

- Although no absolute contraindications are known, the technique may not be ideal for the very elderly or medically unfit patient, for whom recovery of bone stock is unnecessary and a relatively shorter procedure is desirable.
- Although we perform the procedure in two stages in the presence of infection, there are surgeons who have experience with a single-stage revision for infection.[3]
- Where **complete** proximal femoral bone loss exceeds 10 cm, reconstruction with femoral impaction grafting becomes very complex, and other alternatives to femoral reconstruction are recommended.

PREOPERATIVE PLANNING

- Exclusion of infection is carried out in the conventional way. When suspicion of infection is raised by investigations or on clinical grounds, then a preoperative hip aspiration must be performed.
- Preoperative radiographs must be of good quality and must extend to well below the existing stem tip or cement mantle, whichever is most distal.

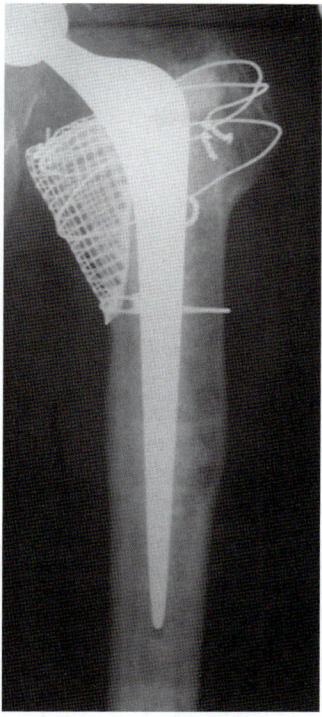

Figure 95-1. Femoral impaction grafting.

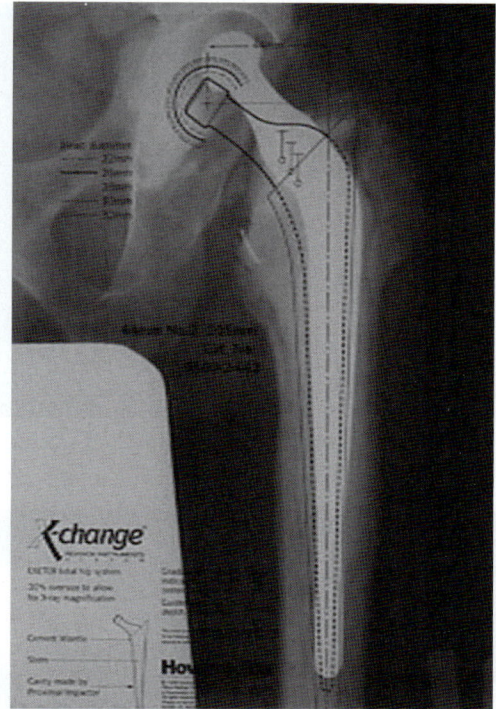

Figure 95-2. Preoperative templating.

- Detailed templating will indicate the stem length, size, and offset, as well as the position of the threaded revision plug, which should be placed 2 cm distal to the tip of the stem. The prosthesis must bypass the most distal major defect, such as a lytic lesion or a cortical defect involving more than 50% of the femoral circumference on two radiographic views, by at least 2 cortical diameters. Femoral impaction grafting system revision instruments allow for implantation of varying offsets and lengths.
- Donor allograft femoral heads or condyles and strut grafts, if necessary, should be ordered in advance from a bone bank. Femoral reconstruction metal mesh, multifilament cables, cerclage wires, and metal plates should be available (Fig. 95-2).

DESCRIPTION OF THE TECHNIQUE

Insertion of Intramedullary Plug

After removal of all debris, the femoral component, and cement, the femoral canal diameter is determined by the largest reamer used during débridement and is checked with a canal sizer (Fig. 95-3). An appropriately sized plug is then fixed to a threaded guide wire (Fig. 95-4) and is inserted down the canal using the revision plug introducer while the plug is positioned to the templated depth. This should be 2 cm distal to the tip of the stem, allowing for a short column of well-impacted graft chips distal to the prosthesis.

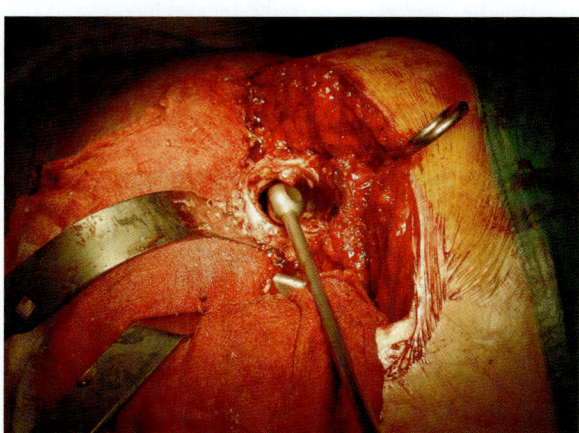

Figure 95-3. Checking femoral canal diameter with a canal sizer.

Sizing of the Femoral Canal

A proximal femoral impactor (phantom) of the templated size, offset, and length is passed over the guide wire. Its shape is that of the definitive prosthesis, but it is oversized to allow for the cement mantle and centralizer (Fig. 95-5). If any resistance is felt, a smaller size should be selected. Before the distal impactors are used, it is important to determine the distance down the canal that each sizer can be passed without jamming in the canal. Driving an impactor distal to this level would cause a femoral fracture. Select a distal impactor

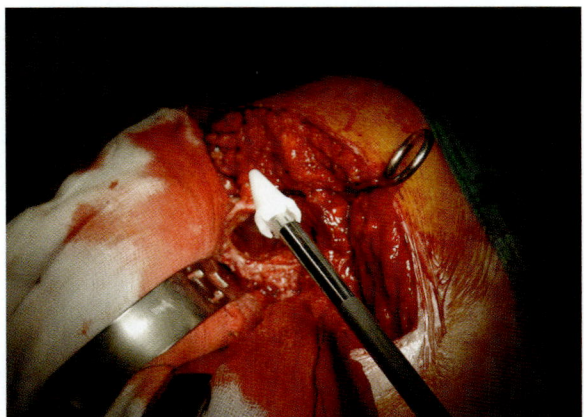

Figure 95-4. Intramedullary plug fixed to threaded guide wire with plug introducer attached.

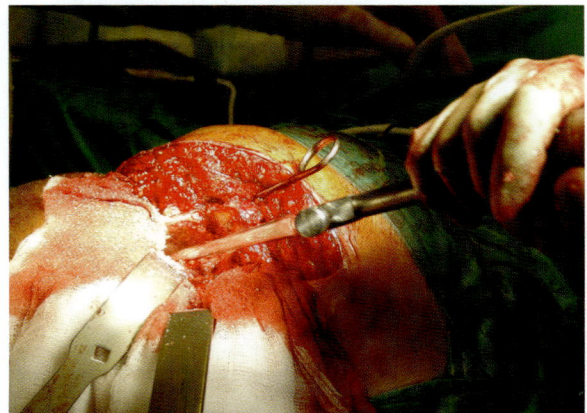

Figure 95-5. Proximal impactor (phantom) is passed over the guide wire, confirming adequate sizing.

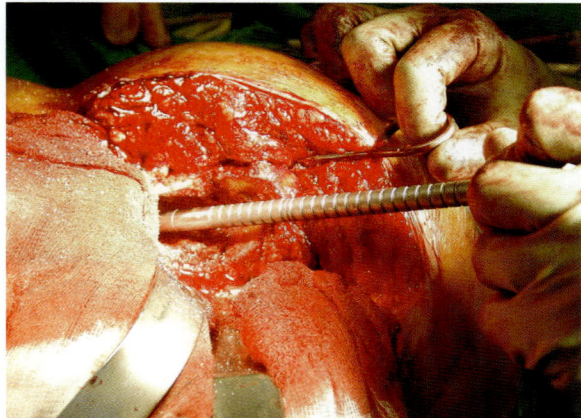

Figure 95-6. Canal sizer one size smaller than the plug diameter used was passed down the guide wire to the plug, and then was retrieved 2 cm for marking.

one size smaller than the diameter of the plug used. This should pass easily down to the plug without resistance (Fig. 95-6). Withdraw the impactor 2 cm from this position, and mark the level against the tip of the greater trochanter with the plastic clip marker. This will allow for the 2-cm column of bone graft distal to the implant

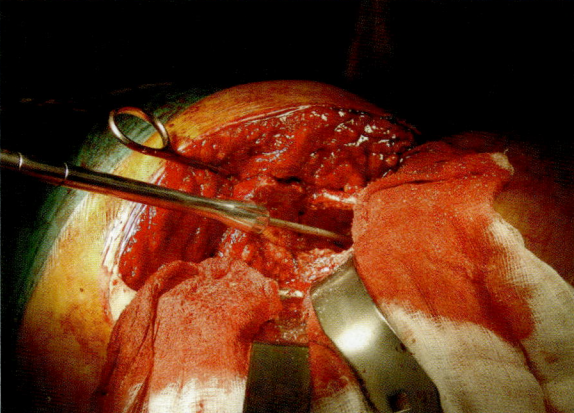

Figure 95-7. Distal impactor of larger diameter introduced over the guide wire as far down the canal as it will pass, and then marked.

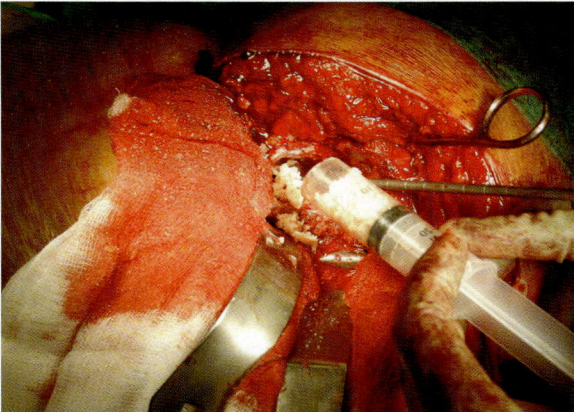

Figure 95-8. Small cancellous bone chips (4 mm) introduced into the canal using an open-ended syringe.

and will reduce the risk that the plug may be driven distally during vigorous impaction. Impactors of larger diameter are sequentially introduced over the guide wire as far down the canal as they will pass (Fig. 95-7) and are marked with a clip. In this way, the maximum depth of insertion allowed for each distal impactor is determined. With impacting bone graft, the impactors must not be driven beyond the marked depth.

Distal Impaction

Small cancellous bone chips (4 mm) are introduced into the canal using an open-ended syringe (Fig. 95-8). Before impaction is started, diaphyseal defects must be repaired with an appropriate wire mesh. Chips are then driven and compacted distally using distal impactors (Fig. 95-9) to the pre-rehearsed depth of the plastic markers. Progressively larger impactors are used as the canal is filled. More chips are firmly compacted until the impactors cannot be driven beyond the distal impaction line. For standard length stems, this line is the transition between polished and ridged sections of the impactors (Fig. 95-10). For longer stems, the distal impaction line is marked accordingly.

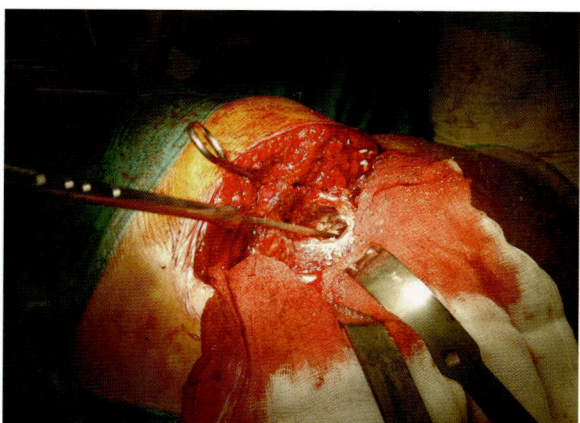

Figure 95-9. Chips driven distally using a distal impactor.

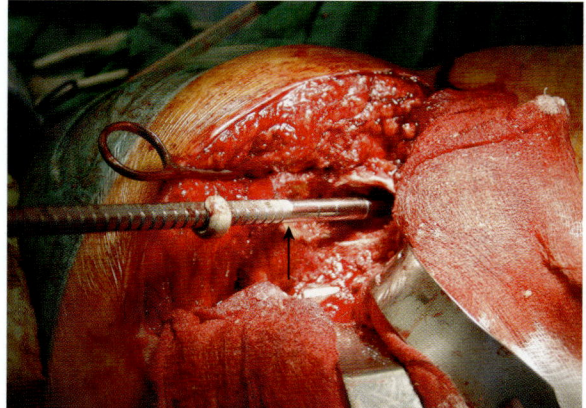

Figure 95-10. Distal impaction line for standard length stems *(arrow)* demonstrating the transition between polished and ridged sections of the impactors.

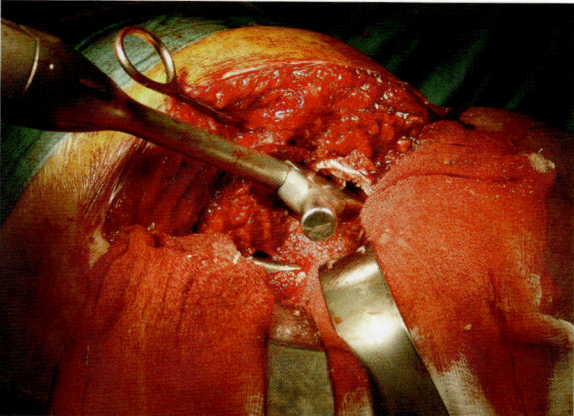

Figure 95-11. The phantom being sequentially driven into the distally impacted bone as more graft is pushed down the canal with handheld impactors.

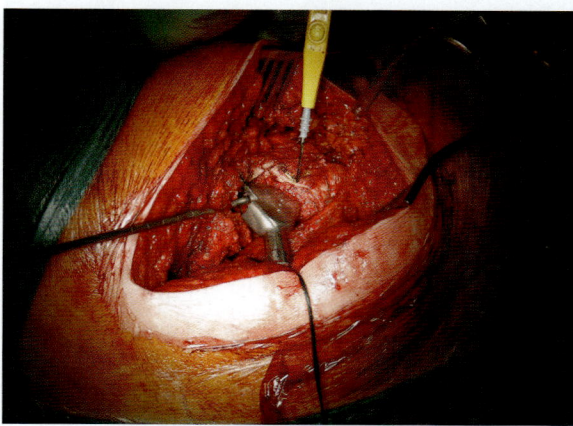

Figure 95-12. The proximal femur marked with diathermy and methylene blue relative to the marks on the phantom for reference when cementing the definitive prosthesis.

Proximal Impaction

The phantom is driven into the distally impacted bone (Fig. 95-11) and then is removed. More graft is pushed down the canal with handheld distal impactors and the phantom reinserted. The procedure is repeated until the phantom is stable enough to allow performance of a trial reduction, when hip stability and leg length can be assessed. The position of the phantom in relation to the proximal femur is marked with diathermy and methylene blue for reference at the time of cementing the stem (Fig. 95-12). The need for reconstruction of a calcar defect is reassessed at this stage, and it is indicated whether less than 1 cm of medial femoral neck is present above the level of the lesser trochanter, or if the most distal leg length mark of the phantom is seen well above cortical bone. The metal mesh is then fixed in position with cables or cerclage wires, avoiding multifilament cables for the most proximal section that will lie within the joint, to minimize the risk of fretting and release of metal debris. The impaction process is repeated until graft is firmly compacted up to within 1 or 2 cm of the top. At this stage, it should be impossible to withdraw the phantom by hand; it can be removed only with the use of the sliding hammer. It should also be impossible to produce any rotational movement of the phantom within the impacted graft. The following steps are the most important part of the procedure and determine the stability of the reconstruction, allowing for transmission of load into the proximal femur and ensuring that subsidence of the stem within the cement mantle is similar to that observed in primary hip arthroplasty. Using dedicated handheld block impactors and large cancellous chips (8 to 10 mm in size), the level of impacted graft is brought up to the top after firm impaction around the phantom (Fig. 95-13). To optimize proximal impaction, the phantom at this final stage should be backed out 1 or 2 cm so that more bone chips can be added; these are firmly impacted and the phantom driven to the correct depth, providing sound stability of the reconstruction. Calcar wires can be further tightened if necessary. The final consistency of the impacted chips should be that of cortical bone. Running out of bone graft material before completing proximal impaction will seriously affect the stability of the reconstruction.

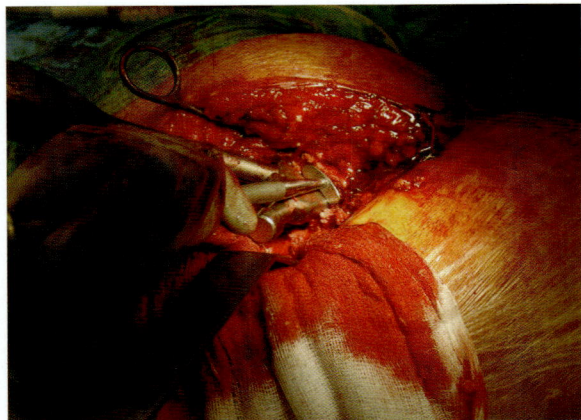

Figure 95-13. Handheld block impactors being used on large cancellous chips, bringing the level of impacted graft up to the top.

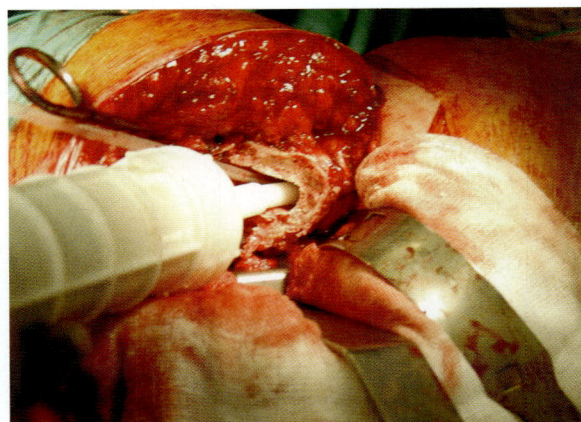

Figure 95-16. Cement being injected in a retrograde fashion, removing the suction catheter as soon as it blocks.

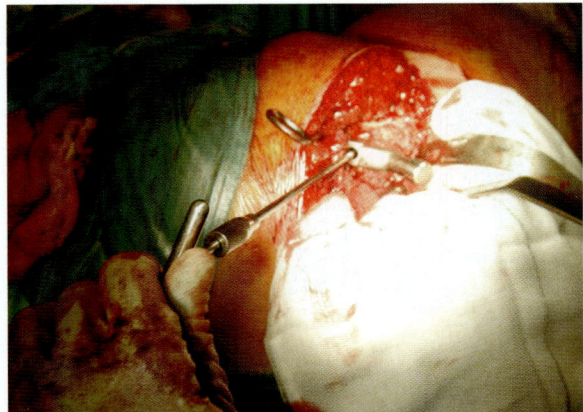

Figure 95-14. Threaded guide wire being unscrewed from the plug and removed.

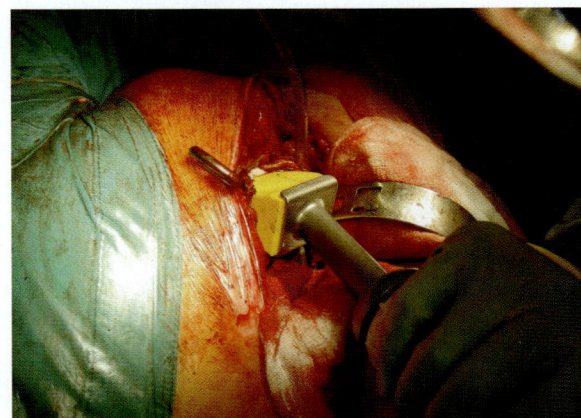

Figure 95-17. Proximal femoral seal firmly applied, ensuring optimal pressurization of cement.

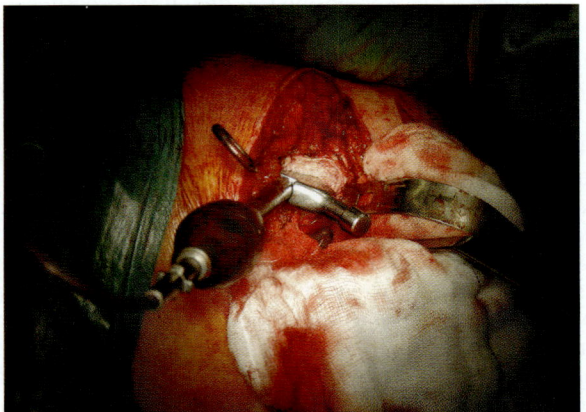

Figure 95-15. Suction catheter inserted down the phantom to suck the canal dry distally.

Cementing and Stem Insertion

The threaded guide wire is unscrewed from the plug and removed (Fig. 95-14) so that a suction catheter can be inserted down the phantom to suck the canal dry distally (Fig. 95-15). Cement is mixed in a cement gun with a dedicated narrow revision spout. The phantom is removed immediately before cement injection and the suction catheter reinserted. Cement is then injected in a retrograde fashion, and the suction catheter is removed as soon as it blocks (Fig. 95-16). A proximal femoral seal is applied to the gun spout, which is cut short. Cement is firmly pressurized (Fig. 95-17). The definitive stem, which is collarless, double-tapered, and polished, attached to a wingless hollow centralizer, is inserted to the marked depth as the viscosity of the cement increases (Fig. 95-18). The introducer is removed and a "horse collar" seal applied until the cement has polymerized (Fig. 95-19). Final tightening of the calcar wires can now be performed. The appropriate femoral head is applied (Fig. 95-20), the hip is reduced, and the short external rotators are repaired. Wound closure is performed by using the surgeon's method of choice. Drains are no longer routinely used, and their requirement is assessed individually. Anteroposterior (AP) and lateral radiographs are obtained postoperatively. Preoperative and postoperative AP views of this case example are shown in Figures 95-21 and 95-22.

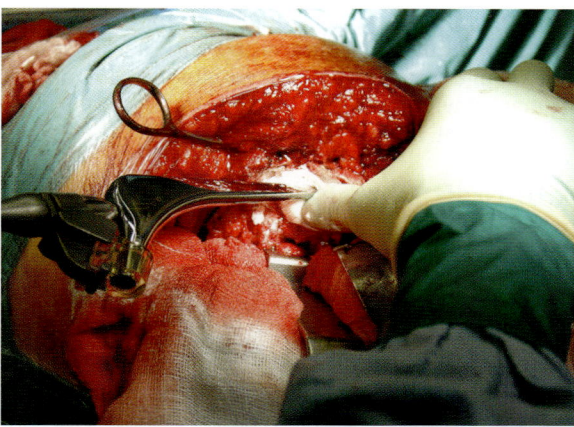

Figure 95-18. Definitive stem being inserted down to the marked depth as the viscosity of the cement increases. Note the surgeon's thumb occluding the cement medially to ensure high pressure of cement.

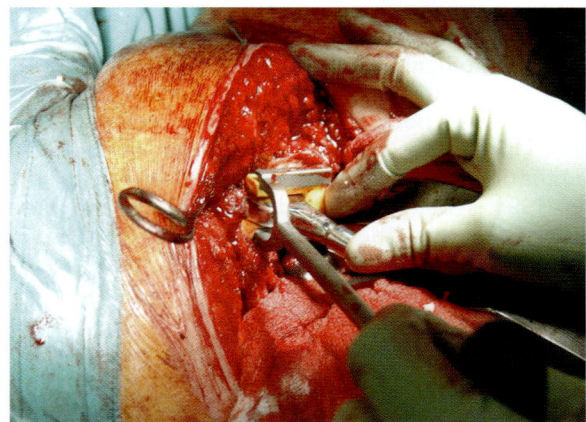

Figure 95-19. "Horse collar" seal applied, maintaining the cement pressure until polymerization.

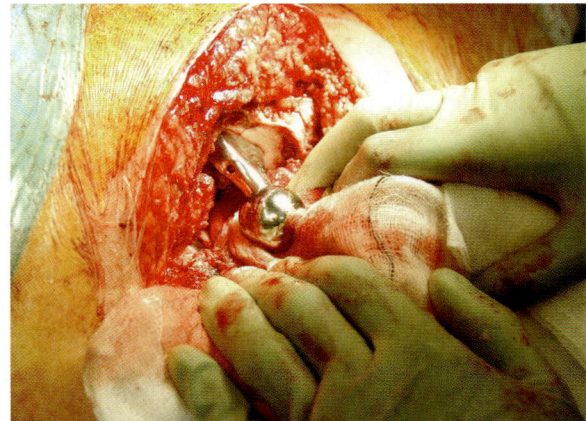

Figure 95-20. Definitive femoral head applied with hip ready for final reduction.

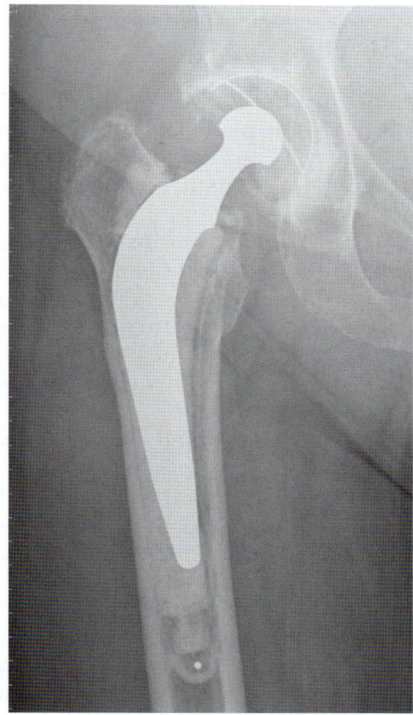

Figure 95-21. Preoperative anteroposterior (AP) view of case example.

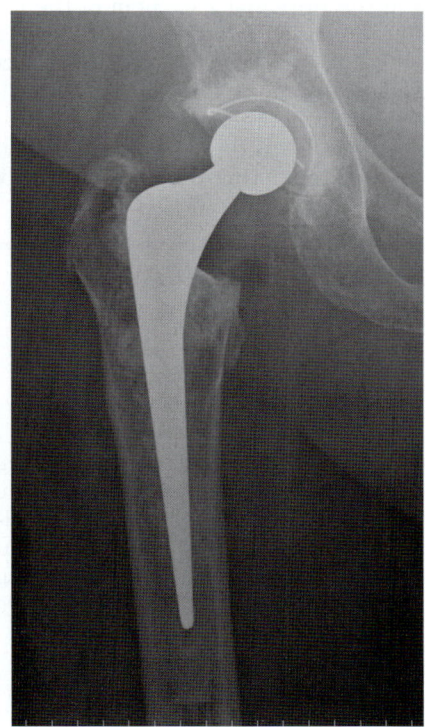

Figure 95-22. Postoperative anteroposterior (AP) view of case example.

TECHNICAL TIPS

- *Presence of significant limb shortening:* The intramedullary plug should be placed a little more distal in the femur in case trial reduction is too tight and the femoral component needs to be inserted deeper than expected.
- *Presence of well-fixed cement distally:* In the absence of infection, when well-fixed distal cement is lying at least 2 cortical diameters beyond the distal-most area of lysis in the femur, the cement can be used as a canal plug by drilling it centrally using a long drill through a distal femoral impactor and screwing a threaded guide wire into it.
- *Increased leg length identified at trial reduction with phantom:* If the leg length is found to be increased or the reduction too tight, and the impacted phantom is so tight that it cannot be driven any deeper, then it should be removed, and a phantom one size smaller should be used. The surgeon then has the option of using the smaller size or driving it deeper than required and reinserting the larger component.
- *Insufficient or excessive buildup of calcar with mesh and impacted graft:* Calcar reconstruction is performed only after the final position of the prosthesis has been determined. First, establish the position for the phantom, then apply the mesh and reconstruct using the phantom as a template. This will prevent overtightening of the mesh and consequently contact between mesh and prosthesis.
- *Bone chips that are too small:* It is very difficult to achieve sound stability with chips that are smaller than 3 to 4 mm in diameter. Larger chips of 8 to 10 mm are used in the proximal 2 to 3 cm of the femur.
- *Inadequate impaction leads to failure:* Firm and tight impaction is the key to success of this procedure.
- *Methylene blue dye mark:* Check that this is still visible because it is sometimes covered by the proximal reconstruction. If not, repeat the trial reduction and re-mark before cementing the definitive implant.

UNUSUAL SITUATIONS/CAVEATS

Templated Plug Position Distal to Isthmus

If the plug is to be inserted to a depth below the level of the isthmus, it will not fix firmly in the canal. A second guide wire is placed externally along the thigh to the same position, indicating the position of the plug, which is then skewered percutaneously with a 2-mm Kirschner wire. This prevents distal migration of the plug during impaction. The Kirschner wire is left protruding through the skin for easy removal at the end of the procedure.

Awareness of Risk of Intraoperative Fracture

During the proximal impaction stage, if the phantom is perceived to offer less resistance as it is inserted than at the previous insertion, a femoral shaft split fracture has occurred and must be treated with cerclage wiring. Use of a longer stem should be considered. Prophylactic fixation with wires or cables before impaction is an easy way to prevent this potential problem.

Risk of Graft Extrusion Through Femoral Cortical Defects

Failure to contain impacted graft by closing cortical defects with metal mesh can cause graft extrusion.

Use of Long Stems

When stems longer than 205 mm are used, an additional step is required before proximal impaction. This involves the use of a coring device, which is passed over the guide wire for removal of only the central part of the distally impacted bone graft, allowing longer phantoms to be inserted down to the correct level to complete the reconstruction.

Combined Use With Extended Trochanteric Osteotomy (ETO)

When indicated, an ETO reduces the risk of compromising the proximal femoral bone stock while it facilitates the removal of both cemented and uncemented prostheses during the revision procedure. In Exeter, the combination of these two techniques has been in use since 1994. When performed appropriately, impaction grafting protects the osteotomy site from cement interposition, leading to a secure union at the osteotomy site.

POSTOPERATIVE CARE

In our hospital, revision total hip arthroplasty is usually carried out under epidural and light general anesthesia. Mobilization is commenced after removal of the epidural catheter, usually at 48 hours. The postoperative weight-bearing regimen is governed by the procedure carried out on the acetabular side. With reasonable host bone stock, full weight bearing is permitted immediately as comfortable. If host bone is flimsy, crutches and restricted weight bearing are encouraged for 6 to 12 weeks. In our experience, the procedure is well tolerated with little early postoperative discomfort.

RESULTS

The initial report by Gie and associates[4] at 44 to 78 months' follow-up of 68 patients in whom revision femoral impaction grafting using a polished, double-tapered, collarless stem had been carried out showed clinical results comparable with those of primary surgery with signs of incorporation and remodeling of bone graft. Results from the same group at 10 years revealed survivorship for aseptic stem loosening of 99.1%.[5] By December 2001, more than 540 cases of femoral impaction bone grafting had been performed in Exeter, and at 15 years' follow-up, survivorship of the stem with reoperation on the femoral side for any reason as the endpoint was 90.6%, and survivorship with aseptic loosening of the stem as the endpoint was 98.5%. In addition, the following results have been published:

- Mikhail and Timperley[6] presented 2- to 6-year results using a stem of similar geometry in 132 patients, showing favorable clinical and radiologic outcomes.
- Elting and colleagues[7] reported on impaction grafting for exchange femoral arthroplasty. Satisfactory results were observed for 67 patients at 2- to 5-year follow-up. The major complication in this series was late femoral fracture.
- Piccaluga and coworkers[8] reported on 59 hips at 57 months' follow-up (2 to 12 years), using the Charnley prosthesis. They found a re-revision rate of 3.5% with low incidence of intraoperative and postoperative complications.
- Ornstein and associates[9] studied stem migration in 18 cases using roentgen stereophotogrammetric analysis. Distal migration at 10 years averaged 2.5 mm. Migration rate decreased with time, with 12 of the stems showing no further migration by 18 months. No clinical failures were observed at 2-year follow-up.
- Ornstein and colleagues[10] most recently reported on a survivorship analysis of 1305 revisions performed between 1989 and 2002 in 30 hospitals in Sweden, with 94% survivorship for all causes at 15 years and 99.1% survivorship for aseptic stem loosening.
- English and coworkers[11] studied 53 hips for which impaction grafting had been used in the second stage of a two-stage revision for infection, with a reinfection rate of 7.5%.
- Buttaro and associates,[12] reporting on 30 hips using vancomycin-loaded allograft in the second stage, reported a reinfection rate of only 3.3%, with no adverse effects on restoration of bone stock.
- Sierra and colleagues[13] studied 42 hips for which impaction bone grafting was performed using long Exeter stems, showing 2 cases of postoperative femoral fracture and highlighting that this is a technically demanding procedure whereby any areas of lysis, cortical perforations, or areas of thinning should be bypassed by long stems.
- Kerboull and coworkers[14] reported on 129 femoral revision hip replacements using the Charnley-Kerboull femoral component, showing 98% survivorship for radiologic failure with no further femoral revision required for up to 16 years.
- Yim and associates[15] studied 56 femoral revisions in 43 South Korean patients at a minimum 39-month follow-up with successful outcomes in patients with smaller femur sizes.
- Wraighte and colleagues,[16] reporting on 75 hips, showed survivorship of 92% at 10.5 years with any further femoral operation as the endpoint.
- Schreurs and coworkers[17] reported on the technique and results of 33 consecutive femoral reconstructions with 100% survivorship for revision of the femoral component at 10.4 years.

- Some reports presented studies with high complication rates, including Meding and associates,[18] Masterson and colleagues,[19] Eldridge and coworkers,[20] and Pekkarinen and associates.[21] Unquestionably, technical issues have played an important role in these varying outcomes.

COMPLICATIONS

Potential complications are the same as for revision hip surgery in general, including thromboembolic episodes, dislocation, sepsis, nerve palsy, leg length discrepancy, femoral fracture, and mortality.

When dealing with significant diaphyseal bone loss, the use of longer stems cannot be overemphasized owing to the increased risk of periprosthetic fracture at the stem tip level. In those cases where the canal is too narrow for a longer stem, use of plates or strut grafts is highly recommended.

The results are technique dependent; therefore significant subsidence and mechanical failure are directly related to the quality of the graft and its impaction, as well as to the stability of the reconstruction and cement pressurization.

CURRENT CONTROVERSIES AND FUTURE CONSIDERATIONS

- When determining the age limit for the use of this technique, physiologic age rather than chronologic age should be considered, as should life expectancy.
- Although undoubtedly the restoration of bone stock is a very desirable effect, the risks of a longer procedure must be considered for each case, depending on the patient's fitness for surgery.

REFERENCES

1. Slooff TJ, Huiskes R, van Horn J, et al: Bone grafting in total hip replacement for acetabular protrusion. Acta Orthop Scand 55:593–596, 1984.
2. Ling RS, Timperley AJ, Linder L: Histology of cancellous impaction grafting in the femur: a case report. J Bone Joint Surg Br 75:693–696, 1993.
3. Rudelli S, Uip D, Honda E, Lima A: One-stage revision of infected total hip arthroplasty with bone graft. J Arthroplasty 23:1165–1177, 2008.
4. Gie GA, Linder L, Ling RSM, et al: Impacted cancellous allografts and cement for revision total hip arthroplasty. J Bone Joint Surg Br 75:14–21, 1993.
5. Halliday BR, English HW, Timperley AJ, et al: Femoral impaction grafting with cement in revision total hip replacement: evolution of the technique and results. J Bone Joint Surg Br 85:809–817, 2003.
6. Mikhail WEM, Timperley AJ: Tight packing of morcellized allograft: new method for managing bone lysis. Orthop Spec Ed 3:21–22, 1994.
7. Elting JJ, Mikhail WEM, Zicat BA: Preliminary report of impaction grafting for exchange femoral arthroplasty. Clin Orthop Relat Res 319:159–167, 1995.
8. Piccaluga F, Della Vale A, Fernandez JC, et al: Revision of the femoral prosthesis with impaction allografting and a Charnley stem. J Bone joint Surg Br 84:544–549, 2002.

9. Ornstein E, Atroshi I, Franzen H, et al: Results of hip revision using the Exeter stem, impacted allograft bone and cement. Clin Orthop Relat Res 389:126–133, 2001.

10. Ornstein E, Linder L, Lewold S, Torper M: Femoral impaction bone grafting with the Exeter stem: the Swedish experience. J Bone Joint Surg Br 91:441–446, 2009.

11. English H, Timperley AJ, Dunlop D, Gie G: Impaction grafting of the femur in two-stage revision for infected total hip replacement. J Bone Joint Surg Br 84:700–705, 2002.

12. Buttaro MA, Pusso R, Piccaluga F: Vancomycin-supplemented impacted bone allografts in infected hip arthroplasty: two-stage revision results. J Bone Joint Surg Br 87:314–319, 2005.

13. Sierra RJ, Charity J, Tsiridis E, et al: The use of long cemented stems for femoral impaction grafting in revision total hip arthoplasty. J Bone Joint Surg Am 90:1330–1336, 2008.

14. Kerboull L, Hamadouche M, Kerboull M: Impaction grafting in association with the Charnley-Kerboull cemented femoral component: operative technique and two- to 16-year follow-up results. J Bone Joint Surg Br 91:304–309, 2009.

15. Yim S, Kim M, Suh Y: Impaction allograft with cement for the revision of the femoral component: a minimum 39-month follow-up study with the use of the Exeter stem in Asian hips. Int Orthop 31:297–302, 2007.

16. Wraighte PJ, Howard PW: Femoral impaction bone allografting with an Exeter cemented, collarless, polished, tapered stem in revision hip replacement: a mean follow-up of 10.5 years. J Bone Joint Surg Br 90:1000–1004, 2008.

17. Schreurs BW, Arts JJ, Verdonschot N, et al: Femoral revision with use of impaction bone-grafting and a cemented polished stem: surgical technique. J Bone Joint Surg Am 88:259–274, 2006.

18. Meding JB, Ritter MA, Keating EM, et al: Impaction bone grafting before insertion of a femoral stem with cement in revision total hip arthroplasty. J Bone Joint Surg Am 79:1834–1841, 1997.

19. Masterson EL, Masri BA, Duncan CP: The cement mantle in the Exeter impaction allografting technqiue: a cause for concern. J Arthroplasty 12:759–764, 1997.

20. Eldridge JD, Smith EJ, Hubble MJ, et al: Massive early subsidence following femoral impaction grafting. J Arthroplasty 12:535–540, 1997.

21. Pekkarinen J, Alho A, Lepistö J: Impaction bone grafting in revision hip surgery: a high incidence of complications. J Bone Joint Surg Br 82:103–107, 2000.

FURTHER READING

1. Bolder SB, Schreurs BW, Verdonschot N, et al: Wire mesh allows more revascularisation than a strut in impaction bone grafting: an animal study in goats. Clin Orthop Relat Res 423:280–286, 2004.
   Medial femoral neck defects were created in goat femora. Reconstruction with medial femoral mesh and impaction grafting or strut grafts were then carried out. Six weeks postoperatively, no revascularization was observed deep to the strut grafts. In the mesh group, fibrous tissue and blood vessels penetrated the mesh, and a superficial zone of revascularised graft was observed.

2. Giesen EB, Lamerights NM, Verdonschot N, et al: Mechanical characteristics of impacted morsellised bone grafts used in revision of total hip arthroplasty. J Bone Joint Surg Br 81:1052–1057, 1999.
   This study documented the time-dependent mechanical properties of morselized bone graft. The conclusion was that in clinical use, bone graft is bound to be subject to permanent deformation postoperatively, and the confined compression modulus was found to be low relative to cancellous bone. Different designs of stems used with impaction grafting must therefore accommodate the viscoelastic properties and permanent deformations in the graft without causing loosening of the interface.

3. Ullmark G, Nilsson O: Impacted cortico-cancellous allografts: recoil and strength. J Arthroplasty 14:1019–1023, 1999.
   In this in vitro study, bone graft was morselized, producing chips of two different sizes, which were impacted with two different impaction forces. Findings were that there was less subsidence with the use of larger bone chips and with the harder impacted graft.

CHAPTER 96

Femoral Revision: Uncemented Extensively Porous-Coated Implants

Bryan P. Springer and William L. Griffin

KEY POINTS

- Managing femoral bone loss in revision total hip arthroplasty is challenging and requires meticulous clinical evaluation and preoperative planning.
- The ideal revision femoral stem is easy to insert, can be used to treat most revision situations, and has reproducible clinical results.
- Extensively porous-coated stems can be used to treat most femoral defects.
- Preoperative planning and surgical technique are essential for success with extensively porous-coated stems.
- Clinical results show excellent midterm to long-term survivorship in the revision setting.

INTRODUCTION

The success of primary total hip arthroplasty is well documented in the literature with survival rates greater than 90% at 15-year follow-up.[1-6] As our population ages, the number of total hip arthroplasties performed is increasing dramatically. Unfortunately, some of these procedures are not successful and require revision. Despite improvements in implant materials and surgical techniques, the number of revisions for failed total hip replacement has not decreased. In addition, expansion of indications to younger, more active patients and improved life expectancy for patients with total hip replacement have increased the number of revisions, and this trend is not expected to decrease. In fact, recent projections indicate that the burden of revision total hip arthroplasty is expected to increase by 137% over the next 25 years.[7] In addition, the cost and resource utilization for revision procedures are substantially higher than those for primary procedures.[8]

The current epidemiology of failed total hip arthroplasty is gathered mainly from large cohort studies and registry data in Europe, Canada, and Australia. These reports indicate that aseptic loosening, osteolysis/wear, and instability are the major causes of failure for total hip arthroplasty.

Springer and associates reviewed a series of 1100 hips that underwent revision total hip arthroplasty over a 20-year period at their institution.[9] The most common reasons for failure of the primary total hip arthroplasty were aseptic loosening and instability. These two diagnoses accounted for 61% of all failed total hip replacements. In addition, instability and aseptic loosening accounted for more than 65% of failures of revision total hip arthroplasty leading to re-revision, indicating an area where improvement is needed.

Dobzyniak and colleagues evaluated early failures of primary total hip arthroplasty defined as those requiring revision within 5 years of the index arthroplasty.[10] Of 745 revision procedures, 39% occurred within the first 5 years following index total hip arthroplasty. Instability (33%) was the major reason for early failure, requiring revision followed by aseptic loosening (30%) and infection (14%).

Utilizing the Nationwide Inpatient Sample, Bozic and coworkers reviewed 51,345 revision total hip arthroplasties performed in the United States over a 1-year period (October 2005 through December 2006).[11] The purpose of this study was to determine the epidemiology of revision total hip arthroplasty. The most common causes of failed total hip arthroplasty requiring revision were instability/dislocation (22.5%), aseptic loosening (19.7%), and infection (14.8%). In addition, full component revision (femoral and acetabular components) was the most common procedure performed to treat failed arthroplasty (41.1%).

Managing the revision femur following failed total hip arthroplasty remains technically challenging. Extensive bone loss from aseptic loosening, sepsis, and osteolysis can lead to a variety of bony defects and a multitude of clinical scenarios. The goals of revision total hip arthroplasty are (1) to obtain rigid initial stability of the implants, (2) to engage the healthy remaining bone proximally or distally with the implant, and (3) to bypass stress risers.

Implant options for the revision femur are numerous and include cemented and cementless fixation. Cemented fixation allows for immediate fixation, is adaptable to a variety of femoral defects, and allows the use of antibiotic-impregnated cemented materials. In many instances, however, a sclerotic endosteal surface leads to poor cement penetration into bone and a decrease in the strength of the bone-cement interface. Clinical results of cemented femoral stems in revision total hip arthroplasty have been poor, with mechanical failure rates as high as 64%.

Cementless stems may engage the proximal metaphysis (proximally coated stems) or may achieve distal fixation in the diaphysis. Femoral revision using proximal fixation with nonmodular, broached systems has met with poor results. Difficulty matching the implant with variable femoral geometry, often with insufficient proximal supports and poor rotational control with lack of distal fixation, has led to high failure rates.[12,13] At 8-year follow-up, Berry reported that only 20% of proximally coated implants were free of aseptic loosening.[14]

In addition, structural allograft (allograft prosthetic composite) or impaction grafting techniques may be utilized in certain clinical circumstances. These implants and techniques are technically demanding, and their use and indications are covered in Chapters 95 and 99.

No one single implant is appropriate for all revision situations, and each case should be considered individually based on the clinical situation and radiographic evaluation. The ideal femoral revision implant would be easy to insert, would have reproducible results, and would be able to handle most revision situations. Extensively porous-coated stems have a long track record of success in revision total hip arthroplasty. These stems are able to handle most femoral defects with reliable clinical results. Meticulous preoperative planning and surgical technique are essential for success. This chapter will focus on the indications, preoperative planning, surgical technique, and results of extensively porous-coated implants in revision total hip arthroplasty.

INDICATIONS FOR EXTENSIVELY POROUS-COATED STEMS

A femoral bone defect classification allows for systematic evaluation of the host bone and the amount of bone loss and assists in standardizing treatment of various femoral defects. Although several classifications exist, the system described by Paprosky and Della Valle is treatment oriented and describes the progression of bony defects.[15] This classification system is based on an evaluation of the bone and available areas for fixation of implants:

- Type 1: minimal bone loss in the metaphysis and an intact diaphysis (Fig. 96-1*A* through *C*)
- Type 2: extensive loss of metaphyseal bone with an intact diaphysis (Fig. 96-2*A* through *C*)
- Type 3A: the metaphysis is damaged and unsupportive; a minimum of 4 cm of intact cortical bone is present in the diaphysis at the isthmus (Fig. 96-3*A* through *C*)
- Type 3B: the metaphysis is damaged and unsupportive; intact cortical bone measuring less than 4 cm is present distal to the isthmus (Fig. 96-4)
- Type 4: extensive metaphyseal and diaphyseal damage; the femoral canal is widened and is not supportive (Fig. 96-5*A* through *C*)

Fully porous-coated stems are indicated for use in the revision femur for Paprosky type 1 through 3A femoral defects. Success is dependent on achieving initial implant stability that will allow adequate bony ingrowth to provide long-term fixation. In general, a minimum of 4 to 6 cm of diaphyseal bone should be available to allow for stable fixation. The term "scratch fit" is used to describe the mechanical fit of the cylindrical stem into the host diaphyseal bone. This scratch fit is dependent on meticulous canal preparation and selection of an appropriately sized implant based on preoperative templating and intraoperative findings.

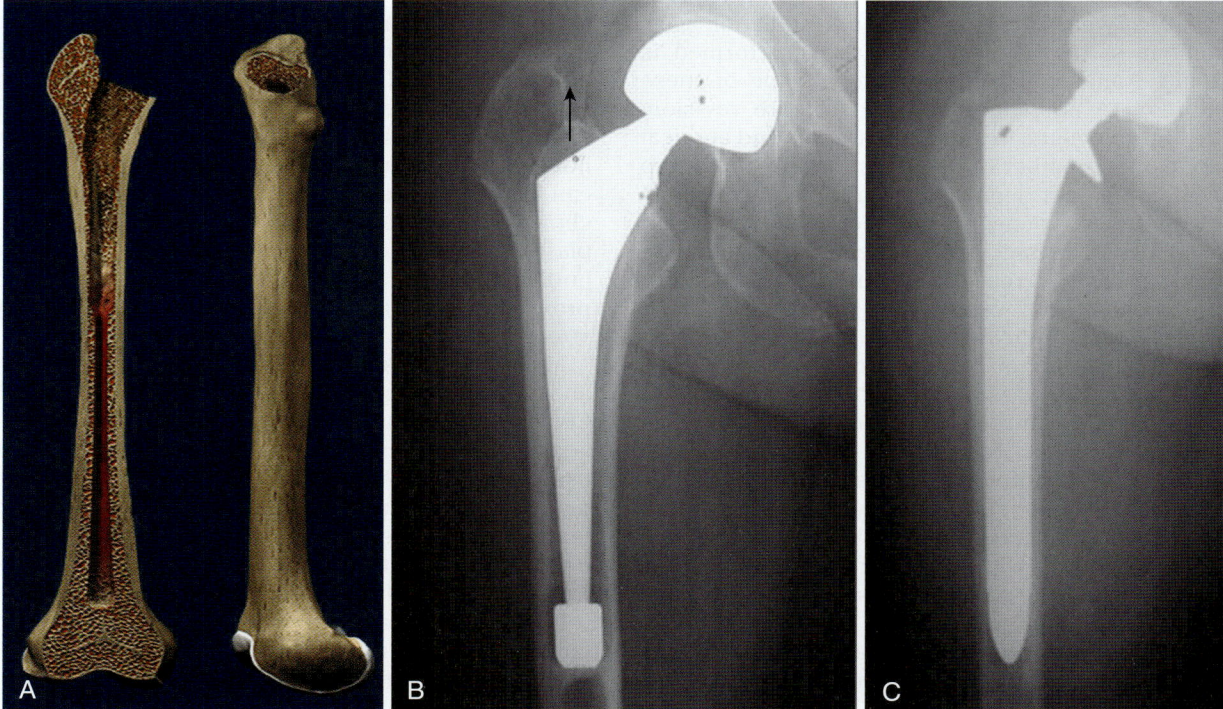

Figure 96-1. Illustration and preoperative and postoperative revision radiographs of a Paprosky type 1 defect treated with a fully porous-coated stem.

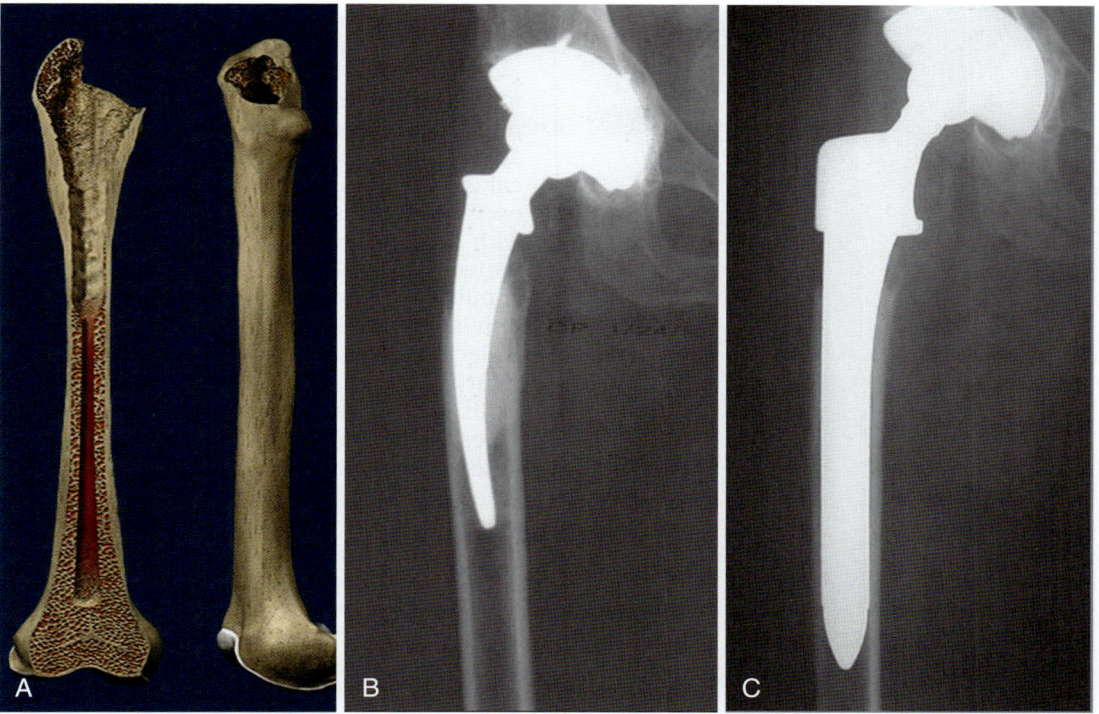

Figure 96-2. Illustration and preoperative and postoperative revision radiographs of a Paprosky type 2 defect treated with a fully porous-coated stem.

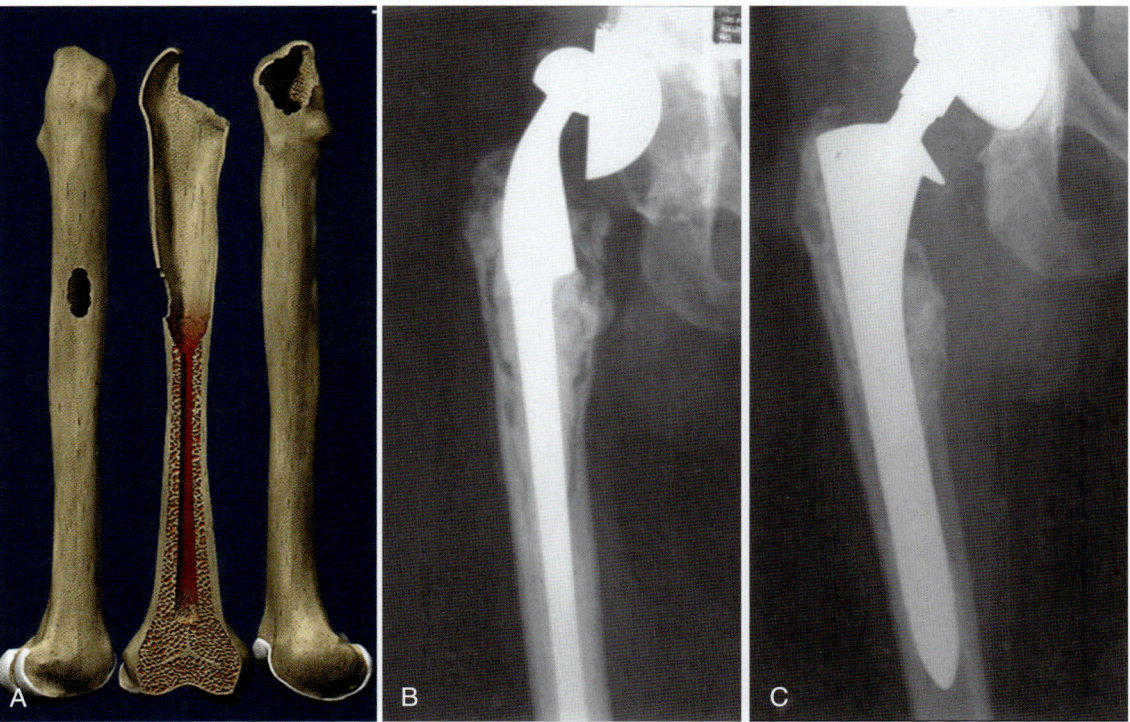

Figure 96-3. Illustration and preoperative and postoperative revision radiographs of a Paprosky type 3A defect treated with a fully porous-coated stem.

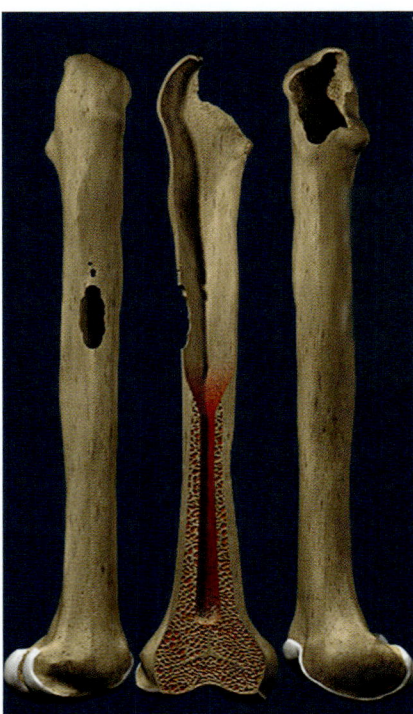

Figure 96-4. Illustration of a Paprosky type 3B defect.

CONTRAINDICATIONS

As with any surgical procedure, revision with a fully porous-coated stem is contraindicated in patients with active and ongoing infection. A thorough history, physical examination, and laboratory testing are required to exclude the possibility of infection before proceeding with revision surgery. In addition, medically infirm patients who are too ill to undergo revision surgery should be medically optimized before surgical intervention is provided.

Because the success of fully porous stems in revision total hip arthroplasty is dependent on achieving intimate fit in the diaphysis over a minimum of 4 cm, these types of stems are contraindicated in patients with severe diaphyseal bone loss. The type 4 femur is characterized by significant diaphyseal damage with a capacious medullary canal. In these situations, attaining initial implant stability to achieve bony ingrowth is difficult, if not impossible. The type 4 femur is best treated with alternative means of reconstruction, including impaction grafting, allograft prosthetic composite, fluted tapered modular stems, and proximal femoral replacement.

Sporer and associates reported on the limits of fully porous-coated stems in revision total hip arthroplasty.[16] In this study, hips reconstructed with fully porous-coated stems in type 3B and 4 femurs were evaluated. Patients with fully porous stems greater than 19 mm in diameter with 3B femoral defects had a mechanical failure rate of 18%. In patients with type 4 femoral defects and stems greater than 19 mm, the mechanical

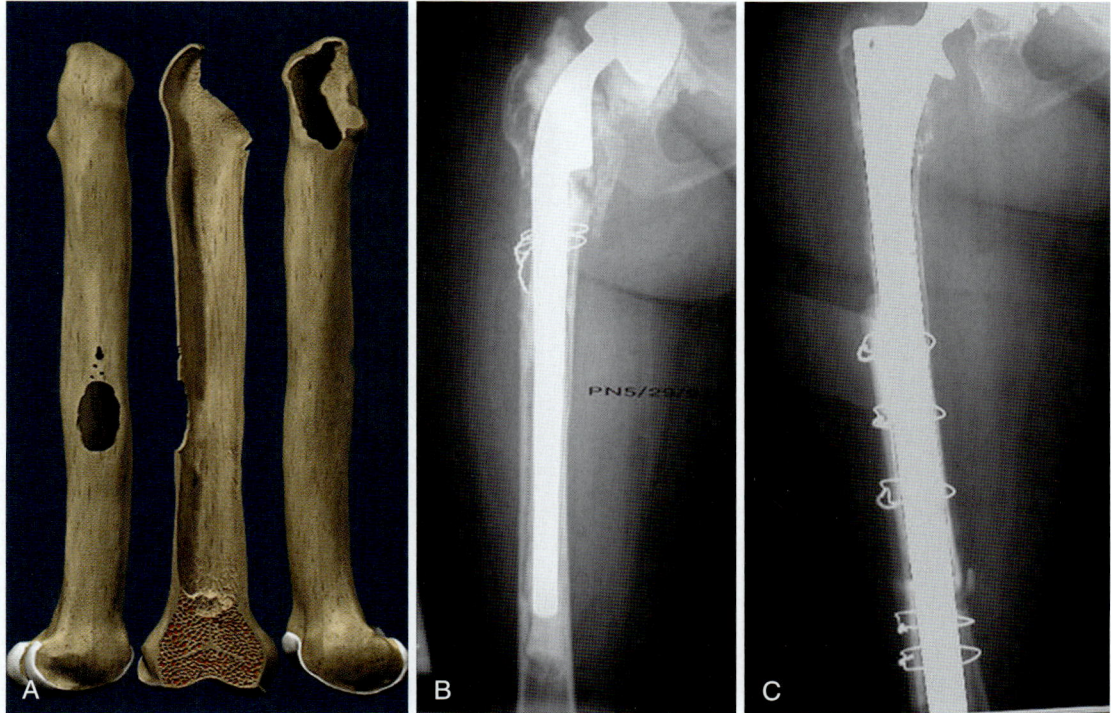

Figure 96-5. Illustration and preoperative and postoperative revision radiographs of a Paprosky type 4 defect treated with a fully porous-coated stem.

failure rate was 37.5%. The authors speculate that these patients with poor bone stock and large canals do not have appropriate bony support to allow for initial axial and rotational stability. In these situations, the authors recommend using alternative techniques for femoral fixation.

PREOPERATIVE PLANNING

A reproducible surgical technique starts with a careful preoperative plan.

Most preoperative planning is performed with x-ray evaluation. However, clinical assessment should include an assessment of leg length discrepancies and prior surgical approaches. Leg lengths should be measured by radiographs but should be confirmed with leg length blocks to ensure that the patient is comfortable with the anticipated leg length. Prior surgical approaches may influence the approach used for revision, but whichever approach is used, it should be easily converted to an extensile approach to the femur if needed.

As with any revision, considerable thought should go into planning for component removal. Use of an extended greater trochanteric osteotomy, removal of well-fixed cementless implants, and osteolysis may influence the amount of bone remaining for fixation and allow identification of the appropriate implant needed.

Preoperative radiographs should include an antero-posterior (AP) x-ray of the femoral component and femur distal to the isthmus, along with a true lateral radiograph to assess the extent of femoral bowing (Fig. 96-6). X-ray technologists need to be instructed in the technique for obtaining a true lateral radiograph of the femur. A Lowenstein lateral of the femur positions the patient with both the ankle and the knee flat on the x-ray table, ensuring a true lateral of the femoral bow. This can be critical when planning for a long canal filling femoral component. Magnification markers allow accurate measurement of the diameter of the endosteal canal of the femur and of component length. These measurements help with predicting the size of the femoral component needed at the time of surgery and facilitate intraoperative decision making regarding fit and length. Templates should be applied to the radiographs with the goal of achieving 4 to 6 cm of intimate endosteal contact "scratch fit." The first step in templating is to select a stem of appropriate diameter to achieve a tight scratch fit. The templated stem is then adjusted axially to provide appropriate leg lengths. The third step is to choose the best stem length to bypass any stress risers and engage the area of scratch fit, while avoiding the anterior cortex of the bowed femur. Stem diameters from 10.5 mm to 21.0 mm and lengths of 6 inches, 8 inches, and 10 inches in straight or bowed configurations are available to best fit the femoral geometry.

DESCRIPTION OF TECHNIQUES

At the time of surgery, the femoral canal should be cleaned of all retained cement and debris. Retained

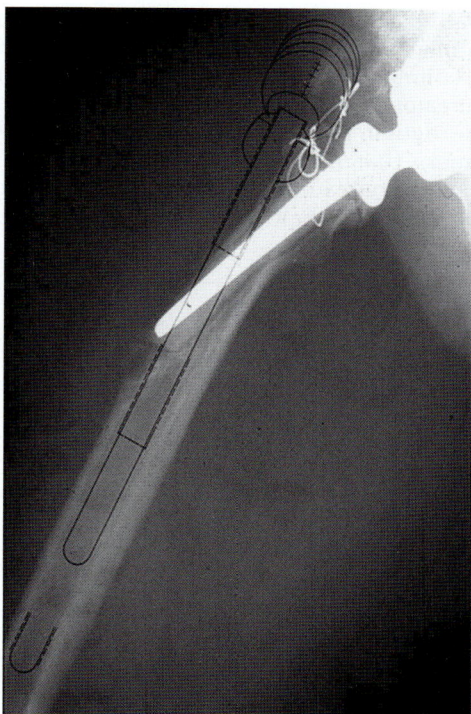

Figure 96-6. Preoperative lateral radiograph should be evaluated and templated to assess the amount of femoral bowing.

cement fragments, when encountered by a tight reamer, can lead to catastrophic femoral fractures. If any question arises as to whether or not all cement has been removed, intraoperative x-rays should be obtained before reaming of the femoral canal. The femoral canal should be reamed to a "tight fit." The canal should be to under-reamed 0.5 mm smaller than the anticipated femoral component (or line-to-line for some longer-bowed stems). The goal is to attain a tight fit over at least a 4- to 6-cm segment, depending on the quality of the bone. Two methods may be used to help determine intraoperatively whether the appropriate amount of scratch fit has been attained. First, once the canal has been reamed to the anticipated size, a reamer of the same size as the final implant is seated into the canal as far as it will go by hand. It should seat at least 4 to 6 cm proud of the final implant to ensure an adequate scratch fit. If the scratch fit is excessive, the appropriate length of scratch fit can be adjusted by incremental reaming with the final same-sized reamer. The second check used to determine whether tight fit within the femoral canal is adequate is to obtain an intraoperative radiograph with the final reamer in place (.5 mm smaller than the final implant) (Fig. 96-7). This intraoperative radiograph can be used to judge appropriate alignment, to ensure that the component is not in varus and that the component will be of appropriate size to fill the endosteal canal, and to check for complete removal of cement. A trial component should be inserted to determine the depth of seating of the implant. The trial components often do not have rotational stability owing to lack of proximal bone; however, this step along with preoperative planning helps determine whether the final optimal leg length is achieved. Before the final implant is impacted, hole gauges are used to measure the final reamer, and the actual implant is used to determine the actual tolerance mismatch (Fig. 96-8*A* and *B*). Reamers that have been in use for several years and have been repeatedly sharpened often lose material and create an envelope of a smaller diameter than

anticipated. Implants have mild variations that may influence the degree of scratch fit that is attained.

In summary, it is a judgment call as to how much is an appropriate scratch fit. Variables encountered include the quality of the bone, the size of the final reamer, the size of the implant, and the potential risk for fracture. It is important to keep in mind that the monoblock extensively coated stem has parallel sides and is not a wedge, and if the endosteum of the femoral canal is adequately prepared, the risk of fracture is low.

There are several critical points at the time of stem impaction. The implant first should be inserted by hand with a twisting motion until tight. The implant then should be impacted with a mallet using moderate force. It should advance roughly 2 mm with each blow. Full impaction within a tight femoral canal can take up to 5 minutes. A trial reduction with the shortest neck length or with no head at all should be attempted roughly 1 cm prior to full seating of the implant. Oftentimes in the revision setting, the soft tissue tension is less than anticipated, and a longer neck length than templated may be required to obtain appropriate soft tissue tension. The goal is to avoid seating the implant too far, so that even the longest neck length does not re-create soft tissue tension.

If the implant suddenly advances during a difficult insertion, be sure to obtain an intraoperative x-ray to check for the possibility of fracture. If a nondisplaced longitudinal fracture is identified on x-ray, this can be treated with protected weight bearing, or if there is significant concern, the fracture may be exposed and secured with wires. If a displaced fracture occurs, it should be treated appropriately with full exposure, wiring, and possibly strut grafts and a longer implant to bypass the defect. After the implant has been fully impacted, the stem should be tested by hand for rotational stability by torquing the proximal end of the implant.

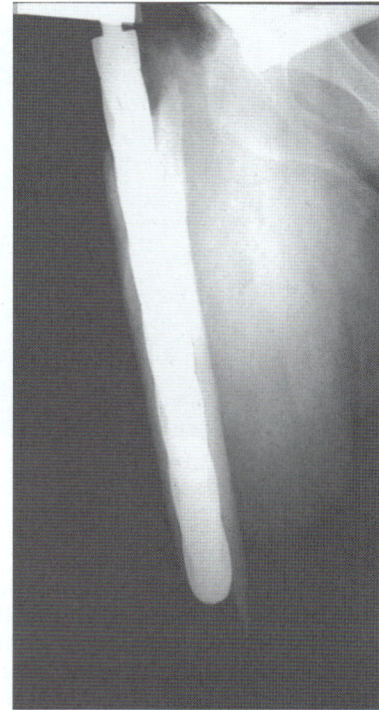

Figure 96-7. An intraoperative radiograph is taken with the reamer left in place to determine the fit and fill of the diaphysis before insertion of the real component.

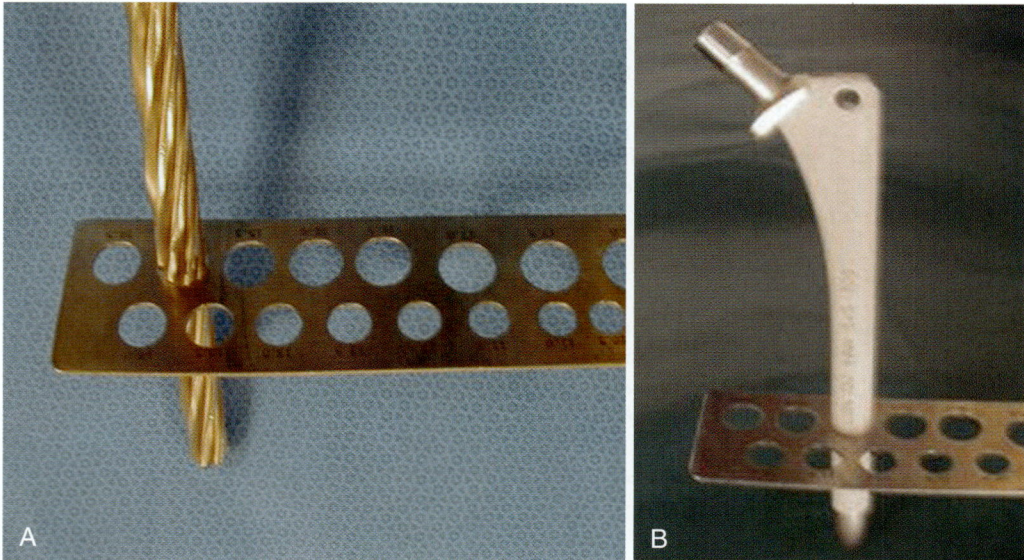

Figure 96-8. A hole gauge is used to adequately determine the size of the reamer and the final implant to be inserted.

VARIATIONS/UNUSUAL SITUATIONS

The most common variable encountered with femoral revision is the degree of femoral bowing or varus remodeling. With monoblock straight stems of 6 to 8 inches, the anterior bow rarely comes into play. However, with longer stems and with patients of short stature, it is imperative to have accurate x-rays and careful planning to avoid perforation of the anterior cortex of the femur. Extended trochanteric osteotomies allow for a straighter trajectory down the distal femur and a better chance of a tight scratch fit when faced with a significant bow. The longer stems have a bowed option that can accommodate a femoral bow but should be implanted in conjunction with a trochanteric osteotomy to allow safer and more precise canal preparation.

POSTOPERATIVE CARE

Postoperative care is dictated by the degree of scratch fit that was attained at the time of surgery, the overall bone quality, the status of acetabular fixation, and the patient's ability to achieve bony ingrowth. All surgical and patient-related factors (such as ability to comply with postoperative restriction) should be taken into consideration when postoperative care is decided.

Six weeks of protected weight bearing (touch toe to 25%) is advisable. Immediate postoperative radiographs should be compared with radiographs taken at the first visit to ensure component stability. Gradual progressive weight bearing then can commence to achieve full weight bearing by approximately 3 months from surgery.

RESULTS

Successful femoral revision requires the use of a component that will be axially and rotationally stable to stresses and will allow for biological ingrowth and fixation. Use of fully porous-coated stems in femoral revision should be considered the gold standard for femoral reconstruction. Several midterm to long-term studies focusing on the use of fully porous-coated stems in femoral revision show excellent results. Table 96-1 lists currently available data on fully porous-coated stems for femoral revision.[17-23]

Weeden and associates reported on 188 consecutive femoral revisions treated between 1984 and 1989 with fully porous-coated stems.[23] A total of 170 patients were followed for 11 to 16 years (mean, 14.2 years). Radiographic evidence of a bone ingrown stem was present in 82% of the hips, stable fibrous fixation was present in 14% of the hips, and 4% of the hips were unstable. Six stems were revised to a larger, fully coated cementless implant. Proximal femoral osteolysis was seen in 23% of femurs but was limited to Gruen zones 1 and 7. No diaphyseal osteolysis was seen. The overall mechanical failure rate in this series was 4.1%. Failure of fixation correlated highly with extent of bone loss present at the time of surgery.

Krishnamurthy and colleagues reported on 297 cementless revision arthroplasties with extensively coated components (Anatomic Medullary Locking femoral component, DePuy, Warsaw, Ind) at 5 to 13 years' follow-up.[17] Patients were evaluated clinically and radiographically at a minimum of 60 months. Clinically, the average Postel-d'Aubigné score improved from 4.8 before surgery to 10.2 after surgery. Definitive radiographic instability was noted in only 7 of 297 hips. Five patients were symptomatic and were revised. The mechanical failure rate was 2.4%. The overall complication rate was 5.7%, with a 2.6% dislocation rate.

At a minimum of 10 years after surgery, Kim and coworkers prospectively evaluated the clinical and radiographic outcomes of revision total hip arthroplasties using cortical strut allografts and fully porous-coated cementless revision femoral components in patients with massive femoral bone deficiency.[24] In all, 21 men and 33 women (54 hips) were included in the series, with patients' mean age at the time of index revision being 54.6 years (range, 36 to 65 years). All femurs had two or three fresh-frozen femoral strut allografts. The Harris hip score improved from a mean of 21 points before revision surgery to a mean of 83 points at the latest case review. Two femoral stems (4%) had aseptic loosening and were revised. All allografts had predictably united to the host femur.

Engh and associates assessed the use of fully porous-coated stems in bypassing weak or absent femoral bone with an extensively porous-coated stem and concluded

Table 96-1. Currently Available Data on Fully Porous-Coated Stems for Femoral Revision

Author	Journal	Year	Stem	No. Hips	Average Follow-up	Results
Reikeras et al[22]	Acta Orthop Scand	2006	Fully porous/HA-coated	66	Minimum 10 years	Only two hips aseptically loose
O'Shea et al[20]	J Bone Joint Surg Br	2005	Fully porous	22	33.7 months	Two aseptically loose
Weeden et al[23]	J Arthroplasty	2002	Fully porous	170	14.2 years	4.1% mechanical failure rate
Mooreland et al[19]	Clin Orthop Relat Res	2001	Fully porous	137	9.2 years	3% revised for aseptic loosening
Paprosky et al[21]	Clin Orthop Relat Res	1999	Fully porous	170	13.2 years	4.1% mechanical failure rate
Krishnamurthy et al[17]	J Arthroplasty	1997	Fully porous	297	Minimum 60 months	2.4% mechanical failure rate
Lawrence et al[18]	J Bone Joint Surg Am	1994	Fully porous	81	5 years	11% mechanical failure rate

that this is an effective reconstructive technique for patients with extensive femoral bone loss.[25] Of 275 femoral revisions done at their institution from 1982 to 1986, investigators identified 34 patients (35 hips) who represented the senior author's (C.A.E., Sr.) most difficult revision cases as a result of extensive femoral bone loss at least 10 cm below the lesser trochanter. Patients were revised with fully porous-coated femoral components of 190 mm or larger. Researchers evaluated 25 patients (26 hips) who had a minimum 10-year follow-up (mean, 13.3 years). Survivorship was 89% at 10 years with femoral revision as the endpoint (Kaplan-Meier). The femoral aseptic loosening rate was 15% (4/26). Three stems were loose but did not warrant reoperation. One stem was revised for aseptic loosening, 1 was revised for septic loosening, and 1 was revised for a fractured femoral component.

More recently, Nadaud and colleagues evaluated the difficult reconstructive challenge of severe proximal femoral bone loss in 46 hips with extensive proximal femoral bone loss that underwent revision total hip arthroplasty using cementless distal fixation without supplemental allograft.[26] All were evaluated with the Harris hip score at a minimum of 2 years. Radiographs were assessed using the Engh fixation scale. At a mean of 6.4 (range, 2 to 12) years, 43 of the 46 prostheses were functioning well. Two patients required revision for symptomatic loosening, and 1 prosthesis remains radiographically loose with a fair clinical score. Mean Harris hip score was 77 at last follow-up. Six intraoperative femur fractures, 9 dislocations, 10 cases of severe stress shielding, and no infections were reported.

COMPLICATIONS

Although the success of fully porous-coated stems in femoral revision is encouraging, unique complications are associated with their use. Failure of osseous integration, thigh pain, and stress shielding are the most common complications. Although thigh pain and stress shielding may be self-limited, each can cause concern for both patients and surgeons. Table 96-2 lists the complications reported in the literature with the use of fully porous-coated stems.

Failure of fully porous-coated stems in revision surgery for mechanical failure due to lack of bone ingrowth is relatively uncommon. The literature would suggest that failure rates range from 0 to 10% for all series and are increased in patients with severe bone loss, most notably type 3B femurs with large stems (>19 mm) and type 4 femurs. A well-ingrown fully porous-coated stem shows characteristic radiographic findings. These include absence of reactive lines around the porous coating, absence of a distal pedestal, spot welds of endosteal bone to the porous coating, and calcar atrophy due to bony ingrowth of the distal stem.[27] Box 96-1 lists the radiographic criteria for a well-fixed and loose fully porous-coated stem.

Fibrous ingrowth appears to be more common than overt loosening with this design category. This occurs when initial stability is not achieved at the time of implantation or a predominance of fibrous tissue grows into the prosthesis rather than bone. Radiographically, these suboptimally fixed stems will show nondivergent radiolucent lines around the porous surface of the implant in the absence of other signs of loosening such as pedestal formation, stem migration, calcar hypertrophy, and divergent lines.

Reactive thigh pain associated with the use of a fully porous-coated femoral component is relatively common and occurs in approximately 10% of patients.[21,28,29] The

---

BOX 96-1. RADIOGRAPHIC CRITERIA FOR FULLY POROUS-COATED STEMS

Well-Fixed Fully Porous-Coated Stem
Absence of reactive lines adjacent to porous coating
Spot welds of new bone contacting the porous surface
Calcar atrophy

Loose Fully Porous-Coated Stems
Migration of the component
Presence of reactive line around the porous surface
Absence of spot welds
Pedestal formation at tip of prosthesis
Calcar atrophy
Particle shedding

Table 96-2. Complications Reported in the Literature With the Use of Fully Porous-Coated Stems

Author	Journal	Year	Stem	No. Hips	Stress Shielding	Clinically Significant Thigh Pain	Intraoperative Fractures
Reikeras et al[22]	Acta Orthop Scand	2006	Fully porous/HA-coated	66	None reported	None	1
Weeden et al[23]	J Arthroplasty	2002	Fully porous	170	21%	9%	8.80%
Mooreland et al[19]	Clin Orthop Relat Res	2001	Fully porous	137	66% mild 22% severe	10%	2 patients
Paprosky et al[21]	Clin Orthop Relat Res	1999	Fully porous	170	21%	10%	8.80%
Krishnamurthy et al[17]	J Arthroplasty	1997	Fully porous	297	29% severe	9%	Not reported
Lawrence et al[18]	J Bone Joint Surg Am	1994	Fully porous	81	Not reported	Not reported	2

proposed cause is a modulus mismatch between the stiff femoral component and the relatively flexible femoral bone. Generally, patients complain of pain located in the anterior and lateral thigh that is activity related. Patients are at increased risk for the development of thigh pain when they lack bony integration (fibrous fixation).

Thigh pain associated with a fully porous-coated stem and caused by stress mismatch is a diagnosis of exclusion. All other possibly causes should be investigated before it is concluded that thigh pain is the source of pain. It is particularly important to investigate the possibility of a loose stem. The patient with thigh pain secondary to a well-fixed fully porous-coated stem should be treated conservatively. For many patients, symptoms will improve over the course of 1 to 2 years with conservative measures. Occasionally, a patient will present with severe thigh pain following surgery; revision will be required, and revision to a different design is indicated.

Stress shielding is a phenomenon that occurs when the proximal femur is relieved of stress, resulting in bony resorption (Fig. 96-9). In contrast to thigh pain, stress shielding occurs in patients with a well-fixed fully porous stem. It is considered a favorable radiographic sign of diaphyseal bony ingrowth. As the implant becomes osteointegrated within the diaphysis, stress on the proximal femur is transferred from the metaphysis to the diaphysis in the area of bony ingrowth.[30-32] As a result of lack of proximal loading, stress-mediated bony resorption occurs.

Stress shielding in the proximal femur is reported to occur in 23% of patients receiving a fully porous-coated stem.[33] Females and patients with larger-diameter stems have been shown to be at increased risk for the development of stress shielding.[34-36] Although the amount of bone loss that may occur with stress shielding can be significant, to date few adverse clinical events have been associated with stress shielding. It has not been shown to increase the risk or incidence of stem failure, osteolysis, or periprosthetic fracture.[36] In fact, patients with stress shielding have been shown to have a lower revision rate than those without.[37]

CURRENT CONTROVERSIES AND FUTURE CONSIDERATIONS

Although the results for fully porous-coated stems in revision surgery are encouraging, even in the setting of significant bone loss, there is certainly room for improvement with regard to implant fixation and thigh pain. Improvements in ingrowth surfaces with porous metals may allow for improvements in fixation. In addition, with a modulus of elasticity similar to bone, newer designs may reduce the incidence of thigh pain associated with rigid cobalt-chrome stems.

With the wide variation in femoral geometries found in the revision setting, the modularity of fully porous-coated stems may provide improved results. Modularity allows for an infinite number of stem lengths and decouples the anteversion of the stem from the anterior bow of the femur. The increased options that modularity provides allow the surgeon to intraoperatively customize the implant to achieve a better fit and improve initial fixation while potentially decreasing the risk for dislocation.

Infection remains one of the most feared complications and is one of the most common causes of implant failure. Novel methods that allow for the elution of antibiotics from the porous surfaces of implants may assist in the prevention and treatment of infection.

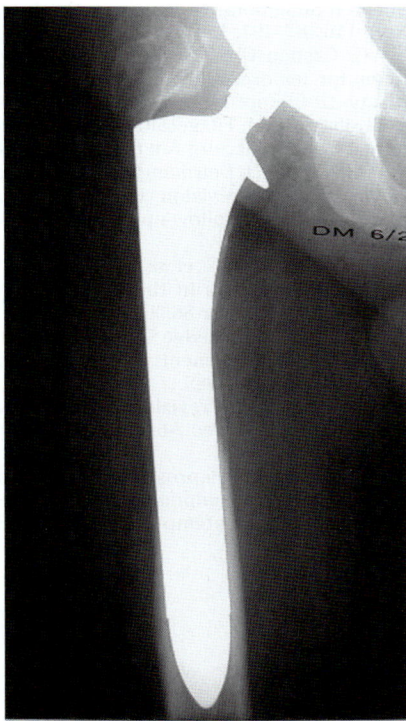

Figure 96-9. Stress shielding of a fully porous-coated stem 10 years postoperatively.

REFERENCES

1. Callaghan JJ, Templeton JE, Liu SS, et al: Results of Charnley total hip arthroplasty at a minimum of thirty years: a concise follow-up of a previous report. J Bone Joint Surg Am 86:690–695, 2004.
2. Callaghan JJ, Tooma GS, Olejniczak JP, et al: Primary hybrid total hip arthroplasty: an interim followup. Clin Orthop Relat Res 333:118–125, 1996.
3. Capello WN, D'Antonio JA, Feinberg JR, Manley MT: Ten-year results with hydroxyapatite-coated total hip femoral components in patients less than fifty years old: a concise follow-up of a previous report. J Bone Joint Surg Am 85:885–889, 2003.
4. Engh CA, Jr, Culpepper WJ, 2nd, Engh CA: Long-term results of use of the anatomic medullary locking prosthesis in total hip arthroplasty. J Bone Joint Surg Am 79:177–184, 1997.
5. Meding JB, Keating EM, Ritter MA, et al: Minimum ten-year follow-up of a straight-stemmed, plasma-sprayed, titanium-alloy, uncemented femoral component in primary total hip arthroplasty. J Bone Joint Surg Am 86:92–97, 2004.
6. Parvizi J, Sullivan T, Duffy G, Cabanela ME: Fifteen-year clinical survivorship of Harris-Galante total hip arthroplasty. J Arthroplasty 19:672–677, 2004.
7. Kurtz S, Ong K, Lau E, et al: Projections of primary and revision hip and knee arthroplasty in the United States from 2005 to 2030. J Bone Joint Surg Am 89:780–785, 2007.

8. Barrack RL, Sawhney J, Hsu J, Cofield RH: Cost analysis of revision total hip arthroplasty: a 5-year followup study. Clin Orthop Relat Res 369:175–178, 1999.

9. Springer BD, Fehring TK, Griffin WL, et al: Why revision total hip arthroplasty fails. Clin Orthop Relat Res 467:166–173, 2009.

10. Dobzyniak M, Fehring TK, Odum S: Early failure in total hip arthroplasty. Clin Orthop Relat Res 447:76–78, 2006.

11. Bozic KJ, Kurtz SM, Lau E, et al: The epidemiology of revision total hip arthroplasty in the United States. J Bone Joint Surg Am 91:128–133, 2009.

12. Hussamy O, Lachiewicz PF: Revision total hip arthroplasty with the BIAS (Biologic Ingrowth Anatomic System) femoral component: three- to six-year results. J Bone Joint Surg Am 76:1137–1148, 1994.

13. Peters CL, Rivero DP, Kull LR, et al: Revision total hip arthroplasty without cement: subsidence of proximally porous-coated femoral components. J Bone Joint Surg Am 77:1217–1226, 1995.

14. Berry DJ, Harmsen WS, Ilstrup D, et al: Survivorship of uncemented proximally porous-coated femoral components. Clin Orthop Relat Res 319:168–177, 1995.

15. Della Valle CJ, Paprosky WG: The femur in revision total hip arthroplasty evaluation and classification. Clin Orthop Relat Res 420:55–62, 2004.

16. Sporer SM, Paprosky WG: Revision total hip arthroplasty: the limits of fully coated stems. Clin Orthop Relat Res 417:203–209, 2003.

17. Krishnamurthy AB, MacDonald SJ, Paprosky WG: 5- to 13-year follow-up study on cementless femoral components in revision surgery. J Arthroplasty 12:839–847, 1997.

18. Lawrence JM, Engh CA, Macalino GE: Revision total hip arthroplasty: long-term results without cement. Orthop Clin North Am 24:635–644, 1993.

19. Moreland JR, Moreno MA: Cementless femoral revision arthroplasty of the hip: minimum 5 years followup. Clin Orthop Relat Res 393:194–201, 2001.

20. O'Shea K, Quinlan JF, Kutty S, et al: The use of uncemented extensively porous-coated femoral components in the management of Vancouver B2 and B3 periprosthetic femoral fractures. J Bone Joint Surg Br 87:1617–1621, 2005.

21. Paprosky WG: Distal fixation with fully coated stems in femoral revision: a 16-year follow-up. Orthopedics 21:993–995, 1998.

22. Reikeras O, Gunderson RB: Excellent results with femoral revision surgery using an extensively hydroxyapatite-coated stem: 59 patients followed for 10-16 years. Acta Orthop 77:98–103, 2006.

23. Weeden SH, Paprosky WG: Minimal 11-year follow-up of extensively porous-coated stems in femoral revision total hip arthroplasty. J Arthroplasty 17(4 Suppl 1):134–137, 2002.

24. Kim YH, Kim JS: Revision hip arthroplasty using strut allografts and fully porous-coated stems. J Arthroplasty 20:454–459, 2005.

25. Engh CA, Jr, Ellis TJ, Koralewicz LM, et al: Extensively porous-coated femoral revision for severe femoral bone loss: minimum 10-year follow-up. J Arthroplasty 17:955–960, 2002.

26. Nadaud MC, Griffin WL, Fehring TK, et al: Cementless revision total hip arthroplasty without allograft in severe proximal femoral defects. J Arthroplasty 20:738–744, 2005.

27. Engh CA, Massin P, Suthers KE: Roentgenographic assessment of the biologic fixation of porous-surfaced femoral components. Clin Orthop Relat Res 257:107–128, 1990.

28. Iorio R, Healy WL, Presutti AH: A prospective outcomes analysis of femoral component fixation in revision total hip arthroplasty. J Arthroplasty 23:662–669, 2008.

29. Moreland JR, Bernstein ML: Femoral revision hip arthroplasty with uncemented, porous-coated stems. Clin Orthop Relat Res 319:141–150, 1995.

30. Huiskes R: The various stress patterns of press-fit, ingrown, and cemented femoral stems. Clin Orthop Relat Res 261:27–38, 1990.

31. Huiskes R, Weinans H, Dalstra M: Adaptive bone remodeling and biomechanical design considerations for noncemented total hip arthroplasty. Orthopedics 12:1255–1267, 1989.

32. Sumner DR, Galante JO: Determinants of stress shielding: design versus materials versus interface. Clin Orthop Relat Res 274:202–212, 1992.

33. Bugbee WD, Culpepper WJ, 2nd, Engh CA, Jr, Engh CA, Sr: Long-term clinical consequences of stress-shielding after total hip arthroplasty without cement. J Bone Joint Surg Am 79:1007–1012, 1997.

34. Engh CA, Jr, McAuley JP, Sychterz CJ, et al: The accuracy and reproducibility of radiographic assessment of stress-shielding: a postmortem analysis. J Bone Joint Surg Am 82:1414–1420, 2000.

35. Engh CA, O'Connor D, Jasty M, et al: Quantification of implant micromotion, strain shielding, and bone resorption with porous-coated anatomic medullary locking femoral prostheses. Clin Orthop Relat Res 285:13–29, 1992.

36. Engh CA, Jr, Young AM, Engh CA, Sr, Hopper RH, Jr: Clinical consequences of stress shielding after porous-coated total hip arthroplasty. Clin Orthop Relat Res 417:157–163, 2003.

37. McAuley JP, Culpepper WJ, Engh CA: Total hip arthroplasty: concerns with extensively porous coated femoral components. Clin Orthop Relat Res 355:182–188, 1998.

38. Bobyn JD, Mortimer ES, Glassman AH, et al: Producing and avoiding stress shielding: laboratory and clinical observations of noncemented total hip arthroplasty. Clin Orthop Relat Res 274:79–96, 1992.

39. Chappell JD, Lachiewicz PF: Fracture of the femur in revision hip arthroplasty with a fully porous-coated component. J Arthroplasty 20:234–238, 2005.

40. Engh CA, Glassman AH, Suthers KE: The case for porous-coated hip implants: the femoral side. Clin Orthop Relat Res 261:63–81, 1990.

41. Estok DM, 2nd, Harris WH: Long-term results of cemented femoral revision surgery using second-generation techniques: an average 11.7-year follow-up evaluation. Clin Orthop Relat Res 299:190–202, 1994.

42. Grunig R, Morscher E, Ochsner PE: Three-to 7-year results with the uncemented SL femoral revision prosthesis. Arch Orthop Trauma Surg 116:187–197, 1997.

43. Hamilton WG, Cashen DV, Ho H, et al: Extensively porous-coated stems for femoral revision: a choice for all seasons. J Arthroplasty 22(4 Suppl 1):106–110, 2007.

44. Kavanagh BF, Ilstrup DM, Fitzgerald RH, Jr: Revision total hip arthroplasty. J Bone Joint Surg Am 67:517–526, 1985.

45. Levine BR, Della Valle CJ, Deirmengian CA, et al: The use of a tripolar articulation in revision total hip arthroplasty: a minimum of 24 months' follow-up. J Arthroplasty 23:1182–1188, 2008.

46. Lie SA, Havelin LI, Furnes ON, et al: Failure rates for 4762 revision total hip arthroplasties in the Norwegian Arthroplasty Register. J Bone Joint Surg Br 86:504–509, 2004.

47. Pellicci PM, Wilson PD, Jr, Sledge CB, et al: Long-term results of revision total hip replacement: a follow-up report. J Bone Joint Surg Am 67:513–516, 1985.

48. Sugimura T, Tohkura A: THA revision with extensively porous-coated stems: 32 hips followed 2-6.5 years. Acta Orthop Scand 69:11–13, 1998.

49. Younger TI, Bradford MS, Paprosky WG: Removal of a well-fixed cementless femoral component with an extended proximal femoral osteotomy. Contemp Orthop 30:375–380, 1995.

CHAPTER 97

Femoral Revision: Uncemented Implants With Bioactive Coatings

Jean-Pierre Vidalain

KEY POINTS

- *Planning:* careful preoperative templating
- *Instruments:* specific and complete instrumentation
- *Implants:* system of fully HA-coated stems
- *Fixation:* as proximal as possible
- *Anchoring:* as distal as necessary

INTRODUCTION

If the choice of cementless versus cemented implants for mild and moderate bone stock loss is still a topic of controversy, cementless femoral revision surgery for cases of severe deficiency has increasingly gained acceptance over the past decade.[1-8]

Revision following major femoral component loosening can be difficult, both in terms of finding a means of stable fixation of the revision implant and in terms of finding viable bone stock. Adequate primary stability must be attained to allow restoration of badly damaged bone around the new implant and to ensure the sound and lasting osteointegration of the new device.[9-13] Stability will be dependent on the preoperative condition of the femur (e.g., granuloma, osteolysis, fracture, implant breakage) and on what happens at revision surgery (e.g., inadvertent perforation, fracture, cortical window, extensive femoral osteotomy). Hydroxyapatite is a naturally occurring mineral form of calcium with the chemical composition $Ca_5(PO_4)_3(OH)$. The crystal form of the material is composed of two crystals, thus yielding the composition $Ca_{10}(PO_8)_6(OH)_2$. Its osteoconductive properties have made it an attractive material for coating both primary and revision total hip arthroplasty components. This has led to successful fixation of hydroxyapatite (HA)-coated implants in the presence of well-vascularized native bone.[14-17]

All these considerations mean that specially designed devices will be required so as to attain the necessary primary stability and to find a solution to the individual patient's needs. A whole system (Fig. 97-1) adapted to the different situations encountered in revision surgery must be considered.[18] Nevertheless, on the femoral side, to accomplish the objective of stable implant fixation, we follow a step-by-step strategy, which with appropriate planning and adequate instrumentation and implants can be summarized as "replacing the initial stem by another with fixation as proximal as possible and as distal as necessary."[19] Although numerous techniques have been described to successfully achieve adequate fixation of the femoral stem in revision total hip arthroplasty (these techniques are covered elsewhere in this book), our preferred techniques utilizes HA-coated implants. The purpose of this chapter is to discuss the use of such implants in revision of the femoral component in revision total hip arthroplasty.

INDICATIONS AND CHOICE OF IMPLANTS

Implant stability is mandatory at the time of surgery: Successful femoral reconstruction with an uncemented stem requires immediate axial and rotational stability, and the implant must have intimate contact with the living host bone to promote osteointegration needed for definitive fixation. Stabilization depends on different bony lesions,[20,21] but also on the shape of the distal femoral canal, where the bone of best quality is located. Three areas can be considered: the proximal part with its funnel-shaped cavity; the medial part with a canal that is more or less cylindrical; and the distal part characterized by gradual widening (Fig. 97-2).

In area 1, a quadrangular implant with a double-tapered geometry will easily find its primary stability and will efficiently resist axial and rotational stresses. In Paprosky type 1 and 2A femurs, a stem designed for primary insertion provides reliable initial fixation. In such situations, our favorite implant is the CORAIL stem (DePuy, Johnson & Johnson, Warsaw, Ind), a grit-blasted straight device of quadrangular cross-section entirely plasma-sprayed with a 150-μm layer of pure HA (Fig. 97-1A). This stem has proved its value in primary hip arthroplasty.[22-24]

In area 2, even a strong diaphyseal fit provides only poor protection against the different forces. In patients with substantial bone loss (Paprosky types 2 and 3A), a longer revision stem, the KAR (DePuy), increases the bioactive area in contact with fresh bone, facilitating osteointegration (Fig. 97-1B). The KAR has the same proximally flared pattern as the CORAIL, but the stem is 25% longer to bridge bone defects or occasional windows. Two distal slots in the sagittal and coronal planes reduce global rigidity and prevent stress risers in the cortex at the tip of the stem.

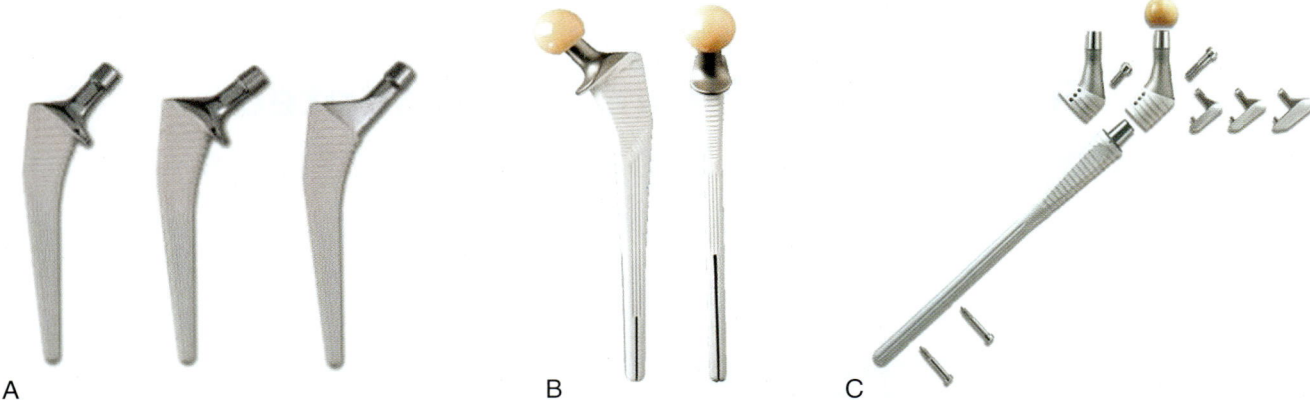

Figure 97-1. The CORAIL Hip System for revision surgery. **A,** The standard CORAIL series with different offset. **B,** The KAR implant with a collar support and two distal slots. **C,** The REEF prosthesis with different modular components and distal interlocking screws.

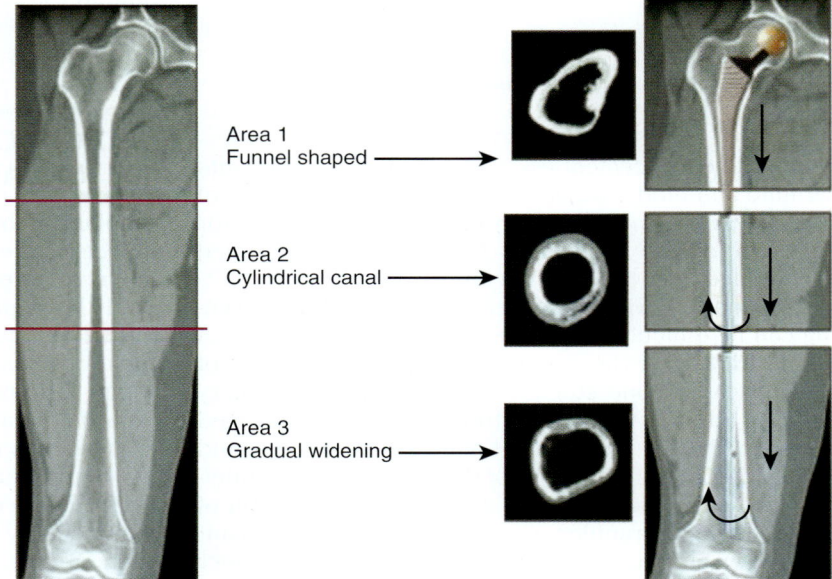

Area 1
Funnel shaped

Area 2
Cylindrical canal

Area 3
Gradual widening

Figure 97-2. The choice of a revision implant according to the stability provided by remaining sound bone.

In area 3, there is no possibility of finding effective mechanical stability through close contact between implant and bone. Interlocking screws must be used.[25,26] The REEF (DePuy) is our dedicated implant for very severe deficiencies (Paprosky types 3B and 4) when very distal fixation is needed (Fig. 97-1C). The REEF is a modular device that is basically composed of two main elements. The first and more distal segment is a metaphyseo-diaphyseal element, conical in its proximal part and cylindrical in its diaphyseal part. The proximal zone is 100 mm high, with horizontal macrostructures to increase the surface of contact and to prevent subsidence. The distal zone, of variable length, has a slight bow to prevent anterior cortical contact, longitudinal grooves to enhance osteointegration, and several horizontal holes for locking with 5-mm diameter screws. The second and more proximal segment is a metaphyseal

component fitted onto the stem with a Morse taper. This neck unit allows the surgeon to fine-tune anteversion within the confines of the existing metaphyseal bone and to restore leg lengths. In addition, this segment has an optional trochanteric claw that can be fixed to stabilize the greater trochanter and to improve the lever arm of the gluteal muscles if required.

The diagnoses that can lead to the use of HA-coated revision implants are not limited to aseptic loosening of different grades (Fig. 97-3); other possible indications are pertrochanteric fracture with cerclage of the greater trochanter, periprosthetic fracture, tumor resection, extensive osteolysis, and reimplantation in one- or two-stage exchange arthroplasty for the treatment of chronic infection at the site of total hip arthroplasty.[27,28] Revision of implants for pain and severe stress shielding has also been discussed by some authors.[18]

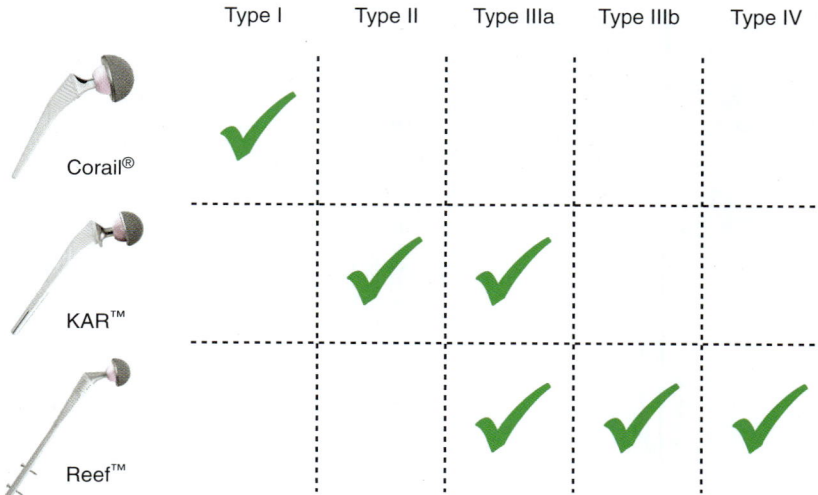

Figure 97-3. Indications algorithm according to types of femoral bone deficiency (Paprosky classification).

PREOPERATIVE PLANNING

Preoperative planning is essential to determine the appropriate size and alignment of the new implant and the length of the femoral neck component. For thorough preoperative planning, the surgeon will need a full set of revision implant templates and the following radiographs: an anteroposterior (AP) film of the entire pelvis and AP and lateral films of the affected femur. Considering the affected femur with its failed implant, successive templates are laid on the AP x-ray of the joint until optimal filling of the medullary canal is achieved and the new stem extends distally beyond damaged femoral bone and at least 2 cortical diameters distal to any osteotomy that is required to remove existing implants. This step determines the type and the size of the implant to be used. Although this is less reliable than in the primary situation, preoperative planning also enables the surgeon to identify any weak zones that will need to be bridged and to assess the quality of diaphyseal filling. Where necessary, the appropriate degree of calcar bone grafting should be established. The level of insertion of the new implant, with the greater or the lesser trochanter as reference, and the calcar height can be determined to ensure equal leg length. If a modular stem seems to be the appropriate implant, templating should assess the combination of components needed to achieve stability of the implant and to restore leg lengths. The location of eventual interlocking screws is also determined, keeping in mind that a minimum distance of 3 cm is needed between the distal extent of damaged bone and the first locking screw.

TECHNIQUE

The surgical approach selected is mainly dependent on the surgeon's preference and experience, keeping in mind that in the great majority of challenging situations, extraction of the failed prosthesis and reconstruction of extensive bone defects are often easier using a posterior approach, which is more extensile and more easily amenable than other approaches to the addition of femoral osteotomies.[29]

The acetabular surgery is usually carried out first, with replacement of the acetabular insert alone or of the entire cup system (the trial implants may be left in position or the final cup may be installed).

The femoral stage of surgery consists of several steps, as described in the following paragraphs.

Removal of the Failed Femoral Stem

This is generally easy if the stem is cemented, or if it is loose and uncemented, but may be more difficult if a well-fixed uncemented implant is in place.[30] The best strategy should allow removal of the stem, cement, membrane, and debris, with minimal additional sacrifice of bone stock. Specific techniques for implant removal are described in detail elsewhere in this book.

Femoral Preparation

In cases of moderate bone loss, with an intact isthmus, the diaphyseal zone is prepared using rigid reamers of increasing diameter to create a femoral canal lumen of at least 11 mm (the distal diameter of all KAR stems). The metaphyseal zone must be reshaped to restore the quadrangular shape that guarantees the rotational stability of the CORAIL or the KAR stem. This is achieved by broaching the sclerotic bone with specific and progressively larger rasps (Fig. 97-4A). In addition, this aggressive broaching exposes more normal bone for osteointegration. The final broach must be longitudinally and rotationally stable in the femoral canal and corresponds to the size of the definitive CORAIL or KAR stem to be implanted. Anteversion must be carefully maintained during this phase to achieve stability of the implant. In case of bone loss distal to the femoral isthmus, or in case of an extended femoral osteotomy, once the bony flap has been opened, the failed implant and the surrounding cement, fibrous tissue, and debris may be removed. The intramedullary canal is cleared

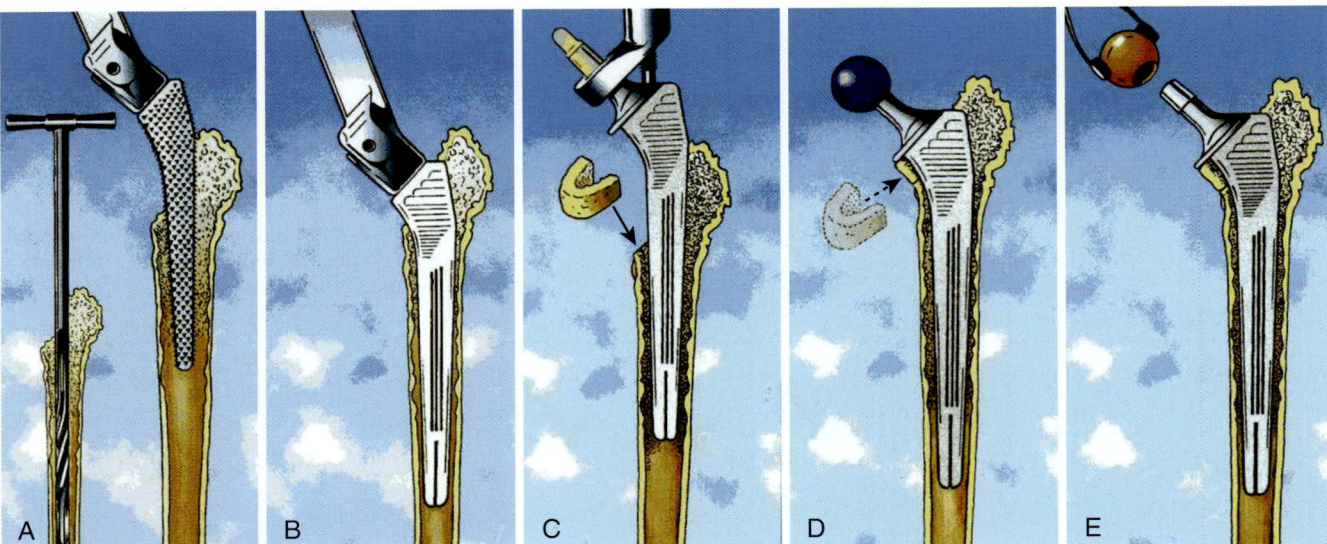

Figure 97-4. Surgical technique for a KAR implantation. **A,** Femoral preparation with rigid reamers and aggressive broaches. **B,** Insertion of the trial stem. **C,** Femoral component insertion. **D,** Calcar allograft stabilized by the collar of the stem and trial reduction. **E,** Definitive head impaction.

and curetted down to healthy bone. The diaphysis may have to be reamed sparingly to ensure that it is of the same diameter as the distal section of the stem chosen during templating. Accurate assessment of defects can now be established. The examination should focus on the condition of the cortices, the actual loss of bone stock, the presence of fractures, and any need for grafting. Decisions made during preoperative planning may be confirmed or altered.

Insertion of the Trial Stem

With the CORAIL or the KAR option, the trial stem of the same size is introduced into the canal with the same anteversion. Similar to the final broach, the trial stem must be axially and rotationally stable (Fig. 97-4B). It should be positioned at the level decided during preoperative planning, relative to the greater or lesser trochanter. If the stem subsides, the femur should be examined for a perforation or a fracture, and if none is found, a larger trial stem should be used. If the stem remains proud of the planned implantation level, it must not be forced in. The trial stem must be removed and the femur broached again, with the final broach size keeping the same anteversion. If a window or a short femoral osteotomy has been made, this can be repaired using two or three cerclage wires before the trial stem is introduced into the femur. With the REEF option, the trial stem is introduced into the medullary canal at the depth estimated during templating (Fig. 97-5C). Stability within the remaining canal is not always perfectly achieved, even with a strong cortical press-fit. Ultimate rotational stability will be achieved after distal interlocking of the definitive implant. Nevertheless, with the stem in place, the chosen trochanteric component is fixed onto the cone of the femoral shaft, and one

of three marks on this component is used to set anteversion.

Mobility and Stability Tests

Then, whatever the implant chosen, a trial head of a diameter matching the acetabular cup liner and a neck length selected during preoperative planning should be fitted on the taper, and a trial reduction carried out. The prosthetic construct is then tested for range of motion, stability of the joint, and tension of the gluteal muscles.

HA-Coated Implants and Bone Grafting

When a femoral revision is performed with HA-coated implants, bone grafting is not essential because the femur has the ability to heal and remodel itself.[31] However, if the surgeon opts for grafting, autografts are preferred to allografts whenever possible,[32] as long as their use does not cause additional morbidity. It must be noted that such grafts should never be used to stabilize the implant[33] but only to fill in gaps around a stable stem and, more specifically, to seal the neck section to prevent the ingress of debris. At the calcar level, the main roles of a horseshoe-shaped cortical graft are to protect all HA coating that remains uncovered by the native bone, and to reduce the risk of HA particle migration into the vicinity of the joint space. Moreover, integration of this graft must not be underevaluated; very often, effective incorporation leads to restoration of normal or near-normal femoral bone stock. The KAR prosthesis is available only with a collar that contributes to stabilization of such a graft (Fig. 97-6). For similar reasons, a collared metaphyseal segment can be used with the REEF stem. To achieve

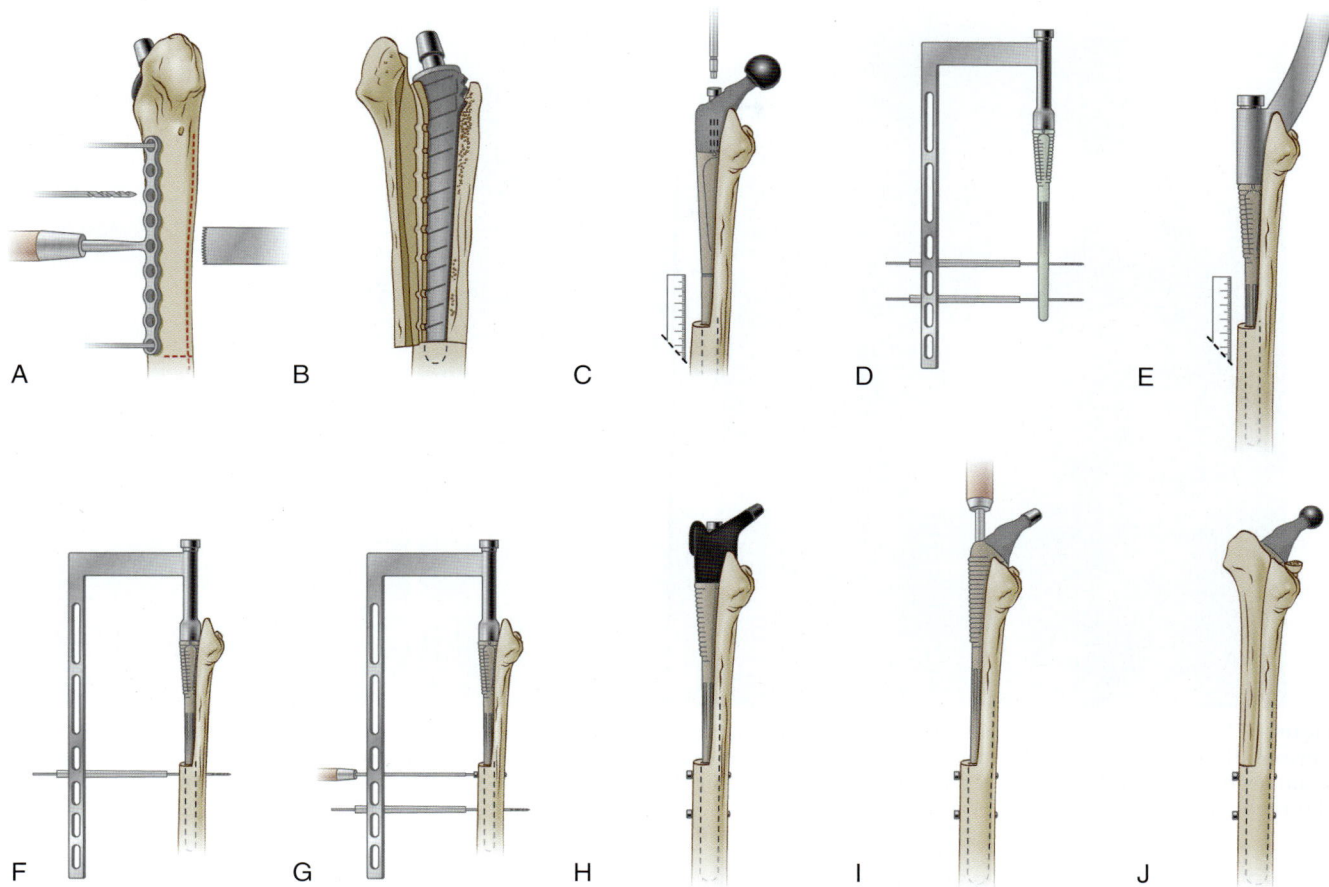

Figure 97-5. Surgical technique for a REEF implantation. **A,** The transfemoral osteotomy combines a posterior saw-cut, a transversal hemisection, and an anterior osteoclasis using a drilling template. **B,** The bony flap is gently opened. **C,** The trial stem is introduced to the depth predetermined during templating. **D,** Alignment of the interlocking holes is checked. **E,** Insertion of the definitive stem at the correct level, and (**F** and **G**) distal screw placement. **H,** Confirmation of the choice of metaphyseal segment. **I,** The definitive proximal body is impacted and fixed onto the stem cone. **J,** Reconstruction of the femoral shaft around the prosthesis.

osteointegration of bioactive implants, the coating of the stem must be in contact with reactive and living bone.[34] Therefore, the CORAIL or the KAR must not be implanted using bone compaction techniques that require the use of compacted allograft. In the case of metaphyseal expansion, it is better to perform a longitudinal reduction osteotomy to move the remaining cortices closer onto the implant surface using cerclage wires, then to fill in the gap with allografts.

Implantation of the Definitive Stem

Once mobility and stability tests have been performed satisfactorily, final implants are confirmed and inserted to replace trial components. The trial stem is replaced with the final implant, which is introduced into the clean femoral cavity. It is important not to irrigate the medullary canal before inserting the definitive device to keep bone fragments in place and to preserve all osteoinductive cells. The CORAIL or the KAR is first introduced by hand, and then is progressively and gently

impacted using a stem holder, which controls anteversion as the stem enters the femur. Before final impaction, it may be necessary to reconstruct the calcar using a crescent-shaped graft (see Fig. 97-4C through E). The collar of the prosthesis is designed to stabilize such grafts; this guarantees the correct impaction level of the stem and contributes to primary vertical stability until osteointegration occurs. If the modular interlocked stem (REEF) is used, distal screw placement is the critical step (see Fig. 97-5D through G). After impaction of the definitive diaphyseal component at the level of reference measured during trial reduction, the targeting device is firmly fitted onto the taper of the stem; this reliable instrumentation allows drilling and positioning of at least two interlocking screws with precision and safety. At that time, trial trochanteric components and trial heads can be used once again to confirm limb length, stability, and version (see Fig. 97-5H). Finally, the definitive proximal body is attached to the stem with the appropriate prosthetic head (see Fig. 97-5I). The final reduction is performed, and reconstruction of the

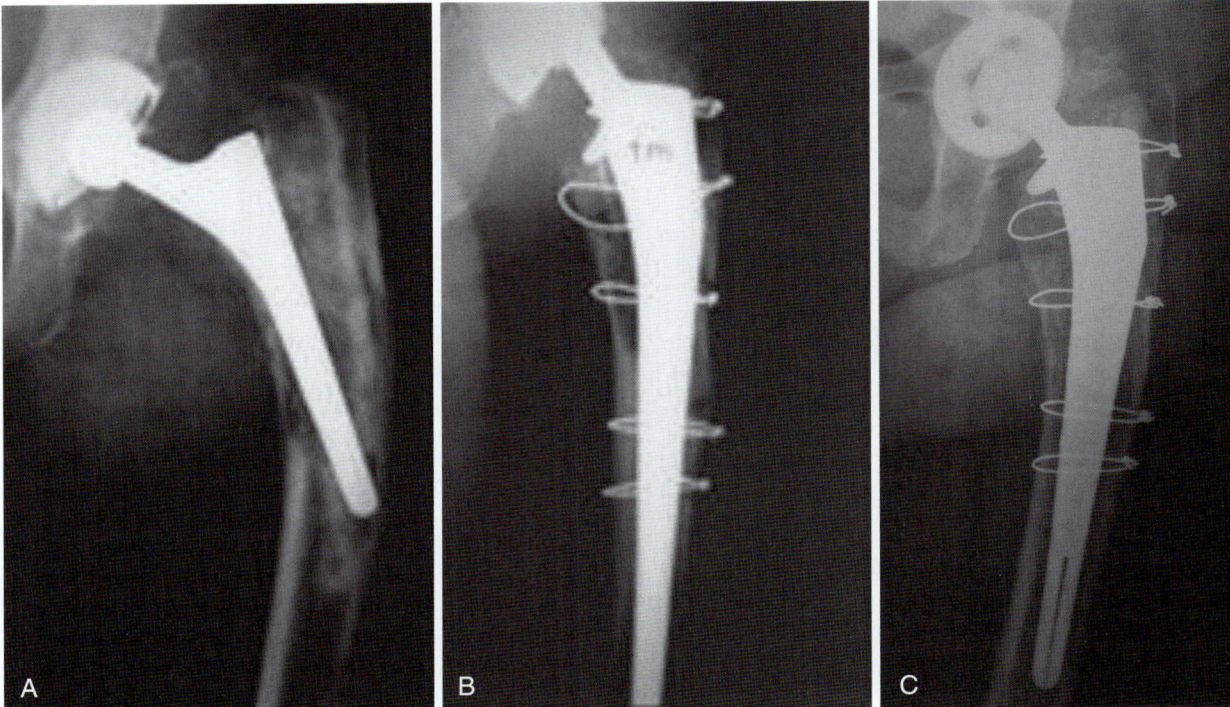

Figure 97-6. A, Revision with KAR prosthesis of an aseptic loosening, type 3A, of a cemented stem, associated with a periprosthetic fracture. **B,** Postoperative control; a horseshoe-shaped graft has been positioned under the collar, but no bone graft augmentation has been used to fill in the other defects. **C,** The last control at 12 years confirms the quality of the reconstruction with normal bone trophicity.

femoral shaft around the prosthetic stem can be undertaken. Reattachment of the flap is achieved by means of cerclage cables (see Fig. 97-5J). As was already mentioned, grafting is not mandatory but may be desirable to rebuild the calcar or to fill cortical defects, and morselized cancellous bone should fill in any remaining cavities. However, it is recommended that the entire HA-coated area of the implant should be covered by native or grafted bone.

RESULTS

The Study

This study comprises three different series (Table 97-1). In the first one, 197 patients were treated between 1991 and 2001, using the KAR prosthesis; in the second one, 77 patients were operated on between 1995 and 2007 and a REEF was implanted. Finally, the third series included 51 patients operated on between 1989 and 2006; they were treated following a so-called *scale-down technique,* and a standard CORAIL was implanted. This nonconventional strategy will be discussed separately. All 325 patients have undergone revision hip surgery as a result of mostly mechanical failure of cemented or cementless femoral components. This study is concerned only with femoral component revisions. Many patients had acetabular revision as well, but they are not the subject of this study. Clinical examination was performed

preoperatively using the Merle d'Aubigné score[35] and the Harris hip score[36] at periodic intervals. Radiologic assessment conducted at each clinical control analyzed the bony lesions[20,21] and their reconstruction in different zones of interest[37] using the Engh criteria,[38] even if they were not specifically developed to assess the integration of bioactive implants. Implant stability was evaluated according to traditional methods.[39] The KAR series included 203 revision stems (197 patients). Average patient age was 64 years at the time of surgery. Five patients died of non–hip-related causes; 3 patients were lost to follow-up. All remaining patients were followed-up clinically and radiographically. Mean follow-up was 10 years. With respect to the Charnley function classification,[40] 59% were in category A, 18% were in category B, and 23% were in category C. The mean preoperative Postel-Merle d'Aubigné (MDA) score of 9.02 and the Harris hip score (HHS) of 50 showed the severity of the patient's disability. The initial radiologic bone defect pattern varied widely; however, most cases were Paprosky types 2 and 3 (1 = 13%, 2 = 60%, 3 and 4 = 26%).

The REEF series included 77 modular and interlocked stems (77 patients). Six patients died in the years after surgery from old age and comorbid conditions. None were lost to follow-up. Mean follow-up was 4 years, but we had 33 cases with follow-up longer than 5 years. Average age of patients was 71 years with a wide range from 17 to 93 years. In terms of Charnley categories, 46% were evaluated A, 38% were B, and 16% were C. In terms of causes, 34 had loose stems, 21 had periprosthetic or

Table 97-1. Overview of Three Series of Femoral Revisions Using Uncemented Implants With Bioactive Coatings

	CORAIL Series	KAR Series	REEF Series
Cohort (patients)	51	197	77
Hips operated	54	203	77
Male/female	21/30	106/91	31/46
Bone lesions	Types I-II (2/3), III (1/3)	I (13%), II (60%), III-IV (26%)	II (39%), III-IV (24%)
Mean FU	10 yr (range, 1-15)	10 yr (range, 4 to15)	4 yr (2-15)
Deceased	0	5	6
Lost to FU	0	3	0
Mean age, yr	62 (range, 28-82)	64 (range, 32-85)	71 (range, 20-80)
Charnley	—	A (59%), B (18%), C (23%)	A (46%), B (38%), C (16%)
Preop MDA score	11.7 (range, 2-18)	9.0 (range, 3-17)	7 (range, 1-15)
Preop HHS score	65 (range, 9-100)	50 (range, 16-100)	32 (range, 6-83)
Postop MDA score	16.2 (range, 5-18)	15.7 (range, 12-18)	14.8 (range, 11-18)
Postop HHS score	90 (range, 50-100)	87 (range, 67-100)	83 (range, 62-100)
Complication rate	5%	7%	22%
Survivorship	100	98.7 (range, 96-100)	94% (range, 85-99)

FU, Follow-up; *HHS,* Harris hip score; *MDA,* Postel-Merle d'Aubigné score.

infraprosthetic fractures associated with implant loosening, 6 had stem breakage associated with severe osteolysis, 6 underwent femoral resection for primary tumor, and the remaining cases involved nonunion or malunion and painful stress shielding. The relatively small cohort of patients showed that the REEF prosthesis was intended only for the management of major deficiencies (Paprosky type 2C = 39%, types 3 and 4 = 24%). The preoperative rating clearly indicated the extent of the disability: Merle d'Aubigné score 7.0, and HHS 32.

Finally, the CORAIL series was probably the least homogeneous because of the great variety of bony lesions treated with a nonconventional implant for relatively severe deficiencies. This strategy, which can be considered today as a bone preserving technique, confirmed the potential, in terms of bone reconstruction, of HA-coated implants, even in very challenging situations. Fifty-four standard CORAIL devices (51 patients) were implanted between 1989 and 2006. Mean age at the date of surgery was 62 years (range, 28 to 84 years). Three patients died with the CORAIL still in place, and no patient had been lost at the last follow-up. Mean follow-up occurred at 10 years, with a range from 1 to 15 years. The average Merle d'Aubigné score was 11.7, and the average HHS was 65. In all, 26 revisions were performed because of aseptic loosening; two thirds corresponded to Paprosky type 1 and 2 defects, and one third to type 3 defects. Nineteen revisions were related to poor biomechanics—unacceptable leg length discrepancy, lack of offset, and instability—and the femoral stem was well-fixed at revision surgery. Eight implant failures (fracture of the stem or the prosthetic neck) and 1 periprosthetic fracture were revised with a standard CORAIL.

Clinical Results

The early disappearance of pain was remarkable, although walking activities might remain restricted for a long period after surgery. The use of crutches was necessary to compensate for limp or other gait disorders in the rehabilitation period. Subjective appreciation from patients after a KAR implantation showed the beneficial effects of the procedure. In all, 73% of patients were satisfied, and 23% were very satisfied; 4% were disappointed because of dislocation or deep infection. None of the patients had thigh pain. This was interpreted as an advantage of the distal slots that prevented stress risers from forming at the tip of the stem. The global Merle d'Aubigné score increased by 6.7, from 9.02 before revision to 15.72 postoperatively (HHS, from 50 to 87). Improvement in the Merle d'Aubigné score was strongly correlated with Charnley's categories: Category A had a mean postoperative Merle d'Aubigné of 16.5, category B 16.3, and category C 14.6. Only 1 patient has been re-revised for 1 cm subsidence related to an underestimated crack during surgery. The other patients were consistently pain-free and had increased range of motion. In this respect, the outcome was comparable with that of primary arthroplasty. With stem extraction as the endpoint, survivorship of the KAR was 98.7% at 10 years. In the REEF series, subjectively, the outcome was assessed as follows: 90% of patients were satisfied, 6% were very satisfied, and 4% who reported dislocation were disappointed. From a functional point of view, the mean global Merle d'Aubigné score went from 7 to 14, but in terms of the pain score, progression from 1 to 5 (HHS, from 32 to 83) was noted. Taking into account the severity of the preoperative status, these results could be considered as satisfactory. With stem extraction for any reason being the endpoint, the survival probability was 94% at 8 years. Last, the CORAIL series provided the best functional outcome, even if the mean Merle d'Aubigné score was 15.8 (HHS, from 65 to 90) at the last control (Merle d'Aubigné range, 7 to 18). The wide range of the function score reflected great variability in terms of indications and was due to complications on the acetabular side (2 cases with instability and 1 case of cup loosening). No patient had to be reoperated because of problems related to the femoral stem. With stem extraction as the endpoint, the survival rate was 100% at 10 years.

Radiologic Results

Three features have been evaluated on serial radiographs: *implant stability* using traditional methods, *osteointegration,* and *bone defect healing.* As was said previously, achievement of stability at surgery is of crucial importance. Where primary stability has been attained, osteointegration is consistently observed, and long-term implant survival is similar to that seen following primary arthroplasty. With the KAR implant, *stability* was excellent; no varus/valgus tilt was seen. In 189 cases with follow-up, only 3 stems had settled at a slightly lower level (<3 mm below the initial level of implantation). One case of 1 cm subsidence required re-revision. In this case, a femoral crack had been overlooked at surgery. With stable implants, *osteointegration* was regularly seen. A change in the bony bed was seen in 65% of cases, with evidence of periprosthetic ossification in 50% of cases. In the space between the implant and the femoral cortices, newly formed bone bridges, similar to the bone trabeculae observed after primary implantation, were noted. No evidence of significant stress shielding or lucent line formation was observed.

Osteopenia in the trochanteric area was infrequent (2%), and calcar remodeling was more often observed (5%), mainly following calcar grafting. Newly formed bone, at the tip of the stem, was seen in 4% of patients. This feature was not considered as a pedestal; it was a healing process with a trabecular pattern and was never associated with other proximal radiographic features of loosening. In 4%, cortical thickening was also observed along the implant stem and was interpreted as restoration of normal bone morphology. Thirty-five percent of cases showed no radiologic changes. *Healing of all bone defects* was a common and important finding. Some of these defects existed before revision as a result of granuloma, osteolysis, or fracture; others were caused at surgery by inadvertent perforation, or when cortical windows or Wagner osteotomies were performed. Cortical windows should be bridged by the implant. Transfemoral osteotomies were found to heal within 3 months, provided the flap was snug against the implant and was held in place with cerclage wires.

Granuloma must be curetted, but grafting has been largely abandoned. The capacity of the femur to rebuild around the implant with the stimulus for bone growth coming from healing of the bony flap was always seen. In terms of cyst reconstruction, we did not find any statistical difference between patients with and without compacted bone grafting (Fig. 97-7). Poor bone stock is a risk factor for femoral revision failure due to loosening. Therefore, a specific analysis of the REEF series was conducted with a special focus on stability and restoration of bone stock. Radiologically, signs of bone stock restoration were seen beyond the second postoperative month. Bone ingrowth was clearly evident in 93% of cases. Two types of new bone formation were noted: periosteal apposition and endosteal ossification. Cortical bone formation was demonstrated by thickening

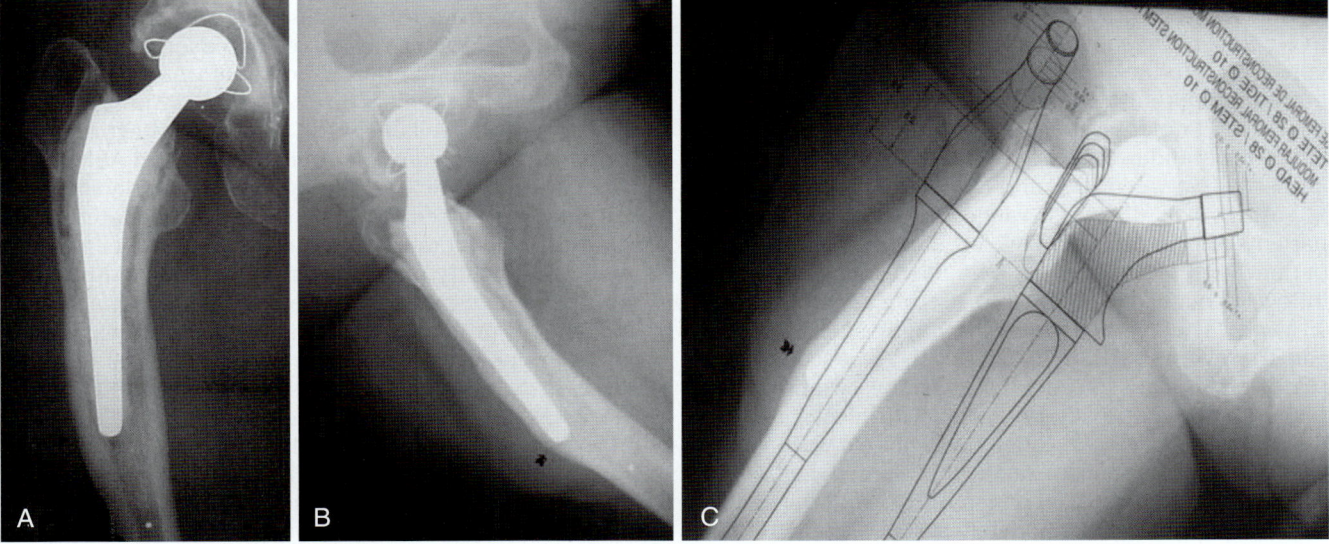

Figure 97-7. A and **B,** Bipolar loosening of a cemented stem, associated with severe deformation of the diaphysis and a distal perforation. **C,** Templating of a modular REEF to restore normal femoral geometry with physiologic hip biomechanics.

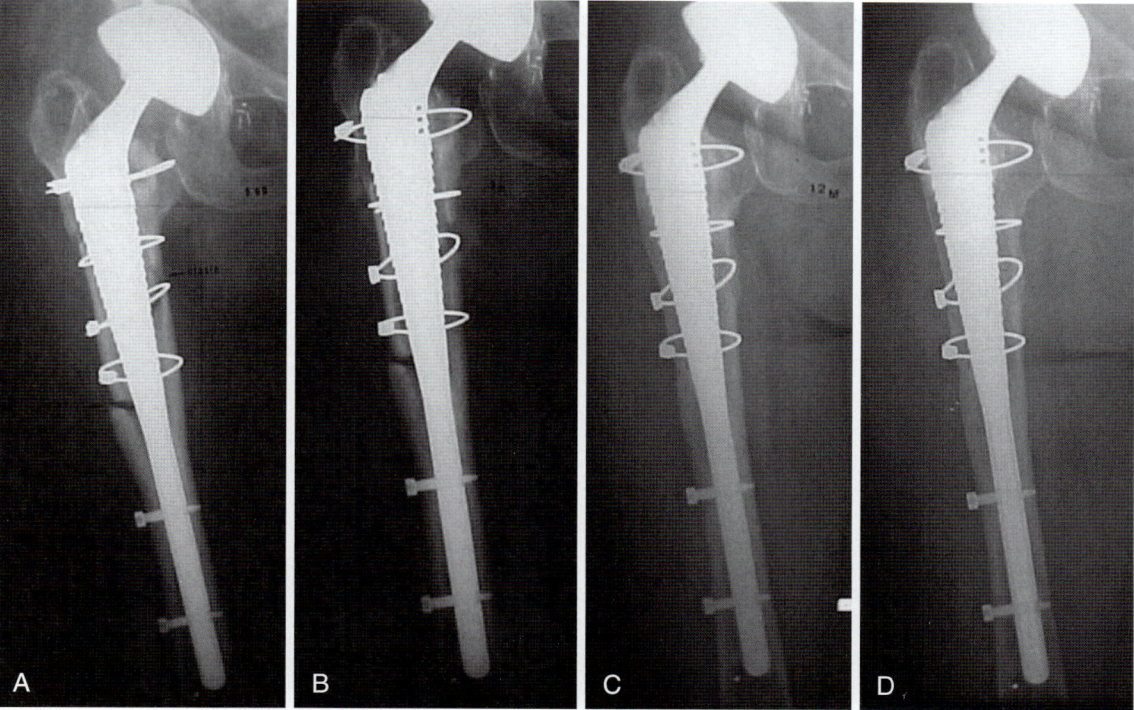

Figure 97-8. Reconstruction around a REEF prosthesis. A transfemoral osteotomy and a medial osteoclasis were performed to remove the failed implant and to restore the axis of the canal. **A,** Immediate postoperative x-ray and successive controls at **(B)** 3 months, **(C)** 1 year, and **(D)** 6 years. Note the rapid healing of the osteotomy and of the fracture, as well as the bone quality of the upper femur.

of the cortex in the diaphysis (32%), and healing of the different bony osteotomies was uniform; in the metaphysis, this cortical reconstruction was not as consistent, and 6 patients with severe trochanteric atrophy prior to revision failed to improve their cortical pattern. All patients were elderly females with severe osteoporosis. However, even in this situation, the cortical defects healed normally. Endosteal ossification was seen in 37% of the radiologic files; thin trabeculae were clearly visible in the sound distal femur. This osteointegration is mainly related to the extent of the coating.[41-43]

A full bioactive coating allows extensive and rapid bone formation with early fixation in the area where the bone of best quality is located. Absence of radiolucent lines was reported in all files (Fig. 97-8). Therefore, permanent stability was always achieved during the first months after surgery; no migration was identified, and unlike in some other reports, no failure of locking screws was identified.[26] When the subgroup of the CORAIL series was examined, integration was found to occur as in primary hip replacement, with the same bone ingrowth pattern. Use of a collared CORAIL increased primary stability and, depending on periprosthetic bone quality and whether a femoral osteotomy was used, full or partial weight bearing was allowed immediately or after a few weeks of restricted activities. At last follow-up, all femoral stems showed positive signs of integration. Femoral fractures, windows, and

osteotomies all healed. No significant migration of the stems could be detected (Fig. 97-9).

COMPLICATIONS

No complications or reoperations were related to HA coating. Dislocation was the most frequent complication: 1.5% in the KAR series, 4% in the REEF series, and 3% in the CORAIL series. No reoperations were related to implant fixation problems. Complications encountered are typical of revision arthroplasty and usually are correlated with the extent of surgery (KAR series: 7 intraoperative perforations, 1 greater trochanter nonunion, 2 deep infections, 1 periprosthetic fracture; REEF series: 3 hematomas, 1 deep vein thrombosis [DVT], 1 fatal pulmonary embolism [PE], 1 stem fracture, 7 periprosthetic fractures; and CORAIL series: 1 preoperative calcar crack, 1 fracture of the greater trochanter). Special extraction techniques were sometimes necessary to reduce different intraoperative bone complications.[44] Extraction of all the cement and of a long cement plug was sometimes difficult. With the distal locking screws of the REEF stem, only one malaligned screw was present. Therefore, checking before insertion that the different holes of the target are correctly aligned with corresponding holes of the definitive stem is always recommended. In the long run, we have never seen any screw-site problems. No distal locking screws had to be

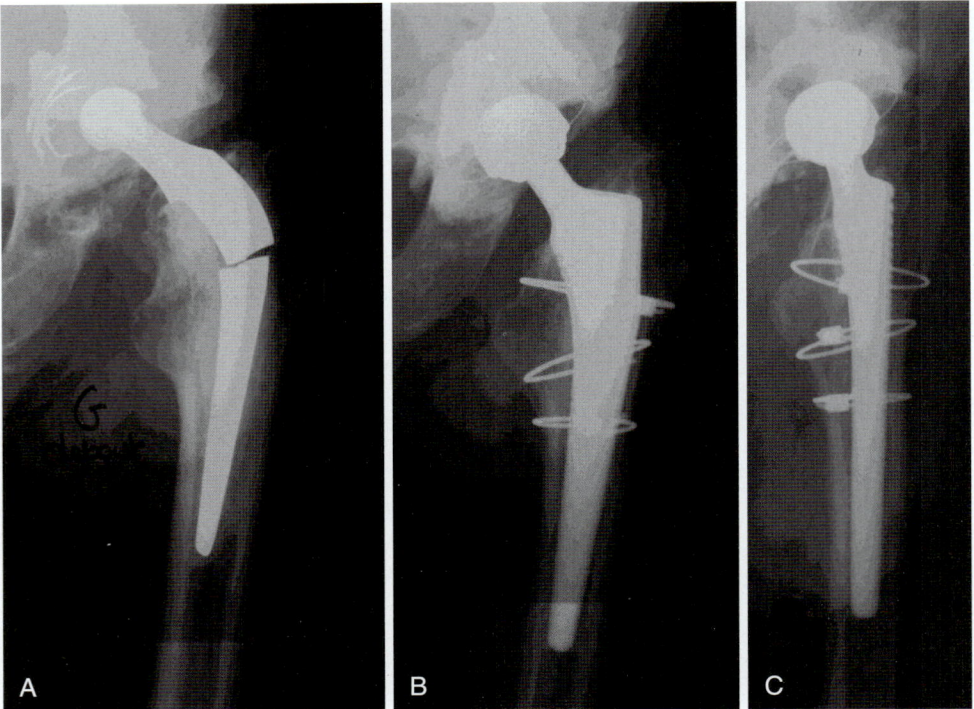

Figure 97-9. A, Treatment of a loosened broken Charnley stem with a standard CORAIL. X-ray assessment at 8-year follow-up. **B,** Anteroposterior (AP) view. **C,** Lateral view.

removed for any reason (e.g., failure, breakage, pain, bone reaction).

CURRENT CONTROVERSIES AND FUTURE CONSIDERATIONS

- Ample literature is available describing hip revision surgery.[45-51] However, comparison between different series is difficult because of lack of homogeneity. In addition, from a clinical point of view, different reported function scores (Merle d'Aubigné or Harris hip score) are influenced by both components of the hip, and it could be hazardous to assert that improvement or deterioration of a score is definitely related to the femoral component or to the acetabular implant. Nevertheless, whatever the grade of femoral loosening, our personal strategy in all cases has been "bioactive" reconstruction of the bone stock; both clinical and radiologic results have been very satisfying after the use of HA-coated implants in femoral revision application.[18,19] However, other solutions have been and are still proposed, such as cemented stem reinsertion, isolated or combined with bone grafting.[52-57] Results of cemented revision of femoral loosening have been poor in the past, but with the use of modern cementing techniques, these results have improved. Literature describes various failure rates, ranging from 6% to 43% at about 12 years.[58,59] Several authors[60-62] confirm this high rate of mechanical failure and suggest that it is probably related to difficulty obtaining good cement interdigitation with

sclerotic bone. Kerboull[54] reports 82% excellent and good results. However, at 5-year follow-up, 32% of cases revealed lucent lines, and 10% were assessed as loose. Furthermore, recurrent loosening is increased relative to the extent of initial bone loss. This point has been underlined by several French authors[63,64] in a multicenter study. Despite progress in terms of cementation techniques, it is recognized[65] that the loosening rate remains higher than 20% at 5 years. Therefore, isolated cemented stem reinsertion is not recommended, particularly in the most severe cases of bone loss. Femoral impaction allografting with cement has the potential to restore bone stock, as demonstrated by Ling[66] and confirmed in several publications,[67,68] which also report, however, subsidence rates of 20% with respect to the cement mantle and the stem itself. Other teams[69] prefer to cement a stem into massive allograft embedded in the living host bone. All these techniques are demanding and time-consuming and are dependent on the availability of massive allograft. At the present time, questions remain regarding the durability of impaction allografting and the rather high rate of complications. On the other hand, cementless revision with extensively porous-coated stems has shown excellent durability, relatively few complications, and good long-term results, as reported by many authors.[70-73] However, concerns regarding proximal stress shielding with extensively coated stems are still reported.[73-75]

- The use of HA coatings in primary cementless hip arthroplasty has led to significantly better results than those attained with previous generations of uncemented implants.[76,77] The biological properties of HA are today well established and well accepted by the whole orthopedic community. Postmortem analyses[76-80] have reported early and extensive bone deposition over the HA layer as compared with porous and grit-blasted coatings. These properties have led to the use of HA coatings in revision surgery. The use of bone graft in conjunction with HA coatings was widely discussed 10 years ago. Bone ingrowth between bone transplant and HA coating remains uncertain. It is of paramount importance that adequate mechanical implant stability be attained at the time of surgery, and the use of bone graft augmentation should not be relied upon to provide the mechanical stability of the construct. Early bone ingrowth fixation is possible only between HA coating and living and vascularized bone, and from his own experience, Geesink, a pioneer in the field of bioactive coating,[4] advocates the use of longer stems with more extensive areas of HA coating when extensive proximal bone deficiencies are present. In a dog model, Geesink had also demonstrated that bone remodeling is always greatly improved in the presence of HA in comparison with a porous surface.[81] From our 25-year experience, we are convinced that HA coating has the potential not only to increase bone ingrowth, but also to minimize stress shielding. A recent clinical report[82] found an overall failure rate of 2% at 2 to 5 years' follow-up with an extensively HA-coated stem in revision surgery. No evidence of stress shielding was seen in 78% of patients.

To summarize, successful femoral reconstruction with an uncemented stem requires immediate stability, and the prosthesis must be in intimate contact with the host bone to promote osteoingration as needed for definitive fixation. HA-coated implants have greatly and quickly enhanced this biological fixation. The tapered design of the stems allows them to gain vertical and rotational stability. When proximal stability cannot be achieved because of the seriousness of the lesions in the upper femur, we must use longer stems designed for distal fixation. Conservative femoral revision can also be considered; standard stems, normally used for primary surgery, allow the preservation of bone stock. This point must be underlined because revisions today are increasingly performed on young and active patients. The relatively simple procedure and the low rate of postoperative complications are of greatest interest. Unfortunately, this strategy is recommended only for patients with limited femoral bone loss. Therefore, we suggest a femoral component to be revised as soon as a loosening is suspected, avoiding progression of osteolysis; clinical and radiologic assessments at periodic and regular intervals are the only way to minimize the complexity of femoral revisions.

REFERENCES

1. Berry DJ, Harmsen WS, Ilstrup D, et al: Survivorship of uncemented proximally porous-coated femoral components. Clin Orthop Relat Res 319:168–177, 1995.
2. Bohm P, Bischel O: Femoral revision with the Wagner SL revision stem: evaluation of one hundred and twenty nine revisions followed for a mean of 4.8 years. J Bone Joint Surg Am 83:1023–1031, 2001.
3. Engh CA, Bobyn JD, Glassman AH: Porous-coated hip replacement: the factors governing bone-ingrowth, stress-shielding and clinical results. J Bone Joint Surg Br 69:45–55, 1987.
4. Geesink RG, Hoefnagels NH: Revision of the femoral component: hydroxyapatite enhancement. In Callaghan JJ, Rosenberg AG, Rubash HE, editors: The adult hip, Philadelphia, 1998, Lippincott-Raven, pp 1537–1547.
5. Harris W: Revision surgery for failed, nonseptic, total hip arthroplasty. Clin Orthop Relat Res 170:8–20, 1982.
6. Kavanagh BF, Ilstrup DM, Fitzgerald RH: Revision total hip arthroplasty. J Bone Joint Surg Am 67:517–526, 1995.
7. Lawrence JM, Engh CA, Macalino GE: Revision total hip arthroplasty: long-term results without cement. Orthop Clin North Am 24:635–644, 1993.
8. Wagner H: A revision prosthesis for the hip joint. Orthopade 18:438–453, 1989.
9. Amstutz HC, Ma SN, Jinnah RH, Mai L: Revision of aseptic loose total hip arthroplasty. Clin Orthop Relat Res 170:21–23, 1982.
10. Berry DJ: Femoral revision: distal fixation with fluted, tapered grit-blasted stems. J Arthroplasty 17(4 Suppl 1):142–146, 2002.
11. Bohm P, Bischel O: The use of tapered stems for femoral revision surgery. Clin Orthop Relat Res 420:148–159, 2004.
12. Boisgard S, Moreau PE, Tixier H, Levai JP: Bone reconstruction, leg length discrepancy and dislocation rate in 52 Wagner revision total hip arthroplasties at 44-month follow-up. Rev Chir Orthop 87:147–154, 2001.
13. Head WC: The Wagner revision prosthesis consistently restores femoral bone structure. Int Orthop 25:63–64, 2001.
14. Coathup MJ, Blunn GW, Flynn N, et al: A comparison of bone remodeling around hydroxyapatite-coated, porous-coated and grit-blasted hip replacements retrieved at post-mortem. J Bone Joint Surg Br 83:118–123, 2001.
15. Raman R, Kamath RP, Parikh A, Angus PD: Revision of cemented hip arthroplasty using a hydroxylapatite ceramic-coated femoral component. J Bone Joint Surg Br 87:1061–1067, 2005.
16. Reikeras O, Gunderson RB: Excellent results with femoral revision surgery using an extensively hydroxyapatite-coated stem. Acta Orthop 77:98–103, 2006.
17. Trikha SP, Singh S, Raynham OW, et al: Hydroxyapatite-ceramic-coated femoral stems in revision hip surgery. J Bone Joint Surg Br 87:1055–1060, 2005.
18. Chatelet JC, Setiey L: Femoral component revision with hydroxyapatite-coated revision stems. In Epinette JA, Manley MT, editors: Fifteen years of clinical experience with hydroxyapatite coatings in joint arthroplasty, Paris, 2004, Springer, pp 385–395.
19. Pinaroli A, Lavoie F, Cartillier JC, et al: Conservative femoral stem revision avoiding therapeutic escalation. J Arthroplasty 24:365–373, 2009.
20. Paprosky W, Lawrence J, Cameron H: Femoral defects classification. Orthop Rev Suppl 9–16, 1990.
21. Della Valle CJ, Paprosky WG: The femur in revision total hip arthroplasty evaluation and classification. Clin Orthop Relat Res 420:55–62, 2004.
22. Froimson MI, Garino J, Machenaud A, Vidalain JP: Minimum 10-year results of a tapered, titanium, hydroxyapatite-coated hip system: an independent review. J Arthroplasty 22:1–7, 2007.
23. Havelin LI, Espehaug B, Vollset SE, et al: Early aseptic loosening of uncemented femoral components in primary total hip replacement: a review based on the Norwegian Arthroplasty Register. J Bone Joint Surg Br 77:1, 1995.
24. Vidalain JP: Corail stem long-term results based upon the 15-year Artro group experience. In Epinette JA, Manley MT, editors: Fifteen years of clinical experience with hydroxyapatite coatings in joint arthroplasty, Paris, 2004, Springer, pp 217–224.
25. Sotereanos N, Sewecke J, Raukar GJ, et al: Revision total hip arthroplasty with a custom cementless stem with distal cross-locking screws: early results in femora with large proximal segmental deficiencies. J Bone Joint Surg Am 88:1079–1084, 2006.

26. Vives P, De Lestang M, Paclot R, Cazeneuve JF: Le descellement aseptique: définitions, classifications—Symposium SOFCOT 1988. Rev Chir Orthop Suppl 75:29–31, 1989.

27. Feldman D, Lonner JH, Desal P, Zucherman J: The role of intraoperative frozen sections in revision total joint arthroplasty. J Bone Joint Surg Am 77:1807–1813, 1995.

28. Vidalain JP: Hydroxyapatite and infection: results of a consecutive series of 49 infected total hip replacements. In Epinette JA, Manley MT, editors: Fifteen years of clinical experience with hydroxyapatite coatings in joint arthroplasty, Paris, 2004, Springer, pp 191–199.

29. Pai VS: A comparison of three lateral approaches in primary total hip replacement. Int Orthop 21:393–398, 1997.

30. Burnstein G, Yoon P, Saleh KJ: Component removal in revision total hip arthroplasty. Clin Orthop Relat Res 420:231–238, 2004.

31. Dujardin F, Mazirt N: Régénération osseuse spontanée—Symposium SOFCOT 1999. Rev Chir Orthop 86(Suppl I):75–77, 2000.

32. Elting JJ, Mikhail WE, Zicat BE: Preliminary report of impaction grafting for exchange femoral arthroplasty. Clin Orthop Relat Res 319:167–169, 1995.

33. Eldridge JD, Smith EJ, Hubble MJ, et al: Massive early subsidence following femoral impaction grafting. J Arthroplasty 12:535–540, 1997.

34. Nadaud MC, Griffin WL, Fehring TK: Cementless revision total hip arthroplasty without allograft in severe proximal femoral defects. J Arthroplasty 20:738–744, 2005.

35. Merle d'Aubigné R: Cotation chiffrée de la fonction de la hanche. Rev Chir Orthop 56:481–486, 1970.

36. Harris WH: Traumatic arthritis of the hip after dislocation and acetabular fractures: treatment by mold arthroplasty: an end-result study using a new method of result evaluation. J Bone Joint Surg Am 51:737–755, 1969.

37. Gruen TA, McNeice GM, Amstutz HC: "Modes of failure" of cemented stem-type femoral components: a radiographic analysis of loosening. Clin Orthop Relat Res 141:17–27, 1979.

38. Engh CA, Massin PH, Suthers KE: Roentgenographic assessment of the biologic fixation of porous-surfaced femoral components. Clin Orthop Relat Res 257:107–128, 1990.

39. Malchau H, Kärrholm J, Xing Wang Y, Herberts P: Accuracy of migration analysis in hip arthroplasty. Acta Orthop Scand 66:418–424, 1995.

40. Charnley J: The long term results of low-friction arthroplasty of the hip as a primary intervention. J Bone Joint Surg Br 54:61, 1972.

41. Berry DJ: Femoral revision: distal fixation with fluted, tapered grit-blasted stems. J Arthroplasty 17(4 Suppl 1), 2002.

42. Woolson ST, Delaney TJ: Failure of proximally porous-coated femoral prosthesis in revision total hip arthroplasty. J Arthroplasty 10:522–528, 1995.

43. Zicat B, Engh CA, Gokcen E: Patterns of osteolysis around total hip component inserted with and without cement. J Bone Joint Surg Am 77:432–439, 1995.

44. Vidalain JP: The mechanical cement extractor: an original device for cement extraction in THA revision. Hip Int 1:6–9, 1996.

45. Haydon CM, Mehin R, Burnett S, et al: Revision total hip arthroplasty with use of a cemented femoral component: results at a mean of ten years. J Bone Joint Surg Am 86:1179–1185, 2004.

46. Mahomey CR, Fehringer E, Kopjar B, Garvin KL: Femoral revision with impaction grafting and a collarless, polished tapered stem. Clin Orthop Relat Res 432:181–187, 2005.

47. McAuley JP, Engh CA, Jr: Femoral fixation in the face of considerable bone loss: cylindrical and extensively coated femoral components. Clin Orthop Relat Res 429:215–221, 2004.

48. Meding JB, Ritter MA, Keating EM, Faris PM: Impaction bone grafting before insertion of a femoral stem with cement in revision total hip arthroplasty: a minimum two-year follow-up study. J Bone Joint Surg Am 79:1834–1841, 1997.

49. Malkani AL, Lewallen DG, Cabanela ME, Wallrichs SL: Femoral component revision using an uncemented proximally coated long stem prosthesis. J Arthroplasty 11:411–418, 1996.

50. Mulliken BD, Rorabeck CH, Bourne RB: Uncemented revision total hip arthroplasty: a 4-to-6 year review. Clin Orthop Relat Res 325:156–162, 1996.

51. Pellicci PM, Wilson PD, Sledge CB, et al: Long-term results of revision total hip replacement: a follow-up report. J Bone Joint Surg Am 67:513–516, 1985.

52. Davis CM, Berry DJ, Harmsen WS: Cemented revision of failed uncemented femoral components of total hip arthroplasty. J Bone Joint Surg Am 85:1264–1269, 2003.

53. Halliday BR, English HW, Timperley AJ, et al: Femoral impaction grafting with cement in revision total hip replacement: evolution of the technique and results. J Bone Joint Surg Br 85:809–817, 2003.

54. Kerboull L, Cullot TH, Kerboull M: Les reprises d'arthroplasties totales non cimentées par une prothèse cimentée. Rev Chir Orthop 80(Suppl I):141, 1994.

55. Leopold SS, Berger RA, Rosenberg AG: Impaction allografting with cement for femoral component revision: minimum four-year follow-up using a precoated femoral stem. J Bone Joint Surg Am 81:1080–1092, 1999.

56. Sinha RK, Kim SY, Rubash HE: Long-stem cemented calcar replacement arthroplasty for proximal bone loss. J Arthroplasty 19:141–150, 2004.

57. Stulberg SD: Impaction grafting: doing it right. J Arthroplasty 17(Suppl I):147–152, 2002.

58. Rubash HE, Harris WH: Revision of nonseptic, loose, cemented femoral components using modern cementing techniques. J Arthroplasty 3:241–248, 1988.

59. Amstutz HC, Nasser S, More RC, Kabo JM: The anthropometric total hip femoral prosthesis: preliminary clinical and roentgenographic findings of exactfit cementless application. Clin Orthop Relat Res 242:104–119, 1989.

60. Katz RP, Callaghan JJ, Sullivan PM, Johnston RC: Results of cemented femoral revision total hip arthroplasty using improved cementing techniques. Clin Orthop Relat Res 319:178–183, 1995.

61. Mulroy WF, Harris WH: Revision total hip arthroplasty with use of so-called second-generation cementing techniques for aseptic loosening of the femoral component: a fifteen-year-average follow-up. J Bone Joint Surg Am 78:325–330, 1996.

62. Hultmark P, Kärrholm J, Strömberg C, et al: Cemented first-time revisions of the femoral component: prospective 7 to 13 years FU using second-generation and third-generation technique. J Arthroplasty 15:551–561, 2000.

63. Huten D, Bouabdallah N, Bassain E, Wodechi PH: Femoral aseptic loosening revision—Symposium SOFCOT 1999. Rev Chir Orthop 86(Suppl I):72–75, 2000.

64. Migaud H, Courpied JP: Femoral aseptic loosening revision: conclusions—Symposium SOFCOT 1999. Rev Chir Orthop 86(Suppl I):86–90, 2000.

65. Pierson JL, Harris WH: Cemented revision for femoral osteolysis in cemented arthroplasties. J Bone Joint Surg Br 76:40–44, 1994.

66. Ling RS, Timperley AJ, Linder L: Histology of cancellous impaction grafting in the femur: a case report. J Bone Joint Surg Br 75:693–696, 1993.

67. Leopold SS, Jacobs JJ, Rosenberg AG, et al: Cancellous allograft in revision total hip arthroplasty: a clinical review. Clin Orthop Relat Res 337:86–97, 2000.

68. Gie GA, Linder L, Ling RS, et al: Impacted cancellous allografts and cement for revision total hip arthroplasty. J Bone Joint Surg Br 75:14–21, 1993.

69. Charrois O, Kerboull L, Vastel L, et al: Femoral reconstruction with massive allograft implanted in a split femur: mid-term results of 18 reconstructions. Rev Chir Orthop 86:801–808, 2000.

70. Moreland AJR, Bernstein ML: Femoral revision hip arthroplasty with uncemented, porous-coated stems. Clin Orthop Relat Res 319:141–150, 1995.

71. Pidhorz LE, Urban RM, Jacobs JJ, et al: A quantitative study of bone and soft tissues in cementless porous-coated acetabular components retrieved at autopsy. J Arthroplasty 8:213–225, 1993.

72. Krishnamurthy AB, McDonald SJ, Paprovsky WG: 5- to 13-year follow-up on cementless femoral components in revision surgery. J Arthroplasty 12:839–847, 1997.

73. Paprovsky WG, Greidanus NV, Antoniou J: Minimum 10-year results of extensively porous-coated stems in revision arthroplasty. Clin Orthop Relat Res 369:230–242, 1999.

74. Engh CA, Jr, Ellis TJ, Koralewicz LM, et al: Extensively porous-coated femoral revision for severe femoral bone loss: minimum 10-year follow-up. J Arthroplasty 17:955–960, 2002.

75. Moreland AJR, Moreno MA: Cementless femoral revision arthroplasty of the hip: minimum 5 years follow-up. Clin Orthop Relat Res 393:194–201, 2001.

76. Furlong RJ: Six years use of the unmodified Furlong hydroxy-apatite ceramic coated total hip replacement. Acta Orthop Belg 59:323–329, 1993.

77. Kärrholm J, Malchau H, Snorrason F, Herberts P: Micromotion of femoral stems in total hip arthroplasty: a randomized study of cemented hydroxyapatite-coated and porous-coated stems with roentgen stereophotogrammetric analysis. J Bone Joint Surg Am 76:1692–1705, 1994.

78. Bauer TW, Geesink RCT, Zimmerman R, McMahon JT: Hydroxyapatite-coated femoral stems: histological analysis of components retrieved at autopsy. J Bone Joint Surg Am 73:1439–1452, 1991.

79. Hardy DCR, Frayssinet P, Guilhem A, et al: Bonding of hydroxyapatite-coated femoral prostheses: histopathology of specimens from four cases. J Bone Joint Surg Br 73:732–740, 1991.

80. Søballe K, Gotfredsen K, Brockstedt-Rasmussen H, et al: Histological analysis of a retrieved hydroxyapatite coated femoral prosthesis. Clin Orthop Relat Res 272:255–258, 1991.

81. Geesink RGT: HA coatings in orthopaedic surgery, New York, 1999, Raven Press.

82. Crawford CH, Malkani AL, Incavo SJ, et al: Femoral component revision using an extensively hydroxyapatite-coated. J Arthroplasty 19:8–13, 2004.

CHAPTER 98

Femoral Revision: Uncemented Tapered Fluted Modular Implants

Christopher R. Gooding, Clive P. Duncan, Bassam A. Masri, and Donald S. Garbuz

KEY POINTS

- The success of revision surgery of the hip can be divided into three parts: the prosthesis design, the surgical technique, and the patient. Surgical technique is probably the most important factor.
- The surgeon should understand the concept of "press-fit" fixation.
- For successful implantation and fixation of the stern, the importance of primary stability and secondary stability and their relevance to uncemented tapered, fluted, modular implants must be appreciated.
- The surgical team should undertake adequate preoperative planning (defined as three distinct steps: radiologic analysis of the femur, surgical strategy, and templating) to identify potential problems and alternative solutions.
- Do not hesitate to perform an osteotomy to allow for a safer revision; this can make a difficult operation much easier and can facilitate a good press-fit construct.

INTRODUCTION

The objective of revising a loose femoral prosthesis is to restore the hip joint to a condition as close to "normal" as possible, that is, to one that is painless and stable and enables the patient to resume a good quality of life. Several concepts have been described for revision of femoral components of a failed hip arthroplasty. Stem stability in the revision setting can be achieved by cemented or cementless fixation. The disadvantage of a cemented revision, in the absence of impacted allograft, lies in the difficulties involved in achieving adequate interdigitation of cement into host bone, because loosening of the primary implant results in enlargement of the femoral canal and causes the cortices to become thinner and sclerotic.

Broadly speaking, cementless revision stems can be divided into stems that are designed to gain fixation in the proximal or in the distal femur. The advantage of achieving fixation in the distal femur is that the bone stock of the proximal femur in the revision setting is often poor. Long-term uncemented fixation in the diaphysis can be achieved by different methods, including extensively porous-coated stems and fluted, tapered

grit-blasted stems. Uncemented, extensively porous-coated stems have long been considered the gold standard of uncemented revision femoral stems in North America[1-13] and are able to gain rotational stability from a scratch fit in the diaphysis. Although this stem design has been successful in the revision setting,[2,5,7] stress shielding remains a concern because of the relative stiffness of the implant.

An alternative method of uncemented diaphyseal stem fixation, used frequently in Europe, requires the use of fluted, tapered, grit-blasted stems. These stems are tapered to gain axial and rotational stability in the diaphysis of the femur. The femur is reamed to a tapered cone. Then a fluted, tapered implant is impacted into the tapered cone of the prepared diaphysis. Essentially, the distal part of the implant, which is cone shaped, is wedged into the diaphysis to achieve primary stability. The purpose of this chapter is to discuss use of these implants, so-called *uncemented modular fluted implants*, in femoral revision during revision total hip arthroplasty.

DESIGN RATIONALE

For fluted, tapered revision femoral stems, Wagner[14] proposed that the contact zone between the implant and the bone needed to measure between 70 and 100 mm for primary stability. However, Beguec and associates[15] believed that a good press fit depends on the quality of the wedging and a contact zone of just 30 mm in excellent bone, but 40 to 50 mm if bone quality is poor. The contact zone between implant and bone can be limited in other ways to help reduce stiffness. Blaimont[16] demonstrated that during hip flexion, tensile forces at the level of the diaphysis occur in the anterior half of the femur and compressive forces in the posterior half. As one moves through the femur in the diaphyseal region from anterior to posterior, these forces gradually become less tensile and more compressive. At a point in this plane, forces are neither compressive nor tensile, and this "zone" is termed the *neutral zone*. An implant that establishes contact with bone in this neutral zone should allow the bone to react and remodel as it would normally, at least partially and theoretically. This can be achieved by using a quadrangular stem or a stem with flutes that contact the femur in the coronal plane, that is, in the neutral zone.

The cross-sectional shape of a press-fit, uncemented stem is also important for rotational stability. A circular cross-section would create a large contact surface while offering little resistance to rotational loading. An implant with a quadrangular cross-section (such as a tapered stem) has been shown to be very successful in resisting rotational torque and achieving good primary fixation.[17,18] A stem with cutting flutes offers further advantages not only in neutralizing any rotational forces but also in preserving a space between implant and bone, which may aid revascularization and subsequent bone regeneration. This also allows the use of a less stiff implant and reduces the stress shielding seen with fully porous-coated cylindrical implants.

These theoretical advantages have been shown in clinical practice using the Wagner stem (a monoblock fluted, tapered titanium stem), as has been reported by several authors.[19-21]

Because these stems depend on a tapered geometry, it is often difficult to predict when they will stabilize as they are being wedged into the femur. For this reason, modularity of the stem, whereby proximal bodies of different lengths to accommodate for the lack of predictability of the exact wedging location of the distal implant, has been developed and is now considered the standard of care for tapered, fluted revision stems. This modularity allows the surgeon to implant the distal segment in the diaphysis for optimal stem rotational stability, with different options for the proximal body that optimize leg length, femoral offset, femoral version, and ultimate stability. However, this poses certain engineering challenges because these stems require a modular junction at a high-stress location of the femoral component. Postak and associates[22] examined the modular junction and found that the structural endurance limit was compatible with good long-term performance.

PREOPERATIVE PLANNING

Before embarking on a revision of the femoral component, the surgeon should evaluate the existing bone stock and anticipate the quality of remaining bone after the implants and cement, if present, are removed. Paprosky[23] described a useful classification system for evaluating femoral bone stock in revision total hip arthroplasty. This classification enables an algorithmic approach as a guide to femoral reconstruction. Although this topic is covered in greater detail elsewhere, a brief summary is provided here:

- Type 1: a well-preserved metaphyseal cancellous bone with an intact diaphysis
- Type 2: considerable loss of metaphyseal cancellous bone but with an intact diaphysis
- Type 3A: severely damaged metaphysis that is unable to support an implant but has more than 4 cm of intact diaphyseal bone available for distal fixation
- Type 3B: severely damaged metaphysis as for type 3A but with less than 4 cm of diaphyseal bone available for distal fixation

When it comes to revising this group, extensively porous-coated implants tend to fail because they are unable to achieve a sufficient scratch fit.[23] However, the modular, cementless, tapered stem with flutes is able to attain a good initial press-fit even in a relatively short isthmus and can also achieve good rotational stability. Good results have been achieved with this stem in this type of revision setting.[24-29]

- Type 4: characterized by considerable damage to both metaphysis and diaphysis associated with a widened femoral canal; may be difficult to get a wedge fit with a tapered stem, which is contraindicated for this degree of femoral bone loss

Preoperative Templating

The aim of preoperative templating in the revision scenario is to determine the following:

1. The location of the new center of rotation of the hip joint and the precise location of the femoral head based on existing leg length inequality; also, the anticipated new location of the acetabular component, if this is being revised
2. The length of stem required to bypass bony defects and to achieve primary stability
3. The length of the extended trochanteric osteotomy (ETO) required to safely remove the implant. Implant removal is covered more thoroughly elsewhere in this book.

The templates are used to identify the diameter and stem required to achieve fixation and to bypass bony defects. At the same time, the length of the osteotomy is determined as the longest possible osteotomy that will allow safe removal of the implants and will also allow an intact femoral tube to achieve at least 5 to 7 cm of fixation into intact bone. The approximate length of the proximal body is then templated, but it has to be kept in mind that this process is fairly inaccurate because the exact length of the proximal body will depend on the ultimate intraoperative seating of the distal stem.

SURGICAL TECHNIQUE

Two methods may be used to implant a modular femoral stem. The surgeon can construct the implant as a two-step procedure or can assemble the implant on the operating room table before final implantation. Whether the surgeon chooses to assemble the implant in situ or on the back table depends on how confident he is about where the final implant will seat based on the use of intraoperative trials. It is much easier to assemble the implant in situ if an ETO had been performed, and this is indeed the case for most of these revisions.

Assembly In Situ With Extended Trochanteric Osteotomy

Wagner was the first to popularize the technique of performing a proximal osteotomy[14] during a revision total hip arthroplasty, although his technique involved creating an osteotomy fragment in the coronal plane consisting of the anterior third of the circumference of the upper femur. This technique has been modified slightly to create an osteotomy fragment in the sagittal plane that consists of the lateral third of the upper femur, including the greater trochanter with attached abductors.

Situations that may require an ETO include revision of a well-fixed uncemented or cemented femoral implant, removal of a loose femoral stem with a well-bonded cement mantle, and correction of a proximal femoral deformity to gain additional acetabular exposure or to assist in dislocation of a failed hip arthroplasty in patients with extensive scarring or heterotopic bone formation.

Potential advantages of this technique include direct access to the distal part of the femoral canal for reaming and removal of distal cement (avoiding the impingement of reamers on the greater trochanter, with inherent risk of fracture), with the added advantages of being able to tension the abductors by trochanteric advancement and reducing the operating time for revisions in which exposure is a problem.[30]

For a tapered stem to function successfully, surface contact between bone and implant must be sufficient, resulting in stable wedging of the prosthesis that eliminates motion to allow sufficient bone ongrowth. If a straight stem is implanted into a femur that is curved in the coronal plane, the areas of contact will be at three points only and will have little capacity to prevent subsidence of the implant or to resist rotational forces, particularly in weak bone. Because conical reamers cannot convert a curved femur into a straight one, this is another indication for performing an osteotomy.

After the osteotomy is performed, the femoral canal is prepared. The first step involves diaphyseal reaming until firm endosteal cortical contact is achieved (Figs. 98-1 through 98-4). The width of the final reamer should be the same as the diameter of the chosen stem. If an osteotomy has been performed, reamers can be placed into the distal bone fragment through the osteotomy site to a depth that matches the final stem placement. In general, with most modular revision systems, it is

possible to complete a trial before insertion of the definitive stem (Fig. 98-5). This is particularly important if one anticipates using the smallest proximal body because with tapered stems, the real prosthesis may not advance as far as the trial implants. Alternatively, the definitive stem can be implanted without a trial, ensuring that it is at least two diaphyseal diameters below a bony defect or the exit site of an osteotomy (Fig. 98-6). With some stem designs, the flutes are not circumferential and are designed to make endosteal contact only in the coronal plane, as was described earlier; therefore, the "bare area" of the stem (area without flutes) is located in the sagittal plane (anteriorly and posteriorly) (Fig. 98-7). Care must be taken at this stage to confirm good "press-fit" or wedging in the

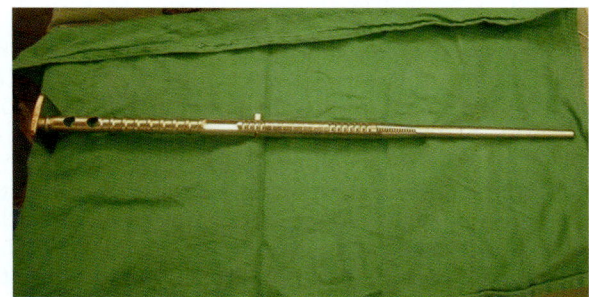

Figure 98-2. Photograph demonstrating the femoral rasp with handle attached.

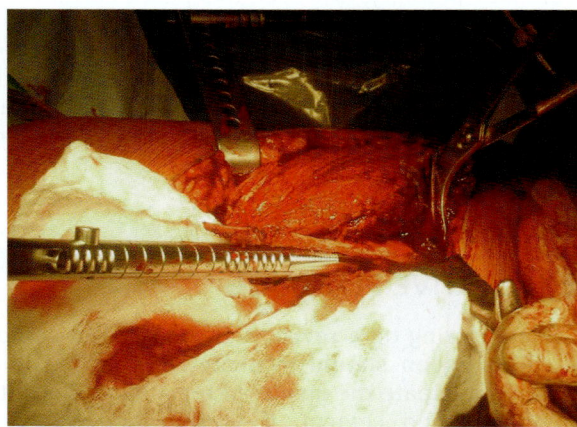

Figure 98-3. Intraoperative photograph demonstrating rasping of the femoral canal to get a good press-fit. The rasp doubles as a distal femoral trial once the rasp handle has been uncoupled.

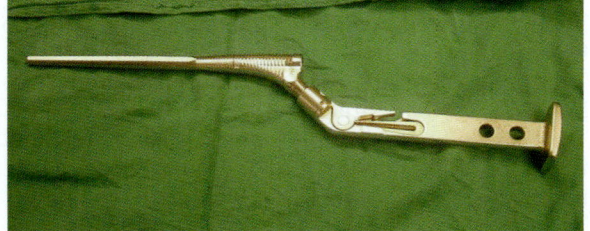

Figure 98-4. Photograph demonstrating the distal rasp attached to the modular proximal body and handle.

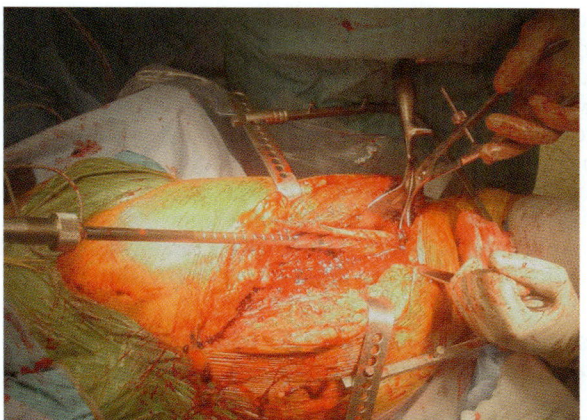

Figure 98-1. Intraoperative photograph of a Vancouver B2 periprosthetic fracture. Reaming of the femoral canal.

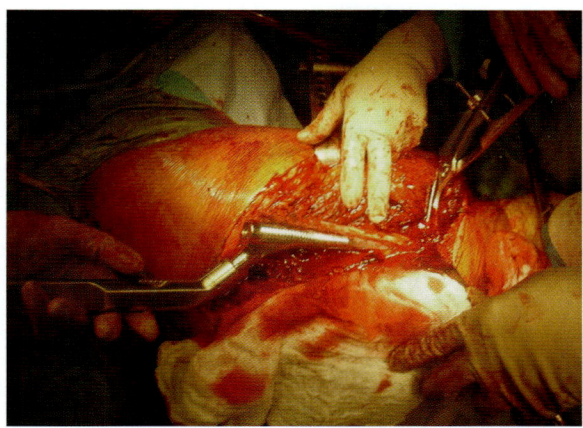

Figure 98-5. Intraoperative photograph demonstrating the siting of the trial component.

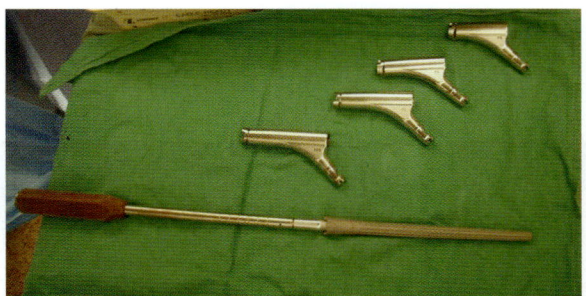

Figure 98-6. Photograph demonstrating the definitive distal implant with a tapered, fluted stem with choices of proximal trial bodies.

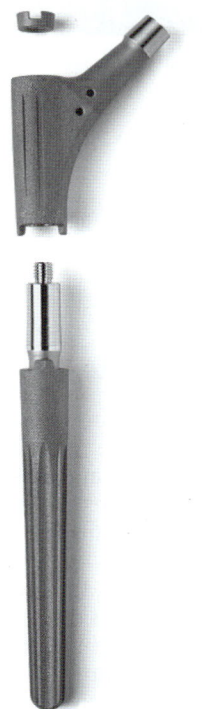

Figure 98-7. Photograph demonstrating the definitive implant, including the distal tapered, fluted stem, along with the proximal body and locking nut. (*Courtesy Zimmer Inc., Mount Laurel, NJ.*)

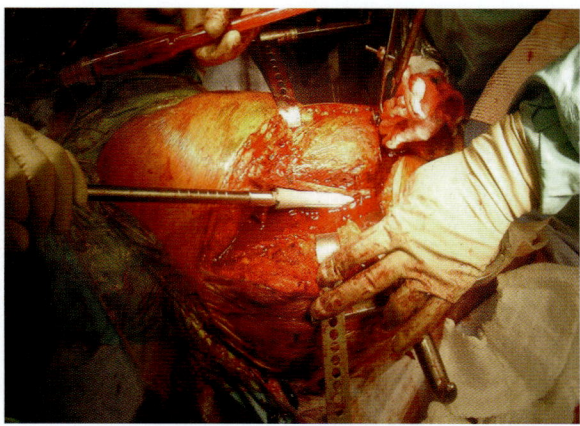

Figure 98-8. Intraoperative photograph demonstrating the siting of the distal stem into the femoral canal. Note the position of the flutes.

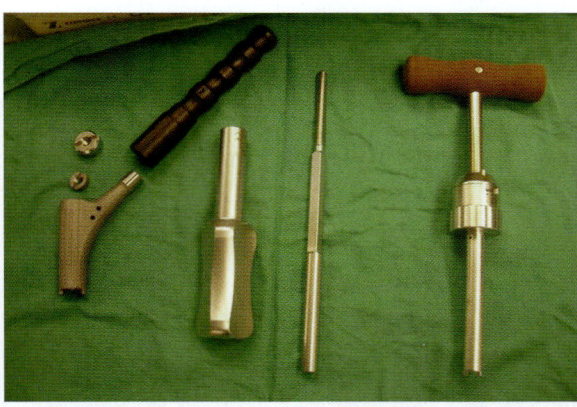

Figure 98-9. Photograph demonstrating instruments for implanting the proximal body (guide rod, impactor, locking nut, and torque screw driver). The definitive proximal body is also shown.

diaphysis (Fig. 98-8). If this is not observed, the definitive implant may subside and subsequently fail. Once the definitive distal stem has been implanted, the surgeon has the choice of a number of proximal bodies of different lengths to restore leg length, depending on the particular system the surgeon is using (Figs. 98-9 through 98-11). Most systems offer the additional option of being able to "dial-in" the appropriate anteversion of ±30 degrees (Fig. 98-12*A* through *C*). The trial proximal prosthesis is then secured to the definitive distal component, usually by means of a nut or screw, of the threaded part of the Morse taper but without direct contact with the Morse taper because of the risk of possibly damaging it. Once the trial body has been secured to the definitive distal implant and a femoral head of appropriate size has been selected, the hip can be reduced and examined for stability, as well as leg lengths. If the hip is not stable at this stage, a proximal component of a different size can be selected to address leg length issues or anteversion changes if the hip is unstable. Once the definitive proximal body is selected, it is secured to the distal segment (Fig. 98-13).

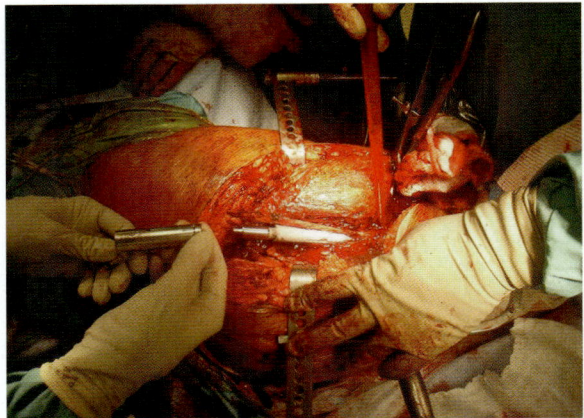

Figure 98-10. Intraoperative photograph showing the distal femoral component, which has been "wedged" into the femoral canal. The trial modular body is about to be located onto the stem.

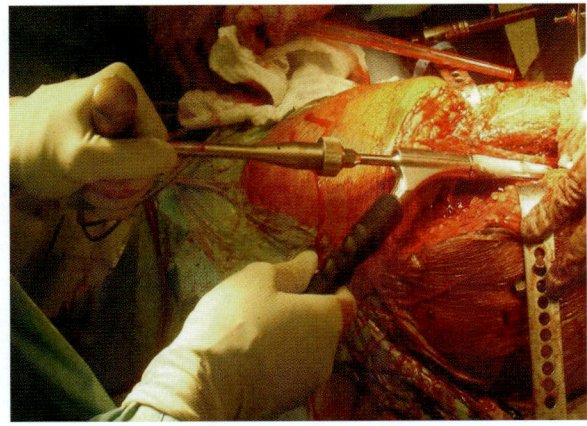

Figure 98-11. Intraoperative photograph demonstrating how the trial body is secured to the distal femoral component.

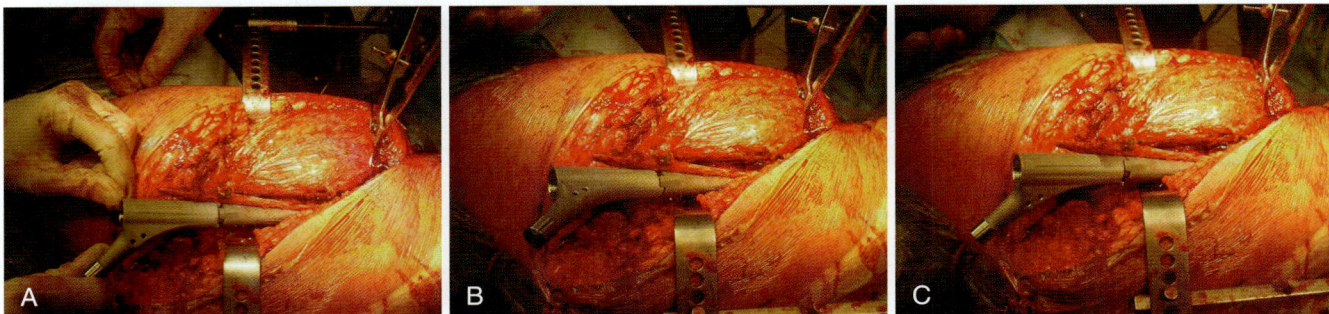

Figure 98-12. Intraoperative photographs demonstrating the modular proximal body and showing how the anteversion can be "dialed-in."

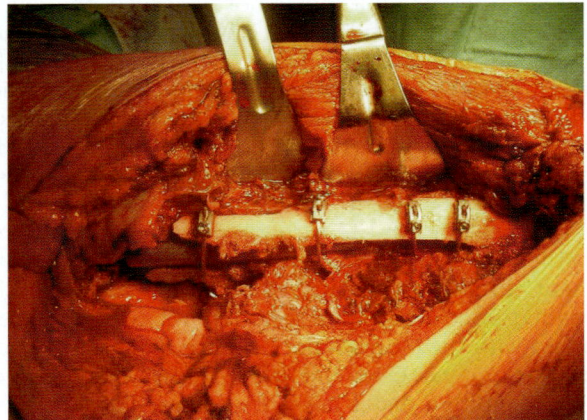

Figure 98-13. Intraoperative photograph demonstrating the definitive implant in situ. The fractured proximal femur has been reduced onto the implant and secured with cables. One additional cable was secured to the femur immediately distal to the distal extent of the femoral fracture to prevent fracture propagation before instrumenting the femoral canal.

Figure 98-14 shows a postoperative radiograph of a similar modular revision femoral stem.

Assembly on the Back Table for the Endofemoral Route

Alternatively, rather than assembling the implant "within the patient," the definitive implant can be assembled on the bench and then implanted into the femur. This is done in cases when an ETO was not performed, but the surgeon may choose to use this technique even with an ETO. Where the femur is straight in the coronal plane with only a slight curve in the sagittal plane and there is good bone stock in a femur that requires a short implant, this is the approach of choice. The surgeon must be comfortable with safely removing any cement from above with this technique. As before, the diaphysis requires reaming until a firm endosteal contact is established. Then modular rasps or proximal reamers, depending on the particular implant system, are used to prepare the proximal femur for the desired

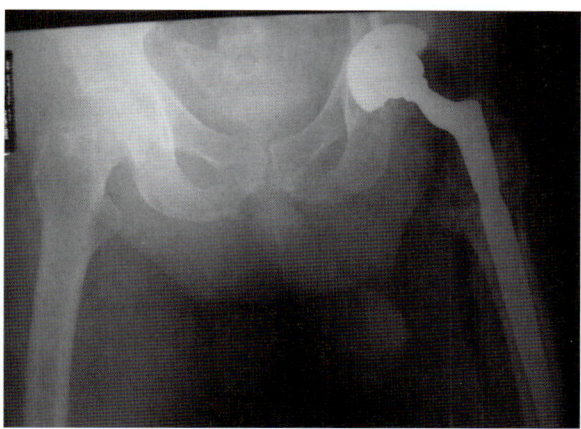

Figure 98-14. Postoperative radiograph demonstrating a ZMR (Zimmer Inc., Warson, Ind) revision femoral stem, which was used to revise a loose femoral implant with considerable proximal bone loss in Gruen zones 1 and 7.

proximal portion of the implant. If rasps are used, they also function as trials, and if reamers are used, dedicated trial components are generally available. After appropriate trials, the correct proximal body is assembled onto the distal segment, using appropriate instrumentation for the system being used. When the implant is assembled, it is critical to ensure that any anterior bevels on the distal stem are correctly oriented anteriorly relative to the femur before final assembly of the stem. In addition, if the flutes are only in the coronal plane, it is important that the implant is assembled with the flutes in the correct orientation. It is also important to assemble the proximal portion with correct anteversion because the distal segment should not be rotated on insertion to achieve correct femoral anteversion. The implant is then impacted into the femur, taking care of the greater trochanter in those patients who have not had an osteotomy because the shoulder of the implant can impinge on it as it is impacted into the femur. When a tapered stem is used, the stem is inserted with multiple small strikes of a mallet until no further advancement is seen and rotational stability is achieved. Further impaction after this point would result in a cortical fracture because of the tapered design. Once the definitive component is implanted, an appropriate trial femoral head can be selected. If leg lengths and stability are satisfactory the definitive femoral head is requested and assembled onto the implant, and the hip is then reduced.

POSTOPERATIVE CARE

If the prosthesis has been wedged perfectly into a femur with good cortical bone and an appropriately conically shaped medullary canal, the construct will be stable. In this situation, the patient can be allowed to bear weight as tolerated with the aid of a walker or crutches. However, in most situations, bone stock is deficient, and for this reason, we generally recommend toe touch weight bearing for a period of 6 to 8 weeks. Apart from general education of safe ambulation and gait progression, we generally do not prescribe prolonged physical therapy immediately postoperatively. Patients should be reviewed at 6 to 8 weeks following surgery for a clinical and radiographic evaluation. The implant should be carefully reviewed at this stage to ensure that it has not subsided and is stable. If this is the case, patients can resume weight bearing as tolerated and can start weaning themselves off their walking aids, if they have sufficient muscle strength at this point. Physical therapy is prescribed at this stage at the discretion of the surgeon, but many patients can rehabilitate with home exercises and do not require a formal physical therapy program.

RESULTS

The first uncemented, tapered, fluted femoral stem was the nonmodular Wagner stem, and despite good overall success,[24] reports have described implant subsidence.[31] Isacson and associates[32] reported that 5 of 22 patients had subsidence of 2 cm or more, Bircher and colleagues[33] reported that 6 of 99 stems subsided enough to require early revision, and Hartwig and coworkers[34] reported that 7 of 41 had subsided. Others have also identified this as a problem.[19-21,31,35] Building on experience with the Wagner stem, the fluted, tapered titanium stem with a proximal modular body was developed. As was already discussed, the modularity allows the surgeon to uncouple the distal segment in the femur from the proximal body. This has the obvious advantage of allowing precision in obtaining a distal fit, as well as in restoring leg lengths and hip stability. However, the solution to one problem can often lead to the creation of another. The very fact that these stems are modular means that they have a junction that is at a high-stress location of the implant. This problem has been addressed with a strong taper junction construct, similar to how the femoral head and neck engage in most hip arthroplasties.[22,35] Despite this taper junction, implant fractures have been seen, and manufacturers have continued to strengthen this junction. For this reason, whenever possible, it is our recommendation to ensure that the medial portion of the junction is supported by bone.

McInnis and associates[25] retrospectively reviewed 70 patients who had undergone revision with a modular fluted, tapered femoral stem with a mean follow-up of 47 months. Combined metaphyseal/diaphyseal bone loss was present preoperatively in 36 (51%) of 70 hips. At final review, 3 of 70 (4.3%) hips had failed and were revised or were awaiting revision. Restoration of proximal bone was noted in 56%. Based on reported results, the authors concluded that this type of implant was equivalent to, or better than, other types of cementless revision femoral stems.

Park and colleagues[27] reviewed patients who had had a revision hip arthroplasty with or without an extended trochanteric osteotomy. A total of 62 revision total hip arthroplasties were performed using a fluted and tapered modular femoral stem. An extended trochanteric osteotomy (ETO) was used in 32 of the 62 hips (52%), whereas no osteotomy was used in the remaining 30 hips. The mean postoperative Harris hip score was 87.3 points with mean follow-up of 4.2 years. With the exception of one reoperation for a deep infection, no femoral revision was performed because of mechanical failure. Postoperative Harris hip scores, femoral component stability, and overall complication rates did not differ whether an ETO was performed or not. However, rates of cortical perforation and stem subsidence greater than 5 mm were significantly higher in the group treated without an ETO.

Mumme and coworkers[26] reviewed 45 patients who underwent revision hip arthroplasty (48 hips) with an uncemented, modular revision stem with a diaphyseal press-fit. Significant improvement was noted in the Harris hip score ($P < .05$), and radiographs showed stable implants without migration in 44 patients. In one patient, the stem needed further revision because of subsidence. Kaplan-Meier survivorship analysis showed survivorship of 97% at 9 years.

Garbuz and associates[28] compared quality of life in 220 patients with two femoral stem designs: a modular, tapered, and fluted titanium stem design, with stem and head-neck modularity; and a cylindrical, extensively coated chrome-cobalt stem with head-neck modularity alone. The median follow-up was 2 years. Outcome assessment and patient satisfaction were measured using the Western Ontario and McMaster University (WOMAC) Osteoarthritis Index, the Oxford Hip Score, the Short Form (SF)-12, and the Arthroplasty Satisfaction Scale. WOMAC pain, function, and overall scores, including patient satisfaction scores, were higher with the fluted titanium stem design. The authors concluded that reduced stiffness of the fluted titanium stem, together with modularity (the advantages of which have been discussed earlier), was responsible for the better outcomes reported with this stem design.

COMPLICATIONS

These are best divided into perioperative, immediate or early postoperative, and late complications. Perioperative complications specific to this type of implant include femoral shaft fractures, which can occur when the rasp or the definitive implant is being impacted into the femoral canal. Fractures of the greater trochanter can also occur when the shoulder of the definitive proximal body and stem construct is being impacted into the femur via the endofemoral route and impinges onto the greater trochanter. If the curve of the femur in the sagittal plane is not fully appreciated and a femoral osteotomy is not performed, then perforation of the anterior cortex can occur when a reamer is used, or when the stem is impacted. This can be avoided with careful preoperative planning and templating, with particular attention to the lateral radiograph in the case of a sagittal bow to the femur.

When a previously cemented femoral stem is revised, incomplete excision of bone cement can lead to malpositioning of the reamer and the stem, with the inherent risk of cortical perforation or fracture. Park and colleagues[27] reported an intraoperative diaphyseal split fracture in 6%, cortical perforation in 6%, and dislocation in 5% following revision hip arthroplasty with or without an extended trochanteric osteotomy.

Immediate or early postoperative complications include dislocation and fracture of the greater trochanter, as mentioned with perioperative complications, as well as stem subsidence. Reasons for dislocations specific to the modular femoral implant may include a proximal body of inadequate length and failure to adequately address femoral neck anteversion. Stem subsidence can also occur as the result of inadequate wedging of the distal component or may be caused by a periprosthetic fracture. Subsidence due to inadequate wedging typically occurs within 1 to 12 months after the operation.[24,35-42] Stem subsidence may present as a dislocation caused by inadequate soft tissue tension or impingement.

McInnis and coworkers[25] reported a mean subsidence of 9.9 mm, dislocation in 7 (10%) of 70 hips, and fracture or cortical perforation in 17 (24.2%) of 70.

SUMMARY AND CONCLUSION

In a revision scenario, bone quality in the proximal femur is often poor, requiring a segmental allograft or a femoral implant that allows stable distal fixation. Although good results have been achieved with fully coated femoral stems, they have shown high rates of failure (up to 21%[43]) in patients with Paprosky types 3B and 4, with large ectatic femoral canals. A modular tapered, fluted implant provides axial and rotational stability through the use of distal flutes, and the proximal body allows independent adjustment of leg length, offset, and anteversion. To conclude, this stem design offers a number of advantages over previous implants in the management of patients requiring revision for a failed hip arthroplasty with poor proximal femoral bone stock. Early results with this implant in cases with large defects are encouraging.

CURRENT CONTROVERSIES AND FUTURE CONSIDERATIONS

- Whether the proximal femur has the ability to reconstitute around a stem of large diameter?
- What is the risk of fatigue fracture through the modular stem junction?
- Is there a need for supplementary onlay cortical allografts?
- To identify the limitations of the press-fit concept (unable to achieve primary stability, such as revising a long-stemmed implant associated with a large osteolytic lesion or a periprosthetic fracture with destruction of the isthmic part of the femur)?
- To identify and address the concerns of stress shielding

REFERENCES

1. Sugimura T, Tohkura A: THA revision with extensively porous-coated stems: 32 hips followed 2-6.5 years. Acta Orthop Scand 69:11–13, 1998.
2. Wu LD, Xiong Y, Yan SG, et al: Femoral component revision using extensively porous-coated cementless stem. Chin J Traumatol 8:358–363, 2005.
3. Paprosky WG, Burnett RS: Extensively porous-coated femoral stems in revision hip arthroplasty: rationale and results. Am J Orthop 31:471–474, 2002.
4. Paprosky WG, Greidanus NV, Antoniou J: Minimum 10-year-results of extensively porous-coated stems in revision hip arthroplasty. Clin Orthop Relat Res 230:42–49, 1999.
5. Weeden SH, Paprosky WG: Minimal 11-year follow-up of extensively porous-coated stems in femoral revision total hip arthroplasty. J Arthroplasty 17:134–137, 2002.
6. Moreland JR, Bernstein ML: Femoral revision hip arthroplasty with uncemented, porous-coated stems. Clin Orthop Relat Res 319:141–150, 1995.
7. Engh CA, Ellis TJ, Koralewicz LM, et al: Extensively porous-coated femoral revision for severe femoral bone loss: minimum 10-year follow-up. J Arthroplasty 17:955–960, 2002.
8. Engh CA, Hopper RH: The odyssey of porous-coated fixation. J Arthroplasty 17:102–107, 2002.
9. Engh CA, Fenwick JA: Extensively porous-coated stems: avoiding modularity. Orthopedics 31:911–912, 2008.
10. Paprosky WG, Weeden SH: Extensively porous-coated stems in femoral revision arthroplasty. Orthopedics 24:871–872, 2001.
11. Engh CA, Hopper RH: Extensively porous-coated stems: a choice for all seasons. Orthopedics 23:951–952, 2000.
12. Nourbash PS, Paprosky WG: Cementless femoral design concerns: rationale for extensive porous coating. Clin Orthop Relat Res 355:189–199, 1998.
13. Sporer SM, Paprosky WG: Extensively coated cementless femoral components in revision total hip arthroplasty: an update. Surg Technol Int 14:265–274, 2005.
14. Wagner H: Prosthese de revision de l'articulation coxo-femorale. Orthopade 18:438–453, 1989.
15. Beguec P, Sieber H: The concept of press-fit: revision of loose femoral prosthesis, Paris, 2007, Springer-Verlag, pp 19–27.
16. Blaimont P, Halleux P, Jedwab J: [Distribution of bony restraints in the femur]. Rev Chir Orthop Reparatrice Appar Mot 54:303–319, 1968.
17. Zweymuller KA, Lintner FK, Semlitsch MF: Biologic fixation of a press-fit titanium hip joint endoprosthesis. Clin Orthop Relat Res 235:195–206, 1988.
18. Kirk KL, Potter BK, Lehman RA, Jr, Xenos JS: Effect of distal stem geometry on interface motion in uncemented revision total hip prostheses. Am J Orthop 36:545–549, 2007.
19. Michelinakis E, Papapolychronlou TF, Vafiadis J: The use of a cementless femoral component for the management of bone loss in revision hip arthroplasty. Bull Hosp Jt Dis 55:28–32, 1996.
20. Rinaldi E, Marenghi PF, Vaienti E: The Wagner prosthesis for femoral reconstruction by transfemoral approach. Chir Organi Mov 79:353–356, 1994.
21. Kolstad KF, Adalberth GF, Mallmin HF, et al: The Wagner revision stem for severe osteolysis: 31 hips followed for 1.5-5 years. Acta Orthop Scand 67:541–544, 1996.
22. Postak PD, Greenwald AS: The influence of modularity on the endurance performance of the Link MP hip stem, Cleveland, 2001, Orthopaedic Research Laboratories.
23. Valle CJ, Paprosky WG: Classification and an algorithmic approach to the reconstruction of femoral deficiency in revision total hip arthroplasty. J Bone Joint Surg Am 85(Suppl 4):1–6, 2003.
24. Weber MF, Hempfing AF, Orler RF, Ganz R: Femoral revision using the Wagner stem: results at 2-9 years. Int Orthop 26:36–39, 2002.
25. Mclnnis DP, Horne GF, Devane PA: Femoral revision with a fluted, tapered, modular stem seventy patients followed for a mean of 3.9 years. J Arthroplasty 21:372–380, 2006.
26. Mumme TF, Muller-Rath RF, Andereya S, Wirtz DC: Uncemented femoral revision arthroplasty using the modular revision prosthesis MRP-TITAN revision stem. Oper Orthop Traumatol 19:56–77, 2007.
27. Park YS, Moon YW, Lim SJ: Revision total hip arthroplasty using a fluted and tapered modular distal fixation stem with and without extended trochanteric osteotomy. J Arthroplasty 22:993–999, 2007.
28. Garbuz DS, Toms AF, Masri BA, Duncan CP: Improved outcome in femoral revision arthroplasty with tapered fluted modular titanium stems. Clin Orthop Relat Res 453:199–202, 2006.
29. Iorio RF, Healy WL, Presutti AH: A prospective outcomes analysis of femoral component fixation in revision total hip arthroplasty. J Arthroplasty 23:662–669, 2008.
30. Dowdy PA, Rorabeck CH, Bourne RB: Uncemented total hip arthroplasty in patients 50 years of age or younger. J Arthroplasty 12:853–862, 1997.
31. Ponziani LF, Rollo GF, Bungaro PF, et al: Revision of the femoral prosthetic component according to the Wagner technique. Chir Organi Mov 80:385–389, 1995.
32. Isacson JF, Stark AF, Wallensten R: The Wagner revision prosthesis consistently restores femoral bone structure. Int Orthop 24:139–142, 2000.
33. Bircher HP, Riede UF, Luem MF, Ochsner PE: [The value of the Wagner SL revision prosthesis for bridging large femoral defects]. Orthopade 30:294–303, 2001.
34. Hartwig CH, Böhm PF, Czech UF, et al: The Wagner revision stem in alloarthroplasty of the hip. Arch Orthop Trauma Surg 115:5–9, 1996.
35. Grunig RF, Morscher E, Ochsner PE: Three to 7 year results with the uncemented SL femoral revision prosthesis. Arch Orthop Trauma Surg 116:187–197, 1997.
36. Christie MJ, DeBoer DK, Trick LW, et al: Primary total hip arthroplasty with use of the modular S-ROM prosthesis: four to seven-year clinical and radiographic results. J Bone Joint Surg Am 81:1707–1716, 1999.
37. Böhm PF, Bischel O: Femoral revision with the Wagner SL revision stem: evaluation of one hundred and twenty-nine revisions followed for a mean of 4.8 years. J Bone Joint Surg Am 83:1023–1031, 2001.
38. Böhm P, Bischel O: The use of tapered stems for femoral revision surgery. Clin Orthop Relat Res 420:148–159, 2004.
39. Gustilo RB, Pasternak HS: Revision total hip arthroplasty with titanium ingrowth prosthesis and bone grafting for failed cemented femoral component loosening. Clin Orthop Relat Res 235:111–119, 1988.
40. Hedley AK, Gruen TA, Ruoff DP: Revision of failed total hip arthroplasties with uncemented porous-coated anatomic components. Clin Orthop Relat Res 235:75–90, 1988.
41. Paprosky WG, Greidanus NV, Antoniou J: Minimum 10 year results of extensively porous-coated stems in revision hip arthroplasty. Clin Orthop Relat Res 369:230–242, 1999.
42. Warren PJ, Thompson PF, Fletcher MD: Transfemoral implantation of the Wagner SL stem: the abolition of subsidence and enhancement of osteotomy union rate using Dall-Miles cables. Arch Orthop Trauma Surg 122:557–560, 2002.
43. Sporer SM, Paprosky WG: Femoral fixation in the face of considerable bone loss: the use of modular stems. Clin Orthop Relat Res 429:227–231, 2004.

FURTHER READING

Berry DJ: Femoral revision: distal fixation with fluted, tapered grit-blasted stems. J Arthroplasty 17:142–146, 2002.
Excellent review article with a good summary of the technical aspects of distal fixation with a tapered, fluted stem.
Garbuz DS, Toms A, Masri BA, Duncan CP: Improved outcome in femoral revision arthroplasty with tapered fluted modular titanium stems. Clin Orthop Relat Res 453:199–202, 2006.
A study comparing a modular tapered and fluted stem with a cylindrical, extensively coated chrome-cobalt stem with single modularity. This study highlights the merits of the modular tapered and fluted stem design over the more traditional cylindrical stem design.
Park YS, Moon YW, Lim SJ: Revision total hip arthroplasty using a fluted and tapered modular distal fixation stem with and without

extended trochanteric osteotomy. J Arthroplasty 22:993–999, 2007.

This study shows that similar results can be obtained with a modular tapered and fluted stem design with or without an extended trochanteric osteotomy.

Sporer SM, Paprosky W: Femoral fixation in the face of considerable bone loss: the use of modular stems. Clin Orthop Relat Res 429:227–231, 2004.

Highlights how a distally fixed, tapered, modular, and fluted stem can provide excellent axial and rotational stability in the presence of considerable proximal femoral bone loss.

Weber MF, Hempfing AF, Orler RF, Ganz R: Femoral revision using the Wagner stem: results at 2-9 years. Int Orthop 26:36–39, 2002.

A study with one of the longest follow-ups reported of the earlier tapered, fluted designs: "the Wagner stem."

CHAPTER 99

Femoral Revision: Allograft Prosthetic Composites and Proximal Femoral Replacement

Paul Tee Hui Lee, Oleg A. Safir, Catherine F. Kellett, David J. Backstein, and Allan E. Gross

KEY POINTS

- Revision of the femoral component in patients with failed total hip replacement with significant proximal femoral bone loss of more than 5 cm distal to the lesser trochanter may be accomplished by the use of APC or PFR.
- The use of proximal allograft aids trochanteric and abductor repairs, resulting in lower rates of abductor impairment, limping, instability, and dislocation compared with PFR. Even when the host greater trochanter is destroyed, the use of proximal femoral allograft incorporated with abductor tendon allograft enables host abductor tendon repair.
- Prerequisites for the use of APC include access to banked bone, expertise in the use of massive structural allograft, patient commitment to a postoperative rehabilitation program, and the ability of the patient to tolerate a prolonged surgical procedure. Failing that, the alternative use of PFR is advised.
- In our current practice, we use APC in younger, higher-demand patients who will potentially require multiple revision surgeries, and reserve the use of PFR for older, lower-demand, and medically frail patients.
- For adequate initial APC implant stability, we use a long reciprocating stepped or oblique cut at the graft-host junction bounded by multiple cerclage wires and reinforced with cortical strut allograft as biological plating. We avoid distal implant cementation, and we believe that distal implant press-fit is not essential for initial implant stability.

INTRODUCTION

Revision total hip replacement (THR) in patients with severe proximal femoral bone loss is difficult. Bone loss extending more than 5 cm distal to the lesser trochanter precludes the use of most conventional THR techniques. Salvage procedures such as excision arthroplasty have shown poor results.[1,2] Arthrodesis is difficult to achieve.[3] Viable options include the use of allograft prosthetic composites, proximal femoral replacements, and impaction bone grafting techniques. The use of allograft prosthetic composites and proximal femoral replacements will be discussed in this chapter.

Proximal femoral replacement (PFR) is defined as a metal femoral implant, proximally connected to a femoral head to articulate with the acetabulum and distally fixed to the host femur. It may be cemented or uncemented, modular or nonmodular. Historically, proximal femoral replacement was used after tumor resection.[4] The initial designs were cobalt-chrome monoblock with segmental length increments cemented into the distal femur. Later developments included modularity to better accommodate leg length and porous coating to promote bony ingrowth at the junction with extracortical bone bridging, although this concept has not been shown to occur with predictability even with bone grafting. Indications recently have been expanded to include non-neoplastic conditions such as failed THR with massive proximal femoral bone loss and periprosthetic fractures.

Allograft prosthetic composite (APC) in revision THR is defined as a long femoral stem prosthesis that is proximally incorporated into a proximal femoral bone allograft. This technique has gained popularity over the past decade with several encouraging longer-term reports.[5-10]

When comparing APC with PFR, the advantages for using PFR include easier availability without the need for access to banked bone, easier implantation without the need for expertise in the use of massive bone allografts, and shorter operative duration with potentially lower blood loss and infection rates. Patients with PFR are generally allowed to bear weight earlier in the postoperative period and have less demanding postoperative rehabilitation programs.

Revision THR with PFR, however, is associated with higher dislocation rates.[11,12] PFR provides poor attachment of host bone and soft tissue, leading to weaker abductors and a higher rate of Trendelenburg limp.[13] There is also the disadvantage of violating the host distal femoral canal with reaming for stem cementation or press-fitting, which is undesirable with regard to bone preservation, especially in younger higher-demand patients. In terms of survivorship, reports have suggested higher rates of loosening and failure with PFR.[13,14]

The use of APC has the potential to restore proximal femoral bone stock and minimize host distal canal violation to preserve bone stock to aid future reconstructions. By avoiding cementing or significant reaming for press-fitting the implant distally, the distal host canal is relatively preserved. The use of proximal allograft aids host bony and soft tissue attachment, in particular the host greater trochanter. When the host greater trochanter is destroyed, the use of proximal femur-abductor tendon allograft facilitates host abductor tendon repair. APCs with trochanteric and abductor repairs have lower rates of abductor impairment, limping, instability, and dislocation compared with PFR.[11-13]

INDICATIONS AND CONTRAINDICATIONS

Indications

The general indication for the use of APC or PFR is significant proximal femoral bone loss of greater than 5 cm distal to the lesser trochanter. Bone loss may be caused by tumor resection, previous THR infection, periprosthetic fracture (e.g., Vancouver B3), or osteolysis.

In general, APC is used in younger, higher-demand patients, who will potentially require multiple revisions.

CONTRAINDICATIONS

Patients with absolute general contraindications to APC and PFR include those who are medically unfit for major surgery, those with unresolved superficial or deep hip infection, and patients who will not be cooperative with the postoperative rehabilitation program. Another contraindication is the ability to reconstruct the femur using alternate techniques, such as modular tapered fluted stems. Relative general contraindications include morbid obesity and poor central or peripheral perfusion. After radiation therapy, APC should not be used because of poor potential for healing at the host-allograft junction. In this setting, PFR is preferred. Finally, lack of familiarity with the technique and limited experience in revision total hip arthroplasty on the part of the surgeon or the surgical team are contraindications to these complex techniques; such cases should be referred to centers with more experience with these techniques.

Of note, prerequisites for the use of APC include access to the bone bank, expertise in the use of massive structural allografts, and patient commitment to the postoperative rehabilitation program. Failing that, the alternative—use of PFR—is advised.

PREOPERATIVE PLANNING

Because the use of PFR is technically similar to that of most distal fixation stems, with the exception of the need for fixation of the hip abductors to the stem, we will focus on the technical details associated with APC.

Allograft Prosthetic Composites

Allograft Availability

We recommend acquiring fresh-frozen allograft from a tissue bank that is accredited by the American Association of Tissue Banks.[15] In general, these allografts are irradiated for sterility and are stored at $-70°$ C.

Preoperative planning is required so the correct sizes of allograft and implant can be ordered. Anteroposterior (AP) pelvis and full femur radiographic views with a calibrated radiographic marker are obtained to estimate the length and diameter of the graft and implant required. The allograft length is estimated from the length of the proximal femoral deficiency. This usually correlates with the distance from the center of rotation of the hip joint to the level in the distal femur where adequate bone stock is present to support the allograft. This estimation should take into account apparent leg length discrepancy due to stem subsidence or periprosthetic fracture. A graft that is substantially longer than estimated is ordered to allow for intraoperative adjustments, and should account for at least a 3- to 5-cm step cut at the allograft host-bone junction. The estimated stem length should be generously longer than the estimated graft length, and the anticipated stem tip is more than 4 to 6 cm away from the knee joint.

The graft canal diameter is usually narrower than the host canal, which is often widened by cortical thinning from osteolysis and cavitation around previous loose femoral components. Avoid choosing a graft with an outer diameter that is substantially narrower than the host to reduce the risk of unstable intussusceptions and uncontrolled subsidence postoperatively. Ideally, the outer diameters of the graft and host should be matched at the distal graft-host junction for optimal junctional stability. However, using a slightly narrower graft to telescope into the host distal femoral canal by 1 to 2 cm and ensuring initial junctional fixation stability may enhance union and long-term stability (Fig. 99-1).

Ruling Out Infection

Preoperative workup should exclude infection using serologic inflammatory markers (C-reactive protein [CRP], erythrocyte sedimentation rate [ESR]). If necessary, other workup as discussed elsewhere in this book may be necessary. The operation should not be booked until the surgeon is reasonably certain that infection is not a cause of failure.

Equipment and Implants

Patients with severe proximal bone loss who requires revision THR usually have multiple previous hip surgeries with poor soft tissue function and increased risks of instability and dislocation. We often consider the potential need for using large bearings or constrained liners. In patients with poor abductor function and destroyed greater trochanter, we would also consider the use of

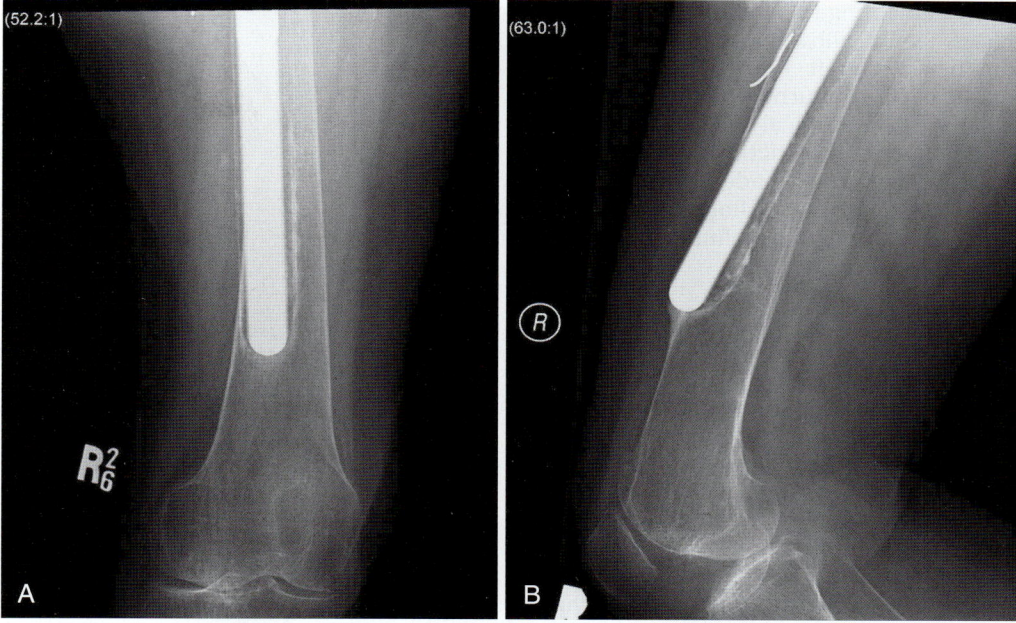

Figure 99-1. Preoperative **(A)** anteroposterior (AP) and **(B)** lateral distal femoral radiographs showing uncontained severe proximal femur bone loss.

proximal femur-abductor tendon allograft for attaching host abductor tendons.

Leg Length Discrepancy

Preoperative assessment for leg length discrepancy will guide the amount of leg lengthening during surgery. Apparent leg length difference measured clinically is correlated with radiographic assessment. Significant fixed flexion or adduction contracture may require release intraoperatively. Our guidelines for safe limb lengthening with regard to risk for sciatic stretch are 4 to 5 cm in previously equal limbs (e.g., before periprosthetic fracture) and 2 to 3 cm in previously unequal limbs (e.g., persistent shortening after THR for severe congenital hip dislocation).

DESCRIPTION OF TECHNIQUE

General Setup

Prophylactic intravenous antibiotics are administered before urinary catheterization is performed. The patient is secured in the lateral decubitus position with protection to pressure areas.

To reduce operative time, the graft is prepared by part of the team on a separate surgical table while the revision surgery is being performed.

Initial Graft Preparation

Microbiological culture specimens are taken before the allograft is thawed in 5% povidone-iodine solution and stripped of soft tissues.

The femur neck is cut just proximal to or even at the base of the lesser trochanter to facilitate implant insertion and version adjustment.

Leg lengthening is affected not by the level at which the neck is cut but by the length of the allograft prosthetic composite, which is determined by the level at which the distal allograft is cut. The allograft should initially be cut long to allow for adjustments.

Because the success of the procedure depends on union at the distal graft-host junction, a stable graft-host junction is crucial. Stability is achieved largely by a stepped or oblique graft-host reciprocating osteotomy. An oblique osteotomy is technically easier to achieve and allows adjustments in rotational alignment without major changes to the osteotomy.

The greater trochanter is excised to allow reattachment of the host greater trochanter. In the absence of host greater trochanter, the allograft greater trochanter is preserved along with a cuff of abductor tendons to which the host abductors can be attached.

The canal is then reamed. We use straight, rigid reamers because we prefer straight stems. Flexible reamers can be used for bowed stems. The canal is reamed just wide enough to accommodate the stem and a 2-mm cement mantle. Care is taken to avoid over-reaming, which leads to disproportionate graft resorption. A thin rim of cancellous bone is preferably preserved for cement-bone interdigitation. We use a long stem, usually 13 to 14 mm in diameter (CRC, Zimmer, Warsaw, Ind), or a modular ZMR (Zimmer) with distal nongrit blasted flutes, which is also proximally narrow. A large-diameter stem for distal press-fit requires excessive graft reaming because the canal is usually narrower than host distal femur. We believe that distal stem press-fit is not essential for construct stability. We achieve stability by cementing the stem to the graft but not the distal host femur, allowing compression and micromotion at the host-graft junction to promote union. The allograft is then returned to the povidone-iodine bath until the main surgical team has finished preparation of the host-femoral junction, at which time a reciprocal and matching cut is made in the allograft at the appropriate location, and the allograft prosthetic construct is trialed, before the definitive stem is cemented into the allograft.

SURGICAL APPROACH

We use a lateral longitudinal skin incision and try to incorporate previous scars. For a loosened stem, a trochanteric slide approach in conjunction with a lateral longitudinal femoral split is usually sufficient for good exposure to the acetabulum and femur. The greater trochanteric-abductor unit can be reattached later to the proximal femoral allograft.

We have modified the trochanteric slide by leaving the posterior 1 cm of the greater trochanter, posterior capsule, and external rotators intact with the shaft to decrease the risk of posterior dislocation.[16]

Because the greater trochanter is usually very thin in the setting of proximal femoral deficiency, care is taken to maintain continuity with the abductors and vastus lateralis to decrease the risk of subsequent trochanteric escape.

The vastus lateralis is then partially detached laterally from the lateral intermuscular septum by blunt dissection to the intended level of distal femoral osteotomy. This level is determined during preoperative planning and intraoperatively by identifying the extent of femoral deficiency where healthy distal femur starts. Care is given to cauterize the perforating vessels away from the septum to avoid vessel retraction, difficult hemostatic control, heavy blood loss, and postoperative hematoma formation.

The trochanteric fragment is then reflected anteriorly and the lateral proximal femur is split longitudinally in the coronal plane to the intended level of the distal femoral osteotomy. At this level, a transverse saw cut is made halfway through the diameter of the femur from lateral to medial, taking care to keep the medial half of the femur intact.

With multiple osteotomes fitted through the lateral longitudinal split and engaging the undersurface of the anterior femoral cortex, the anterolateral proximal femur is pried forward; similarly, the posterolateral proximal femur is pried backward—akin to an open book—from the lateral aspect of the femur. At the level of the transverse cut, care is taken to leave the medial aspect of the femur intact to fashion a step-cut or oblique-cut osteotomy with optimal host bone preservation. The length of the step- or oblique-cut should be at least 2 cm (Figs. 99-2 and 99-3).

Any residual host proximal femur is preserved with soft tissue attached to serve as vascularized autograft for wrapping around the distal allograft-host junction to promote union. Any residual host proximal femur is also

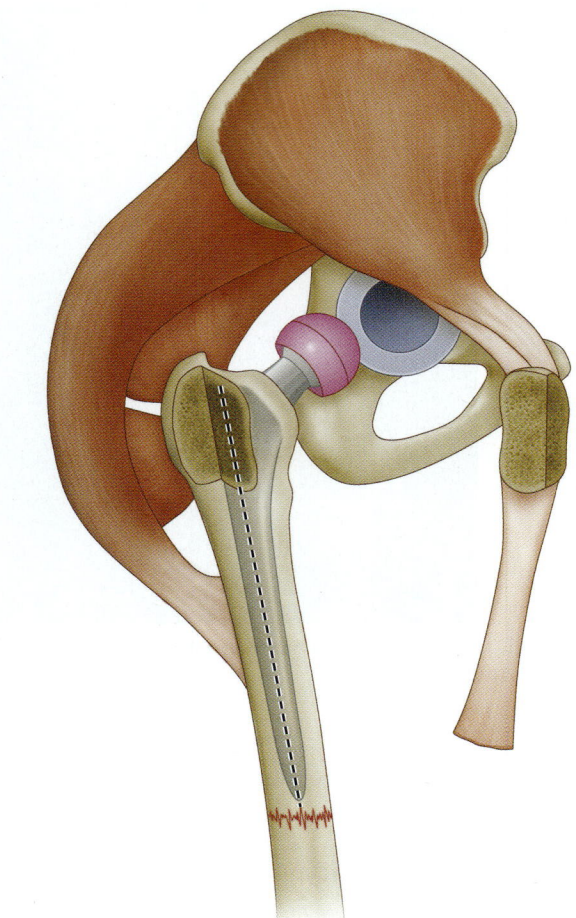

Figure 99-2. The external rotators remain attached to the femur when the posterior 1 cm of the greater trochanter is left attached to the femur. *(Redrawn from Kellett CF, Boscainos PJ, Maury A, et al: Proximal femoral allograft treatment of Vancouver type-B3 periprosthetic femoral fractures after total hip arthroplasty: surgical technique. J Bone Joint Surg Am 89[Suppl 2, Pt 1]:68–79, 2007.)*

wrapped around the proximal allograft. The proximal host femur does not replace the proximal allograft, but union at this interface may reinforce the allograft. The success of the allograft prosthetic composite is determined by the critical union at the distal graft-host junction and not at the host-graft interface proximal to the junction because usually very little proximal host bone is available to wrap around the proximal allograft.

Leg Length Reference and Monitoring

A Steinman pin is inserted over the iliac crest and is referenced to a fixed point in the host distal femur for leg length monitoring during the operation. The distal reference point should be in healthy host bone distal to the allograft and marked by a drill hole. The distance from the Steinman pin to the distal reference point is measured. Preoperative leg length differences can be used to guide leg length adjustments during surgery.

At this point, the hip is dislocated and the old loosened femoral component usually is easily removed.

Preparation of the Host Distal Femur

The shape of the residual host distal femur is assessed to determine the best-suited cut (stepped or oblique) for minimal bone sacrifice to optimize host distal femur bone stock for stem fixation. A stepped cut requires a minimum length of 2 cm and has a usual length of 4 to 5 cm. An oblique cut may be easier to work with, and adjustments in obliquity and orientation can be made more easily without significant changes to the osteotomy. With an oblique osteotomy, rotation of the proximal fragment to obtain optimal anteversion is very difficult. In this case, a modular stem such as the ZMR allows fine-tuning of anteversion, provided a small proximal body is used. Once optimal anteversion is determined, the final stem can be assembled and cemented into the allograft in the correct orientation.

If the graft diameter is narrower than the host such that the graft can be telescoped into the distal femur by 1 to 2 cm with reasonable fit, the host femur can be spared of cuts to optimize bone stock preservation.

The host distal femur is reamed to an extent that is just enough to remove residual cement and granulation tissue. Bony reamings are saved and later are used as morselized autografts at the graft-host junction to enhance union. In addition, any resected bone from the proximal femur and any acetabular reamings can be used as autograft at the junction. When the reaming position or depth within the medullary canal is in doubt, intraoperative radiographic imaging should be employed (Figs. 99-4 and 99-5).

Final Graft Preparation

A trial reduction is performed to estimate graft length as soon as the acetabular bed is sufficiently prepared to seat a trial cup. The trial stem of preplanned length

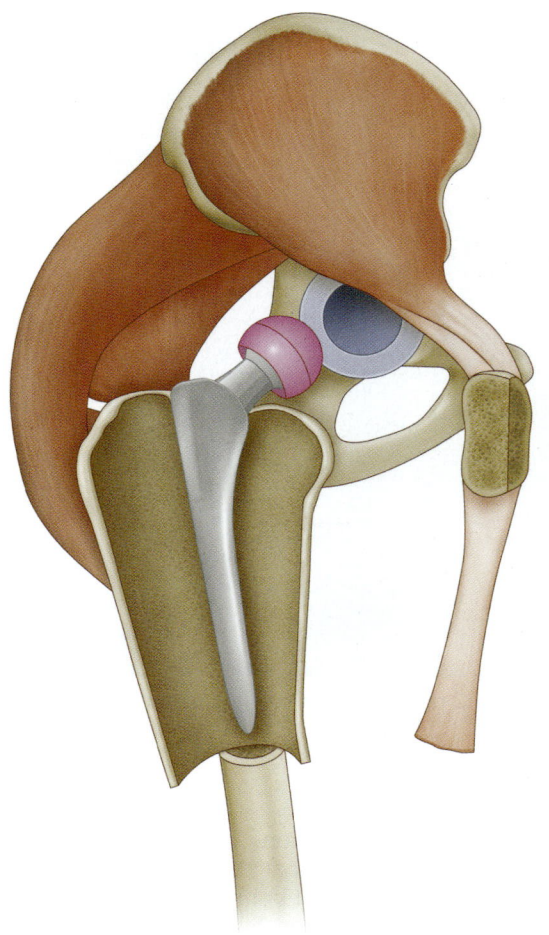

Figure 99-3. Lateral cortex osteotomy of the proximal part of the femur. *(Redrawn from Kellett CF, Boscainos PJ, Maury A, et al: Proximal femoral allograft treatment of Vancouver type-B3 periprosthetic femoral fractures after total hip arthroplasty: surgical technique. J Bone Joint Surg Am 89[Suppl 2, Pt 1]:68–79, 2007.)*

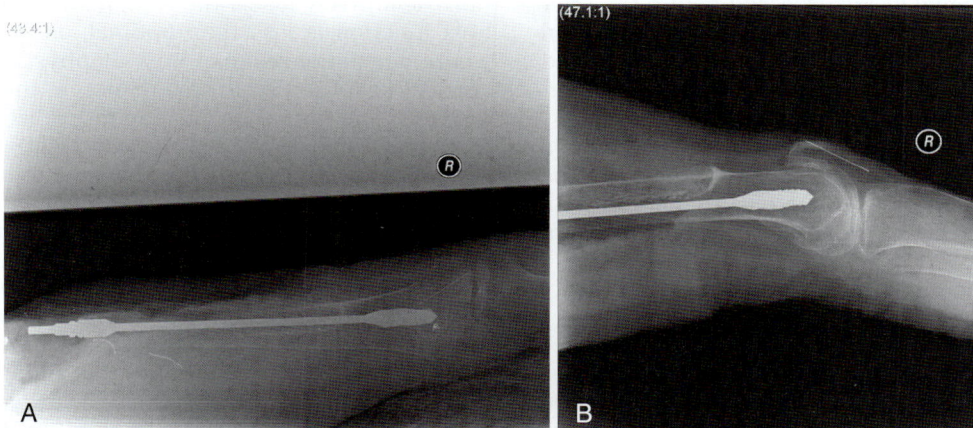

Figure 99-4. Intraoperative **(A)** anteroposterior and **(B)** lateral distal femoral radiographs showing satisfactory alignment and depth of a reaming tip within the medullary canal.

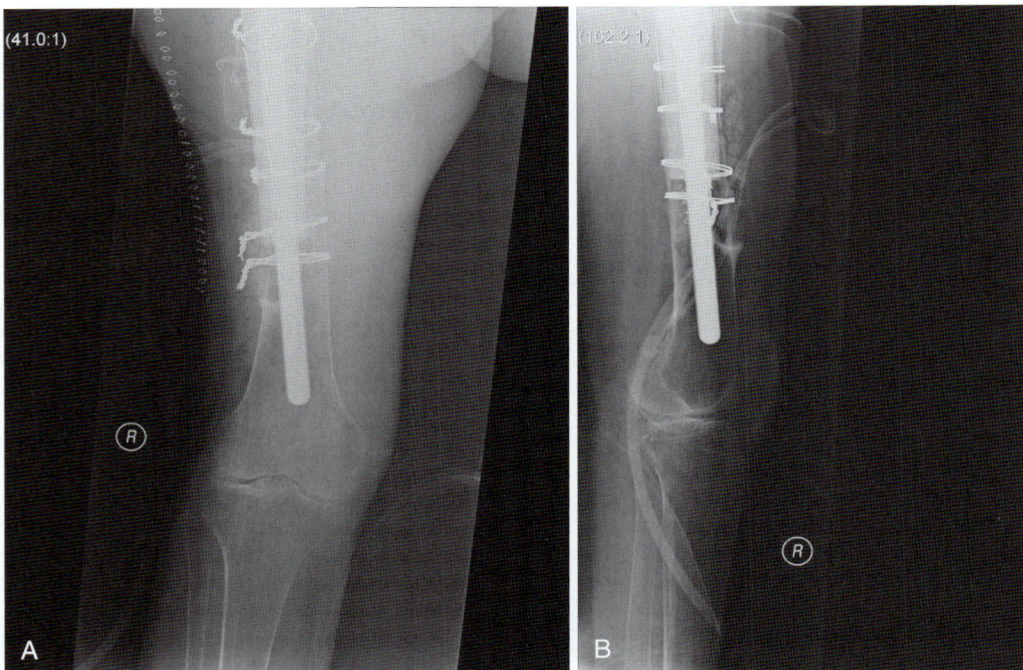

Figure 99-5. Postoperative **(A)** anteroposterior and **(B)** lateral distal femoral radiographs showing alignment and positioning of a definitive implant tip.

is inserted into the host distal femur, and the hip is reduced into the trial cup. Traction is applied to the leg, and the distance from the tip of the host greater trochanter to the host distal femur is taken as an estimate for the graft length. Because graft length determines the amount of leg lengthening, one should take into account the leg length discrepancy due to subsidence or periprosthetic fracture when estimating graft length. The graft is cut to a longer length than the estimated length to allow for adjustments. The shape and rotational orientation of the host femur cut are noted, and the reciprocal cut on the graft is marked with an indelible marker.

The distal end of the graft is cut and the stem is inserted into the graft without cement for another trial reduction. Graft length, with regard to soft tissue tension, and junctional fit are assessed before the graft is re-marked for adjustment cuts. Graft-host rotation alignment and stem neck anteversion are assessed and marked to ensure optimal combined cup-stem anteversion for optimal stability and range of movement.

Adjustment cuts are made on the graft and the whole construct is reduced so that radiographs can be obtained in AP and lateral views to ensure that the stem is central within the host femur and the level of the stem tip is satisfactory.

The stem is cemented into the graft while the acetabular reconstruction is being completed.

Before cementation, the graft is washed with 5% povidone-iodine solution, then with 1% hydrogen peroxide solution, and finally with Bacitracin solution (50,000 units per liter of 0.9% normal saline solution) before it is dried with sponges. During cementation, finger pressurization over the distal canal will optimize

cement-bone interdigitation. Ensure that cement is cleared from the surfaces at the distal end of the graft to allow optimal graft-host bone-to-bone surface contact to enhance junctional union. Similarly, cement is cleared from the graft trochanteric cut surface to enhance host trochanteric reattachment and union.

The allograft prosthetic composite is then trialed with an appropriate neck length to optimize soft tissue tension. Check leg length and confirm satisfactory combined anteversion of neck and cup. Adjust neck length and re-cut graft if necessary (Fig. 99-6).

Final Step

On satisfactory radiologic confirmation of stem position, definitively insert the APC. If stability at the graft-host junction is less than optimal, as in the situation where very little residual host diaphysis is left, use of cortical strut allograft to reinforce the junction is advised. The liberal use of any morselized bony autograft to fill gaps at the graft-host junction is strongly advised. Gel foam sheets may be used to hold the autograft in place. The host cortical shell with soft tissue attachment is pulled down distally to wrap around the distal graft-host junction to act as vascularized autograft. Multiple cerclage wires are used to hold the construct. The host greater trochanter is attached to the proximal allograft with stainless steel wires (16 G or 1.27 mm) with morselized autograft filling any gaps. If the host greater trochanter is destroyed, the host abductor tendon can be attached to the proximal allograft with anchor sutures or to attached abductor tendon allograft if available. Remnants of the host

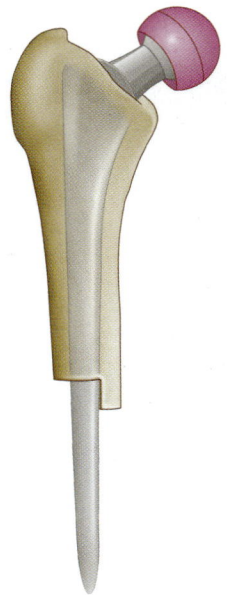

Figure 99-6. The implant is cemented into the allograft and is now ready to be inserted into the host femur. *(Redrawn from Kellett CF, Boscainos PJ, Maury A, et al: Proximal femoral allograft treatment of Vancouver type-B3 periprosthetic femoral fractures after total hip arthroplasty: surgical technique. J Bone Joint Surg Am 89[Suppl 2, Pt 1]:68–79, 2007.)*

proximal cortical shell, usually scarce but preferably still with soft tissue attachment, can be wrapped around the proximal allograft with multiple cerclage wires.

In a proximal femoral replacement, the remnants of the proximal femur from a trochanteric osteotomy or an extended trochanteric osteotomy are attached to or wrapped around the proximal femoral prosthesis with multiple cerclage wires. If the host greater trochanter is destroyed, reconstruction options include the use of a Prolene mesh or Gortex graft to suture the abductor tendons onto the proximal femoral prosthesis (Figs. 99-7 through 99-9).

VARIATIONS/UNUSUAL SITUATIONS

Patients with severe proximal femoral deficiency who require the use of APC for revision THR usually have had multiple previous hip operations and as a result poor abductor function. This increases the risk of instability and dislocation despite best attempts at abductor repair. In such situations, large-diameter bearings and constrained liners may help prevent instability and dislocation. However, the use of large-diameter bearings instead of constrained liners for added stability is preferred when acetabular reconstruction is extensive, especially with concurrent use of acetabular allograft, to avoid acetabular shell pullout risk in the early postoperative period. It has to be kept in mind, however, that large femoral heads cannot be used if the acetabular component is excessively abducted because this may lead to liner fracture.

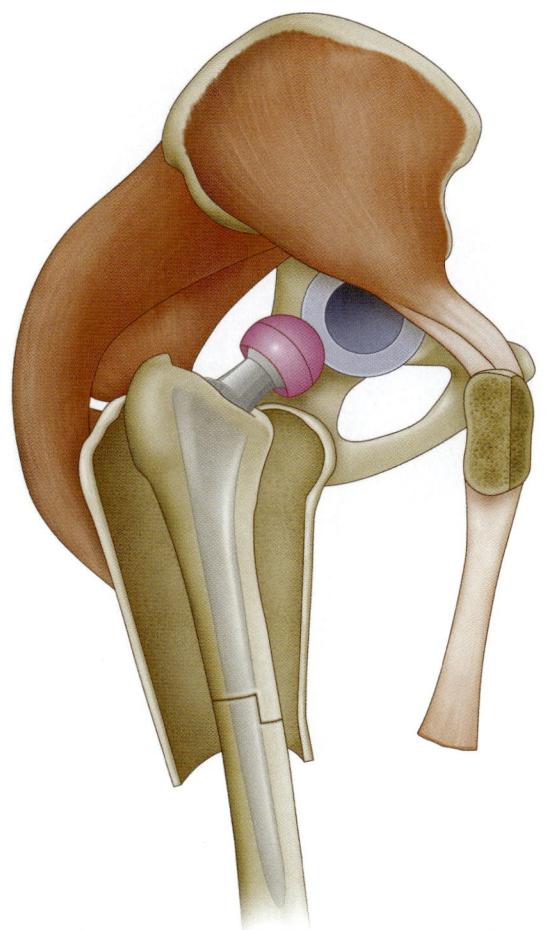

Figure 99-7. The allograft-prosthesis component inserted into the host. *(Redrawn from Kellett CF, Boscainos PJ, Maury A, et al: Proximal femoral allograft treatment of Vancouver type-B3 periprosthetic femoral fractures after total hip arthroplasty: surgical technique. J Bone Joint Surg Am 89[Suppl 2, Pt 1]:68–79, 2007.)*

When limb lengthening is anticipated to be at or beyond the recommended limits, we will plan for an on-table "wake-up test." The anesthetist's cooperation is sought and spinal or epidural anesthesia avoided. Just before general anesthetic induction, the patient is primed to obey instructions for active toe dorsiflexion; the toe dorsiflexes are quickest to be affected when the sciatic nerve is stretched. Intraoperatively, trial reduction of the hip is coordinated with the anesthetist waking the patient up to perform active toe dorsiflexion under the rehearsed instructions. Optimal analgesia is maintained throughout. If dorsiflexion of the toes is absent on the operated leg but present in the unoperated leg, the patient is immediately put back under general anesthesia, the hip re-dislocated, and leg length reduced accordingly.

It is rare for the host canal to be too narrow in comparison with the allograft canal because cortical thinning due to osteolysis and cavitation expands the host canal. The host canal is much more frequently, if not almost always, wider than the graft canal. Occasionally,

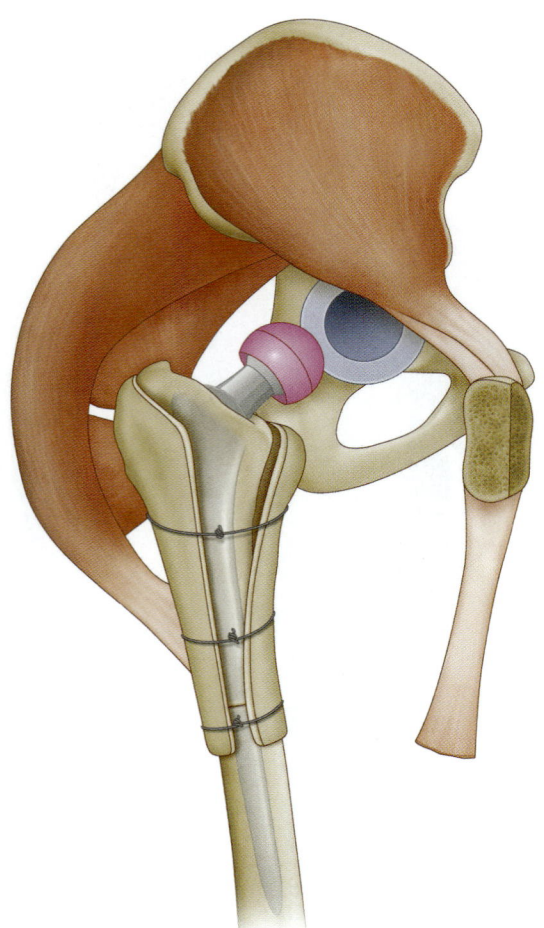

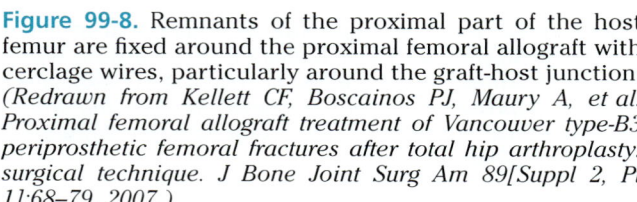

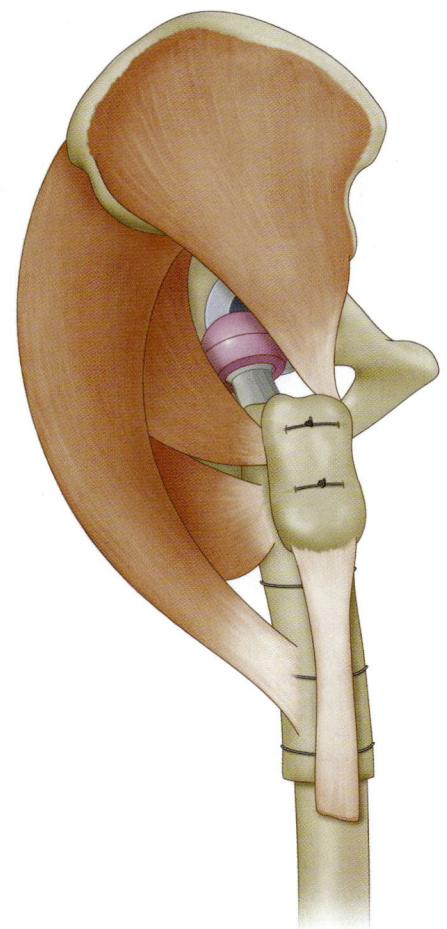

Figure 99-8. Remnants of the proximal part of the host femur are fixed around the proximal femoral allograft with cerclage wires, particularly around the graft-host junction. *(Redrawn from Kellett CF, Boscainos PJ, Maury A, et al: Proximal femoral allograft treatment of Vancouver type-B3 periprosthetic femoral fractures after total hip arthroplasty: surgical technique. J Bone Joint Surg Am 89[Suppl 2, Pt 1]:68–79, 2007.)*

Figure 99-9. Reattachment of the greater trochanter. *(Redrawn from Kellett CF, Boscainos PJ, Maury A, et al: Proximal femoral allograft treatment of Vancouver type-B3 periprosthetic femoral fractures after total hip arthroplasty: surgical technique. J Bone Joint Surg Am 89[Suppl 2, Pt 1]:68–79, 2007.)*

the host canal is wider than the outer diameter of the graft. This may occur when very little residual host distal diaphysis is left, and the relatively softer host cancellous metaphyseal canal easily accepts the distal allograft. Distal allograft telescoping into the distal host canal by 1 to 2 cm may increase initial graft-host bone-to-bone surface contact to enhance healing and union, provided there is initial fixation stability. In the absence of initial fixation stability at the intussuscepting graft-host junction, there is a risk of further uncontrolled subsidence of the APC into the host distal femur in the postoperative period. Subsequently, penetration of the knee joint by the stem tip may present as pseudo-locking at the patellofemoral joint. Initial junctional stabilization achieved by cementing the distal stem into host distal femur may cause stress shielding and proximal allograft resorption and may increase the risks of junctional nonunion and stem fatigue fracture.[7] Plate fixation at the graft-host junction may be an option, but

screws in the proximal allograft may increase the allograft fracture risk.[17] Distal stem press-fit stability is difficult to achieve without over-reaming, possibly detrimentally, of the proximal allograft. In addition, a tight press-fit distally may reduce loading of the allograft host-bone junction, possibly leading to nonunion. If junctional stability is not perfect, we use cortical strut grafts held with multiple cerclage wires to act as biological plates for enhancing junctional stability. This is coupled with delayed weight bearing until radiologic evidence of bony union is seen. Ideally, preoperative templating for ordering of and availability of grafts with compatible diameters would minimize the risk of such difficulties.

POSTOPERATIVE CARE

Antibiotic prophylaxis for infection is continued postoperatively as per each institution's protocol. Urinary catheters are discontinued as quickly as possible. In addition, prophylaxis for thromboembolic disease as per institutional policy is started postoperatively.

Delayed weight-bearing mobilization is advised. Our patients are allowed early postoperative mobilization with crutches but with no weight bearing through the operated leg until radiographic evidence of union (trabecular bridging) is seen at the graft-host junction; this usually occurs between 8 and 12 weeks. Active hip abduction is avoided for 8 weeks to allow union of the host greater trochanter to the allograft. Physical therapy for abductor strengthening and gait training is started at 8 weeks postoperatively.

RESULTS

When comparing outcomes for APC or PFR, one needs to bear in mind that different studies using different techniques with different indications have different lengths of follow-up and employ different outcome measures.

Survivorship

Survivorship for APC ranges from 81% (n = 21 with 6 years' follow-up)[10] to 84% (n = 50 with 16 years'

follow-up)[5] to 90% (n = 30 with 2 years' follow-up).[18] Table 99-1 show survivorships in various studies and includes indication, technique, number of cases, and follow-up in years. Failure for any cause that required re-revision was used as the endpoint. Survivorships for PFR are similarly presented in Table 99-2. Results of comparative studies of PFR versus APC are presented in Table 99-3.

A trend has been noted toward longer survivorship with APC when compared with PFR. Most of these studies were single retrospective series without controls. Three comparative studies examined APC and PFR, and all procedures were performed for reconstruction after tumor resection. All of these studies were nonrandomized retrospective studies with associated limitations and included varying numbers of patients who had received adjuvant chemo/radiotherapy. Farid and associates[13] showed a Kaplan-Meier survivorship of 86% at 10 years for both PFR and APC. Anract and colleagues[14] reported better survivorship with APC compared with PFR (85% vs. 70%) with the same case numbers (18 and 18), but follow-up periods were relatively short and differed between the two groups (4.1 vs. 6 years, respectively). Zehr and coworkers[11] reported better 10-year survivorship with APC compared with PFR (76% vs. 58%).

Table 99-1. Survivorships in Various Studies

Study	Indication	Technique	Number of Hips	Follow-up mean, yr	Survivorship, %
Chandler et al[18]	Non-neoplastic	DPF	30	2	90
Haddad et al[7]	Non-neoplastic	Cemented distally	40	8.8	90
Graham & Stockley[8]	Non-neoplastic	Junction fit/DPF	25	4.4	88
Safir et al[5]	Non-neoplastic	Junction fit/wires	50	16	84
Maury et al[9]	Periprosthetic #	Junction fit/wires	25	5.1	84
Langlais et al[10]	Neoplastic	Cemented distally	21	6	81

DPF, Distal press-fit.

Table 99-2. Survivorships for PFR

Study	Indication	Technique	Number of Hips	Follow-up mean, yr	Survivorship, %
Parvizi et al[19]	Non-neoplastic	Modular PFR	48	3	KM 87%@1 yr; 73%@5 yr
Malkani et al[20]	Non-neoplastic	Cemented distally	32	11.1	KM 64%@12 yr
Klein et al[21]	Periprosthetic #	Cemented distally	21	3.2	90%

KM, Kaplan-Meier survivorship; *PFR*, proximal femoral replacement; *#*, fracture.

Table 99-3. Results of Comparative Studies of PFR Versus APC

Study	Indication	Technique	Number of Hips	Follow-up mean, yr	Survivorship, %
Farid et al[13]	PFR—neoplastic	Cemented distally	52	12.2	KM 6%@10 yr
	APC—neoplastic	Variable/unspecified	20	6.3	KM 86%@10 yr
Zehr et al[11]	PFR—neoplastic	Cemented distally	18	10	58%
	APC—neoplastic	Cemented distally	14	10	76%
Anract et al[14]	PFR—neoplastic	Cemented distally	20	6	70%
	APC—neoplastic	Cemented distally	21	4.1	85%

APC, Allograft prosthetic composite; *KM*, Kaplan-Meier survivorship; *PFR*, proximal femoral replacement.

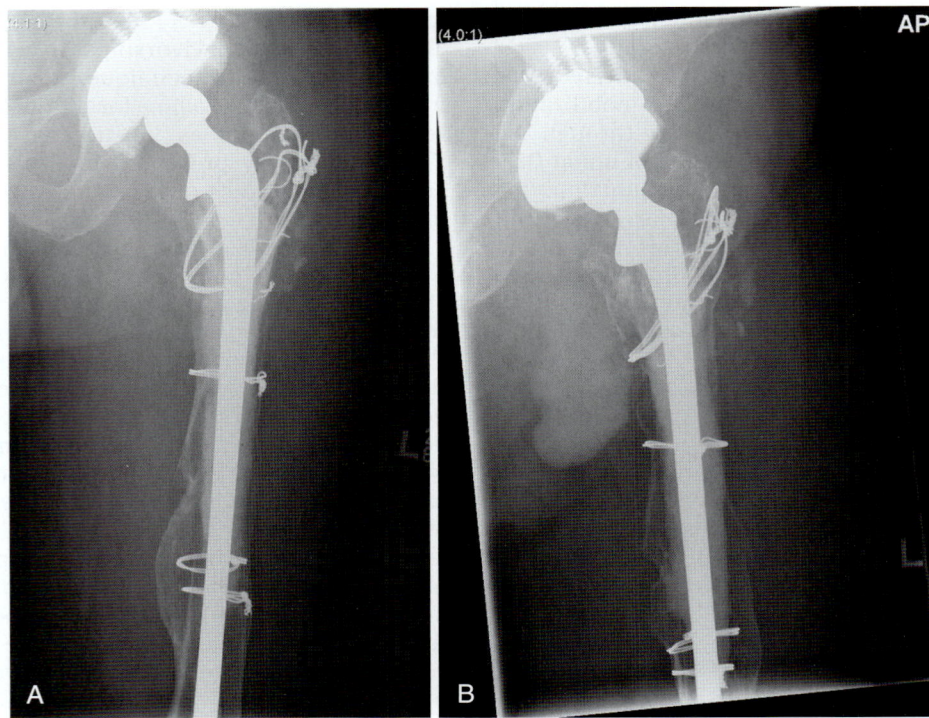

Figure 99-10. A, Anteroposterior and **(B)** lateral hip and proximal femur radiographs. Note intact trochanter and abductor mechanism.

Figure 99-11. A, Anteroposterior and **(B)** lateral distal femoral radiographs. Note healing at the graft-host junction and incorporation of the proximal allograft and cortical struts.

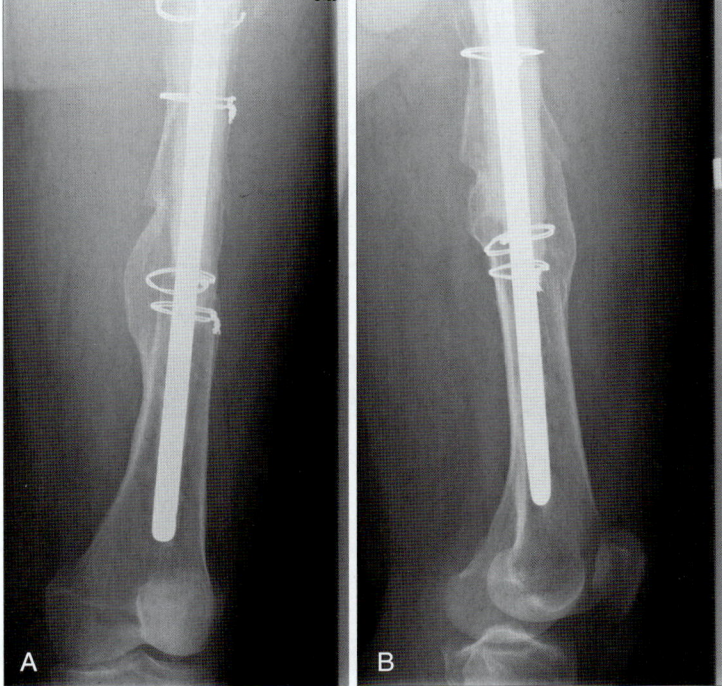

Examples of radiographs of a patient with an APC at 20 years' post surgery are given in Figures 99-10 and 99-11.

Functional Outcomes

Although the functional outcomes of various studies have different outcome measures, a trend has been noted toward better abductor function, hip stability, and walking ability in patients with APC compared with patients with PFR. This trend is observed in studies with reconstruction for neoplastic and non-neoplastic causes. Most authors attribute better functional outcomes to better trochanter-abductor mechanism repair with the use of APC. In all three comparative studies for APC and PFR, superior functional outcomes with APC

Table 99-4. Summary of Functional Outcomes from Various Studies

Study	Limp/Abductor Weakness (%)	Mobility/ Activity, %	Instability, %	Pain, %	Hip Scores (HS)/ Other Scores
APC					
Chandler et al[18]	Troch Migration 10	Independent 40 Cane 47, crutch 13	–	–	Harris HS + 43
Haddad et al[7]	Troch escape 27	Inactive 2.5 Low 17.5, mid 53 High/very high 27	11	55	Harris HS + 40
Graham & Stockley[8]	Troch nonunion 36 Fibrous or bony union 64	–	–	–	Oxford HS 34
Safir et al[5]	Troch migration 26	–	–	–	WOMAC 64.6 SF12 (physical) 34.7 SF12 (mental) 51.4
Maury et al[9]	Mild 75, severe 25 Troch migration 24 Wchair 4	Independent 33 Walking aid 63	–	12	Harris HS 70.8 Trendelenburg 71
Langlais et al[10]	3-4/5 abd power 80 Abd dysfunction 20	Very good 36 Good 46, fair 18	–	–	MTSFS 77
PFR					
Parvizi et al[19]	–	Independent 19 Walking aid 55 Wchair 26	18.6	49	Harris HS + 27.8
Malkani et al[20]	Severe limp 48	Cane/crutch 65 Indoors/Wchair 28	–	27	Harris HS + 30 Mayo Clinic HS + 27
Klein et al[21]	–	Independent 38 Cane 19, crutch 14 Walker 24, Wchair 5	–	5	Harris HS 71
Comparative					
Zehr et al[11]					
PFR	Limp 90 Cane 60	Independent 40	16.7	–	MTSFS 80
APC	Limp 64.3 Cane 43	Independent 57	0	–	MTSFS 87
Farid et al[13]					
PFR	Mean 2.8/5 Trendelenburg 98	MTS gait 2.7	–	–	MTSFS 70
APC	Mean 4.6/5 Trendelenburg <50	MTS gait 3.8	–	–	MTSFS 82
Anract et al[14]					
PFR	Trendelenburg 83	Crutch 39	–	0	MTSFS 75
APC	Trendelenburg 55	Crutch 11	–	0	MTSFS 83

APC, Allograft prosthetic composite; *MTSFS,* Musculoskeletal Tumor Society Function Score; *PFR,* proximal femoral replacement; *SF,* short form; *troch,* trochanter; *Wchair,* wheelchair; *WOMAC,* Western Ontario and McMaster University Osteoarthritis Index.

use have been consistently noted in all modalities for functional comparison: abductor strength, hip stability, walking ability, and Musculoskeletal Tumor Society Function Scores (MTSFS).

Table 99-4 summarizes functional outcomes from various studies.

COMPLICATIONS

Dislocation

In patients undergoing reconstruction for non-neoplastic causes, dislocation rates were generally higher with PFR use (9.5% to 22%) compared with APC use (0 to 16.6%) (see Table 99-5). In patients with reconstruction for neoplastic causes, three comparative studies for APC and PFR showed variable results. Farid and coworkers[13] reported better dislocation rates with PFR use (5.8%) compared with APC use (10%), but different case numbers were reported in each group (52 vs. 20), and patients with pelvic resection were not excluded from the study. Anract and associates[14] showed no difference in dislocation rates between the two groups (5%) with equal case numbers (18 and 18) in each group but did not mention the exclusion of patients with pelvic resection. Zehr and colleagues[11] showed better dislocation rates with APC use (0%) compared with PFR use (28%) with equal case numbers (18 and 18) in each group and exclusion of patients with pelvic resection.

Infection

In patients with reconstruction for non-neoplastic causes, there seems to be a trend toward lower infection rates with APC use (0 to 5%) compared with PFR use (2.3% to 9.5%). In patients with reconstruction for neoplastic causes, the difference in infection rates between APC use (0 to 17%) and PFR use (6% to 11%) is not clear. Heterogeneous use of adjuvant chemotherapy or radiotherapy (immunosuppressants) further complicates assessment.

Nonunion

Nonunion at the distal graft-host junction is a concern for APC use because this may lead to composite instability and failure. The studies reviewed show an incidence between 6% and 28.6%. Junctional nonunion rates did not directly correlate with composite failure rates. Many reports of nonunion were based on radiographic assessment. Radiographic nonunion indicates lack of bony healing at the graft-host junction; of these, a proportion may be asymptomatic fibrous nonunions. In the study by Graham and Stockley,[8] 5 cases (20 %) of radiographic junctional nonunion were noted in their series. Of these, 1 patient was symptomatic with persistent thigh pain. Revision surgery with iliac autograft and plating at the junction facilitated union and resolved the pain. The rest of the patients were asymptomatic with a fibrous nonunion.

Loosening

In patients with reconstruction for non-neoplastic causes, the rates of loosening with PFR use (0 to 13.3%) was comparable with that seen with APC use (0 to 12.5%). In patients undergoing reconstruction for neoplastic causes, the rate of loosening was higher with PFR use (6% to 22%) compared with APC use (0 to 11%). Loosening has been correlated with failure, which required revision surgery.

Resorption

In patients with reconstruction for non-neoplastic causes, the incidence of significant graft resorption with APC use varied between 2% and 24%. Classifications for graft resorption and criteria that constituted significant resorption differed between studies. Bony resorption with PFR use was not commonly noted. Anract and associates[14] noted bony resorption in 24% of cases with PFR use compared with 47% of cases with APC use. The radiologic appearance of significant graft resorption may be worrisome, but in many series with APC use, the extent of graft resorption stabilized after several years and did not correlate with graft failure. Safir and colleagues[5] reported on 50 cases of APC use with a minimum follow-up of 15 years (16.2 years; mean, 15 to 22 years). In all, 29 cases (58%) showed minor resorption without failure and 1 case (2%) showed severe resorption, which led to failure and required revision surgery. Although resorption in PFR per se does not lead to reoperation, another related mechanism of failure with PFR is fracture of the stem. The distal stem remains well fixed within the cement mantle, but the proximal portion of the host bone resorbs because effective extracortical bone bridging does not really occur, and causes

increased stress on the stem in the distal femur. These stems generally are designed with a short solid segment at the proximal end of the stem, with the remainder of the stem having rounded flutes to enhance cement fixation. Stress fractures have been seen at the junction between the proximal solid segment and the fluted portion, particularly with 11-mm or smaller stems. If possible, it is best to avoid these small stems when PFRs are used.

Table 99-5 summarizes the complications reported from various studies.

CURRENT CONTROVERSIES AND FUTURE CONSIDERATIONS

The rate of significant radiologic allograft resorption varies between reports. This may be due to the use of different criteria to define significant resorption in different studies. The extent of graft resorption is affected by surgical technique and loading and stress shielding of the graft. Although the radiologic appearances of severe graft resorption may cause concern, long-term outcomes for this group of patients are still unknown. Safir and coworkers[5] reported long-term results (minimum, 15 years) for APC with very few clinical problems related to graft resorption. A relatively low number of cases (2 of 50, or 2%) presented with severe radiologic graft resorption. This may be related to the uncemented distal fixation technique, which allowed loading of the graft-host junction and avoided stress shielding. In contrast to Haddad and associates,[7] for whom the distal stem was cemented into host femur, a larger number of cases (7 of 40, or 17.5%) of severe resorption were observed. At a mean of 8.8 years after surgery, survivorship was 90%, although 55% of patients reported noticeable pain. Longer-term follow-up is needed to assess the consequences for this subgroup of patients with radiologic severe graft resorption. The incidence of long-term mechanical strength and deterioration of the allograft with increased incidence of stem fatigue fracture is unknown in this subgroup. The effect of bisphophonate use in this setting to prevent graft resorption or restore graft bone density is unknown. And if it does occur, will it affect clinical outcomes?

The rate of dislocation not only reflects the quality of femoral reconstruction in conjunction with abductor repair, it also reflects the quality of the acetabular reconstruction. Hence assessing abductor function or the presence of a Trendelenburg sign or limp may be a better marker for hip instability attributed to femoral reconstruction than assessing dislocation rate alone. Although dislocation rates are generally better with the use of APC compared with PFR, Farid and coworkers[13] showed better dislocation rates in PFR, and Anract and associates[14] reported similar dislocation rates between PFR and APC, given some study limitations. Chandler and colleagues[18] described a relatively high dislocation rate (16.6%) with APC. Although this was not a comparative study, the dislocation rate was higher than in other studies with PFR use. When abductor function and limping are viewed as outcome measures, a clearer

Table 99-5. Summary of Complications from Various Studies

Study	Dislocation, %	Infection, %	Nonunion, %	Loosening, %	Significant Resorption, %	Others, %
APC						
Chandler et al[18]	16.6	3.3	13.6	–	3.3	
Haddad et al[7]	10	5	9	0	17.5	Graft #2.5
Graham[13]	0	4	20	4	8	
						Foot drop 4, Troch Wire removal 8
Safir et al[5]	8	4	6	12	2	Vascular 2, nerve 2
Maury et al[9]	8	0	16	12.5	24	DVT 8, MI 8, CVA 4, Renal failure (fatal) 4
Langlais et al[10]	0	0	28.6	14.3	4.8	
PFR						
Parvizi et al[19]	14	2.3	–	–	–	
Malkani et al[20]	22	6.3	–	13.3	–	Stem #3.3
Klein et al[21]	9.5	9.5	–	0	9.5	Peri-prosthetic Fx 4.8
Comparative						
Zehr et al[11]						
PFR	28	6	–	6	–	Stem Fx 11
APC	–	17	7	–	–	
Farid et al[13]						
PFR	5.8	4	–	10	–	
APC	10	5	10	0	–	
Anract et al[14]						
PFR	5	11	–	22	24	
APC	5	11	14	11	47 (total/partial)	

APC, Allograft prosthetic composite; *CVA,* cerebrovascular accident; *DVT,* deep vein thrombosis; *MI,* myocardial infarction; *PFR,* proximal femoral replacement; *Fx,* fracture.

trend is presented with better results seen with APC use, particularly in comparative studies of PFR versus APC. Recent advances in biologically compatible alloy and porous coat technology for incorporation into PFR may improve trochanteric healing and abductor function, but results are presently preliminary.

The use of PFR in the younger and higher-demand patient is controversial owing to concerns over long-term loosening and failure with further difficulty in revision surgery. With advances in surface metal technology to improve host bony ingrowth and long-term implant fixation, the indications for PFR use in younger and higher-demand patients may evolve.

The use of APC theoretically has the potential to restore proximal femoral bone stock. Controversy arose because this would imply that the bone stock restored by the allograft would aid future femoral reconstruction. Although the proximal femoral allograft may incorporate with graft-host junctional union, unlike morselized allograft, the structural allograft does not convert to host bone and remains as dead bone. Revision surgery for an APC usually involves removing the proximal femoral allograft, and it is difficult to remove a long stem that is cemented into the allograft. Nevertheless, occasional reports[5] have stated that proximal femoral allograft removal was difficult because it was so well incorporated into host bone that the graft was left in place and the femoral stem alone was replaced.

The use of APC may preserve host bone stock by minimizing host distal canal violation to aid future reconstructions. By avoiding significant reaming and canal preparation for cementing or press-fitting the implant distally, the distal host canal is relatively preserved. Distal implant cementation is undesirable because it leads to allograft stress shielding and resorption and increases the risk of distal graft-host junctional nonunion and instability. Distal implant press-fit requires larger-diameter stems and considerable graft canal reaming to accommodate the proximal stem and the cement mantle, leading to cortical thinning and increased graft resorption risks. The proximal graft canal is usually narrower than the distal host canal, which further compounds the problem of proximal reaming to fit a large stem for distal press-fit. We believe that distal implant press-fit is not necessary for distal graft-host union. We employ a long reciprocating stepped or oblique cut at the graft-host junction bounded by multiple cerclage wires and frequently reinforced with cortical strut allograft as biological plating for initial stability.

The use of APC when less than 6 cm of host distal diaphysis remains is technically a more difficult revision compared with when greater than 6 cm of host distal diaphysis is left. This is so because the circumference of the host distal diaphysis widens into the metaphysis with substantially thinner cortices. Initial graft-host junctional stability may be difficult to achieve with short host distal femur. No studies have differentiated the two conditions in terms of the use of APC and have compared results between the two. Theoretically, results for short APC when greater than 6 cm of host distal diaphysis remains would be superior to those for long APC when less than 6 cm of host distal diaphysis is left. If this is true, then previous reports comparing APC use as a whole with PFR use may potentially understate the difference in outcomes between the two. Additional studies may be warranted to compare the use of APC versus PFR in patients in whom the remaining host distal diaphysis is greater than 6 cm. For patients with less than 6 cm host distal femur remaining, alternative treatment includes the use of total femur replacement, especially in neoplastic conditions. It would be interesting to compare the outcomes of APC with total femur replacement in patients with less than 6 cm host distal femur remaining, because both patient groups may be similarly young and active.

It would be difficult to conduct randomized controlled trials to compare results of APC versus PFR use because the patient groups are quite different, and previous studies have suggested better overall outcomes with APC use. In a situation where the patient is young and active with low anesthetic risks, where there is ready access to a bone bank and expertise in the use of APC, most surgeons would opt for the use of APC over PFR at the present time for non-neoplastic indications. This trend may change with advances in implant technology.

REFERENCES

1. Grauer JD, Amstutz HC, O'Carrol PF, Dorey FJ: Resection arthroplasty of the hip. J Bone Joint Surg Am 71:669–678, 1989.
2. Harris WH, White RE, Jr: Resection arthroplasty for nonseptic failure of total hip arthroplasty. Clin Orthop Relat Res 171:62–67, 1982.
3. Kostulk J, Alexander D: Arthrodesis for failed arthroplasty of the hip. Clin Orthop Relat Res 188:173–182, 1984
4. Sim FH, Chao EYS: Hip salvage by proximal femoral replacement. J Bone Joint Surg Am 63:1228–1239, 1981.
5. Safir O, Kellett CF, Flint M, et al: Revision of the deficient proximal femur with a proximal femoral allograft. Clin Orthop Relat Res 467:206–212, 2009.
6. Blackley HRL, Davie AM, Hutchison CR, Gross AE: Proximal femoral allografts for reconstruction of bone stock in revision arthroplasty of the hip. J Bone Joint Surg Am 83:346–354, 2001.
7. Haddad FS, Spangehl MJ, Masri BA, et al: Circumferential allograft replacement of the proximal femur. Clin Orthop Relat Res 371:98–107, 2000.
8. Graham NM, Stockley I: The use of structural proximal femoral allograft in complex revision hip arthroplasty. J Bone Joint Surg Br 86:337–343, 2004.
9. Maury AC, Pressman A, Cayen B, et al: Proximal femoral allograft treatment of Vancouver type-B3 periprosthetic femoral fractures after total hip arthroplasty. J Bone Joint Surg Am 88:953–958, 2006.
10. Langlais F, Lambotte JC, Collin P, Thomazeau H: Long-term results of allograft composite total hip prosthesis for tumor. Clin Orthop Relat Res 414:197–211, 2003.
11. Zehr R, Enneking W, Scarborough M: Allograft-prosthesis composite versus megaprosthesis in proximal femoral reconstruction. Clin Orthop Relat Res 322:207–223, 1996.
12. Mankin HJ, Gebhardt MC, Jennings LC, et al: Long-term results of allograft replacement in the management on bone tumors. Clin Orthop Relat Res 324:86–97, 1996.
13. Farid Y, Lin PP, Lewis VO, Yasko AW: Endoprosthetic and allograft-prosthetic composite reconstruction of the proximal femur for bone neoplasms. Clin Orthop Relat Res 442:223–229, 2006.
14. Anract P, Coste J, Vastel L, et al: Proximal femoral reconstruction with megaprosthesis versus allograft prosthesis composite: a comparative study of functional results, complications and longevity in 41 cases. Rev Orthop Traumatol 86:278, 2000.
15. Tomford WM: Disease transmission, sterilization, and the clinical use of musculoskeletal tissue allografts. In Tomford WM, editor: Musculoskeletal tissue banking, New York, 1993, Raven Press, pp 209–230.
16. Goodman S, Pressman A, Saastamoinen H, Gross A: Modified sliding trochanteric osteotomy in revision total hip arthroplasty. J Arthroplasty 19:1039–1041, 2004.
17. Griffiths HJ, Andersen JR, Thompson RC, et al: Radiographic evaluation of the complications of long bone allografts. Skeletal Radiol 24:283–286, 1995.
18. Chandler H, Clark J, Murphy S, et al: Reconstruction of major segmental loss of the proximal femur in revision total hip arthroplasty. Clin Orthop Relat Res 298:67–74, 1994.
19. Parvizi J, Tarity T, Slenker N, et al: Proximal femoral replacement in patients with non-neoplastic conditions. J Bone Joint Surg Am 89:1036–1043, 2007.
20. Malkani AL, Settecerri JJ, Sim FH, Chao EYS, Wallrichs SL: Long-term results of proximal femoral replacement for non-neoplastic disorders. J Bone Joint Surg 77B(3):351–356, 1995.
21. Klein GR, Parvizi J, Rapuri V, et al: Proximal femoral replacement for the treatment of periprosthetic fractures. J Bone Joint Surg Am 87:1777–1781, 2005.

FURTHER READING

Farid Y, Lin PP, Lewis VO, Yasko AW: Endoprosthetic and allograft-prosthetic composite reconstruction of the proximal femur for bone neoplasms. Clin Orthop Relat Res 442:223–229, 2006.
Aseptic loosening was the most common (10%) late complication for patients with endoprostheses. Nonunion was the most common (10%) complication for patients with allograft prosthetic composite reconstructions. All host-allograft junctions eventually healed after bone grafting. Musculoskeletal Tumor Society scores were similar for patients with endoprostheses (70%) and those with allograft-prosthetic composites (82%). The median hip abductor strength was greater for patients with allograft-prosthetic composite reconstructions (4.6 of 5) than for patients with endoprostheses (2.8 of 5). Kaplan-Meier survivorship of the implant was 86% for both groups at 10 years.

Klein GR, Parvizi J, Rapuri V, et al: Proximal femoral replacement for the treatment of periprosthetic fractures. J Bone Joint Surg Am 87:1777–1781, 2005.
Among 21 patients who had a modular femoral replacement with proximal porous coating at a mean follow-up of 3.2 years, 20 patients were able to walk and had minimal to no pain. Complications included persistent wound drainage that was treated with incision and drainage (two hips), dislocation (two hips), refracture of the femur distal to the stem (one hip), and acetabular cage failure (one hip).

Parvizi J, Tarity T, Slenker N, et al: Proximal femoral replacement in patients with non-neoplastic conditions. J Bone Joint Surg Am 89:1036–1043, 2007.
Among 43 patients with a mean follow-up of 36.5 months, significant improvement was seen in the Harris hip score (P < .05), 22 patients had excellent or good functional outcomes, 10 outcomes were fair, and 11 were poor. Ten patients required reoperation or revision because of at least one complication. Survivorship of the implant was 87% at 1 year and 73% at 5 years with revision as an endpoint.

Safir O, Kellett CF, Flint M, et al: Revision of the deficient proximal femur with a proximal femoral allograft. Clin Orthop Relat Res 467:206–212, 2009.
Among 50 patients who underwent revision hip arthroplasty with a proximal femoral allograft prosthesis composite with average follow-up of 16.2 years (range, 15 to 22 years), 2 had a failed reconstruction due to infection, 6 for aseptic loosening, 3 for nonunion, and 4 for dislocation. Revision of the proximal femoral allograft for all reasons excluding the acetabulum was performed in 7 patients. At last follow-up, 42 patients (84%) had a well-functioning construct.

Zehr R, Enneking W, Scarborough M: Allograft-prosthesis composite versus megaprosthesis in proximal femoral reconstruction. Clin Orthop Relat Res 322:207–223, 1996.
Among 33 patients who underwent proximal femoral resection for primary bone tumor, 16 patients had 18 composites, and 17 patients had 18 megaprostheses. Infection in the composite group and instability in the megaprosthesis group were common causes of failure and removal of reconstructions. The average functional evaluation in surviving patients with composites was 87% of normal, and in those with megaprostheses was 80%. Ten-year survivorship was 76% for patients with composites and 58% for those with megaprostheses.

COMPLICATIONS OF HIP ARTHROPLASTY

CHAPTER 100

Infection

Hany Bedair and Craig J. Della Valle

KEY POINTS

- Periprosthetic infection about a THA occurs at a rate of approximately 0.5% to 1%; the prevalence will increase substantially as the volume for this procedure grows to meet the projected demand.
- Prevention relies on optimizing patient selection and other host factors, improving the surgical suite environment, and administering prophylactic antibiotics.
- The most common infecting organisms are gram-positive cocci (most notably *Staphylococcus* species) but some infections may be polymicrobial.
- Diagnosis is made by a high level of suspicion, a thorough history and physical examination, screening (an erythrocyte sedimentation rate and C-reactive protein) and selected use hip joint aspiration for synovial fluid white blood cell count with differential and culture.
- Successful treatment is predicated upon the duration of the infection; it is reasonable to attempt débridement and component retention in acute postoperative and acute hematogenous infections (although staphylococcal infections seem to do worse with this strategy); chronic infections seem to be best treated by resection arthroplasty and delayed reconstruction (two-stage exchange).

INTRODUCTION

Despite the great success of total hip arthroplasty, deep infection remains one of the most devastating complications. This diagnosis almost inevitably leads to prolonged and complex treatments involving reoperation and ultimately poorer outcomes. The cost to the patient is enormous with regard to the impact on the physical and mental health state. Treatments usually are costly and place significant burden on any healthcare system. In a review of the Healthcare Cost and Utilization Project Nationwide Inpatient Sample, infection was the third most common reason (after instability and loosening) for revision surgery following total hip arthroplasty (THA) and was by far the most common reason for removal of the prosthesis.[1] Although prevention, diagnosis, and treatment have improved as surgical technique and patient management have evolved, the risk of developing this feared complication has not been

eliminated. The unfortunate state is that as the number of total hip arthroplasties expected to be performed in the coming years significantly increases, so too will the prevalence of deep infection.[2]

There exist innumerable factors in infinite permutations that may contribute to or directly result in deep infection following THA. To simplify and thus best address this complex clinical scenario, these factors can be organized into three groups: the host, the local wound environment, and the microbiology.[3] By investigating and addressing how these entities contribute singularly and interact with one another, a better understanding of the disease process and its treatment will emerge.

RISK FACTORS AND PREVENTION

The incidence of deep infection following total hip arthroplasty (THA) in the early experience of Charnley was 9% but fortunately was reduced to 1.3% in his next cohort of patients; this was attributed to air cleanliness and body exhaust attire.[4,5] Although this dramatic reduction was realized over the course of the initial 10 years of his experience into the late 1960s, currently the acknowledged rate of infection is approximately 1% at large-volume centers.[6-10] This relatively small but important improvement in incidence can be attributed to many improvements, including better patient selection, the use of prophylactic antibiotics, and operating room measures.

Improved patient selection has been predicated upon the identification of host risk factors, both systemic and local, predisposing to infection following THA. Although the physiologic stress of surgery[11] itself may predispose to infection, multiple factors should be recognized and, if possible, addressed to reduce risk. Malnutrition and advanced age are independent factors known to affect innate immunity and normal immune response by altering both humeral and cell-mediated immunity, thus increasing infection risk.[12-15] Systemically immunocompromised patients, because of underlying disease or pharmacologic treatment, are at increased risk for infection. Patients with rheumatoid arthritis and those being treated with steroid therapy are at increased risk for infection.[5,13,16,17] Obesity[18] increases the odds of infection 4.2 times. Patients with diabetes mellitus[17,19-21] appear to experience higher rates of infection compared with non-diabetic patients, with some studies suggesting an astonishingly high rate of nearly 11%[22] in matched groups. Improved perioperative glycemic control appears to reduce the risk of infection in thoracic surgery.[23] Although definitive prospective studies have not been completed as of yet, suggestions have been put forth that strict glycemic control in the perioperative period may reduce the rate of infection in THA patients.[24] Chronic renal failure patients on dialysis[25] and those with liver or kidney transplants are at increased risk for infection.[26] Patients with malignancy[19] and those with human immunodeficiency virus, particularly patients with CD4 counts below 240 cells/mm[3],[27] are also at increased risk.

Local host factors that appear to increase the risk of infection include previous infection of the native hip that has not been quiescent for longer than 10 years[28] and revision hip arthroplasty for any cause of failure.[16] Delayed wound healing and persistent wound drainage often lead to infection.[15,29]

Remote sources of infection, including skin lesions,[30,31] dental caries or procedures,[32,33] and urinary retention[34] with subsequent bladder instrumentation can lead to infection at the site of THA. Systemic predispositions should be optimally minimized and potential local and remote sources of infection should be addressed before the time of surgery.

Administration of an appropriate prophylactic antibiotic is considered the single most important factor in reducing postoperative wound infection.[3,7,8,35] The choice of a first-generation cephalosporin is often made on the basis that this agent is bacteriocidal, therapeutic against commonly infecting pathogens, and inexpensive while possessing an appropriate half-life. Antibiotic prophylaxis with cefazolin before and after surgery was demonstrated to reduce the risk of infection after THA compared with placebo from 3.3% to 0.9% in a double-blind controlled study.[36] For patients with hypersensitivity to penicillin, clindamycin or vancomycin should be considered as the alternative.[3] The preoperative dose of prophylactic antibiotic appears to be most effective in reducing infection when administered within 2 hours preceding the incision,[37] and peak bone concentrations are reached within 35 to 40 minutes after intravenous administration.[38] A multicenter prospective trial observed that when the preoperative antibiotic was given within 30 minutes before incision, the rate of surgical site incision was 1.6%, compared with 2.4% when the antibiotic was given between 31 and 60 minutes.[39] In addition, this trial found that intraoperative re-dosing in cases lasting longer than 4 hours appears to reduce the risk of infection. The postoperative duration of prophylactic treatment is debatable; a prospective double-blind multicenter trial found no difference in treatment for 24 hours versus 3 days.[40] Multiple other studies have confirmed that prolonged prophylactic treatment does not appear to be of benefit.[41,42]

Modifications of the surgical suite environment, including limiting operating room personnel or "traffic", surgical time, and the use of iodophor-incorporated drapes, have been shown to reduce the risk of infection.[43-47] Use of ultraclean air operating rooms, vertical laminar flow, and body exhaust suits has been demonstrated to favorably affect the rate of infection; however, these points have been debated.[5,48-51] Gortex gowns may be more appropriate than cotton in preventing dissemination of shed bacteria by the surgical team.[52] The use of double gloves and the choice of the optimal antiseptic remain controversial.[3] Frequent changing of the suction tip may also decrease the introduction of bacteria into the wound.[53] Pulsatile lavage and antibiotic irrigation solutions are effective in reducing the wound bacterial load.[54-56]

Although rates of bacteremia following oral procedures and diagnostic procedures of the genitourinary and gastrointestinal tracts have been documented,[57] and even though bacteremia may lead to bacterial introduction to the hip arthroplasty,[58] antibiotic prophylaxis given before these procedures remains controversial.[3] The most recent statement by the American Academy of Orthopaedic Surgery recommends "antibiotic prophylaxis for all total joint replacement patients prior to any invasive procedure that may cause bacteremia," which includes all dental procedures. The previous treatment limitation period of 2 years postoperatively has been removed, and the current recommendation is for prophylactic treatment of all patients, independent of the time elapsed since surgery. The recommended regimen is 2 g of cephalexin, cephradine, or amoxicillin 1 hour before the dental procedure. Those allergic to penicillin should receive 600 mg of clindamycin 1 hour before the procedure.

MICROBIOLOGY

A thorough understanding of the microbiological environment that leads to infection after total hip arthroplasty is crucial to successful prevention and treatment. The introduction of a biomaterial into the body has been likened to a race to inhabit the surface of the material between host tissue and bacterial pathogens.[59] Should the bacteria win this race, the result is often deep infection of the prosthesis. Introduction of bacteria to the prosthetic interface may occur at the time of surgery through direct inoculation, or it may occur at a later time through hematogenous seeding. Certain bacteria may have a predilection for seeding different biomaterials. For example, *Staphylococcus aureus* seems to preferentially seed metallic implants, and *Staphylococcus epidermidis* shows a preference toward polymers such as polyethylene and polymethylmethacrylate. Many bacteria form a mucopolysaccharide biofilm that isolates and protects organisms from the host immune response, antibiotic penetration, and even mechanical débridement. Even though approximately 75% of cultures in a single study revealed a single organism,[60] retrieval and microbiological analysis have demonstrated that the bacterial glycocalyx may harbor multiple different bacterial species.[61] This makes treatment of such patients difficult without removal of the prosthesis because the appropriate antibiotic regimen cannot be determined. Recent investigation into methods of better diagnosis through molecular diagnostic techniques, as well as more effective antibiotic biofilm penetration, has demonstrated that rifampin appears to improve treatment protocols when used synergistically with other antibiotic agents.[62,63]

In multiple large studies, the most common offending organisms are gram-positive aerobes ranging between 64% and 74% of all infecting organisms following total hip arthroplasty, with the *Staphylococcus* species (mainly *S. epidermidis* and *S. aureus*) representing approximately half of these gram-positive cocci.[7,60,64,65] Other identified gram-positive organisms include *Enterococcus*, *Streptococcus viridans*, and *Streptococcus* groups A, B, and G. There may exist a trend toward an increasing prevalence of cultures positive for *S. epidermidis* and a decrease in gram-negative bacteria.[66] Gram-negative organisms known to cause periprosthetic hip infection range from 11% to 14% of all isolated organisms and include *Pseudomonas aeruginosa, Enterobacter cloacae, Serratia marcescens, Proteus mirabilis, Escherichia coli, Klebsiella pneumoniae,* Acinetobacter species, *Moraxella nonliquefaciens,* and *Salmonella cholerasuis.* Other more rare organisms that have been reported include anaerobes, mycobacterium, and fungi.

A trend that has generated extreme concern has been the emergence of antibiotic-resistant bacterial strains. Over a 5-year period, nosocomial infection rates in intensive care unit (ICU) patients had increased by 31% for methicillin-resistant *S. aureus* and by 55% for vancomycin-resistant *Enterococcus.*[67] Fortunately, these alarming trends have not been observed to this same magnitude in periprosthetic infection of the hip, but they do exist. The rate of methicillin-resistant *S. epidermidis* in hip replacement patients was observed to be as high as 40% of 30 positive cultures[68] and 48% of 56 *S. epidermidis* cultures.[60] In a single study of 35 infected cases following THA, 54% were infected with a resistant organism, and results of treatment for these resistant organisms were far inferior to that given for sensitive organisms, with successful retention of the prosthesis in only 16%.[69] In a second study comparing the treatment of methicillin-resistant and methicillin-sensitive *S. aureus* joint infections, patients with methicillin-resistant organisms had significantly longer hospital stays and higher risks of treatment failure and removal of the prosthesis.[70] This further emphasizes the critical need for accurate diagnosis and identification of the infecting species and its sensitivities in providing optimal care for these patients.

DIAGNOSIS

The diagnosis of infection following total hip arthroplasty requires a high level of suspicion and clinical acumen. These findings should be supplemented with serologic testing, radiographic evaluation (conventional and occasionally advanced imaging), and synovial fluid analysis. Diagnosis should be confirmed by cultures and/or histopathology. The diagnosis should be established expeditiously because the treatment algorithm may shift depending on the chronicity of the infection.

A thorough history should identify any risk factors for infection, including immunocompromised states,

history of prior hip surgery, or history of infection. Persistent wound drainage postoperatively or superficial wound infection raises concern for persistent deep infection. Any abnormalities in the recovery period, including persistent postoperative or even new-onset deep pain, are causes of concern for infection. A history of fever can indicate infection; however, this finding can be unreliable. Any recent procedures that may have caused bacteremia or remote infection should be investigated.

The range of motion of the hip should be determined and compared with previous examination findings. Guarding, pain with passive motion, pain at rest, and diminishing motion are matters of concern regarding infection. A thorough neurovascular examination, as well as examination of the skin for any remote lesions, should be performed. The wound should be carefully examined for drainage, erythema, fluctuance, or an active or healed sinus tract. Wound drainage should not be cultured because these results are highly inconsistent and may only confuse the clinical picture. Empirical antibiotics for wound drainage should be avoided because they only serve to suppress and delay the definitive diagnosis.

Plain radiographs should be evaluated and compared with prior studies for the presence of rapid or progressive loosening, osteolysis, periosteal or endosteal reaction, and osteopenia. These findings, however, may have other causes. Implant loosening or osteolysis within the first 2 years is particularly suspicious for infection (Fig. 100-1). Plain radiographs can be helpful

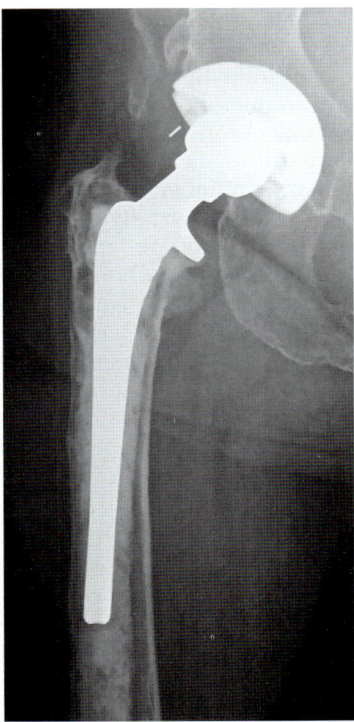

Figure 100-1. Plain radiograph of a total hip arthroplasty (THA) with a cementless acetabular component and a cemented femoral component demonstrating significant osteolysis and implant loosening of the femoral component at 21 months postoperatively, which is highly suggestive of deep infection.

should any of these findings be observed, but the lack of radiographic changes does not exclude infection.

C-reactive protein (CRP) level and erythrocyte sedimentation rate (ESR) should be the initial screening laboratory tests when infection is suspected. In a recent study of preoperative testing for more than 200 revision THAs, 100% specificity for a hip not to be infected was noted when both CRP and ESR were normal.[65] An elevated ESR (>30 mm/hr) was shown to have a sensitivity of 97%, a specificity of 39%, a positive predictive value of 42%, and a negative predictive value of 96%. A CRP value greater than 10 mg/L was shown to have a sensitivity of 94%, a specificity of 71%, a positive predictive value of 59%, and a negative predictive value of 96%. These values are consistent with the findings of previous studies, which additionally showed that when both the ESR and CRP are elevated, the probability of infection was 83%.[71]

If the ESR and CRP are elevated, or if the clinical suspicion for infection is high based on the history and physical examination aspiraiton of the hip is recommended and the fluid obtained is sent for a synovial fluid white blood cell count, differential and culture.[65,72-74] Patients should be off of antibiotics for a minimum of two weeks prior to aspiration to maximize culture yield and accuracy.[71,73] Table 100-1 provides recommended diagnostic criteria from several previously reported studies of periprosthetic infection of the hip and knee using ESR, CRP, synovial WBC, and differential. Although

these synovial tests alone may provide valuable information, the combination of these test results with ESR and CRP results can greatly improve diagnostic accuracy.[65] Bacterial growth on solid media and gross purulence visualized within the joint are generally considered diagnostic for infection,[75] although the clinician should be aware that cultures (even on solid media) can be falsely positive, and alternative causes may be proposed for purulent appearing fluid around a prosthetic hip. These include wear of a polyethylene or metal-on-metal bearing surface; thus the results of multiple tests should be analyzed together to allow the most accurate conclusion to be drawn.

Because serologic markers of inflammation (ESR, CRP), synovial WBC count, and differential are normally elevated in the early postoperative period, these tests may be of debatable utility in the first few weeks after surgery. Recent work by Bedair and associates[76] has revealed in a multicenter, multisurgeon study of almost 12,000 primary total knee arthroplasties that these markers of inflammation can be used reliably in the diagnosis of periprosthetic infection of the knee in the early postoperative period (<6 weeks from surgery), but at threshold levels higher than those previously reported. Specifically, the ESR was not found to be useful in the early postoperative period, but the CRP was useful, with an optimal cutoff value of 95 mg/L. The synovial fluid WBC count was nearly a perfect test at diagnosing infection, with a threshold of less than

Table 100-1. Previously Reported Values for Diagnosis of Periprosthetic Joint Infection

Authors	WBC, cells/μL	PMN, %	CRP, mg/L	ESR, mm/hr	Population	Time from Index Surgery, yr (mean, range)
Spangehl et al[71]	50,000*	80*	10*	30*	202 hips (35 infected)	Mentioned anecdotally, up to 11 years
Mason et al[122]	2500 cells/mL†	60	—	—	86 knees (36 infected)	Not mentioned
Trampuz et al[123]	1700	65	—	—	133 knees (34 infected)	>6 months
Parvizi et al[124]	1760	73	—	—	145 knees (78 infected); 23 hips (16 infected)	Not mentioned
Trampuz et al[125]	1700*	65*	10*	30*	331 joints (207 knees, 124 hips) (79 infected)	Not mentioned
Della Valle et al[126]	3000 cells/mL†	65*	10*	30*	94 knees (41 infected)	Not mentioned
Nilsdotter-Augustinsson et al[127]	1700*	—	10*	30*	85 knees (25 infected)	Uninfected: 9 (1-22) Infected: 3 (0.2-16)
Ghanem et al[128]	1100	64	10*	30*	429 knees (161 infected)	1.2 (0.1-7.8)
Schinsky et al[65]	4200 cells/mL†	80	10*	30*	201 hips (55 infected)	Uninfected: 8 Infected: 4.5 (including 7 <6 weeks)
Parvizi et al[129]	1100	64	10*	30*	296 knees (116 infected)	Not mentioned
Ghanem et al[130]	—	—	20.5	31	479 hips (127 infected)	Not mentioned

*Values not based on independent receiver operating characteristic (ROC) analysis performed for the purpose of the study in question but rather on thresholds set by prior studies.
†Units given in these cases are as reported in source literature.

Table 100-2. Diagnostic Values for Early Postoperative Periprosthetic Joint Infection

Authors	WBC, cells/μL	PMNs, %	CRP, mg/L	ESR, mm/hr	Population	Time from Index Surgery
Bedair et al[76]	27,800	89	95	—	146 knees (19 infected)	<6 weeks
Bedair et al (unpublished, presented at AAOS)	19,200	92	93	—	18 hips (4 infected)	<6 weeks

CRP, C-reactive protein; *ESR,* erythrocyte sedimentation rate; *PMNs,* polymorphonuclear neutrophils; *WBC,* white blood cell.

10,000 WBCs/μL being an excellent "rule-out test," and a threshold of approximately 28,000 WBCs/μL being an excellent "rule-in" test. The differential was also helpful, with an optimal balance of sensitivity and sensitivity at greater than 90% PMNs. Unpublished data from our institution demonstrate similar utility of these tests in the diagnosis of periprosthetic hip infection in the early postoperative period (Table 100-2).

Nuclear medicine tests may aid in the diagnosis of periprosthetic infection. A technetium-99 radioisotope scan may have some value, with a negative test most probably ruling out infection; however, a positive test cannot differentiate septic from aseptic failure.[77,78] The use of an indium-111 leukocyte scan, where host leukocytes are tagged with the radioisotope and reintroduced into the body, has shown some utility, namely, in its negative predictive value of 95%.[79] The differential use of technetium and indium scans may distinguish areas of enhanced metabolic activity and inflammation. When a technetium-99 sulfur colloid marrow scan is combined with an indium scan, accuracy improves to 88%; however, routine use of these studies is debatable, given their high cost and the relative accuracy of synovial fluid WBC count, differential, and culture.[80] Newer nuclear medicine techniques, such as technetium-99 immunoglobulin scintigraphy and 18F positron emission tomography, may provide improved diagnostic accuracy; however, these techniques are not currently in wide use.[81-83]

Unfortunately, there exist many clinical scenarios in which preoperative testing is unable to definitively diagnose or rule out periprosthetic infection. If the clinical picture continues to cause concern for infection, analysis of fluid and tissue around the prosthesis obtained at the time of reoperation is indicated. Gram staining of periprosthetic fluid not only has poor sensitivity but may also generate false-positive results; it should not be done routinely and certainly should not be relied upon as the only method of screening for periprosthetic joint infection.[84-86]

Many authors have investigated the role of histologic analysis of periprosthetic tissue in the diagnosis of infection.[87-91] In these studies, an attempt was made to correlate frozen sections from the time of revision surgery with the diagnosis of infection. Although specific cutoff values are debatable, likely secondary to inconsistencies in sampling, technique, and pathologists, the essence of the findings is that the increased number of neutrophils observed in the tissue surrounding the prosthesis appears to correlate with infection. In an attempt to synthesize this variability, some authors have recommended using the cutoff of at least five neutrophils in each of three 400× high-power microscopic fields to diagnose infection.[75]

Any test for infection will have a given sensitivity and specificity that will not perfectly predict or rule out the presence of infection around a THA, even those tests considered to be "gold standards." Based on Bayesian theory, the predictive values of tests are related to the prevalence of the disease in the given patient population. The burden thus lies upon the treating physician to acquire the relevant data and apply them to a specific patient; the utility of any test will vary based on the specific clinical scenario. We recommend an initial thorough history and physical examination paired with ESR and CRP paired with an ESR and CRP in all patients undergoing revision surgery or who present with a painful or otherwise failed THA. Should the clinical suspicion be high based on the history and physical examination or if the ESR and CRP are elevated, the hip joint should be aspirated and the fluid obtained sent for a synovial fluid WBC count with differential and culture. These results, taken together, should be helpful in establishing the diagnosis in the vast majority of patients.[65,71] If reoperation is indicated, or if the diagnosis remains uncertain, infection can be ruled in or out through additional intraoperative testing, including intraoperative aspiration of the joint for synovial fluid WBC count and differential, an intraoperative frozen section and culture. Given that operative cultures can be both falsely positive and negative, we recommend obtaining multiple cultures (typically three to five sets) from several different sites (including the most suspicious appearing areas) at the time of revision. To perform an aspiration intraoperatively the capsule is exposed and directly visualized as per the surgeon's normal surgical approach, and an 18-gauge spinal needle is used to obtain synovial fluid through the capsule (Fig. 100-2); a result for the synovial fluid WBC count is typically available within 30 minutes, and the differential can take up to 45 minutes to obtain. Advantages of this test include its objective nature, low cost, and availability to surgeons worldwide.

TREATMENT

Once the diagnosis of infection has been established, the duration of symptoms is determined, and the chronicity of the infection can be estimated. Generally, infections should be classified into one of three categories: (1) acute postoperative infection, (2) acute hematogenous infection, or (3) chronic infection.[71,92,93] A fourth category can be considered in which a revision

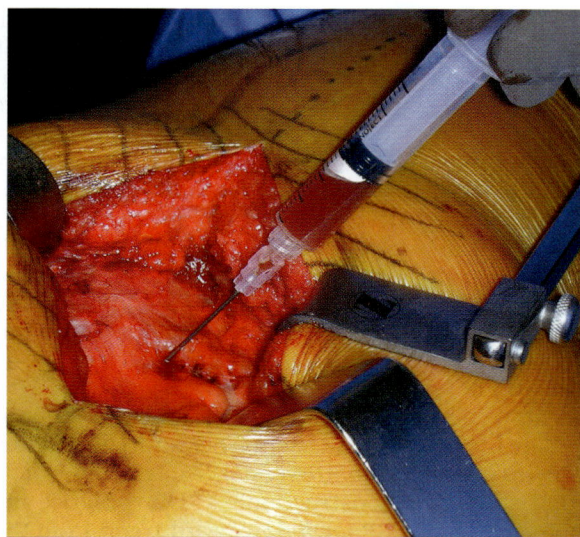

Figure 100-2. Technique for aspirating synovial fluid from the hip joint. The iliotibial band has been incised and is retracted. An 18-gauge spinal needle attached to a 10-mL syringe is used to aspirate fluid through the capsule before the capsulotomy is performed. This technique allows for easy access to the synovial fluid while minimizing potential contamination that can occur when aspirated through the skin or multiple layers of tissue.

arthroplasty is undertaken for diagnosis of aseptic failure, and intraoperative cultures are found to be positive subsequent to the time of surgery.[60] The definition of the acute postoperative period is controversial, but most consider this time period to be within 4 to 6 weeks of the index procedure. An acute hematogenous infection is defined as a scenario wherein the prosthesis had been functioning well for some time with the rapid onset of paid that is typically associated with fever and a distant source of bacteremia such as a dental or cutaneous abscess. A chronic infection is one in which the infection has been present for more than to 6 weeks.

Treatment protocols are generally based on the timing of infection and can be classified as those that retain the original prosthesis and those that involve removal of the prosthesis. Generally speaking, the success rate of retaining the prosthesis is directly correlated with the length of time of infection; infections that develop acutely and are diagnosed and treated expeditiously have more favorable results with component retention, although the infecting pathogen is an important determinant of outcome, and biofilm-producing organisms (such as *Staphylococcus* species) have worse outcomes. Infections that have been present for an extended period are not amenable to attempts at prosthetic retention because success is rarely achieved, and prosthetic removal is generally a more appropriate strategy.

Retention of the Prosthesis

Antibiotic Suppression

Treatment for a periprosthetic infection of the hip with antibiotics alone should be considered only in cases where the patient is unable to tolerate another surgical procedure, the organism in question is sensitive to oral antibiotics, and the patient is not septic. This treatment regimen is intended not to eradicate, but only to suppress the infection. Prolonged antibiotic therapy may lead to the development of resistant organisms, in addition to causing potential adverse systemic effects. In an evaluation of the efficacy of antibiotic suppressive therapy from multiple studies, only 31% of patients ultimately retained their prosthesis.[94] Moreover, most patients underwent surgical débridement in addition to antibiotic therapy. It would be reasonable to speculate that in the absence of this initial débridement, results attained with this strategy would have been even worse.

Irrigation and Débridement

Once the diagnosis of an acute postoperative or acute hematogenous infection has been established, the initial treatment of choice consists of formal open irrigation and débridement of the hip. At this time, the role of arthroscopic débridement is highly controversial[94,95] and, based on reported results, this approach cannot be recommended. As part of open débridement, modular components, such as the femoral head and the acetabular articulating surface, should be removed to facilitate access to all interfaces. All devitalized and necrotic tissue should be excised. If possible, a complete synovectomy should be performed. Irrigation with antibiotic saline solution is advisable. All components should be evaluated for loosening, and, if found to be loose, retention of the prosthesis should be abandoned. Postoperative treatment with intravenous antibiotics follows; however, the duration and type are debatable. Most would consider 4 weeks of intravenous antibiotics to be the minimum prescribed;[60] however, based on many studies and our own experience, we recommend antibiotics for at least 6 weeks.[96] The success rate of this procedure in acute postoperative infection has been reported to range from 14% to 71%.[60,97] However, in the series reporting a 71% success rate, only 2 of 12 (17%) patients with cementless implants had a successful result.[60] Those with an acute hematogenous infection appear to have an approximately 50% success rate based on two independent studies.[60,97] The duration of symptoms before débridement heavily influenced the outcome of this procedure; patients treated with 48 hours of symptoms had a success rate of 56% compared with those treated after more than 48 hours of symptoms, who had a success rate of 13%.[98] As was previously stated, attempted prosthetic retention in the setting of chronic infection is associated with a high rate of failure and should not be attempted in the vast majority of clinical scenarios.

Removal of the Prosthesis

Direct or "One-Stage" Exchange

Direct exchange with cemented implants in the appropriate patient appears to be a reasonably successful treatment, but it has been more popular in Europe than in North America.[99] The infecting organism should be a member of a sensitive gram-positive species, and the patient must be relatively healthy and must not have a draining sinus.[100,101] Although some studies may refute these specific relative contraindications,[102,103] most treating physicians try to reserve this treatment for patients with the highest likelihood of success. The procedure requires meticulous soft tissue débridement with access to all bony interfaces. The use of antibiotic cement at the time of re-implantation appears to be a critical component of a successful outcome, as does a 6-week course of intravenous antibiotics.[96] Several studies that specifically compared a direct exchange with a two-stage procedure have found that the failure rate of the two-stage procedure was significantly lower than that of a one-stage exchange (3.5% to 5.6% vs. 10.1% to 12.4%).[64,104] No published studies have investigated direct exchange with cementless implants.

Delayed or "Two-Stage" Exchange

A two-stage exchange protocol has proved successful in the treatment of the infected THA and has become the standard for treating chronic infections of the hip in North America.[94,95,105-108] At the time of the first stage, all prosthetic material, including residual bone cement, is removed, and a thorough débridement is performed.[60,109-111] An extended trochanteric osteotomy can be used at the time of the first stage, along with fixation of the trochanteric fragment, to facilitate implant removal and canal débridement. Using this approach, we have found high rates of resolution of infection and healing of the osteotomy, which typically does not need to be reopened at the time of the second stage[112] (Fig. 100-3). Insertion of an articulating or static antibiotic-loaded spacer is performed at the time of the first stage of

débridement appears both safe and efficacious,[113] with most authors recommending a minimum of 4 g of antibiotic per 40 g package of cement, although others have described using substantially more antibiotics without systemic effects. The elution rate of the antibiotic from the bone cement is specific to the type of bone cement used and the use of a combination of antibiotics seems to improve elution. A combination of vancomycin and an aminoglycoside is most commonly used as these antibiotics are heat stable, widely available, and provide broad spectrum coverage. Use of a combination of antibiotics seems to be synergistic and improves elution; vancomycin is commonly combined with an aminoglycoside.

Patient are typically treated with a 6-week course of antibiotics; during this time the ESR and CRP are monitored ideally on a weekly basis. The duration of IV antibiotic treatment is controversial, as is timing of the second stage of reconstruction.[96,113] Our practice is to monitor ESR and CRP for a downward trend from their initial levels at the time of diagnosis of infection. After an appropriate response to the antibiotics is seen, the patient is observed for an additional 2 to 6 weeks while off of all antibiotics. At this time, ESR and CRP are repeated, and the patient is brought back to the operating room, where the hip is aspirated intraoperatively as previously described, and a synovial fluid WBC count and differential are obtained, along with an intraoperative frozen section. Any indication of infection warrants a second débridement and placement of a new spacer before prosthetic reimplantation.

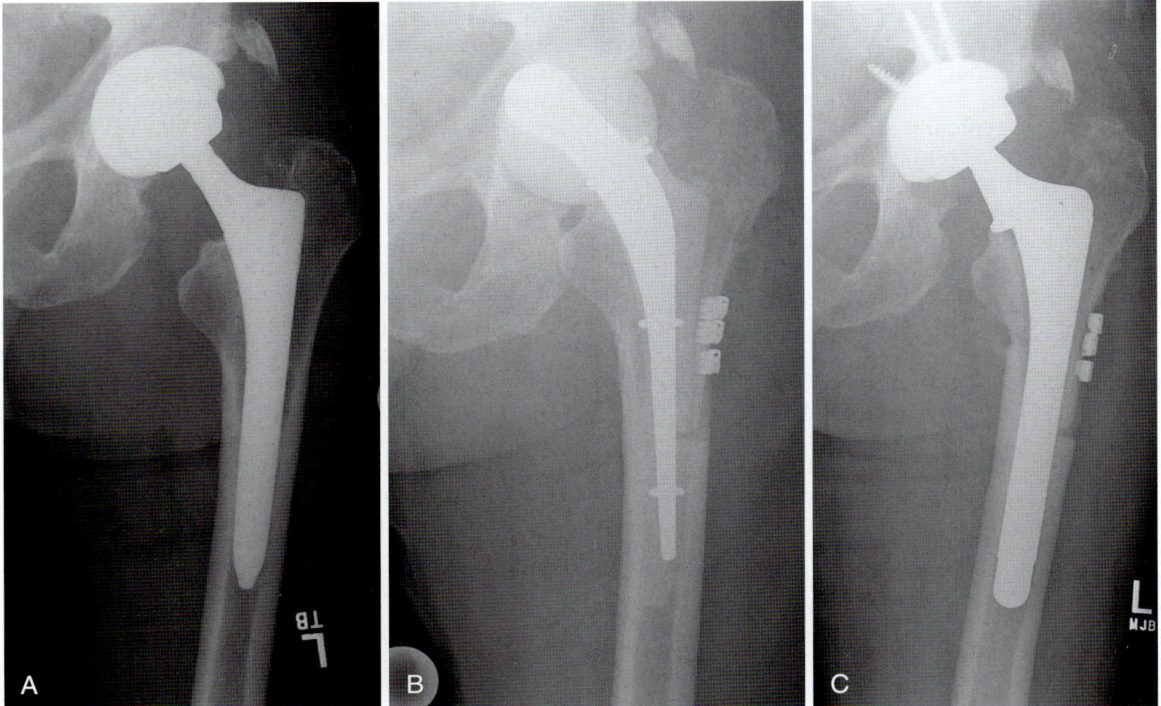

Figure 100-3. Extended trochanteric osteotomy for removal of an infected total hip arthroplasty. **A,** Osteointegrated cementless THA with deep infection. **B,** An extended trochanteric osteotomy was used to remove the ingrown femoral component, and an articulating antibiotic cement spacer has been inserted. The osteotomy has been closed with cables after insertion of the spacer. **C,** At the time of the second-stage reconstruction, the osteotomy was healed. The spacer was removed and the femoral component inserted without repeating the osteotomy.

A recent report from our institution[114] describes a study of 87 hips treated with a two-stage exchange protocol. When compared with preoperative levels, significant decreases in the ESR, CRP, synovial fluid WBC count, and differential were identified. However, despite clinical cure of the infection, the ESR was still greater than 30 mm/hr in nearly two thirds of patients, and the CRP was greater than 10 mg/L in approximately one fourth; unfortunately, discreet values for determining persistent infection could not be identified. Therefore while the ESR and CRP should show a trend toward normalization (particularly after the cessation of antibiotic therapy), they do not necessarily return to normal even if the infection has been successfully eradicated. The synovial fluid WBC count was found to be the best perioperative test, with an optimal cutoff value of 3528 WBCs/μL, which is similar to the cutoff value of 3000 WBCs/μL that we typically recommend.[65]

In a review of multiple studies of two-stage exchange for infection, the success rate appears to vary slightly based on whether reconstruction is performed with cement (with or without antibiotics) and/or local antibiotic delivery is used during the interval between the two stages. The success rate of a two-stage exchange when cementless components were used exclusively for reconstruction was reported to be 92% in two independent studies;[105,106] an antibiotic cement spacer was used between the two stages. Without the antibiotic cement spacer, the success rate was reported to be only 82.3%.[115] Results with the use of a cemented prosthesis with and without antibiotics in the cement were 90% and 82%, respectively.[96] Use of both an antibiotic spacer between stages and the use of antibiotic loaded cement at the time of reimplantation both seem to correlate with successful outcomes. Our preference is to reconstruct the hip with cementless implants and to use an articulating antibiotic cement spacer between the two stages unless the patient has a severe acetabular defect with which an articulating spacer cannot be contained within the acetabulum, or further damage to the host bone stock may occur (Fig. 100-4).

Articulating Spacers

One of the main disadvantages of two-stage reconstruction is the morbidity of the interval period between the two stages when the patient is left without a functioning hip. Many feel that the benefit of avoiding this morbidity through the use of a direct exchange outweighs the risk of a slightly increased failure rate compared with the two-stage exchange. Articulating cement spacers (as opposed to nonarticulating or "static" spacers) are designed to both deliver high dose local antibiotics and to maintain leg length and soft tissue tension which may facilitate the second stage reconstruction. Patient comfort also appears to be increased as leg lengths are maintained, allowing the patients to ambulate more easily and comfortably between stages. The efficacy of a two-stage exchange when such a device is used appears to approach 95%,[107,116,117] which is similar to the success rates reported previously.[105,106] Such devices may have limited use with more extensive femoral and/or acetabular bone loss[94] (see Fig. 100-4). In a study comparing an articulating spacer with traditional cement beads, efficacy rates were comparable, but the articulating spacer group had reduced hospital stays, higher hip scores, and improved function before the second stage, as well as shorter surgical times and less blood loss at the time of reimplantation.

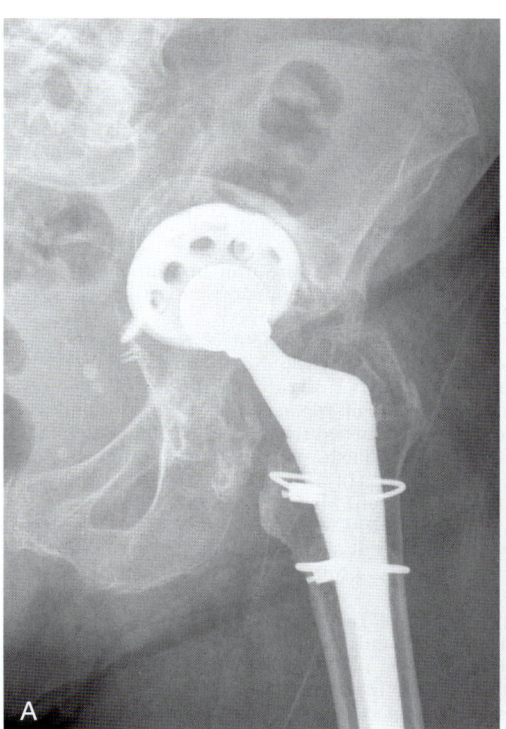
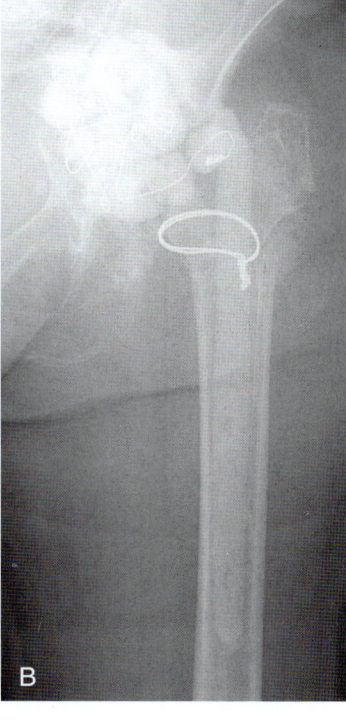

Figure 100-4. A, Infected total hip arthroplasty with significant intrapelvic migration of the acetabular component and severe pelvic bone loss. **B,** An articulating cement spacer is not appropriate in this case; a nonarticulating cement rod for the femur and a string of cement beads for the acetabulum were used instead.

Resection Arthroplasty

Despite the success of a two-stage exchange in most oases, failure inevitably occur. Unfortunately, the results of a second two-stage exchange after failure of an initial two-stage exchange appear to be poor,[118] and based on this single study, a repeat two stage exchange should be attempted with caution. Resection arthroplasty appears to reliably relieve pain and lead to resolution of infection, however the functional result is typically poor.[119-121] Common long-term problems include the need for a walking aid and a significant leg length inequality with many patients becoming nonambulatory.[120] If at some time in the future, the patient is a more suitable host for reimplantation, reconstruction can be carried out. We reserve this treatment for those who have failed all other exhaustive efforts at retaining a well-functioning prosthetic hip.

REFERENCES

1. Bozic KJ, Kurtz SM, Lau E, et al: The epidemiology of revision total hip arthroplasty in the United States. J Bone Joint Surg Am 91:128–133, 2009.
2. Kurtz S, Mowat F, Ong K, et al: Prevalence of primary and revision total hip and knee arthroplasty in the United States from 1990 through 2002. J Bone Joint Surg Am 87:1487–1497, 2005.
3. Hanssen AD, Osmon DR, Nelson CL: Prevention of deep periprosthetic joint infection. Instr Course Lect 46:555–567, 1997.
4. Charnley J: Postoperative infection after total hip replacement with special reference to air contamination in the operating room. Clin Orthop Relat Res 87:167–187, 1972.
5. Charnley J, Eftekhar N: Postoperative infection in total prosthetic replacement arthroplasty of the hip-joint: with special reference to the bacterial content of the air of the operating room. Br J Surg 56:641–649, 1969.
6. Blom AW, Taylor AH, Pattison G, et al: Infection after total hip arthroplasty: the Avon experience. J Bone Joint Surg Br 85:956–959, 2003.
7. Fitzgerald RH, Jr: Total hip arthroplasty sepsis: prevention and diagnosis. Orthop Clin North Am 23:259–264, 1992.
8. Garvin KL, Hanssen AD: Infection after total hip arthroplasty: past, present, and future. J Bone Joint Surg Am 77:1576–1588, 1995.
9. Katz JN, Phillips CB, Baron JA, et al: Association of hospital and surgeon volume of total hip replacement with functional status and satisfaction three years following surgery. Arthritis Rheum 48:560–568, 2003.
10. Phillips CB, Barrett JA, Losina E, et al: Incidence rates of dislocation, pulmonary embolism, and deep infection during the first six months after elective total hip replacement. J Bone Joint Surg Am 85:20–26, 2003.
11. Lennard TW, Shenton BK, Borzotta A, et al: The influence of surgical operations on components of the human immune system. Br J Surg 72:771–776, 1985.
12. Gomez CR, Boehmer ED, Kovacs EJ: The aging innate immune system. Curr Opin Immunol 17:457–462, 2005.
13. Greene KA, Wilde AH, Stulberg BN: Preoperative nutritional status of total joint patients: relationship to postoperative wound complications. J Arthroplasty 6:321–325, 1991.
14. Fernandez MC, Gottlieb M, Menitove JE: Blood transfusion and postoperative infection in orthopedic patients. Transfusion 32:318–322, 1992.
15. Gherini S, Vaughn BK, Lombardi AV, Jr, Mallory TH: Delayed wound healing and nutritional deficiencies after total hip arthroplasty. Clin Orthop Relat Res 293:188–195, 1993.
16. Poss R, Thornhill TS, Ewald FC, et al: Factors influencing the incidence and outcome of infection following total joint arthroplasty. Clin Orthop Relat Res 182:117–126, 1984.
17. Fitzgerald RH, Jr, Nolan DR, Ilstrup DM, et al: Deep wound sepsis following total hip arthroplasty. J Bone Joint Surg Am 59:847–855, 1977.
18. Namba RS, Paxton L, Fithian DC, Stone ML: Obesity and perioperative morbidity in total hip and total knee arthroplasty patients. J Arthroplasty 20(7 Suppl 3):46–50, 2005.
19. Berbari EF, Hanssen AD, Duffy MC, et al: Risk factors for prosthetic joint infection: case-control study. Clin Infect Dis 27:1247–1254, 1998.
20. Menon TJ, Thjellesen D, Wroblewski BM: Charnley low-friction arthroplasty in diabetic patients. J Bone Joint Surg Br 65:580–581, 1983.
21. Moeckel B, Huo MH, Salvati EA, Pellicci PM: Total hip arthroplasty in patients with diabetes mellitus. J Arthroplasty 8:279–284, 1993.
22. Vannini P, Ciavarella A, Olmi R, et al: Diabetes as pro-infective risk factor in total hip replacement. Acta Diabetol Lat 21:275–280, 1984.
23. Furnary AP, Zerr KJ, Grunkemeier GL, Starr A: Continuous intravenous insulin infusion reduces the incidence of deep sternal wound infection in diabetic patients after cardiac surgical procedures. Ann Thorac Surg 67:352–360; discussion 60–62, 1989.
24. Marchant MH, Jr, Viens NA, Cook C, et al: The impact of glycemic control and diabetes mellitus on perioperative outcomes after total joint arthroplasty. J Bone Joint Surg Am 91:1621–1629, 2009.
25. Sunday JM, Guille JT, Torg JS: Complications of joint arthroplasty in patients with end-stage renal disease on hemodialysis. Clin Orthop Relat Res 397:350–355, 2002.
26. Tannenbaum DA, Matthews LS, Grady-Benson JC: Infection around joint replacements in patients who have a renal or liver transplantation. J Bone Joint Surg Am 79:36–43, 1997.
27. Parvizi J, Sullivan TA, Pagnano MW, et al: Total joint arthroplasty in human immunodeficiency virus-positive patients: an alarming rate of early failure. J Arthroplasty 18:259–264, 2003.
28. Kim YH, Oh SH, Kim JS: Total hip arthroplasty in adult patients who had childhood infection of the hip. J Bone Joint Surg Am 85:198–204, 2003.
29. Surin VV, Sundholm K, Backman L: Infection after total hip replacement: with special reference to a discharge from the wound. J Bone Joint Surg Br 65:412–418, 1983.
30. Ainscow DA, Denham RA: The risk of haematogenous infection in total joint replacements. J Bone Joint Surg Br 66:580–582, 1984.
31. Menon TJ, Wroblewski BM: Charnley low-friction arthroplasty in patients with psoriasis. Clin Orthop Relat Res 176:127–128, 1983.
32. Sullivan PM, Johnston RC, Kelley SS: Late infection after total hip replacement, caused by an oral organism after dental manipulation: a case report. J Bone Joint Surg Am 72:121–123, 1990.
33. Rubin R, Salvati EA, Lewis R: Infected total hip replacement after dental procedures. Oral Surg Oral Med Oral Pathol 41:18–23, 1976.
34. Wroblewski BM, del Sel HJ: Urethral instrumentation and deep sepsis in total hip replacement. Clin Orthop Relat Res 146:209–212, 1980.
35. Nasser S: Prevention and treatment of sepsis in total hip replacement surgery. Orthop Clin North Am 23:265–277, 1992.
36. Hill C, Flamant R, Mazas F, Evrard J: Prophylactic cefazolin versus placebo in total hip replacement: report of a multicentre double-blind randomised trial. Lancet 1:795–796, 1981.
37. Classen DC, Evans RS, Pestotnik SL, et al: The timing of prophylactic administration of antibiotics and the risk of surgical-wound infection. N Engl J Med 326:281–286, 1992.
38. Leigh DA, Griggs J, Tighe CM, et al: Pharmacokinetic study of ceftazidime in bone and serum of patients undergoing hip and knee arthroplasty. J Antimicrob Chemother 16:637–642, 1985.
39. Steinberg JP, Braun BI, Hellinger WC, et al: Timing of antimicrobial prophylaxis and the risk of surgical site infections: results from the Trial to Reduce Antimicrobial Prophylaxis Errors. Ann Surg 250:10–16, 2009.
40. Mauerhan DR, Nelson CL, Smith DL, et al: Prophylaxis against infection in total joint arthroplasty: one day of cefuroxime

compared with three days of cefazolin. J Bone Joint Surg Am 76:39–45, 1994.

41. Tang WM, Chiu KY, Ng TP, et al: Efficacy of a single dose of cefazolin as a prophylactic antibiotic in primary arthroplasty. J Arthroplasty 18:714–718, 2003.

42. Wymenga A, van Horn J, Theeuwes A, et al: Cefuroxime for prevention of postoperative coxitis: one versus three doses tested in a randomized multicenter study of 2,651 arthroplasties. Acta Orthop Scand 63:19–24, 1992.

43. Ritter MA: Operating room environment. Clin Orthop Relat Res 369:103–109, 1999.

44. Ritter MA, Campbell ED: Retrospective evaluation of an iodophor-incorporated antimicrobial plastic adhesive wound drape. Clin Orthop Relat Res 228:307–308, 1988.

45. Johnston DH, Fairclough JA, Brown EM, Morris R: Rate of bacterial recolonization of the skin after preparation: four methods compared. Br J Surg 74:64, 1987.

46. Nelson CL: Prevention of sepsis. Clin Orthop Relat Res 222:66–72, 1987.

47. Dalstrom DJ, Venkatarayappa I, Manternach AL, et al: Time-dependent contamination of opened sterile operating-room trays. J Bone Joint Surg Am 90:1022–1025, 2008.

48. Nelson JP, Glassburn AR, Jr, Talbott RD, McElhinney JP: Clean room operating rooms. Clin Orthop Relat Res 96:179–187, 1973.

49. Nelson JP, Glassburn AR, Jr, Talbott RD, McElhinney JP: Horizontal flow operating room clean rooms. Cleve Clin Q 40:191–202, 1973.

50. Lidwell OM, Lowbury EJ, Whyte W, et al: Effect of ultraclean air in operating rooms on deep sepsis in the joint after total hip or knee replacement: a randomised study. Br Med J (Clin Res Ed) 285:10–14, 1982.

51. Marotte JH, Lord GA, Blanchard JP, et al: Infection rate in total hip arthroplasty as a function of air cleanliness and antibiotic prophylaxis: 10-year experience with 2,384 cementless Lord madreporic prostheses. J Arthroplasty 2:77–82, 1987.

52. Whyte W, Bailey PV, Hamblen DL, et al: A bacteriologically occlusive clothing system for use in the operating room. J Bone Joint Surg Br 65:502–506, 1983.

53. Strange-Vognsen HH, Klareskov B: Bacteriologic contamination of suction tips during hip arthroplasty. Acta Orthop Scand 59:410–411, 1988.

54. Hamer ML, Robson MC, Krizek TJ, Southwick WO: Quantitative bacterial analysis of comparative wound irrigations. Ann Surg 181:819–822, 1975.

55. Scherr DD, Dodd TA: In vitro bacteriological evaluation of the effectiveness of antimicrobial irrigating solutions. J Bone Joint Surg Am 58:119–122, 1976.

56. Rosenstein BD, Wilson FC, Funderburk CH: The use of bacitracin irrigation to prevent infection in postoperative skeletal wounds: an experimental study. J Bone Joint Surg Am 71:427–430, 1989.

57. Durack DT: Prevention of infective endocarditis. N Engl J Med 332:38–44, 1995.

58. LaPorte DM, Waldman BJ, Mont MA, Hungerford DS: Infections associated with dental procedures in total hip arthroplasty. J Bone Joint Surg Br 81:56–59, 1999.

59. Gristina AG: Implant failure and the immuno-incompetent fibro-inflammatory zone. Clin Orthop Relat Res 298:106–118, 1994.

60. Tsukayama DT, Estrada R, Gustilo RB: Infection after total hip arthroplasty: a study of the treatment of one hundred and six infections. J Bone Joint Surg Am 78:512–523, 1996.

61. Gristina AG, Costerton JW: Bacterial adherence to biomaterials and tissue: the significance of its role in clinical sepsis. J Bone Joint Surg Am 67:264–273, 1985.

62. Trampuz A, Osmon DR, Hanssen AD, et al: Molecular and antibiofilm approaches to prosthetic joint infection. Clin Orthop Relat Res 414:69–88, 2003.

63. Zimmerli W, Widmer AF, Blatter M, et al: Role of rifampin for treatment of orthopedic implant-related staphylococcal infections: a randomized controlled trial. Foreign-Body Infection (FBI) Study Group. JAMA 279:1537–1541, 1998.

64. Garvin KL, Fitzgerald RH, Jr, Salvati EA, et al: Reconstruction of the infected total hip and knee arthroplasty with gentamicin-impregnated Palacos bone cement. Instr Course Lect 42:293–302, 1993.

65. Schinsky MF, Della Valle CJ, Sporer SM, Paprosky WG: Perioperative testing for joint infection in patients undergoing revision total hip arthroplasty. J Bone Joint Surg Am 90:1869–1875, 2008.

66. Ostendorf M, Johnell O, Malchau H, et al: The epidemiology of total hip replacement in The Netherlands and Sweden: present status and future needs. Acta Orthop Scand 73:282–286, 2002.

67. Garvin KL, Hinrichs SH, Urban JA: Emerging antibiotic-resistant bacteria: their treatment in total joint arthroplasty. Clin Orthop Relat Res 369:110–123, 1999.

68. James PJ, Butcher IA, Gardner ER, Hamblen DL: Methicillin-resistant *Staphylococcus epidermidis* in infection of hip arthroplasties. J Bone Joint Surg Br 76:725–727, 1994.

69. Kilgus DJ, Howe DJ, Strang A: Results of periprosthetic hip and knee infections caused by resistant bacteria. Clin Orthop Relat Res 404:116–124, 2002.

70. Salgado CD, Dash S, Cantey JR, Marculescu CE: Higher risk of failure of methicillin-resistant *Staphylococcus aureus* prosthetic joint infections. Clin Orthop Relat Res 461:48–53, 2007.

71. Spangehl MJ, Masri BA, O'Connell JX, Duncan CP: Prospective analysis of preoperative and intraoperative investigations for the diagnosis of infection at the sites of two hundred and two revision total hip arthroplasties. J Bone Joint Surg Am 81:672–683, 1999.

72. Lachiewicz PF, Rogers GD, Thomason HC: Aspiration of the hip joint before revision total hip arthroplasty: clinical and laboratory factors influencing attainment of a positive culture. J Bone Joint Surg Am 78:749–754, 1996.

73. Barrack RL, Harris WH: The value of aspiration of the hip joint before revision total hip arthroplasty. J Bone Joint Surg Am 75:66–76, 1993.

74. Birmingham P, Helm JM, Manner PA, Tuan RS: Simulated joint infection assessment by rapid detection of live bacteria with real-time reverse transcription polymerase chain reaction. J Bone Joint Surg Am 90:602–608, 2003.

75. Bauer TW, Parvizi J, Kobayashi N, Krebs V: Diagnosis of periprosthetic infection. J Bone Joint Surg Am 88:869–882, 2006.

76. Bedair H, Ting N, Jacovides C, et al: Diagnosis of early postoperative TKA infection using synovial fluid analysis. The Mark Coventry Award. Clin Orthop Relat Res 469:34–40, 2011.

77. Levitsky KA, Hozack WJ, Balderston RA, et al: Evaluation of the painful prosthetic joint: relative value of bone scan, sedimentation rate, and joint aspiration. J Arthroplasty 6:237–244, 1991.

78. Reing CM, Richin PF, Kenmore PI: Differential bone-scanning in the evaluation of a painful total joint replacement. J Bone Joint Surg Am 61:933–936, 1979.

79. Scher DM, Pak K, Lonner JH, et al: The predictive value of indium-111 leukocyte scans in the diagnosis of infected total hip, knee, or resection arthroplasties. J Arthroplasty 15:295–300, 2000.

80. Joseph TN, Mujtaba M, Chen AL, et al: Efficacy of combined technetium-99m sulfur colloid/indium-111 leukocyte scans to detect infected total hip and knee arthroplasties. J Arthroplasty 16:753–758, 2001.

81. Demirkol MO, Adalet I, Unal SN, et al: 99Tc(m)-polyclonal IgG scintigraphy in the detection of infected hip and knee prostheses. Nucl Med Commun 18:543–548, 1997.

82. Zhuang H, Duarte PS, Pourdehnad M, et al: The promising role of 18F-FDG PET in detecting infected lower limb prosthesis implants. J Nucl Med 42:44–48, 2001.

83. Reinartz P, Mumme T, Hermanns B, et al: Radionuclide imaging of the painful hip arthroplasty: positron-emission tomography versus triple-phase bone scanning. J Bone Joint Surg Br 87:465–470, 2005.

84. Atkins BL, Athanasou N, Deeks JJ, et al: Prospective evaluation of criteria for microbiological diagnosis of prosthetic-joint infection at revision arthroplasty. The OSIRIS Collaborative Study Group. J Clin Microbiol 36:2932–2939, 1998.

85. Della Valle CJ, Scher DM, Kim YH, et al: The role of intraoperative Gram stain in revision total joint arthroplasty. J Arthroplasty 14:500–504, 1999.

86. Feldman DS, Lonner JH, Desai P, Zuckerman JD: The role of intraoperative frozen sections in revision total joint arthroplasty. J Bone Joint Surg Am 77:1807–1813, 1995.

87. Mirra JM, Marder RA, Amstutz HC: The pathology of failed total joint arthroplasty. Clin Orthop Relat Res 170:175–183, 1982.

88. Fehring TK, McAlister JA, Jr: Frozen histologic section as a guide to sepsis in revision joint arthroplasty. Clin Orthop Relat Res 304:229–237, 1994.

89. Lonner JH, Desai P, Dicesare PE, et al: The reliability of analysis of intraoperative frozen sections for identifying active infection during revision hip or knee arthroplasty. J Bone Joint Surg Am 78:1553–1558, 1996.

90. Athanasou NA, Pandey R, de Steiger R, et al: Diagnosis of infection by frozen section during revision arthroplasty. J Bone Joint Surg Br 77:28–33, 1995.

91. Banit DM, Kaufer H, Hartford JM: Intraoperative frozen section analysis in revision total joint arthroplasty. Clin Orthop Relat Res 401:230–238, 2002.

92. Coventry MB: Treatment of infections occurring in total hip surgery. Orthop Clin North Am 6:991–1003, 1975.

93. Schmalzried TP, Amstutz HC, Au MK, Dorey FJ: Etiology of deep sepsis in total hip arthroplasty: the significance of hematogenous and recurrent infections. Clin Orthop Relat Res 280:200–207, 1992.

94. Hanssen AD, Spangehl MJ: Treatment of the infected hip replacement. Clin Orthop Relat Res 420:63–71, 2004.

95. Hyman JL, Salvati EA, Laurencin CT, et al: The arthroscopic drainage, irrigation, and débridement of late, acute total hip arthroplasty infections: average 6-year follow-up. J Arthroplasty 14:903–910, 1999.

96. Hanssen AD, Rand JA: Evaluation and treatment of infection at the site of a total hip or knee arthroplasty. Instr Course Lect 48:111–122, 1999.

97. Crockarell JR, Hanssen AD, Osmon DR, Morrey BF: Treatment of infection with débridement and retention of the components following hip arthroplasty. J Bone Joint Surg Am 80:1306–1313, 1998.

98. Brandt CM, Sistrunk WW, Duffy MC, et al: *Staphylococcus aureus* prosthetic joint infection treated with débridement and prosthesis retention. Clin Infect Dis 24:914–919, 1997.

99. Nasser S, Lee Y, Amstutz H: Direct exchange arthroplasty in 30 septic total hip replacements without recurrent infection. Orthop Trans 13:519, 1989.

100. Callaghan JJ, Katz RP, Johnston RC: One-stage revision surgery of the infected hip: a minimum 10-year followup study. Clin Orthop Relat Res 369:139–143, 1999.

101. Ure KJ, Amstutz HC, Nasser S, Schmalzried TP: Direct-exchange arthroplasty for the treatment of infection after total hip replacement: an average ten-year follow-up. J Bone Joint Surg Am 80:961–968, 1998.

102. Raut VV, Siney PD, Wroblewski BM: One-stage revision of infected total hip replacements with discharging sinuses. J Bone Joint Surg Br 76:721–724, 1994.

103. Raut VV, Siney PD, Wroblewski BM: One-stage revision of total hip arthroplasty for deep infection: long-term followup. Clin Orthop Relat Res 321:202–207, 1995.

104. Elson RA: Exchange arthroplasty for infection: perspectives from the United Kingdom. Orthop Clin North Am 24:761–767, 1993.

105. Fehring TK, Calton TF, Griffin WL: Cementless fixation in 2-stage reimplantation for periprosthetic sepsis. J Arthroplasty 14:175–181, 1999.

106. Haddad FS, Muirhead-Allwood SK, Manktelow AR, Bacarese-Hamilton I: Two-stage uncemented revision hip arthroplasty for infection. J Bone Joint Surg Br 82:689–694, 2000.

107. Younger AS, Duncan CP, Masri BA, McGraw RW: The outcome of two-stage arthroplasty using a custom-made interval spacer to treat the infected hip. J Arthroplasty 12:615–623, 1997.

108. Toms AD, Davidson D, Masri BA, Duncan CP: The management of peri-prosthetic infection in total joint arthroplasty. J Bone Joint Surg Br 88:149–155, 2006.

109. Paprosky WG, Weeden SH, Bowling JW, Jr: Component removal in revision total hip arthroplasty. Clin Orthop Relat Res 393:181–193, 2001.

110. Lieberman JR, Callaway GH, Salvati EA, et al: Treatment of the infected total hip arthroplasty with a two-stage reimplantation protocol. Clin Orthop Relat Res 301:205–212, 1994.

111. McDonald DJ, Fitzgerald RH, Jr, Ilstrup DM: Two-stage reconstruction of a total hip arthroplasty because of infection. J Bone Joint Surg Am 71:828–834, 1989.

112. Levine BR, Della Valle CJ, Hamming M, et al: Use of the extended trochanteric osteotomy in treating prosthetic hip infection. J Arthroplasty 24:49–55, 2009.

113. Springer BD, Lee GC, Osmon D, et al: Systemic safety of high-dose antibiotic-loaded cement spacers after resection of an infected total knee arthroplasty. Clin Orthop Relat Res 427:47–51, 2004.

114. Shukla S, Ward JP, Jacofsky MC, et al: Perioperative testing for persistent sepsis following resection arthroplasty of the hip for periprosthetic infection. J Arthroplasty 25:E27, 2010.

115. Nestor BJ, Hanssen AD, Ferrer-Gonzalez R, Fitzgerald RH, Jr: The use of porous prostheses in delayed reconstruction of total hip replacements that have failed because of infection. J Bone Joint Surg Am 76:349–359, 1994.

116. Evans RP: Successful treatment of total hip and knee infection with articulating antibiotic components: a modified treatment method. Clin Orthop Relat Res 427:37–46, 2004.

117. Masri BA, Panagiotopoulos KP, Greidanus NV, et al: Cementless two-stage exchange arthroplasty for infection after total hip arthroplasty. J Arthroplasty 22:72–78, 2007.

118. Pagnano MW, Trousdale RT, Hanssen AD: Outcome after reinfection following reimplantation hip arthroplasty. Clin Orthop Relat Res 338:192–204, 1997.

119. Canner GC, Steinberg ME, Heppenstall RB, Balderston R: The infected hip after total hip arthroplasty. J Bone Joint Surg Am 66:1393–1399, 1984.

120. Castellanos J, Flores X, Llusa M, et al: The Girdlestone pseudarthrosis in the treatment of infected hip replacements. Int Orthop 22:178–181, 1998.

121. Grauer JD, Amstutz HC, O'Carroll PF, Dorey FJ: Resection arthroplasty of the hip. J Bone Joint Surg Am 71:669–678, 1989.

CHAPTER 101

Hip Instability

Michael J. Morris, John J. Callaghan, and Keith R. Berend

KEY POINTS

- Instability is the most common indication for revision THA in the United States.
- The cost burden for treating dislocation is substantial.
- Multiple risk factors for instability are known, including patient-specific (female gender, increasing age, underlying diagnosis of avascular necrosis [AVN] or femoral neck fracture) and surgeon-specific factors (surgical approach, component orientation, head size, proper restoration of leg lengths and offset, and surgical volume).
- Proper treatment of instability requires an understanding of the timing and cause of the dislocation coupled with a thorough physical examination and radiographic evaluation.
- Treatment options include closed reduction, component revision, modular component exchange, increasing femoral head size, soft tissue augmentation, trochanteric advancement, conversion to a bipolar or tripolar arthroplasty, and use of a constrained liner.

INTRODUCTION

Total hip arthroplasty (THA) is an exceptionally cost-effective and successful medical intervention.[1] Dislocation, infection, and osteolysis secondary to wear of the bearing surface are the three most common complications affecting the long-term success of THA.[2] Dislocation rates ranging from 0.3% to 10% of primary THAs and up to 28% for revision THAs have been reported.[3-17] The incidence of dislocation appears to be highest within the first year after the index procedure but rises cumulatively at a rate of about 1% per 5 years to 7% at 25 years postoperatively.[8] Recent population-based estimates have predicted a substantial increase in the future number of primary and revision THA procedures performed in the United States over the next few decades.[18] Despite advances in surgical technique and implant technology, the revision rate for THA has not changed substantially with time.[19] In addition, a recent study evaluating a national database demonstrated that instability/dislocation was the most common diagnosis resulting in revision THA in the United States.[2]

The cost burden for treating dislocations is substantial. Estimates place the hospital costs of treating dislocations following THA at $74,000,000 per year.[20] Investigators have recently reported that dislocations treated by closed methods represent a hospital cost of 19% of the overall cost of an uncomplicated primary THA, and revision surgery results in hospital costs of 148% of an uncomplicated primary THA.[20] These direct costs do not account for patient morbidity or lost work production. This cost burden is expected to increase as the numbers of primary THA and subsequent revision cases for instability increase over the next few decades.

RISK FACTORS FOR INSTABILITY

Multiple factors are correlated with the risk of instability after total hip arthroplasty (THA). Patient-specific risk factors include female gender,[8,10] increasing age,[10,13,21,22] underlying diagnosis (including avascular necrosis [AVN] and femoral neck fracture),[8,12,13,17] and associated comorbidities.[12] Surgeon- and prosthesis-specific variables include surgical approach,[10] component orientation,[4,9,10] femoral head size and prosthetic neck geometry,[12,17] offset,[10] soft tissue integrity, leg length,[23] and impingement and surgeon volume,[13,24] all of which contribute to the risk of dislocation.

Various authors have investigated how gender influences hip stability. Berry and associates in a study of more than 6000 THAs reported a 25-year cumulative risk of dislocation of 8.9% for females compared with 4.5% for males, resulting in a relative risk of dislocation of 2.1 for women.[8] It is hypothesized that greater tissue laxity among females contributes to this reported risk. However, other authors have reported that gender does not play a role in instability risk. Meek and colleagues reviewed more than 14,000 THAs from the Scottish National Arthroplasty Registry, Conroy and coworkers evaluated more than 65,000 THAs from the Australian Orthopaedic Association National Joint Replacement Registry, and Khatod and associates reported on approximately 2000 THAs from a U.S. community registry (Kaiser Permanente Total Joint Registry); none of these authors found gender to be an independent risk factor for dislocation.[12,13,17]

Patient age has also been investigated in relation to hip stability. Berry and colleagues demonstrated a relative risk of dislocation of 1.3 for patients older than 70 years of age.[8] Additional authors have demonstrated a twofold to threefold increased risk of dislocation in the elderly, specifically patients older than 80 years.[10,13,21,22,25] Levy and coworkers explained that predisposing factors in this elderly population that potentially increased their risk of dislocation included cognitive decline, muscle weakness, impaired proprioception, and laxity of the capsular structures.[25] In contrast, other authors could not find a correlation between increasing age and dislocation rate in two large registry databases.[12,17] In addition, a 3.5% dislocation rate was reported by Lachiewicz and associates in a single surgeon review of patients older than 75 years—a dislocation rate that is relatively on par with other reports in the literature, irrespective of age.[26]

Avascular necrosis of the femoral head (AVN), acute fracture or nonunion of the proximal part of the femur, inflammatory arthritis, and previous hip surgery are generally agreed upon risk factors for dislocation. Berry and associates reported that AVN, acute fracture or nonunion of the proximal femur, and inflammatory arthritis had relative rates of dislocation of 1.9, 1.8, and 1.5, respectively, compared with an underlying diagnosis of osteoarthritis, in a study of more than 6000 THAs.[8] In the same report, Berry and colleagues did not find a significantly higher dislocation rate with developmental dysplasia of the hip or posttraumatic arthritis when compared with osteoarthritis.[8] Khatod and coworkers reported a sixfold increased dislocation risk with the underlying diagnosis of rheumatoid arthritis,[12] and Meek and associates reported it as a strong independent risk factor for instability.[13] Zwartele and colleagues described rheumatoid arthritis as an independent risk factor and hypothesized that it resulted from overall poorer soft tissue quality.[27] Lewinnek and coworkers noted a significantly increased dislocation risk in patients with previous hip surgery[4] and suggested the inferior soft tissue envelope as a potential causative factor. The soft tissue insult could also explain the higher dislocation rates reported by various authors for acute femoral neck fracture after total hip arthroplasty.[8,28,29] In addition, the higher combined preoperative range of motion in the nonarthritic hip fracture cohort could contribute to the higher rate of dislocation.[30]

Body mass index (BMI) and medical comorbidities have been studied to evaluate their relationship with instability following THA. Jolles and associates reported a 10-fold increased risk of dislocation with an American Association of Anesthesiologists (ASA) score of 3 or 4.[31] Khatod and colleagues found a 2.3-fold dislocation risk for patients who had ASA scores of 3 or 4 compared with patients with scores of 1 or 2.[12] Khatod and coworkers did not find BMI to be a risk factor for dislocation;[12] this finding is in accordance with most reports in the literature.[32,33] However, a recent study of 2100 primary THAs in male patients from a Swedish Registry determined that BMI was a risk factor for dislocation.[34] In addition, Kim and associates reported a six times higher dislocation risk in the obese patient population in a study of revision THA.[35]

Surgical approach has been described as an additional factor affecting stability and risk of dislocation following THA. Traditionally, the posterior approach has been associated with the highest risk of dislocation compared with transtrochanteric, anterolateral, and anterior-based approaches.[3,6,9,36,37] In a study of more than 21,000 primary THAs, Berry and colleagues reported dislocation rates at 10-year follow-up of 3.1%, 3.4%, and 6.9% for anterolateral, transtrochanteric, and posterolateral approaches, respectively.[36] Masonis and Bourne performed a meta-analysis of the literature and found the posterior approach to have a sixfold higher dislocation rate compared with a direct lateral approach.[37] However, multiple authors have reported that dislocation rates with the posterior approach can be reduced by repair of the capsule and short external rotators.[37-39] Furthermore, Kim and coworkers advocated preserving the external rotators during the posterior approach—a technique that resulted in zero dislocation in one study.[40]

Implant positioning is paramount in optimizing the result of THA and minimizing dislocation risk.[41] Lewinnek and associates defined the "safe zone" of acetabular cup placement as anteversion of 15 ± 10 degrees and abduction of 40 ± 10 degrees, which resulted in a dislocation rate using the posterior approach of 1.5%.[4] Comparatively, when the cup was placed outside of this safe zone, the dislocation rate was 6.1%.[4] McCollum and Gray demonstrated similar dislocation rates using a posterior approach when cup position was maintained within a safe zone of 30 to 50 degrees abduction and 20 to 40 degrees anteversion.[9] However, the accuracy of intraoperative assessment of cup positioning has been shown to be poorer than expected, with 21 of 50 cups unexpectedly falling outside the safe zone when examined radiographically in the postoperative period.[42] In contrast, multiple authors have described intraoperative techniques that focus on specific landmarks to accurately reproduce acetabular cup position and minimize dislocation risk.[43,44] Archbold and associates described using the transverse acetabular ligament to determine cup anteversion, which enabled them to achieve a dislocation rate of 0.6% in 1000 hips treated with a posterior approach.[43] Sotereanos and colleagues advocated using the bony palpable landmarks of the ischium, superior pubic ramus, and superior acetabulum for cup placement and demonstrated both reproducible cup placement and a dislocation rate of less than 1%.[44] Finally, some have advocated for computer-assisted navigation to more accurately reproduce the desired acetabular cup position.[45]

The effect of head size on the stability of THA has been investigated by numerous authors.[36,46-55] "Jump distance" increases as the femoral head diameter increases.[53] Berry and coworkers demonstrated a reduction in dislocation rates for anterolateral, posterolateral, and transtrochanteric hip approaches as the femoral head diameter increased from 22 mm to 28 mm to 32 mm.[36] Smith and associates reported zero dislocations after large head (38 mm) metal-on-metal THA.[46] Dislocation rates for 38-mm versus 28-mm metal-on-metal THAs were zero and 2.5%, respectively, at 3-month follow-up in a study conducted by Cuckler and associates.[47] Peters and colleagues also demonstrated zero

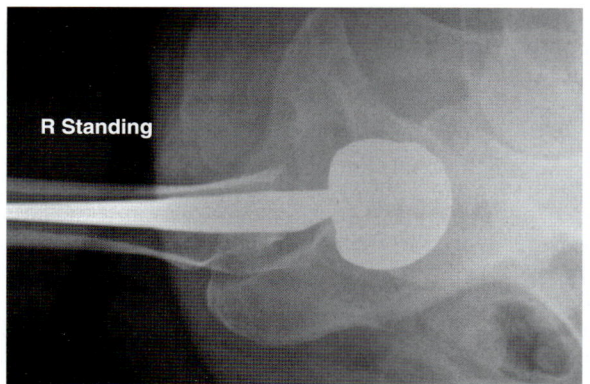

Figure 101-3. Shoot-through lateral radiograph of hip demonstrates proper cup anteversion. *(Courtesy Craig J. Della Valle, MD.)*

reasonably predictable and successful correction of the instability.[14,62-64] However, the condition of the abductors is critical to the success of the operation.[16,63,64]

Component Revision

Rogers and associates corrected instability in 75% and 50%, respectively, of primary and revision THAs requiring revision for dislocation.[64] Stability was achieved in 73% of all cases revised specifically for component malposition.[64] Revision of components for unknown causes of instability resulted in only a 33% success rate.[64] However, when constrained mechanisms were implemented, stability was achieved in 76% and 100% of malpositioned components and cases of unknown causes, respectively.[64] When the abductors were dysfunctional, the success of revision was only 50% regardless of the

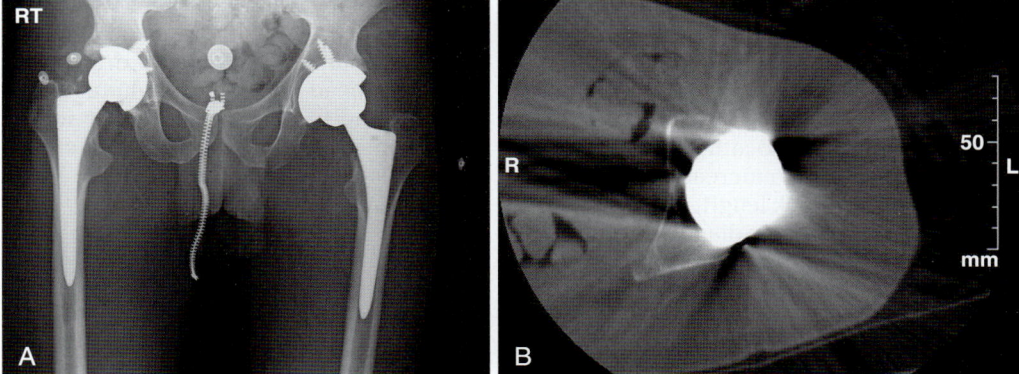

Figure 101-4. A, Anteroposterior radiograph of pelvis for a 32-year-old male patient referred for chronic instability of the left hip. Acetabular inclination is 40 degrees with version that appears neutral or retroverted. Note the limb length inequality with the left side being 1.3 cm longer than the right and with offset that is 1.2 cm greater than the right side. This case illustrates how intraoperative instability can lead to leg length inequality and increased offset in attempts to gain stability; acetabular malposition is usually the underlying cause. *(Reproduced courtesy Joint Implant Surgeons, Inc.)* **B,** Axial computed tomography (CT) scan of the patient, demonstrating acetabular component retroversion. *(Reproduced courtesy Joint Implant Surgeons, Inc.)*

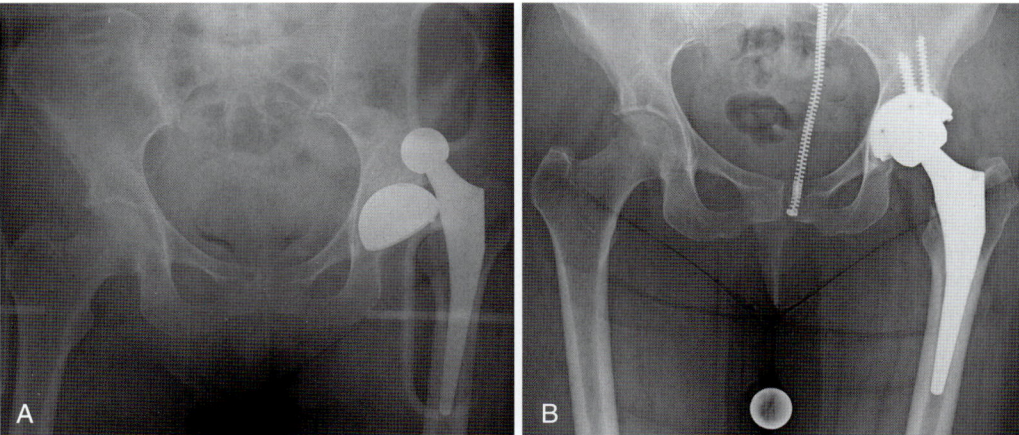

Figure 101-5. A, Anteroposterior radiograph of pelvis in a 65-year-old female referred with recurrent instability of the left hip. Acetabular inclination is 24 degrees with version that appears neutral or retroverted. *(Reproduced courtesy Joint Implant Surgeons, Inc.)* **B,** Anteroposterior radiograph of pelvis following revision surgery, demonstrating inclination of 32 degrees and appropriate anteversion. No further dislocations have occurred 5 years post revision surgery. *(Reproduced courtesy Joint Implant Surgeons, Inc.)*

technique implemented.[64] Alberton and colleagues questioned whether component orientation was an influential factor for instability in the revision setting by showing no difference in abduction and anteversion angles between dislocators and nondislocators following revision surgery.[16] The extent of the soft tissue dissection and specifically the functional condition of the abductors were deemed by these authors to be the most influential factors affecting recurrent instability risk following revision THA.[16,63] Reoperation of the recently unstable hip with malpositioned components usually requires component revision. If dysfunction of the abductors is previously noted, a constrained liner may well need to be added.

Modular Component Exchange

Modular exchange of the femoral head and liner is an attractive, technically straightforward option when recurrent instability is encountered with well-fixed implants. This option is indicated only if the components are reasonably well positioned, and modular components were used in the primary arthroplasty.[65] Toomey and coworkers eliminated recurrent dislocation in 12 of 13 hips despite 3 hips dislocating once during follow-up.[65] Attempts were made to increase the diameter of the femoral head and/or neck length at the time of each revision. Thirty-two-millimeter-diameter femoral heads were used in all revision cases except two, which employed 28-mm diameter heads. These revisions were performed with excision of soft tissue and bony impingement in 10 hips. Nine of the hips were converted to a lipped bearing or a higher-degree lipped bearing.

Other authors have reported on high wall liners to correct instability. McConway and associates reported a 1.6% dislocation rate in 307 revision THA patients treated with a posterior lip augmentation device for recurrent instability.[66] This specific device, however, is more similar to a partially constrained device than to a pure high wall liner and is recommended only for use with Charnley/Charnley Elite systems.[66]

In a series of 22 cases of late instability secondary to polyethylene wear studied by Parvizi and associates, liner exchange in isolation was successful in preventing recurrent dislocation in 11 of 11 patients (100%).[67] Properly oriented well-fixed acetabular components with an adequate locking mechanism were necessary for isolated liner exchange. The other 11 cases had all-polyethylene acetabular components, which required revision with press-fit metal shells. Recurrent dislocations occurred in 4 of 11 cases, which required acetabular revision. Surgical approach was posterolateral in 14 hips and anterolateral in the remaining 8. Femoral heads were upsized to 28-mm diameter in 3 cases, and neck length increased in 3 cases.

Large Femoral Heads

Treatment of instability with large or jumbo femoral heads is based on the principles of optimization of the head-neck ratio to increase range of motion before impingement and increasing the "jump distance" before

the femoral head dislocates. Beaulé and colleagues reported on the use of jumbo femoral heads (40 to 50 mm) in the treatment of 12 recurrent dislocators with reasonable success:[68] More than 90% of the hips showed no further instability at average follow-up of 6.5 years.[68] Five reoperations were performed secondary to various causes, but only one was the result of recurrent instability.[68] Amstutz and coworkers demonstrated an advantage when using large-diameter femoral heads in revision surgery to prevent dislocation for both recurrent instability and other revision causes.[51] However, dislocation prevalence was higher in the revision group treated for recurrent instability than in the revision group for other causes.[51] The dislocation rate was 13% for 29 hips that underwent revision surgery for instability compared with a 1.8% rate of instability in 54 hips that underwent revision surgery for noninstability causes. More modest results were reported by Skeels and associates, who reported a 17% recurrent dislocation rate at average follow-up of 17.2 months in a series of 26 hips revised for instability using femoral heads measuring 36 mm or greater in diameter.[48] Potential drawbacks of the larger-diameter head strategy include the thinner liner required and increased volumetric wear, the long-term significance of which has yet to be elucidated.

Soft Tissue Augmentation

Soft tissue augmentation is an infrequently used treatment option for recurrent instability. Potential options include reinforcement of the abductors or the posterior capsule.[14,69] An Achilles tendon allograft, fascia lata plasty, or synthetic ligament prosthesis has been utilized with modest results.[70-72] Indications might include a deficiency in the abductors or posterior capsule in the setting of well-positioned well-fixed components. More predictable and successful outcomes overall are likely to be achieved by using constrained mechanical devices instead of soft tissue restraints.

Trochanteric Advancement

Trochanteric advancement has been advocated by some authors.[73-75] Indications would include well-positioned and well-fixed implants with recurrent instability in a younger patient. Ekelund[73] and Kaplan and Thomas[74] achieved 80% success in preventing further dislocation using this approach in 21 patients, each with recurrent dislocation and properly oriented components. Nonunion of the greater trochanter is a major concern, and trochanter area hip pain is common. Utilization of this approach should be limited to the young arthroplasty patient with recurrent dislocation in the setting of properly oriented components; otherwise, constrained devices are likely to be more predictable with less potential morbidity.

Conversion to a Bipolar Arthroplasty

Bipolar arthroplasty has been utilized by some authors as a salvage technique for recurrent instability in THA.[76-78] This salvage technique involves placing a bipolar head on the femoral stem and allowing it to articulate with the remaining acetabular bone stock after the cup is removed and any requisite bone grafting is performed. The principal mechanism behind this technique is increasing the overall range of motion by having motion at two different bearing surfaces. This provides a greater safe arc of motion before dislocation occurs. There is also a larger jump distance because the bipolar head is larger than conventional femoral heads. Parvizi and Morrey prevented recurrent dislocation in 81% of 27 revision hips with 5-year follow-up.[76] Attarian[77] and Ries and Wiedel[78] achieved 100% success using this technique in smaller patient samples (six and three, respectively) with shorter follow-up. The major concern with this technique is migration of the prosthesis due to acetabular erosion. In addition, groin pain is not infrequent following this technique.

Unconstrained Tripolar Arthroplasty

Unconstrained tripolar arthroplasty, which uses a bipolar head to articulate with an acetabular shell and liner, has been successful in revision THA for instability (Fig. 101-6).[79-81] Specific indications for this technique include instability with a well-fixed nonmodular femoral

component—a femoral stem with a modular head that does not have a commercially available large-diameter femoral head option—and when trying to minimize shear stresses on the cup during complex acetabular reconstructions, where a constrained liner might otherwise be used (Fig. 101-7A and B).[81] Typically, an

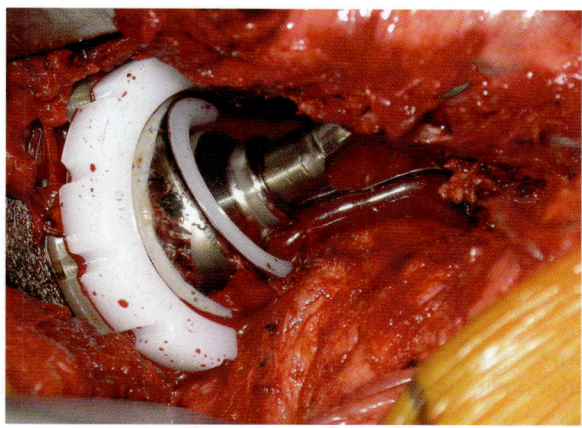

Figure 101-6. Intraoperative photograph of an unconstrained tripolar construct. *(Courtesy Craig J. Della Valle, MD.)*

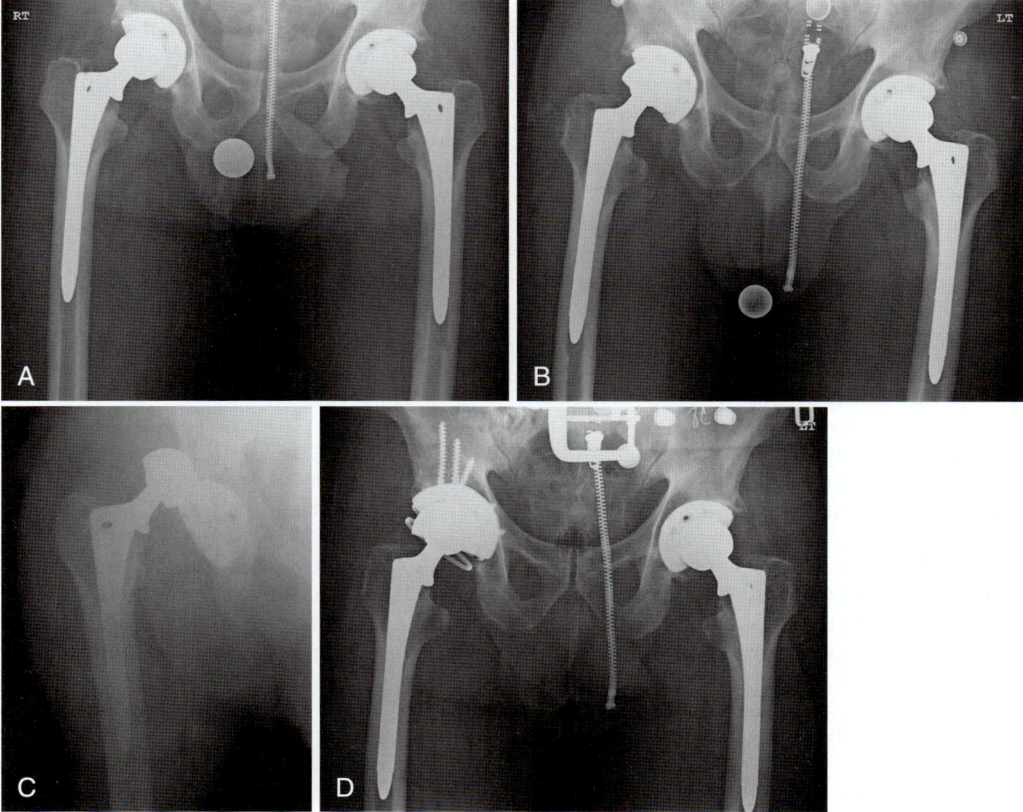

Figure 101-7. A, Anteroposterior radiograph of a 54-year-old male 1 year after primary total hip arthroplasty and multiple dislocations of the right hip. The cup is vertical and appears retroverted. *(Reproduced courtesy Joint Implant Surgeons, Inc.)* **B,** Conversion to an unconstrained tripolar articulation is performed despite malpositioned acetabular shell. *(Reproduced courtesy Joint Implant Surgeons, Inc.)* **C,** Dislocation of the unconstrained tripolar construct. *(Reproduced courtesy Joint Implant Surgeons, Inc.)* **D,** Revision of the acetabular component to improve both inclination and version, along with use of a constrained tripolar construct with resolution of the instability. *(Reproduced courtesy Joint Implant Surgeons, Inc.)*

acetabular revision shell is secured in the acetabulum, and an appropriate 36-, 40-, or 44-mm-inner-diameter liner is inserted. If the acetabular shell is being preserved but the locking mechanism is incompatible with the liner, the polyethylene can be cemented into the acetabular cup. A bipolar head matching the inner diameter of the acetabular liner is then chosen, and a bipolar head can be placed on a modular or nonmodular femoral stem. Trialing should be performed and, when deemed appropriate, the official implants assembled by first locking the bipolar head onto the femoral head and subsequently reducing the construct into the acetabular shell and liner. Originally reported by Grigoris and associates[79] and then updated by Beaulé and colleagues,[80] unconstrained tripolar arthroplasty was successful in treating instability in 95% of cases without compromising acetabular fixation at average follow-up of 5 years in a series of 21 patients with recurrent instability.[79,80] In a more recent series, Levine and coworkers reported on 31 unstable THAs revised using an unconstrained tripolar construct and achieved success in 93% of cases with 38-month follow-up.[81]

Constrained Liners

Constrained acetabular liners provide an option in the salvage of the unstable THA, and their efficacy has been reported by multiple authors.[14,59,82-89] Indications for the use of constrained devices include abductor deficiency, neurologic impairment, low-demand patients with well-fixed components, cases in which the cause of instability cannot be elucidated, and intraoperative instability that cannot be stabilized with other techniques.[14,59,82-86] Concerns with constrained liners include impingement, decreased range of motion, and increased acetabular shear stresses (which could lead to accelerated wear and earlier loosening). It should be noted that all constrained liners are not the same. Constrained liners that lock at the polyethylene rim around the prosthetic head have not been as successful as those that employ a tripolar articulation.[83]

Constrained tripolar arthroplasty is an invaluable salvage tool in revision instability situations, and the implant most commonly studied has been a tripolar constrained device (Fig. 101-7C and D). In the setting of a secure cementless acetabular shell, Callaghan and associates demonstrated no dislocations and only two liner failures (94% success) at short-term follow-up averaging 3.9 years in 31 hips for which a constrained tripolar liner was cemented into the existing cup.[89] One liner failed at the cement-cup interface, and the other liner capturing mechanism fractured.[89] This particular technique has the obvious advantage of decreased morbidity in the setting of a well-fixed and properly oriented acetabular component.[89]

Goetz and colleagues reported a 7% failure rate secondary to recurrent dislocation, osteolysis, or aseptic loosening in 56 constrained tripolar devices at average follow-up of 10.2 years.[82] Bremner and coworkers described similar results with a 6% failure rate secondary to recurrent dislocation or liner failure in 101 tripolar constrained devices at 10.2-year follow-up.[83] Shrader

and associates demonstrated zero dislocations in 110 revision THAs treated with a tripolar constrained device, with short-term follow-up averaging 3.2 years, but noted cup radiolucencies in 14% of cases with radiographic follow-up averaging 2.9 years.[84] However, only two cups had been revised during the study period for aseptic acetabular loosening.[84] Su and Pellici achieved 97.6% success at 4.8-year follow-up in preventing instability in 85 hips treated with a constrained tripolar implant.[85] They did not have problems with loosening or osteolysis in the intermediate follow-up.[85]

Despite the success of these devices, authors are beginning to report on the modes of failure specific to tripolar constrained devices.[90,91] Guyen and colleagues reported on 43 failed tripolar implants at short-term follow-up of 28.4 months.[90] Excluding 12 cases, which were infected, the authors reported on four types of failure specific to the tripolar device, including failure at the bone-implant interface, failure with the mechanism holding the constrained liner to the metal shell, failure of the locking mechanism of the bipolar component, and dislocation of the head at the inner bearing of the bipolar component.[90]

In contrast to the successes of tripolar constrained devices as discussed previously, Berend and coworkers reported on 755 constrained components with primarily a capture mechanism and locking ring.[86] Indications for use of the constrained components included recurrent instability, intraoperative multidirectional instability, neuromuscular and neurologic dysfunction, abductor mechanism dysfunction, and multiple prior revision surgeries.[86] Seventy-five percent of cases were revision THAs, 8% conversion THAs (including previous open reduction and internal fixation, hemiarthroplasty, and hip arthrodesis takedown procedures), 8% primary THAs, 8% reimplantations following two-stage exchange for infection, and 1% procedures performed in the setting of total femoral replacement.[86] Six hundred sixty-seven hips had 10-year follow-up, and the dislocation rate among them was 17.5%.[86] Patients revised for instability or with a history of instability failed, with a recurrent dislocation rate of 28% compared with a rate of 14% in patients without a history of instability.[86] Aseptic loosening of the cup and stem was a major long-term mode of failure, for which reoperation was required.[86] Sixteen cases of acetabular and femoral loosening (2.4%) and 51 cases of acetabular loosening (7.6%) were reported within the follow-up period.[86] These failures could potentially be related to increased constraint of the device, causing higher stresses at bone-implant interfaces.[86] Kaplan-Meier survivorship analysis with revision surgery as an endpoint revealed 68.5% and 51.7% survival at 5 and 10 years, respectively.[86]

In a more recent report, Berend and associates described 98.8% success in preventing recurrent dislocation in 81 THA revisions at an average 9-month follow-up using a novel constrained device (Fig. 101-8A through C).[87] The design incorporates an equatorial flat section at 15 degrees to the vertical axis along the sides of the 36-mm head (Fig. 101-9).[87] A potential advantage of this device is the increased range of motion noted

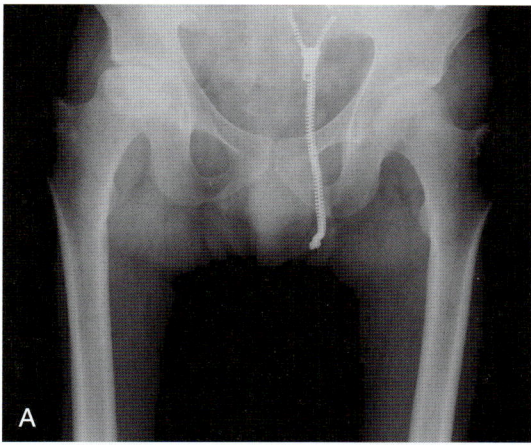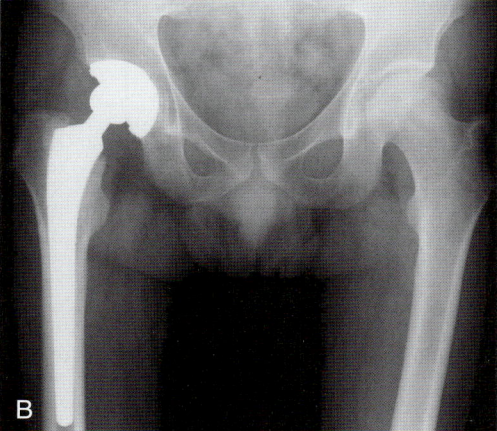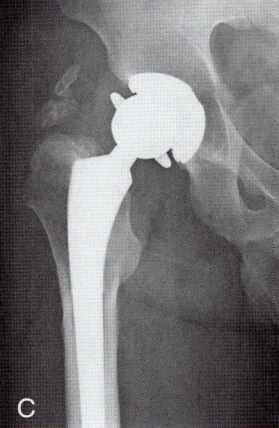

Figure 101-8. A, Preoperative anteroposterior radiograph of a 28-year-old male with alcohol-induced avascular necrosis. *(Reproduced courtesy Joint Implant Surgeons, Inc.)* **B,** Postoperative anteroposterior radiograph noting vertical cup position. The patient developed chronic instability. *(Reproduced courtesy Joint Implant Surgeons, Inc.)* **C,** Anteroposterior radiograph 6 years following revision total hip arthroplasty with conversion to a larger head and a constrained liner. *(Reproduced courtesy Joint Implant Surgeons, Inc.)*

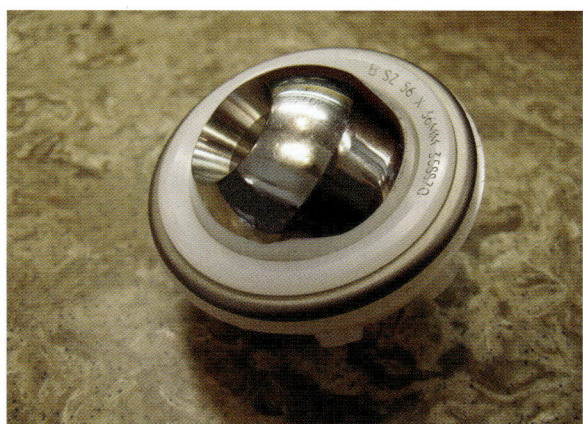

Figure 101-9. Constrained liner and femoral head with flat surfaces. *(Reproduced courtesy Joint Implant Surgeons, Inc.)*

before impingement compared with tripolar constraint and classic capture and locking ring components.[87]

An additional disadvantage of all constrained devices is that dislocation of these revision constructs usually requires open reduction (although a few case reports have described detailed techniques and successes of closed reduction[91-94]). Longer-term follow-up will be required for all constrained devices to elucidate the rate of osteolysis, aseptic loosening, and unique component failure mechanisms.

CONCLUSION

In conclusion, dislocation continues to be a major mode of failure in long-term follow-up of THA. Understanding the risk factors and the causes of instability should help reduce the incidence of this complication. When instability is encountered, an understanding of the treatment

options provides the surgeon with the tools needed to manage this challenging complication.

REFERENCES

1. Chang RW, Pellisier JM, Hazen GB: A cost-effectiveness analysis of total hip arthroplasty for osteoarthritis of the hip. JAMA 275:858–865, 1996.
2. Bozic KJ, Kurtz SM, Lau E, et al: The epidemiology of revision total hip arthroplasty in the United States. J Bone Joint Surg Am 91:128–133, 2009.
3. Eftekhar NS: Dislocation and instability complicating low friction arthroplasty of the hip joint. Clin Orthop Relat Res 121:120–125, 1976.
4. Lewinnek GE, Lewis JL, Tarr R, et al: Dislocations after total hip-replacement arthroplasties. J Bone Joint Surg Am 60:217–220, 1978.
5. Ritter MA: Dislocation and subluxation of the total hip replacement. Clin Orthop Relat Res 121:92–94, 1976.
6. Woo RYG, Morrey BF: Dislocations after total hip arthroplasty. J Bone Joint Surg Am 64:1295–1306, 1982.
7. Heithoff BE, Callaghan JJ, Goetz DD, et al: Dislocation after total hip arthroplasty: a single surgeon's experience. Orthop Clin North Am 32:587, 2001.
8. Berry DJ, von Knoch M, Schleck CD, Harmsen WS: The cumulative long-term risk of dislocation after primary Charnley total hip arthroplasty. J Bone Joint Surg Am 86:9–14, 2004.
9. McCollum DE, Gray WJ: Dislocation after total hip arthroplasty: causes and prevention. Clin Orthop Relat Res 261:159–170, 1990.
10. Morrey BF: Difficult complications after hip joint replacement: dislocation. Clin Orthop Relat Res 344:179–187, 1997.
11. Callaghan JJ, Templeton JE, Liu SS, et al: Results of Charnley total hip arthroplasty at a minimum of thirty years: a concise follow-up of a previous report. J Bone Joint Surg Am 86:690–695, 2004.
12. Khatod M, Barber T, Paxton E, et al: An analysis of the risk of hip dislocation with a contemporary total joint registry. Clin Orthop Relat Res 447:19–23, 2006.
13. Meek RMD, Allan DB, McPhillips G, et al: Epidemiology of dislocation after total hip arthroplasty. Clin Orthop Relat Res 447:9–18, 2006.
14. Parvizi J, Picinic E, Sharkey PF: Revision total hip arthroplasty for instability: surgical techniques and principles. J Bone Joint Surg Am 90:1134–1142, 2008.
15. Phillips CB, Barrett JA, Losina E, et al: Incidence rates of dislocation, pulmonary embolism, and deep infection during the

first six months after elective total hip replacement. J Bone Joint Surg Am 85:20–26, 2003.

16. Alberton GM, High WA, Morrey BF: Dislocation after revision total hip arthroplasty: an analysis of risk factors and treatment options. J Bone Joint Surg Am 84:1788–1792, 2002.

17. Conroy JL, Whitehouse SL, Graves SE, et al: Risk factors for revision for early dislocation in total hip arthroplasty. J Arthroplasty 23:867–872, 2008.

18. Kurtz S, Ong K, Lau E, et al: Projections of primary and revision hip and knee arthroplasty in the United States from 2005 to 2030. J Bone Joint Surg Am 89:780–785, 2007.

19. Bourne RB, Maloney WJ, Wright JG: An AOA critical issue: the outcome of the outcomes movement. J Bone Joint Surg Am 86:633–640, 2004.

20. Sanchez-Sotelo J, Haidukewych GJ, Boberg CJ: Hospital cost of dislocation after primary total hip arthroplasty. J Bone Joint Surg Am 88:290–294, 2006.

21. Morrey BF: Instability after total hip arthroplasty. Orthop Clin North Am 23:237–248, 1992.

22. Ekelund A, Rydell N, Nilsson OS: Total hip arthroplasty in patients 80 years of age and older. Clin Orthop Relat Res 281:101–106, 1992.

23. Parvizi J, Sharkey PF, Bissett GA, et al: Surgical treatment of limb-length discrepancy following total hip arthroplasty. J Bone Joint Surg Am 85:2310–2317, 2003.

24. Katz JN, Losina E, Barrett J, et al: Association between hospital and surgeon procedure volume and outcomes of total hip replacement in the United States Medicare population. J Bone Joint Surg Am 83:1622–1629, 2001.

25. Levy RN, Levy CM, Snyder J, Digiovanni J: Outcome and long-term results following total hip replacement in elderly patients. Clin Orthop Relat Res 316:25–30, 1995.

26. Lachiewicz PF, Soileau ES: Stability of total hip arthroplasty in patients 75 years or older. Clin Orthop Relat Res 405:65–69, 2002.

27. Zwartele RE, Brand R, Doets HC: Increased risk of dislocation after primary total hip arthroplasty in inflammatory arthritis: a prospective observational study of 410 hips. Acta Orthop Scand 75:684–690, 2004.

28. Lee BP, Berry DJ, Harmsen WS, Sim FH: Total hip arthroplasty for the treatment of an acute fracture of the femoral neck: long-term results. J Bone Joint Surg Am 80:70–75, 1998.

29. Mallory TH, Lombardi AV, Jr, Fada RA, et al: Dislocation after total hip arthroplasty using the anterolateral abductor split approach. Clin Orthop Relat Res 358:166–172, 1999.

30. Krenzel BA, Faris PM, Keating EM, et al: High pre-operative range of motion is a significant risk factor for dislocation in primary total hip arthroplasty. Presented at the 19th Annual Meeting of the American Association of Hip and Knee Surgeons, Dallas, November 2009.

31. Jolles BM, Zangeger P, Leyvraz PF: Factors predisposing to dislocation after primary total hip arthroplasty. J Arthroplasty 17:282–288, 2002.

32. Paterno S, Lachiewicz P, Kelley S: The influence of patient-related factors and the position of the acetabular component on the rate of dislocation after total hip replacement. J Bone Joint Surg Am 79:1202–1210, 1997.

33. Jibodh SR, Gurkan I, Wenz JF: In-hospital outcome and resource use in hip arthroplasty: influence of body mass. Orthopedics 27:594–601, 2004.

34. Azodi OS, Adami J, Lindstrom D, et al: High body mass index is associated with increased risk of implant dislocation following primary total hip replacement. Acta Orthop 79:141–147, 2008.

35. Kim Y, Morshed S, Joseph T, et al: Clinical impact of obesity on stability following revision total hip arthroplasty. Clin Orthop Relat Res 453:142–146, 2006.

36. Berry DJ, von Knoch M, Schleck CD, Harmsen WS: Effect of femoral head diameter and operative approach on risk of dislocation after primary total hip arthroplasty. J Bone Joint Surg Am 87:2456–2463, 2005.

37. Masonis JL, Bourne RB: Surgical approach, abductor function, and total hip arthroplasty dislocation. Clin Orthop Relat Res 405:46–53, 2002.

38. Pellicci PM, Bostrom M, Poss R: Posterior approach to total hip replacement using enhanced posterior soft tissue repair. Clin Orthop Relat Res 355:224–228, 1998.

39. Sierra RJ, Raposo JM, Trousdale RT, Cabanela ME: Dislocation of primary THA done through a posterolateral approach in the elderly. Clin Orthop Relat Res 441:262–267, 2005.

40. Kim YS, Kwon SY, Sun DH, et al: Modified posterior approach to total hip arthroplasty to enhance joint stability. Clin Orthop Relat Res 466:294–299, 2008.

41. Biedermann R, Tonin A, Krismer M, et al: Reducing the risk of dislocation after total hip arthroplasty. J Bone Joint Surg Br 87:762–769, 2005.

42. Hassan DM, Johnston GHF, Dust WNC, et al: Accuracy of intra-operative assessment of acetabular prosthesis placement. J Arthroplasty 13:80–84, 1998.

43. Archbold HAP, Mockford B, Molloy D, et al: The transverse acetabular ligament: an aid to orientation of the acetabular component during primary total hip replacement. J Bone Joint Surg Br 88:883–886, 2006.

44. Sotereanos NG, Miller MC, Smith B, et al: Using intraoperative pelvic landmarks for acetabular component placement in total hip arthroplasty. J Arthroplasty 21:832–840, 2006.

45. Honl M, Schwieger K, Salineros M, et al: Orientation of the acetabular component: a comparison of five navigation systems with conventional surgical technique. J Bone Joint Surg Br 88:1401–1405, 2006.

46. Smith TM, Berend KR, Lombardi AV, Jr, et al: Metal-on-metal total hip arthroplasty with large heads may prevent early dislocation. Clin Orthop Relat Res 441:137–142, 2005.

47. Cuckler JM, Moore KD, Lombardi AV, Jr, et al: Large versus small femoral heads in metal-on-metal total hip arthroplasty. J Arthroplasty 19:41–44, 2004.

48. Skeels MD, Berend KR, Lombardi AV, Jr: The dislocator, early and late: the role of large heads. Orthopedics 32:667, 2009.

49. Peters CL, McPherson E, Jackson JD, Erickson JA: Reduction in early dislocation rate with large-diameter femoral heads in primary total hip arthroplasty. J Arthroplasty 22:140–144, 2007.

50. Kung PL, Ries MD: Effect of femoral head size and abductors on dislocation after revision THA. Clin Orthop Relat Res 465:170–174, 2007.

51. Amstutz HC, Le Duff MJ, Beaulé PE: Prevention and treatment of dislocation after total hip replacement using large diameter balls. Clin Orthop Relat Res 429:108–116, 2004.

52. Lachiewicz PF, Soileau ES: Dislocation of primary total hip arthroplasty with 36 and 40-mm femoral heads. Clin Orthop Relat Res 453:153–155, 2006.

53. Sariali E, Lazennec JY, Khiami F, Catonné Y: Mathematical evaluation of jumping distance in total hip arthroplasty: influence of abduction angle, femoral head offset, and head diameter. Acta Orthop 80:277–282, 2009.

54. Smit MJ: Hip stability in primary total hip arthroplasty using an anatomically sized femoral head. Orthopedics 32:489, 2009.

55. Kelley SS, Lachiewicz PF, Hickman JM, Paterno SM: Relationship of femoral head and acetabular size to prevalence of dislocation. Clin Orthop Relat Res 355:163–170, 1998.

56. Scifert CF, Noble PC, Brown TD, et al: Experimental and computational simulation of total hip arthroplasty dislocation. Orthop Clin North Am 32:553–567, 2001.

57. Bourne RB, Rorabeck CH: Soft tissue balancing: the hip. J Arthroplasty 17:17–22, 2002.

58. Parvizi J, Sharkey PF, Bissett GA, et al: Surgical treatment of limb-length discrepancy following total hip arthroplasty. J Bone Joint Surg Am 85:2310–2317, 2003.

59. Cobb TK, Morrey BF, Ilstrup DM: The elevated rim acetabular liner in total hip arthroplasty: relationship to postoperative dislocation. J Bone Joint Surg Am 78:80–86, 2003.

60. Battaglia TC, Mulhall KJ, Brown TE, Saleh KJ: Increased surgical volume is associated with lower THA dislocation rates. Clin Orthop Relat Res 447:28–33, 2006.

61. von Knoch M, Berry DJ, Harmsen WS, Morrey BF: Late dislocation after total hip arthroplasty. J Bone Joint Surg Am 84:1949–1953, 2002.

62. Padgett DE, Warashina H: The unstable total hip replacement. Clin Orthop Relat Res 420:72–79, 2004.

63. Dorr LD, Wan Z: Causes of and treatment protocol for instability of total hip replacement. Clin Orthop Relat Res 355:144–151, 1998.

64. Rogers M, Blom AW, Barnett A, et al: Revision for recurrent dislocation of total hip replacement. Hip Int 19:109–113, 2009.

65. Toomey SD, Hopper RH, Jr, McAuley JP, Engh CA: Modular component exchange for treatment of recurrent dislocation of a total hip replacement in selected patients. J Bone Joint Surg Am 83:1529–1533, 2001.

66. McConway J, O'Brien S, Doran E, et al: The use of a posterior lip augmentation device for a revision of recurrent dislocation after primary cemented Charnley/Charnley Elite total hip replacement: results at a mean follow-up of six years and nine months. J Bone Joint Surg Br 89:1581–1585, 2007.

67. Parvizi J, Wade FA, Rapuri V, et al: Revision hip arthroplasty for late instability secondary to polyethylene wear. Clin Orthop Relat Res 447:66–69, 2006.

68. Beaulé PE, Schmalzried TP, Udomkiat P, Amstutz HC: Jumbo femoral head for the treatment of recurrent dislocation following total hip replacement. J Bone Joint Surg Am 84:256–263, 2002.

69. Lachiewicz PF: Dislocation. In Hozack WJ, Parvizi J, Bender B, editors: Surgical treatment of hip arthritis: reconstruction, replacement, and revision, Philadelphia, 2010, Saunders Elsevier, pp 429–436.

70. Lavigne MJ, Sanchez AA, Coutts RD: Recurrent dislocation after total hip arthroplasty: treatment with an Achilles tendon allograft. J Arthroplasty 16(Suppl 1):13–18, 2001.

71. Stromsoe K, Eikvar K: Fascia lata plasty in recurrent posterior dislocation after total hip arthroplasty. Arch Orthop Trauma Surg 114:292–294, 1995.

72. Barbosa JK, Khan AM, Andrew JG: Treatment of recurrent dislocation of total hip arthroplasty using a ligament prosthesis. J Arthroplasty 19:318–321, 2004.

73. Ekelund A: Trochanteric osteotomy for recurrent dislocation of total hip arthroplasty. J Arthroplasty 8:629–632, 1993.

74. Kaplan SJ, Thomas WH, Poss R: Trochanteric advancement for recurrent dislocation after total hip arthroplasty. J Arthroplasty 2:119–124, 1987.

75. Dennis DA, Lynch CB: Trochanteric osteotomy and advancement: a technique for abductor related hip instability. Orthopedics 27:959–961, 2004.

76. Parvizi J, Morrey BF: Bipolar hip arthroplasty as a salvage treatment for instability of the hip. J Bone Joint Surg Am 82:1132–1139, 2000.

77. Attarian DE: Bipolar arthroplasty for recurrent total hip instability. J South Orthop Assoc 8:249–253, 1999.

78. Ries MD, Wiedel JD: Bipolar hip arthroplasty for recurrent dislocation after total hip arthroplasty: a report of three cases. Clin Orthop Relat Res 278:121–127, 1992.

79. Grigoris P, Grecula MJ, Amstutz HC: Tripolar hip replacement for recurrent prosthetic dislocation. Clin Orthop Relat Res 304:148–155, 1994.

80. Beaulé PE, Roussignol X, Schmalzried TP, et al: Tripolar arthroplasty for recurrent total hip prosthesis dislocation. Rev Chir Orthop Reparatrice Mot 89:242–249, 2003.

81. Levine BR, Della Valle CJ, Deirmengian CA, et al: The use of tripolar articulation in revision total hip arthroplasty: a minimum of 24 months follow-up. J Arthroplasty 23:1182–1188, 2008.

82. Goetz DD, Bremner BRB, Callaghan JJ, et al: Salvage of a recurrently dislocating total hip prosthesis with use of a constrained acetabular component: a concise follow-up of a previous report. J Bone Joint Surg Am 86:2419–2423, 2004.

83. Bremner BRB, Goetz DD, Callaghan JJ, et al: Use of constrained acetabular components for hip instability: an average 10-year follow-up study. J Arthroplasty 18:131–137, 2003.

84. Shrader MW, Parvizi J, Lewallen DG: The use of a constrained acetabular component to treat instability after total hip arthroplasty. J Bone Joint Surg Am 85:2179–2183, 2003.

85. Su EP, Pellicci PM: The role of constrained liners in total hip arthroplasty. Clin Orthop Relat Res 420:122–129, 2004.

86. Berend KR, Lombardi AV, Jr, Mallory TH, et al: The long-term outcome of 755 consecutive constrained acetabular components in total hip arthroplasty: examining the success and failures. J Arthroplasty 20(Suppl 3):93–102, 2003.

87. Berend KR, Lombardi AV, Jr, Welch M, Adams JB: A constrained device with increased range of motion prevents early dislocation. Clin Orthop Relat Res 447:70–75, 2006.

88. Callaghan JJ, O'Rourke MR, Goetz DD, et al: Use of a constrained tripolar acetabular liner to treat intraoperative instability and postoperative dislocation after total hip arthroplasty: a review of our experience. Clin Orthop Relat Res 429:117–123, 2004.

89. Callaghan JJ, Parvizi J, Novak CC, et al: A constrained liner cemented into a secure cementless acetabular shell. J Bone Joint Surg Am 86:2206–2211, 2004.

90. Guyen O, Lewallen DG, Cabanela ME: Modes of failure of osteonics constrained tripolar implants: a retrospective analysis of forty-three failed implants. J Bone Joint Surg Am 90:1153–1160, 2008.

91. Robertson WJ, Mattern CJ, Hur J, et al: Failure mechanisms and closed reduction of a constrained tripolar acetabular liner. J Arthroplasty 242:322e5–322e11, 2009.

92. McPherson EJ, Costigan WM, Gerhardt MB, Norris LR: Closed reduction of dislocated total hip with S-ROM constrained acetabular component. J Arthroplasty 14:882–885, 1999.

93. Miller CW, Zura RD: Closed reduction of a dislocation of a constrained acetabular component. J Arthroplasty 16:504–505, 2001.

94. Harman MK, Hodge WA, Banks SA: Closed reduction of constrained total hip arthroplasty. Clin Orthop Relat Res 414:121–128, 2003.

CHAPTER 102

Periprosthetic Fracture: Prevention/Diagnosis/Treatment

Christopher R. Gooding, Donald S. Garbuz, Bassam A. Masri, and Clive P. Duncan

KEY POINTS

- The diagnosis of periprosthetic fracture is based on the history, physical examination, and radiographic evaluation.
- Use of a classification system for these fractures helps the surgeon better understand the problem, construct a treatment algorithm, and maximize the chances of success.
- Preoperative planning is essential in the management of these fractures, but the surgeon must have the flexibility to change the plan should circumstances change during the course of surgery.
- Secure fixation of the stem to the intact distal fragment is critical for success.

INTRODUCTION

Since the mid-1960s, periprosthetic fractures have posed a difficult surgical problem for orthopedic surgeons.[1,2] Treatment is based on whether the fracture occurred during or after the operation, and whether it involves the acetabulum, the femur, or both.

On the acetabular side, fractures can occur intraoperatively in the course of bone preparation or component insertion (particularly when a press-fit technique is used for a cementless acetabular component), or in the revision situation while implant removal is attempted.[3] Fractures can also occur postoperatively secondary to traumatic injury, or more commonly in association with a loose component that leads to bone loss and a chronic periprosthetic fracture of the acetabulum, where the superior and inferior halves of the hemipelvis are no longer in continuity.[4] The latter, termed *pelvic dissociation* or *discontinuity,* requires careful radiographic and intraoperative evaluation so as to avoid a missed diagnosis because standard revision techniques may not be adequate for reconstruction.

Similarly, on the femoral side, fractures can occur during[5-7] or after surgery.[6,8-14] Missed intraoperative fractures and those treated inappropriately carry a high risk of a poor outcome because of nonunion or malunion. Avoidance of such complications is desirable, and prevention certainly plays a role. It is helpful to classify these fractures to enable the use of a logical treatment algorithm that is based on the stability of the implant (e.g., well fixed or loose) and the bone stock available for reconstruction if a revision procedure is required.

EPIDEMIOLOGY AND RISK FACTORS

The incidence of intraoperative acetabular periprosthetic fracture during cemented total hip arthroplasty (THA) has been reported to be as low as 0.2%.[15] However, with the advent of the cementless acetabular fixation, the incidence has increased.[16-20] A consistent factor in the development of acetabular fractures is under-reaming of the acetabulum in an attempt to gain initial press-fit stability with a cementless component.[3] It has been suggested that under-reaming by as much as 4 mm is acceptable[21]; however, most now agree that 2 mm or less is safer.[22]

Postoperative acetabular fractures are relatively uncommon. Berry and associates reported 0.9% prevalence associated with pelvic discontinuity, which was observed at revision.[4] Risk factors for early postoperative fracture include early weight bearing on pathologic bone, as reported by Sanchez-Sotelo and colleagues.[23]

Another group of patients at risk of developing an early postoperative acetabular fracture includes those who have undergone revision of an acetabular socket to a hemispherical or elliptical, uncemented, trabecular metal shell. Springer and coworkers[24] reported on seven patients who developed a transverse acetabular fracture at a mean postoperative time of 8 months. The authors concluded that the fractures probably occurred as the result of further weakening of the acetabular bone stock caused by the reaming needed to obtain a good press-fit of a large-diameter shell. Once this weakened bone was subjected to weight-bearing, it would fracture. They recommended (1) protecting the columnar support as much as possible during reaming of the socket, and (2) in high-risk patients, limiting early postoperative weight bearing.

The risk of intraoperative femoral fracture appears dependent in part on the method of fixation used. An incidence of 0.1% to 1% has been reported with cemented stems.[25] Berry reported a similar incidence of 0.3% in 20,859 primary cemented stems but 5.4% in 3121 uncemented THAs. This higher incidence in uncemented THAs could be explained by the force sometimes required to achieve primary stem stability.

Revision surgery is associated with an even greater incidence of periprosthetic fracture. Berry reported intraoperative fracture rates of 3.6% of 4813 cemented and 20.9% of 1536 uncemented revision total hip arthroplasties.[8] Meek and associates[26] described a total of 211 patients who underwent revision with a diaphyseal-fitting cementless stem. Sixty-four (30%) patients sustained an intraoperative fracture.

Fredin and colleagues[27] reported 11 (0.56%) periprosthetic fractures following primary total hip arthroplasty in 1961 patients over a 14-year period. Kavanagh[25] suggested that the incidence was closer to 1% after primary and 4.2% after revision hip replacement. Lowenhielm and coworkers[13] reported a similar incidence of 22 (1.5%) fractures out of a total of 1442 total hip replacements, 14 of which were femoral. They also related that the accumulated postoperative risk of femoral fracture over a 15-year period was 25.3 per 1000.

Beals and Tower[28] reviewed 102 revision procedures following 93 periprosthetic fractures. They estimated an incidence of periprosthetic fracture of 1% over the lifetime of the implant. A similar incidence of 1.1% was reported by the Mayo Clinic Joint Registry of postoperative periprosthetic femoral fractures from their large series of almost 24,000 primary THAs.[8] A higher incidence of 4% was associated with revision hip surgery,

after 6349 revision THAs. Table 102-1 summarizes the published incidence/prevalence of periprosthetic hip fracture.

Many reports in the literature indicate that the incidence of late postoperative periprosthetic femoral fractures is increasing.[8,25,29-34] This is to be expected, given the advancing age of our population of individuals who have had a THA, and the fact that the risk of periprosthetic fracture is influenced substantially by the age of the patient at the time of hip replacement.[35] The risk is low for an individual of normal life expectancy who undergoes primary implantation before reaching the age of 70 years. However, patients who are older than 70 years have a 2.9 times greater risk, and those older than 80 years have a 4.4 times greater risk. This increased risk with advancing age is undoubtedly multifactorial.[36]

In their review of the Swedish Registry, Lindahl and associates found that higher risk of periprosthetic fracture was associated with patient age and with every year of aging after the primary procedure.[36] In this study, the risk ratio for fracture was 1.01 per additional year of aging. Investigators also found that the time from the primary hip arthroplasty was a risk factor, perhaps because of osteolysis, as well as implant loosening. This was confirmed in a later study, when it was demonstrated that the younger the patient is at the time

Table 102-1. Summary of the Published Incidence/Prevalence of Periprosthetic Fractures Associated With Total Hip Arthroplasty (THA)

Fracture Type	Author	Incidence	Paper	Sample size
Intraoperative				
Acetabular fractures				
Cemented primary THA	McElfresh[15]	0.2%	McElfresh	5400
Uncemented primary THA	Peterson[16]		Peterson	18630
	Adler[17]		Adler	Estimate
	Curtis[18]	>0.2%	Curtis	Estimate
	MacKenzie[19]		MacKenzie	Estimate
	Stiehl[20]		Stiehl	Estimate
Femoral fractures				
Cemented primary THA	Kavanagh[25]	0.1%-1%	Kavanagh	Sample size not mentioned
	Berry[8]	0.3%	Berry (cemented THA)	20859
Uncemented primary THA	Berry[8]	5.4%	Berry (uncemented THA)	3121
Postoperative				
Acetabular fractures	Peterson[16]	0.07%, including primary and revision hip arthroplasty	Peterson	23850
	Berry[8]	0.9% associated with pelvic discontinuity	Berry (pelvic discontinuity)	3505
Femoral fractures	Berry[8]	1.1%	Berry (femoral fractures)	24000
	Fredin[27]	0.56%	Fredin	1961
	Lowenhielm[13]	1.5% (accumulated risk of femoral fracture over 15-year period = 25.3/1000; 1% over lifetime of implant)	Lowenhielm	1442
	Beals[28]		Beals	102
Revision				
Intraoperative cemented femoral fractures	Berry[8]	3.6%	Berry (intraop cem fem #)	4813
Intraoperative uncemented femoral fractures	Berry[8]	20.9%	Berry (intraop uncem fem #)	1536
	Meek[26]	30%	Meek	211
Postoperative femoral fractures	Berry[8]	4%	Berry (post op # following rev)	6349

of the primary arthroplasty, the greater is the risk for subsequent fracture,[37] although the type of fracture is not influenced by age, gender, or implant type.[38]

Low-energy falls are responsible for a large number of periprosthetic fractures.[39,40] Relatively minor trauma in some studies has accounted for nearly 75% of all periprosthetic fractures.[39] Undoubtedly, a multifactorial element is involved as well, and poor bone stock following numerous revisions has been shown to play a significant role.[39] Falls commonly occur in the home (66%); only a small number occur outdoors (18%).[28]

Female gender has long been thought of as a risk factor for periprosthetic fracture.[5,10,28,34] However, the Finnish Joint Registry showed no difference in fracture rate between sexes.[40] Any perceived risk associated with gender is undoubtedly affected by a number of potential confounding factors, so it is difficult to conclude that gender alone is responsible for an increased fracture rate.

Less controversial is that osteoporosis is a risk factor for periprosthetic femoral fractures post THA.[36,41-43] Beals and associates[28] observed that 38% of patients in their study had previously sustained a fragility fracture such as a vertebral fracture, and many of their patients had osteopenia. Wu and colleagues, using Singh's index for osteoporosis, found that preoperative osteoporosis was a significant predictor of fracture.[35] A large number of periprosthetic fractures occur secondary to low-energy falls, again suggesting that bone fragility plays a role.[36]

Other comorbidities before hip arthroplasty may be associated with the risk of periprosthetic fracture. Rheumatoid arthritis can result in diffuse osteopenia and is over-represented in a number of joint registries among patients who have sustained a periprosthetic femoral fracture.[36,37,40] Patients with a femoral neck fracture who were treated with THA are also at increased risk. The Finnish Registry showed that patients who had sustained a previous hip fracture had twice the risk of a periprosthetic fracture compared with patients who had rheumatoid arthritis[40]; similar observations were made from the Swedish Registry.[36] This increased risk could well be due to poor bone stock, as is present in most patients who have sustained a femoral neck fracture.

Osteolysis also has a role to play in late periprosthetic fractures.[14,34,44] Understanding the pathophysiology is important because it has implications for surgical management of the fracture. Not only must the problem of deficient bone be addressed, as well as the possibility of a loose implant; the issue of the source of wear particles often necessitates revision of bearing surfaces.[29,42]

Aseptic loosening as a risk factor for periprosthetic fracture[34,45] is often the end result of osteolysis secondary to wear particles, causing bone resorption. This is further exacerbated in loose cemented stems by motion at the cement-bone interface.[10] Evidence of loosening before a fracture occurs has been reported in a large number of cases. Bethea and coworkers observed in their series that 75% of patients showed evidence of loosening before fracture.[10] Others have reported that almost half of the patients they reviewed demonstrated evidence of loosening.[11,46] This is supported by one of the largest reviews to date, which demonstrated, in a series of more than 1000 fractures, that 70% were loose before the injury occurred.[39]

Revision surgery is associated with both intraoperative and postoperative periprosthetic fractures.[25,36,47] Poor bone stock is probably the most significant factor in this setting, but the number of revisions also has a role in fracture development.[36] Furthermore, the time between a revision operation and occurrence of fracture appears to diminish with each additional revision surgery.[39]

Various intraoperative factors related to surgical technique can precipitate a fracture. Cortical perforations, such as screw holes, previous hardware, osteotomies, or perforations caused by cement removal or reaming, may result in a stress riser.[44,48] Other risk factors for intraoperative cortical perforation include osteoporosis, poor bone stock, and a narrow medullary canal.[15] Cortical defects can have a significant impact on cortical strength. Animal studies have shown that torsional strength can be adversely affected by 44%,[49] although bypassing the defect by 2 diaphyseal diameters with a long stem can improve bone strength to 84% of the intact contralateral femur. Clinical studies seem to suggest a causal relationship between localized areas of weakened bone and periprosthetic fracture.[2,5,10,50] Meek and associates[26] support this observation. They found that patients with a low ratio of cortical width to femoral diameter were at greatest risk for a diaphyseal fracture. Box 102-1 summarizes the risk factors for periprosthetic hip fracture.

PREVENTION

Prevention of periprosthetic fractures starts from the time of surgery. Particularly in revision surgery, it has been shown that exposure is key to avoidance of complications including periprosthetic fracture. A number of extensile techniques have been developed to help reduce the risk of intraoperative fracture.[51] In the revision setting, a fracture can occur during hip dislocation, cement and implant removal, reaming of the acetabulum and femur, trial reduction, or during final insertion of the implant.[2,7,25,52] During hip dislocation, the risk of fracture is higher in patients who have had previous surgery such as a plate and screws for a femoral fracture, because of stress risers that occur at the old screw holes and stiffness from the prior surgical procedure. One option to help reduce the risk of fracture is to dislocate the hip first if necessary then relocate, before removing the plate.

Patient anatomy may also predispose patients to fracture. From a review of preoperative radiographs, it can be seen that if the trochanter is overhanging the canal in the primary setting or the stem in a revision setting, it would be prudent to provide sufficient clearance of the overhanging bone to allow instrumentation of the femur or removal of a stem without fracturing the greater trochanter (Fig. 102-1). This can be accomplished by creating a channel, or by completing a standard or extended trochanteric osteotomy. Risk of fracture during cement

BOX 102-1. SUMMARY OF RISK FACTORS FOR PERIPROSTHETIC HIP FRACTURE

Intraoperative Risk Factors for Acetabular Fracture
- Osteoporosis
- Poor bone stock
- Uncemented acetabular components
- Under-reaming of the acetabulum

Postoperative Risk Factors for Acetabular Fracture
- Early weight bearing on pathologic bone
- Revision of an acetabular socket to a hemispherical, uncemented trabecular metal shell

Intraoperative Risk Factors for Femoral Fracture
- Cortical perforations and cortical defects
- Osteoporosis
- Poor bone stock
- Uncemented femoral stems
- Revision of a femoral stem, especially if a diaphyseal-fitting stem

Postoperative Risk Factors for Femoral Fracture
- Age (multifactorial)
- Gender (multifactorial)
- Falls (multifactorial)
- Poor bone stock
- Osteoporosis
- Revision arthroplasty
- The greater the time interval between the primary arthroplasty and revision surgery, the greater the risk of fracture
- Rheumatoid arthritis
- Previous fracture neck of femur treated with total hip arthroplasty
- Osteolysis and aseptic loosening

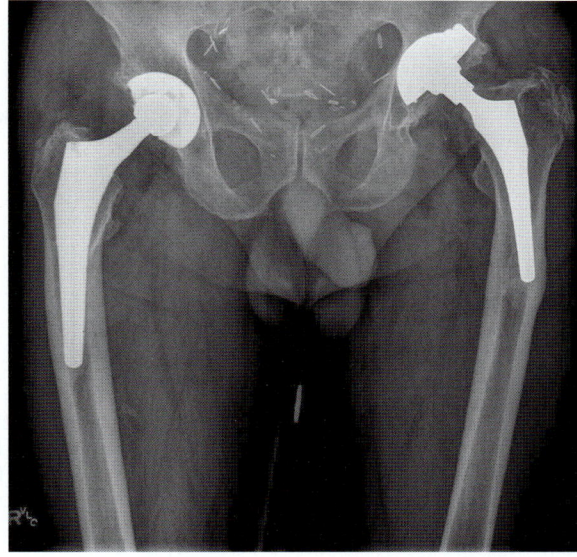

Figure 102-1. Anteroposterior (AP) pelvis radiograph demonstrating a varus deformity of the femur and the greater trochanter overlying the medullary canal, requiring modified exposure to correct the deformity and avoid damage to the trochanter.

removal can be reduced by adequate visualization of the proximal femur; this can be achieved by performing a standard or extended trochanteric osteotomy.[53]

As highlighted by Mitchell and associates,[54] an extended trochanteric osteotomy allows wide exposure, easier cement removal, correct location of the distal medullary canal so as to reduce the risk of cortical perforation, accurate alignment of the revision stem, and correction of the deformity, if required. A cortical window or a controlled perforation of the anterior cortex is another option to assist with implant or cement removal. Sydney and colleagues[55] described a very low rate of subsequent periprosthetic fracture with the latter technique, as long as the perforation is made anteriorly and then is bypassed with a long cementless stem by two diaphyseal diameters. This should be by a minimum distance of two bone diameters at the level of the cortical defect. Another simple measure to help prevent intraoperative fracture in revision surgery is to prepare the acetabulum before the femur. This practice not only reduces blood loss, it also minimizes the risk of weakening the femur and the possibility of fracture during retraction.

Surgeons should be wary of unrecognized cortical perforation at the time of a revision that can be unintentionally made larger during canal preparation; this can predispose the femur to fracture or can create a "false passage" and misplacement of the stem tip outside the canal. The use of guide wires as well as intraoperative fluoroscopy or plain radiographs can help avert such an error.

Excessive force should be avoided when reamers, rasps, or the definitive implant is introduced into the femur. The femoral canal should be meticulously cleared of debris using crochet hooks before femoral reaming; crochet hooks can also act as an extension of the surgeon's hand to ensure that a cortical perforation or a residual pedestal does not exist. Reaming initially by hand or with flexible reamers assists with sizing of the canal and further ensures central positioning within the canal. Further, if an extended trochanteric osteotomy is used, placement of a prophylactic cerclage wire distal to the osteotomy before manipulation of the canal can help to protect the femur from hoop stresses associated with reaming, broaching, and final implant insertion. If considerable resistance to insertion of the broach, trial implant, or final implant occurs, it is advisable to stop and obtain an intraoperative radiograph to confirm appropriate placement.

The danger of under-reaming on the acetabular side has already been highlighted. Similarly, under-reaming on the femoral side is hazardous, particularly if the bone is osteoporotic. If a straight stem is being used, under-reaming by 0.5 mm and no more[54] is considered safe. It is important to recognize that the labeled size of the final implant may vary from the size reported by the manufacturer, and the use of a hole gauge can be invaluable in ensuring that the amount of intended under-reaming is accurate (Fig. 102-2). Ideally these gauges

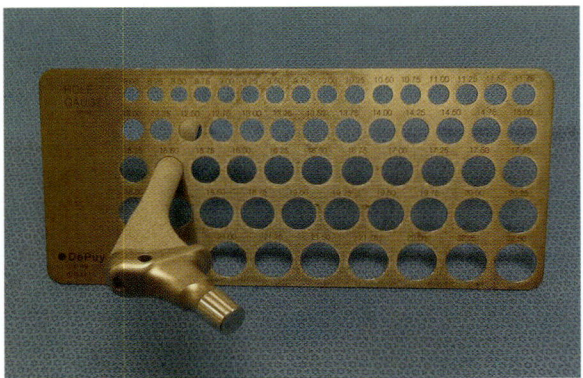

Figure 102-2. Photograph illustrating the use of a hole gauge with a fully porous-coated stem. In this case, the labeled implant size was 15 mm, but measurement of the stem showed it to be 15.5 mm. The femur was subsequently reamed to 15 mm to obtain an appropriate press-fit without increasing the risk of a periprosthetic femur fracture.

should be metallic in construction, rather than the commonly supplied plastic varieties, because the plastic can warp during autoclaving, leading to the risk of mismeasurement.

If cortical defects or osteolytic lesions are present near the tip of the stem, they can be grafted with cortical strut grafts as a prophylactic measure or bypassed with a long stem.* Large osteolytic lesions of the greater trochanter should be packed with bone graft after granulomatous tissue has been excised. If there is any doubt as to the integrity of the greater trochanter, it should be prophylactically reinforced with a cerclage wire or a claw and cable plate system to prevent crack initiation and propagation.[58,59] An intraoperative radiograph should be considered if a fracture is suspected. Finally, postoperative films, including a full-length view of the stem, should be routine, and postoperative management can be modified if necessary.

Anticipation and prevention of intraoperative fractures should form an essential part of preoperative planning. Being aware of possible stress risers in the femur and taking great care with cement removal are essential in avoiding this complication. Postoperatively, the risk of periprosthetic fracture can be reduced by careful supervision and assessment. Clear instructions should be given as to the patient's weight-bearing status and level of activity, and it should be ensured that the patient has suitable accommodations at the time of discharge. Any condition that predisposes to a fall should be identified and treated.

Careful clinical and radiographic follow-up of patients should help in preventing late periprosthetic fractures.[33,36] Radiographs should be assessed for evidence of early osteolysis and aseptic loosening, and if a failing hip arthroplasty is identified, it should be revised.[44] It is difficult to know when to intervene, particularly if the patient is asymptomatic; however, progressive bone loss should be considered as an indication to intervene so as to prevent fracture.[33]

*References 2, 15, 28, 44, 48, 56, and 57.

DIAGNOSIS

The diagnosis of periprosthetic fracture is based on history, as well as on physical and radiographic examinations. Fractures generally can be recognized intraoperatively by direct observation or by radiographs. This is likely to occur during one of the three stages of reconstruction: previous implant removal, bone preparation, or placement of the revision implant. Signs that alert the surgeon to this possibility include a change in pitch while using instruments, a sudden reduction in the force required when a broach or rasp is used, or advancement of the implant beyond the planned level of placement, either in the socket or in the canal.

Postoperative periprosthetic fractures are typically associated with an acute onset of pain and deformity that may or may not follow a history of a fall. However, clinical suspicion of a periprosthetic fracture is necessary in patients with nondescript complaints of pain around their implant, especially if osteolysis is evident. In a review by the Mayo Clinic,[33] as many as 50% of patients with fractures did not have any precipitating traumatic event. Researchers attributed these fractures to implant loosening or osteolysis and highlighted the importance of regular radiographic follow-up of all patients with primary and revision THAs.

Radiographic evaluation of all suspected fractures should be comprehensive, including full-length views of the femur in two planes, an anteroposterior pelvic radiograph, and Judet views to more completely evaluate the floor, roof, and columns of the acetabulum. Comparison with previous radiographs is also helpful. More specialized imaging, such as computed tomography (CT) and magnetic resonance imaging (MRI), has not yet been accepted as standard practice because of difficulty with metal artifact, inconvenience, expense, and unproven cost-benefit. However, these tests may be helpful in selected circumstances of unusual complexity, especially around the acetabulum, and can be combined with three-dimensional reconstruction to assist with preoperative planning. Software packages have been developed for use with CT scanners to help reduce metal artifact, and improvements have been reported with MRI as well.[60,61] Bone scans have been used in the past, but increased uptake is a nonspecific finding; thus their use has been largely superseded by the use of metal artifact–reducing CT scans.

CLASSIFICATION

Undoubtedly the best outcome in the management of periprosthetic fractures is achieved when the surgeon has a thorough understanding of the problem and is appropriately prepared with the necessary implants and instruments. A classification system that combines the anatomy and biomechanics of the fracture type with proven principles of treatment that will lead to the best outcome is critical in achieving this level of understanding and preparedness.

Acetabular Fractures

The classification of periprosthetic acetabular fractures is based on the system developed by Letournel.[62] By defining the anterior and posterior columns, Letournel formed the basis for describing fracture patterns as seen on three plain radiographs: an anteroposterior pelvic view and two 45-degree Judet oblique views. Subsequently, the classification was modified,[63,64] with elementary fractures including posterior wall, posterior column, anterior wall, anterior column, and transverse injuries, and associated fractures including both columns, transverse plus posterior wall, anterior wall/column plus posterior hemitransverse, posterior column plus posterior wall, and T-shaped injuries.

Callaghan and coworkers[65] used a cadaveric model to describe the pattern of acetabular fractures following impaction of acetabular components in under-reamed acetabula. They included anterior wall, transverse, inferior lip, and posterior wall fractures. Peterson[16] modified Letournel's[62-64] system to include fractures of the medial wall. Fractures were also classified according to the stability of the acetabular component: type 1 if stable, and type 2 if not.

Pelvic discontinuity is important to recognize because standard acetabular revision techniques may not be adequate for reconstruction. Berry and associates[4] described the diagnostic features of pelvic discontinuity in their review of 27 patients. On the anteroposterior radiograph, three cardinal features included an obvious fracture line, malalignment of the upper and lower halves of the hemipelvis (usually due to medial displacement of the inferior half), and rotation of the inferior half of the hemipelvis in comparison with the opposite side (observed by comparing the size and shape of the obturator foramina; Fig. 102-3). Investigators emphasized that Judet views can be helpful when implants obscure the normal acetabular anatomy, especially the columns. In some cases, it is still difficult to diagnose a pelvic discontinuity on plain radiographs, and it in this circumstance that a metal artifact–reducing CT scan may be helpful. Furthermore, in every case, it is important to confirm the continuity of the hemipelvis during the revision procedure, regardless of preoperative radiographic findings.

Femoral Fractures

Successful management of these fractures depends on a number of factors, including fracture location and configuration, stability of the implant, quality of host bone, patient physiology and age, and surgeons' experience in managing these fractures.[28] A number of classification schemes have been described,[5,6,25,66,67] but the most widely used is the Vancouver classification.[68] This system is based on the three most important factors that influence outcome: the site of the fracture, the stability of the stem, and the quality of available bone for reconstruction. This system has been validated in two different studies.[69,70]

The three major anatomic types defined by this classification system depend on the location of the fracture: Type A refers to the trochanteric area (one or both trochanters and proximal metaphysis, not extending to the diaphysis); type B refers to a fracture around or just distal to the femoral stem (diaphysis); and type C refers to fractures that are sufficiently distal to the tip of the stem that their treatment can be considered independent of the presence of a total hip arthroplasty (the distal diaphysis and/or metaphysis).

Type A is further subdivided into greater trochanter (A_G; Fig. 102-4) and lesser trochanter (A_L). Type B is also

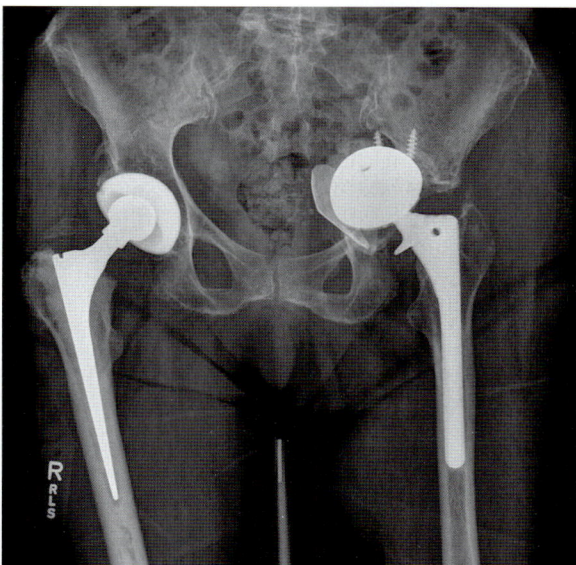

Figure 102-3. Anteroposterior (AP) pelvis radiograph illustrating pelvic dissociation with an absent posterior column, a medially displaced inferior half of the hemipelvis, and asymmetric obturator foramina.

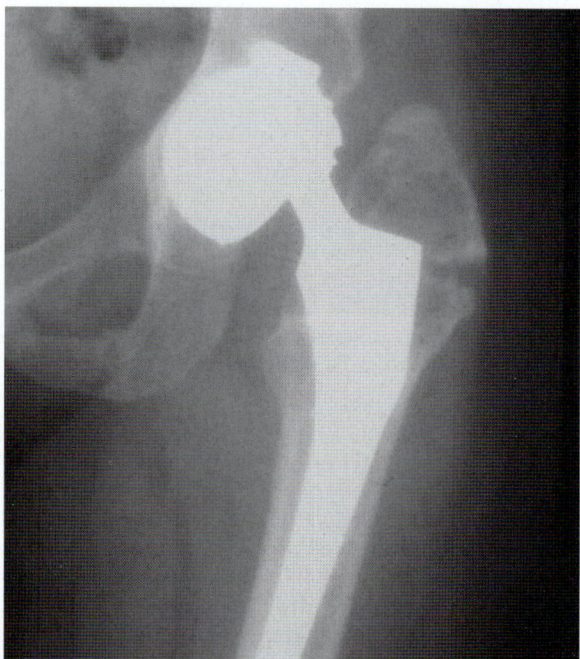

Figure 102-4. Anteroposterior (AP) femoral radiograph demonstrating a Vancouver A_G periprosthetic fracture of the femur secondary to wear debris osteolysis.

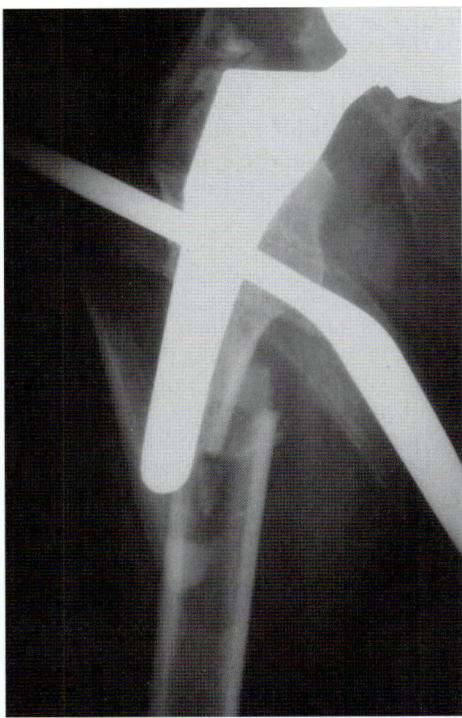

Figure 102-5. Anteroposterior (AP) femoral radiograph demonstrating a Vancouver B_1 periprosthetic fracture.

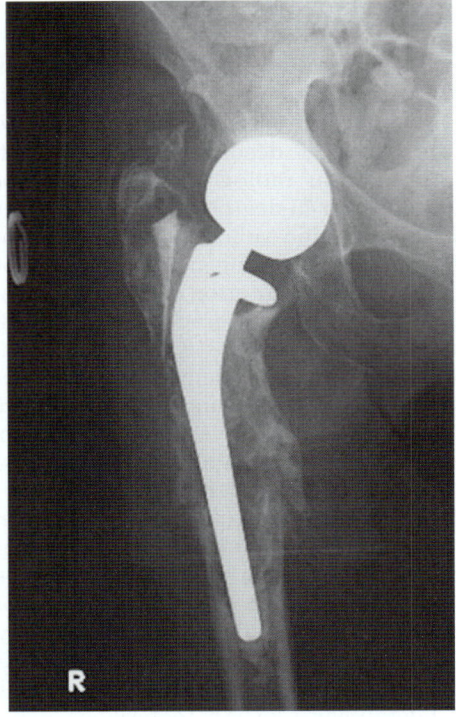

Figure 102-7. Anteroposterior (AP) femoral radiograph demonstrating a Vancouver B_3 periprosthetic fracture.

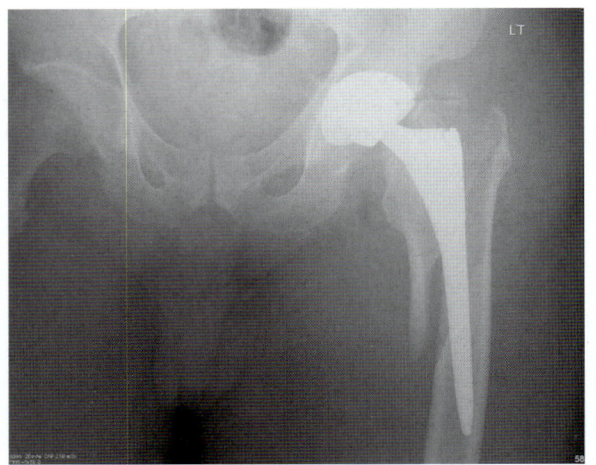

Figure 102-6. Anteroposterior (AP) pelvis radiograph demonstrating a Vancouver B_2 periprosthetic fracture.

subdivided into those where the implant is stable (B_1; Fig. 102-5) and those where the implant is loose (B_2; Fig. 102-6). If a fracture occurs through the cement mantle distal to an otherwise well-fixed cemented stem, this too would be classified as a B_1. Much more commonly, the fracture passes through the cement mantle around the stem, leading to a B_2 fracture, whether or not the stem was well fixed before the fracture. In both of these categories, the bone stock is good. If the femoral bone stock is poor and the implant is loose, the fracture is categorized as a B_3 (Fig. 102-7). An example of a type C fracture is illustrated in Figure 102-8.

Subsequently, the authors modified this system so that it could be applied to intraoperative femoral fractures.[71] The anatomic types A, B, and C are subdivided into three types: subtype 1 represents a simple cortical perforation; subtype 2, an undisplaced linear fracture; and subtype 3, a displaced or unstable fracture (Fig. 102-9).

A rather unique type of fracture, more prevalent in recent years, consists of a fracture of the lesser trochanter with a spike of medial cortex attached, associated with abrupt destabilization of the stem (Fig. 102-10). Characteristically, this occurs within 6 weeks of surgery in the setting of an osteopenic or osteoporotic femur, limited surgical exposure, and a tapered cementless stem.[71a] It can be mistaken for a type A lesser trochanter fracture, but in fact, it is a B_2 with the lesser trochanter attached. Principles of management of the B_2 fracture need to be applied if it is to be successfully managed.

TREATMENT AND RESULTS

Acetabular Fractures

Stable intraoperative acetabular fractures that occur during insertion of an uncemented component require no additional fixation. If considerable motion is noted at the fracture site, additional screw fixation of the shell may be required, followed by a period of non–weight bearing postoperatively. If motion and pelvic dissociation are observed, the posterior column should be

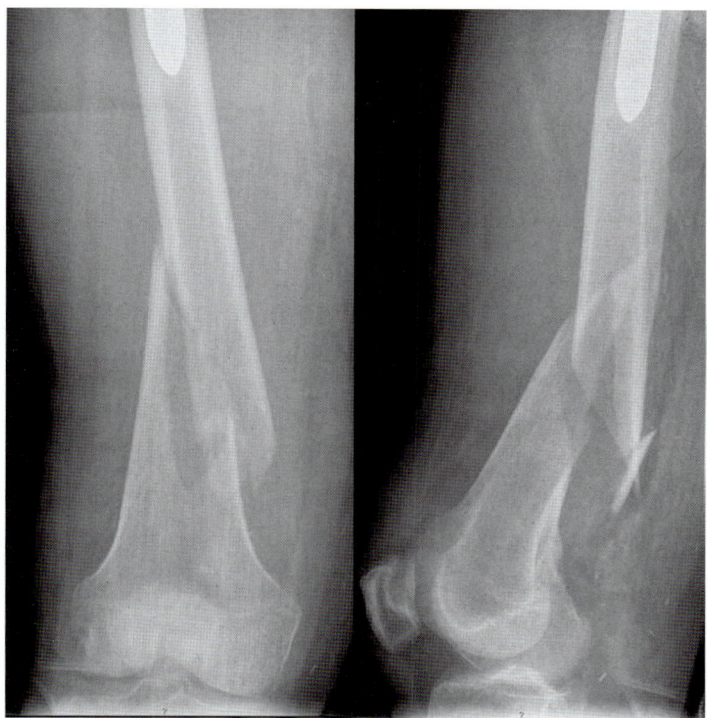

Figure 102-8. Anteroposterior (AP) and lateral femoral radiographs demonstrating a Vancouver C periprosthetic fracture of the femur.

treated with reduction and internal fixation with a pelvic reconstruction plate on the posterior column with or without autograft.[3]

Minimally displaced acetabular fractures discovered soon after operation where the initial fixation of the acetabular component has been augmented with screw fixation, and the implant is judged to be stable, may be treated without further surgical intervention.[65] However, if none of the screws appear to be directed superiorly into the intact pelvis, the implant is at high risk for failure and will likely require revision.[71] If substantial fracture displacement occurs, it will be necessary to revise the component and reduce and stabilize the fracture with a posterior column plate and insertion of an uncemented acetabular component with additional screw fixation.

Fractures that present much later are often associated with considerable osteolysis and bone loss. Callaghan and coworkers advocated allowing minimally displaced fractures to heal before proceeding with revision.[65] Similar to Callaghan, Peterson and associates[16] recommended nonoperative management initially in stable fractures, until the fracture has united. This was based on their review of 11 late-presenting acetabular fractures. Six of 8 stable fractures (type 1) had united. Among patients with an unstable fracture (type 2), 2 out of 3 had undergone revision of the acetabular component without additional plate fixation. The third patient had sustained the fracture from a traumatic episode and subsequently died from a vascular injury related to migration of the acetabular component.

Patients with pelvic discontinuity pose a difficult problem for surgeons. Berry and colleagues[4] at the Mayo clinic treated these fractures with a cemented cup with or without an antiprotrusio cage, or alternatively with an uncemented cup with a posterior column plate to stabilize the pelvis. They reported that 77% of patients with a cage had a satisfactory outcome compared with 56% of patients with an uncemented component. Those who had a cemented acetabular component without a cage did poorly.

If acetabular bone loss is so severe that implant stability cannot be attained with a standard hemispherical uncemented cup, an alternative method of fixation may be required. Such cases have been treated with a porous tantalum shell, which may allow better initial component stability and bone ingrowth.[24] These components can be used in combination with plating of the posterior column, or with a "cup-cage" construct. With this technique, a reconstruction cage is placed within the porous metal shell and is secured to the ischium inferiorly and to the ilium superiorly to augment construct stability. Satisfactory results have been reported with this technique when applied in the revision setting.[24,72] However, to the authors' knowledge, no published results describe use of this technique in the treatment of acute periprosthetic fractures of the acetabulum.

Femoral Fractures

The management of intraoperative femoral fractures as reported in early series was not particularly favorable and was associated with significant morbidity, including high risks for malunion and nonunion, as well as reoperation.[7,73] Later, Fitzgerald and associates[74] reported on their early experience of managing these fractures with cementless femoral stems. Of 40 intraoperative fractures during 630 THAs, all united with the use of various

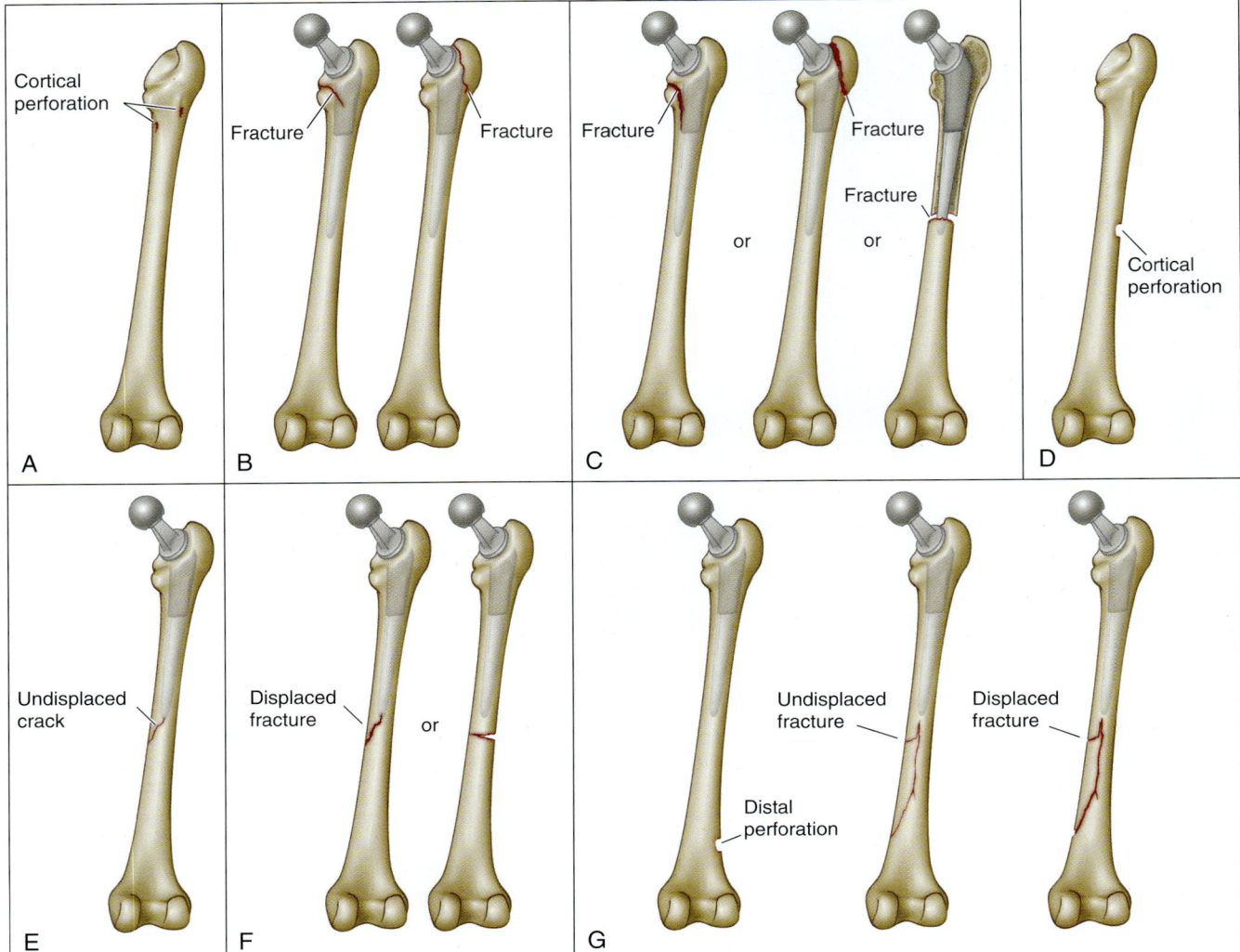

Figure 102-9. Vancouver classification of intraoperative femoral periprosthetic fractures. **A,** Type A$_1$. **B,** Type A$_2$. **C,** Type A$_3$. **D,** Type B$_1$. **E,** Type B$_2$. **F,** Type B$_3$. **G,** Type C$_1$ *(left image),* type C$_2$ *(center image),* and type C$_3$ *(right image). (Redrawn from Greidanus NV, Mitchell PA, Masri BA, et al: Principles of management and results of treating the fractured femur during and after total hip arthroplasty. Instr Course Lect 52:309–322, 2003.)*

treatment options, including Parham bands and cerclage wires with bone graft in most patients. Additionally, patients were managed with protected weight bearing for up to 4 months after surgery.

Schwartz and colleagues[6] reported encouraging results with 39 intraoperative fractures resulting from 1318 THAs, although only half were diagnosed at the time of surgery. Most fractures in this series were stable. Unstable fractures and implants were treated with an extensively porous-coated stem that bypassed the fracture to achieve good distal fixation. Additional cerclage wires were used as required. Patients with incomplete fractures such as cortical perforations that did not involve the posterior femoral cortex, diagnosed postoperatively, were treated in a cast and were protected during weight bearing. For complete fractures, investigators advised open reduction and internal fixation. With this management approach, all fractures united with no adverse consequences.

Increasing use of extensile osteotomies in revision arthroplasty may help to minimize the rate of fracture during femoral revision; however, these approaches have been associated with an increased incidence of proximal femoral fracture related to the creation of the osteotomy fragment.[75] These proximal femoral fractures can be treated successfully with cerclage wires with or without a cortical onlay strut allograft, with little effect on the overall outcome of the revision, so long as the soft tissue attachments are respected.[75] Intraoperative fractures may not be diagnosed until they are recognized on the postoperative radiograph. Usually, these fractures are stable and minimally displaced. Most require no further intervention other than protected weight bearing, and they subsequently go on to unite.[6,26]

Management of intraoperative femoral fractures will be described in accordance with the Vancouver intraoperative classification as outlined earlier.

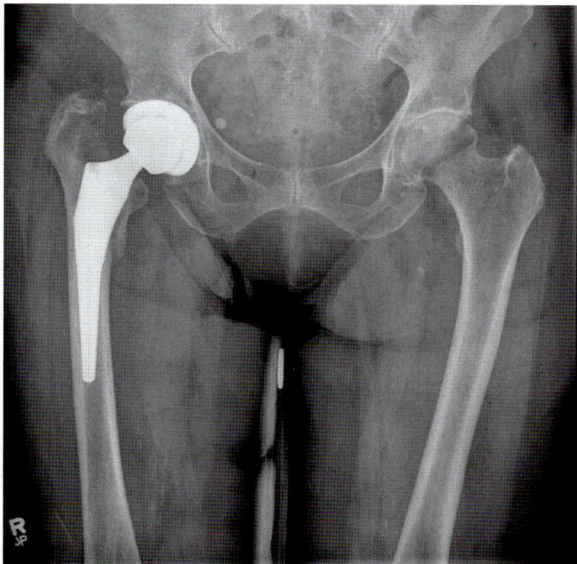

Figure 102-10. Anteroposterior (AP) pelvis radiograph illustrating a Vancouver B_2 variant identified in the early postoperative period. A displaced fracture of the lesser trochanter with attached cortex has destabilized the stem.

Table 102-2. Summary of the Vancouver Classification for Postoperative Periprosthetic Femoral Fractures	
Fracture Type and Subtype	**Location of Fracture**
A_G	Greater trochanteric area
A_L	Lesser trochanteric area
B_1	Around or just distal to the prosthesis; implant stable
B_2	Around or just distal to the prosthesis; implant loose with good bone stock
B_3	Around or just distal to the prosthesis; implant loose with poor bone stock
C	Below the implant

From Duncan CP, Masri BA: Fractures of the femur after hip replacement. Instr Course Lect 44:293–304, 1995.

Type A Intraoperative Fractures of the Greater or Lesser Trochanter

These are further subdivided into A_1 (cortical perforation), A_2 (undisplaced linear crack), and A_3 (displaced or unstable). Cortical perforations can be ignored because they are unlikely to affect the primary fixation of the femoral stem. However, if some acetabular reamings are available, the area can be grafted with some autologous graft.[71]

A nondisplaced linear fracture can be sustained at the time of rasping of the proximal femur or with final stem impaction. With small nondisplaced cracks, a cerclage wire should be sufficient; ideally if such a fracture is identified, the stem should be removed and a cerclage wire applied. The stem should then be reinserted to prevent propagation and to optimize fixation and reduction. If the fracture does propagate and becomes unstable, then a distally fitting diaphyseal stem can be used to bypass the area.[6,66,76]

If a type A_3 involves the calcar and extends medially involving the metaphyseal region of the proximal femur, a diaphyseal-fitting uncemented stem is the implant of choice to bypass the fracture. Displaced fractures of the greater trochanter can be reduced and held with cerclage wires or cables, or with a trochanteric claw plate and cables. Good results have been achieved with this method of fixation, although the fixation hardware may cause discomfort.[77] In the revision setting, with increasing use of a proximal femoral osteotomy,[53,75] a fracture can occur in the medial region of the metaphysis as the result of tension from soft tissues or overzealous retraction. However, in most cases, a diaphyseal-fitting stem is planned, and the fracture will be stabilized when the osteotomy fragment is reduced and held with cables or wires. Following a proximal osteotomy with weakened

bone, an onlay strut allograft can be used to prevent the fixation wire from cutting through and fracturing the weakened osteotomy fragment.[71]

Type B Intraoperative Fractures

Cortical perforations of the diaphysis (B_1) usually occur during cement extraction or reaming of the femoral canal. As with any weakened bone in the diaphyseal cortex, a stem of adequate length should be used to bypass the affected area by a minimum of two cortical diameters.[49] Before stem insertion, a prophylactic cable or cerclage wire can be placed distal to this area to prevent fracture propagation as the stem is impacted into the femur. In those few cases where the perforation extends below the tip of the longest stem, a cortical strut allograft should be used to bypass the area, together with filling of the perforation with bone graft (Table 102-2).

Undisplaced linear fractures (B_2) may occur during rasp or implant insertion. These fractures can be treated with a cerclage wire or cable and the fracture bypassed with a longer stem. If the fracture cannot be bypassed because it is too distal, a cortical strut graft or a plate and screws can be used to bypass the fracture. Cortical strut grafts are favored in the setting of poor bone stock because these types of grafts have been shown to increase cortical strength and are associated with a good clinical outcome.[78,79]

Displaced diaphyseal fractures (B_3) occur when torsional force is applied to weakened bone and are frequently observed during initial dislocation of the hip. For spiral or oblique fractures, they are reduced and held with cerclage wires; for transverse fractures, one or two cortical strut grafts or a plate can be used. Once the fracture has been reduced and fixed, a femoral stem should be implanted that bypasses the fracture by at least two diaphyseal diameters.

Type C Intraoperative Fractures

Cortical perforations (C_1) distal to the tip of the stem are uncommon but may occur during cement removal. Bone grafting and onlay cortical strut grafts are the mainstays of treatment to avoid a possible stress riser and risk of further fracture in the future. Undisplaced linear fractures distal to the tip of the stem can be treated with cerclage wires with or without a cortical strut graft. Displaced fractures that are distal to the stem and that cannot be bypassed by a longer stem should be treated with open reduction and internal fixation. Encouraging results have been published with the use of locking plates. With these devices, unicortical screws can be used proximally at the level of the femoral stem and bicortical screws distally. For additional proximal fixation, cerclage wires or cables can be used to augment the unicortical screw fixation.[80-86]

Postoperative Fractures

When considering revision of a THA with a postoperative periprosthetic fracture, it is prudent to exclude the possibility of infection. Because inflammatory markers (erythrocyte sedimentation rate and C-reactive protein) may be falsely elevated secondary to recent trauma,[87,88] preoperative aspiration of the hip joint with synovial fluid white blood cell count, differential, and culture can be used for diagnosis.[87,88] Intraoperative testing can also be done in the form of frozen section analysis of periprosthetic tissues or intraoperative synovial fluid cell count with differential.[89]

Type A Postoperative Fractures. Fractures of the greater trochanter are usually stable and can be treated nonoperatively if they have displaced less than 2 cm.[90] Patients can be advised to use protected weight bearing and to avoid abduction until evidence indicates that the fracture is uniting; this can take 6 to 12 weeks. If the fracture is displaced by more than 2 cm, or if the patient develops a painful trochanteric nonunion with weak abduction with or without instability or a limp following a period of nonoperative management, these fractures should be reduced and fixed. Fractures of the greater trochanter associated with wear debris osteolysis will require concomitant revision of the bearing surface. If the fracture is minimally displaced, it may be wise to delay intervention until it has united.

Isolated fractures of the lesser trochanter are uncommon. If they are relatively small and the implant is stable, they can be treated nonoperatively. Care must be taken to distinguish them from fractures of the medial femoral cortex with attachment of the lesser trochanter, which has destabilized the stem, as outlined earlier (see Fig. 102-10).

Type B Postoperative Fractures. This is by far the largest group of postoperative fractures associated with hip arthroplasty.

Vancouver B₁ Periprosthetic Fractures. Fractures with a stable implant (B_1) should be treated with a plate and screws, supplemented with cerclage wires or cable fixation if deemed necessary to gain fixation around the stem. An alternative approach is a cortical onlay graft, fixed securely with cerclage wires or cables, often in combination with a plate. In the presence of a stem within the femoral canal, standard plates and screws cannot be used easily without risk of affecting the stability of the implant and damaging the implant-bone interface. However, with the advent of locking plates with

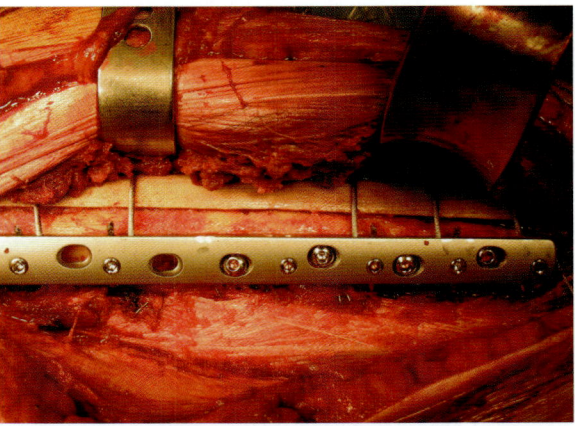

Figure 102-11. Intraoperative photograph showing the unicortical locking plate and cortical strut graft and cables in the management of a Vancouver B_1 fracture.

unicortical screws as well as cerclage wires, this problem has been overcome to a certain extent. These plates can be used on their own or with an anteriorly placed cortical strut allograft[48] (Fig. 102-11). Care must be taken when assessing a periprosthetic B_1 femoral fracture to ensure that the implant is truly stable; early failure can be expected if a B_2 is treated as a B_1.[91]

Ricci and coworkers[92,93] advocated the use of indirect reduction of B_1 fractures while avoiding unnecessary soft tissue stripping. They proposed that careful soft tissue dissection minimized devascularization of bone; in some instances, they utilized a skin bridge centered at the fracture site. Of 41 patients treated with the minimally invasive percutaneous plate osteosynthesis technique (MIPPO), 30 were treated with a 4.5-mm dynamic compression plate (DCP), 8 with a femoral condylar plate, 2 with a blade plate, and 1 with a cable plate. All fractures reported in the study healed satisfactorily at an average of 12 weeks. One patient had a fractured cable, and 2 others sustained a fracture of 1 screw, but all fractures healed without evidence of implant loosening or malalignment. Over the past 5 years, this method of treatment has become the standard of care for B_1 fractures in North America and beyond.[94-96]

Buttaro and associates[97] reviewed 14 Vancouver type B_1 periprosthetic femoral fractures treated with locking compression plates with unicortical screw fixation; however, their results were not as encouraging as those reported by Ricci and colleagues. Five patients had a cortical strut allograft, in addition to the plate. The mean follow-up was 20 months. Eight fractures had united by an average of 5.4 months, 3 constructs had failed with plate fracture within 12 months of surgery, and 3 had failed because of plate pullout. All failures but 1 occurred in constructs in which a cortical strut allograft had not been used. The authors concluded that locking compression plates on their own did not appear to offer any kind of advantage over other plating systems for B_1 fractures. They suggested that if these plates are to be used, they should be supplemented with a strut allograft; however, soft tissue management may have been different leading to devascularization at the fracture site.

A combination of cables and plates is widely used in the treatment of periprosthetic fracture.[71] Venu and coworkers[98] reviewed 12 patients with periprosthetic fractures related to hip arthroplasty, who were treated with the Dall-Miles cable-plate system (Howmedica, Rutherford, NJ). All patients in this series received bone graft, whether it was morselized autograft, allograft, or cortical strut allograft. Three patients went on to nonunion and required further surgery, but 9 went on to unite. Tadross and associates[99] reported on 7 periprosthetic B_1 fractures treated with the Dall-Miles cable plate system. Three patients united with satisfactory results, but 4 failed, because of nonunion in 2 patients and malunion in the other 2. The authors concluded that failure was in part related to the varus positioning of the femoral component, causing distraction at the fracture site. Alternatively, a structural cortical allograft may be helpful for averting such a high rate of failure.

Cortical strut allografts were first reported by Chandler and colleagues in 1989.[100] In a later review,[101] they reported on 19 patients with periprosthetic femoral fractures treated with a cortical strut allograft. By 4.5 months, 16 of the 19 fractures had united, 1 malunion had occurred, and 2 nonunions required further surgery. This problem of malunion or nonunion could possibly be averted by using a combination of a plate on the lateral cortex and a cortical strut allograft anteriorly. Encouraging results have been reported with this technique.[78,102]

Haddad and coworkers[103] reported excellent results with cortical strut allografts with or without a plate and attributed the high union rate to the advantage of being able to customize struts to the morphology of the femur, and also to the fact that the strut shares the same modulus of elasticity as the host bone.

Vancouver B_2 Periprosthetic Fractures. Displaced fractures with a loose implant but good bone stock (B_2) require revision of the femoral component, bypassing the distal extent of the fracture by at least two diaphyseal diameters. Successful outcomes have been achieved with uncemented as well as cemented implants with impaction grafting. If an uncemented stem is used, additional rotational stability can be achieved by using a strut graft with cerclage wires or cables.

To underscore the importance of differentiating a B_1 from a B_2 fracture, Kamineni and coworkers[104] reviewed 15 fractures in the presence of a loose implant that were treated with the cable-plate system. Thirteen patients were treated with the Dall-Miles system, and 2 were treated with the Zimmer cable-ready system (Zimmer, Warsaw, Ind). Four patients required subsequent revision, although 3 were performed after the fracture had united; 1 nonunion was reported. One patient fractured just below the plate and required revision to a longer plate. Results from this study highlight the importance of recognizing a B_2 fracture, and point to the fact that fracture treatment alone when the implant is loose is associated with poor results.

Mont and associates[76] completed a 27-year review of the literature, which included 487 patients, and compared treatment options according to location of fracture. They concluded that mid-stem and distal-stem fractures (B_2/B_3) did better with cerclage cables or wires and bone graft or revision to a longer stem compared with internal fixation with plates and screws or traction. Similar conclusions have been put forth following other studies.[28,50]

In a study by Beal and colleagues[28] of 102 periprosthetic fractures, cemented revisions for Vancouver B_2 fractures had a 62% complication rate, with 38% becoming loose and 24% developing an infection, dislocating, or developing a trochanteric nonunion, whereas uncemented revisions for B_2 fractures had an 18% subsidence rate, with 7% loosening and 9% dislocating, getting infected, or developing a trochanteric nonunion.

More recently, interest in the use of a distally fixed porous-coated stem to provide intramedullary fixation for periprosthetic fractures has been increasing.[50,105-107] The added advantage of this fixation method is that it can be used to bypass any proximal bone deficiency. MacDonald and associates[105] reported on 14 cases of postoperative Vancouver B_2 fractures that were treated with a long cementless stem, which was extensively porous coated. All 14 fractures united. One stem had fibrous stable fixation but had not been revised.

Tower and colleagues[50] looked at the use of a modular prosthesis with a proximal body, which would encourage ingrowth, and a distal fluted stem, which would give good torsional control. In comparison with cemented revisions, this modular stem produced better results. Researchers suggested that if a fully coated diaphyseal stem is used, torsional control can be augmented with a cortical strut allograft and cerclage wires or cables.

Other methods of treating patients with Vancouver type B_2 and type B_3 fractures include the use of impaction grafting. Tsiridis and coworkers[108] reviewed 106 patients who underwent revision surgery for a periprosthetic fracture. Eighty-nine had undergone a cemented revision with impaction grafting with a long or short stem. Seventeen patients had had a cemented revision without impaction grafting. They reported that fractures treated with impaction grafting and a long stem were up to 5 times more likely to unite than those treated with a short stem and impaction grafting. Further, those with a long stem and impaction grafting were significantly more likely to unite than those with a long stem and no impaction grafting. They concluded that impaction grafting had a role to play in these types of fractures, but a long stem should also be used to bypass the distal end of the fracture.

Vancouver B_3 Periprosthetic Fractures. Periprosthetic fracture of the femur associated with a loose implant and compromised proximal femoral poor bone stock (B_3) can often necessitate unique reconstructive techniques that include replacement of the proximal femur with allograft prosthetic composites or a proximal femoral replacing prosthesis. Gross[109] popularized the use of segmental allograft to reconstruct bone deficiency when revising total hip replacements with B_3 fractures. In a review of 15 patients treated with this technique at a mean follow-up of 5 years, it was noted that 13 patients had a good result and 2 patients required further surgery. Of the 2 patients, 1 patient had a nonunion at the allograft host junction and required plating, and the other patient required a revision to a similar construct.

However, the use of segmental allografts has the disadvantage in the elderly population of not enabling patients to bear weight early, while waiting for the allograft point of junction to unite with the distal femur. Therefore, an attractive option in this patient group is to use a proximal femoral replacement or a tumor prosthesis that enables the patient to fully weight bear immediately postoperatively (Fig. 102-12). Proximal femoral replacements have been very successful in this patient group, with up to 64% survivorship reported at 12 years.[89,110,111] However, the use of this type of stem can result in issues of instability caused by lack of abductors. If abductors can be saved with a fragment of the greater trochanter attached, they can be attached to the shoulder of the proximal femoral replacement. A number of these prostheses are designed to facilitate this fixation. However if abductors are absent or cannot be adequately secured to the shoulder of the prosthesis, a constrained liner should be strongly considered to avoid the risk of dislocation postoperatively.

An additional option for treatment of B_3 fractures is to use a distally fixed, fluted, tapered modular stem to bypass the proximal femur, and then to reduce the fracture around the implant proximally to form a stable construct. Provisional results have been encouraging.[112-115] However, this implant design requires an intact isthmus to gain good press-fit fixation. Wagner[116] proposed that the contact zone needs to be between 70 and 100 mm between implant and bone for primary stability. However, Beguec and associates[117] believed that a good press-fit depends on the quality of the wedging and a contact zone of just 30 mm in excellent bone, but 40 to 50 mm if bone quality is poor. Because access to the femoral canal can be difficult to attain in the revision setting, an extended trochanteric osteotomy can be helpful. Levine and colleagues[118] demonstrated that an extended trochanteric osteotomy can provide excellent exposure and can facilitate component implantation in the treatment of Vancouver B_2 and B_3 fractures.

Vancouver Type C Periprosthetic Fractures. Type C periprosthetic fractures are fractures that occur at the level of or distal to the end of the femoral implant. In the past, a number of these patients would be treated without surgery and with a prolonged period of bed rest with or without traction to achieve fracture union.[119] This method of treatment is associated with high rates of nonunion and malunion and with risks associated with prolonged bed rest in an elderly patient population.

Because these fractures are distal to the tip of the femoral component, they can be treated with open reduction and internal fixation in accordance with standard AO principles, as described for intraoperative fractures. Locking plates have considerable potential in the treatment of this type of fracture (Fig. 102-13).

Currall and colleagues[82] performed a retrospective review of Vancouver C periprosthetic fractures treated using the LISS (less invasive skeletal stabilization; Synthes, Solothurn, Switzerland) femoral locking plate.

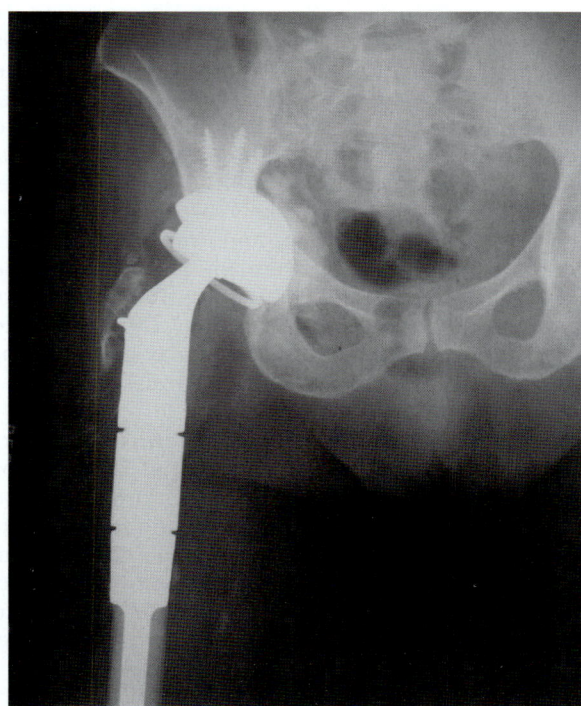

Figure 102-12. Postoperative anteroposterior (AP) pelvis radiograph showing the revision of a Vancouver B₃ periprosthetic fracture with severe segmental bone loss using a proximal femoral replacement in a frail elderly patient.

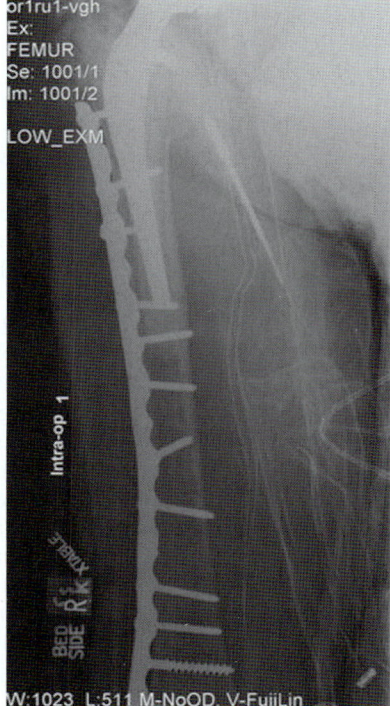

Figure 102-13. Postoperative anteroposterior (AP) femoral radiograph showing the revision of a Vancouver type C periprosthetic fracture with a LISS (less invasive skeletal stabilization) plate.

Table 102-3. Summary of the Results of Different Management Techniques for Vancouver B₁ Fractures

Author	Technique	Results
Ricci[92,93]	MIPPO	All fractures united at a mean of 12 weeks in 41 patients.
Fulkerson[95]	Percutaneous LISS plate	21 of 24 patients went on to unite at a mean of 6.2 months.
Venu[98]	Dall-Miles cable plate system with bone graft	Out of a total of 12 patients, 9 united at a mean of 4.4 months and 3 did not.
Tadross[99]	Dall-Miles cable plate system	Out of 7 patients, 4 failed to unite and 2 developed a malunion.
Chandler[78,102]	Cortical strut allograft	16 out of 19 fractures united by 4.5 months.

LISS, Less invasive skeletal stabilization; MIPPO, minimally invasive percutaneous plate osteosynthesis.

Five patients with a mean age of 87 years with a stable implant were treated with the LISS plate in combination with bone grafting and cables. All fractures united, and 4 of the 5 patients were able to mobilize independently.

Kobbe and coworkers[84] reported on 16 patients with a femoral periprosthetic fracture following total hip replacement, which was managed with a locking plate at a 3-year follow-up. Of the 16 patients, 8 were classified as Vancouver C, 6 Vancouver B₁, 1 B₂, and 1 B₃. The Harris hip score and the Karnofsky activity index averaged 79.5 points and 81%, respectively. Two major complications were attributed to screw pullout, representing a complication rate of 13%. Early results with locking plates are encouraging; however, the series reported to date are small. Larger series with similar fracture patterns are needed to fully evaluate the contribution that a locking plate makes to the management of periprosthetic fractures (Table 102-3).

PROGNOSIS

The prognosis following a periprosthetic fracture very much depends on the type of fracture, the stability of the construct post fixation, the occurrence of postoperative complications, and the patient's age and medical comorbidities. If the biomechanical function of the limb is restored, a good outcome and prognosis can be expected.

Lindahl and coworkers[120] reviewed the Swedish Joint Registry to look at the mortality rates of patients who had sustained a periprosthetic fracture. They concluded that patients with osteoarthritis who had undergone total hip arthroplasty and subsequently sustained a periprosthetic fracture had higher mortality due to the fracture. Mortality decreases over a period of 6 months, but in the 50- to 70-year age group, the risk stays higher than for the general population. In the 70-year and older age group, the mortality risk is the same as for the general population.

When periprosthetic fractures are treated, the stability of the fracture, restoration of mechanical stability, respect for the biological environment, and the flexibility to choose the device that best addresses the fracture configuration are essential in achieving the optimum result for the patient.

CURRENT CONTROVERSIES AND FUTURE CONSIDERATIONS

- Preventative measures need to become a focus of research to reduce the ever rising number of periprosthetic fractures.
- New designs of implants include changes to the femoral stem to share load with the bone and avoid stress shielding of the proximal femur, which can result in bone weakening and increased risk of fracture.
- New plate designs have appeal because limited contact with the underlying bone in theory decreases the risk of stress shielding.
- The role of plates that use unicortical screw fixation in the management of periprosthetic femoral fractures remains controversial. Randomized studies are needed to further elucidate this contribution.
- Minimally invasive osteosynthesis has become an important adjunct in managing the B₁ fracture.
- For B₁ fractures, what is best? Locking plate or standard plates? Are strut allografts necessary?
- For B₂ fractures, full coat versus modular taper.
- For B₃ fractures, proximal femoral replacement with allograft prosthetic construct (APC) versus megaprosthesis. Or are these necessary, and can you use a modular tapered stem in the vast majority of cases?

REFERENCES

1. Charnley J: The healing of human fractures in contact with self-curing acrylic cement. Clin Orthop Relat Res 47:157–163, 1966.
2. Scott RD, Turner RH, Leitzes SM, Aufranc OE: Femoral fractures in conjunction with total hip replacement. J Bone Joint Surg Am 57:494–501, 1975.
3. Sharkey PF, Hozack WJ, Callaghan JJ, et al: Acetabular fracture associated with cementless acetabular component insertion: a report of 13 cases. J Arthroplasty 14:426–431, 1999.
4. Berry DJ, Lewallen DG, Hanssen AD, Cabanela ME: Pelvic discontinuity in revision total hip arthroplasty. J Bone Joint Surg Am 81:1692–1702, 1999.
5. Johansson JE, McBroom RF, Barrington TW, Hunter GA: Fracture of the ipsilateral femur in patients with total hip replacement. J Bone Joint Surg Am 63:1435–1442, 1981.
6. Schwartz JT, Jr, Mayer JG, Engh CA: Femoral fracture during non-cemented total hip arthroplasty. J Bone Joint Surg Am 71:1135–1142, 1989.
7. Taylor MM, Meyers MH, Harvey JP, Jr: Intraoperative femur fractures during total hip replacement. Clin Orthop Relat Res 137:96–103, 1978.
8. Berry DJ: Epidemiology: hip and knee. Orthop Clin North Am 30:183–190, 1999.
9. Adolphson PF, Jonsson UF, Kalen R: Fractures of the ipsilateral femur after total hip arthroplasty. Arch Orthop Trauma Surg 106:353–357, 1987.

10. Bethea JS, III, DeAndrade JR, Fleming LL, et al: Proximal femoral fractures following total hip arthroplasty. Clin Orthop Relat Res 170:95–106, 1982.

11. Fredin H: Late fracture of the femur following perforation during hip arthroplasty: a report of 2 cases. Acta Orthop Scand 59:331–332, 1988.

12. Garcia-Cimbrelo E, Munuera LF, Gil-Garay E: Femoral shaft fractures after cemented total hip arthroplasty. Int Orthop 16:97–100, 1992.

13. Lowenhielm GF, Hansson LI, Karrholm J: Fracture of the lower extremity after total hip replacement. Arch Orthop Trauma Surg 108:141–143, 1989.

14. Pazzaglia UF, Byers PD: Fractured femoral shaft through an osteolytic lesion resulting from the reaction to a prosthesis: a case report. J Bone Joint Surg Br 66:337–339, 1984.

15. McElfresh EC, Coventry MB: Femoral and pelvic fractures after total hip arthroplasty. J Bone Joint Surg Am 56:483–492, 1974.

16. Peterson CA, II, Lewallen DG: Periprosthetic fracture of the acetabulum after total hip arthroplasty. J Bone Joint Surg Am 78:1206–1213, 1996.

17. Adler E, Stuchin SA, Kummer FJ: Stability of press-fit acetabular cups. J Arthroplasty 7:295–301, 1992.

18. Curtis MJ, Jinnah RH, Wilson VD, Hungerford DS: The initial stability of uncemented acetabular components. J Bone Joint Surg Br 74:372–376, 1992.

19. MacKenzie JR, Callaghan JJ, Pedersen DR, Brown TD: Areas of contact and extent of gaps with implantation of oversized acetabular components in total hip arthroplasty. Clin Orthop Relat Res 298:127–136, 1994.

20. Stiehl JB, MacMillan E, Skrade DA: Mechanical stability of porous-coated acetabular components in total hip arthroplasty. J Arthroplasty 6:295–300, 1991.

21. Schmalzried TP, Wessinger SJ, Hill GE, Harris WH: The Harris-Galante porous acetabular component press-fit without screw fixation: five-year radiographic analysis of primary cases. J Arthroplasty 9:235–242, 1994.

22. Kim YS, Callaghan JJ, Ahn PB, Brown TD: Fracture of the acetabulum during insertion of an oversized hemispherical component. J Bone Joint Surg Am 77:111–117, 1995.

23. Sanchez-Sotelo J, McGrory BJ, Berry DJ: Acute periprosthetic fracture of the acetabulum associated with osteolytic pelvic lesions: a report of 3 cases. J Arthroplasty 15:126–130, 2000.

24. Springer BD, Berry DJ, Cabanela ME, et al: Early postoperative transverse pelvic fracture: a new complication related to revision arthroplasty with an uncemented cup. J Bone Joint Surg Am 87:2626–2631, 2005.

25. Kavanagh BF: Femoral fractures associated with total hip arthroplasty. Orthop Clin North Am 23:249–257, 1992.

26. Meek RMD, Garbuz DS, Masri BA, et al: Intraoperative fracture of the femur in revision total hip arthroplasty with a diaphyseal fitting stem. J Bone Joint Surg Am 86:480–485, 2004.

27. Fredin HO, Lindberg HF, Carlsson AS: Femoral fracture following hip arthroplasty. Acta Orthop Scand 58:20–22, 1987.

28. Beals RK, Tower SS: Periprosthetic fractures of the femur: an analysis of 93 fractures. Clin Orthop Relat Res 327:238–246, 1996.

29. Berry DJ: Periprosthetic fractures associated with osteolysis: a problem on the rise. J Arthroplasty 18:107–111, 2003.

30. Malchau HF, Herberts PF, Eisler TF, et al: The Swedish Total Hip Replacement Register. J Bone Joint Surg Am 84(Suppl 2):2–20, 2002.

31. Malchau HF, Herberts PF, Ahnfelt L: Prognosis of total hip replacement in Sweden: follow-up of 92,675 operations performed 1978-1990. Acta Orthop Scand 64:497–506, 1993.

32. Abendschein W: Periprosthetic femur fractures—a growing epidemic. Am J Orthop 32:34–36, 2003.

33. Lewallen DG, Berry DJ: Periprosthetic fracture of the femur after total hip arthroplasty: treatment and results to date. Instr Course Lect 47:243–249, 1998.

34. Tsiridis E, Haddad FS, Gie GA: The management of periprosthetic femoral fractures around hip replacements. Injury 34:95–105, 2003.

35. Wu CC, Au MK, Wu SS, Lin LC: Risk factors for postoperative femoral fracture in cementless hip arthroplasty. J Formos Med Assoc 98:190–194, 1999.

36. Lindahl H, Eisler T, Oden A: Risk factors associated with the late periprosthetic femoral fracture. In Lindahl H, editor: The periprosthetic femur fracture: a study from the Swedish National Hip Arthroplasty Register, Goteberg, 2006, Department of Orthopaedics, Sahlgenska Academy, Goteberg University.

37. Lindahl H, Garellick G, Regner H, et al: Three hundred and twenty-one periprosthetic femoral fractures. J Bone Joint Surg Am 88:1215–1222, 2006.

38. Cook RE, Jenkins PJ, Walmsley PJ, et al: Risk factors for periprosthetic fractures of the hip: a survivorship analysis. Clin Orthop Relat Res 466:1652–1656, 2008.

39. Lindahl H, Malchau H, Herberts P, Garellick G: Periprosthetic femoral fractures: classification and demographics of 1049 periprosthetic femoral fractures from the Swedish National Hip Arthroplasty Register. J Arthroplasty 20:857–865, 2005.

40. Sarvilinna RF, Huhtala HS, Sovelius RT, et al: Factors predisposing to periprosthetic fracture after hip arthroplasty: a case (n = 31)-control study. Acta Orthop Scand 75:16–20, 2004.

41. Haddad FS, Masri BA, Garbuz DS, Duncan CP: The prevention of periprosthetic fractures in total hip and knee arthroplasty. Orthop Clin North Am 30:191–207, 1999.

42. Kelley SS: Periprosthetic femoral fractures. J Am Acad Orthop Surg 2:164–172, 1994.

43. Learmonth ID: The management of periprosthetic fractures around the femoral stem. J Bone Joint Surg Br 86:13–19, 2004.

44. Schmidt AH, Kyle RF: Periprosthetic fractures of the femur. Orthop Clin North Am 33:143–152, ix, 2002.

45. Incavo SJ, Beard DM, Pupparo F, et al: One-stage revision of periprosthetic fractures around loose cemented total hip arthroplasty. Am J Orthop 27:35–41, 1998.

46. Jensen JS, Barfod GF, Hansen DF, et al: Femoral shaft fracture after hip arthroplasty. Acta Orthop Scand 59:9–13, 1988.

47. Lewallen DG, Berry DJ: Instructional course lectures: The American Academy of Orthopaedic Surgeons—Periprosthetic fracture of the femur after total hip arthroplasty: treatment and results to date. J Bone Joint Surg Am 79:1881–1890, 1997.

48. Garbuz DS, Masri BA, Duncan CP: Periprosthetic fractures of the femur: principles of prevention and management. Instr Course Lect 47:237–242, 1998.

49. Larson JE, Chao EY, Fitzgerald RH: Bypassing femoral cortical defects with cemented intramedullary stems. J Orthop Res 9:414–421, 1991.

50. Tower SS, Beals RK: Fractures of the femur after hip replacement: the Oregon experience. Orthop Clin North Am 30:235–247, 1999.

51. Masri BA, Campbell DG, Garbuz DS, Duncan CP: Seven specialized exposures for revision hip and knee replacement. Orthop Clin North Am 29:229–240, 1998.

52. Christensen CM, Seger BM, Schultz RB: Management of intraoperative femur fractures associated with revision hip arthroplasty. Clin Orthop Relat Res 248:177–180, 1989.

53. Younger TI, Bradford MS, Magnus RE, Paprosky WG: Extended proximal femoral osteotomy: a new technique for femoral revision arthroplasty. J Arthroplasty 10:329–338, 1995.

54. Mitchell PA, Greidanus NV, Masri BA, et al: The prevention of periprosthetic fractures of the femur during and after total hip arthroplasty. Instr Course Lect 52:301–308, 2003.

55. Sydney SV, Mallory TH: Controlled perforation: a safe method of cement removal from the femoral canal. Clin Orthop Relat Res 253:168–172, 1990.

56. Missakian ML, Rand JA: Fractures of the femoral shaft adjacent to long stem femoral components of total hip arthroplasty: report of seven cases. Orthopedics 16:149–152, 1993.

57. Talab YA, States JD, Evarts CM: Femoral shaft perforation: a complication of total hip reconstruction. Clin Orthop Relat Res 141:158–165, 1979.

58. Berry DJ: Total hip arthroplasty in patients with proximal femoral deformity. Clin Orthop Relat Res 369:262–272, 1999.

59. Incavo SJ, DiFazio F, Wilder D, et al: Longitudinal crack propagation in bone around femoral prosthesis. Clin Orthop Relat Res 272:175–180, 1991.

60. White LM, Kim JK, Mehta MF, et al: Complications of total hip arthroplasty: MR imaging—initial experience. Radiology 215:254–262, 2000.

61. Olsen RV, Munk PL, Lee MJ, et al: Metal artifact reduction sequence: early clinical applications. Radiographics 20:699–712, 2000.

62. Letournel E: Fractures of the acetabulum: a study of a series of 75 cases (Les fractures du cotyle, etude d'une serie de 75 cas). J Chirurgie 82:47–87, 1961. (Translated and substantially abridged.) J Orthop Trauma 20:S15–S19, 2006.

63. Letournel E: Acetabulum fractures: classification and management. Clin Orthop Relat Res 151:81–106, 1980.

64. Letournel E, Judet RF: Fractures of the acetabulum. In Elson RA, editor: Les fractures du cotyle, New York, 1993, Springer.

65. Callaghan JJ: Instructional Course Lectures, The American Academy of Orthopaedic Surgeons: Periprosthetic fractures of the acetabulum during and following total hip arthroplasty. J Bone Joint Surg Am 79:1416–1421, 1997.

66. Mallory TH, Kraus TJ, Vaughn BK: Intraoperative femoral fractures associated with cementless total hip arthroplasty. Orthopedics 12:231–239, 1989.

67. Stuchin SA: Femoral shaft fracture in porous and press-fit total hip arthroplasty. Orthop Rev 19:153–159, 1990.

68. Duncan CP, Masri BA: Fractures of the femur after hip replacement. Instr Course Lect 44:293–304, 1995.

69. Brady OH, Garbuz DS, Masri BA, Duncan CP: The reliability and validity of the Vancouver classification of femoral fractures after hip replacement. J Arthroplasty 15:59–62, 2000.

70. Rayan F, Dodd M, Haddad FS: European validation of the Vancouver classification of periprosthetic proximal femoral fractures. J Bone Joint Surg Br 90:1576–1579, 2008.

71. Masri BA, Meek RM, Duncan CP: Periprosthetic fractures: evaluation and treatment. Clin Orthop Relat Res 420:80–95, 2004.

71a. Van Houwelengen A, Duncan C: The pseudo plt periprosthetic fracture: It's really a B2. Orthopaedics 34(9):674–675, 2011.

72. Boscainos PJ, Kellett CF, Maury AC, et al: Management of periacetabular bone loss in revision hip arthroplasty. Clin Orthop Relat Res 465:159–165, 2007.

73. Khan MA, O'Driscoll M: Fractures of the femur during total hip replacement and their management. J Bone Joint Surg Br 59:36–41, 1977.

74. Fitzgerald RH, Jr, Brindley GW, Kavanagh BF: The uncemented total hip arthroplasty: intraoperative femoral fractures. Clin Orthop Relat Res 235:61–66, 1988.

75. Chen WM, McAuley JP, Engh CA, Jr, et al: Extended slide trochanteric osteotomy for revision total hip arthroplasty. J Bone Joint Surg Am 82:1215–1219, 2000.

76. Mont MA, Maar DC: Fractures of the ipsilateral femur after hip arthroplasty: a statistical analysis of outcome based on 487 patients. J Arthroplasty 9:511–519, 1994.

77. Zarin JS, Zurakowski DF, Burke DW: Claw plate fixation of the greater trochanter in revision total hip arthroplasty. J Arthroplasty 24:272–280, 2009.

78. Chandler HP, Tigges RG: The role of allografts in the treatment of periprosthetic femoral fractures. Instr Course Lect 47:257–264, 1998.

79. Haddad FS, Duncan CP: Cortical onlay allograft struts in the treatment of periprosthetic femoral fractures. Instr Course Lect 52:291–300, 2003.

80. Large TM, Kellam JF, Bosse MJ, et al: Locked plating of supracondylar periprosthetic femur fractures. J Arthroplasty 23:115–120, 2008.

81. Chakravarthy J, Bansal R, Cooper J: Locking plate osteosynthesis for Vancouver type B1 and type C periprosthetic fractures of femur: a report on 12 patients. Injury 38:725–733, 2007.

82. Currall V, Thomason K, Eastaugh-Waring S, et al: The use of LISS femoral locking plates and cabling in the treatment of periprosthetic fractures around stable proximal femoral implants in elderly patients. Hip Int 18:207–211, 2008.

83. Dennis MG, Simon JA, Kummer FJ, et al: Fixation of periprosthetic femoral shaft fractures occurring at the tip of the stem: a biomechanical study of 5 techniques. J Arthroplasty 15:523–528, 2000.

84. Kobbe P, Klemm R, Reilmann H, Hockertz TJ: Less invasive stabilisation system (LISS) for the treatment of periprosthetic femoral fractures: a 3-year follow-up. Injury 39:472–479, 2008.

85. Panasiuk M, Kmieciak M: [Treatment of periprosthetic fractures of the distal femur with the LISS system]. Chir Narzadow Ruchu Ortop Pol 69:369–371, 2004.

86. Wick M, Muller EJ, Kutscha-Lissberg F, et al: [Periprosthetic supracondylar femoral fractures: LISS or retrograde intramedullary nailing? Problems with the use of minimally invasive technique]. Unfallchirurg 107:181–188, 2004.

87. Spangehl MJ, Masri BA, O'Connell JX, Duncan CP: Prospective analysis of preoperative and intraoperative investigations for the diagnosis of infection at the sites of two hundred and two revision total hip arthroplasties. J Bone Joint Surg Am 81:672–683, 1999.

88. Schinsky MF, Della Valle CJ, Sporer SM, Paprosky WG: Perioperative testing for joint infection in patients undergoing revision total hip arthroplasty. J Bone Joint Surg Am 90:1869–1875, 2008.

89. Sim FH, Chao EY: Hip salvage by proximal femoral replacement. J Bone Joint Surg Am 63:1228–1239, 1981.

90. Pritchett JW: Fracture of the greater trochanter after hip replacement. Clin Orthop Relat Res 390:221–226, 2001.

91. Lindahl H, Malchau H, Oden A, Garellick G: Risk factors for failure after treatment of a periprosthetic fracture of the femur. J Bone Joint Surg Br 88:26–30, 2006.

92. Ricci WM, Bolhofner BR, Loftus T, et al: Indirect reduction and plate fixation, without grafting, for periprosthetic femoral shaft fractures about a stable intramedullary implant. J Bone Joint Surg Am 87:2240–2245, 2005.

93. Ricci WM, Bolhofner BR, Loftus T, et al: Indirect reduction and plate fixation, without grafting, for periprosthetic femoral shaft fractures about a stable intramedullary implant: surgical technique. J Bone Joint Surg Am 88:275–282, 2006.

94. Ebraheim NA, Gomez C, Ramineni SK, Liu J: Fixation of periprosthetic femoral shaft fractures adjacent to a well-fixed femoral stem with reversed distal femoral locking plate. J Trauma 66:1152–1157, 2009.

95. Fulkerson E, Tejwani N, Stuchin S, Egol K: Management of periprosthetic femur fractures with a first generation locking plate. Injury 38:965–972, 2007.

96. Sah AP, Marshall A, Virkus WV, et al: Interprosthetic fractures of the femur: treatment with a single-locked plate. J Arthroplasty 25:280–286, 2008.

97. Buttaro MA, Farfalli G, Nunez MP, et al: Locking compression plate fixation of Vancouver type-B1 periprosthetic femoral fractures. J Bone Joint Surg Am 89:1964–1969, 2007.

98. Venu KM, Koka R, Garikipati R, et al: Dall-Miles cable and plate fixation for the treatment of peri-prosthetic femoral fractures-analysis of results in 13 cases. Injury 32:395–400, 2001.

99. Tadross TS, Nanu AM, Buchanan MJ, Checketts RG: Dall-Miles plating for periprosthetic B1 fractures of the femur. J Arthroplasty 15:47–51, 2000.

100. Chandler HP, Penenberg BL: Bone stock deficiency in total hip replacement: classification and management. In Femoral reconstruction, Thorofare, NJ, 1989, Slack, pp 103–164.

101. Chandler HP, King D, Limbird R, et al: The use of cortical allograft struts for fixation of fractures associated with well-fixed total joint prostheses. Semin Arthroplasty 4:99–107, 1993.

102. Chandler HP, Tigges RG: Instructional course lectures: The American Academy of Orthopaedic Surgeons—The role of allografts in the treatment of periprosthetic femoral fractures. J Bone Joint Surg Am 79:1422–1432, 1997.

103. Haddad FS, Duncan CP, Berry DJ, et al: Periprosthetic femoral fractures around well-fixed implants: use of cortical onlay allografts with or without a plate. J Bone Joint Surg Am 84:945–950, 2002.

104. Kamineni S, Vindlacheruvu RF, Ware HE: Peri-prosthetic femoral shaft fractures treated with plate and cable fixation. Injury 30:261–268, 1999.

105. Macdonald SJ, Paprosky WG, Jablonsky WS, Magnus RG: Periprosthetic femoral fractures treated with a long-stem cementless component. J Arthroplasty 16:379–383, 2001.

106. Moreland JR, Bernstein ML: Femoral revision hip arthroplasty with uncemented, porous-coated stems. Clin Orthop Relat Res 319:141–150, 1995.

107. Paprosky WG, Greidanus NV, Antoniou J: Minimum 10-year-results of extensively porous-coated stems in revision hip arthroplasty. Clin Orthop Relat Res 369:230–242, 1999.

108. Tsiridis E, Narvani AA, Haddad FS, et al: Impaction femoral allografting and cemented revision for periprosthetic femoral fractures. J Bone Joint Surg Br 86:1124–1132, 2004.

109. Gross AE: Revision arthroplasty of the hip using allograft bone. In Czitrom AA, Gross AE, editors: Allografts in orthopaedic practice, Baltimore, 1992, Williams & Wilkins, pp 147–173.

110. Malkani AL, Settecerri JJ, Sim FH, et al: Long-term results of proximal femoral replacement for non-neoplastic disorders. J Bone Joint Surg Br 77:351–356, 1995.

111. Malkani AL, Paiso JM, Sim FH: Proximal femoral replacement with megaprosthesis. Instr Course Lect 49:141–146, 2000.

112. Garbuz DS, Toms AF, Masri BA, Duncan CP: Improved outcome in femoral revision arthroplasty with tapered fluted modular titanium stems. Clin Orthop Relat Res 453:199–202, 2006.

113. McInnis DP, Horne GF, Devane PA: Femoral revision with a fluted, tapered, modular stem: seventy patients followed for a mean of 3.9 years. J Arthroplasty 21:372–380, 2006.

114. Park YS, Moon YW, Lim SJ: Revision total hip arthroplasty using a fluted and tapered modular distal fixation stem with and without extended trochanteric osteotomy. J Arthroplasty 22:993–999, 2007.

115. Mumme TF, Muller-Rath RF, Andereya S, Wirtz DC: Uncemented femoral revision arthroplasty using the modular revision prosthesis MRP-TITAN revision stem. Oper Orthop Traumatol 19:56–77, 2007.

116. Wagner H: Prosthese de revision de l'articulation coxofemorale. Orthopade 18:438–453, 1989.

117. Beguec P, Sieber H: The concept of press-fit revision of loose femoral prosthesis, Paris, 2007, Springer-Verlag, pp 19–27.

118. Levine BR, Della Valle CJ, Lewis P, et al: Extended trochanteric osteotomy for the treatment of Vancouver B2/B3 periprosthetic fractures of the femur. J Arthroplasty 23:527–533, 2008.

119. Somers JF, Suy R, Stuyck J, et al: Conservative treatment of femoral shaft fractures in patients with total hip arthroplasty. J Arthroplasty 13:162–171, 1998.

120. Lindahl H, Oden A, Garellick G, Malchau H: The excess mortality due to periprosthetic femur fracture: a study from the Swedish national hip arthroplasty register. Bone 40:1294–1298, 2007.

CHAPTER 103

Abductor Muscle and Greater Trochanteric Complications

James I. Huddleston III, Jeffrey A. Geller, Dennis W. Burke, and Henrik Malchau

KEY POINTS

- Early detection of intraoperative and postoperative trochanteric problems is important to optimize chances of successful treatment.
- Trochanteric claw plates with locking screws and cables have shown promising results in the fixation of trochanteric fractures and nonunions.
- Trochanteric bursitis after total hip arthroplasty (THA) usually responds well to physical therapy and corticosteroid injections as needed.
- The extended trochanteric osteotomy is most commonly used in revision surgery for removal of well-fixed implants and/or polymethylmethacrylate and has shown low rates of nonunion.
- Constrained liners and/or augmentation with Achilles tendon allograft and calcaneal bone block may be useful for treating instability associated with trochanteric nonunion or tendinous avulsion.

INTRODUCTION

Sir John Charnley strongly advocated for osteotomy of the great trochanter in primary total hip arthroplasty (THA) to optimize soft tissue tensioning and stability.[1,2] The advent of modularity in modern THA systems has enhanced surgeons' ability to restore offset and leg length, as well as to optimize fixation without osteotomizing the greater trochanter. As a result, most contemporary hip surgeons do not routinely use the transtrochanteric approach for uncomplicated primary total hip arthroplasties. Nevertheless, trochanteric osteotomy remains a valuable technique for revision surgery, as well as in primary cases involving severe protrusio acetabuli, ankylosis of the hip joint, heterotopic ossification, femoral deformity associated with dysplasia, and severe periarticular scar.[3-8]

Management of complications associated with the abductor mechanism in total hip arthroplasty can be challenging. These complications are not uncommon and may have a significant impact on a patient's functional status. This chapter reviews the complications associated with osteotomy and fracture of the greater trochanter as well as nerve palsy, avulsion and bursitis of the abducture musculature. Treatment options and results of techniques used to address these complications are discussed as well. Last, the authors present a novel technique for treating tendinous avulsion that has shown early success.

BONY COMPLICATIONS

Nonunion

Nonunion rates of the osteotomized greater trochanter vary and depend on the method of fixation.[9] Numerous first-generation techniques that used stainless steel and cobalt-chrome alloy monofilament wires demonstrated nonunion rates of 0 to 7.9% in studies that ranged in size from 75 to 1162 patients.[10-16] Risk factors for the development of nonunion when wires alone were used include male gender, revision surgery, and a primary diagnosis of rheumatoid arthritis. Technical factors that may predispose to nonunion with this technique include small size of the osteotomy fragment, lack of sufficient wire tension, limited surgical experience, wires placed around the lesser trochanter, and apposition of the trochanter to a bed that is primarily cement.[12,17,18] The need for revision surgery, an antalgic gait, pain, femoral loosening, and lower Charnley hip scores have all been associated with nonunion of the greater trochanter.[16] The development of nonunion after greater trochanteric osteotomy has not been associated with the type of wiring technique or the osteotomy variant used.[19,20] The rate of wire breakage based on a meta-analysis of studies reported from 1978 to 1993 involving 2910 total hip arthroplasties is 22% with various wiring techniques.[10-12,18,20-22]

In 1977, Dall and Miles introduced multifilament cables as the second-generation fixation technique for greater trochanter osteotomy.[23] The major advantages of cables over wires are that they offer greater strength and greater compression at the osteotomy site, while providing greater resistance to deformation.[18,24-31] Despite improvement in mechanical properties, breakage rates for cables have been reported to be as high as 12% (20/160 hips).[22] The use of cables alone in the practice of modern total hip arthroplasty is generally reserved for fixation of extended trochanteric osteotomies (Fig. 103-1). Cables may produce wear debris from micromotion that occurs between filaments, and this debris has been implicated in third-body wear of the

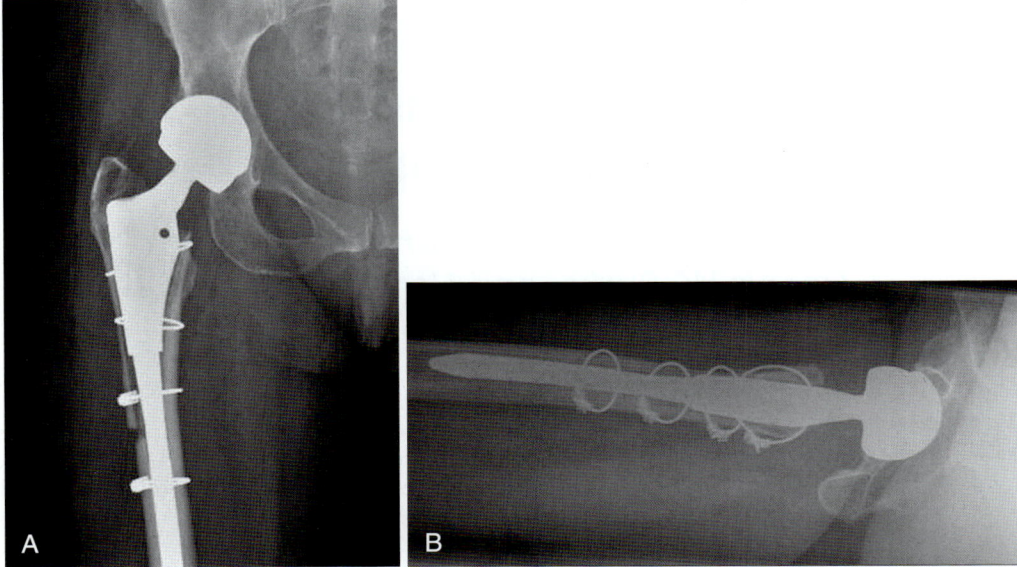

Figure 103-1. A, Anteroposterior (AP) and **(B)** lateral radiographs show an extended trochanteric osteotomy that united with multifilament cables alone.

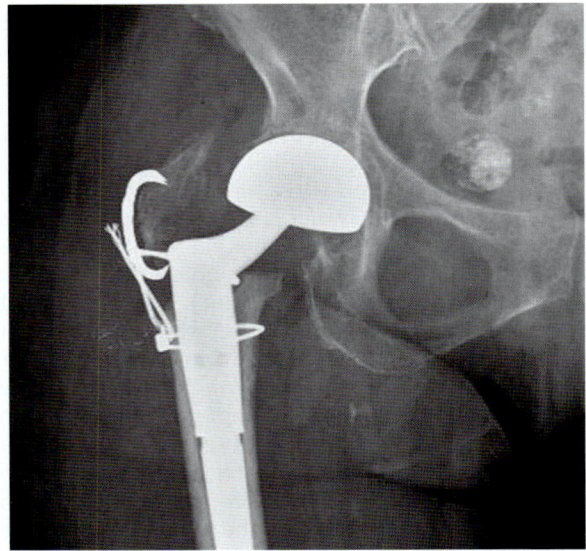

Figure 103-2. Anteroposterior (AP) hip radiograph shows nonunion of an osteotomized greater trochanter fixed with a Dall-Miles cable grip system.

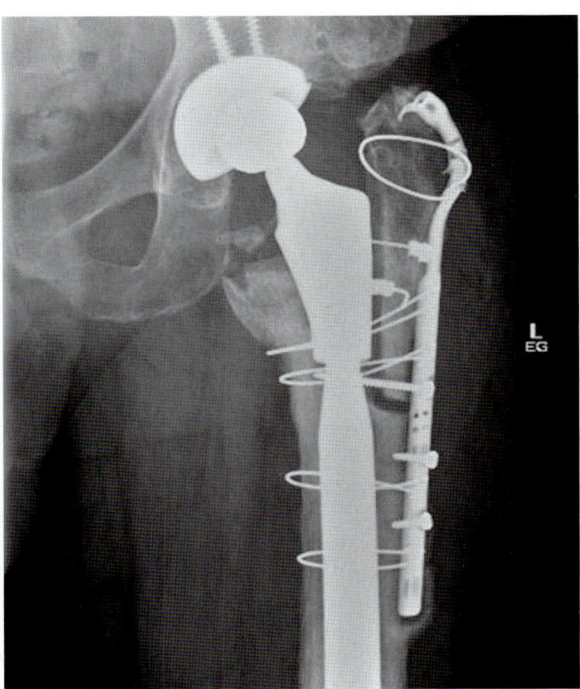

Figure 103-3. Anteroposterior (AP) hip radiograph shows an ununited extended trochanteric osteotomy despite use of a long cable-plate system.

bearing surface, which can affect rates of component loosening.[32,33]

Cable grip systems were introduced to address the shortcomings of wires and cables alone for trochanteric fixation (Fig. 103-2). In 1983, Dall and Miles reported that their new cable grip device was better at capturing the trochanter and prevent trochanteric escape.[23] When compared with wires and cables alone, cable grip systems have been shown to withstand 1.5 times the load to failure and require 2 to 2.5 times the load needed to produce 2-cm of trochanteric displacement.[27] Non-union rates with use of a cable grip system in four series

vary from 0.9% to 38% in series ranging in size from 40 to 321 hips.[23,24,28,30]

Fourth-generation trochanteric fixation implants comprise locking plates that allow for adjuvant cable and/or wire fixation (Fig. 103-3). The ability to extend the length of the construct and retighten the cables is a major advantage of these systems. Early clinical results reported for these constructs are promising.

One study of 42 patients reported significantly lower incidences of cable breakage ($P < .025$) and trochanteric nonunion ($P < .05$) with a 4th generation cable plate when compared with wires and cables alone.[34] A more recent study of four cases describes healing of the fracture or osteotomy with full abductor function and significant improvement in hip scores in all four patients at a minimum of 20 months' follow-up.[35]

The extended trochanteric osteotomy (ETO) was first described by Wagner[36] in 1989 and has been modified and popularized by Paprosky and associates.[37] Wagner's osteotomy is performed in the coronal plane, whereas Paprosky's is a sagittal plane osteotomy. It is most commonly used in revision surgery for removal of well-fixed implants and/or polymethylmethacrylate, although the ability to correct femoral deformity, improve exposure, and potentially improve the accuracy of femoral canal preparations are additional potential benefits. Complications associated with this technique include fracture, malunion, and nonunion. The incidence of ETO nonunion has been reported to be significantly lower when compared with sliding and traditional trochanteric osteotomies.[3,38] In one series of 192 consecutive revision THAs, in which an ETO was used for improved exposure, the authors reported two cases of nonunion (1.2%) and one case of malunion (0.6%) among 166 patients at a minimum of 2 years' follow-up.[8] In another series, the rate of ETO nonunion was 1.4% (1/74). Five of 73 ETOs united with less than 5 mm of migration, and 68 ETOs united with no migration.[39]

Clinical manifestations of trochanteric escape include pain, limp, and reduced abductor strength. Trochanteric migration of 5 to 20 mm has been shown to lead to nonunion and may be associated with development of a Trendelenburg gait pattern.[11,27] Displacement greater than 2 cm has been shown to lead to significant abductor weakness.[40]

Early detection of postoperative trochanteric problems is important to optimize chances of successful treatment. The presence of broken hardware or fragment migration seen on postoperative radiographs is cause for concern, although broken hardware is not pathognomonic for nonunion. Relative indications for revision of the fixation include migration during the first 6 weeks postoperatively, symptomatic nonunion, and symptomatic broken wires, cables, or plates. During revision surgery, all fibrous tissue should be débrided, and bleeding at the bony edges should be ensured when possible. Postoperatively, patients should be placed on trochanteric precautions to include no active abduction and toe touch weight bearing for at least 8 weeks and up to 3 months. Use of a hip abduction orthosis should also be considered.

Instability is a dreaded complication associated with nonunion of an osteotomized greater trochanter. The mechanism is often due to a decrease in abductor tension across the hip[41] but also may be due to trochanteric impingement against the pelvis anteriorly. Although some authors have reported a higher dislocation rate with nonunion, others have not.[42] In a series of 8944 THAs performed via a transtrochanteric approach, Woo and Morrey reported a nonunion rate of 2.2% (194 patients). Most dislocations that they observed occurred in patients who experienced trochanteric migration greater than 2 cm. The dislocation rate was 17.6% in patients with trochanteric nonunion and 2.8% in patients with trochanteric union.[43,44] Although decreased abductor power from nonunion is clearly a contributing factor to instability, component malposition should also be considered.

The use of trochanteric advancement to treat instability is less common today owing to modularity that allows for optimization of leg lengths and femoral offset. If trochanteric advancement is used, the technique described by Chin and Brick, in which the abductors are released from their origins on the outer iliac wing through a separate incision on the iliac crest, may be helpful to gain additional length, thereby decreasing tension on the repair.[45]

Heterotopic Ossification

It is unclear whether heterotopic ossification (HO) is more common with trochanteric osteotomy.[46] After primary THA, one study failed to show a difference in rates of HO among three approaches (posterior, transtrochanteric, and anterolateral).[47] With use of the transtrochanteric approach in routine THA, the rate of HO has been reported at 7% in 1500 low-friction arthroplasties performed by Eftekar.[48] A rate of 90% has been reported when the transtrochanteric approach was used for complicated primary and revision THAs.[49] It is generally accepted that the risk of HO is higher in patients with hypertrophic osteoarthritis, ankylosing spondylitis, closed head injury, or a history of ectopic bone formation. Given this, the surgeon may consider HO prophylaxis in select high-risk cases.

Fracture

It is estimated that periprosthetic fractures occur intraoperatively in approximately 1% to 20% of primary THA cases.[50-55] The incidence of isolated greater trochanter fractures is unknown and has been estimated to be as high as 5%.[56] In a series of primary total hip arthroplasties performed through an anterior approach, the rate of intraoperative greater trochanter fracture was 0.7% (3/437 THAs).[57] The rate of postoperative greater trochanter fractures is unknown. It has been estimated that postoperative periprosthetic femoral fractures occur in less than 1% of primary total hip arthroplasties.[58] Intraoperative fractures should be treated with reduction and internal fixation. Given the relatively high rates of nonunion associated with the use of wires and cables alone, we advocate the use of a cable-plate system. Postoperative greater trochanter fractures with less than 2 cm of displacement have been successfully treated without operative intervention and with 6 to 12 weeks of limited weight bearing and no active abduction exercises until the fracture has united.[56] It is recommended that most fractures with more than 2 cm of displacement be treated with open reduction and internal fixation, if adequate fixation is likely to be achieved.

SOFT TISSUE COMPLICATIONS

Bursitis

The prevalence of trochanteric bursitis after THA ranges from 4% to 17% in series of patients ranging in size from 75 to 1162.[59-63] Although the cause of trochanteric bursitis is multifactorial, the final common pathophysiology likely involves repetitive microtrauma, scar tissue formation, alterations in lower extremity biomechanics, and/or changes in hip mechanics after THA.[64] Risk factors include a direct lateral approach,[60] limb length discrepancy, younger age, and increased lateral offset. Most patients will experience resolution of their symptoms with physical therapy and local corticosteroid injection. In one study, 32 of 689 patients (4.6%) developed trochanteric bursitis after THA. In all, 80% of the 25 patients for whom follow-up was available experienced resolution of their symptoms after corticosteroid injection. A total of 11 of 25 (45%) patients needed multiple injections. The authors commented that nonresponders may benefit from operative treatment to remove trochanteric bursae and local scar tissue.[59]

Trochanteric bursitis after THA is more common in the setting of trochanteric hardware because these devices can easily cause local soft tissue irritation, given that they reside near a bony prominence. Unfortunately, relief of symptoms after removal of hardware is less predictable than desired. In a series of 36 patients with trochanteric bursitis reported by Bernard and Brooks, less than 50% of patients who underwent removal of trochanteric wires reported successful pain relief.[31] Treatment modalities other than hardware removal include stretching, ultrasound, and injections of local anesthetic and corticosteroids.

Nerve Injury

Peripheral nerve injury occurs in 0 to 3% of primary THAs[65-68] and in 2.9% to 7.6% of revision THAs.[65,66,69] The incidence of superior gluteal nerve injury is, however, unknown. Injuries of the superior gluteal nerve can lead to abductor weakness with resultant limp or instability. Splitting of the gluteus medius muscle greater than 5 cm from the tip of the greater trochanter is considered a risk factor for injury to the superior gluteal nerve. This is a concern when the lateral approach to the hip is utilized.[41,60,70]

Tendinous Avulsion

Abductor deficiency secondary to avulsion of the greater trochanter or the abductor insertion is a rare complication after total hip arthroplasty. Patients with this condition suffer from severe pain, a limp, and a general sense of hip dysfunction. The diagnosis, however, can be difficult to make or may be overlooked, and this condition is often misdiagnosed as trochanteric bursitis or postoperative abductor weakness. Little information is available to describe the diagnosis

or treatment of this debilitating problem. One study that looked at the results of a primary repair technique in nine patients with abductor avulsion after total hip arthroplasty found mixed results and inconsistent relief of pain.[71] In one small series of five patients reported on by Kagan, primary repair in this population was reportedly successful at long-term follow-up.[72,73] Use of an Achilles tendon allograft with calcaneal bone block has shown promising early results in treating unstable THAs caused by avulsion of the gluteus medius and minimus tendons.[74]

Constrained liners are an attractive option for treating patients with avulsion of the abductor tendon associated with recurrent instability of the hip. However, they should not be used in cases of implant malposition. Although large femoral heads have been used successfully to treat recurrent hip instability, we do not recommend their use in cases of abductor tendon avulsion.[75]

SURGICAL TECHNIQUES

Surgical options to be considered for abductor complications following THA can be divided into the two categories of intraoperative complications and known preoperative problems. The intraoperative complication most commonly encountered during primary or revision THA is fracture of the greater trochanter. This can occur as an unplanned event, particularly in osteoporotic patients, patients in whom the THA is complex such as those with dysplasia, and patients with overly aggressive retraction. Other instances where this may occur include limited visualization during minimal incision cases and in some types of anterior or anterolateral approaches to the hip where the abductor mechanism is partially detached during the exposure. The other category of abductor muscle and greater trochanteric complications consists of those that occur as a late complication of a hip reconstruction. These may include abductor dysfunction from a prior lateral or anterolateral approach to the hip in which repair of the gluteus medius and/or minimus muscles fails, postoperative greater trochanteric fracture, failure of fixation of a trochanteric advancement, and failure of fixation of an extended trochanteric osteotomy.

In all of these circumstances, the manifestation may be weakened or absent hip abductor support leading to instability, a Trendelenburg gait, pain, or a combination of these manifestations. The techniques for repair will be divided based on the timing of the abductor dysfunction.

Intraoperative Fractures of the Greater Trochanter

If fracture of the greater trochanter occurs during hip reconstruction, repair of the fracture is imperative to avoid long-term abductor problems such as trochanteric escape with hip abductor weakness. Multiple methods of fixation may be used, depending upon the

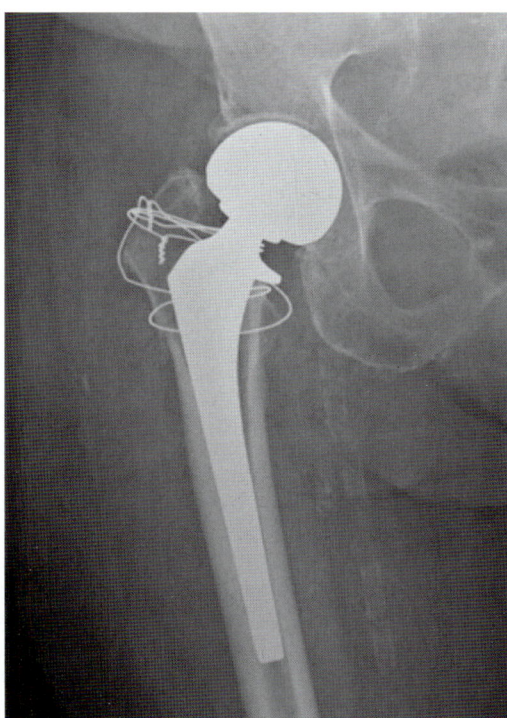

Figure 103-4. Anteroposterior (AP) hip radiograph shows trochanteric wiring of an intraoperative greater trochanter fracture.

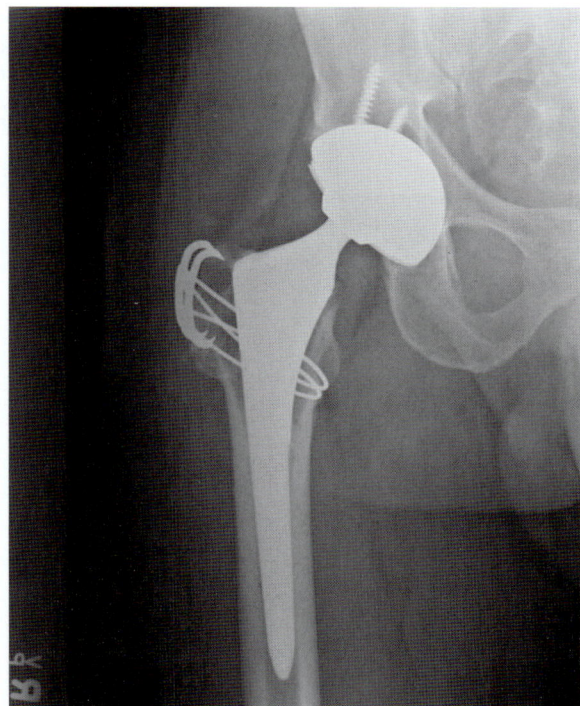

Figure 103-5. Anteroposterior (AP) hip radiograph of a trochanteric claw.

area that has fractured. If the fracture is small and nondisplaced, simple cerclage wiring can be done to stabilize the proximal trochanteric piece. This may be done with metal or polyethylene cables, simple wires, or large-gauge nonabsorbable suture, depending on the size and fracture pattern of the trochanter. In most scenarios, a simple 16- or 18-gauge wire is minimally caustic to surrounding tissues and works well. As with any wiring of the femur, care should be taken to ensure that the wires stay intimately opposed to bone while they are being passed (Fig. 103-4). Additionally, the wires should pass distal to the lesser trochanter to achieve better fixation and compression. Care should be taken to try to avoid passing cables around the neck of the prosthesis because they can fray, leading to particle generation within the effective joint space with possible third-body wear of the hip articulation. Another possible fixation technique involves a trochanteric cable grip system. If the trochanteric fracture is unstable or comminuted, the cable grip system may provide a broader area of fixation and concomitant compression (Fig. 103-5).

Depending on the fracture pattern, it is usually prudent to limit patients to toe touch weight bearing for the first 6 weeks after surgery to promote fracture healing. Additionally, patients should be strictly prohibited from doing any active hip abduction exercises during that time. A hip abduction orthosis may be considered depending upon the stability of the fracture repair. When radiographic evidence of fracture union is noted, patients may be advanced to weight bearing as

tolerated and may begin active hip abduction at that time.

More complex trochanteric fractures where considerable tension is present on the abductor muscle group or the greater trochanteric bone is weakened or osteopenic (as in many revision surgeries) may need a trochanteric plate to achieve stability. Similarly, if bone loss or tension is extensive after an extended trochanteric osteotomy, a similar type of plate may need to be used. These plates are available from a variety of manufacturers in many different sizes. An important concept of use is that the plate chosen should be long enough to impart adequate stability to the fracture—much like what is chosen in a native long-bone fracture. These plates often are best secured to the femur with cerclage cables; however, in certain situations, unicortical screws may be acceptable. The surgeon should try to avoid having the plate end at the same level as the femoral component tip to avoid creating a stress riser in this area (Figs. 103-6 and 103-7).

Placement of this type of plate may be variable, depending upon the clinical scenario. When placed after an unstable ETO, the vastus lateralis may be carefully elevated off of the bony fragment to allow the plate to lie flush on top of the bone. It is then helpful to reapproximate the displaced muscle over the plate to provide as much soft tissue coverage as possible. In the face of an inadvertent fracture of the greater trochanter, a vastus splitting approach to the lateral aspect of the femur allows excellent visualization with relative ease of plate placement. Care should be taken to gently raise a full-thickness flap of muscle with gentle subperiosteal elevation. Similarly, after plate application, the soft tissue can be reapproximated over the plate for soft tissue protection by simply closing the fascial layer overlying the vastus lateralis. Soft tissue coverage is extremely important in this area of the femur: it promotes fracture healing by optimizing blood flow to the region. Furthermore, the hardware may be prominent in this area, leading to tension on the iliotibial band or painful bursitis. This is a very common complication of applying hardware to this area, and quite often after the fracture is healed, the plate may need to be removed.

Technique of Abductor Muscle Reconstruction With Achilles Tendon Allograft

When abductor dysfunction or trochanteric complication leads to pain or an unacceptable gait disturbance, the reconstruction can be more strategically planned. In the event of a greater trochanteric nonunion or escape, the fracture can be exposed and reduced back down to its native position, or it can be advanced enough to put the abductors back down at appropriate muscle tension. Fixation can be achieved using a method similar to that used during an intraoperative fracture (see later). When the abductor muscle attachment is compromised, attempts at primary repair have historically been less successful (Fig. 103-8).[20]

The proximal femur is inspected, as is the status of the abductors. If the tissue appears healthy without signs of infection (based on appearance, intraoperative frozen sections, and/or a synovial fluid white blood cell count), and if an abductor mass is present that can support reconstruction with allograft, the decision is made to proceed. Reconstruction of the abductor mechanism with an achilles tendon allograft and calcaneal bone block is a viable option in this case.

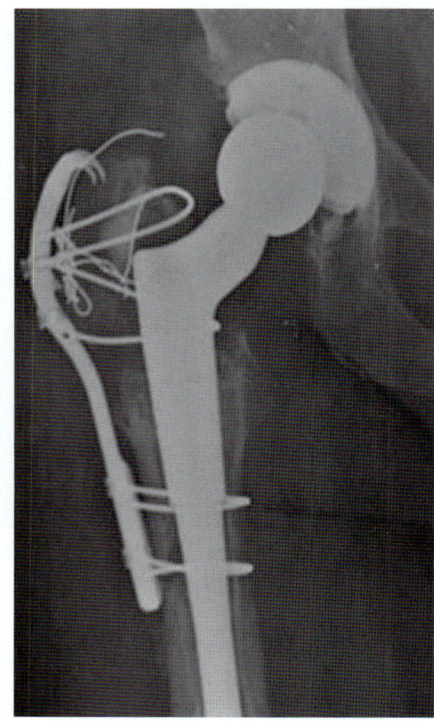

Figure 103-6. Anteroposterior (AP) hip radiograph of a trochanteric cable-plate system that led to a united extended trochanteric osteotomy.

Figure 103-7. A, Preoperative and **(B)** postoperative radiographs show a dislocated revision total hip arthroplasty (THA) with trochanteric fracture treated successfully with acetabular revision and open reduction and internal fixation (ORIF) of the fracture with a trochanteric cable plate.

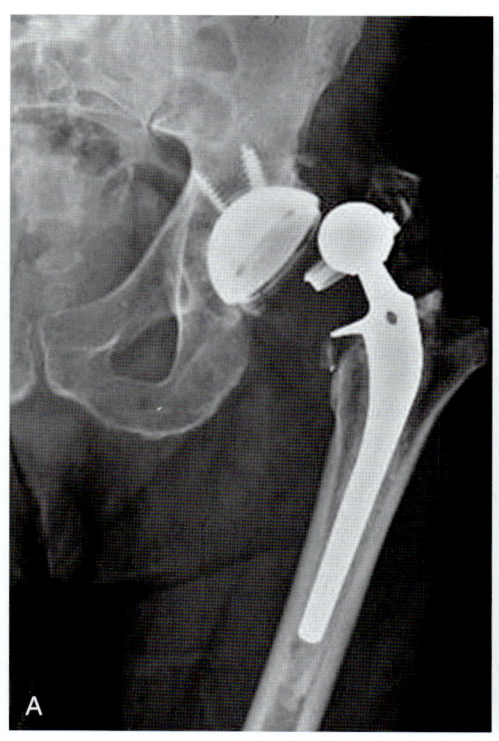
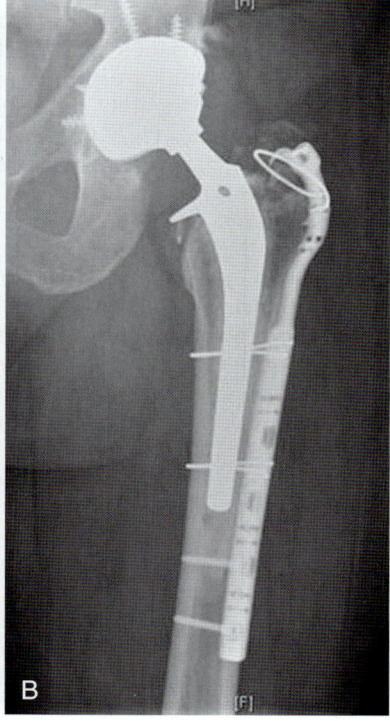

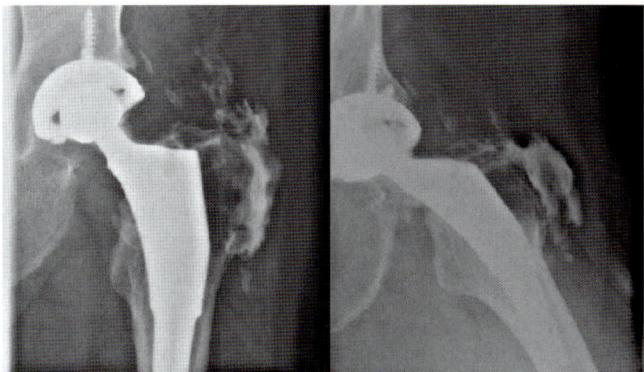

Figure 103-8. Hip arthrogram shows dye extravasation consistent with avulsion of the gluteus medius tendon.

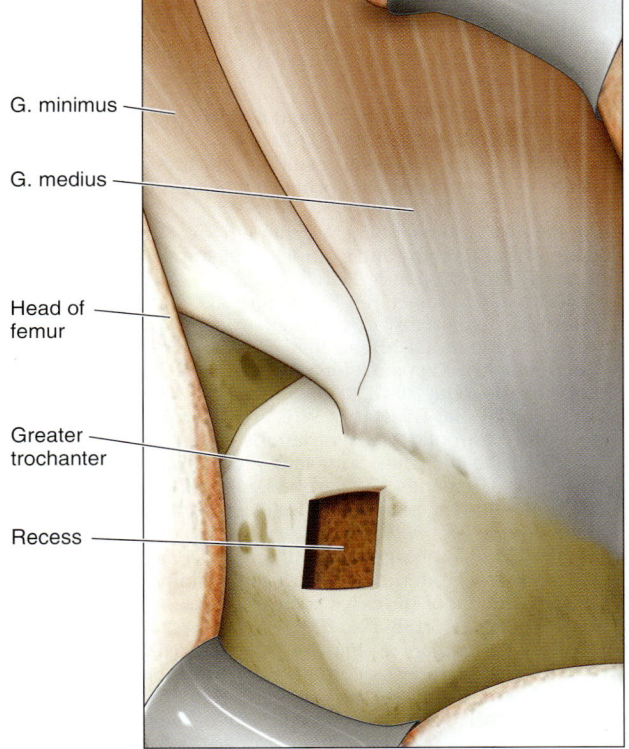

G. minimus

G. medius

Head of femur

Greater trochanter

Recess

Figure 103-9. Drawing depicts the location of the bony trough that will accept the allograft calcaneal bone block. Note the proximal bevel to resist proximal migration.

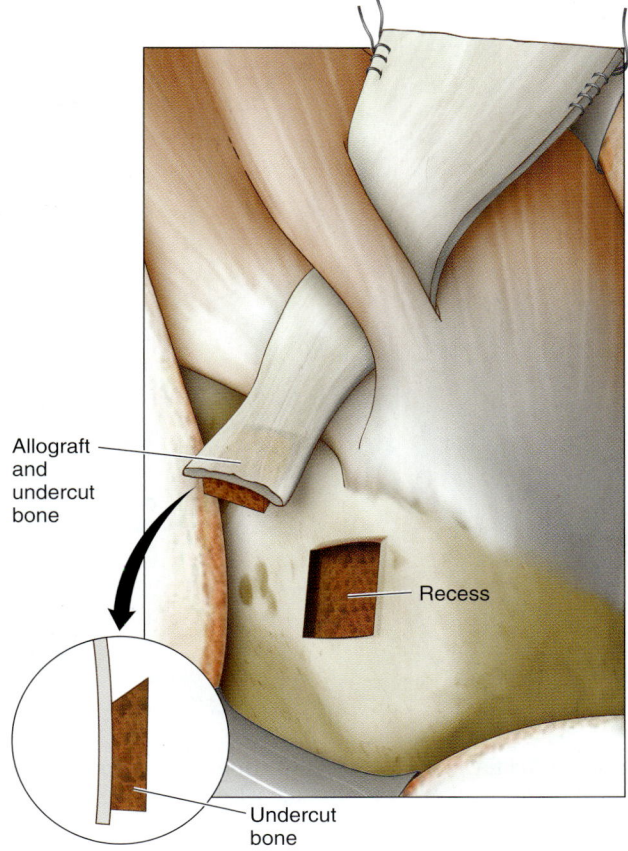

Allograft and undercut bone

Recess

Undercut bone

Figure 103-10. Drawing depicts the allograft Achilles tendon looped through the avulsed gluteus medius tendon and muscle.

Next, the fresh-frozen Achilles tendon allograft with a calcaneal bone block is prepared. The bony block is fashioned with a sagittal saw to be about 2 cm long, 1.5 cm wide, and 0.5 to 1.0 cm deep, with the most proximal cut beveled to hinge into the greater trochanter (Fig. 103-10). To achieve a bony bed for the allograft block to be seated, an appropriate area is selected just below the vastus ridge, approximately 5 to 10 mm distal to the distal extent of the greater trochanter. In this area, a trough is measured to match the size of an allograft block. A sagittal saw and an osteotome are used to create the trough, with specific attention placed on creating a bevel in the proximal cut to resist proximal migration of the bony block from the allograft (Fig. 103-9). Next, the lateral trochanter (area of prior tendinous insertion) is freshened with a high-speed burr to remove all scar tissue and chronic fibrotic tissue until a bleeding bony bed is available for allograft adherence.

The next step involves mobilization of the abductors to identify healthy tissue for repair back to the allograft. To do this, the interval between the gluteus minimus and medius is developed to allow for tension-free translation of the abductors inferiorly. The tendinous portion of the allograft is then passed through intact medius muscle approximately 3 cm above the avulsed end. The allograft is then looped back on itself (Fig. 103-10). The gluteus minimus tendon is usually not incorporated into the repair as it often lacks the structural integrity needed to prevent cut-out of the allograft.

The hip is abducted maximally and is carefully maintained on the surgical stand throughout the remainder of the repair. The bony block is inserted into the trough with a press-fit. Next, a 16-gauge cerclage wire is placed around the bone block and around the proximal femur and is tightened to an appropriate tension and locked into place with a crimper (Fig. 103-11). The tendinous portion of the allograft is repaired anteriorly to the gluteus minimus and the capsule with heavy

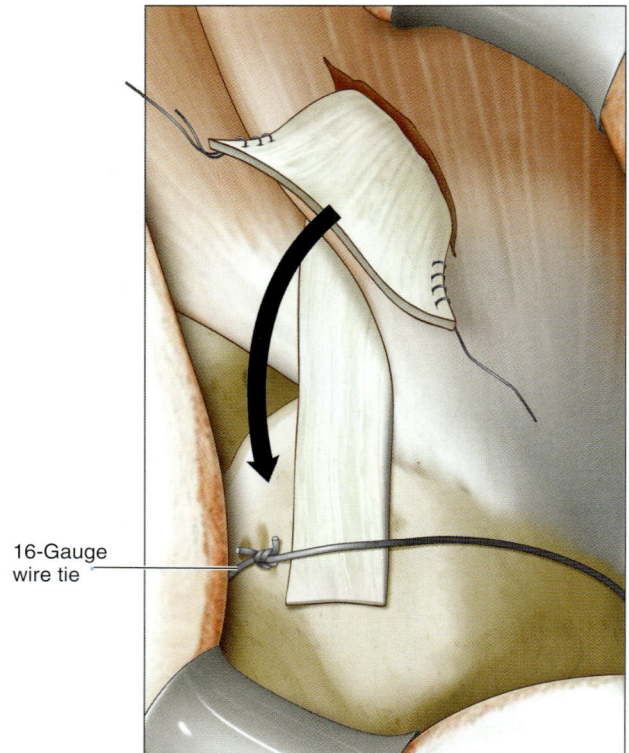

16-Gauge
wire tie

Figure 103-11. Drawing depicts fixation of the allograft calcaneal bone block with a cerclage wire.

nonabsorbable sutures and posteriorly to the intact area of the gluteus medius tendon in similar fashion. The allograft tendon is looped back over onto itself and then is repaired anteriorly again to the gluteus minimus and capsule and posteriorly to the posterior capsule and intact gluteus medius end. Once the repair is completed, the hip is gently ranged and examined for stability of bony fixation and tendinous suture repair.

The hip is maintained in a hip abduction brace with 10 degrees of abduction and 30 degrees of fixed flexion for 6 weeks postoperatively with partial weight-bearing restrictions during this interval. Patients are advanced to a cane at the 6-week follow-up appointment, where follow-up radiographs are obtained.

Our group has recently reported on 2-year outcomes using this technique. From 2003 to 2006, we performed seven abductor reconstructions with Achilles tendon allograft for patients with abductor deficiency after total hip arthroplasty. At a mean of 29 months from the index procedure and before the revision procedure, all seven patients suffered symptoms of lateral hip pain and abductor weakness. At minimum 24-month follow-up after the revision procedure (range, 24 to 48 months), all but one patient showed substantial improvement in both Harris hip scores and pain scores; one patient had only a six-point improvement in hip score. The average Harris Hip Score was 85.9, up from 34.7 preoperatively for an average improvement of 51 points (range, 6 to 65 points). Preoperatively, six patients had marked or severe pain; six had no or slight pain postoperatively. One patient had moderate pain

before surgery and at most recent follow-up. Pain scores improved from an average of 11.4 to 38.9. Six used a walker or a cane full-time before reconstruction. Postoperatively, three did not need assistive devices at all, but two used a cane full-time and two only for long walks. Limp was recorded as severe in five and moderate in two preoperatively. Postoperatively, limp was noted to be absent in two, slight in four, and severe in one patient. Trendelenburg sign, although severe in six patients preoperatively, was not present in two patients and only slight in the remaining five patients after surgery. Side-lying abductor motor strength scores based on a standard 0 to 5 scale measured a mean 2.6 preoperatively and improved to a mean 4.1 postoperatively. Overall, these results have encouraged us to routinely offer this technique to patients who present with abductor insufficiency, having failed all other nonoperative treatment modalities.

REFERENCES

1. Charnley J: Total hip replacement by low-friction arthroplasty. Clin Orthop Relat Res 72:7–21, 1970.
2. Charnley J: The long-term results of low-friction arthroplasty of the hip performed as a primary intervention. J Bone Joint Surg 54:61–76, 1972.
3. Archibeck MJ, Rosenberg AG, Berger RA, Silverton CD: Trochanteric osteotomy and fixation during total hip arthroplasty. J Am Acad Orthop Surg 11:163–173, 2003.
4. Della Valle CJ, Berger RA, Rosenberg AG, et al: Extended trochanteric osteotomy in complex primary total hip arthroplasty: a brief note. J Bone Joint Surg Am 85:2385–2390, 2003.
5. Glassman AH: Exposure for revision: total hip replacement. Clin Orthop Relat Res 420:39–47, 2004.
6. McGrory BJ, Bal BS, Harris WH: Trochanteric osteotomy for total hip arthroplasty: six variations and indications for their use. J Am Acad Orthop Surg 4:258–267, 1996.
7. Meek RM, Greidanus NV, Garbuz DS, et al: Extended trochanteric osteotomy: planning, surgical technique, and pitfalls. Instr Course Lect 53:119–130, 2004.
8. Miner TM, Momberger NG, Chong D, Paprosky WL: The extended trochanteric osteotomy in revision hip arthroplasty: a critical review of 166 cases at mean 3-year, 9-month follow-up. J Arthroplasty 16:188–194, 2001.
9. Jarit GJ, Sathappan SS, Panchal A, et al: Fixation systems of greater trochanteric osteotomies: biomechanical and clinical outcomes. J Am Acad Orthop Surg 15:614–624, 2007.
10. Harris WH, Crothers OD: Reattachment of the greater trochanter in total hip-replacement arthroplasty: a new technique. J Bone Joint Surg Am 60:211–213, 1978.
11. Amstutz HC, Maki S: Complications of trochanteric osteotomy in total hip replacement. J Bone Joint Surg Am 60:214–216, 1978.
12. Boardman KP, Bocco F, Charnley J: An evaluation of a method of trochanteric fixation using three wires in the Charnley low friction arthroplasty. Clin Orthop Relat Res 132:31–38, 1978.
13. Wroblewski BM, Shelley P: Reattachment of the greater trochanter after hip replacement. J Bone Joint Surg 67:736–740, 1985.
14. Jensen NF, Harris WH: A system for trochanteric osteotomy and reattachment for total hip arthroplasty with a ninety-nine percent union rate. Clin Orthop Relat Res 208:174–181, 1986.
15. Peters PC Jr, Head WC, Emerson RH Jr: An extended trochanteric osteotomy for revision total hip replacement. J Bone Joint Surg Am 75:158–159, 1993.
16. Frankel A, Booth RE Jr, Balderston RA, et al: Complications of trochanteric osteotomy: long-term implications. Clin Orthop Relat Res 208:209–213, 1993.
17. Amstutz HC, Mai LL, Schmidt I: Results of interlocking wire trochanteric reattachment and technique refinements to

prevent complications following total hip arthroplasty. Clin Orthop Relat Res 183:82–89, 1984.

18. Schutzer SF, Harris WH: Trochanteric osteotomy for revision total hip arthroplasty: 97% union rate using a comprehensive approach. Clin Orthop Relat Res 227:172–183, 1988.

19. Nercessian OA, Newton PM, Joshi RP, et al: Trochanteric osteotomy and wire fixation: a comparison of 2 techniques. Clin Orthop Relat Res 333:208–216, 1996.

20. Berry DJ, Muller ME: Chevron osteotomy and single wire reattachment of the greater trochanter in primary and revision total hip arthroplasty. Clin Orthop Relat Res 294:155–161, 1993.

21. Clarke RP Jr, Shea WD, Bierbaum ME: Trochanteric osteotomy: analysis of pattern of wire fixation failure and complications. Clin Orthop Relat Res 141:102–110, 1979.

22. Kelley SS, Johnston RC: Debris from cobalt-chrome cable may cause acetabular loosening. Clin Orthop Relat Res 285:140–146, 1992.

23. Dall DM, Miles AW: Re-attachment of the greater trochanter: the use of the trochanter cable-grip system. J Bone Joint Surg Am 65:55–59, 1983.

24. McCarthy JC, Bono JV, Turner RH, et al: The outcome of trochanteric reattachment in revision total hip arthroplasty with a cable grip system: mean 6-year follow-up. J Arthroplasty 14:810–814, 1999.

25. Hop JD, Callaghan JJ, Olejniczak JP, et al: The Frank Stinchfield Award. Contribution of cable debris generation to accelerated polyethylene wear. Clin Orthop Relat Res 344:20–32, 1997.

26. Bauer TW, Ming J, D'Antonio JA, Morawa LG: Abrasive three-body wear of polyethylene caused by broken multifilament cables of a total hip prosthesis: a report of these cases. J Bone Joint Surg Am 78:1244–1247, 1996.

27. Hersh CK, Williams RP, Trick LW, et al: Comparison of the mechanical performance of trochanteric fixation devices. Clin Orthop Relat Res 329:317–325, 1996.

28. Silverton CD, Jacobs JJ, Rosenberg AG, et al: Complications of a cable grip system. J Arthroplasty 11:400–404, 1996.

29. Berman AT, Zamarin R: The use of Dall-Miles cables in total hip arthroplasty. Orthopedics 16:833–835, 1993.

30. Ritter MA, Eizember LE, Keating EM, Faris PM: Trochanteric fixation by cable grip in hip replacement. J Bone Joint Surg Am 73:580–581, 1991.

31. Bernard AA, Brooks S: The role of trochanteric wire revision after total hip replacement. J Bone Joint Surg Am 69:352–354, 1987.

32. Altenburg AJ, Callaghan JJ, Yehyawi TM, et al: Cemented total hip replacement cable debris and acetabular construct durability. J Bone Joint Surg Am 91:1664–1670, 2009.

33. Brown TD, Lundberg HJ, Pedersen DR, Callaghan JJ: 2009 Nicolas Andry Award. Clinical biomechanics of third body acceleration of total hip wear. Clin Orthop Relat Res 467:1885–1897, 2009.

34. Barrack RL, Butler RA: Current status of trochanteric reattachment in complex total hip arthroplasty. Clin Orthop Relat Res 441:237–242, 2005.

35. McGrory BJ, Lucas R: The use of locking plates for greater trochanteric fixation. Orthopedics 32:917–920, 2009.

36. Wagner H: [A revision prosthesis for the hip joint]. Der Orthopade 18:438–453, 1989.

37. Younger TI, Bradford MS, Paprosky WG: Removal of a well-fixed cementless femoral component with an extended proximal femoral osteotomy. Contemp Orthop 30:375–380, 1995.

38. Jando VT, Greidanus NV, Masri BA, et al: Trochanteric osteotomies in revision total hip arthroplasty: contemporary techniques and results. Instr Course Lect 54:143–155, 2005.

39. Mardones R, Gonzalez C, Cabanela ME, et al: Extended femoral osteotomy for revision of hip arthroplasty: results and complications. J Arthroplasty 20:79–83, 2005.

40. Bergstrom B, Lindberg L, Persson BM, Onnerfalt R: Complications after total hip arthroplasty according to Charnley in a Swedish series of cases. Clin Orthop Relat Res 95:91–95, 1973.

41. Baker AS, Bitounis VC: Abductor function after total hip replacement: an electromyographic and clinical review. J Bone Joint Surg Am 71:47–50, 1989.

42. Carlsson AS, Gentz CF: Postoperative dislocation in the Charnley and Brunswik total hip arthroplasty. Clin Orthop Relat Res 125:177–182, 1977.

43. Morrey BF: Instability after total hip arthroplasty. Orthop Clin North Am 23:237–248, 1992.

44. Woo RY, Morrey BF: Dislocations after total hip arthroplasty. J Bone Joint Surg Am 64:1295–1306, 1982.

45. Chin KR, Brick GW: Reattachment of the migrated ununited greater trochanter after revision hip arthroplasty: the abductor slide technique. A review of four cases. J Bone Joint Surg Am 82:401–408, 2000.

46. Errico TJ, Fetto JF, Waugh TR: Heterotopic ossification: incidence and relation to trochanteric osteotomy in 100 total hip arthroplasties. Clin Orthop Relat Res 190:138–141, 1984.

47. Morrey BF, Adams RA, Cabanela ME: Comparison of heterotopic bone after anterolateral, transtrochanteric, and posterior approaches for total hip arthroplasty. Clin Orthop Relat Res 188:160–167, 1984.

48. Eftekar N: Total hip arthroplasty, St Louis, 1993, CV Mosby.

49. Kjaersgaard-Andersen P, Hougaard K, Linde F, et al: Heterotopic bone formation after total hip arthroplasty in patients with primary or secondary coxarthrosis. Orthopedics 13:1211–1217, 1990.

50. Garcia-Cimbrelo E, Munuera L, Gil-Garay E: Femoral shaft fractures after cemented total hip arthroplasty. Int Orthop 16:97–100, 1992.

51. Kelley SS: Periprosthetic femoral fractures. J Am Acad Orthop Surg 2:164–172, 1994.

52. Scott RD, Turner RH, Leitzes SM, Aufranc OE: Femoral fractures in conjunction with total hip replacement. J Bone Joint Surg Am 57:494–501, 1975.

53. Mont MA, Maar DC, Krackow KA, Hungerford DS: Hoop-stress fractures of the proximal femur during hip arthroplasty: management and results in 19 cases. J Bone Joint Surg Am 74:257–260, 1992.

54. Schwartz JT Jr, Mayer JG, Engh CA: Femoral fracture during non-cemented total hip arthroplasty. J Bone Joint Surg Am 71:1135–1142, 1989.

55. Stuchin SA: Femoral shaft fracture in porous and press-fit total hip arthroplasty. Orthop Rev 19:153–159, 1990.

56. Pritchett JW: Fracture of the greater trochanter after hip replacement. Clin Orthop Relat Res 390:221–226, 2001.

57. Matta JM, Ferguson TA: The anterior approach for hip replacement. Orthopedics 28:927–928, 2005.

58. Kavanagh BF: Femoral fractures associated with total hip arthroplasty. Orthop Clin North Am 23:249–257, 1992.

59. Farmer KW, Jones LC, Brownson KE, et al: Trochanteric bursitis after total hip arthroplasty: incidence and evaluation of response to treatment. J Arthroplasty 25:208–212, 2010.

60. Iorio R, Healy WL, Warren PD, Appleby D: Lateral trochanteric pain following primary total hip arthroplasty. J Arthroplasty 21:233–236, 2006.

61. Saito S, Ryu J, Oikawa H, Honda T: Clinical results of Harris-Galante total hip arthroplasty without cement: follow-up study of over five years. Bull Hosp Jt Dis 56:191–196, 1997.

62. Vicar AJ, Coleman CR: A comparison of the anterolateral, transtrochanteric, and posterior surgical approaches in primary total hip arthroplasty. Clin Orthop Relat Res 188:152–159, 1984.

63. Wiesman HJ Jr, Simon SR, Ewald FC, et al: Total hip replacement with and without osteotomy of the greater trochanter: clinical and biomechanical comparisons in the same patients. J Bone Joint Surg Am 60:203–210, 1978.

64. Shbeeb MI, Matteson EL: Trochanteric bursitis (greater trochanter pain syndrome). Mayo Clin Proc 71:565–569, 1996.

65. Edwards BN, Tullos HS, Noble PC: Contributory factors and etiology of sciatic nerve palsy in total hip arthroplasty. Clin Orthop Relat Res 218:136–141, 1987.

66. Johanson NA, Pellicci PM, Tsairis P, Salvati EA: Nerve injury in total hip arthroplasty. Clin Orthop Relat Res 179:214–222, 1983.

67. Solheim LF, Hagen R: Femoral and sciatic neuropathies after total hip arthroplasty. Acta Orthop Scand 51:531–534, 1980.

68. Zechmann JP, Reckling FW: Association of preoperative hip motion and sciatic nerve palsy following total hip arthroplasty. Clin Orthop Relat Res 241:197–199, 1989.

69. Schmalzried TP, Amstutz HC, Dorey FJ: Nerve palsy associated with total hip replacement: risk factors and prognosis. J Bone Joint Surg Am 73:1074–1080, 1991.

70. Hardinge K: The direct lateral approach to the hip. J Bone Joint Surg Am 64:17–19, 1982.

71. Weber M, Berry DJ: Abductor avulsion after primary total hip arthroplasty: results of repair. J Arthroplasty 12:202–206, 1997.

72. Kagan A 2nd: Rotator-cuff tear of the hip. J Bone Joint Surg Am 80:182–183, 1998.

73. Kagan A: Five cases of disruptions of the abductor mechanism of the hip. Orthop Trans 20:329, 1996.

74. McGann WA, Welch RB: Treatment of the unstable total hip arthroplasty using modularity, soft tissue, and allograft reconstruction. J Arthroplasty 16:19–23, 2001.

75. Sikes CV, Lai LP, Schreiber M, et al: Instability after total hip arthroplasty: treatment with large femoral heads vs constrained liners. J Arthroplasty 23:59–63, 2008.

FURTHER READING

Barrack RL, Butler RA: Current status of trochanteric reattachment in complex total hip arthroplasty. Clin Orthop Relat Res 441:237–242, 2005.

The authors performed a retrospective comparative study (therapeutic study, level III) to determine whether a more recent cable fixation device was associated with a higher success rate and a lower incidence of complications compared with early cable devices. Cobalt-chrome cables through holes in a trochanteric cable plate with two or more transversely oriented cables at or below the lesser trochanter were used to resist migration of the trochanteric fragment. Other component features included instrumentation that allowed provisional fixation and measurement of tension in the cables so that cables could be tightened and retightened sequentially to ensure a minimum of 80 inch-pounds of tension in all cables before final crimping. Minimum 2-year follow-up was obtained in 42 patients who had complex arthroplasties (trochanteric nonunions and reattachment to structural grafts) in which such a device was used. Clinical and radiographic results were compared with a series of patients with similar indications in whom wire and/or earlier-generation trochanteric cable fixation devices were used. The cable plate of a more recent design was associated with a possible trend for a lower incidence of limp, use of assistive walking devices, dislocation, and abductor weakness and a significant decrease in the incidence of breakage and trochanteric nonunion.

Jando VT, Greidanus NV, Masri BA, et al: Trochanteric osteotomies in revision total hip arthroplasty: contemporary techniques and results. Instr Course Lect 54:143–155, 2005.

Methods of trochanteric osteotomy can be categorized into three types: the standard trochanteric osteotomy, the trochanteric slide, and the extended trochanteric osteotomy. Although the standard osteotomy and the trochanteric slide osteotomy provide excellent acetabular exposure, in the revision setting they are frequently associated with an unacceptably high rate of nonunion and proximal migration of the trochanteric fragment. The extended trochanteric osteotomy (ETO) has increased in popularity as the number and complexity of revision THAs continue to increase. Two commonly used techniques are the ETO via a posterolateral approach and via a modified direct lateral approach. Both techniques provide wide exposure of the acetabulum, facilitate femoral component exposure and removal, aid in canal preparation and femoral reconstruction, and allow for correction of proximal femoral deformity. The osteotomy fragment is easily secured and may be advanced distally to achieve proper tensioning of the abductors. Recent literature demonstrates that the ETO has a relatively low rate of nonunion and is associated with fewer intraoperative femoral fractures or cortical perforations, as well as decreased surgical time.

CHAPTER 104

Leg Length Inequality: Prevention/Treatment

Saurabh Khakharia and William A. Jiranek

KEY POINTS

- Preoperative assessment of leg length inequality should include a history and physical examination, as well as radiographic evaluation and templating.
- Preoperative education of the patient should include discussion of his or her perception of leg length discrepancy and a discussion of the possibility of a postoperative leg length discrepancy.
- Templating to plan leg length equalization involves planning for socket and stem placement, as well as neck resection levels and offset.
- An intraoperative system is used to assess leg lengths before dislocation of the native hip and after placement of prosthetic components.
- Postoperative management of true and apparent leg length inequality may include physical therapy, lifts, and in rare cases, revision surgery.

INTRODUCTION

True limb length is usually defined as the distance from the anterior superior iliac spine to the medial malleolus. True leg length inequality is defined as lengthening or shortening of the above measurement as compared with the contralateral limb. Apparent leg length is defined as the distance from the umbilicus to the medial malleolus; thus an assessment of the coronal plane equality of the pelvis or spine must be included in the evaluation. Table 104-1 lists the possible combinations of true and apparent leg lengths and their causes.

In 1979, Sir John Charnley[1] stated that overlengthening of up to 1 cm can be justified because "... it permits active rehabilitation ... and patients very soon become adjusted to 1 cm overlengthening." Nonetheless, in most situations with careful preoperative templating and intra-operative trialing, leg length discrepancies can largely be avoided.

INCIDENCE AND PREVALENCE

No precise definition has been put forth for leg length inequality following total hip arthroplasty (THA); therefore, its prevalence following THA remains unknown. Incidence varies from 1% to 27%.[2] Mean leg length discrepancy after hip arthroplasty as reported in the literature ranges from 2.8 to 11.6 mm,[3-6] with some series reporting greater variability (1 to 15.9 mm).[7-12] Leg length inequality is perceived in approximately 32% to 43% of patients with a substantial (defined as greater than 1 cm) limb length discrepancy following THA.[3,7]

Notable leg length inequality may be associated with gait disorders,[13,14] back pain,[15,16] nerve injury,[17] and the need in severe cases for revision surgery.[18] Nerve injury is among the most feared and difficult to manage consequences of leg lengthening, and although some authors have documented an amount of lengthening associated with sciatic nerve palsy, the exact amount by which a limb can be lengthened is unclear. However, the majority of studies show that a range of 2 to 2.5 cm is safe in most patients. (See Chapter 105, "Neurovascular Injuries," for more information.[17]) Leg length inequality can give rise to patient dissatisfaction, which can adversely affect an otherwise good outcome and is a common reason for litigation following THA.

To prevent the previously mentioned problems associated with leg length inequality, the surgeon should take precautionary steps both before and during the operation.

STEPS TO PREVENT AND MINIMIZE LEG LENGTH INEQUALITY

Steps to prevent and minimize leg length inequality should include preoperative and intraoperative assessments of leg length.

Preoperative Assessment

History and Physical Examination

Evaluation should begin with a thorough history and physical examination. Patients should be asked if they perceive any leg length inequality or have any history of unequal hemming of pants or of flexing one knee, preferentially in the stance phase. A history of spinal deformity, hip dysplasia, muscular dystrophy, poliomyelitis, or spinal surgery, including spinal fusion, may be associated with leg length inequality. Physical examination can include an assessment of true and apparent leg length inequality, contractures around the hip joint, spine curvatures, and pelvic obliquity. Clinical methods such as tape measurement and standing blocks can be used as screening tools for measurement of leg lengths.

Measuring True Leg Length Inequality

The "Direct Method": Using a Tape Measure. A tape measure is used to measure the length of the lower extremity by determining the distance from the anterior-superior iliac spine to the medial malleolus; this reflects the actual length of the extremity. The range of error of this measurement has been reported to be .5 to 1.0 cm.[19,20] This is also known as the *direct method* of measuring leg length (Fig. 104-1). However, difficulty in identifying bony prominences, particularly in obese patients, and angular deformities in the lower limb can contribute to error when this clinical measurement tool is used.

Eichler and coworkers[19] described several potential sources of error when measurements are obtained using a tape measure, including poor reproducibility of finding the anterior-superior iliac spine (ASIS) and abduction or adduction contractures of the hip. Beattie and colleagues[20] reported on the reliability of tape measure method (TMM) measurements. They found low reliability (interclass correlation coefficient [ICC] of 0.668; ICC is a descriptive statistic that describes how strongly units in the same group resemble each other) when measurements were obtained by different examiners (interobserver variability). However, when the mean value of paired measurements taken by the same observer was used, intraobserver variability was much lower (ICC, 0.910). Investigators concluded that the reliability of tape measure measurement improved when the means of repeated measurements by the same observer were compared with measurements by other observers.

The Indirect Method: The "Block Test." The use of blocks placed underneath the patient's foot is known as the *indirect clinical method* of assessing leg length inequality. It is helpful in differentiating fixed from flexible pelvis obliquities. Causes of fixed pelvic obliquities include lumbosacral fusion and severe

Table 104-1. Possible Combinations of True and Apparent Leg Lengths and Their Causes

Combination	Cause
TLL and ALL equal	Limb length is equal, pelvis is balanced
TLL and ALL unequal same amount	Limb length is unequal, pelvis is balanced
TLL equal and ALL unequal	Pelvic obliquity exists
TLL unequal and ALL equal	Limb length inequality and compensatory pelvic obliquity are present

ALL, Apparent leg lengths; *TLL,* true leg lengths.

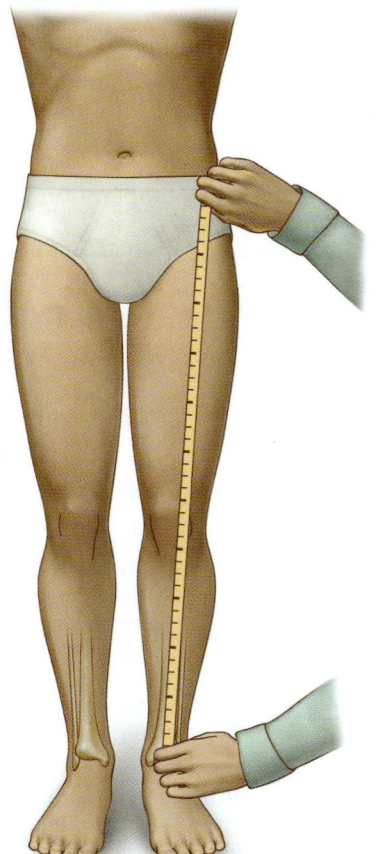
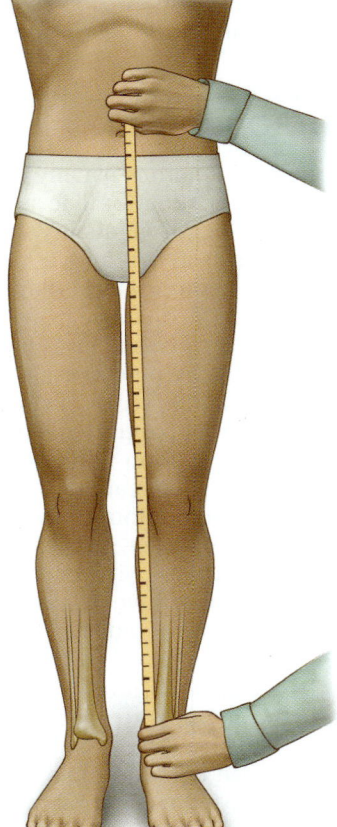

Figure 104-1. Direct tape measurement to assess leg length. **A,** True leg lengths. **B,** Apparent leg lengths.

A

B

lumbar degenerative scoliosis, as well as previous pelvic fracture. The surgeon can inspect and palpate the spinal curvature and the pelvic tilt; then the pelvis should be leveled by placing a series of blocks under the short leg until the spinal curvature and pelvic tilt disappear (Fig. 104-2). If the pelvic tilt corrects, then the pelvic obliquity is flexible; if not, the patient has a fixed pelvic obliquity and will be unable to compensate for any change in leg lengths. Regardless of whether the patient has a fixed or a flexible pelvic obliquity, the height of the block that the patient identifies as making him feel equal indicates the amount of length discrepancy that the surgeon can consider correcting.

Hanada and colleagues[21] studied the reliability and validity of measuring leg length inequality using the *iliac crest palpation and block correction method* in 34 healthy volunteers with simulated leg length inequality; they compared clinical observations with those obtained using standing anteroposterior (AP) pelvis radiographs. Iliac crest palpation underestimated the leg length discrepancy by a mean of 4 mm. Similar findings have been reported by other authors.[22]

Measuring Apparent Leg Length Inequality

When a patient has apparent leg length inequality, despite true leg lengths being equal, the patient feels that one limb is longer. Apparent leg lengths are measured from the umbilicus to the medial malleolus. Apparent leg length measurement takes into account contractures around the hip and lumbar spine pathology, both of which can lead to pelvic obliquity. An abduction contracture of the hip, which is common in the early postoperative period, results in an apparent leg length discrepancy on the involved side, but an adduction contracture of the hip has the opposite effect (Fig. 104-3).

Chronic lumbar spine pathology can produce a fixed pelvic obliquity. Adding blocks underneath the lower extremity in a patient with fixed pelvic obliquity will not level the pelvis and spinal curvature. If a fixed obliquity is recognized preoperatively, the patient can be educated that hip replacement surgery may not equalize an apparent leg length inequality.

Radiographic Assessment. Radiographs may be used to confirm clinical measurements. Radiographic evaluation can include the following:
1. Assessment of leg length inequality on radiographs.
2. Preoperative templating.

Techniques for assessing leg length inequality using radiographs are described in the following section.

AP pelvis radiograph. A low-centered AP radiograph of the pelvis with both femurs in 10 degrees of internal rotation along with a true lateral of the hip is

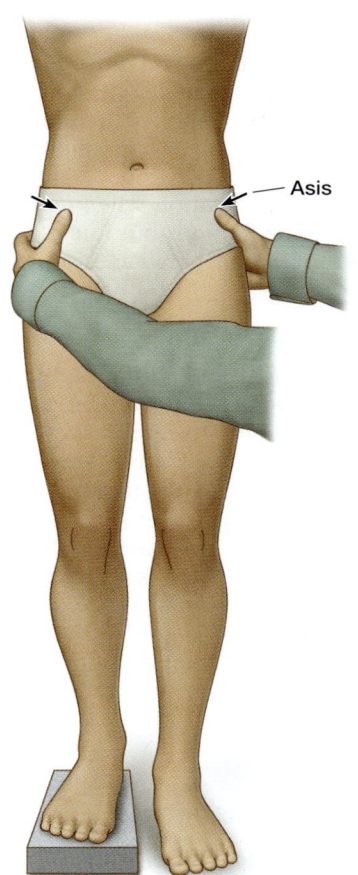

Figure 104-2. Indirect clinical method (block test) used to assess leg length inequality.

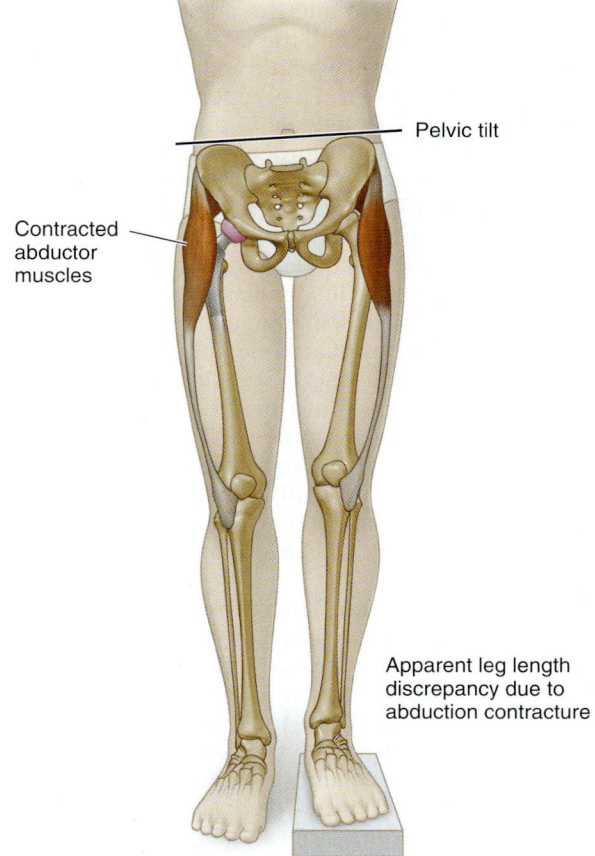

Figure 104-3. An example of apparent leg length inequality due to abduction contracture.

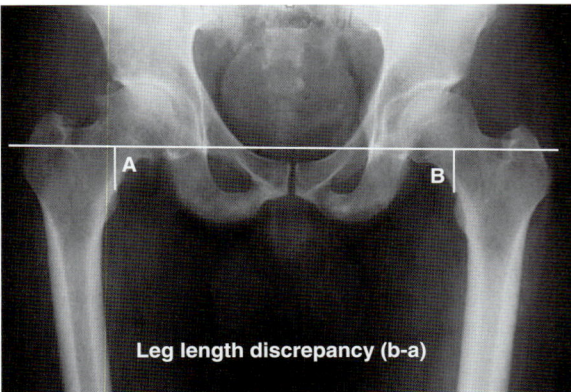

Figure 104-4. Radiographic assessment of leg length inequality using the Woolson technique.

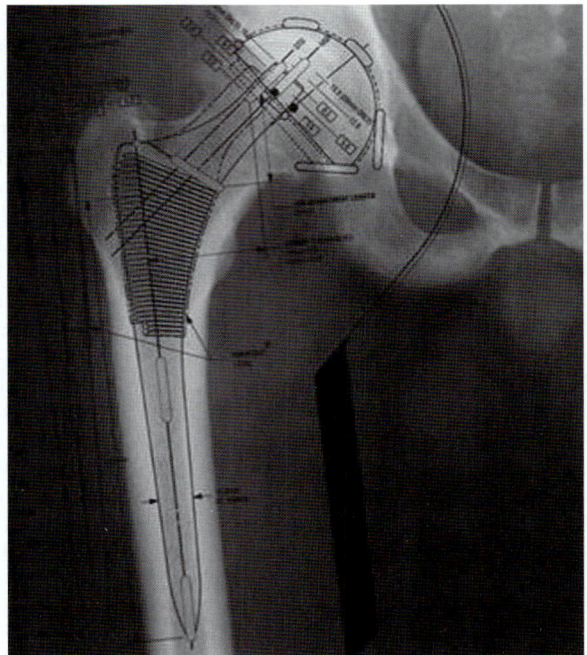

Figure 104-5. Radiograph of anteroposterior (AP) pelvis with superimposed templates. The vertical distance between the planned center of rotation of the acetabular component and the center of the femoral head constitutes the distance by which leg lengths will be adjusted.

optimal for templating. According to Woolson and colleagues,[23] transverse lines are drawn across a pelvic reference point (typically the bottom of the obturator foramen) and a femoral reference point (typically the top of the lesser trochanter). A line is then drawn from each femoral reference point to the perpendicular intersection with the pelvic reference line. This distance between the two reference points is taken as an index of preoperative and postoperative leg length (Fig. 104-4).

Konvyes and coworkers[7] used the inferior margin of the acetabular teardrop and the most prominent point of the lesser trochanter and the center of rotation of the femoral head as reference points and then measured the distances between them. They reported this method of determining leg length inequality due to hip abnormality to be as reliable as orthoroentgenograms and reproducible with a measurement error of ±1 mm.

Full Limb Standing Radiographs. Full limb radiographs are another method used to measure leg lengths. This method helps the surgeon to identify other potential causes of leg length inequality such as prior trauma affecting epiphyseal growth or malunited fractures. Sabharwal and Kumar[24] evaluated the limb length obtained with the use of a full-length standing anteroposterior radiograph of the lower extremities and compared it with lengths obtained with the use of plain radiograph scanograms on 111 patients. Measurement of limb length inequality on a standing anteroposterior radiograph was very similar to that on a scanogram, especially in the absence of substantial mechanical axis deviation.[24]

Beattie and colleagues,[20] in a prospective study, used a plain radiograph scanogram as the gold standard in 19 patients to compare the variability of measurements of true leg lengths performed with a tape measure. The mean value obtained from the two clinical measurements correlated better with the radiographic measurement of leg length inequality than with those obtained during the first and second clinical assessments. The authors concluded that the surgeon should not rely solely on clinical assessment of leg length inequality and encouraged using the average value of two separate measurements when obtaining a tape measurement. In

another study, Cleveland and coworkers[25] compared tape measurements of leg length discrepancy (measured from the anterior-superior iliac spine) of 10 standing patients with standing and supine radiographs. They reported a statistically significant difference and poor to moderate correlation when comparing clinical and radiographic techniques but found no difference in measurements obtained between sitting and standing radiographs.

Preoperative Templating

Based on the clinical and radiographic evaluation, a preoperative plan is determined. One of the main aims of femoral templating is to restore both femoral offset and leg lengths, and preoperative templating should be done to identify the level of the femoral neck osteotomy, neck length, and femoral offset (Fig. 104-5). A low neck cut is typically required in patients with a varus neck shaft angle. A higher neck cut is typically required when the neck shaft angle is valgus, and when lengthening of a short lower extremity is desired. It is important to re-establish hip biomechanics and to minimize leg length inequality. Increased femoral neck offset options allow more accurate soft tissue tensioning without lengthening the leg.

Intraoperative Assessment

Based on preoperative templating, the surgeon can measure the level of the femoral neck osteotomy from the top of the lesser trochanter and can use a trial femoral component with an appropriate amount of

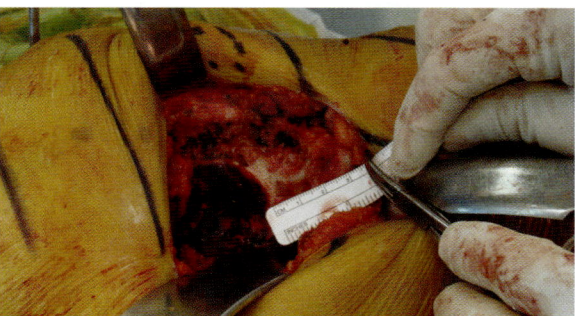

Figure 104-6. Intraoperative photograph of the measurement from the lesser trochanter to the level of the neck osteotomy.

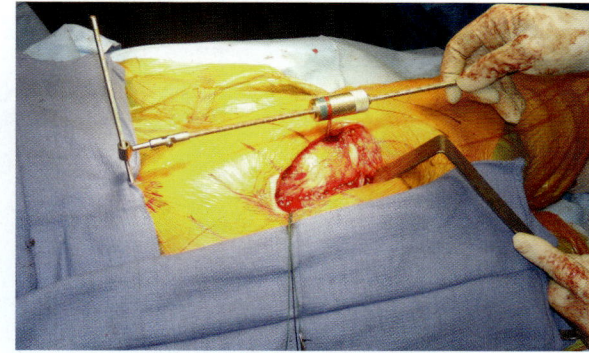

Figure 104-7. Intraoperative photograph showing the use of a leg length caliper for leg length measurement.

offset, combined with a trial femoral head of an appropriate diameter and length as one method to confirm the height of the femoral neck osteotomy.

Before draping of the lower extremity, bony landmarks of the lower extremity and the relative position of the feet and knees can be determined in the lateral decubitus position. After the trial reduction is performed, the surgeon should reassess the relationships of these bony landmarks (feet and knees).

Another method used to intraoperatively assess leg length inequality is to measure the distance between the center of the trial femoral head and the lesser trochanter with a ruler (Fig. 104-6), then select the head in which the measured distance is closest to the distance computed by preoperative templating. Matsuda and colleagues[26] studied 45 cementless hips and compared outcomes with those of a historic control group (47 hips). They calculated the distance between the center of the modular head and the lesser trochanter on a preoperative AP radiograph. During surgery, they measured the lesser trochanter–to–center of femoral head distance and selected the head and neck length that was close to the planned neck length. In the control group, they selected a modular head based on preoperative planning alone. The study group had a smaller mean postoperative limb length discrepancy (2 mm [standard deviation {SD}, 2]) as compared with controls (7 mm [SD, 4]). Gonzalez and associates[27] reported outcomes after cemented and hybrid THAs using the lesser trochanter–to–center of femoral head distance. Their postoperative leg length discrepancy was within 5 mm in 90 of 103 hips.

The intraoperative use of leg length calipers for leg length measurement has also been described. These methods rely on measurement of the distance between fixed points in the femur and in the pelvis. A variety of measuring calipers are available; these articulate with a pin that is placed in the iliac crest and with a stylus with a pointer that slides down to a fixed bony point on the greater trochanter (Fig. 104-7). The change in distance from before dislocation to after trial reduction is the amount of lengthening achieved.

McGee and Scott[28] described using a guide wire in the ilium and then bending the guide wire to act as a pointer to the femur. Mihalko[29] described the use of a

unicortical screw with a screw driver placed proximally in the superior acetabulum and a cautery mark on the vastus tubercle in the greater trochanter. Bose and coworkers[30] reported the use of a leg length caliper in 117 surgeries. They found that the leg was lengthened by more than 12 mm in 5% of hips, compared with 31% of hips in which lengthening was achieved without use of the caliper. All authors emphasize that the relative position of the lower legs should be the same before dislocation and after trial reduction.

Woolson and Harris[31] described a technique of measuring the head and neck removed after femoral neck osteotomy with a caliper and comparing this measurement with the replaced femoral head and neck length. Woolson[32] used this technique of leg length equalization, and the length of the modular femoral head neck was chosen preoperatively, rather than using soft tissue tension across the prosthetic hip joint to determine whether leg lengths were equal. Postoperative leg lengths were determined radiographically in a consecutive series of 351 patients (408 hips). Ninety-seven percent of patients had a postoperative leg length discrepancy of less than 1 cm. The mean discrepancy for these 351 patients was 1 mm. One can also use the relationship of the tip of the greater trochanter with respect to the center of the femoral head, before and after femoral neck osteotomy, to assess restoration of leg length (Fig. 104-8).

The "Shuck test" described by Charnley[1] is affected by various factors and is unreliable for limb length measurement. If the hip seems too lax, this may be the result of soft tissue releases performed during surgery or of muscle relaxation following anesthesia, and it may not reflect leg length inequality.

Most hip surgeons in practice today utilize a combination of methods previously discussed, including preoperative templating, intraoperative palpation, and measurements to minimize leg length inequality. Accurate preoperative templating, appropriate component selection and positioning, and intraoperative diligence in restoring hip anatomy can minimize the chance of leg length inequality. It is important for the patient to understand that a hip replacement does not possess all of the soft tissue restraints that provide stability to a normal hip. Therefore, in some cases, a moderate

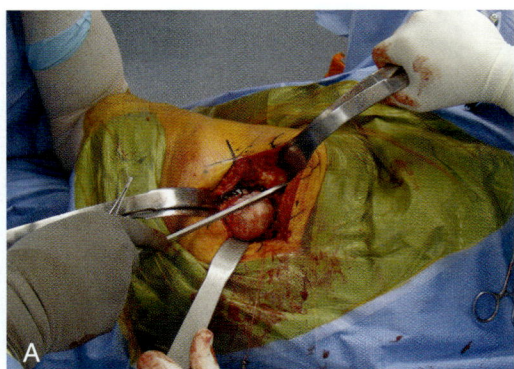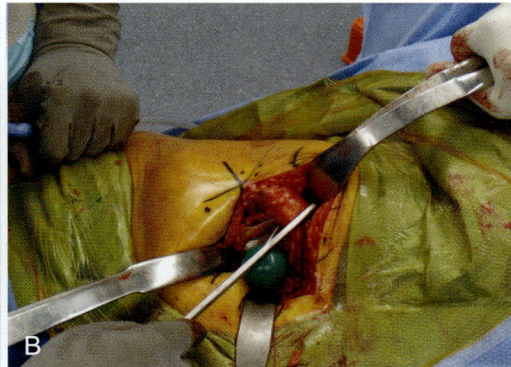

Figure 104-8. Measuring the distance from the center of the femoral head to the tip of the greater trochanter. **A,** Measurement with the native femoral head. **B,** Measurement with the prosthetic femoral head.

amount of limb lengthening may be necessary at the time of total hip arthroplasty to provide optimal hip stability.

LEG LENGTH INEQUALITY FOLLOWING TOTAL HIP ARTHROPLASTY

When a patient is seen following total hip arthroplasty with complaints of leg length inequality, it is important to identify its cause. Physical examination can be used to determine if the leg length inequality is apparent/functional of actual/true.

Apparent Leg Length Inequality

Apparent or functional leg length inequality can be due to lumbosacral scoliosis, pelvic obliquity, periarticular muscular spasm, or a hip contracture that may improve with time. Ranawat and Rodriguez,[33] in their study of 100 consecutive total hip replacement (THR) patients, mentioned that functional limb length inequality resolved in all but 0.5% of their patients by 6 months postoperatively.

Treatment of Apparent Leg Length Inequality

An apparent leg length inequality can be treated with physiotherapy in the form of stretching and abductor strengthening exercises. Most cases of apparent leg length inequality disappear after 3 to 6 months of appropriate physical therapy and rehabilitation. It generally takes 3 months for pelvic obliquity caused by mild abductor contracture to correct, and up to 1 year with severe contracture. The use of corticosteroid or botulinum toxin (Botox) injections[34] has been described in rare recalcitrant cases (corticosteroid into the iliopsoas, and Botox into contracted adductor muscles). With an abduction contracture, the patient feels that the operated leg is longer. Physical therapists should not be allowed to add a shoe lift on the contralateral side because this will perpetuate the pelvic obliquity. In a

Ranawat and Rodriguez[33] review of 100 patients, 14 had pelvic obliquity and apparent leg length inequality 1 month after total hip arthroplasty. At the end of 6 months of physical therapy, no patient complained of leg length inequality.

Preoperatively, the surgeon should inform the patient with fixed coronal plane pelvic obliquity secondary to a lumbosacral condition that surgery may not equalize an apparent leg length inequality. Attempting to achieve this could lead to significant lengthening or shortening of the true leg length. In rare cases of severe hip contracture around total hip arthroplasty, releasing tight tissues or lengthening contracted muscles can be considered.

True Leg Length Inequality

True leg length inequality can occur as a result of component positioning following total hip arthroplasty. The center of rotation of the acetabular component may be moved distally, or the length of the femoral neck and head may be increased over the native length.[35]

Risk Factors for True Leg Length Inequality

Developmental Conditions. It may be technically impossible or may risk neurovascular injury to completely equalize leg lengths when a large preoperative discrepancy is evident with a shorter operated than nonoperated leg. When the leg to be operated is longer than the other before surgery is begun, leg length equalization at surgery usually cannot be achieved without risking hip instability.

Revision Surgery With Soft Tissue Laxity. In revision operations, the soft tissues may be damaged and lax from previous procedures. The surgeon may be forced to use a femoral component with a long neck to more adequately tension slack soft tissues, which will lengthen the leg. An alternative is to use a femoral component with a larger lateral offset. A femoral component with a larger offset will increase soft tissue tension without as much lengthening.

Post-traumatic Conditions. Limb shortening is common with ununited or malunited fractures. In such cases, restoration of leg length at total hip arthroplasty is usually possible, but complete leg length equalization is not always feasible.

Treatment of True Leg Length Inequality After Total Hip Arthroplasty

Leg length inequality of less than 10 mm after total hip replacement often is tolerated because it causes little stretching of the soft tissues and minimal spinal deformity. Physiotherapy has a limited role in the management of true leg length inequality. The simplest treatment is the use of a heel or shoe lift placed on the side that feels short. Freiberg[36] reported on a series of more than 1000 cases and found that adding a shoe lift gave complete relief of symptoms. Occasionally, because of persistent pain, impaired function, and/or a gait disturbance, revision surgery may be considered.[35] Turula and associates[37] found that leg length discrepancy varied from −20 mm (shortened leg) to +15 mm (lengthened leg), with a mean of 2.8 mm. In a consecutive series of 100 patients, Ranawat and Rodriquez[38] demonstrated that the mean leg length discrepancy was 3.4 mm (range, −10 mm to +18 mm). Beard and coworkers[39] reported on 997 patients with primary THA, categorized into two main groups: the no–leg length discrepancy group (discrepancy <10 mm) and the leg length discrepancy group (discrepancy ≥10 mm). At 3 years, the leg length inequality group had a significantly worse Oxford hip score than the no–leg length inequality group ($P = .034$). No significant differences in revision ($P = .389$) or dislocation ($P = .220$) rates were noted between the two groups. Investigators concluded that a postoperative leg length discrepancy of 10 mm or more leads to poorer functional outcomes.

Identification and correction of component malposition that may have hampered stability as assessed intraoperatively at the time of the original reconstruction and restoration of appropriate offset may address the problem in highly selected circumstances where revision is undertaken. Depending on the root cause of leg lengthening, surgical treatment options may include acetabular component revision (to correct version or height), exchange of modular head and liner (including the use of elevated rim, face changing, offset, or constrained liners), or femoral component revision to correct version or to increase offset. Concomitant trochanteric advancement may be required to preserve abductor tension and avoid instability. In cases of instability, trochantric advancement or use of constrained liners may be considered.

Parvizi and coworkers[35] retrospectively reviewed the clinical and radiographic data of 21 patients who underwent revision surgery for symptomatic leg length inequality. Fifteen of the patients had revision of the socket alone, 3 patients had revision of the femur alone, and 3 had revision of both components. Thirteen of the revised acetabular components were felt to have excessive abduction or suboptimal version, and 6 sockets had inferior positioning. The femoral stem was revised secondary to proximal positioning or non anatomic offset in 6 cases. The mean Harris hip score improved significantly from 56.5 to 83.2 points ($P < .005$). All but two patients were satisfied with the outcome of the revision surgery.

STABILITY AND LEG LENGTH INEQUALITY

At times, the surgeon may need to lengthen the leg to obtain acceptable stability of the joint; this possibility should always be discussed with the patient preoperatively. Preoperative discussion with the patient about the risks of leg length inequality can go a long way toward defusing postoperative problems.[40] Discussion with the patient regarding the possibility of not achieving perfectly equal leg lengths particularly in cases of fixed spinal deformity, fixed pelvic obliquity, or intraoperative instability is important. Similarly, the surgeon should be careful to document a preoperative history of leg length inequality and to perform a physical examination that includes leg length measurement.

If intraoperative instability is encountered, the surgeon should look for any signs of impingement and should carefully check femoral and acetabular anteversion. In such situations an intraoperative radiograph may be helpful to confirm the position of the components or trials and if acceptable, the use of elevated rim or offset acetabular liners, as well as larger femoral head sizes or increased femoral offset components, can be considered to improve construct stability. In situations when all of these matters have been addressed, and when the hip joint is unstable, lengthening may be required to achieve stability. Therefore, surgeons should anticipate these problems and should discuss these issues with the patient preoperatively.

CONCLUSION

A thorough history and clinical examination is an important part of the evaluation. Apparent leg length inequality, if present, should be identified preoperatively, and the patient appropriately counseled that it may not be possible to achieve equal leg lengths. Careful preoperative assessment and planning, along with intraoperative attention to detail that optimizes the stability of the construct with measurement of leg lengths before and after trial reduction, can reduce the incidence and magnitude of this problem.

REFERENCES

1. Charnley J: Low friction arthroplasty of the hip: theory and practice, Berlin, 1979, Springer Verlag, pp 246.
2. Khanduja V, Tek V, Scott G: The effect of a neck-retaining femoral implant on leg-length inequality following total hip arthroplasty: a radiological study. J Bone Joint Surg Br 88:712–715, 2006.
3. Edeen J, Sharkey PF, Alexander AH: Clinical significance of leg-length inequality after total hip arthroplasty. Am J Orthop 24:347–351, 1995.
4. Ranawat CS, Rodriquez JA: Functional leg-length inequality following total hip arthroplasty. J Arthroplasty 2:359–364, 1997.
5. Austin MS, Hozack WJ, Sharkey PF: Stability and leg length equality in total hip arthroplasty. J Arthroplasty 18(3 Suppl 1):88–90, 2003.

6. Woolson ST: Leg length equalization during total hip replacement. Orthopedics 13:17–21, 1990.

7. Konyves A, Bannister GC: The importance of leg length discrepancy after total hip arthroplasty. J Bone Joint Surg Br 87:155–157, 2005.

8. Kutty S, Mulqueen D, McCabe JP, Curtin WA: Limb length discrepancy after total hip arthroplasty. J Bone Joint Surg Br 84(Suppl 1):4; 2002.

9. Sarangi PP, Bannister GC: Leg length discrepancy after total hip replacement. Hip 7:121–124, 1997.

10. Williamson JA, Reckling FW: Limb length discrepancy and related problems following total hip joint replacement. Clin Orthop Relat Res 134:135–138, 1978.

11. Turula KB, Friberg O, Lindholm TS, et al: Leg length inequality after total hip arthroplasty. Clin Orthop Relat Res 202:163–168, 1986.

12. Hoikka V, Santavirta S, Eskola A, et al: Methodology for restoring functional leg length in revision total hip arthroplasty. J Arthroplasty 6:189–193, 1991.

13. Lai KA, Lin CJ, Jou IM, Su FC: Gait analysis after total hip arthroplasty with leg length equalization in women with unilateral congenital complete dislocation of the hip: comparison with untreated patients. J Orthop Res 19:1147–1152, 2001.

14. Rosler J, Perka C: The effect of anatomical positional relationships on kinetic parameters after total hip replacement. Int Orthop 24:23–27, 2000.

15. Friberg O: Clinical symptoms and biomechanics of lumbar spine and hip joint in leg length inequality. Spine 8:643–651, 1983.

16. Giles LG, Taylor JR: Low-back pain associated with leg length inequality. Spine 6:510–521, 1981.

17. Hofmann AA, Skrzynski MC: Leg-length inequality and nerve palsy in total hip arthroplasty: a lawyer awaits! Orthopedics 23:943–944, 2000.

18. Woo RYG, Morrey BF: Dislocations after total hip arthroplasty. J Bone Joint Surg Am 64:1295–1306,1982.

19. Eichler J: Methodological errors in documenting leg length and leg length discrepancies. Orthopade 1:14–20, 1972.

20. Beattie P, Rothstein JM, Kopriva L: The clinical reliability of measuring leg length [Abstract]. Phys Ther 68:588, 1988.

21. Hanada ED, Kirby RL, Mitchell ML, Swuste JM: Measuring leg-length discrepancy by the iliac crest palpation and book correction method: reliability and validity. Arch Phys Med Rehabil 82:938–942, 2001.

22. Gross MT, Burns CB, Chapman SW, et al: Reliability and validity of rigid lift and pelvic leveling device method in assessing functional leg length inequality. J Orthop Sports Phys Ther 27:285–294, 1998.

23. Woolson ST, Hartford JM, Sawyer A: Results of a method of leg-length equalization for patients undergoing primary total hip replacement. J Arthroplasty 14:159–164, 1999.

24. Sabharwal S, Kumar A: Methods for assessing leg length discrepancy. Clin Orthop Relat Res 466:2910–2922, 2008.

25. Cleveland RH, Kushner DC, Ogden MC, et al: Determination of leg length discrepancy: a comparison of weight-bearing and supine imaging. Invest Radiol 23:301–304, 1988.

26. Matsuda K, Nakamura S, Matsushita T: A simple method to minimize limb-length discrepancy after hip arthroplasty. Acta Orthop 77:375–379, 2006.

27. Gonzalez Della Valle A, Slullitel G, Piccaluga F, Salvati EA: The precision and usefulness of preoperative planning for cemented and hybrid primary total hip arthroplasty. J Arthroplasty 20:51–58, 2005.

28. McGee JMJ, Scott JHS: A simple method of obtaining equal leg length in total hip arthroplasty. Clin Orthop Relat Res 194:269–270, 1985.

29. Mihalko WM, Phillips MJ, Krackow KA: Acute sciatic and femoral neuritis following total hip arthroplasty: a case report. J Bone Joint Surg Am 83:589–592, 2001.

30. Bose WJ: Accurate limb-length equalization during total hip arthroplasty. Orthopaedics 23:433–436, 2000.

31. Woolson ST, Harris WH: A method of intraoperative limb-length measurement in total hip arthroplasty. Clin Orthop Relat Res 194:207–210, 1985.

32. Woolson ST: Leg length equalization during total hip replacement. Orthopedics 13:17–21, 1990.

33. Ranawat CS, Rao RR, Rodriguez JA, Bhende HS: Correction of limb-length inequality during total hip arthroplasty. J Arthroplasty 16:715–720, 2001.

34. Bhave A, Mont M, Tennis S, et al: Functional problems and treatment solutions after total hip and knee joint arthroplasty. J Bone Joint Surg Am 87(Suppl 2):9–21, 2005.

35. Parvizi J, Sharkey PF, Bissett GA, et al: Surgical treatment of limb-length discrepancy following total hip arthroplasty. J Bone Joint Surg Am 85:2310–2317, 2003.

36. Friberg O: Clinical symptoms and biomechanics of lumbar spine and hip joint in leg length inequality. Spine 8:643–651, 1983.

37. Turula KB, Friberg O, Lindholm TS, et al: Leg length inequality after total hip arthroplasty. Clin Orthop Relat Res 202:163–168, 1986.

38. Ranawat CS, Rodriguez JA: Functional leg-length inequality following total hip arthroplasty. J Arthroplasty 12:359–364, 1997.

39. Beard DJ, Palan J, Andrew JG, et al: Incidence and effect of leg length discrepancy following total hip arthroplasty. Physiotherapy 94:91–96, 2008.

40. Nercessian OA: Intraoperative complications. In Steinberg ME, Garino JP, editors: Revision total hip arthroplasty, Philadelphia, 1999, Lippincott Williams & Wilkins, pp 109–120.

FURTHER READING

Clark CR, Huddleston HD, Schoch EP, 3rd, Thomas BJ: Leg-length discrepancy after total hip arthroplasty. J Am Acad Orthop Surg 14:38–45, 2006.

This article discusses the importance of preoperative assessment and patient preparation in managing leg lengths.

Konyves A, Bannister GC: The importance of leg length discrepancy after total hip arthroplasty. J Bone Joint Surg Br 87:155–157, 2005.

This article provides information on the effect of leg length discrepancy on a common hip rating scale, the Oxford score. It also corroborates the findings of other studies that the number of patients that perceive a leg length discrepancy after THR decreases significantly between 3 and 12 months.

Maloney WJ, Keeney JA: Leg length discrepancy after total hip arthroplasty. J Arthroplasty 19(4 Suppl 1):108–110, 2004.

This article discusses the importance of understanding soft tissue balance as it relates to true and apparent leg lengths.

CHAPTER 105

Neurovascular Injuries

Gregg R. Klein, Scott M. Sporer, and Andrew M. Michael

KEY POINTS

Neurologic Injuries
- Know inherent risks and special considerations for each patient to predict and avoid complications.
- Once inherent risks are known, take intraoperative steps to avoid injury to the nervous or vascular structures at risk.
- Early diagnosis is very important in postoperative nerve palsies. Know the correct physical examination technique used to diagnose nerve palsies, so treatment can commence.
- Once nerve palsy is discovered, know the proper postoperative workup to further delineate the mechanism of injury, so that steps can be taken to resolve the injury.
- Know which palsies can benefit from early surgical intervention and which can benefit from close monitoring. Know the prognosis for each specific injury so you can provide proper patient counseling.

NEUROLOGIC INJURIES

INTRODUCTION

Neurologic injury is an uncommon but devastating complication following total hip arthroplasty (THA) that can delay patient recovery and postoperative physical therapy and can reduce quality of life; it is a leading cause of litigation following THA. With any hip procedure, there will be risk to surrounding neurovascular structures; however, with careful preoperative planning, knowledge of additional risks involved with each individual patient, and meticulous surgical technique, these risks can be minimized. It is important to diagnose and treat neurologic injury early after it has occurred and to know the likely outcomes to facilitate counseling of patients for an optimal recovery.

Neurologic injury can occur in the central or the peripheral nervous system, and it can be acute or delayed. Central nervous system injury following THA is usually the result of a vascular injury and most often is attributed to fat embolism syndrome following manipulation of the femoral canal. Peripheral nervous injury is more common after THA and can occur from a variety of insults intraoperatively, including damage from a retractor, incorrectly placed hardware, limb lengthening, or direct injury. Delayed peripheral nervous injury can be caused by a hematoma, compressive dressings, or patient positioning.[1,2] The peripheral nerves most commonly injured following THA are the sciatic, femoral, superior gluteal, and obturator nerves.

EPIDEMIOLOGY AND RISK FACTORS

Peripheral Nerve Injury

Peripheral neurologic injury following primary total hip arthroplasty (THA) has been reported to have a prevalence that ranges from 0.1% (1 palsy in 1287 cases) to 1.9% (7 palsies in 360 cases).[2-4] The risk of nerve palsy following primary THA is increased if the indication for surgery is congenital hip dislocation or severe hip dysplasia, or if there is otherwise a need for a large degree of leg lengthening. Schmalzried and associates reviewed 3126 consecutive THAs and reported an overall rate of neurologic injury of 1.3% for diagnoses other than hip dysplasia, and 5.2% in patients receiving a primary THA for hip dysplasia (9 palsies in 172 cases).[1] In the same study, nerve injury following a revision THA was reported to be 3.2%; however, this number has been reported to be as high as 7.5% in other series (5 palsies in 66 revision cases).[2,5] Weber and colleagues performed preoperative and early postoperative electromyography (EMG) in 30 hips to determine the incidence of subclinical nerve injury following THA and found that the rate of asymptomatic injury may be as high as 70%.[6]

The nerves most frequently injured following THA are the sciatic, femoral, obturator, and superior gluteal nerves (Box 105-1). Peripheral nerve injuries generally occur in isolation; however, multiple nerve injuries can co-exist. Injury to the sciatic nerve remains the most common, accounting for up to 90% of all post-THA nerve palsies. The peroneal fibers of the sciatic nerve are affected in 94% to 99% of sciatic nerve injuries; up to 41% have tibial nerve involvement as well.[1,2] However, isolated tibial nerve injury is rare, accounting for between 0.5% and 2% of sciatic nerve injuries, and isolated peroneal nerve injury accounts for between 47% and 65% of sciatic nerve injuries. The peroneal nerve is at increased risk owing to a combination of factors, including the density of nerve fibers at the hip, the proximity of the peroneal distribution to retractors (it lies lateral), and susceptibility to tethering or compression.[7,8] Female sex, hip dysplasia, leg lengthening greater than 2.7 cm, revision surgery, a history of lumbar radiculopathy or peripheral neuropathy, excision of heterotopic bone, a deficient posterior wall, a posterior surgical approach, and the use of a cementless femoral implant increase the risk of sciatic nerve injury[1,9-11] (Box 105-2). Lumbar stenosis and radiculopathy are important preoperative risk factors for nerve palsies and should be identified preoperatively because they can exacerbate intraoperative nerve damage through a double-crush phenomenon when impingement to the affected nerve proximally leaves it susceptible to damage at the surgical site.[12] A history of lumbar spine disease should be noted in the preoperative visit because this may change the course or timing of treatment for postoperative nerve palsy.

The femoral nerve is the second most commonly injured nerve following THA, accounting for 13% of all peripheral nerve injuries (32 of 243 palsies).[2] The most common cause of acute injury is thought to be direct compression by aberrant placement of a retractor anterior to the acetabulum. Increased risks of femoral nerve palsy include an anterior surgical approach, deficient anterior acetabular bone, and a previously released or absent psoas tendon. Expanding hematomas are found in up to 11% of patients with diagnosed nerve palsy and are the most common cause of delayed femoral nerve palsy. Schmalzried found that simultaneous femoral and

sciatic nerve injury occurs together in 5.8% of nerve injuries.[2]

Superior gluteal nerve palsies may be increasing in prevalence owing to the use of a gluteal splitting approach for primary THA. The incidence of superior gluteal injury may be as high as 23% when a Hardinge approach is used.[13] The exact incidence of superior gluteal nerve dysfunction is difficult to assess because patients present with abductor weakness or a limp that is common in the early postoperative period following uncomplicated THA.

Obturator nerve injury is extremely rare and accounts for 1.6% of all nerve palsies (4 of 243 palsies) with a prevalence of 0.016% among all cases (4 of 24,469 hips).[2] Obturator nerve injury was probably more common when cemented acetabular components were routinely utilized, and cement that had extravasated into the obturator foramen was the main cause. Difficulty in diagnosis of this entity may contribute to its low reported incidence.

Central Nervous System Injury

Central nervous system injury is much less common than peripheral nervous system injury and is typically associated with fat embolism syndrome (FES). The incidence of FES following THA is not known, but it occurs in as many as 1% to 11% of the trauma population. Fat embolism syndrome is associated with femoral canal manipulation such as reaming, cementing, and implant impaction.[14] In addition to FES, ischemic stroke was noted to occur in 3.9% of patients within 1 year of hip arthroplasty (67 cerebrovascular accidents [CVAs] in 1606 patients) in one large study. Ischemic stroke is associated with a number of factors, including history of atrial fibrillation, hip fracture, and previous history of stroke.[15]

BOX 105-1.   EPIDEMIOLOGY OF NERVE INJURY FOLLOWING TOTAL HIP ARTHROPLASTY

Nerve injured (per all nerve palsies)	Mechanism of injury (per all nerve palsies)
• Peroneal (51.9%)	• Direct trauma (20%)
• Tibial (0.4%)	• Tension (20%)
• Sciatic (27.2%)	• Hematoma (11%)
• Femoral (13.2%)	• Dislocation (2%)
• Obturator (1.6%)	• Unknown (47%)
• Combined femoral and sciatic (5.8%)	**Total:** 260 patients
Total: 243 patients	

Data from Schmalzried TP, Noordin S, Amstutz HC: Update on nerve palsy associated with total hip replacement. Clin Orthop Relat Res 344:188–206, 1997.

PATHOPHYSIOLOGY

Peripheral Nerve Injury

The pathogenesis of neurologic damage following THA differs depending on the nervous structure injured and

---

BOX 105-2.   RISK FACTORS FOR NERVE INJURY FOLLOWING TOTAL HIP ARTHROPLASTY

Sciatic
- Cementless femoral implants
- Deficient posterior wall
- Excessive retraction
- Excision of heterotopic bone
- Female gender
- Hip dysplasia
- Lengthening of the extremity
- Nerve root compression/Lumbar spine disease
- Peripheral neuropathy
- Posterior surgical approach
- Revision surgery

Femoral
- Anterior surgical approach
- Deficient anterior acetabular wall
- Excessive retraction
- Previously released or absent psoas tendon

Superior Gluteal
- Excessive retraction
- Extension of incision >5 cm into gluteus medius
- Lateral surgical approach

Obturator
- Excessive retraction
- Use of cemented acetabular component

the degree of injury (see Box 105-2). Three fundamental degrees of peripheral nerve injury have been identified: neuropraxia, axonotmesis, and neurotmesis. Neuropraxia is defined as loss of conduction in an intact nerve with an intact epineurium and neural sheath. It is often caused by disruption of blood flow or compression to the nerve. Axonotmesis is defined as disrupted axons within an intact sheath. Neurotmesis is defined as disruption of both the axon and the neural sheath. Patients with neuropraxia and axonotmesis often will go on to full recovery, whereas neurotmesis will often lead to partial or no recovery of neural function. Recovery from neuropraxia occurs early, and recovery from the other two is delayed because they must first undergo Wallerian degeneration. Each nerve is susceptible during certain surgical approaches and techniques and has different inherent risk factors that increase the probability of injury. It is crucial for the operating surgeon to anticipate these risks and take the necessary steps to avoid complications and counsel the patient.

Sciatic nerve palsies are the most common nerve injury following THA, and the peroneal division is most commonly affected.[1,2] The likely mechanism of injury to this nerve varies according to the indication for THA, and whether it is a primary or revision procedure. Primary THA performed secondary to developmental dysplasia of the hip frequently results in limb lengthening and subsequent increased strain on the neurovascular structures. It has been conventionally believed that limb lengthening greater than 2.7 cm places the peroneal division at risk, and lengthening greater than 4.4 cm places the entire sciatic nerve at risk for injury.[11] Stretching the nerve just 8% has been shown to reduce the blood supply to the nerve, and 15% stretch causes complete loss of blood flow.[16,17] Stretching of 20% to 35% has been shown to cause functional nerve injury.[17]

Recent studies have shown that lengthening a congenitally shortened limb, as in developmental dysplasia of the hip (DDH), is associated with a higher risk of nerve palsy than a similar amount of lengthening in a patient with an acquired traumatic or degenerative hip who at one point had a limb and a nerve of normal length. This is most likely due to the development of a shortened sciatic nerve in the case of DDH, limiting the amount of leg lengthening that can be attained before excess tension is applied to the nerve.[2] The anatomic location of the peroneal nerve, as well as its microanatomic properties, leaves it more susceptible to injury than the tibial division.

The peroneal division of the sciatic nerve lies lateral to the tibial division, making it more vulnerable to deep retractors during a posterior approach that can damage it by direct compression or increased tension along the nerve. It also has a relatively high density of nerve to connective tissue when compared with the tibial division[2]; this increases its susceptibility to mechanical injury because of the paucity of connective tissue available to absorb these forces. Finally, the peroneal nerve is anatomically susceptible to tension forces owing to its relative tethering at the sciatic notch and the proximal fibula.

Retractor injury to the sciatic nerve can be reduced by placing the posterior acetabular retractor between the bone and the hip capsule to reduce compressive forces to the nerve. Direct trauma can occur with posteroinferior acetabular screw fixation or, rarely, owing to scalpel, suture, or electrocautery injury. A hematoma may result in delayed sciatic nerve palsy caused by excessive internal compression. Excessive external compression from dressings or stockings (particularly at the fibular head) may result in a delayed neurologic injury.

Injury to the femoral nerve is most common during an anterior or lateral approach to the hip.[4] Acetabular retractors must be placed with care owing to the proximity and the sparse protection of the femoral nerve by the tendinous insertion of the iliopsoas. Special attention should be paid to avoid extracapsular or inferior placement of the anterior retractor because this aberrant positioning increases the risk of femoral nerve injury (Fig. 105-1). A deficient or released iliopsoas muscle can predispose the patient to femoral nerve injury through this mechanism. Anteroinferior acetabular screw placement can lead to direct trauma to the femoral nerve as well. Acetabular screws should be placed in the posterosuperior quadrant whenever possible, as described by Wasielewski and colleagues, to prevent nerve impingent secondary to hardware placement (Fig. 105-2).[18] Delayed femoral nerve palsy is often attributed to compression from an expanding hematoma.

Obturator nerve injury is rare and difficult to diagnose. The most common reported cause of injury to this nerve is extravasation of cement through the obturator foramen. Other reported cases of obturator nerve palsy have cited excessive retraction and trauma from acetabular hardware such as anteroinferior screws and acetabular reinforcement rings.[19]

The superior gluteal nerve is susceptible to injury during a lateral approach to the hip, as described by Hardinge.[13] This nerve is at risk for direct trauma when excisions are extended farther than 5 cm into the gluteus medius superior to the greater trochanter (Fig. 105-3). Cadaver studies have shown that the inferior branch of the superior gluteal nerve may be vulnerable to injury as close as 3 cm superior to the greater trochanter.[13] The probability of damaging the superior gluteal nerve in a lateral approach is also increased with excessive retraction. Manual retraction has been shown to be safer than use of a self-retaining retractor.[13,20] The cause of superior gluteal nerve injury is often confounded by normal postoperative abductor weakness, which frequently leads to a delayed diagnosis.

Central Nervous System Injury

Central nervous system injury following THA is most often attributed to fat embolism syndrome. Fat embolism syndrome is caused by embolic fat globules from the bone marrow that travel to the lungs; this can lead to pulmonary failure and acute respiratory distress syndrome (ARDS). Paradoxical emboli are venous thrombi that travel through a patent cardiac septal defect and

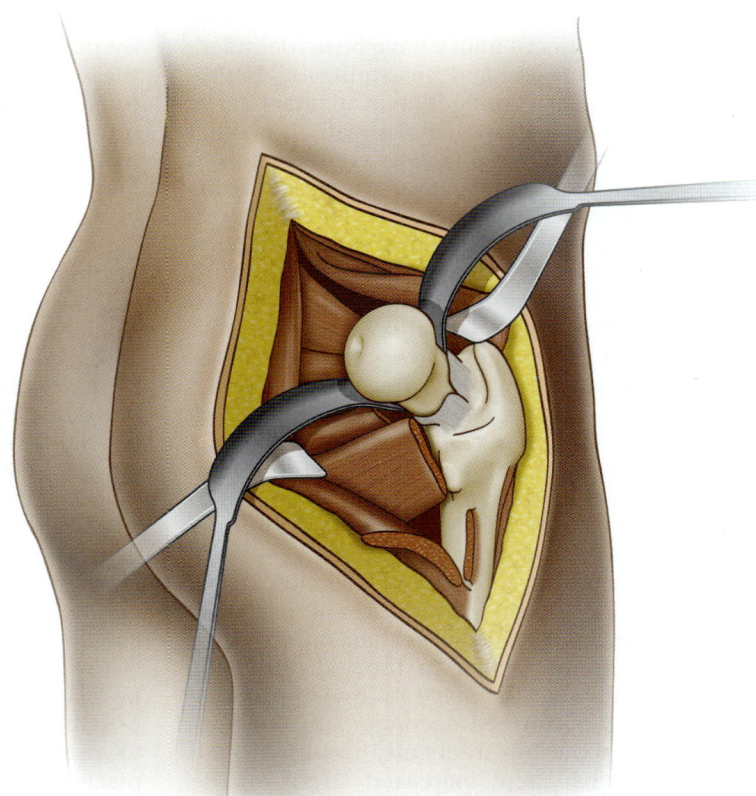

Figure 105-1. Correct acetabular retractor placement: Both anterior and posterior retractors are intracapsular. The anterior retractor is at the 1 o'clock position, and the posterior retractor is at the 7 o'clock position.

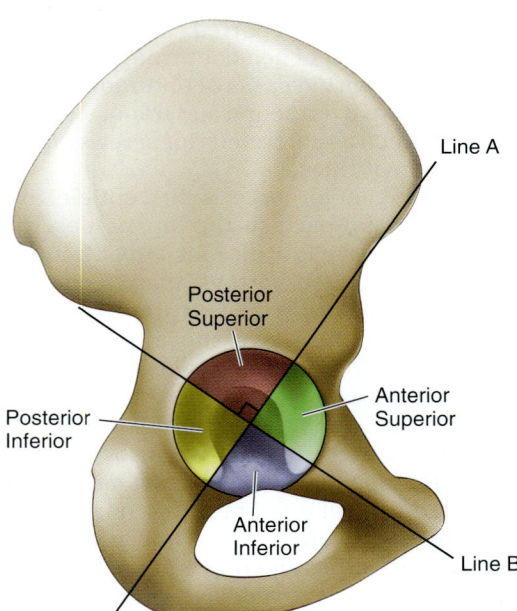

Figure 105-2. Quadrant system for safe placement of acetabular screws. The acetabular quadrant system can be used to identify the "safe zone" for screw fixation. Placing hardware in the posterior-superior quadrant minimizes neurovascular complications and is recommended for routine total hip arthroplasty (THA). *ASIS,* Anterosuperior iliac spine. *(From Wasielewski RC, Cooperstein LA, Kruger MP, Rubash HE: Acetabular anatomy and the transacetabular fixation of screws in total hip arthroplasty. J Bone Joint Surg Am 72:501–508, 1990.)*

cause a cerebrovascular accident.[21] In rare cases, the clot can travel elsewhere, blocking the blood supply to virtually any organ. It is associated most often with trauma but can occur after manipulation of the femoral canal in a THA, as in reaming, cementing, or implant impaction.[22] Increased intramedullary pressure on the femur is a common cause of this entity; care should be taken when manipulating the medullary canal, although no known specific technique has been shown to reduce the incidence of fat embolism.[14,22]

DIAGNOSIS

Peripheral Nerve Injury

Early clinical diagnosis is the key to successful treatment of neurologic injury following THA. A thorough physical examination must be performed, including testing of sensory and motor functions of all extremities and assessment of mental status during the preoperative visit. Preoperative radiographs can be helpful in estimating whether limb lengthening will be needed in the THA, prompting the surgeon to have a higher index of suspicion of nerve injury postoperatively. If excessive limb lengthening (greater than 2.7 cm) is anticipated, the operating surgeon must be prepared to take intraoperative measures to prevent nerve palsy.[11,17] Subtrochanteric shortening may be indicated if the operating

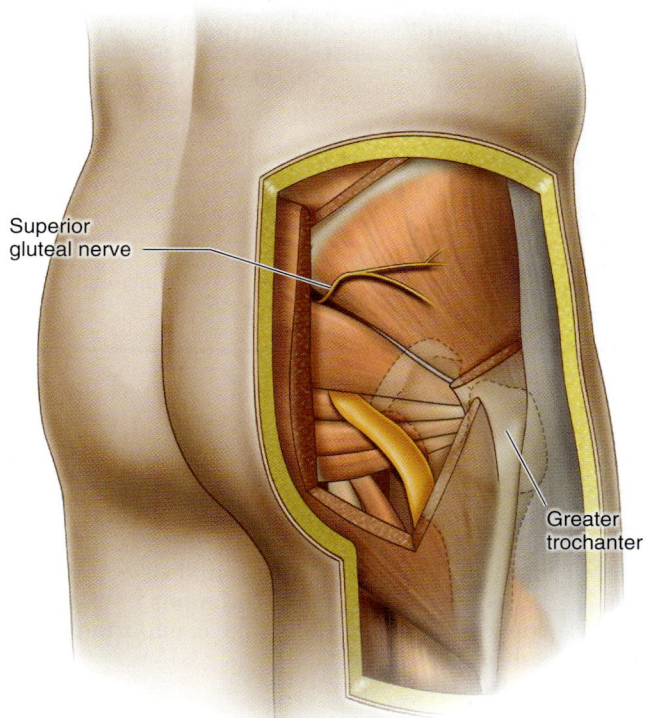

Superior gluteal nerve

Greater trochanter

Figure 105-3. The superior gluteal nerve is susceptible to injury on the lateral approach to the hip if the incision is extended more than 5 cm superior to the greater trochanter.

surgeon believes that tension on the sciatic nerve will be excessive, or if limb lengthening must exceed 2.7 cm to restore the native hip center. Patients who are at high risk for nerve palsies may be educated about the risks of the surgery to guide their postoperative expectations and recovery. Once the patient has recovered from anesthesia, a repeat thorough physical examination should be performed and clearly documented in the medical record. This allows the surgeon to immediately identify a change from the preoperative state and also provides a baseline for evolving neurologic injuries. Use of regional anesthesia may delay postoperative assessment of the operative limb; however, a complete physical examination should still be performed on all extremities in the immediate postoperative period, and again when the regional anesthesia has dissipated. The patient should be examined at least once a day for the remainder of the hospital stay and at follow-up visits to assess for delayed nerve injury. When nerve injury is diagnosed, the surgeon must assess for concomitant damage to other neurovascular structures and must evaluate the patient for a possible compartment syndrome.

Care should be taken to individually assess each nerve at risk when examining a patient (Table 105-1). Tibial and peroneal nerve distributions should be assessed individually when evaluating for sciatic nerve injury. The peroneal nerve can be assessed by placing the ankle in a neutral position and having the patient dorsiflex the ankle and extend the great toe. This must be done from a neutral position against resistance to minimize the confusion of ankle recoil from plantarflexion appearing as dorsiflexion. Patients may also be asked to evert the foot to test the superficial peroneal branch individually. Sensation in the peroneal nerve distribution can be assessed by testing light touch and sharp/dull differentiation to the dorsum of the foot, especially in the first dorsal web space. The tibial nerve can be assessed by once again placing the foot in a neutral position and asking the patient to plantarflex the ankle and flex the great toe. Sensation in the tibial nerve distribution can be tested through light touch and sharp dull differentiation on the plantar surface of the foot.

Femoral nerve function can be examined most accurately by evaluating for knee extensor mechanism weakness and decreased sensation at the anteromedial aspect of the thigh or medial calf. If femoral nerve palsy is found in the immediate postoperative phase, it is most likely a result of retractor injury; however, an expanding hematoma remains the most common cause for delayed femoral nerve palsy.[2] If a hematoma is suspected, serial hemoglobin levels and a coagulation panel should be collected, and the circumference of the upper thigh should be compared with the contralateral limb. Computed tomography (CT) scan or ultrasound may be useful in quantifying the size of the hematoma and in determining whether operative decompression is indicated.

Obturator nerve palsy following THA is difficult to diagnose owing to its rarity, its vague symptoms, and frequently a low index of suspicion. Patients who have consistent groin pain following hip surgery and a radiograph showing cement extravasation or inferior acetabular screws may be further evaluated. These patients may also have hip adductor weakness.

Table 105-1. Physical Examination Findings of Nerve Injury Following Total Hip Arthroplasty

Peripheral Nervous System Injury		Central Nervous System Injury
Sciatic • Inability to dorsiflex ankle (peroneal) • Inability to evert ankle (peroneal) • Numbness over first dorsal web space (peroneal) • Inability to plantarflex ankle (tibial) • Numbness over plantar surface of foot (tibial)	**Femoral** • Quadriceps weakness • Numbness over anteromedial thigh **Obturator** • Adductor weakness • Groin pain or numbness **Superior Gluteal** • Abductor weakness • Trendelenburg gait	**Pulmonary FES** • Respiratory distress • Low oxygen saturation • "ARDS-like picture" **Cerebral FES** • Altered mental state • Paralysis • "CVA-like picture" • Petechiae

ARDS, Adult respiratory distress syndrome; *CVA,* cerebrovascular accident; *FES,* fat embolism syndrome.

The diagnosis of superior gluteal nerve palsy is often confounded because of its similar presentation to normal postoperative limp or abducotr muscle avlusion. On physical examination, the patient will present with abductor weakness and a Trendelenburg gait. Suspicion should be high if these symptoms persist for more than three months postoperatively, particularly if a hardinge type approach to the hip was utilized. Electrophysiologic studies are helpful in confirming the diagnosis in any nerve palsy but are especially helpful when the diagnosis is unclear, as is often the case with obturator or superior gluteal nerve injury. Magnetic resonance imaging (MRI) with metal subtraction algorithms may have a role in differentiating between superior gluteal nerve palsy and abductor avulsion when the cause of the abductor weakness is unknown.

Central Nervous System Injury

Any pulmonary distress, change in mental status, or hemiplegia in a patient following THA should alert the physician to the possibility of FES, pulmonary embolus (PE), or CVA. FES is a clinical diagnosis, and the surgeon should maintain a high index of suspicion in a patient with hypoxemia, altered mental status, or cutaneous petechiae.[23] If the patient is in respiratory distress, initial testing should include a stat arterial blood gas on room air, a complete blood count, a chest x-ray, and an electrocardiogram. A high-resolution CT scan may reveal bilateral ground glass opacities consistent with FES, or it may identify a PE, pneumonia, or another cause of hypoxemia. In a patient with altered mental status, a diffusion-weighted MRI is the most sensitive imaging modality to detect cerebral FES, and a head CT scan is usually negative.[23] Paradoxical cerebral embolus can also occur and presents as an ischemic stroke. This has been described in orthopedic patients when lower extremity or pelvic thrombus passes through a patent foramen ovale and into the cerebral vasculature. If a stroke is suspected, the patient's cardiorespiratory status must be supported, and a neurologic examination should be performed. An emergent CT scan of the head should be ordered without contrast, and the hospital's stroke team activated. If the patient is identified to have had an ischemic stroke

following THA, consideration should be given to concomitant assessment for lower extremity thrombus and PE.[21] A transthoracic echocardiogram (TTE) can assist in diagnosis of a cardiac septal defect or in identification of a cardiac mural thrombus.[24,25] Determining the cause of the ischemic stroke is important in preventing subsequent infarcts.

TREATMENT

A treatment algorithm for neurologic injury is presented in Figure 105-4.

Peripheral Nerve Injuries

Prevention, early diagnosis, and understanding the cause of nerve palsy following THA are the main tenets for successful recovery. Preventing nerve damage requires the surgeon to know the risks of each procedure and to anticipate possible sources of complications in an effort to avoid them. The protective role of somatosensory evoked potentials (SSEPs) remains unclear. Currently, no clear clinical evidence suggests that SSEPs provide benefit in routine THA, although they may confer some benefit in reducing the incidence of nerve palsy in revision surgery, or in cases where significant limb lengthening may occur.[26] Currently, impracticality and cost limit the use of SSEPs for routine THA.

When a nerve injury is diagnosed, the surgeon must search for the inciting factor and must monitor the patient closely for evolving neurovascular complications, including compartment syndrome, because an abnormal neurologic examination in some cases may be the first sign of a compartment syndrome. The patient should immediately be placed in a position that minimizes tension on the affected nerve. When a sciatic nerve injury is encountered, the hip should be extended and the knee flexed (Fig. 105-5). Postoperative radiographs should be compared with preoperative radiographs to determine whether the procedure resulted in leg lengthening. Some studies have suggested that early femoral head exchange to shorten the extremity may result in resolution of symptoms if the palsy is thought to have occurred secondary to excessive limb lengthening.[27,28] Alternatively, subtrochanteric shortening may be used to reduce tension on the sciatic nerve. However, no outcome series are being performed at this time to study the efficacy of early use of this surgical technique in treating nerve palsies.

Mechanical causes of nerve palsy (such as an acetabular fixation screw) can be assessed by CT scan or a Judet view radiograph. The patient should be brought back to the operating room for surgical correction if the palsy is secondary to an identifiable mechanical cause. An expanding hematoma may cause delayed nerve palsy. In these patients, it is important to ensure that anticoagulation is at targeted postoperative levels. Surgical evacuation should be considered for an expanding hematoma with worsening neurologic symptoms once the patient's hemoglobin and coagulation levels have been corrected to desired levels. Decompression of the lumbar spine through laminectomy with partial medial facetectomy and foraminotomy may resolve postoperative symptoms when no identifiable cause for persistent nerve palsy is found in a patient with known lumbar spine disease.[12] This approach has been shown to be particularly effective in demonstrated severe spinal stenosis with persistent nerve injury following THA.

Patients should be closely monitored through serial neurologic checks and should be counseled about their injury to make the medical team aware of evolving neurologic deficits. An ankle-foot orthosis should be prescribed early following a peroneal nerve injury to keep the ankle in a neutral position. Keeping the foot in a neutral position will facilitate ambulation and minimize the chance of developing a plantarflexion contracture. Patients with significant sensory deficit in the sciatic nerve distribution should be counseled about ulcer prevention. Passive range of motion of the ankle by a physiotherapist will assist in preventing ankle stiffness and a plantarflexion contracture.

Electromyography (EMG) or nerve conduction studies (NCSs) may be helpful to further quantify the neurologic dysfunction if a residual deficit persists longer than 1 month postoperatively. Some patients may experience painful dysesthesias following a peripheral nerve injury and may be referred to a pain specialist when such symptoms are identified. Tricyclic antidepressants, gabapentin, or pregabalin may prevent the progression of these dysesthesias to complex regional pain syndrome, and sympathetic blocks may be indicated.

Observation and bracing are the treatment modalities of choice for femoral nerve palsy unless an identifiable cause is known. If the palsy is secondary to a known cause such as impingement from extruded cement, hardware, or an expanding hematoma, surgical intervention should be considered. Because most femoral nerve palsies are attributed to retraction during surgery, the surgeon may opt to observe the patient for recovery. If quadriceps weakness interferes with ambulation, a long leg drop lock brace or knee immobilizer can be beneficial until motor function returns. Obturator and superior gluteal nerve palsies can be treated by close observation unless mechanical impingement is observed. Reoperation in the event of mechanical impingement can help resolve the nerve palsy.

Central Nervous System Injury

Treatment for FES is mainly supportive and should be managed by a critical care specialist, or a neurologist in the case of cerebral FES. Management includes proper maintenance of adequate oxygenation, ventilation, and hydration, as well as pulse oximetry monitoring. Systemic steroids may reduce further inflammatory damage from FES and improve outcomes, but their use remains controversial.[29] Anticoagulation, antiplatelet agents, and thrombolytics are often used in the treatment of thromboembolism and paradoxical cerebral embolism, but these agents have no role in the prevention or treatment of FES. If thromboembolism and paradoxical cerebral embolism are found to be the cause of the patient's neurologic deficit, consideration should be given to therapeutic anticoagulation or to placement of an inferior vena caval filter, if anticoagulation is contraindicated. Treatment of FES, thromboembolism, and stroke may require the assistance of a specialist in internal medicine, critical care, pulmonology, or neurology, depending on the comfort level of the orthopedic surgeon in managing these diagnoses.

PROGNOSIS

The prognosis for individuals sustaining a nerve injury following THA varies by the mechanism and severity of the deficit. Schmalzried and coworkers found that 41% of all patients had complete or near-complete recovery of their deficit. An additional 44% had a continuous mild deficit, and 15% had functionally significant deficits that limited ambulation or presented with a persistent dysesthesia. Good outcomes occurred in most patients when partial motor function was regained within 2 weeks of surgery, and in patients with isolated sensory dysfunction.[2] Poor prognostic factors include increased distance from the site of injury to the end organ, a large zone of injury, and excessive scarring from previous surgery, altering the blood supply to the nerve.[7] Patient-related factors play a role in the prognosis of nerve injury as well. Increased age and comorbidities such as diabetes, spinal stenosis, alcoholism, smoking, and steroid use are all negative prognostic factors.[7] Although limb lengthening is a risk factor for developing nerve palsy, the extent of limb lengthening has not been shown to correlate with recovery. Some studies suggest that femoral nerve palsies may have a higher rate of recovery than sciatic nerve palsies of the same grade, yet the data remain unclear.[2]

CURRENT CONTROVERSIES AND FUTURE CONSIDERATIONS

• Although certain surgical approaches and procedures in THA have been shown to increase the incidence of neurologic injury, more data are needed on specific surgical techniques and intraoperative precautions

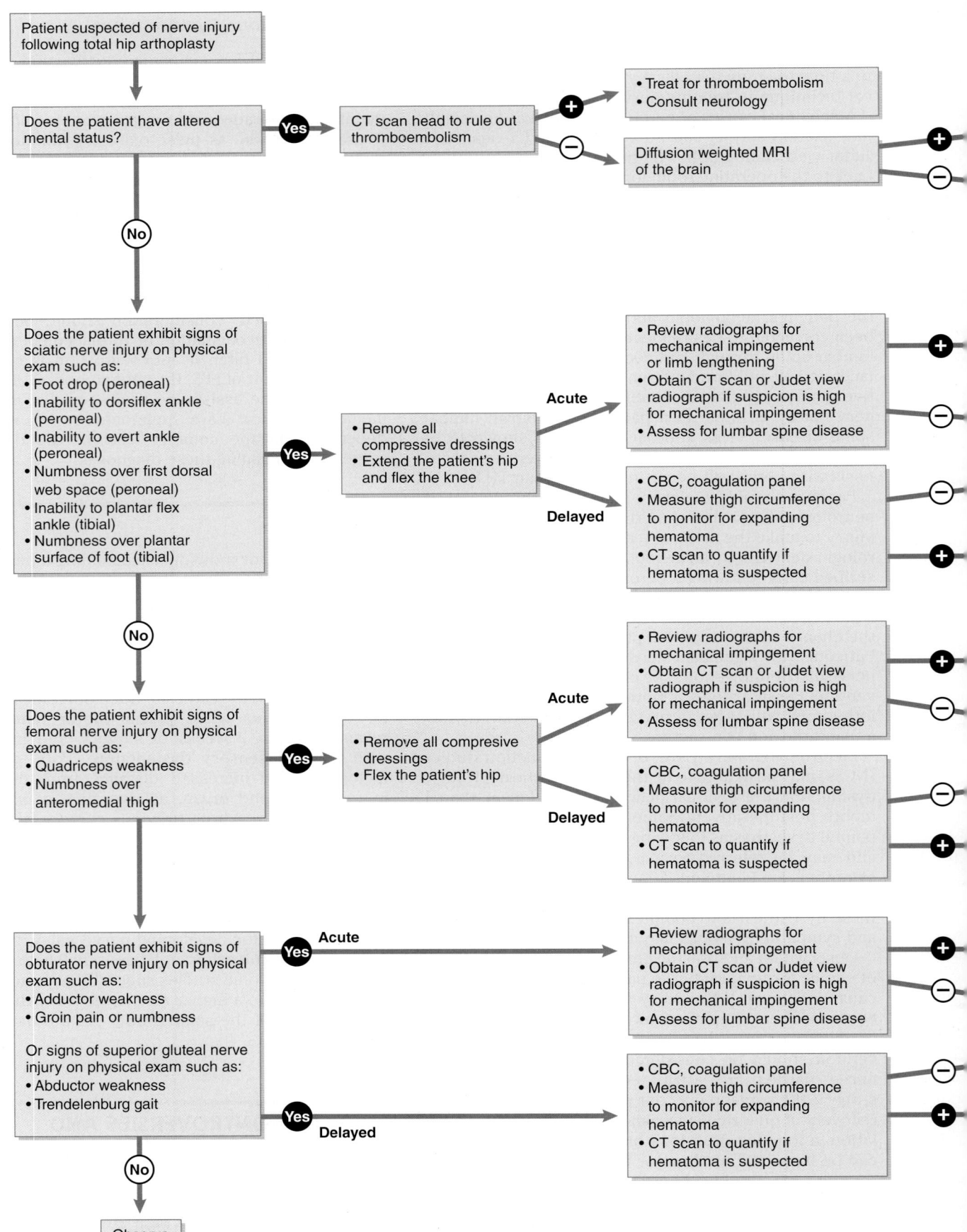

Figure 105-4. Treatment algorithm for suspected nerve injury following total hip arthroplasty.

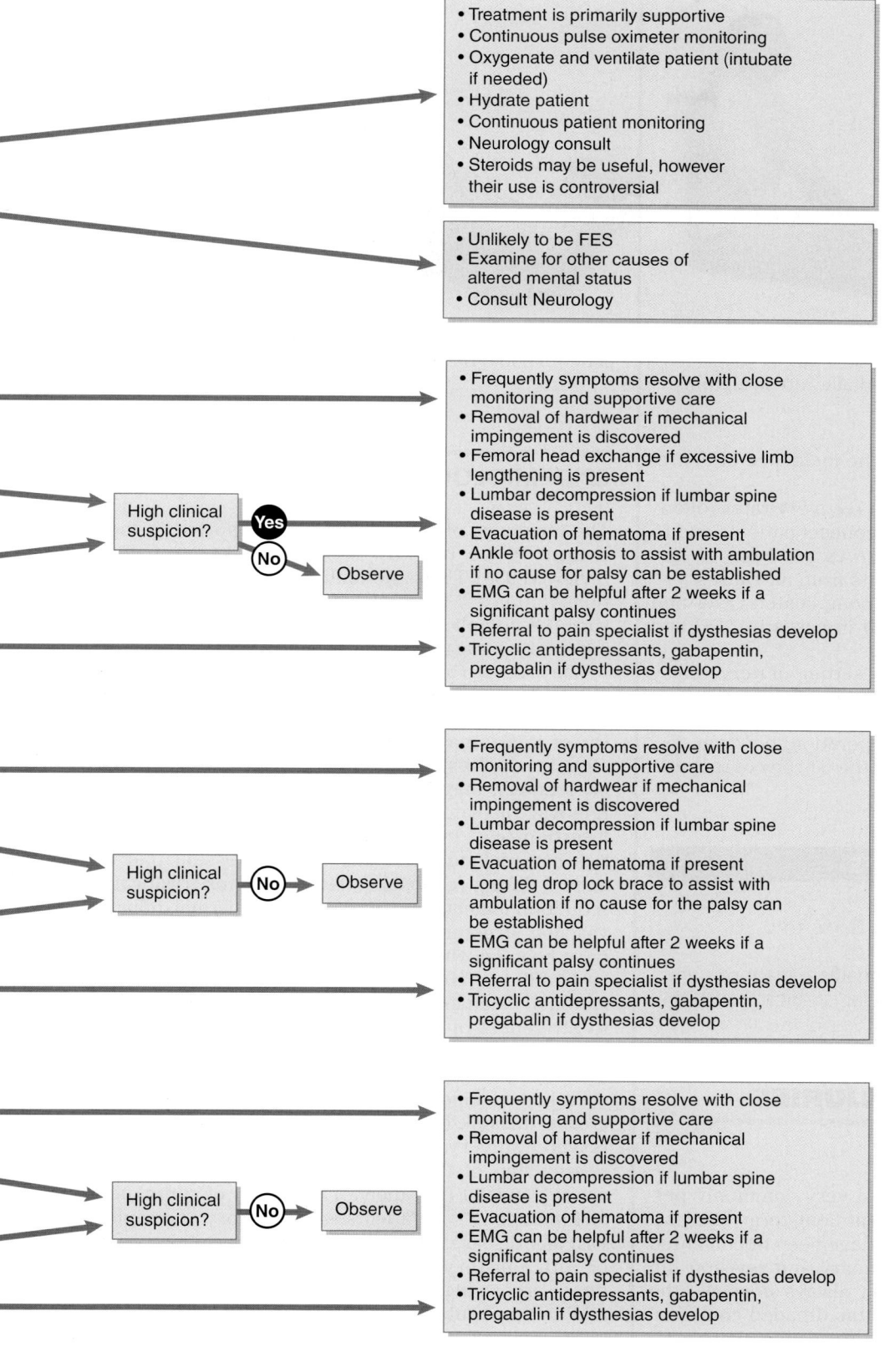

- Treatment is primarily supportive
- Continuous pulse oximeter monitoring
- Oxygenate and ventilate patient (intubate if needed)
- Hydrate patient
- Continuous patient monitoring
- Neurology consult
- Steroids may be useful, however their use is controversial

- Unlikely to be FES
- Examine for other causes of altered mental status
- Consult Neurology

High clinical suspicion? Yes / No → Observe

- Frequently symptoms resolve with close monitoring and supportive care
- Removal of hardwear if mechanical impingement is discovered
- Femoral head exchange if excessive limb lengthening is present
- Lumbar decompression if lumbar spine disease is present
- Evacuation of hematoma if present
- Ankle foot orthosis to assist with ambulation if no cause for palsy can be established
- EMG can be helpful after 2 weeks if a significant palsy continues
- Referral to pain specialist if dysthesias develop
- Tricyclic antidepressants, gabapentin, pregabalin if dysthesias develop

High clinical suspicion? No → Observe

- Frequently symptoms resolve with close monitoring and supportive care
- Removal of hardwear if mechanical impingement is discovered
- Lumbar decompression if lumbar spine disease is present
- Evacuation of hematoma if present
- Long leg drop lock brace to assist with ambulation if no cause for the palsy can be established
- EMG can be helpful after 2 weeks if a significant palsy continues
- Referral to pain specialist if dysthesias develop
- Tricyclic antidepressants, gabapentin, pregabalin if dysthesias develop

High clinical suspicion? No → Observe

- Frequently symptoms resolve with close monitoring and supportive care
- Removal of hardwear if mechanical impingement is discovered
- Lumbar decompression if lumbar spine disease is present
- Evacuation of hematoma if present
- EMG can be helpful after 2 weeks if a significant palsy continues
- Referral to pain specialist if dysthesias develop
- Tricyclic antidepressants, gabapentin, pregabalin if dysthesias develop

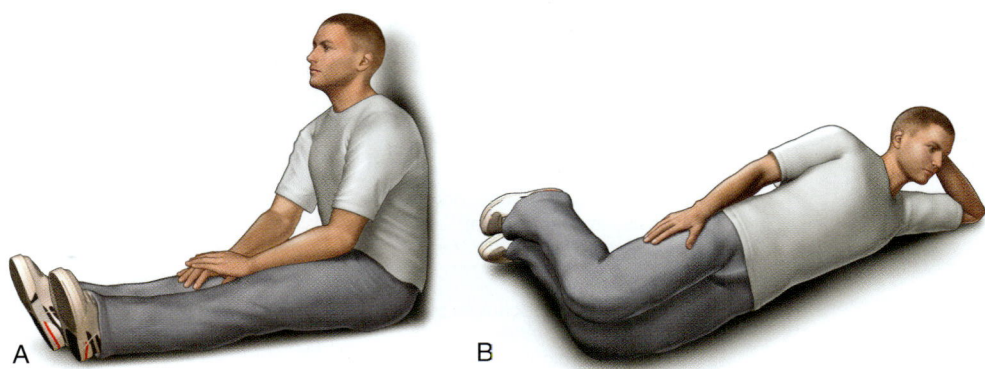

Figure 105-5. A, Placing the patient in an upright sitting position with the leg extended at the knee places tension along the sciatic nerve. **B,** If a sciatic nerve injury is suspected, the patient should be placed in hip extension and knee flexion to reduce sciatic nerve tension and alleviate symptoms.

that can significantly reduce the incidence of neurologic damage.

- Additional data are needed on recovery rates following neurologic injury, both to counsel patients and to determine whether certain nerves are more or less susceptible to long-term deficits from all causes.
- The role of SSEP is unclear in complicated cases and should be explored, especially in cases of DDH and extreme limb lengthening.
- The role of reoperation in the setting of nerve palsy is unclear, and its indications are blurred. Cement extrusion, misplaced hardware, and hematoma formation are indications for reoperation; however, few outcome data are available on the efficacy of reoperation in resolving nerve palsies.

KEY POINTS

Vascular Injuries
- Incidence of vascular injury is 0.1% to 0.3%.
- The best treatment is avoidance.
- If a vascular injury occurs, immediate diagnosis and treatment, including a vascular surgical consultation, are necessary.

VASCULAR INJURIES

INTRODUCTION

Total hip arthroplasty (THA) is a very commonly performed procedure with excellent long-term success. Unfortunately, vascular injuries have been documented during almost every part of primary and revision hip arthroplasty.[30] Although it is not always possible, the best treatment is prevention of this dreaded complication. Thorough knowledge of neurovascular anatomy is essential in minimizing risk to major neurovascular structures. Vascular structures may be injured by direct mechanisms (scalpel, osteotome, retractor, or acetabular reamer) or indirectly as the result of a stretching injury, particularly in patients with atherosclerosis.

EPIDEMIOLOGY AND RISK FACTORS

The incidence of vascular injury is reported in the literature to be between 0.1% and 0.3%.[31-34] Calligaro reviewed 9581 THAs and found acute arterial complications in 0.17%.[31] More recently, Parvizi reported a 0.1% vascular complication rate in 13,517 patients undergoing total joint arthroplasty.[33]

The first step in avoiding vascular injury is identifying patient- or procedure-specific risk factors. Surgical causes of vascular injury may be direct or indirect. Direct injury may result from use of a surgical instrument (scalpel, osteotome, drill bit, retractor, or acetabular reamer), may occur during component or cement removal, or may be noted in the course of component insertion (e.g., cement, screw, cable).[35,36] Indirect injuries can include stretching or compression that may occur during exposure, retraction, or dislocation/reduction maneuvers of the joint. Thermal injury to vascular structures can also occur. Even bulk allografts have been shown to potentially compress neurovascular bundles.[37] THA is a procedure that requires the application of mechanical forces to the joint, which may lead to stretching of the vessels. Complete elimination of force is not realistic or feasible, but force should be minimized.[33]

Patient-specific factors that have been shown to increase the risk of vascular injury include female sex, revision surgery, left-sided procedures (based on the relationship of the aortic bifurcation to the left iliac artery), medial (intrapelvic) migration of components, and infection.[34,38,39] Patients with a history of peripheral vascular disease, with absent or weak peripheral pulses, or with a history of bypass or revascularization procedures are at high risk for vascular complications. In addition, patients with a history of comorbidities (diabetes mellitus, coronary artery disease) that may predispose them to peripheral vascular disease may be at risk for vascular injury. Patients with diabetes or peripheral vascular disease often have calcification of the arterial vessels, which results in noncompliance and noncompressibility of these vessels and could ultimately result in an inaccurate or falsely normal Doppler study such as an ankle-brachial index.[40,41] These patients should undergo a preoperative workup by a vascular surgeon, which may include noninvasive studies (ultrasound or duplex scan) or possibly an arteriogram.

Patients with peripheral bypass grafts such as an aorto-bifemoral graft are particularly at risk for arterial injury. Limb positions such as rotation and adduction may put these grafts at risk.[42,43] Cameron has recommended trochanteric osteotomy in these patients to extreme limb positions.[42]

Components that have migrated medially into the pelvis may adhere to the iliac vessels, and forceful removal of these implants from a traditional lateral hip approach may tear adherent vessels. Intrapelvic cement poses a particularly difficult problem, especially if removal of all of the cement is necessary, as in the case of infection. If infection is not present, removal of all of the intrapelvic cement may not be needed, and removal should be limited to the retained cement that interferes with stability or bone ingrowth of the acetabular component. The timing of when the cement entered the pelvis is critical. Cement that migrated into the pelvis when wet during previous procedures and before its polymerization is more likely to adhere to vessels than cement that has migrated slowly over time, after the cement was fully polymerized.[22] Serial radiographs or an operative report can assist the surgeon before the revision arthroplasty is performed.

Intrapelvic migration of acetabular implants has been frequently associated with infection.[39,44] Infected tissue may adhere to medially migrated components, making removal more difficult and dangerous. This infected tissue usually is more friable and prone to shearing or tearing, especially if in the vicinity of a vascular structure. Wera and colleagues reported on two cases of deep infection and medial migration of the acetabular components, and recommended a preoperative consultation with a vascular surgeon because this combination represents high risk for vascular injury.[44]

If an intrapelvic acetabular component is being revised, contrast-enhanced CT or angiography may be helpful for identifying the relationships of vascular structures to the components being removed[45] (Fig. 105-6). If the components are adhered to neurovascular structures, an intrapelvic or retroperitoneal approach performed by a general or vascular surgeon may be necessary.[46-48]

Wasielewski[18] has described a quadrant system for placement of acetabular screws (see Fig. 105-1). The acetabulum is divided into anterior and posterior halves by a line drawn from the anterior iliac spine to bisect the acetabulum. Another line is drawn perpendicular to this line. The intersection of these two lines creates four quadrants. The safest zone is the posterosuperior quadrant. Screws 35 mm in length may be used in this quadrant because it contains the greatest bone depth. Screws longer than this may injure the sciatic nerve or the superior gluteal artery. The posteroinferior quadrant is the next safest zone. However, the thickness of bone in this quadrant is less, and screws longer than 25 mm

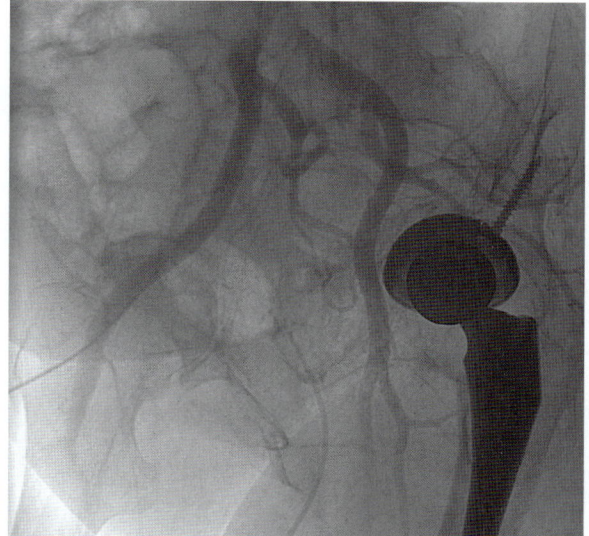

Figure 105-6. Angiogram of the hip showing the relationships of blood vessels to the acetabular hardware.

should be avoided. The inferior gluteal and internal pudendal vessels are at risk in this quadrant. The external iliac vessels are at risk in the anterosuperior quadrant, and the obturator vessels are at risk in the anteroinferior quadrant. If screws may be used in the anterior quadrants, unicortical fixation should be considered.

If a high hip center is used during THA, only the peripheral half of the posterior quadrant is safe for screw placement.[36] In a cadaveric study of acetabular reconstruction cages, Lavernia[49] has reported on a "safe zone" from screw locations and depths. The authors recommended screw sizes of 15 mm for the superior flange and 25 mm for the posterior rim.

PATHOPHYSIOLOGY/ANATOMY

All vascular structures in the vicinity of the hip joint are at risk during THA. These include the femoral, obturator, external iliac, common iliac, profunda femoris, and superior and inferior gluteal vessels.[34] The most commonly injured vessels are the external iliac and common femoral arteries.[38]

The external iliac vessels originate from the L5-S1 region and run down the medial border of the psoas muscle (Fig. 105-7). The psoas muscle runs between the anterior column of the acetabulum and the external iliac vessels. Injuries to the external iliac vessels have been described during most parts of a total hip procedure; thus vessel injury can occur at any time, from patient positioning to implant insertion. External iliac injury may be a direct result of retractor placement over the anterior column of the acetabulum because retractors placed too far medially over the anterior column may directly penetrate, stretch, or tear the vessel. It has been suggested that more proximal placement of the anterior retractor may be safer because

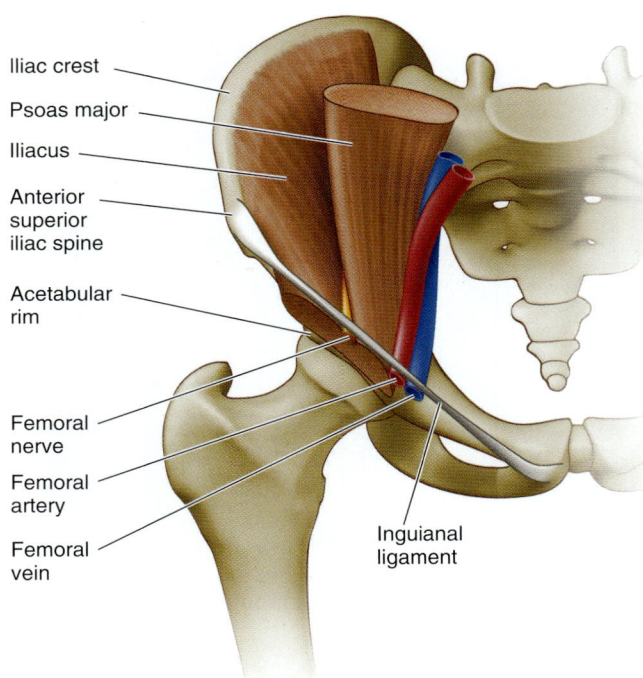

Figure 105-7. The course of the external iliac vessels runs along the medial border of the psoas muscle as they enter the lower limb.

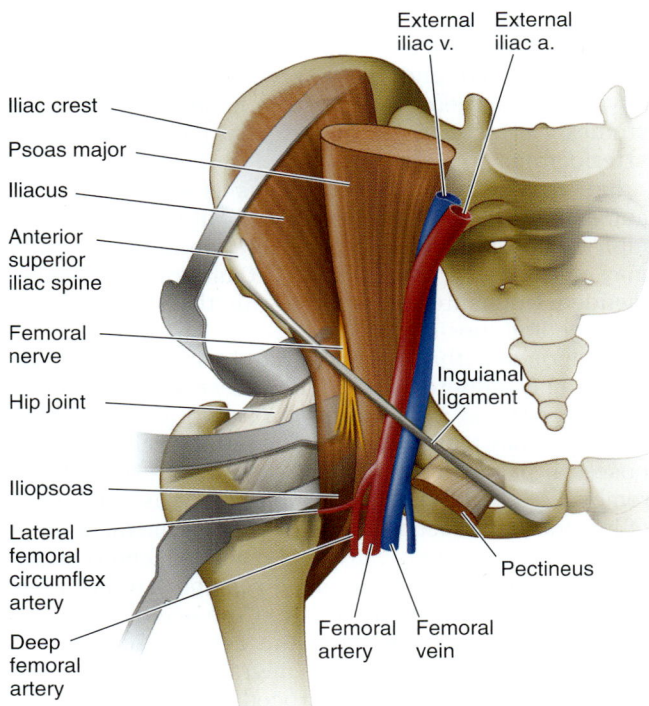

Figure 105-8. The common femoral vessels lie anterior and medial to the hip capsule. Retractors must be placed with care to avoid damage to the femoral vessels, particularly the artery that is lateral to the vein at the level of the acetabulum.

more muscle is present proximally than distally.[30] Iliac vessel injury has also been reported after reaming through the medial wall of the acetabulum.[38,50] Historically, cement intrusion into the pelvis has caused thermal injury to the iliac vessels; however, this is less commonly seen as the use of cemented acetabular components has decreased. More commonly seen today, aberrant screw placement in the anterosuperior quadrant places the iliac artery and vein at risk.[18]

After crossing the inguinal ligament, the external iliac vessels branch into the femoral vessels. The common femoral vessels lie anterior and medial to the hip capsule. At the level of the acetabulum, the artery is more lateral than the vein and is more susceptible to injury (Fig. 105-8). Injury to the common femoral vessels has been reported at multiple points during THA. A variety of hip positioners have been known to cause direct compression of the femoral vessels. Retractor placement too far medially over the anteroinferior acetabulum may directly or indirectly harm the common femoral vessels.[51] Direct injury may occur by placing the retractor tip too far anterior and/or medial, and indirect injury can be caused by levering the retractors, which can stretch or tear the vessel. Overly aggressive resection of anterior osteophytes or the anterior capsule places the femoral vessels at risk.[32] Femoral vessel injury from forceful dislocation and reduction maneuvers has been reported.[38] Although all surgical exposures have been implicated in femoral vessel injury, anterolateral approaches have been shown to have the highest rate of femoral vessel injury.[30]

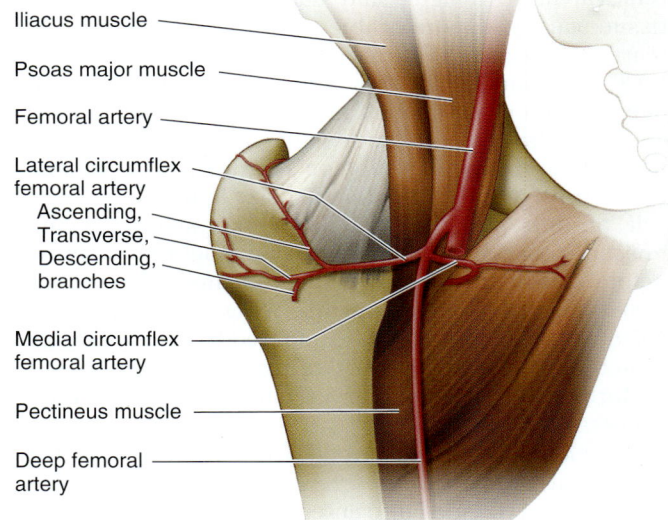

Figure 105-9. The medial and lateral circumflex arteries arise from the profunda femoris. Profunda femoris injury is rare but can occur with aberrant retractor placement.

The profundus femoris artery arises from the lateral aspect of the femoral artery 3.5 cm distal to the inguinal ligament (Fig. 105-9). The lateral circumflex artery then takes off from the lateral side of the profundus femoris artery and further subdivides into ascending and descending branches. The medical circumflex often comes from the profunda femoris artery and courses medially around the femur to the intertrochanteric region, and finally to the upper border of the quadratus femoris. Profunda femoris artery injury is relatively uncommon but has been reported after retractor placement too medially over the anteroinferior quadrant, causing injury to the medial circumflex vessel. Lateral circumflex injuries resulting from removal of a scar or capsule during revision procedures have been reported.[30,38,52] Damage to the medial and lateral circumflex vessels may occur with aberrant retractor placement around the femoral neck.

The obturator neurovascular bundle (Fig. 105-10) runs along the quadrilateral surface of the acetabulum, and the obturator internus muscle lies between the vessels and the anteroinferior bony acetabulum. Although less common, injury to these vessels may be the result of retractor placement under the transverse acetabular ligament or may be caused by screws placed in the anteroinferior quadrant of the acetabulum.[18]

The superior gluteal vessels are branches of the internal iliac artery and exit through the superior aspect of the sciatic notch (Fig. 105-11). They may be injured during posterior retractor placement or by screws placed into the sciatic notch. The inferior gluteal vessels branch from the internal iliac artery and are at risk when excessively long screws are placed in the posteroinferior quadrant.[18]

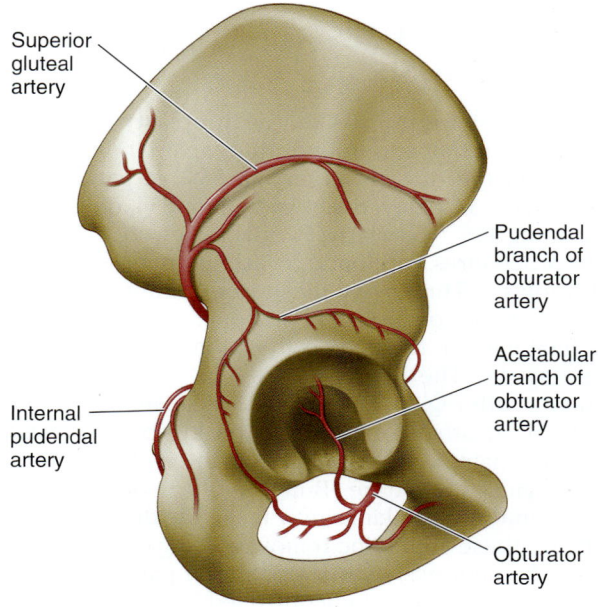

Figure 105-10. The obturator neurovascular bundle runs along the quadrilateral surface of the acetabulum, and the obturator internus muscle lies between the vessels and the anteroinferior bony acetabulum.

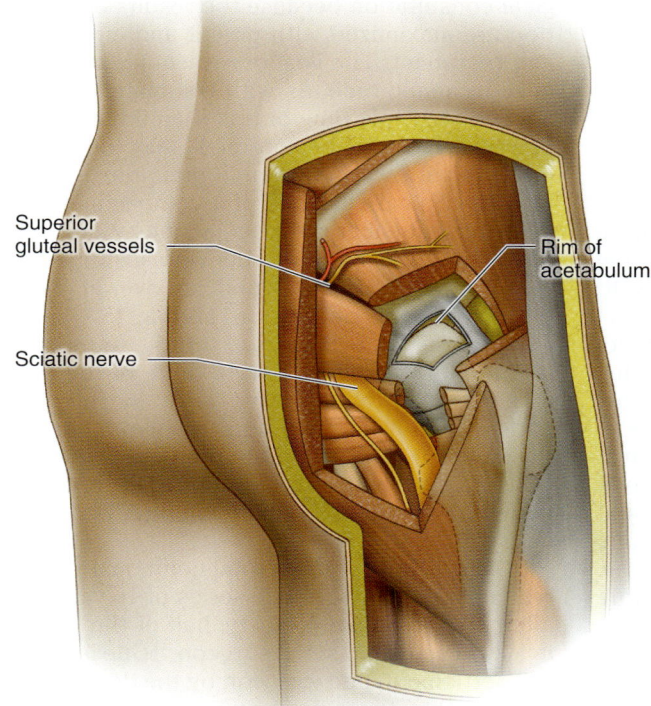

Figure 105-11. The superior gluteal vessels are shown exiting through the superior portion of the sciatic notch between the piriformis and the superior gemellus. These vessels can be injured through aberrant retractor placement or excessively long screw placement.

CLINICAL FEATURES AND DIAGNOSIS

Calligaro reviewed 23,199 knee arthroplasty procedures and 9581 THAs and found that arterial injury was diagnosed the day of surgery in 56% of patients, but diagnosis was delayed between 1 and 4 days in the remaining 44%.[31] Similarly, Parvizi reviewed 13,517 total joint procedures and found 5 vascular injuries after hip arthroplasty. Three were diagnosed intraoperatively, in 1 the diagnosis occurred on postoperative day 1, and in the final patient, the diagnosis was made on postoperative day 4.[33] The diagnosis may be delayed in some patients with regional anesthesia because the effects of epidural anesthesia can mask the symptoms of ischemic rest pain. In addition, pain is often attributable to the surgical procedure. Bulky surgical dressings and antithrombotic stockings may make the diagnosis more difficult; these should be removed if any concern arises about the neurovascular status of the patient. Vascular injury may manifest as uncontrolled bleeding, thrombosis, arteriovenous fistula, compartment syndrome, or false aneurysm formation.[34]

TREATMENT

A treatment algorithm for vascular injury is given in Figure 105-12.

The best treatment for vascular injury is prevention, especially when a revision procedure is anticipated. A thorough preoperative evaluation is necessary to identify the risk factors described earlier. Previous operative reports should be obtained to ascertain whether a previous vascular issue occurred. A preoperative consultation by a vascular surgeon is recommended if the patient has any of the previously described risk factors. Often noninvasive studies or angiograms, which may ultimately result in preoperative corrective procedures such as angioplasty, stenting, or bypass, may be needed.

Gentle surgical technique is desirable; however, the nature of the surgical procedure makes manipulation of the limb necessary. Forceful dislocation or reduction of the joint should be avoided. Retractors should be placed directly on bone with vigilance to avoid soft tissue interposition (which may contain a neurovascular structure). The anterior acetabular retractor should be placed with the hip flexed because this will relax the femoral neurovascular bundle. Assistants holding the retractors should be watched vigilantly by the surgeon to avoid overzealous retraction. Once the acetabulum is exposed, forceful removal of the components even if grossly loose should be avoided because this may result in shearing or tearing of friable tissue. The acetabulum should be reamed carefully to avoid penetration of the medial wall.[50] Careful screw insertion with a thorough understanding of the quadrant system and accurate measurement of screw lengths is essential.

In the event of intraoperative bleeding, an attempt should be made to identify the source of bleeding. Local control and hemostasis should be attempted, but if not possible, direct pressure should be applied to the area of bleeding. If the source of bleeding is not controllable or identifiable, the wound should be packed, and an emergent intraoperative vascular surgical consultation should be obtained. The hemodynamic status of the patient should be vigilantly monitored by the surgeon and the anesthesiologist. Fluid resuscitation, including packed red blood cells and relevant blood factors, should start immediately because a common error in revision surgery is to fall behind on blood and factor replacement.

If the vascular surgeon is unable to control bleeding from the surgical hip wound, the wound should be packed and provisionally closed so the patient can be positioned and prepared for a laparotomy and exposure of the iliac vessels or direct anterior exposure of the femoral vessels. Vessel repair, bypass, and/or embolization may be necessary. Once hemostasis is attained, the patient may be repositioned to continue the hip procedure, or this may be performed at a later time, when the patient is more stable. It is important to be aware that retroperitoneal or intrapelvic bleeding may not always be visualized. A sudden drop in blood pressure or tachycardia after a risky maneuver should alert the surgeon to a possible vascular injury. If suspected, an intraoperative vascular surgery consultation is imperative.

PROGNOSIS

The prognosis varies considerably in this patient population because vascular injury is rare and often occurs in patients with multiple comorbidities. The surgeon should have a low threshold to obtain a vascular surgical consultation because the results of this complication are maximized with urgent and efficient diagnosis and treatment. The goal of revascularization is to minimize ischemic time. As with traumatic vascular injury, a warm ischemic time of less than 6 hours is optimal.[53] Lower extremity fasciotomies may be necessary in patients with warm ischemia time longer than 6 hours or with clinical evidence of a compartment syndrome. The consequences of vascular injury are great. Shoenfeld reported on 68 patients who sustained a vascular injury after THA and found an overall 7% mortality in this patient population and a 15% incidence of amputation.[38] In Parvizi's series, four-compartment fasciotomy was performed in three of the five patients with vascular injury after THA. In this group, one patient died from multiorgan system failure related to the vascular injury, and another had wound complications related to the fasciotomy. The remaining three patients were not adversely affected by their vascular injury.[33]

Vascular injury after total joint arthroplasty often results in litigation. In one series of 16 vascular injuries after total joint arthroplasty, half of the cases resulted in a legal suit against the surgeon.[33] One lawsuit resulted in a settlement, one was won by the defendant, one was dismissed by the judge, and the others are still pending at the time of publication.

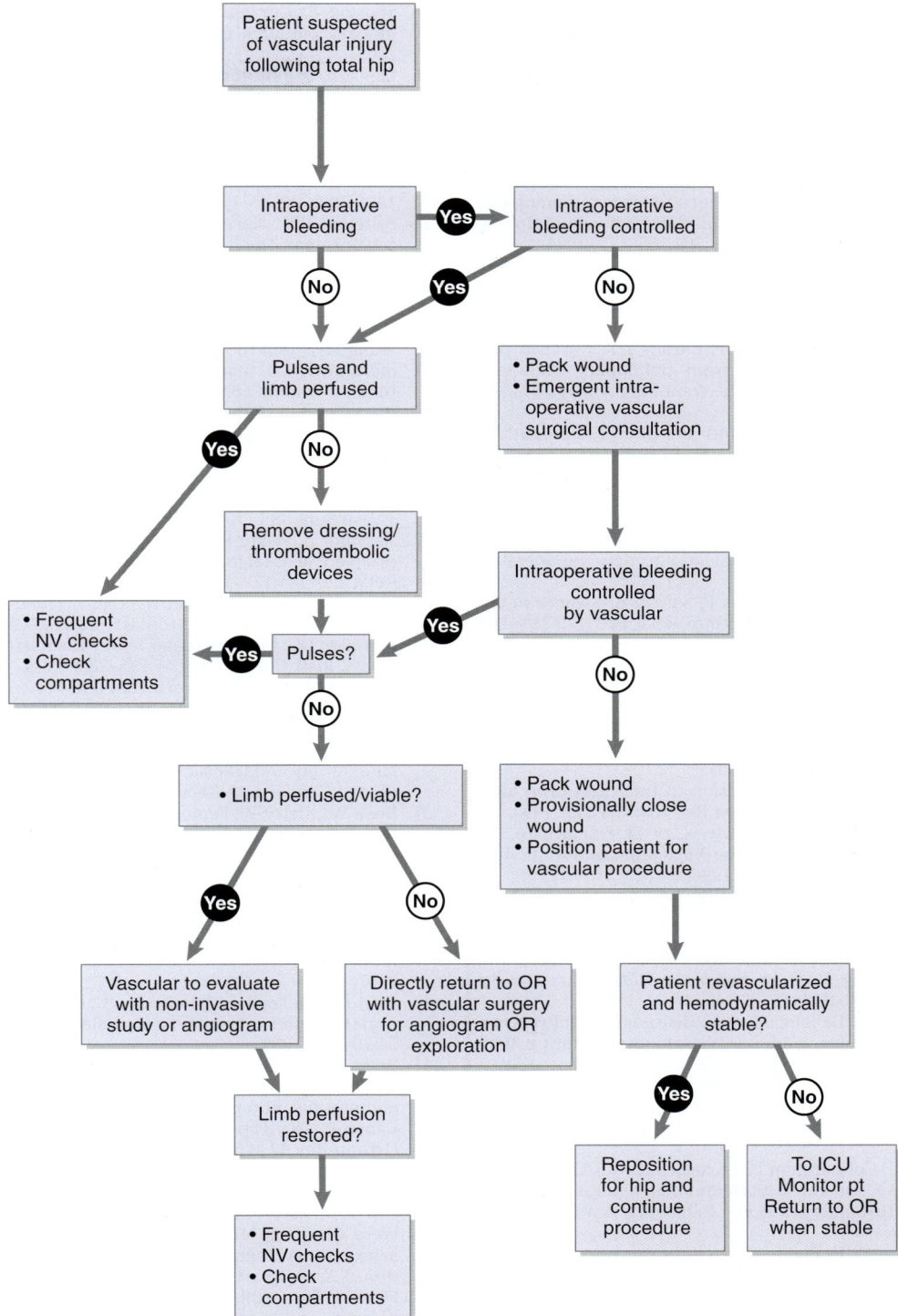

Figure 105-12. Treatment algorithm for suspected vascular injury following total hip arthroplasty.

REFERENCES

1. Schmalzried TP, Amstutz HC, Dorey FJ: Nerve palsy associated with total hip replacement: risk factors and prognosis. J Bone Joint Surg Am 73:1074–1080, 1991.
2. Schmalzried TP, Noordin S, Amstutz HC: Update on nerve palsy associated with total hip replacement. Clin Orthop Relat Res 344:188–206, 1997.
3. Nercessian OA, Piccoluga F, Eftekhar NS: Postoperative sciatic and femoral nerve palsy with reference to leg lengthening and medialization/lateralization of the hip joint following total hip arthroplasty. Clin Orthop Relat Res 304:165–171, 1994.
4. Simmons C, Jr, Izant TH, Rothman RH, et al: Femoral neuropathy following total hip arthroplasty: anatomic study, case reports, and literature review. J Arthroplasty 6(Suppl):S57–S66, 1991.
5. Amstutz HC, Friscia DA, Dorney F, Carney BT: Warfarin prophylaxis to prevent mortality from pulmonary embolism after total hip replacement. J Bone Joint Surg Am 71:321–326, 1989.
6. Weber ER, Daube JR, Coventry MB: Peripheral neuropathies associated with total hip arthroplasty. J Bone Joint Surg Am 58:66–69, 1976.
7. DeHart MM, Riley LH Jr: Nerve injuries in total hip arthroplasty. J Am Acad Orthop Surg 7:101–111, 1999.
8. Hurd JL, Potter HG, Dua V, Ranawat CS: Sciatic nerve palsy after primary total hip arthroplasty: a new perspective. J Arthroplasty 21:796–802, 2006.
9. Johanson NA, Pellicci PM, Tsairis P, Salvati EA: Nerve injury in total hip arthroplasty. Clin Orthop Relat Res 179:214–222, 1983.
10. Farrell CM, Springer BD, Haidukewych GJ, Morrey BF: Motor nerve palsy following primary total hip arthroplasty. J Bone Joint Surg Am 87:2619–2625, 2005.
11. Edwards BN, Tullos HS, Noble PC: Contributory factors and etiology of sciatic nerve palsy in total hip arthroplasty. Clin Orthop Relat Res 218:136–141, 1987.
12. Pritchett JW: Lumbar decompression to treat foot drop after hip arthroplasty. Clin Orthop Relat Res 303:173–177, 1994.
13. Ramesh M, O'Byrne JM, McCarthy N, et al: Damage to the superior gluteal nerve after the Hardinge approach to the hip. J Bone Joint Surg Br 78:903–906, 1996.
14. Memtsoudis SG, Rosenberger P, Walz JM: Critical care issues in the patient after major joint replacement. J Intensive Care Med 22:92–104, 2007.
15. Popa AS, Rabinstein AA, Huddleston PM, et al: Predictors of ischemic stroke after hip operation: a population-based study. J Hosp Med 4:298–303, 2009.
16. Ippolito E, Peretti G, Bellocci M, et al: Histology and ultrastructure of arteries, veins, and peripheral nerves during limb lengthening. Clin Orthop Relat Res 308:54–62, 1994.
17. Eggli S, Hankemayer S, Muller ME: Nerve palsy after leg lengthening in total replacement arthroplasty for developmental dysplasia of the hip. J Bone Joint Surg Br 81:843–845, 1999.
18. Wasielewski RC, Cooperstein LA, Kruger MP, Rubash HE: Acetabular anatomy and the transacetabular fixation of screws in total hip arthroplasty. J Bone Joint Surg Am 72:501–508, 1990.
19. Fricker RM, Troeger H, Pfeiffer KM: Obturator nerve palsy due to fixation of an acetabular reinforcement ring with transacetabular screws: a case report. J Bone Joint Surg Am 79:444–446, 1997.
20. Kenny P, O'Brien CP, Synnott K, Walsh MG: Damage to the superior gluteal nerve after two different approaches to the hip. J Bone Joint Surg Br 81:979–981, 1999.
21. Della Valle CJ, Jazrawi LM, Di Cesare PE, Steiger DJ: Paradoxical cerebral embolism complicating a major orthopaedic operation: a report of two cases. J Bone Joint Surg Am 81:108–110, 1999.
22. Barrack RL, Butler RA: Avoidance and management of neurovascular injuries in total hip arthroplasty. Instr Course Lect 52:267–274, 2003.
23. Georgopoulos D, Bouros D: Fat embolism syndrome: clinical examination is still the preferable diagnostic method. Chest 123:982–983, 2003.
24. Sharma R, Curzen NP: Caught in the act: paradoxical pulmonary embolus captured in transit. Eur J Neurol 16:e111, 2009.
25. Loscalzo J: Paradoxical embolism: clinical presentation, diagnostic strategies, and therapeutic options. Am Heart J 112:141–145, 1986.
26. Nercessian OA, Gonzalez EG, Stinchfield FE: The use of somatosensory evoked potential during revision or reoperation for total hip arthroplasty. Clin Orthop Relat Res 243:138–142, 1989.
27. Pritchett JW: Nerve injury and limb lengthening after hip replacement: treatment by shortening. Clin Orthop Relat Res 418:168–171, 2004.
28. Silbey MB, Callaghan JJ: Sciatic nerve palsy after total hip arthroplasty: treatment by modular neck shortening. Orthopedics 14:351–352, 1991.
29. Wong MW, Tsui HF, Yung SH, et al: Continuous pulse oximeter monitoring for inapparent hypoxemia after long bone fractures. J Trauma 56:356–362, 2004.
30. Wasielewski RC, Crossett LS, Rubash HE: Neural and vascular injury in total hip arthroplasty. Orthop Clin North Am 23:219–235, 1992.
31. Calligaro KD, Dougherty MJ, Ryan S, Booth RE: Acute arterial complications associated with total hip and knee arthroplasty. J Vasc Surg 38:1170–1177, 2003.
32. Nachbur B, Meyer RP, Verkkala K, Kürcher R: The mechanisms of severe arterial injury in surgery of the hip joint. Clin Orthop Relat Res 141:122–133, 1979.
33. Parvizi J, Pulido L, Slenker N, et al: Vascular injuries after total joint arthroplasty. J Arthroplasty 23:1115–1121, 2008.
34. Lewallen DG: Neurovascular injury associated with hip arthroplasty. Instr Course Lect 47:275–283, 1998.
35. Mehta V, Finn HA: Femoral artery and vein injury after cerclage wiring of the femur: a case report. J Arthroplasty 20:811–814, 2005.
36. Wasielewski RC, Galat DD, Sheridan KC, Rubash HE: Acetabular anatomy and transacetabular screw fixation at the high hip center. Clin Orthop Relat Res 438:171–176, 2005.
37. Bose WJ, Petty W: Femoral artery and nerve compression by bulk allograft used for acetabular reconstruction: an unreported complication. J Arthroplasty 11:348–350, 1996.
38. Shoenfeld NA, Stuchin SA, Pearl R, Haveson S: The management of vascular injuries associated with total hip arthroplasty. J Vasc Surg 11:549–555, 1990.
39. Stiehl JB: Acetabular prosthetic protrusion and sepsis: case report and review of the literature. J Arthroplasty 22:283–288, 2007.
40. Goss DE, de Trafford J, Roberts VC, et al: Raised ankle/brachial pressure index in insulin-treated diabetic patients. Diabet Med 6:576–578, 1989.
41. Wyss CR, Harrington RM, Burgess EM, Matsen FA 3rd: Transcutaneous oxygen tension as a predictor of success after an amputation. J Bone Joint Surg Am 70:203–207, 1988.
42. Cameron HU: Hip surgery in aortofemoral bypass patients. Orthop Rev 17:195–197, 1988.
43. Trousdale RT, Donnelly RS, Hallett JW: Thrombosis of an aortobifemoral bypass graft after total hip arthroplasty. J Arthroplasty 14:386–390, 1990.
44. Wera GD, Ting NT, Della Valle CJ, Sporer SM: External iliac artery injury complicating prosthetic hip resection for infection. J Arthroplasty 25:660.e1–e4, 2010.
45. Fehring TK, Guilford WB, Baron J: Assessment of intrapelvic cement and screws in revision total hip arthroplasty. J Arthroplasty 7:509–518, 1992.
46. al-Salman M, Taylor DC, Beauchamp CP, Duncan CP: Prevention of vascular injuries in revision total hip replacement. Can J Surg 35:261–264, 1992.
47. Eftekhar NS, Nercessian O: Intrapelvic migration of total hip prostheses: operative treatment. J Bone Joint Surg Am 71:1480–1486, 1989.
48. Petrera P, Trakru S, Mehta S, et al: Revision total hip arthroplasty with a retroperitoneal approach to the iliac vessels. J Arthroplasty 11:704–708, 1996.
49. Lavernia CJ, Cook CC, Hernandez RA, et al: Neurovascular injuries in acetabular reconstruction cage surgery: an anatomical study. J Arthroplasty 22:124–132, 2007.

50. Mallory TH: Rupture of the common iliac vein from reaming the acetabulum during total hip replacement: a case report. J Bone Joint Surg Am 54:276–277, 1972.

51. Riouallon G, Zilber S, Allain J: Common femoral artery intimal injury following total hip replacement: a case report and literature review. Orthop Traumatol Surg Res 95:154–158, 2009.

52. Aust JC, Bredenberg CE, Murray DG: Mechanisms of arterial injuries associated with total hip replacement. Arch Surg 116:345–349, 1981.

53. Graves M, Cole PA: Diagnosis of peripheral vascular injury in extremity trauma. Orthopedics 29:35–37, 2006.

CHAPTER 106

Wound Complications

*Yeukkei Cheung, Derek F. Amanatullah,
and Paul E. Di Cesare*

KEY POINTS

- Choice of anticoagulation, body mass index, and high drain output are significant risk factors for persistent wound drainage and subsequent infection.
- Irrigation and débridement of hip wounds with persistent drainage within 14 days of the index total hip arthroplasty can eradicate superficial infection and prevent further deep infection.
- It is critical to identify malnourished patients with a low serum albumin, serum transferrin, or total lymphocyte count to minimize their wound healing deficits.
- Preoperative antibiotics can reduce the risk of wound infection.
- Erythrocyte sedimentation rate, serum C-reactive protein level, and serum interleukin-6 level are valuable markers of periprosthetic wound infection.
- The diagnosis of deep infection is a critical decision in the course of treating an infected THA.

INTRODUCTION

Although managing the surgical wound is not the main goal of a total hip arthroplasty, it is critically important as prolonged postoperative surgical wound drainage has been associated with increased wound complications. Among the many potential causes of wound drainage include obesity, bleeding associated with various anti-coagulation regimens, and high closed suction drain output. Other factors that may be important include the nutritional status of the patient. The goal of this chapter is to provide the clinician with a practical guide to wound management including ways to avoid wound healing problems, guidelines to differentiate superficial from deeper wound problems, and strategies to manage the problematic wound.

WOUND DRAINAGE IN TOTAL HIP ARTHROPLASTY

Understanding the potential causes of and methods to prevent wound drainage is important because prolonged postoperative surgical wound drainage has been associated with increased risk of deep infection, increased morbidity, and longer postoperative hospitalization after total hip arthroplasty (THA).[1-3] No strict definition of "prolonged" or "persistent" wound drainage has been put forth. Some authors have defined prolonged or persistent wound drainage as wound drainage occurring or continuing 48 hours after the operative procedure.[4] The overall incidence of superficial infection, defined as infection superficial to the fascia lata, in one series of 183 THAs was approximately 17%, and the overall incidence of deep wound infection within 6 weeks was slightly above 1%.[5] However, the rate of deep wound infection increases from 1.3% to 50% with prolonged wound drainage.[2,3,6,7]

A retrospective review of 10,000 patients after THA or total knee arthroplasty (TKA) over a 5-year period identified 300 patients with wound drainage occurring more than 48 hours postoperatively.[4] Persistent wound drainage stopped after 2 to 4 days in 217 patients (72.3%) when treated with a standardized initial treatment protocol of local wound care, which involved cleaning the wound with sterile saline solution followed by application of povidone-iodine solution and oral prophylactic antibiotics.

The remaining 83 patients (27.7%) with persistent wound drainage who failed the standardized protocol were treated with surgical irrigation and débridement performed 2 to 37 days postoperatively. Deep irrigation and débridement was performed when the deep fascia had not sealed. Surgical irrigation and débridement (performed 4 to 32 days postoperatively) was successful (no further intervention required) in 63 patients (75.9%). The remaining 20 patients (24.1%), who failed the initial surgical irrigation and débridement, were treated with removal of hardware, two-stage exchange arthroplasty with an antibiotic spacer, or long-term antibiotic suppression.[4] Critical evaluation of the 83 patients necessitating surgical irrigation and débridement revealed that surgical irrigation and débridement was significantly more successful in patients who received surgical irrigation and débridement within 14 days from the index arthroplasty.[4] In addition, an association was found between malnutrition (defined as serum transferrin less than 200 mg/dL, serum albumin less than 3.5 g/dL, or total lymphocyte count less than 1500 per mL) and failure of the initial surgical irrigation and débridement.[4] All of the other variables evaluated, including age, gender, surgical blood loss, operative time, and diabetes mellitus, were not statistically significant risk factors for failure of initial surgical irrigation and débridement.

A similar retrospective study involving 1211 THAs identified risk factors associated with wound drainage 15 days after THA. Obesity (i.e., a body mass index greater than 35), use of low-molecular-weight heparin (LMWH) as venous thromboembolism prophylaxis, and high closed suction drain output were associated with prolonged wound drainage and higher rates of postoperative infection.[1] It should be noted that in this study, use of LMWH was associated with earlier postoperative wound drainage compared with use of aspirin with intermittent compression devices or warfarin, but the time to a dry surgical wound between LMWH and warfarin equalized on postoperative day 8.

A meta-analysis comparing deep venous thrombosis prophylaxis with warfarin, low-dose unfractionated heparin, LMWH, and aspirin and pneumatic compression found that minor wound bleeding was greatest with LMWH and low-dose unfractionated heparin.[8] However, LMWH does not requiring monitoring, hence its ease of use may outweigh the risk of a longer time to a dry surgical wound.[9] Low-dose unfractionated heparin was also associated with a higher risk of major bleeding requiring surgical evacuation.[8] Unfortunately, no randomized clinical trials have examined factor Xa inhibitors (e.g., fondaparinux) and their effects on surgical wound drainage. Appropriate deep vein thrombosis prophylaxis is important, and although many agents have been shown to be effective, some studies suggest that LMWH produces more wound drainage than Coumadin.

Use of a Closed Suction Drain

The routine use of a closed suction drain in THA remains controversial. Recent data demonstrate that rates of wound infection, postoperative hematoma, and reoperation are the same with or without a drain.[10] One hypothesis is that a closed suction drain prevents hematoma formation, decreases wound tension, and subsequently prevents infection.[10,11] Another hypothesis is that a closed suction drain may itself be a source of infection by acting as a conduit for entry of bacteria into the wound.[12] A meta-analysis evaluating the use of closed suction drains during THA or TKA concluded that, although many studies have showed the pros and cons of closed suction drains, most lacked the appropriate methods or included an underpowered sample size.[13] Often infection was used as a primary endpoint. However, the rate of infection after primary THA is low, hence most studies lack the power to support or refute the use of a closed suction drain in THA.

More recent data suggest that a closed suction drain does not decrease wound drainage, and that wounds without a closed suction drain require fewer dressing changes and dry faster.[14,15] In one report, a high volume of closed suction drain output was correlated with prolonged wound drainage and a higher rate of postoperative infection in THA.[1] Further, patients with a closed suction drain tended to require a greater number of postoperative blood transfusions.

One prospective study evaluated the effect of a closed suction drain on hematoma volume via nuclear medicine erythrocyte scintigraphy after THA.[16] No statistically significant difference in volume of postoperative hematoma was noted after THA in either group at 22 hours. However, patients with closed suction drains had an increased need for postoperative blood transfusions. These studies show that it is important to tailor the placement of closed suction drains according to the needs of each individual, bearing in mind that data are available to support a higher rate of postoperative blood transfusion when closed suction drains are used, and that significant controversy continues about whether closed suction drains prevent infection after THA.

EARLY PLASTIC SURGERY CONSULTATION

Few studies have focused on the management of complex infected wounds (e.g., those with exposed endoprosthetic implants or bone) (Fig. 106-1A and B). In a retrospective review of 10 patients with infected THA wounds, early plastic surgery consultation was evaluated for the management of these complex wounds. Plastic surgery intervention within 5 to 7 days of the index THA resulted in endoprosthetic salvage in 6 of 10 (60%) THAs when a deep wound infection was present.[17]

Prior studies have supported the finding that early recognition, aggressive surgical irrigation and débridement, and stable wound coverage (primary or with a muscle flap) may result in endoprosthetic salvage.[18-20] Vastus lateralis, rectus femoris, and rectus abdominis flaps have been advocated for coverage and salvage of THA.[20-22] However, there remains no consensus regarding optimal management of an infected deep hip wound for endoprosthetic salvage. Although many wounds can be managed via local wound care, use of vacuum-assisted dressing, or delayed wound closure, muscular flaps remain an option because they enhance the blood supply to regional tissues, improving the delivery of antibiotics and reducing dead space.

SERUM MARKERS OF MALNUTRITION

It is important to recognize and identify malnourished patients preoperatively to optimize their postoperative wound healing potential. Many studies have shown that the process of postoperative wound healing is directly related to nutritional status (Fig. 106-2).[4,23,24] Laboratory animals with protein malnutrition have less tensile wound strength, suggesting that protein malnutrition may increase the incidence of wound dehiscence in the early postoperative period.[25] A prospective study evaluated the ability of serum albumin, serum transferrin,

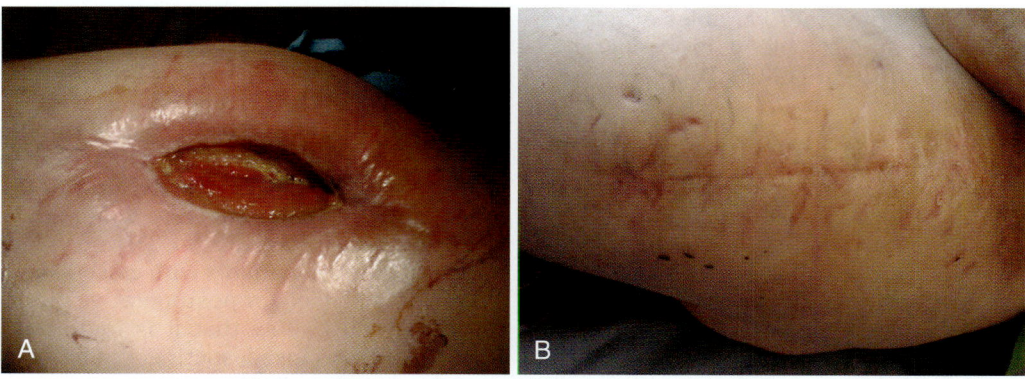

Figure 106-1. A, An example of an infected wound after total hip arthroplasty. **B,** Same wound after prosthesis removal and delayed primary closure.

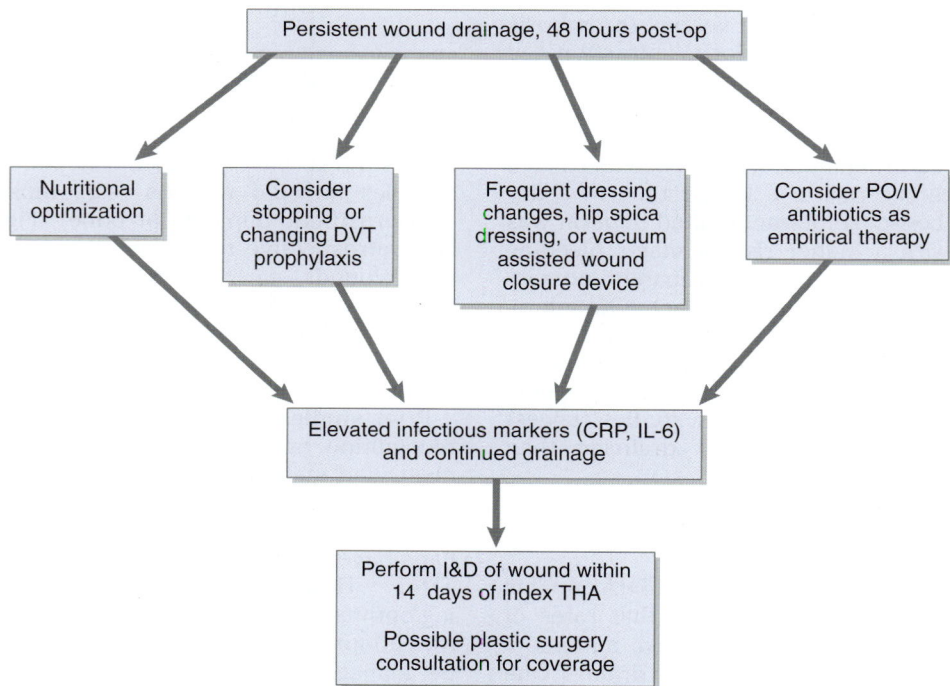

Figure 106-2. Treatment algorithm for persistent wound drainage. *CRP,* C-reactive protein; *DVT,* deep vein thrombosis; *IL-6,* interleukin-6; *I&D,* irrigation and débridement; *postop,* postoperatively; *THA,* total hip arthroplasty.

hematocrit, platelet count, prothrombin time (PT), partial thromboplastin time (PTT), erythrocyte sedimentation rate (ESR), and total lymphocyte count (TLC) to predict malnutrition and wound complications in 103 THAs. Low preoperative serum transferrin and albumin were observed in 34 (33.0%) patients with delayed wound healing. All measured nutritional markers were significantly lower in the immediate postoperative period. Each marker began to increase slowly on postoperative day 6. In the same study, patients who underwent single-stage, bilateral THAs had significantly lower serum transferrin and albumin levels on postoperative days 2, 4, and 6, and had higher rates of wound healing

complications than patients who underwent unilateral THA.[26]

Another prospective study that evaluated the mini-nutritional assessment (MNA), as well as preoperative serum albumin, serum transferrin, and TLC, in 207 patients with femoral neck and intertrochanteric fractures who underwent THA reported delayed wound healing in 46 (22.2%) patients. Preoperative serum transferrin, TLC, and MNA score were significantly lower for patients who subsequently developed wound complications.[27] In summary, if malnutrition is suspected in a THA patient, serum transferrin, serum albumin, and total lymphocyte count should be checked, and nutrition consultation should be considered to optimize the patient's nutrition status before an elective surgery is performed.

THE DIAGNOSIS OF ACUTE POSTSURGICAL INFECTION

Various markers, including peripheral white blood cell (WBC) count, erythrocyte sedimentation rate (ESR), and C-reactive protein (CRP) levels, have been used to aid in the diagnosis of acute orthopedic wound infection. WBC count suffers from low sensitivity and low specificity in diagnosing acute wound infection.[28,29] Typically, the ESR peaks 5 to 7 days postoperatively, then slowly returns to normal more than 3 months postoperatively, making it more useful in the diagnosis of chronic infection and in monitoring the treatment of infection than in diagnosing an acute postoperative infection.[30,31] CRP levels, on the other hand, is an acute phase reactant that peaks 3 days postoperatively and returns to baseline level in approximately 3 weeks.[32-34] CRP has gained wide acceptance in the orthopedic community in recent years, facilitating the diagnosis of more acute infectious processes in total joint arthroplasty.[35] Despite their utility in diagnosing chronic infection, little is known specifically about the value of ESR and CRP in the early postoperative period after THA. One recent study[36] showed CRP to be useful in the early postoperative period for diagnosing deep infection following TKA, with an optimal cutoff value of 95 mg/L.

Interleukin-6 (IL-6) has been suggested as a more sensitive indicator of acute infection.[37] IL-6 is a cytokine produced by activated macrophages and monocytes. The normal serum concentration of IL-6 is 1 pg/mL. However, it surges during periods of stress and inflammation. Postoperatively, IL-6 concentration peaks within the first 6 to 12 hours and rapidly returns to normal within 48 to 72 hours, making persistent elevation of serum IL-6 concentration an excellent marker of acute postsurgical wound infection.[38] Despite this promise, only a few studies have validated the use of serum IL-6 concentration to monitor wound infection. Additionally, IL-6 levels may not be available in all hospitals.

The diagnosis of deep infection is a critical decision in the course of treating an infected THA. However, few studies are available on the diagnosis of an acute deep wound infection in the early postoperative period. In general, aspiration of the hip for culture and synovial fluid WBC count has been shown to be an accurate method of diagnosing periprosthetic joint infection.[35] Because timely treatment of an early postoperative wound infection is important, culture results may not be as valuable given the delay in obtaining a final result.

Bedair and associates evaluated the utility of synovial fluid, white blood cell count, and differential in the early postoperative period.[36] Although this study examined the diagnosis of early periprosthetic joint infection following total knee arthroplasty, lessons learned can assist in evaluating the potentially infected THA. In this multicenter retrospective study of nearly 12,000 primary

TKAs, 146 were identified that had undergone aspiration within the first 6 weeks postoperatively. The mean synovial fluid WBC count in infected cases was 92,600/μL compared with 4200/μL; the optimal cutoff value for diagnosing infection based on receiver operator curves was 27,800/μL, with all but one noninfected case having a synovial fluid WBC count less than 10,000/μL. The differential was found to be helpful, with an optimal cut off value of 89% polymorphonuclear cells. Correction of the number of red blood cells in synovial fluid did not improve overall testing performance. Based on these data, aspiration in the early postoperative period should be considered for diagnosis; however, optimal cutoff values are higher than generally recommended for diagnosis of a chronic infection (approximately 3000 WBCs/μL). If aspiration shows more than 27,800 WBCs/μL and the differential is greater than 90% polymorphonuclear cells, infection is likely; similarly, a synovial fluid WBC count of less than 10,000 seems unlikely to be infected. In cases where the clinician is unsure whether a deep infection is present based on these values, antibiotics can be initiated after the synovial fluid culture has been obtained, and culture results can be relied on in most cases for a final diagnosis.

Reducing the Probability of Infection

Most THAs performed on healthy individuals are considered clean surgical procedures, hence the primary sources of bacterial organisms causing wound infections can be traced to the patient's endogenous skin flora or to airborne microorganisms in the operating theater.[39] Studies have shown that gram-positive organisms (e.g., *Staphylococcus aureus, Staphylococcus epidermidis*) are the main sources of wound infection in THA.[40,41] These organisms are often found on the patient's skin and can directly inoculate the surgical wound site, causing superficial or deep infection. The judicious use of perioperative prophylactic antibiotics can decrease the bacterial burden at the surgical wound site.

According to recommendations put forth by the American Academy of Orthopaedic Surgeons, cefazolin and cefuroxime are preferred first-line prophylactic antibiotics for routine orthopedic procedures. However, the use of vancomycin should be considered in case of a documented local outbreak of methicillin-resistant *Staphylococcus aureus* (MRSA), as well as in cases involving patients who are colonized with MRSA or are institutionalized.[42] Prophylactic perioperative antibiotics should be given within 1 hour before incision.[43] The routine use of perioperative prophylactic antibiotics is an inexpensive and effective way to prevent wound infection in THA, and the surgeon should work with his or her operative staff to implement antibiotic administration into the surgical pause following a standardized protocol for dosage, choice of drugs, timing, and duration of antibiotic use. Typically, two to three additional doses of cefazolin or cefuroxime are administered after the initial preoperative dose, and if vancomycin was utilized for prophylaxis two additional doses are administered postoperatively. Lack of appropriate antibiotic prophylaxis during THA has been shown to increase the relative risk of postoperative infection by fivefold.[2]

WOUND CLOSURE AND COSMESIS

The effects of direct closure of subcutaneous tissue on wound complications and infection have been evaluated. Closure of subcutaneous tissues in the presence of a closed suction drain (in both superficial and deep layers) has been shown to significantly decrease wound drainage without increasing fat necrosis.[44] Closure of subcutaneous tissues without a drain has been evaluated in a prospective cohort study of 44 hemiarthroplasties in which subcutaneous tissues were closed directly and 35 hemiarthroplasties without subcutaneous wound closure.[45] A 33% incidence of wound complications was reported without subcutaneous wound closure—fivefold higher than with subcutaneous wound closure. Specifically, a 20% incidence of wound infection and an 11% incidence of wound dehiscence were noted in the group without subcutaneous wound closure compared with 2% and 0%, respectively, with subcutaneous wound closure.[45] These data support the close apposition of subcutaneous tissues to avoid tension on the superficial closure and minimization of dead space for fluid accumulation and possible infection.

Three common methods of final wound closure may be used. All three—staples, suture, and skin adhesive (e.g., 2-octylcyanoarcylate)—hold the skin edges together while it heals. Staples and nonabsorbable sutures are removed after 10 to 21 days; absorbable sutures and skin adhesive do not require dedicated removal. Additionally, skin adhesive avoids the trauma associated with staples or needles.[46] A small clinical trial of 102 THA patients randomized to final closure with staples, Monocryl subcuticular suture, or skin adhesive demonstrated no significant difference in wound complications (i.e., drainage or infection), length of stay, incision length, or patient satisfaction.[47] However, a sixfold decrease in blood strike-through onto the dressing was noted with skin adhesive, and a threefold to fivefold decrease in application time was reported with staples in THA.[47] Another small clinical trial with 90 THA patients randomized to final closure with staples or skin adhesive revealed no significant difference in cosmetic scar appearance after plastic and orthopedic surgeon evaluation; in addition, no difference in incidence of wound complications (i.e., drainage or dehiscence) or in patient satisfaction at 3 months was noted.[48] Both methods are effective in attaining final closure; however, the cost of skin adhesive was more than five times greater than the cost of staples.[48] Nonetheless, both of these small trials were underpowered, making it difficult for investigators to arrive at definitive recommendations on final wound closure.

Scar cosmesis and patient satisfaction have been proposed as benefits of the mini-incision THA.[49-51] Mini-incision THA (Fig. 106-3) is often defined as an incision less than 10 cm in length.[52] A 30% incidence of poor scar formation was observed when mini-incision THA scars

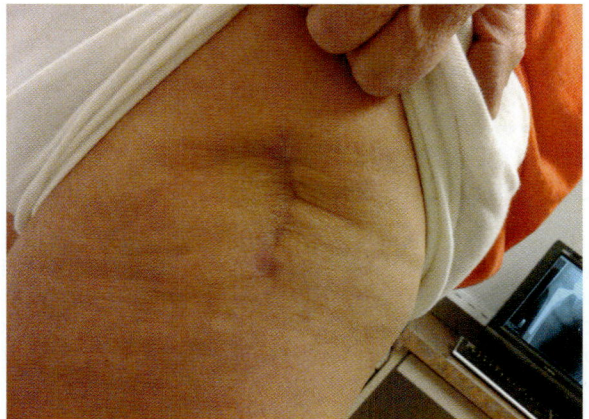

Figure 106-3. An example of a healed mini-posterior incision.

were evaluated by plastic surgeons blinded to the length of the incision. The incidence of poor scar formation was sixfold greater than the incidence in standard incision THA.[53] Increased discoloration, subcutaneous necrosis, and skin curling were associated with the mini-incision THA, likely from force applied to the subcutaneous tissues during retraction.[52,54] Mini-incision THA patients gave their incisions a higher cosmetic appearance score than was assigned by those who had standard incision THA, indicating that patients subjectively felt happier with a shorter scar. However, despite these cosmetic differences, all patients rated their scars as acceptable.[53] One questionnaire study reported optimal cosmesis in 74% of patients undergoing a standard incision and in 62% of patients undergoing a mini-incision THA.[54] Hence, the decision to choose a mini-incision THA should be based on the surgeon's technical skills in executing a THA with a small window into the hip joint without causing surrounding skin and soft tissue breakdown. Ultimately, this is a complex and individualized decision that balances the needs of the surgeon and the expectations of the patient.

REFERENCES

1. Patel VP, Walsh M, Sehgal B, et al: Factors associated with prolonged wound drainage after primary total hip and knee arthroplasty. J Bone Joint Surg Am 89:33–38, 2007.
2. Eveillard M, Mertl P, Canarelli B, et al: [Risk of deep infection in first-intention total hip replacement: evaluation concerning a continuous series of 790 cases]. Presse Med 30:1868–1875, 2001.
3. Saleh K, Olson M, Resig S, et al: Predictors of wound infection in hip and knee joint replacement: results from a 20 year surveillance program. J Orthop Res 20:506–515, 2002.
4. Jaberi FM, Parvizi J, Haytmanek CT, et al: Procrastination of wound drainage and malnutrition affect the outcome of joint arthroplasty. Clin Orthop Relat Res 466:1368–1371, 2008.
5. Gaine WJ, Ramamohan NA, Hussein NA, et al: Wound infection in hip and knee arthroplasty. J Bone Joint Surg Br 82:561–565, 2000.
6. Surin VV, Sundholm K, Backman L: Infection after total hip replacement: with special reference to a discharge from the wound. J Bone Joint Surg Br 65:412–418, 1983.

7. Masterson EL, Masri BA, Duncan CP: Treatment of infection at the site of total hip replacement. Instr Course Lect 47:297–306, 1998.

8. Freedman KB, Brookenthal KR, Fitzgerald RH Jr, et al: A meta-analysis of thromboembolic prophylaxis following elective total hip arthroplasty. J Bone Joint Surg Am 82:929–938, 2000.

9. American Academy of Orthopaedic Surgeons: Prevention of pulmonary embolism in patients undergoing total hip or knee arthroplasty, 2007 (updated 2007; cited) (http://www.aaos.org/research/guidelines/PE_guideline.pdf).

10. Cobb JP: Why use drains? J Bone Joint Surg Br 72:993–995, 1990.

11. Alexander JW, Korelitz J, Alexander NS: Prevention of wound infections: a case for closed suction drainage to remove wound fluids deficient in opsonic proteins. Am J Surg 132:59–63, 1976.

12. Willett KM, Simmons CD, Bentley G: The effect of suction drains after total hip replacement. J Bone Joint Surg Br 70:607–610, 1988.

13. Parker MJ, Roberts CP, Hay D: Closed suction drainage for hip and knee arthroplasty: a meta-analysis. J Bone Joint Surg Am 86:1146–1152, 2004.

14. Dora C, von Campe A, Mengiardi B, et al: Simplified wound care and earlier wound recovery without closed suction drainage in elective total hip arthroplasty: a prospective randomized trial in 100 operations. Arch Orthop Trauma Surg 127:919–923, 2007.

15. Strahovnik A, Fokter SK, Kotnik M: Comparison of drainage techniques on prolonged serous drainage after total hip arthroplasty: a prospective, randomized study. J Arthroplasty 25:244–248, 2010.

16. Widman J, Jacobsson H, Larsson SA, Isacson J: No effect of drains on the postoperative hematoma volume in hip replacement surgery: a randomized study using scintigraphy. Acta Orthop Scand 73:625–629, 2002.

17. Gusenoff JA, Hungerford DS, Orlando JC, Nahabedian MY: Outcome and management of infected wounds after total hip arthroplasty. Ann Plast Surg 49:587–592, 2002.

18. Arnold PG, Witzke DJ: Management of failed total hip arthroplasty with muscle flaps. Ann Plast Surg 11:474–478, 1983.

19. Jones NF, Eadie P, Johnson PC, Mears DC: Treatment of chronic infected hip arthroplasty wounds by radical débridement and obliteration with pedicled and free muscle flaps. Plast Reconstr Surg 88:95–101, 1991.

20. Meland NB, Arnold PG, Weiss HC: Management of the recalcitrant total-hip arthroplasty wound. Plast Reconstr Surg 88:681–685, 1991.

21. Collins DN, Garvin KL, Nelson CL: The use of the vastus lateralis flap in patients with intractable infection after resection arthroplasty following the use of a hip implant. J Bone Joint Surg Am 69:510–516, 1987.

22. Bentivegna PE, Greenberg BM: Use of an inferiorly based rectus muscle flap in flank wound coverage. Ann Plast Surg 29:261–262, 1992.

23. Irvin TT: Effects of malnutrition and hyperalimentation on wound healing. Surg Gynecol Obstet 146:33–37, 1978.

24. Greene KA, Wilde AH, Stulberg BN: Preoperative nutritional status of total joint patients: relationship to postoperative wound problems. Presented at the American Academy of Orthopaedic Surgeons 56th Annual Meeting, Las Vegas, February 9, 1989.

25. Kobak MW, Benditt EP, Wissler RW, Steffee CH: Relation of protein deficiency to experimental wound healing. Surg Gynecol Obstet 85:751, 1947.

26. Gherini S, Vaughn BK, Lombardi AV Jr, Mallory TH: Delayed wound healing and nutritional deficiencies after total hip arthroplasty. Clin Orthop Relat Res 293:188–195, 1993.

27. Guo JJ, Yang H, Qian H, et al: The effects of different nutritional measurements on delayed wound healing after hip fracture in the elderly. J Surg Res 159:503–508, 2010.

28. Canner GC, Steinberg ME, Heppenstall RB, Balderston R: The infected hip after total hip arthroplasty. J Bone Joint Surg Am 66:1393–1399, 1984.

29. Spangehl MJ, Masri BA, O'Connell JX, Duncan CP: Prospective analysis of preoperative and intraoperative investigations for the diagnosis of infection at the sites of two hundred and two revision total hip arthroplasties. J Bone Joint Surg Am 81:672–683, 1999.

30. Bilgen O, Atici T, Durak K, Karaeminogullari Bilgen MS: C-reactive protein values and erythrocyte sedimentation rates after total hip and total knee arthroplasty. J Int Med Res 29:7–12, 2001.

31. Shih LY, Wu JJ, Yang DJ: Erythrocyte sedimentation rate and C-reactive protein values in patients with total hip arthroplasty. Clin Orthop Relat Res 225:238–246, 1987.

32. Di Cesare PE, Chang E, Preston CF, Liu CJ: Serum interleukin-6 as a marker of periprosthetic infection following total hip and knee arthroplasty. J Bone Joint Surg Am 87:1921–1927, 2005.

33. Moreschini O, Greggi G, Giordano MC, et al: Postoperative physiopathological analysis of inflammatory parameters in patients undergoing hip or knee arthroplasty. Int J Tissue React 23:151–154, 2001.

34. White J, Kelly M, Dunsmuir R: C-reactive protein level after total hip and total knee replacement. J Bone Joint Surg Br 80:909–911, 1998.

35. Schinsky MF, Della Valle CJ, Sporer SM, Paprosky WG: Perioperative testing for joint infection in patients undergoing revision total hip arthroplasty. J Bone Joint Surg Am 90:1869–1875, 2008.

36. Bedair H, Ting N, Moric M, et al, editors: Diagnosis of infection in the early post-operative period following primary total knee arthroplasty: the utility of synovial fluid white blood cell count. Presented at American Academy of Orthopaedic Surgeons Annual Meeting, New Orleans, March 9, 2010.

37. Kragsbjerg P, Holmberg H, Vikerfors T: Serum concentrations of interleukin-6, tumour necrosis factor-alpha, and C-reactive protein in patients undergoing major operations. Eur J Surg 161:17–22, 1995.

38. Wirtz DC, Heller KD, Miltner O, et al: Interleukin-6: a potential inflammatory marker after total joint replacement. Int Orthop 24:194–196, 2000.

39. Meehan J, Jamali AA, Nguyen H: Prophylactic antibiotics in hip and knee arthroplasty. J Bone Joint Surg Am 91:2480–2490, 2009.

40. Fulkerson E, Valle CJ, Wise B, et al: Antibiotic susceptibility of bacteria infecting total joint arthroplasty sites. J Bone Joint Surg Am 88:1231–1237, 2006.

41. Mahomed NN, Barrett JA, Katz JN, et al: Rates and outcomes of primary and revision total hip replacement in the United States Medicare population. J Bone Joint Surg Am 85:27–32, 2003.

42. Prokuski L: Prophylactic antibiotics in orthopaedic surgery. J Am Acad Orthop Surg 16:283–293, 2008.

43. Classen DC, Evans RS, Pestotnik SL, et al: The timing of prophylactic administration of antibiotics and the risk of surgical-wound infection. N Engl J Med 326:281–286, 1992.

44. Ferris BD, Wickens D, Bhamra M, et al: To stitch or not to stitch the fat? Ann R Coll Surg Engl 71:115–116, 1989.

45. Lemon M, Bali SL, Ibery N, et al: Is a fat stitch required when closing a hip hemiarthroplasty wound without a drain? Injury 37:190–193, 2006.

46. Singer AJ, Quinn JV, Clark RE, Hollander JE; TraumaSeal Study G: Closure of lacerations and incisions with octylcyanoacrylate: a multicenter randomized controlled trial. Surgery 131:270–276, 2002.

47. Khan RJ, Fick D, Yao F, et al: A comparison of three methods of wound closure following arthroplasty: a prospective, randomised, controlled trial. J Bone Joint Surg Br 88:238–242, 2006.

48. Livesey C, Wylde V, Descamps S, et al: Skin closure after total hip replacement: a randomised controlled trial of skin adhesive versus surgical staples. J Bone Joint Surg Br 91:725–729, 2009.

49. Goldstein WM, Branson JJ, Berland KA, Gordon AC: Minimal-incision total hip arthroplasty. J Bone Joint Surg Am 85(Suppl 4):33–38, 2003.

50. Howell JR, Masri BA, Duncan CP: Minimally invasive versus standard incision anterolateral hip replacement: a comparative study. Orthop Clin North Am 35:153–162, 2004.

51. Wright JM, Crockett HC, Delgado S, et al: Mini-incision for total hip arthroplasty: a prospective, controlled investigation

with 5-year follow-up evaluation. J Arthroplasty 19:538–545, 2004.

52. Woolson ST, Mow CS, Syquia JF, et al: Comparison of primary total hip replacements performed with a standard incision or a mini-incision. J Bone Joint Surg Am 86:1353–1358, 2004.

53. Mow CS, Woolson ST, Ngarmukos SG, et al: Comparison of scars from total hip replacements done with a standard

or a mini-incision. Clin Orthop Relat Res 441:80–85, 2005.

54. Goldstein WM, Ali R, Branson JJ, Berland KA: Comparison of patient satisfaction with incision cosmesis after standard and minimally invasive total hip arthroplasty. Orthopedics 31:368, 2008.

CHAPTER 107

Heterotopic Ossification

Oliver O. Tannous and Vincent Pellegrini, Jr.

KEY POINTS

- Although the causes of heterotopic ossification (HO) are diverse, it most commonly occurs through a process of endochondral ossification after operative procedures about the hip.
- Heterotopic ossification is typically only a radiographic finding without clinical consequences; however, clinically meaningful stiffness may result from extensive ectopic bone formation in 8% to 10% of patients after total hip arthroplasty.
- Patients at greatest risk for HO are (1) those in whom heterotopic bone has developed after prior hip surgery; (2) patients who have hypertrophic osteoarthritis, ankylosing spondylitis, diffuse idiopathic skeletal hyperostosis, or Parkinson's disease; and (3) male patients.
- Effective prophylaxis of high-risk patients with nonsteroidal anti-inflammatory agents or external beam radiation must be instituted within 5 days of operation.
- When surgical excision of HO is necessary to restore function, recurrence is the rule, unless prophylaxis is administered in the early postoperative period.

INTRODUCTION

Heterotopic ossification is the process by which aberrant bone is formed in the soft connective tissues, joint capsule, or skeletal muscle outside the normal confines of the skeleton. Several causes of heterotopic ossification are known; these are generally grouped as neurologic, genetic, and traumatic, with orthopedic procedures included in the latter. This pathologic process most often occurs about the hip and typically is incited by surgical procedures such as total hip arthroplasty, repair of acetabular fractures, pelvic osteotomy, and intramedullary nailing of femoral shaft fractures. Heterotopic ossification also occurs about other joints, such as the shoulder, elbow, and knee. It can appear in conjunction with other nonsurgical events such as head injury, cerebrovascular accident, burns, and genetic disorders such as fibrodysplasia ossificans progressiva (FOP). Most recently, owing to armed conflicts and the use of improvised explosive devices (IEDs), heterotopic

ossification has appeared in the residual limbs of up to two thirds of combat-related amputees after blast injury.[1] Nonetheless, it most often manifests clinically as ectopic bone formation in the abductor musculature after total hip arthroplasty. Factors intrinsic to the patient, injury to the abductor musculature, surgical approach, hemorrhage, and bone debris remaining in the soft tissues all contribute to the overall risk of heterotopic ossification in any individual patient.

As a radiographic phenomenon without accompanying symptoms, heterotopic ossification has been reported to occur in as many as 90% of patients who have undergone total hip arthroplasty. In this setting, it manifests as small islands of bone in the soft tissues about the hip, or as bony outgrowths from the margin of the acetabulum or the proximal femur, measuring less than 1 cm in length. However, in 8% to 10% of patients, ectopic bone formation after total hip arthroplasty occurs to such an extent or in such a location that it results in clinical manifestations of pain soon after operation and late restrictions in motion that are of consequence to the patient. In the most extreme cases, resulting symptoms of pain and stiffness replace those that prompted the patient to seek surgery in the first place and may actually negate the beneficial effect of the arthroplasty.

EPIDEMIOLOGY AND RISK FACTORS

Patients judged to be at increased risk for development of heterotopic bone should receive some form of prophylaxis for heterotopic ossification; this group constitutes less than 20% of those undergoing total hip arthroplasty in the author's practice. Classically, these "high-risk" patients include those with a diagnosis of hypertrophic osteoarthritis and prominent marginal osteophytes (Fig. 107-1A and B), diffuse idiopathic skeletal hyperostosis, or ankylosing spondylitis, and those in whom heterotopic bone has formed after a previous procedure or injury about the hip (Box 107-1). Nearly all patients in whom heterotopic bone has formed after undergoing surgery about the hip will develop bone again, usually to a greater degree, after reoperation on the involved hip or primary operation on the contralateral hip. Men are generally twice as likely as women to form heterotopic bone, but women in these high-risk categories develop ectopic bone at rates comparable with those of men. It is increasingly recognized that

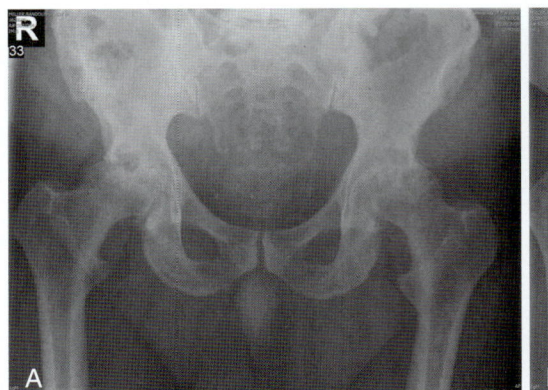
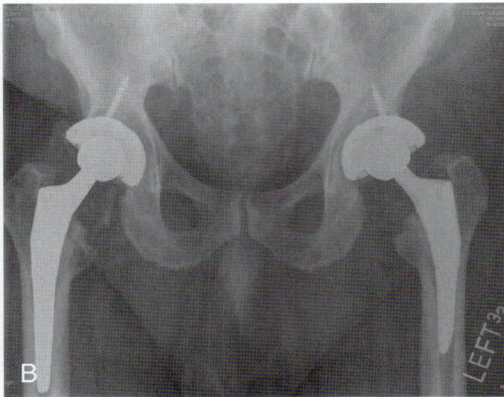

Figure 107-1. A, Radiograph of a 66-year-old male patient with primary osteoarthritis and diffuse hypertrophic skeletal hyperostosis. "Whiskering" of periosteal new bone about the ischial tuberosity and the iliac crest is evident. Stigmata of enthesopathy are seen as calcification in the tendinous insertion of the iliopsoas on the lesser trochanter. **B,** Postoperative radiograph after bilateral total hip arthroplasty, staged 1 year apart. Grade III heterotopic ossification is evident on the right after the initial hip replacement. No HO developed on the left following postoperative radiation prophylaxis administered after total hip arthroplasty.

BOX 107-1. RISK FACTORS FOR DEVELOPING HO FOLLOWING THA

Prior heterotopic bone formation after hip surgery or trauma
Hypertrophic osteoarthritis with prominent osteophytosis
Diffuse idiopathic skeletal hyperostosis (DISH)
Ankylosing spondylitis
Male gender
CNS disorders: Parkinson's disease, perioperative stroke, traumatic brain injury

CNS, Central nervous system; *HO,* heterotopic ossification; *THA,* total hip arthroplasty.

---

central nervous system disorders, specifically Parkinson's disease (Fig. 107-2), spinal cord injury, and perioperative cerebrovascular accident, substantially predispose patients to heterotopic ossification about the hip.

PATHOPHYSIOLOGY

In 1975, Chalmers and associates postulated that three requisite conditions must be met to allow heterotopic bone formation: (1) the presence of an inducing agent, (2) an osteogenic precursor cell, and (3) an environment conducive to osteogenesis.[2] The causes of heterotopic bone formation are generally classified as neurologic, genetic, and traumatic. Over the past decade, much research has been done to identify the osteogenic precursor cell, as well as the molecular signals that stimulate pluripotent mesenchymal stem cell differentiation down osteogenic cell lines (Fig. 107-3). Although the specific osteogenic precursor remains unknown, much progress has been made in our

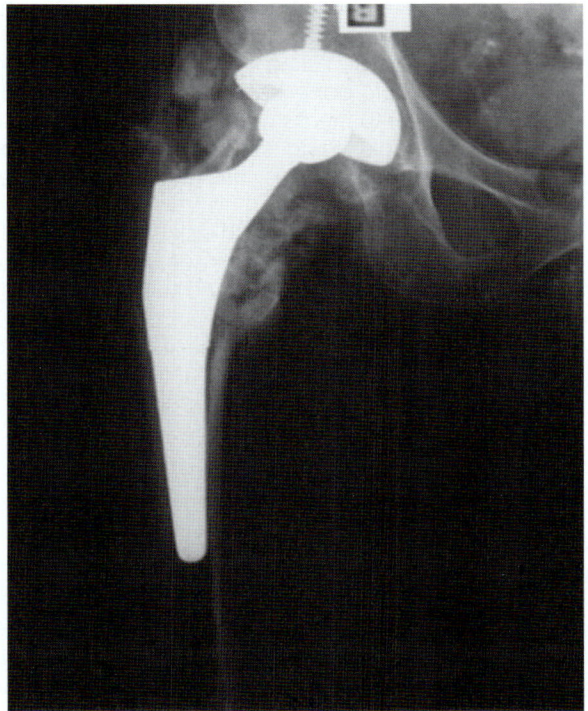

Figure 107-2. Radiograph of a 72-year-old male with a history of Parkinson's disease following total hip replacement without radiation prophylaxis. Grade IV heterotopic ossification is apparent, and the patient's hip was clinically ankylosed; he ultimately came to surgical resection and received adjunctive postoperative radiation to an expanded field with no recurrence of ossification and a good functional result.

understanding of the inductive role of bone morphogenetic protein (BMP) signaling.

Several bone morphogenic proteins have been identified, and "bone dust" (particulate bone fragments resulting from reaming or machining of bone with power

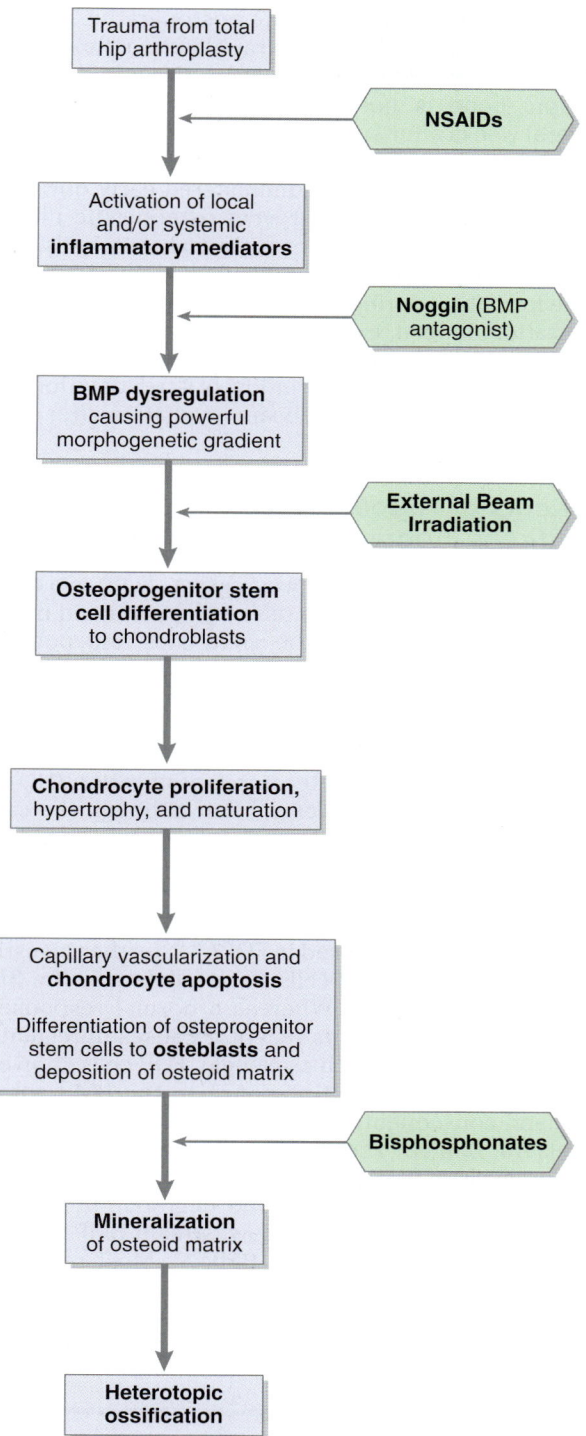

Figure 107-3. Basic schematic of the pathophysiology of heterotopic ossification and the points of prophylactic intervention along the pathway. *(Modified from Balboni TA, Gobezie R, Mamon HJ: Heterotopic ossification: pathophysiology, clinical features, and the role of radiotherapy for prophylaxis. Int J Radiat Oncol Biol Phys 65:1292, 2006.)*

instruments) recovered from patients who formed heterotopic bone has been shown to stimulate proliferation of isolated bone progenitor cells in culture at a rate sixfold greater than similar material extracted from patients who did not form bone. It is suggested that induction of pro-osteogenic pathways occurs through dysregulation of BMP signaling in the presence of inflammatory triggers. In the local environment, BMPs are overexpressed,[3-9] and, in combination with underexpression of antagonists,[10-13] a powerful morphogenetic gradient is created. Inflammatory factors such as interleukin-1β and prostaglandin E1 and E2 have been shown to enhance the expression of BMPs and ultimately the appearance of heterotopic bone.[14-16] The role of these inflammatory signals is further supported by known inhibitory effects of nonsteroidal antiinflammatory drugs on heterotopic ossification.[17,18] Attesting to the metabolic hyperactivity of this tissue, histomorphometric and biochemical data have shown that heterotopic bone contains more than twice the number of active osteoclasts and has a rate of appositional new bone formation nearly three times that of normal age-matched bone.[19]

Central to the issue of heterotopic ossification is the question of the anatomic origin of pluripotential mesenchymal cells participating in the process of bone formation within soft tissues. Transformation of local cells into bone-producing elements has been proposed by many investigators. Moreover, the demonstrated efficacy of preoperative radiation in preventing heterotopic ossification provides strong circumstantial evidence in support of a local source of osteoprogenitor cells, resulting in ectopic ossification. Trauma to muscle leads to hemorrhage, muscle degeneration, and proliferation of perivascular connective tissue, culminating in the production of heterotopic bone. Studies in an animal model using hydrogen-3–labeled thymidine and uridine have shown that local soft tissue fibroblasts adjacent to an implanted demineralized bone fragment were induced to transform into pluripotential mesenchymal cells that differentiated into osteoblasts.[20] Pluripotential mesenchymal stem cells are ubiquitous in the soft tissues about the hip, and it is postulated that these cell lines may be induced to undergo atypical differentiation into osteogenic stem cells capable of participating in the process of heterotopic ossification. Maturation of these cells down osteoblastic or chondroblastic stem cell lines could then lead to the formation of ectopic bone. Increasing evidence suggests that the pathologic process of heterotopic ossification proceeds through a pathway of secondary bone formation, first passing through an intermediate phase of cartilage model bone, which then undergoes ossification to mature lamellar bone[29] (Fig. 107-4).

Several groups have identified stem cells with osteogenic capacities. One candidate is a muscle-derived stem cell isolated from skeletal muscle that has been shown to commit to an osteogenic lineage in response to BMP-2 and BMP-4.[21-24] Another potential source is a vascular endothelial precursor cell known to respond to an inflammatory trigger that forms heterotopic bone in response to overactive BMP signaling.[25] Yet another

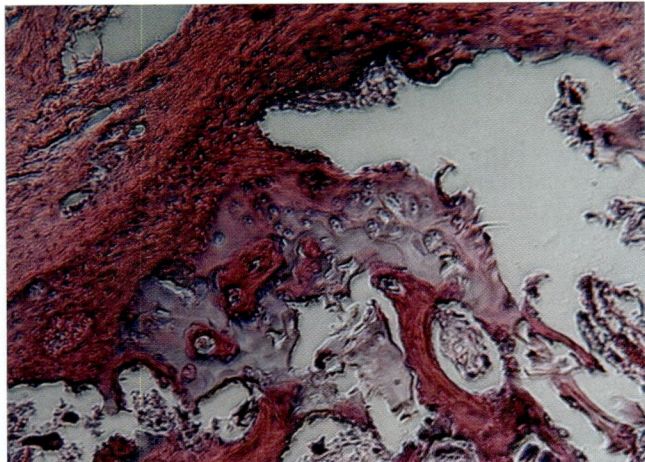

Figure 107-4. Histologic section of heterotopic bone from a rabbit animal model 12 weeks after hip surgery. Periosteal new bone is appearing from the cortical surface. Chondroid tissue is giving rise to islands of lamellar bone through a process of calcification of hypertrophic cartilage, reminiscent of the growth plate.

group has recently identified mesenchymal progenitor cells (MPCs) obtained from the traumatized muscle of combatants with extensive soft tissue extremity wounds; these cells function as osteoprogenitor cells in the appropriate biochemical environment.[26] It is conceivable that several cell populations have the potential to form bone by following the proper signals.

Alternatively, it is possible that distant migratory hematopoietic stem cells may be essential for inducing local connective tissue elements to form heterotopic bone. Pluripotential mesenchymal cells and osteocytes are liberated from the marrow space of the ilium and femoral canal during hip arthroplasty surgery and likely are present in the local hematoma. They may contribute to the process of heterotopic ossification directly by bone formation or indirectly via stimulation of local cells to express osteogenic phenotypes. Distant hematopoietic stem cells transported to the wound by virtue of the normal response to surgical injury also possess the capability to mature along osteogenic cell lines under the influence of mitogenic stimuli in the wound environment.

Regardless of the site of origin of these pluripotential mesenchymal stem cells, heterotopic ossification seems to be clearly dependent on cellular differentiation down osteoprogenitor cell lines. Ionizing radiation is known to exert its greatest influence on rapidly dividing cells by interfering with the normal production of nuclear deoxyribonucleic acid. One study has shown that ionizing radiation in doses from 0 to 20 Gy reduces the formation of the BMP-2/BMP receptor complex in a dose-dependent fashion.[27] The authors of this study postulate that ionizing radiation acts to downregulate the BMP receptor. Tonna and Cronkite demonstrated in mice that differentiation of pluripotential mesenchymal cells into osteoblasts began 16 hours after fracture of the femur and peaked at approximately 32 hours.[20] In their model, the critical events of cellular differentiation

occurred during the immediate postoperative period. A similar chronology may be extrapolated to the sequence of heterotopic ossification, even though the actual ectopic bone is not detectable radiographically for several weeks after surgery. Therefore, to be most effective, it seems essential that irradiation or other prophylactic measures must be administered early during the postoperative period to prevent osteoblastic differentiation of pluripotential mesenchymal stem cells, effectively arresting osteoid and subsequent heterotopic bone formation during the initial phases of cellular reorganization. Indeed, experience with postoperative radiation therapy for prevention of heterotopic ossification has empirically defined a window of 4 to 5 days for effective institution of external beam irradiation after operation about the hip.

Genetics of Fibrodysplasia Ossificans Progressiva

Fibrodysplasia ossificans progressiva (FOP) is a heritable disorder of connective tissue characterized by congenital malformation of the great toes and postnatal formation of heterotopic ossification.[28] Over the past decade, much progress has been made in our understanding of the pathophysiology of FOP. Heterotopic bone in FOP undergoes an endochondral process of ossification similar to heterotopic ossification (HO) following total hip arthroplasty,[29] and although the cause of HO in FOP is different from that following THA, study of this rare genetic disorder may provide some insight into the condition following surgery about the hip. It was first discovered that BMP-4 mRNA and protein are specifically overexpressed in FOP[6,30-32]; further investigation revealed that FOP cells have a defect in the BMP-antagonist response.[11] Whereas a normal response to BMP-4 activation onto its receptor causes upregulation of BMP antagonists such as Noggin, FOP cells showed a dramatically attenuated response to the BMP antagonist, and consequently an accumulation of much higher levels of BMP-4. These cells also have significantly higher levels of BMP-R1A cell surface receptors, marked reduction of internalization and degradation of receptors,[33] and dysregulation of downstream BMP signaling and hyperresponsiveness to BMP.[34-37] Most recently, a mutation in the activation domain of the activin A type 1 receptor (ACVR1), a BMP type 1 receptor, has been shown to enhance receptor signaling.[38]

CLINICAL FEATURES AND DIAGNOSIS

Radiographic Staging

A radiographic classification system popularized by Brooker and associates[39] is most commonly used to describe the pattern and extent of ossification on the anteroposterior pelvic radiograph: stage I, islands of bone appearing in the soft tissues; stage II, bone spurs arising from the pelvis or proximal femur with greater than 1 cm between adjacent bone surfaces; stage III, bone spurs arising from the pelvis or proximal femur with less than 1 cm between adjacent bone surfaces; and stage IV, confluent bone bridging the pelvis and proximal femur and apparent bony ankylosis of the hip.

Further description of the radiographic *extent* of ossification correlates with the degree of functional impairment attributed to ectopic bone formation. One grading system describes the proportion of the area involved in the triangle defined by the base of the greater trochanter, the anterior iliac spine, and the inferior aspect of the ischium. Grade A bone involves 33% or less of this area, grade B involves 34% to 66%, and grade C involves 67% to 100%. Greater extent of involvement was correlated with more clinically significant limitation of motion about the hip.

Clinical Presentation

Vague discomfort or frank pain in the region of the hip is thought to be the direct result of the inflammatory process that is involved in the process of heterotopic ossification. It is characteristically present at rest, is unaffected by activity, and often interferes with sleep. This pain typically occurs during the first 6 months after surgery and spontaneously resolves as the biological activity of the process subsides and the radiographic appearance of the bone matures. The extent of radiographic ossification is variable at this point in time and is difficult to assess because symptoms often occur before the bone is well mineralized; ultimately, grade III or IV bone formation is apparent in those patients with clinically bothersome restriction of motion. Nonsteroidal anti-inflammatory medications or non-narcotic analgesics are the cornerstone of treatment until the inflammatory process runs its self-limited course.

Greater trochanteric bursitis may occur in association with small bone spurs (stage II) originating from the base or lateral surface of the greater trochanter. Although not extensive, the strategic location of these spurs at the prominence of the greater trochanter beneath the iliotibial band may provoke troublesome irritation of the bursa located in this area. Symptoms are aggravated by postoperative gluteal abductor weakness secondary to disuse during a prolonged period of arthritic disease before surgery. Effective treatment typically consists of nonsteroidal anti-inflammatory medications and a gluteal abductor strengthening program. Occasionally, a steroid injection into the region of the bursa and the offending bone spur is necessary to break the cycle of symptoms for the patient. Symptoms usually resolve over a period of several months, but the bursitis associated with these spurs of ectopic bone can be particularly troublesome and refractory to usual treatment measures. A series of several steroid injections may be indicated and, rarely, surgical removal of the spurs might be considered in conjunction with postoperative measures to prevent recurrence.

Stiffness about the hip is the most problematic long-term consequence of heterotopic ossification occurring after total hip arthroplasty and typically is present only when grade III or IV bone is evident on the radiograph. Most commonly, the operating surgeon finds it remarkable that rather prominent radiographic ossification is accompanied by a modest decrease in range of motion with comparatively little, if any, functional restriction in most patients. The degree of loss of range of motion necessary to compromise function varies from patient to patient and is dependent on the individual patient's needs for mobility during daily activities, in addition to the degree of arthritic disease of adjacent joints and the low back. Considering that the lumbar spine is most often called upon to compensate for a stiff hip, high-grade heterotopic ossification is most problematic in patients with concurrent lumbar spondylosis and spinal stenosis. In such patients, a hip flexion contracture resulting from heterotopic ossification results in compensatory exaggeration of the lumbar lordosis, which, in turn, aggravates the symptoms of lumbar spondylosis and claudication associated with spinal stenosis. Typical limitations occur secondary to restricted rotation and flexion ranges of the hip, producing compromised sitting ability, donning of shoes and socks, and foot hygiene. Neither medication nor injection therapy is effective in restoring range of motion once radiographs show evidence of ectopic bone, or clinical restriction of motion is present. Although relatively few patients seek surgery to restore lost mobility secondary to heterotopic ossification after total hip arthroplasty, surgical excision of the offending bone is the only effective intervention once restricted motion is clinically evident. Surgery is rarely indicated for less than radiographic stage III or IV ossification. Moreover, adjunctive prophylactic measures such as radiation or nonsteroidal anti-inflammatory medication are essential in conjunction with surgical excision to prevent postoperative recurrence of bone formation to the same or an even greater degree. Because of this fact, the development of effective methods of prophylaxis has attracted even more attention than the surgical management of this problem.

DIFFERENTIAL DIAGNOSIS

In its early stages, the clinical presentation of pain associated with the inflammatory phase of heterotopic ossification is most often mistaken for infection. Patients typically report persistent postoperative pain, and physical examination may reveal swelling, warmth, and tenderness about the hip. Some patients may even experience fevers associated with the inflammatory response. Given that the diagnosis of heterotopic ossification is confirmed by radiographic evaluation, it may be several weeks before a definitive diagnosis can be made, when the osteoid matrix mineralizes and heterotopic bone becomes evident on routine radiographs.

TREATMENT

Prophylaxis of Heterotopic Ossification

Recognition of early initiation of osteoblastic cell differentiation at the time of surgical insult, coupled with the understanding that this process is not easily arrested once begun, has made *prevention* of heterotopic ossification the cornerstone of management of this condition. External beam irradiation and nonsteroidal anti-inflammatory agents, particularly indomethacin, are the most thoroughly studied and widely used interventions for prophylaxis. Bisphosphonates have been previously used for this purpose; however, their use was abandoned after it was recognized that these agents only *delay* the appearance of heterotopic ossification by blocking mineralization of osteoid matrix, which proceeds normally after discontinuation of the drug.

Indications

Patients with known risk factors for heterotopic ossification should receive perioperative prophylaxis. In addition to the risk factors previously mentioned, the surgical approach to the hip also conditions the risk of heterotopic ossification, reflecting the extent to which the abductor musculature is violated or injured during the procedure. Although specific frequencies of occurrence vary among authors, the modified Hardinge or related transgluteal approaches are credited with the highest rates of severe ossification,[40] followed by the transtrochanteric, anterolateral, and posterolateral approaches. The posterolateral approach has the lowest rate of heterotopic ossification after arthroplasty of the hip. Similarly, after acetabular fracture repair, the ilioinguinal approach has the lowest incidence of heterotopic bone formation, followed by the posterolateral and transtrochanteric approaches. The extended iliofemoral approach strips the abductors from the iliac wing and has the greatest risk of heterotopic ossification.

Contraindications

Contraindications to prophylaxis are dependent on the specific modality used for prevention. Although external beam irradiation in doses less than 3000 rad delivered over 3 weeks has not been shown to result in local sarcoma formation,[41] patients receiving treatment specifically for heterotopic ossification have only recently been followed long enough (and not yet in sufficient numbers) to permit this analysis. More specifically, in one series, radiation-induced sarcoma of bone was not observed as long as 25 years after less than 1000 rad was administered in the treatment of patients with childhood cancers.[42] Typically, radiation-induced sarcoma has a latency period of 20 to 25 years. Given that longer life expectancy provides greater opportunity for development of this complication, patients of younger age (particularly those younger than 40 years) present a relative contraindication to radiation prophylaxis. Women of childbearing age should not receive radiation prophylaxis for heterotopic ossification. Patients who have received previous radiation therapy for a cancer diagnosis, such as Hodgkin's disease, require special consideration to avoid a cumulative effective radiation dose in the toxic range. Use of nonsteroidal anti-inflammatory medications should be avoided for patients with a history of peptic ulcer disease; specifically, previous gastrointestinal bleeding is a contraindication to this form of prophylaxis. In one

study, more than one third of patients receiving indomethacin prophylaxis for heterotopic ossification after total hip arthroplasty experienced gastrointestinal symptoms that precluded completion of the prescribed 6-week course.[43]

Both external beam irradiation and nonsteroidal anti-inflammatory medications have been shown in the laboratory to *delay* bone ingrowth into cementless devices intended for biological fixation. Radiation fields have been successfully limited to exclude ingrowth surfaces of prosthetic hip implants, such that areas 1 cm outside the intended treatment portal receive less than 5% of the prescribed dose delivered to the specified area.[44,45] In contrast, indomethacin causes a systemic effect from which the hip prosthesis cannot be effectively protected. Nonetheless, to date, no clinical hip arthroplasty failures have been attributed to lack of component fixation related to irradiation or indomethacin prophylaxis for heterotopic bone formation.

Treatment Alternatives and Results

Prophylaxis. External beam irradiation and nonsteroidal anti-inflammatory medications, specifically, indomethacin or ibuprofen, have been used most widely in the clinical setting to prevent ectopic bone formation. *External beam irradiation* is the author's preferred method of prophylaxis and has been shown to be effective in single doses of 700 or 800 rad, provided that treatment is delivered before the fifth postoperative day.[46-53] Notwithstanding other complicating medical conditions, the patient typically is treated on the first or second day after surgery. Historically, divided doses of 2000 and 1000 rad have been delivered in ten and five fractions, respectively, but single-dose regimens have demonstrated comparable efficacy and have rendered fractionated protocols obsolete because of greater ease of treatment.[51,54] A single-dose regimen of 550 rad has been shown to be ineffective.[50] *Preoperative* single-dose administration of 800 rad within 6 hours of surgery has been shown to provide efficacy comparable with postoperative treatment with greater patient convenience and comfort, while eliminating the complications associated with transport of the patient, such as dislocation, soon after total hip arthroplasty.[49] Other studies have confirmed that preoperative single-dose irradiation administered within 24 hours *before* operation is as effective as postoperative irradiation given within 72 hours after surgery.[55-58] Limited treatment fields, usually an obliquely oriented rectangular portal centered over the joint space and oriented parallel to the acetabular component, have effectively prevented heterotopic ossification while excluding ingrowth surfaces of hip components from the adverse effects of radiation and have eliminated concern regarding impairment of bone ingrowth needed for fixation[51] (Fig. 107-5). The addition of a small lateral treatment area over the greater trochanter, converting the rectangle into an L-shaped treatment portal, has reduced the incidence of greater trochanteric bursitis associated with extra-field ossification at the vastus lateralis ridge.[51] Appropriate use of radiation prophylaxis has nearly eliminated clinically significant (grades III and IV) heterotopic ossification,

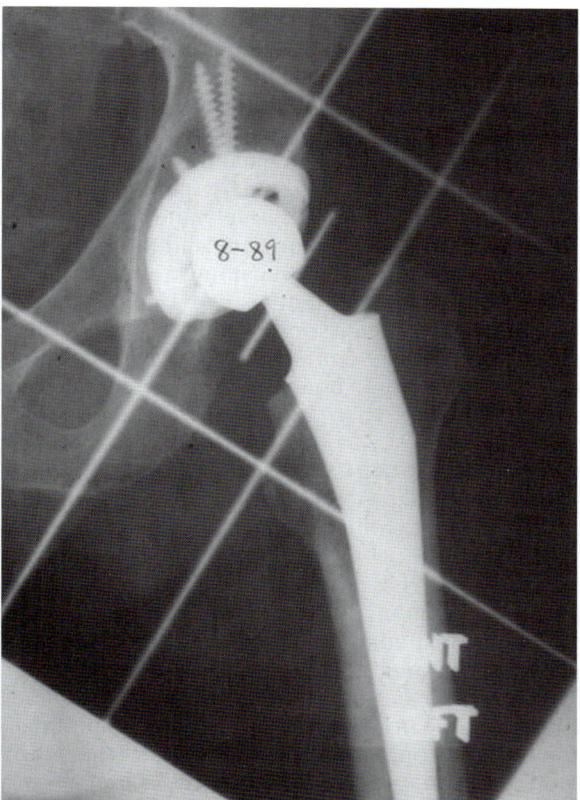

Figure 107-5. Standard radiation prophylaxis treatment portal. Primary total hip arthroplasty with obliquely oriented limited field portal aligned approximately parallel to the horizontal opening angle of the acetabular component, covering an approximately 2- to 4-cm-wide strip that excludes ingrowth surfaces of the femoral stem and the acetabular cup.

while reducing the occurrence of grade I and II ectopic bone to 10% to 20% in the high-risk patients studied.

Several nonsteroidal anti-inflammatory drugs have been found to reduce heterotopic bone formation, including indomethacin, ibuprofen, diclofenac, and naproxen.[59-65] Indomethacin, however, is the drug that has been studied most extensively; it has been shown to be effective in reducing the prevalence of heterotopic ossification compared with control agents.[18,66,67] Historically, 6 weeks of indomethacin at doses of 25 mg administered three times a day effectively prevented clinically meaningful heterotopic bone formation.[43,68,69] More recently, a divided daily dose of 75 mg (25 mg three times a day) administered for 7, 10, or 14 days has been shown to be effective in eliminating grade III and IV ossification, while reducing the occurrence of grade I and II bone to less than 10% among patients studied.[70-72] Conversely, a higher daily dose of 150 mg (50 mg three times a day) administered over only 3 days has been shown to be *in*effective in preventing ectopic bone formation.[72] Although prospective controlled clinical trials have failed to demonstrate a statistically significant difference between single-dose postoperative radiation and indomethacin administered in a divided daily dose of 75 mg in preventing heterotopic ossification after surgery about the hip, as much as twofold greater efficacy has been observed with radiation prophylaxis.[47,73-75]

Complications

Adverse events associated with prophylactic regimens directed against heterotopic ossification have been few. Although the risk of radiation-induced malignancy is ever-present, as previously noted, no cases have been reported in association with doses as low as those used for heterotopic ossification prophylaxis. No wound complications of any kind, including skin erythema, pigmentation, and delay in wound healing, have been observed about the hip. Parenthetically, the authors have observed increased skin pigmentation about the elbow after radiation prophylaxis for heterotopic ossification after takedown of post-traumatic bony ankylosis.

As previously noted, nonsteroidal anti-inflammatory medications in general, and indomethacin in particular, are associated with gastrointestinal bleeding complications. This propensity for bleeding is further exaggerated perioperatively in patients undergoing total joint arthroplasty who have preexisting comorbidities. Concurrent use of nonsteroidal medications with anticoagulant agents for prophylaxis of venous thromboembolic disease further complicates the management of bleeding complications in these patients. One study noted doubling of the rate of bleeding complications in patients receiving indomethacin for prevention of heterotopic ossification while receiving warfarin for prophylaxis of deep vein thrombosis after total hip arthroplasty.[76]

Excision of Heterotopic Bone

Once heterotopic bone is apparent on radiographs of the hip, nonoperative measures are ineffective in retarding progression of bone formation or removing the offending bone from the region of the hip.

Indications

Surgical excision of heterotopic bone about the hip is rarely necessary. Severe restriction of functional range of motion is the primary indication for operation. In its mildest form, this may consist of difficulty in reaching the feet for personal hygiene and dressing; in more severe cases, inability to sit secondary to bony ankylosis of the hip may occur. Problems with sitting posture and balance, adversely affecting ability to independently achieve transfers, may pose a serious threat to functional independence in the spinal cord– or head-injured patient. Not uncommonly, stiffness about the hip aggravates pathology of the low back that may present as symptoms of spinal stenosis or lumbar spondylosis owing to the inability of the diseased lumbar spine to tolerate the stiff hip. Infrequently, impingement of more modest degrees of heterotopic bone may contribute to recurrent instability of the hip replacement, requiring surgical excision. More commonly, however, the patient with heterotopic ossification about the hip has restricted range of motion with a stable prosthetic hip joint, and other reasons for the instability should be sought.

The timing of surgical excision of heterotopic bone is a matter of ongoing discussion. Based on a high rate of recurrence when excision is undertaken at an earlier interval, conventional wisdom has held that 12 to 24 months should pass from the index operation before an attempt is made to excise ectopic bone. Bone scan and serum alkaline phosphatase levels have traditionally been used to monitor activity of the pathologic process of bone formation; it has been recommended that surgical excision should be deferred until these studies have returned to normal, often requiring 2 years after the index operation. With increasing appreciation of the necessity for and efficacy of adjunctive measures such as perioperative irradiation or indomethacin in reducing the recurrence of heterotopic ossification, the importance of an extended period of waiting for maturation of ectopic bone before attempting excision is less clear. A 6-month interval before excision may be more reasonable; it will allow radiographic maturation of the bone sufficient to judge its extent and functional significance, and it may encourage formation of the surrounding fibrous membrane, which facilitates blunt dissection during the surgical procedure.

Finally, it should be emphasized that pain about the hip is not an indication for excision of radiographically apparent heterotopic bone. The pain associated with heterotopic ossification is transient and occurs while the inflammatory process is active and the bone is immature. Other sources for continued pain about the hip should be sought when heterotopic bone is radiographically mature and metabolically quiescent, as judged by serum alkaline phosphatase levels and bone scan. Clinical results have generally been poor when the primary indication for excision of ectopic bone about the hip has been pain.

Contraindications

Substantial amounts of ectopic bone are surprisingly well tolerated by most patients, so that the simple radiographic presence of extensive heterotopic ossification is not, in and of itself, an indication for operation. Sufficient time should pass after the index procedure to allow for functional accommodation by the patient and a reliable determination of the true clinical importance of radiographic bone and its related restriction of motion. Likewise, excision of ectopic bone before radiographic maturation sufficient to determine its extent and therefore the correct surgical approach is a relative contraindication to the procedure. A minimum of 6 months should elapse from the index procedure before surgical excision of heterotopic bone is undertaken; in practice, it is unusual for the author to undertake resection of ectopic ossification within 1 year after the inciting operation or injury. Similarly, because the procedure is accompanied by considerable blood loss, coagulopathies should be corrected and anticoagulants reversed before such an operation is undertaken.

It should be clearly understood by the patient and the operating surgeon that pathologic ectopic bone arises most commonly from the gluteal abductor muscle mass.

Therefore, the larger the amount of heterotopic bone, the smaller is the mass of functional abductor muscle that remains to stabilize the hip. The implication is that excision of large amounts of heterotopic bone is accompanied by risk of destabilizing the hip and imparting a gluteal limp secondary to weak and inadequate remaining abductor muscle mass. The patient should be apprised of this risk preoperatively and must be willing to use a cane indefinitely, or until abductor strength is regained, in exchange for regaining range of motion. Unwillingness of the patient to use a cane postoperatively, especially when one was not needed before surgery, is a relative contraindication to surgical excision of the heterotopic bone that stiffens, and stabilizes, the hip.

Treatment Alternatives and Results

Preoperative Judet views of the pelvis and computed tomography are helpful in defining soft tissue structures that are displaced by the mass of ectopic bone and therefore are at risk during the dissection, particularly when the bone is medial to the hip center (Fig. 107-6A through C). Most commonly, the ectopic bone *displaces* adjacent structures and does not invade neighboring soft tissue planes; a fibrous plane usually exists at the periphery of the bone mass that facilitates blunt dissection of the ectopic bone. Nevertheless, the mass of ectopic bone may occasionally *encircle* major peripheral nerves or named vessels, and special caution is indicated in these circumstances. Accordingly, although the bone often must be divided ultimately with an osteotome, sharp dissection of the bone mass should be avoided.

The surgical approach used for excision of heterotopic bone is most commonly the same approach used for the index procedure that resulted in bone formation. Occasionally, in the event of extensive circumferential ectopic ossification, osteotomy of the greater trochanter greatly facilitates the surgical approach, preservation of the remaining abductor mass, and protection of critical soft tissue structures (Fig. 107-7A through E). Blunt dissection of normal soft tissue structures at the periphery of the ectopic bone, resulting in isolation of the pathologic bone mass, should be the operative strategy; commencement of the dissection in normal tissues proximal and distal to the ectopic bone is advised. Sharp dissection should be avoided; an elevator is the instrument of choice in dissecting the periphery of the ectopic bone. Final separation and removal of the bone mass may require a mallet and osteotome. Radical circumferential excision of the hip capsule or pseudocapsule, ultimately allowing for dislocation of the hip arthroplasty, typically is necessary to maximize improvement in range of motion. It is unrealistic to expect that a "limited" resection of strategic portions of the ectopic bone will impart any meaningful improvement in motion about the hip; it should be the goal of the operating surgeon to restore the normal margins of the femur and pelvis as much as practically possible.

Adjunctive radiation or indomethacin treatment is *essential* to avoid reactivation of the process of heterotopic ossification; without some form of effective

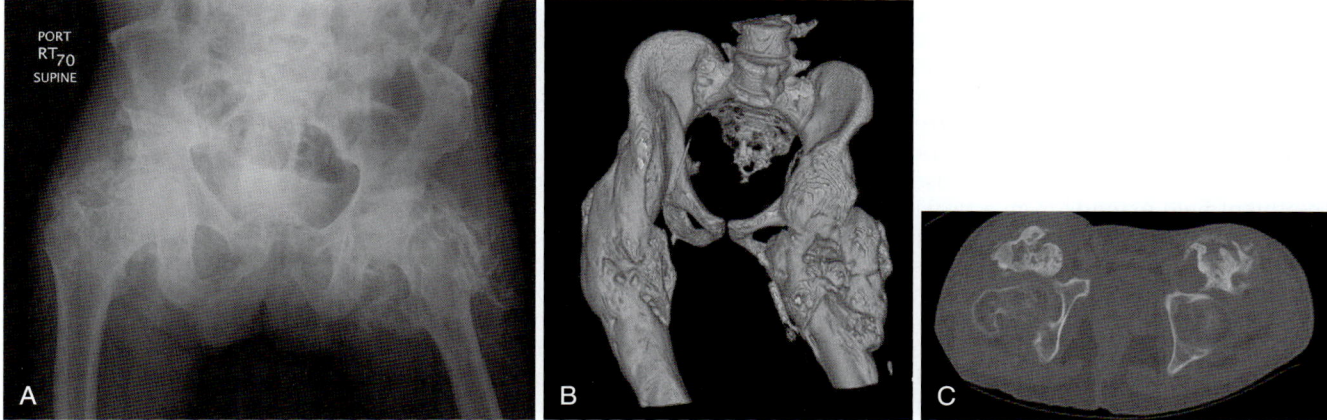

Figure 107-6. A, Fifty-six-year-old male, 5 years out from a fall resulting in traumatic T8 paraplegia with extensive heterotopic ossification of both hips in a windswept position with deformities that limited effective sitting posture and precluded independent sliding board transfer. **B,** Three-dimensional reconstruction of computed tomography (CT) images demonstrating confluent and circumferential ectopic ossification about both hips. **C,** Axial CT cuts demonstrating medial displacement, rather than circumferential envelopment, of femoral nerve within its sheath by the mass of ectopic bone.

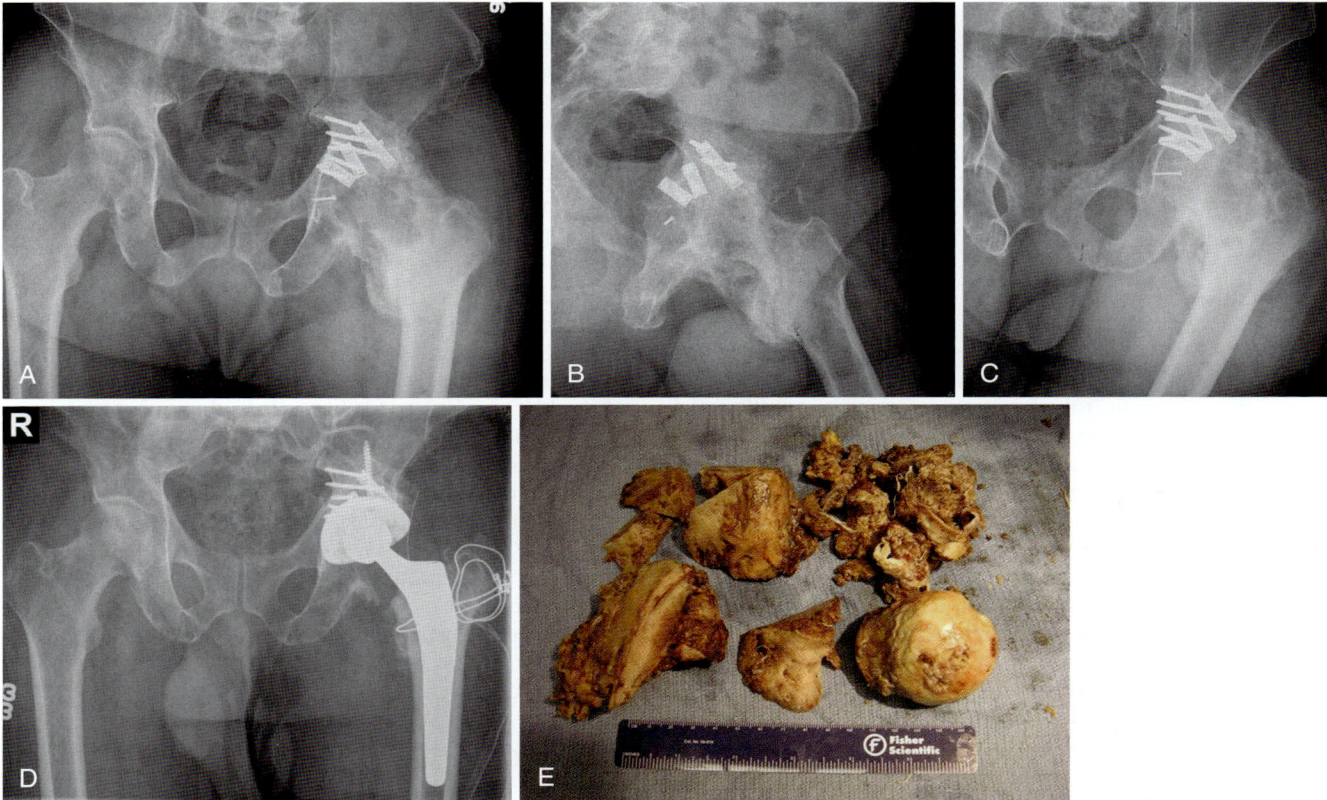

Figure 107-7. A, Fifty-four-year-old male sustained a complex high posterior wall fracture with a high-grade sciatic nerve palsy in a motor vehicle accident. He underwent open reduction and internal fixation of the fracture with three spring plates and developed grade IV heterotopic ossification that precluded functional hip motion. **B,** Judet views; iliac oblique, demonstrating modest bone along the posterior column. **C,** Judet views; obturator oblique, demonstrating heavy ossification along the posterior wall and in the space behind the hip. **D,** Postoperative radiographs after conversion to total hip arthroplasty through a transtrochanteric approach that allowed optimal preservation of remaining abductor muscle mass and exploration and neurolysis of the sciatic nerve. **E,** Operative specimen of resected ectopic bone. Note the channel in which the sciatic nerve was encased in bone and liberated by blunt dissection with a Cobb elevator before resection of bone mass. Sciatic function recovered to grade IV postoperatively.

prophylaxis, recurrence is almost guaranteed, often to a greater extent than that which prompted the effort at excision. The author prefers radiation for prophylaxis after resection of ankylosing heterotopic bone. If ectopic bone is excised without concurrent revision of the arthroplasty, and if well-fixed components are retained, an expanded field of radiation is used. This rectangular treatment field extends from a proximal point cephalad to the acetabulum to a distal point at the midshaft of the femoral component and includes a symmetrical area medial and lateral to the hip center, encompassing the entire abductor musculature. Such an expanded field both minimizes the risk of ectopic bone recurrence at the margins of the treatment portal, as is occasionally seen after primary radiation prophylaxis following total hip arthroplasty.

Excision of heterotopic bone formation, accompanied by expanded field radiation or indomethacin prophylaxis, reliably provides an increase in functional range of hip motion but does not restore normal mobility. Published results report an average increase in flexion range of 34 to 45 degrees and approximately 25 degrees of abduction. The greatest functional gain is evident in those hips with the most severe preoperative limitation in motion. Pain is not reliably relieved by excision of heterotopic bone.

Complications

Recurrence of ectopic bone is the most common complication, especially in the absence of adjunctive measures such as indomethacin or irradiation. Recovery of less than full range of motion is the rule and reflects the dense connective tissue that replaces the excised bone mass, even in the absence of recurrence of the ossification.

Gluteal abductor weakness is a common occurrence after this procedure if a large amount of bone (and replaced abductor muscle mass) is excised. Use of a cane is often necessary for 6 to 12 months postoperatively, if not indefinitely. In severe cases, instability of the prosthetic hip may result, and thus the surgeon might consider using a large femoral head (>32mm) at the time of revision and in selected cases (where much of the abductor mass is compromised), use of a constrained liner may be necessary.

Massive blood loss from the raw surfaces of excised ectopic bone is common, and liberal transfusion of blood in conjunction with crystalloid is the rule to prevent problematic hypovolemia. Clotting factor replacement with fresh-frozen plasma, calcium repletion after banked blood transfusion, correction of critical thrombocytopenia, maintenance of body temperature, and vigilant monitoring of impending coagulopathy are routine components of postoperative care of these patients. Nerve palsy and blood vessel injury may result from difficult dissection of soft tissue or from removal of ectopic bone encircling these structures. In general, in the setting of previous nerve palsy or imaging evidence of encasement of a major peripheral nerve by ectopic bone, the involved nerve should be identified in normal tissue proximal and distal to the ectopic bone before neurolysis and resection of the offending bone. In short, these major surgical procedures should be undertaken only by experienced hip surgeons supported by full-service institutions capable of providing care for the critically ill surgical patient.

PROGNOSIS

In general, following radical excision of the offending ectopic bone and timely delivery of effective prophylaxis, substantial recovery of hip motion is noted, along with a functional improvement that is gratifying for both patient and surgeon. Radiographic recurrence of a small amount of ectopic bone at the margins of the treatment field is not uncommon, but with an expanded radiation field, this does not compromise the functional result.

CURRENT CONTROVERSIES AND FUTURE CONSIDERATIONS

Noggin is a protein that binds to and antagonizes the function of BMPs, including BMP-2 and BMP-4, which are the factors believed to play a role in heterotopic bone development. Noggin plays a critical role during embryonal development and limb morphogenesis through its antagonistic effects on BMPs.[77,78] By binding to BMP, Noggin prevents subsequent interaction of BMP with its receptor.[79] Over the past decade, several studies have investigated the use of Noggin as an inhibitor of heterotopic ossification. Aspenberg and associates found that both human Noggin (hNog) and Noggin mutein (hNogΔB2) were engineered for higher bioavailability and inhibited bone growth into a titanium bone chamber screwed into the rat tibia.[80] Hanallah and colleagues, using a mouse model for HO through hindlimb BMP-4 implantation, inhibited HO by implanting muscle-derived stem cells transduced with a retroviral vector carrying the gene encoding hNog.[12] They found that Noggin reduced HO by 53% to 99% in a dose-dependent manner. Glaser and coworkers, using a mouse model for HO through abdominal muscle injections of BMP-4, found that both local administration of hNog and systemic administration of hNogΔB2 inhibited heterotopic bone formation.[81] These studies imply the use of Noggin as a potential therapeutic agent for HO, but further study is needed to understand the effects of BMP antagonists on bone and other normal tissues before a clear therapeutic role for Noggin in prevention of heterotopic ossification after total hip arthroplasty can be delineated.

REFERENCES

1. Potter BK, Burns TC, Lacap AP, et al: Heterotopic ossification following traumatic and combat-related amputations: prevalence, risk factors, and preliminary results of excision. J Bone Joint Surg Am 89:476–486, 2007.
2. Chalmers J, Gray DH, Rush J: Observations on the induction of bone in soft tissues. J Bone Joint Surg Br 57:36–45, 1975.
3. Urist MR: Bone: formation by autoinduction. Science 150:893–899, 1965.
4. Wozney JM, Rosen V, Celeste AJ, et al: Novel regulators of bone formation: molecular clones and activities. Science 242:1528–1534, 1988.

5. Reddi AH: Bone morphogenetic proteins, bone marrow stromal cells, and mesenchymal stem cells: Maureen Owen revisited. Clin Orthop Relat Res 313:115–119, 1995.

6. Shafritz AB, Shore EM, Gannon FH, et al: Overexpression of an osteogenic morphogen in fibrodysplasia ossificans progressiva. N Engl J Med 335:555–561, 1996.

7. Kaplan FS, Groppe J, Pignolo RJ, Shore EM: Morphogen receptor genes and metamorphogenes: skeleton keys to metamorphosis. Ann N Y Acad Sci 1116:113–133, 2007.

8. Lieberman JR, Le LQ, Wu L, et al: Regional gene therapy with a BMP-2-producing murine stromal cell line induces heterotopic and orthotopic bone formation in rodents. J Orthop Res 16:330–339, 1998.

9. Bosch P, Musgrave D, Ghivizzani S, et al: The efficiency of muscle-derived cell-mediated bone formation. Cell Transplant 9:463–470, 2000.

10. Brunet LJ, McMahon JA, McMahon AP, Harland RM: Noggin, cartilage morphogenesis, and joint formation in the mammalian skeleton. Science 280:1455–1457, 1998.

11. Ahn J, Serrano de la Pena L, Shore EM, Kaplan FS: Paresis of a bone morphogenetic protein-antagonist response in a genetic disorder of heterotopic skeletogenesis. J Bone Joint Surg Am 85:667–674, 2003.

12. Hannallah D, Peng H, Young B, et al: Retroviral delivery of Noggin inhibits the formation of heterotopic ossification induced by BMP-4, demineralized bone matrix, and trauma in an animal model. J Bone Joint Surg Am 86:80–91, 2004.

13. Gazzerro E, Canalis E: Bone morphogenetic proteins and their antagonists. Rev Endocr Metab Disord 7:51–65, 2006.

14. Mahy PR, Urist MR: Experimental heterotopic bone formation induced by bone morphogenetic protein and recombinant human interleukin-1B. Clin Orthop Relat Res 237:236–244, 1988.

15. Ono I, Inoue M, Kuboki Y: Promotion of the osteogenetic activity of recombinant human bone morphogenetic protein by prostaglandin E1. Bone 19:581–588, 1996.

16. Arikawa T, Omura K, Morita I: Regulation of bone morphogenetic protein-2 expression by endogenous prostaglandin E2 in human mesenchymal stem cells. J Cell Physiol 200:400–406, 2004.

17. DiCesare PE, Nimni ME, Peng L, et al: Effects of indomethacin on demineralized bone-induced heterotopic ossification in the rat. J Orthop Res 9:855–861, 1991.

18. Neal BC, Rodgers A, Clark T, et al: A systematic survey of 13 randomized trials of non-steroidal anti-inflammatory drugs for the prevention of heterotopic bone formation after major hip surgery. Acta Orthop Scand 71:122–128, 2000.

19. Puzas JE, Miller MD, Rosier RN: Pathologic bone formation. Clin Orthop Relat Res 245:269–281, 1989.

20. Tonna EA, Cronkite EP: Autoradiographic studies of cell proliferation in the periosteum of intact and fractured femora of mice utilizing DNA labeling with H3-thymidine. Proc Soc Exp Biol Med 107:719–721, 1961.

21. Bosch P, Musgrave DS, Lee JY, et al: Osteoprogenitor cells within skeletal muscle. J Orthop Res 18:933–944, 2000.

22. Musgrave DS, Pruchnic R, Wright V, et al: The effect of bone morphogenetic protein-2 expression on the early fate of skeletal muscle-derived cells. Bone 28:499–506, 2001.

23. Wright V, Peng H, Usas A, et al: BMP4-expressing muscle-derived stem cells differentiate into osteogenic lineage and improve bone healing in immunocompetent mice. Mol Ther 6:169–178, 2002.

24. Cao B, Huard J: Muscle-derived stem cells. Cell Cycle 3:104–107, 2004.

25. Lounev VY, Ramachandran R, Wosczyna MN, et al: Identification of progenitor cells that contribute to heterotopic skeletogenesis. J Bone Joint Surg Am 91:652–663, 2009.

26. Jackson WM, Aragon AB, Bulken-Hoover JD, et al: Putative heterotopic ossification progenitor cells derived from traumatized muscle. J Orthop Res 27:1645–1651, 2009.

27. Pohl F, Hassel S, Nohe A, et al: Radiation-induced suppression of the Bmp2 signal transduction pathway in the pluripotent mesenchymal cell line C2C12: an in vitro model for prevention of heterotopic ossification by radiotherapy. Radiat Res 159:345–350, 2003.

28. Shore EM, Kaplan FS: Insights from a rare genetic disorder of extra-skeletal bone formation, fibrodysplasia ossificans progressiva (FOP). Bone 43:427–433, 2008.

29. Stall AC, Tannous O, Griffith C, et al: Histological characterization of heterotopic ossification about the hip: an animal model in the rabbit. Presented at the 6th Combined Meeting of the Orthopaedic Research Society; Honolulu, October 2007.

30. Gannon FH, Kaplan FS, Olmsted E, et al: Bone morphogenetic protein 2/4 in early fibromatous lesions of fibrodysplasia ossificans progressiva. Hum Pathol 28:339–343, 1997.

31. Lanchoney TF, Olmsted EA, Shore EM, et al: Characterization of bone morphogenetic protein 4 receptor in fibrodysplasia ossificans progressiva. Clin Orthop Relat Res 346:38–45, 1998.

32. Olmsted EA, Kaplan FS, Shore EM: Bone morphogenetic protein-4 regulation in fibrodysplasia ossificans progressiva. Clin Orthop Relat Res 408:331–343, 2003.

33. de la Pena LS, Billings PC, Fiori JL, et al: Fibrodysplasia ossificans progressiva (FOP), a disorder of ectopic osteogenesis, misregulates cell surface expression and trafficking of BMPRIA. J Bone Miner Res 20:1168–1176, 2005.

34. Fiori JL, Billings PC, de la Pena LS, et al: Dysregulation of the BMP-p38 MAPK signaling pathway in cells from patients with fibrodysplasia ossificans progressiva (FOP). J Bone Miner Res 21:902–909, 2006.

35. Kaplan FS, Fiori J, Ahn J, et al: Dysregulation of the BMP-4 signaling pathway in fibrodysplasia ossificans progressiva. Ann N Y Acad Sci 1068:54–65, 2006.

36. O'Connell MP, Billings PC, Fiori JL, et al: HSPG modulation of BMP signaling in fibrodysplasia ossificans progressiva cells. J Cell Biochem 102:1493–1503, 2007.

37. Billings PC, Fiori JL, Bentwood JL, et al: Dysregulated BMP signaling and enhanced osteogenic differentiation of connective tissue progenitor cells from patients with fibrodysplasia ossificans progressiva (FOP). J Bone Miner Res 23:305–313, 2008.

38. Shore EM, Xu M, Feldman GJ, et al: A recurrent mutation in the BMP type I receptor ACVR1 causes inherited and sporadic fibrodysplasia ossificans progressiva. Nat Genet 38:525–527, 2006.

39. Brooker AF, Bowerman JW, Robinson RA, Riley LH, Jr: Ectopic ossification following total hip replacement: incidence and a method of classification. J Bone Joint Surg Am 55:1629–1632, 1973.

40. Pai VS: Heterotopic ossification in total hip arthroplasty: the influence of the approach. J Arthroplasty 9:199–202, 1994.

41. Kim JH, Chu FC, Woodard HQ, et al: Radiation-induced soft-tissue and bone sarcoma. Radiology 129:501–508, 1978.

42. Tucker MA, D'Angio GJ, Boice JD, Jr, et al: Bone sarcomas linked to radiotherapy and chemotherapy in children. N Engl J Med 317:588–593, 1987.

43. Cella JP, Salvati EA, Sculco TP: Indomethacin for the prevention of heterotopic ossification following total hip arthroplasty: effectiveness, contraindications, and adverse effects. J Arthroplasty 3:229–234, 1988.

44. Konski A, Weiss C, Rosier R, et al: The use of postoperative irradiation for the prevention of heterotopic bone after total hip replacement with biologic fixation (porous coated) prosthesis: an animal model. Int J Radiat Oncol Biol Phys 18:861–865, 1990.

45. Ayers DC, Pellegrini VD, Jr, Evarts CM: Prevention of heterotopic ossification in high-risk patients by radiation therapy. Clin Orthop Relat Res 263:87–93, 1991.

46. Knelles D, Barthel T, Karrer A, et al: Prevention of heterotopic ossification after total hip replacement: a prospective, randomised study using acetylsalicylic acid, indomethacin and fractional or single-dose irradiation. J Bone Joint Surg Br 79:596–602, 1997.

47. Burd TA, Lowry KJ, Anglen JO: Indomethacin compared with localized irradiation for the prevention of heterotopic ossification following surgical treatment of acetabular fractures. J Bone Joint Surg Am 83:1783–1788, 2001.

48. Schneider DJ, Moulton MJ, Singapuri K, et al: The Frank Stinchfield Award. Inhibition of heterotopic ossification with radiation therapy in an animal model. Clin Orthop Relat Res 355:35–46, 1998.

49. Pellegrini VD, Jr, Gregoritch SJ: Preoperative irradiation for prevention of heterotopic ossification following total hip arthroplasty. J Bone Joint Surg Am 78:870–881, 1996.

50. Healy WL, Lo TC, DeSimone AA, et al: Single-dose irradiation for the prevention of heterotopic ossification after total hip arthroplasty: a comparison of doses of five hundred and fifty and seven hundred centigray. J Bone Joint Surg Am 77:590–595, 1995.

51. Pellegrini VD, Jr, Konski AA, Gastel JA, et al: Prevention of heterotopic ossification with irradiation after total hip arthroplasty: radiation therapy with a single dose of eight hundred centigray administered to a limited field. J Bone Joint Surg Am 74:186–200, 1992.

52. Pellegrini VD, Jr, Evarts CM: Radiation prophylaxis of heterotopic bone formation following total hip arthroplasty: current status. Semin Arthroplasty 3:156–166, 1992.

53. Pellegrini VD, Jr: Radiation prophylaxis of heterotopic ossification. Int J Radiat Oncol Biol Phys 30:743–744, 1994.

54. Coventry MB, Scanlon PW: The use of radiation to discourage ectopic bone: a nine-year study in surgery about the hip. J Bone Joint Surg Am 63:201–208, 1991.

55. Roth A, Fuller J, Fahrmann M, et al: Prophylaxis of heterotopic bone formation by radiotherapy—a comparison between pre- and postsurgical activity. Acta Chir Orthop Traumatol Cech 72:38–41, 2005.

56. Seegenschmiedt MH, Keilholz L, Martus P, et al: Prevention of heterotopic ossification about the hip: final results of two randomized trials in 410 patients using either preoperative or postoperative radiation therapy. Int J Radiat Oncol Biol Phys 39:161–171, 1997.

57. Seegenschmiedt MH, Makoski HB, Micke O: Radiation prophylaxis for heterotopic ossification about the hip joint—a multicenter study. Int J Radiat Oncol Biol Phys 51:756–765, 2001.

58. Rumi MN, Deol GS, Bergandi JA, et al: Optimal timing of preoperative radiation for prophylaxis against heterotopic ossification: a rabbit hip model. J Bone Joint Surg Am 87:366–373, 2005.

59. Vielpeau C, Joubert JM, Hulet C: Naproxen in the prevention of heterotopic ossification after total hip replacement. Clin Orthop Relat Res 369:279–288, 1999.

60. Persson PE, Sodemann B, Nilsson OS: Preventive effects of ibuprofen on periarticular heterotopic ossification after total hip arthroplasty: a randomized double-blind prospective study of treatment time. Acta Orthop Scand 69:111–115, 1998.

61. Jockheck M, Willms R, Volkmann R, et al: Prevention of periarticular heterotopic ossification after endoprosthetic hip joint replacement by means of diclofenac. Arch Orthop Trauma Surg 117:337–340, 1998.

62. Gebuhr P, Wilbek H, Soelberg M: Naproxen for 8 days can prevent heterotopic ossification after hip arthroplasty. Clin Orthop Relat Res 314:166–169, 1995.

63. Reis HJ, Kussweter W, Schellinger T: The suppression of heterotopic ossification after total hip arthroplasty. Int Orthop 16:140–145, 1992.

64. Wahlstrom O, Risto O, Djerf K, Hammerby S: Heterotopic bone formation prevented by diclofenac: prospective study of 100 hip arthroplasties. Acta Orthop Scand 62:419–421, 1991.

65. Gebuhr P, Soelberg M, Orsnes T, Wilbek H: Naproxen prevention of heterotopic ossification after hip arthroplasty: a prospective control study of 55 patients. Acta Orthop Scand 62:226–229, 1991.

66. Fransen M, Neal B: Non-steroidal anti-inflammatory drugs for preventing heterotopic bone formation after hip arthroplasty. Cochrane Database Syst Rev (3):CD001160, 2004.

67. Fijn R, Koorevaar RT, Brouwers JR: Prevention of heterotopic ossification after total hip replacement with NSAIDs. Pharm World Sci 25:138–145, 2003.

68. Ritter MA, Sieber JM: Prophylactic indomethacin for the prevention of heterotopic bone formation following total hip arthroplasty. Clin Orthop Relat Res 196:217–225, 1985.

69. Schmidt SA, Kjaersgaard-Andersen P, Pedersen NW, et al: The use of indomethacin to prevent the formation of heterotopic bone after total hip replacement: a randomized, double-blind clinical trial. J Bone Joint Surg Am 70:834–838, 1988.

70. Kjaersgaard-Andersen P, Nafei A, Teichert G, et al: Indomethacin for prevention of heterotopic ossification: a randomized controlled study in 41 hip arthroplasties. Acta Orthop Scand 64:639–642, 1993.

71. Amstutz HC, Fowble VA, Schmalzried TP, Dorey FJ: Short-course indomethacin prevents heterotopic ossification in a high-risk population following total hip arthroplasty. J Arthroplasty 12:126–132, 1997.

72. van der Heide HJ, Koorevaar RT, Schreurs BW, et al: Indomethacin for 3 days is not effective as prophylaxis for heterotopic ossification after primary total hip arthroplasty. J Arthroplasty 14:796–799, 1999.

73. Pakos EE, Ioannidis JP: Radiotherapy vs. nonsteroidal anti-inflammatory drugs for the prevention of heterotopic ossification after major hip procedures: a meta-analysis of randomized trials. Int J Radiat Oncol Biol Phys 60:888–895, 2004.

74. Vavken P, Castellani L, Sculco TP: Prophylaxis of heterotopic ossification of the hip: systematic review and meta-analysis. Clin Orthop Relat Res 467:3283–3289, 2009.

75. Blokhuis TJ, Frolke JP: Is radiation superior to indomethacin to prevent heterotopic ossification in acetabular fractures? A systematic review. Clin Orthop Relat Res 467:526–530, 2009.

76. Gallay S, Waddell JP, Cardella P, Morton J: A short course of low-molecular-weight heparin to prevent deep venous thrombosis after elective total hip replacement. Can J Surg 40:119–123, 1997.

77. Capdevila J, Johnson RL: Endogenous and ectopic expression of noggin suggests a conserved mechanism for regulation of BMP function during limb and somite patterning. Dev Biol 197:205–217, 1998.

78. Merino R, Ganan Y, Macias D, et al: Morphogenesis of digits in the avian limb is controlled by FGFs, TGFbetas, and noggin through BMP signaling. Dev Biol 200:35–45, 1998.

79. Zimmerman LB, De Jesus-Escobar JM, Harland RM: The Spemann organizer signal noggin binds and inactivates bone morphogenetic protein 4. Cell 86:599–606, 1996.

80. Aspenberg P, Jeppsson C, Economides AN: The bone morphogenetic proteins antagonist Noggin inhibits membranous ossification. J Bone Miner Res 16:497–500, 2001.

81. Glaser DL, Economides AN, Wang L, et al: In vivo somatic cell gene transfer of an engineered Noggin mutein prevents BMP4-induced heterotopic ossification. J Bone Joint Surg Am 85:2332–2342, 2003.

FURTHER READINGS

Neal BC, Rodgers A, Clark T, et al: A systematic survey of 13 randomized trials of non-steroidal anti-inflammatory drugs for the prevention of heterotopic bone formation after major hip surgery. Acta Orthop Scand 71:122–128, 2000.
A review of clinical trials with nonsteroidal anti-inflammatory drugs (NSAIDs) used as prophylaxis of heterotopic ossification after surgery about the hip.

Pakos EE, Ioannidis JP: Radiotherapy vs. nonsteroidal anti-inflammatory drugs for the prevention of heterotopic ossification after major hip procedures: a meta-analysis of randomized trials. Int J Radiat Oncol Biol Phys 60:888–895, 2004.
A review of comparative trials investigating efficacy of radiation versus nonsteroidal anti-inflammatory drugs (NSAIDs) for prophylaxis of heterotopic ossification.

Pellegrini VD, Jr, Evarts CM: Radiation prophylaxis of heterotopic bone formation following total hip arthroplasty: current status. Semin Arthroplasty 3:156–166, 1992.
A useful historical review of the evolution and development of current radiation protocols used in prophylaxis of heterotopic ossification.

Pellegrini VD, Jr, Gregoritch SJ: Preoperative irradiation for prevention of heterotopic ossification following total hip arthroplasty. J Bone Joint Surg Am 78:870–881, 1996.
Clinical trial comparing preoperative versus postoperative radiation for prevention of heterotopic ossification after total hip replacement.

Index

Page numbers followed by "f" indicate figures, "t" indicate tables, and "b" indicate boxes.